200

ICD•9•CM

Expert for Hospitals
Volumes 1, 2, and 3

International Classification of Diseases
9th Revision
Clinical Modification

Sixth Edition

Effective October 1, 2002–September 30, 2003

Edited by:
Anita C. Hart, RHIA, CCS, CCS-P
Catherine A. Hopkins, CPC

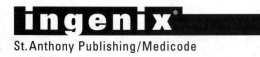
St. Anthony Publishing/Medicode

3539/IHEU/U503

Copyright © 2002 Ingenix, Inc.
All Rights Reserved

First Printing — August 2002

This book, or parts hereof, may not be reproduced in any form without permission.

Additional copies may be ordered from:
Your local bookstore
or
1.800.INGENIX (464-3649)

IHES ISBN 1-56329-878-3
IHEU ISBN 1-56329-879-1

DISCLAIMER

All the codes, indexes and other material in the ICD-9-CM are compiled from official ICD-9-CM codes and instructions as well as the Medicare regulations and manuals issued or authorized by the Centers for Medicare and Medicaid Services. The code book is designed to provide accurate and authoritative information in regard to the subject covered, and every reasonable effort has been made to ensure the accuracy of the information within these pages. However, the ultimate responsibility for correct coding lies with the provider of services.

Ingenix, Inc., its employees, agents and staff make no representation, warranty or guarantee that this compilation of codes and narratives is error-free or that the use of this code book will prevent differences of opinion or disputes with Medicare or other third-party payers as to the codes that are accepted or the amounts that will be paid to providers of services, and will bear no responsibility or liability for the results or consequences of the use of this code book.

SPECIAL REPORTS AND ANNOUNCEMENTS

Purchase of this publication entitles you to Special Reports and announcements via e-mail. Please call customer service at 800 INGENIX (464-3649) or contact your bookstore to take advantage of this exciting new free service that will keep you abreast of important code changes and regulatory developments.

Review, download, and print the Special Reports in .pdf format. Log on to
http://www.ingenixonline.com/content/2003I9Expert

American Academy of Professional Coders (AAPC)
Continuing Education Units Credits: 5 CEUs
Contact AAPC directly for credits: 1.800.626.CODE

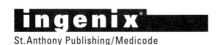

St. Anthony Publishing/Medicode

2525 Lake Park Boulevard • Salt Lake City, UT 84120
11410 Isaac Newton Square • Reston, VA 20190

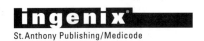

September 2002

Dear Ingenix Customer:

St. Anthony Publishing and Medicode joined their expertise and after intense research involving real-world coders developed a new and innovative code book. Your *2003 ICD-9-CM Expert for Hospitals, Volumes 1, 2 & 3*, is the result of this effort. Designed by coders for coders, we are certain you will find the new page design and intuitive symbols will improve coding accuracy and efficiency.

If you have purchased the updateable *ICD-9-CM Expert for Hospitals, Volumes 1, 2 & 3*, binder with subscription service, please follow the arch-ring binder instructions and the assembly instructions carefully.

The codes contained in this book are the official code set issued by the U.S. Department of Health and Human Services, effective October 1, 2002 through September 30, 2003.

Your new *2003 ICD-9-CM Expert for Hospitals, Volumes 1, 2 & 3*, features:

- **New! FREE set of tabs for the Volume 2, Disease Index**
- New! Chapter 00, Procedures and Interventions, NEC, in Volume 3 Procedures
- New! ICD-9-CM convention — Code, if applicable any causal condition first
- fiscal year 2003 official ICD-9-CM codes
- summary of code changes for 2003
- symbols indicating code changes and pages are dated to indicate when the changes occurred
- 1st (2nd quarter Coding Clinic was delayed, therefore, the references were not available at press time) *2002 AHA Coding Clinic* for ICD-9-CM references
- updated CC principal diagnosis exclusion list with each CC condition
- clinically-oriented illustrations and comprehensive definitions
- check fourth- and fifth-digit symbols in the index and tabular sections
- age and sex edit symbols
- exclusive color coding and symbols for all major Medicare code edits
- complex cardiovascular diagnosis alert
- major cardiovascular complication condition alert
- HIV major related condition notations
- symbols identify all the major Medicare edits pertaining to procedures

.......PLUS the accuracy and quality you expect from the leaders!

In addition to the features listed above, the *2003 ICD-9-CM Expert for Hospitals, Volumes 1, 2 & 3*, includes:

- special reports and regulatory information delivered via e-mail
- complete Dx/MDC/DRG list
- listing of the common drugs and pharmacology considerations to link treatment with disease
- an updated complications and comorbidity (CC) condition list that affect DRG assignment
- valid three-digit code list as a quick reference to speed auditing of claims

Note: The ICD-9-CM Coordination and Maintenance Committee has undertaken the task of completely revising the official coding guidelines. At the time of press the guidelines had not yet been finalized. The new guidelines build upon the current set and therefore, the guidance provided by the current set is still valid. Release of the revised guidelines is expected before the effective date of October 1, 2002. We have created a web site specifically to provide you with the revised guidelines once they are released. You will be able to log on to www.ingenixonline.com/I9guidelines toward the end of September to view and print the new ICD-9-CM official coding guidelines.

We appreciate your choosing Ingenix/St. Anthony Publishing/Medicode/ to meet your coding needs. If you have any questions or comments concerning your *2003 ICD-9-CM Expert for Hospitals, Volumes 1, 2 & 3*, please do not hesitate to call our customer service department. The toll free number is 1.800.INGENIX (464-3649).

Cordially,

Elizabeth Boudrie

Elizabeth Boudrie
Vice President, Regulatory Services

2003 ICD•9•CM EXPERT FOR HOSPITALS, VOLUMES 1, 2, AND 3

If you have purchased the updateable *ICD-9-CM Expert for Hospitals, Volumes 1, 2, & 3* binder with subscription service, please follow the arch-ring binder instructions and the assembly instructions below.

Step One: Operating your binder mechanism

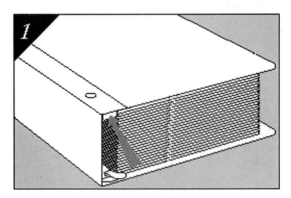

- **To Unlock binder**—Push in locking channel
- **To Lock binder**—Pull out locking channel

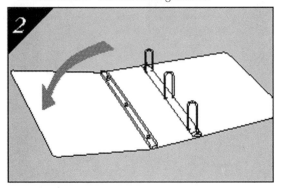

- Lay front cover flat

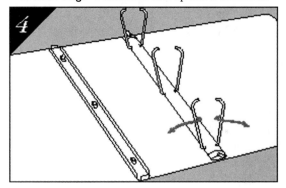

- **To Unlock rings**—Push metal tabs down and away from book
- **To Lock rings**—Push metal tabs up and toward book

- **To Open rings**—Pull the rings apart

Step Two
Insert the pages behind the appropriate divider tabs.

Step Three
Securly lock the binder and rings. Your *ICD-9-CM Expert for Hospitals* is now ready to use.

If you have any questions or comments regarding your book, please call our customer service department at 1.800.INGENIX (464.3649).

2003 Publications

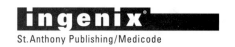

The ICD-9-CM System is Changing!

ICD-9-CM Professional for Hospitals, Vols. 1, 2 & 3

Softbound
ISBN: 1-56329-876-7   Item No. 3654   **$74.95**
Available: September 2002

Compact
ISBN: 1-56329-877-5   Item No. 3662   **$74.95**
Available: September 2002

ICD-9-CM Expert for Hospitals, Vols. 1, 2 & 3

Spiral
ISBN: 1-56329-878-3   Item No. 3656   **$94.95**
Available: September 2002

Updateable Binder
ISBN: 1-56329-879-1   Item No. 3539   **$154.95**

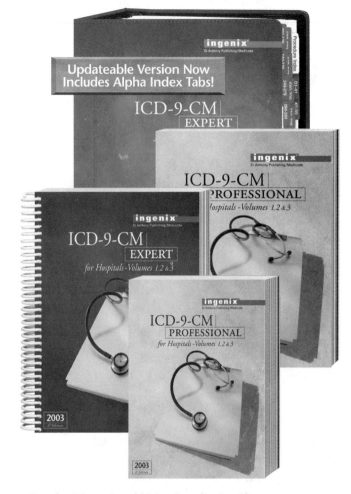

This year, a chapter on New Technologies and Medical Services has been added to the ICD-9-CM code books for Hospitals, and code changes that affect nearly every chapter! Last year, our newly designed pages, featuring intuitive symbols, exclusive color-coding, and additional resources, demonstrated why our customers consider these codes books the BEST!

Professional and Expert editions of ICD-9-CM for Hospitals Feature:

- New and Revised Code Symbols
- Fourth-and Fifth-digit Requirement Alerts
- Complete Official Coding Guidelines
- AHA's *Coding Clinic for ICD-9-CM* References
- Illustrations and Definitions
- Age and Sex Edits
- Nonspecific and Unacceptable Primary Diagnosis Alerts
- Medicare as Secondary Payer Indicators
- Manifestation Code Alerts
- Complex Diagnosis and Major Complication Alerts
- HIV Major Related Diagnosis Alerts
- CC Principal Diagnosis Exclusion List
- CC Diagnosis Symbol
- Crucial Medicare Procedure Code Edits

Expert Editions Also Include These Enhancements:

- Special Reports Via E-mail.
- Complete Principal Diagnosis/MDC/DRG Listing
- Pharmacological List
- CC Code List
- Valid Three-digit Code List

The Expert Updateable Binder Subscriptions Feature:

- Money Saving Update Service
- Three Updates per Year [October (full text), January and July]

Call Toll-Free 1.877.INGENIX (464.3649) or Shop Online at www.IngenixOnline.com

Also Available from your Medical Bookstore or Distributor

2003 Publications

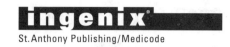

2003 ICD-9-CM Code Books for Physicians Volumes 1 & 2

ICD-9-CM Professional for Physicians, Vols. 1 & 2

Softbound
ISBN: 1-56329-872-4   Item No. 3650 **$64.95**
Available: September 2002

Compact
ISBN: 1-56329-873-2   Item No. 3661 **$64.95**
Available: September 2002

ICD-9-CM Expert for Physicians, Vols. 1 & 2

Spiral
ISBN: 1-56329-874-0   Item No. 3652 **$84.95**
Available: September 2002

Updateable Binder
ISBN: 1-56329-875-9   Item No. 3534 **$144.95**

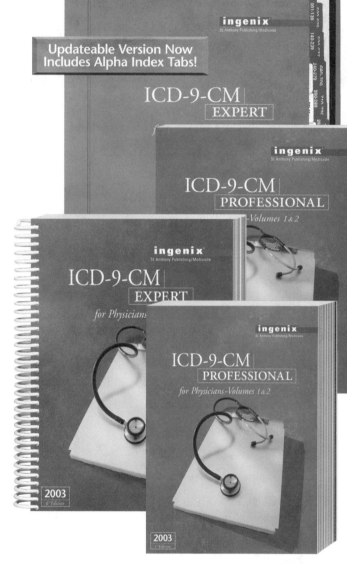

Our page design, featuring intuitive symbols, exclusive color-coding, and additional resources provides a new approach to pertinent coding and reimbursement information. New codes and changes to the ICD-9-CM make our 2003 code books a must buy! Order today and keep currenton all changes!

Professional and Expert Editions of ICD-9-CM for Physicians Feature:
- New and Revised Code Symbols
- Fourth-and Fifth-digit Requirement Alerts
- Complete Official Coding Guidelines
- Age and Sex Edits
- Clinically Oriented Definitions and Illustrations
- Medicare as Secondary Payer Indicators
- Manifestation Code Alerts
- "Other" and "Unspecified" Diagnosis Alerts
- Symbols Identifying V Codes Designated for only Primary or only Secondary Diagnosis Use

Expert **Editions Also Include These Enhancements:**
- Special Reports Via E-mail.
- Code Tables--Complex coding issues are simplified in coding tables, as developed for I-9 Express
- Valid Three-digit Category List

The *Expert* Updateable Binder Subscriptions Feature:
- Money Saving Update Service
- Three Updates per Year [October (full text), January and July]

Call Toll-Free 1.877.INGENIX (464.3649) or Shop Online at www.IngenixOnline.com

Also Available from your Medical Bookstore or Distributor

2003 Publications

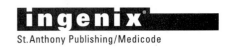
St. Anthony Publishing/Medicode

An Exceptional Code Book! An Exceptional Year for ICD-9-CM!

2003 ICD-9-CM Expert for Home Health Services, Nursing Facilities & Hospices, Volumes 1, 2 & 3

Softbound
ISBN: 1-56329-880-5   Item No. 3658   **$129.95**
Available: September 2002

In the healthcare marketplace, this is the only ICD-9-CM code book designed specifically for the needs of the home health, nursing home, and hospice coder. This enhanced code book now includes features that will take the coder to the next level of coding. Code quickly and accurately using this resource filled with important alerts and references specific to each facility type. No other code book exists that explains each prospective payment system in detail or that can serve as a reference for specific coding guidelines.

Inside You Will Find:

- **New Chapter in Volume 3 for New Technologies and Medical Services**
- Illustrations and Definitions
- **Exclusive**—E-mail delivered Special Reports
- Additional Digit Requirement Alerts in the Index and the Tabular Sections

- "10 Steps to Correct Coding" Tutorial
- Excerpts from the Home Health Agency Prospective Payment System (HHA PPS) and Symbols Identifying Clinical Dimension Diagnoses
- Medicare Home Health Manual Section on Coverage Qualifications
- Explanation of the SNF Prospective Payment System (SNF PPS) and Color-coding Indicating ICD-9-CM Codes Associated with Specific RUG-III Categories
- Color-coding and Criteria for Acceptable Non-cancer Diagnoses for Hospice Coverage
- Complete Official Coding Guidelines, Including LTC Guidelines
- Symbols Identifying V Codes Designated for only Primary or only Secondary Diagnosis Use

Call Toll-Free 1.877.INGENIX (464.3649) or Shop Online at www.IngenixOnline.com

Also Available from your Medical Bookstore or Distributor

060102

2003 Publications

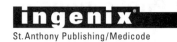
St. Anthony Publishing/Medicode

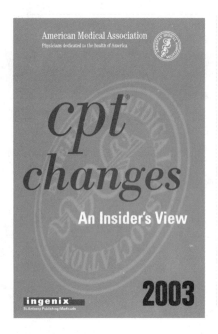

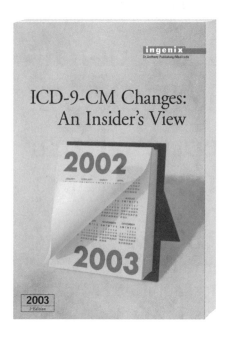

NEW!
CPT® Changes 2003: An Insider's View

7" x 10" Perfect Bound

The American Medical Association and Ingenix Publishing present **CPT® Changes 2003: An Insider's View**, a must-have resource for Physicians' Current Procedural Terminology (CPT®) Professional users! This book serves as a reference tool to understanding each of the CPT® code changes found in CPT® 2003.

In both books you'll find:

- **Every new, revised and deleted code change**—Listed along with a detailed rationale for the change. Index changes, convention changes and instructional note changes are also explained.

- **Organized by ICD-9-CM and CPT® code section and code number**—Includes a separate section that discusses index changes.

- **Illustrated**—Helps orient you to change in code.

- **Clinical Examples/Diagnostic or Procedural Descriptions**—Helps you understand the practical application of the code.

CPT is a registered trademark of the American Medical Association

NEW!
ICD-9-CM Changes 2003: An Insider's View

7" x 10" Perfect Bound
Item No. 4951 **$54.95**
Available: November 2002

A must have resource for ICD-9-CM users! **ICD-9-CM Changes 2003: An Insider's View** serves as a reference tool to understanding each of the ICD-9-CM code changes found in ICD-9-CM 2003.

CPT® Changes for 2003:
- 204 New Codes
- 23 Deleted Codes
- 203 Revised Codes
- Place of Service section added to appendices

ICD-9-CM Changes for 2003:
- 163 New Diagnosis Codes
- 23 Revised Diagnosis Codes
- 25 New Procedure Codes
- 3 Revised Procedure Codes
- New chapter on New Technology and Medical Services in Volume 3
- Changes to conventions and to the index

Call Toll-Free 1.877.INGENIX (1.877.464.3649) or Shop Online at www.IngenixOnLine.com
Also Available from your Medical Bookstore or Distributor

2003 Publications

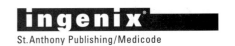
St. Anthony Publishing/Medicode

DRG System Changes Impact 12 of the Top 25 DRGs!

2003 DRG Expert
(formerly called the DRG Guidebook)

Compact, Spiral
ISBN: 1-56329-891-0   Item No. 3575   **$99.95**
Available: September 2002

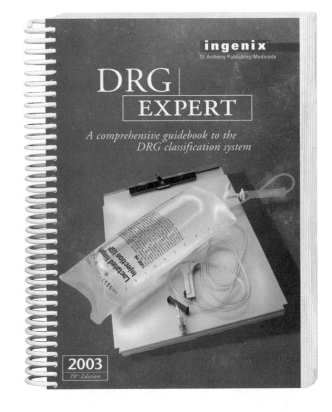

Trust the nation's DRG experts to bring you the DRG guidebook designed specifically for those who need a comprehensive resource for accurate assignment of DRGs, concurrently and retrospectively. The most trusted and comprehensive guidebook to the DRG classification system for 19 years should be your guide to navigate the changes in the DRG system!

NEW—Exclusive Color Coding Helps Hospitals to:
- See at a glance surgical/medical partitioning
- Know if CCs must be assigned and when age limits apply
- Know when certain qualifications for principal or secondary diagnosis must be met
- Identify DRGs targeted for audits

Other Features Include:
- **Organized by Major Diagnositic Category (MDC)**
- **Transfer DRG Alert**—Indicates a DRG selected as a qualified discharge that may be paid by per diem rate
- **Main Term Code Search**—Customized code descriptions that list main conditions or operative terms first
- **Average National Payment**—Listed with every DRG for quick benchmark comparisons
- **Surgical Hierarchy Table**—Quickly shows DRG hierarchy for multiple procedure cases
- **Invalid DRG Conversion Table**—Easily track the reassignment of codes to the new DRG
- **Full Listing of All Dx Within a MDC**
- **Numeric and Alphabetic ICD-9-CM Indexes**
- **Current CMS Rate Structure** (RW, AMLOS, GMLOS)
- **QuickFlip Color Tabs**—Find the right code in half the time of traditional thumb tabs

Call Toll-Free 1.877.INGENIX (464.3649) or Shop Online at www.IngenixOnline.com
Also Available from your Medical Bookstore or Distributor

2003 Publications

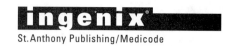
St. Anthony Publishing/Medicode

New! DRG Desk Reference— The Book You've Been Requesting!

DRG Desk Reference

Compact, Softbound
ISBN: 1-56329-929-1   Item No. 4282   **$199.95**
Available: September 2002

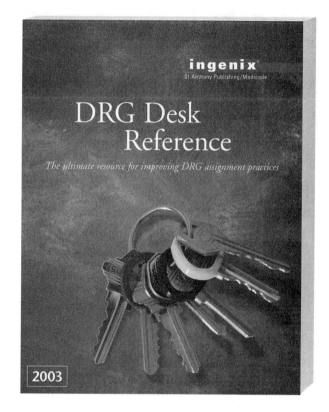

A truly comprehensive resource that creates an inpatient coding resource that functions to work efficiently and effectively with either *DRG Expert* or *DRG Guidebook*.

A must-have resource for anyone who assigns DRGs or audits claims for inpatient cases!

DRG Desk Reference **will bring you:**

- **Optimal Reimbursement Indicators**—Quickly identify the top ICD-9-CM diagnosis or procedure codes and key indicators for each DRG to ensure optimal payment while ensuring compliance.

- **Tips for the Encoder User**—Many decisions faced by coders using grouper software, or encoder, have significant impact on final DRG assignment. Tips are provided on how to avoid making the wrong decisions.

- **New Technology and Medical Services**—Descriptions of the new technology and medical services and which services will receive add-on payment under the Medicare inpatient prospective payment system.

- **Key Abstracting Field Items**—An in-depth look at the significance of key abstracting fields for DRG assignment and the impact on reimbursement.

- **DRG Assignment Tutorial**—This tutorial will explain the DRG assignment process in clear and understandable language.

- **Coding and Documentation Guidelines for DRG Validation**—Uncover potential coding problems and ensure the accuracy and validity of DRG assignment.

- **Key Complication and Comorbidity Condition (CC) Indicators:**
  Drug Usage and Treatment
  Durable Medical Equipment
  Noninvasive Diagnostic Test Outcomes
  Abnormal EKG Findings
  Abnormal Laboratory Values
  Major Cardiovascular Complications
  Complex Diagnoses
  Organisms

- **DRG Decision Trees**

- **Complete CC List**

- **CC Principal Diagnosis Exclusion List**

- **Relative Weights of Valid DRG**

Call Toll-Free 1.877.INGENIX (464.3649) or Shop Online at www.IngenixOnline.com
Also Available from your Medical Bookstore or Distributor

2003 Publications

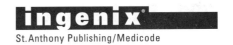
St. Anthony Publishing/Medicode

Take Charge of Your Chargemaster

Hospital Chargemaster Guide—2003

ISBN: 1-56329-870-8 Item No. 4302 **$199.95**

Available: December 2002

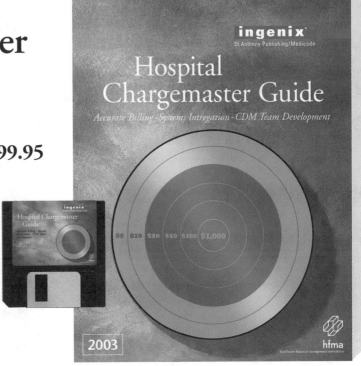

This "consultant in a book" provides step-by-step guidance for implementing and maintaining an accurate hospital chargemaster from a coding, billing, and reimbursement perspective. The *Hospital Chargemaster* provides the HCPCS/Physicians' Current Procedural Terminology (CPT®) codes, applicable revenue codes, Medicare compliance and fraud issues, payment guidelines, and claim submission procedures by clinical department for all chargemaster-driven hospital-based procedures.

- **Step-by-step Guidance to Setting Up and Maintaining an Accurate Charge Description Master.** Helps improve billing accuracy and compliance throughout your facility. Also helps establish a process for reviewing and maintaining the CDM on an annual basis, and makes educating and training clinical department heads and your CDM team easier.

- **Provides Relevant CPT®/HCPCS Code and Revenue Code Combinations for Each Clinical Department.** Takes the guesswork out of assigning revenue codes to each line item on your chargemaster.

- **APC Payment Status Indicators.** Identify how each line item charge should be billed and how it will be reimbursed under APCs or other payment methodology.

- **Easy-to-use Diskette.** Provides templates with recommendations on procedure codes, and descriptions for radiology, laboratory, and other clinical areas to eliminate confusion over code selection.

- **Easy-to-use Tables within each Clinical Department Section.**

- **Recommendations as to How Each HCPCS Code Should Be Described in the CDM.**

- **Department-specific Billing Information and Tips.**

- **Expanded Modifier Section.**

- **Regulations and Reimbursement Information.** Provides new regulatory and reimbursement information for pharmacy, supplies, observation services, and more.

- **Co-published with HFMA.**

CPT is a registered trademark of the American Medical Association

Call Toll-Free 1.877.INGENIX (464.3649) or Shop Online at www.IngenixOnline.com

Also Available from your Medical Bookstore or Distributor

2003 Publications

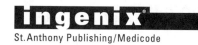

Look to the Source Most People Trust for UB-92 Billing Perfection

UB-92 Editor

Item No. 4787 **$269.95**
*Call for CD multi-user pricing

Available: Now

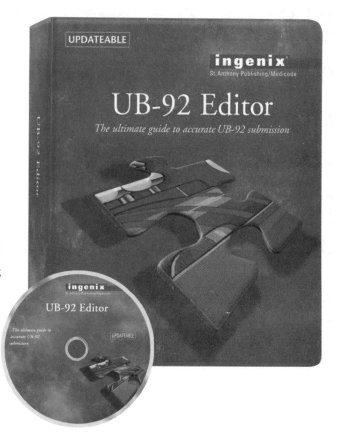

This one-of-a-kind book, published by "the experts" in UB-92 billing for Medicare, enables you to minimize billing and payment delays. The *UB-92 Editor* walks you through the UB-92 claim form for billing Medicare inpatient and outpatient services. It helps you understand the requirements of each form locator (FL) and revenue code, and provides detailed billing and coding tips for accurate claim submission.

- **EXCLUSIVE — Links HCPCS and Physicians' Current Procedural Terminology (CPT®) Codes to Applicable Revenue Codes.** Helps prevent the most common reasons for rejections(mismatched revenue codes and CPT® or HCPCS codes. Updated to include the latest billing and coding rules for OPPS.

- **EXCLUSIVE — Step-by-step Instructions for Completing the UB-92 Claim Form.** Gives you the most current Medicare billing and coding information for each data element on the UB-92 claim form and ensures accurate submission of inpatient and outpatient claims.

- **Addresses Home Health and SNF Issues, Consolidated Billing, Use of HIPPS Rate Codes and Modifiers.** Increases efficiency and accuracy, ensuring timely payment.

- **CD-ROM with Hypertext and Jump Links.** Provides all of the information available in the hard-copy book with jump links to revenue codes, other form locators, condition codes, occurrence codes, and value codes. Use it to ensure that your claims are submitted accurately to Medicare the first time.

- **Quarterly Updates — Fully Indexed and Tabbed.** New coding and billing tips are highlighted with an arrow, so you know what changed from update to update. Eliminates billing with outdated information. It's easy to find and use the information necessary to bill Medicare.

- **Earn 5 CEUS from AAPC.**

CPT is a registered trademark of the American Medical Association

Call Toll-Free 1.877.INGENIX (464.3649) or Shop Online at www.IngenixOnline.com
Also Available from your Medical Bookstore or Distributor

2003 Publications

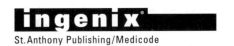
St. Anthony Publishing/Medicode

Solutions for PFS operational and compliance challenges with proven policies and procedures!

Hospital Toolkit for Patient Financial Services

ISBN: 1-56329-812-0   Item No. 3017   **$249.95**

Available: Now

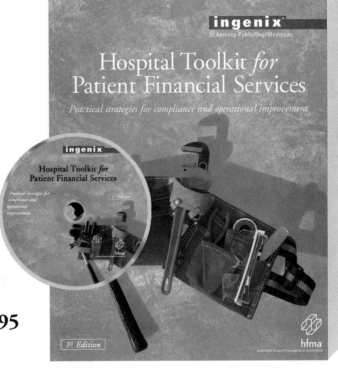

This is the first all-in-one guide to managing patient financial services and ensuring Medicare compliance. It offers practical guidance to reduce A/R days, streamline operations, and ensure compliance with Medicare regulations. The *Hospital Toolkit for Patient Financial Services* has been developed by a PFS professional with more than 20 years of experience in hospitals, managing the same challenges you face every day. Inside you will find strategies you can trust!

- **Expert Management Strategies and Compliance Guidance—Specifically for Your PFS Team.** Combines leading-edge strategies with best practices to reduce AR and increase efficiency. Will help you prevent mistakes that can lead to accounts receivable problems, trigger a compliance audit, or put you under a corporate integrity agreement.

- **Solutions to Patient Accounting and Compliance Problems.** Use proven strategies to establish an effective compliance program, streamline billing, and ensure low levels of accounts receivable.

- **Organized by Function within Patient Financial Services/Patient Accounts.** Presents billing and compliance problems by functional area. Allows you to tackle compliance issues at each stage of the billing process.

- **Templates, Checklists, Procedures, and Worksheets on CD.** Develop procedures for your department, analyze errors, identify risk areas, record results, document actions, and more.

- **Addresses Interdepartmental Issues Central to Patient Accounts Management.** Helps to improve billing accuracy and compliance throughout your facility.

- **Deals with Fraud and Abuse Issues Specific to Patient Accounts.** Calls attention to the compliance issues pertinent to each function within PFS. Incorporates the OIG's compliance guidance for hospitals and the latest high-risk issues identified in the annual OIG work plan.

- **Co-published with HFMA.**

Call Toll-Free 1.877.INGENIX (464.3649) or Shop Online at www.IngenixOnline.com

Also Available from your Medical Bookstore or Distributor

2003 Publications

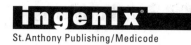
St. Anthony Publishing/Medicode

You Can Depend on Us for Answers to All Your Inpatient and Outpatient Billing Compliance Questions

Medicare Billing Compliance Guide

Item No. 2446 **$279.95**
*Call for CD multi-user pricing

Available: Now

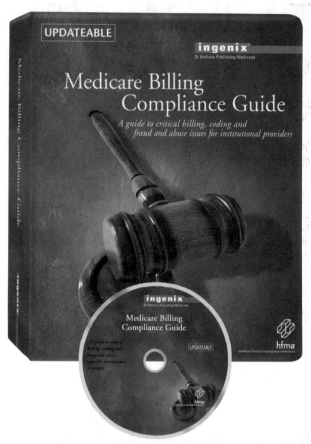

Since 1996 the *Medicare Billing Compliance Guide* has been providing guidance and interpretation of Medicare inpatient and outpatient billing and coding rules for hospitals and institutional providers in a language that your entire staff can understand.

This reliable guide will take you step by step through the Medicare maze of inpatient and outpatient billing and coding issues. Only the *Medicare Billing Compliance Guide* interprets Medicare requirements and translates them into easy-to-understand language, ensuring that you and your staff understand what you must to do stay in compliance.

- **Interpret Medicare Billing Rules and Fraud Issues.** Get easy-to-understand explanations, examples, and interpretations of Medicare billing rules, fraud issues, and OIG compliance program guidance. Plus, get answers to high-risk and complex billing questions affecting your hospital or facility.

- **Complete Coverage of Hospital Billing Rules and Targeted Fraud and Abuse Issues.** Includes complete information on Medicare fraud and abuse, corporate integrity agreements, fraud alerts, compliance program guidance, and OIG hot issues affecting hospitals. Ensures that your billing and coding practices are in compliance with Medicare program requirements. Helps you stay up to date on all of the OIG fraud and abuse initiatives and investigations.

- **A to Z Billing, Coding, and Coverage Rules— Fully Indexed.** Provides a quick, easy-to-use format to find important billing, coding, and coverage issues. Helps you easily find answers to your most pressing billing and coding questions, such as modifiers, medical coverage, observation services, emergency room, medical necessity and local medical review policies.

- **Updates for One Full Year.** Keeps you current with the regulatory changes that affect the accuracy of claim submission and billing operations at your facility.

- **Full Text of Product on CD-ROM in PDF Format.** Electronic solution for researching billing and fraud and abuse issues or problems. The jump links and search capabilities allow you to get the information you need quickly.

- **Co-published with HFMA.**

- **Earn 5 CEUS from AAPC.**

Call Toll-Free 1.877.INGENIX (464.3649) or Shop Online at www.IngenixOnline.com

Also Available from your Medical Bookstore or Distributor

060102

2003 Publications

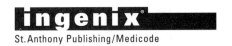
St. Anthony Publishing/Medicode

Take the Mystery Out of Medicare Coverage and Issuing ABNs

Complete Guide to Medicare Coverage Issues

Item No. 3036 **$279.95**
*Call for CD multi-user pricing

Available: Now

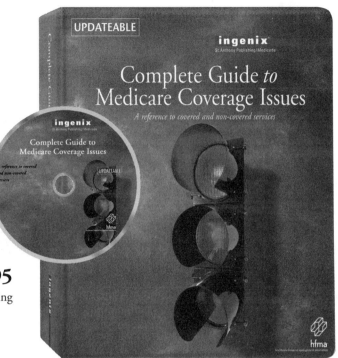

Know exactly which services and items Medicare will pay for, and which it won't, before you submit a claim.

This one-of-a-kind, updateable guide details Medicare's national coverage policies using CMS's official source documents. For any site of service, know what Medicare will and will not cover before submitting claims. Your subscription includes a CD-ROM with the full text of the manual and a newsletter with information about new and existing Medicare coverage for both Part A and Part B services.

- **New — Now Includes Pending National Decisions.**
  You'll have pending decisions available in one resource to help you and your staff manage all national coverage issues affecting Part A and Part B services.

- **Exclusive — Color-coded Coverage Prompts.**
  Know at a glance whether an item or procedure has restricted coverage, enabling you to make accurate coverage decisions promptly and submit bills correctly the first time. Helps prevent costly denials and claim resubmissions. Provides guidance regarding proper documentation for medical necessity, and helps you know when to issue an advance beneficiary notice for noncovered services. Also helps health plans understand Medicare coverage policies.

- **Fully Indexed.** Easily locate a specific item or service.

- **Updates and Coverage Alert Newsletter.** Keep you up to date on all new national Medicare coverage policies and revisions to existing policies.

- **Full Text of Manual on CD-ROM in PDF Format.**
  Electronic solution for researching national coverage decisions and medical necessity issues. Allows you to find key coverage issues and/or specific items and services with the click of a mouse. Other easy-to-use features include hypertext links and electronic bookmarks to take you quickly to the sections of the manual that you use the most.

- **Physicians' Current Procedural Terminology (CPT®) Codes and HCPCS Codes Assigned to National Issues.**
  Helps you identify coverage issues by CPT® or HCPCS code. Includes coverage issues pertaining to medical equipment, devices, procedures, clinical trials, and more!

- **Co-published with HFMA.**

- **Earn 5 CEUS from AAPC.**

CPT is a registered trademark of the American Medical Association

Call Toll-Free 1.877.INGENIX (464.3649) or Shop Online at www.IngenixOnline.com
Also Available from your Medical Bookstore or Distributor

4 Easy Ways to Order

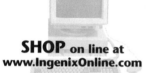

CALL toll-free
**1.800.INGENIX
(464.3649)**
and mention the
Source Code: FOBA3

SHOP on line at
www.IngenixOnline.com

MAIL this form with
payment and/or purchase
order to:
PO Box 27116
Salt Lake City, UT 84127-0116

FAX this order form with
credit card information and /or
purchase order to 801.982.4033

100% Money Back Guarantee

If our merchandise* ever fails to meet your expectations, please contact our Customer Service Department toll-free at 1.800.INGENIX (464.3649) for an immediate response. We will resolve any concern without hesitation.

*Software: Credit will be granted for unopened packages only.

| Shipping and Handling ||
No. of Items	Fee
1	$9.95
2-4	$11.95
5-7	$14.95
8-10	$19.95
11+	Call

PUBLICATION ORDER AND FAX FORM

FOBA

Customer No._____ Contact No._____

Purchase Order No._____ Source Code_____
(Attach copy of Purchase Order)

Contact Name _____ Title_____

Company_____

Address _____
(no P.O. Boxes, please)

City_____ State_____ Zip_____

Phone (____)_____ Fax (____)_____
(in case we have questions about your order)

IMPORTANT: E-MAIL REQUIRED FOR ORDER CONFIRMATION AND SELECT PRODUCT DELIVERY.
E-mail _____

☐ YES, I WANT TO RECEIVE SPECIAL REPORTS AND INFORMATION VIA E-MAIL.
☐ YES, I WANT TO RECEIVE NEW PRODUCT ANNOUNCEMENTS VIA E-MAIL.

Item #	Qty	Item Description	Price	Total
~~4025~~	~~1~~	~~(SAMPLE) DRG Guidebook~~	~~$89.95~~	~~$89.95~~
			Sub Total	
		TX, UT, OH, and VA residents please add applicable sales tax		
		Shipping & handling (see chart)		
		(11 plus items, foreign and Canadian orders, please call for shipping costs)		
		Total enclosed		

Payment Options

☐ Check enclosed. (Make payable to Ingenix, Inc.)
☐ Charge my: ☐ MasterCard ☐ VISA ☐ AMEX ☐ Discover
Card # | | | | | | | | | | | | | | | | Exp. Date: | | |
                                                                    MM YR
☐ Bill Me P.O.#_____
Signature _____

©2002 Ingenix, Inc. All prices subject to change without notice.

Preface

Since the federal government implemented diagnosis-related groups (DRGs) on October 1, 1983, medical record professionals and others have had to refer to many sources for ICD-9-CM codes and coding and reimbursement principles.

ICD-9-CM for Hospitals, Volumes 1, 2, and 3, has been designed with the hospital coder in mind. All three volumes of the most recent official government version of ICD-9-CM have been combined into one book.

Our technical experts have drawn upon their extensive hands-on experience to enhance the government's book with valuable features essential to correct coding and reimbursement. Without these enhancements, health information management departments would spend hours locating the information required to code each record accurately. Because of the thoroughness, accuracy, timeliness and ease of use of *ICD-9-CM for Hospitals,* health information departments nationwide have turned to them for their coding needs.

ICD-9-CM for Hospitals includes many of the enhancements described below in direct response to requests from our subscribers. As you review the content, you'll find the following:

- the complete ICD-9-CM official guidelines for coding and reporting, published by the U.S. Department of Health and Human Services and approved by the cooperating parties (American Hospital Association, American Health Information Management Association, Health Care Financing Administration and National Center for Health Statistics)
- all the official ICD-9-CM codes, indexes, notes, footnotes and symbols
- color-highlighted illustrations and clearly worded definitions integrated in the tabular, provide important clinical information
- exclusive color coding, symbols, and footnotes that alert coders to coding and reimbursement issues, including the majority of the Medicare code edits and identification of conditions that significantly affect DRG assignment of cardiovascular and HIV cases.
- the complication and comorbidity (CC) exclusion list, integrated beneath the applicable codes makes it easier to determine complications and comorbidities excluded with a particular principal diagnosis
- the American Hospital Association (AHA's) *Coding Clinic for ICD-9-CM references*, integrated beneath the applicable codes to provide easy reference to official coding advice as designated by the four cooperating parties (AHA, AHIMA, CMS, and NCHS)
- compliance symbol identifying diagnosis codes associated with DRGs targeted by the government for audit
- check fourth- and fifth-digit symbols identify codes that require the addition of a fourth or fifth digit for code specificity and validity
- symbols identify new codes and text revisions and pages are dated to indicate when the changes were made
- synopsis of the code changes for the current year
- color coding and symbol legend at the bottom of each page
- exclusive QuickFlip Color Tabs for quick, easy location of terms and codes in the index and tabular list

Please review "How to Use *ICD-9-CM for Hospital's (Volumes 1, 2, and 3)*" in this section to learn about the features that will help you assign and report correct codes, ensuring appropriate reimbursement.

USE OF OFFICIAL SOURCES

The *ICD-9-CM for Hospitals* contains the official U.S. Department of Health and Human Services, Ninth Revision, Sixth Edition ICD-9-CM codes, effective for the current year.

The color-coding, footnotes and symbols, which identify coding and reimbursement issues, are derived from official federal government sources, including the Medicare code edit (MCE), Version 20.0.

The American Hospital Association (AHA) Coding Clinic for ICD-9-CM references are used with permission of the AHA.

In addition to the editors, the following people have contributed to this book:

Stacy Perry, Desktop Publishing Manager
Kerrie Hornsby, Desktop Publishing Manger
Tracy Betzler, Desktop Publishing Specialist
Irene Day, Desktop Publishing Specialist
Paul Driscoll, Illustrator
Sheri Bernard, Director of Essential Regulatory Products
Lynn Speirs, Managing Editor

IMPORTANT INFORMATION ABOUT YOUR SUBSCRIPTION SERVICE

If you have purchased the updateable *ICD-9-CM Expert for Hospitals,* your subscription includes an updating service throughout the year to keep the code book current and accurate. The January update includes new illustrations and definitions, *AHA Coding Clinic* references for third and fourth quarter, the latest MCEs, and official errata changes. In July you will receive a list of all new, revised, and invalid codes for the upcoming year.

TECHNICAL EDITORS

Anita C. Hart, RHIA, CCS, CCS-P
Product Manager
Ingenix, Inc
Reston, VA

Ms. Hart's experience includes fifteen years conducting and publishing research in clinical medicine and human genetics for Yale University, Massachusetts General Hospital, and Massachusetts Institute of Technology. In addition, Ms. Hart has supervised medical records management, health information management, coding and reimbursement, and worker's compensation issues as the office manager for a physical therapy rehabilitation clinic. Ms. Hart is an expert in physician and facility coding, reimbursement systems, and compliance issues. Ms. Hart developed the *Complete Coding Tutor*, an advanced self-study guide for ICD-9-CM, CPT, and HCPCS Level II coding and served as technical consultant for numerous other publications for hospital and physician practices. Currrently, Ms. Hart is the Product Manager for the ICD-9-CM and DRG product lines.

Catherine A. Hopkins, CPC
Technical Consultant
Ingenix, Inc.
Reston, VA

Ms. Hopkins has 17 years of experience in the healthcare field. Her experience includes six years as office manager and senior coding specialist for a large multi-specialty practice. Ms. Hopkins has written several coding manuals and newsletters and has taught seminars on CPT, HCPCS, and ICD-9-CM coding. She also serves as technical support for various software products.

PRODUCT REVIEW PANEL

DeAnne Bloomquist, RHIT, CCS, Consultant and President, Mid-Continent Coding, Inc

Lori J. Date Daun, RHIT, Coder/Abstractor-OPDQ, Allina-Mercy Hospital

Nan-Jean Dobrowski, RHIT, CCs, Director, Medical Records, Delnor-Community Hospital

Corella Marie Fenwick, CCP, Compliance Auditor/Fiscal Coordinator, GWU, Dept. of Medicine

Gwen Kalor, RHIT, HIM Specialist, Coding, North Memorial Medical Center

Jo Ann Steigerwald, RHIT, Senior Healthcare Consultant, The Wellington Group

Denise Von Dohren, Manager, Reimbursement Planning, Merck & Co.

Carol Wojcik, MS, RHIA, CCS, CCS-P, Coding Supervisor, Central DuPage Hospital

Laura C. Zeranski, RHIA, Consultant, Laura Zeranski and Associates

WHAT TO DO IF YOU HAVE QUESTIONS

If you have any questions about your subscription, call our customer service department toll free at (800) INGENIX (464-3649).

If you have comments on the content of this book, please address them in writing to:
Product Manager, Ingenix, Inc.
11410 Isaac Newton Square,
Reston, VA 20190
Tel no.:(800) 464-3649;
Fax no.: (801) 982-4033

ADDITIONAL COPIES

Contact the customer service order department toll free at (800) INGENIX (464-3649).

Introduction

HISTORY AND FUTURE OF ICD•9

The International Classification of Diseases, Ninth Revision, Clinical Modification (ICD-9-CM) is based on the official version of the World Health Organization's Ninth Revision, International Classification of Diseases (ICD-9). ICD-9 classifies morbidity and mortality information for statistical purposes, and for the indexing of hospital records by disease and operations, for data storage and retrieval.

This modification of ICD-9 supplants the Eighth Revision International Classification of Diseases, Adapted for Use in the United States (ICDA-8) and the Hospital Adaptation of ICDA (H-ICDA).

The concept of extending the International Classification of Diseases for use in hospital indexing was originally developed in response to a need for a more efficient basis for storage and retrieval of diagnostic data. In 1950, the U.S. Public Health Service and the Veterans Administration began independent tests of the International Classification of Diseases for hospital indexing purposes. The following year, the Columbia Presbyterian Medical Center in New York City adopted the International Classification of Diseases, Sixth Revision, with some modifications for use in its medical record department. A few years later, the Commission on Professional and Hospital Activities (CPHA) in Ann Arbor, Mich., adopted the International Classification of Diseases with similar modifications for use in hospitals participating in the Professional Activity Study.

The problem of adapting ICD for indexing hospital records was taken up by the U.S. National Committee on Vital and Health Statistics through its subcommittee on hospital statistics. The subcommittee reviewed the modifications made by the various users of ICD and proposed that uniform changes be made. This was done by a small working party.

In view of the growing interest in the use of the International Classification of Diseases for hospital indexing, a study was undertaken in 1956 by the American Hospital Association and the American Medical Record Association (then the American Association of Medical Record Librarians) of the relative efficiencies of coding systems for diagnostic indexing. This study indicated the International Classification of Diseases provided a suitable and efficient framework for indexing hospital records. The major users of the International Classification of Diseases for hospital indexing purposes then consolidated their experiences, and an adaptation was first published in December 1959. A revision was issued in 1962 and the first "Classification of Operations and Treatments" was included.

In 1966, the international conference for revising the International Classification of Diseases noted the eighth revision of ICD had been constructed with hospital indexing in mind and considered the revised classification suitable, in itself, for hospital use in some countries. However, it was recognized that the basic classification might provide inadequate detail for diagnostic indexing in other countries.

A group of consultants was asked to study the eighth revision of ICD (ICD-8) for applicability to various users in the United States. This group recommended that further detail be provided for coding of hospital and morbidity data. The American Hospital Association was requested to develop the needed adaptation proposals. This was done by an advisory committee (the Advisory Committee to the Central Office on ICDA). In 1968 the United States Public Health Service published the product, Eighth Revision International Classification of Diseases, Adapted for Use in the United States. This became commonly known as ICDA-8, and beginning in 1968 it served as the basis for coding diagnostic data for both official morbidity and mortality statistics in the United States.

In 1968, the CPHA published the Hospital Adaptation of ICDA (H-ICDA) based on both the original ICD-8 and ICDA-8. In 1973, CPHA published a revision of H-ICDA, referred to as H-ICDA-2. Hospitals throughout the United States were divided in their use of these classifications until January 1979, when ICD-9-CM was made the single classification intended primarily for use in the United States, replacing these earlier related, but somewhat dissimilar, classifications.

Physicians have been required by law to submit diagnosis codes for Medicare reimbursement since the passage of the Medicare Catastrophic Coverage Act of 1988. This act requires physician offices to include the appropriate diagnosis codes when billing for services provided to Medicare beneficiaries on or after April 1, 1989. The Health Care Financing Administration designated ICD-9-CM as the coding system physicians must use.

In 1993 the World Health Organization published the newest version of International Classification of Diseases, Tenth Revision, ICD-10. This version contains the greatest number of changes in the history of ICD. There are more codes (5,500 more than ICD-9) to allow more specific reporting of diseases and newly recognized conditions. ICD-10 consists of three volumes; tabular list (volume I), instructions (volume 2) and the alphabetic index (volume 3). It contains 21 chapters including two supplementary ones. The codes are alphanumeric (A00–T98, V01–Y98 and Z00–Z99). Currently ICD-10 is being used in some European countries with implementation expected after the year 2000 in the United States.

ICD-9-CM BACKGROUND

In February 1977, a steering committee was convened by the National Center for Health Statistics to provide advice and counsel in developing a clinical modification of ICD-9. The organizations represented on the steering committee included the following:

- American Association of Health Data Systems
- American Hospital Association
- American Medical Record Association
- Association for Health Records

- Council on Clinical Classifications
- Centers for Medicare and Medicaid Services (formerly known as Health Care Financing Administration,) Department of Health and Human Services
- WHO Center for Classification of Diseases for North America, sponsored by the National Center for Health Statistics, Department of Health and Human Services

The Council on Clinical Classifications was sponsored by the following:

- American Academy of Pediatrics
- American College of Obstetricians and Gynecologists
- American College of Physicians
- American College of Surgeons
- American Psychiatric Association
- Commission on Professional and Hospital Activities

The steering committee met periodically in 1977. Clinical guidance and technical input were provided by task forces on classification from the Council on Clinical Classification's sponsoring organizations.

ICD-9-CM is a clinical modification of the World Health Organization's ICD-9. The term "clinical" is used to emphasize the modification's intent: to serve as a useful tool to classify morbidity data for indexing medical records, medical care review, and ambulatory and other medical care programs, as well as for basic health statistics. To describe the clinical picture of the patient, the codes must be more precise than those needed only for statistical groupings and trend analysis.

CHARACTERISTICS OF ICD-9-CM

ICD-9-CM far exceeds its predecessors in the number of codes provided. The disease classification has been expanded to include health-related conditions and to provide greater specificity at the fifth-digit level of detail. These fifth digits are not optional; they are intended for use in recording the information substantiated in the clinical record.

Volume I (tabular list) of ICD-9-CM contains five appendices:

Appendix A:	Morphology of Neoplasms
Appendix B:	Glossary of Mental Disorders
Appendix C:	Classification of Drugs by American Hospital Formulary Service List Number and Their ICD-9-CM Equivalents
Appendix D:	Classification of Industrial Accidents According to Agency
Appendix E:	List of Three-Digit Categories

These appendices are included as a reference to provide further information about the patient's clinical picture, to further define a diagnostic statement, to aid in classifying new drugs or to reference three-digit categories.

Volume 2 (alphabetic index) of ICD-9-CM contains many diagnostic terms that do not appear in Volume I since the index includes most diagnostic terms currently in use.

Volume 3 (procedure index and procedure tabular) of ICD-9-CM contains codes for operations and procedures. The format for the tabular is the same as Volume 1 disease tabular, except the codes consist of two digits with one or two digits following the decimal point. Conventions in the index follow Volume 2 conventions except some subterms appear immediately below the main term rather than following alphabetizing rules

THE DISEASE CLASSIFICATION

ICD-9-CM is totally compatible with its parent system, ICD-9, thus meeting the need for comparability of morbidity and mortality statistics at the international level. A few fourth-digit codes were created in existing three-digit rubrics only when the necessary detail could not be accommodated by the use of a fifth-digit subclassification. To ensure that each rubric of ICD-9-CM collapses back to its ICD-9 counterpart the following specifications governed the ICD-9-CM disease classification:

Specifications for the tabular list:

1. Three-digit rubrics and their contents are unchanged from ICD-9.
2. The sequence of three-digit rubrics is unchanged from ICD-9.
3. Three-digit rubrics are not added to the main body of the classification.
4. Unsubdivided three-digit rubrics are subdivided where necessary to
   - add clinical detail
   - isolate terms for clinical accuracy
5. The modification in ICD-9-CM is accomplished by adding a fifth digit to existing ICD-9 rubrics, except as noted under #7 below.
6. The optional dual classification in ICD-9 is modified.
   - Duplicate rubrics are deleted:
     - four-digit manifestation categories duplicating etiology entries
     - manifestation inclusion terms duplicating etiology entries
   - Manifestations of disease are identified, to the extent possible, by creating five-digit codes in the etiology rubrics.
   - When the manifestation of a disease cannot be included in the etiology rubrics, provision for its identification is made by retaining the ICD-9 rubrics used for classifying manifestations of disease.
7. The format of ICD-9-CM is revised from that used in ICD-9.
   - American spelling of medical terms is used.
   - Inclusion terms are indented beneath the titles of codes.
   - Codes not to be used for primary tabulation of disease are printed in italics with the notation, "code first underlying disease."

Specifications for the alphabetic index:

1. The format of the alphabetic index follows that of ICD-9.
2. When two codes are required to indicate etiology and manifestation, the manifestation code appears in brackets (e.g., diabetic cataract 250.5 [*366.41*]).

How to Use the ICD•9•CM for Hospitals (Volumes 1, 2, & 3)

This *ICD-9-CM for Hospitals* is based on the official version of the International Classification of Diseases, Ninth Revision, Clinical Modification, Sixth Edition, issued by the U.S. Department of Health and Human Services. Annual code changes are implemented by the government and are effective Oct. 1 and valid through Sept. 30 of the following year.

The code book is totally compatible with its parent system, ICD-9, thus meeting the need for comparability of morbidity and mortality statistics at the international level.

This book is consistent with the content of the government's version of ICD-9-CM. However, to accommodate the coder's approach to coding, the alphabetic index has been placed before the tabular list in both the disease and procedure classifications. This allows the user to locate the correct codes in a logical, natural manner by locating the term in the index, then confirming the accuracy of the code in the tabular list.

STEPS TO CORRECT CODING

1. Look up the main term in the alphabetic index and scan the subterm entries as appropriate. Follow any cross-references such as "*see*" and "*see also.*" Do not code from the alphabetic index without verifying the accuracy of the code in the tabular list.
2. Locate the code in the numerically arranged tabular list.
3. Observe the punctuation, footnotes, cross-references, color-coded prompts and other conventions described in the 'Conventions' section.
4. To determine the appropriateness of the code selection, read all instructional material:
   - "includes" and "*excludes*" notes
   - "*see,*" "*see also*" and "*see category*" cross-references
   - "use additional code" and "*code first underlying disease*" instructions
   - "code also" and "*omit code*" notes
   - fourth- and fifth-digit requirements
   - CC exclusions
5. Consult definitions, relevant illustrations, CC exclusions, color coding and reimbursement prompts, the check fourth- and fifth-digit, age and sex symbols. Refer to the color/symbol legend at the bottom of each page for symbols. Refer to the list of footnotes that is included in the "Additional Conventions" section of this book for a full explanation of a footnote associated with a code.
6. Consult the official ICD-9-CM guidelines for coding and reporting, and refer to the AHA's *Coding Clinic for ICD-9-CM* for coding guidelines governing the use of specific codes.
7. Confirm and transcribe the correct code.

ORGANIZATION

Introduction
The introductory material in this book includes the history and future of ICD-9-CM as well as an overview of the classification system

Official ICD-9-CM Conventions
This section provides a full explanation of all the official footnotes, symbols, instructional notes, and conventions found in the official government version

Additional Conventions
Exclusive color-coding, symbols, and notations have been included in the *ICD-9-CM for Hospitals, Volumes 1, 2 & 3*, to alert coders to important coding and reimbursement issues. This section provides a full explanation of the additional conventions used throughout this book.

Coding Guidelines
Included in this book are the official ICD-9-CM coding guidelines as approved by the four cooperating parties of the ICD-9-CM Coordination and Maintenance Committee. Failure to comply with the official coding guidelines may result in denied or delayed claims.

Synopsis of Code Changes
This section includes a complete listing of all new code changes for the current year.

Disease Classification: Alphabetic Index to Diseases
The Alphabetic Index to Diseases is separated by tabs labeled with the letters of the alphabet, contains diagnostic terms for illnesses, injuries and reasons for encounters with health care professionals. The Table of Drugs and Chemicals is easily located with the tab in this section.

Disease Classification: Tabular List of Diseases
The Tabular List of Diseases arranges the ICD-9-CM codes and descriptors numerically. Tabs divide this section into chapters, identified by the code range on the tab.

The tabular list includes two supplementary classifications:

- V Codes—Supplementary Classification of Factors Influencing Health Status and Contact with Health Services (V01–V83)
- E Codes—Supplementary Classification of External Causes of Injury and Poisoning (E800–E999)

ICD-9-CM includes five official appendixes.

- Appendix A Morphology of Neoplasms
- Appendix B Glossary of Mental Disorders
- Appendix C Classification of Drugs by AHFS List
- Appendix D Classification of Industrial Accidents According to Agency
- Appendix E List of Three-digit Categories

These appendices are included as a reference to provide further information about the patient's circumstances, help further define a diagnostic statement, maintain a tumor registry and aid in classifying new drugs.

Procedure Classification: Alphabetic Index to Procedures
The Alphabetic Index to Procedures lists common surgical and procedural terminology.

Procedure Classification: Tabular List of Procedures
The Tabular List of Procedures numerically arranges the procedure codes and their descriptors.

RESOURCES
Listed below are the exclusive resources found ONLY in the *ICD-9-CM Expert for Hospitals, Volumes 1, 2 & 3* books.

Dx/MDC/DRG List
Provides the complete list of diagnosis codes and the MDC and DRG to which they group, except when a secondary diagnosis affects DRG assignment for a quick audit.

CC Condition List
A complete list of all codes considered CC (Complications and Comorbidities) that will affect DRG assignment. This an essential auditing tool for assigning the most appropriate DRG.

Pharmacological Listings
The most common generic and brand names of drugs are linked with the disease processes to assist in the identification of CC, thereby improving DRG assignment practices.

Valid Three-digit Code Table
ICD-9-CM is composed of codes with either 3, 4, or 5 digits. A code is invalid if it has not been coded to the full number of digits required for that code. There are a certain number codes that are valid for reporting as three digit codes. A list of the valid three-digit code is included as a convenient reference when auditing claims.

ICD-9-CM Official Conventions

ICD-9-CM FOOTNOTES, SYMBOLS, INSTRUCTIONAL NOTES AND CONVENTIONS

This *ICD-9-CM for Hospitals* preserves all the footnotes, symbols, instructional notes and conventions found in the government's official version. Accurate coding depends upon understanding the meaning of these elements.

The following appear in the disease tabular list, unless otherwise noted.

OFFICIAL GOVERNMENT SYMBOLS

§ The section mark preceding a code denotes a footnote on the page. This symbol is used in the Tabular List of Diseases and in the Tabular List of Procedures.

ICD-9-CM CONVENTIONS USED IN THE TABULAR LIST

In addition to the symbols and footnotes above, the ICD-9-CM disease tabular has certain abbreviations, punctuation, symbols and other conventions. Our *ICD-9-CM for Hospitals* preserves these conventions. Proper use of the conventions will lead to efficient and accurate coding.

Abbreviations

NEC Not elsewhere classifiable

This abbreviation is used when the ICD-9-CM system does not provide a code specific for the patient's condition.

NOS Not otherwise specified

This abbreviation is the equivalent of 'unspecified' and is used only when the coder lacks the information necessary to code to a more specific four-digit subcategory.

[ ] Brackets enclose synonyms, alternative terminology or explanatory phrases:

482.2 Pneumonia due to Hemophilus influenzae [H. influenzae]

Brackets that appear beneath a code indicate the fifth digits that are considered valid fifth digits for the code. This convention is applied for those instances in ICD-9-CM where not all common fifth digits are considered valid for each subcategory within a category.

715.0 Osteoarthrosis, generalized
[0,4,9]

Generalized arthrosis can only be assigned in cases for which the degenerative joint disease involves multiple joints. Therefore, this code is considered for arthrosis in the sites described as unspecified, hand (which consists of multiple joints), or multiple sites. Therefore, only fifth digits 0, 4, and 9 are valid with subcategory 715.0.

( ) Parentheses enclose supplementary words, called nonessential modifiers, that may be present in the narrative description of a disease without affecting the code assignment:

198.4 Other parts of nervous system
   Meninges (cerebral) (spinal)

: Colons are used in the tabular list after an incomplete term that needs one or more of the modifiers that follow in order to make it assignable to a given category:

021.1 Enteric tularemia
   Tularemia:
      cryptogenic
      intestinal
      typhoidal

} Braces enclose a series of terms, each of which is modified by the statement appearing to the right of the brace:

560.2 Volvulus
   Knotting
   Strangulation } of intestine, bowel, or
   Torsion   colon
   Twist

OTHER CONVENTIONS

Boldface Boldface type is used for all codes and titles in the tabular list.

Italicized Italicized type is used for all exclusion notes and to identify codes that should not be used for describing the primary diagnosis.

INSTRUCTIONAL NOTES

These notes appear only in the Tabular List of Diseases

Includes An includes note further defines or clarifies the content of the chapter, subchapter, category, subcategory or subclassification. The includes note in the example below applies only to category 461.

Excludes Terms following the word "*Excludes*" are not classified to the chapter, subchapter, category, subcategory or specific subclassification code under which it is found. The note also may provide the location of the excluded diagnosis. Excludes notes are italicized.

461 Acute sinusitis

INCLUDES abscess
empyema
infection   acute, of sinus
inflammation   (accessory)
suppuration   (nasal)

EXCLUDES *chronic or unspecified sinusitis (473.0-473.9)*

Use additional code:

This instruction signals the coder that an additional code should be used if the information is available to provide a more complete picture of that diagnosis.

330 Cerebral degenerations usually manifest in childhood

Use additional code to identify associated mental retardation

Code first underlying disease:

This instruction is used in those categories not intended for primary tabulation of disease. These codes, called manifestation codes, may never be used alone or indicated as the primary diagnosis (i.e., sequenced first). They must always be preceded by another code.

The code and its descriptor appear in italics in the tabular list. The instruction "*Code first underlying disease*" is usually followed by the code or codes for the most common underlying disease (etiology). Record the code for the etiology or origin of the disease, and then record the italicized manifestation code in the next position.

590.81 Pyelitis or pyelonephritis in diseases classified elsewhere

Code first underlying disease as:
tuberculosis (016.0)

Code, if applicable, any causal condition first:

A code with this note may be principal if no causal condition is applicable or known.

590.0 Chronic pyelonephritis
Chronic pyelitis
Chronic pyonephrosis
Code, if applicable, any causal condition first

Omit code

"*Omit code*" is used to instruct the coder that no code is to be assigned. When this instruction is found in the Alphabetic Index to Diseases the medical term should not be coded as a diagnosis.

Metaplasia
cervix—*omit code*

When used in Volume 3, 'omit code' is meant to indicate procedures that do not merit separate code assignments, such as minor procedures preformed in conjunction with more extensive procedures or procedures that represent an operative approach.

Arthrotomy 80.10
as operative approach—*omit code*

Additional Conventions

NEW AND REVISED TEXT SYMBOLS

● A bullet at a code or line of text indicates that that the entry is new.

▲ A triangle in the Tabular List indicates that the code title is revised. In the Alphabetic Index the triangle indicates that a code has changed.

►◄ These symbols appear at the beginning and at the end of a section of new or revised text.

When these symbols appear on a page there will be a date on the lower outside corner of the page indicating the date of the change, (e.g., October 2002).

ADDITIONAL DIGITS REQUIRED

√3rd This symbol indicates that the code requires a third digit.

√4th This symbol indicates that the code requires a fourth digit.

√5th This symbol indicates that a code requires a fifth digit.

DEFINITIONS

DEF: This symbol indicates a definition of disease or procedure term. The definition will appear in blue type in the Disease and Procedure Tabular Lists.

AHA *CODING CLINIC FOR ICD-9-CM* REFERENCES

The four cooperating parties have designated the AHA's *Coding Clinic for ICD-9-CM* as the official publication for coding guidelines. The references are identified by the notation AHA: followed by the issue, year and page number.

In the example below, AHA *Coding Clinic for ICD-9-CM*, third quarter 1991, page 15, contains a discussion on code assignment for vitreous hemorrhage:

> 379.23 **Vitreous hemorrhage**
> AHA: 3Q, '91, 15

The table below explains the abbreviations in the *Coding Clinic* references:

J-F	January/February
M-A	March/April
M-J	May/June
J-A	July/August
S-O	September/October
N-D	November/December
1Q	First quarter
2Q	Second quarter
3Q	Third quarter
4Q	Fourth quarter

MEDICARE CODE EDITS

Fiscal intermediaries use the Medicare Code Editor (MCE) to check the coding accuracy on claims. The Medicare code edits are listed below:

1. Invalid diagnosis or procedure code
2. E-code as principal diagnosis
3. Duplicate of principal diagnosis (PDx) (as applied to a secondary diagnosis)
* 4. Age conflict
* 5. Sex conflict
* 6. Manifestation code as principal diagnosis
* 7. Nonspecific principal diagnosis
* 8. Questionable admission
*9. Unacceptable principal diagnosis
*10. Nonspecific OR procedure
*11. Noncovered procedure
12. Open biopsy check
*13. Bilateral procedure
14. Invalid age
15. Invalid sex
16. Invalid discharge status

Starred edits are identified by colors, symbols or footnotes as described on the next page.

Age and Sex Edit Symbols

The age edits below address MCE edits and are used to detect inconsistencies between the patient's age and diagnosis. They appear in the Tabular List of Diseases to the right of the code description.

Newborn Age: 0
These diagnoses are intended for newborns and neonates and the patient's age must be 0 years

Pediatric Age: 0-17
These diagnoses are intended for children and the patient's age must between 0 and 17 years

Maternity Age: 12-55
These diagnoses are intended for the patients between the age of 12 and 55 years

Adult Age: 15-124
These diagnoses are intended for the patients between the age of 15 and 124 years.

The sex symbols below address MCE edits and are used to detect inconsistencies between the patient's sex and diagnosis. They appear in the Tabular Lists to the right of the code description:

♂ **Male diagnosis only**

This symbol appears to the right of the code description. This reference appears in the disease tabular list.

♀ **Female diagnosis only**

This symbol appears to the right of the code description. This reference appears in the disease tabular list.

Color Coding

For a quick reference to the color codes and their meaning, refer to the color/symbol legend located at the bottom of each page.

To alert the coder to important reimbursement issues affected by the code assignment, color bars have been added. The colors represent Medicare code edits as well as other reimbursement issues.

Color coding appears in both tabular lists. Some codes carry more than one color. Please note that the same color may appear in the disease and procedure tabular lists, but with different meanings.

Disease Tabular List
Manifestation Code

These codes will appear in italic type as well as with a blue color bar over the code title. A manifestation code is not allowed to be reported as a primary diagnosis because each describes a manifestation of some other underlying disease, not the disease itself. This is also referred to as mandatory multiple coding. Code the underlying disease first. A *'Code first underlying disease'* instructional note will appear with underlying disease codes identified. In the Alphabetic Index these codes are listed as the secondary code in slanted bracket with the code for the underlying disease listed first. Medicare code edit (MCE) 6

Unacceptable PDx

These codes will appear with a gray color bar over the code title. These codes do not describe a current illness or injury, but a circumstance which influences a patient's health status. These are considered an unacceptable principal diagnosis for inpatient admission. Medicare code edit (MCE) 9

Questionable Admission

These codes will also appear with a gray color bar over the code title. These codes identify a condition that usually is insufficient justification for hospital admission. Since these codes are considered an unacceptable principal diagnoses for inpatient admission, they are color coded in the same manner as the "unacceptable PDx codes". Medicare code edit (MCE) 8

Nonspecific PDx

These codes will have a yellow color bar over the code title. While these codes are considered valid ICD-9-CM codes, for inpatients discharged alive, a more specific principal diagnosis should be assigned. These codes are used when the neither the diagnostic statement nor the documentation provides enough information to assign a more specified diagnosis code. These codes may be stated as "Unspecified" or "Not otherwise specified (NOS)." Medicare code edit (MCE) 7

Procedure Tabular List
Non-specific OR Procedure

While this code is a valid unspecific or not otherwise specified (NOS) procedure code, a more precise code should be used. The code is recognized as a nonspecific operating room procedure ONLY if ALL OR procedures performed are coded NOS. Medicare Code Edit (MCE 10)

Valid OR

A procedure that triggers a change in DRG assignment.

Non-OR Procedure

A non-operating room procedure that affects DRG assignment.

Footnotes

All footnotes are identified by a numerical superscript that appears to the upper left of the code:

[1]**718.5 Ankylosis of joint**

The footnote 1 indicates "Nonspecific PDx = 0". This means that when code 718.50, Ankylosis of the joint, site unspecified, the diagnosis is considered a nonspecific principal diagnosis. While this code may be valid according to ICD-9-CM, a more precise diagnosis should be used for the principal diagnosis for inpatient admission.

The following list identifies the meaning of each footnote number and the classification in which the footnote appears:

Disease Tabular
1. Nonspecific PDx = 0
2. Nonspecific PDx = 9
3. These V codes may be used as principal diagnosis on Medicare patients.
4. This V code, with the fourth digit of 1 or 2, is unacceptable as a principal diagnosis.
5. These codes, with the fourth digit of 0 or 1, may be used as a principal diagnosis for Medicare patients.
6. Rehabilitation codes acceptable as a principal diagnosis when accompanied by a secondary diagnosis reflecting the condition treated.
7. These V codes are acceptable as principal diagnosis when accompanied by a diagnosis of personal history of malignancy. These codes group to DRG 465.
8. Questionable admission = 0
9. The codes with fifth-digit of 1 are considered a major complication condition that causes DRG assignment from DRG 121 to DRG 122.

Procedure Tabular
10. Valid OR procedure code if accompanied by one of the following codes: 37.80, 37.81, 37.82, 37.85, 37.86, 37.87.
11. Valid OR procedure code if accompanied by one of the following codes: 37.80, 37.83.
12. Valid OR procedure code if accompanied by one of the following codes: 37.80, 37.85, 37.86, 37.87.
13. Valid OR procedure code if accompanied by any one of the following codes: 37.80, 37.81, 37.82, 37.83, 37.85, 37.86, 37.87.

14 Valid OR procedure code if accompanied by any other pacemaker procedure except 37.72, 37.76.

15 Valid OR procedure code if accompanied by any other pacemaker procedure except 37.70, 37.71, 37.73, 37.76.

16 Nonspecific OR procedure = 0.

17 Noncovered procedure only if none of the following codes are present as either a principal or secondary diagnosis: 200.00-202.08, 202.80-202.98, 204.01, 205.01, 206.01, 207.01, 208.01.

18 Noncovered procedure only if none of the following codes are present as either a principal or secondary diagnosis: 204.00-208.91, 279.12, 279.2, 284.0-284.9

19 Noncovered procedure unless diagnosis code is present from 250.00–250.93 and 585, V42.0 or V43.89

Other Notations

Disease Tabular
CC Exclusion List

A exclusive feature of *ICD-9-CM for Hospitals* is the integration of the government's CC exclusion list with each affected code.

The CC exclusion list indicates secondary diagnosis codes that are excluded as CC conditions with certain principal diagnoses. This exclusion occurs because the cited conditions are inherent to the disease process of the principal diagnosis.

Listed below each code that is considered a complication or comorbidity (CC) diagnosis, are the codes or code ranges of principal diagnosis with which the CC code cannot be used.

In the example below, code 254.1 is normally a CC condition. However, the CC exclusion (CC Excl:) notation indicates that if a code from the listed code ranges is assigned as the principal diagnosis, the secondary diagnosis of 254.0 will not be recognized as a CC condition in DRG assignment.

> **254.1 Abscess of thymus**
> CC Excl: 254.0-254.1, 254.8-254.9, 259.8-259.9

CC Condition

A complication or comorbidity diagnosis that may change DRG assignment. A complication is defined as a condition that arises during the hospital stay that extends the length of stay by at least one day in 75 percent of the cases. A comorbidity is a pre-existing condition that will, because of its presence with a specific principal diagnosis, that extends the length of stay by at least one day in 75 percent of the cases.

CC listed with a digit or range of digits indicates the fifth-digit assignments for that code that are considered CC conditions. Example: code 250.1 has a symbol CC 1-3 which means that only 250.11, 250.12, and 250.13 are considered CC conditions. Code 251.0 is not a CC condition.

Major Cardiovascular Complication

A complication that causes the DRG to change from DRG 122 to DRG 121.

Complex Diagnosis

A diagnosis that causes the DRG assignment of a case to change from DRG 125 to DRG 124.

Medicare as Secondary Payer

Specific trauma diagnoses are identified that alert fiscal intermediaries (FIs) that another carrier should be billed first and Medicare billed second if payment from the first payer does not equal or exceed the amount Medicare would pay.

DRG

This symbol indicates the diagnosis is assigned to a diagnosis related group (DRG) that has been targeted for audit. The condition must be thoroughly documented in the medical record to prevent inappropriate coding or "upcoding."

HIV

This symbol indicates that the condition is considered a major HIV related diagnosis. When the condition is coded in combination with a diagnosis of human immunodeficiency virus (HIV), code 042, the case will move from DRG 490 to DRG 489.

Procedure Tabular
Noncovered procedure

A procedure not covered by Medicare. In some instances this procedure may also be identified as a valid operating room (OR) procedure that may trigger a DRG assignment. Even if a DRG assignment is made, Medicare may not reimburse for the noncovered procedure. (MCE 11)

Bilateral Edit

Due to the lack of laterality in ICD-9-CM, there are certain lower extremity joint procedure codes that do not accurately reflect procedures that are performed in one admission on two or more different bilateral joints. To group to DRG 471, Bilateral or Multiple Joint Procedures of Lower Extremity, a case must be coded with a combination of two or more different major lower extremity joint procedures. The bilateral procedure symbol identifies those procedure codes that when coded twice represent the same procedure performed on both of the same bilateral joints of the lower extremity. Otherwise, a code edit will instruct the fiscal intermediary to verify that the two different procedures were performed on two different bilateral joints. (MCE 13)

Summary of Code Changes

DISEASE TABULAR LIST (VOLUME 1)

038	Excludes term added
● 040.82	Toxic shock syndrome Use additional code note added
062.8	Excludes note added
066.3	Includes term deleted
● 066.4	West Nile fever Includes notes added
256.2	Use additional code note added Excludes term deleted
256.3	Use additional code note revised
277.00	Includes note added
● 277.02	Cystic fibrosis with pulmonary manifestations Includes note added Use additional code note added
● 277.03	Cystic fibrosis with gastrointestinal manifestations Excludes note added
● 277.09	Cystic fibrosis with other manifestations
277.7	Use additional code note revised
337.3	Use additional code note revised
357.8	Includes note deleted
● 357.81	Chronic inflammatory demyelinating polyneuritis
● 357.82	Critical illness polyneuropathy Includes note added
● 357.89	Other inflammatory and toxic neuropathy
● 359.81	Critical illness myopathy Includes note added
● 359.89	Other myopathies
● 365.83	Aqueous misdirection Includes note added
368.6	Includes term deleted
402	Use additional code note added
▲ 402.00	Hypertensive heart disease, malignant, without congestive heart failure
▲ 402.01	Hypertensive heart disease, malignant, with congestive heart failure
▲ 402.10	Hypertensive heart disease, benign, without congestive heart failure
▲ 402.11	Hypertensive heart disease, benign, with congestive heart failure
▲ 402.90	Hypertensive heart disease, unspecified, without congestive heart failure
▲ 402.91	Hypertensive heart disease, unspecified, with congestive heart failure
404	Use additional code note added Fifth-digit code definitions revised 0 without mention of congestive heart failure or renal failure 1 with congestive heart failure 2 with congestive heart failure and renal failure
▲ 404.00	Hypertensive heart and renal disease, malignant, without mention of congestive heart failure or renal failure
▲ 404.01	Hypertensive heart and renal disease, malignant, with congestive heart failure
▲ 404.03	Hypertensive heart and renal disease, malignant, with congestive heart failure and renal failure
▲ 404.10	Hypertensive heart and renal disease, benign, without mention of congestive heart failure or renal failure
▲ 404.11	Hypertensive heart and renal disease, benign, with congestive heart failure
▲ 404.13	Hypertensive heart and renal disease, benign, with congestive heart failure and renal failure
▲ 404.90	Hypertensive heart and renal disease, unspecified, without mention of congestive heart failure or renal failure
▲ 404.91	Hypertensive heart and renal disease, unspecified, with congestive heart failure
▲ 404.93	Hypertensive heart and renal disease, unspecified, with congestive heart failure and renal failure
411.81	Excludes terms revised
● 414.06	Coronary atherosclerosis of coronary artery of transplanted heart
▲ 414.1	Aneurysm ►and dissection◄ of heart
▲ 414.10	►Aneurysm◄ of heart (wall)
▲ 414.11	►Aneurysm◄ of coronary vessels
● 414.12	Dissection of coronary artery
▲ 414.19	Other ►aneurysm of heart◄
427.89	Excludes terms added
428	Excludes term deleted Code, if applicable, note added
▲ 428.0	Congestive heart failure, ►unspecified◄ Excludes note added
● 428.2	Systolic heart failure Excludes note added
● 428.20	Systolic heart failure, unspecified
● 428.21	Systolic heart failure, acute
● 428.22	Systolic heart failure, chronic
● 428.23	Systolic heart failure, acute on chronic
● 428.3	Diastolic heart failure Excludes note added
● 428.30	Diastolic heart failure, unspecified
● 428.31	Diastolic heart failure, acute
● 428.32	Diastolic heart failure, chronic
● 428.33	Diastolic heart failure, acute on chronic
● 428.4	Combined systolic and diastolic heart failure
● 428.40	Combined systolic and diastolic heart failure, unspecified
● 428.41	Combined systolic and diastolic heart failure, acute
● 428.42	Combined systolic and diastolic heart failure, chronic
● 428.43	Combined systolic and diastolic heart failure, acute on chronic
(430-438)	Cerebrovascular Disease section Excludes term added
436	Excludes term added
● 438.6	Late effects of cerebrovascular disease, alterations of sensations Use additional code note added
● 438.7	Late effects of cerebrovascular disease, disturbances of vision Use additional code note added
● 438.83	Other late effects of cerebrovascular disease, facial weakness Includes term added
● 438.84	Other late effects of cerebrovascular disease, ataxia
● 438.85	Other late effects of cerebrovascular disease, vertigo
440	Excludes term added
440.8	Excludes term revised
441.0	Includes note deleted
● 443.2	Other arterial dissection Excludes note added
● 443.21	Dissection of carotid artery
● 443.22	Dissection of iliac artery
● 443.23	Dissection of renal artery
● 443.24	Dissection of vertebral artery
● 443.29	Dissection of other artery
444	Excludes term added
● 445	Atheroembolism Includes note added
● 445.0	Atheroembolism, of extermities
● 445.01	Atheroembolism, upper extermity
● 445.02	Atheroembolism, lower extremity
● 445.8	Atheroembolism, of other sites
● 445.81	Atheroembolism, kidney Use additional code note added
● 445.89	Atheroembolism, other site
447.6	Excludes term revised
● 454.8	Varicose veins of the lower extremities, with other complications Includes note added

►◄ Revised Text ● New Code ▲ Revised Code Title

▲ 454.9	Varicose veins of lower extremities, ~~without mention of ulcer or inflammation~~ ▶asymptomatic varicose veins◀ Includes term added
459.1	Includes note added Excludes note added
● 459.10	Postphlebetic syndrome without complications Includes note added
● 459.11	Postphlebetic syndrome with ulcer
● 459.12	Postphlebetic syndrome with inflammation
● 459.13	Postphlebetic syndrome with ulcer and inflammation
● 459.19	Postphlebetic syndrome with other complication
● 459.3	Chronic venous hypertension (idiopathic) Includes note added Excludes note added
● 459.30	Chronic venous hypertension without complications Includes note added
● 459.31	Chronic venous hypertension with ulcer
● 459.32	Chronic venous hypertension with inflammation
● 459.33	Chronic venous hypertension with ulcer and inflammation
● 459.39	Chronic venous hypertension with other complication
491.2	Includes term deleted
491.20	Includes term deleted
491.21	Includes term deleted
493.2	Includes term added Excludes term deleted
518.81	Excludes term revised
518.82	Excludes term revised
● 537.84	Dieulafoy lesion (hemorrhagic) of stomach and duodenum
● 569.86	Dieulafoy lesion (hemorrhagic) of intestine
577.8	Excludes term revised
590.0	Code first note deleted Code, if applicable, note added
593.7	Use additional code note deleted
599.0	Excludes term added
602.3	Includes terms revised Excludes terms revised
622.1	Includes terms added
▲ 627.2	▶Symptomatic◀ menopausal or female climacteric states
▲ 627.4	▶Symptomatic◀ states associated with artificial menopause
629.0	Excludes term revised
● 633.00	Abdominal pregnancy without intrauterine pregnancy
● 633.01	Abdominal pregnancy with intrauterine pregnancy
● 633.10	Tubal pregnancy without intrauterine pregnancy
● 633.11	Tubal pregnancy with intrauterine pregnancy
● 633.20	Ovarian pregnancy without intrauterine pregnancy
● 633.21	Ovarian pregnancy with intrauterine pregnancy
● 633.80	Other ectopic pregnancy without intrauterine pregnancy
● 633.81	Other ectopic pregnancy with intrauterine pregnancy
● 633.90	Unspecified ectopic pregnancy without intrauterine pregnancy
● 633.91	Unspecified ectopic pregnancy with intrauterine pregnancy
646.6	Includes term revised
647.1	Excludes note added
707.1	Code first note revised Code, if applicable, terms added
710	Use additional code note deleted
710.1	Use additional code note added
718.7	Excludes terms deleted Excludes terms added
723.5	Excludes term added
730.1	Includes term deleted
733.4	Excludes term deleted
● 747.83	Persistent fetal circulation Includes note added
751.7	Excludes term revised
753.0	Code first note deleted
753.15	Code first note deleted
(764-779)	Other conditions originating in the perinatal period section Fifth-digit subclassification instructions revised
▲ 765	Disorders relating to short gestation and low birthweight
765.0	Instructional note revised Use additional code note added
765.1	Instrucitonal note revised Use additional code note added
● 765.2	Disorders relating to short gestation and low birthweight, weeks of gestation
● 765.20	Unspecified weeks of gestation
● 765.21	Less than 24 completed weeks of gestation
● 765.22	24 completed weeks of gestation
● 765.23	25-26 completed weeks of gestation
● 765.24	27-28 completed weeks of gestation
● 765.25	29-30 completed weeks of gestation
● 765.26	31-32 completed weeks of gestation
● 765.27	33-34 completed weeks of gestation
● 765.28	35-36 completed weeks of gestation
● 765.29	37 or more completed weeks of gestation
770.8	Includes note deleted
● 770.81	Primary apnea of newborn Includes note added
● 770.82	Other apnea of newborn Includes note added
● 770.83	Cyanotic attacks of newborn
● 770.84	Respiratory failure of newborn Excludes note added
● 770.89	Other respiratory problems after birth
771.8	Includes note deleted Use additional code note added
● 771.81	Septicemia [sepsis] of newborn
● 771.82	Urinary tract infection of newborn
● 771.83	Bacteremia of newborn
● 771.89	Other infections specific to the perinatal period Includes note added
774.5	Code first term revised
● 779.81	Neonatal bradycardia Excludes note added
● 779.82	Neonatal tachycardia Excludes note added
● 779.89	Other specified conditions originating in the perinatal period
780.9	Includes note deleted
● 780.91	Fussy infant (baby)
● 780.92	Excessive crying of infant (baby)
● 780.99	Other general symptoms Includes note added
● 781.93	Ocular torticollis
782.5	Excludes note revised
785.0	Excludes note added
786.03	Excludes term added
786.09	Excludes terms revised
788.3	Code first note deleted Code, if applicable, note added
790.7	Excludes term added
795.0	Includes note deleted Excludes note added
● 795.00	Nonspecific abnormal Papanicolaou smear of cervix, unspecified
● 795.01	Atypical squamous cell changes of undetermined significance favor benign (ASCUS favor benign) Includes note added
● 795.02	Atypical squamous cell changes of undetermined significance favor dysplasia (ASCUS favor dysplasia) Includes note added
● 795.09	Other nonspecific abnormal Papanicolaou smear of cervix Includes note added
● 795.31	Nonspecific positive findings for anthrax Includes term added
● 795.39	Other nonspecific positive culture findings
799.1	Excludes terms revised
(800-829)	Fractures section Instructional note revised
● 813.45	Torus fracture of radius
● 823.4	Fracture of tibia and fibula, torus fracture
959.01	Excludes term added
991.6	Excludes term revised
995.0	Code first note deleted
● 995.9	Systemic inflammatory response syndrome (SIRS)
● 995.90	Systemic inflammatory response syndrome, unspecified Includes note added

▶◀ Revised Text ● New Code ▲ Revised Code Title

● 995.91	Systemic inflammatory response syndrome due to infectious process without organ dysfunction	● V54.22	Aftercare for healing pathologic fracture of lower arm	● V71.83	Observation and evaluation for suspected exposure to other biological agent	
● 995.92	Systemic inflammatory response syndrome due to infectious process with organ dysfunction Includes note added Use additional code note added	● V54.23	Aftercare for healing pathologic fracture of hip	● V83.8	Other genetic carrier status	
		● V54.24	Aftercare for healing pathologic fracture of leg, unspecified	● V83.81	Cystic fibrosis gene carrier	
		● V54.25	Aftercare for healing pathologic fracture of upper leg Excludes note added	● V83.89	Other genetic carrier status	
● 995.93	Systemic inflammatory response syndrome due to non-infectious process without organ dysfunction			● E885.0	Fall from (nonmotorized) scooter	
		● V54.26	Aftercare for healing pathologic fracture of lower leg	● E922.5	Accident caused by firearm, and air gun missle, paintball gun	
● 995.94	Systemic inflammatory response syndrome due to non-infectious process with organ dysfunction Use additional code note added	● V54.27	Aftercare for healing pathologic fracture of vertebrae	● E955.7	Suicide and self-inflicted injury by firearms, air guns and explosives, paintball gun	
		● V54.29	Aftercare for healing pathologic fracture of other bone	E960-E969	Homicide and injury purposely inflicted by other persons section Excludes term added	
996.72	Excludes note revised	V54.8	Includes note deleted	● (E979)	Terrorism (E979) new section	
● 998.31	Disruption of internal operation wound	● V54.81	Aftercare following joint replacement Use additional code note added	● E979	Terrorism Instructional note added	
● 998.32	Disruption of external operation wound Includes note added			● E979.0	Terrorism involving explosion of marine weapons Includes note added	
		● V54.89	Other orthopedic aftercare Includes note added			
● V01.81	Contact with or exposure to anthrax	V58.4	Instructional note added	● E979.1	Terrorism involving destruction of aircraft Includes note added	
		● V58.42	Aftercare following surgery for neoplasm Includes note added			
● V01.89	Contact with or exposure to other communicable diseases			● E979.2	Terrorism involving other explosions and fragments Includes note added	
		● V58.43	Aftercare following surgery for injury and trauma Includes note added Excludes note added			
● V13.21	Personal history of pre-term labor Excludes note added			● E979.3	Terrorism involving fires, conflagration and hot substances Includes note added	
● V13.29	Personal history of other genital system and obstetric disorders					
		● V58.7	Aftercare following surgery to specified body systems, not elsewhere classified Instructional note added	● E979.4	Terrorism involving firearms Includes note added	
● V23.41	Pregnancy with history of pre-term labor					
● V23.49	Pregnancy with other poor obstetric history			● E979.5	Terrorism involving nuclear weapons Includes note added	
		● V58.71	Aftercare following surgery of the sense organs, NEC Includes note added			
● V46.2	Other dependence on machines, supplemental oxygen Includes note added			● E979.6	Terrorism involving biological weapons Includes note added	
		● V58.72	Aftercare following surgery of the nervous system, NEC Includes note added Excludes note added			
▲ V49.81	▶Asymptomatic◀ postmenopausal status (age-related) (natural)			● E979.7	Terrorism involving chemical weapons Includes note added	
V54.0	Excludes term revised					
● V54.1	Aftercare for healing traumatic fracture	● V58.73	Aftercare following surgery of the circulatory system, NEC Includes note added	● E979.8	Terrorism involving other means Includes note added	
● V54.10	Aftercare for healing traumatic fracture of arm, unspecified					
● V54.11	Aftercare for healing traumatic fracture of upper arm	● V58.74	Aftercare following surgery of the respiratory system, NEC Includes note added	● E979.9	Terrorism, secondary effects Instructional note added Excludes note added	
● V54.12	Aftercare for healing traumatic fracture of lower arm					
		● V58.75	Aftercare following surgery of the teeth, oral cavity and digestive system, NEC Includes note added	● E985.7	Injury by paintball gun, undetermined whether accidentally or purposely inflicted	
● V54.13	Aftercare for healing traumatic fracture of hip					
● V54.14	Aftercare for healing traumatic fracture of leg, unspecified			▲ E999	Late effect of injury due to war operations ▶and terrorism◀ Instructional note revised	
		● V58.76	Aftercare following surgery of the genitourinary system, NEC Includes note added Excludes note added			
● V54.15	Aftercare for healing traumatic fracture of upper leg Excludes note added			● E999.0	Late effect of injury due to war operations	
		● V58.77	Aftercare following surgery of the skin and subcutaneous tissue, NEC Includes note added	● E999.1	Late effect of injury due to terrorism	
● V54.16	Aftercare for healing traumatic fracture of lower leg					
● V54.17	Aftercare for healing traumatic fracture of vertebrae			**PROCEDURE TABULAR LIST (VOLUME 3)**		
● V54.19	Aftercare for healing traumatic fracture of other bone	● V58.78	Aftercare following surgery of the musculoskeletal system, NEC Includes note added			
● V54.2	Aftercare for healing pathologic fracture			● 00	Procedures and interventions, not elsewhere classified	
		V58.83	Use additional code note added	● 00.0	Therapeutic ultrasound	
● V54.20	Aftercare for healing pathologic fracture of arm, unspecified	▲ V71.8	Observation ▶and evaluation◀ for other specified suspected conditions	● 00.01	Therapeutic ultrasound of vessels of head and neck Includes note added Excludes note added	
● V54.21	Aftercare for healing pathologic fracture of upper arm					
		● V71.82	Observation and evaluation for suspected exposure to anthrax			

▶◀ Revised Text ● New Code ▲ Revised Code Title

● 00.02	Therapeutic ultrasound of heart Includes note added Excludes note added	33.99 ▲ 36.06	Includes note added Insertion of ►non-drug-eluting◄ coronary artery stent(s) Includes terms added Includes term revised Excludes note added	54.95 55 56 57 58 59	Includes term added Code also note added Code also note added Code also note added Code also note added Code also note added
● 00.03	Therapeutic ultrasound of peripheral vascular vessels Includes note added Excludes note added				
● 00.09	Other therapeutic ultrasound Excludes note added	● 36.07	Insertion of drug-eluting coronary artery stent(s) Includes note added Code also note added Excludes note added	60 65 66 67	Code also note added Code also note added Code also note added Code also note added
● 00.1	Pharmaceuticals				
● 00.10	Implantation of chemotherapeutic agent Includes note added Excludes note added	37.26 37.7 37.79	Includes term added Excludes note added Includes term revised	68 69 70	Code also note added Code also note added Code also note added
● 00.11	Infusion of drotrecogin alfa (activated) Includes note added	37.8 37.89	Excludes note added Includes term added Excludes note added	71 81.0 81.3	Code also note added Code also notes added Includes terms added Code also notes added
● 00.12	Administration of inhaled nitric oxide Includes note added	37.94 37.96 37.98	Excludes note added Excludes note added Excludes note added	● 81.6 ● 81.61	Other procedures on spine 360 degree spinal fusion, single incision approach Includes note added Code also notes added
● 00.13	Injection or infusion of nesiritide Includes note added	37.99 38 38.9	Includes terms added Code also note added Excludes note revised		
● 00.14	Injection or infusion of oxazolidinone class of antibiotics Includes note added	39.53 ● 39.72	Excludes term revised Endovascular repair or occlusion of head and neck vessels Includes note added	● 84.5	Implantation of other musculoskeletal devices and substances
● 00.5	Other cardiovascular procedures				
● 00.50	Implantation of cardiac resynchronization pacemaker without mention of defibrillation, total system [CRT-P] Includes note added Excludes note added	▲ 39.79	Other endovascular graft repair of aneurysm ►of other vessels◄ Includes note deleted Includes note added Excludes note added	● 84.51	Insertion of interbody spinal fusion device Includes note added Code also notes added
		▲ 39.90	Insertion of ►non-drug-eluting,◄ non-coronary artery stent(s) or stents Includes terms added Excludes term added	● 84.52	Insertion of recombinant bone morphogenetic protein Includes note added Code also note added
● 00.51	Implantation of cardiac resynchronization defibrillator, total system [CRT-D] Includes note added Excludes note added			86.28 86.65 88.7 88.91	Includes note added Excludes note added Excludes note added Excludes note added
● 00.52	Implantation or replacement of transvenous lead [electrode] into left ventricular coronary venous system Excludes note added	41.4 41.5 41.9 43	Code also note added Code also note added Code also note added Code also note added	● 88.96	Other intraoperative magnetic resonance imaging Includes note added
● 00.53	Implantation or replacement of cardiac resynchronization pacemaker pulse generator only [CRT-P] Includes note added Excludes note added	44 44.32 45 46 46.32 46.79	Code also note added Includes note added Code also note added Code also note added Includes note deleted Includes note added	● 89.60	Continuous intra-arterial blood gas monitoring Includes note added
				89.65 93.57 93.98	Excludes note added Includes term added Includes term deleted Excludes note added
● 00.54	Implantation or replacement of cardiac resynchronization defibrillator pulse generator device only [CRT-D] Includes note added Excludes note added	47 48 49 ● 49.75	Code also note added Code also note added Code also note added Implantation or revision of artificial anal sphincter Includes note added	96.56 99.19 99.21 99.22 99.25 99.28 99.29 99.71	Excludes note added Excludes note added Excludes note added Excludes note added Excludes term added Includes terms added Excludes terms added Excludes note added
● 00.55	Insertion of drug-eluting non-coronary artery stent(s) Includes note added Code also note added Excludes note added	● 49.76	Removal of artificial anal sphincter Includes note added Excludes note added		
		50 51 51.01 51.37	Code also note added Code also note added Includes note added Includes note added	● 99.76	Extracorporeal immunoadsorption Includes note added
▲ 02.41	Irrigation ►and exploration◄ of ventricular shunt Includes note added			● 99.77	Application or administration of adhesion barrier substance
03	Code also note added	52	Code also note added	99.99	Includes note added
03.09	Includes term added	53	Code also note added		
04.2	Includes term added	54	Code also note added		
33.24	Includes term added Excludes term added				

►◄ Revised Text   ● New Code   ▲ Revised Code Title

Coding Guidelines

OFFICIAL ICD-9-CM GUIDELINES FOR CODING AND REPORTING

The Public Health Service and the Centers for Medicare and Medicaid (formerly know as Health Care Financing Administration) of the U.S. Department of Health and Human Services present the following guidelines for coding and reporting using the International Classification of Diseases, 9th Revision, Clinical Modification (ICD-9-CM). These guidelines should be used as a companion document to the official versions of the ICD-9-CM.

These guidelines for coding and reporting have been developed and approved by the cooperating parties for ICD-9-CM: American Hospital Association, American Health Information Management Association, Center for Medicare and Medicaid Services and the National Center for Health Statistics. These guidelines previously appeared in the Coding Clinic for ICD-9-CM, published by the American Hospital Association.

These guidelines have been developed to assist the user in coding and reporting in situations where the ICD-9-CM manual does not provide direction. Coding and sequencing instructions in the three ICD-9-CM manuals take precedence over any guidelines.

These guidelines are not exhaustive. The cooperating parties are continuing to conduct review of these guidelines and develop new guidelines as needed. Users of the ICD-9-CM should be aware that only guidelines approved by the cooperating parties are official. Revision of these guidelines and new guidelines will be published by the U.S. Department of Health and Human Services when they are approved by the cooperating parties.

OUTPATIENT SERVICES

(Hospital-Based and Physician Office)

Table of Contents
Introduction . . . .
Code Range. . . . . A
Accurate Reporting . . . . B
Code Selection. C
Symptoms, Signs and Ill-defined Conditions . . . . D
Circumstances other than Disease or Injury . . . . E
Code Specificity. . . . . F
Code Sequence . . . . G
Uncertain Diagnosis . . . . H
Chronic Disease I
Coexisting Conditions I
Ancillary Diagnostic Services . . . . K
Ancillary Therapeutic Services L
Preoperative Evaluations . . . . N
Ambulatory Surgery . . . . O

INPATIENT SERVICES

Table of Contents
Adverse Effects and Poisoning 9
   Adverse Effect 9.1
   Poisoning 9.2
External Causes of Diseases and Injuries 11
   Child and Adult Abuse 11.5
   General Coding guidelines 11.1
   Late effects 11.8
   Misadventures and complications of care 11.9
   Multiple external causes. 11.4
   Place of occurrence 11.2
   Poisonings and adverse effects of drugs. 11.3
   Undetermined cause 11.7
   Unknown intent. 11.6
General Inpatient Coding Guidelines 1
   Acute and Chronic Conditions 1.4; 2.3
   Combination Code 1.5
   Impending or Threatened Condition 1.9
   Late Effect. 1.7
   Level of Specificity in Coding 1.2
   Multiple Coding of Diagnoses 1.6
   Other and Unspecified (NOS) Code Titles 1.3
   Uncertain Diagnosis 1.8
   Use of Alphabetic Index and Tabular List 1.1
Human Immunodeficiency Virus (HIV) Infections 10
   Asymptomatic HIV Infection 10.6
   Confirmed Cases of HIV Infection/Illness 10.1
   HIV Infection in Pregnancy, Childbirth and
      the Puerperium 10.5
   Inconclusive Lab Test for HIV 10.7
   Previously Diagnosed HIV-related Illness 10.3
   Selection of HIV Code. 10.2
   Sequencing 10.4
   Testing for HIV 10.8
Hypertension 4
   Controlled Hypertension. 4.9
   Elevated Blood Pressure 4.11
   Essential Hypertension 4.1
   Hypertension with Heart Disease 4.2
   Hypertensive Cardiovascular Disease 4.5
   Hypertensive Heart and Renal Disease 4.4
   Hypertensive Renal Disease with Chronic Renal
      Failure 4.3
   Hypertensive Retinopathy. 4.6
   Secondary Hypertension. 4.7
   Transient Hypertension 4.8
   Uncontrolled Hypertension 4.10
Newborn Coding 6
   Category V29. . . . . 6.3

Congenital Anomalies. 6.5
Maternal Causes of Perinatal Morbidity. 6.4
Newborn Transfers. 6.2
Other (Additional) Diagnoses 6.6
Prematurity and Fetal Growth Retardation 6.7
Use of Codes V30-V39 . . . . 6.1
Obstetrics 5
General Rules 5.1
Selection of Principal Diagnosis 5.2
Chapter 11 Fifth-digits. 5.3
Fetal Conditions Affecting Managment of Mother . . 5.4
Normal Delivery 650 . . . . 5.5
Procedure Codes 5.6
Postpartum Period. 5.7
Abortions 5.8
Late Effects of Complications of Pregnancy,
 Childbirth and the Puerperium 5.9
Reporting Other (Additional) Diagnoses 3
Abnormal Findings 3.5
Conditions Integral to a Disease Process 3.3
Conditions Not Integral to a Disease Process 3.4
Diagnoses Not Listed in Final Diagnostic Statement 3.2
Previous Conditions. 3.1
Selection of Principal Diagnosis 2
Acute and Chronic Conditions 2.3; 1.4
Codes from V71.0-V71.9, Observation and
 Evaluation for Suspected Conditions, not found 2.8
Complications of Pregnancy 2.16
Complications of Surgery and Other
 Medical Care. 2.15
Codes in Brackets in the Alphabetic Index 2.2
Multiple Burns 2.11; 8.3
Multiple Injuries 2.12
Neoplasms. 2.13
Original Treatment Plan Not Carried Out. 2.9
Poisoning 2.14
Residual Condition or Nature of Late Effect 2.10
Symptoms, Signs, and Ill-defined Conditions. 2.1
Symptom Followed by Contrasting/
 Comparative Diagnoses 2.7
Two or More Interrelated Conditions 2.4
Two or More Equally Meet Definition. 2.5
Two or More Comparative or Contrasting
 Conditions 2.6
Septicemia and Shock 7
Trauma 8
Current Burns and Encounters for Late Effects
 of Burns. 8.3
Debridement of Wound, Infection or Burn 8.4
Multiple Fractures. 8.2
Multiple Injuries 8.1

OFFICIAL GUIDELINES FOR CODING AND REPORTING OUTPATIENT SERVICES (HOSPITAL-BASED AND PHYSICIAN OFFICE)

Introduction

These revised coding guidelines for outpatient diagnoses have been approved for use by hospitals/physicians in coding and reporting hospital-based outpatient services and physician office visits.

The terms encounter and visit are often used interchangeably in describing outpatient service contacts and, therefore, appear together in these guidelines without distinguishing one from the other.

Coding guidelines for outpatient and physician reporting of diagnoses will vary in a number of instances from those for inpatient diagnoses, recognizing that:

The Uniform Hospital Discharge Data Set (UHDDS) definition of principal diagnosis applies only to inpatients in acute, short-term, general hospitals.

Coding guidelines for inconclusive diagnoses (probable, suspected, rule out, etc.) were developed for inpatient reporting and do not apply to outpatients.

Diagnoses often are not established at the time of the initial encounter/visit. It may take two or more visits before the diagnosis is confirmed.

The most critical rule involves beginning the search for the correct code assignment through the Alphabetic Index. Never begin searching initially in the Tabular List as this will lead to coding errors.

Basic Coding Guidelines for Outpatient Services

A. Code Range

   The appropriate code or codes from 001.0 through V82.9 must be used to identify diagnoses, symptoms, conditions, problems, complaints, or other reason(s) for the encounter/visit.

B. Accurate Reporting

   For accurate reporting of ICD-9-CM diagnosis codes, the documentation should describe the patient's condition, using terminology which includes specific diagnoses as well as symptoms, problems, or reasons for the encounter. There are ICD-9-CM codes to describe all of these.

C. Code Selection

   The selection of codes 001.0 through 999.9 will frequently be used to describe the reason for the encounter. These codes are from the section of ICD-9-CM for the classification of diseases and injuries (e.g. infectious and parasitic diseases; neoplasms; symptoms, signs, and ill-defined conditions, etc.).

D. Symptoms, Signs and Ill-defined Conditions

Codes that describe symptoms and signs, as opposed to diagnoses, are acceptable for reporting purposes when an established diagnosis has not been diagnosed (confirmed) by the physician. Chapter 16 of ICD-9-CM, Symptoms, Signs, and Ill-defined conditions (codes 780.0 - 799.9) contain many, but not all codes for symptoms.

E. Circumstances other than Disease or Injury

ICD-9-CM provides codes to deal with encounters for circumstances other than a disease or injury. The Supplementary Classification of factors Influencing Health Status and Contact with Health Services (V01.0- V82.9) is provided to deal with occasions when circumstances other than a disease or injury are recorded as diagnosis or problems. The V codes should be used for encounters of this type. For example, the correct code for a cancer patient who is seen solely for radiotherapy is V58.0, radiotherapy session.

Example:

Discharge diagnosis: Open-angle glaucoma

Reason for visit code: 365.10

Discharge diagnosis: Follow-up examination after surgery

Reason for visit code: V67.0

F. Code Specificity

ICD-9-CM is composed of codes with either 3, 4, or 5 digits. Codes with 3 digits are included in ICD-9-CM as the heading of a category of codes that may be further subdivided by the use of fourth and/or fifth digits which provide greater specificity. A code is invalid if it has not been coded to the full number of digits required for that code.

- Assign three-digit codes only if there are no four-digit codes within that code category.
- Assign four-digit codes only if there is no fifth-digit subclassification for that subcategory.
- Assign the fifth-digit subclassification code for those subcategories where it exists.

Example:

Diagnosis: Acute tonsillitis

Correct code: 463

Diagnosis: Benign neoplasm of colon

Incorrect code: 211

Correct code: 211.3

G. Code Sequence

List first the ICD-9-CM code for the diagnosis, condition, problem, or other reason for encounter/visit shown in the medical record to be chiefly responsible for the services provided. List additional codes that describe any coexisting conditions.

H. Uncertain Diagnosis

Do not code diagnoses documented as "probable", "suspected," "questionable," "rule out," or working diagnosis. Rather, code the condition(s) to the highest degree of certainty for that encounter/visit, such as symptoms, signs, abnormal test results, or other reason for the visit.

Coders should be aware that this is contrary to the coding practices used by health information management departments for coding the diagnoses of hospital inpatients. For inpatient coding, all discharge diagnoses listed as "probable," "suspected," "questionable" or "rule out" would be coded as if the condition existed. Further, coding symptoms for inpatients is generally unacceptable, particularly when there is an established diagnosis. A requirement that conditions listed as "probable," "suspected," "questionable" or "rule out" be coded in the outpatient setting as if the condition existed would lead to significant over-reporting of conditions. Therefore codes for symptoms and signs are appropriate and acceptable for hospital outpatient reporting.

Example:

Reason for visit: Chest pain, code 786.50

Discharge diagnosis: Rule out angina, code 413.9

Correct code: 786.50

Comment: Do not code angina as if it were established; code the reason for the visit.

I. Chronic Disease

Chronic diseases treated on an ongoing basis may be coded and reported as many times as the patient receives treatment and care for the condition(s).

Example:

History of illness: Patient is seen for monthly lumbar epidural block with steroid injection.

Discharge diagnosis: Chronic low back pain, code 724.2

Comment: Report code 724.2, low back pain, for each visit during which the patient receives lumbar-block treatment, regardless of the number or frequency of visits.

J. Coexisting Conditions

Code all documented conditions that coexist at the time of the encounter/visit, and require or affect patient care treatment or management. Do not code conditions that were previously treated and no longer exist. However, history codes (V10- V19) may be used as secondary codes if the historical condition or family history has an impact on current care or influences treatment.

Coders are advised to exercise care in identifying (a) conditions presently existing, (b) conditions no longer existing, (c) residuals (late effects) of conditions no longer existing, and (d) certain postoperative status conditions that require consideration in managing patient care and that warrant coding. Some physicians add to the list of conditions currently being treated any previous surgery or conditions that no longer exist to provide easy reference of the patient's history for recapitulation in the ongoing care of the patient. These conditions should not be coded unless they require or affect patient care treatment or management.

Example:

Chief complaint: Uncontrolled diabetes mellitus, 250.02

Review of systems: Patient has congestive heart failure (428.0) and is curently on Lasix.

Medical history: Patient is status three months post right inguinal herniorrherapy for incarcerated inguinal hernia.

Comment: First code "uncontrolled diabetes mellitus" as the reason for the visit, followed by "congestive heart failure" as a coexisting condition. Do not code the incarcerated inguinal hernia; it was treated successfully.

Code sequence: 250.02, 428.0

K. Ancillary Diagnostic Services

For patients receiving diagnostic services only during an encounter/visit, sequence first the diagnosis, condition, problem, or other reason for encounter/visit shown in the medical record to be chiefly responsible for the outpatient services provided during the encounter/visit. Codes for other diagnoses (e.g., chronic conditions) may be sequenced as additional diagnoses.

Example:

Chief complaint: Hematuria, code 599.7

Laboratory studies: Intravenous pyelogram, code V72.5

History of illness: Patient was referred to hospital outpatient clinic for intravenous pyelogram only. Will provide patient's physician with the results.

Code sequence: 599.7

L. Ancillary Therapeutic Services

For patients receiving therapeutic services only during an encounter/visit, sequence first the diagnosis, condition, problem, or other reason for encounter/visit shown in the medical record to be chiefly responsible for the outpatient services provided during the encounter/visit. Codes for other diagnoses (e.g., chronic conditions) may be sequenced as additional diagnoses.

Example:

Chief complaint: Chronic renal failure, code 585

Procedure performed: Hemodialysis, code V56.0

History of illness: Patient is being seen for hemodialysis treatment.

Code sequence: 585

NOTE: The appropriate V code can be listed first for patients receiving the following (the diagnosis or problem for which the service is being performed should be listed second):

- chemotherapy
- radiation therapy
- rehabilitation.

Example:

Chief complaint: Trigone bladder cancer, code 188.0

Procedure performed: Chemotherapy infusion, code V58.1

History of illness: Patient is being seen for second course of five chemotherapy infusions.

Code sequence: V58.1, 188.0

M. [Guideline M-deleted in the official guidelines]

N. Preoperative Evaluations

For patient's receiving preoperative evaluations only, sequence a code from category V72.8, Other specified examinations, to describe the pre-op consultations. Assign a code for the condition to describe the reason for the surgery as an additional diagnosis. Code also any findings related to the pre-op evaluation.

Example:

Chief complaint: Rhegmatogenous retinal detachment in left eye, code 361.00

Procedure performed: Preoperative cardiovascular examination, V72.81

History of illness: Patient is being seen for preoperative cardiovascular examination, due to history of myocardial infarction 1 year ago. Patient is scheduled for a repair of his retinal detachment next week.

Code sequence: V72.81, 361.00

O. Ambulatory Surgery

For ambulatory surgery, code the diagnosis for which the surgery was performed. If the postoperative diagnosis is known to be different from the preoperative diagnosis at the time the diagnosis is confirmed, select the postoperative diagnosis for coding, since it is the most definitive.

Example:

Preoperative diagnosis: Breast mass, code 611.72

Postoperative diagnosis: Fibrocystic breast disease, code 610.3

Comment: Code 610.3 as the reason for the visit because it is the postoperative diagnosis.

OFFICIAL GUIDELINES FOR CODING AND REPORTING INPATIENT SERVICES

1. GENERAL INPATIENT CODING GUIDELINES

   1.1. Use of Both Alphabetic Index and Tabular List

   A. Use both the Alphabetic Index and the Tabular List when locating and assigning a code. Reliance on only the Alphabetic Index or the Tabular List leads to errors in code assignments and less specificity in code selection.

   B. Locate each term in the Alphabetic Index and verify the code selected in the Tabular List. Read and be guided by instructional notations that appear in both the Alphabetic Index and the Tabular List.

   1.2. Level of Specificity in Coding

   Diagnostic and procedure codes are to be used at their highest level of specificity:

   - Assign three-digit codes only if there are no four-digit codes within that code category.
   - Assign four-digit codes only if there is no fifth-digit subclassification for that category.
   - Assign the fifth-digit subclassification code for those categories where it exists.

   1.3. Other (NEC) and Unspecified (NOS) Code Titles

   Codes labeled "other specified" (NEC—not elsewhere classified) or "unspecified" (NOS—not otherwise specified) are used only when neither the diagnostic statement nor a thorough review of the medical record provides adequate information to permit assignment of a more specific code.

   - Use the code assignment for "other" or NEC when the information at hand specifies a condition but no separate code for that condition is provided.
   - Use "unspecified" (NOS) when the information at hand does not permit either a more specific or "other" code assignment.
   - When the Alphabetic Index assigns a code to a category labeled "other (NEC)" or to a category labeled "unspecified (NOS)", refer to the Tabular List and review the titles and inclusion terms in the subdivisions under that particular three-digit category (or subdivision under the four-digit code) to determine if the information at hand can be appropriately assigned to a more specific code.

   1.4. Acute and Chronic Conditions

   If the same condition is described as both acute (subacute) and chronic and separate subentries exist in the Alphabetic Index at the same indentation level, code both and sequence the acute (subacute) code first.

   1.5. Combination Code

   A single code used to classify two diagnoses or a diagnosis with an associated secondary process (manifestation) or an associated complication is called a combination code. Combination codes are identified by referring to subterm entries in the Alphabetic Index and by reading the inclusion and exclusion notes in the Tabular List.

   Assign only the combination code when that code fully identifies the diagnostic conditions involved or when the Alphabetic Index so directs. Multiple coding should not be used when the classification provides a combination code that clearly identifies all of the elements documented in the diagnosis. When the combination code lacks necessary specificity in describing the manifestation or complication, an additional code may be used as a secondary code.

   1.6. Multiple Coding of Diagnoses

   Multiple coding is required for certain conditions not subject to the rules for combination codes.

   Instruction for conditions that require multiple coding appear in the Alphabetic Index and the Tabular List.

   A. Alphabetic Index: Codes for both etiology and manifestation of a disease appear following the subentry term, with the second code in brackets. Assign both codes in the same sequence in which they appear in the Alphabetic Index.

   B. Tabular List: Instructional terms, such as "Code first...," "Use additional code for any...," and "Note...," indicate when to use more than one code.

   - "Code first underlying disease" - Assign the codes for both the manifestation and underlying cause. The codes for manifestations cannot be used (designated) as principal diagnosis.
   - "Use additional code, to identify manifestation, as ..." - Assign also the code that identifies the manifestation, such as, but not limited to, the examples listed. The codes for manifestations cannot be used (designated) as principal diagnosis.

   C. Apply multiple coding instructions throughout the classification where appropriate, whether or not multiple coding directions appear in the Alphabetic Index or the Tabular List. Avoid indiscriminate multiple coding or irrelevant information, such as symptoms or signs characteristic of the diagnosis.

Coding Guidelines—Inpatient

1.7. Late Effect

A late effect is the residual effect (condition produced) after the acute phase of an illness or injury has terminated. There is no time limit on when a late effect code can be used. The residual may be apparent early, such as in cerebrovascular accident cases, or it may occur months or years later, such as that due to a previous injury.

Coding of late effects requires two codes:

- The residual condition or nature of the late effect
- The cause of the late effect

The residual condition or nature of the late effect is sequenced first, followed by the cause of the late effect, except in those few instances where the code for late effect is followed by a manifestation code identified in the Tabular List and title or the late effect code has been expanded (at the fourth and fifth-digit levels) to include the manifestation(s).

The code for the acute phase of an illness or injury that led to the late effect is never used with a code for the cause of the late effect.

A. Late Effects of Cerebrovascular Disease

Category 438 is used to indicate conditions classifiable to categories 430-437 as the causes of late effects (neurologic deficits), themselves classified elsewhere. These "late effects" include neurologic deficits that persist after initial onset of conditions classifiable to 430-437. The neurologic deficits caused by cerebrovascular disease may be present from the onset or may arise at any time after the onset of the condition classifiable to 430–437.

- Codes from category 438 may be assigned on a health care record with codes from 430–437, if the patient has a current CVA and deficits from an old CVA.
- Assign code V12.59 (and not a code from category 438) as an additional code for history of cerebrovascular disease when no neurologic deficits are present.

1.8. Uncertain Diagnosis

If the diagnosis documented at the time of discharge is qualified as "probable", "suspected", "likely", "questionable", "possible", or "still to be ruled out", code the condition as if it existed or was established. The bases for this guidelines are the diagnostic workup, arrangements for further workup or observation, and initial therapeutic approach that correspond most closely with the established diagnosis.

1.9. Impending or Threatened Condition

Code any condition described at the time of discharge as "impending" or "threatened" as follows:

If it did occur, code as confirmed diagnosis.

If it did not occur, reference the Alphabetic Index to determine if the condition has a subentry term for "impending" or "threatened" and also reference main term entries for Impending and for Threatened.

- If the subterms are listed, assign the given code.
- If the subterms are not listed, code the existing forerunner condition(s) and not the condition described as impending or threatened.

2. SELECTION OF PRINCIPAL DIAGNOSIS

The circumstances of inpatient admission always govern the selection of principal diagnosis. The principal diagnosis is defined in the Uniform Hospital Discharge Data Set (UHDDS) as "that condition established after study to be chiefly responsible for occasioning the admission of the patient to the hospital for care".

In determining principal diagnosis the coding directives in the ICD-9-CM manuals, Volumes I, II, and III, take precedence over all other guidelines.

The importance of consistent, complete documentation in the medical record cannot be overemphasized. Without such documentation the application of all coding guidelines is a difficult, if not impossible, task.

2.1. Codes for symptoms, signs, and ill-defined conditions

Codes for symptoms, signs, and ill-defined conditions from Chapter 16 are not to be used as principal diagnosis when a related definitive diagnosis has been established.

2.2. Codes in brackets

Codes in brackets in the Alphabetic Index can never be sequenced as principal diagnosis. Coding directives require that the codes in brackets be sequenced in the order as they appear in the Alphabetic Index.

2.3. Acute and chronic conditions

If the same condition is described as both acute (subacute) and chronic and separate subentries exist in the Alphabetic Index at the same indentation level, code both and sequence the acute (subacute) code first.

2.4. Two or more interrelated conditions, each potentially meeting the definition for principal diagnosis

When there are two or more interrelated conditions (such as diseases in the same ICD-9-CM chapter or manifestations characteristically associated with a certain disease) potentially meeting the definition of principal diagnosis, either condition may be sequenced first, unless the circumstances of the admission, the therapy provided, the Tabular List, or the Alphabetic Index indicate otherwise.

2.5. Two or more diagnoses that equally meet the definition for principal diagnosis

In the unusual instance when two or more diagnoses equally meet the criteria for principal diagnosis as determined by the circumstances of admission, diagnostic workup and/or therapy provided, and the Alphabetic Index, Tabular List, or another coding guidelines does not provide sequencing direction, any one of the diagnoses may be sequenced first.

2.6. Two or more comparative or contrasting conditions

In those rare instances when two or more contrasting or comparative diagnoses are documented as "either/or" (or similar terminology), they are coded as if the diagnoses were confirmed and the diagnoses are sequenced according to the circumstances of the admission. If no further determination can be made as to which diagnosis should be principal, either diagnosis may be sequenced first.

2.7. A symptom(s) followed by contrasting/comparative diagnoses

When a symptom(s) is followed by contrasting/comparative diagnoses, the symptom code is sequenced first. All the contrasting/comparative diagnoses should be coded as suspected conditions.

2.8. Codes from the V71.0-V71.9 series, Observation and evaluation for suspected conditions

Codes from the V71.0-V71.9 series are assigned as principal diagnoses for encounters or admissions to evaluate the patient's condition when there is some evidence to suggest the existence of an abnormal condition or following an accident or other incident that ordinarily results in a health problem, and where no supporting evidence for the suspected condition is found and no treatment is currently required. The fact that the patient may be scheduled for continuing observation in the office/clinic setting following discharge does not limit the use of this category.

2.9. Original treatment plan not carried out

Sequence as the principal diagnosis the condition which after study occasioned the admission to the hospital, even though treatment may not have been carried out due to unforeseen circumstances.

2.10. Residual condition or nature of late effect

The residual condition or nature of the late effect is sequenced first, followed by the late effect code for the cause of the residual condition, except in a few instances where the Alphabetic Index or Tabular List directs otherwise.

2.11. Multiple burns

Sequence first the code that reflects the highest degree of burn when more than one burn is present. (See also Burns guideline 8.3)

2.12. Multiple injuries

When multiple injuries exist, the code for the most severe injury as determined by the attending physician is sequenced first.

2.13. Neoplasms

A. If the treatment is directed at the malignancy, designate the malignancy as the principal diagnosis, except when the purpose of the encounter or hospital admission is for radiotherapy session(s), V58.0, or for chemotherapy session(s), V58.1, in which instance the malignancy is coded and sequenced second.

B. When a patient is admitted for the purpose of radiotherapy or chemotherapy and develops complications such as uncontrolled nausea and vomiting or dehydration, the principal diagnosis is Encounter for radiotherapy, V58.0, or Encounter for chemotherapy, V58.1.

C. When an episode of inpatient care involves surgical removal of a primary site or secondary site malignancy followed by adjunct chemotherapy or radiotherapy, code the malignancy as the principal diagnosis, using codes in the 140-198 series or where appropriate in the 200-203 series.

D. When the reason for admission is to determine the extent of the malignancy, or for a procedure such as paracentesis or thoracentesis, the primary malignancy or appropriate metastatic site is designated as the principal diagnosis, even though chemotherapy or radiotherapy is administered.

E. When the primary malignancy has been previously excised or eradicated from its site and there is not adjunct treatment directed to that site and no evidence of any remaining malignancy at the primary site, use the appropriate code from the V10 series to indicate the former site of primary malignancy. Any mention of extension, invasion, or metastasis to a nearby structure or organ or to a distant site is coded as a secondary malignant neoplasm to that site and may be the principal diagnosis in the absence of the primary site.

F. When a patient is admitted because of a primary neoplasm with metastasis and treatment is directed toward the secondary site only, the secondary neoplasm is designated as the principal diagnosis even though the primary malignancy is still present.

G. Symptoms, signs, and ill-defined conditions listed in Chapter 16 characteristic of, or associated with, an existing primary or secondary site malignancy cannot be used to replace the malignancy as principal diagnosis, regardless of the number of admissions or encounters for treatment and care of the neoplasm.

H. Coding and sequencing of complications associated with the malignant neoplasm or with the therapy thereof are subject to the following guidelines:

- When admission is for management of an anemia associated with the malignancy, and the treatment is only for anemia, the anemia is designated at the principal diagnosis and is followed by the appropriate code(s) for the malignancy.
- When the admission is for management of an anemia associated with chemotherapy or radiotherapy and the only treatment is for the anemia, the anemia is designated as the principal diagnosis followed by the appropriate code(s) for the malignancy.
- When the admission is for management of dehydration due to the malignancy or the therapy, or a combination of both, and only the dehydration is being treated (intravenous rehydration), the dehydration is designated as the principal diagnosis, followed by the code(s) for the malignancy.
- When the admission is for treatment of a complication resulting from a surgical procedure performed for the treatment of an intestinal malignancy, designate the complication as the principal diagnosis if treatment is directed at resolving the complication.

2.14. Poisoning

When coding a poisoning or reaction to the improper use of a medication (e.g., wrong dose, wrong substance, wrong route of administration) the poisoning code is sequenced first, followed by a code for the manifestation. If there is also a diagnosis of drug abuse or dependence to the substance, the abuse or dependence is coded as an additional code.

2.15. Complications of surgery and other medical care

When the admission is for treatment of a complication resulting from surgery or other medical care, the complication code is sequenced as the principal diagnosis. If the complication is classified to the 996-999 series, an additional code for the specific complication may be assigned.

2.16. Complication of pregnancy

When a patient is admitted because of a condition that is either a complication pregnancy or that is complicating the pregnancy, the code for the obstetric complication is the principal diagnosis. An additional code may be assigned as needed to provide specificity.

3. REPORTING OTHER (ADDITIONAL) DIAGNOSES

A joint effort between the attending physician and coder is essential to achieve complete and accurate documentation, code assignment, and reporting of diagnoses and procedures.

These guidelines have been developed and approved by the Cooperating Parties to assure both the physician and the coder in identifying those diagnoses that are to be reported in addition to the principal diagnosis. Hospitals may record other diagnoses as needed for internal data use.

The UHDDS definitions are used by acute care short-term hospitals to report inpatient data elements in a standardized manner. These data elements and their definitions can be found in the July 31, 1985, Federal Register (Vol. 50, No, 147), pp. 31038-40.

The UHDDS item #11-b defines Other Diagnoses as "all conditions that coexist at the time of admission, that develop subsequently, or that affect the treatment received and/or the length of stay. Diagnoses that relate to an earlier episode which have no bearing on the current hospital stay are to be excluded".

General Rule

For reporting purposes the definition for "other diagnoses" is interpreted as additional conditions that affect patient care in terms of requiring:

- clinical evaluation; or
- therapeutic treatment; or
- diagnostic procedures; or
- extended length of hospital stay; or
- increased nursing care and/or monitoring.

The following guidelines are to be applied in designating "other diagnoses" when neither the Alphabetic Index nor the Tabular List in ICD-9-CM provide direction.

The listing of the diagnoses on the attestation statement is the responsibility of the attending physician.

3.1. Previous conditions

If the physician has included a diagnosis in the final diagnostic statement, such as the discharge summary or the face sheet, it should ordinarily be coded. Some physicians include in the diagnostic statement resolved conditions or diagnoses and status-post procedures from previous admission that have no bearing on the current stay. Such conditions are not to be reported and are coded only if required by hospital policy.

However, history codes (V10-V19) may be used as secondary codes if the historical condition or family history has an impact on current care or influences treatment.

3.2. Diagnoses not listed in the final diagnostic statement

When the physician has documented what appears to be a current diagnosis in the body of the record, but has not included the diagnosis in the final diagnostic statement, the physician should be asked whether the diagnosis should be added.

3.3. Conditions that are an integral part of a disease process

Conditions that are integral to the disease process should not be assigned as additional codes.

3.4. Conditions that are not an integral part of a disease process

Additional conditions that may not be associated routinely with a disease process should be coded when present.

3.5. Abnormal findings

Abnormal findings (laboratory, x-ray, pathologic, and other diagnostic results) are not coded and reported unless the physician indicates their clinical significance. If the findings are outside the normal range and the physician has ordered other tests to evaluate the condition or prescribed treatment, it is appropriate to ask the physician whether the diagnosis should be added.

4. HYPERTENSION

4.1. Hypertension, Essential, or NOS

Assign hypertension (arterial) (essential) (primary) (systemic) (NOS) to category code 401 with the appropriate fourth digit to indicate malignant (.0), benign (.1), or unspecified (.9). Do not use either .0 malignant or .1 benign unless medical record documentation supports such a designation.

4.2. Hypertension with Heart Disease

Certain heart conditions (425.8, 428, 429.0-429.3, 429.8, 429.9) are assigned to a code from category 402 when a causal relationship is stated (due to hypertension) or implied (hypertensive). Use only the code from category 402.

The same heart conditions (425.8, 428, 429.0-429.3, 429.8, 429.9) with hypertension, but without a stated casual relationship, are coded separately. Sequence according to the circumstances of the admission.

4.3. Hypertensive Renal Disease with Chronic Renal Failure

Assign codes from category 403, Hypertensive renal disease, when conditions classified to categories 585-587 are present. Unlike hypertension with heart disease, ICD-9-CM presumes a cause-and-effect relationship and classifies renal failure with hypertension as hypertensive renal disease.

4.4. Hypertensive Heart and Renal Disease

Assign codes from combination category 404, Hypertensive heart and renal disease, when both hypertensive renal disease and hypertensive heart disease are stated in the diagnosis. Assume a relationship between the hypertension and the renal disease, whether or not the condition is so designated.

4.5. Hypertensive Cerebrovascular Disease.

First assign codes from 430-438, Cerebrovascular disease, then the appropriate hypertension code from categories 401-405.

4.6. Hypertensive Retinopathy

Two codes are necessary to identify the condition. First assign the code from subcategory 362.11, Hypertensive retinopathy, then the appropriate code from categories 401-405 to indicate the type of hypertension.

4.7. Hypertension, Secondary

Two codes are required: one to identify the underlying condition and one from category 405 to identify the hypertension. Sequencing of codes is determined by the reason for admission to the hospital.

4.8. Hypertension, Transient

Assign code 796.2, Elevated blood pressure reading without diagnosis of hypertension, unless patient has an established diagnosis of hypertension. Assign code 642.3x for transient hypertension of pregnancy.

4.9. Hypertension, Controlled

Assign appropriate code from categories 401-405. This diagnostic statement usually refers to an existing state of hypertension under control by therapy.

4.10. Hypertension, Uncontrolled

Uncontrolled hypertension may refer to untreated hypertension or hypertension not responding to current therapeutic regimen. In either case. assign the appropriate code from categories 401-405 to designate the stage and type of hypertension. Code to the type of hypertension.

4.11. Elevated Blood Pressure

For a statement of elevated blood pressure without further specificity, assign code 796.2, Elevated blood pressure reading without diagnosis of hypertension, rather than a code from category 401.

5. OBSTETRICS

Introduction

These guidelines have been developed and approved by the Cooperating Parties in conjunction with the Editorial Advisory Board of Coding Clinic and the American College of Obstetricians and Gynecologists, to assist the coder in coding and reporting obstetric cases. Where feasible, previously published advice has been incorporated. Some advice in these new guidelines may supersede previous advice. The guidelines are provided for reporting purposes. Health care facilities may record additional diagnoses as needed for internal data needs.

5.1. General Rules

A. Obstetric cases require codes from chapter 11, codes in the range 630-677, Complications of Pregnancy, Childbirth, and the Puerperium. Should the physician document that the pregnancy is incidental to the encounter then code V22.2 should be used in place of any chapter 11 codes. It is the physician's responsibility to state that the condition being treated is not affecting the pregnancy.

B. Chapter 11 codes have sequencing priority over codes from other chapters. Additional codes from other chapters may be used in conjunction with chapter 11 codes to further specify conditions.

C. Chapter 11 codes are to be used only on the maternal record, never on the record of the newborn.

D. An outcome of delivery code, V27.0-V27.9, should be included on every maternal record when a delivery has occurred. These codes are not to be used on subsequent records or on the newborn record.

5.2. Selection of Principal Diagnosis

A. The circumstances of the encounter govern the selection of the principal diagnosis.

B. In episodes when no delivery occurs the principal diagnosis should correspond to the principal complication of the pregnancy which necessitated the encounter. Should more than one complication exist, all of which are treated or monitored, any of the complications codes may be sequenced first.

C. When a delivery occurs the principal diagnosis should correspond to the main circumstances or complication of the delivery. In cases of cesarean deliveries, the principal diagnosis should correspond to the reason the cesarean was performed, unless the reason for admission was unrelated to the condition resulting in the cesarean delivery.

D. For routine prenatal visits when no complications are present codes V22.0, Supervision of normal first pregnancy, and V22.1, Supervision of other normal pregnancy, should be used as principal diagnoses. These codes should not be used in conjunction with chapter 11 codes.

E. For prenatal outpatient visits for patients with high-risk pregnancies, a code from category V23, Supervision of high-risk pregnancy, should be used as the principal diagnosis. Secondary chapter 11 codes may be used in conjunction with these codes if appropriate. A thorough review of any pertinent excludes note is necessary to be certain that these V codes are being used properly.

5.3. Chapter 11 Fifth-digits

A. Categories 640-648, 651-676 have required fifth-digits which indicate whether the encounter is antepartum, postpartum and whether a delivery has also occurred.

B. The fifth-digits which are appropriate for each code number are listed in brackets under each code. The fifth-digits on each code should all be consistent with each other. That is, should a delivery occur all of the fifth-digits should indicate the delivery.

5.4. Fetal Conditions Affecting the Management of the Mother.

Codes from category 655, Known or suspected fetal abnormality affecting management of the mother, and category 656, Other fetal and placental problems affecting the management of the mother, are assigned only when the fetal condition is actually responsible for modifying the management of the mother, i.e., by requiring diagnostic studies, additional observation, special care, or termination of pregnancy. The fact that the fetal condition exists does not justify assigning a code from this series to the mother's record.

5.5. Normal Delivery, 650

A. Code 650 is for use in cases when a woman is admitted for a full-term normal delivery and delivers a single, healthy infant without any complications antepartum, during the delivery, or postpartum during the delivery episode.

B. 650 may be used if the patient had a complications at some point during her pregnancy but the complication is not present at the time of the admission for delivery.

C. Code 650 is always a principal diagnosis. It is not to be used if any other code from chapter 11 is needed to describe a current complication of the antenatal, delivery, or perinatal period. Additional codes from other chapters may be used with code 650 if they are not related to or are in any way complicating the pregnancy.

D. V27.0, Single liveborn, is the only outcome of delivery code appropriate for use with 650.

5.6. Procedure Codes

A. In cases of cesarean delivery, the selection of the principal diagnosis should correspond to the reason the cesarean delivery was performed unless the reason for admission was unrelated to the condition resulting in the cesarean delivery.

B. A delivery procedure code should not be used for a woman who has delivered prior to admission to the hospital. Any postpartum repairs should be coded.

5.7. The Postpartum Period

A. The postpartum period begins immediately after delivery and continues for 6 weeks following delivery.

B. A postpartum complication is any complication occurring within the 6 week period.

C. Chapter 11 codes may also be used to describe pregnancy-related complications after the 6 week period should the physician document that a condition is pregnancy related.

D. Postpartum complications that occur during the same admission as the delivery are identified with a fifth digit of "2". Subsequent admissions for postpartum complications should identified with a fifth digit of "4".

E. When the mother delivers outside the hospital prior to admission and is admitted for routine postpartum care and no complications are noted, code V24.0, Postpartum care and examination immediately after delivery, should be assigned as the principal diagnosis.

5.8. Abortions

A. Fifth-digits are required for abortion categories 634-637. Fifth-digit 1, incomplete, indicates that all of the products of conception have not been expelled from the uterus. Fifth-digit 2, complete, indicates that all products of conception have been expelled from the uterus prior to the episode of care.

B. A code from categories 640-648 and 651-657 may be used as additional codes with an abortion code to indicate the complication leading to the abortion.

Fifth digit 3 is assigned with codes from these categories when used with an abortion code because the other fifth digits will not apply. Codes from the 660-669 series are not to be used for complications of abortion.

C. Code 639 is to be used for all complications following abortion. Code 639 cannot be assigned with codes from categories 634-638.

D. Abortion with Liveborn Fetus. When an attempted termination of pregnancy results in a liveborn fetus assign code 644.21, Early onset of delivery, with an appropriate code from category V27, Outcome of Delivery. The procedure code for the attempted termination of pregnancy should also be assigned.

E. Retained Products of Conception following an abortion. Subsequent admissions for retained products of conception following a spontaneous or legally induced abortion are assigned the appropriate code from category 634, Spontaneous abortion, or legally induced abortion, with a fifth digit of "1" (incomplete). This advice is appropriate even when the patient was discharged previously with a discharge diagnosis of complete abortion.

5.9. Code 677, Late effect of complication of pregnancy, childbirth, and the puerperium

A. Code 677, Late effect of complication of pregnancy, childbirth, and the puerperium is for use in those cases when an initial complication of a pregnancy develops a sequelae requiring care or treatment at a future date.

B. This code may be used at any time after the initial postpartum period.

C. This code, like all late effect codes, is to be sequenced following the code describing the sequelae of the complication.

6. **NEWBORN GUIDELINES**

   Definition

   The newborn period is defined as beginning at birth and lasting through the 28th day following birth.

   The following guidelines are provided for reporting purposes. Hospitals may record other diagnoses as needed for internal data use.

   General Rule

   All clinically significant conditions noted on routine newborn examination should be coded. A condition is clinically significant if it requires:

   - clinical evaluation; or
   - therapeutic treatment; or
   - diagnostic procedures; or
   - extended length of hospital stay; or
   - increased nursing care and/or monitoring; or
   - has implications for future health care needs.

   Note: The newborn guidelines listed above are the same as the general coding guidelines for "other diagnoses," except for the final bullet regarding implications for future health care needs. Whether or not a condition is clinically significant can only be determined by the physician.

   6.1. Use of Codes V30-V39

   When coding the birth of an infant, assign a code from categories V30-V39, according to the type of birth. A code from this series is assigned as a principal diagnosis, and assigned only once to a newborn at the time of birth.

   6.2. Newborn Transfers

   If the newborn is transferred to another institution, the V30 series is not used.

   6.3. Use of Category V29

   A. Assign a code from category V29, Observation and evaluation of newborns and infants for suspected conditions not found, to identify those instances when a healthy newborn is evaluated for a suspected condition that is determined after study not to be present. Do not use a code from category V29 when the patient has identified signs or symptoms of a suspected problem; in such cases, code the sign or symptom.

   B. A V29 code is to be used as a secondary code after the V30, Outcome of delivery, code. It may also be assigned as a principal code for readmissions or encounters when the V30 code no longer applies. It is for use only for healthy newborns and infants for which no condition after study is found to be present.

   6.4. Maternal Causes of Perinatal Morbidity

   Codes from categories 760-763, Maternal causes of perinatal morbidity and mortality, are assigned only when the maternal condition has actually affected the fetus or newborn. The fact that the mother has an associated medical condition or experiences some complication of pregnancy, labor or delivery does not justify the routine assignment of codes from these categories to the newborn record.

   6.5. Congenital Anomalies

   Assign an appropriate code from categories 740-759, Congenital Anomalies, when a specific abnormality is diagnosed for an infant. Such abnormalities may occur as a set of symptoms or multiple malformations. A code should be assigned for each presenting manifestation of the syndrome if the syndrome is not specifically indexed in ICD-9-CM.

   6.6. Coding of Other (Additional) Diagnoses

   A. Assign codes for conditions that require treatment or further investigation, prolong the length of stay, or require resource utilization.

   B. Assign codes for conditions that have been specified by the physician as having implications for future health care needs.

   NOTE: This guideline should not be used for adult patients.

   C. Assign a code for Newborn conditions originating in the perinatal period (categories 760-779), as well as complications arising during the current episode of care classified in other chapters, only if the diagnoses have been documented by the responsible physician at the time of transfer or discharge as having affected the fetus or newborn.

   D. Insignificant conditions or signs or symptoms that resolve without treatment are not coded.

   6.7. Prematurity and Fetal Growth Retardation

   Codes from categories 764 and 765 should not be assigned based solely on recorded birthweight or estimated gestational age, but upon the attending physician's clinical assessment of maturity of the infant.

   NOTE: Since physicians may utilize different criteria in determining prematurity, do not code the diagnosis of prematurity unless the physician documents this condition.

7. **SEPTICEMIA AND SEPTIC SHOCK**

   When the diagnosis of septicemia with shock or the diagnosis of general sepsis with septic shock is documented, code and list the septicemia first and report the septic shock code as a secondary condition. The septicemia code assignment should identify the type of bacteria if it is known.

   Sepsis and septic shock associated with abortion, ectopic pregnancy, and molar pregnancy are classified to category codes in Chapter 11 (630-639).

Negative or inconclusive blood cultures do not preclude a diagnosis of septicemia in patients with clinical evidence of the condition.

8. TRAUMA

   8.1. Coding for Multiple Injuries

   When coding multiple injuries such as fracture of tibia and fibula, assign separate codes for each injury unless a combination code is provided, in which case the combination code is assigned. Multiple injury codes are provided in ICD-9-CM, but should not be assigned unless information for a more specific code is not available.

   A. The code for the most serious injury, as determined by the physician, is sequenced first.

   B. Superficial injuries such as abrasions or contusions are not coded when associated with more severe injuries of the same site.

   C. When a primary injury results in minor damage to peripheral nerves or blood vessels, the primary injury is sequenced first with additional code(s) from categories 950-957, Injury to nerves and spinal cord, and/or 900-904, Injury to blood vessels. When the primary injury is to the blood vessels or nerves, that injury should be sequenced first.

   8.2. Coding for Multiple Fractures

   The principle of multiple coding of injuries should be followed in coding multiple fractures. Multiple fractures of specified sites are coded individually by site in accordance with both the provisions within categories 800-829 and the level of detail furnished by medical record content. Combination categories for multiple fractures are provided for use when there is insufficient detail in the medical record (such as trauma cases transferred to another hospital), when the reporting form limits the number of codes that can be used in reporting pertinent clinical data, or when there is insufficient specificity at the fourth-digit or fifth-digit level. More specific guidelines are as follows:

   A. Multiple fractures of same limb classifiable to the same three-digit or four-digit category are coded to that category.

   B. Multiple unilateral or bilateral fractures of same bone(s) but classified to different fourth-digit subdivisions (bone part) within the same three-digit category are coded individually by site.

   C. Multiple fracture categories 819 and 828 classify bilateral fractures of both upper limbs (819) and both lower limbs (828), but without any detail at the fourth-digit level other than open and closed type of fractures.

   D. Multiple fractures are sequenced in accordance with the severity of the fracture and the physician should be asked to list the fracture diagnoses in the order of severity.

   8.3. Current Burns and Encounters for Late Effects of Burns

   Current burns (940-948) are classified by depth, extent and, if desired, by agent (E code). By depth burns are classified as first degree (erythema), second degree (blistering), and third degree (full-thickness involvement).

   A. All burns are coded with the highest degree of burn sequenced first.

   B. Classify burns of the same local site (three-digit category level, (940-947) but of different degrees to the subcategory identifying the highest degree recorded in the diagnosis.

   C. Non-healing burns are coded as acute burns. Necrosis of burned skin should be coded as a non-healed burn.

   D. Assign code 958.3, Posttraumatic wound infection, not elsewhere classified, as an additional code for any documented infected burn site.

   E. When coding multiple burns, assign separate codes for each burn site. Category 946 Burns of Multiple specified sites, should only be used if the location of the burns are not documented. Category 949, Burn, unspecified, is extremely vague and should rarely be used.

   F. Assign codes from category 948, Burns classified according to extent of body surface involved, when the site of the burn is not specified or when there is a need for additional data. It is advisable to use category 948 as additional coding when needed to provide data for evaluating burn mortality, such as that needed by burn units. It is also advisable to use category 948 as an additional code for reporting purposes when there is mention of a third-degree burn involving 20 percent or more of the body surface. In assigning a code from category 948:

   - Four-digit codes are used to identify the percentage of total body surface involved in a burn (all degree).
   - Fifth-digits are assigned to identify the percentage of body surface involved in third-degree burn.
   - Fifth-digit zero (0) is assigned when less than 10 percent or when no

body surface is involved in a third-degree burn.

Category 948 is based on the classic "rule of nines" in estimating body surface involved: head and neck are assigned nine percent, each arm nine percent, each leg 18 percent, the anterior trunk 18 percent, posterior trunk 18 percent, and genitalia one percent. Physicians may change these percentage assignments where necessary to accommodate infants and children who have proportionately larger heads than adults and patients who have large buttocks, thighs, or abdomen that involve burns.

G. Encounters for the treatment of the late effects of burns (i.e., scars or joint contractures) should be coded to the residual condition (sequelae) followed by the appropriate late effect code (906.5-906.9). A late effect E code may also be used, if desired.

H. When appropriate, both a sequelae with a late effect code, and a current burn code may be assigned on the same record.

8.4. Debridement of Wound, Infection, or Burn

A. For coding purposes, excisional debridement, 86.22, is assigned only when the procedure is performed by a physician.

B. For coding purposes, nonexcisional debridement performed by the physician or nonphysician health care professional is assigned to 86.28. Any "excisional" type procedure performed by a nonphysician is assigned to 86. 28.

9. ADVERSE EFFECTS AND POISONING

The properties of certain drugs, medicinal and biological substances or combinations of such substances, may cause toxic reactions. The occurrence of drug toxicity is classified in ICD-9-CM as follows:

9.1. Adverse Effect

When the drug was correctly prescribed and properly administered, code the reaction plus the appropriate code from the E930-E949 series.

Adverse effects of therapeutic substances correctly prescribed and properly administered (toxicity, synergistic reaction, side effect, and idiosyncratic reaction) may be due to (1) differences among patients, such as age, sex, disease, and genetic factors, and (2) drug-related factors, such as type of drug, route of administration, duration of therapy, dosage, and bioavailability.

Codes from the E930-E949 series must be used to identify the causative substance for an adverse effect of drug, medicinal and biological substances, correctly prescribed and properly administered. The effect, such as tachycardia, delirium, gastrointestinal hemorrhaging, vomiting, hypokalemia, hepatitis, renal failure, or respiratory failure, is coded and followed by the appropriate code from the E930-E949 series.

9.2. Poisoning

Poisoning when an error was made in drug prescription or in the administration of the drug by physician, nurse, patient, or other person, use the appropriate code from the 960-979 series. If an overdose of a drug was intentionally taken or administered and resulted in drug toxicity, it would be coded as a poisoning (960-979 series). If a nonprescribed drug or medicinal agent was taken in combination with a correctly prescribed and properly administered drug, any drug toxicity or other reaction resulting from the interaction of the two drugs would be classified as a poisoning.

10. HUMAN IMMUNODEFICIENCY VIRUS (HIV) INFECTIONS

10.1. Code only confirmed cases of HIV infection/illness.

This is an exception to guideline 1.8 which states "If the diagnosis documented at the time of discharge is qualified as 'probable,' 'suspected,' 'likely,' 'questionable,' 'possible,' or 'still to be ruled out,' code the condition as if it existed or was established..."

In this context, "confirmation" does not require documentation of positive serology or culture for HIV; the physician's diagnostic statement that the patient is HIV positive, or has an HIV-related illness is sufficient.

10.2. Selection of HIV code

042 Human Immunodeficiency Virus [HIV] Disease

Patients with an HIV-related illness should be coded to 042, Human Immunodeficiency Virus [HIV] Disease.

V08 Asymptomatic Human Immunodeficiency Virus [HIV] Infection

Patients with physician-documented asymptomatic HIV infections who have never had an HIV-related illness should be coded to V08, Asymptomatic Human Immunodeficiency Virus [HIV] Infection.

795.71 Nonspecific Serologic Evidence of Human Immunodeficiency Virus [HIV]

Code 795.71, Nonspecific serologic evidence of human immunodeficiency virus [HIV], should be used for patients (including infants) with inconclusive HIV test results.

10.3. Previously diagnosed HIV-related illness

Patients with any known prior diagnosis of an HIV-related illness should be coded to 042. Once a patient had developed an HIV-related illness, the patient should always be assigned code 042 on every subsequent admission. Patients previously diagnosed with any HIV illness (042) should never be assigned to 795.71 or V 08.

10.4. Sequencing

The sequencing of diagnoses for patients with HIV-related illnesses follows guideline 2 for selection of principal diagnosis. That is, the circumstances of admission govern the selection of principal diagnosis, "that condition established after study to be chiefly responsible for occasioning the admission of the patient to the hospital for care."

Patients who are admitted for an HIV-related illness should be assigned a minimum of two codes: first assign code 042 to identify the HIV disease and then sequence additional codes to identify the other diagnoses. If a patient is admitted for an HIV-related condition, the principal diagnosis should be 042, followed by additional diagnosis codes for all reported HIV-related conditions.

If a patient with HIV disease is admitted for an unrelated condition (such as a traumatic injury), the code for the unrelated condition (e.g., the nature of injury code) should be the principal diagnosis. Other diagnoses would be 042 followed by additional diagnosis codes for all reported HIV-related conditions.

Whether the patient is newly diagnosed or has had previous admissions for HIV conditions (or has expired) is irrelevant to the sequencing decision.

10.5. HIV Infection in Pregnancy, Childbirth and the Puerperium

During pregnancy, childbirth or the puerperium, a patient admitted because of an HIV-related illness should receive a principal diagnosis of 647.6X, Other specified infectious and parasitic diseases in the mother classifiable elsewhere, but complicating the pregnancy, childbirth or the puerperium, followed by 042 and the code(s) for the HIV-related illness(es). This is an exception to the sequencing rule found in 10.4 above.

Patients with asymptomatic HIV infection status admitted during pregnancy, childbirth, or the puerperium should receive codes of 647.6X and V08.

10.6. Asymptomatic HIV Infection

V08 Asymptomatic human immunodeficiency virus [HIV] infection, is to be applied when the patient without any documentation of symptoms is listed as being "HIV positive," "known HIV," "HIV test positive," or similar terminology. Do not use this code if the term "AIDS" is used or if the patient is treated for any HIV-related illness or is described as having any condition(s) resulting from his/her HIV positive status; use 042 in these cases.

10.7. Inconclusive Laboratory Test for HIV

Patients with inconclusive HIV serology, but no definitive diagnosis or manifestations of the illness may be assigned code 795.71.Inconclusive serologic test for Human Immunodeficiency Virus [HIV]

10.8. Testing for HIV

If the patient is asymptomatic but wishes to know his/her HIV status, use code V73.89, Screening for other specified viral disease. Use code V69.8, Other problems related to lifestyle, as a secondary code if an asymptomatic patient is in a known high-risk group for HIV. Should a patient with signs or symptoms or illness, or a confirmed HIV related diagnosis be tested for HIV code the signs and symptoms or the diagnosis. An additional counseling code V65.44 may be used if counseling is provided during the encounter for the test.

When the patient returns to be informed of his/her HIV test results use code V65.44, HIV counseling, if the results of the test are negative. If the results are positive but the patient is asymptomatic use code V08, Asymptomatic HIV infection. If the results are positive and the patient is symptomatic use code 042, HIV infection, with codes for the HIV related symptoms or diagnosis. The HIV counseling code may also be used if counseling is provided for patients with positive test results.

11. GUIDELINES FOR CODING EXTERNAL CAUSES OF INJURIES, POISONINGS AND ADVERSE EFFECTS OF DRUGS (E Codes)

Introduction

These guidelines are provided for those who are currently collecting E codes in order that there will be standardization in the process. If your institution plans to begin collecting E codes, these guidelines are to be applied. The use of E codes are supplemental to the application of basic ICD-9-CM codes. E codes are never to be recorded as principal diagnosis (first listed in the outpatient setting) and are not required for reporting to the Health Care Financing Administration.

Injuries are a major cause of mortality, morbidity and disability. In the United States, the care of patients who suffer intentional and unintentional injuries and poisonings contributes significantly to the increase in medical care costs. External causes of injury and poisoning codes (E codes) are intended to provide data for injury research and evaluation of injury prevention strategies. E codes capture how the injury or poisoning happened (cause), the intent (unintentional or accidental; or intentional, such as suicide or assault), and the place where the event occurred. Some major categories of E codes include:

- transport accidents
- poisoning and adverse effects of drugs, medicinal substances and biologicals
- accidental falls
- accidents caused by fire and flames
- accidents due to natural and environmental factors
- late effects of accidents, assaults or self injury
- assaults or purposely inflicted injury
- suicide or self inflicted injury

These guidelines apply for the coding and collection of E code from records in hospitals, outpatient clinics, emergency departments, other ambulatory care settings and physician offices except when other specific guidelines apply. (See Reporting Diagnostic Guidelines for Hospital-based Outpatient Services/Reporting Requirements for Physician Billing.)

11.1. General E Code Coding Guidelines

    A. An E code may be used with any code in the range of 001-V83.89 which indicates an injury, poisoning, or adverse effect due to an external cause.

    B. Assign the appropriate E-code for all initial treatments of an injury, poisoning, or adverse effect of drugs.

    C. Use a late effect E code for subsequent visits when a late effect of the initial injury or poisoning is being treated. There is no late effect E code for adverse effects of drugs.

    D. Use the full range of E codes to completely describe the cause, the intent and the place of occurrence, if applicable, for all injuries, poisonings, and adverse effects of drugs.

    E. Assign as many E codes as necessary to fully explain each cause. If only one E code can be recorded, assign the E code most related to the principal diagnosis.

    F. The selection of the appropriate E code is guided by the Index to External Causes which is located after the alphabetical index to diseases and by Inclusion and Exclusion notes in the Tabular List.

    G. An E code can never be a principal (first listed) diagnosis.

11.2. Place of Occurrence Guideline

Use an additional code from category E849 to indicate the Place of Occurrence for injuries and poisonings. The Place of Occurrence describes the place where the event occurred and not the patient's activity at the time of the event.

Do not use E849.9 if the place of occurrence is not stated.

11.3. Poisonings and Adverse Effects of Drugs, Medicinal and Biological Substances Guidelines

    A. Do not code directly from the Table of Drugs and Chemicals. Always refer back to the Tabular List.

    B. Use as many codes as necessary to describe completely all drugs, medicinal or biological substances.

    C. If the same E code would describe the causative agent for more than one adverse reaction, assign the code only once.

    D. If two or more drugs, medicinal or biological substances are reported, code each individually unless the combination code is listed in the Table of Drugs and Chemicals. In that case, assign the E code for the combination.

    E. When a reaction results from the interaction of a drug(s) and alcohol, use poisoning codes and E codes for both.

    F. If the reporting format limits the number of E codes that can be used in reporting clinical data, code the one most related to the principal diagnosis. Include at least one from each category (cause, intent, place) if possible.

- If there are different fourth digit codes in the same three digit category, use the code for "Other specified" of that category. If there is no "Other specified" code in that category, use the appropriate "Unspecified" code in that category.
- If the codes are in different three digit categories, assign the appropriate E code for other multiple drugs and medicinal substances.

11.4. Multiple Cause E Code Coding Guidelines

If two or more events cause separate injuries, an E code should be assigned for each cause. The first listed E code will be selected in the following order:

- E codes for child and adult abuse take priority over all other E code—see Child and Adult abuse guidelines
- E codes for cataclysmic events take priority over all other E codes except child and adult abuse
- E codes for transport accidents take priority over all other E codes except cataclysmic events and child and adult abuse

The first listed E code should correspond to the cause of the most serious diagnosis due to an assault, accident, or self-harm, following the order of hierarchy listed above.

11.5. Child and Adult Abuse Guideline

  A. When the cause of an injury or neglect is intentional child or adult abuse, the first listed E code should be assigned from categories E960-E968, Homicide and injury purposely inflicted by other persons, (except category E967). An E code from category E967, Child and adult battering and other maltreatment, should be added as an additional code to identify the perpetrator, if known.

  B. In cases of neglect when the intent is determined to be accidental E code E904.0, Abandonment or neglect of infant and helpless person, should be the first listed E code.

11.6. Unknown or Suspected Intent Guideline

  A. If the intent (accident, self-harm, assault) of the cause of an injury or poisoning is unknown or unspecified, code the intent as undetermined E980-E989.

  B. If the intent (accident, self-harm, assault) of the cause of an injury or poisoning is questionable, probable or suspected, code the intent as undetermined E980-E989.

11.7. Undetermined Cause

When the intent of an injury or poisoning is known, but the cause is unknown, use codes: E928.9, Unspecified accident, E958.9, Suicide and self-inflicted injury by unspecified means, and E968.9, Assault by unspecified means.

These E codes should rarely be used as the documentation in the medical record, in both the inpatient and outpatient settings, should normally provide sufficient detail to determine the cause of the injury.

11.8. Late Effects of External Cause Guidelines

  A. Late effect E codes exist for injuries and poisonings but not for adverse effects of drugs, misadventures and surgical complications.

  B. A late effect E code (E929, E959, E969, E977, E989, or E999) should be used with any report of a late effect or sequela resulting from a previous injury or poisoning (905-909).

  C. A late effect E code should never be used with a related current nature of injury code.

11.9. Misadventures and Complications of Care Guidelines

  A. Assign a code in the range of E870-E876 if misadventures are stated by the physician.

  B. Assign a code in the range of E878-E879 if the physician attributes an abnormal reaction or later complication to a surgical or medical procedure, but does not mention misadventure at the time of the procedure as the cause of the reaction.

Index to Diseases

A

AAV (disease) (illness) (infection) — see Human immunodeficiency virus (disease) (illness) (infection)
Abactio — see Abortion, induced
Abactus venter — see Abortion, induced
Abarognosis 781.99
Abasia (-astasia) 307.9
   atactica 781.3
   choreic 781.3
   hysterical 300.11
   paroxysmal trepidant 781.3
   spastic 781.3
   trembling 781.3
   trepidans 781.3
Abderhalden-Kaufmann-Lignac syndrome (cystinosis) 270.0
Abdomen, abdominal — see also condition
   accordion 306.4
   acute 789.0
   angina 557.1
   burst 868.00
   convulsive equivalent (see also Epilepsy) 345.5
   heart 746.87
   muscle deficiency syndrome 756.79
   obstipum 756.79
Abdominalgia 789.0
   periodic 277.3
Abduction contracture, hip or other joint — see Contraction, joint
Abercrombie's syndrome (amyloid degeneration) 277.3
Aberrant (congenital) — see also Malposition, congenital
   adrenal gland 759.1
   blood vessel NEC 747.60
     arteriovenous NEC 747.60
     cerebrovascular 747.81
     gastrointestinal 747.61
     lower limb 747.64
     renal 747.62
     spinal 747.82
     upper limb 747.63
   breast 757.6
   endocrine gland NEC 759.2
   gastrointestinal vessel (peripheral) 747.61
   hepatic duct 751.69
   lower limb vessel (peripheral) 747.64
   pancreas 751.7
   parathyroid gland 759.2
   peripheral vascular vessel NEC 747.60
   pituitary gland (pharyngeal) 759.2
   renal blood vessel 747.62
   sebaceous glands, mucous membrane, mouth 750.26
   spinal vessel 747.82
   spleen 759.0
   testis (descent) 752.51
   thymus gland 759.2
   thyroid gland 759.2
   upper limb vessel (peripheral) 747.63
Aberratio
   lactis 757.6
   testis 752.51
Aberration — see also Anomaly
   chromosome — see Anomaly, chromosome(s)
   distantial 368.9
   mental (see also Disorder, mental, nonpsychotic) 300.9
Abetalipoproteinemia 272.5
Abionarce 780.79
Abiotrophy 799.8
Ablatio
   placentae — see Placenta, ablatio
   retinae (see also Detachment, retina) 361.9
Ablation
   pituitary (gland) (with hypofunction) 253.7
   placenta — see Placenta, ablatio
   uterus 621.8
Ablepharia, ablepharon, ablephary 743.62
Ablepsia — see Blindness
Ablepsy — see Blindness

Ablutomania 300.3
Abnormal, abnormality, abnormalities — see also Anomaly
   acid-base balance 276.4
     fetus or newborn — see Distress, fetal
   adaptation curve, dark 368.63
   alveolar ridge 525.9
   amnion 658.9
     affecting fetus or newborn 762.9
   anatomical relationship NEC 759.9
   apertures, congenital, diaphragm 756.6
   auditory perception NEC 388.40
   autosomes NEC 758.5
     13 758.1
     18 758.2
     21 or 22 758.0
     D_1 758.1
     E_3 758.2
     G 758.0
   ballistocardiogram 794.39
   basal metabolic rate (BMR) 794.7
   biosynthesis, testicular androgen 257.2
   blood level (of)
     cobalt 790.6
     copper 790.6
     iron 790.6
     lithium 790.6
     magnesium 790.6
     mineral 790.6
     zinc 790.6
   blood pressure
     elevated (without diagnosis of hypertension) 796.2
     low (see also Hypotension) 458.9
       reading (incidental) (isolated) (nonspecific) 796.3
   bowel sounds 787.5
   breathing behavior — see Respiration
   caloric test 794.19
   cervix (acquired) NEC 622.9
     congenital 752.40
     in pregnancy or childbirth 654.6
       causing obstructed labor 660.2
         affecting fetus or newborn 763.1
   chemistry, blood NEC 790.6
   chest sounds 786.7
   chorion 658.9
     affecting fetus or newborn 762.9
   chromosomal NEC 758.89
     analysis, nonspecific result 795.2
     autosomes (see also Abnormal, autosomes NEC) 758.5
     fetal, (suspected) affecting management of pregnancy 655.1
     sex 758.81
   clinical findings NEC 796.4
   communication — see Fistula
   configuration of pupils 379.49
   coronary
     artery 746.85
     vein 746.9
   cortisol-binding globulin 255.8
   course, Eustachian tube 744.24
   dentofacial NEC 524.9
     functional 524.5
     specified type NEC 524.8
   development, developmental NEC 759.9
     bone 756.9
     central nervous system 742.9
   direction, teeth 524.3
   Dynia (see also Defect, coagulation) 286.9
   Ebstein 746.2
   echocardiogram 793.2
   echoencephalogram 794.01
   echogram NEC — see Findings, abnormal, structure
   electrocardiogram (ECG) (EKG) 794.31
   electroencephalogram (EEG) 794.02
   electromyogram (EMG) 794.17
     ocular 794.14
   electro-oculogram (EOG) 794.12
   electroretinogram (ERG) 794.11
   erythrocytes 289.9
     congenital, with perinatal jaundice 282.9 [774.0]
   Eustachian valve 746.9
   excitability under minor stress 301.9

Abnormal, abnormality, abnormalities — see also Anomaly — continued
   fat distribution 782.9
   feces 787.7
   fetal heart rate — see Distress, fetal
   fetus NEC
     affecting management of pregnancy — see Pregnancy, management affected by, fetal
     causing disproportion 653.7
       affecting fetus or newborn 763.1
       causing obstructed labor 660.1
         affecting fetus or newborn 763.1
   findings without manifest disease — see Findings, abnormal
   fluid
     amniotic 792.3
     cerebrospinal 792.0
     peritoneal 792.9
     pleural 792.9
     synovial 792.9
     vaginal 792.9
   forces of labor NEC 661.9
     affecting fetus or newborn 763.7
   form, teeth 520.2
   function studies
     auditory 794.15
     bladder 794.9
     brain 794.00
     cardiovascular 794.30
     endocrine NEC 794.6
     kidney 794.4
     liver 794.8
     nervous system
       central 794.00
       peripheral 794.19
     oculomotor 794.14
     pancreas 794.9
     placenta 794.9
     pulmonary 794.2
     retina 794.11
     special senses 794.19
     spleen 794.9
     thyroid 794.5
     vestibular 794.16
   gait 781.2
     hysterical 300.11
   gastrin secretion 251.5
   globulin
     cortisol-binding 255.8
     thyroid-binding 246.8
   glucagon secretion 251.4
   glucose tolerance test 790.2
     in pregnancy, childbirth, or puerperium 648.8
     fetus or newborn 775.0
   gravitational (G) forces or states 994.9
   hair NEC 704.2
   hard tissue formation in pulp 522.3
   head movement 781.0
   heart
     rate
       fetus, affecting liveborn infant
         before the onset of labor 763.81
         during labor 763.82
         unspecified as to time of onset 763.83
       intrauterine
         before the onset of labor 763.81
         during labor 763.82
         unspecified as to time of onset 763.83
       newborn
         before the onset of labor 763.81
         during labor 763.82
         unspecified as to time of onset 763.83
     shadow 793.2
     sounds NEC 785.3
   hemoglobin (see also Disease, hemoglobin) 282.7
     trait — see Trait, hemoglobin, abnormal
   hemorrhage, uterus — see Hemorrhage, uterus
   histology NEC 795.4
   increase
     in
       appetite 783.6
       development 783.9
   involuntary movement 781.0
   jaw closure 524.5

Abnormal, abnormality, abnormalities

Abnormal, abnormality, abnormalities — see also Anomaly — continued
- karyotype 795.2
- knee jerk 796.1
- labor NEC 661.9 ✓5
  - affecting fetus or newborn 763.7
- laboratory findings — see Findings, abnormal
- length, organ or site, congenital — see Distortion
- loss of height 781.91
- loss of weight 783.21
- lung shadow 793.1
- mammogram 793.80
  - microcalcification 793.81
- Mantoux test 795.5
- membranes (fetal)
  - affecting fetus or newborn 762.9
  - complicating pregnancy 658.8 ✓5
- menstruation — see Menstruation
- metabolism (see also condition) 783.9
- movement 781.0
  - disorder NEC 333.90
    - specified NEC 333.99
  - head 781.0
  - involuntary 781.0
  - specified type NEC 333.99
- muscle contraction, localized 728.85
- myoglobin (Aberdeen) (Annapolis) 289.9
- narrowness, eyelid 743.62
- optokinetic response 379.57
- organs or tissues of pelvis NEC
  - in pregnancy or childbirth 654.9 ✓5
    - affecting fetus or newborn 763.89
    - causing obstructed labor 660.2 ✓5
      - affecting fetus or newborn 763.1
- origin — see Malposition, congenital
- palmar creases 757.2
- Papanicolaou (smear)
  - cervix 795.00 ▲
    - atypical squamous cell changes of undetermined significance ●
      - favor benign (ASCUS favor benign) 795.01 ●
      - favor dysplasia (ASCUS favor dysplasia) 795.02 ●
    - nonspecific finding NEC 795.09 ●
  - other site 795.1
- parturition
  - affecting fetus or newborn 763.9
  - mother — see Delivery, complicated
- pelvis (bony) — see Deformity, pelvis
- percussion, chest 786.7
- periods (grossly) (see also Menstruation) 626.9
- phonocardiogram 794.39
- placenta — see Placenta, abnormal
- plantar reflex 796.1
- plasma protein — see Deficiency, plasma, protein
- pleural folds 748.8
- position — see also Malposition
  - gravid uterus 654.4 ✓5
    - causing obstructed labor 660.2 ✓5
      - affecting fetus or newborn 763.1
- posture NEC 781.92
- presentation (fetus) — see Presentation, fetus, abnormal
- product of conception NEC 631
- puberty — see Puberty
- pulmonary
  - artery 747.3
  - function, newborn 770.89 ▲
  - test results 794.2
  - ventilation, newborn 770.89 ▲
    - hyperventilation 786.01
- pulsations in neck 785.1
- pupil reflexes 379.40
- quality of milk 676.8 ✓5
- radiological examination 793.9
  - abdomen NEC 793.6
  - biliary tract 793.3
  - breast 793.89
    - mammogram NOS 793.80
      - mammographic microcalcification 793.81
  - gastrointestinal tract 793.4
  - genitourinary organs 793.5
  - head 793.0
  - intrathoracic organ NEC 793.2

Abnormal, abnormality, abnormalities — see also Anomaly — continued
- radiological examination — continued
  - lung (field) 793.1
  - musculoskeletal system 793.7
  - retroperitoneum 793.6
  - skin and subcutaneous tissue 793.9
  - skull 793.0
- red blood cells 790.09
  - morphology 790.09
  - volume 790.09
- reflex NEC 796.1
- renal function test 794.4
- respiration signs — see Respiration
- response to nerve stimulation 794.10
- retinal correspondence 368.34
- rhythm, heart — see also Arrhythmia
  - fetus — see Distress, fetal
- saliva 792.4
- scan
  - brain 794.09
  - kidney 794.4
  - liver 794.8
  - lung 794.2
  - thyroid 794.5
- secretion
  - gastrin 251.5
  - glucagon 251.4
- semen 792.2
- serum level (of)
  - acid phosphatase 790.5
  - alkaline phosphatase 790.5
  - amylase 790.5
  - enzymes NEC 790.5
  - lipase 790.5
- shape
  - cornea 743.41
  - gallbladder 751.69
  - gravid uterus 654.4 ✓5
    - affecting fetus or newborn 763.89
    - causing obstructed labor 660.2 ✓5
      - affecting fetus or newborn 763.1
  - head (see also Anomaly, skull) 756.0
  - organ or site, congenital NEC — see Distortion
- sinus venosus 747.40
- size
  - fetus, complicating delivery 653.5 ✓5
    - causing obstructed labor 660.1 ✓5
  - gallbladder 751.69
  - head (see also Anomaly, skull) 756.0
  - organ or site, congenital NEC — see Distortion
  - teeth 520.2
- skin and appendages, congenital NEC 757.9
- soft parts of pelvis — see Abnormal, organs or tissues of pelvis
- spermatozoa 792.2
- sputum (amount) (color) (excessive) (odor) (purulent) 786.4
- stool NEC 787.7
  - bloody 578.1
    - occult 792.1
  - bulky 787.7
  - color (dark) (light) 792.1
  - content (fat) (mucus) (pus) 792.1
  - occult blood 792.1
- synchondrosis 756.9
- test results without manifest disease — see Findings, abnormal
- thebesian valve 746.9
- thermography — see Findings, abnormal, structure
- threshold, cones or rods (eye) 368.63
- thyroid-binding globulin 246.8
- thyroid product 246.8
- toxicology (findings) NEC 796.0
- tracheal cartilage (congenital) 748.3
- transport protein 273.8
- ultrasound results — see Findings, abnormal, structure
- umbilical cord
  - affecting fetus or newborn 762.6
  - complicating delivery 663.9 ✓5
  - specified NEC 663.8 ✓5
- union
  - cricoid cartilage and thyroid cartilage 748.3
  - larynx and trachea 748.3

Abnormal, abnormality, abnormalities — see also Anomaly — continued
- union — continued
  - thyroid cartilage and hyoid bone 748.3
- urination NEC 788.69
  - psychogenic 306.53
  - stream
    - intermittent 788.61
    - slowing 788.62
    - splitting 788.61
    - weak 788.62
- urine (constituents) NEC 791.9
- uterine hemorrhage (see also Hemorrhage, uterus) 626.9
  - climacteric 627.0
  - postmenopausal 627.1
- vagina (acquired) (congenital)
  - in pregnancy or childbirth 654.7 ✓5
    - affecting fetus or newborn 763.89
    - causing obstructed labor 660.2 ✓5
      - affecting fetus or newborn 763.1
- vascular sounds 785.9
- vectorcardiogram 794.39
- visually evoked potential (VEP) 794.13
- vulva (acquired) (congenital)
  - in pregnancy or childbirth 654.8 ✓5
    - affecting fetus or newborn 763.89
    - causing obstructed labor 660.2 ✓5
      - affecting fetus or newborn 763.1
- weight
  - gain 783.1
    - of pregnancy 646.1 ✓5
      - with hypertension — see Toxemia, of pregnancy
  - loss 783.21
- x-ray examination — see Abnormal, radiological examination

Abnormally formed uterus — see Anomaly, uterus

Abnormity (any organ or part) — see Anomaly

ABO
- hemolytic disease 773.1
- incompatibility reaction 999.6

Abocclusion 524.2

Abolition, language 784.69

Aborter, habitual or recurrent NEC
- without current pregnancy 629.9
- current abortion (see also Abortion, spontaneous) 634.9 ✓5
  - affecting fetus or newborn 761.8
- observation in current pregnancy 646.3 ✓5

Abortion (complete) (incomplete) (inevitable) (with retained products of conception) 637.9 ✓5

> Note — Use the following fifth-digit subclassification with categories 634–637:
>
> 0   unspecified
> 1   incomplete
> 2   complete

- with
  - complication(s) (any) following previous abortion — see category 639 ✓4
  - damage to pelvic organ (laceration) (rupture) (tear) 637.2 ✓5
  - embolism (air) (amniotic fluid) (blood clot) (pulmonary) (pyemic) (septic) (soap) 637.6 ✓5
  - genital tract and pelvic infection 637.0 ✓5
  - hemorrhage, delayed or excessive 637.1 ✓5
  - metabolic disorder 637.4 ✓5
  - renal failure (acute) 637.3 ✓5
  - sepsis (genital tract) (pelvic organ) 637.0 ✓5
    - urinary tract 637.7 ✓5
  - shock (postoperative) (septic) 637.5 ✓5
  - specified complication NEC 637.7 ✓5
  - toxemia 637.3 ✓5
  - unspecified complication(s) 637.8 ✓5
  - urinary tract infection 637.7 ✓5
- accidental — see Abortion, spontaneous
- artificial — see Abortion, induced
- attempted (failed) — see Abortion, failed
- criminal — see Abortion, illegal
- early — see Abortion, spontaneous
- elective — see Abortion, legal

Index to Diseases

Abortion — *continued*
  failed (legal) 638.9
    with
      damage to pelvic organ (laceration)
          (rupture) (tear) 638.2
      embolism (air) (amniotic fluid) (blood clot)
          (pulmonary) (pyemic) (septic) (soap)
          638.6
      genital tract and pelvic infection 638.0
      hemorrhage, delayed or excessive 638.1
      metabolic disorder 638.4
      renal failure (acute) 638.3
      sepsis (genital tract) (pelvic organ) 638.0
        urinary tract 638.7
      shock (postoperative) (septic) 638.5
      specified complication NEC 638.7
      toxemia 638.3
      unspecified complication(s) 638.8
      urinary tract infection 638.7
  fetal indication — *see* Abortion, legal
  fetus 779.6
  following threatened abortion — *see* Abortion,
      by type
  habitual or recurrent (care during pregnancy)
      646.3
    with current abortion (*see also* Abortion,
        spontaneous) 634.9
      affecting fetus or newborn 761.8
    without current pregnancy 629.9
  homicidal — *see* Abortion, illegal
  illegal 636.9
    with
      damage to pelvic organ (laceration)
          (rupture) (tear) 636.2
      embolism (air) (amniotic fluid) (blood clot)
          (pulmonary) (pyemic) (septic) (soap)
          636.6
      genital tract and pelvic infection
          636.0
      hemorrhage, delayed or excessive
          636.1
      metabolic disorder 636.4
      renal failure 636.3
      sepsis (genital tract) (pelvic organ)
          636.0
        urinary tract 636.7
      shock (postoperative) (septic) 636.5
      specified complication NEC 636.7
      toxemia 636.3
      unspecified complication(s) 636.8
      urinary tract infection 636.7
    fetus 779.6
  induced 637.9
    illegal — *see* Abortion, illegal
    legal indications — *see* Abortion, legal
    medical indications — *see* Abortion, legal
    therapeutic — *see* Abortion, legal
  late — *see* Abortion, spontaneous
  legal (legal indication) (medical indication)
      (under medical supervision) 635.9
    with
      damage to pelvic organ (laceration)
          (rupture) (tear) 635.2
      embolism (air) (amniotic fluid) (blood clot)
          (pulmonary) (pyemic) (septic) (soap)
          635.6
      genital tract and pelvic infection
          635.0
      hemorrhage, delayed or excessive
          635.1
      metabolic disorder 635.4
      renal failure (acute) 635.3
      sepsis (genital tract) (pelvic organ)
          635.0
        urinary tract 635.7
      shock (postoperative) (septic) 635.5
      specified complication NEC 635.7
      toxemia 635.3
      unspecified complication(s) 635.8
      urinary tract infection 635.7
    fetus 779.6
  medical indication — *see* Abortion, legal
  mental hygiene problem — *see* Abortion, legal
  missed 632
  operative — *see* Abortion, legal
  psychiatric indication — *see* Abortion, legal

Abortion — *continued*
  recurrent — *see* Abortion, spontaneous
  self-induced — *see* Abortion, illegal
  septic — *see* Abortion, by type, with sepsis
  spontaneous 634.9
    with
      damage to pelvic organ (laceration)
          (rupture) (tear) 634.2
      embolism (air) (amniotic fluid) (blood clot)
          (pulmonary) (pyemic) (septic) (soap)
          634.6
      genital tract and pelvic infection
          634.0
      hemorrhage, delayed or excessive
          634.1
      metabolic disorder 634.4
      renal failure 634.3
      sepsis (genital tract) (pelvic organ)
          634.0
        urinary tract 634.7
      shock (postoperative) (septic) 634.5
      specified complication NEC 634.7
      toxemia 634.3
      unspecified complication(s) 634.8
      urinary tract infection 634.7
    fetus 761.8
    threatened 640.0
      affecting fetus or newborn 762.1
  surgical — *see* Abortion, legal
  therapeutic — *see* Abortion, legal
  threatened 640.0
    affecting fetus or newborn 762.1
  tubal — *see* Pregnancy, tubal
  voluntary — *see* Abortion, legal
Abortus fever 023.9
Aboulomania 301.6
Abrachia 755.20
Abrachiatism 755.20
Abrachiocephalia 759.89
Abrachiocephalus 759.89
Abrami's disease (acquired hemolytic jaundice)
    283.9
Abramov-Fiedler myocarditis (acute isolated
    myocarditis) 422.91
Abrasion — *see also* Injury, superficial, by site
  cornea 918.1
  dental 521.2
  teeth, tooth (dentifrice) (habitual) (hard tissues)
      (occupational) (ritual) (traditional) (wedge
      defect) 521.2
Abrikossov's tumor (M9580/0) — *see also*
    Neoplasm, connective tissue, benign
  malignant (M9580/3) — *see* Neoplasm,
      connective tissue, malignant
Abrism 988.8
Abruption, placenta — *see* Placenta, abruptio
Abruptio placentae — *see* Placenta, abruptio
Abscess (acute) (chronic) (infectional)
    (lymphangitic) (metastatic) (multiple)
    (pyogenic) (septic) (with lymphangitis) (*see
    also* Cellulitis) 682.9
  abdomen, abdominal
    cavity — *see* Abscess, peritoneum
    wall 682.2
  abdominopelvic — *see* Abscess, peritoneum
  accessory sinus (chronic) (*see also* Sinusitis)
      473.9
  adrenal (capsule) (gland) 255.8
  alveolar 522.5
    with sinus 522.7
  amebic 006.3
    bladder 006.8
    brain (with liver or lung abscess) 006.5
    liver (without mention of brain or lung
        abscess) 006.3
      with
        brain abscess (and lung abscess)
            006.5
        lung abscess 006.4
    lung (with liver abscess) 006.4
      with brain abscess 006.5
    seminal vesicle 006.8
    specified site NEC 006.8
    spleen 006.8

Abscess (*see also* Cellulitis) — *continued*
  anaerobic 040.0
  ankle 682.6
  anorectal 566
  antecubital space 682.3
  antrum (chronic) (Highmore) (*see also* Sinusitis,
      maxillary) 473.0
  anus 566
  apical (tooth) 522.5
    with sinus (alveolar) 522.7
  appendix 540.1
  areola (acute) (chronic) (nonpuerperal) 611.0
    puerperal, postpartum 675.1
  arm (any part, above wrist) 682.3
  artery (wall) 447.2
  atheromatous 447.2
  auditory canal (external) 380.10
  auricle (ear) (staphylococcal) (streptococcal)
      380.10
  axilla, axillary (region) 682.3
    lymph gland or node 683
  back (any part) 682.2
  Bartholin's gland 616.3
    with
      abortion — *see* Abortion, by type, with
          sepsis
      ectopic pregnancy (*see also* categories
          633.0-633.9) 639.0
      molar pregnancy (*see also* categories 630-
          632) 639.0
    complicating pregnancy or puerperium
        646.6
    following
      abortion 639.0
      ectopic or molar pregnancy 639.0
  bartholinian 616.3
  Bezold's 383.01
  bile, biliary, duct or tract (*see also*
      Cholecystitis) 576.8
  bilharziasis 120.1
  bladder (wall) 595.89
    amebic 006.8
  bone (subperiosteal) (*see also* Osteomyelitis)
      730.0
    accessory sinus (chronic) (*see also* Sinusitis)
        473.9
    acute 730.0
    chronic or old 730.1
    jaw (lower) (upper) 526.4
    mastoid — *see* Mastoiditis, acute
    petrous (*see also* Petrositis) 383.20
    spinal (tuberculous) (*see also* Tuberculosis)
        015.0 [730.88]
    nontuberculous 730.08
  bowel 569.5
  brain (any part) 324.0
    amebic (with liver or lung abscess) 006.5
    cystic 324.0
    late effect — *see* category 326
    otogenic 324.0
    tuberculous (*see also* Tuberculosis)
        013.3
  breast (acute) (chronic) (nonpuerperal) 611.0
    newborn 771.5
    puerperal, postpartum 675.1
    tuberculous (*see also* Tuberculosis)
        017.9
  broad ligament (chronic) (*see also* Disease,
      pelvis, inflammatory) 614.4
    acute 614.3
  Brodie's (chronic) (localized) (*see also*
      Osteomyelitis) 730.1
  bronchus 519.1
  buccal cavity 528.3
  bulbourethral gland 597.0
  bursa 727.89
    pharyngeal 478.29
  buttock 682.5
  canaliculus, breast 611.0
  canthus 372.20
  cartilage 733.99
  cecum 569.5
    with appendicitis 540.1
  cerebellum, cerebellar 324.0
    late effect — *see* category 326
  cerebral (embolic) 324.0
    late effect — *see* category 326

Abscess (*see also* Cellulitis) — *continued*
  cervical (neck region) 682.1
    lymph gland or node 683
    stump (*see also* Cervicitis) 616.0
  cervix (stump) (uteri) (*see also* Cervicitis) 616.0
  cheek, external 682.0
    inner 528.3
  chest 510.9
    with fistula 510.0
    wall 682.2
  chin 682.0
  choroid 363.00
  ciliary body 364.3
  circumtonsillar 475
  cold (tuberculous) — *see also* Tuberculosis, abscess
    articular — *see* Tuberculosis, joint
  colon (wall) 569.5
  colostomy or enterostomy 569.61
  conjunctiva 372.00
  connective tissue NEC 682.9
  cornea 370.55
    with ulcer 370.00
  corpus
    cavernosum 607.2
    luteum (*see also* Salpingo-oophoritis) 614.2
  Cowper's gland 597.0
  cranium 324.0
  cul-de-sac (Douglas') (posterior) (*see also* Disease, pelvis, inflammatory) 614.4
    acute 614.3
  dental 522.5
    with sinus (alveolar) 522.7
  dentoalveolar 522.5
    with sinus (alveolar) 522.7
  diaphragm, diaphragmatic — *see* Abscess, peritoneum
  digit NEC 681.9
  Douglas' cul-de-sac or pouch (*see also* Disease, pelvis, inflammatory) 614.4
    acute 614.3
  Dubois' 090.5
  ductless gland 259.8
  ear
    acute 382.00
    external 380.10
    inner 386.30
    middle — *see* Otitis media
  elbow 682.3
  endamebic — *see* Abscess, amebic
  entamebic — *see* Abscess, amebic
  enterostomy 569.61
  epididymis 604.0
  epidural 324.9
    brain 324.0
    late effect — *see* category 326
    spinal cord 324.1
  epiglottis 478.79
  epiploon, epiploic — *see* Abscess, peritoneum
  erysipelatous (*see also* Erysipelas) 035
  esophagus 530.19
  ethmoid (bone) (chronic) (sinus) (*see also* Sinusitis, ethmoidal) 473.2
  external auditory canal 380.10
  extradural 324.9
    brain 324.0
    late effect — *see* category 326
    spinal cord 324.1
  extraperitoneal — *see* Abscess, peritoneum
  eye 360.00
  eyelid 373.13
  face (any part, except eye) 682.0
  fallopian tube (*see also* Salpingo-oophoritis) 614.2
  fascia 728.89
  fauces 478.29
  fecal 569.5
  femoral (region) 682.6
  filaria, filarial (*see also* Infestation, filarial) 125.9
  finger (any) (intrathecal) (periosteal) (subcutaneous) (subcuticular) 681.00
  fistulous NEC 682.9
  flank 682.2
  foot (except toe) 682.7
  forearm 682.3
  forehead 682.0

Abscess (*see also* Cellulitis) — *continued*
  frontal (sinus) (chronic) (*see also* Sinusitis, frontal) 473.1
  gallbladder (*see also* Cholecystitis, acute) 575.0
  gastric 535.0 ✓5ᵗʰ
  genital organ or tract NEC
    female 616.9
      with
        abortion — *see* Abortion, by type, with sepsis
        ectopic pregnancy (*see also* categories 633.0-633.9) 639.0
        molar pregnancy (*see also* categories 630-632) 639.0
      following
        abortion 639.0
        ectopic or molar pregnancy 639.0
      puerperal, postpartum, childbirth 670 ✓5ᵗʰ
    male 608.4
  genitourinary system, tuberculous (*see also* Tuberculosis) 016.9 ✓5ᵗʰ
  gingival 523.3
  gland, glandular (lymph) (acute) NEC 683
  glottis 478.79
  gluteal (region) 682.5
  gonorrheal NEC (*see also* Gonococcus) 098.0
  groin 682.2
  gum 523.3
  hand (except finger or thumb) 682.4
  head (except face) 682.8
  heart 429.89
  heel 682.7
  helminthic (*see also* Infestation, by specific parasite) 128.9
  hepatic 572.0
    amebic (*see also* Abscess, liver, amebic) 006.3
    duct 576.8
  hip 682.6
    tuberculous (active) (*see also* Tuberculosis) 015.1 ✓5ᵗʰ
  ileocecal 540.1
  ileostomy (bud) 569.61
  iliac (region) 682.2
    fossa 540.1
  iliopsoas (tuberculous) (*see also* Tuberculosis) 015.0 ✓5ᵗʰ [730.88]
    nontuberculous 728.89
  infraclavicular (fossa) 682.3
  inguinal (region) 682.2
    lymph gland or node 683
  intersphincteric (anus) 566
  intestine, intestinal 569.5
    rectal 566
  intra-abdominal (*see also* Abscess, peritoneum) 567.2
    postoperative 998.59
  intracranial 324.0
    late effect — *see* category 326
  intramammary — *see* Abscess, breast
  intramastoid (*see also* Mastoiditis, acute) 383.00
  intraorbital 376.01
  intraperitoneal — *see* Abscess, peritoneum
  intraspinal 324.1
    late effect — *see* category 326
  intratonsillar 475
  iris 364.3
  ischiorectal 566
  jaw (bone) (lower) (upper) 526.4
    skin 682.0
  joint (*see also* Arthritis, pyogenic) 711.0 ✓5ᵗʰ
    vertebral (tuberculous) (*see also* Tuberculosis) 015.0 ✓5ᵗʰ [730.88]
    nontuberculous 724.8
  kidney 590.2
    with
      abortion — *see* Abortion, by type, with urinary tract infection
      calculus 592.0
      ectopic pregnancy (*see also* categories 633.0-633.9) 639.8
      molar pregnancy (*see also* categories 630-632) 639.8

Abscess (*see also* Cellulitis) — *continued*
  kidney — *continued*
    complicating pregnancy or puerperium 646.6 ✓5ᵗʰ
      affecting fetus or newborn 760.1
    following
      abortion 639.8
      ectopic or molar pregnancy 639.8
  knee 682.6
    joint 711.06
    tuberculous (active) (*see also* Tuberculosis) 015.2 ✓5ᵗʰ
  labium (majus) (minus) 616.4
    complicating pregnancy, childbirth, or puerperium 646.6 ✓5ᵗʰ
  lacrimal (passages) (sac) (*see also* Dacryocystitis) 375.30
    caruncle 375.30
    gland (*see also* Dacryoadenitis) 375.00
  lacunar 597.0
  larynx 478.79
  lateral (alveolar) 522.5
    with sinus 522.7
  leg, except foot 682.6
  lens 360.00
  lid 373.13
  lingual 529.0
    tonsil 475
  lip 528.5
  Littre's gland 597.0
  liver 572.0
    amebic 006.3
      with
        brain abscess (and lung abscess) 006.5
        lung abscess 006.4
      due to Entamoeba histolytica 006.3
      dysenteric (*see also* Abscess, liver, amebic) 006.3
    pyogenic 572.0
    tropical (*see also* Abscess, liver, amebic) 006.3
  loin (region) 682.2
  lumbar (tuberculous) (*see also* Tuberculosis) 015.0 ✓5ᵗʰ [730.88]
    nontuberculous 682.2
  lung (miliary) (putrid) 513.0
    amebic (with liver abscess) 006.4
      with brain abscess 006.5
  lymph, lymphatic, gland or node (acute) 683
    any site, except mesenteric 683
    mesentery 289.2
  lymphangitic, acute — *see* Cellulitis
  malar 526.4
  mammary gland — *see* Abscess, breast
  marginal (anus) 566
  mastoid (process) (*see also* Mastoiditis, acute) 383.00
    subperiosteal 383.01
  maxilla, maxillary 526.4
    molar (tooth) 522.5
      with sinus 522.7
    premolar 522.5
    sinus (chronic) (*see also* Sinusitis, maxillary) 473.0
  mediastinum 513.1
  meibomian gland 373.12
  meninges (*see also* Meningitis) 320.9
  mesentery, mesenteric — *see* Abscess, peritoneum
  mesosalpinx (*see also* Salpingo-oophoritis) 614.2
  milk 675.1 ✓5ᵗʰ
  Monro's (psoriasis) 696.1
  mons pubis 682.2
  mouth (floor) 528.3
  multiple sites NEC 682.9
  mural 682.2
  muscle 728.89
  myocardium 422.92
  nabothian (follicle) (*see also* Cervicitis) 616.0
  nail (chronic) (with lymphangitis) 681.9
    finger 681.02
    toe 681.11
  nasal (fossa) (septum) 478.1
    sinus (chronic) (*see also* Sinusitis) 473.9
  nasopharyngeal 478.29

Index to Diseases

Abscess

Abscess (see also Cellulitis) — continued
- nates 682.5
- navel 682.2
  - newborn NEC 771.4
- neck (region) 682.1
  - lymph gland or node 683
- nephritic (see also Abscess, kidney) 590.2
- nipple 611.0
  - puerperal, postpartum 675.0 ✓5ᵗʰ
- nose (septum) 478.1
  - external 682.0
- omentum — see Abscess, peritoneum
- operative wound 998.59
- orbit, orbital 376.01
- ossifluent — see Abscess, bone
- ovary, ovarian (corpus luteum) (see also Salpingo-oophoritis) 614.2
- oviduct (see also Salpingo-oophoritis) 614.2
- palate (soft) 528.3
  - hard 526.4
- palmar (space) 682.4
- pancreas (duct) 577.0
- paradontal 523.3
- parafrenal 607.2
- parametric, parametrium (chronic) (see also Disease, pelvis, inflammatory) 614.4
  - acute 614.3
- paranephric 590.2
- parapancreatic 577.0
- parapharyngeal 478.22
- pararectal 566
- parasinus (see also Sinusitis) 473.9
- parauterine (see also Disease, pelvis, inflammatory) 614.4
  - acute 614.3
- paravaginal (see also Vaginitis) 616.10
- parietal region 682.8
- parodontal 523.3
- parotid (duct) (gland) 527.3
  - region 528.3
- parumbilical 682.2
  - newborn 771.4
- pectoral (region) 682.2
- pelvirectal — see Abscess, peritoneum
- pelvis, pelvic
  - female (chronic) (see also Disease, pelvis, inflammatory) 614.4
    - acute 614.3
  - male, peritoneal (cellular tissue) — see Abscess, peritoneum
  - tuberculous (see also Tuberculosis) 016.9 ✓5ᵗʰ
- penis 607.2
  - gonococcal (acute) 098.0
    - chronic or duration of 2 months or over 098.2
- perianal 566
- periapical 522.5
  - with sinus (alveolar) 522.7
- periappendiceal 540.1
- pericardial 420.99
- pericecal 540.1
- pericemental 523.3
- pericholecystic (see also Cholecystitis, acute) 575.0
- pericoronal 523.3
- peridental 523.3
- perigastric 535.0 ✓5ᵗʰ
- perimetric (see also Disease, pelvis, inflammatory) 614.4
  - acute 614.3
- perinephric, perinephritic (see also Abscess, kidney) 590.2
- perineum, perineal (superficial) 682.2
  - deep (with urethral involvement) 597.0
  - urethra 597.0
- periodontal (parietal) 523.3
  - apical 522.5
- periosteum, periosteal (see also Periostitis) 730.3 ✓5ᵗʰ
  - with osteomyelitis (see also Osteomyelitis) 730.2 ✓5ᵗʰ
    - acute or subacute 730.0 ✓5ᵗʰ
    - chronic or old 730.1 ✓5ᵗʰ
- peripleuritic 510.9
  - with fistula 510.0
- periproctic 566
- periprostatic 601.2

Abscess (see also Cellulitis) — continued
- perirectal (staphylococcal) 566
- perirenal (tissue) (see also Abscess, kidney) 590.2
- perisinuous (nose) (see also Sinusitis) 473.9
- peritoneum, peritoneal (perforated) (ruptured) 567.2
  - with
    - abortion — see Abortion, by type, with sepsis
    - appendicitis 540.1
    - ectopic pregnancy (see also categories 633.0-633.9) 639.0
    - molar pregnancy (see also categories 630-632) 639.0
  - following
    - abortion 639.0
    - ectopic or molar pregnancy 639.0
  - pelvic, female (see also Disease, pelvis, inflammatory) 614.4
    - acute 614.3
  - postoperative 998.59
  - puerperal, postpartum, childbirth 670 ✓4ᵗʰ
  - tuberculous (see also Tuberculosis) 014.0 ✓5ᵗʰ
- peritonsillar 475
- perityphlic 540.1
- periureteral 593.89
- periurethral 597.0
  - gonococcal (acute) 098.0
    - chronic or duration of 2 months or over 098.2
- periuterine (see also Disease, pelvis, inflammatory) 614.4
  - acute 614.3
- perivesical 595.89
- pernicious NEC 682.9
- petrous bone — see Petrositis
- phagedenic NEC 682.9
  - chancroid 099.0
- pharynx, pharyngeal (lateral) 478.29
- phlegmonous NEC 682.9
- pilonidal 685.0
- pituitary (gland) 253.8
- pleura 510.9
  - with fistula 510.0
- popliteal 682.6
- postanal 566
- postcecal 540.1
- postlaryngeal 478.79
- postnasal 478.1
- postpharyngeal 478.24
- posttonsillar 475
- posttyphoid 002.0
- Pott's (see also Tuberculosis) 015.0 ✓5ᵗʰ [730.88]
- pouch of Douglas (chronic) (see also Disease, pelvis, inflammatory) 614.4
- premammary — see Abscess, breast
- prepatellar 682.6
- prostate (see also Prostatitis) 601.2
  - gonococcal (acute) 098.12
    - chronic or duration of 2 months or over 098.32
- psoas (tuberculous) (see also Tuberculosis) 015.0 ✓5ᵗʰ [730.88]
  - nontuberculous 728.89
- pterygopalatine fossa 682.8
- pubis 682.2
- puerperal — Puerperal, abseess, by site
- pulmonary — see Abscess, lung
- pulp, pulpal (dental) 522.0
  - finger 681.01
  - toe 681.10
- pyemic — see Septicemia
- pyloric valve 535.0 ✓5ᵗʰ
- rectovaginal septum 569.5
- rectovesical 595.89
- rectum 566
- regional NEC 682.9
- renal (see also Abscess, kidney) 590.2
- retina 363.00
- retrobulbar 376.01
- retrocecal — see Abscess, peritoneum
- retrolaryngeal 478.79
- retromammary — see Abscess, breast
- retroperineal 682.2

Abscess (see also Cellulitis) — continued
- retroperitoneal — see Abscess, peritoneum
- retropharyngeal 478.24
  - tuberculous (see also Tuberculosis) 012.8 ✓5ᵗʰ
- retrorectal 566
- retrouterine (see also Disease, pelvis, inflammatory) 614.4
  - acute 614.3
- retrovesical 595.89
- root, tooth 522.5
  - with sinus (alveolar) 522.7
- round ligament (see also Disease, pelvis, inflammatory) 614.4
  - acute 614.3
- rupture (spontaneous) NEC 682.9
- sacrum (tuberculous) (see also Tuberculosis) 015.0 ✓5ᵗʰ [730.88]
  - nontuberculous 730.08
- salivary duct or gland 527.3
- scalp (any part) 682.8
- scapular 730.01
- sclera 379.09
- scrofulous (see also Tuberculosis) 017.2 ✓5ᵗʰ
- scrotum 608.4
- seminal vesicle 608.0
  - amebic 006.8
- septal, dental 522.5
  - with sinus (alveolar) 522.7
- septum (nasal) 478.1
- serous (see also Periostitis) 730.3 ✓5ᵗʰ
- shoulder 682.3
- side 682.2
- sigmoid 569.5
- sinus (accessory) (chronic) (nasal) (see also Sinusitis) 473.9
  - intracranial venous (any) 324.0
    - late effect — see category 326
- Skene's duct or gland 597.0
- skin NEC 682.9
  - tuberculous (primary) (see also Tuberculosis) 017.0 ✓5ᵗʰ
- sloughing NEC 682.9
- specified site NEC 682.8
  - amebic 006.8
- spermatic cord 608.4
- sphenoidal (sinus) (see also Sinusitis, sphenoidal) 473.3
- spinal
  - cord (any part) (staphylococcal) 324.1
    - tuberculous (see also Tuberculosis) 013.5 ✓5ᵗʰ
  - epidural 324.1
- spine (column) (tuberculous) (see also Tuberculosis) 015.0 ✓5ᵗʰ [730.88]
  - nontuberculous 730.08
- spleen 289.59
  - amebic 006.8
- staphylococcal NEC 682.9
- stitch 998.59
- stomach (wall) 535.0 ✓5ᵗʰ
- strumous (tuberculous) (see also Tuberculosis) 017.2 ✓5ᵗʰ
- subarachnoid 324.9
  - brain 324.0
  - cerebral 324.0
  - late effect — see category 326
  - spinal cord 324.1
- subareolar — see also Abscess, breast
  - puerperal, postpartum 675.1 ✓5ᵗʰ
- subcecal 540.1
- subcutaneous NEC 682.9
- subdiaphragmatic — see Abscess, peritoneum
- subdorsal 682.2
- subdural 324.9
  - brain 324.0
  - late effect — see category 326
  - spinal cord 324.1
- subgaleal 682.8
- subhepatic — see Abscess, peritoneum
- sublingual 528.3
  - gland 527.3
- submammary — see Abscess, breast
- submandibular (region) (space) (triangle) 682.0
  - gland 527.3
- submaxillary (region) 682.0
  - gland 527.3

Abscess

Abscess (see also Cellulitis) — continued
- submental (pyogenic) 682.0
  - gland 527.3
- subpectoral 682.2
- subperiosteal — see Abscess, bone
- subperitoneal — see Abscess, peritoneum
- subphrenic — see also Abscess, peritoneum
  - postoperative 998.59
- subscapular 682.2
- subungual 681.9
- suburethral 597.0
- sudoriparous 705.89
- suppurative NEC 682.9
- supraclavicular (fossa) 682.3
- suprahepatic — see Abscess, peritoneum
- suprapelvic (see also Disease, pelvis, inflammatory) 614.4
  - acute 614.3
- suprapubic 682.2
- suprarenal (capsule) (gland) 255.8
- sweat gland 705.89
- syphilitic 095.8
- teeth, tooth (root) 522.5
  - with sinus (alveolar) 522.7
  - supporting structures NEC 523.3
- temple 682.0
- temporal region 682.0
- temporosphenoidal 324.0
  - late effect — see category 326
- tendon (sheath) 727.89
- testicle — see Orchitis
- thecal 728.89
- thigh (acquired) 682.6
- thorax 510.9
  - with fistula 510.0
- throat 478.29
- thumb (intrathecal) (periosteal) (subcutaneous) (subcuticular) 681.00
- thymus (gland) 254.1
- thyroid (gland) 245.0
- toe (any) (intrathecal) (periosteal) (subcutaneous) (subcuticular) 681.10
- tongue (staphylococcal) 529.0
- tonsil(s) (lingual) 475
- tonsillopharyngeal 475
- tooth, teeth (root) 522.5
  - with sinus (alveolar) 522.7
  - supporting structure NEC 523.3
- trachea 478.9
- trunk 682.2
- tubal (see also Salpingo-oophoritis) 614.2
- tuberculous — see Tuberculosis, abscess
- tubo-ovarian (see also Salpingo-oophoritis) 614.2
- tunica vaginalis 608.4
- umbilicus NEC 682.2
  - newborn 771.4
- upper arm 682.3
- upper respiratory 478.9
- urachus 682.2
- urethra (gland) 597.0
- urinary 597.0
- uterus, uterine (wall) (see also Endometritis) 615.9
  - ligament (see also Disease, pelvis, inflammatory) 614.4
    - acute 614.3
  - neck (see also Cervicitis) 616.0
- uvula 528.3
- vagina (wall) (see also Vaginitis) 616.10
- vaginorectal (see also Vaginitis) 616.10
- vas deferens 608.4
- vermiform appendix 540.1
- vertebra (column) (tuberculous) (see also Tuberculosis) 015.0 [730.88]
  - nontuberculous 730.0
- vesical 595.89
- vesicouterine pouch (see also Disease, pelvis, inflammatory) 614.4
- vitreous (humor) (pneumococcal) 360.04
- vocal cord 478.5
- von Bezold's 383.01
- vulva 616.4
  - complicating pregnancy, childbirth, or puerperium 646.6
- vulvovaginal gland (see also Vaginitis) 616.3
- web-space 682.4
- wrist 682.4

Absence (organ or part) (complete or partial)
- acoustic nerve 742.8
- adrenal (gland) (congenital) 759.1
  - acquired V45.79
- albumin (blood) 273.8
- alimentary tract (complete) (congenital) (partial) 751.8
  - lower 751.5
  - upper 750.8
- alpha-fucosidase 271.8
- alveolar process (acquired) 525.8
  - congenital 750.26
- anus, anal (canal) (congenital) 751.2
- aorta (congenital) 747.22
- aortic valve (congenital) 746.89
- appendix, congenital 751.2
- arm (acquired) V49.60
  - above elbow V49.66
  - below elbow V49.65
  - congenital (see also Deformity, reduction, upper limb) 755.20
    - lower — see Absence, forearm, congenital
    - upper (complete) (partial) (with absence of distal elements, incomplete) 755.24
      - with
        - complete absence of distal elements 755.21
        - forearm (incomplete) 755.23
- artery (congenital) (peripheral) NEC (see also Anomaly, peripheral vascular system) 747.60
  - brain 747.81
  - cerebral 747.81
  - coronary 746.85
  - pulmonary 747.3
  - umbilical 747.5
- atrial septum 745.69
- auditory canal (congenital) (external) 744.01
- auricle (ear) (with stenosis or atresia of auditory canal), congenital 744.01
- bile, biliary duct (common) or passage (congenital) 751.61
- bladder (acquired) V45.74
  - congenital 753.8
- bone (congenital) NEC 756.9
  - marrow 284.9
    - acquired (secondary) 284.8
    - congenital 284.0
    - hereditary 284.0
    - idiopathic 284.9
  - skull 756.0
- bowel sounds 787.5
- brain 740.0
  - specified part 742.2
- breast(s) (acquired) V45.71
  - congenital 757.6
- broad ligament (congenital) 752.19
- bronchus (congenital) 748.3
- calvarium, calvaria (skull) 756.0
- canaliculus lacrimalis, congenital 743.65
- carpal(s) (congenital) (complete) (partial) (with absence of distal elements, incomplete) (see also Deformity, reduction, upper limb) 755.28
  - with complete absence of distal elements 755.21
- cartilage 756.9
- caudal spine 756.13
- cecum (acquired) (postoperative) (posttraumatic) V45.72
  - congenital 751.2
- cementum 520.4
- cerebellum (congenital) (vermis) 742.2
- cervix (acquired) (uteri) V45.77
  - congenital 752.49
- chin, congenital 744.89
- cilia (congenital) 743.63
  - acquired 374.89
- circulatory system, part NEC 747.89
- clavicle 755.51
- clitoris (congenital) 752.49
- coccyx, congenital 756.13
- cold sense (see also Disturbance, sensation) 782.0
- colon (acquired) (postoperative) V45.72
  - congenital 751.2

Absence — continued
- congenital
  - lumen — see Atresia
  - organ or site NEC — see Agenesis
  - septum — see Imperfect, closure
- corpus callosum (congenital) 742.2
- cricoid cartilage 748.3
- diaphragm (congenital) (with hernia) 756.6
  - with obstruction 756.6
- digestive organ(s) or tract, congenital (complete) (partial) 751.8
  - acquired V45.79
  - lower 751.5
  - upper 750.8
- ductus arteriosus 747.89
- duodenum (acquired) (postoperative) V45.72
  - congenital 751.1
- ear, congenital 744.09
  - acquired V45.79
  - auricle 744.01
  - external 744.01
  - inner 744.05
  - lobe, lobule 744.21
  - middle, except ossicles 744.03
    - ossicles 744.04
  - ossicles 744.04
- ejaculatory duct (congenital) 752.8
- endocrine gland NEC (congenital) 759.2
- epididymis (congenital) 752.8
  - acquired V45.77
- epiglottis, congenital 748.3
- epileptic (atonic) (typical) (see also Epilepsy) 345.0
- erythrocyte 284.9
- erythropoiesis 284.9
  - congenital 284.0
- esophagus (congenital) 750.3
- Eustachian tube (congenital) 744.24
- extremity (acquired)
  - congenital (see also Deformity, reduction) 755.4
  - lower V49.70
  - upper V49.60
- extrinsic muscle, eye 743.69
- eye (acquired) V45.78
  - adnexa (congenital) 743.69
  - congenital 743.00
  - muscle (congenital) 743.69
- eyelid (fold), congenital 743.62
  - acquired 374.89
- face
  - bones NEC 756.0
  - specified part NEC 744.89
- fallopian tube(s) (acquired) V45.77
  - congenital 752.19
- femur, congenital (complete) (partial) (with absence of distal elements, incomplete) (see also Deformity, reduction, lower limb) 755.34
  - with
    - complete absence of distal elements 755.31
    - tibia and fibula (incomplete) 755.33
- fibrin 790.92
- fibrinogen (congenital) 286.3
  - acquired 286.6
- fibula, congenital (complete) (partial) (with absence of distal elements, incomplete) (see also Deformity, reduction, lower limb) 755.37
  - with
    - complete absence of distal elements 755.31
    - tibia 755.35
      - with
        - complete absence of distal elements 755.31
        - femur (incomplete) 755.33
          - with complete absence of distal elements 755.31
- finger (acquired) V49.62
  - congenital (complete) (partial) (see also Deformity, reduction, upper limb) 755.29
    - meaning all fingers (complete) (partial) 755.21
    - transverse 755.21

Index to Diseases

Absence — continued

fissures of lungs (congenital) 748.5
foot (acquired) V49.73
    congenital (complete) 755.31
forearm (acquired) V49.65
    congenital (complete) (partial) (with absence of distal elements, incomplete) (*see also* Deformity, reduction, upper limb) 755.25
      with
        complete absence of distal elements (hand and fingers) 755.21
        humerus (incomplete) 755.23
fovea centralis 743.55
fucosidase 271.8
gallbladder (acquired) V45.79
    congenital 751.69
gamma globulin (blood) 279.00
genital organs
    acquired V45.77
    congenital
      female 752.8
        external 752.49
        internal NEC 752.8
      male 752.8
        penis 752.69
genitourinary organs, congenital NEC 752.8
glottis 748.3
gonadal, congenital NEC 758.6
hair (congenital) 757.4
    acquired — *see* Alopecia
hand (acquired) V49.63
    congenital (complete) (*see also* Deformity, reduction, upper limb) 755.21
heart (congenital) 759.89
    acquired — *see* Status, organ replacement
heat sense (*see also* Disturbance, sensation) 782.0
humerus, congenital (complete) (partial) (with absence of distal elements, incomplete) (*see also* Deformity, reduction, upper limb) 755.24
    with
      complete absence of distal elements 755.21
      radius and ulna (incomplete) 755.23
hymen (congenital) 752.49
ileum (acquired) (postoperative) (posttraumatic) V45.72
    congenital 751.1
immunoglobulin, isolated NEC 279.03
    IgA 279.01
    IgG 279.03
    IgM 279.02
incus (acquired) 385.24
    congenital 744.04
internal ear (congenital) 744.05
intestine (acquired) (small) V45.72
    congenital 751.1
      large 751.2
    large V45.72
      congenital 751.2
iris (congenital) 743.45
jaw — *see* Absence, mandible
jejunum (acquired) V45.72
    congenital 751.1
joint, congenital NEC 755.8
kidney(s) (acquired) V45.73
    congenital 753.0
labium (congenital) (majus) (minus) 752.49
labyrinth, membranous 744.05
lacrimal apparatus (congenital) 743.65
larynx (congenital) 748.3
leg (acquired) V49.70
    above knee V49.76
    below knee V49.75
    congenital (partial) (unilateral) (*see also* Deformity, reduction, lower limb) 755.31
      lower (complete) (partial) (with absence of distal elements, incomplete) 755.35
        with
          complete absence of distal elements (foot and toes) 755.31
          thigh (incomplete) 755.33
            with complete absence of distal elements 755.31

Absence — continued

leg — *continued*
    congenital — *continued*
      upper — *see* Absence, femur
lens (congenital) 743.35
    acquired 379.31
ligament, broad (congenital) 752.19
limb (acquired)
    congenital (complete) (partial) (*see also* Deformity, reduction) 755.4
      lower 755.30
        complete 755.31
        incomplete 755.32
        longitudinal — *see* Deficiency, lower limb, longitudinal
        transverse 755.31
      upper 755.20
        complete 755.21
        incomplete 755.22
        longitudinal — *see* Deficiency, upper limb, longitudinal
        transverse 755.21
    lower NEC V49.70
    upper NEC V49.60
lip 750.26
liver (congenital) (lobe) 751.69
lumbar (congenital) (vertebra) 756.13
    isthmus 756.11
    pars articularis 756.11
lumen — *see* Atresia
lung (bilateral) (congenital) (fissure) (lobe) (unilateral) 748.5
    acquired (any part) V45.76
mandible (congenital) 524.09
maxilla (congenital) 524.09
menstruation 626.0
metacarpal(s), congenital (complete) (partial) (with absence of distal elements, incomplete) (*see also* Deformity, reduction, upper limb) 755.28
    with all fingers, complete 755.21
metatarsal(s), congenital (complete) (partial) (with absence of distal elements, incomplete) (*see also* Deformity, reduction, lower limb) 755.38
    with complete absence of distal elements 755.31
muscle (congenital) (pectoral) 756.81
    ocular 743.69
musculoskeletal system (congenital) NEC 756.9
nail(s) (congenital) 757.5
neck, part 744.89
nerve 742.8
nervous system, part NEC 742.8
neutrophil 288.0
nipple (congenital) 757.6
nose (congenital) 748.1
    acquired 738.0
nuclear 742.8
ocular muscle (congenital) 743.69
organ
    of Corti (congenital) 744.05
    or site
      acquired V45.79
      congenital NEC 759.89
osseous meatus (ear) 744.03
ovary (acquired) V45.77
    congenital 752.0
oviduct (acquired) V45.77
    congenital 752.19
pancreas (congenital) 751.7
    acquired (postoperative) (posttraumatic) V45.79
parathyroid gland (congenital) 759.2
parotid gland(s) (congenital) 750.21
patella, congenital 755.64
pelvic girdle (congenital) 755.69
penis (congenital) 752.69
    acquired V45.77
pericardium (congenital) 746.89
perineal body (congenital) 756.81
phalange(s), congenital 755.4
    lower limb (complete) (intercalary) (partial) (terminal) (*see also* Deformity, reduction, lower limb) 755.39
      meaning all toes (complete) (partial) 755.31

Absence — continued

phalange(s), congenital — *continued*
    lower limb (*see also* Deformity, reduction, lower limb) — *continued*
      transverse 755.31
    upper limb (complete) (intercalary) (partial) (terminal) (*see also* Deformity, reduction, upper limb) 755.29
      meaning all digits (complete) (partial) 755.21
      transverse 755.21
pituitary gland (congenital) 759.2
postoperative — *see* Absence, by site, acquired
prostate (congenital) 752.8
    acquired V45.77
pulmonary
    artery 747.3
    trunk 747.3
    valve (congenital) 746.01
    vein 747.49
punctum lacrimale (congenital) 743.65
radius, congenital (complete) (partial) (with absence of distal elements, incomplete) 755.26
    with
      complete absence of distal elements 755.21
      ulna 755.25
        with
          complete absence of distal elements 755.21
          humerus (incomplete) 755.23
ray, congenital 755.4
    lower limb (complete) (partial) (*see also* Deformity, reduction, lower limb) 755.38
      meaning all rays 755.31
      transverse 755.31
    upper limb (complete) (partial) (*see also* Deformity, reduction, upper limb) 755.28
      meaning all rays 755.21
      transverse 755.21
rectum (congenital) 751.2
    acquired V45.79
red cell 284.9
    acquired (secondary) 284.8
    congenital 284.0
    hereditary 284.0
    idiopathic 284.9
respiratory organ (congenital) NEC 748.9
rib (acquired) 738.3
    congenital 756.3
roof of orbit (congenital) 742.0
round ligament (congenital) 752.8
sacrum, congenital 756.13
salivary gland(s) (congenital) 750.21
scapula 755.59
scrotum, congenital 752.8
seminal tract or duct (congenital) 752.8
    acquired V45.77
septum (congenital) — *see also* Imperfect, closure, septum
    atrial 745.69
      and ventricular 745.7
    between aorta and pulmonary artery 745.0
    ventricular 745.3
      and atrial 745.7
sex chromosomes 758.81
shoulder girdle, congenital (complete) (partial) 755.59
skin (congenital) 757.39
skull bone 756.0
    with
      anencephalus 740.0
      encephalocele 742.0
      hydrocephalus 742.3
        with spina bifida (*see also* Spina bifida) 741.0
      microcephalus 742.1
spermatic cord (congenital) 752.8
spinal cord 742.59
spine, congenital 756.13
spleen (congenital) 759.0
    acquired V45.79
sternum, congenital 756.3

Absence

Absence — continued
- stomach (acquired) (partial) (postoperative) V45.75
  - with postgastric surgery syndrome 564.2
  - congenital 750.7
- submaxillary gland(s) (congenital) 750.21
- superior vena cava (congenital) 747.49
- tarsal(s), congenital (complete) (partial) (with absence of distal elements, incomplete) (see also Deformity, reduction, lower limb) 755.38
- teeth, tooth (congenital) 520.0
  - with abnormal spacing 524.3
  - acquired 525.10
    - with malocclusion 524.3
    - due to
      - caries 525.13
      - extraction 525.10
      - periodontal disease 525.12
      - trauma 525.11
- tendon (congenital) 756.81
- testis (congenital) 752.8
  - acquired V45.77
- thigh (acquired) 736.89
- thumb (acquired) V49.61
  - congenital 755.29
- thymus gland (congenital) 759.2
- thyroid (gland) (surgical) 246.8
  - with hypothyroidism 244.0
  - cartilage, congenital 748.3
  - congenital 243
- tibia, congenital (complete) (partial) (with absence of distal elements, incomplete) (see also Deformity, reduction, lower limb) 755.36
  - with
    - complete absence of distal elements 755.31
    - fibula 755.35
      - with
        - complete absence of distal elements 755.31
        - femur (incomplete) 755.33
          - with complete absence of distal elements 755.31
- toe (acquired) V49.72
  - congenital (complete) (partial) 755.39
    - meaning all toes 755.31
    - transverse 755.31
  - great V49.71
- tongue (congenital) 750.11
- tooth, teeth, (congenital) 520.0
  - with abnormal spacing 524.3
  - acquired 525.10
    - with malocclusion 524.3
    - due to
      - caries 525.13
      - extraction 525.10
      - periodontal disease 525.12
      - trauma 525.11
- trachea (cartilage) (congenital) (rings) 748.3
- transverse aortic arch (congenital) 747.21
- tricuspid valve 746.1
- ulna, congenital (complete) (partial) (with absence of distal elements, incomplete) (see also Deformity, reduction, upper limb) 755.27
  - with
    - complete absence of distal elements 755.21
    - radius 755.25
      - with
        - complete absence of distal elements 755.21
        - humerus (incomplete) 755.23
- umbilical artery (congenital) 747.5
- ureter (congenital) 753.4
  - acquired V45.74
- urethra, congenital 753.8
  - acquired V45.74
- urinary system, part NEC, congenital 753.8
  - acquired V45.74
- uterus (acquired) V45.77
  - congenital 752.3
- uvula (congenital) 750.26
- vagina, congenital 752.49
  - acquired V45.77

Absence — continued
- vas deferens (congenital) 752.8
  - acquired V45.77
- vein (congenital) (peripheral) NEC (see also Anomaly, peripheral vascular system) 747.60
  - brain 747.81
  - great 747.49
  - portal 747.49
  - pulmonary 747.49
- vena cava (congenital) (inferior) (superior) 747.49
- ventral horn cell 742.59
- ventricular septum 745.3
- vermis of cerebellum 742.2
- vertebra, congenital 756.13
- vulva, congenital 752.49

Absentia epileptica (see also Epilepsy) 345.0
Absinthemia (see also Dependence) 304.6
Absinthism (see also Dependence) 304.6
Absorbent system disease 459.89
Absorption
- alcohol, through placenta or breast milk 760.71
- antibiotics, through placenta or breast milk 760.74
- anti-infective, through placenta or breast milk 760.74
- chemical NEC 989.9
  - specified chemical or substance — see Table of Drugs and Chemicals
  - through placenta or breast milk (fetus or newborn) 760.70
    - alcohol 760.71
    - anti-infective agents 760.74
    - cocaine 760.75
    - "crack" 760.75
    - diethylstilbestrol [DES] 760.76
    - hallucinogenic agents 760.73
    - medicinal agents NEC 760.79
    - narcotics 760.72
    - obstetric anesthetic or analgesic drug 763.5
    - specified agent NEC 760.79
  - suspected, affecting management of pregnancy 655.5
- cocaine, through placenta or breast milk 760.75
- drug NEC (see also Reaction, drug)
  - through placenta or breast milk (fetus or newborn) 760.70
    - alcohol 760.71
  - through placenta or breast milk (fetus or newborn) — continued
    - anti-infective agents 760.74
    - cocaine 760.75
    - "crack" 760.75
    - diethylstilbestrol [DES] 760.76
    - hallucinogenic agents 760.73
    - medicinal agents NEC 760.79
    - narcotics 760.72
    - obstetric anesthetic or analgesic drug 763.5
    - specified agent NEC 760.79
  - suspected, affecting management of pregnancy 655.5
- fat, disturbance 579.8
- hallucinogenic agents, through placenta or breast milk 760.73
- immune sera, through placenta or breast milk 760.79
- lactose defect 271.3
- medicinal agents NEC, through placenta or breast milk 760.79
- narcotics, through placenta or breast milk 760.72
- noxious substance, — see Absorption, chemical
- protein, disturbance 579.8
- pus or septic, general — see Septicemia
- quinine, through placenta or breast milk 760.74
- toxic substance, — see Absorption, chemical
- uremic — see Uremia

Abstinence symptoms or syndrome
- alcohol 291.81
- drug 292.0

Abt-Letterer-Siwe syndrome (acute histiocytosis X) (M9722/3) 202.5
Abulia 799.8
Abulomania 301.6
Abuse
- adult 995.80
  - emotional 995.82
  - multiple forms 995.85
  - neglect (nutritional) 995.84
  - physical 995.81
  - psychological 995.82
  - sexual 995.83
- alcohol (see also Alcoholism) 305.0
  - dependent 303.9
  - non-dependent 305.0
- child 995.50
  - counseling
    - perpetrator
      - non-parent V62.83
      - parent V61.22
    - victim V61.21
  - emotional 995.51
  - multiple forms 995.59
  - neglect (nutritional) 995.52
  - psychological 995.51
  - physical 995.54
    - shaken infant syndrome 995.55
  - sexual 995.53
- drugs, nondependent 305.9

Note — Use the following fifth-digit subclassification with the following codes: 305.0, 305.2-305.9:

| 0 | unspecified | 2 | episodic |
| 1 | continuous | 3 | in remission |

- amphetamine type 305.7
- antidepressants 305.8
- barbiturates 305.4
- caffeine 305.9
- cannabis 305.2
- cocaine type 305.6
- hallucinogens 305.3
- hashish 305.2
- LSD 305.3
- marijuana 305.2
- mixed 305.9
- morphine type 305.5
- opioid type 305.5
- phencyclidine (PCP) 305.9
- specified NEC 305.9
- tranquilizers 305.4
- spouse 995.80
- tobacco 305.1

Acalcerosis 275.40
Acalcicosis 275.40
Acalculia 784.69
- developmental 315.1

Acanthocheilonemiasis 125.4
Acanthocytosis 272.5
Acanthokeratodermia 701.1
Acantholysis 701.8
- bullosa 757.39

Acanthoma (benign) (M8070/0) — see also Neoplasm, by site, benign
- malignant (M8070/3) — see Neoplasm, by site, malignant

Acanthosis (acquired) (nigricans) 701.2
- adult 701.2
- benign (congenital) 757.39
- congenital 757.39
- glycogenic
  - esophagus 530.89
- juvenile 701.2
- tongue 529.8

Acanthrocytosis 272.5
Acapnia 276.3
Acarbia 276.2
Acardia 759.89
Acardiacus amorphus 759.89
Acardiotrophia 429.1
Acardius 759.89

Index to Diseases

Acariasis 133.9
  sarcoptic 133.0
Acaridiasis 133.9
Acarinosis 133.9
Acariosis 133.9
Acarodermatitis 133.9
  urticarioides 133.9
Acarophobia 300.29
Acatalasemia 277.8
Acatalasia 277.8
Acatamathesia 784.69
Acataphasia 784.5
Acathisia 781.0
  due to drugs 333.99
Acceleration, accelerated
  atrioventricular conduction 426.7
  idioventricular rhythm 427.89
Accessory (congenital)
  adrenal gland 759.1
  anus 751.5
  appendix 751.5
  atrioventricular conduction 426.7
  auditory ossicles 744.04
  auricle (ear) 744.1
  autosome(s) NEC 758.5
    21 or 22 758.0
  biliary duct or passage 751.69
  bladder 753.8
  blood vessels (peripheral) (congenital) NEC (*see also* Anomaly, peripheral vascular system) 747.60
    cerebral 747.81
    coronary 746.85
  bone NEC 756.9
    foot 755.67
  breast tissue, axilla 757.6
  carpal bones 755.56
  cecum 751.5
  cervix 752.49
  chromosome(s) NEC 758.5
    13-15 758.1
    16-18 758.2
    21 or 22 758.0
    autosome(s) NEC 758.5
    D_1 758.1
    E_3 758.2
    G 758.0
    sex 758.81
  coronary artery 746.85
  cusp(s), heart valve NEC 746.89
    pulmonary 746.09
  cystic duct 751.69
  digits 755.00
  ear (auricle) (lobe) 744.1
  endocrine gland NEC 759.2
  external os 752.49
  eyelid 743.62
  eye muscle 743.69
  face bone(s) 756.0
  fallopian tube (fimbria) (ostium) 752.19
  fingers 755.01
  foreskin 605
  frontonasal process 756.0
  gallbladder 751.69
  genital organ(s)
    female 752.8
      external 752.49
      internal NEC 752.8
    male NEC 752.8
      penis 752.69
  genitourinary organs NEC 752.8
  heart 746.89
    valve NEC 746.89
      pulmonary 746.09
  hepatic ducts 751.69
  hymen 752.49
  intestine (large) (small) 751.5
  kidney 753.3
  lacrimal canal 743.65
  leaflet, heart valve NEC 746.89
    pulmonary 746.09
  ligament, broad 752.19
  liver (duct) 751.69
  lobule (ear) 744.1
  lung (lobe) 748.69

Accessory — *continued*
  muscle 756.82
  navicular of carpus 755.56
  nervous system, part NEC 742.8
  nipple 757.6
  nose 748.1
  organ or site NEC — *see* Anomaly, specified type NEC
  ovary 752.0
  oviduct 752.19
  pancreas 751.7
  parathyroid gland 759.2
  parotid gland (and duct) 750.22
  pituitary gland 759.2
  placental lobe — *see* Placenta, abnormal
  preauricular appendage 744.1
  prepuce 605
  renal arteries (multiple) 747.62
  rib 756.3
    cervical 756.2
  roots (teeth) 520.2
  salivary gland 750.22
  sesamoids 755.8
  sinus — *see* condition
  skin tags 757.39
  spleen 759.0
  sternum 756.3
  submaxillary gland 750.22
  tarsal bones 755.67
  teeth, tooth 520.1
    causing crowding 524.3
  tendon 756.89
  thumb 755.01
  thymus gland 759.2
  thyroid gland 759.2
  toes 755.02
  tongue 750.13
  tragus 744.1
  ureter 753.4
  urethra 753.8
  urinary organ or tract NEC 753.8
  uterus 752.2
  vagina 752.49
  valve, heart NEC 746.89
    pulmonary 746.09
  vertebra 756.19
  vocal cords 748.3
  vulva 752.49
Accident, accidental — *see also* condition
  birth NEC 767.9
  cardiovascular (*see also* Disease, cardiovascular) 429.2
  cerebral (*see also* Disease, cerebrovascular, acute) 436
  cerebrovascular (current) (CVA) (*see also* Disease, cerebrovascular, acute) 436
    healed or old V12.59
    impending 435.9
    late effect — *see* Late effect(s) (of) cerebrovascular disease
    postoperative 997.02 ●
  coronary (*see also* Infarct, myocardium) 410.9 ✓5ᵗʰ
  craniovascular (*see also* Disease, cerebrovascular, acute) 436
  during pregnancy, to mother
    affecting fetus or newborn 760.5
  heart, cardiac (*see also* Infarct, myocardium) 410.9 ✓5ᵗʰ
  intrauterine 779.89 ▲
  vascular — *see* Disease, cerebrovascular, acute
Accommodation
  disorder of 367.51
    drug-induced 367.89
    toxic 367.89
  insufficiency of 367.4
  paralysis of 367.51
    hysterical 300.11
  spasm of 367.53
Accouchement — *see* Delivery
Accreta placenta (without hemorrhage) 667.0 ✓5ᵗʰ
  with hemorrhage 666.0 ✓5ᵗʰ
Accretio cordis (nonrheumatic) 423.1
Accretions on teeth 523.6
Accumulation secretion, prostate 602.8
Acephalia, acephalism, acephaly 740.0

Acidemia

Acephalic 740.0
Acephalobrachia 759.89
Acephalocardia 759.89
Acephalocardius 759.89
Acephalochiria 759.89
Acephalochirus 759.89
Acephalogaster 759.89
Acephalostomus 759.89
Acephalothorax 759.89
Acephalus 740.0
Acetonemia 790.6
  diabetic 250.1 ✓5ᵗʰ
Acetonglycosuria 982.8
Acetonuria 791.6
Achalasia 530.0
  cardia 530.0
  digestive organs congenital NEC 751.8
  esophagus 530.0
  pelvirectal 751.3
  psychogenic 306.4
  pylorus 750.5
  sphincteral NEC 564.89
Achard-Thiers syndrome (adrenogenital) 255.2
Ache(s) — *see* Pain
Acheilia 750.26
Acheiria 755.21
Achillobursitis 726.71
Achillodynia 726.71
Achlorhydria, achlorhydric 536.0
  anemia 280.9
  diarrhea 536.0
  neurogenic 536.0
  postvagotomy 564.2
  psychogenic 306.4
  secondary to vagotomy 564.2
Achloroblepsia 368.52
Achloropsia 368.52
Acholia 575.8
Acholuric jaundice (familial) (splenomegalic) (*see also* Spherocytosis) 282.0
  acquired 283.9
Achondroplasia 756.4
Achrestic anemia 281.8
Achroacytosis, lacrimal gland 375.00
  tuberculous (*see also* Tuberculosis) 017.3 ✓5ᵗʰ
Achroma, cutis 709.00
Achromate (congenital) 368.54
Achromatopia 368.54
Achromatopsia (congenital) 368.54
Achromia
  congenital 270.2
  parasitica 111.0
  unguium 703.8
Achylia
  gastrica 536.8
    neurogenic 536.3
    psychogenic 306.4
  pancreatica 577.1
Achylosis 536.8
Acid
  burn — *see also* Burn, by site
    from swallowing acid — *see* Burn, internal organs
  deficiency
    amide nicotinic 265.2
    amino 270.9
    ascorbic 267
    folic 266.2
    nicotinic (amide) 265.2
    pantothenic 266.2
  intoxication 276.2
  peptic disease 536.8
  stomach 536.8
    psychogenic 306.4
Acidemia 276.2
  arginosuccinic 270.6
  fetal
    affecting management of pregnancy 656.3 ✓5ᵗʰ
    before onset of labor, in liveborn infant 768.2

Acidemia — *continued*
  fetal — *continued*
    during labor, in liveborn infant 768.3
    intrauterine — *see* Distress, fetal 656.3
    unspecified as to time of onset, in liveborn infant 768.4
  pipecolic 270.7
Acidity, gastric (high) (low) 536.8
  psychogenic 306.4
Acidocytopenia 288.0
Acidocytosis 288.3
Acidopenia 288.0
Acidosis 276.2
  diabetic 250.1
  fetal, affecting management of pregnancy 756.8
  fetal, affecting newborn 768.9
  kidney tubular 588.8
  lactic 276.2
  metabolic NEC 276.2
    with respiratory acidosis 276.4
    late, of newborn 775.7
  renal
    hyperchloremic 588.8
    tubular (distal) (proximal) 588.8
  respiratory 276.2
    complicated by
      metabolic acidosis 276.4
      metabolic alkalosis 276.4
Aciduria 791.9
  arginosuccinic 270.6
  beta-aminoisobutyric (BAIB) 277.2
  glycolic 271.8
  methylmalonic 270.3
    with glycinemia 270.7
  organic 270.9
  orotic (congenital) (hereditary) (pyrimidine deficiency) 281.4
Acladiosis 111.8
  skin 111.8
Aclasis
  diaphyseal 756.4
  tarsoepiphyseal 756.59
Acleistocardia 745.5
Aclusion 524.4
Acmesthesia 782.0
Acne (pustular) (vulgaris) 706.1
  agminata (*see also* Tuberculosis) 017.0
  artificialis 706.1
  atrophica 706.0
  cachecticorum (Hebra) 706.1
  conglobata 706.1
  conjunctiva 706.1
  cystic 706.1
  decalvans 704.09
  erythematosa 695.3
  eyelid 706.1
  frontalis 706.0
  indurata 706.1
  keloid 706.1
  lupoid 706.0
  necrotic, necrotica 706.0
    miliaris 704.8
  nodular 706.1
  occupational 706.1
  papulosa 706.1
  rodens 706.0
  rosacea 695.3
  scorbutica 267
  scrofulosorum (Bazin) (*see also* Tuberculosis) 017.0
  summer 692.72
  tropical 706.1
  varioliformis 706.0
Acneiform drug eruptions 692.3
Acnitis (primary) (*see also* Tuberculosis) 017.0
Acomia 704.00
Acontractile bladder 344.61
Aconuresis (*see also* Incontinence) 788.30
Acosta's disease 993.2
Acousma 780.1
Acoustic — *see* condition
Acousticophobia 300.29

Acquired — *see* condition
Acquired immune deficiency syndrome — *see* Human immunodeficiency virus (disease) (illness) (infection)
Acquired immunodeficiency syndrome — *see* Human immunodeficiency virus (disease) (illness) (infection)
Acragnosis 781.99
Acrania 740.0
Acroagnosis 781.99
Acroasphyxia, chronic 443.89
Acrobrachycephaly 756.0
Acrobystiolith 608.89
Acrobystitis 607.2
Acrocephalopolysyndactyly 755.55
Acrocephalosyndactyly 755.55
Acrocephaly 756.0
Acrochondrohyperplasia 759.82
Acrocyanosis 443.89
  newborn 770.83
Acrodermatitis 686.8
  atrophicans (chronica) 701.8
  continua (Hallopeau) 696.1
  enteropathica 686.8
  Hallopeau's 696.1
  perstans 696.1
  pustulosa continua 696.1
  recalcitrant pustular 696.1
Acrodynia 985.0
Acrodysplasia 755.55
Acrohyperhidrosis 780.8
Acrokeratosis verruciformis 757.39
Acromastitis 611.0
Acromegaly, acromegalia (skin) 253.0
Acromelalgia 443.89
Acromicria acromikria 756.59
Acronyx 703.0
Acropachy, thyroid (*see also* Thyrotoxicosis) 242.9
Acropachyderma 757.39
Acroparesthesia 443.89
  simple (Schultz's type) 443.89
  vasomotor (Nothnagel's type) 443.89
Acropathy thyroid (*see also* Thyrotoxicosis) 242.9
Acrophobia 300.29
Acroposthitis 607.2
Acroscleriasis (*see also* Scleroderma) 710.1
Acroscleroderma (*see also* Scleroderma) 710.1
Acrosclerosis (*see also* Scleroderma) 710.1
Acrosphacelus 785.4
Acrosphenosyndactylia 755.55
Acrospiroma, eccrine (M8402/0) — *see* Neoplasm, skin, benign
Acrostealgia 732.9
Acrosyndactyly (*see also* Syndactylism) 755.10
Acrotrophodynia 991.4
Actinic — *see also* condition
  cheilitis (due to sun) 692.72
    chronic NEC 692.74
    due to radiation, except from sun 692.82
  conjunctivitis 370.24
  dermatitis (due to sun) (*see also* Dermatitis, actinic) 692.70
    due to
      roentgen rays or radioactive substance 692.82
      ultraviolet radiation, except from sun 692.82
      sun NEC 692.70
  elastosis solare 692.74
  granuloma 692.73
  keratitis 370.24
  ophthalmia 370.24
  reticuloid 692.73
Actinobacillosis, general 027.8
Actinobacillus
  lignieresii 027.8
  mallei 024
  muris 026.1

Actinocutitis NEC (*see also* Dermatitis, actinic) 692.70
Actinodermatitis NEC (*see also* Dermatitis, actinic) 692.70
Actinomyces
  israelii (infection) — *see* Actinomycosis
  muris-ratti (infection) 026.1
Actinomycosis, actinomycotic 039.9
  with
    pneumonia 039.1
  abdominal 039.2
  cervicofacial 039.3
  cutaneous 039.0
  pulmonary 039.1
  specified site NEC 039.8
  thoracic 039.1
Actinoneuritis 357.89
Action, heart
  disorder 427.9
    postoperative 997.1
  irregular 427.9
    postoperative 997.1
    psychogenic 306.2
Active — *see* condition
Activity decrease, functional 780.99
Acute — *see also* condition
  abdomen NEC 789.0
  gallbladder (*see also* Cholecystitis, acute) 575.0
Acyanoblepsia 368.53
Acyanopsia 368.53
Acystia 753.8
Acystinervia — *see* Neurogenic, bladder
Acystineuria — *see* Neurogenic, bladder
Adactylia, adactyly (congenital) 755.4
  lower limb (complete) (intercalary) (partial) (terminal) (*see also* Deformity, reduction, lower limb) 755.39
    meaning all digits (complete) (partial) 755.31
    transverse (complete) (partial) 755.31
  upper limb (complete) (intercalary) (partial) (terminal) (*see also* Deformity, reduction, upper limb) 755.29
    meaning all digits (complete) (partial) 755.21
    transverse (complete) (partial) 755.21
Adair-Dighton syndrome (brittle bones and blue sclera, deafness) 756.51
Adamantinoblastoma (M9310/0) — *see* Ameloblastoma
Adamantinoma (M9310/0) — *see* Ameloblastoma
Adamantoblastoma (M9310/0) — *see* Ameloblastoma
Adams-Stokes (-Morgagni) disease or syndrome (syncope with heart block) 426.9
Adaptation reaction (*see also* Reaction, adjustment) 309.9
Addiction — *see also* Dependence
  absinthe 304.6
  alcoholic (ethyl) (methyl) (wood) 303.9
    complicating pregnancy, childbirth, or puerperium 648.4
      affecting fetus or newborn 760.71
    suspected damage to fetus affecting management of pregnancy 655.4
  drug (*see also* Dependence) 304.9
  ethyl alcohol 303.9
  heroin 304.0
  hospital 301.51
  methyl alcohol 303.9
  methylated spirit 303.9
  morphine (-like substances) 304.0
  nicotine 305.1
  opium 304.0
  tobacco 305.1
  wine 303.9
Addison's
  anemia (pernicious) 281.0
  disease (bronze) (primary adrenal insufficiency) 255.4
    tuberculous (*see also* Tuberculosis) 017.6
  keloid (morphea) 701.0
  melanoderma (adrenal cortical hypofunction) 255.4

Index to Diseases

Addison-Biermer anemia (pernicious) 281.0
Addison-Gull disease — *see* Xanthoma
Addisonian crisis or melanosis (acute adrenocortical insufficiency) 255.4
Additional — *see also* Accessory
   chromosome(s) 758.5
      13-15 758.1
      16-18 758.2
      21 758.0
      autosome(s) NEC 758.5
      sex 758.81
Adduction contracture, hip or other joint — *see* Contraction, joint
Adenasthenia gastrica 536.0
Aden fever 061
Adenitis (*see also* Lymphadenitis) 289.3
   acute, unspecified site 683
      epidemic infectious 075
   axillary 289.3
      acute 683
      chronic or subacute 289.1
   Bartholin's gland 616.8
   bulbourethral gland (*see also* Urethritis) 597.89
   cervical 289.3
      acute 683
      chronic or subacute 289.1
   chancroid (Ducrey's bacillus) 099.0
   chronic (any lymph node, except mesenteric) 289.1
      mesenteric 289.2
   Cowper's gland (*see also* Urethritis) 597.89
   epidemic, acute 075
   gangrenous 683
   gonorrheal NEC 098.89
   groin 289.3
      acute 683
      chronic or subacute 289.1
   infectious 075
   inguinal (region) 289.3
      acute 683
      chronic or subacute 289.1
   lymph gland or node, except mesenteric 289.3
      acute 683
      chronic or subacute 289.1
      mesenteric (acute) (chronic) (nonspecific) (subacute) 289.2
   mesenteric (acute) (chronic) (nonspecific) (subacute) 289.2
      due to Pasteurella multocida (P. septica) 027.2
   parotid gland (suppurative) 527.2
   phlegmonous 683
   salivary duct or gland (any) (recurring) (suppurative) 527.2
   scrofulous (*see also* Tuberculosis) 017.2 ✓5ᵗʰ
   septic 289.3
   Skene's duct or gland (*see also* Urethritis) 597.89
   strumous, tuberculous (*see also* Tuberculosis) 017.2 ✓5ᵗʰ
   subacute, unspecified site 289.1
   sublingual gland (suppurative) 527.2
   submandibular gland (suppurative) 527.2
   submaxillary gland (suppurative) 527.2
   suppurative 683
   tuberculous — *see* Tuberculosis, lymph gland
   urethral gland (*see also* Urethritis) 597.89
   venereal NEC 099.8
   Wharton's duct (suppurative) 527.2
Adenoacanthoma (M8570/3) — *see* Neoplasm, by site, malignant
Adenoameloblastoma (M9300/0) 213.1
   upper jaw (bone) 213.0

Adenocarcinoma

Adenocarcinoma (M8140/3) — *see also* Neoplasm, by site, malignant

> *Note* — The following list of adjectival modifiers is not exhaustive. A description of adenocarcinoma that does not appear in this list should be coded in the same manner as carcinoma with that description. Thus, "mixed acidophil-basophil adenocarcinoma," should be coded in the same manner as "mixed acidophil-basophil carcinoma," which appears in the list under "Carcinoma."
>
> Except where otherwise indicated, the morphological varieties of adenocarcinoma in the list should be coded by site as for "Neoplasm, malignant."

   with
      apocrine metaplasia (M8573/3)
      cartilaginous (and osseous) metaplasia (M8571/3)
      osseous (and cartilaginous) metaplasia (M8571/3)
      spindle cell metaplasia (M8572/3)
      squamous metaplasia (M8570/3)
   acidophil (M8280/3)
      specified site — *see* Neoplasm, by site, malignant
      unspecified site 194.3
   acinar (M8550/3)
   acinic cell (M8550/3)
   adrenal cortical (M8370/3) 194.0
   alveolar (M8251/3)
      and
         epidermoid carcinoma, mixed (M8560/3)
         squamous cell carcinoma, mixed (M8560/3)
   apocrine (M8401/3)
      breast — *see* Neoplasm, breast, malignant
      specified site NEC — *see* Neoplasm, skin, malignant
      unspecified site 173.9
   basophil (M8300/3)
      specified site — *see* Neoplasm, by site, malignant
      unspecified site 194.3
   bile duct type (M8160/3)
      liver 155.1
      specified site NEC — *see* Neoplasm, by site, malignant
      unspecified site 155.1
   bronchiolar (M8250/3) — *see* Neoplasm, lung, malignant
   ceruminous (M8420/3) 173.2
   chromophobe (M8270/3)
      specified site — *see* Neoplasm, by site, malignant
      unspecified site 194.3
   clear cell (mesonephroid type) (M8310/3)
   colloid (M8480/3)
   cylindroid type (M8200/3)
   diffuse type (M8145/3)
      specified site — *see* Neoplasm, by site, malignant
      unspecified site 151.9
   duct (infiltrating) (M8500/3)
      with Paget's disease (M8541/3) — *see* Neoplasm, breast, malignant
      specified site — *see* Neoplasm, by site, malignant
      unspecified site 174.9
   embryonal (M9070/3)
   endometrioid (M8380/3) — *see* Neoplasm, by site, malignant
   eosinophil (M8280/3)
      specified site — *see* Neoplasm, by site malignant
      unspecified site 194.3
   follicular (M8330/3)
      and papillary (M8340/3) 193
      moderately differentiated type (M8332/3) 193
      pure follicle type (M8331/3) 193
      specified site — *see* Neoplasm, by site, malignant
      trabecular type (M8332/3) 193
      unspecified type 193
      well differentiated type (M8331/3) 193
   gelatinous (M8480/3)

Adenocarcinoma — *see also* Neoplasm, by site, malignant — *continued*
   granular cell (M8320/3)
   Hürthle cell (M8290/3) 193
   in
      adenomatous
         polyp (M8210/3)
         polyposis coli (M8220/3) 153.9
      polypoid adenoma (M8210/3)
      tubular adenoma (M8210/3)
      villous adenoma (M8261/3)
   infiltrating duct (M8500/3)
      with Paget's disease (M8541/3) — *see* Neoplasm, breast, malignant
      specified site — *see* Neoplasm, by site, malignant
      unspecified site 174.9
   inflammatory (M8530/3)
      specified site — *see* Neoplasm, by site, malignant
      unspecified site 174.9
   in situ (M8140/2) — *see* Neoplasm, by site, in situ
   intestinal type (M8144/3)
      specified site — *see* Neoplasm, by site, malignant
      unspecified site 151.9
   intraductal (noninfiltrating) (M8500/2)
      papillary (M8503/2)
         specified site — *see* Neoplasm, by site, in situ
         unspecified site 233.0
      specified site — *see* Neoplasm, by site, in situ
      unspecified site 233.0
   islet cell (M8150/3)
      and exocrine, mixed (M8154/3)
         specified site — *see* Neoplasm, by site, malignant
         unspecified site 157.9
      pancreas 157.4
      specified site NEC — *see* Neoplasm, by site, malignant
      unspecified site 157.4
   lobular (M8520/3)
      specified site — *see* Neoplasm, by site, malignant
      unspecified site 174.9
   medullary (M8510/3)
   mesonephric (M9110/3)
   mixed cell (M8323/3)
   mucinous (M8480/3)
   mucin-producing (M8481/3)
   mucoid (M8480/3) — *see also* Neoplasm, by site, malignant
      cell (M8300/3)
         specified site — *see* Neoplasm, by site, malignant
         unspecified site 194.3
   nonencapsulated sclerosing (M8350/3) 193
   oncocytic (M8290/3)
   oxyphilic (M8290/3)
   papillary (M8260/3)
      and follicular (M8340/3) 193
      intraductal (noninfiltrating) (M8503/2)
         specified site — *see* Neoplasm, by site, in situ
         unspecified site 233.0
      serous (M8460/3)
         specified site — *see* Neoplasm, by site, malignant
         unspecified site 183.0
   papillocystic (M8450/3)
      specified site — *see* Neoplasm, by site, malignant
      unspecified site 183.0
   pseudomucinous (M8470/3)
      specified site — *see* Neoplasm, by site, malignant
      unspecified site 183.0
   renal cell (M8312/3) 189.0
   sebaceous (M8410/3)
   serous (M8441/3) — *see also* Neoplasm, by site, malignant
      papillary
         specified site — *see* Neoplasm, by site malignant

Adenocarcinoma

Adenocarcinoma — see also Neoplasm, by site, malignant — continued
- serous — see also Neoplasm, by site, malignant — continued
  - papillary — continued
    - unspecified site 183.0
  - signet ring cell (M8490/3)
  - superficial spreading (M8143/3)
  - sweat gland (M8400/3) — see Neoplasm, skin, malignant
  - trabecular (M8190/3)
  - tubular (M8211/3)
  - villous (M8262/3)
  - water-clear cell (M8322/3) 194.1

Adenofibroma (M9013/0)
- clear cell (M8313/0) — see Neoplasm, by site, benign
- endometrioid (M8381/0) 220
  - borderline malignancy (M8381/1) 236.2
  - malignant (M8381/3) 183.0
- mucinous (M9015/0)
  - specified site — see Neoplasm, by site, benign
  - unspecified site 220
- prostate 600.2
- serous (M9014/0)
  - specified site — see Neoplasm, by site, benign
  - unspecified site 220
- specified site — see Neoplasm, by site, benign
- unspecified site 220

Adenofibrosis
- breast 610.2
- endometrioid 617.0

Adenoiditis 474.01
- acute 463
- chronic 474.01
  - with chronic tonsillitis 474.02

Adenoids (congenital) (of nasal fossa) 474.9
- hypertrophy 474.12
- vegetations 474.2

Adenolipomatosis (symmetrical) 272.8

Adenolymphoma (M8561/0)
- specified site — see Neoplasm, by site, benign
- unspecified 210.2

Adenoma (sessile) (M8140/0) — see also Neoplasm, by site, benign

> Note — Except where otherwise indicated, the morphological varieties of adenoma in the list below should be coded by site as for "Neoplasm, benign."

- acidophil (M8280/0)
  - specified site — see Neoplasm, by site, benign
  - unspecified site 227.3
- acinar (cell) (M8550/0)
- acinic cell (M8550/0)
- adrenal (cortex) (cortical) (functioning) (M8370/0) 227.0
  - clear cell type (M8373/0) 227.0
  - compact cell type (M8371/0) 227.0
  - glomerulosa cell type (M8374/0) 227.0
  - heavily pigmented variant (M8372/0) 227.0
  - mixed cell type (M8375/0) 227.0
- alpha cell (M8152/0)
  - pancreas 211.7
  - specified site NEC — see Neoplasm, by site, benign
  - unspecified site 211.7
- alveolar (M8251/0)
- apocrine (M8401/0)
  - breast 217
  - specified site NEC — see Neoplasm, skin, benign
  - unspecified site 216.9
- basal cell (M8147/0)
- basophil (M8300/0)
  - specified site — see Neoplasm, by site, benign
  - unspecified site 227.3
- beta cell (M8151/0)
  - pancreas 211.7

Adenoma — see also Neoplasm, by site, benign — continued
- beta cell — continued
  - specified site NEC — see Neoplasm, by site, benign
  - unspecified site 211.7
- bile duct (M8160/0) 211.5
- black (M8372/0) 227.0
- bronchial (M8140/1) 235.7
  - carcinoid type (M8240/3) — see Neoplasm, lung, malignant
  - cylindroid type (M8200/3) — see Neoplasm, lung, malignant
- ceruminous (M8420/0) 216.2
- chief cell (M8321/0) 227.1
- chromophobe (M8270/0)
  - specified site — see Neoplasm, by site, benign
  - unspecified site 227.3
- clear cell (M8310/0)
- colloid (M8334/0)
  - specified site — see Neoplasm, by site, benign
  - unspecified site 226
- cylindroid type, bronchus (M8200/3) — see Neoplasm, lung, malignant
- duct (M8503/0)
- embryonal (M8191/0)
- endocrine, multiple (M8360/1)
  - single specified site — see Neoplasm, by site, uncertain behavior
  - two or more specified sites 237.4
  - unspecified site 237.4
- endometrioid (M8380/0) — see also Neoplasm, by site, benign
  - borderline malignancy (M8380/1) — see Neoplasm, by site, uncertain behavior
- eosinophil (M8280/0)
  - specified site — see Neoplasm, by site, benign
  - unspecified site 227.3
- fetal (M8333/0)
  - specified site — see Neoplasm, by site, benign
  - unspecified site 226
- follicular (M8330/0)
  - specified site — see Neoplasm, by site, benign
  - unspecified site 226
- hepatocellular (M8170/0) 211.5
- Hürthle cell (M8290/0) 226
- intracystic papillary (M8504/0)
- islet cell (functioning) (M8150/0)
  - pancreas 211.7
  - specified site NEC — see Neoplasm, by site, benign
  - unspecified site 211.7
- liver cell (M8170/0) 211.5
- macrofollicular (M8334/0)
  - specified site NEC — see Neoplasm, by site, benign
  - unspecified site 226
- malignant, malignum (M8140/3) — see Neoplasm, by site, malignant
- mesonephric (M9110/0)
- microfollicular (M8333/0)
  - specified site — see Neoplasm, by site, benign
  - unspecified site 226
- mixed cell (M8323/0)
- monomorphic (M8146/0)
- mucinous (M8480/0)
- mucoid cell (M8300/0)
  - specified site — see Neoplasm, by site, benign
  - unspecified site 227.3
- multiple endocrine (M8360/1)
  - single specified site — see Neoplasm, by site, uncertain behavior
  - two or more specified sites 237.4
  - unspecified site 237.4
- nipple (M8506/0) 217
- oncocytic (M8290/0)
- oxyphilic (M8290/0)
- papillary (M8260/0) — see also Neoplasm, by site, benign
  - intracystic (M8504/0)
- papillotubular (M8263/0)

Adenoma — see also Neoplasm, by site, benign — continued
- Pick's tubular (M8640/0)
  - specified site — see Neoplasm, by site, benign
  - unspecified site
    - female 220
    - male 222.0
- pleomorphic (M8940/0)
- polypoid (M8210/0)
- prostate (benign) 600.2
- rete cell 222.0
- sebaceous, sebaceum (gland) (senile) (M8410/0) — see also Neoplasm, skin, benign
  - disseminata 759.5
- Sertoli cell (M8640/0)
  - specified site — see Neoplasm, by site, benign
  - unspecified site
    - female 220
    - male 222.0
- skin appendage (M8390/0) — see Neoplasm, skin, benign
- sudoriferous gland (M8400/0) — see Neoplasm, skin, benign
- sweat gland or duct (M8400/0) — see Neoplasm, skin, benign
- testicular (M8640/0)
  - specified site — see Neoplasm, by site, benign
  - unspecified site
    - female 220
    - male 222.0
- thyroid 226
- trabecular (M8190/0)
- tubular (M8211/0) — see also Neoplasm, by site, benign
  - papillary (M8460/3)
  - Pick's (M8640/0)
    - specified site — see Neoplasm, by site, benign
    - unspecified site
      - female 220
      - male 222.0
- tubulovillous (M8263/0)
- villoglandular (M8263/0)
- villous (M8261/1) — see Neoplasm, by site, uncertain behavior
- water-clear cell (M8322/0) 227.1
- wolffian duct (M9110/0)

Adenomatosis (M8220/0)
- endocrine (multiple) (M8360/1)
  - single specified site — see Neoplasm, by site, uncertain behavior
  - two or more specified sites 237.4
  - unspecified site 237.4
- erosive of nipple (M8506/0) 217
- pluriendocrine — see Adenomatosis, endocrine
- pulmonary (M8250/1) 235.7
  - malignant (M8250/3) — see Neoplasm, lung, malignant
- specified site — see Neoplasm, by site, benign
- unspecified site 211.3

Adenomatous
- cyst, thyroid (gland) — see Goiter, nodular
- goiter (nontoxic) (see also Goiter, nodular) 241.9
- toxic or with hyperthyroidism 242.3

Adenomyoma (M8932/0) — see also Neoplasm, by site, benign
- prostate 600.2

Adenomyometritis 617.0

Adenomyosis (uterus) (internal) 617.0

Adenopathy (lymph gland) 785.6
- inguinal 785.6
- mediastinal 785.6
- mesentery 785.6
- syphilitic (secondary) 091.4
- tracheobronchial 785.6
  - tuberculous (see also Tuberculosis) 012.1
    - primary, progressive 010.8
  - tuberculous (see also Tuberculosis, lymph gland) 017.2
    - tracheobronchial 012.1
      - primary, progressive 010.8

Adenopharyngitis 462
Adenophlegmon 683
Adenosalpingitis 614.1
Adenosarcoma (M8960/3) 189.0
Adenosclerosis 289.3
Adenosis
   breast (sclerosing) 610.2
   vagina, congenital 752.49
Adentia (complete) (partial) (see also Absence,
      teeth) 520.0
Adherent
   labium (minus) 624.4
   pericardium (nonrheumatic) 423.1
      rheumatic 393
   placenta 667.0
      with hemorrhage 666.0
   prepuce 605
   scar (skin) NEC 709.2
   tendon in scar 709.2
Adhesion(s), adhesive (postinfectional)
      (postoperative)
   abdominal (wall) (see also Adhesions,
      peritoneum) 568.0
   amnion to fetus 658.8
      affecting fetus or newborn 762.8
   appendix 543.9
   arachnoiditis — see Meningitis
   auditory tube (Eustachian) 381.89
   bands — see also Adhesions, peritoneum
      cervix 622.3
      uterus 621.5
   bile duct (any) 576.8
   bladder (sphincter) 596.8
   bowel (see also Adhesions, peritoneum) 568.0
   cardiac 423.1
      rheumatic 398.99
   cecum (see also Adhesions, peritoneum) 568.0
   cervicovaginal 622.3
      congenital 752.49
      postpartal 674.8
         old 622.3
   cervix 622.3
   clitoris 624.4
   colon (see also Adhesions, peritoneum) 568.0
   common duct 576.8
   congenital — see also Anomaly, specified type
      NEC
      fingers (see also Syndactylism, fingers)
         755.11
      labium (majus) (minus) 752.49
      omental, anomalous 751.4
      ovary 752.0
      peritoneal 751.4
      toes (see also Syndactylism, toes) 755.13
      tongue (to gum or roof of mouth) 750.12
   conjunctiva (acquired) (localized) 372.62
      congenital 743.63
      extensive 372.63
   cornea — see Opacity, cornea
   cystic duct 575.8
   diaphragm (see also Adhesions, peritoneum)
      568.0
   due to foreign body — see Foreign body
   duodenum (see also Adhesions, peritoneum)
      568.0
      with obstruction 537.3
   ear, middle — see Adhesions, middle ear
   epididymis 608.89
   epidural — see Adhesions, meninges
   epiglottis 478.79
   Eustachian tube 381.89
   eyelid 374.46
      postoperative 997.99
         surgically created V45.69
   gallbladder (see also Disease, gallbladder)
      575.8
   globe 360.89
   heart 423.1
      rheumatic 398.99
   ileocecal (coil) (see also Adhesions, peritoneum)
      568.0
   ileum (see also Adhesions, peritoneum) 568.0
   intestine (postoperative) (see also Adhesions,
      peritoneum) 568.0

Adhesion(s), adhesive — continued
   intestine (see also Adhesions, peritoneum) —
      continued
      with obstruction 560.81
         with hernia — see also Hernia, by site,
            with obstruction
            gangrenous — see Hernia, by site,
               with gangrene
   intra-abdominal (see also Adhesions,
      peritoneum) 568.0
   iris 364.70
      to corneal graft 996.79
   joint (see also Ankylosis) 718.5
   kidney 593.89
   labium (majus) (minus), congenital 752.49
   liver 572.8
   lung 511.0
   mediastinum 519.3
   meninges 349.2
      cerebral (any) 349.2
         congenital 742.4
      congenital 742.8
      spinal (any) 349.2
         congenital 742.59
      tuberculous (cerebral) (spinal) (see also
         Tuberculosis, meninges) 013.0
   mesenteric (see also Adhesions, peritoneum)
      568.0
   middle ear (fibrous) 385.10
      drum head 385.19
         to
            incus 385.11
            promontorium 385.13
            stapes 385.12
      specified NEC 385.19
   nasal (septum) (to turbinates) 478.1
   nerve NEC 355.9
      spinal 355.9
         root 724.9
            cervical NEC 723.4
            lumbar NEC 724.4
            lumbosacral 724.4
            thoracic 724.4
   ocular muscle 378.60
   omentum (see also Adhesions, peritoneum)
      568.0
   organ or site, congenital NEC — see Anomaly,
      specified type NEC
   ovary 614.6
      congenital (to cecum, kidney, or omentum)
         752.0
   parauterine 614.6
   parovarian 614.6
   pelvic (peritoneal)
      female (postoperative) (postinfection) 614.6
      male (postoperative) (postinfection) (see also
         Adhesions, peritoneum) 568.0
      postpartal (old) 614.6
      tuberculous (see also Tuberculosis)
         016.9
   penis to scrotum (congenital) 752.69
   periappendiceal (see also Adhesions,
      peritoneum) 568.0
   pericardium (nonrheumatic) 423.1
      rheumatic 393
      tuberculous (see also Tuberculosis)
         017.9 [420.0]
   pericholecystic 575.8
   perigastric (see also Adhesions, peritoneum)
      568.0
   periovarian 614.6
   periprostatic 602.8
   perirectal (see also Adhesions, peritoneum)
      568.0
   perirenal 593.89
   peritoneum, peritoneal (fibrous) (postoperative)
      568.0
      with obstruction (intestinal) 560.81
         with hernia — see also Hernia, by site,
            with obstruction
            gangrenous — see Hernia, by site,
               with gangrene
         duodenum 537.3
      congenital 751.4
      female (postoperative) (postinfective) 614.6
      pelvic, female 614.6
      pelvic, male 568.0
      postpartal, pelvic 614.6

Adhesion(s), adhesive — continued
   peritoneum, peritoneal — continued
      to uterus 614.6
   peritubal 614.6
   periureteral 593.89
   periuterine 621.5
   perivesical 596.8
   perivesicular (seminal vesicle) 608.89
   pleura, pleuritic 511.0
      tuberculous (see also Tuberculosis, pleura)
         012.0
   pleuropericardial 511.0
   postoperative (gastrointestinal tract) (see also
      Adhesions, peritoneum) 568.0
      eyelid 997.99
         surgically created V45.69
      pelvic female 614.9
      pelvic male 568.0
      urethra 598.2
   postpartal, old 624.4
   preputial, prepuce 605
   pulmonary 511.0
   pylorus (see also Adhesions, peritoneum) 568.0
   Rosenmüller's fossa 478.29
   sciatic nerve 355.0
   seminal vesicle 608.89
   shoulder (joint) 726.0
   sigmoid flexure (see also Adhesions,
      peritoneum) 568.0
   spermatic cord (acquired) 608.89
      congenital 752.8
   spinal canal 349.2
      nerve 355.9
         root 724.9
            cervical NEC 723.4
            lumbar NEC 724.4
            lumbosacral 724.4
            thoracic 724.4
   stomach (see also Adhesions, peritoneum)
      568.0
   subscapular 726.2
   tendonitis 726.90
      shoulder 726.0
   testicle 608.89
   tongue (congenital) (to gum or roof of mouth)
      750.12
      acquired 529.8
   trachea 519.1
   tubo-ovarian 614.6
   tunica vaginalis 608.89
   ureter 593.89
   uterus 621.5
      to abdominal wall 614.6
         in pregnancy or childbirth 654.4
            affecting fetus or newborn 763.89
   vagina (chronic) (postoperative) (postradiation)
      623.2
   vaginitis (congenital) 752.49
   vesical 596.8
   vitreous 379.29
Adie (-Holmes) syndrome (tonic pupillary
      reaction) 379.46
Adiponecrosis neonatorum 778.1
Adiposa dolorosa 272.8
Adiposalgia 272.8
Adiposis
   cerebralis 253.8
   dolorosa 272.8
   tuberosa simplex 272.8
Adiposity 278.00
   heart (see also Degeneration, myocardial) 429.1
   localized 278.1
Adiposogenital dystrophy 253.8
Adjustment
   prosthesis or other device — see Fitting of
   reaction — see Reaction, adjustment
Administration, prophylactic
   antibiotics V07.39
   antitoxin, any V07.2
   antivenin V07.2
   chemotherapeutic agent NEC V07.39
   chemotherapy V07.39
   diphtheria antitoxin V07.2
   fluoride V07.31
   gamma globulin V07.2
   immune sera (gamma globulin) V07.2

Administration, prophylactic

Administration, prophylactic — *continued*
  passive immunization agent V07.2
  RhoGAM V07.2

Admission (encounter)
  as organ donor — *see* Donor
  by mistake V68.9
  for
    adequacy testing (for)
      hemodialysis V56.31
      peritoneal dialysis V56.32
    adjustment (of)
      artificial
        arm (complete) (partial) V52.0
        eye V52.2
        leg (complete) (partial) V52.1
      brain neuropacemaker V53.02
      breast
        implant V52.4
        prosthesis V52.4
      cardiac device V53.39
        defibrillator, automatic implantable V53.32
        pacemaker V53.31
          carotid sinus V53.39
      catheter
        non-vascular V58.82
        vascular V58.81
      cerebral ventricle (communicating) shunt V53.01
      colostomy belt V55.3
      contact lenses V53.1
      cystostomy device V53.6
      dental prosthesis V52.3
      device NEC V53.9
        abdominal V53.5
        cardiac V53.39
          defibrillator, automatic implantable V53.32
          pacemaker V53.31
        carotid sinus V53.39
        cerebral ventricle (communicating) shunt V53.01
        intrauterine contraceptive V25.1
        nervous system V53.09
        orthodontic V53.4
        prosthetic V52.9
          breast V52.4
          dental V52.3
          eye V52.2
          specified type NEC V52.8
        special senses V53.09
        substitution
          auditory V53.09
          nervous system V53.09
          visual V53.09
        urinary V53.6
      dialysis catheter
        extracorporeal V56.1
        peritoneal V56.2
      diaphragm (contraceptive) V25.02
      hearing aid V53.2
      ileostomy device V55.2
      intestinal appliance or device NEC V53.5
      intrauterine contraceptive device V25.1
      neuropacemaker (brain) (peripheral nerve) (spinal cord) V53.02
      orthodontic device V53.4
      orthopedic (device) V53.7
        brace V53.7
        cast V53.7
        shoes V53.7
      pacemaker
        brain V53.02
        cardiac V53.31
        carotid sinus V53.39
        peripheral nerve V53.02
        spinal cord V53.02
      prosthesis V52.9
        arm (complete) (partial) V52.0
        breast V52.4
        dental V52.3
        eye V52.2
        leg (complete) (partial) V52.1
        specified type NEC V52.8
      spectacles V53.1
      wheelchair V53.8

Admission — *continued*
  for — *continued*
    adoption referral or proceedings V68.89
    aftercare (*see also* Aftercare) V58.9
      cardiac pacemaker V53.31
      chemotherapy V58.1
      dialysis
        extracorporeal (renal) V56.0
        peritoneal V56.8
        renal V56.0
      fracture (*see also* Aftercare, fracture) V54.9
      medical NEC V58.89
      orthopedic V54.9
        specified care NEC V54.89 ▲
      pacemaker device
        brain V53.02
        cardiac V53.31
        carotid sinus V53.39
        nervous system V53.02
        spinal cord V53.02
      postoperative NEC V58.49
        wound closure, planned V58.41
      postpartum
        immediately after delivery V24.0
        routine follow-up V24.2
      postradiation V58.0
      radiation therapy V58.0
      removal of
        non-vascular catheter V58.82
        vascular catheter V58.81
      specified NEC V58.89
      surgical NEC V58.49
        wound closure, planned V58.41
    artificial insemination V26.1
    attention to artificial opening (of) V55.9
      artificial vagina V55.7
      colostomy V55.3
      cystostomy V55.5
      enterostomy V55.4
      gastrostomy V55.1
      ileostomy V55.2
      jejunostomy V55.4
      nephrostomy V55.6
      specified site NEC V55.8
        intestinal tract V55.4
        urinary tract V55.6
      tracheostomy V55.0
      ureterostomy V55.6
      urethrostomy V55.6
    battery replacement
      cardiac pacemaker V53.31
    boarding V65.0
    breast
      augmentation or reduction V50.1
      removal, prophylactic V50.41
    change of
      cardiac pacemaker (battery) V53.31
      carotid sinus pacemaker V53.39
      catheter in artificial opening — *see* Attention to, artificial, opening
      dressing V58.3
      fixation device
        external V54.89 ▲
        internal V54.0
      Kirschner wire V54.89 ▲
      neuropacemaker device (brain) (peripheral nerve) (spinal cord) V53.02
      pacemaker device
        brain V53.02
        cardiac V53.31
        carotid sinus V53.39
        nervous system V53.02
      plaster cast V54.89 ▲
      splint, external V54.89 ▲
      Steinmann pin V54.89 ▲
      surgical dressing V58.3
      traction device V54.89 ▲
    checkup only V70.0
    chemotherapy V58.1
    circumcision, ritual or routine (in absence of medical indication) V50.2
    clinical research investigation (control) (normal comparison) (participant) V70.7

Admission — *continued*
  for — *continued*
    closure of artificial opening — *see* Attention to, artificial, opening
    contraceptive
      counseling V25.09
      management V25.9
        specified type NEC V25.8
    convalescence following V66.9
      chemotherapy V66.2
      psychotherapy V66.3
      radiotherapy V66.1
      surgery V66.0
      treatment (for) V66.5
        combined V66.6
        fracture V66.4
        mental disorder NEC V66.3
        specified condition NEC V66.5
    cosmetic surgery NEC V50.1
      following healed injury or operation V51
    counseling (*see also* Counseling) V65.40
      without complaint or sickness V65.49
      contraceptive management V25.09
      dietary V65.3
      exercise V65.41
      for
        nonattending third party V65.1
        victim of abuse
          child V61.21
          partner or spouse V61.11
      genetic V26.3
      gonorrhea V65.45
      HIV V65.44
      human immunodeficiency virus V65.44
      injury prevention V65.43
      procreative management V26.4
      sexually transmitted disease NEC V65.45
        HIV V65.44
      specified reason NEC V65.49
      substance use and abuse V65.42
      syphilis V65.45
      victim of abuse
        child V61.21
        partner or spouse V61.11
    desensitization to allergens V07.1
    dialysis V56.0
      catheter
        fitting and adjustment
          extracorporeal V56.1
          peritoneal V56.2
        removal or replacement
          extracorporeal V56.1
          peritoneal V56.2
      extracorporeal (renal) V56.0
      peritoneal V56.8
      renal V56.0
    dietary surveillance and counseling V65.3
    drug monitoring, therapeutic V58.83
    ear piercing V50.3
    elective surgery V50.9
      breast
        augmentation or reduction V50.1
        removal, prophylactic V50.41
      circumcision, ritual or routine (in absence of medical indication) V50.2
      cosmetic NEC V50.1
        following healed injury or operation V51
      ear piercing V50.3
      face-lift V50.1
      hair transplant V50.0
      plastic
        cosmetic NEC V50.1
        following healed injury or operation V51
      prophylactic organ removal V50.49
        breast V50.41
        ovary V50.42
      repair of scarred tissue (following healed injury or operation) V51
      specified type NEC V50.8
    end-of-life care V66.7
    examination (*see also* Examination) V70.9
      administrative purpose NEC V70.3
      adoption V70.3

Index to Diseases

Admission — *continued*
  for — *continued*
    examination (*see also* Examination) — *continued*
      allergy V72.7
      at health care facility V70.0
      athletic team V70.3
      camp V70.3
      cardiovascular, preoperative V72.81
      clinical research investigation (control) (participant) V70.7
      dental V72.2
      developmental testing (child) (infant) V20.2
      donor (potential) V70.8
      driver's license V70.3
      ear V72.1
      employment V70.5
      eye V72.0
      follow-up (routine) — *see* Examination, follow-up
      for admission to
        old age home V70.3
        school V70.3
      general V70.9
        specified reason NEC V70.8
      gynecological V72.3
      health supervision (child) (infant) V20.2
      hearing V72.1
      immigration V70.3
      insurance certification V70.3
      laboratory V72.6
      marriage license V70.3
      medical (general) (*see also* Examination, medical) V70.9
      medicolegal reasons V70.4
      naturalization V70.3
      pelvic (annual) (periodic) V72.3
      postpartum checkup V24.2
      pregnancy (possible) (unconfirmed) V72.4
      preoperative V72.84
        cardiovascular V72.81
        respiratory V72.82
        specified NEC V72.83
      prison V70.3
      psychiatric (general) V70.2
        requested by authority V70.1
      radiological NEC V72.5
      respiratory, preoperative V72.82
      school V70.3
      screening — *see* Screening
      skin hypersensitivity V72.7
      specified type NEC V72.85
      sport competition V70.3
      vision V72.0
      well baby and child care V20.2
    exercise therapy V57.1
    face-lift, cosmetic reason V50.1
    fitting (of)
      artificial
        arm (complete) (partial) V52.0
        eye V52.2
        leg (complete) (partial) V52.1
      biliary drainage tube V58.82
      brain neuropacemaker V53.02
      breast V52.4
        implant V52.4
        prosthesis V52.4
      cardiac pacemaker V53.31
      catheter
        non-vascular V58.82
        vascular V58.81
      cerebral ventricle (communicating) shunt V53.01
      chest tube V58.82
      colostomy belt V55.2
      contact lenses V53.1
      cystostomy device V53.6
      dental prosthesis V52.3
      device NEC V53.9
        abdominal V53.5
        cerebral ventricle (communicating) shunt V53.01
        intrauterine contraceptive V25.1
        nervous system V53.09
        orthodontic V53.4

Admission — *continued*
  for — *continued*
    fitting — *continued*
      device NEC — *continued*
        prosthetic V52.9
          breast V52.4
          dental V52.3
          eye V52.2
        special senses V53.09
        substitution
          auditory V53.09
          nervous system V53.09
          visual V53.09
      diaphragm (contraceptive) V25.02
      fistula (sinus tract) drainage tube V58.82
      hearing aid V53.2
      ileostomy device V55.2
      intestinal appliance or device NEC V53.5
      intrauterine contraceptive device V25.1
      neuropacemaker (brain) (peripheral nerve) (spinal cord) V53.02
      orthodontic device V53.4
      orthopedic (device) V53.7
        brace V53.7
        cast V53.7
        shoes V53.7
      pacemaker
        brain V53.02
        cardiac V53.31
        carotid sinus V53.39
        spinal cord V53.02
      pleural drainage tube V58.82
      prosthesis V52.9
        arm (complete) (partial) V52.0
        breast V52.4
        dental V52.3
        eye V52.2
        leg (complete) (partial) V52.1
        specified type NEC V52.8
      spectacles V53.1
      wheelchair V53.8
    follow-up examination (routine) (following) V67.9
      cancer chemotherapy V67.2
      chemotherapy V67.2
      high-risk medication NEC V67.51
      injury NEC V67.59
      psychiatric V67.3
      psychotherapy V67.3
      radiotherapy V67.1
      specified surgery NEC V67.09
      surgery V67.00
        vaginal pap smear V67.01
      treatment (for) V67.9
        combined V67.6
        fracture V67.4
        involving high-risk medication NEC V67.51
        mental disorder V67.3
        specified NEC V67.59
    hair transplant, for cosmetic reason V50.0
    health advice, education, or instruction V65.4
    hospice care V66.7
    insertion (of)
      subdermal implantable contraceptive V25.5
    intrauterine device
      insertion V25.1
      management V25.42
    investigation to determine further disposition V63.8
    isolation V07.0
    issue of
      medical certificate NEC V68.0
      repeat prescription NEC V68.1
        contraceptive device NEC V25.49
    kidney dialysis V56.0
    mental health evaluation V70.2
      requested by authority V70.1
    nonmedical reason NEC V68.89
    nursing care evaluation V63.8
    observation (without need for further medical care) (*see also* Observation) V71.9
      accident V71.4

Admission — *continued*
  for — *continued*
    observation (*see also* Observation) — *continued*
      alleged rape or seduction V71.5
      criminal assault V71.6
      following accident V71.4
        at work V71.3
      foreign body ingestion V71.89
      growth and development variations, childhood V21.0
      inflicted injury NEC V71.6
      ingestion of deleterious agent or foreign body V71.89
      injury V71.6
      malignant neoplasm V71.1
      mental disorder V71.09
      newborn — *see* Observation, suspected, condition, newborn
      rape V71.5
      specified NEC V71.89
      suspected disorder V71.9
        abuse V71.81
        accident V71.4
          at work V71.3
        benign neoplasm V71.89
        cardiovascular V71.7
        exposure ●
          anthrax V71.82 ●
          biological agent NEC V71.83 ●
        heart V71.7
        inflicted injury NEC V71.6
        malignant neoplasm V71.1
        mental NEC V71.09
        neglect V71.81
        specified condition NEC V71.89
        tuberculosis V71.2
      tuberculosis V71.2
    occupational therapy V57.21
    organ transplant, donor — *see* Donor
    ovary, ovarian removal, prophylactic V50.42
    palliative care V66.7
    Papanicolaou smear
      cervix V76.2
        for suspected malignant neoplasm V76.2
        no disease found V71.1
        routine, as part of gynecological examination V72.3
      vaginal V76.47
        following hysterectomy for malignant condition V67.01
    passage of sounds or bougie in artificial opening — *see* Attention to, artificial, opening
    paternity testing V70.4
    peritoneal dialysis V56.32
    physical therapy NEC V57.1
    plastic surgery
      cosmetic NEC V50.1
      following healed injury or operation V51
    postmenopausal hormone replacement therapy V07.4
    postpartum observation
      immediately after delivery V24.0
      routine follow-up V24.2
    poststerilization (for restoration) V26.0
    procreative management V26.9
      specified type NEC V26.8
    prophylactic
      administration of
        antibiotics V07.39
        antitoxin, any V07.2
        antivenin V07.2
        chemotherapeutic agent NEC V07.39
        chemotherapy NEC V07.39
        diphtheria antitoxin V07.2
        fluoride V07.31
        gamma globulin V07.2
        immune sera (gamma globulin) V07.2
        RhoGAM V07.2
        tetanus antitoxin V07.2
      breathing exercises V57.0
      chemotherapy NEC V07.39
        fluoride V07.31
      measure V07.9
        specified type NEC V07.8

Admission

Admission — *continued*
  for — *continued*
    prophylactic — *continued*
      organ removal V50.49
        breast V50.41
        ovary V50.42
    psychiatric examination (general) V70.2
      requested by authority V70.1
    radiation management V58.0
    radiotherapy V58.0
    reforming of artificial opening — *see* Attention to, artificial, opening
    rehabilitation V57.9
      multiple types V57.89
      occupational V57.21
      orthoptic V57.4
      orthotic V57.81
      physical NEC V57.1
      specified type NEC V57.89
      speech V57.3
      vocational V57.22
    removal of
      cardiac pacemaker V53.31
      cast (plaster) V54.89 ▲
      catheter from artificial opening — *see* Attention to, artificial, opening
      cerebral ventricle (communicating) shunt V53.01
      cystostomy catheter V55.5
      device
        cerebral ventricle (communicating) shunt V53.01
        fixation
          external V54.89 ▲
          internal V54.0
        intrauterine contraceptive V25.42
        traction, external V54.89 ▲
      dressing V58.3
      fixation device
        external V54.89 ▲
        internal V54.0
      intrauterine contraceptive device V25.42
      Kirschner wire V54.89 ▲
      neuropacemaker (brain) (peripheral nerve) (spinal cord) V53.02
      orthopedic fixation device
        external V54.89 ▲
        internal V54.0
      pacemaker device
        brain V53.02
        cardiac V53.31
        carotid sinus V53.39
        nervous system V53.02
      plaster cast V54.89 ▲
      plate (fracture) V54.0
      rod V54.0
      screw (fracture) V54.0
      splint, traction V54.89 ▲
      Steinmann pin V54.89 ▲
      subdermal implantable contraceptive V25.43
      surgical dressing V58.3
      sutures V58.3
      traction device, external V54.89 ▲
      ureteral stent V53.6
    repair of scarred tissue (following healed injury or operation) V51
    reprogramming of cardiac pacemaker V53.31
    restoration of organ continuity (poststerilization) (tuboplasty) (vasoplasty) V26.0
    sensitivity test — *see also* Test, skin
      allergy NEC V72.7
      bacterial disease NEC V74.9
      Dick V74.8
      Kveim V82.89
      Mantoux V74.1
      mycotic infection NEC V75.4
      parasitic disease NEC V75.8
      Schick V74.3
      Schultz-Charlton V74.8
    social service (agency) referral or evaluation V63.8
    speech therapy V57.3
    sterilization V25.2

Admission — *continued*
  for — *continued*
    suspected disorder (ruled out) (without need for further care) — *see* Observation
    terminal care V66.7
    tests only — *see* Test
    therapeutic drug monitoring V58.83
    therapy
      blood transfusion, without reported diagnosis V58.2
      breathing exercises V57.0
      chemotherapy V58.1
        prophylactic NEC V07.39
          fluoride V07.31
      dialysis (intermittent) (treatment)
        extracorporeal V56.0
        peritoneal V56.8
        renal V56.0
        specified type NEC V56.8
      exercise (remedial) NEC V57.1
        breathing V57.0
      long-term (current) drug use NEC V58.69
        antibiotics V58.62
        anticoagulant V58.61
      occupational V57.21
      orthoptic V57.4
      physical NEC V57.1
      radiation V58.0
      speech V57.3
      vocational V57.22
    toilet or cleaning
      of artificial opening — *see* Attention to, artificial, opening
      of non-vascular catheter V58.82
      of vascular catheter V58.81
    tubal ligation V25.2
    tuboplasty for previous sterilization V26.0
    vaccination, prophylactic (against)
      arthropod-borne virus, viral NEC V05.1
        disease NEC V05.1
        encephalitis V05.0
      Bacille Calmette Guérin (BCG) V03.2
      BCG V03.2
      chickenpox V05.4
      cholera alone V03.0
        with typhoid-paratyphoid (cholera + TAB) V06.0
      common cold V04.7
      dengue V05.1
      diphtheria alone V03.5
      diphtheria-tetanus [Td] without pertussis V06.5
      diphtheria-tetanus-pertussis (DTP) V06.1
        with
          poliomyelitis (DTP + polio) V06.3
          typhoid-paratyphoid (DTP + TAB) V06.2
      disease (single) NEC V05.9
        bacterial NEC V03.9
          specified type NEC V03.89
        combinations NEC V06.9
          specified type NEC V06.8
        specified type NEC V05.8
      encephalitis, viral, arthropod-borne V05.0
      Hemophilus infuenzae, type B [Hib] V03.81
      hepatitis, viral V05.3
      immune sera (gamma globulin) V07.2
      influenza V04.8
        with
          Streptococcus pneumoniae [pneumococcus] V06.6
      Leishmaniasis V05.2
      measles alone V04.2
      measles-mumps-rubella (MMR) V06.4
      mumps alone V04.6
        with measles and rubella (MMR) V06.4
      not done because of contraindication V64.0
      pertussis alone V03.6
      plague V03.3
      pneumonia V03.82
      poliomyelitis V04.0
        with diphtheria-tetanus-pertussis (DTP+ polio) V06.3
      rabies V04.5

Admission — *continued*
  for — *continued*
    vaccination, prophylactic — *continued*
      rubella alone V04.3
        with measles and mumps (MMR) V06.4
      smallpox V04.1
      specified type NEC V05.8
      Streptococcus pneumoniae [pneumococcus] V03.82
        with
          influenza V06.6
      tetanus toxoid alone V03.7
        with diphtheria [Td] V06.5
          and pertussis (DTP) V06.1
      tuberculosis (BCG) V03.2
      tularemia V03.4
      typhoid alone V03.1
        with diphtheria-tetanus-pertussis (TAB + DTP) V06.2
      typhoid-paratyphoid alone (TAB) V03.1
      typhus V05.8
      varicella (chicken pox) V05.4
      viral encephalitis, arthropod-borne V05.0
      viral hepatitis V05.3
      yellow fever V04.4
    vasectomy V25.2
    vasoplasty for previous sterilization V26.0
    vision examination V72.0
    vocational therapy V57.22
    waiting period for admission to other facility V63.2
      undergoing social agency investigation V63.8
    well baby and child care V20.2
    x-ray of chest
      for suspected tuberculosis V71.2
      routine V72.5

Adnexitis (suppurative) (*see also* Salpingo-oophoritis) 614.2
Adolescence NEC V21.2
Adoption
  agency referral V68.89
  examination V70.3
  held for V68.89
Adrenal gland — *see* condition
Adrenalism 255.9
  tuberculous (*see also* Tuberculosis) 017.6 ✓5ᵗʰ
Adrenalitis, adrenitis 255.8
  meningococcal hemorrhagic 036.3
Adrenarche, precocious 259.1
Adrenocortical syndrome 255.2
Adrenogenital syndrome (acquired) (congenital) 255.2
  iatrogenic, fetus or newborn 760.79
Adventitious bursa — *see* Bursitis
Adynamia (episodica) (hereditary) (periodic) 359.3
Adynamic
  ileus or intestine (*see also* Ileus) 560.1
  ureter 753.22
Aeration lung, imperfect, newborn 770.5
Aerobullosis 993.3
Aerocele — *see* Embolism, air
Aerodermectasia
  subcutaneous (traumatic) 958.7
    surgical 998.81
  surgical 998.81
Aerodontalgia 993.2
Aeroembolism 993.3
Aerogenes capsulatus infection (*see also* Gangrene, gas) 040.0
Aero-otitis media 993.0
Aerophagy, aerophagia 306.4
  psychogenic 306.4
Aerosinusitis 993.1
Aerotitis 993.0
Affection, affections — *see also* Disease
  sacroiliac (joint), old 724.6
  shoulder region NEC 726.2
Afibrinogenemia 286.3
  acquired 286.6
  congenital 286.3

Index to Diseases

Afibrinogenemia — *continued*
  postpartum 666.3 ✓5ᵗʰ

African
  sleeping sickness 086.5
  tick fever 087.1
  trypanosomiasis 086.5
    Gambian 086.3
    Rhodesian 086.4

Aftercare V58.9
  artificial openings — *see* Attention to, artificial, opening
  blood transfusion without reported diagnosis V58.2
  breathing exercise V57.0
  cardiac device V53.39
    defibrillator, automatic implantable V53.32
    pacemaker V53.31
      carotid sinus V53.39
  carotid sinus pacemaker V53.39
  cerebral ventricle (communicating) shunt V53.01
  chemotherapy session (adjunctive) (maintenance) V58.1
  defibrillator, automatic implantable cardiac V53.32
  exercise (remedial) (therapeutic) V57.1
    breathing V57.0
  extracorporeal dialysis (intermittent) (treatment) V56.0
  following surgery NEC V58.49
    for
      injury V58.43
      neoplasm V58.42
      trauma V58.43
    joint replacement V58.81
    of
      circulatory system V58.73
      digestive system V58.75
      genital organs V58.76
      genitourinary system V58.76
      musculoskeletal system V58.78
      nervous system V58.72
      oral cavity V58.75
      respiratory system V58.74
      sense organs V58.71
      skin V58.77
      subcutaneous tissue V58.77
      teeth V58.75
      urinary system V58.76
    wound closure, planned V58.41
  fracture V54.9
    healing V54.89
      pathologic
        arm V54.20
          lower V54.22
          upper V54.21
        hip V54.23
        leg V54.24
          lower V54.26
          upper V54.25
        specified site NEC V54.29
        vertebrae V54.27
      traumatic
        arm V54.10
          lower V54.12
          upper V54.11
        hip V54.13
        leg V54.14
          lower V54.16
          upper V54.15
        specified site NEC V54.19
        vertebrae V54.17
    removal of
      external fixation device V54.89 ▲
      internal fixation device V54.0
    specified care NEC V54.89 ▲
  gait training V57.1
    for use of artificial limb(s) V57.81
  involving
    dialysis (intermittent) (treatment)
      extracorporeal V56.0
      peritoneal V56.8
      renal V56.0
    gait training V57.1
      for use of artificial limb(s) V57.81
    orthoptic training V57.4

Aftercare — *continued*
  involving — *continued*
    orthotic training V57.81
    radiotherapy session V58.0
    removal of
      dressings V58.3
      fixation device
        external V54.89 ▲
        internal V54.0
      fracture plate V54.0
      pins V54.0
      plaster cast V54.89 ▲
      rods V54.0
      screws V54.0
      surgical dressings V58.3
      sutures V58.3
      traction device, external V54.89 ▲
    neuropacemaker (brain) (peripheral nerve) (spinal cord) V53.02
    occupational therapy V57.21
    orthodontic V58.5
    orthopedic V54.9
      change of external fixation or traction device V54.89 ▲
      following joint replacement V54.81 ●
      removal of fixation device
        external V54.89 ▲
        internal V54.0
      specified care NEC V54.89 ▲
    orthoptic training V57.4
    orthotic training V57.81
    pacemaker
      brain V53.02
      cardiac V53.31
      carotid sinus V53.39
      peripheral nerve V53.02
      spinal cord V53.02
    peritoneal dialysis (intermittent) (treatment) V56.8
    physical therapy NEC V57.1
      breathing exercises V57.0
    radiotherapy session V58.0
    rehabilitation procedure V57.9
      breathing exercises V57.0
      multiple types V57.89
      occupational V57.21
      orthoptic V57.4
      orthotic V57.81
      physical therapy NEC V57.1
      remedial exercises V57.1
      specified type NEC V57.89
      speech V57.3
      therapeutic exercises V57.1
      vocational V57.22
    renal dialysis (intermittent) (treatment) V56.0
    specified type NEC V58.89
      removal of non-vascular catheter V58.82
      removal of vascular catheter V58.81
    speech therapy V57.3
    vocational rehabilitation V57.22

After-cataract 366.50
  obscuring vision 366.53
  specified type, not obscuring vision 366.52

Agalactia 676.4 ✓5ᵗʰ

Agammaglobulinemia 279.00
  with lymphopenia 279.2
  acquired (primary) (secondary) 279.06
  Bruton's X-linked 279.04
  infantile sex-linked (Bruton's) (congenital) 279.04
  Swiss-type 279.2

Aganglionosis (bowel) (colon) 751.3

AGCUS (atypical glandular cell changes of undetermined significance)
  favor benign 795.01
  favor dysplasia 795.02

Age (old) (*see also* Senile) 797

Agenesis — *see also* Absence, by site, congenital
  acoustic nerve 742.8
  adrenal (gland) 759.1
  alimentary tract (complete) (partial) NEC 751.8
    lower 751.2
    upper 750.8
  anus, anal (canal) 751.2
  aorta 747.22
  appendix 751.2

Agenesis — *see also* Absence, by site, congenital — *continued*
  arm (complete) (partial) (*see also* Deformity, reduction, upper limb) 755.20
  artery (peripheral) NEC (*see also* Anomaly, peripheral vascular system) 747.60
    brain 747.81
    coronary 746.85
    pulmonary 747.3
    umbilical 747.5
  auditory (canal) (external) 744.01
  auricle (ear) 744.01
  bile, biliary duct or passage 751.61
  bone NEC 756.9
  brain 740.0
    specified part 742.2
  breast 757.6
  bronchus 748.3
  canaliculus lacrimalis 743.65
  carpus NEC (*see also* Deformity, reduction, upper limb) 755.28
  cartilage 756.9
  cecum 751.2
  cerebellum 742.2
  cervix 752.49
  chin 744.89
  cilia 743.63
  circulatory system, part NEC 747.89
  clavicle 755.51
  clitoris 752.49
  coccyx 756.13
  colon 751.2
  corpus callosum 742.2
  cricoid cartilage 748.3
  diaphragm (with hernia) 756.6
  digestive organ(s), or tract (complete) (partial) NEC 751.8
    lower 751.2
    upper 750.8
  ductus arteriosus 747.89
  duodenum 751.1
  ear NEC 744.09
    auricle 744.01
    lobe 744.21
  ejaculatory duct 752.8
  endocrine (gland) NEC 759.2
  epiglottis 748.3
  esophagus 750.3
  Eustachian tube 744.24
  extrinsic muscle, eye 743.69
  eye 743.00
    adnexa 743.69
  eyelid (fold) 743.62
  face
    bones NEC 756.0
    specified part NEC 744.89
  fallopian tube 752.19
  femur NEC (*see also* Absence, femur, congenital) 755.34
  fibula NEC (*see also* Absence, fibula, congenital) 755.37
  finger NEC (*see also* Absence, finger, congenital) 755.29
  foot (complete) (*see also* Deformity, reduction, lower limb) 755.31
  gallbladder 751.69
  gastric 750.8
  genitalia, genital (organ)
    female 752.8
      external 752.49
      internal NEC 752.8
    male 752.8
      penis 752.69
  glottis 748.3
  gonadal 758.6
  hair 757.4
  hand (complete) (*see also* Deformity, reduction, upper limb) 755.21
  heart 746.89
    valve NEC 746.89
      aortic 746.89
      mitral 746.89
      pulmonary 746.01
  hepatic 751.69
  humerus NEC (*see also* Absence, humerus, congenital) 755.24
  hymen 752.49
  ileum 751.1

Agenesis

Agenesis — see also Absence, by site, congenital — continued
  incus 744.04
  intestine (small) 751.1
    large 751.2
  iris (dilator fibers) 743.45
  jaw 524.09
  jejunum 751.1
  kidney(s) (partial) (unilateral) 753.0
  labium (majus) (minus) 752.49
  labyrinth, membranous 744.05
  lacrimal apparatus (congenital) 743.65
  larynx 748.3
  leg NEC (see also Deformity, reduction, lower limb) 755.30
  lens 743.35
  limb (complete) (partial) (see also Deformity, reduction) 755.4
    lower NEC 755.30
    upper 755.20
  lip 750.26
  liver 751.69
  lung (bilateral) (fissures) (lobe) (unilateral) 748.5
  mandible 524.09
  maxilla 524.09
  metacarpus NEC 755.28
  metatarsus NEC 755.38
  muscle (any) 756.81
  musculoskeletal system NEC 756.9
  nail(s) 757.5
  neck, part 744.89
  nerve 742.8
  nervous system, part NEC 742.8
  nipple 757.6
  nose 748.1
  nuclear 742.8
  organ
    of Corti 744.05
    or site not listed — see Anomaly, specified type NEC
  osseous meatus (ear) 744.03
  ovary 752.0
  oviduct 752.19
  pancreas 751.7
  parathyroid (gland) 759.2
  patella 755.64
  pelvic girdle (complete) (partial) 755.69
  penis 752.69
  pericardium 746.89
  perineal body 756.81
  pituitary (gland) 759.2
  prostate 752.8
  pulmonary
    artery 747.3
    trunk 747.3
    vein 747.49
  punctum lacrimale 743.65
  radioulnar NEC (see also Absence, forearm, congenital) 755.25
  radius NEC (see also Absence, radius, congenital) 755.26
  rectum 751.2
  renal 753.0
  respiratory organ NEC 748.9
  rib 756.3
  roof of orbit 742.0
  round ligament 752.8
  sacrum 756.13
  salivary gland 750.21
  scapula 755.59
  scrotum 752.8
  seminal duct or tract 752.8
  septum
    atrial 745.69
    between aorta and pulmonary artery 745.0
    ventricular 745.3
  shoulder girdle (complete) (partial) 755.59
  skull (bone) 756.0
    with
      anencephalus 740.0
      encephalocele 742.0
      hydrocephalus 742.3
        with spina bifida (see also Spina bifida) 741.0 ☑5ᵗʰ
      microcephalus 742.1
  spermatic cord 752.8
  spinal cord 742.59

Agenesis — see also Absence, by site, congenital — continued
  spine 756.13
    lumbar 756.13
      isthmus 756.11
      pars articularis 756.11
  spleen 759.0
  sternum 756.3
  stomach 750.7
  tarsus NEC 755.38
  tendon 756.81
  testicular 752.8
  testis 752.8
  thymus (gland) 759.2
  thyroid (gland) 243
    cartilage 748.3
  tibia NEC (see also Absence, tibia, congenital) 755.36
  tibiofibular NEC 755.35
  toe (complete) (partial) (see also Absence, toe, congenital) 755.39
  tongue 750.11
  trachea (cartilage) 748.3
  ulna NEC (see also Absence, ulna, congenital) 755.27
  ureter 753.4
  urethra 753.8
  urinary tract NEC 753.8
  uterus 752.3
  uvula 750.26
  vagina 752.49
  vas deferens 752.8
  vein(s) (peripheral) NEC (see also Anomaly, peripheral vascular system) 747.60
    brain 747.81
    great 747.49
    portal 747.49
    pulmonary 747.49
  vena cava (inferior) (superior) 747.49
  vermis of cerebellum 742.2
  vertebra 756.13
    lumbar 756.13
      isthmus 756.11
      pars articularis 756.11
  vulva 752.49

Ageusia (see also Disturbance, sensation) 781.1
Aggressiveness 301.3
Aggressive outburst (see also Disturbance, conduct) 312.0 ☑5ᵗʰ
  in children and adolescents 313.9
Aging skin 701.8
Agitated — see condition
Agitation 307.9
  catatonic (see also Schizophrenia) 295.2 ☑5ᵗʰ
Aglossia (congenital) 750.11
Aglycogenosis 271.0
Agnail (finger) (with lymphangitis) 681.02
Agnosia (body image) (tactile) 784.69
  verbal 784.69
    auditory 784.69
      secondary to organic lesion 784.69
    developmental 315.8
      secondary to organic lesion 784.69
    visual 784.69
      developmental 315.8
      secondary to organic lesion 784.69
  visual 368.16
    developmental 315.31
Agoraphobia 300.22
  with panic attacks 300.21
Agrammatism 784.69
Agranulocytopenia 288.0
Agranulocytosis (angina) (chronic) (cyclical) (genetic) (infantile) (periodic) (pernicious) 288.0
Agraphia (absolute) 784.69
  with alexia 784.61
  developmental 315.39
Agrypnia (see also Insomnia) 780.52
Ague (see also Malaria) 084.6
  brass-founders' 985.8
  dumb 084.6
  tertian 084.1
Agyria 742.2

Ahumada-del Castillo syndrome (nonpuerperal galactorrhea and amenorrhea) 253.1
AIDS 042
AIDS-associated retrovirus (disease) (illness) 042
  infection — see Human immunodeficiency virus, infection
AIDS-associated virus (disease) (illness) 042
  infection — see Human immunodeficiency virus, infection
AIDS-like disease (illness) (syndrome) 042
AIDS-related complex 042
AIDS-related conditions 042
AIDS-related virus (disease) (illness) 042
  infection — see Human immunodeficiency virus, infection
AIDS virus (disease) (illness) 042
  infection — see Human immunodeficiency virus, infection
Ailment, heart — see Disease, heart
Ailurophobia 300.29
Ainhum (disease) 136.0
Air
  anterior mediastinum 518.1
  compressed, disease 993.3
  embolism (any site) (artery) (cerebral) 958.0
    with
      abortion — see Abortion, by type, with embolism
      ectopic pregnancy (see also categories 633.0-633.9) 639.6
      molar pregnancy (see also categories 630-632) 639.6
      due to implanted device — see Complications, due to (presence of) any device, implant, or graft classified to 996.0-996.5 NEC
    following
      abortion 639.6
      ectopic or molar pregnancy 639.6
    infusion, perfusion, or transfusion 999.1
    in pregnancy, childbirth, or puerperium 673.0 ☑5ᵗʰ
    traumatic 958.0
  hunger 786.09
    psychogenic 306.1
  leak (lung) (pulmonary) (thorax) 512.8
    iatrogenic 512.1
    postoperative 512.1
  rarefied, effects of — see Effect, adverse, high altitude
  sickness 994.6
Airplane sickness 994.6
Akathisia, acathisia 781.0
  due to drugs 333.99
Akinesia algeria 352.6
Akiyami 100.89
Akureyri disease (epidemic neuromyasthenia) 049.8
Alacrima (congenital) 743.65
Alactasia (hereditary) 271.3
Alalia 784.3
  developmental 315.31
    receptive-expressive 315.32
  secondary to organic lesion 784.3
Alaninemia 270.8
Alastrim 050.1
Albarrán's disease (colibacilluria) 791.9
Albers-Schönberg's disease (marble bones) 756.52
Albert's disease 726.71
Albinism, albino (choroid) (cutaneous) (eye) (generalized) (isolated) (ocular) (oculocutaneous) (partial) 270.2
Albinismus 270.2
Albright (-Martin) (-Bantam) disease (pseudohypoparathyroidism) 275.49
Albright (-McCune) (-Sternberg) syndrome (osteitis fibrosa disseminata) 756.59
Albuminous — see condition
Albuminuria, albuminuric (acute) (chronic) (subacute) 791.0

Index to Diseases

Albuminuria, albuminuric — continued
- Bence-Jones 791.0
- cardiac 785.9
- complicating pregnancy, childbirth, or puerperium 646.2 ✓5th
  - with hypertension — see Toxemia, of pregnancy
  - affecting fetus or newborn 760.1
- cyclic 593.6
- gestational 646.2 ✓5th
- gravidarum 646.2 ✓5th
  - with hypertension — see Toxemia, of pregnancy
  - affecting fetus or newborn 760.1
- heart 785.9
- idiopathic 593.6
- orthostatic 593.6
- postural 593.6
- pre-eclamptic (mild) 642.4 ✓5th
  - affecting fetus or newborn 760.0
  - severe 642.5 ✓5th
    - affecting fetus or newborn 760.0
- recurrent physiologic 593.6
- scarlatinal 034.1

Albumosuria 791.0
- Bence-Jones 791.0
- myelopathic (M9730/3) 203.0 ✓5th

Alcaptonuria 270.2

Alcohol, alcoholic
- abstinence 291.81
- acute intoxication 305.0 ✓5th
  - with dependence 303.0 ✓5th
- addiction (see also Alcoholism) 303.9 ✓5th
  - maternal
    - with suspected fetal damage affecting management of pregnancy 655.4 ✓5th
    - affecting fetus or newborn 760.71
- amnestic disorder, persisting 291.1
- anxiety 291.89
- brain syndrome, chronic 291.2
- cardiopathy 425.5
- chronic (see also Alcoholism) 303.9 ✓5th
- cirrhosis (liver) 571.2
- delirium 291.0
  - acute 291.0
  - chronic 291.1
  - tremens 291.0
  - withdrawal 291.0
- dementia NEC 291.2
- deterioration 291.2
- drunkenness (simple) 305.0 ✓5th
- hallucinosis (acute) 291.3
- insanity 291.9
- intoxication (acute) 305.0 ✓5th
  - with dependence 303.0 ✓5th
  - pathological 291.4
- jealousy 291.5
- Korsakoff's, Korsakov's, Korsakow's 291.1
- liver NEC 571.3
  - acute 571.1
  - chronic 571.2
- mania (acute) (chronic) 291.9
- mood 291.89
- paranoia 291.5
- paranoid (type) psychosis 291.5
- pellagra 265.2
- poisoning, accidental (acute) NEC 980.9
  - specified type of alcohol — see Table of Drugs and Chemicals
- psychosis (see also Psychosis, alcoholic) 291.9
  - Korsakoff's, Korsakov's, Korsakow's 291.1
  - polyneuritic 291.1
    - with
      - delusions 291.5
      - hallucinations 291.3
- withdrawal symptoms, syndrome NEC 291.81
  - delirium 291.0
  - hallucinosis 291.3

Alcoholism 303.9 ✓5th

> Note — Use the following fifth-digit subclassification with category 303:
> 0   unspecified
> 1   continuous
> 2   episodic
> 3   in remission

- with psychosis (see also Psychosis, alcoholic) 291.9
- acute 303.0 ✓5th
- chronic 303.9 ✓5th
  - with psychosis 291.9
- complicating pregnancy, childbirth, or puerperium 648.4 ✓5th
  - affecting fetus or newborn 760.71
- history V11.3
- Korsakoff's, Korsakov's, Korsakow's 291.1
- suspected damage to fetus affecting management of pregnancy 655.4 ✓5th

Alder's anomaly or syndrome (leukocyte granulation anomaly) 288.2

Alder-Reilly anomaly (leukocyte granulation) 288.2

Aldosteronism (primary) (secondary) 255.1
- congenital 255.1

Aldosteronoma (M8370/1) 237.2

Aldrich (-Wiskott) syndrome (eczema-thrombocytopenia) 279.12

Aleppo boil 085.1

Aleukemic — see condition

Aleukia
- congenital 288.0
- hemorrhagica 284.9
  - acquired (secondary) 284.8
  - congenital 284.0
  - idiopathic 284.9
- splenica 289.4

Alexia (congenital) (developmental) 315.01
- secondary to organic lesion 784.61

Algoneurodystrophy 733.7

Algophobia 300.29

Alibert's disease (mycosis fungoides) (M9700/3) 202.1 ✓5th

Alibert-Bazin disease (M9700/3) 202.1 ✓5th

Alice in Wonderland syndrome 293.89

Alienation, mental (see also Psychosis) 298.9

Alkalemia 276.3

Alkalosis 276.3
- metabolic 276.3
  - with respiratory acidosis 276.4
- respiratory 276.3

Alkaptonuria 270.2

Allen-Masters syndrome 620.6

Allergic bronchopulmonary aspergillosis 518.6

Allergy, allergic (reaction) 995.3
- air-borne substance (see also Fever, hay) 477.9
  - specified allergen NEC 477.8
- alveolitis (extrinsic) 495.9
  - due to
    - Aspergillus clavatus 495.4
    - cryptostroma corticale 495.6
    - organisms (fungal, thermophilic actinomycete, other) growing in ventilation (air conditioning systems) 495.7
  - specified type NEC 495.8
- anaphylactic shock 999.4
  - due to food — see Anaphylactic shock, due to, food
- angioneurotic edema 995.1
- animal (dander) (epidermal) (hair) 477.8
- arthritis (see also Arthritis, allergic) 716.2 ✓5th
- asthma — see Asthma
- bee sting (anaphylactic shock) 989.5
- biological — see Allergy, drug
- bronchial asthma — see Asthma
- conjunctivitis (eczematous) 372.14
- dander (animal) 477.8
- dandruff 477.8
- dermatitis (venenata) — see Dermatitis

Allergy, allergic — continued
- diathesis V15.09
- drug, medicinal substance, and biological (any) (correct medicinal substance properly administered) (external) (internal) 995.2
  - wrong substance given or taken NEC 977.9
  - specified drug or substance — see Table of Drugs and Chemicals
- dust (house) (stock) 477.8
- eczema — see Eczema
- endophthalmitis 360.19
- epidermal (animal) 477.8
- feathers 477.8
- food (any) (ingested) 693.1
  - atopic 691.8
  - in contact with skin 692.5
- gastritis 535.4 ✓5th
- gastroenteritis 558.3
- gastrointestinal 558.3
- grain 477.0
- grass (pollen) 477.0
  - asthma (see also Asthma) 493.0 ✓5th
  - hay fever 477.0
- hair (animal) 477.8
- hay fever (grass) (pollen) (ragweed) (tree) (see also Fever, hay) 477.9
- history (of) V15.09
  - to
    - eggs V15.03
    - food additives V15.05
    - insect bite V15.06
    - latex V15.07
    - milk products V15.02
    - nuts V15.05
      - peanuts V15.01
    - radiographic dye V15.08
    - seafood V15.04
    - specified food NEC V15.05
    - spider bite V15.06
- horse serum — see Allergy, serum
- inhalant 477.9
  - dust 477.8
  - pollen 477.0
  - specified allergen other than pollen 477.8
- kapok 477.8
- medicine — see Allergy, drug
- migraine 346.2 ✓5th
- pannus 370.62
- pneumonia 518.3
- pollen (any) (hay fever) 477.0
  - asthma (see also Asthma) 493.0 ✓5th
- primrose 477.0
- primula 477.0
- purpura 287.0
- ragweed (pollen) (Senecio jacobae) 477.0
  - asthma (see also Asthma) 493.0 ✓5th
  - hay fever 477.0
- respiratory (see also Allergy, inhalant) 477.9
  - due to
    - drug — see Allergy, drug
    - food — see Allergy, food
- rhinitis (see also Fever, hay) 477.9
  - due to food 477.1
- rose 477.0
- Senecio jacobae 477.0
- serum (prophylactic) (therapeutic) 999.5
  - anaphylactic shock 999.4
- shock (anaphylactic) (due to adverse effect of correct medicinal substance properly administered) 995.0
  - food — see Anaphylactic shock, due to, food
  - from serum or immunization 999.5
    - anaphylactic 999.4
- sinusitis (see also Fever, hay) 477.9
- skin reaction 692.9
  - specified substance — see Dermatitis, due to
- tree (any) (hay fever) (pollen) 477.0
  - asthma (see also Asthma) 493.0 ✓5th
- upper respiratory (see also Fever, hay) 477.9
- urethritis 597.89
- urticaria 708.0
- vaccine — see Allergy, serum

Allescheriosis 117.6

Alligator skin disease (ichthyosis congenita) 757.1
- acquired 701.1

Allocheiria, allochiria (see also Disturbance, sensation) 782.0
Almeida's disease (Brazilian blastomycosis) 116.1
Alopecia (atrophicans) (pregnancy) (premature) (senile) 704.00
   adnata 757.4
   areata 704.01
   celsi 704.01
   cicatrisata 704.09
   circumscripta 704.01
   congenital, congenitalis 757.4
   disseminata 704.01
   effluvium (telogen) 704.02
   febrile 704.09
   generalisata 704.09
   hereditaria 704.09
   marginalis 704.01
   mucinosa 704.09
   postinfectional 704.09
   seborrheica 704.09
   specific 091.82
   syphilitic (secondary) 091.82
   telogen effluvium 704.02
   totalis 704.09
   toxica 704.09
   universalis 704.09
   x-ray 704.09
Alpers' disease 330.8
Alpha-lipoproteinemia 272.4
Alpha thalassemia 282.4
Alphos 696.1
Alpine sickness 993.2
Alport's syndrome (hereditary hematurianephropathy-deafness) 759.89
Alteration (of), altered
   awareness 780.09
      transient 780.02
   consciousness 780.09
      persistent vegetative state 780.03
      transient 780.02
   mental status 780.99 ▲
Alternaria (infection) 118
Alternating — see condition
Altitude, high (effects) — see Effect, adverse, high altitude
Aluminosis (of lung) 503
Alvarez syndrome (transient cerebral ischemia) 435.9
Alveolar capillary block syndrome 516.3
Alveolitis
   allergic (extrinsic) 495.9
      due to organisms (fungal, thermophilic actinomycete, other) growing in ventilation (air conditioning systems) 495.7
      specified type NEC 495.8
   due to
      Aspergillus clavatus 495.4
      Cryptostroma corticale 495.6
   fibrosing (chronic) (cryptogenic) (lung) 516.3
      idiopathic 516.3
      rheumatoid 714.81
   jaw 526.5
   sicca dolorosa 526.5
Alveolus, alveolar — see condition
Alymphocytosis (pure) 279.2
Alymphoplasia, thymic 279.2
Alzheimer's
   dementia (senile)
      with behavioral disturbance 331.0 [294.11]
      without behavioral disturbance 331.0 [294.10]
   disease or sclerosis 331.0
      with dementia — see Alzheimer's, dementia
Amastia (see also Absence, breast) 611.8
Amaurosis (acquired) (congenital) (see also Blindness) 369.00
   fugax 362.34
   hysterical 300.11
   Leber's (congenital) 362.76
   tobacco 377.34
   uremic — see Uremia

Amaurotic familial idiocy (infantile) (juvenile) (late) 330.1
Ambisexual 752.7
Amblyopia (acquired) (congenital) (partial) 368.00
   color 368.59
      acquired 368.55
   deprivation 368.02
   ex anopsia 368.00
   hysterical 300.11
   nocturnal 368.60
      vitamin A deficiency 264.5
   refractive 368.03
   strabismic 368.01
   suppression 368.01
   tobacco 377.34
   toxic NEC 377.34
   uremic — see Uremia
Ameba, amebic (histolytica) — see also Amebiasis
   abscess 006.3
      bladder 006.8
      brain (with liver and lung abscess) 006.5
      liver 006.3
         with
            brain abscess (and lung abscess) 006.5
            lung abscess 006.4
      lung (with liver abscess) 006.4
         with brain abscess 006.5
      seminal vesicle 006.8
      spleen 006.8
   carrier (suspected of) V02.2
   meningoencephalitis
      due to Naegleria (gruberi) 136.2
      primary 136.2
Amebiasis NEC 006.9
   with
      brain abscess (with liver or lung abscess) 006.5
      liver abscess (without mention of brain or lung abscess) 006.3
      lung abscess (with liver abscess) 006.4
         with brain abscess 006.5
   acute 006.0
   bladder 006.8
   chronic 006.1
   cutaneous 006.6
   cutis 006.6
   due to organism other than Entamoeba histolytica 007.8
   hepatic (see also Abscess, liver, amebic) 006.3
   nondysenteric 006.2
   seminal vesicle 006.8
   specified
      organism NEC 007.8
      site NEC 006.8
Ameboma 006.8
Amelia 755.4
   lower limb 755.31
   upper limb 755.21
Ameloblastoma (M9310/0) 213.1
   jaw (bone) (lower) 213.1
      upper 213.0
   long bones (M9261/3) — see Neoplasm, bone, malignant
   malignant (M9310/3) 170.1
      jaw (bone) (lower) 170.1
         upper 170.0
   mandible 213.1
   tibial (M9261/3) 170.7
Amelogenesis imperfecta 520.5
   nonhereditaria (segmentalis) 520.4
Amenorrhea (primary) (secondary) 626.0
   due to ovarian dysfunction 256.8
   hyperhormonal 256.8
Amentia (see also Retardation, mental) 319
   Meynert's (nonalcoholic) 294.0
      alcoholic 291.1
   nevoid 759.6
American
   leishmaniasis 085.5
   mountain tick fever 066.1
   trypanosomiasis — see Trypanosomiasis, American
Ametropia (see also Disorder, accommodation) 367.9

Amianthosis 501
Amimia 784.69
Amino acid
   deficiency 270.9
      anemia 281.4
   metabolic disorder (see also Disorder, amino acid) 270.9
Aminoaciduria 270.9
   imidazole 270.5
Amnesia (retrograde) 780.99 ▲
   auditory 784.69
      developmental 315.31
      secondary to organic lesion 784.69
   hysterical or dissociative type 300.12
   psychogenic 300.12
   transient global 437.7
Amnestic (confabulatory) syndrome 294.0
   alcohol induced 291.1
   drug-induced 292.83
   posttraumatic 294.0
Amniocentesis screening (for) V28.2
   alphafetoprotein level, raised V28.1
   chromosomal anomalies V28.0
Amnion, amniotic — see also condition
   nodosum 658.8 ✓5ᵗʰ
Amnionitis (complicating pregnancy) 658.4 ✓5ᵗʰ
   affecting fetus or newborn 762.7
Amoral trends 301.7
Amotio retinae (see also Detachment, retina) 361.9
Ampulla
   lower esophagus 530.89
   phrenic 530.89
Amputation
   any part of fetus, to facilitate delivery 763.89
   cervix (supravaginal) (uteri) 622.8
      in pregnancy or childbirth 654.6 ✓5ᵗʰ
         affecting fetus or newborn 763.89
   clitoris — see Wound, open, clitoris
   congenital
      lower limb 755.31
      upper limb 755.21
   neuroma (traumatic) — see also Injury, nerve, by site
   surgical complication (late) 997.61
   penis — see Amputation, traumatic, penis
   status (without complication) — see Absence, by site, acquired
   stump (surgical) (posttraumatic)
      abnormal, painful, or with complication (late) 997.61
      healed or old NEC — see also Absence, by site, acquired
      lower V49.70
      upper V49.60
   traumatic (complete) (partial)

> Note — "Complicated" includes traumatic amputation with delayed healing, delayed treatment, foreign body, or infection.

      arm 887.4
         at or above elbow 887.2
            complicated 887.3
         below elbow 887.0
            complicated 887.1
         both (bilateral) (any level(s)) 887.6
            complicated 887.7
         complicated 887.5
      finger(s) (one or both hands) 886.0
         with thumb(s) 885.0
            complicated 885.1
         complicated 886.1
      foot (except toe(s) only) 896.0
         and other leg 897.6
            complicated 897.7
         both (bilateral) 896.2
            complicated 896.3
         complicated 896.1
         toe(s) only (one or both feet) 895.0
            complicated 895.1
      genital organ(s) (external) NEC 878.8
         complicated 878.9
      hand (except finger(s) only) 887.0
         and other arm 887.6

Index to Diseases

Amputation — *continued*
traumatic — *continued*
  hand — *continued*
    and other arm — *continued*
      complicated 887.7
    both (bilateral) 887.6
      complicated 887.7
    complicated 887.1
    finger(s) (one or both hands) 886.0
      with thumb(s) 885.0
        complicated 885.1
      complicated 886.1
    thumb(s) (with fingers of either hand) 885.0
      complicated 885.1
  head 874.9
  late effect — *see* Late, effects (of), amputation
  leg 897.4
    and other foot 897.6
      complicated 897.7
    at or above knee 897.2
      complicated 897.3
    below knee 897.0
      complicated 897.1
    both (bilateral) 897.6
      complicated 897.7
    complicated 897.5
  lower limb(s) except toe(s) — *see* Amputation, traumatic, leg
  nose — *see* Wound, open, nose
  penis 878.0
    complicated 878.1
  sites other than limbs — *see* Wound, open, by site
  thumb(s) (with finger(s) of either hand) 885.0
    complicated 885.1
  toe(s) (one or both feet) 895.0
    complicated 895.1
  upper limb(s) — *see* Amputation, traumatic, arm

Amputee (bilateral) (old) — *see also* Absence, by site, acquired V49.70

Amusia 784.69
  developmental 315.39
  secondary to organic lesion 784.69

Amyelencephalus 740.0

Amyelia 742.59

Amygdalitis — *see* Tonsillitis

Amygdalolith 474.8

Amyloid disease or degeneration 277.3
  heart 277.3 [425.7]

Amyloidosis (familial) (general) (generalized) (genetic) (primary) (secondary) 277.3
  with lung involvement 277.3 [517.8]
  heart 277.3 [425.7]
  nephropathic 277.3 [583.81]
  neuropathic (Portuguese) (Swiss) 277.3 [357.4]
  pulmonary 277.3 [517.8]
  systemic, inherited 277.3

Amylopectinosis (brancher enzyme deficiency) 271.0

Amylophagia 307.52

Amyoplasia, congenita 756.89

Amyotonia 728.2
  congenita 358.8

Amyotrophia, amyotrophy, amyotrophic 728.2
  congenita 756.89
  diabetic 250.6 [358.1]
  lateral sclerosis (syndrome) 335.20
  neuralgic 353.5
  sclerosis (lateral) 335.20
  spinal progressive 335.21

Anacidity, gastric 536.0
  psychogenic 306.4

▲ **Anaerosis of newborn** 768.9

Analbuminemia 273.8

Analgesia (*see also* Anesthesia) 782.0

Analphalipoproteinemia 272.5

Anaphylactic shock or reaction (correct substance properly administered) 995.0
  due to
    food 995.60
      additives 995.66
      crustaceans 995.62
      eggs 995.68
      fish 995.65
      fruits 995.63
      milk products 995.67
      nuts (tree) 995.64
      peanuts 995.61
      seeds 995.64
      specified NEC 995.69
      tree nuts 995.64
      vegetables 995.63
    immunization 999.4
    overdose or wrong substance given or taken 977.9
    specified drug — *see* Table of Drugs and Chemicals
    serum 999.4
  following sting(s) 989.5
  purpura 287.0
  serum 999.4

Anaphylactoid shock or reaction — *see* Anaphylactic shock

Anaphylaxis — *see* Anaphylactic shock

Anaplasia, cervix 622.1

Anarthria 784.5

Anarthritic rheumatoid disease 446.5

Anasarca 782.3
  cardiac (*see also* Failure, heart) 428.0
  fetus or newborn 778.0
  lung 514
  nutritional 262
  pulmonary 514
  renal (*see also* Nephrosis) 581.9

Anaspadias 752.62

Anastomosis
  aneurysmal — *see* Aneurysm
  arteriovenous, congenital NEC (*see also* Anomaly, arteriovenous) 747.60
    ruptured, of brain (*see also* Hemorrhage, subarachnoid) 430
  intestinal 569.89
    complicated NEC 997.4
      involving urinary tract 997.5
  retinal and choroidal vessels 743.58
  acquired 362.17

Anatomical narrow angle (glaucoma) 365.02

Ancylostoma (infection) (infestation) 126.9
  americanus 126.1
  braziliense 126.2
  caninum 126.8
  ceylanicum 126.3
  duodenale 126.0
  Necator americanus 126.1

Ancylostomiasis (intestinal) 126.9
  Ancylostoma
    americanus 126.1
    caninum 126.8
    ceylanicum 126.3
    duodenale 126.0
    braziliense 126.2
    Necator americanus 126.1

Anders' disease or syndrome (adiposis tuberosa simplex) 272.8

Andersen's glycogen storage disease 271.0

Anderson's disease 272.7

Andes disease 993.2

Andrews' disease (bacterid) 686.8

Androblastoma (M8630/1)
  benign (M8630/0)
    specified site — *see* Neoplasm, by site, benign
    unspecified site
      female 220
      male 222.0
  malignant (M8630/3)
    specified site — *see* Neoplasm, by site, malignant
    unspecified site
      female 183.0

Androblastoma — *continued*
malignant — *continued*
  unspecified site — *continued*
    male 186.9
specified site — *see* Neoplasm, by site, uncertain behavior
tubular (M8640/0)
  with lipid storage (M8641/0)
    specified site — *see* Neoplasm, by site, benign
    unspecified site
      female 220
      male 222.0
  specified site — *see* Neoplasm, by site, benign
  unspecified site
    female 220
    male 222.0
unspecified site
  female 236.2
  male 236.4

Android pelvis 755.69
  with disproportion (fetopelvic) 653.3 ✓5ᵗʰ
    affecting fetus or newborn 763.1
  causing obstructed labor 660.1 ✓5ᵗʰ
    affecting fetus or newborn 763.1

Anectasis, pulmonary (newborn or fetus) 770.5

Anemia 285.9
  with
    disorder of
      anaerobic glycolysis 282.3
      pentose phosphate pathway 282.2
    koilonychia 280.9
    6-phosphogluconic dehydrogenase deficiency 282.2
  achlorhydric 280.9
  achrestic 281.8
  Addison's (pernicious) 281.0
  Addison-Biermer (pernicious) 281.0
  agranulocytic 288.0
  amino acid deficiency 281.4
  aplastic 284.9
    acquired (secondary) 284.8
    congenital 284.0
    constitutional 284.0
    due to
      chronic systemic disease 284.8
      drugs 284.8
      infection 284.8
      radiation 284.8
    idiopathic 284.9
    myxedema 244.9
    of or complicating pregnancy 648.2 ✓5ᵗʰ
    red cell (acquired) (pure) (with thymoma) 284.8
      congenital 284.0
    specified type NEC 284.8
    toxic (paralytic) 284.8
  aregenerative 284.9
    congenital 284.0
  asiderotic 280.9
  atypical (primary) 285.9
  autohemolysis of Selwyn and Dacie (type I) 282.2
  autoimmune hemolytic 283.0
  Baghdad Spring 282.2
  Balantidium coli 007.0
  Biermer's (pernicious) 281.0
  blood loss (chronic) 280.0
    acute 285.1
  bothriocephalus 123.4
  brickmakers' (*see also* Ancylostomiasis) 126.9
  cerebral 437.8
  childhood 285.9
  chlorotic 280.9
  chronica congenita aregenerativa 284.0
  chronic simple 281.9
  combined system disease NEC 281.0 [336.2]
    due to dietary deficiency 281.1 [336.2]
  complicating pregnancy or childbirth 648.2 ✓5ᵗʰ
  congenital (following fetal blood loss) 776.5
    aplastic 284.0
    due to isoimmunization NEC 773.2
    Heinz-body 282.7
    hereditary hemolytic NEC 282.9
    nonspherocytic
      Type I 282.2

Anemia

Anemia — *continued*
  congenital — *continued*
    nonspherocytic — *continued*
      Type II 282.3
    pernicious 281.0
    spherocytic (*see also* Spherocytosis) 282.0
  Cooley's (erythroblastic) 282.4
  crescent — *see* Disease, sickle-cell
  cytogenic 281.0
  Dacie's (nonspherocytic)
    type I 282.2
    type II 282.3
  Davidson's (refractory) 284.9
  deficiency 281.9
    2, 3 diphosphoglycurate mutase 282.3
    2, 3 PG 282.3
    6-PGD 282.2
    6-phosphogluronic dehydrogenase 282.2
    amino acid 281.4
    combined B_{12} and folate 281.3
    enzyme, drug-induced (hemolytic) 282.2
    erythrocytic glutathione 282.2
    folate 281.2
      dietary 281.2
      drug-induced 281.2
    folic acid 281.2
      dietary 281.2
      drug-induced 281.2
    G-6-PD 282.2
    GGS-R 282.2
    glucose-6-phosphate dehydrogenase (G-6-PD) 282.2
    glucose-phosphate isomerase 282.3
    glutathione peroxidase 282.2
    glutathione reductase 282.2
    glyceraldehyde phosphate dehydrogenase 282.3
    GPI 282.3
    G SH 282.2
    hexokinase 282.3
    iron (Fe) 280.9
      specified NEC 280.8
    nutritional 281.9
      with
        poor iron absorption 280.9
        specified deficiency NEC 281.8
      due to inadequate dietary iron intake 280.1
      specified type NEC 281.8
    of or complicating pregnancy 648.2 ✓5
    pentose phosphate pathway 282.2
    PFK 282.3
    phosphofructo-aldolase 282.3
    phosphofructokinase 282.3
    phosphoglycerate kinase 282.3
    PK 282.3
    protein 281.4
    pyruvate kinase (PK) 282.3
    TPI 282.3
    triosephosphate isomerase 282.3
    vitamin B_{12} NEC 281.1
      dietary 281.1
      pernicious 281.0
  Diamond-Blackfan (congenital hypoplastic) 284.0
  dibothriocephalus 123.4
  dimorphic 281.9
  diphasic 281.8
  diphtheritic 032.89
  Diphyllobothrium 123.4
  drepanocytic (*see also* Disease, sickle-cell) 282.60
  due to
    blood loss (chronic) 280.0
      acute 285.1
    defect of Embden-Meyerhof pathway glycolysis 282.3
    disorder of glutathione metabolism 282.2
    fetal blood loss 776.5
    fish tapeworm (D. latum) infestation 123.4
    glutathione metabolism disorder 282.2
    hemorrhage (chronic) 280.0
      acute 285.1
    hexose monophosphate (HMP) shunt deficiency 282.2
    impaired absorption 280.9

Anemia — *continued*
  due to — *continued*
    loss of blood (chronic) 280.0
      acute 285.1
    myxedema 244.9
    Necator americanus 126.1
    prematurity 776.6
    selective vitamin B_{12} malabsorption with proteinuria 281.1
  Dyke-Young type (secondary) (symptomatic) 283.9
  dyserythropoietic (congenital) (types I, II, III) 285.8
  dyshemopoietic (congenital) 285.8
  Egypt (*see also* Ancylostomiasis) 126.9
  elliptocytosis (*see also* Elliptocytosis) 282.1
  enzyme deficiency, drug-induced 282.2
  epidemic (*see also* Ancylostomiasis) 126.9
  erythroblastic
    familial 282.4
    fetus or newborn (*see also* Disease, hemolytic) 773.2
      late 773.5
  erythrocytic glutathione deficiency 282.2
  essential 285.9
  Faber's (achlorhydric anemia) 280.9
  factitious (self-induced blood letting) 280.0
  familial erythroblastic (microcytic) 282.4
  Fanconi's (congenital pancytopenia) 284.0
  favism 282.2
  fetal, following blood loss 776.5
  fetus or newborn
    due to
      ABO
        antibodies 773.1
        incompatibility, maternal/fetal 773.1
        isoimmunization 773.1
      Rh
        antibodies 773.0
        incompatibility, maternal/fetal 773.0
        isoimmunization 773.0
    following fetal blood loss 776.5
  fish tapeworm (D. latum) infestation 123.4
  folate (folic acid) deficiency 281.2
    dietary 281.2
    drug-induced 281.2
  folate malabsorption, congenital 281.2
  folic acid deficiency 281.2
    dietary 281.2
    drug-induced 281.2
  G-6-PD 282.2
  general 285.9
  glucose-6-phosphate dehydrogenase deficiency 282.2
  glutathione-reductase deficiency 282.2
  goat's milk 281.2
  granulocytic 288.0
  Heinz-body, congenital 282.7
  hemoglobin deficiency 285.9
  hemolytic 283.9
    acquired 283.9
      with hemoglobinuria NEC 283.2
      autoimmune (cold type) (idiopathic) (primary) (secondary) (symptomatic) (warm type) 283.0
      due to
        cold reactive antibodies 283.0
        drug exposure 283.0
        warm reactive antibodies 283.0
      fragmentation 283.19
      idiopathic (chronic) 283.9
      infectious 283.19
        autoimmune 283.0
      non-autoimmune NEC 283.10
      toxic 283.19
      traumatic cardiac 283.19
    acute 283.9
      due to enzyme deficiency NEC 282.3
      fetus or newborn (*see also* Disease, hemolytic) 773.2
        late 773.5
      Lederer's (acquired infectious hemolytic anemia) 283.19
    autoimmune (acquired) 283.0
    chronic 282.9
      idiopathic 283.9
    cold type (secondary) (symptomatic) 283.0

Anemia — *continued*
  hemolytic — *continued*
    congenital (spherocytic) (*see also* Spherocytosis) 282.0
      nonspherocytic — *see* Anemia, hemolytic, nonspherocytic, congenital
    drug-induced 283.0
      enzyme deficiency 282.2
    due to
      cardiac conditions 283.19
      drugs 283.0
      enzyme deficiency NEC 282.3
        drug-induced 282.2
      presence of shunt or other internal prosthetic device 283.19
      thrombotic thrombocytopenic purpura 446.6
    elliptocytotic (*see also* Elliptocytosis) 282.1
    familial 282.9
    hereditary 282.9
      due to enzyme deficiency NEC 282.3
      specified NEC 282.8
    idiopathic (chronic) 283.9
    infectious (acquired) 283.19
    mechanical 283.19
    microangiopathic 283.19
    non-autoimmune NEC 283.10
    nonspherocytic
      congenital or hereditary NEC 282.3
        glucose-6-phosphate dehydrogenase deficiency 282.2
        pyruvate kinase (PK) deficiency 282.3
        type I 282.2
        type II 282.3
      type I 282.2
      type II 282.3
    of or complicating pregnancy 648.2 ✓5
    resulting from presence of shunt or other internal prosthetic device 283.19
    secondary 283.19
      autoimmune 283.0
    sickle-cell — *see* Disease, sickle-cell
    Stransky-Regala type (Hb-E) (*see also* Disease, hemoglobin) 282.7
    symptomatic 283.19
      autoimmune 283.0
    toxic (acquired) 283.19
    uremic (adult) (child) 283.11
    warm type (secondary) (symptomatic) 283.0
  hemorrhagic (chronic) 280.0
    acute 285.1
  HEMPAS 285.8
  hereditary erythroblast multinuclearity-positive acidified serum test 285.8
  Herrick's (hemoglobin S disease) 282.61
  hexokinase deficiency 282.3
  high A_2 282.4
  hookworm (*see also* Ancylostomiasis) 126.9
  hypochromic (idiopathic) (microcytic) (normoblastic) 280.9
    with iron loading 285.0
    due to blood loss (chronic) 280.0
      acute 285.1
    familial sex linked 285.0
    pyridoxine-responsive 285.0
  hypoplasia, red blood cells 284.8
    congenital or familial 284.0
  hypoplastic (idiopathic) 284.9
    congenital 284.0
    familial 284.0
    of childhood 284.0
  idiopathic 285.9
    hemolytic, chronic 283.9
  in
    chronic illness NEC 285.29
    end-stage renal disease 285.21
    neoplastic disease 285.22
  infantile 285.9
  infective, infectional 285.9
  intertropical (*see also* Ancylostomiasis) 126.9
  iron (Fe) deficiency 280.9
    due to blood loss (chronic) 280.0
      acute 285.1
    of or complicating pregnancy 648.2 ✓5
    specified NEC 280.8
  Jaksch's (pseudoleukemia infantum) 285.8

Anemia — *continued*
  Joseph-Diamond-Blackfan (congenital hypoplastic) 284.0
  labyrinth 386.50
  Lederer's (acquired infectious hemolytic anemia) 283.19
  leptocytosis (hereditary) 282.4
  leukoerythroblastic 285.8
  macrocytic 281.9
    nutritional 281.2
    of or complicating pregnancy 648.2
    tropical 281.2
  malabsorption (familial), selective B_{12} with proteinuria 281.1
  malarial (*see also* Malaria) 084.6
  malignant (progressive) 281.0
  malnutrition 281.9
  marsh (*see also* Malaria) 084.6
  Mediterranean (with hemoglobinopathy) 282.4
  megaloblastic 281.9
    combined B_{12} and folate deficiency 281.3
    nutritional (of infancy) 281.2
    of infancy 281.2
    of or complicating pregnancy 648.2
    refractory 281.3
    specified NEC 281.3
  megalocytic 281.9
  microangiopathic hemolytic 283.19
  microcytic (hypochromic) 280.9
    due to blood loss (chronic) 280.0
      acute 285.1
    familial 282.4
    hypochromic 280.9
  microdrepanocytosis 282.4
  miners' (*see also* Ancylostomiasis) 126.9
  myelopathic 285.8
  myelophthisic (normocytic) 285.8
  newborn (*see also* Disease, hemolytic) 773.2
    due to isoimmunization (*see also* Disease, hemolytic) 773.2
    late, due to isoimmunization 773.5
    posthemorrhagic 776.5
  nonregenerative 284.9
  nonspherocytic hemolytic — *see* Anemia, hemolytic, nonspherocytic
  normocytic (infectional) (not due to blood loss) 285.9
    due to blood loss (chronic) 280.0
      acute 285.1
    myelophthisic 284.8
  nutritional (deficiency) 281.9
    with
      poor iron absorption 280.9
      specified deficiency NEC 281.8
    due to inadequate dietary iron intake 280.1
    megaloblastic (of infancy) 281.2
  of childhood (*see also* Thalassemia) 282.4
  of chronic illness NEC 285.29
  of or complicating pregnancy 648.2
    affecting fetus or newborn 760.8
  of prematurity 776.6
  orotic aciduric (congenital) (hereditary) 281.4
  osteosclerotic 289.8
  ovalocytosis (hereditary) (*see also* Elliptocytosis) 282.1
  paludal (*see also* Malaria) 084.6
  pentose phosphate pathway deficiency 282.2
  pernicious (combined system disease) (congenital) (dorsolateral spinal degeneration) (juvenile) (myelopathy) (neuropathy) (posterior sclerosis) (primary) (progressive) (spleen) 281.0
    of or complicating pregnancy 648.2
  pleochromic 285.9
    of sprue 281.8
  portal 285.8
  posthemorrhagic (chronic) 280.0
    acute 285.1
    newborn 776.5
  pressure 285.9
  primary 285.9
  profound 285.9
  progressive 285.9
    malignant 281.0
    pernicious 281.0
  protein-deficiency 281.4
  pseudoleukemica infantum 285.8
  puerperal 648.2

Anemia — *continued*
  pure red cell 284.8
    congenital 284.0
  pyridoxine-responsive (hypochromic) 285.0
  pyruvate kinase (PK) deficiency 282.3
  refractoria sideroblastica 285.0
  refractory (primary) 284.9
    with hemochromatosis 285.0
    megaloblastic 281.3
    sideroblastic 285.0
    sideropenic 280.9
  Rietti-Greppi-Micheli (thalassemia minor) 282.4
  scorbutic 281.8
  secondary (to) 285.9
    blood loss (chronic) 280.0
      acute 285.1
    hemorrhage 280.0
      acute 285.1
    inadequate dietary iron intake 280.1
  semiplastic 284.9
  septic 285.9
  sickle-cell (*see also* Disease, sickle-cell) 282.60
  sideroachrestic 285.0
  sideroblastic (acquired) (any type) (congenital) (drug-induced) (due to disease) (hereditary) (primary) (refractory) (secondary) (sex-linked hypochromic) (vitamin B_6 responsive) 285.0
  sideropenic (refractory) 280.9
    due to blood loss (chronic) 280.0
      acute 285.1
  simple chronic 281.9
  specified type NEC 285.8
  spherocytic (hereditary) (*see also* Spherocytosis) 282.0
  splenic 285.8
    familial (Gaucher's) 272.7
  splenomegalic 285.8
  stomatocytosis 282.8
  syphilitic 095.8
  target cell (oval) 282.4
  thalassemia 282.4
  thrombocytopenic (*see also* Thrombocytopenia) 287.5
  toxic 284.8
  triosephosphate isomerase deficiency 282.3
  tropical, macrocytic 281.2
  tuberculous (*see also* Tuberculosis) 017.9
  vegan's 281.1
  vitamin
    B_6-responsive 285.0
    B_{12} deficiency (dietary) 281.1
      pernicious 281.0
  von Jaksch's (pseudoleukemia infantum) 285.8
  Witts' (achlorhydric anemia) 280.9
  Zuelzer (-Ogden) (nutritional megaloblastic anemia) 281.2

Anencephalus, anencephaly 740.0
  fetal, affecting management of pregnancy 655.0

Anergasia (*see also* Psychosis, organic) 294.9
  senile 290.0

Anesthesia, anesthetic 782.0
  complication or reaction NEC 995.2
    due to
      correct substance properly administered 995.2
      overdose or wrong substance given 968.4
      specified anesthetic — *see* Table of Drugs and Chemicals
  cornea 371.81
  death from
    correct substance properly administered 995.4
    during delivery 668.9
    overdose or wrong substance given 968.4
    specified anesthetic — *see* Table of Drugs and Chemicals
  eye 371.81
  functional 300.11
  hyperesthetic, thalamic 348.8
  hysterical 300.11
  local skin lesion 782.0
  olfactory 781.1
  sexual (psychogenic) 302.72

Anesthesia, anesthetic — *continued*
  shock
    due to
      correct substance properly administered 995.4
      overdose or wrong substance given 968.4
      specified anesthetic — *see* Table of Drugs and Chemicals
  skin 782.0
  tactile 782.0
  testicular 608.9
  thermal 782.0

Anetoderma (maculosum) 701.3

Aneuploidy NEC 758.5

Aneurin deficiency 265.1

Aneurysm (anastomotic) (artery) (cirsoid) (diffuse) (false) (fusiform) (multiple) (ruptured) (saccular) (varicose) 442.9
  abdominal (aorta) 441.4
    ruptured 441.3
    syphilitic 093.0
  aorta, aortic (nonsyphilitic) 441.9
    abdominal 441.4
      dissecting 441.02
      ruptured 441.3
      syphilitic 093.0
    arch 441.2
      ruptured 441.1
    arteriosclerotic NEC 441.9
      ruptured 441.5
    ascending 441.2
      ruptured 441.1
    congenital 747.29
    descending 441.9
      abdominal 441.4
        ruptured 441.3
      ruptured 441.5
      thoracic 441.2
        ruptured 441.1
    dissecting 441.00
      abdominal 441.02
      thoracic 441.01
      thoracoabdominal 441.03
    due to coarctation (aorta) 747.10
    ruptured 441.5
    sinus, right 747.29
    syphilitic 093.0
    thoracoabdominal 441.7
      ruptured 441.6
    thorax, thoracic (arch) (nonsyphilitic) 441.2
      dissecting 441.01
      ruptured 441.1
      syphilitic 093.0
    transverse 441.2
      ruptured 441.1
    valve (heart) (*see also* Endocarditis, aortic) 424.1
  arteriosclerotic NEC 442.9
    cerebral 437.3
      ruptured (*see also* Hemorrhage, subarachnoid) 430
  arteriovenous (congenital) (peripheral) NEC (*see also* Anomaly, arteriovenous) 747.60
    acquired NEC 447.0
    brain 437.3
      ruptured (*see also* Hemorrhage, subarachnoid) 430
    coronary 414.11
    pulmonary 417.0
    brain (cerebral) 747.81
      ruptured (*see also* Hemorrhage, subarachnoid) 430
    coronary 746.85
    pulmonary 747.3
    retina 743.58
    specified site NEC 747.89
      acquired 447.0
    traumatic (*see also* Injury, blood vessel, by site) 904.9
  basal — *see* Aneurysm, brain
  berry (congenital) (ruptured) (*see also* Hemorrhage, subarachnoid) 430
  brain 437.3
    arteriosclerotic 437.3
      ruptured (*see also* Hemorrhage, subarachnoid) 430

Aneurysm — *continued*
  brain — *continued*
    arteriovenous 747.81
      acquired 437.3
        ruptured (*see also* Hemorrhage, subarachnoid) 430
      ruptured (*see also* Hemorrhage, subarachnoid) 430
    berry (congenital) (ruptured) (*see also* Hemorrhage, subarachnoid) 430
    congenital 747.81
      ruptured (*see also* Hemorrhage, subarachnoid) 430
    meninges 437.3
      ruptured (*see also* Hemorrhage, subarachnoid) 430
    miliary (congenital) (ruptured) (*see also* Hemorrhage, subarachnoid) 430
    mycotic 421.0
      ruptured (*see also* Hemorrhage, subarachnoid) 430
    nonruptured 437.3
    ruptured (*See also* Hemorrhage, subarachnoid) 430
      syphilitic 094.87
    syphilitic (hemorrhage) 094.87
    traumatic — *see* Injury, intracranial
  cardiac (false) (*see also* Aneurysm, heart) 414.10
  carotid artery (common) (external) 442.81
    internal (intracranial portion) 437.3
      extracranial portion 442.81
      ruptured into brain (*see also* Hemorrhage, subarachnoid) 430
    syphilitic 093.89
      intracranial 094.87
  cavernous sinus (*see also* Aneurysm, brain) 437.3
    arteriovenous 747.81
      ruptured (*see also* Hemorrhage, subarachnoid) 430
    congenital 747.81
      ruptured (*see also* Hemorrhage, subarachnoid) 430
  celiac 442.84
  central nervous system, syphilitic 094.89
  cerebral — *see* Aneurysm, brain
  chest — *see* Aneurysm, thorax
  circle of Willis (*see also* Aneurysm, brain) 437.3
    congenital 747.81
      ruptured (*see also* Hemorrhage, subarachnoid) 430
    ruptured (*see also* Hemorrhage, subarachnoid) 430
  common iliac artery 442.2
  congenital (peripheral) NEC 747.60
    brain 747.81
      ruptured (*see also* Hemorrhage, subarachnoid) 430
    cerebral — *see* Aneurysm, brain, congenital
    coronary 746.85
    gastrointestinal 747.61
    lower limb 747.64
    pulmonary 747.3
    renal 747.62
    retina 743.58
    specified site NEC 747.89
    spinal 747.82
    upper limb 747.63
  conjunctiva 372.74
  conus arteriosus (*see also* Aneurysm, heart) 414.10
  coronary (arteriosclerotic) (artery) (vein) (*see also* Aneurysm, heart) 414.11
    arteriovenous 746.85
    congenital 746.85
    syphilitic 093.89
  cylindrical 441.9
    ruptured 441.5
    syphilitic 093.9
  dissecting 442.9
    aorta (any part) 441.00
      abdominal 441.02
      thoracic 441.01
      thoracoabdominal 441.03
    syphilitic 093.9

Aneurysm — *continued*
  ductus arteriosus 747.0
  embolic — *see* Embolism, artery
  endocardial, infective (any valve) 421.0
  femoral 442.3
  gastroduodenal 442.84
  gastroepiploic 442.84
  heart (chronic or with a stated duration of over 8 weeks) (infectional) (wall) 414.10
    acute or with a stated duration of 8 weeks or less (*see also* Infarct, myocardium) 410.9
    congenital 746.89
    valve — *see* Endocarditis
  hepatic 442.84
  iliac (common) 442.2
  infective (any valve) 421.0
  innominate (nonsyphilitic) 442.89
    syphilitic 093.89
  interauricular septum (*see also* Aneurysm, heart) 414.10
  interventricular septum (*see also* Aneurysm, heart) 414.10
  intracranial — *see* Aneurysm, brain
  intrathoracic (nonsyphilitic) 441.2
    ruptured 441.1
    syphilitic 093.0
  jugular vein 453.8
  lower extremity 442.3
  lung (pulmonary artery) 417.1
  malignant 093.9
  mediastinal (nonsyphilitic) 442.89
    syphilitic 093.89
  miliary (congenital) (ruptured) (*see also* Hemorrhage, subarachnoid) 430
  mitral (heart) (valve) 424.0
  mural (arteriovenous) (heart) (*see also* Aneurysm, heart) 414.10
  mycotic, any site 421.0
    ruptured, brain (*see also* Hemorrhage, subarachnoid) 430
  myocardium (*see also* Aneurysm, heart) 414.10
  neck 442.81
  pancreaticoduodenal 442.84
  patent ductus arteriosus 747.0
  peripheral NEC 442.89
    congenital NEC (*see also* Aneurysm, congenital) 747.60
  popliteal 442.3
  pulmonary 417.1
    arteriovenous 747.3
      acquired 417.0
    syphilitic 093.89
    valve (heart) (*see also* Endocarditis, pulmonary) 424.3
  racemose 442.9
    congenital (peripheral) NEC 747.60
  radial 442.0
  Rasmussen's (*see also* Tuberculosis) 011.2
  renal 442.1
  retinal (acquired) 362.17
    congenital 743.58
    diabetic 250.5 [362.01]
  sinus, aortic (of Valsalva) 747.29
  specified site NEC 442.89
  spinal (cord) 442.89
    congenital 747.82
    syphilitic (hemorrhage) 094.89
  spleen, splenic 442.83
  subclavian 442.82
    syphilitic 093.89
  superior mesenteric 442.84
  syphilitic 093.9
    aorta 093.0
    central nervous system 094.89
    congenital 090.5
    spine, spinal 094.89
  thoracoabdominal 441.7
    ruptured 441.6
  thorax, thoracic (arch) (nonsyphilitic) 441.2
    dissecting 441.0
    ruptured 441.1
    syphilitic 093.0
  traumatic (complication) (early) — *see* Injury, blood vessel, by site
  tricuspid (heart) (valve) — *see* Endocarditis, tricuspid
  ulnar 442.0

Aneurysm — *continued*
  upper extremity 442.0
  valve, valvular — *see* Endocarditis
  venous 456.8
    congenital NEC (*see also* Aneurysm, congenital) 747.60
  ventricle (arteriovenous) (*see also* Aneurysm, heart) 414.10
  visceral artery NEC 442.84

Angiectasis 459.89
Angiectopia 459.9
Angiitis 447.6
  allergic granulomatous 446.4
  hypersensitivity 446.20
    Goodpasture's syndrome 446.21
    specified NEC 446.29
  necrotizing 446.0
  Wegener's (necrotizing respiratory granulomatosis) 446.4

Angina (attack) (cardiac) (chest) (effort) (heart) (pectoris) (syndrome) (vasomotor) 413.9
  abdominal 557.1
  agranulocytic 288.0
  aphthous 074.0
  catarrhal 462
  crescendo 411.1
  croupous 464.4
  cruris 443.9
    due to atherosclerosis NEC (*see also* Arteriosclerosis, extremities) 440.20
  decubitus 413.0
  diphtheritic (membranous) 032.0
  erysipelatous 034.0
  erythematous 462
  exudative, chronic 476.0
  faucium 478.29
  gangrenous 462
    diphtheritic 032.0
  infectious 462
  initial 411.1
  intestinal 557.1
  ludovici 528.3
  Ludwig's 528.3
  malignant 462
    diphtheritic 032.0
  membranous 464.4
    diphtheritic 032.0
  mesenteric 557.1
  monocytic 075
  nocturnal 413.0
  phlegmonous 475
    diphtheritic 032.0
  preinfarctional 411.1
  Prinzmetal's 413.1
  progressive 411.1
  pseudomembranous 101
  psychogenic 306.2
  pultaceous, diphtheritic 032.0
  scarlatinal 034.1
  septic 034.0
  simple 462
  stable NEC 413.9
  staphylococcal 462
  streptococcal 034.0
  stridulous, diphtheritic 032.3
  syphilitic 093.9
    congenital 090.5
  tonsil 475
  trachealis 464.4
  unstable 411.1
  variant 413.1
  Vincent's 101

Angioblastoma (M9161/1) — *see* Neoplasm, connective tissue, uncertain behavior
Angiocholecystitis (*see also* Cholecystitis, acute) 575.0
Angiocholitis (*see also* Cholecystitis, acute) 576.1
Angiodysgensis spinalis 336.1
Angiodysplasia (intestinalis) (intestine) 569.84
  with hemorrhage 569.85
  duodenum 537.82
    with hemorrhage 537.83
  stomach 537.82
    with hemorrhage 537.83

Angioedema (allergic) (any site) (with urticaria) 995.1
  hereditary 277.6
Angioendothelioma (M9130/1) — see also Neoplasm, by site, uncertain behavior
  benign (M9130/0) (see also Hemangioma, by site) 228.00
    bone (M9260/3) — see Neoplasm, bone, malignant
    Ewing's (M9260/3) — see Neoplasm, bone, malignant
    nervous system (M9130/0) 228.09
Angiofibroma (M9160/0) — see also Neoplasm, by site, benign
  juvenile (M9160/0) 210.7
    specified site — see Neoplasm, by site, benign
    unspecified site 210.7
Angiohemophilia (A) (B) 286.4
Angioid streaks (choroid) (retina) 363.43
Angiokeratoma (M9141/0) — see also Neoplasm, skin, benign
  corporis diffusum 272.7
Angiokeratosis
  diffuse 272.7
Angioleiomyoma (M8894/0) — see Neoplasm, connective tissue, benign
Angioleucitis 683
Angiolipoma (M8861/0) (see also Lipoma, by site) 214.9
  infiltrating (M8861/1) — see Neoplasm, connective tissue, uncertain behavior
Angioma (M9120/0) (see also Hemangioma, by site) 228.00
  capillary 448.1
  hemorrhagicum hereditaria 448.0
  malignant (M9120/3) — see Neoplasm, connective tissue, malignant
  pigmentosum et atrophicum 757.33
  placenta — see Placenta, abnormal
  plexiform (M9131/0) — see Hemangioma, by site
  senile 448.1
  serpiginosum 709.1
  spider 448.1
  stellate 448.1
Angiomatosis 757.32
  bacillary 083.8
  corporis diffusum universale 272.7
  cutaneocerebral 759.6
  encephalocutaneous 759.6
  encephalofacial 759.6
  encephalotrigeminal 759.6
  hemorrhagic familial 448.0
  hereditary familial 448.0
  heredofamilial 448.0
  meningo-oculofacial 759.6
  multiple sites 228.09
  neuro-oculocutaneous 759.6
  retina (Hippel's disease) 759.6
  retinocerebellosa 759.6
  retinocerebral 759.6
  systemic 228.09
Angiomyolipoma (M8860/0)
  specified site — see Neoplasm, connective tissue, benign
  unspecified site 223.0
Angiomyoliposarcoma (M8860/3) — see Neoplasm, connective tissue, malignant
Angiomyoma (M8894/0) — see Neoplasm, connective tissue, benign
Angiomyosarcoma (M8894/3) — see Neoplasm, connective tissue, malignant
Angioneurosis 306.2
Angioneurotic edema (allergic) (any site) (with urticaria) 995.1
  hereditary 277.6
Angiopathia, angiopathy 459.9
  diabetic (peripheral) 250.7 ✓5 [443.81]
  peripheral 443.9
    diabetic 250.7 ✓5 [443.81]
    specified type NEC 443.89
  retinae syphilitica 093.89

Angiopathia, angiopathy — continued
  retinalis (juvenilis) 362.18
    background 362.10
    diabetic 250.5 ✓5 [362.01]
    proliferative 362.29
    tuberculous (see also Tuberculosis) 017.3 ✓5 [362.18]
Angiosarcoma (M9120/3) — see Neoplasm, connective tissue, malignant
Angiosclerosis — see Arteriosclerosis
Angioscotoma, enlarged 368.42
Angiospasm 443.9
  brachial plexus 353.0
  cerebral 435.9
  cervical plexus 353.2
  nerve
    arm 354.9
      axillary 353.0
      median 354.1
      ulnar 354.2
    autonomic (see also Neuropathy, peripheral, autonomic) 337.9
    axillary 353.0
    leg 355.8
      plantar 355.6
    lower extremity — see Angiospasm, nerve, leg
    median 354.1
    peripheral NEC 355.9
    spinal NEC 355.9
    sympathetic (see also Neuropathy, peripheral, autonomic) 337.9
    ulnar 354.2
    upper extremity — see Angiospasm, nerve, arm
  peripheral NEC 443.9
  traumatic 443.9
    foot 443.9
    leg 443.9
  vessel 443.9
Angiospastic disease or edema 443.9
Anguillulosis 127.2
Angulation
  cecum (see also Obstruction, intestine) 560.9
  coccyx (acquired) 738.6
    congenital 756.19
  femur (acquired) 736.39
    congenital 755.69
  intestine (large) (small) (see also Obstruction, intestine) 560.9
  sacrum (acquired) 738.5
    congenital 756.19
  sigmoid (flexure) (see also Obstruction, intestine) 560.9
  spine (see also Curvature, spine) 737.9
  tibia (acquired) 736.89
    congenital 755.69
  ureter 593.3
  wrist (acquired) 736.09
    congenital 755.59
Angulus infectiosus 686.8
Anhedonia 302.72
Anhidrosis (lid) (neurogenic) (thermogenic) 705.0
Anhydration 276.5
  with
    hypernatremia 276.0
    hyponatremia 276.1
Anhydremia 276.5
  with
    hypernatremia 276.0
    hyponatremia 276.1
Anidrosis 705.0
Aniridia (congenital) 743.45
Anisakiasis (infection) (infestation) 127.1
Anisakis larva infestation 127.1
Aniseikonia 367.32
Anisocoria (pupil) 379.41
  congenital 743.46
Anisocytosis 790.09
Anisometropia (congenital) 367.31
Ankle — see condition
Ankyloblepharon (acquired) (eyelid) 374.46
  filiforme (adnatum) (congenital) 743.62

Ankyloblepharon — continued
  total 743.62
Ankylodactly (see also Syndactylism) 755.10
Ankyloglossia 750.0
Ankylosis (fibrous) (osseous) 718.50
  ankle 718.57
  any joint, produced by surgical fusion V45.4
  cricoarytenoid (cartilage) (joint) (larynx) 478.79
  dental 521.6
  ear ossicle NEC 385.22
    malleus 385.21
  elbow 718.52
  finger 718.54
  hip 718.55
  incostapedial joint (infectional) 385.22
  joint, produced by surgical fusion NEC V45.4
  knee 718.56
  lumbosacral (joint) 724.6
  malleus 385.21
  multiple sites 718.59
  postoperative (status) V45.4
  sacroiliac (joint) 724.6
  shoulder 718.51
  specified site NEC 718.58
  spine NEC 724.9
  surgical V45.4
  teeth, tooth (hard tissues) 521.6
  temporomandibular joint 524.61
  wrist 718.53
Ankylostoma — see Ancylostoma
Ankylostomiasis (intestinal) — see Ancylostomiasis
Ankylurethria (see also Stricture, urethra) 598.9
Annular — see also condition
  detachment, cervix 622.8
  organ or site, congenital NEC — see Distortion
  pancreas (congenital) 751.7
Anodontia (complete) (partial) (vera) 520.0
  with abnormal spacing 524.3
  acquired 525.10
    causing malocclusion 524.3
    due to
      caries 525.13
      extraction 525.10
      periodontal disease 525.12
      trauma 525.11
Anomaly, anomalous (congenital) (unspecified type) 759.9
  abdomen 759.9
  abdominal wall 756.70
  acoustic nerve 742.9
  adrenal (gland) 759.1
  Alder (-Reilly) (leukocyte granulation) 288.2
  alimentary tract 751.9
    lower 751.5
    specified type NEC 751.8
    upper (any part, except tongue) 750.9
      tongue 750.10
        specified type NEC 750.19
  alveolar ridge (process) 525.8
  ankle (joint) 755.69
  anus, anal (canal) 751.5
  aorta, aortic 747.20
    arch 747.21
    coarctation (postductal) (preductal) 747.10
    cusp or valve NEC 746.9
    septum 745.0
    specified type NEC 747.29
  aorticopulmonary septum 745.0
  apertures, diaphragm 756.6
  appendix 751.5
  aqueduct of Sylvius 742.3
    with spina bifida (see also Spina bifida) 741.0 ✓5
  arm 755.50
    reduction (see also Deformity, reduction, upper limb) 755.20
  arteriovenous (congenital) (peripheral) NEC 747.60
    brain 747.81
    cerebral 747.81
    coronary 746.85
    gastrointestinal 747.61
    lower limb 747.64
    renal 747.62
    specified site NEC 747.69

Anomaly, anomalous — continued
- arteriovenous — continued
  - spinal 747.82
  - upper limb 747.63
- artery (see also Anomaly, peripheral vascular system) NEC 747.60
  - brain 747.81
  - cerebral 747.81
  - coronary 746.85
  - eye 743.9
  - pulmonary 747.3
  - renal 747.62
  - retina 743.9
  - umbilical 747.5
- arytenoepiglottic folds 748.3
- atrial
  - bands 746.9
  - folds 746.9
  - septa 745.5
- atrioventricular
  - canal 745.69
  - common 745.69
  - conduction 426.7
  - excitation 426.7
  - septum 745.4
- atrium — see Anomaly, atrial
- auditory canal 744.3
  - specified type NEC 744.29
    - with hearing impairment 744.02
- auricle
  - ear 744.3
    - causing impairment of hearing 744.02
  - heart 746.9
    - septum 745.5
- autosomes, autosomal NEC 758.5
- Axenfeld's 743.44
- back 759.9
- band
  - atrial 746.9
  - heart 746.9
  - ventricular 746.9
- Bartholin's duct 750.9
- biliary duct or passage 751.60
  - atresia 751.61
- bladder (neck) (sphincter) (trigone) 753.9
  - specified type NEC 753.8
- blood vessel 747.9
  - artery — see Anomaly, artery
  - peripheral vascular — see Anomaly, peripheral vascular system
  - vein — see Anomaly, vein
- bone NEC 756.9
  - ankle 755.69
  - arm 755.50
  - chest 756.3
  - cranium 756.0
  - face 756.0
  - finger 755.50
  - foot 755.67
  - forearm 755.50
  - frontal 756.0
  - head 756.0
  - hip 755.63
  - leg 755.60
  - lumbosacral 756.10
  - nose 748.1
  - pelvic girdle 755.60
  - rachitic 756.4
  - rib 756.3
  - shoulder girdle 755.50
  - skull 756.0
    - with
      - anencephalus 740.0
      - encephalocele 742.0
      - hydrocephalus 742.3
        - with spina bifida (see also Spina bifida) 741.0
      - microcephalus 742.1
  - toe 755.66
- brain 742.9
  - multiple 742.4
  - reduction 742.2
  - specified type NEC 742.4
  - vessel 747.81
- branchial cleft NEC 744.49
  - cyst 744.42
  - fistula 744.41

Anomaly, anomalous — continued
- branchial cleft NEC — continued
  - persistent 744.41
  - sinus (external) (internal) 744.41
- breast 757.9
- broad ligament 752.10
  - specified type NEC 752.19
- bronchus 748.3
- bulbar septum 745.0
- bulbus cordis 745.9
  - persistent (in left ventricle) 745.8
- bursa 756.9
- canal of Nuck 752.9
- canthus 743.9
- capillary NEC (see also Anomaly, peripheral vascular system) 747.60
- cardiac 746.9
  - septal closure 745.9
    - acquired 429.71
  - valve NEC 746.9
    - pulmonary 746.00
    - specified type NEC 746.89
- cardiovascular system 746.9
  - complicating pregnancy, childbirth, or puerperium 648.5
- carpus 755.50
- cartilage, trachea 748.3
- cartilaginous 756.9
- caruncle, lacrimal, lachrymal 743.9
- cascade stomach 750.7
- cauda equina 742.59
- cecum 751.5
- cerebral — see also Anomaly, brain vessels 747.81
- cerebrovascular system 747.81
- cervix (uterus) 752.40
  - with doubling of vagina and uterus 752.2
  - in pregnancy or childbirth 654.6
    - affecting fetus or newborn 763.89
  - causing obstructed labor 660.2
    - affecting fetus or newborn 763.1
- Chédiak-Higashi (-Steinbrinck) (congenital gigantism of peroxidase granules) 288.2
- cheek 744.9
- chest (wall) 756.3
- chin 744.9
  - specified type NEC 744.89
- chordae tendineae 746.9
- choroid 743.9
  - plexus 742.9
- chromosomes, chromosomal 758.9
  - 13 (13-15) 758.1
  - 18 (16-18) 758.2
  - 21 or 22 758.0
  - autosomes NEC (see also Abnormality, autosomes) 758.5
    - deletion 758.3
  - Christchurch 758.3
  - D_1 758.1
  - E_3 758.2
  - G 758.0
  - mitochondrial 758.9
  - mosaics 758.89
  - sex 758.81
    - complement, XO 758.6
    - complement, XXX 758.81
    - complement, XXY 758.7
    - complement, XYY 758.81
    - gonadal dysgenesis 758.6
    - Klinefelter's 758.7
    - Turner's 758.6
  - trisomy 21 758.0
- cilia 743.9
- circulatory system 747.9
  - specified type NEC 747.89
- clavicle 755.51
- clitoris 752.40
- coccyx 756.10
- colon 751.5
- common duct 751.60
- communication
  - coronary artery 746.85
  - left ventricle with right atrium 745.4
- concha (ear) 744.3
- connection
  - renal vessels with kidney 747.62
  - total pulmonary venous 747.41

Anomaly, anomalous — continued
- connective tissue 756.9
  - specified type NEC 756.89
- cornea 743.9
  - shape 743.41
  - size 743.41
  - specified type NEC 743.49
- coronary
  - artery 746.85
  - vein 746.89
- cranium — see Anomaly, skull
- cricoid cartilage 748.3
- cushion, endocardial 745.60
  - specified type NEC 745.69
- cystic duct 751.60
- dental arch relationship 524.2
- dentition 520.6
- dentofacial NEC 524.9
  - functional 524.5
  - specified type NEC 524.8
- dermatoglyphic 757.2
- Descemet's membrane 743.9
  - specified type NEC 743.49
- development
  - cervix 752.40
  - vagina 752.40
  - vulva 752.40
- diaphragm, diaphragmatic (apertures) NEC 756.6
- digestive organ(s) or system 751.9
  - lower 751.5
  - specified type NEC 751.8
  - upper 750.9
- distribution, coronary artery 746.85
- ductus
  - arteriosus 747.0
  - Botalli 747.0
- duodenum 751.5
- dura 742.9
  - brain 742.4
  - spinal cord 742.59
- ear 744.3
  - causing impairment of hearing 744.00
    - specified type NEC 744.09
  - external 744.3
    - causing impairment of hearing 744.02
    - specified type NEC 744.29
  - inner (causing impairment of hearing) 744.05
  - middle, except ossicles (causing impairment of hearing) 744.03
    - ossicles 744.04
  - ossicles 744.04
  - prominent auricle 744.29
  - specified type NEC 744.29
    - with hearing impairment 744.09
- Ebstein's (heart) 746.2
  - tricuspid valve 746.2
- ectodermal 757.9
- ejaculatory duct 752.9
  - specified type NEC 752.8
- elbow (joint) 755.50
- endocardial cushion 745.60
  - specified type NEC 745.69
- endocrine gland NEC 759.2
- epididymis 752.9
- epiglottis 748.3
- esophagus 750.9
  - specified type NEC 750.4
- Eustachian tube 744.3
  - specified type NEC 744.24
- eye (any part) 743.9
  - adnexa 743.9
    - specified type NEC 743.69
  - anophthalmos 743.00
  - anterior
    - chamber and related structures 743.9
      - angle 743.9
        - specified type NEC 743.44
      - specified type NEC 743.44
    - segment 743.9
      - combined 743.48
      - multiple 743.48
      - specified type NEC 743.49
  - cataract (see also Cataract) 743.30
  - glaucoma (see also Buphthalmia) 743.20

Index to Diseases

Anomaly, anomalous — *continued*
  eye — *continued*
    lid 743.9
      specified type NEC 743.63
    microphthalmos (*see also* Microphthalmos) 743.10
    posterior segment 743.9
      specified type NEC 743.59
      vascular 743.58
      vitreous 743.9
        specified type NEC 743.51
    ptosis (eyelid) 743.61
    retina 743.9
      specified type NEC 743.59
    sclera 743.9
      specified type NEC 743.47
    specified type NEC 743.8
  eyebrow 744.89
  eyelid 743.9
    specified type NEC 743.63
  face (any part) 744.9
    bone(s) 756.0
    specified type NEC 744.89
  fallopian tube 752.10
    specified type NEC 752.19
  fascia 756.9
    specified type NEC 756.89
  femur 755.60
  fibula 755.60
  finger 755.50
    supernumerary 755.01
    webbed (*see also* Syndactylism, fingers) 755.11
  fixation, intestine 751.4
  flexion (joint) 755.9
    hip or thigh (*see also* Dislocation, hip, congenital) 754.30
  folds, heart 746.9
  foot 755.67
  foramen
    Botalli 745.5
    ovale 745.5
  forearm 755.50
  forehead (*see also* Anomaly, skull) 756.0
  form, teeth 520.2
  fovea centralis 743.9
  frontal bone (*see also* Anomaly, skull) 756.0
  gallbladder 751.60
  Gartner's duct 752.11
  gastrointestinal tract 751.9
    specified type NEC 751.8
    vessel 747.61
  genitalia, genital organ(s) or system
    female 752.9
      external 752.40
        specified type NEC 752.49
      internal NEC 752.9
    male (external and internal) 752.9
      epispadias 752.62
      hidden penis 752.65
      hydrocele, congenital 778.6
      hypospadias 752.61
      micropenis 752.64
      testis, undescended 752.51
        retractile 752.52
    specified type NEC 752.8
  genitourinary NEC 752.9
  Gerbode 745.4
  globe (eye) 743.9
  glottis 748.3
  granulation or granulocyte, genetic 288.2
    constitutional 288.2
    leukocyte 288.2
  gum 750.9
  gyri 742.9
  hair 757.9
    specified type NEC 757.4
  hand 755.50
  hard tissue formation in pulp 522.3
  head (*see also* Anomaly, skull) 756.0
  heart 746.9
    auricle 746.9
    bands 746.9
    fibroelastosis cordis 425.3
    folds 746.9
    malposition 746.87
    maternal, affecting fetus or newborn 760.3

Anomaly, anomalous — *continued*
  heart — *continued*
    obstructive NEC 746.84
    patent ductus arteriosus (Botalli) 747.0
    septum 745.9
      acquired 429.71
      aortic 745.0
      aorticopulmonary 745.0
      atrial 745.5
      auricular 745.5
      between aorta and pulmonary artery 745.0
      endocardial cushion type 745.60
        specified type NEC 745.69
      interatrial 745.5
      interventricular 745.4
        with pulmonary stenosis or atresia, dextraposition of aorta, and hypertrophy of right ventricle 745.2
        acquired 429.71
      specified type NEC 745.8
      ventricular 745.4
        with pulmonary stenosis or atresia, dextraposition of aorta, and hypertrophy of right ventricle 745.2
        acquired 429.71
    specified type NEC 746.89
    tetralogy of Fallot 745.2
    valve NEC 746.9
      aortic 746.9
        atresia 746.89
        bicuspid valve 746.4
        insufficiency 746.4
        specified type NEC 746.89
        stenosis 746.3
          subaortic 746.81
          supravalvular 747.22
      mitral 746.9
        atresia 746.89
        insufficiency 746.6
        specified type NEC 746.89
        stenosis 746.5
      pulmonary 746.00
        atresia 746.01
        insufficiency 746.09
        stenosis 746.02
          infundibular 746.83
          subvalvular 746.83
      tricuspid 746.9
        atresia 746.1
        stenosis 746.1
    ventricle 746.9
  heel 755.67
  Hegglin's 288.2
  hemianencephaly 740.0
  hemicephaly 740.0
  hemicrania 740.0
  hepatic duct 751.60
  hip (joint) 755.63
  hourglass
    bladder 753.8
    gallbladder 751.69
    stomach 750.7
  humerus 755.50
  hymen 752.40
  hypersegmentation of neutrophils, hereditary 288.2
  hypophyseal 759.2
  ileocecal (coil) (valve) 751.5
  ileum (intestine) 751.5
  ilium 755.60
  integument 757.9
    specified type NEC 757.8
  intervertebral cartilage or disc 756.10
  intestine (large) (small) 751.5
    fixational type 751.4
  iris 743.9
    specified type NEC 743.46
  ischium 755.60
  jaw NEC 524.9
    closure 524.5
    size (major) NEC 524.00
    specified type NEC 524.8
  jaw-cranial base relationship 524.10
    specified NEC 524.19

Anomaly, anomalous — *continued*
  jejunum 751.5
  joint 755.9
    hip
      dislocation (*see also* Dislocation, hip, congenital) 754.30
      predislocation (*see also* Subluxation, congenital, hip) 754.32
      preluxation (*see also* Subluxation, congenital, hip) 754.32
      subluxation (*see also* Subluxation, congenital, hip) 754.32
    lumbosacral 756.10
      spondylolisthesis 756.12
      spondylosis 756.11
    multiple arthrogryposis 754.89
    sacroiliac 755.69
  Jordan's 288.2
  kidney(s) (calyx) (pelvis) 753.9
    vessel 747.62
  Klippel-Feil (brevicollis) 756.16
  knee (joint) 755.64
  labium (majus) (minus) 752.40
  labyrinth, membranous (causing impairment of hearing) 744.05
  lacrimal
    apparatus, duct or passage 743.9
      specified type NEC 743.65
    gland 743.9
      specified type NEC 743.64
  Langdon Down (mongolism) 758.0
  larynx, laryngeal (muscle) 748.3
    web, webbed 748.2
  leg (lower) (upper) 755.60
    reduction NEC (*see also* Deformity, reduction, lower limb) 755.30
  lens 743.9
    shape 743.36
    specified type NEC 743.39
  leukocytes, genetic 288.2
    granulation (constitutional) 288.2
  lid (fold) 743.9
  ligament 756.9
    broad 752.10
    round 752.9
  limb, except reduction deformity 755.9
    lower 755.60
      reduction deformity (*see also* Deformity, reduction, lower limb) 755.30
      specified type NEC 755.69
    upper 755.50
      reduction deformity (*see also* Deformity, reduction, upper limb) 755.20
      specified type NEC 755.59
  lip 750.9
    harelip (*see also* Cleft, lip) 749.10
    specified type NEC 750.26
  liver (duct) 751.60
    atresia 751.69
  lower extremity 755.60
    vessel 747.64
  lumbosacral (joint) (region) 756.10
  lung (fissure) (lobe) NEC 748.60
    agenesis 748.5
    specified type NEC 748.69
  lymphatic system 759.9
  Madelung's (radius) 755.54
  mandible 524.9
    size NEC 524.00
  maxilla 524.9
    size NEC 524.00
  May (-Hegglin) 288.2
  meatus urinarius 753.9
    specified type NEC 753.8
  meningeal bands or folds, constriction of 742.8
  meninges 742.9
    brain 742.4
    spinal 742.59
  meningocele (*see also* Spina bifida) 741.9
  mesentery 751.9
  metacarpus 755.50
  metatarsus 755.67
  middle ear, except ossicles (causing impairment of hearing) 744.03
    ossicles 744.04
  mitral (leaflets) (valve) 746.9
    atresia 746.89

Anomaly, anomalous — continued
- mitral — continued
  - insufficiency 746.6
  - specified type NEC 746.89
  - stenosis 746.5
- mouth 750.9
  - specified type NEC 750.26
- multiple NEC 759.7
  - specified type NEC 759.89
- muscle 756.9
  - eye 743.9
    - specified type NEC 743.69
  - specified type NEC 756.89
- musculoskeletal system, except limbs 756.9
  - specified type NEC 756.9
- nail 757.9
  - specified type NEC 757.5
- narrowness, eyelid 743.62
- nasal sinus or septum 748.1
- neck (any part) 744.9
  - specified type NEC 744.89
- nerve 742.9
  - acoustic 742.9
    - specified type NEC 742.8
  - optic 742.9
    - specified type NEC 742.8
  - specified type NEC 742.8
- nervous system NEC 742.9
  - brain 742.9
    - specified type NEC 742.4
  - specified type NEC 742.8
- neurological 742.9
- nipple 757.9
- nonteratogenic NEC 754.89
- nose, nasal (bone) (cartilage) (septum) (sinus) 748.1
- ocular muscle 743.9
- omphalomesenteric duct 751.0
- opening, pulmonary veins 747.49
- optic
  - disc 743.9
    - specified type NEC 743.57
  - nerve 742.9
- opticociliary vessels 743.9
- orbit (eye) 743.9
  - specified type NEC 743.66
- organ
  - of Corti (causing impairment of hearing) 744.05
  - or site 759.9
    - specified type NEC 759.89
- origin
  - both great arteries from same ventricle 745.11
  - coronary artery 746.85
  - innominate artery 747.69
  - left coronary artery from pulmonary artery 746.85
  - pulmonary artery 747.3
  - renal vessels 747.62
  - subclavian artery (left) (right) 747.21
- osseous meatus (ear) 744.03
- ovary 752.0
- oviduct 752.10
- palate (hard) (soft) 750.9
  - cleft (see also Cleft, palate) 749.00
- pancreas (duct) 751.7
- papillary muscles 746.9
- parathyroid gland 759.2
- paraurethral ducts 753.9
- parotid (gland) 750.9
- patella 755.64
- Pelger-Huët (hereditary hyposegmentation) 288.2
- pelvic girdle 755.60
  - specified type NEC 755.69
- pelvis (bony) 755.60
  - complicating delivery 653.0 ✓5ᵗʰ
    - rachitic 268.1
      - fetal 756.4
- penis (glans) 752.69
- pericardium 746.89
- peripheral vascular system NEC 747.60
  - gastrointestinal 747.61
  - lower limb 747.64
  - renal 747.62
  - specified site NEC 747.69

Anomaly, anomalous — continued
- peripheral vascular system NEC — continued
  - spinal 747.82
  - upper limb 747.63
- Peter's 743.44
- pharynx 750.9
  - branchial cleft 744.41
  - specified type NEC 750.29
- Pierre Robin 756.0
- pigmentation NEC 709.00
  - congenital 757.33
- pituitary (gland) 759.2
- pleural folds 748.8
- portal vein 747.40
- position tooth, teeth 524.3
- preauricular sinus 744.46
- prepuce 752.9
- prostate 752.9
- pulmonary 748.60
  - artery 747.3
  - circulation 747.3
  - specified type NEC 748.69
  - valve 746.00
    - atresia 746.01
    - insufficiency 746.09
    - specified type NEC 746.09
    - stenosis 746.02
      - infundibular 746.83
      - subvalvular 746.83
  - vein 747.40
  - venous
    - connection 747.49
      - partial 747.42
      - total 747.41
    - return 747.49
      - partial 747.42
      - total (TAPVR) (complete) (subdiaphragmatic) (supradiaphrag-matic) 747.41
- pupil 743.9
- pylorus 750.9
  - hypertrophy 750.5
  - stenosis 750.5
- rachitic, fetal 756.4
- radius 755.50
- rectovaginal (septum) 752.40
- rectum 751.5
- refraction 367.9
- renal 753.9
  - vessel 747.62
- respiratory system 748.9
  - specified type NEC 748.8
- rib 756.3
  - cervical 756.2
- Rieger's 743.44
- rings, trachea 748.3
- rotation — see also Malrotation
  - hip or thigh (see also Subluxation, congenital, hip) 754.32
- round ligament 752.9
- sacroiliac (joint) 755.69
- sacrum 756.10
- saddle
  - back 754.2
  - nose 754.0
    - syphilitic 090.5
- salivary gland or duct 750.9
  - specified type NEC 750.26
- scapula 755.50
- sclera 743.9
  - specified type NEC 743.47
- scrotum 752.9
- sebaceous gland 757.9
- seminal duct or tract 752.9
- sense organs 742.9
  - specified type NEC 742.8
- septum
  - heart — see Anomaly, heart, septum
  - nasal 748.1
- sex chromosomes NEC (see also Anomaly, chromosomes) 758.81
- shoulder (girdle) (joint) 755.50
  - specified type NEC 755.59
- sigmoid (flexure) 751.5
- sinus of Valsalva 747.29
- site NEC 759.9
- skeleton generalized NEC 756.50

Anomaly, anomalous — continued
- skin (appendage) 757.9
  - specified type NEC 757.39
- skull (bone) 756.0
  - with
    - anencephalus 740.0
    - encephalocele 742.0
    - hydrocephalus 742.3
      - with spina bifida (see also Spina bifida) 741.0 ✓5ᵗʰ
    - microcephalus 742.1
- specified type NEC
  - adrenal (gland) 759.1
  - alimentary tract (complete) (partial) 751.8
    - lower 751.5
    - upper 750.8
  - ankle 755.69
  - anus, anal (canal) 751.5
  - aorta, aortic 747.29
    - arch 747.21
  - appendix 751.5
  - arm 755.59
  - artery (peripheral) NEC (see also Anomaly, peripheral vascular system) 747.60
    - brain 747.81
    - coronary 746.85
    - eye 743.58
    - pulmonary 747.3
    - retinal 743.58
    - umbilical 747.5
  - auditory canal 744.29
    - causing impairment of hearing 744.02
  - bile duct or passage 751.69
  - bladder 753.8
    - neck 753.8
  - bone(s) 756.9
    - arm 755.59
    - face 756.0
    - leg 755.69
    - pelvic girdle 755.69
    - shoulder girdle 755.59
    - skull 756.0
      - with
        - anencephalus 740.0
        - encephalocele 742.0
        - hydrocephalus 742.3
          - with spina bifida (see also Spina bifida) 741.0 ✓5ᵗʰ
        - microcephalus 742.1
  - brain 742.4
  - breast 757.6
  - broad ligament 752.19
  - bronchus 748.3
  - canal of Nuck 752.8
  - cardiac septal closure 745.8
  - carpus 755.59
  - cartilaginous 756.9
  - cecum 751.5
  - cervix 752.49
  - chest (wall) 756.3
  - chin 744.89
  - ciliary body 743.46
  - circulatory system 747.89
  - clavicle 755.51
  - clitoris 752.49
  - coccyx 756.19
  - colon 751.5
  - common duct 751.69
  - connective tissue 756.89
  - cricoid cartilage 748.3
  - cystic duct 751.69
  - diaphragm 756.6
  - digestive organ(s) or tract 751.8
    - lower 751.5
    - upper 750.8
  - duodenum 751.5
  - ear 744.29
    - auricle 744.29
      - causing impairment of hearing 744.02
    - causing impairment of hearing 744.09
    - inner (causing impairment of hearing) 744.05
    - middle, except ossicles 744.03
      - ossicles 744.04
  - ejaculatory duct 752.8
  - endocrine 759.2
  - epiglottis 748.3

Index to Diseases

Anomaly, anomalous — *continued*
specified type NEC — *continued*
esophagus 750.4
Eustachian tube 744.24
eye 743.8
lid 743.63
muscle 743.69
face 744.89
bone(s) 756.0
fallopian tube 752.19
fascia 756.89
femur 755.69
fibula 755.69
finger 755.59
foot 755.67
fovea centralis 743.55
gallbladder 751.69
Gartner's duct 752.8
gastrointestinal tract 751.8
genitalia, genital organ(s)
female 752.8
external 752.49
internal NEC 752.8
male 752.8
penis 752.69
genitourinary tract NEC 752.8
glottis 748.3
hair 757.4
hand 755.59
heart 746.89
valve NEC 746.89
pulmonary 746.09
hepatic duct 751.69
hydatid of Morgagni 752.8
hymen 752.49
integument 757.8
intestine (large) (small) 751.5
fixational type 751.4
iris 743.46
jejunum 751.5
joint 755.8
kidney 753.3
knee 755.64
labium (majus) (minus) 752.49
labyrinth, membranous 744.05
larynx 748.3
leg 755.69
lens 743.39
limb, except reduction deformity 755.8
lower 755.69
reduction deformity (*see also* Deformity, reduction, lower limb) 755.30
upper 755.59
reduction deformity (*see also* Deformity, reduction, upper limb) 755.20
lip 750.26
liver 751.69
lung (fissure) (lobe) 748.69
meatus urinarius 753.8
metacarpus 755.59
mouth 750.26
muscle 756.89
eye 743.69
musculoskeletal system, except limbs 756.9
nail 757.5
neck 744.89
nerve 742.8
acoustic 742.8
optic 742.8
nervous system 742.8
nipple 757.6
nose 748.1
organ NEC 759.89
of Corti 744.05
osseous meatus (ear) 744.03
ovary 752.0
oviduct 752.19
pancreas 751.7
parathyroid 759.2
patella 755.64
pelvic girdle 755.69
penis 752.69
pericardium 746.89

Anomaly, anomalous — *continued*
specified type NEC — *continued*
peripheral vascular system NEC (*see also* Anomaly, peripheral vascular system) 747.60
pharynx 750.29
pituitary 759.2
prostate 752.8
radius 755.59
rectum 751.5
respiratory system 748.8
rib 756.3
round ligament 752.8
sacrum 756.19
salivary duct or gland 750.26
scapula 755.59
sclera 743.47
scrotum 752.8
seminal duct or tract 752.8
shoulder girdle 755.59
site NEC 759.89
skin 757.39
skull (bone(s)) 756.0
with
anencephalus 740.0
encephalocele 742.0
hydrocephalus 742.3
with spina bifida (*see also* Spina bifida) 741.0 ✓5ᵗʰ
microcephalus 742.1
specified organ or site NEC 759.89
spermatic cord 752.8
spinal cord 742.59
spine 756.19
spleen 759.0
sternum 756.3
stomach 750.7
tarsus 755.67
tendon 756.89
testis 752.8
thorax (wall) 756.3
thymus 759.2
thyroid (gland) 759.2
cartilage 748.3
tibia 755.69
toe 755.66
tongue 750.19
trachea (cartilage) 748.3
ulna 755.59
urachus 753.7
ureter 753.4
obstructive 753.29
urethra 753.8
obstructive 753.6
urinary tract 753.8
uterus 752.3
uvula 750.26
vagina 752.49
vascular NEC (*see also* Anomaly, peripheral vascular system) 747.60
brain 747.81
vas deferens 752.8
vein(s) (peripheral) NEC (*see also* Anomaly, peripheral vascular system) 747.60
brain 747.81
great 747.49
portal 747.49
pulmonary 747.49
vena cava (inferior) (superior) 747.49
vertebra 756.19
vulva 752.49
spermatic cord 752.9
spine, spinal 756.10
column 756.10
cord 742.9
meningocele (*see also* Spina bifida) 741.9 ✓5ᵗʰ
specified type NEC 742.59
spina bifida (*see also* Spina bifida) 741.9 ✓5ᵗʰ
vessel 747.82
meninges 742.59
nerve root 742.9
spleen 759.0
Sprengel's 755.52
sternum 756.3

Anomaly, anomalous — *continued*
stomach 750.9
specified type NEC 750.7
submaxillary gland 750.9
superior vena cava 747.40
talipes — *see* Talipes
tarsus 755.67
with complete absence of distal elements 755.31
teeth, tooth NEC 520.9
position 524.3
spacing 524.3
tendon 756.9
specified type NEC 756.89
termination
coronary artery 746.85
testis 752.9
thebesian valve 746.9
thigh 755.60
flexion (*see also* Subluxation, congenital, hip) 754.32
thorax (wall) 756.3
throat 750.9
thumb 755.50
supernumerary 755.01
thymus gland 759.2
thyroid (gland) 759.2
cartilage 748.3
tibia 755.60
saber 090.5
toe 755.66
supernumerary 755.02
webbed (*see also* Syndactylism, toes) 755.13
tongue 750.10
specified type NEC 750.19
trachea, tracheal 748.3
cartilage 748.3
rings 748.3
tragus 744.3
transverse aortic arch 747.21
trichromata 368.59
trichromatopsia 368.59
tricuspid (leaflet) (valve) 746.9
atresia 746.1
Ebstein's 746.2
specified type NEC 746.89
stenosis 746.1
trunk 759.9
Uhl's (hypoplasia of myocardium, right ventricle) 746.84
ulna 755.50
umbilicus 759.9
artery 747.5
union, trachea with larynx 748.3
unspecified site 759.9
upper extremity 755.50
vessel 747.63
urachus 753.7
specified type NEC 753.7
ureter 753.9
obstructive 753.20
specified type NEC 753.4
obstructive 753.29
urethra (valve) 753.9
obstructive 753.6
specified type NEC 753.8
urinary tract or system (any part, except urachus) 753.9
specified type NEC 753.8
urachus 753.7
uterus 752.3
with only one functioning horn 752.3
in pregnancy or childbirth 654.0 ✓5ᵗʰ
affecting fetus or newborn 763.89
causing obstructed labor 660.2 ✓5ᵗʰ
affecting fetus or newborn 763.1
uvula 750.9
vagina 752.40
valleculae 748.3
valve (heart) NEC 746.9
formation, ureter 753.29
pulmonary 746.00
specified type NEC 746.89
vascular NEC (*see also* Anomaly, peripheral vascular system) 747.60
ring 747.21
vas deferens 752.9

Anomaly, anomalous — continued
- vein(s) (peripheral) NEC (see also Anomaly, peripheral vascular system) 747.60
  - brain 747.81
  - cerebral 747.81
  - coronary 746.89
  - great 747.40
    - specified type NEC 747.49
  - portal 747.40
  - pulmonary 747.40
  - retina 743.9
  - vena cava (inferior) (superior) 747.40
- venous return (pulmonary) 747.49
  - partial 747.42
  - total 747.41
- ventricle, ventricular (heart) 746.9
  - bands 746.9
  - folds 746.9
  - septa 745.4
- vertebra 756.19
- vesicourethral orifice 753.9
- vessels NEC (see also Anomaly, peripheral vascular system) 747.60
  - optic papilla 743.9
- vitelline duct 751.0
- vitreous humor 743.9
  - specified type NEC 743.51
- vulva 752.40
- wrist (joint) 755.50

Anomia 784.69
Anonychia 757.5
- acquired 703.8

Anophthalmos, anophthalmus (clinical) (congenital) (globe) 743.00
- acquired V45.78

Anopsia (altitudinal) (quadrant) 368.46
Anorchia 752.8
Anorchism, anorchidism 752.8
Anorexia 783.0
- hysterical 300.11
- nervosa 307.1

Anosmia (see also Disturbance, sensation) 781.1
- hysterical 300.11
- postinfectional 478.9
- psychogenic 306.7
- traumatic 951.8

Anosognosia 780.99
Anosphrasia 781.1
Anosteoplasia 756.50
Anotia 744.09
Anovulatory cycle 628.0
Anoxemia 799.0
- newborn 768.9

Anoxia 799.0
- altitude 993.2
- cerebral 348.1
  - with
    - abortion — see Abortion, by type, with specified complication NEC
    - ectopic pregnancy (see also categories 633.0-633.9) 639.8
    - molar pregnancy (see also categories 630-632) 639.8
  - complicating
    - delivery (cesarean) (instrumental) 669.4
    - ectopic or molar pregnancy 639.8
    - obstetric anesthesia or sedation 668.2
  - during or resulting from a procedure 997.01
  - following
    - abortion 639.8
    - ectopic or molar pregnancy 639.8
  - newborn (see also Distress, fetal, liveborn infant) 768.9
- due to drowning 994.1
- fetal, affecting newborn 768.9
- heart — see Insufficiency, coronary
- high altitude 993.2
- intrauterine
  - fetal death (before onset of labor) 768.0
    - during labor 768.1
  - liveborn infant — see Distress, fetal, liveborn infant

Anoxia — continued
- myocardial — see Insufficiency, coronary
- newborn 768.9
  - mild or moderate 768.6
  - severe 768.5
- pathological 799.0

Anteflexion — see Anteversion
Antenatal
- care, normal pregnancy V22.1
  - first V22.0
- screening (for) V28.9
  - based on amniocentesis NEC V28.2
    - chromosomal anomalies V28.0
    - raised alphafetoprotein levels V28.1
  - chromosomal anomalies V28.0
  - fetal growth retardation using ultrasonics V28.4
  - isoimmunization V28.5
  - malformations using ultrasonics V28.3
  - raised alphafetoprotein levels in amniotic fluid V28.1
  - specified condition NEC V28.8
  - Streptococcus B V28.6

Antepartum — see condition
Anterior — see also condition
- spinal artery compression syndrome 721.1

Antero-occlusion 524.2
Anteversion
- cervix (see also Anteversion, uterus) 621.6
- femur (neck), congenital 755.63
- uterus, uterine (cervix) (postinfectional) (postpartal, old) 621.6
  - congenital 752.3
  - in pregnancy or childbirth 654.4
    - affecting fetus or newborn 763.89
    - causing obstructed labor 660.2
      - affecting fetus or newborn 763.1

Anthracosilicosis (occupational) 500
Anthracosis (lung) (occupational) 500
- lingua 529.3

Anthrax 022.9
- with pneumonia 022.1 [484.5]
- colitis 022.2
- cutaneous 022.0
- gastrointestinal 022.2
- intestinal 022.2
- pulmonary 022.1
- respiratory 022.1
- septicemia 022.3
- specified manifestation NEC 022.8

Anthropoid pelvis 755.69
- with disproportion (fetopelvic) 653.2
  - affecting fetus or newborn 763.1
  - causing obstructed labor 660.1
    - affecting fetus or newborn 763.1

Anthropophobia 300.29
Antibioma, breast 611.0
Antibodies
- maternal (blood group) (see also Incompatibility) 656.2
- anti-D, cord blood 656.1
- fetus or newborn 773.0

Antibody deficiency syndrome
- agammaglobulinemic 279.00
- congenital 279.04
- hypogammaglobulinemic 279.00

Anticoagulant, circulating (see also Circulating anticoagulants) 286.5
Antimongolism syndrome 758.3
Antimonial cholera 985.4
Antisocial personality 301.7
Antithrombinemia (see also Circulating anticoagulants) 286.5
Antithromboplastinemia (see also Circulating anticoagulants) 286.5
Antithromboplastinogenemia (see also Circulating anticoagulants) 286.5
Antitoxin complication or reaction — see Complications, vaccination
Anton (-Babinski) syndrome (hemiasomatognosia) 307.9
Antritis (chronic) 473.0
- acute 461.0

Antrum, antral — see condition
Anuria 788.5
- with
  - abortion — see Abortion, by type, with renal failure
  - ectopic pregnancy (see also categories 633.0-633.9) 639.3
  - molar pregnancy (see also categories 630-632) 639.3
- calculus (impacted) (recurrent) 592.9
  - kidney 592.0
  - ureter 592.1
- congenital 753.3
- due to a procedure 997.5
- following
  - abortion 639.3
  - ectopic or molar pregnancy 639.3
- newborn 753.3
- postrenal 593.4
- puerperal, postpartum, childbirth 669.3
- specified as due to a procedure 997.5
- sulfonamide
  - correct substance properly administered 788.5
  - overdose or wrong substance given or taken 961.0
- traumatic (following crushing) 958.5

Anus, anal — see condition
Anusitis 569.49
Anxiety (neurosis) (reaction) (state) 300.00
- alcohol-induced 291.89
- depression 300.4
- drug-induced 292.89
- due to or associated with physical condition 293.84
- generalized 300.02
- hysteria 300.20
- in
  - acute stress reaction 308.0
  - transient adjustment reaction 309.24
- panic type 300.01
- separation, abnormal 309.21
- syndrome (organic) (transient) 293.84

Aorta, aortic — see condition
Aortectasia 441.9
Aortitis (nonsyphilitic) 447.6
- arteriosclerotic 440.0
- calcific 447.6
- Döhle-Heller 093.1
- luetic 093.1
- rheumatic (see also Endocarditis, acute, rheumatic) 391.1
- rheumatoid — see Arthritis, rheumatoid
- specific 093.1
- syphilitic 093.1
  - congenital 090.5

Apethetic thyroid storm (see also Thyrotoxicosis) 242.9
Apepsia 536.8
- achlorhydric 536.0
- psychogenic 306.4

Aperistalsis, esophagus 530.0
Apert's syndrome (acrocephalosyndactyly) 755.55
Apert-Gallais syndrome (adrenogenital) 255.2
Apertognathia 524.2
Aphagia 787.2
- psychogenic 307.1

Aphakia (acquired) (bilateral) (postoperative) (unilateral) 379.31
- congenital 743.35

Aphalangia (congenital) 755.4
- lower limb (complete) (intercalary) (partial) (terminal) 755.39
  - meaning all digits (complete) (partial) 755.31
  - transverse 755.31
- upper limb (complete) (intercalary) (partial) (terminal) 755.29
  - meaning all digits (complete) (partial) 755.21
  - transverse 755.21

Aphasia (amnestic) (ataxic) (auditory) (Broca's) (choreatic) (classic) (expressive) (global) (ideational) (ideokinetic) (ideomotor) (jargon) (motor) (nominal) (receptive) (semantic) (sensory) (syntactic) (verbal) (visual) (Wernicke's) 784.3
    developmental 315.31
    syphilis, tertiary 094.89
    uremic — see Uremia
Aphemia 784.3
    uremic — see Uremia
Aphonia 784.41
    clericorum 784.49
    hysterical 300.11
    organic 784.41
    psychogenic 306.1
Aphthae, aphthous — see also condition
    Bednar's 528.2
    cachectic 529.0
    epizootic 078.4
    fever 078.4
    oral 528.2
    stomatitis 528.2
    thrush 112.0
    ulcer (oral) (recurrent) 528.2
        genital organ(s) NEC
            female 629.8
            male 608.89
        larynx 478.79
Apical — see condition
Aplasia — see also Agenesis
    alveolar process (acquired) 525.8
        congenital 750.26
    aorta (congenital) 747.22
    aortic valve (congenital) 746.89
    axialis extracorticalis (congenital) 330.0
    bone marrow (myeloid) 284.9
        acquired (secondary) 284.8
        congenital 284.0
        idiopathic 284.9
    brain 740.0
        specified part 742.2
    breast 757.6
    bronchus 748.3
    cementum 520.4
    cerebellar 742.2
    congenital pure red cell 284.0
    corpus callosum 742.2
    erythrocyte 284.8
        congenital 284.0
    extracortical axial 330.0
    eye (congenital) 743.00
    fovea centralis (congenital) 743.55
    germinal (cell) 606.0
    iris 743.45
    labyrinth, membranous 744.05
    limb (congenital) 755.4
        lower NEC 755.30
        upper NEC 755.20
    lung (bilateral) (congenital) (unilateral) 748.5
    nervous system NEC 742.8
    nuclear 742.8
    ovary 752.0
    Pelizaeus-Merzbacher 330.0
    prostate (congenital) 752.8
    red cell (pure) (with thymoma) 284.8
        acquired (secondary) 284.8
        congenital 284.0
        hereditary 284.0
        of infants 284.0
        primary 284.0
    round ligament (congenital) 752.8
    salivary gland 750.21
    skin (congenital) 757.39
    spinal cord 742.59
    spleen 759.0
    testis (congenital) 752.8
    thymic, with immunodeficiency 279.2
    thyroid 243
    uterus 752.3
    ventral horn cell 742.59
Apleuria 756.3
Apnea, apneic (spells) 786.03
    newborn, neonatorum 770.81
        essential 770.81

Apnea, apneic — continued
    newborn, neonatorum — continued
        obstructive 770.82
        primary 770.81
        sleep 770.81
        specified NEC 770.82
    psychogenic 306.1
    sleep NEC 780.57
        with
            hypersomnia 780.53
            hyposomnia 780.51
            insomnia 780.51
        sleep disturbance NEC 780.57
Apneumatosis newborn 770.4
Apodia 755.31
Apophysitis (bone) (see also Osteochondrosis) 732.9
    calcaneus 732.5
    juvenile 732.6
Apoplectiform convulsions (see also Disease, cerebrovascular, acute) 436
Apoplexia, apoplexy, apoplectic (see also Disease, cerebrovascular, acute) 436
    abdominal 569.89
    adrenal 036.3
    attack 436
    basilar (see also Disease, cerebrovascular, acute) 436
    brain (see also Disease, cerebrovascular, acute) 436
    bulbar (see also Disease, cerebrovascular, acute) 436
    capillary (see also Disease, cerebrovascular, acute) 436
    cardiac (see also Infarct, myocardium) 410.9
    cerebral (see also Disease, cerebrovascular, acute) 436
    chorea (see also Disease, cerebrovascular, acute) 436
    congestive (see also Disease, cerebrovascular, acute) 436
        newborn 767.4
    embolic (see also Embolism, brain) 434.1
    fetus 767.0
    fit (see also Disease, cerebrovascular, acute) 436
    healed or old V12.59
    heart (auricle) (ventricle) (see also Infarct, myocardium) 410.9
    heat 992.0
    hemiplegia (see also Disease, cerebrovascular, acute) 436
    hemorrhagic (stroke) (see also Hemorrhage, brain) 432.9
    ingravescent (see also Disease, cerebrovascular, acute) 436
    late effect — see Late effect(s) (of) cerebrovascular disease
    lung — see Embolism, pulmonary
    meninges, hemorrhagic (see also Hemorrhage, subarachnoid) 430
    neonatorum 767.0
    newborn 767.0
    pancreatitis 577.0
    placenta 641.2
    progressive (see also Disease, cerebrovascular, acute) 436
    pulmonary (artery) (vein) — see Embolism, pulmonary
    sanguineous (see also Disease, cerebrovascular, acute) 436
    seizure (see also Disease, cerebrovascular, acute) 436
    serous (see also Disease, cerebrovascular, acute) 436
    spleen 289.59
    stroke (see also Disease, cerebrovascular, acute) 436
    thrombotic (see also Thrombosis, brain) 434.0
    uremic — see Uremia
    uteroplacental 641.2
Appendage
    fallopian tube (cyst of Morgagni) 752.11
    intestine (epiploic) 751.5

Appendage — continued
    preauricular 744.1
    testicular (organ of Morgagni) 752.8
Appendicitis 541
    with
        perforation, peritonitis (generalized), or rupture 540.0
            with peritoneal abscess 540.1
        peritoneal abscess 540.1
    acute (catarrhal) (fulminating) (gangrenous) (inflammatory) (obstructive) (retrocecal) (suppurative) 540.9
        with
            perforation, peritonitis, or rupture 540.0
                with peritoneal abscess 540.1
            peritoneal abscess 540.1
    amebic 006.8
    chronic (recurrent) 542
    exacerbation — see Appendicitis, acute
    fulminating — see Appendicitis, acute
    gangrenous — see Appendicitis, acute
    healed (obliterative) 542
    interval 542
    neurogenic 542
    obstructive 542
    pneumococcal 541
    recurrent 542
    relapsing 542
    retrocecal 541
    subacute (adhesive) 542
    subsiding 542
    suppurative — see Appendicitis, acute
    tuberculous (see also Tuberculosis) 014.8
Appendiclausis 543.9
Appendicolithiasis 543.9
Appendicopathia oxyurica 127.4
Appendix, appendicular — see also condition
    Morgagni (male) 752.8
        fallopian tube 752.11
Appetite
    depraved 307.52
    excessive 783.6
        psychogenic 307.51
    lack or loss (see also Anorexia) 783.0
        nonorganic origin 307.59
    perverted 307.52
        hysterical 300.11
Apprehension, apprehensiveness (abnormal) (state) 300.00
    specified type NEC 300.09
Approximal wear 521.1
Apraxia (classic) (ideational) (ideokinetic) (ideomotor) (motor) 784.69
    oculomotor, congenital 379.51
    verbal 784.69
Aptyalism 527.7
Aqueous misdirection 365.83
Arabicum elephantiasis (see also Infestation, filarial) 125.9
Arachnidism 989.5
Arachnitis — see Meningitis
Arachnodactyly 759.82
Arachnoidism 989.5
Arachnoiditis (acute) (adhesive) (basic) (brain) (cerebrospinal) (chiasmal) (chronic) (spinal) (see also Meningitis) 322.9
    meningococcal (chronic) 036.0
    syphilitic 094.2
    tuberculous (see also Tuberculosis meninges) 013.0
Araneism 989.5
Arboencephalitis, Australian 062.4
Arborization block (heart) 426.6
Arbor virus, arbovirus (infection) NEC 066.9
ARC 042
Arches — see condition
Arcuatus uterus 752.3
Arcus (cornea)
    juvenilis 743.43
        interfering with vision 743.42
    senilis 371.41
Arc-welders' lung 503

Arc-welders' syndrome (photokeratitis) 370.24
Areflexia 796.1
Areola — *see* condition
Argentaffinoma (M8241/1) — *see also* Neoplasm, by site, uncertain behavior
   benign (M8241/0) — *See* Neoplasm, by site, benign
   malignant (M8241/3) — *see* Neoplasm, by site, malignant
   syndrome 259.2
Argentinian hemorrhagic fever 078.7
Arginosuccinicaciduria 270.6
Argonz-Del Castillo syndrome (nonpuerperal galactorrhea and amenorrhea) 253.1
Argyll-Robertson phenomenon, pupil, or syndrome (syphilitic) 094.89
   atypical 379.45
   nonluetic 379.45
   nonsyphilitic 379.45
   reversed 379.45
Argyria, argyriasis NEC 985.8
   conjunctiva 372.55
   cornea 371.16
   from drug or medicinal agent
      correct substance properly administered 709.09
      overdose or wrong substance given or taken 961.2
Arhinencephaly 742.2
Arias-Stella phenomenon 621.3
Ariboflavinosis 266.0
Arizona enteritis 008.1
Arm — *see* condition
Armenian disease 277.3
Arnold-Chiari obstruction or syndrome (*see also* Spina bifida) 741.0 ✓5ᵗʰ
   type I 348.4
   type II (*see also* Spina bifida) 741.0 ✓5ᵗʰ
   type III 742.0
   type IV 742.2
Arrest, arrested
   active phase of labor 661.1 ✓5ᵗʰ
      affecting fetus or newborn 763.7
   any plane in pelvis
      complicating delivery 660.1 ✓5ᵗʰ
         affecting fetus or newborn 763.1
   bone marrow (*see also* Anemia, aplastic) 284.9
   cardiac 427.5
      with
         abortion — *see* Abortion, by type, with specified complication NEC
         ectopic pregnancy (*see also* categories 633.0-633.9) 639.8
         molar pregnancy (*see also* categories 630-632) 639.8
      complicating
         anesthesia
            correct substance properly administered 427.5
            obstetric 668.1 ✓5ᵗʰ
            overdose or wrong substance given 968.4
            specified anesthetic — *see* Table of Drugs and Chemicals
         delivery (cesarean) (instrumental) 669.4 ✓5ᵗʰ
         ectopic or molar pregnancy 639.8
         surgery (nontherapeutic) (therapeutic) 997.1
      fetus or newborn 779.89 ▲
      following
         abortion 639.8
         ectopic or molar pregnancy 639.8
      postoperative (immediate) 997.1
      long-term effect of cardiac surgery 429.4
   cardiorespiratory (*see also* Arrest, cardiac) 427.5
   deep transverse 660.3 ✓5ᵗʰ
      affecting fetus or newborn 763.1
   development or growth
      bone 733.91
      child 783.40

Arrest, arrested — *continued*
   development or growth — *continued*
      fetus 764.9 ✓5ᵗʰ
         affecting management of pregnancy 656.5 ✓5ᵗʰ
      tracheal rings 748.3
   epiphyseal 733.91
   granulopoiesis 288.0
   heart — *see* Arrest, cardiac
   respiratory 799.1
      newborn 770.89 ▲
   sinus 426.6
   transverse (deep) 660.3 ✓5ᵗʰ
      affecting fetus or newborn 763.1
Arrhenoblastoma (M8630/1)
   benign (M8630/0)
      specified site — *see* Neoplasm, by site, benign
      unspecified site
         female 220
         male 222.0
   malignant (M8630/3)
      specified site — *see* Neoplasm, by site, malignant
      unspecified site
         female 183.0
         male 186.9
   specified site — *see* Neoplasm, by site, uncertain behavior
   unspecified site
      female 236.2
      male 236.4
Arrhinencephaly 742.2
   due to
      trisomy 13 (13-15) 758.1
      trisomy 18 (16-18) 758.2
Arrhythmia (auricle) (cardiac) (cordis) (gallop rhythm) (juvenile) (nodal) (reflex) (sinus) (supraventricular) (transitory) (ventricle) 427.9
   bigeminal rhythm 427.89
   block 426.9
   bradycardia 427.89
   contractions, premature 427.60
   coronary sinus 427.89
   ectopic 427.89
   extrasystolic 427.60
   postoperative 997.1
   psychogenic 306.2
   vagal 780.2
Arrillaga-Ayerza syndrome (pulmonary artery sclerosis with pulmonary hypertension) 416.0
Arsenical
   dermatitis 692.4
   keratosis 692.4
   pigmentation 985.1
      from drug or medicinal agent
         correct substance properly administered 709.09
         overdose or wrong substance given or taken 961.1
Arsenism 985.1
   from drug or medicinal agent
      correct substance properly administered 692.4
      overdose or wrong substance given or taken 961.1
Arterial — *see* condition
Arteriectasis 447.8
Arteriofibrosis — *see* Arteriosclerosis
Arteriolar sclerosis — *see* Arteriosclerosis
Arteriolith — *see* Arteriosclerosis
Arteriolitis 447.6
   necrotizing, kidney 447.5
   renal — *see* Hypertension, kidney
Arteriolosclerosis — *see* Arteriosclerosis
Arterionephrosclerosis (*see also* Hypertension, kidney) 403.90
Arteriopathy 447.9
Arteriosclerosis, arteriosclerotic (artery) (deformans) (diffuse) (disease) (endarteritis) (general) (obliterans) (obliterative) (occlusive) (senile) (with calcification) 440.9

Arteriosclerosis, arteriosclerotic — *continued*
   with
      gangrene 440.24
      psychosis (*see also* Psychosis, arteriosclerotic) 290.40
      ulceration 440.23
   aorta 440.0
   arteries of extremities — *see* Arteriosclerosis, extremities
   basilar (artery) (*see also* Occlusion, artery, basilar) 433.0 ✓5ᵗʰ
   brain 437.0
   bypass graft
      coronary artery 414.05
         autologous artery (gastroepiploic) (internal mammary) 414.04
         autologous vein 414.02
         nonautologous biological 414.03
      extremity 440.30
         autologous vein 440.31
         nonautologous biological 440.32
   cardiac — *see* Arteriosclerosis, coronary
   cardiopathy — *see* Arteriosclerosis, coronary
   cardiorenal (*see also* Hypertension, cardiorenal) 404.90
   cardiovascular (*see also* Disease, cardiovascular) 429.2
   carotid (artery) (common) (internal) (*see also* Occlusion, artery, carotid) 433.1 ✓5ᵗʰ
   central nervous system 437.0
   cerebral 437.0
      late effect — *see* Late effect(s) (of) cerebrovascular disease
   cerebrospinal 437.0
   cerebrovascular 437.0
   coronary (artery) 414.00
      graft — *see* Arteriosclerosis, bypass graft
      native artery 414.01
      of transplanted heart 414.06 ●
   extremities (native artery) NEC 440.20
      bypass graft 440.30
         autologous vein 440.31
         nonautologous biological 440.32
      claudication (intermittent) 440.21
      and
         gangrene 440.24
         rest pain 440.22
            and
               gangrene 440.24
               ulceration 440.23
                   and gangrene 440.24
         ulceration 440.23
            and gangrene 440.24
      gangrene 440.24
      rest pain 440.22
      and
         gangrene 440.24
         ulceration 440.23
            and gangrene 440.24
      specified site NEC 440.29
      ulceration 440.23
         and gangrene 440.24
   heart (disease) — *see also* Arteriosclerosis, coronary
      valve 424.99
         aortic 424.1
         mitral 424.0
         pulmonary 424.3
         tricuspid 424.2
   kidney (*see also* Hypertension, kidney) 403.90
   labyrinth, labyrinthine 388.00
   medial NEC 440.20
   mesentery (artery) 557.1
   Mönckeberg's 440.20
   myocarditis 429.0
   nephrosclerosis (*see also* Hypertension, kidney) 403.90
   peripheral (of extremities) — *see* Arteriosclerosis, extremities
   precerebral 433.9 ✓5ᵗʰ
      specified artery NEC 433.8 ✓5ᵗʰ
   pulmonary (idiopathic) 416.0
   renal (*see also* Hypertension, kidney) 403.90
      arterioles (*see also* Hypertension, kidney) 403.90
      artery 440.1
   retinal (vascular) 440.8 *[362.13]*

Index to Diseases

Arteriosclerosis, arteriosclerotic — *continued*
specified artery NEC 440.8
with gangrene 440.8 *[785.4]*
spinal (cord) 437.0
vertebral (artery) (*see also* Occlusion, artery, vertebral) 433.2 ✓5ᵗʰ
Arteriospasm 443.9
Arteriovenous — *see* condition
Arteritis 447.6
allergic (*see also* Angiitis, hypersensitivity) 446.20
aorta (nonsyphilitic) 447.6
syphilitic 093.1
aortic arch 446.7
brachiocephalica 446.7
brain 437.4
syphilitic 094.89
branchial 446.7
cerebral 437.4
late effect — *see* Late effect(s) (of) cerebrovascular disease
syphilitic 094.89
coronary (artery) — *see also* Arteriosclerosis, coronary
rheumatic 391.9
chronic 398.99
syphilitic 093.89
cranial (left) (right) 446.5
deformans — *see* Arteriosclerosis
giant cell 446.5
necrosing or necrotizing 446.0
nodosa 446.0
obliterans — *see also* Arteriosclerosis
subclaviocarotica 446.7
pulmonary 417.8
retina 362.18
rheumatic — *see* Fever, rheumatic
senile — *see* Arteriosclerosis
suppurative 447.2
syphilitic (general) 093.89
brain 094.89
coronary 093.89
spinal 094.89
temporal 446.5
young female, syndrome 446.7
Artery, arterial — *see* condition
Arthralgia (*see also* Pain, joint) 719.4 ✓5ᵗʰ
allergic (*see also* Pain, joint) 719.4 ✓5ᵗʰ
in caisson disease 993.3
psychogenic 307.89
rubella 056.71
Salmonella 003.23
temporomandibular joint 524.62
Arthritis, arthritic (acute) (chronic) (subacute) 716.9 ✓5ᵗʰ
meaning Osteoarthritis — *see* Osteoarthrosis

> Note — Use the following fifth-digit subclassification with categories 711-712, 715-716:
>
> 0 site unspecified
> 1 shoulder region
> 2 upper arm
> 3 forearm
> 4 hand
> 5 pelvic region and thigh
> 6 lower leg
> 7 ankle and foot
> 8 other specified sites
> 9 multiple sites

allergic 716.2 ✓5ᵗʰ
ankylosing (crippling) (spine) 720.0
sites other than spine 716.9 ✓5ᵗʰ
atrophic 714.0
spine 720.9
back (*see also* Arthritis, spine) 721.90
Bechterew's (ankylosing spondylitis) 720.0
blennorrhagic 098.50
cervical, cervicodorsal (*see also* Spondylosis, cervical) 721.0
Charcôt's 094.0 *[713.5]*
diabetic 250.6 ✓5ᵗʰ *[713.5]*
syringomyelic 336.0 *[713.5]*

Arthritis, arthritic — *continued*
Charcôt's — *continued*
tabetic 094.0 *[713.5]*
chylous (*see also* Filariasis) 125.9 *[711.7]* ✓5ᵗʰ
climacteric NEC 716.3 ✓5ᵗʰ
coccyx 721.8
cricoarytenoid 478.79
crystal (-induced) — *see* Arthritis, due to crystals
deformans (*see also* Osteoarthrosis) 715.9 ✓5ᵗʰ
spine 721.90
with myelopathy 721.91
degenerative (*see also* Osteoarthrosis) 715.9 ✓5ᵗʰ
idiopathic 715.09
polyarticular 715.09
spine 721.90
with myelopathy 721.91
dermatoarthritis, lipoid 272.8 *[713.0]*
due to or associated with
acromegaly 253.0 *[713.0]*
actinomycosis 039.8 *[711.4]* ✓5ᵗʰ
amyloidosis 277.3 *[713.7]*
bacterial disease NEC 040.89 *[711.4]* ✓5ᵗʰ
Behçet's syndrome 136.1 *[711.2]* ✓5ᵗʰ
blastomycosis 116.0 *[711.6]* ✓5ᵗʰ
brucellosis (*see also* Brucellosis) 023.9 *[711.4]* ✓5ᵗʰ
caisson disease 993.3
coccidioidomycosis 114.3 *[711.6]* ✓5ᵗʰ
coliform (Escherichia coli) 711.0 ✓5ᵗʰ
colitis, ulcerative (*see also* Colitis, ulcerative) 556.9 *[713.1]*
cowpox 051.0 *[711.5]* ✓5ᵗʰ
crystals — *see also* Gout
dicalcium phosphate 275.49 *[712.1]*
pyrophosphate 275.49 *[712.2]*
specified NEC 275.49 *[712.8]*
dermatoarthritis, lipoid 272.8 *[713.0]*
dermatological disorder NEC 709.9 *[713.3]*
diabetes 250.6 ✓5ᵗʰ *[713.5]*
diphtheria 032.89 *[711.4]* ✓5ᵗʰ
dracontiasis 125.7 *[711.7]* ✓5ᵗʰ
dysentery 009.0 *[711.3]* ✓5ᵗʰ
endocrine disorder NEC 259.9 *[713.0]*
enteritis NEC 009.1 *[711.3]* ✓5ᵗʰ
infectious (*see also* Enteritis, infectious) 009.0 *[711.3]* ✓5ᵗʰ
specified organism NEC 008.8 *[711.3]* ✓5ᵗʰ
regional (*see also* Enteritis, regional) 555.9 *[713.1]*
specified organism NEC 008.8 *[711.3]* ✓5ᵗʰ
epiphyseal slip, nontraumatic (old) 716.8 ✓5ᵗʰ
erysipelas 035 *[711.4]* ✓5ᵗʰ
erythema
epidemic 026.1
multiforme 695.1 *[713.3]*
nodosum 695.2 *[713.3]*
Escherichia coli 711.0 ✓5ᵗʰ
filariasis NEC 125.9 *[711.7]* ✓5ᵗʰ
gastrointestinal condition NEC 569.9 *[713.1]*
glanders 024 *[711.4]* ✓5ᵗʰ
Gonococcus 098.50
gout 274.0
H. influenzae 711.0 ✓5ᵗʰ
helminthiasis NEC 128.9 *[711.7]* ✓5ᵗʰ
hematological disorder NEC 289.9 *[713.2]*
hemochromatosis 275.0 *[713.0]*
hemoglobinopathy NEC (*see also* Disease, hemoglobin) 282.7 *[713.2]*
hemophilia (*see also* Hemophilia) 286.0 *[713.2]*
Hemophilus influenzae (H. influenzae) 711.0 ✓5ᵗʰ
Henoch (-Schönlein) purpura 287.0 *[713.6]*
histoplasmosis NEC (*see also* Histoplasmosis) 115.99 *[711.6]* ✓5ᵗʰ
hyperparathyroidism 252.0 *[713.0]*
hypersensitivity reaction NEC 995.3 *[713.6]*
hypogammaglobulinemia (*see also* Hypogamma-globulinemia) 279.00 *[713.0]*
hypothyroidism NEC 244.9 *[713.0]*
infection (*see also* Arthritis, infectious) 711.9 ✓5ᵗʰ

Arthritis, arthritic — *continued*
due to or associated with — *continued*
infectious disease NEC 136.9 *[711.8]* ✓5ᵗʰ
leprosy (*see also* Leprosy) 030.9 *[711.4]* ✓5ᵗʰ
leukemia NEC (M9800/3) 208.9 ✓5ᵗʰ *[713.2]*
lipoid dermatoarthritis 272.8 *[713.0]*
Lyme disease 088.81 *[711.8]* ✓5ᵗʰ
Mediterranean fever, familial 277.3 *[713.7]*
meningococcal infection 036.82
metabolic disorder NEC 277.9 *[713.0]*
multiple myelomatosis (M9730/3) 203.0 ✓5ᵗʰ *[713.2]*
mumps 072.79 *[711.5]* ✓5ᵗʰ
mycobacteria 031.8 *[711.4]* ✓5ᵗʰ
mycosis NEC 117.9 *[711.6]* ✓5ᵗʰ
neurological disorder NEC 349.9 *[713.5]*
ochronosis 270.2 *[713.0]*
O'Nyong Nyong 066.3 *[711.5]* ✓5ᵗʰ
parasitic disease NEC 136.9 *[711.8]* ✓5ᵗʰ
paratyphoid fever (*see also* Fever, paratyphoid) 002.9 *[711.3]* ✓5ᵗʰ
Pneumococcus 711.0 ✓5ᵗʰ
poliomyelitis (*see also* Poliomyelitis) 045.9 ✓5ᵗʰ *[711.5]* ✓5ᵗʰ
Pseudomonas 711.0 ✓5ᵗʰ
psoriasis 696.0
pyogenic organism (E. coli) (H. influenzae) (Pseudomonas) (Streptococcus) 711.0 ✓5ᵗʰ
rat-bite fever 026.1 *[711.4]* ✓5ᵗʰ
regional enteritis (*see also* Enteritis, regional) 555.9 *[713.1]*
Reiter's disease 099.3 *[711.1]* ✓5ᵗʰ
respiratory disorder NEC 519.9 *[713.4]*
reticulosis, malignant (M9720/3) 202.3 ✓5ᵗʰ *[713.2]*
rubella 056.71
salmonellosis 003.23
sarcoidosis 135 *[713.7]*
serum sickness 999.5 *[713.6]*
Staphylococcus 711.0 ✓5ᵗʰ
Streptococcus 711.0 ✓5ᵗʰ
syphilis (*see also* Syphilis) 094.0 *[711.4]* ✓5ᵗʰ
syringomyelia 336.0 *[713.5]*
thalassemia 282.4 *[713.2]*
tuberculosis (*see also* Tuberculosis, arthritis) 015.9 ✓5ᵗʰ *[711.4]* ✓5ᵗʰ
typhoid fever 002.0 *[711.3]* ✓5ᵗʰ
ulcerative colitis (*see also* Colitis, ulcerative) 556.9 *[713.1]*
urethritis
nongonococcal (*see also* Urethritis, nongonococcal) 099.40 *[711.1]* ✓5ᵗʰ
nonspecific (*see also* Urethritis, nongonococcal) 099.40 *[711.1]* ✓5ᵗʰ
Reiter's 099.3 *[711.1]* ✓5ᵗʰ
viral disease NEC 079.99 *[711.5]* ✓5ᵗʰ
erythema epidemic 026.1
gonococcal 098.50
gouty (acute) 274.0
hypertrophic (*see also* Osteoarthrosis) 715.9 ✓5ᵗʰ
spine 721.90
with myelopathy 721.91
idiopathic, blennorrheal 099.3
in caisson disease 993.3 *[713.8]*
infectious or infective (acute) (chronic) (subacute) NEC 711.9 ✓5ᵗʰ
nonpyogenic 711.9 ✓5ᵗʰ
spine 720.9
inflammatory NEC 714.9
juvenile rheumatoid (chronic) (polyarticular) 714.30
acute 714.31
monoarticular 714.33
pauciarticular 714.32
lumbar (*see also* Spondylosis, lumbar) 721.3
meningococcal 036.82
menopausal NEC 716.3 ✓5ᵗʰ
migratory — *see* Fever, rheumatic
neuropathic (Charcôt's) 094.0 *[713.5]*
diabetic 250.6 ✓5ᵗʰ *[713.5]*
nonsyphilitic NEC 349.9 *[713.5]*
syringomyelic 336.0 *[713.5]*
tabetic 094.0 *[713.5]*
nodosa (*see also* Osteoarthrosis) 715.9 ✓5ᵗʰ
spine 721.90
with myelopathy 721.91

Arthritis, arthritic

Arthritis, arthritic — continued
- nonpyogenic NEC 716.9 ✓5
  - spine 721.90
    - with myelopathy 721.91
- ochronotic 270.2 [713.0]
- palindromic (see also Rheumatism, palindromic) 719.3 ✓5
- pneumococcal 711.0 ✓5
- postdysenteric 009.0 [711.3] ✓5
- postrheumatic, chronic (Jaccoud's) 714.4
- primary progressive 714.0
  - spine 720.9
- proliferative 714.0
  - spine 720.0
- psoriatic 696.0
- purulent 711.0 ✓5
- pyogenic or pyemic 711.0 ✓5
- rheumatic 714.0
  - acute or subacute — see Fever, rheumatic
  - chronic 714.0
  - spine 720.9
- rheumatoid (nodular) 714.0
  - with
    - splenoadenomegaly and leukopenia 714.1
    - visceral or systemic involvement 714.2
  - aortitis 714.89
  - carditis 714.2
  - heart disease 714.2
  - juvenile (chronic) (polyarticular) 714.30
    - acute 714.31
    - monoarticular 714.33
    - pauciarticular 714.32
  - spine 720.0
- rubella 056.71
- sacral, sacroiliac, sacrococcygeal (see also Spondylosis, sacral) 721.3
- scorbutic 267
- senile or senescent (see also Osteoarthrosis) 715.9 ✓5
  - spine 721.90
    - with myelopathy 721.91
- septic 711.0 ✓5
- serum (nontherapeutic) (therapeutic) 999.5 [713.6]
- specified form NEC 716.8 ✓5
- spine 721.90
  - with myelopathy 721.91
  - atrophic 720.9
  - degenerative 721.90
    - with myelopathy 721.91
  - hypertrophic (with deformity) 721.90
    - with myelopathy 721.91
  - infectious or infective NEC 720.9
  - Marie-Strümpell 720.0
  - nonpyogenic 721.90
    - with myelopathy 721.91
  - pyogenic 720.9
  - rheumatoid 720.0
  - traumatic (old) 721.7
  - tuberculous (see also Tuberculosis) 015.0 ✓5 [720.81]
- staphylococcal 711.0 ✓5
- streptococcal 711.0 ✓5
- suppurative 711.0 ✓5
- syphilitic 094.0 [713.5]
  - congenital 090.49 [713.5]
- syphilitica deformans (Charcôt) 094.0 [713.5]
- temporomandibular joint 524.69
- thoracic (see also Spondylosis, thoracic) 721.2
- toxic of menopause 716.3 ✓5
- transient 716.4 ✓5
- traumatic (chronic) (old) (post) 716.1 ✓5
  - current injury — see nature of injury
- tuberculous (see also Tuberculosis, arthritis) 015.9 ✓5 [711.4] ✓5
- urethritica 099.3 [711.1] ✓5
- urica, uratic 274.0
- venereal 099.3 [711.1] ✓5
- vertebral (see also Arthritis, spine) 721.90
- villous 716.8 ✓5
- von Bechterew's 720.0

Arthrocele (see also Effusion, joint) 719.0 ✓5
Arthrochondritis — see Arthritis
Arthrodesis status V45.4
Arthrodynia (see also Pain, joint) 719.4 ✓5
- psychogenic 307.89

Arthrodysplasia 755.9
Arthrofibrosis, joint (see also Ankylosis) 718.5 ✓5
Arthrogryposis 728.3
- multiplex, congenita 754.89

Arthrokatadysis 715.35
Arthrolithiasis 274.0
Arthro-onychodysplasia 756.89
Arthro-osteo-onychodysplasia 756.89
Arthropathy (see also Arthritis) 716.9 ✓5

> Note — Use the following fifth-digit subclassification with categories 711-712, 716:
>
> 0 site unspecified
> 1 shoulder region
> 2 upper arm
> 3 forearm
> 4 hand
> 5 pelvic region and thigh
> 6 lower leg
> 7 ankle and foot
> 8 other specified sites
> 9 multiple sites

- Behçets 136.1 [711.2] ✓5
- Charcôt's 094.0 [713.5]
  - diabetic 250.6 ✓5 [713.5]
  - syringomyelic 336.0 [713.5]
  - tabetic 094.0 [713.5]
- crystal (-induced) — see Arthritis, due to crystals
- gouty 274.0
- neurogenic, neuropathic (Charcôt's) (tabetic) 094.0 [713.5]
  - diabetic 250.6 ✓5 [713.5]
  - nonsyphilitic NEC 349.9 [713.5]
  - syringomyelic 336.0 [713.5]
- postdysenteric NEC 009.0 [711.3] ✓5
- postrheumatic, chronic (Jaccoud's) 714.4
- psoriatic 696.0
- pulmonary 731.2
- specified NEC 716.8 ✓5
- syringomyelia 336.0 [713.5]
- tabes dorsalis 094.0 [713.5]
- tabetic 094.0 [713.5]
- transient 716.4 ✓5
- traumatic 716.1 ✓5
- uric acid 274.0

Arthophyte (see also Loose, body, joint) 718.1 ✓5
Arthrophytis 719.80
- ankle 719.87
- elbow 719.82
- foot 719.87
- hand 719.84
- hip 719.85
- knee 719.86
- multiple sites 719.89
- pelvic region 719.85
- shoulder (region) 719.81
- specified site NEC 719.88
- wrist 719.83

Arthropyosis (see also Arthritis, pyogenic) 711.0 ✓5
Arthrosis (deformans) (degenerative) (see also Osteoarthrosis) 715.9 ✓5
- Charcôt's 094.0 [713.5]
- polyarticular 715.09
- spine (see also Spondylosis) 721.90

Arthus' phenomenon 995.2
- due to
  - correct substance properly administered 995.2
  - overdose or wrong substance given or taken 977.9
    - specified drug — see Table of Drugs and Chemicals
  - serum 999.5

Articular — see also condition
- disc disorder (reducing or non-reducing) 524.63
- spondylolisthesis 756.12

Index to Diseases

Artificial
- device (prosthetic) — see Fitting, device
- insemination V26.1
- menopause (states) (symptoms) (syndrome) 627.4
- opening status (functioning) (without complication) V44.9
  - anus (colostomy) V44.3
  - colostomy V44.3
  - cystostomy V44.50
    - appendico-vesicostomy V44.52
    - cutaneous-vesicostomy V44.51
    - specified type NEC V44.59
  - enterostomy V44.4
  - gastrostomy V44.1
  - ileostomy V44.2
  - intestinal tract NEC V44.4
  - jejunostomy V44.4
  - nephrostomy V44.6
  - specified site NEC V44.8
  - tracheostomy V44.0
  - ureterostomy V44.6
  - urethrostomy V44.6
  - urinary tract NEC V44.6
  - vagina V44.7
- vagina status V44.7

ARV (disease) (illness) (infection) — see Human immunodeficiency virus (disease) (illness) (infection)

Arytenoid — see condition
Asbestosis (occupational) 501
Asboe-Hansen's disease (incontinentia pigmenti) 757.33
Ascariasis (intestinal) (lung) 127.0
Ascaridiasis 127.0
Ascaris 127.0
- lumbricoides (infestation) 127.0
- pneumonia 127.0

Ascending — see condition
Aschoff's bodies (see also Myocarditis, rheumatic) 398.0
Ascites 789.5
- abdominal NEC 789.5
- cancerous (M80000/6) 197.6
- cardiac 428.0
- chylous (nonfilarial) 457.8
  - filarial (see also Infestation, filarial) 125.9
- congenital 778.0
- due to S. japonicum 120.2
- fetal, causing fetopelvic disproportion 653.7 ✓5
- heart 428.0
- joint (see also Effusion, joint) 719.0 ✓5
- malignant (M8000/6) 197.6
- pseudochylous 789.5
- syphilitic 095.2
- tuberculous (see also Tuberculosis) 014.0 ✓5

Ascorbic acid (vitamin C) **deficiency** (scurvy) 267
ASCUS (atypical squamous cell changes of undetermined significance) ●
- favor benign 795.01 ●
- favor dysplasia 795.02 ●

ASCVD (arteriosclerotic cardiovascular disease) 429.2

Aseptic — see condition
Asherman's syndrome 621.5
Asialia 527.7
Asiatic cholera (see also Cholera) 001.9 ▶◀
Asocial personality or trends 301.7
Asomatognosia 781.8
Aspergillosis 117.3
- with pneumonia 117.3 [484.6]
- allergic bronchopulmonary 518.6
- nonsyphilitic NEC 117.3

Aspergillus (flavus) (fumigatus) (infection) (terreus) 117.3
Aspermatogenesis 606.0
Aspermia (testis) 606.0
Asphyxia, asphyxiation (by) 799.0
- antenatal — see Distress, fetal
- bedclothes 994.7
- birth (see also Ashpyxia, newborn) 768.9
- bunny bag 994.7
- carbon monoxide 986

Index to Diseases

Asphyxia, asphyxiation — *continued*
  caul (*see also* Asphyxia, newborn)
  cave-in 994.7
    crushing — *see* Injury, internal, intrathoracic organs
  constriction 994.7
  crushing — *see* Injury, internal, intrathoracic organs
  drowning 994.1
  fetal, affecting newborn 768.9 ▲
  food or foreign body (in larynx) 933.1
    bronchioles 934.8
    bronchus (main) 934.1
    lung 934.8
    nasopharynx 933.0
    nose, nasal passages 932
    pharynx 933.0
    respiratory tract 934.9
      specified part NEC 934.8
    throat 933.0
    trachea 934.0
  gas, fumes, or vapor NEC 987.9
    specified — *see* Table of Drugs and Chemicals
  gravitational changes 994.7
  hanging 994.7
  inhalation — *see* Inhalation
  intrauterine
    fetal death (before onset of labor) 768.0
      during labor 768.1
    liveborn infant — *see* Distress, fetal, liveborn infant
  local 443.0
  mechanical 994.7
    during birth (*see also* Distress, fetal) 768.9 ▲
  mucus 933.1
    bronchus (main) 934.1
    larynx 933.1
    lung 934.8
    nasal passages 932
    newborn 770.1
    pharynx 933.0
    respiratory tract 934.9
      specfied part NEC 934.8
    throat 933.0
    trachea 934.0
    vaginal (fetus or newborn) 770.1
  newborn 768.9
    blue 768.6
    livida 768.6
    mild or moderate 768.6
    pallida 768.5
    severe 768.5
    white 768.5
  pathological 799.0
  plastic bag 994.7
  postnatal (*see also* Asphyxia, newborn) 768.9
    mechanical 994.7
  pressure 994.7
  reticularis 782.61
  strangulation 994.7
  submersion 994.1
  traumatic NEC — *see* Injury, internal, intrathoracic organs
  vomiting, vomitus — *see* Asphyxia, food or foreign body

Aspiration
  acid pulmonary (syndrome) 997.3
    obstetric 668.0 ✓5ᵗʰ
  amniotic fluid 770.1
  bronchitis 507.0
  contents of birth canal 770.1
  fetal pneumonitis 770.1
  food, foreign body, or gasoline (with asphyxiation) — *see* Asphyxia, food or foreign body
  meconium 770.1
  mucus 933.1
    into
      bronchus (main) 934.1
      lung 934.8
      respiratory tract 934.9
        specified part NEC 934.8
      trachea 934.0
    newborn 770.1
    vaginal (fetus or newborn) 770.1

Aspiration — *continued*
  newborn 770.1
  pneumonia 507.0
  pneumonitis 507.0
    fetus or newborn 770.1
    obstetric 668.0 ✓5ᵗʰ
  syndrome of newborn (massive) (meconium) 770.1
  vernix caseosa 770.1

Asplenia 759.0
  with mesocardia 746.87

Assam fever 085.0

Assimilation, pelvis
  with disproportion 653.2 ✓5ᵗʰ
    affecting fetus or newborn 763.1
    causing obstructed labor 660.1 ✓5ᵗʰ
      affecting fetus or newborn 763.1

Assmann's focus (*see also* Tuberculosis) 011.0 ✓5ᵗʰ

Astasia (-asbasia) 307.9
  hysterical 300.11

Asteatosis 706.8
  cutis 706.8

Astereognosis 780.99 ▲

Asterixis 781.3
  in liver disease 572.8

Asteroid hyalitis 379.22

Asthenia, asthenic 780.79
  cardiac (*see also* Failure, heart) 428.9
    psychogenic 306.2
  cardiovascular (*see also* Failure, heart) 428.9
    psychogenic 306.2
  heart (*see also* Failure, heart) 428.9
    psychogenic 306.2
  hysterical 300.11
  myocardial (*see also* Failure, heart) 428.9
    psychogenic 306.2
  nervous 300.5
  neurocirculatory 306.2
  neurotic 300.5
  psychogenic 300.5
  psychoneurotic 300.5
  psychophysiologic 300.5
  reaction, psychoneurotic 300.5
  senile 797
  Stiller's 780.79
  tropical anhidrotic 705.1

Asthenopia 368.13
  accommodative 367.4
  hysterical (muscular) 300.11
  psychogenic 306.7

Asthenospermia 792.2

Asthma, asthmatic (bronchial) (catarrh) (spasmodic) 493.9 ✓5ᵗʰ

Note — Use the following fifth-digit subclassification with category 493:

  0 *without mention of status asthmaticus or acute exacerbation or unspecified*
  1 *with status asthmaticus*
  2 *with acute exacerbation*

  with
    chronic obstructive pulmonary disease (COPD) 493.2 ✓5ᵗʰ
    hay fever 493.0 ✓5ᵗʰ
    rhinitis, allergic 493.0 ✓5ᵗʰ
  allergic 493.9 ✓5ᵗʰ
    stated cause (external allergen) 493.0 ✓5ᵗʰ
  atopic 493.0 ✓5ᵗʰ
  cardiac (*see also* Failure, ventricular, left) 428.1
  cardiobronchial (*see also* Failure, ventricular, left) 428.1
  cardiorenal (*see also* Hypertension, cardiorenal) 404.90
  childhood 493.0 ✓5ᵗʰ
  colliers' 500
  croup 493.9 ✓5ᵗʰ
  detergent 507.8
  due to
    detergent 507.8
    inhalation of fumes 506.3
    internal immunological process 493.0 ✓5ᵗʰ
  endogenous (intrinsic) 493.1 ✓5ᵗʰ

Asthma, asthmatic — *continued*
  eosinophilic 518.3
  exogenous (cosmetics) (dander or dust) (drugs) (dust) (feathers) (food) (hay) (platinum) (pollen) 493.0 ✓5ᵗʰ
  extrinsic 493.0 ✓5ᵗʰ
  grinders' 502
  hay 493.0 ✓5ᵗʰ
  heart (*see also* Failure, ventricular, left) 428.1
  IgE 493.0 ✓5ᵗʰ
  infective 493.1 ✓5ᵗʰ
  intrinsic 493.1 ✓5ᵗʰ
  Kopp's 254.8
  late-onset 493.1 ✓5ᵗʰ
  meat-wrappers' 506.9
  Millar's (laryngismus stridulus) 478.75
  millstone makers' 502
  miners' 500
  Monday morning 504
  New Orleans (epidemic) 493.0 ✓5ᵗʰ
  platinum 493.0 ✓5ᵗʰ
  pneumoconiotic (occupational) NEC 505
  potters' 502
  psychogenic 316 [493.9] ✓5ᵗʰ
  pulmonary eosinophilic 518.3
  red cedar 495.8
  Rostan's (*see also* Failure, ventricular, left) 428.1
  sandblasters' 502
  sequoiosis 495.8
  stonemasons' 502
  thymic 254.8
  tuberculous (*see also* Tuberculosis, pulmonary) 011.9 ✓5ᵗʰ
  Wichmann's (laryngismus stridulus) 478.75
  wood 495.8

Astigmatism (compound) (congenital) 367.20
  irregular 367.22
  regular 367.21

Astroblastoma (M9430/3)
  nose 748.1
  specified site — *see* Neoplasm, by site, malignant
  unspecified site 191.9

Astrocytoma (cystic) (M9400/3)
  anaplastic type (M9401/3)
    specified site — *see* Neoplasm, by site, malignant
    unspecified site 191.9
  fibrillary (M9420/3)
    specified site — *see* Neoplasm, by site, malignant
    unspecified site 191.9
  fibrous (M9420/3)
    specified site — *see* Neoplasm, by site, malignant
    unspecified site 191.9
  gemistocytic (M9411/3)
    specified site — *see* Neoplasm, by site, malignant
    unspecified site 191.9
  juvenile (M9421/3)
    specified site — *see* Neoplasm, by site, malignant
    unspecified site 191.9
  nose 748.1
  pilocytic (M9421/3)
    specified site — *see* Neoplasm, by site, malignant
    unspecified site 191.9
  piloid (M9421/3)
    specified site — *see* Neoplasm, by site, malignant
    unspecified site 191.9
  protoplasmic (M9410/3)
    specified site — *see* Neoplasm, by site, malignant
    unspecified site 191.9
  specified site — *see* Neoplasm, by site, malignant
  subependymal (M9383/1) 237.5
    giant cell (M9384/1) 237.5
  unspecified site 191.9

Astroglioma (M9400/3)
  nose 748.1
  specified site — *see* Neoplasm, by site, malignant
  unspecified site 191.9

Asymbolia

Asymbolia 784.60
Asymmetrical breathing 786.09
Asymmetry — *see also* Distortion
    chest 786.9
    face 754.0
    jaw NEC 524.12
        maxillary 524.11
    pelvis with disproportion 653.0 ✓5ᵗʰ
        affecting fetus or newborn 763.1
        causing obstructed labor 660.1 ✓5ᵗʰ
            affecting fetus or newborn 763.1
Asynergia 781.3
Asynergy 781.3
    ventricular 429.89
Asystole (heart) (*see also* Arrest, cardiac) 427.5
Ataxia, ataxy, ataxic 781.3
    acute 781.3
    brain 331.89
    cerebellar 334.3
        hereditary (Marie's) 334.2
        in
            alcoholism 303.9 ✓5ᵗʰ [334.4]
            myxedema (*see also* Myxedema) 244.9 [334.4]
            neoplastic disease NEC 239.9 [334.4]
    cerebral 331.89
    family, familial 334.2
        cerebral (Marie's) 334.2
        spinal (Friedreich's) 334.0
    Friedreich's (heredofamilial) (spinal) 334.0
    frontal lobe 781.3
    gait 781.2
        hysterical 300.11
    general 781.3
    hereditary NEC 334.2
        cerebellar 334.2
        spastic 334.1
        spinal 334.0
    heredofamilial (Marie's) 334.2
    hysterical 300.11
    locomotor (progressive) 094.0
        diabetic 250.6 ✓5ᵗʰ [337.1]
    Marie's (cerebellar) (heredofamilial) 334.2
    nonorganic origin 307.9
    partial 094.0
    postchickenpox 052.7
    progressive locomotor 094.0
    psychogenic 307.9
    Sanger-Brown's 334.2
    spastic 094.0
        hereditary 334.1
        syphilitic 094.0
    spinal
        hereditary 334.0
        progressive locomotor 094.0
    telangiectasia 334.8
Ataxia-telangiectasia 334.8
Atelectasis (absorption collapse) (complete) (compression) (massive) (partial) (postinfective) (pressure collapse) (pulmonary) (relaxation) 518.0
    newborn (congenital) (partial) 770.5
        primary 770.4
    primary 770.4
    tuberculous (*see also* Tuberculosis, pulmonary) 011.9 ✓5ᵗʰ
Ateleiosis, ateliosis 253.3
Atelia — *see* Distortion
Ateliosis 253.3
Atelocardia 746.9
Atelomyelia 742.59
Athelia 757.6
Atheroembolism
    extremity
        lower 445.02
        upper 445.01
    kidney 445.81
    specified site NEC 445.89
Atheroma, atheromatous (*see also* Arteriosclerosis) 440.9
    aorta, aortic 440.0
        valve (*see also* Endocarditis, aortic) 424.1
    artery — *see* Arteriosclerosis

Atheroma, atheromatous (*see also* Arteriosclerosis) — *continued*
    basilar (artery) (*see also* Occlusion, artery, basilar) 433.0 ✓5ᵗʰ
    carotid (artery) (common) (internal) (*see also* Occlusion, artery, carotid) 433.1 ✓5ᵗʰ
    cerebral (arteries) 437.0
    coronary (artery) — *see* Arteriosclerosis, coronary
    degeneration — *see* Arteriosclerosis
    heart, cardiac — *see* Arteriosclerosis, coronary
    mitral (valve) 424.0
    myocardium, myocardial — *see* Arteriosclerosis, coronary
    pulmonary valve (heart) (*see also* Endocarditis, pulmonary) 424.3
    skin 706.2
    tricuspid (heart) (valve) 424.2
    valve, valvular — *see* Endocarditis
    vertebral (artery) (*see also* Occlusion, artery, vertebral) 433.2 ✓5ᵗʰ
Atheromatosis — *see also* Arteriosclerosis
    arterial, congenital 272.8
Atherosclerosis — *see* Arteriosclerosis
Athetosis (acquired) 781.0
    bilateral 333.7
    congenital (bilateral) 333.7
    double 333.7
    unilateral 781.0
Athlete's
    foot 110.4
    heart 429.3
Athletic team examination V70.3
Athrepsia 261
Athyrea (acquired) (*see also* Hypothyroidism) 244.9
    congenital 243
Athyreosis (congenital) 243
    acquired — *see* Hypothyroidism
Athyroidism (acquired) (*see also* Hypothyroidism) 244.9
    congenital 243
Atmospheric pyrexia 992.0
Atonia, atony, atonic
    abdominal wall 728.2
    bladder (sphincter) 596.4
        neurogenic NEC 596.54
            with cauda equina syndrome 344.61
    capillary 448.9
    cecum 564.89
        psychogenic 306.4
    colon 564.89
        psychogenic 306.4
    congenital 779.89
    dyspepsia 536.3
        psychogenic 306.4
    intestine 564.89
        psychogenic 306.4
    stomach 536.3
        neurotic or psychogenic 306.4
        psychogenic 306.4
    uterus 666.1 ✓5ᵗʰ
        affecting fetus or newborn 763.7
    vesical 596.4
Atopy NEC V15.09
Atransferrinemia, congenital 273.8
Atresia, atretic (congenital) 759.89
    alimentary organ or tract NEC 751.8
        lower 751.2
        upper 750.8
    ani, anus, anal (canal) 751.2
    aorta 747.22
        with hypoplasia of ascending aorta and defective development of left ventricle (with mitral valve atresia) 746.7
        arch 747.11
        ring 747.21
    aortic (orifice) (valve) 746.89
        arch 747.11
    aqueduct of Sylvius 742.3
        with spina bifida (*see also* Spina bifida) 741.0 ✓5ᵗʰ
    artery NEC (*see also* Atresia, blood vessel) 747.60
        cerebral 747.81

Atresia, atretic — *continued*
    artery NEC (*see also* Atresia, blood vessel) — *continued*
        coronary 746.85
        eye 743.58
        pulmonary 747.3
        umbilical 747.5
    auditory canal (external) 744.02
    bile, biliary duct (common) or passage 751.61
        acquired (*see also* Obstruction, biliary) 576.2
    bladder (neck) 753.6
    blood vessel (peripheral) NEC 747.60
        cerebral 747.81
        gastrointestinal 747.61
        lower limb 747.64
        pulmonary artery 747.3
        renal 747.62
        spinal 747.82
        upper limb 747.63
    bronchus 748.3
    canal, ear 744.02
    cardiac
        valve 746.89
            aortic 746.89
            mitral 746.89
            pulmonary 746.01
            tricuspid 746.1
    cecum 751.2
    cervix (acquired) 622.4
        congenital 752.49
        in pregnancy or childbirth 654.6 ✓5ᵗʰ
            affecting fetus or newborn 763.89
            causing obstructed labor 660.2 ✓5ᵗʰ
                affecting fetus or newborn 763.1
    choana 748.0
    colon 751.2
    cystic duct 751.61
        acquired 575.8
            with obstruction (*see also* Obstruction, gallbladder) 575.2
    digestive organs NEC 751.8
    duodenum 751.1
    ear canal 744.02
    ejaculatory duct 752.8
    epiglottis 748.3
    esophagus 750.3
    Eustachian tube 744.24
    fallopian tube (acquired) 628.2
        congenital 752.19
    follicular cyst 620.0
    foramen of
        Luschka 742.3
            with spina bifida (*see also* Spina bifida) 741.0 ✓5ᵗʰ
        Magendie 742.3
            with spina bifida (*see also* Spina bifida) 741.0 ✓5ᵗʰ
    gallbladder 751.69
    genital organ
        external
            female 752.49
            male NEC 752.8
                penis 752.69
        internal
            female 752.8
            male 752.8
    glottis 748.3
    gullet 750.3
    heart
        valve NEC 746.89
            aortic 746.89
            mitral 746.89
            pulmonary 746.01
            tricuspid 746.1
    hymen 752.42
        acquired 623.3
        postinfective 623.3
    ileum 751.1
    intestine (small) 751.1
        large 751.2
    iris, filtration angle (*see also* Buphthalmia) 743.20
    jejunum 751.1
    kidney 753.3
    lacrimal, apparatus 743.65
        acquired — *see* Stenosis, lacrimal

Index to Diseases

Atresia, atretic — continued
- larynx 748.3
- ligament, broad 752.19
- lung 748.5
- meatus urinarius 753.6
- mitral valve 746.89
  - with atresia or hypoplasia of aortic orifice or valve, with hypoplasia of ascending aorta and defective development of left ventricle 746.7
- nares (anterior) (posterior) 748.0
- nasolacrimal duct 743.65
- nasopharynx 748.8
- nose, nostril 748.0
  - acquired 738.0
- organ or site NEC — see Anomaly, specified type NEC
- osseous meatus (ear) 744.03
- oviduct (acquired) 628.2
  - congenital 752.19
- parotid duct 750.23
  - acquired 527.8
- pulmonary (artery) 747.3
  - valve 746.01
  - vein 747.49
- pulmonic 746.01
- pupil 743.46
- rectum 751.2
- salivary duct or gland 750.23
  - acquired 527.8
- sublingual duct 750.23
  - acquired 527.8
- submaxillary duct or gland 750.23
  - acquired 527.8
- trachea 748.3
- tricuspid valve 746.1
- ureter 753.29
- ureteropelvic junction 753.21
- ureterovesical orifice 753.22
- urethra (valvular) 753.6
- urinary tract NEC 753.29
- uterus 752.3
  - acquired 621.8
- vagina (acquired) 623.2
  - congenital 752.49
  - postgonococcal (old) 098.2
  - postinfectional 623.2
  - senile 623.2
- vascular NEC (see also Atresia, blood vessel) 747.60
  - cerebral 747.81
- vas deferens 752.8
- vein NEC (see also Atresia, blood vessel) 747.60
  - cardiac 746.89
  - great 747.49
  - portal 747.49
  - pulmonary 747.49
- vena cava (inferior) (superior) 747.49
- vesicourethral orifice 753.6
- vulva 752.49
  - acquired 624.8

Atrichia, atrichosis 704.00
- congenital (universal) 757.4

Atrioventricularis commune 745.69

Atrophia — see also Atrophy
- alba 709.09
- cutis 701.8
  - idiopathica progressiva 701.8
  - senilis 701.8
- dermatological, diffuse (idiopathic) 701.8
- flava hepatis (acuta) (subacuta) (see also Necrosis, liver) 570
- gyrata of choroid and retina (central) 363.54
  - generalized 363.57
- senilis 797
  - dermatological 701.8
- unguium 703.8
  - congenita 757.5

Atrophoderma, atrophodermia 701.9
- diffusum (idiopathic) 701.8
- maculatum 701.3
  - et striatum 701.3
    - due to syphilis 095.8
    - syphilitic 091.3
- neuriticum 701.8
- pigmentosum 757.33
- reticulatum symmetricum faciei 701.8

Atrophoderma, atrophodermia — continued
- senile 701.8
- symmetrical 701.8
- vermiculata 701.8

Atrophy, atrophic
- adrenal (autoimmune) (capsule) (cortex) (gland) 255.4
  - with hypofunction 255.4
- alveolar process or ridge (edentulous) 525.2
- appendix 543.9
- Aran-Duchenne muscular 335.21
- arm 728.2
- arteriosclerotic — see Arteriosclerosis
- arthritis 714.0
  - spine 720.9
- bile duct (any) 576.8
- bladder 596.8
- blanche (of Milian) 701.3
- bone (senile) 733.99
  - due to
    - disuse 733.7
    - infection 733.99
    - tabes dorsalis (neurogenic) 094.0
  - posttraumatic 733.99
- brain (cortex) (progressive) 331.9
  - with dementia 290.10
  - Alzheimer's 331.0
    - with dementia — see Alzheimer's, dementia
  - circumscribed (Pick's) 331.1
    - with dementia
      - with behavioral disturbance 331.1 [294.11]
      - without behavioral disturbance 331.1 [294.10]
  - congenital 742.4
  - hereditary 331.9
  - senile 331.2
- breast 611.4
  - puerperal, postpartum 676.3
- buccal cavity 528.9
- cardiac (brown) (senile) (see also Degeneration, myocardial) 429.1
- cartilage (infectional) (joint) 733.99
- cast, plaster of Paris 728.2
- cerebellar — see Atrophy, brain
- cerebral — see Atrophy, brain
- cervix (endometrium) (mucosa) (myometrium) (senile) (uteri) 622.8
  - menopausal 627.8
- Charcôt-Marie-Tooth 356.1
- choroid 363.40
  - diffuse secondary 363.42
  - hereditary (see also Dystrophy, choroid) 363.50
  - gyrate
    - central 363.54
    - diffuse 363.57
    - generalized 363.57
  - senile 363.41
- ciliary body 364.57
- colloid, degenerative 701.8
- conjunctiva (senile) 372.89
- corpus cavernosum 607.89
- cortical (see also Atrophy, brain) 331.9
- Cruveilhier's 335.21
- cystic duct 576.8
- dacryosialadenopathy 710.2
- degenerative
  - colloid 701.3
  - senile 701.3
- Déjérine-Thomas 333.0
- diffuse idiopathic, dermatological 701.8
- disuse
  - bone 733.7
  - muscle 728.2
- Duchenne-Aran 335.21
- ear 388.9
- edentulous alveolar ridge 525.2
- emphysema, lung 492.8
- endometrium (senile) 621.8
  - cervix 622.8
- enteric 569.89
- epididymis 608.3
- eyeball, cause unknown 360.41
- eyelid (senile) 374.50
- facial (skin) 701.9

Atrophy, atrophic — continued
- facioscapulohumeral (Landouzy-Déjérine) 359.1
- fallopian tube (senile), acquired 620.3
- fatty, thymus (gland) 254.8
- gallbladder 575.8
- gastric 537.89
- gastritis (chronic) 535.1
- gastrointestinal 569.89
- genital organ, male 608.89
- glandular 289.3
- globe (phthisis bulbi) 360.41
- gum 523.2
- hair 704.2
- heart (brown) (senile) (see also Degeneration, myocardial) 429.1
- hemifacial 754.0
  - Romberg 349.89
- hydronephrosis 591
- infantile 261
  - paralysis, acute (see also Poliomyelitis, with paralysis) 045.1
- intestine 569.89
- iris (generalized) (postinfectional) (sector shaped) 364.59
  - essential 364.51
  - progressive 364.51
  - sphincter 364.54
- kidney (senile) (see also Sclerosis, renal) 587
  - with hypertension (see also Hypertension, kidney) 403.90
  - congenital 753.0
  - hydronephrotic 591
  - infantile 753.0
- lacrimal apparatus (primary) 375.13
  - secondary 375.14
- Landouzy-Déjérine 359.1
- laryngitis, infection 476.0
- larynx 478.79
- Leber's optic 377.16
- lip 528.5
- liver (acute) (subacute) (see also Necrosis, liver) 570
  - chronic (yellow) 571.8
  - yellow (congenital) 570
    - with
      - abortion — see Abortion, by type, with specified complication NEC
      - ectopic pregnancy (see also categories 633.0-633.9) 639.8
      - molar pregnancy (see also categories 630-632) 639.8
    - chronic 571.8
    - complicating pregnancy 646.7
    - following
      - abortion 639.8
      - ectopic or molar pregnancy 639.8
    - from injection, inoculation or transfusion (onset within 8 months after administration) — see Hepatitis, viral
    - healed 571.5
    - obstetric 646.7
    - postabortal 639.8
    - postimmunization — see Hepatitis, viral
    - posttransfusion — see Hepatitis, viral
    - puerperal, postpartum 674.8
- lung 518.89
  - congenital 748.69
- macular (dermatological) 701.3
  - syphilitic, skin 091.3
  - striated 095.8
- muscle, muscular 728.2
  - disuse 728.2
  - Duchenne-Aran 335.21
  - extremity (lower) (upper) 728.2
  - familial spinal 335.11
  - general 728.2
  - idiopathic 728.2
  - infantile spinal 335.0
  - myelopathic (progressive) 335.10
  - myotonic 359.2
  - neuritic 356.1
  - neuropathic (peroneal) (progressive) 356.1
  - peroneal 356.1
  - primary (idiopathic) 728.2
  - progressive (familial) (hereditary) (pure) 335.21

Atrophy, atrophic

Atrophy, atrophic — *continued*
  muscle, muscular — *continued*
    progressive — *continued*
      adult (spinal) 335.19
      infantile (spinal) 335.0
      juvenile (spinal) 335.11
      spinal 335.10
        adult 335.19
        Aran-Duchenne 335.10
        hereditary or familial 335.11
        infantile 335.0
      pseudohypertrophic 359.1
      spinal (progressive) 335.10
        adult 335.19
        Aran-Duchenne 335.21
        familial 335.11
        hereditary 335.11
        infantile 335.0
        juvenile 335.11
      syphilitic 095.6
    myocardium (*see also* Degeneration, myocardial) 429.1
    myometrium (senile) 621.8
      cervix 622.8
    myotatic 728.2
    myotonia 359.2
  nail 703.8
    congenital 757.5
  nasopharynx 472.2
  nerve — *see also* Disorder, nerve
    abducens 378.54
    accessory 352.4
    acoustic or auditory 388.5
    cranial 352.9
      first (olfactory) 352.0
      second (optic) (*see also* Atrophy, optic nerve) 377.10
      third (oculomotor)(partial) 378.51
        total 378.52
      fourth (trochlear) 378.53
      fifth (trigeminal) 350.8
      sixth (abducens) 378.54
      seventh (facial) 351.8
      eighth (auditory) 388.5
      ninth (glossopharyngeal) 352.2
      tenth (pneumogastric) (vagus) 352.3
      eleventh (accessory) 352.4
      twelfth (hypoglossal) 352.5
    facial 351.8
    glossopharyngeal 352.2
    hypoglossal 352.5
    oculomotor (partial) 378.51
      total 378.52
    olfactory 352.0
    peripheral 355.9
    pneumogastric 352.3
    trigeminal 350.8
    trochlear 378.53
    vagus (pneumogastric) 352.3
  nervous system, congenital 742.8
  neuritic (*see also* Disorder, nerve) 355.9
  neurogenic NEC 355.9
    bone
      tabetic 094.0
  nutritional 261
  old age 797
  olivopontocerebellar 333.0
  optic nerve (ascending) (descending) (infectional) (nonfamilial) (papillomacular bundle) (postretinal) (secondary NEC) (simple) 377.10
    associated with retinal dystrophy 377.13
    dominant hereditary 377.16
    glaucomatous 377.14
    hereditary (dominant) (Leber's) 377.16
    Leber's (hereditary) 377.16
    partial 377.15
    postinflammatory 377.12
    primary 377.11
    syphilitic 094.84
      congenital 090.49
      tabes dorsalis 094.0
  orbit 376.45
  ovary (senile), acquired 620.3
  oviduct (senile), acquired 620.3
  palsy, diffuse 335.20
  pancreas (duct) (senile) 577.8

Atrophy, atrophic — *continued*
  papillary muscle 429.81
  paralysis 355.9
  parotid gland 527.0
  patches skin 701.3
    senile 701.8
  penis 607.89
  pharyngitis 472.1
  pharynx 478.29
  pluriglandular 258.8
  polyarthritis 714.0
  prostate 602.2
  pseudohypertrophic 359.1
  renal (*see also* Sclerosis, renal) 587
  reticulata 701.8
  retina (*see also* Degeneration, retina) 362.60
    hereditary (*see also* Dystrophy, retina) 362.70
  rhinitis 472.0
  salivary duct or gland 527.0
  scar NEC 709.2
  sclerosis, lobar (of brain) 331.0
    with dementia
      with behavioral disturbance 331.1 [294.11]
      without behavioral disturbance 331.1 [294.10]
  scrotum 608.89
  seminal vesicle 608.89
  senile 797
    degenerative, of skin 701.3
  skin (patches) (senile) 701.8
  spermatic cord 608.89
  spinal (cord) 336.8
    acute 336.8
    muscular (chronic) 335.10
      adult 335.19
      familial 335.11
      juvenile 335.10
    paralysis 335.10
      acute (*see also* Poliomyelitis, with paralysis) 045.1 ✓5ᵗʰ
  spine (column) 733.99
  spleen (senile) 289.59
  spots (skin) 701.3
    senile 701.8
  stomach 537.89
  striate and macular 701.3
    syphilitic 095.8
  subcutaneous 701.9
    due to injection 999.9
  sublingual gland 527.0
  submaxillary gland 527.0
  Sudeck's 733.7
  suprarenal (autoimmune) (capsule) (gland) 255.4
    with hypofunction 255.4
  tarso-orbital fascia, congenital 743.66
  testis 608.3
  thenar, partial 354.0
  throat 478.29
  thymus (fat) 254.8
  thyroid (gland) 246.8
    with
      cretinism 243
      myxedema 244.9
      congenital 243
  tongue (senile) 529.8
    papillae 529.4
    smooth 529.4
  trachea 519.1
  tunica vaginalis 608.89
  turbinate 733.99
  tympanic membrane (nonflaccid) 384.82
    flaccid 384.81
  ulcer (*see also* Ulcer, skin) 707.9
  upper respiratory tract 478.9
  uterus, uterine (acquired) (senile) 621.8
    cervix 622.8
    due to radiation (intended effect) 621.8
  vagina (senile) 627.3
  vascular 459.89
  vas deferens 608.89
  vertebra (senile) 733.99
  vulva (primary) (senile) 624.1
  Werdnig-Hoffmann 335.0

Atrophy, atrophic — *continued*
  yellow (acute) (congenital) (liver) (subacute) (*see also* Necrosis, liver) 570
    chronic 571.8
    resulting from administration of blood, plasma, serum, or other biological substance (within 8 months of administration) — *see* Hepatitis, viral

Attack
  akinetic (*see also* Epilepsy) 345.0 ✓5ᵗʰ
  angina — *see* Angina
  apoplectic (*see also* Disease, cerebrovascular, acute) 436
  benign shuddering 333.93
  bilious — *see* Vomiting
  cataleptic 300.11
  cerebral (*see also* Disease, cerebrovascular, acute) 436
  coronary (*see also* Infarct, myocardium) 410.9 ✓5ᵗʰ
  cyanotic, newborn 770.83 ▲
  epileptic (*see also* Epilepsy) 345.9 ✓5ᵗʰ
  epileptiform 780.39
  heart (*see also* Infarct, myocardium) 410.9 ✓5ᵗʰ
  hemiplegia (*see also* Disease, cerebrovascular, acute) 436
  hysterical 300.11
  jacksonian (*see also* Epilepsy) 345.5 ✓5ᵗʰ
  myocardium, myocardial (*see also* Infarct, myocardium) 410.9 ✓5ᵗʰ
  myoclonic (*see also* Epilepsy) 345.1 ✓5ᵗʰ
  panic 300.01
  paralysis (*see also* Disease, cerebrovascular, acute) 436
  paroxysmal 780.39
  psychomotor (*see also* Epilepsy) 345.4 ✓5ᵗʰ
  salaam (*see also* Epilepsy) 345.6 ✓5ᵗʰ
  schizophreniform (*see also* Schizophrenia) 295.4 ✓5ᵗʰ
  sensory and motor 780.39
  syncope 780.2
  toxic, cerebral 780.39
  transient ischemic (TIA) 435.9
  unconsciousness 780.2
    hysterical 300.11
  vasomotor 780.2
  vasovagal (idiopathic) (paroxysmal) 780.2

Attention to
  artificial opening (of) V55.9
    digestive tract NEC V55.4
    specified site NEC V55.8
    urinary tract NEC V55.6
    vagina V55.7
  colostomy V55.3
  cystostomy V55.5
  gastrostomy V55.1
  ileostomy V55.2
  jejunostomy V55.4
  nephrostomy V55.6
  surgical dressings V58.3
  sutures V58.3
  tracheostomy V55.0
  ureterostomy V55.6
  urethrostomy V55.6

Attrition
  gum 523.2
  teeth (excessive) (hard tissues) 521.1

Atypical — *see also* condition
  distribution, vessel (congenital) (peripheral) NEC 747.60
  endometrium 621.9
  glandular cell changes of undetermined significance ●
    favor benign (AGCUS favor benign) 795.01 ●
    favor dysplasia (AGCUS favor dysplasia) 795.02 ●
  kidney 593.89
  squamous cell changes of undetermined significance ●
    favor benign (ASCUS favor benign) 795.01 ●
    favor dysplasia (ASCUS favor dysplasia) 795.02 ●

Atypism, cervix 622.1
Audible tinnitus (*see also* Tinnitus) 388.30

Auditory — see condition
Audry's syndrome (acropachyderma) 757.39
Aujeszky's disease 078.89
Aura, jacksonian (see also Epilepsy) 345.5
Aurantiasis, cutis 278.3
Auricle, auricular — see condition
Auriculotemporal syndrome 350.8
Australian
 Q fever 083.0
 X disease 062.4
Autism, autistic (child) (infantile) 299.0
Autodigestion 799.8
Autoerythrocyte sensitization 287.2
Autographism 708.3
Autoimmune
 cold sensitivity 283.0
 disease NEC 279.4
 hemolytic anemia 283.0
 thyroiditis 245.2
Autoinfection, septic — see Septicemia
Autointoxication 799.8
Automatism 348.8
 epileptic (see also Epilepsy) 345.4
 paroxysmal, idiopathic (see also Epilepsy) 345.4
Autonomic, autonomous
 bladder 596.54
  neurogenic NEC 596.54
   with cauda equina 344.61
 dysreflexia 337.3
 faciocephalalgia (see also Neuropathy, peripheral, autonomic) 337.9
 hysterical seizure 300.11
 imbalance (see also Neuropathy, peripheral, autonomic) 337.9
Autophony 388.40
Autosensitivity, erythrocyte 287.2
Autotopagnosia 780.99
Autotoxemia 799.8
Autumn — see condition
Avellis' syndrome 344.89
Aviators
 disease or sickness (see also Effect, adverse, high altitude) 993.2
 ear 993.0
 effort syndrome 306.2
Avitaminosis (multiple NEC) (see also Deficiency, vitamin) 269.2
 A 264.9
 B 266.9
  with
   beriberi 265.0
   pellagra 265.2
 B_1 265.1
 B_2 266.0
 B_6 266.1
 B_{12} 266.2
 C (with scurvy) 267
 D 268.9
  with
   osteomalacia 268.2
   rickets 268.0
 E 269.1
 G 266.0
 H 269.1
 K 269.0
 multiple 269.2
 nicotinic acid 265.2
 P 269.1
Avulsion (traumatic) 879.8
 blood vessel — see Injury, blood vessel, by site
 cartilage — see also Dislocation, by site
  knee, current (see also Tear, meniscus) 836.2
  symphyseal (inner), complicating delivery 665.6
 complicated 879.9
 diaphragm — see Injury, internal, diaphragm
 ear — see Wound, open, ear
 epiphysis of bone — see Fracture, by site
 external site other than limb — see Wound, open, by site
 eye 871.3

Avulsion — continued
 fingernail — see Wound, open, finger
 fracture — see Fracture, by site
 genital organs, external — see Wound, open, genital organs
 head (intracranial) NEC — see also Injury, intracranial, with open intracranial wound
  complete 874.9
  external site NEC 873.8
   complicated 873.9
 internal organ or site — see Injury, internal, by site
 joint — see also Dislocation, by site
  capsule — see Sprain, by site
  ligament — see Sprain, by site
 limb — see also Amputation, traumatic, by site
  skin and subcutaneous tissue — see Wound, open, by site
 muscle — see Sprain, by site
 nerve (root) — see Injury, nerve, by site
 scalp — see Wound, open, scalp
 skin and subcutaneous tissue — see Wound, open, by site
 symphyseal cartilage (inner), complicating delivery 665.6
 tendon — see also Sprain, by site
  with open wound — see Wound, open, by site
 toenail — see Wound, open, toe(s)
 tooth 873.63
  complicated 873.73
Awareness of heart beat 785.1
Axe grinders' disease 502
Axenfeld's anomaly or syndrome 743.44
Axilla, axillary — see also condition
 breast 757.6
Axonotmesis — see Injury, nerve, by site
Ayala's disease 756.89
Ayerza's disease or syndrome (pulmonary artery sclerosis with pulmonary hypertension) 416.0
Azoospermia 606.0
Azotemia 790.6
 meaning uremia (see also Uremia) 586
Aztec ear 744.29
Azorean disease (of the nervous system) 334.8
Azygos lobe, lung (fissure) 748.69

B

Baader's syndrome (erythema multiforme exudativum) 695.1
Baastrup's syndrome 721.5
Babesiasis 088.82
Babesiosis 088.82
Babington's disease (familial hemorrhagic telangiectasia) 448.0
Babinski's syndrome (cardiovascular syphilis) 093.89
Babinski-Fröhlich syndrome (adiposogenital dystrophy) 253.8
Babinski-Nageotte syndrome 344.89
Bacillary — see condition
Bacilluria 791.9
 asymptomatic, in pregnancy or puerperium 646.5
 tuberculous (see also Tuberculosis) 016.9
Bacillus — see also Infection, bacillus
 abortus infection 023.1
 anthracis infection 022.9
 coli
  infection 041.4
   generalized 038.42
   intestinal 008.00
  pyemia 038.42
  septicemia 038.42
 Flexner's 004.1
 fusiformis infestation 101
 mallei infection 024
 Shiga's 004.0
 suipestifer infection (see also Infection, Salmonella) 003.9

Back — see condition
Backache (postural) 724.5
 psychogenic 307.89
 sacroiliac 724.6
Backflow (pyelovenous) (see also Disease, renal) 593.9
Backknee (see also Genu, recurvatum) 736.5
Bacteremia 790.7
 with
  sepsis — see Septicemia
 during
  labor 659.3
  pregnancy 647.8
 newborn 771.83
Bacteria
 in blood (see also Bacteremia) 790.7
 in urine (see also Bacteriuria) 599.0
Bacterial — see condition
Bactericholia (see also Cholecystitis, acute) 575.0
Bacterid, bacteride (Andrews' pustular) 686.8
Bacteriuria, bacteruria 791.9
 with
  urinary tract infection 599.0
  asymptomatic 791.9
   in pregnancy or puerperium 646.5
    affecting fetus or newborn 760.1
Bad
 breath 784.9
 heart — see Disease, heart
 trip (see also Abuse, drugs, nondependent) 305.3
Baehr-Schiffrin disease (thrombotic thrombocytopenic purpura) 446.6
Baelz's disease (cheilitis glandularis apostematosa) 528.5
Baerensprung's disease (eczema marginatum) 110.3
Bagassosis (occupational) 495.1
Baghdad boil 085.1
Bagratuni's syndrome (temporal arteritis) 446.5
Baker's
 cyst (knee) 727.51
  tuberculous (see also Tuberculosis) 015.2
 itch 692.82
Bakwin-Krida syndrome (craniometaphyseal dysplasia) 756.89
Balanitis (circinata) (gangraenosa) (infectious) (vulgaris) 607.1
 amebic 006.8
 candidal 112.2
 chlamydial 099.53
 due to Ducrey's bacillus 099.0
 erosiva circinata et gangraenosa 607.1
 gangrenous 607.1
 gonococcal (acute) 098.0
  chronic or duration of 2 months or over 098.2
 nongonococcal 607.1
 phagedenic 607.1
 venereal NEC 099.8
 xerotica obliterans 607.81
Balanoposthitis 607.1
 chlamydial 099.53
 gonococcal (acute) 098.0
  chronic or duration of 2 months or over 098.2
 ulcerative NEC 099.8
Balanorrhagia — see Balanitis
Balantidiasis 007.0
Balantidiosis 007.0
Balbuties, balbutio 307.0
Bald
 patches on scalp 704.00
 tongue 529.4
Baldness (see also Alopecia) 704.00
Balfour's disease (chloroma) 205.3
Balint's syndrome (psychic paralysis of visual fixation) 368.16
Balkan grippe 083.0

Ball

Ball
    food 938
    hair 938
Ballantyne (-Runge) syndrome (postmaturity) 766.2
Balloon disease (see also Effect, adverse, high altitude) 993.2
Ballooning posterior leaflet syndrome 424.0
Baló's disease or concentric sclerosis 341.1
Bamberger's disease (hypertrophic pulmonary osteoarthropathy) 731.2
Bamberger-Marie disease (hypertrophic pulmonary osteoarthropathy) 731.2
Bamboo spine 720.0
Bancroft's filariasis 125.0
Band(s)
    adhesive (see also Adhesions, peritoneum) 568.0
    amniotic 658.8 ✓5ᵗʰ
        affecting fetus or newborn 762.8
    anomalous or congenital — see also Anomaly, specified type NEC
        atrial 746.9
        heart 746.9
        intestine 751.4
        omentum 751.4
        ventricular 746.9
    cervix 622.3
    gallbladder (congenital) 751.69
    intestinal (adhesive) (see also Adhesions, peritoneum) 568.0
        congenital 751.4
    obstructive (see also Obstruction, intestine) 560.81
    periappendiceal (congenital) 751.4
    peritoneal (adhesive) (see also Adhesions, peritoneum) 568.0
        with intestinal obstruction 560.81
        congenital 751.4
    uterus 621.5
    vagina 623.2
Bandl's ring (contraction)
    complicating delivery 661.4 ✓5ᵗʰ
        affecting fetus or newborn 763.7
Bang's disease (Brucella abortus) 023.1
Bangkok hemorrhagic fever 065.4
Bannister's disease 995.1
Bantam-Albright-Martin disease (pseudohypoparathyroidism) 275.49
Banti's disease or syndrome (with cirrhosis) (with portal hypertension) — see Cirrhosis, liver
Bar
    calcaneocuboid 755.67
    calcaneonavicular 755.67
    cubonavicular 755.67
    prostate 600.9
    talocalcaneal 755.67
Baragnosis 780.99 ▲
Barasheh, barashek 266.2
Barcoo disease or rot (see also Ulcer, skin) 707.9
Bard-Pic syndrome (carcinoma, head of pancreas) 157.0
Bärensprung's disease (eczema marginatum) 110.3
Baritosis 503
Barium lung disease 503
Barlow's syndrome (meaning mitral valve prolapse) 424.0
Barlow (-Möller) disease or syndrome (meaning infantile scurvy) 267
Barodontalgia 993.2
Baron Münchausen syndrome 301.51
Barosinusitis 993.1
Barotitis 993.0
Barotrauma 993.2
    odontalgia 993.2
    otitic 993.0
    sinus 993.1
Barraquer's disease or syndrome (progressive lipodystrophy) 272.6

Barré-Guillain syndrome 357.0
Barré-Liéou syndrome (posterior cervical sympathetic) 723.2
Barrel chest 738.3
Barrett's syndrome or ulcer (chronic peptic ulcer of esophagus) 530.2
Bársony-Polgár syndrome (corkscrew esophagus) 530.5
Bársony-Teschendorf syndrome (corkscrew esophagus) 530.5
Bartholin's
    adenitis (see also Bartholinitis) 616.8
    gland — see condition
Bartholinitis (suppurating) 616.8
    gonococcal (acute) 098.0
        chronic or duration of 2 months or over 098.2
Bartonellosis 088.0
Bartter's syndrome (secondary hyperaldosteronism with juxtaglomerular hyperplasia) 255.1
Basal — see condition
Basan's (hidrotic) ectodermal dysplasia 757.31
Baseball finger 842.13
Basedow's disease or syndrome (exophthalmic goiter) 242.0 ✓5ᵗʰ
Basic — see condition
Basilar — see condition
Bason's (hidrotic) ectodermal dysplasia 757.31
Basopenia 288.0
Basophilia 288.8
Basophilism (corticoadrenal) (Cushing's) (pituitary) (thymic) 255.0
Bassen-Kornzweig syndrome (abetalipoproteinemia) 272.5
Bat ear 744.29
Bateman's
    disease 078.0
    purpura (senile) 287.2
Bathing cramp 994.1
Bathophobia 300.23
Batten's disease, retina 330.1 [362.71]
Batten-Mayou disease 330.1 [362.71]
Batten-Steinert syndrome 359.2
Battered
    adult (syndrome) 995.81
    baby or child (syndrome) 995.54
    spouse (syndrome) 995.81
Battey mycobacterium infection 031.0
Battledore placenta — see Placenta, abnormal
Battle exhaustion (see also Reaction, stress, acute) 308.9
Baumgarten-Cruveilhier (cirrhosis) disease, or syndrome 571.5
Bauxite
    fibrosis (of lung) 503
    workers' disease 503
Bayle's disease (dementia paralytica) 094.1
Bazin's disease (primary) (see also Tuberculosis) 017.1 ✓5ᵗʰ
Beach ear 380.12
Beaded hair (congenital) 757.4
Beard's disease (neurasthenia) 300.5
Bearn-Kunkel (-Slater) syndrome (lupoid hepatitis) 571.49
Beat
    elbow 727.2
    hand 727.2
    knee 727.2
Beats
    ectopic 427.60
    escaped, heart 427.60
        postoperative 997.1
    premature (nodal) 427.60
        atrial 427.61
        auricular 427.61
        postoperative 997.1
        specified type NEC 427.69

Beats — continued
    premature (nodal) — continued
        supraventricular 427.61
        ventricular 427.69
Beau's
    disease or syndrome (see also Degeneration, myocardial) 429.1
    lines (transverse furrows on fingernails) 703.8
Bechterew's disease (ankylosing spondylitis) 720.0
Bechterew-Strümpell-Marie syndrome (ankylosing spondylitis) 720.0
Beck's syndrome (anterior spinal artery occlusion) 433.8 ✓5ᵗʰ
Becker's
    disease (idiopathic mural endomyocardial disease) 425.2
    dystrophy 359.1
Beckwith (-Wiedemann) syndrome 759.89
Bedclothes, asphyxiation or suffocation by 994.7
Bednar's aphthae 528.2
Bedsore 707.0
    with gangrene 707.0 [785.4]
Bedwetting (see also Enuresis) 788.36
Beer-drinkers' heart (disease) 425.5
Bee sting (with allergic or anaphylactic shock) 989.5
Begbie's disease (exophthalmic goiter) 242.0 ✓5ᵗʰ
Behavior disorder, disturbance — see also Disturbance, conduct
    antisocial, without manifest psychiatric disorder
        adolescent V71.02
        adult V71.01
        child V71.02
    dyssocial, without manifest psychiatric disorder
        adolescent V71.02
        adult V71.01
        child V71.02
    high risk — see Problem
Behçet's syndrome 136.1
Behr's disease 362.50
Beigel's disease or morbus (white piedra) 111.2
Bejel 104.0
Bekhterev's disease (ankylosing spondylitis) 720.0
Bekhterev-Strümpell-Marie syndrome (ankylosing spondylitis) 720.0
Belching (see also Eructation) 787.3
Bell's
    disease (see also Psychosis, affective) 296.0 ✓5ᵗʰ
    mania (see also Psychosis, affective) 296.0 ✓5ᵗʰ
    palsy, paralysis 351.0
        infant 767.5
        newborn 767.5
        syphilitic 094.89
    spasm 351.0
Bence-Jones albuminuria, albuminosuria, or proteinuria 791.0
Bends 993.3
Benedikt's syndrome (paralysis) 344.89
Benign — see also condition
    cellular changes, cervix 795.09 ●
    prostate
        hyperplasia 600.0
        neoplasm 222.2
Bennett's
    disease (leukemia) 208.9 ✓5ᵗʰ
    fracture (closed) 815.01
        open 815.11
Benson's disease 379.22
Bent
    back (hysterical) 300.11
    nose 738.0
        congenital 754.0
Bereavement V62.82
    as adjustment reaction 309.0
Berger's paresthesia (lower limb) 782.0
Bergeron's disease (hysteroepilepsy) 300.11

Beriberi (acute) (atrophic) (chronic) (dry) (subacute) (wet) 265.0
 with polyneuropathy 265.0 [357.4]
  heart (disease) 265.0 [425.7]
  leprosy 030.1
  neuritis 265.0 [357.4]
Berlin's disease or edema (traumatic) 921.3
Berloque dermatitis 692.72
Bernard-Horner syndrome (see also Neuropathy, peripheral, autonomic) 337.9
Bernard-Sergent syndrome (acute adrenocortical insufficiency) 255.4
Bernard-Soulier disease or thrombopathy 287.1
Bernhardt's disease or paresthesia 355.1
Bernhardt-Roth disease or syndrome (paresthesia) 355.1
Bernheim's syndrome (see also Failure, heart) 428.0
Bertielliasis 123.8
Bertolotti's syndrome (sacralization of fifth lumbar vertebra) 756.15
Berylliosis (acute) (chronic) (lung) (occupational) 503
Besnier's
 lupus pernio 135
 prurigo (atopic dermatitis) (infantile eczema) 691.8
Besnier-Boeck disease or sarcoid 135
Besnier-Boeck-Schaumann disease (sarcoidosis) 135
Best's disease 362.76
Bestiality 302.1
Beta-adrenergic hyperdynamic circulatory state 429.82
Beta-aminoisobutyric aciduria 277.2
Beta-mercaptolactate-cysteine disulfiduria 270.0
Beta thalassemia (major) (minor) (mixed) 282.4
Beurmann's disease (sporotrichosis) 117.1
Bezoar 938
 intestine 936
 stomach 935.2
Bezold's abscess (see also Mastoiditis) 383.01
Bianchi's syndrome (aphasia-apraxia-alexia) 784.69
Bicornuate or bicornis uterus 752.3
 in pregnancy or childbirth 654.0
  with obstructed labor 660.2
   affecting fetus or newborn 763.1
  affecting fetus or newborn 763.89
Bicuspid aortic valve 746.4
Biedl-Bardet syndrome 759.89
Bielschowsky's disease 330.1
Bielschowsky-Jansky
 amaurotic familial idiocy 330.1
 disease 330.1
Biemond's syndrome (obesity, polydactyly, and mental retardation) 759.89
Biermer's anemia or disease (pernicious anemia) 281.0
Biett's disease 695.4
Bifid (congenital) — see also Imperfect, closure
 apex, heart 746.89
 clitoris 752.49
 epiglottis 748.3
 kidney 753.3
 nose 748.1
 patella 755.64
 scrotum 752.8
 toe 755.66
 tongue 750.13
 ureter 753.4
 uterus 752.3
 uvula 749.02
  with cleft lip (see also Cleft, palate, with cleft lip) 749.20
Biforis uterus (suprasimplex) 752.3
Bifurcation (congenital) — see also Imperfect, closure
 gallbladder 751.69
 kidney pelvis 753.3

Bifurcation — see also Imperfect, closure — continued
 renal pelvis 753.3
 rib 756.3
 tongue 750.13
 trachea 748.3
 ureter 753.4
 urethra 753.8
 uvula 749.02
  with cleft lip (see also Cleft, palate, with cleft lip) 749.20
 vertebra 756.19
Bigeminal pulse 427.89
Bigeminy 427.89
Big spleen syndrome 289.4
Bilateral — see condition
Bile duct — see condition
Bile pigments in urine 791.4
Bilharziasis (see also Schistosomiasis) 120.9
 chyluria 120.0
 cutaneous 120.3
 galacturia 120.0
 hematochyluria 120.0
 intestinal 120.1
 lipemia 120.9
 lipuria 120.0
 Oriental 120.2
 piarhemia 120.9
 pulmonary 120.2
 tropical hematuria 120.0
 vesical 120.0
Biliary — see condition
Bilious (attack) — see also Vomiting
 fever, hemoglobinuric 084.8
Bilirubinuria 791.4
Biliuria 791.4
Billroth's disease
 meningocele (see also Spina bifida) 741.9
Bilobate placenta — see Placenta, abnormal
Bilocular
 heart 745.7
 stomach 536.8
Bing-Horton syndrome (histamine cephalgia) 346.2
Binswanger's disease or dementia 290.12
Biörck (-Thorson) syndrome (malignant carcinoid) 259.2
Biparta, bipartite — see also Imperfect, closure
 carpal scaphoid 755.59
 patella 755.64
 placenta — see Placenta, abnormal
 vagina 752.49
Bird
 face 756.0
 fanciers' lung or disease 495.2
Bird's disease (oxaluria) 271.8
Birth
 abnormal fetus or newborn 763.9
 accident, fetus or newborn — see Birth, injury
 complications in mother — see Delivery, complicated
 compression during NEC 767.9
 defect — see Anomaly
 delayed, fetus 763.9
 difficult NEC, affecting fetus or newborn 763.9
 dry, affecting fetus or newborn 761.1
 forced, NEC, affecting fetus or newborn 763.89
 forceps, affecting fetus or newborn 763.2
 hematoma of sternomastoid 767.8
 immature 765.1
  extremely 765.0
 inattention, after or at 995.52
 induced, affecting fetus or newborn 763.89
 infant — see Newborn
 injury NEC 767.9
  adrenal gland 767.8
  basal ganglia 767.0
  brachial plexus (paralysis) 767.6
  brain (compression) (pressure) 767.0
  cerebellum 767.0
  cerebral hemorrhage 767.0
  conjunctiva 767.8
  eye 767.8

Birth — continued
 injury NEC — continued
  fracture
   bone, any except clavicle or spine 767.3
   clavicle 767.2
   femur 767.3
   humerus 767.3
   long bone 767.3
   radius and ulna 767.3
   skeleton NEC 767.3
   skull 767.3
   spine 767.4
   tibia and fibula 767.3
  hematoma 767.8
   liver (subcapsular) 767.8
   mastoid 767.8
   skull 767.1
   sternomastoid 767.8
   testes 767.8
   vulva 767.8
  intracranial (edema) 767.0
  laceration
   brain 767.0
   by scalpel 767.8
   peripheral nerve 767.7
  liver 767.8
  meninges
   brain 767.0
   spinal cord 767.4
  nerves (cranial, peripheral) 767.7
   brachial plexus 767.6
   facial 767.5
  paralysis 767.7
   brachial plexus 767.6
   Erb (-Duchenne) 767.6
   facial nerve 767.5
   Klumpke (-Déjérine) 767.6
   radial nerve 767.6
   spinal (cord) (hemorrhage) (laceration) (rupture) 767.4
  rupture
   intracranial 767.0
   liver 767.8
   spinal cord 767.4
   spleen 767.8
   viscera 767.8
  scalp 767.1
  scalpel wound 767.8
  skeleton NEC 767.3
  specified NEC 767.8
  spinal cord 767.4
  spleen 767.8
  subdural hemorrhage 767.0
  tentorial, tear 767.0
  testes 767.8
  vulva 767.8
 instrumental, NEC, affecting fetus or newborn 763.2
 lack of care, after or at 995.52
 multiple
  affected by maternal complications of pregnancy 761.5
  healthy liveborn — see Newborn, multiple
 neglect, after or at 995.52
 newborn — see Newborn
 palsy or paralysis NEC 767.7
 precipitate, fetus or newborn 763.6
 premature (infant) 765.1
 prolonged, affecting fetus or newborn 763.9
 retarded, fetus or newborn 763.9
 shock, newborn 779.89
 strangulation or suffocation
  due to aspiration of amniotic fluid 770.1
  mechanical 767.8
 trauma NEC 767.9
 triplet
  affected by maternal complications of pregnancy 761.5
  healthy liveborn — see Newborn, multiple
 twin
  affected by maternal complications of pregnancy 761.5
  healthy liveborn — see Newborn, twin
 ventouse, affecting fetus or newborn 763.3
Birthmark 757.32
Bisalbuminemia 273.8

Biskra button 085.1
Bite(s)
  with intact skin surface — see Contusion
  animal — see Wound, open, by site
    intact skin surface — see Contusion
  centipede 989.5
  chigger 133.8
  fire ant 989.5
  flea — see Injury, superficial, by site
  human (open wound) — see also Wound, open, by site
    intact skin surface — see Contusion
  insect
    nonvenomous — see Injury, superficial, by site
    venomous 989.5
  mad dog (death from) 071
  poisonous 989.5
  red bug 133.8
  reptile 989.5
    nonvenomous — see Wound, open, by site
  snake 989.5
    nonvenomous — see Wound, open, by site
  spider (venomous) 989.5
    nonvenomous — see Injury, superficial, by site
  venomous 989.5
Biting
  cheek or lip 528.9
  nail 307.9
Black
  death 020.9
  eye NEC 921.0
  hairy tongue 529.3
  lung disease 500
Blackfan-Diamond anemia or syndrome (congenital hypoplastic anemia) 284.0
Blackhead 706.1
Blackout 780.2
Blackwater fever 084.8
Bladder — see condition
Blast
  blindness 921.3
  concussion — see Blast, injury
  injury 869.0
    with open wound into cavity 869.1
    abdomen or thorax — see Injury, internal, by site
    brain (see also Concussion, brain) 850.9
      with skull fracture — see Fracture, skull
    ear (acoustic nerve trauma) 951.5
      with perforation, tympanic membrane — see Wound, open, ear, drum
    lung (see also Injury, internal, lung) 861.20
    otitic (explosive) 388.11
Blastomycosis, blastomycotic (chronic) (cutaneous) (disseminated) (lung) (pulmonary) (systemic) 116.0
  Brazilian 116.1
  European 117.5
  keloidal 116.2
  North American 116.0
  primary pulmonary 116.0
  South American 116.1
Bleb(s) 709.8
  emphysematous (bullous) (diffuse) (lung) (ruptured) (solitary) 492.0
  filtering, eye (postglaucoma) (status) V45.69
    with complication 997.99
      postcataract extraction (complication) 997.99
  lung (ruptured) 492.0
    congenital 770.5
  subpleural (emphysematous) 492.0
Bleeder (familial) (hereditary) (see also Defect, coagulation) 286.9
  nonfamilial 286.9
Bleeding (see also Hemorrhage) 459.0
  anal 569.3
  anovulatory 628.0
  atonic, following delivery 666.1 ✓5ᵗʰ
  capillary 448.9
  due to subinvolution 621.1
    puerperal 666.2 ✓5ᵗʰ
  ear 388.69

Bleeding (see also Hemorrhage) — continued
  excessive, associated with menopausal onset 627.0
  familial (see also Defect, coagulation) 286.9
  following intercourse 626.7
  gastrointestinal 578.9
  gums 523.8
  hemorrhoids — see Hemorrhoids, bleeding
  intermenstrual
    irregular 626.6
    regular 626.5
  intraoperative 998.11
  irregular NEC 626.4
  menopausal 627.0
  mouth 528.9
  nipple 611.79
  nose 784.7
  ovulation 626.5
  postclimacteric 627.1
  postcoital 626.7
  postmenopausal 627.1
    following induced menopause 627.4
  postoperative 998.11
  preclimacteric 627.0
  puberty 626.3
    excessive, with onset of menstrual periods 626.3
  rectum, rectal 569.3
  tendencies (see also Defect, coagulation) 286.9
  throat 784.8
  umbilical stump 772.3
  umbilicus 789.9
  unrelated to menstrual cycle 626.6
  uterus, uterine 626.9
    climacteric 627.0
    dysfunctional 626.8
    functional 626.8
    unrelated to menstrual cycle 626.6
  vagina, vaginal 623.8
    functional 626.8
  vicarious 625.8
Blennorrhagia, blennorrhagic — see Blennorrhea
Blennorrhea (acute) 098.0
  adultorum 098.40
  alveolaris 523.4
  chronic or duration of 2 months or over 098.2
  gonococcal (neonatorum) 098.40
  inclusion (neonatal) (newborn) 771.6
  neonatorum 098.40
Blepharelosis (see also Entropion) 374.00
Blepharitis (eyelid) 373.00
  angularis 373.01
  ciliaris 373.00
    with ulcer 373.01
  marginal 373.00
    with ulcer 373.01
  scrofulous (see also Tuberculosis) 017.3 ✓5ᵗʰ [373.00]
  squamous 373.02
  ulcerative 373.01
Blepharochalasis 374.34
  congenital 743.62
Blepharoclonus 333.81
Blepharoconjunctivitis (see also Conjunctivitis) 372.20
  angular 372.21
  contact 372.22
Blepharophimosis (eyelid) 374.46
  congenital 743.62
Blepharoplegia 374.89
Blepharoptosis 374.30
  congenital 743.61
Blepharopyorrhea 098.49
Blepharospasm 333.81
Blessig's cyst 362.62
Blighted ovum 631
Blind
  bronchus (congenital) 748.3
  eye — see also Blindness
    hypertensive 360.42
    hypotensive 360.41
  loop syndrome (postoperative) 579.2
  sac, fallopian tube (congenital) 752.19
  spot, enlarged 368.42
  tract or tube (congenital) NEC — see Atresia

Blindness (acquired) (congenital) (both eyes) 369.00
  blast 921.3
    with nerve injury — see Injury, nerve, optic
  Bright's — see Uremia
  color (congenital) 368.59
    acquired 368.55
    blue 368.53
    green 368.52
    red 368.51
    total 368.54
  concussion 950.9
  cortical 377.75
  day 368.10 ▲
    acquired 368.10 ▲
    congenital 368.10 ▲
    hereditary 368.10 ▲
    specified type NEC 368.10 ▲
  due to
    injury NEC 950.9
    refractive error — see Error, refractive
  eclipse (total) 363.31
  emotional 300.11
  hysterical 300.11
  legal (both eyes) (USA definition) 369.4
    with impairment of better (less impaired) eye
      near-total 369.02
        with
          lesser eye impairment 369.02
          near-total 369.04
          total 369.03
      profound 369.05
        with
          lesser eye impairment 369.05
          near-total 369.07
          profound 369.08
          total 369.06
      severe 369.21
        with
          lesser eye impairment 369.21
          blind 369.11
          near-total 369.13
          profound 369.14
          severe 369.22
          total 369.12
      total
        with lesser eye impairment
          total 369.01
  mind 784.69
  moderate
    both eyes 369.25
      with impairment of lesser eye (specified as)
        blind, not further specified 369.15
        low vision, not further specified 369.23
        near-total 369.17
        profound 369.18
        severe 369.24
        total 369.16
    one eye 369.74
      with vision of other eye (specified as)
        near-normal 369.75
        normal 369.76
  near-total
    both eyes 369.04
      with impairment of lesser eye (specified as)
        blind, not further specified 369.02
        total 369.03
    one eye 369.64
      with vision of other eye (specified as)
        near-normal 369.65
        normal 369.66
  night 368.60
    acquired 368.62
    congenital (Japanese) 368.61
    hereditary 368.61
    specified type NEC 368.69
    vitamin A deficiency 264.5
  nocturnal — see Blindness, night
  one eye 369.60
    with low vision of other eye 369.10
  profound
    both eyes 369.08
      with impairment of lesser eye (specified as)
        blind, not further specified 369.05

Blindness — continued
- profound — continued
  - both eyes — continued
    - with impairment of lesser eye (specified as) — continued
      - near-total 369.07
      - total 369.06
  - one eye 369.67
    - with vision of other eye (specified as)
      - near-normal 369.68
      - normal 369.69
- psychic 784.69
- severe
  - both eyes 369.22
    - with impairment of lesser eye (specified as)
      - blind, not further specified 369.11
      - low vision, not further specified 369.21
      - near-total 369.13
      - profound 369.14
      - total 369.12
  - one eye 369.71
    - with vision of other eye (specified as)
      - near-normal 369.72
      - normal 369.73
- snow 370.24
- sun 363.31
- temporary 368.12
- total
  - both eyes 369.01
  - one eye 369.61
    - with vision of other eye (specified as)
      - near-normal 369.62
      - normal 369.63
- transient 368.12
- traumatic NEC 950.9
- word (developmental) 315.01
  - acquired 784.61
  - secondary to organic lesion 784.61

Blister — see also Injury, superficial, by site
- beetle dermatitis 692.89
- due to burn — see Burn, by site, second degree
- fever 054.9
- multiple, skin, nontraumatic 709.8

Bloating 787.3

Bloch-Siemens syndrome (incontinentia pigmenti) 757.33

Bloch-Stauffer dyshormonal dermatosis 757.33

Bloch-Sulzberger disease or syndrome (incontinentia pigmenti) (melanoblastosis) 757.33

Block
- alveolar capillary 516.3
- arborization (heart) 426.6
- arrhythmic 426.9
- atrioventricular (AV) (incomplete) (partial) 426.10
  - with
    - 2:1 atrioventricular response block 426.13
    - atrioventricular dissociation 426.0
  - first degree (incomplete) 426.11
  - second degree (Mobitz type I) 426.13
    - Mobitz (type) II 426.12
  - third degree 426.0
  - complete 426.0
    - congenital 746.86
  - congenital 746.86
  - Mobitz (incomplete)
    - type I (Wenckebach's) 426.13
    - type II 426.12
  - partial 426.13
- auriculoventricular (see also Block, atrioventricular) 426.10
  - complete 426.0
    - congenital 746.86
  - congenital 746.86
- bifascicular (cardiac) 426.53
- bundle branch (complete) (false) (incomplete) 426.50
  - bilateral 426.53
  - left (complete) (main stem) 426.3
    - with right bundle branch block 426.53

Block — continued
- bundle branch — continued
  - left — continued
    - anterior fascicular 426.2
      - with
        - posterior fascicular block 426.3
        - right bundle branch block 426.52
    - hemiblock 426.2
    - incomplete 426.2
      - with right bundle branch block 426.53
    - posterior fascicular 426.2
      - with
        - anterior fascicular block 426.3
        - right bundle branch block 426.51
  - right 426.4
    - with
      - left bundle branch block (incomplete) (main stem) 426.53
      - left fascicular block 426.53
        - anterior 426.52
        - posterior 426.51
  - Wilson's type 426.4
- cardiac 426.9
- conduction 426.9
  - complete 426.0
- Eustachian tube (see also Obstruction, Eustachian tube) 381.60
- fascicular (left anterior) (left posterior) 426.2
- foramen Magendie (acquired) 331.3
  - congenital 742.3
    - with spina bifida (see also Spina bifida) 741.0 ✓5ᵗʰ
- heart 426.9
  - first degree (atrioventricular) 426.11
  - second degree (atrioventricular) 426.13
  - third degree (atrioventricular) 426.0
  - bundle branch (complete) (false) (incomplete) 426.50
    - bilateral 426.53
    - left (see also Block, bundle branch, left) 426.3
    - right (see also Block, bundle branch, right) 426.4
  - complete (atrioventricular) 426.0
    - congenital 746.86
  - incomplete 426.13
  - intra-atrial 426.6
  - intraventricular NEC 426.6
  - sinoatrial 426.6
  - specified type NEC 426.6
- hepatic vein 453.0
- intraventricular (diffuse) (myofibrillar) 426.6
  - bundle branch (complete) (false) (incomplete) 426.50
    - bilateral 426.53
    - left (see also Block, bundle branch, left) 426.3
    - right (see also Block, bundle branch, right) 426.4
- kidney (see also Disease, renal) 593.9
  - postcystoscopic 997.5
- myocardial (see also Block, heart) 426.9
- nodal 426.10
- optic nerve 377.49
- organ or site (congenital) NEC — see Atresia
- parietal 426.6
- peri-infarction 426.6
- portal (vein) 452
- sinoatrial 426.6
- sinoauricular 426.6
- spinal cord 336.9
- trifascicular 426.54
- tubal 628.2
- vein NEC 453.9

Blocq's disease or syndrome (astasia-abasia) 307.9

Blood
- constituents, abnormal NEC 790.6
- disease 289.9
  - specified NEC 289.8
- donor V59.01
  - other blood components V59.09
  - stem cells V59.02
  - whole blood V59.01

Blood — continued
- dyscrasia 289.9
  - with
    - abortion — see Abortion, by type, with hemorrhage, delayed or excessive
    - ectopic pregnancy (see also categories 633.0-633.9) 639.1
    - molar pregnancy (see also categories 630-632) 639.1
  - fetus or newborn NEC 776.9
  - following
    - abortion 639.1
    - ectopic or molar pregnancy 639.1
  - puerperal, postpartum 666.3 ✓5ᵗʰ
- flukes NEC (see also Infestation, Schistosoma) 120.9
- in
  - feces (see also Melena) 578.1
    - occult 792.1
  - urine (see also Hematuria) 599.7
- mole 631
- occult 792.1
- poisoning (see also Septicemia) 038.9
- pressure
  - decreased, due to shock following injury 958.4
  - fluctuating 796.4
  - high (see also Hypertension) 401.9
    - incidental reading (isolated) (nonspecific), without diagnosis of hypertension 796.2
  - low (see also Hypotension) 458.9
    - incidental reading (isolated) (nonspecific), without diagnosis of hypotension 796.3
- spitting (see also Hemoptysis) 786.3
- staining cornea 371.12
- transfusion
  - without reported diagnosis V58.2
  - donor V59.01
    - stem cells V59.02
  - reaction or complication — see Complications, transfusion
- tumor — see Hematoma
- vessel rupture — see Hemorrhage
- vomiting (see also Hematemesis) 578.0

Blood-forming organ disease 289.9

Bloodgood's disease 610.1

Bloodshot eye 379.93

Bloom (-Machacek) (-Torre) syndrome 757.39

Blotch, palpebral 372.55

Blount's disease (tibia vara) 732.4

Blount-Barber syndrome (tibia vara) 732.4

Blue
- baby 746.9
- bloater 491.20
  - with acute bronchitis or exacerbation 491.21
- diaper syndrome 270.0
- disease 746.9
- dome cyst 610.0
- drum syndrome 381.02
- sclera 743.47
  - with fragility of bone and deafness 756.51
- toe syndrome — see Atherosclerosis

Blueness (see also Cyanosis) 782.5

Blurring, visual 368.8

Blushing (abnormal) (excessive) 782.62

Boarder, hospital V65.0
- infant V65.0

Bockhart's impetigo (superficial folliculitis) 704.8

Bodechtel-Guttmann disease (subacute sclerosing panencephalitis) 046.2

Boder-Sedgwick syndrome (ataxia-telangiectasia) 334.8

Body, bodies
- Aschoff (see also Myocarditis, rheumatic) 398.0
- asteroid, vitreous 379.22
- choroid, colloid (degenerative) 362.57
  - hereditary 362.77
- cytoid (retina) 362.82
- drusen (retina) (see also Drusen) 362.57
  - optic disc 377.21
- fibrin, pleura 511.0

Body, bodies — continued
  foreign — see Foreign body
  Hassall-Henle 371.41
  loose
    joint (see also Loose, body, joint) 718.1 ✓5th
      knee 717.6
    knee 717.6
    sheath, tendon 727.82
  Mallory's 034.1
  Mooser 081.0
  Negri 071
  rice (joint) (see also Loose, body, joint) 718.1 ✓5th
    knee 717.6
  rocking 307.3
Boeck's
  disease (sarcoidosis) 135
  lupoid (miliary) 135
  sarcoid 135
Boerhaave's syndrome (spontaneous esophageal rupture) 530.4
Boggy
  cervix 622.8
  uterus 621.8
Boil (see also Carbuncle) 680.9
  abdominal wall 680.2
  Aleppo 085.1
  ankle 680.6
  anus 680.5
  arm (any part, above wrist) 680.3
  auditory canal, external 680.0
  axilla 680.3
  back (any part) 680.2
  Baghdad 085.1
  breast 680.2
  buttock 680.5
  chest wall 680.2
  corpus cavernosum 607.2
  Delhi 085.1
  ear (any part) 680.0
  eyelid 373.13
  face (any part, except eye) 680.0
  finger (any) 680.4
  flank 680.2
  foot (any part) 680.7
  forearm 680.3
  Gafsa 085.1
  genital organ, male 608.4
  gluteal (region) 680.5
  groin 680.2
  hand (any part) 680.4
  head (any part, except face) 680.8
  heel 680.7
  hip 680.6
  knee 680.6
  labia 616.4
  lacrimal (see also Dacryocystitis) 375.30
    gland (see also Dacryoadenitis) 375.00
    passages (duct) (sac) (see also Dacryocystitis) 375.30
  leg, any part except foot 680.6
  multiple sites 680.9
  natal 085.1
  neck 680.1
  nose (external) (septum) 680.0
  orbit, orbital 376.01
  partes posteriores 680.5
  pectoral region 680.2
  penis 607.2
  perineum 680.2
  pinna 680.0
  scalp (any part) 680.8
  scrotum 608.4
  seminal vesicle 608.0
  shoulder 680.3
  skin NEC 680.9
  specified site NEC 680.8
  spermatic cord 608.4
  temple (region) 680.0
  testis 608.4
  thigh 680.6
  thumb 680.4
  toe (any) 680.7
  tropical 085.1
  trunk 680.2
  tunica vaginalis 608.4
  umbilicus 680.2

Boil (see also Carbuncle) — continued
  upper arm 680.3
  vas deferens 608.4
  vulva 616.4
  wrist 680.4
Bold hives (see also Urticaria) 708.9
Bolivian hemorrhagic fever 078.7
Bombé, iris 364.74
Bomford-Rhoads anemia (refractory) 284.9
Bone — see condition
Bonnevie-Ullrich syndrome 758.6
Bonnier's syndrome 386.19
Bonvale Dam fever 780.79
Bony block of joint 718.80
  ankle 718.87
  elbow 718.82
  foot 718.87
  hand 718.84
  hip 718.85
  knee 718.86
  multiple sites 718.89
  pelvic region 718.85
  shoulder (region) 718.81
  specified site NEC 718.88
  wrist 718.83
Borderline
  intellectual functioning V62.89
  pelvis 653.1 ✓5th
    with obstruction during labor 660.1 ✓5th
      affecting fetus or newborn 763.1
  psychosis (see also Schizophrenia) 295.5 ✓5th
    of childhood (see also Psychosis, childhood) 299.8 ✓5th
  schizophrenia (see also Schizophrenia) 295.5 ✓5th
Borna disease 062.9
Bornholm disease (epidemic pleurodynia) 074.1
Borrelia vincentii (mouth) (pharynx) (tonsils) 101
Bostock's catarrh (see also Fever, hay) 477.9
Boston exanthem 048
Botalli, ductus (patent) (persistent) 747.0
Bothriocephalus latus infestation 123.4
Botulism 005.1
Bouba (see also Yaws) 102.9
Bouffée délirante 298.3
Bouillaud's disease or syndrome (rheumatic heart disease) 391.9
Bourneville's disease (tuberous sclerosis) 759.5
Boutonneuse fever 082.1
Boutonniere
  deformity (finger) 736.21
  hand (intrinsic) 736.21
Bouveret (-Hoffmann) disease or syndrome (paroxysmal tachycardia) 427.2
Bovine heart — see Hypertrophy, cardiac
Bowel — see condition
Bowen's
  dermatosis (precancerous) (M8081/2) — see Neoplasm, skin, in situ
  disease (M8081/2) — see Neoplasm, skin, in situ
  epithelioma (M8081/2) — see Neoplasm, skin, in situ
  type
    epidermoid carcinoma in situ (M8081/2) — see Neoplasm, skin, in situ
    intraepidermal squamous cell carcinoma (M8081/2) — see Neoplasm, skin, in situ
Bowing
  femur 736.89
    congenital 754.42
  fibula 736.89
    congenital 754.43
  forearm 736.09
    away from midline (cubitus valgus) 736.01
    toward midline (cubitus varus) 736.02
  leg(s), long bones, congenital 754.44
  radius 736.09
    away from midline (cubitus valgus) 736.01
    toward midline (cubitus varus) 736.02

Bowing — continued
  tibia 736.89
    congenital 754.43
Bowleg(s) 736.42
  congenital 754.44
  rachitic 268.1
Boyd's dysentery 004.2
Brachial — see condition
Brachman-de Lange syndrome (Amsterdam dwarf, mental retardation, and brachycephaly) 759.89
Brachycardia 427.89
Brachycephaly 756.0
Brachymorphism and ectopia lentis 759.89
Bradley's disease (epidemic vomiting) 078.82
Bradycardia 427.89
  chronic (sinus) 427.81
  newborn 779.81
  nodal 427.89
  postoperative 997.1
  reflex 337.0
  sinoatrial 427.89
    with paroxysmal tachyarrhythmia or tachycardia 427.81
    chronic 427.81
  sinus 427.89
    with paroxysmal tachyarrhythmia or tachycardia 427.81
    chronic 427.81
    persistent 427.81
    severe 427.81
  tachycardia syndrome 427.81
  vagal 427.89
Bradypnea 786.09
Brailsford's disease 732.3
  radial head 732.3
  tarsal scaphoid 732.5
Brailsford-Morquio disease or syndrome (mucopolysac-charidosis IV) 277.5
Brain — see also condition
  death 348.8
  syndrome (acute) (chronic) (nonpsychotic) (organic) (with neurotic reaction) (with behavioral reaction) (see also Syndrome, brain) 310.9
    with
      presenile brain disease 290.10
      psychosis, psychotic reaction (see also Psychosis, organic) 294.9
    congenital (see also Retardation, mental) 319
Branched-chain amino-acid disease 270.3
Branchial — see condition
Branchopulmonitis — see Pneumonia, broncho-
Brandt's syndrome (acrodermatitis enteropathica) 686.8
Brash (water) 787.1
Brass-founders', ague 985.8
Bravais-Jacksonian epilepsy (see also Epilepsy) 345.5 ✓5th
Braxton Hicks contractions 644.1 ✓5th
Braziers' disease 985.8
Brazilian
  blastomycosis 116.1
  leishmaniasis 085.5
Break
  cardiorenal — see Hypertension, cardiorenal
  retina (see also Defect, retina) 361.30
Breakbone fever 061
Breakdown
  device, implant, or graft — see Complications, mechanical
  nervous (see also Disorder, mental, nonpsychotic) 300.9
  perineum 674.2 ✓5th
Breast — see condition
Breast feeding difficulties 676.8 ✓5th
Breath
  foul 784.9
  holder, child 312.81
  holding spells 786.9
  shortness 786.05

Breathing
  asymmetrical 786.09
  bronchial 786.09
  exercises V57.0
  labored 786.09
  mouth 784.9
  periodic 786.09
  tic 307.20
Breathlessness 786.09
Breda's disease (see also Yaws) 102.9
Breech
  delivery, affecting fetus or newborn 763.0
  extraction, affecting fetus or newborn 763.0
  presentation (buttocks) (complete) (frank) 652.2 ✓5ᵗʰ
    with successful version 652.1 ✓5ᵗʰ
    before labor, affecting fetus or newborn 761.7
    during labor, affecting fetus or newborn 763.0
Breisky's disease (kraurosis vulvae) 624.0
Brennemann's syndrome (acute mesenteric lymphadenitis) 289.2
Brenner's
  tumor (benign) (M9000/0) 220
    borderline malignancy (M9000/1) 236.2
    malignant (M9000/3) 183.0
    proliferating (M9000/1) 236.2
Bretonneau's disease (diphtheritic malignant angina) 032.0
Breus' mole 631
Brevicollis 756.16
Bricklayers' itch 692.89
Brickmakers' anemia 126.9
Bridge
  myocardial 746.85
Bright's
  blindness — see Uremia
  disease (see also Nephritis) 583.9
    arteriosclerotic (see also Hypertension, kidney) 403.90
Brill's disease (recrudescent typhus) 081.1
  flea-borne 081.0
  louse-borne 081.1
Brill-Symmers disease (follicular lymphoma) (M9690/3) 202.0 ✓5ᵗʰ
Brill-Zinsser disease (recrudescent typhus) 081.1
Brinton's disease (linitis plastica) (M8142/3) 151.9
Brion-Kayser disease (see also Fever, paratyphoid) 002.9
Briquet's disorder or syndrome 300.81
Brissaud's
  infantilism (infantile myxedema) 244.9
  motor-verbal tic 307.23
Brissaud-Meige syndrome (infantile myxedema) 244.9
Brittle
  bones (congenital) 756.51
  nails 703.8
    congenital 757.5
Broad — see also condition
  beta disease 272.2
  ligament laceration syndrome 620.6
Brock's syndrome (atelectasis due to enlarged lymph nodes) 518.0
Brocq's disease 691.8
  atopic (diffuse) neurodermatitis 691.8
  lichen simplex chronicus 698.3
  parakeratosis psoriasiformis 696.2
  parapsoriasis 696.2
Brocq-Duhring disease (dermatitis herpetiformis) 694.0
Brodie's
  abscess (localized) (chronic) (see also Osteomyelitis) 730.1 ✓5ᵗʰ
  disease (joint) (see also Osteomyelitis) 730.1 ✓5ᵗʰ
Broken
  arches 734
    congenital 755.67

Broken — continued
  back — see Fracture, vertebra, by site
  bone — see Fracture, by site
  compensation — see Disease, heart
  implant or internal device — see listing under Complications, mechanical
  neck — see Fracture, vertebra, cervical
  nose 802.0
    open 802.1
  tooth, teeth 873.63
    complicated 873.73
Bromhidrosis 705.89
Bromidism, bromism
  acute 967.3
    correct substance properly administered 349.82
    overdose or wrong substance given or taken 967.3
  chronic (see also Dependence) 304.1 ✓5ᵗʰ
Bromidrosiphobia 300.23
Bromidrosis 705.89
Bronchi, bronchial — see condition
Bronchiectasis (cylindrical) (diffuse) (fusiform) (localized) (moniliform) (postinfectious) (recurrent) (saccular) 494.0
  with acute exacerbation 494.1
  congenital 748.61
  tuberculosis (see also Tuberculosis) 011.5 ✓5ᵗʰ
Bronchiolectasis — see Bronchiectasis
Bronchiolitis (acute) (infectious) (subacute) 466.19
  with
    bronchospasm or obstruction 466.19
    influenza, flu, or grippe 487.1
  catarrhal (acute) (subacute) 466.19
  chemical 506.0
    chronic 506.4
  chronic (obliterative) 491.8
  due to external agent — see Bronchitis, acute, due to
  fibrosa obliterans 491.8
  influenzal 487.1
  obliterans 491.8
    with organizing pneumonia (B.O.O.P.) 516.8
    status post lung transplant 996.84
  obliterative (chronic) (diffuse) (subacute) 491.8
    due to fumes or vapors 506.4
  respiratory syncytial virus 466.11
  vesicular — see Pneumonia, broncho-
Bronchitis (diffuse) (hypostatic) (infectious) (inflammatory) (simple) 490
  with
    emphysema — see Emphysema
    influenza, flu, or grippe 487.1
    obstruction airway, chronic 491.20
      with acute exacerbation 491.21
    tracheitis 490
      acute or subacute 466.0
        with bronchospasm or obstruction 466.0
      chronic 491.8
  acute or subacute 466.0
    with
      bronchospasm 466.0
      chronic
        bronchitis (obstructive) 491.21
        obstructive pulmonary disease (COPD) 491.21
      obstruction 466.0
      tracheitis 466.0
    chemical (due to fumes or vapors) 506.0
    due to
      fumes or vapors 506.0
      radiation 508.8
  allergic (acute) (see also Asthma) 493.9 ✓5ᵗʰ
  arachidic 934.1
  aspiration 507.0
    due to fumes or vapors 506.0
  asthmatic (acute) 493.90
    with
      acute exacerbation 493.92
      status asthmaticus 493.91
    chronic 493.2 ✓5ᵗʰ ▲
  capillary 466.19
    with bronchospasm or obstruction 466.19

Bronchitis — continued
  capillary — continued
    chronic 491.8
  caseous (see also Tuberculosis) 011.3 ✓5ᵗʰ
  Castellani's 104.8
  catarrhal 490
    acute — see Bronchitis, acute
    chronic 491.0
  chemical (acute) (subacute) 506.0
    chronic 506.4
    due to fumes or vapors (acute) (subacute) 506.0
      chronic 506.4
  chronic 491.9
    with
      tracheitis (chronic) 491.8
      asthmatic 493.2 ✓5ᵗʰ ▲
    catarrhal 491.0
    chemical (due to fumes and vapors) 506.4
    due to
      fumes or vapors (chemical) (inhalation) 506.4
      radiation 508.8
      tobacco smoking 491.0
    mucopurulent 491.1
    obstructive 491.20
      with acute bronchitis or acute exacerbation 491.21
    purulent 491.1
    simple 491.0
    specified type NEC 491.8
  croupous 466.0
    with bronchospasm or obstruction 466.0
    due to fumes or vapors 506.0
  emphysematous 491.20
    with acute bronchitis or acute exacerbation 491.21
  exudative 466.0
  fetid (chronic) (recurrent) 491.1
  fibrinous, acute or subacute 466.0
    with bronchospasm or obstruction 466.0
  grippal 487.1
  influenzal 487.1
  membranous, acute or subacute 466.0
    with bronchospasm or obstruction 466.0
  moulders' 502
  mucopurulent (chronic) (recurrent) 491.1
    acute or subacute 466.0
  non-obstructive 491.0
  obliterans 491.8
  obstructive (chronic) 491.20
    with acute bronchitis or acute exacerbation 491.21
  pituitous 491.1
  plastic (inflammatory) 466.0
  pneumococcal, acute or subacute 466.0
    with bronchospasm or obstruction 466.0
  pseudomembranous 466.0
  purulent (chronic) (recurrent) 491.1
    acute or subacute 466.0
      with bronchospasm or obstruction 466.0
  putrid 491.1
  scrofulous (see also Tuberculosis) 011.3 ✓5ᵗʰ
  senile 491.9
  septic, acute or subacute 466.0
    with bronchospasm or obstruction 466.0
  smokers' 491.0
  spirochetal 104.8
  suffocative, acute or subacute 466.0
  summer (see also Asthma) 493.9 ✓5ᵗʰ
  suppurative (chronic) 491.1
    acute or subacute 466.0
  tuberculous (see also Tuberculosis) 011.3 ✓5ᵗʰ
  ulcerative 491.8
    Vincent's 101
  Vincent's 101
  viral, acute or subacute 466.0
Bronchoalveolitis 485
Bronchoaspergillosis 117.3
Bronchocele
  meaning
    dilatation of bronchus 519.1
    goiter 240.9
Bronchogenic carcinoma 162.9
Bronchohemisporosis 117.9

Broncholithiasis 518.89
   tuberculous (see also Tuberculosis) 011.3 ✓5ᵗʰ
Bronchomalacia 748.3
Bronchomoniliasis 112.89
Bronchomycosis 112.89
Bronchonocardiosis 039.1
Bronchopleuropneumonia — see Pneumonia, broncho-
Bronchopneumonia — see Pneumonia, broncho-
Bronchopneumonitis — see Pneumonia, broncho-
Bronchopulmonary — see condition
Bronchorrhagia 786.3
   newborn 770.3
   tuberculous (see also Tuberculosis) 011.3 ✓5ᵗʰ
Bronchorrhea (chronic) (purulent) 491.0
   acute 466.0
Bronchospasm 519.1
   with
      asthma — see Asthma
      bronchiolitis
         due to respiratory syncytial virus 466.11
      bronchitis — see Bronchitis
      chronic obstructive pulmonary disease (COPD) 496
      emphysema — see Emphysema
         due to external agent — see Condition, respiratory, acute, due to
Bronchospirochetosis 104.8
Bronchostenosis 519.1
Bronchus — see condition
Bronze, bronzed
   diabetes 275.0
   disease (Addison's) (skin) 255.4
      tuberculous (see also Tuberculosis) 017.6 ✓5ᵗʰ
Brooke's disease or tumor (M8100/0) — see Neoplasm, skin, benign
Brown's tendon sheath syndrome 378.61
Brown enamel of teeth (hereditary) 520.5
Brown-Séquard's paralysis (syndrome) 344.89
Brow presentation complicating delivery 652.4 ✓5ᵗʰ
Brucella, brucellosis (infection) 023.9
   abortus 023.1
   canis 023.3
   dermatitis, skin 023.9
   melitensis 023.0
   mixed 023.8
   suis 023.2
Bruck's disease 733.99
Bruck-de Lange disease or syndrome (Amsterdam dwarf, mental retardation, and brachycephaly) 759.89
Brugada syndrome 746.89
Brugsch's syndrome (acropachyderma) 757.39
Brug's filariasis 125.1
Bruhl's disease (splenic anemia with fever) 285.8
Bruise (skin surface intact) — see also Contusion
   with
      fracture — see Fracture, by site
      open wound — see Wound, open, by site
      internal organ (abdomen, chest, or pelvis) — see Injury, internal, by site
   umbilical cord 663.6 ✓5ᵗʰ
      affecting fetus or newborn 762.6
Bruit 785.9
   arterial (abdominal) (carotid) 785.9
   supraclavicular 785.9
Brushburn — see Injury, superficial, by site
Bruton's X-linked agammaglobulinemia 279.04
Bruxism 306.8
Bubbly lung syndrome 770.7
Bubo 289.3
   blennorrhagic 098.89
   chancroidal 099.0
   climatic 099.1
   due to Hemophilus ducreyi 099.0
   gonococcal 098.89
   indolent NEC 099.8
   inguinal NEC 099.8

Bubo — continued
   inguinal NEC — continued
      chancroidal 099.0
      climatic 099.1
      due to H. ducreyi 099.0
   scrofulous (see also Tuberculosis) 017.2 ✓5ᵗʰ
   soft chancre 099.0
   suppurating 683
   syphilitic 091.0
      congenital 090.0
   tropical 099.1
   venereal NEC 099.8
   virulent 099.0
Bubonic plague 020.0
Bubonocele — see Hernia, inguinal
Buccal — see condition
Buchanan's disease (juvenile osteochondrosis of iliac crest) 732.1
Buchem's syndrome (hyperostosis corticalis) 733.3
Buchman's disease (osteochondrosis, juvenile) 732.1
Bucket handle fracture (semilunar cartilage) (see also Tear, meniscus) 836.2
Budd-Chiari syndrome (hepatic vein thrombosis) 453.0
Budgerigar-fanciers' disease or lung 495.2
Büdinger-Ludloff-Läwen disease 717.89
Buerger's disease (thromboangiitis obliterans) 443.1
Bulbar — see condition
Bulbus cordis 745.9
   persistent (in left ventricle) 745.8
Bulging fontanels (congenital) 756.0
Bulimia 783.6
   nonorganic origin 307.51
Bulky uterus 621.2
Bulla(e) 709.8
   lung (emphysematous) (solitary) 492.0
Bullet wound — see also Wound, open, by site
   fracture — see Fracture, by site, open
   internal organ (abdomen, chest, or pelvis) — see Injury, internal, by site, with open wound
   intracranial — see Laceration, brain, with open wound
Bullis fever 082.8
Bullying (see also Disturbance, conduct) 312.0 ✓5ᵗʰ
Bundle
   branch block (complete) (false) (incomplete) 426.50
      bilateral 426.53
      left (see also Block, bundle branch, left) 426.3
         hemiblock 426.2
      right (see also Block, bundle branch, right) 426.4
   of His — see condition
   of Kent syndrome (anomalous atrioventricular excitation) 426.7
Bungpagga 040.81
Bunion 727.1
Bunionette 727.1
Bunyamwera fever 066.3
Buphthalmia, buphthalmos (congenital) 743.20
   associated with
      keratoglobus, congenital 743.22
      megalocornea 743.22
      ocular anomalies NEC 743.22
   isolated 743.21
   simple 743.21
Bürger-Grütz disease or syndrome (essential familial hyperlipemia) 272.3
Buried roots 525.3
Burke's syndrome 577.8
Burkitt's
   tumor (M9750/3) 200.2 ✓5ᵗʰ
   type malignant, lymphoma, lymphoblastic, or undifferentiated (M9750/3) 200.2 ✓5ᵗʰ

Burn (acid) (cathode ray) (caustic) (chemical) (electric heating appliance) (electricity) (fire) (flame) (hot liquid or object) (irradiation) (lime) (radiation) (steam) (thermal) (x-ray) 949.0

Note — Use the following fifth-digit subclassification with category 948 to indicate the percent of body surface with third degree burn:	
0	Less than 10% or unspecified
1	10–19%
2	20–29%
3	30–39%
4	40–49%
5	50–59%
6	60–69%
7	70–79%
8	80–89%
9	90% or more of body surface

   with
      blisters — see Burn, by site, second degree
      erythema — see Burn, by site, first degree
      skin loss (epidermal) — see also Burn, by site, second degree
      full thickness — see also Burn, by site, third degree
         with necrosis of underlying tissues — see Burn, by site, third degree, deep
   first degree — see Burn, by site, first degree
   second degree — see Burn, by site, second degree
   third degree — see Burn, by site, third degree
      deep — see Burn, by site, third degree, deep
   abdomen, abdominal (muscle) (wall) 942.03
      with
         trunk — see Burn, trunk, multiple sites
      first degree 942.13
      second degree 942.23
      third degree 942.33
         deep 942.43
            with loss of body part 942.53
   ankle 945.03
      with
         lower limb(s) — see Burn, leg, multiple sites
      first degree 945.13
      second degree 945.23
      third degree 945.33
         deep 945.43
            with loss of body part 945.53
   anus — see Burn, trunk, specified site NEC
   arm(s) 943.00
      first degree 943.10
      second degree 943.20
      third degree 943.30
         deep 943.40
            with loss of body part 943.50
      lower — see Burn, forearm(s)
      multiple sites, except hand(s) or wrist(s) 943.09
      first degree 943.19
      second degree 943.29
      third degree 943.39
         deep 943.49
            with loss of body part 943.59
      upper 943.03
      first degree 943.13
      second degree 943.23
      third degree 943.33
         deep 943.43
            with loss of body part 943.53
   auditory canal (external) — see Burn, ear
   auricle (ear) — see Burn, ear
   axilla 943.04
      with
         upper limb(s) except hand(s) or wrist(s) — see Burn, arm(s), multiple sites
      first degree 943.14
      second degree 943.24
      third degree 943.34
         deep 943.44
            with loss of body part 943.54

Index to Diseases

Burn

Burn — *continued*
- back 942.04
  - with
    - trunk — *see* Burn, trunk, multiple sites
  - first degree 942.14
  - second degree 942.24
  - third degree 942.34
    - deep 942.44
      - with loss of body part 942.54
- biceps
  - brachii — *see* Burn, arm(s), upper
  - femoris — *see* Burn, thigh
- breast(s) 942.01
  - with
    - trunk — *see* Burn, trunk, multiple sites
  - first degree 942.11
  - second degree 942.21
  - third degree 942.31
    - deep 942.41
      - with loss of body part 942.51
- brow — *see* Burn, forehead
- buttock(s) — *see* Burn, back
- canthus (eye) 940.1
  - chemical 940.0
- cervix (uteri) 947.4
- cheek (cutaneous) 941.07
  - with
    - face or head — *see* Burn, head, multiple sites
  - first degree 941.17
  - second degree 941.27
  - third degree 941.37
    - deep 941.47
      - with loss of body part 941.57
- chest wall (anterior) 942.02
  - with
    - trunk — *see* Burn, trunk, multiple sites
  - first degree 942.12
  - second degree 942.22
  - third degree 942.32
    - deep 942.42
      - with loss of body part 942.52
- chin 941.04
  - with
    - face or head — *see* Burn, head, multiple sites
  - first degree 941.14
  - second degree 941.24
  - third degree 941.34
    - deep 941.44
      - with loss of body part 941.54
- clitoris — *see* Burn, genitourinary organs, external
- colon 947.3
- conjunctiva (and cornea) 940.4
  - chemical
    - acid 940.3
    - alkaline 940.2
- cornea (and conjunctiva) 940.4
  - chemical
    - acid 940.3
    - alkaline 940.2
- costal region — *see* Burn, chest wall
- due to ingested chemical agent — *see* Burn, internal organs
- ear (auricle) (canal) (drum) (external) 941.01
  - with
    - face or head — *see* Burn, head, multiple sites
  - first degree 941.11
  - second degree 941.21
  - third degree 941.31
    - deep 941.41
      - with loss of a body part 941.51
- elbow 943.02
  - with
    - hand(s) and wrist(s) — *see* Burn, multiple specified sites
    - upper limb(s) except hand(s) or wrist(s) — *see also* Burn, arm(s), multiple sites
  - first degree 943.12
  - second degree 943.22
  - third degree 943.32
    - deep 943.42
      - with loss of body part 943.52

Burn — *continued*
- electricity, electric current — *See* Burn, by site
- entire body — *see* Burn, multiple, specified sites
- epididymis — *see* Burn, genitourinary organs, external
- epigastric region — *see* Burn, abdomen
- epiglottis 947.1
- esophagus 947.2
- extent (percent of body surface)
  - less than 10 percent 948.0 ✓5ᵗʰ
  - 10-19 percent 948.1 ✓5ᵗʰ
  - 20-29 percent 948.2 ✓5ᵗʰ
  - 30-39 percent 948.3 ✓5ᵗʰ
  - 40-49 percent 948.4 ✓5ᵗʰ
  - 50-59 percent 948.5 ✓5ᵗʰ
  - 60-69 percent 948.6 ✓5ᵗʰ
  - 70-79 percent 948.7 ✓5ᵗʰ
  - 80-89 percent 948.8 ✓5ᵗʰ
  - 90 percent or more 948.9 ✓5ᵗʰ
- extremity
  - lower — *see* Burn, leg
  - upper — *see* Burn, arm(s)
- eye(s) (and adnexa) (only) 940.9
  - with
    - face, head, or neck 941.02
      - first degree 941.12
      - second degree 941.22
      - third degree 941.32
        - deep 941.42
          - with loss of body part 941.52
    - other sites (classifiable to more than one category in 940-945) — *see* Burn, multiple, specified sites
    - resulting rupture and destruction of eyeball 940.5
  - specified part — *see* Burn, by site
- eyeball — *see also* Burn, eye with resulting rupture and destruction of eyeball 940.5
- eyelid(s) 940.1
  - chemical 940.0
- face — *see* Burn, head
- finger (nail) (subungual) 944.01
  - with
    - hand(s) — *see* Burn, hand(s), multiple sites
    - other sites — *see* Burn, multiple, specified sites
    - thumb 944.04
      - first degree 944.14
      - second degree 944.24
      - third degree 944.34
        - deep 944.44
          - with loss of body part 944.54
  - first degree 944.11
  - second degree 944.21
  - third degree 944.31
    - deep 944.41
      - with loss of body part 944.51
  - multiple (digits) 944.03
    - with thumb — *see* Burn, finger, with thumb
    - first degree 944.13
    - second degree 944.23
    - third degree 944.33
      - deep 944.43
        - with loss of body part 944.53
- flank — *see* Burn, abdomen
- foot 945.02
  - with
    - lower limb(s) — *see* Burn, leg, multiple sites
  - first degree 945.12
  - second degree 945.22
  - third degree 945.32
    - deep 945.42
      - with loss of body part 945.52
- forearm(s) 943.01
  - with
    - upper limb(s) except hand(s) or wrist(s) — *see* Burn, arm(s), multiple sites
  - first degree 943.11
  - second degree 943.21
  - third degree 943.31
    - deep 943.41
      - with loss of body part 943.51

Burn — *continued*
- forehead 941.07
  - with
    - face or head — *see* Burn, head, multiple sites
  - first degree 941.17
  - second degree 941.27
  - third degree 941.37
    - deep 941.47
      - with loss of body part 941.57
- fourth degree — *see* Burn, by site, third degree, deep
- friction — *see* Injury, superficial, by site
- from swallowing caustic or corrosive substance NEC — *see* Burn, internal organs
- full thickness — *see* Burn, by site, third degree
- gastrointestinal tract 947.3
- genitourinary organs
  - external 942.05
    - with
      - trunk — *see* Burn, trunk, multiple sites
    - first degree 942.15
    - second degree 942.25
    - third degree 942.35
      - deep 942.45
        - with loss of body part 942.55
  - internal 947.8
- globe (eye) — *see* Burn, eyeball
- groin — *see* Burn, abdomen
- gum 947.0
- hand(s) (phalanges) (and wrist) 944.00
  - first degree 944.10
  - second degree 944.20
  - third degree 944.30
    - deep 944.40
      - with loss of body part 944.50
  - back (dorsal surface) 944.06
    - first degree 944.16
    - second degree 944.26
    - third degree 944.36
      - deep 944.46
        - with loss of body part 944.56
  - multiple sites 944.08
    - first degree 944.18
    - second degree 944.28
    - third degree 944.38
      - deep 944.48
        - with loss of body part 944.58
- head (and face) 941.00
  - eye(s) only 940.9
    - specified part — *see* Burn, by site
  - first degree 941.10
  - second degree 941.20
  - third degree 941.30
    - deep 941.40
      - with loss of body part 941.50
  - multiple sites 941.09
    - with eyes — *see* Burn, eyes, with face, head, or neck
    - first degree 941.19
    - second degree 941.29
    - third degree 941.39
      - deep 941.49
        - with loss of body part 941.59
- heel — *see* Burn, foot
- hip — *see* Burn, trunk, specified site NEC
- iliac region — *see* Burn, trunk, specified site NEC
- infected 958.3
- inhalation (*see also* Burn, internal organs) 947.9
- internal organs 947.9
  - from caustic or corrosive substance (swallowing) NEC 947.9
  - specified NEC (*see also* Burn, by site) 947.8
- interscapular region — *see* Burn, back
- intestine (large) (small) 947.3
- iris — *see* Burn, eyeball
- knee 945.05
  - with
    - lower limb(s) — *see* Burn, leg, multiple sites
  - first degree 945.15
  - second degree 945.25

Burn — continued
- knee — continued
  - third degree 945.35
    - deep 945.45
      - with loss of body part 945.55
- labium (majorus) (minus) — see Burn, genitourinary organs, external
- lacrimal apparatus, duct, gland, or sac 940.1
  - chemical 940.0
- larynx 947.1
- late effect — see Late, effects (of), burn
- leg 945.00
  - first degree 945.10
  - second degree 945.20
  - third degree 945.30
    - deep 945.40
      - with loss of body part 945.50
  - lower 945.04
    - with other part(s) of lower limb(s) — see Burn, leg, multiple sites
    - first degree 945.14
    - second degree 945.24
    - third degree 945.34
      - deep 945.44
        - with loss of body part 945.54
  - multiple sites 945.09
    - first degree 945.19
    - second degree 945.29
    - third degree 945.39
      - deep 945.49
        - with loss of body part 945.59
  - upper — see Burn, thigh
- lightning — see Burn, by site
- limb(s)
  - lower (including foot or toe(s)) — see Burn, leg
  - upper (except wrist and hand) — see Burn, arm(s)
- lip(s) 941.03
  - with
    - face or head — see Burn, head, multiple sites
  - first degree 941.13
  - second degree 941.23
  - third degree 941.33
    - deep 941.43
      - with loss of body part 941.53
- lumbar region — see Burn, back
- lung 947.1
- malar region — see Burn, cheek
- mastoid region — see Burn, scalp
- membrane, tympanic — see Burn, ear
- midthoracic region — see Burn, chest wall
- mouth 947.0
- multiple (see also Burn, unspecified) 949.0
  - specified sites classifiable to more than one category in 940-945 946.0
    - first degree 946.1
    - second degree 946.2
    - third degree 946.3
      - deep 946.4
        - with loss of body part 946.5
- muscle, abdominal — see Burn, abdomen
- nasal (septum) — see Burn, nose
- neck 941.08
  - with
    - face or head — see Burn, head, multiple sites
  - first degree 941.18
  - second degree 941.28
  - third degree 941.38
    - deep 941.48
      - with loss of body part 941.58
- nose (septum) 941.05
  - with
    - face or head — see Burn, head, multiple sites
  - first degree 941.15
  - second degree 941.25
  - third degree 941.35
    - deep 941.45
      - with loss of body part 941.55
- occipital region — see Burn, scalp
- orbit region 940.1
  - chemical 940.0
- oronasopharynx 947.0
- palate 947.0

Burn — continued
- palm(s) 944.05
  - with
    - hand(s) and wrist(s) — see Burn, hand(s), multiple sites
  - first degree 944.15
  - second degree 944.25
  - third degree 944.35
    - deep 944.45
      - with loss of a body part 944.55
- parietal region — see Burn, scalp
- penis — see Burn, genitourinary organs, external
- perineum — see Burn, genitourinary organs, external
- periocular area 940.1
  - chemical 940.0
- pharynx 947.0
- pleura 947.1
- popliteal space — see Burn, knee
- prepuce — see Burn, genitourinary organs, external
- pubic region — see Burn, genitourinary organs, external
- pudenda — see Burn, genitourinary organs, external
- rectum 947.3
- sac, lacrimal 940.1
  - chemical 940.0
- sacral region — see Burn, back
- salivary (ducts) (glands) 947.0
- scalp 941.06
  - with
    - face or neck — see Burn, head, multiple sites
  - first degree 941.16
  - second degree 941.26
  - third degree 941.36
    - deep 941.46
      - with loss of body part 941.56
- scapular region 943.06
  - with
    - upper limb(s), except hand(s) or wrist(s) — see Burn, arm(s), multiple sites
  - first degree 943.16
  - second degree 943.26
  - third degree 943.36
    - deep 943.46
      - with loss of body part 943.56
- sclera — see Burn, eyeball
- scrotum — see Burn, genitourinary organs, external
- septum, nasal — see Burn, nose
- shoulder(s) 943.05
  - with
    - hand(s) and wrist(s) — see Burn, multiple, specified sites
    - upper limb(s), except hand(s) or wrist(s) — see Burn, arm(s), multiple sites
  - first degree 943.15
  - second degree 943.25
  - third degree 943.35
    - deep 943.45
      - with loss of body part 943.55
- skin NEC (see also Burn, unspecified) 949.0
- skull — see Burn, head
- small intestine 947.3
- sternal region — see Burn, chest wall
- stomach 947.3
- subconjunctival — see Burn, conjunctiva
- subcutaneous — see Burn, by site, third degree
- submaxillary region — see Burn, head
- submental region — see Burn, chin
- sun — see Sunburn
- supraclavicular fossa — see Burn, neck
- supraorbital — see Burn, forehead
- temple — see Burn, scalp
- temporal region — see Burn, scalp
- testicle — see Burn, genitourinary organs, external
- testis — see Burn, genitourinary organs, external
- thigh 945.06
  - with
    - lower limb(s) — see Burn, leg, multiple sites

Burn — continued
- thigh — continued
  - first degree 945.16
  - second degree 945.26
  - third degree 945.36
    - deep 945.46
      - with loss of body part 945.56
- thorax (external) — see Burn, chest wall
- throat 947.0
- thumb(s) (nail) (subungual) 944.02
  - with
    - finger(s) — see Burn, finger, with other sites, thumb
    - hand(s) and wrist(s) — see Burn, hand(s), multiple sites
  - first degree 944.12
  - second degree 944.22
  - third degree 944.32
    - deep 944.42
      - with loss of body part 944.52
- toe (nail) (subungual) 945.01
  - with
    - lower limb(s) — see Burn, leg, multiple sites
  - first degree 945.11
  - second degree 945.21
  - third degree 945.31
    - deep 945.41
      - with loss of body part 945.51
- tongue 947.0
- tonsil 947.0
- trachea 947.1
- trunk 942.00
  - first degree 942.10
  - second degree 942.20
  - third degree 942.30
    - deep 942.40
      - with loss of body part 942.50
  - multiple sites 942.09
    - first degree 942.19
    - second degree 942.29
    - third degree 942.39
      - deep 942.49
        - with loss of body part 942.59
  - specified site NEC 942.09
    - first degree 942.19
    - second degree 942.29
    - third degree 942.39
      - deep 942.49
        - with loss of body part 942.59
- tunica vaginalis — see Burn, genitourinary organs, external
- tympanic membrane — see Burn, ear
- tympanum — see Burn, ear
- ultraviolet 692.82
- unspecified site (multiple) 949.0
  - with extent of body surface involved specified
    - less than 10 percent 948.0 ✓5ᵗʰ
    - 10-19 percent 948.1 ✓5ᵗʰ
    - 20-29 percent 948.2 ✓5ᵗʰ
    - 30-39 percent 948.3 ✓5ᵗʰ
    - 40-49 percent 948.4 ✓5ᵗʰ
    - 50-59 percent 948.5 ✓5ᵗʰ
    - 60-69 percent 948.6 ✓5ᵗʰ
    - 70-79 percent 948.7 ✓5ᵗʰ
    - 80-89 percent 948.8 ✓5ᵗʰ
    - 90 percent or more 948.9 ✓5ᵗʰ
  - first degree 949.1
  - second degree 949.2
  - third degree 949.3
    - deep 949.4
      - with loss of body part 949.5
- uterus 947.4
- uvula 947.0
- vagina 947.4
- vulva — see Burn, genitourinary organs, external
- wrist(s) 944.07
  - with
    - hand(s) — see Burn, hand(s), multiple sites
  - first degree 944.17
  - second degree 944.27
  - third degree 944.37
    - deep 944.47
      - with loss of body part 944.57

Burnett's syndrome (milk-alkali) 999.9
Burnier's syndrome (hypophyseal dwarfism) 253.3
Burning
  feet syndrome 266.2
  sensation (*see also* Disturbance, sensation) 782.0
  tongue 529.6
Burns' disease (osteochondrosis, lower ulna) 732.3
Bursa — *see also* condition
  pharynx 478.29
Bursitis NEC 727.3
  Achilles tendon 726.71
  adhesive 726.90
    shoulder 726.0
  ankle 726.79
  buttock 726.5
  calcaneal 726.79
  collateral ligament
    fibular 726.63
    tibial 726.62
  Duplay's 726.2
  elbow 726.33
  finger 726.8
  foot 726.79
  gonococcal 098.52
  hand 726.4
  hip 726.5
  infrapatellar 726.69
  ischiogluteal 726.5
  knee 726.60
  occupational NEC 727.2
  olecranon 726.33
  pes anserinus 726.61
  pharyngeal 478.29
  popliteal 727.51
  prepatellar 726.65
  radiohumeral 727.3
  scapulohumeral 726.19
    adhesive 726.0
  shoulder 726.10
    adhesive 726.0
  subacromial 726.19
    adhesive 726.0
  subcoracoid 726.19
  subdeltoid 726.19
    adhesive 726.0
  subpatellar 726.69
  syphilitic 095.7
  Thornwaldt's, Tornwaldt's (pharyngeal) 478.29
  toe 726.79
  trochanteric area 726.5
  wrist 726.4
Burst stitches or sutures (complication of surgery) ▶(external)◀ 998.32 ▲
  internal 998.31 ●
Buruli ulcer 031.1
Bury's disease (erythema elevatum diutinum) 695.89
Buschke's disease or scleredema (adultorum) 710.1
Busquet's disease (osteoperiostitis) (*see also* Osteomyelitis) 730.1 ✓5ᵗʰ
Busse-Buschke disease (cryptococcosis) 117.5
Buttock — *see* condition
Button
  Biskra 085.1
  Delhi 085.1
  oriental 085.1
Buttonhole hand (intrinsic) 736.21
Bwamba fever (encephalitis) 066.3
Byssinosis (occupational) 504
Bywaters' syndrome 958.5

C

Cacergasia 300.9
Cachexia 799.4
  cancerous (M8000/3) 199.1
  cardiac — *see* Disease, heart
Cachexia — *continued*
  dehydration 276.5
    with
      hypernatremia 276.0
      hyponatremia 276.1
    due to malnutrition 261
  exophthalmic 242.0 ✓5ᵗʰ
  heart — *see* Disease, heart
  hypophyseal 253.2
  hypopituitary 253.2
  lead 984.9
    specified type of lead — *see* Table of Drugs and Chemicals
  malaria 084.9
  malignant (M8000/3) 199.1
  marsh 084.9
  nervous 300.5
  old age 797
  pachydermic — *see* Hypothyroidism
  paludal 084.9
  pituitary (postpartum) 253.2
  renal (*see also* Disease, renal) 593.9
  saturnine 984.9
    specified type of lead — *see* Table of Drugs and Chemicals
  senile 797
  Simmonds' (pituitary cachexia) 253.2
  splenica 289.59
  strumipriva (*see also* Hypothyroidism) 244.9
  tuberculous NEC (*see also* Tuberculosis) 011.9 ✓5ᵗʰ
Café au lait spots 709.09
Caffey's disease or syndrome (infantile cortical hyperostosis) 756.59
Caisson disease 993.3
Caked breast (puerperal, postpartum) 676.2 ✓5ᵗʰ
Cake kidney 753.3
Calabar swelling 125.2
Calcaneal spur 726.73
Calcaneoapophysitis 732.5
Calcaneonavicular bar 755.67
Calcareous — *see* condition
Calcicosis (occupational) 502
Calciferol (vitamin D) deficiency 268.9
  with
    osteomalacia 268.2
    rickets (*see also* Rickets) 268.0
Calcification
  adrenal (capsule) (gland) 255.4
    tuberculous (*see also* Tuberculosis) 017.6 ✓5ᵗʰ
  aorta 440.0
  artery (annular) — *see* Arteriosclerosis
  auricle (ear) 380.89
  bladder 596.8
    due to S. hematobium 120.0
  brain (cortex) — *see* Calcification, cerebral
  bronchus 519.1
  bursa 727.82
  cardiac (*see also* Degeneration, myocardial) 429.1
  cartilage (postinfectional) 733.99
  cerebral (cortex) 348.8
    artery 437.0
  cervix (uteri) 622.8
  choroid plexus 349.2
  conjunctiva 372.54
  corpora cavernosa (penis) 607.89
  cortex (brain) — *see* Calcification, cerebral
  dental pulp (nodular) 522.2
  dentinal papilla 520.4
  disc, intervertebral 722.90
    cervical, cervicothoracic 722.91
    lumbar, lumbosacral 722.93
    thoracic, thoracolumbar 722.92
  fallopian tube 620.8
  falx cerebri — *see* Calcification, cerebral
  fascia 728.89
  gallbladder 575.8
  general 275.40
  heart (*see also* Degeneration, myocardial) 429.1
    valve — *see* Endocarditis
  intervertebral cartilage or disc (postinfectional) 722.90
    cervical, cervicothoracic 722.91
Calcification — *continued*
  intervertebral cartilage or disc — *continued*
    lumbar, lumbosacral 722.93
    thoracic, thoracolumbar 722.92
  intracranial — *see* Calcification, cerebral
  intraspinal ligament 728.89
  joint 719.80
    ankle 719.87
    elbow 719.82
    foot 719.87
    hand 719.84
    hip 719.85
    knee 719.86
    multiple sites 719.89
    pelvic region 719.85
    shoulder (region) 719.81
    specified site NEC 719.88
    wrist 719.83
  kidney 593.89
    tuberculous (*see also* Tuberculosis) 016.0 ✓5ᵗʰ
  larynx (senile) 478.79
  lens 366.8
  ligament 728.89
    intraspinal 728.89
    knee (medial collateral) 717.89
  lung 518.89
    active 518.89
    postinfectional 518.89
    tuberculous (*see also* Tuberculosis, pulmonary) 011.9 ✓5ᵗʰ
  lymph gland or node (postinfectional) 289.3
    tuberculous (*see also* Tuberculosis, lymph gland) 017.2 ✓5ᵗʰ
  massive (paraplegic) 728.10
  medial NEC (*see also* Arteriosclerosis, extremities) 440.20
  meninges (cerebral) 349.2
  metastatic 275.40
  Mönckeberg's — *see* Arteriosclerosis
  muscle 728.10
    heterotopic, postoperative 728.13
  myocardium, myocardial (*see also* Degeneration, myocardial) 429.1
  ovary 620.8
  pancreas 577.8
  penis 607.89
  periarticular 728.89
  pericardium (*see also* Pericarditis) 423.8
  pineal gland 259.8
  pleura 511.0
    postinfectional 518.89
    tuberculous (*see also* Tuberculosis, pleura) 012.0 ✓5ᵗʰ
  pulp (dental) (nodular) 522.2
  renal 593.89
  Rider's bone 733.99
  sclera 379.16
  semilunar cartilage 717.89
  spleen 289.59
  subcutaneous 709.3
  suprarenal (capsule) (gland) 255.4
  tendon (sheath) 727.82
    with bursitis, synovitis or tenosynovitis 727.82
  trachea 519.1
  ureter 593.89
  uterus 621.8
  vitreous 379.29
Calcified — *see also* Calcification
  hematoma NEC 959.9
Calcinosis (generalized) (interstitial) (tumoral) (universalis) 275.49
  circumscripta 709.3
  cutis 709.3
  intervertebralis 275.49 [722.90]
  Raynaud's
    phenomenonsclerodactyltelangiectasis (CRST) 710.1
Calcium
  blood
    high (*see also* Hypercalcemia) 275.42
    low (*see also* Hypocalcemia) 275.41
  deposits — *see also* Calcification, by site
    in bursa 727.82

Calcium

Calcium — *continued*
  deposits — *see also* Calcification, by site — *continued*
    in tendon (sheath) 727.82
      with bursitis, synovitis or tenosynovitis 727.82
    salts or soaps in vitreous 379.22
Calciuria 791.9
Calculi — *see* Calculus
Calculosis, intrahepatic — *see* Choledocholithiasis
Calculus, calculi, calculous 592.9
  ampulla of Vater — *see* Choledocholithiasis
  anuria (impacted) (recurrent) 592.0
  appendix 543.9
  bile duct (any) — *see* Choledocholithiasis
  biliary — *see* Cholelithiasis
  bilirubin, multiple — *see* Cholelithiasis
  bladder (encysted) (impacted) (urinary) 594.1
    diverticulum 594.0
  bronchus 518.89
  calyx (kidney) (renal) 592.0
    congenital 753.3
  cholesterol (pure) (solitary) — *see* Cholelithiasis
  common duct (bile) — *see* Choledocholithiasis
  conjunctiva 372.54
  cystic 594.1
    duct — *see* Cholelithiasis
  dental 523.6
    subgingival 523.6
    supragingival 523.6
  epididymis 608.89
  gallbladder — *see also* Cholelithiasis
    congenital 751.69
  hepatic (duct) — *see* Choledocholithiasis
  intestine (impaction) (obstruction) 560.39
  kidney (impacted) (multiple) (pelvis) (recurrent) (staghorn) 592.0
    congenital 753.3
  lacrimal (passages) 375.57
  liver (impacted) — *see* Choledocholithiasis
  lung 518.89
  nephritic (impacted) (recurrent) 592.0
  nose 478.1
  pancreas (duct) 577.8
  parotid gland 527.5
  pelvis, encysted 592.0
  prostate 602.0
  pulmonary 518.89
  renal (impacted) (recurrent) 592.0
    congenital 753.3
  salivary (duct) (gland) 527.5
  seminal vesicle 608.89
  staghorn 592.0
  Stensen's duct 527.5
  sublingual duct or gland 527.5
    congenital 750.26
  submaxillary duct, gland, or region 527.5
  suburethral 594.8
  tonsil 474.8
  tooth, teeth 523.6
  tunica vaginalis 608.89
  ureter (impacted) (recurrent) 592.1
  urethra (impacted) 594.2
  urinary (duct) (impacted) (passage) (tract) 592.9
    lower tract NEC 594.9
      specified site 594.8
  vagina 623.8
  vesical (impacted) 594.1
  Wharton's duct 527.5
Caliectasis 593.89
California
  disease 114.0
  encephalitis 062.5
Caligo cornea 371.03
Callositas, callosity (infected) 700
Callus (infected) 700
  bone 726.91
  excessive, following fracture — *see also* Late, effect (of), fracture
Calvé (-Perthes) disease (osteochondrosis, femoral capital) 732.1
Calvities (*see also* Alopecia) 704.00
Cameroon fever (*see also* Malaria) 084.6
Camptocormia 300.11

Camptodactyly (congenital) 755.59
Camurati-Engelmann disease (diaphyseal sclerosis) 756.59
Canal — *see* condition
Canaliculitis (lacrimal) (acute) 375.31
  Actinomyces 039.8
  chronic 375.41
Canavan's disease 330.0
Cancer (M8000/3) — *see also* Neoplasm, by site, malignant

> Note — The term "cancer" when modified by an adjective or adjectival phrase indicating a morphological type should be coded in the same manner as "carcinoma" with that adjective or phrase. Thus, "squamous-cell cancer" should be coded in the same manner as "squamous-cell carcinoma," which appears in the list under "Carcinoma."

  bile duct type (M8160/3), liver 155.1
  hepatocellular (M8170/3) 155.0
Cancerous (M8000/3) — *see* Neoplasm, by site, malignant
Cancerphobia 300.29
Cancrum oris 528.1
Candidiasis, candidal 112.9
  with pneumonia 112.4
  balanitis 112.2
  congenital 771.7
  disseminated 112.5
  endocarditis 112.81
  esophagus 112.84
  intertrigo 112.3
  intestine 112.85
  lung 112.4
  meningitis 112.83
  mouth 112.0
  nails 112.3
  neonatal 771.7
  onychia 112.3
  otitis externa 112.82
  otomycosis 112.82
  paronychia 112.3
  perionyxis 112.3
  pneumonia 112.4
  pneumonitis 112.4
  skin 112.3
  specified site NEC 112.89
  systemic 112.5
  urogenital site NEC 112.2
  vagina 112.1
  vulva 112.1
  vulvovaginitis 112.1
Candidiosis — *see* Candidiasis
Candiru infection or infestation 136.8
Canities (premature) 704.3
  congenital 757.4
Canker (mouth) (sore) 528.2
  rash 034.1
Cannabinosis 504
Canton fever 081.9
Cap
  cradle 690.11
Capillariasis 127.5
Capillary — *see* condition
Caplan's syndrome 714.81
Caplan-Colinet syndrome 714.81
Capsule — *see* condition
Capsulitis (joint) 726.90
  adhesive (shoulder) 726.0
  hip 726.5
  knee 726.60
  labyrinthine 387.8
  thyroid 245.9
  wrist 726.4
Caput
  crepitus 756.0
  medusae 456.8
  succedaneum 767.1
Carapata disease 087.1
Carate — *see* Pinta

Carboxyhemoglobinemia 986
Carbuncle 680.9
  abdominal wall 680.2
  ankle 680.6
  anus 680.5
  arm (any part, above wrist) 680.3
  auditory canal, external 680.0
  axilla 680.3
  back (any part) 680.2
  breast 680.2
  buttock 680.5
  chest wall 680.2
  corpus cavernosum 607.2
  ear (any part) (external) 680.0
  eyelid 373.13
  face (any part except eye) 680.0
  finger (any) 680.4
  flank 680.2
  foot (any part) 680.7
  forearm 680.3
  genital organ (male) 608.4
  gluteal (region) 680.5
  groin 680.2
  hand (any part) 680.4
  head (any part except face) 680.8
  heel 680.7
  hip 680.6
  kidney (*see also* Abscess, kidney) 590.2
  knee 680.6
  labia 616.4
  lacrimal
    gland (*see also* Dacryoadenitis) 375.00
    passages (duct) (sac) (*see also* Dacryocystitis) 375.30
  leg, any part except foot 680.6
  lower extremity, any part except foot 680.6
  malignant 022.0
  multiple sites 680.9
  neck 680.1
  nose (external) (septum) 680.0
  orbit, orbital 376.01
  partes posteriores 680.5
  pectoral region 680.2
  penis 607.2
  perineum 680.2
  pinna 680.0
  scalp (any part) 680.8
  scrotum 608.4
  seminal vesicle 608.0
  shoulder 680.3
  skin NEC 680.9
  specified site NEC 680.8
  spermatic cord 608.4
  temple (region) 680.0
  testis 608.4
  thigh 680.6
  thumb 680.4
  toe (any) 680.7
  trunk 680.2
  tunica vaginalis 608.4
  umbilicus 680.2
  upper arm 680.3
  urethra 597.0
  vas deferens 608.4
  vulva 616.4
  wrist 680.4
Carbunculus (*see also* Carbuncle) 680.9
Carcinoid (tumor) (M8240/1) — *see also* Neoplasm, by site, uncertain behavior
  and struma ovarii (M9091/1) 236.2
  argentaffin (M8241/1) — *see* Neoplasm, by site, uncertain behavior
    malignant (M8241/3) — *see* Neoplasm, by site, malignant
  benign (M9091/0) 220
  composite (M8244/3) — *see* Neoplasm, by site, malignant
  goblet cell (M8243/3) — *see* Neoplasm, by site, malignant
  malignant (M8240/3) — *see* Neoplasm, by site, malignant
  nonargentaffin (M8242/1) — *see also* Neoplasm, by site, uncertain behavior
    malignant (M8242/3) — *see* Neoplasm, by site, malignant
  strumal (M9091/1) 236.2
  syndrome (intestinal) (metastatic) 259.2

Index to Diseases

Carcinoid — *see also* Neoplasm, by site, uncertain behavior — *continued*
   type bronchial adenoma (M8240/3) — *see* Neoplasm, lung, malignant

Carcinoidosis 259.2

Carcinoma (M8010/3) — *see also* Neoplasm, by site, malignant

> Note — Except where otherwise indicated, the morphological varieties of carcinoma in the list below should be coded by site as for "Neoplasm, malignant."

  with
    apocrine metaplasia (M8573/3)
    cartilaginous (and osseous) metaplasia (M8571/3)
    osseous (and cartilaginous) metaplasia (M8571/3)
    productive fibrosis (M8141/3)
    spindle cell metaplasia (M8572/3)
    squamous metaplasia (M8570/3)
  acidophil (M8280/3)
    specified site — *see* Neoplasm, by site, malignant
    unspecified site 194.3
  acidophil-basophil, mixed (M8281/3)
    specified site — *see* Neoplasm, by site, malignant
    unspecified site 194.3
  acinar (cell) (M8550/3)
  acinic cell (M8550/3)
  adenocystic (M8200/3)
  adenoid
    cystic (M8200/3)
    squamous cell (M8075/3)
  adenosquamous (M8560/3)
  adnexal (skin) (M8390/3) — *see* Neoplasm, skin, malignant
  adrenal cortical (M8370/3) 194.0
  alveolar (M8251/3)
    cell (M8250/3) — *see* Neoplasm, lung, malignant
  anaplastic type (M8021/3)
  apocrine (M8401/3)
    breast — *see* Neoplasm, breast, malignant
    specified site NEC — *see* Neoplasm, skin, malignant
    unspecified site 173.9
  basal cell (pigmented) (M8090/3) — *see also* Neoplasm, skin, malignant
    fibro-epithelial type (M8093/3) — *see* Neoplasm, skin, malignant
    morphea type (M8092/3) — *see* Neoplasm, skin, malignant
    multicentric (M8091/3) — *see* Neoplasm, skin, malignant
  basaloid (M8123/3)
  basal-squamous cell, mixed (M8094/3) — *see* Neoplasm, skin, malignant
  basophil (M8300/3)
    specified site — *see* Neoplasm, by site, malignant
    unspecified site 194.3
  basophil-acidophil, mixed (M8281/3)
    specified site — *see* Neoplasm, by site, malignant
    unspecified site 194.3
  basosquamous (M8094/3) — *see* Neoplasm, skin, malignant
  bile duct type (M8160/3)
    and hepatocellular, mixed (M8180/3) 155.0
    liver 155.1
    specified site NEC — *see* Neoplasm, by site, malignant
    unspecified site 155.1
  branchial or branchiogenic 146.8
  bronchial or bronchogenic — *see* Neoplasm, lung, malignant
  bronchiolar (terminal) (M8250/3) — *see* Neoplasm, lung, malignant
  bronchiolo-alveolar (M8250/3) — *see* Neoplasm, lung, malignant
  bronchogenic (epidermoid) 162.9
  C cell (M8510/3)
    specified site — *see* Neoplasm, by site, malignant
    unspecified site 193

Carcinoma — *see also* Neoplasm, by site, malignant — *continued*
  ceruminous (M8420/3) 173.2
  chorionic (M9100/3)
    specified site — *see* Neoplasm, by site, malignant
    unspecified site
      female 181
      male 186.9
  chromophobe (M8270/3)
    specified site — *see* Neoplasm, by site, malignant
    unspecified site 194.3
  clear cell (mesonephroid type) (M8310/3)
  cloacogenic (M8124/3)
    specified site — *see* Neoplasm, by site, malignant
    unspecified site 154.8
  colloid (M8480/3)
  cribriform (M8201/3)
  cylindroid type (M8200/3)
  diffuse type (M8145/3)
    specified site — *see* Neoplasm, by site, malignant
    unspecified site 151.9
  duct (cell) (M8500/3)
    with Paget's disease (M8541/3) — *see* Neoplasm, breast, malignant
    infiltrating (M8500/3)
      specified site — *see* Neoplasm, by site, malignant
      unspecified site 174.9
  ductal (M8500/3)
  ductular, infiltrating (M8521/3)
  embryonal (M9070/3)
    and teratoma, mixed (M9081/3)
    combined with choriocarcinoma (M9101/3) — *see* Neoplasm, by site, malignant
    infantile type (M9071/3)
    liver 155.0
    polyembryonal type (M9072/3)
  endometrioid (M8380/3)
  eosinophil (M8280/3)
    specified site — *see* Neoplasm, by site, malignant
    unspecified site 194.3
  epidermoid (M8070/3) — *see also* Carcinoma, squamous cell
    and adenocarcinoma, mixed (M8560/3)
    in situ, Bowen's type (M8081/2) — *see* Neoplasm, skin, in situ
    intradermal — *see* Neoplasm, skin, in situ
  fibroepithelial type basal cell (M8093/3) — *see* Neoplasm, skin, malignant
  follicular (M8330/3)
    and papillary (mixed) (M8340/3) 193
    moderately differentiated type (M8332/3) 193
    pure follicle type (M8331/3) 193
    specified site — *see* Neoplasm, by site, malignant
    trabecular type (M8332/3) 193
    unspecified site 193
    well differentiated type (M8331/3) 193
  gelatinous (M8480/3)
  giant cell (M8031/3)
    and spindle cell (M8030/3)
  granular cell (M8320/3)
  granulosa cell (M8620/3) 183.0
  hepatic cell (M8170/3) 155.0
  hepatocellular (M8170/3) 155.0
    and bile duct, mixed (M8180/3) 155.0
  hepatocholangiolitic (M8180/3) 155.0
  Hürthle cell (thyroid) 193
  hypernephroid (M8311/3)
  in
    adenomatous
      polyp (M8210/3)
      polyposis coli (M8220/3) 153.9
    pleomorphic adenoma (M8940/3)
    polypoid adenoma (M8210/3)
    situ (M8010/3) — *see* Carcinoma, in situ
    tubular adenoma (M8210/3)
    villous adenoma (M8261/3)
  infiltrating duct (M8500/3)
    with Paget's disease (M8541/3) — *see* Neoplasm, breast, malignant

Carcinoma — *see also* Neoplasm, by site, malignant — *continued*
  infiltrating duct — *continued*
    specified site — *see* Neoplasm, by site, malignant
    unspecified site 174.9
  inflammatory (M8530/3)
    specified site — *see* Neoplasm, by site, malignant
    unspecified site 174.9
  in situ (M8010/2) — *see also* Neoplasm, by site, in situ
    epidermoid (M8070/2) — *see also* Neoplasm, by site, in situ
      with questionable stromal invasion (M8076/2)
      specified site — *see* Neoplasm, by site, in situ
      unspecified site 233.1
    Bowen's type (M8081/2) — *see* Neoplasm, skin, in situ
    intraductal (M8500/2)
      specified site — *see* Neoplasm, by site, in situ
      unspecified site 233.0
    lobular (M8520/2)
      specified site — *see* Neoplasm, by site, in situ
      unspecified site 233.0
    papillary (M8050/2) — *see* Neoplasm, by site, in situ
    squamous cell (M8070/2) — *see also* Neoplasm, by site, in situ
      with questionable stromal invasion (M8076/2)
      specified site — *see* Neoplasm, by site, in situ
      unspecified site 233.1
    transitional cell (M8120/2) — *see* Neoplasm, by site, in situ
  intestinal type (M8144/3)
    specified site — *see* Neoplasm, by site, malignant
    unspecified site 151.9
  intraductal (noninfiltrating) (M8500/2)
    papillary (M8503/2)
      specified site — *see* Neoplasm, by site, in situ
      unspecified site 233.0
    specified site — *see* Neoplasm, by site, in situ
    unspecified site 233.0
  intraepidermal (M8070/2) — *see also* Neoplasm, skin, in situ
    squamous cell, Bowen's type (M8081/2) — *see* Neoplasm, skin, in situ
  intraepithelial (M8010/2) — *see also* Neoplasm, by site, in situ
    squamous cell (M8072/2) — *see* Neoplasm, by site, in situ
  intraosseous (M9270/3) 170.1
    upper jaw (bone) 170.0
  islet cell (M8150/3)
    and exocrine, mixed (M8154/3)
      specified site — *see* Neoplasm, by site, malignant
      unspecified site 157.9
    pancreas 157.4
    specified site NEC — *see* Neoplasm, by site, malignant
    unspecified site 157.4
  juvenile, breast (M8502/3) — *see* Neoplasm, breast, malignant
  Kulchitsky's cell (carcinoid tumor of intestine) 259.2
  large cell (M8012/3)
    squamous cell, nonkeratinizing type (M8072/3)
  Leydig cell (testis) (M8650/3)
    specified site — *see* Neoplasm, by site, malignant
    unspecified site 186.9
      female 183.0
      male 186.9
  liver cell (M8170/3) 155.0

Carcinoma — see also Neoplasm, by site, malignant — continued
- lobular (infiltrating) (M8520/3)
  - non-infiltrating (M8520/3)
    - specified site — see Neoplasm, by site, in situ
    - unspecified site 233.0
  - specified site — see Neoplasm, by site, malignant
  - unspecified site 174.9
- lymphoepithelial (M8082/3)
- medullary (M8510/3)
  - with
    - amyloid stroma (M8511/3)
      - specified site — see Neoplasm, by site, malignant
      - unspecified site 193
    - lymphoid stroma (M8512/3)
      - specified site — see Neoplasm, by site, malignant
      - unspecified site 174.9
- mesometanephric (M9110/3)
- mesonephric (M9110/3)
- metastatic (M8010/6) — see Metastasis, cancer
- metatypical (M8095/3) — see Neoplasm, skin, malignant
- morphea type basal cell (M8092/3) — see Neoplasm, skin, malignant
- mucinous (M8480/3)
- mucin-producing (M8481/3)
- mucin-secreting (M8481/3)
- mucoepidermoid (M8430/3)
- mucoid (M8480/3)
  - cell (M8300/3)
    - specified site — see Neoplasm, by site, malignant
    - unspecified site 194.3
- mucous (M8480/3)
- nonencapsulated sclerosing (M8350/3) 193
- noninfiltrating
  - intracystic (M8504/2) — see Neoplasm, by site, in situ
  - intraductal (M8500/2)
    - papillary (M8503/2)
      - specified site — see Neoplasm, by site, in situ
      - unspecified site 233.0
    - specified site — see Neoplasm, by site, in situ
    - unspecified site 233.0
  - lobular (M8520/2)
    - specified site — see Neoplasm, by site, in situ
    - unspecified site 233.0
- oat cell (M8042/3)
  - specified site — see Neoplasm, by site, malignant
  - unspecified site 162.9
- odontogenic (M9270/3) 170.1
  - upper jaw (bone) 170.0
- onocytic (M8290/3)
- oxyphilic (M8290/3)
- papillary (M8050/3)
  - and follicular (mixed) (M8340/3) 193
  - epidermoid (M8052/3)
  - intraductal (noninfiltrating) (M8503/2)
    - specified site — see Neoplasm, by site, in situ
    - unspecified site 233.0
  - serous (M8460/3)
    - specified site — see Neoplasm, by site, malignant
    - surface (M8461/3)
      - specified site — see Neoplasm, by site, malignant
      - unspecified site 183.0
    - unspecified site 183.0
  - squamous cell (M8052/3)
  - transitional cell (M8130/3)
- papillocystic (M8450/3)
  - specified site — see Neoplasm, by site, malignant
  - unspecified site 183.0
- parafollicular cell (M8510/3)
  - specified site — see Neoplasm, by site, malignant
  - unspecified site 193

Carcinoma — see also Neoplasm, by site, malignant — continued
- pleomorphic (M8022/3)
- polygonal cell (M8034/3)
- prickle cell (M8070/3)
- pseudoglandular, squamous cell (M8075/3)
- pseudomucinous (M8470/3)
  - specified site — see Neoplasm, by site, malignant
  - unspecified site 183.0
- pseudosarcomatous (M8033/3)
- regaud type (M8082/3) — see Neoplasm, nasopharynx, malignant
- renal cell (M8312/3) 189.0
- reserve cell (M8041/3)
- round cell (M8041/3)
- Schmincke (M8082/3) — see Neoplasm, nasopharynx, malignant
- Schneiderian (M8121/3)
  - specified site — see Neoplasm, by site, malignant
  - unspecified site 160.0
- scirrhous (M8141/3)
- sebaceous (M8410/3) — see Neoplasm, skin, malignant
- secondary (M8010/6) — see Neoplasm, by site, malignant, secondary
- secretory, breast (M8502/3) — see Neoplasm, breast, malignant
- serous (M8441/3)
  - papillary (M8460/3)
    - specified site — see Neoplasm, by site, malignant
    - unspecified site 183.0
  - surface, papillary (M8461/3)
    - specified site — see Neoplasm, by site, malignant
    - unspecified site 183.0
- Sertoli cell (M8640/3)
  - specified site — see Neoplasm, by site, malignant
  - unspecified site 186.9
- signet ring cell (M8490/3)
  - metastatic (M8490/6) — see Neoplasm, by site, secondary
- simplex (M8231/3)
- skin appendage (M8390/3) — see Neoplasm, skin, malignant
- small cell (M8041/3)
  - fusiform cell type (M8043/3)
  - squamous cell, non-keratinizing type (M8073/3)
- solid (M8230/3)
  - with amyloid stroma (M8511/3)
    - specified site — see Neoplasm, by site, malignant
    - unspecified site 193
- spheroidal cell (M8035/3)
- spindle cell (M8032/3)
  - and giant cell (M8030/3)
- spinous cell (M8070/3)
- squamous (cell) (M8070/3)
  - adenoid type (M8075/3)
  - and adenocarcinoma, mixed (M8560/3)
  - intraepidermal, Bowen's type — see Neoplasm, skin, in situ
  - keratinizing type (large cell) (M8071/3)
  - large cell, non-keratinizing type (M8072/3)
  - microinvasive (M8076/3)
    - specified site — see Neoplasm, by site, malignant
    - unspecified site 180.9
  - non-keratinizing type (M8072/3)
  - papillary (M8052/3)
  - pseudoglandular (M8075/3)
  - small cell, non-keratinizing type (M8073/3)
  - spindle cell type (M8074/3)
  - verrucous (M8051/3)
- superficial spreading (M8143/3)
- sweat gland (M8400/3) — see Neoplasm, skin, malignant
- theca cell (M8600/3) 183.0
- thymic (M8580/3) 164.0
- trabecular (M8190/3)
- transitional (cell) (M8120/3)
  - papillary (M8130/3)
  - spindle cell type (M8122/3)

Carcinoma — see also Neoplasm, by site, malignant — continued
- tubular (M8211/3)
- undifferentiated type (M8020/3)
- urothelial (M8120/3)
- ventriculi 151.9
- verrucous (epidermoid) (squamous cell) (M8051/3)
- villous (M8262/3)
- water-clear cell (M8322/3) 194.1
- wolffian duct (M9110/3)

Carcinomaphobia 300.29

Carcinomatosis
- peritonei (M8010/6) 197.6
- specified site NEC (M8010/3) — see Neoplasm, by site, malignant
- unspecified site (M8010/6) 199.0

Carcinosarcoma (M8980/3) — see also Neoplasm, by site, malignant
- embryonal type (M8981/3) — see Neoplasm, by site, malignant

Cardia, cardial — see condition

Cardiac — see also condition
- death — see Disease, heart
- device
  - defibrillator, automatic implantable V45.02
  - in situ NEC V45.00
  - pacemaker
    - cardiac
      - fitting or adjustment V53.31
      - in situ V45.01
    - carotid sinus
      - fitting or adjustment V53.39
      - in situ V45.09
- pacemaker — see Cardiac, device, pacemaker
- tamponade 423.9

Cardialgia (see also Pain, precordial) 786.51

Cardiectasis — see Hypertrophy, cardiac

Cardiochalasia 530.81

Cardiomalacia (see also Degeneration, myocardial) 429.1

Cardiomegalia glycogenica diffusa 271.0

Cardiomegaly (see also Hypertrophy, cardiac) 429.3
- congenital 746.89
- glycogen 271.0
- hypertensive (see also Hypertension, heart) 402.90
- idiopathic 429.3

Cardiomyolipsis (see also Degeneration, myocardial) 429.1

Cardiomyopathy (congestive) (constrictive) (familial) (infiltrative) (obstructive) (restrictive) (sporadic) 425.4
- alcoholic 425.5
- amyloid 277.3 [425.7]
- beriberi 265.0 [425.7]
- cobalt-beer 425.5
- congenital 425.3
- due to
  - amyloidosis 277.3 [425.7]
  - beriberi 265.0 [425.7]
  - cardiac glycogenosis 271.0 [425.7]
  - Chagas' disease 086.0
  - Friedreich's ataxia 334.0 [425.8]
  - hypertension —see Hypertension, with, heart involvement
  - mucopolysaccharidosis 277.5 [425.7]
  - myotonia atrophica 359.2 [425.8]
  - progressive muscular dystrophy 359.1 [425.8]
  - sarcoidosis 135 [425.8]
- glycogen storage 271.0 [425.7]
- hypertensive — see Hypertension, with, heart involvement
- hypertrophic
  - nonobstructive 425.4
  - obstructive 425.1
    - congenital 746.84
- idiopathic (concentric) 425.4
- in
  - Chagas' disease 086.0
  - sarcoidosis 135 [425.8]
- ischemic 414.8

Index to Diseases

Cardiomyopathy — *continued*
  metabolic NEC 277.9 *[425.7]*
    amyloid 277.3 *[425.7]*
    thyrotoxic (*see also* Thyrotoxicosis) 242.9 ✓5th *[425.7]*
    thyrotoxicosis (*see also* Thyrotoxicosis) 242.9 ✓5th *[425.7]*
  nutritional 269.9 *[425.7]*
    beriberi 265.0 *[425.7]*
  obscure of Africa 425.2
  postpartum 674.8 ✓5th
  primary 425.4
  secondary 425.9
  thyrotoxic (*see also* Thyrotoxicosis) 242.9 ✓5th *[425.7]*
  toxic NEC 425.9
  tuberculous (*see also* Tuberculosis) 017.9 ✓5th *[425.8]*
Cardionephritis — *see* Hypertension, cardiorenal
Cardionephropathy — *see* Hypertension, cardiorenal
Cardionephrosis — *see* Hypertension, cardiorenal
Cardioneurosis 306.2
Cardiopathia nigra 416.0
Cardiopathy (*see also* Disease, heart) 429.9
  hypertensive (*see also* Hypertension, heart) 402.90
  idiopathic 425.4
  mucopolysaccharidosis 277.5 *[425.7]*
Cardiopericarditis (*see also* Pericarditis) 423.9
Cardiophobia 300.29
Cardioptosis 746.87
Cardiorenal — *see* condition
Cardiorrhexis (*see also* Infarct, myocardium) 410.9 ✓5th
Cardiosclerosis — *see* Arteriosclerosis, coronary
Cardiosis — *see* Disease, heart
Cardiospasm (esophagus) (reflex) (stomach) 530.0
  congenital 750.7
Cardiostenosis — *see* Disease, heart
Cardiosymphysis 423.1
Cardiothyrotoxicosis — *see* Hyperthyroidism
Cardiovascular — *see* condition
Carditis (acute) (bacterial) (chronic) (subacute) 429.89
  Coxsackie 074.20
  hypertensive (*see also* Hypertension, heart) 402.90
  meningococcal 036.40
  rheumatic — *see* Disease, heart, rheumatic
  rheumatoid 714.2
Care (of)
  child (routine) V20.1
  convalescent following V66.9
    chemotherapy V66.2
    medical NEC V66.5
    psychotherapy V66.3
    radiotherapy V66.1
    surgery V66.0
    surgical NEC V66.0
    treatment (for) V66.5
      combined V66.6
      fracture V66.4
      mental disorder NEC V66.3
      specified type NEC V66.5
  end-of-life V66.7
  family member (handicapped) (sick)
    creating problem for family V61.49
    provided away from home for holiday relief V60.5
    unavailable, due to
      absence (person rendering care) (sufferer) V60.4
      inability (any reason) of person rendering care V60.4
  holiday relief V60.5
  hospice V66.7
  lack of (at or after birth) (infant) (child) 995.52
    adult 995.84
  lactation of mother V24.1
  palliative V66.7
  postpartum
    immediately after delivery V24.0
    routine follow-up V24.2

Care (of) — *continued*
  prenatal V22.1
    first pregnancy V22.0
    high risk pregnancy V23.9
      specified problem NEC V23.89
  terminal V66.7
  unavailable, due to
    absence of person rendering care V60.4
    inability (any reason) of person rendering care V60.4
  well baby V20.1
Caries (bone) (*see also* Tuberculosis, bone) 015.9 ✓5th *[730.8]* ✓5th
  arrested 521.04
  cementum 521.03
  cerebrospinal (tuberculous) 015.0 ✓5th *[730.88]*
  dental (acute) (chronic) (incipient) (infected) 521.09
    with pulp exposure 521.03
    extending to
      dentine 521.02
      pulp 521.03
    other specified NEC 521.09
  dentin (acute) (chronic) 521.02
  enamel (acute) (chronic) (incipient) 521.01
  external meatus 380.89
  hip (*see also* Tuberculosis) 015.1 ✓5th *[730.85]*
  knee 015.2 ✓5th *[730.86]*
  labyrinth 386.8
  limb NEC 015.7 ✓5th *[730.88]*
  mastoid (chronic) (process) 383.1
  middle ear 385.89
  nose 015.7 ✓5th *[730.88]*
  orbit 015.7 ✓5th *[730.88]*
  ossicle 385.24
  petrous bone 383.20
  sacrum (tuberculous) 015.0 ✓5th *[730.88]*
  spine, spinal (column) (tuberculous) 015.0 ✓5th *[730.88]*
  syphilitic 095.5
    congenital 090.0 *[730.8]* ✓5th
  teeth (internal) 521.00
    initial 521.01
  vertebra (column) (tuberculous) 015.0 ✓5th *[730.88]*
Carini's syndrome (ichthyosis congenita) 757.1
Carious teeth 521.00
Carneous mole 631
Carnosinemia 270.5
Carotid body or sinus syndrome 337.0
Carotidynia 337.0
Carotenemia (dietary) 278.3
Carotinosis (cutis) (skin) 278.3
Carpal tunnel syndrome 354.0
Carpenter's syndrome 759.89
Carpopedal spasm (*see also* Tetany) 781.7
Carpoptosis 736.05
Carrier (suspected) of
  amebiasis V02.2
  bacterial disease (meningococcal, staphylococcal, streptococcal) NEC V02.59
  cholera V02.0
  cystic fibrosis gene V83.81 ●
  defective gene V83.89 ▲
  diphtheria V02.4
  dysentery (bacillary) V02.3
    amebic V02.2
  Endamoeba histolytica V02.2
  gastrointestinal pathogens NEC V02.3
  genetic defect V83.89 ▲
  gonorrhea V02.7
  group B streptococcus V02.51
  HAA (hepatitis Australian-antigen) V02.61
  hemophilia A (asymptomatic) V83.01
    symptomatic V83.02
  hepatitis V02.60
    Australian-antigen (HAA) V02.61
    B V02.61
    C V02.62
    serum V02.61
    specified type NEC V02.69
    viral V02.60
  infective organism NEC V02.9
  malaria V02.9

Cataract

Carrier (suspected) **of** — *continued*
  paratyphoid V02.3
  Salmonella V02.3
    typhosa V02.1
  serum hepatitis V02.61
  Shigella V02.3
  Staphylococcus NEC V02.59
  Streptococcus NEC V02.52
    group B V02.51
  typhoid V02.1
  venereal disease NEC V02.8
Carrión's disease (Bartonellosis) 088.0
Car sickness 994.6
Carter's
  relapsing fever (Asiatic) 087.0
Cartilage — *see* condition
Caruncle (inflamed)
  abscess, lacrimal (*see also* Dacryocystitis) 375.30
  conjunctiva 372.00
    acute 372.00
  eyelid 373.00
  labium (majus) (minus) 616.8
  lacrimal 375.30
  urethra (benign) 599.3
  vagina (wall) 616.8
Cascade stomach 537.6
Caseation lymphatic gland (*see also* Tuberculosis) 017.2 ✓5th
Caseous
  bronchitis — *see* Tuberculosis, pulmonary
  meningitis 013.0 ✓5th
  pneumonia — *see* Tuberculosis, pulmonary
Cassidy (-Scholte) syndrome (malignant carcinoid) 259.2
Castellani's bronchitis 104.8
Castleman's tumor or lymphoma (mediastinal lymph node hyperplasia) 785.6
Castration, traumatic 878.2
  complicated 878.3
Casts in urine 791.7
Cat's ear 744.29
Catalepsy 300.11
  catatonic (acute) (*see also* Schizophrenia) 295.2 ✓5th
  hysterical 300.11
  schizophrenic (*see also* Schizophrenia) 295.2 ✓5th
Cataphasia 307.0
Cataplexy (idiopathic) 347
Cataract (anterior cortical) (anterior polar) (black) (capsular) (central) (cortical) (hypermature) (immature) (incipient) (mature) 366.9
  anterior
    and posterior axial embryonal 743.33
    pyramidal 743.31
    subcapsular polar
      infantile, juvenile, or presenile 366.01
      senile 366.13
  associated with
    calcinosis 275.40 *[366.42]*
    craniofacial dysostosis 756.0 *[366.44]*
    galactosemia 271.1 *[366.44]*
    hypoparathyroidism 252.1 *[366.42]*
    myotonic disorders 359.2 *[366.43]*
    neovascularization 366.33
  blue dot 743.39
  cerulean 743.39
  complicated NEC 366.30
  congenital 743.30
    capsular or subcapsular 743.31
    cortical 743.32
    nuclear 743.33
    specified type NEC 743.39
    total or subtotal 743.34
    zonular 743.32
  coronary (congenital) 743.39
    acquired 366.12
  cupuliform 366.14
  diabetic 250.5 ✓5th *[366.41]*
  drug-induced 366.45
  due to
    chalcosis 360.24 *[366.34]*

Cataract

Cataract — *continued*
  due to — *continued*
    chronic choroiditis (*see also* Choroiditis) 363.20 *[366.32]*
    degenerative myopia 360.21 *[366.34]*
    glaucoma (*see also* Glaucoma) 365.9 *[366.31]*
    infection, intraocular NEC 366.32
    inflammatory ocular disorder NEC 366.32
    iridocyclitis, chronic 364.10 *[366.33]*
    pigmentary retinal dystrophy 362.74 *[366.34]*
    radiation 366.46
  electric 366.46
  glassblowers' 366.46
  heat ray 366.46
  heterochromic 366.33
  in eye disease NEC 366.30
  infantile (*see also* Cataract, juvenile) 366.00
  intumescent 366.12
  irradiational 366.46
  juvenile 366.00
    anterior subcapsular polar 366.01
    combined forms 366.09
    cortical 366.03
    lamellar 366.03
    nuclear 366.04
    posterior subcapsular polar 366.02
    specified NEC 366.09
    zonular 366.03
  lamellar 743.32
    infantile, juvenile, or presenile 366.03
  morgagnian 366.18
  myotonic 359.2 *[366.43]*
  myxedema 244.9 *[366.44]*
  nuclear 366.16
  posterior, polar (capsular) 743.31
    infantile, juvenile, or presenile 366.02
    senile 366.14
  presenile (*see also* Cataract, juvenile) 366.00
  punctate
    acquired 366.12
    congenital 743.39
  secondary (membrane) 366.50
    obscuring vision 366.53
    specified type, not obscuring vision 366.52
  senile 366.10
    anterior subcapsular polar 366.13
    combined forms 366.19
    cortical 366.15
    hypermature 366.18
    immature 366.12
    incipient 366.12
    mature 366.17
    nuclear 366.16
    posterior subcapsular polar 366.14
    specified NEC 366.19
    total or subtotal 366.17
  snowflake 250.5 *[366.41]*
  specified NEC 366.8
  subtotal (senile) 366.17
    congenital 743.34
  sunflower 360.24 *[366.34]*
  tetanic NEC 252.1 *[366.42]*
  total (mature) (senile) 366.17
    congenital 743.34
    localized 366.21
    traumatic 366.22
  toxic 366.45
  traumatic 366.20
    partially resolved 366.23
    total 366.22
  zonular (perinuclear) 743.32
    infantile, juvenile, or presenile 366.03

Cataracta 366.10
  brunescens 366.16
  cerulea 743.39
  complicata 366.30
  congenita 743.30
  coralliformis 743.39
  coronaria (congenital) 743.39
    acquired 366.12
  diabetica 250.5 *[366.41]*
  floriformis 360.24 *[366.34]*
  membranacea
    accreta 366.50
    congenita 743.39
  nigra 366.16

Catarrh, catarrhal (inflammation) (*see also* condition) 460
  acute 460
  asthma, asthmatic (*see also* Asthma) 493.9
  Bostock's (*see also* Fever, hay) 477.9
  bowel — *see* Enteritis
  bronchial 490
    acute 466.0
    chronic 491.0
    subacute 466.0
  cervix, cervical (canal) (uteri) — *see* Cervicitis
  chest (*see also* Bronchitis) 490
  chronic 472.0
  congestion 472.0
  conjunctivitis 372.03
  due to syphilis 095.9
    congenital 090.0
  enteric — *see* Enteritis
  epidemic 487.1
  Eustachian 381.50
  eye (acute) (vernal) 372.03
  fauces (*see also* Pharyngitis) 462
  febrile 460
  fibrinous acute 466.0
  gastroenteric — *see* Enteritis
  gastrointestinal — *see* Enteritis
  gingivitis 523.0
  hay (*see also* Fever, hay) 477.9
  infectious 460
  intestinal — *see* Enteritis
  larynx (*see also* Laryngitis, chronic) 476.0
  liver 070.1
    with hepatic coma 070.0
  lung (*see also* Bronchitis) 490
    acute 466.0
    chronic 491.0
  middle ear (chronic) — *see* Otitis media, chronic
  mouth 528.0
  nasal (chronic) (*see also* Rhinitis) 472.0
    acute 460
  nasobronchial 472.2
  nasopharyngeal (chronic) 472.2
    acute 460
  nose — *see* Catarrh, nasal
  ophthalmia 372.03
  pneumococcal, acute 466.0
  pulmonary (*see also* Bronchitis) 490
    acute 466.0
    chronic 491.0
  spring (eye) 372.13
  suffocating (*see also* Asthma) 493.9
  summer (hay) (*see also* Fever, hay) 477.9
  throat 472.1
  tracheitis 464.10
    with obstruction 464.11
  tubotympanal 381.4
    acute (*see also* Otitis media, acute, nonsuppurative) 381.00
    chronic 381.10
  vasomotor (*see also* Fever, hay) 477.9
  vesical (bladder) — *see* Cystitis

Catarrhus aestivus (*see also* Fever, hay) 477.9

Catastrophe, cerebral (*see also* Disease, cerebrovascular, acute) 436

Catatonia, catatonic (acute) 781.99
  with
    affective psychosis — *see* Psychosis, affective
  agitation 295.2
  Churg-Strauss syndrome 446.4
  dementia (praecox) 295.2
  due to or associated with physical condition 293.89
  excitation 295.2
  excited type 295.2
  schizophrenia 295.2
  stupor 295.2

Cat-scratch — *see also* Injury, superficial disease or fever 078.3

Cauda equina — *see also* condition
  syndrome 344.60

Cauliflower ear 738.7

Caul over face 768.9

Causalgia 355.9
  lower limb 355.71
  upper limb 354.4

Cause
  external, general effects NEC 994.9
  not stated 799.9
  unknown 799.9

Caustic burn — *see also* Burn, by site
  from swallowing caustic or corrosive substance — *see* Burn, internal organs

Cavare's disease (familial periodic paralysis) 359.3

Cave-in, injury
  crushing (severe) (*see also* Crush, by site) 869.1
  suffocation 994.7

Cavernitis (penis) 607.2
  lymph vessel — *see* Lymphangioma

Cavernositis 607.2

Cavernous — *see* condition

Cavitation of lung (*see also* Tuberculosis) 011.2
  nontuberculous 518.89
  primary, progressive 010.8

Cavity
  lung — *see* Cavitation of lung
  optic papilla 743.57
  pulmonary — *see* Cavitation of lung
  teeth 521.00
  vitreous (humor) 379.21

Cavovarus foot, congenital 754.59

Cavus foot (congenital) 754.71
  acquired 736.73

Cazenave's
  disease (pemphigus) NEC 694.4
  lupus (erythematosus) 695.4

Cecitis — *see* Appendicitis

Cecocele — *see* Hernia

Cecum — *see* condition

Celiac
  artery compression syndrome 447.4
  disease 579.0
  infantilism 579.0

Cell, cellular — *see also* condition
  anterior chamber (eye) (positive aqueous ray) 364.04

Cellulitis (diffuse) (with lymphangitis) (*see also* Abscess) 682.9
  abdominal wall 682.2
  anaerobic (*see also* Gas gangrene) 040.0
  ankle 682.6
  anus 566
  areola 611.0
  arm (any part, above wrist) 682.3
  auditory canal (external) 380.10
  axilla 682.3
  back (any part) 682.2
  breast 611.0
    postpartum 675.1
  broad ligament (*see also* Disease, pelvis, inflammatory) 614.4
    acute 614.3
  buttock 682.5
  cervical (neck region) 682.1
  cervix (uteri) (*see also* Cervicitis) 616.0
  cheek, external 682.0
    internal 528.3
  chest wall 682.2
  chronic NEC 682.9
  corpus cavernosum 607.2
  digit 681.9
  Douglas' cul-de-sac or pouch (chronic) (*see also* Disease, pelvis, inflammatory) 614.4
    acute 614.3
  drainage site (following operation) 998.59
  ear, external 380.10
  enterostomy 569.61
  erysipelar (*see also* Erysipelas) 035
  eyelid 373.13
  face (any part, except eye) 682.0
  finger (intrathecal) (periosteal) (subcutaneous) (subcuticular) 681.00
  flank 682.2
  foot (except toe) 682.7

Index to Diseases

Cellulitis (*see also* Abscess) — *continued*
  forearm 682.3
  gangrenous (*see also* Gangrene) 785.4
  genital organ NEC
    female — *see* Abscess, genital organ, female
    male 608.4
  glottis 478.71
  gluteal (region) 682.5
  gonococcal NEC 098.0
  groin 682.2
  hand (except finger or thumb) 682.4
  head (except face) NEC 682.8
  heel 682.7
  hip 682.6
  jaw (region) 682.0
  knee 682.6
  labium (majus) (minus) (*see also* Vulvitis) 616.10
  larynx 478.71
  leg, except foot 682.6
  lip 528.5
  mammary gland 611.0
  mouth (floor) 528.3
  multiple sites NEC 682.9
  nasopharynx 478.21
  navel 682.2
    newborn NEC 771.4
  neck (region) 682.1
  nipple 611.0
  nose 478.1
    external 682.0
  orbit, orbital 376.01
  palate (soft) 528.3
  pectoral (region) 682.2
  pelvis, pelvic
    with
      abortion — *see* Abortion, by type, with sepsis
      ectopic pregnancy (*see also* categories 633.0–633.9) 639.0
      molar pregnancy (*see also* categories 630–632) 639.0
    female (*see also* Disease, pelvis, inflammatory) 614.4
      acute 614.3
    following
      abortion 639.0
      ectopic or molar pregnancy 639.0
    male (*see also* Abscess, peritoneum) 567.2
    puerperal, postpartum, childbirth 670 ✓4ᵗʰ
  penis 607.2
  perineal, perineum 682.2
  perirectal 566
  peritonsillar 475
  periurethral 597.0
  periuterine (*see also* Disease, pelvis, inflammatory) 614.4
    acute 614.3
  pharynx 478.21
  phlegmonous NEC 682.9
  rectum 566
  retromammary 611.0
  retroperitoneal (*see also* Peritonitis) 567.2
  round ligament (*see also* Disease, pelvis, inflammatory) 614.4
    acute 614.3
  scalp (any part) 682.8
    dissecting 704.8
  scrotum 608.4
  seminal vesicle 608.0
  septic NEC 682.9
  shoulder 682.3
  specified sites NEC 682.8
  spermatic cord 608.4
  submandibular (region) (space) (triangle) 682.0
    gland 527.3
  submaxillary 528.3
    gland 527.3
  submental (pyogenic) 682.0
    gland 527.3
  suppurative NEC 682.9
  testis 608.4
  thigh 682.6
  thumb (intrathecal) (periosteal) (subcutaneous) (subcuticular) 681.00
  toe (intrathecal) (periosteal) (subcutaneous) (subcuticular) 681.10

Cellulitis (*see also* Abscess) — *continued*
  tonsil 475
  trunk 682.2
  tuberculous (primary) (*see also* Tuberculosis) 017.0 ✓5ᵗʰ
  tunica vaginalis 608.4
  umbilical 682.2
    newborn NEC 771.4
  vaccinal 999.3
  vagina — *see* Vaginitis
  vas deferens 608.4
  vocal cords 478.5
  vulva (*see also* Vulvitis) 616.10
  wrist 682.4
Cementoblastoma, benign (M9273/0) 213.1
  upper jaw (bone) 213.0
Cementoma (M9273/0) 213.1
  gigantiform (M9276/0) 213.1
    upper jaw (bone) 213.0
  upper jaw (bone) 213.0
Cementoperiostitis 523.4
Cephalgia, cephalagia (*see also* Headache) 784.0
  histamine 346.2 ✓5ᵗʰ
  nonorganic origin 307.81
  psychogenic 307.81
  tension 307.81
Cephalhematocele, cephalematocele
  due to birth injury 767.1
  fetus or newborn 767.1
  traumatic (*see also* Contusion, head) 920
Cephalhematoma, cephalematoma (calcified)
  due to birth injury 767.1
  fetus or newborn 767.1
  traumatic (*see also* Contusion, head) 920
Cephalic — *see* condition
Cephalitis — *see* Encephalitis
Cephalocele 742.0
Cephaloma — *see* Neoplasm, by site, malignant
Cephalomenia 625.8
Cephalopelvic — *see* condition
Cercomoniasis 007.3
Cerebellitis — *see* Encephalitis
Cerebellum (cerebellar) — *see* condition
Cerebral — *see* condition
Cerebritis — *see* Encephalitis
Cerebrohepatorenal syndrome 759.89
Cerebromacular degeneration 330.1
Cerebromalacia (*see also* Softening, brain) 434.9 ✓5ᵗʰ
Cerebrosidosis 272.7
Cerebrospasticity — *see* Palsy, cerebral
Cerebrospinal — *see* condition
Cerebrum — *see* condition
Ceroid storage disease 272.7
Cerumen (accumulation) (impacted) 380.4
Cervical — *see also* condition
  auricle 744.43
  rib 756.2
Cervicalgia 723.1
Cervicitis (acute) (chronic) (nonvenereal) (subacute) (with erosion or ectropion) 616.0
  with
    abortion — *see* Abortion, by type, with sepsis
    ectopic pregnancy (*see also* categories 633.0-633.9) 639.0
    molar pregnancy (*see also* categories 630-632) 639.0
    ulceration 616.0
  chlamydial 099.53
  complicating pregnancy or puerperium 646.6 ✓5ᵗʰ
    affecting fetus or newborn 760.8
  following
    abortion 639.0
    ectopic or molar pregnancy 639.0
  gonococcal (acute) 098.15
    chronic or duration of 2 months or more 098.35
  senile (atrophic) 616.0
  syphilitic 095.8
  trichomonal 131.09

Cervicitis — *continued*
  tuberculous (*see also* Tuberculosis) 016.7 ✓5ᵗʰ
Cervicoaural fistula 744.49
Cervicocolpitis (emphysematosa) (*see also* Cervicitis) 616.0
Cervix — *see* condition
Cesarean delivery, operation or section NEC 669.7 ✓5ᵗʰ
  affecting fetus or newborn 763.4
  post mortem, affecting fetus or newborn 761.6
  previous, affecting management of pregnancy 654.2 ✓5ᵗʰ
Céstan's syndrome 344.89
Céstan-Chenais paralysis 344.89
Céstan-Raymond syndrome 433.8 ✓5ᵗʰ
Cestode infestation NEC 123.9
  specified type NEC 123.8
Cestodiasis 123.9
Chabert's disease 022.9
Chacaleh 266.2
Chafing 709.8
Chagas' disease (*see also* Trypanosomiasis, American) 086.2
  with heart involvement 086.0
Chagres fever 084.0
Chalasia (cardiac sphincter) 530.81
Chalazion 373.2
Chalazoderma 757.39
Chalcosis 360.24
  cornea 371.15
  crystalline lens 360.24 [366.34]
  retina 360.24
Chalicosis (occupational) (pulmonum) 502
Chancre (any genital site) (hard) (indurated) (infecting) (primary) (recurrent) 091.0
  congenital 090.0
  conjunctiva 091.2
  Ducrey's 099.0
  extragenital 091.2
  eyelid 091.2
  Hunterian 091.0
  lip (syphilis) 091.2
  mixed 099.8
  nipple 091.2
  Nisbet's 099.0
  of
    carate 103.0
    pinta 103.0
    yaws 102.0
  palate, soft 091.2
  phagedenic 099.0
  Ricord's 091.0
  Rollet's (syphilitic) 091.0
  seronegative 091.0
  seropositive 091.0
  simple 099.0
  soft 099.0
    bubo 099.0
  urethra 091.0
  yaws 102.0
Chancriform syndrome 114.1
Chancroid 099.0
  anus 099.0
  penis (Ducrey's bacillus) 099.0
  perineum 099.0
  rectum 099.0
  scrotum 099.0
  urethra 099.0
  vulva 099.0
Chandipura fever 066.8
Chandler's disease (osteochondritis dissecans, hip) 732.7
Change(s) (of) — *see also* Removal of
  arteriosclerotic — *see* Arteriosclerosis
  battery
    cardiac pacemaker V53.31
  bone 733.90
    diabetic 250.8 ✓5ᵗʰ [731.8]
    in disease, unknown cause 733.90
  bowel habits 787.99

Change(s) (of)

Change(s) (of) — see also Removal of — continued
  cardiorenal (vascular) (see also Hypertension, cardiorenal) 404.90
  cardiovascular — see Disease, cardiovascular
  circulatory 459.9
  cognitive or personality change of other type, nonpsychotic 310.1
  color, teeth, tooth
    during formation 520.8
    posteruptive 521.7
  contraceptive device V25.42
  cornea, corneal
    degenerative NEC 371.40
    membrane NEC 371.30
    senile 371.41
  coronary (see also Ischemia, heart) 414.9
  degenerative
    chamber angle (anterior) (iris) 364.56
    ciliary body 364.57
    spine or vertebra (see also Spondylosis) 721.90
  dental pulp, regressive 522.2
  dressing V58.3
  fixation device V54.89 ▲
    external V54.89 ▲
    internal V54.0
  heart — see also Disease, heart
  hip joint 718.95
  hyperplastic larynx 478.79
  hypertrophic
    nasal sinus (see also Sinusitis) 473.9
    turbinate, nasal 478.0
    upper respiratory tract 478.9
  inflammatory — see Inflammation
  joint (see also Derangement, joint) 718.90
    sacroiliac 724.6
  Kirschner wire V54.89 ▲
  knee 717.9
  macular, congenital 743.55
  malignant (M—— /3) — see also Neoplasm, by site, malignant

> Note — for malignant change occurring in a neoplasm, use the appropriate M code with behavior digit /3 e.g., malignant change in uterine fibroid — M8890/3. For malignant change occurring in a nonneoplastic condition (e.g., gastric ulcer) use the M code M8000/3.

  mental (status) NEC 780.99 ▲
    due to or associated with physical condition — see Syndrome, brain
  myocardium, myocardial — see Degeneration, myocardial
  of life (see also Menopause) 627.2
  pacemaker battery (cardiac) V53.31
  peripheral nerve 355.9
  personality (nonpsychotic) NEC 310.1
  plaster cast V54.89 ▲
  refractive, transient 367.81
  regressive, dental pulp 522.2
  retina 362.9
    myopic (degenerative) (malignant) 360.21
    vascular appearance 362.13
  sacroiliac joint 724.6
  scleral 379.19
    degenerative 379.16
  senile (see also Senility) 797
  sensory (see also Disturbance, sensation) 782.0
  skin texture 782.8
  spinal cord 336.9
  splint, external V54.89 ▲
  subdermal implantable contraceptive V25.5
  suture V58.3
  traction device V54.89 ▲
  trophic 355.9
    arm NEC 354.9
    leg NEC 355.8
    lower extremity NEC 355.8
    upper extremity NEC 354.9
  vascular 459.9
  vasomotor 443.9
  voice 784.49
    psychogenic 306.1

Changing sleep-work schedule, affecting sleep 307.45

Changuinola fever 066.0

Chapping skin 709.8

Character
  depressive 301.12

Charcôt's
  arthropathy 094.0 [713.5]
  cirrhosis — see Cirrhosis, biliary
  disease 094.0
    spinal cord 094.0
  fever (biliary) (hepatic) (intermittent) — see Choledocholithiasis
  joint (disease) 094.0 [713.5]
    diabetic 250.6 ✓5ᵗʰ [713.5]
    syringomyelic 336.0 [713.5]
  syndrome (intermittent claudication) 443.9
    due to atherosclerosis 440.21

Charcôt-Marie-Tooth disease, paralysis, or syndrome 356.1

Charleyhorse (quadriceps) 843.8
  muscle, except quadriceps — see Sprain, by site

Charlouis' disease (see also Yaws) 102.9

Chauffeur's fracture — see Fracture, ulna, lower end

Cheadle (-Möller) (-Barlow) disease or syndrome (infantile scurvy) 267

Checking (of)
  contraceptive device (intrauterine) V25.42
  device
    fixation V54.89 ▲
      external V54.89 ▲
      internal V54.0
    traction V54.89 ▲
  Kirschner wire V54.89 ▲
  plaster cast V54.89 ▲
  splint, external V54.89 ▲

Checkup
  following treatment — see Examination
  health V70.0
  infant (not sick) V20.2
  pregnancy (normal) V22.1
    first V22.0
    high risk pregnancy V23.9
      specified problem NEC V23.89

Chédiak-Higashi (-Steinbrinck) anomaly, disease, or syndrome (congenital gigantism of peroxidase granules) 288.2

Cheek — see also condition
  biting 528.9

Cheese itch 133.8

Cheese washers' lung 495.8

Cheilitis 528.5
  actinic (due to sun) 692.72
    chronic NEC 692.72
      due to radiation, except from sun 692.82
    due to radiation, except from sun 692.82
  acute 528.5
  angular 528.5
  catarrhal 528.5
  chronic 528.5
  exfoliative 528.5
  gangrenous 528.5
  glandularis apostematosa 528.5
  granulomatosa 351.8
  infectional 528.5
  membranous 528.5
  Miescher's 351.8
  suppurative 528.5
  ulcerative 528.5
  vesicular 528.5

Cheilodynia 528.5

Cheilopalatoschisis (see also Cleft, palate, with cleft lip) 749.20

Cheilophagia 528.5

Cheiloschisis (see also Cleft, lip) 749.10

Cheilosis 528.5
  with pellagra 265.2
  angular 528.5
  due to
    dietary deficiency 266.0
    vitamin deficiency 266.0

Cheiromegaly 729.89

Cheiropompholyx 705.81

Cheloid (see also Keloid) 701.4

Chemical burn — see also Burn, by site
  from swallowing chemical — see Burn, internal organs

Chemodectoma (M8693/1) — see Paraganglioma, nonchromaffin

Chemoprophylaxis NEC V07.39

Chemosis, conjunctiva 372.73

Chemotherapy
  convalescence V66.2
  encounter (for) V58.1
  maintenance V58.1
  prophylactic NEC V07.39
    fluoride V07.31

Cherubism 526.89

Chest — see condition

Cheyne-Stokes respiration (periodic) 786.04

Chiari's
  disease or syndrome (hepatic vein thrombosis) 453.0
  malformation
    type I 348.4
    type II (see also Spina bifida) 741.0 ✓5ᵗʰ
    type III 742.0
    type IV 742.2
  network 746.89

Chiari-Frommel syndrome 676.6 ✓5ᵗʰ

Chicago disease (North American blastomycosis) 116.0

Chickenpox (see also Varicella) 052.9
  vaccination and inoculation (prophylactic) V05.4

Chiclero ulcer 085.4

Chiggers 133.8

Chignon 111.2
  fetus or newborn (from vacuum extraction) 767.1

Chigoe disease 134.1

Chikungunya fever 066.3

Chilaiditi's syndrome (subphrenic displacement, colon) 751.4

Chilblains 991.5
  lupus 991.5

Child
  behavior causing concern V61.20

Childbed fever 670 ✓4ᵗʰ

Childbirth — see also Delivery
  puerperal complications — see Puerperal

Childhood, period of rapid growth V21.0

Chill(s) 780.99 ▲
  with fever 780.6
  congestive 780.99 ▲
    in malarial regions 084.6
  septic — see Septicemia
  urethral 599.84

Chilomastigiasis 007.8

Chin — see condition

Chinese dysentery 004.9

Chiropractic dislocation (see also Lesion, nonallopathic, by site) 739.9

Chitral fever 066.0

Chlamydia, chlamydial — see condition

Chloasma 709.09
  cachecticorum 709.09
  eyelid 374.52
    congenital 757.33
    hyperthyroid 242.0 ✓5ᵗʰ
  gravidarum 646.8 ✓5ᵗʰ
  idiopathic 709.09
  skin 709.09
  symptomatic 709.09

Chloroma (M9930/3) 205.3 ✓5ᵗʰ

Chlorosis 280.9
  Egyptian (see also Ancylostomiasis) 126.9
  miners (see also Ancylostomiasis) 126.9

Chlorotic anemia 280.9

Chocolate cyst (ovary) 617.1

Choked
  disk or disc — see Papilledema
  on food, phlegm, or vomitus NEC (see also Asphyxia, food) 933.1
  phlegm 933.1

Index to Diseases — Chorea

Choked — continued
  while vomiting NEC (see also Asphyxia, food) 933.1
Chokes (resulting from bends) 993.3
Choking sensation 784.9
Cholangiectasis (see also Disease, gallbladder) 575.8
Cholangiocarcinoma (M8160/3)
  and hepatocellular carcinoma, combined (M8180/3) 155.0
  liver 155.1
  specified site NEC — see Neoplasm, by site, malignant
  unspecified site 155.1
Cholangiohepatitis 575.8
  due to fluke infestation 121.1
Cholangiohepatoma (M8180/3) 155.0
Cholangiolitis (acute) (chronic) (extrahepatic) (gangrenous) 576.1
  intrahepatic 575.8
  paratyphoidal (see also Fever, paratyphoid) 002.9
  typhoidal 002.0
Cholangioma (M8160/0) 211.5
  malignant — see Cholangiocarcinoma
Cholangitis (acute) (ascending) (catarrhal) (chronic) (infective) (malignant) (primary) (recurrent) (sclerosing) (secondary) (stenosing) (suppurative) 576.1
  chronic nonsuppurative destructive 571.6
  nonsuppurative destructive (chronic) 571.6
Cholecystdocholithiasis — see Choledocholithiasis
Cholecystitis 575.10
  with
    calculus, stones in
      bile duct (common) (hepatic) — see Choledocholithiasis
      gallbladder — see Cholelithiasis
  acute 575.0
  acute and chronic 575.12
  chronic 575.11
  emphysematous (acute) (see also Cholecystitis, acute) 575.0
  gangrenous (see also Cholecystitis, acute) 575.0
  paratyphoidal, current (see also Fever, paratyphoid) 002.9
  suppurative (see also Cholecystitis, acute) 575.0
  typhoidal 002.0
Choledochitis (suppurative) 576.1
Choledocholith — see Choledocholithiasis
Choledocholithiasis 574.5 ✓5ᵗʰ

> Note — Use the following fifth-digit subclassification with category 574:
> 0 without mention of obstruction
> 1 with obstruction

  with
    cholecystitis 574.4 ✓5ᵗʰ
      acute 574.3 ✓5ᵗʰ
      chronic 574.4 ✓5ᵗʰ
    cholelithiasis 574.9 ✓5ᵗʰ
      with
        cholecystitis 574.7 ✓5ᵗʰ
          acute 574.6 ✓5ᵗʰ
            and chronic 574.8 ✓5ᵗʰ
          chronic 574.7 ✓5ᵗʰ
Cholelithiasis (impacted) (multiple) 574.2 ✓5ᵗʰ

> Note — Use the following fifth-digit subclassification with category 574:
> 0 without mention of obstruction
> 1 with obstruction

  with
    cholecystitis 574.1 ✓5ᵗʰ
      acute 574.0 ✓5ᵗʰ
      chronic 574.1 ✓5ᵗʰ

Cholelithiasis — continued
  with — continued
    choledocholithiasis 574.9 ✓5ᵗʰ
      with
        cholecystitis 574.7 ✓5ᵗʰ
          acute 574.6 ✓5ᵗʰ
            and chronic 574.8 ✓5ᵗʰ
          chronic cholecystitis 574.7 ✓5ᵗʰ
Cholemia (see also Jaundice) 782.4
  familial 277.4
  Gilbert's (familial nonhemolytic) 277.4
Cholemic gallstone — see Cholelithiasis
Choleperitoneum, choleperitonitis (see also Disease, gallbladder) 567.8
Cholera (algid) (Asiatic) (asphyctic) (epidemic) (gravis) (Indian) (malignant) (morbus) (pestilential) (spasmodic) 001.9
  antimonial 985.4
  carrier (suspected) of V02.0
  classical 001.0
  contact V01.0
  due to
    Vibrio
      cholerae (Inaba, Ogawa, Hikojima serotypes) 001.0
      El Tor 001.1
  El Tor 001.1
  exposure to V01.0
  vaccination, prophylactic (against) V03.0
Cholerine (see also Cholera) 001.9
Cholestasis 576.8
Cholesteatoma (ear) 385.30
  attic (primary) 385.31
  diffuse 385.35
  external ear (canal) 380.21
  marginal (middle ear) 385.32
    with involvement of mastoid cavity 385.33
    secondary (with middle ear involvement) 385.33
  mastoid cavity 385.30
  middle ear (secondary) 385.32
    with involvement of mastoid cavity 385.33
  postmastoidectomy cavity (recurrent) 383.32
  primary 385.31
  recurrent, postmastoidectomy cavity 383.32
  secondary (middle ear) 385.32
    with involvement of mastoid cavity 385.33
Cholesteatosis (middle ear) (see also Cholesteatoma) 385.30
  diffuse 385.35
Cholesteremia 272.0
Cholesterin
  granuloma, middle ear 385.82
  in vitreous 379.22
Cholesterol
  deposit
    retina 362.82
    vitreous 379.22
  imbibition of gallbladder (see also Disease, gallbladder) 575.6
Cholesterolemia 272.0
  essential 272.0
  familial 272.0
  hereditary 272.0
Cholesterosis, cholesterolosis (gallbladder) 575.6
  with
    cholecystitis — see Cholecystitis
    cholelithiasis — see Cholelithiasis
  middle ear (see also Cholesteatoma) 385.30
Cholocolic fistula (see also Fistula, gallbladder) 575.5
Choluria 791.4
Chondritis (purulent) 733.99
  costal 733.6
    Tietze's 733.6
  patella, posttraumatic 717.7
  posttraumatica patellae 717.7
  tuberculous (active) (see also Tuberculosis) 015.9 ✓5ᵗʰ
    intervertebral 015.0 ✓5ᵗʰ [730.88]
Chondroangiopathia calcarea seu punctate 756.59

Chondroblastoma (M9230/0) — see also Neoplasm, bone, benign
  malignant (M9230/3) — see Neoplasm, bone, malignant
Chondrocalcinosis (articular) (crystal deposition) (dihydrate) (see also Arthritis, due to, crystals) 275.49 [712.3] ✓5ᵗʰ
  due to
    calcium pyrophosphate 275.49 [712.2] ✓5ᵗʰ
    dicalcium phosphate crystals 275.49 [712.1] ✓5ᵗʰ
    pyrophosphate crystals 275.49 [712.2] ✓5ᵗʰ
Chondrodermatitis nodularis helicis 380.00
Chondrodysplasia 756.4
  angiomatose 756.4
  calcificans congenita 756.59
  epiphysialis punctata 756.59
  hereditary deforming 756.4
Chondrodystrophia (fetalis) 756.4
  calcarea 756.4
  calcificans congenita 756.59
  fetalis hypoplastica 756.59
  hypoplastica calcinosa 756.59
  punctata 756.59
  tarda 277.5
Chondrodystrophy (familial) (hypoplastic) 756.4
Chondroectodermal dysplasia 756.55
Chondrolysis 733.99
Chondroma (M9220/0) — see also Neoplasm, cartilage, benign
  juxtacortical (M9221/0) — see Neoplasm, bone, benign
  periosteal (M9221/0) — see Neoplasm, bone, benign
Chondromalacia 733.92
  epiglottis (congenital) 748.3
  generalized 733.92
  knee 717.7
  larynx (congenital) 748.3
  localized, except patella 733.92
  patella, patellae 717.7
  systemic 733.92
  tibial plateau 733.92
  trachea (congenital) 748.3
Chondromatosis (M9220/1) — see Neoplasm, cartilage, uncertain behavior
Chondromyxosarcoma (M9220/3) — see Neoplasm, cartilage, malignant
Chondro-osteodysplasia (Morquio-Brailsford type) 277.5
Chondro-osteodystrophy 277.5
Chondro-osteoma (M9210/0) — see Neoplasm, bone, benign
Chondropathia tuberosa 733.6
Chondrosarcoma (M9220/3) — see also Neoplasm, cartilage, malignant
  juxtacortical (M9221/3) — see Neoplasm, bone, malignant
  mesenchymal (M9240/3) — see Neoplasm, connective tissue, malignant
Chordae tendineae rupture (chronic) 429.5
Chordee (nonvenereal) 607.89
  congenital 752.63
  gonococcal 098.2
Chorditis (fibrinous) (nodosa) (tuberosa) 478.5
Chordoma (M9370/3) — see Neoplasm, by site, malignant
Chorea (gravis) (minor) (spasmodic) 333.5
  with
    heart involvement — see Chorea with rheumatic heart disease
    rheumatic heart disease (chronic, inactive, or quiescent) (conditions classifiable to 393-398) — see also Rheumatic heart condition involved
      active or acute (conditions classifiable to 391) 392.0
  acute — see Chorea, Sydenham's
  apoplectic (see also Disease, cerebrovascular, acute) 436
  chronic 333.4
  electric 049.8
  gravidarum — see Eclampsia, pregnancy

Chorea

Chorea — *continued*
  habit 307.22
  hereditary 333.4
  Huntington's 333.4
  posthemiplegic 344.89
  pregnancy — *see* Eclampsia, pregnancy
  progressive 333.4
    chronic 333.4
    hereditary 333.4
  rheumatic (chronic) 392.9
    with heart disease or involvement — *see* Chorea, with rheumatic heart disease
  senile 333.5
  Sydenham's 392.9
    with heart involvement — *see* Chorea, with rheumatic heart disease
    nonrheumatic 333.5
  variabilis 307.23
Choreoathetosis (paroxysmal) 333.5
Chorioadenoma (destruens) (M9100/1) 236.1
Chorioamnionitis 658.4 ✓5
  affecting fetus or newborn 762.7
Chorioangioma (M9120/0) 219.8
Choriocarcinoma (M9100/3)
  combined with
    embryonal carcinoma (M9101/3) — *see* Neoplasm, by site, malignant
    teratoma (M9101/3) — *see* Neoplasm, by site, malignant
  specified site — *see* Neoplasm, by site, malignant
  unspecified site
    female 181
    male 186.9
Chorioencephalitis, lymphocytic (acute) (serous) 049.0
Chorioepithelioma (M9100/3) — *see* Choriocarcinoma
Choriomeningitis (acute) (benign) (lymphocytic) (serous) 049.0
Chorionepithelioma (M9100/3) — *see* Choriocarcinoma
Chorionitis (*see also* Scleroderma) 710.1
Chorioretinitis 363.20
  disseminated 363.10
    generalized 363.13
    in
      neurosyphilis 094.83
      secondary syphilis 091.51
    peripheral 363.12
    posterior pole 363.11
    tuberculous (*see also* Tuberculosis) 017.3 ✓5 [363.13]
  due to
    histoplasmosis (*see also* Histoplasmosis) 115.92
    toxoplasmosis (acquired) 130.2
      congenital (active) 771.2
  focal 363.00
    juxtapapillary 363.01
    peripheral 363.04
    posterior pole NEC 363.03
  juxtapapillaris, juxtapapillary 363.01
  progressive myopia (degeneration) 360.21
  syphilitic (secondary) 091.51
    congenital (early) 090.0 [363.13]
    late 090.5 [363.13]
    late 095.8 [363.13]
  tuberculous (*see also* Tuberculosis) 017.3 ✓5 [363.13]
Choristoma — *see* Neoplasm, by site, benign
Choroid — *see* condition
Choroideremia, choroidermia (initial stage) (late stage) (partial or total atrophy) 363.55
Choroiditis (*see also* Chorioretinitis) 363.20
  leprous 030.9 [363.13]
  senile guttate 363.41
  sympathetic 360.11
  syphilitic (secondary) 091.51
    congenital (early) 090.0 [363.13]
      late 090.5 [363.13]
      late 095.8 [363.13]
  Tay's 363.41
  tuberculous (*see also* Tuberculosis) 017.3 ✓5 [363.13]

Choroidopathy NEC 363.9
  degenerative (*see also* Degeneration, choroid) 363.40
  hereditary (*see also* Dystrophy, choroid) 363.50
  specified type NEC 363.8
Choroidoretinitis — *see* Chorioretinitis
Choroidosis, central serous 362.41
Choroidretinopathy, serous 362.41
Christian's syndrome (chronic histiocytosis X) 277.8
Christian-Weber disease (nodular nonsuppurative panniculitis) 729.30
Christmas disease 286.1
Chromaffinoma (M8700/0) — *see also* Neoplasm, by site, benign
  malignant (M8700/3) — *see* Neoplasm, by site, malignant
Chromatopsia 368.59
Chromhidrosis, chromidrosis 705.89
Chromoblastomycosis 117.2
Chromomycosis 117.2
Chromophytosis 111.0
Chromotrichomycosis 111.8
Chronic — *see* condition
Churg-Strauss syndrome 446.4
Chyle cyst, mesentery 457.8
Chylocele (nonfilarial) 457.8
  filarial (*see also* Infestation, filarial) 125.9
  tunica vaginalis (nonfilarial) 608.84
    filarial (*see also* Infestation, filarial) 125.9
Chylomicronemia (fasting) (with hyperprebetalipoproteinemia) 272.3
Chylopericardium (acute) 420.90
Chylothorax (nonfilarial) 457.8
  filarial (*see also* Infestation, filarial) 125.9
Chylous
  ascites 457.8
  cyst of peritoneum 457.8
  hydrocele 603.9
  hydrothorax (nonfilarial) 457.8
    filarial (*see also* Infestation, filarial) 125.9
Chyluria 791.1
  bilharziasis 120.0
  due to
    Brugia (malayi) 125.1
    Wuchereria (bancrofti) 125.0
    malayi 125.1
  filarial (*see also* Infestation, filarial) 125.9
  filariasis (*see also* Infestation, filarial) 125.9
  nonfilarial 791.1
Cicatricial (deformity) — *see* Cicatrix
Cicatrix (adherent) (contracted) (painful) (vicious) 709.2
  adenoid 474.8
  alveolar process 525.8
  anus 569.49
  auricle 380.89
  bile duct (*see also* Disease, biliary) 576.8
  bladder 596.8
  bone 733.99
  brain 348.8
  cervix (postoperative) (postpartal) 622.3
    in pregnancy or childbirth 654.6 ✓5
      causing obstructed labor 660.2 ✓5
  chorioretinal 363.30
    disseminated 363.35
    macular 363.32
    peripheral 363.34
    posterior pole NEC 363.33
  choroid — *see* Cicatrix, chorioretinal
  common duct (*see also* Disease, biliary) 576.8
  congenital 757.39
  conjunctiva 372.64
  cornea 371.00
    tuberculous (*see also* Tuberculosis) 017.3 ✓5 [371.05]
  duodenum (bulb) 537.3
  esophagus 530.3
  eyelid 374.46
    with
      ectropion — *see* Ectropion
      entropion — *see* Entropion
  hypopharynx 478.29

Cicatrix — *continued*
  knee, semilunar cartilage 717.5
  lacrimal
    canaliculi 375.53
    duct
      acquired 375.56
      neonatal 375.55
    punctum 375.52
    sac 375.54
  larynx 478.79
  limbus (cystoid) 372.64
  lung 518.89
  macular 363.32
    disseminated 363.35
    peripheral 363.34
  middle ear 385.89
  mouth 528.9
  muscle 728.89
  nasolacrimal duct
    acquired 375.56
    neonatal 375.55
  nasopharynx 478.29
  palate (soft) 528.9
  penis 607.89
  prostate 602.8
  rectum 569.49
  retina 363.30
    disseminated 363.35
    macular 363.32
    peripheral 363.34
    posterior pole NEC 363.33
  semilunar cartilage — *see* Derangement, meniscus
  seminal vesicle 608.89
  skin 709.2
    infected 686.8
    postinfectional 709.2
    tuberculous (*see also* Tuberculosis) 017.0 ✓5
  specified site NEC 709.2
  throat 478.29
  tongue 529.8
  tonsil (and adenoid) 474.8
  trachea 478.9
  tuberculous NEC (*see also* Tuberculosis) 011.9 ✓5
  ureter 593.89
  urethra 599.84
  uterus 621.8
  vagina 623.4
    in pregnancy or childbirth 654.7 ✓5
      causing obstructed labor 660.2 ✓5
  vocal cord 478.5
  wrist, constricting (annular) 709.2
CIN I [cervical intraepithelial neoplasia I] 622.1
CIN II [cervical intraepithelial neoplasia II] 622.1
CIN III [cervical intraepithelial neoplasia III] 233.1
Cinchonism
  correct substance properly administered 386.9
  overdose or wrong substance given or taken 961.4
Circine herpes 110.5
Circle of Willis — *see* condition
Circular — *see also* condition
  hymen 752.49
Circulating anticoagulants 286.5
  following childbirth 666.3 ✓5
  postpartum 666.3 ✓5
Circulation
  collateral (venous), any site 459.89
  defective 459.9
    congenital 747.9
    lower extremity 459.89
  embryonic 747.9
  failure 799.8
    fetus or newborn 779.89 ▲
    peripheral 785.59
  fetal, persistent 747.83 ▲
  heart, incomplete 747.9
Circulatory system — *see* condition
Circulus senilis 371.41
Circumcision
  in absence of medical indication V50.2
  ritual V50.2
  routine V50.2

Circumscribed — see condition
Circumvallata placenta — see Placenta, abnormal
Cirrhosis, cirrhotic 571.5
  with alcoholism 571.2
  alcoholic (liver) 571.2
  atrophic (of liver) — see Cirrhosis, portal
  Baumgarten-Cruveilhier 571.5
  biliary (cholangiolitic) (cholangitic) (cholestatic) (extrahepatic) (hypertrophic) (intrahepatic) (nonobstructive) (obstructive) (pericholangiolitic) (posthepatic) (primary) (secondary) (xanthomatous) 571.6
    due to
      clonorchiasis 121.1
      flukes 121.3
  brain 331.9
  capsular — see Cirrhosis, portal
  cardiac 571.5
    alcoholic 571.2
  central (liver) — see Cirrhosis, liver
  Charcôt's 571.6
  cholangiolitic — see Cirrhosis, biliary
  cholangitic — see Cirrhosis, biliary
  cholestatic — see Cirrhosis, biliary
  clitoris (hypertrophic) 624.2
  coarsely nodular 571.5
  congestive (liver) — see Cirrhosis, cardiac
  Cruveilhier-Baumgarten 571.5
  cryptogenic (of liver) 571.5
    alcoholic 571.2
  dietary (see also Cirrhosis, portal) 571.5
    due to
      bronzed diabetes 275.0
      congestive hepatomegaly — see Cirrhosis, cardiac
      cystic fibrosis 277.00
      hemochromatosis 275.0
      hepatolenticular degeneration 275.1
      passive congestion (chronic) — see Cirrhosis, cardiac
      Wilson's disease 275.1
      xanthomatosis 272.2
  extrahepatic (obstructive) — see Cirrhosis, biliary
  fatty 571.8
    alcoholic 571.0
  florid 571.2
  Glisson's — see Cirrhosis, portal
  Hanot's (hypertrophic) — see Cirrhosis, biliary
  hepatic — see Cirrhosis, liver
  hepatolienal — see Cirrhosis, liver
  hobnail — see Cirrhosis, portal
  hypertrophic — see also Cirrhosis, liver
    biliary — see Cirrhosis, biliary
    Hanot's — see Cirrhosis, biliary
  infectious NEC — see Cirrhosis, portal
  insular — see Cirrhosis, portal
  intrahepatic (obstructive) (primary) (secondary) — see Cirrhosis, biliary
  juvenile (see also Cirrhosis, portal) 571.5
  kidney (see also Sclerosis, renal) 587
  Laennec's (of liver) 571.2
    nonalcoholic 571.5
  liver (chronic) (hepatolienal) (hypertrophic) (nodular) (splenomegalic) (unilobar) 571.5
    with alcoholism 571.2
    alcoholic 571.2
    congenital (due to failure of obliteration of umbilical vein) 777.8
    cryptogenic 571.5
      alcoholic 571.2
    fatty 571.8
      alcoholic 571.0
    macronodular 571.5
      alcoholic 571.2
    micronodular 571.5
      alcoholic 571.2
    nodular, diffuse 571.5
      alcoholic 571.2
    pigmentary 275.0
    portal 571.5
      alcoholic 571.2
    postnecrotic 571.5
      alcoholic 571.2
    syphilitic 095.3

Cirrhosis, cirrhotic — continued
  lung (chronic) (see also Fibrosis, lung) 515
  macronodular (of liver) 571.5
    alcoholic 571.2
  malarial 084.9
  metabolic NEC 571.5
  micronodular (of liver) 571.5
    alcoholic 571.2
  monolobular — see Cirrhosis, portal
  multilobular — see Cirrhosis, portal
  nephritis (see also Sclerosis, renal) 587
  nodular — see Cirrhosis, liver
  nutritional (fatty) 571.5
  obstructive (biliary) (extrahepatic) (intrahepatic) — see Cirrhosis, biliary
  ovarian 620.8
  paludal 084.9
  pancreas (duct) 577.8
  pericholangiolitic — see Cirrhosis, biliary
  periportal — see Cirrhosis, portal
  pigment, pigmentary (of liver) 275.0
  portal (of liver) 571.5
    alcoholic 571.2
  posthepatitic (see also Cirrhosis, postnecrotic) 571.5
  postnecrotic (of liver) 571.5
    alcoholic 571.2
  primary (intrahepatic) — see Cirrhosis, biliary
  pulmonary (see also Fibrosis, lung) 515
  renal (see also Sclerosis, renal) 587
  septal (see also Cirrhosis, postnecrotic) 571.5
  spleen 289.51
  splenomegalic (of liver) — see Cirrhosis, liver
  stasis (liver) — see Cirrhosis, liver
  stomach 535.4 ✓5ᵗʰ
  Todd's (see also Cirrhosis, biliary) 571.6
  toxic (nodular) — see Cirrhosis, postnecrotic
  trabecular — see Cirrhosis, postnecrotic
  unilobar — see Cirrhosis, liver
  vascular (of liver) — see Cirrhosis, liver
  xanthomatous (biliary) (see also Cirrhosis, biliary) 571.6
    due to xanthomatosis (familial) (metabolic) (primary) 272.2
Cistern, subarachnoid 793.0
Citrullinemia 270.6
Citrullinuria 270.6
Ciuffini-Pancoast tumor (M8010/3) (carcinoma, pulmonary apex) 162.3
Civatte's disease or poikiloderma 709.09
Clam diggers' itch 120.3
Clap — see Gonorrhea
Clark's paralysis 343.9
Clarke-Hadfield syndrome (pancreatic infantilism) 577.8
Clastothrix 704.2
Claude's syndrome 352.6
Claude Bernard-Horner syndrome (see also Neuropathy, peripheral, autonomic) 337.9
Claudication, intermittent 443.9
  cerebral (artery) (see also Ischemia, cerebral, transient) 435.9
  due to atherosclerosis 440.21
  spinal cord (arteriosclerotic) 435.1
    syphilitic 094.89
  spinalis 435.1
  venous (axillary) 453.8
Claudicatio venosa intermittens 453.8
Claustrophobia 300.29
Clavus (infected) 700
Clawfoot (congenital) 754.71
  acquired 736.74
Clawhand (acquired) 736.06
  congenital 755.59
Clawtoe (congenital) 754.71
  acquired 735.5
Clay eating 307.52
Clay shovelers' fracture — see Fracture, vertebra, cervical
Cleansing of artificial opening (see also Attention to artificial opening) V55.9
Cleft (congenital) — see also Imperfect, closure
  alveolar process 525.8

Cleft — see also Imperfect, closure — continued
  branchial (persistent) 744.41
    cyst 744.42
  clitoris 752.49
  cricoid cartilage, posterior 748.3
  facial (see also Cleft, lip) 749.10
  lip 749.10
    with cleft palate 749.20
      bilateral (lip and palate) 749.24
        with unilateral lip or palate 749.25
        complete 749.23
        incomplete 749.24
      unilateral (lip and palate) 749.22
        with bilateral lip or palate 749.25
        complete 749.21
        incomplete 749.22
    bilateral 749.14
      with cleft palate, unilateral 749.25
      complete 749.13
      incomplete 749.14
    unilateral 749.12
      with cleft palate, bilateral 749.25
      complete 749.11
      incomplete 749.12
  nose 748.1
  palate 749.00
    with cleft lip 749.20
      bilateral (lip and palate) 749.24
        with unilateral lip or palate 749.25
        complete 749.23
        incomplete 749.24
      unilateral (lip and palate) 749.22
        with bilateral lip or palate 749.25
        complete 749.21
        incomplete 749.22
    bilateral 749.04
      with cleft lip, unilateral 749.25
      complete 749.03
      incomplete 749.04
    unilateral 749.02
      with cleft lip, bilateral 749.25
      complete 749.01
      incomplete 749.02
  penis 752.69
  posterior, cricoid cartilage 748.3
  scrotum 752.8
  sternum (congenital) 756.3
  thyroid cartilage (congenital) 748.3
  tongue 750.13
  uvula 749.02
    with cleft lip (see also Cleft, lip, with cleft palate) 749.20
  water 366.12
Cleft hand (congenital) 755.58
Cleidocranial dysostosis 755.59
Cleidotomy, fetal 763.89
Cleptomania 312.32
Clérambault's syndrome 297.8
  erotomania 302.89
Clergyman's sore throat 784.49
Click, clicking
  systolic syndrome 785.2
Clifford's syndrome (postmaturity) 766.2
Climacteric (see also Menopause) 627.2
  arthritis NEC (see also Arthritis, climacteric) 716.3 ✓5ᵗʰ
  depression (see also Psychosis, affective) 296.2 ✓5ᵗʰ
  disease 627.2
    recurrent episode 296.3 ✓5ᵗʰ
    single episode 296.2 ✓5ᵗʰ
  female (symptoms) 627.2
  male (symptoms) (syndrome) 608.89
  melancholia (see also Psychosis, affective) 296.2 ✓5ᵗʰ
    recurrent episode 296.3 ✓5ᵗʰ
    single episode 296.2 ✓5ᵗʰ
  paranoid state 297.2
  paraphrenia 297.2
  polyarthritis NEC 716.39
    male 608.89
  symptoms (female) 627.2
Clinical research investigation (control) (participant) V70.7
Clinodactyly 755.59

Clitoris — see condition
Cloaca, persistent 751.5
Clonorchiasis 121.1
Clonorchiosis 121.1
Clonorchis infection, liver 121.1
Clonus 781.0
Closed bite 524.2
Closure
  artificial opening (see also Attention to artificial opening) V55.9
  congenital, nose 748.0
  cranial sutures, premature 756.0
  defective or imperfect NEC — see Imperfect, closure
  fistula, delayed — see Fistula
  fontanelle, delayed 756.0
  foramen ovale, imperfect 745.5
  hymen 623.3
  interauricular septum, defective 745.5
  interventricular septum, defective 745.4
  lacrimal duct 375.56
    congenital 743.65
    neonatal 375.55
  nose (congenital) 748.0
    acquired 738.0
  vagina 623.2
  valve — see Endocarditis
  vulva 624.8
Clot (blood)
  artery (obstruction) (occlusion) (see also Embolism) 444.9
  bladder 596.7
  brain (extradural or intradural) (see also Thrombosis, brain) 434.0 ✓5ᵗʰ
    late effects — see Late effect(s) (of) cerebrovascular disease
  circulation 444.9
  heart (see also Infarct, myocardium) 410.9 ✓5ᵗʰ
  vein (see also Thrombosis) 453.9
Clotting defect NEC (see also Defect, coagulation) 286.9
Clouded state 780.09
  epileptic (see also Epilepsy) 345.9 ✓5ᵗʰ
  paroxysmal (idiopathic) (see also Epilepsy) 345.9 ✓5ᵗʰ
Clouding
  corneal graft 996.51
Cloudy
  antrum, antra 473.0
  dialysis effluent 792.5
Clouston's (hidrotic) ectodermal dysplasia 757.31
Clubbing of fingers 781.5
Clubfinger 736.29
  acquired 736.29
  congenital 754.89
Clubfoot (congenital) 754.70
  acquired 736.71
  equinovarus 754.51
  paralytic 736.71
Club hand (congenital) 754.89
  acquired 736.07
Clubnail (acquired) 703.8
  congenital 757.5
Clump kidney 753.3
Clumsiness 781.3
  syndrome 315.4
Cluttering 307.0
Clutton's joints 090.5
Coagulation, intravascular (diffuse) (disseminated) (see also Fibrinolysis) 286.6
  newborn 776.2
Coagulopathy (see also Defect, coagulation) 286.9
  consumption 286.6
  intravascular (disseminated) NEC 286.6
    newborn 776.2
Coalition
  calcaneoscaphoid 755.67
  calcaneus 755.67
  tarsal 755.67
Coal miners'
  elbow 727.2
  lung 500

Coal workers' lung or pneumoconiosis 500
Coarctation
  aorta (postductal) (preductal) 747.10
  pulmonary artery 747.3
Coated tongue 529.3
Coats' disease 362.12
Cocainism (see also Dependence) 304.2 ✓5ᵗʰ
Coccidioidal granuloma 114.3
Coccidioidomycosis 114.9
  with pneumonia 114.0
  cutaneous (primary) 114.1
  disseminated 114.3
  extrapulmonary (primary) 114.1
  lung 114.5
    acute 114.0
    chronic 114.4
    primary 114.0
  meninges 114.2
  primary (pulmonary) 114.0
    acute 114.0
  prostate 114.3
  pulmonary 114.5
    acute 114.0
    chronic 114.4
    primary 114.0
  specified site NEC 114.3
Coccidioidosis 114.9
  lung 114.5
    acute 114.0
    chronic 114.4
    primary 114.0
  meninges 114.2
Coccidiosis (colitis) (diarrhea) (dysentery) 007.2
Cocciuria 791.9
Coccus in urine 791.9
Coccydynia 724.79
Coccygodynia 724.79
Coccyx — see condition
Cochin-China
  diarrhea 579.1
    anguilluliasis 127.2
  ulcer 085.1
Cock's peculiar tumor 706.2
Cockayne's disease or syndrome (microcephaly and dwarfism) 759.89
Cockayne-Weber syndrome (epidermolysis bullosa) 757.39
Cocked-up toe 735.2
Codman's tumor (benign chondroblastoma) (M9230/0) — see Neoplasm, bone, benign
Coenurosis 123.8
Coffee workers' lung 495.8
Cogan's syndrome 370.52
  congenital oculomotor apraxia 379.51
  nonsyphilitic interstitial keratitis 370.52
Coiling, umbilical cord — see Complications, umbilical cord
Coitus, painful (female) 625.0
  male 608.89
  psychogenic 302.76
Cold 460
  with influenza, flu, or grippe 487.1
  abscess — see also Tuberculosis, abscess
    articular — see Tuberculosis, joint
  agglutinin
    disease (chronic) or syndrome 283.0
    hemoglobinuria 283.0
      paroxysmal (cold) (nocturnal) 283.2
  allergic (see also Fever, hay) 477.9
  bronchus or chest — see Bronchitis
    with grippe or influenza 487.1
  common (head) 460
    vaccination, prophylactic (against) V04.7
  deep 464.10
  effects of 991.9
    specified effect NEC 991.8
  excessive 991.9
    specified effect NEC 991.8
  exhaustion from 991.8
  exposure to 991.9
    specified effect NEC 991.8
  grippy 487.1
  head 460

Cold — continued
  injury syndrome (newborn) 778.2
  intolerance 780.99 ▲
  on lung — see Bronchitis
  rose 477.0
  sensitivity, autoimmune 283.0
  virus 460
Coldsore (see also Herpes, simplex) 054.9
Colibacillosis 041.4
  generalized 038.42
Colibacilluria 791.9
Colic (recurrent) 789.0 ✓5ᵗʰ
  abdomen 789.0 ✓5ᵗʰ
    psychogenic 307.89
  appendicular 543.9
  appendix 543.9
  bile duct — see Choledocholithiasis
  biliary — see Cholelithiasis
  bilious — see Cholelithiasis
  common duct — see Choledocholithiasis
  Devonshire NEC 984.9
    specified type of lead — see Table of Drugs and Chemicals
  flatulent 787.3
  gallbladder or gallstone — see Cholelithiasis
  gastric 536.8
  hepatic (duct) — see Choledocholithiasis
  hysterical 300.11
  infantile 789.0 ✓5ᵗʰ
  intestinal 789.0 ✓5ᵗʰ
  kidney 788.0
  lead NEC 984.9
    specified type of lead — see Table of Drugs and Chemicals
  liver (duct) — see Choledocholithiasis
  mucous 564.9
    psychogenic 316 [564.9]
  nephritic 788.0
  painter's NEC 984.9
  pancreas 577.8
  psychogenic 306.4
  renal 788.0
  saturnine NEC 984.9
    specified type of lead — see Table of Drugs and Chemicals
  spasmodic 789.0 ✓5ᵗʰ
  ureter 788.0
  urethral 599.84
    due to calculus 594.2
  uterus 625.8
    menstrual 625.3
  vermicular 543.9
  virus 460
  worm NEC 128.9
Colicystitis (see also Cystitis) 595.9
Colitis (acute) (catarrhal) (croupous) (cystica superficialis) (exudative) (hemorrhagic) (noninfectious) (phlegmonous) (presumed noninfectious) 558.9
  adaptive 564.9
  allergic 558.3
  amebic (see also Amebiasis) 006.9
    nondysenteric 006.2
  anthrax 022.2
  bacillary (see also Infection, Shigella) 004.9
  balantidial 007.0
  chronic 558.9
    ulcerative (see also Colitis, ulcerative) 556.9
  coccidial 007.2
  dietetic 558.9
  due to radiation 558.1
  functional 558.9
  gangrenous 009.0
  giardial 007.1
  granulomatous 555.1
  gravis (see also Colitis, ulcerative) 556.9
  infectious (see also Enteritis, due to, specific organism) 009.0
    presumed 009.1
  ischemic 557.9
    acute 557.0
    chronic 557.1
    due to mesenteric artery insufficiency 557.1
  membranous 564.9
    psychogenic 316 [564.9]

Colitis — continued
- mucous 564.9
    - psychogenic 316 *[564.9]*
- necrotic 009.0
- polyposa (*see also* Colitis, ulcerative) 556.9
- protozoal NEC 007.9
- pseudomembranous 008.45
- pseudomucinous 564.9
- regional 555.1
- segmental 555.1
- septic (*see also* Enteritis, due to, specific organism) 009.0
- spastic 564.9
    - psychogenic 316 *[564.9]*
- staphylococcus 008.41
    - food 005.0
- thromboulcerative 557.0
- toxic 558.2
- transmural 555.1
- trichomonal 007.3
- tuberculous (ulcerative) 014.8 ✓5
- ulcerative (chronic) (idiopathic) (nonspecific) 556.9
    - entero- 556.0
    - fulminant 557.0
    - ileo- 556.1
    - left-sided 556.5
    - procto- 556.2
    - proctosigmoid 556.3
    - psychogenic 316 *[556]* ✓4
    - specified NEC 556.8
    - universal 556.6

Collagen disease NEC 710.9
- nonvascular 710.9
- vascular (allergic) (*see also* Angiitis, hypersensitivity) 446.20

Collagenosis (*see also* Collagen disease) 710.9
- cardiovascular 425.4
- mediastinal 519.3

Collapse 780.2
- adrenal 255.8
- cardiorenal (*see also* Hypertension, cardiorenal) 404.90
- cardiorespiratory 785.51
    - fetus or newborn 779.89 ▲
- cardiovascular (*see also* Disease, heart) 785.51
    - fetus or newborn 779.89 ▲
- circulatory (peripheral) 785.59
    - with
        - abortion — *see* Abortion, by type, with shock
        - ectopic pregnancy (*see also* categories 633.0-633.9) 639.5
        - molar pregnancy (*see also* categories 630-632) 639.5
    - during or after labor and delivery 669.1 ✓5
    - fetus or newborn 779.89 ▲
    - following
        - abortion 639.5
        - ectopic or molar pregnancy 639.5
    - during or after labor and delivery 669.1 ✓5
    - fetus or newborn 779.89 ▲
- external ear canal 380.50
    - secondary to
        - inflammation 380.53
        - surgery 380.52
        - trauma 380.51
- general 780.2
- heart — *see* Disease, heart
- heat 992.1
- hysterical 300.11
- labyrinth, membranous (congenital) 744.05
- lung (massive) (*see also* Atelectasis) 518.0
    - pressure, during labor 668.0 ✓5
- myocardial — *see* Disease, heart
- nervous (*see also* Disorder, mental, nonpsychotic) 300.9
- neurocirculatory 306.2
- nose 738.0
- postoperative (cardiovascular) 998.0
- pulmonary (*see also* Atelectasis) 518.0
    - fetus or newborn 770.5
        - partial 770.5
        - primary 770.4
- thorax 512.8
    - iatrogenic 512.1
    - postoperative 512.1

Collapse — continued
- trachea 519.1
- valvular — *see* Endocarditis
- vascular (peripheral) 785.59
    - with
        - abortion — *see* Abortion, by type, with shock
        - ectopic pregnancy (*see also* categories 633.0-633.9) 639.5
        - molar pregnancy (*see also* categories 630-632) 639.5
    - cerebral (*see also* Disease, cerebrovascular, acute) 436
    - during or after labor and delivery 669.1 ✓5
    - fetus or newborn 779.89 ▲
    - following
        - abortion 639.5
        - ectopic or molar pregnancy 639.5
- vasomotor 785.59
- vertebra 733.13

Collateral — *see also* condition
- circulation (venous) 459.89
- dilation, veins 459.89

Colles' fracture (closed) (reversed) (separation) 813.41
- open 813.51

Collet's syndrome 352.6
Collet-Sicard syndrome 352.6
Colliculitis urethralis (*see also* Urethritis) 597.89
Colliers'
- asthma 500
- lung 500
- phthisis (*see also* Tuberculosis) 011.4 ✓5

Collodion baby (ichthyosis congenita) 757.1
Colloid milium 709.3
Coloboma NEC 743.49
- choroid 743.59
- fundus 743.52
- iris 743.46
- lens 743.36
- lids 743.62
- optic disc (congenital) 743.57
    - acquired 377.23
- retina 743.56
- sclera 743.47

Coloenteritis — *see* Enteritis
Colon — *see* condition
Coloptosis 569.89
Color
- amblyopia NEC 368.59
    - acquired 368.55
- blindness NEC (congenital) 368.59
    - acquired 368.55

Colostomy
- attention to V55.3
- fitting or adjustment V53.5
- malfunctioning 569.62
- status V44.3

Colpitis (*see also* Vaginitis) 616.10
Colpocele 618.6
Colpocystitis (*see also* Vaginitis) 616.10
Colporrhexis 665.4 ✓5
Colpospasm 625.1
Column, spinal, vertebral — *see* condition
Coma 780.01
- apoplectic (*see also* Disease, cerebrovascular, acute) 436
- diabetic (with ketoacidosis) 250.3 ✓5
    - hyperosmolar 250.2 ✓5
- eclamptic (*see also* Eclampsia) 780.39
- epileptic 345.3
- hepatic 572.2
- hyperglycemic 250.2 ✓5
- hyperosmolar (diabetic) (nonketotic) 250.2 ✓5
- hypoglycemic 251.0
    - diabetic 250.3 ✓5
- insulin 250.3 ✓5
    - hypersmolar 250.2 ✓5
    - non-diabetic 251.0
    - organic hyperinsulinism 251.0
- Kussmaul's (diabetic) 250.3 ✓5
- liver 572.2
- newborn 779.2

Coma — continued
- prediabetic 250.2 ✓5
- uremic — *see* Uremia

Combat fatigue (*see also* Reaction, stress, acute) 308.9
Combined — *see* condition
Comedo 706.1
Comedocarcinoma (M8501/3) — *see also* Neoplasm, breast, malignant
- noninfiltrating (M8501/2)
    - specified site — *see* Neoplasm, by site, in situ
    - unspecified site 233.0

Comedomastitis 610.4
Comedones 706.1
- lanugo 757.4

Comma bacillus, carrier (suspected) of V02.3
Comminuted fracture — *see* Fracture, by site
Common
- aortopulmonary trunk 745.0
- atrioventricular canal (defect) 745.69
- atrium 745.69
- cold (head) 460
    - vaccination, prophylactic (against) V04.7
- truncus (arteriosus) 745.0
- ventricle 745.3

Commotio (current)
- cerebri (*see also* Concussion, brain) 850.9
    - with skull fracture — *see* Fracture, skull, by site
- retinae 921.3
- spinalis — *see* Injury, spinal, by site

Commotion (current)
- brain (without skull fracture) (*see also* Concussion, brain) 850.9
    - with skull fracture — *see* Fracture, skull, by site
- spinal cord — *see* Injury, spinal, by site

Communication
- abnormal — *see also* Fistula
    - between
        - base of aorta and pulmonary artery 745.0
        - left ventricle and right atrium 745.4
        - pericardial sac and pleural sac 748.8
        - pulmonary artery and pulmonary vein 747.3
        - congenital, between uterus and anterior abdominal wall 752.3
            - bladder 752.3
            - intestine 752.3
            - rectum 752.3
    - left ventricular— right atrial 745.4
    - pulmonary artery— pulmonary vein 747.3

Compensation
- broken — *see* Failure, heart
- failure — *see* Failure, heart
- neurosis, psychoneurosis 300.11

Complaint — *see also* Disease
- bowel, functional 564.9
    - psychogenic 306.4
- intestine, functional 564.9
    - psychogenic 306.4
- kidney (*see also* Disease, renal) 593.9
- liver 573.9
- miners' 500

Complete — *see* condition
Complex
- cardiorenal (*see also* Hypertension, cardiorenal) 404.90
- castration 300.9
- Costen's 524.60
- ego-dystonic homosexuality 302.0
- Eisenmenger's (ventricular septal defect) 745.4
- homosexual, ego-dystonic 302.0
- hypersexual 302.89
- inferiority 301.9
- jumped process
    - spine — *see* Dislocation, vertebra
- primary, tuberculosis (*see also* Tuberculosis) 010.0 ✓5
- Taussig-Bing (transposition, aorta and overriding pulmonary artery) 745.11

Complications

Complications
- abortion NEC — *see* categories 634-639
- accidental puncture or laceration during a procedure 998.2
- amputation stump (late) (surgical) 997.60
  - traumatic — *see* Amputation, traumatic
- anastomosis (and bypass) NEC — *see also* Complications, due to (presence of) any device, implant, or graft classified to 996.0-996.5 NEC
  - hemorrhage NEC 998.11
  - intestinal (internal) NEC 997.4
    - involving urinary tract 997.5
  - mechanical — *see* Complications, mechanical, graft
  - urinary tract (involving intestinal tract) 997.5
- anesthesia, anesthetic NEC (*see also* Anesthesia, complication) 995.2
  - in labor and delivery 668.9 ☑5ᵗʰ
    - affecting fetus or newborn 763.5
    - cardiac 668.1 ☑5ᵗʰ
    - central nervous system 668.2 ☑5ᵗʰ
    - pulmonary 668.0 ☑5ᵗʰ
    - specified type NEC 668.8 ☑5ᵗʰ
- aortocoronary (bypass) graft 996.03
  - atherosclerosis — *see* Arteriosclerosis, coronary
  - embolism 996.72
  - occlusion NEC 996.72
  - thrombus 996.72
- arthroplasty 996.4
- artificial opening
  - cecostomy 569.60
  - colostomy 569.60
  - cystostomy 997.5
  - enterostomy 569.60
  - gastrostomy 536.40
  - ileostomy 569.60
  - jejunostomy 569.60
  - nephrostomy 997.5
  - tracheostomy 519.00
  - ureterostomy 997.5
  - urethrostomy 997.5
- bile duct implant (prosthetic) NEC 996.79
  - infection or inflammation 996.69
  - mechanical 996.59
- bleeding (intraoperative) (postoperative) 998.11
- blood vessel graft 996.1
  - aortocoronary 996.03
    - atherosclerosis — *see* Arteriosclerosis, coronary
    - embolism 996.72
    - occlusion NEC 996.72
    - thrombus 996.72
  - atherosclerosis — *see* Arteriosclerosis, extremities
  - embolism 996.74
  - occlusion NEC 996.74
  - thrombus 996.74
- bone growth stimulator 996.78
  - infection or inflammation 996.67
- bone marrow transplant 996.85
- breast implant (prosthetic) NEC 996.79
  - infection or inflammation 996.69
  - mechanical 996.54
- bypass — *see also* Complications, anastomosis
  - aortocoronary 996.03
    - atherosclerosis — *see* Arteriosclerosis, coronary
    - embolism 996.72
    - occlusion NEC 996.72
    - thrombus 996.72
  - carotid artery 996.1
    - atherosclerosis — *see* Arteriosclerosis, extremities
    - embolism 996.74
    - occulsion NEC 996.74
    - thrombus 996.74
- cardiac (*see also* Disease, heart) 429.9
  - device, implant, or graft NEC 996.72
    - infection or inflammation 996.61
    - long-term effect 429.4
    - mechanical (*see also* Complications, mechanical, by type) 996.00
      - valve prosthesis 996.71
        - infection or inflammation 996.61

Complications — *continued*
- cardiac (*see also* Disease, heart) — *continued*
  - postoperative NEC 997.1
    - long-term effect 429.4
- cardiorenal (*see also* Hypertension, cardiorenal) 404.90
- carotid artery bypass graft 996.1
  - atherosclerosis — *see* Arteriosclerosis, extremities
  - embolism 996.74
  - occlusion NEC 996.74
  - thrombus 996.74
- cataract fragments in eye 998.82
- catheter device NEC — *see also* Complications, due to (presence of) any device, implant, or graft classified to 996.0-996.5 NEC
  - mechanical — *see* Complications, mechanical, catheter
- cecostomy 569.60
- cesarean section wound 674.3 ☑5ᵗʰ
- chin implant (prosthetic) NEC 996.79
  - infection or inflammation 996.69
  - mechanical 996.59
- colostomy (enterostomy) 569.60
  - specified type NEC 569.69
- contraceptive device, intrauterine NEC 996.76
  - infection 996.65
  - inflammation 996.65
  - mechanical 996.32
- cord (umbilical) — *see* Complications, umbilical cord
- cornea
  - due to
    - contact lens 371.82
- coronary (artery) bypass (graft) NEC 996.03
  - atherosclerosis — *see* Arterio-sclerosis, coronary
  - embolism 996.72
  - infection or inflammation 996.61
  - mechanical 996.03
  - occlusion NEC 996.72
  - specified type NEC 996.72
  - thrombus 996.72
- cystostomy 997.5
- delivery 669.9 ☑5ᵗʰ
  - procedure (instrumental) (manual) (surgical) 669.4 ☑5ᵗʰ
  - specified type NEC 669.8 ☑5ᵗʰ
- dialysis (hemodialysis) (peritoneal) (renal) NEC 999.9
  - catheter NEC — *see also* Complications, due to (presence of) any device, implant or graft classified to 996.0-996.5 NEC
    - infection or inflammation 996.62
      - peritoneal 996.68
    - mechanical 996.1
      - peritoneal 996.56
  - due to (presence of) any device, implant, or graft classified to 996.0-996.5 NEC 996.70
    - with infection or inflammation — *see* Complications, infection or inflammation, due to (presence of) any device, implant, or graft classified to 996.0-996.5 NEC
    - arterial NEC 996.74
      - coronary NEC 996.03
        - atherosclerosis — *see* Arteriosclerosis, coronary
        - embolism 996.72
        - occlusion NEC 996.72
        - specified type NEC 996.72
        - thrombus 996.72
      - renal dialysis 996.73
    - arteriovenous fistula or shunt NEC 996.74
    - bone growth stimulator 996.78
    - breast NEC 996.70
    - cardiac NEC 996.72
      - defibrillator 996.72
      - pacemaker 996.72
      - valve prosthesis 996.71
    - catheter NEC 996.79
      - spinal 996.75
      - urinary, indwelling 996.76
      - vascular NEC 996.74
        - renal dialysis 996.73
      - ventricular shunt 996.75

Complications — *continued*
- due to (presence of) any device, implant, or graft classified to 996.0-996.5 NEC — *continued*
  - coronary (artery) bypass (graft) NEC 996.03
    - atherosclerosis — *see* Arteriosclerosis, coronary
    - embolism 996.72
    - occlusion NEC 996.72
    - thrombus 996.72
  - electrodes
    - brain 996.75
    - heart 996.72
  - gastrointestinal NEC 996.79
  - genitourinary NEC 996.76
  - heart valve prosthesis NEC 996.71
  - infusion pump 996.74
  - internal
    - joint prosthesis 996.77
    - orthopedic NEC 996.78
    - specified type NEC 996.79
  - intrauterine contraceptive device NEC 996.76
  - joint prosthesis, internal NEC 996.77
  - mechanical — *see* Complications, mechanical
  - nervous system NEC 996.75
  - ocular lens NEC 996.79
  - orbital NEC 996.79
  - orthopedic NEC 996.78
    - joint, internal 996.77
  - renal dialysis 996.73
  - specified type NEC 996.79
  - urinary catheter, indwelling 996.76
  - vascular NEC 996.74
  - ventricular shunt 996.75
- during dialysis NEC 999.9
- ectopic or molar pregnancy NEC 639.9
- electroshock therapy NEC 999.9
- enterostomy 569.60
  - specified type NEC 569.69
- external (fixation) device with internal component(s) NEC 996.78
  - infection or inflammation 996.67
  - mechanical 996.4
- extracorporeal circulation NEC 999.9
- eye implant (prosthetic) NEC 996.79
  - infection or inflammation 996.69
  - mechanical
    - ocular lens 996.53
    - orbital globe 996.59
- gastrointestinal, postoperative NEC (*see also* Complications, surgical procedures) 997.4
- gastrostomy 536.40
  - specified type NEC 536.49
- genitourinary device, implant or graft NEC 996.76
  - infection or inflammation 996.65
    - urinary catheter, indwelling 996.64
  - mechanical (*see also* Complications, mechanical, by type) 996.30
  - specified NEC 996.39
- graft (bypass) (patch) NEC — *see also* Complications, due to (presence of) any device, implant, or graft classified to 996.0-996.5 NEC
  - bone marrow 996.85
  - corneal NEC 996.79
    - infection or inflammation 996.69
    - rejection or reaction 996.51
  - mechanical — *see* Complications, mechanical, graft
  - organ (immune or nonimmune cause) (partial) (total) 996.80
    - bone marrow 996.85
    - heart 996.83
    - intestines 996.87
    - kidney 996.81
    - liver 996.82
    - lung 996.84
    - pancreas 996.86
    - specified NEC 996.89
  - skin NEC 996.79
    - infection or inflammation 996.69

Complications

Complications — *continued*
- graft (bypass) (patch) NEC — *see also* Complications, due to (presence of) any device, implant, or graft classified to 996.0-996.5 NEC — *continued*
  - skin NEC — *continued*
    - rejection 996.52
      - artificial 996.55
      - decellularized allodermis 996.55
  - heart — *see also* Disease, heart transplant (immune or nonimmune cause) 996.83
  - hematoma (intraoperative) (postoperative) 998.12
  - hemorrhage (intraoperative) (postoperative) 998.11
  - hyperalimentation therapy NEC 999.9
  - immunization (procedure) — *see* Complications, vaccination
  - implant — *see also* Complications, due to (presence of) any device, implant, or graft classified to 996.0-996.5 NEC
    - mechanical — *see* Complications, mechanical, implant
  - infection and inflammation
    - due to (presence of) any device, implant or graft classified to 996.0-996.5 NEC 996.60
      - arterial NEC 996.62
        - coronary 996.61
        - renal dialysis 996.62
      - arteriovenous fistula or shunt 996.62
      - bone growth stimulator 996.67
      - breast 996.69
      - cardiac 996.61
      - catheter NEC 996.69
        - peritoneal 996.68
        - spinal 996.63
        - urinary, indwelling 996.64
        - vascular NEC 996.62
        - ventricular shunt 996.63
      - coronary artery bypass 996.61
      - electrodes
        - brain 996.63
        - heart 996.61
      - gastrointestinal NEC 996.69
      - genitourinary NEC 996.65
        - indwelling urinary catheter 996.64
      - heart valve 996.61
      - infusion pump 996.62
      - intrauterine contraceptive device 996.65
      - joint prosthesis, internal 996.66
      - ocular lens 996.69
      - orbital (implant) 996.69
      - orthopedic NEC 996.67
        - joint, internal 996.66
      - specified type NEC 996.69
      - urinary catheter, indwelling 996.64
      - ventricular shunt 996.63
  - infusion (procedure) 999.9
    - blood — *see* Complications, transfusion
    - infection NEC 999.3
    - sepsis NEC 999.3
  - inhalation therapy NEC 999.9
  - injection (procedure) 999.9
    - drug reaction (*see also* Reaction, drug) 995.2
    - infection NEC 999.3
    - sepsis NEC 999.3
    - serum (prophylactic) (therapeutic) — *see* Complications, vaccination
    - vaccine (any) — *see* Complications, vaccination
  - inoculation (any) — *see* Complications, vaccination
  - internal device (catheter) (electronic) (fixation) (prosthetic) NEC — *see also* Complications, due to (presence of) any device, implant, or graft classified to 996.0-996.5 NEC
    - mechanical — *see* Complications, mechanical
  - intestinal transplant (immune or nonimmune cause) 996.87
  - intraoperative bleeding or hemorrhage 998.11
  - intrauterine contraceptive device 996.76 — *see also* Complications, contraceptive device
    - with fetal damage affecting management of pregnancy 655.8 ✓5ᵗʰ

Complications — *continued*
- intrauterine contraceptive device 996.76 — *see also* Complications, contraceptive device — *continued*
  - infection or inflammation 996.65
- jejunostomy 569.60
- kidney transplant (immune or nonimmune cause) 996.81
- labor 669.9 ✓5ᵗʰ
  - specified condition NEC 669.8 ✓5ᵗʰ
- liver transplant (immune or nonimmune cause) 996.82
- lumbar puncture 349.0
- mechanical
  - anastomosis — *see* Complications, mechanical, graft
  - bypass — *see* Complications, mechanical, graft
  - catheter NEC 996.59
    - cardiac 996.09
    - cystostomy 996.39
    - dialysis (hemodialysis) 996.1
      - peritoneal 996.56
    - during a procedure 998.2
    - urethral, indwelling 996.31
  - colostomy 569.62
  - device NEC 996.59
    - balloon (counterpulsation), intra-aortic 996.1
    - cardiac 996.00
      - automatic implantable defibrillator 996.04
      - long-term effect 429.4
      - specified NEC 996.09
    - contraceptive, intrauterine 996.32
    - counterpulsation, intra-aortic 996.1
    - fixation, external, with internal components 996.4
    - fixation, internal (nail, rod, plate) 996.4
    - genitourinary 996.30
      - specified NEC 996.39
    - nervous system 996.2
    - orthopedic, internal 996.4
    - prosthetic NEC 996.59
    - umbrella, vena cava 996.1
    - vascular 996.1
  - dorsal column stimulator 996.2
  - electrode NEC 996.59
    - brain 996.2
    - cardiac 996.01
    - spinal column 996.2
  - enterostomy 569.62
  - fistula, arteriovenous, surgically created 996.1
  - gastrostomy 536.42
  - graft NEC 996.52
    - aortic (bifurcation) 996.1
    - aortocoronary bypass 996.03
    - blood vessel NEC 996.1
    - bone 996.4
    - cardiac 996.00
    - carotid artery bypass 996.1
    - cartilage 996.4
    - corneal 996.51
    - coronary bypass 996.03
    - decellularized allodermis 996.55
    - genitourinary 996.30
      - specified NEC 996.39
    - muscle 996.4
    - nervous system 996.2
    - organ (immune or nonimmune cause) 996.80
      - heart 996.83
      - intestines 996.87
      - kidney 996.81
      - liver 996.82
      - lung 996.84
      - pancreas 996.86
      - specified NEC 996.89
    - orthopedic, internal 996.4
    - peripheral nerve 996.2
    - prosthetic NEC 996.59
    - skin 996.52
      - artificial 996.55
    - specified NEC 996.59
    - tendon 996.4

Complications — *continued*
- mechanical — *continued*
  - graft NEC — *continued*
    - tissue NEC 996.52
    - tooth 996.59
    - ureter, without mention of resection 996.39
    - vascular 996.1
  - heart valve prosthesis 996.02
    - long-term effect 429.4
  - implant NEC 996.59
    - cardiac 996.00
      - automatic implantable defibrillator 996.04
      - long-term effect 429.4
      - specified NEC 996.09
    - electrode NEC 996.59
      - brain 996.2
      - cardiac 996.01
      - spinal column 996.2
    - genitourinary 996.30
    - nervous system 996.2
    - orthopedic, internal 996.4
    - prosthetic NEC 996.59
      - in
        - bile duct 996.59
        - breast 996.54
        - chin 996.59
        - eye
          - ocular lens 996.53
          - orbital globe 996.59
    - vascular 996.1
  - nonabsorbable surgical material 996.59
  - pacemaker NEC 996.59
    - brain 996.2
    - cardiac 996.01
    - nerve (phrenic) 996.2
  - patch — *see* Complications, mechanical, graft
  - prosthesis NEC 996.59
    - bile duct 996.59
    - breast 996.54
    - chin 996.59
    - ocular lens 996.53
    - reconstruction, vas deferens 996.39
  - reimplant NEC 996.59
    - extremity (*see also* Complications, reattached, extremity) 996.90
    - organ (*see also* Complications, transplant, organ, by site) 996.80
  - repair — *see* Complications, mechanical, graft
  - shunt NEC 996.59
    - arteriovenous, surgically created 996.1
    - ventricular (communicating) 996.2
  - stent NEC 996.59
  - tracheostomy 519.02
  - vas deferens reconstruction 996.39
- medical care NEC 999.9
  - cardiac NEC 997.1
  - gastrointestinal NEC 997.4
  - nervous system NEC 997.00
  - peripheral vascular NEC 997.2
  - respiratory NEC 997.3
  - urinary NEC 997.5
  - vascular
    - mesenteric artery 997.71
    - other vessels 997.79
    - peripheral vessels 997.2
    - renal artery 997.72
- nephrostomy 997.5
- nervous system
  - device, implant, or graft NEC 349.1
    - mechanical 996.2
  - postoperative NEC 997.00
- obstetric 669.9 ✓5ᵗʰ
  - procedure (instrumental) (manual) (surgical) 669.4 ✓5ᵗʰ
  - specified NEC 669.8 ✓5ᵗʰ
  - surgical wound 674.3 ✓5ᵗʰ
- ocular lens implant NEC 996.79
  - infection or inflammation 996.69
  - mechanical 996.53
- organ transplant — *see* Complications, transplant, organ, by site

Complications

Complications — *continued*
  orthopedic device, implant, or graft
    internal (fixation) (nail) (plate) (rod) NEC
        996.78
      infection or inflammation 996.67
      joint prosthesis 996.77
        infection or inflammation 996.66
      mechanical 996.4
    pacemaker (cardiac) 996.72
      infection or inflammation 996.61
      mechanical 996.01
    pancreas transplant (immune or nonimmune
        cause) 996.86
  perfusion NEC 999.9
  perineal repair (obstetrical) 674.3 ✓5ᵗʰ
    disruption 674.2 ✓5ᵗʰ
  pessary (uterus) (vagina) — *see* Complications,
      contraceptive device
  phototherapy 990
  postcystoscopic 997.5
  postmastoidectomy NEC 383.30
  postoperative — *see* Complications, surgical
      procedures
  pregnancy NEC 646.9 ✓5ᵗʰ
    affecting fetus or newborn 761.9
  prosthetic device, internal NEC — *see also*
      Complications, due to (presence of) any
      device, implant or graft classified to
      996.0-996.5 NEC
    mechanical NEC (*see also* Complications,
        mechanical) 996.59
  puerperium NEC (*see also* Puerperal) 674.9 ✓5ᵗʰ
  puncture, spinal 349.0
  pyelogram 997.5
  radiation 990
  radiotherapy 990
  reattached
    body part, except extremity 996.99
    extremity (infection) (rejection) 996.90
      arm(s) 996.94
      digit(s) (hand) 996.93
        foot 996.95
      finger(s) 996.93
      foot 996.95
      forearm 996.91
      hand 996.92
      leg 996.96
      lower NEC 996.96
      toe(s) 996.95
      upper NEC 996.94
  reimplant NEC — *see also* Complications, to
      (presence of) any device, implant, or graft
      classified to 996.0-996.5 NEC
    bone marrow 996.85
    extremity (*see also* Complications,
        reattached, extremity) 996.90
      due to infection 996.90
    mechanical — *see* Complications,
        mechanical, reimplant
    organ (immune or nonimmune cause)
        (partial) (total) (*see also* Complications,
        transplant, organ, by site) 996.80
  renal allograft 996.81
  renal dialysis — *see* Complications, dialysis
  respiratory 519.9
    device, implant or graft NEC 996.79
      infection or inflammation 996.69
      mechanical 996.59
    distress syndrome, adult, following trauma
        or surgery 518.5
    insufficiency, acute, postoperative 518.5
    postoperative NEC 997.3
    therapy NEC 999.9
  sedation during labor and delivery 668.9 ✓5ᵗʰ
    affecting fetus or newborn 763.5
    cardiac 668.1 ✓5ᵗʰ
    central nervous system 668.2 ✓5ᵗʰ
    pulmonary 668.0 ✓5ᵗʰ
    specified type NEC 668.8 ✓5ᵗʰ
  seroma (intraoperative) (postoperative)
      (noninfected) 998.13
    infected 998.51
  shunt NEC — *see also* Complications, due to
      (presence of) any device, implant, or graft
      classified to 996.0-996.5 NEC
    mechanical — *see* Complications,
        mechanical, shunt

Complications — *continued*
  specified body system NEC
    device, implant, or graft NEC — *see*
        Complications, due to (presence of)
        any device, implant, or graft classified
        to 996.0-996.5 NEC
    postoperative NEC 997.99
  spinal puncture or tap 349.0
  stoma, external
    gastrointestinal tract
      colostomy 569.60
      enterostomy 569.60
      gastrostomy 536.40
    urinary tract 997.5
  surgical procedures 998.9
    accidental puncture or laceration 998.2
    amputation stump (late) 997.60
    anastomosis — *see* Complications,
        anastomosis
    burst stitches or sutures ▶(external)◀   ▲
        998.32
      internal 998.31   ●
    cardiac 997.1
      long-term effect following cardiac surgery
          429.4
    cataract fragments in eye 998.82
    catheter device — *see* Complications,
        catheter device
    cecostomy malfunction 569.62
    colostomy malfunction 569.62
    cystostomy malfunction 997.5
    dehiscence (of incision) ▶(external)◀   ▲
        998.32
      internal 998.31   ●
    dialysis NEC (*see also* Complications,
        dialysis) 999.9
    disruption
      anastomosis (internal) — *see*
          Complications, mechanical, graft
      internal suture (line) 998.31   ▲
      wound ▶(external)◀ 998.32   ▲
        internal 998.31   ●
    dumping syndrome (postgastrectomy) 564.2
    elephantiasis or lymphedema 997.99
      postmastectomy 457.0
    emphysema (surgical) 998.81
    enterostomy malfunction 569.62
    evisceration 998.32   ▲
    fistula (persistent postoperative) 998.6
    foreign body inadvertently left in wound
        (sponge) (suture) (swab) 998.4
    from nonabsorbable surgical material
        (Dacron) (mesh) (permanent suture)
        (reinforcing) (Teflon) — *see*
        Complications, due to (presence of)
        any device, implant, or graft classified
        to 996.0-996.5 NEC
    gastrointestinal NEC 997.4
    gastrostomy malfunction 536.42
    hematoma 998.12
    hemorrhage 998.11
    ileostomy malfunction 569.62
    internal prosthetic device NEC (*see also*
        Complications, internal device) 996.70
      hemolytic anemia 283.19
      infection or inflammation 996.60
      malfunction — *see* Complications,
          mechanical
      mechanical complication — *see*
          Complications, mechanical
      thrombus 996.70
    jejunostomy malfunction 569.62
    nervous system NEC 997.00
    obstruction, internal anastomosis — *see*
        Complications, mechanical, graft
    other body system NEC 997.99
    peripheral vascular NEC 997.2
    postcardiotomy syndrome 429.4
    postcholecystectomy syndrome 576.0
    postcommissurotomy syndrome 429.4
    postgastrectomy dumping syndrome 564.2
    postmastectomy lymphedema syndrome
        457.0
    postmastoidectomy 383.30
      cholesteatoma, recurrent 383.32
      cyst, mucosal 383.31
      granulation 383.33

Complications — *continued*
  surgical procedures — *continued*
    postmastoidectomy — *continued*
      inflammation, chronic 383.33
    postvagotomy syndrome 564.2
    postvalvulotomy syndrome 429.4
    reattached extremity (infection) (rejection)
        (*see also* Complications, reattached,
        extremity) 996.90
    respiratory NEC 997.3
    seroma 998.13
    shock (endotoxic) (hypovolemic) (septic)
        998.0
    shunt, prosthetic (thrombus) — *see also*
        Complications, due to (presence of)
        any device, implant, or graft classified
        to 996.0-996.5 NEC
      hemolytic anemia 283.19
    specified complication NEC 998.89
    stitch abscess 998.59
    transplant — *see* Complications, graft
    ureterostomy malfunction 997.5
    urethrostomy malfunction 997.5
    urinary NEC 997.5
    vascular
      mesenteric artery 997.71
      other vessels 997.79
      peripheral vessels 997.2
      renal artery 997.72
    wound infection 998.59
  therapeutic misadventure NEC 999.9
    surgical treatment 998.9
  tracheostomy 519.00
  transfusion (blood) (lymphocytes) (plasma) NEC
      999.8
    atrophy, liver, yellow, subacute (within 8
        months of administration) — *see*
        Hepatitis, viral
    bone marrow 996.85
    embolism
      air 999.1
      thrombus 999.2
    hemolysis NEC 999.8
      bone marrow 996.85
    hepatitis (serum) (type B) (within 8 months
        after administration) — *see* Hepatitis,
        viral
    incompatibility reaction (ABO) (blood group)
        999.6
      Rh (factor) 999.7
    infection 999.3
    jaundice (serum) (within 8 months after
        administration) — *see* Hepatitis, viral
    sepsis 999.3
    shock or reaction NEC 999.8
      bone marrow 996.85
    subacute yellow atrophy of liver (within 8
        months after administration) — *see*
        Hepatitis, viral
    thromboembolism 999.2
  transplant NEC — *see also* Complications, due
      to (presence of) any device, implant, or
      graft classified to 996.0-996.5 NEC
    bone marrow 996.85
    organ (immune or nonimmune cause)
        (partial) (total) 996.80
      bone marrow 996.85
      heart 996.83
      intestines 996.87
      kidney 996.81
      liver 996.82
      lung 996.84
      pancreas 996.86
      specified NEC 996.89
  trauma NEC (early) 958.8
  ultrasound therapy NEC 999.9
  umbilical cord
    affecting fetus or newborn 762.6
    complicating delivery 663.9 ✓5ᵗʰ
      affecting fetus or newborn 762.6
    specified type NEC 663.8 ✓5ᵗʰ
  urethral catheter NEC 996.76
    infection or inflammation 996.64
    mechanical 996.31
  urinary, postoperative NEC 997.5
  vaccination 999.9
    anaphylaxis NEC 999.4

Complications — *continued*
  vaccination — *continued*
    cellulitis 999.3
    encephalitis or encephalomyelitis 323.5
    hepatitis (serum) (type B) (within 8 months after administration) — *see* Hepatitis, viral
    infection (general) (local) NEC 999.3
    jaundice (serum) (within 8 months after administration) — *see* Hepatitis, viral
    meningitis 997.09 [321.8]
    myelitis 323.5
    protein sickness 999.5
    reaction (allergic) 999.5
      Herxheimer's 995.0
      serum 999.5
    sepsis 999.3
    serum intoxication, sickness, rash, or other serum reaction NEC 999.5
    shock (allergic) (anaphylactic) 999.4
    subacute yellow atrophy of liver (within 8 months after administration) — *see* Hepatitis, viral
    vaccinia (generalized) 999.0
      localized 999.3
  vascular
    device, implant, or graft NEC 996.74
      infection or inflammation 996.62
      mechanical NEC 996.1
        cardiac (*see also* Complications, mechanical, by type) 996.00
    following infusion, perfusion, or transfusion 999.2
    postoperative NEC 997.2
      mesenteric artery 997.71
      other vessels 997.79
      peripheral vessels 997.2
      renal artery 997.72
  ventilation therapy NEC 999.9
Compound presentation, complicating delivery 652.8 ✓5ᵗʰ
  causing obstructed labor 660.0 ✓5ᵗʰ
Compressed air disease 993.3
Compression
  with injury — *see* specific injury
  arm NEC 354.9
  artery 447.1
    celiac, syndrome 447.4
  brachial plexus 353.0
  brain (stem) 348.4
    due to
      contusion, brain — *see* Contusion, brain
      injury NEC — *see also* Hemorrhage, brain, traumatic
        birth — *see* Birth, injury, brain
        laceration, brain — *see* Laceration, brain
      osteopathic 739.0
  bronchus 519.1
  by cicatrix — *see* Cicatrix
  cardiac 423.9
  cauda equina 344.60
    with neurogenic bladder 344.61
  celiac (artery) (axis) 447.4
  cerebral — *see* Compression, brain
  cervical plexus 353.2
  cord (umbilical) — *see* Compression, umbilical cord
  cranial nerve 352.9
    second 377.49
    third (partial) 378.51
      total 378.52
    fourth 378.53
    fifth 350.8
    sixth 378.54
    seventh 351.8
  divers' squeeze 993.3
  duodenum (external) (*see also* Obstruction, duodenum) 537.3
  during birth 767.9
  esophagus 530.3
    congenital, external 750.3
  Eustachian tube 381.63
  facies (congenital) 754.0
  fracture — *see* Fracture, by site
  heart — *see* Disease, heart

Compression — *continued*
  intestine (*see also* Obstruction, intestine) 560.9
    with hernia — *see* Hernia, by site, with obstruction
  laryngeal nerve, recurrent 478.79
  leg NEC 355.8
  lower extremity NEC 355.8
  lumbosacral plexus 353.1
  lung 518.89
  lymphatic vessel 457.1
  medulla — *see* Compression, brain
  nerve NEC — *see also* Disorder, nerve
    arm NEC 354.9
    autonomic nervous system (*see also* Neuropathy, peripheral, autonomic) 337.9
    axillary 353.0
    cranial NEC 352.9
    due to displacement of intervertebral disc 722.2
      with myelopathy 722.70
      cervical 722.0
        with myelopathy 722.71
      lumbar, lumbosacral 722.10
        with myelopathy 722.73
      thoracic, thoracolumbar 722.11
        with myelopathy 722.72
    iliohypogastric 355.79
    ilioinguinal 355.79
    leg NEC 355.8
    lower extremity NEC 355.8
    median (in carpal tunnel) 354.0
    obturator 355.79
    optic 377.49
    plantar 355.6
    posterior tibial (in tarsal tunnel) 355.5
    root (by scar tissue) NEC 724.9
      cervical NEC 723.4
      lumbar NEC 724.4
      lumbosacral 724.4
      thoracic 724.4
    saphenous 355.79
    sciatic (acute) 355.0
    sympathetic 337.9
    traumatic — *see* Injury, nerve
    ulnar 354.2
    upper extremity NEC 354.9
  peripheral — *see* Compression, nerve
  spinal (cord) (old or nontraumatic) 336.9
    by displacement of intervertebral disc — *see* Displacement, intervertebral disc
    nerve
      root NEC 724.9
        postoperative 722.80
          cervical region 722.81
          lumbar region 722.83
          thoracic region 722.82
        traumatic — *see* Injury, nerve, spinal
      traumatic — *see* Injury, nerve, spinal
    spondylogenic 721.91
      cervical 721.1
      lumbar, lumbosacral 721.42
      thoracic 721.41
    traumatic — *see also* Injury, spinal, by site
      with fracture, vertebra — *see* Fracture, vertebra, by site, with spinal cord injury
  spondylogenic — *see* Compression, spinal cord, spondylogenic
  subcostal nerve (syndrome) 354.8
  sympathetic nerve NEC 337.9
  syndrome 958.5
  thorax 512.8
    iatrogenic 512.1
    postoperative 512.1
  trachea 519.1
    congenital 748.3
  ulnar nerve (by scar tissue) 354.2
  umbilical cord
    affecting fetus or newborn 762.5
      cord prolapsed 762.4
    complicating delivery 663.2 ✓5ᵗʰ
      cord around neck 663.1 ✓5ᵗʰ
      cord prolapsed 663.0 ✓5ᵗʰ
  upper extremity NEC 354.9
  ureter 593.3
  urethra — *see* Stricture, urethra

Compression — *continued*
  vein 459.2
  vena cava (inferior) (superior) 459.2
  vertebral NEC — *see* Compression, spinal (cord)
Compulsion, compulsive
  eating 307.51
  neurosis (obsessive) 300.3
  personality 301.4
  states (mixed) 300.3
  swearing 300.3
    in Gilles de la Tourette's syndrome 307.23
  tics and spasms 307.22
  water drinking NEC (syndrome) 307.9
Concato's disease (pericardial polyserositis) 423.2
  peritoneal 568.82
  pleural — *see* Pleurisy
Concavity, chest wall 738.3
Concealed
  hemorrhage NEC 459.0
  penis 752.65
Concentric fading 368.12
Concern (normal) about sick person in family V61.49
Concrescence (teeth) 520.2
Concretio cordis 423.1
  rheumatic 393
Concretion — *see also* Calculus
  appendicular 543.9
  canaliculus 375.57
  clitoris 624.8
  conjunctiva 372.54
  eyelid 374.56
  intestine (impaction) (obstruction) 560.39
  lacrimal (passages) 375.57
  prepuce (male) 605
    female (clitoris) 624.8
  salivary gland (any) 527.5
  seminal vesicle 608.89
  stomach 537.89
  tonsil 474.8
Concussion (current) 850.9
  with
    loss of consciousness 850.5
      brief (less than one hour) 850.1
      moderate (1-24 hours) 850.2
      prolonged (more than 24 hours) (with complete recovery) (with return to pre-existing conscious level) 850.3
        without return to pre-existing conscious level 850.4
    mental confusion or disorientation (without loss of consciousness) 850.0
      with loss of consciousness — *see* Concussion, with, loss of consciousness
  without loss of consciousness 850.0
  blast (air) (hydraulic) (immersion) (underwater) 869.0
    with open wound into cavity 869.1
    abdomen or thorax — *see* Injury, internal, by site
    brain — *see* Concussion, brain
    ear (acoustic nerve trauma) 951.5
      with perforation, tympanic membrane — *see* Wound, open, ear drum
    thorax — *see* Injury, internal, intrathoracic organs NEC
  brain or cerebral (without skull fracture) 850.9
    with
      loss of consciousness 850.5
        brief (less than one hour) 850.1
        moderate (1-24 hours) 850.2
        prolonged (more than 24 hours) (with complete recovery) (with return to pre-existing conscious level) 850.3
          without return to pre-existing conscious level 850.4
      mental confusion or disorientation (without loss of consciousness) 850.0
        with loss of consciousness — *see* Concussion, brain, with, loss of consciousness

Concussion

Concussion — continued
- brain or cerebral — continued
    - with — continued
        - skull fracture — see Fracture, skull, by site
    - without loss of consciousness 850.0
- cauda equina 952.4
- cerebral — see Concussion, brain
- conus medullaris (spine) 952.4
- hydraulic — see Concussion, blast
- internal organs — see Injury, internal, by site
- labyrinth — see Injury, intracranial
- ocular 921.3
- osseous labyrinth — see Injury, intracranial
- spinal (cord) — see also Injury, spinal, by site
    - due to
        - broken
            - back — see Fracture, vertebra, by site, with spinal cord injury
            - neck — see Fracture, vertebra, cervical, with spinal cord injury
        - fracture, fracture dislocation, or compression fracture of spine or vertebra — see Fracture, vertebra, by site, with spinal cord injury
- syndrome 310.2
- underwater blast — see Concussion, blast

Condition — see also Disease
- psychiatric 298.9
- respiratory NEC 519.9
    - acute or subacute NEC 519.9
        - due to
            - external agent 508.9
                - specified type NEC 508.8
            - fumes or vapors (chemical) (inhalation) 506.3
            - radiation 508.0
    - chronic NEC 519.9
        - due to
            - external agent 508.9
                - specified type NEC 508.8
            - fumes or vapors (chemical) (inhalation) 506.4
            - radiation 508.1
    - due to
        - external agent 508.9
            - specified type NEC 508.8
        - fumes or vapors (chemical) (inhalation) 506.9

Conduct disturbance (see also Disturbance, conduct) 312.9
- adjustment reaction 309.3
- hyperkinetic 314.2

Condyloma NEC 078.10
- acuminatum 078.11
- gonorrheal 098.0
- latum 091.3
- syphilitic 091.3
    - congenital 090.0
- venereal, syphilitic 091.3

Confinement — see Delivery

Conflagration — see also Burn, by site
- asphyxia (by inhalation of smoke, gases, fumes, or vapors) 987.9
    - specified agent — see Table of Drugs and Chemicals

Conflict
- family V61.9
    - specified circumstance NEC V61.8
- interpersonal NEC V62.81
- marital V61.10
    - involving divorce or estrangement V61.0
- parent-child V61.20
- partner V61.10

Confluent — see condition

Confusion, confused (mental) (state) (see also State, confusional) 298.9
- acute 293.0
- epileptic 293.0
- postoperative 293.9
- psychogenic 298.2
- reactive (from emotional stress, psychological trauma) 298.2
- subacute 293.1

Congelation 991.9

Congenital — see also condition
- aortic septum 747.29
- intrinsic factor deficiency 281.0
- malformation — see Anomaly

Congestion, congestive (chronic) (passive)
- asphyxia, newborn 768.9
- bladder 596.8
- bowel 569.89
- brain (see also Disease, cerebrovascular NEC) 437.8
    - malarial 084.9
- breast 611.79
- bronchi 519.1
- bronchial tube 519.1
- catarrhal 472.0
- cerebral — see Congestion, brain
- cerebrospinal — see Congestion, brain
- chest 514
- chill 780.99 ▲
    - malarial (see also Malaria) 084.6
- circulatory NEC 459.9
- conjunctiva 372.71
- due to disturbance of circulation 459.9
- duodenum 537.3
- enteritis — see Enteritis
- eye 372.71
- fibrosis syndrome (pelvic) 625.5
- gastroenteritis — see Enteritis
- general 799.8
- glottis 476.0
- heart (see also Failure, heart) 428.0
- hepatic 573.0
- hypostatic (lung) 514
- intestine 569.89
- intracranial — see Congestion, brain
- kidney 593.89
- labyrinth 386.50
- larynx 476.0
- liver 573.0
- lung 514
    - active or acute (see also Pneumonia) 486
        - congenital 770.0
    - chronic 514
    - hypostatic 514
    - idiopathic, acute 518.5
    - passive 514
- malaria, malarial (brain) (fever) (see also Malaria) 084.6
- medulla — see Congestion, brain
- nasal 478.1
- orbit, orbital 376.33
    - inflammatory (chronic) 376.10
        - acute 376.00
- ovary 620.8
- pancreas 577.8
- pelvic, female 625.5
- pleural 511.0
- prostate (active) 602.1
- pulmonary — see Congestion, lung
- renal 593.89
- retina 362.89
- seminal vesicle 608.89
- spinal cord 336.1
- spleen 289.51
    - chronic 289.51
- stomach 537.89
- trachea 464.11
- urethra 599.84
- uterus 625.5
    - with subinvolution 621.1
- viscera 799.8

Congestive — see Congestion

Conical
- cervix 622.6
- cornea 371.60
- teeth 520.2

Conjoined twins 759.4
- causing disproportion (fetopelvic) 653.7 ✓5ᵗʰ

Conjugal maladjustment V61.10
- involving divorce or estrangement V61.0

Conjunctiva — see condition

Conjunctivitis (exposure) (infectious) (nondiphtheritic) (pneumococcal) (pustular) (staphylococcal) (streptococcal) NEC 372.30
- actinic 370.24
- acute 372.00

Conjunctivitis NEC — continued
- acute — continued
    - atopic 372.05
    - contagious 372.03
    - follicular 372.02
    - hemorrhagic (viral) 077.4
- adenoviral (acute) 077.3
- allergic (chronic) 372.14
    - with hay fever 372.05
- anaphylactic 372.05
- angular 372.03
- Apollo (viral) 077.4
- atopic 372.05
- blennorrhagic (neonatorum) 098.40
- catarrhal 372.03
- chemical 372.05
- chlamydial 077.98
    - due to
        - Chlamydia trachomatis — see Trachoma
    - paratrachoma 077.0
- chronic 372.10
    - allergic 372.14
    - follicular 372.12
    - simple 372.11
    - specified type NEC 372.14
    - vernal 372.13
- diphtheritic 032.81
- due to
    - dust 372.05
    - enterovirus type 70 077.4
    - erythema multiforme 695.1 [372.33]
    - filariasis (see also Filiariasis) 125.9 [372.15]
    - mucocutaneous
        - disease NEC 372.33
        - leishmaniasis 085.5 [372.15]
    - Reiter's disease 099.3 [372.33]
    - syphilis 095.8 [372.10]
    - toxoplasmosis (acquired) 130.1
        - congenital (active) 771.2
    - trachoma — see Trachoma
- dust 372.05
- eczematous 370.31
- epidemic 077.1
    - hemorrhagic 077.4
- follicular (acute) 372.02
    - adenoviral (acute) 077.3
    - chronic 372.12
- glare 370.24
- gonococcal (neonatorum) 098.40
- granular (trachomatous) 076.1
    - late effect 139.1
- hemorrhagic (acute) (epidemic) 077.4
- herpetic (simplex) 054.43
    - zoster 053.21
- inclusion 077.0
- infantile 771.6
- influenzal 372.03
- Koch-Weeks 372.03
- light 372.05
- medicamentosa 372.05
- membranous 372.04
- meningococcic 036.89
- Morax-Axenfeld 372.02
- mucopurulent NEC 372.03
- neonatal 771.6
    - gonococcal 098.40
- Newcastle's 077.8
- nodosa 360.14
- of Beal 077.3
- parasitic 372.15
    - filariasis (see also Filiariasis) 125.9 [372.15]
    - mucocutaneous leishmaniasis 085.5 [372.15]
- Parinaud's 372.02
- petrificans 372.39
- phlyctenular 370.31
- pseudomembranous 372.04
    - diphtheritic 032.81
- purulent 372.03
- Reiter's 099.3 [372.33]
- rosacea 695.3 [372.31]
- serous 372.01
    - viral 077.99
- simple chronic 372.11
- specified NEC 372.39
- sunlamp 372.04
- swimming pool 077.0

Index to Diseases

Conjunctivitis NEC — *continued*
  trachomatous (follicular) 076.1
    acute 076.0
    late effect 139.1
  traumatic NEC 372.39
  tuberculous (*see also* Tuberculosis) 017.3 ✓5ᵗʰ
    [370.31]
  tularemic 021.3
  tularensis 021.3
  vernal 372.13
    limbar 372.13 [370.32]
  viral 077.99
    acute hemorrhagic 077.4
    specified NEC 077.8
Conjunctivochalasis 372.81
Conjunctoblepharitis — *see* Conjunctivitis
Conn (-Louis) syndrome (primary aldosteronism) 255.1
Connective tissue — *see* condition
Conradi (-Hünermann) syndrome or disease (chondrodysplasia calcificans congenita) 756.59
Consanguinity V19.7
Consecutive — *see* condition
Consolidated lung (base) — *see* Pneumonia, lobar
Constipation 564.00
  atonic 564.09
  drug induced
    correct substance properly administered 564.09
    overdose or wrong substance given or taken 977.9
      specified drug — *see* Table of Drugs and Chemicals
  neurogenic 564.09
  other specified NEC 564.09
  outlet dysfunction 564.02
  psychogenic 306.4
  simple 564.00
  slow transit 564.01
  spastic 564.09
Constitutional — *see also* condition
  arterial hypotension (*see also* Hypotension) 458.9
  obesity 278.00
    morbid 278.01
  psychopathic state 301.9
  short stature in childhood 783.43
  state, developmental V21.9
    specified development NEC V21.8
  substandard 301.6
Constitutionally substandard 301.6
Constriction
  anomalous, meningeal bands or folds 742.8
  aortic arch (congenital) 747.10
  asphyxiation or suffocation by 994.7
  bronchus 519.1
  canal, ear (*see also* Stricture, ear canal, acquired) 380.50
  duodenum 537.3
  gallbladder (*see also* Obstruction, gallbladder) 575.2
    congenital 751.69
  intestine (*see also* Obstruction, intestine) 560.9
  larynx 478.74
    congenital 748.3
  meningeal bands or folds, anomalous 742.8
  organ or site, congenital NEC — *see* Atresia
  prepuce (congenital) 605
  pylorus 537.0
    adult hypertrophic 537.0
    congenital or infantile 750.5
    newborn 750.5
  ring (uterus) 661.4 ✓5ᵗʰ
    affecting fetus or newborn 763.7
  spastic — *see also* Spasm
    ureter 593.3
    urethra — *see* Stricture, urethra
  stomach 537.89
  ureter 593.3
  urethra — *see* Stricture, urethra
  visual field (functional) (peripheral) 368.45
Constrictive — *see* condition

Consultation
  medical — *see also* Counseling, medical
  specified reason NEC V65.8
  without complaint or sickness V65.9
    feared complaint unfounded V65.5
    specified reason NEC V65.8
Consumption — *see* Tuberculosis
Contact
  with
    AIDS virus V01.7
    anthrax V01.81 ●
    cholera V01.0
    communicable disease V01.9
      specified type NEC V01.89 ▲
      viral NEC V01.7
    German measles V01.4
    gonorrhea V01.6
    HIV V01.7
    human immunodeficiency virus V01.7
    parasitic disease NEC V01.89 ▲
    poliomyelitis V01.2
    rabies V01.5
    rubella V01.4
    smallpox V01.3
    syphilis V01.6
    tuberculosis V01.1
    venereal disease V01.6
    viral disease NEC V01.7
  dermatitis — *see* Dermatitis
Contamination, food (*see also* Poisoning, food) 005.9
Contraception, contraceptive
  advice NEC V25.09
    family planning V25.09
    fitting of diaphragm V25.02
    prescribing or use of
      oral contraceptive agent V25.01
      specified agent NEC V25.02
  counseling NEC V25.09
    family planning V25.09
    fitting of diaphragm V25.02
    prescribing or use of
      oral contraceptive agent V25.01
      specified agent NEC V25.02
  device (in situ) V45.59
    causing menorrhagia 996.76
    checking V25.42
    complications 996.32
    insertion V25.1
    intrauterine V45.51
    reinsertion V25.42
    removal V25.42
    subdermal V45.52
  fitting of diaphragm V25.02
  insertion
    intrauterine contraceptive device V25.1
    subdermal implantable V25.5
  maintenance V25.40
    examination V25.40
      subdermal implantable V25.43
        intrauterine device V25.42
      oral contraceptive V25.41
      specified method NEC V25.49
    intrauterine device V25.42
    oral contraceptive V25.41
    specified method NEC V25.49
    subdermal implantable V25.43
  management NEC V25.49
  prescription
    oral contraceptive agent V25.01
      repeat V25.41
    specified agent NEC V25.02
      repeat V25.49
  sterilization V25.2
  surveillance V25.40
    intrauterine device V25.42
    oral contraceptive agent V25.41
    subdermal implantable V25.43
    specified method NEC V25.49
Contraction, contracture, contracted
  Achilles tendon (*see also* Short, tendon, Achilles) 727.81
  anus 564.89
  axilla 729.9
  bile duct (*see also* Disease, biliary) 576.8

Contraction, contracture, contracted — *continued*
  bladder 596.8
    neck or sphincter 596.0
  bowel (*see also* Obstruction, intestine) 560.9
  Braxton Hicks 644.1 ✓5ᵗʰ
  bronchus 519.1
  burn (old) — *see* Cicatrix
  cecum (*see also* Obstruction, intestine) 560.9
  cervix (*see also* Stricture, cervix) 622.4
    congenital 752.49
  cicatricial — *see* Cicatrix
  colon (*see also* Obstruction, intestine) 560.9
  conjunctiva trachomatous, active 076.1
    late effect 139.1
  Dupuytren's 728.6
  eyelid 374.41
  eye socket (after enucleation) 372.64
  face 729.9
  fascia (lata) (postural) 728.89
    Dupuytren's 728.6
    palmar 728.6
    plantar 728.71
  finger NEC 736.29
    congenital 755.59
    joint (*see also* Contraction, joint) 718.44
  flaccid, paralytic
    joint (*see also* Contraction, joint) 718.4 ✓5ᵗʰ
    muscle 728.85
    ocular 378.50
  gallbladder (*see also* Obstruction, gallbladder) 575.2
  hamstring 728.89
    tendon 727.81
  heart valve — *see* Endocarditis
  Hicks' 644.1 ✓5ᵗʰ
  hip (*see also* Contraction, joint) 718.4 ✓5ᵗʰ
  hourglass
    bladder 596.8
      congenital 753.8
    gallbladder (*see also* Obstruction, gallbladder) 575.2
      congenital 751.69
    stomach 536.8
      congenital 750.7
      psychogenic 306.4
    uterus 661.4 ✓5ᵗʰ
      affecting fetus or newborn 763.7
  hysterical 300.11
  infantile (*see also* Epilepsy) 345.6 ✓5ᵗʰ
  internal os (*see also* Stricture, cervix) 622.4
  intestine (*see also* Obstruction, intestine) 560.9
  joint (abduction) (acquired) (adduction) (flexion) (rotation) 718.40
    ankle 718.47
    congenital NEC 755.8
      generalized or multiple 754.89
        lower limb joints 754.89
      hip (*see also* Subluxation, congenital, hip) 754.32
      lower limb (including pelvic girdle) not involving hip 754.89
      upper limb (including shoulder girdle) 755.59
    elbow 718.42
    foot 718.47
    hand 718.44
    hip 718.45
    hysterical 300.11
    knee 718.46
    multiple sites 718.49
    pelvic region 718.45
    shoulder (region) 718.41
    specified site NEC 718.48
    wrist 718.43
  kidney (granular) (secondary) (*see also* Sclerosis, renal) 587
    congenital 753.3
    hydronephritic 591
    pyelonephritic (*see also* Pyelitis, chronic) 590.00
    tuberculous (*see also* Tuberculosis) 016.0 ✓5ᵗʰ
  ligament 728.89
    congenital 756.89
  liver — *see* Cirrhosis, liver
  muscle (postinfectional) (postural) NEC 728.85

Contraction, contracture, contracted — *continued*
- muscle NEC — *continued*
  - congenital 756.89
    - sternocleidomastoid 754.1
  - extraocular 378.60
  - eye (extrinsic) (*see also* Strabismus) 378.9
    - paralytic (*see also* Strabismus, paralytic) 378.50
  - flaccid 728.85
  - hysterical 300.11
  - ischemic (Volkmann's) 958.6
  - paralytic 728.85
  - posttraumatic 958.6
  - psychogenic 306.0
    - specified as conversion reaction 300.11
- myotonic 728.85
- neck (*see also* Torticollis) 723.5
  - congenital 754.1
  - psychogenic 306.0
- ocular muscle (*see also* Strabismus) 378.9
  - paralytic (*see also* Strabismus, paralytic) 378.50
- organ or site, congenital NEC — *see* Atresia
- outlet (pelvis) — *see* Contraction, pelvis
- palmar fascia 728.6
- paralytic
  - joint (*see also* Contraction, joint) 718.4 ✓5ᵗʰ
  - muscle 728.85
    - ocular (*see also* Strabismus, paralytic) 378.50
- pelvis (acquired) (general) 738.6
  - affecting fetus or newborn 763.1
  - complicating delivery 653.1 ✓5ᵗʰ
    - causing obstructed labor 660.1 ✓5ᵗʰ
    - generally contracted 653.1 ✓5ᵗʰ
      - causing obstructed labor 660.1 ✓5ᵗʰ
    - inlet 653.2 ✓5ᵗʰ
      - causing obstructed labor 660.1 ✓5ᵗʰ
    - midpelvic 653.8 ✓5ᵗʰ
      - causing obstructed labor 660.1 ✓5ᵗʰ
    - midplane 653.8 ✓5ᵗʰ
      - causing obstructed labor 660.1 ✓5ᵗʰ
    - outlet 653.3 ✓5ᵗʰ
      - causing obstructed labor 660.1 ✓5ᵗʰ
- plantar fascia 728.71
- premature
  - atrial 427.61
  - auricular 427.61
  - auriculoventricular 427.61
  - heart (junctional) (nodal) 427.60
  - supraventricular 427.61
  - ventricular 427.69
- prostate 602.8
- pylorus (*see also* Pylorospasm) 537.81
- rectosigmoid (*see also* Obstruction, intestine) 560.9
- rectum, rectal (sphincter) 564.89
  - psychogenic 306.4
- ring (Bandl's) 661.4 ✓5ᵗʰ
  - affecting fetus or newborn 763.7
- scar — *see* Cicatrix
- sigmoid (*see also* Obstruction, intestine) 560.9
- socket, eye 372.64
- spine (*see also* Curvature, spine) 737.9
- stomach 536.8
  - hourglass 536.8
    - congenital 750.7
    - psychogenic 306.4
  - psychogenic 306.4
- tendon (sheath) (*see also* Short, tendon) 727.81
- toe 735.8
- ureterovesical orifice (postinfectional) 593.3
- urethra 599.84
- uterus 621.8
  - abnormal 661.9 ✓5ᵗʰ
    - affecting fetus or newborn 763.7
  - clonic, hourglass or tetanic 661.4 ✓5ᵗʰ
    - affecting fetus or newborn 763.7
  - dyscoordinate 661.4 ✓5ᵗʰ
    - affecting fetus or newborn 763.7
  - hourglass 661.4 ✓5ᵗʰ
    - affecting fetus or newborn 763.7
  - hypotonic NEC 661.2 ✓5ᵗʰ
    - affecting fetus or newborn 763.7
  - incoordinate 661.4 ✓5ᵗʰ
    - affecting fetus or newborn 763.7

Contraction, contracture, contracted — *continued*
- uterus — *continued*
  - inefficient or poor 661.2 ✓5ᵗʰ
    - affecting fetus or newborn 763.7
  - irregular 661.2 ✓5ᵗʰ
    - affecting fetus or newborn 763.7
  - tetanic 661.4 ✓5ᵗʰ
    - affecting fetus or newborn 763.7
- vagina (outlet) 623.2
- vesical 596.8
  - neck or urethral orifice 596.0
- visual field, generalized 368.45
- Volkmann's (ischemic) 958.6

Contusion (skin surface intact) 924.9
- with
  - crush injury — *see* Crush
  - dislocation — *see* Dislocation, by site
  - fracture — *see* Fracture, by site
  - internal injury — *see also* Injury, internal, by site
    - heart — *see* Contusion, cardiac
    - kidney — *see* Contusion, kidney
    - liver — *see* Contusion, liver
    - lung — *see* Contusion, lung
    - spleen — *see* Contusion, spleen
  - intracranial injury — *see* Injury, intracranial
  - nerve injury — *see* Injury, nerve
  - open wound — *see* Wound, open, by site
- abdomen, abdominal (muscle) (wall) 922.2
  - organ(s) NEC 868.00
- adnexa, eye NEC 921.9
- ankle 924.21
  - with other parts of foot 924.20
- arm 923.9
  - lower (with elbow) 923.10
  - upper 923.03
    - with shoulder or axillary region 923.09
- auditory canal (external) (meatus) (and other part(s) of neck, scalp, or face, except eye) 920
- auricle, ear (and other part(s) of neck, scalp, or face except eye) 920
- axilla 923.02
  - with shoulder or upper arm 923.09
- back 922.31
- bone NEC 924.9
- brain (cerebral) (membrane) (with hemorrhage) 851.8 ✓5ᵗʰ

> *Note* — Use the following fifth-digit subclassification with categories 851-854:
>
> 0   unspecified state of consciousness
> 1   with no loss of consciousness
> 2   with brief [less than one hour] loss of consciousness
> 3   with moderate [1-24 hours] loss of consciousness
> 4   with prolonged [more than 24 hours] loss of consciousness and return to pre-existing conscious level
> 5   with prolonged [more than 24 hours] loss of consciousness, without return to pre-existing conscious level
>
> Use fifth-digit to designate when a patient is unconscious and dies before regaining consciousness, regardless of the duration of the loss of consciousness
>
> 6   with loss of consciousness of unspecified duration
> 9   with concussion, unspecified

- with
  - open intracranial wound 851.9 ✓5ᵗʰ
  - skull fracture — *see* Fracture, skull, by site
- cerebellum 851.4 ✓5ᵗʰ
  - with open intracranial wound 851.5 ✓5ᵗʰ
- cortex 851.0 ✓5ᵗʰ
  - with open intracranial wound 851.1 ✓5ᵗʰ
- occipital lobe 851.4 ✓5ᵗʰ
  - with open intracranial wound 851.5 ✓5ᵗʰ

Contusion — *continued*
- brain — *continued*
  - stem 851.4 ✓5ᵗʰ
    - with open intracranial wound 851.5 ✓5ᵗʰ
- breast 922.0
- brow (and other part(s) of neck, scalp, or face, except eye) 920
- buttock 922.32
- canthus 921.1
- cardiac 861.01
  - with open wound into thorax 861.11
- cauda equina (spine) 952.4
- cerebellum — *see* Contusion, brain, cerebellum
- cerebral — *see* Contusion, brain
- cheek(s) (and other part(s) of neck, scalp, or face, except eye) 920
- chest (wall) 922.1
- chin (and other part(s) of neck, scalp, or face, except eye) 920
- clitoris 922.4
- conjunctiva 921.1
- conus medullaris (spine) 952.4
- cornea 921.3
- corpus cavernosum 922.4
- cortex (brain) (cerebral) — *see* Contusion, brain, cortex
- costal region 922.1
- ear (and other part(s) of neck, scalp, or face except eye) 920
- elbow 923.11
  - with forearm 923.10
- epididymis 922.4
- epigastric region 922.2
- eye NEC 921.9
- eyeball 921.3
- eyelid(s) (and periocular area) 921.1
- face (and neck, or scalp, any part except eye) 920
- femoral triangle 922.2
- fetus or newborn 772.6
- finger(s) (nail) (subungual) 923.3
- flank 922.2
- foot (with ankle) (excluding toe(s)) 924.20
- forearm (and elbow) 923.10
- forehead (and other part(s) of neck, scalp, or face, except eye) 920
- genital organs, external 922.4
- globe (eye) 921.3
- groin 922.2
- gum(s) (and other part(s) of neck, scalp, or face, except eye) 920
- hand(s) (except fingers alone) 923.20
- head (any part, except eye) (and face) (and neck) 920
- heart — *see* Contusion, cardiac
- heel 924.20
- hip 924.01
  - with thigh 924.00
- iliac region 922.2
- inguinal region 922.2
- internal organs (abdomen, chest, or pelvis) NEC — *see* Injury, internal, by site
- interscapular region 922.33
- iris (eye) 921.3
- kidney 866.01
  - with open wound into cavity 866.11
- knee 924.11
  - with lower leg 924.10
- labium (majus) (minus) 922.4
- lacrimal apparatus, gland, or sac 921.1
- larynx (and other part(s) of neck, scalp, or face, except eye) 920
- late effect — *see* Late, effects (of), contusion
- leg 924.5
  - lower (with knee) 924.10
- lens 921.3
- lingual (and other part(s) of neck, scalp, or face, except eye) 920
- lip(s) (and other part(s) of neck, scalp, or face, except eye) 920
- liver 864.01
  - with
    - laceration — *see* Laceration, liver
    - open wound into cavity 864.11
- lower extremity 924.5
  - multiple sites 924.4
- lumbar region 922.31

Index to Diseases

Contusion — *continued*
　lung 861.21
　　with open wound into thorax 861.31
　malar region (and other part(s) of neck, scalp, or face, except eye) 920
　mandibular joint (and other part(s) of neck, scalp, or face, except eye) 920
　mastoid region (and other part(s) of neck, scalp. or face, except eye) 920
　membrane, brain — *see* Contusion, brain
　midthoracic region 922.1
　mouth (and other part(s) of neck, scalp, or face, except eye) 920
　multiple sites (not classifiable to same three-digit category) 924.8
　　lower limb 924.4
　　trunk 922.8
　　upper limb 923.8
　muscle NEC 924.9
　myocardium — *see* Contusion, cardiac
　nasal (septum) (and other part(s) of neck, scalp, or face, except eye) 920
　neck (and scalp, or face any part, except eye) 920
　nerve — *see* Injury, nerve, by site
　nose (and other part(s) of neck, scalp, or face, except eye) 920
　occipital region (scalp) (and neck or face, except eye) 920
　　lobe — *see* Contusion, brain, occipital lobe
　orbit (region) (tissues) 921.2
　palate (soft) (and other part(s) of neck, scalp, or face, except eye) 920
　parietal region (scalp) (and neck, or face, except eye) 920
　　lobe — *see* Contusion, brain
　penis 922.4
　pericardium — *see* Contusion, cardiac
　perineum 922.4
　periocular area 921.1
　pharynx (and other part(s) of neck, scalp, or face, except eye) 920
　popliteal space (*see also* Contusion, knee) 924.11
　prepuce 922.4
　pubic region 922.4
　pudenda 922.4
　pulmonary — *see* Contusion, lung
　quadriceps femoralis 924.00
　rib cage 922.1
　sacral region 922.32
　salivary ducts or glands (and other part(s) of neck, scalp, or face, except eye) 920
　scalp (and neck, or face any part, except eye) 920
　scapular region 923.01
　　with shoulder or upper arm 923.09
　sclera (eye) 921.3
　scrotum 922.4
　shoulder 923.00
　　with upper arm or axillar regions 923.09
　skin NEC 924.9
　skull 920
　spermatic cord 922.4
　spinal cord — *see also* Injury, spinal, by site
　　cauda equina 952.4
　　conus medullaris 952.4
　spleen 865.01
　　with open wound into cavity 865.11
　sternal region 922.1
　stomach — *see* Injury, internal, stomach
　subconjunctival 921.1
　subcutaneous NEC 924.9
　submaxillary region (and other part(s) of neck, scalp, or face, except eye) 920
　submental region (and other part(s) of neck, scalp, or face, except eye) 920
　subperiosteal NEC 924.9
　supraclavicular fossa (and other part(s) of neck, scalp, or face, except eye) 920
　supraorbital (and other part(s) of neck, scalp, or face, except eye) 920
　temple (region) (and other part(s) of neck, scalp, or face, except eye) 920
　testis 922.4
　thigh (and hip) 924.00

Contusion — *continued*
　thorax 922.1
　　organ — *see* Injury, internal, intrathoracic
　throat (and other part(s) of neck, scalp, or face, except eye) 920
　thumb(s) (nail) (subungual) 923.3
　toe(s) (nail) (subungual) 924.3
　tongue (and other part(s) of neck, scalp, or face, except eye) 920
　trunk 922.9
　　multiple sites 922.8
　　specified site — *see* Contusion, by site
　tunica vaginalis 922.4
　tympanum (membrane) (and other part(s) of neck, scalp, or face, except eye) 920
　upper extremity 923.9
　　multiple sites 923.8
　uvula (and other part(s) of neck, scalp, or face, except eye) 920
　vagina 922.4
　vocal cord(s) (and other part(s) of neck, scalp, or face, except eye) 920
　vulva 922.4
　wrist 923.21
　　with hand(s), except finger(s) alone 923.20
Conus (any type) (congenital) 743.57
　acquired 371.60
　medullaris syndrome 336.8
Convalescence (following) V66.9
　chemotherapy V66.2
　medical NEC V66.5
　psychotherapy V66.3
　radiotherapy V66.1
　surgery NEC V66.0
　treatment (for) NEC V66.5
　　combined V66.6
　　fracture V66.4
　　mental disorder NEC V66.3
　　specified disorder NEC V66.5
Conversion
　hysteria, hysterical, any type 300.11
　laparoscopic surgical procedure to open procedure V64.4
　neurosis, any 300.11
　reaction, any 300.11
Converter, tuberculosis (test reaction) 795.5
Convulsions (idiopathic) 780.39
　apoplectiform (*see also* Disease, cerebrovascular, acute) 436
　brain 780.39
　cerebral 780.39
　cerebrospinal 780.39
　due to trauma NEC — *see* Injury, intracranial
　eclamptic (*see also* Eclampsia) 780.39
　epileptic (*see also* Epilepsy) 345.9 ✓5ᵗʰ
　epileptiform (*see also* Seizure, epileptiform) 780.39
　epileptoid (*see also* Seizure, epileptiform) 780.39
　ether
　　anesthetic
　　　correct substance properly administered 780.39
　　　overdose or wrong substance given 968.2
　　other specified type — *see* Table of Drugs and Chemicals
　febrile 780.31
　generalized 780.39
　hysterical 300.11
　infantile 780.39
　　epilepsy — *see* Epilepsy
　internal 780.39
　jacksonian (*see also* Epilepsy) 345.5 ✓5ᵗʰ
　myoclonic 333.2
　newborn 779.0
　paretic 094.1
　pregnancy (nephritic) (uremic) — *see* Eclampsia, pregnancy
　psychomotor (*see also* Epilepsy) 345.4 ✓5ᵗʰ
　puerperal, postpartum — *see* Eclampsia, pregnancy
　recurrent 780.39
　　epileptic — *see* Epilepsy
　reflex 781.0
　repetitive 780.39
　　epileptic — *see* Epilepsy

Convulsions — *continued*
　salaam (*see also* Epilepsy) 345.6 ✓5ᵗʰ
　scarlatinal 034.1
　spasmodic 780.39
　tetanus, tetanic (*see also* Tetanus) 037
　thymic 254.8
　uncinate 780.39
　uremic 586
Convulsive — *see also* Convulsions
　disorder or state 780.39
　　epileptic — *see* Epilepsy
　equivalent, abdominal (*see also* Epilepsy) 345.5 ✓5ᵗʰ
Cooke-Apert-Gallais syndrome (adrenogenital) 255.2
Cooley's anemia (erythroblastic) 282.4
Coolie itch 126.9
Cooper's
　disease 610.1
　hernia — *see* Hernia, Cooper's
Coordination disturbance 781.3
Copper wire arteries, retina 362.13
Copra itch 133.8
Coprolith 560.39
Coprophilia 302.89
Coproporphyria, hereditary 277.1
Coprostasis 560.39
　with hernia — *see also* Hernia, by site, with obstruction
　　gangrenous — *see* Hernia, by site, with gangrene
Cor
　biloculare 745.7
　bovinum — *see* Hypertrophy, cardiac
　bovis — *see* Hypertrophy, cardiac
　pulmonale (chronic) 416.9
　　acute 415.0
　triatriatum, triatrium 746.82
　triloculare 745.8
　　biatriatum 745.3
　　biventriculare 745.69
Corbus' disease 607.1
Cord — *see also* condition
　around neck (tightly) (with compression)
　　affecting fetus or newborn 762.5
　　complicating delivery 663.1 ✓5ᵗʰ
　　　without compression 663.3 ✓5ᵗʰ
　　　　affecting fetus or newborn 762.6
　bladder NEC 344.61
　　tabetic 094.0
　prolapse
　　affecting fetus or newborn 762.4
　　complicating delivery 663.0 ✓5ᵗʰ
Cord's angiopathy (*see also* Tuberculosis) 017.3 ✓5ᵗʰ *[362.18]*
Cordis ectopia 746.87
Corditis (spermatic) 608.4
Corectopia 743.46
Cori type glycogen storage disease — *see* Disease, glycogen storage
Cork-handlers' disease or lung 495.3
Corkscrew esophagus 530.5
Corlett's pyosis (impetigo) 684
Corn (infected) 700
Cornea — *see also* condition
　donor V59.5
　guttata (dystrophy) 371.57
　plana 743.41
Cornelia de Lange's syndrome (Amsterdam dwarf, mental retardation, and brachycephaly) 759.89
Cornual gestation or pregnancy — *see* Pregnancy, cornual
Cornu cutaneum 702.8
Coronary (artery) — *see also* condition
　arising from aorta or pulmonary trunk 746.85
Corpora — *see also* condition
　amylacea (prostate) 602.8
　cavernosa — *see* condition
Corpulence (*see also* Obesity) 278.0 ✓5ᵗʰ
Corpus — *see* condition

Corrigan's disease — see Insufficiency, aortic
Corrosive burn — see Burn, by site
Corsican fever (see also Malaria) 084.6
Cortical — see also condition
  blindness 377.75
  necrosis, kidney (bilateral) 583.6
Corticoadrenal — see condition
Corticosexual syndrome 255.2
Coryza (acute) 460
  with grippe or influenza 487.1
  syphilitic 095.8
    congenital (chronic) 090.0
Costen's syndrome or complex 524.60
Costiveness (see also Constipation) 564.00
Costochondritis 733.6
Cotard's syndrome (paranoia) 297.1
Cot death 798.0
Cotungo's disease 724.3
Cough 786.2
  with hemorrhage (see also Hemoptysis) 786.3
  affected 786.2
  bronchial 786.2
    with grippe or influenza 487.1
  chronic 786.2
  epidemic 786.2
  functional 306.1
  hemorrhagic 786.3
  hysterical 300.11
  laryngeal, spasmodic 786.2
  nervous 786.2
  psychogenic 306.1
  smokers' 491.0
  tea tasters' 112.89
Counseling NEC V65.40
  without complaint or sickness V65.49
  abuse victim NEC V62.89
    child V61.21
    partner V61.11
    spouse V61.11
  child abuse, maltreatment, or neglect V61.21
  contraceptive NEC V25.09
    device (intrauterine) V25.02
    maintenance V25.40
      intrauterine contraceptive device V25.42
      oral contraceptive (pill) V25.41
      specified type NEC V25.49
      subdermal implantable V25.43
    management NEC V25.9
    oral contraceptive (pill) V25.01
    prescription NEC V25.02
      oral contraceptive (pill) V25.01
        repeat prescription V25.41
      repeat prescription V25.40
    subdermal implantable V25.43
    surveillance NEC V25.40
  dietary V65.3
  excercise V65.41
  explanation of
    investigation finding NEC V65.49
    medication NEC V65.49
  family planning V25.09
  for nonattending third party V65.1
  genetic V26.3
  gonorrhea V65.45
  health (advice) (education) (instruction) NEC V65.49
  HIV V65.44
  human immunodeficiency virus V65.44
  injury prevention V65.43
  marital V61.10
  medical (for) V65.9
    boarding school resident V60.6
    condition not demonstrated V65.5
    feared complaint and no disease found V65.5
    institutional resident V60.6
    on behalf of another V65.1
    person living alone V60.3
  parent-child conflict V61.20
    specified problem NEC V61.29
  partner abuse
    perpetrator V61.12
    victim V61.11

Counseling NEC — continued
  perpetrator of
    child abuse V62.83
      parental V61.22
    partner abuse V61.12
    spouse abuse V61.12
  procreative V65.49
  sex NEC V65.49
    transmitted disease NEC V65.45
      HIV V65.44
  specified reason NEC V65.49
  spousal abuse
    perpetrator V61.12
    victim V61.11
  substance use and abuse V65.42
  syphilis V65.45
  victim (of)
    abuse NEC V62.89
    child abuse V61.21
    partner abuse V61.11
    spousal abuse V61.11
Coupled rhythm 427.89
Couvelaire uterus (complicating delivery) — see Placenta, separation
Cowper's gland — see condition
Cowperitis (see also Urethritis) 597.89
  gonorrheal (acute) 098.0
    chronic or duration of 2 months or over 098.2
Cowpox (abortive) 051.0
  due to vaccination 999.0
  eyelid 051.0 [373.5]
    postvaccination 999.0 [373.5]
Coxa
  plana 732.1
  valga (acquired) 736.31
    congenital 755.61
    late effect of rickets 268.1
  vara (acquired) 736.32
    congenital 755.62
    late effect of rickets 268.1
Coxae malum senilis 715.25
Coxalgia (nontuberculous) 719.45
  tuberculous (see also Tuberculosis) 015.1 ✓5ᵗʰ [730.85]
Coxalgic pelvis 736.30
Coxitis 716.65
Coxsackie (infection) (virus) 079.2
  central nervous system NEC 048
  endocarditis 074.22
  enteritis 008.67
  meningitis (aseptic) 047.0
  myocarditis 074.23
  pericarditis 074.21
  pharyngitis 074.0
  pleurodynia 074.1
  specific disease NEC 074.8
Crabs, meaning pubic lice 132.2
Crack baby 760.75
Cracked nipple 611.2
  puerperal, postpartum 676.1 ✓5ᵗʰ
Cradle cap 690.11
Craft neurosis 300.89
Craigiasis 007.8
Cramp(s) 729.82
  abdominal 789.0 ✓5ᵗʰ
  bathing 994.1
  colic 789.0 ✓5ᵗʰ
    psychogenic 306.4
  due to immersion 994.1
  extremity (lower) (upper) NEC 729.82
  fireman 992.2
  heat 992.2
  hysterical 300.11
  immersion 994.1
  intestinal 789.0 ✓5ᵗʰ
    psychogenic 306.4
  linotypist's 300.89
    organic 333.84
  muscle (extremity) (general) 729.82
    due to immersion 994.1
    hysterical 300.11
  occupational (hand) 300.89
    organic 333.84

Cramp(s) — continued
  psychogenic 307.89
  salt depletion 276.1
  stoker 992.2
  stomach 789.0 ✓5ᵗʰ
  telegraphers' 300.89
    organic 333.84
  typists' 300.89
    organic 333.84
  uterus 625.8
    menstrual 625.3
  writers' 333.84
    organic 333.84
    psychogenic 300.89
Cranial — see condition
Cranioclasis, fetal 763.89
Craniocleidodysostosis 755.59
Craniofenestria (skull) 756.0
Craniolacunia (skull) 756.0
Craniopagus 759.4
Craniopathy, metabolic 733.3
Craniopharyngeal — see condition
Craniopharyngioma (M9350/1) 237.0
Craniorachischisis (totalis) 740.1
Cranioschisis 756.0
Craniostenosis 756.0
Craniosynostosis 756.0
Craniotabes (cause unknown) 733.3
  rachitic 268.1
  syphilitic 090.5
Craniotomy, fetal 763.89
Cranium — see condition
Craw-craw 125.3
Creaking joint 719.60
  ankle 719.67
  elbow 719.62
  foot 719.67
  hand 719.64
  hip 719.65
  knee 719.66
  multiple sites 719.69
  pelvic region 719.65
  shoulder (region) 719.61
  specified site NEC 719.68
  wrist 719.63
Creeping
  eruption 126.9
  palsy 335.21
  paralysis 335.21
Crenated tongue 529.8
Creotoxism 005.9
Crepitus
  caput 756.0
  joint 719.60
    ankle 719.67
    elbow 719.62
    foot 719.67
    hand 719.64
    hip 719.65
    knee 719.66
    multiple sites 719.69
    pelvic region 719.65
    shoulder (region) 719.61
    specified site NEC 719.68
    wrist 719.63
Crescent or conus choroid, congenital 743.57
Cretin, cretinism (athyrotic) (congenital) (endemic) (metabolic) (nongoitrous) (sporadic) 243
  goitrous (sporadic) 246.1
  pelvis (dwarf type) (male type) 243
    with disproportion (fetopelvic) 653.1 ✓5ᵗʰ
      affecting fetus or newborn 763.1
      causing obstructed labor 660.1 ✓5ᵗʰ
        affecting fetus or newborn 763.1
  pituitary 253.3
Cretinoid degeneration 243
Creutzfeldt-Jakob disease (syndrome) 046.1
  with dementia
    with behavioral disturbance 046.1 [294.11]
    without behavioral disturbance 046.1 [294.10]

Index to Diseases

Crib death 798.0
Cribriform hymen 752.49
Cri-du-chat syndrome 758.3
Crigler-Najjar disease or syndrome (congenital hyperbilirubinemia) 277.4
Crimean hemorrhagic fever 065.0
Criminalism 301.7
Crisis
 abdomen 789.0 ✓5ᵗʰ
 addisonian (acute adrenocortical insufficiency) 255.4
 adrenal (cortical) 255.4
 asthmatic — see Asthma
 brain, cerebral (see also Disease, cerebrovascular, acute) 436
 celiac 579.0
 Dietl's 593.4
 emotional NEC 309.29
  acute reaction to stress 308.0
  adjustment reaction 309.9
  specific to childhood and adolescence 313.9
 gastric (tabetic) 094.0
 glaucomatocyclitic 364.22
 heart (see also Failure, heart) 428.9
 hypertensive — see Hypertension
 nitritoid
  correct substance properly administered 458.2
  overdose or wrong substance given or taken 961.1
 oculogyric 378.87
  psychogenic 306.7
 Pel's 094.0
 psychosexual identity 302.6
 rectum 094.0
 renal 593.81
 sickle cell 282.62
 stomach (tabetic) 094.0
 tabetic 094.0
 thyroid (see also Thyrotoxicosis) 242.9 ✓5ᵗʰ
 thyrotoxic (see also Thyrotoxicosis) 242.9 ✓5ᵗʰ
 vascular — see Disease, cerebrovascular, acute
Crocq's disease (acrocyanosis) 443.89
Crohn's disease (see also Enteritis, regional) 555.9
Cronkhite-Canada syndrome 211.3
Crooked septum, nasal 470
Cross
 birth (of fetus) complicating delivery 652.3 ✓5ᵗʰ
  with successful version 652.1 ✓5ᵗʰ
  causing obstructed labor 660.0 ✓5ᵗʰ
 bite, anterior or posterior 524.2
 eye (see also Esotropia) 378.00
Crossed ectopia of kidney 753.3
Crossfoot 754.50
Croup, croupous (acute) (angina) (catarrhal) (infective) (inflammatory) (laryngeal) (membranous) (nondiphtheritic) (pseudomembranous) 464.4
 asthmatic (see also Asthma) 493.9 ✓5ᵗʰ
 bronchial 466.0
 diphtheritic (membranous) 032.3
 false 478.75
 spasmodic 478.75
  diphtheritic 032.3
 stridulous 478.75
  diphtheritic 032.3
Crouzon's disease (craniofacial dysostosis) 756.0
Crowding, teeth 524.3
CRST syndrome (cutaneous systemic sclerosis) 710.1
Cruchet's disease (encephalitis lethargica) 049.8
Cruelty in children (see also Disturbance, conduct) 312.9
Crural ulcer (see also Ulcer, lower extremity) 707.10
Crush, crushed, crushing (injury) 929.9
 with
  fracture — see Fracture, by site
 abdomen 926.19
  internal — see Injury, internal, abdomen
 ankle 928.21
  with other parts of foot 928.20

Crush, crushed, crushing — continued
 arm 927.9
  lower (and elbow) 927.10
  upper 927.03
   with shoulder or axillary region 927.09
 axilla 927.02
  with shoulder or upper arm 927.09
 back 926.11
 breast 926.19
 buttock 926.12
 cheek 925.1
 chest — see Injury, internal, chest
 ear 925.1
 elbow 927.11
  with forearm 927.10
 face 925.1
 finger(s) 927.3
  with hand(s) 927.20
   and wrist(s) 927.21
 flank 926.19
 foot, excluding toe(s) alone (with ankle) 928.20
 forearm (and elbow) 927.10
 genitalia, external (female) (male) 926.0
  internal — see Injury, internal, genital organ NEC
 hand, except finger(s) alone (and wrist) 927.20
 head — see Fracture, skull, by site
 heel 928.20
 hip 928.01
  with thigh 928.00
 internal organ (abdomen, chest, or pelvis) — see Injury, internal, by site
 knee 928.11
  with leg, lower 928.10
 labium (majus) (minus) 926.0
 larynx 925.2
 late effect — see Late, effects (of), crushing
 leg 928.9
  lower 928.10
   and knee 928.11
  upper 928.00
 limb
  lower 928.9
   multiple sites 928.8
  upper 927.9
   multiple sites 927.8
 multiple sites NEC 929.0
 neck 925.2
 nerve — see Injury, nerve, by site
 nose 802.0
  open 802.1
 penis 926.0
 pharynx 925.2
 scalp 925.1
 scapular region 927.01
  with shoulder or upper arm 927.09
 scrotum 926.0
 shoulder 927.00
  with upper arm or axillary region 927.09
 skull or cranium — see Fracture, skull, by site
 spinal cord — see Injury, spinal, by site
 syndrome (complication of trauma) 958.5
 testis 926.0
 thigh (with hip) 928.00
 throat 925.2
 thumb(s) (and fingers) 927.3
 toe(s) 928.3
  with foot 928.20
   and ankle 928.21
 tonsil 925.2
 trunk 926.9
  chest — see Injury, internal, intrathoracic organs NEC
  internal organ — see Injury, internal, by site
  multiple sites 926.8
  specified site NEC 926.19
 vulva 926.0
 wrist 927.21
  with hand(s), except fingers alone 927.20
Crusta lactea 690.11
Crusts 782.8
Crutch paralysis 953.4
Cruveilhier's disease 335.21
Cruveilhier-Baumgarten cirrhosis, disease, or syndrome 571.5

Cruz-Chagas disease (see also Trypanosomiasis) 086.2
Cryoglobulinemia (mixed) 273.2
Crypt (anal) (rectal) 569.49
Cryptitis (anal) (rectal) 569.49
Cryptococcosis (European) (pulmonary) (systemic) 117.5
Cryptococcus 117.5
 epidermicus 117.5
 neoformans, infection by 117.5
Cryptopapillitis (anus) 569.49
Cryptophthalmos (eyelid) 743.06
Cryptorchid, cryptorchism, cryptorchidism 752.51
Cryptosporidiosis 007.4
Cryptotia 744.29
Crystallopathy
 calcium pyrophosphate (see also Arthritis) 275.49 [712.2]
 dicalcium phosphate (see also Arthritis) 275.49 [712.1]
 gouty 274.0
 pyrophosphate NEC (see also Arthritis) 275.49 [712.2]
 uric acid 274.0
Crystalluria 791.9
Csillag's disease (lichen sclerosus or atrophicus) 701.0
Cuban itch 050.1
Cubitus
 valgus (acquired) 736.01
  congenital 755.59
  late effect of rickets 268.1
 varus (acquired) 736.02
  congenital 755.59
  late effect of rickets 268.1
Cultural deprivation V62.4
Cupping of optic disc 377.14
Curling's ulcer — see Ulcer, duodenum
Curling esophagus 530.5
Curschmann (-Batten) (-Steinert) disease or syndrome 359.2
Curvature
 organ or site, congenital NEC — see Distortion
 penis (lateral) 752.69
 Pott's (spinal) (see also Tuberculosis) 015.0 ✓5ᵗʰ [737.43]
 radius, idiopathic, progressive (congenital) 755.54
 spine (acquired) (angular) (idiopathic) (incorrect) (postural) 737.9
  congenital 754.2
  due to or associated with
   Charcôt-Marie-Tooth disease 356.1 [737.40]
   mucopolysaccharidosis 277.5 [737.40]
   neurofibromatosis 237.71 [737.40]
   osteitis
    deformans 731.0 [737.40]
    fibrosa cystica 252.0 [737.40]
   osteoporosis (see also Osteoporosis) 733.00 [737.40]
   poliomyelitis (see also Poliomyelitis) 138 [737.40]
   tuberculosis (Pott's curvature) (see also Tuberculosis) 015.0 ✓5ᵗʰ [737.43]
  kyphoscoliotic (see also Kyphoscoliosis) 737.30
  kyphotic (see also Kyphosis) 737.10
  late effect of rickets 268.1 [737.40]
  Pott's 015.0 ✓5ᵗʰ [737.40]
  scoliotic (see also Scoliosis) 737.30
  specified NEC 737.8
  tuberculous 015.0 ✓5ᵗʰ [737.40]
Cushing's
 basophilism, disease, or syndrome (iatrogenic) (idiopathic) (pituitary basophilism) (pituitary dependent) 255.0
 ulcer — see Ulcer, peptic
Cushingoid due to steroid therapy
 correct substance properly administered 255.0
 overdose or wrong substance given or taken 962.0

Cut

Cut (external) — see Wound, open, by site
Cutaneous — see also condition
    hemorrahage 782.7
    horn (cheek) (eyelid) (mouth) 702.8
    larva migrans 126.9
Cutis — see also condition
    hyperelastic 756.83
        acquired 701.8
    laxa 756.83
        senilis 701.8
    marmorata 782.61
    osteosis 709.3
    pendula 756.83
        acquired 701.8
    rhomboidalis nuchae 701.8
    verticis gyrata 757.39
        acquired 701.8
Cyanopathy, newborn 770.83 ▲
Cyanosis 782.5
    autotoxic 289.7
    common atrioventricular canal 745.69
    congenital 770.83 ▲
    conjunctiva 372.71
    due to
        endocardial cushion defect 745.60
        nonclosure, foramen botalli 745.5
        patent foramen botalli 745.5
        persistent foramen ovale 745.5
    enterogenous 289.7
    fetus or newborn 770.83 ▲
    ostium primum defect 745.61
    paroxysmal digital 443.0
    retina, retinal 362.10
Cycle
    anovulatory 628.0
    menstrual, irregular 626.4
Cyclencephaly 759.89
Cyclical vomiting 536.2
    psychogenic 306.4
Cyclitic membrane 364.74
Cyclitis (see also Iridocyclitis) 364.3
    acute 364.00
        primary 364.01
        recurrent 364.02
    chronic 364.10
        in
            sarcoidosis 135 [364.11]
            tuberculosis (see also Tuberculosis)
                017.3 ✓5ᵗʰ [364.11]
    Fuchs' heterochromic 364.21
    granulomatous 364.10
    lens induced 364.23
    nongranulomatous 364.00
    posterior 363.21
    primary 364.01
    recurrent 364.02
    secondary (noninfectious) 364.04
        infectious 364.03
    subacute 364.00
        primary 364.01
        recurrent 364.02
Cyclokeratitis — see Keratitis
Cyclophoria 378.44
Cyclopia, cyclops 759.89
Cycloplegia 367.51
Cyclospasm 367.53
Cyclosporiasis 007.5
Cyclothymia 301.13
Cyclothymic personality 301.13
Cyclotropia 378.33
Cyesis — see Pregnancy
Cylindroma (M8200/3) — see also Neoplasm, by site, malignant
    eccrine dermal (M8200/0) — see Neoplasm, skin, benign
    skin (M8200/0) — see Neoplasm, skin, benign
Cylindruria 791.7
Cyllosoma 759.89
Cynanche
    diphtheritic 032.3
    tonsillaris 475
Cynorexia 783.6
Cyphosis — see Kyphosis

Cyprus fever (see also Brucellosis) 023.9
Cyriax's syndrome (slipping rib) 733.99
Cyst (mucus) (retention) (serous) (simple)

> Note — In general, cysts are not neoplastic and are classified to the approriate category for disease of the specified anatomical site. This generalization does not apply to certain types of cysts which are neoplastic in nature, for example, dermoid, nor does it apply to cysts of certain structures, for example, branchial cleft, which are classified as developmental anomalies.
>
> The following listing includes some of the most frequently reported sites of cysts as well as qualifiers which indicate the type of cyst. The latter qualifiers usually are not repeated under the anatomical sites. Since the code assignment for a given site may vary depending upon the type of cyst, the coder should refer to the listings under the specified type of cyst before consideration is given to the site.

    accessory, fallopian tube 752.11
    adenoid (infected) 474.8
    adrenal gland 255.8
        congenital 759.1
    air, lung 518.89
    allantoic 753.7
    alveolar process (jaw bone) 526.2
    amnion, amniotic 658.8 ✓5ᵗʰ
    anterior chamber (eye) 364.60
        exudative 364.62
        implantation (surgical) (traumatic) 364.61
        parasitic 360.13
    anterior nasopalatine 526.1
    antrum 478.1
    anus 569.49
    apical (periodontal) (tooth) 522.8
    appendix 543.9
    arachnoid, brain 348.0
    arytenoid 478.79
    auricle 706.2
    Baker's (knee) 727.51
        tuberculous (see also Tuberculosis)
            015.2 ✓5ᵗʰ
    Bartholin's gland or duct 616.2
    bile duct (see also Disease, biliary) 576.8
    bladder (multiple) (trigone) 596.8
    Blessig's 362.62
    blood, endocardial (see also Endocarditis) 424.90
    blue dome 610.0
    bone (local) 733.20
        aneurysmal 733.22
        jaw 526.2
            developmental (odontogenic) 526.0
            fissural 526.1
            latent 526.89
        solitary 733.21
        unicameral 733.21
    brain 348.0
        congenital 742.4
        hydatid (see also Echinococcus) 122.9
        third ventricle (colloid) 742.4
    branchial (cleft) 744.42
    branchiogenic 744.42
    breast (benign) (blue dome) (pedunculated) (solitary) (traumatic) 610.0
        involution 610.4
        sebaceous 610.8
    broad ligament (benign) 620.8
        embryonic 752.11
    bronchogenic (mediastinal) (sequestration) 518.89
        congenital 748.4
    buccal 528.4
    bulbourethral gland (Cowper's) 599.89
    bursa, bursal 727.49
        pharyngeal 478.26
    calcifying odontogenic (M9301/0) 213.1
        upper jaw (bone) 213.0
    canal of Nuck (acquired) (serous) 629.1
        congenital 752.41
    canthus 372.75

Cyst — continued
    carcinomatous (M8010/3) — see Neoplasm, by site, malignant
    cartilage (joint) — see Derangement, joint
    cauda equina 336.8
    cavum septi pellucidi NEC 348.0
    celomic (pericardium) 746.89
    cerebellopontine (angle) — see Cyst, brain
    cerebellum — see Cyst, brain
    cerebral — see Cyst, brain
    cervical lateral 744.42
    cervix 622.8
        embryonal 752.41
        nabothian (gland) 616.0
    chamber, anterior (eye) 364.60
        exudative 364.62
        implantation (surgical) (traumatic) 364.61
        parasitic 360.13
    chiasmal, optic NEC (see also Lesion, chiasmal) 377.54
    chocolate (ovary) 617.1
    choledochal (congenital) 751.69
        acquired 576.8
    choledochus 751.69
    chorion 658.8 ✓5ᵗʰ
    choroid plexus 348.0
    chyle, mesentery 457.8
    ciliary body 364.60
        exudative 364.64
        implantation 364.61
        primary 364.63
    clitoris 624.8
    coccyx (see also Cyst, bone) 733.20
    colloid
        third ventricle (brain) 742.4
        thyroid gland — see Goiter
    colon 569.89
    common (bile) duct (see also Disease, biliary) 576.8
    congenital NEC 759.89
        adrenal glands 759.1
        epiglottis 748.3
        esophagus 750.4
        fallopian tube 752.11
        kidney 753.10
            multiple 753.19
            single 753.11
        larynx 748.3
        liver 751.62
        lung 748.4
        mediastinum 748.8
        ovary 752.0
        oviduct 752.11
        pancreas 751.7
        periurethral (tissue) 753.8
        prepuce NEC 752.69
            penis 752.69
        sublingual 750.26
        submaxillary gland 750.26
        thymus (gland) 759.2
        tongue 750.19
        ureterovesical orifice 753.4
        vulva 752.41
    conjunctiva 372.75
    cornea 371.23
    corpora quadrigemina 348.0
    corpus
        albicans (ovary) 620.2
        luteum (ruptured) 620.1
    Cowper's gland (benign) (infected) 599.89
    cranial meninges 348.0
    craniobuccal pouch 253.8
    craniopharyngeal pouch 253.8
    cystic duct (see also Disease, gallbladder) 575.8
    Cysticercus (any site) 123.1
    Dandy-Walker 742.3
        with spina bifida (see also Spina bifida) 741.0 ✓5ᵗʰ
    dental 522.8
        developmental 526.0
        eruption 526.0
        lateral periodontal 526.0
        primordial (keratocyst) 526.0
        root 522.8
    dentigerous 526.0
        mandible 526.0
        maxilla 526.0

Index to Diseases

Cyst — *continued*
- dermoid (M9084/0) — *see also* Neoplasm, by site, benign
  - with malignant transformation (M9084/3) 183.0
  - implantation
    - external area or site (skin) NEC 709.8
    - iris 364.61
    - skin 709.8
    - vagina 623.8
    - vulva 624.8
  - mouth 528.4
  - oral soft tissue 528.4
  - sacrococcygeal 685.1
    - with abscess 685.0
- developmental of ovary, ovarian 752.0
- dura (cerebral) 348.0
  - spinal 349.2
- ear (external) 706.2
- echinococcal (*see also* Echinococcus) 122.9
- embryonal
  - cervix uteri 752.41
  - genitalia, female external 752.41
  - uterus 752.3
  - vagina 752.41
- endometrial 621.8
  - ectopic 617.9
- endometrium (uterus) 621.8
  - ectopic — *see* Endometriosis
- enteric 751.5
- enterogenous 751.5
- epidermal (inclusion) (*see also* Cyst, skin) 706.2
- epidermoid (inclusion) (*see also* Cyst, skin) 706.2
  - mouth 528.4
  - not of skin — *see* Cyst, by site
  - oral soft tissue 528.4
- epididymis 608.89
- epiglottis 478.79
- epiphysis cerebri 259.8
- epithelial (inclusion) (*see also* Cyst, skin) 706.2
- epoophoron 752.11
- eruption 526.0
- esophagus 530.89
- ethmoid sinus 478.1
- eye (retention) 379.8
  - congenital 743.03
  - posterior segment, congenital 743.54
- eyebrow 706.2
- eyelid (sebaceous) 374.84
  - infected 373.13
  - sweat glands or ducts 374.84
- falciform ligament (inflammatory) 573.8
- fallopian tube 620.8
- female genital organs NEC 629.8
- fimbrial (congenital) 752.11
- fissural (oral region) 526.1
- follicle (atretic) (graafian) (ovarian) 620.0
  - nabothian (gland) 616.0
- follicular (atretic) (ovarian) 620.0
  - dentigerous 526.0
- frontal sinus 478.1
- gallbladder or duct 575.8
- ganglion 727.43
- Gartner's duct 752.11
- gas, of mesentery 568.89
- gingiva 523.8
- gland of moll 374.84
- globulomaxillary 526.1
- graafian follicle 620.0
- granulosal lutein 620.2
- hemangiomatous (M9121/0) (*see also* Hemangioma) 228.00
- hydatid (*see also* Echinococcus) 122.9
  - fallopian tube (Morgagni) 752.11
  - liver NEC 122.8
  - lung NEC 122.9
  - Morgagni 752.8
    - fallopian tube 752.11
  - specified site NEC 122.9
- hymen 623.8
  - embryonal 752.41
- hypopharynx 478.26
- hypophysis, hypophyseal (duct) (recurrent) 253.8
  - cerebri 253.8

Cyst — *continued*
- implantation (dermoid)
  - anterior chamber (eye) 364.61
  - external area or site (skin) NEC 709.8
  - iris 364.61
  - vagina 623.8
  - vulva 624.8
- incisor, incisive canal 526.1
- inclusion (epidermal) (epithelial) (epidermoid) (mucous) (squamous) (*see also* Cyst, skin) 706.2
  - not of skin — *see* Neoplasm, by site, benign
- intestine (large) (small) 569.89
- intracranial — *see* Cyst, brain
- intraligamentous 728.89
  - knee 717.89
- intrasellar 253.8
- iris (idiopathic) 364.60
  - exudative 364.62
  - implantation (surgical) (traumatic) 364.61
  - miotic pupillary 364.55
  - parasitic 360.13
- Iwanoff's 362.62
- jaw (bone) (aneurysmal) (extravasation) (hemorrhagic) (traumatic) 526.2
  - developmental (odontogenic) 526.0
  - fissural 526.1
- keratin 706.2
- kidney (congenital) 753.10
  - acquired 593.2
  - calyceal (*see also* Hydronephrosis) 591
  - multiple 753.19
  - pyelogenic (*see also* Hydronephrosis) 591
  - simple 593.2
  - single 753.11
  - solitary (not congenital) 593.2
- labium (majus) (minus) 624.8
  - sebaceous 624.8
- lacrimal
  - apparatus 375.43
  - gland or sac 375.12
- larynx 478.79
- lens 379.39
  - congenital 743.39
- lip (gland) 528.5
- liver 573.8
  - congenital 751.62
  - hydatid (*see also* Echinococcus) 122.8
    - granulosis 122.0
    - multilocularis 122.5
- lung 518.89
  - congenital 748.4
  - giant bullous 492.0
- lutein 620.1
- lymphangiomatous (M9173/0) 228.1
- lymphoepithelial
  - mouth 528.4
  - oral soft tissue 528.4
- macula 362.54
- malignant (M8000/3) — *see* Neoplasm, by site, malignant
- mammary gland (sweat gland) (*see also* Cyst, breast) 610.0
- mandible 526.2
  - dentigerous 526.0
  - radicular 522.8
- maxilla 526.2
  - dentigerous 526.0
  - radicular 522.8
- median
  - anterior maxillary 526.1
  - palatal 526.1
- mediastinum (congenital) 748.8
- meibomian (gland) (retention) 373.2
  - infected 373.12
- membrane, brain 348.0
- meninges (cerebral) 348.0
  - spinal 349.2
- meniscus knee 717.5
- mesentery, mesenteric (gas) 568.89
  - chyle 457.8
  - gas 568.89
- mesonephric duct 752.8
- mesothelial
  - peritoneum 568.89
  - pleura (peritoneal) 569.89
- milk 611.5

Cyst — *continued*
- miotic pupillary (iris) 364.55
- Morgagni (hydatid) 752.8
  - fallopian tube 752.11
- mouth 528.4
- mullerian duct 752.8
- multilocular (ovary) (M8000/1) 239.5
- myometrium 621.8
- nabothian (follicle) (ruptured) 616.0
- nasal sinus 478.1
- nasoalveolar 528.4
- nasolabial 528.4
- nasopalatine (duct) 526.1
  - anterior 526.1
- nasopharynx 478.26
- neoplastic (M8000/1) — *see also* Neoplasm, by site, unspecified nature
  - benign (M8000/0) — *see* Neoplasm, by site, benign
  - uterus 621.8
- nervous system — *see* Cyst, brain
- neuroenteric 742.59
- neuroepithelial ventricle 348.0
- nipple 610.0
- nose 478.1
  - skin of 706.2
- odontogenic, developmental 526.0
- omentum (lesser) 568.89
  - congenital 751.8
- oral soft tissue (dermoid) (epidermoid) (lymphoepithelial) 528.4
- ora serrata 361.19
- orbit 376.81
- ovary, ovarian (twisted) 620.2
  - adherent 620.2
  - chocolate 617.1
  - corpus
    - albicans 620.2
    - luteum 620.1
  - dermoid (M9084/0) 220
  - developmental 752.0
  - due to failure of involution NEC 620.2
  - endometrial 617.1
  - follicular (atretic) (graafian) (hemorrhagic) 620.0
  - hemorrhagic 620.2
  - in pregnancy or childbirth 654.4
    - affecting fetus or newborn 763.89
    - causing obstructed labor 660.2
      - affecting fetus or newborn 763.1
  - multilocular (M8000/1) 239.5
  - pseudomucinous (M8470/0) 220
  - retention 620.2
  - serous 620.2
  - theca lutein 620.2
  - tuberculous (*see also* Tuberculosis) 016.6
  - unspecified 620.2
- oviduct 620.8
- palatal papilla (jaw) 526.1
- palate 526.1
  - fissural 526.1
  - median (fissural) 526.1
- palatine, of papilla 526.1
- pancreas, pancreatic 577.2
  - congenital 751.7
  - false 577.2
  - hemorrhagic 577.2
  - true 577.2
- paranephric 593.2
- para ovarian 752.11
- paraphysis, cerebri 742.4
- parasitic NEC 136.9
- parathyroid (gland) 252.8
- paratubal (fallopian) 620.8
- paraurethral duct 599.89
- paroophoron 752.11
- parotid gland 527.6
  - mucous extravasation or retention 527.6
- parovarian 752.11
- pars planus 364.60
  - exudative 364.64
  - primary 364.63

Cyst — continued
  pelvis, female
    in pregnancy or childbirth 654.4 ✓5
      affecting fetus or newborn 763.89
      causing obstructed labor 660.2 ✓5
        affecting fetus or newborn 763.1
  penis (sebaceous) 607.89
  periapical 522.8
  pericardial (congenital) 746.89
    acquired (secondary) 423.8
  pericoronal 526.0
  perineural (Tarlov's) 355.9
  periodontal 522.8
    lateral 526.0
  peripancreatic 577.2
  peripelvic (lymphatic) 593.2
  peritoneum 568.89
    chylous 457.8
  pharynx (wall) 478.26
  pilonidal (infected) (rectum) 685.1
    with abscess 685.0
    malignant (M9084/3) 173.5
  pituitary (duct) (gland) 253.8
  placenta (amniotic) — see Placenta, abnormal
  pleura 519.8
  popliteal 727.51
  porencephalic 742.4
    acquired 348.0
  postanal (infected) 685.1
    with abscess 685.0
  posterior segment of eye, congenital 743.54
  postmastoidectomy cavity 383.31
  preauricular 744.47
  prepuce 607.89
    congenital 752.69
  primordial (jaw) 526.0
  prostate 600.3
  pseudomucinous (ovary) (M8470/0) 220
  pudenda (sweat glands) 624.8
  pupillary, miotic 364.55
    sebaceous 624.8
  radicular (residual) 522.8
  radiculodental 522.8
  ranular 527.6
  Rathke's pouch 253.8
  rectum (epithelium) (mucous) 569.49
  renal — see Cyst, kidney
  residual (radicular) 522.8
  retention (ovary) 620.2
  retina 361.19
    macular 362.54
    parasitic 360.13
    primary 361.13
    secondary 361.14
  retroperitoneal 568.89
  sacrococcygeal (dermoid) 685.1
    with abscess 685.0
  salivary gland or duct 527.6
    mucous extravasation or retention 527.6
  Sampson's 617.1
  sclera 379.19
  scrotum (sebaceous) 706.2
    sweat glands 706.2
  sebaceous (duct) (gland) 706.2
    breast 610.8
    eyelid 374.84
    genital organ NEC
      female 629.8
      male 608.89
    scrotum 706.2
  semilunar cartilage (knee) (multiple) 717.5
  seminal vesicle 608.89
  serous (ovary) 620.2
  sinus (antral) (ethmoidal) (frontal) (maxillary) (nasal) (sphenoidal) 478.1
  Skene's gland 599.89
  skin (epidermal) (epidermoid, inclusion) (epithelial) (inclusion) (retention) (sebaceous) 706.2
    breast 610.8
    eyelid 374.84
    genital organ NEC
      female 629.8
      male 608.89
    neoplastic 216.3
    scrotum 706.2
    sweat gland or duct 705.89

Cyst — continued
  solitary
    bone 733.21
    kidney 593.2
  spermatic cord 608.89
  sphenoid sinus 478.1
  spinal meninges 349.2
  spine (see also Cyst, bone) 733.20
  spleen NEC 289.59
    congenital 759.0
    hydatid (see also Echinococcus) 122.9
  spring water (pericardium) 746.89
  subarachnoid 348.0
    intrasellar 793.0
  subdural (cerebral) 348.0
    spinal cord 349.2
  sublingual gland 527.6
    mucous extravasation or retention 527.6
  submaxillary gland 527.6
    mucous extravasation or retention 527.6
  suburethral 599.89
  suprarenal gland 255.8
  suprasellar — see Cyst, brain
  sweat gland or duct 705.89
  sympathetic nervous system 337.9
  synovial 727.40
    popliteal space 727.51
  Tarlov's 355.9
  tarsal 373.2
  tendon (sheath) 727.42
  testis 608.89
  theca-lutein (ovary) 620.2
  Thornwaldt's, Tornwaldt's 478.26
  thymus (gland) 254.8
  thyroglossal (duct) (infected) (persistent) 759.2
  thyroid (gland) 246.2
    adenomatous — see Goiter, nodular
    colloid (see also Goiter) 240.9
  thyrolingual duct (infected) (persistent) 759.2
  tongue (mucous) 529.8
  tonsil 474.8
  tooth (dental root) 522.8
  tubo-ovarian 620.8
    inflammatory 614.1
  tunica vaginalis 608.89
  turbinate (nose) (see also Cyst, bone) 733.20
  Tyson's gland (benign) (infected) 607.89
  umbilicus 759.89
  urachus 753.7
  ureter 593.89
  ureterovesical orifice 593.89
    congenital 753.4
  urethra 599.84
  urethral gland (Cowper's) 599.89
  uterine
    ligament 620.8
      embryonic 752.11
    tube 620.8
  uterus (body) (corpus) (recurrent) 621.8
    embryonal 752.3
  utricle (ear) 386.8
    prostatic 599.89
  utriculus masculinus 599.89
  vagina, vaginal (squamous cell) (wall) 623.8
    embryonal 752.41
    implantation 623.8
    inclusion 623.8
  vallecula, vallecular 478.79
  ventricle, neuroepithelial 348.0
  verumontanum 599.89
  vesical (orifice) 596.8
  vitreous humor 379.29
  vulva (sweat glands) 624.8
    congenital 752.41
    implantation 624.8
    inclusion 624.8
    sebaceous gland 624.8
  vulvovaginal gland 624.8
  wolffian 752.8

Cystadenocarcinoma (M8440/3) — see also Neoplasm, by site, malignant
  bile duct type (M8161/3) 155.1
  endometrioid (M8380/3) — see Neoplasm, by site, malignant

Cystadenocarcinoma — see also Neoplasm, by site, malignant — continued
  mucinous (M8470/3)
    papillary (M8471/3)
      specified site — see Neoplasm, by site, malignant
      unspecified site 183.0
    specified site — see Neoplasm, by site, malignant
    unspecified site 183.0
  papillary (M8450/3)
    mucinous (M8471/3)
      specified site — see Neoplasm, by site, malignant
      unspecified site 183.0
    pseudomucinous (M8471/3)
      specified site — see Neoplasm, by site, malignant
      unspecified site 183.0
    serous (M8460/3)
      specified site — see Neoplasm, by site, malignant
      unspecified site 183.0
    specified site — see Neoplasm, by site, malignant
    unspecified site 183.0
  pseudomucinous (M8470/3)
    papillary (M8471/3)
      specified site — see Neoplasm, by site, malignant
      unspecified site 183.0
    specified site — see Neoplasm, by site, malignant
    unspecified site 183.0
  serous (M8441/3)
    papillary (M8460/3)
      specified site — see Neoplasm, by site, malignant
      unspecified site 183.0
    specified site — see Neoplasm, by site, malignant
    unspecified site 183.0

Cystadenofibroma (M9013/0)
  clear cell (M8313/0) — see Neoplasm, by site, benign
  endometrioid (M8381/0) 220
    borderline malignancy (M8381/1) 236.2
    malignant (M8381/3) 183.0
  mucinous (M9015/0)
    specified site — see Neoplasm, by site, benign
    unspecified site 220
  serous (M9014/0)
    specified site — see Neoplasm, by site, benign
    unspecified site 220
  specified site — see Neoplasm, by site, benign
  unspecified site 220

Cystadenoma (M8440/0) — see also Neoplasm, by site, benign
  bile duct (M8161/0) 211.5
  endometrioid (M8380/0) — see also Neoplasm, by site, benign
    borderline malignancy (M8380/1) — see Neoplasm, by site, uncertain behavior
    malignant (M8440/3) — see Neoplasm, by site, malignant
  mucinous (M8470/0)
    borderline malignancy (M8470/1)
      specified site — see Neoplasm, uncertain behavior
      unspecified site 236.2
    papillary (M8471/0)
      borderline malignancy (M8471/1)
        specified site — see Neoplasm, by site, uncertain behavior
        unspecified site 236.2
      specified site — see Neoplasm, by site, benign
      unspecified site 220
    specified site — see Neoplasm, by site, benign
    unspecified site 220
  papillary (M8450/0)
    borderline malignancy (M8450/1)
      specified site — see Neoplasm, by site, uncertain behavior

Index to Diseases

Cystadenoma — see also Neoplasm, by site, benign — continued
  papillary — continued
    borderline malignancy — continued
      unspecified site 236.2
    lymphomatosum (M8561/0) 210.2
    mucinous (M8471/0)
      borderline malignancy (M8471/1)
        specified site — see Neoplasm, by site, uncertain behavior
        unspecified site 236.2
      specified site — see Neoplasm, by site, benign
      unspecified site 220
    pseudomucinous (M8471/0)
      borderline malignancy (M8471/1)
        specified site — see Neoplasm, by site, uncertain behavior
        unspecified site 236.2
      specified site — see Neoplasm, by site, benign
      unspecified site 220
    serous (M8460/0)
      borderline malignancy (M8460/1)
        specified site — see Neoplasm, by site, uncertain behavior
        unspecified site 236.2
      specified site — see Neoplasm, by site, benign
      unspecified site 220
    specified site — see Neoplasm, by site, benign
    unspecified site 220
  pseudomucinous (M8470/0)
    borderline malignancy (M8470/1)
      specified site — see Neoplasm, by site, uncertain behavior
      unspecified site 236.2
    papillary (M8471/0)
      borderline malignancy (M8471/1)
        specified site — see Neoplasm, by site, uncertain behavior
        unspecified site 236.2
      specified site — see Neoplasm, by site, benign
      unspecified site 220
    specified site — see Neoplasm, by site, benign
    unspecified site 220
  serous (M8441/0)
    borderline malignancy (M8441/1)
      specified site — see Neoplasm, by site, uncertain behavior
      unspecified site 236.2
    papillary (M8460/0)
      borderline malignancy (M8460/1)
        specified site — see Neoplasm, by site, uncertain behavior
        unspecified site 236.2
      specified site — see Neoplasm, by site, benign
      unspecified site 220
    specified site — see Neoplasm, by site, benign
    unspecified site 220
  thyroid 226

Cystathioninemia 270.4

Cystathioninuria 270.4

Cystic — see also condition
  breast, chronic 610.1
  corpora lutea 620.1
  degeneration, congenital
    brain 742.4
    kidney 753.10
  disease
    breast, chronic 610.1
    kidney, congenital 753.10
      medullary 753.16
      multiple 753.19
      polycystic — see Polycystic, kidney
      single 753.11
      specified NEC 753.19
    liver, congenital 751.62
    lung 518.89
      congenital 748.4

Cystic — see also condition — continued
  disease — continued
    pancreas, congenital 751.7
    semilunar cartilage 717.5
  duct — see condition
  eyeball, congenital 743.03
  fibrosis (pancreas) 277.00
    with ●
      manifestations ●
        gastrointestinal 277.03 ●
        pulmonary 277.02 ●
        specified NEC 277.09 ●
      meconium ileus 277.01 ●
      pulmonary exacerbation 277.02 ●
  hygroma (M9173/0) 228.1
  kidney, congenital 753.10
    medullary 753.16
    multiple 753.19
    polycystic — see Polycystic, kidney
    single 753.11
    specified NEC 753.19
  liver, congenital 751.62
  lung 518.89
    congenital 748.4
  mass — see Cyst
  mastitis, chronic 610.1
  ovary 620.2
  pancreas, congenital 751.7

Cysticerciasis 123.1

Cysticercosis (mammary) (subretinal) 123.1

Cysticercus 123.1
  cellulosae infestation 123.1

Cystinosis (malignant) 270.0

Cystinuria 270.0

Cystitis (bacillary) (colli) (diffuse) (exudative) (hemorrhagic) (purulent) (recurrent) (septic) (suppurative) (ulcerative) 595.9
  with
    abortion — see Abortion, by type, with urinary tract infection
    ectopic pregnancy (see also categories 633.0-633.9) 639.8
    fibrosis 595.1
    leukoplakia 595.1
    malakoplakia 595.1
    metaplasia 595.1
    molar pregnancy (see also categories 630-632) 639.8
  actinomycotic 039.8 [595.4]
  acute 595.0
    of trigone 595.3
  allergic 595.89
  amebic 006.8 [595.4]
  bilharzial 120.9 [595.4]
  blennorrhagic (acute) 098.11
    chronic or duration of 2 months or more 098.31
  bullous 595.89
  calculous 594.1
    chlamydial 099.53
  chronic 595.2
    interstitial 595.1
    of trigone 595.3
  complicating pregnancy, childbirth, or puerperium 646.6 ✓5th
    affecting fetus or newborn 760.1
  cystic(a) 595.81
  diphtheritic 032.84
  echinococcal
    granulosus 122.3 [595.4]
    multilocularis 122.6 [595.4]
  emphysematous 595.89
  encysted 595.81
  follicular 595.3
  following
    abortion 639.8
    ectopic or molar pregnancy 639.8
  gangrenous 595.89
  glandularis 595.89
  gonococcal (acute) 098.11
    chronic or duration of 2 months or more 098.31
  incrusted 595.89
  interstitial 595.1
  irradiation 595.82
  irritation 595.89

Cystitis — continued
  malignant 595.89
  monilial 112.2
  of trigone 595.3
  panmural 595.1
  polyposa 595.89
  prostatic 601.3
  radiation 595.82
  Reiter's (abacterial) 099.3
  specified NEC 595.89
  subacute 595.2
  submucous 595.1
  syphilitic 095.8
  trichomoniasis 131.09
  tuberculous (see also Tuberculosis) 016.1 ✓5th
  ulcerative 595.1

Cystocele (-rectocele)
  female (without uterine prolapse) 618.0
    with uterine prolapse 618.4
      complete 618.3
      incomplete 618.2
  in pregnancy or childbirth 654.4 ✓5th
    affecting fetus or newborn 763.89
    causing obstructed labor 660.2 ✓5th
      affecting fetus or newborn 763.1
  male 596.8

Cystoid
  cicatrix limbus 372.64
  degeneration macula 362.53

Cystolithiasis 594.1

Cystoma (M8440/0) — see also Neoplasm, by site, benign
  endometrial, ovary 617.1
  mucinous (M8470/0)
    specified site — see Neoplasm, by site, benign
    unspecified site 220
  serous (M8441/0)
    specified site — see Neoplasm, by site, benign
    unspecified site 220
  simple (ovary) 620.2

Cystoplegia 596.53

Cystoptosis 596.8

Cystopyelitis (see also Pyelitis) 590.80

Cystorrhagia 596.8

Cystosarcoma phyllodes (M9020/1) 238.3
  benign (M9020/0) 217
  malignant (M9020/3) — see Neoplasm, breast, malignant

Cystostomy status V44.50
  appendico-vesicostomy V44.52
  cutaneous-vesicostomy V44.51
  specified type NEC V44.59
  with complication 997.5

Cystourethritis (see also Urethritis) 597.89

Cystourethrocele (see also Cystocele)
  female (without uterine prolapse) 618.0
    with uterine prolapse 618.4
      complete 618.3
      incomplete 618.2
  male 596.8

Cytomegalic inclusion disease 078.5
  congenital 771.1

Cytomycosis, reticuloendothelial (see also Histoplasmosis, American) 115.00

Index to Diseases

D

Daae (-Finsen) disease (epidemic pleurodynia) 074.1
Dabney's grip 074.1
Da Costa's syndrome (neurocirculatory asthenia) 306.2
Dacryoadenitis, dacryadenitis 375.00
  acute 375.01
  chronic 375.02
Dacryocystitis 375.30
  acute 375.32
  chronic 375.42
  neonatal 771.6
  phlegmonous 375.33
  syphilitic 095.8
    congenital 090.0
  trachomatous, active 076.1
    late effect 139.1
  tuberculous (see also Tuberculosis) 017.3
Dacryocystoblenorrhea 375.42
Dacryocystocele 375.43
Dacryolith, dacryolithiasis 375.57
Dacryoma 375.43
Dacryopericystitis (acute) (subacute) 375.32
  chronic 375.42
Dacryops 375.11
Dacryosialadenopathy, atrophic 710.2
Dacryostenosis 375.56
  congenital 743.65
Dactylitis 686.9
  bone (see also Osteomyelitis) 730.2
  sickle cell 282.61
  syphilitic 095.5
  tuberculous (see also Tuberculosis) 015.5
Dactylolysis opontaned 136.0
Dactylosymphysis (see also Syndactylism) 755.10
Damage
  arteriosclerotic — see Arteriosclerosis
  brain 348.9
    anoxic, hypoxic 348.1
      during or resulting from a procedure 997.01
    child NEC 343.9
    due to birth injury 767.0
    minimal (child) (see also Hyperkinesia) 314.9
    newborn 767.0
  cardiac — see also Disease, heart
  cardiorenal (vascular) (see also Hypertension, cardiorenal) 404.90
  central nervous system — see Damage, brain
  cerebral NEC — see Damage, brain
  coccyx, complicating delivery 665.6
  coronary (see also Ischemia, heart) 414.9
  eye, birth injury 767.0
  heart — see also Disease, heart
    valve — see Endocarditis
  hypothalamus NEC 348.9
  liver 571.9
    alcoholic 571.3
  myocardium (see also Degeneration, myocardial) 429.1
  pelvic
    joint or ligament, during delivery 665.6
    organ NEC
      with
        abortion — see Abortion, by type, with damage to pelvic organs
        ectopic pregnancy (see also categories 633.0-633.9) 639.2
        molar pregnancy (see also categories 630-632) 639.2
      during delivery 665.5
      following
        abortion 639.2
        ectopic or molar pregnancy 639.2
  renal (see also Disease, renal) 593.9
  skin, solar 692.79
    acute 692.72
    chronic 692.74
  subendocardium, subendocardial (see also Degeneration, myocardial) 429.1
  vascular 459.9

Dameshek's syndrome (erythroblastic anemia) 282.4
Dana-Putnam syndrome (subacute combined sclerosis with pernicious anemia) 281.0 [336.2]
Danbolt (-Closs) syndrome (acrodermatitis enteropathica) 686.8
Dandruff 690.18
Dandy fever 061
Dandy-Walker deformity or syndrome (atresia, foramen of Magendie) 742.3
  with spina bifida (see also Spina bifida) 741.0
Dangle foot 736.79
Danielssen's disease (anesthetic leprosy) 030.1
Danlos' syndrome 756.83
Darier's disease (congenital) (keratosis follicularis) 757.39
  due to vitamin A deficiency 264.8
  meaning erythema annulare centrifugum 695.0
Darier-Roussy sarcoid 135
Darling's
  disease (see also Histoplasmosis, American) 115.00
  histoplasmosis (see also Histoplasmosis, American) 115.00
Dartre 054.9
Darwin's tubercle 744.29
Davidson's anemia (refractory) 284.9
Davies' disease 425.0
Davies-Colley syndrome (slipping rib) 733.99
Dawson's encephalitis 046.2
Day blindness (see also Blindness, day) 368.60
Dead
  fetus
    retained (in utero) 656.4
      early pregnancy (death before 22 completed weeks gestation) 632
      late (death after 22 completed weeks gestation) 656.4
    syndrome 641.3
  labyrinth 386.50
  ovum, retained 631
Deaf and dumb NEC 389.7
Deaf mutism (acquired) (congenital) NEC 389.7
  endemic 243
  hysterical 300.11
  syphilitic, congenital 090.0
Deafness (acquired) (bilateral) (both ears) (complete) (congenital) (hereditary) (middle ear) (partial) (unilateral) 389.9
  with blue sclera and fragility of bone 756.51
  auditory fatigue 389.9
  aviation 993.0
    nerve injury 951.5
  boilermakers' 951.5
  central 389.14
    with conductive hearing loss 389.2
  conductive (air) 389.00
    with sensorineural hearing loss 389.2
    combined types 389.08
    external ear 389.01
    inner ear 389.04
    middle ear 389.03
    multiple types 389.08
    tympanic membrane 389.02
  emotional (complete) 300.11
  functional (complete) 300.11
  high frequency 389.8
  hysterical (complete) 300.11
  injury 951.5
  low frequency 389.8
  mental 784.69
  mixed conductive and sensorineural 389.2
  nerve 389.12
    with conductive hearing loss 389.2
  neural 389.12
    with conductive hearing loss 389.2
  noise-induced 388.12
    nerve injury 951.5
  nonspeaking 389.7

Deafness — continued
  perceptive 389.10
    with conductive hearing loss 389.2
    central 389.14
    combined types 389.18
    multiple types 389.18
    neural 389.12
    sensory 389.11
  psychogenic (complete) 306.7
  sensorineural (see also Deafness, perceptive) 389.10
  sensory 389.11
    with conductive hearing loss 389.2
  specified type NEC 389.8
  sudden NEC 388.2
  syphilitic 094.89
  transient ischemic 388.02
  transmission — see Deafness, conductive
  traumatic 951.5
  word (secondary to organic lesion) 784.69
    developmental 315.31
Death
  after delivery (cause not stated) (sudden) 674.9
  anesthetic
    due to
      correct substance properly administered 995.4
      overdose or wrong substance given 968.4
      specified anesthetic — see Table of Drugs and Chemicals
    during delivery 668.9
  brain 348.8
  cardiac — see Disease, heart
  cause unknown 798.2
  cot (infant) 798.0
  crib (infant) 798.0
  fetus, fetal (cause not stated) (intrauterine) 779.9
    early, with retention (before 22 completed weeks gestation) 632
    from asphyxia or anoxia (before labor) 768.0
      during labor 768.1
    late, affecting management of pregnancy (after 22 completed weeks gestation) 656.4
  from pregnancy NEC 646.9
  instantaneous 798.1
  intrauterine (see also Death, fetus) 779.9
    complicating pregnancy 656.4
  maternal, affecting fetus or newborn 761.6
  neonatal NEC 779.9
  sudden (cause unknown) 798.1
    during delivery 669.9
      under anesthesia NEC 668.9
    infant, syndrome (SIDS) 798.0
    puerperal, during puerperium 674.9
  unattended (cause unknown) 798.9
  under anesthesia NEC
    due to
      correct substance properly administered 995.4
      overdose or wrong substance given 968.4
      specified anesthetic — see Table of Drugs and Chemicals
    during delivery 668.9
  violent 798.1
de Beurmann-Gougerot disease (sporotrichosis) 117.1
Debility (general) (infantile) (postinfectional) 799.3
  with nutritional difficulty 269.9
  congenital or neonatal NEC 779.9
  nervous 300.5
  old age 797
  senile 797
Débove's disease (splenomegaly) 789.2
Decalcification
  bone (see also Osteoporosis) 733.00
  teeth 521.8
Decapitation 874.9
  fetal (to facilitate delivery) 763.89
Decapsulation, kidney 593.89
Decay
  dental 521.00
  senile 797
  tooth, teeth 521.00

Decensus, uterus

Decensus, uterus — see Prolapse, uterus
Deciduitis (acute)
  with
    abortion — see Abortion, by type, with sepsis
    ectopic pregnancy (see also categories 633.0-633.9) 639.0
    molar pregnancy (see also categories 630-632) 639.0
  affecting fetus or newborn 760.8
  following
    abortion 639.0
    ectopic or molar pregnancy 639.0
  in pregnancy 646.6
  puerperal, postpartum 670
Deciduoma malignum (M9100/3) 181
Deciduous tooth (retained) 520.6
Decline (general) (see also Debility) 799.3
Decompensation
  cardiac (acute) (chronic) (see also Disease, heart) 429.9
    failure — see Failure, heart
  cardiorenal (see also Hypertension, cardiorenal) 404.90
  cardiovascular (see also Disease, cardiovascular) 429.2
  heart (see also Disease, heart) 429.9
    failure — see Failure, heart
  hepatic 572.2
  myocardial (acute) (chronic) (see also Disease, heart) 429.9
    failure — see Failure, heart
  respiratory 519.9
Decompression sickness 993.3
Decrease, decreased
  blood
    platelets (see also Thrombocytopenia) 287.5
    pressure 796.3
      due to shock following
        injury 958.4
        operation 998.0
  cardiac reserve — see Disease, heart
  estrogen 256.39
    postablative 256.2
  fetal movements 655.7
  fragility of erythrocytes 289.8
  function
    adrenal (cortex) 255.4
      medulla 255.5
    ovary in hypopituitarism 253.4
    parenchyma of pancreas 577.8
    pituitary (gland) (lobe) (anterior) 253.2
      posterior (lobe) 253.8
  functional activity 780.99 ▲
  glucose 790.2
  haptoglobin (serum) NEC 273.8
  platelets (see also Thrombocytopenia) 287.5
  pulse pressure 785.9
  respiration due to shock following injury 958.4
  tear secretion NEC 375.15
  tolerance
    fat 579.8
    glucose 790.2
    salt and water 276.9
  vision NEC 369.9
Decubital gangrene 707.0 [785.4]
Decubiti (see also Decubitus) 707.0
Decubitus (ulcer) 707.0
  with gangrene 707.0 [785.4]
Deepening acetabulum 718.85
Defect, defective 759.9
  3-beta-hydroxysteroid dehydrogenase 255.2
  11-hydroxylase 255.2
  21-hydroxylase 255.2
  abdominal wall, congenital 756.70
  aorticopulmonary septum 745.0
  aortic septal 745.0
  atrial septal (ostium secundum type) 745.5
    acquired 429.71
    ostium primum type 745.61
    sinus venosus 745.8
  atrioventricular
    canal 745.69
    septum 745.4
      acquired 429.71

Defect, defective — continued
  atrium secundum 745.5
    acquired 429.71
  auricular septal 745.5
    acquired 429.71
  bilirubin excretion 277.4
  biosynthesis, testicular androgen 257.2
  bulbar septum 745.0
  butanol-insoluble iodide 246.1
  chromosome — see Anomaly, chromosome
  circulation (acquired) 459.9
    congenital 747.9
    newborn 747.9
  clotting NEC (see also Defect, coagulation) 286.9
  coagulation (factor) (see also Deficiency, coagulation factor) 286.9
    with
      abortion — see Abortion, by type, with hemorrhage
      ectopic pregnancy (see also categories 634-638) 639.1
      molar pregnancy (see also categories 630-632) 639.1
    acquired (any) 286.7
    antepartum or intrapartum 641.3
      affecting fetus or newborn 762.1
    causing hemorrhage of pregnancy or delivery 641.3
    due to
      liver disease 286.7
      vitamin K deficiency 286.7
    newborn, transient 776.3
    postpartum 666.3
    specified type NEC 286.3
  conduction (heart) 426.9
    bone (see also Deafness, conductive) 389.00
  congenital, organ or site NEC — see also Anomaly
    circulation 747.9
    Descemet's membrane 743.9
      specified type NEC 743.49
    diaphragm 756.6
    ectodermal 757.9
    esophagus 750.9
    pulmonic cusps — see Anomaly, heart valve
    respiratory system 748.9
      specified type NEC 748.8
  cushion endocardial 745.60
  dentin (hereditary) 520.5
  Descemet's membrane (congenital) 743.9
    acquired 371.30
    specific type NEC 743.49
  deutan 368.52
  developmental — see also Anomaly, by site
    cauda equina 742.59
    left ventricle 746.9
      with atresia or hypoplasia of aortic orifice or valve, with hypoplasia of ascending aorta 746.7
      in hypoplastic left heart syndrome 746.7
    testis 752.9
    vessel 747.9
  diaphragm
    with elevation, eventration, or hernia — see Hernia, diaphragm
    congenital 756.6
      with elevation, eventration, or hernia 756.6
      gross (with elevation, eventration, or hernia) 756.6
  ectodermal, congenital 757.9
  Eisenmenger's (ventricular septal defect) 745.4
  endocardial cushion 745.60
    specified type NEC 745.69
  esophagus, congenital 750.9
  extensor retinaculum 728.9
  fibrin polymerization (see also Defect, coagulation) 286.3
  filling
    biliary tract 793.3
    bladder 793.5
    gallbladder 793.3
    kidney 793.5
    stomach 793.4
    ureter 793.5
  fossa ovalis 745.5

Defect, defective — continued
  gene, carrier (suspected) of V83.89 ▲
  Gerbode 745.4
  glaucomatous, without elevated tension 365.89
  Hageman (factor) (see also Defect, coagulation) 286.3
  hearing (see also Deafness) 389.9
  high grade 317
  homogentisic acid 270.2
  interatrial septal 745.5
    acquired 429.71
  interauricular septal 745.5
    acquired 429.71
  interventricular septal 745.4
    with pulmonary stenosis or atresia, dextraposition of aorta, and hypertrophy of right ventricle 745.2
    acquired 429.71
    in tetralogy of Fallot 745.2
  iodide trapping 246.1
  iodotyrosine dehalogenase 246.1
  kynureninase 270.2
  learning, specific 315.2
  mental (see also Retardation, mental) 319
  osteochondral NEC 738.8
  ostium
    primum 745.61
    secundum 745.5
  pericardium 746.89
  peroxidase-binding 246.1
  placental blood supply — see Placenta, insufficiency
  platelet (qualitative) 287.1
    constitutional 286.4
  postural, spine 737.9
  protan 368.51
  pulmonic cusps, congenital 746.00
  renal pelvis 753.9
    obstructive 753.29
    specified type NEC 753.3
  respiratory system, congenital 748.9
    specified type NEC 748.8
  retina, retinal 361.30
    with detachment (see also Detachment, retina, with retinal defect) 361.00
    multiple 361.33
      with detachment 361.02
    nerve fiber bundle 362.85
    single 361.30
      with detachment 361.01
  septal (closure) (heart) NEC 745.9
    acquired 429.71
    atrial 745.5
    specified type NEC 745.8
  speech NEC 784.5
    developmental 315.39
    secondary to organic lesion 784.5
  Taussig-Bing (transposition, aorta and overriding pulmonary artery) 745.11
  teeth, wedge 521.2
  thyroid hormone synthesis 246.1
  tritan 368.53
  ureter 753.9
    obstructive 753.29
  vascular (acquired) (local) 459.9
    congenital (peripheral) NEC 747.60
      gastrointestinal 747.61
      lower limb 747.64
      renal 747.62
      specified NEC 747.69
      spinal 747.82
      upper limb 747.63
  ventricular septal 745.4
    with pulmonary stenosis or atresia, dextraposition of aorta, and hypertrophy of right ventricle 745.2
    acquired 429.71
    atrioventricular canal type 745.69
    between infundibulum and anterior portion 745.4
    in tetralogy of Fallot 745.2
    isolated anterior 745.4
  vision NEC 369.9
  visual field 368.40
    arcuate 368.43
    heteronymous, bilateral 368.47
    homonymous, bilateral 368.46

Index to Diseases

Defect, defective — *continued*
- visual field — *continued*
  - localized NEC 368.44
  - nasal step 368.44
  - peripheral 368.44
  - sector 368.43
- voice 784.40
- wedge, teeth (abrasion) 521.2

Defeminization syndrome 255.2

Deferentitis 608.4
- gonorrheal (acute) 098.14
  - chronic or duration of 2 months or over 098.34

Defibrination syndrome (*see also* Fibrinolysis) 286.6

Deficiency, deficient
- 3-beta-hydroxysteroid dehydrogenase 255.2
- 6-phosphogluconic dehydrogenase (anemia) 282.2
- 11-beta-hydroxylase 255.2
- 17-alpha-hydroxylase 255.2
- 18-hydroxysteroid dehydrogenase 255.2
- 20-alpha-hydroxylase 255.2
- 21-hydroxylase 255.2
- abdominal muscle syndrome 756.79
- accelerator globulin (Ac G) (blood) (*see also* Defect, coagulation) 286.3
- AC globulin (congenital) (*see also* Defect, coagulation) 286.3
  - acquired 286.7
- activating factor (blood) (*see also*, Defect, coagulation) 286.3
- adenohypophyseal 253.2
- adenosine deaminase 277.2
- aldolase (hereditary) 271.2
- alpha-1-antitrypsin 277.6
- alpha-1-trypsin inhibitor 277.6
- alpha-fucosidase 271.8
- alpha-lipoprotein 272.5
- alpha-mannosidase 271.8
- amino acid 270.9
- anemia — *see* Anemia, deficiency
- aneurin 265.1
  - with beriberi 265.0
- antibody NEC 279.00
- antidiuretic hormone 253.5
- antihemophilic
  - factor (A) 286.0
    - B 286.1
    - C 286.2
  - globulin (AHG) NEC 286.0
- antitrypsin 277.6
- argininosuccinate synthetase or lyase 270.6
- ascorbic acid (with scurvy) 267
- autoprothrombin
  - I (*see also* Defect, coagulation) 286.3
  - II 286.1
  - C (*see also* Defect, coagulation) 286.3
- bile salt 579.8
- biotin 266.2
- biotinidase 277.6
- bradykinase-1 277.6
- brancher enzyme (amylopectinosis) 271.0
- calciferol 268.9
  - with
    - osteomalacia 268.2
    - rickets (*see also* Rickets) 268.0
- calcium 275.40
  - dietary 269.3
- calorie, severe 261
- carbamyl phosphate synthetase 270.6
- cardiac (*see also* Insufficiency, myocardial) 428.0
- carnitine palmityl transferase 791.3
- carotene 264.9
- Carr factor (*see also* Defect, coagulation) 286.9
- central nervous system 349.9
- ceruloplasmin 275.1
- cevitamic acid (with scurvy) 267
- choline 266.2
- Christmas factor 286.1
- chromium 269.3
- citrin 269.1
- clotting (blood) (*see also* Defect, coagulation) 286.9

Deficiency, deficient — *continued*
- coagulation factor NEC 286.9
  - with
    - abortion — *see* Abortion, by type, with hemorrhage
    - ectopic pregnancy (*see also* categories 634-638) 639.1
    - molar pregnancy (*see also* categories 630-632) 639.1
  - acquired (any) 286.7
  - antepartum or intrapartum 641.3 ✓5ᵗʰ
    - affecting fetus or newborn 762.1
  - due to
    - liver disease 286.7
    - vitamin K deficiency 286.7
  - newborn, transient 776.3
  - postpartum 666.3 ✓5ᵗʰ
  - specified type NEC 286.3
- color vision (congenital) 368.59
  - acquired 368.55
- combined, two or more coagulation factors (*see also* Defect, coagulation) 286.9
- complement factor NEC 279.8
- contact factor (*see also* Defect, coagulation) 286.3
- copper NEC 275.1
- corticoadrenal 255.4
- craniofacial axis 756.0
- cyanocobalamin (vitamin B₁₂) 266.2
- debrancher enzyme (limit dextrinosis) 271.0
- desmolase 255.2
- diet 269.9
- dihydrofolate reductase 281.2
- dihydropteridine reductase 270.1
- disaccharidase (intestinal) 271.3
- disease NEC 269.9
- ear(s) V48.8
- edema 262
- endocrine 259.9
- enzymes, circulating NEC (*see also* Deficiency, by specific enzyme) 277.6
- ergosterol 268.9
  - with
    - osteomalacia 268.2
    - rickets (*see also* Rickets) 268.0
- erythrocytic glutathione (anemia) 282.2
- eyelid(s) V48.8
- factor (*See also* Defect, coagulation) 286.9
  - I (congenital) (fibrinogen) 286.3
    - antepartum or intrapartum 641.3 ✓5ᵗʰ
      - affecting fetus or newborn 762.1
    - newborn, transient 776.3
    - postpartum 666.3 ✓5ᵗʰ
  - II (congenital) (prothrombin) 286.3
  - V (congenital) (labile) 286.3
  - VII (congenital) (stable) 286.3
  - VIII (congenital) (functional) 286.0
    - with
      - functional defect 286.0
      - vascular defect 286.4
  - IX (Christmas) (congenital) (functional) 286.1
  - X (congenital) (Stuart-Prower) 286.3
  - XI (congenital) (plasma thromboplastin antecedent) 286.2
  - XII (congenital) (Hageman) 286.3
  - XIII (congenital) (fibrin stabilizing) 286.3
  - Hageman 286.3
  - multiple (congenital) 286.9
    - acquired 286.7
- fibrinase (*see also* Defect, coagulation) 286.3
- fibrinogen (congenital) (*see also* Defect, coagulation) 286.3
  - acquired 286.6
- fibrin-stabilizing factor (congenital) (*see also* Defect, coagulation) 286.3
- finger — *see* Absence, finger
- fletcher factor (*see also* Defect, coagulation) 286.9
- fluorine 269.3
- folate, anemia 281.2
- folic acid (vitamin B₉) 266.2
  - anemia 281.2
- fructokinase 271.2
- fructose-1, 6-diphosphate 271.2
- fructose-1-phosphate aldolase 271.2
- FSH (follicle-stimulating hormone) 253.4
- fucosidase 271.8

Deficiency, deficient — *continued*
- galactokinase 271.1
- galactose-1-phosphate uridyl transferase 271.1
- gamma globulin in blood 279.00
- glass factor (*see also* Defect, coagulation) 286.3
- glucocorticoid 255.4
- glucose-6-phosphatase 271.0
- glucose-6-phosphate dehydrogenase anemia 282.2
- glucuronyl transferase 277.4
- glutathione-reductase (anemia) 282.2
- glycogen synthetase 271.0
- growth hormone 253.3
- Hageman factor (congenital) (*see also* Defect, coagulation) 286.3
- head V48.0
- hemoglobin (*see also* Anemia) 285.9
- hepatophosphorylase 271.0
- hexose monophosphate (HMP) shunt 282.2
- HGH (human growth hormone) 253.3
- HG-PRT 277.2
- homogentisic acid oxidase 270.2
- hormone — *see also* Deficiency, by specific hormone
  - anterior pituitary (isolated) (partial) NEC 253.4
    - growth (human) 253.3
  - follicle-stimulating 253.4
  - growth (human) (isolated) 253.3
  - human growth 253.3
  - interstitial cell-stimulating 253.4
  - luteinizing 253.4
  - melanocyte-stimulating 253.4
  - testicular 257.2
- human growth hormone 253.3
- humoral 279.00
  - with
    - hyper-IgM 279.05
      - autosomal recessive 279.05
      - X-linked 279.05
      - increased IgM 279.05
    - congenital hypogammaglobulinemia 279.04
    - non-sex-linked 279.06
    - selective immunoglobulin NEC 279.03
      - IgA 279.01
      - IgG 279.03
      - IgM 279.02
      - increased 279.05
    - specified NEC 279.09
- hydroxylase 255.2
- hypoxanthine-guanine phosphoribosyltransferase (HG-PRT) 277.2
- ICSH (interstitial cell-stimulating hormone) 253.4
- immunity NEC 279.3
  - cell-mediated 279.10
    - with
      - hyperimmunoglob-ulinemia 279.2
      - thrombocytopenia and eczema 279.12
    - specified NEC 279.19
  - combined (severe) 279.2
    - syndrome 279.2
  - common variable 279.06
  - humoral NEC 279.00
  - IgA (secretory) 279.01
  - IgG 279.03
  - IgM 279.02
- immunoglobulin, selective NEC 279.03
  - IgA 279.01
  - IgG 279.03
  - IgM 279.02
- inositol (B complex) 266.2
- interferon 279.4
- internal organ V47.0
- interstitial cell-stimulating hormone (ICSH) 253.4
- intrinsic factor (Castle's) (congenital) 281.0
- intrinsic (urethral) sphincter (ISD) 599.82
- invertase 271.3
- iodine 269.3
- iron, anemia 280.9
- labile factor (congenital) (*see also* Defect, coagulation) 286.3
  - acquired 286.7
- lacrimal fluid (acquired) 375.15
  - congenital 743.64
- lactase 271.3

Deficiency, deficient

Deficiency, deficient — *continued*
- Laki-Lorand factor (*see also* Defect, coagulation) 286.3
- lecithin-cholesterol acyltranferase 272.5
- LH (luteinizing hormone) 253.4
- limb V49.0
  - lower V49.0
    - congenital (*see also* Deficiency, lower limb, congenital) 755.30
  - upper V49.0
    - congenital (*see also* Deficiency, upper limb, congenital) 755.20
- lipocaic 577.8
- lipoid (high-density) 272.5
- lipoprotein (familial) (high density) 272.5
- liver phosphorylase 271.0
- lower limb V49.0
  - congenital 755.30
    - with complete absence of distal elements 755.31
    - longitudinal (complete) (partial) (with distal deficiencies, incomplete) 755.32
      - with complete absence of distal elements 755.31
      - combined femoral, tibial, fibular (incomplete) 755.33
      - femoral 755.34
      - fibular 755.37
      - metatarsal(s) 755.38
      - phalange(s) 755.39
        - meaning all digits 755.31
      - tarsal(s) 755.38
      - tibia 755.36
      - tibiofibular 755.35
    - transverse 755.31
- luteinizing hormone (LH) 253.4
- lysosomal alpha-1, 4 glucosidase 271.0
- magnesium 275.2
- mannosidase 271.8
- melanocyte-stimulating hormone (MSH) 253.4
- menadione (vitamin K) 269.0
  - newborn 776.0
- mental (familial) (hereditary) (*see also* Retardation, mental) 319
- mineral NEC 269.3
- molybdenum 269.3
- moral 301.7
- multiple, syndrome 260
- myocardial (*see also* Insufficiency myocardial) 428.0
- myophosphorylase 271.0
- NADH (DPNH)-methemoglobin-reductase (congenital) 289.7
- NADH-diaphorase or reductase (congenital) 289.7
- neck V48.1
- niacin (amide) (-tryptophan) 265.2
- nicotinamide 265.2
- nicotinic acid (amide) 265.2
- nose V48.8
- number of teeth (*see also* Anodontia) 520.0
- nutrition, nutritional 269.9
  - specified NEC 269.8
- ornithine transcarbamylase 270.6
- ovarian 256.39
- oxygen (*see also* Anoxia) 799.0
- pantothenic acid 266.2
- parathyroid (gland) 252.1
- phenylalanine hydroxylase 270.1
- phosphofructokinase 271.2
- phosphoglucomutase 271.0
- phosphohexosisomerase 271.0
- phosphorylase kinase, liver 271.0
- pituitary (anterior) 253.2
  - posterior 253.5
- placenta — *see* Placenta, insufficiency
- plasma
  - cell 279.00
    - protein (paraproteinemia) (pyroglobulinemia) 273.8
      - gamma globulin 279.00
  - thrombosplastin
    - antecedent (PTA) 286.2
    - component (PTC) 286.1
- platelet NEC 287.1
  - constitutional 286.4

Deficiency, deficient — *continued*
- polyglandular 258.9
- potassium (K) 276.8
- proaccelerin (congenital) (*see also* Defect, congenital) 286.3
  - acquired 286.7
- proconvertin factor (congenital) (*see also* Defect, coagulation) 286.3
  - acquired 286.7
- prolactin 253.4
- protein 260
  - anemia 281.4
  - plasma — *see* Deficiency, plasma protein
- prothrombin (congenital) (*see also* Defect coagulation) 286.3
  - acquired 286.7
- Prower factor (*see also* Defect, coagulation) 286.3
- PRT 277.2
- pseudocholinesterase 289.8
- psychobiological 301.6
- PTA 286.2
- PTC 286.1
- purine nucleoside phosphorylase 277.2
- pyracin (alpha) (Beta) 266.1
- pyridoxal 266.1
- pyridoxamine 266.1
- pyridoxine (derivatives) 266.1
- pyruvate kinase (PK) 282.3
- riboflavin (vitamin B_2) 266.0
- saccadic eye movements 379.57
- salivation 527.7
- salt 276.1
- secretion
  - ovary 256.39
  - salivary gland (any) 527.7
  - urine 788.5
- selenium 269.3
- serum
  - antitrypsin, familial 277.6
  - protein (congenital) 273.8
- smooth pursuit movements (eye) 379.58
- sodium (Na) 276.1
- SPCA (*see also* Defect, coagulation) 286.3
- specified NEC 269.8
- stable factor (congenital) (*see also* Defect, coagulation) 286.3
  - acquired 286.7
- Stuart (-Prower) factor (*see also* Defect, coagulation) 286.3
- sucrase 271.3
- sucrase-isomaltase 271.3
- sulfite oxidase 270.0
- syndrome, multiple 260
- thiamine, thiaminic (chloride) 265.1
- thrombokinase (*see also* Defect, coagulation) 286.3
  - newborn 776.0
- thrombopoieten 287.3
- thymolymphatic 279.2
- thyroid (gland) 244.9
- tocopherol 269.1
- toe — *see* Absence, toe
- tooth bud (*see also* Anodontia) 520.0
- trunk V48.1
- UDPG-glycogen transferase 271.0
- upper limb V49.0
  - congenital 755.20
    - with complete absence of distal elements 755.21
    - longitudinal (complete) (partial) (with distal deficiencies, incomplete) 755.22
      - carpal(s) 755.28
      - combined humeral, radial, ulnar (incomplete) 755.23
      - humeral 755.24
      - metacarpal(s) 755.28
      - phalange(s) 755.29
        - meaning all digits 755.21
      - radial 755.26
      - radioulnar 755.25
      - ulnar 755.27
    - transverse (complete) (partial) 755.21
- vascular 459.9
- vasopressin 253.5
- viosterol (*see also* Deficiency, calciferol) 268.9

Deficiency, deficient — *continued*
- vitamin (multiple) NEC 269.2
  - A 264.9
    - with
      - Bitôt's spot 264.1
        - corneal 264.2
          - with corneal ulceration 264.3
      - keratomalacia 264.4
      - keratosis, follicular 264.8
      - night blindness 264.5
      - scar of cornea, xerophthalmic 264.6
      - specified manifestation NEC 264.8
      - ocular 264.7
      - xeroderma 264.8
      - xerophthalmia 264.7
      - xerosis
        - conjunctival 264.0
          - with Bitôt's spot 264.1
        - corneal 264.2
          - with corneal ulceraton 264.3
  - B (complex) NEC 266.9
    - with
      - beriberi 265.0
      - pellagra 265.2
    - specified type NEC 266.2
  - B_1 NEC 265.1
    - beriberi 265.0
  - B_2 266.0
  - B_6 266.1
  - B_{12} 266.2
  - B_9 (folic acid) 266.2
  - C (ascorbic acid) (with scurvy) 267
  - D (calciferol) (ergosterol) 268.9
    - with
      - osteomalacia 268.2
      - rickets (*see also* Rickets) 268.0
  - E 269.1
  - folic acid 266.2
  - G 266.0
  - H 266.2
  - K 269.0
    - of newborn 776.0
  - nicotinic acid 265.2
  - P 269.1
  - PP 265.2
  - specified NEC 269.1
- zinc 269.3

Deficient — *see also* Deficiency
- blink reflex 374.45
- craniofacial axis 756.0
- number of teeth (*see also* Anodontia) 520.0
- secretion of urine 788.5

Deficit
- neurologic NEC 781.99
  - due to
    - cerebrovascular lesion (*see also* Disease, cerebrovascular, acute) 436
      - late effect — *see* Late effect(s) (of) cerebrovascular disease
    - transient ischemic attack 435.9
- oxygen 799.0

Deflection
- radius 736.09
- septum (acquired) (nasal) (nose) 470
- spine — *see* Curvature, spine
- turbinate (nose) 470

Defluvium
- capillorum (*see also* Alopecia) 704.00
- ciliorum 374.55
- unguium 703.8

Deformity 738.9
- abdomen, congental 759.9
- abdominal wall
  - acquired 738.8
  - congenital 756.70
  - muscle deficiency syndrome 756.79
- acquired (unspecified site) 738.9
  - specified site NEC 738.8
- adrenal gland (congenital) 759.1
- alimentary tract, congenital 751.9
  - lower 751.5
  - specified type NEC 751.8
  - upper (any part, except tongue) 750.9
    - specified type NEC 750.8
    - tongue 750.10
      - specified type NEC 750.19

Index to Diseases

Deformity — continued
- ankle (joint) (acquired) 736.70
  - abduction 718.47
  - congenital 755.69
  - contraction 718.47
  - specified NEC 736.79
- anus (congenital) 751.5
  - acquired 569.49
- aorta (congenital) 747.20
  - acquired 447.8
  - arch 747.21
    - acquired 447.8
  - coarctation 747.10
- aortic
  - arch 747.21
    - acquired 447.8
  - cusp or valve (congenital) 746.9
    - acquired (see also Endocarditis, aortic) 424.1
  - ring 747.21
- appendix 751.5
- arm (acquired) 736.89
  - congenital 755.50
- arteriovenous (congenital) (peripheral) NEC 747.60
  - gastrointestinal 747.61
  - lower limb 747.64
  - renal 747.62
  - specified NEC 747.69
  - spinal 747.82
  - upper limb 747.63
- artery (congenital) (peripheral) NEC (see also Deformity, vascular) 747.60
  - acquired 447.8
  - cerebral 747.81
  - coronary (congenital) 746.85
    - acquired (see also Ischemia, heart) 414.9
  - retinal 743.9
  - umbilical 747.5
- atrial septal (congenital) (heart) 745.5
- auditory canal (congenital) (external) (see also Deformity, ear) 744.3
  - acquired 380.50
- auricle
  - ear (congenital) (see also Deformity, ear) 744.3
    - acquired 380.32
  - heart (congenital) 746.9
- back (acquired) — see Deformity, spine
- Bartholin's duct (congenital) 750.9
- bile duct (congenital) 751.60
  - acquired 576.8
    - with calculus, choledocholithiasis, or stones — see Choledocholithiasis
- biliary duct or passage (congenital) 751.60
  - acquired 576.8
    - with calculus, choledocholithiasis, or stones — see Choledocholithiasis
- bladder (neck) (spincter) (trigone) (acquired) 596.8
  - congenital 753.9
- bone (acquired) NEC 738.9
  - congenital 756.9
  - turbinate 738.0
- boutonniere (finger) 736.21
- brain (congenital) 742.9
  - acquired 348.8
  - multiple 742.4
  - reduction 742.2
  - vessel (congenital) 747.81
- breast (acquired) 611.8
  - congenital 757.9
- bronchus (congenital) 748.3
  - acquired 519.1
- bursa, congenital 756.9
- canal of Nuck 752.9
- canthus (congenital) 743.9
  - acquired 374.89
- capillary (acquired) 448.9
  - congenital NEC (see also Deformity, vascular) 747.60
- cardiac — see Deformity, heart
- cardiovascular system (congenital) 746.9
- caruncle, lacrimal (congenital) 743.9
  - acquired 375.69
- cascade, stomach 537.6
- cecum (congenital) 751.5
  - acquired 569.89

Deformity — continued
- cerebral (congenital) 742.9
  - acquired 348.8
- cervix (acquired) (uterus) 622.8
  - congenital 752.40
- cheek (acquired) 738.19
  - congenital 744.9
- chest (wall) (acquired) 738.3
  - congenital 754.89
  - late effect of rickets 268.1
- chin (acquired) 738.19
  - congenital 744.9
- choroid (congenital) 743.9
  - acquired 363.8
  - plexus (congenital) 742.9
    - acquired 349.2
- cicatricial — see Cicatrix
- cilia (congenital) 743.9
  - acquired 374.89
- circulatory system (congenital) 747.9
- clavicle (acquired) 738.8
  - congenital 755.51
- clitoris (congenital) 752.40
  - acquired 624.8
- clubfoot — see Clubfoot
- coccyx (acquired) 738.6
  - congenital 756.10
- colon (congenital) 751.5
  - acquired 569.89
- concha (ear) (congenital) (see also Deformity, ear) 744.3
  - acquired 380.32
- congenital, organ or site not listed (see also Anomaly) 759.9
- cornea (congenital) 743.9
  - acquired 371.70
- coronary artery (congenital) 746.85
  - acquired (see also Ischemia, heart) 414.9
- cranium (acquired) 738.19
  - congenital (see also Deformity, skull, congenital) 756.0
- cricoid cartilage (congenital) 748.3
  - acquired 478.79
- cystic duct (congenital) 751.60
  - acquired 575.8
- Dandy-Walker 742.3
  - with spina bifida (see also Spina bifida) 741.0 ✓5ᵗʰ
- diaphragm (congenital) 756.6
  - acquired 738.8
- digestive organ(s) or system (congenital) NEC 751.9
  - specified type NEC 751.8
- ductus arteriosus 747.0
- duodenal bulb 537.89
- duodenum (congenital) 751.5
  - acquired 537.89
- dura (congenital) 742.9
  - brain 742.4
    - acquired 349.2
  - spinal 742.59
    - acquired 349.2
- ear (congenital) 744.3
  - acquired 380.32
  - auricle 744.3
    - causing impairment of hearing 744.02
  - causing impairment of hearing 744.00
  - external 744.3
    - causing impairment of hearing 744.02
  - internal 744.05
  - lobule 744.3
  - middle 744.03
    - ossicles 744.04
  - ossicles 744.04
- ectodermal (congenital) NEC 757.9
  - specified type NEC 757.8
- ejaculatory duct (congenital) 752.9
  - acquired 608.89
- elbow (joint) (acquired) 736.00
  - congenital 755.50
  - contraction 718.42
- endocrine gland NEC 759.2
- epididymis (congenital) 752.9
  - acquired 608.89
  - torsion 608.2
- epiglottis (congenital) 748.3
  - acquired 478.79

Deformity — continued
- esophagus (congenital) 750.9
  - acquired 530.89
- Eustachian tube (congenital) NEC 744.3
  - specified type NEC 744.24
- extremity (acquired) 736.9
  - congenital, except reduction deformity 755.9
    - lower 755.60
    - upper 755.50
  - reduction — see Deformity, reduction
- eye (congenital) 743.9
  - acquired 379.8
  - muscle 743.9
- eyebrow (congenital) 744.89
- eyelid (congenital) 743.9
  - acquired 374.89
  - specified type NEC 743.62
- face (acquired) 738.19
  - congenital (any part) 744.9
    - due to intrauterine malposition and pressure 754.0
- fallopian tube (congenital) 752.10
  - acquired 620.8
- femur (acquired) 736.89
  - congenital 755.60
- fetal
  - with fetopelvic disproportion 653.7 ✓5ᵗʰ
    - affecting fetus or newborn 763.1
  - causing obstructed labor 660.1 ✓5ᵗʰ
    - affecting fetus or newborn 763.1
  - known or suspected, affecting management of pregnancy 655.9 ✓5ᵗʰ
- finger (acquired) 736.20
  - boutonniere type 736.21
  - congenital 755.50
  - flexion contracture 718.44
  - swan neck 736.22
- flexion (joint) (acquired) 736.9
  - congenital NEC 755.9
  - hip or thigh (acquired) 736.39
    - congenital (see also Subluxation, congenital, hip) 754.32
- foot (acquired) 736.70
  - cavovarus 736.75
  - congenital 754.59
  - congenital NEC 754.70
    - specified type NEC 754.79
  - valgus (acquired) 736.79
    - congenital 754.60
      - specified type NEC 754.69
  - varus (acquired) 736.79
    - congenital 754.59
      - specified type NEC 754.59
- forearm (acquired) 736.00
  - congenital 755.50
- forehead (acquired) 738.19
  - congenital (see also Deformity, skull, congenital) 756.0
- frontal bone (acquired) 738.19
  - congenital (see also Deformity, skull, congenital) 756.0
- gallbladder (congenital) 751.60
  - acquired 575.8
- gastrointestinal tract (congenital) NEC 751.9
  - acquired 569.89
  - specified type NEC 751.8
- genitalia, genital organ(s) or system NEC
  - congenital 752.9
  - female (congenital) 752.9
    - acquired 629.8
    - external 752.40
    - internal 752.9
  - male (congenital) 752.9
    - acquired 608.89
- globe (eye) (congenital) 743.9
  - acquired 360.89
- gum (congenital) 750.9
  - acquired 523.9
- gunstock 736.02
- hand (acquired) 736.00
  - claw 736.06
  - congenital 755.50
  - minus (and plus) (intrinsic) 736.09
  - pill roller (intrinsic) 736.09
  - plus (and minus) (intrinsic) 736.09
  - swan neck (intrinsic) 736.09

Deformity

Deformity — continued
- head (acquired) 738.10
  - congenital (see also Deformity, skull congenital) 756.0
  - specified NEC 738.19
- heart (congenital) 746.9
  - auricle (congenital) 746.9
  - septum 745.9
    - auricular 745.5
    - specified type NEC 745.8
    - ventricular 745.4
  - valve (congenital) NEC 746.9
    - acquired — see Endocarditis
    - pulmonary (congenital) 746.00
    - specified type NEC 746.89
  - ventricle (congenital) 746.9
- heel (acquired) 736.76
  - congenital 755.67
- hepatic duct (congenital) 751.60
  - acquired 576.8
    - with calculus, choledocholithiasis, or stones — see Choledocholithiasis
- hip (joint) (acquired) 736.30
  - congenital NEC 755.63
  - flexion 718.45
    - congenital (see also Subluxation, congenital, hip) 754.32
- hourglass — see Contraction, hourglass
- humerus (acquired) 736.89
  - congenital 755.50
- hymen (congenital) 752.40
- hypophyseal (congenital) 759.2
- ileocecal (coil) (valve) (congenital) 751.5
  - acquired 569.89
- ileum (intestine) (congenital) 751.5
  - acquired 569.89
- ilium (acquired) 738.6
  - congenital 755.60
- integument (congenital) 757.9
- intervertebral cartilage or disc (acquired) — see also Displacement, intervertebral disc
  - congenital 756.10
- intestine (large) (small) (congenital) 751.5
  - acquired 569.89
- iris (acquired) 364.75
  - congenital 743.9
  - prolapse 364.8
- ischium (acquired) 738.6
  - congenital 755.60
- jaw (acquired) (congenital) NEC 524.9
  - due to intrauterine malposition and pressure 754.0
- joint (acquired) NEC 738.8
  - congenital 755.9
  - contraction (abduction) (adduction) (extension) (flexion) — see Contraction, joint
- kidney(s) (calyx) (pelvis) (congenital) 753.9
  - acquired 593.89
  - vessel 747.62
    - acquired 459.9
- Klippel-Feil (brevicollis) 756.16
- knee (acquired) NEC 736.6
  - congenital 755.64
- labium (majus) (minus) (congenital) 752.40
  - acquired 624.8
- lacrimal apparatus or duct (congenital) 743.9
  - acquired 375.69
- larynx (muscle) (congenital) 748.3
  - acquired 478.79
  - web (glottic) (subglottic) 748.2
- leg (lower) (upper) (acquired) NEC 736.89
  - congenital 755.60
    - reduction — see Deformity, reduction, lower limb
- lens (congenital) 743.9
  - acquired 379.39
- lid (fold) (congenital) 743.9
  - acquired 374.89
- ligament (acquired) 728.9
  - congenital 756.9
- limb (acquired) 736.9
  - congenital, except reduction deformity 755.9
    - lower 755.60
      - reduction (see also Deformity, reduction, lower limb) 755.30

Deformity — continued
- limb — continued
  - congenital, except reduction deformity — continued
    - upper 755.50
      - reduction (see also Deformity, reduction, upper limb) 755.20
    - specified NEC 736.89
- lip (congenital) NEC 750.9
  - acquired 528.5
  - specified type NEC 750.26
- liver (congenital) 751.60
  - acquired 573.8
  - duct (congenital) 751.60
    - acquired 576.8
      - with calculus, choledocholithiasis, or stones — see Choledocholithiasis
- lower extremity — see Deformity, leg
- lumbosacral (joint) (region) (congenital) 756.10
  - acquired 738.5
- lung (congenital) 748.60
  - acquired 518.89
  - specified type NEC 748.69
- lymphatic system, congenital 759.9
- Madelung's (radius) 755.54
- maxilla (acquired) (congenital) 524.9
- meninges or membrane (congenital) 742.9
  - brain 742.4
    - acquired 349.2
  - spinal (cord) 742.59
    - acquired 349.2
- mesentery (congenital) 751.9
  - acquired 568.89
- metacarpus (acquired) 736.00
  - congenital 755.50
- metatarsus (acquired) 736.70
  - congenital 754.70
- middle ear, except ossicles (congenital) 744.03
  - ossicles 744.04
- mitral (leaflets) (valve) (congenital) 746.9
  - acquired — see Endocarditis, mitral
  - Ebstein's 746.89
  - parachute 746.5
  - specified type NEC 746.89
  - stenosis, congenital 746.5
- mouth (acquired) 528.9
  - congenital NEC 750.9
    - specified type NEC 750.26
- multiple, congenital NEC 759.7
  - specified type NEC 759.89
- muscle (acquired) 728.9
  - congenital 756.9
    - specified type NEC 756.89
    - sternocleidomastoid (due to intrauterine malposition and pressure) 754.1
- musculoskeletal system, congenital NEC 756.9
  - specified type NEC 756.9
- nail (acquired) 703.9
  - congenital 757.9
- nasal — see Deformity, nose
- neck (acquired) NEC 738.2
  - congenital (any part) 744.9
    - sternocleidomastoid 754.1
- nervous system (congenital) 742.9
- nipple (congenital) 757.9
  - acquired 611.8
- nose, nasal (cartilage) (acquired) 738.0
  - bone (turbinate) 738.0
  - congenital 748.1
    - bent 754.0
    - squashed 754.0
  - saddle 738.0
    - syphilitic 090.5
  - septum 470
    - congenital 748.1
  - sinus (wall) (congenital) 748.1
    - acquired 738.0
  - syphilitic (congenital) 090.5
    - late 095.8
- ocular muscle (congenital) 743.9
  - acquired 378.60
- opticociliary vessels (congenital) 743.9
- orbit (congenital) (eye) 743.9
  - acquired NEC 376.40
    - associated with craniofacial deformities 376.44

Deformity — continued
- orbit — continued
  - acquired NEC — continued
    - due to
      - bone disease 376.43
      - surgery 376.47
      - trauma 376.47
- organ of Corti (congenital) 744.05
- ovary (congenital) 752.0
  - acquired 620.8
- oviduct (congenital) 752.10
  - acquired 620.8
- palate (congenital) 750.9
  - acquired 526.89
  - cleft (congenital) (see also Cleft, palate) 749.00
  - hard, acquired 526.89
  - soft, acquired 528.9
- pancreas (congenital) 751.7
  - acquired 577.8
- parachute, mitral valve 746.5
- parathyroid (gland) 759.2
- parotid (gland) (congenital) 750.9
  - acquired 527.8
- patella (acquired) 736.6
  - congenital 755.64
- pelvis, pelvic (acquired) (bony) 738.6
  - with disproportion (fetopelvic) 653.0
    - affecting fetus or newborn 763.1
    - causing obstructed labor 660.1
      - affecting fetus or newborn 763.1
  - congenital 755.60
  - rachitic (late effect) 268.1
- penis (glans) (congenital) 752.9
  - acquired 607.89
- pericardium (congenital) 746.9
  - acquired — see Pericarditis
- pharynx (congenital) 750.9
  - acquired 478.29
- Pierre Robin (congenital) 756.0
- pinna (acquired) 380.32
  - congenital 744.3
- pituitary (congenital) 759.2
- pleural folds (congenital) 748.8
- portal vein (congenital) 747.40
- posture see Curvature, spine
- prepuce (congenital) 752.9
  - acquired 607.89
- prostate (congenital) 752.9
  - acquired 602.8
- pulmonary valve — see Endocarditis, pulmonary
- pupil (congenital) 743.9
  - acquired 364.75
- pylorus (congenital) 750.9
  - acquired 537.89
- rachitic (acquired), healed or old 268.1
- radius (acquired) 736.00
  - congenital 755.50
    - reduction — see Deformity, reduction, upper limb
- rectovaginal septum (congenital) 752.40
  - acquired 623.8
- rectum (congenital) 751.5
  - acquired 569.49
- reduction (extremity) (limb) 755.4
  - brain 742.2
  - lower limb 755.30
    - with complete absence of distal elements 755.31
    - longitudinal (complete) (partial) (with distal deficiencies, incomplete) 755.32
      - with complete absence of distal elements 755.31
      - combined femoral, tibial, fibular (incomplete) 755.33
      - femoral 755.34
      - fibular 755.37
      - metatarsal(s) 755.38
      - phalange(s) 755.39
        - meaning all digits 755.31
      - tarsal(s) 755.38
      - tibia 755.36
      - tibiofibular 755.35
    - transverse 755.31

Index to Diseases

Deformity — *continued*
  reduction — *continued*
    upper limb 755.20
      with complete absence of distal elements 755.21
      longitudinal (complete) (partial) (with distal deficiencies, incomplete) 755.22
        with complete absence of distal elements 755.21
        carpal(s) 755.28
        combined humeral, radial, ulnar (incomplete) 755.23
        humeral 755.24
        metacarpal(s) 755.28
        phalange(s) 755.29
          meaning all digits 755.21
        radial 755.26
        radioulnar 755.25
        ulnar 755.27
      transverse (complete) (partial) 755.21
  renal — *see* Deformity, kidney
  respiratory system (congenital) 748.9
    specified type NEC 748.8
  rib (acquired) 738.3
    congenital 756.3
      cervical 756.2
  rotation (joint) (acquired) 736.9
    congenital 755.9
    hip or thigh 736.39
      congenital (*see also* Subluxation, congenital, hip) 754.32
  sacroiliac joint (congenital) 755.69
    acquired 738.5
  sacrum (acquired) 738.5
    congenital 756.10
  saddle
    back 737.8
    nose 738.0
      syphilitic 090.5
  salivary gland or duct (congenital) 750.9
    acquired 527.8
  scapula (acquired) 736.89
    congenital 755.50
  scrotum (congenital) 752.9
    acquired 608.89
  sebaceous gland, acquired 706.8
  seminal tract or duct (congenital) 752.9
    acquired 608.89
  septum (nasal) (acquired) 470
    congenital 748.1
  shoulder (joint) (acquired) 736.89
    congenital 755.50
      specified type NEC 755.59
    contraction 718.41
  sigmoid (flexure) (congenital) 751.5
    acquired 569.89
  sinus of Valsalva 747.29
  skin (congenital) 757.9
    acquired NEC 709.8
  skull (acquired) 738.19
    congenital 756.0
      with
        anencephalus 740.0
        encephalocele 742.0
        hydrocephalus 742.3
          with spina bifida (*see also* Spina bifida) 741.0 ✓5ᵗʰ
        microcephalus 742.1
      due to intrauterine malposition and pressure 754.0
  soft parts, organs or tissues (of pelvis)
    in pregnancy or childbirth NEC 654.9 ✓5ᵗʰ
      affecting fetus or newborn 763.89
      causing obstructed labor 660.2 ✓5ᵗʰ
        affecting fetus or newborn 763.1
  spermatic cord (congenital) 752.9
    acquired 608.89
      torsion 608.2
  spinal
    column — *see* Deformity, spine
    cord (congenital) 742.9
      acquired 336.8
      vessel (congenital) 747.82
    nerve root (congenital) 742.9
      acquired 724.9

Deformity — *continued*
  spine (acquired) NEC 738.5
    congenital 756.10
      due to intrauterine malposition and pressure 754.2
    kyphoscoliotic (*see also* Kyphoscoliosis) 737.30
    kyphotic (*see also* Kyphosis) 737.10
    lordotic (*see also* Lordosis) 737.20
    rachitic 268.1
    scoliotic (*see also* Scoliosis) 737.30
  spleen
    acquired 289.59
    congenital 759.0
  Sprengel's (congenital) 755.52
  sternum (acquired) 738.3
    congenital 756.3
  stomach (congenital) 750.9
    acquired 537.89
  submaxillary gland (congenital) 750.9
    acquired 527.8
  swan neck (acquired)
    finger 736.22
    hand 736.09
  talipes — *see* Talipes
  teeth, tooth NEC 520.9
  testis (congenital) 752.9
    acquired 608.89
    torsion 608.2
  thigh (acquired) 736.89
    congenital 755.60
  thorax (acquired) (wall) 738.3
    congenital 754.89
    late effect of rickets 268.1
  thumb (acquired) 736.20
    congenital 755.50
  thymus (tissue) (congenital) 759.2
  thyroid (gland) (congenital) 759.2
    cartilage 748.3
      acquired 478.79
  tibia (acquired) 736.89
    congenital 755.60
    saber 090.5
  toe (acquired) 735.9
    congenital 755.66
    specified NEC 735.8
  tongue (congenital) 750.10
    acquired 529.8
  tooth, teeth NEC 520.9
  trachea (rings) (congenital) 748.3
    acquired 519.1
  transverse aortic arch (congenital) 747.21
  tricuspid (leaflets) (valve) (congenital) 746.9
    acquired — *see* Endocarditis, tricuspid
    atresia or stenosis 746.1
    specified type NEC 746.89
  trunk (acquired) 738.3
    congenital 759.9
  ulna (acquired) 736.00
    congenital 755.50
  upper extremity — *see* Deformity, arm
  urachus (congenital) 753.7
  ureter (opening) (congenital) 753.9
    acquired 593.89
  urethra (valve) (congenital) 753.9
    acquired 599.84
  urinary tract or system (congenital) 753.9
    urachus 753.7
  uterus (congenital) 752.3
    acquired 621.8
  uvula (congenital) 750.9
    acquired 528.9
  vagina (congenital) 752.40
    acquired 623.8
  valve, valvular (heart) (congenital) 746.9
    acquired — *see* Endocarditis
    pulmonary 746.00
    specified type NEC 746.89
  vascular (congenital) (peripheral) NEC 747.60
    acquired 459.9
  vas deferens (congenital) 752.9
    acquired 608.89
  vein (congenital) NEC (*see also* Deformity, vascular) 747.60
    brain 747.81
    coronary 746.9
    great 747.40

Deformity — *continued*
  vena cava (inferior) (superior) (congenital) 747.40
  vertebra — *see* Deformity, spine
  vesicourethral orifice (acquired) 596.8
    congenital NEC 753.9
      specified type NEC 753.8
  vessels of optic papilla (congenital) 743.9
  visual field (contraction) 368.45
  vitreous humor (congenital) 743.9
    acquired 379.29
  vulva (congenital) 752.40
    acquired 624.8
  wrist (joint) (acquired) 736.00
    congenital 755.50
    contraction 718.43
    valgus 736.03
      congenital 755.59
    varus 736.04
      congenital 755.59

Degeneration, degenerative
  adrenal (capsule) (gland) 255.8
    with hypofunction 255.4
    fatty 255.8
    hyaline 255.8
    infectional 255.8
    lardaceous 277.3
  amyloid (any site) (general) 277.3
  anterior cornua, spinal cord 336.8
  aorta, aortic 440.0
    fatty 447.8
    valve (heart) (*see also* Endocarditis, aortic) 424.1
  arteriovascular — *see* Arteriosclerosis
  artery, arterial (atheromatous) (calcareous) — *see also* Arteriosclerosis
    amyloid 277.3
    lardaceous 277.3
    medial NEC (*see also* Arteriosclerosis, extremities) 440.20
  articular cartilage NEC (*see also* Disorder, cartilage, articular) 718.0 ✓5ᵗʰ
    elbow 718.02
    knee 717.5
    patella 717.7
    shoulder 718.01
    spine (*see also* Spondylosis) 721.90
  atheromatous — *see* Arteriosclerosis
  bacony (any site) 277.3
  basal nuclei or ganglia NEC 333.0
  bone 733.90
  brachial plexus 353.0
  brain (cortical) (progressive) 331.9
    arteriosclerotic 437.0
    childhood 330.9
      specified type NEC 330.8
    congenital 742.4
    cystic 348.0
      congenital 742.4
    familial NEC 331.89
    grey matter 330.8
    heredofamilial NEC 331.89
    in
      alcoholism 303.9 ✓5ᵗʰ *[331.7]*
      beriberi 265.0 *[331.7]*
      cerebrovascular disease 437.9 *[331.7]*
      congenital hydrocephalus 742.3 *[331.7]*
        with spina bifida (*see also* Spina bifida) 741.0 ✓5ᵗʰ *[331.7]*
      Fabry's disease 272.7 *[330.2]*
      Gaucher's disease 272.7 *[330.2]*
      Hunter's disease or syndrome 277.5 *[330.3]*
      lipidosis
        cerebral 330.1
        generalized 272.7 *[330.2]*
      mucopolysaccharidosis 277.5 *[330.3]*
      myxedema (*see also* Myxedema) 244.9 *[331.7]*
      neoplastic disease NEC (M8000/1) 239.9 *[331.7]*
      Niemann-Pick disease 272.7 *[330.2]*
      sphingolipidosis 272.7 *[330.2]*
      vitamin B_{12} deficiency 266.2 *[331.7]*
    motor centers 331.89
    senile 331.2
    specified type NEC 331.89

Degeneration, degenerative — continued

- breast — see Disease, breast
- Bruch's membrane 363.40
- bundle of His 426.50
  - left 426.3
  - right 426.4
- calcareous NEC 275.49
- capillaries 448.9
  - amyloid 277.3
  - fatty 448.9
  - lardaceous 277.3
- cardiac (brown) (calcareous) (fatty) (fibrous) (hyaline) (mural) (muscular) (pigmentary) (senile) (with arteriosclerosis) (see also Degeneration, myocardial) 429.1
  - valve, valvular — see Endocarditis
- cardiorenal (see also Hypertension, cardiorenal) 404.90
- cardiovascular (see also Disease, cardiovascular) 429.2
  - renal (see also Hypertension, cardiorenal) 404.90
- cartilage (joint) — see Derangement, joint
- cerebellar NEC 334.9
  - primary (hereditary) (sporadic) 334.2
- cerebral — see Degeneration, brain
- cerebromacular 330.1
- cerebrovascular 437.1
  - due to hypertension 437.2
  - late effect — see Late effect(s) (of) cerebrovascular disease
- cervical plexus 353.2
- cervix 622.8
  - due to radiation (intended effect) 622.8
    - adverse effect or misadventure 622.8
- changes, spine or vertebra (see also Spondylosis) 721.90
- chitinous 277.3
- chorioretinal 363.40
  - congenital 743.53
  - hereditary 363.50
- choroid (colloid) (drusen) 363.40
  - hereditary 363.50
  - senile 363.41
    - diffuse secondary 363.42
- cochlear 386.8
- collateral ligament (knee) (medial) 717.82
  - lateral 717.81
- combined (spinal cord) (subacute) 266.2 [336.2]
  - with anemia (pernicious) 281.0 [336.2]
    - due to dietary deficiency 281.1 [336.2]
  - due to vitamin B₁₂ deficiency anemia (dietary) 281.1 [336.2]
- conjunctiva 372.50
  - amyloid 277.3 [372.50]
- cornea 371.40
  - calcerous 371.44
  - familial (hereditary) (see also Dystrophy, cornea) 371.50
    - macular 371.55
    - reticular 371.54
  - hyaline (of old scars) 371.41
  - marginal (Terrien's) 371.48
  - mosaic (shagreen) 371.41
  - nodular 371.46
  - peripheral 371.48
  - senile 371.41
- cortical (cerebellar) (parenchymatous) 334.2
  - alcoholic 303.9 [334.4]
  - diffuse, due to arteriopathy 437.0
- corticostriatal-spinal 334.8
- cretinoid 243
- cruciate ligament (knee) (posterior) 717.84
  - anterior 717.83
- cutis 709.3
  - amyloid 277.3
- dental pulp 522.2
- disc disease — see Degeneration, intervertebral disc
- dorsolateral (spinal cord) — see Degeration, combined
- endocardial 424.90
- extrapyramidal NEC 333.90
- eye NEC 360.40
  - macular (see also Degeneration, macula) 362.50
    - congenital 362.75
    - hereditary 362.76

Degeneration, degenerative — continued

- fatty (diffuse) (general) 272.8
  - liver 571.8
    - alcoholic 571.0
  - localized site — see Degeneration, by site, fatty
  - placenta — see Placenta, abnormal
- globe (eye) NEC 360.40
  - macular — see Degeneration, macula
- grey matter 330.8
- heart (brown) (calcareous) (fatty) (fibrous) (hyaline) (mural) (muscular) (pigmentary) (senile) (with arteriosclerosis) (see also Degeneration, myocardial) 429.1
  - amyloid 277.3 [425.7]
  - atheromatous — see Arteriosclerosis, coronary
  - gouty 274.82
  - hypertensive (see also Hypertension, heart) 402.90
  - ischemic 414.9
  - valve, valvular — see Endocarditis
- hepatolenticular (Wilson's) 275.1
- hepatorenal 572.4
- heredofamilial
  - brain NEC 331.89
  - spinal cord NEC 336.8
- hyaline (diffuse) (generalized) 728.9
  - localized — see also Degeneration, by site
  - cornea 371.41
  - keratitis 371.41
- hypertensive vascular — see Hypertension
- infrapatellar fat pad 729.31
- internal semilunar cartilage 717.3
- intervertebral disc 722.6
  - with myelopathy 722.70
  - cervical, cervicothoracic 722.4
    - with myelopathy 722.71
  - lumbar, lumbosacral 722.52
    - with myelopathy 722.73
  - thoracic, thoracolumbar 722.51
    - with myelopathy 722.72
- intestine 569.89
  - amyloid 277.3
  - lardaceous 277.3
- iris (generalized) (see also Atrophy, iris) 364.59
  - pigmentary 364.53
  - pupillary margin 364.54
- ischemic — see Ischemia
- joint disease (see also Osteoarthrosis) 715.9 ✓5ᵗʰ
  - multiple sites 715.09
  - spine (see also Spondylosis) 721.90
- kidney (see also Sclerosis, renal) 587
  - amyloid 277.3 [583.81]
  - cyst, cystic (multiple) (solitary) 593.2
    - congenital (see also Cystic, disease, kidney) 753.10
  - fatty 593.89
  - fibrocystic (congenital) 753.19
  - lardaceous 277.3 [583.81]
  - polycystic (congenital) 753.12
    - adult type (APKD) 753.13
    - autosomal dominant 753.13
    - autosomal recessive 753.14
    - childhood type (CPKD) 753.14
    - infantile type 753.14
  - waxy 277.3 [583.81]
- Kuhnt-Junius (retina) 362.52
- labyrinth, osseous 386.8
- lacrimal passages, cystic 375.12
- lardaceous (any site) 277.3
- lateral column (posterior), spinal cord (see also Degeneration, combined) 266.2 [336.2]
- lattice 362.63
- lens 366.9
  - infantile, juvenile, or presenile 366.00
  - senile 366.10
- lenticular (familial) (progressive) (Wilson's) (with cirrhosis of liver) 275.1
- striate artery 437.0
- lethal ball, prosthetic heart valve 996.02
- ligament
  - collateral (knee) (medial) 717.82
    - lateral 717.81
  - cruciate (knee) (posterior) 717.84
    - anterior 717.83

Degeneration, degenerative — continued

- liver (diffuse) 572.8
  - amyloid 277.3
  - congenital (cystic) 751.62
  - cystic 572.8
    - congenital 751.62
  - fatty 571.8
    - alcoholic 571.0
  - hypertrophic 572.8
  - lardaceous 277.3
  - parenchymatous, acute or subacute (see also Necrosis, liver) 570
  - pigmentary 572.8
  - toxic (acute) 573.8
  - waxy 277.3
- lung 518.89
- lymph gland 289.3
  - hyaline 289.3
  - lardaceous 277.3
- macula (acquired) (senile) 362.50
  - atrophic 362.51
  - Best's 362.76
  - congenital 362.75
  - cystic 362.54
  - cystoid 362.53
  - disciform 362.52
  - dry 362.51
  - exudative 362.52
  - familial pseudoinflammatory 362.77
  - hereditary 362.76
  - hole 362.54
  - juvenile (Stargardt's) 362.75
  - nonexudative 362.51
  - pseudohole 362.54
  - wet 362.52
- medullary — see Degeneration, brain
- membranous labyrinth, congenital (causing impairment of hearing) 744.05
- meniscus — see Derangement, joint
- microcystoid 362.62
- mitral — see Insufficiency, mitral
- Mönckeberg's (see also Arteriosclerosis, extremities) 440.20
- moral 301.7
- motor centers, senile 331.2
- mural (see also Degeneration, myocardial) 429.1
  - heart, cardiac (see also Degeneration, myocardial) 429.1
  - myocardium, myocardial (see also Degeneration, myocardial) 429.1
- muscle 728.9
  - fatty 728.9
  - fibrous 728.9
  - heart (see also Degeneration, myocardial) 429.1
  - hyaline 728.9
- muscular progressive 728.2
- myelin, central nervous system NEC 341.9
- myocardium, myocardial (brown) (calcareous) (fatty) (fibrous) (hyaline) (mural) (muscular) (pigmentary) (senile) (with arteriosclerosis) 429.1
  - with rheumatic fever (conditions classifiable to 390) 398.0
    - active, acute, or subacute 391.2
      - with chorea 392.0
    - inactive or quiescent (with chorea) 398.0
  - amyloid 277.3 [425.7]
  - congenital 746.89
  - fetus or newborn 779.89 ▲
  - gouty 274.82
  - hypertensive (see also Hypertension, heart) 402.90
  - ischemic 414.8
  - rheumatic (see also Degeneration, myocardium, with rheumatic fever) 398.0
  - syphilitic 093.82
- nasal sinus (mucosa) (see also Sinusitis) 473.9
  - frontal 473.1
  - maxillary 473.0
- nerve — see Disorder, nerve
- nervous system 349.89
  - amyloid 277.3 [357.4]
  - autonomic (see also Neuropathy, peripheral, autonomic) 337.9
  - fatty 349.89

Degeneration, degenerative — *continued*
  nervous system — *continued*
    peripheral autonomic NEC (*see also* Neuropathy, peripheral, autonomic) 337.9
  nipple 611.9
  nose 478.1
  oculoacousticocerebral, congenital (progressive) 743.8
  olivopontocerebellar (familial) (hereditary) 333.0
  osseous labyrinth 386.8
  ovary 620.8
    cystic 620.2
    microcystic 620.2
  pallidal, pigmentary (progressive) 333.0
  pancreas 577.8
    tuberculous (*see also* Tuberculosis) 017.9 ✓5ᵗʰ
  papillary muscle 429.81
  paving stone 362.61
  penis 607.89
  peritoneum 568.89
  pigmentary (diffuse) (general)
    localized — *see* Degeneration, by site
    pallidal (progressive) 333.0
    secondary 362.65
  pineal gland 259.8
  pituitary (gland) 253.8
  placenta (fatty) (fibrinoid) (fibroid) — *see* Placenta, abnormal
  popliteal fat pad 729.31
  posterolateral (spinal cord) (*see also* Degeneration, combined) 266.2 [336.2]
  pulmonary valve (heart) (*see also* Endocarditis, pulmonary) 424.3
  pulp (tooth) 522.2
  pupillary margin 364.54
  renal (*see also* Sclerosis, renal) 587
    fibrocystic 753.19
    polycystic 753.12
      adult type (APKD) 753.13
      autosomal dominant 753.13
      autosomal recessive 753.14
      childhood type (CPKD) 753.14
      infantile type 753.14
  reticuloendothelial system 289.8
  retina (peripheral) 362.60
    with retinal defect (*see also* Detachment, retina, with retinal defect) 361.00
    cystic (senile) 362.50
    cystoid 362.53
    hereditary (*see also* Dystrophy, retina) 362.70
      cerebroretinal 362.71
      congenital 362.75
      juvenile (Stargardt's) 362.75
      macula 362.76
    Kuhnt-Junius 362.52
    lattice 362.63
    macular (*see also* Degeneration, macula) 362.50
    microcystoid 362.62
    palisade 362.63
    paving stone 362.61
    pigmentary (primary) 362.74
      secondary 362.65
    posterior pole (*see also* Degeneration, macula) 362.50
    secondary 362.66
    senile 362.60
      cystic 362.53
      reticular 362.64
  saccule, congenital (causing impairment of hearing) 744.05
  sacculocochlear 386.8
  senile 797
    brain 331.2
    cardiac, heart, or myocardium (*see also* Degeneration, myocardial) 429.1
    motor centers 331.2
    reticule 362.64
    retina, cystic 362.50
    vascular — *see* Arteriosclerosis
  silicone rubber poppet (prosthetic valve) 996.02
  sinus (cystic) (*see also* Sinusitis) 473.9
    polypoid 471.1

Degeneration, degenerative — *continued*
  skin 709.3
    amyloid 277.3
    colloid 709.3
  spinal (cord) 336.8
    amyloid 277.3
    column 733.90
    combined (subacute) (*see also* Degeneration, combined) 266.2 [336.2]
      with anemia (pernicious) 281.0 [336.2]
    dorsolateral (*see also* Degeneration, combined) 266.2 [336.2]
    familial NEC 336.8
    fatty 336.8
    funicular (*see also* Degeneration, combined) 266.2 [336.2]
    heredofamilial NEC 336.8
    posterolateral (*see also* Degeneration, combined) 266.2 [336.2]
    subacute combined — *see* Degeneration, combined
    tuberculous (*see also* Tuberculosis) 013.8 ✓5ᵗʰ
  spine 733.90
  spleen 289.59
    amyloid 277.3
    lardaceous 277.3
  stomach 537.89
    lardaceous 277.3
  strionigral 333.0
  sudoriparous (cystic) 705.89
  suprarenal (capsule) (gland) 255.8
    with hypofunction 255.4
  sweat gland 705.89
  synovial membrane (pulpy) 727.9
  tapetoretinal 362.74
    adult or presenile form 362.50
  testis (postinfectional) 608.89
  thymus (gland) 254.8
    fatty 254.8
    lardaceous 277.3
  thyroid (gland) 246.8
  tricuspid (heart) (valve) *see* Endocarditis, tricuspid
  tuberculous NEC (*see also* Tuberculosis) 011.9 ✓5ᵗʰ
  turbinate 733.90
  uterus 621.8
    cystic 621.8
  vascular (senile) — *see also* Arteriosclerosis
    hypertensive — *see* Hypertension
  vitreoretinal (primary) 362.73
    secondary 362.66
  vitreous humor (with infiltration) 379.21
  wallerian NEC — *see* Disorder, nerve
  waxy (any site) 277.3
  Wilson's hepatolenticular 275.1

Deglutition
  paralysis 784.9
    hysterical 300.11
  pneumonia 507.0

Degos' disease or syndrome 447.8

Degradation disorder, branched-chain amino acid 270.3

Dehiscence
  anastomosis — *see* Complications, anastomosis
  cesarean wound 674.1 ✓5ᵗʰ
  episiotomy 674.2 ✓5ᵗʰ
  operation wound 998.32 ▲
    internal 998.31 ●
  perineal wound (postpartum) 674.2 ✓5ᵗʰ
  postoperative 998.32 ▲
    abdomen 998.32 ▲
      internal 998.31 ●
    internal 998.31 ●
  uterine wound 674.1 ✓5ᵗʰ

Dehydration (cachexia) 276.5
  with
    hypernatremia 276.0 ●
    hyponatremia 276.1 ●
  newborn 775.5

Deiters' nucleus syndrome 386.19

Déjérine's disease 356.0

Déjérine-Klumpke paralysis 767.6

Déjérine-Roussy syndrome 348.8

Déjérine-Sottas disease or neuropathy (hypertrophic) 356.0

Déjérine-Thomas atrophy or syndrome 333.0

de Lange's syndrome (Amsterdam dwarf, mental retardation, and brachycephaly) 759.89

Delay, delayed
  adaptation, cones or rods 368.63
  any plane in pelvis
    affecting fetus or newborn 763.1
    complicating delivery 660.1 ✓5ᵗʰ
  birth or delivery NEC 662.1 ✓5ᵗʰ
    affecting fetus or newborn 763.89
    second twin, triplet, or multiple mate 662.3 ✓5ᵗʰ
  closure — *see also* Fistula
    cranial suture 756.0
    fontanel 756.0
  coagulation NEC 790.92
  conduction (cardiac) (ventricular) 426.9
  delivery NEC 662.1 ✓5ᵗʰ
    second twin, triplet, etc. 662.3 ✓5ᵗʰ
      affecting fetus or newborn 763.89
  development
    in childhood 783.40
      physiological 783.40
    intellectual NEC 315.9
    learning NEC 315.2
    reading 315.00
    sexual 259.0
    speech 315.39
      associated with hyperkinesis 314.1
    spelling 315.09
  gastric emptying 536.8
  menarche 256.39
    due to pituitary hypofunction 253.4
  menstruation (cause unknown) 626.8
  milestone in childhood 783.42
  motility — *see* Hypomotility
  passage of meconium (newborn) 777.1
  primary respiration 768.9
  puberty 259.0
  sexual maturation, female 259.0

Del Castillo's syndrome (germinal aplasia) 606.0

Déleage's disease 359.89 ▲

Delhi (boil) (button) (sore) 085.1

Delinquency (juvenile) 312.9
  group (*see also* Disturbance, conduct) 312.2 ✓5ᵗʰ
  neurotic 312.4

Delirium, delirious 780.09
  acute (psychotic) 293.0
  alcoholic 291.0
    acute 291.0
    chronic 291.1
  alcoholicum 291.0
  chronic (*see also* Psychosis) 293.89
    due to or associated with physical condition — *see* Psychosis, organic
  drug-induced 292.81
  eclamptic (*see also* Eclampsia) 780.39
  exhaustion (*see also* Reaction, stress, acute) 308.9
  hysterical 300.11
  in
    presenile dementia 290.11
    senile dementia 290.3
  induced by drug 292.81
  manic, maniacal (acute) (*see also* Psychosis, affective) 296.0 ✓5ᵗʰ
    recurrent episode 296.1 ✓5ᵗʰ
    single episode 296.0 ✓5ᵗʰ
  puerperal 293.9
  senile 290.3
  subacute (psychotic) 293.1
  thyroid (*see also* Thyrotoxicosis) 242.9 ✓5ᵗʰ
  traumatic — *see also* Injury, intracranial
    with
      lesion, spinal cord — *see* Injury, spinal, by site
      shock, spinal — *see* Injury, spinal, by site
  tremens (impending) 291.0
  uremic — *see* Uremia
  withdrawal
    alcoholic (acute) 291.0
      chronic 291.1
    drug 292.0

Delivery

Delivery

Note — Use the following fifth-digit subclassification with categories 640-648, 651-676:

- 0 unspecified as to episode of care
- 1 delivered, with or without mention of antepartum condition
- 2 delivered, with mention of postpartum complication
- 3 antepartum condition or complication
- 4 postpartum condition or complication

- breech (assisted) (spontaneous) 652.2 ✓5ᵗʰ
  - affecting fetus or newborn 763.0
  - extraction NEC 669.6 ✓5ᵗʰ
- cesarean (for) 669.7 ✓5ᵗʰ
  - abnormal
    - cervix 654.6 ✓5ᵗʰ
    - pelvic organs or tissues 654.9 ✓5ᵗʰ
    - pelvis (bony) (major) NEC 653.0 ✓5ᵗʰ
    - presentation or position 652.9 ✓5ᵗʰ
      - in multiple gestation 652.6 ✓5ᵗʰ
    - size, fetus 653.5 ✓5ᵗʰ
    - soft parts (of pelvis) 654.9 ✓5ᵗʰ
    - uterus, congenital 654.0 ✓5ᵗʰ
    - vagina 654.7 ✓5ᵗʰ
    - vulva 654.8 ✓5ᵗʰ
  - abruptio placentae 641.2 ✓5ᵗʰ
  - acromion presentation 652.8 ✓5ᵗʰ
  - affecting fetus or newborn 763.4
  - anteversion, cervix or uterus 654.4 ✓5ᵗʰ
  - atony, uterus 666.1 ✓5ᵗʰ
  - bicornis or bicornuate uterus 654.0 ✓5ᵗʰ
  - breech presentation 652.2 ✓5ᵗʰ
  - brow presentation 652.4 ✓5ᵗʰ
  - cephalopelvic disproportion (normally formed fetus) 653.4 ✓5ᵗʰ
  - chin presentation 652.4 ✓5ᵗʰ
  - cicatrix of cervix 654.6 ✓5ᵗʰ
  - contracted pelvis (general) 653.1 ✓5ᵗʰ
    - inlet 653.2 ✓5ᵗʰ
    - outlet 653.3 ✓5ᵗʰ
  - cord presentation or prolapse 663.0 ✓5ᵗʰ
  - cystocele 654.4 ✓5ᵗʰ
  - deformity (acquired) (congenital)
    - pelvic organs or tissues NEC 654.9 ✓5ᵗʰ
    - pelvis (bony) NEC 653.0 ✓5ᵗʰ
  - displacement, uterus NEC 654.4 ✓5ᵗʰ
  - disproportion NEC 653.9 ✓5ᵗʰ
  - distress
    - fetal 656.8 ✓5ᵗʰ
    - maternal 669.0 ✓5ᵗʰ
  - eclampsia 642.6 ✓5ᵗʰ
  - face presentation 652.4 ✓5ᵗʰ
  - failed
    - forceps 660.7 ✓5ᵗʰ
    - trial of labor NEC 660.6 ✓5ᵗʰ
    - vacuum extraction 660.7 ✓5ᵗʰ
    - ventouse 660.7 ✓5ᵗʰ
  - fetal deformity 653.7 ✓5ᵗʰ
  - fetal-maternal hemorrhage 656.0 ✓5ᵗʰ
  - fetus, fetal
    - distress 656.8 ✓5ᵗʰ
    - prematurity 656.8 ✓5ᵗʰ
  - fibroid (tumor) (uterus) 654.1 ✓5ᵗʰ
  - footling 652.8 ✓5ᵗʰ
    - with successful version 652.1 ✓5ᵗʰ
  - hemorrhage (antepartum) (intrapartum) NEC 641.9 ✓5ᵗʰ
  - hydrocephalic fetus 653.6 ✓5ᵗʰ
  - incarceration of uterus 654.3 ✓5ᵗʰ
  - incoordinate uterine action 661.4 ✓5ᵗʰ
  - inertia, uterus 661.2 ✓5ᵗʰ
    - primary 661.0 ✓5ᵗʰ
    - secondary 661.1 ✓5ᵗʰ
  - lateroversion, uterus or cervix 654.4 ✓5ᵗʰ
  - mal lie 652.9 ✓5ᵗʰ
  - malposition
    - fetus 652.9 ✓5ᵗʰ
      - in multiple gestation 652.6 ✓5ᵗʰ
    - pelvic organs or tissues NEC 654.9 ✓5ᵗʰ
    - uterus NEC or cervix 654.4 ✓5ᵗʰ
  - malpresentation NEC 652.9 ✓5ᵗʰ
    - in multiple gestation 652.6 ✓5ᵗʰ

Delivery — continued
- cesarean — continued
  - maternal
    - diabetes mellitus 648.0 ✓5ᵗʰ
    - heart disease NEC 648.6 ✓5ᵗʰ
  - meconium in liquor 656.8 ✓5ᵗʰ
    - staining only 792.3
  - oblique presentation 652.3 ✓5ᵗʰ
  - oversize fetus 653.5 ✓5ᵗʰ
  - pelvic tumor NEC 654.9 ✓5ᵗʰ
  - placental insufficiency 656.5 ✓5ᵗʰ
  - placenta previa 641.0 ✓5ᵗʰ
    - with hemorrhage 641.1 ✓5ᵗʰ
  - poor dilation, cervix 661.0 ✓5ᵗʰ
  - preeclampsia 642.4 ✓5ᵗʰ
    - severe 642.5 ✓5ᵗʰ
  - previous
    - cesarean delivery 654.2 ✓5ᵗʰ
    - surgery (to)
      - cervix 654.6 ✓5ᵗʰ
      - gynecological NEC 654.9 ✓5ᵗʰ
      - uterus NEC 654.9 ✓5ᵗʰ
        - previous cesarean delivery 654.2 ✓5ᵗʰ
      - vagina 654.7 ✓5ᵗʰ
  - prolapse
    - arm or hand 652.7 ✓5ᵗʰ
    - uterus 654.4 ✓5ᵗʰ
  - prolonged labor 662.1 ✓5ᵗʰ
  - rectocele 654.4 ✓5ᵗʰ
  - retroversion, uterus or cervix 654.3 ✓5ᵗʰ
  - rigid
    - cervix 654.6 ✓5ᵗʰ
    - pelvic floor 654.4 ✓5ᵗʰ
    - perineum 654.8 ✓5ᵗʰ
    - vagina 654.7 ✓5ᵗʰ
    - vulva 654.8 ✓5ᵗʰ
  - sacculation, pregnant uterus 654.4 ✓5ᵗʰ
  - scar(s)
    - cervix 654.6 ✓5ᵗʰ
    - cesarean delivery 654.2 ✓5ᵗʰ
    - uterus NEC 654.9 ✓5ᵗʰ
      - due to previous cesarean delivery 654.2 ✓5ᵗʰ
  - Shirodkar suture in situ 654.5 ✓5ᵗʰ
  - shoulder presentation 652.8 ✓5ᵗʰ
  - stenosis or stricture, cervix 654.6 ✓5ᵗʰ
  - transverse presentation or lie 652.3 ✓5ᵗʰ
  - tumor, pelvic organs or tissues NEC 654.4 ✓5ᵗʰ
  - umbilical cord presentation or prolapse 663.0 ✓5ᵗʰ
- completely normal case — see category 650
- complicated (by) NEC 669.9 ✓5ᵗʰ
  - abdominal tumor, fetal 653.7 ✓5ᵗʰ
    - causing obstructed labor 660.1 ✓5ᵗʰ
  - abnormal, abnormality of
    - cervix 654.6 ✓5ᵗʰ
      - causing obstructed labor 660.2 ✓5ᵗʰ
    - forces of labor 661.9 ✓5ᵗʰ
    - formation of uterus 654.0 ✓5ᵗʰ
    - pelvic organs or tissues 654.9 ✓5ᵗʰ
      - causing obstructed labor 660.2 ✓5ᵗʰ
    - pelvis (bony) (major) NEC 653.0 ✓5ᵗʰ
      - causing obstructed labor 660.1 ✓5ᵗʰ
    - presentation or position NEC 652.9 ✓5ᵗʰ
      - causing obstructed labor 660.0 ✓5ᵗʰ
    - size, fetus 653.5 ✓5ᵗʰ
      - causing obstructed labor 660.1 ✓5ᵗʰ
    - soft parts (of pelvis) 654.9 ✓5ᵗʰ
      - causing obstructed labor 660.2 ✓5ᵗʰ
    - uterine contractions NEC 661.9 ✓5ᵗʰ
    - uterus (formation) 654.0 ✓5ᵗʰ
      - causing obstructed labor 660.2 ✓5ᵗʰ
    - vagina 654.7 ✓5ᵗʰ
      - causing obstructed labor 660.2 ✓5ᵗʰ
  - abnormally formed uterus (any type) (congenital) 654.0 ✓5ᵗʰ
    - causing obstructed labor 660.2 ✓5ᵗʰ
  - acromion presentation 652.8 ✓5ᵗʰ
    - causing obstructed labor 660.0 ✓5ᵗʰ
  - adherent placenta 667.0 ✓5ᵗʰ
    - with hemorrhage 666.0 ✓5ᵗʰ
  - adhesions, uterus (to abdominal wall) 654.4 ✓5ᵗʰ

Delivery — continued
- complicated (by) NEC — continued
  - advanced maternal age NEC 659.6 ✓5ᵗʰ
    - multigravida 659.6 ✓5ᵗʰ
    - primigravida 659.5 ✓5ᵗʰ
  - air embolism 673.0 ✓5ᵗʰ
  - amnionitis 658.4 ✓5ᵗʰ
  - amniotic fluid embolism 673.1 ✓5ᵗʰ
  - anesthetic death 668.9 ✓5ᵗʰ
  - annular detachment, cervix 665.3 ✓5ᵗʰ
  - antepartum hemorrhage — see Delivery, complicated, hemorrhage
  - anteversion, cervix or uterus 654.4 ✓5ᵗʰ
    - causing obstructed labor 660.2 ✓5ᵗʰ
  - apoplexy 674.0 ✓5ᵗʰ
    - placenta 641.2 ✓5ᵗʰ
  - arrested active phase 661.1 ✓5ᵗʰ
  - asymmetrical pelvis bone 653.0 ✓5ᵗʰ
    - causing obstructed labor 660.1 ✓5ᵗʰ
  - atony, uterus (hypotonic) (inertia) 666.1 ✓5ᵗʰ
    - hypertonic 661.4 ✓5ᵗʰ
  - Bandl's ring 661.4 ✓5ᵗʰ
  - battledore placenta — see Placenta, abnormal
  - bicornis or bicornuate uterus 654.0 ✓5ᵗʰ
    - causing obstructed labor 660.2 ✓5ᵗʰ
  - birth injury to mother NEC 665.9 ✓5ᵗʰ
  - bleeding (see also Delivery, complicated, hemorrhage) 641.9 ✓5ᵗʰ
  - breech presentation (assisted) (buttocks) (complete) (frank) (spontaneous) 652.2 ✓5ᵗʰ
    - with successful version 652.1 ✓5ᵗʰ
  - brow presentation 652.4 ✓5ᵗʰ
  - cephalopelvic disproportion (normally formed fetus) 653.4 ✓5ᵗʰ
    - causing obstructed labor 660.1 ✓5ᵗʰ
  - cerebral hemorrhage 674.0 ✓5ᵗʰ
  - cervical dystocia 661.0 ✓5ᵗʰ
  - chin presentation 652.4 ✓5ᵗʰ
    - causing obstructed labor 660.0 ✓5ᵗʰ
  - cicatrix
    - cervix 654.6 ✓5ᵗʰ
      - causing obstructed labor 660.2 ✓5ᵗʰ
    - vagina 654.7 ✓5ᵗʰ
      - causing obstructed labor 660.2 ✓5ᵗʰ
  - colporrhexis 665.4 ✓5ᵗʰ
    - with perineal laceration 664.0 ✓5ᵗʰ
  - compound presentation 652.8 ✓5ᵗʰ
    - causing obstructed labor 660.0 ✓5ᵗʰ
  - compression of cord (umbilical) 663.2 ✓5ᵗʰ
    - around neck 663.1 ✓5ᵗʰ
    - cord prolapsed 663.0 ✓5ᵗʰ
  - contraction, contracted pelvis 653.1 ✓5ᵗʰ
    - causing obstructed labor 660.1 ✓5ᵗʰ
    - general 653.1 ✓5ᵗʰ
      - causing obstructed labor 660.1 ✓5ᵗʰ
    - inlet 653.2 ✓5ᵗʰ
      - causing obstructed labor 660.1 ✓5ᵗʰ
    - midpelvic 653.8 ✓5ᵗʰ
      - causing obstructed labor 660.1 ✓5ᵗʰ
    - midplane 653.8 ✓5ᵗʰ
      - causing obstructed labor 660.1 ✓5ᵗʰ
    - outlet 653.3 ✓5ᵗʰ
      - causing obstructed labor 660.1 ✓5ᵗʰ
  - contraction ring 661.4 ✓5ᵗʰ
  - cord (umbilical) 663.9 ✓5ᵗʰ
    - around neck, tightly or with compression 663.1 ✓5ᵗʰ
      - without compression 663.3 ✓5ᵗʰ
    - bruising 663.6 ✓5ᵗʰ
    - complication NEC 663.9 ✓5ᵗʰ
      - specified type NEC 663.8 ✓5ᵗʰ
    - compression NEC 663.2 ✓5ᵗʰ
    - entanglement NEC 663.3 ✓5ᵗʰ
      - with compression 663.2 ✓5ᵗʰ
    - forelying 663.0 ✓5ᵗʰ
    - hematoma 663.6 ✓5ᵗʰ
    - marginal attachment 663.8 ✓5ᵗʰ
    - presentation 663.0 ✓5ᵗʰ
    - prolapse (complete) (occult) (partial) 663.0 ✓5ᵗʰ
    - short 663.4 ✓5ᵗʰ
    - specified complication NEC 663.8 ✓5ᵗʰ
    - thrombosis (vessels) 663.6 ✓5ᵗʰ
    - vascular lesion 663.6 ✓5ᵗʰ

Index to Diseases

Delivery — *continued*
  complicated (by) NEC — *continued*
    cord — *continued*
      velamentous insertion 663.8 ✓5ᵗʰ
    Couvelaire uterus 641.2 ✓5ᵗʰ
    cretin pelvis (dwarf type) (male type) 653.1 ✓5ᵗʰ
      causing obstructed labor 660.1 ✓5ᵗʰ
    crossbirth 652.3 ✓5ᵗʰ
      with successful version 652.1 ✓5ᵗʰ
      causing obstructed labor 660.0 ✓5ᵗʰ
    cyst (Gartner's duct) 654.7 ✓5ᵗʰ
    cystocele 654.4 ✓5ᵗʰ
      causing obstructed labor 660.2 ✓5ᵗʰ
    death of fetus (near term) 656.4 ✓5ᵗʰ
      early (before 22 completed weeks gestation) 632
    deformity (acquired) (congenital)
      fetus 653.7 ✓5ᵗʰ
        causing obstructed labor 660.1 ✓5ᵗʰ
      pelvic organs or tissues NEC 654.9 ✓5ᵗʰ
        causing obstructed labor 660.2 ✓5ᵗʰ
      pelvis (bony) NEC 653.0 ✓5ᵗʰ
        causing obstructed labor 660.1 ✓5ᵗʰ
    delay, delayed
      delivery in multiple pregnancy 662.3 ✓5ᵗʰ
        due to locked mates 660.5 ✓5ᵗʰ
      following rupture of membranes (spontaneous) 658.2 ✓5ᵗʰ
        artificial 658.3 ✓5ᵗʰ
    depressed fetal heart tones 659.7 ✓5ᵗʰ
    diastasis recti 665.8 ✓5ᵗʰ
    dilation
      bladder 654.4 ✓5ᵗʰ
        causing obstructed labor 660.2 ✓5ᵗʰ
      cervix, incomplete, poor or slow 661.0 ✓5ᵗʰ
    diseased placenta 656.7 ✓5ᵗʰ
    displacement uterus NEC 654.4 ✓5ᵗʰ
      causing obstructed labor 660.2 ✓5ᵗʰ
    disproportion NEC 653.9 ✓5ᵗʰ
      causing obstructed labor 660.1 ✓5ᵗʰ
    disruptio uteri — *see* Delivery, complicated, rupture, uterus
    distress
      fetal 656.8 ✓5ᵗʰ
      maternal 669.0 ✓5ᵗʰ
    double uterus (congenital) 654.0 ✓5ᵗʰ
      causing obstructed labor 660.2 ✓5ᵗʰ
    dropsy amnion 657 ✓4ᵗʰ
    dysfunction, uterus 661.9 ✓5ᵗʰ
      hypertonic 661.4 ✓5ᵗʰ
      hypotonic 661.2 ✓5ᵗʰ
        primary 661.0 ✓5ᵗʰ
        secondary 661.1 ✓5ᵗʰ
      incoordinate 661.4 ✓5ᵗʰ
    dystocia
      cervical 661.0 ✓5ᵗʰ
      fetal — *see* Delivery, complicated, abnormal presentation
      maternal — *see* Delivery, complicated, prolonged labor
      pelvic — *see* Delivery, complicated, contraction pelvis
      positional 652.8 ✓5ᵗʰ
      shoulder girdle 660.4 ✓5ᵗʰ
    eclampsia 642.6 ✓5ᵗʰ
    ectopic kidney 654.4 ✓5ᵗʰ
      causing obstructed labor 660.2 ✓5ᵗʰ
    edema, cervix 654.6 ✓5ᵗʰ
      causing obstructed labor 660.2 ✓5ᵗʰ
    effusion, amniotic fluid 658.1 ✓5ᵗʰ
    elderly multigravida 659.6 ✓5ᵗʰ
    elderly primigravida 659.5 ✓5ᵗʰ
    embolism (pulmonary) 673.2 ✓5ᵗʰ
      air 673.0 ✓5ᵗʰ
      amniotic fluid 673.1 ✓5ᵗʰ
      blood clot 673.2 ✓5ᵗʰ
      cerebral 674.0 ✓5ᵗʰ
      fat 673.8 ✓5ᵗʰ
      pyemic 673.3 ✓5ᵗʰ
      septic 673.3 ✓5ᵗʰ
    entanglement, umbilical cord 663.3 ✓5ᵗʰ
      with compression 663.2 ✓5ᵗʰ
        around neck (with compression) 663.1 ✓5ᵗʰ
    eversion, cervix or uterus 665.2 ✓5ᵗʰ

Delivery — *continued*
  complicated (by) NEC — *continued*
    excessive
      fetal growth 653.5 ✓5ᵗʰ
        causing obstructed labor 660.1 ✓5ᵗʰ
      size of fetus 653.5 ✓5ᵗʰ
        causing obstructed labor 660.1 ✓5ᵗʰ
    face presentation 652.4 ✓5ᵗʰ
      causing obstructed labor 660.0 ✓5ᵗʰ
      to pubes 660.3 ✓5ᵗʰ
    failure, fetal head to enter pelvic brim 652.5 ✓5ᵗʰ
      causing obstructed labor 660.0 ✓5ᵗʰ
    fetal
      acid-base balance 656.8 ✓5ᵗʰ
      death (near term) NEC 656.4 ✓5ᵗʰ
        early (before 22 completed weeks gestation) 632
      deformity 653.7 ✓5ᵗʰ
        causing obstructed labor 660.1 ✓5ᵗʰ
      distress 656.8 ✓5ᵗʰ
      heart rate or rhythm 659.7 ✓5ᵗʰ
    fetopelvic disproportion 653.4 ✓5ᵗʰ
      causing obstructed labor 660.1 ✓5ᵗʰ
    fever during labor 659.2 ✓5ᵗʰ
    fibroid (tumor) (uterus) 654.1 ✓5ᵗʰ
      causing obstructed labor 660.2 ✓5ᵗʰ
    fibromyomata 654.1 ✓5ᵗʰ
      causing obstructed labor 660.2 ✓5ᵗʰ
    forelying umbilical cord 663.0 ✓5ᵗʰ
    fracture of coccyx 665.6 ✓5ᵗʰ
    hematoma 664.5 ✓5ᵗʰ
      broad ligament 665.7 ✓5ᵗʰ
      ischial spine 665.7 ✓5ᵗʰ
      pelvic 665.7 ✓5ᵗʰ
      perineum 664.5 ✓5ᵗʰ
      soft tissues 665.7 ✓5ᵗʰ
      subdural 674.0 ✓5ᵗʰ
      umbilical cord 663.6 ✓5ᵗʰ
      vagina 665.7 ✓5ᵗʰ
      vulva or perineum 664.5 ✓5ᵗʰ
    hemorrhage (uterine) (antepartum) (intrapartum) (pregnancy) 641.9 ✓5ᵗʰ
      accidental 641.2 ✓5ᵗʰ
      associated with
        afibrinogenemia 641.3 ✓5ᵗʰ
        coagulation defect 641.3 ✓5ᵗʰ
          hyperfibrinolysis 641.3 ✓5ᵗʰ
          hypofibrinogenemia 641.3 ✓5ᵗʰ
      cerebral 674.0 ✓5ᵗʰ
      due to
        low-lying placenta 641.1 ✓5ᵗʰ
        placenta previa 641.1 ✓5ᵗʰ
        premature separation of placenta (normally implanted) 641.2 ✓5ᵗʰ
        retained placenta 666.0 ✓5ᵗʰ
        trauma 641.8 ✓5ᵗʰ
        uterine leiomyoma 641.8 ✓5ᵗʰ
      marginal sinus rupture 641.2 ✓5ᵗʰ
      placenta NEC 641.9 ✓5ᵗʰ
      postpartum (atonic) (immediate) (within 24 hours) 666.1 ✓5ᵗʰ
        with retained or trapped placenta 666.0 ✓5ᵗʰ
        delayed 666.2 ✓5ᵗʰ
        secondary 666.2 ✓5ᵗʰ
        third stage 666.0 ✓5ᵗʰ
    hourglass contraction, uterus 661.4 ✓5ᵗʰ
    hydramnios 657 ✓5ᵗʰ
    hydrocephalic fetus 653.6 ✓5ᵗʰ
      causing obstructed labor 660.1 ✓5ᵗʰ
    hydrops fetalis 653.7 ✓5ᵗʰ
      causing obstructed labor 660.1 ✓5ᵗʰ
    hypertension — *see* Hypertension, complicating pregnancy
    hypertonic uterine dysfunction 661.4 ✓5ᵗʰ
    hypotonic uterine dysfunction 661.2 ✓5ᵗʰ
    impacted shoulders 660.4 ✓5ᵗʰ
    incarceration, uterus 654.3 ✓5ᵗʰ
      causing obstructed labor 660.2 ✓5ᵗʰ
    incomplete dilation (cervix) 661.0 ✓5ᵗʰ
    incoordinate uterus 661.4 ✓5ᵗʰ
    indication NEC 659.9 ✓5ᵗʰ
      specified type 659.8 ✓5ᵗʰ
    inertia, uterus 661.2 ✓5ᵗʰ
      hypertonic 661.4 ✓5ᵗʰ

Delivery — *continued*
  complicated (by) NEC — *continued*
    inertia, uterus — *continued*
      hypotonic 661.2 ✓5ᵗʰ
      primary 661.0 ✓5ᵗʰ
      secondary 661.1 ✓5ᵗʰ
    infantile
      genitalia 654.4 ✓5ᵗʰ
        causing obstructed labor 660.2 ✓5ᵗʰ
      uterus (os) 654.4 ✓5ᵗʰ
        causing obstructed labor 660.2 ✓5ᵗʰ
    injury (to mother) NEC 665.9 ✓5ᵗʰ
    intrauterine fetal death (near term) NEC 656.4 ✓5ᵗʰ
      early (before 22 completed weeks gestation) 632
    inversion, uterus 665.2 ✓5ᵗʰ
    kidney, ectopic 654.4 ✓5ᵗʰ
      causing obstructed labor 660.2 ✓5ᵗʰ
    knot (true), umbilical cord 663.2 ✓5ᵗʰ
    labor, premature (before 37 completed weeks gestation) 644.2 ✓5ᵗʰ
    laceration 664.9 ✓5ᵗʰ
      anus (spincter) 664.2 ✓5ᵗʰ
        with mucosa 664.3 ✓5ᵗʰ
      bladder (urinary) 665.5 ✓5ᵗʰ
      bowel 665.5 ✓5ᵗʰ
      central 664.4 ✓5ᵗʰ
      cervix (uteri) 665.3 ✓5ᵗʰ
      fourchette 664.0 ✓5ᵗʰ
      hymen 664.0 ✓5ᵗʰ
      labia (majora) (minora) 664.0 ✓5ᵗʰ
      pelvic
        floor 664.1 ✓5ᵗʰ
        organ NEC 665.5 ✓5ᵗʰ
      perineum, perineal 664.4 ✓5ᵗʰ
        first degree 664.0 ✓5ᵗʰ
        second degree 664.1 ✓5ᵗʰ
        third degree 664.2 ✓5ᵗʰ
        fourth degree 664.3 ✓5ᵗʰ
        central 664.4 ✓5ᵗʰ
        extensive NEC 664.4 ✓5ᵗʰ
        muscles 664.1 ✓5ᵗʰ
        skin 664.0 ✓5ᵗʰ
        slight 664.0 ✓5ᵗʰ
      peritoneum 665.5 ✓5ᵗʰ
      periurethral tissue 665.5 ✓5ᵗʰ
      rectovaginal (septum) (without perineal laceration) 665.4 ✓5ᵗʰ
        with perineum 664.2 ✓5ᵗʰ
          with anal rectal mucosa 664.3 ✓5ᵗʰ
      skin (perineum) 664.0 ✓5ᵗʰ
      specified site or type NEC 664.8 ✓5ᵗʰ
      sphincter ani 664.2 ✓5ᵗʰ
        with mucosa 664.3 ✓5ᵗʰ
      urethra 665.5 ✓5ᵗʰ
      uterus 665.1 ✓5ᵗʰ
        before labor 665.0 ✓5ᵗʰ
      vagina, vaginal (deep) (high) (sulcus) (wall) (without perineal laceration) 665.4 ✓5ᵗʰ
        with perineum 664.0 ✓5ᵗʰ
        muscles, with perineum 664.1 ✓5ᵗʰ
      vulva 664.0 ✓5ᵗʰ
    lateroversion, uterus or cervix 654.4 ✓5ᵗʰ
      causing obstructed labor 660.2 ✓5ᵗʰ
    locked mates 660.5 ✓5ᵗʰ
    low implantation of placenta — *see* Delivery, complicated, placenta, previa
    mal lie 652.9 ✓5ᵗʰ
    malposition
      fetus NEC 652.9 ✓5ᵗʰ
        causing obstructed labor 660.0 ✓5ᵗʰ
      pelvic organs or tissues NEC 654.9 ✓5ᵗʰ
        causing obstructed labor 660.2 ✓5ᵗʰ
      placenta 641.1 ✓5ᵗʰ
        without hemorrhage 641.0 ✓5ᵗʰ
      uterus NEC or cervix 654.4 ✓5ᵗʰ
        causing obstructed labor 660.2 ✓5ᵗʰ
    malpresentation 652.9 ✓5ᵗʰ
      causing obstructed labor 660.0 ✓5ᵗʰ
    marginal sinus (bleeding) (rupture) 641.2 ✓5ᵗʰ
    maternal hypotension syndrome 669.2 ✓5ᵗʰ
    meconium in liquor 656.8 ✓5ᵗʰ

Delivery

Delivery — *continued*
  complicated (by) NEC — *continued*
    membranes, retained — *see* Delivery, complicated, placenta, retained
    mentum presentation 652.4 ✓5ᵗʰ
      causing obstructed labor 660.0 ✓5ᵗʰ
    metrorrhagia (myopathia) — *see* Delivery, complicated, hemorrhage
    metrorrhexis — *see* Delivery, complicated, rupture, uterus
    multiparity (grand) 659.4 ✓5ᵗʰ
    myelomeningocele, fetus 653.7 ✓5ᵗʰ
      causing obstructed labor 660.1 ✓5ᵗʰ
    Nägele's pelvis 653.0 ✓5ᵗʰ
      causing obstructed labor 660.1 ✓5ᵗʰ
    nonengagement, fetal head 652.5 ✓5ᵗʰ
      causing obstructed labor 660.0 ✓5ᵗʰ
    oblique presentation 652.3 ✓5ᵗʰ
      causing obstructed labor 660.0 ✓5ᵗʰ
    obstetric
      shock 669.1 ✓5ᵗʰ
      trauma NEC 665.9 ✓5ᵗʰ
    obstructed labor 660.9 ✓5ᵗʰ
      due to
        abnormality pelvic organs or tissues (conditions classifiable to 654.0-654.9) 660.2 ✓5ᵗʰ
        deep transverse arrest 660.3 ✓5ᵗʰ
        impacted shoulders 660.4 ✓5ᵗʰ
        locked twins 660.5 ✓5ᵗʰ
        malposition and malpresentation of fetus (conditions classifiable to 652.0-652.9) 660.0 ✓5ᵗʰ
        persistent occipitoposterior 660.3 ✓5ᵗʰ
        shoulder dystocia 660.4 ✓5ᵗʰ
    occult prolapse of umbilical cord 663.0 ✓5ᵗʰ
    oversize fetus 653.5 ✓5ᵗʰ
      causing obstructed labor 660.1 ✓5ᵗʰ
    pathological retraction ring, uterus 661.4 ✓5ᵗʰ
    pelvic
      arrest (deep) (high) (of fetal head) (transverse) 660.3 ✓5ᵗʰ
      deformity (bone) — *see also* Deformity, pelvis, with disproportion
      soft tissue 654.9 ✓5ᵗʰ
        causing obstructed labor 660.2 ✓5ᵗʰ
      tumor NEC 654.9 ✓5ᵗʰ
        causing obstructed labor 660.2 ✓5ᵗʰ
    penetration, pregnant uterus by instrument 665.1 ✓5ᵗʰ
    perforation — *see* Delivery, complicated, laceration
    persistent
      hymen 654.8 ✓5ᵗʰ
        causing obstructed labor 660.2 ✓5ᵗʰ
      occipitoposterior 660.3 ✓5ᵗʰ
    placenta, placental
      ablatio 641.2 ✓5ᵗʰ
      abnormality 656.7 ✓5ᵗʰ
        with hemorrhage 641.2 ✓5ᵗʰ
      abruptio 641.2 ✓5ᵗʰ
      accreta 667.0 ✓5ᵗʰ
        with hemorrhage 666.0 ✓5ᵗʰ
      adherent (without hemorrhage) 667.0 ✓5ᵗʰ
        with hemorrhage 666.0 ✓5ᵗʰ
      apoplexy 641.2 ✓5ᵗʰ
      battledore placenta — *see* Placenta, abnormal 663.8 ✓5ᵗʰ
      detachment (premature) 641.2 ✓5ᵗʰ
      disease 656.7 ✓5ᵗʰ
      hemorrhage NEC 641.9 ✓5ᵗʰ
      increta (without hemorrhage) 667.0 ✓5ᵗʰ
        with hemorrhage 666.0 ✓5ᵗʰ
      low (implantation) 641.0 ✓5ᵗʰ
        without hemorrhage 641.0 ✓5ᵗʰ
      malformation 656.7 ✓5ᵗʰ
        with hemorrhage 641.2 ✓5ᵗʰ
      malposition 641.1 ✓5ᵗʰ
        without hemorrhage 641.0 ✓5ᵗʰ
      marginal sinus rupture 641.2 ✓5ᵗʰ
      percreta 667.0 ✓5ᵗʰ
        with hemorrhage 666.0 ✓5ᵗʰ
      premature separation 641.2 ✓5ᵗʰ
      previa (central) (lateral) (marginal) partial) 641.1 ✓5ᵗʰ

Delivery — *continued*
  complicated (by) NEC — *continued*
    placenta, placental — *continued*
      previa — *continued*
        without hemorrhage 641.0 ✓5ᵗʰ
      retained (with hemorrhage) 666.0 ✓5ᵗʰ
        without hemorrhage 667.0 ✓5ᵗʰ
      rupture of marginal sinus 641.2 ✓5ᵗʰ
      separation (premature) 641.2 ✓5ᵗʰ
      trapped 666.0 ✓5ᵗʰ
        without hemorrhage 667.0 ✓5ᵗʰ
      vicious insertion 641.1 ✓5ᵗʰ
    polyhydramnios 657 ✓4ᵗʰ
    polyp, cervix 654.6 ✓5ᵗʰ
      causing obstructed labor 660.2 ✓5ᵗʰ
    precipitate labor 661.3 ✓5ᵗʰ
    premature
      labor (before 37 completed weeks gestation) 644.2 ✓5ᵗʰ
      rupture, membranes 658.1 ✓5ᵗʰ
        delayed delivery following 658.2 ✓5ᵗʰ
    presenting umbilical cord 663.0 ✓5ᵗʰ
    previous
      cesarean delivery 654.2 ✓5ᵗʰ
      surgery
        cervix 654.6 ✓5ᵗʰ
          causing obstructed labor 660.2 ✓5ᵗʰ
        gynecological NEC 654.9 ✓5ᵗʰ
          causing obstructed labor 660.2 ✓5ᵗʰ
        perineum 654.8 ✓5ᵗʰ
        uterus NEC 654.9 ✓5ᵗʰ
          due to previous cesarean delivery 654.2 ✓5ᵗʰ
        vagina 654.7 ✓5ᵗʰ
          causing obstructed labor 660.2 ✓5ᵗʰ
        vulva 654.8 ✓5ᵗʰ
    primary uterine inertia 661.0 ✓5ᵗʰ
    primipara, elderly or old 659.5 ✓5ᵗʰ
    prolapse
      arm or hand 652.7 ✓5ᵗʰ
        causing obstructed labor 660.0 ✓5ᵗʰ
      cord (umbilical) 663.0 ✓5ᵗʰ
      fetal extremity 652.8 ✓5ᵗʰ
      foot or leg 652.8 ✓5ᵗʰ
        causing obstructed labor 660.0 ✓5ᵗʰ
      umbilical cord (complete) (occult) (partial) 663.0 ✓5ᵗʰ
      uterus 654.4 ✓5ᵗʰ
        causing obstructed labor 660.2 ✓5ᵗʰ
    prolonged labor 662.1 ✓5ᵗʰ
      first stage 662.0 ✓5ᵗʰ
      second stage 662.2 ✓5ᵗʰ
      active phase 661.2 ✓5ᵗʰ
      due to
        cervical dystocia 661.0 ✓5ᵗʰ
        contraction ring 661.4 ✓5ᵗʰ
        tetanic uterus 661.4 ✓5ᵗʰ
        uterine inertia 661.2 ✓5ᵗʰ
          primary 661.0 ✓5ᵗʰ
          secondary 661.1 ✓5ᵗʰ
      latent phase 661.0 ✓5ᵗʰ
    pyrexia during labor 659.2 ✓5ᵗʰ
    rachitic pelvis 653.2 ✓5ᵗʰ
      causing obstructed labor 660.1 ✓5ᵗʰ
    rectocele 654.4 ✓5ᵗʰ
      causing obstructed labor 660.2 ✓5ᵗʰ
    retained membranes or portions of placenta 666.2 ✓5ᵗʰ
      without hemorrhage 667.1 ✓5ᵗʰ
    retarded (prolonged) birth 662.1 ✓5ᵗʰ
    retention secundines (with hemorrhage) 666.2 ✓5ᵗʰ
      without hemorrhage 667.1 ✓5ᵗʰ
    retroversion, uterus or cervix 654.3 ✓5ᵗʰ
      causing obstructed labor 660.2 ✓5ᵗʰ
    rigid
      cervix 654.6 ✓5ᵗʰ
        causing obstructed labor 660.2 ✓5ᵗʰ
      pelvic floor 654.4 ✓5ᵗʰ
        causing obstructed labor 660.2 ✓5ᵗʰ
      perineum or vulva 654.8 ✓5ᵗʰ
        causing obstructed labor 660.2 ✓5ᵗʰ
      vagina 654.7 ✓5ᵗʰ
        causing obstructed labor 660.2 ✓5ᵗʰ
    Robert's pelvis 653.0 ✓5ᵗʰ
      causing obstructed labor 660.1 ✓5ᵗʰ

Delivery — *continued*
  complicated (by) NEC — *continued*
    rupture — *see also* Delivery, complicated, laceration
      bladder (urinary) 665.5 ✓5ᵗʰ
      cervix 665.3 ✓5ᵗʰ
      marginal sinus 641.2 ✓5ᵗʰ
      membranes, premature 658.1 ✓5ᵗʰ
      pelvic organ NEC 665.5 ✓5ᵗʰ
      perineum (without mention of other laceration) — *see* Delivery, complicated, laceration, perineum
      peritoneum 665.5 ✓5ᵗʰ
      urethra 665.5 ✓5ᵗʰ
      uterus (during labor) 665.1 ✓5ᵗʰ
        before labor 665.0 ✓5ᵗʰ
    sacculation, pregnant uterus 654.4 ✓5ᵗʰ
    sacral teratomas, fetal 653.7 ✓5ᵗʰ
      causing obstructed labor 660.1 ✓5ᵗʰ
    scar(s)
      cervix 654.6 ✓5ᵗʰ
        causing obstructed labor 660.2 ✓5ᵗʰ
      cesarean delivery 654.2 ✓5ᵗʰ
        causing obstructed labor 660.2 ✓5ᵗʰ
      perineum 654.8 ✓5ᵗʰ
        causing obstructed labor 660.2 ✓5ᵗʰ
      uterus NEC 654.9 ✓5ᵗʰ
        causing obstructed labor 660.2 ✓5ᵗʰ
        due to previous cesarean delivery 654.2 ✓5ᵗʰ
      vagina 654.7 ✓5ᵗʰ
        causing obstructed labor 660.2 ✓5ᵗʰ
      vulva 654.8 ✓5ᵗʰ
        causing obstructed labor 660.2 ✓5ᵗʰ
    scoliotic pelvis 653.0 ✓5ᵗʰ
      causing obstructed labor 660.1 ✓5ᵗʰ
    secondary uterine inertia 661.1 ✓5ᵗʰ
    secundines, retained — *see* Delivery, complicated, placenta, retained
    separation
      placenta (premature) 641.2 ✓5ᵗʰ
      pubic bone 665.6 ✓5ᵗʰ
      symphysis pubis 665.6 ✓5ᵗʰ
    septate vagina 654.7 ✓5ᵗʰ
      causing obstructed labor 660.2 ✓5ᵗʰ
    shock (birth) (obstetric) (puerperal) 669.1 ✓5ᵗʰ
    short cord syndrome 663.4 ✓5ᵗʰ
    shoulder
      girdle dystocia 660.4 ✓5ᵗʰ
      presentation 652.8 ✓5ᵗʰ
        causing obstructed labor 660.0 ✓5ᵗʰ
    Siamese twins 653.7 ✓5ᵗʰ
      causing obstructed labor 660.1 ✓5ᵗʰ
    slow slope active phase 661.2 ✓5ᵗʰ
    spasm
      cervix 661.4 ✓5ᵗʰ
      uterus 661.4 ✓5ᵗʰ
    spondylolisthesis, pelvis 653.3 ✓5ᵗʰ
      causing obstructed labor 660.1 ✓5ᵗʰ
    spondylolysis (lumbosacral) 653.3 ✓5ᵗʰ
      causing obstructed labor 660.1 ✓5ᵗʰ
    spondylosis 653.0 ✓5ᵗʰ
      causing obstructed labor 660.1 ✓5ᵗʰ
    stenosis or stricture
      cervix 654.6 ✓5ᵗʰ
        causing obstructed labor 660.2 ✓5ᵗʰ
      vagina 654.7 ✓5ᵗʰ
        causing obstructed labor 660.2 ✓5ᵗʰ
    sudden death, unknown cause 669.9 ✓5ᵗʰ
    tear (pelvic organ) (*see also* Delivery, complicated, laceration) 664.9 ✓5ᵗʰ
    teratomas, sacral, fetal 653.7 ✓5ᵗʰ
      causing obstructed labor 660.1 ✓5ᵗʰ
    tetanic uterus 661.4 ✓5ᵗʰ
    tipping pelvis 653.0 ✓5ᵗʰ
      causing obstructed labor 660.1 ✓5ᵗʰ
    transverse
      arrest (deep) 660.3 ✓5ᵗʰ
      presentation or lie 652.3 ✓5ᵗʰ
        with successful version 652.1 ✓5ᵗʰ
        causing obstructed labor 660.0 ✓5ᵗʰ
    trauma (obstetrical) NEC 665.9 ✓5ᵗʰ
    tumor
      abdominal, fetal 653.7 ✓5ᵗʰ
        causing obstructed labor 660.1 ✓5ᵗʰ

Delivery — *continued*
complicated (by) NEC — *continued*
tumor — *continued*
pelvic organs or tissues NEC 654.9 ✓5
causing obstructed labor 660.2 ✓5
umbilical cord (*see also* Delivery,
complicated, cord) 663.9 ✓5
around neck tightly, or with compression
663.1 ✓5
entanglement NEC 663.3 ✓5
with compression 663.2 ✓5
prolapse (complete) (occult) (partial)
663.0 ✓5
unstable lie 652.0 ✓5
causing obstructed labor 660.0 ✓5
uterine
inertia (*see also* Delivery, complicated,
inertia, uterus) 661.2 ✓5
spasm 661.4 ✓5
vasa previa 663.5 ✓5
velamentous insertion of cord 663.8 ✓5
young maternal age 659.8 ✓5
delayed NEC 662.1 ✓5
following rupture of membranes
(spontaneous) 658.2 ✓5
artificial 658.3 ✓5
second twin, triplet, etc. 662.3 ✓5
difficult NEC 669.9 ✓5
previous, affecting management of
pregnancy or childbirth V23.49 ▲
specified type NEC 669.8 ✓5
early onset (spontaneous) 644.2 ✓5
footling 652.8 ✓5
with successful version 652.1 ✓5
forceps NEC 669.5 ✓5
affecting fetus or newborn 763.2
missed (at or near term) 656.4 ✓5
multiple gestation NEC 651.9 ✓5
with fetal loss and retention of one or more
fetus(es) 651.6 ✓5
specified type NEC 651.8 ✓5
with fetal loss and retention of one or
more fetus(es) 651.6 ✓5
nonviable infant 656.4 ✓5
normal — *see* category 650
precipitate 661.3 ✓5
affecting fetus or newborn 763.6
premature NEC (before 37 completed weeks
gestation) 644.2 ✓5
previous, affecting management of
pregnancy V23.41 ▲
quadruplet NEC 651.2 ✓5
with fetal loss and retention of one or more
fetus(es) 651.5 ✓5
quintuplet NEC 651.8 ✓5
with fetal loss and retention of one or more
fetus(es) 651.6 ✓5
sextuplet NEC 651.8 ✓5
with fetal loss and retention of one or more
fetus(es) 651.6 ✓5
specified complication NEC 669.8 ✓5
stillbirth (near term) NEC 656.4 ✓5
early (before 22 completed weeks gestation)
632
term pregnancy (live birth) NEC — *see* category
650
stillbirth NEC 656.4 ✓5
threatened premature 644.2 ✓5
triplets NEC 651.1 ✓5
with fetal loss and retention of one or more
fetus(es) 651.4 ✓5
delayed delivery (one or more mates)
662.3 ✓5
locked mates 660.5 ✓5
twins NEC 651.0 ✓5
with fetal loss and retention of one fetus
651.3 ✓5
delayed delivery (one or more mates)
662.3 ✓5
locked mates 660.5 ✓5
uncomplicated — *see* category 650
vacuum extractor NEC 669.5 ✓5
affecting fetus or newborn 763.3
ventouse NEC 669.5 ✓5
affecting fetus or newborn 763.3
Dellen, cornea 371.41

Delusions (paranoid) 297.9
grandiose 297.1
parasitosis 300.29
systematized 297.1
Dementia 294.8
alcoholic (*see also* Psychosis, alcoholic) 291.2
Alzheimer's — *see* Alzheimer's dementia
arteriosclerotic (simple type) (uncomplicated)
290.40
with
acute confusional state 290.41
delirium 290.41
delusional features 290.42
depressive features 290.43
depressed type 290.43
paranoid type 290.42
Binswanger's 290.12
catatonic (acute) (*see also* Schizophrenia)
295.2 ✓5
congenital (*see also* Retardation, mental) 319
degenerative 290.9
presenile-onset — *see* Dementia, presenile
senile-onset — *see* Dementia, senile
developmental (*see also* Schizophrenia)
295.9 ✓5
dialysis 294.8
transient 293.9
due to or associated with condition(s) classified
elsewhere
Alzheimer's
with behavioral disturbance
331.0 [294.11]
without behavioral disturbance
331.0 [294.10]
cerebral lipidoses
with behavioral disturbance
330.1 [294.11]
without behavioral disturbance
330.1 [294.10]
epilepsy
with behavioral disturbance
345.9 ✓5 [294.11]
without behavioral disturbance
345.9 ✓5 [294.10]
hepatolenticular degeneration
with behavioral disturbance
275.1 [294.11]
without behavioral disturbance
275.1 [294.10]
HIV
with behavioral disturbance 042 [294.11]
without behavioral disturbance
042 [294.10]
Huntington's chorea
with behavioral disturbance
333.4 [294.11]
without behavioral disturbance
333.4 [294.10]
Jakob-Creutzfeldt disease
with behavioral disturbance
046.1 [294.11]
without behavioral disturbance
046.1 [294.10]
multiple sclerosis
with behavioral disturbance 340 [294.11]
without behavioral disturbance
340 [294.10]
neurosyphilis
with behavioral disturbance
094.9 [294.11]
without behavioral disturbance
094.9 [294.10]
Pelizaeus-Merzbacher disease
with behavioral disturbance
333.0 [294.11]
without behavioral disturbance
333.0 [294.10]
Pick's disease
with behavioral disturbance
331.1 [294.11]
without behavioral disturbance
331.1 [294.10]
polyarteritis nodosa
with behavioral disturbance
446.0 [294.11]

Dementia — *continued*
due to or associated with condition(s) classified
elsewhere — *continued*
polyarteritis nodosa — *continued*
without behavioral disturbance
446.0 [294.10]
syphilis
with behavioral disturbance
094.1 [294.11]
without behavioral disturbance
094.1 [294.10]
Wilson's disease
with behavioral disturbance
275.1 [294.11]
without behavioral disturbance
275.1 [294.10]
hebephrenic (acute) 295.1 ✓5
Heller's (infantile psychosis) (*see also*
Psychosis, childhood) 299.1 ✓5
idiopathic 290.9
presenile-onset — *see* Dementia, presenile
senile-onset — *see* Dementia, senile
in
arteriosclerotic brain disease 290.40
senility 290.0
induced by drug 292.82
infantile, infantilia (*see also* Psychosis,
childhood) 299.0 ✓5
multi-infarct (cerebrovascular) (*see also*
Dementia, arteriosclerotic) 290.40
old age 290.0
paralytica, paralytic 094.1
juvenilis 090.40
syphilitic 094.1
congenital 090.40
tabetic form 094.1
paranoid (*see also* Schizophrenia) 295.3 ✓5
paraphrenic (*see also* Schizophrenia) 295.3 ✓5
paretic 094.1
praecox (*see also* Schizophrenia) 295.9 ✓5
presenile 290.10
with
acute confusional state 290.11
delirium 290.11
delusional features 290.12
depressive features 290.13
depressed type 290.13
paranoid type 290.12
simple type 290.10
uncomplicated 290.10
primary (acute) (*see also* Schizophrenia)
295.0 ✓5
progressive, syphilitic 094.1
puerperal — *see* Psychosis, puerperal
schizophrenic (*see also* Schizophrenia)
295.9 ✓5
senile 290.0
with
acute confusional state 290.3
delirium 290.3
delusional features 290.20
depressive features 290.21
depressed type 290.21
exhaustion 290.0
paranoid type 290.20
simple type (acute) (*see also* Schizophrenia)
295.0 ✓5
simplex (acute) (*see also* Schizophrenia)
295.0 ✓5
syphilitic 094.1
uremic — *see* Uremia
vascular 290.40
Demerol dependence (*see also* Dependence)
304.0 ✓5
Demineralization, ankle (*see also* Osteoporosis)
733.00
Demodex folliculorum (infestation) 133.8
de Morgan's spots (senile angiomas) 448.1
Demyelinating
polyneuritis, chronic inflammatory 357.81 ▲
Demyelination, demyelinization
central nervous system 341.9
specified NEC 341.8
corpus callosum (central) 341.8
global 340

Dengue (fever) 061
- sandfly 061
- vaccination, prophylactic (against) V05.1
- virus hemorrhagic fever 065.4

Dens
- evaginatus 520.2
- in dente 520.2
- invaginatus 520.2

Density
- increased, bone (disseminated) (generalized) (spotted) 733.99
- lung (nodular) 518.89

Dental — *see also* condition
- examination only V72.2

Dentia praecox 520.6

Denticles (in pulp) 522.2

Dentigerous cyst 526.0

Dentin
- irregular (in pulp) 522.3
- opalescent 520.5
- secondary (in pulp) 522.3
- sensitive 521.8

Dentinogenesis imperfecta 520.5

Dentinoma (M9271/0) 213.1
- upper jaw (bone) 213.0

Dentition 520.7
- abnormal 520.6
- anomaly 520.6
- delayed 520.6
- difficult 520.7
- disorder of 520.6
- precocious 520.6
- retarded 520.6

Denture sore (mouth) 528.9

Dependence

> Note — Use the following fifth-digit subclassification with category 304:
>
> 0   unspecified
> 1   continuous
> 2   episodic
> 3   in remission

- with
  - withdrawal symptoms
    - alcohol 291.81
    - drug 292.0
- 14-hydroxy-dihydromorphinone 304.0
- absinthe 304.6
- acemorphan 304.0
- acetanilid(e) 304.6
- acetophenetidin 304.6
- acetorphine 304.0
- acetyldihydrocodeine 304.0
- acetyldihydrocodeinone 304.0
- Adalin 304.1
- Afghanistan black 304.3
- agrypnal 304.1
- alcohol, alcoholic (ethyl) (methyl) (wood) 303.9
  - maternal, with suspected fetal damage affecting management of pregnancy 655.4
- allobarbitone 304.1
- allonal 304.1
- allylisopropylacetylurea 304.1
- alphaprodine (hydrochloride) 304.0
- Alurate 304.1
- Alvodine 304.0
- amethocaine 304.6
- amidone 304.0
- amidopyrine 304.6
- aminopyrine 304.6
- amobarbital 304.1
- amphetamine(s) (type) (drugs classifiable to 969.7) 304.4
- amylene hydrate 304.6
- amylobarbitone 304.1
- amylocaine 304.6
- Amytal (sodium) 304.1
- analgesic (drug) NEC 304.6
  - synthetic with morphine-like effect 304.0

Dependence — *continued*
- anesthetic (agent) (drug) (gas) (general) (local) NEC 304.6
- Angel dust 304.6
- anileridine 304.0
- antipyrine 304.6
- aprobarbital 304.1
- aprobarbitone 304.1
- atropine 304.6
- Avertin (bromide) 304.6
- barbenyl 304.1
- barbital(s) 304.1
- barbitone 304.1
- barbiturate(s) (compounds) (drugs classifiable to 967.0) 304.1
- barbituric acid (and compounds) 304.1
- benzedrine 304.4
- benzylmorphine 304.0
- Beta-chlor 304.1
- bhang 304.3
- blue velvet 304.0
- Brevital 304.1
- bromal (hydrate) 304.1
- bromide(s) NEC 304.1
- bromine compounds NEC 304.1
- bromisovalum 304.1
- bromoform 304.1
- Bromo-seltzer 304.1
- bromural 304.1
- butabarbital (sodium) 304.1
- butabarpal 304.1
- butallylonal 304.1
- butethal 304.1
- buthalitone (sodium) 304.1
- Butisol 304.1
- butobarbitone 304.1
- butyl chloral (hydrate) 304.1
- caffeine 304.4
- cannabis (indica) (sativa) (resin) (derivatives) (type) 304.3
- carbamazepine 304.6
- Carbrital 304.1
- carbromal 304.1
- carisoprodol 304.6
- Catha (edulis) 304.4
- chloral (betaine) (hydrate) 304.1
- chloralamide 304.1
- chloralformamide 304.1
- chloralose 304.1
- chlordiazepoxide 304.1
- Chloretone 304.1
- chlorobutanol 304.1
- chlorodyne 304.1
- chloroform 304.6
- Cliradon 304.0
- coca (leaf) and derivatives 304.2
- cocaine 304.2
  - hydrochloride 304.2
  - salt (any) 304.2
- codeine 304.0
- combination of drugs (excluding morphine or opioid type drug) NEC 304.8
  - morphine or opioid type drug with any other drug 304.7
- croton-chloral 304.1
- cyclobarbital 304.1
- cyclobarbitone 304.1
- dagga 304.3
- Delvinal 304.1
- Demerol 304.0
- desocodeine 304.0
- desomorphine 304.0
- desoxyephedrine 304.4
- DET 304.5
- dexamphetamine 304.4
- dexedrine 304.4
- dextromethorphan 304.0
- dextromoramide 304.0
- dextronorpseudoephedrine 304.4
- dextrorphan 304.0
- diacetylmorphine 304.0
- Dial 304.1
- diallylbarbituric acid 304.1
- diamorphine 304.0
- diazepam 304.1
- dibucaine 304.6
- dichloroethane 304.6
- diethyl barbituric acid 304.1

Dependence — *continued*
- diethylsulfone-diethylmethane 304.1
- difencloxazine 304.0
- dihydrocodeine 304.0
- dihydrocodeinone 304.0
- dihydrohydroxycodeinone 304.0
- dihydroisocodeine 304.0
- dihydromorphine 304.0
- dihydromorphinone 304.0
- dihydroxcodeinone 304.0
- Dilaudid 304.0
- dimenhydrinate 304.6
- dimethylmeperidine 304.0
- dimethyltriptamine 304.5
- Dionin 304.0
- diphenoxylate 304.6
- dipipanone 304.0
- d-lysergic acid diethylamide 304.5
- DMT 304.5
- Dolophine 304.0
- DOM 304.2
- Doriden 304.1
- dormiral 304.1
- Dormison 304.1
- Dromoran 304.0
- drug NEC 304.9
  - analgesic NEC 304.6
  - combination (excluding morphine or opioid type drug) NEC 304.8
    - morphine or opioid type drug with any other drug 304.7
  - complicating pregnancy, childbirth, or puerperium 648.3
    - affecting fetus or newborn 779.5
  - hallucinogenic 304.5
  - hypnotic NEC 304.1
  - narcotic NEC 304.9
  - psychostimulant NEC 304.4
  - sedative 304.1
  - soporific NEC 304.1
  - specified type NEC 304.6
  - suspected damage to fetus affecting management of pregnancy 655.5
  - synthetic, with morphine-like effect 304.0
  - tranquilizing 304.1
- duboisine 304.6
- ectylurea 304.1
- Endocaine 304.6
- Equanil 304.1
- Eskabarb 304.1
- ethchlorvynol 304.1
- ether (ethyl) (liquid) (vapor) (vinyl) 304.6
- ethidene 304.6
- ethinamate 304.1
- ethoheptazine 304.6
- ethyl
  - alcohol 303.9
  - bromide 304.6
  - carbamate 304.6
  - chloride 304.6
  - morphine 304.0
- ethylene (gas) 304.6
  - dichloride 304.6
- ethylidene chloride 304.6
- etilfen 304.1
- etorphine 304.0
- etoval 304.1
- eucodal 304.0
- euneryl 304.1
- Evipal 304.1
- Evipan 304.1
- fentanyl 304.0
- ganja 304.3
- gardenal 304.1
- gardenpanyl 304.1
- gelsemine 304.6
- Gelsemium 304.6
- Gemonil 304.1
- glucochloral 304.1
- glue (airplane) (sniffing) 304.6
- glutethimide 304.1
- hallucinogenics 304.5
- hashish 304.3
- headache powder NEC 304.6
- Heavenly Blue 304.5
- hedonal 304.1
- hemp 304.3

Index to Diseases

Dependence — *continued*
- heptabarbital 304.1 ✓5ᵗʰ
- Heptalgin 304.0 ✓5ᵗʰ
- heptobarbitone 304.1 ✓5ᵗʰ
- heroin 304.0 ✓5ᵗʰ
  - salt (any) 304.0 ✓5ᵗʰ
- hexethal (sodium) 304.1 ✓5ᵗʰ
- hexobarbital 304.1 ✓5ᵗʰ
- Hycodan 304.0 ✓5ᵗʰ
- hydrocodone 304.0 ✓5ᵗʰ
- hydromorphinol 304.0 ✓5ᵗʰ
- hydromorphinone 304.0 ✓5ᵗʰ
- hydromorphone 304.0 ✓5ᵗʰ
- hydroxycodeine 304.0 ✓5ᵗʰ
- hypnotic NEC 304.1 ✓5ᵗʰ
- Indian hemp 304.3 ✓5ᵗʰ
- intranarcon 304.1 ✓5ᵗʰ
- Kemithal 304.1 ✓5ᵗʰ
- ketobemidone 304.0 ✓5ᵗʰ
- khat 304.4 ✓5ᵗʰ
- kif 304.3 ✓5ᵗʰ
- Lactuca (virosa) extract 304.1 ✓5ᵗʰ
- lactucarium 304.1 ✓5ᵗʰ
- laudanum 304.0 ✓5ᵗʰ
- Lebanese red 304.3 ✓5ᵗʰ
- Leritine 304.0 ✓5ᵗʰ
- lettuce opium 304.1 ✓5ᵗʰ
- Levanil 304.1 ✓5ᵗʰ
- Levo-Dromoran 304.0 ✓5ᵗʰ
- levo-iso-methadone 304.0 ✓5ᵗʰ
- levorphanol 304.0 ✓5ᵗʰ
- Librium 304.1 ✓5ᵗʰ
- Lomotil 304.6 ✓5ᵗʰ
- Lotusate 304.1 ✓5ᵗʰ
- LSD (-25) (and derivatives) 304.5 ✓5ᵗʰ
- Luminal 304.1 ✓5ᵗʰ
- lysergic acid 304.5 ✓5ᵗʰ
  - amide 304.5 ✓5ᵗʰ
- maconha 304.3 ✓5ᵗʰ
- magic mushroom 304.5 ✓5ᵗʰ
- marihuana 304.3 ✓5ᵗʰ
- MDA (methylene dioxyamphetamine) 304.4 ✓5ᵗʰ
- Mebaral 304.1 ✓5ᵗʰ
- Medinal 304.1 ✓5ᵗʰ
- Medomin 304.1 ✓5ᵗʰ
- megahallucinogenics 304.5 ✓5ᵗʰ
- meperidine 304.0 ✓5ᵗʰ
- mephobarbital 304.1 ✓5ᵗʰ
- meprobamate 304.1 ✓5ᵗʰ
- mescaline 304.5 ✓5ᵗʰ
- methadone 304.0 ✓5ᵗʰ
- methamphetamine(s) 304.4 ✓5ᵗʰ
- methaqualone 304.1 ✓5ᵗʰ
- metharbital 304.1 ✓5ᵗʰ
- methitural 304.1 ✓5ᵗʰ
- methobarbitone 304.1 ✓5ᵗʰ
- methohexital 304.1 ✓5ᵗʰ
- methopholine 304.6 ✓5ᵗʰ
- methyl
  - alcohol 303.9 ✓5ᵗʰ
  - bromide 304.6 ✓5ᵗʰ
  - morphine 304.0 ✓5ᵗʰ
  - sulfonal 304.1 ✓5ᵗʰ
- methylated spirit 303.9 ✓5ᵗʰ
- methylbutinol 304.6 ✓5ᵗʰ
- methyldihydromorphinone 304.0 ✓5ᵗʰ
- methylene
  - chloride 304.6 ✓5ᵗʰ
  - dichloride 304.6 ✓5ᵗʰ
  - dioxyamphetamine (MDA) 304.4 ✓5ᵗʰ
- methylaparafynol 304.1 ✓5ᵗʰ
- methylphenidate 304.4 ✓5ᵗʰ
- methyprylone 304.1 ✓5ᵗʰ
- metopon 304.0 ✓5ᵗʰ
- Miltown 304.1 ✓5ᵗʰ
- morning glory *seed*s 304.5 ✓5ᵗʰ
- morphinan(s) 304.0 ✓5ᵗʰ
- morphine (sulfate) (sulfite) (type) (drugs classifiable to 965.00-965.09) 304.0 ✓5ᵗʰ
- morphine or opioid type drug (drugs classifiable to 965.00-965.09) with any other drug 304.7 ✓5ᵗʰ
- morphinol(s) 304.0 ✓5ᵗʰ
- morphinon 304.0 ✓5ᵗʰ
- morpholinylethylmorphine 304.0 ✓5ᵗʰ
- mylomid 304.1 ✓5ᵗʰ
- myristicin 304.5 ✓5ᵗʰ
- narcotic (drug) NEC 304.9 ✓5ᵗʰ

Dependence — *continued*
- nealbarbital 304.1 ✓5ᵗʰ
- nealbarbitone 304.1 ✓5ᵗʰ
- Nembutal 304.1 ✓5ᵗʰ
- Neonal 304.1 ✓5ᵗʰ
- Neraval 304.1 ✓5ᵗʰ
- Neravan 304.1 ✓5ᵗʰ
- neurobarb 304.1 ✓5ᵗʰ
- nicotine 305.1
- Nisentil 304.0 ✓5ᵗʰ
- nitrous oxide 304.6 ✓5ᵗʰ
- Noctec 304.1 ✓5ᵗʰ
- Noludar 304.1 ✓5ᵗʰ
- nonbarbiturate sedatives and tranquilizers with similar effect 304.1 ✓5ᵗʰ
- noptil 304.1 ✓5ᵗʰ
- normorphine 304.0 ✓5ᵗʰ
- noscapine 304.0 ✓5ᵗʰ
- Novocaine 304.6 ✓5ᵗʰ
- Numorphan 304.0 ✓5ᵗʰ
- nunol 304.1 ✓5ᵗʰ
- Nupercaine 304.6 ✓5ᵗʰ
- Oblivon 304.1 ✓5ᵗʰ
- on
  - aspirator V46.0
  - hyperbaric chamber V46.8
  - iron lung V46.1
  - machine (enabling) V46.9
    - specified type NEC V46.8
  - Possum (Patient-Operated-Selector-Mechanism) V46.8
  - renal dialysis machine V45.1
  - respirator V46.1
  - supplemental oxygen V46.2 ●
- opiate 304.0 ✓5ᵗʰ
- opioids 304.0 ✓5ᵗʰ
- opioid type drug 304.0 ✓5ᵗʰ
  - with any other drug 304.7 ✓5ᵗʰ
- opium (alkaloids) (derivatives) (tincture) 304.0 ✓5ᵗʰ
- ortal 304.1 ✓5ᵗʰ
- Oxazepam 304.1 ✓5ᵗʰ
- oxycodone 304.0 ✓5ᵗʰ
- oxymorphone 304.0 ✓5ᵗʰ
- Palfium 304.0 ✓5ᵗʰ
- Panadol 304.6 ✓5ᵗʰ
- pantopium 304.0 ✓5ᵗʰ
- pantopon 304.0 ✓5ᵗʰ
- papaverine 304.0 ✓5ᵗʰ
- paracetamol 304.6 ✓5ᵗʰ
- paracodin 304.0 ✓5ᵗʰ
- paraldehyde 304.1 ✓5ᵗʰ
- paregoric 304.0 ✓5ᵗʰ
- Parzone 304.0 ✓5ᵗʰ
- PCP (phencyclidine) 304.6 ✓5ᵗʰ
- Pearly Gates 304.5 ✓5ᵗʰ
- pentazocine 304.0 ✓5ᵗʰ
- pentobarbital 304.1 ✓5ᵗʰ
- pentobarbitone (sodium) 304.1 ✓5ᵗʰ
- Pentothal 304.1 ✓5ᵗʰ
- Percaine 304.6 ✓5ᵗʰ
- Percodan 304.0 ✓5ᵗʰ
- Perichlor 304.1 ✓5ᵗʰ
- Pernocton 304.1 ✓5ᵗʰ
- Pernoston 304.1 ✓5ᵗʰ
- peronine 304.0 ✓5ᵗʰ
- pethidine (hydrochloride) 304.0 ✓5ᵗʰ
- petrichloral 304.1 ✓5ᵗʰ
- peyote 304.5 ✓5ᵗʰ
- Phanodron 304.1 ✓5ᵗʰ
- phenacetin 304.6 ✓5ᵗʰ
- phenadoxone 304.0 ✓5ᵗʰ
- phenaglycodol 304.1 ✓5ᵗʰ
- phenazocine 304.0 ✓5ᵗʰ
- phencyclidine 304.6 ✓5ᵗʰ
- phenmetrazine 304.4 ✓5ᵗʰ
- phenobal 304.1 ✓5ᵗʰ
- phenobarbital 304.1 ✓5ᵗʰ
- phenobarbitone 304.1 ✓5ᵗʰ
- phenomorphan 304.0 ✓5ᵗʰ
- phenonyl 304.1 ✓5ᵗʰ
- phenoperidine 304.0 ✓5ᵗʰ
- pholcodine 304.0 ✓5ᵗʰ
- piminodine 304.0 ✓5ᵗʰ
- Pipadone 304.0 ✓5ᵗʰ
- Pitkin's solution 304.6 ✓5ᵗʰ
- Placidyl 304.1 ✓5ᵗʰ
- polysubstance 304.8 ✓5ᵗʰ

Dependence — *continued*
- Pontocaine 304.6 ✓5ᵗʰ
- pot 304.3 ✓5ᵗʰ
- potassium bromide 304.1 ✓5ᵗʰ
- Preludin 304.4 ✓5ᵗʰ
- Prinadol 304.0 ✓5ᵗʰ
- probarbital 304.1 ✓5ᵗʰ
- procaine 304.6 ✓5ᵗʰ
- propanal 304.1 ✓5ᵗʰ
- propoxyphene 304.6 ✓5ᵗʰ
- psilocibin 304.5 ✓5ᵗʰ
- psilocin 304.5 ✓5ᵗʰ
- psilocybin 304.5 ✓5ᵗʰ
- psilocyline 304.5 ✓5ᵗʰ
- psilocyn 304.5 ✓5ᵗʰ
- psychedelic agents 304.5 ✓5ᵗʰ
- psychostimulant NEC 304.4 ✓5ᵗʰ
- psychotomimetic agents 304.5 ✓5ᵗʰ
- pyrahexyl 304.3 ✓5ᵗʰ
- Pyramidon 304.6 ✓5ᵗʰ
- quinalbarbitone 304.1 ✓5ᵗʰ
- racemoramide 304.0 ✓5ᵗʰ
- racemorphan 304.0 ✓5ᵗʰ
- Rela 304.6 ✓5ᵗʰ
- scopolamine 304.6 ✓5ᵗʰ
- secobarbital 304.1 ✓5ᵗʰ
- Seconal 304.1 ✓5ᵗʰ
- sedative NEC 304.1 ✓5ᵗʰ
  - nonbarbiturate with barbiturate effect 304.1 ✓5ᵗʰ
- Sedormid 304.1 ✓5ᵗʰ
- sernyl 304.1 ✓5ᵗʰ
- sodium bromide 304.1 ✓5ᵗʰ
- Soma 304.6 ✓5ᵗʰ
- Somnal 304.1 ✓5ᵗʰ
- Somnos 304.1 ✓5ᵗʰ
- Soneryl 304.1 ✓5ᵗʰ
- soporific (drug) NEC 304.1 ✓5ᵗʰ
- specified drug NEC 304.6 ✓5ᵗʰ
- speed 304.4 ✓5ᵗʰ
- spinocaine 304.6 ✓5ᵗʰ
- Stovaine 304.6 ✓5ᵗʰ
- STP 304.5 ✓5ᵗʰ
- stramonium 304.6 ✓5ᵗʰ
- Sulfonal 304.1 ✓5ᵗʰ
- sulfonethylmethane 304.1 ✓5ᵗʰ
- sulfonmethane 304.1 ✓5ᵗʰ
- Surital 304.1 ✓5ᵗʰ
- synthetic drug with morphine-like effect 304.0 ✓5ᵗʰ
- talbutal 304.1 ✓5ᵗʰ
- tetracaine 304.6 ✓5ᵗʰ
- tetrahydrocannabinol 304.3 ✓5ᵗʰ
- tetronal 304.1 ✓5ᵗʰ
- THC 304.3 ✓5ᵗʰ
- thebacon 304.0 ✓5ᵗʰ
- thebaine 304.0 ✓5ᵗʰ
- thiamil 304.1 ✓5ᵗʰ
- thiamylal 304.1 ✓5ᵗʰ
- thiopental 304.1 ✓5ᵗʰ
- tobacco 305.1
- toluene, toluol 304.6 ✓5ᵗʰ
- tranquilizer NEC 304.1 ✓5ᵗʰ
  - nonbarbiturate with barbiturate effect 304.1 ✓5ᵗʰ
- tribromacetaldehyde 304.6 ✓5ᵗʰ
- tribromethanol 304.6 ✓5ᵗʰ
- tribromomethane 304.6 ✓5ᵗʰ
- trichloroethanol 304.6 ✓5ᵗʰ
- trichroethyl phosphate 304.1 ✓5ᵗʰ
- triclofos 304.1 ✓5ᵗʰ
- Trional 304.1 ✓5ᵗʰ
- Tuinal 304.1 ✓5ᵗʰ
- Turkish Green 304.3 ✓5ᵗʰ
- urethan(e) 304.6 ✓5ᵗʰ
- Valium 304.1 ✓5ᵗʰ
- Valmid 304.1 ✓5ᵗʰ
- veganin 304.0 ✓5ᵗʰ
- veramon 304.1 ✓5ᵗʰ
- Veronal 304.1 ✓5ᵗʰ
- versidyne 304.6 ✓5ᵗʰ
- vinbarbital 304.1 ✓5ᵗʰ
- vinbarbitone 304.1 ✓5ᵗʰ
- vinyl bitone 304.1 ✓5ᵗʰ
- vitamin B_6 266.1
- wine 303.9 ✓5ᵗʰ
- Zactane 304.6 ✓5ᵗʰ

Dependency

Dependency
- passive 301.6
- reactions 301.6

Depersonalization (episode, in neurotic state) (neurotic) (syndrome) 300.6

Depletion
- carbohydrates 271.9
- complement factor 279.8
- extracellular fluid 276.5
- plasma 276.5
- potassium 276.8
  - nephropathy 588.8
- salt or sodium 276.1
  - causing heat exhaustion or prostration 992.4
  - nephropathy 593.9
- volume 276.5
  - extracellular fluid 276.5
  - plasma 276.5

Deposit
- argentous, cornea 371.16
- bone, in Boeck's sarcoid 135
- calcareous, calcium — see Calcification
- cholesterol
  - retina 362.82
  - skin 709.3
  - vitreous (humor) 379.22
- conjunctival 372.56
- cornea, corneal NEC 371.10
  - argentous 371.16
  - in
    - cystinosis 270.0 [371.15]
    - mucopolysaccharidosis 277.5 [371.15]
- crystalline, vitreous (humor) 379.22
- hemosiderin, in old scars of cornea 371.11
- metallic, in lens 366.45
- skin 709.3
- teeth, tooth (betel) (black) (green) (materia alba) (orange) (soft) (tobacco) 523.6
- urate, in kidney (see also Disease, renal) 593.9

Depraved appetite 307.52

Depression 311
- acute (see also Psychosis, affective) 296.2 ✓5
  - recurrent episode 296.3 ✓5
  - single episode 296.2 ✓5
- agitated (see also Psychosis, affective) 296.2 ✓5
  - recurrent episode 296.3 ✓5
  - single episode 296.2 ✓5
- anaclitic 309.21
- anxiety 300.4
- arches 734
  - congenital 754.61
- autogenous (see also Psychosis, affective) 296.2 ✓5
  - recurrent episode 296.3 ✓5
  - single episode 296.2 ✓5
- basal metabolic rate (BMR) 794.7
- bone marrow 289.9
- central nervous system 799.1
  - newborn 779.2
- cerebral 331.9
  - newborn 779.2
- cerebrovascular 437.8
  - newborn 779.2
- chest wall 738.3
- endogenous (see also Psychosis, affective) 296.2 ✓5
  - recurrent episode 296.3 ✓5
  - single episode 296.2 ✓5
- functional activity 780.99 ▲
- hysterical 300.11
- involutional, climacteric, or menopausal (see also Psychosis, affective) 296.2 ✓5
  - recurrent episode 296.3 ✓5
  - single episode 296.2 ✓5
- manic (see also Psychosis, affective) 296.80
- medullary 348.8
  - newborn 779.2
- mental 300.4
- metatarsal heads — see Depression, arches
- metatarsus — see Depression, arches
- monopolar (see also Psychosis, affective) 296.2 ✓5
  - recurrent episode 296.3 ✓5
  - single episode 296.2 ✓5
- nervous 300.4

Depression — continued
- neurotic 300.4
- nose 738.0
- postpartum 648.4 ✓5
- psychogenic 300.4
  - reactive 298.0
- psychoneurotic 300.4
- psychotic (see also Psychosis, affective) 296.2 ✓5
  - reactive 298.0
  - recurrent episode 296.3 ✓5
  - single episode 296.2 ✓5
- reactive 300.4
  - neurotic 300.4
  - psychogenic 298.0
  - psychoneurotic 300.4
  - psychotic 298.0
- recurrent 296.3 ✓5
- respiratory center 348.8
  - newborn 770.89 ▲
- scapula 736.89
- senile 290.21
- situational (acute) (brief) 309.0
  - prolonged 309.1
- skull 754.0
- sternum 738.3
- visual field 368.40

Depressive reaction — see also Reaction, depressive
- acute (transient) 309.0
  - with anxiety 309.28
  - prolonged 309.1
- situational (acute) 309.0
  - prolonged 309.1

Deprivation
- cultural V62.4
- emotional V62.89
  - affecting
    - adult 995.82
    - infant or child 995.51
- food 994.2
  - specific substance NEC 269.8
- protein (familial) (kwashiorkor) 260
- social V62.4
  - affecting
    - adult 995.82
    - infant or child 995.51
- symptoms, syndrome
  - alcohol 291.81
  - drug 292.0
- vitamins (see also Deficiency, vitamin) 269.2
- water 994.3

de Quervain's
- disease (tendon sheath) 727.04
- thyroiditis (subacute granulomatous thyroiditis) 245.1

Derangement
- ankle (internal) 718.97
  - current injury (see also Dislocation, ankle) 837.0
  - recurrent 718.37
- cartilage (articular) NEC (see also Disorder, cartilage, articular) 718.0 ✓5
  - knee 717.9
    - recurrent 718.36
  - recurrent 718.3 ✓5
- collateral ligament (knee) (medial) (tibial) 717.82
  - current injury 844.1
    - lateral (fibular) 844.0
  - lateral (fibular) 717.81
    - current injury 844.0
- cruciate ligament (knee) (posterior) 717.84
  - anterior 717.83
    - current injury 844.2
  - current injury 844.2
- elbow (internal) 718.92
  - current injury (see also Dislocation, elbow) 832.00
  - recurrent 718.32
- gastrointestinal 536.9
- heart — see Disease, heart
- hip (joint) (internal) (old) 718.95
  - current injury (see also Dislocation, hip) 835.00
  - recurrent 718.35

Derangement — continued
- intervertebral disc — see Displacement, intervertebral disc
- joint (internal) 718.90
  - ankle 718.97
    - current injury — see also Dislocation, by site
    - knee, meniscus or cartilage (see also Tear, meniscus) 836.2
  - elbow 718.92
  - foot 718.97
  - hand 718.94
  - hip 718.95
  - knee 717.9
  - multiple sites 718.99
  - pelvic region 718.95
  - recurrent 718.30
    - ankle 718.37
    - elbow 718.32
    - foot 718.37
    - hand 718.34
    - hip 718.35
    - knee 718.36
    - multiple sites 718.39
    - pelvic region 718.35
    - shoulder (region) 718.31
    - specified site NEC 718.38
    - temporomandibular (old) 524.69
    - wrist 718.33
  - shoulder (region) 718.91
  - specified site NEC 718.98
  - spine NEC 724.9
  - temporomandibular 524.69
  - wrist 718.93
- knee (cartilage) (internal) 717.9
  - current injury (see also Tear, meniscus) 836.2
  - ligament 717.89
    - capsular 717.85
    - collateral — see Derangement, collateral ligament
    - cruciate — see Derangement, cruciate ligament
    - specified NEC 717.85
  - recurrent 718.36
- low back NEC 724.9
- meniscus NEC (knee) 717.5
  - current injury (see also Tear, meniscus) 836.2
  - lateral 717.40
    - anterior horn 717.42
    - posterior horn 717.43
    - specified NEC 717.49
  - medial 717.3
    - anterior horn 717.1
    - posterior horn 717.2
  - recurrent 718.3 ✓5
  - site other than knee — see Disorder, cartilage, articular
- mental (see also Psychosis) 298.9
- rotator cuff (recurrent) (tear) 726.10
  - current 840.4
- sacroiliac (old) 724.6
  - current — see Dislocation, sacroiliac
- semilunar cartilage (knee) 717.5
  - current injury 836.2
    - lateral 836.1
    - medial 836.0
  - recurrent 718.3 ✓5
- shoulder (internal) 718.91
  - current injury (see also Dislocation, shoulder) 831.00
  - recurrent 718.31
- spine (recurrent) NEC 724.9
  - current — see Dislocation, spine
- temporomandibular (internal) (joint) (old) 524.69
  - current — see Dislocation, jaw

Dercum's disease or syndrome (adiposis dolorosa) 272.8

Derealization (neurotic) 300.6

Dermal — see condition

Dermaphytid — see Dermatophytosis

Dermatergosis — see Dermatitis

Index to Diseases

Dermatitis

Dermatitis (allergic) (contact) (occupational) (venenata) 692.9
- ab igne 692.82
- acneiform 692.9
- actinic (due to sun) 692.70
  - acute 692.72
  - chronic NEC 692.74
  - other than from sun NEC 692.82
- ambustionis
  - due to
    - burn or scald — see Burn, by site
    - sunburn (see also Sunburn) 692.71
- amebic 006.6
- ammonia 691.0
- anaphylactoid NEC 692.9
- arsenical 692.4
- artefacta 698.4
  - psychogenic 316 [698.4]
- asthmatic 691.8
- atopic (allergic) (intrinsic) 691.8
  - psychogenic 316 [691.8]
- atrophicans 701.8
  - diffusa 701.8
  - maculosa 701.3
- berlock, berloque 692.72
- blastomycetic 116.0
- blister beetle 692.89
- Brucella NEC 023.9
- bullosa 694.9
  - striata pratensis 692.6
- bullous 694.9
  - mucosynechial, atrophic 694.60
    - with ocular involvement 694.61
  - seasonal 694.8
- calorica
  - due to
    - burn or scald — see Burn, by site
    - cold 692.89
    - sunburn (see also Sunburn) 692.71
- caterpillar 692.89
- cercarial 120.3
- combustionis
  - due to
    - burn or scald — see Burn, by site
    - sunburn (see also Sunburn) 692.71
- congelationis 991.5
- contusiformis 695.2
- diabetic 250.8 ✓5ᵗʰ
- diaper 691.0
- diphtheritica 032.85
- due to
  - acetone 692.2
  - acids 692.4
  - adhesive plaster 692.4
  - alcohol (skin contact) (substances classifiable to 980.0-980.9) 692.4
    - taken internally 693.8
  - alkalis 692.4
  - allergy NEC 692.9
  - ammonia (household) (liquid) 692.4
  - arnica 692.3
  - arsenic 692.4
    - taken internally 693.8
  - blister beetle 692.89
  - cantharides 692.3
  - carbon disulphide 692.2
  - caterpillar 692.89
  - caustics 692.4
  - cereal (ingested) 693.1
    - contact with skin 692.5
  - chemical(s) NEC 692.4
    - internal 693.8
    - irritant NEC 692.4
    - taken internally 693.8
  - chlorocompounds 692.2
  - coffee (ingested) 693.1
    - contact with skin 692.5
  - cold weather 692.89
  - cosmetics 692.81
  - cyclohexanes 692.2
  - deodorant 692.81
  - detergents 692.0
  - dichromate 692.4

Dermatitis — continued
- due to — continued
  - drugs and medicinals (correct substance properly administered) (internal use) 693.0
    - external (in contact with skin) 692.3
      - wrong substance given or taken 976.9
      - specified substance — see Table of Drugs and Chemicals
    - wrong substance given or taken 977.9
      - specified substance — see Table of Drugs and Chemicals
  - dyes 692.89
    - hair 692.89
  - epidermophytosis — see Dermatophytosis
  - esters 692.2
  - external irritant NEC 692.9
    - specified agent NEC 692.89
  - eye shadow 692.81
  - fish (ingested) 693.1
    - contact with skin 692.5
  - flour (ingested) 693.1
    - contact with skin 692.5
  - food (ingested) 693.1
    - in contact with skin 692.5
  - fruit (ingested) 693.1
    - contact with skin 692.5
  - fungicides 692.3
  - furs 692.89
  - glycols 692.2
  - greases NEC 692.1
  - hair dyes 692.89
  - hot
    - objects and materials — see Burn, by site
    - weather or places 692.89
  - hydrocarbons 692.2
  - infrared rays, except from sun 692.82
    - solar NEC (see also Dermatitis, due to, sun) 692.70
  - ingested substance 693.9
    - drugs and medicinals (see also Dermatitis, due to, drugs and medicinals) 693.0
    - food 693.1
    - specified substance NEC 693.8
  - ingestion or injection of chemical 693.8
    - drug (correct substance properly administered) 693.0
    - wrong substance given or taken 977.9
      - specified substance — see Table of Drugs and Chemicals
  - insecticides 692.4
  - internal agent 693.9
    - drugs and medicinals (see also Dermatitis, due to, drugs and medicinals) 693.0
    - food (ingested) 693.1
      - in contact with skin 692.5
    - specified agent NEC 693.8
  - iodine 692.3
  - iodoform 692.3
  - irradiation 692.82
  - jewelry 692.83
  - keratolytics 692.3
  - ketones 692.2
  - lacquer tree (Rhus verniciflua) 692.6
  - light NEC (see also Dermatitis, due to, sun) 692.70
    - other 692.82
  - low temperature 692.89
  - mascara 692.81
  - meat (ingested) 693.1
    - contact with skin 692.5
  - mercury, mercurials 692.3
  - metals 692.83
  - milk (ingested) 693.1
    - contact with skin 692.5
  - Neomycin 692.3
  - nylon 692.4
  - oils NEC 692.1
  - paint solvent 692.2
  - pediculocides 692.3
  - petroleum products (substances classifiable to 981) 692.4
  - phenol 692.3

Dermatitis — continued
- due to — continued
  - photosensitiveness, photosensitivity (sun) 692.72
    - other light 692.82
  - plants NEC 692.6
  - plasters, medicated (any) 692.3
  - plastic 692.4
  - poison
    - ivy (Rhus toxicodendron) 692.6
    - oak (Rhus diversiloba) 692.6
    - plant or vine 692.6
    - sumac (Rhus venenata) 692.6
    - vine (Rhus radicans) 692.6
  - preservatives 692.89
  - primrose (primula) 692.6
  - primula 692.6
  - radiation 692.82
    - sun NEC (see also Dermatitis, due to, sun) 692.70
    - tanning bed 692.82
  - radioactive substance 692.82
  - radium 692.82
  - ragweed (Senecio jacobae) 692.6
  - Rhus (diversiloba) (radicans) (toxicodendron) (venenata) (verniciflua) 692.6
  - rubber 692.4
  - scabicides 692.3
  - Senecio jacobae 692.6
  - solar radiation — see Dermatitis, due to, sun
  - solvents (any) (substances classifiable to 982.0-982.8) 692.2
    - chlorocompound group 692.2
    - cyclohexane group 692.2
    - ester group 692.2
    - glycol group 692.2
    - hydrocarbon group 692.2
    - ketone group 692.2
    - paint 692.2
  - specified agent NEC 692.89
  - sun 692.70
    - acute 692.72
    - chronic NEC 692.74
    - specified NEC 692.79
  - sunburn (see also Sunburn) 692.71
  - sunshine NEC (see also Dermatitis, due to, sun) 692.70
  - tanning bed 692.82
  - tetrachlorethylene 692.2
  - toluene 692.2
  - topical medications 692.3
  - turpentine 692.2
  - ultraviolet rays, except from sun 692.82
    - sun NEC (see also Dermatitis, due to, sun) 692.82
  - vaccine or vaccination (correct substance properly administered) 693.0
    - wrong substance given or taken
      - bacterial vaccine 978.8
        - specified — see Table of Drugs and Chemicals
      - other vaccines NEC 979.9
        - specified — see Table of Drugs and Chemicals
  - varicose veins (see also Varicose, vein, inflamed or infected) 454.1
  - x-rays 692.82
- dyshydrotic 705.81
- dysmenorrheica 625.8
- eczematoid NEC 692.9
  - infectious 690.8
- eczematous NEC 692.9
- epidemica 695.89
- erysipelatosa 695.81
- escharotica — see Burn, by site
- exfoliativa, exfoliative 695.89
  - generalized 695.89
  - infantum 695.81
  - neonatorum 695.81
- eyelid 373.31
  - allergic 373.32
  - contact 373.32
  - eczematous 373.31
  - herpes (zoster) 053.20
    - simplex 054.41

Dermatitis

Dermatitis — *continued*
  eyelid — *continued*
    infective 373.5
      due to
        actinomycosis 039.3 *[373.5]*
        herpes
          simplex 054.41
          zoster 053.20
        impetigo 684 *[373.5]*
        leprosy (*see also* Leprosy)
          030.0 *[373.4]*
        lupus vulgaris (tuberculous) (*see also*
          Tuberculosis) 017.0 ☑5ᵗʰ *[373.4]*
        mycotic dermatitis (*see also*
          Dermatomycosis) 111.9 *[373.5]*
        vaccinia 051.0 *[373.5]*
          postvaccination 999.0 *[373.5]*
        yaws (*see also* Yaws) 102.9 *[373.4]*
  facta, factitia 698.4
    psychogenic 316 *[698.4]*
  ficta 698.4
    psychogenic 316 *[698.4]*
  flexural 691.8
  follicularis 704.8
  friction 709.8
  fungus 111.9
    specified type NEC 111.8
  gangrenosa, gangrenous (infantum) (*see also*
    Gangrene) 785.4
  gestationis 646.8 ☑5ᵗʰ
  gonococcal 098.89
  gouty 274.89
  harvest mite 133.8
  heat 692.89
  herpetiformis (bullous) (erythematous)
    (pustular) (vesicular) 694.0
    juvenile 694.2
    senile 694.5
  hiemalis 692.89
  hypostatic, hypostatica 454.1
    with ulcer 454.2
  impetiginous 684
  infantile (acute) (chronic) (intertriginous)
    (intrinsic) (seborrheic) 690.12
  infectiosa eczematoides 690.8
  infectious (staphylococcal) (streptococcal) 686.9
    eczematoid 690.8
  infective eczematoid 690.8
  Jacquet's (diaper dermatitis) 691.0
  leptus 133.8
  lichenified NEC 692.9
  lichenoid, chronic 701.0
  lichenoides purpurica pigmentosa 709.1
  meadow 692.6
  medicamentosa (correct substance properly
    administered) (internal use) (*see also*
    Dermatitis, due to, drugs, or medicinals)
    693.0
    due to contact with skin 692.3
  mite 133.8
  multiformis 694.0
    juvenile 694.2
    senile 694.5
  napkin 691.0
  neuro 698.3
  neurotica 694.0
  nummular NEC 692.9
  osteatosis, osteatotic 706.8
  papillaris capillitii 706.1
  pellagrous 265.2
  perioral 695.3
  perstans 696.1
  photosensitivity (sun) 692.72
    other light 692.82
  pigmented purpuric lichenoid 709.1
  polymorpha dolorosa 694.0
  primary irritant 692.9
  pruriginosa 694.0
  pruritic NEC 692.9
  psoriasiform nodularis 696.2
  psychogenic 316
  purulent 686.00
  pustular contagious 051.2
  pyococcal 686.00
  pyocyaneus 686.09
  pyogenica 686.00
  radiation 692.82

Dermatitis — *continued*
  repens 696.1
  Ritter's (exfoliativa) 695.81
  Schamberg's (progressive pigmentary
    dermatosis) 709.09
  schistosome 120.3
  seasonal bullous 694.8
  seborrheic 690.10
    infantile 690.12
  sensitization NEC 692.9
  septic (*see also* Septicemia) 686.00
    gonococcal 098.89
  solar, solare NEC (*see also* Dermatitis, due to,
    sun) 692.70
  stasis 459.81
    due to
      postphlebitic syndrome 459.12 ▲
        with ulcer 459.13 ●
      varicose veins — *see* Varicose
      ulcerated or with ulcer (varicose) 454.2
  sunburn (*see also* Sunburn) 692.71
  suppurative 686.00
  traumatic NEC 709.8
  trophoneurotica 694.0
  ultraviolet, except from sun 692.82
    due to sun NEC (*see also* Dermatitis, due to,
      sun) 692.70
  varicose 454.1
    with ulcer 454.2
  vegetans 686.8
  verrucosa 117.2
  xerotic 706.8

Dermatoarthritis, lipoid 272.8 *[713.0]*
Dermatochalasia, dermatochalasis 374.87
Dermatofibroma (lenticulare) (M8832/0) — *see*
  also Neoplasm, skin, benign
  protuberans (M8832/1) — *see* Neoplasm, skin,
    uncertain behavior
Dermatofibrosarcoma (protuberans) (M8832/3)
  — *see* Neoplasm, skin, malignant
Dermatographia 708.3
Dermatolysis (congenital) (exfoliativa) 757.39
  acquired 701.8
  eyelids 374.34
  palpebrarum 374.34
  senile 701.8
Dermatomegaly NEC 701.8
Dermatomucomyositis 710.3
Dermatomycosis 111.9
  furfuracea 111.0
  specified type NEC 111.8
Dermatomyositis (acute) (chronic) 710.3
Dermatoneuritis of children 985.0
Dermatophiliasis 134.1
Dermatophytide — *see* Dermatophytosis
Dermatophytosis (Epidermophyton) (infection)
  (microsporum) (tinea) (Trichophyton) 110.9
  beard 110.0
  body 110.5
  deep seated 110.6
  fingernails 110.1
  foot 110.4
  groin 110.3
  hand 110.2
  nail 110.1
  perianal (area) 110.3
  scalp 110.0
  scrotal 110.8
  specified site NEC 110.8
  toenails 110.1
  vulva 110.8
Dermatopolyneuritis 985.0
Dermatorrhexis 756.83
  acquired 701.8
Dermatosclerosis (*see also* Scleroderma) 710.1
  localized 701.0
Dermatosis 709.9
  Andrews' 686.8
  atopic 691.8
  Bowen's (M8081/2) — *see* Neoplasm, skin, in
    situ
  bullous 694.9
    specified type NEC 694.8
  erythematosquamous 690.8

Dermatosis — *continued*
  exfoliativa 695.89
  factitial 698.4
  gonococcal 098.89
  herpetiformis 694.0
    juvenile 694.2
    senile 694.5
  hysterical 300.11
  Linear IgA 694.8   ●
  menstrual NEC 709.8
  neutrophilic, acute febrile 695.89
  occupational (*see also* Dermatitis) 692.9
  papulosa nigra 709.8
  pigmentary NEC 709.00
    progressive 709.09
    Schamberg's 709.09
    Siemens-Bloch 757.33
  progressive pigmentary 709.09
  psychogenic 316
  pustular subcorneal 694.1
  Schamberg's (progressive pigmentary) 709.09
  senile NEC 709.3
  Unna's (seborrheic dermatitis) 690.10
Dermographia 708.3
Dermographism 708.3
Dermoid (cyst) (M9084/0) — *see also* Neoplasm,
  by site, benign
  with malignant transformation (M9084/3)
    183.0
Dermopathy
  infiltrative, with throtoxicosis 242.0 ☑5ᵗʰ
  senile NEC 709.3
Dermophytosis — *see* Dermatophytosis
Descemet's membrane — *see* condition
Descemetocele 371.72
Descending — *see* condition
Descensus uteri (complete) (incomplete) (partial)
  (without vaginal wall prolapse) 618.1
  with mention of vaginal wall proplapse — *see*
    Prolapse, uterovaginal
Desensitization to allergens V07.1
Desert
  rheumatism 114.0
  sore (*see also* Ulcer, skin) 707.9
Desertion (child) (newborn) 995.52
  adult 995.84
Desmoid (extra-abdominal) (tumor) (M8821/1) —
  see also Neoplasm, connective tissue,
  uncertain behavior
  abdominal (M8822/1) — *see* Neoplasm,
    connective tissue, uncertain behavior
Despondency 300.4
Desquamative dermatitis NEC 695.89
Destruction
  articular facet (*see also* Derangement, joint)
    718.9 ☑5ᵗʰ
    vertebra 724.9
  bone 733.90
    syphilitic 095.5
  joint (*see also* Derangement, joint) 718.9 ☑5ᵗʰ
    sacroiliac 724.6
  kidney 593.89
  live fetus to facilitate birth NEC 763.89
  ossicles (ear) 385.24
  rectal sphincter 569.49
  septum (nasal) 478.1
  tuberculous NEC (*see also* Tuberculosis)
    011.9 ☑5ᵗʰ
  tympanic membrane 384.82
  tympanum 385.89
  vertebral disc — *see* Degeneration,
    intervertebral disc
Destructiveness (*see also* Disturbance, conduct)
  312.9
  adjustment reaction 309.3
Detachment
  cartilage — *see also* Sprain, by site
    knee — *see* Tear, meniscus
  cervix, annular 622.8
    complicating delivery 665.3 ☑5ᵗʰ
  choroid (old) (postinfectional) (simple)
    (spontaneous) 363.70
    hemorrhagic 363.72

Index to Diseases

Detachment — *continued*
  choroid — *continued*
    serous 363.71
  knee, medial meniscus (old) 717.3
    current injury 836.0
  ligament — *see* Sprain, by site
  placenta (premature) — *see* Placenta, separation
  retina (recent) 361.9
    with retinal defect (rhegmatogenous) 361.00
      giant tear 361.03
      multiple 361.02
      partial
        with
          giant tear 361.03
          multiple defects 361.02
          retinal dialysis (juvenile) 361.04
          single defect 361.01
        retinal dialysis (juvenile) 361.04
        single 361.01
        subtotal 361.05
        total 361.05
    delimited (old) (partial) 361.06
    old
      delimited 361.06
      partial 361.06
      total or subtotal 361.07
    pigment epithelium (RPE) (serous) 362.42
      exudative 362.42
      hemorrhagic 362.43
    rhegmatogenous (*see also* Detachment, retina, with retinal defect) 361.00
    serous (without retinal defect) 361.2
    specified type NEC 361.89
    traction (with vitreoretinal organization) 361.81
  vitreous humor 379.21
Detergent asthma 507.8
Deterioration
  epileptic
    with behavioral disturbance 345.9 [294.11]
    without behavioral disturbance 345.9 [294.10]
  heart, cardiac (*see also* Degeneration, myocardial) 429.1
  mental (*see also* Psychosis) 298.9
  myocardium, myocardial (*see also* Degeneration, myocardial) 429.1
  senile (simple) 797
  transplanted organ — *see* Complications, transplant, organ, by site
de Toni-Fanconi syndrome (cystinosis) 270.0
Deuteranomaly 368.52
Deuteranopia (anomalous trichromat) (complete) (incomplete) 368.52
Deutschländer's disease — *see* Fracture, foot
Development
  abnormal, bone 756.9
  arrested 783.40
    bone 733.91
    child 783.40
    due to malnutrition (protein-calorie) 263.2
    fetus or newborn 764.9 ✓5ᵗʰ
    tracheal rings (congenital) 748.3
  defective, congenital — *see also* Anomaly
    cauda equina 742.59
    left ventricle 746.9
      with atresia or hypoplasia of aortic orifice or valve with hypoplasia of ascending aorta 746.7
      in hypoplastic left heart syndrome 746.7
  delayed (*see also* Delay, development) 783.40
    arithmetical skills 315.1
    language (skills) 315.31
      expressive 315.31
      mixed receptive-expressive 315.32
    learning skill, specified NEC 315.2
    mixed skills 315.5
    motor coordination 315.4
    reading 315.00
    specified
      learning skill NEC 315.2
      type NEC, except learning 315.8
    speech 315.39
      associated with hyperkinesia 314.1
      phonological 315.39

Development — *continued*
  delayed (*see also* Delay, development) — *continued*
    spelling 315.09
  imperfect, congenital — *see also* Anomaly
    heart 746.9
    lungs 748.60
  improper (fetus or newborn) 764.9 ✓5ᵗʰ
  incomplete (fetus or newborn) 764.9 ✓5ᵗʰ
    affecting management of pregnancy 656.5 ✓5ᵗʰ
    bronchial tree 748.3
    organ or site not listed — *see* Hypoplasia
    respiratory system 748.9
  sexual, precocious NEC 259.1
  tardy, mental (*see also* Retardation, mental) 319
  written expression 315.2
Developmental — *see* condition
Devergie's disease (pityriasis rubra pilaris) 696.4
Deviation
  conjugate (eye) 378.87
    palsy 378.81
    spasm, spastic 378.82
  esophagus 530.89
  eye, skew 378.87
  midline (jaw) (teeth) 524.2
    specified site NEC — *see* Malposition
  organ or site, congenital NEC — *see* Malposition, congenital
  septum (acquired) (nasal) 470
    congenital 754.0
  sexual 302.9
    bestiality 302.9
    coprophilia 302.89
    ego-dystonic
      homosexuality 302.0
      lesbianism 302.0
    erotomania 302.89
      Clérambault's 297.8
    exhibitionism (sexual) 302.4
    fetishism 302.81
      transvestic 302.3
    frotteurism 302.89
    homosexuality, ego-dystonic 302.0
      pedophilic 302.2
    lesbianism, ego-dystonic 302.0
    masochism 302.83
    narcissism 302.89
    necrophilia 302.89
    nymphomania 302.89
    pederosis 302.2
    pedophilia 302.2
    sadism 302.84
    sadomasochism 302.84
    satyriasis 302.89
    specified type NEC 302.89
    transvestic fetishism 302.3
    transvestism 302.3
    voyeurism 302.82
    zoophilia (erotica) 302.1
  teeth, midline 524.2
  trachea 519.1
  ureter (congenital) 753.4
Devic's disease 341.0
Device
  cerebral ventricle (communicating) in situ V45.2
  contraceptive — *see* Contraceptive, device
  drainage, cerebrospinal fluid V45.2
Devil's
  grip 074.1
  pinches (purpura simplex) 287.2
Devitalized tooth 522.9
Devonshire colic 984.9
  specified type of lead — *see* Table of Drugs and Chemicals
Dextraposition, aorta 747.21
  with ventricular septal defect, pulmonary stenosis or atresia, and hypertrophy of right ventricle 745.2
  in tetralogy of Fallot 745.2
Dextratransposition, aorta 745.11
Dextrinosis, limit (debrancher enzyme deficiency) 271.0

Dextrocardia (corrected) (false) (isolated) (secondary) (true) 746.87
  with
    complete transposition of viscera 759.3
    situs inversus 759.3
Dextroversion, kidney (left) 753.3
Dhobie itch 110.3
Diabetes, diabetic (brittle) (congenital) (familial) (mellitus) (severe) (slight) (without complication) 250.0 ✓5ᵗʰ

> Note — Use the following fifth-digit subclassification with category 250:
>
> 0 type II [non-insulin dependent type] [NIDDM type] [adult-onset type] or unspecified type, not stated as uncontrolled
>
> 1 type I [insulin dependent type] [IDDM type] [juvenile type], not stated as uncontrolled
>
> 2 type II [non-insulin dependent type] [NIDDM type] [adult-onset type] or unspecified type, uncontrolled
>
> 3 type I [insulin dependent type] [IDDM type] [juvenile type], uncontrolled

  with
    coma (with ketoacidosis) 250.3 ✓5ᵗʰ
      hyperosmolar (nonketotic) 250.2 ✓5ᵗʰ
    complication NEC 250.9 ✓5ᵗʰ
      specified NEC 250.8 ✓5ᵗʰ
    gangrene 250.7 ✓5ᵗʰ [785.4]
    hyperosmolarity 250.2 ✓5ᵗʰ
    ketosis, ketoacidosis 250.1 ✓5ᵗʰ
    osteomyelitis 250.8 ✓5ᵗʰ [731.8]
    specified manifestations NEC 250.8 ✓5ᵗʰ
  acetonemia 250.1 ✓5ᵗʰ
  acidosis 250.1 ✓5ᵗʰ
  amyotrophy 250.6 ✓5ᵗʰ [358.1]
  angiopathy, peripheral 250.7 ✓5ᵗʰ [443.81]
  asymptomatic 790.2
  autonomic neuropathy (peripheral) 250.6 ✓5ᵗʰ [337.1]
  bone change 250.8 ✓5ᵗʰ [731.8]
  bronze, bronzed 275.0
  cataract 250.5 ✓5ᵗʰ [366.41]
  chemical 790.2
    complicating pregnancy, childbirth, or puerperium 648.8 ✓5ᵗʰ
  coma (with ketoacidosis) 250.3 ✓5ᵗʰ
    hyperglycemic 250.3 ✓5ᵗʰ
    hyperosmolar (nonketotic) 250.2 ✓5ᵗʰ
    hypoglycemic 250.3 ✓5ᵗʰ
    insulin 250.3 ✓5ᵗʰ
  complicating pregnancy, childbirth, or puerperium (maternal) 648.0 ✓5ᵗʰ
    affecting fetus or newborn 775.0
  complication NEC 250.9 ✓5ᵗʰ
    specified NEC 250.8 ✓5ᵗʰ
  dorsal sclerosis 250.6 ✓5ᵗʰ [340] ✓5ᵗʰ
  dwarfism-obesity syndrome 258.1
  gangrene 250.7 ✓5ᵗʰ [785.4]
  gastroparesis 250.6 ✓5ᵗʰ [536.3]
  gestational 648.8 ✓5ᵗʰ
    complicating pregnancy, childbirth, or puerperium 648.8 ✓5ᵗʰ
  glaucoma 250.5 ✓5ᵗʰ [365.44]
  glomerulosclerosis (intercapillary) 250.4 ✓5ᵗʰ [581.81]
  glycogenosis, secondary 250.8 ✓5ᵗʰ [259.8]
  hemochromatosis 275.0
  hyperosmolar coma 250.2 ✓5ᵗʰ
  hyperosmolarity 250.2 ✓5ᵗʰ
  hypertension-nephrosis syndrome 250.4 ✓5ᵗʰ [581.81]
  hypoglycemia 250.8 ✓5ᵗʰ
  hypoglycemic shock 250.8 ✓5ᵗʰ
  insipidus 253.5
    nephrogenic 588.1
    pituitary 253.5
    vasopressin-resistant 588.1
  intercapillary glomerulosclerosis 250.4 ✓5ᵗʰ [581.81]
  iritis 250.5 ✓5ᵗʰ [364.42]
  ketosis, ketoacidosis 250.1 ✓5ᵗʰ

Diabetes — Difficulty

Diabetes, diabetic — *continued*
- Kimmelstiel (-Wilson) disease or syndrome (intercapillary glomerulosclerosis) 250.4 ✓5 *[581.81]*
- Lancereaux's (diabetes mellitus with marked emaciation) 250.8 ✓5 *[261]*
- latent (chemical) 790.2
  - complicating pregnancy, childbirth, or puerperium 648. ✓5
- lipoidosis 250.8 ✓5 *[272.7]*
- macular edema 250.5 ✓5 *[362.01]*
- maternal
  - with manifest disease in the infant 775.1
  - affecting fetus or newborn 775.0
- microaneurysms, retinal 250.5 ✓5 *[362.01]*
- mononeuropathy 250.6 ✓5 *[355.9]*
- neonatal, transient 775.1
- nephropathy 250.4 ✓5 *[583.81]*
- nephrosis (syndrome) 250.4 ✓5 *[581.81]*
- neuralgia 250.6 ✓5 *[357.2]*
- neuritis 250.6 ✓5 *[357.2]*
- neurogenic arthropathy 250.6 ✓5 *[713.5]*
- neuropathy 250.6 ✓5 *[357.2]*
- nonclinical 790.2
- osteomyelitis 250.8 ✓5 *[731.8]*
- peripheral autonomic neuropathy 250.6 ✓5 *[337.1]*
- phosphate 275.3
- polyneuropathy 250.6 ✓5 *[357.2]*
- renal (true) 271.4
- retinal
  - edema 250.5 ✓5 *[362.01]*
  - hemorrhage 250.5 ✓5 *[362.01]*
  - microaneurysms 250.5 ✓5 *[362.01]*
- retinitis 250.5 ✓5 *[362.01]*
- retinopathy 250.5 ✓5 *[362.01]*
  - background 250.5 ✓5 *[362.01]*
  - proliferative 250.5 ✓5 *[362.02]*
- steroid induced
  - correct substance properly administered 251.8
  - overdose or wrong substance given or taken 962.0
- stress 790.2
- subclinical 790.2
- subliminal 790.2
- sugar 250.0 ✓5
- ulcer (skin) 250.8 ✓5 *[707.9]*
  - lower extremity 250.8 ✓5 *[707.10]*
    - ankle 250.8 *[707.13]*
    - calf 250.8 *[707.12]*
    - foot 250.8 *[707.15]*
    - heel 250.8 *[707.14]*
    - knee 250.8 *[707.19]*
    - specified site NEC 250.8 *[707.19]*
    - thigh 250.8 *[707.11]*
    - toes 250.8 *[707.15]*
  - specified site NEC 250.8 ✓5 *[707.8]*
- xanthoma 250.8 ✓5 *[272.2]*

Diacyclothrombopathia 287.1
Diagnosis deferred 799.9
Dialysis (intermittent) (treatment)
- anterior retinal (juvenile) (with detachment) 361.04
- extracorporeal V56.0
- peritoneal V56.8
- renal V56.0
  - status only V45.1
- specified type NEC V56.8

Diamond-Blackfan anemia or syndrome (congenital hypoplastic anemia) 284.0
Diamond-Gardner syndrome (autoerythrocyte sensitization) 287.2
Diaper rash 691.0
Diaphoresis (excessive) NEC 780.8
Diaphragm — *see* condition
Diaphragmalgia 786.52
Diaphragmitis 519.4
Diaphyseal aclasis 756.4
Diaphysitis 733.99

Diarrhea, diarrheal (acute) (autumn) (bilious) (bloody) (catarrhal) (choleraic) (chronic) (gravis) (green) (infantile) (lienteric) (noninfectious) (presumed noninfectious) (putrefactive) (secondary) (sporadic) (summer) (symptomatic) (thermic) 787.91
- achlorhydric 536.0
- allergic 558.3
- amebic (*see also* Amebiasis) 006.9
  - with abscess — *see* Abscess, amebic
  - acute 006.0
  - chronic 006.1
  - nondysenteric 006.2
- bacillary — *see* Dysentery, bacillary
- bacterial NEC 008.5
- balantidial — 007.0
- bile salt-induced 579.8
- cachectic NEC 787.91
- chilomastix 007.8
- choleriformis 001.1
- coccidial 007.2
- Cochin-China 579.1
  - anguilluliasis 127.2
  - psilosis 579.1
- Dientamoeba 007.8
- dietetic 787.91
- due to
  - achylia gastrica 536.8
  - Aerobacter aerogenes 008.2 ✓5
  - Bacillus coli — *see* Enteritis, E. coli
  - bacteria NEC 008.5
  - bile salts 579.8
  - Capillaria
    - hepatica 128.8
    - philippinensis 127.5
  - Clostridium perfringens (C) (F) 008.46
  - Enterobacter aerogenes 008.2 ✓5
  - enterococci 008.49
  - Escherichia coli — *see* Enteritis, E. coli
  - Giardia lamblia 007.1
  - Heterophyes heterophyes 121.6
  - irritating foods 787.91
  - Metagonimus yokogawai 121.5
  - Necator americanus 126.1
  - Paracolobactrum arizonae 008.1
  - Paracolon bacillus NEC 008.47
    - Arizona 008.1
  - Proteus (bacillus) (mirabilis) (Morganii) 008.3
  - Pseudomonas aeruginosa 008.42
  - S. japonicum 120.2
  - specified organism NEC 008.8
    - bacterial 008.49
    - viral NEC 008.69
  - Staphylococcus 008.41
  - Streptococcus 008.49
    - anaerobic 008.46
  - Strongyloides stercoralis 127.2
  - Trichuris trichiuria 127.3
  - virus NEC (*see also* Enteritis, viral) 008.69
- dysenteric 009.2
  - due to specified organism NEC 008.8
- dyspeptic 787.91
- endemic 009.3
  - due to specified organism NEC 008.8
- epidemic 009.2
  - due to specified organism NEC 008.8
- fermentative 787.91
- flagellate 007.9
- Flexner's (ulcerative) 004.1
- functional 564.5
  - following gastrointestinal surgery 564.4
  - psychogenic 306.4
- giardial 007.1
- Giardia lamblia 007.1
- hill 579.1
- hyperperistalsis (nervous) 306.4
- infectious 009.2
  - due to specified organism NEC 008.8
  - presumed 009.3
- inflammatory 787.91
  - due to specified organism NEC 008.8
- malarial (*see also* Malaria) 084.6
- mite 133.8
- mycotic 117.9
- nervous 306.4
- neurogenic 564.5
- parenteral NEC 009.2

Diarrhea, diarrheal — *continued*
- postgastrectomy 564.4
- postvagotomy 564.4
- prostaglandin induced 579.8
- protozoal NEC 007.9
- psychogenic 306.4
- septic 009.2
  - due to specified organism NEC 008.8
- specified organism NEC 008.8
  - bacterial 008.49
  - viral NEC 008.69
- Staphylococcus 008.41
- Streptococcus 008.49
  - anaerobic 008.46
- toxic 558.2
- travelers' 009.2
  - due to specified organism NEC 008.8
- trichomonal 007.3
- tropical 579.1
- tuberculous 014.8 ✓5
- ulcerative (chronic) (*see also* Colitis, ulcerative) 556.9
- viral (*see also* Enteritis, viral) 008.8
- zymotic NEC 009.2

Diastasis
- cranial bones 733.99
  - congenital 756.0
- joint (traumatic) — *see* Dislocation, by site
- muscle 728.84
  - congenital 756.89
- recti (abdomen) 728.84
  - complicating delivery 665.8 ✓5
  - congenital 756.79

Diastema, teeth, tooth 524.3
Diastematomyelia 742.51
Diataxia, cerebral, infantile 343.0
Diathesis
- allergic V15.09
- bleeding (familial) 287.9
- cystine (familial) 270.0
- gouty 274.9
- hemorrhagic (familial) 287.9
  - newborn NEC 776.0
- oxalic 271.8
- scrofulous (*see also* Tuberculosis) 017.2 ✓5
- spasmophilic (*see also* Tetany) 781.7
- ulcer 536.9
- uric acid 274.9

Diaz's disease or osteochondrosis 732.5
Dibothriocephaliasis 123.4
- larval 123.5
Dibothriocephalus (infection) (infestation) (latus) 123.4
- larval 123.5
Dicephalus 759.4
Dichotomy, teeth 520.2
Dichromat, dichromata (congenital) 368.59
Dichromatopsia (congenital) 368.59
Dichuchwa 104.0
Dicroceliasis 121.8
Didelphys, didelphic (*see also* Double uterus) 752.2
Didymitis (*see also* Epididymitis) 604.90
Died — *see also* Death
- without
  - medical attention (cause unknown) 798.9
  - sign of disease 798.2
Dientamoeba diarrhea 007.8
Dietary
- inadequacy or deficiency 269.9
- surveillance and counseling V65.3
Dietl's crisis 593.4
Dieulafoy ▶lesion◀ (hemorrhagic)
- of
  - duodenum 537.84
  - intestine 569.86
  - stomach 537.84
Difficult
- birth, affecting fetus or newborn 763.9
- delivery NEC 669.9 ✓5
Difficulty
- feeding 783.3
  - breast 676.8 ✓5

Index to Diseases

Difficulty — continued
feeding — continued
- newborn 779.3
- nonorganic (infant) NEC 307.59
- mechanical, gastroduodenal stoma 537.89
- reading 315.00
- specific, spelling 315.09
- swallowing (see also Dysphagia) 787.2
- walking 719.7 ✓5th

Diffuse — see condition

Diffused ganglion 727.42

DiGeorge's syndrome (thymic hypoplasia) 279.11

Digestive — see condition

Di Guglielmo's disease or syndrome (M9841/3) 207.0 ✓5th

Diktyoma (M9051/3) — see Neoplasm, by site, malignant

Dilaceration, tooth 520.4

Dilatation
- anus 564.89
  - venule — see Hemorrhoids
- aorta (focal) (general) (see also Aneurysm, aorta) 441.9
  - congenital 747.29
  - infectional 093.0
  - ruptured 441.5
  - syphilitic 093.0
- appendix (cystic) 543.9
- artery 447.8
- bile duct (common) (cystic) (congenital) 751.69
  - acquired 576.8
- bladder (sphincter) 596.8
  - congenital 753.8
  - in pregnancy or childbirth 654.4 ✓5th
    - causing obstructed labor 660.2 ✓5th
      - affecting fetus or newborn 763.1
- blood vessel 459.89
- bronchus, bronchi 494.0
  - with acute exacerbation 494.1
- calyx (due to obstruction) 593.89
- capillaries 448.9
- cardiac (acute) (chronic) (see also Hypertrophy, cardiac) 429.3
  - congenital 746.89
    - valve NEC 746.89
      - pulmonary 746.09
  - hypertensive (see also Hypertension, heart) 402.90
- cavum septi pellucidi 742.4
- cecum 564.89
  - psychogenic 306.4
- cervix (uteri) — see also Incompetency, cervix
  - incomplete, poor, slow
    - affecting fetus or newborn 763.7
    - complicating delivery 661.0 ✓5th
      - affecting fetus or newborn 763.7
- colon 564.7
  - congenital 751.3
  - due to mechanical obstruction 560.89
  - psychogenic 306.4
- common bile duct (congenital) 751.69
  - acquired 576.8
    - with calculus, choledocholithiasis, or stones — see Choledocholithiasis
- cystic duct 751.69
  - acquired (any bile duct) 575.8
- duct, mammary 610.4
- duodenum 564.89
- esophagus 530.89
  - congenital 750.4
  - due to
    - achalasia 530.0
    - cardiospasm 530.0
- Eustachian tube, congenital 744.24
- fontanel 756.0
- gallbladder 575.8
  - congenital 751.69
- gastric 536.8
  - acute 536.1
  - psychogenic 306.4
- heart (acute) (chronic) (see also Hypertrophy, cardiac) 429.3
  - congenital 746.89
  - hypertensive (see also Hypertension, heart) 402.90

Dilatation — continued
heart (see also Hypertrophy, cardiac) — continued
- valve — see also Endocarditis
  - congenital 746.89
- ileum 564.89
  - psychogenic 306.4
- inguinal rings — see Hernia, inguinal
- jejunum 564.89
  - psychogenic 306.4
- kidney (calyx) (collecting structures) (cystic) (parenchyma) (pelvis) 593.89
- lacrimal passages 375.69
- lymphatic vessel 457.1
- mammary duct 610.4
- Meckel's diverticulum (congenital) 751.0
- meningeal vessels, congenital 742.8
- myocardium (acute) (chronic) (see also Hypertrophy, cardiac) 429.3
- organ or site, congenital NEC — see Distortion
- pancreatic duct 577.8
- pelvis, kidney 593.89
- pericardium — see Pericarditis
- pharynx 478.29
- prostate 602.8
- pulmonary
  - artery (idiopathic) 417.8
    - congenital 747.3
  - valve, congenital 746.09
- pupil 379.43
- rectum 564.89
- renal 593.89
- saccule vestibularis, congenital 744.05
- salivary gland (duct) 527.8
- sphincter ani 564.89
- stomach 536.8
  - acute 536.1
  - psychogenic 306.4
- submaxillary duct 527.8
- trachea, congenital 748.3
- ureter (idiopathic) 593.89
  - congenital 753.20
  - due to obstruction 593.5
- urethra (acquired) 599.84
- vasomotor 443.9
- vein 459.89
- ventricular, ventricle (acute) (chronic) (see also Hypertrophy, cardiac) 429.3
  - cerebral, congenital 742.4
  - hypertensive (see also Hypertension, heart) 402.90
- venule 459.89
  - anus — see Hemorrhoids
- vesical orifice 596.8

Dilated, dilation — see Dilatation

Diminished
- hearing (acuity) (see also Deafness) 389.9
- pulse pressure 785.9
- vision NEC 369.9
- vital capacity 794.2

Diminuta taenia 123.6

Diminution, sense or sensation (cold) (heat) (tactile) (vibratory) (see also Disturbance, sensation) 782.0

Dimitri-Sturge-Weber disease (encephalocutaneous angiomatosis) 759.6

Dimple
- parasacral 685.1
  - with abscess 685.0
- pilonidal 685.1
  - with abscess 685.0
- postanal 685.1
  - with abscess 685.0

Dioctophyma renale (infection) (infestation) 128.8

Dipetalonemiasis 125.4

Diphallus 752.69

Diphtheria, diphtheritic (gangrenous) (hemorrhagic) 032.9
- carrier (suspected) of V02.4
- cutaneous 032.85
- cystitis 032.84
- faucial 032.0
- infection of wound 032.85
- inoculation (anti) (not sick) V03.5
- laryngeal 032.3
- myocarditis 032.82

Discoloration

Diphtheria, diphtheritic — continued
- nasal anterior 032.2
- nasopharyngeal 032.1
- neurological complication 032.89
- peritonitis 032.83
- specified site NEC 032.89

Diphyllobothriasis (intestine) 123.4
- larval 123.5

Diplacusis 388.41

Diplegia (upper limbs) 344.2
- brain or cerebral 437.8
- congenital 343.0
- facial 351.0
  - congenital 352.6
- infantile or congenital (cerebral) (spastic) (spinal) 343.0
- lower limbs 344.1
- syphilitic, congenital 090.49

Diplococcus, diplococcal — see condition

Diplomyelia 742.59

Diplopia 368.2
- refractive 368.15

Dipsomania (see also Alcoholism) 303.9 ✓5th
- with psychosis (see also Psychosis, alcoholic) 291.9

Dipylidiasis 123.8
- intestine 123.8

Direction, teeth, abnormal 524.3

Dirt-eating child 307.52

Disability
- heart — see Disease, heart
- learning NEC 315.2
- special spelling 315.09

Disarticulation (see also Derangement, joint) 718.9 ✓5th
- meaning
  - amputation
    - status — see Absence, by site
    - traumatic — see Amputation, traumatic
  - dislocation, traumatic or congenital — see Dislocation

Disaster, cerebrovascular (see also Disease, cerebrovascular, acute) 436

Discharge
- anal NEC 787.99
- breast (female) (male) 611.79
- conjunctiva 372.89
- continued locomotor idiopathic (see also Epilepsy) 345.5 ✓5th
- diencephalic autonomic idiopathic (see also Epilepsy) 345.5 ✓5th
- ear 388.60
  - blood 388.69
  - cerebrospinal fluid 388.61
- excessive urine 788.42
- eye 379.93
- nasal 478.1
- nipple 611.79
- patterned motor idiopathic (see also Epilepsy) 345.5 ✓5th
- penile 788.7
- postnasal — see Sinusitis
- sinus, from mediastinum 510.0
- umbilicus 789.9
- urethral 788.7
  - bloody 599.84
- vaginal 623.5

Discitis 722.90
- cervical, cervicothoracic 722.91
- lumbar, lumbosacral 722.93
- thoracic, thoracolumbar 722.92

Discogenic syndrome — see Displacement, intervertebral disc

Discoid
- kidney 753.3
- meniscus, congenital 717.5
- semilunar cartilage 717.5

Discoloration
- mouth 528.9
- nails 703.8
- teeth 521.7
  - due to
    - drugs 521.7

Discoloration

Discoloration — continued
  teeth — continued
    due to — continued
      metals (copper) (silver) 521.7
      pulpal bleeding 521.7
    during formation 520.8
    posteruptive 521.7
Discomfort
  chest 786.59
  visual 368.13
Discomycosis — see Actinomycosis
Discontinuity, ossicles, ossicular chain 385.23
Discrepancy
  leg length (acquired) 736.81
    congenital 755.30
  uterine size-date 646.8 ✓5
Discrimination
  political V62.4
  racial V62.4
  religious V62.4
  sex V62.4
Disease, diseased — see also Syndrome
  Abrami's (acquired hemolytic jaundice) 283.9
  absorbent system 459.89
  accumulation — see Thesaurismosis
  acid-peptic 536.8
  Acosta's 993.2
  Adams-Stokes (-Morgagni) (syncope with heart block) 426.9
  Addison's (bronze) (primary adrenal insufficiency) 255.4
    anemia (pernicious) 281.0
    tuberculous (see also Tuberculosis) 017.6 ✓5
  Addison-Gull — see Xanthoma
  adenoids (and tonsils) (chronic) 474.9
  adrenal (gland) (capsule) (cortex) 255.9
    hyperfunction 255.3
    hypofunction 255.4
    specified type NEC 255.8
  ainhum (dactylolysis spontanea) 136.0
  akamushi (scrub typhus) 081.2
  Akureyri (epidemic neuromyasthenia) 049.8
  Albarrán's (colibacilluria) 791.9
  Albers-Schönberg's (marble bones) 756.52
  Albert's 726.71
  Albright (-Martin) (-Bantam) 275.49
  Alibert's (mycosis fungoides) (M9700/3) 202.1 ✓5
  Alibert-Bazin (M9700/3) 202.1 ✓5
  alimentary canal 569.9
  alligator skin (ichthyosis congenita) 757.1
    acquired 701.1
  Almeida's (Brazilian blastomycosis) 116.1
  Alpers' 330.8
  alpine 993.2
  altitude 993.2
  alveoli, teeth 525.9
  Alzheimer's — see Alzheimer's
  amyloid (any site) 277.3
  anarthritic rheumatoid 446.5
  Anders' (adiposis tuberosa simplex) 272.8
  Andersen's (glycogenosis IV) 271.0
  Anderson's (angiokeratoma corporis diffusum) 272.7
  Andes 993.2
  Andrews' (bacterid) 686.8
  angiospastic, angiospasmodic 443.9
    cerebral 435.9
      with transient neurologic deficit 435.9
    vein 459.89
  anterior
    chamber 364.9
    horn cell 335.9
      specified type NEC 335.8
  antral (chronic) 473.0
    acute 461.0
  anus NEC 569.49
  aorta (nonsyphilitic) 447.9
    syphilitic NEC 093.89
  aortic (heart) (valve) (see also Endocarditis, aortic) 424.1
  apollo 077.4
  aponeurosis 726.90
  appendix 543.9
  aqueous (chamber) 364.9

Disease, diseased — see also Syndrome — continued
  arc-welders' lung 503
  Armenian 277.3
  Arnold-Chiari (see also Spina bifida) 741.0 ✓5
  arterial 447.9
    occlusive (see also Occlusion, by site) 444.22
      with embolus or thrombus — see Occlusion, by site
    due to stricture or stenosis 447.1
    specified type NEC 447.8
  arteriocardiorenal (see also Hypertension, cardiorenal) 404.90
  arteriolar (generalized) (obliterative) 447.9
    specified type NEC 447.8
  arteriorenal — see Hypertension, kidney
  arteriosclerotic — see also Arteriosclerosis
    cardiovascular 429.2
    coronary — see Arteriosclerosis, coronary
    heart — see Arteriosclerosis, coronary
    vascular — see Arteriosclerosis
  artery 447.9
    cerebral 437.9
    coronary — see Arteriosclerosis, coronary
    specified type NEC 447.8
  arthropod-borne NEC 088.9
    specified type NEC 088.89
  Asboe-Hansen's (incontinentia pigmenti) 757.33
  atticoantral, chronic (with posterior or superior marginal perforation of ear drum) 382.2
  auditory canal, ear 380.9
  Aujeszky's 078.89
  auricle, ear NEC 380.30
  Australian X 062.4
  autoimmune NEC 279.4
    hemolytic (cold type) (warm type) 283.0
    parathyroid 252.1
    thyroid 245.2
  aviators' (see also Effect, adverse, high altitude) 993.2
  ax(e)-grinders' 502
  Ayala's 756.89
  Ayerza's (pulmonary artery sclerosis with pulmonary hypertension) 416.0
  Azorean (of the nervous system) 334.8
  Babington's (familial hemorrhagic telangiectasia) 448.0
  back bone NEC 733.90
  bacterial NEC 040.89
    zoonotic NEC 027.9
      specified type NEC 027.8
  Baehr-Schiffrin (thrombotic thrombocytopenic purpura) 446.6
  Baelz's (cheilitis glandularis apostematosa) 528.5
  Baerensprung's (eczema marginatum) 110.3
  Balfour's (chloroma) 205.3 ✓5
  balloon (see also Effect, adverse, high altitude) 993.2
  Baló's 341.1
  Bamberger (-Marie) (hypertrophic pulmonary osteoarthropathy) 731.2
  Bang's (Brucella abortus) 023.1
  Bannister's 995.1
  Banti's (with cirrhosis) (with portal hypertension) — see Cirrhosis, liver
  Barcoo (see also Ulcer, skin) 707.9
  barium lung 503
  Barlow (-Möller) (infantile scurvy) 267
  barometer makers' 985.0
  Barraquer (-Simons) (progressive lipodystrophy) 272.6
  basal ganglia 333.90
    degenerative NEC 333.0
    specified NEC 333.89
  Basedow's (exophthalmic goiter) 242.0 ✓5
  basement membrane NEC 583.89
    with
      pulmonary hemorrhage (Goodpasture's syndrome) 446.21 [583.81]
  Bateman's 078.0
    purpura (senile) 287.2
  Batten's 330.1 [362.71]
  Batten-Mayou (retina) 330.1 [362.71]
  Batten-Steinert 359.2
  Battey 031.0

Disease, diseased — see also Syndrome — continued
  Baumgarten-Cruveilhier (cirrhosis of liver) 571.5
  bauxite-workers' 503
  Bayle's (dementia paralytica) 094.1
  Bazin's (primary) (see also Tuberculosis) 017.1 ✓5
  Beard's (neurasthenia) 300.5
  Beau's (see also Degeneration, myocardial) 429.1
  Bechterew's (ankylosing spondylitis) 720.0
  Becker's (idiopathic mural endomyocardial disease) 425.2
  Begbie's (exophthalmic goiter) 242.0 ✓5
  Behr's 362.50
  Beigel's (white piedra) 111.2
  Bekhterev's (ankylosing spondylitis) 720.0
  Bell's (see also Psychosis, affective) 296.0 ✓5
  Bennett's (leukemia) 208.9 ✓5
  Benson's 379.22
  Bergeron's (hysteroepilepsy) 300.11
  Berlin's 921.3
  Bernard-Soulier (thrombopathy) 287.1
  Bernhardt (-Roth) 355.1
  beryllium 503
  Besnier-Boeck (-Schaumann) (sarcoidosis) 135
  Best's 362.76
  Beurmann's (sporotrichosis) 117.1
  Bielschowsky (-Jansky) 330.1
  Biermer's (pernicious anemia) 281.0
  Biett's (discoid lupus erythematosus) 695.4
  bile duct (see also Disease, biliary) 576.9
  biliary (duct) (tract) 576.9
    with calculus, choledocholithiasis, or stones — see Choledocholithiasis
  Billroth's (meningocele) (see also Spina bifida) 741.9 ✓5
  Binswanger's 290.12
  Bird's (oxaluria) 271.8
  bird fanciers' 495.2
  black lung 500
  bladder 596.9
    specified NEC 596.8
  bleeder's 286.0
  Bloch-Sulzberger (incontinentia pigmenti) 757.33
  Blocq's (astasia-abasia) 307.9
  blood (-forming organs) 289.9
    specified NEC 289.8
    vessel 459.9
  Bloodgood's 610.1
  Blount's (tibia vara) 732.4
  blue 746.9
  Bodechtel-Guttmann (subacute sclerosing panencephalitis) 046.2
  Boeck's (sarcoidosis) 135
  bone 733.90
    fibrocystic NEC 733.29
      jaw 526.2
    marrow 289.9
    Paget's (osteitis deformans) 731.0
    specified type NEC 733.99
    von Rechlinghausen's (osteitis fibrosa cystica) 252.0
  Bonfils' — see Disease, Hodgkin's
  Borna 062.9
  Bornholm (epidemic pleurodynia) 074.1
  Bostock's (see also Fever, hay) 477.9
  Bouchard's (myopathic dilatation of the stomach) 536.1
  Bouillaud's (rheumatic heart disease) 391.9
  Bourneville (-Brissaud) (tuberous sclerosis) 759.5
  Bouveret (-Hoffmann) (paroxysmal tachycardia) 427.2
  bowel 569.9
    functional 564.9
      psychogenic 306.4
  Bowen's (M8081/2) — see Neoplasm, skin, in situ
  Bozzolo's (multiple myeloma) (M973/3) 203.0 ✓5
  Bradley's (epidemic vomiting) 078.82
  Brailsford's 732.3
    radius, head 732.3
    tarsal, scaphoid 732.5

Index to Diseases

Disease, diseased — *see also* Syndrome — *continued*
- Brailsford-Morquio (mucopolysaccharidosis IV) 277.5
- brain 348.9
  - Alzheimer's 331.0
    - with dementia — *see* Alzheimer's, dementia
  - arterial, artery 437.9
  - arteriosclerotic 437.0
  - congenital 742.9
  - degenerative — *see* Degeneration, brain
  - inflammatory — *see also* Encephalitis
    - late effect — *see* category 326
  - organic 348.9
    - arteriosclerotic 437.0
  - parasitic NEC 123.9
  - Pick's 331.1
    - with dementia
      - with behavioral disturbance 331.1 [294.11]
      - without behavioral disturbance 331.1 [294.10]
  - senile 331.2
- brazier's 985.8
- breast 611.9
  - cystic (chronic) 610.1
  - fibrocystic 610.1
  - inflammatory 611.0
  - Paget's (M8540/3) 174.0
  - puerperal, postpartum NEC 676.3 ✓5ᵗʰ
  - specified NEC 611.8
- Breda's (*see also* Yaws) 102.9
- Breisky's (kraurosis vulvae) 624.0
- Bretonneau's (diphtheritic malignant angina) 032.0
- Bright's (*see also* Nephritis) 583.9
  - arteriosclerotic (*see also* Hypertension, kidney) 403.90
- Brill's (recrudescent typhus) 081.1
  - flea-borne 081.0
  - louse-borne 081.1
- Brill-Symmers (follicular lymphoma) (M9690/3) 202.0 ✓5ᵗʰ
- Brill-Zinsser (recrudescent typhus) 081.1
- Brinton's (leather bottle stomach) (M8142/3) 151.9
- Brion-Kayser (*see also* Fever, paratyphoid) 002.9
- broad
  - beta 272.2
  - ligament, noninflammatory 620.9
    - specified NEC 620.8
- Brocq's 691.8
  - meaning
    - atopic (diffuse) neurodermatitis 691.8
    - dermatitis herpetiformis 694.0
    - lichen simplex chronicus 698.3
    - parapsoriasis 696.2
    - prurigo 698.2
- Brocq-Duhring (dermatitis herpetiformis) 694.0
- Brodie's (joint) (*see also* Osteomyelitis) 730.1 ✓5ᵗʰ
- bronchi 519.1
- bronchopulmonary 519.1
- bronze (Addison's) 255.4
  - tuberculous (*see also* Tuberculosis) 017.6 ✓5ᵗʰ
- Brown-Séquard 344.89
- Bruck's 733.99
- Bruck-de Lange (Amsterdam dwarf, mental retardation and brachycephaly) 759.89
- Bruhl's (splenic anemia with fever) 285.8
- Bruton's (X-linked agammaglobulinemia) 279.04
- buccal cavity 528.9
- Buchanan's (juvenile osteochondrosis, iliac crest) 732.1
- Buchman's (osteochondrosis juvenile) 732.1
- Budgerigar-fanciers' 495.2
- Büdinger-Ludloff-Läwen 717.89
- Buerger's (thromboangiitis obliterans) 443.1
- Bürger-Grütz (essential familial hyperlipemia) 272.3
- Burns' (lower ulna) 732.3
- bursa 727.9
- Bury's (erythema elevatum diutinum) 695.89

Disease, diseased — *see also* Syndrome — *continued*
- Buschke's 710.1
- Busquet's (*see also* Osteomyelitis) 730.1 ✓5ᵗʰ
- Busse-Buschke (cryptococcosis) 117.5
- C₂ (*see also* Alcoholism) 303.9 ✓5ᵗʰ
- Caffey's (infantile cortical hyperostosis) 756.59
- caisson 993.3
- calculous 592.9
- California 114.0
- Calvé (-Perthes) (osteochondrosis, femoral capital) 732.1
- Camurati-Engelmann (diaphyseal sclerosis) 756.59
- Canavan's 330.0
- capillaries 448.9
- Carapata 087.1
- cardiac — *see* Disease, heart
- cardiopulmonary, chronic 416.9
- cardiorenal (arteriosclerotic) (hepatic) (hypertensive) (vascular) (*see also* Hypertension, cardiorenal) 404.90
- cardiovascular (arteriosclerotic) 429.2
  - congenital 746.9
  - hypertensive (*see also* Hypertension, heart) 402.90
    - benign 402.10
    - malignant 402.00
  - renal (*see also* Hypertension, cardiorenal) 404.90
  - syphilitic (asymptomatic) 093.9
- carotid gland 259.8
- Carrión's (Bartonellosis) 088.0
- cartilage NEC 733.90
  - specified NEC 733.99
- Castellani's 104.8
- cat-scratch 078.3
- Cavare's (familial periodic paralysis) 359.3
- Cazenave's (pemphigus) 694.4
- cecum 569.9
- celiac (adult) 579.0
  - infantile 579.0
- cellular tissue NEC 709.9
- central core 359.0
- cerebellar, cerebellum — *see* Disease, brain
- cerebral (*see also* Disease, brain) 348.9
  - arterial, artery 437.9
  - degenerative — *see* Degeneration, brain
- cerebrospinal 349.9
- cerebrovascular NEC 437.9
  - acute 436
    - embolic — *see* Embolism, brain
    - late effect — *see* Late effect(s) (of) cerebrovascular disease
    - puerperal, postpartum, childbirth 674.0 ✓5ᵗʰ
    - thrombotic — *see* Thrombosis, brain
  - arteriosclerotic 437.0
  - embolic — *see* Embolism, brain
  - ischemic, generalized NEC 437.1
  - late effect — *see* Late effect(s) (of) cerebrovascular disease
  - occlusive 437.1
  - puerperal, postpartum, childbirth 674.0 ✓5ᵗʰ
  - specified type NEC 437.8
  - thrombotic — *see* Thrombosis, brain
- ceroid storage 272.7
- cervix (uteri)
  - inflammatory 616.9
    - specified NEC 616.8
  - noninflammatory 622.9
    - specified NEC 622.8
- Chabert's 022.9
- Chagas' (*see also* Trypanosomiasis, American) 086.2
- Chandler's (osteochondritis dissecans, hip) 732.7
- Charcots' (joint) 094.0 [713.5]
  - spinal cord 094.0
- Charcôt-Marie-Tooth 356.1
- Charlouis' (*see also* Yaws) 102.9
- Cheadle (-Möller) (-Barlow) (infantile scurvy) 267
- Chédiak-Steinbrinck (-Higashi) (congenital gigantism of peroxidase granules) 288.2
- cheek, inner 528.9
- chest 519.9

Disease, diseased — *see also* Syndrome — *continued*
- Chiari's (hepatic vein thrombosis) 453.0
- Chicago (North American blastomycosis) 116.0
- chignon (white piedra) 111.2
- chigoe, chigo (jigger) 134.1
- childhood granulomatous 288.1
- Chinese liver fluke 121.1
- chlamydial NEC 078.88
- cholecystic (*see also* Disease, gallbladder) 575.9
- choroid 363.9
  - degenerative (*see also* Degeneration, choroid) 363.40
  - hereditary (*see also* Dystrophy, choroid) 363.50
  - specified type NEC 363.8
- Christian's (chronic histiocytosis X) 277.8
- Christian-Weber (nodular nonsuppurative panniculitis) 729.30
- Christmas 286.1
- ciliary body 364.9
- circulatory (system) NEC 459.9
  - chronic, maternal, affecting fetus or newborn 760.3
  - specified NEC 459.89
  - syphilitic 093.9
    - congenital 090.5
- Civatte's (poikiloderma) 709.09
- climacteric 627.2
  - male 608.89
- coagulation factor deficiency (congenital) (*see also* Defect, coagulation) 286.9
- Coats' 362.12
- coccidiodal pulmonary 114.5
  - acute 114.0
  - chronic 114.4
  - primary 114.0
  - residual 114.4
- Cockayne's (microcephaly and dwarfism) 759.89
- Cogan's 370.52
- cold
  - agglutinin 283.0
    - or hemoglobinuria 283.0
      - paroxysmal (cold) (nocturnal) 283.2
  - hemagglutinin (chronic) 283.0
- collagen NEC 710.9
  - nonvascular 710.9
  - specified NEC 710.8
  - vascular (allergic) (*see also* Angiitis, hypersensitivity) 446.20
- colon 569.9
  - functional 564.9
    - congenital 751.3
  - ischemic 557.0
- combined system (of spinal cord) 266.2 [336.2]
  - with anemia (pernicious) 281.0 [336.2]
- compressed air 993.3
- Concato's (pericardial polyserositis) 423.2
  - peritoneal 568.82
  - pleural — *see* Pleurisy
- congenital NEC 799.8
- conjunctiva 372.9
  - chlamydial 077.98
    - specified NEC 077.8
  - specified type NEC 372.89
  - viral 077.99
    - specified NEC 077.8
- connective tissue, diffuse (*see also* Disease, collagen) 710.9
- Conor and Bruch's (boutonneuse fever) 082.1
- Conradi (-Hünermann) 756.59
- Cooley's (erythroblastic anemia) 282.4
- Cooper's 610.1
- Corbus' 607.1
- cork-handlers' 495.3
- cornea (*see also* Keratopathy) 371.9
- coronary (*see also* Ischemia, heart) 414.9
  - congenital 746.85
  - ostial, syphilitic 093.20
    - aortic 093.22
    - mitral 093.21
    - pulmonary 093.24
    - tricuspid 093.23
- Corrigan's — *see* Insufficiency, aortic
- Cotugno's 724.3
- Coxsackie (virus) NEC 074.8

Disease, diseased — see also Syndrome — continued
  cranial nerve NEC 352.9
  Creutzfeldt-Jakob 046.1
    with dementia
      with behavioral disturbance
            046.1 [294.11]
      without behavioral disturbance
            046.1 [294.10]
  Crigler-Najjar (congenital hyperbilirubinemia) 277.4
  Crocq's (acrocyanosis) 443.89
  Crohn's (intestine) (see also Enteritis, regional) 555.9
  Crouzon's (craniofacial dysostosis) 756.0
  Cruchet's (encephalitis lethargica) 049.8
  Cruveilhier's 335.21
  Cruz-Chagas (see also Trypanosomiasis, American) 086.2
  crystal deposition (see also Arthritis, due to, crystals) 712.9 ✓5ᵗʰ
  Csillag's (lichen sclerosus et atrophicus) 701.0
  Curschmann's 359.2
  Cushing's (pituitary basophilism) 255.0
  cystic
    breast (chronic) 610.1
    kidney, congenital (see also Cystic, disease, kidney) 753.10
    liver, congenital 751.62
    lung 518.89
      congenital 748.4
    pancreas 577.2
      congenital 751.7
    renal, congenital (see also Cystic, disease, kidney) 753.10
    semilunar cartilage 717.5
  cysticercus 123.1
  cystine storage (with renal sclerosis) 270.0
  cytomegalic inclusion (generalized) 078.5
    with
      pneumonia 078.5 [484.1]
      congenital 771.1
  Daae (-Finsen) (epidemic pleurodynia) 074.1
  dancing 297.8
  Danielssen's (anesthetic leprosy) 030.1
  Darier's (congenital) (keratosis follicularis) 757.39
    erythema annulare centrifugum 695.0
    vitamin A deficiency 264.8
  Darling's (histoplasmosis) (see also Histoplasmosis, American) 115.00
  Davies' 425.0
  de Beurmann-Gougerot (sporotrichosis) 117.1
  Débove's (splenomegaly) 789.2
  deer fly (see also Tularemia) 021.9
  deficiency 269.9
  degenerative — see also Degeneration
    disc — see Degeneration, intervertebral disc
  Degos' 447.8
  Déjérine (-Sottas) 356.0
  Déleage's 359.89 ▲
  demyelinating, demyelinizating (brain stem) (central nervous system) 341.9
    multiple sclerosis 340
    specified NEC 341.8
  de Quervain's (tendon sheath) 727.04
    thyroid (subacute granulomatous thyroiditis) 245.1
  Dercum's (adiposis dolorosa) 272.8
  Deutschländer's — see Fracture, foot
  Devergie's (pityriasis rubra pilaris) 696.4
  Devic's 341.0
  diaphorase deficiency 289.7
  diaphragm 519.4
  diarrheal, infectious 009.2
  diatomaceous earth 502
  Diaz's (osteochondrosis astragalus) 732.5
  digestive system 569.9
  Di Guglielmo's (erythemic myelosis) (M9841/3) 207.0 ✓5ᵗʰ
  Dimitri-Sturge-Weber (encephalocutaneous angiomatosis) 759.6
  disc, degenerative — see Degeneration, intervertebral disc
  discogenic (see also Disease, intervertebral disc) 722.90
  diverticular — see Diverticula
  Down's (mongolism) 758.0

Disease, diseased — see also Syndrome — continued
  Dubini's (electric chorea) 049.8
  Dubois' (thymus gland) 090.5
  Duchenne's 094.0
    locomotor ataxia 094.0
    muscular dystrophy 359.1
    paralysis 335.22
    pseudohypertrophy, muscles 359.1
  Duchenne-Griesinger 359.1
  ductless glands 259.9
  Duhring's (dermatitis herpetiformis) 694.0
  Dukes (-Filatov) 057.8
  duodenum NEC 537.9
    specified NEC 537.89
  Duplay's 726.2
  Dupré's (meningism) 781.6
  Dupuytren's (muscle contracture) 728.6
  Durand-Nicolas-Favre (climatic bubo) 099.1
  Duroziez' (congenital mitral stenosis) 746.5
  Dutton's (trypanosomiasis) 086.9
  Eales' 362.18
  ear (chronic) (inner) NEC 388.9
    middle 385.9
      adhesive (see also Adhesions, middle ear) 385.10
      specified NEC 385.89
  Eberth's (typhoid fever) 002.0
  Ebstein's
    heart 746.2
    meaning diabetes 250.4 ✓5ᵗʰ [581.81]
  Echinococcus (see also Echinococcus) 122.9
  ECHO virus NEC 078.89
  Economo's (encephalitis lethargica) 049.8
  Eddowes' (brittle bones and blue sclera) 756.51
  Edsall's 992.2
  Eichstedt's (pityriasis versicolor) 111.0
  Ellis-van Creveld (chondroectodermal dysplasia) 756.55
  endocardium — see Endocarditis
  endocrine glands or system NEC 259.9
    specified NEC 259.8
  endomyocardial, idiopathic mural 425.2
  Engel-von Recklinghausen (osteitis fibrosa cystica) 252.0
  Engelmann's (diaphyseal sclerosis) 756.59
  English (rickets) 268.0
  Engman's (infectious eczematoid dermatitis) 690.8
  enteroviral, enterovirus NEC 078.89
    central nervous system NEC 048
  epidemic NEC 136.9
  epididymis 608.9
  epigastric, functional 536.9
    psychogenic 306.4
  Erb (-Landouzy) 359.1
  Erb-Goldflam 358.0
  Erichsen's (railway spine) 300.16
  esophagus 530.9
    functional 530.5
    psychogenic 306.4
  Eulenburg's (congenital paramyotonia) 359.2
  Eustachian tube 381.9
  Evans' (thrombocytopenic purpura) 287.3
  external auditory canal 380.9
  extrapyramidal NEC 333.90
  eye 379.90
    anterior chamber 364.9
    inflammatory NEC 364.3
    muscle 378.9
  eyeball 360.9
  eyelid 374.9
  eyeworm of Africa 125.2
  Fabry's (angiokeratoma corporis diffusum) 272.7
  facial nerve (seventh) 351.9
    newborn 767.5
  Fahr-Volhard (malignant nephrosclerosis) 403.00
  fallopian tube, noninflammatory 620.9
    specified NEC 620.8
  familial periodic 277.3
    paralysis 359.3
  Fanconi's (congenital pancytopenia) 284.0
  Farber's (disseminated lipogranulomatosis) 272.8
  fascia 728.9
    inflammatory 728.9

Disease, diseased — see also Syndrome — continued
  Fauchard's (periodontitis) 523.4
  Favre-Durand-Nicolas (climatic bubo) 099.1
  Favre-Racouchot (elastoidosis cutanea nodularis) 701.8
  Fede's 529.0
  Feer's 985.0
  Felix's (juvenile osteochondrosis, hip) 732.1
  Fenwick's (gastric atrophy) 537.89
  Fernels' (aortic aneurysm) 441.9
  fibrocaseous, of lung (see also Tuberculosis, pulmonary) 011.9 ✓5ᵗʰ
  fibrocystic — see also Fibrocystic, disease
    newborn 277.01
  Fiedler's (leptospiral jaundice) 100.0
  fifth 057.0
  Filatoff's (infectious mononucleosis) 075
  Filatov's (infectious mononucleosis) 075
  file-cutters' 984.9
    specified type of lead — see Table of Drugs and Chemicals
  filterable virus NEC 078.89
  fish skin 757.1
    acquired 701.1
  Flajani (-Basedow) (exophthalmic goiter) 242.0 ✓5ᵗʰ
  Flatau-Schilder 341.1
  flax-dressers' 504
  Fleischner's 732.3
  flint 502
  fluke — see Infestation, fluke
  Følling's (phenylketonuria) 270.1
  foot and mouth 078.4
  foot process 581.3
  Forbes' (glycogenosis III) 271.0
  Fordyce's (ectopic sebaceous glands) (mouth) 750.26
  Fordyce-Fox (apocrine miliaria) 705.82
  Fothergill's
    meaning scarlatina anginosa 034.1
    neuralgia (see also Neuralgia, trigeminal) 350.1
  Fournier's 608.83
  fourth 057.8
  Fox (-Fordyce) (apocrine miliaria) 705.82
  Francis' (see also Tularemia) 021.9
  Franklin's (heavy chain) 273.2
  Frei's (climatic bubo) 099.1
  Freiberg's (flattening metarsal) 732.5
  Friedländer's (endarteritis obliterans) — see Arteriosclerosis
  Friedreich's
    combined systemic or ataxia 334.0
    facial hemihypertrophy 756.0
    myoclonia 333.2
  Fröhlich's (adiposogenital dystrophy) 253.8
  Frommel's 676.6 ✓5ᵗʰ
  frontal sinus (chronic) 473.1
    acute 461.1
  Fuller's earth 502
  fungus, fungous NEC 117.9
  Gaisböck's (polycythemia hypertonica) 289.0
  gallbladder 575.9
    congenital 751.60
  Gamna's (siderotic splenomegaly) 289.51
  Gamstorp's (adynamia episodica hereditaria) 359.3
  Gandy-Nanta (siderotic splenomegaly) 289.51
  gannister (occupational) 502
  Garré's (see also Osteomyelitis) 730.1 ✓5ᵗʰ
  gastric (see also Disease, stomach) 537.9
  gastrointestinal (tract) 569.9
    amyloid 277.3
    functional 536.9
      psychogenic 306.4
  Gaucher's (adult) (cerebroside lipidosis) (infantile) 272.7
  Gayet's (superior hemorrhagic polioencephalitis) 265.1
  Gee (-Herter) (-Heubner) (-Thaysen) (nontropical sprue) 579.0
  generalized neoplastic (M8000/6) 199.0
  genital organs NEC
    female 629.9
      specified NEC 629.8
    male 608.9
  Gerhardt's (erythromelalgia) 443.89

Index to Diseases

Disease, diseased

Disease, diseased — see also Syndrome — continued
- Gerlier's (epidemic vertigo) 078.81
- Gibert's (pityriasis rosea) 696.3
- Gibney's (perispondylitis) 720.9
- Gierke's (glycogenosis I) 271.0
- Gilbert's (familial nonhemolytic jaundice) 277.4
- Gilchrist's (North American blastomycosis) 116.0
- Gilford (-Hutchinson) (progeria) 259.8
- Gilles de la Tourette's (motor-verbal tic) 307.23
- Giovannini's 117.9
- gland (lymph) 289.9
- Glanzmann's (hereditary hemorrhagic thrombasthenia) 287.1
- glassblowers' 527.1
- Glénard's (enteroptosis) 569.89
- Glisson's (see also Rickets) 268.0
- glomerular
  - membranous, idiopathic 581.1
  - minimal change 581.3
- glycogen storage (Andersen's) (Cori types 1-7) (Forbes') (McArdle-Schmid-Pearson) (Pompe's) (types I-VII) 271.0
  - cardiac 271.0 [425.7]
  - generalized 271.0
  - glucose-6-phosphatase deficiency 271.0
  - heart 271.0 [425.7]
  - hepatorenal 271.0
  - liver and kidneys 271.0
  - myocardium 271.0 [425.7]
  - von Gierke's (glycogenosis I) 271.0
- Goldflam-Erb 358.0
- Goldscheider's (epidermolysis bullosa) 757.39
- Goldstein's (familial hemorrhagic telangiectasia) 448.0
- gonococcal NEC 098.0
- Goodall's (epidemic vomiting) 078.82
- Gordon's (exudative enteropathy) 579.8
- Gougerot's (trisymptomatic) 709.1
- Gougerot-Carteaud (confluent reticulate papillomatosis) 701.8
- Gougerot-Hailey-Hailey (benign familial chronic pemphigus) 757.39
- graft-versus-host (bone marrow) 996.85
  - due to organ transplant NEC — see Complications, transplant, organ
- grain-handlers' 495.8
- Grancher's (splenopneumonia) — see Pneumonia
- granulomatous (childhood) (chronic) 288.1
- graphite lung 503
- Graves' (exophthalmic goiter) 242.0 ✓5ᵗʰ
- Greenfield's 330.0
- green monkey 078.89
- Griesinger's (see also Ancylostomiasis) 126.9
- grinders' 502
- Grisel's 723.5
- Gruby's (tinea tonsurans) 110.0
- Guertin's (electric chorea) 049.8
- Guillain-Barré 357.0
- Guinon's (motor-verbal tic) 307.23
- Gull's (thyroid atrophy with myxedema) 244.8
- Gull and Sutton's — see Hypertension, kidney
- gum NEC 523.9
- Günther's (congenital erythropoietic porphyria) 277.1
- gynecological 629.9
  - specified NEC 629.8
- H 270.0
- Haas' 732.3
- Habermann's (acute parapsoriasis varioliformis) 696.2
- Haff 985.1
- Hageman (congenital factor XII deficiency) (see also Defect, congenital) 286.3
- Haglund's (osteochondrosis os tibiale externum) 732.5
- Hagner's (hypertrophic pulmonary osteoarthropathy) 731.2
- Hailey-Hailey (benign familial chronic pemphigus) 757.39
- hair (follicles) NEC 704.9
  - specified type NEC 704.8
- Hallervorden-Spatz 333.0
- Hallopeau's (lichen sclerosus et atrophicus) 701.0

Disease, diseased — see also Syndrome — continued
- Hamman's (spontaneous mediastinal emphysema) 518.1
- hand, foot, and mouth 074.3
- Hand-Schüller-Christian (chronic histiocytosis X) 277.8
- Hanot's — see Cirrhosis, biliary
- Hansen's (leprosy) 030.9
  - benign form 030.1
  - malignant form 030.0
- Harada's 363.22
- Harley's (intermittent hemoglobinuria) 283.2
- Hart's (pellagra-cerebellar ataxia renal aminoaciduria) 270.0
- Hartnup (pellagra-cerebellar ataxia renal aminoaciduria) 270.0
- Hashimoto's (struma lymphomatosa) 245.2
- Hb — see Disease, hemoglobin
- heart (organic) 429.9
  - with
    - acute pulmonary edema (see also Failure, ventricular, left) 428.1
      - hypertensive 402.91
        - with renal failure 404.91
        - benign 402.11
          - with renal failure 404.11
        - malignant 402.01
          - with renal failure 404.01
    - kidney disease — see Hypertension, cardiorenal
    - rheumatic fever (conditions classifiable to 390)
      - active 391.9
        - with chorea 392.0
      - inactive or quiescent (with chorea) 398.90
  - amyloid 277.3 [425.7]
  - aortic (valve) (see also Endocarditis, aortic) 424.1
  - arteriosclerotic or sclerotic (minimal) (senile) — see Arteriosclerosis, coronary
  - artery — see Arteriosclerosis, coronary
  - atherosclerotic — see Arteriosclerosis, coronary
  - beer drinkers' 425.5
  - beriberi 265.0 [425.7]
  - black 416.0
  - congenital NEC 746.9
    - cyanotic 746.9
    - maternal, affecting fetus or newborn 760.3
    - specified type NEC 746.89
  - congestive (see also Failure, heart) 428.0
  - coronary 414.9
  - cryptogenic 429.9
  - due to
    - amyloidosis 277.3 [425.7]
    - beriberi 265.0 [425.7]
    - cardiac glycogenosis 271.0 [425.7]
    - Friedreich's ataxia 334.0 [425.8]
    - gout 274.82
    - mucopolysaccharidosis 277.5 [425.7]
    - myotonia atrophica 359.2 [425.8]
    - progressive muscular dystrophy 359.1 [425.8]
    - sarcoidosis 135 [425.8]
  - fetal 746.9
    - inflammatory 746.89
  - fibroid (see also Myocarditis) 429.0
  - functional 427.9
    - postoperative 997.1
    - psychogenic 306.2
  - glycogen storage 271.0 [425.7]
  - gonococcal NEC 098.85
  - gouty 274.82
  - hypertensive (see also Hypertension, heart) 402.90
    - benign 402.10
    - malignant 402.00
  - hyperthyroid (see also Hyperthyroidism) 242.9 ✓5ᵗʰ [425.7]
  - incompletely diagnosed — see Disease, heart
  - ischemic (chronic) (see also Ischemia, heart) 414.9

Disease, diseased — see also Syndrome — continued
- heart — continued
  - ischemic (see also Ischemia, heart) — continued
    - acute (see also Infarct, myocardium)
      - without myocardial infarction 411.89
        - with coronary (artery) occlusion 411.81
    - asymptomatic 412
    - diagnosed on ECG or other special investigation but currently presenting no symptoms 412
  - kyphoscoliotic 416.1
  - mitral (see also Endocarditis, mitral) 394.9
  - muscular (see also Degeneration, myocardial) 429.1
  - postpartum 674.8 ✓5ᵗʰ
  - psychogenic (functional) 306.2
  - pulmonary (chronic) 416.9
    - acute 415.0
    - specified NEC 416.8
  - rheumatic (chronic) (inactive) (old) (quiescent) (with chorea) 398.90
    - active or acute 391.9
      - with chorea (active) (rheumatic) (Sydenham's) 392.0
    - specified type NEC 391.8
    - maternal, affecting fetus or newborn 760.3
  - rheumatoid — see Arthritis, rheumatoid
  - sclerotic — see Arteriosclerosis, coronary
  - senile (see also Myocarditis) 429.0
  - specified type NEC 429.89
  - syphilitic 093.89
    - aortic 093.1
    - aneurysm 093.0
    - asymptomatic 093.89
    - congenital 090.5
  - thyroid (gland) (see also Hyper-thyroidism) 242.9 ✓5ᵗʰ [425.7]
  - thyrotoxic (see also Thyrotoxicosis) 242.9 ✓5ᵗʰ [425.7]
  - tuberculous (see also Tuberculosis) 017.9 ✓5ᵗʰ [425.8]
  - valve, valvular (obstructive) (regurgitant) — see also Endocarditis
    - congenital NEC (see also Anomaly, heart, valve) 746.9
    - pulmonary 746.00
    - specified type NEC 746.89
  - vascular — see Disease, cardiovascular
- heavy-chain (gamma G) 273.2
- Heberden's 715.04
- Hebra's
  - dermatitis exfoliativa 695.89
  - erythema multiforme exudativum 695.1
  - pityriasis
    - maculata et circinata 696.3
    - rubra 695.89
    - pilaris 696.4
  - prurigo 698.2
- Heerfordt's (uveoparotitis) 135
- Heidenhain's 290.10
  - with dementia 290.10
- Heilmeyer-Schöner (M9842/3) 207.1 ✓5ᵗʰ
- Heine-Medin (see also Poliomyelitis) 045.9 ✓5ᵗʰ
- Heller's (see also Psychosis, childhood) 299.1 ✓5ᵗʰ
- Heller-Döhle (syphilitic aortitis) 093.1
- hematopoietic organs 289.9
- hemoglobin (Hb) 282.7
  - with thalassemia 282.4
  - abnormal (mixed) NEC 282.7
    - with thalassemia 282.4
  - AS genotype 282.5
  - Bart's 282.7
  - C (Hb-C) 282.7
    - with other abnormal hemoglobin NEC 282.7
  - elliptocytosis 282.7
  - Hb-S 282.63
  - sickle-cell 282.63
  - thalassemia 282.4
  - constant spring 282.7

Disease, diseased — see also Syndrome — continued
  hemoglobin — continued
    D (Hb-D) 282.7
      with other abnormal hemoglobin NEC 282.7
      Hb-S 282.69
      sickle-cell 282.69
      thalassemia 282.4
    E (Hb-E) 282.7
      with other abnormal hemoglobin NEC 282.7
      Hb-S 282.69
      sickle-cell 282.69
      thalassemia 282.4
    elliptocytosis 282.7
    F (Hb-F) 282.7
    G (Hb-G) 282.7
    H (Hb-H) 282.4
    hereditary persistence, fetal (HPFH) ("Swiss variety") 282.7
    high fetal gene 282.7
    I thalassemia 282.4
    M 289.7
    S — see Disease, sickle-cell, Hb-S
    spherocytosis 282.7
    unstable, hemolytic 282.7
    Zurich (Hb-Zurich) 282.7
  hemolytic (fetus) (newborn) 773.2
    autoimmune (cold type) (warm type) 283.0
    due to or with
      incompatibility
        ABO (blood group) 773.1
        blood (group) (Duffy) (Kell) (Kidd) (Lewis) (M) (S) NEC 773.2
        Rh (blood group) (factor) 773.0
      Rh negative mother 773.0
    unstable hemoglobin 282.7
  hemorrhagic 287.9
    newborn 776.0
  Henoch (-Schönlein) (purpura nervosa) 287.0
  hepatic — see Disease, liver
  hepatolenticular 275.1
  heredodegenerative NEC
    brain 331.89
    spinal cord 336.8
  Hers' (glycogenosis VI) 271.0
  Herter (-Gee) (-Heubner) (nontropical sprue) 579.0
  Herxheimer's (diffuse idiopathic cutaneous atrophy) 701.8
  Heubner's 094.89
  Heubner-Herter (nontropical sprue) 579.0
  high fetal gene or hemoglobin thalassemia 282.4
  Hildenbrand's (typhus) 081.9
  hip (joint) NEC 719.95
    congenital 755.63
    suppurative 711.05
    tuberculous (see also Tuberculosis) 015.1 ✓5ᵗʰ [730.85]
  Hippel's (retinocerebral angiomatosis) 759.6
  Hirschfield's (acute diabetes mellitus) (see also Diabetes) 250.0 ✓5ᵗʰ
  Hirschsprung's (congenital megacolon) 751.3
  His (-Werner) (trench fever) 083.1
  HIV 042
  Hodgkin's (M9650/3) 201.9 ✓5ᵗʰ

> *Note* — *Use the following fifth-digit subclassification with category 201:*
>
> 0   *unspecifed site*
> 1   *lymph nodes of head, face, and neck*
> 2   *intrathoracic lymp nodes*
> 3   *intra-abdominal lymph nodes*
> 4   *lymph nodes of axilla and upper limb*
> 5   *lymph nodes of inguinal region and lower limb*
> 6   *intrapelvic lymph nodes*
> 7   *spleen*
> 8   *lymph nodes of multiple sites*

Disease, diseased — see also Syndrome — continued
  Hodgkin's — continued
    lymphocytic
      depletion (M9653/3) 201.7 ✓5ᵗʰ
        diffuse fibrosis (M9654/3) 201.7 ✓5ᵗʰ
        reticular type (M9655/3) 201.7 ✓5ᵗʰ
      predominance (M9651/3) 201.4 ✓5ᵗʰ
    lymphocytic-histiocytic predominance (M9651/3) 201.4 ✓5ᵗʰ
    mixed cellularity (M9652/3) 201.6 ✓5ᵗʰ
    nodular sclerosis (M9656/3) 201.5 ✓5ᵗʰ
      cellular phase (M9657/3) 201.5 ✓5ᵗʰ
  Hodgson's 441.9
    ruptured 441.5
  Hoffa (-Kastert) (liposynovitis prepatellaris) 272.8
  Holla (see also Spherocytosis) 282.0
  homozygous-Hb-S 282.61
  hoof and mouth 078.4
  hookworm (see also Ancylostomiasis) 126.9
  Horton's (temporal arteritis) 446.5
  host-versus-graft (immune or nonimmune cause) 996.80
    bone marrow 996.85
    heart 996.83
    intestines 996.87
    kidney 996.81
    liver 996.82
    lung 996.84
    pancreas 996.86
    specified NEC 996.89
  HPFH (hereditary persistence of fetal hemoglobin) ("Swiss variety") 282.7
  Huchard's (continued arterial hypertension) 401.9
  Huguier's (uterine fibroma) 218.9
  human immunodeficiency (virus) 042
  hunger 251.1
  Hunt's
    dyssynergia cerebellaris myoclonica 334.2
    herpetic geniculate ganglionitis 053.11
  Huntington's 333.4
  Huppert's (multiple myeloma) (M9730/3) 203.0 ✓5ᵗʰ
  Hurler's (mucopolysaccharidosis I) 277.5
  Hutchinson's, meaning
    angioma serpiginosum 709.1
    cheiropompholyx 705.81
    prurigo estivalis 692.72
  Hutchinson-Boeck (sarcoidosis) 135
  Hutchinson-Gilford (progeria) 259.8
  hyaline (diffuse) (generalized) 728.9
    membrane (lung) (newborn) 769
  hydatid (see also Echinococcus) 122.9
  Hyde's (prurigo nodularis) 698.3
  hyperkinetic (see also Hyperkinesia) 314.9
    heart 429.82
  hypertensive (see also Hypertension) 401.9
  hypophysis 253.9
    hyperfunction 253.1
    hypofunction 253.2
  Iceland (epidemic neuromyasthenia) 049.8
  I cell 272.7
  ill-defined 799.8
  immunologic NEC 279.9
  immunoproliferative 203.8 ✓5ᵗʰ
  inclusion 078.5
    salivary gland 078.5
  infancy, early NEC 779.9
  infective NEC 136.9
  inguinal gland 289.9
  internal semilunar cartilage, cystic 717.5
  intervertebral disc 722.90
    with myelopathy 722.70
    cervical, cervicothoracic 722.91
      with myelopathy 722.71
    lumbar, lumbosacral 722.93
      with myelopathy 722.73
    thoracic, thoracolumbar 722.92
      with myelopathy 722.72
  intestine 569.9
    functional 564.9
      congenital 751.3
      psychogenic 306.4
    lardaceous 277.3

Disease, diseased — see also Syndrome — continued
  intestine — continued
    organic 569.9
    protozoal NEC 007.9
  iris 364.9
  iron
    metabolism 275.0
    storage 275.0
  Isambert's (see also Tuberculosis, larynx) 012.3 ✓5ᵗʰ
  Iselin's (osteochondrosis, fifth metatarsal) 732.5
  Island (scrub typhus) 081.2
  itai-itai 985.5
  Jadassohn's (maculopapular erythroderma) 696.2
  Jadassohn-Pellizari's (anetoderma) 701.3
  Jakob-Creutzfeldt 046.1
    with dementia
      with behavioral disturbance 046.1 [294.11]
      without behavioral disturbance 046.1 [294.10]
  Jaksch (-Luzet) (pseudoleukemia infantum) 285.8
  Janet's 300.89
  Jansky-Bielschowsky 330.1
  jaw NEC 526.9
    fibrocystic 526.2
  Jensen's 363.05
  Jeune's (asphyxiating thoracic dystrophy) 756.4
  jigger 134.1
  Johnson-Stevens (erythema multiforme exudativum) 695.1
  joint NEC 719.9 ✓5ᵗʰ
    ankle 719.97
    Charcôt 094.0 [713.5]
    degenerative (see also Osteoarthrosis) 715.9 ✓5ᵗʰ
      multiple 715.09
      spine (see also Spondylosis) 721.90
    elbow 719.92
    foot 719.97
    hand 719.94
    hip 719.95
    hypertrophic (chronic) (degenerative) (see also Osteoarthrosis) 715.9 ✓5ᵗʰ
      spine (see also Spondylosis) 721.90
    knee 719.96
    Luschka 721.90
    multiple sites 719.99
    pelvic region 719.95
    sacroiliac 724.6
    shoulder (region) 719.91
    specified site NEC 719.98
    spine NEC 724.9
      pseudarthrosis following fusion 733.82
      sacroiliac 724.6
    wrist 719.93
  Jourdain's (acute gingivitis) 523.0
  Jüngling's (sarcoidosis) 135
  Kahler (-Bozzolo) (multiple myeloma) (M9730/3) 203.0 ✓5ᵗʰ
  Kalischer's 759.6
  Kaposi's 757.33
    lichen ruber 697.8
      acuminatus 696.4
      moniliformis 697.8
    xeroderma pigmentosum 757.33
  Kaschin-Beck (endemic polyarthritis) 716.00
    ankle 716.07
    arm 716.02
      lower (and wrist) 716.03
      upper (and elbow) 716.02
    foot (and ankle) 716.07
    forearm (and wrist) 716.03
    hand 716.04
    leg 716.06
      lower 716.06
      upper 716.05
    multiple sites 716.09
    pelvic region (hip) (thigh) 716.05
    shoulder region 716.01
    specified site NEC 716.08
  Katayama 120.2
  Kawasaki 446.1
  Kedani (scrub typhus) 081.2

Index to Diseases

Disease, diseased — see also Syndrome — continued
- kidney (functional) (pelvis) (see also Disease, renal) 593.9
  - cystic (congenital) 753.10
    - multiple 753.19
    - single 753.11
    - specified NEC 753.19
  - fibrocystic (congenital) 753.19
  - in gout 274.10
  - polycystic (congenital) 753.12
    - adult type (APKD) 753.13
    - autosomal dominant 753.13
    - autosomal recessive 753.14
    - childhood type (CPKD) 753.14
    - infantile type 753.14
- Kienböck's (carpal lunate) (wrist) 732.3
- Kimmelstiel (-Wilson) (intercapillary glomerulosclerosis) 250.4 ✓5 [581.81]
- Kinnier Wilson's (hepatolenticular degeneration) 275.1
- kissing 075
- Kleb's (see also Nephritis) 583.9
- Klinger's 446.4
- Klippel's 723.8
- Klippel-Feil (brevicollis) 756.16
- knight's 911.1
- Köbner's (epidermolysis bullosa) 757.39
- Koenig-Wichmann (pemphigus) 694.4
- Köhler's
  - first (osteoarthrosis juvenilis) 732.5
  - second (Freiberg's infraction, metatarsal head) 732.5
  - patellar 732.4
  - tarsal navicular (bone) (osteoarthrosis juvenilis) 732.5
- Köhler-Freiberg (infraction, metatarsal head) 732.5
- Köhler-Mouchet (osteoarthrosis juvenilis) 732.5
- Köhler-Pellegrini-Stieda (calcification, knee joint) 726.62
- König's (osteochondritis dissecans) 732.7
- Korsakoff's (nonalcoholic) 294.0
  - alcoholic 291.1
- Kostmann's (infantile genetic agranulocytosis) 288.0
- Krabbe's 330.0
- Kraepelin-Morel (see also Schizophrenia) 295.9 ✓5
- Kraft-Weber-Dimitri 759.6
- Kufs' 330.1
- Kugelberg-Welander 335.11
- Kuhnt-Junius 362.52
- Kümmell's (-Verneuil) (spondylitis) 721.7
- Kundrat's (lymphosarcoma) 200.1 ✓5
- kuru 046.0
- Kussmaul (-Meier) (polyarteritis nodosa) 446.0
- Kyasanur Forest 065.2
- Kyrle's (hyperkeratosis follicularis in cutem penetrans) 701.1
- labia
  - inflammatory 616.9
    - specified NEC 616.8
  - noninflammatory 624.9
    - specified NEC 624.8
- labyrinth, ear 386.8
- lacrimal system (apparatus) (passages) 375.9
  - gland 375.00
  - specified NEC 375.89
- Lafora's 333.2
- Lagleyze-von Hippel (retinocerebral angiomatosis) 759.6
- Lancereaux-Mathieu (leptospiral jaundice) 100.0
- Landry's 357.0
- Lane's 569.89
- lardaceous (any site) 277.3
- Larrey-Weil (leptospiral jaundice) 100.0
- Larsen (-Johansson) (juvenile osteopathia patellae) 732.4
- larynx 478.70
- Lasègue's (persecution mania) 297.9
- Leber's 377.16
- Lederer's (acquired infectious hemolytic anemia) 283.19
- Legg's (capital femoral osteochondrosis) 732.1

Disease, diseased — see also Syndrome — continued
- Legg-Calvé-Perthes (capital femoral osteochondrosis) 732.1
- Legg-Calvé-Waldenström (femoral capital osteochondrosis) 732.1
- Legg-Perthes (femoral capital osteochrondosis) 732.1
- Legionnaires' 482.84
- Leigh's 330.8
- Leiner's (exfoliative dermatitis) 695.89
- Leloir's (lupus erythematosus) 695.4
- Lenegre's 426.0
- lens (eye) 379.39
- Leriche's (osteoporosis, post-traumatic) 733.7
- Letterer-Siwe (acute histiocytosis X) (M9722/3) 202.5 ✓5
- Lev's (acquired complete heart block) 426.0
- Lewandowski's (see also Tuberculosis) 017.0 ✓5
- Lewandowski-Lutz (epidermodysplasia verruciformis) 078.19
- Leyden's (periodic vomiting) 536.2
- Libman-Sacks (verrucous endocarditis) 710.0 [424.91]
- Lichtheim's (subacute combined sclerosis with pernicious anemia) 281.0 [336.2]
- ligament 728.9
- light chain 203.0 ✓5
- Lightwood's (renal tubular acidosis) 588.8
- Lignac's (cystinosis) 270.0
- Lindau's (retinocerebral angiomatosis) 759.6
- Lindau-von Hippel (angiomatosis retinocerebellosa) 759.6
- lip NEC 528.5
- lipidosis 272.7
- lipoid storage NEC 272.7
- Lipschütz's 616.50
- Little's — see Palsy, cerebral
- liver 573.9
  - alcoholic 571.3
    - acute 571.1
    - chronic 571.3
  - chronic 571.9
    - alcoholic 571.3
  - cystic, congenital 751.62
  - drug-induced 573.3
  - due to
    - chemicals 573.3
    - fluorinated agents 573.3
    - hypersensitivity drugs 573.3
    - isoniazids 573.3
  - fibrocystic (congenital) 751.62
  - glycogen storage 271.0
  - organic 573.9
  - polycystic (congenital) 751.62
- Lobo's (keloid blastomycosis) 116.2
- Lobstein's (brittle bones and blue sclera) 756.51
- locomotor system 334.9
- Lorain's (pituitary dwarfism) 253.3
- Lou Gehrig's 335.20
- Lucas-Championnière (fibrinous bronchitis) 466.0
- Ludwig's (submaxillary cellulitis) 528.3
- luetic — see Syphilis
- lumbosacral region 724.6
- lung NEC 518.89
  - black 500
  - congenital 748.60
  - cystic 518.89
    - congenital 748.4
  - fibroid (chronic) (see also Fibrosis, lung) 515
  - fluke 121.2
    - Oriental 121.2
  - in
    - amyloidosis 277.3 [517.8]
    - polymyositis 710.4 [517.8]
    - sarcoidosis 135 [517.8]
    - Sjögren's syndrome 710.2 [517.8]
    - syphilis 095.1
    - systemic lupus erythematosus 710.0 [517.8]
    - systemic sclerosis 710.1 [517.2]
  - interstitial (chronic) 515
    - acute 136.3
  - nonspecific, chronic 496

Disease, diseased — see also Syndrome — continued
- lung NEC — continued
  - obstructive (chronic) (COPD) 496
    - with
      - acute exacerbation NEC 491.21
      - alveolitis, allergic (see also Alveolitis, allergic) 495.9
      - asthma (chronic) (obstructive) 493.2 ✓5
      - bronchiectasis 494.0
        - with acute exacerbation 494.1
      - bronchitis (chronic) 491.20
        - with acute exacerbation 491.21
      - emphysema NEC 492.8
    - diffuse (with fibrosis) 496
  - polycystic 518.89
    - asthma (chronic) (obstructive) 493.2 ✓5
    - congenital 748.4
    - purulent (cavitary) 513.0
    - restrictive 518.89
    - rheumatoid 714.81
      - diffuse interstitial 714.81
    - specified NEC 518.89
- Lutembacher's (atrial septal defect with mitral stenosis) 745.5
- Lutz-Miescher (elastosis perforans serpiginosa) 701.1
- Lutz-Splendore-de Almeida (Brazilian blastomycosis) 116.1
- Lyell's (toxic epidermal necrolysis) 695.1
  - due to drug
    - correct substance properly administered 695.1
    - overdose or wrong substance given or taken 977.9
      - specific drug — see Table of Drugs and Chemicals
- Lyme 088.81
- lymphatic (gland) (system) 289.9
  - channel (noninfective) 457.9
  - vessel (noninfective) 457.9
  - specified NEC 457.8
- lymphoproliferative (chronic) (M9970/1) 238.7
- Machado-Joseph 334.8
- Madelung's (lipomatosis) 272.8
- Madura (actinomycotic) 039.9
  - mycotic 117.4
- Magitot's 526.4
- Majocchi's (purpura annularis telangiectodes) 709.1
- malarial (see also Malaria) 084.6
- Malassez's (cystic) 608.89
- Malibu 919.8
  - infected 919.9
- malignant (M8000/3) — see also Neoplasm, by site, malignant
  - previous, affecting management of pregnancy V23.8 ✓5
- Manson's 120.1
- maple bark 495.6
- maple syrup (urine) 270.3
- Marburg (virus) 078.89
- Marchiafava (-Bignami) 341.8
- Marfan's 090.49
  - congenital syphilis 090.49
  - meaning Marfan's syndrome 759.82
- Marie-Bamberger (hypertrophic pulmonary osteoarthropathy) (secondary) 731.2
  - primary or idiopathic (acropachyderma) 757.39
  - pulmonary (hypertrophic osteoarthropathy) 731.2
- Marie-Strümpell (ankylosing spondylitis) 720.0
- Marion's (bladder neck obstruction) 596.0
- Marsh's (exophthalmic goiter) 242.0 ✓5
- Martin's 715.27
- mast cell 757.33
  - systemic (M9741/3) 202.6 ✓5
- mastoid (see also Mastoiditis) 383.9
  - process 385.9
- maternal, unrelated to pregnancy NEC, affecting fetus or newborn 760.9
- Mathieu's (leptospiral jaundice) 100.0
- Mauclaire's 732.3
- Mauriac's (erythema nodosum syphiliticum) 091.3 ✓5

Disease, diseased — see also Syndrome — continued
  Maxcy's 081.0
  McArdle (-Schmid-Pearson) (glycogenosis V) 271.0
  mediastinum NEC 519.3
  Medin's (see also Poliomyelitis) 045.9 ✓5ᵗʰ
  Mediterranean (with hemoglobinopathy) 282.4
  medullary center (idiopathic) (respiratory) 348.8
  Meige's (chronic hereditary edema) 757.0
  Meleda 757.39
  Ménétrier's (hypertrophic gastritis) 535.2 ✓5ᵗʰ
  Ménière's (active) 386.00
    cochlear 386.02
    cochleovestibular 386.01
    inactive 386.04
    in remission 386.04
    vestibular 386.03
  meningeal — see Meningitis
  mental (see also Psychosis) 298.9
  Merzbacher-Pelizaeus 330.0
  mesenchymal 710.9
  mesenteric embolic 557.0
  metabolic NEC 277.9
  metal polishers' 502
  metastatic — see Metastasis
  Mibelli's 757.39
  microdrepanocytic 282.4
  Miescher's 709.3
  Mikulicz's (dryness of mouth, absent or decreased lacrimation) 527.1
  Milkman (-Looser) (osteomalacia with pseudofractures) 268.2
  Miller's (osteomalacia) 268.2
  Mills' 335.29
  Milroy's (chronic hereditary edema) 757.0
  Minamata 985.0
  Minor's 336.1
  Minot's (hemorrhagic disease, newborn) 776.0
  Minot-von Willebrand-Jürgens (angiohemophilia) 286.4
  Mitchell's (erythromelalgia) 443.89
  mitral — see Endocarditis, mitral
  Mljet (mal de Meleda) 757.39
  Möbius', Moebius' 346.8 ✓5ᵗʰ
  Moeller's 267
  Möller (-Barlow) (infantile scurvy) 267
  Mönckeberg's (see also Arteriosclerosis, extremities) 440.20
  Mondor's (thrombophlebitis of breast) 451.89
  Monge's 993.2
  Morel-Kraepelin (see also Schizophrenia) 295.9 ✓5ᵗʰ
  Morgagni's (syndrome) (hyperostosis frontalis interna) 733.3
  Morgagni-Adams-Stokes (syncope with heart block) 426.9
  Morquio (-Brailsford) (-Ullrich) (mucopolysaccharidosis IV) 277.5
  Morton's (with metatarsalgia) 355.6
  Morvan's 336.1
  motor neuron (bulbar) (mixed type) 335.20
  Mouchet's (juvenile osteochondrosis, foot) 732.5
  mouth 528.9
  Moyamoya 437.5
  Mucha's (acute parapsoriasis varioliformis) 696.2
  mu-chain 273.2
  mucolipidosis (I) (II) (III) 272.7
  Münchmeyer's (exostosis luxurians) 728.11
  Murri's (intermittent hemoglobinuria) 283.2
  muscle 359.9
    inflammatory 728.9
    ocular 378.9
  musculoskeletal system 729.9
  mushroom workers' 495.5
  Myà's (congenital dilation, colon) 751.3
  mycotic 117.9
  myeloproliferative (chronic) (M9960/1) 238.7
  myocardium, myocardial (see also Degeneration, myocardial) 429.1
    hypertensive (see also Hypertension, heart) 402.90
    primary (idiopathic) 425.4
  myoneural 358.9
  Naegeli's 287.1

Disease, diseased — see also Syndrome — continued
  nail 703.9
    specified type NEC 703.8
  Nairobi sheep 066.1
  nasal 478.1
    cavity NEC 478.1
    sinus (chronic) — see Sinusitis
  navel (newborn) NEC 779.89 ▲
  nemaline body 359.0
  neoplastic, generalized (M8000/6) 199.0
  nerve — see Disorder, nerve
  nervous system (central) 349.9
    autonomic, peripheral (see also Neuropathy, peripheral, autonomic) 337.9
    congenital 742.9
    inflammatory — see Encephalitis
    parasympathetic (see also Neuropathy, peripheral, autonomic) 337.9
    peripheral NEC 355.9
    specified NEC 349.89
    sympathetic (see also Neuropathy, peripheral, autonomic) 337.9
    vegetative (see also Neuropathy, peripheral, autonomic) 337.9
  Nettleship's (urticaria pigmentosa) 757.33
  Neumann's (pemphigus vegetans) 694.4
  neurologic (central) NEC (see also Disease, nervous system) 349.9
    peripheral NEC 355.9
  neuromuscular system NEC 358.9
  Newcastle 077.8
  Nicolas (-Durand) — Favre (climatic bubo) 099.1
  Niemann-Pick (lipid histiocytosis) 272.7
  nipple 611.9
    Paget's (M8540/3) 174.0
  Nishimoto (-Takeuchi) 437.5
  nonarthropod-borne NEC 078.89
    central nervous system NEC 049.9
    enterovirus NEC 078.89
  non-autoimmune hemolytic NEC 283.10
  Nonne-Milroy-Meige (chronic hereditary edema) 757.0
  Norrie's (congenital progressive oculoacousticocerebral degeneration) 743.8
  nose 478.1
  nucleus pulposus — see Disease, intervertebral disc
  nutritional 269.9
    maternal, affecting fetus or newborn 760.4
  oasthouse, urine 270.2
  obliterative vascular 447.1
  Odelberg's (juvenile osteochondrosis) 732.1
  Oguchi's (retina) 368.61
  Ohara's (see also Tularemia) 021.9
  Ollier's (chondrodysplasia) 756.4
  Opitz's (congestive splenomegaly) 289.51
  Oppenheim's 358.8
  Oppenheim-Urbach (necrobiosis lipoidica diabeticorum) 250.8 ✓5ᵗʰ [709.3]
  optic nerve NEC 377.49
  orbit 376.9
    specified NEC 376.89
  Oriental liver fluke 121.1
  Oriental lung fluke 121.2
  Ormond's 593.4
  Osgood's tibia (tubercle) 732.4
  Osgood-Schlatter 732.4
  Osler (-Vaquez) (polycythemia vera) (M9950/1) 238.4
  Osler-Rendu (familial hemorrhagic telangiectasia) 448.0
  osteofibrocystic 252.0
  Otto's 715.35
  outer ear 380.9
  ovary (noninflammatory) NEC 620.9
    cystic 620.2
    polycystic 256.4
    specified NEC 620.8
  Owren's (congenital) (see also Defect, coagulation) 286.3
  Paas' 756.59
  Paget's (osteitis deformans) 731.0
    with infiltrating duct carcinoma of the breast (M8541/3) — see Neoplasm, breast, malignant

Disease, diseased — see also Syndrome — continued
  Paget's — continued
    bone 731.0
      osteosarcoma in (M9184/3) — see Neoplasm, bone, malignant
    breast (M8540/3) 174.0
    extramammary (M8542/3) — see also Neoplasm, skin, malignant
      anus 154.3
      skin 173.5
    malignant (M8540/3)
      breast 174.0
      specified site NEC (M8542/3) — see Neoplasm, skin, malignant
      unspecified site 174.0
    mammary (M8540/3) 174.0
    nipple (M8540/3) 174.0
  palate (soft) 528.9
  Paltauf-Sternberg 201.9 ✓5ᵗʰ
  pancreas 577.9
    cystic 577.2
      congenital 751.7
    fibrocystic 277.00
  Panner's 732.3
    capitellum humeri 732.3
    head of humerus 732.3
    tarsal navicular (bone) (osteochondrosis) 732.5
  panvalvular — see Endocarditis, mitral
  parametrium 629.9
  parasitic NEC 136.9
    cerebral NEC 123.9
    intestinal NEC 129
    mouth 112.0
    skin NEC 134.9
    specified type — see Infestation
    tongue 112.0
  parathyroid (gland) 252.9
    specified NEC 252.8
  Parkinson's 332.0
  parodontal 523.9
  Parrot's (syphilitic osteochondritis) 090.0
  Parry's (exophthalmic goiter) 242.0 ✓5ᵗʰ
  Parson's (exophthalmic goiter) 242.0 ✓5ᵗʰ
  Pavy's 593.6
  Paxton's (white piedra) 111.2
  Payr's (splenic flexure syndrome) 569.89
  pearl-workers' (chronic osteomyelitis) (see also Osteomyelitis) 730.1 ✓5ᵗʰ
  Pel-Ebstein — see Disease, Hodgkin's
  Pelizaeus-Merzbacher 330.0
    with dementia
      with behavioral disturbance 330.0 [294.11]
      without behavioral disturbance 330.0 [294.10]
  Pellegrini-Stieda (calcification, knee joint) 726.62
  pelvis, pelvic
    female NEC 629.9
      specified NEC 629.8
    gonococcal (acute) 098.19
      chronic or duration of 2 months or over 098.39
    infection (see also Disease, pelvis, inflammatory) 614.9
    inflammatory (female) (PID) 614.9
      with
        abortion — see Abortion, by type, with sepsis
        ectopic pregnancy (see also categories (633.0-633.9) 639.0
        molar pregnancy (see also categories 630-632) 639.0
      acute 614.3
      chronic 614.4
      complicating pregnancy 646.6 ✓5ᵗʰ
        affecting fetus or newborn 760.8
      following
        abortion 639.0
        ectopic or molar pregnancy 639.0
      peritonitis (acute) 614.5
        chronic NEC 614.7
      puerperal, postpartum, childbirth 670 ✓4ᵗʰ
      specified NEC 614.8

Disease, diseased — see also Syndrome — continued
  pelvis, pelvic — continued
    organ, female NEC 629.9
      specified NEC 629.8
    peritoneum, female NEC 629.9
      specified NEC 629.8
  penis 607.9
    inflammatory 607.2
  peptic NEC 536.9
    acid 536.8
  periapical tissues NEC 522.9
  pericardium 423.9
    specified type NEC 423.8
  perineum
    female
      inflammatory 616.9
        specified NEC 616.8
      noninflammatory 624.9
        specified NEC 624.8
    male (inflammatory) 682.2
  periodic (familial) (Reimann's) NEC 277.3
    paralysis 359.3
  periodontal NEC 523.9
    specified NEC 523.8
  periosteum 733.90
  peripheral
    arterial 443.9
    autonomic nervous system (see also Neuropathy, autonomic) 337.9
    nerve NEC (see also Neuropathy) 356.9
      multiple — see Polyneuropathy
    vascular 443.9
      specified type NEC 443.89
  peritoneum 568.9
    pelvic, female 629.9
      specified NEC 629.8
  Perrin-Ferraton (snapping hip) 719.65
  persistent mucosal (middle ear) (with posterior or superior marginal perforation of ear drum) 382.2
  Perthes' (capital femoral osteochondrosis) 732.1
  Petit's (see also Hernia, lumbar) 553.8
  Peutz-Jeghers 759.6
  Peyronie's 607.89
  Pfeiffer's (infectious mononucleosis) 075
  pharynx 478.20
  Phocas' 610.1
  photochromogenic (acid-fast bacilli) (pulmonary) 031.0
    nonpulmonary 031.9
  Pick's
    brain 331.1
      with dementia
        with behavioral disturbance 331.1 [294.11]
        without behavioral disturbance 331.1 [294.10]
    cerebral atrophy 331.1
      with dementia
        with behavioral disturbance 331.1 [294.11]
        without behavioral disturbance 331.1 [294.10]
    lipid histiocytosis 272.7
    liver (pericardial pseudocirrhosis of liver) 423.2
    pericardium (pericardial pseudocirrhosis of liver) 423.2
    polyserositis (pericardial pseudocirrhosis of liver) 423.2
  Pierson's (osteochondrosis) 732.1
  pigeon fanciers' or breeders' 495.2
  pineal gland 259.8
  pink 985.0
  Pinkus' (lichen nitidus) 697.1
  pinworm 127.4
  pituitary (gland) 253.9
    hyperfunction 253.1
    hypofunction 253.2
  pituitary snuff-takers' 495.8
  placenta
    affecting fetus or newborn 762.2
    complicating pregnancy or childbirth 656.7 ✓5ᵗʰ
  pleura (cavity) (see also Pleurisy) 511.0
  Plummer's (toxic nodular goiter) 242.3 ✓5ᵗʰ

Disease, diseased — see also Syndrome — continued
  pneumatic
    drill 994.9
    hammer 994.9
  policeman's 729.2
  Pollitzer's (hidradenitis suppurativa) 705.83
  polycystic (congenital) 759.89
    kidney or renal 753.12
      adult type (APKD) 753.13
      autosomal dominant 753.13
      autosomal recessive 753.14
      childhood type (CPKD) 753.14
      infantile type 753.14
    liver or hepatic 751.62
    lung or pulmonary 518.89
      congenital 748.4
    ovary, ovaries 256.4
    spleen 759.0
  Pompe's (glycogenosis II) 271.0
  Poncet's (tuberculous rheumatism) (see also Tuberculosis) 015.9 ✓5ᵗʰ
  Posada-Wernicke 114.9
  Potain's (pulmonary edema) 514
  Pott's (see also Tuberculosis) 015.0 ✓5ᵗʰ [730.88]
    osteomyelitis 015.0 ✓5ᵗʰ [730.88]
    paraplegia 015.0 ✓5ᵗʰ [730.88]
    spinal curvature 015.0 ✓5ᵗʰ [737.43]
    spondylitis 015.0 ✓5ᵗʰ [720.81]
  Potter's 753.0
  Poulet's 714.2
  pregnancy NEC (see also Pregnancy) 646.9 ✓5ᵗʰ
  Preiser's (osteoporosis) 733.09
  Pringle's (tuberous sclerosis) 759.5
  Profichet's 729.9
  prostate 602.9
    specified type NEC 602.8
  protozoal NEC 136.8
    intestine, intestinal NEC 007.9
  pseudo-Hurler's (mucolipidosis III) 272.7
  psychiatric (see also Psychosis) 298.9
  psychotic (see also Psychosis) 298.9
  Puente's (simple glandular cheilitis) 528.5
  puerperal NEC (see also Puerperal) 674.9 ✓5ᵗʰ
  pulmonary — see also Disease, lung
    amyloid 277.3 [517.8]
    artery 417.9
    circulation, circulatory 417.9
      specified NEC 417.8
    diffuse obstructive (chronic) 496
      with
        acute exacerbation NEC 491.21
        asthma (chronic) (obstructive) 493.2 ✓5ᵗʰ
    heart (chronic) 416.9
      specified NEC 416.8
    hypertensive (vascular) 416.0
      cardiovascular 416.0
    obstructive diffuse (chronic) 496
      with
        acute exacerbation NEC 491.21
        asthma (chronic) (obstructive) 493.2 ✓5ᵗʰ
        bronchitis (chronic) 491.20
          with acute exacerbation 491.21
    valve (see also Endocarditis, pulmonary) 424.3
  pulp (dental) NEC 522.9
  pulseless 446.7
  Putnam's (subacute combined sclerosis with pernicious anemia) 281.0 [336.2]
  Pyle (-Cohn) (craniometaphyseal dysplasia) 756.89
  pyramidal tract 333.90
  Quervain's
    tendon sheath 727.04
    thyroid (subacute granulomatous thyroiditis) 245.1
  Quincke's — see Edema, angioneurotic
  Quinquaud (acne decalvans) 704.09
  rag sorters' 022.1
  Raynaud's (paroxysmal digital cyanosis) 443.0
  reactive airway — see Asthma
  Recklinghausen's (M9540/1) 237.71
    bone (osteitis fibrosa cystica) 252.0
  Recklinghausen-Applebaum (hemochromatosis) 275.0

Disease, diseased — see also Syndrome — continued
  Reclus' (cystic) 610.1
  rectum NEC 569.49
  Refsum's (heredopathia atactica polyneuritiformis) 356.3
  Reichmann's (gastrosuccorrhea) 536.8
  Reimann's (periodic) 277.3
  Reiter's 099.3
  renal (functional) (pelvis) 593.9
    with
      edema (see also Nephrosis) 581.9
      exudative nephritis 583.89
      lesion of interstitial nephritis 583.89
      stated generalized cause — see Nephritis
    acute — see Nephritis, acute
    basement membrane NEC 583.89
      with
        pulmonary hemorrhage (Goodpasture's syndrome) 446.21 [583.81]
    chronic — see Nephritis, chronic
    complicating pregnancy or puerperium NEC 646.2 ✓5ᵗʰ
      with hypertension — see Toxemia, of pregnancy
    cystic, congenital (see also Cystic, disease, kidney) 753.10
    diabetic 250.4 ✓5ᵗʰ [583.81]
    due to
      amyloidosis 277.3 [583.81]
      diabetes mellitus 250.4 ✓5ᵗʰ [583.81]
      systemic lupus erythematosis 710.0 [583.81]
    end-stage 585
    exudative 583.89
    fibrocystic (congenital) 753.19
    gonococcal 098.19 [583.81]
    gouty 274.10
    hypertensive (see also Hypertension, kidney) 403.90
    immune complex NEC 583.89
    interstitial (diffuse) (focal) 583.89
    lupus 710.0 [583.81]
    maternal, affecting fetus or newborn 760.1
      hypertensive 760.0
    phosphate-losing (tubular) 588.0
    polycystic (congenital) 753.12
      adult type (APKD) 753.13
      autosomal dominant 753.13
      autosomal recessive 753.14
      childhood type (CPKD) 753.14
      infantile type 753.14
    specified lesion or cause NEC (see also Glomerulonephritis) 583.89
    subacute 581.9
    syphilitic 095.4
    tuberculous (see also Tuberculosis) 016.0 ✓5ᵗʰ [583.81]
    tubular (see also Nephrosis, tubular) 584.5
  Rendu-Osler-Weber (familial hemorrhagic telangiectasia) 448.0
  renovascular (arteriosclerotic) (see also Hypertension, kidney) 403.90
  respiratory (tract) 519.9
    acute or subacute (upper) NEC 465.9
      due to fumes or vapors 506.3
      multiple sites NEC 465.8
      noninfectious 478.9
      streptococcal 034.0
    chronic 519.9
      arising in the perinatal period 770.7
      due to fumes or vapors 506.4
    due to
      aspiration of liquids or solids 508.9
      external agents NEC 508.9
        specified NEC 508.8
      fumes or vapors 506.9
        acute or subacute NEC 506.3
        chronic 506.4
    fetus or newborn NEC 770.9
    obstructive 496
    specified type NEC 519.8
    upper (acute) (infectious) NEC 465.9
      multiple sites NEC 465.8
      noninfectious NEC 478.9
      streptococcal 034.0

Disease, diseased — see also Syndrome — continued
    retina, retinal NEC 362.9
        Batten's or Batten-Mayou 330.1 [362.71]
        degeneration 362.89
        vascular lesion 362.17
    rheumatic (see also Arthritis) 716.8
        heart — see Disease, heart, rheumatic
    rheumatoid (heart) — see Arthritis, rheumatoid
    rickettsial NEC 083.9
        specified type NEC 083.8
    Riedel's (ligneous thyroiditis) 245.3
    Riga (-Fede) (cachectic aphthae) 529.0
    Riggs' (compound periodontitis) 523.4
    Ritter's 695.81
    Rivalta's (cervicofacial actinomycosis) 039.3
    Robles' (onchocerciasis) 125.3 [360.13]
    Roger's (congenital interventricular septal defect) 745.4
    Rokitansky's (see also Necrosis, liver) 570
    Romberg's 349.89
    Rosenthal's (factor XI deficiency) 286.2
    Rossbach's (hyperchlorhydria) 536.8
        psychogenic 306.4
    Roth (-Bernhardt) 355.1
    Runeberg's (progressive pernicious anemia) 281.0
    Rust's (tuberculous spondylitis) (see also Tuberculosis) 015.0 [720.81]
    Rustitskii's (multiple myeloma) (M9730/3) 203.0
    Ruysch's (Hirschsprung's disease) 751.3
    Sachs (-Tay) 330.1
    sacroiliac NEC 724.6
    salivary gland or duct NEC 527.9
        inclusion 078.5
            streptococcal 034.0
        virus 078.5
    Sander's (paranoia) 297.1
    Sandhoff's 330.1
    sandworm 126.9
    Savill's (epidemic exfoliative dermatitis) 695.89
    Schamberg's (progressive pigmentary dermatosis) 709.09
    Schaumann's (sarcoidosis) 135
    Schenck's (sporotrichosis) 117.1
    Scheuermann's (osteochondrosis) 732.0
    Schilder (-Flatau) 341.1
    Schimmelbusch's 610.1
    Schlatter's tibia (tubercle) 732.4
    Schlatter-Osgood 732.4
    Schmorl's 722.30
        cervical 722.39
        lumbar, lumbosacral 722.32
        specified region NEC 722.39
        thoracic, thoracolumbar 722.31
    Scholz's 330.0
    Schönlein (-Henoch) (purpura rheumatica) 287.0
    Schottmüller's (see also Fever, paratyphoid) 002.9
    Schüller-Christian (chronic histiocytosis X) 277.8
    Schultz's (agranulocytosis) 288.0
    Schwalbe-Ziehen-Oppenheimer 333.6
    Schweninger-Buzzi (macular atrophy) 701.3
    sclera 379.19
    scrofulous (see also Tuberculosis) 017.2
    scrotum 608.9
    sebaceous glands NEC 706.9
    Secretan's (posttraumatic edema) 782.3
    semilunar cartilage, cystic 717.5
    seminal vesicle 608.9
    Senear-Usher (pemphigus erythematosus) 694.4
    serum NEC 999.5
    Sever's (osteochondrosis calcaneum) 732.5
    Sézary's (reticulosis) (M9701/3) 202.2
    Shaver's (bauxite pneumoconiosis) 503
    Sheehan's (postpartum pituitary necrosis) 253.2
    shimamushi (scrub typus) 081.2
    shipyard 077.1
    sickle cell 282.60
        with
            crisis 282.62
            Hb-S disease 282.61

Disease, diseased — see also Syndrome — continued
    sickle cell — continued
        with — continued
            other abnormal hemoglobin (Hb-D) (Hb-E) (Hb-G) (Hb-J) (Hb-K) (Hb-O) (Hb-P) (high fetal gene) 282.69
        elliptocytosis 282.60
        Hb-C 282.63
        Hb-S 282.61
            with
                crisis 282.62
                Hb-C 282.63
                other abnormal hemoglobin (Hb-D) (Hb-E) (Hb-G) (Hb-J) (Hb-K) (Hb-O) (Hb-P) (high fetal gene) 282.69
        spherocytosis 282.60
        thalassemia 282.4
    Siegal-Cattan-Mamou (periodic) 277.3
    silo fillers' 506.9
    Simian B 054.3
    Simmonds' (pituitary cachexia) 253.2
    Simons' (progressive lipodystrophy) 272.6
    Sinding-Larsen (juvenile osteopathia patellae) 732.4
    sinus — see also Sinusitis
        brain 437.9
        specified NEC 478.1
    Sirkari's 085.0
    sixth 057.8
    Sjögren (-Gougerot) 710.2
        with lung involvement 710.2 [517.8]
    Skevas-Zerfus 989.5
    skin NEC 709.9
        due to metabolic disorder 277.9
        specified type NEC 709.8
    sleeping 347
        meaning sleeping sickness (see also Trypanosomiasis) 086.5
    small vessel 443.9
    Smith-Strang (oasthouse urine) 270.2
    Sneddon-Wilkinson (subcorneal pustular dermatosis) 694.1
    South African creeping 133.8
    Spencer's (epidemic vomiting) 078.82
    Spielmeyer-Stock 330.1
    Spielmeyer-Vogt 330.1
    spine, spinal 733.90
        combined system (see also Degeneration, combined) 266.2 [336.2]
            with pernicious anemia 281.0 [336.2]
        cord NEC 336.9
            congenital 742.9
        demyelinating NEC 341.8
        joint (see also Disease, joint, spine) 724.9
        tuberculous 015.0 [730.8]
    spinocerebellar 334.9
        specified NEC 334.8
    spleen (organic) (postinfectional) 289.50
        amyloid 277.3
        lardaceous 277.3
        polycystic 759.0
        specified NEC 289.59
    sponge divers' 989.5
    Stanton's (melioidosis) 025
    Stargardt's 362.75
    Steinert's 359.2
    Sternberg's — see Disease, Hodgkin's
    Stevens-Johnson (erythema multiforme exudativum) 695.1
    Sticker's (erythema infectiosum) 057.0
    Stieda's (calcification, knee joint) 726.62
    Still's (juvenile rheumatoid arthritis) 714.30
    Stiller's (asthenia) 780.79
    Stokes' (exophthalmic goiter) 242.0
    Stokes-Adams (syncope with heart block) 426.9
    Stokvis (-Talma) (enterogenous cyanosis) 289.7
    stomach NEC (organic) 537.9
        functional 536.9
            psychogenic 306.4
        lardaceous 277.3
    stonemasons' 502
    storage
        glycogen (see also Disease, glycogen storage) 271.0
        lipid 272.7
        mucopolysaccharide 277.5

Disease, diseased — see also Syndrome — continued
    striatopallidal system 333.90
        specified NEC 333.89
    Strümpell-Marie (ankylosing spondylitis) 720.0
    Stuart's (congenital factor X deficiency) (see also Defect, coagulation) 286.3
    Stuart-Prower (congenital factor X deficiency) (see also Defect, coagulation) 286.3
    Sturge (-Weber) (-Dimitri) (encephalocutaneous angiomatosis) 759.6
    Stuttgart 100.89
    Sudeck's 733.7
    supporting structures of teeth NEC 525.9
    suprarenal (gland) (capsule) 255.9
        hyperfunction 255.3
        hypofunction 255.4
    Sutton's 709.09
    Sutton and Gull's — see Hypertension, kidney
    sweat glands NEC 705.9
        specified type NEC 705.89
    sweating 078.2
    Sweeley-Klionsky 272.4
    Swift (-Feer) 985.0
    swimming pool (bacillus) 031.1
    swineherd's 100.89
    Sylvest's (epidemic pleurodynia) 074.1
    Symmers (follicular lymphoma) (M9690/3) 202.0
    sympathetic nervous system (see also Neuropathy, peripheral, autonomic) 337.9
    synovium 727.9
    syphilitic — see Syphilis
    systemic tissue mast cell (M9741/3) 202.6
    Taenzer's 757.4
    Takayasu's (pulseless) 446.7
    Talma's 728.85
    Tangier (familial high-density lipoprotein deficiency) 272.5
    Tarral-Besnier (pityriasis rubra pilaris) 696.4
    Tay-Sachs 330.1
    Taylor's 701.8
    tear duct 375.69
    teeth, tooth 525.9
        hard tissues NEC 521.9
        pulp NEC 522.9
    tendon 727.9
        inflammatory NEC 727.9
    terminal vessel 443.9
    testis 608.9
    Thaysen-Gee (nontropical sprue) 579.0
    Thomsen's 359.2
    Thomson's (congenital poikiloderma) 757.33
    Thornwaldt's, Tornwaldt's (pharyngeal bursitis) 478.29
    throat 478.20
        septic 034.0
    thromboembolic (see also Embolism) 444.9
    thymus (gland) 254.9
        specified NEC 254.8
    thyroid (gland) NEC 246.9
        heart (see also Hyperthyroidism) 242.9 [425.7]
        lardaceous 277.3
        specified NEC 246.8
    Tietze's 733.6
    Tommaselli's
        correct substance properly administered 599.7
        overdose or wrong substance given or taken 961.4
    tongue 529.9
    tonsils, tonsillar (and adenoids) (chronic) 474.9
        specified NEC 474.8
    tooth, teeth 525.9
        hard tissues NEC 521.9
        pulp NEC 522.9
    Tornwaldt's (pharyngeal bursitis) 478.29
    Tourette's 307.23
    trachea 519.1
    tricuspid — see Endocarditis, tricuspid
    triglyceride-storage, type I, II, III 272.7
    triple vessel (coronary arteries) — see Arteriosclerosis, coronary
    trisymptomatic, Gougerot's 709.1
    trophoblastic (see also Hydatidiform mole) 630
        previous, affecting management of pregnancy V23.1

Index to Diseases

Disease, diseased — *see also* Syndrome — *continued*
  tsutsugamushi (scrub typhus) 081.2
  tube (fallopian), noninflammatory 620.9
    specified NEC 620.8
  tuberculous NEC (*see also* Tuberculosis) 011.9 ✓5ᵗʰ
  tubo-ovarian
    inflammatory (*see also* Salpingo-oophoritis) 614.2
    noninflammatory 620.9
      specified NEC 620.8
  tubotympanic, chronic (with anterior perforation of ear drum) 382.1
  tympanum 385.9
  Uhl's 746.84
  umbilicus (newborn) NEC 779.89 ▲
  Underwood's (sclerema neonatorum) 778.1
  undiagnosed 799.9
  Unna's (seborrheic dermatitis) 690.18
  unstable hemoglobin hemolytic 282.7
  Unverricht (-Lundborg) 333.2
  Urbach-Oppenheim (necrobiosis lipoidica diabeticorum) 250.8 ✓5ᵗʰ [709.3]
  Urbach-Wiethe (lipoid proteinosis) 272.8
  ureter 593.9
  urethra 599.9
    specified type NEC 599.84
  urinary (tract) 599.9
    bladder 596.9
      specified NEC 596.8
    maternal, affecting fetus or newborn 760.1
  Usher-Senear (pemphigus erythematosus) 694.4
  uterus (organic) 621.9
    infective (*see also* Endometritis) 615.9
    inflammatory (*see also* Endometritis) 615.9
    noninflammatory 621.9
      specified type NEC 621.8
  uveal tract
    anterior 364.9
    posterior 363.9
  vagabonds' 132.1
  vagina, vaginal
    inflammatory 616.9
      specified NEC 616.8
    noninflammatory 623.9
      specified NEC 623.8
  Valsuani's (progressive pernicious anemia, puerperal) 648.2 ✓5ᵗʰ
    complicating pregnancy or puerperium 648.2 ✓5ᵗʰ
  valve, valvular — *see* Endocarditis
  van Bogaert-Nijssen (-Peiffer) 330.0
  van Creveld-von Gierke (glycogenosis I) 271.0
  van den Bergh's (enterogenous cyanosis) 289.7
  van Neck's (juvenile osteochondrosis) 732.1
  Vaquez (-Osler) (polycythemia vera) (M9950/1) 238.4
  vascular 459.9
    arteriosclerotic — *see* Arteriosclerosis
    hypertensive — *see* Hypertension
    obliterative 447.1
      peripheral 443.9
    occlusive 459.9
    peripheral (occlusive) 443.9
      in diabetes mellitus 250.7 ✓5ᵗʰ [443.81]
      specified type NEC 443.89
  vas deferens 608.9
  vasomotor 443.9
  vasopastic 443.9
  vein 459.9
  venereal 099.9
    chlamydial NEC 099.50
      anus 099.52
      bladder 099.53
      cervix 099.53
      epididymis 099.54
      genitourinary NEC 099.55
        lower 099.53
        specified NEC 099.54
      pelvic inflammatory disease 099.54
      perihepatic 099.56
      peritoneum 099.56
      pharynx 099.51
      rectum 099.52
      specified site NEC 099.54

Disease, diseased — *see also* Syndrome — *continued*
  venereal — *continued*
    chlamydial NEC — *continued*
      testis 099.54
      vagina 099.53
      vulva 099.53
    fifth 099.1
    sixth 099.1
    complicating pregnancy, childbirth, or puerperium 647.2 ✓5ᵗʰ
    specified nature or type NEC 099.8
      chlamydial — *see* Disease, venereal, chlamydial
  Verneuil's (syphilitic bursitis) 095.7
  Verse's (calcinosis intervertebralis) 275.49 [722.90]
  vertebra, vertebral NEC 733.90
    disc — *see* Disease, Intervertebral disc
  vibration NEC 994.9
  Vidal's (lichen simplex chronicus) 698.3
  Vincent's (trench mouth) 101
  Virchow's 733.99
  virus (filterable) NEC 078.89
    arbovirus NEC 066.9
    arthropod-borne NEC 066.9
    central nervous system NEC 049.9
      specified type NEC 049.8
    complicating pregnancy, childbirth, or puerperium 647.6 ✓5ᵗʰ
    contact (with) V01.7
    exposure to V01.7
    Marburg 078.89
    maternal
      with fetal damage affecting management of pregnancy 655.3 ✓5ᵗʰ
    nonarthropod-borne NEC 078.89
      central nervous sytem NEC 049.9
        specified NEC 049.8
  vitreous 379.29
  vocal cords NEC 478.5
  Vogt's (Cecile) 333.7
  Vogt-Spielmeyer 330.1
  Volhard-Fahr (malignant nephrosclerosis) 403.00
  Volkmann's
    acquired 958.6
  von Bechterew's (ankylosing spondylitis) 720.0
  von Economo's (encephalitis lethargica) 049.8
  von Eulenburg's (congenital paramyotonia) 359.2
  von Gierke's (glycogenosis I) 271.0
  von Graefe's 378.72
  von Hippel's (retinocerebral angiomatosis) 759.6
  von Hippel-Lindau (angiomatosis retinocerebellosa) 759.6
  von Jaksch's (pseudoleukemia infantum) 285.8
  von Recklinghausen's (M9540/1) 237.71
    bone (osteitis fibrosa cystica) 252.0
  von Recklinghausen-Applebaum (hemochromatosis) 275.0
  von Willebrand (-Jürgens) (angiohemophilia) 286.4
  von Zambusch's (lichen sclerosus et atrophicus) 701.0
  Voorhoeve's (dyschondroplasia) 756.4
  Vrolik's (osteogenesis imperfecta) 756.51
  vulva
    noninflammatory 624.9
      specified NEC 624.8
  Wagner's (colloid milium) 709.3
  Waldenström's (osteochondrosis capital femoral) 732.1
  Wallgren's (obstruction of splenic vein with collateral circulation) 459.89
  Wardrop's (with lymphangitis) 681.9
    finger 681.02
    toe 681.11
  Wassilieff's (leptospiral jaundice) 100.0
  wasting NEC 799.4
    due to malnutrition 261
    paralysis 335.21
  Waterhouse-Friderichsen 036.3
  waxy (any site) 277.3
  Weber-Christian (nodular nonsuppurative panniculitis) 729.30

Disease, diseased — *see also* Syndrome — *continued*
  Wegner's (syphilitic osteochondritis) 090.0
  Weil's (leptospral jaundice) 100.0
    of lung 100.0
  Weir Mitchell's (erythromelalgia) 443.89
  Werdnig-Hoffmann 335.0
  Werlhof's (*see also* Purpura, thrombocytopenic) 287.3
  Wermer's 258.0
  Werner's (progeria adultorum) 259.8
  Werner-His (trench fever) 083.1
  Werner-Schultz (agranulocytosis) 288.0
  Wernicke's (superior hemorrhagic polioencephalitis) 265.1
  Wernicke-Posadas 114.9
  Whipple's (intestinal lipodystrophy) 040.2
  whipworm 127.3
  white
    blood cell 288.9
      specified NEC 288.8
    spot 701.0
  White's (congenital) (keratosis follicularis) 757.39
  Whitmore's (melioidosis) 025
  Widal-Abrami (acquired hemolytic jaundice) 283.9
  Wilkie's 557.1
  Wilkinson-Sneddon (subcorneal pustular dermatosis) 694.1
  Willis' (diabetes mellitus) (*see also* Diabetes) 250.0 ✓5ᵗʰ
  Wilson's (hepatolenticular degeneration) 275.1
  Wilson-Brocq (dermatitis exfoliativa) 695.89
  winter vomiting 078.82
  Wise's 696.2
  Wohlfart-Kugelberg-Welander 335.11
  Woillez's (acute idiopathic pulmonary congestion) 518.5
  Wolman's (primary familial xanthomatosis) 272.7
  wool-sorters' 022.1
  Zagari's (xerostomia) 527.7
  Zahorsky's (exanthem subitum) 057.8
  Ziehen-Oppenheim 333.6
  zoonotic, bacterial NEC 027.9
    specified type NEC 027.8

Disfigurement (due to scar) 709.2
  head V48.6
  limb V49.4
  neck V48.7
  trunk V48.7

Disgerminoma — *see* Dysgerminoma

Disinsertion, retina 361.04

Disintegration, complete, of the body 799.8
  traumatic 869.1

Disk kidney 753.3

Dislocatable hip, congenital (*see also* Dislocation, hip, congenital) 754.30

Dislocation (articulation) (closed) (displacement) (simple) (subluxation) 839.8

> Note — "Closed" includes simple, complete, partial, uncomplicated, and unspecified dislocation.
>
> "Open" includes dislocation specified as infected or compound and dislocation with foreign body.
>
> "Chronic," "habitual," "old," or "recurrent" dislocations should be coded as indicated under the entry "Dislocation, recurrent," and "pathological" as indicated under the entry "Dislocation, pathological."
>
> For late effect of dislocation see Late, effect, dislocation.

  with fracture — *see* Fracture, by site
  acromioclavicular (joint) (closed) 831.04
    open 831.14
  anatomical site (closed)
    specified NEC 839.69
      open 839.79
    unspecified or ill-defined 839.8
      open 839.9

Dislocation

Dislocation — *continued*
- ankle (scaphoid bone) (closed) 837.0
  - open 837.1
- arm (closed) 839.8
  - open 839.9
- astragalus (closed) 837.0
  - open 837.1
- atlanto-axial (closed) 839.01
  - open 839.11
- atlas (closed) 839.01
  - open 839.11
- axis (closed) 839.02
  - open 839.12
- back (closed) 839.8
  - open 839.9
- Bell-Daly 723.8
- breast bone (closed) 839.61
  - open 839.71
- capsule, joint — *see* Dislocation, by site
- carpal (bone) — *see* Dislocation, wrist
- carpometacarpal (joint) (closed) 833.04
  - open 833.14
- cartilage (joint) — *see also* Dislocation, by site
  - knee — *see* Tear, meniscus
- cervical, cervicodorsal, or cervicothoracic (spine) (vertebra) — *see* Dislocation, vertebra, cervical
- chiropractic (*see also* Lesion, nonallopathic) 739.9
- chondrocostal — *see* Dislocation, costochondral
- chronic — *see* Dislocation, recurrent
- clavicle (closed) 831.04
  - open 831.14
- coccyx (closed) 839.41
  - open 839.51
- collar bone (closed) 831.04
  - open 831.14
- compound (open) NEC 839.9
- congenital NEC 755.8
  - hip (*see also* Dislocation, hip, congenital) 754.30
  - lens 743.37
  - rib 756.3
  - sacroiliac 755.69
  - spine NEC 756.19
  - vertebra 756.19
- coracoid (closed) 831.09
  - open 831.19
- costal cartilage (closed) 839.69
  - open 839.79
- costochondral (closed) 839.69
  - open 839.79
- cricoarytenoid articulation (closed) 839.69
  - open 839.79
- cricothyroid (cartilage) articulation (closed) 839.69
  - open 839.79
- dorsal vertebrae (closed) 839.21
  - open 839.31
- ear ossicle 385.23
- elbow (closed) 832.00
  - anterior (closed) 832.01
    - open 832.11
  - congenital 754.89
  - divergent (closed) 832.09
    - open 832.19
  - lateral (closed) 832.04
    - open 832.14
  - medial (closed) 832.03
    - open 832.13
  - open 832.10
  - posterior (closed) 832.02
    - open 832.12
  - recurrent 718.32
  - specified type NEC 832.09
    - open 832.19
- eye 360.81
  - lateral 376.36
- eyeball 360.81
  - lateral 376.36
- femur
  - distal end (closed) 836.50
    - anterior 836.52
      - open 836.62
    - lateral 836.53
      - open 836.63

Dislocation — *continued*
- femur — *continued*
  - distal end — *continued*
    - medial 836.54
      - open 836.64
    - open 836.60
    - posterior 836.51
      - open 836.61
  - proximal end (closed) 835.00
    - anterior (pubic) 835.03
      - open 835.13
    - obturator 835.02
      - open 835.12
    - open 835.10
    - posterior 835.01
      - open 835.11
- fibula
  - distal end (closed) 837.0
    - open 837.1
  - proximal end (closed) 836.59
    - open 836.69
- finger(s) (phalanx) (thumb) (closed) 834.00
  - interphalangeal (joint) 834.02
    - open 834.12
  - metacarpal (bone), distal end 834.01
    - open 834.11
  - metacarpophalangeal (joint) 834.01
    - open 834.11
  - open 834.10
  - recurrent 718.34
- foot (closed) 838.00
  - open 838.10
  - recurrent 718.37
- forearm (closed) 839.8
  - open 839.9
- fracture — *see* Fracture, by site
- glenoid (closed) 831.09
  - open 831.19
- habitual — *see* Dislocation, recurrent
- hand (closed) 839.8
  - open 839.9
- hip (closed) 835.00
  - anterior 835.03
    - obturator 835.02
      - open 835.12
    - open 835.13
  - congenital (unilateral) 754.30
    - with subluxation of other hip 754.35
    - bilateral 754.31
  - developmental 718.75
  - open 835.10
  - posterior 835.01
    - open 835.11
  - recurrent 718.35
- humerus (closed) 831.00
  - distal end (*see also* Dislocation, elbow) 832.00
  - open 831.10
  - proximal end (closed) 831.00
    - anterior (subclavicular) (subcoracoid) (subglenoid) (closed) 831.01
      - open 831.11
    - inferior (closed) 831.03
      - open 831.13
    - open 831.10
    - posterior (closed) 831.02
      - open 831.12
- implant — *see* Complications, mechanical
- incus 385.23
- infracoracoid (closed) 831.01
  - open 831.11
- innominate (pubic juntion) (sacral junction) (closed) 839.69
  - acetabulum (*see also* Dislocation, hip) 835.00
  - open 839.79
- interphalangeal (joint)
  - finger or hand (closed) 834.02
    - open 834.12
  - foot or toe (closed) 838.06
    - open 838.16
- jaw (cartilage) (meniscus) (closed) 830.0
  - open 830.1
  - recurrent 524.69
- joint NEC (closed) 839.8
  - developmental 718.7 ✓5ᵗʰ
  - open 839.9

Dislocation — *continued*
- joint NEC — *continued*
  - pathological — *see* Dislocation, pathological
  - recurrent — *see* Dislocation, recurrent
- knee (closed) 836.50
  - anterior 836.51
    - open 836.61
  - congenital (with genu recurvatum) 754.41
  - habitual 718.36
  - lateral 836.54
    - open 836.64
  - medial 836.53
    - open 836.63
  - old 718.36
  - open 836.60
  - posterior 836.52
    - open 836.62
  - recurrent 718.36
  - rotatory 836.59
    - open 836.69
- lacrimal gland 375.16
- leg (closed) 839.8
  - open 839.9
- lens (crystalline) (complete) (partial) 379.32
  - anterior 379.33
  - congenital 743.37
  - ocular implant 996.53
  - posterior 379.34
  - traumatic 921.3
- ligament — *see* Dislocation, by site
- lumbar (vertebrae) (closed) 839.20
  - open 839.30
- lumbosacral (vertebrae) (closed) 839.20
  - congenital 756.19
  - open 839.30
- mandible (closed) 830.0
  - open 830.1
- maxilla (inferior) (closed) 830.0
  - open 830.1
- meniscus (knee) — *see also* Tear, meniscus
  - other sites — *see* Dislocation, by site
- metacarpal (bone)
  - distal end (closed) 834.01
    - open 834.11
  - proximal end (closed) 833.05
    - open 833.15
- metacarpophalangeal (joint) (closed) 834.01
  - open 834.11
- metatarsal (bone) (closed) 838.04
  - open 838.14
- metatarsophalangeal (joint) (closed) 838.05
  - open 838.15
- midcarpal (joint) (closed) 833.03
  - open 833.13
- midtarsal (joint) (closed) 838.02
  - open 838.12
- Monteggia's — *see* Dislocation, hip
- multiple locations (except fingers only or toes only) (closed) 839.8
  - open 839.9
- navicular (bone) foot (closed) 837.0
  - open 837.1
- neck (*see also* Dislocation, vertebra, cervical) 839.00
- Nélaton's — *see* Dislocation, ankle
- nontraumatic (joint) — *see* Dislocation, pathological
- nose (closed) 839.69
  - open 839.79
- not recurrent, not current injury — *see* Dislocation, pathological
- occiput from atlas (closed) 839.01
  - open 839.11
- old — *see* Dislocation, recurrent
- open (compound) NEC 839.9
- ossicle, ear 385.23
- paralytic (flaccid) (spastic) — *see* Dislocation, pathological
- patella (closed) 836.3
  - congenital 755.64
  - open 836.4
- pathological NEC 718.20
  - ankle 718.27
  - elbow 718.22
  - foot 718.27
  - hand 718.24
  - hip 718.25
  - knee 718.26

Index to Diseases

Dislocation — *continued*
  pathological NEC — *continued*
    lumbosacral joint 724.6
    multiple sites 718.29
    pelvic region 718.25
    sacroiliac 724.6
    shoulder (region) 718.21
    specified site NEC 718.28
    spine 724.8
      sacroiliac 724.6
    wrist 718.23
  pelvis (closed) 839.69
    acetabulum (*see also* Dislocation, hip) 835.00
    open 839.79
  phalanx
    foot or toe (closed) 838.09
      open 838.19
    hand or finger (*see also* Dislocation, finger) 834.00
  postpoliomyelitic — *see* Dislocation, pathological
  prosthesis, internal — *see* Complications, mechanical
  radiocarpal (joint) (closed) 833.02
    open 833.12
  radioulnar (joint)
    distal end (closed) 833.01
      open 833.11
    proximal end (*see also* Dislocation, elbow) 832.00
  radius
    distal end (closed) 833.00
      open 833.10
    proximal end (closed) 832.01
      open 832.11
  recurrent (*see also* Derangement, joint, recurrent) 718.3
    elbow 718.32
    hip 718.35
    joint NEC 718.38
    knee 718.36
    lumbosacral (joint) 724.6
    patella 718.36
    sacroiliac 724.6
    shoulder 718.31
    temporomandibular 524.69
  rib (cartilage) (closed) 839.69
    congenital 756.3
    open 839.79
  sacrococcygeal (closed) 839.42
    open 839.52
  sacroiliac (joint) (ligament) (closed) 839.42
    congenital 755.69
    open 839.52
    recurrent 724.6
  sacrum (closed) 839.42
    open 839.52
  scaphoid (bone)
    ankle or foot (closed) 837.0
      open 837.1
    wrist (closed) (*see also* Dislocation, wrist) 833.00
      open 833.10
  scapula (closed) 831.09
    open 831.19
  semilunar cartilage, knee — *see* Tear, meniscus
  septal cartilage (nose) (closed) 839.69
    open 839.79
  septum (nasal) (old) 470
  sesamoid bone — *see* Dislocation, by site
  shoulder (blade) (ligament) (closed) 831.00
    anterior (subclavicular) (subcoracoid) (subglenoid) (closed) 831.01
      open 831.11
    chronic 718.31
    inferior 831.03
      open 831.13
    open 831.10
    posterior (closed) 831.02
      open 831.12
    recurrent 718.31
  skull — *see* Injury, intracranial
  Smith's — *see* Dislocation, foot
  spine (articular process) (*see also* Dislocation, vertebra) (closed) 839.40
    atlanto-axial (closed) 839.01

Dislocation — *continued*
  spine (*see also* Dislocation, vertebra) — *continued*
    atlanto-axial — *continued*
      open 839.11
      recurrent 723.8
    cervical, cervicodorsal, cervicothoracic (closed) (*see also* Dislocation, vertebrae, cervical) 839.00
      open 839.10
      recurrent 723.8
    coccyx 839.41
      open 839.51
    congenital 756.19
    due to birth trauma 767.4
    open 839.50
    recurrent 724.9
    sacroiliac 839.42
      recurrent 724.6
    sacrum (sacrococcygeal) (sacroiliac) 839.42
      open 839.52
  spontaneous — *see* Dislocation, pathological
  sternoclavicular (joint) (closed) 839.61
    open 839.71
  sternum (closed) 839.61
    open 839.71
  subastragalar — *see* Dislocation, foot
  subglenoid (closed) 831.01
    open 831.11
  symphysis
    jaw (closed) 830.0
      open 830.1
    mandibular (closed) 830.0
      open 830.1
    pubis (closed) 839.69
      open 839.79
  tarsal (bone) (joint) 838.01
    open 838.11
  tarsometatarsal (joint) 838.03
    open 838.13
  temporomandibular (joint) (closed) 830.0
    open 830.1
    recurrent 524.69
  thigh
    distal end (*see also* Dislocation, femur, distal end) 836.50
    proximal end (*see also* Dislocation, hip) 835.00
  thoracic (vertebrae) (closed) 839.21
    open 839.31
  thumb(s) (*see also* Dislocation, finger) 834.00
  thyroid cartilage (closed) 839.69
    open 839.79
  tibia
    distal end (closed) 837.0
      open 837.1
    proximal end (closed) 836.50
      anterior 836.51
        open 836.61
      lateral 836.54
        open 836.64
      medial 836.53
        open 836.63
      open 836.60
      posterior 836.52
        open 836.62
      rotatory 836.59
        open 836.69
  tibiofibular
    distal (closed) 837.0
      open 837.1
    superior (closed) 836.59
      open 836.69
  toe(s) (closed) 838.09
    open 838.19
  trachea (closed) 839.69
    open 839.79
  ulna
    distal end (closed) 833.09
      open 833.19
    proximal end — *see* Dislocation, elbow
  vertebra (articular process) (body) (closed) 839.40
    cervical, cervicodorsal or cervicothoracic (closed) 839.00
      first (atlas) 839.01
        open 839.11

Dislocation — *continued*
  vertebra — *continued*
    cervical, cervicodorsal or cervicothoracic — *continued*
      second (axis) 839.02
        open 839.12
      third 839.03
        open 839.13
      fourth 839.04
        open 839.14
      fifth 839.05
        open 839.15
      sixth 839.06
        open 839.16
      seventh 839.07
        open 839.17
      congenital 756.19
      multiple sites 839.08
        open 839.18
      open 839.10
    congenital 756.19
    dorsal 839.21
      open 839.31
      recurrent 724.9
    lumbar, lumbosacral 839.20
      open 839.30
      open NEC 839.50
      recurrent 724.9
      specified region NEC 839.49
        open 839.59
    thoracic 839.21
      open 839.31
  wrist (carpal bone) (scaphoid) (semilunar) (closed) 833.00
    carpometacarpal (joint) 833.04
      open 833.14
    metacarpal bone, proximal end 833.05
      open 833.15
    midcarpal (joint) 833.03
      open 833.13
    open 833.10
    radiocarpal (joint) 833.02
      open 833.12
    radioulnar (joint) 833.01
      open 833.11
    recurrent 718.33
    specified site NEC 833.09
      open 833.19
  xiphoid cartilage (closed) 839.61
    open 839.71

Dislodgement
  artificial skin graft 996.55
  decellularized allodermis graft 996.55

Disobedience, hostile (covert) (overt) (*see also* Disturbance, conduct) 312.0

Disorder — *see also* Disease
  academic underachievement, childhood and adolescence 313.83
  accommodation 367.51
    drug-induced 367.89
    toxic 367.89
  adjustment (*see also* Reaction, adjustment) 309.9
  adrenal (capsule) (cortex) (gland) 255.9
    specified type NEC 255.8
  adrenogenital 255.2
  affective (*see also* Psychosis, affective) 296.90
    atypical 296.81
  aggressive, unsocialized (*see also* Disturbance, conduct) 312.0
  alcohol, alcoholic (*see also* Alcohol) 291.9
  allergic — *see* Allergy
  amnestic (*see also* Amnestic syndrome) 294.0
  amino acid (metabolic) (*see also* Disturbance, metabolism, amino acid) 270.9
    albinism 270.2
    alkaptonuria 270.2
    argininosuccinicaciduria 270.6
    beta-amino-isobutyricaciduria 277.2
    cystathioninuria 270.4
    cystinosis 270.0
    cystinuria 270.0
    glycinuria 270.0
    homocystinuria 270.4
    imidazole 270.5
    maple syrup (urine) disease 270.3

Disorder — see also Disease — continued
- amino acid (see also Disturbance, metabolism, amino acid) — continued
  - neonatal, transitory 775.8
  - oasthouse urine disease 270.2
  - ochronosis 270.2
  - phenylketonuria 270.1
  - phenylpyruvic oligophrenia 270.1
  - purine NEC 277.2
  - pyrimidine NEC 277.2
  - renal transport NEC 270.0
  - specified type NEC 270.8
  - transport NEC 270.0
    - renal 270.0
  - xanthinuria 277.2
- anaerobic glycolysis with anemia 282.3
- anxiety (see also Anxiety) 300.00
  - due to or associated with physical condition 293.84
- arteriole 447.9
  - specified type NEC 447.8
- artery 447.9
  - specified type NEC 447.8
- articulation — see Disorder, joint
- Asperger's 299.8
- attachment of infancy 313.89
- attention deficit 314.00
  - with hyperactivity 314.01
  - predominantly
    - combined hyperactive/inattentive 314.01
    - hyperactive/impulsive 314.01
    - inattentive 314.00
  - residual type 314.8
- autoimmune NEC 279.4
  - hemolytic (cold type) (warm type) 283.0
  - parathyroid 252.1
  - thyroid 245.2
- autistic 299.0
- avoidant, childhood or adolescence 313.21
- balance
  - acid-base 276.9
    - mixed (with hypercapnia) 276.4
  - electrolyte 276.9
  - fluid 276.9
- behavior NEC (see also Disturbance, conduct) 312.9
- bilirubin excretion 277.4
- bipolar (affective) (alternating) (type I) (see also Psychosis, affective) 296.7
  - atypical 296.7
  - currently
    - depressed 296.5
    - hypomanic 296.4
    - manic 296.4
  - mixed 296.6
  - type II (recurrent major depressive episodes with hypomania) 296.89
- bladder 596.9
  - functional NEC 596.59
  - specified NEC 596.8
- bone NEC 733.90
  - specified NEC 733.99
- brachial plexus 353.0
- branched-chain amino-acid degradation 270.3
- breast 611.9
  - puerperal, postpartum 676.3
  - specified NEC 611.8
- Briquet's 300.81
- bursa 727.9
  - shoulder region 726.10
- carbohydrate metabolism, congenital 271.9
- cardiac, functional 427.9
  - postoperative 997.1
  - psychogenic 306.2
- cardiovascular, psychogenic 306.2
- cartilage NEC 733.90
  - articular 718.00
    - ankle 718.07
    - elbow 718.02
    - foot 718.07
    - hand 718.04
    - hip 718.05
    - knee 717.9
    - multiple sites 718.09
    - pelvic region 718.05
    - shoulder region 718.01

Disorder — see also Disease — continued
- cartilage NEC — continued
  - articular — continued
    - specified
      - site NEC 718.08
      - type NEC 733.99
    - wrist 718.03
- catatonic — see Catatonia
- cervical region NEC 723.9
- cervical root (nerve) NEC 353.2
- character NEC (see also Disorder, personality) 301.9
- coagulation (factor) (see also Defect, coagulation) 286.9
  - factor VIII (congenital) (functional) 286.0
  - factor IX (congenital) (functional) 286.1
  - neonatal, transitory 776.3
- coccyx 724.70
  - specified NEC 724.79
- colon 569.9
  - functional 564.9
  - congenital 751.3
- cognitive 294.9
- conduct (see also Disturbance, conduct) 312.9
  - adjustment reaction 309.3
  - adolescent onset type 312.82
  - childhood onset type 312.81
  - compulsive 312.30
    - specified type NEC 312.39
  - hyperkinetic 314.2
  - socialized (type) 312.20
    - aggressive 312.23
    - unaggressive 312.21
  - specified NEC 312.89
- conduction, heart 426.9
  - specified NEC 426.89
- convulsive (secondary) (see also Convulsions) 780.39
  - due to injury at birth 767.0
  - idiopathic 780.39
- coordination 781.3
- cornea NEC 371.89
  - due to contact lens 371.82
- corticosteroid metabolism NEC 255.2
- cranial nerve — see Disorder, nerve, cranial
- cyclothymic 301.13
- degradation, branched-chain amino acid 270.3
- delusional 297.9
- dentition 520.6
- depressive NEC 311
  - atypical 296.82
  - major (see also Psychosis, affective) 296.2
    - recurrent episode 296.3
    - single episode 296.2
- development, specific 315.9
  - associated with hyperkinesia 314.1
  - language 315.31
  - learning 315.2
    - arithmetical 315.1
    - reading 315.00
  - mixed 315.5
  - motor coordination 315.4
  - specified type NEC 315.8
  - speech 315.39
- diaphragm 519.4
- digestive 536.9
  - fetus or newborn 777.9
    - specified NEC 777.8
  - psychogenic 306.4
- disintegrative (childhood) 299.1
- dissociative 300.14
  - identity 300.14
- dysmorphic body 300.7
- dysthymic 300.4
- ear 388.9
  - degenerative NEC 388.00
  - external 380.9
    - specified 380.89
  - pinna 380.30
  - specified type NEC 388.8
  - vascular NEC 388.00
- eating NEC 307.50
- electrolyte NEC 276.9
  - with
    - abortion — see Abortion, by type, with metabolic disorder

Disorder — see also Disease — continued
- electrolyte NEC — continued
  - with — continued
    - ectopic pregnancy (see also categories 633.0-633.9) 639.4
    - molar pregnancy (see also categories 630-632) 639.4
  - acidosis 276.2
    - metabolic 276.2
    - respiratory 276.2
  - alkalosis 276.3
    - metabolic 276.3
    - respiratory 276.3
  - following
    - abortion 639.4
    - ectopic or molar pregnancy 639.4
  - neonatal, transitory NEC 775.5
- emancipation as adjustment reaction 309.22
- emotional (see also Disorder, mental, nonpsychotic) V40.9
- endocrine 259.9
  - specified type NEC 259.8
- esophagus 530.9
  - functional 530.5
  - psychogenic 306.4
- explosive
  - intermittent 312.34
  - isolated 312.35
- expressive language 315.31
- eye 379.90
  - globe — see Disorder, globe
  - ill-defined NEC 379.99
  - limited duction NEC 378.63
  - specified NEC 379.8
- eyelid 374.9
  - degenerative 374.50
  - sensory 374.44
  - specified type NEC 374.89
  - vascular 374.85
- factitious — see Illness, factitious
- factor, coagulation (see also Defect, coagulation) 286.9
  - VIII (congenital) (functional) 286.0
  - IX (congenital) (funcitonal) 286.1
- fascia 728.9
- feeding — see Feeding
- female sexual arousal 302.72
- fluid NEC 276.9
- gastric (functional) 536.9
  - motility 536.8
  - psychogenic 306.4
  - secretion 536.8
- gastrointestinal (functional) NEC 536.9
  - newborn (neonatal) 777.9
    - specified NEC 777.8
  - psychogenic 306.4
- gender (child) 302.6
  - adult 302.85
- gender identity (childhood) 302.6
  - adult-life 302.85
- genitourinary system, psychogenic 306.50
- globe 360.9
  - degenerative 360.20
    - specified NEC 360.29
  - specified type NEC 360.89
- hearing — see also Deafness
  - conductive type (air) (see also Deafness, conductive) 389.00
  - mixed conductive and sensorineural 389.2
  - nerve 389.12
  - perceptive (see also Deafness, perceptive) 389.10
  - sensorineural type NEC (see also Deafness, perceptive) 389.10
- heart action 427.9
  - postoperative 997.1
- hematological, transient neonatal 776.9
  - specified type NEC 776.8
- hematopoietic organs 289.9
- hemorrhagic NEC 287.9
  - due to circulating anticoagulants 286.5
  - specified type NEC 287.8
- hemostasis (see also Defect, coagulation) 286.9
- homosexual conflict 302.0
- hypomanic (chronic) 301.11

Index to Diseases

Disorder — see also Disease — continued
  identity
    childhood and adolescence 313.82
      gender 302.6
    gender 302.6
  immune mechanism (immunity) 279.9
    single complement (C-C) 279.8
    specified type NEC 279.8
  impulse control (see also Disturbance, conduct, compulsive) 312.30
  infant sialic acid storage 271.8
  integument, fetus or newborn 778.9
    specified type NEC 778.8
  interactional psychotic (childhood) (see also Psychosis, childhood) 299.1 ✓5ᵗʰ
  intermittent explosive 312.34
  intervertebral disc 722.90
    cervical, cervicothoracic 722.91
    lumbar, lumbosacral 722.93
    thoracic, thoracolumbar 722.92
  intestinal 569.9
    functional NEC 564.9
      congenital 751.3
      postoperative 564.4
    psychogenic 306.4
  introverted, of childhood and adolescence 313.22
  iron, metabolism 275.0
  isolated explosive 312.35
  joint NEC 719.90
    ankle 719.97
    elbow 719.92
    foot 719.97
    hand 719.94
    hip 719.95
    knee 719.96
    multiple sites 719.99
    pelvic region 719.95
    psychogenic 306.0
    shoulder (region) 719.91
    specified site NEC 719.98
    temporomandibular 524.60
      specified NEC 524.69
    wrist 719.93
  kidney 593.9
    functional 588.9
      specified NEC 588.8
  labyrinth, labyrinthine 386.9
    specified type NEC 386.8
  lactation 676.9 ✓5ᵗʰ
  language (developmental) (expressive) 315.31
    mixed (receptive) (receptive-expressive) 315.32
  ligament 728.9
  ligamentous attachments, peripheral — see also Enthesopathy
    spine 720.1
  limb NEC 729.9
    psychogenic 306.0
  lipid
    metabolism, congenital 272.9
    storage 272.7
  lipoprotein deficiency (familial) 272.5
  low back NEC 724.9
    psychogenic 306.0
  lumbosacral
    plexus 353.1
    root (nerve) NEC 353.4
  lymphoproliferative (chronic) NEC (M9970/1) 238.7
  male erectile 302.72
    organic origin 607.84
  major depressive (see also Psychosis, affective) 296.2 ✓5ᵗʰ
    recurrent episode 296.3 ✓5ᵗʰ
    single episode 296.2 ✓5ᵗʰ
  manic (see also Psychosis, affective) 296.0 ✓5ᵗʰ
    atypical 296.81
  meniscus NEC (see also Disorder, cartilage, articular) 718.0 ✓5ᵗʰ
  menopausal 627.9
    specified NEC 627.8
  menstrual 626.9
    psychogenic 306.52
    specified NEC 626.8
  mental (nonpsychotic) 300.9
    affecting management of pregnancy, childbirth, or puerperium 648.4 ✓5ᵗʰ

Disorder — see also Disease — continued
  mental — continued
    drug-induced 292.9
      hallucinogen persisting perception 292.89
      specified type NEC 292.89
    due to or associated with
      alcoholism 291.9
      drug consumption NEC 292.9
        specified type NEC 292.89
      physical condition NEC 293.9
    induced by drug 292.9
      specified type NEC 292.89
    neurotic (see also Neurosis) 300.9
    presenile 310.1
      psychotic NEC 290.10
    previous, affecting management of pregnancy V23.8 ✓5ᵗʰ
    psychoneurotic (see also Neurosis) 300.9
    psychotic (see also Psychosis) 298.9
      senile 290.20
    specific, following organic brain damage 310.9
      cognitive or personality change of other type 310.1
      frontal lobe syndrome 310.0
      postconcussional syndrome 310.2
      specified type NEC 310.8
  metabolism NEC 277.9
    with
      abortion — see Abortion, by type with metabolic disorder
      ectopic pregnancy (see also categories 633.0-633.9) 639.4
      molar pregnancy (see also categories 630-632) 639.4
    alkaptonuria 270.2
    amino acid (see also Disorder, amino acid) 270.9
      specified type NEC 270.8
    ammonia 270.6
    arginine 270.6
    argininosuccinic acid 270.6
    basal 794.7
    bilirubin 277.4
    calcium 275.40
    carbohydrate 271.9
      specified type NEC 271.8
    cholesterol 272.9
    citrulline 270.6
    copper 275.1
    corticosteroid 255.2
    cystine storage 270.0
    cystinuria 270.0
    fat 272.9
    following
      abortion 639.4
      ectopic or molar pregnancy 639.4
    fructosemia 271.2
    fructosuria 271.2
    fucosidosis 271.8
    galactose-1-phosphate uridyl transferase 271.1
    glutamine 270.7
    glycine 270.7
    glycogen storage NEC 271.0
      hepatorenal 271.0
    hemochromatosis 275.0
    in labor and delivery 669.0 ✓5ᵗʰ
    iron 275.0
    lactose 271.3
    lipid 272.9
      specified type NEC 272.8
      storage 272.7
    lipoprotein — see also Hyperlipemia
      deficiency (familial) 272.5
    lysine 270.7
    magnesium 275.2
    mannosidosis 271.8
    mineral 275.9
      specified type NEC 275.8
    mucopolysaccharide 277.5
    nitrogen 270.9
    ornithine 270.6
    oxalosis 271.8
    pentosuria 271.8
    phenylketonuria 270.1
    phosphate 275.3

Disorder — see also Disease — continued
  metabolism NEC — continued
    phosphorous 275.3
    plasma protein 273.9
      specified type NEC 273.8
    porphyrin 277.1
    purine 277.2
    pyrimidine 277.2
    serine 270.7
    sodium 276.9
    specified type NEC 277.8
    steroid 255.2
    threonine 270.7
    urea cycle 270.6
    xylose 271.8
  micturition NEC 788.69
    psychogenic 306.53
  misery and unhappiness, of childhood and adolescence 313.1
  mitral valve 424.0
  mood — see Psychosis, affective
  motor tic 307.20
    chronic 307.22
    transient, childhood 307.21
  movement NEC 333.90
    hysterical 300.11
    specified type NEC 333.99
    stereotypic 307.3
  mucopolysaccharide 277.5
  muscle 728.9
    psychogenic 306.0
    specified type NEC 728.3
  muscular attachments, peripheral — see also Enthesopathy
    spine 720.1
  musculoskeletal system NEC 729.9
    psychogenic 306.0
  myeloproliferative (chronic) NEC (M9960/1) 238.7
  myoneural 358.9
    due to lead 358.2
    specified type NEC 358.8
    toxic 358.2
  myotonic 359.2
  neck region NEC 723.9
  nerve 349.9
    abducens NEC 378.54
    accessory 352.4
    acoustic 388.5
    auditory 388.5
    auriculotemporal 350.8
    axillary 353.0
    cerebral — see Disorder, nerve, cranial
    cranial 352.9
      first 352.0
      second 377.49
      third
        partial 378.51
        total 378.52
      fourth 378.53
      fifth 350.9
      sixth 378.54
      seventh NEC 351.9
      eighth 388.5
      ninth 352.2
      tenth 352.3
      eleventh 352.4
      twelfth 352.5
      multiple 352.6
    entrapment — see Neuropathy, entrapment
    facial 351.9
      specified NEC 351.8
    femoral 355.2
    glossopharyngeal NEC 352.2
    hypoglossal 352.5
    iliohypogastric 355.79
    ilioinguinal 355.79
    intercostal 353.8
    lateral
      cutaneous of thigh 355.1
      popliteal 355.3
    lower limb NEC 355.8
    medial, popliteal 355.4
    median NEC 354.1
    obturator 355.79

Disorder — see also Disease — continued
- nerve — continued
  - oculomotor
    - partial 378.51
    - total 378.52
  - olfactory 352.0
  - optic 377.49
    - ischemic 377.41
    - nutritional 377.33
    - toxic 377.34
  - peroneal 355.3
  - phrenic 354.8
  - plantar 355.6
  - pneumogastric 352.3
  - posterior tibial 355.5
  - radial 354.3
  - recurrent laryngeal 352.3
  - root 353.9
    - specified NEC 353.8
  - saphenous 355.79
  - sciatic NEC 355.0
  - specified NEC 355.9
    - lower limb 355.79
    - upper limb 354.8
  - spinal 355.9
  - sympathetic NEC 337.9
  - trigeminal 350.9
    - specified NEC 350.8
  - trochlear 378.53
  - ulnar 354.2
  - upper limb NEC 354.9
  - vagus 352.3
- nervous system NEC 349.9
  - autonomic (peripheral) (see also Neuropathy, peripheral, autonomic) 337.9
  - cranial 352.9
  - parasympathetic (see also Neuropathy, peripheral, autonomic) 337.9
  - specified type NEC 349.89
  - sympathetic (see also Neuropathy, peripheral, autonomic) 337.9
  - vegetative (see also Neuropathy, peripheral, autonomic) 337.9
- neurohypophysis NEC 253.6
- neurological NEC 781.99
  - peripheral NEC 355.9
- neuromuscular NEC 358.9
  - hereditary NEC 359.1
  - specified NEC 358.8
  - toxic 358.2
- neurotic 300.9
  - specified type NEC 300.89
- neutrophil, polymorphonuclear (functional) 288.1
- obsessive-compulsive 300.3
- oppositional, childhood and adolescence 313.81
- optic
  - chiasm 377.54
    - associated with
      - inflammatory disorders 377.54
      - neoplasm NEC 377.52
        - pituitary 377.51
      - pituitary disorders 377.51
      - vascular disorders 377.53
  - nerve 377.49
  - radiations 377.63
  - tracts 377.63
- orbit 376.9
  - specified NEC 376.89
- overanxious, of childhood and adolescence 313.0
- pancreas, internal secretion (other than diabetes mellitus) 251.9
  - specified type NEC 251.8
- panic 300.01
  - with agoraphobia 300.21
- papillary muscle NEC 429.81
- paranoid 297.9
  - induced 297.3
  - shared 297.3
- parathyroid 252.9
  - specified type NEC 252.8
- paroxysmal, mixed 780.39
- pentose phosphate pathway with anemia 282.2
- personality 301.9
  - affective 301.10
  - aggressive 301.3

Disorder — see also Disease — continued
- personality — continued
  - amoral 301.7
  - anancastic, anankastic 301.4
  - antisocial 301.7
  - asocial 301.7
  - asthenic 301.6
  - boderline 301.83
  - compulsive 301.4
  - cyclothymic 301.13
  - dependent-passive 301.6
  - dyssocial 301.7
  - emotional instability 301.59
  - epileptoid 301.3
  - explosive 301.3
  - following organic brain damage 310.1
  - histrionic 301.50
  - hyperthymic 301.11
  - hypomanic (chronic) 301.11
  - hypothymic 301.12
  - hysterical 301.50
  - immature 301.89
  - inadequate 301.6
  - introverted 301.21
  - labile 301.59
  - moral deficiency 301.7
  - obsessional 301.4
  - obsessive (-compulsive) 301.4
  - overconscientious 301.4
  - paranoid 301.0
  - passive (-dependent) 301.6
  - passive-aggressive 301.84
  - pathological NEC 301.9
  - pseudosocial 301.7
  - psychopathic 301.9
  - schizoid 301.20
    - introverted 301.21
    - schizotypal 301.22
  - schizotypal 301.22
  - seductive 301.59
  - type A 301.4
  - unstable 301.59
- pervasive developmental, childhood-onset 299.8 ✓5ᵗʰ
- pigmentation, choroid (congenital) 743.53
- pinna 380.30
  - specified type NEC 380.39
- pituitary, thalamic 253.9
  - anterior NEC 253.4
  - iatrogenic 253.7
  - postablative 253.7
  - specified NEC 253.8
- pityriasis-like NEC 696.8
- platelets (blood) 287.1
- polymorphonuclear neutrophils (functional) 288.1
- porphyrin metabolism 277.1
- postmenopausal 627.9
  - specified type NEC 627.8
- posttraumatic stress 309.81
  - acute 308.3
  - brief 308.3
  - chronic 309.81
- premenstrual dysphoric 625.4 ●
- psoriatic-like NEC 696.8
- psychic, with diseases classified elsewhere 316
- psychogenic NEC (see also condition) 300.9
  - allergic NEC
    - respiratory 306.1
  - anxiety 300.00
    - atypical 300.00
    - generalized 300.02
  - appetite 307.50
  - articulation, joint 306.0
  - asthenic 300.5
  - blood 306.8
  - cardiovascular (system) 306.2
  - compulsive 300.3
  - cutaneous 306.3
  - depressive 300.4
  - digestive (system) 306.4
  - dysmenorrheic 306.52
  - dyspneic 306.1
  - eczematous 306.3
  - endocrine (system) 306.6
  - eye 306.7
  - feeding 307.59
  - functional NEC 306.9

Disorder — see also Disease — continued
- psychogenic NEC (see also condition) — continued
  - gastric 306.4
  - gastrointestinal (system) 306.4
  - genitourinary (system) 306.50
  - heart (function) (rhythm) 306.2
  - hemic 306.8
  - hyperventilatory 306.1
  - hypochondriacal 300.7
  - hysterical 300.10
  - intestinal 306.4
  - joint 306.0
  - learning 315.2
  - limb 306.0
  - lymphatic (system) 306.8
  - menstrual 306.52
  - micturition 306.53
  - monoplegic NEC 306.0
  - motor 307.9
  - muscle 306.0
  - musculoskeletal 306.0
  - neurocirculatory 306.2
  - obsessive 300.3
  - occupational 300.89
  - organ or part of body NEC 306.9
  - organs of special sense 306.7
  - paralytic NEC 306.0
  - phobic 300.20
  - physical NEC 306.9
  - pruritic 306.3
  - rectal 306.4
  - respiratory (system) 306.1
  - rheumatic 306.0
  - sexual (function) 302.70
    - specified type NEC 302.79
  - skin (allergic) (eczematous) (pruritic) 306.3
  - sleep 307.40
    - initiation or maintenance 307.41
      - persistent 307.42
      - transient 307.41
    - specified type NEC 307.49
  - specified part of body NEC 306.8
  - stomach 306.4
- psychomotor NEC 307.9
  - hysterical 300.11
- psychoneurotic (see also Neurosis) 300.9
  - mixed NEC 300.89
- psychophysiologic (see also Disorder, psychosomatic) 306.9
- psychosexual identity (childhood) 302.6
  - adult-life 302.85
- psychosomatic NEC 306.9
  - allergic NEC
    - respiratory 306.1
  - articulation, joint 306.0
  - cardiovascular (system) 306.2
  - cutaneous 306.3
  - digestive (system) 306.4
  - dysmenorrheic 306.52
  - dyspneic 306.1
  - endocrine (system) 306.6
  - eye 306.7
  - gastric 306.4
  - gastrointestinal (system) 306.4
  - genitourinary (system) 306.50
  - heart (functional) (rhythm) 306.2
  - hyperventilatory 306.1
  - intestinal 306.4
  - joint 306.0
  - limb 306.0
  - lymphatic (system) 306.8
  - menstrual 306.52
  - micturition 306.53
  - monoplegic NEC 306.0
  - muscle 306.0
  - musculoskeletal 306.0
  - neurocirculatory 306.2
  - organs of special sense 306.7
  - paralytic NEC 306.0
  - pruritic 306.3
  - rectal 306.4
  - respiratory (system) 306.1
  - rheumatic 306.0
  - sexual (function) 302.70
    - specified type NEC 302.79
  - skin 306.3
  - specified part of body NEC 306.8

Index to Diseases

Disorder — see also Disease — continued
- psychosomatic NEC — continued
  - stomach 306.4
- psychotic — see Psychosis
- purine metabolism NEC 277.2
- pyrimidine metabolism NEC 277.2
- reactive attachment (of infancy or early childhood) 313.89
- reading, developmental 315.00
- reflex 796.1
- renal function, impaired 588.9
  - specified type NEC 588.8
- renal transport NEC 588.8
- respiration, respiratory NEC 519.9
  - due to
    - aspiration of liquids or solids 508.9
    - inhalation of fumes or vapors 506.9
  - psychogenic 306.1
- retina 362.9
  - specified type NEC 362.89
- sacroiliac joint NEC 724.6
- sacrum 724.6
- schizo-affective (see also Schizophrenia) 295.7
- schizoid, childhood or adolescence 313.22
- schizophreniform 295.4
- schizotypal personality 301.22
- secretion, thyrocalcitonin 246.0
- seizure 780.39
  - recurrent 780.39
    - epileptic — see Epilepsy
- sense of smell 781.1
  - psychogenic 306.7
- separation anxiety 309.21
- sexual (see also Deviation, sexual) 302.9
  - function, psychogenic 302.70
- shyness, of childhood and adolescence 313.21
- single complement (C-C) 279.8
- skin NEC 709.9
  - fetus or newborn 778.9
    - specified type 778.8
  - psychogenic (allergic) (eczematous) (pruritic) 306.3
  - specified type NEC 709.8
  - vascular 709.1
- sleep 780.50
  - with apnea — see Apnea, sleep
  - circadian rhythm 307.45
  - initiation or maintenance (see also Insomnia) 780.52
    - nonorganic origin (transient) 307.41
      - persistent 307.42
  - nonorganic origin 307.40
    - specified type NEC 307.49
  - specified NEC 780.59
- social, of childhood and adolescence 313.22
  - specified NEC 780.59
- soft tissue 729.9
- somatization 300.81
- somatoform (atypical) (undifferentiated) 300.82
  - severe 300.81
- speech NEC 784.5
  - nonorganic origin 307.9
- spine NEC 724.9
  - ligamentous or muscular attachments, peripheral 720.1
- steroid metabolism NEC 255.2
- stomach (functional) (see also Disorder, gastric) 536.9
  - psychogenic 306.4
- storage, iron 275.0
- stress (see also Reaction, stress, acute) 308.9
  - posttraumatic
    - acute 308.3
    - brief 308.3
    - chronic 309.81
- substitution 300.11
- suspected — see Observation
- synovium 727.9
- temperature regulation, fetus or newborn 778.4
- temporomandibular joint NEC 524.60
  - specified NEC 524.69
- tendon 727.9
  - shoulder region 726.10
- thoracic root (nerve) NEC 353.3
- thyrocalcitonin secretion 246.0

Disorder — see also Disease — continued
- thyroid (gland) NEC 246.9
  - specified type NEC 246.8
- tic 307.20
  - chronic (motor or vocal) 307.22
  - motor-verbal 307.23
  - organic origin 333.1
  - transient of childhood 307.21
- tooth NEC 525.9
  - development NEC 520.9
    - specified type NEC 520.8
  - eruption 520.6
    - with abnormal position 524.3
  - specified type NEC 525.8
- transport, carbohydrate 271.9
  - specified type NEC 271.8
- tubular, phosphate-losing 588.0
- tympanic membrane 384.9
- unaggressive, unsocialized (see also Disturbance, conduct) 312.1
- undersocialized, unsocialized (see also Disturbance, conduct)
  - aggressive (type) 312.0
  - unaggressive (type) 312.1
- vision, visual NEC 368.9
  - binocular NEC 368.30
  - cortex 377.73
    - associated with
      - inflammatory disorders 377.73
      - neoplasms 377.71
      - vascular disorders 377.72
  - pathway NEC 377.63
    - associated with
      - inflammatory disorders 377.63
      - neoplasms 377.61
      - vascular disorders 377.62
- wakefulness (see also Hypersomnia) 780.54
  - nonorganic origin (transient) 307.43
    - persistent 307.44

Disorganized globe 360.29

Displacement, displaced

> Note — For acquired displacement of bones, cartilage, joints, tendons, due to injury, see also Dislocation.
>
> Displacements at ages under one year should be considered congenital, provided there is no indication the condition was acquired after birth.

- acquired traumatic of bone, cartilage, joint, tendon NEC (without fracture) (see also Dislocation) 839.8
  - with fracture — see Fracture, by site
- adrenal gland (congenital) 759.1
- appendix, retrocecal (congenital) 751.5
- auricle (congenital) 744.29
- bladder (acquired) 596.8
  - congenital 753.8
- brachial plexus (congenital) 742.8
- brain stem, caudal 742.4
- canaliculus lacrimalis 743.65
- cardia, through esophageal hiatus 750.6
- cerebellum, caudal 742.4
- cervix (see also Malposition, uterus) 621.6
- colon (congenital) 751.4
- device, implant, or graft — see Complications, mechanical
- epithelium
  - columnar of cervix 622.1
  - cuboidal, beyond limits of external os (uterus) 752.49
- esophageal mucosa into cardia of stomach, congenital 750.4
- esophagus (acquired) 530.89
  - congenital 750.4
- eyeball (acquired) (old) 376.36
  - congenital 743.8
  - current injury 871.3
  - lateral 376.36
- fallopian tube (acquired) 620.4
  - congenital 752.19
  - opening (congenital) 752.19
- gallbladder (congenital) 751.69

Displacement, displaced — continued
- gastric mucosa 750.7
  - into
    - duodenum 750.7
    - esophagus 750.7
    - Meckel's diverticulum, congenital 750.7
- globe (acquired) (lateral) (old) 376.36
  - current injury 871.3
- graft
  - artificial skin graft 996.55
  - decellularized allodermis graft 996.55
- heart (congenital) 746.87
  - acquired 429.89
- hymen (congenital) (upward) 752.49
- internal prothesis NEC — see Complications, mechanical
- intervertebral disc (with neuritis, radiculutis, sciatica, or other pain) 722.2
  - with myelopathy 722.70
  - cervical, cervicodorsal, cervicothoracic 722.0
    - with myelopathy 722.71
    - due to major trauma — see Dislocation, vertebra, cervical
  - due to major trauma — see Dislocation, vertebra
- intervertebral disc
  - lumbar, lumbosacral 722.10
    - with myelopathy 722.73
    - due to major trauma — see Dislocation, vertebra, lumbar
  - thoracic, thoracolumbar 722.11
    - with myelopathy 722.72
    - due to major trauma — see Dislocation, vertebra, thoracic
- intrauterine device 996.32
- kidney (acquired) 593.0
  - congenital 753.3
- lacrimal apparatus or duct (congenital) 743.65
- macula (congenital) 743.55
- Meckel's diverticulum (congenital) 751.0
- nail (congenital) 757.5
  - acquired 703.8
- opening of Wharton's duct in mouth 750.26
- organ or site, congenital NEC — see Malposition, congenital
- ovary (acquired) 620.4
  - congenital 752.0
  - free in peritoneal cavity (congenital) 752.0
  - into hernial sac 620.4
- oviduct (acquired) 620.4
  - congenital 752.19
- parathyroid (gland) 252.8
- parotid gland (congenital) 750.26
- punctum lacrimale (congenital) 743.65
- sacroiliac (congenital) (joint) 755.69
  - current injury — see Dislocation, sacroiliac
  - old 724.6
- spine (congenital) 756.19
- spleen, congenital 759.0
- stomach (congenital) 750.7
  - acquired 537.89
- subglenoid (closed) 831.01
- sublingual duct (congenital) 750.26
- teeth, tooth 524.3
- tongue (congenital) (downward) 750.19
- trachea (congenital) 748.3
- ureter or ureteric opening or orifice (congenital) 753.4
- uterine opening of oviducts or fallopian tubes 752.19
- uterus, uterine (see also Malposition, uterus) 621.6
  - congenital 752.3
- ventricular septum 746.89
  - with rudimentary ventricle 746.89
- xyphoid bone (process) 738.3

Disproportion 653.9
- affecting fetus or newborn 763.1
- caused by
  - conjoined twins 653.7
  - contraction, pelvis (general) 653.1
    - inlet 653.2
    - midpelvic 653.8
    - midplane 653.8
    - outlet 653.3
  - fetal
    - ascites 653.7
    - hydrocephalus 653.6

Disproportion

Disproportion — *continued*
- caused by — *continued*
  - fetal — *continued*
    - hydrops 653.7 ✓5ᵗʰ
    - meningomyelocele 653.7 ✓5ᵗʰ
    - sacral teratoma 653.7 ✓5ᵗʰ
    - tumor 653.7 ✓5ᵗʰ
  - hydrocephalic fetus 653.6 ✓5ᵗʰ
  - pelvis, pelvic, abnormality (bony) NEC 653.0 ✓5ᵗʰ
  - unusually large fetus 653.5 ✓5ᵗʰ
- causing obstructed labor 660.1 ✓5ᵗʰ
- cephalopelvic, normally formed fetus 653.4 ✓5ᵗʰ
  - causing obstructed labor 660.1 ✓5ᵗʰ
- fetal NEC 653.5 ✓5ᵗʰ
  - causing obstructed labor 660.1 ✓5ᵗʰ
- fetopelvic, normally formed fetus 653.4 ✓5ᵗʰ
  - causing obstructed labor 660.1 ✓5ᵗʰ
- mixed maternal and fetal origin, normally formed fetus 653.4 ✓5ᵗʰ
- pelvis, pelvic (bony) NEC 653.1 ✓5ᵗʰ
  - causing obstructed labor 660.1 ✓5ᵗʰ
- specified type NEC 653.8 ✓5ᵗʰ

Disruption
- cesarean wound 674.1 ✓5ᵗʰ
- family V61.0
- gastrointestinal anastomosis 997.4
- ligament(s) — *see also* Sprain
  - knee
    - current injury — *see* Dislocation knee
    - old 717.89
      - capsular 717.85
      - collateral (medial) 717.82
        - lateral 717.81
      - cruciate (posterior) 717.84
        - anterior 717.83
      - specified site NEC 717.85
- marital V61.10
  - involving divorce or estrangement V61.0
- operation wound ►(external)◄ 998.32 ▲
  - internal 998.31 ●
- organ transplant, anastomosis site — *see* Complications, transplant, organ, by site
- ossicles, ossicular chain 385.23
  - traumatic — *see* Fracture, skull, base
- parenchyma
  - liver (hepatic) — *see* Laceration, liver, major
  - spleen — *see* Laceration, spleen, parenchyma, massive
- phase-shift, of 24-hour sleep-wake cycle 780.55
  - nonorganic origin 307.45
- sleep-wake cycle (24-hour) 780.55
  - circadian rhythm 307.45
  - nonorganic origin 307.45
- suture line (external) 998.32 ▲
  - internal 998.31 ▲
- wound
  - cesarean operation 674.1 ✓5ᵗʰ
  - episiotomy 674.2 ✓5ᵗʰ
  - operation 998.32 ▲
    - cesarean 674.1 ✓5ᵗʰ
    - internal 998.31 ●
  - perineal (obstetric) 674.2 ✓5ᵗʰ
  - uterine 674.1 ✓5ᵗʰ

Disruptio uteri — *see also* Rupture, uterus
- complicating delivery — *see* Delivery, complicated, rupture, uterus

Dissatisfaction with
- employment V62.2
- school environment V62.3

Dissecting — *see* condition

Dissection
- aorta 441.00
  - abdominal 441.02
  - thoracic 441.01
  - thoracoabdominal 441.03
- artery, arterial ●
  - carotid 443.21 ●
  - coronary 414.12 ●
  - iliac 443.22 ●
  - renal 443.23 ●
  - specified NEC 443.29 ●
  - vertebral 443.24 ●
- vascular 459.9
- wound — *see* Wound, open, by site

Disseminated — *see* condition

Dissociated personality NEC 300.15

Dissociation
- auriculoventricular or atrioventricular (any degree) (AV) 426.89
  - with heart block 426.0
- interference 426.89
- isorhythmic 426.89
- rhythm
  - atrioventricular (AV) 426.89
  - interference 426.89

Dissociative
- identity disorder 300.14
- reaction NEC 300.15

Dissolution, vertebra (*see also* Osteoporosis) 733.00

Distention
- abdomen (gaseous) 787.3
- bladder 596.8
- cecum 569.89
- colon 569.89
- gallbladder 575.8
- gaseous (abdomen) 787.3
- intestine 569.89
- kidney 593.89
- liver 573.9
- seminal vesicle 608.89
- stomach 536.8
  - acute 536.1
  - psychogenic 306.4
- ureter 593.5
- uterus 621.8

Distichia, distichiasis (eyelid) 743.63

Distoma hepaticum infestation 121.3

Distomiasis 121.9
- bile passages 121.3
  - due to Clonorchis sinensis 121.1
- hemic 120.9
- hepatic (liver) 121.3
  - due to Clonorchis sinensis (clonorchiasis) 121.1
- intestinal 121.4
- liver 121.3
  - due to Clonorchis sinensis 121.1
- lung 121.2
- pulmonary 121.2

Distomolar (fourth molar) 520.1
- causing crowding 524.3

Disto-occlusion 524.2

Distortion (congenital)
- adrenal (gland) 759.1
- ankle (joint) 755.69
- anus 751.5
- aorta 747.29
- appendix 751.5
- arm 755.59
- artery (peripheral) NEC (*see also* Distortion, peripheral vascular system) 747.60
  - cerebral 747.81
  - coronary 746.85
  - pulmonary 747.3
  - retinal 743.58
  - umbilical 747.5
- auditory canal 744.29
  - causing impairment of hearing 744.02
- bile duct or passage 751.69
- bladder 753.8
- brain 742.4
- bronchus 748.3
- cecum 751.5
- cervix (uteri) 752.49
- chest (wall) 756.3
- clavicle 755.51
- clitoris 752.49
- coccyx 756.19
- colon 751.5
- common duct 751.69
- cornea 743.41
- cricoid cartilage 748.3
- cystic duct 751.69
- duodenum 751.5
- ear 744.29
  - auricle 744.29
    - causing impairment of hearing 744.02
    - causing impairment of hearing 744.09
  - external 744.29
    - causing impairment of hearing 744.02

Distortion — *continued*
- ear — *continued*
  - inner 744.05
  - middle, except ossicles 744.03
    - ossicles 744.04
  - ossicles 744.04
- endocrine (gland) NEC 759.2
- epiglottis 748.3
- Eustachian tube 744.24
- eye 743.8
  - adnexa 743.69
- face bone(s) 756.0
- fallopian tube 752.19
- femur 755.69
- fibula 755.69
- finger(s) 755.59
- foot 755.67
- gallbladder 751.69
- genitalia, genital organ(s)
  - female 752.8
    - external 752.49
    - internal NEC 752.8
  - male 752.8
    - penis 752.69
- glottis 748.3
- gyri 742.4
- hand bone(s) 755.59
- heart (auricle) (ventricle) 746.89
  - valve (cusp) 746.89
- hepatic duct 751.69
- humerus 755.59
- hymen 752.49
- ileum 751.5
- intestine (large) (small) 751.5
  - with anomalous adhesions, fixation or malrotation 751.4
- jaw NEC 524.8
- jejunum 751.5
- kidney 753.3
- knee (joint) 755.64
- labium (majus) (minus) 752.49
- larynx 748.3
- leg 755.69
- lens 743.36
- liver 751.69
- lumbar spine 756.19
  - with disproportion (fetopelvic) 653.0 ✓5ᵗʰ
    - affecting fetus or newborn 763.1
    - causing obstructed labor 660.1 ✓5ᵗʰ
- lumbosacral (joint) (region) 756.19
- lung (fissures) (lobe) 748.69
- nerve 742.8
- nose 748.1
- organ
  - of Corti 744.05
  - or site not listed — *see* Anomaly, specified type NEC
- ossicles, ear 744.04
- ovary 752.0
- oviduct 752.19
- pancreas 751.7
- parathyroid (gland) 759.2
- patella 755.64
- peripheral vascular system NEC 747.60
  - gastrointestinal 747.61
  - lower limb 747.64
  - renal 747.62
  - spinal 747.82
  - upper limb 747.63
- pituitary (gland) 759.2
- radius 755.59
- rectum 751.5
- rib 756.3
- sacroiliac joint 755.69
- sacrum 756.19
- scapula 755.59
- shoulder girdle 755.59
- site not listed — *see* Anomaly, specified type NEC
- skull bone(s) 756.0
  - with
    - anencephalus 740.0
    - encephalocele 742.0
    - hydrocephalus 742.3
      - with spina bifida (*see also* Spina bifida) 741.0 ✓5ᵗʰ
    - microcephalus 742.1

Index to Diseases

Distortion — *continued*
  spinal cord 742.59
  spine 756.19
  spleen 759.0
  sternum 756.3
  thorax (wall) 756.3
  thymus (gland) 759.2
  thyroid (gland) 759.2
    cartilage 748.3
  tibia 755.69
  toe(s) 755.66
  tongue 750.19
  trachea (cartilage) 748.3
  ulna 755.59
  ureter 753.4
    causing obstruction 753.20
  urethra 753.8
    causing obstruction 753.6
  uterus 752.3
  vagina 752.49
  vein (peripheral) NEC (*see also* Distortion, peripheral vascular system) 747.60
    great 747.49
    portal 747.49
    pulmonary 747.49
  vena cava (inferior) (superior) 747.49
  vertebra 756.19
  visual NEC 368.15
    shape or size 368.14
  vulva 752.49
  wrist (bones) (joint) 755.59

Distress
  abdomen 789.0 ✓5ᵗʰ
  colon 789.0 ✓5ᵗʰ
  emotional V40.9
  epigastric 789.0 ✓5ᵗʰ
  fetal (syndrome) 768.4
    affecting management of pregnancy or childbirth 656.8 ✓5ᵗʰ ▲
    liveborn infant 768.4
      first noted
        before onset of labor 768.2
        during labor or delivery 768.3
      stillborn infant (death before onset of labor) 768.0
      death during labor 768.1
  gastrointestinal (functional) 536.9
    psychogenic 306.4
  intestinal (functional) NEC 564.9
    psychogenic 306.4
  intrauterine — *see* Distress, fetal
  leg 729.5
  maternal 669.0 ✓5ᵗʰ
  mental V40.9
  respiratory 786.09
    acute (adult) 518.82
    adult syndrome (following shock, surgery, or trauma) 518.5
      specified NEC 518.82
    fetus or newborn 770.89 ▲
    syndrome (idiopathic) (newborn) 769
  stomach 536.9
    psychogenic 306.4

Distribution vessel, atypical NEC 747.60
  coronary artery 746.85
  spinal 747.82

Districhiasis 704.2

Disturbance — *see also* Disease
  absorption NEC 579.9
    calcium 269.3
    carbohydrate 579.8
    fat 579.8
    protein 579.8
    specified type NEC 579.8
    vitamin (*see also* Deficiency, vitamin) 269.2
  acid-base equilibrium 276.9
  activity and attention, simple, with hyperkinesis 314.01
  amino acid (metabolic) (*see also* Disorder, amino acid) 270.9
    imidazole 270.5
    maple syrup (urine) disease 270.3
    transport 270.0
  assimilation, food 579.9
  attention, simple 314.00
    with hyperactivity 314.01

Disturbance — *see also* Disease — *continued*
  auditory, nerve, except deafness 388.5
  behavior (*see also* Disturbance, conduct) 312.9
  blood clotting (hypoproteinemia) (mechanism) (*see also* Defect, coagulation) 286.9
  central nervous system NEC 349.9
  cerebral nerve NEC 352.9
  circulatory 459.9
  conduct 312.9
    adjustment reaction 309.3
    adolescent onset type 312.82
    childhood onset type 312.81

> Note — Use the following fifth-digit subclassification with categories 312.0–312.2:
>
> 0 unspecified
> 1 mild
> 2 moderate
> 3 severe

    compulsive 312.30
      intermittent explosive disorder 312.34
      isolated explosive disorder 312.35
      kleptomania 312.32
      pathological gambling 312.31
      pyromania 312.33
    hyperkinetic 314.2
    intermittent explosive 312.34
    isolated explosive 312.35
    mixed with emotions 312.4
    socialized (type) 312.20
      aggressive 312.23
      unaggressive 312.21
    specified type NEC 312.89
    undersocialized, unsocialized
      aggressive (type) 312.0 ✓5ᵗʰ
      unaggressive (type) 312.1 ✓5ᵗʰ
  coordination 781.3
  cranial nerve NEC 352.9
  deep sensibility — *see* Disturbance, sensation
  digestive 536.9
    psychogenic 306.4
  electrolyte — *see* Imbalance, electrolyte
  emotions specific to childhood and adolescence 313.9
    with
      academic underachievement 313.83
      anxiety and fearfulness 313.0
      elective mutism 313.23
      identity disorder 313.82
      jealousy 313.3
      misery and unhappiness 313.1
      oppositional disorder 313.81
      overanxiousness 313.0
      sensitivity 313.21
      shyness 313.21
      social withdrawal 313.22
      withdrawal reaction 313.22
    involving relationship problems 313.3
    mixed 313.89
    specified type NEC 313.89
  endocrine (gland) 259.9
    neonatal, transitory 775.9
      specified NEC 775.8
  equilibrium 780.4
  feeding (elderly) (infant) 783.3
    newborn 779.3
    nonorganic origin NEC 307.59
    psychogenic NEC 307.59
  fructose metabolism 271.2
  gait 781.2
    hysterical 300.11
  gastric (functional) 536.9
    motility 536.8
    psychogenic 306.4
    secretion 536.8
  gastrointestinal (functional) 536.9
    psychogenic 306.4
  habit, child 307.9
  hearing, except deafness 388.40
  heart, functional (conditions classifiable to 426, 427, 428)
    due to presence of (cardiac) prosthesis 429.4
    postoperative (immediate) 997.1
      long-term effect of cardiac surgery 429.4

Disturbance — *see also* Disease — *continued*
  heart, functional — *continued*
    psychogenic 306.2
  hormone 259.9
  innervation uterus, sympathetic, parasympathetic 621.8
  keratinization NEC
    gingiva 523.1
    lip 528.5
    oral (mucosa) (soft tissue) 528.7
    tongue 528.7
  labyrinth, labyrinthine (vestibule) 386.9
  learning, specific NEC 315.2
  memory (*see also* Amnesia) 780.99 ▲
    mild, following organic brain damage 310.1
  mental (*see also* Disorder, mental) 300.9
    associated with diseases classified elsewhere 316
  metabolism (acquired) (congenital) (*see also* Disorder, metabolism) 277.9
    with
      abortion — *see* Abortion, by type, with metabolic disorder
      ectopic pregnancy (*see also* categories 633.0-633.9) 639.4
      molar pregnancy (*see also* categories 630-632) 639.4
    amino acid (*see also* Disorder, amino acid) 270.9
      aromatic NEC 270.2
      branched-chain 270.3
      specified type NEC 270.8
      straight-chain NEC 270.7
      sulfur-bearing 270.4
      transport 270.0
    ammonia 270.6
    arginine 270.6
    argininosuccinic acid 270.6
    carbohydrate NEC 271.9
    cholesterol 272.9
    citrulline 270.6
    cystathionine 270.4
    fat 272.9
    following
      abortion 639.4
      ectopic or molar pregnancy 639.4
    general 277.9
      carbohydrate 271.9
      iron 275.0
      phosphate 275.3
      sodium 276.9
    glutamine 270.7
    glycine 270.7
    histidine 270.5
    homocystine 270.4
    in labor or delivery 669.0 ✓5ᵗʰ
    iron 275.0
    isoleucine 270.3
    leucine 270.3
    lipoid 272.9
      specified type NEC 272.8
    lysine 270.7
    methionine 270.4
    neonatal, transitory 775.9
      specified type NEC 775.8
    nitrogen 788.9
    ornithine 270.6
    phosphate 275.3
    phosphatides 272.7
    serine 270.7
    sodium NEC 276.9
    threonine 270.7
    tryptophan 270.2
    tyrosine 270.2
    urea cycle 270.6
    valine 270.3
  motor 796.1
  nervous functional 799.2
  neuromuscular mechanism (eye) due to syphilis 094.84
  nutritional 269.9
    nail 703.8
  ocular motion 378.87
    psychogenic 306.7
  oculogyric 378.87
    psychogenic 306.7

Disturbance

Disturbance — see also Disease — continued
  oculomotor NEC 378.87
    psychogenic 306.7
  olfactory nerve 781.1
  optic nerve NEC 377.49
  oral epithelium, including tongue 528.7
  personality (pattern) (trait) (see also Disorder, personality) 301.9
    following organic brain damage 310.1
  polyglandular 258.9
  psychomotor 307.9
  pupillary 379.49
  reflex 796.1
  rhythm, heart 427.9
    postoperative (immediate) 997.1
      long-term effect of cardiac surgery 429.4
    psychogenic 306.2
  salivary secretion 527.7
  sensation (cold) (heat) (localization) (tactile discrimination localization) (texture) (vibratory) NEC 782.0
    hysterical 300.11
    skin 782.0
    smell 781.1
    taste 781.1
  sensory (see also Disturbance, sensation) 782.0
    innervation 782.0
  situational (transient) (see also Reaction, adjustment) 309.9
    acute 308.3
  sleep 780.50
    with apnea — see Apnea, sleep
    initiation or maintenance (see also Insomnia) 780.52
      nonorganic origin 307.41
    nonorganic origin 307.40
      specified type NEC 307.49
    specified NEC 780.59
      nonorganic origin 307.49
    wakefulness (see also Hypersomnia) 780.54
      nonorganic origin 307.43
  sociopathic 301.7
  speech NEC 784.5
    developmental 315.39
      associated with hyperkinesis 314.1
    secondary to organic lesion 784.5
  stomach (functional) (see also Disturbance, gastric) 536.9
  sympathetic (nerve) (see also Neuropathy, peripheral, autonomic) 337.9
  temperature sense 782.0
    hysterical 300.11
  tooth
    eruption 520.6
    formation 520.4
    structure, hereditary NEC 520.5
  touch (see also Disturbance, sensation) 782.0
  vascular 459.9
    arteriosclerotic — see Arteriosclerosis
  vasomotor 443.9
  vasospastic 443.9
  vestibular labyrinth 386.9
  vision, visual NEC 368.9
    psychophysical 368.16
    specified NEC 368.8
    subjective 368.10
  voice 784.40
  wakefulness (initiation or maintenance) (see also Hypersomnia) 780.54
    nonorganic origin 307.43

Disulfiduria, beta-mercaptolactate-cysteine 270.0

Disuse atrophy, bone 733.7

Ditthomska syndrome 307.81

Diuresis 788.42

Divers'
  palsy or paralysis 993.3
  squeeze 993.3

Diverticula, diverticulosis, diverticulum (acute) (multiple) (perforated) (ruptured) 562.10
  with diverticulitis 562.11
  aorta (Kommerell's) 747.21
  appendix (noninflammatory) 543.9
  bladder (acquired) (sphincter) 596.3
    congenital 753.8
  broad ligament 620.8

Diverticula, diverticulosis, diverticulum — continued
  bronchus (congenital) 748.3
    acquired 494.0
      with acute exacerbation 494.1
  calyx, calyceal (kidney) 593.89
  cardia (stomach) 537.1
  cecum 562.10
    with
      diverticulitis 562.11
        with hemorrhage 562.13
      hemorrhage 562.12
    congenital 751.5
  colon (acquired) 562.10
    with
      diverticulitis 562.11
        with hemorrhage 562.13
      hemorrhage 562.12
    congenital 751.5
  duodenum 562.00
    with
      diverticulitis 562.01
        with hemorrhage 562.03
      hemorrhage 562.02
    congenital 751.5
  epiphrenic (esophagus) 530.6
  esophagus (congenital) 750.4
    acquired 530.6
    epiphrenic 530.6
    pulsion 530.6
    traction 530.6
    Zenker's 530.6
  Eustachian tube 381.89
  fallopian tube 620.8
  gallbladder (congenital) 751.69
  gastric 537.1
  heart (congenital) 746.89
  ileum 562.00
    with
      diverticulitis 562.01
        with hemorrhage 562.03
      hemorrhage 562.02
  intestine (large) 562.10
    with
      diverticulitis 562.11
        with hemorrhage 562.13
      hemorrhage 562.12
    congenital 751.5
    small 562.00
      with
        diverticulitis 562.01
          with hemorrhage 562.03
        hemorrhage 562.02
      congenital 751.5
  jejunum 562.00
    with
      diverticulitis 562.01
        with hemorrhage 562.03
      hemorrhage 562.02
  kidney (calyx) (pelvis) 593.89
    with calculus 592.0
  Kommerell's 747.21
  laryngeal ventricle (congenital) 748.3
  Meckel's (displaced) (hypertrophic) 751.0
  midthoracic 530.6
  organ or site, congenital NEC — see Distortion
  pericardium (congenital) (cyst) 746.89
    acquired (true) 423.8
  pharyngoesophageal (pulsion) 530.6
  pharynx (congenital) 750.27
  pulsion (esophagus) 530.6
  rectosigmoid 562.10
    with
      diverticulitis 562.11
        with hemorrhage 562.13
      hemorrhage 562.12
    congenital 751.5
  rectum 562.10
    with
      diverticulitis 562.11
        with hemorrhage 562.13
      hemorrhage 562.12
  renal (calyces) (pelvis) 593.89
    with calculus 592.0
  Rokitansky's 530.6
  seminal vesicle 608.0

Diverticula, diverticulosis, diverticulum — continued
  sigmoid 562.10
    with
      diverticulitis 562.11
        with hemorrhage 562.13
      hemorrhage 562.12
    congenital 751.5
  small intestine 562.00
    with
      diverticulitis 562.01
        with hemorrhage 562.03
      hemorrhage 562.02
  stomach (cardia) (juxtacardia) (juxtapyloric) (acquired) 537.1
    congenital 750.7
  subdiaphragmatic 530.6
  trachea (congenital) 748.3
    acquired 519.1
  traction (esophagus) 530.6
  ureter (acquired) 593.89
    congenital 753.4
  ureterovesical orifice 593.89
  urethra (acquired) 599.2
    congenital 753.8
  ventricle, left (congenital) 746.89
  vesical (urinary) 596.3
    congenital 753.8
  Zenker's (esophagus) 530.6

Diverticulitis (acute) (see also Diverticula) 562.11
  with hemorrhage 562.13
  bladder (urinary) 596.3
  cecum (perforated) 562.11
    with hemorrhage 562.13
  colon (perforated) 562.11
    with hemorrhage 562.13
  duodenum 562.01
    with hemorrhage 562.03
  esophagus 530.6
  ileum (perforated) 562.01
    with hemorrhage 562.03
  intestine (large) (perforated) 562.11
    with hemorrhage 562.13
    small 562.01
      with hemorrhage 562.03
  jejunum (perforated) 562.01
    with hemorrhage 562.03
  Meckel's (perforated) 751.0
  pharyngoesophageal 530.6
  rectosigmoid (perforated) 562.11
    with hemorrhage 562.13
  rectum 562.11
    with hemorrhage 562.13
  sigmoid (old) (perforated) 562.11
    with hemorrhage 562.13
  small intestine (perforated) 562.01
    with hemorrhage 562.03
  vesical (urinary) 596.3

Diverticulosis — see Diverticula

Division
  cervix uteri 622.8
    external os into two openings by frenum 752.49
  external (cervical) into two openings by frenum 752.49
  glans penis 752.69
  hymen 752.49
  labia minora (congenital) 752.49
  ligament (partial or complete) (current) — see also Sprain, by site
    with open wound — see Wound, open, by site
  muscle (partial or complete) (current) — see also Sprain, by site
    with open wound — see Wound, open, by site
  nerve — see Injury, nerve, by site
  penis glans 752.69
  spinal cord — see Injury, spinal, by site
  vein 459.9
    traumatic — see Injury, vascular, by site

Divorce V61.0

Dix-Hallpike neurolabyrinthitis 386.12

Dizziness 780.4
  hysterical 300.11
  psychogenic 306.9

Index to Diseases

Doan-Wiseman syndrome (primary splenic neutropenia) 288.0
Dog bite — see Wound, open, by site
Döhle-Heller aortitis 093.1
Döhle body-panmyelopathic syndrome 288.2
Dolichocephaly, dolichocephalus 754.0
Dolichocolon 751.5
Dolichostenomelia 759.82
Donohue's syndrome (leprechaunism) 259.8
Donor
    blood V59.01
        other blood components V59.09
        stem cells V59.02
        whole blood V59.01
    bone V59.2
        marrow V59.3
    cornea V59.5
    heart V59.8
    kidney V59.4
    liver V59.6
    lung V59.8
    lymphocyte V59.8
    organ V59.9
        specified NEC V59.8
    potential, examination of V70.8
    skin V59.1
    specified organ or tissue NEC V59.8
    stem cells V59.02
    tissue V59.9
        specified type NEC V59.8
Donovanosis (granuloma venereum) 099.2
DOPS (diffuse obstructive pulmonary syndrome) 496
Double
    albumin 273.8
    aortic arch 747.21
    auditory canal 744.29
    auricle (heart) 746.82
    bladder 753.8
    external (cervical) os 752.49
    kidney with double pelvis (renal) 753.3
    larynx 748.3
    meatus urinarius 753.8
    organ or site NEC — see Accessory
    orifice
        heart valve NEC 746.89
            pulmonary 746.09
    outlet, right ventricle 745.11
    pelvis (renal) with double ureter 753.4
    penis 752.69
    tongue 750.13
    ureter (one or both sides) 753.4
        with double pelvis (renal) 753.4
    urethra 753.8
    urinary meatus 753.8
    uterus (any degree) 752.2
        with doubling of cervix and vagina 752.2
            in pregnancy or childbirth 654.0
                affecting fetus or newborn 763.89
    vagina 752.49
        with doubling of cervix and uterus 752.2
    vision 368.2
    vocal cords 748.3
    vulva 752.49
    whammy (syndrome) 360.81
Douglas' pouch, cul-de-sac — see condition
Down's disease or syndrome (mongolism) 758.0
Down-growth, epithelial (anterior chamber) 364.61
Dracontiasis 125.7
Dracunculiasis 125.7
Dracunculosis 125.7
Drainage
    abscess (spontaneous) — see Abscess
    anomalous pulmonary veins to hepatic veins or right atrium 747.41
    stump (amputation) (surgical) 997.62
    suprapubic, bladder 596.8
Dream state, hysterical 300.13
Drepanocytic anemia (see also Disease, sickle cell) 282.60
Dresbach's syndrome (elliptocytosis) 282.1

Dreschlera (infection) 118
    hawaiiensis 117.8
Dressler's syndrome (postmyocardial infarction) 411.0
Dribbling (post-void) 788.35
Drift, ulnar 736.09
Drinking (alcohol) — see also Alcoholism
    excessive, to excess NEC (see also Abuse, drugs, nondependent) 305.0
        bouts, periodic 305.0
        continual 303.9
        episodic 305.0
        habitual 303.9
        periodic 305.0
Drip, postnasal (chronic) — see Sinusitis
Drivers' license examination V70.3
Droop
    Cooper's 611.8
    facial 781.99
Drop
    finger 736.29
    foot 736.79
    hematocrit (precipitous) 790.01
    toe 735.8
    wrist 736.05
Dropped
    dead 798.1
    heart beats 426.6
Dropsy, dropsical (see also Edema) 782.3
    abdomen 789.5
    amnion (see also Hydramnios) 657
    brain — see Hydrocephalus
    cardiac (see also Failure, heart) 428.0
    cardiorenal (see also Hypertension, cardiorenal) 404.90
    chest 511.9
    fetus or newborn 778.0
        due to isoimmunization 773.3
    gangrenous (see also Gangrene) 785.4
    heart (see also Failure, heart) 428.0
    hepatic — see Cirrhosis, liver
    infantile — see Hydrops, fetalis
    kidney (see also Nephrosis) 581.9
    liver — see Cirrhosis, liver
    lung 514
    malarial (see also Malaria) 084.9
    neonatorum — see Hydrops, fetalis
    nephritic 581.9
    newborn — see Hydrops, fetalis
    nutritional 269.9
    ovary 620.8
    pericardium (see also Pericarditis) 423.9
    renal (see also Nephrosis) 581.9
    uremic — see Uremia
Drowned, drowning 994.1
    lung 518.5
Drowsiness 780.09
Drug — see also condition
    addiction (see also listing under Dependence) 304.9
    adverse effect NEC, correct substance properly administered 995.2
    dependence (see also listing under Dependence) 304.9
    habit (see also listing under Dependence) 304.9
    overdose — see Table of Drugs and Chemicals
    poisoning — see Table of Drugs and Chemicals
    therapy (maintenance) status NEC V58.1
        anticoagulant V58.61
        long-term (current) use V58.69
            antibiotics V58.62
    wrong substance given or taken in error — see Table of Drugs and Chemicals
Drunkenness (see also Abuse, drugs, nondependent) 305.0
    acute in alcoholism (see also Alcoholism) 303.0
    chronic (see also Alcoholism) 303.9
    pathologic 291.4
    simple (acute) 305.0
        in alcoholism 303.0
    sleep 307.47

Drusen
    optic disc or papilla 377.21
    retina (colloid) (hyaloid degeneration) 362.57
        hereditary 362.77
Drusenfieber 075
Dry, dryness — see also condition
    eye 375.15
        syndrome 375.15
    larynx 478.79
    mouth 527.7
    nose 478.1
    skin syndrome 701.1
    socket (teeth) 526.5
    throat 478.29
DSAP (disseminated superficial actinic porokeratosis) 692.75
Duane's retraction syndrome 378.71
Duane-Stilling-Türk syndrome (ocular retraction syndrome) 378.71
Dubin-Johnson disease or syndrome 277.4
Dubini's disease (electric chorea) 049.8
Dubois' abscess or disease 090.5
Duchenne's
    disease 094.0
        locomotor ataxia 094.0
        muscular dystrophy 359.1
        pseudohypertrophy, muscles 359.1
    paralysis 335.22
    syndrome 335.22
Duchenne-Aran myelopathic, muscular atrophy (nonprogressive) (progressive) 335.21
Duchenne-Griesinger disease 359.1
Ducrey's
    bacillus 099.0
    chancre 099.0
    disease (chancroid) 099.0
Duct, ductus — see condition
Duengero 061
Duhring's disease (dermatitis herpetiformis) 694.0
Dukes (-Filatov) disease 057.8
Dullness
    cardiac (decreased) (increased) 785.3
Dumb ague (see also Malaria) 084.6
Dumbness (see also Aphasia) 784.3
Dumdum fever 085.0
Dumping syndrome (postgastrectomy) 564.2
    nonsurgical 536.8
Duodenitis (nonspecific) (peptic) 535.60
    with hemorrhage 535.61
    due to
        Strongyloides stercoralis 127.2
Duodenocholangitis 575.8
Duodenum, duodenal — see condition
Duplay's disease, periarthritis, or syndrome 726.2
Duplex — see also Accessory
    kidney 753.3
    placenta — see Placenta, abnormal
    uterus 752.2
Duplication — see also Accessory
    anus 751.5
    aortic arch 747.21
    appendix 751.5
    biliary duct (any) 751.69
    bladder 753.8
    cecum 751.5
        and appendix 751.5
    clitoris 752.49
    cystic duct 751.69
    digestive organs 751.8
    duodenum 751.5
    esophagus 750.4
    fallopian tube 752.19
    frontonasal process 756.0
    gallbladder 751.69
    ileum 751.5
    intestine (large) (small) 751.5
    jejunum 751.5
    kidney 753.3
    liver 751.69
    nose 748.1

Duplication — *see also* Accessory — *continued*
  pancreas 751.7
  penis 752.69
  respiratory organs NEC 748.9
  salivary duct 750.22
  spinal cord (incomplete) 742.51
  stomach 750.7
  ureter 753.4
  vagina 752.49
  vas deferens 752.8
  vocal cords 748.3
Dupré's disease or syndrome (meningism) 781.6
Dupuytren's
  contraction 728.6
  disease (muscle contracture) 728.6
  fracture (closed) 824.4
    ankle (closed) 824.4
      open 824.5
    fibula (closed) 824.4
      open 824.5
    open 824.5
    radius (closed) 813.42
      open 813.52
  muscle contracture 728.6
Durand-Nicolas-Favre disease (climatic bubo) 099.1
Duroziez's disease (congenital mitral stenosis) 746.5
Dust
  conjunctivitis 372.05
  reticulation (occupational) 504
Dutton's
  disease (trypanosomiasis) 086.9
  relapsing fever (West African) 087.1
Dwarf, dwarfism 259.4
  with infantilism (hypophyseal) 253.3
  achondroplastic 756.4
  Amsterdam 759.89
  bird-headed 759.89
  congenital 259.4
  constitutional 259.4
  hypophyseal 253.3
  infantile 259.4
  Levi type 253.3
  Lorain-Levi (pituitary) 253.3
  Lorain type (pituitary) 253.3
  metatropic 756.4
  nephrotic-glycosuric, with hypophosphatemic rickets 270.0
  nutritional 263.2
  ovarian 758.6
  pancreatic 577.8
  pituitary 253.3
  polydystrophic 277.5
  primordial 253.3
  psychosocial 259.4
  renal 588.0
    with hypertension — *see* Hypertension, kidney
  Russell's (uterine dwarfism and craniofacial dysostosis) 759.89
Dyke-Young anemia or syndrome (acquired macrocytic hemolytic anemia) (secondary) (symptomatic) 283.9
Dynia abnormality (*see also* Defect, coagulation) 286.9
Dysacousis 388.40
Dysadrenocortism 255.9
  hyperfunction 255.3
  hypofunction 255.4
Dysarthria 784.5
Dysautonomia (*see also* Neuropathy, peripheral, autonomic) 337.9
  familial 742.8
Dysbarism 993.3
Dysbasia 719.7
  angiosclerotica intermittens 443.9
    due to atherosclerosis 440.21
  hysterical 300.11
  lordotica (progressiva) 333.6
  nonorganic origin 307.9
  psychogenic 307.9
Dysbetalipoproteinemia (familial) 272.2
Dyscalculia 315.1

Dyschezia (*see also* Constipation) 564.00
Dyschondroplasia (with hemangiomata) 756.4
  Voorhoeve's 756.4
Dyschondrosteosis 756.59
Dyschromia 709.00
Dyscollagenosis 710.9
Dyscoria 743.41
Dyscraniopyophalangy 759.89
Dyscrasia
  blood 289.9
    with antepartum hemorrhage 641.3
    fetus or newborn NEC 776.9
    hemorrhage, subungual 287.8
    puerperal, postpartum 666.3
  ovary 256.8
  plasma cell 273.9
  pluriglandular 258.9
  polyglandular 258.9
Dysdiadochokinesia 781.3
Dysectasia, vesical neck 596.8
Dysendocrinism 259.9
Dysentery, dysenteric (bilious) (catarrhal) (diarrhea) (epidemic) (gangrenous) (hemorrhagic) (infectious) (sporadic) (tropical) (ulcerative) 009.0
  abscess, liver (*see also* Abscess, amebic) 006.3
  amebic (*see also* Amebiasis) 006.9
    with abscess — *see* Abscess, amebic
    acute 006.0
    carrier (suspected) of V02.2
    chronic 006.1
  arthritis (*see also* Arthritis, due to, dysentery) 009.0 [711.3]
    bacillary 004.9 [711.3]
  asylum 004.9
  bacillary 004.9
    arthritis 004.9 [711.3]
    Boyd 004.2
    Flexner 004.1
    Schmitz (-Stutzer) 004.0
    Shiga 004.0
    Shigella 004.9
      group A 004.0
      group B 004.1
      group C 004.2
      group D 004.3
      specified type NEC 004.8
    Sonne 004.3
    specified type NEC 004.8
  bacterium 004.9
  balantidial 007.0
  Balantidium coli 007.0
  Boyd's 004.2
  Chilomastix 007.8
  Chinese 004.9
  choleriform 001.1
  coccidial 007.2
  Dientamoeba fragilis 007.8
  due to specified organism NEC — *see* Enteritis, due to, by organism
  Embadomonas 007.8
  Endolimax nana — *see* Dysentery, amebic
  Entamoba, entamebic — *see* Dysentery, amebic
  Flexner's 004.1
  Flexner-Boyd 004.2
  giardial 007.1
  Giardia lamblia 007.1
  Hiss-Russell 004.1
  lamblia 007.1
  leishmanial 085.0
  malarial (*see also* Malaria) 084.6
  metazoal 127.9
  Monilia 112.89
  protozoal NEC 007.9
  Russell's 004.8
  salmonella 003.0
  schistosomal 120.1
  Schmitz (-Stutzer) 004.0
  Shiga 004.0
  Shigella NEC (*see also* Dysentery, bacillary) 004.9
    boydii 004.2
    dysenteriae 004.0
      Schmitz 004.0
      Shiga 004.0

Dysentery, dysenteric — *continued*
  Shigella NEC (*see also* Dysentery, bacillary) — *continued*
    flexneri 004.1
    Group A 004.0
    Group B 004.1
    Group C 004.2
    Group D 004.3
    Schmitz 004.0
    Shiga 004.0
    Sonnei 004.3
  Sonne 004.3
  strongyloidiasis 127.2
  trichomonal 007.3
  tuberculous (*see also* Tuberculosis) 014.8
  viral (*see also* Enteritis, viral) 008.8
Dysequilibrium 780.4
Dysesthesia 782.0
  hysterical 300.11
Dysfibrinogenemia (congenital) (*see also* Defect, coagulation) 286.3
Dysfunction
  adrenal (cortical) 255.9
    hyperfunction 255.3
    hypofunction 255.4
  associated with sleep stages or arousal from sleep 780.56
    nonorganic origin 307.47
  bladder NEC 596.59
  bleeding, uterus 626.8
  brain, minimal (*see also* Hyperkinesia) 314.9
  cerebral 348.3
  colon 564.9
    psychogenic 306.4
  colostomy or enterostomy 569.62
  cystic duct 575.8
  diastolic 429.9
    with heart failure — *see* Failure, heart
    due to
      cardiomyopathy — *see* Cardiomyopathy
      hypertension — *see* Hypertension, heart
  endocrine NEC 259.9
  endometrium 621.8
  enteric stoma 569.62
  enterostomy 569.62
  Eustachian tube 381.81
  gallbladder 575.8
  gastrointestinal 536.9
  gland, glandular NEC 259.9
  heart 427.9
    postoperative (immediate) 997.1
      long-term effect of cardiac surgery 429.4
  hemoglobin 288.8
  hepatic 573.9
  hepatocellular NEC 573.9
  hypophysis 253.9
    hyperfunction 253.1
    hypofunction 253.2
    posterior lobe 253.6
      hypofunction 253.5
  kidney (*see also* Disease, renal) 593.9
  labyrinthine 386.50
    specified NEC 386.58
  liver 573.9
    constitutional 277.4
  minimal brain (child) (*see also* Hyperkinesia) 314.9
  ovary, ovarian 256.9
    hyperfunction 256.1
      estrogen 256.0
    hypofunction 256.39
      postablative 256.2
    postablative 256.2
    specified NEC 256.8
  papillary muscle 429.81
    with myocardial infarction 410.8
  parathyroid 252.8
    hyperfunction 252.0
    hypofunction 252.1
  pineal gland 259.8
  pituitary (gland) 253.9
    hyperfunction 253.1
    hypofunction 253.2
    posterior 253.6
      hypofunction 253.5
  placental — *see* Placenta, insufficiency
  platelets (blood) 287.1

Index to Diseases

Dysfunction — *continued*
  polyglandular 258.9
    specified NEC 258.8
  psychosexual 302.70
    with
      dyspareunia (functional) (psychogenic) 302.76
      frigidity 302.72
      impotence 302.72
      inhibition
        orgasm
          female 302.73
          male 302.74
        sexual
          desire 302.71
          excitement 302.72
      premature ejaculation 302.75
      sexual aversion 302.79
      specified disorder NEC 302.79
      vaginismus 306.51
  pylorus 537.9
  rectum 564.9
    psychogenic 306.4
  segmental (*see also* Dysfunction, somatic) 739.9
  senile 797
  sinoatrial node 427.81
  somatic 739.9
    abdomen 739.9
    acromioclavicular 739.7
    cervical 739.1
    cervicothoracic 739.1
    costochondral 739.8
    costovertebral 739.8
    extremities
      lower 739.6
      upper 739.7
    head 739.0
    hip 739.5
    lumbar, lumbosacral 739.3
    occipitocervical 739.0
    pelvic 739.5
    pubic 739.5
    rib cage 739.8
    sacral 739.4
    sacrococcygeal 739.4
    sacroiliac 739.4
    specified site NEC 739.9
    sternochondral 739.8
    sternoclavicular 739.7
    temporomandibular 739.0
    thoracic, thoracolumbar 739.2
  stomach 536.9
    psychogenic 306.4
  suprarenal 255.9
    hyperfunction 255.3
    hypofunction 255.4
  symbolic NEC 784.60
    specified type NEC 784.69
  temporomandibular (joint) (joint-pain-syndrome) NEC 524.60
    specified NEC 524.69
  testicular 257.9
    hyperfunction 257.0
    hypofunction 257.2
    specified type NEC 257.8
  thymus 254.9
  thyroid 246.9
    complicating pregnancy, childbirth or puerperium 648.1 ✓5ᵗʰ
    hyperfunction — *see* Hyperthyroidism
    hypofunction — *see* Hypothyroidism
  uterus, complicating delivery 661.9 ✓5ᵗʰ
    affecting fetus or newborn 763.7
    hypertonic 661.4 ✓5ᵗʰ
    hypotonic 661.2 ✓5ᵗʰ
      primary 661.0 ✓5ᵗʰ
      secondary 661.1 ✓5ᵗʰ
  velopharyngeal (acquired) 528.9
    congenital 750.29
  ventricular 429.9
    with congestive heart failure (*see also* Failure, heart) 428.0
    due to
      cardiomyopathy — *see* Cardiomyopathy
      hypertension — *see* Hypertension, heart
  vesicourethral NEC 596.59

Dysfunction — *continued*
  vestibular 386.50
    specified type NEC 386.58
Dysgammaglobulinemia 279.06
Dysgenesis
  gonadal (due to chromosomal anomaly) 758.6
    pure 752.7
  kidney(s) 753.0
  ovarian 758.6
  renal 753.0
  reticular 279.2
  seminiferous tubules 758.6
  tidal platelet 287.3
Dysgerminoma (M9060/3)
  specified site — *see* Neoplasm, by site, malignant
  unspecified site
    female 183.0
    male 186.9
Dysgeusia 781.1
Dysgraphia 781.3
Dyshidrosis 705.81
Dysidrosis 705.81
Dysinsulinism 251.8
Dyskaryotic cervical smear 795.09 ▲
Dyskeratosis (*see also* Keratosis) 701.1
  bullosa hereditaria 757.39
  cervix 622.1
  congenital 757.39
  follicularis 757.39
    vitamin A deficiency 264.8
  gingiva 523.8
  oral soft tissue NEC 528.7
  tongue 528.7
  uterus NEC 621.8
Dyskinesia 781.3
  biliary 575.8
  esophagus 530.5
  hysterical 300.11
  intestinal 564.89
  nonorganic origin 307.9
  orofacial 333.82
  psychogenic 307.9
  tardive (oral) 333.82
Dyslalia 784.5
  developmental 315.39
Dyslexia 784.61
  developmental 315.02
  secondary to organic lesion 784.61
Dysmaturity (*see also* Immaturity) 765.1 ✓5ᵗʰ
  lung 770.4
  pulmonary 770.4
Dysmenorrhea (essential) (exfoliative) (functional) (intrinsic) (membranous) (primary) (secondary) 625.3
  psychogenic 306.52
Dysmetabolic syndrome X 277.7
Dysmetria 781.3
Dysmorodystrophia mesodermalis congenita 759.82
Dysnomia 784.3
Dysorexia 783.0
  hysterical 300.11
Dysostosis
  cleidocranial, cleidocranialis 755.59
  craniofacial 756.0
  Fairbank's (idiopathic familial generalized osteophytosis) 756.50
  mandibularis 756.0
  mandibulofacial, incomplete 756.0
  multiplex 277.5
  orodigitofacial 759.89
Dyspareunia (female) 625.0
  male 608.89
  psychogenic 302.76
Dyspepsia (allergic) (congenital) (fermentative) (flatulent) (functional) (gastric) (gastrointestinal) (neurogenic) (occupational) (reflex) 536.8
  acid 536.8
  atonic 536.3
    psychogenic 306.4

Dyspepsia — *continued*
  diarrhea 787.91
    psychogenic 306.4
  intestinal 564.89
    psychogenic 306.4
  nervous 306.4
  neurotic 306.4
  psychogenic 306.4
Dysphagia 787.2
  functional 300.11
  hysterical 300.11
  nervous 300.11
  psychogenic 306.4
  sideropenic 280.8
  spastica 530.5
Dysphagocytosis, congenital 288.1
Dysphasia 784.5
Dysphonia 784.49
  clericorum 784.49
  functional 300.11
  hysterical 300.11
  psychogenic 306.1
  spastica 478.79
Dyspigmentation — *see also* Pigmentation
  eyelid (acquired) 374.52
Dyspituitarism 253.9
  hyperfunction 253.1
  hypofunction 253.2
  posterior lobe 253.6
Dysplasia — *see also* Anomaly
  artery
    fibromuscular NEC 447.8
      carotid 447.8
      renal 447.3
  bladder 596.8
  bone (fibrous) NEC 733.29
    diaphyseal, progressive 756.59
    jaw 526.89
    monostotic 733.29
    polyostotic 756.54
    solitary 733.29
  brain 742.9
  bronchopulmonary, fetus or newborn 770.7
  cervix (uteri) 622.1
    cervical intraepithelial neoplasia I [CIN I] 622.1
    cervical intraepithelial neoplasia II [CIN II] 622.1
    cervical intraepithelial neoplasia III [CIN III] 233.1
    CIN I 622.1
    CIN II 622.1
    CIN III 233.1
  chondroectodermal 756.55
  chondromatose 756.4
  craniocarpotarsal 759.89
  craniometaphyseal 756.89
  dentinal 520.5
  diaphyseal, progressive 756.59
  ectodermal (anhidrotic) (Bason) (Clouston's) (congenital) (Feinmesser) (hereditary) (hidrotic) (Marshall) (Robinson's) 757.31
  epiphysealis 756.9
    multiplex 756.56
    punctata 756.59
  epiphysis 756.9
    multiple 756.56
  epithelial
    epiglottis 478.79
    uterine cervix 622.1
  erythroid NEC 289.8
  eye (*see also* Microphthalmos) 743.10
  familial metaphyseal 756.89
  fibromuscular, artery NEC 447.8
    carotid 447.8
    renal 447.3
  fibrous
    bone NEC 733.29
    diaphyseal, progressive 756.59
    jaw 526.89
    monostotic 733.29
    polyostotic 756.54
    solitary 733.29
  high grade squamous intraepithelial (HGSIL) 622.1 ●
                                                     ●

Dysplasia

Dysplasia — see also Anomaly — continued
- hip (congenital) 755.63
  - with dislocation (see also Dislocation, hip, congenital) 754.30
- hypohidrotic ectodermal 757.31
- joint 755.8
- kidney 753.15
- leg 755.69
- linguofacialis 759.89
- low grade squamous intraepithelial (LGSIL) 622.1 ●
- lung 748.5
- macular 743.55
- mammary (benign) (gland) 610.9
  - cystic 610.1
  - specified type NEC 610.8
- metaphyseal 756.9
  - familial 756.89
- monostotic fibrous 733.29
- muscle 756.89
- myeloid NEC 289.8
- nervous system (general) 742.9
- neuroectodermal 759.6
- oculoauriculovertebral 756.0
- oculodentodigital 759.89
- olfactogenital 253.4
- osteo-onycho-arthro (hereditary) 756.89
- periosteum 733.99
- polyostotic fibrous 756.54
- progressive diaphyseal 756.59
- prostate 602.3
  - intraepithelial neoplasia I [PIN I] 602.3
  - intraepithelial neoplasia II [PIN II] 602.3
  - intraepithelial neoplasia III [PIN III] 233.4
- renal 753.15
- renofacialis 753.0
- retinal NEC 743.56
- retrolental 362.21
- spinal cord 742.9
- thymic, with immunodeficiency 279.2
- vagina 623.0
- vocal cord 478.5
- vulva 624.8
  - intraepithelial neoplasia I [VIN I] 624.8
  - intraepithelial neoplasia II [VIN II] 624.8
  - intraepithelial neoplasia III [VIN III] 233.3
  - VIN I 624.8
  - VIN II 624.8
  - VIN III 233.3

Dyspnea (nocturnal) (paroxysmal) 786.09
- asthmatic (bronchial) (see also Asthma) 493.9 ✓5ᵗʰ
  - with bronchitis (see also Asthma) 493.9 ✓5ᵗʰ
    - chronic 493.2 ✓5ᵗʰ ▲
  - cardiac (see also Failure, ventricular, left) 428.1
- cardiac (see also Failure, ventricular, left) 428.1
- functional 300.11
- hyperventilation 786.01
- hysterical 300.11
- Monday morning 504
- newborn 770.89 ▲
- psychogenic 306.1
- uremic — see Uremia

Dyspraxia 781.3
- syndrome 315.4

Dysproteinemia 273.8
- transient with copper deficiency 281.4

Dysprothrombinemia (constitutional) (see also Defect, coagulation) 286.3

Dysreflexia, autonomic 337.3

Dysrhythmia
- cardiac 427.9
  - postoperative (immediate) 997.1
    - long-term effect of cardiac surgery 429.4
  - specified type NEC 427.89
- cerebral or cortical 348.3

Dyssecretosis, mucoserous 710.2

Dyssocial reaction, without manifest psychiatric disorder
- adolescent V71.02
- adult V71.01
- child V71.02

Dyssomnia NEC 780.56
- nonorganic origin 307.47

Dyssplenism 289.4

Dyssynergia
- biliary (see also Disease, biliary) 576.8
- cerebellaris myoclonica 334.2
- detrusor sphincter (bladder) 596.55
- ventricular 429.89

Dystasia, hereditary areflexic 334.3

Dysthymia 300.4

Dysthymic disorder 300.4

Dysthyroidism 246.9

Dystocia 660.9 ✓5ᵗʰ
- affecting fetus or newborn 763.1
- cervical 661.0 ✓5ᵗʰ
  - affecting fetus or newborn 763.7
- contraction ring 661.4 ✓5ᵗʰ
  - affecting fetus or newborn 763.7
- fetal 660.9 ✓5ᵗʰ
  - abnormal size 653.5 ✓5ᵗʰ
    - affecting fetus or newborn 763.1
  - deformity 653.7 ✓5ᵗʰ
- maternal 660.9 ✓5ᵗʰ
  - affecting fetus or newborn 763.1
- positional 660.0 ✓5ᵗʰ
  - affecting fetus or newborn 763.1
- shoulder (girdle) 660.4 ✓5ᵗʰ
  - affecting fetus or newborn 763.1
- uterine NEC 661.4 ✓5ᵗʰ
  - affecting fetus or newborn 763.7

Dystonia
- deformans progressiva 333.6
- due to drugs 333.7
- lenticularis 333.6
- musculorum deformans 333.6
- torsion (idiopathic) 333.6
  - fragments (of) 333.89
  - symptomatic 333.7

Dystonic
- movements 781.0

Dystopia kidney 753.3

Dystrophy, dystrophia 783.9
- adiposogenital 253.8
- asphyxiating thoracic 756.4
- Becker's type 359.1
- brevicollis 756.16
- Bruch's membrane 362.77
- cervical (sympathetic) NEC 337.0
- chondro-osseus with punctate epiphyseal dysplasia 756.59
- choroid (hereditary) 363.50
  - central (areolar) (partial) 363.53
    - total (gyrate) 363.54
  - circinate 363.53
  - circumpapillary (partial) 363.51
    - total 363.52
  - diffuse
    - partial 363.56
    - total 363.57
  - generalized
    - partial 363.56
    - total 363.57
  - gyrate
    - central 363.54
    - generalized 363.57
  - helicoid 363.52
  - peripapillary — see Dystrophy, choroid, circumpapillary
  - serpiginous 363.54
- cornea (hereditary) 371.50
  - anterior NEC 371.52
  - Cogan's 371.52
  - combined 371.57
  - crystalline 371.56
  - endothelial (Fuchs') 371.57
  - epithelial 371.50
    - juvenile 371.51
    - microscopic cystic 371.52
  - granular 371.53
  - lattice 371.54
  - macular 371.55
  - marginal (Terrien's) 371.48
  - Meesman's 371.51
  - microscopic cystic (epithelial) 371.52
  - nodular, Salzmann's 371.46
  - polymorphous 371.58
  - posterior NEC 371.58
  - ring-like 371.52
  - Salzmann's nodular 371.46

Dystrophy, dystrophia — continued
- cornea — continued
  - stromal NEC 371.56
- dermatochondrocorneal 371.50
- Duchenne's 359.1
- due to malnutrition 263.9
- Erb's 359.1
- familial
  - hyperplastic periosteal 756.59
  - osseous 277.5
- foveal 362.77
- Fuchs', cornea 371.57
- Gowers' muscular 359.1
- hair 704.2
- hereditary, progressive muscular 359.1
- hypogenital, with diabetic tendency 759.81
- Landouzy-Déjérine 359.1
- Leyden-Möbius 359.1
- mesodermalis congenita 759.82
- muscular 359.1
  - congenital (hereditary) 359.0
    - myotonic 359.2
  - distal 359.1
  - Duchenne's 359.1
  - Erb's 359.1
  - fascioscapulohumeral 359.1
  - Gowers' 359.1
  - hereditary (progressive) 359.1
  - Landouzy-Déjérine 359.1
  - limb-girdle 359.1
  - myotonic 359.2
  - progressive (hereditary) 359.1
    - Charcôt-Marie-Tooth 356.1
  - pseudohypertrophic (infantile) 359.1
- myocardium, myocardial (see also Degeneration, myocardial) 429.1
- myotonic 359.2
- myotonica 359.2
- nail 703.8
  - congenital 757.5
- neurovascular (traumatic) (see also Neuropathy, peripheral, autonomic) 337.9
- nutritional 263.9
- ocular 359.1
- oculocerebrorenal 270.8
- oculopharyngeal 359.1
- ovarian 620.8
- papillary (and pigmentary) 701.1
- pelvicrural atrophic 359.1
- pigmentary (see also Acanthosis) 701.2
- pituitary (gland) 253.8
- polyglandular 258.8
- posttraumatic sympathetic — see Dystrophy, sympathetic
- progressive ophthalmoplegic 359.1
- retina, retinal (hereditary) 362.70
  - albipunctate 362.74
  - Bruch's membrane 362.77
  - cone, progressive 362.75
  - hyaline 362.77
  - in
    - Bassen-Kornzweig syndrome 272.5 [362.72]
    - cerebroretinal lipidosis 330.1 [362.71]
    - Refsum's disease 356.3 [362.72]
    - systemic lipidosis 272.7 [362.71]
  - juvenile (Stargardt's) 362.75
  - pigmentary 362.74
  - pigment epithelium 362.76
  - progressive cone (-rod) 362.75
  - pseudoinflammatory foveal 362.77
  - rod, progressive 362.75
  - sensory 362.75
  - vitelliform 362.76
- Salzmann's nodular 371.46
- scapuloperoneal 359.1
- skin NEC 709.9
- sympathetic (posttraumatic) (reflex) 337.20
  - lower limb 337.22
  - specified NEC 337.29
  - upper limb 337.21
- tapetoretinal NEC 362.74
- thoracic asphyxiating 756.4
- unguium 703.8
  - congenital 757.5
- vitreoretinal (primary) 362.73
  - secondary 362.66
- vulva 624.0

Dysuria 788.1
  psychogenic 306.53

E

Eagle-Barrett syndrome 756.71
Eales' disease (syndrome) 362.18
Ear — *see also* condition
  ache 388.70
    otogenic 388.71
    referred 388.72
  lop 744.29
  piercing V50.3
  swimmers' acute 380.12
  tank 380.12
  tropical 111.8 *[380.15]*
  wax 380.4
Earache 388.70
  otogenic 388.71
  referred 388.72
Eaton-Lambert syndrome (*see also* Neoplasm, by site, malignant) 199.1 *[358.1]*
Eberth's disease (typhoid fever) 002.0
Ebstein's
  anomaly or syndrome (downward displacement, tricuspid valve into right ventricle) 746.2
  disease (diabetes) 250.4 ✓5ᵗʰ *[581.81]*
Eccentro-osteochondrodysplasia 277.5
Ecchondroma (M9210/0) — *see* Neoplasm, bone, benign
Ecchondrosis (M9210/1) 238.0
Ecchordosis physaliphora 756.0
Ecchymosis (multiple) 459.89
  conjunctiva 372.72
  eye (traumatic) 921.0
  eyelids (traumatic) 921.1
  newborn 772.6
  spontaneous 782.7
  traumatic — *see* Contusion
Echinococciasis — *see* Echinococcus
Echinococcosis — *see* Echinococcus
Echinococcus (infection) 122.9
  granulosus 122.4
    liver 122.0
    lung 122.1
    orbit 122.3 *[376.13]*
    specified site NEC 122.3
    thyroid 122.2
  liver NEC 122.8
    granulosus 122.0
    multilocularis 122.5
  lung NEC 122.9
    granulosus 122.1
    multilocularis 122.6
  multilocularis 122.7
    liver 122.5
    specified site NEC 122.6
  orbit 122.9 *[376.13]*
    granulosus 122.3 *[376.13]*
    multilocularis 122.6 *[376.13]*
  specified site NEC 122.9
    granulosus 122.3
    multilocularis 122.6 *[376.13]*
  thyroid NEC 122.9
    granulosus 122.2
    multilocularis 122.6
Echinorhynchiasis 127.7
Echinostomiasis 121.8
Echolalia 784.69
ECHO virus infection NEC 079.1
Eclampsia, eclamptic (coma) (convulsions) (delirium) 780.39
  female, child-bearing age NEC — *see* Eclampsia, pregnancy
  gravidarum — *see* Eclampsia, pregnancy
  male 780.39
  not associated with pregnancy or childbirth 780.39
  pregnancy, childbirth, or puerperium 642.6 ✓5ᵗʰ
    with pre-existing hypertension 642.7 ✓5ᵗʰ
    affecting fetus or newborn 760.0
  uremic 586
Eclipse blindness (total) 363.31

Economic circumstance affecting care V60.9
  specified type NEC V60.8
Economo's disease (encephalitis lethargica) 049.8
Ectasia, ectasis
  aorta (*see also* Aneurysm, aorta) 441.9
    ruptured 441.5
  breast 610.4
  capillary 448.9
  cornea (marginal) (postinfectional) 371.71
  duct (mammary) 610.4
  kidney 593.89
  mammary duct (gland) 610.4
  papillary 448.9
  renal 593.89
  salivary gland (duct) 527.8
  scar, cornea 371.71
  sclera 379.11
Ecthyma 686.8
  contagiosum 051.2
  gangrenosum 686.09
  infectiosum 051.2
Ectocardia 746.87
Ectodermal dysplasia, congenital 757.31
Ectodermosis erosiva pluriorificialis 695.1
Ectopic, ectopia (congenital) 759.89
  abdominal viscera 751.8
    due to defect in anterior abdominal wall 756.79
  ACTH syndrome 255.0
  adrenal gland 759.1
  anus 751.5
  auricular beats 427.61
  beats 427.60
  bladder 753.5
  bone and cartilage in lung 748.69
  brain 742.4
  breast tissue 757.6
  cardiac 746.87
  cerebral 742.4
  cordis 746.87
  endometrium 617.9
  gallbladder 751.69
  gastric mucosa 750.7
  gestation — *see* Pregnancy, ectopic
  heart 746.87
  hormone secretion NEC 259.3
  hyperparathyroidism 259.3
  kidney (crossed) (intrathoracic) (pelvis) 753.3
    in pregnancy or childbirth 654.4 ✓5ᵗʰ
      causing obstructed labor 660.2 ✓5ᵗʰ
  lens 743.37
  lentis 743.37
  mole — *see* Pregnancy, ectopic
  organ or site NEC — *see* Malposition, congenital
  ovary 752.0
  pancreas, pancreatic tissue 751.7
  pregnancy — *see* Pregnancy, ectopic
  pupil 364.75
  renal 753.3
  sebaceous glands of mouth 750.26
  secretion
    ACTH 255.0
    adrenal hormone 259.3
    adrenalin 259.3
    adrenocorticotropin 255.0
    antidiuretic hormone (ADH) 259.3
    epinephrine 259.3
    hormone NEC 259.3
    norepinephrine 259.3
    pituitary (posterior) 259.3
  spleen 759.0
  testis 752.51
  thyroid 759.2
  ureter 753.4
  ventricular beats 427.69
  vesicae 753.5
Ectrodactyly 755.4
  finger (*see also* Absence, finger, congenital) 755.29
  toe (*see also* Absence, toe, congenital) 755.39
Ectromelia 755.4
  lower limb 755.30
  upper limb 755.20
Ectropion 374.10
  anus 569.49

Ectropion — *continued*
  cervix 622.0
    with mention of cervicitis 616.0
  cicatricial 374.14
  congenital 743.62
  eyelid 374.10
    cicatricial 374.14
    congenital 743.62
    mechanical 374.12
    paralytic 374.12
    senile 374.11
    spastic 374.13
  iris (pigment epithelium) 364.54
  lip (congenital) 750.26
    acquired 528.5
  mechanical 374.12
  paralytic 374.12
  rectum 569.49
  senile 374.11
  spastic 374.13
  urethra 599.84
  uvea 364.54
Eczema (acute) (allergic) (chronic) (erythematous) (fissum) (occupational) (rubrum) (squamous) 692.9
  asteatotic 706.8
  atopic 691.8
  contact NEC 692.9
  dermatitis NEC 692.9
  due to specified cause — *see* Dermatitis, due to
  dyshidrotic 705.81
  external ear 380.22
  flexural 691.8
  gouty 274.89
  herpeticum 054.0
  hypertrophicum 701.8
  hypostatic — *see* Varicose, vein
  impetiginous 684
  infantile (acute) (chronic) (due to any substance) (intertriginous) (seborrheic) 690.12
  intertriginous NEC 692.9
    infantile 690.12
  intrinsic 691.8
  lichenified NEC 692.9
  marginatum 110.3
  nummular 692.9
  pustular 686.8
  seborrheic 690.18
    infantile 690.12
  solare 692.72
  stasis (lower extremity) 454.1
    ulcerated 454.2
  vaccination, vaccinatum 999.0
  varicose (lower extremity) — *see* Varicose, vein
  verrucosum callosum 698.3
Eczematoid, exudative 691.8
Eddowes' syndrome (brittle bone and blue sclera) 756.51
Edema, edematous 782.3
  with nephritis (*see also* Nephrosis) 581.9
  allergic 995.1
  angioneurotic (allergic) (any site) (with urticaria) 995.1
    hereditary 277.6
  angiospastic 443.9
  Berlin's (traumatic) 921.3
  brain 348.5
    due to birth injury 767.8
    fetus or newborn 767.8
  cardiac (*see also* Failure, heart) 428.0
  cardiovascular (*see also* Failure, heart) 428.0
  cerebral — *see* Edema, brain
  cerebrospinal vessel — *see* Edema, brain
  cervix (acute) (uteri) 622.8
    puerperal, postpartum 674.8 ✓5ᵗʰ
  chronic hereditary 757.0
  circumscribed, acute 995.1
    hereditary 277.6
  complicating pregnancy (gestational) 646.1 ✓5ᵗʰ
    with hypertension — *see* Toxemia, of pregnancy
  conjunctiva 372.73
  connective tissue 782.3
  cornea 371.20
    due to contact lenses 371.24
    idiopathic 371.21

Edema, edematous

Edema, edematous — *continued*
- cornea — *continued*
  - secondary 371.22
  - due to
    - lymphatic obstruction — *see* Edema, lymphatic
    - salt retention 276.0
  - epiglottis — *see* Edema, glottis
- essential, acute 995.1
  - hereditary 277.6
- extremities, lower — *see* Edema, legs
- eyelid NEC 374.82
- familial, hereditary (legs) 757.0
- famine 262
- fetus or newborn 778.5
- genital organs
  - female 629.8
  - male 608.86
- gestational 646.1 ✓5th
  - with hypertension — *see* Toxemia, of pregnancy
- glottis, glottic, glottides (obstructive) (passive) 478.6
  - allergic 995.1
    - hereditary 277.6
  - due to external agent — *see* Condition, respiratory, acute, due to specified agent
- heart (*see also* Failure, heart) 428.0
  - newborn 779.89 ▲
- heat 992.7
- hereditary (legs) 757.0
- inanition 262
- infectious 782.3
- intracranial 348.5
  - due to injury at birth 767.8
- iris 364.8
- joint (*see also* Effusion, joint) 719.0 ✓5th
- larynx (*see also* Edema, glottis) 478.6
- legs 782.3
  - due to venous obstruction 459.2
  - hereditary 757.0
- localized 782.3
  - due to venous obstruction 459.2
  - lower extremity 459.2
- lower extremities — *see* Edema, legs
- lung 514
  - acute 518.4
    - with heart disease or failure (*see also* Failure, ventricular, left) 428.1
      - congestive 428.0
    - chemical (due to fumes or vapors) 506.1
    - due to
      - external agent(s) NEC 508.9
        - specified NEC 508.8
      - fumes and vapors (chemical) (inhalation) 506.1
      - radiation 508.0
  - chemical (acute) 506.1
    - chronic 506.4
  - chronic 514
    - chemical (due to fumes or vapors) 506.4
    - due to
      - external agent(s) NEC 508.9
        - specified NEC 508.8
      - fumes or vapors (chemical) (inhalation) 506.4
      - radiation 508.1
  - due to
    - external agent 508.9
      - specified NEC 508.8
    - high altitude 993.2
    - near drowning 994.1
  - postoperative 518.4
  - terminal 514
- lymphatic 457.1
  - due to mastectomy operation 457.0
- macula 362.83
  - cystoid 362.53
  - diabetic 250.5 ✓5th [362.01]
- malignant (*see also* Gangrene, gas) 040.0
- Milroy's 757.0
- nasopharynx 478.25
- neonatorum 778.5
- nutritional (newborn) 262
  - with dyspigmentation, skin and hair 260
- optic disc or nerve — *see* Papilledema

Edema, edematous — *continued*
- orbit 376.33
  - circulatory 459.89
- palate (soft) (hard) 528.9
- pancrease 577.8
- penis 607.83
- periodic 995.1
  - hereditary 277.6
- pharynx 478.25
- pitting 782.3
- pulmonary — *see* Edema, lung
- Quincke's 995.1
  - hereditary 277.6
- renal (*see also* Nephrosis) 581.9
- retina (localized) (macular) (perepheral) 362.83
  - cystoid 362.53
  - diabetic 250.5 ✓5th [362.01]
- salt 276.0
- scrotum 608.86
- seminal vesicle 608.86
- spermatic cord 608.86
- spinal cord 336.1
- starvation 262
- stasis (*see also* Hypertension, venous) 459.30 ●
- subconjunctival 372.73
- subglottic (*see also* Edema, glottis) 478.6
- supraglottic (*see also* Edema, glottis) 478.6
- testis 608.86
- toxic NEC 782.3
- traumatic NEC 782.3
- tunica vaginalis 608.86
- vas deferens 608.86
- vocal cord — *see* Edema, glottis
- vulva (acute) 624.8

Edentia (complete) (partial) (*see also* Absence, tooth) 520.0
- acquired 525.10
  - due to
    - caries 525.13
    - extraction 525.10
    - periodontal disease 525.12
    - specified NEC 525.19
    - trauma 525.11
- causing malocclusion 524.3
- congenital (deficiency of tooth buds) 520.0

Edentulism 525.10

Edsall's disease 992.2

Educational handicap V62.3

Edwards' syndrome 758.2

Effect, adverse NEC
- abnormal gravitation (G) forces or states 994.9
- air pressure — *see* Effect, adverse, atmospheric pressure
- altitude (high) — *see* Effect, adverse, high altitude
- anesthetic
  - in labor and delivery NEC 668.9 ✓5th
    - affecting fetus or newborn 763.5
- antitoxin — *see* Complications, vaccination
- atmospheric pressure 993.9
  - due to explosion 993.4
  - high 993.3
  - low — *see* Effect, adverse, high altitude
  - specified effect NEC 993.8
- biological, correct substance properly administered (*see also* Effect, adverse, drug) 995.2
- blood (derivatives) (serum) (transfusion) — *see* Complications, transfusion
- chemical substance NEC 989.9
  - specified — *see* Table of Drugs and Chemicals
- cobalt, radioactive (*see also* Effect, adverse, radioactive substance) 990
- cold (temperature) (weather) 991.9
  - chilblains 991.5
  - frostbite — *see* Frostbite
  - specified effect NEC 991.8
- drugs and medicinals NEC 995.2
  - correct substance properly administered 995.2
  - overdose or wrong substance given or taken 977.9
  - specified drug — *see* Table of Drugs and Chemicals

Effect, adverse NEC — *continued*
- electric current (shock) 994.8
  - burn — *see* Burn, by site
- electricity (electrocution) (shock) 994.8
  - burn — *see* Burn, by site
- exertion (excessive) 994.5
- exposure 994.9
  - exhaustion 994.4
- external cause NEC 994.9
- fallout (radioactive) NEC 990
- fluoroscopy NEC 990
- foodstuffs
  - allergic reaction (*see also* Allergy, food) 693.1
  - anaphylactic shock due to food NEC 995.60
  - noxious 988.9
    - specified type NEC (*see also* Poisoning, by name of noxious foodstuff) 988.8
- gases, fumes, or vapors — *see* Table of Drugs and Chemicals
- glue (airplane) sniffing 304.6 ✓5th
- heat — *see* Heat
- high altitude NEC 993.2
  - anoxia 993.2
  - on
    - ears 993.0
    - sinuses 993.1
  - polycythemia 289.0
- hot weather — *see* Heat
- hunger 994.2
- immersion, foot 991.4
- immunization — *see* Complications, vaccination
- immunological agents — *see* Complications, vaccination
- implantation (removable) of isotope or radium NEC 990
- infrared (radiation) (rays) NEC 990
  - burn — *see* Burn, by site
  - dermatitis or eczema 692.82
- infusion — *see* Complications, infusion
- ingestion or injection of isotope (therapeutic) NEC 990
- irradiation NEC (*see also* Effect, adverse, radiation) 990
- isotope (radioactive) NEC 990
- lack of care (child) (infant) (newborn) 995.52
  - adult 995.84
- lightning 994.0
  - burn — *see* Burn, by site
- Lirugin — *see* Complications, vaccination
- medicinal substance, correct, properly administered (*see also* Effect, adverse, drugs) 995.2
- mesothorium NEC 990
- motion 994.6
- noise, inner ear 388.10
- overheated places — *see* Heat
- polonium NEC 990
- psychosocial, of work environment V62.1
- radiation (diagnostic) (fallout) (infrared) (natural source) (therapeutic) (tracer) (ultraviolet) (x-ray) NEC 990
  - with pulmonary manifestations
    - acute 508.0
    - chronic 508.1
  - dermatitis or eczema 692.82
    - due to sun NEC (*see also* Dermatitis, due to, sun) 692.70
  - fibrosis of lungs 508.1
  - maternal with suspected damage to fetus affecting management of pregnancy 655.6 ✓5th
  - pneumonitis 508.0
- radioactive substance NEC 990
  - dermatitis or eczema 692.82
- radioactivity NEC 990
- radiotherapy NEC 990
  - dermatitis or eczema 692.82
- radium NEC 990
- reduced temperature 991.9
  - frostbite — *see* Frostbite
  - immersion, foot (hand) 991.4
  - specified effect NEC 991.8
- roentgenography NEC 990
- roentgenoscopy NEC 990

Index to Diseases — Embolism

Effect, adverse NEC — *continued*
  roentgen rays NEC 990
  serum (prophylactic) (therapeutic) NEC 999.5
  specified NEC 995.89
    external cause NEC 994.9
  strangulation 994.7
  submersion 994.1
  teletherapy NEC 990
  thirst 994.3
  transfusion — *see* Complications, transfusion
  ultraviolet (radiation) (rays) NEC 990
    burn — *see also* Burn, by site
      from sun (*see also* Sunburn) 692.71
    dermatitis or eczema 692.82
      due to sun NEC (*see also* Dermatitis, due to, sun) 692.70
  uranium NEC 990
  vaccine (any) — *see* Complications, vaccination
  weightlessness 994.9
  whole blood — *see also* Complications, transfusion
    overdose or wrong substance given (*see also* Table of Drugs and Chemicals) 964.7
  working environment V62.1
  x-rays NEC 990
    dermatitis or eczema 692.82
Effects, late — *see* Late, effect (of)
Effect, remote
  of cancer — *see* condition
Effluvium, telogen 704.02
Effort
  intolerance 306.2
  syndrome (aviators) (psychogenic) 306.2
Effusion
  amniotic fluid (*see also* Rupture, membranes, premature) 658.1
  brain (serous) 348.5
  bronchial (*see also* Bronchitis) 490
  cerebral 348.5
  cerebrospinal (*see also* Meningitis) 322.9
    vessel 348.5
  chest — *see* Effusion, pleura
  intracranial 348.5
  joint 719.00
    ankle 719.07
    elbow 719.02
    foot 719.07
    hand 719.04
    hip 719.05
    knee 719.06
    multiple sites 719.09
    pelvic region 719.05
    shoulder (region) 719.01
    specified site NEC 719.08
    wrist 719.03
  meninges (*see also* Meningitis) 322.9
  pericardium, pericardial (*see also* Pericarditis) 423.9
    acute 420.90
  peritoneal (chronic) 568.82
  pleura, pleurisy, pleuritic, pleuropericardial 511.9
    bacterial, nontuberculous 511.1
    fetus or newborn 511.9
    malignant 197.2
    nontuberculous 511.9
      bacterial 511.1
    pneumococcal 511.1
    staphylococcal 511.1
    streptococcal 511.1
    traumatic 862.29
      with open wound 862.39
    tuberculous (*see also* Tuberculosis, pleura) 012.0
      primary progressive 010.1
  pulmonary — *see* Effusion, pleura
  spinal (*see also* Meningitis) 322.9
  thorax, thoracic — *see* Effusion, pleura
Eggshell nails 703.8
  congenital 757.5
Ego-dystonic
  homosexuality 302.0
  lesbianism 302.0
Egyptian splenomegaly 120.1
Ehlers-Danlos syndrome 756.83

Ehrlichiosis 082.40
  chaffeensis 082.41
  specified type NEC 082.49
Eichstedt's disease (pityriasis versicolor) 111.0
Eisenmenger's complex or syndrome (ventricular septal defect) 745.4
Ejaculation, semen
  painful 608.89
    psychogenic 306.59
  premature 302.75
  retrograde 608.87
Ekbom syndrome (restless legs) 333.99
Ekman's syndrome (brittle bones and blue sclera) 756.51
Elastic skin 756.83
  acquired 701.8
Elastofibroma (M8820/0) — *see* Neoplasm, connective tissue, benign
Elastoidosis
  cutanea nodularis 701.8
  cutis cystica et comedonica 701.8
Elastoma 757.39
  juvenile 757.39
  Miescher's (elastosis perforans serpiginosa) 701.1
Elastomyofibrosis 425.3
Elastosis 701.8
  atrophicans 701.8
  perforans serpiginosa 701.1
  reactive perforating 701.1
  senilis 701.8
  solar (actinic) 692.74
Elbow — *see* condition
Electric
  current, electricity, effects (concussion) (fatal) (nonfatal) (shock) 994.8
  burn — *see* Burn, by site
  feet (foot) syndrome 266.2
Electrocution 994.8
Electrolyte imbalance 276.9
  with
    abortion — *see* Abortion, by type with metabolic disorder
    ectopic pregnancy (*see also* categories 633.0-633.9) 639.4
    hyperemesis gravidarum (before 22 completed weeks gestation) 643.1
    molar pregnancy (*see also* categories 630-632) 639.4
  following
    abortion 639.4
    ectopic or molar pregnancy 639.4
Elephant man syndrome 237.71
Elephantiasis (nonfilarial) 457.1
  arabicum (*see also* Infestation, filarial) 125.9
  congenita hereditaria 757.0
  congenital (any site) 757.0
  due to
    Brugia (malayi) 125.1
    mastectomy operation 457.0
    Wuchereria (bancrofti) 125.0
      malayi 125.1
  eyelid 374.83
  filarial (*see also* Infestation, filarial) 125.9
  filariensis (*see also* Infestation, filarial) 125.9
  gingival 523.8
  glandular 457.1
  graecorum 030.9
  lymphangiectatic 457.1
  lymphatic vessel 457.1
    due to mastectomy operation 457.0
  neuromatosa 237.71
  postmastectomy 457.0
  scrotum 457.1
  streptococcal 457.1
  surgical 997.99
    postmastectomy 457.0
  telangiectodes 457.1
  vulva (nonfilarial) 624.8
Elevated — *see* Elevation
Elevation
  17-ketosteroids 791.9
  acid phosphatase 790.5
  alkaline phosphatase 790.5

Elevation — *continued*
  amylase 790.5
  antibody titers 795.79
  basal metabolic rate (BMR) 794.7
  blood pressure (*see also* Hypertension) 401.9
    reading (incidental) (isolated) (nonspecific), no diagnosis or hypertension 796.2
  body temperature (of unknown origin) (*see also* Pyrexia) 780.6
  conjugate, eye 378.81
  diaphragm, congenital 756.6
  immunoglobulin level 795.79
  indolacetic acid 791.9
  lactic acid dehydrogenase (LDH) level 790.4
  lipase 790.5
  prostate specific antigen (PSA) 790.93
  renin 790.99
    in hypertension (*see also* Hypertension, renovascular) 405.91
  Rh titer 999.7
  scapula, congenital 755.52
  sedimentation rate 790.1
  SGOT 790.4
  SGPT 790.4
  transaminase 790.4
  vanillylmandelic acid 791.9
  venous pressure 459.89
  VMA 791.9
Elliptocytosis (congenital) (hereditary) 282.1
  Hb-C (disease) 282.7
  hemoglobin disease 282.7
  sickle-cell (disease) 282.60
  trait 282.5
Ellis-van Creveld disease or syndrome (chondroectodermal dysplasia) 756.55
Ellison-Zollinger syndrome (gastric hypersecretion with pancreatic islet cell tumor) 251.5
Elongation, elongated (congenital) — *see also* Distortion
  bone 756.9
  cervix (uteri) 752.49
    acquired 622.6
    hypertrophic 622.6
  colon 751.5
  common bile duct 751.69
  cystic duct 751.69
  frenulum, penis 752.69
  labia minora, acquired 624.8
  ligamentum patellae 756.89
  petiolus (epiglottidis) 748.3
  styloid bone (process) 733.99
  tooth, teeth 520.2
  uvula 750.26
    acquired 528.9
Elschnig bodies or pearls 366.51
El Tor cholera 001.1
Emaciation (due to malnutrition) 261
Emancipation disorder 309.22
Embadomoniasis 007.8
Embarrassment heart, cardiac — *see* Disease, heart
Embedded tooth, teeth 520.6
  with abnormal position (same or adjacent tooth) 524.3
  root only 525.3
Embolic — *see* conditon
Embolism 444.9
  with
    abortion — *see* Abortion, by type, with embolism
    ectopic pregnancy (*see also* categories 633.0-633.9) 639.6
    molar pregnancy (*see also* categories 630-632) 639.6
  air (any site) 958.0
    with
      abortion — *see* Abortion, by type, with embolism
      ectopic pregnancy (*see also* categories 633.0-633.9) 639.6
      molar pregnancy (*see also* categories 630-632) 639.6

Embolism

Embolism — *continued*
  air — *continued*
    due to implanted device — *see* Complications, due to (presence of) any device, implant, or graft classified to 996.0-996.5 NEC
    following
      abortion 639.6
      ectopic or molar pregnancy 639.6
      infusion, perfusion, or transfusion 999.1
    in pregnancy, childbirth, or puerperium 673.0 ✓5ᵗʰ
    traumatic 958.0
  amniotic fluid (pulmonary) 673.1 ✓5ᵗʰ
    with
      abortion — *see* Abortion, by type, with embolism
      ectopic pregnancy (*see also* categories 633.0-633.9) 639.6
      molar pregnancy (*see also* categories 630-632) 639.6
    following
      abortion 639.6
      ectopic or molar pregnancy 639.6
  aorta, aortic 444.1
    abdominal 444.0
    bifurcation 444.0
    saddle 444.0
    thoracic 444.1
  artery 444.9
    auditory, internal 433.8 ✓5ᵗʰ
    basilar (*see also* Occlusion, artery, basilar) 433.0 ✓5ᵗʰ
    bladder 444.89
    carotid (common) (internal) (*see also* Occlusion, artery, carotid) 433.1 ✓5ᵗʰ
    cerebellar (anterior inferior) (posterior inferior) (superior) 433.8 ✓5ᵗʰ
    cerebral (*see also* Embolism, brain) 434.1 ✓5ᵗʰ
    choroidal (anterior) 433.8 ✓5ᵗʰ
    communicating posterior 433.8 ✓5ᵗʰ
    coronary (*see also* Infarct, myocardium) 410.9 ✓5ᵗʰ
      without myocardial infarction 411.81
    extremity 444.22
      lower 444.22
      upper 444.21
    hypophyseal 433.8 ✓5ᵗʰ
    mesenteric (with gangrene) 557.0
    ophthalmic (*see also* Occlusion, retina) 362.30
    peripheral 444.22
    pontine 433.8 ✓5ᵗʰ
    precerebral NEC — *see* Occlusion, artery, precerebral
    pulmonary — *see* Embolism, pulmonary
    renal 593.81
    retinal (*see also* Occlusion, retina) 362.30
    specified site NEC 444.89
    vertebral (*see also* Occlusion, artery, vertebral) 433.2 ✓5ᵗʰ
  auditory, internal 433.8 ✓5ᵗʰ
  basilar (artery) (*see also* Occlusion, artery, basilar) 433.0 ✓5ᵗʰ
  birth, mother — *see* Embolism, obstetrical
  blood-clot
    with
      abortion — *see* Abortion, by type, with embolism
      ectopic pregnancy (*see also* categories 633.0-633.9) 639.6
      molar pregnancy (*see also* categories 630-632) 639.6
    following
      abortion 639.6
      ectopic or molar pregnancy 639.6
    in pregnancy, childbirth, or puerperium 673.2 ✓5ᵗʰ
  brain 434.1 ✓5ᵗʰ
    with
      abortion — *see* Abortion, by type, with embolism
      ectopic pregnancy (*see also* categories 633.0-633.9) 639.6
      molar pregnancy (*see also* categories 630-632) 639.6

Embolism — *continued*
  brain — *continued*
    following
      abortion 639.6
      ectopic or molar pregnancy 639.6
    late effect — *see* Late effect(s) (of) cerebrovascular disease
    puerperal, postpartum, childbirth 674.0 ✓5ᵗʰ
  capillary 448.9
  cardiac (*see also* Infarct, myocardium) 410.9 ✓5ᵗʰ
  carotid (artery) (common) (internal) (*see also* Occlusion, artery, carotid) 433.1 ✓5ᵗʰ
  cavernous sinus (venous) — *see* Embolism, intracranial venous sinus
  cerebral (*see also* Embolism, brain) 434.1 ✓5ᵗʰ
  cholesterol — *see* Atheroembolism ●
  choroidal (anterior) (artery) 433.8 ✓5ᵗʰ
  coronary (artery or vein) (systemic) (*see also* Infarct, myocardium) 410.9 ✓5ᵗʰ
    without myocardial infarction 411.81
  due to (presence of) any device, implant, or graft classifiable to 996.0-996.5 — *see* Complications, due to (presence of) any device, implant, or graft classified to 996.0-996.5 NEC
  encephalomalacia (*see also* Embolism, brain) 434.1 ✓5ᵗʰ
  extremities 444.22
    lower 444.22
    upper 444.21
  eye 362.30
  fat (cerebral) (pulmonary) (systemic) 958.1
    with
      abortion — *see* Abortion, by type, with embolism
      ectopic pregnancy (*see also* categories 633.0-633.9) 639.6
      molar pregnancy (*see also* categories 630-632) 639.6
    complicating delivery or puerperium 673.8 ✓5ᵗʰ
    following
      abortion 639.6
      ectopic or molar pregnancy 639.6
    in pregnancy, childbirth, or the puerperium 673.8 ✓5ᵗʰ
  femoral (artery) 444.22
    vein 453.8
  following
    abortion 639.6
    ectopic or molar pregnancy 639.6
    infusion, perfusion, or transfusion
      air 999.1
      thrombus 999.2
  heart (fatty) (*see also* Infarct, myocardium) 410.9 ✓5ᵗʰ
  hepatic (vein) 453.0
  iliac (artery) 444.81
  iliofemoral 444.81
  in pregnancy, childbirth, or puerperium (pulmonary) — *see* Embolism, obstetrical
  intestine (artery) (vein) (with gangrene) 557.0
  intracranial (*see also* Embolism, brain) 434.1 ✓5ᵗʰ
    venous sinus (any) 325
      late effect — *see* category 326
      nonpyogenic 437.6
        in pregnancy or puerperium 671.5 ✓5ᵗʰ
  kidney (artery) 593.81
  lateral sinus (venous) — *see* Embolism, intracranial venous sinus
  longitudinal sinus (venous) — *see* Embolism, intracranial venous sinus
  lower extremity 444.22
  lung (massive) — *see* Embolism, pulmonary
  meninges (*see also* Embolism, brain) 434.1 ✓5ᵗʰ
  mesenteric (artery) (with gangrene) 557.0
  multiple NEC 444.9
  obstetrical (pulmonary) 673.2 ✓5ᵗʰ
    air 673.0 ✓5ᵗʰ
    amniotic fluid (pulmonary) 673.1 ✓5ᵗʰ
    blood-clot 673.2 ✓5ᵗʰ
    cardiac 674.8 ✓5ᵗʰ
    fat 673.8 ✓5ᵗʰ
    heart 674.8 ✓5ᵗʰ
    pyemic 673.3 ✓5ᵗʰ

Embolism — *continued*
  obstetrical — *continued*
    septic 673.3 ✓5ᵗʰ
    specified NEC 674.8 ✓5ᵗʰ
  ophthalmic (*see also* Occlusion, retina) 362.30
  paradoxical NEC 444.9
  penis 607.82
  peripheral arteries NEC 444.22
    lower 444.22
    upper 444.21
  pituitary 253.8
  popliteal (artery) 444.22
  portal (vein) 452
  postoperative NEC 997.2
    cerebral 997.02
    mesenteric artery 997.71
    other vessels 997.79
    peripheral vascular 997.2
    pulmonary 415.11
    renal artery 997.72
  precerebral artery (*see also* Occlusion, artery, precerebral) 433.9 ✓5ᵗʰ
  puerperal — *see* Embolism, obstetrical
  pulmonary (artery) (vein) 415.1 ✓5ᵗʰ
    with
      abortion — *see* Abortion, by type, with embolism
      ectopic pregnancy (*see also* categories 633.0-633.9) 639.6
      molar pregnancy (*see also* categories 630-632) 639.6
    following
      abortion 639.6
      ectopic or molar pregnancy 639.6
    iatrogenic 415.11
    in pregnancy, childbirth, or puerperium — *see* Embolism, obstetrical
    postoperative 415.11
  pyemic (multiple) 038.9
    with
      abortion — *see* Abortion, by type, with embolism
      ectopic pregnancy (*see also* categories 633.0-633.9) 639.6
      molar pregnancy (*see also* categories 630-632) 639.6
    Aerobacter aerogenes 038.49
    enteric gram-negative bacilli 038.40
    Enterobacter aerogenes 038.49
    Escherichia coli 038.42
    following
      abortion 639.6
      ectopic or molar pregnancy 639.6
    Hemophilus influenzae 038.41
    pneumococcal 038.2
    Proteus vulgaris 038.49
    Pseudomonas (aeruginosa) 038.43
    puerperal, postparztum, childbirth (any organism) 673.3 ✓5ᵗʰ
    Serratia 038.44
    specified organism NEC 038.8
    staphylococcal 038.10
      aureus 038.11
      specified organism NEC 038.19
    streptococcal 038.0
  renal (artery) 593.81
    vein 453.3
  retina, retinal (*see also* Occlusion, retina) 362.30
  saddle (aorta) 444.0
  septicemic — *see* Embolism, pyemic
  sinus — *see* Embolism, intracranial venous sinus
  soap
    with
      abortion — *see* Abortion, by type, with embolism
      ectopic pregnancy (*see also* categories 633.0-633.9) 639.6
      molar pregnancy (*see also* categories 630-632) 639.6
    following
      abortion 639.6
      ectopic or molar pregnancy 639.6
  spinal cord (nonpyogenic) 336.1
    in pregnancy or puerperium 671.5 ✓5ᵗʰ

Index to Diseases

Embolism — continued
spinal cord — continued
  pyogenic origin 324.1
  late effect — see category 326
spleen, splenic (artery) 444.89
thrombus (thromboembolism) following
  infusion, perfusion, or transfusion 999.2
upper extremity 444.21
vein 453.9
  with inflammation or phlebitis — see
    Thrombophlebitis
  cerebral (see also Embolism, brain)
    434.1 ✓5ᵗʰ
  coronary (see also Infarct, myocardium)
    410.9 ✓5ᵗʰ
    without myocardial infarction 411.81
  hepatic 453.0
  mesenteric (with gangrene) 557.0
  portal 452
  pulmonary — see Embolism, pulmonary
  renal 453.3
  specified NEC 453.8
    with inflammation or phlebitis — see
      Thrombophlebitis
  vena cava (inferior) (superior) 453.2
vessels of brain (see also Embolism, brain)
  434.1 ✓5ᵗʰ

Embolization — see Embolism
Embolus — see Embolism
Embryoma (M9080/1) — see also Neoplasm, by
  site, uncertain behavior
  benign (M9080/0) — see Neoplasm, by site,
    benign
    kidney (M8960/3) 189.0
    liver (M8970/3) 155.0
  malignant (M9080/3) — see also Neoplasm, by
    site, malignant
    kidney (M8960/3) 189.0
    liver (M8970/3) 155.0
    testis (M9070/3) 186.9
      undescended 186.0
  testis (M9070/3) 186.9
    undescended 186.0

Embryonic
  circulation 747.9
  heart 747.9
  vas deferens 752.8

Embryopathia NEC 759.9
Embryotomy, fetal 763.89
Embryotoxon 743.43
  interfering with vision 743.42
Emesis — see Vomiting
  gravidarum — see Hyperemesis, gravidarum
Emissions, nocturnal (semen) 608.89
Emotional
  crisis — see Crisis, emotional
  disorder (see also Disorder, mental) 300.9
  instability (excessive) 301.3
  overlay — see Reaction, adjustment
  upset 300.9
Emotionality, pathological 301.3
Emotogenic disease (see also Disorder,
  psychogenic) 306.9
Emphysema (atrophic) (centriacinar)
  (centrilobular) (chronic) (diffuse) (essential)
  (hypertrophic) (interlobular) (lung)
  (obstructive) (panlobular) (paracicatricial)
  (paracinar) (postural) (pulmonary) (senile)
  (subpleural) (traction) (unilateral)
  (unilobular) (vesicular) 492.8
  with
    bronchitis
      acute and chronic 491.21
      chronic 491.20
        with acute bronchitis or acute
          exacerbation 491.21
  bullous (giant) 492.0
  cellular tissue 958.7
    surgical 998.81
  compensatory 518.2
  congenital 770.2
  conjunctiva 372.89
  connective tissue 958.7
    surgical 998.81

Emphysema — continued
due to fumes or vapors 506.4
eye 376.89
eyelid 374.85
  surgical 998.81
  traumatic 958.7
fetus or newborn (interstitial) (mediastinal)
  (unilobular) 770.2
heart 416.9
interstitial 518.1
  congenital 770.2
  fetus or newborn 770.2
laminated tissue 958.7
  surgical 998.81
mediastinal 518.1
  fetus or newborn 770.2
newborn (interstitial) (mediastinal) (unilobular)
  770.2
obstructive diffuse with fibrosis 492.8
orbit 376.89
subcutaneous 958.7
  due to trauma 958.7
  nontraumatic 518.1
  surgical 998.81
surgical 998.81
thymus (gland) (congenital) 254.8
traumatic 958.7
tuberculous (see also Tuberculosis, pulmonary)
  011.9 ✓5ᵗʰ

Employment examination (certification) V70.5
Empty sella (turcica) syndrome 253.8
Empyema (chest) (diaphragmatic) (double)
  (encapsulated) (general) (interlobar) (lung)
  (medial) (necessitatis) (perforating chest wall)
  (pleura) (pneumococcal) (residual)
  (sacculated) (streptococcal)
  (supradiaphragmatic) 510.9
  with fistula 510.0
  accessory sinus (chronic) (see also Sinusitis)
    473.9
  acute 510.9
    with fistula 510.0
  antrum (chronic) (see also Sinusitis, maxillary)
    473.0
  brain (any part) (see also Abcess, brain) 324.0
  ethmoidal (sinus) (chronic) (see also Sinusitis,
    ethmoidal) 473.2
  extradural (see also Abscess, extradural) 324.9
  frontal (sinus) (chronic) (see also Sinusitis,
    frontal) 473.1
  gallbladder (see also Cholecystitis, acute) 575.0
  mastoid (process) (acute) (see also Mastoiditis,
    acute) 383.00
  maxilla, maxillary 526.4
    sinus (chronic) (see also Sinusitis, maxillary)
      473.0
  nasal sinus (chronic) (see also Sinusitis) 473.9
  sinus (accessory) (nasal) (see also Sinusitis)
    473.9
  sphenoidal (chronic) (sinus) (see also Sinusitis,
    sphenoidal) 473.3
  subarachnoid (see also Abscess, extradural)
    324.9
  subdural (see also Abscess, extradural) 324.9
  tuberculous (see also Tuberculosis, pleura)
    012.0 ✓5ᵗʰ
  ureter (see also Ureteritis) 593.89
  ventricular (see also Abscess, brain) 324.0
Enameloma 520.2
Encephalitis (bacterial) (chronic) (hemorrhagic)
  (idiopathic) (nonepidemic) (spurious)
  (subacute) 323.9
  acute — see also Encephalitis, viral
    disseminated (postinfectious) NEC
      136.9 [323.6]
      postimmunization or postvaccination
        323.5
    inclusional 049.8
    inclusion body 049.8
    necrotizing 049.8
  arboviral, arbovirus NEC 064
  arthropod-borne (see also Encephalitis, viral,
    arthropod-borne) 064
  Australian X 062.4
  Bwamba fever 066.3
  California (virus) 062.5
  Central European 063.2

Encephalitis — continued
Czechoslovakian 063.2
Dawson's (inclusion body) 046.2
diffuse sclerosing 046.2
due to
  actinomycosis 039.8 [323.4]
  cat-scratch disease 078.3 [323.0]
  infectious mononucleosis 075 [323.0]
  malaria (see also Malaria) 084.6 [323.2]
  Negishi virus 064
  ornithosis 073.7 [323.0]
  prophylactic inoculation against smallpox
    323.5
  rickettsiosis (see also Rickettsiosis)
    083.9 [323.1]
  rubella 056.01
  toxoplasmosis (acquired) 130.0
    congenital (active) 771.2 [323.4]
  typhus (fever) (see also Typhus)
    081.9 [323.1]
  vaccination (smallpox) 323.5
Eastern equine 062.2
endemic 049.8
epidemic 049.8
equine (acute) (infectious) (viral) 062.9
  Eastern 062.2
  Venezuelan 066.2
  Western 062.1
Far Eastern 063.0
following vaccination or other immunization
  procedure 323.5
herpes 054.3
Ilheus (virus) 062.8
inclusion body 046.2
infectious (acute) (virus) NEC 049.8
influenzal 487.8 [323.4]
  lethargic 049.8
Japanese (B type) 062.0
La Crosse 062.5
Langat 063.8
late effect — see Late, effect, encephalitis
lead 984.9 [323.7]
lethargic (acute) (infectious) (influenzal) 049.8
lethargica 049.8
louping ill 063.1
lupus 710.0 [323.8]
lymphatica 049.0
Mengo 049.8
meningococcal 036.1
mumps 072.2
Murray Valley 062.4
myoclonic 049.8
Negishi virus 064
otitic NEC 382.4 [323.4]
parasitic NEC 123.9 [323.4]
periaxialis (concentrica) (diffusa) 341.1
postchickenpox 052.0
postexanthematous NEC 057.9 [323.6]
postimmunization 323.5
postinfectious NEC 136.9 [323.6]
postmeasles 055.0
posttraumatic 323.8
postvaccinal (smallpox) 323.5
postvaricella 052.0
postviral NEC 079.99 [323.6]
  postexanthematous 057.9 [323.6]
  specified NEC 057.8 [323.6]
Powassan 063.8
progressive subcortical (Binswanger's) 290.12
Rio Bravo 049.8
rubella 056.01
Russian
  autumnal 062.0
  spring-summer type (taiga) 063.0
saturnine 984.9 [323.7]
Semliki Forest 062.8
serous 048
slow-acting virus NEC 046.8
specified cause NEC 323.8
St. Louis type 062.3
subacute sclerosing 046.2
subcorticalis chronica 290.12
summer 062.0
suppurative 324.0
syphilitic 094.81
  congenital 090.41
tick-borne 063.9
torula, torular 117.5 [323.4]

Encephalitis

Encephalitis — *continued*
- toxic NEC 989.9 *[323.7]*
- toxoplasmic (acquired) 130.0
  - congenital (active) 771.2 *[323.4]*
- trichinosis 124 *[323.4]*
- Trypanosomiasis (*see also* Trypanosomiasis) 086.9 *[323.2]*
- tuberculous (*see also* Tuberculosis) 013.6 ✓5ᵗʰ
- type B (Japanese) 062.0
- type C 062.3
- van Bogaert's 046.2
- Venezuelan 066.2
- Vienna type 049.8
- viral, virus 049.9
  - arthropod-borne NEC 064
    - mosquito-borne 062.9
      - Australian X disease 062.4
      - California virus 062.5
      - Eastern equine 062.2
      - Ilheus virus 062.8
      - Japanese (B type) 062.0
      - Murray Valley 062.4
      - specified type NEC 062.8
      - St. Louis 062.3
      - type B 062.0
      - type C 062.3
      - Western equine 062.1
    - tick-borne 063.9
      - biundulant 063.2
      - Central European 063.2
      - Czechoslovakian 063.2
      - diphasic meningoencephalitis 063.2
      - Far Eastern 063.0
      - Langat 063.8
      - louping ill 063.1
      - Powassan 063.8
      - Russian spring-summer (taiga) 063.0
      - specified type NEC 063.8
    - vector unknown 064
  - slow acting NEC 046.8
  - specified type NEC 049.8
  - vaccination, prophylactic (against) V05.0
- von Economo's 049.8
- Western equine 062.1
- West Nile type 066.4 ▲

Encephalocele 742.0
- orbit 376.81

Encephalocystocele 742.0

Encephalomalacia (brain) (cerebellar) (cerebral) (cerebrospinal) (*see also* Softening, brain) 434.9 ✓5ᵗʰ
- due to
  - hemorrhage (*see also* Hemorrhage, brain) 431
  - recurrent spasm of artery 435.9
- embolic (cerebral) (*see also* Embolism, brain) 434.1 ✓5ᵗʰ
- subcorticalis chronicus arteriosclerotica 290.12
- thrombotic (*see also* thrombosis, brain) 434.0 ✓5ᵗʰ

Encephalomeningitis — *see* Meningoencephalitis

Encephalomeningocele 742.0

Encephalomeningomyelitis — *see* Meningoencephalitis

Encephalomeningopathy (*see also* Meningoencephalitis) 349.9

Encephalomyelitis (chronic) (granulomatous) (hemorrhagic necrotizing, acute) (myalgic, benign) (*see also* Encephalitis) 323.9
- abortive disseminated 049.8
- acute disseminated (postinfectious) 136.9 *[323.6]*
  - postimmunization 323.5
- due to or resulting from vaccination (any) 323.5
- equine (acute) (infectious) 062.9
  - Eastern 062.2
  - Venezuelan 066.2
  - Western 062.1
- funicularis infectiosa 049.8
- late effect — *see* Late, effect, encephalitis
- Munch-Peterson's 049.8
- postchickenpox 052.0
- postimmunization 323.5
- postmeasles 055.0
- postvaccinal (smallpox) 323.5

Encephalomyelitis (*see also* Encephalitis) — *continued*
- rubella 056.01
- specified cause NEC 323.8
- syphilitic 094.81

Encephalomyelocele 742.0

Encephalomyelomeningitis — *see* Meningoencephalitis

Encephalomyeloneuropathy 349.9

Encephalomyelopathy 349.9
- subacute necrotizing (infantile) 330.8

Encephalomyeloradiculitis (acute) 357.0

Encephalomyeloradiculoneuritis (acute) 357.0

Encephalomyeloradiculopathy 349.9

Encephalomyocarditis 074.23

Encephalopathia hyperbilirubinemica, newborn 774.7
- due to isoimmunization (conditions classifiable to 773.0-773.2) 773.4

Encephalopathy (acute) 348.3
- alcoholic 291.2
- anoxic — *see* Damage, brain, anoxic
- arteriosclerotic 437.0
  - late effect — *see* Late effect(s) (of) cerebrovascular disease
- bilirubin, newborn 774.7
  - due to isoimmunization 773.4
- congenital 742.9
- demyelinating (callosal) 341.8
- due to
  - birth injury (intracranial) 767.8
  - dialysis 294.8
    - transient 293.9
  - hyperinsulinism — *see* Hyperinsulinism
  - influenza (virus) 487.8
  - lack of vitamin (*see also* Deficiency, vitamin) 269.2
  - nicotinic acid deficiency 291.2
  - serum (nontherapeutic) (therapeutic) 999.5
  - syphilis 094.81
  - trauma (postconcussional) 310.2
    - current (*see also* Concussion, brain) 850.9
      - with skull fracture — *see* Fracture, skull, by site, with intracranial injury
  - vaccination 323.5
- hepatic 572.2
- hyperbilirubinemic, newborn 774.7
  - due to isoimmunization (conditions classifiable to 773.0-773.2) 773.4
- hypertensive 437.2
- hypoglycemic 251.2
- hypoxic — *see* Damage, brain, anoxic
- infantile cystic necrotizing (congenital) 341.8
- lead 984.9 *[323.7]*
- leukopolio 330.0
- metabolic (toxic) — *see* Delirium
- necrotizing, subacute 330.8
- pellagrous 265.2
- portal-systemic 572.2
- postcontusional 310.2
- posttraumatic 310.2
- saturnine 984.9 *[323.7]*
- spongioform, subacute (viral) 046.1
- subacute
  - necrotizing 330.8
  - spongioform 046.1
  - viral, spongioform 046.1
- subcortical progressive (Schilder) 341.1
  - chronic (Binswanger's) 290.12
- toxic 349.82
  - metabolic — *see* Delirium
- traumatic (postconcussional) 310.2
  - current (*see also* Concussion, brain) 850.9
    - with skull fracture — *see* Fracture, skull, by site, with intracranial injury
- vitamin B deficiency NEC 266.9
- Wernicke's (superior hemorrhagic polioencephalitis) 265.1

Encephalorrhagia (*see also* Hemorrhage, brain) 432.9
- healed or old V12.59
- late effect — *see* Late effect(s) (of) cerebrovascular disease

Encephalosis, posttraumatic 310.2

Enchondroma (M9220/0) — *see also* Neoplasm, bone, benign
- multiple, congenital 756.4

Enchondromatosis (cartilaginous) (congenital) (multiple) 756.4

Enchondroses, multiple (cartilaginous) (congenital) 756.4

Encopresis (*see also* Incontinence, feces) 787.6
- nonorganic origin 307.7

Encounter for — *see also* Admission for
- administrative purpose only V68.9
  - referral of patient without examination or treatment V68.81
  - specified purpose NEC V68.89
- chemotherapy V58.1
- end-of-life care V66.7
- hospice care V66.7
- palliative care V66.7
- paternity testing V70.4
- radiotherapy V58.0
- screening mammogram NEC V76.12
  - for high-risk patient V76.11
- terminal care V66.7

Encystment — *see* Cyst

End-of-life care V66.7

Endamebiasis — *see* Amebiasis

Endamoeba — *see* Amebiasis

Endarteritis (bacterial, subacute) (infective) (septic) 447.6
- brain, cerebral or cerebrospinal 437.4
  - late effect — *see* Late effect(s) (of) cerebrovascular disease
- coronary (artery) — *see* Arteriosclerosis, coronary
- deformans — *see* Arteriosclerosis
- embolic (*see also* Embolism) 444.9
- obliterans — *see also* Arteriosclerosis
  - pulmonary 417.8
- pulmonary 417.8
- retina 362.18
- senile — *see* Arteriosclerosis
- syphilitic 093.89
  - brain or cerebral 094.89
  - congenital 090.5
  - spinal 094.89
- tuberculous (*see also* Tuberculosis) 017.9 ✓5ᵗʰ

Endemic — *see* condition

Endocarditis (chronic) (indeterminate) (interstitial) (marantis) (nonbacterial thrombotic) (residual) (sclerotic) (sclerous) (senile) (valvular) 424.90
- with
  - rheumatic fever (conditions classifiable to 390)
    - active — *see* Endocarditis, acute, rheumatic
    - inactive or quiescent (with chorea) 397.9
- acute or subacute 421.9
  - rheumatic (aortic) (mitral) (pulmonary) (tricuspid) 391.1
    - with chorea (acute) (rheumatic) (Sydenham's) 392.0
- aortic (heart) (nonrheumatic) (valve) 424.1
  - with
    - mitral (valve) disease 396.9
      - active or acute 391.1
        - with chorea (acute) (rheumatic) (Sydenham's) 392.0
    - rheumatic fever (conditions classifiable to 390)
      - active — *see* Endocarditis, acute, rheumatic
      - inactive or quiescent (with chorea) 395.9
        - with mitral disease 396.9
  - acute or subacute 421.9
  - arteriosclerotic 424.1
  - congenital 746.89
  - hypertensive 424.1
  - rheumatic (chronic) (inactive) 395.9
    - with mitral (valve) disease 396.9
      - active or acute 391.1
        - with chorea (acute) (rheumatic) (Sydenham's) 392.0

Index to Diseases

Endocarditis — *continued*
  aortic — *continued*
    rheumatic — *continued*
      active or acute 391.1
        with chorea (acute) (rheumatic) (Sydenham's) 392.0
      specified cause, except rheumatic 424.1
      syphilitic 093.22
    arteriosclerotic or due to arteriosclerosis 424.99
    atypical verrucous (Libman-Sacks) 710.0 *[424.91]*
  bacterial (acute) (any valve) (chronic) (subacute) 421.0
  blastomycotic 116.0 *[421.1]*
  candidal 112.81
  congenital 425.3
  constrictive 421.0
  Coxsackie 074.22
  due to
    blastomycosis 116.0 *[421.1]*
    candidiasis 112.81
    Coxsackie (virus) 074.22
    disseminated lupus erythematosus 710.0 *[424.91]*
    histoplasmosis (*see also* Histoplasmosis) 115.94
    hypertension (benign) 424.99
    moniliasis 112.81
    prosthetic cardiac valve 996.61
    Q fever 083.0 *[421.1]*
    serratia marcescens 421.0
    typhoid (fever) 002.0 *[421.1]*
  fetal 425.3
  gonococcal 098.84
  hypertensive 424.99
  infectious or infective (acute) (any valve) (chronic) (subacute) 421.0
  lenta (acute) (any valve) (chronic) (subacute) 421.0
  Libman-Sacks 710.0 *[424.91]*
  Loeffler's (parietal fibroplastic) 421.0
  malignant (acute) (any valve) (chronic) (subacute) 421.0
  meningococcal 036.42
  mitral (chronic) (double) (fibroid) (heart) (inactive) (valve) (with chorea) 394.9
    with
      aortic (valve) disease 396.9
        active or acute 391.1
          with chorea (acute) (rheumatic) (Sydenham's) 392.0
        rheumatic fever (conditions classifiable to 390)
          active — *see* Endocarditis, acute, rheumatic
          inactive or quiescent (with chorea) 394.9
            with aortic valve disease 396.9
    active or acute 391.1
      with chorea (acute) (rheumatic) (Sydenham's) 392.0
      bacterial 421.0
    arteriosclerotic 424.0
    congenital 746.89
    hypertensive 424.0
    nonrheumatic 424.0
      acute or subacute 421.9
    syphilitic 093.21
  monilial 112.81
  mycotic (acute) (any valve) (chronic) (subacute) 421.0
  pneumococcic (acute) (any valve) (chronic) (subacute) 421.0
  pulmonary (chronic) (heart) (valve) 424.3
    with
      rheumatic fever (conditions classifiable to 390)
        active — *see* Endocarditis, acute, rheumatic
        inactive or quiescent (with chorea) 397.1
      acute or subacute 421.9
        rheumatic 391.1
          with chorea (acute) (rheumatic) (Sydenham's) 392.0

Endocarditis — *continued*
  pulmonary — *continued*
    arteriosclerotic or due to arteriosclerosis 424.3
    congenital 746.09
    hypertensive or due to hypertension (benign) 424.3
    rheumatic (chronic) (inactive) (with chorea) 397.1
      active or acute 391.1
        with chorea (acute) (rheumatic) (Sydenham's) 392.0
      syphilitic 093.24
  purulent (acute) (any valve) (chronic) (subacute) 421.0
  rheumatic (chronic) (inactive) (with chorea) 397.9
    active or acute (aortic) (mitral) (pulmonary) (tricuspid) 391.1
      with chorea (acute) (rheumatic) (Sydenham's) 392.0
  septic (acute) (any valve) (chronic) (subacute) 421.0
  specified cause, except rheumatic 424.99
  streptococcal (acute) (any valve) (chronic) (subacute) 421.0
  subacute — *see* Endocarditis, acute
  suppurative (any valve) (acute) (chronic) (subacute) 421.0
  syphilitic NEC 093.20
  toxic (*see also* Endocarditis, acute) 421.9
  tricuspid (chronic) (heart) (inactive) (rheumatic) (valve) (with chorea) 397.0
    with
      rheumatic fever (conditions classifiable to 390)
        active — *see* Endocarditis, acute, rheumatic
        inactive or quiescent (with chorea) 397.0
      active or acute 391.1
        with chorea (acute) (rheumatic) (Sydenham's) 392.0
    arteriosclerotic 424.2
    congenital 746.89
    hypertensive 424.2
    nonrheumatic 424.2
      acute or subacute 421.9
    specified cause, except rheumatic 424.2
    syphilitic 093.23
  tuberculous (*see also* Tuberculosis) 017.9 ☑5ᵗʰ *[424.91]*
  typhoid 002.0 *[421.1]*
  ulcerative (acute) (any valve) (chronic) (subacute) 421.0
  vegetative (acute) (any valve) (chronic) (subacute) 421.0
  verrucous (acute) (any valve) (chronic) (subacute) NEC 710.0 *[424.91]*
    nonbacterial 710.0 *[424.91]*
    nonrheumatic 710.0 *[424.91]*

Endocardium, endocardial — *see also* condition
  cushion defect 745.60
    specified type NEC 745.69

Endocervicitis (*see also* Cervicitis) 616.0
  due to
    intrauterine (contraceptive) device 996.65
  gonorrheal (acute) 098.15
    chronic or duration of 2 months or over 098.35
  hyperplastic 616.0
  syphilitic 095.8
  trichomonal 131.09
  tuberculous (*see also* Tuberculosis) 016.7 ☑5ᵗʰ

Endocrine — *see* condition

Endocrinopathy, pluriglandular 258.9

Endodontitis 522.0

Endomastoiditis (*see also* Mastoiditis) 383.9

Endometrioma 617.9

Endometriosis 617.9
  appendix 617.5
  bladder 617.8
  bowel 617.5
  broad ligament 617.3
  cervix 617.0
  colon 617.5

Endometriosis — *continued*
  cul-de-sac (Douglas') 617.3
  exocervix 617.0
  fallopian tube 617.2
  female genital organ NEC 617.8
  gallbladder 617.8
  in scar of skin 617.6
  internal 617.0
  intestine 617.5
  lung 617.8
  myometrium 617.0
  ovary 617.1
  parametrium 617.3
  pelvic peritoneum 617.3
  peritoneal (pelvic) 617.3
  rectovaginal septum 617.4
  rectum 617.5
  round ligament 617.3
  skin 617.6
  specified site NEC 617.8
  stromal (M8931/1) 236.0
  umbilicus 617.8
  uterus 617.0
    internal 617.0
  vagina 617.4
  vulva 617.8

Endometritis (nonspecific) (purulent) (septic) (suppurative) 615.9
  with
    abortion — *see* Abortion, by type, with sepsis
    ectopic pregnancy (*see also* categories 633.0-633.9) 639.0
    molar pregnancy (*see also* categories 630-632) 639.0
  acute 615.0
  blennorrhagic 098.16
    acute 098.16
    chronic or duration of 2 months or over 098.36
  cervix, cervical (*see also* Cervicitis) 616.0
    hyperplastic 616.0
  chronic 615.1
  complicating pregnancy 646.6 ☑5ᵗʰ
    affecting fetus or newborn 760.8
  decidual 615.9
  following
    abortion 639.0
    ectopic or molar pregnancy 639.0
  gonorrheal (acute) 098.16
    chronic or duration of 2 months or over 098.36
  hyperplastic 621.3
    cervix 616.0
  polypoid — *see* Endometritis, hyperplastic
  puerperal, postpartum, childbirth 670 ☑4ᵗʰ
  senile (atrophic) 615.9
  subacute 615.0
  tuberculous (*see also* Tuberculosis) 016.7 ☑5ᵗʰ

Endometrium — *see* condition

Endomyocardiopathy, South African 425.2

Endomyocarditis — *see* Endocarditis

Endomyofibrosis 425.0

Endomyometritis (*see also* Endometritis) 615.9

Endopericarditis — *see* Endocarditis

Endoperineuritis — *see* Disorder, nerve

Endophlebitis (*see also* Phlebitis) 451.9
  leg 451.2
    deep (vessels) 451.19
    superficial (vessels) 451.0
  portal (vein) 572.1
  retina 362.18
  specified site NEC 451.89
  syphilitic 093.89

Endophthalmia (*see also* Endophthalmitis) 360.00
  gonorrheal 098.42

Endophthalmitis (globe) (infective) (metastatic) (purulent) (subacute) 360.00
  acute 360.01
  chronic 360.03
  parasitis 360.13
  phacoanaphylactic 360.19
  specified type NEC 360.19
  sympathetic 360.11

Endosalpingioma

Endosalpingioma (M9111/1) 236.2
Endosteitis — see Osteomyelitis
Endothelioma, bone (M9260/3) — see Neoplasm, bone, malignant
Endotheliosis 287.8
    hemorrhagic infectional 287.8
Endotoxic shock 785.59
Endotrachelitis (see also Cervicitis) 616.0
Enema rash 692.89
Engel-von Recklinghausen disease or syndrome (osteitis fibrosa cystica) 252.0
Engelmann's disease (diaphyseal sclerosis) 756.9
English disease (see also Rickets) 268.0
Engman's disease (infectious eczematoid dermatitis) 690.8
Engorgement
    breast 611.79
        newborn 778.7
        puerperal, postpartum 676.2 ✓5th
    liver 573.9
    lung 514
    pulmonary 514
    retina, venous 362.37
    stomach 536.8
    venous, retina 362.37
Enlargement, enlarged — see also Hypertrophy
    abdomen 789.3 ✓5th
    adenoids 474.12
        and tonsils 474.10
    alveolar process or ridge 525.8
    apertures of diaphragm (congenital) 756.6
    blind spot, visual field 368.42
    gingival 523.8
    heart, cardiac (see also Hypertrophy, cardiac) 429.3
    lacrimal gland, chronic 375.03
    liver (see also Hypertrophy, liver) 789.1
    lymph gland or node 785.6
    orbit 376.46
    organ or site, congenital NEC — see Anomaly, specified type NEC
    parathyroid (gland) 252.0
    pituitary fossa 793.0
    prostate ▶(simple) (soft)◀ 600.0
    sella turcica 793.0
    spleen (see also Splenomegaly) 789.2
        congenital 759.0
    thymus (congenital) (gland) 254.0
    thyroid (gland) (see also Goiter) 240.9
    tongue 529.8
    tonsils 474.11
        and adenoids 474.10
    uterus 621.2
Enophthalmos 376.50
    due to
        atrophy of orbital tissue 376.51
        surgery 376.52
        trauma 376.52
Enostosis 526.89
Entamebiasis — see Amebiasis
Entamebic — see Amebiasis
Entanglement, umbilical cord(s) 663.3 ✓5th
    with compression 663.2 ✓5th
    affecting fetus or newborn 762.5
    around neck with compression 663.1 ✓5th
    twins in monoamniotic sac 663.2 ✓5th
Enteralgia 789.0 ✓5th
Enteric — see condition
Enteritis (acute) (catarrhal) (choleraic) (chronic) (congestive) (diarrheal) (exudative) (follicular) (hemorrhagic) (infantile) (lienteric) (noninfectious) (perforative) (phlegmonous) (presumed noninfectious) (pseudomembranous) 558.9
    adaptive 564.9
    aertrycke infection 003.0
    allergic 558.3
    amebic (see also Amebiasis) 006.9
        with abscess — see Abscess, amebic
        acute 006.0
            with abscess — see Abscess, amebic
            nondysenteric 006.2

Enteritis — continued
    amebic (see also Amebiasis) — continued
        chronic 006.1
            with abscess — see Abscess, amebic
            nondysenteric 006.2
        nondysenteric 006.2
    anaerobic (cocci) (gram-negative) (gram-positive) (mixed) NEC 008.46
    bacillary NEC 004.9
    bacterial NEC 008.5
        specified NEC 008.49
    Bacteroides (fragilis) (melaninogeniscus) (oralis) 008.46
    Butyrivibrio (fibriosolvens) 008.46
    Campylobacter 008.43
    Candida 112.85
    Chilomastix 007.8
    choleriformis 001.1
    chronic 558.9
        ulcerative (see also Colitis, ulcerative) 556.9
    cicatrizing (chronic) 555.0
    Clostridium
        botulinum 005.1
        difficile 008.45
        haemolyticum 008.46
        novyi 008.46
        perfringens (C) (F) 008.46
        specified type NEC 008.46
    coccidial 007.2
    dietetic 558.9
    due to
        achylia gastrica 536.8
        adenovirus 008.62
        Aerobacter aerogenes 008.2 ✓5th
        anaerobes — see Enteritis, anaerobic
        Arizona (bacillus) 008.1
        astrovirus 008.66
        Bacillus coli — see Enteritis, E. coli 008.0 ✓5th
        bacteria NEC 008.5
            specified NEC 008.49
        Bacteroides 008.46
        Butyrivibrio (fibriosolvens)
        Calcivirus 008.65
        Camplyobacter 008.43
        Clostridium — see Enteritis, Clostridium
        Cockle agent 008.64
        Coxsackie (virus) 008.67
        Ditchling agent 008.64
        ECHO virus 008.67
        Enterobacter aerogenes 008.2 ✓5th
        enterococci 008.49
        enterovirus NEC 008.67
        Escherichia coli — see Enteritis, E. coli 008.0 ✓5th
        Eubacterium 008.46
        Fusobacterium (nucleatum) 008.46
        gram-negative bacteria NEC 008.47
            anaerobic NEC 008.46
        Hawaii agent 008.63
        irritating foods 558.9
        Klebsiella aerogenes 008.47
        Marin County agent 008.66
        Montgomery County agent 008.63
        Norwalk-like agent 008.63
        Norwalk virus 008.63
        Otofuke agent 008.63
        Paracolobactrum arizonae 008.1
        paracolon bacillus NEC 008.47
            Arizona 008.1
        Paramatta agent 008.64
        Peptococcus 008.46
        Peptostreptococcus 008.46
        Proprionibacterium 008.46
        Proteus (bacillus) (mirabilis) (morganii) 008.3
        Pseudomonas aeruginosa 008.42
        Rotavirus 008.61
        Sapporo agent 008.63
        small round virus (SRV) NEC 008.64
            featureless NEC 008.63
            structured NEC 008.63
        Snow Mountain (SM) agent 008.63
        specified
            bacteria NEC 008.49
            organism, nonbacterial NEC 008.8
            virus (NEC) 008.69
        Staphylococcus 008.41

Enteritis — continued
    due to — continued
        Streptococcus 008.49
            anaerobic 008.46
        Taunton agent 008.63
        Torovirus 008.69
        Treponema 008.46
        Veillonella 008.46
        virus 008.8
            specified type NEC 008.69
        Wollan (W) agent 008.64
        Yersinia enterocolitica 008.44
    dysentery — see Dysentery
    E. coli 008.00
        enterohemorrhagic 008.04
        enteroinvasive 008.03
        enteropathogenic 008.01
        enterotoxigenic 008.02
        specified type NEC 008.09
    el tor 001.1
    embadomonial 007.8
    epidemic 009.0
    Eubacterium 008.46
    fermentative 558.9
    fulminant 557.0
    Fusobacterium (nucleatum) 008.46
    gangrenous (see also Enteritis, due to, by organism) 009.0
    giardial 007.1
    gram-negative bacteria NEC 008.47
        anaerobic NEC 008.46
    infectious NEC (see also Enteritis, due to, by organism) 009.0
        presumed 009.1
    influenzal 487.8
    ischemic 557.9
        acute 557.0
        chronic 557.1
        due to mesenteric artery insufficiency 557.1
    membranous 564.9
    mucous 564.9
    myxomembranous 564.9
    necrotic (see also Enteritis, due to, by organism) 009.0
    necroticans 005.2
    necrotizing of fetus or newborn 777.5
    neurogenic 564.9
    newborn 777.8
        necrotizing 777.5
    parasitic NEC 129
    paratyphoid (fever) (see also Fever, paratyphoid) 002.9
    Peptococcus 008.46
    Peptostreptococcus 008.46
    Proprionibacterium 008.46
    protozoal NEC 007.9
    radiation 558.1
    regional (of) 555.9
        intestine
            large (bowel, colon, or rectum) 555.1
                with small intestine 555.2
            small (duodenum, ileum, or jejunum) 555.0
                with large intestine 555.2
    Salmonella infection 003.0
    salmonellosis 003.0
    segmental (see also Enteritis, regional) 555.9
    septic (see also Enteritis, due to, by organism) 009.0
    Shigella 004.9
    simple 558.9
    spasmodic 564.9
    spastic 564.9
    staphylococcal 008.41
        due to food 005.0
    streptococcal 008.49
        anaerobic 008.46
    toxic 558.2
    Treponema (denticola) (macrodentium) 008.46
    trichomonal 007.3
    tuberculous (see also Tuberculosis) 014.8 ✓5th
    typhosa 002.0
    ulcerative (chronic) (see also Colitis, ulcerative) 556.9
    Veillonella 008.46
    viral 008.8
        adenovirus 008.62

Index to Diseases

Enteritis — *continued*
  viral — *continued*
    enterovirus 008.67
    specified virus NEC 008.69
    Yersinia enterocolitica 008.44
    zymotic 009.0
Enteroarticular syndrome 099.3
Enterobiasis 127.4
Enterobius vermicularis 127.4
Enterocele (*see also* Hernia) 553.9
  pelvis, pelvic (acquired) (congenital) 618.6
  vagina, vaginal (acquired) (congenital) 618.6
Enterocolitis — *see also* Enteritis
  fetus or newborn 777.8
    necrotizing 777.5
  fulminant 557.0
  granulomatous 555.2
  hemorrhagic (acute) 557.0
    chronic 557.1
  necrotizing (acute) (membranous) 557.0
  primary necrotizing 777.5
  pseudomembranous 008.45
  radiation 558.1
    newborn 777.5
  ulcerative 556.0
Enterocystoma 751.5
Enterogastritis — *see* Enteritis
Enterogenous cyanosis 289.7
Enterolith, enterolithiasis (impaction) 560.39
  with hernia — *see also* Hernia, by site, with obstruction
    gangrenous — *see* Hernia, by site, with gangrene
Enteropathy 569.9
  exudative (of Gordon) 579.8
  gluten 579.0
  hemorrhagic, terminal 557.0
  protein-losing 579.8
Enteroperitonitis (*see also* Peritonitis) 567.9
Enteroptosis 569.89
Enterorrhagia 578.9
Enterospasm 564.9
  psychogenic 306.4
Enterostenosis (*see also* Obstruction, intestine) 560.9
Enterostomy status V44.4
  with complication 569.60
Enthesopathy 726.39
  ankle and tarsus 726.70
  elbow region 726.30
    specified NEC 726.39
  hip 726.5
  knee 726.60
  peripheral NEC 726.8
  shoulder region 726.10
    adhesive 726.0
  spinal 720.1
  wrist and carpus 726.4
Entrance, air into vein — *see* Embolism, air
Entrapment, nerve — *see* Neuropathy, entrapment
Entropion (eyelid) 374.00
  cicatricial 374.04
  congenital 743.62
  late effect of trachoma (healed) 139.1
  mechanical 374.02
  paralytic 374.02
  senile 374.01
  spastic 374.03
Enucleation of eye (current) (traumatic) 871.3
Enuresis 788.30
  habit disturbance 307.6
  nocturnal 788.36
    psychogenic 307.6
  nonorganic origin 307.6
  psychogenic 307.6
Enzymopathy 277.9
Eosinopenia 288.0
Eosinophilia 288.3
  allergic 288.3
  hereditary 288.3
  idiopathic 288.3

Eosinophilia — *continued*
  infiltrative 518.3
  Loeffler's 518.3
  myalgia syndrome 710.5
  pulmonary (tropical) 518.3
  secondary 288.3
  tropical 518.3
Eosinophilic — *see also* condition
  fasciitis 728.89
  granuloma (bone) 277.8
  infiltration lung 518.3
Ependymitis (acute) (cerebral) (chronic) (granular) (*see also* Meningitis) 322.9
Ependymoblastoma (M9392/3)
  specified site — *see* Neoplasm, by site, malignant
  unspecified site 191.9
Ependymoma (epithelial) (malignant) (M9391/3)
  anaplastic type (M9392/3)
    specified site — *see* Neoplasm, by site, malignant
    unspecified site 191.9
  benign (M9391/0)
    specified site — *see* Neoplasm, by site, benign
    unspecified site 225.0
  myxopapillary (M9394/1) 237.5
  papillary (M9393/1) 237.5
  specified site — *see* Neoplasm, by site, malignant
  unspecified site 191.9
Ependymopathy 349.2
  spinal cord 349.2
Ephelides, ephelis 709.09
Ephemeral fever (*see also* Pyrexia) 780.6
Epiblepharon (congenital) 743.62
Epicanthus, epicanthic fold (congenital) (eyelid) 743.63
Epicondylitis (elbow) (lateral) 726.32
  medial 726.31
Epicystitis (*see also* Cystitis) 595.9
Epidemic — *see* condition
Epidermidalization, cervix — *see* condition
Epidermidization, cervix — *see* condition
Epidermis, epidermal — *see* condition
Epidermization, cervix — *see* condition
Epidermodysplasia verruciformis 078.19
Epidermoid
  cholesteatoma — *see* Cholesteatoma
  inclusion (*see also* Cyst, skin) 706.2
Epidermolysis
  acuta (combustiformis) (toxica) 695.1
  bullosa 757.39
  necroticans combustiformis 695.1
    due to drug
      correct substance properly administered 695.1
      overdose or wrong substance given or taken 977.9
        specified drug — *see* Table of Drugs and Chemicals
Epidermophytid — *see* Dermatophytosis
Epidermophytosis (infected) — *see* Dermatophytosis
Epidermosis, ear (middle) (*see also* Cholesteatoma) 385.30
Epididymis — *see* condition
Epididymitis (nonvenereal) 604.90
  with abscess 604.0
  acute 604.99
  blennorrhagic (acute) 098.0
    chronic or duration of 2 months or over 098.2
  caseous (*see also* Tuberculosis) 016.4
  chlamydial 099.54
  diphtheritic 032.89 [604.91]
  filarial 125.9 [604.91]
  gonococcal (acute) 098.0
    chronic or duration of 2 months or over 098.2
  recurrent 604.99
  residual 604.99
  syphilitic 095.8 [604.91]

Epididymitis — *continued*
  tuberculous (*see also* Tuberculosis) 016.4
Epididymo-orchitis (*see also* Epididymitis) 604.90
  with abscess 604.0
  chlamydial 099.54
  gonococcal (acute) 098.13
    chronic or duration of 2 months or over 098.33
Epidural — *see* condition
Epigastritis (*see also* Gastritis) 535.5
Epigastrium, epigastric — *see* condition
Epigastrocele (*see also* Hernia, epigastric) 553.29
Epiglottiditis (acute) 464.30
  with obstruction 464.31
  chronic 476.1
  viral 464.30
    with obstruction 464.31
Epiglottis — *see* condition
Epiglottitis (acute) 464.30
  with obstruction 464.31
  chronic 476.1
  viral 464.30
    with obstruction 464.31
Epignathus 759.4
Epilepsia
  partialis continua (*see also* Epilepsy) 345.7
  procursiva (*see also* Epilepsy) 345.8
Epilepsy, epileptic (idiopathic) 345.9

> *Note* — *use the following fifth-digit subclassification with categories 345.0, 345.1, 345.4–345.9:*
>   0 *without mention of intractable epilepsy*
>   1 *with intractable epilepsy*

  abdominal 345.5
  absence (attack) 345.0
  akinetic 345.0
    psychomotor 345.4
  automatism 345.4
  autonomic diencephalic 345.5
  brain 345.9
  Bravais-Jacksonian 345.5
  cerebral 345.9
  climacteric 345.9
  clonic 345.1
  clouded state 345.9
  coma 345.3
  communicating 345.4
  congenital 345.9
  convulsions 345.9
  cortical (focal) (motor) 345.5
  cursive (running) 345.8
  cysticercosis 123.1
  deterioration
    with behavioral disturbance 345.9 [294.11]
    without behavioral disturbance 345.9 [294.10]
  due to syphilis 094.89
  equivalent 345.5
  fit 345.9
  focal (motor) 345.5
  gelastic 345.8
  generalized 345.9
    convulsive 345.1
    flexion 345.1
    nonconvulsive 345.0
  grand mal (idiopathic) 345.1
  Jacksonian (motor) (sensory) 345.5
  Kojevnikoff's, Kojevnikov's, Kojewnikoff's 345.7
  laryngeal 786.2
  limbic system 345.4
  major (motor) 345.1
  minor 345.0
  mixed (type) 345.9
  motor partial 345.5
  musicogenic 345.1
  myoclonus, myoclonic 345.1
    progressive (familial) 333.2
  nonconvulsive, generalized 345.0
  parasitic NEC 123.9

Epilepsy, epileptic

Epilepsy, epileptic — *continued*
   partial (focalized) 345.5 ✓5th
      with
         impairment of consciousness 345.4 ✓5th
         memory and ideational disturbances 345.4 ✓5th
      abdominal type 345.5 ✓5th
      motor type 345.5 ✓5th
      psychomotor type 345.4 ✓5th
      psychosensory type 345.4 ✓5th
      secondarily generalized 345.4 ✓5th
      sensory type 345.5 ✓5th
      somatomotor type 345.5 ✓5th
      somatosensory type 345.5 ✓5th
      temporal lobe type 345.4 ✓5th
      visceral type 345.5 ✓5th
      visual type 345.5 ✓5th
   peripheral 345.9 ✓5th
   petit mal 345.0 ✓5th
   photokinetic 345.8 ✓5th
   progressive myoclonic (familial) 333.2
   psychic equivalent 345.5 ✓5th
   psychomotor 345.4 ✓5th
   psychosensory 345.4 ✓5th
   reflex 345.1 ✓5th
   seizure 345.9 ✓5th
   senile 345.9 ✓5th
   sensory-induced 345.5 ✓5th
   sleep 347
   somatomotor type 345.5 ✓5th
   somatosensory 345.5 ✓5th
   specified type NEC 345.8 ✓5th
   status (grand mal) 345.3
      focal motor 345.7 ✓5th
      petit mal 345.2
      psychomotor 345.7 ✓5th
      temporal lobe 345.7 ✓5th
   symptomatic 345.9 ✓5th
   temporal lobe 345.4 ✓5th
   tonic (-clonic) 345.1 ✓5th
   traumatic (injury unspecified) 907.0
      injury specified — *see* Late, effect (of) specified injury
   twilight 293.0
   uncinate (gyrus) 345.4 ✓5th
   Unverricht (-Lundborg) (familial myoclonic) 333.2
   visceral 345.5 ✓5th
   visual 345.5 ✓5th
Epileptiform
   convulsions 780.39
   seizure 780.39
Epiloia 759.5
Epimenorrhea 626.2
Epipharyngitis (*see also* Nasopharyngitis) 460
Epiphora 375.20
   due to
      excess lacrimation 375.21
      insufficient drainage 375.22
Epiphyseal arrest 733.91
   femoral head 732.2
Epiphyseolysis, epiphysiolysis (*see also* Osteochondrosis) 732.9
Epiphysitis (*see also* Osteochondrosis) 732.9
   juvenile 732.6
   marginal (Scheuermann's) 732.0
   os calcis 732.5
   syphilitic (congenital) 090.0
   vertebral (Scheuermann's) 732.0
Epiplocele (*see also* Hernia) 553.9
Epiploitis (*see also* Peritonitis) 567.9
Epiplosarcomphalocele (*see also* Hernia, umbilicus) 553.1
Episcleritis 379.00
   gouty 274.89 [379.09]
   nodular 379.02
   periodica fugax 379.01
      angioneurotic — *see* Edema, angioneurotic
   specified NEC 379.09
   staphylococcal 379.00
   suppurative 379.00
   syphilitic 095.0
   tuberculous (*see also* Tuberculosis) 017.3 ✓5th [379.09]

Episode
   brain (*see also* Disease, cerebrovascular, acute) 436
   cerebral (*see also* Disease, cerebrovascular, acute) 436
   depersonalization (in neurotic state) 300.6
   hyporesponsive 780.09
   psychotic (*see also* Psychosis) 298.9
      organic, transient 293.9
   schizophrenic (acute) NEC (*see also* Schizophrenia) 295.4 ✓5th
Epispadias
   female 753.8
   male 752.62
Episplenitis 289.59
Epistaxis (multiple) 784.7
   hereditary 448.0
   vicarious menstruation 625.8
Epithelioma (malignant) (M8011/3) — *see also* Neoplasm, by site, malignant
   adenoides cysticum (M8100/0) — *see* Neoplasm, skin, benign
   basal cell (M8090/3) — *see* Neoplasm, skin, malignant
   benign (M8011/0) — *see* Neoplasm, by site, benign
   Bowen's (M8081/2) — *see* Neoplasm, skin, in situ
   calcifying (benign) (Malherbe's) (M8110/0) — *see* Neoplasm, skin, benign
   external site — *see* Neoplasm, skin, malignant
   intraepidermal, Jadassohn (M8096/0) — *see* Neoplasm, skin, benign
   squamous cell (M8070/3) — *see* Neoplasm, by site, malignant
Epitheliopathy
   pigment, retina 363.15
   posterior multifocal placoid (acute) 363.15
Epithelium, epithelial — *see* condition
Epituberculosis (allergic) (with atelectasis) (*see also* Tuberculosis) 010.8 ✓5th
Eponychia 757.5
Epstein's
   nephrosis or syndrome (*see also* Nephrosis) 581.9
   pearl (mouth) 528.4
Epstein-Barr infection (viral) 075
   chronic 780.79 [139.8]
Epulis (giant cell) (gingiva) 523.8
Equinia 024
Equinovarus (congenital) 754.51
   acquired 736.71
Equivalent
   convulsive (abdominal) (*see also* Epilepsy) 345.5 ✓5th
   epileptic (psychic) (*see also* Epilepsy) 345.5 ✓5th
Erb's
   disease 359.1
   palsy, paralysis (birth) (brachial) (newborn) 767.6
      spinal (spastic) syphilitic 094.89
   pseudohypertrophic muscular dystrophy 359.1
Erb (-Duchenne) paralysis (birth injury) (newborn) 767.6
Erb-Goldflam disease or syndrome 358.0
Erdheim's syndrome (acromegalic macrospondylitis) 253.0
Erection, painful (persistent) 607.3
Ergosterol deficiency (vitamin D) 268.9
   with
      osteomalacia 268.2
      rickets (*see also* Rickets) 268.0
Ergotism (ergotized grain) 988.2
   from ergot used as drug (migraine therapy)
      correct substance properly administered 349.82
      overdose or wrong substance given or taken 975.0
Erichsen's disease (railway spine) 300.16
Erlacher-Blount syndrome (tibia vara) 732.4
Erosio interdigitalis blastomycetica 112.3

Erosion
   artery NEC 447.2
      without rupture 447.8
   arteriosclerotic plaque — *see* Arteriosclerosis, by site
   bone 733.99
   bronchus 519.1
   cartilage (joint) 733.99
   cervix (uteri) (acquired) (chronic) (congenital) 622.0
      with mention of cervicitis 616.0
   cornea (recurrent) (*see also* Keratitis) 371.42
      traumatic 918.1
   dental (idiopathic) (occupational) 521.3
   duodenum, postpyloric — *see* Ulcer, duodenum
   esophagus 530.89
   gastric 535.4 ✓5th
   intestine 569.89
   lymphatic vessel 457.8
   pylorus, pyloric (ulcer) 535.4 ✓5th
   sclera 379.16
   spine, aneurysmal 094.89
   spleen 289.59
   stomach 535.4 ✓5th
   teeth (idiopathic) (occupational) 521.3
      due to
         medicine 521.3
         persistent vomiting 521.3
   urethra 599.84
   uterus 621.8
   vertebra 733.99
Erotomania 302.89
   Clérambault's 297.8
Error
   in diet 269.9
   refractive 367.9
      astigmatism (*see also* Astigmatism) 367.20
      drug-induced 367.89
      hypermetropia 367.0
      hyperopia 367.0
      myopia 367.1
      presbyopia 367.4
      toxic 367.89
Eructation 787.3
   nervous 306.4
   psychogenic 306.4
Eruption
   creeping 126.9
   drug — *see* Dermatitis, due to, drug
   Hutchinson, summer 692.72
   Kaposi's varicelliform 054.0
   napkin (psoriasiform) 691.0
   polymorphous
      light (sun) 692.72
         other source 692.82
   psoriasiform, napkin 691.0
   recalcitrant pustular 694.8
   ringed 695.89
   skin (*see also* Dermatitis) 782.1
      creeping (meaning hookworm) 126.9
      due to
         chemical(s) NEC 692.4
            internal use 693.8
         drug — *see* Dermatitis, due to, drug
         prophylactic inoculation or vaccination against disease — *see* Dermatitis, due to, vaccine
         smallpox vaccination NEC — *see* Dermatitis, due to, vaccine
      erysipeloid 027.1
      feigned 698.4
      Hutchinson, summer 692.72
      Kaposi's, varicelliform 054.0
         vaccinia 999.0
      lichenoid, axilla 698.3
      polymorphous, due to light 692.72
      toxic NEC 695.0
      vesicular 709.8
   teeth, tooth
      accelerated 520.6
      delayed 520.6
      difficult 520.6
      disturbance of 520.6
      in abnormal sequence 520.6
      incomplete 520.6
      late 520.6

Index to Diseases

Eruption — *continued*
  teeth, tooth — *continued*
    natal 520.6
    neonatal 520.6
    obstructed 520.6
    partial 520.6
    persistent primary 520.6
    premature 520.6
  vesicular 709.8
Erysipelas (gangrenous) (infantile) (newborn) (phlegmonous) (suppurative) 035
  external ear 035 *[380.13]*
  puerperal, postpartum, childbirth 670 ✓5ᵗʰ
Erysipelatoid (Rosenbach's) 027.1
Erysipeloid (Rosenbach's) 027.1
Erythema, erythematous (generalized) 695.9
  ab igne — *see* Burn, by site, first degree
  annulare (centrifugum) (rheumaticum) 695.0
  arthriticum epidemicum 026.1
  brucellum (*see also* Brucellosis) 023.9
  bullosum 695.1
  caloricum — *see* Burn, by site, first degree
  chronicum migrans 088.81
    chronicum 088.81
  circinatum 695.1
  diaper 691.0
  due to
    chemical (contact) NEC 692.4
      internal 693.8
    drug (internal use) 693.0
      contact 692.3
  elevatum diutinum 695.89
  endemic 265.2
  epidemic, arthritic 026.1
  figuratum perstans 695.0
  gluteal 691.0
  gyratum (perstans) (repens) 695.1
  heat — *see* Burn, by site, first degree
  ichthyosiforme congenitum 757.1
  induratum (primary) (scrofulosorum) (*see also* Tuberculosis) 017.1 ✓5ᵗʰ
    nontuberculous 695.2
  infantum febrile 057.8
  infectional NEC 695.9
  infectiosum 057.0
  inflammation NEC 695.9
  intertrigo 695.89
  iris 695.1
  lupus (discoid) (localized) (*see also* Lupus erythematosus) 695.4
  marginatum 695.0
    rheumaticum — *see* Fever, rheumatic
  medicamentosum — *see* Dermatitis, due to, drug
  migrans 529.1
    chronicum 088.81
  multiforme 695.1
    bullosum 695.1
    conjunctiva 695.1
    exudativum (Hebra) 695.1
    pemphigoides 694.5
  napkin 691.0
  neonatorum 778.8
  nodosum 695.2
    tuberculous (*see also* Tuberculosis) 017.1 ✓5ᵗʰ
  nummular, nummulare 695.1
  palmar 695.0
  palmaris hereditarium 695.0
  pernio 991.5
  perstans solare 692.72
  rash, newborn 778.8
  scarlatiniform (exfoliative) (recurrent) 695.0
  simplex marginatum 057.8
  solare (*see also* Sunburn) 692.71
  streptogenes 696.5
  toxic, toxicum NEC 695.0
    newborn 778.8
  tuberculous (primary) (*see also* Tuberculosis) 017.0 ✓5ᵗʰ
  venenatum 695.0
Erythematosus — *see* condition
Erythematous — *see* condition
Erythermalgia (primary) 443.89
Erythralgia 443.89
Erythrasma 039.0

Erythredema 985.0
  polyneuritica 985.0
  polyneuropathy 985.0
Erythremia (acute) (M9841/3) 207.0 ✓5ᵗʰ
  chronic (M9842/3) 207.1 ✓5ᵗʰ
  secondary 289.0
Erythroblastopenia (acquired) 284.8
  congenital 284.0
Erythroblastophthisis 284.0
Erythroblastosis (fetalis) (newborn) 773.2
  due to
    ABO
      antibodies 773.1
      incompatibility, maternal/fetal 773.1
      isoimmunization 773.1
    Rh
      antibodies 773.0
      incompatibility, maternal/fetal 773.0
      isoimmunization 773.0
Erythrocyanosis (crurum) 443.89
Erythrocythemia — *see* Erythremia
Erythrocytopenia 285.9
Erythrocytosis (megalosplenic)
  familial 289.6
  oval, hereditary (*see also* Elliptocytosis) 282.1
  secondary 289.0
  stress 289.0
Erythroderma (*see also* Erythema) 695.9
  desquamativa (in infants) 695.89
  exfoliative 695.89
  ichthyosiform, congenital 757.1
  infantum 695.89
  maculopapular 696.2
  neonatorum 778.8
  psoriaticum 696.1
  secondary 695.9
Erythrogenesis imperfecta 284.0
Erythroleukemia (M9840/3) 207.0 ✓5ᵗʰ
Erythromelalgia 443.89
Erythromelia 701.8
Erythropenia 285.9
Erythrophagocytosis 289.9
Erythrophobia 300.23
Erythroplakia
  oral mucosa 528.7
  tongue 528.7
Erythroplasia (Queyrat) (M8080/2)
  specified site — *see* Neoplasm, skin, in situ
  unspecified site 233.5
Erythropoiesis, idiopathic ineffective 285.0
Escaped beats, heart 427.60
  postoperative 997.1
Esoenteritis — *see* Enteritis
Esophagalgia 530.89
Esophagectasis 530.89
  due to cardiospasm 530.0
Esophagismus 530.5
Esophagitis (alkaline) (chemical) (chronic) (infectional) (necrotic) (peptic) (postoperative) (regurgitant) 530.10
  acute 530.12
  candidal 112.84
  reflux 530.11
  specified NEC 530.19
  tuberculous (*see also* Tuberculosis) 017.8 ✓5ᵗʰ
  ulcerative 530.19
Esophagocele 530.6
Esophagodynia 530.89
Esophagomalacia 530.89
Esophagoptosis 530.89
Esophagospasm 530.5
Esophagostenosis 530.3
Esophagostomiasis 127.7
Esophagotracheal — *see* condition
Esophagus — *see* condition
Esophoria 378.41
  convergence, excess 378.84
  divergence, insufficiency 378.85
Esotropia (nonaccommodative) 378.00
  accommodative 378.35

Esotropia — *continued*
  alternating 378.05
    with
      A pattern 378.06
      specified noncomitancy NEC 378.08
      V pattern 378.07
      X pattern 378.08
      Y pattern 378.08
    intermittent 378.22
  intermittent 378.20
    alternating 378.22
    monocular 378.21
  monocular 378.01
    with
      A pattern 378.02
      specified noncomitancy NEC 378.04
      V pattern 378.03
      X pattern 378.04
      Y pattern 378.04
    intermittent 378.21
Espundia 085.5
Essential — *see* condition
Esterapenia 289.8
Esthesioneuroblastoma (M9522/3) 160.0
Esthesioneurocytoma (M9521/3) 160.0
Esthesioneuroepithelioma (M9523/3) 160.0
Esthiomene 099.1
Estivo-autumnal
  fever 084.0
  malaria 084.0
Estrangement V61.0
Estriasis 134.0
Ethanolaminuria 270.8
Ethanolism (*see also* Alcoholism) 303.9 ✓5ᵗʰ
Ether dependence, dependency (*see also* Dependence) 304.6 ✓5ᵗʰ
Etherism (*see also* Dependence) 304.6 ✓5ᵗʰ
Ethmoid, ethmoidal — *see* condition
Ethmoiditis (chronic) (nonpurulent) (purulent) (*see also* Sinusitis, ethmoidal) 473.2
  influenzal 487.1
  Woakes' 471.1
Ethylism (*see also* Alcoholism) 303.9 ✓5ᵗʰ
Eulenburg's disease (congenital paramyotonia) 359.2
Eunuchism 257.2
Eunuchoidism 257.2
  hypogonadotropic 257.2
European blastomycosis 117.5
Eustachian — *see* condition
Euthyroid sick syndrome 790.94
Euthyroidism 244.9
Evaluation
  fetal lung maturity 659.8
  for suspected condition (*see also* Observation) V71.9
    abuse V71.81
    exposure
      anthrax V71.82
      biologic agent NEC V71.83
    neglect V71.81
    newborn — *see* Observation, suspected, condition, newborn
    specified condition NEC V71.89
  mental health V70.2
    requested by authority V70.1
  nursing care V63.8
  social service V63.8
Evan's syndrome (thrombocytopenic purpura) 287.3
Eventration
  colon into chest — *see* Hernia, diaphragm
  diaphragm (congenital) 756.6
Eversion
  bladder 596.8
  cervix (uteri) 622.0
    with mention of cervicitis 616.0
  foot NEC 736.79
    congenital 755.67
  lacrimal punctum 375.51
  punctum lacrimale (postinfectional) (senile) 375.51

Eversion

Eversion — *continued*
- ureter (meatus) 593.89
- urethra (meatus) 599.84
- uterus 618.1
  - complicating delivery 665.2 ✓5ᵗʰ
    - affecting fetus or newborn 763.89
  - puerperal, postpartum 674.8 ✓5ᵗʰ

Evisceration
- birth injury 767.8
- bowel (congenital) — see Hernia, ventral
- congenital (see also Hernia, ventral) 553.29
- operative wound 998.32 ▲
- traumatic NEC 869.1
  - eye 871.3

Evulsion — see Avulsion

Ewing's
- angioendothelioma (M9260/3) — see Neoplasm, bone, malignant
- sarcoma (M9260/3) — see Neoplasm, bone, malignant
- tumor (M9260/3) — see Neoplasm, bone, malignant

Exaggerated lumbosacral angle (with impinging spine) 756.12

Examination (general) (routine) (of) (for) V70.9
- allergy V72.7
- annual V70.0
- cardiovascular preoperative V72.81
- cervical Papanicolaou smear V76.2
  - as a part of routine gynecological examination V72.3
- child care (routine) V20.2
- clinical research investigation (normal control patient) (participant) V70.7
- dental V72.2
- developmental testing (child) (infant) V20.2
- donor (potential) V70.8
- ear V72.1
- eye V72.0
- following
  - accident (motor vehicle) V71.4
  - alleged rape or seduction (victim or culprit) V71.5
  - inflicted injury (victim or culprit) NEC V71.6
  - rape or seduction, alleged (victim or culprit) V71.5
  - treatment (for) V67.9
    - combined V67.6
    - fracture V67.4
    - involving high-risk medication NEC V67.51
    - mental disorder V67.3
    - specified condition NEC V67.59
- follow-up (routine) (following) V67.9
  - cancer chemotherapy V67.2
  - chemotherapy V67.2
  - disease NEC V67.59
  - high-risk medication NEC V67.51
  - injury NEC V67.59
  - population survey V70.6
  - postpartum V24.2
  - psychiatric V67.3
  - psychotherapy V67.3
  - radiotherapy V67.1
  - specified surgery NEC V67.09
  - surgery V67.00
    - vaginal pap smear V67.01
- gynecological V72.3
  - for contraceptive maintenance V25.40
    - intrauterine device V25.42
    - pill V25.41
    - specified method NEC V25.49
- health (of)
  - armed forces personnel V70.5
  - checkup V70.0
  - child, routine V20.2
  - defined subpopulation NEC V70.5
  - inhabitants of institutions V70.5
  - occupational V70.5
  - pre-employment screening V70.5
  - preschool children V70.5
    - for admission to school V70.3
  - prisoners V70.5
    - for entrance into prison V70.3
  - prostitutes V70.5
  - refugees V70.5

Examination — *continued*
- health — *continued*
  - school children V70.5
  - students V70.5
- hearing V72.1
- infant V20.2
- laboratory V72.6
- lactating mother V24.1
- medical (for) (of) V70.9
  - administrative purpose NEC V70.3
  - admission to
    - old age home V70.3
    - prison V70.3
    - school V70.3
  - adoption V70.3
  - armed forces personnel V70.5
  - at health care facility V70.0
  - camp V70.3
  - child, routine V20.2
  - clinical research investigation (control) (normal comparison) (participant) V70.7
  - defined subpopulation NEC V70.5
  - donor (potential) V70.8
  - driving license V70.3
  - general V70.9
    - routine V70.0
    - specified reason NEC V70.8
  - immigration V70.3
  - inhabitants of institutions V70.5
  - insurance certification V70.3
  - marriage V70.3
  - medicolegal reasons V70.4
  - naturalization V70.3
  - occupational V70.5
  - population survey V70.6
  - pre-employment V70.5
  - preschool children V70.5
    - for admission to school V70.3
  - prison V70.3
  - prisoners V70.5
    - for entrance into prison V70.3
  - prostitutes V70.5
  - refugees V70.5
  - school children V70.5
  - specified reason NEC V70.8
  - sport competition V70.3
  - students V70.5
- medicolegal reason V70.4
- pelvic (annual) (periodic) V72.3
- periodic (annual) (routine) V70.0
- postpartum
  - immediately after delivery V24.0
  - routine follow-up V24.2
- pregnancy (unconfirmed) (possible) V72.4
- prenatal V22.1
  - first pregnancy V22.0
  - high-risk pregnancy V23.9
    - specified problem NEC V23.8 ✓5ᵗʰ
- preoperative V72.84
  - cardiovascular V72.81
  - respiratory V72.82
  - specified NEC V72.83
- psychiatric V70.2
  - follow-up not needing further care V67.3
  - requested by authority V70.1
- radiological NEC V72.5
- respiratory preoperative V72.82
- screening — see Screening
- sensitization V72.7
- skin V72.7
  - hypersensitivity V72.7
- special V72.9
- specified type or reason NEC V72.85
  - preoperative V72.83
  - specified NEC V72.83
- teeth V72.2
- victim or culprit following
  - alleged rape or seduction V71.5
  - inflicted injury NEC V71.6
- vaginal Papanicolaou smear V76.47
  - following hysterectomy for malignant condition V67.01
- vision V72.0
- well baby V20.2

Exanthem, exanthema (see also Rash) 782.1
- Boston 048
- epidemic, with meningitis 048
- lichenoid psoriasiform 696.2
- subitum 057.8
- viral, virus NEC 057.9
  - specified type NEC 057.8

Excess, excessive, excessively
- alcohol level in blood 790.3
- carbohydrate tissue, localized 278.1
- carotene (dietary) 278.3
- cold 991.9
  - specified effect NEC 991.8
- convergence 378.84
- crying of infant (baby) 780.92 ●
- development, breast 611.1
- diaphoresis 780.8
- divergence 378.85
- drinking (alcohol) NEC (see also Abuse, drugs, nondependent) 305.0 ✓5ᵗʰ
  - continual (see also Alcoholism) 303.9 ✓5ᵗʰ
  - habitual (see also Alcoholism) 303.9 ✓5ᵗʰ
- eating 783.6
- eyelid fold (congenital) 743.62
- fat 278.00
  - in heart (see also Degeneration, myocardial) 429.1
  - tissue, localized 278.1
- foreskin 605
- gas 787.3
- gastrin 251.5
- glucagon 251.4
- heat (see also Heat) 992.9
- large
  - colon 564.7
    - congenital 751.3
  - fetus or infant 766.0
    - with obstructed labor 660.1 ✓5ᵗʰ
      - affecting management of pregnancy 656.6 ✓5ᵗʰ
    - causing disproportion 653.5 ✓5ᵗʰ
  - newborn (weight of 4500 grams or more) 766.0
  - organ or site, congenital NEC — see Anomaly, specified type NEC
- lid fold (congenital) 743.62
- long
  - colon 751.5
  - organ or site, congenital NEC — see Anomaly, specified type NEC
  - umbilical cord (entangled)
    - affecting fetus or newborn 762.5
    - in pregnancy or childbirth 663.3 ✓5ᵗʰ
      - with compression 663.2 ✓5ᵗʰ
- menstruation 626.2
- number of teeth 520.1
  - causing crowding 524.3
- nutrients (dietary) NEC 783.6
- potassium (K) 276.7
- salivation (see also Ptyalism) 527.7
- secretion — see also Hypersecretion
  - milk 676.6 ✓5ᵗʰ
  - sputum 786.4
  - sweat 780.8
- short
  - organ or site, congenital NEC — see Anomaly, specified type NEC
  - umbilical cord
    - affecting fetus or newborn 762.6
    - in pregnancy or childbirth 663.4 ✓5ᵗʰ
- skin NEC 701.9
  - eyelid 743.62
    - acquired 374.30
- sodium (Na) 276.0
- sputum 786.4
- sweating 780.8
- tearing (ducts) (eye) (see also Epiphora) 375.20
- thirst 783.5
  - due to deprivation of water 994.3
- vitamin
  - A (dietary) 278.2
    - administered as drug (chronic) (prolonged excessive intake) 278.2
    - reaction to sudden overdose 963.5

Index to Diseases

Excess, excessive, excessively — *continued*
  vitamin — *continued*
    D (dietary) 278.4
      administered as drug (chronic) (prolonged excessive intake) 278.4
      reaction to sudden overdose 963.5
  weight 278.00
    gain 783.1
      of pregnancy 646.1 ✓5ᵗʰ
    loss 783.21

Excitability, abnormal, under minor stress 309.29

Excitation
  catatonic (*see also* Schizophrenia) 295.2 ✓5ᵗʰ
  psychogenic 298.1
  reactive (from emotional stress, psychological trauma) 298.1

Excitement
  manic (*see also* Psychosis, affective) 296.0 ✓5ᵗʰ
    recurrent episode 296.1 ✓5ᵗʰ
    single episode 296.0 ✓5ᵗʰ
  mental, reactive (from emotional stress, psychological trauma) 298.1
  state, reactive (from emotional stress, psychological trauma) 298.1

Excluded pupils 364.76

Excoriation (traumatic) (*see also* Injury, superficial, by site) 919.8
  neurotic 698.4

Excyclophoria 378.44

Excyclotropia 378.33

Exencephalus, exencephaly 742.0

Exercise
  breathing V57.0
  remedial NEC V57.1
  therapeutic NEC V57.1

Exfoliation, teeth due to systemic causes 525.0

Exfoliative — *see also* condition dermatitis 695.89

Exhaustion, exhaustive (physical NEC) 780.79
  battle (*see also* Reaction, stress, acute) 308.9
  cardiac (*see also* Failure, heart) 428.9
  delirium (*see also* Reaction, stress, acute) 308.9
  due to
    cold 991.8
    excessive exertion 994.5
    exposure 994.4
  fetus or newborn 779.89 ▲
  heart (*see also* Failure, heart) 428.9
  heat 992.5
    due to
      salt depletion 992.4
      water depletion 992.3
  manic (*see also* Psychosis, affective) 296.0 ✓5ᵗʰ
    recurrent episode 296.1 ✓5ᵗʰ
    single episode 296.0 ✓5ᵗʰ
  maternal, complicating delivery 669.8 ✓5ᵗʰ
    affecting fetus or newborn 763.89
  mental 300.5
  myocardium, myocardial (*see also* Failure, heart) 428.9
  nervous 300.5
  old age 797
  postinfectional NEC 780.79
  psychogenic 300.5
  psychosis (*see also* Reaction, stress, acute) 308.9
  senile 797
    dementia 290.0

Exhibitionism (sexual) 302.4

Exomphalos 756.79

Exophoria 378.42
  convergence, insufficiency 378.83
  divergence, excess 378.85

Exophthalmic
  cachexia 242.0 ✓5ᵗʰ
  goiter 242.0 ✓5ᵗʰ
  ophthalmoplegia 242.0 ✓5ᵗʰ [376.22]

Exophthalmos 376.30
  congenital 743.66
  constant 376.31
  endocrine NEC 259.9 [376.22]
  hyperthyroidism 242.0 ✓5ᵗʰ [376.21]

Exophthalmos — *continued*
  intermittent NEC 376.34
  malignant 242.0 ✓5ᵗʰ [376.21]
  pulsating 376.35
    endocrine NEC 259.9 [376.22]
  thyrotoxic 242.0 ✓5ᵗʰ [376.21]

Exostosis 726.91
  cartilaginous (M9210/0) — *see* Neoplasm, bone, benign
  congenital 756.4
  ear canal, external 380.81
  gonococcal 098.89
  hip 726.5
  intracranial 733.3
  jaw (bone) 526.81
  luxurians 728.11
  multiple (cancellous) (congenital) (hereditary) 756.4
  nasal bones 726.91
  orbit, orbital 376.42
  osteocartilaginous (M9210/0) — *see* Neoplasm, bone, benign
  spine 721.8
    with spondylosis — *see* Spondylosis
  syphilitic 095.5
  wrist 726.4

Exotropia 378.10
  alternating 378.15
    with
      A pattern 378.16
      specified noncomitancy NEC 378.18
      V pattern 378.17
      X pattern 378.18
      Y pattern 378.18
    intermittent 378.24
  intermittent 378.20
    alternating 378.24
    monocular 378.23
  monocular 378.11
    with
      A pattern 378.12
      specified noncomitancy NEC 378.14
      V pattern 378.13
      X pattern 378.14
      Y pattern 378.14
    intermittent 378.23

Explanation of
  investigation finding V65.4
  medication V65.4

Exposure 994.9
  cold 991.9
    specified effect NEC 991.8
  effects of 994.9
  exhaustion due to 994.4
  to
    AIDS virus V01.7
    anthrax V01.81 ●
    asbestos V15.84
    body fluids (hazardous) V15.85
    cholera V01.0
    communicable disease V01.9
      specified type NEC V01.89 ▲
    German measles V01.4
    gonorrhea V01.6
    hazardous body fluids V15.85
    HIV V01.7
    human immunodeficiency virus V01.7
    lead V15.86
    parasitic disease V01.89 ▲
    poliomyelitis V01.2
    potentially hazardous body fluids V15.85
    rabies V01.5
    rubella V01.4
    smallpox V01.3
    syphilis V01.6
    tuberculosis V01.1
    venereal disease V01.6
    viral disease NEC V01.7

Exsanguination, fetal 772.0

Exstrophy
  abdominal content 751.8
  bladder (urinary) 753.5

Extensive — *see* condition

Extra — *see also* Accessory
  rib 756.3
    cervical 756.2

Failure, failed

Extraction
  with hook 763.89
  breech NEC 669.6 ✓5ᵗʰ
    affecting fetus or newborn 763.0
  cataract postsurgical V45.61
  manual NEC 669.8 ✓5ᵗʰ
    affecting fetus or newborn 763.89

Extrasystole 427.60
  atrial 427.61
  postoperative 997.1
  ventricular 427.69

Extrauterine gestation or pregnancy — *see* Pregnancy, ectopic

Extravasation
  blood 459.0
    lower extremity 459.0
  chyle into mesentery 457.8
  pelvicalyceal 593.4
  pyelosinus 593.4
  urine 788.8
    from ureter 788.8

Extremity — *see* condition

Extrophy — *see* Exstrophy

Extroversion
  bladder 753.5
  uterus 618.1
    complicating delivery 665.2 ✓5ᵗʰ
      affecting fetus or newborn 763.89
    postpartal (old) 618.1

Extrusion
  breast implant (prosthetic) 996.54
  device, implant, or graft — *see* Complications, mechanical
  eye implant (ball) (globe) 996.59
  intervertebral disc — *see* Displacement, intervertebral disc
  lacrimal gland 375.43
  mesh (reinforcing) 996.59
  ocular lens implant 996.53
  prosthetic device NEC — *see* Complications, mechanical
  vitreous 379.26

Exudate, pleura — *see* Effusion, pleura

Exudates, retina 362.82

Exudative — *see* condition

Eye, eyeball, eyelid — *see* condition

Eyestrain 368.13

Eyeworm disease of Africa 125.2

F

Faber's anemia or syndrome (achlorhydric anemia) 280.9

Fabry's disease (angiokeratoma corporis diffusum) 272.7

Face, facial — *see* condition

Facet of cornea 371.44

Faciocephalalgia, autonomic (*see also* Neuropathy, peripheral, autonomic) 337.9

Facioscapulohumeral myopathy 359.1

Factitious disorder, illness — *see* Illness, factitious

Factor
  deficiency — *see* Deficiency, factor
  psychic, associated with diseases classified elsewhere 316
  risk — *see* Problem

Fahr-Volhard disease (malignant nephrosclerosis) 403.00

Failure, failed
  adenohypophyseal 253.2
  attempted abortion (legal) (*see also* Abortion, failed) 638.9
  bone marrow (anemia) 284.9
    acquired (secondary) 284.8
    congenital 284.0
    idiopathic 284.9
  cardiac (*see also* Failure, heart) 428.9
    newborn 779.89 ▲
  cardiorenal (chronic) 428.9
    hypertensive (*see also* Hypertension, cardiorenal) 404.93

Failure, failed

Failure, failed — continued
- cardiorespiratory 799.1
  - specified during or due to a procedure 997.1
    - long-term effect of cardiac surgery 429.4
- cardiovascular (chronic) 428.9
- cerebrovascular 437.8
- cervical dilatation in labor 661.0 ✓5
  - affecting fetus or newborn 763.7
- circulation, circulatory 799.8
  - fetus or newborn 779.89
  - peripheral 785.50
- compensation — see Disease, heart
- congestive (see also Failure, heart) 428.0
- coronary (see also Insufficiency, coronary) 411.89
- descent of head (at term) 652.5 ✓5
  - affecting fetus or newborn 763.1
  - in labor 660.0 ✓5
    - affecting fetus or newborn 763.1
- device, implant, or graft — see Complications, mechanical
- engagement of head NEC 652.5 ✓5
  - in labor 660.0 ✓5
    - affecting fetus or newborn 763.1
- extrarenal 788.9
- fetal head to enter pelvic brim 652.5 ✓5
  - affecting fetus or newborn 763.1
  - in labor 660.0 ✓5
    - affecting fetus or newborn 763.1
- forceps NEC 660.7 ✓5
  - affecting fetus or newborn 763.1
- fusion (joint) (spinal) 996.4
- growth in childhood 783.43
- heart (acute) (sudden) 428.9
  - with
    - abortion — see Abortion, by type, with specified complication NEC
    - acute pulmonary edema (see also Failure, ventricular, left) 428.1
      - with congestion ▶(see also Failure, heart)◀ 428.0
    - decompensation (see also Failure, heart) 428.0
    - dilation — see Disease, heart
    - ectopic pregnancy (see also categories 633.0-633.9) 639.8
    - molar pregnancy (see also categories 630-632) 639.8
  - arteriosclerotic 440.9
  - combined left-right sided 428.0
  - combined systolic and diastolic 428.40 ●
    - acute 428.41 ●
    - acute on chronic 428.43 ●
    - chronic 428.42 ●
  - compensated (see also Failure, heart) 428.0
  - complicating
    - abortion — see Abortion, by type, with specified complication NEC
    - delivery (cesarean) (instrumental) 669.4 ✓5
    - ectopic pregnancy (see also categories 633.0-633.9) 639.8
    - molar pregnancy (see also categories 630-632) 639.8
    - obstetric anesthesia or sedation 668.1 ✓5
    - surgery 997.1
  - congestive (compensated) (decompensated) ▶(see also Failure, heart)◀ 428.0
    - with rheumatic fever (conditions classifiable to 390)
      - active 391.8
      - inactive or quiescent (with chorea) 398.91
  - fetus or newborn 779.89
  - hypertensive (see also Hypertension, heart) 402.90
    - with renal disease (see also Hypertension, cardiorenal) 404.91
      - with renal failure 404.93
    - benign 402.11
    - malignant 402.01
  - rheumatic (chronic) (inactive) (with chorea) 398.91
    - active or acute 391.8
      - with chorea (Sydenham's) 392.0

Failure, failed — continued
- heart — continued
  - decompensated (see also Failure, heart) 428.0
  - degenerative (see also Degeneration, myocardial) 429.1
  - diastolic 428.30 ●
    - acute 428.31 ●
    - acute on chronic 428.33 ●
    - chronic 428.32 ●
  - due to presence of (cardiac) prosthesis 429.4
  - fetus or newborn 779.89 ▲
  - following
    - abortion 639.8
    - cardiac surgery 429.4
    - ectopic or molar pregnancy 639.8
  - high output NEC 428.9
  - hypertensive (see also Hypertension, heart) 402.91
    - with renal disease (see also Hypertension, cardiorenal) 404.91
      - with renal failure 404.93
    - benign 402.11
    - malignant 402.01
  - left (ventricular) (see also Failure, ventricular, left) 428.1
    - with right-sided failure ▶(see also Failure, heart)◀ 428.0
  - low output (syndrome) NEC 428.9
  - organic — see Disease, heart
  - postoperative (immediate) 997.1
    - long term effect of cardiac surgery 429.4
  - rheumatic (chronic) (congestive) (inactive) 398.91
  - right (secondary to left heart failure, conditions classifiable to 428.1) (ventricular) (see also Failure, heart) 428.0
  - senile 797
  - specified during or due to a procedure 997.1
    - long-term effect of cardiac surgery 429.4
  - systolic 428.20 ●
    - acute 428.21 ●
    - acute on chronic 428.23 ●
    - chronic 428.22 ●
  - thyrotoxic (see also Thyrotoxicosis) 242.9 ✓5 [425.7]
  - valvular — see Endocarditis
- hepatic 572.8
  - acute 570
  - due to a procedure 997.4
- hepatorenal 572.4
- hypertensive heart (see also Hypertension, heart) 402.91
  - benign 402.11
  - malignant 402.01
- induction (of labor) 659.1 ✓5
  - abortion (legal) (see also Abortion, failed) 638.9
  - affecting fetus or newborn 763.89
  - by oxytocic drugs 659.1 ✓5
  - instrumental 659.0 ✓5
  - mechanical 659.0 ✓5
  - medical 659.1 ✓5
  - surgical 659.0 ✓5
- initial alveolar expansion, newborn 770.4
- involution, thymus (gland) 254.8
- kidney — see Failure, renal
- lactation 676.4 ✓5
- Leydig's cell, adult 257.2
- liver 572.8
  - acute 570
- medullary 799.8
- mitral — see Endocarditis, mitral
- myocardium, myocardial (see also Failure, heart) 428.9
  - chronic (see also Failure, heart) 428.0
  - congestive (see also Failure, heart) 428.0
- ovarian (primary) 256.39
  - iatrogenic 256.2
  - postablative 256.2
  - postirradiation 256.2
  - postsurgical 256.2
- ovulation 628.0
- prerenal 788.9

Failure, failed — continued
- renal 586
  - with
    - abortion — see Abortion, by type, with renal failure
    - ectopic pregnancy (see also categories 633.0-633.9) 639.3
    - edema (see also Nephrosis) 581.9
    - hypertension (see also Hypertension, kidney) 403.91
    - hypertensive heart disease (conditions classifiable to 402) 404.92
      - with heart failure 404.93
      - benign 404.12
        - with heart failure 404.13
      - malignant 404.02
        - with heart failure 404.03
    - molar pregnancy (see also categories 630-632) 639.3
    - tubular necrosis (acute) 584.5
  - acute 584.9
    - with lesion of
      - necrosis
        - cortical (renal) 584.6
        - medullary (renal) (papillary) 584.7
        - tubular 584.5
      - specified pathology NEC 584.8
  - chronic 585
    - hypertensive or with hypertension (see also Hypertension, kidney) 403.91
  - due to a procedure 997.5
  - following
    - abortion 639.3
    - crushing 958.5
    - ectopic or molar pregnancy 639.3
    - labor and delivery (acute) 669.3 ✓5
  - hypertensive (see also Hypertension, kidney) 403.91
  - puerperal, postpartum 669.3 ✓5
- respiration, respiratory 518.81
  - acute 518.81
  - acute and chronic 518.84
  - center 348.8
    - newborn 770.84 ▲
  - chronic 518.83
  - due to trauma, surgery or shock 518.5
  - newborn 770.84 ▲
- rotation
  - cecum 751.4
  - colon 751.4
  - intestine 751.4
  - kidney 753.3
- segmentation — see also Fusion
  - fingers (see also Syndactylism, fingers) 755.11
  - toes (see also Syndactylism, toes) 755.13
- seminiferous tubule, adult 257.2
- senile (general) 797
  - with psychosis 290.20
- testis, primary (seminal) 257.2
- to progress 661.2 ✓5
- to thrive
  - adult 783.7
  - child 783.41
- transplant 996.80
  - bone marrow 996.85
  - organ (immune or nonimmune cause) 996.80
    - bone marrow 996.85
    - heart 996.83
    - intestines 996.87
    - kidney 996.81
    - liver 996.82
    - lung 996.84
    - pancreas 996.86
    - specified NEC 996.89
  - skin 996.52
    - artificial 996.55
    - decellularized allodermis 996.55
    - temporary allograft or pigskin graft — omit code
- trial of labor NEC 660.6 ✓5
  - affecting fetus or newborn 763.1
- urinary 586
- vacuum extraction
  - abortion — see Abortion, failed
  - delivery NEC 660.7 ✓5

Index to Diseases

Failure, failed — *continued*
  vacuum extraction — *continued*
    delivery NEC — *continued*
      affecting fetus or newborn 763.1
    ventouse NEC 660.7 ✓5ᵗʰ
      affecting fetus or newborn 763.1
  ventricular (*see also* Failure, heart) 428.9
    left 428.1
      with rheumatic fever (conditions classifiable to 390)
        active 391.8
          with chorea 392.0
        inactive or quiescent (with chorea) 398.91
      hypertensive (*see also* Hypertension, heart) 402.91
        benign 402.11
        malignant 402.01
      rheumatic (chronic) (inactive) (with chorea) 398.91
        active or acute 391.8
          with chorea 392.0
    right (*see also* Failure, heart) 428.0
  vital centers, fetus or newborn 779.8
  weight gain in childhood 783.41
Fainting (fit) (spell) 780.2
Falciform hymen 752.49
Fall, maternal, affecting fetus or newborn 760.5
Fallen arches 734
Falling, any organ or part — *see* Prolapse
Fallopian
  insufflation
    fertility testing V26.21
    following sterilization reversal V26.22
  tube — *see* condition
Fallot's
  pentalogy 745.2
  tetrad or tetralogy 745.2
  triad or trilogy 746.09
Fallout, radioactive (adverse effect) NEC 990
False — *see also* condition
  bundle branch block 426.50
  bursa 727.89
  croup 478.75
  joint 733.82
  labor (pains) 644.1 ✓5ᵗʰ
  opening, urinary, male 752.69
  passage, urethra (prostatic) 599.4
  positive
    serological test for syphilis 795.6
    Wassermann reaction 795.6
  pregnancy 300.11
Family, familial — *see also* condition
  disruption V61.0
  planning advice V25.09
  problem V61.9
    specified circumstance NEC V61.8
Famine 994.2
  edema 262
Fanconi's anemia (congenital pancytopenia) 284.0
Fanconi (-de Toni) (-Debré) syndrome (cystinosis) 270.0
Farber (-Uzman) syndrome or disease (disseminated lipogranulomatosis) 272.8
Farcin 024
Farcy 024
Farmers'
  lung 495.0
  skin 692.74
Farsightedness 367.0
Fascia — *see* condition
Fasciculation 781.0
Fasciculitis optica 377.32
Fasciitis 729.4
  eosinophilic 728.89
  necrotizing 728.86
  nodular 728.79
  perirenal 593.4
  plantar 728.71
  pseudosarcomatous 728.79

Fasciitis — *continued*
  traumatic (old) NEC 728.79
    current — *see* Sprain, by site
Fasciola hepatica infestation 121.3
Fascioliasis 121.3
Fasciolopsiasis (small intestine) 121.4
Fasciolopsis (small intestine) 121.4
Fast pulse 785.0
Fat
  embolism (cerebral) (pulmonary) (systemic) 958.1
    with
      abortion — *see* Abortion, by type, with embolism
      ectopic pregnancy (*see also* categories 633.0-633.9) 639.6
      molar pregnancy (*see also* categories 630-632) 639.6
    complicating delivery or puerperium 673.8 ✓5ᵗʰ
    following
      abortion 639.6
      ectopic or molar pregnancy 639.6
    in pregnancy, childbirth, or the puerperium 673.8 ✓5ᵗʰ
  excessive 278.00
    in heart (*see also* Degeneration, myocardial) 429.1
  general 278.00
  hernia, herniation 729.30
    eyelid 374.34
    knee 729.31
    orbit 374.34
    retro-orbital 374.34
    retropatellar 729.31
    specified site NEC 729.39
  indigestion 579.8
  in stool 792.1
  localized (pad) 278.1
    heart (*see also* Degeneration, myocardial) 429.1
    knee 729.31
    retropatellar 729.31
  necrosis — *see also* Fatty, degeneration breast (aseptic)
    (segmental) 611.3
    mesentery 567.8
    omentum 567.8
  pad 278.1
Fatal syncope 798.1
Fatigue 780.79
  auditory deafness (*see also* Deafness) 389.9
  chronic 780.7 ✓5ᵗʰ
  chronic, syndrome 780.71
  combat (*see also* Reaction, stress, acute) 308.9
  during pregnancy 646.8 ✓5ᵗʰ
  general 780.79
    psychogenic 300.5
  heat (transient) 992.6
  muscle 729.89
  myocardium (*see also* Failure, heart) 428.9
  nervous 300.5
  neurosis 300.5
  operational 300.89
  postural 729.89
  posture 729.89
  psychogenic (general) 300.5
  senile 797
  syndrome NEC 300.5
    chronic 780.71
  undue 780.79
  voice 784.49
Fatness 278.00
Fatty — *see also* condition
  apron 278.1
  degeneration (diffuse) (general) NEC 272.8
    localized — *see* Degeneration, by site, fatty
    placenta — *see* Placenta, abnormal
  heart (enlarged) (*see also* Degeneration, myocardial) 429.1
  infiltration (diffuse) (general) (*see also* Degeneration, by site, fatty) 272.8
    heart (enlarged) (*see also* Degeneration, myocardial) 429.1
  liver 571.8
    alcoholic 571.0

Fatty — *see also* condition — *continued*
  necrosis — *see* Degeneration, fatty
  phanerosis 272.8
Fauces — *see* condition
Fauchard's disease (periodontitis) 523.4
Faucitis 478.29
Faulty — *see also* condition
  position of teeth 524.3
Favism (anemia) 282.2
Favre-Racouchot disease (elastoidosis cutanea nodularis) 701.8
Favus 110.9
  beard 110.0
  capitis 110.0
  corporis 110.5
  eyelid 110.8
  foot 110.4
  hand 110.2
  scalp 110.0
  specified site NEC 110.8
Fear, fearfullness (complex) (reaction) 300.20
  child 313.0
  of
    animals 300.29
    closed spaces 300.29
    crowds 300.29
    eating in public 300.23
    heights 300.29
    open spaces 300.22
      with panic attacks 300.21
    public speaking 300.23
    streets 300.22
      with panic attacks 300.21
    travel 300.22
      with panic attacks 300.21
    washing in public 300.23
  transient 308.0
Feared complaint unfounded V65.5
Febricula (continued) (simple) (*see also* Pyrexia) 780.6
Febrile (*see also* Pyrexia) 780.6
  convulsion 780.31
  seizure 780.31
Febris (*see also* Fever) 780.6
  aestiva (*see also* Fever, hay) 477.9
  flava (*see also* Fever, yellow) 060.9
  melitensis 023.0
  pestis (*see also* Plague) 020.9
  puerperalis 672 ✓5ᵗʰ
  recurrens (*see also* Fever, relapsing) 087.9
    pediculo vestimenti 087.0
  rubra 034.1
  typhoidea 002.0
  typhosa 002.0
Fecal — *see* condition
Fecalith (impaction) 560.39
  with hernia — *see also* Hernia, by site, with obstruction
    gangrenous — *see* Hernia, by site, with gangrene
  appendix 543.9
  congenital 777.1
Fede's disease 529.0
Feeble-minded 317
Feeble rapid pulse due to shock following injury 958.4
Feeding
  faulty (elderly) (infant) 783.3
    newborn 779.3
  formula check V20.2
  improper (elderly) (infant) 783.3
    newborn 779.3
  problem (elderly) (infant) 783.3
    newborn 779.3
    nonorganic origin 307.59
Feer's disease 985.0
Feet — *see* condition
Feigned illness V65.2
Feil-Klippel syndrome (brevicollis) 756.16
Feinmesser's (hidrotic) **ectodermal dysplasia** 757.31

Felix's disease (juvenile osteochondrosis, hip) 732.1
Felon (any digit) (with lymphangitis) 681.01
    herpetic 054.6
Felty's syndrome (rheumatoid arthritis with splenomegaly and leukopenia) 714.1
Feminism in boys 302.6
Feminization, testicular 257.8
    with pseudohermaphroditism, male 257.8
Femoral hernia — see Hernia, femoral
Femora vara 736.32
Femur, femoral — see condition
Fenestrata placenta — see Placenta, abnormal
Fenestration, fenestrated — see also Imperfect, closure
    aorta-pulmonary 745.0
    aorticopulmonary 745.0
    aortopulmonary 745.0
    cusps, heart valve NEC 746.89
        pulmonary 746.09
    hymen 752.49
    pulmonic cusps 746.09
Fenwick's disease 537.89
Fermentation (gastric) (gastrointestinal) (stomach) 536.8
    intestine 564.89
        psychogenic 306.4
    psychogenic 306.4
Fernell's disease (aortic aneurysm) 441.9
Fertile eunuch syndrome 257.2
Fertility, meaning multiparity — see Multiparity
Fetal alcohol syndrome 760.71
Fetalis uterus 752.3
Fetid
    breath 784.9
    sweat 705.89
Fetishism 302.81
    transvestic 302.3
Fetomaternal hemorrhage
    affecting management of pregnancy 656.0
    fetus or newborn 772.0
Fetus, fetal — see also condition
    papyraceous 779.89
    type lung tissue 770.4
Fever 780.6
    with chills 780.6
        in malarial regions (see also Malaria) 084.6
    abortus NEC 023.9
    Aden 061
    African tick-borne 087.1
    American
        mountain tick 066.1
        spotted 082.0
    and ague (see also Malaria) 084.6
    aphthous 078.4
    arbovirus hemorrhagic 065.9
    Assam 085.0
    Australian A or Q 083.0
    Bangkok hemorrhagic 065.4
    biliary, Charcôt's intermittent — see Choledocholithiasis
    bilious, hemoglobinuric 084.8
    blackwater 084.8
    blister 054.9
    Bonvale Dam 780.79
    boutonneuse 082.1
    brain 323.9
        late effect — see category 326
    breakbone 061
    Bullis 082.8
    Bunyamwera 066.3
    Burdwan 085.0
    Bwamba (encephalitis) 066.3
    Cameroon (see also Malaria) 084.6
    Canton 081.9
    catarrhal (acute) 460
        chronic 472.0
    cat-scratch 078.3
    cerebral 323.9
        late effect — see category 326
    cerebrospinal (meningococcal) (see also Meningitis, cerebrospinal) 036.0
    Chagres 084.0

Fever — continued
    Chandipura 066.8
    changuinola 066.0
    Charcôt's (biliary) (hepatic) (intermittent) see Choledocholithiasis
    Chikungunya (viral) 066.3
        hemorrhagic 065.4
    childbed 670
    Chitral 066.0
    Colombo (see also Fever, paratyphoid) 002.9
    Colorado tick (virus) 066.1
    congestive
        malarial (see also Malaria) 084.6
        remittent (see also Malaria) 084.6
    Congo virus 065.0
    continued 780.6
        malarial 084.0
    Corsican (see also Malaria) 084.6
    Crimean hemorrhagic 065.0
    Cyprus (see also Brucellosis) 023.9
    dandy 061
    deer fly (see also Tularemia) 021.9
    dehydration, newborn 778.4
    dengue (virus) 061
        hemorrhagic 065.4
    desert 114.0
    due to heat 992.0
    Dumdum 085.0
    enteric 002.0
    ephemeral (of unknown origin) (see also Pyrexia) 780.6
    epidemic, hemorrhagic of the Far East 065.0
    erysipelatous (see also Erysipelas) 035
    estivo-autumnal (malarial) 084.0
    etiocholanolone 277.3
    famine — see also Fever, relapsing
        meaning typhus — see Typhus
    Far Eastern hemorrhagic 065.0
    five day 083.1
    Fort Bragg 100.89
    gastroenteric 002.0
    gastromalarial (see also Malaria) 084.6
    Gibraltar (see also Brucellosis) 023.9
    glandular 075
    Guama (viral) 066.3
    Haverhill 026.1
    hay (allergic) (with rhinitis) 477.9
        with
            asthma (bronchial) (see also Asthma) 493.0
        due to
            dander 477.8
            dust 477.8
            fowl 477.8
            pollen, any plant or tree 477.0
            specified allergen other than pollen 477.8
    heat (effects) 992.0
    hematuric, bilious 084.8
    hemoglobinuric (malarial) 084.8
        bilious 084.8
    hemorrhagic (arthropod-borne) NEC 065.9
        with renal syndrome 078.6
        arenaviral 078.7
        Argentine 078.7
        Bangkok 065.4
        Bolivian 078.7
        Central Asian 065.0
        chikungunya 065.4
        Crimean 065.0
        dengue (virus) 065.4
        Ebola 065.8
        epidemic 078.6
            of Far East 065.0
        Far Eastern 065.0
        Junin virus 078.7
        Korean 078.6
        Kyasanur forest 065.2
        Machupo virus 078.7
        mite-borne NEC 065.8
        mosquito-borne 065.4
        Omsk 065.1
        Philippine 065.4
        Russian (Yaroslav) 078.6
        Singapore 065.4
        Southeast Asia 065.4
        Thailand 065.4
        tick-borne NEC 065.3

Fever — continued
    hepatic (see also Cholecystitis) 575.8
        intermittent (Charcôt's) — see Choledocholithiasis
    herpetic (see also Herpes) 054.9
    Hyalomma tick 065.0
    icterohemorrhagic 100.0
    inanition 780.6
        newborn 778.4
    infective NEC 136.9
    intermittent (bilious) (see also Malaria) 084.6
        hepatic (Charcôt) — see Choledocholithiasis
        of unknown origin (see also Pyrexia) 780.6
        pernicious 084.0
    iodide
        correct substance properly administered 780.6
        overdose or wrong substance given or taken 975.5
    Japanese river 081.2
    jungle yellow 060.0
    Junin virus, hemorrhagic 078.7
    Katayama 120.2
    Kedani 081.2
    Kenya 082.1
    Korean hemorrhagic 078.6
    Lassa 078.89
    Lone Star 082.8
    lung — see Pneumonia
    Machupo virus, hemorrhagic 078.7
    malaria, malarial (see also Malaria) 084.6
    Malta (see also Brucellosis) 023.9
    Marseilles 082.1
    marsh (see also Malaria) 084.6
    Mayaro (viral) 066.3
    Mediterranean (see also Brucellosis) 023.9
        familial 277.3
        tick 082.1
    meningeal — see Meningitis
    metal fumes NEC 985.8
    Meuse 083.1
    Mexican — see Typhus, Mexican
    Mianeh 087.1
    miasmatic (see also Malaria) 084.6
    miliary 078.2
    milk, female 672
    mill 504
    mite-borne hemorrhagic 065.8
    Monday 504
    mosquito-borne NEC 066.3
        hemorrhagic NEC 065.4
    mountain 066.1
        meaning
            Rocky Mountain spotted 082.0
            undulant fever (see also Brucellosis) 023.9
        tick (American) 066.1
    Mucambo (viral) 066.3
    mud 100.89
    Neapolitan (see also Brucellosis) 023.9
    neutropenic 288.0
    nine-mile 083.0
    nonexanthematous tick 066.1
    North Asian tick-borne typhus 082.2
    Omsk hemorrhagic 065.1
    O'nyong-nyong (viral) 066.3
    Oropouche (viral) 066.3
    Oroya 088.0
    paludal (see also Malaria) 084.6
    Panama 084.0
    pappataci 066.0
    paratyphoid 002.9
        A 002.1
        B (Schottmüller's) 002.2
        C (Hirschfeld) 002.3
    parrot 073.9
    periodic 277.3
    pernicious, acute 084.0
    persistent (of unknown origin) (see also Pyrexia) 780.6
    petechial 036.0
    pharyngoconjunctival 077.2
        adenoviral type 3 077.2
    Philippine hemorrhagic 065.4
    phlebotomus 066.0
    Piry 066.8
    Pixuna (viral) 066.3
    Plasmodium ovale 084.3

Index to Diseases

Fever — *continued*
  pleural (*see also* Pleurisy) 511.0
  pneumonic — *see* Pneumonia
  polymer fume 987.8
  postoperative 998.89
    due to infection 998.59
  pretibial 100.89
  puerperal, postpartum 672 ✓4ᵗʰ
  putrid — *see* Septicemia
  pyemic — *see* Septicemia
  Q 083.0
    with pneumonia 083.0 [484.8]
  quadrilateral 083.0
  quartan (malaria) 084.2
  Queensland (coastal) 083.0
    seven-day 100.89
  Quintan (A) 083.1
  quotidian 084.0
  rabbit (*see also* Tularemia) 021.9
  rat-bite 026.9
    due to
      Spirillum minor or minus 026.0
      Spirochaeta morsus muris 026.0
      Streptobacillus moniliformis 026.1
  recurrent — *see* Fever, relapsing
  relapsing 087.9
    Carter's (Asiatic) 087.0
    Dutton's (West African) 087.1
    Koch's 087.9
    louse-borne (epidemic) 087.0
    Novy's (American) 087.1
    Obermeyer's (European) 087.0
    spirillum NEC 087.9
    tick-borne (endemic) 087.1
  remittent (bilious) (congestive) (gastric) (*see also* Malaria) 084.6
  rheumatic (active) (acute) (chronic) (subacute) 390
    with heart involvement 391.9
      carditis 391.9
      endocarditis (aortic) (mitral) (pulmonary) (tricuspid) 391.1
      multiple sites 391.8
      myocarditis 391.2
      pancarditis, acute 391.8
      pericarditis 391.0
      specified type NEC 391.8
      valvulitis 391.1
    inactive or quiescent with cardiac hypertrophy 398.99
      carditis 398.90
      endocarditis 397.9
        aortic (valve) 395.9
          with mitral (valve) disease 396.9
        mitral (valve) 394.9
          with aortic (valve) disease 396.9
        pulmonary (valve) 397.1
        tricuspid (valve) 397.0
      heart conditions (classifiable to 429.3, 429.6, 429.9) 398.99
        failure (congestive) (conditions classifiable to 428.0, 428.9) 398.91
          left ventricular failure (conditions classifiable to 428.1) 398.91
        myocardial degeneration (conditions classifiable to 429.1) 398.0
        myocarditis (conditions classifiable to 429.0) 398.0
      pancarditis 398.99
      pericarditis 393
  Rift Valley (viral) 066.3
  Rocky Mountain spotted 082.0
  rose 477.0
  Ross river (viral) 066.3
  Russian hemorrhagic 078.6
  sandfly 066.0
  San Joaquin (valley) 114.0
  São Paulo 082.0
  scarlet 034.1
  septic — *see* Septicemia
  seven-day 061
    Japan 100.89
    Queensland 100.89
  shin bone 083.1
  Singapore hemorrhagic 065.4
  solar 061

Fever — *continued*
  sore 054.9
  South African tick-bite 087.1
  Southeast Asia hemorrhagic 065.4
  spinal — *see* Meningitis
  spirillary 026.0
  splenic (*see also* Anthrax) 022.9
  spotted (Rocky Mountain) 082.0
    American 082.0
    Brazilian 082.0
    Colombian 082.0
    meaning
      cerebrospinal meningitis 036.0
      typhus 082.9
  spring 309.23
  steroid
    correct substance properly administered 780.6
    overdose or wrong substance given or taken 962.0
  streptobacillary 026.1
  subtertian 084.0
  Sumatran mite 081.2
  sun 061
  swamp 100.89
  sweating 078.2
  swine 003.8
  sylvatic yellow 060.0
  Tahyna 062.5
  tertian — *see* Malaria, tertian
  Thailand hemorrhagic 065.4
  thermic 992.0
  three day 066.0
    with Coxsackie exanthem 074.8
  tick
    American mountain 066.1
    Colorado 066.1
    Kemerovo 066.1
    Mediterranean 082.1
    mountain 066.1
    nonexanthematous 066.1
    Quaranfil 066.1
  tick-bite NEC 066.1
  tick-borne NEC 066.1
    hemorrhagic NEC 065.3
  transitory of newborn 778.4
  trench 083.1
  tsutsugamushi 081.2
  typhogastric 002.0
  typhoid (abortive) (ambulant) (any site) (hemorrhagic) (infection) (intermittent) (malignant) (rheumatic) 002.0
  typhomalarial (*see also* Malaria) 084.6
  typhus — *see* Typhus
  undulant (*see also* Brucellosis) 023.9
  unknown origin (*see also* Pyrexia) 780.6
  uremic — *see* Uremia
  uveoparotid 135
  valley (Coccidioidomycosis) 114.0
  Venezuelan equine 066.2
  Volhynian 083.1
  Wesselsbron (viral) 066.3
  West
    African 084.8
    Nile (viral) 066.4 ▲
  Whitmore's 025
  Wolhynian 083.1
  worm 128.9
  Yaroslav hemorrhagic 078.6
  yellow 060.9
    jungle 060.0
    sylvatic 060.0
    urban 060.1
    vaccination, prophylactic (against) V04.4
  Zika (viral) 066.3
Fibrillation
  atrial (established) (paroxysmal) 427.31
  auricular (atrial) (established) 427.31
  cardiac (ventricular) 427.41
  coronary (*see also* Infarct, myocardium) 410.9 ✓5ᵗʰ
  heart (ventricular) 427.41
  muscular 728.9
  postoperative 997.1
  ventricular 427.41

Fibrin
  ball or bodies, pleural (sac) 511.0
  chamber, anterior (eye) (gelatinous exudate) 364.04
Fibrinogenolysis (hemorrhagic) — *see* Fibrinolysis
Fibrinogenopenia (congenital) (hereditary) (*see also* Defect, coagulation) 286.3
  acquired 286.6
Fibrinolysis (acquired) (hemorrhagic) (pathologic) 286.6
  with
    abortion — *see* Abortion, by type, with hemorrhage, delayed or excessive
    ectopic pregnancy (*see also* categories 633.0-633.9) 639.1
    molar pregnancy (*see also* categories 630-632) 639.1
  antepartum or intrapartum 641.3 ✓5ᵗʰ
    affecting fetus or newborn 762.1
  following
    abortion 639.1
    ectopic or molar pregnancy 639.1
  newborn, transient 776.2
  postpartum 666.3 ✓5ᵗʰ
Fibrinopenia (hereditary) (*see also* Defect, coagulation) 286.3
  acquired 286.6
Fibrinopurulent — *see* condition
Fibrinous — *see* condition
Fibroadenoma (M9010/0) 217
  cellular intracanalicular (M9020/0) 217
  giant (intracanalicular) (M9020/0) 217
  intracanalicular (M9011/0)
    cellular (M9020/0) 217
    giant (M9020/0) 217
    specified site — *see* Neoplasm, by site, benign
    unspecified site 217
  juvenile (M9030/0) 217
  pericanicular (M9012/0)
    specified site — *see* Neoplasm, by site, benign
    unspecified site 217
  phyllodes (M9020/0) 217
  prostate 600.2
  specified site — *see* Neoplasm, by site, benign
  unspecified site 217
Fibroadenosis, breast (chronic) (cystic) (diffuse) (periodic) (segmental) 610.2
Fibroangioma (M9160/0) — *see also* Neoplasm, by site, benign
  juvenile (M9160/0)
    specified site — *see* Neoplasm, by site, benign
    unspecified site 210.7
Fibrocellulitis progressiva ossificans 728.11
Fibrochondrosarcoma (M9220/3) — *see* Neoplasm, cartilage, malignant
Fibrocystic
  disease 277.00
    bone NEC 733.29
    breast 610.1
    jaw 526.2
    kidney (congenital) 753.19
    liver 751.62
    lung 518.89
      congenital 748.4
    pancreas 277.00
  kidney (congenital) 753.19
Fibrodysplasia ossificans multiplex (progressiva) 728.11
Fibroelastosis (cordis) (endocardial) (endomyocardial) 425.3
Fibroid (tumor) (M8890/0) — *see also* Neoplasm, connective tissue, benign
  disease, lung (chronic) (*see also* Fibrosis, lung) 515
  heart (disease) (*see also* Myocarditis) 429.0
  induration, lung (chronic) (*see also* Fibrosis, lung) 515
  in pregnancy or childbirth 654.1 ✓5ᵗʰ
    affecting fetus or newborn 763.89
    causing obstructed labor 660.2 ✓5ᵗʰ
      affecting fetus or newborn 763.1

✓4ᵗʰ Fourth-digit Required   ✓5ᵗʰ Fifth-digit Required   ▶◀ Revised Text   ● New Line   ▲ Revised Code

Fibroid — *see also* Neoplasm, connective tissue, benign — *continued*
  liver — *see* Cirrhosis, liver
  lung (*see also* Fibrosis, lung) 515
  pneumonia (chronic) (*see also* Fibrosis, lung) 515
  uterus (M8890/0) (*see also* Leiomyoma, uterus) 218.9
Fibrolipoma (M8851/0) (*see also* Lipoma, by site) 214.9
Fibroliposarcoma (M8850/3) — *see* Neoplasm, connective tissue, malignant
Fibroma (M8810/0) — *see also* Neoplasm, connective tissue, benign
  ameloblastic (M9330/0) 213.1
    upper jaw (bone) 213.0
  bone (nonossifying) 733.99
    ossifying (M9262/0) — *see* Neoplasm, bone, benign
  cementifying (M9274/0) — *see* Neoplasm, bone, benign
  chondromyxoid (M9241/0) — *see* Neoplasm, bone, benign
  desmoplastic (M8823/1) — *see* Neoplasm, connective tissue, uncertain behavior
  facial (M8813/0) — *see* Neoplasm, connective tissue, benign
  invasive (M8821/1) — *see* Neoplasm, connective tissue, uncertain behavior
  molle (M8851/0) (*see also* Lipoma, by site) 214.9
  myxoid (M8811/0) — *see* Neoplasm, connective tissue, benign
  nasopharynx, nasopharyngeal (juvenile) (M9160/0) 210.7
  nonosteogenic (nonossifying) — *see* Dysplasia, fibrous
  odontogenic (M9321/0) 213.1
    upper jaw (bone) 213.0
  ossifying (M9262/0) — *see* Neoplasm, bone, benign
  periosteal (M8812/0) — *see* Neoplasm, bone, benign
  prostate 600.2
  soft (M8851/0) (*see also* Lipoma, by site) 214.9
Fibromatosis
  abdominal (M8822/1) — *see* Neoplasm, connective tissue, uncertain behavior
  aggressive (M8821/1) — *see* Neoplasm, connective tissue, uncertain behavior
  Dupuytren's 728.6
  gingival 523.8
  plantar fascia 728.71
  proliferative 728.79
  pseudosarcomatous (proliferative) (subcutaneous) 728.79
  subcutaneous pseudosarcomatous (proliferative) 728.79
Fibromyalgia 729.1
Fibromyoma (M8890/0) — *see also* Neoplasm, connective tissue, benign
  uterus (corpus) (*see also* Leiomyoma, uterus) 218.9
    in pregnancy or childbirth 654.1
      affecting fetus or newborn 763.89
      causing obstructed labor 660.2
        affecting fetus or newborn 763.1
Fibromyositis (*see also* Myositis) 729.1
  scapulohumeral 726.2
Fibromyxolipoma (M8852/0) (*see also* Lipoma, by site) 214.9
Fibromyxoma (M8811/0) — *see* Neoplasm, connective tissue, benign
Fibromyxosarcoma (M8811/3) — *see* Neoplasm, connective tissue, malignant
Fibro-odontoma, ameloblastic (M9290/0) 213.1
  upper jaw (bone) 213.0
Fibro-osteoma (M9262/0) — *see* Neoplasm, bone, benign
Fibroplasia, retrolental 362.21
Fibropurulent — *see* condition
Fibrosarcoma (M8810/3) — *see also* Neoplasm, connective tissue, malignant
  ameloblastic (M9330/3) 170.1
    upper jaw (bone) 170.0

Fibrosarcoma — *see also* Neoplasm, connective tissue, malignant — *continued*
  congenital (M8814/3) — *see* Neoplasm, connective tissue, malignant
  fascial (M8813/3) — *see* Neoplasm, connective tissue, malignant
  infantile (M8814/3) — *see* Neoplasm, connective tissue, malignant
  odontogenic (M9330/3) 170.1
    upper jaw (bone) 170.0
  periosteal (M8812/3) — *see* Neoplasm, bone, malignant
Fibrosclerosis
  breast 610.3
  corpora cavernosa (penis) 607.89
  familial multifocal NEC 710.8
  multifocal (idiopathic) NEC 710.8
  penis (corpora cavernosa) 607.89
Fibrosis, fibrotic
  adrenal (gland) 255.8
  alveolar (diffuse) 516.3
  amnion 658.8
  anal papillae 569.49
  anus 569.49
  appendix, appendiceal, noninflammatory 543.9
  arteriocapillary — *see* Arteriosclerosis
  bauxite (of lung) 503
  biliary 576.8
    due to Clonorchis sinensis 121.1
  bladder 596.8
    interstitial 595.1
    localized submucosal 595.1
    panmural 595.1
  bone, diffuse 756.59
  breast 610.3
  capillary — *see also* Arteriosclerosis
    lung (chronic) (*see also* Fibrosis, lung) 515
  cardiac (*see also* Myocarditis) 429.0
  cervix 622.8
  chorion 658.8
  corpus cavernosum 607.89
  cystic (of pancreas) 277.00
    with
      manifestations
        gastrointestinal 277.03
        pulmonary 277.02
        specified NEC 277.09
      meconium ileus 277.01
      pulmonary exacerbation 277.02
  due to (presence of) any device, implant, or graft — *see* Complications, due to (presence of) any device, implant, or graft classified to 996.0-996.5 NEC
  ejaculatory duct 608.89
  endocardium (*see also* Endocarditis) 424.90
  endomyocardial (African) 425.0
  epididymis 608.89
  eye muscle 378.62
  graphite (of lung) 503
  heart (*see also* Myocarditis) 429.0
  hepatic — *see also* Cirrhosis, liver due to Clonorchis sinensis 121.1
  hepatolienal — *see* Cirrhosis, liver
  hepatosplenic — *see* Cirrhosis, liver
  infrapatellar fat pad 729.31
  interstitial pulmonary, newborn 770.7
  intrascrotal 608.89
  kidney (*see also* Sclerosis, renal) 587
  liver — *see* Cirrhosis, liver
  lung (atrophic) (capillary) (chronic) (confluent) (massive) (perialveolar) (peribronchial) 515
    with
      anthracosilicosis (occupational) 500
      anthracosis (occupational) 500
      asbestosis (occupational) 501
      bagassosis (occupational) 495.1
      bauxite 503
      berylliosis (occupational) 503
      byssinosis (occupational) 504
      calcicosis (occupational) 502
      chalicosis (occupational) 502
      dust reticulation (occupational) 504
      farmers' lung 495.0
      gannister disease (occupational) 502
      graphite 503
      pneumoconiosis (occupational) 505

Fibrosis, fibrotic — *continued*
  lung — *continued*
    with — *continued*
      pneumosiderosis (occupational) 503
      siderosis (occupational) 503
      silicosis (occupational) 502
      tuberculosis (*see also* Tuberculosis) 011.4
    diffuse (idiopathic) (interstitial) 516.3
    due to
      bauxite 503
      fumes or vapors (chemical) inhalation) 506.4
      graphite 503
    following radiation 508.1
    postinflammatory 515
    silicotic (massive) (occupational) 502
    tuberculous (*see also* Tuberculosis) 011.4
  lymphatic gland 289.3
  median bar 600.9
  mediastinum (idiopathic) 519.3
  meninges 349.2
  muscle NEC 728.2
    iatrogenic (from injection) 999.9
  myocardium, myocardial (*see also* Myocarditis) 429.0
  oral submucous 528.8
  ovary 620.8
  oviduct 620.8
  pancreas 577.8
    cystic 277.00
      with ●
        manifestations ●
          gastrointestinal 277.03 ●
          pulmonary 277.02 ●
          specified NEC 277.09 ●
        meconium ileus 277.01 ●
        pulmonary exacerbation 277.02 ●
  penis 607.89
  periappendiceal 543.9
  periarticular (*see also* Ankylosis) 718.5
  pericardium 423.1
  perineum, in pregnancy or childbirth 654.8
    affecting fetus or newborn 763.89
    causing obstructed labor 660.2
      affecting fetus or newborn 763.1
  perineural NEC 355.9
    foot 355.6
  periureteral 593.89
  placenta — *see* Placenta, abnormal
  pleura 511.0
  popliteal fat pad 729.31
  preretinal 362.56
  prostate (chronic) 600.9
  pulmonary (chronic) (*see also* Fibrosis, lung) 515
    alveolar capillary block 516.3
    interstitial
      diffuse (idiopathic) 516.3
      newborn 770.7
  radiation — *see* Effect, adverse, radiation
  rectal sphincter 569.49
  retroperitoneal, idiopathic 593.4
  scrotum 608.89
  seminal vesicle 608.89
  senile 797
  skin NEC 709.2
  spermatic cord 608.89
  spleen 289.59
    bilharzial (*see also* Schistosomiasis) 120.9
  subepidermal nodular (M8832/0) — *see* Neoplasm, skin, benign
  submucous NEC 709.2
    oral 528.8
    tongue 528.8
  syncytium — *see* Placenta, abnormal
  testis 608.89
    chronic, due to syphilis 095.8
  thymus (gland) 254.8
  tunica vaginalis 608.89
  ureter 593.89
  urethra 599.84
  uterus (nonneoplastic) 621.8
    bilharzial (*see also* Schistosomiasis) 120.9
    neoplastic (*see also* Leiomyoma, uterus) 218.9

Index to Diseases

Fibrosis, fibrotic — *continued*
  vagina 623.8
  valve, heart (*see also* Endocarditis) 424.90
  vas deferens 608.89
  vein 459.89
    lower extremities 459.89
  vesical 595.1

Fibrositis (periarticular) (rheumatoid) 729.0
  humeroscapular region 726.2
  nodular, chronic
    Jaccoud's 714.4
    rheumatoid 714.4
  ossificans 728.11
  scapulohumeral 726.2

Fibrothorax 511.0

Fibrotic — *see* Fibrosis

Fibrous — *see* condition

Fibroxanthoma (M8831/0) — *see also* Neoplasm, connective tissue, benign
  atypical (M8831/1) — *see* Neoplasm, connective tissue, uncertain behavior
  malignant (M8831/3) — *see* Neoplasm, connective tissue, malignant

Fibroxanthosarcoma (M8831/3) — *see* Neoplasm, connective tissue, malignant

Fiedler's
  disease (leptospiral jaundice) 100.0
  myocarditis or syndrome (acute isolated myocarditis) 422.91

Fiessinger-Leroy (-Reiter) syndrome 099.3

Fiessinger-Rendu syndrome (erythema muliforme exudativum) 695.1

Fifth disease (eruptive) 057.0
  venereal 099.1

Filaria, filarial — *see* Infestation, filarial

Filariasis (*see also* Infestation, filarial) 125.9
  bancroftian 125.0
  Brug's 125.1
  due to
    bancrofti 125.0
    Brugia (Wuchereria) (malayi) 125.1
    Loa loa 125.2
    malayi 125.1
    organism NEC 125.6
    Wuchereria (bancrofti) 125.0
      malayi 125.1
  Malayan 125.1
  ozzardi 125.1
  specified type NEC 125.6

Filatoff's, Filatov's, Filatow's disease (infectious mononucleosis) 075

File-cutters' disease 984.9
  specified type of lead — *see* Table of Drugs and Chemicals

Filling defect
  biliary tract 793.3
  bladder 793.5
  duodenum 793.4
  gallbladder 793.3
  gastrointestinal tract 793.4
  intestine 793.4
  kidney 793.5
  stomach 793.4
  ureter 793.5

Filtering bleb, eye (postglaucoma) (status) V45.69
  with complication or rupture 997.99
  postcataract extraction (complication) 997.99

Fimbrial cyst (congenital) 752.11

Fimbriated hymen 752.49

Financial problem affecting care V60.2

Findings, abnormal, without diagnosis (examination) (laboratory test) 796.4
  17-ketosteroids, elevated 791.9
  acetonuria 791.6
  acid phosphatase 790.5
  albumin-globulin ratio 790.99
  albuminuria 791.0
  alcohol in blood 790.3
  alkaline phosphatase 790.5
  amniotic fluid 792.3
  amylase 790.5
  anisocytosis 790.09
  antenatal screening 796.5

Findings, abnormal, without diagnosis — *continued*
  anthrax, positive 795.31 ●
  antibody titers, elevated 795.79
  anticardiolipin antibody 795.79
  antigen-antibody reaction 795.79
  antiphospholipid antibody 795.79
  bacteriuria 791.9
  ballistocardiogram 794.39
  bicarbonate 276.9
  bile in urine 791.4
  bilirubin 277.4
  bleeding time (prolonged) 790.92
  blood culture, positive 790.7
  blood gas level 790.91
  blood sugar level 790.2
    high 790.2
    low 251.2
  calcium 275.40
  carbonate 276.9
  casts, urine 791.7
  catecholamines 791.9
  cells, urine 791.7
  cerebrospinal fluid (color) (content) (pressure) 792.0
  chloride 276.9
  cholesterol 272.9
  chromosome analysis 795.2
  chyluria 791.1
  circulation time 794.39
  cloudy dialysis effluent 792.5
  cloudy urine 791.9
  coagulation study 790.92
  cobalt, blood 790.6
  color of urine (unusual) NEC 791.9
  copper, blood 790.6
  crystals, urine 791.9
  culture, positive NEC 795.39 ▲
    blood 790.7
    HIV V08
    human immunodeficiency virus V08
    nose 795.39 ▲
    skin lesion NEC 795.39 ▲
    spinal fluid 792.0
    sputum 795.39 ▲
    stool 792.1
    throat 795.39 ▲
    urine 791.9
    viral
      human immunodeficiency V08
    wound 795.39 ▲
  echocardiogram 793.2
  echoencephalogram 794.01
  echogram NEC — *see* Findings, abnormal, structure
  electrocardiogram (ECG) (EKG) 794.31
  electroencephalogram (EEG) 794.02
  electrolyte level, urinary 791.9
  electromyogram (EMG) 794.17
    ocular 794.14
  electro-oculogram (EOG) 794.12
  electroretinogram (ERG) 794.11
  enzymes, serum NEC 790.5
  fibrinogen titer coagulation study 790.92
  filling defect — *see* Filling defect
  function study NEC 794.9
    auditory 794.15
    bladder 794.9
    brain 794.00
    cardiac 794.30
    endocrine NEC 794.6
      thyroid 794.5
    kidney 794.4
    liver 794.8
    nervous system
      central 794.00
      peripheral 794.19
    oculomotor 794.14
    pancreas 794.9
    placenta 794.9
    pulmonary 794.2
    retina 794.11
    special senses 794.19
    spleen 794.9
    vestibular 794.16
  gallbladder, nonvisualization 793.3
  glucose 790.2
    tolerance test 790.2

Findings, abnormal, without diagnosis — *continued*
  glycosuria 791.5
  heart
    shadow 793.2
    sounds 785.3
  hematinuria 791.2
  hematocrit
    drop (precipitous) 790.01
    elevated 282.7
    low 285.9
  hematologic NEC 790.99
  hematuria 599.7
  hemoglobin
    elevated 282.7
    low 285.9
  hemoglobinuria 791.2
  histological NEC 795.4
  hormones 259.9
  immunoglobulins, elevated 795.79
  indolacetic acid, elevated 791.9
  iron 790.6
  karyotype 795.2
  ketonuria 791.6
  lactic acid dehydrogenase (LDH) 790.4
  lipase 790.5
  lipids NEC 272.9
  lithium, blood 790.6
  lung field (coin lesion) (shadow) 793.1
  magnesium, blood 790.6
  mammogram 793.80
    microcalcification 793.81
  mediastinal shift 793.2
  melanin, urine 791.9
  microbiologic NEC 795.39 ▲
  mineral, blood NEC 790.6
  myoglobinuria 791.3
  nasal swab, anthrax 795.31 ●
  nitrogen derivatives, blood 790.6
  nonvisualization of gallbladder 793.3
  nose culture, positive 795.39 ▲
  odor of urine (unusual) NEC 791.9
  oxygen saturation 790.91
  Papanicolaou (smear) 795.1
    cervix 795.00 ▲
      atypical squamous cell changes of undetermined significance ●
        favor benign (ASCUS favor benign) 795.01 ●
        favor dysplasia (ASCUS favor dysplasia) 795.02 ●
      dyskaryotic 795.09 ●
      nonspecific finding NEC 795.09 ●
    other site 795.1
  peritoneal fluid 792.9
  phonocardiogram 794.39
  phosphorus 275.3
  pleural fluid 792.9
  pneumoencephalogram 793.0
  PO$_2$-oxygen ratio 790.91
  poikilocytosis 790.09
  potassium
    deficiency 276.8
    excess 276.7
  PPD 795.5
  prostate specific antigen (PSA) 790.93
  protein, serum NEC 790.99
  proteinuria 791.0
  prothrombin time (partial) (prolonged) (PT) (PTT) 790.92
  pyuria 791.9
  radiologic (x-ray) 793.9
    abdomen 793.6
    biliary tract 793.3
    breast 793.89
      abnormal mammogram NOS 793.80
      mammographic microcalcification 793.81
    gastrointestinal tract 793.4
    genitourinary organs 793.5
    head 793.0
    intrathoracic organs NEC 793.2
    lung 793.1
    musculoskeletal 793.7
    placenta 793.9
    retroperitoneum 793.6
    skin 793.9
    skull 793.0

Findings, abnormal, without diagnosis — *continued*
  radiologic — *continued*
    subcutaneous tissue 793.9
  red blood cell 790.09
    count 790.09
    morphology 790.09
    sickling 790.09
    volume 790.09
  saliva 792.4
  scan NEC 794.9
    bladder 794.9
    bone 794.9
    brain 794.09
    kidney 794.4
    liver 794.8
    lung 794.2
    pancreas 794.9
    placental 794.9
    spleen 794.9
    thyroid 794.5
  sedimentation rate, elevated 790.1
  semen 792.2
  serological (for)
    human immunodeficiency virus (HIV)
      inconclusive 795.71
      positive V08
    syphilis — *see* Findings, serology for syphilis
  serology for syphilis
    false positive 795.6
    positive 097.1
      false 795.6
      follow-up of latent syphilis — *see* Syphilis, latent
      only finding — *see* Syphilis, latent
  serum 790.99
    blood NEC 790.99
    enzymes NEC 790.5
    proteins 790.99
  SGOT 790.4
  SGPT 790.4
  sickling of red blood cells 790.09
  skin test, positive 795.79
    tuberculin (without active tuberculosis) 795.5
  sodium 790.6
    deficiency 276.1
    excess 276.0
  spermatozoa 792.2
  spinal fluid 792.0
    culture, positive 792.0
  sputum culture, positive 795.39 ▲
    for acid-fast bacilli 795.39 ▲
  stool NEC 792.1
    bloody 578.1
      occult 792.1
    color 792.1
    culture, positive 792.1
    occult blood 792.1
  structure, body (echogram) (thermogram) (ultrasound) (x-ray) NEC 793.9
    abdomen 793.6
    breast 793.89
      abnormal mammogram 793.80
      mammographic microcalcification 793.81
    gastrointestinal tract 793.4
    genitourinary organs 793.5
    head 793.0
      echogram (ultrasound) 794.01
    intrathoracic organs NEC 793.2
    lung 793.1
    musculoskeletal 793.7
    placenta 793.9
    retroperitoneum 793.6
    skin 793.9
    subcutaneous tissue NEC 793.9
  synovial fluid 792.9
  thermogram — *see* Finding, abnormal, structure
  throat culture, positive 795.39 ▲
  thyroid (function) 794.5
    metabolism (rate) 794.5
    scan 794.5
    uptake 794.5
  total proteins 790.99
  toxicology (drugs) (heavy metals) 796.0
  transaminase (level) 790.4

Findings, abnormal, without diagnosis — *continued*
  triglycerides 272.9
  tuberculin skin test (without active tuberculosis) 795.5
  ultrasound — *see also* Finding, abnormal, structure
    cardiogram 793.2
  uric acid, blood 790.6
  urine, urinary constituents 791.9
    acetone 791.6
    albumin 791.0
    bacteria 791.9
    bile 791.4
    blood 599.7
    casts or cells 791.7
    chyle 791.1
    culture, positive 791.9
    glucose 791.5
    hemoglobin 791.2
    ketone 791.6
    protein 791.0
    pus 791.9
    sugar 791.5
  vaginal fluid 792.9
  vanillylmandelic acid, elevated 791.9
  vectorcardiogram (VCG) 794.39
  ventriculogram (cerebral) 793.0
  VMA, elevated 791.9
  Wassermann reaction
    false positive 795.6
    positive 097.1
      follow-up of latent syphilis — *see* Syphilis, latent
      only finding — *see* Syphilis, latent
  white blood cell 288.9
    count 288.9
      elevated 288.8
      low 288.0
    differential 288.9
    morphology 288.9
  wound culture 795.39 ▲
  xerography 793.89
  zinc, blood 790.6

Finger — *see* condition
Fire, St. Anthony's (*see also* Erysipelas) 035
Fish
  hook stomach 537.89
  meal workers' lung 495.8
Fisher's syndrome 357.0
Fissure, fissured
  abdominal wall (congenital) 756.79
  anus, anal 565.0
    congenital 751.5
  buccal cavity 528.9
  clitoris (congenital) 752.49
  ear, lobule (congenital) 744.29
  epiglottis (congenital) 748.3
  larynx 478.79
    congenital 748.3
  lip 528.5
    congenital (*see also* Cleft, lip) 749.10
  nipple 611.2
    puerperal, postpartum 676.1 ✓5ᵗʰ
  palate (congenital) (*see also* Cleft, palate) 749.00
  postanal 565.0
  rectum 565.0
  skin 709.8
    streptococcal 686.9
  spine (congenital) (*see also* Spina bifida) 741.9 ✓5ᵗʰ
  sternum (congenital) 756.3
  tongue (acquired) 529.5
    congenital 750.13
Fistula (sinus) 686.9
  abdomen (wall) 569.81
    bladder 596.2
    intestine 569.81
    ureter 593.82
    uterus 619.2
  abdominorectal 569.81
  abdominosigmoidal 569.81
  abdominothoracic 510.0
  abdominouterine 619.2
    congenital 752.3

Fistula — *continued*
  abdominovesical 596.2
  accessory sinuses (*see also* Sinusitis) 473.9
  actinomycotic — *see* Actinomycosis
  alveolar
    antrum (*see also* Sinusitis, maxillary) 473.0
    process 522.7
  anorectal 565.1
  antrobuccal (*see also* Sinusitis, maxillary) 473.0
  antrum (*see also* Sinusitis, maxillary) 473.0
  anus, anal (infectional) (recurrent) 565.1
    congenital 751.5
    tuberculous (*see also* Tuberculosis) 014.8 ✓5ᵗʰ
  aortic sinus 747.29
  aortoduodenal 447.2
  appendix, appendicular 543.9
  arteriovenous (acquired) 447.0
    brain 437.3
      congenital 747.81
        ruptured (*see also* Hemorrhage, subarachnoid) 430
      ruptured (*see also* Hemorrhage, subarachnoid) 430
    cerebral 437.3
      congenital 747.81
    congenital (peripheral) 747.60
      brain — *see* Fistula, arteriovenous, brain, congenital
      coronary 746.85
      gastrointestinal 747.61
      lower limb 747.64
      pulmonary 747.3
      renal 747.62
      specified NEC 747.69
      upper limb 747.63
    coronary 414.19
      congenital 746.85
    heart 414.19
    pulmonary (vessels) 417.0
      congenital 747.3
    surgically created (for dialysis) V45.1
      complication NEC 996.73
        atherosclerosis — *see* Arteriosclerosis, extremities
        embolism 996.74
        infection or inflammation 996.62
        mechanical 996.1
        occlusion NEC 996.74
        thrombus 996.74
    traumatic — *see* Injury, blood vessel, by site
  artery 447.2
  aural 383.81
    congenital 744.49
  auricle 383.81
    congenital 744.49
  Bartholin's gland 619.8
  bile duct (*see also* Fistula, biliary) 576.4
  biliary (duct) (tract) 576.4
    congenital 751.69
  bladder (neck) (sphincter) 596.2
    into seminal vesicle 596.2
  bone 733.99
  brain 348.8
    arteriovenous — *see* Fistula, arteriovenous, brain
  branchial (cleft) 744.41
  branchiogenous 744.41
  breast 611.0
    puerperal, postpartum 675.1 ✓5ᵗʰ
  bronchial 510.0
  bronchocutaneous, bronchomediastinal, bronchopleural, bronchopleuromediastinal (infective) 510.0
    tuberculous (*see also* Tuberculosis) 011.3 ✓5ᵗʰ
  bronchoesophageal 530.89
    congenital 750.3
  buccal cavity (infective) 528.3
  canal, ear 380.89
  carotid-cavernous
    congenital 747.81
      with hemorrhage 430

Fistula

Fistula — *continued*
- carotid-cavernous — *continued*
  - traumatic 900.82
    - with hemorrhage (*see also* Hemorrhage, brain, traumatic) 853.0
      - late effect 908.3
- cecosigmoidal 569.81
- cecum 569.81
- cerebrospinal (fluid) 349.81
- cervical, lateral (congenital) 744.41
- cervicoaural (congenital) 744.49
- cervicosigmoidal 619.1
- cervicovesical 619.0
- cervix 619.8
- chest (wall) 510.0
- cholecystocolic (*see also* Fistula, gallbladder) 575.5
- cholecystocolonic (*see also* Fistula, gallbladder) 575.5
- cholecystoduodenal (*see also* Fistula, gallbladder) 575.5
- cholecystoenteric (*see also* Fistula, gallbladder) 575.5
- cholecystogastric (*see also* Fistula, gallbladder) 575.5
- cholecystointestinal (*see also* Fistula, gallbladder) 575.5
- choledochoduodenal 576.4
- cholocolic (*see also* Fistula, gallbladder) 575.5
- coccyx 685.1
  - with abscess 685.0
- colon 569.81
- colostomy 569.69
- colovaginal (acquired) 619.1
- common duct (bile duct) 576.4
- congenital, NEC — *see* Anomaly, specified type NEC
- cornea, causing hypotony 360.32
- coronary, arteriovenous 414.19
  - congenital 746.85
- costal region 510.0
- cul-de-sac, Douglas' 619.8
- cutaneous 686.9
- cystic duct (*see also* Fistula, gallbladder) 575.5
  - congenital 751.69
- dental 522.7
- diaphragm 510.0
  - bronchovisceral 510.0
  - pleuroperitoneal 510.0
  - pulmonoperitoneal 510.0
- duodenum 537.4
- ear (canal) (external) 380.89
- enterocolic 569.81
- enterocutaneous 569.81
- enteroenteric 569.81
- entero-uterine 619.1
  - congenital 752.3
- enterovaginal 619.1
  - congenital 752.49
- enterovesical 596.1
- epididymis 608.89
  - tuberculous (*see also* Tuberculosis) 016.4
- esophagobronchial 530.89
  - congenital 750.3
- esophagocutaneous 530.89
- esophagopleurocutaneous 530.89
- esophagotracheal 530.84
  - congenital 750.3
- esophagus 530.89
  - congenital 750.4
- ethmoid (*see also* Sinusitis, ethmoidal) 473.2
- eyeball (cornea) (sclera) 360.32
- eyelid 373.11
- fallopian tube (external) 619.2
- fecal 569.81
  - congenital 751.5
- from periapical lesion 522.7
- frontal sinus (*see also* Sinusitis, frontal) 473.1
- gallbladder 575.5
  - with calculus, cholelithiasis, stones (*see also* Cholelithiasis) 574.2
  - congenital 751.69
- gastric 537.4
- gastrocolic 537.4
  - congenital 750.7
  - tuberculous (*see also* Tuberculosis) 014.8

Fistula — *continued*
- gastroenterocolic 537.4
- gastroesophageal 537.4
- gastrojejunal 537.4
- gastrojejunocolic 537.4
- genital
  - organs
    - female 619.9
      - specified site NEC 619.8
    - male 608.89
  - tract-skin (female) 619.2
- hepatopleural 510.0
- hepatopulmonary 510.0
- horseshoe 565.1
- ileorectal 569.81
- ileosigmoidal 569.81
- ileostomy 569.69
- ileovesical 596.1
- ileum 569.81
- in ano 565.1
  - tuberculous (*see also* Tuberculosis) 014.8
- inner ear (*see also* Fistula, labyrinth) 386.40
- intestine 569.81
- intestinocolonic (abdominal) 569.81
- intestinoureteral 593.82
- intestinouterine 619.1
- intestinovaginal 619.1
  - congenital 752.49
- intestinovesical 596.1
- involving female genital tract 619.9
  - digestive-genital 619.1
  - genital tract-skin 619.2
  - specified site NEC 619.8
  - urinary-genital 619.0
- ischiorectal (fossa) 566
- jejunostomy 569.69
- jejunum 569.81
- joint 719.89
  - ankle 719.87
  - elbow 719.82
  - foot 719.87
  - hand 719.84
  - hip 719.85
  - knee 719.86
  - multiple sites 719.89
  - pelvic region 719.85
  - shoulder (region) 719.81
  - specified site NEC 719.88
  - tuberculous — *see* Tuberculosis, joint
  - wrist 719.83
- kidney 593.89
- labium (majus) (minus) 619.8
- labyrinth, labyrinthine NEC 386.40
  - combined sites 386.48
  - multiple sites 386.48
  - oval window 386.42
  - round window 386.41
  - semicircular canal 386.43
- lacrimal, lachrymal (duct) (gland) (sac) 375.61
- lacrimonasal duct 375.61
- laryngotracheal 748.3
- larynx 478.79
- lip 528.5
  - congenital 750.25
- lumbar, tuberculous (*see also* Tuberculosis) 015.0 [730.8]
- lung 510.0
- lymphatic (node) (vessel) 457.8
- mamillary 611.0
- mammary (gland) 611.0
  - puerperal, postpartum 675.1
- mastoid (process) (region) 383.1
- maxillary (*see also* Sinusitis, maxillary) 473.0
- mediastinal 510.0
- mediastinobronchial 510.0
- mediastinocutaneous 510.0
- middle ear 385.89
- mouth 528.3
- nasal 478.1
  - sinus (*see also* Sinusitis) 473.9
- nasopharynx 478.29
- nipple — *see* Fistula, breast
- nose 478.1
- oral (cutaneous) 528.3
  - maxillary (*see also* Sinusitis, maxillary) 473.0

Fistula — *continued*
- oral — *continued*
  - nasal (with cleft palate) (*see also* Cleft, palate) 749.00
- orbit, orbital 376.10
- oro-antral (*see also* Sinusitis, maxillary) 473.0
- oval window (internal ear) 386.42
- oviduct (external) 619.2
- palate (hard) 526.89
  - soft 528.9
- pancreatic 577.8
- pancreaticoduodenal 577.8
- parotid (gland) 527.4
  - region 528.3
- pelvoabdominointestinal 569.81
- penis 607.89
- perianal 565.1
- pericardium (pleura) (sac) (*see also* Pericarditis) 423.8
- pericecal 569.81
- perineal — *see* Fistula, perineum
- perineorectal 569.81
- perineosigmoidal 569.81
- perineo-urethroscrotal 608.89
- perineum, perineal (with urethral involvement) NEC 599.1
  - tuberculous (*see also* Tuberculosis) 017.9
  - ureter 593.82
- perirectal 565.1
  - tuberculous (*see also* Tuberculosis) 014.8
- peritoneum (*see also* Peritonitis) 567.2
- periurethral 599.1
- pharyngo-esophageal 478.29
- pharynx 478.29
  - branchial cleft (congenital) 744.41
- pilonidal (infected) (rectum) 685.1
  - with abscess 685.0
- pleura, pleural, pleurocutaneous, pleuroperitoneal 510.0
  - stomach 510.0
  - tuberculous (*see also* Tuberculosis) 012.0
- pleuropericardial 423.8
- postauricular 383.81
- postoperative, persistent 998.6
- preauricular (congenital) 744.46
- prostate 602.8
- pulmonary 510.0
  - arteriovenous 417.0
    - congenital 747.3
  - tuberculous (*see also* Tuberculosis, pulmonary) 011.9
- pulmonoperitoneal 510.0
- rectolabial 619.1
- rectosigmoid (intercommunicating) 569.81
- rectoureteral 593.82
- rectourethral 599.1
  - congenital 753.8
- rectouterine 619.1
  - congenital 752.3
- rectovaginal 619.1
  - congenital 752.49
  - old, postpartal 619.1
  - tuberculous (*see also* Tuberculosis) 014.8
- rectovesical 596.1
  - congenital 753.8
- rectovesicovaginal 619.1
- rectovulvar 619.1
  - congenital 752.49
- rectum (to skin) 565.1
  - tuberculous (*see also* Tuberculosis) 014.8
- renal 593.89
- retroauricular 383.81
- round window (internal ear) 386.41
- salivary duct or gland 527.4
  - congenital 750.24
- sclera 360.32
- scrotum (urinary) 608.89
  - tuberculous (*see also* Tuberculosis) 016.5
- semicircular canals (internal ear) 386.43
- sigmoid 569.81
  - vesicoabdominal 596.1

Fistula — *continued*
  sigmoidovaginal 619.1
    congenital 752.49
  skin 686.9
    ureter 593.82
    vagina 619.2
  sphenoidal sinus (*see also* Sinusitis, sphenoidal) 473.3
  splenocolic 289.59
  stercoral 569.81
  stomach 537.4
  sublingual gland 527.4
    congenital 750.24
  submaxillary
    gland 527.4
      congenital 750.24
    region 528.3
  thoracic 510.0
    duct 457.8
  thoracicoabdominal 510.0
  thoracicogastric 510.0
  thoracicointestinal 510.0
  thoracoabdominal 510.0
  thoracogastric 510.0
  thorax 510.0
  thyroglossal duct 759.2
  thyroid 246.8
  trachea (congenital) (external) (internal) 748.3
  tracheoesophageal 530.84
    congenital 750.3
    following tracheostomy 519.09
  traumatic
    arteriovenous (*see also* Injury, blood vessel, by site) 904.9
      brain — *see* Injury, intracranial
  tuberculous — *see* Tuberculosis, by site
  typhoid 002.0
  umbilical 759.89
  umbilico-urinary 753.8
  urachal, urachus 753.7
  ureter (persistent) 593.82
  ureteroabdominal 593.82
  ureterocervical 593.82
  ureterorectal 593.82
  ureterosigmoido-abdominal 593.82
  ureterovaginal 619.0
  ureterovesical 596.2
  urethra 599.1
    congenital 753.8
    tuberculous (*see also* Tuberculosis) 016.3 ✓5ᵗʰ
  urethroperineal 599.1
  urethroperineovesical 596.2
  urethrorectal 599.1
    congenital 753.8
  urethroscrotal 608.89
  urethrovaginal 619.0
  urethrovesical 596.2
  urethrovesicovaginal 619.0
  urinary (persistent) (recurrent) 599.1
  uteroabdominal (anterior wall) 619.2
    congenital 752.3
  uteroenteric 619.1
  uterofecal 619.1
  uterointestinal 619.1
    congenital 752.3
  uterorectal 619.1
    congenital 752.3
  uteroureteric 619.0
  uterovaginal 619.8
  uterovesical 619.0
    congenital 752.3
  uterus 619.8
  vagina (wall) 619.8
    postpartal, old 619.8
  vaginocutaneous (postpartal) 619.2
  vaginoileal (acquired) 619.1
  vaginoperineal 619.2
  vesical NEC 596.2
  vesicoabdominal 596.2
  vesicocervicovaginal 619.0
  vesicocolic 596.1
  vesicocutaneous 596.2
  vesicoenteric 596.1
  vesicointestinal 596.1
  vesicometrorectal 619.1
  vesicoperineal 596.2

Fistula — *continued*
  vesicorectal 596.1
    congenital 753.8
  vesicosigmoidal 596.1
  vesicosigmoidovaginal 619.1
  vesicoureteral 596.2
  vesicoureterovaginal 619.0
  vesicourethral 596.2
  vesicourethrorectal 596.1
  vesicouterine 619.0
    congenital 752.3
  vesicovaginal 619.0
  vulvorectal 619.1
    congenital 752.49

Fit 780.39
  apoplectic (*see also* Disease, cerebrovascular, acute) 436
    late effect — *see* Late effect(s) (of) cerebrovascular disease
  epileptic (*see also* Epilepsy) 345.9 ✓5ᵗʰ
  fainting 780.2
  hysterical 300.11
  newborn 779.0

Fitting (of)
  artificial
    arm (complete) (partial) V52.0
    breast V52.4
    eye(s) V52.2
    leg(s) (complete) (partial) V52.1
  brain neuropacemaker V53.02
  cardiac pacemaker V53.31
  carotid sinus pacemaker V53.39
  cerebral ventricle (communicating) shunt V53.01
  colostomy belt V53.5
  contact lenses V53.1
  cystostomy device V53.6
  defibrillator, automatic implantable cardiac V53.32
  dentures V52.3
  device NEC V53.9
    abdominal V53.5
    cardiac
      defibrillator, automatic implantable V53.32
      pacemaker V53.31
      specified NEC V53.39
    cerebral ventricle (communicating) shunt V53.01
    intrauterine contraceptive V25.1
    nervous system V53.09
    orthodontic V53.4
    orthoptic V53.1
    prosthetic V52.9
      breast V52.4
      dental V52.3
      eye V52.2
      specified type NEC V52.8
    special senses V53.09
    substitution
      auditory V53.09
      nervous system V53.09
      visual V53.09
    urinary V53.6
  diaphragm (contraceptive) V25.02
  glasses (reading) V53.1
  hearing aid V53.2
  ileostomy device V53.5
  intestinal appliance or device NEC V53.5
  intrauterine contraceptive device V25.1
  neuropacemaker (brain) (peripheral nerve) (spinal cord) V53.02
  orthodontic device V53.4
  orthopedic (device) V53.7
    brace V53.7
    cast V53.7
    corset V53.7
    shoes V53.7
  pacemaker (cardiac) V53.31
    brain V53.02
    carotid sinus V53.39
    peripheral nerve V53.02
    spinal cord V53.02
  prosthesis V52.9
    arm (complete) (partial) V52.0
    breast V52.4
    dental V52.3

Fitting — *continued*
  prosthesis — *continued*
    eye V52.2
    leg (complete) (partial) V52.1
    specified type NEC V52.8
  spectacles V53.1
  wheelchair V53.8

Fitz's syndrome (acute hemorrhagic pancreatitis) 577.0

Fitz-Hugh and Curtis syndrome (gonococcal peritonitis) 098.86

Fixation
  joint — *see* Ankylosis
  larynx 478.79
  pupil 364.76
  stapes 385.22
    deafness (*see also* Deafness, conductive) 389.04
  uterus (acquired) — *see* Malposition, uterus
  vocal cord 478.5

Flaccid — *see also* condition
  foot 736.79
  forearm 736.09
  palate, congenital 750.26

Flail
  chest 807.4
    newborn 767.3
  joint (paralytic) 718.80
    ankle 718.87
    elbow 718.82
    foot 718.87
    hand 718.84
    hip 718.85
    knee 718.86
    multiple sites 718.89
    pelvic region 718.85
    shoulder (region) 718.81
    specified site NEC 718.88
    wrist 718.83

Flajani (-Basedow) syndrome or disease (exophthalmic goiter) 242.0 ✓5ᵗʰ

Flap, liver 572.8

Flare, anterior chamber (aqueous) (eye) 364.04

Flashback phenomena (drug) (hallucinogenic) 292.89

Flat
  chamber (anterior) (eye) 360.34
  chest, congenital 754.89
  electroencephalogram (EEG) 348.8
  foot (acquired) (fixed type) (painful) (postural) (spastic) 734
    congenital 754.61
      rocker bottom 754.61
      vertical talus 754.61
    rachitic 268.1
    rocker bottom (congenital) 754.61
    vertical talus, congenital 754.61
  organ or site, congenital NEC — *see* Anomaly, specified type NEC
  pelvis 738.6
    with disproportion (fetopelvic) 653.2 ✓5ᵗʰ
      affecting fetus or newborn 763.1
      causing obstructed labor 660.1 ✓5ᵗʰ
        affecting fetus or newborn 763.1
    congenital 755.69

Flatau-Schilder disease 341.1

Flattening
  head, femur 736.39
  hip 736.39
  lip (congenital) 744.89
  nose (congenital) 754.0
    acquired 738.0

Flatulence 787.3

Flatus 787.3
  vaginalis 629.8

Flax dressers' disease 504

Flea bite — *see* Injury, superficial, by site

Fleischer (-Kayser) ring (corneal pigmentation) 275.1 [371.14]

Fleischner's disease 732.3

Fleshy mole 631

Flexibilitas cerea (*see also* Catalepsy) 300.11

Flexion
- cervix (see also Malposition, uterus) 621.6
- contracture, joint (see also Contraction, joint) 718.4 ✓5ᵗʰ
- deformity, joint (see also Contraction, joint) 718.4 ✓5ᵗʰ
  - hip, congenital (see also Subluxation, congenital, hip) 754.32
- uterus (see also Malposition, uterus) 621.6

Flexner's
- bacillus 004.1
- diarrhea (ulcerative) 004.1
- dysentery 004.1

Flexner-Boyd dysentery 004.2

Flexure — see condition

Floater, vitreous 379.24

Floating
- cartilage (joint) (see also Disorder, cartilage, articular) 718.0 ✓5ᵗʰ
  - knee 717.6
- gallbladder (congenital) 751.69
- kidney 593.0
  - congenital 753.3
- liver (congenital) 751.69
- rib 756.3
- spleen 289.59

Flooding 626.2

Floor — see condition

Floppy
- infant NEC 781.99
- valve syndrome (mitral) 424.0

Flu — see also Influenza
- gastric NEC 008.8

Fluctuating blood pressure 796.4

Fluid
- abdomen 789.5
- chest (see also Pleurisy, with effusion) 511.9
- heart (see also Failure, heart) 428.0
- joint (see also Effusion, joint) 719.0 ✓5ᵗʰ
- loss (acute) 276.5
  - with
    - hypernatremia 276.0
    - hyponatremia 276.1
- lung — see also Edema, lung encysted 511.8
- peritoneal cavity 789.5
- pleural cavity (see also Pleurisy, with effusion) 511.9
- retention 276.6

Flukes NEC (see also Infestation, fluke) 121.9
- blood NEC (see also Infestation, Schistosoma) 120.9
- liver 121.3

Fluor (albus) (vaginalis) 623.5
- trichomonal (Trichomonas vaginalis) 131.00

Fluorosis (dental) (chronic) 520.3

Flushing 782.62
- menopausal 627.2

Flush syndrome 259.2

Flutter
- atrial or auricular 427.32
- heart (ventricular) 427.42
  - atrial 427.32
  - impure 427.32
  - postoperative 997.1
  - ventricular 427.42

Flux (bloody) (serosanguineous) 009.0

Focal — see condition

Fochier's abscess — see Abscess, by site

Focus, Assmann's (see also Tuberculosis) 011.0 ✓5ᵗʰ

Fogo selvagem 694.4

Foix-Alajouanine syndrome 336.1

Folds, anomalous — see also Anomaly, specified type NEC
- Bowman's membrane 371.31
- Descemet's membrane 371.32
- epicanthic 743.63
- heart 746.89
- posterior segment of eye, congenital 743.54

Folie à deux 297.3

Follicle
- cervix (nabothian) (ruptured) 616.0
- graafian, ruptured, with hemorrhage 620.0

Follicle — continued
- nabothian 616.0

Folliclis (primary) (see also Tuberculosis) 017.0 ✓5ᵗʰ

Follicular — see also condition
- cyst (atretic) 620.0

Folliculitis 704.8
- abscedens et suffodiens 704.8
- decalvans 704.09
- gonorrheal (acute) 098.0
  - chronic or duration of 2 months or more 098.2
- keloid, keloidalis 706.1
- pustular 704.8
- ulerythematosa reticulata 701.8

Folliculosis, conjunctival 372.02

Følling's disease (phenylketonuria) 270.1

Follow-up (examination) (routine) (following) V67.9
- cancer chemotherapy V67.2
- chemotherapy V67.2
- fracture V67.4
- high-risk medication V67.51
- injury NEC V67.59
- postpartum
  - immediately after delivery V24.0
  - routine V24.2
- psychiatric V67.3
- psychotherapy V67.3
- radiotherapy V67.1
- specified condition NEC V67.59
- specified surgery NEC V67.09
- surgery V67.00
  - vaginal pap smear V67.01
- treatment V67.9
  - combined NEC V67.6
  - fracture V67.4
  - involving high-risk medication NEC V67.51
  - mental disorder V67.3
  - specified NEC V67.59

Fong's syndrome (hereditary osteoonychodysplasia) 756.89

Food
- allergy 693.1
- anaphylactic shock — see Anaphylactic shock, due to, food
- asphyxia (from aspiration or inhalation) (see also Asphyxia, food) 933.1
- choked on (see also Asphyxia, food) 933.1
- deprivation 994.2
  - specified kind of food NEC 269.8
- intoxication (see also Poisoning, food) 005.9
- lack of 994.2
- poisoning (see also Poisoning, food) 005.9
- refusal or rejection NEC 307.59
- strangulation or suffocation (see also Asphyxia, food) 933.1
- toxemia (see also Poisoning, food) 005.9

Foot — see also condition
- and mouth disease 078.4
- process disease 581.3

Foramen ovale (nonclosure) (patent) (persistent) 745.5

Forbes' (glycogen storage) disease 271.0

Forbes-Albright syndrome (nonpuerperal amenorrhea and lactation associated with pituitary tumor) 253.1

Forced birth or delivery NEC 669.8 ✓5ᵗʰ
- affecting fetus or newborn NEC 763.89

Forceps
- delivery NEC 669.6 ✓5ᵗʰ
  - affecting fetus or newborn 763.2

Fordyce's disease (ectopic sebaceous glands) (mouth) 750.26

Fordyce-Fox disease (apocrine miliaria) 705.82

Forearm — see condition

Foreign body

> Note — For foreign body with open wound or other injury, see Wound, open, or the type of injury specified.

- accidentally left during a procedure 998.4

Foreign body — continued
- anterior chamber (eye) 871.6
  - magnetic 871.5
    - retained or old 360.51
  - retained or old 360.61
- ciliary body (eye) 871.6
  - magnetic 871.5
    - retained or old 360.52
  - retained or old 360.62
- entering through orifice (current) (old)
  - accessory sinus 932
  - air passage (upper) 933.0
    - lower 934.8
  - alimentary canal 938
  - alveolar process 935.0
  - antrum (Highmore) 932
  - anus 937
  - appendix 936
  - asphyxia due to (see also Asphyxia, food) 933.1
  - auditory canal 931
  - auricle 931
  - bladder 939.0
  - bronchioles 934.8
  - bronchus (main) 934.1
  - buccal cavity 935.0
  - canthus (inner) 930.1
  - cecum 936
  - cervix (canal) uterine 939.1
  - coil, ileocecal 936
  - colon 936
  - conjunctiva 930.1
  - conjunctival sac 930.1
  - cornea 930.0
  - digestive organ or tract NEC 938
  - duodenum 936
  - ear (external) 931
  - esophagus 935.1
  - eye (external) 930.9
    - combined sites 930.8
    - intraocular — see Foreign body, by site
    - specified site NEC 930.8
  - eyeball 930.8
    - intraocular — see Foreign body, intraocular
  - eyelid 930.1
    - retained or old 374.86
  - frontal sinus 932
  - gastrointestinal tract 938
  - genitourinary tract 939.9
  - globe 930.8
    - penetrating 871.6
      - magnetic 871.5
        - retained or old 360.50
      - retained or old 360.60
  - gum 935.0
  - Highmore's antrum 932
  - hypopharynx 933.0
  - ileocecal coil 936
  - ileum 936
  - inspiration (of) 933.1
  - intestine (large) (small) 936
  - lacrimal apparatus, duct, gland, or sac 930.2
  - larynx 933.1
  - lung 934.8
  - maxillary sinus 932
  - mouth 935.0
  - nasal sinus 932
  - nasopharynx 933.0
  - nose (passage) 932
  - nostril 932
  - oral cavity 935.0
  - palate 935.0
  - penis 939.3
  - pharynx 933.0
  - pyriform sinus 933.0
  - rectosigmoid 937
    - junction 937
  - rectum 937
  - respiratory tract 934.9
    - specified part NEC 934.8
  - sclera 930.1
  - sinus 932
    - accessory 932
    - frontal 932
    - maxillary 932

Foreign body — *continued*
- entering through orifice — *continued*
  - sinus — *continued*
    - nasal 932
    - pyriform 933.0
  - small intestine 936
  - stomach (hairball) 935.2
  - suffocation by (*see also* Asphyxia, food) 933.1
  - swallowed 938
    - tongue 933.0
  - tear ducts or glands 930.2
  - throat 933.0
  - tongue 935.0
    - swallowed 933.0
  - tonsil, tonsillar 933.0
    - fossa 933.0
  - trachea 934.0
  - ureter 939.0
  - urethra 939.0
  - uterus (any part) 939.1
  - vagina 939.2
  - vulva 939.2
  - wind pipe 934.0
- granuloma (old) 728.82
  - bone 733.99
  - in operative wound (inadvertently left) 998.4
    - due to surgical material intentionally left — *see* Complications, due to (presence of) any device, implant, or graft classified to 996.0-996.5 NEC
  - muscle 728.82
  - skin 709.4
  - soft tissue 709.4
  - subcutaneous tissue 709.4
- in
  - bone (residual) 733.99
  - open wound — *see* Wound, open, by site complicated
  - soft tissue (residual) 729.6
- inadvertently left in operation wound (causing adhesions, obstruction, or perforation) 998.4
- ingestion, ingested NEC 938
- inhalation or inspiration (*see also* Asphyxia, food) 933.1
- internal organ, not entering through an orifice — *see* Injury, internal, by site, with open wound
- intraocular (nonmagnetic 871.6
  - combined sites 871.6
    - magnetic 871.5
      - retained or old 360.59
    - retained or old 360.69
  - magnetic 871.5
    - retained or old 360.50
  - retained or old 360.60
  - specified site NEC 871.6
    - magnetic 871.5
      - retained or old 360.59
    - retained or old 360.69
  - iris (nonmagnetic) 871.6
    - magnetic 871.5
      - retained or old 360.52
    - retained or old 360.62
  - lens (nonmagnetic) 871.6
    - magnetic 871.5
      - retained or old 360.53
    - retained or old 360.63
- lid, eye 930.1
- ocular muscle 870.4
  - retained or old 376.6
- old or residual
  - bone 733.99
  - eyelid 374.86
  - middle ear 385.83
  - muscle 729.6
    - ocular 376.6
  - retrobulbar 376.6
  - skin 729.6
    - with granuloma 709.4
  - soft tissue 729.6
    - with granuloma 709.4
  - subcutaneous tissue 729.6
    - with granuloma 709.4
- operation wound, left accidentally 998.4

Foreign body — *continued*
- orbit 870.4
  - retained or old 376.6
- posterior wall, eye 871.6
  - magnetic 871.5
    - retained or old 360.55
  - retained or old 360.65
- respiratory tree 934.9
  - specified site NEC 934.8
- retained (old) (nonmagnetic) (in)
  - anterior chamber (eye) 360.61
    - magnetic 360.51
  - ciliary body 360.62
    - magnetic 360.52
  - eyelid 374.86
  - globe 360.60
    - magnetic 360.50
  - intraocular 360.60
    - magnetic 360.50
    - specified site NEC 360.69
      - magnetic 360.59
  - iris 360.62
    - magnetic 360.52
  - lens 360.63
    - magnetic 360.53
  - muscle 729.6
  - orbit 376.6
  - posterior wall of globe 360.65
    - magnetic 360.55
  - retina 360.65
    - magnetic 360.55
  - retrobulbar 376.6
  - soft tissue 729.6
  - vitreous 360.64
    - magnetic 360.54
  - skin 729.6
    - with granuloma 709.4
  - soft tissue 729.6
    - with granuloma 709.4
  - subcutaneous tissue 729.6
    - with granuloma 709.4
- retina 871.6
  - magnetic 871.5
    - retained or old 360.55
  - retained or old 360.65
- superficial, without major open wound (*see also* Injury, superficial, by site) 919.6
- swallowed NEC 938
- vitreous (humor) 871.6
  - magnetic 871.5
    - retained or old 360.54
  - retained or old 360.64

Forking, aqueduct of Sylvius 742.3
- with spina bifida (*see also* Spina bifida) 741.0

Formation
- bone in scar tissue (skin) 709.3
- connective tissue in vitreous 379.25
- Elschnig pearls (postcataract extraction) 366.51
- hyaline in cornea 371.49
- sequestrum in bone (due to infection) (*see also* Osteomyelitis) 730.1
- valve
  - colon, congenital 751.5
  - ureter (congenital) 753.29

Formication 782.0
Fort Bragg fever 100.89
Fossa — *see also* condition
- pyriform — *see* condition

Foster-Kennedy syndrome 377.04
Fothergill's
- disease, meaning scarlatina anginosa 034.1
- neuralgia (*see also* Neuralgia, trigeminal) 350.1

Foul breath 784.9
Found dead (cause unknown) 798.9
Foundling V20.0
Fournier's disease (idiopathic gangrene) 608.83
Fourth
- cranial nerve — *see* condition
- disease 057.8
- molar 520.1

Foville's syndrome 344.89

Fox's
- disease (apocrine miliaria) 705.82
- impetigo (contagiosa) 684

Fox-Fordyce disease (apocrine miliaria) 705.82

Fracture (abduction) (adduction) (avulsion) (compression) (crush) (dislocation) (oblique) (separation) (closed) 829.0

> Note — For fracture of any of the following sites with fracture of other bones — see Fracture, multiple.
> "Closed" includes the following descriptions of fractures, with or without delayed healing, unless they are specified as open or compound:
>
> | | |
> |---|---|
> | comminuted | linear |
> | depressed | simple |
> | elevated | slipped epiphysis |
> | fissured | spiral |
> | greenstick | unspecified |
> | impacted | |
>
> "Open" includes the following descriptions of fractures, with or without delayed healing:
>
> | | |
> |---|---|
> | compound | puncture |
> | infected | with foreign body |
> | missile | |
>
> For late effect of fracture, see Late, effect, fracture, by site.

- with
  - internal injuries in same region (conditions classifiable to 860-869) — *see also* Injury, internal, by site pelvic region — *see* Fracture, pelvis
- acetabulum (with visceral injury) (closed) 808.0
  - open 808.1
- acromion (process) (closed) 811.01
  - open 811.11
- alveolus (closed) 802.8
  - open 802.9
- ankle (malleolus) (closed) 824.8
  - bimalleolar (Dupuytren's) (Pott's) 824.4
    - open 824.5
  - bone 825.21
    - open 825.31
  - lateral malleolus only (fibular) 824.2
    - open 824.3
  - medial malleolus only (tibial) 824.0
    - open 824.1
  - open 824.9
  - pathologic 733.16
  - talus 825.21
    - open 825.31
  - trimalleolar 824.6
    - open 824.7
- antrum — *see* Fracture, skull, base
- arm (closed) 818.0
  - and leg(s) (any bones) 828.0
    - open 828.1
  - both (any bones) (with rib(s)) (with sternum) 819.0
    - open 819.1
  - lower 813.80
    - open 813.90
  - open 818.1
  - upper — *see* Fracture, humerus
- astragalus (closed) 825.21
  - open 825.31
- atlas — *see* Fracture, vertebra, cervical, first
- axis — *see* Fracture, vertebra, cervical, second
- back — *see* Fracture, vertebra, by site
- Barton's — *see* Fracture, radius, lower end
- basal (skull) — *see* Fracture, skull, base
- Bennett's (closed) 815.01
  - open 815.11
- bimalleolar (closed) 824.4
  - open 824.5
- bone (closed) NEC 829.0
  - birth injury NEC 767.3
  - open 829.1
  - pathologic NEC (*see also* Fracture, pathologic) 733.10
  - stress NEC (*see also* Fracture, stress) 733.95
- boot top — *see* Fracture, fibula
- boxers' — *see* Fracture, metacarpal bone(s)
- breast bone — *see* Fracture, sternum

Index to Diseases

Fracture — *continued*
  bucket handle (semilunar cartilage) — *see* Tear, meniscus
  bursting — *see* Fracture, phalanx, hand, distal
  calcaneus (closed) 825.0
    open 825.1
  capitate (bone) (closed) 814.07
    open 814.17
  capitellum (humerus) (closed) 812.49
    open 812.59
  carpal bone(s) (wrist NEC) (closed) 814.00
    open 814.10
    specified site NEC 814.09
      open 814.19
  cartilage, knee (semilunar) — *see* Tear, meniscus
  cervical — *see* Fracture, vertebra, cervical
  chauffeur's — *see* Fracture, ulna, lower end
  chisel — *see* Fracture, radius, upper end
  clavicle (interligamentous part) (closed) 810.00
    acromial end 810.03
      open 810.13
    due to birth trauma 767.2
    open 810.10
    shaft (middle third) 810.02
      open 810.12
    sternal end 810.01
      open 810.11
  clayshovelers' — *see* Fracture, vertebra, cervical
  coccyx — *see also* Fracture, vertebra, coccyx
    complicating delivery 665.6
  collar bone — *see* Fracture, clavicle
  Colles' (reversed) (closed) 813.41
    open 813.51
  comminuted — *see* Fracture, by site
  compression — *see also* Fracture, by site
    nontraumatic — *see* Fracture, pathologic
  congenital 756.9
  coracoid process (closed) 811.02
    open 811.12
  coronoid process (ulna) (closed) 813.02
    mandible (closed) 802.23
      open 802.33
    open 813.12
  costochondral junction — *see* Fracture, rib
  costosternal junction — *see* Fracture, rib
  cranium — *see* Fracture, skull, by site
  cricoid cartilage (closed) 807.5
    open 807.6
  cuboid (ankle) (closed) 825.23
    open 825.33
  cuneiform
    foot (closed) 825.24
      open 825.34
    wrist (closed) 814.03
      open 814.13
  due to
    birth injury — *see* Birth injury, fracture
    gunshot — *see* Fracture, by site, open
    neoplasm — *see* Fracture, pathologic
    osteoporosis — *see* Fracture, pathologic
  Dupuytren's (ankle) (fibula) (closed) 824.4
    open 824.5
    radius 813.42
      open 813.52
  Duverney's — *see* Fracture, ilium
  elbow — *see also* Fracture, humerus, lower end
    olecranon (process) (closed) 813.01
      open 813.11
    supracondylar (closed) 812.41
      open 812.51
  ethmoid (bone) (sinus) — *see* Fracture, skull, base
  face bone(s) (closed) NEC 802.8
    with
      other bone(s) — *see* Fracture, multiple, skull
      skull — *see also* Fracture, skull
        involving other bones — *see* Fracture, multiple, skull
    open 802.9
  fatigue — *see* Fracture, march
  femur, femoral (closed) 821.00
    cervicotrochanteric 820.03
      open 820.13
    condyles, epicondyles 821.21
      open 821.31

Fracture — *continued*
  femur, femoral — *continued*
    distal end — *see* Fracture, femur, lower end
    epiphysis (separation)
      capital 820.01
        open 820.11
      head 820.01
        open 820.11
      lower 821.22
        open 821.32
      trochanteric 820.01
        open 820.11
      upper 820.01
        open 820.11
    head 820.09
      open 820.19
    lower end or extremity (distal end) (closed) 821.20
      condyles, epicondyles 821.21
        open 821.31
      epiphysis (separation) 821.22
        open 821.32
      multiple sites 821.29
        open 821.39
      open 821.30
      specified site NEC 821.29
        open 821.39
      supracondylar 821.23
        open 821.33
      T-shaped 821.21
        open 821.31
    neck (closed) 820.8
      base (cervicotrochanteric) 820.03
        open 820.13
      extracapsular 820.20
        open 820.30
      intertrochanteric (section) 820.21
        open 820.31
      intracapsular 820.00
        open 820.10
      intratrochanteric 820.21
        open 820.31
      midcervical 820.02
        open 820.12
      open 820.9
      pathologic 733.14
        specified part NEC 733.15
      specified site NEC 820.09
        open 820.19
      transcervical 820.02
        open 820.12
      transtrochanteric 820.20
        open 820.30
    open 821.10
    pathologic 733.14
      specified part NEC 733.15
    peritrochanteric (section) 820.20
      open 820.30
    shaft (lower third) (middle third) (upper third) 821.01
      open 821.11
    subcapital 820.09
      open 820.19
    subtrochanteric (region) (section) 820.22
      open 820.32
    supracondylar 821.23
      open 821.33
    transepiphyseal 820.01
      open 820.11
    trochanter (greater) (lesser) (*see also* Fracture, femur, neck, by site) 820.20
      open 820.30
    T-shaped, into knee joint 821.21
      open 821.31
    upper end 820.8
      open 820.9
  fibula (closed) 823.81
    with tibia 823.82
      open 823.92
    distal end 824.8
      open 824.9
    epiphysis
      lower 824.8
        open 824.9
      upper — *see* Fracture, fibula, upper end

Fracture — *continued*
  fibula — *continued*
    head — *see* Fracture, fibula, upper end
    involving ankle 824.2
      open 824.3
    lower end or extremity 824.8
      open 824.9
    malleolus (external) (lateral) 824.2
      open 824.3
    open NEC 823.91
    pathologic 733.16
    proximal end — *see* Fracture, fibula, upper end
    shaft 823.21
      with tibia 823.22
        open 823.32
      open 823.31
    stress 733.93
    torus 823.41 ●
      with tibia 823.42 ●
    upper end or extremity (epiphysis) (head) (proximal end) (styloid) 823.01
      with tibia 823.02
        open 823.12
      open 823.11
  finger(s), of one hand (closed) (*see also* Fracture, phalanx, hand) 816.00
    with
      metacarpal bone(s), of same hand 817.0
        open 817.1
      thumb of same hand 816.03
        open 816.13
    open 816.10
  foot, except toe(s) alone (closed) 825.20
    open 825.30
  forearm (closed) NEC 813.80
    lower end (distal end) (lower epiphysis) 813.40
      open 813.50
    open 813.90
    shaft 813.20
      open 813.30
    upper end (proximal end) (upper epiphysis) 813.00
      open 813.10
  fossa, anterior, middle, or posterior — *see* Fracture, skull, base
  frontal (bone) — *see also* Fracture, skull, vault
    sinus — *see* Fracture, skull, base
  Galeazzi's — *see* Fracture, radius, lower end
  glenoid (cavity) (fossa) (scapula) (closed) 811.03
    open 811.13
  Gosselin's — *see* Fracture, ankle
  greenstick — *see* Fracture, by site
  grenade-throwers' — *see* Fracture, humerus, shaft
  gutter — *see* Fracture, skull, vault
  hamate (closed) 814.08
    open 814.18
  hand, one (closed) 815.00
    carpals 814.00
      open 814.10
      specified site NEC 814.09
        open 814.19
    metacarpals 815.00
      open 815.10
    multiple, bones of one hand 817.0
      open 817.1
    open 815.10
    phalanges (*see also* Fracture, phalanx, hand) 816.00
      open 816.10
  healing
    aftercare ▶(*see also* Aftercare, fracture)◀ V54.89 ▲
    change of cast V54.89 ▲
    complications — *see* condition
    convalescence V66.4 ●
    removal of
      cast V54.89 ▲
      fixation device
        external V54.89 ▲
        internal V54.0
  heel bone (closed) 825.0
    open 825.1
  hip (closed) (*see also* Fracture, femur, neck) 820.8

Fracture

Fracture — *continued*
  hip (*see also* Fracture, femur, neck) — *continued*
    open 820.9
    pathologic 733.14
  humerus (closed) 812.20
    anatomical neck 812.02
      open 812.12
    articular process (*see also* Fracture humerus, condyle(s)) 812.44
      open 812.54
    capitellum 812.49
      open 812.59
    condyle(s) 812.44
      lateral (external) 812.42
        open 812.52
      medial (internal epicondyle) 812.43
        open 812.53
      open 812.54
    distal end — *see* Fracture, humerus, lower end
    epiphysis
      lower (*see also* Fracture, humerus, condyle(s)) 812.44
        open 812.54
      upper 812.09
        open 812.19
    external condyle 812.42
      open 812.52
    great tuberosity 812.03
      open 812.13
    head 812.09
      open 812.19
    internal epicondyle 812.43
      open 812.53
    lesser tuberosity 812.09
      open 812.19
    lower end or extremity (distal end) (*see also* Fracture, humerus, by site) 812.40
      multiple sites NEC 812.49
        open 812.59
      open 812.50
      specified site NEC 812.49
        open 812.59
    neck 812.01
      open 812.11
    open 812.30
    pathologic 733.11
    proximal end — *see* Fracture, humerus, upper end
    shaft 812.21
      open 812.31
    supracondylar 812.41
      open 812.51
    surgical neck 812.01
      open 812.11
    trochlea 812.49
      open 812.59
    T-shaped 812.44
      open 812.54
    tuberosity — *see* Fracture, humerus, upper end
    upper end or extremity (proximal end) (*see also* Fracture, humerus, by site) 812.00
      open 812.10
      specified site NEC 812.09
        open 812.19
  hyoid bone (closed) 807.5
    open 807.6
  hyperextension — *see* Fracture, radius, lower end
  ilium (with visceral injury) (closed) 808.41
    open 808.51
  impaction, impacted — *see* Fracture, by site
  incus — *see* Fracture, skull, base
  innominate bone (with visceral injury) (closed) 808.49
    open 808.59
  instep, of one foot (closed) 825.20
    with toe(s) of same foot 827.0
      open 827.1
    open 825.30
  internal
    ear — *see* Fracture, skull, base
    semilunar cartilage, knee — *see* Tear, meniscus, medial

Fracture — *continued*
  intertrochanteric — *see* Fracture, femur, neck, intertrochanteric
  ischium (with visceral injury) (closed) 808.42
    open 808.52
  jaw (bone) (lower) (closed) (*see also* Fracture, mandible) 802.20
    angle 802.25
      open 802.35
    open 802.30
    upper — *see* Fracture, maxilla
  knee
    cap (closed) 822.0
      open 822.1
    cartilage (semilunar) — *see* Tear, meniscus
  labyrinth (osseous) — *see* Fracture, skull, base
  larynx (closed) 807.5
    open 807.6
  late effect — *see* Late, effects (of), fracture
  Le Fort's — *see* Fracture, maxilla
  leg (closed) 827.0
    with rib(s) or sternum 828.0
      open 828.1
    both (any bones) 828.0
      open 828.1
    lower — *see* Fracture, tibia
      open 827.1
    upper — *see* Fracture, femur
  limb
    lower (multiple) (closed) NEC 827.0
      open 827.1
    upper (multiple) (closed) NEC 818.0
      open 818.1
  long bones, due to birth trauma — *see* Birth injury, fracture
  lumbar — *see* Fracture, vertebra, lumbar
  lunate bone (closed) 814.02
    open 814.12
  malar bone (closed) 802.4
    open 802.5
  Malgaigne's (closed) 808.43
    open 808.53
  malleolus (closed) 824.8
    bimalleolar 824.4
      open 824.5
    lateral 824.2
      and medial — *see also* Fracture, malleolus, bimalleolar
        with lip of tibia — *see* Fracture, malleolus, trimalleolar
      open 824.3
    medial (closed) 824.0
      and lateral — *see also* Fracture, malleolus, bimalleolar
        with lip of tibia — *see* Fracture, malleolus, trimalleolar
      open 824.1
    open 824.9
    trimalleolar (closed) 824.6
      open 824.7
  malleus — *see* Fracture, skull, base
  malunion 733.81
  mandible (closed) 802.20
    angle 802.25
      open 802.35
    body 802.28
      alveolar border 802.27
        open 802.37
      open 802.38
      symphysis 802.26
        open 802.36
    condylar process 802.21
      open 802.31
    coronoid process 802.23
      open 802.33
    multiple sites 802.29
      open 802.39
    open 802.30
    ramus NEC 802.24
      open 802.34
    subcondylar 802.22
      open 802.32
  manubrium — *see* Fracture, sternum
  march 733.95 ▲
    fibula 733.94 ●
    metatarsals 733.94 ●
    tibia 733.94 ●

Fracture — *continued*
  maxilla, maxillary (superior) (upper jaw) (closed) 802.4
    inferior — *see* Fracture, mandible
    open 802.5
  meniscus, knee — *see* Tear, meniscus
  metacarpus, metacarpal (bone(s)), of one hand (closed) 815.00
    with phalanx, phalanges, hand (finger(s)) (thumb) of same hand 817.0
      open 817.1
    base 815.02
      first metacarpal 815.01
        open 815.11
      open 815.12
      thumb 815.01
        open 815.11
    multiple sites 815.09
      open 815.19
    neck 815.04
      open 815.14
    open 815.10
    shaft 815.03
      open 815.13
  metatarsus, metatarsal (bone(s)), of one foot (closed) 825.25
    with tarsal bone(s) 825.29
      open 825.39
    open 825.35
  Monteggia's (closed) 813.03
    open 813.13
  Moore's — *see* Fracture, radius, lower end
  multangular bone (closed)
    larger 814.05
      open 814.15
    smaller 814.06
      open 814.16
  multiple (closed) 829.0

> Note — Multiple fractures of sites classifiable to the same three- or four-digit category are coded to that category, except for sites classifiable to 810-818 or 820-827 in different limbs.
> Multiple fractures of sites classifiable to different fourth-digit subdivisions within the same three-digit category should be dealt with according to coding rules.
> Multiple fractures of sites classifiable to different three-digit categories (identifiable from the listing under "Fracture"), and of sites classifiable to 810-818 or 820-827 in different limbs should be coded according to the following list, which should be referred to in the following priority order: skull or face bones, pelvis or vertebral column, legs, arms.

  arm (multiple bones in same arm except in hand alone) (sites classifiable to 810-817 with sites classifiable to a different three-digit category in 810-817 in same arm) (closed) 818.0
    open 818.1
  arms, both or arm(s) with rib(s) or sternum (sites classifiable to 810-818 with sites classifiable to same range of categories in other limb or to 807) (closed) 819.0
    open 819.1
  bones of trunk NEC (closed) 809.0
    open 809.1
  hand, metacarpal bone(s) with phalanx or phalanges of same hand (sites classifiable to 815 with sites classifiable to 816 in same hand) (closed) 817.0
    open 817.1
  leg (multiple bones in same leg) (sites classifiable to 820-826 with sites classifiable to a different three-digit category in that range in same leg) (closed) 827.0
    open 827.1
  legs, both or leg(s) with arm(s), rib(s), or sternum (sites classifiable to 820-827 with sites classifiable to same range of categories in other leg or to 807 or 810-819) (closed) 828.0
    open 828.1

Index to Diseases

Fracture — *continued*
  Moore's — *see* Fracture, radius, lower end
  multangular bone — *continued*
    open 829.1
    pelvis with other bones except skull or face bones (sites classifiable to 808 with sites classifiable to 805-807 or 810-829) (closed) 809.0
      open 809.1
    skull, specified or unspecified bones, or face bone(s) with any other bone(s) (sites classifiable to 800-803 with sites classifiable to 805-829) (closed) 804.0 ✓5ᵗʰ

> Note — Use the following fifth-digit subclassification with categories 800, 801, 803, and 804:
>
> 0   unspecified state of consciousness
> 1   with no loss of consciousness
> 2   with brief [less than one hour] loss of consciousness
> 3   with moderate [1-24 hours] loss of consciousness
> 4   with prolonged [more than 24 hours] loss of consciousness and return to pre-existing conscious level
> 5   with prolonged [more than 24 hours] loss of consciousness, without return to pre-existing conscious level
>
> Use fifth-digit 5 to designate when a patient is unconscious and dies before regaining consciousness, regardless of the duration of the loss of consciousness
>
> 6   with loss of consciousness of unspecified duration
> 9   with concussion, unspecified

    with
      contusion, cerebral 804.1 ✓5ᵗʰ
      epidural hemorrhage 804.2 ✓5ᵗʰ
      extradural hemorrhage 804.2 ✓5ᵗʰ
      hemorrhage (intracranial) NEC 804.3 ✓5ᵗʰ
      intracranial injury NEC 804.4 ✓5ᵗʰ
      laceration, cerebral 804.1 ✓5ᵗʰ
      subarachnoid hemorrhage 804.2 ✓5ᵗʰ
      subdural hemorrhage 804.2 ✓5ᵗʰ
    open 804.5 ✓5ᵗʰ
      with
        contusion, cerebral 804.6 ✓5ᵗʰ
        epidural hemorrhage 804.7 ✓5ᵗʰ
        extradural hemorrhage 804.7 ✓5ᵗʰ
        hemorrhage (intracranial) NEC 804.8 ✓5ᵗʰ
        intracranial injury NEC 804.9 ✓5ᵗʰ
        laceration, cerebral 804.6 ✓5ᵗʰ
        subarachnoid hemorrhage 804.7 ✓5ᵗʰ
        subdural hemorrhage 804.7 ✓5ᵗʰ
    vertebral column with other bones, except skull or face bones (sites classifiable to 805 or 806 with sites classifiable to 807-808 or 810-829) (closed) 809.0
      open 809.1
  nasal (bone(s)) (closed) 802.0
    open 802.1
    sinus — *see* Fracture, skull, base
  navicular
    carpal (wrist) (closed) 814.01
      open 814.11
    tarsal (ankle) (closed) 825.22
      open 825.32
  neck — *see* Fracture, vertebra, cervical
  neural arch — *see* Fracture, vertebra, by site
  nonunion 733.82
  nose, nasal, (bone) (septum) (closed) 802.0
    open 802.1
  occiput — *see* Fracture, skull, base
  odontoid process — *see* Fracture, vertebra, cervical
  olecranon (process) (ulna) (closed) 813.01
    open 813.11
  open 829.1

Fracture — *continued*
  orbit, orbital (bone) (region) (closed) 802.8
    floor (blow-out) 802.6
      open 802.7
    open 802.9
    roof — *see* Fracture, skull, base
    specified part NEC 802.8
      open 802.9
  os
    calcis (closed) 825.0
      open 825.1
    magnum (closed) 814.07
      open 814.17
    pubis (with visceral injury) (closed) 808.2
      open 808.3
    triquetrum (closed) 814.03
      open 814.13
  osseous
    auditory meatus — *see* Fracture, skull, base
    labyrinth — *see* Fracture, skull, base
      ossicles, auditory (incus) (malleus) (stapes) — *see* Fracture, skull, base
  osteoporotic — *see* Fracture, pathologic
  palate (closed) 802.8
    open 802.9
  paratrooper — *see* Fracture, tibia, lower end
  parietal bone — *see* Fracture, skull, vault
  parry — *see* Fracture, Monteggia's
  patella (closed) 822.0
    open 822.1
  pathologic (cause unknown) 733.10
    ankle 733.16
    femur (neck) 733.14
      specified NEC 733.15
    fibula 733.16
    hip 733.14
    humerus 733.11
    radius 733.12
    specified site NEC 733.19
    tibia 733.16
    ulna 733.12
    vertebrae (collapse) 733.13
    wrist 733.12
  pedicle (of vertebral arch) — *see* Fracture, vertebra, by site
  pelvis, pelvic (bone(s)) (with visceral injury) (closed) 808.8
    multiple (with disruption of pelvic circle) 808.43
      open 808.53
    open 808.9
    rim (closed) 808.49
      open 808.59
  peritrochanteric (closed) 820.20
    open 820.30
  phalanx, phalanges, of one
    foot (closed) 826.0
      with bone(s) of same lower limb 827.0
        open 827.1
      open 826.1
    hand (closed) 816.00
      with metacarpal bone(s) of same hand 817.0
        open 817.1
      distal 816.02
        open 816.12
      middle 816.01
        open 816.11
      multiple sites NEC 816.03
        open 816.13
      open 816.10
      proximal 816.01
        open 816.11
  pisiform (closed) 814.04
    open 814.14
  pond — *see* Fracture, skull, vault
  Pott's (closed) 824.4
    open 824.5
  prosthetic device, internal — *see* Complications, mechanical
  pubis (with visceral injury) (closed) 808.2
    open 808.3
  Quervain's (closed) 814.01
    open 814.11
  radius (alone) (closed) 813.81
    with ulna NEC 813.83
      open 813.93

Fracture — *continued*
  radius — *continued*
    distal end — *see* Fracture, radius, lower end
    epiphysis
      lower — *see* Fracture, radius, lower end
      upper — *see* Fracture, radius, upper end
    head — *see* Fracture, radius, upper end
    lower end or extremity (distal end) (lower epiphysis) 813.42
      with ulna (lower end) 813.44
        open 813.54
      torus 813.45 ●
      open 813.52
    neck — *see* Fracture, radius, upper end
    open NEC 813.91
    pathologic 733.12
    proximal end — *see* Fracture, radius, upper end
    shaft (closed) 813.21
      with ulna (shaft) 813.23
        open 813.33
      open 813.31
    upper end 813.07
      with ulna (upper end) 813.08
        open 813.18
      epiphysis 813.05
        open 813.15
      head 813.05
        open 813.15
      multiple sites 813.07
        open 813.17
      neck 813.06
        open 813.16
      open 813.17
      specified site NEC 813.07
        open 813.17
  ramus
    inferior or superior (with visceral injury) (closed) 808.2
      open 808.3
    ischium — *see* Fracture, ischium
    mandible 802.24
      open 802.34
  rib(s) (closed) 807.0

> Note — Use the following fifth-digit subclassification with categories 807.0-807.1:
>
> 0   rib(s), unspecified
> 1   one rib
> 2   two ribs
> 3   three ribs
> 4   four ribs
> 5   five ribs
> 6   six ribs
> 7   seven ribs
> 8   eight or more ribs
> 9   multiple ribs, unspecified

    with flail chest (open) 807.4
    open 807.1 ✓5ᵗʰ
  root, tooth 873.63
    complicated 873.73
  sacrum — *see* Fracture, vertebra, sacrum
  scaphoid
    ankle (closed) 825.22
      open 825.32
    wrist (closed) 814.01
      open 814.11
  scapula (closed) 811.00
    acromial, acromion (process) 811.01
      open 811.11
    body 811.09
      open 811.19
    coracoid process 811.02
      open 811.12
    glenoid (cavity) (fossa) 811.03
      open 811.13
    neck 811.03
      open 811.13
    open 811.10
  semilunar
    bone, wrist (closed) 814.02
      open 814.12

Fracture

Fracture — continued
  semilunar — continued
    cartilage (interior) (knee) — see Tear, meniscus
  sesamoid bone — see Fracture, by site
  Shepherd's (closed) 825.21
    open 825.31
  shoulder — see also Fracture, humerus, upper end
    blade — see Fracture, scapula
  silverfork — see Fracture, radius, lower end
  sinus (ethmoid) (frontal) (maxillary) (nasal) (sphenoidal) — see Fracture, skull, base
  Skillern's — see Fracture, radius, shaft
  skull (multiple NEC) (with face bones) (closed) 803.0 ✓5ᵗʰ

> Note — Use the following fifth digit subclassification with categories 800, 801, 803, and 804:
>
> 0 unspecified state of consciousness
> 1 with no loss of consciousness
> 2 with brief [less than one hour] loss of consciousness
> 3 with moderate [1-24 hours] loss of consciousness
> 4 with prolonged [more than 24 hours] loss of consciousness and return to pre-existing conscious level
> 5 with prolonged [more than 24 hours] loss of consciousness, without return to pre-existing conscious level
>
> Use fifth-digit 5 to designate when a patient is unconscious and dies before regaining consciousness, regardless of the duration of loss of consciousness
>
> 6 with loss of consciousness of unspecified duration
> 9 with concussion, unspecified

    with
      contusion, cerebral 803.1 ✓5ᵗʰ
      epidural hemorrhage 803.2 ✓5ᵗʰ
      extradural hemorrhage 803.2 ✓5ᵗʰ
      hemorrhage (intracranial) NEC 803.3 ✓5ᵗʰ
      intracranial injury NEC 803.4 ✓5ᵗʰ
      laceration, cerebral 803.1 ✓5ᵗʰ
      other bones — see Fracture, multiple, skull
      subarachnoid hemorrhage 803.2 ✓5ᵗʰ
      subdural hemorrhage 803.2 ✓5ᵗʰ
    base (antrum) (ethmoid bone) (fossa) (internal ear) (nasal sinus) (occiput) (sphenoid) (temporal bone) (closed) 801.0 ✓5ᵗʰ
      with
        contusion, cerebral 801.1 ✓5ᵗʰ
        epidural hemorrhage 801.2 ✓5ᵗʰ
        extradural hemorrhage 801.2 ✓5ᵗʰ
        hemorrhage (intracranial) NEC 801.3 ✓5ᵗʰ
        intracranial injury NEC 801.4 ✓5ᵗʰ
        laceration, cerebral 801.1 ✓5ᵗʰ
        subarachnoid hemorrhage 801.2 ✓5ᵗʰ
        subdural hemorrhage 801.2 ✓5ᵗʰ
      open 801.5 ✓5ᵗʰ
        with
          contusion, cerebral 801.6 ✓5ᵗʰ
          epidural hemorrhage 801.7 ✓5ᵗʰ
          extradural hemorrhage 801.7 ✓5ᵗʰ
          hemorrhage (intracranial) NEC 801.8 ✓5ᵗʰ
          intracranial injury NEC 801.9 ✓5ᵗʰ
          laceration, cerebral 801.6 ✓5ᵗʰ
          subarachnoid hemorrhage 801.7 ✓5ᵗʰ
          subdural hemorrhage 801.7 ✓5ᵗʰ
    birth injury 767.3
    face bones — see Fracture, face bones
    open 803.5 ✓5ᵗʰ
      with
        contusion, cerebral 803.6 ✓5ᵗʰ
        epidural hemorrhage 803.7 ✓5ᵗʰ
        extradural hemorrhage 803.7 ✓5ᵗʰ

Fracture — continued
  skull — continued
    open — continued
      with — continued
        hemorrhage (intracranial) NEC 803.8 ✓5ᵗʰ
        intracranial injury NEC 803.9 ✓5ᵗʰ
        laceration, cerebral 803.6 ✓5ᵗʰ
        subarachnoid hemorrhage 803.7 ✓5ᵗʰ
        subdural hemorrhage 803.7 ✓5ᵗʰ
    vault (frontal bone) (parietal bone) (vertex) (closed) 800.0 ✓5ᵗʰ
      with
        contusion, cerebral 800.1 ✓5ᵗʰ
        epidural hemorrhage 800.2 ✓5ᵗʰ
        extradural hemorrhage 800.2 ✓5ᵗʰ
        hemorrhage (intracranial) NEC 800.3 ✓5ᵗʰ
        intracranial injury NEC 800.4 ✓5ᵗʰ
        laceration, cerebral 800.1 ✓5ᵗʰ
        subarachnoid hemorrhage 800.2 ✓5ᵗʰ
        subdural hemorrhage 800.2 ✓5ᵗʰ
      open 800.5 ✓5ᵗʰ
        with
          contusion, cerebral 800.6 ✓5ᵗʰ
          epidural hemorrhage 800.7 ✓5ᵗʰ
          extradural hemorrhage 800.7 ✓5ᵗʰ
          hemorrhage (intracranial) NEC 800.8 ✓5ᵗʰ
          intracranial injury NEC 800.9 ✓5ᵗʰ
          laceration, cerebral 800.6 ✓5ᵗʰ
          subarachnoid hemorrhage 800.7 ✓5ᵗʰ
          subdural hemorrhage 800.7 ✓5ᵗʰ
  Smith's 813.41
    open 813.51
  sphenoid (bone) (sinus) — see Fracture, skull, base
  spine — see also Fracture, vertebra, by site due to birth trauma 767.4
  spinous process — see Fracture, vertebra, by site
  spontaneous — see Fracture, pathologic
  sprinters' — see Fracture, ilium
  stapes — see Fracture, skull, base
  stave — see also Fracture, metacarpus, metacarpal bone(s)
    spine — see Fracture, tibia, upper end
  sternum (closed) 807.2
    with flail chest (open) 807.4
    open 807.3
  Stieda's — see Fracture, femur, lower end
  stress 733.95
    fibula 733.93
    metatarsals 733.94
    specified site NEC 733.95
    tibia 733.93
  styloid process
    metacarpal (closed) 815.02
      open 815.12
    radius — see Fracture, radius, lower end
    temporal bone — see Fracture, skull, base
    ulna — see Fracture, ulna, lower end
  supracondylar, elbow 812.41
    open 812.51
  symphysis pubis (with visceral injury) (closed) 808.2
    open 808.3
  talus (ankle bone) (closed) 825.21
    open 825.31
  tarsus, tarsal bone(s) (with metatarsus) of one foot (closed) NEC 825.29
    open 825.39
  temporal bone (styloid) — see Fracture, skull, base
  tendon — see Sprain, by site
  thigh — see Fracture, femur, shaft
  thumb (and finger(s)) of one hand (closed) (see also Fracture, phalanx, hand) 816.00
    with metacarpal bone(s) of same hand 817.0
    open 817.1
    metacarpal(s) — see Fracture, metacarpus
    open 816.10
  thyroid cartilage (closed) 807.5
    open 807.6

Fracture — continued
  tibia (closed) 823.80
    with fibula 823.82
      open 823.92
    condyles — see Fracture, tibia, upper end
    distal end 824.8
      open 824.9
    epiphysis
      lower 824.8
        open 824.9
      upper — see Fracture, tibia, upper end
    head (involving knee joint) — see Fracture, tibia, upper end
    intercondyloid eminence — see Fracture, tibia, upper end
    involving ankle 824.0
      open 824.9
    malleolus (internal) (medial) 824.0
      open 824.1
    open NEC 823.90
    pathologic 733.16
    proximal end — see Fracture, tibia, upper end
    shaft 823.20
      with fibula 823.22
        open 823.32
      open 823.30
    spine — see Fracture, tibia, upper end
    stress 733.93
    torus 823.40 •
      with tibia 823.42 •
    tuberosity — see Fracture, tibia, upper end
    upper end or extremity (condyle) (epiphysis) (head) (spine) (proximal end) (tuberosity) 823.00
      with fibula 823.02
        open 823.12
      open 823.10
  toe(s), of one foot (closed) 826.0
    with bone(s) of same lower limb 827.0
      open 827.1
    open 826.1
  tooth (root) 873.63
    complicated 873.73
  torus •
    fibula 823.41 •
      with tibia 823.42 •
    radius 813.45 •
    tibia 823.40 •
      with fibula 823.42 •
  trachea (closed) 807.5
    open 807.6
  transverse process — see Fracture, vertebra, by site
  trapezium (closed) 814.05
    open 814.15
  trapezoid bone (closed) 814.06
    open 814.16
  trimalleolar (closed) 824.6
    open 824.7
  triquetral (bone) (closed) 814.03
    open 814.13
  trochanter (greater) (lesser) (closed) (see also Fracture, femur, neck, by site) 820.20
    open 820.30
  trunk (bones) (closed) 809.0
    open 809.1
  tuberosity (external) — see Fracture, by site
  ulna (alone) (closed) 813.82
    with radius NEC 813.83
      open 813.93
    coronoid process (closed) 813.02
      open 813.12
    distal end — see Fracture, ulna, lower end
    epiphysis
      lower — see Fracture, ulna, lower end
      upper — see Fracture, ulna, upper end
    head — see Fracture, ulna, lower end
    lower end (distal end) (head) (lower epiphysis) (styloid process) 813.43
      with radius (lower end) 813.44
        open 813.54
      open 813.53
    olecranon process (closed) 813.01
      open 813.11
    open NEC 813.92

Index to Diseases

Fracture — *continued*
  ulna — *continued*
    pathologic 733.12
    proximal end — *see* Fracture, ulna, upper end
    shaft 813.22
      with radius (shaft) 813.23
        open 813.33
      open 813.32
    styloid process — *see* Fracture, ulna, lower end
    transverse — *see* Fracture, ulna, by site
    upper end (epiphysis) 813.04
      with radius (upper end) 813.08
        open 813.18
      multiple sites 813.04
        open 813.14
      specified site NEC 813.04
        open 813.14
  unciform (closed) 814.08
    open 814.18
  vertebra, vertebral (back) (body) (column) (neural arch) (pedicle) (spine) (spinous process) (transverse process) (closed) 805.8
    with
      hematomyelia — *see* Fracture, vertebra, by site, with spinal cord injury
      injury to
        cauda equina — *see* Fracture, vertebra, sacrum, with spinal cord injury
        nerve — *see* Fracture, vertebra, by site, with spinal cord injury
      paralysis — *see* Fracture, vertebra, by site, with spinal cord injury
      paraplegia — *see* Fracture, vertebra, by site, with spinal cord injury
      quadriplegia — *see* Fracture, vertebra, by site, with spinal cord injury
      spinal concussion — *see* Fracture, vertebra, by site, with spinal cord injury
      spinal cord injury (closed) NEC 806.8

Note — Use the following fifth-digit subclassification with categories 806.0-806.3:

C_1-C_4 or unspecified level and D_1-D_6 (T_1-T_6) or unspecified level with

  0 *unspecified spinal cord injury*
  1 *complete lesion of cord*
  2 *anterior cord syndrome*
  3 *central cord syndrome*
  4 *specified injury NEC*

C_5-C_7 level and D_7-D_{12} level with:

  5 *unspecified spinal cord injury*
  6 *complete lesion of cord*
  7 *anterior cord syndrome*
  8 *central cord syndrome*
  9 *specified injury NEC*

      cervical 806.0 ✓5ᵗʰ
        open 806.1 ✓5ᵗʰ
      dorsal, dorsolumbar 806.2 ✓5ᵗʰ
        open 806.3 ✓5ᵗʰ
      open 806.9
      thoracic, thoracolumbar 806.2 ✓5ᵗʰ
        open 806.3 ✓5ᵗʰ
    atlanto-axial — *see* Fracture, vertebra, cervical
    cervical (hangman) (teardrop) (closed) 805.00
      with spinal cord injury — *see* Fracture, vertebra, with spinal cord injury, cervical
      first (atlas) 805.01
        open 805.11
      second (axis) 805.02
        open 805.12
      third 805.03
        open 805.13
      fourth 805.04
        open 805.14

Fracture — *continued*
  vertebra, vertebral — *continued*
    cervical — *continued*
      fifth 805.05
        open 805.15
      sixth 805.06
        open 805.16
      seventh 805.07
        open 805.17
      multiple sites 805.08
        open 805.18
      open 805.10
    coccyx (closed) 805.6
      with spinal cord injury (closed) 806.60
        cauda equina injury 806.62
          complete lesion 806.61
            open 806.71
          open 806.72
        open 806.70
        specified type NEC 806.69
          open 806.79
      open 805.7
    collapsed 733.13
    compression, not due to trauma 733.13
    dorsal (closed) 805.2
      with spinal cord injury — *see* Fracture, vertebra, with spinal cord injury, dorsal
      open 805.3
    dorsolumbar (closed) 805.2
      with spinal cord injury — *see* Fracture, vertebra, with spinal cord injury, dorsal
      open 805.3
    due to osteoporosis 733.13
    fetus or newborn 767.4
    lumbar (closed) 805.4
      with spinal cord injury (closed) 806.4
        open 806.5
      open 805.5
    nontraumatic 733.13
    open NEC 805.9
    pathologic (any site) 733.13
    sacrum (closed) 805.6
      with spinal cord injury 806.60
        cauda equina injury 806.62
          complete lesion 806.61
            open 806.71
          open 806.72
        open 806.70
        specified type NEC 806.69
          open 806.79
      open 805.7
    site unspecified (closed) 805.8
      with spinal cord injury (closed) 806.8
        open 806.9
      open 805.9
    stress (any site) 733.95
    thoracic (closed) 805.2
      with spinal cord injury — *see* Fracture, vertebra, with spinal cord injury, thoracic
      open 805.3
  vertex — *see* Fracture, skull, vault
  vomer (bone) 802.0
    open 802.1
  Wagstaffe's — *see* Fracture, ankle
  wrist (closed) 814.00
    open 814.10
    pathologic 733.12
  xiphoid (process) — *see* Fracture, sternum
  zygoma (zygomatic arch) (closed) 802.4
    open 802.5

Fragile X syndrome 759.83

Fragilitas
  crinium 704.2
  hair 704.2
  ossium 756.51
    with blue sclera 756.51
  unguium 703.8
    congenital 757.5

Fragility
  bone 756.51
    with deafness and blue sclera 756.51
  capillary (hereditary) 287.8

Fragility — *continued*
  hair 704.2
  nails 703.8

Fragmentation — *see* Fracture, by site

Frambesia, frambesial (tropica) (*see also* Yaws) 102.9
  initial lesion or ulcer 102.0
  primary 102.0

Frambeside
  gummatous 102.4
  of early yaws 102.2

Frambesioma 102.1

Franceschetti's syndrome (mandibulofacial dysotosis) 756.0

Francis' disease (*see also* Tularemia) 021.9

Frank's essential thrombocytopenia (*see also* Purpura, thrombocytopenic) 287.3

Franklin's disease (heavy chain) 273.2

Fraser's syndrome 759.89

Freckle 709.09
  malignant melanoma in (M8742/3) — *see* Melanoma
  melanotic (of Hutchinson) (M8742/2) — *see* Neoplasm, skin, in situ

Freeman-Sheldon syndrome 759.89

Freezing 991.9
  specified effect NEC 991.8

Frei's disease (climatic bubo) 099.1

Freiberg's
  disease (osteochondrosis, second metatarsal) 732.5
  infraction of metatarsal head 732.5
  osteochondrosis 732.5

Fremitus, friction, cardiac 785.3

Frenulum linguae 750.0

Frenum
  external os 752.49
  tongue 750.0

Frequency (urinary) NEC 788.41
  micturition 788.41
  nocturnal 788.43
  psychogenic 306.53

Frey's syndrome (auriculotemporal syndrome) 350.8

Friction
  burn (*see also* Injury, superficial, by site) 919.0
  fremitus, cardiac 785.3
  precordial 785.3
  sounds, chest 786.7

Friderichsen-Waterhouse syndrome or disease 036.3

Friedländer's
  B (bacillus) NEC (*see also* condition) 041.3
  sepsis or septicemia 038.49
  disease (endarteritis obliterans) — *see* Arteriosclerosis

Friedreich's
  ataxia 334.0
  combined systemic disease 334.0
  disease 333.2
    combined systemic 334.0
  myoclonia 333.2
  sclerosis (spinal cord) 334.0

Friedrich-Erb-Arnold syndrome (acropachyderma) 757.39

Frigidity 302.72
  psychic or psychogenic 302.72

Fröhlich's disease or syndrome (adiposogenital dystrophy) 253.8

Froin's syndrome 336.8

Frommel's disease 676.6 ✓5ᵗʰ

Frommel-Chiari syndrome 676.6 ✓5ᵗʰ

Frontal — *see also* condition
  lobe syndrome 310.0

Frostbite 991.3
  face 991.0
  foot 991.2
  hand 991.1
  specified site NEC 991.3

Frotteurism 302.89

Frozen 991.9
- pelvis 620.8
- shoulder 726.0

Fructosemia 271.2
Fructosuria (benign) (essential) 271.2
Fuchs'
- black spot (myopic) 360.21
- corneal dystrophy (endothelial) 371.57
- heterochromic cyclitis 364.21

Fucosidosis 271.8
Fugue 780.99
- hysterical (dissociative) 300.13
- reaction to exceptional stress (transient) 308.1

Fuller Albright's syndrome (osteitis fibrosa disseminata) 756.59
Fuller's earth disease 502
Fulminant, fulminating — see condition
Functional — see condition
Fundus — see also condition
- flavimaculatus 362.76

Fungemia 117.9
Fungus, fungous
- cerebral 348.8
- disease NEC 117.9
- infection — see Infection, fungus
- testis (see also Tuberculosis) 016.5 [608.81]

Funiculitis (acute) 608.4
- chronic 608.4
- endemic 608.4
- gonococcal (acute) 098.14
  - chronic or duration of 2 months or over 098.34
- tuberculous (see also Tuberculosis) 016.5

Funnel
- breast (acquired) 738.3
  - congenital 754.81
  - late effect of rickets 268.1
- chest (acquired) 738.3
  - congenital 754.81
  - late effect of rickets 268.1
- pelvis (acquired) 738.6
  - with disproportion (fetopelvic) 653.3
    - affecting fetus or newborn 763.1
    - causing obstructed labor 660.1
      - affecting fetus or newborn 763.1
  - congenital 755.69
  - tuberculous (see also Tuberculosis) 016.9

F.U.O. (see also Pyrexia) 780.6
Furfur 690.18
- microsporon 111.0

Furor, paroxysmal (idiopathic) (see also Epilepsy) 345.8
Furriers' lung 495.8
Furrowed tongue 529.5
- congenital 750.13

Furrowing nail(s) (transverse) 703.8
- congenital 757.5

Furuncle 680.9
- abdominal wall 680.2
- ankle 680.6
- anus 680.5
- arm (any part, above wrist) 680.3
- auditory canal, external 680.0
- axilla 680.3
- back (any part) 680.2
- breast 680.2
- buttock 680.5
- chest wall 680.2
- corpus cavernosum 607.2
- ear (any part) 680.0
- eyelid 373.13
- face (any part, except eye) 680.0
- finger (any) 680.4
- flank 680.2
- foot (any part) 680.7
- forearm 680.3
- gluteal (region) 680.5
- groin 680.2
- hand (any part) 680.4
- head (any part, except face) 680.8
- heel 680.7

Furuncle — continued
- hip 680.6
- kidney (see also Abscess, kidney) 590.2
- knee 680.6
- labium (majus) (minus) 616.4
- lacrimal
  - gland (see also Dacryoadenitis) 375.00
  - passages (duct) (sac) (see also Dacryocystitis) 375.30
- leg, any part except foot 680.6
- malignant 022.0
- multiple sites 680.9
- neck 680.1
- nose (external) (septum) 680.0
- orbit 376.01
- partes posteriores 680.5
- pectoral region 680.2
- penis 607.2
- perineum 680.2
- pinna 680.0
- scalp (any part) 680.8
- scrotum 608.4
- seminal vesicle 608.0
- shoulder 680.3
- skin NEC 680.9
- specified site NEC 680.8
- spermatic cord 608.4
- temple (region) 680.0
- testis 604.90
- thigh 680.6
- thumb 680.4
- toe (any) 680.7
- trunk 680.2
- tunica vaginalis 608.4
- umbilicus 680.2
- upper arm 680.3
- vas deferens 608.4
- vulva 616.4
- wrist 680.4

Furunculosis (see also Furuncle) 680.9
- external auditory meatus 680.0 [380.13]

Fusarium (infection) 118
Fusion, fused (congenital)
- anal (with urogenital canal) 751.5
- aorta and pulmonary artery 745.0
- astragaloscaphoid 755.67
- atria 745.5
- atrium and ventricle 745.69
- auditory canal 744.02
- auricles, heart 745.5
- binocular, with defective stereopsis 368.33
- bone 756.9
- cervical spine — see Fusion, spine
- choanal 748.0
- commissure, mitral valve 746.5
- cranial sutures, premature 756.0
- cusps, heart valve NEC 746.89
  - mitral 746.5
  - tricuspid 746.89
- ear ossicles 744.04
- fingers (see also Syndactylism, fingers) 755.11
- hymen 752.42
- hymeno-urethral 599.89
  - causing obstructed labor 660.1
    - affecting fetus or newborn 763.1
- joint (acquired) — see also Ankylosis
  - congenital 755.8
- kidneys (incomplete) 753.3
- labium (majus) (minus) 752.49
- larynx and trachea 748.3
- limb 755.8
  - lower 755.69
  - upper 755.59
- lobe, lung 748.5
- lumbosacral (acquired) 724.6
  - congenital 756.15
  - surgical V45.4
- nares (anterior) (posterior) 748.0
- nose, nasal 748.0
- nostril(s) 748.0
- organ or site NEC — see Anomaly, specified type NEC
- ossicles 756.9
  - auditory 744.04
- pulmonary valve segment 746.02

Fusion, fused — continued
- pulmonic cusps 746.02
- ribs 756.3
- sacroiliac (acquired) (joint) 724.6
  - congenital 755.69
  - surgical V45.4
- skull, imperfect 756.0
- spine (acquired) 724.9
  - arthrodesis status V45.4
  - congenital (vertebra) 756.15
  - postoperative status V45.4
- sublingual duct with submaxillary duct at opening in mouth 750.26
- talonavicular (bar) 755.67
- teeth, tooth 520.2
- testes 752.8
- toes (see also Syndactylism, toes) 755.13
- trachea and esophagus 750.3
- twins 759.4
- urethral-hymenal 599.89
- vagina 752.49
- valve cusps — see Fusion, cusps, heart valve
- ventricles, heart 745.4
- vertebra (arch) — see Fusion, spine
- vulva 752.49

Fusospirillosis (mouth) (tongue) (tonsil) 101
Fussy infant (baby) 780.91

G

Gafsa boil 085.1
Gain, weight (abnormal) (excessive) (*see also* Weight, gain) 783.1
Gaisböck's disease or syndrome (polycythemia hypertonica) 289.0
Gait
 abnormality 781.2
  hysterical 300.11
 ataxic 781.2
  hysterical 300.11
 disturbance 781.2
  hysterical 300.11
 paralytic 781.2
 scissor 781.2
 spastic 781.2
 staggering 781.2
  hysterical 300.11
Galactocele (breast) (infected) 611.5
 puerperal, postpartum 676.8
Galactophoritis 611.0
 puerperal, postpartum 675.2
Galactorrhea 676.6
 not associated with childbirth 611.6
Galactosemia (classic) (congenital) 271.1
Galactosuria 271.1
Galacturia 791.1
 bilharziasis 120.0
Galen's vein — *see* condition
Gallbladder — *see also* condition
 acute (*see also* Disease, gallbladder) 575.0
Gall duct — *see* condition
Gallop rhythm 427.89
Gallstone (cholemic) (colic) (impacted) — *see also* Cholelithiasis
 causing intestinal obstruction 560.31
Gambling, pathological 312.31
Gammaloidosis 277.3
Gammopathy 273.9
 macroglobulinemia 273.3
 monoclonal (benign) (essential) (idiopathic) (with lymphoplasmacytic dyscrasia) 273.1
Gamna's disease (siderotic splenomegaly) 289.51
Gampsodactylia (congenital) 754.71
Gamstorp's disease (adynamia episodica hereditaria) 359.3
Gandy-Nanta disease (siderotic splenomegaly) 289.51
Gang activity, without manifest psychiatric disorder V71.09
 adolescent V71.02
 adult V71.01
 child V71.02
Gangliocytoma (M9490/0) — *see* Neoplasm, connective tissue, benign
Ganglioglioma (M9505/1) — *see* Neoplasm, by site, uncertain behavior
Ganglion 727.43
 joint 727.41
 of yaws (early) (late) 102.6
 periosteal (*see also* Periostitis) 730.3
 tendon sheath (compound) (diffuse) 727.42
 tuberculous (*see also* Tuberculosis) 015.9
Ganglioneuroblastoma (M9490/3) — *see* Neoplasm, connective tissue, malignant
Ganglioneuroma (M9490/0) — *see also* Neoplasm, connective tissue, benign
 malignant (M9490/3) — *see* Neoplasm, connective tissue, malignant
Ganglioneuromatosis (M9491/0) — *see* Neoplasm, connective tissue, benign
Ganglionitis
 fifth nerve (*see also* Neuralgia, trigeminal) 350.1
 gasserian 350.1
 geniculate 351.1
  herpetic 053.11
  newborn 767.5
 herpes zoster 053.11
 herpetic geniculate (Hunt's syndrome) 053.11
Gangliosidosis 330.1

Gangosa 102.5
Gangrene, gangrenous (anemia) (artery) (cellulitis) (dermatitis) (dry) (infective) (moist) (pemphigus) (septic) (skin) (stasis) (ulcer) 785.4
 with
  arteriosclerosis (native artery) 440.24
   bypass graft 440.30
    autologous vein 440.31
    nonautologous biological 440.32
  diabetes (mellitus) 250.7 [785.4]
 abdomen (wall) 785.4
  arteriosclerosis 440.29 [785.4]
 adenitis 683
 alveolar 526.5
 angina 462
  diphtheritic 032.0
 anus 569.49
 appendices epiploicae — *see* Gangrene, mesentery
 appendix — *see* Appendicitis, acute
 arteriosclerotic — *see* Arteriosclerosis, with, gangrene
 auricle 785.4
 Bacillus welchii (*see also* Gangrene, gas) 040.0
 bile duct (*see also* Cholangitis) 576.8
 bladder 595.89
 bowel — *see* Gangrene, intestine
 cecum — *see* Gangrene, intestine
 Clostridium perfringens or welchii (*see also* Gangrene, gas) 040.0
 colon — *see* Gangrene, intestine
 connective tissue 785.4
 cornea 371.40
 corpora cavernosa (infective) 607.2
  noninfective 607.89
 cutaneous, spreading 785.4
 decubital 707.0 [785.4]
 diabetic (any site) 250.7 [785.4]
 dropsical 785.4
 emphysematous (*see also* Gangrene, gas) 040.0
 epidemic (ergotized grain) 988.2
 epididymis (infectional) (*see also* Epididymitis) 604.99
 erysipelas (*see also* Erysipelas) 035
 extremity (lower) (upper) 785.4
 gallbladder or duct (*see also* Cholecystitis, acute) 575.0
 gas (bacillus) 040.0
  with
   abortion — *see* Abortion, by type, with sepsis
   ectopic pregnancy (*see also* categories 633.0-633.9) 639.0
   molar pregnancy (*see also* categories 630-632) 639.0
  following
   abortion 639.0
   ectopic or molar pregnancy 639.0
  puerperal, postpartum, childbirth 670
 glossitis 529.0
 gum 523.8
 hernia — *see* Hernia, by site, with gangrene
 hospital noma 528.1
 intestine, intestinal (acute) (hemorrhagic) (massive) 557.0
  with
   hernia — *see* Hernia, by site, with gangrene
   mesenteric embolism or infarction 557.0
   obstruction (*see also* Obstruction, intestine) 560.9
 laryngitis 464.00
  with obstruction 464.01
 liver 573.8
 lung 513.0
  spirochetal 104.8
 lymphangitis 457.2
 Meleney's (cutaneous) 686.09
 mesentery 557.0
  with
   embolism or infarction 557.0
   intestinal obstruction (*see also* Obstruction, intestine) 560.9
 mouth 528.1
 noma 528.1
 orchitis 604.90

Gangrene, gangrenous — *continued*
 ovary (*see also* Salpingo-oophoritis) 614.2
 pancreas 577.0
 penis (infectional) 607.2
  noninfective 607.89
 perineum 785.4
 pharynx 462
 septic 034.0
 pneumonia 513.0
 Pott's 440.24
 presenile 443.1
 pulmonary 513.0
 pulp, tooth 522.1
 quinsy 475
 Raynaud's (symmetric gangrene) 443.0 [785.4]
 rectum 569.49
 retropharyngeal 478.24
 rupture — *see* Hernia, by site, with gangrene
 scrotum 608.4
  noninfective 608.83
 senile 440.24
 sore throat 462
 spermatic cord 608.4
  noninfective 608.89
 spine 785.4
 spirochetal NEC 104.8
 spreading cutaneous 785.4
 stomach 537.89
 stomatitis 528.1
 symmetrical 443.0 [785.4]
 testis (infectional) (*see also* Orchitis) 604.99
  noninfective 608.89
 throat 462
  diphtheritic 032.0
 thyroid (gland) 246.8
 tonsillitis (acute) 463
 tooth (pulp) 522.1
 tuberculous NEC (*see also* Tuberculosis) 011.9
 tunica vaginalis 608.4
  noninfective 608.89
 umbilicus 785.4
 uterus (*see also* Endometritis) 615.9
 uvulitis 528.3
 vas deferens 608.4
  noninfective 608.89
 vulva (*see also* Vulvitis) 616.10
Gannister disease (occupational) 502
 with tuberculosis — *see* Tuberculosis, pulmonary
Ganser's syndrome, hysterical 300.16
Gardner-Diamond syndrome (autoerythrocyte sensitization) 287.2
Gargoylism 277.5
Garré's
 disease (*see also* Osteomyelitis) 730.1
 osteitis (sclerosing) (*see also* Osteomyelitis) 730.1
 osteomyelitis (*see also* Osteomyelitis) 730.1
Garrod's pads, knuckle 728.79
Gartner's duct
 cyst 752.11
 persistent 752.11
Gas
 asphyxia, asphyxiation, inhalation, poisoning, suffocation NEC 987.9
  specified gas — *see* Table of Drugs and Chemicals
 bacillus gangrene or infection — *see* Gas, gangrene
 cyst, mesentery 568.89
 excessive 787.3
 gangrene 040.0
  with
   abortion — *see* Abortion, by type, with sepsis
   ectopic pregnancy (*see also* categories 633.0-633.9) 639.0
   molar pregnancy (*see also* categories 630-632) 639.0
  following
   abortion 639.0
   ectopic or molar pregnancy 639.0
  puerperal, postpartum, childbirth 670
 on stomach 787.3
 pains 787.3

Gastradenitis

Gastradenitis 535.0 E
Gastralgia 536.8
   psychogenic 307.89
Gastrectasis, gastrectasia 536.1
   psychogenic 306.4
Gastric — *see* condition
Gastrinoma (M8153/1)
   malignant (M8153/3)
     pancreas 157.4
     specified site NEC — *see* Neoplasm, by site, malignant
     unspecified site 157.4
   specified site — *see* Neoplasm, by site, uncertain behavior
   unspecified site 235.5
Gastritis 535.5 ✓5ᵗʰ

> Note — Use the following fifth-digit subclassification for category 535:
> 0   without mention of hemorrhage
> 1   with hemorrhage

   acute 535.0 ✓5ᵗʰ
   alcoholic 535.3 ✓5ᵗʰ
   allergic 535.4 ✓5ᵗʰ
   antral 535.4 ✓5ᵗʰ
   atrophic 535.1 ✓5ᵗʰ
   atrophic-hyperplastic 535.1 ✓5ᵗʰ
   bile-induced 535.4 ✓5ᵗʰ
   catarrhal 535.0 ✓5ᵗʰ
   chronic (atrophic) 535.1 ✓5ᵗʰ
   cirrhotic 535.4 ✓5ᵗʰ
   corrosive (acute) 535.4 ✓5ᵗʰ
   dietetic 535.4 ✓5ᵗʰ
   due to diet deficiency 269.9 [535.4]
   eosinophilic 535.4 ✓5ᵗʰ
   erosive 535.4 ✓5ᵗʰ
   follicular 535.4 ✓5ᵗʰ
     chronic 535.1 ✓5ᵗʰ
   giant hypertrophic 535.2 ✓5ᵗʰ
   glandular 535.4 ✓5ᵗʰ
     chronic 535.1 ✓5ᵗʰ
   hypertrophic (mucosa) 535.2 ✓5ᵗʰ
     chronic giant 211.1
   irritant 535.4 ✓5ᵗʰ
   nervous 306.4
   phlegmonous 535.0 ✓5ᵗʰ
   psychogenic 306.4
   sclerotic 535.4 ✓5ᵗʰ
   spastic 536.8
   subacute 535.0 ✓5ᵗʰ
   superficial 535.4 ✓5ᵗʰ
   suppurative 535.0 ✓5ᵗʰ
   toxic 535.4 ✓5ᵗʰ
   tuberculous (*see also* Tuberculosis) 017.9 ✓5ᵗʰ
Gastrocarcinoma (M8010/3) 151.9
Gastrocolic — *see* condition
Gastrocolitis — *see* Enteritis
Gastrodisciasis 121.8
Gastroduodenitis (*see also* Gastritis) 535.5 ✓5ᵗʰ
   catarrhal 535.0 ✓5ᵗʰ
   infectional 535.0 ✓5ᵗʰ
   virus, viral 008.8
     specified type NEC 008.69
Gastrodynia 536.8
Gastroenteritis (acute) (catarrhal) (congestive) (hemorrhagic) (noninfectious) (*see also* Enteritis) 558.9
   aertrycke infection 003.0
   allergic 558.3
   chronic 558.9
     ulcerative (*see also* Colitis, ulcerative) 556.9
   dietetic 558.9
   due to
     food poisoning (*see also* Poisoning, food) 005.9
     radiation 558.1
   epidemic 009.0
   functional 558.9
   infectious (*see also* Enteritis, due to, by organism) 009.0
     presumed 009.1
   salmonella 003.0
   septic (*see also* Enteritis, due to, by organism) 009.0

Gastroenteritis — *continued*
   toxic 558.2
   tuberculous (*see also* Tuberculosis) 014.8 ✓5ᵗʰ
   ulcerative (*see also* Colitis, ulcerative) 556.9
   viral NEC 008.8
     specified type NEC 008.69
   zymotic 009.0
Gastroenterocolitis — *see* Enteritis
Gastroenteropathy, protein-losing 579.8
Gastroenteroptosis 569.89
Gastroesophageal laceration-hemorrhage syndrome 530.7
Gastroesophagitis 530.19
Gastrohepatitis (*see also* Gastritis) 535.5 ✓5ᵗʰ
Gastrointestinal — *see* condition
Gastrojejunal — *see* condition
Gastrojejunitis (*see also* Gastritis) 535.5 ✓5ᵗʰ
Gastrojejunocolic — *see* condition
Gastroliths 537.89
Gastromalacia 537.89
Gastroparalysis 536.8
   diabetic 250.6 ✓5ᵗʰ [536.3]
Gastroparesis 536.3
   diabetic 250.6 ✓5ᵗʰ [536.3]
Gastropathy, exudative 579.8
Gastroptosis 537.5
Gastrorrhagia 578.0
Gastorrhea 536.8
   psychogenic 306.4
Gastroschisis (congenital) 756.79
   acquired 569.89
Gastrospasm (neurogenic) (reflex) 536.8
   neurotic 306.4
   psychogenic 306.4
Gastrostaxis 578.0
Gastrostenosis 537.89
Gastrostomy
   attention to V55.1
   complication 536.40
     specified type 536.49
   infection 536.41
   malfunctioning 536.42
   status V44.1
Gastrosuccorrhea (continous) (intermittent) 536.8
   neurotic 306.4
   psychogenic 306.4
Gaucher's
   disease (adult) (cerebroside lipidosis) (infantile) 272.7
   hepatomegaly 272.7
   splenomegaly (cerebroside lipidosis) 272.7
Gayet's disease (superior hemorrhagic polioencephalitis) 265.1
Gayet-Wernicke's syndrome (superior hemorrhagic polioencephalitis) 265.1
Gee (-Herter) (-Heubner) (-Thaysen) disease or syndrome (nontropical sprue) 579.0
Gélineau's syndrome 347
Gemination, teeth 520.2
Gemistocytoma (M9411/3)
   specified site — *see* Neoplasm, by site, malignant
   unspecified site 191.9
General, generalized — *see* condtion
Genital — *see* condition
Genito-anorectal syndrome 099.1
Genitourinary system — *see* condition
Genu
   congenital 755.64
   extrorsum (acquired) 736.42
     congenital 755.64
     late effects of rickets 268.1
   introrsum (acquired) 736.41
     congenital 755.64
     late effects of rickets 268.1
   rachitic (old) 268.1
   recurvatum (acquired) 736.5
     congenital 754.40
       with dislocation of knee 754.41
     late effects or rickets 268.1

Genu — *continued*
   valgum (acquired) (knock-knee) 736.41
     congenital 755.64
     late effects of rickets 268.1
   varum (acquired) (bowleg) 736.42
     congenital 755.64
     late effect of rickets 268.1
Geographic tongue 529.1
Geophagia 307.52
Geotrichosis 117.9
   intestine 117.9
   lung 117.9
   mouth 117.9
Gephyrophobia 300.29
Gerbode defect 745.4
Gerhardt's
   disease (erythromelalgia) 443.89
   syndrome (vocal cord paralysis) 478.30
Gerlier's disease (epidemic vertigo) 078.81
German measles 056.9
   exposure to V01.4
Germinoblastoma (diffuse) (M9614/3) 202.8 ✓5ᵗʰ
   follicular (M9692/3) 202.0 ✓5ᵗʰ
Germinoma (M9064/3) — *see* Neoplasm, by site, malignant
Gerontoxon 371.41
Gerstmann's syndrome (finger agnosia) 784.69
Gestation (period) — *see also* Pregnancy
   ectopic NEC (*see also* Pregnancy, ectopic) 633.90 ▲
     with intrauterine pregnancy 633.91 ●
Gestational proteinuria 646.2 ✓5ᵗʰ
   with hypertension — *see* Toxemia, of pregnancy
Ghon tubercle primary infection (*see also* Tuberculosis) 010.0 ✓5ᵗʰ
Ghost
   teeth 520.4
   vessels, cornea 370.64
Ghoul hand 102.3
Giant
   cell
     epulis 523.8
     peripheral (gingiva) 523.8
     tumor, tendon sheath 727.02
   colon (congenital) 751.3
   esophagus (congenital) 750.4
   kidney 753.3
   urticaria 995.1
     hereditary 277.6
Giardia lamblia infestation 007.1
Giardiasis 007.1
Gibert's disease (pityriasis rosea) 696.3
Gibraltar fever — *see* Brucellosis
Giddiness 780.4
   hysterical 300.11
   psychogenic 306.9
Gierke's disease (glycogenosis I) 271.0
Gigantism (cerebral) (hypophyseal) (pituitary) 253.0
Gilbert's disease or cholemia (familial nonhemolytic jaundice) 277.4
Gilchrist's disease (North American blastomycosis) 116.0
Gilford (-Hutchinson) disease or syndrome (progeria) 259.8
Gilles de la Tourette's disease (motor-verbal tic) 307.23
Gillespie's syndrome (dysplasia oculodentodigitalis) 759.89
Gingivitis 523.1
   acute 523.0
     necrotizing 101
   catarrhal 523.0
   chronic 523.1
   desquamative 523.1
   expulsiva 523.4
   hyperplastic 523.1
   marginal, simple 523.1
   necrotizing, acute 101
   pellagrous 265.2
   ulcerative 523.1
     acute necrotizing 101

Index to Diseases

Gingivitis — *continued*
  Vincent's 101
Gingivoglossitis 529.0
Gingivopericementitis 523.4
Gingivosis 523.1
Gingivostomatitis 523.1
  herpetic 054.2
Giovannini's disease 117.9
Gland, glandular — *see* condition
Glanders 024
Glanzmann (-Naegeli) disease or thrombasthenia 287.1
Glassblowers' disease 527.1
Glaucoma (capsular) (inflammatory) (noninflammatory) (primary) 365.9
  with increased episcleral venous pressure 365.82
  absolute 360.42
  acute 365.22
    narrow angle 365.22
    secondary 365.60
  angle closure 365.20
    acute 365.22
    chronic 365.23
    intermittent 365.21
    interval 365.21
    residual stage 365.24
    subacute 365.21
  borderline 365.00
  chronic 365.11
    noncongestive 365.11
    open angle 365.11
    simple 365.11
  closed angle — *see* Glaucoma, angle closure
  congenital 743.20
    associated with other eye anomalies 743.22
    simple 743.21
  congestive — *see* Glaucoma, narrow angle
  corticosteroid-induced (glaucomatous stage) 365.31
    residual stage 365.32
  hemorrhagic 365.60
  hypersecretion 365.81
  in or with
    aniridia 743.45 [365.42]
    Axenfeld's anomaly 743.44 [365.41]
    concussion of globe 921.3 [365.65]
    congenital syndromes NEC 759.89 [365.44]
    dislocation of lens
      anterior 379.33 [365.59]
      posterior 379.34 [365.59]
    disorder of lens NEC 365.59
    epithelial down-growth 364.61 [365.64]
    glaucomatocyclitic crisis 364.22 [365.62]
    hypermature cataract 366.18 [365.51]
    hyphema 364.41 [365.63]
    inflammation, ocular 365.62
    iridocyclitis 364.3 [365.62]
    iris
      anomalies NEC 743.46 [365.42]
      atrophy, essential 364.51 [365.42]
      bombé 364.74 [365.61]
      rubeosis 364.42 [365.63]
    microcornea 743.41 [365.43]
    neurofibromatosis 237.71 [365.44]
    ocular
      cysts NEC 365.64
      disorders NEC 365.60
      trauma 365.65
      tumors NEC 365.64
    postdislocation of lens
      anterior 379.33 [365.59]
      posterior 379.34 [365.59]
    pseudoexfoliation of capsule 366.11 [365.52]
    pupillary block or seclusion 364.74 [365.61]
    recession of chamber angle 364.77 [365.65]
    retinal vein occlusion 362.35 [365.63]
    Rieger's anomaly or syndrome 743.44 [365.41]
    rubeosis of iris 364.42 [365.63]
    seclusion of pupil 364.74 [365.61]
    spherophakia 743.36 [365.59]
    Sturge-Weber (-Dimitri) syndrome 759.6 [365.44]
    systemic syndrome NEC 365.44

Glaucoma — *continued*
  in or with — *continued*
    tumor of globe 365.64
    vascular disorders NEC 365.63
  infantile 365.14
    congenital 743.20
      associated with other eye anomalies 743.22
      simple 743.21
  juvenile 365.14
  low tension 365.12
  malignant 365.83 ▲
  narrow angle (primary) 365.20
    acute 365.22
    chronic 365.23
    intermittent 365.21
    interval 365.21
    residual stage 365.24
    subacute 365.21
  newborn 743.20
    associated with other eye anomalies 743.22
    simple 743.21
  noncongestive (chronic) 365.11
  nonobstructive (chronic) 365.11
  obstructive 365.60
    due to lens changes 365.59
  open angle 365.10
    with
      borderline intraocular pressure 365.01
      cupping of optic discs 365.01
    primary 365.11
    residual stage 365.15
  phacolytic 365.51
    with hypermature cataract 366.18 [365.51]
  pigmentary 365.13
  postinfectious 365.60
  pseudoexfoliation 365.52
    with pseudoexfoliation of capsule 366.11 [365.52]
  secondary NEC 365.60
  simple (chronic) 365.11
  simplex 365.11
  steroid responders 365.03
  suspect 365.00
  syphilitic 095.8
  traumatic NEC 365.65
    newborn 767.8
  tuberculous (*see also* Tuberculosis) 017.3 ✓4ᵗʰ [365.62]
  wide angle (*see also* Glaucoma, open angle) 365.10

Glaucomatous flecks (subcapsular) 366.31
Glazed tongue 529.4
Gleet 098.2
Glénard's disease or syndrome (enteroptosis) 569.89
Glinski-Simmonds syndrome (pituitary cachexia) 253.2
Glioblastoma (multiforme) (M9440/3)
  with sarcomatous component (M9442/3)
    specified site — *see* Neoplasm, by site, malignant
    unspecified site 191.9
  giant cell (M9441/3)
    specified site — *see* Neoplasm, by site, malignant
    unspecified site 191.9
  specified site — *see* Neoplasm, by site, malignant
  unspecified site 191.9
Glioma (malignant) (M9380/3)
  astrocytic (M9400/3)
    specified site — *see* Neoplasm, by site, malignant
    unspecified site 191.9
  mixed (M9382/3)
    specified site — *see* Neoplasm, by site, malignant
    unspecified site 191.9
  nose 748.1
  specified site NEC — *see* Neoplasm, by site, malignant
  subependymal (M9383/1) 237.5
  unspecified site 191.9
Gliomatosis cerebri (M9381/3) 191.0

Glioneuroma (M9505/1) — *see* Neoplasm, by site, uncertain behavior
Gliosarcoma (M9380/3)
  specified site — *see* Neoplasm, by site, malignant
  unspecified site 191.9
Gliosis (cerebral) 349.89
  spinal 336.0
Glisson's
  cirrhosis — *see* Cirrhosis, portal
  disease (*see also* Rickets) 268.0
Glissonitis 573.3
Globinuria 791.2
Globus 306.4
  hystericus 300.11
Glomangioma (M8712/0) (*see also* Hemangioma) 228.00
Glomangiosarcoma (M8710/3) — *see* Neoplasm, connective tissue, malignant
Glomerular nephritis (*see also* Nephritis) 583.9
Glomerulitis (*see also* Nephritis) 583.9
Glomerulonephritis (*see also* Nephritis) 583.9
  with
    edema (*see also* Nephrosis) 581.9
    lesion of
      exudative nephritis 583.89
      interstitial nephritis (diffuse) (focal) 583.89
      necrotizing glomerulitis 583.4
        acute 580.4
        chronic 582.4
      renal necrosis 583.9
        cortical 583.6
        medullary 583.7
      specified pathology NEC 583.89
        acute 580.89
        chronic 582.89
    necrosis, renal 583.9
      cortical 583.6
      medullary (papillary) 583.7
    specified pathology or lesion NEC 583.89
  acute 580.9
    with
      exudative nephritis 580.89
      interstitial nephritis (diffuse) (focal) 580.89
      necrotizing glomerulitis 580.4
      extracapillary with epithelial crescents 580.4
    poststreptococcal 580.0
    proliferative (diffuse) 580.0
    rapidly progressive 580.4
    specified pathology NEC 580.89
  arteriolar (*see also* Hypertension, kidney) 403.90
  arteriosclerotic (*see also* Hypertension, kidney) 403.90
  ascending (*see also* Pyelitis) 590.80
  basement membrane NEC 583.89
    with
      pulmonary hemorrhage (Goodpasture's syndrome) 446.21 [583.81]
  chronic 582.9
    with
      exudative nephritis 582.89
      interstitial nephritis (diffuse) (focal) 582.89
      necrotizing glomerulitis 582.4
      specified pathology or lesion NEC 582.89
  endothelial 582.2
  extracapillary with epithelial crescents 582.4
  hypocomplementemic persistent 582.2
  lobular 582.2
  membranoproliferative 582.2
  membranous 582.1
    and proliferative (mixed) 582.2
    sclerosing 582.1
  mesangiocapillary 582.2
  mixed membranous and proliferative 582.2
  proliferative (diffuse) 582.0
  rapidly progressive 582.4
  sclerosing 582.1
  cirrhotic — *see* Sclerosis, renal
  desquamative — *see* Nephrosis

Glomerulonephritis

Glomerulonephritis (see also Nephritis) — continued
  due to or associated with
    amyloidosis 277.3 [583.81]
      with nephrotic syndrome 277.3 [581.81]
        chronic 277.3 [582.81]
    diabetes mellitus 250.4 ✓5ᵗʰ [583.81]
      with nephrotic syndrome
        250.4 ✓5ᵗʰ [581.81]
    diphtheria 032.89 [580.81]
    gonococcal infection (acute) 098.19 [583.81]
      chronic or duration of 2 months or over
        098.39 [583.81]
    infectious hepatitis 070.9 [580.81]
    malaria (with nephrotic syndrome)
      084.9 [581.81]
    mumps 072.79 [580.81]
    polyarteritis (nodosa) (with nephrotic
      syndrome) 446.0 [581.81]
    specified pathology NEC 583.89
      acute 580.89
      chronic 582.89
    streptotrichosis 039.8 [583.81]
    subacute bacterial endocarditis
      421.0 [580.81]
    syphilis (late) 095.4
      congenital 090.5 [583.81]
      early 091.69 [583.81]
    systemic lupus erythematosus 710.0 [583.81]
      with nephrotic syndrome 710.0 [581.81]
        chronic 710.0 [582.81]
    tuberculosis (see also Tuberculosis)
      016.0 ✓5ᵗʰ [583.81]
    typhoid fever 002.0 [580.81]
  extracapillary with epithelial crescents 583.4
    acute 580.4
    chronic 582.4
  exudative 583.89
    acute 580.89
    chronic 582.89
  focal (see also Nephritis) 583.9
    embolic 580.4
  granular 582.89
  granulomatous 582.89
  hydremic (see also Nephrosis) 581.9
  hypocomplementemic persistent 583.2
    with nephrotic syndrome 581.2
      chronic 582.2
  immune complex NEC 583.89
  infective (see also Pyelitis) 590.80
  interstitial (diffuse) (focal) 583.89
    with nephrotic syndrome 581.89
      acute 580.89
      chronic 582.89
  latent or quiescent 582.9
  lobular 583.2
    with nephrotic syndrome 581.2
      chronic 582.2
  membranoproliferative 583.2
    with nephrotic syndrome 581.2
      chronic 582.2
  membranous 583.1
    with nephrotic syndrome 581.1
    and proliferative (mixed) 583.2
      with nephrotic syndrome 581.2
        chronic 582.2
    chronic 582.1
    sclerosing 582.1
      with nephrotic syndrome 581.1
  mesangiocapillary 583.2
    with nephrotic syndrome 581.2
      chronic 582.2
  minimal change 581.3
  mixed membranous and proliferative 583.2
    with nephrotic syndrome 581.2
      chronic 582.2
  necrotizing 583.4
    acute 580.4
    chronic 582.4
  nephrotic (see also Nephrosis) 581.9
  old — see Glomerulonephritis, chronic
  parenchymatous 581.89
  poststreptococcal 580.0
  proliferative (diffuse) 583.0
    with nephrotic syndrome 581.0
      acute 580.0
      chronic 582.0

Glomerulonephritis (see also Nephritis) — continued
  purulent (see also Pyelitis) 590.80
  quiescent — see Nephritis, chronic
  rapidly progressive 583.4
    acute 580.4
    chronic 582.4
  sclerosing membranous (chronic) 582.1
    with nephrotic syndrome 581.1
  septic (see also Pyelitis) 590.80
  specified pathology or lesion NEC 583.89
    with nephrotic syndrome 581.89
    acute 580.89
    chronic 582.89
  suppurative (acute) (disseminated) (see also
    Pyelitis) 590.80
  toxic — see Nephritis, acute
  tubal, tubular — see Nephrosis, tubular
  type II (Ellis) — see Nephrosis
  vascular — see Hypertension, kidney
Glomerulosclerosis (see also Sclerosis, renal) 587
  focal 582.1
    with nephrotic syndrome 581.1
  intercapillary (nodular) (with diabetes)
    250.4 ✓5ᵗʰ [581.81]
Glossagra 529.6
Glossalgia 529.6
Glossitis 529.0
  areata exfoliativa 529.1
  atrophic 529.4
  benign migratory 529.1
  gangrenous 529.0
  Hunter's 529.4
  median rhomboid 529.2
  Moeller's 529.4
  pellagrous 265.2
Glossocele 529.8
Glossodynia 529.6
  exfoliativa 529.4
Glossoncus 529.8
Glossophytia 529.3
Glossoplegia 529.8
Glossoptosis 529.8
Glossopyrosis 529.6
Glossotrichia 529.3
Glossy skin 710.9
Glottis — see condition
Glottitis — see Glossitis
Glucagonoma (M8152/0)
  malignant (M8152/3)
    pancreas 157.4
    specified site NEC — see Neoplasm, by site,
      malignant
    unspecified site 157.4
  pancreas 211.7
  specified site NEC — see Neoplasm, by site,
    benign
  unspecified site 211.7
Glucoglycinuria 270.7
Glue ear syndrome 381.20
Glue sniffing (airplane glue) (see also
    Dependence) 304.6 ✓5ᵗʰ
Glycinemia (with methylmalonic acidemia) 270.7
Glycinuria (renal) (with ketosis) 270.0
Glycogen
  infiltration (see also Disease, glycogen storage)
    271.0
  storage disease (see also Disease, glycogen
    storage) 271.0
Glycogenosis (see also Disease, glycogen storage)
    271.0
  cardiac 271.0 [425.7]
  Cori, types I-VII 271.0
  diabetic, secondary 250.8 ✓5ᵗʰ [259.8]
  diffuse (with hepatic cirrhosis) 271.0
  generalized 271.0
  glucose-6-phosphatase deficiency 271.0
  hepatophosphorylase deficiency 271.0
  hepatorenal 271.0
  myophosphorylase deficiency 271.0
Glycopenia 251.2
Glycoprolinuria 270.8

Glycosuria 791.5
  renal 271.4
Gnathostoma (spinigerum) (infection) (infestation)
    128.1
  wandering swellings from 128.1
Gnathostomiasis 128.1
Goiter (adolescent) (colloid) (diffuse) (dipping) (due
    to iodine deficiency) (endemic) (euthyroid)
    (heart) (hyperplastic) (internal)
    (intrathoracic) (juvenile) (mixed type)
    (nonendemic) (parenchymatous) (plunging)
    (sporadic) (subclavicular) (substernal) 240.9
  with
    hyperthyroidism (recurrent) (see also Goiter,
      toxic) 242.0 ✓5ᵗʰ
    thyrotoxicosis (see also Goiter, toxic)
      242.0 ✓5ᵗʰ
  adenomatous (see also Goiter, nodular) 241.9
  cancerous (M8000/3) 193
  complicating pregnancy, childbirth, or
    puerperium 648.1 ✓5ᵗʰ
  congenital 246.1
  cystic (see also Goiter, nodular) 241.9
  due to enzyme defect in synthesis of thyroid
    hormone (butane-insoluble iodine)
    (coupling) (deiodinase) (iodide trapping or
    organificaiton) (iodotyrosine
    dehalogenase) (peroxidase) 246.1
  dyshormonogenic 246.1
  exophthalmic (see also Goiter, toxic) 242.0 ✓5ᵗʰ
  familial (with deaf-mutism) 243
  fibrous 245.3
  lingual 759.2
  lymphadenoid 245.2
  malignant (M8000/3) 193
  multinodular (nontoxic) 241.1
    toxic or with hyperthyroidism (see also
      Goiter, toxic) 242.2 ✓5ᵗʰ
  nodular (nontoxic) 241.9
    with
      hyperthyroidism (see also Goiter, toxic)
        242.3 ✓5ᵗʰ
      thyrotoxicosis (see also Goiter, toxic)
        242.3 ✓5ᵗʰ
    endemic 241.9
    exophthalmic (diffuse) (see also Goiter, toxic)
      242.0 ✓5ᵗʰ
    multinodular (nontoxic) 241.1
    sporadic 241.9
    toxic (see also Goiter, toxic) 242.3 ✓5ᵗʰ
    uninodular (nontoxic) 241.0
  nontoxic (nodular) 241.9
    multinodular 241.1
    uninodular 241.0
  pulsating (see also Goiter, toxic) 242.0 ✓5ᵗʰ
  simple 240.0
  toxic 242.0 ✓5ᵗʰ

> Note — Use the following fifth-digit
> subclassification with category 242:
>
> 0   without mention of thyrotoxic crisis or
>   storm
> 1   with mention of thyrotoxic crisis or
>   storm

    adenomatous 242.3 ✓5ᵗʰ
      multinodular 242.2 ✓5ᵗʰ
      uninodular 242.1 ✓5ᵗʰ
    multinodular 242.2 ✓5ᵗʰ
    nodular 242.3 ✓5ᵗʰ
      multinodular 242.2 ✓5ᵗʰ
      uninodular 242.1 ✓5ᵗʰ
    uninodular 242.1 ✓5ᵗʰ
  uninodular (nontoxic) 241.0
    toxic or with hyperthyroidism (see also
      Goiter, toxic) 242.1 ✓5ᵗʰ
Goldberg (-Maxwell) (-Morris) syndrome
    (testicular feminization) 257.8
Goldblatt's
  hypertension 440.1
  kidney 440.1
Goldenhar's syndrome (oculoauriculovertebral
    dysplasia) 756.0
Goldflam-Erb disease or syndrome 358.0
Goldscheider's disease (epidermolysis bullosa)
    757.39

Goldstein's disease (familial hemorrhagic telangiectasia) 448.0
Golfer's elbow 726.32
Goltz-Gorlin syndrome (dermal hypoplasia) 757.39
Gonadoblastoma (M9073/1)
  specified site — see Neoplasm, by site uncertain behavior
  unspecified site
    female 236.2
    male 236.4
Gonecystitis (see also Vesiculitis) 608.0
Gongylonemiasis 125.6
  mouth 125.6
Goniosynechiae 364.73
Gonococcemia 098.89
Gonococcus, gonococcal (disease) (infection) (see also condition) 098.0
  anus 098.7
  bursa 098.52
  chronic NEC 098.2
  complicating pregnancy, childbirth, or puerperium 647.1 ✓5ᵗʰ
    affecting fetus or newborn 760.2
  conjunctiva, conjunctivitis (neonatorum) 098.40
  dermatosis 098.89
  endocardium 098.84
  epididymo-orchitis 098.13
    chronic or duration of 2 months or over 098.33
  eye (newborn) 098.40
  fallopian tube (chronic) 098.37
    acute 098.17
  genitourinary (acute) (organ) (system) (tract) (see also Gonnorrhea) 098.0
    lower 098.0
      chronic 098.2
    upper 098.10
      chronic 098.30
  heart NEC 098.85
  joint 098.50
  keratoderma 098.81
  keratosis (blennorrhagica) 098.81
  lymphatic (gland) (node) 098.89
  meninges 098.82
  orchitis (acute) 098.13
    chronic or duration of 2 months or over 098.33
  pelvis (acute) 098.19
    chronic or duration of 2 months or over 098.39
  pericarditis 098.83
  peritonitis 098.86
  pharyngitis 098.6
  pharynx 098.6
  proctitis 098.7
  pyosalpinx (chronic) 098.37
    acute 098.17
  rectum 098.7
  septicemia 098.89
  skin 098.89
  specified site NEC 098.89
  synovitis 098.51
  tendon sheath 098.51
  throat 098.6
  urethra (acute) 098.0
    chronic or duration of 2 months or over 098.2
  vulva (acute) 098.0
    chronic or duration of 2 months or over 098.2
Gonocytoma (M9073/1)
  specified site — see Neoplasm, by site, uncertain behavior
  unspecified site
    female 236.2
    male 236.4
Gonorrhea 098.0
  acute 098.0
  Bartholin's gland (acute) 098.0
    chronic or duration of 2 months or over 098.2
  bladder (acute) 098.11
    chronic or duration of 2 months or over 098.31

Gonorrhea — continued
  carrier (suspected of) V02.7
  cervix (acute) 098.15
    chronic or duration of 2 months or over 098.35
  chronic 098.2
  complicating pregnancy, childbirth, or puerperium 647.1 ✓5ᵗʰ
    affecting fetus or newborn 760.2
  conjunctiva, conjunctivitis (neonatorum) 098.40
  contact V01.6
  Cowper's gland (acute) 098.0
    chronic or duration of 2 months or over 098.2
  duration of two months or over 098.2
  exposure to V01.6
  fallopian tube (chronic) 098.37
    acute 098.17
  genitourinary (acute) (organ) (system) (tract) 098.0
    chronic 098.2
    duration of two months or over 098.2
  kidney (acute) 098.19
    chronic or duration of 2 months or over 098.39
  ovary (acute) 098.19
    chronic or duration of 2 months or over 098.39
  pelvis (acute) 098.19
    chronic or duration of 2 months or over 098.39
  penis (acute) 098.0
    chronic or duration of 2 months or over 098.2
  prostate (acute) 098.12
    chronic or duration of 2 months or over 098.32
  seminal vesicle (acute) 098.14
    chronic or duration of 2 months or over 098.34
  specified site NEC — see Gonococcus
  spermatic cord (acute) 098.14
    chronic or duration of 2 months or over 098.34
  urethra (acute) 098.0
    chronic or duration of 2 months or over 098.2
  vagina (acute) 098.0
    chronic or duration of 2 months or over 098.2
  vas deferens (acute) 098.14
    chronic or duration of 2 months or over 098.34
  vulva (acute) 098.0
    chronic or duration of 2 months or over 098.2
Goodpasture's syndrome (pneumorenal) 446.21
Gopalan's syndrome (burning feet) 266.2
Gordon's disease (exudative enteropathy) 579.8
Gorlin-Chaudhry-Moss syndrome 759.89
Gougerot's syndrome (trisymptomatic) 709.1
Gougerot-Blum syndrome (pigmented purpuric lichenoid dermatitis) 709.1
Gougerot-Carteaud disease or syndrome (confluent reticulate papillomatosis) 701.8
Gougerot-Hailey-Hailey disease (benign familial chronic pemphigus) 757.39
Gougerot (-Houwer) - Sjögren syndrome (keratoconjunctivitis sicca) 710.2
Gouley's syndrome (constrictive pericarditis) 423.2
Goundou 102.6
Gout, gouty 274.9
  with specified manifestations NEC 274.89
  arthritis (acute) 274.0
  arthropathy 274.0
  degeneration, heart 274.82
  diathesis 274.9
  eczema 274.89
  episcleritis 274.89 [379.09]
  external ear (tophus) 274.81
  glomerulonephritis 274.10
  iritis 274.89 [364.11]
  joint 274.0

Gout, gouty — continued
  kidney 274.10
  lead 984.9
    specified type of lead — see Table of Drugs and Chemicals
  nephritis 274.10
  neuritis 274.89 [357.4]
  phlebitis 274.89 [451.9]
  rheumatic 714.0
  saturnine 984.9
    specified type of lead — see Table of Drugs and Chemicals
  spondylitis 274.0
  synovitis 274.0
  syphilitic 095.8
  tophi 274.0
    ear 274.81
    heart 274.82
    specified site NEC 274.82
Gowers'
  muscular dystrophy 359.1
  syndrome (vasovagal attack) 780.2
Gowers-Paton-Kennedy syndrome 377.04
Gradenigo's syndrome 383.02
Graft-versus-host disease (bone marrow) 996.85
  due to organ transplant NEC — see Complications, transplant, organ
Graham Steell's murmur (pulmonic regurgitation) (see also Endocarditis, pulmonary) 424.3
Grain-handlers' disease or lung 495.8
Grain mite (itch) 133.8
Grand
  mal (idiopathic) (see also Epilepsy) 345.1 ✓5ᵗʰ
    hysteria of Charcôt 300.11
    nonrecurrent or isolated 780.39
  multipara
    affecting management of labor and delivery 659.4 ✓5ᵗʰ
    status only (not pregnant) V61.5
Granite workers' lung 502
Granular — see also condition
  inflammation, pharynx 472.1
  kidney (contracting) (see also Sclerosis, renal) 587
  liver — see Cirrhosis, liver
  nephritis — see Nephritis
Granulation tissue, abnormal — see also Granuloma
  abnormal or excessive 701.5
  postmastoidectomy cavity 383.33
  postoperative 701.5
  skin 701.5
Granulocytopenia, granulocytopenic (primary) 288.0
  malignant 288.0
Granuloma NEC 686.1
  abdomen (wall) 568.89
    skin (pyogenicum) 686.1
      from residual foreign body 709.4
  annulare 695.89
  anus 569.49
  apical 522.6
  appendix 543.9
  aural 380.23
  beryllium (skin) 709.4
    lung 503
  bone (see also Osteomyelitis) 730.1 ✓5ᵗʰ
    eosinophilic 277.8
    from residual foreign body 733.99
  canaliculus lacrimalis 375.81
  cerebral 348.8
  cholesterin, middle ear 385.82
  coccidioidal (progressive) 114.3
    lung 114.4
    meninges 114.2
    primary (lung) 114.0
  colon 569.89
  conjunctiva 372.61
  dental 522.6
  ear, middle (cholesterin) 385.82
    with otitis media — see Otitis media
  eosinophilic 277.8
    bone 277.8
    lung 277.8

Granuloma

Granuloma NEC — *continued*
  eosinophilic — *continued*
    oral mucosa 528.9
  exuberant 701.5
  eyelid 374.89
  facial
    lethal midline 446.3
    malignant 446.3
  faciale 701.8
  fissuratum (gum) 523.8
  foot NEC 686.1
  foreign body (in soft tissue) NEC 728.82
    bone 733.99
    in operative wound 998.4
    muscle 728.82
    skin 709.4
    subcutaneous tissue 709.4
  fungoides 202.1 ✓5ᵗʰ
  gangraenescens 446.3
  giant cell (central) (jaw) (reparative) 526.3
    gingiva 523.8
    peripheral (gingiva) 523.8
  gland (lymph) 289.3
  Hodgkin's (M9661/3) 201.1 ✓5ᵗʰ
  ileum 569.89
  infectious NEC 136.9
  inguinale (Donovan) 099.2
    venereal 099.2
  intestine 569.89
  iridocyclitis 364.10
  jaw (bone) 526.3
    reparative giant cell 526.3
  kidney (*see also* Infection, kidney) 590.9
  lacrimal sac 375.81
  larynx 478.79
  lethal midline 446.3
  lipid 277.8
  lipoid 277.8
  liver 572.8
  lung (infectious) (*see also* Fibrosis, lung) 515
    coccidioidal 114.4
    eosinophilic 277.8
  lymph gland 289.3
  Majocchi's 110.6
  malignant, face 446.3
  mandible 526.3
  mediastinum 519.3
  midline 446.3
  monilial 112.3
  muscle 728.82
    from residual foreign body 728.82
  nasal sinus (*see also* Sinusitis) 473.9
  operation wound 998.59
    foreign body 998.4
    stitch (external) 998.89
      internal organ 996.7 ✓5ᵗʰ
      internal wound 998.89
    talc 998.7
  oral mucosa, eosinophilic or pyogenic 528.9
  orbit, orbital 376.11
  paracoccidiodal 116.1
  penis, venereal 099.2
  periapical 522.6
  peritoneum 568.89
    due to ova of helminths NEC (*see also* Helminthiasis) 128.9
  postmastoidectomy cavity 383.33
  postoperative — *see* Granuloma, operation wound
  prostate 601.8
  pudendi (ulcerating) 099.2
  pudendorum (ulcerative) 099.2
  pulp, internal (tooth) 521.4
  pyogenic, pyogenicum (skin) 686.1
    maxillary alveolar ridge 522.6
    oral mucosa 528.9
  rectum 569.49
  reticulohistiocytic 277.8
  rubrum nasi 705.89
  sarcoid 135
  Schistosoma 120.9
  septic (skin) 686.1
  silica (skin) 709.4
  sinus (accessory) (infectional) (nasal) (*see also* Sinusitis) 473.9
  skin (pyogenicum) 686.1
    from foreign body or material 709.4
  sperm 608.89

Granuloma NEC — *continued*
  spine
    syphilitic (epidural) 094.89
    tuberculous (*see also* Tuberculosis) 015.0 ✓5ᵗʰ *[730.88]*
  stitch (postoperative) 998.89
    internal wound 998.89
  suppurative (skin) 686.1
  suture (postoperative) 998.89
    internal wound 998.89
  swimming pool 031.1
  talc 728.82
    in operation wound 998.7
  telangiectaticum (skin) 686.1
  trichophyticum 110.6
  tropicum 102.4
  umbilicus 686.1
    newborn 771.4
  urethra 599.84
  uveitis 364.10
  vagina 099.2
  venereum 099.2
  vocal cords 478.5
  Wegener's (necrotizing respiratory granulomatosis) 446.4
Granulomatosis NEC 686.1
  disciformis chronica et progressiva 709.3
  infantiseptica 771.2
  lipoid 277.8
  lipohagic, intestinal 040.2
  miliary 027.0
  necrotizing, respiratory 446.4
  progressive, septic 288.1
  Wegener's (necrotizing respiratory) 446.4
Granulomatous tissue — *see* Granuloma
Granulosis rubra nasi 705.89
Graphite fibrosis (of lung) 503
Graphospasm 300.89
  organic 333.84
Grating scapula 733.99
Gravel (urinary) (*see also* Calculus) 592.9
Graves' disease (exophthalmic goiter) (*see also* Goiter, toxic) 242.0 ✓5ᵗʰ
Gravis — *see* condition
Grawitz's tumor (hypernephroma) (M8312/3) 189.0
Grayness, hair (premature) 704.3
  congenital 757.4
Gray or grey syndrome (chloramphenicol) (newborn) 779.4
Greenfield's disease 330.0
Green sickness 280.9
Greenstick fracture — *see* Fracture, by site
Greig's syndrome (hypertelorism) 756.0
Griesinger's disease (*see also* Ancylostomiasis) 126.9
Grinders'
  asthma 502
  lung 502
  phthisis (*see also* Tuberculosis) 011.4 ✓5ᵗʰ
Grinding, teeth 306.8
Grip
  Dabney's 074.1
  devil's 074.1
Grippe, grippal — *see also* Influenza
  Balkan 083.0
  intestinal 487.8
  summer 074.8
Grippy cold 487.1
Grisel's disease 723.5
Groin — *see* condition
Grooved
  nails (transverse) 703.8
  tongue 529.5
    congenital 750.13
Ground itch 126.9
Growing pains, children 781.99
Growth (fungoid) (neoplastic) (new) (M8000/1) — *see also* Neoplasm, by site, unspecified nature
  adenoid (vegetative) 474.12

Growth — *see also* Neoplasm, by site, unspecified nature — *continued*
  benign (M8000/0) — *see* Neoplasm, by site, benign
  fetal, poor 764.9 ✓5ᵗʰ
    affecting management of pregnancy 656.5 ✓5ᵗʰ
  malignant (M8000/3) — *see* Neoplasm, by site, malignant
  rapid, childhood V21.0
  secondary (M8000/6) — *see* Neoplasm, by site, malignant, secondary
Gruber's hernia — *see* Hernia, Gruber's
Gruby's disease (tinea tonsurans) 110.0
G-trisomy 758.0
Guama fever 066.3
Gubler (-Millard) paralysis or syndrome 344.89
Guérin-Stern syndrome (arthorgryposis multiplex congenita) 754.89
Guertin's disease (electric chorea) 049.8
Guillain-Barré disease or syndrome 357.0
Guinea worms (infection) (infestation) 125.7
Guinon's disease (motor-verbal tic) 307.23
Gull's disease (thyroid atrophy with myxedema) 244.8
Gull and Sutton's disease — *see* Hypertension, kidney
Gum — *see* condition
Gumboil 522.7
Gumma (syphilitic) 095.9
  artery 093.89
    cerebral or spinal 094.89
  bone 095.5
    of yaws (late) 102.6
  brain 094.89
  cauda equina 094.89
  central nervous system NEC 094.9
  ciliary body 095.8 *[364.11]*
  congenital 090.5
    testis 090.5
  eyelid 095.8 *[373.5]*
  heart 093.89
  intracranial 094.89
  iris 095.8 *[364.11]*
  kidney 095.4
  larynx 095.8
  leptomeninges 094.2
  liver 095.3
  meninges 094.2
  myocardium 093.82
  nasopharynx 095.8
  neurosyphilitic 094.9
  nose 095.8
  orbit 095.8
  palate (soft) 095.8
  penis 095.8
  pericardium 093.81
  pharynx 095.8
  pituitary 095.8
  scrofulous (*see also* Tuberculosis) 017.0 ✓5ᵗʰ
  skin 095.8
  specified site NEC 095.8
  spinal cord 094.89
  tongue 095.8
  tonsil 095.8
  trachea 095.8
  tuberculous (*see also* Tuberculosis) 017.0 ✓5ᵗʰ
  ulcerative due to yaws 102.4
  ureter 095.8
  yaws 102.4
    bone 102.6
Gunn's syndrome (jaw-winking syndrome) 742.8
Gunshot wound — *see also* Wound, open, by site
  fracture — *see* Fracture, by site, open
  internal organs (abdomen, chest, or pelvis) — *see* Injury, internal, by site, with open wound
  intracranial — *see* Laceration, brain, with open intracranial wound
Günther's disease or syndrome (congenital erythropoietic porphyria) 277.1
Gustatory hallucination 780.1
Gynandrism 752.7

Index to Diseases

Gynanadroblastoma (M8632/1)
  specified site — see Neoplasm, by site, uncertain behavior
  unspecified site
    female 236.2
    male 236.4
Gynandromorphism 752.7
Gynatresia (congenital) 752.49
Gynecoid pelvis, male 738.6
Gynecological examination V72.3
  for contraceptive maintenance V25.40
Gynecomastia 611.1
Gynephobia 300.29
Gyrate scalp 757.39

H

Haas' disease (osteochondrosis head of humerus) 732.3
Habermann's disease (acute parapsoriasis varioliformis) 696.2
Habit, habituation
  chorea 307.22
  disturbance, child 307.9
  drug (see also Dependence) 304.9 ✓5ᵗʰ
  laxative (see also Abuse, drugs, nondependent) 305.9 ✓5ᵗʰ
  spasm 307.20
    chronic 307.22
    transient of childhood 307.21
  tic 307.20
    chronic 307.22
    transient of childhood 307.21
  use of
    nonprescribed drugs (see also Abuse, drugs, nondependent) 305.9 ✓5ᵗʰ
    patent medicines (see also Abuse, drugs, nondependent) 305.9 ✓5ᵗʰ
  vomiting 536.2
Hadfield-Clarke syndrome (pancreatic infantilism) 577.8
Haff disease 985.1
Hageman factor defect, deficiency, or disease (see also Defect, coagulation) 286.3
Haglund's disease (osteochondrosis os tibiale externum) 732.5
Haglund-Läwen-Fründ syndrome 717.89
Hagner's disease (hypertrophic pulmonary osteoarthropathy) 731.2
Hag teeth, tooth 524.3
Hailey-Hailey disease (benign familial chronic pemphigus) 757.39
Hair — see also condition
  plucking 307.9
Hairball in stomach 935.2
Hairy black tongue 529.3
Half vertebra 756.14
Halitosis 784.9
Hallermann-Streiff syndrome 756.0
Hallervorden-Spatz disease or syndrome 333.0
Hallopeau's
  acrodermatitis (continua) 696.1
  disease (lichen sclerosis et atrophicus) 701.0
Hallucination (auditory) (gustatory) (olfactory) (tactile) 780.1
  alcoholic 291.3
  drug-induced 292.12
  visual 368.16
Hallucinosis 298.9
  alcoholic (acute) 291.3
  drug-induced 292.12
Hallus — see Hallux
Hallux 735.9
  malleus (acquired) 735.3
  rigidus (acquired) 735.2
    congenital 755.66
    late effects of rickets 268.1
  valgus (acquired) 735.0
    congenital 755.66
  varus (acquired) 735.1
    congenital 755.66

Halo, visual 368.15
Hamartoblastoma 759.6
Hamartoma 759.6
  epithelial (gingival), odontogenic, central, or peripheral (M9321/0) 213.1
    upper jaw (bone) 213.0
  vascular 757.32
Hamartosis, hamartoses NEC 759.6
Hamman's disease or syndrome (spontaneous mediastinal emphysema) 518.1
Hamman-Rich syndrome (diffuse interstitial pulmonary fibrosis) 516.3
Hammer toe (acquired) 735.4
  congenital 755.66
  late effects of rickets 268.1
Hand — see condition
Hand-Schüller-Christian disease or syndrome (chronic histiocytosis x) 277.8
Hand-foot syndrome 282.61
Hanging (asphyxia) (strangulation) (suffocation) 994.7
Hangnail (finger) (with lymphangitis) 681.02
Hangover (alcohol) (see also Abuse, drugs, nondependent) 305.0 ✓5ᵗʰ
Hanot's cirrhosis or disease — see Cirrhosis, biliary
Hanot-Chauffard (-Troisier) syndrome (bronze diabetes) 275.0
Hansen's disease (leprosy) 030.9
  benign form 030.1
  malignant form 030.0
Harada's disease or syndrome 363.22
Hard chancre 091.0
Hard firm prostate 600.1
Hardening
  artery — see Arteriosclerosis
  brain 348.8
  liver 571.8
Hare's syndrome (M8010/3) (carcinoma, pulmonary apex) 162.3
Harelip (see also Cleft, lip) 749.10
Harkavy's syndrome 446.0
Harlequin (fetus) 757.1
  color change syndrome 779.89 ▲
Harley's disease (intermittent hemoglobinuria) 283.2
Harris'
  lines 733.91
  syndrome (organic hyperinsulinism) 251.1
Hart's disease or syndrome (pellagra-cerebellar ataxia-renal aminoaciduria) 270.0
Hartmann's pouch (abnormal sacculation of gallbladder neck) 575.8
  of intestine V44.3
    attention to V55.3
Hartnup disease (pellagra-cerebellar ataxia-renal aminoaciduria) 270.0
Harvester lung 495.0
Hashimoto's disease or struma (struma lymphomatosa) 245.2
Hassell-Henle bodies (corneal warts) 371.41
Haut mal (see also Epilepsy) 345.1 ✓5ᵗʰ
Haverhill fever 026.1
Hawaiian wood rose dependence 304.5 ✓5ᵗʰ
Hawkins' keloid 701.4
Hay
  asthma (see also Asthma) 493.0 ✓5ᵗʰ
  fever (allergic) (with rhinitis) 477.9
    with asthma (bronchial) (see also Asthma) 493.0 ✓5ᵗʰ
    allergic, due to grass, pollen, ragweed, or tree 477.0
    conjunctivitis 372.05
    due to
      dander 477.8
      dust 477.8
      fowl 477.8
      pollen 477.0
    specified allergen other than pollen 477.8

Hayem-Faber syndrome (achlorhydric anemia) 280.9
Hayem-Widal syndrome (acquired hemolytic jaundice) 283.9
Haygarth's nodosities 715.04
Hazard-Crile tumor (M8350/3) 193
Hb (abnormal)
  disease — see Disease, hemoglobin
  trait — see Trait
H disease 270.0
Head — see also condition
  banging 307.3
Headache 784.0
  allergic 346.2 ✓5ᵗʰ
  cluster 346.2 ✓5ᵗʰ
  due to
    loss, spinal fluid 349.0
    lumbar puncture 349.0
    saddle block 349.0
  emotional 307.81
  histamine 346.2 ✓5ᵗʰ
  lumbar puncture 349.0
  menopausal 627.2
  migraine 346.9 ✓5ᵗʰ
  nonorganic origin 307.81
  postspinal 349.0
  psychogenic 307.81
  psychophysiologic 307.81
  sick 346.1 ✓5ᵗʰ
  spinal 349.0
    complicating labor and delivery 668.8 ✓5ᵗʰ ●
    postpartum 668.8 ✓5ᵗʰ ●
  spinal fluid loss 349.0
  tension 307.81
  vascular 784.0
    migraine type 346.9 ✓5ᵗʰ
  vasomotor 346.9 ✓5ᵗʰ
Health
  advice V65.4
  audit V70.0
  checkup V70.0
  education V65.4
  hazard (see also History of) V15.9
    specified cause NEC V15.89
  instruction V65.4
  services provided because (of)
    boarding school residence V60.6
    holiday relief for person providing home care V60.5
    inadequate
      housing V60.1
      resources V60.2
    lack of housing V60.0
    no care available in home V60.4
    person living alone V60.3
    poverty V60.3
    residence in institution V60.6
    specified cause NEC V60.8
    vacation relief for person providing home care V60.5
Healthy
  donor (see also Donor) V59.9
  infant or child
    accompanying sick mother V65.0
    receiving care V20.1
  person
    accompanying sick relative V65.0
    admitted for sterilization V25.2
    receiving prophylactic inoculation or vaccination (see also Vaccination, prophylactic) V05.9
Hearing examination V72.1
Heart — see condition
Heartburn 787.1
  psychogenic 306.4
Heat (effects) 992.9
  apoplexy 992.0
  burn — see also Burn, by site
    from sun (see also Sunburn) 692.71
  collapse 992.1
  cramps 992.2
  dermatitis or eczema 692.89
  edema 992.7
  erythema — see Burn, by site

Heat

Heat — *continued*
- excessive 992.9
  - specified effect NEC 992.8
- exhaustion 992.5
  - anhydrotic 992.3
  - due to
    - salt (and water) depletion 992.4
    - water depletion 992.3
- fatigue (transient) 992.6
- fever 992.0
- hyperpyrexia 992.0
- prickly 705.1
- prostration — *see* Heat, exhaustion
- pyrexia 992.0
- rash 705.1
- specified effect NEC 992.8
- stroke 992.0
- sunburn (*see also* Sunburn) 692.71
- syncope 992.1

Heavy-chain disease 273.2

Heavy-for-dates (fetus or infant) 766.1
- 4500 grams or more 766.0
- exceptionally 766.0

Hebephrenia, hebephrenic (acute) (*see also* Schizophrenia) 295.1 ✓5ᵗʰ
- dementia (praecox) (*see also* Schizophrenia) 295.1 ✓5ᵗʰ
- schizophrenia (*see also* Schizophrenia) 295.1 ✓5ᵗʰ

Heberden's
- disease or nodes 715.04
- syndrome (angina pectoris) 413.9

Hebra's disease
- dermatitis exfoliativa 695.89
- erythema multiforme exudativum 695.1
- pityriasis 695.89
  - maculata et circinata 696.3
  - rubra 695.89
    - pilaris 696.4
- prurigo 698.2

Hebra, nose 040.1

Hedinger's syndrome (malignant carcinoid) 259.2

Heel — *see* condition

Heerfordt's disease or syndrome (uveoparotitis) 135

Hegglin's anomaly or syndrome 288.2

Heidenhain's disease 290.10
- with dementia 290.10

Heilmeyer-Schöner disease (M9842/3) 207.1 ✓5ᵗʰ

Heine-Medin disease (*see also* Poliomyelitis) 045.9 ✓5ᵗʰ

Heinz-body anemia, congenital 282.7

Heller's disease or syndrome (infantile psychosis) (*see also* Psychosis, childhood) 299.1 ✓5ᵗʰ

H.E.L.L.P 642.5 ✓5ᵗʰ

Helminthiasis (*see also* Infestation, by specific parasite) 128.9
- Ancylostoma (*see also* Ancylostoma) 126.9
- intestinal 127.9
  - mixed types (types classifiable to more than one of the titles 120.0-127.7) 127.8
  - specified type 127.7
- mixed types (intestinal) (types classifiable to more than one of the titles 120.0-127.7) 127.8
- Necator americanus 126.1
- specified type NEC 128.8
- Trichinella 124

Heloma 700

Hemangioblastoma (M9161/1) — *see also* Neoplasm, connective tissue, uncertain behavior
- malignant (M9161/3) — *see* Neoplasm, connective tissue, malignant

Hemangioblastomatosis, cerebelloretinal 759.6

Hemangioendothelioma (M9130/1) — *see also* Neoplasm, by site, uncertain behavior
- benign (M9130/0) 228.00
- bone (diffuse) (M9130/3) — *see* Neoplasm, bone, malignant
- malignant (M9130/3) — *see* Neoplasm, connective tissue, malignant

Hemangioendothelioma — *see also* Neoplasm, by site, uncertain behavior — *continued*
- nervous system (M9130/0) 228.09

Hemangioendotheliosarcoma (M9130/3) — *see* Neoplasm, connective tissue, malignant

Hemangiofibroma (M9160/0) — *see* Neoplasm, by site, benign

Hemangiolipoma (M8861/0) — *see* Lipoma

Hemangioma (M9120/0) 228.00
- arteriovenous (M9123/0) — *see* Hemangioma, by site
- brain 228.02
- capillary (M9131/0) — *see* Hemangioma, by site
- cavernous (M9121/0) — *see* Hemangioma, by site
- central nervous system NEC 228.09
- choroid 228.09
- heart 228.09
- infantile (M9131/0) — *see* Hemangioma, by site
- intra-abdominal structures 228.04
- intracranial structures 228.02
- intramuscular (M9132/0) — *see* Hemangioma, by site
- iris 228.09
- juvenile (M9131/0) — *see* Hemangioma, by site
- malignant (M9120/3) — *see* Neoplasm, connective tissue, malignant
- meninges 228.09
  - brain 228.02
  - spinal cord 228.09
- peritoneum 228.04
- placenta — *see* Placenta, abnormal
- plexiform (M9131/0) — *see* Hemangioma, by site
- racemose (M9123/0) — *see* Hemangioma, by site
- retina 228.03
- retroperitoneal tissue 228.04
- sclerosing (M8832/0) — *see* Neoplasm, skin, benign
- simplex (M9131/0) — *see* Hemangioma, by site
- skin and subcutaneous tissue 228.01
- specified site NEC 228.09
- spinal cord 228.09
- venous (M9122/0) — *see* Hemangioma, by site
- verrucous keratotic (M9142/0) — *see* Hemangioma, by site

Hemangiomatosis (systemic) 757.32
- involving single site — *see* Hemangioma

Hemangiopericytoma (M9l50/1) — *see also* Neoplasm, connective tissue, uncertain behavior
- benign (M9150/0) — *see* Neoplasm, connective tissue, benign
- malignant (M9150/3) — *see* Neoplasm, connective tissue, malignant

Hemangiosarcoma (M9120/3) — *see* Neoplasm, connective tissue, malignant

Hemarthrosis (nontraumatic) 719.10
- ankle 719.17
- elbow 719.12
- foot 719.17
- hand 719.14
- hip 719.15
- knee 719.16
- multiple sites 719.19
- pelvic region 719.15
- shoulder (region) 719.11
- specified site NEC 719.18
- traumatic — *see* Sprain, by site
- wrist 719.13

Hematemesis 578.0
- with ulcer — *see* Ulcer, by site, with hemorrhage
- due to S. japonicum 120.2
- Goldstein's (familial hemorrhagic telangiectasia) 448.0
- newborn 772.4
  - due to swallowed maternal blood 777.3

Hematidrosis 705.89

Hematinuria (*see also* Hemoglobinuria) 791.2
- malarial 084.8
- paroxysmal 283.2

Hematite miners' lung 503

Hematobilia 576.8

Hematocele (congenital) (diffuse) (idiopathic) 608.83
- broad ligament 620.7
- canal of Nuck 629.0
- cord male 608.83
- fallopian tube 620.8
- female NEC 629.0
- ischiorectal 569.89
- male NEC 608.83
- ovary 629.0
- pelvis, pelvic
  - female 629.0
    - with ectopic pregnancy (*see also* Pregnancy, ectopic) 633.90 ▲
      - with intrauterine pregnancy 633.91 ●
  - male 608.83
- periuterine 629.0
- retrouterine 629.0
- scrotum 608.83
- spermatic cord (diffuse) 608.83
- testis 608.84
- traumatic — *see* Injury, internal, pelvis
- tunica vaginalis 608.83
- uterine ligament 629.0
- uterus 621.4
- vagina 623.6
- vulva 624.5

Hematocephalus 742.4

Hematochezia (*see also* Melena) 578.1

Hematochyluria (*see also* Infestation, filarial) 125.9

Hematocolpos 626.8

Hematocornea 371.12

Hematogenous — *see* condition

Hematoma (skin surface intact) (traumatic) — *see also* Contusion

> Note — Hematomas are coded according to origin and the nature and site of the hematoma or the accompanying injury. Hematomas of unspecified origin are coded as injuries of the sites involved, except:
>
> (a) hematomas of genital organs which are coded as diseases of the organ involved unless they complicate pregnancy or delivery
>
> (b) hematomas of the eye which are coded as diseases of the eye.
>
> For late effect of hematoma classifiable to 920-924 see Late, effect, contusion.

with
- crush injury — *see* Crush
- fracture — *see* Fracture, by site
- injury of internal organs — *see also* Injury, internal, by site
  - kidney — *see* Hematoma, kidney traumatic
  - liver — *see* Hematoma, liver, traumatic
  - spleen — *see* Hematoma, spleen
- nerve injury — *see* Injury, nerve
- open wound — *see* Wound, open, by site
- skin surface intact — *see* Contusion
- abdomen (wall) — *see* Contusion, abdomen
- amnion 658.8 ✓5ᵗʰ
- aorta, dissecting 441.00
  - abdominal 441.02
  - thoracic 441.01
  - thoracoabdominal 441.03
- arterial (complicating trauma) 904.9
  - specified site — *see* Injury, blood vessel, by site
- auricle (ear) 380.31
- birth injury 767.8
  - skull 767.1

Index to Diseases

Hematoma — *see also* Contusion — *continued*
  brain (traumatic) 853.0 ✓5ᵗʰ

> *Note* — *Use the following fifth-digit subclassification with categories 851-854:*
>
> 0   *unspecified state of consciousness*
> 1   *with no loss of consciousness*
> 2   *with brief [less than one hour] loss of consciousness*
> 3   *with moderate [1-24 hours] loss of consciousness*
> 4   *with prolonged [more than 24 hours] loss of consciousness and return to pre-existing conscious level*
> 5   *with prolonged [more than 24 hours] loss of consciousness, without return to pre-existing conscious level*
>
> *Use fifth-digit 5 to designate when a patient is unconscious and dies before regaining consciousness, regardless of the duration of the loss of consciousness*
>
> 6   *with loss of consciousness of unspecified duration*
> 9   *with concussion, unspecified*

  with
    cerebral
      contusion — *see* Contusion, brain
      laceration — *see* Laceration, brain
    open intracranial wound 853.1 ✓5ᵗʰ
    skull fracture — *see* Fracture, skull, by site
  extradural or epidural 852.4 ✓5ᵗʰ
    with open intracranial wound 852.5 ✓5ᵗʰ
    fetus or newborn 767.0
    nontraumatic 432.0
  fetus or newborn NEC 767.0
  nontraumatic (*see also* Hemorrhage, brain) 431
    epidural or extradural 432.0
    newborn NEC 772.8
    subarachnoid, arachnoid, or meningeal (*see also* Hemorrhage, subarachnoid) 430
    subdural (*see also* Hemorrhage, subdural) 432.1
  subarachnoid, arachnoid, or meningeal 852.0 ✓5ᵗʰ
    with open intracranial wound 852.1 ✓5ᵗʰ
    fetus or newborn 772.2
    nontraumatic (*see also* Hemorrhage, subarachnoid) 430
  subdural 852.2 ✓5ᵗʰ
    with open intracranial wound 852.3 ✓5ᵗʰ
    fetus or newborn (localized) 767.0
    nontraumatic (*see also* Hemorrhage, subdural) 432.1
breast (nontraumatic) 611.8
broad ligament (nontraumatic) 620.7
  complicating delivery 665.7 ✓5ᵗʰ
  traumatic — *see* Injury, internal, broad ligament
calcified NEC 959.9
capitis 920
  due to birth injury 767.1
  newborn 767.1
cerebral — *see* Hematoma, brain
cesarean section wound 674.3 ✓5ᵗʰ
chorion — *see* Placenta, abnormal
complicating delivery (perineum) (vulva) 664.5 ✓5ᵗʰ
  pelvic 665.7 ✓5ᵗʰ
  vagina 665.7 ✓5ᵗʰ
corpus
  cavernosum (nontraumatic) 607.82
  luteum (nontraumatic) (ruptured) 620.1
dura (mater) — *see* Hematoma, brain, subdural
epididymis (nontraumatic) 608.83
epidural (traumatic) — *see also* Hematoma, brain, extradural
  spinal — *see* Injury, spinal, by site
episiotomy 674.3 ✓5ᵗʰ
external ear 380.31

Hematoma — *see also* Contusion — *continued*
extradural — *see also* Hematoma, brain, extradural
  fetus or newborn 767.0
  nontraumatic 432.0
    fetus or newborn 767.0
fallopian tube 620.8
genital organ (nontraumatic)
  female NEC 629.8
  male NEC 608.83
  traumatic (external site) 922.4
    internal — *see* Injury, internal, genital organ
graafian follicle (ruptured) 620.0
internal organs (abdomen, chest, or pelvis) — *see also* Injury, internal, by site
  kidney — *see* Hematoma, kidney, traumatic
  liver — *see* Hematoma, liver, traumatic
  spleen — *see* Hematoma, brain
intracrainal — *see* Hematoma, brain
kidney, cystic 593.81
  traumatic 866.01
    with open wound into cavity 866.11
labia (nontraumatic) 624.5
lingual (and other parts of neck, scalp, or face, except eye) 920
liver (subcapsular) 573.8
  birth injury 767.8
  fetus or newborn 767.8
  traumatic NEC 864.01
    with
      laceration — *see* Laceration, liver
      open wound into cavity 864.11
mediastinum — *see* Injury, internal, mediastinum
meninges, meningeal (brain) — *see also* Hematoma, brain, subarachnoid
  spinal — *see* Injury, spinal, by site
mesosalpinx (nontraumatic) 620.8
  traumatic — *see* Injury, internal, pelvis
muscle (traumatic — *see* Contusion, by site
nasal (septum) (and other part(s) of neck, scalp, or face, except eye) 920
obstetrical surgical wound 674.3 ✓5ᵗʰ
orbit, orbital (nontraumatic) 376.32
  traumatic 921.2
ovary (corpus luteum) (nontraumatic) 620.1
  traumatic — *see* Injury, internal, ovary
pelvis (female) (nontraumatic) 629.8
  complicating delivery 665.7 ✓5ᵗʰ
  male 608.83
  traumatic — *see also* Injury, internal, pelvis
    specified organ NEC (*see also* Injury, internal, pelvis) 867.6
penis (nontraumatic) 607.82
pericranial (and neck, or face any part, except eye) 920
  due to injury at birth 767.1
perineal wound (obstetrical) 674.3 ✓5ᵗʰ
  complicating delivery 664.5 ✓5ᵗʰ
perirenal, cystic 593.81
pinna 380.31
placenta — *see* Placenta, abnormal
postoperative 998.12
retroperitoneal (nontraumatic) 568.81
  traumatic — *see* Injury, internal, retroperitoneum
retropubic, male 568.81
scalp (and neck, or face any part, except eye) 920
  fetus or newborn 767.1
scrotum (nontraumatic) 608.83
  traumatic 922.4
seminal vesicle (nontraumatic) 608.83
  traumatic — *see* Injury, internal, seminal, vesicle
spermatic cord — *see also* Injury, internal, spermatic cord
  nontraumatic 608.83
spinal (cord) (meninges) — *see also* Injury, spinal, by site
  fetus or newborn 767.4
  nontraumatic 336.1
spleen 865.01
  with
    laceration — *see* Laceration, spleen
    open wound into cavity 865.11

Hematoma — *see also* Contusion — *continued*
sternocleidomastoid, birth injury 767.8
sternomastoid, birth injury 767.8
subarachnoid — *see also* Hematoma, brain, subarachnoid
  fetus or newborn 772.2
  nontraumatic (*see also* Hemorrhage, subarachnoid) 430
  newborn 772.2
subdural — *see also* Hematoma, brain, subdural
  fetus or newborn (localized) 767.0
  nontraumatic (*see also* Hemorrhage, subdural) 432.1
subperiosteal (syndrome) 267
  traumatic — *see* Hematoma, by site
superficial, fetus or newborn 772.6
syncytium — *see* Placenta, abnormal
testis (nontraumatic) 608.83
  birth injury 767.8
  traumatic 922.4
tunica vaginalis (nontraumatic) 608.83
umbilical cord 663.6 ✓5ᵗʰ
  affecting fetus or newborn 762.6
uterine ligament (nontraumatic) 620.7
  traumatic — *see* Injury, internal, pelvis
uterus 621.4
  traumatic — *see* Injury, internal, pelvis
vagina (nontraumatic) (ruptured) 623.6
  complicating delivery 665.7 ✓5ᵗʰ
  traumatic 922.4
vas deferens (nontraumatic) 608.83
  traumatic — *see* Injury, internal, vas deferens
vitreous 379.23
vocal cord 920
vulva (nontraumatic) 624.5
  complicating delivery 664.5 ✓5ᵗʰ
  fetus or newborn 767.8
  traumatic 922.4
Hematometra 621.4
Hematomyelia 336.1
  with fracture of vertebra (*see also* Fracture, vertebra, by site, with spinal cord injury) 806.8
  fetus or newborn 767.4
Hematomyelitis 323.9
  late effect — *see* category 326
Hematoperitoneum (*see also* Hemoperitoneum) 568.81
Hematopneumothorax (*see also* Hemothorax) 511.8
Hematoporphyria (acquired) (congenital) 277.1
Hematoporphyrinuria (acquired) (congenital) 277.1
Hematorachis, hematorrhachis 336.1
  fetus or newborn 767.4
Hematosalpinx 620.8
  with
    ectopic pregnancy (*see also* categories 633.0-633.9) 639.2
    molar pregnancy (*see also* categories 630-632) 639.2
    infectional (*see also* Salpingo-oophoritis) 614.2
Hematospermia 608.82
Hematothorax (*see also* Hemothorax) 511.8
Hematotympanum 381.03
Hematuria (benign) (essential) (idiopathic) 599.7
  due to S. hematobium 120.0
  endemic 120.0
  intermittent 599.7
  malarial 084.8
  paroxysmal 599.7
  sulfonamide
    correct substance properly administered 599.7
    overdose or wrong substance given or taken 961.0
  tropical (bilharziasis) 120.0
  tuberculous (*see also* Tuberculosis) 016.9 ✓5ᵗʰ
Hematuric bilious fever 084.8
Hemeralopia 368.10 ▲

Hemiabiotrophy 799.8
Hemi-akinesia 781.8
Hemianalgesia (see also Disturbance, sensation) 782.0
Hemianencephaly 740.0
Hemianesthesia (see also Disturbance, sensation) 782.0
Hemianopia, hemianopsia (altitudinal) (homonymous) 368.46
    binasal 368.47
    bitemporal 368.47
    heteronymous 368.47
    syphilitic 095.8
Hemiasomatognosia 307.9
Hemiathetosis 781.0
Hemiatrophy 799.8
    cerebellar 334.8
    face 349.89
        progressive 349.89
    fascia 728.9
    leg 728.2
    tongue 529.8
Hemiballism(us) 333.5
Hemiblock (cardiac) (heart) (left) 426.2
Hemicardia 746.89
Hemicephalus, hemicephaly 740.0
Hemichorea 333.5
Hemicrania 346.9
    congenital malformation 740.0
Hemidystrophy — see Hemiatrophy
Hemiectromelia 755.4
Hemihypalgesia (see also Disturbance, sensation) 782.0
Hemihypertrophy (congenital) 759.89
    cranial 756.0
Hemihypesthesia (see also Disturbance, sensation) 782.0
Hemi-inattention 781.8
Hemimelia 755.4
    lower limb 755.30
        paraxial (complete) (incomplete) (intercalary) (terminal) 755.32
            fibula 755.37
            tibia 755.36
        transverse (complete) (partial) 755.31
    upper limb 755.20
        paraxial (complete) (incomplete) (intercalary) (terminal) 755.22
            radial 755.26
            ulnar 755.27
        transverse (complete) (partial) 755.21
Hemiparalysis (see also Hemiplegia) 342.9
Hemiparesis (see also Hemiplegia) 342.9
Hemiparesthesia (see also Disturbance, sensation) 782.0
Hemiplegia 342.9
    acute (see also Disease, cerebrovascular, acute) 436
    alternans facialis 344.89
    apoplectic (see also Disease, cerebrovascular, acute) 436
        late effect or residual
            affecting
                dominant side 438.21
                nondominant side 438.22
                unspecified side 438.20
    arteriosclerotic 437.0
        late effect or residual
            affecting
                dominant side 438.21
                nondominant side 438.22
                unspecified side 438.20
    ascending (spinal) NEC 344.89
    attack (see also Disease, cerebrovascular, acute) 436
    brain, cerebral (current episode) 437.8
        congenital 343.1
    cerebral — see Hemiplegia, brain
    congenital (cerebral) (spastic) (spinal) 343.1
    conversion neurosis (hysterical) 300.11

Hemiplegia — continued
    cortical — see Hemiplegia, brain
    due to
        arteriosclerosis 437.0
            late effect or residual
                affecting
                    dominant side 438.21
                  nondominant side 438.22
                  unspecified side 438.20
        cerebrovascular lesion (see also Disease, cerebrovascular, acute) 436
            late effect
                affecting
                  dominant side 438.21
                  nondominant side 438.22
                  unspecified side 438.20
    embolic (current) (see also Embolism, brain) 434.1
        late effect
            affecting
                dominant side 438.21
                nondominant side 438.22
                unspecified side 438.20
    flaccid 342.0
    hypertensive (current episode) 437.8
    infantile (postnatal) 343.4
    late effect
        birth injury, intracranial or spinal 343.4
        cerebrovascular lesion — see Late effect(s) (of) cerebrovascular disease
        viral encephalitis 139.0
    middle alternating NEC 344.89
    newborn NEC 767.0
    seizure (current episode) (see also Disease, cerebrovascular, acute) 436
    spastic 342.1
        congenital or infantile 343.1
    specified NEC 342.8
    thrombotic (current) (see also Thrombosis, brain) 434.0
        late effect — see Late effect(s) (of) cerebrovascular disease
Hemisection, spinal cord — see Fracture, vertebra, by site, with spinal cord injury
Hemispasm 781.0
    facial 781.0
Hemispatial neglect 781.8
Hemisporosis 117.9
Hemitremor 781.0
Hemivertebra 756.14
Hemobilia 576.8
Hemocholecyst 575.8
Hemochromatosis (acquired) (diabetic) (hereditary) (liver) (myocardium) (primary idiopathic) (secondary) 275.0
    with refractory anemia 285.0
Hemodialysis V56.0
Hemoglobin — see also condition
    abnormal (disease) — see Disease, hemoglobin
    AS genotype 282.5
    fetal, hereditary persistence 282.7
    high-oxygen-affinity 289.0
    low NEC 285.9
    S (Hb-S), heterozygous 282.5
Hemoglobinemia 283.2
    due to blood transfusion NEC 999.8
        bone marrow 996.85
    paroxysmal 283.2
Hemoglobinopathy (mixed) (see also Disease, hemoblobin) 282.7
    with thalassemia 282.4
    sickle-cell 282.60
        with thalassemia 282.4
Hemoglobinuria, hemoglobinuric 791.2
    with anemia, hemolytic, acquired (chronic) NEC 283.2
    cold (agglutinin) (paroxysmal) (with Raynaud's syndrome) 283.2
    due to
        exertion 283.2
        hemolysis (from external causes) NEC 283.2
    exercise 283.2
    fever (malaria) 084.8
    infantile 791.2

Hemoglobinuria, hemoglobinuric — continued
    intermittent 283.2
    malarial 084.8
    march 283.2
    nocturnal (paroxysmal) 283.2
    paroxysmal (cold) (nocturnal) 283.2
Hemolymphangioma (M9175/0) 228.1
Hemolysis
    fetal — see Jaundice, fetus or newborn
    intravascular (disseminated) NEC 286.6
        with
            abortion — see Abortion, by type, with hemorrhage, delayed or excessive
            ectopic pregnancy (see also categories 633.0-633.9) 639.1
            hemorrhage of pregnancy 641.3
                affecting fetus or newborn 762.1
            molar pregnancy (see also categories 630-632) 639.1
        acute 283.2
        following
            abortion 639.1
            ectopic or molar pregnancy 639.1
        neonatal — see Jaundice, fetus or newborn
        transfusion NEC 999.8
            bone marrow 996.85
Hemolytic — see also condition
    anemia — see Anemia, hemolytic
    uremic syndrome 283.11
Hemometra 621.4
Hemopericardium (with effusion) 423.0
    newborn 772.8
    traumatic (see also Hemothorax, traumatic) 860.2
        with open wound into thorax 860.3
Hemoperitoneum 568.81
    infectional (see also Peritonitis) 567.2
    traumatic — see Injury, internal, peritoneum
Hemophilia (familial) (hereditary) 286.0
    A 286.0
        carrier (asymptomatic) V83.01
            symptomatic V83.02
    acquired 286.5 ●
    B (Leyden) 286.1
    C 286.2
    calcipriva (see also Fibrinolysis) 286.7
    classical 286.0
    nonfamilial 286.7
    vascular 286.4
Hemophilus influenzae NEC 041.5
    arachnoiditis (basic) (brain) (spinal) 320.0
        late effect — see category 326
    bronchopneumonia 482.2
    cerebral ventriculitis 320.0
        late effect — see category 326
    cerebrospinal inflammation 320.0
        late effect — see category 326
    infection NEC 041.5
    leptomeningitis 320.0
        late effect — see category 326
    meningitis (cerebral) (cerebrospinal) (spinal) 320.0
        late effect — see category 326
    meningomyelitis 320.0
        late effect — see category 326
    pachymeningitis (adhesive) (fibrous) (hemorrhagic) (hypertrophic) (spinal) 320.0
        late effect — see category 326
    pneumonia (broncho-) 482.2
Hemophthalmos 360.43
Hemopneumothorax (see also Hemothorax) 511.8
    traumatic 860.4
        with open wound into thorax 860.5
Hemoptysis 786.3
    due to Paragonimus (westermani) 121.2
    newborn 770.3
    tuberculous (see also Tuberculosis, pulmonary) 011.9
Hemorrhage, hemorrhagic (nontraumatic) 459.0
    abdomen 459.0
    accidental (antepartum) 641.2
        affecting fetus or newborn 762.1
    adenoid 474.8

Index to Diseases

Hemorrhage, hemorrhagic — continued

adrenal (capsule) (gland) (medulla) 255.4
    newborn 772.5
after labor — see Hemorrhage, postpartum
alveolar
    lung, newborn 770.3
    process 525.8
alveolus 525.8
amputation stump (surgical) 998.11
    secondary, delayed 997.69
anemia (chronic) 280.0
    acute 285.1
antepartum — see Hemorrhage, pregnancy
anus (sphincter) 569.3
apoplexy (stroke) 432.9
arachnoid — see Hemorrhage, subarachnoid
artery NEC 459.0
    brain (see also Hemorrhage, brain) 431
    middle meningeal — see Hemorrhage, subarachnoid
basilar (ganglion) (see also Hemorrhage, brain) 431
bladder 596.8
blood dyscrasia 289.9
bowel 578.9
    newborn 772.4
brain (miliary) (nontraumatic) 431
    with
        birth injury 767.0
        arachnoid — see Hemorrhage, subarachnoid
        due to
            birth injury 767.0
            rupture of aneurysm (congenital) (see also Aneurysm, subarachnoid) 430
            mycotic 431
            syphilis 094.89
    epidural or extradural — see Hemorrhage, extradural
    fetus or newborn (anoxic) (hypoxic) (due to birth trauma) (nontraumatic) 767.0
        intraventricular 772.10
            grade I 772.11
            grade II 772.12
            grade III 772.13
            grade IV 772.14
    iatrogenic 997.02
    postoperative 997.02
    puerperal, postpartum, childbirth 674.0
    stem 431
    subarachnoid, arachnoid, or meningeal — see Hemorrhage, subarachnoid
    subdural — see Hemorrhage, subdural
    traumatic NEC 853.0

> Note — Use the following fifth-digit subclassification with categories 851-854:
>
> 0   unspecified state of consciousness
> 1   with no loss of consciousness
> 2   with brief [less than one hour] loss of consciousness
> 3   with moderate [1-24 hours] loss of consciousness
> 4   with prolonged [more than 24 hours] loss of consciousness and return to pre-existing conscious level
> 5   with prolonged [more than 24 hours] loss of consciousness, without return to pre-existing conscious level
>
> Use fifth-digit 5 to designate when a patient is unconscious and dies before regaining consciousness, regardless of the duration of the loss of consciousness
>
> 6   with loss of consciousness of unspecified duration
> 9   with concussion, unspecified

        with
            cerebral
                contusion — see Contusion, brain
                laceration — see Laceration, brain
            open intracranial wound 853.1
            skull fracture — see Fracture, skull, by site

Hemorrhage, hemorrhagic — continued

brain — continued
    traumatic NEC — continued
        extradural or epidural 852.4
            with open intracranial wound 852.5
        subarachnoid 852.0
            with open intracranial wound 852.1
        subdural 852.2
            with open intracranial wound 852.3
breast 611.79
bronchial tube — see Hemorrhage, lung
bronchopulmonary — see Hemorrhage, lung
bronchus (cause unknown) (see also Hemorrhage, lung) 786.3
bulbar (see also Hemorrhage, brain) 431
bursa 727.89
capillary 448.9
    primary 287.8
capsular — see Hemorrhage, brain
cardiovascular 429.89
cecum 578.9
cephalic (see also Hemorrhage, brain) 431
cerebellar (see also Hemorrhage, brain) 431
cerebellum (see also Hemorrhage, brain) 431
cerebral (see also Hemorrhage, brain) 431
    fetus or newborn (anoxic) (traumatic) 767.0
cerebromeningeal (see also Hemorrhage, brain) 431
cerebrospinal (see also Hemorrhage, brain) 431
cerebrum (see also Hemorrhage, brain) 431
cervix (stump) (uteri) 622.8
cesarean section wound 674.3
chamber, anterior (eye) 364.41
childbirth — see Hemorrhage, complicating, delivery
choroid 363.61
    expulsive 363.62
ciliary body 364.41
cochlea 386.8
colon — see Hemorrhage, intestine
complicating
    delivery 641.9
        affecting fetus or newborn 762.1
        associated with
            afibrinogenemia 641.3
                affecting fetus or newborn 763.89
            coagulation defect 641.3
                affecting fetus or newborn 763.89
            hyperfibrinolysis 641.3
                affecting fetus or newborn 763.89
            hypofibrinogenemia 641.3
                affecting fetus or newborn 763.89
        due to
            low-lying placenta 641.1
                affecting fetus or newborn 762.0
            placenta previa 641.1
                affecting fetus or newborn 762.0
            premature separation of placenta 641.2
                affecting fetus or newborn 762.1
            retained
                placenta 666.0
                secundines 666.2
            trauma 641.8
                affecting fetus or newborn 763.89
            uterine leiomyoma 641.8
                affecting fetus or newborn 763.89
    surgical procedure 998.11
concealed NEC 459.0
congenital 772.9
conjunctiva 372.72
    newborn 772.8
cord, newborn 772.0
    slipped ligature 772.3
    stump 772.3
corpus luteum (ruptured) 620.1
cortical (see also Hemorrhage, brain) 431
cranial 432.9
cutaneous 782.7
    newborn 772.6
cyst, pancreas 577.2
cystitis — see Cystitis

Hemorrhage, hemorrhagic — continued

delayed
    with
        abortion — see Abortion, by type, with hemorrhage, delayed or excessive
        ectopic pregnancy (see also categories 633.0-633.9) 639.1
        molar pregnancy (see also categories 630-632) 639.1
    following
        abortion 639.1
        ectopic or molar pregnancy 639.1
    postpartum 666.2
diathesis (familial) 287.9
    newborn 776.0
disease 287.9
    newborn 776.0
    specified type NEC 287.8
disorder 287.9
    due to circulating anticoagulants 286.5
    specified type NEC 287.8
due to
    any device, implant or graft (presence of) classifiable to 996.0-996.5 — see Complications, due to (presence of) any device, implant, or graft classified to 996.0-996.5 NEC
    circulating anticoagulant 286.5
duodenum, duodenal 537.89
    ulcer — see Ulcer, duodenum, with hemorrhage
dura mater — see Hemorrhage, subdural
endotracheal — see Hemorrhage, lung
epidural — see Hemorrhage, extradural
episiotomy 674.3
esophagus 530.82
    varix (see also Varix, esophagus, bleeding) 456.0
excessive
    with
        abortion — see Abortion, by type, with hemorrhage, delayed or excessive
        ectopic pregnancy (see also categories 633.0-633.9) 639.1
        molar pregnancy (see also categories 630-632) 639.1
    following
        abortion 639.1
        ectopic or molar pregnancy 639.1
external 459.0
extradural (traumatic) — see also Hemorrhage, brain, traumatic, extradural
    birth injury 767.0
    fetus or newborn (anoxic) (traumatic) 767.0
    nontraumatic 432.0
eye 360.43
    chamber (anterior) (aqueous) 364.41
    fundus 362.81
eyelid 374.81
fallopian tube 620.8
fetomaternal 772.0
    affecting management of pregnancy or puerperium 656.0
fetus, fetal 772.0
    from
        cut end of co-twin's cord 772.0
        placenta 772.0
        ruptured cord 772.0
        vasa previa 772.0
    into
        co-twin 772.0
        mother's circulation 772.0
            affecting management of pregnancy or puerperium 656.0
fever (see also Fever, hemorrhagic) 065.9
    with renal syndrome 078.6
    arthropod-borne NEC 065.9
    Bangkok 065.4
    Crimean 065.0
    dengue virus 065.4
    epidemic 078.6
    Junin virus 078.7
    Korean 078.6
    Machupo virus 078.7
    mite-borne 065.8
    mosquito-borne 065.4
    Philippine 065.4

Hemorrhage, hemorrhagic — *continued*
- fever (*see also* Fever, hemorrhagic) — *continued*
  - Russian (Yaroslav) 078.6
  - Singapore 065.4
  - southeast Asia 065.4
  - Thailand 065.4
  - tick-borne NEC 065.3
- fibrinogenolysis (*see also* Fibrinolysis) 286.6
- fibrinolytic (acquired) (*see also* Fibrinolysis) 286.6
- fontanel 767.1
- from tracheostomy stoma 519.09
- fundus, eye 362.81
- funis
  - affecting fetus or newborn 772.0
  - complicating delivery 663.8 ✓5ᵗʰ
- gastric (*see also* Hemorrhage, stomach) 578.9
- gastroenteric 578.9
  - newborn 772.4
- gastrointestinal (tract) 578.9
  - newborn 772.4
- genitourinary (tract) NEC 599.89
- gingiva 523.8
- globe 360.43
- gravidarum — *see* Hemorrhage, pregnancy
- gum 523.8
- heart 429.89
- hypopharyngeal (throat) 784.8
- intermenstrual 626.6
  - irregular 626.6
  - regular 626.5
- internal (organs) 459.0
  - capsule (*see also* Hemorrhage, brain) 431
  - ear 386.8
  - newborn 772.8
- intestine 578.9
  - congenital 772.4
  - newborn 772.4
- into
  - bladder wall 596.7
  - bursa 727.89
  - corpus luysii (*see also* Hemorrhage, brain) 431
- intra-abdominal 459.0
  - during or following surgery 998.11
- intra-alveolar, newborn (lung) 770.3
- intracerebral (*see also* Hemorrhage, brain) 431
- intracranial NEC 432.9
  - puerperal, postpartum, childbirth 674.0 ✓5ᵗʰ
  - traumatic — *see* Hemorrhage, brain, traumatic
- intramedullary NEC 336.1
- intraocular 360.43
- intraoperative 998.11
- intrapartum — *see* Hemorrhage, complicating, delivery
- intrapelvic
  - female 629.8
  - male 459.0
- intraperitoneal 459.0
- intrapontine (*see also* Hemorrhage, brain) 431
- intrauterine 621.4
  - complicating delivery — *see* Hemorrhage, complicating, delivery
  - in pregnancy or childbirth — *see* Hemorrhage, pregnancy
  - postpartum (*see also* Hemorrhage, postpartum) 666.1 ✓5ᵗʰ
- intraventricular (*see also* Hemorrhage, brain) 431
  - fetus or newborn (anoxic) (traumatic) 772.10
    - grade I 772.11
    - grade II 772.12
    - grade III 772.13
    - grade IV 772.14
- intravesical 596.7
- iris (postinfectional) (postinflammatory) (toxic) 364.41
- joint (nontraumatic) 719.10
  - ankle 719.17
  - elbow 719.12
  - foot 719.17
  - forearm 719.13
  - hand 719.14
  - hip 719.15
  - knee 719.16
  - lower leg 719.16
  - multiple sites 719.19

Hemorrhage, hemorrhagic — *continued*
- joint — *continued*
  - pelvic region 719.15
  - shoulder (region) 719.11
  - specified site NEC 719.18
  - thigh 719.15
  - upper arm 719.12
  - wrist 719.13
- kidney 593.81
- knee (joint) 719.16
- labyrinth 386.8
- leg NEC 459.0
- lenticular striate artery (*see also* Hemorrhage, brain) 431
- ligature, vessel 998.11
- liver 573.8
- lower extremity NEC 459.0
- lung 786.3
  - newborn 770.3
  - tuberculous (*see also* Tuberculosis, pulmonary) 011.9 ✓5ᵗʰ
- malaria 084.8
- marginal sinus 641.2 ✓5ᵗʰ
- massive subaponeurotic, birth injury 767.1
- maternal, affecting fetus or newborn 762.1
- mediastinum 786.3
- medulla (*see also* Hemorrhage, brain) 431
- membrane (brain) (*see also* Hemorrhage, subarachnoid) 430
  - spinal cord — *see* Hemorrhage, spinal cord
- meninges, meningeal (brain) (middle) (*see also* Hemorrhage, subarachnoid) 430
  - spinal cord — *see* Hemorrhage, spinal cord
- mesentery 568.81
- metritis 626.8
- midbrain (*see also* Hemorrhage, brain) 431
- mole 631
- mouth 528.9
- mucous membrane NEC 459.0
  - newborn 728.8 ✓5ᵗʰ
- muscle 728.89
- nail (subungual) 703.8
- nasal turbinate 784.7
  - newborn 772.8
- nasopharynx 478.29
- navel, newborn 772.3
- newborn 772.9
  - adrenal 772.5
  - alveolar (lung) 770.3
  - brain (anoxic) (hypoxic) (due to birth trauma) 767.0
  - cerebral (anoxic) (hypoxic) (due to birth trauma) 767.0
  - conjunctiva 772.8
  - cutaneous 772.6
  - diathesis 776.0
    - due to vitamin K deficiency 776.0
  - gastrointestinal 772.4
  - internal (organs) 772.8
  - intestines 772.4
  - intra-alveolar (lung) 770.3
  - intracranial (from any perinatal cause) 767.0
  - intraventricular (from any perinatal cause) 772.10
    - grade I 772.11
    - grade II 772.12
    - grade III 772.13
    - grade IV 772.14
  - lung 770.3
  - pulmonary (massive) 770.3
  - spinal cord, traumatic 767.4
  - stomach 772.4
  - subaponeurotic (massive) 767.1
  - subarachnoid (from any perinatal cause) 772.2
  - subconjunctival 772.8
  - umbilicus 772.0
    - slipped ligature 772.3
    - vasa previa 772.0
- nipple 611.79
- nose 784.7
  - newborn 772.8
- obstetrical surgical wound 674.3 ✓5ᵗʰ
- omentum 568.89
  - newborn 772.4
- optic nerve (sheath) 377.42
- orbit 376.32
- ovary 620.1

Hemorrhage, hemorrhagic — *continued*
- oviduct 620.8
- pancreas 577.8
- parathyroid (gland) (spontaneous) 252.8
- parturition — *see* Hemorrhage, complicating, delivery
- penis 607.82
- pericardium, paricarditis 423.0
- perineal wound (obstetrical) 674.3 ✓5ᵗʰ
- peritoneum, peritoneal 459.0
- peritonsillar tissue 474.8
  - after operation on tonsils 998.11
  - due to infection 475
- petechial 782.7
- pituitary (gland) 253.8
- placenta NEC 641.9 ✓5ᵗʰ
  - affecting fetus or newborn 762.1
  - from surgical or instrumental damage 641.8 ✓5ᵗʰ
    - affecting fetus or newborn 762.1
  - previa 641.8 ✓5ᵗʰ
    - affecting fetus or newborn 762.0
- pleura — *see* Hemorrhage, lung
- polioencephalitis, superior 265.1
- polymyositis — *see* Polymyositis
- pons (*see also* Hemorrhage, brain) 431
- pontine (*see also* Hemorrhage, brain) 431
- popliteal 459.0
- postcoital 626.7
- postextraction (dental) 998.11
- postmenopausal 627.1
- postnasal 784.7
- postoperative 998.11
- postpartum (atonic) (following delivery of placenta) 666. ✓5ᵗʰ
  - delayed or secondary (after 24 hours) 666.2 ✓5ᵗʰ
  - retained placenta 666.0 ✓5ᵗʰ
  - third stage 666.0 ✓5ᵗʰ
- pregnancy (concealed) 641.9 ✓5ᵗʰ
  - accidental 641.2 ✓5ᵗʰ
    - affecting fetus or newborn 762.1
  - affecting fetus or newborn 762.1
  - before 22 completed weeks gestation 640.9 ✓5ᵗʰ
    - affecting fetus or newborn 762.1
  - due to
    - abruptio placenta 641.2 ✓5ᵗʰ
      - affecting fetus or newborn 762.1
    - afibrinogenemia or other coagulation defect (conditions classifiable to 286.0-286.9) 641.3 ✓5ᵗʰ
      - affecting fetus or newborn 762.1
    - coagulation defect 641.3 ✓5ᵗʰ
      - affecting fetus or newborn 762.1
    - hyperfibrinolysis 641.3 ✓5ᵗʰ
      - affecting fetus or newborn 762.1
    - hypofibrinogenemia 641.3 ✓5ᵗʰ
      - affecting fetus or newborn 762.1
    - leiomyoma, uterus 641.8 ✓5ᵗʰ
      - affecting fetus or newborn 762.1
    - low-lying placenta 641.1 ✓5ᵗʰ
      - affecting fetus or newborn 762.1
    - marginal sinus (rupture) 641.2 ✓5ᵗʰ
      - affecting fetus or newborn 762.1
    - placenta previa 641.1 ✓5ᵗʰ
      - affecting fetus or newborn 762.0
    - premature separation of placenta (normally implanted) 641.2 ✓5ᵗʰ
      - affecting fetus or newborn 762.1
    - threatend abortion 640.0 ✓5ᵗʰ
      - affecting fetus or newborn 762.1
    - trauma 641.8 ✓5ᵗʰ
      - affecting fetus or newborn 762.1
  - early (before 22 completed weeks gestation) 640.9 ✓5ᵗʰ
    - affecting fetus or newborn 762.1
  - previous, affecting management of pregnancy or childbirth V23.49 ▲
  - unavoidable — *see* Hemorrhage, pregnancy, due to placenta previa
- prepartum (mother) — *see* Hemorrhage, pregnancy
- preretinal, cause unspecified 362.81
- prostate 602.1
- puerperal (*see also* Hemorrhage, postpartum) 666.1 ✓5ᵗʰ

Hemorrhage, hemorrhagic — *continued*
  pulmonary — *see also* Hemorrhage, lung
    newborn (massive) 770.3
    renal syndrome 446.21
  purpura (primary) (*see also* Purpura, thrombocytopenic) 287.3
  rectum (sphincter) 569.3
  recurring, following initial hemorrhage at time of injury 958.2
  renal 593.81
    pulmonary syndrome 446.21
  respiratory tract (*see also* Hemorrhage, lung) 786.3
  retina, retinal (deep) (superficial) (vessels) 362.81
    diabetic 250.5 ✓5ᵗʰ [362.01]
    due to birth injury 772.8
  retrobulbar 376.89
  retroperitoneal 459.0
  retroplacental (*see also* Placenta, separation) 641.2 ✓5ᵗʰ
  scalp 459.0
    due to injury at birth 767.1
  scrotum 608.83
  secondary (nontraumatic) 459.0
    following initial hemorrhage at time of injury 958.2
  seminal vesicle 608.83
  skin 782.7
    newborn 772.6
  spermatic cord 608.83
  spinal (cord) 336.1
    aneurysm (ruptured) 336.1
      syphilitic 094.89
    due to birth injury 767.4
    fetus or newborn 767.4
  spleen 289.59
  spontaneous NEC 459.0
    petechial 782.7
  stomach 578.9
    newborn 772.4
    ulcer — *see* Ulcer, stomach, with hemorrhage
  subaponeurotic, newborn 767.1
    massive (birth injury) 767.1
  subarachnoid (nontraumatic) 430
    fetus or newborn (anoxic) (traumatic) 772.2
    puerperal, postpartum, childbirth 674.0 ✓5ᵗʰ
    traumatic — *see* Hemorrhage, brain, traumatic, subarachnoid
  subconjunctival 372.72
    due to birth injury 772.8
    newborn 772.8
  subcortical (*see also* Hemorrhage, brain) 431
  subcutaneous 782.7
  subdiaphragmatic 459.0
  subdural (nontraumatic) 432.1
    due to birth injury 767.0
    fetus or newborn (anoxic) (hypoxic) (due to birth trauma) 767.0
    puerperal, postpartum, childbirth 674.0 ✓5ᵗʰ
    spinal 336.1
    traumatic — *see* Hemorrhage, brain, traumatic, subdural
  subhyaloid 362.81
  subperiosteal 733.99
  subretinal 362.81
  subtentorial (*see also* Hemorrhage, subdural) 432.1
  subungual 703.8
    due to blood dyscrasia 287.8
  suprarenal (capsule) (gland) 255.4
    fetus or newborn 772.5
  tentorium (traumatic) — *see also* Hemorrhage, brain, traumatic
    fetus or newborn 767.0
    nontraumatic — *see* Hemorrhage, subdural
  testis 608.83
  thigh 459.0
  third stage 666.0 ✓5ᵗʰ
  thorax — *see* Hemorrhage, lung
  throat 784.8
  thrombocythemia 238.7
  thymus (gland) 254.8
  thyroid (gland) 246.3
    cyst 246.3
  tongue 529.8

Hemorrhage, hemorrhagic — *continued*
  tonsil 474.8
    postoperative 998.11
  tooth socket (postextraction) 998.11
  trachea — *see* Hemorrhage, lung
  traumatic — *see also* nature of injury
    brain — *see* Hemorrhage, brain, traumatic
    recurring or secondary (following initial hemorrhage at time of injury) 958.2
  tuberculous NEC (*see also* Tuberculosis, pulmonary) 011.9 ✓5ᵗʰ
  tunica vaginalis 608.83
  ulcer — *see* Ulcer, by site, with hemorrhage
  umbilicus, umbilical cord 772.0
    after birth, newborn 772.3
    complicating delivery 663.8 ✓5ᵗʰ
      affecting fetus or newborn 772.0
    slipped ligature 772.3
    stump 772.3
  unavoidable (due to placenta previa) 641.1 ✓5ᵗʰ
    affecting fetus or newborn 762.0
  upper extremity 459.0
  urethra (idiopathic) 599.84
  uterus, uterine (abnormal) 626.9
    climacteric 627.0
    complicating delivery — *see* Hemorrhage, complicating delivery
    due to
      intrauterine contraceptive device 996.76
        perforating uterus 996.32
    functional or dysfunctional 626.8
    in pregnancy — *see* Hemorrhage, pregnancy
    intermenstrual 626.6
      irregular 626.6
      regular 626.5
    postmenopausal 627.1
    postpartum (*see also* Hemorrhage, postpartum) 666.1 ✓5ᵗʰ
    prepubertal 626.8
    pubertal 626.3
    puerperal (immediate) 666.1 ✓5ᵗʰ
  vagina 623.8
  vasa previa 663.5 ✓5ᵗʰ
    affecting fetus or newborn 772.0
  vas deferens 608.83
  ventricular (*see also* Hemorrhage, brain) 431
  vesical 596.8
  viscera 459.0
    newborn 772.8
  vitreous (humor) (intraocular) 379.23
  vocal cord 478.5
  vulva 624.8

Hemorrhoids (anus) (rectum) (without complication) 455.6
  bleeding, prolapsed, strangulated, or ulcerated NEC 455.8
    external 455.5
    internal 455.2
  complicated NEC 455.8
  complicating pregnancy and puerperium 671.8 ✓5ᵗʰ
  external 455.3
    with complication NEC 455.5
    bleeding, prolapsed, strangulated, or ulcerated 455.5
    thrombosed 455.4
  internal 455.0
    with complication NEC 455.2
    bleeding, prolapsed, strangulated, or ulcerated 455.2
    thrombosed 455.1
  residual skin tag 455.9
  sentinel pile 455.9
  thrombosed NEC 455.7
    external 455.4
    internal 455.1

Hemosalpinx 620.8
Hemosiderosis 275.0
  dietary 275.0
  pulmonary (idiopathic) 275.0 [516.1]
  transfusion NEC 999.8
    bone marrow 996.85
Hemospermia 608.82
Hemothorax 511.8
  bacterial, nontuberculous 511.1
  newborn 772.8

Hemothorax — *continued*
  nontuberculous 511.8
    bacterial 511.1
  pneumococcal 511.1
  postoperative 998.11
  staphylococcal 511.1
  streptococcal 511.1
  traumatic 860.2
    with
      open wound into thorax 860.3
      pneumothorax 860.4
        with open wound into thorax 860.5
  tuberculous (*see also* Tuberculosis, pleura) 012.0 ✓5ᵗʰ
Hemotympanum 385.89
Hench-Rosenberg syndrome (palindromic arthritis) (*see also* Rheumatism, palindromic) 719.3 ✓5ᵗʰ
Henle's warts 371.41
Henoch (-Schönlein)
  disease or syndrome (allergic purpura) 287.0
  purpura (allergic) 287.0
Henpue, henpuye 102.6
Heparitinuria 277.5
Hepar lobatum 095.3
Hepatalgia 573.8
Hepatic — *see also* conditon
  flexure syndrome 569.89
Hepatitis 573.3
  acute (*see also* Necrosis, liver) 570
    alcoholic 571.1
    infective 070.1
      with hepatic coma 070.0
  alcoholic 571.1
  amebic — *see* Abscess, liver, amebic
  anicteric (acute) — *see* Hepatitis, viral
  antigen-associated (HAA) — *see* Hepatitis, viral, type B
  Australian antigen (positive) — *see* Hepatitis, viral, type B
  catarrhal (acute) 070.1
    with hepatic coma 070.0
    chronic 571.40
    newborn 070.1
      with hepatic coma 070.0
  chemical 573.3
  cholangiolitic 573.8
  cholestatic 573.8
  chronic 571.40
    active 571.49
      viral — *see* Hepatitis, viral
    aggressive 571.49
    persistent 571.41
    viral — *see* Hepatitis, viral
  cytomegalic inclusion virus 078.5 [573.1]
  diffuse 573.3
  "dirty needle" — *see* Hepatitis, viral
    with hepatic coma 070.2 ✓5ᵗʰ
  drug-induced 573.3
  due to
    Coxsackie 074.8 [573.1]
    cytomegalic inclusion virus 078.5 [573.1]
    infectious mononucleosis 075 [573.1]
    malaria 084.9 [573.2]
    mumps 072.71
    secondary syphilis 091.62
    toxoplasmosis (acquired) 130.5
      congenital (active) 771.2
  epidemic — *see* Hepatitis, viral, type A
  fetus or newborn 774.4
  fibrous (chronic) 571.49
    acute 570
  from injection, inoculation, or transfusion (blood) (other substance) (plasma) serum) (onset within 8 months after administration) — *see* Hepatitis, viral
  fulminant (viral) (*see also* Hepatitis, viral) 070.9
    with hepatic coma 070.6
    type A 070.1
      with hepatic coma 070.0
    type B — *see* Hepatitis, viral, type B
  giant cell (neonatal) 774.4
  hemorrhagic 573.8
  homologous serum — *see* Hepatitis, viral
  hypertrophic (chronic) 571.49
    acute 570

Hepatitis

Hepatitis — *continued*
- infectious, infective (acute) (chronic) (subacute) 070.1
  - with hepatic coma 070.0
- inoculation — *see* Hepatitis, viral
- interstitial (chronic) 571.49
  - acute 570
- lupoid 571.49
- malarial 084.9 *[573.2]*
- malignant (*see also* Necrosis, liver) 570
- neonatal (toxic) 774.4
- newborn 774.4
- parenchymatous (acute) (*see also* Necrosis, liver) 570
- peliosis 573.3
- persistent, chronic 571.41
- plasma cell 571.49
- postimmunization — *see* Hepatitis, viral
- postnecrotic 571.49
- posttransfusion — *see* Hepatitis, viral
- recurrent 571.49
- septic 573.3
- serum — *see* Hepatitis, viral
  - carrier (suspected of) V02.61
- subacute (*see also* Necrosis, liver) 570
- suppurative (diffuse) 572.0
- syphilitic (late) 095.3
  - congenital (early) 090.0 *[573.2]*
    - late 090.5 *[573.2]*
  - secondary 091.62
- toxic (noninfectious) 573.3
  - fetus or newborn 774.4
- tuberculous (*see also* Tuberculosis) 017.9 ✓5ᵗʰ
- viral (acute) (anicteric) (cholangiolitic) (cholestatic) (chronic) (subacute) 070.9
  - with hepatic coma 070.6
  - AU-SH type virus — *see* Hepatitis, viral, type B
  - Australian antigen — *see* Hepatitis, viral, type B
  - B-antigen — *see* Hepatitis, viral, type B
  - Coxsackie 074.8 *[573.1]*
  - cytomegalic inclusion 078.5 *[573.1]*
  - IH (virus) — *see* Hepatitis, viral, type A
  - infectious hepatitis, viral, type A
  - serum hepatitis virus — *see* Hepatitis, viral, type B
  - SH — *see* Hepatitis, viral, type B
  - specified type NEC 070.59
    - with hepatic coma 070.49
  - type A 070.1
    - with hepatic coma 070.0
  - type B (acute) 070.30
    - with
      - hepatic coma 070.20
        - with hepatitis delta 070.21
      - hepatitis delta 070.31
        - with hepatic coma 070.21
    - carrier status V02.61
    - chronic 070.32
      - with
        - hepatic coma 070.22
          - with hepatitis delta 070.23
        - hepatitis delta 070.33
          - with hepatic coma 070.23
  - type C (acute) 070.51
    - with hepatic coma 070.41
    - carrier status V02.62
    - chronic 070.54
      - with hepatic coma 070.44
  - type delta (with hepatitis B carrier state) 070.52
    - with
      - active hepatitis B disease — *see* Hepatitis, viral, type B
      - hepatic coma 070.42
  - type E 070.53
    - with hepatic coma 070.43
  - vaccination and inoculation (prophylactic) V05.3
- Waldenstrom's (lupoid hepatitis) 571.49

Hepatization, lung (acute) — *see also* Pneumonia, lobar
- chronic (*see also* Fibrosis, lung) 515

Hepatoblastoma (M8970/3) 155.0
Hepatocarcinoma (M8170/3) 155.0
Hepatocholangiocarcinoma (M8180/3) 155.0
Hepatocholangioma, benign (M8180/0) 211.5
Hepatocholangitis 573.8
Hepatocystitis (*see also* Cholecystitis) 575.10
Hepatodystrophy 570
Hepatolenticular degeneration 275.1
Hepatolithiasis — *see* Choledocholithiasis
Hepatoma (malignant) (M8170/3) 155.0
- benign (M8170/0) 211.5
- congenital (M8970/3) 155.0
- embryonal (M8970/3) 155.0

Hepatomegalia glycogenica diffusa 271.0
Hepatomegaly (*see also* Hypertrophy, liver) 789.1
- congenital 751.69
  - syphilitic 090.0
- due to Clonorchis sinensis 121.1
- Gaucher's 272.7
- syphilitic (congenital) 090.0

Hepatoptosis 573.8
Hepatorrhexis 573.8
Hepatosis, toxic 573.8
Hepatosplenomegaly 571.8
- due to S. japonicum 120.2
- hyperlipemic (Burger-Grutz type) 272.3

Herald patch 696.3
Hereditary — *see* condition
Heredodegeneration 330.9
- macular 362.70

Heredopathia atactica polyneuritiformis 356.3
Heredosyphilis (*see also* Syphilis, congenital) 090.9 ✓5ᵗʰ

Hermaphroditism (true) 752.7
- with specified chromosomal anomaly — *see* Anomaly, chromosomes, sex

Hernia, hernial (acquired) (recurrent) 553.9
- with
  - gangrene (obstructed) NEC 551.9
  - obstruction NEC 552.9
    - and gangrene 551.9
- abdomen (wall) — *see* Hernia, ventral
- abdominal, specified site NEC 553.8
  - with
    - gangrene (obstructed) 551.8
    - obstruction 552.8
      - and gangrene 551.8
- appendix 553.8
  - with
    - gangrene (obstructed) 551.8
    - obstruction 552.8
      - and gangrene 551.8
- bilateral (inguinal) — *see* Hernia, inguinal
- bladder (sphincter)
  - congenital (female) (male) 756.71
  - female 618.0
  - male 596.8
- brain 348.4
  - congenital 742.0
- broad ligament 553.8
- cartilage, vertebral — *see* Displacement, intervertebral disc
- cerebral 348.4
  - congenital 742.0
  - endaural 742.0
- ciliary body 364.8
  - traumatic 871.1
- colic 553.9
  - with
    - gangrene (obstructed) 551.9
    - obstruction 552.9
      - and gangrene 551.9
- colon 553.9
  - with
    - gangrene (obstructed) 551.9
    - obstruction 552.9
      - and gangrene 551.9
- colostomy (stoma) 569.69
- Cooper's (retroperitoneal) 553.8
  - with
    - gangrene (obstructed) 551.8
    - obstruction 552.8
      - and gangrene 551.8
- crural — *see* Hernia, femoral

Hernia, hernial — *continued*
- diaphragm, diaphragmatic 553.3
  - with
    - gangrene (obstructed) 551.3
    - obstruction 552.3
      - and gangrene 551.3
  - congenital 756.6
  - due to gross defect of diaphragm 756.6
  - traumatic 862.0
    - with open wound into cavity 862.1
- direct (inguinal) — *see* Hernia, inguinal
- disc, intervetebral — *see* Displacement, intervertebral disc
- diverticulum, intestine 553.9
  - with
    - gangrene (obstructed) 551.9
    - obstruction 552.9
      - and gangrene 551.9
- double (inguinal) — *see* Hernia, inguinal
- duodenojejunal 553.8
  - with
    - gangrene (obstructed) 551.8
    - obstruction 552.8
      - and gangrene 551.8
- en glissade — *see* Hernia, inguinal
- enterostomy (stoma) 569.69
- epigastric 553.29
  - with
    - gangrene (obstruction) 551.29
    - obstruction 552.29
      - and gangrene 551.29
  - recurrent 553.21
    - with
      - gangrene (obstructed) 551.21
      - obstruction 552.21
        - and gangrene 551.21
- esophageal hiatus (sliding) 553.3
  - with
    - gangrene (obstructed) 551.3
    - obstruction 552.3
      - and gangrene 551.3
  - congenital 750.6
- external (inguinal) — *see* Hernia, inguinal
- fallopian tube 620.4
- fascia 728.89
- fat 729.30
  - eyelid 374.34
  - orbital 374.34
  - pad 729.30
    - eye, eyelid 374.34
    - knee 729.31
    - orbit 374.34
    - popliteal (space) 729.31
    - specified site NEC 729.39
- femoral (unilateral) 553.00
  - with
    - gangrene (obstructed) 551.00
    - obstruction 552.00
      - with gangrene 551.0 ✓5ᵗʰ
  - bilateral 553.02
    - gangrenous (obstructed) 551.02
    - obstructed 552.02
      - with gangrene 551.02
    - recurrent 553.03
      - gangrenous (obstructed) 551.03
      - obstructed 552.03
        - with gangrene 551.03
  - recurrent (unilateral) 553.01
    - bilateral 553.03
      - gangrenous (obstructed) 551.03
      - obstructed 552.03
        - with gangrene 551.03
    - gangrenous (obstructed) 551.01
    - obstructed 552.01
      - with gangrene
- foramen
  - Bochdalek 553.3
    - with
      - gangrene (obstructed) 551.3
      - obstruction 552.3
        - and gangrene 551.3
    - congenital 756.6
  - magnum 348.4
  - Morgagni, Morgagnian 553.3
    - with
      - gangrene 551.3

Index to Diseases

Hernia, hernial — *continued*
  foramen — *continued*
    Morgagni, Morgagnian — *continued*
      with — *continued*
        obstruction 552.3
          and gangrene 551.3
      congenital 756.6
  funicular (umbilical) 553.1
    with
      gangrene (obstructed) 551.1
      obstruction 552.1
        and gangrene 551.1
    spermatic cord — *see* Hernia, inguinal
  gangrenous — *see* Hernia, by site, with gangrene
  gastrointestinal tract 553.9
    with
      gangrene (obstructed) 551.9
      obstruction 552.9
        and gangrene 551.9
  gluteal — *see* Hernia, femoral
  Gruber's (internal mesogastric) 553.8
    with
      gangrene (obstructed) 551.8
      obstruction 552.8
        and gangrene 551.8
  Hesselbach's 553.8
    with
      gangrene (obstructed) 551.8
      obstruction 552.8
        and gangrene 551.8
  hiatal (esophageal) (sliding) 553.3
    with
      gangrene (obstructed) 551.3
      obstruction 552.3
        and gangrene 551.3
    congenital 750.6
  incarcerated (*see also* Hernia, by site, with obstruction) 552.9
    gangrenous (*see also* Hernia, by site, with gangrene) 551.9
  incisional 553.21
    with
      gangrene (obstructed) 551.21
      obstruction 552.21
        and gangrene 551.21
    lumbar — *see* Hernia, lumbar
    recurrent 553.21
      with
        gangrene (obstructed) 551.21
        obstruction 552.21
          and gangrene 551.21
  indirect (inguinal) — *see* Hernia, inguinal
  infantile — *see* Hernia, inguinal
  infrapatellar fat pad 729.31
  inguinal (direct) (double) (encysted) (external) (funicular) (indirect) (infantile) (internal) (interstitial) (oblique) (scrotal) (sliding) 550.9

> *Note* — *Use the following fifth-digit subclassification with category 550:*
>
> 0   unilateral or unspecified (not specified as recurrent)
> 1   unilateral or unspecified, recurrent
> 2   bilateral (not specified as recurrent)
> 3   bilateral, recurrent

    with
      gangrene (obstructed) 550.0
      obstruction 550.1
        and gangrene 550.0
    internal 553.8
      with
        gangrene (obstructed) 551.8
        obstruction 552.8
          and gangrene 551.8
    inguinal — *see* Hernia, inguinal
  interstitial 553.9
    with
      gangrene (obstructed) 551.9
      obstruction 552.9
        and gangrene 551.9
    inguinal — *see* Hernia, inguinal
  intervertebral cartilage or disc — *see* Displacement, intervertebral disc
  intestine, intestinal 553.9
    with
      gangrene (obstructed) 551.9
      obstruction 552.9
        and gangrene 551.9
  intra-abdominal 553.9
    with
      gangrene (obstructed) 551.9
      obstruction 552.9
        and gangrene 551.9
  intraparietal 553.9
    with
      gangrene (obstructed) 551.9
      obstruction 552.9
        and gangrene 551.9
  iris 364.8
    traumatic 871.1
  irreducible (*see also* Hernia, by site, with obstruction) 552.9
    gangrenous (with obstruction) (*see also* Hernia, by site, with gangrene) 551.9
  ischiatic 553.8
    with
      gangrene (obstructed) 551.8
      obstruction 552.8
        and gangrene 551.8
  ischiorectal 553.8
    with
      gangrene (obstructed) 551.8
      obstruction 552.8
        and gangrene 551.8
  lens 379.32
    traumatic 871.1
  linea
    alba — *see* Hernia, epigastric
    semilunaris — *see* Hernia, spigelian
  Littre's (diverticular) 553.9
    with
      gangrene (obstructed) 551.9
      obstruction 552.9
        and gangrene 551.9
  lumbar 553.8
    with
      gangrene (obstructed) 551.8
      obstruction 552.8
        and gangrene 551.8
    intervertebral disc 722.10
  lung (subcutaneous) 518.89
    congenital 748.69
  mediastinum 519.3
  mesenteric (internal) 553.8
    with
      gangrene (obstructed) 551.8
      obstruction 552.8
        and gangrene 551.8
  mesocolon 553.8
    with
      gangrene (obstructed) 551.8
      obstruction 552.8
        and gangrene 551.8
  muscle (sheath) 728.89
  nucleus pulposus — *see* Displacement, intervertebral disc
  oblique (inguinal) — *see* Hernia, inguinal
  obstructive (*see also* Hernia, by site, with obstruction) 552.9
    gangrenous (with obstruction) (*see also* Hernia, by site, with gangrene) 551.9
  obturator 553.8
    with
      gangrene (obstructed) 551.8
      obstruction 552.8
        and gangrene 551.8
  omental 553.8
    with
      gangrene (obstructed) 551.8
      obstruction 552.8
        and gangrene 551.8
  orbital fat (pad) 374.34
  ovary 620.4
  oviduct 620.4
  paracolostomy (stoma) 569.69
  paraduodenal 553.8
    with
      gangrene (obstructed) 551.8
      obstruction 552.8
        and gangrene 551.8
  paraesophageal 553.3
    with
      gangrene (obstructed) 551.3
      obstruction 552.3
        and gangrene 551.3
    congenital 750.6
  parahiatal 553.3
    with
      gangrene (obstructed) 551.3
      obstruction 552.3
        and gangrene 551.3
  paraumbilical 553.1
    with
      gangrene (obstructed) 551.1
      obstruction 552.1
        and gangrene 551.1
  parietal 553.9
    with
      gangrene (obstructed) 551.9
      obstruction 552.9
        and gangrene 551.9
  perineal 553.8
    with
      gangrene (obstructed) 551.8
      obstruction 552.8
        and gangrene 551.8
  peritoneal sac, lesser 553.8
    with
      gangrene (obstructed) 551.8
      obstruction 552.8
        and gangrene 551.8
  popliteal fat pad 729.31
  postoperative 553.21
    with
      gangrene (obstructed) 551.21
      obstruction 552.21
        and gangrene 551.21
  pregnant uterus 654.4
  prevesical 596.8
  properitoneal 553.8
    with
      gangrene (obstructed) 551.8
      obstruction 552.8
        and gangrene 551.8
  pudendal 553.8
    with
      gangrene (obstructed) 551.8
      obstruction 552.8
        and gangrene 551.8
  rectovaginal 618.6
  retroperitoneal 553.8
    with
      gangrene (obstructed) 551.8
      obstruction 552.8
        and gangrene 551.8
  Richter's (parietal) 553.9
    with
      gangrene (obstructed) 551.9
      obstruction 552.9
        and gangrene 551.9
  Rieux's, Riex's (retrocecal) 553.8
    with
      gangrene (obstructed) 551.8
      obstruction 552.8
        and gangrene 551.8
  sciatic 553.8
    with
      gangrene (obstructed) 551.8
      obstruction 552.8
        and gangrene 551.8
  scrotum, scrotal — *see* Hernia, inguinal
  sliding (inguinal) — *see also* Hernia, inguinal
    hiatus — *see* Hernia, hiatal
  spigelian 553.29
    with
      gangrene (obstructed) 551.29
      obstruction 552.29
        and gangrene 551.29
  spinal (*see also* Spina bifida) 741.9
    with hydrocephalus 741.0
  strangulated (*see also* Hernia, by site, with obstruction) 552.9
    gangrenous (with obstruction) (*see also* Hernia, by site, with gangrene) 551.9
  supraumbilicus (linea alba) — *see* Hernia, epigastric

Hernia, hernial — *continued*
  tendon 727.9
  testis (nontraumatic) 550.9
    meaning
      scrotal hernia 550.9
      symptomatic late syphilis 095.8
    Treitz's (fossa) 553.8
      with
        gangrene (obstructed) 551.8
        obstruction 552.8
          and gangrene 551.8
    tunica
      albuginea 608.89
      vaginalis 752.8
    umbilicus, umbilical 553.1
      with
        gangrene (obstructed) 551.1
        obstruction 552.1
          and gangrene 551.1
    ureter 593.89
      with obstruction 593.4
    uterus 621.8
      pregnant 654.4 ✓5ᵗʰ
    vaginal (posterior) 618.6
    Velpeau's (femoral) (*see also* Hernia, femoral) 553.00
    ventral 553.20
      with
        gangrene (obstructed) 551.20
        obstruction 552.20
          and gangrene 551.20
      recurrent 553.21
        with
          gangrene (obstructed) 551.21
          obstruction 552.21
            and gangrene 551.21
    vesical
      congenital (female) (male) 756.71
      female 618.0
      male 596.8
    vitreous (into anterior chamber) 379.21
      traumatic 871.1
Herniation — *see also* Hernia
  brain (stem) 348.4
  cerebral 348.4
  gastric mucosa (into duodenal bulb) 537.89
  mediastinum 519.3
  nucleus pulposus — *see* Displacement, intervertebral disc
Herpangina 074.0
Herpes, herpetic 054.9
  auricularis (zoster) 053.71
    simplex 054.73
  blepharitis (zoster) 053.20
    simplex 054.41
  circinate 110.5
  circinatus 110.5
    bullous 694.5
  conjunctiva (simplex) 054.43
    zoster 053.21
  cornea (simplex) 054.43
    disciform (simplex) 054.43
      zoster 053.21
  encephalitis 054.3
  eye (zoster) 053.29
    simplex 054.40
  eyelid (zoster) 053.20
    simplex 054.41
  febrilis 054.9
  fever 054.9
  geniculate ganglionitis 053.11
  genital, genitalis 054.10
    specified site NEC 054.19
  gestationis 646.8 ✓5ᵗʰ
  gingivostomatitis 054.2
  iridocyclitis (simplex) 054.44
    zoster 053.22
  iris (any site) 695.1
  iritis (simplex) 054.44
  keratitis (simplex) 054.43
    dendritic 054.42
    disciform 054.43
    interstitial 054.43
      zoster 053.21
  keratoconjunctivitis (simplex) 054.43
    zoster 053.21

Herpes, herpetic — *continued*
  labialis 054.9
    meningococcal 036.89
  lip 054.9
  meningitis (simplex) 054.72
    zoster 053.0
  ophthalmicus (zoster) 053.20
    simplex 054.40
  otitis externa (zoster) 053.71
    simplex 054.73
  penis 054.13
  perianal 054.10
  pharyngitis 054.79
  progenitalis 054.10
  scrotum 054.19
  septicemia 054.4 ✓5ᵗʰ
  simplex 054.9
    complicated 054.8
      ophthalmic 054.40
        specified NEC 054.49
      specified NEC 054.79
    congenital 771.2
    external ear 054.73
    keratitis 054.43
      dendritic 054.42
    meningitis 054.72
    neuritis 054.79
    specified complication NEC 054.79
      ophthalmic 054.49
    visceral 054.71
  stomatitis 054.2
  tonsurans 110.0
    maculosus (of Hebra) 696.3
  visceral 054.71
  vulva 054.12
  vulvovaginitis 054.11
  whitlow 054.6
  zoster 053.9
    auricularis 053.71
    complicated 053.8
      specified NEC 053.79
    conjunctiva 053.21
    cornea 053.21
    ear 053.71
    eye 053.29
    geniculate 053.11
    keratitis 053.21
      interstitial 053.21
    neuritis 053.10
    ophthalmicus(a) 053.20
    oticus 053.71
    otitis externa 053.71
    specified complication NEC 053.79
    specified site NEC 053.9
  zosteriform, intermediate type 053.9
Herrick's
  anemia (hemoglobin S disease) 282.61
  syndrome (hemoglobin S disease) 282.61
Hers' disease (glycogenosis VI) 271.0
Herter's infantilism (nontropical sprue) 579.0
Herter (-Gee) disease or syndrome (nontropical sprue) 579.0
Herxheimer's disease (diffuse idiopathic cutaneous atrophy) 701.8
Herxheimer's reaction 995.0
Hesselbach's hernia — *see* Hernia, Hesselbach's
Heterochromia (congenital) 743.46
  acquired 364.53
  cataract 366.33
  cyclitis 364.21
  hair 704.3
  iritis 364.21
  retained metallic foreign body 360.62
    magnetic 360.52
  uveitis 364.21
Heterophoria 378.40
  alternating 378.45
  vertical 378.43
Heterophyes, small intestine 121.6
Heterophyiasis 121.6
Heteropsia 368.8
Heterotopia, heterotopic — *see also* Malposition, congenital
  cerebralis 742.4
  pancreas, pancreatic 751.7

Heterotopia, heterotopic — *see also* Malposition, congenital — *continued*
  spinalis 742.59
Heterotropia 378.30
  intermittent 378.20
    vertical 378.31
  vertical (constant) (intermittent) 378.31
Heubner's disease 094.89
Heubner-Herter disease or syndrome (nontropical sprue) 579.0
Hexadactylism 755.0 ✓5ᵗʰ
Heyd's syndrome (hepatorenal) 572.4
HGSIL (high grade squamous intraepithelial dysplasia) 622.1 ●
Hibernoma (M8880/0) — *see* Lipoma
Hiccough 786.8
  epidemic 078.89
  psychogenic 306.1
Hiccup (*see also* Hiccough) 786.8
Hicks (-Braxton) contractures 644.1 ✓5ᵗʰ
Hidden penis 752.65
Hidradenitis (axillaris) (suppurative) 705.83
Hidradenoma (nodular) (M8400/0) — *see also* Neoplasm, skin, benign
  clear cell (M8402/0) — *see* Neoplasm, skin, benign
  papillary (M8405/0) — *see* Neoplasm, skin, benign
Hidrocystoma (M8404/0) — *see* Neoplasm, skin, benign
High
  A_2 anemia 282.4
  altitude effects 993.2
    anoxia 993.2
    on
      ears 993.0
      sinuses 993.1
    polycythemia 289.0
  arch
    foot 755.67
    palate 750.26
  artery (arterial) tension (*see also* Hypertension) 401.9
    without diagnosis of hypertension 796.2
  basal metabolic rate (BMR) 794.7
  blood pressure (*see also* Hypertension) 401.9
    incidental reading (isolated) (nonspecific), no diagnosis of hypertension 796.2
  compliance bladder 596.4
  diaphragm (congenital) 756.6
  frequency deafness (congenital) (regional) 389.8
  head at term 652.5 ✓5ᵗʰ
    affecting fetus or newborn 763.1
  output failure (cardiac) (*see also* Failure, heart) 428.9
  oxygen-affinity hemoglobin 289.0
  palate 750.26
  risk
    behavior — *see* Problem
    family situation V61.9
      specified circumstance NEC V61.8
    individual NEC V62.89
    infant NEC V20.1
    patient taking drugs (prescribed) V67.51
      nonprescribed (*see also* Abuse, drugs, nondependent) 305.9 ✓5ᵗʰ
    pregnancy V23.9
      inadequate prenatal care V23.7
      specified problem NEC V23.8 ✓5ᵗʰ
  temperature (of unknown origin) (*see also* Pyrexia) 780.6
  thoracic rib 756.3
Hildenbrand's disease (typhus) 081.9
Hilger's syndrome 337.0
Hill diarrhea 579.1
Hilliard's lupus (*see also* Tuberculosis) 017.0 ✓5ᵗʰ
Hilum — *see* condition
Hip — *see* condition
Hippel's disease (retinocerebral angiomatosis) 759.6
Hippus 379.49
Hirschfeld's disease (acute diabetes mellitus) (*see also* Diabetes) 250.0 ✓5ᵗʰ

Hirschsprung's disease or megacolon (congenital) 751.3
Hirsuties (see also Hypertrichosis) 704.1
Hirsutism (see also Hypertrichosis) 704.1
Hirudiniasis (external) (internal) 134.2
His-Werner disease (trench fever) 083.1
Hiss-Russell dysentery 004.1
Histamine cephalgia 346.2 ✓5
Histidinemia 270.5
Histidinuria 270.5
Histiocytoma (M8832/0) — see also Neoplasm, skin, benign
  fibrous (M8830/0) — see also Neoplasm, skin, benign
    atypical (M8830/1) — see Neoplasm, connective tissue, uncertain behavior
    malignant (M8830/3) — see Neoplasm, connective tissue, malignant
Histiocytosis (acute) (chronic) (subacute) 277.8
  acute differentiated progressive (M9722/3) 202.5 ✓5
  cholesterol 277.8
  essential 277.8
  lipid, lipoid (essential) 272.7
  lipochrome (familial) 288.1
  malignant (M9720/3) 202.3 ✓5
  X (chronic) 277.8
    acute (progressive) (M9722/3) 202.5 ✓5
Histoplasmosis 115.90
  with
    endocarditis 115.94
    meningitis 115.91
    pericarditis 115.93
    pneumonia 115.95
    retinitis 115.92
    specified manifestation NEC 115.99
  African (due to Histoplasma duboisii) 115.10
    with
      endocarditis 115.14
      meningitis 115.11
      pericarditis 115.13
      pneumonia 115.15
      retinitis 115.12
      specified manifestation NEC 115.19
  American (due to Histoplasma capsulatum) 115.00
    with
      endocarditis 115.04
      meningitis 115.01
      pericarditis 115.03
      pneumonia 115.05
      retinitis 115.02
      specified manifestation NEC 115.09
  Darling's — see Histoplasmosis, American
  large form (see also Histoplasmosis, African) 115.10
  lung 115.05
  small form (see also Histoplasmosis, American) 115.00
History (personal) of
  abuse
    emotional V15.42
    neglect V15.42
    physical V15.41
    sexual V15.41
  affective psychosis V11.1
  alcoholism V11.3
    specified as drinking problem (see also Abuse, drugs, nondependent) 305.0 ✓5
  allergy to
    analgesic agent NEC V14.6
    anesthetic NEC V14.4
    antibiotic agent NEC V14.1
      penicillin V14.0
    anti-infective agent NEC V14.3
    diathesis V15.09
    drug V14.9
      specified type NEC V14.8
    eggs V15.03
    food additives V15.05
    insect bite V15.06
    latex V15.07
    medicinal agents V14.9
      specified type NEC V14.8

History (personal) of — continued
  allergy to — continued
    milk products V15.02
    narcotic agent NEC V14.5
    nuts V15.05
      peanuts V15.01
    penicillin V14.0
    radiographic dye V15.08
    seafood V15.04
    serum V14.7
    specified food NEC V15.05
    specified nonmedicinal agents NEC V15.09
    spider bite V15.06
    sulfa V14.2
    sulfonamides V14.2
    therapeutic agent NEC V15.09
    vaccine V14.7
  anemia V12.3
  arthritis V13.4
  benign neoplasm of brain V12.41
  blood disease V12.3
  calculi, urinary V13.01
  cardiovascular disease V12.50
    myocardial infarction 412
  child abuse V15.41
  cigarette smoking V15.82
  circulatory system disease V12.50
    myocardial infarction 412
  congenital malformation V13.69
  contraception V15.7
  diathesis, allergic V15.09
  digestive system disease V12.70
    peptic ulcer V12.71
    polyps, colonic V12.72
    specified NEC V12.79
  disease (of) V13.9
    blood V12.3
    blood-forming organs V12.3
    cardiovascular system V12.50
    circulatory system V12.50
    digestive system V12.70
      peptic ulcer V12.71
      polyps, colonic V12.72
      specified NEC V12.79
    infectious V12.00
      malaria V12.03
      poliomyelitis V12.02
      specified NEC V12.09
      tuberculosis V12.01
    parasitic V12.00
      specified NEC V12.09
    respiratory system V12.6
    skin V13.3
    specified site NEC V13.8
    subcutaneous tissue V13.3
    trophoblastic V13.1
      affecting management of pregnant V23.1
  disorder (of) V13.9
    endocrine V12.2
    genital system V13.29 ▲
    hematological V12.3
    immunity V12.2
    mental V11.9
      affective type V11.1
      manic-depressive V11.1
      neurosis V11.2
      schizophrenia V11.0
      specified type NEC V11.8
    metabolic V12.2
    musculoskeletal NEC V13.5
    nervous system V12.40
      specified type NEC V12.49
    obstetric V13.29 ▲
      affecting management of current pregnancy V23.49 ▲
      pre-term labor V23.41 ●
      pre-term labor V13.21 ●
    sense organs V12.40
      specified type NEC V12.49
    specified site NEC V13.8
    urinary system V13.00
      calculi V13.01
      specified NEC V13.09
  drug use
    nonprescribed (see also Abuse, drugs, nondependent) 305.9 ✓5

History (personal) of — continued
  drug use — continued
    patent (see also Abuse, drugs, nondependent) 305.9 ✓5
  effect NEC of external cause V15.89
  embolism (pulmonary) V12.51
  emotional abuse V15.42
  endocrine disorder V12.2
  family
    allergy V19.6
    anemia V18.2
    arteriosclerosis V17.4
    arthritis V17.7
    asthma V17.5
    blindness V19.0
    blood disorder NEC V18.3
    cardiovascular disease V17.4
    cerebrovascular disease V17.1
    chronic respiratory condition NEC V17.6
    congenital anomalies V19.5
    consanguinity V19.7
    coronary artery disease V17.3
    cystic fibrosis V18.1
    deafness V19.2
    diabetes mellitus V18.0
    digestive disorders V18.5
    disease or disorder (of)
      allergic V19.6
      blood NEC V18.3
      cardiovascular NEC V17.4
      cerebrovascular V17.1
      coronary artery V17.3
      digestive V18.5
      ear NEC V19.3
      endocrine V18.1
      eye NEC V19.1
      genitourinary NEC V18.7
      hypertensive V17.4
      infectious V18.8
      ischemic heart V17.3
      kidney V18.69
        polycystic V18.61
      mental V17.0
      metabolic V18.1
      musculoskeletal NEC V17.8
      neurological NEC V17.2
      parasitic V18.8
      psychiatric condition V17.0
      skin condition V19.4
    ear disorder NEC V19.3
    endocrine disease V18.1
    epilepsy V17.2
    eye disorder NEC V19.1
    genitourinary disease NEC V18.7
    glomerulonephritis V18.69
    gout V18.1
    hay fever V17.6
    hearing loss V19.2
    hematopoietic neoplasia V16.7
    Hodgkin's disease V16.7
    Huntington's chorea V17.2
    hydrocephalus V19.5
    hypertension V17.4
    hypospadias V13.61
    infectious disease V18.8
    ischemia heart disease V17.3
    kidney disease V18.69
      polycystic V18.61
    leukemia V16.6
    lymphatic malignant neoplasia NEC V16.7
    malignant neoplasm (of) NEC V16.9
      anorectal V16.0
      anus V16.0
      appendix V16.0
      bladder V16.59
      bone V16.8
      brain V16.8
      breast V16.3
        male V16.8
      bronchus V16.1
      cecum V16.0
      cervix V16.49
      colon V16.0
      duodenum V16.0
      esophagus V16.0
      eye V16.8
      gallbladder V16.0

History (personal) of — *continued*
  family — *continued*
    malignant neoplasm (of) NEC — *continued*
      gastrointestinal tract V16.0
      genital organs V16.40
      hemopoietic NEC V16.7
      ileum V16.0
      ilium V16.8
      intestine V16.0
      intrathoracic organs NEC V16.2
      kidney V16.51
      larynx V16.2
      liver V16.0
      lung V16.1
      lymphatic NEC V16.7
      ovary V16.41
      oviduct V16.41
      pancreas V16.0
      penis V16.49
      prostate V16.42
      rectum V16.0
      respiratory organs NEC V16.2
      skin V16.8
      specified site NEC V16.8
      stomach V16.0
      testis V16.43
      trachea V16.1
      ureter V16.59
      urethra V16.59
      urinary organs V16.59
      uterus V16.49
      vagina V16.49
      vulva V16.49
    mental retardation V18.4
    metabolic disease NEC V18.1
    mongolism V19.5
    multiple myeloma V16.7
    musculoskeletal disease NEC V17.8
    nephritis V18.69
    nephrosis V18.69
    parasitic disease V18.8
    polycystic kidney disease V18.61
    psychiatric disorder V17.0
    psychosis V17.0
    retardation, mental V18.4
    retinitis pigmentosa V19.1
    schizophrenia V17.0
    skin conditions V19.4
    specified condition NEC V19.8
    stroke (cerebrovascular) V17.1
    visual loss V19.0
  genital system disorder V13.29 ▲
    pre-term labor V13.21 ●
  health hazard V15.9
    specified cause NEC V15.89
  Hodgkin's disease V10.72
  immunity disorder V12.2
  infectious disease V12.00
    malaria V12.03
    poliomyelitis V12.02
    specified NEC V12.09
    tuberculosis V12.01
  injury NEC V15.5
  insufficient prenatal care V23.7
  irradiation V15.3
  leukemia V10.60
    lymphoid V10.61
    monocytic V10.63
    myeloid V10.62
    specified type NEC V10.69
  little or no prenatal care V23.7
  low birth weight (*see also* Status, low birth weight) V21.30
  lymphosarcoma V10.71
  malaria V12.03
  malignant neoplasm (of) V10.9
    accessory sinus V10.22
    adrenal V10.88
    anus V10.06
    bile duct V10.09
    bladder V10.51
    bone V10.81
    brain V10.85
    breast V10.3
    bronchus V10.11
    cervix uteri V10.41
    colon V10.05

History (personal) of — *continued*
  malignant neoplasm (of) — *continued*
    connective tissue NEC V10.89
    corpus uteri V10.42
    digestive system V10.00
      specified part NEC V10.09
    duodenum V10.09
    endocrine gland NEC V10.88
    epididymis V10.48
    esophagus V10.03
    eye V10.84
    fallopian tube V10.44
    female genital organ V10.40
      specified site NEC V10.44
    gallbladder V10.09
    gastrointestinal tract V10.00
    gum V10.02
    hematopoietic NEC V10.79
    hypopharynx V10.02
    ileum V10.09
    intrathoracic organs NEC V10.20
    jejunum V10.09
    kidney V10.52
    large intestine V10.05
    larynx V10.21
    lip V10.02
    liver V10.07
    lung V10.11
    lymphatic NEC V10.79
    lymph glands or nodes NEC V10.79
    male genital organ V10.45
      specified site NEC V10.49
    mediastinum V10.29
    melanoma (of skin) V10.82
    middle ear V10.22
    mouth V10.02
      specified part NEC V10.02
    nasal cavities V10.22
    nasopharynx V10.02
    nervous system NEC V10.86
    nose V10.22
    oropharynx V10.02
    ovary V10.43
    pancreas V10.09
    parathyroid V10.88
    penis V10.49
    pharynx V10.02
    pineal V10.88
    pituitary V10.88
    placenta V10.44
    pleura V10.29
    prostate V10.46
    rectosigmoid junction V10.06
    rectum V10.06
    renal pelvis V10.53
    respiratory organs NEC V10.20
    salivary gland V10.02
    skin V10.83
      melanoma V10.82
    small intestine NEC V10.09
    soft tissue NEC V10.89
    specified site NEC V10.89
    stomach V10.04
    testis V10.47
    thymus V10.29
    thyroid V10.87
    tongue V10.01
    trachea V10.12
    ureter V10.59
    urethra V10.59
    urinary organ V10.50
    uterine adnexa V10.44
    uterus V10.42
    vagina V10.44
    vulva V10.44
  manic-depressive psychosis V11.1
  mental disorder V11.9
    affective type V11.1
    manic-depressive V11.1
    neurosis V11.2
    schizophrenia V11.0
    specified type NEC V11.8
  metabolic disorder V12.2
  musculoskeletal disorder NEC V13.5
  myocardial infarction 412
  neglect (emotional) V15.42
  nervous system disorder V12.40
    specified type NEC V12.49

History (personal) of — *continued*
  neurosis V11.2
  noncompliance with medical treatment V15.81
  nutritional deficiency V12.1
  obstetric disorder V13.29 ●
    affecting management of current
      pregnancy V23.49 ▲
      pre-term labor V23.41 ●
    pre-term labor V13.41 ●
  parasitic disease V12.00
    specified NEC V12.09
  perinatal problems V13.7
    low birth weight (*see also* Status, low birth weight) V21.30
  physical abuse V15.41
  poisoning V15.6
  poliomyelitis V12.02
  polyps, colonic V12.72
  poor obstetric V13.49 ▲
    affecting management of current ●
      pregnancy V23.49
      pre-term labor V23.41 ●
    pre-term labor V13.41 ●
  psychiatric disorder V11.9
    affective type V11.1
    manic-depressive V11.1
    neurosis V11.2
    schizophrenia V11.0
    specified type NEC V11.8
  psychological trauma V15.49
    emotional abuse V15.42
    neglect V15.42
    physical abuse V15.41
    rape V15.41
  psychoneurosis V11.2
  radiation therapy V15.3
  rape V15.41
  respiratory system disease V12.6
  reticulosarcoma V10.71
  schizophrenia V11.0
  skin disease V13.3
  smoking (tobacco) V15.82
  subcutaneous tissue disease V13.3
  surgery (major) to
    great vessels V15.1
    heart V15.1
    major organs NEC V15.2
  thrombophlebitis V12.52
  thrombosis V12.51
  tobacco use V15.82
  trophoblastic disease V13.1
    affecting management of pregnancy V23.1
  tuberculosis V12.01
  ulcer, peptic V12.71
  urinary system disorder V13.00
    calculi V13.01
    specified NEC V13.09

HIV infection (disease) (illness) — *see* Human immunodeficiency virus (disease) (illness) (infection)
Hives (bold) (*see also* Urticaria) 708.9
Hoarseness 784.49
Hobnail liver — *see* Cirrhosis, portal
Hobo, hoboism V60.0
Hodgkins
  disease (M9650/3) 201.9 ✓5ᵗʰ
    lymphocytic
      depletion (M9653/3) 201.7 ✓5ᵗʰ
        diffuse fibrosis (M9654/3) 201.7 ✓5ᵗʰ
        reticular type (M9655/3) 201.7 ✓5ᵗʰ
      predominance (M9651/3) 201.4 ✓5ᵗʰ
    lymphocytic-histiocytic predominance (M9651/3) 201.4 ✓5ᵗʰ
    mixed cellularity (M9652/3) 201.6 ✓5ᵗʰ
    nodular sclerosis (M9656/3) 201.5 ✓5ᵗʰ
      cellular phase (M9657/3) 201.5 ✓5ᵗʰ
  granuloma (M9661/3) 201.1 ✓5ᵗʰ
  lymphogranulomatosis (M9650/3) 201.9 ✓5ᵗʰ
  lymphoma (M9650/3) 201.9 ✓5ᵗʰ
  lymphosarcoma (M9650/3) 201.9 ✓5ᵗʰ
  paragranuloma (M9660/3) 201.0 ✓5ᵗʰ
  sarcoma (M9662/3) 201.2 ✓5ᵗʰ
Hodgson's disease (aneurysmal dilatation of aorta) 441.9
  ruptured 441.5
Hodi-potsy 111.0

Hoffa (-Kastert) disease or syndrome
(liposynovitis prepatellaris) 272.8
Hoffman's syndrome 244.9 [359.5]
Hoffmann-Bouveret syndrome (paroxysmal tachycardia) 427.2
Hole
   macula 362.54
   optic disc, crater-like 377.22
   retina (macula) 362.54
      round 361.31
         with detachment 361.01
Holla disease (see also Spherocytosis) 282.0
Holländer-Simons syndrome (progressive lipodystrophy) 272.6
Hollow foot (congenital) 754.71
   acquired 736.73
Holmes' syndrome (visual disorientation) 368.16
Holoprosencephaly 742.2
   due to
      trisomy 13 758.1
      trisomy 18 758.2
Holthouse's hernia — see Hernia, inguinal
Homesickness 309.89
Homocystinemia 270.4
Homocystinuria 270.4
Homologous serum jaundice (prophylactic) (therapeutic) — see Hepatitis, viral
Homosexuality — omit code
   ego-dystonic 302.0
   pedophilic 302.2
   problems with 302.0
Homozygous Hb-S disease 282.61
Honeycomb lung 518.89
   congenital 748.4
Hong Kong ear 117.3
HOOD (hereditary osteo-onychodysplasia) 756.89
Hooded
   clitoris 752.49
   penis 752.69
Hookworm (anemia) (disease) (infestation) — see Ancylostomiasis
Hoppe-Goldflam syndrome 358.0
Hordeolum (external) (eyelid) 373.11
   internal 373.12
Horn
   cutaneous 702.8
      cheek 702.8
      eyelid 702.8
      penis 702.8
   iliac 756.89
   nail 703.8
      congenital 757.5
   papillary 700
Horner's
   syndrome (see also Neuropathy, peripheral, autonomic) 337.9
      traumatic 954.0
   teeth 520.4
Horseshoe kidney (congenital) 753.3
Horton's
   disease (temporal arteritis) 446.5
   headache or neuralgia 346.2
Hospice care V66.7
Hospitalism (in children) NEC 309.83
Hourglass contraction, contracture
   bladder 596.8
   gallbladder 575.2
      congenital 751.69
   stomach 536.8
      congenital 750.7
      psychogenic 306.4
   uterus 661.4
      affecting fetus or newborn 763.7
Household circumstance affecting care V60.9
   specified type NEC V60.8
Housemaid's knee 727.2
Housing circumstance affecting care V60.9
   specified type NEC V60.8
Huchard's disease (continued arterial hypertension) 401.9

Hudson-Stähli lines 371.11
Huguier's disease (uterine fibroma) 218.9
Hum, venous — omit code
Human bite (open wound) — see also Wound, open, by site
   intact skin surface — see Contusion
Human immunodeficiency virus (disease) (illness) 042
   infection V08
      with symptoms, symptomatic 042
Human immunodeficiency virus-2 infection 079.53
Human immunovirus (disease) (illness) (infection) — see Human immunodeficiency virus (disease) (illness) (infection)
Human papillomavirus 079.4
Human T-cell lymphotrophic virus-I infection 079.51
Human T-cell lymphotrophic virus-II infection 079.52
Human T-cell lymphotrophic virus-III (disease) (illness) (infection) — see Human immunodeficiency virus (disease) (illness) (infection)
HTLV-I infection 079.51
HTLV-II infection 079.52
HTLV-III (disease) (illness) (infection) — see Human immunodeficiency virus (disease) (illness) (infection)
HTLV-III/LAV (disease) (illness) (infection) — see Human immunodeficiency virus (disease) (illness) (infection)
Humpback (acquired) 737.9
   congenital 756.19
Hunchback (acquired) 737.9
   congenital 756.19
Hunger 994.2
   air, psychogenic 306.1
   disease 251.1
Hunner's ulcer (see also Cystitis) 595.1
Hunt's
   neuralgia 053.11
   syndrome (herpetic geniculate ganglionitis) 053.11
      dyssynergia cerebellaris myoclonica 334.2
Hunter's glossitis 529.4
Hunter (-Hurler) syndrome (mucopolysaccharidosis II) 277.5
Hunterian chancre 091.0
Huntington's
   chorea 333.4
   disease 333.4
Huppert's disease (multiple myeloma) (M9730/3) 203.0
Hurler (-Hunter) disease or syndrome (mucopolysaccharidosis II) 277.5
Hürthle cell
   adenocarcinoma (M8290/3) 193
   adenoma (M8290/0) 226
   carcinoma (M8290/3) 193
   tumor (M8290/0) 226
Hutchinson's
   disease meaning
      angioma serpiginosum 709.1
      cheiropompholyx 705.81
      prurigo estivalis 692.72
      summer eruption, or summer prurigo 692.72
   incisors 090.5
   melanotic freckle (M8742/2) — see also Neoplasm, skin, in situ
      malignant melanoma in (M8742/3) — see Melanoma
   teeth or incisors (congenital syphilis) 090.5
Hutchinson-Boeck disease or syndrome (sarcoidosis) 135
Hutchinson-Gilford disease or syndrome (progeria) 259.8
Hyaline
   degeneration (diffuse) (generalized) 728.9
   localized — see Degeneration, by site

Hyaline — continued
   membrane (disease) (lung) (newborn) 769
Hyalinosis cutis et mucosae 272.8
Hyalin plaque, sclera, senile 379.16
Hyalitis (asteroid) 379.22
   syphilitic 095.8
Hydatid
   cyst or tumor — see also Echinococcus
      fallopian tube 752.11
   mole — see Hydatidiform mole
   Morgagni (congenital) 752.8
      fallopian tube 752.11
Hydatidiform mole (benign) (complicating pregnancy) (delivered) (undelivered) 630
   invasive (M9100/1) 236.1
   malignant (M9100/1) 236.1
   previous, affecting management of pregnancy V23.1
Hydatidosis — see Echinococcus
Hyde's disease (prurigo nodularis) 698.3
Hydradenitis 705.83
Hydradenoma (M8400/0) — see Hidradenoma
Hydralazine lupus or syndrome
   correct substance properly administered 695.4
   overdose or wrong substance given or taken 972.6
Hydramnios 657
   affecting fetus or newborn 761.3
Hydrancephaly 742.3
   with spina bifida (see also Spina bifida) 741.0
Hydranencephaly 742.3
   with spina bifida (see also Spina bifida) 741.0
Hydrargyrism NEC 985.0
Hydrarthrosis (see also Effusion, joint) 719.0
   gonococcal 098.50
   intermittent (see also Rheumatism, palindromic) 719.3
   of yaws (early) (late) 102.6
   syphilitic 095.8
      congenital 090.5
Hydremia 285.9
Hydrencephalocele (congenital) 742.0
Hydrencephalomeningocele (congenital) 742.0
Hydroa 694.0
   aestivale 692.72
   gestationis 646.8
   herpetiformis 694.0
   pruriginosa 694.0
   vacciniforme 692.72
Hydroadenitis 705.83
Hydrocalycosis (see also Hydronephrosis) 591
   congenital 753.29
Hydrocalyx (see also Hydronephrosis) 591
Hydrocele (calcified) (chylous) (idiopathic) (infantile) (inguinal canal) (recurrent) (senile) (spermatic cord) (testis) (tunica vaginalis) 603.9
   canal of Nuck (female) 629.1
      male 603.9
   congenital 778.6
   encysted 603.0
      congenital 778.6
   female NEC 629.8
   infected 603.1
   round ligament 629.8
   specified type NEC 603.8
      congenital 778.6
   spinalis (see also Spina bifida) 741.9
   vulva 624.8
Hydrocephalic fetus
   affecting management or pregnancy 655.0
   causing disproportion 653.6
      with obstructed labor 660.1
      affecting fetus or newborn 763.1
Hydrocephalus (acquired) (external) (internal) (malignant) (noncommunicating) (obstructive) (recurrent) 331.4
   aqueduct of Sylvius structure 742.3
   with spina bifida (see also Spina bifida) 741.0

Hydrocephalus — continued
  chronic 742.3
    with spina bifida (see also Spina bifida) 741.0 ✓5ᵗʰ
  communicating 331.3
  congenital (external) (internal) 742.3
    with spina bifida (see also Spina bifida) 741.0 ✓5ᵗʰ
  due to
    structure of aqueduct of Sylvius 742.3
      with spina bifida (see also Spina bifida) 741.0 ✓5ᵗʰ
    toxoplasmosis (congenital) 771.2
  fetal affecting management of pregnancy 655.0 ✓5ᵗʰ
  foramen Magendie block (acquired) 331.3
    congenital 742.3
      with spina bifida (see also Spina bifida) 741.0 ✓5ᵗʰ
  newborn 742.3
    with spina bifida (see also Spina bifida) 741.0 ✓5ᵗʰ
  otitic 331.4
  syphilitic, congenital 090.49
  tuberculous (see also Tuberculosis) 013.8 ✓5ᵗʰ
Hydrocolpos (congenital) 623.8
Hydrocystoma (M8404/0) — see Neoplasm, skin, benign
Hydroencephalocele (congenital) 742.0
Hydroencephalomeningocele (congenital) 742.0
Hydrohematopneumothorax (see also Hemothorax) 511.8
Hydromeningitis — see Meningitis
Hydromeningocele (spinal) (see also Spina bifida) 741.9 ✓5ᵗʰ
  cranial 742.0
Hydrometra 621.8
Hydrometrocolpos 623.8
Hydromicrocephaly 742.1
Hydromphalus (congenital) (since birth) 757.39
Hydromyelia 742.53
Hydromyelocele (see also Spina bifida) 741.9 ✓5ᵗʰ
Hydronephrosis 591
  atrophic 591
  congenital 753.29
  due to S. hematobium 120.0
  early 591
  functionless (infected) 591
  infected 591
  intermittent 591
  primary 591
  secondary 591
  tuberculous (see also Tuberculosis) 016.0 ✓5ᵗʰ
Hydropericarditis (see also Pericarditis) 423.9
Hydropericardium (see also Pericarditis) 423.9
Hydroperitoneum 789.5
Hydrophobia 071
Hydrophthalmos (see also Buphthalmia) 743.20
Hydropneumohemothorax (see also Hemothorax) 511.8
Hydropneumopericarditis (see also Pericarditis) 423.9
Hydropneumopericardium (see also Pericarditis) 423.9
Hydropneumothorax 511.8
  nontuberculous 511.8
    bacterial 511.1
    pneumococcal 511.1
    staphylococcal 511.1
    streptococcal 511.1
  traumatic 860.0
    with open wound into thorax 860.1
  tuberculous (see also Tuberculosis, pleura) 012.0 ✓5ᵗʰ
Hydrops 782.3
  abdominis 789.5
  amnii (complicating pregnancy) (see also Hydramnios) 657 ✓4ᵗʰ
  articulorum intermittens (see also Rheumatism, palindromic) 719.3 ✓5ᵗʰ
  cardiac (see also Failure, heart) 428.0
  congenital — see Hydrops, fetalis

Hydrops — continued
  endolymphatic (see also Disease, Ménière's) 386.00
  fetal(is) or newborn 778.0
    due to isoimmunization 773.3
    not due to isoimmunization 778.0
  gallbladder 575.3
  idiopathic (fetus or newborn) 778.0
  joint (see also Effusion, joint) 719.0 ✓5ᵗʰ
  labyrinth (see also Disease, Ménière's) 386.00
  meningeal NEC 331.4
  nutritional 262
  pericardium — see Pericarditis
  pleura (see also Hydrothorax) 511.8
  renal (see also Nephrosis) 581.9
  spermatic cord (see also Hydrocele) 603.9
Hydropyonephrosis (see also Pyelitis) 590.80
  chronic 590.00
Hydrorachis 742.53
Hydrorrhea (nasal) 478.1
  gravidarum 658.1 ✓5ᵗʰ
  pregnancy 658.1 ✓5ᵗʰ
Hydrosadenitis 705.83
Hydrosalpinx (fallopian tube) (follicularis) 614.1
Hydrothorax (double) (pleural) 511.8
  chylous (nonfilarial) 457.8
    filaria (see also Infestation, filarial) 125.9
  nontuberculous 511.8
    bacterial 511.1
    pneumococcal 511.1
    staphylococcal 511.1
    streptococcal 511.1
  traumatic 862.29
    with open wound into thorax 862.39
  tuberculous (see also Tuberculosis, pleura) 012.0 ✓5ᵗʰ
Hydroureter 593.5
  congenital 753.22
Hydroureteronephrosis (see also Hydronephrosis) 591
Hydrourethra 599.84
Hydroxykynureninuria 270.2
Hydroxyprolinemia 270.8
Hydroxyprolinuria 270.8
Hygroma (congenital) (cystic) (M9173/0) 228.1
  prepatellar 727.3
  subdural — see Hematoma, subdural
Hymen — see condition
Hymenolepiasis (diminuta) (infection) (infestation) (nana) 123.6
Hymenolepis (diminuta) (infection) (infestation) (nana) 123.6
Hypalgesia (see also Disturbance, sensation) 782.0
Hyperabduction syndrome 447.8
Hyperacidity, gastric 536.8
  psychogenic 306.4
Hyperactive, hyperactivity
  basal cell, uterine cervix 622.1
  bladder 596.51
  bowel (syndrome) 564.9
    sounds 787.5
  cervix epithelial (basal) 622.1
  child 314.01
  colon 564.9
  gastrointestinal 536.8
    psychogenic 306.4
  intestine 564.9
  labyrinth (unilateral) 386.51
    with loss of labyrinthine reactivity 386.58
    bilateral 386.52
  nasal mucous membrane 478.1
  stomach 536.8
  thyroid (gland) (see also Thyrotoxicosis) 242.9 ✓5ᵗʰ
Hyperacusis 388.42
Hyperadrenalism (cortical) 255.3
  medullary 255.6
Hyperadrenocorticism 255.3
  congenital 255.2
  iatrogenic
    correct substance properly administered 255.3

Hyperadrenocorticism — continued
  iatrogenic — continued
    overdose or wrong substance given or taken 962.0
Hyperaffectivity 301.11
Hyperaldosteronism (atypical) (hyperplastic) (normoaldosteronal) (normotensive) (primary) (secondary) 255.1
Hyperalgesia (see also Disturbance, sensation) 782.0
Hyperalimentation 783.6
  carotene 278.3
  specified NEC 278.8
  vitamin A 278.2
  vitamin D 278.4
Hyperaminoaciduria 270.9
  arginine 270.6
  citrulline 270.6
  cystine 270.0
  glycine 270.0
  lysine 270.7
  ornithine 270.6
  renal (types I, II, III) 270.0
Hyperammonemia (congenital) 270.6
Hyperamnesia 780.99 ▲
Hyperamylasemia 790.5
Hyperaphia 782.0
Hyperazotemia 791.9
Hyperbetalipoproteinemia (acquired) (essential) (familial) (hereditary) (primary) (secondary) 272.2
  with prebetalipoproteinemia 272.2
Hyperbilirubinemia 782.4
  congenital 277.4
  constitutional 277.4
  neonatal (transient) (see also Jaundice, fetus or newborn) 774.6
  of prematurity 774.2
Hyperbilirubinemica encephalopathia, newborn 774.7
  due to isoimmunization 773.4
Hypercalcemia, hypercalcemic (idiopathic) 275.42
  nephropathy 588.8
Hypercalciuria 275.40
Hypercapnia 786.09
  with mixed acid-base disorder 276.4
  fetal, affecting newborn 770.89 ▲
Hypercarotinemia 278.3
Hypercementosis 521.5
Hyperchloremia 276.9
Hyperchlorhydria 536.8
  neurotic 306.4
  psychogenic 306.4
Hypercholesterinemia — see Hypercholesterolemia
Hypercholesterolemia 272.0
  with hyperglyceridemia, endogenous 272.2
  essential 272.0
  familial 272.0
  hereditary 272.0
  primary 272.0
  pure 272.0
Hypercholesterolosis 272.0
Hyperchylia gastrica 536.8
  psychogenic 306.4
Hyperchylomicronemia (familial) (with hyperbetalipoproteinemia) 272.3
Hypercoagulation syndrome 289.8
Hypercorticosteronism
  correct substance properly administered 255.3
  overdose or wrong substance given or taken 962.0
Hypercortisonism
  correct substance properly administered 255.3
  overdose or wrong substance given or taken 962.0
Hyperdynamic beta-adrenergic state or syndrome (circulatory) 429.82
Hyperelectrolytemia 276.9

Index to Diseases

Hyperemesis 536.2
  arising during pregnancy — see Hyperemesis, gravidarum
  gravidarum (mild) (before 22 completed weeks gestation) 643.0 ✓5ᵗʰ
    with
      carbohydrate depletion 643.1 ✓5ᵗʰ
      dehydration 643.1 ✓5ᵗʰ
      electrolyte imbalance 643.1 ✓5ᵗʰ
      metabolic disturbance 643.1 ✓5ᵗʰ
    affecting fetus or newborn 761.8
    severe (with metabolic disturbance) 643.1 ✓5ᵗʰ
  psychogenic 306.4
Hyperemia (acute) 780.99 ▲
  anal mucosa 569.49
  bladder 596.7
  cerebral 437.8
  conjunctiva 372.71
  ear, internal, acute 386.30
  enteric 564.89
  eye 372.71
  eyelid (active) (passive) 374.82
  intestine 564.89
  iris 364.41
  kidney 593.81
  labyrinth 386.30
  liver (active) (passive) 573.8
  lung 514
  ovary 620.8
  passive 780.99 ▲
  pulmonary 514
  renal 593.81
  retina 362.89
  spleen 289.59
  stomach 537.89
Hyperesthesia (body surface) (see also Disturbance, sensation) 782.0
  larynx (reflex) 478.79
    hysterical 300.11
  pharynx (reflex) 478.29
Hyperestrinism 256.0
Hyperestrogenism 256.0
Hyperestrogenosis 256.0
Hyperextension, joint 718.80
  ankle 718.87
  elbow 718.82
  foot 718.87
  hand 718.84
  hip 718.85
  knee 718.86
  multiple sites 718.89
  pelvic region 718.85
  shoulder (region) 718.81
  specified site NEC 718.88
  wrist 718.83
Hyperfibrinolysis — see Fibrinolysis
Hyperfolliculinism 256.0
Hyperfructosemia 271.2
Hyperfunction
  adrenal (cortex) 255.3
    androgenic, acquired benign 255.3
    medulla 255.6
    virilism 255.2
  corticoadrenal NEC 255.3
  labyrinth — see Hyperactive, labyrinth
  medulloadrenal 255.6
  ovary 256.1
    estrogen 256.0
  pancreas 577.8
  parathyroid (gland) 252.0
  pituitary (anterior) (gland) (lobe) 253.1
  testicular 257.0
Hypergammaglobulinemia 289.8
  monoclonal, benign (BMH) 273.1
  polyclonal 273.0
  Waldenström's 273.0
Hyperglobulinemia 273.8
Hyperglycemia 790.6
  maternal
    affecting fetus or newborn 775.0
      manifest diabetes in infant 775.1
  postpancreatectomy (complete) (partial) 251.3

Hyperglyceridemia 272.1
  endogenous 272.1
  essential 272.1
  familial 272.1
  hereditary 272.1
  mixed 272.3
  pure 272.1
Hyperglycinemia 270.7
Hypergonadism
  ovarian 256.1
  testicular (infantile) (primary) 257.0
Hyperheparinemia (see also Circulating anticoagulants) 286.5
Hyperhidrosis, hyperidrosis 780.8
  psychogenic 306.3
Hyperhistidinemia 270.5
Hyperinsulinism (ectopic) (functional) (organic) NEC 251.1
  iatrogenic 251.0
  reactive 251.2
  spontaneous 251.2
  therapeutic misadventure (from administration of insulin) 962.3
Hyperiodemia 276.9
Hyperirritability (cerebral), in newborn 779.1
Hyperkalemia 276.7
Hyperkeratosis (see also Keratosis) 701.1
  cervix 622.1
  congenital 757.39
  cornea 371.89
  due to yaws (early) (late) (palmar or plantar) 102.3
  eccentrica 757.39
  figurata centrifuga atrophica 757.39
  follicularis 757.39
    in cutem penetrans 701.1
  limbic (cornea) 371.89
  palmoplantaris climacterica 701.1
  pinta (carate) 103.1
  senile (with pruritus) 702.0
  tongue 528.7
  universalis congenita 757.1
  vagina 623.1
  vocal cord 478.5
  vulva 624.0
Hyperkinesia, hyperkinetic (disease) (reaction) (syndrome) 314.9
  with
    attention deficit — see Disorder, attention deficit
    conduct disorder 314.2
    developmental delay 314.1
    simple disturbance of activity and attention 314.01
    specified manifestation NEC 314.8
  heart (disease) 429.82
  of childhood or adolescence NEC 314.9
Hyperlacrimation (see also Epiphora) 375.20
Hyperlipemia (see also Hyperlipidemia) 272.4
Hyperlipidemia 272.4
  carbohydrate-induced 272.1
  combined 272.4
  endogenous 272.1
  exogenous 272.3
  fat-induced 272.3
  group
    A 272.0
    B 272.1
    C 272.2
    D 272.3
  mixed 272.2
  specified type NEC 272.4
Hyperlipidosis 272.7
  hereditary 272.7
Hyperlipoproteinemia (acquired) (essential) (familial) (hereditary) (primary) (secondary) 272.4
  Fredrickson type
    I 272.3
    IIa 272.0
    IIb 272.2
    III 272.2
    IV 272.1
    V 272.3

Hyperlipoproteinemia — continued
  low-density-lipoid-type (LDL) 272.0
  very-low-density-lipoid-type (VLDL) 272.1
Hyperlucent lung, unilateral 492.8
Hyperluteinization 256.1
Hyperlysinemia 270.7
Hypermagnesemia 275.2
  neonatal 775.5
Hypermaturity (fetus or newborn) 766.2
Hypermenorrhea 626.2
Hypermetabolism 794.7
Hypermethioninemia 270.4
Hypermetropia (congenital) 367.0
Hypermobility
  cecum 564.9
  coccyx 724.71
  colon 564.9
    psychogenic 306.4
  ileum 564.89
  joint (acquired) 718.80
    ankle 718.87
    elbow 718.82
    foot 718.87
    hand 718.84
    hip 718.85
    knee 718.86
    multiple sites 718.89
    pelvic region 718.85
    shoulder (region) 718.81
    specified site NEC 718.88
    wrist 718.83
  kidney, congenital 753.3
  meniscus (knee) 717.5
  scapula 718.81
  stomach 536.8
    psychogenic 306.4
  syndrome 728.5
  testis, congenital 752.52
  urethral 599.81
Hypermotility
  gastrointestinal 536.8
  intestine 564.9
    psychogenic 306.4
  stomach 536.8
Hypernasality 784.49
Hypernatremia 276.0
  with water depletion 276.0
Hypernephroma (M8312/3) 189.0
Hyperopia 367.0
Hyperorexia 783.6
Hyperornithinemia 270.6
Hyperosmia (see also Disturbance, sensation) 781.1
Hyperosmolality 276.0
Hyperosteogenesis 733.99
Hyperostosis 733.99
  calvarial 733.3
  cortical 733.3
    infantile 756.59
  frontal, internal of skull 733.3
  interna frontalis 733.3
  monomelic 733.99
  skull 733.3
    congenital 756.0
  vertebral 721.8
    with spondylosis — see Spondylosis
  ankylosing 721.6
Hyperovarianism 256.1
Hyperovarism, hyperovaria 256.1
Hyperoxaluria (primary) 271.8
Hyperoxia 987.8
Hyperparathyroidism 252.0
  ectopic 259.3
  secondary, of renal origin 588.8
Hyperpathia (see also Disturbance, sensation) 782.0
  psychogenic 307.80
Hyperperistalsis 787.4
  psychogenic 306.4
Hyperpermeability, capillary 448.9
Hyperphagia 783.6

Hyperphenylalaninemia 270.1
Hyperphoria 378.40
   alternating 378.45
Hyperphosphatemia 275.3
Hyperpiesia (see also Hypertension) 401.9
Hyperpiesis (see also Hypertension) 401.9
Hyperpigmentation — see Pigmentation
Hyperpinealism 259.8
Hyperpipecolatemia 270.7
Hyperpituitarism 253.1
Hyperplasia, hyperplastic
   adenoids (lymphoid tissue) 474.12
     and tonsils 474.10
   adrenal (capsule) (cortex) (gland) 255.8
     with
       sexual precocity (male) 255.2
       virilism, adrenal 255.2
       virilization (female) 255.2
     congenital 255.2
     due to excess ACTH (ectopic) (pituitary) 255.0
     medulla 255.8
   alpha cells (pancreatic)
     with
       gastrin excess 251.5
       glucagon excess 251.4
   appendix (lymphoid) 543.0
   artery, fibromuscular NEC 447.8
     carotid 447.8
     renal 447.3
   bone 733.99
     marrow 289.9
   breast (see also Hypertrophy, breast) 611.1
   carotid artery 447.8
   cementation, cementum (teeth) (tooth) 521.5
   cervical gland 785.6
   cervix (uteri) 622.1
     basal cell 622.1
     congenital 752.49
     endometrium 622.1
     polypoid 622.1
   chin 524.05
   clitoris, congenital 752.49
   dentin 521.5
   endocervicitis 616.0
   endometrium, endometrial (adenomatous) (atypical) (cystic) (glandular) (polypoid) (uterus) 621.3
     cervix 622.1
   epithelial 709.8
     focal, oral, including tongue 528.7
     mouth (focal) 528.7
     nipple 611.8
     skin 709.8
     tongue (focal) 528.7
     vaginal wall 623.0
   erythroid 289.9
   fascialis ossificans (progressiva) 728.11
   fibromuscular, artery NEC 447.8
     carotid 447.8
     renal 447.3
   genital
     female 629.8
     male 608.89
   gingiva 523.8
   glandularis
     cystica uteri 621.3
     endometrium (uterus) 621.3
     interstitialis uteri 621.3
   granulocytic 288.8
   gum 523.8
   hymen, congenital 752.49
   islands of Langerhans 251.1
   islet cell (pancreatic) 251.9
     alpha cells
       with excess
         gastrin 251.5
         glucagon 251.4
     beta cells 251.1
   juxtaglomerular (complex) (kidney) 593.89
   kidney (congenital) 753.3
   liver (congenital) 751.69
   lymph node (gland) 785.6
   lymphoid (diffuse) (nodular) 785.6
     appendix 543.0

Hyperplasia, hyperplastic — continued
   lymphoid — continued
     intestine 569.89
   mandibular 524.02
     alveolar 524.72
     unilateral condylar 526.89
   Marchand multiple nodular (liver) — see Cirrhosis, postnecrotic
   maxillary 524.01
     alveolar 524.71
   medulla, adrenal 255.8
   myometrium, myometrial 621.2
   nose (lymphoid) (polypoid) 478.1
   oral soft tissue (inflammatory) (irritative) (mucosa) NEC 528.9
     gingiva 523.8
     tongue 529.8
   organ or site, congenital NEC — see Anomaly, specified type NEC
   ovary 620.8
   palate, papillary 528.9
   pancreatic islet cells 251.9
     alpha
       with excess
         gastrin 251.5
         glucagon 251.4
     beta 251.1
   parathyroid (gland) 252.0
   persistent, vitreous (primary) 743.51
   pharynx (lymphoid) 478.29
   prostate 600.9 ▲
     adenofibromatous 600.2
     nodular 600.1
   renal artery (fibromuscular) 447.3
   reticuloendothelial (cell) 289.9
   salivary gland (any) 527.1
   Schimmelbusch's 610.1
   suprarenal (capsule) (gland) 255.8
   thymus (gland) (persistent) 254.0
   thyroid (see also Goiter) 240.9
     primary 242.0 ✓5th
     secondary 242.2 ✓5th
   tonsil (lymphoid tissue) 474.11
     and adenoids 474.10
   urethrovaginal 599.89
   uterus, uterine (myometrium) 621.2
     endometrium 621.3
   vitreous (humor), primary persistent 743.51
   vulva 624.3
   zygoma 738.11
Hyperpnea (see also Hyperventilation) 786.01
Hyperpotassemia 276.7
Hyperprebetalipoproteinemia 272.1
   with chylomicronemia 272.3
   familial 272.1
Hyperprolactinemia 253.1
Hyperprolinemia 270.8
Hyperproteinemia 273.8
Hyperprothrombinemia 289.8
Hyperpselaphesia 782.0
Hyperpyrexia 780.6
   heat (effects of) 992.0
   malarial (see also Malaria) 084.6
   malignant, due to anesthetic 995.86
   rheumatic — see Fever, rheumatic
   unknown origin (see also Pyrexia) 780.6
Hyperreactor, vascular 780.2
Hyperreflexia 796.1
   bladder, autonomic 596.54
     with cauda equina 344.61
   detrusor 344.61
Hypersalivation (see also Ptyalism) 527.7
Hypersarcosinemia 270.8
Hypersecretion
   ACTH 255.3
   androgens (ovarian) 256.1
   calcitonin 246.0
   corticoadrenal 255.3
   cortisol 255.0
   estrogen 256.0
   gastric 536.8
     psychogenic 306.4
   gastrin 251.5
   glucagon 251.4

Hypersecretion — continued
   hormone
     ACTH 255.3
     anterior pituitary 253.1
     growth NEC 253.0
     ovarian androgen 256.1
     testicular 257.0
     thyroid stimulating 242.8 ✓5th
   insulin — see Hyperinsulinism
   lacrimal glands (see also Epiphora) 375.20
   medulloadrenal 255.6
   milk 676.6 ✓5th
   ovarian androgens 256.1
   pituitary (anterior) 253.1
   salivary gland (any) 527.7
   testicular hormones 257.0
   thyrocalcitonin 246.0
   upper respiratory 478.9
Hypersegmentation, hereditary 288.2
   eosinophils 288.2
   neutrophil nuclei 288.2
Hypersensitive, hypersensitiveness, hypersensitivity — see also Allergy
   angiitis 446.20
     specified NEC 446.29
   carotid sinus 337.0
   colon 564.9
     psychogenic 306.4
   DNA (deoxyribonucleic acid) NEC 287.2
   drug (see also Allergy, drug) 995.2
   esophagus 530.89
   insect bites — see Injury, superficial, by site
   labyrinth 386.58
   pain (see also Disturbance, sensation) 782.0
   pneumonitis NEC 495.9
   reaction (see also Allergy) 995.3
     upper respiratory tract NEC 478.8
   stomach (allergic) (nonallergic) 536.8
     psychogenic 306.4
Hypersomatotropism (classic) 253.0
Hypersomnia 780.54
   with sleep apnea 780.53
   nonorganic origin 307.43
     persistent (primary) 307.44
     transient 307.43
Hypersplenia 289.4
Hypersplenism 289.4
Hypersteatosis 706.3
Hyperstimulation, ovarian 256.1
Hypersuprarenalism 255.3
Hypersusceptibility — see Allergy
Hyper-TBG-nemia 246.8
Hypertelorism 756.0
   orbit, orbital 376.41

Index to Diseases

Hypertension, hypertensive

	Malignant	Benign	Unspecified
Hypertension, hypertensive (arterial) (arteriolar) (crisis) (degeneration) (disease) (essential) (fluctuating) (idiopathic) (intermittent) (labile) (low renin) (orthostatic) (paroxysmal) (primary) (systemic) (uncontrolled) (vascular)	401.0	401.1	401.9
with			
heart involvement (conditions classifiable to 425.8, 428, 429.0-429.3, 429.8, 429.9 due to hypertension) (see also Hypertension, heart)	402.00	402.10	402.90
with kidney involvement — see Hypertension, cardiorenal			
renal involvement (only conditions classifiable to 585, 586, 587) (excludes conditions classifiable to 584) (see also Hypertension, kidney)	403.00	403.10	403.90
renal sclerosis or failure	403.00	403.10	403.90
with heart involvement — see Hypertension, cardiorenal			
failure (and sclerosis) (see also Hypertension, kidney)	403.01	403.11	403.91
sclerosis without failure (see also Hypertension, kidney)	403.00	403.10	403.90
accelerated — (see also Hypertension, by type, malignant)	401.0	—	—
antepartum — see Hypertension, complicating pregnancy, childbirth, or the puerperium			
cardiorenal (disease)	404.00	404.10	404.90
with			
heart failure	404.01	404.11	404.91
and renal failure	404.03	404.13	404.93
renal failure	404.02	404.12	404.92
and heart failure	404.03	404.13	404.93
cardiovascular disease (arteriosclerotic) (sclerotic)	402.00	402.10	402.90
with			
heart failure	402.01	402.11	402.91
renal involvement (conditions classifiable to 403) (see also Hypertension, cardiorenal)	404.00	404.10	404.90
cardiovascular renal (disease) (sclerosis) (see also Hypertension, cardiorenal)	404.00	404.10	404.90
cerebrovascular disease NEC	437.2	437.2	437.2
complicating pregnancy, childbirth, or the puerperium	642.2 ✓5ᵗʰ	642.0	642.9 ✓5ᵗʰ
with			
albuminuria (and edema) (mild)	—	—	642.4 ✓5ᵗʰ
severe	—	—	642.5 ✓5ᵗʰ
edema (mild)	—	—	642.4 ✓5ᵗʰ
severe	—	—	642.5 ✓5ᵗʰ
heart disease	642.2 ✓5ᵗʰ	642.2 ✓5ᵗʰ	642.2 ✓5ᵗʰ
and renal disease	642.2 ✓5ᵗʰ	642.2 ✓5ᵗʰ	642.2 ✓5ᵗʰ
renal disease	642.2 ✓5ᵗʰ	642.2 ✓5ᵗʰ	642.2 ✓5ᵗʰ
and heart disease	642.2 ✓5ᵗʰ	642.2 ✓5ᵗʰ	642.2 ✓5ᵗʰ
chronic	642.2 ✓5ᵗʰ	642.0 ✓5ᵗʰ	642.0 ✓5ᵗʰ
with pre-eclampsia or eclampsia	642.7 ✓5ᵗʰ	642.7 ✓5ᵗʰ	642.7 ✓5ᵗʰ
fetus or newborn	760.0	760.0	760.0
essential	—	642.0	642.0 ✓5ᵗʰ
with pre-eclampsia or eclampsia	—	642.7 ✓5ᵗʰ	642.7 ✓5ᵗʰ
fetus or newborn	760.0	760.0	760.0
fetus or newborn	760.0	760.0	760.0
gestational	—	—	642.3 ✓5ᵗʰ
pre-existing	642.2 ✓5ᵗʰ	642.0	642.0 ✓5ᵗʰ
with pre-eclampsia or eclampsia	642.7 ✓5ᵗʰ	642.7 ✓5ᵗʰ	642.7 ✓5ᵗʰ
fetus or newborn	760.0	760.0	760.0
secondary to renal disease	642.1 ✓5ᵗʰ	642.1 ✓5ᵗʰ	642.1 ✓5ᵗʰ
with pre-eclampsia or eclampsia	642.7 ✓5ᵗʰ	642.7 ✓5ᵗʰ	642.7 ✓5ᵗʰ
fetus or newborn	760.0	760.0	760.0
transient	—	—	642.3 ✓5ᵗʰ
due to			
aldosteronism, primary	405.09	405.19	405.99
brain tumor	405.09	405.19	405.99
bulbar poliomyelitis	405.09	405.19	405.99
calculus			
kidney	405.09	405.19	405.99
ureter	405.09	405.19	405.99
coarctation, aorta	405.09	405.19	405.99
Cushing's disease	405.09	405.19	405.99
glomerulosclerosis (see also Hypertension, kidney)	403.00	403.10	403.90
periarteritis nodosa	405.09	405.19	405.99
pheochromocytoma	405.09	405.19	405.99
polycystic kidney(s)	405.09	405.19	405.99

✓4ᵗʰ Fourth-digit Required   ✓5ᵗʰ Fifth-digit Required   ▶◀ Revised Text   ● New Line   ▲ Revised Code

Hypertension, hypertensive

	Malignant	Benign	Unspecified
Hypertension, hypertensive — *continued*			
due to — *continued*			
polycythemia	405.09	405.19	405.99
porphyria	405.09	405.19	405.99
pyelonephritis	405.09	405.19	405.99
renal (artery)			
aneurysm	405.01	405.11	405.91
anomaly	405.01	405.11	405.91
embolism	405.01	405.11	405.91
fibromuscular hyperplasia	405.01	405.11	405.91
occlusion	405.01	405.11	405.91
stenosis	405.01	405.11	405.91
thrombosis	405.01	405.11	405.91
encephalopathy	437.2	437.2	437.2
gestational (transient) NEC	—	—	642.3 ✓5ᵗʰ
Goldblatt's	440.1	440.1	440.1
heart (disease) (conditions classifiable to 425.8, 428, 429.0-429.3, 429.8, 429.9 due to hypertension)	402.00	402.10	402.90
with heart failure	402.01	402.11	402.91
hypertensive kidney disease (conditions classifiable to 403) (*see also* Hypertension, cardiorenal)	404.00	404.10	404.90
renal sclerosis (*see also* Hypertension, cardiorenal)	404.00	404.10	404.90
intracranial, benign	—	348.2	—
intraocular	—	—	365.04
kidney	403.00	403.10	403.90
with			
heart involvement (conditions classifiable to 425.8, 428, 429.0-429.3, 429.8, 429.9 due to hypertension) (*see also* Hypertension, cardiorenal)	404.00	404.10	404.90
hypertensive heart (disease) (conditions classifiable to 402) (*see also* Hypertension, cardiorenal)	404.00	404.10	404.90
lesser circulation	—	—	416.0
necrotizing	401.0	—	—
ocular	—	—	365.04
portal (due to chronic liver disease)	—	—	572.3
postoperative	—	—	997.91
psychogenic	—	—	306.2
puerperal, postpartum — *see* Hypertension, complicating pregnancy, childbirth, or the puerperium			
pulmonary (artery)	—	—	416.8
with cor pulmonale (chronic)	—	—	416.8
acute	—	—	415.0
idiopathic	—	—	416.0
primary	—	—	416.0
of newborn	—	—	747.83 ●
secondary	—	—	416.8
renal (disease) (*see also* Hypertension, kidney)	403.00	403.10	403.90
renovascular NEC	405.01	405.11	405.91
secondary NEC	405.09	405.19	405.99
due to			
aldosteronism, primary	405.09	405.19	405.99
brain tumor	405.09	405.19	405.99
bulbar poliomyelitis	405.09	405.19	405.99
calculus			
kidney	405.09	405.19	405.99
ureter	405.09	405.19	405.99
coarctation, aorta	405.09	405.19	405.99
Cushing's disease	405.09	405.19	405.99
glomerulosclerosis (*see also* Hypertension, kidney)	403.00	403.10	403.90
periarteritis nodosa	405.09	405.19	405.99
pheochromocytoma	405.09	405.19	405.99
polycystic kidney(s)	405.09	405.19	405.99
polycythemia	405.09	405.19	405.99
porphyria	405.09	405.19	405.99
pyelonephritis	405.09	405.19	405.99
renal (artery)			
aneurysm	405.01	405.11	405.91
anomaly	405.01	405.11	405.91
embolism	405.01	405.11	405.91
fibromuscular hyperplasia	405.01	405.11	405.91
occlusion	405.01	405.11	405.91
stenosis	405.01	405.11	405.91
thrombosis	405.01	405.11	405.91
transient	—	—	796.2
of pregnancy	—	—	642.3 ✓5ᵗʰ

✓4ᵗʰ Fourth-digit Required   ✓5ᵗʰ Fifth-digit Required   ▶◀ Revised Text   ● New Line   ▲ Revised Code

Index to Diseases

Hypertrophy, hypertrophic

	Malignant	Benign	Unspecified
Hypertension, hypertensive — *continued*			
venous, chronic (asymptomatic) (idiopathic)	—	—	459.30 ●
due to			●
deep vein thrombosis (see also Syndrome, postphlebetic)	—	—	459.10 ●
with			●
complication, NEC	—	—	459.39 ●
inflammation	—	—	459.32 ●
with ulcer	—	—	459.33 ●
ulcer	—	—	459.31 ●
with inflammation	—	—	459.33 ●

Hyperthecosis, ovary 256.8
Hyperthermia (of unknown origin) (*see also* Pyrexia) 780.6
  malignant (due to anesthesia) 995.86
  newborn 778.4
Hyperthymergasia (*see also* Psychosis, affective) 296.0 ✓5th
  reactive (from emotional stress, psychological trauma) 298.1
  recurrent episode 296.1 ✓5th
  single episode 296.0 ✓5th
Hyperthymism 254.8
Hyperthyroid (recurrent) — *see* Hyperthyroidism
Hyperthyroidism (latent) (preadult) (recurrent) (without goiter) 242.9 ✓5th

> Note — Use the following fifth-digit subclassification with category 242:
>
> 0   without mention of thyrotoxic crisis or storm
> 1   with mention of thyrotoxic crisis or storm

  with
    goiter (diffuse) 242.0 ✓5th
      adenomatous 242.3 ✓5th
        multinodular 242.2 ✓5th
        uninodular 242.1 ✓5th
      nodular 242.3 ✓5th
        multinodular 242.2 ✓5th
        uninodular 242.1 ✓5th
      thyroid nodule 242.1 ✓5th
    complicating pregnancy, childbirth, or puerperium 648.1 ✓5th
  neonatal (transient) 775.3
Hypertonia — *see* Hypertonicity
Hypertonicity
  bladder 596.51
  fetus or newborn 779.89 ▲
  gastrointestinal (tract) 536.8
  infancy 779.89 ▲
    due to electrolyte imbalance 779.89 ▲
  muscle 728.85
  stomach 536.8
    psychogenic 306.4
  uterus, uterine (contractions) 661.4 ✓5th
    affecting fetus or newborn 763.7
Hypertony — *see* Hypertonicity
Hypertransaminemia 790.4
Hypertrichosis 704.1
  congenital 757.4
  eyelid 374.54
  lanuginosa 757.4
    acquired 704.1
Hypertriglyceridemia, essential 272.1
Hypertrophy, hypertrophic
  adenoids (infectional) 474.12
    and tonsils (faucial) (infective) (lingual) (lymphoid) 474.10
  adrenal 255.8
  alveolar process or ridge 525.8
  anal papillae 569.49
  apocrine gland 705.82
  artery NEC 447.8
    carotid 447.8
      congenital (peripheral) NEC 747.60
        gastrointestinal 747.61
        lower limb 747.64
        renal 747.62
        specified NEC 747.69
        spinal 747.82
        upper limb 747.63
  arthritis (chronic) (*see also* Osteoarthrosis) 715.9 ✓5th
    spine (*see also* Spondylosis) 721.90
  arytenoid 478.79
  asymmetrical (heart) 429.9
  auricular — *see* Hypertrophy, cardiac
  Bartholin's gland 624.8
  bile duct 576.8
  bladder (sphincter) (trigone) 596.8
  blind spot, visual field 368.42
  bone 733.99

Hypertrophy, hypertrophic — *continued*
- brain 348.8
- breast 611.1
  - cystic 610.1
  - fetus or newborn 778.7
  - fibrocystic 610.1
  - massive pubertal 611.1
  - puerperal, postpartum 676.3 ✓5ᵗʰ
  - senile (parenchymatous) 611.1
- cardiac (chronic) (idiopathic) 429.3
  - with
    - rheumatic fever (conditions classifiable to 390)
      - active 391.8
        - with chorea 392.0
      - inactive or quiescent (with chorea) 398.99
  - congenital NEC 746.89
  - fatty (*see also* Degeneration, myocardial) 429.1
  - hypertensive (*see also* Hypertension, heart) 402.90
  - rheumatic (with chorea) 398.99
    - active or acute 391.8
      - with chorea 392.0
  - valve (*see also* Endocarditis) 424.90
    - congenital NEC 746.89
- cartilage 733.99
- cecum 569.89
- cervix (uteri) 622.6
  - congenital 752.49
  - elongation 622.6
- clitoris (cirrhotic) 624.2
  - congenital 752.49
- colon 569.89
  - congenital 751.3
- conjunctiva, lymphoid 372.73
- cornea 371.89
- corpora cavernosa 607.89
- duodenum 537.89
- endometrium (uterus) 621.3
  - cervix 622.6
- epididymis 608.89
- esophageal hiatus (congenital) 756.6
  - with hernia — *see* Hernia, diaphragm
- eyelid 374.30
- falx, skull 733.99
- fat pad 729.30
  - infrapatellar 729.31
  - knee 729.31
  - orbital 374.34
  - popliteal 729.31
  - prepatellar 729.31
  - retropatellar 729.31
  - specified site NEC 729.39
- foot (congenital) 755.67
- frenum, frenulum (tongue) 529.8
  - linguae 529.8
  - lip 528.5
- gallbladder or cystic duct 575.8
- gastric mucosa 535.2 ✓5ᵗʰ
- gingiva 523.8
- gland, glandular (general) NEC 785.6
- gum (mucous membrane) 523.8
- heart (idiopathic) — *see also* Hypertrophy, cardiac
  - valve — *see also* Endocarditis
  - congenital NEC 746.89
- hemifacial 754.0
- hepatic — *see* Hypertrophy, liver
- hiatus (esophageal) 756.6
- hilus gland 785.6
- hymen, congenital 752.49
- ileum 569.89
- infrapatellar fat pad 729.31
- intestine 569.89
- jejunum 569.89
- kidney (compensatory) 593.1
  - congenital 753.3
- labial frenulum 528.5
- labium (majus) (minus) 624.3
- lacrimal gland, chronic 375.03
- ligament 728.9
  - spinal 724.8
- linguae frenulum 529.8
- lingual tonsil (infectional) 474.11

Hypertrophy, hypertrophic — *continued*
- lip (frenum) 528.5
  - congenital 744.81
- liver 789.1
  - acute 573.8
  - cirrhotic — *see* Cirrhosis, liver
  - congenital 751.69
  - fatty — *see* Fatty, liver
- lymph gland 785.6
  - tuberculous — *see* Tuberculosis, lymph gland
- mammary gland — *see* Hypertrophy, breast
- maxillary frenulum 528.5
- Meckel's diverticulum (congenital) 751.0
- medial meniscus, acquired 717.3
- median bar 600.9
- mediastinum 519.3
- meibomian gland 373.2
- meniscus, knee, congenital 755.64
- metatarsal head 733.99
- metatarsus 733.99
- mouth 528.9
- mucous membrane
  - alveolar process 523.8
  - nose 478.1
  - turbinate (nasal) 478.0
- muscle 728.9
- muscular coat, artery NEC 447.8
  - carotid 447.8
  - renal 447.3
- myocardium (*see also* Hypertrophy, cardiac) 429.3
  - idiopathic 425.4
- myometrium 621.2
- nail 703.8
  - congenital 757.5
- nasal 478.1
  - alae 478.1
  - bone 738.0
  - cartilage 478.1
  - mucous membrane (septum) 478.1
  - sinus (*see also* Sinusitis) 473.9
  - turbinate 478.0
- nasopharynx, lymphoid (infectional) (tissue) (wall) 478.29
- neck, uterus 622.6
- nipple 611.1
- normal aperture diaphragm (congenital) 756.6
- nose (*see also* Hypertrophy, nasal) 478.1
- orbit 376.46
- organ or site, congenital NEC — *see* Anomaly, specified type NEC
- osteoarthropathy (pulmonary) 731.2
- ovary 620.8
- palate (hard) 526.89
  - soft 528.9
- pancreas (congenital) 751.7
- papillae
  - anal 569.49
  - tongue 529.3
- parathyroid (gland) 252.0
- parotid gland 527.1
- penis 607.89
- phallus 607.89
  - female (clitoris) 624.2
- pharyngeal tonsil 474.12
- pharyngitis 472.1
- pharynx 478.29
  - lymphoid (infectional) (tissue) (wall) 478.29
- pituitary (fossa) (gland) 253.8
- popliteal fat pad 729.31
- preauricular (lymph) gland (Hampstead) 785.6
- prepuce (congenital) 605
  - female 624.2
- prostate (asymptomatic) (early) (recurrent) 600.9
  - adenofibromatous 600.2
  - benign 600.0
  - congenital 752.8
- pseudoedematous hypodermal 757.0
- pseudomuscular 359.1
- pylorus (muscle) (sphincter) 537.0
  - congenital 750.5
  - infantile 750.5
- rectal sphincter 569.49
- rectum 569.49
- renal 593.1
- rhinitis (turbinate) 472.0

Hypertrophy, hypertrophic — *continued*
- salivary duct or gland 527.1
  - congenital 750.26
- scaphoid (tarsal) 733.99
- scar 701.4
- scrotum 608.89
- sella turcica 253.8
- seminal vesicle 608.89
- sigmoid 569.89
- skin condition NEC 701.9
- spermatic cord 608.89
- spinal ligament 728.9
- spleen — *see* Splenomegaly
- spondylitis (spine) (*see also* Spondylosis) 721.90
- stomach 537.89
- subaortic stenosis (idiopathic) 425.1
- sublingual gland 527.1
  - congenital 750.26
- submaxillary gland 527.1
- suprarenal (gland) 255.8
- tendon 727.9
- testis 608.89
  - congenital 752.8
- thymic, thymus (congenital) (gland) 254.0
- thyroid (gland) (*see also* Goiter) 240.9
  - primary 242.0 ✓5ᵗʰ
  - secondary 242.2 ✓5ᵗʰ
- toe (congenital) 755.65
  - acquired 735.8
- tongue 529.8
  - congenital 750.15
  - frenum 529.8
  - papillae (foliate) 529.3
- tonsil (faucial) (infective) (lingual) (lymphoid) 474.11
  - with
    - adenoiditis 474.01
    - tonsillitis 474.00
      - and adenoiditis 474.02
  - and adenoids 474.10
- tunica vaginalis 608.89
- turbinate (mucous membrane) 478.0
- ureter 593.89
- urethra 599.84
- uterus 621.2
  - puerperal, postpartum 674.8 ✓5ᵗʰ
- uvula 528.9
- vagina 623.8
- vas deferens 608.89
- vein 459.89
- ventricle, ventricular (heart) (left) (right) — *see also* Hypertrophy, cardiac
  - congenital 746.89
  - due to hypertension (left) (right) (*see also* Hypertension, heart) 402.90
    - benign 402.10
    - malignant 402.00
  - right with ventricular septal defect, pulmonary stenosis or atresia, and dextraposition of aorta 745.2
- verumontanum 599.89
- vesical 596.8
- vocal cord 478.5
- vulva 624.3
  - stasis (nonfilarial) 624.3

Hypertropia (intermittent) (periodic) 378.31
Hypertyrosinemia 270.2
Hyperuricemia 790.6
Hypervalinemia 270.3
Hyperventilation (tetany) 786.01
- hysterical 300.11
- psychogenic 306.1
- syndrome 306.1

Hyperviscidosis 277.00
Hyperviscosity (of serum) (syndrome) NEC 273.3
- polycythemic 289.0
- sclerocythemic 282.8

Hypervitaminosis (dietary) NEC 278.8
- A (dietary) 278.2
- D (dietary) 278.4
- from excessive administration or use of vitamin preparations (chronic) 278.8
  - reaction to sudden overdose 963.5

Index to Diseases

Hypervitaminosis (dietary) NEC
  from excessive administration or use of vitamin preparations — *continued*
    vitamin A 278.2
      reaction to sudden overdose 963.5
    vitamin D 278.4
      reaction to sudden overdose 963.5
    vitamin K
      correct substance properly administered 278.8
      overdose or wrong substance given or taken 964.3
Hypervolemia 276.6
Hypesthesia (*see also* Disturbance, sensation) 782.0
  cornea 371.81
Hyphema (anterior chamber) (ciliary body) (iris) 364.41
  traumatic 921.3
Hyphemia — *see* Hyphema
Hypoacidity, gastric 536.8
  psychogenic 306.4
Hypoactive labyrinth (function) — *see* Hypofunction, labyrinth
Hypoadrenalism 255.4
  tuberculous (*see also* Tuberculosis) 017.6
Hypoadrenocorticism 255.4
  pituitary 253.4
Hypoalbuminemia 273.8
Hypoalphalipoproteinemia 272.5
Hypobarism 993.2
Hypobaropathy 993.2
Hypobetalipoproteinemia (familial) 272.5
Hypocalcemia 275.41
  cow's milk 775.4
  dietary 269.3
  neonatal 775.4
  phosphate-loading 775.4
Hypocalcification, teeth 520.4
Hypochloremia 276.9
Hypochlorhydria 536.8
  neurotic 306.4
  psychogenic 306.4
Hypocholesteremia 272.5
Hypochondria (reaction) 300.7
Hypochondriac 300.7
Hyponchondriasis 300.7
Hypochromasia blood cells 280.9
Hypochromic anemia 280.9
  due to blood loss (chronic) 280.0
    acute 285.1
  microcytic 280.9
Hypocoagulability (*see also* Defect, coagulation) 286.9
Hypocomplementemia 279.8
Hypocythemia (progressive) 284.9
Hypodontia (*see also* Anodontia) 520.0
Hypoeosinophilia 288.8
Hypoesthesia (*see also* Disturbance, sensation) 782.0
  cornea 371.81
  tactile 782.0
Hypoestrinism 256.39
Hypoestrogenism 256.39
Hypoferremia 280.9
  due to blood loss (chronic) 280.0
Hypofertility
  female 628.9
  male 606.1
Hypofibrinogenemia 286.3
  acquired 286.6
  congenital 286.3
Hypofunction
  adrenal (gland) 255.4
    cortex 255.4
    medulla 255.5
    specified NEC 255.5
  cerebral 331.9
  corticoadrenal NEC 255.4
  intestinal 564.89

Hypofunction — *continued*
  labyrinth (unilateral) 386.53
    with loss of labyrinthine reactivity 386.55
    bilateral 386.54
      with loss of labyrinthine reactivity 386.56
  Leydig cell 257.2
  ovary 256.39
    postablative 256.2
  pituitary (anterior) (gland) (lobe) 253.2
    posterior 253.5
  testicular 257.2
    iatrogenic 257.1
    postablative 257.1
    postirradiation 257.1
    postsurgical 257.1
Hypogammaglobulinemia 279.00
  acquired primary 279.06
  non-sex-linked, congenital 279.06
  sporadic 279.06
  transient of infancy 279.09
Hypogenitalism (congenital) (female) (male) 752.8
  penis 752.69
Hypoglycemia (spontaneous) 251.2
  coma 251.0
    diabetic 250.3
  diabetic 250.8
  due to insulin 251.0
    therapeutic misadventure 962.3
  familial (idiopathic) 251.2
  following gastrointestinal surgery 579.3
  infantile (idiopathic) 251.2
  in infant of diabetic mother 775.0
  leucine-induced 270.3
  neonatal 775.6
  reactive 251.2
  specified NEC 251.1
Hypoglycemic shock 251.0
  diabetic 250.8
  due to insulin 251.0
  functional (syndrome) 251.1
Hypogonadism
  female 256.39
  gonadotrophic (isolated) 253.4
  hypogonadotropic (isolated) (with anosmia) 253.4
  isolated 253.4
  male 257.2
  ovarian (primary) 256.39
  pituitary (secondary) 253.4
  testicular (primary) (secondary) 257.2
Hypohidrosis 705.0
Hypohidrotic ectodermal dysplasia 757.31
Hypoidrosis 705.0
Hypoinsulinemia, postsurgical 251.3
  postpancreatectomy (complete) (partial) 251.3
Hypokalemia 276.8
Hypokinesia 780.99 ▲
Hypoleukia splenica 289.4
Hypoleukocytosis 288.8
Hypolipidemia 272.5
Hypolipoproteinemia 272.5
Hypomagnesemia 275.2
  neonatal 775.4
Hypomania, hypomanic reaction (*see also* Psychosis, affective) 296.0
  recurrent episode 296.1
  single episode 296.0
Hypomastia (congenital) 757.6
Hypomenorrhea 626.1
Hypometabolism 783.9
Hypomotility
  gastrointestinal tract 536.8
    psychogenic 306.4
  intestine 564.89
    psychogenic 306.4
  stomach 536.8
    psychogenic 306.4
Hyponasality 784.49
Hyponatremia 276.1
Hypo-ovarianism 256.39
Hypo-ovarism 256.39

Hypoparathyroidism (idiopathic) (surgically induced) 252.1
  neonatal 775.4
Hypopharyngitis 462
Hypophoria 378.40
Hypophosphatasia 275.3
Hypophosphatemia (acquired) (congenital) (familial) 275.3
  renal 275.3
Hypophyseal, hypophysis — *see also* condition
  dwarfism 253.3
  gigantism 253.0
  syndrome 253.8
Hypophyseothalamic syndrome 253.8
Hypopiesis — *see* Hypotension
Hypopigmentation 709.00
  eyelid 374.53
Hypopinealism 259.8
Hypopituitarism (juvenile) (syndrome) 253.2
  due to
    hormone therapy 253.7
    hypophysectomy 253.7
    radiotherapy 253.7
  postablative 253.7
  postpartum hemorrhage 253.2
Hypoplasia, hypoplasis 759.89
  adrenal (gland) 759.1
  alimentary tract 751.8
    lower 751.2
    upper 750.8
  anus, anal (canal) 751.2
  aorta 747.22
  aortic
    arch (tubular) 747.10
    orifice or valve with hypoplasia of ascending aorta and defective development of left ventricle (with mitral valve atresia) 746.7
  appendix 751.2
  areola 757.6
  arm (*see also* Absence, arm, congenital) 755.20
  artery (congenital) (peripheral) NEC 747.60
    brain 747.81
    cerebral 747.81
    coronary 746.85
    gastrointestinal 747.61
    lower limb 747.64
    pulmonary 747.3
    renal 747.62
    retinal 743.58
    specified NEC 747.69
    spinal 747.82
    umbilical 747.5
    upper limb 747.63
  auditory canal 744.29
    causing impairment of hearing 744.02
  biliary duct (common) or passage 751.61
  bladder 753.8
  bone NEC 756.9
    face 756.0
    malar 756.0
    mandible 524.04
      alveolar 524.74
    marrow 284.9
      acquired (secondary) 284.8
      congenital 284.0
      idiopathic 284.9
    maxilla 524.03
      alveolar 524.73
    skull (*see also* Hypoplasia, skull) 756.0
  brain 742.1
    gyri 742.2
    specified part 742.2
  breast (areola) 757.6
  bronchus (tree) 748.3
  cardiac 746.89
    valve — *see* Hypoplasia, heart, valve
    vein 746.89
  carpus (*see also* Absence, carpal, congenital) 755.28
  cartilaginous 756.9
  cecum 751.2
  cementum 520.4
    hereditary 520.5
  cephalic 742.1

Hypoplasia, hypoplasis — *continued*
- cerebellum 742.2
- cervix (uteri) 752.49
- chin 524.06
- clavicle 755.51
- coccyx 756.19
- colon 751.2
- corpus callosum 742.2
- cricoid cartilage 748.3
- dermal, focal (Goltz) 757.39
- digestive organ(s) or tract NEC 751.8
  - lower 751.2
  - upper 750.8
- ear 744.29
  - auricle 744.23
  - lobe 744.29
  - middle, except ossicles 744.03
    - ossicles 744.04
  - ossicles 744.04
- enamel of teeth (neonatal) (postnatal) (prenatal) 520.4
  - hereditary 520.5
- endocrine (gland) NEC 759.2
- endometrium 621.8
- epididymis 752.8
- epiglottis 748.3
- erythroid, congenital 284.0
- erythropoietic, chronic acquired 284.8
- esophagus 750.3
- Eustachian tube 744.24
- eye (*see also* Microphthalmos) 743.10
  - lid 743.62
- face 744.89
  - bone(s) 756.0
- fallopian tube 752.19
- femur (*see also* Absence, femur, congenital) 755.34
- fibula (*see also* Absence, fibula, congenital) 755.37
- finger (*see also* Absence, finger, congenital) 755.29
- focal dermal 757.39
- foot 755.31
- gallbladder 751.69
- genitalia, genital organ(s)
  - female 752.8
    - external 752.49
    - internal NEC 752.8
  - in adiposogenital dystrophy 253.8
  - male 752.8
    - penis 752.69
- glottis 748.3
- hair 757.4
- hand 755.21
- heart 746.89
  - left (complex) (syndrome) 746.7
  - valve NEC 746.89
    - pulmonary 746.01
- humerus (*see also* Absence, humerus, congenital) 755.24
- hymen 752.49
- intestine (small) 751.1
  - large 751.2
- iris 743.46
- jaw 524.09
- kidney(s) 753.0
- labium (majus) (minus) 752.49
- labyrinth, membranous 744.05
- lacrimal duct (apparatus) 743.65
- larynx 748.3
- leg (*see also* Absence, limb, congenital, lower) 755.30
- limb 755.4
  - lower (*see also* Absence, limb, congenital, lower) 755.30
  - upper (*see also* Absence, limb, congenital, upper) 755.20
- liver 751.69
- lung (lobe) 748.5
- mammary (areolar) 757.6
- mandibular 524.04
  - alveolar 524.74
  - unilateral condylar 526.89
- maxillary 524.03
  - alveolar 524.73
- medullary 284.9
- megakaryocytic 287.3

Hypoplasia, hypoplasis — *continued*
- metacarpus (*see also* Absence, metacarpal, congenital) 755.28
- metatarsus (*see also* Absence, metatarsal, congenital) 755.38
- muscle 756.89
  - eye 743.69
- myocardium (congenital) (Uhl's anomaly) 746.84
- nail(s) 757.5
- nasolacrimal duct 743.65
- nervous system NEC 742.8
- neural 742.8
- nose, nasal 748.1
- ophthalmic (*see also* Microphthalmos) 743.10
- organ
  - of Corti 744.05
  - or site NEC — *see* Anomaly, by site
- osseous meatus (ear) 744.03
- ovary 752.0
- oviduct 752.19
- pancreas 751.7
- parathyroid (gland) 759.2
- parotid gland 750.26
- patella 755.64
- pelvis, pelvic girdle 755.69
- penis 752.69
- peripheral vascular system (congenital) NEC 747.60
  - gastrointestinal 747.61
  - lower limb 747.64
  - renal 747.62
  - specified NEC 747.69
  - spinal 747.82
  - upper limb 747.63
- pituitary (gland) 759.2
- pulmonary 748.5
  - arteriovenous 747.3
  - artery 747.3
  - valve 746.01
- punctum lacrimale 743.65
- radioulnar (*see also* Absence, radius, congenital, with ulna) 755.25
- radius (*see also* Absence, radius, congenital) 755.26
- rectum 751.2
- respiratory system NEC 748.9
- rib 756.3
- sacrum 756.19
- scapula 755.59
- shoulder girdle 755.59
- skin 757.39
- skull (bone) 756.0
  - with
    - anencephalus 740.0
    - encephalocele 742.0
    - hydrocephalus 742.3
      - with spina bifida (*see also* Spina bifida) 741.0 ✓5ᵗʰ
    - microcephalus 742.1
- spinal (cord) (ventral horn cell) 742.59
  - vessel 747.82
- spine 756.19
- spleen 759.0
- sternum 756.3
- tarsus (*see also* Absence, tarsal, congenital) 755.38
- testis, testicle 752.8
- thymus (gland) 279.11
- thyroid (gland) 243
  - cartilage 748.3
- tibiofibular (*see also* Absence, tibia, congenital, with fibula) 755.35
- toe (*see also* Absence, toe, congenital) 755.39
- tongue 750.16
- trachea (cartilage) (rings) 748.3
- Turner's (tooth) 520.4
- ulna (*see also* Absence, ulna, congenital) 755.27
- umbilical artery 747.5
- ureter 753.29
- uterus 752.3
- vagina 752.49
- vascular (peripheral) NEC (*see also* Hypoplasia, peripheral vascular system) 747.60
  - brain 747.81

Hypoplasia, hypoplasis — *continued*
- vein(s) (peripheral) NEC (*see also* Hypoplasia, peripheral vascular system) 747.60
  - brain 747.81
  - cardiac 746.89
  - great 747.49
  - portal 747.49
  - pulmonary 747.49
  - vena cava (inferior) (superior) 747.49
- vertebra 756.19
- vulva 752.49
- zonule (ciliary) 743.39
- zygoma 738.12

Hypopotassemia 276.8
Hypoproaccelerinemia (*see also* Defect, coagulation) 286.3
Hypoproconvertinemia (congenital) (*see also* Defect, coagulation) 286.3
Hypoproteinemia (essential) (hypermetabolic) (idiopathic) 273.8
Hypoproteinosis 260
Hypoprothrombinemia (congenital) (hereditary) (idiopathic) (*see also* Defect, coagulation) 286.3
- acquired 286.7
- newborn 776.3

Hypopselaphesia 782.0
Hypopyon (anterior chamber) (eye) 364.05
- iritis 364.05
- ulcer (cornea) 370.04

Hypopyrexia 780.99 ▲
Hyporeflex 796.1
Hyporeninemia, extreme 790.99
- in primary aldosteronism 255.1

Hyporesponsive episode 780.09
Hyposecretion
- ACTH 253.4
- ovary 256.39
  - postblative 256.2
- salivary gland (any) 527.7

Hyposegmentation of neutrophils, hereditary 288.2
Hyposiderinemia 280.9
Hyposmolality 276.1
- syndrome 276.1

Hyposomatotropism 253.3
Hyposomnia (*see also* Insomnia) 780.52
Hypospadias (male) 752.61
- female 753.8

Hypospermatogenesis 606.1
Hyposphagma 372.72
Hyposplenism 289.59
Hypostasis, pulmonary 514
Hypostatic — *see* condition
Hyposthenuria 593.89
Hyposuprarenalism 255.4
Hypo-TBG-nemia 246.8
Hypotension (arterial) (constitutional) 458.9
- chronic 458.1
- iatrogenic 458.2
- maternal, syndrome (following labor and delivery) 669.2 ✓5ᵗʰ
- orthostatic (chronic) 458.0
  - dysautonomic-dyskinetic syndrome 333.0
- permanent idiopathic 458.1
- postoperative 458.2
- postural 458.0
- specified type NEC 458.8
- transient 796.3

Hypothermia (accidental) 991.6
- anesthetic 995.89
- newborn NEC 778.3
- not associated with low environmental temperature 780.99 ▲

Hypothymergasia (*see also* Psychosis, affective) 296.2 ✓5ᵗʰ
- recurrent episode 296.3 ✓5ᵗʰ
- single episode 296.2 ✓5ᵗʰ

Hypothyroidism (acquired) 244.9
- complicating pregnancy, childbirth, or puerperium 648.1 ✓5ᵗʰ
- congenital 243

Hypothyroidism — *continued*
  due to
    ablation 244.1
      radioactive iodine 244.1
        surgical 244.0
    iodine (administration) (ingestion) 244.2
      radioactive 244.1
    irradiation therapy 244.1
    p-aminosalicylic acid (PAS) 244.3
    phenylbutazone 244.3
    resorcinol 244.3
    specified cause NEC 244.8
    surgery 244.0
  goitrous (sporadic) 246.1
  iatrogenic NEC 244.3
  iodine 244.2
  pituitary 244.8
  postablative NEC 244.1
  postsurgical 244.0
  primary 244.9
  secondary NEC 244.8
  specified cause NEC 244.8
  sporadic goitrous 246.1
Hypotonia, hypotonicity, hypotony 781.3
  benign congenital 358.8
  bladder 596.4
  congenital 779.89 ▲
    benign 358.8
  eye 360.30
    due to
      fistula 360.32
        ocular disorder NEC 360.33
    following loss of aqueous or vitreous 360.33
    primary 360.31
  infantile muscular (benign) 359.0
  muscle 728.9
  uterus, uterine (contractions) — *see* Inertia, uterus
Hypotrichosis 704.09
  congenital 757.4
  lid (congenital) 757.4
    acquired 374.55
  postinfectional NEC 704.09
Hypotropia 378.32
Hypoventilation 786.09
Hypovitaminosis (*see also* Deficiency, vitamin) 269.2
Hypovolemia 276.5
  surgical shock 998.0
  traumatic (shock) 958.4
Hypoxemia (*see also* Anoxia) 799.0
Hypoxia (*see also* Anoxia) 799.0
  cerebral 348.1
    during or resulting from a procedure 997.01
    newborn 768.9
      mild or moderate 768.6
      severe 768.5
  fetal, affecting newborn 768.9 ▲
  intrauterine — *see* Distress, fetal
  myocardial (*see also* Insufficiency, coronary) 411.89
    arteriosclerotic — *see* Arteriosclerosis, coronary
  newborn 768.9 ▲
Hypsarrhythmia (*see also* Epilepsy) 345.6 ✓5ᵗʰ
Hysteralgia, pregnant uterus 646.8 ✓5ᵗʰ
Hysteria, hysterical 300.10
  anxiety 300.20
  Charcôt's gland 300.11
  conversion (any manifestation) 300.11
  dissociative type NEC 300.15
  psychosis, acute 298.1
Hysteroepilepsy 300.11
Hysterotomy, affecting fetus or newborn 763.89

I

Iatrogenic syndrome of excess cortisol 255.0
Iceland disease (epidemic neuromyasthenia) 049.8
Ichthyosis (congenita) 757.1
  acquired 701.1
  fetalis gravior 757.1

Ichthyosis — *continued*
  follicularis 757.1
  hystrix 757.39
  lamellar 757.1
  lingual 528.6
  palmaris and plantaris 757.39
  simplex 757.1
  vera 757.1
  vulgaris 757.1
Ichthyotoxism 988.0
  bacterial (*see also* Poisoning, food) 005.9
Icteroanemia, hemolytic (acquired) 283.9
  congenital (*see also* Spherocytosis) 282.0
Icterus (*see also* Jaundice) 782.4
  catarrhal — *see* Icterus, infectious
  conjunctiva 782.4
    newborn 774.6
  epidemic — *see* Icterus, infectious
  febrilis — *see* Icterus, infectious
  fetus or newborn — *see* Jaundice, fetus or newborn
  gravis (*see also* Necrosis, liver) 570
    complicating pregnancy 646.7 ✓5ᵗʰ
      affecting fetus or newborn 760.8
    fetus or newborn NEC 773.0
    obstetrical 646.7 ✓5ᵗʰ
      affecting fetus or newborn 760.8
  hematogenous (acquired) 283.9
  hemolytic (acquired) 283.9
    congenital (*see also* Spherocytosis) 282.0
  hemorrhagic (acute) 100.0
    leptospiral 100.0
    newborn 776.0
    spirochetal 100.0
  infectious 070.1
    with hepatic coma 070.0
    leptospiral 100.0
    spirochetal 100.0
  intermittens juvenilis 277.4
  malignant (*see also* Necrosis, liver) 570
  neonatorum (*see also* Jaundice, fetus or newborn) 774.6
  pernicious (*see also* Necrosis, liver) 570
  spirochetal 100.0
Ictus solaris, solis 992.0
Identity disorder 313.82
  dissociative 300.14
  gender role (child) 302.6
    adult 302.85
  psychosexual (child) 302.6
    adult 302.85
Idioglossia 307.9
Idiopathic — *see* condition
Idiosyncrasy (*see also* Allergy) 995.3
  drug, medicinal substance, and biological — *see* Allergy, drug
Idiot, idiocy (congenital) 318.2
  amaurotic (Bielschowsky) (-Jansky) (family) (infantile (late)) (juvenile (late)) (Vogt-Spielmeyer) 330.1
  microcephalic 742.1
  Mongolian 758.0
  oxycephalic 756.0
Id reaction (due to bacteria) 692.89
IgE asthma 493.0 ✓5ᵗʰ
Ileitis (chronic) (*see also* Enteritis) 558.9
  infectious 009.0
  noninfectious 558.9
  regional (ulcerative) 555.0
    with large intestine 555.2
  segmental 555.0
    with large intestine 555.2
  terminal (ulcerative) 555.0
    with large intestine 555.2
Ileocolitis (*see also* Enteritis) 558.9
  infectious 009.0
  regional 555.2
  ulcerative 556.1
Ileostomy status V44.2
  with complication 569.60
Ileotyphus 002.0
Ileum — *see* condition

Ileus (adynamic) (bowel) (colon) (inhibitory) (intestine) (neurogenic) (paralytic) 560.1
  arteriomesenteric duodenal 537.2
  due to gallstone (in intestine) 560.31
  duodenal, chronic 537.2
  following gastrointestinal surgery 997.4
  gallstone 560.31
  mechanical (*see also* Obstruction, intestine) 560.9
  meconium 777.1
    due to cystic fibrosis 277.01
  myxedema 564.89
  postoperative 997.4
  transitory, newborn 777.4
Iliac — *see* condition
Iliotibial band friction syndrome 728.89
Ill, louping 063.1
Illegitimacy V61.6
Illness — *see also* Disease
  factitious 300.19
    with
      combined physical and psychological symptoms 300.19
      physical symptoms 300.19
      psychological symptoms 300.16
    chronic (with physical symptoms) 301.51
  heart — *see* Disease, heart
  manic-depressive (*see also* Psychosis, affective) 296.80
  mental (*see also* Disorder, mental) 300.9
Imbalance 781.2
  autonomic (*see also* Neuropathy, peripheral, autonomic) 337.9
  electrolyte 276.9
    with
      abortion — *see* Abortion, by type, with metabolic disorder
      ectopic pregnancy (*see also* categories 633.0-633.9) 639.4
      hyperemesis gravidarum (before 22 completed weeks gestation) 643.1 ✓5ᵗʰ
      molar pregnancy (*see also* categories 630-632) 639.4
    following
      abortion 639.4
      ectopic or molar pregnancy 639.4
    neonatal, transitory NEC 775.5
  endocrine 259.9
  eye muscle NEC 378.9
    heterophoria — *see* Heterophoria
  glomerulotubular NEC 593.89
  hormone 259.9
  hysterical (*see also* Hysteria) 300.10
  labyrinth NEC 386.50
  posture 729.9
  sympathetic (*see also* Neuropathy, peripheral, autonomic) 337.9
Imbecile, imbecility 318.0
  moral 301.7
  old age 290.9
  senile 290.9
  specified IQ — *see* IQ
  unspecified IQ 318.0
Imbedding, intrauterine device 996.32
Imbibition, cholesterol (gallbladder) 575.6
Imerslund (-Gräsbeck) syndrome (anemia due to familial selective vitamin B_{12} malabsorption) 281.1
Iminoacidopathy 270.8
Iminoglycinuria, familial 270.8
Immature — *see also* Immaturity
  personality 301.89
Immaturity 765.1 ✓5ᵗʰ
  extreme 765.0 ✓5ᵗʰ
  fetus or infant light-for-dates — *see* Light-for-dates
  lung, fetus or newborn 770.4
  organ or site NEC — *see* Hypoplasia
  pulmonary, fetus or newborn 770.4
  reaction 301.89
  sexual (female) (male) 259.0

Immersion 994.1
- foot 991.4
- hand 991.4

Immobile, immobility
- intestine 564.89
- joint — see Ankylosis
- syndrome (paraplegic) 728.3

Immunization
- ABO
  - affecting management of pregnancy 656.2 ✓5ᵗʰ
    - fetus or newborn 773.1
  - complication — see Complications, vaccination
- Rh factor
  - affecting management of pregnancy 656.1 ✓5ᵗʰ
    - fetus or newborn 773.0
  - from transfusion 999.7

Immunodeficiency 279.3
- with
  - adenosine-deaminase deficiency 279.2
  - defect, predominant
    - B-cell 279.00
    - T-cell 279.10
  - hyperimmunoglobulinemia 279.2
  - lymphopenia, hereditary 279.2
  - thrombocytopenia and eczema 279.12
  - thymic
    - aplasia 279.2
    - dysplasia 279.2
- autosomal recessive, Swiss-type 279.2
- common variable 279.06
- severe combined (SCID) 279.2
- to Rh factor
  - affecting management of pregnancy 656.1 ✓5ᵗʰ
    - fetus or newborn 773.0
- X-linked, with increased IgM 279.05

Immunotherapy, prophylactic V07.2

Impaction, impacted
- bowel, colon, rectum 560.30
  - with hernia — see also Hernia, by site, with obstruction
    - gangrenous — see Hernia, by site, with gangrene
  - by
    - calculus 560.39
    - gallstone 560.31
  - fecal 560.39
  - specified type NEC 560.39
- calculus — see Calculus
- cerumen (ear) (external) 380.4
- cuspid 520.6
  - with abnormal position (same or adjacent tooth) 524.3
- dental 520.6
  - with abnormal position (same or adjacent tooth) 524.3
- fecal, feces 560.39
  - with hernia — see also Hernia, by site, with obstruction
    - gangrenous — see Hernia, by site, with gangrene
- fracture — see Fracture, by site
- gallbladder — see Cholelithiasis
- gallstone(s) — see Cholelithiasis
  - in intestine (any part) 560.31
- intestine(s) 560.30
  - with hernia — see also Hernia, by site, with obstruction
    - grangrenous — see Hernia, by site, with gangrene
  - by
    - calculus 560.39
    - gallstone 560.31
  - fecal 560.39
  - specified type NEC 560.39
- intrauterine device (IUD) 996.32
- molar 520.6
  - with abnormal position (same or adjacent tooth) 524.3
- shoulder 660.4 ✓5ᵗʰ
  - affecting fetus or newborn 763.1
- tooth, teeth 520.6
  - with abnormal position (same or adjacent tooth) 524.3

Impaction, impacted — continued
- turbinate 733.99

Impaired, impairment (function)
- arm V49.1
  - movement, involving
    - musculoskeletal system V49.1
    - nervous system V49.2
- auditory discrimination 388.43
- back V48.3
- body (entire) V49.89
- hearing (see also Deafness) 389.9
- heart — see Disease, heart
- kidney (see also Disease, renal) 593.9
  - disorder resulting from 588.9
    - specified NEC 588.8
- leg V49.1
  - movement, involving
    - musculoskeletal system V49.1
    - nervous system V49.2
- limb V49.1
  - movement, involving
    - musculoskeletal system V49.1
    - nervous system V49.2
- liver 573.8
- mastication 524.9
- mobility
  - ear ossicles NEC 385.22
  - incostapedial joint 385.22
  - malleus 385.21
- myocardium, myocardial (see also Insufficiency, myocardial) 428.0
- neuromusculoskeletal NEC V49.89
  - back V48.3
  - head V48.2
  - limb V49.2
  - neck V48.3
  - spine V48.3
  - trunk V48.3
- rectal sphincter 787.99
- renal (see also Disease, renal) 593.9
  - disorder resulting from 588.9
    - specified NEC 588.8
- spine V48.3
- vision NEC 369.9
  - both eyes NEC 369.3
  - moderate 369.74
    - both eyes 369.25
      - with impairment of lesser eye (specified as)
        - blind, not further specified 369.15
        - low vision, not further specified 369.23
        - near-total 369.17
        - profound 369.18
        - severe 369.24
        - total 369.16
    - one eye 369.74
      - with vision of other eye (specified as)
        - near-normal 369.75
        - normal 369.76
  - near-total 369.64
    - both eyes 369.04
      - with impairment of lesser eye (specified as)
        - blind, not further specified 369.02
        - total 369.03
    - one eye 369.64
      - with vision of other eye (specified as)
        - near normal 369.65
        - normal 369.66
  - one eye 369.60
    - with low vision of other eye 369.10
  - profound 369.67
    - both eyes 369.08
      - with impairment of lesser eye (specified as)
        - blind, not further specified 369.05
        - near-total 369.07
        - total 369.06
    - one eye 369.67
      - with vision of other eye (specified as)
        - near-normal 369.68
        - normal 369.69

Impaired, impairment — continued
- vision NEC — continued
  - severe 369.71
    - both eyes 369.22
      - with impairment of lesser eye (specified as)
        - blind, not further specified 369.11
        - low vision, not further specified 369.21
        - near-total 369.13
        - profound 369.14
        - total 369.12
    - one eye 369.71
      - with vision of other eye (specified as)
        - near-normal 369.72
        - normal 369.73
  - total
    - both eyes 369.01
    - one eye 369.61
      - with vision of other eye (specified as)
        - near-normal 369.62
        - normal 369.63

Impaludism — see Malaria

Impediment, speech NEC 784.5
- psychogenic 307.9
- secondary to organic lesion 784.5

Impending
- cerebrovascular accident or attack 435.9
- coronary syndrome 411.1
- delirium tremens 291.0
- myocardial infarction 411.1

Imperception, auditory (acquired) (congenital) 389.9

Imperfect
- aeration, lung (newborn) 770.5
- closure (congenital)
  - alimentary tract NEC 751.8
    - lower 751.5
    - upper 750.8
  - atrioventricular ostium 745.69
  - atrium (secundum) 745.5
    - primum 745.61
  - branchial cleft or sinus 744.41
  - choroid 743.59
  - cricoid cartilage 748.3
  - cusps, heart valve NEC 746.89
    - pulmonary 746.09
  - ductus
    - arteriosus 747.0
    - Botalli 747.0
  - ear drum 744.29
    - causing impairment of hearing 744.03
  - endocardial cushion 745.60
  - epiglottis 748.3
  - esophagus with communication to bronchus or trachea 750.3
  - Eustachian valve 746.89
  - eyelid 743.62
  - face, facial (see also Cleft, lip) 749.10
  - foramen
    - Botalli 745.5
    - ovale 745.5
  - genitalia, genital organ(s) or system
    - female 752.8
      - external 752.49
      - internal NEC 752.8
      - uterus 752.3
    - male 752.8
      - penis 752.69
  - glottis 748.3
  - heart valve (cusps) NEC 746.89
  - interatrial ostium or septum 745.5
  - interauricular ostium or septum 745.5
  - interventricular ostium or septum 745.4
  - iris 743.46
  - kidney 753.3
  - larynx 748.3
  - lens 743.36
  - lip (see also Cleft, lip) 749.10
  - nasal septum or sinus 748.1
  - nose 748.1
  - omphalomesenteric duct 751.0
  - optic nerve entry 743.57
  - organ or site NEC — see Anomaly, specified type, by site

Imperfect — *continued*
  closure — *continued*
    ostium
      interatrial 745.5
      interauricular 745.5
      interventricular 745.4
    palate (*see also* Cleft, palate) 749.00
    preauricular sinus 744.46
    retina 743.56
    roof of orbit 742.0
    sclera 743.47
    septum
      aortic 745.0
      aorticopulmonary 745.0
      atrial (secundum) 745.5
        primum 745.61
      between aorta and pulmonary artery 745.0
      heart 745.9
      interatrial (secundum) 745.5
        primum 745.61
      interauricular (secundum) 745.5
        primum 745.61
      interventricular 745.4
        with pulmonary stenosis or atresia, dextraposition of aorta, and hypertrophy of right ventricle 745.2
          in tetralogy of Fallot 745.2
      nasal 748.1
      ventricular 745.4
        with pulmonary stenosis or atresia, dextraposition of aorta, and hypertrophy of right ventricle 745.2
          in tetralogy of Fallot 745.2
    skull 756.0
      with
        anencephalus 740.0
        encephalocele 742.0
        hydrocephalus 742.3
          with spina bifida (*see also* Spina bifida) 741.0 ✓5ᵗʰ
        microcephalus 742.1
    spine (with meningocele) (*see also* Spina bifida) 741.90
    thyroid cartilage 748.3
    trachea 748.3
    tympanic membrane 744.29
      causing impairment of hearing 744.03
    uterus (with communication to bladder, intestine, or rectum) 752.3
    uvula 749.02
      with cleft lip (*see also* Cleft, palate, with cleft lip) 749.20
    vitelline duct 751.0
  development — *see* Anomaly, by site
  erection 607.84
  fusion — *see* Imperfect, closure
  inflation lung (newborn) 770.5
  intestinal canal 751.5
  poise 729.9
  rotation — *see* Malrotation
  septum, ventricular 745.4
Imperfectly descended testis 752.51
Imperforate (congenital) — *see also* Atresia
  anus 751.2
  bile duct 751.61
  cervix (uteri) 752.49
  esophagus 750.3
  hymen 752.42
  intestine (small) 751.1
    large 751.2
  jejunum 751.1
  pharynx 750.29
  rectum 751.2
  salivary duct 750.23
  urethra 753.6
  urinary meatus 753.6
  vagina 752.49
Impervious (congenital) — *see also* Atresia
  anus 751.2
  bile duct 751.61
  esophagus 750.3
  intestine (small) 751.1
    large 751.5
  rectum 751.2
  urethra 753.6

Impetiginization of other dermatoses 684
Impetigo (any organism) (any site) (bullous) (circinate) (contagiosa) (neonatorum) (simplex) 684
  Bockhart's (superficial folliculitis) 704.8
  external ear 684 [380.13]
  eyelid 684 [373.5]
  Fox's (contagiosa) 684
  furfuracea 696.5
  herpetiformis 694.3
    nonobstetrical 694.3
  staphylococcal infection 684
  ulcerative 686.8
  vulgaris 684
Impingement, soft tissue between teeth 524.2
Implant, endometrial 617.9
Implantation
  anomalous — *see also* Anomaly, specified type, by site
    ureter 753.4
  cyst
    external area or site (skin) NEC 709.8
    iris 364.61
    vagina 623.8
    vulva 624.8
  dermoid (cyst)
    external area or site (skin) NEC 709.8
    iris 364.61
    vagina 623.8
    vulva 624.8
  placenta, low or marginal — *see* Placenta previa
Impotence (sexual) (psychogenic) 302.72
  organic origin NEC 607.84
Impoverished blood 285.9
Impression, basilar 756.0
Imprisonment V62.5
Improper
  development, infant 764.9 ✓5ᵗʰ
Improperly tied umbilical cord (causing hemorrhage) 772.3
Impulses, obsessional 300.3
Impulsive neurosis 300.3
Inaction, kidney (*see also* Disease, renal) 593.9
Inactive — *see* condition
Inadequate, inadequacy
  biologic 301.6
  cardiac and renal — *see* Hypertension, cardiorenal
  constitutional 301.6
  development
    child 783.40
    fetus 764.9 ✓5ᵗʰ
      affecting management of pregnancy 656.5 ✓5ᵗʰ
    genitalia
      after puberty NEC 259.0
      congenital — *see* Hypoplasia, genitalia
    lungs 748.5
    organ or site NEC — *see* Hypoplasia, by site
  dietary 269.9
  education V62.3
  environment
    economic problem V60.2
    household condition NEC V60.1
    poverty V60.2
    unemployment V62.0
  functional 301.6
  household care, due to
    family member
      handicapped or ill V60.4
      temporarily away from home V60.4
        on vacation V60.5
    technical defects in home V60.1
    temporary absence from home of person rendering care V60.4
  housing (heating) (space) V60.1
  material resources V60.2
  mental (*see also* Retardation, mental) 319
  nervous system 799.2
  personality 301.6
  prenatal care in current pregnancy V23.7
  pulmonary
    function 786.09
      newborn 770.89 ▲
    ventilation, newborn 770.89 ▲

Inadequate, inadequacy — *continued*
  respiration 786.09
    newborn 770.89 ▲
  social 301.6
Inanition 263.9
  with edema 262
  due to
    deprivation of food 994.2
    malnutrition 263.9
  fever 780.6
Inappropriate secretion
  ACTH 255.0
  antidiuretic hormone (ADH) (excessive) 253.6
    deficiency 253.5
  ectopic hormone NEC 259.3
  pituitary (posterior) 253.6
Inattention after or at birth 995.52
Inborn errors of metabolism — *see* Disorder, metabolism
Incarceration, incarcerated
  bubonocele — *see also* Hernia, inguinal, with obstruction
    gangrenous — *see* Hernia, inguinal, with gangrene
  colon (by hernia) — *see also* Hernia, by site with obstruction
    gangrenous — *see* Hernia, by site, with gangrene
  enterocele 552.9
    gangrenous 551.9
  epigastrocele 552.29
    gangrenous 551.29
  epiplocele 552.9
    gangrenous 551.9
  exomphalos 552.1
    gangrenous 551.1
  fallopian tube 620.8
  hernia — *see also* Hernia, by site, with obstruction
    gangrenous — *see* Hernia, by site, with gangrene
  iris, in wound 871.1
  lens, in wound 871.1
  merocele — *see also* Hernia, femoral, with obstruction) 552.00
  omentum (by hernia) — *see also* Hernia, by site, with obstruction
    gangrenous — *see* Hernia, by site, with gangrene
  omphalocele 756.79
  rupture (meaning hernia) (*see also* Hernia, by site, with obstruction) 552.9
    gangrenous (*see also* Hernia, by site, with gangrene) 551.9
  sarcoepiplocele 552.9
    gangrenous 551.9
  sarcoepiplomphalocele 552.1
    with gangrene 551.1
  uterus 621.8
    gravid 654.3 ✓5ᵗʰ
      causing obstructed labor 660.2 ✓5ᵗʰ
        affecting fetus or newborn 763.1
Incident, cerebrovascular (*see also* Disease, cerebrovascular, acute) 436
Incineration (entire body) (from fire, conflagration, electricity, or lightning) — *see* Burn, multiple, specified sites
Incised wound
  external — *see* Wound, open, by site
  internal organs (abdomen, chest, or pelvis) — *see* Injury, internal, by site, with open wound
Incision, incisional
  hernia — *see* Hernia, incisional
  surgical, complication — *see* Complications, surgical procedures
  traumatic
    external — *see* Wound, open, by site
    internal organs (abdomen, chest, or pelvis) — *see* Injury, internal, by site, with open wound
Inclusion
  azurophilic leukocytic 288.2
  blennorrhea (neonatal) (newborn) 771.6
  cyst — *see* Cyst, skin
  gallbladder in liver (congenital) 751.69

Incompatibility
  ABO
    affecting management of pregnancy 656.2 ✓5ᵗʰ
    fetus or newborn 773.1
    infusion or transfusion reaction 999.6
  blood (group) (Duffy) (E) (K(ell)) (Kidd) (Lewis) (M) (N) (P) (S) NEC
    affecting management of pregnancy 656.2 ✓5ᵗʰ
    fetus or newborn 773.2
    infusion or transfusion reaction 999.6
  marital V61.10
    involving divorce or estrangement V61.0
  Rh (blood group) (factor)
    affecting management of pregnancy 656.1 ✓5ᵗʰ
    fetus or newborn 773.0
    infusion or transfusion reaction 999.7
  Rhesus — see Incompatibility, Rh

Incompetency, incompetence, incompetent
  annular
  aortic (valve) (see also Insufficiency, aortic) 424.1
  mitral (valve) — (see also Insufficiency, mitral) 424.0
  pulmonary valve (heart) (see also Endocarditis, pulmonary) 424.3
  aortic (valve) (see also Insufficiency, aortic) 424.1
    syphilitic 093.22
  cardiac (orifice) 530.0
    valve — see Endocarditis
  cervix, cervical (os) 622.5
    in pregnancy 654.5 ✓5ᵗʰ
      affecting fetus or newborn 761.0
  esophagogastric (junction) (sphincter) 530.0
  heart valve, congenital 746.89
  mitral (valve) — see Insufficiency, mitral
  papillary muscle (heart) 429.81
  pelvic fundus 618.8
  pulmonary valve (heart) (see also Endocarditis, pulmonary) 424.3
    congenital 746.09
  tricuspid (annular) (rheumatic) (valve) (see also Endocarditis, tricuspid) 397.0
  valvular — see Endocarditis
  vein, venous (saphenous) (varicose) (see also Varicose, vein) 454.9
  velopharyngeal (closure)
    acquired 528.9
    congenital 750.29

Incomplete — see also condition
  bladder emptying 788.21
  expansion lungs (newborn) 770.5
  gestation (liveborn) — see Immaturity
  rotation — see Malrotation

Incontinence 788.30
  without sensory awareness 788.34
  anal sphincter 787.6
  continuous leakage 788.37
  feces 787.6
    due to hysteria 300.11
    nonorganic origin 307.7
  hysterical 300.11
  mixed (male) (female) (urge and stress) 788.33
  overflow 788.39
  paradoxical 788.39
  rectal 787.6
  specified NEC 788.39
  stress (female) 625.6
    male NEC 788.32
  urethral sphincter 599.84
  urge 788.31
    and stress (male) (female) 788.33
  urine 788.30
    active 788.30
    male 788.30
      stress 788.32
        and urge 788.33
      neurogenic 788.39
      nonorganic origin 307.6
      stress (female) 625.6
        male NEC 788.32
      urge 788.31
        and stress 788.33

Incontinentia pigmenti 757.33

Incoordinate
  uterus (action) (contractions) 661.4 ✓5ᵗʰ
    affecting fetus or newborn 763.7

Incoordination
  esophageal-pharyngeal (newborn) 787.2
  muscular 781.3
  papillary muscle 429.81

Increase, increased
  abnormal, in development 783.9
  androgens (ovarian) 256.1
  anticoagulants (antithrombin) (anti-VIIIa) (anti-IXa) (anti-Xa) (anti-XIa) 286.5
    postpartum 666.3 ✓5ᵗʰ
  cold sense (see also Disturbance, sensation) 782.0
  estrogen 256.0
  function
    adrenal (cortex) 255.3
      medulla 255.6
    pituitary (anterior) (gland) (lobe) 253.1
      posterior 253.6
  heat sense (see also Disturbance, sensation) 782.0
  intracranial pressure 781.99
    injury at birth 767.8
  light reflex of retina 362.13
  permeability, capillary 448.9
  pressure
    intracranial 781.99
      injury at birth 767.8
    intraocular 365.00
  pulsations 785.9
  pulse pressure 785.9
  sphericity, lens 743.36
  splenic activity 289.4
  venous pressure 459.89
    portal 572.3

Incrustation, cornea, lead or zinc 930.0
Incyclophoria 378.44
Incyclotropia 378.33
Indeterminate sex 752.7
India rubber skin 756.83
Indicanuria 270.2
Indigestion (bilious) (functional) 536.8
  acid 536.8
  catarrhal 536.8
  due to decomposed food NEC 005.9
  fat 579.8
  nervous 306.4
  psychogenic 306.4

Indirect — see condition
Indolent bubo NEC 099.8
Induced
  abortion — see Abortion, induced
  birth, affecting fetus or newborn 763.89
  delivery — see Delivery
  labor — see Delivery

Induration, indurated
  brain 348.8
  breast (fibrous) 611.79
    puerperal, postpartum 676.3 ✓5ᵗʰ
  broad ligament 620.8
  chancre 091.0
    anus 091.1
    congenital 090.0
    extragenital NEC 091.2
  corpora cavernosa (penis) (plastic) 607.89
  liver (chronic) 573.8
    acute 573.8
  lung (black) (brown) (chronic) (fibroid) (see also Fibrosis, lung) 515
    essential brown 275.0 [516.1]
  penile 607.89
  phlebitic — see Phlebitis
  skin 782.8
  stomach 537.89

Induratio penis plastica 607.89
Industrial — see condition
Inebriety (see also Abuse, drugs, nondependent) 305.0 ✓5ᵗʰ
Inefficiency
  kidney (see also Disease, renal) 593.9
  thyroid (acquired) (gland) 244.9

Inelasticity, skin 782.8

Inequality, leg (acquired) (length) 736.81
  congenital 755.30

Inertia
  bladder 596.4
    neurogenic 596.54
      with cauda equina syndrome 344.61
  stomach 536.8
    psychogenic 306.4
  uterus, uterine 661.2 ✓5ᵗʰ
    affecting fetus or newborn 763.7
    primary 661.0 ✓5ᵗʰ
    secondary 661.1 ✓5ᵗʰ
  vesical 596.4
    neurogenic 596.54
      with cauda equina 344.61

Infant — see also condition
  excessive crying of 780.92 ●
  fussy (baby) 780.91 ●
  held for adoption V68.89
  newborn — see Newborn
  syndrome of diabetic mother 775.0

"Infant Hercules" syndrome 255.2

Infantile — see also condition
  genitalia, genitals 259.0
    in pregnancy or childbirth NEC 654.4 ✓5ᵗʰ
      affecting fetus or newborn 763.89
      causing obstructed labor 660.2 ✓5ᵗʰ
        affecting fetus or newborn 763.1
  heart 746.9
  kidney 753.3
  lack of care 995.52
  macula degeneration 362.75
  melanodontia 521.05
  os, uterus (see also Infantile, genitalia) 259.0
  pelvis 738.6
    with disproportion (fetopelvic) 653.1 ✓5ᵗʰ
      affecting fetus or newborn 763.1
      causing obstructed labor 660.1 ✓5ᵗʰ
        affecting fetus or newborn 763.1
  penis 259.0
  testis 257.2
  uterus (see also Infantile, genitalia) 259.0
  vulva 752.49

Infantilism 259.9
  with dwarfism (hypophyseal) 253.3
  Brissaud's (infantile myxedema) 244.9
  celiac 579.0
  Herter's (nontropical sprue) 579.0
  hypophyseal 253.3
  hypothalamic (with obesity) 253.8
  idiopathic 259.9
  intestinal 579.0
  pancreatic 577.8
  pituitary 253.3
  renal 588.0
  sexual (with obesity) 259.0

Infants, healthy liveborn — see Newborn
Infarct, infarction
  adrenal (capsule) (gland) 255.4
  amnion 658.8 ✓5ᵗʰ
  anterior (with contiguous portion of intraventricular septum) NEC (see also Infarct, myocardium) 410.1 ✓5ᵗʰ
  appendices epiploicae 557.0
  bowel 557.0
  brain (stem) 434.91
    embolic (see also Embolism, brain) 434.11
    healed or old without residuals V12.59
    iatrogenic 997.02
    postoperative 997.02
    puerperal, postpartum, childbirth 674.0 ✓5ᵗʰ
    thrombotic (see also Thrombosis, brain) 434.01
  breast 611.8
  Brewer's (kidney) 593.81
  cardiac (see also Infarct, myocardium) 410.9 ✓5ᵗʰ
  cerebellar (see also Infarct, brain) 434.91
    embolic (see also Embolism, brain) 434.11
  cerebral (see also Infarct, brain) 434.91
    embolic (see also Embolism, brain) 434.11
  chorion 658.8 ✓5ᵗʰ
  colon (acute) (agnogenic) (embolic) (hemorrhagic) (nonocclusive) (nonthrombotic) (occlusive) (segmental) (thrombotic) (with gangrene) 557.0

Index to Diseases

Infarct, infarction — continued

coronary artery (see also Infarct, myocardium) 410.9 ✓5
embolic (see also Embolism) 444.9
fallopian tube 620.8
gallbladder 575.8
heart (see also Infarct, myocardium) 410.9 ✓5
hepatic 573.4
hypophysis (anterior lobe) 253.8
impending (myocardium) 411.1
intestine (acute) (agnogenic) (embolic) (hemorrhagic) (nonocclusive) (nonthrombotic) (occlusive) (thrombotic) (with gangrene) 557.0
kidney 593.81
liver 573.4
lung (embolic) (thrombotic) 415.1 ✓5
  with
    abortion — see Abortion, by type, with embolism
    ectopic pregnancy (see also categories 633.0-633.9) 639.6
    molar pregnancy (see also categories 630-632) 639.6
  following
    abortion 639.6
    ectopic or molar pregnancy 639.6
  iatrogenic 415.11
  in pregnancy, childbirth, or puerperium — see Embolism, obstetrical
  postoperative 415.11
lymph node or vessel 457.8
medullary (brain) — see Infarct, brain
meibomian gland (eyelid) 374.85
mesentary, mesenteric (embolic) (thrombotic) (with gangrene) 557.0
midbrain — see Infarct, brain
myocardium, myocardial (acute or with a stated duration of 8 weeks or less) (with hypertension) 410.9 ✓5

Note — Use the following fifth-digit subclassification with category 410:

  0   episode unspecified
  1   initial episode
  2   subsequent episode without recurrence

  with symptoms after 8 weeks from date of infarction 414.8
  anterior (wall) (with contiguous portion of intraventricular septum) NEC 410.1 ✓5
  anteroapical (with contiguous portion of intraventricular septum) 410.1 ✓5
  anterolateral (wall) 410.0 ✓5
  anteroseptal (with contiguous portion of intraventricular septum) 410.1 ✓5
  apical-lateral 410.8 ✓5
  atrial 410.8 ✓5
  basal-lateral 410.5 ✓5
  chronic (with symptoms after 8 weeks from date of infarction) 414.8
  diagnosed on ECG, but presenting no symptoms 412
  diaphragmatic wall (with contiguous portion of intraventricular septum) 410.4 ✓5
  healed or old, currently presenting no symptoms 412
  high lateral 410.5 ✓5
  impending 411.1
  inferior (wall) (with contiguous portion of intraventricular septum) 410.4 ✓5
  inferolateral (wall) 410.2 ✓5
  inferoposterior wall 410.3 ✓5
  lateral wall 410.5 ✓5
  nontransmural 410.7 ✓5
  papillary muscle 410.8 ✓5
  past (diagnosed on ECG or other special investigation, but currently presenting no symptoms) 412
    with symptoms NEC 414.8
  posterior (strictly) (true) (wall) 410.6 ✓5
  posterobasal 410.6 ✓5
  posteroinferior 410.3 ✓5
  posterolateral 410.5 ✓5

Infarct, infarction — continued

myocardium, myocardial — continued
  previous, currently presenting no symptoms 412
  septal 410.8 ✓5
  specified site NEC 410.8 ✓5
  subendocardial 410.7 ✓5
  syphilitic 093.82
nontransmural 410.7 ✓5
omentum 557.0
ovary 620.8
pancreas 577.8
papillary muscle (see also Infarct, myocardium) 410.8 ✓5
parathyroid gland 252.8
pituitary (gland) 253.8
placenta (complicating pregnancy) 656.7 ✓5
  affecting fetus or newborn 762.2
pontine — see Infarct, brain
posterior NEC (see also Infarct, myocardium) 410.6 ✓5
prostate 602.8
pulmonary (artery) (hemorrhagic) (vein) 415.1 ✓5
  with
    abortion — see Abortion, by type, with embolism
    ectopic pregnancy (see also categories 633.0-633.9) 639.6
    molar pregnancy (see also categories 630-632) 639.6
  following
    abortion 639.6
    ectopic or molar pregnancy 639.6
  iatrogenic 415.11
  in pregnancy, childbirth, or puerperium — see Embolism, obstetrical
  postoperative 415.11
renal 593.81
  embolic or thrombotic 593.81
retina, retinal 362.84
  with occlusion — see Occlusion, retina
spinal (acute) (cord) (embolic) (nonembolic) 336.1
spleen 289.59
  embolic or thrombotic 444.89
subchorionic — see Infarct, placenta
subendocardial (see also Infarct, myocardium) 410.7 ✓5
suprarenal (capsule) (gland) 255.4
syncytium — see Infarct, placenta
testis 608.83
thrombotic (see also Thrombosis) 453.9
  artery, arterial — see Embolism
thyroid (gland) 246.3
ventricle (heart) (see also Infarct, myocardium) 410.9 ✓5

Infecting — see condition

Infection, infected, infective (opportunistic) 136.9

with lymphangitis — see Lymphangitis
abortion — see Abortion, by type, with sepsis
abscess (skin) — see Abscess, by site
Absidia 117.7
Acanthocheilonema (perstans) 125.4
  streptocerca 125.6
accessory sinus (chronic) (see also Sinusitis) 473.9
Achorion — see Dermatophytosis
Acremonium falciforme 117.4
acromioclavicular (joint) 711.91
actinobacillus
  lignieresii 027.8
  mallei 024
  muris 026.1
actinomadura — see Actinomycosis
Actinomyces (israelii) — see also Actinomycosis
  muris-ratti 026.1
Actinomycetales (actinomadura) (Actinomyces) (Nocardia) (Streptomyces) — see Actinomycosis
actinomycotic NEC (see also Actinomycosis) 039.9
adenoid (chronic) 474.01
  acute 463
  and tonsil (chronic) 474.02
    acute or subacute 463

Infection, infected, infective — continued

adenovirus NEC 079.0
  in diseases classified elsewhere — see category 079 ✓4
  unspecified nature or site 079.0
Aerobacter aerogenes NEC 041.85
  enteritis 008.2
aerogenes capsulatus (see also Gangrene, gas) 040.0
aertrycke (see also Infection, Salmonella) 003.9
ajellomyces dermatitidis 116.0
alimentary canal NEC (see also Enteritis, due to, by organism) 009.0
Allescheria boydii 117.6
Alternaria 118
alveolus, alveolar (process) (pulpal origin) 522.4
ameba, amebic (histolytica) (see also Amebiasis) 006.9
  acute 006.0
  chronic 006.1
  free-living 136.2
  hartmanni 007.8
  specified
    site NEC 006.8
    type NEC 007.8
amniotic fluid or cavity 658.4 ✓5
  affecting fetus or newborn 762.7
anaerobes (cocci) (gram-negative) (gram-positive) (mixed) NEC 041.84
anal canal 569.49
Ancylostoma braziliense 126.2
Angiostrongylus cantonensis 128.8
anisakiasis 127.1
Anisakis larva 127.1
anthrax (see also Anthrax) 022.9
antrum (chronic) (see also Sinusitis, maxillary) 473.0
anus (papillae) (sphincter) 569.49
arbor virus NEC 066.9
arbovirus NEC 066.9
argentophil-rod 027.0
Ascaris lumbricoides 127.0
ascomycetes 117.4
Aspergillus (flavus) (fumigatus) (terreus) 117.3
atypical
  acid-fast (bacilli) (see also Mycobacterium, atypical) 031.9
  mycobacteria (see also Mycobacterium, atypical) 031.9
auditory meatus (circumscribed) (diffuse) (external) (see also Otitis, externa) 380.10
auricle (ear) (see also Otitis, externa) 380.10
axillary gland 683
Babesiasis 088.82
Babesiosis 088.82
Bacillus NEC 041.89
  abortus 023.1
  anthracis (see also Anthrax) 022.9
  cereus (food poisoning) 005.89
  coli — see Infection, Escherichia coli
  coliform NEC 041.85
  Ducrey's (any location) 099.0
  Flexner's 004.1
  fragilis NEC 041.82
  Friedländer's NEC 041.3
  fusiformis 101
  gas (gangrene) (see also Gangrene, gas) 040.0
  mallei 024
  melitensis 023.0
  paratyphoid, paratyphosus 002.9
    A 002.1
    B 002.2
    C 002.3
  Schmorl's 040.3
  Shiga 004.0
  suipestifer (see also Infection, Salmonella) 003.9
  swimming pool 031.1
  typhosa 002.0
  welchii (see also Gangrene, gas) 040.0
  Whitmore's 025
bacterial NEC 041.9
  specified NEC 041.89
    anaerobic NEC 041.84
    gram-negative NEC 041.85
      anaerobic NEC 041.84

Infection, infected, infective — continued
  Bacterium
    paratyphosum 002.9
      A 002.1
      B 002.2
      C 002.3
    typhosum 002.0
  Bacteroides (fragilis) (melaninogenicus) (oralis) NEC 041.84
  balantidium coli 007.0
  Bartholin's gland 616.8
  Basidiobolus 117.7
  Bedsonia 079.98
    specified NEC 079.88
  bile duct 576.1
  bladder (see also Cystitis) 595.9
  Blastomyces, blastomycotic 116.0
    brasiliensis 116.1
    dermatitidis 116.0
    European 117.5
    Loboi 116.2
    North American 116.0
    South American 116.1
  blood stream — see Septicemia
  bone 730.9 ✓5ᵗʰ
    specified — see Osteomyelitis
  Bordetella 033.9
    bronchiseptica 033.8
    parapertussis 033.1
    pertussis 033.0
  Borrelia
    bergdorfi 088.81
    vincentii (mouth) (pharynx) (tonsil) 101
  brain (see also Encephalitis) 323.9
    late effect — see category 326
    membranes — (see also Meningitis) 322.9
    septic 324.0
      late effect — see category 326
    meninges (see also Meningitis) 320.9
  branchial cyst 744.42
  breast 611.0
    puerperal, postpartum 675.2 ✓5ᵗʰ
      with nipple 675.9 ✓5ᵗʰ
        specified type NEC 675.8 ✓5ᵗʰ
      nonpurulent 675.2 ✓5ᵗʰ
      purulent 675.1 ✓5ᵗʰ
  bronchus (see also Bronchitis) 490
    fungus NEC 117.9
  Brucella 023.9
    abortus 023.1
    canis 023.3
    melitensis 023.0
    mixed 023.8
    suis 023.2
  Brugia (Wuchereria) malayi 125.1
  bursa — see Bursitis
  buttocks (skin) 686.9
  Candida (albicans) (tropicalis) (see also Candidiasis) 112.9
    congenital 771.7
  Candiru 136.8
  Capillaria
    hepatica 128.8
    philippinensis 127.5
  cartilage 733.99
  cat liver fluke 121.0
  cellulitis — see Cellulitis, by site
  Cephalosporum falciforme 117.4
  Cercomonas hominis (intestinal) 007.3
  cerebrospinal (see also Meningitis) 322.9
    late effect — see category 326
  cervical gland 683
  cervix (see also Cervicitis) 616.0
  cesarean section wound 674.3 ✓5ᵗʰ
  Chilomastix (intestinal) 007.8
  Chlamydia 079.98
    specified NEC 079.88
  cholera (see also Cholera) 001.9
  chorionic plate 658.8 ✓5ᵗʰ
  Cladosporium
    bantianum 117.8
    carrionii 117.2
    mansoni 111.1
    trichoides 117.8
    wernecki 111.1
  Clonorchis (sinensis) (liver) 121.1

Infection, infected, infective — continued
  Clostridium (haemolyticum) (novyi) NEC 041.84
    botulinum 005.1
    congenital 771.89 ▲
    histolyticum (see also Gangrene, gas) 040.0
    oedematiens (see also Gangrene, gas) 040.0
    perfringens 041.83
      due to food 005.2
    septicum (see also Gangrene, gas) 040.0
    sordellii (see also Gangrene, gas) 040.0
    welchii (see also Gangrene, gas) 040.0
      due to food 005.2
  Coccidioides (immitis) (see also Coccidioidomycosis) 114.9
  coccus NEC 041.89
  colon (see also Enteritis, due to, by organism) 009.0
    bacillus — see Infection, Escherichia coli
  colostomy or enterostomy 569.61
  common duct 576.1
  complicating pregnancy, childbirth, or puerperium NEC 647.9 ✓5ᵗʰ
    affecting fetus or newborn 760.2
  Condiobolus 117.7
  congenital NEC 771.89 ▲
    Candida albicans 771.7
    chronic 771.2
    clostridial 771.89 ▲
    cytomegalovirus 771.1
    Escherichia coli 771.89 ▲
    hepatitis, viral 771.2
    herpes simplex 771.2
    listeriosis 771.2
    malaria 771.2
    poliomyelitis 771.2
    rubella 771.0
    Salmonella 771.89 ▲
    streptococcal 771.89 ▲
    toxoplasmosis 771.2
    tuberculosis 771.2
    urinary (tract) 771.82 ▲
    vaccinia 771.2
  corpus luteum (see also Salpingo-oophoritis) 614.2
    chronic 614.2
  Corynebacterium diphtheriae — see Diphtheria
  Coxsackie (see also Coxsackie) 079.2
    endocardium 074.22
    heart NEC 074.20
    in diseases classified elsewhere — see category 079 ✓5ᵗʰ
    meninges 047.0
    myocardium 074.23
    pericardium 074.21
    pharynx 074.0
    specified disease NEC 074.8
    unspecified nature or site 079.2
  Cryptococcus neoformans 117.5
  Cryptosporidia 007.4
  Cunninghamella 117.7
  cyst — see Cyst
  Cysticercus cellulosae 123.1
  cytomegalovirus 078.5
    congenital 771.1
  dental (pulpal origin) 522.4
  deuteromycetes 117.4
  Dicrocoelium dendriticum 121.8
  Dipetalonema (perstans) 125.4
    streptocerca 125.6
  diphtherial — see Diphtheria
  Diphyllobothrium (adult) (latum) (pacificum) 123.4
    larval 123.5
  Diplogonoporus (grandis) 123.8
  Dipylidium (caninum) 123.8
  Dirofilaria 125.6
  dog tapeworm 123.8
  Dracunculus medinensis 125.7
  Dreschlera 118
    hawaiiensis 117.8
  Ducrey's bacillus (any site) 099.0
  due to or resulting from
    device, implant, or graft (any) (presence of) — see Complications, infection and inflammation, due to (presence of) any device, implant, or graft classified to 996.0-996.5 NEC

Infection, infected, infective — continued
  due to or resulting from — continued
    injection, inoculation, infusion, transfusion, or vaccination (prophylactic) (therapeutic) 999.3
    injury NEC — see Wound, open, by site, complicated
    surgery 998.59
  duodenum 535.6 ✓5ᵗʰ
  ear — see also Otitis
    external (see also Otitis, externa) 380.10
    inner (see also Labyrinthitis) 386.30
    middle — see Otitis, media
  Eaton's agent NEC 041.81
  Eberthella typhosa 002.0
  Ebola 065.8
  echinococcosis 122.9
  Echinococcus (see also Echinococcus) 122.9
  Echinostoma 121.8
  ECHO virus 079.1
    in diseases classified elsewhere — see category 079 ✓4ᵗʰ
    unspecified nature or site 079.1
  Ehrlichiosis 082.40
    chaffeensis 082.41
    specified type NEC 082.49
  Endamoeba — see Infection, ameba
  endocardium (see also Endocarditis) 421.0
  endocervix (see also Cervicitis) 616.0
  Entamoeba — see Infection, ameba
  enteric (see also Enteritis, due to, by organism) 009.0
  Enterobacter aerogenes NEC 041.85
  Enterobius vermicularis 127.4
  enterococcus NEC 041.04
  enterovirus NEC 079.89
    central nervous system NEC 048
    enteritis 008.67
    meningitis 047.9
  Entomophthora 117.7
  Epidermophyton — see Dermatophytosis
  epidermophytosis — see Dermatophytosis
  episiotomy 674.3 ✓5ᵗʰ
  Epstein-Barr virus 075
    chronic 780.79 [139.8]
  erysipeloid 027.1
  Erysipelothrix (insidiosa) (rhusiopathiae) 027.1
  erythema infectiosum 057.0
  Escherichia coli NEC 041.4
    congenital 771.89 ▲
    enteritis — see Enteritis, E. coli
    generalized 038.42
    intestinal — see Enteritis, E. coli
  ethmoidal (chronic) (sinus) (see also Sinusitis, ethmoidal) 473.2
  Eubacterium 041.84
  Eustachian tube (ear) 381.50
    acute 381.51
    chronic 381.52
  exanthema subitum 057.8
  external auditory canal (meatus) (see also Otitis, externa) 380.10
  eye NEC 360.00
  eyelid 373.9
    specified NEC 373.8
  fallopian tube (see also Salpingo-oophoritis) 614.2
  fascia 728.89
  Fasciola
    gigantica 121.3
    hepatica 121.3
  Fasciolopsis (buski) 121.4
  fetus (intra-amniotic) — see Infection, congenital
  filarial — see Infestation, filarial
  finger (skin) 686.9
    abscess (with lymphangitis) 681.00
      pulp 681.01
    cellulitis (with lymphangitis) 681.00
    distal closed space (with lymphangitis) 681.00
    nail 681.02
      fungus 110.1
  fish tapeworm 123.4
    larval 123.5
  flagellate, intestinal 007.9
  fluke — see Infestation, fluke

Index to Diseases

Infection, infected, infective — *continued*
focal
  teeth (pulpal origin) 522.4
  tonsils 474.00
    and adenoids 474.02
Fonsecaea
  compactum 117.2
  pedrosoi 117.2
food (*see also* Poisoning, food) 005.9
foot (skin) 686.9
  fungus 110.4
Francisella tularensis (*see also* Tularemia) 021.9
frontal sinus (chronic) (*see also* Sinusitis, frontal) 473.1
fungus NEC 117.9
  beard 110.0
  body 110.5
  dermatiacious NEC 117.8
  foot 110.4
  groin 110.3
  hand 110.2
  nail 110.1
  pathogenic to compromised host only 118
  perianal (area) 110.3
  scalp 110.0
  scrotum 110.8
  skin 111.9
    foot 110.4
    hand 110.2
  toenails 110.1
  trachea 117.9
Fusarium 118
Fusobacterium 041.84
gallbladder (*see also* Cholecystitis, acute) 575.0
Gardnerella vaginalis 041.89 ●
gas bacillus (*see also* Gas, gangrene) 040.0
gastric (*see also* Gastritis) 535.5 ✓5ᵗʰ
Gastrodiscoides hominis 121.8
gastroenteric (*see also* Enteritis, due to, by organism) 009.0
gastrointestinal (*see also* Enteritis, due to, by organism) 009.0
gastrostomy 536.41
generalized NEC (*see also* Septicemia) 038.9
genital organ or tract NEC
  female 614.9
    with
      abortion — *see* Abortion, by type, with sepsis
      ectopic pregnancy (*see also* categories 633.0-633.9) 639.0
      molar pregnancy (*see also* categories 630-632) 639.0
    complicating pregnancy 646.6 ✓5ᵗʰ
      affecting fetus or newborn 760.8
    following
      abortion 639.0
      ectopic or molar pregnancy 639.0
    puerperal, postpartum, childbirth 670 ✓4ᵗʰ
      minor or localized 646.6 ✓5ᵗʰ
        affecting fetus or newborn 760.8
  male 608.4
genitourinary tract NEC 599.0
Ghon tubercle, primary (*see also* Tuberculosis) 010.0 ✓5ᵗʰ
Giardia lamblia 007.1
gingival (chronic) 523.1
  acute 523.0
  Vincent's 101
glanders 024
Glenosporopsis amazonica 116.2
Gnathostoma spinigerum 128.1
Gongylonema 125.6
gonococcal NEC (*see also* Gonococcus) 098.0
gram-negative bacilli NEC 041.85
  anaerobic 041.84
guinea worm 125.7
gum (*see also* Infection, gingival) 523.1
Hantavirus 079.81
heart 429.89
Helicobacter pylori (H. pylori) 041.86
helminths NEC 128.9
  intestinal 127.9
    mixed (types classifiable to more than one category in 120.0-127.7) 127.8

Infection, infected, infective — *continued*
helminths NEC — *continued*
  intestinal — *continued*
    specified type NEC 127.7
  specified type NEC 128.8
Hemophilus influenzae NEC 041.5
  generalized 038.41
herpes (simplex) (*see also* Herpes, simplex) 054.9
  congenital 771.2
  zoster (*see also* Herpes, zoster) 053.9
    eye NEC 053.29
Heterophyes heterophyes 121.6
Histoplasma (*see also* Histoplasmosis) 115.90
  capsulatum (*see also* Histoplasmosis, American) 115.00
  duboisii (*see also* Histoplasmosis, African) 115.10
HIV V08
  with symptoms, symptomatic 042
hookworm (*see also* Ancylostomiasis) 126.9
human immunodeficiency virus V08
  with symptoms, symptomatic 042
human papillomavirus 079.4
hydrocele 603.1
hydronephrosis 591
Hymenolepis 123.6
hypopharynx 478.29
inguinal glands 683
  due to soft chancre 099.0
intestine, intestinal (*see also* Enteritis, due to, by organism) 009.0
intrauterine (*see also* Endometritis) 615.9
  complicating delivery 646.6 ✓5ᵗʰ
isospora belli or hominis 007.2
Japanese B encephalitis 062.0
jaw (bone) (acute) (chronic) (lower) (subacute) (upper) 526.4
joint — *see* Arthritis, infectious or infective
kidney (cortex) (hematogenous) 590.9
  with
    abortion — *see* Abortion, by type, with urinary tract infection
    calculus 592.0
    ectopic pregnancy (*see also* categories 633.0-633.9) 639.8
    molar pregnancy (*see also* categories 630-632) 639.8
  complicating pregnancy or puerperium 646.6 ✓5ᵗʰ
    affecting fetus or newborn 760.1
  following
    abortion 639.8
    ectopic or molar pregnancy 639.8
  pelvis and ureter 590.3
Klebsiella pneumoniae NEC 041.3
knee (skin) NEC 686.9
  joint — *see* Arthritis, infectious
Koch's (*see also* Tuberculosis, pulmonary) 011.9 ✓5ᵗʰ
labia (majora) (minora) (*see also* Vulvitis) 616.10
lacrimal
  gland (*see also* Dacryoadenitis) 375.00
  passages (duct) (sac) (*see also* Dacryocystitis) 375.30
larynx NEC 478.79
leg (skin) NEC 686.9
Leishmania (*see also* Leishmaniasis) 085.9
  braziliensis 085.5
  donovani 085.0
  Ethiopica 085.3
  furunculosa 085.1
  infantum 085.0
  mexicana 085.4
  tropica (minor) 085.1
    major 085.2
Leptosphaeria senegalensis 117.4
leptospira (*see also* Leptospirosis) 100.9
  Australis 100.89
  Bataviae 100.89
  pyrogenes 100.89
  specified type NEC 100.89
leptospirochetal NEC (*see also* Leptospirosis) 100.9
Leptothrix — *see* Actinomycosis

Infection, infected, infective — *continued*
Listeria monocytogenes (listeriosis) 027.0
  congenital 771.2
liver fluke — *see* Infestation, fluke, liver
Loa loa 125.2
  eyelid 125.2 [373.6]
Loboa loboi 116.2
local, skin (staphylococcal) (streptococcal) NEC 686.9
  abscess — *see* Abscess, by site
  cellulitis — *see* Cellulitis, by site
  ulcer (*see also* Ulcer, skin) 707.9
Loefflerella
  mallei 024
  whitmori 025
lung 518.89
  atypical Mycobacterium 031.0
    tuberculous (*see also* Tuberculosis, pulmonary) 011.9 ✓5ᵗʰ
  basilar 518.89
  chronic 518.89
  fungus NEC 117.9
  spirochetal 104.8
  virus — *see* Pneumonia, virus
lymph gland (axillary) (cervical) (inguinal) 683
  mesenteric 289.2
lymphoid tissue, base of tongue or posterior pharynx, NEC 474.00
madurella
  grisea 117.4
  mycetomii 117.4
major
  with
    abortion — *see* Abortion, by type, with sepsis
    ectopic pregnancy (*see also* categories 633.0-633.9) 639.0
    molar pregnancy (*see also* categories 630-632) 639.0
  following
    abortion 639.0
    ectopic or molar pregnancy 639.0
  puerperal, postpartum, childbirth 670 ✓4ᵗʰ
Malassezia furfur 111.0
Malleomyces
  mallei 024
  pseudomallei 025
mammary gland 611.0
  puerperal, postpartum 675.2 ✓5ᵗʰ
Mansonella (ozzardi) 125.5
mastoid (suppurative) — *see* Mastoiditis
maxilla, maxillary 526.4
  sinus (chronic) (*see also* Sinusitis, maxillary) 473.0
mediastinum 519.2
medina 125.7
meibomian
  cyst 373.12
  gland 373.12
melioidosis 025
meninges (*see also* Meningitis) 320.9
meningococcal (*see also* condition) 036.9
  brain 036.1
  cerebrospinal 036.0
  endocardium 036.42
  generalized 036.2
  meninges 036.0
  meningococcemia 036.2
  specified site NEC 036.89
mesenteric lymph nodes or glands NEC 289.2
Metagonimus 121.5
metatarsophalangeal 711.97
microorganism resistant to drugs — *see* Resistance (to), drugs by microorganisms
Microsporidia 136.8
microsporum, microsporic — *see* Dermatophytosis
Mima polymorpha NEC 041.85
mixed flora NEC 041.89
Monilia (*see also* Candidiasis) 112.9
  neonatal 771.7
Monosporium apiospermum 117.6
mouth (focus) NEC 528.9
  parasitic 112.0
Mucor 117.7
muscle NEC 728.89

Infection, infected, infective — continued
  mycelium NEC 117.9
  mycetoma
    actinomycotic NEC (see also Actinomycosis) 039.9
    mycotic NEC 117.4
  Mycobacterium, mycobacterial (see also Mycobacterium) 031.9
  mycoplasma NEC 041.81
  mycotic NEC 117.9
    pathogenic to compromised host only 118
    skin NEC 111.9
    systemic 117.9
  myocardium NEC 422.90
  nail (chronic) (with lymphangitis) 681.9
    finger 681.02
      fungus 110.1
    ingrowing 703.0
    toe 681.11
      fungus 110.1
  nasal sinus (chronic) (see also Sinusitis) 473.9
  nasopharynx (chronic) 478.29
    acute 460
  navel 686.9
    newborn 771.4
  Neisserian — see Gonococcus
  Neotestudina rosatii 117.4
  newborn, generalized 771.89 ▲
  nipple 611.0
    puerperal, postpartum 675.0 ✓5ᵗʰ
      with breast 675.9 ✓5ᵗʰ
        specified type NEC 675.8 ✓5ᵗʰ
  Nocardia — see Actinomycosis
  nose 478.1
  nostril 478.1
  obstetrical surgical wound 674.3 ✓5ᵗʰ
  Oesophagostomum (apiostomum) 127.7
  Oestrus ovis 134.0
  Oidium albicans (see also Candidiasis) 112.9
  Onchocerca (volvulus) 125.3
    eye 125.3 [360.13]
    eyelid 125.3 [373.6]
  operation wound 998.59
  Opisthorchis (felineus) (tenuicollis) (viverrini) 121.0
  orbit 376.00
    chronic 376.10
  ovary (see also Salpingo-oophoritis) 614.2
  Oxyuris vermicularis 127.4
  pancreas 577.0
  Paracoccidioides brasiliensis 116.1
  Paragonimus (westermani) 121.2
  parainfluenza virus 079.89
  parameningococcus NEC 036.9
    with meningitis 036.0
  parasitic NEC 136.9
  paratyphoid 002.9
    Type A 002.1
    Type B 002.2
    Type C 002.3
  paraurethral ducts 597.89
  parotid gland 527.2
  Pasteurella NEC 027.2
    multocida (cat-bite) (dog-bite) 027.2
    pestis (see also Plague) 020.9
    pseudotuberculosis 027.2
    septica (cat-bite) (dog-bite) 027.2
    tularensis (see also Tularemia) 021.9
  pelvic, female (see also Disease, pelvis, inflammatory) 614.9
  penis (glans) (retention) NEC 607.2
    herpetic 054.13
  Peptococcus 041.84
  Peptostreptococcus 041.84
  periapical (pulpal origin) 522.4
  peridental 523.3
  perineal wound (obstetrical) 674.3 ✓5ᵗʰ
  periodontal 523.3
  periorbital 376.00
    chronic 376.10
  perirectal 569.49
  perirenal (see also Infection, kidney) 590.9
  peritoneal (see also Peritonitis) 567.9
  periureteral 593.89
  periurethral 597.89
  Petriellidium boydii 117.6

Infection, infected, infective — continued
  pharynx 478.29
    Coxsackievirus 074.0
    phlegmonous 462
    posterior, lymphoid 474.00
  Phialophora
    gougerotii 117.8
    jeanselmei 117.8
    verrucosa 117.2
  Piedraia hortai 111.3
  pinna, acute 380.11
  pinta 103.9
    intermediate 103.1
    late 103.2
    mixed 103.3
    primary 103.0
  pinworm 127.4
  pityrosporum furfur 111.0
  pleuropneumonia-like organisms NEC (PPLO) 041.81
  pneumococcal NEC 041.2
    generalized (purulent) 038.2
  Pneumococcus NEC 041.2
  postoperative wound 998.59
  posttraumatic NEC 958.3
  postvaccinal 999.3
  prepuce NEC 607.1
  Proprionibacterium 041.84
  prostate (capsule) (see also Prostatitis) 601.9
  Proteus (mirabilis) (morganii) (vulgaris) NEC 041.6
    enteritis 008.3
  protozoal NEC 136.8
    intestinal NEC 007.9
  Pseudomonas NEC 041.7
    mallei 024
    pneumonia 482.1
    pseudomallei 025
  psittacosis 073.9
  puerperal, postpartum (major) 670 ✓4ᵗʰ
    minor 646.6 ✓5ᵗʰ
  pulmonary — see Infection, lung
  purulent — see Abscess
  putrid, generalized — see Septicemia
  pyemic — see Septicemia
  Pyrenochaeta romeroi 117.4
  Q fever 083.0
  rabies 071
  rectum (sphincter) 569.49
  renal (see also Infection, kidney) 590.9
    pelvis and ureter 590.3
  resistant to drugs — see Resistance (to), drugs by microorganisms
  respiratory 519.8
    chronic 519.8
    influenzal (acute) (upper) 487.1
    lung 518.89
    rhinovirus 460
    syncytial virus 079.6
    upper (acute) (infectious) NEC 465.9
      with flu, grippe, or influenza 487.1
      influenzal 487.1
      multiple sites NEC 465.8
      streptococcal 034.0
      viral NEC 465.9
  respiratory syncytial virus (RSV) 079.6
  resulting from presence of shunt or other internal prosthetic device — see Complications, infection and inflammation, due to (presence of) any device, implant, or graft classified to 996.0-996.5 NEC
  retrovirus 079.50
    human immunodeficiency virus type 2 [HIV 2] 079.53
    human T-cell lymphotrophic virus type I [HTLV-I] 079.51
    human T-cell lymphotrophic virus type II [HTLV-II] 079.52
    specified NEC 079.59
  Rhinocladium 117.1
  Rhinosporidium (seeberi) 117.0
  rhinovirus
    in diseases classified elsewhere — see category 079 ✓4ᵗʰ
    unspecified nature or site 079.3
  Rhizopus 117.7
  rickettsial 083.9

Infection, infected, infective — continued
  rickettsialpox 083.2
  rubella (see also Rubella) 056.9
    congenital 771.0
  Saccharomyces (see also Candidiasis) 112.9
  Saksenaea 117.7
  salivary duct or gland (any) 527.2
  Salmonella (aertrycke) (callinarum) (choleraesuis) (enteritidis) (suipestifer) (typhimurium) 003.9
    with
      arthritis 003.23
      gastroenteritis 003.0
      localized infection 003.20
        specified type NEC 003.29
      meningitis 003.21
      osteomyelitis 003.24
      pneumonia 003.22
      septicemia 003.1
      specified manifestation NEC 003.8
    congenital 771.89 ▲
    due to food (poisoning) (any serotype) (see also Poisoning, food, due to, Salmonella)
    hirschfeldii 002.3
    localized 003.20
      specified type NEC 003.29
    paratyphi 002.9
      A 002.1
      B 002.2
      C 002.3
    schottmuelleri 002.2
    specified type NEC 003.8
    typhi 002.0
    typhosa 002.0
  saprophytic 136.8
  Sarcocystis, lindemanni 136.5
  scabies 133.0
  Schistosoma — see Infestation, Schistosoma
  Schmorl's bacillus 040.3
  scratch or other superficial injury — see Injury, superficial, by site
  scrotum (acute) NEC 608.4
  secondary, burn or open wound (dislocation) (fracture) 958.3
  seminal vesicle (see also Vesiculitis) 608.0
  septic
    generalized — see Septicemia
    localized, skin (see also Abscess) 682.9
  septicemic — see Septicemia
  seroma 998.51
  Serratia (marcescens) 041.85
    generalized 038.44
  sheep liver fluke 121.3
  Shigella 004.9
    boydii 004.2
    dysenteriae 004.0
    flexneri 004.1
    group
      A 004.0
      B 004.1
      C 004.2
      D 004.3
    Schmitz (-Stutzer) 004.0
    schmitzii 004.0
    shiga 004.0
    sonnei 004.3
    specified type NEC 004.8
  Sin Nombre virus 079.81
  sinus (see also Sinusitis) 473.9
    pilonidal 685.1
      with abscess 685.0
    skin NEC 686.9
  Skene's duct or gland (see also Urethritis) 597.89
  skin (local) (staphylococcal) (streptococcal) NEC 686.9
    abscess — see Abscess, by site
    cellulitis — see Cellulitis, by site
    due to fungus 111.9
      specified type NEC 111.8
    mycotic 111.9
      specified type NEC 111.8
    ulcer (see also Ulcer, skin) 707.9
  slow virus 046.9
    specified condition NEC 046.8
  Sparganum (mansoni) (proliferum) 123.5

Index to Diseases

Infection, infected, infective — *continued*
- spermatic cord NEC 608.4
- sphenoidal (chronic) (sinus) (*see also* Sinusitis, sphenoidal 473.3)
- Spherophorus necrophorus 040.3
- spinal cord NEC (*see also* Encephalitis) 323.9
  - abscess 324.1
    - late effect — *see* category 326
  - late effect — *see* category 326
  - meninges — *see* Meningitis
  - streptococcal 320.2
- Spirillum
  - minus or minor 026.0
  - morsus muris 026.0
  - obermeieri 087.0
- spirochetal NEC 104.9
  - lung 104.8
  - specified nature or site NEC 104.8
- spleen 289.59
- Sporothrix schenckii 117.1
- Sporotrichum (schenckii) 117.1
- Sporozoa 136.8
- staphylococcal NEC 041.10
  - aureus 041.11
  - food poisoning 005.0
  - generalized (purulent) 038.10
    - aureus 038.11
    - specified organism NEC 038.19
  - pneumonia 482.40
    - aureus 482.41
    - specified type NEC 482.49
  - septicemia 038.10
    - aureus 038.11
    - specified organism NEC 038.19
  - specified NEC 041.19
- steatoma 706.2
- Stellantchasmus falcatus 121.6
- Streptobacillus moniliformis 026.1
- streptococcal NEC 041.00
  - congenital 771.89 ▲
  - generalized (purulent) 038.0
  - Group
    - A 041.01
    - B 041.02
    - C 041.03
    - D [enterococcus] 041.04
    - G 041.05
  - pneumonia — *see* Pneumonia, streptococcal 482.3 ✓5ᵗʰ
  - septicemia 038.0
  - sore throat 034.0
  - specified NEC 041.09
- Streptomyces — *see* Actinomycosis
- streptotrichosis — *see* Actinomycosis
- Strongyloides (stercoralis) 127.2
- stump (amputation) (posttraumatic) (surgical) 997.62
  - traumatic — *see* Amputation, traumatic, by site, complicated
- subcutaneous tissue, local NEC 686.9
- submaxillary region 528.9
- suipestifer (*see also* Infection, Salmonella) 003.9
- swimming pool bacillus 031.1
- syphilitic — *see* Syphilis
- systemic — *see* Septicemia
- Taenia — *see* Infestation, Taenia
- Taeniarhynchus saginatus 123.2
- tapeworm — *see* Infestation, tapeworm
- tendon (sheath) 727.89
- Ternidens diminutus 127.7
- testis (*see also* Orchitis) 604.90
- thigh (skin) 686.9
- threadworm 127.4
- throat 478.29
  - pneumococcal 462
  - staphylococcal 462
  - streptococcal 034.0
  - viral NEC (*see also* Pharyngitis) 462
- thumb (skin) 686.9
  - abscess (with lymphangitis) 681.00
    - pulp 681.01
  - cellulitis (with lymphangitis) 681.00
  - nail 681.02
- thyroglossal duct 529.8
- toe (skin) 686.9
  - abscess (with lymphangitis) 681.10

Infection, infected, infective — *continued*
- toe — *continued*
  - cellulitis (with lymphangitis) 681.10
  - nail 681.11
    - fungus 110.1
- tongue NEC 529.0
  - parasitic 112.0
- tonsil (faucial) (lingual) (pharyngeal) 474.00
  - acute or subacute 463
  - and adenoid 474.02
  - tag 474.00
- tooth, teeth 522.4
  - periapical (pulpal origin) 522.4
  - peridental 523.3
  - periodontal 523.3
  - pulp 522.0
  - socket 526.5
- Torula histolytica 117.5
- Toxocara (cani) (cati) (felis) 128.0
- Toxoplasma gondii (*see also* Toxoplasmosis) 130.9
- trachea, chronic 491.8
  - fungus 117.9
- traumatic NEC 958.3
- trematode NEC 121.9
- trench fever 083.1
- Treponema
  - denticola 041.84
  - macrodenticum 041.84
  - pallidum (*see also* Syphillis) 097.9
- Trichinella (spiralis) 124
- Trichomonas 131.9
  - bladder 131.09
  - cervix 131.09
  - hominis 007.3
  - intestine 007.3
  - prostate 131.03
  - specified site NEC 131.8
  - urethra 131.02
  - urogenitalis 131.00
  - vagina 131.01
  - vulva 131.01
- Trichophyton, trichophytid — *see* Dermatophytosis
- Trichosporon (beigelii) cutaneum 111.2
- Trichostrongylus 127.6
- Trichuris (trichiuria) 127.3
- Trombicula (irritans) 133.8
- Trypanosoma (*see also* Trypanosomiasis) 086.9
  - cruzi 086.2
- tubal (*see also* Salpingo-oophoritis) 614.2
- tuberculous NEC (*see also* Tuberculosis) 011.9 ✓5ᵗʰ
- tubo-ovarian (*see also* Salpingo-oophoritis) 614.2
- tunica vaginalis 608.4
- tympanic membrane — *see* Myringitis
- typhoid (abortive) (ambulant) (bacillus) 002.0
- typhus 081.9
  - flea-borne (endemic) 081.0
  - louse-borne (epidemic) 080
  - mite-borne 081.2
  - recrudescent 081.1
  - tick-borne 082.9
    - African 082.1
    - North Asian 082.2
- umbilicus (septic) 686.9
  - newborn NEC 771.4
- ureter 593.89
- urethra (*see also* Urethritis) 597.80
- urinary (tract) NEC 599.0
  - with
    - abortion — *see* Abortion, by type, with urinary tract infection
    - ectopic pregnancy (*see also* categories 633.0-633.9) 639.8
    - molar pregnancy (*see also* categories 630-632) 639.8
  - candidal 112.2
  - complicating pregnancy, childbirth, or puerperium 646.6 ✓5ᵗʰ
    - affecting fetus or newborn 760.1
  - asymptomatic 646.5 ✓5ᵗʰ
    - affecting fetus or newborn 760.1
  - diplococcal (acute) 098.0
    - chronic 098.2

Infection, infected, infective — *continued*
- urinary (tract) NEC — *continued*
  - due to Trichomonas (vaginalis) 131.00
  - following
    - abortion 639.8
    - ectopic or molar pregnancy 639.8
  - gonococcal (acute) 098.0
    - chronic or duration of 2 months or over 098.2
  - newborn 771.82 ▲
  - trichomonal 131.00
  - tuberculous (*see also* Tuberculosis) 016.3 ✓5ᵗʰ
- uterus, uterine (*see also* Endometritis) 615.9
- utriculus masculinus NEC 597.89
- vaccination 999.3
- vagina (granulation tissue) (wall) (*see also* Vaginitis) 616.10
- varicella 052.9
- varicose veins — *see* Varicose, veins
- variola 050.9
  - major 050.0
  - minor 050.1
- vas deferens NEC 608.4
- Veillonella 041.84
- verumontanum 597.89
- vesical (*see also* Cystitis) 595.9
- Vibrio
  - cholerae 001.0
    - El Tor 001.1
  - parahaemolyticus (food poisoning) 005.4
  - vulnificus 041.85
- Vincent's (gums) (mouth) (tonsil) 101
- virus, viral 079.99
  - adenovirus
    - in diseases classified elsewhere — *see* category 079 ✓4ᵗʰ
    - unspecified nature or site 079.0
  - central nervous system NEC 049.9
    - enterovirus 048
      - meningitis 047.9
      - specified type NEC 047.8
    - slow virus 046.9
      - specified condition NEC 046.8
  - chest 519.8
  - conjunctivitis 077.99
    - specified type NEC 077.8
  - Coxsackie (*see also* Infection, Coxsackie) 079.2
  - Ebola 065.8
  - ECHO
    - in diseases classified elsewhere — *see* category 079 ✓4ᵗʰ
    - unspecified nature or site 079.1
  - encephalitis 049.9
    - arthropod-borne NEC 064
    - tick-borne 063.9
      - specified type NEC 063.8
  - enteritis NEC (*see also* Enteritis, viral) 008.8
  - exanthem NEC 057.9
  - Hantavirus 079.81
  - human papilloma 079.4
    - in diseases classified elsewhere — *see* category 079 ✓4ᵗʰ
  - intestine (*see also* Enteritis, viral) 008.8
  - lung — *see* Pneumonia, viral
  - respiratory syncytial (RSV) 079.6
  - retrovirus 079.50
  - rhinovirus
    - in diseases classified elsewhere — *see* category 079 ✓4ᵗʰ
    - unspecified nature or site 079.3
  - salivary gland disease 078.5
  - slow 046.9
    - specified condition NEC 046.8
  - specified type NEC 079.89
    - in diseases classified elsewhere — *see* category 079 ✓4ᵗʰ
  - unspecified nature or site 079.99
  - warts NEC 078.10
- vulva (*see also* Vulvitis) 616.10
- whipworm 127.3
- Whitmore's bacillus 025
- wound (local) (posttraumatic) NEC 958.3
  - with
    - dislocation — *see* Dislocation, by site, open

Infection, infected, infective — continued
    wound — continued
        with — continued
            fracture — see Fracture, by site, open
            open wound — see Wound, open, by site, complicated
        postoperative 998.59
        surgical 998.59
    Wuchereria 125.0
        bancrofti 125.0
        malayi 125.1
    yaws — see Yaws
    yeast (see also Candidiasis) 112.9
    yellow fever (see also Fever, yellow) 060.9
    Yersinia pestis (see also Plague) 020.9
    Zeis' gland 373.12
    zoonotic bacterial NEC 027.9
    Zopfia senegalensis 117.4
Infective, infectious — see condition
Inferiority complex 301.9
    constitutional psychopathic 301.9
Infertility
    female 628.9
        associated with
            adhesions, peritubal 614.6 [628.2]
            anomaly
                cervical mucus 628.4
                congenital
                    cervix 628.4
                    fallopian tube 628.2
                    uterus 628.3
                    vagina 628.4
            anovulation 628.0
            dysmucorrhea 628.4
            endometritis, tuberculous (see also Tuberculosis) 016.7 ✓5ᵗʰ [628.3]
            Stein-Leventhal syndrome 256.4 [628.0]
        due to
            adiposogenital dystrophy 253.8 [628.1]
            anterior pituitary disorder NEC 253.4 [628.1]
                hyperfunction 253.1 [628.1]
            cervical anomaly 628.4
            fallopian tube anomaly 628.2
            ovarian failure 256.39 [628.0]
            Stein-Leventhal syndrome 256.4 [628.0]
            uterine anomaly 628.3
            vaginal anomaly 628.4
        nonimplantation 628.3
        origin
            cervical 628.4
            pituitary-hypothalamus NEC 253.8 [628.1]
                anterior pituitary NEC 253.4 [628.1]
                    hyperfunction NEC 253.1 [628.1]
                dwarfism 253.3 [628.1]
                panhypopituitarism 253.2 [628.1]
            specified NEC 628.8
            tubal (block) (occlusion) (stenosis) 628.2
                adhesions 614.6 [628.2]
            uterine 628.3
            vaginal 628.4
        previous, requiring supervision of pregnancy V23.0
    male 606.9
        absolute 606.0
        due to
            azoospermia 606.0
            drug therapy 606.8
            extratesticular cause NEC 606.8
            germinal cell
                aplasia 606.0
                desquamation 606.1
            hypospermatogenesis 606.1
            infection 606.8
            obstruction, afferent ducts 606.8
            oligospermia 606.1
            radiation 606.8
            spermatogenic arrest (complete) 606.0
                incomplete 606.1
            systemic disease 606.8
Infestation 134.9
    Acanthocheilonema (perstans) 125.4
        streptocerca 125.6
    Acariasis 133.9
        demodex folliculorum 133.8

Infestation — continued
    Acariasis — continued
        Sarcoptes scabiei 133.0
        trombiculae 133.8
    Agamofilaria streptocerca 125.6
    Ancylostoma, Ankylostoma 126.9
        americanum 126.1
        braziliense 126.2
        canium 126.8
        ceylanicum 126.3
        duodenale 126.0
        new world 126.1
        old world 126.0
    Angiostrongylus cantonensis 128.8
    anisakiasis 127.1
    Anisakis larva 127.1
    arthropod NEC 134.1
    Ascaris lumbricoides 127.0
    Bacillus fusiformis 101
    Balantidium coli 007.0
    beef tapeworm 123.2
    Bothriocephalus (latus) 123.4
        larval 123.5
    broad tapeworm 123.4
        larval 123.5
    Brugia malayi 125.1
    Candiru 136.8
    Capillaria
        hepatica 128.8
        philippinensis 127.5
    cat liver fluke 121.0
    Cercomonas hominis (intestinal) 007.3
    cestodes 123.9
        specified type NEC 123.8
    chigger 133.8
    chigoe 134.1
    Chilomastix 007.8
    Clonorchis (sinensis) (liver) 121.1
    coccidia 007.2
    complicating pregnancy, childbirth, or puerperium 647.9 ✓5ᵗʰ
        affecting fetus or newborn 760.8
    Cysticercus cellulosae 123.1
    Demodex folliculorum 133.8
    Dermatobia (hominis) 134.0
    Dibothriocephalus (latus) 123.4
        larval 123.5
    Dicrocoelium dendriticum 121.8
    Diphyllobothrium (adult) (intestinal) (latum) (pacificum) 123.4
        larval 123.5
    Diplogonoporus (grandis) 123.8
    Dipylidium (caninum) 123.8
    Distoma hepaticum 121.3
    dog tapeworm 123.8
    Dracunculus medinensis 125.7
    dragon worm 125.7
    dwarf tapeworm 123.6
    Echinococcus (see also Echinococcus) 122.9
    Echinostoma ilocanum 121.8
    Embadomonas 007.8
    Endamoeba (histolytica) — see Infection, ameba
    Entamoeba (histolytica) — see Infection, ameba
    Enterobius vermicularis 127.4
    Epidermophyton — see Dermatophytosis
    eyeworm 125.2
    Fasciola
        gigantica 121.3
        hepatica 121.3
    Fasciolopsis (buski) (small intestine) 121.4
        filarial 125.9
            due to
                Acanthocheilonema (perstans) 125.4
                    streptocerca 125.6
                Brugia (Wuchereria) malayi 125.1
                Dracunculus medinensis 125.7
                guinea worms 125.7
                Mansonella (ozzardi) 125.5
                Onchocerca volvulus 125.3
                    eye 125.3 [360.13]
                    eyelid 125.3 [373.6]
                Wuchereria (bancrofti) 125.0
                    malayi 125.1
            specified type NEC 125.6
    fish tapeworm 123.4
        larval 123.5

Infestation — continued
    Fasciolopsis — continued
        fluke 121.9
        blood NEC (see also Schistosomiasis) 120.9
        cat liver 121.0
        intestinal (giant) 121.4
        liver (sheep) 121.3
            cat 121.0
            Chinese 121.1
            clonorchiasis 121.1
            fascioliasis 121.3
            Oriental 121.1
        lung (oriental) 121.2
        sheep liver 121.3
    fly larva 134.0
    Gasterophilus (intestinalis) 134.0
    Gastrodiscoides hominis 121.8
    Giardia lamblia 007.1
    Gnathostoma (spinigerum) 128.1
    Gongylonema 125.6
    guinea worm 125.7
    helminth NEC 128.9
        intestinal 127.9
            mixed (types classifiable to more than one category in 120.0-127.7) 127.8
            specified type NEC 127.7
        specified type NEC 128.8
    Heterophyes heterophyes (small intestine) 121.6
    hookworm (see also Infestation, ancylostoma) 126.9
    Hymenolepis (diminuta) (nana) 123.6
    intestinal NEC 129
    leeches (aquatic) (land) 134.2
    Leishmania — see Leishmaniasis
    lice (see also Infestation, pediculus) 132.9
    Linguatulidae, linguatula (pentastoma) (serrata) 134.1
    Loa loa 125.2
        eyelid 125.2 [373.6]
    louse (see also Infestation, pediculus) 132.9
        body 132.1
        head 132.0
        pubic 132.2
    maggots 134.0
    Mansonella (ozzardi) 125.5
    medina 125.7
    Metagonimus yokogawai (small intestine) 121.5
    Microfilaria streptocerca 125.3
        eye 125.3 [360.13]
        eyelid 125.3 [373.6]
    Microsporon furfur 111.0
    microsporum — see Dermatophytosis
    mites 133.9
        scabic 133.0
        specified type NEC 133.8
    Monilia (albicans) (see also Candidiasis) 112.9
        vagina 112.1
        vulva 112.1
    mouth 112.0
    Necator americanus 126.1
    nematode (intestinal) 127.9
        Ancylostoma (see also Ancylostoma) 126.9
        Ascaris lumbricoides 127.0
        conjunctiva NEC 128.9
        Dioctophyma 128.8
        Enterobius vermicularis 127.4
        Gnathostoma spinigerum 128.1
        Oesophagostomum (apiostomum) 127.7
        Physaloptera 127.4
        specified type NEC 127.7
        Strongyloides stercoralis 127.2
        Ternidens diminutus 127.7
        Trichinella spiralis 124
        Trichostrongylus 127.6
        Trichuris (trichiuria) 127.3
    Oesophagostomum (apiostomum) 127.7
    Oestrus ovis 134.0
    Onchocerca (volvulus) 125.3
        eye 125.3 [360.13]
        eyelid 125.3 [373.6]
    Opisthorchis (felineus) (tenuicollis) (viverrini) 121.0
    Oxyuris vermicularis 127.4
    Paragonimus (westermani) 121.2
    parasite, parasitic NEC 136.9
        eyelid 134.9 [373.6]

Index to Diseases

Infestation — continued
  parasite, parasitic NEC — continued
    intestinal 129
    mouth 112.0
    orbit 376.13
    skin 134.9
    tongue 112.0
  pediculus 132.9
    capitis (humanus) (any site) 132.0
    corporis (humanus) (any site) 132.1
    eyelid 132.0 [373.6]
    mixed (classifiable to more than one category in 132.0-132.2) 132.3
    pubis (any site) 132.2
  phthirus (pubis) (any site) 132.2
    with any infestation classifiable to 132.0, 132.1 and 132.3
  pinworm 127.4
  pork tapeworm (adult) 123.0
  protozoal NEC 136.8
  pubic louse 132.2
  rat tapeworm 123.6
  red bug 133.8
  roundworm (large) NEC 127.0
  sand flea 134.1
  saprophytic NEC 136.8
  Sarcoptes scabiei 133.0
  scabies 133.0
  Schistosoma 120.9
    bovis 120.8
    cercariae 120.3
    hematobium 120.0
    intercalatum 120.8
    japonicum 120.2
    mansoni 120.1
    mattheii 120.8
    specified
      site — see Schistosomiasis
      type NEC 120.8
    spindale 120.8
  screw worms 134.0
  skin NEC 134.9
  Sparganum (mansoni) (proliferum) 123.5
    larval 123.5
  specified type NEC 134.8
  Spirometra larvae 123.5
  Sporozoa NEC 136.8
  Stellantchasmus falcatus 121.6
  Strongyloides 127.2
  Strongylus (gibsoni) 127.7
  Taenia 123.3
    diminuta 123.6
    Echinococcus (see also Echinococcus) 122.9
    mediocanellata 123.2
    nana 123.6
    saginata (mediocanellata) 123.2
    solium (intestinal form) 123.0
      larval form 123.1
  Taeniarhynchus saginatus 123.2
  tapeworm 123.9
    beef 123.2
    broad 123.4
      larval 123.5
    dog 123.8
    dwarf 123.6
    fish 123.4
      larval 123.5
    pork 123.0
    rat 123.6
  Ternidens diminutus 127.7
  Tetranychus molestissimus 133.8
  threadworm 127.4
  tongue 112.0
  Toxocara (cani) (cati) (felis) 128.0
  trematode(s) NEC 121.9
  Trichina spiralis 124
  Trichinella spiralis 124
  Trichocephalus 127.3
  Trichomonas 131.9
    bladder 131.09
    cervix 131.09
    intestine 007.3
    prostate 131.03
    specified site NEC 131.8
    urethra (female) (male) 131.02
    urogenital 131.00

Infestation — continued
  Trichomonas — continued
    vagina 131.01
    vulva 131.01
  Trichophyton — see Dermatophytosis
  Trichostrongylus instabilis 127.6
  Trichuris (trichiuria) 127.3
  Trombicula (irritans) 133.8
  Trypanosoma — see Trypanosomiasis
  Tunga penetrans 134.1
  Uncinaria americana 126.1
  whipworm 127.3
  worms NEC 128.9
    intestinal 127.9
  Wuchereria 125.0
    bancrofti 125.0
    malayi 125.1

Infiltrate, infiltration
  with an iron compound 275.0
  amyloid (any site) (generalized) 277.3
  calcareous (muscle) NEC 275.49
    localized — see Degeneration, by site
  calcium salt (muscle) 275.49
  corneal (see also Edema, cornea) 371.20
  eyelid 373.9
  fatty (diffuse) (generalized) 272.8
    localized — see Degeneration, by site, fatty
  glycogen, glycogenic (see also Disease, glycogen storage) 271.0
  heart, cardiac
    fatty (see also Degeneration, myocardial) 429.1
    glycogenic 271.0 [425.7]
  inflammatory in vitreous 379.29
  kidney (see also Disease, renal) 593.9
  leukemic (M9800/3) — see Leukemia
  liver 573.8
    fatty — see Fatty, liver
    glycogen (see also Disease, glycogen storage) 271.0
  lung (see also Infiltrate, pulmonary) 518.3
    eosinophilic 518.3
    x-ray finding only 793.1
  lymphatic (see also Leukemia, lymphatic) 204.9 ✓5th
    gland, pigmentary 289.3
  muscle, fatty 728.9
  myelogenous (see also Leukemia, myeloid) 205.9 ✓5th
  myocardium, myocardial
    fatty (see also Degeneration, myocardial) 429.1
    glycogenic 271.0 [425.7]
  pulmonary 518.3
    with
      eosinophilia 518.3
      pneumonia — see Pneumonia, by type
    x-ray finding only 793.1
  Ranke's primary (see also Tuberculosis) 010.0 ✓5th
  skin, lymphocytic (benign) 709.8
  thymus (gland) (fatty) 254.8
  urine 788.8
  vitreous humor 379.29

Infirmity 799.8
  senile 797

Inflammation, inflamed, inflammatory (with exudation)
  abducens (nerve) 378.54
  accessory sinus (chronic) (see also Sinusitis) 473.9
  adrenal (gland) 255.8
  alimentary canal — see Enteritis
  alveoli (teeth) 526.5
    scorbutic 267
  amnion — see Amnionitis
  anal canal 569.49
  antrum (chronic) (see also Sinusitis, maxillary) 473.0
  anus 569.49
  appendix (see also Appendicitis) 541
  arachnoid — see Meningitis
  areola 611.0
    puerperal, postpartum 675.0 ✓5th
  areolar tissue NEC 686.9
  artery — see Arteritis

Inflammation, inflamed, inflammatory — continued
  auditory meatus (external) (see also Otitis, externa) 380.10
  Bartholin's gland 616.8
  bile duct or passage 576.1
  bladder (see also Cystitis) 595.9
  bone — see Osteomyelitis
  bowel (see also Enteritis) 558.9
  brain (see also Encephalitis) 323.9
    late effect — see category 326
    membrane — see Meningitis
  breast 611.0
    puerperal, postpartum 675.2 ✓5th
  broad ligament (see also Disease, pelvis, inflammatory) 614.4
    acute 614.3
  bronchus — see Bronchitis
  bursa — see Bursitis
  capsule
    liver 573.3
    spleen 289.59
  catarrhal (see also Catarrh) 460
    vagina 616.10
  cecum (see also Appendicitis) 541
  cerebral (see also Encephalitis) 323.9
    late effect — see category 326
    membrane — see Meningitis
  cerebrospinal (see also Meningitis) 322.9
    late effect — see category 326
    meningococcal 036.0
    tuberculous (see also Tuberculosis) 013.6 ✓5th
  cervix (uteri) (see also Cervicitis) 616.0
  chest 519.9
  choroid NEC (see also Choroiditis) 363.20
  cicatrix (tissue) — see Cicatrix
  colon (see also Enteritis) 558.9
    granulomatous 555.1
    newborn 558.9
  connective tissue (diffuse) NEC 728.9
  cornea (see also Keratitis) 370.9
    with ulcer (see also Ulcer, cornea) 370.00
  corpora cavernosa (penis) 607.2
  cranial nerve — see Disorder, nerve, cranial
  diarrhea — see Diarrhea
  disc (intervertebral) (space) 722.90
    cervical, cervicothoracic 722.91
    lumbar, lumbosacral 722.93
    thoracic, thoracolumbar 722.92
  Douglas' cul-de-sac or pouch (chronic) (see also Disease, pelvis, inflammatory) 614.4
    acute 614.3
  due to (presence of) any device, implant, or graft classifiable to 996.0-996.5 — see Complications, infection and inflammation, due to (presence of) any device, implant, or graft classified to 996.0-996.5 NEC
  duodenum 535.6 ✓5th
  dura mater — see Meningitis
  ear — see also Otitis
    external (see also Otitis, externa) 380.10
    inner (see also Labyrinthitis) 386.30
    middle — see Otitis media
  esophagus 530.10
  ethmoidal (chronic) (sinus) (see also Sinusitis, ethmoidal) 473.2
  Eustachian tube (catarrhal) 381.50
    acute 381.51
    chronic 381.52
  extrarectal 569.49
  eye 379.99
  eyelid 373.9
    specified NEC 373.8
  fallopian tube (see also Salpingo-oophoritis) 614.2
  fascia 728.9
  fetal membranes (acute) 658.4 ✓5th
    affecting fetus or newborn 762.7
  follicular, pharynx 472.1
  frontal (chronic) (sinus) (see also Sinusitis, frontal) 473.1
  gallbladder (see also Cholecystitis, acute) 575.0
  gall duct (see also Cholecystitis) 575.10
  gastrointestinal (see also Enteritis) 558.9

Inflammation, inflamed, inflammatory

Inflammation, inflamed, inflammatory — *continued*
- genital organ (diffuse) (internal)
  - female 614.9
    - with
      - abortion — *see* Abortion, by type, with sepsis
      - ectopic pregnancy (*see also* categories 633.0-633.9) 639.0
      - molar pregnancy (*see also* categories 630-632) 639.0
      - complicating pregnancy, childbirth, or puerperium 646.6 ✓5ᵗʰ
        - affecting fetus or newborn 760.8
      - following
        - abortion 639.0
        - ectopic or molar pregnancy 639.0
    - male 608.4
- gland (lymph) (*see also* Lymphadenitis) 289.3
- glottis (*see also* Laryngitis) 464.00
  - with obstruction 464.01
- granular, pharynx 472.1
- gum 523.1
- heart (*see also* Carditis) 429.89
- hepatic duct 576.8
- hernial sac — *see* Hernia, by site
- ileum (*see also* Enteritis) 558.9
  - terminal or regional 555.0
    - with large intestine 555.2
- intervertebral disc 722.90
  - cervical, cervicothoracic 722.91
  - lumbar, lumbosacral 722.93
  - thoracic, thoracolumbar 722.92
- intestine (*see also* Enteritis) 558.9
- jaw (acute) (bone) (chronic) (lower) (suppurative) (upper) 526.4
- jejunum — *see* Enteritis
- joint NEC (*see also* Arthritis) 716.9 ✓5ᵗʰ
  - sacroiliac 720.2
- kidney (*see also* Nephritis) 583.9
- knee (joint) 716.66
  - tuberculous (active) (*see also* Tuberculosis) 015.2 ✓5ᵗʰ
- labium (majus) (minus) (*see also* Vulvitis) 616.10
- lacrimal
  - gland (*see also* Dacryoadenitis) 375.00
  - passages (duct) (sac) (*see also* Dacryocystitis) 375.30
- larynx (*see also* Laryngitis) 464.00
  - with obstruction 464.01
  - diphtheritic 032.3
- leg NEC 686.9
- lip 528.5
- liver (capsule) (*see also* Hepatitis) 573.3
  - acute 570
  - chronic 571.40
  - suppurative 572.0
- lung (acute) (*see also* Pneumonia) 486
  - chronic (interstitial) 518.89
- lymphatic vessel (*see also* Lymphangitis) 457.2
- lymph node or gland (*see also* Lymphadenitis) 289.3
- mammary gland 611.0
  - puerperal, postpartum 675.2 ✓5ᵗʰ
- maxilla, maxillary 526.4
  - sinus (chronic) (*see also* Sinusitis, maxillary) 473.0
- membranes of brain or spinal cord — *see* Meningitis
- meninges — *see* Meningitis
- mouth 528.0
- muscle 728.9
- myocardium (*see also* Myocarditis) 429.0
- nasal sinus (chronic) (*see also* Sinusitis) 473.9
- nasopharynx — *see* Nasopharyngitis
- navel 686.9
  - newborn NEC 771.4
- nerve NEC 729.2
- nipple 611.0
  - puerperal, postpartum 675.0 ✓5ᵗʰ
- nose 478.1
  - suppurative 472.0
- oculomotor nerve 378.51
- optic nerve 377.30
- orbit (chronic) 376.10
  - acute 376.00

Inflammation, inflamed, inflammatory — *continued*
- orbit — *continued*
  - chronic 376.10
- ovary (*see also* Salpingo-oophoritis) 614.2
- oviduct (*see also* Salpingo-oophoritis) 614.2
- pancreas — *see* Pancreatitis
- parametrium (chronic) (*see also* Disease, pelvis, inflammatory) 614.4
  - acute 614.3
- parotid region 686.9
  - gland 527.2
- pelvis, female (*see also* Disease, pelvis, inflammatory) 614.9
- penis (corpora cavernosa) 607.2
- perianal 569.49
- pericardium (*see also* Pericarditis) 423.9
- perineum (female) (male) 686.9
- perirectal 569.49
- peritoneum (*see also* Peritonitis) 567.9
- periuterine (*see also* Disease, pelvis, inflammatory) 614.9
- perivesical (*see also* Cystitis) 595.9
- petrous bone (*see also* Petrositis) 383.20
- pharynx (*see also* Pharyngitis) 462
  - follicular 472.1
  - granular 472.1
- pia mater — *see* Meningitis
- pleura — *see* Pleurisy
- postmastoidectomy cavity 383.30
  - chronic 383.33
- prostate (*see also* Prostatitis) 601.9
- rectosigmoid — *see* Rectosigmoiditis
- rectum (*see also* Proctitis) 569.49
- respiratory, upper (*see also* Infection, respiratory, upper) 465.9
  - chronic, due to external agent — *see* Condition, respiratory, chronic, due to, external agent
  - due to
    - fumes or vapors (chemical) (inhalation) 506.2
    - radiation 508.1
- retina (*see also* Retinitis) 363.20
- retrocecal (*see also* Appendicitis) 541
- retroperitoneal (*see also* Peritonitis) 567.9
- salivary duct or gland (any) (suppurative) 527.2
- scorbutic, alveoli, teeth 267
- scrotum 608.4
- sigmoid — *see* Enteritis
- sinus (*see also* Sinusitis) 473.9
- Skene's duct or gland (*see also* Urethritis) 597.89
- skin 686.9
- spermatic cord 608.4
- sphenoidal (sinus) (*see also* Sinusitis, sphenoidal) 473.3
- spinal
  - cord (*see also* Encephalitis) 323.9
    - late effect — *see* category 326
  - membrane — *see* Meningitis
  - nerve — *see* Disorder, nerve
- spine (*see also* Spondylitis) 720.9
- spleen (capsule) 289.59
- stomach — *see* Gastritis
- stricture, rectum 569.49
- subcutaneous tissue NEC 686.9
- suprarenal (gland) 255.8
- synovial (fringe) (membrane) — *see* Bursitis
- tendon (sheath) NEC 726.90
- testis (*see also* Orchitis) 604.90
- thigh 686.9
- throat (*see also* Sore throat) 462
- thymus (gland) 254.8
- thyroid (gland) (*see also* Thyroiditis) 245.9
- tongue 529.0
- tonsil — *see* Tonsillitis
- trachea — *see* Tracheitis
- trochlear nerve 378.53
- tubal (*see also* Salpingo-oophoritis) 614.2
- tuberculous NEC (*see also* Tuberculosis) 011.9 ✓5ᵗʰ
- tubo-ovarian (*see also* Salpingo-oophoritis) 614.2
- tunica vaginalis 608.4
- tympanic membrane — *see* Myringitis
- umbilicus, umbilical 686.9
  - newborn NEC 771.4

Inflammation, inflamed, inflammatory — *continued*
- uterine ligament (*see also* Disease, pelvis, inflammatory) 614.4
  - acute 614.3
- uterus (catarrhal) (*see also* Endometritis) 615.9
- uveal tract (anterior) (*see also* Iridocyclitis) 364.3
  - posterior — *see* Chorioretinitis
  - sympathetic 360.11
- vagina (*see also* Vaginitis) 616.10
- vas deferens 608.4
- vein (*see also* Phlebitis) 451.9
  - thrombotic 451.9
    - cerebral (*see also* Thrombosis, brain) 434.0 ✓5ᵗʰ
    - leg 451.2
      - deep (vessels) NEC 451.19
      - superficial (vessels) 451.0
    - lower extremity 451.2
      - deep (vessels) NEC 451.19
      - superficial (vessels) 451.0
- vocal cord 478.5
- vulva (*see also* Vulvitis) 616.10

Inflation, lung imperfect (newborn) 770.5

Influenza, influenzal 487.1
- with
  - bronchitis 487.1
  - bronchopneumonia 487.0
  - cold (any type) 487.1
  - digestive manifestations 487.8
  - hemoptysis 487.1
  - involvement of
    - gastrointestinal tract 487.8
    - nervous system 487.8
  - laryngitis 487.1
  - manifestations NEC 487.8
    - respiratory 487.1
      - pneumonia 487.0
  - pharyngitis 487.1
  - pneumonia (any form classifiable to 480-483, 485-486) 487.0
  - respiratory manifestations NEC 487.1
  - sinusitis 487.1
  - sore throat 487.1
  - tonsillitis 487.1
  - tracheitis 487.1
  - upper respiratory infection (acute) 487.1
- abdominal 487.8
- Asian 487.1
- bronchial 487.1
- bronchopneumonia 487.0
- catarrhal 487.1
- epidemic 487.1
- gastric 487.8
- intestinal 487.8
- laryngitis 487.1
- maternal affecting fetus or newborn 760.2
  - manifest influenza in infant 771.2
- pharyngitis 487.1
- pneumonia (any form) 487.0
- respiratory (upper) 487.1
- stomach 487.8
- vaccination, prophylactic (against) V04.8

Influenza-like disease 487.1

Infraction, Freiberg's (metatarsal head) 732.5

Infusion complication, misadventure, or reaction — *see* Complication, infusion

Ingestion
- chemical — *see* Table of Drugs and Chemicals
- drug or medicinal substance
  - overdose or wrong substance given or taken 977.9
  - specified drug — *see* Table of Drugs and Chemicals
- foreign body NEC (*see also* Foreign body) 938

Ingrowing
- hair 704.8
- nail (finger) (toe) (infected) 703.0

Inguinal — *see also* condition
- testis 752.51

Inhalation
- carbon monoxide 986
- flame
  - mouth 947.0

Index to Diseases

Inhalation — *continued*
  flame — *continued*
    lung 947.1
  food or foreign body (*see also* Asphyxia, food or foreign body) 933.1
  gas, fumes, or vapor (noxious) 987.9
    specified agent — *see* Table of Drugs and Chemicals
  liquid or vomitus (*see also* Asphyxia, food or foreign body) 933.1
    lower respiratory tract NEC 934.9
  meconium (fetus or newborn) 770.1
  mucus (*see also* Asphyxia, mucus) 933.1
  oil (causing suffocation) (*see also* Asphyxia, food or foreign body) 933.1
  pneumonia — *see* Pneumonia, aspiration
  smoke 987.9
  steam 987.9
  stomach contents or secretions (*see also* Asphyxia, food or foreign body) 933.1
    in labor and delivery 668.0

Inhibition, inhibited
  academic as adjustment reaction 309.23
  orgasm
    female 302.73
    male 302.74
  sexual
    desire 302.71
    excitement 302.72
  work as adjustment reaction 309.23

Inhibitor, systemic lupus erythematosus (presence of) 286.5

Iniencephalus, iniencephaly 740.2

Injected eye 372.74

Injury 959.9

> *Note* — For abrasion, insect bite (nonvenomous), blister, or scratch, see Injury, superficial.
>
> For laceration, traumatic rupture, tear, or penetrating wound of internal organs, such as heart, lung, liver, kidney, pelvic organs, whether or not accompanied by open wound in the same region, see Injury, internal.
>
> For nerve injury, see Injury, nerve.
>
> For late effect of injuries classifiable to 850-854, 860-869, 900-919, 950-959, see Late, effect, injury, by type.

  abdomen, abdominal (viscera) — *see also* Injury, internal, abdomen
    muscle or wall 959.1
  acoustic, resulting in deafness 951.5
  adenoid 959.09
  adrenal (gland) — *see* Injury, internal, adrenal
  alveolar (process) 959.09
  ankle (and foot) (and knee) (and leg, except thigh) 959.7
  anterior chamber, eye 921.3
  anus 959.1
  aorta (thoracic) 901.0
    abdominal 902.0
  appendix — *see* Injury, internal, appendix
  arm, upper (and shoulder) 959.2
  artery (complicating trauma) (*see also* Injury, blood vessel, by site) 904.9
    cerebral or meningeal (*see also* Hemorrhage, brain, traumatic, subarachnoid) 852.0
  auditory canal (external) (meatus) 959.09
  auricle, auris, ear 959.09
  axilla 959.2
  back 959.1
  bile duct — *see* Injury, internal, bile duct
  birth — *see also* Birth, injury
    canal NEC, complicating delivery 665.9
  bladder (sphincter) — *see* Injury, internal, bladder
  blast (air) (hydraulic) (immersion) (underwater) NEC 869.0
    with open wound into cavity NEC 869.1
    abdomen or thorax — *see* Injury, internal, by site
    brain — *see* Concussion, brain

Injury — *continued*
  blast — *continued*
    ear (acoustic nerve trauma) 951.5
      with perforation of tympanic membrane — *see* Wound, open, ear, drum
  blood vessel NEC 904.9
    abdomen 902.9
      multiple 902.87
      specified NEC 902.89
    aorta (thoracic) 901.0
      abdominal 902.0
    arm NEC 903.9
    axillary 903.00
      artery 903.01
      vein 903.02
    azygos vein 901.89
    basilic vein 903.1
    brachial (artery) (vein) 903.1
    bronchial 901.89
    carotid artery 900.00
      common 900.01
      external 900.02
      internal 900.03
    celiac artery 902.20
      specified branch NEC 902.24
    cephalic vein (arm) 903.1
    colica dextra 902.26
    cystic
      artery 902.24
      vein 902.39
    deep plantar 904.6
    digital (artery) (vein) 903.5
    due to accidental puncture or laceration during procedure 998.2
    extremity
      lower 904.8
        multiple 904.7
        specified NEC 904.7
      upper 903.9
        multiple 903.8
        specified NEC 903.8
    femoral
      artery (superficial) 904.1
        above profunda origin 904.0
        common 904.0
      vein 904.2
    gastric
      artery 902.21
      vein 902.39
    head 900.9
      intracranial — *see* Injury, intracranial
      multiple 900.82
      specified NEC 900.89
    hemiazygos vein 901.89
    hepatic
      artery 902.22
      vein 902.11
    hypogastric 902.59
      artery 902.51
      vein 902.52
    ileocolic
      artery 902.26
      vein 902.31
    iliac 902.50
      artery 902.53
      specified branch NEC 902.59
      vein 902.54
    innominate
      artery 901.1
      vein 901.3
    intercostal (artery) (vein) 901.81
    jugular vein (external) 900.81
      internal 900.1
    leg NEC 904.8
    mammary (artery) (vein) 901.82
    mesenteric
      artery 902.20
        inferior 902.27
        specified branch NEC 902.29
        superior (trunk) 902.25
          branches, primary 902.26
      vein 902.39
        inferior 902.32
        superior (and primary subdivisions) 902.31

Injury — *continued*
  blood vessel NEC — *continued*
    neck 900.9
      multiple 900.82
      specified NEC 900.89
    ovarian 902.89
      artery 902.81
      vein 902.82
    palmar artery 903.4
    pelvis 902.9
      multiple 902.87
      specified NEC 902.89
    plantar (deep) (artery) (vein) 904.6
    popliteal 904.40
      artery 904.41
      vein 904.42
    portal 902.33
    pulmonary 901.40
      artery 901.41
      vein 901.42
    radial (artery) (vein) 903.2
    renal 902.40
      artery 902.41
      specified NEC 902.49
      vein 902.42
    saphenous
      artery 904.7
      vein (greater) (lesser) 904.3
    splenic
      artery 902.23
      vein 902.34
    subclavian
      artery 901.1
      vein 901.3
    suprarenal 902.49
    thoracic 901.9
      multiple 901.83
      specified NEC 901.89
    tibial 904.50
      artery 904.50
        anterior 904.51
        posterior 904.53
      vein 904.50
        anterior 904.52
        posterior 904.54
    ulnar (artery) (vein) 903.3
    uterine 902.59
      artery 902.55
      vein 902.56
    vena cava
      inferior 902.10
        specified branches NEC 902.19
      superior 901.2
  brachial plexus 953.4
    newborn 767.6
  brain NEC (*see also* Injury, intracranial) 854.0
  breast 959.1
  broad ligament — *see* Injury, internal, broad ligament
  bronchus, bronchi — *see* Injury, internal, bronchus
  brow 959.09
  buttock 959.1
  canthus, eye 921.1
  cathode ray 990
  cauda equina 952.4
    with fracture, vertebra — *see* Fracture, vertebra, sacrum
  cavernous sinus (*see also* Injury, intracranial) 854.0
  cecum — *see* Injury, internal, cecum
  celiac ganglion or plexus 954.1
  cerebellum (*see also* Injury, intracranial) 854.0
  cervix (uteri) — *see* Injury, internal, cervix
  cheek 959.09
  chest — *see also* Injury, internal, chest
    wall 959.1
  childbirth — *see also* Birth, injury
    maternal NEC 665.9
  chin 959.09
  choroid (eye) 921.3
  clitoris 959.1
  coccyx 959.1
    complicating delivery 665.6
  colon — *see* Injury, internal, colon

Injury — continued
- common duct — *see* Injury, internal, common duct
- conjunctiva 921.1
  - superficial 918.2
- cord
  - spermatic — *see* Injury, internal, spermatic cord
  - spinal — *see* Injury, spinal, by site
- cornea 921.3
  - abrasion 918.1
  - due to contact lens 371.82
  - penetrating — *see* Injury, eyeball, penetrating
  - superficial 918.1
    - due to contact lens 371.82
- cortex (cerebral) (*see also* Injury, intracranial) 854.0 ☑5ᵗʰ
  - visual 950.3
- costal region 959.1
- costochondral 959.1
- cranial
  - bones — *see* Fracture, skull, by site
  - cavity (*see also* Injury, intracranial) 854.0 ☑5ᵗʰ
  - nerve — *see* Injury, nerve, cranial
- crushing — *see* Crush
- cutaneous sensory nerve
  - lower limb 956.4
  - upper limb 955.5 ☑5ᵗʰ
- delivery — *see also* Birth, injury
  - maternal NEC 665.9 ☑5ᵗʰ
- Descemet's membrane — *see* Injury, eyeball, penetrating
- diaphragm — *see* Injury, internal, diaphragm
- duodenum — *see* Injury, internal, duodenum
- ear (auricle) (canal) (drum) (external) 959.09
- elbow (and forearm) (and wrist) 959.3
- epididymis 959.1
- epigastric region 959.1
- epiglottis 959.09
- epiphyseal, current — *see* Fracture, by site
- esophagus — *see* Injury, internal, esophagus
- Eustachian tube 959.09
- extremity (lower) (upper) NEC 959.8
- eye 921.9
  - penetrating eyeball — *see* Injury, eyeball, penetrating
  - superficial 918.9
- eyeball 921.3
  - penetrating 871.7
    - with
      - partial loss (of intraocular tissue) 871.2
      - prolapse or exposure (of intraocular tissue) 871.1
      - without prolapse 871.0
      - foreign body (nonmagnetic) 871.6
        - magnetic 871.5
  - superficial 918.9
- eyebrow 959.09
- eyelid(s) 921.1
  - laceration — *see* Laceration, eyelid
  - superficial 918.0
- face (and neck) 959.09
- fallopian tube — *see* Injury, internal, fallopian tube
- finger(s) (nail) 959.5
- flank 959.1
- foot (and ankle) (and knee) (and leg except thigh) 959.7
- forceps NEC 767.9
  - scalp 767.1
- forearm (and elbow) (and wrist) 959.3
- forehead 959.09
- gallbladder — *see* Injury, internal, gallbladder
- gasserian ganglion 951.2
- gastrointestinal tract — *see* Injury, internal, gastrointestinal tract
- genital organ(s)
  - with
    - abortion — *see* Abortion, by type, with damage to pelvic organs
    - ectopic pregnancy (*see also* categories 633.0-633.9) 639.2
    - molar pregnancy (*see also* categories 630-632) 639.2

Injury — continued
- genital organ(s) — continued
  - external 959.1
  - following
    - abortion 639.2
    - ectopic or molar pregnancy 639.2
  - internal — *see* Injury, internal, genital organs
  - obstetrical trauma NEC 665. ☑5ᵗʰ
    - affecting fetus or newborn 763.89
- gland
  - lacrimal 921.1
    - laceration 870.8
  - parathyroid 959.09
  - salivary 959.09
  - thyroid 959.09
- globe (eye) (*see also* Injury, eyeball) 921.3
- grease gun — *see* Wound, open, by site, complicated
- groin 959.1
- gum 959.09
- hand(s) (except fingers) 959.4
- head NEC 959.01
  - with
    - loss of consciousness 850.5 ●
    - skull fracture — *see* Fracture, skull, by site
- heart — *see* Injury, internal, heart
- heel 959.7
- hip (and thigh) 959.6
- hymen 959.1
- hyperextension (cervical) (vertebra) 847.0
- ileum — *see* Injury, internal, ileum
- iliac region 959.1
- infrared rays NEC 990
- instrumental (during surgery) 998.2
  - birth injury — *see* Birth, injury
  - nonsurgical (*see also* Injury, by site) 959.9
  - obstetrical 665.9 ☑5ᵗʰ
    - affecting fetus or newborn 763.89
    - bladder 665.5 ☑5ᵗʰ
    - cervix 665.3 ☑5ᵗʰ
    - high vaginal 665.4 ☑5ᵗʰ
    - perineal NEC 664.9 ☑5ᵗʰ
    - urethra 665.5 ☑5ᵗʰ
    - uterus 665.5 ☑5ᵗʰ
- internal 869.0

> Note — For injury of internal organ(s) by foreign body entering through a natural orifice (e.g., inhaled, ingested, or swallowed) — *see* Foreign body, entering through orifice.
>
> For internal injury of any of the following sites with internal injury of any other of the sites — *see* Injury, internal, multiple.

  - with
    - fracture
      - open wound into cavity 869.1
      - pelvis — *see* Fracture, pelvis
      - specified site, except pelvis — *see* Injury, internal, by site
    - abdomen, abdominal (viscera) NEC 868.00
      - with
        - fracture, pelvis — *see* Fracture, pelvis
        - open wound into cavity 868.10
      - specified site NEC 868.09
        - with open wound into cavity 868.19
    - adrenal (gland) 868.01
      - with open wound into cavity 868.11
    - aorta (thoracic) 901.0
      - abdominal 902.0
    - appendix 863.85
      - with open wound into cavity 863.95
    - bile duct 868.02
      - with open wound into cavity 868.12
    - bladder (sphincter) 867.0
      - with
        - abortion — *see* Abortion, by type, with damage to pelvic organs
        - ectopic pregnancy (*see also* categories 633.0-633.9) 639.2
        - molar pregnancy (*see also* categories 630-632) 639.2
        - open wound into cavity 867.1

Injury — continued
- internal — continued
  - bladder — continued
    - following
      - abortion 639.2
      - ectopic or molar pregnancy 639.2
    - obstetrical trauma 665.5 ☑5ᵗʰ
      - affecting fetus or newborn 763.89
  - blood vessel — *see* Injury, blood vessel, by site
  - broad ligament 867.6
    - with open wound into cavity 867.7
  - bronchus, bronchi 862.21
    - with open wound into cavity 862.31
  - cecum 863.89
    - with open wound into cavity 863.99
  - cervix (uteri) 867.4
    - with
      - abortion — *see* Abortion, by type, with damage to pelvic organs
      - ectopic pregnancy (*see also* categories 633.0-633.9) 639.2
      - molar pregnancy (*see also* categories 630-632) 639.2
      - open wound into cavity 867.5
    - following
      - abortion 639.2
      - ectopic or molar pregnancy 639.2
    - obstetrical trauma 665.3 ☑5ᵗʰ
      - affecting fetus or newborn 763.89
  - chest (*see also* Injury, internal, intrathoracic organs) 862.8
    - with open wound into cavity 862.9
  - colon 863.40
    - with
      - open wound into cavity 863.50
      - rectum 863.46
        - with open wound into cavity 863.56
    - ascending (right) 863.41
      - with open wound into cavity 863.51
    - descending (left) 863.43
      - with open wound into cavity 863.53
    - multiple sites 863.46
      - with open wound into cavity 863.56
    - sigmoid 863.44
      - with open wound into cavity 863.54
    - specified site NEC 863.49
      - with open wound into cavity 863.59
    - transverse 863.42
      - with open wound into cavity 863.52
  - common duct 868.02
    - with open wound into cavity 868.12
  - complicating delivery 665.9 ☑5ᵗʰ
    - affecting fetus or newborn 763.89
  - diaphragm 862.0
    - with open wound into cavity 862.1
  - duodenum 863.21
    - with open wound into cavity 863.31
  - esophagus (intrathoracic) 862.22
    - with open wound into cavity 862.32
    - cervical region 874.4
      - complicated 874.5
  - fallopian tube 867.6
    - with open wound into cavity 867.7
  - gallbladder 868.02
    - with open wound into cavity 868.12
  - gastrointestinal tract NEC 863.80
    - with open wound into cavity 863.90
  - genital organ NEC 867.6
    - with open wound into cavity 867.7
  - heart 861.00
    - with open wound into thorax 861.10
  - ileum 863.29
    - with open wound into cavity 863.39
  - intestine NEC 863.89
    - with open wound into cavity 863.99
    - large NEC 863.40
      - with open wound into cavity 863.50
    - small NEC 863.20
      - with open wound into cavity 863.30
  - intra-abdominal (organ) 868.00
    - with open wound into cavity 868.10
    - multiple sites 868.09
      - with open wound into cavity 868.19
    - specified site NEC 868.09
      - with open wound into cavity 868.19

Index to Diseases

Injury — continued
  internal — continued
    intrathoracic organs (multiple) 862.8
      with open wound into cavity 862.9
      diaphragm (only) — see Injury, internal, diaphragm
      heart (only) — see Injury, internal, heart
      lung (only) — see Injury, internal, lung
      specified site NEC 862.29
        with open wound into cavity 862.39
    intrauterine (see also Injury, internal, uterus) 867.4
      with open wound into cavity 867.5
    jejunum 863.29
      with open wound into cavity 863.39
    kidney (subcapsular) 866.00
      with
        disruption of parenchyma (complete) 866.03
          with open wound into cavity 866.13
        hematoma (without rupture of capsule) 866.01
          with open wound into cavity 866.11
        laceration 866.02
          with open wound into cavity 866.12
        open wound into cavity 866.10
    liver 864.00
      with
        contusion 864.01
          with open wound into cavity 864.11
        hematoma 864.01
          with open wound into cavity 864.11
        laceration 864.05
          with open wound into cavity 864.15
          major (disruption of hepatic parenchyma) 864.04
            with open wound into cavity 864.14
          minor (capsule only) 864.02
            with open wound into cavity 864.12
          moderate (involving parenchyma) 864.03
            with open wound into cavity 864.13
          multiple 864.04
          stellate 864.04
            with open wound into cavity 864.14
        open wound into cavity 864.10
    lung 861.20
      with open wound into thorax 861.30
      hemopneumothorax — see Hemopneumothorax, traumatic
      hemothorax — see Hemothorax, traumatic
      pneumohemothorax — see Pneumohemothorax, traumatic
      pneumothorax — see Pneumothorax, traumatic
    mediastinum 862.29
      with open wound into cavity 862.39
    mesentery 863.89
      with open wound into cavity 863.99
    mesosalpinx 867.6
      with open wound into cavity 867.7
    multiple 869.0

> Note — Multiple internal injuries of sites classifiable to the same three- or four-digit category should be classified to that category.
>
> Multiple injuries classifiable to different fourth-digit subdivisions of 861 (heart and lung injuries) should be dealt with according to coding rules.

      internal
        with open wound into cavity 869.1
        intra-abdominal organ (sites classifiable to 863-868)
          with
            intrathoracic organ(s) (sites classifiable to 861-862) 869.0
              with open wound into cavity 869.1

Injury — continued
  internal — continued
    multiple — continued
      intra-abdominal organ — continued
        with — continued
          other intra-abdominal organ(s) (sites classifiable to 863-868, except where classifiable to the same three-digit category) 868.09
            with open wound into cavity 868.19
      intrathoracic organ (sites classifiable to 861-862)
        with
          intra-abdominal organ(s) (sites classifiable to 863-868) 869.0
            with open wound into cavity 869.1
          other intrathoracic organ(s) (sites classifiable to 861-862, except where classifiable to the same three-digit category) 862.8
            with open wound into cavity 862.9
    myocardium — see Injury, internal, heart
    ovary 867.6
      with open wound into cavity 867.7
    pancreas (multiple sites) 863.84
      with open wound into cavity 863.94
      body 863.82
        with open wound into cavity 863.92
      head 863.81
        with open wound into cavity 863.91
      tail 863.83
        with open wound into cavity 863.93
    pelvis, pelvic (organs) (viscera) 867.8
      with
        fracture, pelvis — see Fracture, pelvis
        open wound into cavity 867.9
      specified site NEC 867.6
        with open wound into cavity 867.7
    peritoneum 868.03
      with open wound into cavity 868.13
    pleura 862.29
      with open wound into cavity 862.39
    prostate 867.6
      with open wound into cavity 867.7
    rectum 863.45
      with
        colon 863.46
          with open wound into cavity 863.56
        open wound into cavity 863.55
    retroperitoneum 868.04
      with open wound into cavity 868.14
    round ligament 867.6
      with open wound into cavity 867.7
    seminal vesicle 867.6
      with open wound into cavity 867.7
    spermatic cord 867.6
      with open wound into cavity 867.7
      scrotal — see Wound, open, spermatic cord
    spleen 865.00
      with
        disruption of parenchyma (massive) 865.04
          with open wound into cavity 865.14
        hematoma (without rupture of capsule) 865.01
          with open wound into cavity 865.11
        open wound into cavity 865.10
        tear, capsular 865.02
          with open wound into cavity 865.12
          extending into parenchyma 865.03
            with open wound into cavity 865.13
    stomach 863.0
      with open wound into cavity 863.1
    suprarenal gland (multiple) 868.01
      with open wound into cavity 868.11
    thorax, thoracic (cavity) (organs) (multiple) (see also Injury, internal, intrathoracic organs) 862.8
      with open wound into cavity 862.9
    thymus (gland) 862.29
      with open wound into cavity 862.39

Injury — continued
  internal — continued
    trachea (intrathoracic) 862.29
      with open wound into cavity 862.39
      cervical region (see also Wound, open, trachea) 874.02
    ureter 867.2
      with open wound into cavity 867.3
    urethra (sphincter) 867.0
      with
        abortion — see Abortion, by type, with damage to pelvic organs
        ectopic pregnancy (see also categories 633.0-633.9) 639.2
        molar pregnancy (see also categories 630-632) 639.2
        open wound into cavity 867.1
      following
        abortion 639.2
        ectopic or molar pregnancy 639.2
      obstetrical trauma 665.5
        affecting fetus or newborn 763.89
    uterus 867.4
      with
        abortion — see Abortion, by type, with damage to pelvic organs
        ectopic pregnancy (see also categories 633.0-633.9) 639.2
        molar pregnancy (see also categories 630-632) 639.2
        open wound into cavity 867.5
      following
        abortion 639.2
        ectopic or molar pregnancy 639.2
      obstetrical trauma NEC 665.5
        affecting fetus or newborn 763.89
    vas deferens 867.6
      with open wound into cavity 867.7
    vesical (sphincter) 867.0
      with open wound into cavity 867.1
    viscera (abdominal) (see also Injury, internal, multiple) 868.00
      with
        fracture, pelvis — see Fracture, pelvis
        open wound into cavity 868.10
      thoracic NEC (see also Injury, internal, intrathoracic organs) 862.8
        with open wound into cavity 862.9
  interscapular region 959.1
  intervertebral disc 959.1
  intestine — see Injury, internal, intestine
  intra-abdominal (organs) NEC — see Injury, internal, intra-abdominal
  intracranial 854.0

> Note — Use the following fifth-digit subclassification with categories 851-854:
>
> 0   unspecified state of consciousness
> 1   with no loss of consciousness
> 2   with brief [less than one hour] loss of consciousness
> 3   with moderate [1-24 hours] loss of consciousness
> 4   with prolonged [more than 24 hours] loss of consciousness and return to pre-existing conscious level
> 5   with prolonged [more than 24 hours] loss of consciousness, without return to pre-existing conscious level
>
> Use fifth-digit 5 to designate when a patient is unconscious and dies before regaining consciousness, regardless of the duration of the loss of consciousness
>
> 6   with loss of consciousness of unspecified duration
> 9   with concussion, unspecified

    with
      open intracranial wound 854.1
      skull fracture — see Fracture, skull, by site
    contusion 851.8
      with open intracranial wound 851.9

Injury

Injury — *continued*
  intracranial — *continued*
    contusion — *continued*
      brain stem 851.4 ✓5th
        with open intracranial wound 851.5 ✓5th
      cerebellum 851.4 ✓5th
        with open intracranial wound 851.5 ✓5th
      cortex (cerebral) 851.0 ✓5th
        with open intracranial wound 851.2 ✓5th
    hematoma — *see* Injury, intracranial, hemorrhage
    hemorrhage 853.0 ✓5th
      with
        laceration — *see* Injury, intracranial, laceration
        open intracranial wound 853.1 ✓5th
      extradural 852.4 ✓5th
        with open intracranial wound 852.5 ✓5th
      subarachnoid 852.0 ✓5th
        with open intracranial wound 852.1 ✓5th
      subdural 852.2 ✓5th
        with open intracranial wound 852.3 ✓5th
    laceration 851.8 ✓5th
      with open intracranial wound 851.9 ✓5th
      brain stem 851.6 ✓5th
        with open intracranial wound 851.7 ✓5th
      cerebellum 851.6 ✓5th
        with open intracranial wound 851.7 ✓5th
      cortex (cerebral) 851.2 ✓5th
        with open intracranial wound 851.3 ✓5th
  intraocular — *see* Injury, eyeball, penetrating
  intrathoracic organs (multiple) — *see* Injury, internal, intrathoracic organs
  intrauterine — *see* Injury, internal, intrauterine
  iris 921.3
    penetrating — *see* Injury, eyeball, penetrating
  jaw 959.09
  jejunum — *see* Injury, internal, jejunum
  joint NEC 959.9
    old or residual 718.80
      ankle 718.87
      elbow 718.82
      foot 718.87
      hand 718.84
      hip 718.85
      knee 718.86
      multiple sites 718.89
      pelvic region 718.85
      shoulder (region) 718.81
      specified site NEC 718.88
      wrist 718.83
  kidney — *see* Injury, internal, kidney
  knee (and ankle) (and foot) (and leg, except thigh) 959.7
  labium (majus) (minus) 959.1
  labyrinth, ear 959.09
  lacrimal apparatus, gland, or sac 921.1
    laceration 870.8
  larynx 959.09
  late effect — *see* Late, effects (of), injury
  leg except thigh (and ankle) (and foot) (and knee) 959.7
    upper or thigh 959.6
  lens, eye 921.3
    penetrating — *see* Injury, eyeball, penetrating
  lid, eye — *see* Injury, eyelid
  lip 959.09
  liver — *see* Injury, internal, liver
  lobe, parietal — *see* Injury, intracranial
  lumbar (region) 959.1
    plexus 953.5
  lumbosacral (region) 959.1
    plexus 953.5
  lung — *see* Injury, internal, lung
  malar region 959.09
  mastoid region 959.09

Injury — *continued*
  maternal, during pregnancy, affecting fetus or newborn 760.5
  maxilla 959.09
  mediastinum — *see* Injury, internal, mediastinum
  membrane
    brain (*see also* Injury, intracranial) 854.0 ✓5th
    tympanic 959.09
  meningeal artery — *see* Hemorrhage, brain, traumatic, subarachnoid
  meninges (cerebral) — *see* Injury, intracranial
  mesenteric
    artery — *see* Injury, blood vessel, mesenteric, artery
    plexus, inferior 954.1
    vein — *see* Injury, blood vessel, mesenteric, vein
  mesentery — *see* Injury, internal, mesentery
  mesosalpinx — *see* Injury, internal, mesosalpinx
  middle ear 959.09
  midthoracic region 959.1
  mouth 959.09
  multiple (sites not classifiable to the same four-digit category in 959.0-959.7) 959.8
    internal 869.0
      with open wound into cavity 869.1
  musculocutaneous nerve 955.4
  nail
    finger 959.5
    toe 959.7
  nasal (septum) (sinus) 959.09
  nasopharynx 959.09
  neck (and face) 959.09
  nerve 957.9
    abducens 951.3
    abducent 951.3
    accessory 951.6
    acoustic 951.5
    ankle and foot 956.9
    anterior crural, femoral 956.1
    arm (*see also* Injury, nerve, upper limb) 955.9
    auditory 951.5
    axillary 955.0
    brachial plexus 953.4
    cervical sympathetic 954.0
    cranial 951.9
      first or olfactory 951.8
      second or optic 950.0
      third or oculomotor 951.0
      fourth or trochlear 951.1
      fifth or trigeminal 951.2
      sixth or abducens 951.3
      seventh or facial 951.4
      eighth, acoustic, or auditory 951.5
      ninth or glossopharyngeal 951.8
      tenth, pneumogastric, or vagus 951.8
      eleventh or accessory 951.6
      twelfth or hypoglossal 951.7
      newborn 767.7
    cutaneous sensory
      lower limb 956.4
      upper limb 955.5 ✓5th
    digital (finger) 955.6
      toe 956.5
    facial 951.4
      newborn 767.5
    femoral 956.1
    finger 955.9
    foot and ankle 956.9
    forearm 955.9
    glossopharyngeal 951.8
    hand and wrist 955.9
    head and neck, superficial 957.0
    hypoglossal 951.7
    involving several parts of body 957.8
    leg (*see also* Injury, nerve, lower limb) 956.9
    lower limb 956.9
      multiple 956.8
      specified site NEC 956.5
    lumbar plexus 953.5
    lumbosacral plexus 953.5
    median 955.1
      forearm 955.1

Injury — *continued*
  nerve — *continued*
    median — *continued*
      wrist and hand 955.1
    multiple (in several parts of body) (sites not classifiable to the same three-digit category) 957.8
    musculocutaneous 955.4
    musculospiral 955.3
      upper arm 955.3
    oculomotor 951.0
    olfactory 951.8
    optic 950.0
    pelvic girdle 956.9
      multiple sites 956.8
      specified site NEC 956.5
    peripheral 957.9
      multiple (in several regions) (sites not classifiable to the same three-digit category) 957.8
      specified site NEC 957.1
    peroneal 956.3
      ankle and foot 956.3
      lower leg 956.3
    plantar 956.5
    plexus 957.9
      celiac 954.1
      mesenteric, inferior 954.1
      spinal 953.9
        brachial 953.4
        lumbosacral 953.5
        multiple sites 953.8
      sympathetic NEC 954.1
    pneumogastric 951.8
    radial 955.3
      wrist and hand 955.3
    sacral plexus 953.5
    sciatic 956.0
      thigh 956.0
    shoulder girdle 955.9
      multiple 955.8
      specified site NEC 955.7
    specified site NEC 957.1
    spinal 953.9
      plexus — *see* Injury, nerve, plexus, spinal
      root 953.9
        cervical 953.0
        dorsal 953.1
        lumbar 953.2
        multiple sites 953.8
        sacral 953.3
    splanchnic 954.1
    sympathetic NEC 954.1
      cervical 954.0
    thigh 956.9
    tibial 956.5
      ankle and foot 956.2
      lower leg 956.5
      posterior 956.2
    toe 956.9
    trigeminal 951.2
    trochlear 951.1
    trunk, excluding shoulder and pelvic girdles 954.9
      specified site NEC 954.8
      sympathetic NEC 954.1
    ulnar 955.2
      forearm 955.2
      wrist (and hand) 955.2
    upper limb 955.9
      multiple 955.8
      specified site NEC 955.7
    vagus 951.8
    wrist and hand 955.9
  nervous system, diffuse 957.8
  nose (septum) 959.09
  obstetrical NEC 665.9 ✓5th
    affecting fetus or newborn 763.89
  occipital (region) (scalp) 959.09
    lobe (*see also* Injury, intracranial) 854.0 ✓5th
  optic 950.9
    chiasm 950.1
    cortex 950.3
    nerve 950.0
    pathways 950.2

Index to Diseases

Injury — continued

orbit, orbital (region) 921.2
    penetrating 870.3
        with foreign body 870.4
ovary — see Injury, internal, ovary
paint-gun — see Wound, open, by site, complicated
palate (soft) 959.09
pancreas — see Injury, internal, pancreas
parathyroid (gland) 959.09
parietal (region) (scalp) 959.09
    lobe — see Injury, intracranial
pelvic
    floor 959.1
        complicating delivery 664.1 ✓5ᵗʰ
            affecting fetus or newborn 763.89
    joint or ligament, complicating delivery 665.6 ✓5ᵗʰ
        affecting fetus or newborn 763.89
    organs — see also Injury, internal, pelvis
        with
            abortion — see Abortion, by type, with damage to pelvic organs
            ectopic pregnancy (see also categories 633.0-633.9) 639.2
            molar pregnancy (see also categories 633.0-633.9) 639.2
        following
            abortion 639.2
            ectopic or molar pregnancy 639.2
        obstetrical trauma 665.5 ✓5ᵗʰ
            affecting fetus or newborn 763.89
pelvis 959.1
penis 959.1
perineum 959.1
peritoneum — see Injury, internal, peritoneum
periurethral tissue
    with
        abortion — see Abortion, by type, with damage to pelvic organs
        ectopic pregnancy (see also categories 633.0-633.9) 639.2
        molar pregnancy (see also categories 630-632) 639.2
    complicating delivery 665.5 ✓5ᵗʰ
        affecting fetus or newborn 763.89
    following
        abortion 639.2
        ectopic or molar pregnancy 639.2
phalanges
    foot 959.7
    hand 959.5
pharynx 959.09
pleura — see Injury, internal, pleura
popliteal space 959.7
prepuce 959.1
prostate — see Injury, internal, prostate
pubic region 959.1
pudenda 959.1
radiation NEC 990
radioactive substance or radium NEC 990
rectovaginal septum 959.1
rectum — see Injury, internal, rectum
retina 921.3
    penetrating — see Injury, eyeball, penetrating
retroperitoneal — see Injury, internal, retroperitoneum
roentgen rays NEC 990
round ligament — see Injury, internal, round ligament
sacral (region) 959.1
    plexus 953.5
sacroiliac ligament NEC 959.1
sacrum 959.1
salivary ducts or glands 959.09
scalp 959.09
    due to birth trauma 767.1
    fetus or newborn 767.1
scapular region 959.2
sclera 921.3
    penetrating — see Injury, eyeball, penetrating
    superficial 918.2
scrotum 959.1
seminal vesicle — see Injury, internal, seminal vesicle
shoulder (and upper arm) 959.2

Injury — continued

sinus
    cavernous (see also Injury, intracranial) 854.0 ✓5ᵗʰ
    nasal 959.09
skeleton NEC, birth injury 767.3
skin NEC 959.9
skull — see Fracture, skull, by site
soft tissue (of external sites) (severe) — see Wound, open, by site
specified site NEC 959.8
spermatic cord — see Injury, internal, spermatic cord
spinal (cord) 952.9
    with fracture, vertebra — see Fracture, vertebra, by site, with spinal cord injury
    cervical (C_1-C_4) 952.00
        with
            anterior cord syndrome 952.02
            central cord syndrome 952.03
            complete lesion of cord 952.01
            incomplete lesion NEC 952.04
            posterior cord syndrome 952.04
        C_5-C_7 level 952.05
            with
                anterior cord syndrome 952.07
                central cord syndrome 952.08
                complete lesion of cord 952.06
                incomplete lesion NEC 952.09
                posterior cord syndrome 952.09
            specified type NEC 952.09
        specified type NEC 952.04
    dorsal (D_1-D_6) (T_1-T_6) (thoracic) 952.10
        with
            anterior cord syndrome 952.12
            central cord syndrome 952.13
            complete lesion of cord 952.11
            incomplete lesion NEC 952.14
            posterior cord syndrome 952.14
        D_7-D_{12} level (T_7-T_{12}) 952.15
            with
                anterior cord syndrome 952.17
                central cord syndrome 952.18
                complete lesion of cord 952.16
                incomplete lesion NEC 952.19
                posterior cord syndrome 952.19
            specified type NEC 952.19
        specified type NEC 952.14
    lumbar 952.2
    multiple sites 952.8
    nerve (root) NEC — see Injury, nerve, spinal, root
    plexus 953.9
        brachial 953.4
        lumbosacral 953.5
        multiple sites 953.8
    sacral 952.3
    thoracic (see also Injury, spinal, dorsal) 952.10
spleen — see Injury, internal, spleen
stellate ganglion 954.1
sternal region 959.1
stomach — see Injury, internal, stomach
subconjunctival 921.1
subcutaneous 959.9
subdural — see Injury, intracranial
submaxillary region 959.09
submental region 959.09
subungual
    fingers 959.5
    toes 959.7
superficial 919 ✓4ᵗʰ

Injury — continued

superficial — continued

> Note — Use the following fourth-digit subdivisions with categories 910-919:
>
> 0   Abrasion or friction burn without mention of infection
> 1   Abrasion or friction burn, infected
> 2   Blister without mention of infection
> 3   Blister, infected
> 4   Insect bite, nonvenomous, without mention of infection
> 5   Insect bite, nonvenomous, infected
> 6   Superficial foreign body (splinter) without major open wound and without mention of infection
> 7   Superficial foreign body (splinter) without major open wound, infected
> 8   Other and unspecified superficial injury without mention of infection
> 9   Other and unspecified superficial injury, infected
>
> For late effects of superficial injury, see category 906.2.

abdomen, abdominal (muscle) (wall) (and other part(s) of trunk) 911 ✓4ᵗʰ
ankle (and hip, knee, leg, or thigh) 916 ✓4ᵗʰ
anus (and other part(s) of trunk) 911 ✓4ᵗʰ
arm 913 ✓4ᵗʰ
    upper (and shoulder) 912 ✓4ᵗʰ
auditory canal (external) (meatus) (and other part(s) of face, neck, or scalp, except eye) 910 ✓4ᵗʰ
axilla (and upper arm) 912 ✓4ᵗʰ
back (and other part(s) of trunk) 911 ✓4ᵗʰ
breast (and other part(s) of trunk) 911 ✓4ᵗʰ
brow (and other part(s) of face, neck, or scalp, except eye) 910 ✓4ᵗʰ
buttock (and other part(s) of trunk) 911 ✓4ᵗʰ
canthus, eye 918.0
cheek(s) (and other part(s) of face, neck, or scalp, except eye) 910 ✓4ᵗʰ
chest wall (and other part(s) of trunk) 911 ✓4ᵗʰ
chin (and other part(s) of face, neck, or scalp, except eye) 910 ✓4ᵗʰ
clitoris (and other part(s) of trunk) 911 ✓4ᵗʰ
conjunctiva 918.2
cornea 918.1
    due to contact lens 371.82
costal region (and other part(s) of trunk) 911 ✓4ᵗʰ
ear(s) (auricle) (canal) (drum) (external) (and other part(s) of face, neck, or scalp, except eye) 910 ✓4ᵗʰ
elbow (and forearm) (and wrist) 913 ✓4ᵗʰ
epididymis (and other part(s) of trunk) 911 ✓4ᵗʰ
epigastric region (and other part(s) of trunk) 911 ✓4ᵗʰ
epiglottis (and other part(s) of face, neck, or scalp, except eye) 910 ✓4ᵗʰ
eye(s) (and adnexa) NEC 918.9
eyelid(s) (and periocular area) 918.0
face (any part(s), except eye) (and neck or scalp) 910 ✓4ᵗʰ
finger(s) (nail) (any) 915 ✓4ᵗʰ
flank (and other part(s) of trunk) 911 ✓4ᵗʰ
foot (phalanges) (and toe(s)) 917 ✓4ᵗʰ
forearm (and elbow) (and wrist) 913 ✓4ᵗʰ
forehead (and other part(s) of face, neck, or scalp, except eye) 910 ✓4ᵗʰ
globe (eye) 918.9
groin (and other part(s) of trunk) 911 ✓4ᵗʰ
gum(s) (and other part(s) of face, neck, or scalp, except eye) 910 ✓4ᵗʰ
hand(s) (except fingers alone) 914 ✓4ᵗʰ
head (and other part(s) of face, neck, or scalp, except eye) 910 ✓4ᵗʰ
heel (and foot or toe) 917 ✓4ᵗʰ
hip (and ankle, knee, leg, or thigh) 916 ✓4ᵗʰ
iliac region (and other part(s) of trunk) 911 ✓4ᵗʰ

Injury

Injury — *continued*
  superficial — *continued*
    interscapular region (and other part(s) of trunk) 911 ✓4ᵗʰ
    iris 918.9
    knee (and ankle, hip, leg, or thigh) 916 ✓4ᵗʰ
    labium (majus) (minus) (and other part(s) of trunk) 911 ✓4ᵗʰ
    lacrimal (apparatus) (gland) (sac) 918.0
    leg (lower) (upper) (and ankle, hip, knee, or thigh) 916 ✓4ᵗʰ
    lip(s) (and other part(s) of face, neck, or scalp, except eye) 910 ✓4ᵗʰ
    lower extremity (except foot) 916 ✓4ᵗʰ
    lumbar region (and other part(s) of trunk) 911 ✓4ᵗʰ
    malar region (and other part(s) of face, neck, or scalp, except eye) 910 ✓4ᵗʰ
    mastoid region (and other part(s) of face, neck, or scalp, except eye) 910 ✓4ᵗʰ
    midthoracic region (and other part(s) of trunk) 911 ✓4ᵗʰ
    mouth (and other part(s) of face, neck, or scalp, except eye) 910 ✓4ᵗʰ
    multiple sites (not classifiable to the same three-digit category) 919 ✓4ᵗʰ
    nasal (septum) (and other part(s) of face, neck, or scalp, except eye) 910 ✓4ᵗʰ
    neck (and face or scalp, any part(s), except eye) 910 ✓4ᵗʰ
    nose (septum) (and other part(s) of face, neck, or scalp, except eye) 910 ✓4ᵗʰ
    occipital region (and other part(s) of face, neck, or scalp, except eye) 910 ✓4ᵗʰ
    orbital region 918.0
    palate (soft) (and other part(s) of face, neck, or scalp, except eye) 910 ✓4ᵗʰ
    parietal region (and other part(s) of face, neck, or scalp, except eye) 910 ✓4ᵗʰ
    penis (and other part(s) of trunk) 911 ✓4ᵗʰ
    perineum (and other part(s) of trunk) 911 ✓4ᵗʰ
    periocular area 918.0
    pharynx (and other part(s) of face, neck, or scalp, except eye) 910 ✓4ᵗʰ
    popliteal space (and ankle, hip, leg, or thigh) 916 ✓4ᵗʰ
    prepuce (and other part(s) of trunk) 911 ✓4ᵗʰ
    pubic region (and other part(s) of trunk) 911 ✓4ᵗʰ
    pudenda (and other part(s) of trunk) 911 ✓4ᵗʰ
    sacral region (and other part(s) of trunk) 911 ✓4ᵗʰ
    salivary (ducts) (glands) (and other part(s) of face, neck, or scalp, except eye) 910 ✓4ᵗʰ
    scalp (and other part(s) of face or neck, except eye) 910 ✓4ᵗʰ
    scapular region (and upper arm) 912 ✓4ᵗʰ
    sclera 918.2
    scrotum (and other part(s) of trunk) 911 ✓4ᵗʰ
    shoulder (and upper arm) 912 ✓4ᵗʰ
    skin NEC 919 ✓4ᵗʰ
    specified site(s) NEC 919 ✓4ᵗʰ
    sternal region (and other part(s) of trunk) 911 ✓4ᵗʰ
    subconjunctival 918.2
    subcutaneous NEC 919 ✓4ᵗʰ
    submaxillary region (and other part(s) of face, neck, or scalp, except eye) 910 ✓4ᵗʰ
    submental region (and other part(s) of face, neck, or scalp, except eye) 910 ✓4ᵗʰ
    supraclavicular fossa (and other part(s) of face, neck or scalp, except eye) 910 ✓4ᵗʰ
    supraorbital 918.0
    temple (and other part(s) of face, neck, or scalp, except eye) 910 ✓4ᵗʰ
    temporal region (and other part(s) of face, neck, or scalp, except eye) 910 ✓4ᵗʰ
    testis (and other part(s) of trunk) 911 ✓4ᵗʰ
    thigh (and ankle, hip, knee, or leg) 916 ✓4ᵗʰ
    thorax, thoracic (external) (and other part(s) of trunk) 911 ✓4ᵗʰ
    throat (and other part(s) of face, neck, or scalp, except eye) 910 ✓4ᵗʰ
    thumb(s) (nail) 915 ✓4ᵗʰ

Injury — *continued*
  superficial — *continued*
    toe(s) (nail) (subungual) (and foot) 917 ✓4ᵗʰ
    tongue (and other part(s) of face, neck, or scalp, except eye) 910 ✓4ᵗʰ
    tooth, teeth 521.2
    trunk (any part(s)) 911 ✓4ᵗʰ
    tunica vaginalis (and other part(s) of trunk) 911 ✓4ᵗʰ
    tympanum, tympanic membrane (and other part(s) of face, neck, or scalp, except eye) 910 ✓4ᵗʰ
    upper extremity NEC 913 ✓4ᵗʰ
    uvula (and other part(s) of face, neck, or scalp, except eye) 910 ✓4ᵗʰ
    vagina (and other part(s) of trunk) 911 ✓4ᵗʰ
    vulva (and other part(s) of trunk) 911 ✓4ᵗʰ
    wrist (and elbow) (and forearm) 913 ✓4ᵗʰ
  supraclavicular fossa 959.1
  supraorbital 959.09
  surgical complication (external or internal site) 998.2
  symphysis pubis 959.1
    complicating delivery 665.6 ✓5ᵗʰ
      affecting fetus or newborn 763.89
  temple 959.09
  temporal region 959.09
  testis 959.1
  thigh (and hip) 959.6
  thorax, thoracic (external) 959.1
    cavity — *see* Injury, internal, thorax
    internal — *see* Injury, internal, intrathoracic organs
  throat 959.09
  thumb(s) (nail) 959.5
  thymus — *see* Injury, internal, thymus
  thyroid (gland) 959.09
  toe (nail) (any) 959.7
  tongue 959.09
  tonsil 959.09
  tooth NEC 873.63
    complicated 873.73
  trachea — *see* Injury, internal, trachea
  trunk 959.1
  tunica vaginalis 959.1
  tympanum, tympanic membrane 959.09
  ultraviolet rays NEC 990
  ureter — *see* Injury, internal, ureter
  urethra (sphincter) — *see* Injury, internal, urethra
  uterus — *see* Injury, internal, uterus
  uvula 959.09
  vagina 959.1
  vascular — *see* Injury, blood vessel
  vas deferens — *see* Injury, internal, vas deferens
  vein (*see also* Injury, blood vessel, by site) 904.9
  vena cava
    inferior 902.10
    superior 901.2
  vesical (sphincter) — *see* Injury, internal, vesical
  viscera (abdominal) — *see also* Injury, internal, viscera
    with fracture, pelvis — *see* Fracture, pelvis
  visual 950.9
    cortex 950.3
  vitreous (humor) 871.2
  vulva 959.1
  whiplash (cervical spine) 847.0
  wringer — *see* Crush, by site
  wrist (and elbow) (and forearm) 959.3
  x-ray NEC 990

Inoculation — *see also* Vaccination
  complication or reaction — *see* Complication, vaccination

Insanity, insane (*see also* Psychosis) 298.9
  adolescent (*see also* Schizophrenia) 295.9 ✓5ᵗʰ
  alternating (*see also* Psychosis, affective, circular) 296.7
  confusional 298.9
    acute 293.0
    subacute 293.1
  delusional 298.9

Insanity, insane (*see also* Psychosis) — *continued*
  paralysis, general 094.1
    progressive 094.1
  paresis, general 094.1
  senile 290.20

Insect
  bite — *see* Injury, superficial, by site
  venomous, poisoning by 989.5

Insemination, artificial V26.1

Insertion
  cord (umbilical) lateral or velamentous 663.8 ✓5ᵗʰ
    affecting fetus or newborn 762.6
  intrauterine contraceptive device V25.1
  placenta, vicious — *see* Placenta, previa
  subdermal implantable contraceptive V25.5
  velamentous, umbilical cord 663.8 ✓5ᵗʰ
    affecting fetus or newborn 762.6

Insolation 992.0
  meaning sunstroke 992.0

Insomnia 780.52
  with sleep apnea 780.51
  nonorganic origin 307.41
    persistent (primary) 307.42
    transient 307.41
  subjective complaint 307.49

Inspiration
  food or foreign body (*see also* Asphyxia, food or foreign body) 933.1
  mucus (*see also* Asphyxia, mucus) 933.1

Inspissated bile syndrome, newborn 774.4

Instability
  detrusor 596.59
  emotional (excessive) 301.3
  joint (posttraumatic) 718.80
    ankle 718.87
    elbow 718.82
    foot 718.87
    hand 718.84
    hip 718.85
    knee 718.86
    lumbosacral 724.6
    multiple sites 718.89
    pelvic region 718.85
    sacroiliac 724.6
    shoulder (region) 718.81
    specified site NEC 718.88
    wrist 718.83
  lumbosacral 724.6
  nervous 301.89
  personality (emotional) 301.59
  thyroid, paroxysmal 242.9 ✓5ᵗʰ
  urethral 599.83
  vasomotor 780.2

Insufficiency, insufficient
  accommodation 367.4
  adrenal (gland) (acute) (chronic) 255.4
    medulla 255.5
    primary 255.4
    specified NEC 255.5
  adrenocortical 255.4
  anus 569.49
  aortic (valve) 424.1
    with
      mitral (valve) disease 396.1
        insufficiency, incompetence, or regurgitation 396.3
        stenosis or obstruction 396.1
      stenosis or obstruction 424.1
        with mitral (valve) disease 396.8
    congenital 746.4
    rheumatic 395.1
      with
        mitral (valve) disease 396.1
          insufficiency, incompetence, or regurgitation 396.3
          stenosis or obstruction 396.1
        stenosis or obstruction 395.2
          with mitral (valve) disease 396.8
    specified cause NEC 424.1
    syphilitic 093.22
  arterial 447.1
    basilar artery 435.0
    carotid artery 435.8
    cerebral 437.1
    coronary (acute or subacute) 411.89

Insufficiency, insufficient — *continued*
  arterial — *continued*
    mesenteric 557.1
    peripheral 443.9
    precerebral 435.9
    vertebral artery 435.1
    vertebrobasilar 435.3
  arteriovenous 459.9
  basilar artery 435.0
  biliary 575.8
  cardiac (*see also* Insufficiency, myocardial) 428.0
    complicating surgery 997.1
    due to presence of (cardiac) prosthesis 429.4
    postoperative 997.1
      long-term effect of cardiac surgery 429.4
    specified during or due to a procedure 997.1
      long-term effect of cardiac surgery 429.4
  cardiorenal (*see also* Hypertension, cardiorenal) 404.90
  cardiovascular (*see also* Disease, cardiovascular) 429.2
    renal (*see also* Hypertension, cardiorenal) 404.90
  carotid artery 435.8
  cerebral (vascular) 437.9
  cerebrovascular 437.9
    with transient focal neurological signs and symptoms 435.9
    acute 437.1
      with transient focal neurological signs and symptoms 435.9
  circulatory NEC 459.9
    fetus or newborn 779.89 ▲
  convergence 378.83
  coronary (acute or subacute) 411.89
    chronic or with a stated duration of over 8 weeks 414.8
  corticoadrenal 255.4
  dietary 269.9
  divergence 378.85
  food 994.2
  gastroesophageal 530.89
  gonadal
    ovary 256.39
    testis 257.2
  gonadotropic hormone secretion 253.4
  heart — *see also* Insufficiency, myocardial
    fetus or newborn 779.89 ▲
    valve (*see also* Endocarditis) 424.90
      congenital NEC 746.89
  hepatic 573.8
  idiopathic autonomic 333.0
  kidney ▶(acute) (chronic)◀ 593.9
  labyrinth, labyrinthine (function) 386.53
    bilateral 386.54
    unilateral 386.53
  lacrimal 375.15
  liver 573.8
  lung (acute) (*see also* Insufficiency, pulmonary) 518.82
    following trauma, surgery, or shock 518.5
    newborn 770.89 ▲
  mental (congenital) (*see also* Retardation, mental) 319
  mesenteric 557.1
  mitral (valve) 424.0
    with
      aortic (valve) disease 396.3
        insufficiency, incompetence, or regurgitation 396.3
        stenosis or obstruction 396.2
      obstruction or stenosis 394.2
        with aortic valve disease 396.8
      congenital 746.6
      rheumatic 394.1
        with
          aortic (valve) disease 396.3
            insufficiency, incompetence, or regurgitation 396.3
            stenosis or obstruction 396.2
          obstruction or stenosis 394.2
            with aortic valve disease 396.8
          active or acute 391.1
            with chorea, rheumatic (Sydenham's) 392.0
        specified cause, except rheumatic 424.0

Insufficiency, insufficient — *continued*
  muscle
    heart — *see* Insufficiency, myocardial
    ocular (*see also* Strabismus) 378.9
  myocardial, myocardium (with arteriosclerosis) 428.0
    with rheumatic fever (conditions classifiable to 390)
      active, acute, or subacute 391.2
        with chorea 392.0
      inactive or quiescent (with chorea) 398.0
    congenital 746.89
    due to presence of (cardiac) prosthesis 429.4
    fetus or newborn 779.89 ▲
    following cardiac surgery 429.4
    hypertensive (*see also* Hypertension, heart) 402.91
      benign 402.11
      malignant 402.01
    postoperative 997.1
      long-term effect of cardiac surgery 429.4
    rheumatic 398.0
      active, acute, or subacute 391.2
        with chorea (Sydenham's) 392.0
    syphilitic 093.82
  nourishment 994.2
  organic 799.8
  ovary 256.39
    postablative 256.2
  pancreatic 577.8
  parathyroid (gland) 252.1
  peripheral vascular (arterial) 443.9
  pituitary (anterior) 253.2
    posterior 253.5
  placental — *see* Placenta, insufficiency
  platelets 287.5
  prenatal care in current pregnancy V23.7
  progressive pluriglandular 258.9
  pseudocholinesterase 289.8
  pulmonary (acute) 518.82
    following
      shock 518.5
      surgery 518.5
      trauma 518.5
    newborn 770.89 ▲
    valve (*see also* Endocarditis, pulmonary) 424.3
      congenital 746.09
  pyloric 537.0
  renal ▶(acute) (chronic)◀ 593.9
    due to a procedure 997.5
  respiratory 786.09
    acute 518.82
      following shock, surgery, or trauma 518.5
    newborn 770.89 ▲
  rotation — *see* Malrotation
  suprarenal 255.4
    medulla 255.5
  tarso-orbital fascia, congenital 743.66
  tear film 375.15
  testis 257.2
  thyroid (gland) (acquired) — *see also* Hypothyroidism
    congenital 243
  tricuspid (*see also* Endocarditis, tricuspid) 397.0
    congenital 746.89
    syphilitic 093.23
  urethral sphincter 599.84
  valve, valvular (heart) (*see also* Endocarditis) 424.90
  vascular 459.9
    intestine NEC 557.9
    mesenteric 557.1
    peripheral 443.9
    renal (*see also* Hypertension, kidney) 403.90
  velopharyngeal
    acquired 528.9
    congenital 750.29
  venous (peripheral) 459.81
  ventricular — *see* Insufficiency, myocardial
  vertebral artery 435.1
  vertebrobasilar artery 435.3
  weight gain during pregnancy 646.8 ✓5ᵗʰ
  zinc 269.3

Insufflation
  fallopian
    fertility testing V26.21
    following sterilization reversal V26.22
  meconium 770.1
Insular — *see* condition
Insulinoma (M8151/0)
  malignant (M8151/3)
    pancreas 157.4
    specified site — *see* Neoplasm, by site, malignant
    unspecified site 157.4
  pancreas 211.7
  specified site — *see* Neoplasm, by site, benign
  unspecified site 211.7
Insuloma — *see* Insulinoma
Insult
  brain 437.9
    acute 436
  cerebral 437.9
    acute 436
  cerebrovascular 437.9
    acute 436
  vascular NEC 437.9
    acute 436
Insurance examination (certification) V70.3
Intemperance (*see also* Alcoholism) 303.9 ✓5ᵗʰ
Interception of pregnancy (menstrual extraction) V25.3
Intermenstrual
  bleeding 626.6
    irregular 626.6
    regular 626.5
  hemorrhage 626.6
    irregular 626.6
    regular 626.5
  pain(s) 625.2
Intermittent — *see* condition
Internal — *see* condition
Interproximal wear 521.1
Interruption
  aortic arch 747.11
  bundle of His 426.50
  fallopian tube (for sterilization) V25.2
  phase-shift, sleep cycle 307.45
  repeated REM-sleep 307.48
  sleep
    due to perceived environmental disturbances 307.48
    phase-shift, of 24-hour sleep-wake cycle 307.45
    repeated REM-sleep type 307.48
  vas deferens (for sterilization) V25.2
Intersexuality 752.7
Interstitial — *see* condition
Intertrigo 695.89
  labialis 528.5
Intervertebral disc — *see* condition
Intestine, intestinal — *see also* condition
  flu 487.8
Intolerance
  carbohydrate NEC 579.8
  cardiovascular exercise, with pain (at rest) (with less than ordinary activity) (with ordinary activity) V47.2
  cold 780.99 ▲
  dissacharide (hereditary) 271.3
  drug
    correct substance properly administered 995.2
    wrong substance given or taken in error 977.9
    specified drug — *see* Table of Drugs and Chemicals
  effort 306.2
  fat NEC 579.8
  foods NEC 579.8
  fructose (hereditary) 271.2
  glucose (-galactose) (congenital) 271.3
  gluten 579.0
  lactose (hereditary) (infantile) 271.3
  lysine (congenital) 270.7
  milk NEC 579.8
  protein (familial) 270.7
  starch NEC 579.8

Intolerance

Intolerance — continued
  sucrose (-isomaltose) (congenital) 271.3
Intoxicated NEC (see also Alcoholism) 305.0 ✓5th
Intoxication
  acid 276.2
  acute
    alcoholic 305.0 ✓5th
      with alcoholism 303.0 ✓5th
        hangover effects 305.0 ✓5th
      caffeine 305.9 ✓5th
      hallucinogenic (see also Abuse, drugs, nondependent) 305.3 ✓5th
    alcohol (acute) 305.0 ✓5th
      with alcoholism 303.0 ✓5th
        hangover effects 305.0 ✓5th
      idiosyncratic 291.4
      pathological 291.4
  alimentary canal 558.2
  ammonia (hepatic) 572.2
  chemical — see also Table of Drugs and Chemicals
    via placenta or breast milk 760.70
      alcohol 760.71
      anti-infective agents 760.74
      cocaine 760.75
      "crack" 760.75
      hallucinogenic agents NEC 760.73
      medicinal agents NEC 760.79
  chemical — see also Table of Drugs and Chemicals — continued
    via placenta or breast milk — continued
      narcotics 760.72
      obstetric anesthetic or analgesic drug 763.5
      specified agent NEC 760.79
      suspected, affecting management of pregnancy 655.5 ✓5th
  cocaine, through placenta or breast milk 760.75
  delirium
    alcohol 291.0
    drug 292.81
  drug
    with delirium 292.81
    correct substance properly administered (see also Allergy, drug) 995.2
    newborn 779.4
    obstetric anesthetic or sedation 668.9 ✓5th
      affecting fetus or newborn 763.5
    overdose or wrong substance given or taken — see Table of Drugs and Chemicals
    pathologic 292.2
    specific to newborn 779.4
    via placenta or breast milk 760.70
      alcohol 760.71
      anti-infective agents 760.74
      cocaine 760.75
      "crack" 760.75
      hallucinogenic agents 760.73
      medicinal agents NEC 760.79
      narcotics 760.72
      obstetric anesthetic or analgesic drug 763.5
      specified agent NEC 760.79
      suspected, affecting management of pregnancy 655.5 ✓5th
  enteric — see Intoxication, intestinal
  fetus or newborn, via placenta or breast milk 760.70
    alcohol 760.71
    anti-infective agents 760.74
    cocaine 760.75
    "crack" 760.75
    hallucinogenic agents 760.73
    medicinal agents NEC 760.79
    narcotics 760.72
    obstetric anesthetic or analgesic drug 763.5
    specified agent NEC 760.79
    suspected, affecting management of pregnancy 655.5 ✓5th
  food — see Poisoning, food
  gastrointestinal 558.2
  hallucinogenic (acute) 305.3 ✓5th
  hepatocerebral 572.2
  idiosyncratic alcohol 291.4
  intestinal 569.89
    due to putrefaction of food 005.9

Intoxication — continued
  methyl alcohol (see also Alcoholism) 305.0 ✓5th
    with alcoholism 303.0 ✓5th
  pathologic 291.4
    drug 292.2
  potassium (K) 276.7
  septic
    with
      abortion — see Abortion, by type, with sepsis
      ectopic pregnancy (see also categories 633.0-633.9) 639.0
      molar pregnancy (see also categories 630-632) 639.0
    during labor 659.3 ✓5th
    following
      abortion 639.0
      ectopic or molar pregnancy 639.0
    generalized — see Septicemia
    puerperal, postpartum, childbirth 670 ✓4th
  serum (prophylactic) (therapeutic) 999.5
  uremic — see Uremia
  water 276.6
Intracranial — see condition
Intrahepatic gallbladder 751.69
Intraligamentous — see also condition
  pregnancy — see Pregnancy, cornual
Intraocular — see also condition
  sepsis 360.00
Intrathoracic — see also condition
  kidney 753.3
  stomach — see Hernia, diaphragm
Intrauterine contraceptive device
  checking V25.42
  insertion V25.1
  in situ V45.51
  management V25.42
  prescription V25.02
    repeat V25.42
  reinsertion V25.42
  removal V25.42
Intraventricular — see condition
Intrinsic deformity — see Deformity
Intrusion, repetitive, of sleep (due to environmental disturbances) (with atypical polysomnographic features) 307.48
Intumescent, lens (eye) NEC 366.9
  senile 366.12
Intussusception (colon) (enteric) (intestine) (rectum) 560.0
  appendix 543.9
  congenital 751.5
  fallopian tube 620.8
  ileocecal 560.0
  ileocolic 560.0
  ureter (with obstruction) 593.4
Invagination
  basilar 756.0
  colon or intestine 560.0
Invalid (since birth) 799.8
Invalidism (chronic) 799.8
Inversion
  albumin-globulin (A-G) ratio 273.8
  bladder 596.8
  cecum (see also Intussusception) 560.0
  cervix 622.8
  nipple 611.79
    congenital 757.6
    puerperal, postpartum 676.3 ✓5th
  optic papilla 743.57
  organ or site, congenital NEC — see Anomaly, specified type NEC
  sleep rhythm 780.55
    nonorganic origin 307.45
  testis (congenital) 752.51
  uterus (postinfectional) (postpartal, old) 621.7
    chronic 621.7
    complicating delivery 665.2 ✓5th
      affecting fetus or newborn 763.89
  vagina — see Prolapse, vagina
Investigation
  allergens V72.7
  clinical research (control) (normal comparison) (participant) V70.7

Inviability — see Immaturity
Involuntary movement, abnormal 781.0
Involution, involutional — see also condition
  breast, cystic or fibrocystic 610.1
  depression (see also Psychosis, affective) 296.2 ✓5th
    recurrent episode 296.3 ✓5th
    single episode 296.2 ✓5th
  melancholia (see also Psychosis, affective) 296.2 ✓5th
    recurrent episode 296.3 ✓5th
    single episode 296.2 ✓5th
  ovary, senile 620.3
  paranoid state (reaction) 297.2
  paraphrenia (climacteric) (menopause) 297.2
  psychosis 298.8
  thymus failure 254.8
IQ
  under 20 318.2
  20-34 318.1
  35-49 318.0
  50-70 317
IRDS 769
Irideremia 743.45
Iridis rubeosis 364.42
  diabetic 250.5 ✓5th [364.42]
Iridochoroiditis (panuveitis) 360.12
Iridocyclitis NEC 364.3
  acute 364.00
    primary 364.01
    recurrent 364.02
  chronic 364.10
    in
      lepromatous leprosy 030.0 [364.11]
      sarcoidosis 135 [364.11]
      tuberculosis (see also Tuberculosis) 017.3 ✓5th [364.11]
  due to allergy 364.04
  endogenous 364.01
  gonococcal 098.41
  granulomatous 364.10
  herpetic (simplex) 054.44
    zoster 053.22
  hypopyon 364.05
  lens induced 364.23
  nongranulomatous 364.00
  primary 364.01
  recurrent 364.02
  rheumatic 364.10
  secondary 364.04
    infectious 364.03
    noninfectious 364.04
  subacute 364.00
    primary 364.01
    recurrent 364.02
  sympathetic 360.11
  syphilitic (secondary) 091.52
  tuberculous (chronic) (see also Tuberculosis) 017.3 ✓5th [364.11]
Iridocyclochoroiditis (panuveitis) 360.12
Iridodialysis 364.76
Iridodonesis 364.8
Iridoplegia (complete) (partial) (reflex) 379.49
Iridoschisis 364.52
Iris — see condition
Iritis 364.3
  acute 364.00
    primary 364.01
    recurrent 364.02
  chronic 364.10
    in
      sarcoidosis 135 [364.11]
      tuberculosis (see also Tuberculosis) 017.3 ✓5th [364.11]
  diabetic 250.5 ✓5th [364.42]
  due to
    allergy 364.04
    herpes simplex 054.44
    leprosy 030.0 [364.11]
  endogenous 364.01
  gonococcal 098.41
  gouty 274.89 [364.11]
  granulomatous 364.10
  hypopyon 364.05
  lens induced 364.23

Iritis — continued
- nongranulomatous 364.00
- papulosa 095.8 [364.11]
- primary 364.01
- recurrent 364.02
- rheumatic 364.10
- secondary 364.04
  - infectious 364.03
  - noninfectious 364.04
- subacute 364.00
  - primary 364.01
  - recurrent 364.02
- sympathetic 360.11
- syphilitic (secondary) 091.52
  - congenital 090.0 [364.11]
  - late 095.8 [364.11]
- tuberculous (see also Tuberculosis) 017.3 ✓5th [364.11]
- uratic 274.89 [364.11]

Iron
- deficiency anemia 280.9
- metabolism disease 275.0
- storage disease 275.0

Iron-miners' lung 503

Irradiated enamel (tooth, teeth) 521.8

Irradiation
- burn — see Burn, by site
- effects, adverse 990

Irreducible, irreducibility — see condition

Irregular, irregularity
- action, heart 427.9
- alveolar process 525.8
- bleeding NEC 626.4
- breathing 786.09
- colon 569.89
- contour of cornea 743.41
  - acquired 371.70
- dentin in pulp 522.3
- eye movements NEC 379.59
- menstruation (cause unknown) 626.4
- periods 626.4
- prostate 602.9
- pupil 364.75
- respiratory 786.09
- septum (nasal) 470
- shape, organ or site, congenital NEC — see Distortion
- sleep-wake rhythm (non-24-hour) 780.55
  - nonorganic origin 307.45
- vertebra 733.99

Irritability (nervous) 799.2
- bladder 596.8
  - neurogenic 596.54
    - with cauda equina syndrome 344.61
- bowel (syndrome) 564.1
- bronchial (see also Bronchitis) 490
- cerebral, newborn 779.1
- colon 564.1
  - psychogenic 306.4
- duodenum 564.89
- heart (psychogenic) 306.2
- ileum 564.89
- jejunum 564.89
- myocardium 306.2
- rectum 564.89
- stomach 536.9
  - psychogenic 306.4
- sympathetic (nervous system) (see also Neuropathy, peripheral, autonomic) 337.9
- urethra 599.84
- ventricular (heart) (psychogenic) 306.2

Irritable — see Irritability

Irritation
- anus 569.49
- axillary nerve 353.0
- bladder 596.8
- brachial plexus 353.0
- brain (traumatic) (see also Injury, intracranial) 854.0 ✓5th
  - nontraumatic — see Encephalitis
- bronchial (see also Bronchitis) 490
- cerebral (traumatic) (see also Injury, intracranial) 854.0 ✓5th
  - nontraumatic — see Encephalitis
- cervical plexus 353.2
- cervix (see also Cervicitis) 616.0

Irritation — continued
- choroid, sympathetic 360.11
- cranial nerve — see Disorder, nerve, cranial
- digestive tract 536.9
  - psychogenic 306.4
- gastric 536.9
  - psychogenic 306.4
- gastrointestinal (tract) 536.9
  - functional 536.9
  - psychogenic 306.4
- globe, sympathetic 360.11
- intestinal (bowel) 564.9
- labyrinth 386.50
- lumbosacral plexus 353.1
- meninges (traumatic) (see also Injury, intracranial) 854.0 ✓5th
  - nontraumatic — see Meningitis
- myocardium 306.2
- nerve — see Disorder, nerve
- nervous 799.2
- nose 478.1
- penis 607.89
- perineum 709.9
- peripheral
  - autonomic nervous system (see also Neuropathy, peripheral, autonomic) 337.9
  - nerve — see Disorder, nerve
- peritoneum (see also Peritonitis) 567.9
- pharynx 478.29
- plantar nerve 355.6
- spinal (cord) (traumatic) — see also Injury, spinal, by site
  - nerve — see also Disorder, nerve
  - root NEC 724.9
  - traumatic — see Injury, nerve, spinal
  - nontraumatic — see Myelitis
- stomach 536.9
  - psychogenic 306.4
- sympathetic nerve NEC (see also Neuropathy, peripheral, autonomic) 337.9
- ulnar nerve 354.2
- vagina 623.9

Isambert's disease 012.3 ✓5th

Ischemia, ischemic 459.9
- basilar artery (with transient neurologic deficit) 435.0
- bone NEC 733.40
- bowel (transient) 557.9
  - acute 557.0
  - chronic 557.1
  - due to mesenteric artery insufficiency 557.1
- brain — see also Ischemia, cerebral
  - recurrent focal 435.9
- cardiac (see also Ischemia, heart) 414.9
- cardiomyopathy 414.8
- carotid artery (with transient neurologic deficit) 435.9
- cerebral (chronic) (generalized) 437.1
  - arteriosclerotic 437.0
  - intermittent (with transient neurologic deficit) 435.9
  - puerperal, postpartum, childbirth 674.0 ✓5th
  - recurrent focal (with transient neurologic deficit) 435.9
  - transient (with transient neurologic deficit) 435.9
- colon 557.9
  - acute 557.0
  - chronic 557.1
  - due to mesenteric artery insufficiency 557.1
- coronary (chronic) (see also Ischemia, heart) 414.9
- heart (chronic or with a stated duration of over 8 weeks) 414.9
  - acute or with a stated duration of 8 weeks or less (see also Infarct, myocardium) 410.9 ✓5th
    - without myocardial infarction 411.89
      - with coronary (artery) occlusion 411.81
  - subacute 411.89
- intestine (transient) 557.9
  - acute 557.0
  - chronic 557.1
  - due to mesenteric artery insufficiency 557.1
- kidney 593.81

Ischemia, ischemic — continued
- labyrinth 386.50
- muscles, leg 728.89
- myocardium, myocardial (chronic or with a stated duration of over 8 weeks) 414.8
  - acute (see also Infarct, myocardium) 410.9 ✓5th
    - without myocardial infarction 411.89
      - with coronary (artery) occlusion 411.81
- renal 593.81
- retina, retinal 362.84
- small bowel 557.9
  - acute 557.0
  - chronic 557.1
  - due to mesenteric artery insufficiency 557.1
- spinal cord 336.1
- subendocardial (see also Insufficiency, coronary) 411.89
- vertebral artery (with transient neurologic deficit) 435.1

Ischialgia (see also Sciatica) 724.3

Ischiopagus 759.4

Ischium, ischial — see condition

Ischomenia 626.8

Ischuria 788.5

Iselin's disease or osteochondrosis 732.5

Islands of
- parotid tissue in
  - lymph nodes 750.26
  - neck structures 750.26
- submaxillary glands in
  - fascia 750.26
  - lymph nodes 750.26
  - neck muscles 750.26

Islet cell tumor, pancreas (M8150/0) 211.7

Isoimmunization NEC (see also Incompatibility) 656.2 ✓5th
- fetus or newborn 773.2
  - ABO blood groups 773.1
  - Rhesus (Rh) factor 773.0

Isolation V07.0
- social V62.4

Isosporosis 007.2

Issue
- medical certificate NEC V68.0
  - cause of death V68.0
  - fitness V68.0
  - incapacity V68.0
- repeat prescription NEC V68.1
  - appliance V68.1
  - contraceptive V25.40
    - device NEC V25.49
      - intrauterine V25.42
      - specified type NEC V25.49
    - pill V25.41
  - glasses V68.1
  - medicinal substance V68.1

Itch (see also Pruritus) 698.9
- bakers' 692.89
- barbers' 110.0
- bricklayers' 692.89
- cheese 133.8
- clam diggers' 120.3
- coolie 126.9
- copra 133.8
- Cuban 050.1
- dew 126.9
- dhobie 110.3
- eye 379.99
- filarial (see also Infestation, filarial) 125.9
- grain 133.8
- grocers' 133.8
- ground 126.9
- harvest 133.8
- jock 110.3
- Malabar 110.9
  - beard 110.0
  - foot 110.4
  - scalp 110.0
- meaning scabies 133.0
- Norwegian 133.0
- perianal 698.0
- poultrymen's 133.8

Itch (see also Pruritus) — continued
- sarcoptic 133.0
- scrub 134.1
- seven year V61.10
  - meaning scabies 133.0
- straw 133.8
- swimmers' 120.3
- washerwoman's 692.4
- water 120.3
- winter 698.8

Itsenko-Cushing syndrome (pituitary basophilism) 255.0

Ivemark's syndrome (asplenia with congenital heart disease) 759.0

Ivory bones 756.52

Ixodes 134.8

Ixodiasis 134.8

J

Jaccoud's nodular fibrositis, chronic (Jaccoud's syndrome) 714.4
Jackson's
　membrane 751.4
　paralysis or syndrome 344.89
　veil 751.4
Jacksonian
　epilepsy (see also Epilepsy) 345.5 ✓5ᵗʰ
　seizures (focal) (see also Epilepsy) 345.5 ✓5ᵗʰ
Jacob's ulcer (M8090/3) — see Neoplasm, skin, malignant, by site
Jacquet's dermatitis (diaper dermatitis) 691.0
Jadassohn's
　blue nevus (M8780/0) — see Neoplasm, skin, benign
　disease (maculopapular erythroderma) 696.2
　intraepidermal epithelioma (M8096/0) — see Neoplasm, skin, benign
Jadassohn-Lewandowski syndrome (pachyonychia congenita) 757.5
Jadassohn-Pellizari's disease (anetoderma) 701.3
Jadassohn-Tièche nevus (M8780/0) — see Neoplasm, skin, benign
Jaffe-Lichtenstein (-Uehlinger) syndrome 252.0
Jahnke's syndrome (encephalocutaneous angiomatosis) 759.6
Jakob-Creutzfeldt disease or syndrome 046.1
　with dementia
　　with behavioral disturbance 046.1 [294.11]
　　without behavioral disturbance 046.1 [294.10]
Jaksch (-Luzet) disease or syndrome (pseudoleukemia infantum) 285.8
Jamaican
　neuropathy 349.82
　paraplegic tropical ataxic-spastic syndrome 349.82
Janet's disease (psychasthenia) 300.89
Janiceps 759.4
Jansky-Bielschowsky amaurotic familial idiocy 330.1
Japanese
　B type encephalitis 062.0
　river fever 081.2
　seven-day fever 100.89
Jaundice (yellow) 782.4
　acholuric (familial) (splenomegalic) (see also Spherocytosis) 282.0
　acquired 283.9
　breast milk 774.39
　catarrhal (acute) 070.1
　　with hepatic coma 070.0
　　chronic 571.9
　　epidemic — see Jaundice, epidemic
　cholestatic (benign) 782.4
　chronic idiopathic 277.4
　epidemic (catarrhal) 070.1
　　with hepatic coma 070.0
　　leptospiral 100.0
　　spirochetal 100.0
　febrile (acute) 070.1
　　with hepatic coma 070.0
　　leptospiral 100.0
　　spirochetal 100.0
　fetus or newborn 774.6
　　due to or associated with
　　　ABO
　　　　antibodies 773.1
　　　　incompatibility, maternal/fetal 773.1
　　　　isoimmunization 773.1
　　　absence or deficiency of enzyme system for bilirubin conjugation (congenital) 774.39
　　　blood group incompatibility NEC 773.2
　　　breast milk inhibitors to conjugation 774.39
　　　　associated with preterm delivery 774.2
　　　bruising 774.1
　　　Crigler-Najjar syndrome 277.4 [774.31]
　　　delayed conjugation 774.30
　　　　associated with preterm delivery 774.2
　　　　development 774.39

Jaundice — continued
　fetus or newborn — continued
　　due to or associated with — continued
　　　drugs or toxins transmitted from mother 774.1
　　　G-6-PD deficiency 282.2 [774.0]
　　　galactosemia 271.1 [774.5]
　　　Gilbert's syndrome 277.4 [774.31]
　　　hepatocellular damage 774.4
　　　hereditary hemolytic anemia (see also Anemia, hemolytic) 282.9 [774.0]
　　　hypothyroidism, congenital 243 [774.31]
　　　incompatibility, maternal/fetal NEC 773.2
　　　infection 774.1
　　　inspissated bile syndrome 774.4
　　　isoimmunization NEC 773.2
　　　mucoviscidosis 277.01 [774.5]
　　　obliteration of bile duct, congenital 751.61 [774.5]
　　　polycythemia 774.1
　　　preterm delivery 774.2
　　　red cell defect 282.9 [774.0]
　　　Rh
　　　　antibodies 773.0
　　　　incompatibility, maternal/fetal 773.0
　　　　isoimmunization 773.0
　　　spherocytosis (congenital) 282.0 [774.0]
　　　swallowed maternal blood 774.1
　　physiological NEC 774.6
　from injection, inoculation, infusion, or transfusion (blood) (plasma) (serum) (other substance) (onset within 8 months after administration) — see Hepatitis, viral
　Gilbert's (familial nonhemolytic) 277.4
　hematogenous 283.9
　hemolytic (acquired) 283.9
　　congenital (see also Spherocytosis) 282.0
　hemorrhagic (acute) 100.0
　　leptospiral 100.0
　　newborn 776.0
　hemorrhagic
　　spirochetal 100.0
　hepatocellular 573.8
　homologous (serum) — see Hepatitis, viral
　idiopathic, chronic 277.4
　infectious (acute) (subacute) 070.1
　　with hepatic coma 070.0
　　leptospiral 100.0
　　spirochetal 100.0
　leptospiral 100.0
　malignant (see also Necrosis, liver) 570
　newborn (physiological) (see also Jaundice, fetus or newborn) 774.6
　nonhemolytic, congenital familial (Gilbert's) 277.4
　nuclear, newborn (see also Kernicterus of newborn) 774.7
　obstructive NEC (see also Obstruction, biliary) 576.8
　postimmunization — see Hepatitis, viral
　posttransfusion — see Hepatitis, viral
　regurgitation (see also Obstruction, biliary) 576.8
　serum (homologous) (prophylactic) (therapeutic) — see Hepatitis, viral
　spirochetal (hemorrhagic) 100.0
　symptomatic 782.4
　　newborn 774.6
Jaw — see condition
Jaw-blinking 374.43
　congenital 742.8
Jaw-winking phenomenon or syndrome 742.8
Jealousy
　alcoholic 291.5
　childhood 313.3
　sibling 313.3
Jejunitis (see also Enteritis) 558.9
Jejunostomy status V44.4
Jejunum, jejunal — see condition
Jensen's disease 363.05
Jericho boil 085.1
Jerks, myoclonic 333.2

Jeune's disease or syndrome (asphyxiating thoracic dystrophy) 756.4
Jigger disease 134.1
Job's syndrome (chronic granulomatous disease) 288.1
Jod-Basedow phenomenon 242.8 ✓5ᵗʰ
Johnson-Stevens disease (erythema multiforme exudativum) 695.1
Joint — see also condition
　Charcôt's 094.0 [713.5]
　false 733.82
　flail — see Flail, joint
　mice — see Loose, body, joint, by site
　sinus to bone 730.9 ✓5ᵗʰ
　von Gies' 095.8
Jordan's anomaly or syndrome 288.2
Josephs-Diamond-Blackfan anemia (congenital hypoplastic) 284.0
Joubert syndrome 759.89
Jumpers' knee 727.2
Jungle yellow fever 060.0
Jüngling's disease (sarcoidosis) 135
Junin virus hemorrhagic fever 078.7
Juvenile — see also condition
　delinquent 312.9
　　group (see also Disturbance, conduct) 312.2 ✓5ᵗʰ
　neurotic 312.4

K

Kahler (-Bozzolo) disease (multiple myeloma) (M9730/3) 203.0 ✓5ᵗʰ
Kakergasia 300.9
Kakke 265.0
Kala-azar (Indian) (infantile) (Mediterranean) (Sudanese) 085.0
Kalischer's syndrome (encephalocutaneous angiomatosis) 759.6
Kallmann's syndrome (hypogonadotropic hypogonadism with anosmia) 253.4
Kanner's syndrome (autism) (see also Psychosis, childhood) 299.0 ✓5ᵗʰ
Kaolinosis 502
Kaposi's
　disease 757.33
　　lichen ruber 696.4
　　　acuminatus 696.4
　　　moniliformis 697.8
　　xeroderma pigmentosum 757.33
　sarcoma (M9140/3) 176.9
　　adipose tissue 176.1
　　aponeurosis 176.1
　　artery 176.1
　　blood vessel 176.1
　　bursa 176.1
　　connective tissue 176.1
　　external genitalia 176.8
　　fascia 176.1
　　fatty tissue 176.1
　　fibrous tissue 176.1
　　gastrointestinal tract NEC 176.3
　　ligament 176.1
　　lung 176.4
　　lymph
　　　gland(s) 176.5
　　　node(s) 176.5
　　lymphatic(s) NEC 176.1
　　muscle (skeletal) 176.1
　　oral cavity NEC 176.8
　　palate 176.2
　　scrotum 176.8
　　skin 176.0
　　soft tissue 176.1
　　specified site NEC 176.8
　　subcutaneous tissue 176.1
　　synovia 176.1
　　tendon (sheath) 176.1
　　vein 176.1
　　vessel 176.1
　　viscera NEC 176.9
　　vulva 176.8

Kaposi's — continued
  varicelliform eruption 054.0
    vaccinia 999.0
Kartagener's syndrome or triad (sinusitis, bronchiectasis, situs inversus) 759.3
Kasabach-Merritt syndrome (capillary hemangioma associated with thrombocytopenic purpura) 287.3
Kaschin-Beck disease (endemic polyarthritis) — see Disease, Kaschin-Beck
Kast's syndrome (dyschondroplasia with hemangiomas) 756.4
Katatonia (see also Schizophrenia) 295.2 ✓5ᵗʰ
Katayama disease or fever 120.2
Kathisophobia 781.0
Kawasaki disease 446.1
Kayser-Fleischer ring (cornea) (pseudosclerosis) 275.1 [371.14]
Kaznelson's syndrome (congenital hypoplastic anemia) 284.0
Kedani fever 081.2
Kelis 701.4
Kelly (-Patterson) syndrome (sideropenic dysphagia) 280.8
Keloid, cheloid 701.4
  Addison's (morphea) 701.0
  cornea 371.00
  Hawkins' 701.4
  scar 701.4
Keloma 701.4
Kenya fever 082.1
Keratectasia 371.71
  congenital 743.41
Keratitis (nodular) (nonulcerative) (simple) (zonular) NEC 370.9
  with ulceration (see also Ulcer, cornea) 370.00
  actinic 370.24
  arborescens 054.42
  areolar 370.22
  bullosa 370.8
  deep — see Keratitis, interstitial
  dendritic(a) 054.42
  desiccation 370.34
  diffuse interstitial 370.52
  disciform(is) 054.43
    varicella 052.7 [370.44]
  epithelialis vernalis 372.13 [370.32]
  exposure 370.34
  filamentary 370.23
  gonococcal (congenital) (prenatal) 098.43
  herpes, herpetic (simplex) NEC 054.43
    zoster 053.21
  hypopyon 370.04
  in
    chickenpox 052.7 [370.44]
    exanthema (see also Exanthem) 057.9 [370.44]
    paravaccinia (see also Paravaccinia) 051.9 [370.44]
    smallpox (see also Smallpox) 050.9 [370.44]
    vernal conjunctivitis 372.13 [370.32]
  interstitial (nonsyphilitic) 370.50
    with ulcer (see also Ulcer, cornea) 370.00
    diffuse 370.52
    herpes, herpetic (simplex) 054.43
      zoster 053.21
    syphilitic (congenital) (hereditary) 090.3
    tuberculous (see also Tuberculosis) 017.3 ✓5ᵗʰ [370.59]
  lagophthalmic 370.34
  macular 370.22
  neuroparalytic 370.35
  neurotrophic 370.35
  nummular 370.22
  oyster-shuckers' 370.8
  parenchymatous — see Keratitis, interstitial
  petrificans 370.8
  phlyctenular 370.31
  postmeasles 055.71
  punctata, punctate 370.21
    leprosa 030.0 [370.21]
    profunda 090.3
    superficial (Thygeson's) 370.21
  purulent 370.8

Keratitis — continued
  pustuliformis profunda 090.3
  rosacea 695.3 [370.49]
  sclerosing 370.54
  specified type NEC 370.8
  stellate 370.22
  striate 370.22
  superficial 370.20
    with conjunctivitis (see also Keratoconjunctivitis) 370.40
    punctate (Thygeson's) 370.21
  suppurative 370.8
  syphilitic (congenital) (prenatal) 090.3
  trachomatous 076.1
    late effect 139.1
  tuberculous (phlyctenular) (see also Tuberculosis) 017.3 ✓5ᵗʰ [370.31]
  ulcerated (see also Ulcer, cornea) 370.00
  vesicular 370.8
  welders' 370.24
  xerotic (see also Keratomalacia) 371.45
    vitamin A deficiency 264.4
Keratoacanthoma 238.2
Keratocele 371.72
Keratoconjunctivitis (see also Keratitis) 370.40
  adenovirus type 8 077.1
  epidemic 077.1
  exposure 370.34
  gonococcal 098.43
  herpetic (simplex) 054.43
    zoster 053.21
  in
    chickenpox 052.7 [370.44]
    exanthema (see also Exanthem) 057.9 [370.44]
    paravaccinia (see also Paravaccinia) 051.9 [370.44]
    smallpox (see also Smallpox) 050.9 [370.44]
  infectious 077.1
  neurotrophic 370.35
  phlyctenular 370.31
  postmeasles 055.71
  shipyard 077.1
  sicca (Sjögren's syndrome) 710.2
    not in Sjögren's syndrome 370.33
  specified type NEC 370.49
  tuberculous (phlyctenular) (see also Tuberculosis) 017.3 ✓5ᵗʰ [370.31]
Keratoconus 371.60
  acute hydrops 371.62
  congenital 743.41
  stable 371.61
Keratocyst (dental) 526.0
Keratoderma, keratodermia (congenital) (palmaris et plantaris) (symmetrical) 757.39
  acquired 701.1
  blennorrhagica 701.1
    gonococcal 098.81
  climacterium 701.1
  eccentrica 757.39
  gonorrheal 098.81
  punctata 701.1
  tylodes, progressive 701.1
Keratodermatocele 371.72
Keratoglobus 371.70
  congenital 743.41
    associated with buphthalmos 743.22
Keratohemia 371.12
Keratoiritis (see also Iridocyclitis) 364.3
  syphilitic 090.3
  tuberculous (see also Tuberculosis) 017.3 ✓5ᵗʰ [364.11]
Keratolysis exfoliativa (congenital) 757.39
  acquired 695.89
  neonatorum 757.39
Keratoma 701.1
  congenital 757.39
  malignum congenitale 757.1
  palmaris et plantaris hereditarium 757.39
  senile 702.0
Keratomalacia 371.45
  vitamin A deficiency 264.4
Keratomegaly 743.41
Keratomycosis 111.1
  nigricans (palmaris) 111.1

Keratopathy 371.40
  band (see also Keratitis) 371.43
  bullous (see also Keratitis) 371.23
  degenerative (see also Degeneration, cornea) 371.40
    hereditary (see also Dystrophy, cornea) 371.50
  discrete colliquative 371.49
Keratoscleritis, tuberculous (see also Tuberculosis) 017.3 ✓5ᵗʰ [370.31]
Keratosis 701.1
  actinic 702.0
  arsenical 692.4
  blennorrhagica 701.1
    gonococcal 098.81
  congenital (any type) 757.39
  ear (middle) (see also Cholesteatoma) 385.30
  female genital (external) 629.8
  follicular, vitamin A deficiency 264.8
  follicularis 757.39
    acquired 701.1
    congenital (acneiformis) (Siemens') 757.39
    spinulosa (decalvans) 757.39
    vitamin A deficiency 264.8
  gonococcal 098.81
  larynx, laryngeal 478.79
  male genital (external) 608.89
  middle ear (see also Cholesteatoma) 385.30
  nigricans 701.2
    congenital 757.39
  obturans 380.21
  palmaris et plantaris (symmetrical) 757.39
  penile 607.89
  pharyngeus 478.29
  pilaris 757.39
    acquired 701.1
  punctata (palmaris et plantaris) 701.1
  scrotal 608.89
  seborrheic 702.19
    inflamed 702.11
  senilis 702.0
  solar 702.0
  suprafollicularis 757.39
  tonsillaris 478.29
  vagina 623.1
  vegetans 757.39
  vitamin A deficiency 264.8
Kerato-uveitis (see also Iridocyclitis) 364.3
Keraunoparalysis 994.0
Kerion (celsi) 110.0
Kernicterus of newborn (not due to isoimmunization) 774.7
  due to isoimmunization (conditions classifiable to 773.0-773.2) 773.4
Ketoacidosis 276.2
  diabetic 250.1 ✓5ᵗʰ
Ketonuria 791.6
  branched-chain, intermittent 270.3
Ketosis 276.2
  diabetic 250.1 ✓5ᵗʰ
Kidney — see condition
Kienböck's
  disease 732.3
    adult 732.8
  osteochondrosis 732.3
Kimmelstiel (-Wilson) disease or syndrome (intercapillary glomerulosclerosis) 250.4 ✓5ᵗʰ [581.81]
Kink, kinking
  appendix 543.9
  artery 447.1
  cystic duct, congenital 751.61
  hair (acquired) 704.2
  ileum or intestine (see also Obstruction, intestine) 560.9
  Lane's (see also Obstruction, intestine) 560.9
  organ or site, congenital NEC — see Anomaly, specified type NEC, by site
  ureter (pelvic junction) 593.3
    congenital 753.20
  vein(s) 459.2
    caval 459.2
    peripheral 459.2
Kinnier Wilson's disease (hepatolenticular degeneration) 275.1

Index to Diseases

Kissing
   osteophytes 721.5
   spine 721.5
   vertebra 721.5
Klauder's syndrome (erythema multiforme, exudativum) 695.1
Klebs' disease (see also Nephritis) 583.9
Klein-Waardenburg syndrome (ptosisepicanthus) 270.2
Kleine-Levin syndrome 349.89
Kleptomania 312.32
Klinefelter's syndrome 758.7
Klinger's disease 446.4
Klippel's disease 723.8
Klippel-Feil disease or syndrome (brevicollis) 756.16
Klippel-Trenaunay syndrome 759.89
Klumpke (-Déjérine) palsy, paralysis (birth) (newborn) 767.6
Klüver-Bucy (-Terzian) syndrome 310.0
Knee — see condition
Knifegrinders' rot (see also Tuberculosis) 011.4 ✓5ᵗʰ
Knock-knee (acquired) 736.41
   congenital 755.64
Knot
   intestinal, syndrome (volvulus) 560.2
   umbilical cord (true) 663.2 ✓5ᵗʰ
      affecting fetus or newborn 762.5
Knots, surfer 919.8
   infected 919.9
Knotting (of)
   hair 704.2
   intestine 560.2
Knuckle pads (Garrod's) 728.79
Köbner's disease (epidermolysis bullosa) 757.39
Koch's
   infection (see also Tuberculosis, pulmonary) 011.9 ✓5ᵗʰ
   relapsing fever 087.9
Koch-Weeks conjunctivitis 372.03
Koenig-Wichman disease (pemphigus) 694.4
Köhler's disease (osteochondrosis) 732.5
   first (osteochondrosis juvenilis) 732.5
   second (Freiburg's infarction, metatarsal head) 732.5
   patellar 732.4
   tarsal navicular (bone) (osteoarthrosis juvenilis) 732.5
Köhler-Mouchet disease (osteoarthrosis juvenilis) 732.5
Köhler-Pellegrini-Stieda disease or syndrome (calcification, knee joint) 726.62
Koilonychia 703.8
   congenital 757.5
Kojevnikov's, Kojewnikoff's epilepsy (see also Epilepsy) 345.7 ✓5ᵗʰ
König's
   disease (osteochondritis dissecans) 732.7
   syndrome 564.89
Koniophthisis (see also Tuberculosis) 011.4 ✓5ᵗʰ
Koplik's spots 055.9
Kopp's asthma 254.8
Korean hemorrhagic fever 078.6
Korsakoff (-Wernicke) disease, psychosis, or syndrome (nonalcoholic) 294.0
   alcoholic 291.1
Korsakov's disease — see Korsakoff's disease
Korsakow's disease — see Korsakoff's disease
Kostmann's disease or syndrome (infantile genetic agranulocytosis) 288.0
Krabbe's
   disease (leukodystrophy) 330.0
   syndrome
      congenital muscle hypoplasia 756.89
      cutaneocerebral angioma 759.6
Kraepelin-Morel disease (see also Schizophrenia) 295.9 ✓5ᵗʰ
Kraft-Weber-Dimitri disease 759.6

Kraurosis
   ani 569.49
   penis 607.0
   vagina 623.8
   vulva 624.0
Kreotoxism 005.9
Krukenberg's
   spindle 371.13
   tumor (M8490/6) 198.6
Kufs' disease 330.1
Kugelberg-Welander disease 335.11
Kuhnt-Junius degeneration or disease 362.52
Kulchitsky's cell carcinoma (carcinoid tumor of intestine) 259.2
Kümmell's disease or spondylitis 721.7
Kundrat's disease (lymphosarcoma) 200.1 ✓5ᵗʰ
Kunekune — see Dermatophytosis
Kunkel syndrome (lupoid hepatitis) 571.49
Kupffer cell sarcoma (M9124/3) 155.0
Kuru 046.0
Kussmaul's
   coma (diabetic) 250.3 ✓5ᵗʰ
   disease (polyarteritis nodosa) 446.0
   respiration (air hunger) 786.09
Kwashiorkor (marasmus type) 260
Kyasanur Forest disease 065.2
Kyphoscoliosis, kyphoscoliotic (acquired) (see also Scoliosis) 737.30
   congenital 756.19
   due to radiation 737.33
   heart (disease) 416.1
   idiopathic 737.30
      infantile
         progressive 737.32
         resolving 737.31
   late effect of rickets 268.1 [737.43]
   specified NEC 737.39
   thoracogenic 737.34
   tuberculous (see also Tuberculosis) 015.0 ✓5ᵗʰ [737.43]
Kyphosis, kyphotic (acquired) (postural) 737.10
   adolescent postural 737.0
   congenital 756.19
   dorsalis juvenilis 732.0
   due to or associated with
      Charcôt-Marie-Tooth disease 356.1 [737.41]
      mucopolysaccharidosis 277.5 [737.41]
      neurofibromatosis 237.71 [737.41]
      osteitis
         deformans 731.0 [737.41]
         fibrosa cystica 252.0 [737.41]
      osteoporosis (see also Osteoporosis) 733.0 ✓5ᵗʰ [737.41]
      poliomyelitis (see also Poliomyelitis) 138 [737.41]
      radiation 737.11
      tuberculosis (see also Tuberculosis) 015.0 ✓5ᵗʰ [737.41]
   Kümmell's 721.7
   late effect of rickets 268.1 [737.41]
   Morquio-Brailsford type (spinal) 277.5 [737.41]
   pelvis 738.6
   postlaminectomy 737.12
   specified cause NEC 737.19
   syphilitic, congenital 090.5 [737.41]
   tuberculous (see also Tuberculosis) 015.0 ✓5ᵗʰ [737.41]
Kyrle's disease (hyperkeratosis follicularis in cutem penetrans) 701.1

L

Labia, labium — see condition
Labiated hymen 752.49
Labile
   blood pressure 796.2
   emotions, emotionality 301.3
   vasomotor system 443.9
Labioglossal paralysis 335.22
Labium leporinum (see also Cleft, lip) 749.10
Labor (see also Delivery)
   with complications — see Delivery, complicated

Laceration

Labor (see also Delivery) — continued
   abnormal NEC 661.9 ✓5ᵗʰ
      affecting fetus or newborn 763.7
   arrested active phase 661.1 ✓5ᵗʰ
      affecting fetus or newborn 763.7
   desultory 661.2 ✓5ᵗʰ
      affecting fetus or newborn 763.7
   dyscoordinate 661.4 ✓5ᵗʰ
      affecting fetus or newborn 763.7
   early onset (22-36 weeks gestation) 644.2 ✓5ᵗʰ
   failed
      induction 659.1 ✓5ᵗʰ
         mechanical 659.0 ✓5ᵗʰ
         medical 659.1 ✓5ᵗʰ
         surgical 659.0 ✓5ᵗʰ
      trial (vaginal delivery) 660.6 ✓5ᵗʰ
   false 644.1 ✓5ᵗʰ
   forced or induced, affecting fetus or newborn 763.89
   hypertonic 661.4 ✓5ᵗʰ
      affecting fetus or newborn 763.7
   hypotonic 661.2 ✓5ᵗʰ
      affecting fetus or newborn 763.7
      primary 661.0 ✓5ᵗʰ
         affecting fetus or newborn 763.7
      secondary 661.1 ✓5ᵗʰ
         affecting fetus or newborn 763.7
   incoordinate 661.4 ✓5ᵗʰ
      affecting fetus or newborn 763.7
   irregular 661.2 ✓5ᵗʰ
      affecting fetus or newborn 763.7
   long — see Labor, prolonged
   missed (at or near term) 656.4 ✓5ᵗʰ
   obstructed NEC 660.9 ✓5ᵗʰ
      affecting fetus or newborn 763.1
      specified cause NEC 660.8 ✓5ᵗʰ
         affecting fetus or newborn 763.1
   pains, spurious 644.1 ✓5ᵗʰ
   precipitate 661.3 ✓5ᵗʰ
      affecting fetus or newborn 763.6
   premature 644.2 ✓5ᵗʰ
      threatened 644.0 ✓5ᵗʰ
   prolonged or protracted 662.1 ✓5ᵗʰ
      affecting fetus or newborn 763.89
      first stage 662.0 ✓5ᵗʰ
         affecting fetus or newborn 763.89
      second stage 662.2 ✓5ᵗʰ
         affecting fetus or newborn 763.89
   threatened NEC 644.1 ✓5ᵗʰ
   undelivered 644.1 ✓5ᵗʰ
Labored breathing (see also Hyperventilation) 786.09
Labyrinthitis (inner ear) (destructive) (latent) 386.30
   circumscribed 386.32
   diffuse 386.31
   focal 386.32
   purulent 386.33
   serous 386.31
   suppurative 386.33
   syphilitic 095.8
   toxic 386.34
   viral 386.35
Laceration — see also Wound, open, by site
   accidental, complicating surgery 998.2
   Achilles tendon 845.09
      with open wound 892.2
   anus (sphincter) 863.89
      with
         abortion — see Abortion, by type, with damage to pelvic organs
         ectopic pregnancy (see also categories 633.0-633.9) 639.2
         molar pregnancy (see also categories 630-632) 639.2
      complicating delivery 664.2 ✓5ᵗʰ
         with laceration of anal or rectal mucosa 664.3 ✓5ᵗʰ
      following
         abortion 639.2
         ectopic or molar pregnancy 639.2
      nontraumatic, nonpuerperal 565.0
   bladder (urinary)
      with
         abortion — see Abortion, by type, with damage to pelvic organs

Laceration — *see also* Wound, open, by site — *continued*
- bladder (urinary) — *continued*
  - with — *continued*
    - ectopic pregancy (*see also* categories 633.0-633.9) 639.2
    - molar pregnancy (*see also* categories 630-632) 639.2
  - following
    - abortion 639.2
    - ectopic or molar pregnancy 639.2
  - obstetrical trauma 665.5 ✓5ᵗʰ
- blood vessel — *see* Injury, blood vessel, by site
- bowel
  - with
    - abortion — *see* Abortion, by type, with damage to pelvic organs
    - ectopic pregnancy (*see also* categories 633.0-633.9) 639.2
    - molar pregnancy (*see also* categories 630-632) 639.2
  - following
    - abortion 639.2
    - ectopic or molar pregnancy 639.2
  - obstetrical trauma 665.5 ✓5ᵗʰ
- brain (with hemorrhage) (cerebral) (membrane) 851.8 ✓5ᵗʰ
- brain (cerebral) (membrane) 851.8 ✓5ᵗʰ

> *Note* — Use the following fifth-digit subclassification with categories 851–854:
> 0   unspecified state of consciousness
> 1   with no loss of consciousness
> 2   with brief [less than one hour] loss of consciousness
> 3   with moderate [1-24 hours] loss of consciousness
> 4   with prolonged [more than 24 hours] loss of consciousness and return to pre-existing conscious level
> 5   with prolonged [more than 24 hours] loss of consciousness, without return to pre-existing conscious level
> Use fifth-digit 5 to designate when a patient is unconscious and dies before regaining consciousness, regardless of the duration of the loss of consciousness
> 6   with loss of consciousness of unspecified duration
> 9   with concussion, unspecified

- with
  - open intracranial wound 851.9 ✓5ᵗʰ
  - skull fracture — *see* Fracture, skull, by site
- cerebellum 851.6 ✓5ᵗʰ
  - with open intracranial wound 851.7 ✓5ᵗʰ
- cortex 851.2 ✓5ᵗʰ
  - with open intracranial wound 851.3 ✓5ᵗʰ
- during birth 767.0
- stem 851.6 ✓5ᵗʰ
  - with open intracranial wound 851.7 ✓5ᵗʰ
- broad ligament
  - with
    - abortion — *see* Abortion, by type, with damage to pelvic organs
    - ectopic pregnancy (*see also* categories 633.0-633.9) 639.2
    - molar pregnancy (*see also* categories 630-632) 639.2
  - following
    - abortion 639.2
    - ectopic or molar pregnancy 639.2
  - nontraumatic 620.6
  - obstetrical trauma 665.6 ✓5ᵗʰ
  - syndrome (nontraumatic) 620.6
- capsule, joint — *see* Sprain, by site
- cardiac — *see* Laceration, heart
- causing eversion of cervix uteri (old) 622.0
- central, complicating delivery 664.4 ✓5ᵗʰ
- cerebellum — *see* Laceration, brain, cerebellum
- cerebral — *see also* Laceration, brain during birth 767.0

Laceration — *see also* Wound, open, by site — *continued*
- cervix (uteri)
  - with
    - abortion — *see* Abortion, by type, with damage to pelvic organs
    - ectopic pregnancy (*see also* categories 633.0-633.9) 639.2
    - molar pregnancy (*see also* categories 630-632) 639.2
  - following
    - abortion 639.2
    - ectopic or molar pregnancy 639.2
  - nonpuerperal, nontraumatic 622.3
  - obstetrical trauma (current) 665.3 ✓5ᵗʰ
  - old (postpartal) 622.3
  - traumatic — *see* Injury, internal, cervix
- chordae heart 429.5
- complicated 879.9
- cornea — *see* Laceration, eyeball
  - superficial 918.1
- cortex (cerebral) — *see* Laceration, brain, cortex
- esophagus 530.89
- eye(s) — *see* Laceration, ocular
- eyeball NEC 871.4
  - with prolapse or exposure of intraocular tissue 871.1
  - penetrating — *see* Penetrating wound, eyeball
  - specified as without prolapse of intraocular tissue 871.0
- eyelid NEC 870.8
  - full thickness 870.1
    - involving lacrimal passages 870.2
  - skin (and periocular area) 870.0
    - penetrating — *see* Penetrating wound, orbit
- fourchette
  - with
    - abortion — *see* Abortion, by type, with damage to pelvic organs
    - ectopic pregnancy (*see also* categories 633.0-633.9) 639.2
    - molar pregnancy (*see also* categories 630-632) 639.2
  - complicating delivery 664.0 ✓5ᵗʰ
  - following
    - abortion 639.2
    - ectopic or molar pregnancy 639.2
- heart (without penetration of heart chambers) 861.02
  - with
    - open wound into thorax 861.12
    - penetration of heart chambers 861.03
      - with open wound into thorax 861.13
- hernial sac — *see* Hernia, by site
- internal organ (abdomen) (chest) (pelvis) NEC — *see* Injury, internal, by site
- kidney (parenchyma) 866.02
  - with
    - complete disruption of parenchyma (rupture) 866.03
      - with open wound into cavity 866.13
    - open wound into cavity 866.12
- labia
  - complicating delivery 664.0 ✓5ᵗʰ
- ligament — *see also* Sprain, by site
  - with open wound — *see* Wound, open, by site
- liver 864.05
  - with open wound into cavity 864.15
  - major (disruption of hepatic parenchyma) 864.04
    - with open wound into cavity 864.14
  - minor (capsule only) 864.02
    - with open wound into cavity 864.12
  - moderate (involving parenchyma without major disruption) 864.03
    - with open wound into cavity 864.13
  - multiple 864.04
    - with open wound into cavity 864.14
  - stellate 864.04
    - with open wound into cavity 864.14
- lung 861.22
  - with open wound into thorax 861.32
- meninges — *see* Laceration, brain

Laceration — *see also* Wound, open, by site — *continued*
- meniscus (knee) (*see also* Tear, meniscus) 836.2
  - old 717.5
  - site other than knee — *see also* Sprain, by site
    - old NEC (*see also* Disorder, cartilage, articular) 718.0 ✓5ᵗʰ
- muscle — *see also* Sprain, by site
  - with open wound — *see* Wound, open, by site
- myocardium — *see* Laceration, heart
- nerve — *see* Injury, nerve, by site
- ocular NEC (*see also* Laceration, eyeball) 871.4
  - adnexa NEC 870.8
    - penetrating 870.3
      - with foreign body 870.4
- orbit (eye) 870.8
  - penetrating 870.3
    - with foreign body 870.4
- pelvic
  - floor (muscles)
    - with
      - abortion — *see* Abortion, by type, with damage to pelvic organs
      - ectopic pregnancy (*see also* categories 633.0-633.9) 639.2
      - molar pregnancy (*see also* categories 630-632) 639.2
    - complicating delivery 664.1 ✓5ᵗʰ
    - following
      - abortion 639.2
      - ectopic or molar pregnancy 639.2
    - nonpuerperal 618.7
    - old (postpartal) 618.7
  - organ NEC
    - with
      - abortion — *see* Abortion, by type, with damage to pelvic organs
      - ectopic pregnancy (*see also* categories 633.0-633.9) 639.2
      - molar pregnancy (*see also* categories 630-632) 639.2
    - complicating delivery 665.5 ✓5ᵗʰ
      - affecting fetus or newborn 763.89
    - following
      - abortion 639.2
      - ectopic or molar pregnancy 639.2
    - obstetrical trauma 665.5 ✓5ᵗʰ
- perineum, perineal (old) (postpartal) 618.7
  - with
    - abortion — *see* Abortion, by type, with damage to pelvic floor
    - ectopic pregnancy (*see also* categories 633.0-633.9) 639.2
    - molar pregnancy (*see also* categories 630-632) 639.2
  - complicating delivery 664.4 ✓5ᵗʰ
    - first degree 664.0 ✓5ᵗʰ
    - second degree 664.1 ✓5ᵗʰ
    - third degree 664.2 ✓5ᵗʰ
    - fourth degree 664.3 ✓5ᵗʰ
    - central 664.4 ✓5ᵗʰ
    - involving
      - anal sphincter 664.2 ✓5ᵗʰ
      - fourchette 664.0 ✓5ᵗʰ
      - hymen 664.0 ✓5ᵗʰ
      - labia 664.0 ✓5ᵗʰ
      - pelvic floor 664.1 ✓5ᵗʰ
      - perineal muscles 664.1 ✓5ᵗʰ
      - rectovaginal septum 664.2 ✓5ᵗʰ
        - with anal mucosa 664.3 ✓5ᵗʰ
      - skin 664.0 ✓5ᵗʰ
      - sphincter (anal) 664.2 ✓5ᵗʰ
        - with anal mucosa 664.3 ✓5ᵗʰ
      - vagina 664.0 ✓5ᵗʰ
      - vaginal muscles 664.1 ✓5ᵗʰ
      - vulva 664.0 ✓5ᵗʰ
    - secondary 674.2 ✓5ᵗʰ
  - following
    - abortion 639.2
    - ectopic or molar pregnancy 639.2
  - male 879.6
  - complicated 879.7
  - muscles, complicating delivery 664.1 ✓5ᵗʰ

Index to Diseases

Laceration — *see also* Wound, open, by site — *continued*
- perineum, perineal — *continued*
  - nonpuerperal, current injury 879.6
    - complicated 879.7
  - secondary (postpartal) 674.2 ✓5ᵗʰ
- peritoneum
  - with
    - abortion — *see* Abortion, by type, with damage to pelvic organs
    - ectopic pregnancy (*see also* categories 633.0-633.9) 639.2
    - molar pregnancy (*see also* categories 630-632) 639.2
  - following
    - abortion 639.2
    - ectopic or molar pregnancy 639.2
  - obstetrical trauma 665.5 ✓5ᵗʰ
- periurethral tissue
  - with
    - abortion — *see* Abortion, by type, with damage to pelvic organs
    - ectopic pregnancy (*see also* categories 633.0-633.9) 639.2
    - molar pregnancy (*see also* categories 630-632) 639.2
  - following
    - abortion 639.2
    - ectopic or molar pregnancy 639.2
  - obstetrical trauma 665.5 ✓5ᵗʰ
- rectovaginal (septum)
  - with
    - abortion — *see* Abortion, by type, with damage to pelvic organs
    - ectopic pregnancy (*see also* categories 633.0-633.9) 639.2
    - molar pregnancy (*see also* categories 630-632) 639.2
  - complicating delivery 665.4 ✓5ᵗʰ
    - with perineum 664.2 ✓5ᵗʰ
      - involving anal or rectal mucosa 664.3 ✓5ᵗʰ
  - following
    - abortion 639.2
    - ectopic or molar pregnancy 639.2
  - nonpuerperal 623.4
  - old (postpartal) 623.4
- spinal cord (meninges) — *see also* Injury, spinal, by site
  - due to injury at birth 767.4
  - fetus or newborn 767.4
- spleen 865.09
  - with
    - disruption of parenchyma (massive) 865.04
      - with open wound into cavity 865.14
    - open wound into cavity 865.19
    - capsule (without disruption of parenchyma) 865.02
      - with open wound into cavity 865.12
    - parenchyma 865.03
      - with open wound into cavity 865.13
      - massive disruption (rupture) 865.04
        - with open wound into cavity 865.14
- tendon 848.9
  - with open wound — *see* Wound, open, by site
  - Achilles 845.09
    - with open wound 892.2
  - lower limb NEC 844.9
    - with open wound NEC 894.2
  - upper limb NEC 840.9
    - with open wound NEC 884.2
- tentorium cerebelli — *see* Laceration, brain, cerebellum
- tongue 873.64
  - complicated 873.74
- urethra
  - with
    - abortion — *see* Abortion, by type, with damage to pelvic organs
    - ectopic pregnancy (*see also* categories 633.0-633.9) 639.2
    - molar pregnancy (*see also* categories 630-632) 639.2

Laceration — *see also* Wound, open, by site — *continued*
- urethra — *continued*
  - following
    - abortion 639.2
    - ectopic or molar pregnancy 639.2
  - nonpuerperal, nontraumatic 599.84
  - obstetrical trauma 665.5 ✓5ᵗʰ
- uterus
  - with
    - abortion — *see* Abortion, by type, with damage to pelvic organs
    - ectopic pregnancy (*see also* categories 633.0-633.9) 639.2
    - molar pregnancy (*see also* categories 630-632) 639.2
  - following
    - abortion 639.2
    - ectopic or molar pregnancy 639.2
  - nonpuerperal, nontraumatic 621.8
  - obstetrical trauma NEC 665.8 ✓5ᵗʰ ▲
  - old (postpartal) 621.8
- vagina
  - with
    - abortion — *see* Abortion, by type, with damage to pelvic organs
    - ectopic pregnancy (*see also* categories 633.0-633.9) 639.2
    - molar pregnancy (*see also* categories 630-632) 639.2
  - perineal involvement, complicating delivery 664.0 ✓5ᵗʰ
  - complicating delivery 665.4 ✓5ᵗʰ
    - first degree 664.0 ✓5ᵗʰ
    - second degree 664.1 ✓5ᵗʰ
    - third degree 664.2 ✓5ᵗʰ
    - fourth degree 664.3 ✓5ᵗʰ
    - high 665.4 ✓5ᵗʰ
    - muscles 664.1 ✓5ᵗʰ
    - sulcus 665.4 ✓5ᵗʰ
    - wall 665.4 ✓5ᵗʰ
  - following
    - abortion 639.2
    - ectopic or molar pregnancy 639.2
  - nonpuerperal, nontraumatic 623.4
  - old (postpartal) 623.4
- valve, heart — *see* Endocarditis
- vulva
  - with
    - abortion — *see* Abortion, by type, with damage to pelvic organs,
    - ectopic pregnancy (*see also* categories 633.0-633.9) 639.2
    - molar pregnancy (*see also* categories 630-632) 639.2
  - complicating delivery 664.0 ✓5ᵗʰ
  - following
    - abortion 639.2
    - ectopic or molar pregnancy 639.2
  - nonpuerperal, nontraumatic 624.4
  - old (postpartal) 624.4

Lachrymal — *see* condition

Lachrymonasal duct — *see* condition

Lack of
- appetite (*see also* Anorexia) 783.0
- care
  - in home V60.4
  - of adult 995.84
  - of infant (at or after birth) 995.52
- coordination 781.3
- development — *see also* Hypoplasia
  - physiological in childhood 783.40
- education V62.3
- energy 780.79
- financial resources V60.2
- food 994.2
  - in environment V60.8
- growth in childhood 783.43
- heating V60.1
- housing (permanent) (temporary) V60.0
  - adequate V60.1
- material resources V60.2
- medical attention 799.8
- memory (*see also* Amnesia) 780.99 ▲
  - mild, following organic brain damage 310.1
- ovulation 628.0

Lack of — *continued*
- person able to render necessary care V60.4
- physical exercise V69.0
- physiologic development in childhood 783.40
- prenatal care in current pregnancy V23.7
- shelter V60.0
- water 994.3

Lacrimal — *see* condition

Lacrimation, abnormal (*see also* Epiphora) 375.20

Lacrimonasal duct — *see* condition

Lactation, lactating (breast) (puerperal) (postpartum)
- defective 676.4 ✓5ᵗʰ
- disorder 676.9 ✓5ᵗʰ
  - specified type NEC 676.8 ✓5ᵗʰ
- excessive 676.6 ✓5ᵗʰ
- failed 676.4 ✓5ᵗʰ
- mastitis NEC 675.2 ✓5ᵗʰ
- mother (care and/or examination) V24.1
- nonpuerperal 611.6
- suppressed 676.5 ✓5ᵗʰ

Lacticemia 271.3
- excessive 276.2

Lactosuria 271.3

Lacunar skull 756.0

Laennec's cirrhosis (alcoholic) 571.2
- nonalcoholic 571.5

Lafora's disease 333.2

Lag, lid (nervous) 374.41

Lagleyze-von Hippel disease (retinocerebral angiomatosis) 759.6

Lagophthalmos (eyelid) (nervous) 374.20
- cicatricial 374.23
- keratitis (*see also* Keratitis) 370.34
- mechanical 374.22
- paralytic 374.21

La grippe — *see* Influenza

Lahore sore 085.1

Lakes, venous (cerebral) 437.8

Laki-Lorand factor deficiency (*see also* Defect, coagulation) 286.3

Lalling 307.9

Lambliasis 007.1

Lame back 724.5

Lancereaux's diabetes (diabetes mellitus with marked emaciation) 250.8 ✓5ᵗʰ [261]

Landouzy-Déjérine dystrophy (fascioscapulohumeral atrophy) 359.1

Landry's disease or paralysis 357.0

Landry-Guillain-Barré syndrome 357.0

Lane's
- band 751.4
- disease 569.89
- kink (*see also* Obstruction, intestine) 560.9

Langdon Down's syndrome (mongolism) 758.0

Language abolition 784.69

Lanugo (persistent) 757.4

Laparoscopic surgical procedure converted to open procedure V64.4

Lardaceous
- degeneration (any site) 277.3
- disease 277.3
- kidney 277.3 [583.81]
- liver 277.3

Large
- baby (regardless of gestational age) 766.1
  - exceptionally (weight of 4500 grams or more) 766.0
  - of diabetic mother 775.0
- ear 744.22
- fetus — *see also* Oversize, fetus
  - causing disproportion 653.5 ✓5ᵗʰ
    - with obstructed labor 660.1 ✓5ᵗʰ
  - for dates
    - fetus or newborn (regardless of gestational age) 766.1
      - affecting management of pregnancy 656.6 ✓5ᵗʰ
      - exceptionally (weight of 4500 grams or more) 766.0

Large

Large — *continued*
   physiological cup 743.57
   waxy liver 277.3
   white kidney — *see* Nephrosis
Larsen's syndrome (flattened facies and multiple congenital dislocations) 755.8
Larsen-Johansson disease (juvenile osteopathia patellae) 732.4
Larva migrans
   cutaneous NEC 126.9
      ancylostoma 126.9
   of Diptera in vitreous 128.0
   visceral NEC 128.0
Laryngeal — *see also* condition syncope 786.2
Laryngismus (acute) (infectious) (stridulous) 478.75
   congenital 748.3
   diphtheritic 032.3
Laryngitis (acute) (edematous) (fibrinous) (gangrenous) (infective) (infiltrative) (malignant) (membranous) (phlegmonous) (pneumococcal) (pseudomembranous) (septic) (subglottic) (suppurative) (ulcerative) (viral) 464.00
   with
      influenza, flu, or grippe 487.1
      obstruction 464.01
      tracheitis (*see also* Laryngotracheitis) 464.20
         with obstruction 464.21
         acute 464.20
            with obstruction 464.21
         chronic 476.1
   atrophic 476.0
   Borrelia vincentii 101
   catarrhal 476.0
   chronic 476.0
      with tracheitis (chronic) 476.1
      due to external agent — *see* Condition, respiratory, chronic, due to
   diphtheritic (membranous) 032.3
   due to external agent — *see* Inflammation, respiratory, upper, due to
   H. influenzae 464.00
      with obstruction 464.01
   Hemophilus influenzae 464.00
      wtih obstruction 464.01
   hypertrophic 476.0
   influenzal 487.1
   pachydermic 478.79
   sicca 476.0
   spasmodic 478.75
      acute 464.00
         with obstruction 464.01
   streptococcal 034.0
   stridulous 478.75
   syphilitic 095.8
      congenital 090.5
   tuberculous (*see also* Tuberculosis, larynx) 012.3 ✓5ᵗʰ
   Vincent's 101
Laryngocele (congenital) (ventricular) 748.3
Laryngofissure 478.79
   congenital 748.3
Laryngomalacia (congenital) 748.3
Laryngopharyngitis (acute) 465.0
   chronic 478.9
      due to external agent — *see* Condition, respiratory, chronic, due to
   due to external agent — *see* Inflammation, respiratory, upper, due to
   septic 034.0
Laryngoplegia (*see also* Paralysis, vocal cord) 478.30
Laryngoptosis 478.79
Laryngospasm 478.75
   due to external agent — *see* Condition, respiratory, acute, due to
Laryngostenosis 478.74
   congenital 748.3
Laryngotracheitis (acute) (infectional) (viral) (*see also* Laryngitis) 464.20
   with obstruction 464.21
   atrophic 476.1
   Borrelia vincenti 101

Laryngotracheitis (*see also* Laryngitis) — *continued*
   catarrhal 476.1
   chronic 476.1
      due to external agent — *see* Condition, respiratory, chronic, due to
   diphtheritic (membranous) 032.3
   due to external agent — *see* Inflammation, respiratory, upper, due to
   H. influenzae 464.20
      with obstruction 464.21
   hypertrophic 476.1
   influenzal 487.1
   pachydermic 478.75
   sicca 476.1
   spasmodic 478.75
      acute 464.20
         with obstruction 464.21
   streptococcal 034.0
   stridulous 478.75
   syphilitic 095.8
      congenital 090.5
   tuberculous (*see also* Tuberculosis, larynx) 012.3 ✓5ᵗʰ
   Vincent's 101
Laryngotracheobronchitis (*see also* Bronchitis) 490
   acute 466.0
   chronic 491.8
   viral 466.0
Laryngotracheobronchopneumonitis — *see* Pneumonia, broncho-
Larynx, laryngeal — *see* condition
Lasègue's disease (persecution mania) 297.9
Lassa fever 078.89
Lassitude (*see also* Weakness) 780.79
Late — *see also* condition
   effect(s) (of) — *see also* condition
      abscess
         intracranial or intraspinal (conditions classifiable to 324) — *see* category 326
      adverse effect of drug, medicinal or biological substance 909.5
      amputation
         postoperative (late) 997.60
         traumatic (injury classifiable to 885-887 and 895-897) 905.9
      burn (injury classifiable to 948-949) 906.9
         extremities NEC (injury classifiable to 943 or 945) 906.7
         hand or wrist (injury classifiable to 944) 906.6
         eye (injury classifiable to 940) 906.5
         face, head, and neck (injury classifiable to 941) 906.5
         specified site NEC (injury classifiable to 942 and 946-947) 906.8
      cerebrovascular disease (conditions classifiable to 430-437) 438.9
         with
            alterations of sensations 438.6 •
            aphasia 438.11
            apraxia 438.81
            ataxia 438.84 •
            cognitive deficits 438.0
            disturbances of vision 438.7 •
            dysphagia 438.82
            dysphasia 438.12
            facial droop 438.83 •
            facial weakness 438.83 •
            hemiplegia/hemiparesis
               affecting
                  dominant side 438.21
                  nondominant side 438.22
                  unspecified side 438.20
            monoplegia of lower limb
               affecting
                  dominant side 438.41
                  nondominant side 438.42
                  unspecified side 438.40
            monoplegia of upper limb
               affecting
                  dominant side 438.31

Late — *see also* condition — *continued*
   effect(s) (of) — *see also* condition — *continued*
      cerebrovascular disease — *continued*
         with — *continued*
            monoplegia of upper limb — *continued*
               affecting — *continued*
                  nondominant side 438.32
                  unspecified side 438.30
            paralytic syndrome NEC
               affecting
                  bilateral 438.53
                  dominant side 438.51
                  nondominant side 438.52
                  unspecified side 438.50
            speech and language deficit 438.10
            vertigo 438.85 •
         specified type NEC 438.89
      childbirth complication(s) 677
      complication(s) of
         childbirth 677
         delivery 677
         pregnancy 677
         puerperium 677
         surgical and medical care (conditions classifiable to 996-999) 909.3
      complication(s) of — *continued*
         trauma (conditions classifiable to 958) 908.6
      contusion (injury classifiable to 920-924) 906.3
      crushing (injury classifiable to 925-929) 906.4
      delivery complication(s) 677
      dislocation (injury classifiable to 830-839) 905.6
      encephalitis or encephalomyelitis (conditions classifiable to 323) — *see* category 326
         in infectious diseases 139.8
            viral (conditions classifiable to 049.8, 049.9, 062-064) 139.0
      external cause NEC (conditions classifiable to 995) 909.9
      certain conditions classifiable to categories 991-994 909.4
      foreign body in orifice (injury classifiable to 930-939) 908.5
      fracture (multiple) (injury classifiable to 828-829) 905.5
         extremity
            lower (injury classifiable to 821-827) 905.4
               neck of femur (injury classifiable to 820) 905.3
            upper (injury classifiable to 810-819) 905.2
         face and skull (injury classifiable to 800-804) 905.0
         skull and face (injury classifiable to 800-804) 905.0
         spine and trunk (injury classifiable to 805 and 807-809) 905.1
            with spinal cord lesion (injury classifiable to 806) 907.2
      infection
         pyogenic, intracranial — *see* category 326
      infectious diseases (conditions classifiable to 001-136) NEC 139.8
      injury (injury classifiable to 959) 908.9
         blood vessel 908.3
            abdomen and pelvis (injury classifiable to 902) 908.4
            extremity (injury classifiable to 903-904) 908.3
            head and neck (injury classifiable to 900) 908.3
               intracranial (injury classifiable to 850-854) 907.0
                  with skull fracture 905.0
            thorax (injury classifiable to 901) 908.4
         internal organ NEC (injury classifiable to 867 and 869) 908.2
            abdomen (injury classifiable to 863-866 and 868) 908.1
            thorax (injury classifiable to 860-862) 908.0

Late — *see also* condition — *continued*
  effect(s) (of) — *see also* condition — *continued*
    injury — *continued*
      intracranial (injury classifiable to 850-854) 907.0
        with skull fracture (injury classifiable to 800-801 and 803-804) 905.0
      nerve NEC (injury classifiable to 957) 907.9
        cranial (injury classifiable to 950-951) 907.1
        peripheral NEC (injury classifiable to 957) 907.9
          lower limb and pelvic girdle (injury classifiable to 956) 907.5
          upper limb and shoulder girdle (injury classifiable to 955) 907.4
        roots and plexus(es), spinal (injury classifiable to 953) 907.3
        trunk (injury classifiable to 954) 907.3
      spinal
        cord (injury classifiable to 806 and 952) 907.2
        nerve root(s) and plexus(es) (injury classifiable to 953) 907.3
      superficial (injury classifiable to 910-919) 906.2
      tendon (tendon injury classifiable to 840-848, 880-884 with .2, and 890-894 with .2) 905.8
    meningitis
      bacterial (conditions classifiable to 320) — *see* category 326
      unspecified cause (conditions classifiable to 322) — *see* category 326
    myelitis (*see also* Late, effect(s) (of), encephalitis) — *see* category 326
    parasitic diseases (conditions classifiable to 001-136 NEC) 139.8
    phlebitis or thrombophlebitis of intracranial venous sinuses (conditions classifiable to 325) — *see* category 326
    poisoning due to drug, medicinal or biological substance (conditions classifiable to 960-979) 909.0
    poliomyelitis, acute (conditions classifiable to 045) 138
    pregnancy complication(s) 677
    puerperal complication(s) 677
    radiation (conditions classifiable to 990) 909.2
    rickets 268.1
    sprain and strain without mention of tendon injury (injury classifiable to 840-848, except tendon injury) 905.7
      tendon involvement 905.8
    toxic effect of
      drug, medicinal or biological substance (conditions classifiable to 960-979) 909.0
      nonmedical substance (conditions classifiable to 980-989) 909.1
    trachoma (conditions classifiable to 076) 139.1
    tuberculosis 137.0
      bones and joints (conditions classifiable to 015) 137.3
      central nervous system (conditions classifiable to 013) 137.1
      genitourinary (conditions classifiable to 016) 137.2
      pulmonary (conditions classifiable to 010-012) 137.0
      specified organs NEC (conditions classifiable to 014, 017-018) 137.4
    viral encephalitis (conditions classifiable to 049.8, 049.9, 062-064) 139.0
    wound, open
      extremity (injury classifiable to 880-884 and 890-894, except .2) 906.1
        tendon (injury classifiable to 880-884 with .2 and 890-894 with.2) 905.8
      head, neck, and trunk (injury classifiable to 870-879) 906.0

Latent — *see* condition
Lateral — *see* condition
Laterocession — *see* Lateroversion
Lateroflexion — *see* Lateroversion
Lateroversion
  cervix — *see* Lateroversion, uterus
  uterus, uterine (cervix) (postinfectional) (postpartal, old) 621.6
    congenital 752.3
    in pregnancy or childbirth 654.4
      affecting fetus or newborn 763.89
Lathyrism 988.2
Launois' syndrome (pituitary gigantism) 253.0
Launois-Bensaude's lipomatosis 272.8
Launois-Cléret syndrome (adiposogenital dystrophy) 253.8
Laurence-Moon-Biedl syndrome (obesity, polydactyly, and mental retardation) 759.89
LAV (disease) (illness) (infection) — *see* Human immunodeficiency virus (disease) (illness) (infection)
LAV/HTLV-III (disease) (illness) (infection) — *see* Human immunodeficiency virus (disease) (illness) (infection)
Lawford's syndrome (encephalocutaneous angiomatosis) 759.6
Lax, laxity — *see also* Relaxation
  ligament 728.4
  skin (acquired) 701.8
    congenital 756.83
Laxative habit (*see also* Abuse, drugs, nondependent) 305.9
Lazy leukocyte syndrome 288.0
Lead — *see also* condition
  exposure to V15.86
  incrustation of cornea 371.15
  poisoning 984.9
    specified type of lead — *see* Table of Drugs and Chemicals
Lead miners' lung 503
Leakage
  amniotic fluid 658.1
    with delayed delivery 658.2
    affecting fetus or newborn 761.1
  bile from drainage tube (T tube) 997.4
  blood (microscopic), fetal, into maternal circulation 656.0
    affecting management of pregnancy or puerperium 656.0
  device, implant, or graft — *see* Complications, mechanical
  spinal fluid at lumbar puncture site 997.09
  urine, continuous 788.37
Leaky heart — *see* Endocarditis
Learning defect, specific NEC (strephosymbolia) 315.2
Leather bottle stomach (M8142/3) 151.9
Leber's
  congenital amaurosis 362.76
  optic atrophy (hereditary) 377.16
Lederer's anemia or disease (acquired infectious hemolytic anemia) 283.19
Lederer-Brill syndrome (acquired infectious hemolytic anemia) 283.19
Leeches (aquatic) (land) 134.2
Left-sided neglect 781.8
Leg — *see* condition
Legal investigation V62.5
Legg (-Calvé) -Perthes disease or syndrome (osteochondrosis, femoral capital) 732.1
Legionnaires' disease 482.84
Leigh's disease 330.8
Leiner's disease (exfoliative dermatitis) 695.89
Leiofibromyoma (M8890/0) — *see also* Leiomyoma
  uterus (cervix) (corpus) (*see also* Leiomyoma, uterus) 218.9
Leiomyoblastoma (M8891/1) — *see* Neoplasm, connective tissue, uncertain behavior

Leiomyofibroma (M8890/0) — *see also* Neoplasm, connective tissue, benign
  uterus (cervix) (corpus) (*see also* Leiomyoma, uterus) 218.9
Leiomyoma (M8890/0) — *see also* Neoplasm, connective tissue, benign
  bizarre (M8893/0) — *see* Neoplasm, connective tissue, benign
  cellular (M8892/1) — *see* Neoplasm, connective tissue, uncertain behavior
  epithelioid (M8891/1) — *see* Neoplasm, connective tissue, uncertain behavior
  prostate (polypoid) 600.2
  uterus (cervix) (corpus) 218.9
    interstitial 218.1
    intramural 218.1
    submucous 218.0
    subperitoneal 218.2
    subserous 218.2
  vascular (M8894/0) — *see* Neoplasm, connective tissue, benign
Leiomyomatosis (intravascular) (M8890/1) — *see* Neoplasm, connective tissue, uncertain behavior
Leiomyosarcoma (M8890/3) — *see also* Neoplasm, connective tissue, malignant
  epithelioid (M8891/3) — *see* Neoplasm, connective tissue, malignant
Leishmaniasis 085.9
  American 085.5
    cutaneous 085.4
    mucocutaneous 085.5
  Asian desert 085.2
  Brazilian 085.5
  cutaneous 085.9
    acute necrotizing 085.2
    American 085.4
    Asian desert 085.2
    diffuse 085.3
    dry form 085.1
    Ethiopian 085.3
    eyelid 085.5 [373.6]
    late 085.1
    lepromatous 085.3
    recurrent 085.1
    rural 085.2
    ulcerating 085.1
    urban 085.1
    wet form 085.2
    zoonotic form 085.2
  dermal — *see also* Leishmaniasis, cutaneous
    post kala-azar 085.0
  eyelid 085.5 [373.6]
  infantile 085.0
  Mediterranean 085.0
  mucocutaneous (American) 085.5
  naso-oral 085.5
  nasopharyngeal 085.5
  Old World 085.1
  tegumentaria diffusa 085.4
  vaccination, prophylactic (against) V05.2
  visceral (Indian) 085.0
Leishmanoid, dermal — *see also* Leishmaniasis, cutaneous
  post kala-azar 085.0
Leloir's disease 695.4
Lenegre's disease 426.0
Lengthening, leg 736.81
Lennox's syndrome (*see also* Epilepsy) 345.0
Lens — *see* condition
Lenticonus (anterior) (posterior) (congenital) 743.36
Lenticular degeneration, progressive 275.1
Lentiglobus (posterior) (congenital) 743.36
Lentigo (congenital) 709.09
  juvenile 709.09
  Maligna (M8742/2) — *see also* Neoplasm, skin, in situ
    melanoma (M8742/3) — *see* Melanoma
  senile 709.09
Leonine leprosy 030.0
Leontiasis
  ossium 733.3
  syphilitic 095.8
    congenital 090.5

Léopold-Lévi's syndrome (paroxysmal thyroid instability) 242.9 ✓5ᵗʰ
Lepore hemoglobin syndrome 282.4
Lepothrix 039.0
Lepra 030.9
    Willan's 696.1
Leprechaunism 259.8
Lepromatous leprosy 030.0
Leprosy 030.9
    anesthetic 030.1
    beriberi 030.1
    borderline (group B) (infiltrated) (neuritic) 030.3
    cornea (see also Leprosy, by type) 030.9 [371.89]
    dimorphous (group B) (infiltrated) (lepromatous) (neuritic) (tuberculoid) 030.3
    eyelid 030.0 [373.4]
    indeterminate (group I) (macular) (neuritic) (uncharacteristic) 030.2
    leonine 030.0
    lepromatous (diffuse) (infiltrated) (macular) (neuritic) (nodular) (type L) 030.0
    macular (early) (neuritic) (simple) 030.2
    maculoanesthetic 030.1
    mixed 030.0
    neuro 030.1
    nodular 030.0
    primary neuritic 030.3
    specified type or group NEC 030.8
    tubercular 030.1
    tuberculoid (macular) (maculoanesthetic) (major) (minor) (neuritic) (type T) 030.1
Leptocytosis, hereditary 282.4
Leptomeningitis (chronic) (circumscribed) (hemorrhagic) (nonsuppurative) (see also Meningitis) 322.9
    aseptic 047.9
        adenovirus 049.1
        Coxsackie virus 047.0
        ECHO virus 047.1
        enterovirus 047.9
        lymphocytic choriomeningitis 049.0
    epidemic 036.0
    late effect — see category 326
    meningococcal 036.0
    pneumococcal 320.1
    syphilitic 094.2
    tuberculous (see also Tuberculosis, meninges) 013.0 ✓5ᵗʰ
Leptomeningopathy (see also Meningitis) 322.9
Leptospiral — see condition
Leptospirochetal — see condition
Leptospirosis 100.9
    autumnalis 100.89
    canicula 100.89
    grippotyphosa 100.89
    hebdomidis 100.89
    icterohemorrhagica 100.0
    nanukayami 100.89
    pomona 100.89
    Weil's disease 100.0
Leptothricosis — see Actinomycosis
Leptothrix infestation — see Actinomycosis
Leptotricosis — see Actinomycosis
Leptus dermatitis 133.8
Léris pleonosteosis 756.89
Léri-Weill syndrome 756.59
Leriche's syndrome (aortic bifurcation occlusion) 444.0
Lermoyez's syndrome (see also Disease, Ménière's) 386.00
Lesbianism — omit code
    ego-dystonic 302.0
    problems with 302.0
Lesch-Nyhan syndrome (hypoxanthineguanine-phosphoribosyltransferase deficiency) 277.2
Lesion
    abducens nerve 378.54
    alveolar process 525.8
    anorectal 569.49
    aortic (valve) — see Endocarditis, aortic
    auditory nerve 388.5
    basal ganglion 333.90

Lesion — continued
    bile duct (see also Disease, biliary) 576.8
    bladder 596.9
    bone 733.90
    brachial plexus 353.0
    brain 348.8
        congenital 742.9
        vascular (see also Lesion, cerebrovascular) 437.9
            degenerative 437.1
            healed or old without residuals V12.59
            hypertensive 437.2
            late effect — see Late effect(s) (of) cerebrovascular disease
    buccal 528.9
    calcified — see Calcification
    canthus 373.9
    carate — see Pinta, lesions
    cardia 537.89
    cardiac — see also Disease, heart
        congenital 746.9
        valvular — see Endocarditis
    cauda equina 344.60
        with neurogenic bladder 344.61
    cecum 569.89
    cerebral — see Lesion, brain
    cerebrovascular (see also Disease, cerebrovascular NEC) 437.9
        degenerative 437.1
        healed or old without residuals V12.59
        hypertensive 437.2
        specified type NEC 437.8
    cervical root (nerve) NEC 353.2
    chiasmal 377.54
        associated with
            inflammatory disorders 377.54
            neoplasm NEC 377.52
                pituitary 377.51
            pituitary disorders 377.51
            vascular disorders 377.53
    chorda tympani 351.8
    coin, lung 793.1
    colon 569.89
    congenital — see Anomaly
    conjunctiva 372.9
    coronary artery (see also Ischemia, heart) 414.9
    cranial nerve 352.9
        first 352.0
        second 377.49
        third
            partial 378.51
            total 378.52
        fourth 378.53
        fifth 350.9
        sixth 378.54
        seventh 351.9
        eighth 388.5
        ninth 352.2
        tenth 352.3
        eleventh 352.4
        twelfth 352.5
    cystic — see Cyst
    degenerative — see Degeneration
    dermal (skin) 709.9
    Dieulafoy (hemorrhagic) ●
        of
            duodenum 537.84 ●
            intestine 569.86 ●
            stomach 537.84 ●
    duodenum 537.89
        with obstruction 537.3
    eyelid 373.9
    gasserian ganglion 350.8
    gastric 537.89
    gastroduodenal 537.89
    gastrointestinal 569.89
    glossopharyngeal nerve 352.2
    heart (organic) — see also Disease, heart
        vascular — see Disease, cardiovascular
    helix (ear) 709.9
    hyperchromic, due to pinta (carate) 103.1
    hyperkeratotic (see also Hyperkeratosis) 701.1
    hypoglossal nerve 352.5
    hypopharynx 478.29
    hypothalamic 253.9
    ileocecal coil 569.89
    ileum 569.89

Lesion — continued
    iliohypogastric nerve 355.79
    ilioinguinal nerve 355.79
    in continuity — see Injury, nerve, by site
    inflammatory — see Inflammation
    intestine 569.89
    intracerebral — see Lesion, brain
    intrachiasmal (optic) (see also Lesion, chiasmal) 377.54
    intracranial, space-occupying NEC 784.2
    joint 719.90
        ankle 719.97
        elbow 719.92
        foot 719.97
        hand 719.94
        hip 719.95
        knee 719.96
        multiple sites 719.99
        pelvic region 719.95
        sacroiliac (old) 724.6
        shoulder (region) 719.91
        specified site NEC 719.98
        wrist 719.93
    keratotic (see also Keratosis) 701.1
    kidney (see also Disease, renal) 593.9
    laryngeal nerve (recurrent) 352.3
    leonine 030.0
    lip 528.5
    liver 573.8
    lumbosacral
        plexus 353.1
        root (nerve) NEC 353.4
    lung 518.89
        coin 793.1
    maxillary sinus 473.0
    mitral — see Endocarditis, mitral
    motor cortex 348.8
    nerve (see also Disorder, nerve) 355.9
    nervous system 349.9
        congenital 742.9
    nonallopathic NEC 739.9
        in region (of)
            abdomen 739.9
            acromioclavicular 739.7
            cervical, cervicothoracic 739.1
            costochondral 739.8
            costovertebral 739.8
            extremity
                lower 739.6
                upper 739.7
            head 739.0
            hip 739.5
            lower extremity 739.6
            lumbar, lumbosacral 739.3
            occipitocervical 739.0
            pelvic 739.5
            pubic 739.5
            rib cage 739.8
            sacral, sacrococcygeal, sacroiliac 739.4
            sternochondral 739.8
            sternoclavicular 739.7
            thoracic, thoracolumbar 739.2
            upper extremity 739.7
    nose (internal) 478.1
    obstructive — see Obstruction
    obturator nerve 355.79
    occlusive
        artery — see Embolism, artery
    organ or site NEC — see Disease, by site
    osteolytic 733.90
    paramacular, of retina 363.32
    peptic 537.89
    periodontal, due to traumatic occlusion 523.8
    perirectal 569.49
    peritoneum (granulomatous) 568.89
    pigmented (skin) 709.00
    pinta — see Pinta, lesions
    polypoid — see Polyp
    prechiasmal (optic) (see also Lesion, chiasmal) 377.54
    primary — see also Syphilis, primary
        carate 103.0
        pinta 103.0
        yaws 102.0
    pulmonary 518.89
        valve (see also Endocarditis, pulmonary) 424.3

Index to Diseases

Lesion — *continued*
  pylorus 537.89
  radiation NEC 990
  radium NEC 990
  rectosigmoid 569.89
  retina, retinal — *see also* Retinopathy
    vascular 362.17
  retroperitoneal 568.89
  romanus 720.1
  sacroiliac (joint) 724.6
  salivary gland 527.8
    benign lymphoepithelial 527.8
  saphenous nerve 355.79
  secondary — *see* Syphilis, secondary
  sigmoid 569.89
  sinus (accessory) (nasal) (*see also* Sinusitis) 473.9
  skin 709.9
    suppurative 686.00
  SLAP (superior glenoid labrum) 840.7
  space-occupying, intracranial NEC 784.2
  spinal cord 336.9
    congenital 742.9
    traumatic (complete) (incomplete) (transverse) — *see also* Injury, spinal, by site
      with
        broken
          back — *see* Fracture, vertebra, by site, with spinal cord injury
          neck — *see* Fracture, vertebra, cervical, with spinal cord injury
        fracture, vertebra — *see* Fracture, vertebra, by site, with spinal cord injury
  spleen 289.50
  stomach 537.89
  superior glenoid labrum (SLAP) 840.7
  syphilitic — *see* Syphilis
  tertiary — *see* Syphilis, tertiary
  thoracic root (nerve) 353.3
  tonsillar fossa 474.9
  tooth, teeth 525.8
    white spot 521.01
  traumatic NEC (*see also* nature and site of injury) 959.9
  tricuspid (valve) — *see* Endocarditis, tricuspid
  trigeminal nerve 350.9
  ulcerated or ulcerative — *see* Ulcer
  uterus NEC 621.9
  vagina 623.8
  vagus nerve 352.3
  valvular — *see* Endocarditis
  vascular 459.9
    affecting central nervous system (*see also* Lesion, cerebrovascular) 437.9
    following trauma (*see also* Injury, blood vessel, by site) 904.9
    retina 362.17
    traumatic — *see* Injury, blood vessel, by site
    umbilical cord 663.6 ✓5ᵗʰ
      affecting fetus or newborn 762.6
  visual
    cortex NEC (*see also* Disorder, visual, cortex) 377.73
    pathway NEC (*see also* Disorder, visual, pathway) 377.63
  warty — *see* Verruca
  white spot, on teeth 521.01
  x-ray NEC 990
Lethargic — *see* condition
Lethargy 780.79
Letterer-Siwe disease (acute histiocytosis X) (M9722/3) 202.5 ✓5ᵗʰ
Leucinosis 270.3
Leucocoria 360.44
Leucosarcoma (M9850/3) 207.8 ✓5ᵗʰ
Leukasmus 270.2

Leukemia, leukemic (congenital) (M9800/3) 208.9 ✓5ᵗʰ

> *Note* — Use the following fifth-digit subclassification for categories 203–208:
> 0 without mention of remission
> 1 with remission

  acute NEC (M9801/3) 208.0 ✓5ᵗʰ
  aleukemic NEC (M9804/3) 208.8 ✓5ᵗʰ
    granulocytic (M9864/3) 205.8 ✓5ᵗʰ
  basophilic (M9870/3) 205.1 ✓5ᵗʰ
  blast (cell) (M9801/3) 208.0 ✓5ᵗʰ
  blastic (M9801/3) 208.0 ✓5ᵗʰ
    granulocytic (M9861/3) 205.0 ✓5ᵗʰ
  chronic NEC (M9803/3) 208.1 ✓5ᵗʰ
  compound (M9810/3) 207.8 ✓5ᵗʰ
  eosinophilic (M9880/3) 205.1 ✓5ᵗʰ
  giant cell (M9910/3) 207.2 ✓5ᵗʰ
  granulocytic (M9860/3) 205.9 ✓5ᵗʰ
    acute (M9861/3) 205.0 ✓5ᵗʰ
    aleukemic (M9864/3) 205.8 ✓5ᵗʰ
    blastic (M9861/3) 205.0 ✓5ᵗʰ
    chronic (M9863/3) 205.1 ✓5ᵗʰ
    subacute (M9862/3) 205.2 ✓5ᵗʰ
    subleukemic (M9864/3) 205.8 ✓5ᵗʰ
  hairy cell (M9940/3) 202.4 ✓5ᵗʰ
  hemoblastic (M9801/3) 208.0 ✓5ᵗʰ
  histiocytic (M9890/3) 206.9 ✓5ᵗʰ
  lymphatic (M9820/3) 204.9 ✓5ᵗʰ
    acute (M9821/3) 204.0 ✓5ᵗʰ
    aleukemic (M9824/3) 204.8 ✓5ᵗʰ
    chronic (M9823/3) 204.1 ✓5ᵗʰ
    subacute (M9822/3) 204.2 ✓5ᵗʰ
    subleukemic (M9824/3) 204.8 ✓5ᵗʰ
  lymphoblastic (M9821/3) 204.0 ✓5ᵗʰ
  lymphocytic (M9820/3) 204.9 ✓5ᵗʰ
    acute (M9821/3) 204.0 ✓5ᵗʰ
    aleukemic (M9824/3) 204.8 ✓5ᵗʰ
    chronic (M9823/3) 204.1 ✓5ᵗʰ
    subacute (M9822/3) 204.2 ✓5ᵗʰ
    subleukemic (M9824/3) 204.8 ✓5ᵗʰ
  lymphogenous (M9820/3) — *see* Leukemia, lymphoid
  lymphoid (M9820/3) 204.9 ✓5ᵗʰ
    acute (M9821/3) 204.0 ✓5ᵗʰ
    aleukemic (M9824/3) 204.8 ✓5ᵗʰ
    blastic (M9821/3) 204.0 ✓5ᵗʰ
    chronic (M9823/3) 204.1 ✓5ᵗʰ
    subacute (M9822/3) 204.2 ✓5ᵗʰ
    subleukemic (M9824/3) 204.8 ✓5ᵗʰ
  lymphosarcoma cell (M9850/3) 207.8 ✓5ᵗʰ
  mast cell (M9900/3) 207.8 ✓5ᵗʰ
  megakaryocytic (M9910/3) 207.2 ✓5ᵗʰ
  megakaryocytoid (M9910/3) 207.2 ✓5ᵗʰ
  mixed (cell) (M9810/3) 207.8 ✓5ᵗʰ
  monoblastic (M9891/3) 206.0 ✓5ᵗʰ
  monocytic (Schilling-type) (M9890/3) 206.9 ✓5ᵗʰ
    acute (M9891/3) 206.0 ✓5ᵗʰ
    aleukemic (M9894/3) 206.8 ✓5ᵗʰ
    chronic (M9893/3) 206.1 ✓5ᵗʰ
    Naegeli-type (M9863/3) 205.1 ✓5ᵗʰ
    subacute (M9892/3) 206.2 ✓5ᵗʰ
    subleukemic (M9894/3) 206.8 ✓5ᵗʰ
  monocytoid (M9890/3) 206.9 ✓5ᵗʰ
    acute (M9891/3) 206.0 ✓5ᵗʰ
    aleukemic (M9894/3) 206.8 ✓5ᵗʰ
    chronic (M9893/3) 206.1 ✓5ᵗʰ
    myelogenous (M9863/3) 205.1 ✓5ᵗʰ
    subacute (M9892/3) 206.2 ✓5ᵗʰ
    subleukemic (M9894/3) 206.8 ✓5ᵗʰ
  monomyelocytic (M9860/3) — *see* Leukemia, myelomonocytic
  myeloblastic (M9861/3) 205.0 ✓5ᵗʰ
  myelocytic (M9863/3) 205.1 ✓5ᵗʰ
    acute (M9861/3) 205.0 ✓5ᵗʰ
  myelogenous (M9860/3) 205.9 ✓5ᵗʰ
    acute (M9861/3) 205.0 ✓5ᵗʰ
    aleukemic (M9864/3) 205.8 ✓5ᵗʰ
    chronic (M9863/3) 205.1 ✓5ᵗʰ
    monocytoid (M9863/3) 205.1 ✓5ᵗʰ
    subacute (M9862/3) 205.2 ✓5ᵗʰ
    subleukemic (M9864) 205.8 ✓5ᵗʰ
  myeloid (M9860/3) 205.9 ✓5ᵗʰ
    acute (M9861/3) 205.0 ✓5ᵗʰ
    aleukemic (M9864/3) 205.8 ✓5ᵗʰ
    chronic (M9863/3) 205.1 ✓5ᵗʰ

Leukemia, leukemic — *continued*
  myeloid — *continued*
    subacute (M9862/3) 205.2 ✓5ᵗʰ
    subleukemic (M9864/3) 205.8 ✓5ᵗʰ
  myelomonocytic (M9860/3) 205.9 ✓5ᵗʰ
    acute (M9861/3) 205.0 ✓5ᵗʰ
    chronic (M9863/3) 205.1 ✓5ᵗʰ
  Naegeli type monocytic (M9863/3) 205.1 ✓5ᵗʰ
  neutrophilic (M9865/3) 205.1 ✓5ᵗʰ
  plasma cell (M9830/3) 203.1 ✓5ᵗʰ
  plasmacytic (M9830/3) 203.1 ✓5ᵗʰ
  prolymphocytic (M9825/3) — *see* Leukemia, lymphoid
  promyelocytic, acute (M9866/3) 205.0 ✓5ᵗʰ
  Schilling-type monocytic (M9890/3) — *see* Leukemia, monocytic
  stem cell (M9801/3) 208.0 ✓5ᵗʰ
  subacute NEC (M9802/3) 208.2 ✓5ᵗʰ
  subleukemic NEC (M9804/3) 208.8 ✓5ᵗʰ
  thrombocytic (M9910/3) 207.2 ✓5ᵗʰ
  undifferentiated (M9801/3) 208.0 ✓5ᵗʰ
Leukemoid reaction (lymphocytic) (monocytic) (myelocytic) 288.8
Leukoclastic vasculitis 446.29
Leukocoria 360.44
Leukocythemia — *see* Leukemia
Leukocytosis 288.8
  basophilic 288.8
  eosinophilic 288.3
  lymphocytic 288.8
  monocytic 288.8
  neutrophilic 288.8
Leukoderma 709.09
  syphilitic 091.3
    late 095.8
Leukodermia (*see also* Leukoderma) 709.09
Leukodystrophy (cerebral) (globoid cell) (metachromatic) (progressive) (sudanophilic) 330.0
Leukoedema, mouth or tongue 528.7
Leukoencephalitis
  acute hemorrhagic (postinfectious) NEC 136.9 *[323.6]*
  postimmunization or postvaccinal 323.5
  subacute sclerosing 046.2
    van Bogaert's 046.2
  van Bogaert's (sclerosing) 046.2
Leukoencephalopathy (*see also* Encephalitis) 323.9
  acute necrotizing hemorrhagic (postinfectious) 136.9 *[323.6]*
  postimmunization or postvaccinal 323.5
  metachromatic 330.0
  multifocal (progressive) 046.3
  progressive multifocal 046.3
Leukoerythroblastosis 289.0
Leukoerythrosis 289.0
Leukokeratosis (*see also* Leukoplakia) 702.8
  mouth 528.6
  nicotina palati 528.7
  tongue 528.6
Leukokoria 360.44
Leukokraurosis vulva, vulvae 624.0
Leukolymphosarcoma (M9850/3) 207.8 ✓5ᵗʰ
Leukoma (cornea) (interfering with central vision) 371.03
  adherent 371.04
Leukomalacia, periventricular 779.7
Leukomelanopathy, hereditary 288.2
Leukonychia (punctata) (striata) 703.8
  congenital 757.5
Leukopathia
  unguium 703.8
    congenital 757.5
Leukopenia 288.0
  cyclic 288.0
  familial 288.0
  malignant 288.0
  periodic 288.0
  transitory neonatal 776.7
Leukopenic — *see* condition
Leukoplakia 702.8
  anus 569.49

Leukoplakia

Leukoplakia — *continued*
  bladder (postinfectional) 596.8
  buccal 528.6
  cervix (uteri) 622.2
  esophagus 530.83
  gingiva 528.6
  kidney (pelvis) 593.89
  larynx 478.79
  lip 528.6
  mouth 528.6
  oral soft tissue (including tongue) (mucosa) 528.6
  palate 528.6
  pelvis (kidney) 593.89
  penis (infectional) 607.0
  rectum 569.49
  syphilitic 095.8
  tongue 528.6
  tonsil 478.29
  ureter (postinfectional) 593.89
  urethra (postinfectional) 599.84
  uterus 621.8
  vagina 623.1
  vesical 596.8
  vocal cords 478.5
  vulva 624.0
Leukopolioencephalopathy 330.0
Leukorrhea (vagina) 623.5
  due to trichomonas (vaginalis) 131.00
  trichomonal (Trichomonas vaginalis) 131.00
Leukosarcoma (M9850/3) 207.8 ✓5ᵗʰ
Leukosis (M9800/3) — *see* Leukemia
Lev's disease or syndrome (acquired complete heart block) 426.0
Levi's syndrome (pituitary dwarfism) 253.3
Levocardia (isolated) 746.87
  with situs inversus 759.3
Levulosuria 271.2
Lewandowski's disease (primary) (*see also* Tuberculosis) 017.0 ✓5ᵗʰ
Lewandowski-Lutz disease (epidermodysplasia verruciformis) 078.19
Leyden's disease (periodic vomiting) 536.2
Leyden-Möbius dystrophy 359.1
Leydig cell
  carcinoma (M8650/3)
    specified site — *see* Neoplasm, by site, malignant
    unspecified site
      female 183.0
      male 186.9
  tumor (M8650/1)
    benign (M8650/0)
      specified site — *see* Neoplasm, by site, benign
      unspecified site
        female 220
        male 222.0
    malignant (M8650/3)
      specified site — *see* Neoplasm, by site, malignant
      unspecified site
        female 183.0
        male 186.9
    specified site — *see* Neoplasm, by site, uncertain behavior
    unspecified site
      female 236.2
      male 236.4
Leydig-Sertoli cell tumor (M8631/0)
  specified site — *see* Neoplasm, by site, benign
  unspecified site
    female 220
    male 222.0
LGSIL (low grade squamous intraepithelial dysplasia) 622.1 ●
Liar, pathologic 301.7
Libman-Sacks disease or syndrome 710.0 [424.91]
Lice (infestation) 132.9
  body (pediculus corporis) 132.1
  crab 132.2
  head (pediculus capitis) 132.0

Lice — *continued*
  mixed (classifiable to more than one of the categories 132.0-132.2) 132.3
  pubic (pediculus pubis) 132.2
Lichen 697.9
  albus 701.0
  annularis 695.89
  atrophicus 701.0
  corneus obtusus 698.3
  myxedematous 701.8
  nitidus 697.1
  pilaris 757.39
    acquired 701.1
  planopilaris 697.0
  planus (acute) (chronicus) (hypertrophic) (verrucous) 697.0
    morphoeicus 701.0
    sclerosus (et atrophicus) 701.0
  ruber 696.4
    acuminatus 696.4
    moniliformis 697.8
    obtusus corneus 698.3
    of Wilson 697.0
    planus 697.0
  selerosus (et atrophicus) 701.0
  scrofulosus (primary) (*see also* Tuberculosis) 017.0 ✓5ᵗʰ
  simplex (Vidal's) 698.3
    chronicus 698.3
    circumscriptus 698.3
  spinulosus 757.39
    mycotic 117.9
  striata 697.8
  urticatus 698.2
Lichenification 698.3
  nodular 698.3
Lichenoides tuberculosis (primary) (*see also* Tuberculosis) 017.0 ✓5ᵗʰ
Lichtheim's disease or syndrome (subacute combined sclerosis with pernicious anemia) 281.0 [336.2]
Lien migrans 289.59
Lientery (*see also* Diarrhea) 787.91
  infectious 009.2
Life circumstance problem NEC V62.89
Li-Fraumeni cancer syndrome 758.3
Ligament — *see* condition
Light-for-dates (infant) 764.0 ✓5ᵗʰ
  with signs of fetal malnutrition 764.1 ✓5ᵗʰ
  affecting management of pregnancy 656.5 ✓5ᵗʰ
Light-headedness 780.4
Lightning (effects) (shock) (stroke) (struck by) 994.0
  burn — *see* Burn, by site
  foot 266.2
Lightwood's disease or syndrome (renal tubular acidosis) 588.8
Lignac's disease (cystinosis) 270.0
Lignac (-de Toni) (-Fanconi) (-Debré) syndrome (cystinosis) 270.0
Lignac (-Fanconi) syndrome (cystinosis) 270.0
Ligneous thyroiditis 245.3
Likoff's syndrome (angina in menopausal women) 413.9
Limb — *see* condition
Limitation of joint motion (*see also* Stiffness, joint) 719.5 ✓5ᵗʰ
  sacroiliac 724.6
Limit dextrinosis 271.0
Limited
  cardiac reserve — *see* Disease, heart
  duction, eye NEC 378.63
Lindau's disease (retinocerebral angiomatosis) 759.6
Lindau (-von Hippel) disease (angiomatosis retinocerebellosa) 759.6
Linea corneae senilis 371.41
Lines
  Beau's (transverse furrows on fingernails) 703.8
  Harris' 733.91
  Hudson-Stähli 371.11
  Stähli's 371.11

Lingua
  geographical 529.1
  nigra (villosa) 529.3
  plicata 529.5
    congenital 750.13
  tylosis 528.6
Lingual (tongue) — *see also* condition
  thyroid 759.2
Linitis (gastric) 535.4 ✓5ᵗʰ
  plastica (M8142/3) 151.9
Lioderma essentialis (cum melanosis et telangiectasia) 757.33
Lip — *see also* condition
  biting 528.9
Lipalgia 272.8
Lipedema — *see* Edema
Lipemia (*see also* Hyperlipidemia) 272.4
  retina, retinalis 272.3
Lipidosis 272.7
  cephalin 272.7
  cerebral (infantile) (juvenile) (late) 330.1
  cerebroretinal 330.1 [362.71]
  cerebroside 272.7
  cerebrospinal 272.7
  chemically-induced 272.7
  cholesterol 272.7
  diabetic 250.8 ✓5ᵗʰ [272.7]
  dystopic (hereditary) 272.7
  glycolipid 272.7
  hepatosplenomegalic 272.3
  hereditary, dystopic 272.7
  sulfatide 330.0
Lipoadenoma (M8324/0) — *see* Neoplasm, by site, benign
Lipoblastoma (M8881/0) — *see* Lipoma, by site
Lipoblastomatosis (M8881/0) — *see* Lipoma, by site
Lipochondrodystrophy 277.5
Lipochrome histiocytosis (familial) 288.1
Lipodystrophia progressiva 272.6
Lipodystrophy (progressive) 272.6
  insulin 272.6
  intestinal 040.2
Lipofibroma (M8851/0) — *see* Lipoma, by site
Lipoglycoproteinosis 272.8
Lipogranuloma, sclerosing 709.8
Lipogranulomatosis (disseminated) 272.8
  kidney 272.8
Lipoid — *see also* condition
  histiocytosis 272.7
    essential 272.7
  nephrosis (*see also* Nephrosis) 581.3
  proteinosis of Urbach 272.8
Lipoidemia (*see also* Hyperlipidemia) 272.4
Lipoidosis (*see also* Lipidosis) 272.7
Lipoma (M8850/0) 214.9
  breast (skin) 214.1
  face 214.0
  fetal (M8881/0) — *see also* Lipoma, by site
    fat cell (M8880/0) — *see* Lipoma, by site
  infiltrating (M8856/0) — *see* Lipoma, by site
  intra-abdominal 214.3
  intramuscular (M8856/0) — *see* Lipoma, by site
  intrathoracic 214.2
  kidney 214.3
  mediastinum 214.2
  muscle 214.8
  peritoneum 214.3
  retroperitoneum 214.3
  skin 214.1
    face 214.0
  spermatic cord 214.4
  spindle cell (M8857/0) — *see* Lipoma, by site
  stomach 214.3
  subcutaneous tissue 214.1
    face 214.0
  thymus 214.2
  thyroid gland 214.2
Lipomatosis (dolorosa) 272.8
  epidural 214.8
  fetal (M8881/0) — *see* Lipoma, by site

Index to Diseases

Lipomatosis — *continued*
  Launois-Bensaude's 272.8
Lipomyohemangioma (M8860/0)
  specified site — *see* Neoplasm, connective tissue, benign
  unspecified site 223.0
Lipomyoma (M8860/0)
  specified site — *see* Neoplasm, connective tissue, benign
  unspecified site 223.0
Lipomyxoma (M8852/0) — *see* Lipoma, by site
Lipomyxosarcoma (M8852/3) — *see* Neoplasm, connective tissue, malignant
Lipophagocytosis 289.8
Lipoproteinemia (alpha) 272.4
  broad-beta 272.2
  floating-beta 272.2
  hyper-pre-beta 272.1
Lipoproteinosis (Rössle-Urbach-Wiethe) 272.8
Liposarcoma (M8850/3) — *see also* Neoplasm, connective tissue, malignant
  differentiated type (M8851/3) — *see* Neoplasm, connective tissue, malignant
  embryonal (M8852/3) — *see* Neoplasm, connective tissue, malignant
  mixed type (M8855/3) — *see* Neoplasm, connective tissue, malignant
  myxoid (M8852/3) — *see* Neoplasm, connective tissue, malignant
  pleomorphic (M8854/3) — *see* Neoplasm, connective tissue, malignant
  round cell (M8853/3) — *see* Neoplasm, connective tissue, malignant
  well differentiated type (M8851/3) — *see* Neoplasm, connective tissue, malignant
Lipsynovitis prepatellaris 272.8
Lipping
  cervix 622.0
  spine (*see also* Spondylosis) 721.90
  vertebra (*see also* Spondylosis) 721.90
Lip pits (mucus), congenital 750.25
Lipschütz disease or ulcer 616.50
Lipuria 791.1
  bilharziasis 120.0
Liquefaction, vitreous humor 379.21
Lisping 307.9
Lissauer's paralysis 094.1
Lissencephalia, lissencephaly 742.2
Listerellose 027.0
Listeriose 027.0
Listeriosis 027.0
  congenital 771.2
  fetal 771.2
  suspected fetal damage affecting management of pregnancy 655.4 ✓5ᵗʰ
Listlessness 780.79
Lithemia 790.6
Lithiasis — *see also* Calculus
  hepatic (duct) — *see* Choledocholithiasis
  urinary 592.9
Lithopedion 779.9
  affecting management of pregnancy 656.8 ✓5ᵗʰ
Lithosis (occupational) 502
  with tuberculosis — *see* Tuberculosis, pulmonary
Lithuria 791.9
Litigation V62.5
Little
  league elbow 718.82
  stroke syndrome 435.9
Little's disease — *see* Palsy, cerebral
Littre's
  gland — *see* condition
  hernia — *see* Hernia, Littre's
Littritis (*see also* Urethritis) 597.89
Livedo 782.61
  annularis 782.61
  racemose 782.61
  reticularis 782.61
Live flesh 781.0

Liver — *see also* condition
  donor V59.6
Livida, asphyxia
  newborn 768.6
Living
  alone V60.3
    with handicapped person V60.4
Lloyd's syndrome 258.1
Loa loa 125.2
Loasis 125.2
Lobe, lobar — *see* condition
Lobo's disease or blastomycosis 116.2
Lobomycosis 116.2
Lobotomy syndrome 310.0
Lobstein's disease (brittle bones and blue sclera) 756.51
Lobster-claw hand 755.58
Lobulation (congenital) — *see also* Anomaly, specified type NEC, by site
  kidney, fetal 753.3
  liver, abnormal 751.69
  spleen 759.0
Lobule, lobular — *see* condition
Local, localized — *see* condition
Locked bowel or intestine (*see also* Obstruction, intestine) 560.9
Locked-in state 344.81
Locked twins 660.5 ✓5ᵗʰ
  affecting fetus or newborn 763.1
Locking
  joint (*see also* Derangement, joint) 718.90
  knee 717.9
Lockjaw (*see also* Tetanus) 037
Locomotor ataxia (progressive) 094.0
Löffler's
  endocarditis 421.0
  eosinophilia or syndrome 518.3
  pneumonia 518.3
  syndrome (eosinophilic pneumonitis) 518.3
Löfgren's syndrome (sarcoidosis) 135
Loiasis 125.2
  eyelid 125.2 [373.6]
Loneliness V62.89
Lone star fever 082.8
Long labor 662.1 ✓5ᵗʰ
  affecting fetus or newborn 763.89
  first stage 662.0 ✓5ᵗʰ
  second stage 662.2 ✓5ᵗʰ
Longitudinal stripes or grooves, nails 703.8
  congenital 757.5
Long-term (current) drug use V58.69
  antibiotics V58.62
  anticoagulants V58.61
Loop
  intestine (*see also* Volvulus) 560.2
  intrascleral nerve 379.29
  vascular on papilla (optic) 743.57
Loose — *see also* condition
  body
    in tendon sheath 727.82
    joint 718.10
      ankle 718.17
      elbow 718.12
      foot 718.17
      hand 718.14
      hip 718.15
      knee 717.6
      multiple sites 718.19
      pelvic region 718.15
      prosthetic implant — *see* Complications, mechanical
      shoulder (region) 718.11
      specified site NEC 718.18
      wrist 718.13
  cartilage (joint) (*see also* Loose, body, joint) 718.1 ✓5ᵗʰ
    knee 717.6
  facet (vertebral) 724.9
  prosthetic implant — *see* Complications, mechanical

Loose — *see also* condition — *continued*
  sesamoid, joint (*see also* Loose, body, joint) 718.1 ✓5ᵗʰ
  tooth, teeth 525.8
Loosening epiphysis 732.9
Looser (-Debray) -Milkman syndrome (osteomalacia with pseudofractures) 268.2
Lop ear (deformity) 744.29
Lorain's disease or syndrome (pituitary dwarfism) 253.3
Lorain-Levi syndrome (pituitary dwarfism) 253.3
Lordosis (acquired) (postural) 737.20
  congenital 754.2
  due to or associated with
    Charcôt-Marie-Tooth disease 356.1 [737.42]
    mucopolysaccharidosis 277.5 [737.42]
    neurofibromatosis 237.71 [737.42]
    osteitis
      deformans 731.0 [737.42]
      fibrosa cystica 252.0 [737.42]
    osteoporosis (*see also* Osteoporosis) 733.00 [737.42]
    poliomyelitis (*see also* Poliomyelitis) 138 [737.42]
    tuberculosis (*see also* Tuberculosis) 015.0 ✓5ᵗʰ [737.42]
  late effect of rickets 268.1 [737.42]
  postlaminectomy 737.21
  postsurgical NEC 737.22
  rachitic 268.1 [737.42]
  specified NEC 737.29
  tuberculous (*see also* Tuberculosis) 015.0 ✓5ᵗʰ [737.42]
Loss
  appetite 783.0
    hysterical 300.11
    nonorganic origin 307.59
    psychogenic 307.59
  blood — *see* Hemorrhage
  central vision 368.41
  consciousness 780.09
    transient 780.2
  control, sphincter, rectum 787.6
    nonorganic origin 307.7
  ear ossicle, partial 385.24
  elasticity, skin 782.8
  extremity or member, traumatic, current — *see* Amputation, traumatic
  fluid (acute) 276.5
    with
      hypernatremia 276.0
      hyponatremia 276.1
    fetus or newborn 775.5
  hair 704.00
  hearing — *see also* Deafness
    central 389.14
    conductive (air) 389.00
      with sensorineural hearing loss 389.2
      combined types 389.08
      external ear 389.01
      inner ear 389.04
      middle ear 389.03
      multiple types 389.08
      tympanic membrane 389.02
    mixed type 389.2
    nerve 389.12
    neural 389.12
    noise-induced 388.12
    perceptive NEC (*see also* Loss, hearing, sensorineural) 389.10
    sensorineural 389.10
      with conductive hearing loss 389.2
      central 389.14
      combined types 389.18
      multiple types 389.18
      neural 389.12
      sensory 389.11
    sensory 389.11
    specified type NEC 389.8
    sudden NEC 388.2
  height 781.91
  labyrinthine reactivity (unilateral) 386.55
    bilateral 386.56
  memory (*see also* Amnesia) 780.99 ▲
    mild, following organic brain damage 310.1

Loss

Loss — *continued*
  mind (*see also* Psychosis) 298.9
  organ or part — *see* Absence, by site, acquired
  sensation 782.0
  sense of
    smell (*see also* Disturbance, sensation) 781.1
    taste (*see also* Disturbance, sensation) 781.1
    touch (*see also* Disturbance, sensation) 781.1
  sight (acquired) (complete) (congenital) *see* Blindness
  spinal fluid
    headache 349.0
  substance of
    bone (*see also* Osteoporosis) 733.00
    cartilage 733.99
    ear 380.32
    vitreous (humor) 379.26
  tooth, teeth
    acquired 525.10
      due to
        caries 525.13
        extraction 525.10
        periodontal disease 525.12
        specified NEC 525.19
        trauma 525.11
  vision, visual (*see also* Blindness) 369.9
    both eyes (*see also* Blindness, both eyes) 369.3
    complete (*see also* Blindness, both eyes) 369.00
    one eye 369.8
    sudden 368.11
    transient 368.12
  vitreous 379.26
  voice (*see also* Aphonia) 784.41
  weight (cause unknown) 783.21
Lou Gehrig's disease 335.20
Louis-Bar syndrome (ataxia-telangiectasia) 334.8
Louping ill 063.1
Lousiness — *see* Lice
Low
  back syndrome 724.2
  basal metabolic rate (BMR) 794.7
  birthweight 765.1 ✓5ᵗʰ
    extreme (less than 1000 grams) 765.0 ✓5ᵗʰ
    for gestational age 764.0 ✓5ᵗʰ
    status (*see also* Status, low birth weight) V21.30
  bladder compliance 596.52
  blood pressure (*see also* Hypotension) 458.9
    reading (incidental) (isolated) (nonspecific) 796.3
  cardiac reserve — *see* Disease, heart
  compliance bladder 596.52
  frequency deafness — *see* Disorder, hearing
  function — *see* Hypofunction
    kidney (*see also* Disease, renal) 593.9
    liver 573.9
  hemoglobin 285.9
  implantation, placenta — *see* Placenta, previa
  insertion, placenta — *see* placenta, previa
  lying
    kidney 593.0
    organ or site, congenital — *see* Malposition, congenital
    placenta — *see* Placenta, previa
  output syndrome (cardiac) (*see also* Failure, heart) 428.9
  platelets (blood) (*see also* Thrombocytopenia) 287.5
  reserve, kidney (*see also* Disease, renal) 593.9
  salt syndrome 593.9
  tension glaucoma 365.12
  vision 369.9
    both eyes 369.20
    one eye 369.70
Lowe (-Terrey-MacLachlan) syndrome (oculocerebrorenal dystrophy) 270.8
Lower extremity — *see* condition
Lown (-Ganong) -Levine syndrome (short P-R interval, normal QRS complex, and paroxysmal supraventricular tachycardia) 426.81

LSD reaction (*see also* Abuse, drugs, nondependent) 305.3 ✓5ᵗʰ
L-shaped kidney 753.3
Lucas-Championnière disease (fibrinous bronchitis) 466.0
Lucey-Driscoll syndrome (jaundice due to delayed conjugation) 774.30
Ludwig's
  angina 528.3
  disease (submaxillary cellulitis) 528.3
Lues (venerea), luetic — *see* Syphilis
Luetscher's syndrome (dehydration) 276.5
Lumbago 724.2
  due to displacement, intervertebral disc 722.10
Lumbalgia 724.2
  due to displacement, intervertebral disc 722.10
Lumbar — *see* condition
Lumbarization, vertebra 756.15
Lumbermen's itch 133.8
Lump — *see also* Mass
  abdominal 789.3 ✓5ᵗʰ
  breast 611.72
  chest 786.6
  epigastric 789.3 ✓5ᵗʰ
  head 784.2
  kidney 753.3
  liver 789.1
  lung 786.6
  mediastinal 786.6
  neck 784.2
  nose or sinus 784.2
  pelvic 789.3 ✓5ᵗʰ
  skin 782.2
  substernal 786.6
  throat 784.2
  umbilicus 789.3 ✓5ᵗʰ
Lunacy (*see also* Psychosis) 298.9
Lunatomalacia 732.3
Lung — *see also* condition
  donor V59.8
  drug addict's 417.8
  mainliners' 417.8
  vanishing 492.0
Lupoid (miliary) **of Boeck** 135
Lupus 710.0
  Cazenave's (erythematosus) 695.4
  discoid (local) 695.4
  disseminated 710.0
  erythematosus (discoid) (local) 695.4
    disseminated 710.0
    eyelid 373.34
    systemic 710.0
      with
        encephalitis 710.0 [323.8]
        lung involvement 710.0 [517.8]
        inhibitor (presence of) 286.5
  exedens 017.0 ✓5ᵗʰ
  eyelid (*see also* Tuberculosis) 017.0 ✓5ᵗʰ [373.4]
  Hilliard's 017.0 ✓5ᵗʰ
  hydralazine
    correct substance properly administered 695.4
    overdose or wrong substance given or taken 972.6
  miliaris disseminatus faciei 017.0 ✓5ᵗʰ
  nephritis 710.0 [583.81]
    acute 710.0 [580.81]
    chronic 710.0 [582.81]
  nontuberculous, not disseminated 695.4
  pernio (Besnier) 135
  tuberculous (*see also* Tuberculosis) 017.0 ✓5ᵗʰ
    eyelid (*see also* Tuberculosis) 017.0 ✓5ᵗʰ [373.4]
  vulgaris 017.0 ✓5ᵗʰ
Luschka's joint disease 721.90
Luteinoma (M8610/0) 220
Lutembacher's disease or syndrome (atrial septal defect with mitral stenosis) 745.5
Luteoma (M8610/0) 220
Lutz-Miescher disease (elastosis perforans serpiginosa) 701.1
Lutz-Splendore-de Almeida disease (Brazilian blastomycosis) 116.1

Luxatio
  bulbi due to birth injury 767.8
  coxae congenita (*see also* Dislocation, hip, congenital) 754.30
  erecta — *see* Dislocation, shoulder
  imperfecta — *see* Sprain, by site
  perinealis — *see* Dislocation, hip
Luxation — *see also* Dislocation, by site
  eyeball 360.81
    due to birth injury 767.8
    lateral 376.36
  genital organs (external) NEC — *see* Wound, open, genital organs
  globe (eye) 360.81
    lateral 376.36
  lacrimal gland (postinfectional) 375.16
  lens (old) (partial) 379.32
    congenital 743.37
    syphilitic 090.49 [379.32]
    Marfan's disease 090.49
    spontaneous 379.32
  penis — *see* Wound, open, penis
  scrotum — *see* Wound, open, scrotum
  testis — *see* Wound, open, testis
L-xyloketosuria 271.8
Lycanthropy (*see also* Psychosis) 298.9
Lyell's disease or syndrome (toxic epidermal necrolysis) 695.1
  due to drug
    correct substance properly administered 695.1
    overdose or wrong substance given or taken 977.9
      specified drug — *see* Table of Drugs and Chemicals
Lyme disease 088.81
Lymph
  gland or node — *see* condition
  scrotum (*see also* Infestation, filarial) 125.9
Lymphadenitis 289.3
  with
    abortion — *see* Abortion, by type, with sepsis
    ectopic pregnancy (*see also* categories 633.0-633.9) 639.0
    molar pregnancy (*see also* categories 630-632) 639.0
  acute 683
    mesenteric 289.2
  any site, except mesenteric 289.3
    acute 683
    chronic 289.1
    mesenteric (acute) (chronic) (nonspecific) (subacute) 289.2
    subacute 289.1
      mesenteric 289.2
  breast, puerperal, postpartum 675.2 ✓5ᵗʰ
  chancroidal (congenital) 099.0
  chronic 289.1
    mesenteric 289.2
  dermatopathic 695.89
  due to
    anthracosis (occupational) 500
    Brugia (Wuchereria) malayi 125.1
    diphtheria (toxin) 032.89
    lymphogranuloma venereum 099.1
    Wuchereria bancrofti 125.0
  following
    abortion 639.0
    ectopic or molar pregnancy 639.0
  generalized 289.3
  gonorrheal 098.89
  granulomatous 289.1
  infectional 683
  mesenteric (acute) (chronic) (nonspecific) (subacute) 289.2
    due to Bacillus typhi 002.0
    tuberculous (*see also* Tuberculosis) 014.8 ✓5ᵗʰ
  mycobacterial 031.8
  purulent 683
  pyogenic 683
  regional 078.3
  septic 683
  streptococcal 683
  subacute, unspecified site 289.1

Index to Diseases

Lymphadenitis — continued
- suppurative 683
- syphilitic (early) (secondary) 091.4
  - late 095.8
- tuberculous — see Tuberculosis, lymph gland
- venereal 099.1

Lymphadenoid goiter 245.2

Lymphadenopathy (general) 785.6
- due to toxoplasmosis (acquired) 130.7
  - congenital (active) 771.2

Lymphadenopathy-associated virus (disease) (illness) (infection) — see Human immunodeficiency virus (disease) (illness) (infection)

Lymphadenosis 785.6
- acute 075

Lymphangiectasis 457.1
- conjunctiva 372.89
- postinfectional 457.1
- scrotum 457.1

Lymphangiectatic elephantiasis, nonfilarial 457.1

Lymphangioendothelioma (M9170/0) 228.1
- malignant (M9170/3) — see Neoplasm, connective tissue, malignant

Lymphangioma (M9170/0) 228.1
- capillary (M9171/0) 228.1
- cavernous (M9172/0) 228.1
- cystic (M9173/0) 228.1
- malignant (M9170/3) — see Neoplasm, connective tissue, malignant

Lymphangiomyoma (M9174/0) 228.1

Lymphangiomyomatosis (M9174/1) — see Neoplasm, connective tissue, uncertain behavior

Lymphangiosarcoma (M9170/3) — see Neoplasm, connective tissue, malignant

Lymphangitis 457.2
- with
  - abortion — see Abortion, by type, with sepsis
  - abscess — see Abscess, by site
  - cellulitis — see Abscess, by site
  - ectopic pregnancy (see also categories 633.0-633.9) 639.0
  - molar pregnancy (see also categories 630-632) 639.0
- acute (with abscess or cellulitis) 682.9
  - specified site — see Abscess, by site
- breast, puerperal, postpartum 675.2 ✓5ᵗʰ
- chancroidal 099.0
- chronic (any site) 457.2
- due to
  - Brugia (Wuchereria) malayi 125.1
  - Wuchereria bancrofti 125.0
- following
  - abortion 639.0
  - ectopic or molar pregnancy 639.0
- gangrenous 457.2
- penis
  - acute 607.2
  - gonococcal (acute) 098.0
    - chronic or duration of 2 months or more 098.2
- puerperal, postpartum, childbirth 670 ✓4ᵗʰ
- strumous, tuberculous (see also Tuberculosis) 017.2 ✓5ᵗʰ
- subacute (any site) 457.2
- tuberculous — see Tuberculosis, lymph gland

Lymphatic (vessel) — see condition

Lymphatism 254.8
- scrofulous (see also Tuberculosis) 017.2 ✓5ᵗʰ

Lymphectasia 457.1

Lymphedema (see also Elephantiasis) 457.1
- acquired (chronic) 457.1
- chronic hereditary 757.0
- congenital 757.0
- idiopathic hereditary 757.0
- praecox 457.1
- secondary 457.1
- surgical NEC 997.99
  - postmastectomy (syndrome) 457.0

Lymph-hemangioma (M9120/0) — see Hemangioma, by site

Lymphoblastic — see condition

Lymphoblastoma (diffuse) (M9630/3) 200.1 ✓5ᵗʰ
- giant follicular (M9690/3) 202.0 ✓5ᵗʰ
- macrofollicular (M9690/3) 202.0 ✓5ᵗʰ

Lymphoblastosis, acute benign 075

Lymphocele 457.8

Lymphocythemia 288.8

Lymphocytic — see also condition
- chorioencephalitis (acute) (serous) 049.0
- choriomeningitis (acute) (serous) 049.0

Lymphocytoma (diffuse) (malignant) (M9620/3) 200.1 ✓5ᵗʰ

Lymphocytomatosis (M9620/3) 200.1 ✓5ᵗʰ

Lymphocytopenia 288.8

Lymphocytosis (symptomatic) 288.8
- infectious (acute) 078.89

Lymphoepithelioma (M8082/3) — see Neoplasm, by site, malignant

Lymphogranuloma (malignant) (M9650/3) 201.9 ✓5ᵗʰ
- inguinale 099.1
- venereal (any site) 099.1
  - with stricture of rectum 099.1
- venereum 099.1

Lymphogranulomatosis (malignant) (M9650/3) 201.9 ✓5ᵗʰ
- benign (Boeck's sarcoid) (Schaumann's) 135
- Hodgkin's (M9650/3) 201.9 ✓5ᵗʰ

Lymphoid — see condition

Lympholeukoblastoma (M9850/3) 207.8 ✓5ᵗʰ

Lympholeukosarcoma (M9850/3) 207.8 ✓5ᵗʰ

Lymphoma (malignant) (M9590/3) 202.8 ✓5ᵗʰ

> Note — Use the following fifth-digit subclassification with categories 200–202:
>
> 0 unspecified site
> 1 lymph nodes of head, face, and neck
> 2 intrathoracic lymph nodes
> 3 intra-abdominal lymph nodes
> 4 lymph nodes of axilla and upper limb
> 5 lymph nodes of inguinal region and lower limb
> 6 intrapelvic lymph nodes
> 7 spleen
> 8 lymph nodes of multiple sites

- benign (M9590/0) — see Neoplasm, by site, benign
- Burkitt's type (lymphoblastic) (undifferentiated) (M9750/3) 200.2 ✓5ᵗʰ
- Castleman's (mediastinal lymph node hyperplasia) 785.6
- centroblastic-centrocytic
  - diffuse (M9614/3) 202.8 ✓5ᵗʰ
  - follicular (M9692/3) 202.0 ✓5ᵗʰ
- centroblastic type (diffuse) (M9632/3) 202.8 ✓5ᵗʰ
  - follicular (M9697/3) 202.0 ✓5ᵗʰ
- centrocytic (M9622/3) 202.8 ✓5ᵗʰ
- compound (M9613/3) 200.8 ✓5ᵗʰ
- convoluted cell type (lymphoblastic) (M9602/3) 202.8 ✓5ᵗʰ
- diffuse NEC (M9590/3) 202.8 ✓5ᵗʰ
- follicular (giant) (M9690/3) 202.0 ✓5ᵗʰ
  - center cell (diffuse) (M9615/3) 202.8 ✓5ᵗʰ
  - cleaved (diffuse) (M9623/3) 202.8 ✓5ᵗʰ
    - follicular (M9695/3) 202.0 ✓5ᵗʰ
  - non-cleaved (diffuse) (M9633/3) 202.8 ✓5ᵗʰ
    - follicular (M9698/3) 202.0 ✓5ᵗʰ
  - centroblastic-centrocytic (M9692/3) 202.0 ✓5ᵗʰ
  - centroblastic type (M9697/3) 202.0 ✓5ᵗʰ
  - lymphocytic
    - intermediate differentiation (M9694/3) 202.0 ✓5ᵗʰ
    - poorly differentiated (M9696/3) 202.0 ✓5ᵗʰ
  - mixed (cell type) (lymphocytic-histiocytic) (small cell and large cell) (M9691/3) 202.0 ✓5ᵗʰ

Lymphoma — continued
- germinocytic (M9622/3) 202.8 ✓5ᵗʰ
- giant, follicular or follicle (M9690/3) 202.0 ✓5ᵗʰ
- histiocytic (diffuse) (M9640/3) 200.0 ✓5ᵗʰ
  - nodular (M9642/3) 200.0 ✓5ᵗʰ
  - pleomorphic cell type (M9641/3) 200.0 ✓5ᵗʰ
- Hodgkin's (M9650/3) (see also Disease, Hodgkin's) 201.9 ✓5ᵗʰ
- immunoblastic (type) (M9612/3) 200.8 ✓5ᵗʰ
- large cell (M9640/3) 200.0 ✓5ᵗʰ
  - nodular (M9642/3) 200.0 ✓5ᵗʰ
  - pleomorphic cell type (M9641/3) 200.0 ✓5ᵗʰ
- lymphoblastic (diffuse) (M9630/3) 200.1 ✓5ᵗʰ
  - Burkitt's type (M9750/3) 200.2 ✓5ᵗʰ
  - convoluted cell type (M9602/3) 202.8 ✓5ᵗʰ
- lymphocytic (cell type) (diffuse) (M9620/3) 200.1 ✓5ᵗʰ
  - with plasmacytoid differentiation, diffuse (M9611/3) 200.8 ✓5ᵗʰ
  - intermediate differentiation (diffuse) (M9621/3) 200.1 ✓5ᵗʰ
    - follicular (M9694/3) 202.0 ✓5ᵗʰ
    - nodular (M9694/3) 202.0 ✓5ᵗʰ
  - nodular (M9690/3) 202.0 ✓5ᵗʰ
  - poorly differentiated (diffuse) (M9630/3) 200.1 ✓5ᵗʰ
    - follicular (M9696/3) 202.0 ✓5ᵗʰ
    - nodular (M9696/3) 202.0 ✓5ᵗʰ
  - well differentiated (diffuse) (M9620/3) 200.1 ✓5ᵗʰ
    - follicular (M9693/3) 202.0 ✓5ᵗʰ
    - nodular (M9693/3) 202.0 ✓5ᵗʰ
- lymphocytic-histiocytic, mixed (diffuse) (M9613/3) 200.8 ✓5ᵗʰ
  - follicular (M9691/3) 202.0 ✓5ᵗʰ
  - nodular (M9691/3) 202.0 ✓5ᵗʰ
- lymphoplasmacytoid type (M9611/3) 200.8 ✓5ᵗʰ
- lymphosarcoma type (M9610/3) 200.1 ✓5ᵗʰ
- macrofollicular (M9690/3) 202.0 ✓5ᵗʰ
- mixed cell type (diffuse) (M9613/3) 200.8 ✓5ᵗʰ
  - follicular (M9691/3) 202.0 ✓5ᵗʰ
  - nodular (M9691/3) 202.0 ✓5ᵗʰ
- nodular (M9690/3) 202.0 ✓5ᵗʰ
  - histiocytic (M9642/3) 200.0 ✓5ᵗʰ
  - lymphocytic (M9690/3) 202.0 ✓5ᵗʰ
    - intermediate differentiation (M9694/3) 202.0 ✓5ᵗʰ
    - poorly differentiated (M9696/3) 202.0 ✓5ᵗʰ
  - mixed (cell type) (lymphocytic-histiocytic) (small cell and large cell) (M9691/3) 202.0 ✓5ᵗʰ
- non-Hodgkin's type NEC (M9591/3) 202.8 ✓5ᵗʰ
- reticulum cell (type) (M9640/3) 200.0 ✓5ᵗʰ
- small cell and large cell, mixed (diffuse) (M9613/3) 200.8 ✓5ᵗʰ
  - follicular (M9691/3) 202.0 ✓5ᵗʰ
  - nodular (9691/3) 202.0 ✓5ᵗʰ
- stem cell (type) (M9601/3) 202.8 ✓5ᵗʰ
- T-cell 202.1 ✓5ᵗʰ
- undifferentiated (cell type) (non-Burkitt's) (M9600/3) 202.8 ✓5ᵗʰ
  - Burkitt's type (M9750/3) 200.2 ✓5ᵗʰ

Lymphomatosis (M9590/3) — see also Lymphoma
- granulomatous 099.1

Lymphopathia
- venereum 099.1
- veneris 099.1

Lymphopenia 288.8
- familial 279.2

Lymphoreticulosis, benign (of inoculation) 078.3

Lymphorrhea 457.8

Lymphosarcoma (M9610/3) 200.1 ✓5ᵗʰ
- diffuse (M9610/3) 200.1 ✓5ᵗʰ
  - with plasmacytoid differentiation (M9611/3) 200.8 ✓5ᵗʰ
  - lymphoplasmacytic (M9611/3) 200.8 ✓5ᵗʰ
- follicular (giant) (M9690/3) 202.0 ✓5ᵗʰ
  - lymphoblastic (M9696/3) 202.0 ✓5ᵗʰ
  - lymphocytic, intermediate differentiation (M9694/3) 202.0 ✓5ᵗʰ
  - mixed cell type (M9691/3) 202.0 ✓5ᵗʰ
- giant follicular (M9690/3) 202.0 ✓5ᵗʰ
- Hodgkin's (M9650/3) 201.9 ✓5ᵗʰ
- immunoblastic (M9612/3) 200.8 ✓5ᵗʰ

Lymphosarcoma

Lymphosarcoma — *continued*
- lymphoblastic (diffuse) (M9630/3) 200.1 ✓5ᵗʰ
  - follicular (M9696/3) 202.0 ✓5ᵗʰ
  - nodular (M9696/3) 202.0 ✓5ᵗʰ
- lymphocytic (diffuse) (M9620/3) 200.1 ✓5ᵗʰ
  - intermediate differentiation (diffuse) (M9621/3) 200.1 ✓5ᵗʰ
    - follicular (M9694/3) 202.0 ✓5ᵗʰ
    - nodular (M9694/3) 202.0 ✓5ᵗʰ
- mixed cell type (diffuse) (M9613/3) 200.8 ✓5ᵗʰ
  - follicular (M9691/3) 202.0 ✓5ᵗʰ
  - nodular (M9691/3) 202.0 ✓5ᵗʰ
- nodular (M9690/3) 202.0 ✓5ᵗʰ
  - lymphoblastic (M9696/3) 202.0 ✓5ᵗʰ
  - lymphocytic, intermediate differentiation (M9694/3) 202.0 ✓5ᵗʰ
  - mixed cell type (M9691/3) 202.0 ✓5ᵗʰ
- prolymphocytic (M9631/3) 200.1 ✓5ᵗʰ
- reticulum cell (M9640/3) 200.0 ✓5ᵗʰ

Lymphostasis 457.8
Lypemania (*see also* Melancholia) 296.2 ✓5ᵗʰ
Lyssa 071

M

Macacus ear 744.29
Maceration
- fetus (cause not stated) 779.9
- wet feet, tropical (syndrome) 991.4

Machado-Joseph disease 334.8
Machupo virus hemorrhagic fever 078.7
Macleod's syndrome (abnormal transradiancy, one lung) 492.8
Macrocephalia, macrocephaly 756.0
Macrocheilia (congenital) 744.81
Macrochilia (congenital) 744.81
Macrocolon (congenital) 751.3
Macrocornea 743.41
- associated with buphthalmos 743.22

Macrocytic — *see* condition
Macrocytosis 289.8
Macrodactylia, macrodactylism (fingers) (thumbs) 755.57
- toes 755.65

Macrodontia 520.2
Macroencephaly 742.4
Macrogenia 524.05
Macrogenitosomia (female) (male) (praecox) 255.2
Macrogingivae 523.8
Macroglobulinemia (essential) (idiopathic) (monoclonal) (primary) (syndrome) (Waldenström's) 273.3
Macroglossia (congenital) 750.15
- acquired 529.8

Macrognathia, macrognathism (congenital) 524.00
- mandibular 524.02
  - alveolar 524.72
- maxillary 524.01
  - alveolar 524.71

Macrogyria (congenital) 742.4
Macrohydrocephalus (*see also* Hydrocephalus) 331.4
Macromastia (*see also* Hypertrophy, breast) 611.1
Macropsia 368.14
Macrosigmoid 564.7
- congenital 751.3

Macrospondylitis, acromegalic 253.0
Macrostomia (congenital) 744.83
Macrotia (external ear) (congenital) 744.22
Macula
- cornea, corneal
  - congenital 743.43
    - interfering with vision 743.42
    - interfering with central vision 371.03
    - not interfering with central vision 371.02
  - degeneration (*see also* Degeneration, macula) 362.50
  - hereditary (*see also* Dystrophy, retina) 362.70

Macula — *continued*
- edema, cystoid 362.53

Maculae ceruleae 132.1
Macules and papules 709.8
Maculopathy, toxic 362.55
Madarosis 374.55
Madelung's
- deformity (radius) 755.54
- disease (lipomatosis) 272.8
- lipomatosis 272.8

Madness (*see also* Psychosis) 298.9
- myxedema (acute) 293.0
  - subacute 293.1

Madura
- disease (actinomycotic) 039.9
  - mycotic 117.4
- foot (actinomycotic) 039.4
  - mycotic 117.4

Maduromycosis (actinomycotic) 039.9
- mycotic 117.4

Maffucci's syndrome (dyschondroplasia with hemangiomas) 756.4
Magenblase syndrome 306.4
Main en griffe (acquired) 736.06
- congenital 755.59

Maintenance
- chemotherapy regimen or treatment V58.1
- dialysis regimen or treatment
  - extracorporeal (renal) V56.0
  - peritoneal V56.8
  - renal V56.0
- drug therapy or regimen V58.1
- external fixation NEC V54.89 ▲
- radiotherapy V58.0
- traction NEC V54.89 ▲

Majocchi's
- disease (purpura annularis telangiectodes) 709.1
- granuloma 110.6

Major — *see* condition
Mal
- cerebral (idiopathic) (*see also* Epilepsy) 345.9 ✓5ᵗʰ
- comital (*see also* Epilepsy) 345.9 ✓5ᵗʰ
- de los pintos (*see also* Pinta) 103.9
- de Meleda 757.39
- de mer 994.6
- lie — *see* Presentation, fetal
- perforant (*see also* Ulcer, lower extremity) 707.15

Malabar itch 110.9
- beard 110.0
- foot 110.4
- scalp 110.0

Malabsorption 579.9
- calcium 579.8
- carbohydrate 579.8
- disaccharide 271.3
- drug-induced 579.8
- due to bacterial overgrowth 579.8
- fat 579.8
- folate, congenital 281.2
- galactose 271.1
- glucose-galactose (congenital) 271.3
- intestinal 579.9
- isomaltose 271.3
- lactose (hereditary) 271.3
- methionine 270.4
- monosaccharide 271.8
- postgastrectomy 579.3
- postsurgical 579.3
- protein 579.8
- sucrose (-isomaltose) (congenital) 271.3
- syndrome 579.9
  - postgastrectomy 579.3
  - postsurgical 579.3

Malacia, bone 268.2
- juvenile (*see also* Rickets) 268.0
- Kienböck's (juvenile) (lunate) (wrist) 732.3
  - adult 732.8

Malacoplakia
- bladder 596.8
- colon 569.89
- pelvis (kidney) 593.89

Malacoplakia — *continued*
- ureter 593.89
- urethra 599.84

Malacosteon 268.2
- juvenile (*see also* Rickets) 268.0

Maladaptation — *see* Maladjustment
Maladie de Roger 745.4
Maladjustment
- conjugal V61.10
  - involving divorce or estrangement V61.0
- educational V62.3
- family V61.9
  - specified circumstance NEC V61.8
- marital V61.10
  - involving divorce or estrangement V61.0
- occupational V62.2
- simple, adult (*see also* Reaction, adjustment) 309.9
- situational acute (*see also* Reaction, adjustment) 309.9
- social V62.4

Malaise 780.79
Malakoplakia — *see* Malacoplakia
Malaria, malarial (fever) 084.6
- algid 084.9
- any type, with
  - algid malaria 084.9
  - blackwater fever 084.8
  - fever
    - blackwater 084.8
    - hemoglobinuric (bilious) 084.8
  - hemoglobinuria, malarial 084.8
  - hepatitis 084.9 [573.2]
  - nephrosis 084.9 [581.81]
  - pernicious complication NEC 084.9
    - cardiac 084.9
    - cerebral 084.9
- cardiac 084.9
- carrier (suspected) of V02.9
- cerebral 084.9
- complicating pregnancy, childbirth, or puerperium 647.4 ✓5ᵗʰ
- congenital 771.2
- congestion, congestive 084.6
  - brain 084.9
- continued 084.0
- estivo-autumnal 084.0
- falciparum (malignant tertian) 084.0
- hematinuria 084.8
- hematuria 084.8
- hemoglobinuria 084.8
- hemorrhagic 084.6
- induced (therapeutically) 084.7
  - accidental — *see* Malaria, by type
- liver 084.9 [573.2]
- malariae (quartan) 084.2
- malignant (tertian) 084.0
- mixed infections 084.5
- monkey 084.4
- ovale 084.3
- pernicious, acute 084.0
- Plasmodium, P.
  - falciparum 084.0
  - malariae 084.2
  - ovale 084.3
  - vivax 084.1
- quartan 084.2
- quotidian 084.0
- recurrent 084.6
  - induced (therapeutically) 084.7
    - accidental — *see* Malaria, by type
- remittent 084.6
- specified types NEC 084.4
- spleen 084.6
- subtertian 084.0
- tertian (benign) 084.1
  - malignant 084.0
- tropical 084.0
- typhoid 084.6
- vivax (benign tertian) 084.1

Malassez's disease (testicular cyst) 608.89
Malassimilation 579.9
Maldescent, testis 752.51

Index to Diseases

Maldevelopment — see also Anomaly, by site
- brain 742.9
- colon 751.5
- hip (joint) 755.63
  - congenital dislocation (see also Dislocation, hip, congenital) 754.30
  - mastoid process 756.0
- middle ear, except ossicles 744.03
  - ossicles 744.04
- newborn (not malformation) 764.9 ✓5th
- ossicles, ear 744.04
- spine 756.10
- toe 755.66

Male type pelvis 755.69
- with disproportion (fetopelvic) 653.2 ✓5th
  - affecting fetus or newborn 763.1
  - causing obstructed labor 660.1 ✓5th
    - affecting fetus or newborn 763.1

Malformation (congenital) — see also Anomaly
- bone 756.9
- bursa 756.9
- circulatory system NEC 747.9
  - specified type NEC 747.89
- Chiari
  - type I 348.4
  - type II (see also Spina bifida) 741.0 ✓5th
  - type III 742.0
  - type IV 742.2
- cochlea 744.05
- digestive system NEC 751.9
  - lower 751.5
  - specified type NEC 751.8
  - upper 750.9
- eye 743.9
- gum 750.9
- heart NEC 746.9
  - specified type NEC 746.89
  - valve 746.9
- internal ear 744.05
- joint NEC 755.9
  - specified type NEC 755.8
- Mondini's (congenital) (malformation, cochlea) 744.05
- muscle 756.9
- nervous system (central) 742.9
- pelvic organs or tissues
  - in pregnancy or childbirth 654.9 ✓5th
    - affecting fetus or newborn 763.89
    - causing obstructed labor 660.2 ✓5th
      - affecting fetus or newborn 763.1
- placenta (see also Placenta, abnormal) 656.7 ✓5th
- respiratory organs 748.9
  - specified type NEC 748.8
- Rieger's 743.44
- sense organs NEC 742.9
  - specified type NEC 742.8
- skin 757.9
  - specified type NEC 757.8
- spinal cord 742.9
- teeth, tooth NEC 520.9
- tendon 756.9
- throat 750.9
- umbilical cord (complicating delivery) 663.9 ✓5th
  - affecting fetus or newborn 762.6
- umbilicus 759.9
- urinary system NEC 753.9
  - specified type NEC 753.8

Malfunction — see also Dysfunction
- arterial graft 996.1
- cardiac pacemaker 996.01
- catheter device — see Complications, mechanical, catheter
- colostomy 569.62
- cystostomy 997.5
- device, implant, or graft NEC — see Complications, mechanical
- enteric stoma 569.62
- enterostomy 569.62
- gastroenteric 536.8
- gastrostomy 536.42
- nephrostomy 997.5
- pacemaker — see Complications, mechanical, pacemaker
- prosthetic device, internal — see Complications, mechanical
- tracheostomy 519.02

Malfunction — see also Dysfunction — continued
- vascular graft or shunt 996.1

Malgaigne's fracture (closed) 808.43
- open 808.53

Malherbe's
- calcifying epithelioma (M8110/0) — see Neoplasm, skin, benign
- tumor (M8110/0) — see Neoplasm, skin, benign

Malibu disease 919.8
- infected 919.9

Malignancy (M8000/3) — see Neoplasm, by site, malignant

Malignant — see condition

Malingerer, malingering V65.2

Mallet, finger (acquired) 736.1
- congenital 755.59
- late effect of rickets 268.1

Malleus 024

Mallory's bodies 034.1

Mallory-Weiss syndrome 530.7

Malnutrition (calorie) 263.9
- complicating pregnancy 648.9 ✓5th
- degree
  - first 263.1
  - second 263.0
  - third 262
  - mild 263.1
  - moderate 263.0
  - severe 261
    - protein-calorie 262
- fetus 764.2 ✓5th
  - "light-for-dates" 764.1 ✓5th
- following gastrointestinal surgery 579.3
- intrauterine or fetal 764.2 ✓5th
  - fetus or infant "light-for-dates" 764.1 ✓5th
- lack of care, or neglect (child) (infant) 995.52
  - adult 995.84
- malignant 260
- mild 263.1
- moderate 263.0
- protein 260
- protein-calorie 263.9
  - severe 262
  - specified type NEC 263.8
- severe 261
  - protein-calorie NEC 262

Malocclusion (teeth) 524.4
- due to
  - abnormal swallowing 524.5
  - accessory teeth (causing crowding) 524.3
  - dentofacial abnormality NEC 524.8
  - impacted teeth (causing crowding) 524.3
  - missing teeth 524.3
  - mouth breathing 524.5
  - supernumerary teeth (causing crowding) 524.3
  - thumb sucking 524.5
  - tongue, lip, or finger habits 524.5
- temporomandibular (joint) 524.69

Malposition
- cardiac apex (congenital) 746.87
- cervix — see Malposition, uterus
- congenital
  - adrenal (gland) 759.1
  - alimentary tract 751.8
    - lower 751.5
    - upper 750.8
  - aorta 747.21
  - appendix 751.5
  - arterial trunk 747.29
  - artery (peripheral) NEC (see also Malposition, congenital, peripheral vascular system) 747.60
    - coronary 746.85
    - pulmonary 747.3
  - auditory canal 744.29
    - causing impairment of hearing 744.02
  - auricle (ear) 744.29
    - causing impairment of hearing 744.02
    - cervical 744.43
  - biliary duct or passage 751.69
  - bladder (mucosa) 753.8
    - exteriorized or extroverted 753.5
  - brachial plexus 742.8

Malposition — continued
- congenital — continued
  - brain tissue 742.4
  - breast 757.6
  - bronchus 748.3
  - cardiac apex 746.87
  - cecum 751.5
  - clavicle 755.51
  - colon 751.5
  - digestive organ or tract NEC 751.8
    - lower 751.5
    - upper 750.8
  - ear (auricle) (external) 744.29
    - ossicles 744.04
  - endocrine (gland) NEC 759.2
  - epiglottis 748.3
  - Eustachian tube 744.24
  - eye 743.8
  - facial features 744.89
  - fallopian tube 752.19
  - finger(s) 755.59
    - supernumerary 755.01
  - foot 755.67
  - gallbladder 751.69
  - gastrointestinal tract 751.8
  - genitalia, genital organ(s) or tract
    - female 752.8
      - external 752.49
      - internal NEC 752.8
    - male 752.8
      - penis 752.69
  - glottis 748.3
  - hand 755.59
  - heart 746.87
    - dextrocardia 746.87
      - with complete transposition of viscera 759.3
  - hepatic duct 751.69
  - hip (joint) (see also Dislocation, hip, congenital) 754.30
  - intestine (large) (small) 751.5
    - with anomalous adhesions, fixation, or malrotation 751.4
  - joint NEC 755.8
  - kidney 753.3
  - larynx 748.3
  - limb 755.8
    - lower 755.69
    - upper 755.59
  - liver 751.69
  - lung (lobe) 748.69
  - nail(s) 757.5
  - nerve 742.8
  - nervous system NEC 742.8
  - nose, nasal (septum) 748.1
  - organ or site NEC — see Anomaly, specified type NEC, by site
  - ovary 752.0
  - pancreas 751.7
  - parathyroid (gland) 759.2
  - patella 755.64
  - peripheral vascular system 747.60
    - gastrointestinal 747.61
    - lower limb 747.64
    - renal 747.62
    - specified NEC 747.69
    - spinal 747.82
    - upper limb 747.63
  - pituitary (gland) 759.2
  - respiratory organ or system NEC 748.9
  - rib (cage) 756.3
    - supernumerary in cervical region 756.2
  - scapula 755.59
  - shoulder 755.59
  - spinal cord 742.59
  - spine 756.19
  - spleen 759.0
  - sternum 756.3
  - stomach 750.7
  - symphysis pubis 755.69
  - testis (undescended) 752.51
  - thymus (gland) 759.2
  - thyroid (gland) (tissue) 759.2
    - cartilage 748.3
  - toe(s) 755.66
    - supernumerary 755.02
  - tongue 750.19

Malposition

Malposition — *continued*
  congenital — *continued*
    trachea 748.3
    uterus 752.3
    vein(s) (peripheral) NEC (*see also* Malposition, congenital, peripheral vascular system) 747.60
      great 747.49
      portal 747.49
      pulmonary 747.49
      vena cava (inferior) (superior) 747.49
  device, implant, or graft — *see* Complications, mechanical
  fetus NEC — (*see also* Presentation, fetal) 652.9 ✓5ᵗʰ
    with successful version 652.1 ✓5ᵗʰ
    affecting fetus or newborn 763.1
    before labor, affecting fetus or newborn 761.7
    causing obstructed labor 660.0 ✓5ᵗʰ
    in multiple gestation (one fetus or more) 652.6 ✓5ᵗʰ
      with locking 660.5 ✓5ᵗʰ
    causing obstructed labor 660.0 ✓5ᵗʰ
  gallbladder — (*see also* Disease, gallbladder) 575.8
  gastrointestinal tract 569.89
    congenital 751.8
  heart (*see also* Malposition, congenital, heart) 746.87
  intestine 569.89
    congenital 751.5
  pelvic organs or tissues
    in pregnancy or childbirth 654.4 ✓5ᵗʰ
      affecting fetus or newborn 763.89
      causing obstructed labor 660.2 ✓5ᵗʰ
        affecting fetus or newborn 763.1
  placenta — *see* Placenta, previa
  stomach 537.89
    congenital 750.7
  tooth, teeth (with impaction) 524.3
  uterus or cervix (acquired) (acute) (adherent) (any degree) (asymptomatic) (postinfectional) (postpartal, old) 621.6
    anteflexion or anteversion (*see also* Anteversion, uterus) 621.6
    congenital 752.3
    flexion 621.6
      lateral (*see also* Lateroversion, uterus) 621.6
      in pregnancy or childbirth 654.4 ✓5ᵗʰ
        affecting fetus or newborn 763.89
        causing obstructed labor 660.2 ✓5ᵗʰ
          affecting fetus or newborn 763.1
    inversion 621.6
    lateral (flexion) (version) (*see also* Lateroversion, uterus) 621.6
    lateroflexion (*see also* Lateroversion, uterus) 621.6
    lateroversion (*see also* Lateroversion, uterus) 621.6
    retroflexion or retroversion (*see also* Retroversion, uterus) 621.6

Malposture 729.9

Malpresentation, fetus — (*see also* Presentation, fetal) 652.9 ✓5ᵗʰ

Malrotation
  cecum 751.4
  colon 751.4
  intestine 751.4
  kidney 753.3

Malta fever (*see also* Brucellosis) 023.9

Maltosuria 271.3

Maltreatment (of)
  adult 995.80
    emotional 995.82
    multiple forms 995.85
    neglect (nutritional) 995.84
    physical 995.81
    psychological 995.82
    sexual 995.83
  child 995.50
    emotional 995.51
    multiple forms 995.59
    neglect (nutritional) 995.52

Maltreatment — *continued*
  child — *continued*
    physical 995.54
      shaken infant syndrome 995.55
    psychological 995.51
    sexual 995.53
  spouse 995.80 — (*see also* Maltreatment, adult)

Malt workers' lung 495.4

Malum coxae senilis 715.25

Malunion, fracture 733.81

Mammillitis (*see also* Mastitis) 611.0
  puerperal, postpartum 675.2 ✓5ᵗʰ

Mammitis (*see also* Mastitis) 611.0
  puerperal, postpartum 675.2 ✓5ᵗʰ

Mammographic microcalcification 793.81

Mammoplasia 611.1

Management
  contraceptive V25.9
    specified type NEC V25.8
  procreative V26.9
    specified type NEC V26.8

Mangled NEC (*see also* nature and site of injury) 959.9

Mania (monopolar) — (*see also* Psychosis, affective) 296.0 ✓5ᵗʰ
  alcoholic (acute) (chronic) 291.9
  Bell's — *see* Mania, chronic
  chronic 296.0 ✓5ᵗʰ
    recurrent episode 296.1 ✓5ᵗʰ
    single episode 296.0 ✓5ᵗʰ
  compulsive 300.3
  delirious (acute) 296.0 ✓5ᵗʰ
    recurrent episode 296.1 ✓5ᵗʰ
    single episode 296.0 ✓5ᵗʰ
  epileptic (*see also* Epilepsy) 345.4 ✓5ᵗʰ
  hysterical 300.10
  inhibited 296.89
  puerperal (after delivery) 296.0 ✓5ᵗʰ
    recurrent episode 296.1 ✓5ᵗʰ
    single episode 296.0 ✓5ᵗʰ
  recurrent episode 296.1 ✓5ᵗʰ
  senile 290.8
  single episode 296.0 ✓5ᵗʰ
  stupor 296.89
  stuporous 296.89
  unproductive 296.89

Manic-depressive insanity, psychosis, reaction, or syndrome (*see also* Psychosis, affective) 296.80
  circular (alternating) 296.7
    currently
      depressed 296.5 ✓5ᵗʰ
      episode unspecified 296.7
      hypomanic, previously depressed 296.4 ✓5ᵗʰ
      manic 296.4 ✓5ᵗʰ
      mixed 296.6 ✓5ᵗʰ
  depressed (type), depressive 296.2 ✓5ᵗʰ
    atypical 296.82
    recurrent episode 296.3 ✓5ᵗʰ
    single episode 296.2 ✓5ᵗʰ
  hypomanic 296.0 ✓5ᵗʰ
    recurrent episode 296.1 ✓5ᵗʰ
    single episode 296.0 ✓5ᵗʰ
  manic 296.0 ✓5ᵗʰ
    atypical 296.81
    recurrent episode 296.1 ✓5ᵗʰ
    single episode 296.0 ✓5ᵗʰ
  mixed NEC 296.89
  perplexed 296.89
  stuporous 296.89

Manifestations, rheumatoid
  lungs 714.81
  pannus — *see* Arthritis, rheumatoid
  subcutaneous nodules — *see* Arthritis, rheumatoid

Mankowsky's syndrome (familial dysplastic osteopathy) 731.2

Mannoheptulosuria 271.8

Mannosidosis 271.8

Manson's
  disease (schistosomiasis) 120.1
  pyosis (pemphigus contagiosus) 684
  schistosomiasis 120.1

Index to Diseases

Mansonellosis 125.5

Manual — *see* condition

Maple bark disease 495.6

Maple bark-strippers' lung 495.6

Maple syrup (urine) disease or syndrome 270.3

Marable's syndrome (celiac artery compression) 447.4

Marasmus 261
  brain 331.9
  due to malnutrition 261
  intestinal 569.89
  nutritional 261
  senile 797
  tuberculous NEC (*see also* Tuberculosis) 011.9 ✓5ᵗʰ

Marble
  bones 756.52
  skin 782.61

Marburg disease (virus) 078.89

March ▲
  foot 733.94
  hemoglobinuria 283.2

Marchand multiple nodular hyperplasia (liver) 571.5

Marchesani (-Weill) syndrome (brachymorphism and ectopia lentis) 759.89

Marchiafava (-Bignami) disease or syndrome 341.8

Marchiafava-Micheli syndrome (paroxysmal nocturnal hemoglobinuria) 283.2

Marcus Gunn's syndrome (jaw-winking syndrome) 742.8

Marfan's
  congenital syphilis 090.49
  disease 090.49
  syndrome (arachnodactyly) 759.82
    meaning congenital syphilis 090.49
      with luxation of lens 090.49 [379.32]

Marginal
  implantation, placenta — *see* Placenta, previa
  placenta — *see* Placenta, previa
  sinus (hemorrhage) (rupture) 641.2 ✓5ᵗʰ
    affecting fetus or newborn 762.1

Marie's
  cerebellar ataxia 334.2
  syndrome (acromegaly) 253.0

Marie-Bamberger disease or syndrome (hypertrophic) (pulmonary) (secondary) 731.2
  idiopathic (acropachyderma) 757.39
  primary (acropachyderma) 757.39

Marie-Charcôt-Tooth neuropathic atrophy, muscle 356.1

Marie-Strümpell arthritis or disease (ankylosing spondylitis) 720.0

Marihuana, marijuana
  abuse (*see also* Abuse, drugs, nondependent) 305.2 ✓5ᵗʰ
  dependence (*see also* Dependence) 304.3 ✓5ᵗʰ

Marion's disease (bladder neck obstruction) 596.0

Marital conflict V61.10

Mark
  port wine 757.32
  raspberry 757.32
  strawberry 757.32
  stretch 701.3
  tattoo 709.09

Maroteaux-Lamy syndrome (mucopolysaccharidosis VI) 277.5

Marriage license examination V70.3

Marrow (bone)
  arrest 284.9
  megakaryocytic 287.3
  poor function 289.9

Marseilles fever 082.1

Marsh's disease (exophthalmic goiter) 242.0 ✓5ᵗʰ

Marshall's (hidrotic) **ectodermal dysplasia** 757.31

Marsh fever (*see also* Malaria) 084.6

Martin's disease 715.27

Index to Diseases

Martin-Albright syndrome
(pseudohypoparathyroidism) 275.49
Martorell-Fabre syndrome (pulseless disease) 446.7
Masculinization, female, with adrenal hyperplasia 255.2
Masculinovoblastoma (M8670/0) 220
Masochism 302.83
Masons' lung 502
Mass
- abdominal 789.3 ✓5ᵗʰ
- anus 787.99
- bone 733.90
- breast 611.72
- cheek 784.2
- chest 786.6
- cystic — see Cyst
- ear 388.8
- epigastric 789.3 ✓5ᵗʰ
- eye 379.92
- female genital organ 625.8
- gum 784.2
- head 784.2
- intracranial 784.2
- joint 719.60
  - ankle 719.67
  - elbow 719.62
  - foot 719.67
  - hand 719.64
  - hip 719.65
  - knee 719.66
  - multiple sites 719.69
  - pelvic region 719.65
  - shoulder (region) 719.61
  - specified site NEC 719.68
  - wrist 719.63
- kidney (see also Disease, kidney) 593.9
- lung 786.6
- lymph node 785.6
- malignant (M8000/3) — see Neoplasm, by site, malignant
- mediastinal 786.6
- mouth 784.2
- muscle (limb) 729.89
- neck 784.2
- nose or sinus 784.2
- palate 784.2
- pelvis, pelvic 789.3 ✓5ᵗʰ
- penis 607.89
- perineum 625.8
- rectum 787.99
- scrotum 608.89
- skin 782.2
- specified organ NEC — see Disease of specified organ or site
- splenic 789.2
- substernal 786.6
  - thyroid (see also Goiter) 240.9
- superficial (localized) 782.2
- testes 608.89
- throat 784.2
- tongue 784.2
- umbilicus 789.3 ✓5ᵗʰ
- uterus 625.8
- vagina 625.8
- vulva 625.8

Massive — see condition
Mastalgia 611.71
- psychogenic 307.89
Mast cell
- disease 757.33
  - systemic (M9741/3) 202.6 ✓5ᵗʰ
- leukemia (M9900/3) 207.8 ✓5ᵗʰ
- sarcoma (M9742/3) 202.6 ✓5ᵗʰ
- tumor (M9740/1) 238.5
  - malignant (M9740/3) 202.6 ✓5ᵗʰ
Masters-Allen syndrome 620.6
Mastitis (acute) (adolescent) (diffuse) (interstitial) (lobular) (nonpuerperal) (nonsuppurative) (parenchymatous) (phlegmonous) (simple) (subacute) (suppurative) 611.0
- chronic (cystic) (fibrocystic) 610.1
- cystic 610.1
  - Schimmelbusch's type 610.1
- fibrocystic 610.1

Mastitis — continued
- infective 611.0
- lactational 675.2 ✓5ᵗʰ
- lymphangitis 611.0
- neonatal (noninfective) 778.7
  - infective 771.5
- periductal 610.4
- plasma cell 610.4
- puerperal, postpartum, (interstitial) (nonpurulent) (parenchymatous) 675.2 ✓5ᵗʰ
  - purulent 675.1 ✓5ᵗʰ
  - stagnation 676.2 ✓5ᵗʰ
- puerperalis 675.2 ✓5ᵗʰ
- retromammary 611.0
  - puerperal, postpartum 675.1 ✓5ᵗʰ
- submammary 611.0
  - puerperal, postpartum 675.1 ✓5ᵗʰ
Mastocytoma (M9740/1) 238.5
- malignant (M9740/3) 202.6 ✓5ᵗʰ
Mastocytosis 757.33
- malignant (M9741/3) 202.6 ✓5ᵗʰ
- systemic (M9741/3) 202.6 ✓5ᵗʰ
Mastodynia 611.71
- psychogenic 307.89
Mastoid — see condition
Mastoidalgia (see also Otalgia) 388.70
Mastoiditis (coalescent) (hemorrhagic) (pneumococcal) (streptococcal) (suppurative) 383.9
- acute or subacute 383.00
  - with
    - Gradenigo's syndrome 383.02
    - petrositis 383.02
    - specified complication NEC 383.02
    - subperiosteal abscess 383.01
- chronic (necrotic) (recurrent) 383.1
- tuberculous (see also Tuberculosis) 015.6 ✓5ᵗʰ
Mastopathy, mastopathia 611.9
- chronica cystica 610.1
- diffuse cystic 610.1
- estrogenic 611.8
- ovarian origin 611.8
Mastoplasia 611.1
Masturbation 307.9
Maternal condition, affecting fetus or newborn
- acute yellow atrophy of liver 760.8
- albuminuria 760.1
- anesthesia or analgesia 763.5
- blood loss 762.1
- chorioamnionitis 762.7
- circulatory disease, chronic (conditions classifiable to 390-459, 745-747) 760.3
- congenital heart disease (conditions classifiable to 745-746) 760.3
- cortical necrosis of kidney 760.1
- death 761.6
- diabetes mellitus 775.0
  - manifest diabetes in the infant 775.1
- disease NEC 760.9
  - circulatory system, chronic (conditions classifiable to 390-459, 745-747) 760.3
  - genitourinary system (conditions classifiable to 580-599) 760.1
  - respiratory (conditions classifiable to 490-519, 748) 760.3
- eclampsia 760.0
- hemorrhage NEC 762.1
- hepatitis acute, malignant, or subacute 760.8
- hyperemesis (gravidarum) 761.8
- hypertension (arising during pregnancy) (conditions classifiable to 642) 760.0
- infection
  - disease classifiable to 001-136 760.2
  - genital tract NEC 760.8
  - urinary tract 760.1
- influenza 760.2
  - manifest influenza in the infant 771.2
- injury (conditions classifiable to 800-996) 760.5
- malaria 760.2
  - manifest malaria in infant or fetus 771.2
- malnutrition 760.4
- necrosis of liver 760.8
- nephritis (conditions classifiable to 580-583) 760.1

Maternal condition, affecting fetus or newborn — continued
- nephrosis (conditions classifiable to 581) 760.1
- noxious substance transmitted via breast milk or placenta 760.70
  - alcohol 760.71
  - anti-infective agents 760.74
  - cocaine 760.75
  - "crack" 760.75
  - diethylstilbestrol [DES] 760.76
  - hallucinogenic agents 760.73
  - medicinal agents NEC 760.79
  - narcotics 760.72
  - obstetric anesthetic or analgesic drug 760.72
  - specified agent NEC 760.79
- nutritional disorder (conditions classifiable to 260-269) 760.4
- operation unrelated to current delivery 760.6
- preeclampsia 760.0
- pyelitis or pyelonephritis, arising during pregnancy (conditions classifiable to 590) 760.1
- renal disease or failure 760.1
- respiratory disease, chronic (conditions classifiable to 490-519, 748) 760.3
- rheumatic heart disease (chronic) (conditions classifiable to 393-398) 760.3
- rubella (conditions classifiable to 056) 760.2
  - manifest rubella in the infant or fetus 771.0
- surgery unrelated to current delivery 760.6
  - to uterus or pelvic organs 763.89
- syphilis (conditions classifiable to 090-097) 760.2
  - manifest syphilis in the infant or fetus 090.0
- thrombophlebitis 760.3
- toxemia (of pregnancy) 760.0
  - preeclamptic 760.0
- toxoplasmosis (conditions classifiable to 130) 760.2
  - manifest toxoplasmosis in the infant or fetus 771.2
- transmission of chemical substance through the placenta 760.70
  - alcohol 760.71
  - anti-infective 760.74
  - cocaine 760.75
  - "crack" 760.75
  - diethylstilbestrol [DES] 760.76
  - hallucinogenic agents 760.73
  - narcotics 760.72
  - specified substance NEC 760.79
- uremia 760.1
- urinary tract conditions (conditions classifiable to 580-599) 760.1
- vomiting (pernicious) (persistent) (vicious) 761.8

Maternity — see Delivery
Matheiu's disease (leptospiral jaundice) 100.0
Mauclaire's disease or osteochondrosis 732.3
Maxcy's disease 081.0
Maxilla, maxillary — see condition
May (-Hegglin) anomaly or syndrome 288.2
Mayaro fever 066.3
Mazoplasia 610.8
MBD (minimal brain dysfunction), child (see also Hyperkinesia) 314.9
McArdle (-Schmid-Pearson) disease or syndrome (glycogenosis V) 271.0
McCune-Albright syndrome (osteitis fibrosa disseminata) 756.59
MCLS (mucocutaneous lymph node syndrome) 446.1
McQuarrie's syndrome (idiopathic familial hypoglycemia) 251.2
Measles (black) (hemorrhagic) (suppressed) 055.9
- with
  - encephalitis 055.0
  - keratitis 055.71
  - keratoconjunctivitis 055.71
  - otitis media 055.2
  - pneumonia 055.1
- complication 055.8
  - specified type NEC 055.79
- encephalitis 055.0

Measles

Measles — *continued*
  French 056.9
  German 056.9
  keratitis 055.71
  keratoconjunctivitis 055.71
  liberty 056.9
  otitis media 055.2
  pneumonia 055.1
  specified complications NEC 055.79
  vaccination, prophylactic (against) V04.2
Meatitis, urethral (*see also* Urethritis) 597.89
Meat poisoning — *see* Poisoning, food
Meatus, meatal — *see* condition
Meat-wrappers' asthma 506.9
Meckel's
  diverticulitis 751.0
  diverticulum (displaced) (hypertrophic) 751.0
Meconium
  aspiration 770.1
  delayed passage in newborn 777.1
  ileus 777.1
    due to cystic fibrosis 277.01
  in liquor 792.3
    noted during delivery 656.8 ✓5ᵗʰ
  insufflation 770.1
  obstruction
    fetus or newborn 777.1
      in mucoviscidosis 277.01
  passage of 792.3
    noted during delivery — *omit code*
  peritonitis 777.6
  plug syndrome (newborn) NEC 777.1
Median — *see also* condition
  arcuate ligament syndrome 447.4
  bar (prostate) 600.9
    vesical orifice 600.9
  rhomboid glossitis 529.2
Mediastinal shift 793.2
Mediastinitis (acute) (chronic) 519.2
  actinomycotic 039.8
  syphilitic 095.8
  tuberculous (*see also* Tuberculosis) 012.8 ✓5ᵗʰ
Mediastinopericarditis (*see also* Pericarditis) 423.9
  acute 420.90
  chronic 423.8
    rheumatic 393
  rheumatic, chronic 393
Mediastinum, mediastinal — *see* condition
Medical services provided for — *see* Health, services provided because (of)
Medicine poisoning (by overdose) (wrong substance given or taken in error) 977.9
  specified drug or substance — *see* Table of Drugs and Chemicals
Medin's disease (poliomyelitis) 045.9 ✓5ᵗʰ
Mediterranean
  anemia (with other hemoglobinopathy) 282.4
  disease or syndrome (hemipathic) 282.4
  fever (*see also* Brucellosis) 023.9
    familial 277.3
  kala-azar 085.0
  leishmaniasis 085.0
  tick fever 082.1
Medulla — *see* condition
Medullary
  cystic kidney 753.16
  sponge kidney 753.17
Medullated fibers
  optic (nerve) 743.57
  retina 362.85
Medulloblastoma (M9470/3)
  desmoplastic (M9471/3) 191.6
  specified site — *see* Neoplasm, by site, malignant
  unspecified site 191.6
Medulloepithelioma (M9501/3) — *see also* Neoplasm, by site, malignant
  teratoid (M9502/3) — *see* Neoplasm, by site, malignant
Medullomyoblastoma (M9472/3)
  specified site — *see* Neoplasm, by site, malignant

Medullomyoblastoma — *continued*
  unspecified site 191.6
Meekeren-Ehlers-Danlos syndrome 756.83
Megacaryocytic — *see* condition
Megacolon (acquired) (functional) (not Hirschsprung's disease) 564.7
  aganglionic 751.3
  congenital, congenitum 751.3
  Hirschsprung's (disease) 751.3
  psychogenic 306.4
  toxic (*see also* Colitis, ulcerative) 556.9
Megaduodenum 537.3
Megaesophagus (functional) 530.0
  congenital 750.4
Megakaryocytic — *see* condition
Megalencephaly 742.4
Megalerythema (epidermicum) (infectiosum) 057.0
Megalia, cutis et ossium 757.39
Megaloappendix 751.5
Megalocephalus, megalocephaly NEC 756.0
Megalocornea 743.41
  associated with buphthalmos 743.22
Megalocytic anemia 281.9
Megalodactylia (fingers) (thumbs) 755.57
  toes 755.65
Megaloduodenum 751.5
Megaloesophagus (functional) 530.0
  congenital 750.4
Megalogastria (congenital) 750.7
Megalomania 307.9
Megalophthalmos 743.8
Megalopsia 368.14
Megalosplenia (*see also* Splenomegaly) 789.2
Megaloureter 593.89
  congenital 753.22
Megarectum 569.49
Megasigmoid 564.7
  congenital 751.3
Megaureter 593.89
  congenital 753.22
Megrim 346.9 ✓5ᵗʰ
Meibomian
  cyst 373.2
    infected 373.12
  gland — *see* condition
  infarct (eyelid) 374.85
  stye 373.11
Meibomitis 373.12
Meige
  -Milroy disease (chronic hereditary edema) 757.0
  syndrome (blepharospasm-oromandibular dystonia) 333.82
Melalgia, nutritional 266.2
Melancholia (*see also* Psychosis, affective) 296.90
  climacteric 296.2 ✓5ᵗʰ
    recurrent episode 296.3 ✓5ᵗʰ
    single episode 296.2 ✓5ᵗʰ
  hypochondriac 300.7
  intermittent 296.2 ✓5ᵗʰ
    recurrent episode 296.3 ✓5ᵗʰ
    single episode 296.2 ✓5ᵗʰ
  involutional 296.2 ✓5ᵗʰ
    recurrent episode 296.3 ✓5ᵗʰ
    single episode 296.2 ✓5ᵗʰ
  menopausal 296.2 ✓5ᵗʰ
    recurrent episode 296.3 ✓5ᵗʰ
    single episode 296.2 ✓5ᵗʰ
  puerperal 296.2 ✓5ᵗʰ
  reactive (from emotional stress, psychological trauma) 298.0
  recurrent 296.3 ✓5ᵗʰ
  senile 290.21
  stuporous 296.2 ✓5ᵗʰ
    recurrent episode 296.3 ✓5ᵗʰ
    single episode 296.2 ✓5ᵗʰ
Melanemia 275.0
Melanoameloblastoma (M9363/0) — *see* Neoplasm, bone, benign
Melanoblastoma (M8720/3) — *see* Melanoma

Index to Diseases

Melanoblastosis
  Block-Sulzberger 757.33
  cutis linearis sive systematisata 757.33
Melanocarcinoma (M8720/3) — *see* Melanoma
Melanocytoma, eyeball (M8726/0) 224.0
Melanoderma, melanodermia 709.09
  Addison's (primary adrenal insufficiency) 255.4
Melanodontia, infantile 521.05
Melanodontoclasia 521.05
Melanoepithelioma (M8720/3) — *see* Melanoma
Melanoma (malignant) (M8720/3) 172.9

> Note — Except where otherwise indicated, the morphological varieties of melanoma in the list below should be coded by site as for "Melanoma (malignant)". Internal sites should be coded to malignant neoplasm of those sites.

  abdominal wall 172.5
  ala nasi 172.3
  amelanotic (M8730/3) — *see* Melanoma, by site
  ankle 172.7
  anus, anal 154.3
    canal 154.2
  arm 172.6
  auditory canal (external) 172.2
  auricle (ear) 172.2
  auricular canal (external) 172.2
  axilla 172.5
  axillary fold 172.5
  back 172.5
  balloon cell (M8722/3) — *see* Melanoma, by site
  benign (M8720/0) — *see* Neoplasm, skin, benign
  breast (female) (male) 172.5
  brow 172.3
  buttock 172.5
  canthus (eye) 172.1
  cheek (external) 172.3
  chest wall 172.5
  chin 172.3
  choroid 190.6
  conjunctiva 190.3
  ear (external) 172.2
  epithelioid cell (M8771/3) — *see also* Melanoma, by site
    and spindle cell, mixed (M8775/3) — *see* Melanoma, by site
  external meatus (ear) 172.2
  eye 190.9
  eyebrow 172.3
  eyelid (lower) (upper) 172.1
  face NEC 172.3
  female genital organ (external) NEC 184.4
  finger 172.6
  flank 172.5
  foot 172.7
  forearm 172.6
  forehead 172.3
  foreskin 187.1
  gluteal region 172.5
  groin 172.5
  hand 172.6
  heel 172.7
  helix 172.2
  hip 172.7
  in
    giant pigmented nevus (M8761/3) — *see* Melanoma, by site
    Hutchinson's melanotic freckle (M8742/3) — *see* Melanoma, by site
    junctional nevus (M8740/3) — *see* Melanoma, by site
    precancerous melanosis (M8741/3) — *see* Melanoma, by site
  interscapular region 172.5
  iris 190.0
  jaw 172.3
  juvenile (M8770/0) — *see* Neoplasm, skin, benign
  knee 172.7
  labium
    majus 184.1
    minus 184.2

Index to Diseases

Melanoma — *continued*
  lacrimal gland 190.2
  leg 172.7
  lip (lower) (upper) 172.0
  liver 197.7
  lower limb NEC 172.7
  male genital organ (external) NEC 187.9
  meatus, acoustic (external) 172.2
  meibomian gland 172.1
  metastatic
    of or from specified site — *see* Melanoma, by site
    site not of skin — *see* Neoplasm, by site, malignant, secondary
    to specified site — *see* Neoplasm, by site, malignant, secondary
    unspecified site 172.9
  nail 172.9
    finger 172.6
    toe 172.7
  neck 172.4
  nodular (M8721/3) — *see* Melanoma, by site
  nose, external 172.3
  orbit 190.1
  penis 187.4
  perianal skin 172.5
  perineum 172.5
  pinna 172.2
  popliteal (fossa) (space) 172.7
  prepuce 187.1
  pubes 172.5
  pudendum 184.4
  retina 190.5
  scalp 172.4
  scrotum 187.7
  septum nasal (skin) 172.3
  shoulder 172.6
  skin NEC 172.8
  spindle cell (M8772/3) — *see also* Melanoma, by site
    type A (M8773/3) 190.0
    type B (M8774/3) 190.0
  submammary fold 172.5
  superficial spreading (M8743/3) — *see* Melanoma, by site
  temple 172.3
  thigh 172.7
  toe 172.7
  trunk NEC 172.5
  umbilicus 172.5
  upper limb NEC 172.6
  vagina vault 184.0
  vulva 184.4
Melanoplakia 528.9
Melanosarcoma (M8720/3) — *see also* Melanoma
  epithelioid cell (M8771/3) — *see* Melanoma
Melanosis 709.09
  addisonian (primary adrenal insufficiency) 255.4
    tuberculous (*see also* Tuberculosis) 017.6
  adrenal 255.4
  colon 569.89
  conjunctiva 372.55
    congenital 743.49
  corii degenerativa 757.33
  cornea (presenile) (senile) 371.12
    congenital 743.43
      interfering with vision 743.42
    prenatal 743.43
      interfering with vision 743.42
  eye 372.55
    congenital 743.49
  jute spinners' 709.09
  lenticularis progressiva 757.33
  liver 573.8
  precancerous (M8741/2) — *see also* Neoplasm, skin, in situ
    malignant melanoma in (M8741/3) — *see* Melanoma
  Riehl's 709.09
  sclera 379.19
    congenital 743.47
  suprarenal 255.4
  tar 709.09
  toxic 709.09
Melanuria 791.9

MELAS 758.89
Melasma 709.09
  adrenal (gland) 255.4
  suprarenal (gland) 255.4
Melena 578.1
  due to
    swallowed maternal blood 777.3
    ulcer — *see* Ulcer, by site, with hemorrhage
  newborn 772.4
    due to swallowed maternal blood 777.3
Meleney's
  gangrene (cutaneous) 686.09
  ulcer (chronic undermining) 686.09
Melioidosis 025
Melitensis, febris 023.0
Melitococcosis 023.0
Melkersson (-Rosenthal) syndrome 351.8
Mellitus, diabetes — *see* Diabetes
Melorheostosis (bone) (leri) 733.99
Meloschisis 744.83
Melotia 744.29
Membrana
  capsularis lentis posterior 743.39
  epipapillaris 743.57
Membranacea placenta — *see* Placenta, abnormal
Membranaceous uterus 621.8
Membrane, membranous — *see also* condition
  folds, congenital — *see* Web
  Jackson's 751.4
  over face (causing asphyxia), fetus or newborn 768.9
  premature rupture — *see* Rupture, membranes, premature
  pupillary 364.74
    persistent 743.46
  retained (complicating delivery) (with hemorrhage) 666.2
    without hemorrhage 667.1
  secondary (eye) 366.50
  unruptured (causing asphyxia) 768.9
  vitreous humor 379.25
Membranitis, fetal 658.4
  affecting fetus or newborn 762.7
Memory disturbance, loss or lack (*see also* Amnesia) 780.99 ▲
  mild, following organic brain damage 310.1
Menadione (vitamin K) deficiency 269.0
Menarche, precocious 259.1
Mendacity, pathologic 301.7
Mende's syndrome (ptosis-epicanthus) 270.2
Mendelson's syndrome (resulting from a procedure) 997.3
  obstetric 668.0
Ménétrier's disease or syndrome (hypertrophic gastritis) 535.2
Ménière's disease, syndrome, or vertigo 386.00
  cochlear 386.02
  cochleovestibular 386.01
  inactive 386.04
  in remission 386.04
  vestibular 386.03
Meninges, meningeal — *see* condition
Meningioma (M9530/0) — *see also* Neoplasm, meninges, benign
  angioblastic (M9535/0) — *see* Neoplasm, meninges, benign
  angiomatous (M9534/0) — *see* Neoplasm, meninges, benign
  endotheliomatous (M9531/0) — *see* Neoplasm, meninges, benign
  fibroblastic (M9532/0) — *see* Neoplasm, meninges, benign
  fibrous (M9532/0) — *see* Neoplasm, meninges, benign
  hemangioblastic (M9535/0) — *see* Neoplasm, meninges, benign
  hemangiopericytic (M9536/0) — *see* Neoplasm, meninges, benign
  malignant (M9530/3) — *see* Neoplasm, meninges, malignant
  meningiothelial (M9531/0) — *see* Neoplasm, meninges, benign

Meningioma — *see also* Neoplasm, meninges, benign — *continued*
  meningotheliomatous (M9531/0) — *see* Neoplasm, meninges, benign
  mixed (M9537/0) — *see* Neoplasm, meninges, benign
  multiple (M9530/1) 237.6
  papillary (M9538/1) 237.6
  psammomatous (M9533/0) — *see* Neoplasm, meninges, benign
  syncytial (M9531/0) — *see* Neoplasm, meninges, benign
  transitional (M9537/0) — *see* Neoplasm, meninges, benign
Meningiomatosis (diffuse) (M9530/1) 237.6
Meningism (*see also* Meningismus) 781.6
Meningismus (infectional) (pneumococcal) 781.6
  due to serum or vaccine 997.09 [321.8]
  influenzal NEC 487.8
Meningitis (basal) (basic) (basilar) (brain) (cerebral) (cervical) (congestive) (diffuse) (hemorrhagic) (infantile) (membranous) (metastatic) (nonspecific) (pontine) (progressive) (simple) (spinal) (subacute) (sympathetica) (toxic) 322.9
  abacterial NEC (*see also* Meningitis, aseptic) 047.9
  actinomycotic 039.8 [320.7]
  adenoviral 049.1
  Aerobacter aerogenes 320.82
  anaerobes (cocci) (gram-negative) (gram-positive) (mixed) (NEC) 320.81
  arbovirus NEC 066.9 [321.2]
    specified type NEC 066.8 [321.2]
  aseptic (acute) NEC 047.9
    adenovirus 049.1
    Coxsackievirus 047.0
    due to
      adenovirus 049.1
      Coxsackievirus 047.0
      ECHO virus 047.1
      enterovirus 047.9
      mumps 072.1
      poliovirus (*see also* Poliomyelitis) 045.2 [321.2]
    ECHO virus 047.1
    herpes (simplex) virus 054.72
      zoster 053.0
    leptospiral 100.81
    lymphocytic choriomeningitis 049.0
    noninfective 322.0
  Bacillus pyocyaneus 320.89
  bacterial NEC 320.9
    anaerobic 320.81
    gram-negative 320.82
      anaerobic 320.81
  Bacteroides (fragilis) (oralis) (melaninogenicus) 320.81
  cancerous (M8000/6) 198.4
  candidal 112.83
  carcinomatous (M8010/6) 198.4
  caseous (*see also* Tuberculosis, meninges) 013.0
  cerebrospinal (acute) (chronic) (diplococcal) (endemic) (epidemic) (fulminant) (infectious) (malignant) (meningococcal) (sporadic) 036.0
    carrier (suspected) of V02.59
  chronic NEC 322.2
  clear cerebrospinal fluid NEC 322.0
  Clostridium (haemolyticum) (novyi) NEC 320.81
  coccidioidomycosis 114.2
  Coxsackievirus 047.0
  cryptococcal 117.5 [321.0]
  diplococcal 036.0
    gram-negative 036.0
    gram-positive 320.1
  Diplococcus pneumoniae 320.1
  due to
    actinomycosis 039.8 [320.7]
    adenovirus 049.1
    coccidiomycosis 114.2
    enterovirus 047.9
      specified NEC 047.8
    histoplasmosis (*see also* Histoplasmosis) 115.91
    Listerosis 027.0 [320.7]

Meningitis

Meningitis — continued
   due to — continued
      Lyme disease 088.81 *[320.7]*
      moniliasis 112.83
      mumps 072.1
      neurosyphilis 094.2
      nonbacterial organisms NEC 321.8
      oidiomycosis 112.83
      poliovirus (*see also* Poliomyelitis)
         045.2 ✓5ᵗʰ *[321.2]*
      preventive immunization, inoculation, or vaccination 997.09 *[321.8]*
      sarcoidosis 135 *[321.4]*
      sporotrichosis 117.1 *[321.1]*
      syphilis 094.2
         acute 091.81
         congenital 090.42
         secondary 091.81
      trypanosomiasis (*see also* Trypanosomiasis) 086.9 *[321.3]*
      whooping cough 033.9 *[320.7]*
   E. coli 320.82
   ECHO virus 047.1
   endothelial-leukocytic, benign, recurrent 047.9
   Enterobacter aerogenes 320.82
   enteroviral 047.9
      specified type NEC 047.8
   enterovirus 047.9
      specified NEC 047.8
   eosinophilic 322.1
   epidemic NEC 036.0
   Escherichia coli (E. coli) 320.82
   Eubacterium 320.81
   fibrinopurulent NEC 320.9
      specified type NEC 320.89
   Friedländer (bacillus) 320.82
   fungal NEC 117.9 *[321.1]*
   Fusobacterium 320.81
   gonococcal 098.82
   gram-negative bacteria NEC 320.82
      anaerobic 320.81
      cocci 036.0
         specified NEC 320.82
   gram-negative cocci NEC 036.0
      specified NEC 320.82
   gram-positive cocci NEC 320.9
   H. influenzae 320.0
   herpes (simplex) virus 054.72
      zoster 053.0
   infectious NEC 320.9
   influenzal 320.0
   Klebsiella pneumoniae 320.82
   late effect — *see* Late, effect, meningitis
   leptospiral (aseptic) 100.81
   Listerella (monocytogenes) 027.0 *[320.7]*
   Listeria monocytogenes 027.0 *[320.7]*
   lymphocytic (acute) (benign) (serous) 049.0
      choriomeningitis virus 049.0
   meningococcal (chronic) 036.0
   Mima polymorpha 320.82
   Mollaret's 047.9
   monilial 112.83
   mumps (virus) 072.1
   mycotic NEC 117.9 *[321.1]*
   Neisseria 036.0
   neurosyphilis 094.2
   nonbacterial NEC (*see also* Meningitis, aseptic) 047.9
   nonpyogenic NEC 322.0
   oidiomycosis 112.83
   ossificans 349.2
   Peptococcus 320.81
   Peptostreptococcus 320.81
   pneumococcal 320.1
   poliovirus (*see also* Poliomyelitis) 045.2 ✓5ᵗʰ *[321.2]*
   Proprionibacterium 320.81
   Proteus morganii 320.82
   Pseudomonas (aeruginosa) (pyocyaneus) 320.82
   purulent NEC 320.9
      specified organism NEC 320.89
   pyogenic NEC 320.9
      specified organism NEC 320.89
   Salmonella 003.21
   septic NEC 320.9
      specified organism NEC 320.89
   serosa circumscripta NEC 322.0

Meningitis — continued
   serous NEC (*see also* Meningitis, aseptic) 047.9
      lymphocytic 049.0
      syndrome 348.2
   Serratia (marcescens) 320.82
   specified organism NEC 320.89
   sporadic cerebrospinal 036.0
   sporotrichosis 117.1 *[321.1]*
   staphylococcal 320.3
   sterile 997.09
   streptococcal (acute) 320.2
   suppurative 320.9
      specified organism NEC 320.89
   syphilitic 094.2
      acute 091.81
      congenital 090.42
      secondary 091.81
   torula 117.5 *[321.0]*
   traumatic (complication of injury) 958.8
   Treponema (denticola) (Macrodenticum) 320.81
   trypanosomiasis 086.1 *[321.3]*
   tuberculous (*see also* Tuberculosis, meninges) 013.0 ✓5ᵗʰ
   typhoid 002.0 *[320.7]*
   Veillonella 320.81
   Vibrio vulnificus 320.82
   viral, virus NEC (*see also* Meningitis, aseptic) 047.9
   Wallgren's (*see also* Meningitis, aseptic) 047.9
Meningocele (congenital) (spinal) (*see also* Spina bifida) 741.9 ✓5ᵗʰ
   acquired (traumatic) 349.2
   cerebral 742.0
   cranial 742.0
Meningocerebritis — *see* Meningoencephalitis
Meningococcemia (acute) (chronic) 036.2
Meningococcus, meningococcal (*see also* condition) 036.9
   adrenalitis, hemorrhagic 036.3
   carditis 036.40
   carrier (suspected) of V02.59
   cerebrospinal fever 036.0
   encephalitis 036.1
   endocarditis 036.42
   infection NEC 036.9
   meningitis (cerebrospinal) 036.0
   myocarditis 036.43
   optic neuritis 036.81
   pericarditis 036.41
   septicemia (chronic) 036.2
Meningoencephalitis (*see also* Encephalitis) 323.9
   acute NEC 048
   bacterial, purulent, pyogenic, or septic — *see* Meningitis
   chronic NEC 094.1
   diffuse NEC 094.1
   diphasic 063.2
   due to
      actinomycosis 039.8 *[320.7]*
      blastomycosis NEC (*see also* Blastomycosis) 116.0 *[323.4]*
      free-living amebae 136.2
      Listeria monocytogenes 027.0 *[320.7]*
      Lyme disease 088.81 *[320.7]*
      mumps 072.2
      Naegleria (amebae) (gruberi) (organisms) 136.2
      rubella 056.01
      sporotrichosis 117.1 *[321.1]*
      toxoplasmosis (acquired) 130.0
         congenital (active) 771.2 *[323.4]*
      Trypanosoma 086.1 *[323.2]*
   epidemic 036.0
   herpes 054.3
   herpetic 054.3
   H. influenzae 320.0
   infectious (acute) 048
   influenzal 320.0
   late effect — *see* category 326
   Listeria monocytogenes 027.0 *[320.7]*
   lymphocytic (serous) 049.0
   mumps 072.2
   parasitic NEC 123.9 *[323.4]*
   pneumococcal 320.1
   primary amebic 136.2
   rubella 056.01

Meningoencephalitis (*see also* Encephalitis) — continued
   serous 048
      lymphocytic 049.0
   specific 094.2
   staphylococcal 320.3
   streptococcal 320.2
   syphilitic 094.2
   toxic NEC 989.9 *[323.7]*
      due to
         carbon tetrachloride 987.8 *[323.7]*
         hydroxyquinoline derivatives poisoning 961.3 *[323.7]*
         lead 984.9 *[323.7]*
         mercury 985.0 *[323.7]*
         thallium 985.8 *[323.7]*
   toxoplasmosis (acquired) 130.0
   trypanosomic 086.1 *[323.2]*
   tuberculous (*see also* Tuberculosis, meninges) 013.0 ✓5ᵗʰ
   virus NEC 048
Meningoencephalocele 742.0
   syphilitic 094.89
   congenital 090.49
Meningoencephalomyelitis (*see also* Meningoencephalitis) 323.9
   acute NEC 048
      disseminated (postinfectious) 136.9 *[323.6]*
         postimmunization or postvaccination 323.5
   due to
      actinomycosis 039.8 *[320.7]*
      torula 117.5 *[323.4]*
      toxoplasma or toxoplasmosis (acquired) 130.0
         congenital (active) 771.2 *[323.4]*
   late effect — *see* category 326
Meningoencephalomyelopathy (*see also* Meningoencephalomyelitis) 349.9
Meningoencephalopathy (*see also* Meningoencephalitis) 348.3
Meningoencephalopoliomyelitis (*see also* Poliomyelitis, bulbar) 045.0 ✓5ᵗʰ
   late effect 138
Meningomyelitis (*see also* Meningoencephalitis) 323.9
   blastomycotic NEC (*see also* Blastomycosis) 116.0 *[323.4]*
   due to
      actinomycosis 039.8 *[320.7]*
      blastomycosis (*see also* Blastomycosis) 116.0 *[323.4]*
      Meningococcus 036.0
      sporotrichosis 117.1 *[323.4]*
      torula 117.5 *[323.4]*
   late effect — *see* category 326
   lethargic 049.8
   meningococcal 036.0
   syphilitic 094.2
   tuberculous (*see also* Tuberculosis, meninges) 013.0 ✓5ᵗʰ
Meningomyelocele (*see also* Spina bifida) 741.9 ✓5ᵗʰ
   syphilitic 094.89
Meningomyeloneuritis — *see* Meningoencephalitis
Meningoradiculitis — *see* Meningitis
Meningovascular — *see* condition
Meniscocytosis 282.60
Menkes' syndrome — *see* Syndrome, Menkes'
Menolipsis 626.0
Menometrorrhagia 626.2
Menopause, menopausal (symptoms) (syndrome) 627.2
   arthritis (any site) NEC 716.3 ✓5ᵗʰ
   artificial 627.4
   bleeding 627.0
   crisis 627.2
   depression (*see also* Psychosis, affective) 296.2 ✓5ᵗʰ
      agitated 296.2 ✓5ᵗʰ
         recurrent episode 296.3 ✓5ᵗʰ
         single episode 296.2 ✓5ᵗʰ

Menopause, menopausal — *continued*
  depression (*see also* Psychosis, affective) — *continued*
    psychotic 296.2 ✓5ᵗʰ
      recurrent episode 296.3 ✓5ᵗʰ
        single episode 296.2 ✓5ᵗʰ
      recurrent episode 296.3 ✓5ᵗʰ
      single episode 296.2 ✓5ᵗʰ
    melancholia (*see also* Psychosis, affective) 296.2 ✓5ᵗʰ
      recurrent episode 296.3 ✓5ᵗʰ
      single episode 296.2 ✓5ᵗʰ
  paranoid state 297.2
  paraphrenia 297.2
  postsurgical 627.4
  premature 256.31
    postirradiation 256.2
    postsurgical 256.2
  psychoneurosis 627.2
  psychosis NEC 298.8
  surgical 627.4
  toxic polyarthritis NEC 716.39
Menorrhagia (primary) 626.2
  climacteric 627.0
  menopausal 627.0
  postclimacteric 627.1
  postmenopausal 627.1
  preclimacteric 627.0
  premenopausal 627.0
  puberty (menses retained) 626.3
Menorrhalgia 625.3
Menoschesis 626.8
Menostaxis 626.2
Menses, retention 626.8
Menstrual — *see also* Menstruation
  cycle, irregular 626.4
  disorders NEC 626.9
  extraction V25.3
  fluid, retained 626.8
  molimen 625.4
  period, normal V65.5
  regulation V25.3
Menstruation
  absent 626.0
  anovulatory 628.0
  delayed 626.8
  difficult 625.3
  disorder 626.9
    psychogenic 306.52
    specified NEC 626.8
  during pregnancy 640.8 ✓5ᵗʰ
  excessive 626.2
  frequent 626.2
  infrequent 626.1
  irregular 626.4
  latent 626.8
  membranous 626.8
  painful (primary) (secondary) 625.3
    psychogenic 306.52
  passage of clots 626.2
  precocious 626.8
  protracted 626.8
  retained 626.8
  retrograde 626.8
  scanty 626.1
  suppression 626.8
  vicarious (nasal) 625.8
Mentagra (*see also* Sycosis) 704.8
Mental — *see also* condition
  deficiency (*see also* Retardation, mental) 319
  deterioration (*see also* Psychosis) 298.9
  disorder (*see also* Disorder, mental) 300.9
  exhaustion 300.5
  insufficiency (congenital) (*see also* Retardation, mental) 319
  observation without need for further medical care NEC V71.09
  retardation (*see also* Retardation, mental) 319
  subnormality (*see also* Retardation, mental) 319
    mild 317
    moderate 318.0
    profound 318.2
    severe 318.1
  upset (*see also* Disorder, mental) 300.9

Meralgia paresthetica 355.1
Mercurial — *see* condition
Mercurialism NEC 985.0
Merergasia 300.9
MERFF 758.89
Merkel cell tumor — *see* Neoplasm, by site, malignant
Merocele (*see also* Hernia, femoral) 553.00
Meromelia 755.4
  lower limb 755.30
    intercalary 755.32
      femur 755.34
        tibiofibular (complete) (incomplete) 755.33
      fibula 755.37
      metatarsal(s) 755.38
      tarsal(s) 755.38
      tibia 755.36
      tibiofibular 755.35
    terminal (complete) (partial) (transverse) 755.31
      longitudinal 755.32
        metatarsal(s) 755.38
        phalange(s) 755.39
        tarsal(s) 755.38
      transverse 755.31
  upper limb 755.20
    intercalary 755.22
      carpal(s) 755.28
      humeral 755.24
        radioulnar (complete) (incomplete) 755.23
      metacarpal(s) 755.28
      phalange(s) 755.29
      radial 755.26
      radioulnar 755.25
      ulnar 755.27
    terminal (complete) (partial) (transverse) 755.21
      longitudinal 755.22
        carpal(s) 755.28
        metacarpal(s) 755.28
        phalange(s) 755.29
      transverse 755.21
Merosmia 781.1
Merycism — *see also* Vomiting
  psychogenic 307.53
Merzbacher-Pelizaeus disease 330.0
Mesaortitis — *see* Aortitis
Mesarteritis — *see* Arteritis
Mesencephalitis (*see also* Encephalitis) 323.9
  late effect — *see* category 326
Mesenchymoma (M8990/1) — *see also* Neoplasm, connective tissue, uncertain behavior
  benign (M8990/0) — *see* Neoplasm, connective tissue, benign
  malignant (M8990/3) — *see* Neoplasm, connective tissue, malignant
Mesentery, mesenteric — *see* condition
Mesiodens, mesiodentes 520.1
  causing crowding 524.3
Mesio-occlusion 524.2
Mesocardia (with asplenia) 746.87
Mesocolon — *see* condition
Mesonephroma (malignant) (M9110/3) — *see also* Neoplasm, by site, malignant
  benign (M9110/0) — *see* Neoplasm, by site, benign
Mesophlebitis — *see* Phlebitis
Mesostromal dysgenesis 743.51
Mesothelioma (malignant) (M9050/3) — *see also* Neoplasm, by site, malignant
  benign (M9050/0) — *see* Neoplasm, by site, benign
  biphasic type (M9053/3) — *see also* Neoplasm, by site, malignant
    benign (M9053/0) — *see* Neoplasm, by site, benign
  epithelioid (M9052/3) — *see also* Neoplasm, by site, malignant
    benign (M9052/0) — *see* Neoplasm, by site, benign

Mesothelioma — *see also* Neoplasm, by site, malignant — *continued*
  fibrous (M9051/3) — *see also* Neoplasm, by site, malignant
  benign (M9051/0) — *see* Neoplasm, by site, benign
Metabolism disorder 277.9
  specified type NEC 277.8
Metagonimiasis 121.5
Metagonimus infestation (small intestine) 121.5
Metal
  pigmentation (skin) 709.00
  polishers' disease 502
Metalliferous miners' lung 503
Metamorphopsia 368.14
Metaplasia
  bone, in skin 709.3
  breast 611.8
  cervix — *omit code*
  endometrium (squamous) 621.8
  intestinal, of gastric mucosa 537.89
  kidney (pelvis) (squamous) (*see also* Disease, renal) 593.89
  myelogenous 289.8
  myeloid (agnogenic) (megakaryocytic) 289.8
  spleen 289.59
  squamous cell
    amnion 658.8 ✓5ᵗʰ
    bladder 596.8
    cervix — *see* condition
    trachea 519.1
    tracheobronchial tree 519.1
    uterus 621.8
      cervix — *see* condition
Metastasis, metastatic
  abscess — *see* Abscess
  calcification 275.40
  cancer, neoplasm, or disease
    from specified site (M8000/3) — *see* Neoplasm, by site, malignant
    to specified site (M8000/6) — *see* Neoplasm, by site, secondary
  deposits (in) (M8000/6) — *see* Neoplasm, by site, secondary
  pneumonia 038.8 [484.8]
  spread (to) (M8000/6) — *see* Neoplasm, by site, secondary
Metatarsalgia 726.70
  anterior 355.6
  due to Freiberg's disease 732.5
  Morton's 355.6
Metatarsus, metatarsal — *see also* condition
  abductus valgus (congenital) 754.60
  adductus varus (congenital) 754.53
  primus varus 754.52
  valgus (adductus) (congenital) 754.60
  varus (abductus) (congenital) 754.53
    primus 754.52
Methemoglobinemia 289.7
  acquired (with sulfhemoglobinemia) 289.7
  congenital 289.7
  enzymatic 289.7
  Hb-M disease 289.7
  hereditary 289.7
  toxic 289.7
Methemoglobinuria (*see also* Hemoglobinuria) 791.2
Methioninemia 270.4
Metritis (catarrhal) (septic) (suppurative) (*see also* Endometritis) 615.9
  blennorrhagic 098.16
    chronic or duration of 2 months or over 098.36
  cervical (*see also* Cervicitis) 616.0
  gonococcal 098.16
    chronic or duration of 2 months or over 098.36
  hemorrhagic 626.8
  puerperal, postpartum, childbirth 670 ✓5ᵗʰ
  tuberculous (*see also* Tuberculosis) 016.7 ✓5ᵗʰ
Metropathia hemorrhagica 626.8
Metroperitonitis (*see also* Peritonitis, pelvic, female) 614.5

Metrorrhagia

Metrorrhagia 626.6
  arising during pregnancy — *see* Hemorrhage, pregnancy
  postpartum NEC 666.2 ✓5ᵗʰ
  primary 626.6
  psychogenic 306.59
  puerperal 666.2 ✓5ᵗʰ
Metrorrhexis — *see* Rupture, uterus
Metrosalpingitis (*see also* Salpingo-oophoritis) 614.2
Metrostaxis 626.6
Metrovaginitis (*see also* Endometritis) 615.9
  gonococcal (acute) 098.16
    chronic or duration of 2 months or over 098.36
Mexican fever — *see* Typhus, Mexican
Meyenburg-Altherr-Uehlinger syndrome 733.99
Meyer-Schwickerath and Weyers syndrome (dysplasia oculodentodigitalis) 759.89
Meynert's amentia (nonalcoholic) 294.0
  alcoholic 291.1
Mibelli's disease 757.39
Mice, joint (*see also* Loose, body, joint) 718.1 ✓5ᵗʰ
  knee 717.6
Micheli-Rietti syndrome (thalassemia minor) 282.4
Michotte's syndrome 721.5
Micrencephalon, micrencephaly 742.1
Microaneurysm, retina 362.14
  diabetic 250.5 ✓5ᵗʰ [362.01]
Microangiopathy 443.9
  diabetic (peripheral) 250.7 ✓5ᵗʰ [443.81]
    retinal 250.5 ✓5ᵗʰ [362.01]
  peripheral 443.9
    diabetic 250.7 ✓5ᵗʰ [443.81]
  retinal 362.18
    diabetic 250.5 ✓5ᵗʰ [362.01]
  thrombotic 446.6
    Moschcowitz's (thrombotic thrombocytopenic purpura) 446.6
Microcalcification, mammographic 793.81
Microcephalus, microcephalic, microcephaly 742.1
  due to toxoplasmosis (congenital) 771.2
Microcheilia 744.82
Microcolon (congenital) 751.5
Microcornea (congenital) 743.41
Microcytic — *see* condition
Microdontia 520.2
Microdrepanocytosis (thalassemia-Hb-S disease) 282.4
Microembolism
  atherothrombotic — *see* Atheroembolism
  retina 362.33
Microencephalon 742.1
Microfilaria streptocerca infestation 125.3
Microgastria (congenital) 750.7
Microgenia 524.0 ✓5ᵗʰ
Microgenitalia (congenital) 752.8
  penis 752.64
Microglioma (M9710/3)
  specified site — *see* Neoplasm, by site, malignant
  unspecified site 191.9
Microglossia (congenital) 750.16
Micrognathia, micrognathism (congenital) 524.00
  mandibular 524.04
    alveolar 524.74
  maxillary 524.03
    alveolar 524.73
Microgyria (congenital) 742.2
Microinfarct, heart (*see also* Insufficiency, coronary) 411.89
Microlithiasis, alveolar, pulmonary 516.2
Micromyelia (congenital) 742.59
Micropenis 752.64
Microphakia (congenital) 743.36
Microphthalmia (congenital) (*see also* Microphthalmos) 743.10

Microphthalmos (congenital) 743.10
  associated with eye and adnexal anomalies NEC 743.12
  due to toxoplasmosis (congenital) 771.2
  isolated 743.11
  simple 743.11
  syndrome 759.89
Micropsia 368.14
Microsporidiosis 136.8
Microsporon furfur infestation 111.0
Microsporosis (*see also* Dermatophytosis) 110.9
  nigra 111.1
Microstomia (congenital) 744.84
Microthelia 757.6
Microthromboembolism — *see* Embolism
Microtia (congenital) (external ear) 744.23
Microtropia 378.34
Micturition
  disorder NEC 788.69
    psychogenic 306.53
  frequency 788.41
    psychogenic 306.53
  nocturnal 788.43
  painful 788.1
    psychogenic 306.53
Middle
  ear — *see* condition
  lobe (right) syndrome 518.0
Midplane — *see* condition
Miescher's disease 709.3
  cheilitis 351.8
  granulomatosis disciformis 709.3
Miescher-Leder syndrome or granulomatosis 709.3
Mieten's syndrome 759.89
Migraine (idiopathic) 346.9 ✓5ᵗʰ
  with aura 346.0 ✓5ᵗʰ
  abdominal (syndrome) 346.2 ✓5ᵗʰ
  allergic (histamine) 346.2 ✓5ᵗʰ
  atypical 346.1 ✓5ᵗʰ
  basilar 346.2 ✓5ᵗʰ
  classical 346.0 ✓5ᵗʰ
  common 346.1 ✓5ᵗʰ
  hemiplegic 346.8 ✓5ᵗʰ
  lower-half 346.2 ✓5ᵗʰ
  menstrual 625.4
  ophthalmic 346.8 ✓5ᵗʰ
  ophthalmoplegic 346.8 ✓5ᵗʰ
  retinal 346.2 ✓5ᵗʰ
  variant 346.2 ✓5ᵗʰ
Migrant, social V60.0
Migratory, migrating — *see also* condition
  person V60.0
  testis, congenital 752.52
Mikulicz's disease or syndrome (dryness of mouth, absent or decreased lacrimation) 527.1
Milian atrophia blanche 701.3
Miliaria (crystallina) (rubra) (tropicalis) 705.1
  apocrine 705.82
Miliary — *see* condition
Milium (*see also* Cyst, sebaceous) 706.2
  colloid 709.3
  eyelid 374.84
Milk
  crust 690.11
  excess secretion 676.6 ✓5ᵗʰ
  fever, female 672 ✓5ᵗʰ
  poisoning 988.8
  retention 676.2 ✓5ᵗʰ
  sickness 988.8
  spots 423.1
Milkers' nodes 051.1
Milk-leg (deep vessels) 671.4 ✓5ᵗʰ
  complicating pregnancy 671.3 ✓5ᵗʰ
  nonpuerperal 451.19
  puerperal, postpartum, childbirth 671.4 ✓5ᵗʰ
Milkman (-Looser) disease or syndrome (osteomalacia with pseudofractures) 268.2
Milky urine (*see also* Chyluria) 791.1
Millar's asthma (laryngismus stridulus) 478.75
Millard-Gubler paralysis or syndrome 344.89

Index to Diseases

Millard-Gubler-Foville paralysis 344.89
Miller's disease (osteomalacia) 268.2
Miller Fisher's syndrome 357.0
Milles' syndrome (encephalocutaneous angiomatosis) 759.6
Mills' disease 335.29
Millstone makers' asthma or lung 502
Milroy's disease (chronic hereditary edema) 757.0
Miners' — *see also* condition
  asthma 500
  elbow 727.2
  knee 727.2
  lung 500
  nystagmus 300.89
  phthisis (*see also* Tuberculosis) 011.4 ✓5ᵗʰ
  tuberculosis (*see also* Tuberculosis) 011.4 ✓5ᵗʰ
Minkowski-Chauffard syndrome (*see also* Spherocytosis) 282.0
Minor — *see* condition
Minor's disease 336.1
Minot's disease (hemorrhagic disease, newborn) 776.0
Minot-von Willebrand (-Jürgens) disease or syndrome (angiohemophilia) 286.4
Minus (and plus) hand (intrinsic) 736.09
Miosis (persistent) (pupil) 379.42
Mirizzi's syndrome (hepatic duct stenosis) (*see also* Obstruction, biliary) 576.2
  with calculus, cholelithiasis, or stones — *see* Choledocholithiasis
Mirror writing 315.09
  secondary to organic lesion 784.69
Misadventure (prophylactic) (therapeutic) (*see also* Complications) 999.9
  administration of insulin 962.3
  infusion — *see* Complications, infusion
  local applications (of fomentations, plasters, etc.) 999.9
    burn or scald — *see* Burn, by site
  medical care (early) (late) NEC 999.9
    adverse effect of drugs or chemicals — *see* Table of Drugs and Chemicals
    burn or scald — *see* Burn, by site
  radiation NEC 990
  radiotherapy NEC 990
  surgical procedure (early) (late) — *see* Complications, surgical procedure
  transfusion — *see* Complications, transfusion
  vaccination or other immunological procedure — *see* Complications, vaccination
Misanthropy 301.7
Miscarriage — *see* Abortion, spontaneous
Mischief, malicious, child (*see also* Disturbance, conduct) 312.0 ✓5ᵗʰ
Misdirection
  aqueous 365.83
Mismanagement, feeding 783.3
Misplaced, misplacement
  kidney (*see also* Disease, renal) 593.0
    congenital 753.3
  organ or site, congenital NEC — *see* Malposition, congenital
Missed
  abortion 632
  delivery (at or near term) 656.4 ✓5ᵗʰ
  labor (at or near term) 656.4 ✓5ᵗʰ
Missing — *see also* Absence
  teeth (acquired) 525.10
    congenital (*see also* Anodontia) 520.0
    due to
      caries 525.13
      extraction 525.10
      periodontal disease 525.12
      specified NEC 525.19
      trauma 525.11
  vertebrae (congenital) 756.13
Misuse of drugs NEC (*see also* Abuse, drug, nondependent) 305.9 ✓5ᵗʰ
Mitchell's disease (erythromelalgia) 443.89
Mite(s)
  diarrhea 133.8
  grain (itch) 133.8

Mite(s) — continued
  hair follicle (itch) 133.8
  in sputum 133.8
Mitral — see condition
Mittelschmerz 625.2
Mixed — see condition
Mljet disease (mal de Meleda) 757.39
Mobile, mobility
  cecum 751.4
  coccyx 733.99
  excessive — see Hypermobility
  gallbladder 751.69
  kidney 593.0
    congenital 753.3
  organ or site, congenital NEC — see Malposition, congenital
  spleen 289.59
Mobitz heart block (atrioventricular) 426.10
  type I (Wenckebach's) 426.13
  type II 426.12
Möbius'
  disease 346.8 ✓5ᵗʰ
  syndrome
    congenital oculofacial paralysis 352.6
    ophthalmoplegic migraine 346.8 ✓5ᵗʰ
Moeller (-Barlow) disease (infantile scurvy) 267
  glossitis 529.4
Mohr's syndrome (types I and II) 759.89
Mola destruens (M9100/1) 236.1
Molarization, premolars 520.2
Molar pregnancy 631
  hydatidiform (delivered) (undelivered) 630
Mold(s)
  in vitreous 117.9
Molding, head (during birth) 767.3
Mole (pigmented) (M8720/0) — see also Neoplasm, skin, benign
  blood 631
  Breus' 631
  cancerous (M8720/3) — see Melanoma
  carneous 631
  destructive (M9100/1) 236.1
  ectopic — see Pregnancy, ectopic
  fleshy 631
  hemorrhagic 631
  hydatid, hydatidiform (benign) (complicating pregnancy) (delivered) (undelivered) (see also Hydatidiform mole) 630
    invasive (M9100/1) 236.1
    malignant (M9100/1) 236.1
    previous, affecting management of pregnancy V23.1
  invasive (hydatidiform) (M9100/1) 236.1
  malignant
    meaning
      malignant hydatidiform mole (9100/1) 236.1
      melanoma (M8720/3) — see Melanoma
  nonpigmented (M8730/0) — see Neoplasm, skin, benign
  pregnancy NEC 631
  skin (M8720/0) — see Neoplasm, skin, benign
  tubal — see Pregnancy, tubal
  vesicular (see also Hydatidiform mole) 630
Molimen, molimina (menstrual) 625.4
Mollaret's meningitis 047.9
Mollities (cerebellar) (cerebral) 437.8
  ossium 268.2
Molluscum
  contagiosum 078.0
  epitheliale 078.0
  fibrosum (M8851/0) — see Lipoma, by site
  pendulum (M8851/0) — see Lipoma, by site
Mönckeberg's arteriosclerosis, degeneration, disease, or sclerosis (see also Arteriosclerosis, extremities) 440.20
Monday fever 504
Monday morning dyspnea or asthma 504
Mondini's malformation (cochlea) 744.05
Mondor's disease (thrombophlebitis of breast) 451.89

Mongolian, mongolianism, mongolism, mongoloid 758.0
  spot 757.33
Monilethrix (congenital) 757.4
Monilia infestation — see Candidiasis
Moniliasis — see also Candidiasis
  neonatal 771.7
  vulvovaginitis 112.1
Monoarthritis 716.60
  ankle 716.67
  arm 716.62
    lower (and wrist) 716.63
    upper (and elbow) 716.62
  foot (and ankle) 716.67
  forearm (and wrist) 716.63
  hand 716.64
  leg 716.66
    lower 716.66
    upper 716.65
  pelvic region (hip) (thigh) 716.65
  shoulder (region) 716.61
  specified site NEC 716.68
Monoblastic — see condition
Monochromatism (cone) (rod) 368.54
Monocytic — see condition
Monocytosis (symptomatic) 288.8
Monofixation syndrome 378.34
Monomania (see also Psychosis) 298.9
Mononeuritis 355.9
  cranial nerve — see Disorder, nerve, cranial
  femoral nerve 355.2
  lateral
    cutaneous nerve of thigh 355.1
    popliteal nerve 355.3
  lower limb 355.8
    specified nerve NEC 355.79
  medial popliteal nerve 355.4
  median nerve 354.1
  multiplex 354.5
  plantar nerve 355.6
  posterior tibial nerve 355.5
  radial nerve 354.3
  sciatic nerve 355.0
  ulnar nerve 354.2
  upper limb 354.9
    specified nerve NEC 354.8
  vestibular 388.5
Mononeuropathy (see also Mononeuritis) 355.9
  diabetic NEC 250.6 ✓5ᵗʰ [355.9]
    lower limb 250.6 ✓5ᵗʰ [355.8]
    upper limb 250.6 ✓5ᵗʰ [354.9]
  iliohypogastric 355.79
  ilioinguinal 355.79
  obturator 355.79
  saphenous 355.79
Mononucleosis, infectious 075
  with hepatitis 075 [573.1]
Monoplegia 344.5
  brain (current episode) (see also Paralysis, brain) 437.8
    fetus or newborn 767.8
  cerebral (current episode) (see also Paralysis, brain) 437.8
  congenital or infantile (cerebral) (spastic) (spinal) 343.3
  embolic (current) (see also Embolism, brain) 434.1 ✓5ᵗʰ
    late effect — see Late effect(s) (of) cerebrovascular disease
  infantile (cerebral) (spastic) (spinal) 343.3
  lower limb 344.30
    affecting
      dominant side 344.31
      nondominant side 344.32
    due to late effect of cerebrovascular accident — see Late effect(s) (of) cerebrovascular accident
  newborn 767.8
  psychogenic 306.0
    specified as conversion reaction 300.11
  thrombotic (current) (see also Thrombosis, brain) 434.0 ✓5ᵗʰ
    late effect — see Late effect(s) (of) cerebrovascular disease
  transient 781.4

Monoplegia — continued
  upper limb 344.40
    affecting
      dominant side 344.41
      nondominant side 344.42
    due to late effect of cerebrovascular accident — see Late effect(s) (of) cerebrovascular accident
Monorchism, monorchidism 752.8
Monster, monstrosity — see Anomaly
Monteggia's fracture (closed) 813.03
  open 813.13
Mood swings
  brief compensatory 296.99
  rebound 296.99
Moore's syndrome (see also Epilepsy) 345.5 ✓5ᵗʰ
Mooren's ulcer (cornea) 370.07
Mooser-Neill reaction 081.0
Mooser bodies 081.0
Moral
  deficiency 301.7
  imbecility 301.7
Morax-Axenfeld conjunctivitis 372.03
Morbilli (see also Measles) 055.9
Morbus
  anglicus, anglorum 268.0
  Beigel 111.2
  caducus (see also Epilepsy) 345.9 ✓5ᵗʰ
  caeruleus 746.89
  celiacus 579.0
  comitialis (see also Epilepsy) 345.9 ✓5ᵗʰ
  cordis — see also Disease, heart
    valvulorum — see Endocarditis
  coxae 719.95
    tuberculous (see also Tuberculosis) 015.1 ✓5ᵗʰ
  hemorrhagicus neonatorum 776.0
  maculosus neonatorum 772.6
  renum 593.0
  senilis (see also Osteoarthrosis) 715.9 ✓5ᵗʰ
Morel-Kraepelin disease (see also Schizophrenia) 295.9 ✓5ᵗʰ
Morel-Moore syndrome (hyperostosis frontalis interna) 733.3
Morel-Morgagni syndrome (hyperostosis frontalis interna) 733.3
Morgagni
  cyst, organ, hydatid, or appendage 752.8
    fallopian tube 752.11
  disease or syndrome (hyperostosis frontalis interna) 733.3
Morgagni-Adams-Stokes syndrome (syncope with heart block) 426.9
Morgagni-Stewart-Morel syndrome (hyperostosis frontalis interna) 733.3
Moria (see also Psychosis) 298.9
Morning sickness 643.0 ✓5ᵗʰ
Moron 317
Morphea (guttate) (linear) 701.0
Morphine dependence (see also Dependence) 304.0 ✓5ᵗʰ
Morphinism (see also Dependence) 304.0 ✓5ᵗʰ
Morphinomania (see also Dependence) 304.0 ✓5ᵗʰ
Morphoea 701.0
Morquio (-Brailsford) (-Ullrich) disease or syndrome (mucopolysaccharidosis IV) 277.5
  kyphosis 277.5
Morris syndrome (testicular feminization) 257.8
Morsus humanus (open wound) — see also Wound, open, by site
  skin surface intact — see Contusion
Mortification (dry) (moist) (see also Gangrene) 785.4
Morton's
  disease 355.6
  foot 355.6
  metatarsalgia (syndrome) 355.6
  neuralgia 355.6
  neuroma 355.6
  syndrome (metatarsalgia) (neuralgia) 355.6
  toe 355.6

Morvan's disease 336.0
Mosaicism, mosaic (chromosomal) 758.9
　autosomal 758.5
　sex 758.81
Moschcowitz's syndrome (thrombotic thrombocytopenic purpura) 446.6
Mother yaw 102.0
Motion sickness (from travel, any vehicle) (from roundabouts or swings) 994.6
Mottled teeth (enamel) (endemic) (nonendemic) 520.3
Mottling enamel (endemic) (nonendemic) (teeth) 520.3
Mouchet's disease 732.5
Mould(s) (in vitreous) 117.9
Moulders'
　bronchitis 502
　tuberculosis (see also Tuberculosis) 011.4 ✓5ᵗʰ
Mounier-Kuhn syndrome 494.0
　with acute exacerbation 494.1
Mountain
　fever — see Fever, mountain
　sickness 993.2
　　with polycythemia, acquired 289.0
　　acute 289.0
　tick fever 066.1
Mouse, joint (see also Loose, body, joint) 718.1 ✓5ᵗʰ
　knee 717.6
Mouth — see condition
Movable
　coccyx 724.71
　kidney (see also Disease, renal) 593.0
　　congenital 753.3
　organ or site, congenital NEC — see Malposition, congenital
　spleen 289.59
Movement
　abnormal (dystonic) (involuntary) 781.0
　decreased fetal 655.7 ✓5ᵗʰ
　paradoxical facial 374.43
Moya Moya disease 437.5
Mozart's ear 744.29
Mucha's disease (acute parapsoriasis varioliformis) 696.2
Mucha-Haberman syndrome (acute parapsoriasis varioliformis) 696.2
Mu-chain disease 273.2
Mucinosis (cutaneous) (papular) 701.8
Mucocele
　appendix 543.9
　buccal cavity 528.9
　gallbladder (see also Disease, gallbladder) 575.3
　lacrimal sac 375.43
　orbit (eye) 376.81
　salivary gland (any) 527.6
　sinus (accessory) (nasal) 478.1
　turbinate (bone) (middle) (nasal) 478.1
　uterus 621.8
Mucocutaneous lymph node syndrome (acute) (febrile) (infantile) 446.1
Mucoenteritis 564.9
Mucolipidosis I, II, III 272.7
Mucopolysaccharidosis (types 1-6) 277.5
　cardiopathy 277.5 [425.7]
Mucormycosis (lung) 117.7
Mucositis — see also Inflammation by site
　necroticans agranulocytica 288.0
Mucous — see also condition
　patches (syphilitic) 091.3
　　congenital 090.0
Mucoviscidosis 277.00
　with meconium obstruction 277.01
Mucus
　asphyxia or suffocation (see also Asphyxia, mucus) 933.1
　　newborn 770.1
　in stool 792.1
　plug (see also Asphyxia, mucus) 933.1
　　aspiration, of newborn 770.1

Mucus — continued
　plug (see also Asphyxia, mucus) — continued
　　tracheobronchial 519.1
　　　newborn 770.1
Muguet 112.0
Mulberry molars 090.5
Mullerian mixed tumor (M8950/3) — see Neoplasm, by site, malignant
Multicystic kidney 753.19
Multilobed placenta — see Placenta, abnormal
Multinodular prostate 600.1
Multiparity V61.5
　affecting
　　fetus or newborn 763.89
　　management of
　　　labor and delivery 659.4 ✓5ᵗʰ
　　　pregnancy V23.3
　requiring contraceptive management (see also Contraception) V25.9
Multipartita placenta — see Placenta, abnormal
Multiple, multiplex — see also condition
　birth
　　affecting fetus or newborn 761.5
　　healthy liveborn — see Newborn, multiple
　digits (congenital) 755.00
　　fingers 755.01
　　toes 755.02
　organ or site NEC — see Accessory
　personality 300.14
　renal arteries 747.62
Mumps 072.9
　with complication 072.8
　　specified type NEC 072.79
　encephalitis 072.2
　hepatitis 072.71
　meningitis (aseptic) 072.1
　meningoencephalitis 072.2
　oophoritis 072.79
　orchitis 072.0
　pancreatitis 072.3
　polyneuropathy 072.72
　vaccination, prophylactic (against) V04.6
Mumu (see also Infestation, filarial) 125.9
Münchausen syndrome 301.51
Münchmeyer's disease or syndrome (exostosis luxurians) 728.11
Mural — see condition
Murmur (cardiac) (heart) (nonorganic) (organic) 785.2
　abdominal 787.5
　aortic (valve) (see also Endocarditis, aortic) 424.1
　benign — omit code
　cardiorespiratory 785.2
　diastolic — see condition
　Flint (see also Endocarditis, aortic) 424.1
　functional — omit code
　Graham Steell (pulmonic regurgitation) (see also Endocarditis, pulmonary) 424.3
　innocent — omit code
　insignificant — omit code
　midsystolic 785.2
　mitral (valve) — see Stenosis, mitral
　physiologic — see condition
　presystolic, mitral — see Insufficiency, mitral
　pulmonic (valve) (see also Endocarditis, pulmonary) 424.3
　Still's (vibratory) — omit code
　systolic (valvular) — see condition
　tricuspid (valve) — see Endocarditis, tricuspid
　undiagnosed 785.2
　valvular — see condition
　vibratory — omit code
Murri's disease (intermittent hemoglobinuria) 283.2
Muscae volitantes 379.24
Muscle, muscular — see condition
Musculoneuralgia 729.1
Mushrooming hip 718.95
Mushroom workers' (pickers') lung 495.5
Mutism (see also Aphasia) 784.3
　akinetic 784.3
　deaf (acquired) (congenital) 389.7

Mutism (see also Aphasia) — continued
　elective (selective) 313.23
　　adjustment reaction 309.83
　hysterical 300.11
Myà's disease (congenital dilation, colon) 751.3
Myalgia (intercostal) 729.1
　eosinophilia syndrome 710.5
　epidemic 074.1
　　cervical 078.89
　psychogenic 307.89
　traumatic NEC 959.9
Myasthenia, myasthenic 358.0
　cordis — see Failure, heart
　gravis 358.0
　　neonatal 775.2
　　pseudoparalytica 358.0
　stomach 536.8
　　psychogenic 306.4
　syndrome
　　in
　　　botulism 005.1 [358.1]
　　　diabetes mellitus 250.6 ✓5ᵗʰ [358.1]
　　　hypothyroidism (see also Hypothyroidism) 244.9 [358.1]
　　　malignant neoplasm NEC 199.1 [358.1]
　　　pernicious anemia 281.0 [358.1]
　　　thyrotoxicosis (see also Thyrotoxicosis) 242.9 ✓5ᵗʰ [358.1]
Mycelium infection NEC 117.9
Mycetismus 988.1
Mycetoma (actinomycotic) 039.9
　bone 039.8
　　mycotic 117.4
　foot 039.4
　　mycotic 117.4
　madurae 039.9
　　mycotic 117.4
　maduromycotic 039.9
　　mycotic 117.4
　mycotic 117.4
　nocardial 039.9
Mycobacteriosis — see Mycobacterium
Mycobacterium, mycobacterial (infection) 031.9
　acid-fast (bacilli) 031.9
　anonymous (see also Mycobacterium, atypical) 031.9
　atypical (acid-fast bacilli) 031.9
　　cutaneous 031.1
　　pulmonary 031.0
　　　tuberculous (see also Tuberculosis, pulmonary) 011.9 ✓5ᵗʰ
　　specified site NEC 031.8
　avium 031.0
　　intracellulare complex bacteremia (MAC) 031.2
　balnei 031.1
　Battey 031.0
　cutaneous 031.1
　disseminated 031.2
　　avium-intracellulare complex (DMAC) 031.2
　fortuitum 031.0
　intracellulare (battey bacillus) 031.0
　kakerifu 031.8
　kansasii 031.0
　kasongo 031.8
　leprae — see Leprosy
　luciflavum 031.0
　marinum 031.1
　pulmonary 031.0
　　tuberculous (see also Tuberculosis, pulmonary) 011.9 ✓5ᵗʰ
　scrofulaceum 031.1
　tuberculosis (human, bovine) — see also Tuberculosis
　　avian type 031.0
　ulcerans 031.1
　xenopi 031.0
Mycosis, mycotic 117.9
　cutaneous NEC 111.9
　ear 111.8 [380.15]
　fungoides (M9700/3) 202.1 ✓5ᵗʰ
　mouth 112.0
　pharynx 117.9
　skin NEC 111.9
　stomatitis 112.0
　systemic NEC 117.9

Mycosis, mycotic — *continued*
  tonsil 117.9
  vagina, vaginitis 112.1
Mydriasis (persistent) (pupil) 379.43
Myelatelia 742.59
Myelinoclasis, perivascular, acute
    (postinfectious) NEC 136.9 *[323.6]*
  postimmunization or postvaccinal 323.5
Myelinosis, central pontine 341.8
Myelitis (acute) (ascending) (cerebellar)
    (childhood) (chronic) (descending) (diffuse)
    (disseminated) (pressure) (progressive)
    (spinal cord) (subacute) (transverse) (*see also*
    Encephalitis) 323.9
  late effect — *see* category 326
  optic neuritis in 341.0
  postchickenpox 052.7
  postvaccinal 323.5
  syphilitic (transverse) 094.89
  tuberculous (*see also* Tuberculosis) 013.6 ✓5ᵗʰ
  virus 049.9
Myeloblastic — *see* condition
Myelocele (*see also* Spina bifida) 741.9 ✓5ᵗʰ
  with hydrocephalus 741.0 ✓5ᵗʰ
Myelocystocele (*see also* Spina bifida) 741.9 ✓5ᵗʰ
Myelocytic — *see* condition
Myelocytoma 205.1 ✓5ᵗʰ
Myelodysplasia (spinal cord) 742.59
  meaning myelodysplastic syndrome — *see*
    Syndrome, myelodysplastic
Myeloencephalitis — *see* Encephalitis
Myelofibrosis (osteosclerosis) 289.8
Myelogenous — *see* condition
Myeloid — *see* condition
Myelokathexis 288.0
Myeloleukodystrophy 330.0
Myelolipoma (M8870/0) — *see* Neoplasm, by site,
    benign
Myeloma (multiple) (plasma cell) (plasmacytic)
    (M9730/3) 203.0 ✓5ᵗʰ
  monostotic (M9731/1) 238.6
  solitary (M9731/1) 238.6
Myelomalacia 336.8
Myelomata, multiple (M9730/3) 203.0 ✓5ᵗʰ
Myelomatosis (M9730/3) 203.0 ✓5ᵗʰ
Myelomeningitis — *see* Meningoencephalitis
Myelomeningocele (spinal cord) (*see also* Spina
    bifida) 741.9 ✓5ᵗʰ
  fetal, causing fetopelvic disproportion 653.7 ✓5ᵗʰ
Myelo-osteo-musculodysplasia hereditaria
    756.89
Myelopathic — *see* condition
Myelopathy (spinal cord) 336.9
  cervical 721.1
  diabetic 250.6 ✓5ᵗʰ *[336.3]*
  drug-induced 336.8
  due to or with
    carbon tetrachloride 987.8 *[323.7]*
    degeneration or displacement, intervertebral
      disc 722.70
        cervical, cervicothoracic 722.71
        lumbar, lumbosacral 722.73
        thoracic, thoracolumbar 722.72
    hydroxyquinoline derivatives 961.3 *[323.7]*
    infection — *see* Encephalitis
    intervertebral disc disorder 722.70
      cervical, cervicothoracic 722.71
      lumbar, lumbosacral 722.73
      thoracic, thoracolumbar 722.72
    lead 984.9 *[323.7]*
    mercury 985.0 *[323.7]*
    neoplastic disease (*see also* Neoplasm, by
      site) 239.9 *[336.3]*
    pernicious anemia 281.0 *[336.3]*
    spondylosis 721.91
      cervical 721.1
      lumbar, lumbosacral 721.42
      thoracic 721.41
    thallium 985.8 *[323.7]*
  lumbar, lumbosacral 721.42
  necrotic (subacute) 336.1
  radiation-induced 336.8

Myelopathy — *continued*
  spondylogenic NEC 721.91
    cervical 721.1
    lumbar, lumbosacral 721.42
    thoracic 721.41
  toxic NEC 989.9 *[323.7]*
  transverse (*see also* Encephalitis) 323.9
  vascular 336.1
Myeloproliferative disease (M9960/1) 238.7
Myeloradiculitis (*see also* Polyneuropathy) 357.0
Myeloradiculodysplasia (spinal) 742.59
Myelosarcoma (M9930/3) 205.3 ✓5ᵗʰ
Myelosclerosis 289.8
  with myeloid metaplasia (M9961/1) 238.7
  disseminated, of nervous system 340
  megakaryocytic (M9961/1) 238.7
Myelosis (M9860/3) (*see also* Leukemia, myeloid)
    205.9 ✓5ᵗʰ
  acute (M9861/3) 205.0 ✓5ᵗʰ
  aleukemic (M9864/3) 205.8 ✓5ᵗʰ
  chronic (M9863/3) 205.1 ✓5ᵗʰ
  erythremic (M9840/3) 207.0 ✓5ᵗʰ
    acute (M9841/3) 207.0 ✓5ᵗʰ
  megakaryocytic (M9920/3) 207.2 ✓5ᵗʰ
  nonleukemic (chronic) 288.8
  subacute (M9862/3) 205.2 ✓5ᵗʰ
Myesthenia — *see* Myasthenia
Myiasis (cavernous) 134.0
  orbit 134.0 *[376.13]*
Myoadenoma, prostate 600.2
Myoblastoma
  granular cell (M9580/0) — *see also* Neoplasm,
    connective tissue, benign
  malignant (M9580/3) — *see* Neoplasm,
    connective tissue, malignant
  tongue (M9580/0) 210.1
Myocardial — *see* condition
Myocardiopathy (congestive) (constrictive)
    (familial) (hypertrophic nonobstructive)
    (idiopathic) (infiltrative) (obstructive)
    (primary) (restrictive) (sporadic) 425.4
  alcoholic 425.5
  amyloid 277.3 *[425.7]*
  beriberi 265.0 *[425.7]*
  cobalt-beer 425.5
  due to
    amyloidosis 277.3 *[425.7]*
    beriberi 265.0 *[425.7]*
    cardiac glycogenosis 271.0 *[425.7]*
    Chagas' disease 086.0
    Friedreich's ataxia 334.0 *[425.8]*
    influenza 487.8 *[425.8]*
    mucopolysaccharidosis 277.5 *[425.7]*
    myotonia atrophica 359.2 *[425.8]*
    progressive muscular dystrophy 359.1
      [425.8]
    sarcoidosis 135 *[425.8]*
  glycogen storage 271.0 *[425.7]*
  hypertrophic obstructive 425.1
  metabolic NEC 277.9 *[425.7]*
  nutritional 269.9 *[425.7]*
  obscure (African) 425.2
  postpartum 674.8 ✓5ᵗʰ
  secondary 425.9
  thyrotoxic (*see also* Thyrotoxicosis)
    242.9 ✓5ᵗʰ *[425.7]*
  toxic NEC 425.9
Myocarditis (fibroid) (interstitial) (old)
    (progressive) (senile) (with arteriosclerosis)
    429.0
  with
    rheumatic fever (conditions classifiable to
      390) 398.0
      active (*see also* Myocarditis, acute,
        rheumatic) 391.2
      inactive or quiescent (with chorea) 398.0
  active (nonrheumatic) 422.90
    rheumatic 391.2
      with chorea (acute) (rheumatic)
        (Sydenham's) 392.0
  acute or subacute (interstitial) 422.90
    due to Streptococcus (beta-hemolytic) 391.2
    idiopathic 422.91

Myocarditis — *continued*
  acute or subacute — *continued*
    rheumatic 391.2
      with chorea (acute) (rheumatic)
        (Sydenham's) 392.0
    specified type NEC 422.99
  aseptic of newborn 074.23
  bacterial (acute) 422.92
  chagasic 086.0
  chronic (interstitial) 429.0
  congenital 746.89
  constrictive 425.4
  Coxsackie (virus) 074.23
  diphtheritic 032.82
  due to or in
    Coxsackie (virus) 074.23
    diphtheria 032.82
    epidemic louse-borne typhus 080 *[422.0]*
    influenza 487.8 *[422.0]*
    Lyme disease 088.81 *[422.0]*
    scarlet fever 034.1 *[422.0]*
    toxoplasmosis (acquired) 130.3
    tuberculosis (*see also* Tuberculosis)
      017.9 ✓5ᵗʰ *[422.0]*
    typhoid 002.0 *[422.0]*
    typhus NEC 081.9 *[422.0]*
  eosinophilic 422.91
  epidemic of newborn 074.23
  Fiedler's (acute) (isolated) (subacute) 422.91
  giant cell (acute) (subacute) 422.91
  gonococcal 098.85
  granulomatous (idiopathic) (isolated)
    (nonspecific) 422.91
  hypertensive (*see also* Hypertension, heart)
    402.90
  idiopathic 422.91
    granulomatous 422.91
  infective 422.92
  influenzal 487.8 *[422.0]*
  isolated (diffuse) (granulomatous) 422.91
  malignant 422.99
  meningococcal 036.43
  nonrheumatic, active 422.90
  parenchymatous 422.90
  pneumococcal (acute) (subacute) 422.92
  rheumatic (chronic) (inactive) (with chorea)
    398.0
    active or acute 391.2
      with chorea (acute) (rheumatic)
        (Sydenham's) 392.0
  septic 422.92
  specific (giant cell) (productive) 422.91
  staphylococcal (acute) (subacute) 422.92
  suppurative 422.92
  syphilitic (chronic) 093.82
  toxic 422.93
    rheumatic (*see also* Myocarditis, acute
      rheumatic) 391.2
  tuberculous (*see also* Tuberculosis)
    017.9 ✓5ᵗʰ *[422.0]*
  typhoid 002.0 *[422.0]*
  valvular — *see* Endocarditis
  viral, except Coxsackie 422.91
    Coxsackie 074.23
    of newborn (Coxsackie) 074.23
Myocardium, myocardial — *see* condition
Myocardosis (*see also* Cardiomyopathy) 425.4
Myoclonia (essential) 333.2
  epileptica 333.2
  Friedrich's 333.2
  massive 333.2
Myoclonic
  epilepsy, familial (progressive) 333.2
  jerks 333.2
Myoclonus (familial essential) (multifocal)
    (simplex) 333.2
  facial 351.8
  massive (infantile) 333.2
  pharyngeal 478.29
Myodiastasis 728.84
Myoendocarditis — *see also* Endocarditis
  acute or subacute 421.9
Myoepithelioma (M8982/0) — *see* Neoplasm, by
    site, benign
Myofascitis (acute) 729.1
  low back 724.2

Myofibroma

Myofibroma (M8890/0) — see also Neoplasm, connective tissue, benign
   uterus (cervix) (corpus) (see also Leiomyoma) 218.9
Myofibrosis 728.2
   heart (see also Myocarditis) 429.0
   humeroscapular region 726.2
   scapulohumeral 726.2
Myofibrositis (see also Myositis) 729.1
   scapulohumeral 726.2
Myogelosis (occupational) 728.89
Myoglobinuria 791.3
Myoglobulinuria, primary 791.3
Myokymia — see also Myoclonus
   facial 351.8
Myolipoma (M8860/0)
   specified site — see Neoplasm, connective tissue, benign
   unspecified site 223.0
Myoma (M8895/0) — see also Neoplasm, connective tissue, benign
   cervix (stump) (uterus) (see also Leiomyoma) 218.9
   malignant (M8895/3) — see Neoplasm, connective tissue, malignant
   prostate 600.2
   uterus (cervix) (corpus) (see also Leiomyoma) 218.9
      in pregnancy or childbirth 654.1 ✓5ᵗʰ
         affecting fetus or newborn 763.89
         causing obstructed labor 660.2 ✓5ᵗʰ
            affecting fetus or newborn 763.1
Myomalacia 728.9
   cordis, heart (see also Degeneration, myocardial) 429.1
Myometritis (see also Endometritis) 615.9
Myometrium — see condition
Myonecrosis, clostridial 040.0
Myopathy 359.9
   alcoholic 359.4
   amyloid 277.3 [359.6]
   benign congenital 359.0
   central core 359.0
   centronuclear 359.0
   congenital (benign) 359.0
   critical illness 359.81 ●
   distal 359.1
   due to drugs 359.4
   endocrine 259.9 [359.5]
      specified type NEC 259.8 [359.5]
   extraocular muscles 376.82
   facioscapulohumeral 359.1
   in
      Addison's disease 255.4 [359.5]
      amyloidosis 277.3 [359.6]
      cretinism 243 [359.5]
      Cushing's syndrome 255.0 [359.5]
      disseminated lupus erythematosus 710.0 [359.6]
      giant cell arteritis 446.5 [359.6]
      hyperadrenocorticism NEC 255.3 [359.5]
      hyperparathyroidism 252.0 [359.5]
      hypopituitarism 253.2 [359.5]
      hypothyroidism (see also Hypothyroidism) 244.9 [359.5]
      malignant neoplasm NEC (M8000/3) 199.1 [359.6]
      myxedema (see also Myxedema) 244.9 [359.5]
      polyarteritis nodosa 446.0 [359.6]
      rheumatoid arthritis 714.0 [359.6]
      sarcoidosis 135 [359.6]
      scleroderma 710.1 [359.6]
      Sjögren's disease 710.2 [359.6]
      thyrotoxicosis (see also Thyrotoxicosis) 242.9 ✓5ᵗʰ [359.5]
   inflammatory 359.89 ▲
   intensive care (ICU) 359.81 ●
   limb-girdle 359.1
   myotubular 359.0
   necrotizing, acute 359.81 ●
   nemaline 359.0
   ocular 359.1
   oculopharyngeal 359.1
   of critical illness 359.81 ●

Myopathy — continued
   primary 359.89 ▲
   progressive NEC 359.89 ▲
   quadriplegic, acute 359.81 ●
   rod body 359.0
   scapulohumeral 359.1
   specified type NEC 359.89 ▲
   toxic 359.4
Myopericarditis (see also Pericarditis) 423.9
Myopia (axial) (congenital) (increased curvature or refraction, nucleus of lens) 367.1
   degenerative, malignant 360.21
   malignant 360.21
   progressive high (degenerative) 360.21
Myosarcoma (M8895/3) — see Neoplasm, connective tissue, malignant
Myosis (persistent) 379.42
   stromal (endolymphatic) (M8931/1) 236.0
Myositis 729.1
   clostridial 040.0
   due to posture 729.1
   epidemic 074.1
   fibrosa or fibrous (chronic) 728.2
      Volkmann's (complicating trauma) 958.6
   infective 728.0
   interstitial 728.81
   multiple — see Polymyositis
   occupational 729.1
   orbital, chronic 376.12
   ossificans 728.12
      circumscribed 728.12
      progressive 728.11
      traumatic 728.12
   progressive fibrosing 728.11
   purulent 728.0
   rheumatic 729.1
   rheumatoid 729.1
   suppurative 728.0
   syphilitic 095.6
   traumatic (old) 729.1
Myospasia impulsiva 307.23
Myotonia (acquisita) (intermittens) 728.85
   atrophica 359.2
   congenita 359.2
   dystrophica 359.2
Myotonic pupil 379.46
Myriapodiasis 134.1
Myringitis
   with otitis media — see Otitis media
   acute 384.00
      specified type NEC 384.09
   bullosa hemorrhagica 384.01
   bullous 384.01
   chronic 384.1
Mysophobia 300.29
Mytilotoxism 988.0
Myxadenitis labialis 528.5
Myxedema (adult) (idiocy) (infantile) (juvenile) (thyroid gland) (see also Hypothyroidism) 244.9
   circumscribed 242.9 ✓5ᵗʰ
   congenital 243
   cutis 701.8
   localized (pretibial) 242.9 ✓5ᵗʰ
   madness (acute) 293.0
      subacute 293.1
   papular 701.8
   pituitary 244.8
   postpartum 674.8 ✓5ᵗʰ
   pretibial 242.9 ✓5ᵗʰ
   primary 244.9
Myxochondrosarcoma (M9220/3) — see Neoplasm, cartilage, malignant
Myxofibroma (M8811/0) — see also Neoplasm, connective tissue, benign
   odontogenic (M9320/0) 213.1
   upper jaw (bone) 213.0
Myxofibrosarcoma (M8811/3) — see Neoplasm, connective tissue, malignant
Myxolipoma (M8852/0) (see also Lipoma, by site) 214.9
Myxoliposarcoma (M8852/3) — see Neoplasm, connective tissue, malignant

Myxoma (M8840/0) — see also Neoplasm, connective tissue, benign
   odontogenic (M9320/0) 213.1
   upper jaw (bone) 213.0
Myxosarcoma (M8840/3) — see Neoplasm, connective tissue, malignant

N

Naegeli's
   disease (hereditary hemorrhagic thrombasthenia) 287.1
   leukemia, monocytic (M9863/3) 205.1 ✓5ᵗʰ
   syndrome (incontinentia pigmenti) 757.33
Naffziger's syndrome 353.0
Naga sore (see also Ulcer, skin) 707.9
Nägele's pelvis 738.6
   with disproportion (fetopelvic) 653.0 ✓5ᵗʰ
      affecting fetus or newborn 763.1
      causing obstructed labor 660.1 ✓5ᵗʰ
         affecting fetus or newborn 763.1
Nager-de Reynier syndrome (dysostosis mandibularis) 756.0
Nail — see also condition
   biting 307.9
   patella syndrome (hereditary osteoonychodysplasia) 756.89
Nanism, nonosomia (see also Dwarfism) 259.4
   hypophyseal 253.3
   pituitary 253.3
   renis, renalis 588.0
Nanukayami 100.89
Napkin rash 691.0
Narcissism 301.81
Narcolepsy 347
Narcosis
   carbon dioxide (respiratory) 786.09
   due to drug
      correct substance properly administered 780.09
      overdose or wrong substance given or taken 977.9
         specified drug — see Table of Drugs and Chemicals
Narcotism (chronic) (see also listing under Dependence) 304.9 ✓5ᵗʰ
   acute
      correct substance properly administered 349.82
      overdose or wrong substance given or taken 967.8
         specified drug — see Table of Drugs and Chemicals
Narrow
   anterior chamber angle 365.02
   pelvis (inlet) (outlet) — see Contraction, pelvis
Narrowing
   artery NEC 447.1
      auditory, internal 433.8 ✓5ᵗʰ
      basilar 433.0 ✓5ᵗʰ
         with other precerebral artery 433.3 ✓5ᵗʰ
         bilateral 433.3 ✓5ᵗʰ
      carotid 433.1 ✓5ᵗʰ
         with other precerebral artery 433.3 ✓5ᵗʰ
         bilateral 433.3 ✓5ᵗʰ
      cerebellar 433.8 ✓5ᵗʰ
      choroidal 433.8 ✓5ᵗʰ
      communicating posterior 433.8 ✓5ᵗʰ
      coronary — see also Arteriosclerosis, coronary
         congenital 746.85
         due to syphilis 090.5
      hypophyseal 433.8 ✓5ᵗʰ
      pontine 433.8 ✓5ᵗʰ
      precerebral NEC 433.9 ✓5ᵗʰ
         multiple or bilateral 433.3 ✓5ᵗʰ
         specified NEC 433.8 ✓5ᵗʰ
      vertebral 433.2 ✓5ᵗʰ
         with other precerebral artery 433.3 ✓5ᵗʰ
         bilateral 433.3 ✓5ᵗʰ
   auditory canal (external) (see also Stricture, ear canal, acquired) 380.50
   cerebral arteries 437.0
   cicatricial — see Cicatrix

Narrowing — *continued*
  congenital — *see* Anomaly, congenital
  coronary artery — *see* Narrowing, artery, coronary
  ear, middle 385.22
  Eustachian tube (*see also* Obstruction, Eustachian tube) 381.60
  eyelid 374.46
    congenital 743.62
  intervertebral disc or space NEC — *see* Degeneration, intervertebral disc
  joint space, hip 719.85
  larynx 478.74
  lids 374.46
    congenital 743.62
  mesenteric artery (with gangrene) 557.0
  palate 524.8
  palpebral fissure 374.46
  retinal artery 362.13
  ureter 593.3
  urethra (*see also* Stricture, urethra) 598.9
Narrowness, abnormal, eyelid 743.62
Nasal — *see* condition
Nasolacrimal — *see* condition
Nasopharyngeal — *see also* condition
  bursa 478.29
  pituitary gland 759.2
  torticollis 723.5
Nasopharyngitis (acute) (infective) (subacute) 460
  chronic 472.2
    due to external agent — *see* Condition, respiratory, chronic, due to
  due to external agent — *see* Condition, respiratory, due to
  septic 034.0
  streptococcal 034.0
  suppurative (chronic) 472.2
  ulcerative (chronic) 472.2
Nasopharynx, nasopharyngeal — *see* condition
Natal tooth, teeth 520.6
Nausea (*see also* Vomiting) 787.02
  with vomiting 787.01
  epidemic 078.82
  gravidarum — *see* Hyperemesis, gravidarum
  marina 994.6
Navel — *see* condition
Neapolitan fever (*see also* Brucellosis) 023.9
Nearsightedness 367.1
Near-syncope 780.2
Nebécourt's syndrome 253.3
Nebula, cornea (eye) 371.01
  congenital 743.43
    interfering with vision 743.42
Necator americanus infestation 126.1
Necatoriasis 126.1
Neck — *see* condition
Necrencephalus (*see also* Softening, brain) 437.8
Necrobacillosis 040.3
Necrobiosis 799.8
  brain or cerebral (*see also* Softening, brain) 437.8
  lipoidica 709.3
    diabeticorum 250.8 [709.3]
Necrodermolysis 695.1
Necrolysis, toxic epidermal 695.1
  due to drug
    correct substance properly administered 695.1
    overdose or wrong substance given or taken 977.9
      specified drug — *see* Table of Drugs and Chemicals
Necrophilia 302.89
Necrosis, necrotic
  adrenal (capsule) (gland) 255.8
  antrum, nasal sinus 478.1
  aorta (hyaline) (*see also* Aneurysm, aorta) 441.9
    cystic medial 441.00
      abdominal 441.02
      thoracic 441.01
      thoracoabdominal 441.03
    ruptured 441.5

Necrosis, necrotic — *continued*
  arteritis 446.0
  artery 447.5
  aseptic, bone 733.40
    femur (head) (neck) 733.42
      medial condyle 733.43
    humoral head 733.41
    medial femoral condyle 733.43
    specific site NEC 733.49
    talus 733.44
  avascular, bone NEC (*see also* Necrosis, aseptic, bone) 733.40
  bladder (aseptic) (sphincter) 596.8
  bone (*see also* Osteomyelitis) 730.1
    acute 730.0
    aseptic or avascular 733.40
      femur (head) (neck) 733.42
        medial condyle 733.43
      humoral head 733.41
      medial femoral condyle 733.43
      specified site NEC 733.49
      talus 733.44
    ethmoid 478.1
    ischemic 733.40
    jaw 526.4
    marrow 289.8
    Paget's (osteitis deformans) 731.0
    tuberculous — *see* Tuberculosis, bone
  brain (softening) (*see also* Softening, brain) 437.8
  breast (aseptic) (fat) (segmental) 611.3
  bronchus, bronchi 519.1
  central nervous system NEC (*see also* Softening, brain) 437.8
  cerebellar (*see also* Softening, brain) 437.8
  cerebral (softening) (*see also* Softening, brain) 437.8
  cerebrospinal (softening) (*see also* Softening, brain) 437.8
  cornea (*see also* Keratitis) 371.40
  cortical, kidney 583.6
  cystic medial (aorta) 441.00
    abdominal 441.02
    thoracic 441.01
    thoracoabdominal 441.03
  dental 521.09
    pulp 522.1
  due to swallowing corrosive substance — *see* Burn, by site
  ear (ossicle) 385.24
  esophagus 530.89
  ethmoid (bone) 478.1
  eyelid 374.50
  fat, fatty (generalized) (*see also* Degeneration, fatty) 272.8
    breast (aseptic) (segmental) 611.3
    intestine 569.89
    localized — *see* Degeneration, by site, fatty
    mesentery 567.8
    omentum 567.8
    pancreas 577.8
    peritoneum 567.8
    skin (subcutaneous) 709.3
      newborn 778.1
  femur (aseptic) (avascular) 733.42
    head 733.42
    medial condyle 733.43
    neck 733.42
  gallbladder (*see also* Cholecystitis, acute) 575.0
  gangrenous 785.4
  gastric 537.89
  glottis 478.79
  heart (myocardium) — *see* Infarct, myocardium
  hepatic (*see also* Necrosis, liver) 570
  hip (aseptic) (avascular) 733.42
  intestine (acute) (hemorrhagic) (massive) 557.0
  ischemic 785.4
  jaw 526.4
  kidney (bilateral) 583.9
    acute 584.9
    cortical 583.6
      acute 584.6
        with
          abortion — *see* Abortion, by type, with renal failure
          ectopic pregnancy (*see also* categories 633.0-633.9) 639.3

Necrosis, necrotic — *continued*
  kidney — *continued*
    cortical — *continued*
      acute — *continued*
        with — *continued*
          molar pregnancy (*see also* categories 630-632) 639.3
        complicating pregnancy 646.2
          affecting fetus or newborn 760.1
        following labor and delivery 669.3
    medullary (papillary) (*see also* Pyelitis) 590.80
      in
        acute renal failure 584.7
        nephritis, nephropathy 583.7
    papillary (*see also* Pyelitis) 590.80
      in
        acute renal failure 584.7
        nephritis, nephropathy 583.7
    tubular 584.5
      with
        abortion — *see* Abortion, by type, with renal failure
        ectopic pregnancy (*see also* categories 633.0-633.9) 639.3
        molar pregnancy (*see also* categories 630-632) 639.3
      complicating
        abortion 639.3
        ectopic or molar pregnancy 639.3
        pregnancy 646.2
          affecting fetus or newborn 760.1
        following labor and delivery 669.3
      traumatic 958.5
  larynx 478.79
  liver (acute) (congenital) (diffuse) (massive) (subacute) 570
    with
      abortion — *see* Abortion, by type, with specified complication NEC
      ectopic pregnancy (*see also* categories 633.0-633.9) 639.8
      molar pregnancy (*see also* categories 630-632) 639.8
    complicating pregnancy 646.7
      affecting fetus or newborn 760.8
    following
      abortion 639.8
      ectopic or molar pregnancy 639.8
    obstetrical 646.7
    postabortal 639.8
    puerperal, postpartum 674.8
    toxic 573.3
  lung 513.0
  lymphatic gland 683
  mammary gland 611.3
  mastoid (chronic) 383.1
  mesentery 557.0
    fat 567.8
  mitral valve — *see* Insufficiency, mitral
  myocardium, myocardial — *see* Infarct, myocardium
  nose (septum) 478.1
  omentum 557.0
    with mesenteric infarction 557.0
    fat 567.8
  orbit, orbital 376.10
  ossicles, ear (aseptic) 385.24
  ovary (*see also* Salpingo-oophoritis) 614.2
  pancreas (aseptic) (duct) (fat) 577.8
    acute 577.0
    infective 577.0
  papillary, kidney (*see also* Pyelitis) 590.80
  peritoneum 557.0
    with mesenteric infarction 557.0
    fat 567.8
  pharynx 462
    in granulocytopenia 288.0
  phosphorus 983.9
  pituitary (gland) (postpartum) (Sheehan) 253.2
  placenta (*see also* Placenta, abnormal) 656.7
  pneumonia 513.0
  pulmonary 513.0
  pulp (dental) 522.1
  pylorus 537.89
  radiation — *see* Necrosis, by site

Necrosis, necrotic — continued
    radium — *see* Necrosis, by site
    renal — *see* Necrosis, kidney
    sclera 379.19
    scrotum 608.89
    skin or subcutaneous tissue 709.8
        due to burn — *see* Burn, by site
        gangrenous 785.4
    spine, spinal (column) 730.18
        acute 730.18
        cord 336.1
    spleen 289.59
    stomach 537.89
    stomatitis 528.1
    subcutaneous fat 709.3
        fetus or newborn 778.1
    subendocardial — *see* Infarct, myocardium
    suprarenal (capsule) (gland) 255.8
    teeth, tooth 521.09
    testis 608.89
    thymus (gland) 254.8
    tonsil 474.8
    trachea 519.1
    tuberculous NEC — *see* Tuberculosis
    tubular (acute) (anoxic) (toxic) 584.5
        due to a procedure 997.5
    umbilical cord, affecting fetus or newborn 762.6
    vagina 623.8
    vertebra (lumbar) 730.18
        acute 730.18
        tuberculous (*see also* Tuberculosis) 015.0 [730.8]
    vesical (aseptic) (bladder) 596.8
    x-ray — *see* Necrosis, by site

Necrospermia 606.0

Necrotizing angiitis 446.0

Negativism 301.7

Neglect (child) (newborn) NEC 995.52
    adult 995.84
    after or at birth 995.52
    hemispatial 781.8
    left-sided 781.8
    sensory 781.8
    visuospatial 781.8

Negri bodies 071

Neill-Dingwall syndrome (microcephaly and dwarfism) 759.89

Neisserian infection NEC — *see* Gonococcus

Nematodiasis NEC (*see also* Infestation, Nematode) 127.9
    ancylostoma (*see also* Ancylostomiasis) 126.9

Neoformans cryptococcus infection 117.5

Neonatal — *see also* condition
    teeth, tooth 520.6

Neonatorum — *see* condition

Index to Diseases — Neoplasm, arachnoid

	Malignant			Benign	Uncertain Behavior	Unspecified
	Primary	Secondary	Ca in situ			
Neoplasm, neoplastic	199.1	199.1	234.9	229.9	238.9	239.9

Notes — 1. The list below gives the code numbers for neoplasms by anatomical site. For each site there are six possible code numbers according to whether the neoplasm in question is malignant, benign, in situ, of uncertain behavior, or of unspecified nature. The description of the neoplasm will often indicate which of the six columns is appropriate; e.g., malignant melanoma of skin, benign fibroadenoma of breast, carcinoma in situ of cervix uteri.

Where such descriptors are not present, the remainder of the Index should be consulted where guidance is given to the appropriate column for each morphological (histological) variety listed; e.g., Mesonephroma — see Neoplasm, malignant; Embryoma — see also Neoplasm, uncertain behavior; Disease, Bowen's — see Neoplasm, skin, in situ. However, the guidance in the Index can be overridden if one of the descriptors mentioned above is present; e.g., malignant adenoma of colon is coded to 153.9 and not to 211.3 as the adjective "malignant" overrides the Index entry "Adenoma — see also Neoplasm, benign."

2. Sites marked with the sign * (e.g., face NEC*) should be classified to malignant neoplasm of skin of these sites if the variety of neoplasm is a squamous cell carcinoma or an epidermoid carcinoma, and to benign neoplasm of skin of these sites if the variety of neoplasm is a papilloma (any type).

Site	Primary	Secondary	Ca in situ	Benign	Uncertain Behavior	Unspecified
abdomen, abdominal	195.2	198.89	234.8	229.8	238.8	239.8
cavity	195.2	198.89	234.8	229.8	238.8	239.8
organ	195.2	198.89	234.8	229.8	238.8	239.8
viscera	195.2	198.89	234.8	229.8	238.8	239.8
wall	173.5	198.2	232.5	216.5	238.2	239.2
connective tissue	171.5	198.89	—	215.5	238.1	239.2
abdominopelvic	195.8	198.89	234.8	229.8	238.8	239.8
accessory sinus — see Neoplasm, sinus						
acoustic nerve	192.0	198.4	—	225.1	237.9	239.7
acromion (process)	170.4	198.5	—	213.4	238.0	239.2
adenoid (pharynx) (tissue)	147.1	198.89	230.0	210.7	235.1	239.0
adipose tissue (see also Neoplasm, connective tissue)	171.9	198.89	—	215.9	238.1	239.2
adnexa (uterine)	183.9	198.82	233.3	221.8	236.3	239.5
adrenal (cortex) (gland) (medulla)	194.0	198.7	234.8	227.0	237.2	239.7
ala nasi (external)	173.3	198.2	232.3	216.3	238.2	239.2
alimentary canal or tract NEC	159.9	197.8	230.9	211.9	235.5	239.0
alveolar	143.9	198.89	230.0	210.4	235.1	239.0
mucosa	143.9	198.89	230.0	210.4	235.1	239.0
lower	143.1	198.89	230.0	210.4	235.1	239.0
upper	143.0	198.89	230.0	210.4	235.1	239.0
ridge or process	170.1	198.5	—	213.1	238.0	239.2
carcinoma	143.9	—	—	—	—	—
lower	143.1	—	—	—	—	—
upper	143.0	—	—	—	—	—
lower	170.1	198.5	—	213.1	238.0	239.2
mucosa	143.9	198.89	230.0	210.4	235.1	239.0
lower	143.1	198.89	230.0	210.4	235.1	239.0
upper	143.0	198.89	230.0	210.4	235.1	239.0
upper	170.0	198.5	—	213.0	238.0	239.2
sulcus	145.1	198.89	230.0	210.4	235.1	239.0
alveolus	143.9	198.89	230.0	210.4	235.1	239.0
lower	143.1	198.89	230.0	210.4	235.1	239.0
upper	143.0	198.89	230.0	210.4	235.1	239.0
ampulla of Vater	156.2	197.8	230.8	211.5	235.3	239.0
ankle NEC*	195.5	198.89	232.7	229.8	238.8	239.8
anorectum, anorectal (junction)	154.8	197.5	230.7	211.4	235.2	239.0
antecubital fossa or space*	195.4	198.89	232.6	229.8	238.8	239.8
antrum (Highmore) (maxillary)	160.2	197.3	231.8	212.0	235.9	239.1
pyloric	151.2	197.8	230.2	211.1	235.2	239.0
tympanicum	160.1	197.3	231.8	212.0	235.9	239.1
anus, anal	154.3	197.5	230.6	211.4	235.5	239.0
canal	154.2	197.5	230.5	211.4	233.5	239.0
contiguous sites with rectosigmoid junction or rectum	154.8	—	—	—	—	—
margin	173.5	198.2	232.5	216.5	238.2	239.2
skin	173.5	198.2	232.5	216.5	238.2	239.2
sphincter	154.2	197.5	230.5	211.4	235.5	239.0
aorta (thoracic)	171.4	198.89	—	215.4	238.1	239.2
abdominal	171.5	198.89	—	215.5	238.1	239.2
aortic body	194.6	198.89	—	227.6	237.3	239.7
aponeurosis	171.9	198.89	—	215.9	238.1	239.2
palmar	171.2	198.89	—	215.2	238.1	239.2
plantar	171.3	198.89	—	215.3	238.1	239.2
appendix	153.5	197.5	230.3	211.3	235.2	239.0
arachnoid (cerebral)	192.1	198.4	—	225.2	237.6	239.7
spinal	192.3	198.4	—	225.4	237.6	239.7

Neoplasm, areola

Index to Diseases

	Malignant			Benign	Uncertain Behavior	Unspecified
	Primary	Secondary	Ca in situ			
Neoplasm, neoplastic — *continued*						
areola (female)	174.0	198.81	233.0	217	238.3	239.3
male	175.0	198.81	233.0	217	238.3	239.3
arm NEC*	195.4	198.89	232.6	229.8	238.8	239.8
artery — *see* Neoplasm, connective tissue						
aryepiglottic fold	148.2	198.89	230.0	210.8	235.1	239.0
hypopharyngeal aspect	148.2	198.89	230.0	210.8	235.1	239.0
laryngeal aspect	161.1	197.3	231.0	212.1	235.6	239.1
marginal zone	148.2	198.89	230.0	210.8	235.1	239.0
arytenoid (cartilage)	161.3	197.3	231.0	212.1	235.6	239.1
fold — *see* Neoplasm, aryepiglottic						
atlas	170.2	198.5	—	213.2	238.0	239.2
atrium, cardiac	164.1	198.89	—	212.7	238.8	239.8
auditory						
canal (external) (skin)	173.2	198.2	232.2	216.2	238.2	239.2
internal	160.1	197.3	231.8	212.0	235.9	239.1
nerve	192.0	198.4	—	225.1	237.9	239.7
tube	160.1	197.3	231.8	212.0	235.9	239.1
opening	147.2	198.89	230.0	210.7	235.1	239.0
auricle, ear	173.2	198.2	232.2	216.2	238.2	239.2
cartilage	171.0	198.89	—	215.0	238.1	239.2
auricular canal (external)	173.2	198.2	232.2	216.2	238.2	239.2
internal	160.1	197.3	231.8	212.0	235.9	239.1
autonomic nerve or nervous system NEC	171.9	198.89	—	215.9	238.1	239.2
axilla, axillary	195.1	198.89	234.8	229.8	238.8	239.8
fold	173.5	198.2	232.5	216.5	238.2	239.2
back NEC*	195.8	198.89	232.5	229.8	238.8	239.8
Bartholin's gland	184.1	198.82	233.3	221.2	236.3	239.5
basal ganglia	191.0	198.3	—	225.0	237.5	239.6
basis pedunculi	191.7	198.3	—	225.0	237.5	239.6
bile or biliary (tract)	156.9	197.8	230.8	211.5	235.3	239.0
canaliculi (biliferi) (intrahepatic)	155.1	197.8	230.8	211.5	235.3	239.0
canals, interlobular	155.1	197.8	230.8	211.5	235.3	239.0
contiguous sites	156.8	—	—	—	—	—
duct or passage (common) (cystic) (extrahepatic)	156.1	197.8	230.8	211.5	235.3	239.0
contiguous sites with gallbladder	156.8	—	—	—	—	—
interlobular	155.1	197.8	230.8	211.5	235.3	239.0
intrahepatic	155.1	197.8	230.8	211.5	235.3	239.0
and extrahepatic	156.9	197.8	230.8	211.5	235.3	239.0
bladder (urinary)	188.9	198.1	233.7	223.3	236.7	239.4
contiguous sites	188.8	—	—	—	—	—
dome	188.1	198.1	233.7	223.3	236.7	239.4
neck	188.5	198.1	233.7	223.3	236.7	239.4
orifice	188.9	198.1	233.7	223.3	236.7	239.4
ureteric	188.6	198.1	233.7	223.3	236.7	239.4
urethral	188.5	198.1	233.7	223.3	236.7	239.4
sphincter	188.8	198.1	233.7	223.3	236.7	239.4
trigone	188.0	198.1	233.7	223.3	236.7	239.4
urachus	188.7	—	233.7	223.3	236.7	239.4
wall	188.9	198.1	233.7	223.3	236.7	239.4
anterior	188.3	198.1	233.7	223.3	236.7	239.4
lateral	188.2	198.1	233.7	223.3	236.7	239.4
posterior	188.4	198.1	233.7	223.3	236.7	239.4
blood vessel — *see* Neoplasm, connective tissue						
bone (periosteum)	170.9	198.5	—	213.9	238.0	239.2

Note — Carcinomas and adenocarcinomas, of any type other than intraosseous or odontogenic, of the sites listed under "Neoplasm, bone" should be considered as constituting metastatic spread from an unspecified primary site and coded to 198.5 for morbidity coding and to 199.1 for underlying cause of death coding.

acetabulum	170.6	198.5	—	213.6	238.0	239.2
acromion (process)	170.4	198.5	—	213.4	238.0	239.2
ankle	170.8	198.5	—	213.8	238.0	239.2
arm NEC	170.4	198.5	—	213.4	238.0	239.2
astragalus	170.8	198.5	—	213.8	238.0	239.2
atlas	170.2	198.5	—	213.2	238.0	239.2
axis	170.2	198.5	—	213.2	238.0	239.2
back NEC	170.2	198.5	—	213.2	238.0	239.2
calcaneus	170.8	198.5	—	213.8	238.0	239.2

Index to Diseases — Neoplasm, bone

	Malignant			Benign	Uncertain Behavior	Unspecified
	Primary	Secondary	Ca in situ			
Neoplasm, neoplastic — *continued*						
bone — *continued*						
calvarium	170.0	198.5	—	213.0	238.0	239.2
carpus (any)	170.5	198.5	—	213.5	238.0	239.2
cartilage NEC	170.9	198.5	—	213.9	238.0	239.2
clavicle	170.3	198.5	—	213.3	238.0	239.2
clivus	170.0	198.5	—	213.0	238.0	239.2
coccygeal vertebra	170.6	198.5	—	213.6	238.0	239.2
coccyx	170.6	198.5	—	213.6	238.0	239.2
costal cartilage	170.3	198.5	—	213.3	238.0	239.2
costovertebral joint	170.3	198.5	—	213.3	238.0	239.2
cranial	170.0	198.5	—	213.0	238.0	239.2
cuboid	170.8	198.5	—	213.8	238.0	239.2
cuneiform	170.9	198.5	—	213.9	238.0	239.2
ankle	170.8	198.5	—	213.8	238.0	239.2
wrist	170.5	198.5	—	213.5	238.0	239.2
digital	170.9	198.5	—	213.9	238.0	239.2
finger	170.5	198.5	—	213.5	238.0	239.2
toe	170.8	198.5	—	213.8	238.0	239.2
elbow	170.4	198.5	—	213.4	238.0	239.2
ethmoid (labyrinth)	170.0	198.5	—	213.0	238.0	239.2
face	170.0	198.5	—	213.0	238.0	239.2
lower jaw	170.1	198.5	—	213.1	238.0	239.2
femur (any part)	170.7	198.5	—	213.7	238.0	239.2
fibula (any part)	170.7	198.5	—	213.7	238.0	239.2
finger (any)	170.5	198.5	—	213.5	238.0	239.2
foot	170.8	198.5	—	213.8	238.0	239.2
forearm	170.4	198.5	—	213.4	238.0	239.2
frontal	170.0	198.5	—	213.0	238.0	239.2
hand	170.5	198.5	—	213.5	238.0	239.2
heel	170.8	198.5	—	213.8	238.0	239.2
hip	170.6	198.5	—	213.6	238.0	239.2
humerus (any part)	170.4	198.5	—	213.4	238.0	239.2
hyoid	170.0	198.5	—	213.0	238.0	239.2
ilium	170.6	198.5	—	213.6	238.0	239.2
innominate	170.6	198.5	—	213.6	238.0	239.2
intervertebral cartilage or disc	170.2	198.5	—	213.2	238.0	239.2
ischium	170.6	198.5	—	213.6	238.0	239.2
jaw (lower)	170.1	198.5	—	213.1	238.0	239.2
upper	170.0	198.5	—	213.0	238.0	239.2
knee	170.7	198.5	—	213.7	238.0	239.2
leg NEC	170.7	198.5	—	213.7	238.0	239.2
limb NEC	170.9	198.5	—	213.9	238.0	239.2
lower (long bones)	170.7	198.5	—	213.7	238.0	239.2
short bones	170.8	198.5	—	213.8	238.0	239.2
upper (long bones)	170.4	198.5	—	213.4	238.0	239.2
short bones	170.5	198.5	—	213.5	238.0	239.2
long	170.9	198.5	—	213.9	238.0	239.2
lower limbs NEC	170.7	198.5	—	213.7	238.0	239.2
upper limbs NEC	170.4	198.5	—	213.4	238.0	239.2
malar	170.0	198.5	—	213.0	238.0	239.2
mandible	170.1	198.5	—	213.1	238.0	239.2
marrow NEC	202.9 ✓5ᵗʰ	198.5	—	—	—	238.7
mastoid	170.0	198.5	—	213.0	238.0	239.2
maxilla, maxillary (superior)	170.0	198.5	—	213.0	238.0	239.2
inferior	170.1	198.5	—	213.1	238.0	239.2
metacarpus (any)	170.5	198.5	—	213.5	238.0	239.2
metatarsus (any)	170.8	198.5	—	213.8	238.0	239.2
navicular (ankle)	170.8	198.5	—	213.8	238.0	239.2
hand	170.5	198.5	—	213.5	238.0	239.2
nose, nasal	170.0	198.5	—	213.0	238.0	239.2
occipital	170.0	198.5	—	213.0	238.0	239.2
orbit	170.0	198.5	—	213.0	238.0	239.2
parietal	170.0	198.5	—	213.0	238.0	239.2
patella	170.8	198.5	—	213.8	238.0	239.2
pelvic	170.6	198.5	—	213.6	238.0	239.2

Neoplasm, bone

Index to Diseases

	Malignant			Benign	Uncertain Behavior	Unspecified
	Primary	Secondary	Ca in situ			
Neoplasm, neoplastic — *continued*						
bone — *continued*						
phalanges	170.9	198.5	—	213.9	238.0	239.2
foot	170.8	198.5	—	213.8	238.0	239.2
hand	170.5	198.5	—	213.5	238.0	239.2
pubic	170.6	198.5	—	213.6	238.0	239.2
radius (any part)	170.4	198.5	—	213.4	238.0	239.2
rib	170.3	198.5	—	213.3	238.0	239.2
sacral vertebra	170.6	198.5	—	213.6	238.0	239.2
sacrum	170.6	198.5	—	213.6	238.0	239.2
scaphoid (of hand)	170.5	198.5	—	213.5	238.0	239.2
of ankle	170.8	198.5	—	213.8	238.0	239.2
scapula (any part)	170.4	198.5	—	213.4	238.0	239.2
sella turcica	170.0	198.5	—	213.0	238.0	239.2
short	170.9	198.5	—	213.9	238.0	239.2
lower limb	170.8	198.5	—	213.8	238.0	239.2
upper limb	170.5	198.5	—	213.5	238.0	239.2
shoulder	170.4	198.5	—	213.4	238.0	239.2
skeleton, skeletal NEC	170.9	198.5	—	213.9	238.0	239.2
skull	170.0	198.5	—	213.0	238.0	239.2
sphenoid	170.0	198.5	—	213.0	238.0	239.2
spine, spinal (column)	170.2	198.5	—	213.2	238.0	239.2
coccyx	170.6	198.5	—	213.6	238.0	239.2
sacrum	170.6	198.5	—	213.6	238.0	239.2
sternum	170.3	198.5	—	213.3	238.0	239.2
tarsus (any)	170.8	198.5	—	213.8	238.0	239.2
temporal	170.0	198.5	—	213.0	238.0	239.2
thumb	170.5	198.5	—	213.5	238.0	239.2
tibia (any part)	170.7	198.5	—	213.7	238.0	239.2
toe (any)	170.8	198.5	—	213.8	238.0	239.2
trapezium	170.5	198.5	—	213.5	238.0	239.2
trapezoid	170.5	198.5	—	213.5	238.0	239.2
turbinate	170.0	198.5	—	213.0	238.0	239.2
ulna (any part)	170.4	198.5	—	213.4	238.0	239.2
unciform	170.5	198.5	—	213.5	238.0	239.2
vertebra (column)	170.2	198.5	—	213.2	238.0	239.2
coccyx	170.6	198.5	—	213.6	238.0	239.2
sacrum	170.6	198.5	—	213.6	238.0	239.2
vomer	170.0	198.5	—	213.0	238.0	239.2
wrist	170.5	198.5	—	213.5	238.0	239.2
xiphoid process	170.3	198.5	—	213.3	238.0	239.2
zygomatic	170.0	198.5	—	213.0	238.0	239.2
book-leaf (mouth)	145.8	198.89	230.0	210.4	235.1	239.0
bowel — *see* Neoplasm, intestine						
brachial plexus	171.2	198.89	—	215.2	238.1	239.2
brain NEC	191.9	198.3	—	225.0	237.5	239.6
basal ganglia	191.0	198.3	—	225.0	237.5	239.6
cerebellopontine angle	191.6	198.3	—	225.0	237.5	239.6
cerebellum NOS	191.6	198.3	—	225.0	237.5	239.6
cerebrum	191.0	198.3	—	225.0	237.5	239.6
choroid plexus	191.5	198.3	—	225.0	237.5	239.6
contiguous sites	191.8	—	—	—	—	—
corpus callosum	191.8	198.3	—	225.0	237.5	239.6
corpus striatum	191.0	198.3	—	225.0	237.5	239.6
cortex (cerebral)	191.0	198.3	—	225.0	237.5	239.6
frontal lobe	191.1	198.3	—	225.0	237.5	239.6
globus pallidus	191.0	198.3	—	225.0	237.5	239.6
hippocampus	191.2	198.3	—	225.0	237.5	239.6
hypothalamus	191.0	198.3	—	225.0	237.5	239.6
internal capsule	191.0	198.3	—	225.0	237.5	239.6
medulla oblongata	191.7	198.3	—	225.0	237.5	239.6
meninges	192.1	198.4	—	225.2	237.6	239.7
midbrain	191.7	198.3	—	225.0	237.5	239.6
occipital lobe	191.4	198.3	—	225.0	237.5	239.6
parietal lobe	191.3	198.3	—	225.0	237.5	239.6
peduncle	191.7	198.3	—	225.0	237.5	239.6
pons	191.7	198.3	—	225.0	237.5	239.6

Index to Diseases

Neoplasm, cardiac orifice

	Malignant			Benign	Uncertain Behavior	Unspecified
	Primary	Secondary	Ca in situ			
Neoplasm, neoplastic — *continued*						
brain NEC — *continued*						
stem	191.7	198.3	—	225.0	237.5	239.6
tapetum	191.8	198.3	—	225.0	237.5	239.6
temporal lobe	191.2	198.3	—	225.0	237.5	239.6
thalamus	191.0	198.3	—	225.0	237.5	239.6
uncus	191.2	198.3	—	225.0	237.5	239.6
ventricle (floor)	191.5	198.3	—	225.0	237.5	239.6
branchial (cleft) (vestiges)	146.8	198.89	230.0	210.6	235.1	239.0
breast (connective tissue) (female) (glandular tissue) (soft parts)	174.9	198.81	233.0	217	238.3	239.3
areola	174.0	198.81	233.0	217	238.3	239.3
male	175.0	198.81	233.0	217	238.3	239.3
axillary tail	174.6	198.81	233.0	217	238.3	239.3
central portion	174.1	198.81	233.0	217	238.3	239.3
contiguous sites	174.8	—	—	—	—	—
ectopic sites	174.8	198.81	233.0	217	238.3	239.3
inner	174.8	198.81	233.0	217	238.3	239.3
lower	174.8	198.81	233.0	217	238.3	239.3
lower-inner quadrant	174.3	198.81	233.0	217	238.3	239.3
lower-outer quadrant	174.5	198.81	233.0	217	238.3	239.3
male	175.9	198.81	233.0	217	238.3	239.3
areola	175.0	198.81	233.0	217	238.3	239.3
ectopic tissue	175.9	198.81	233.0	217	238.3	239.3
nipple	175.0	198.81	233.0	217	238.3	239.3
mastectomy site (skin)	173.5	198.2	—	—	—	—
specified as breast tissue	174.8	198.81	—	—	—	—
midline	174.8	198.81	233.0	217	238.3	239.3
nipple	174.0	198.81	233.0	217	238.3	239.3
male	175.0	198.81	233.0	217	238.3	239.3
outer	174.8	198.81	233.0	217	238.3	239.3
skin	173.5	198.2	232.5	216.5	238.2	239.2
tail (axillary)	174.6	198.81	233.0	217	238.3	239.3
upper	174.8	198.81	233.0	217	238.3	239.3
upper-inner quadrant	174.2	198.81	233.0	217	238.3	239.3
upper-outer quadrant	174.4	198.81	233.0	217	238.3	239.3
broad ligament	183.3	198.82	233.3	221.0	236.3	239.5
bronchiogenic, bronchogenic (lung)	162.9	197.0	231.2	212.3	235.7	239.1
bronchiole	162.9	197.0	231.2	212.3	235.7	239.1
bronchus	162.9	197.0	231.2	212.3	235.7	239.1
carina	162.2	197.0	231.2	212.3	235.7	239.1
contiguous sites with lung or trachea	162.8	—	—	—	—	—
lower lobe of lung	162.5	197.0	231.2	212.3	235.7	239.1
main	162.2	197.0	231.2	212.3	235.7	239.1
middle lobe of lung	162.4	197.0	231.2	212.3	235.7	239.1
upper lobe of lung	162.3	197.0	231.2	212.3	235.7	239.1
brow	173.3	198.2	232.3	216.3	238.2	239.2
buccal (cavity)	145.9	198.89	230.0	210.4	235.1	239.0
commissure	145.0	198.89	230.0	210.4	235.1	239.0
groove (lower) (upper)	145.1	198.89	230.0	210.4	235.1	239.0
mucosa	145.0	198.89	230.0	210.4	235.1	239.0
sulcus (lower) (upper)	145.1	198.89	230.0	210.4	235.1	239.0
bulbourethral gland	189.3	198.1	233.9	223.81	236.99	239.5
bursa — *see* Neoplasm, connective tissue						
buttock NEC*	195.3	198.89	232.5	229.8	238.8	239.8
calf*	195.5	198.89	232.7	229.8	238.8	239.8
calvarium	170.0	198.5	—	213.0	238.0	239.2
calyx, renal	189.1	198.0	233.9	223.1	236.91	239.5
canal						
anal	154.2	197.5	230.5	211.4	235.5	239.0
auditory (external)	173.2	198.2	232.2	216.2	238.2	239.2
auricular (external)	173.2	198.2	232.2	216.2	238.2	239.2
canaliculi, biliary (biliferi) (intrahepatic)	155.1	197.8	230.8	211.5	235.3	239.0
canthus (eye) (inner) (outer)	173.1	198.2	232.1	216.1	238.2	239.2
capillary — *see* Neoplasm, connective tissue						
caput coli	153.4	197.5	230.3	211.3	235.2	239.0
cardia (gastric)	151.0	197.8	230.2	211.1	235.2	239.0
cardiac orifice (stomach)	151.0	197.8	230.2	211.1	235.2	239.0

	Malignant			Benign	Uncertain Behavior	Unspecified
	Primary	Secondary	Ca in situ			
Neoplasm, neoplastic — *continued*						
cardio-esophageal junction	151.0	197.8	230.2	211.1	235.2	239.0
cardio-esophagus	151.0	197.8	230.2	211.1	235.2	239.0
carina (trachea) (bronchus)	162.2	197.0	231.2	212.3	235.7	239.1
carotid (artery)	171.0	198.89	—	215.0	238.1	239.2
body	194.5	198.89	—	227.5	237.3	239.7
carpus (any bone)	170.5	198.5	—	213.5	238.0	239.2
cartilage (articular) (joint) NEC — *see also* Neoplasm, bone	170.9	198.5	—	213.9	238.0	239.2
arytenoid	161.3	197.3	231.0	212.1	235.6	239.1
auricular	171.0	198.89	—	215.0	238.1	239.2
bronchi	162.2	197.3	—	212.3	235.7	239.1
connective tissue — *see* Neoplasm, connective tissue						
costal	170.3	198.5	—	213.3	238.0	239.2
cricoid	161.3	197.3	231.0	212.1	235.6	239.1
cuneiform	161.3	197.3	231.0	212.1	235.6	239.1
ear (external)	171.0	198.89	—	215.0	238.1	239.2
ensiform	170.3	198.5	—	213.3	238.0	239.2
epiglottis	161.1	197.3	231.0	212.1	235.6	239.1
anterior surface	146.4	198.89	230.0	210.6	235.1	239.0
eyelid	171.0	198.89	—	215.0	238.1	239.2
intervertebral	170.2	198.5	—	213.2	238.0	239.2
larynx, laryngeal	161.3	197.3	231.0	212.1	235.6	239.1
nose, nasal	160.0	197.3	231.8	212.0	235.9	239.1
pinna	171.0	198.89	—	215.0	238.1	239.2
rib	170.3	198.5	—	213.3	238.0	239.2
semilunar (knee)	170.7	198.5	—	213.7	238.0	239.2
thyroid	161.3	197.3	231.0	212.1	235.6	239.1
trachea	162.0	197.3	231.1	212.2	235.7	239.1
cauda equina	192.2	198.3	—	225.3	237.5	239.7
cavity						
buccal	145.9	198.89	230.0	210.4	235.1	239.0
nasal	160.0	197.3	231.8	212.0	235.9	239.1
oral	145.9	198.89	230.0	210.4	235.1	239.0
peritoneal	158.9	197.6	—	211.8	235.4	239.0
tympanic	160.1	197.3	231.8	212.0	235.9	239.1
cecum	153.4	197.5	230.3	211.3	235.2	239.0
central						
nervous system — *see* Neoplasm, nervous system						
white matter	191.0	198.3	—	225.0	237.5	239.6
cerebellopontine (angle)	191.6	198.3	—	225.0	237.5	239.6
cerebellum, cerebellar	191.6	198.3	—	225.0	237.5	239.6
cerebrum, cerebral (cortex) (hemisphere) (white matter)	191.0	198.3	—	225.0	237.5	239.6
meninges	192.1	198.4	—	225.2	237.6	239.7
peduncle	191.7	198.3	—	225.0	237.5	239.6
ventricle (any)	191.5	198.3	—	225.0	237.5	239.6
cervical region	195.0	198.89	234.8	229.8	238.8	239.8
cervix (cervical) (uteri) (uterus)	180.9	198.82	233.1	219.0	236.0	239.5
canal	180.0	198.82	233.1	219.0	236.0	239.5
contiguous sites	180.8	—	—	—	—	—
endocervix (canal) (gland)	180.0	198.82	233.1	219.0	236.0	239.5
exocervix	180.1	198.82	233.1	219.0	236.0	239.5
external os	180.1	198.82	233.1	219.0	236.0	239.5
internal os	180.0	198.82	233.1	219.0	236.0	239.5
nabothian gland	180.0	198.82	233.1	219.0	236.0	239.5
squamocolumnar junction	180.8	198.82	233.1	219.0	236.0	239.5
stump	180.8	198.82	233.1	219.0	236.0	239.5
cheek	195.0	198.89	234.8	229.8	238.8	239.8
external	173.3	198.2	232.3	216.3	238.2	239.2
inner aspect	145.0	198.89	230.0	210.4	235.1	239.0
internal	145.0	198.89	230.0	210.4	235.1	239.0
mucosa	145.0	198.89	230.0	210.4	235.1	239.0
chest (wall) NEC	195.1	198.89	234.8	229.8	238.8	239.8
chiasma opticum	192.0	198.4	—	225.1	237.9	239.7
chin	173.3	198.2	232.3	216.3	238.2	239.2
choana	147.3	198.89	230.0	210.7	235.1	239.0
cholangiole	155.1	197.8	230.8	211.5	235.3	239.0
choledochal duct	156.1	197.8	230.8	211.5	235.3	239.0

Index to Diseases — Neoplasm, connective tissue

	Malignant			Benign	Uncertain Behavior	Unspecified
	Primary	Secondary	Ca in situ			
Neoplasm, neoplastic — *continued*						
choroid	190.6	198.4	234.0	224.6	238.8	239.8
plexus	191.5	198.3	—	225.0	237.5	239.6
ciliary body	190.0	198.4	234.0	224.0	238.8	239.8
clavicle	170.3	198.5	—	213.3	238.0	239.2
clitoris	184.3	198.82	233.3	221.2	236.3	239.5
clivus	170.0	198.5	—	213.0	238.0	239.2
cloacogenic zone	154.8	197.5	230.7	211.4	235.5	239.0
coccygeal						
body or glomus	194.6	198.89	—	227.6	237.3	239.7
vertebra	170.6	198.5	—	213.6	238.0	239.2
coccyx	170.6	198.5	—	213.6	238.0	239.2
colon — *see also* Neoplasm, intestine, large						
and rectum	154.0	197.5	230.4	211.4	235.2	239.0
column, spinal — *see* Neoplasm, spine						
columnella	173.3	198.2	232.3	216.3	238.2	239.2
commissure						
labial, lip	140.6	198.89	230.0	210.4	235.1	239.0
laryngeal	161.0	197.3	231.0	212.1	235.6	239.1
common (bile) duct	156.1	197.8	230.8	211.5	235.3	239.0
concha	173.2	198.2	232.2	216.2	238.2	239.2
nose	160.0	197.3	231.8	212.0	235.9	239.1
conjunctiva	190.3	198.4	234.0	224.3	238.8	239.8
connective tissue NEC	171.9	198.89	—	215.9	238.1	239.2

Note — For neoplasms of connective tissue (blood vessel, bursa, fascia, ligament, muscle, peripheral nerves, sympathetic and parasympathetic nerves and ganglia, synovia, tendon, etc.) or of morphological types that indicate connective tissue, code according to the list under "Neoplasm, connective tissue"; for sites that do not appear in this list, code to neoplasm of that site; e.g.,

> liposarcoma, shoulder 171.2
> leiomyosarcoma, stomach 151.9
> neurofibroma, chest wall 215.4

Morphological types that indicate connective tissue appear in the proper place in the alphabetic index with the instruction "*see* Neoplasm, connective tissue..."

	Primary	Secondary	Ca in situ	Benign	Uncertain Behavior	Unspecified
abdomen	171.5	198.89	—	215.5	238.1	239.2
abdominal wall	171.5	198.89	—	215.5	238.1	239.2
ankle	171.3	198.89	—	215.3	238.1	239.2
antecubital fossa or space	171.2	198.89	—	215.2	238.1	239.2
arm	171.2	198.89	—	215.2	238.1	239.2
auricle (ear)	171.0	198.89	—	215.0	238.1	239.2
axilla	171.4	198.89	—	215.4	238.1	239.2
back	171.7	198.89	—	215.7	238.1	239.2
breast (female) (*see also* Neoplasm, breast)	174.9	198.81	233.0	217	238.3	239.3
male	175.9	198.81	233.0	217	238.3	239.3
buttock	171.6	198.89	—	215.6	238.1	239.2
calf	171.3	198.89	—	215.3	238.1	239.2
cervical region	171.0	198.89	—	215.0	238.1	239.2
cheek	171.0	198.89	—	215.0	238.1	239.2
chest (wall)	171.4	198.89	—	215.4	238.1	239.2
chin	171.0	198.89	—	215.0	238.1	239.2
contiguous sites	171.8	—	—	—	—	—
diaphragm	171.4	198.89	—	215.4	238.1	239.2
ear (external)	171.0	198.89	—	215.0	238.1	239.2
elbow	171.2	198.89	—	215.2	238.1	239.2
extrarectal	171.6	198.89	—	215.6	238.1	239.2
extremity	171.8	198.89	—	215.8	238.1	239.2
lower	171.3	198.89	—	215.3	238.1	239.2
upper	171.2	198.89	—	215.2	238.1	239.2
eyelid	171.0	198.89	—	215.0	238.1	239.2
face	171.0	198.89	—	215.0	238.1	239.2
finger	171.2	198.89	—	215.2	238.1	239.2
flank	171.7	198.89	—	215.7	238.1	239.2
foot	171.3	198.89	—	215.3	238.1	239.2
forearm	171.2	198.89	—	215.2	238.1	239.2
forehead	171.0	198.89	—	215.0	238.1	239.2
gluteal region	171.6	198.89	—	215.6	238.1	239.2
great vessels NEC	171.4	198.89	—	215.4	238.1	239.2
groin	171.6	198.89	—	215.6	238.1	239.2
hand	171.2	198.89	—	215.2	238.1	239.2
head	171.0	198.89	—	215.0	238.1	239.2

Neoplasm, connective tissue

		Malignant			Benign	Uncertain Behavior	Unspecified
		Primary	Secondary	Ca in situ			
Neoplasm, neoplastic — *continued*							
connective tissue NEC — *continued*							
	heel	171.3	198.89	—	215.3	238.1	239.2
	hip	171.3	198.89	—	215.3	238.1	239.2
	hypochondrium	171.5	198.89	—	215.5	238.1	239.2
	iliopsoas muscle	171.6	198.89	—	215.5	238.1	239.2
	infraclavicular region	171.4	198.89	—	215.4	238.1	239.2
	inguinal (canal) (region)	171.6	198.89	—	215.6	238.1	239.2
	intrathoracic	171.4	198.89	—	215.4	238.1	239.2
	ischorectal fossa	171.6	198.89	—	215.6	238.1	239.2
	jaw	143.9	198.89	230.0	210.4	235.1	239.0
	knee	171.3	198.89	—	215.3	238.1	239.2
	leg	171.3	198.89	—	215.3	238.1	239.2
	limb NEC	171.9	198.89	—	215.8	238.1	239.2
	lower	171.3	198.89	—	215.3	238.1	239.2
	upper	171.2	198.89	—	215.2	238.1	239.2
	nates	171.6	198.89	—	215.6	238.1	239.2
	neck	171.0	198.89	—	215.0	238.1	239.2
	orbit	190.1	198.4	234.0	224.1	238.8	239.8
	pararectal	171.6	198.89	—	215.6	238.1	239.2
	para-urethral	171.6	198.89	—	215.6	238.1	239.2
	paravaginal	171.6	198.89	—	215.6	238.1	239.2
	pelvis (floor)	171.6	198.89	—	215.6	238.1	239.2
	pelvo-abdominal	171.8	198.89	—	215.8	238.1	239.2
	perineum	171.6	198.89	—	215.6	238.1	239.2
	perirectal (tissue)	171.6	198.89	—	215.6	238.1	239.2
	periurethral (tissue)	171.6	198.89	—	215.6	238.1	239.2
	popliteal fossa or space	171.3	198.89	—	215.3	238.1	239.2
	presacral	171.6	198.89	—	215.6	238.1	239.2
	psoas muscle	171.5	198.89	—	215.5	238.1	239.2
	pterygoid fossa	171.0	198.89	—	215.0	238.1	239.2
	rectovaginal septum or wall	171.6	198.89	—	215.6	238.1	239.2
	rectovesical	171.6	198.89	—	215.6	238.1	239.2
	retroperitoneum	158.0	197.6	—	211.8	235.4	239.0
	sacrococcygeal region	171.6	198.89	—	215.6	238.1	239.2
	scalp	171.0	198.89	—	215.0	238.1	239.2
	scapular region	171.4	198.89	—	215.4	238.1	239.2
	shoulder	171.2	198.89	—	215.2	238.1	239.2
	skin (dermis) NEC	173.9	198.2	232.9	216.9	238.2	239.2
	submental	171.0	198.89	—	215.0	238.1	239.2
	supraclavicular region	171.0	198.89	—	215.0	238.1	239.2
	temple	171.0	198.89	—	215.0	238.1	239.2
	temporal region	171.0	198.89	—	215.0	238.1	239.2
	thigh	171.3	198.89	—	215.3	238.1	239.2
	thoracic (duct) (wall)	171.4	198.89	—	215.4	238.1	239.2
	thorax	171.4	198.89	—	215.4	238.1	239.2
	thumb	171.2	198.89	—	215.2	238.1	239.2
	toe	171.3	198.89	—	215.3	238.1	239.2
	trunk	171.7	198.89	—	215.7	238.1	239.2
	umbilicus	171.5	198.89	—	215.5	238.1	239.2
	vesicorectal	171.6	198.89	—	215.6	238.1	239.2
	wrist	171.2	198.89	—	215.2	238.1	239.2
conus medullaris		192.2	198.3	—	225.3	237.5	239.7
cord (true) (vocal)		161.0	197.3	231.0	212.1	235.6	239.1
	false	161.1	197.3	231.0	212.1	235.6	239.1
	spermatic	187.6	198.82	233.6	222.8	236.6	239.5
	spinal (cervical) (lumbar) (thoracic)	192.2	198.3	—	225.3	237.5	239.7
cornea (limbus)		190.4	198.4	234.0	224.4	238.8	239.8
corpus							
	albicans	183.0	198.6	233.3	220	236.2	239.5
	callosum, brain	191.8	198.3	—	225.0	237.5	239.6
	cavernosum	187.3	198.82	233.5	222.1	236.6	239.5
	gastric	151.4	197.8	230.2	211.1	235.2	239.0
	penis	187.3	198.82	233.5	222.1	236.6	239.5
	striatum, cerebrum	191.0	198.3	—	225.0	237.5	239.6
	uteri	182.0	198.82	233.2	219.1	236.0	239.5
	isthmus	182.1	198.82	233.2	219.1	236.0	239.5

	Malignant			Benign	Uncertain Behavior	Unspecified
	Primary	Secondary	Ca in situ			
Neoplasm, neoplastic — *continued*						
cortex						
adrenal	194.0	198.7	234.8	227.0	237.2	239.7
cerebral	191.0	198.3	—	225.0	237.5	239.6
costal cartilage	170.3	198.5	—	213.3	238.0	239.2
costovertebral joint	170.3	198.5	—	213.3	238.0	239.2
Cowper's gland	189.3	198.1	233.9	223.81	236.99	239.5
cranial (fossa, any)	191.9	198.3	—	225.0	237.5	239.6
meninges	192.1	198.4	—	225.2	237.6	239.7
nerve (any)	192.0	198.4	—	225.1	237.9	239.7
craniobuccal pouch	194.3	198.89	234.8	227.3	237.0	239.7
craniopharyngeal (duct) (pouch)	194.3	198.89	234.8	227.3	237.0	239.7
cricoid	148.0	198.89	230.0	210.8	235.1	239.0
cartilage	161.3	197.3	231.0	212.1	235.6	239.1
cricopharynx	148.0	198.89	230.0	210.8	235.1	239.0
crypt of Morgagni	154.8	197.5	230.7	211.4	235.2	239.0
crystalline lens	190.0	198.4	234.0	224.0	238.8	239.8
cul-de-sac (Douglas')	158.8	197.6	—	211.8	235.4	239.0
cuneiform cartilage	161.3	197.3	231.0	212.1	235.6	239.1
cutaneous — *see* Neoplasm, skin						
cutis — *see* Neoplasm, skin						
cystic (bile) duct (common)	156.1	197.8	230.8	211.5	235.3	239.0
dermis — *see* Neoplasm, skin						
diaphragm	171.4	198.89	—	215.4	238.1	239.2
digestive organs, system, tube, or tract NEC	159.9	197.8	230.9	211.9	235.5	239.0
contiguous sites with peritoneum	159.8	—	—	—	—	—
disc, intervertebral	170.2	198.5	—	213.2	238.0	239.2
disease, generalized	199.0	199.0	234.9	229.9	238.9	199.0
disseminated	199.0	199.0	234.9	229.9	238.9	199.0
Douglas' cul-de-sac or pouch	158.8	197.6	—	211.8	235.4	239.0
duodenojejunal junction	152.8	197.4	230.7	211.2	235.2	239.0
duodenum	152.0	197.4	230.7	211.2	235.2	239.0
dura (cranial) (mater)	192.1	198.4	—	225.2	237.6	239.7
cerebral	192.1	198.4	—	225.2	237.6	239.7
spinal	192.3	198.4	—	225.4	237.6	239.7
ear (external)	173.2	198.2	232.2	216.2	238.2	239.2
auricle or auris	173.2	198.2	232.2	216.2	238.2	239.2
canal, external	173.2	198.2	232.2	216.2	238.2	239.2
cartilage	171.0	198.89	—	215.0	238.1	239.2
external meatus	173.2	198.2	232.2	216.2	238.2	239.2
inner	160.1	197.3	231.8	212.0	235.9	239.8 ▲
lobule	173.2	198.2	232.2	216.2	238.2	239.2
middle	160.1	197.3	231.8	212.0	235.9	239.8 ▲
contiguous sites with accessory sinuses or nasal cavities	160.8	—	—	—	—	—
skin	173.2	198.2	232.2	216.2	238.2	239.2
earlobe	173.2	198.2	232.2	216.2	238.2	239.2
ejaculatory duct	187.8	198.82	233.6	222.8	236.6	239.5
elbow NEC*	195.4	198.89	232.6	229.8	238.8	239.8
endocardium	164.1	198.89	—	212.7	238.8	239.8
endocervix (canal) (gland)	180.0	198.82	233.1	219.0	236.0	239.5
endocrine gland NEC	194.9	198.89	—	227.9	237.4	239.7
pluriglandular NEC	194.8	198.89	234.8	227.8	237.4	239.7
endometrium (gland) (stroma)	182.0	198.82	233.2	219.1	236.0	239.5
ensiform cartilage	170.3	198.5	—	213.3	238.0	239.2
enteric — *see* Neoplasm, intestine						
ependyma (brain)	191.5	198.3	—	225.0	237.5	239.6
epicardium	164.1	198.89	—	212.7	238.8	239.8
epididymis	187.5	198.82	233.6	222.3	236.6	239.5
epidural	192.9	198.4	—	225.9	237.9	239.7
epiglottis	161.1	197.3	231.0	212.1	235.6	239.1
anterior aspect or surface	146.4	198.89	230.0	210.6	235.1	239.0
cartilage	161.3	197.3	231.0	212.1	235.6	239.1
free border (margin)	146.4	198.89	230.0	210.6	235.1	239.0
junctional region	146.5	198.89	230.0	210.6	235.1	239.0
posterior (laryngeal) surface	161.1	197.3	231.0	212.1	235.6	239.1
suprahyoid portion	161.1	197.3	231.0	212.1	235.6	239.1
esophagogastric junction	151.0	197.8	230.2	211.1	235.2	239.0

Neoplasm, esophagus Index to Diseases

	Malignant			Benign	Uncertain Behavior	Unspecified
	Primary	Secondary	Ca in situ			
Neoplasm, neoplastic — *continued*						
esophagus	150.9	197.8	230.1	211.0	235.5	239.0
abdominal	150.2	197.8	230.1	211.0	235.5	239.0
cervical	150.0	197.8	230.1	211.0	235.5	239.0
contiguous sites	150.8	—	—	—	—	—
distal (third)	150.5	197.8	230.1	211.0	235.5	239.0
lower (third)	150.5	197.8	230.1	211.0	235.5	239.0
middle (third)	150.4	197.8	230.1	211.0	235.5	239.0
proximal (third)	150.3	197.8	230.1	211.0	235.5	239.0
specified part NEC	150.8	197.8	230.1	211.0	235.5	239.0
thoracic	150.1	197.8	230.1	211.0	235.5	239.0
upper (third)	150.3	197.8	230.1	211.0	235.5	239.0
ethmoid (sinus)	160.3	197.3	231.8	212.0	235.9	239.1
bone or labyrinth	170.0	198.5	—	213.0	238.0	239.2
Eustachian tube	160.1	197.3	231.8	212.0	235.9	239.1
exocervix	180.1	198.82	233.1	219.0	236.0	239.5
external						
meatus (ear)	173.2	198.2	232.2	216.2	238.2	239.2
os, cervix uteri	180.1	198.82	233.1	219.0	236.0	239.5
extradural	192.9	198.4	—	225.9	237.9	239.7
extrahepatic (bile) duct	156.1	197.8	230.8	211.5	235.3	239.0
contiguous sites with gallbladder	156.8	—	—	—	—	—
extraocular muscle	190.1	198.4	234.0	224.1	238.8	239.8
extrarectal	195.3	198.89	234.8	229.8	238.8	239.8
extremity*	195.8	198.89	232.8	229.8	238.8	239.8
lower*	195.5	198.89	232.7	229.8	238.8	239.8
upper*	195.4	198.89	232.6	229.8	238.8	239.8
eye NEC	190.9	198.4	234.0	224.9	238.8	239.8
contiguous sites	190.8	—	—	—	—	—
specified sites NEC	190.8	198.4	234.0	224.8	238.8	239.8
eyeball	190.0	198.4	234.0	224.0	238.8	239.8
eyebrow	173.3	198.2	232.3	216.3	238.2	239.2
eyelid (lower) (skin) (upper)	173.1	198.2	232.1	216.1	238.2	239.2
cartilage	171.0	198.89	—	215.0	238.1	239.2
face NEC*	195.0	198.89	232.3	229.8	238.8	239.8
fallopian tube (accessory)	183.2	198.82	233.3	221.0	236.3	239.5
falx (cerebelli) (cerebri)	192.1	198.4	—	225.2	237.6	239.7
fascia — *see also* Neoplasm, connective tissue						
palmar	171.2	198.89	—	215.2	238.1	239.2
plantar	171.3	198.89	—	215.3	238.1	239.2
fatty tissue — *see* Neoplasm, connective tissue						
fauces, faucial NEC	146.9	198.89	230.0	210.6	235.1	239.0
pillars	146.2	198.89	230.0	210.6	235.1	239.0
tonsil	146.0	198.89	230.0	210.5	235.1	239.0
femur (any part)	170.7	198.5	—	213.7	238.0	239.2
fetal membrane	181	198.82	233.2	219.8	236.1	239.5
fibrous tissue — *see* Neoplasm, connective tissue						
fibula (any part)	170.7	198.5	—	213.7	238.0	239.2
filum terminale	192.2	198.3	—	225.3	237.5	239.7
finger NEC*	195.4	198.89	232.6	229.8	238.8	239.8
flank NEC*	195.8	198.89	232.5	229.8	238.8	239.8
follicle, nabothian	180.0	198.82	233.1	219.0	236.0	239.5
foot NEC*	195.5	198.89	232.7	229.8	238.8	239.8
forearm NEC*	195.4	198.89	232.6	229.8	238.8	239.8
forehead (skin)	173.3	198.2	232.3	216.3	238.2	239.2
foreskin	187.1	198.82	233.5	222.1	236.6	239.5
fornix						
pharyngeal	147.3	198.89	230.0	210.7	235.1	239.0
vagina	184.0	198.82	233.3	221.1	236.3	239.5
fossa (of)						
anterior (cranial)	191.9	198.3	—	225.0	237.5	239.6
cranial	191.9	198.3	—	225.0	237.5	239.6
ischiorectal	195.3	198.89	234.8	229.8	238.8	239.8
middle (cranial)	191.9	198.3	—	225.0	237.5	239.6
pituitary	194.3	198.89	234.8	227.3	237.0	239.7
posterior (cranial)	191.9	198.3	—	225.0	237.5	239.6
pterygoid	171.0	198.89	—	215.0	238.1	239.2

Index to Diseases

Neoplasm, hand

	Malignant			Benign	Uncertain Behavior	Unspecified
	Primary	Secondary	Ca in situ			
Neoplasm, neoplastic — *continued*						
fossa (of) — *continued*						
pyriform	148.1	198.89	230.0	210.8	235.1	239.0
Rosenmüller	147.2	198.89	230.0	210.7	235.1	239.0
tonsillar	146.1	198.89	230.0	210.6	235.1	239.0
fourchette	184.4	198.82	233.3	221.2	236.3	239.5
frenulum						
labii — *see* Neoplasm, lip, internal						
linguae	141.3	198.89	230.0	210.1	235.1	239.0
frontal						
bone	170.0	198.5	—	213.0	238.0	239.2
lobe, brain	191.1	198.3	—	225.0	237.5	239.6
meninges	192.1	198.4	—	225.2	237.6	239.7
pole	191.1	198.3	—	225.0	237.5	239.6
sinus	160.4	197.3	231.8	212.0	235.9	239.1
fundus						
stomach	151.3	197.8	230.2	211.1	235.2	239.0
uterus	182.0	198.82	233.2	219.1	236.0	239.5
gall duct (extrahepatic)	156.1	197.8	230.8	211.5	235.3	239.0
intrahepatic	155.1	197.8	230.8	211.5	235.3	239.0
gallbladder	156.0	197.8	230.8	211.5	235.3	239.0
contiguous sites with extrahepatic bile ducts	156.8	—	—	—	—	—
ganglia (*see also* Neoplasm, connective tissue)	171.9	198.89	—	215.9	238.1	239.2
basal	191.0	198.3	—	225.0	237.5	239.6
ganglion (*see also* Neoplasm, connective tissue)	171.9	198.89	—	215.9	238.1	239.2
cranial nerve	192.0	198.4	—	225.1	237.9	239.7
Gartner's duct	184.0	198.82	233.3	221.1	236.3	239.5
gastric — *see* Neoplasm, stomach						
gastrocolic	159.8	197.8	230.9	211.9	235.5	239.0
gastroesophageal junction	151.0	197.8	230.2	211.1	235.2	239.0
gastrointestinal (tract) NEC	159.9	197.8	230.9	211.9	235.5	239.0
generalized	199.0	199.0	234.9	229.9	238.9	199.0
genital organ or tract						
female NEC	184.9	198.82	233.3	221.9	236.3	239.5
contiguous sites	184.8	—	—	—	—	—
specified site NEC	184.8	198.82	233.3	221.8	236.3	239.5
male NEC	187.9	198.82	233.6	222.9	236.6	239.5
contiguous sites	187.8	—	—	—	—	—
specified site NEC	187.8	198.82	233.6	222.8	236.6	239.5
genitourinary tract						
female	184.9	198.82	233.3	221.9	236.3	239.5
male	187.9	198.82	233.6	222.9	236.6	239.5
gingiva (alveolar) (marginal)	143.9	198.89	230.0	210.4	235.1	239.0
lower	143.1	198.89	230.0	210.4	235.1	239.0
mandibular	143.1	198.89	230.0	210.4	235.1	239.0
maxillary	143.0	198.89	230.0	210.4	235.1	239.0
upper	143.0	198.89	230.0	210.4	235.1	239.0
gland, glandular (lymphatic) (system) — *see also* Neoplasm, lymph gland						
endocrine NEC	194.9	198.89	—	227.9	237.4	239.7
salivary — *see* Neoplasm, salivary, gland						
glans penis	187.2	198.82	233.5	222.1	236.6	239.5
globus pallidus	191.0	198.3	—	225.0	237.5	239.6
glomus						
coccygeal	194.6	198.89	—	227.6	237.3	239.7
jugularis	194.6	198.89	—	227.6	237.3	239.7
glosso-epiglottic fold(s)	146.4	198.89	230.0	210.6	235.1	239.0
glossopalatine fold	146.2	198.89	230.0	210.6	235.1	239.0
glossopharyngeal sulcus	146.1	198.89	230.0	210.6	235.1	239.0
glottis	161.0	197.3	231.0	212.1	235.6	239.1
gluteal region*	195.3	198.89	232.5	229.8	238.8	239.8
great vessels NEC	171.4	198.89	—	215.4	238.1	239.2
groin NEC*	195.3	198.89	232.5	229.8	238.8	239.8
gum	143.9	198.89	230.0	210.4	235.1	239.0
contiguous sites	143.8	—	—	—	—	—
lower	143.1	198.89	230.0	210.4	235.1	239.0
upper	143.0	198.89	230.0	210.4	235.1	239.0
hand NEC*	195.4	198.89	232.6	229.8	238.8	239.8

Neoplasm, head Index to Diseases

	Malignant			Benign	Uncertain Behavior	Unspecified
	Primary	Secondary	Ca in situ			
Neoplasm, neoplastic — *continued*						
head NEC*	195.0	198.89	232.4	229.8	238.8	239.8
heart	164.1	198.89	—	212.7	238.8	239.8
contiguous sites with mediastinum or thymus	164.8	—	—	—	—	—
heel NEC*	195.5	198.89	232.7	229.8	238.8	239.8
helix	173.2	198.2	232.2	216.2	238.2	239.2
hematopoietic, hemopoietic tissue NEC	202.8 ✓5ᵗʰ	198.89	—	—	—	238.7
hemisphere, cerebral	191.0	198.3	—	225.0	237.5	239.6
hemorrhoidal zone	154.2	197.5	230.5	211.4	235.5	239.0
hepatic	155.2	197.7	230.8	211.5	235.3	239.0
duct (bile)	156.1	197.8	230.8	211.5	235.3	239.0
flexure (colon)	153.0	197.5	230.3	211.3	235.2	239.0
primary	155.0	—	—	—	—	—
hilus of lung	162.2	197.0	231.2	212.3	235.7	239.1
hip NEC*	195.5	198.89	232.7	229.8	238.8	239.8
hippocampus, brain	191.2	198.3	—	225.0	237.5	239.6
humerus (any part)	170.4	198.5	—	213.4	238.0	239.2
hymen	184.0	198.82	233.3	221.1	236.3	239.5
hypopharynx, hypopharyngeal NEC	148.9	198.89	230.0	210.8	235.1	239.0
contiguous sites	148.8	—	—	—	—	—
postcricoid region	148.0	198.89	230.0	210.8	235.1	239.0
posterior wall	148.3	198.89	230.0	210.8	235.1	239.0
pyriform fossa (sinus)	148.1	198.89	230.0	210.8	235.1	239.0
specified site NEC	148.8	198.89	230.0	210.8	235.1	239.0
wall	148.9	198.89	230.0	210.8	235.1	239.0
posterior	148.3	198.89	230.0	210.8	235.1	239.0
hypophysis	194.3	198.89	234.8	227.3	237.0	239.7
hypothalamus	191.0	198.3	—	225.0	237.5	239.6
ileocecum, ileocecal (coil) (junction) (valve)	153.4	197.5	230.3	211.3	235.2	239.0
ileum	152.2	197.4	230.7	211.2	235.2	239.0
ilium	170.6	198.5	—	213.6	238.0	239.2
immunoproliferative NEC	203.8 ✓5ᵗʰ	—	—	—	—	—
infraclavicular (region)*	195.1	198.89	232.5	229.8	238.8	239.8
inguinal (region)*	195.3	198.89	232.5	229.8	238.8	239.8
insula	191.0	198.3	—	225.0	237.5	239.6
insular tissue (pancreas)	157.4	197.8	230.9	211.7	235.5	239.0
brain	191.0	198.3	—	225.0	237.5	239.6
interarytenoid fold	148.2	198.89	230.0	210.8	235.1	239.0
hypopharyngeal aspect	148.2	198.89	230.0	210.8	235.1	239.0
laryngeal aspect	161.1	197.3	231.0	212.1	235.6	239.1
marginal zone	148.2	198.89	230.0	210.8	235.1	239.0
interdental papillae	143.9	198.89	230.0	210.4	235.1	239.0
lower	143.1	198.89	230.0	210.4	235.1	239.0
upper	143.0	198.89	230.0	210.4	235.1	239.0
internal						
capsule	191.0	198.3	—	225.0	237.5	239.6
os (cervix)	180.0	198.82	233.1	219.0	236.0	239.5
intervertebral cartilage or disc	170.2	198.5	—	213.2	238.0	239.2
intestine, intestinal	159.0	197.8	230.7	211.9	235.2	239.0
large	153.9	197.5	230.3	211.3	235.2	239.0
appendix	153.5	197.5	230.3	211.3	235.2	239.0
caput coli	153.4	197.5	230.3	211.3	235.2	239.0
cecum	153.4	197.5	230.3	211.3	235.2	239.0
colon	153.9	197.5	230.3	211.3	235.2	239.0
and rectum	154.0	197.5	230.4	211.4	235.2	239.0
ascending	153.6	197.5	230.3	211.3	235.2	239.0
caput	153.4	197.5	230.3	211.3	235.2	239.0
contiguous sites	153.8	—	—	—	—	—
descending	153.2	197.5	230.3	211.3	235.2	239.0
distal	153.2	197.5	230.3	211.3	235.2	239.0
left	153.2	197.5	230.3	211.3	235.2	239.0
pelvic	153.3	197.5	230.3	211.3	235.2	239.0
right	153.6	197.5	230.3	211.3	235.2	239.0
sigmoid (flexure)	153.3	197.5	230.3	211.3	235.2	239.0
transverse	153.1	197.5	230.3	211.3	235.2	239.0
contiguous sites	153.8	—	—	—	—	—

	Malignant			Benign	Uncertain Behavior	Unspecified
	Primary	Secondary	Ca in situ			
Neoplasm, neoplastic — *continued*						
intestine, intestinal — *continued*						
large — *continued*						
hepatic flexure	153.0	197.5	230.3	211.3	235.2	239.0
ileocecum, ileocecal (coil) (valve)	153.4	197.5	230.3	211.3	235.2	239.0
sigmoid flexure (lower) (upper)	153.3	197.5	230.3	211.3	235.2	239.0
splenic flexure	153.7	197.5	230.3	211.3	235.2	239.0
small	152.9	197.4	230.7	211.2	235.2	239.0
contiguous sites	152.8	—	—	—	—	—
duodenum	152.0	197.4	230.7	211.2	235.2	239.0
ileum	152.2	197.4	230.7	211.2	235.2	239.0
jejunum	152.1	197.4	230.7	211.2	235.2	239.0
tract NEC	159.0	197.8	230.7	211.9	235.2	239.0
intra-abdominal	195.2	198.89	234.8	229.8	238.8	239.8
intracranial NEC	191.9	198.3	—	225.0	237.5	239.6
intrahepatic (bile) duct	155.1	197.8	230.8	211.5	235.3	239.0
intraocular	190.0	198.4	234.0	224.0	238.8	239.8
intraorbital	190.1	198.4	234.0	224.1	238.8	239.8
intrasellar	194.3	198.89	234.8	227.3	237.0	239.7
intrathoracic (cavity) (organs NEC)	195.1	198.89	234.8	229.8	238.8	239.8
contiguous sites with respiratory organs	165.8	—	—	—	—	—
iris	190.0	198.4	234.0	224.0	238.8	239.8
ischiorectal (fossa)	195.3	198.89	234.8	229.8	238.8	239.8
ischium	170.6	198.5	—	213.6	238.0	239.2
island of Reil	191.0	198.3	—	225.0	237.5	239.6
islands or islets of Langerhans	157.4	197.8	230.9	211.7	235.5	239.0
isthmus uteri	182.1	198.82	233.2	219.1	236.0	239.5
jaw	195.0	198.89	234.8	229.8	238.8	239.8
bone	170.1	198.5	—	213.1	238.0	239.2
carcinoma	143.9	—	—	—	—	—
lower	143.1	—	—	—	—	—
upper	143.0	—	—	—	—	—
lower	170.1	198.5	—	213.1	238.0	239.2
upper	170.0	198.5	—	213.0	238.0	239.2
carcinoma (any type) (lower) (upper)	195.0	—	—	—	—	—
skin	173.3	198.2	232.3	216.3	238.2	239.2
soft tissues	143.9	198.89	230.0	210.4	235.1	239.0
lower	143.1	198.89	230.0	210.4	235.1	239.0
upper	143.0	198.89	230.0	210.4	235.1	239.0
jejunum	152.1	197.4	230.7	211.2	235.2	239.0
joint NEC (*see also* Neoplasm, bone)	170.9	198.5	—	213.9	238.0	239.2
acromioclavicular	170.4	198.5	—	213.4	238.0	239.2
bursa or synovial membrane — *see* Neoplasm, connective tissue						
costovertebral	170.3	198.5	—	213.3	238.0	239.2
sternocostal	170.3	198.5	—	213.3	238.0	239.2
temporomandibular	170.1	198.5	—	213.1	238.0	239.2
junction						
anorectal	154.8	197.5	230.7	211.4	235.5	239.0
cardioesophageal	151.0	197.8	230.2	211.1	235.2	239.0
esophagogastric	151.0	197.8	230.2	211.1	235.2	239.0
gastroesophageal	151.0	197.8	230.2	211.1	235.2	239.0
hard and soft palate	145.5	198.89	230.0	210.4	235.1	239.0
ileocecal	153.4	197.5	230.3	211.3	235.2	239.0
pelvirectal	154.0	197.5	230.4	211.4	235.2	239.0
pelviureteric	189.1	198.0	233.9	223.1	236.91	239.5
rectosigmoid	154.0	197.5	230.4	211.4	235.2	239.0
squamocolumnar, of cervix	180.8	198.82	233.1	219.0	236.0	239.5
kidney (parenchyma)	189.0	198.0	233.9	223.0	236.91	239.5
calyx	189.1	198.0	233.9	223.1	236.91	239.5
hilus	189.1	198.0	233.9	223.1	236.91	239.5
pelvis	189.1	198.0	233.9	223.1	236.91	239.5
knee NEC*	195.5	198.89	232.7	229.8	238.8	239.8
labia (skin)	184.4	198.82	233.3	221.2	236.3	239.5
majora	184.1	198.82	233.3	221.2	236.3	239.5
minora	184.2	198.82	233.3	221.2	236.3	239.5
labial — *see also* Neoplasm, lip						
sulcus (lower) (upper)	145.1	198.89	230.0	210.4	235.1	239.0

Neoplasm, labium

	Malignant			Benign	Uncertain Behavior	Unspecified
	Primary	Secondary	Ca in situ			
Neoplasm, neoplastic — *continued*						
labium (skin)	184.4	198.82	233.3	221.2	236.3	239.5
majus	184.1	198.82	233.3	221.2	236.3	239.5
minus	184.2	198.82	233.3	221.2	236.3	239.5
lacrimal						
canaliculi	190.7	198.4	234.0	224.7	238.8	239.8
duct (nasal)	190.7	198.4	234.0	224.7	238.8	239.8
gland	190.2	198.4	234.0	224.2	238.8	239.8
punctum	190.7	198.4	234.0	224.7	238.8	239.8
sac	190.7	198.4	234.0	224.7	238.8	239.8
Langerhans, islands or islets	157.4	197.8	230.9	211.7	235.5	239.0
laryngopharynx	148.9	198.89	230.0	210.8	235.1	239.0
larynx, laryngeal NEC	161.9	197.3	231.0	212.1	235.6	239.1
aryepiglottic fold	161.1	197.3	231.0	212.1	235.6	239.1
cartilage (arytenoid) (cricoid) (cuneiform) (thyroid)	161.3	197.3	231.0	212.1	235.6	239.1
commissure (anterior) (posterior)	161.0	197.3	231.0	212.1	235.6	239.1
contiguous sites	161.8	—	—	—	—	—
extrinsic NEC	161.1	197.3	231.0	212.1	235.6	239.1
meaning hypopharynx	148.9	198.89	230.0	210.8	235.1	239.0
interarytenoid fold	161.1	197.3	231.0	212.1	235.6	239.1
intrinsic	161.0	197.3	231.0	212.1	235.6	239.1
ventricular band	161.1	197.3	231.0	212.1	235.6	239.1
leg NEC*	195.5	198.89	232.7	229.8	238.8	239.8
lens, crystalline	190.0	198.4	234.0	224.0	238.8	239.8
lid (lower) (upper)	173.1	198.2	232.1	216.1	238.2	239.2
ligament — *see also* Neoplasm, connective tissue						
broad	183.3	198.82	233.3	221.0	236.3	239.5
Mackenrodt's	183.8	198.82	233.3	221.8	236.3	239.5
non-uterine — *see* Neoplasm, connective tissue						
round	183.5	198.82	—	221.0	236.3	239.5
sacro-uterine	183.4	198.82	—	221.0	236.3	239.5
uterine	183.4	198.82	—	221.0	236.3	239.5
utero-ovarian	183.8	198.82	233.3	221.8	236.3	239.5
uterosacral	183.4	198.82	—	221.0	236.3	239.5
limb*	195.8	198.89	232.8	229.8	238.8	239.8
lower*	195.5	198.89	232.7	229.8	238.8	239.8
upper*	195.4	198.89	232.6	229.8	238.8	239.8
limbus of cornea	190.4	198.4	234.0	224.4	238.8	239.8
lingual NEC (*see also* Neoplasm, tongue)	141.9	198.89	230.0	210.1	235.1	239.0
lingula, lung	162.3	197.0	231.2	212.3	235.7	239.1
lip (external) (lipstick area) (vermillion border)	140.9	198.89	230.0	210.0	235.1	239.0
buccal aspect — *see* Neoplasm, lip, internal						
commissure	140.6	198.89	230.0	210.4	235.1	239.0
contiguous sites	140.8	—	—	—	—	—
with oral cavity or pharynx	149.8	—	—	—	—	—
frenulum — *see* Neoplasm, lip, internal						
inner aspect — *see* Neoplasm, lip, internal						
internal (buccal) (frenulum) (mucosa) (oral)	140.5	198.89	230.0	210.0	235.1	239.0
lower	140.4	198.89	230.0	210.0	235.1	239.0
upper	140.3	198.89	230.0	210.0	235.1	239.0
lower	140.1	198.89	230.0	210.0	235.1	239.0
internal (buccal) (frenulum) (mucosa) (oral)	140.4	198.89	230.0	210.0	235.1	239.0
mucosa — *see* Neoplasm, lip, internal						
oral aspect — *see* Neoplasm, lip, internal						
skin (commissure) (lower) (upper)	173.0	198.2	232.0	216.0	238.2	239.2
upper	140.0	198.89	230.0	210.0	235.1	239.0
internal (buccal) (frenulum) (mucosa) (oral)	140.3	198.89	230.0	210.0	235.1	239.0
liver	155.2	197.7	230.8	211.5	235.3	239.0
primary	155.0	—	—	—	—	—
lobe						
azygos	162.3	197.0	231.2	212.3	235.7	239.1
frontal	191.1	198.3	—	225.0	237.5	239.6
lower	162.5	197.0	231.2	212.3	235.7	239.1
middle	162.4	197.0	231.2	212.3	235.7	239.1
occipital	191.4	198.3	—	225.0	237.5	239.6
parietal	191.3	198.3	—	225.0	237.5	239.6

Index to Diseases

Neoplasm, lymph

	Malignant			Benign	Uncertain Behavior	Unspecified
	Primary	Secondary	Ca in situ			
Neoplasm, neoplastic — *continued*						
lobe — *continued*						
temporal	191.2	198.3	—	225.0	237.5	239.6
upper	162.3	197.0	231.2	212.3	235.7	239.1
lumbosacral plexus	171.6	198.4	—	215.6	238.1	239.2
lung	162.9	197.0	231.2	212.3	235.7	239.1
azgos lobe	162.3	197.0	231.2	212.3	235.7	239.1
carina	162.2	197.0	231.2	212.3	235.7	239.1
contiguous sites with bronchus or trachea	162.8	—	—	—	—	—
hilus	162.2	197.0	231.2	212.3	235.7	239.1
lingula	162.3	197.0	231.2	212.3	235.7	239.1
lobe NEC	162.9	197.0	231.2	212.3	235.7	239.1
lower lobe	162.5	197.0	231.2	212.3	235.7	239.1
main bronchus	162.2	197.0	231.2	212.3	235.7	239.1
middle lobe	162.4	197.0	231.2	212.3	235.7	239.1
upper lobe	162.3	197.0	231.2	212.3	235.7	239.1
lymph, lymphatic						
channel NEC (*see also* Neoplasm, connective tissue)	171.9	198.89	—	215.9	238.1	239.2
gland (secondary)	—	196.9	—	229.0	238.8	239.8
abdominal	—	196.2	—	229.0	238.8	239.
aortic	—	196.2	—	229.0	238.8	239.8
arm	—	196.3	—	229.0	238.8	239.8
auricular (anterior) (posterior)	—	196.0	—	229.0	238.8	239.8
axilla, axillary	—	196.3	—	229.0	238.8	239.8
brachial	—	196.3	—	229.0	238.8	239.8
bronchial	—	196.1	—	229.0	238.8	239.8
bronchopulmonary	—	196.1	—	229.0	238.8	239.8
celiac	—	196.2	—	229.0	238.8	239.8
cervical	—	196.0	—	229.0	238.8	239.8
cervicofacial	—	196.0	—	229.0	238.8	239.8
Cloquet	—	196.5	—	229.0	238.8	239.8
colic	—	196.2	—	229.0	238.8	239.8
common duct	—	196.2	—	229.0	238.8	239.8
cubital	—	196.3	—	229.0	238.8	239.8
diaphragmatic	—	196.1	—	229.0	238.8	239.8
epigastric, inferior	—	196.6	—	229.0	238.8	239.8
epitrochlear	—	196.3	—	229.0	238.8	239.8
esophageal	—	196.1	—	229.0	238.8	239.8
face	—	196.0	—	229.0	238.8	239.8
femoral	—	196.5	—	229.0	238.8	239.8
gastric	—	196.2	—	229.0	238.8	239.8
groin	—	196.5	—	229.0	238.8	239.8
head	—	196.0	—	229.0	238.8	239.8
hepatic	—	196.2	—	229.0	238.8	239.8
hilar (pulmonary)	—	196.1	—	229.0	238.8	239.8
splenic	—	196.2	—	229.0	238.8	239.8
hypogastric	—	196.6	—	229.0	238.8	239.8
ileocolic	—	196.2	—	229.0	238.8	239.8
iliac	—	196.6	—	229.0	238.8	239.8
infraclavicular	—	196.3	—	229.0	238.8	239.8
inguina, inguinal	—	196.5	—	229.0	238.8	239.8
innominate	—	196.1	—	229.0	238.8	239.8
intercostal	—	196.1	—	229.0	238.8	239.8
intestinal	—	196.2	—	229.0	238.8	239.8
intra-abdominal	—	196.2	—	229.0	238.8	239.8
intrapelvic	—	196.6	—	229.0	238.8	239.8
intrathoracic	—	196.1	—	229.0	238.8	239.9
jugular	—	196.0	—	229.0	238.8	239.8
leg	—	196.5	—	229.0	238.8	239.8
limb						
lower	—	196.5	—	229.0	238.8	239.8
upper	—	196.3	—	229.0	238.8	239.8
lower limb	—	196.5	—	229.0	238.8	238.9
lumbar	—	196.2	—	229.0	238.8	239.8
mandibular	—	196.0	—	229.0	238.8	239.8
mediastinal	—	196.1	—	229.0	238.8	239.8
mesenteric (inferior) (superior)	—	196.2	—	229.0	238.8	239.8

Neoplasm, lymph

Index to Diseases

	Malignant			Benign	Uncertain Behavior	Unspecified
	Primary	Secondary	Ca in situ			
Neoplasm, neoplastic — *continued*						
lymph, lymphatic — *continued*						
gland — *continued*						
midcolic	—	196.2	—	229.0	238.8	239.8
multiple sites in categories 196.0-196.6	—	196.8	—	229.0	238.8	239.8
neck	—	196.0	—	229.0	238.8	239.8
obturator	—	196.6	—	229.0	238.8	239.8
occipital	—	196.0	—	229.0	238.8	239.8
pancreatic	—	196.2	—	229.0	238.8	239.8
para-aortic	—	196.2	—	229.0	238.8	239.8
paracervical	—	196.6	—	229.0	238.8	239.8
parametrial	—	196.6	—	229.0	238.8	239.8
parasternal	—	196.1	—	229.0	238.8	239.8
parotid	—	196.0	—	229.0	238.8	239.8
pectoral	—	196.3	—	229.0	238.8	239.8
pelvic	—	196.6	—	229.0	238.8	239.8
peri-aortic	—	196.2	—	229.0	238.8	239.8
peripancreatic	—	196.2	—	229.0	238.8	239.8
popliteal	—	196.5	—	229.0	238.8	239.8
porta hepatis	—	196.2	—	229.0	238.8	239.8
portal	—	196.2	—	229.0	238.8	239.8
preauricular	—	196.0	—	229.0	238.8	239.8
prelaryngeal	—	196.0	—	229.0	238.8	239.8
presymphysial	—	196.6	—	229.0	238.8	239.8
pretracheal	—	196.0	—	229.0	238.8	239.8
primary (any site) NEC	202.9 ✓5ᵗʰ	—	—	—	—	—
pulmonary (hiler)	—	196.1	—	229.0	238.8	239.8
pyloric	—	196.2	—	229.0	238.8	239.8
retroperitoneal	—	196.2	—	229.0	238.8	239.8
retropharyngeal	—	196.0	—	229.0	238.8	239.8
Rosenmüller's	—	196.5	—	229.0	238.8	239.8
sacral	—	196.6	—	229.0	238.8	239.8
scalene	—	196.0	—	229.0	238.8	239.8
site NEC	—	196.9	—	229.0	238.8	239.8
splenic (hilar)	—	196.2	—	229.0	238.8	239.8
subclavicular	—	196.3	—	229.0	238.8	239.8
subinguinal	—	196.5	—	229.0	238.8	239.8
sublingual	—	196.0	—	229.0	238.8	239.8
submandibular	—	196.0	—	229.0	238.8	239.8
submaxillary	—	196.0	—	229.0	238.8	239.8
submental	—	196.0	—	229.0	238.8	239.8
subscapular	—	196.3	—	229.0	238.8	239.8
supraclavicular	—	196.0	—	229.0	238.8	239.8
thoracic	—	196.1	—	229.0	238.8	239.8
tibial	—	196.5	—	229.0	238.8	239.8
tracheal	—	196.1	—	229.0	238.8	239.8
tracheobronchial	—	196.1	—	229.0	238.8	239.8
upper limb	—	196.3	—	229.0	238.8	239.8
Virchow's	—	196.0	—	229.0	238.8	239.8
node — *see also* Neoplasm, lymph gland						
primary NEC	202.9 ✓5ᵗʰ	—	—	—	—	—
vessel (*see also* Neoplasm, connective tissue)	171.9	198.89	—	215.9	238.1	239.2
Nackenrodt's ligament	183.8	198.82	233.3	221.8	236.3	239.5
malar	170.0	198.5	—	213.0	238.0	239.2
region — *see* Neoplasm, cheek						
mammary gland — *see* Neoplasm, breast						
mandible	170.1	198.5	—	213.1	238.0	239.2
alveolar						
mucose	143.1	198.89	230.0	210.4	235.1	239.0
ridge or process	170.1	198.5	—	213.1	238.0	239.2
carcinoma	143.1	—	—	—	—	—
carcinoma	143.1	—	—	—	—	—
marrow (bone) NEC	202.9 ✓5ᵗʰ	198.5	—	—	—	238.7
mastectomy site (skin)	173.5	198.2	—	—	—	—
specified as breast tissue	174.8	198.81	—	—	—	—
mastoid (air cells) (antrum) (cavity)	160.1	197.3	231.8	212.0	235.9	239.1
bone or process	170.0	198.5	—	213.0	238.0	239.2

Index to Diseases — Neoplasm, myocardium

	Malignant			Benign	Uncertain Behavior	Unspecified
	Primary	Secondary	Ca in situ			
Neoplasm, neoplastic — *continued*						
maxilla, maxillary (superior)	170.0	198.5	—	213.0	238.0	239.2
alveolar						
mucosa	143.0	198.89	230.0	210.4	235.1	239.0
ridge or process	170.0	198.5	—	213.0	238.0	239.2
carcinoma	143.0	—	—	—	—	—
antrum	160.2	197.3	231.8	212.0	235.9	239.1
carcinoma	143.0	—	—	—	—	—
inferior — *see* Neoplasm, mandible						
sinus	160.2	197.3	231.8	212.0	235.9	239.1
meatus						
external (ear)	173.2	198.2	232.2	216.2	238.2	239.2
Meckel's diverticulum	152.3	197.4	230.7	211.2	235.2	239.0
mediastinum, mediastinal	164.9	197.1	—	212.5	235.8	239.8
anterior	164.2	197.1	—	212.5	235.8	239.8
contiguous sites with heart and thymus	164.8	—	—	—	—	—
posterior	164.3	197.1	—	212.5	235.8	239.8
medulla						
adrenal	194.0	198.7	234.8	227.0	237.2	239.7
oblongata	191.7	198.3	—	225.0	237.5	239.6
meibomian gland	173.1	198.2	232.1	216.1	238.2	239.2
melanoma — *see* Melanoma						
meninges (brain) (cerebral) (cranial) (intracranial)	192.1	198.4	—	225.2	237.6	239.7
spinal (cord)	192.3	198.4	—	225.4	237.6	239.7
meniscus, knee joint (lateral) (medial)	170.7	198.5	—	213.7	238.0	239.2
mesentery, mesenteric	158.8	197.6	—	211.8	235.4	239.0
mesoappendix	158.8	197.6	—	211.8	235.4	239.0
mesocolon	158.8	197.6	—	211.8	235.4	239.0
mesopharynx — *see* Neoplasm, oropharynx						
mesosalpinx	183.3	198.82	233.3	221.0	236.3	239.5
mesovarium	183.3	198.82	233.3	221.0	236.3	239.5
metacarpus (any bone)	170.5	198.5	—	213.5	238.0	239.2
metastatic NEC — *see also* Neoplasm, by site, secondary	—	199.1	—	—	—	—
metatarsus (any bone)	170.8	198.5	—	213.8	238.0	239.2
midbrain	191.7	198.3	—	225.0	237.5	239.6
milk duct — *see* Neoplasm, breast						
mons						
pubis	184.4	198.82	233.3	221.2	236.3	239.5
veneris	184.4	198.82	233.3	221.2	236.3	239.5
motor tract	192.9	198.4	—	225.9	237.9	239.7
brain	191.9	198.3	—	225.0	237.5	239.6
spinal	192.2	198.3	—	225.3	237.5	239.7
mouth	145.9	198.89	230.0	210.4	235.1	239.0
contiguous sites	145.8	—	—	—	—	—
floor	144.9	198.89	230.0	210.3	235.1	239.0
anterior portion	144.0	198.89	230.0	210.3	235.1	239.0
contiguous sites	144.8	—	—	—	—	—
lateral portion	144.1	198.89	230.0	210.3	235.1	239.0
roof	145.5	198.89	230.0	210.4	235.1	239.0
specified part NEC	145.8	198.89	230.0	210.4	235.1	239.0
vestibule	145.1	198.89	230.0	210.4	235.1	239.0
mucosa						
alveolar (ridge or process)	143.9	198.89	230.0	210.4	235.1	239.0
lower	143.1	198.89	230.0	210.4	235.1	239.0
upper	143.0	198.89	230.0	210.4	235.1	239.0
buccal	145.0	198.89	230.0	210.4	235.1	239.0
cheek	145.0	198.89	230.0	210.4	235.1	239.0
lip — *see* Neoplasm, lip, internal						
nasal	160.0	197.3	231.8	212.0	235.9	239.1
oral	145.0	198.89	230.0	210.4	235.1	239.0
Müllerian duct						
female	184.8	198.82	233.3	221.8	236.3	239.5
male	187.8	198.82	233.6	222.8	236.6	239.5
multiple sites NEC	199.0	199.0	234.9	229.9	238.9	199.0
muscle — *see also* Neoplasm, connective tissue						
extraocular	190.1	198.4	234.0	224.1	238.8	239.8
myocardium	164.1	198.89	—	212.7	238.8	239.8

	Malignant			Benign	Uncertain Behavior	Unspecified
	Primary	Secondary	Ca in situ			
Neoplasm, neoplastic — *continued*						
myometrium	182.0	198.82	233.2	219.1	236.0	239.5
myopericardium	164.1	198.89	—	212.7	238.8	239.8
nabothian gland (follicle)	180.0	198.82	233.1	219.0	236.0	239.5
nail	173.9	198.2	232.9	216.9	238.2	239.2
finger	173.6	198.2	232.6	216.6	238.2	239.2
toe	173.7	198.2	232.7	216.7	238.2	239.2
nares, naris (anterior) (posterior)	160.0	197.3	231.8	212.0	235.9	239.1
nasal — *see* Neoplasm, nose						
nasolabial groove	173.3	198.2	232.3	216.3	238.2	239.2
nasolacrimal duct	190.7	198.4	234.0	224.7	238.8	239.8
nasopharynx, nasopharyngeal	147.9	198.89	230.0	210.7	235.1	239.0
contiguous sites	147.8	—	—	—	—	—
floor	147.3	198.89	230.0	210.7	235.1	239.0
roof	147.0	198.89	230.0	210.7	235.1	239.0
specified site NEC	147.8	198.89	230.0	210.7	235.1	239.0
wall	147.9	198.89	230.0	210.7	235.1	239.0
anterior	147.3	198.89	230.0	210.7	235.1	239.0
lateral	147.2	198.89	230.0	210.7	235.1	239.0
posterior	147.1	198.89	230.0	210.7	235.1	239.0
superior	147.0	198.89	230.0	210.7	235.1	239.0
nates	173.5	198.2	232.5	216.5	238.2	239.2
neck NEC*	195.0	198.89	234.8	229.8	238.8	239.8*
nerve (autonomic) (ganglion) (parasympathetic) (peripheral) (sympathetic) — *see also* Neoplasm, connective tissue						
abducens	192.0	198.4	—	225.1	237.9	239.7
accessory (spinal)	192.0	198.4	—	225.1	237.9	239.7
acoustic	192.0	198.4	—	225.1	237.9	239.7
auditory	192.0	198.4	—	225.1	237.9	239.7
brachial	171.2	198.89	—	215.2	238.1	239.2
cranial (any)	192.0	198.4	—	225.1	237.9	239.7
facial	192.0	198.4	—	225.1	237.9	239.7
femoral	171.3	198.89	—	215.3	238.1	239.2
glossopharyngeal	192.0	198.4	—	225.1	237.9	239.7
hypoglossal	192.0	198.4	—	225.1	237.9	239.7
intercostal	171.4	198.89	—	215.4	238.1	239.2
lumbar	171.7	198.89	—	215.7	238.1	239.2
median	171.2	198.89	—	215.2	238.1	239.2
obturator	171.3	198.89	—	215.3	238.1	239.2
oculomotor	192.0	198.4	—	225.1	237.9	239.7
olfactory	192.0	198.4	—	225.1	237.9	239.7
optic	192.0	198.4	—	225.1	237.9	239.7
peripheral NEC	171.9	198.89	—	215.9	238.1	239.2
radial	171.2	198.89	—	215.2	238.1	239.2
sacral	171.6	198.89	—	215.6	238.1	239.2
sciatic	171.3	198.89	—	215.3	238.1	239.2
spinal NEC	171.9	198.89	—	215.9	238.1	239.2
trigeminal	192.0	198.4	—	225.1	237.9	239.7
trochlear	192.0	198.4	—	225.1	237.9	239.7
ulnar	171.2	198.89	—	215.2	238.1	239.2
vagus	192.0	198.4	—	225.1	237.9	239.7
nervous system (central) NEC	192.9	198.4	—	225.9	237.9	239.7
autonomic NEC	171.9	198.89	—	215.9	238.1	239.2
brain — *see also* Neoplasm, brain						
membrane or meninges	192.1	198.4	—	225.2	237.6	239.7
contiguous sites	192.8	—	—	—	—	—
parasympathetic NEC	171.9	198.89	—	215.9	238.1	239.2
sympathetic NEC	171.9	198.89	—	215.9	238.1	239.2
nipple (female)	174.0	198.81	233.0	217	238.3	239.3
male	175.0	198.81	233.0	217	238.3	239.3
nose, nasal	195.0	198.89	234.8	229.8	238.8	239.8
ala (external)	173.3	198.2	232.3	216.3	238.2	239.2
bone	170.0	198.5	—	213.0	238.0	239.2
cartilage	160.0	197.3	231.8	212.0	235.9	239.1
cavity	160.0	197.3	231.8	212.0	235.9	239.1
contiguous sites with accessory sinuses or middle ear	160.8	—	—	—	—	—
choana	147.3	198.89	230.0	210.7	235.1	239.0

Index to Diseases — Neoplasm, pancreas

	Malignant			Benign	Uncertain Behavior	Unspecified
	Primary	Secondary	Ca in situ			
Neoplasm, neoplastic — *continued*						
nose, nasal — *continued*						
external (skin)	173.3	198.2	232.3	216.3	238.2	239.2
fossa	160.0	197.3	231.8	212.0	235.9	239.1
internal	160.0	197.3	231.8	212.0	235.9	239.1
mucosa	160.0	197.3	231.8	212.0	235.9	239.1
septum	160.0	197.3	231.8	212.0	235.9	239.1
posterior margin	147.3	198.89	230.0	210.7	235.1	239.0
sinus — *see* Neoplasm, sinus						
skin	173.3	198.2	232.3	216.3	238.2	239.2
turbinate (mucosa)	160.0	197.3	231.8	212.0	235.9	239.1
bone	170.0	198.5	—	213.0	238.0	239.2
vestibule	160.0	197.3	231.8	212.0	235.9	239.1
nostril	160.0	197.3	231.8	212.0	235.9	239.1
nucleus pulposus	170.2	198.5	—	213.2	238.0	239.2
occipital						
bone	170.0	198.5	—	213.0	238.0	239.2
lobe or pole, brain	191.4	198.3	—	225.0	237.5	239.6
odontogenic — *see* Neoplasm, jaw bone						
oesophagus — *see* Neoplasm, esophagus						
olfactory nerve or bulb	192.0	198.4	—	225.1	237.9	239.7
olive (brain)	191.7	198.3	—	225.0	237.5	239.6
omentum	158.8	197.6	—	211.8	235.4	239.0
operculum (brain)	191.0	198.3	—	225.0	237.5	239.6
optic nerve, chiasm, or tract	192.0	198.4	—	225.1	237.9	239.7
oral (cavity)	145.9	198.89	230.0	210.4	235.1	239.0
contiguous sites with lip or pharynx	149.8	—	—	—	—	—
ill-defined	149.9	198.89	230.0	210.4	235.1	239.0
mucosa	145.9	198.89	230.0	210.4	235.1	239.0
orbit	190.1	198.4	234.0	224.1	238.8	239.8
bone	170.0	198.5	—	213.0	238.0	239.2
eye	190.1	198.4	234.0	224.1	238.8	239.8
soft parts	190.1	198.4	234.0	224.1	238.8	239.8
organ of Zuckerkandl	194.6	198.89	—	227.6	237.3	239.7
oropharynx	146.9	198.89	230.0	210.6	235.1	239.0
branchial cleft (vestige)	146.8	198.89	230.0	210.6	235.1	239.0
contiguous sites	146.8	—	—	—	—	—
junctional region	146.5	198.89	230.0	210.6	235.1	239.0
lateral wall	146.6	198.89	230.0	210.6	235.1	239.0
pillars of fauces	146.2	198.89	230.0	210.6	235.1	239.0
posterior wall	146.7	198.89	230.0	210.6	235.1	239.0
specified part NEC	146.8	198.89	230.0	210.6	235.1	239.0
vallecula	146.3	198.89	230.0	210.6	235.1	239.0
os						
external	180.1	198.82	233.1	219.0	236.0	239.5
internal	180.0	198.82	233.1	219.0	236.0	239.5
ovary	183.0	198.6	233.3	220	236.2	239.5
oviduct	183.2	198.82	233.3	221.0	236.3	239.5
palate	145.5	198.89	230.0	210.4	235.1	239.0
hard	145.2	198.89	230.0	210.4	235.1	239.0
junction of hard and soft palate	145.5	198.89	230.0	210.4	235.1	239.0
soft	145.3	198.89	230.0	210.4	235.1	239.0
nasopharyngeal surface	147.3	198.89	230.0	210.7	235.1	239.0
posterior surface	147.3	198.89	230.0	210.7	235.1	239.0
superior surface	147.3	198.89	230.0	210.7	235.1	239.0
palatoglossal arch	146.2	198.89	230.0	210.6	235.1	239.0
palatopharyngeal arch	146.2	198.89	230.0	210.6	235.1	239.0
pallium	191.0	198.3	—	225.0	237.5	239.6
palpebra	173.1	198.2	232.1	216.1	238.2	239.2
pancreas	157.9	197.8	230.9	211.6	235.5	239.0
body	157.1	197.8	230.9	211.6	235.5	239.0
contiguous sites	157.8	—	—	—	—	—
duct (of Santorini) (of Wirsung)	157.3	197.8	230.9	211.6	235.5	239.0
ectopic tissue	157.8	197.8	230.9	211.6	235.5	239.0
head	157.0	197.8	230.9	211.6	235.5	239.0
islet cells	157.4	197.8	230.9	211.7	235.5	239.0

Neoplasm, pancreas

	Malignant			Benign	Uncertain Behavior	Unspecified
	Primary	Secondary	Ca in situ			
Neoplasm, neoplastic — *continued*						
pancreas — *continued*						
neck	157.8	197.8	230.9	211.6	235.5	239.0
tail	157.2	197.8	230.9	211.6	235.5	239.0
para-aortic body	194.6	198.89	—	227.6	237.3	239.7
paraganglion NEC	194.6	198.89	—	227.6	237.3	239.7
parametrium	183.4	198.82	—	221.0	236.3	239.5
paranephric	158.0	197.6	—	211.8	235.4	239.0
pararectal	195.3	198.89	—	229.8	238.8	239.8
parasagittal (region)	195.0	198.89	234.8	229.8	238.8	239.8
parasellar	192.9	198.4	—	225.9	237.9	239.7
parathyroid (gland)	194.1	198.89	234.8	227.1	237.4	239.7
paraurethral	195.3	198.89	—	229.8	238.8	239.8
gland	189.4	198.1	233.9	223.89	236.99	239.5
paravaginal	195.3	198.89	—	229.8	238.8	239.8
parenchyma, kidney	189.0	198.0	233.9	223.0	236.91	239.5
parietal						
bone	170.0	198.5	—	213.0	238.0	239.2
lobe, brain	191.3	198.3	—	225.0	237.5	239.6
paroophoron	183.3	198.82	233.3	221.0	236.3	239.5
parotid (duct) (gland)	142.0	198.89	230.0	210.2	235.0	239.0
parovarium	183.3	198.82	233.3	221.0	236.3	239.5
patella	170.8	198.5	—	213.8	238.0	239.2
peduncle, cerebral	191.7	198.3	—	225.0	237.5	239.6
pelvirectal junction	154.0	197.5	230.4	211.4	235.2	239.0
pelvis, pelvic	195.3	198.89	234.8	229.8	238.8	239.8
bone	170.6	198.5	—	213.6	238.0	239.2
floor	195.3	198.89	234.8	229.8	238.8	239.8
renal	189.1	198.0	233.9	223.1	236.91	239.5
viscera	195.3	198.89	234.8	229.8	238.8	239.8
wall	195.3	198.89	234.8	229.8	238.8	239.8
pelvo-abdominal	195.8	198.89	234.8	229.8	238.8	239.8
penis	187.4	198.82	233.5	222.1	236.6	239.5
body	187.3	198.82	233.5	222.1	236.6	239.5
corpus (cavernosum)	187.3	198.82	233.5	222.1	236.6	239.5
glans	187.2	198.82	233.5	222.1	236.6	239.5
skin NEC	187.4	198.82	233.5	222.1	236.6	239.5
periadrenal (tissue)	158.0	197.6	—	211.8	235.4	239.0
perianal (skin)	173.5	198.2	232.5	216.5	238.2	239.2
pericardium	164.1	198.89	—	212.7	238.8	239.8
perinephric	158.0	197.6	—	211.8	235.4	239.0
perineum	195.3	198.89	234.8	229.8	238.8	239.8
periodontal tissue NEC	143.9	198.89	230.0	210.4	235.1	239.0
periosteum — *see* Neoplasm, bone						
peripancreatic	158.0	197.6	—	211.8	235.4	239.0
peripheral nerve NEC	171.9	198.89	—	215.9	238.1	239.2
perirectal (tissue)	195.3	198.89	—	229.8	238.8	239.8
perirenal (tissue)	158.0	197.6	—	211.8	235.4	239.0
peritoneum, peritoneal (cavity)	158.9	197.6	—	211.8	235.4	239.0
contiguous sites	158.8	—	—	—	—	—
with digestive organs	159.8	—	—	—	—	—
parietal	158.8	197.6	—	211.8	235.4	239.0
pelvic	158.8	197.6	—	211.8	235.4	239.0
specified part NEC	158.8	197.6	—	211.8	235.4	239.0
peritonsillar (tissue)	195.0	198.89	234.8	229.8	238.8	239.8
periurethral tissue	195.3	198.89	—	229.8	238.8	239.8
phalanges	170.9	198.5	—	213.9	238.0	239.2
foot	170.8	198.5	—	213.8	238.0	239.2
hand	170.5	198.5	—	213.5	238.0	239.2
pharynx, pharyngeal	149.0	198.89	230.0	210.9	235.1	239.0
bursa	147.1	198.89	230.0	210.7	235.1	239.0
fornix	147.3	198.89	230.0	210.7	235.1	239.0
recess	147.2	198.89	230.0	210.7	235.1	239.0
region	149.0	198.89	230.0	210.9	235.1	239.0
tonsil	147.1	198.89	230.0	210.7	235.1	239.0
wall (lateral) (posterior)	149.0	198.89	230.0	210.9	235.1	239.0

Index to Diseases

	Malignant			Benign	Uncertain Behavior	Unspecified
	Primary	Secondary	Ca in situ			
Neoplasm, neoplastic — continued						
pia mater (cerebral) (cranial)	192.1	198.4	—	225.2	237.6	239.7
spinal	192.3	198.4	—	225.4	237.6	239.7
pillars of fauces	146.2	198.89	230.0	210.6	235.1	239.0
pineal (body) (gland)	194.4	198.89	234.8	227.4	237.1	239.7
pinna (ear) NEC	173.2	198.2	232.2	216.2	238.2	239.2
cartilage	171.0	198.89	—	215.0	238.1	239.2
piriform fossa or sinus	148.1	198.89	230.0	210.8	235.1	239.0
pituitary (body) (fossa) (gland) (lobe)	194.3	198.89	234.8	227.3	237.0	239.7
placenta	181	198.82	233.2	219.8	236.1	239.5
pleura, pleural (cavity)	163.9	197.2	—	212.4	235.8	239.1
contiguous sites	163.8	—	—	—	—	—
parietal	163.0	197.2	—	212.4	235.8	239.1
visceral	163.1	197.2	—	212.4	235.8	239.1
plexus						
brachial	171.2	198.89	—	215.2	238.1	239.2
cervical	171.0	198.89	—	215.0	238.1	239.2
choroid	191.5	198.3	—	225.0	237.5	239.6
lumbosacral	171.6	198.89	—	215.6	238.1	239.2
sacral	171.6	198.89	—	215.6	238.1	239.2
pluri-endocrine	194.8	198.89	234.8	227.8	237.4	239.7
pole						
frontal	191.1	198.3	—	225.0	237.5	239.6
occipital	191.4	198.3	—	225.0	237.5	239.6
pons (varolii)	191.7	198.3	—	225.0	237.5	239.6
popliteal fossa or space*	195.5	198.89	234.8	229.8	238.8	239.8
postcricoid (region)	148.0	198.89	230.0	210.8	235.1	239.0
posterior fossa (cranial)	191.6	198.3	—	225.0	237.5	239.6
postnasal space	147.9	198.89	230.0	210.7	235.1	239.0
prepuce	187.1	198.82	233.5	222.1	236.6	239.5
prepylorus	151.1	197.8	230.2	211.1	235.2	239.0
presacral (region)	195.3	198.89	—	229.8	238.8	239.8
prostate (gland)	185	198.82	233.4	222.2	236.5	239.5
utricle	189.3	198.1	233.9	223.81	236.99	239.5
pterygoid fossa	171.0	198.89	—	215.0	238.1	239.2
pubic bone	170.6	198.5	—	213.6	238.0	239.2
pudenda, pudendum (female)	184.4	198.82	233.3	221.2	236.3	239.5
pulmonary	162.9	197.0	231.2	212.3	235.7	239.1
putamen	191.0	198.3	—	225.0	237.5	239.6
pyloric						
antrum	151.2	197.8	230.2	211.1	235.2	239.0
canal	151.1	197.8	230.2	211.1	235.2	239.0
pylorus	151.1	197.8	230.2	211.1	235.2	239.0
pyramid (brain)	191.7	198.3	—	225.0	237.5	239.6
pyriform fossa or sinus	148.1	198.89	230.0	210.8	235.1	239.0
radius (any part)	170.4	198.5	—	213.4	238.0	239.2
Rathke's pouch	194.3	198.89	234.8	227.3	237.0	239.7
rectosigmoid (colon) (junction)	154.0	197.5	230.4	211.4	235.2	239.0
contiguous sites with anus or rectum	154.8	—	—	—	—	—
rectouterine pouch	158.8	197.6	—	211.8	235.4	239.0
rectovaginal septum or wall	195.3	198.89	234.8	229.8	238.8	239.8
rectovesical septum	195.3	198.89	234.8	229.8	238.8	239.8
rectum (ampulla)	154.1	197.5	230.4	211.4	235.2	239.0
and colon	154.0	197.5	230.4	211.4	235.2	239.0
contiguous sites with anus or rectosigmoid junction	154.8	—	—	—	—	—
renal	189.0	198.0	233.9	223.0	236.91	239.5
calyx	189.1	198.0	233.9	223.1	236.91	239.5
hilus	189.1	198.0	233.9	223.1	236.91	239.5
parenchyma	189.0	198.0	233.9	223.0	236.91	239.5
pelvis	189.1	198.0	233.9	223.1	236.91	239.5
respiratory						
organs or system NEC	165.9	197.3	231.9	212.9	235.9	239.1
contiguous sites with intrathoracic organs	165.8	—	—	—	—	—
specified sites NEC	165.8	197.3	231.8	212.8	235.9	239.1
tract NEC	165.9	197.3	231.9	212.9	235.9	239.1
upper	165.0	197.3	231.9	212.9	235.9	239.1
retina	190.5	198.4	234.0	224.5	238.8	239.8

Fourth-digit Required Fifth-digit Required ▶◀ Revised Text ● New Line ▲ Revised Code

	Malignant			Benign	Uncertain Behavior	Unspecified
	Primary	Secondary	Ca in situ			
Neoplasm, neoplastic — *continued*						
retrobulbar	190.1	198.4	—	224.1	238.8	239.8
retrocecal	158.0	197.6	—	211.8	235.4	239.0
retromolar (area) (triangle) (trigone)	145.6	198.89	230.0	210.4	235.1	239.0
retro-orbital	195.0	198.89	234.8	229.8	238.8	239.8
retroperitoneal (space) (tissue)	158.0	197.6	—	211.8	235.4	239.0
contiguous sites	158.8	—	—	—	—	—
retroperitoneum	158.0	197.6	—	211.8	235.4	239.0
contiguous sites	158.8	—	—	—	—	—
retropharyngeal	149.0	198.89	230.0	210.9	235.1	239.0
retrovesical (septum)	195.3	198.89	234.8	229.8	238.8	239.8
rhinencephalon	191.0	198.3	—	225.0	237.5	239.6
rib	170.3	198.5	—	213.3	238.0	239.2
Rosenmüller's fossa	147.2	198.89	230.0	210.7	235.1	239.0
round ligament	183.5	198.82	—	221.0	236.3	239.5
sacrococcyx, sacrococcygeal	170.6	198.5	—	213.6	238.0	239.2
region	195.3	198.89	234.8	229.8	238.8	239.8
sacrouterine ligament	183.4	198.82	—	221.0	236.3	239.5
sacrum, sacral (vertebra)	170.6	198.5	—	213.6	238.0	239.2
salivary gland or duct (major)	142.9	198.89	230.0	210.2	235.0	239.0
contiguous sites	142.8	—	—	—	—	—
minor NEC	145.9	198.89	230.0	210.4	235.1	239.0
parotid	142.0	198.89	230.0	210.2	235.0	239.0
pluriglandular	142.8	198.89	230.0	210.2	235.0	239.0
sublingual	142.2	198.89	230.0	210.2	235.0	239.0
submandibular	142.1	198.89	230.0	210.2	235.0	239.0
submaxillary	142.1	198.89	230.0	210.2	235.0	239.0
salpinx (uterine)	183.2	198.82	233.3	221.0	236.3	239.5
Santorini's duct	157.3	197.8	230.9	211.6	235.5	239.0
scalp	173.4	198.2	232.4	216.4	238.2	239.2
scapula (any part)	170.4	198.5	—	213.4	238.0	239.2
scapular region	195.1	198.89	234.8	229.8	238.8	239.8
scar NEC (*see also* Neoplasm, skin)	173.9	198.2	232.9	216.9	238.2	239.2
sciatic nerve	171.3	198.89	—	215.3	238.1	239.2
sclera	190.0	198.4	234.0	224.0	238.8	239.8
scrotum (skin)	187.7	198.82	233.6	222.4	236.6	239.5
sebaceous gland — *see* Neoplasm, skin						
sella turcica	194.3	198.89	234.8	227.3	237.0	239.7
bone	170.0	198.5	—	213.0	238.0	239.2
semilunar cartilage (knee)	170.7	198.5	—	213.7	238.0	239.2
seminal vesicle	187.8	198.82	233.6	222.8	236.6	239.5
septum						
nasal	160.0	197.3	231.8	212.0	235.9	239.1
posterior margin	147.3	198.89	230.0	210.7	235.1	239.0
rectovaginal	195.3	198.89	234.8	229.8	238.8	239.8
rectovesical	195.3	198.89	234.8	229.8	238.8	239.8
urethrovaginal	184.9	198.82	233.3	221.9	236.3	239.5
vesicovaginal	184.9	198.82	233.3	221.9	236.3	239.5
shoulder NEC*	195.4	198.89	232.6	229.8	238.8	239.8
sigmoid flexure (lower) (upper)	153.3	197.5	230.3	211.3	235.2	239.0
sinus (accessory)	160.9	197.3	231.8	212.0	235.9	239.1
bone (any)	170.0	198.5	—	213.0	238.0	239.2
contiguous sites with middle ear or nasal cavities	160.8	—	—	—	—	—
ethmoidal	160.3	197.3	231.8	212.0	235.9	239.1
frontal	160.4	197.3	231.8	212.0	235.9	239.1
maxillary	160.2	197.3	231.8	212.0	235.9	239.1
nasal, paranasal NEC	160.9	197.3	231.8	212.0	235.9	239.1
pyriform	148.1	198.89	230.0	210.8	235.1	239.0
sphenoidal	160.5	197.3	231.8	212.0	235.9	239.1
skeleton, skeletal NEC	170.9	198.5	—	213.9	238.0	239.2
Skene's gland	189.4	198.1	233.9	223.89	236.99	239.5
skin NEC	173.9	198.2	232.9	216.9	238.2	239.2
abdominal wall	173.5	198.2	232.5	216.5	238.2	239.2
ala nasi	173.3	198.2	232.3	216.3	238.2	239.2
ankle	173.7	198.2	232.7	216.7	238.2	239.2
antecubital space	173.6	198.2	232.6	216.6	238.2	239.2
anus	173.5	198.2	232.5	216.5	238.2	239.2

Index to Diseases — Neoplasm, skin

	Malignant			Benign	Uncertain Behavior	Unspecified
	Primary	**Secondary**	**Ca in situ**			
Neoplasm, neoplastic — *continued*						
skin NEC — *continued*						
arm	173.6	198.2	232.6	216.6	238.2	239.2
auditory canal (external)	173.2	198.2	232.2	216.2	238.2	239.2
auricle (ear)	173.2	198.2	232.2	216.2	238.2	239.2
auricular canal (external)	173.2	198.2	232.2	216.2	238.2	239.2
axilla, axillary fold	173.5	198.2	232.5	216.5	238.2	239.2
back	173.5	198.2	232.5	216.5	238.2	239.2
breast	173.5	198.2	232.5	216.5	238.2	239.2
brow	173.3	198.2	232.3	216.3	238.2	239.2
buttock	173.5	198.2	232.5	216.5	238.2	239.2
calf	173.7	198.2	232.7	216.7	238.2	239.2
canthus (eye) (inner) (outer)	173.1	198.2	232.1	216.1	238.2	239.2
cervical region	173.4	198.2	232.4	216.4	238.2	239.2
cheek (external)	173.3	198.2	232.3	216.3	238.2	239.2
chest (wall)	173.5	198.2	232.5	216.5	238.2	239.2
chin	173.3	198.2	232.3	216.3	238.2	239.2
clavicular area	173.5	198.2	232.5	216.5	238.2	239.2
clitoris	184.3	198.82	233.3	221.2	236.3	239.5
columnella	173.3	198.2	232.3	216.3	238.2	239.2
concha	173.2	198.2	232.2	216.2	238.2	239.2
contiguous sites	173.8	—	—	—	—	—
ear (external)	173.2	198.2	232.2	216.2	238.2	239.2
elbow	173.6	198.2	232.6	216.6	238.2	239.2
eyebrow	173.3	198.2	232.3	216.3	238.2	239.2
eyelid	173.1	198.2	232.1	216.1	238.2	239.2
face NEC	173.3	198.2	232.3	216.3	238.2	239.2
female genital organs (external)	184.4	198.82	233.3	221.2	236.3	239.5
clitoris	184.3	198.82	233.3	221.2	236.3	239.5
labium NEC	184.4	198.82	233.3	221.2	236.3	239.5
majus	184.1	198.82	233.3	221.2	236.3	239.5
minus	184.2	198.82	233.3	221.2	236.3	239.5
pudendum	184.4	198.82	233.3	221.2	236.3	239.5
vulva	184.4	198.82	233.3	221.2	236.3	239.5
finger	173.6	198.2	232.6	216.6	238.2	239.2
flank	173.5	198.2	232.5	216.5	238.2	239.2
foot	173.7	198.2	232.7	216.7	238.2	239.2
forearm	173.6	198.2	232.6	216.6	238.2	239.2
forehead	173.3	198.2	232.3	216.3	238.2	239.2
glabella	173.3	198.2	232.3	216.3	238.2	239.2
gluteal region	173.5	198.2	232.5	216.5	238.2	239.2
groin	173.5	198.2	232.5	216.5	238.2	239.2
hand	173.6	198.2	232.6	216.6	238.2	239.2
head NEC	173.4	198.2	232.4	216.4	238.2	239.2
heel	173.7	198.2	232.7	216.7	238.2	239.2
helix	173.2	198.2	232.2	216.2	238.2	239.2
hip	173.7	198.2	232.7	216.7	238.2	239.2
infraclavicular region	173.5	198.2	232.5	216.5	238.2	239.2
inguinal region	173.5	198.2	232.5	216.5	238.2	239.2
jaw	173.3	198.2	232.3	216.3	238.2	239.2
knee	173.7	198.2	232.7	216.7	238.2	239.2
labia						
majora	184.1	198.82	233.3	221.2	236.3	239.5
minora	184.2	198.82	233.3	221.2	236.3	239.5
leg	173.7	198.2	232.7	216.7	238.2	239.2
lid (lower) (upper)	173.1	198.2	232.1	216.1	238.2	239.2
limb NEC	173.9	198.2	232.9	216.9	238.2	239.5
lower	173.7	198.2	232.7	216.7	238.2	239.2
upper	173.6	198.2	232.6	216.6	238.2	239.2
lip (lower) (upper)	173.0	198.2	232.0	216.0	238.2	239.2
male genital organs	187.9	198.82	233.6	222.9	236.6	239.5
penis	187.4	198.82	233.5	222.1	236.6	239.5
prepuce	187.1	198.82	233.5	222.1	236.6	239.5
scrotum	187.7	198.82	233.6	222.4	236.6	239.5
mastectomy site	173.5	198.2	—	—	—	—
specified as breast tissue	174.8	198.81	—	—	—	—
meatus, acoustic (external)	173.2	198.2	232.2	216.2	238.2	239.2

✓4ᵗʰ Fourth-digit Required   ✓5ᵗʰ Fifth-digit Required   ▶◀ Revised Text   ● New Line   ▲ Revised Code

Neoplasm, skin

	Malignant			Benign	Uncertain Behavior	Unspecified
	Primary	Secondary	Ca in situ			
Neoplasm, neoplastic — *continued*						
skin NEC — *continued*						
melanoma — *see* Melanoma						
nates	173.5	198.2	232.5	216.5	238.2	239.0
neck	173.4	198.2	232.4	216.4	238.2	239.2
nose (external)	173.3	198.2	232.3	216.3	238.2	239.2
palm	173.6	198.2	232.6	216.6	238.2	239.2
palpebra	173.1	198.2	232.1	216.1	238.2	239.2
penis NEC	187.4	198.82	233.5	222.1	236.6	239.5
perianal	173.5	198.2	232.5	216.5	238.2	239.2
perineum	173.5	198.2	232.5	216.5	238.2	239.2
pinna	173.2	198.2	232.2	216.2	238.2	239.2
plantar	173.7	198.2	232.7	216.7	238.2	239.2
popliteal fossa or space	173.7	198.2	232.7	216.7	238.2	239.2
prepuce	187.1	198.82	233.5	222.1	236.6	239.5
pubes	173.5	198.2	232.5	216.5	238.2	239.2
sacrococcygeal region	173.5	198.2	232.5	216.5	238.2	239.2
scalp	173.4	198.2	232.4	216.4	238.2	239.2
scapular region	173.5	198.2	232.5	216.5	238.2	239.2
scrotum	187.7	198.82	233.6	222.4	236.6	239.5
shoulder	173.6	198.2	232.6	216.6	238.2	239.2
sole (foot)	173.7	198.2	232.7	216.7	238.2	239.2
specified sites NEC	173.8	198.2	232.8	216.8	232.8	239.2
submammary fold	173.5	198.2	232.5	216.5	238.2	239.2
supraclavicular region	173.4	198.2	232.4	216.4	238.2	239.2
temple	173.3	198.2	232.3	216.3	238.2	239.2
thigh	173.7	198.2	232.7	216.7	238.2	239.2
thoracic wall	173.5	198.2	232.5	216.5	238.2	239.2
thumb	173.6	198.2	232.6	216.6	238.2	239.2
toe	173.7	198.2	232.7	216.7	238.2	239.2
tragus	173.2	198.2	232.2	216.2	238.2	239.2
trunk	173.5	198.2	232.5	216.5	238.2	239.2
umbilicus	173.5	198.2	232.5	216.5	238.2	239.2
vulva	184.4	198.82	233.3	221.2	236.3	239.5
wrist	173.6	198.2	232.6	216.6	238.2	239.2
skull	170.0	198.5	—	213.0	238.0	239.2
soft parts or tissues — *see* Neoplasm, connective tissue						
specified site NEC	195.8	198.89	234.8	229.8	238.8	239.8
spermatic cord	187.6	198.82	233.6	222.8	236.6	239.5
sphenoid	160.5	197.3	231.8	212.0	235.9	239.1
bone	170.0	198.5	—	213.0	238.0	239.2
sinus	160.5	197.3	231.8	212.0	235.9	239.1
sphincter						
anal	154.2	197.5	230.5	211.4	235.5	239.0
of Oddi	156.1	197.8	230.8	211.5	235.3	239.0
spine, spinal (column)	170.2	198.5	—	213.2	238.0	239.2
bulb	191.7	198.3	—	225.0	237.5	239.6
coccyx	170.6	198.5	—	213.6	238.0	239.2
cord (cervical) (lumbar) (sacral) (thoracic)	192.2	198.3	—	225.3	237.5	239.7
dura mater	192.3	198.4	—	225.4	237.6	239.7
lumbosacral	170.2	198.5	—	213.2	238.0	239.2
membrane	192.3	198.4	—	225.4	237.6	239.7
meninges	192.3	198.4	—	225.4	237.6	239.7
nerve (root)	171.9	198.89	—	215.9	238.1	239.2
pia mater	192.3	198.4	—	225.4	237.6	239.7
root	171.9	198.89	—	215.9	238.1	239.2
sacrum	170.6	198.5	—	213.6	238.0	239.2
spleen, splenic NEC	159.1	197.8	230.9	211.9	235.5	239.0
flexure (colon)	153.7	197.5	230.3	211.3	235.2	239.0
stem, brain	191.7	198.3	—	225.0	237.5	239.6
Stensen's duct	142.0	198.89	230.0	210.2	235.0	239.0
sternum	170.3	198.5	—	213.3	238.0	239.2
stomach	151.9	197.8	230.2	211.1	235.2	239.0
antrum (pyloric)	151.2	197.8	230.2	211.1	235.2	239.0
body	151.4	197.8	230.2	211.1	235.2	239.0
cardia	151.0	197.8	230.2	211.1	235.2	239.0
cardiac orifice	151.0	197.8	230.2	211.1	235.2	239.0

Index to Diseases

Neoplasm, tongue

	Malignant			Benign	Uncertain Behavior	Unspecified
	Primary	Secondary	Ca in situ			
Neoplasm, neoplastic — *continued*						
stomach — *continued*						
contiguous sites	151.8	—	—	—	—	—
corpus	151.4	197.8	230.2	211.1	235.2	239.0
fundus	151.3	197.8	230.2	211.1	235.2	239.0
greater curvature NEC	151.6	197.8	230.2	211.1	235.2	239.0
lesser curvature NEC	151.5	197.8	230.2	211.1	235.2	239.0
prepylorus	151.1	197.8	230.2	211.1	235.2	239.0
pylorus	151.1	197.8	230.2	211.1	235.2	239.0
wall NEC	151.9	197.8	230.2	211.1	235.2	239.0
anterior NEC	151.8	197.8	230.2	211.1	235.2	239.0
posterior NEC	151.8	197.8	230.2	211.1	235.2	239.0
stroma, endometrial	182.0	198.82	233.2	219.1	236.0	239.5
stump, cervical	180.8	198.82	233.1	219.0	236.0	239.5
subcutaneous (nodule) (tissue) NEC — *see* Neoplasm, connective tissue						
subdural	192.1	198.4	—	225.2	237.6	239.7
subglottis, subglottic	161.2	197.3	231.0	212.1	235.6	239.1
sublingual	144.9	198.89	230.0	210.3	235.1	239.0
gland or duct	142.2	198.89	230.0	210.2	235.0	239.0
submandibular gland	142.1	198.89	230.0	210.2	235.0	239.0
submaxillary gland or duct	142.1	198.89	230.0	210.2	235.0	239.0
submental	195.0	198.89	234.8	229.8	238.8	239.8
subpleural	162.9	197.0	—	212.3	235.7	239.1
substernal	164.2	197.1	—	212.5	235.8	239.8
sudoriferous, sudoriparous gland, site unspecified	173.9	198.2	232.9	216.9	238.2	239.2
specified site — *see* Neoplasm, skin						
supraclavicular region	195.0	198.89	234.8	229.8	238.8	239.8
supraglottis	161.1	197.3	231.0	212.1	235.6	239.1
suprarenal (capsule) (cortex) (gland) (medulla)	194.0	198.7	234.8	227.0	237.2	239.7
suprasellar (region)	191.9	198.3	—	225.0	237.5	239.6
sweat gland (apocrine) (eccrine), site unspecified	173.9	198.2	232.9	216.9	238.2	239.2
specified site — *see* Neoplasm, skin						
sympathetic nerve or nervous system NEC	171.9	198.89	—	215.9	238.1	239.2
symphysis pubis	170.6	198.5	—	213.6	238.0	239.2
synovial membrane — *see* Neoplasm, connective tissue						
tapetum, brain	191.8	198.3	—	225.0	237.5	239.6
tarsus (any bone)	170.8	198.5	—	213.8	238.0	239.2
temple (skin)	173.3	198.2	232.3	216.3	238.2	239.2
temporal						
bone	170.0	198.5	—	213.0	238.0	239.2
lobe or pole	191.2	198.3	—	225.0	237.5	239.6
region	195.0	198.89	234.8	229.8	238.8	239.8
skin	173.3	198.2	232.3	216.3	238.2	239.2
tendon (sheath) — *see* Neoplasm, connective tissue						
tentorium (cerebelli)	192.1	198.4	—	225.2	237.6	239.7
testis, testes (descended) (scrotal)	186.9	198.82	233.6	222.0	236.4	239.5
ectopic	186.0	198.82	233.6	222.0	236.4	239.5
retained	186.0	198.82	233.6	222.0	236.4	239.5
undescended	186.0	198.82	233.6	222.0	236.4	239.5
thalamus	191.0	198.3	—	225.0	237.5	239.6
thigh NEC*	195.5	198.89	234.8	229.8	238.8	239.8
thorax, thoracic (cavity) (organs NEC)	195.1	198.89	234.8	229.8	238.8	239.8
duct	171.4	198.89	—	215.4	238.1	239.2
wall NEC	195.1	198.89	234.8	229.8	238.8	239.8
throat	149.0	198.89	230.0	210.9	235.1	239.0
thumb NEC*	195.4	198.89	232.6	229.8	238.8	239.8
thymus (gland)	164.0	198.89	—	212.6	235.8	239.8
contiguous sites with heart and mediastinum	164.8	—	—	—	—	—
thyroglossal duct	193	198.89	234.8	226	237.4	239.7
thyroid (gland)	193	198.89	234.8	226	237.4	239.7
cartilage	161.3	197.3	231.0	212.1	235.6	239.1
tibia (any part)	170.7	198.5	—	213.7	238.0	239.2
toe NEC*	195.5	198.89	232.7	229.8	238.8	239.8
tongue	141.9	198.89	230.0	210.1	235.1	239.0
anterior (two-thirds) NEC	141.4	198.89	230.0	210.1	235.1	239.0
dorsal surface	141.1	198.89	230.0	210.1	235.1	239.0
ventral surface	141.3	198.89	230.0	210.1	235.1	239.0

	Malignant			Benign	Uncertain Behavior	Unspecified
	Primary	Secondary	Ca in situ			
Neoplasm, neoplastic — *continued*						
tongue — *continued*						
base (dorsal surface)	141.0	198.89	230.0	210.1	235.1	239.0
border (lateral)	141.2	198.89	230.0	210.1	235.1	239.0
contiguous sites	141.8	—	—	—	—	—
dorsal surface NEC	141.1	198.89	230.0	210.1	235.1	239.0
fixed part NEC	141.0	198.89	230.0	210.1	235.1	239.0
foreamen cecum	141.1	198.89	230.0	210.1	235.1	239.0
frenulum linguae	141.3	198.89	230.0	210.1	235.1	239.0
junctional zone	141.5	198.89	230.0	210.1	235.1	239.0
margin (lateral)	141.2	198.89	230.0	210.1	235.1	239.0
midline NEC	141.1	198.89	230.0	210.1	235.1	239.0
mobile part NEC	141.4	198.89	230.0	210.1	235.1	239.0
posterior (third)	141.0	198.89	230.0	210.1	235.1	239.0
root	141.0	198.89	230.0	210.1	235.1	239.0
surface (dorsal)	141.1	198.89	230.0	210.1	235.1	239.0
base	141.0	198.89	230.0	210.1	235.1	239.0
ventral	141.3	198.89	230.0	210.1	235.1	239.0
tip	141.2	198.89	230.0	210.1	235.1	239.0
tonsil	141.6	198.89	230.0	210.1	235.1	239.0
tonsil	146.0	198.89	230.0	210.5	235.1	239.0
fauces, faucial	146.0	198.89	230.0	210.5	235.1	239.0
lingual	141.6	198.89	230.0	210.1	235.1	239.0
palatine	146.0	198.89	230.0	210.5	235.1	239.0
pharyngeal	147.1	198.89	230.0	210.7	235.1	239.0
pillar (anterior) (posterior)	146.2	198.89	230.0	210.6	235.1	239.0
tonsillar fossa	146.1	198.89	230.0	210.6	235.1	239.0
tooth socket NEC	143.9	198.89	230.0	210.4	235.1	239.0
trachea (cartilage) (mucosa)	162.0	197.3	231.1	212.2	235.7	239.1
contiguous sites with bronchus or lung	162.8	—	—	—	—	—
tracheobronchial	162.8	197.3	231.1	212.2	235.7	239.1
contiguous sites with lung	162.8	—	—	—	—	—
tragus	173.2	198.2	232.2	216.2	238.2	239.2
trunk NEC*	195.8	198.89	232.5	229.8	238.8	239.8
tubo-ovarian	183.8	198.82	233.3	221.8	236.3	239.5
tunica vaginalis	187.8	198.82	233.6	222.8	236.6	239.5
turbinate (bone)	170.0	198.5	—	213.0	238.0	239.2
nasal	160.0	197.3	231.8	212.0	235.9	239.1
tympanic cavity	160.1	197.3	231.8	212.0	235.9	239.1
ulna (any part)	170.4	198.5	—	213.4	238.0	239.2
umbilicus, umbilical	173.5	198.2	232.5	216.5	238.2	239.2
uncus, brain	191.2	198.3	—	225.0	237.5	239.6
unknown site or unspecified	199.1	199.1	234.9	229.9	238.9	239.9
urachus	188.7	198.1	233.7	223.3	236.7	239.4
ureter, ureteral	189.2	198.1	233.9	223.2	236.91	239.5
orifice (bladder)	188.6	198.1	233.7	223.3	236.7	239.4
ureter-bladder junction)	188.6	198.1	233.7	223.3	236.7	239.4
urethra, urethral (gland)	189.3	198.1	233.9	223.81	236.99	239.5
orifice, internal	188.5	198.1	233.7	223.3	236.7	239.4
urethrovaginal (septum)	184.9	198.82	233.3	221.9	236.3	239.5
urinary organ or system NEC	189.9	198.1	233.9	223.9	236.99	239.5
bladder — *see* Neoplasm, bladder						
contiguous sites	189.8	—	—	—	—	—
specified sites NEC	189.8	198.1	233.9	223.89	236.99	239.5
utero-ovarian	183.8	198.82	233.3	221.8	236.3	239.5
ligament	183.3	198.82	—	221.0	236.3	239.5
uterosacral ligament	183.4	198.82	—	221.0	236.3	239.5
uterus, uteri, uterine	179	198.82	233.2	219.9	236.0	239.5
adnexa NEC	183.9	198.82	233.3	221.8	236.3	239.5
contiguous sites	183.8	—	—	—	—	—
body	182.0	198.82	233.2	219.1	236.0	239.5
contiguous sites	182.8	—	—	—	—	—
cervix	180.9	198.82	233.1	219.0	236.0	239.5
tornu	182.0	198.82	233.2	219.1	236.0	239.5
corpus	182.0	198.82	233.2	219.1	236.0	239.5
endocervix (canal) (gland)	180.0	198.82	233.1	219.0	236.0	239.5
endometrium	182.0	198.82	233.2	219.1	236.0	239.5

Index to Diseases

	Malignant			Benign	Uncertain Behavior	Unspecified
	Primary	Secondary	Ca in situ			
Neoplasm, neoplastic — *continued*						
uterus, uteri, uterine — *continued*						
exocervix	180.1	198.82	233.1	219.0	236.0	239.5
external os	180.1	198.82	233.1	219.0	236.0	239.5
fundus	182.0	198.82	233.2	219.1	236.0	239.5
internal os	180.0	198.82	233.1	219.0	236.0	239.5
isthmus	182.1	198.82	233.2	219.1	236.0	239.5
ligament	183.4	198.82	—	221.0	236.3	239.5
broad	183.3	198.82	233.3	221.0	236.3	239.5
round	183.5	198.82	—	221.0	236.3	239.5
lower segment	182.1	198.82	233.2	219.1	236.0	239.5
myometrium	182.0	198.82	233.2	219.1	236.0	239.5
squamocolumnar junction	180.8	198.82	233.1	219.0	236.0	239.5
tube	183.2	198.82	233.3	221.0	236.3	239.5
utricle, prostatic	189.3	198.1	233.9	223.81	236.99	239.5
uveal tract	190.0	198.4	234.0	224.0	238.8	239.8
uvula	145.4	198.89	230.0	210.4	235.1	239.0
vagina, vaginal (fornix) (vault) (wall)	184.0	198.82	233.3	221.1	236.3	239.5
vaginovesical	184.9	198.82	233.3	221.9	236.3	239.5
septum	194.9	198.82	233.3	221.9	236.3	239.5
vallecula (epiglottis)	146.3	198.89	230.0	210.6	235.1	239.0
vascular — *see* Neoplasm, connective tissue						
vas deferens	187.6	198.82	233.6	222.8	236.6	239.5
Vater's ampulla	156.2	197.8	230.8	211.5	235.3	239.0
vein, venous — *see* Neoplasm, connective tissue						
vena cava (abdominal) (inferior)	171.5	198.89	—	215.5	238.1	239.2
superior	171.4	198.89	—	215.4	238.1	239.2
ventricle (cerebral) (floor) (fourth) (lateral) (third)	191.5	198.3	—	225.0	237.5	239.6
cardiac (left) (right)	164.1	198.89	—	212.7	238.8	239.8
ventricular band of larynx	161.1	197.3	231.0	212.1	235.6	239.1
ventriculus — *see* Neoplasm, stomach						
vermillion border — *see* Neoplasm, lip						
vermis, cerebellum	191.6	198.3	—	225.0	237.5	239.6
vertebra (column)	170.2	198.5	—	213.2	238.0	239.2
coccyx	170.6	198.5	—	213.6	238.0	239.2
sacrum	170.6	198.5	—	213.6	238.0	239.2
vesical — *see* Neoplasm, bladder						
vesicle, seminal	187.8	198.82	233.6	222.8	236.6	239.5
vesicocervical tissue	184.9	198.82	233.3	221.9	236.3	239.5
vesicorectal	195.3	198.89	234.8	229.8	238.8	239.8
vesicovaginal	184.9	198.82	233.3	221.9	236.3	239.5
septum	184.9	198.82	233.3	221.9	236.3	239.5
vessel (blood) — *see* Neoplasm, connective tissue						
vestibular gland, greater	184.1	198.82	233.3	221.2	236.3	239.5
vestibule						
mouth	145.1	198.89	230.0	210.4	235.1	239.0
nose	160.0	197.3	231.8	212.0	235.9	239.1
Virchow's gland	—	196.0	—	229.0	238.8	239.8
viscera NEC	195.8	198.89	234.8	229.8	238.8	239.8
vocal cords (true)	161.0	197.3	231.0	212.1	235.6	239.1
false	161.1	197.3	231.0	212.1	235.6	239.1
vomer	170.0	198.5	—	213.0	238.0	239.2
vulva	184.4	198.82	233.3	221.2	236.3	239.5
vulvovaginal gland	184.4	198.82	233.3	221.2	236.3	239.5
Waldeyer's ring	149.1	198.89	230.0	210.9	235.1	239.0
Wharton's duct	142.1	198.89	230.0	210.2	235.0	239.0
white matter (central) (cerebral)	191.0	198.3	—	225.0	237.5	239.6
windpipe	162.0	197.3	231.1	212.2	235.7	239.1
Wirsung's duct	157.3	197.8	230.9	211.6	235.5	239.0
wolffian (body) (duct)						
female	184.8	198.82	233.3	221.8	236.3	239.5
male	187.8	198.82	233.6	222.8	236.6	239.5
womb — *see* Neoplasm, uterus						
wrist NEC*	195.4	198.89	232.6	229.8	238.8	239.8
xiphoid process	170.3	198.5	—	213.3	238.0	239.2
Zuckerkandl's organ	194.6	198.89	—	227.6	237.3	239.7

Neovascularization
- choroid 362.16
- ciliary body 364.42
- cornea 370.60
  - deep 370.63
  - localized 370.61
- iris 364.42
- retina 362.16
- subretinal 362.16

Nephralgia 788.0

Nephritis, nephritic (albuminuric) (azotemic) (congenital) (degenerative) (diffuse) (disseminated) (epithelial) (familial) (focal) (granulomatous) (hemorrhagic) (infantile) (nonsuppurative, excretory) (uremic) 583.9
- with
  - edema — see Nephrosis
  - lesion of
    - glomerulonephritis
      - hypocomplementemic persistent 583.2
        - with nephrotic syndrome 581.2
        - chronic 582.2
      - lobular 583.2
        - with nephrotic syndrome 581.2
        - chronic 582.2
      - membranoproliferative 583.2
        - with nephrotic syndrome 581.2
        - chronic 582.2
      - membranous 583.1
        - with nephrotic syndrome 581.1
        - chronic 582.1
      - mesangiocapillary 583.2
        - with nephrotic syndrome 581.2
        - chronic 582.2
      - mixed membranous and proliferative 583.2
        - with nephrotic syndrome 581.2
        - chronic 582.2
      - proliferative (diffuse) 583.0
        - with nephrotic syndrome 581.0
        - acute 580.0
        - chronic 582.0
      - rapidly progressive 583.4
        - acute 580.4
        - chronic 582.4
    - interstitial nephritis (diffuse) (focal) 583.89
      - with nephrotic syndrome 581.89
      - acute 580.89
      - chronic 582.89
    - necrotizing glomerulitis 583.4
      - acute 580.4
      - chronic 582.4
    - renal necrosis 583.9
      - cortical 583.6
      - medullary 583.7
    - specified pathology NEC 583.89
      - with nephrotic syndrome 581.89
      - acute 580.89
      - chronic 582.89
  - necrosis, renal 583.9
    - cortical 583.6
    - medullary (papillary) 583.7
  - nephrotic syndrome (see also Nephrosis) 581.9
  - papillary necrosis 583.7
  - specified pathology NEC 583.89
- acute 580.9
  - extracapillary with epithelial crescents 580.4
  - hypertensive (see also Hypertension, kidney) 403.90
  - necrotizing 580.4
  - poststreptococcal 580.0
  - proliferative (diffuse) 580.0
  - rapidly progressive 580.4
  - specified pathology NEC 580.89
- amyloid 277.3 [583.81]
  - chronic 277.3 [582.81]
- arteriolar (see also Hypertension, kidney) 403.90
- arteriosclerotic (see also Hypertension, kidney) 403.90
- ascending (see also Pyelitis) 590.80
- atrophic 582.9

Nephritis, nephritic — continued
- basement membrane NEC 583.89
  - with
    - pulmonary hemorrhage (Goodpasture's syndrome) 446.21 [583.81]
- calculous, calculus 592.0
- cardiac (see also Hypertension, kidney) 403.90
- cardiovascular (see also Hypertension, kidney) 403.90
- chronic 582.9
  - arteriosclerotic (see also Hypertension, kidney) 403.90
  - hypertensive (see also Hypertension, kidney) 403.90
- cirrhotic (see also Sclerosis, renal) 587
- complicating pregnancy, childbirth, or puerperium 646.2 ✓5
  - with hypertension 642.1 ✓5
  - affecting fetus or newborn 760.0
  - affecting fetus or newborn 760.1
- croupous 580.9
- desquamative — see Nephrosis
- due to
  - amyloidosis 277.3 [583.81]
    - chronic 277.3 [582.81]
  - arteriosclerosis (see also Hypertension, kidney) 403.90
  - diabetes mellitus 250.4 ✓5 [583.81]
    - with nephrotic syndrome 250.4 ✓5 [581.81]
  - diphtheria 032.89 [580.81]
  - gonococcal infection (acute) 098.19 [583.81]
    - chronic or duration of 2 months or over 098.39 [583.81]
  - gout 274.10
  - infectious hepatitis 070.9 [580.81]
  - mumps 072.79 [580.81]
  - specified kidney pathology NEC 583.89
    - acute 580.89
    - chronic 582.89
  - streptotrichosis 039.8 [583.81]
  - subacute bacterial endocarditis 421.0
  - systemic lupus erythematosus 710.0 [583.81]
    - chronic 710.0 [582.81]
  - typhoid fever 002.0 [580.81]
- endothelial 582.2
- end stage (chronic) (terminal) NEC 585
- epimembranous 581.1
- exudative 583.89
  - with nephrotic syndrome 581.89
  - acute 580.89
  - chronic 582.89
- gonococcal (acute) 098.19 [583.81]
  - chronic or duration of 2 months or over 098.39 [583.81]
- gouty 274.10
- hereditary (Alport's syndrome) 759.89
- hydremic — see Nephrosis
- hypertensive (see also Hypertension, kidney) 403.90
- hypocomplementemic persistent 583.2
  - with nephrotic syndrome 581.2
  - chronic 582.2
- immune complex NEC 583.89
- infective (see also Pyelitis) 590.80
- interstitial (diffuse) (focal) 583.89
  - with nephrotic syndrome 581.89
  - acute 580.89
  - chronic 582.89
- latent or quiescent — see Nephritis, chronic
- lead 984.9
  - specified type of lead — see Table of Drugs and Chemicals
- lobular 583.2
  - with nephrotic syndrome 581.2
  - chronic 582.2
- lupus 710.0 [583.81]
  - acute 710.0 [580.81]
  - chronic 710.0 [582.81]
- membranoproliferative 583.2
  - with nephrotic syndrome 581.2
  - chronic 582.2
- membranous 583.1
  - with nephrotic syndrome 581.1
  - chronic 582.1

Nephritis, nephritic — continued
- mesangiocapillary 583.2
  - with nephrotic syndrome 581.2
  - chronic 582.2
- minimal change 581.3
- mixed membranous and proliferative 583.2
  - with nephrotic syndrome 581.2
  - chronic 582.2
- necrotic, necrotizing 583.4
  - acute 580.4
  - chronic 582.4
- nephrotic — see Nephrosis
- old — see Nephritis, chronic
- parenchymatous 581.89
- polycystic 753.12
  - adult type (APKD) 753.13
  - autosomal dominant 753.13
  - autosomal recessive 753.14
  - childhood type (CPKD) 753.14
  - infantile type 753.14
- poststreptococcal 580.0
- pregnancy — see Nephritis, complicating pregnancy
- proliferative 583.0
  - with nephrotic syndrome 581.0
  - acute 580.0
  - chronic 582.0
- purulent (see also Pyelitis) 590.80
- rapidly progressive 583.4
  - acute 580.4
  - chronic 582.4
- salt-losing or salt-wasting (see also Disease, renal) 593.9
- saturnine 984.9
  - specified type of lead — see Table of Drugs and Chemicals
- septic (see also Pyelitis) 590.80
- specified pathology NEC 583.89
  - acute 580.89
  - chronic 582.89
- staphylococcal (see also Pyelitis) 590.80
- streptotrichosis 039.8 [583.81]
- subacute (see also Nephrosis) 581.9
- suppurative (see also Pyelitis) 590.80
- syphilitic (late) 095.4
  - congenital 090.5 [583.81]
  - early 091.69 [583.81]
- terminal (chronic) (end-stage) NEC 585
- toxic — see Nephritis, acute
- tubal, tubular — see Nephrosis, tubular
- tuberculous (see also Tuberculosis) 016.0 ✓5 [583.81]
- type II (Ellis) — see Nephrosis
- vascular — see Hypertension, kidney
- war 580.9

Nephroblastoma (M8960/3) 189.0
- epithelial (M8961/3) 189.0
- mesenchymal (M8962/3) 189.0

Nephrocalcinosis 275.49

Nephrocystitis, pustular (see also Pyelitis) 590.80

Nephrolithiasis (congenital) (pelvis) (recurrent) 592.0
- uric acid 274.11

Nephroma (M8960/3) 189.0
- mesoblastic (M8960/1) 236.9 ✓5

Nephronephritis (see also Nephrosis) 581.9

Nephronopthisis 753.16

Nephropathy (see also Nephritis) 583.9
- with
  - exudative nephritis 583.89
  - interstitial nephritis (diffuse) (focal) 583.89
  - medullary necrosis 583.7
  - necrosis 583.9
    - cortical 583.6
    - medullary or papillary 583.7
  - papillary necrosis 583.7
  - specified lesion or cause NEC 583.89
- analgesic 583.89
  - with medullary necrosis, acute 584.7
- arteriolar (see also Hypertension, kidney) 403.90
- arteriosclerotic (see also Hypertension, kidney) 403.90
- complicating pregnancy 646.2 ✓5
- diabetic 250.4 ✓5 [583.81]

Index to Diseases

Nephropathy (see also Nephritis) — continued
- gouty 274.10
  - specified type NEC 274.19
- hypercalcemic 588.8
- hypertensive (see also Hypertension, kidney) 403.90
- hypokalemic (vacuolar) 588.8
- obstructive 593.89
  - congenital 753.20
- phenacetin 584.7
- phosphate-losing 588.0
- potassium depletion 588.8
- proliferative (see also Nephritis, proliferative) 583.0
- protein-losing 588.8
- salt-losing or salt-wasting (see also Disease, renal) 593.9
- sickle-cell (see also Disease, sickle-cell) 282.60 [583.81]
- toxic 584.5
- vasomotor 584.5
- water-losing 588.8

Nephroptosis (see also Disease, renal) 593.0
- congenital (displaced) 753.3

Nephropyosis (see also Abscess, kidney) 590.2

Nephrorrhagia 593.81

Nephrosclerosis (arteriolar) (arteriosclerotic) (chronic) (hyaline) (see also Hypertension, kidney) 403.90
- gouty 274.10
- hyperplastic (arteriolar) (see also Hypertension, kidney) 403.90
- senile (see also Sclerosis, renal) 587

Nephrosis, nephrotic (Epstein's) (syndrome) 581.9
- with
  - lesion of
    - focal glomerulosclerosis 581.1
    - glomerulonephritis
      - endothelial 581.2
      - hypocomplementemic persistent 581.2
      - lobular 581.2
      - membranoproliferative 581.2
      - membranous 581.1
      - mesangiocapillary 581.2
      - minimal change 581.3
      - mixed membranous and proliferative 581.2
      - proliferative 581.0
      - segmental hyalinosis 581.1
      - specified pathology NEC 581.89
- acute — see Nephrosis, tubular
- anoxic — see Nephrosis, tubular
- arteriosclerotic (see also Hypertension, kidney) 403.90
- chemical — see Nephrosis, tubular
- cholemic 572.4
- complicating pregnancy, childbirth, or puerperium — see Nephritis, complicating pregnancy
- diabetic 250.4 [581.81]
- hemoglobinuric — see Nephrosis, tubular
- in
  - amyloidosis 277.3 [581.81]
  - diabetes mellitus 250.4 [581.81]
  - epidemic hemorrhagic fever 078.6
  - malaria 084.9 [581.81]
  - polyarteritis 446.0 [581.81]
  - systemic lupus erythematosus 710.0 [581.81]
- ischemic — see Nephrosis, tubular
- lipoid 581.3
- lower nephron — see Nephrosis, tubular
- lupoid 710.0 [581.81]
- lupus 710.0 [581.81]
- malarial 084.9 [581.81]
- minimal change 581.3
- necrotizing — see Nephrosis, tubular
- osmotic (sucrose) 588.8
- polyarteritic 446.0 [581.81]
- radiation 581.9
- specified lesion or cause NEC 581.89
- syphilitic 095.4
- toxic — see Nephrosis, tubular

Nephrosis, nephrotic — continued
- tubular (acute) 584.5
  - due to a procedure 997.5
  - radiation 581.9

Nephrosonephritis hemorrhagic (endemic) 078.6

Nephrostomy status V44.6
- with complication 997.5

Nerve — see condition

Nerves 799.2

Nervous (see also condition) 799.2
- breakdown 300.9
- heart 306.2
- stomach 306.4
- tension 799.2

Nervousness 799.2

Nesidioblastoma (M8150/0)
- pancreas 211.7
- specified site NEC — see Neoplasm, by site, benign
- unspecified site 211.7

Netherton's syndrome (ichthyosiform erythroderma) 757.1

Nettle rash 708.8

Nettleship's disease (urticaria pigmentosa) 757.33

Neumann's disease (pemphigus vegetans) 694.4

Neuralgia, neuralgic (acute) (see also Neuritis) 729.2
- accessory (nerve) 352.4
- acoustic (nerve) 388.5
- ankle 355.8
- anterior crural 355.8
- anus 787.99
- arm 723.4
- auditory (nerve) 388.5
- axilla 353.0
- bladder 788.1
- brachial 723.4
- brain — see Disorder, nerve, cranial
- broad ligament 625.9
- cerebral — see Disorder, nerve, cranial
- ciliary 346.2
- cranial nerve — see also Disorder, nerve, cranial
  - fifth or trigeminal (see also Neuralgia, trigeminal) 350.1
- ear 388.71
  - middle 352.1
- facial 351.8
- finger 354.9
- flank 355.8
- foot 355.8
- forearm 354.9
- Fothergill's (see also Neuralgia, trigeminal) 350.1
  - postherpetic 053.12
- glossopharyngeal (nerve) 352.1
- groin 355.8
- hand 354.9
- heel 355.8
- Horton's 346.2
- Hunt's 053.11
- hypoglossal (nerve) 352.5
- iliac region 355.8
- infraorbital (see also Neuralgia, trigeminal) 350.1
- inguinal 355.8
- intercostal (nerve) 353.8
  - postherpetic 053.19
- jaw 352.1
- kidney 788.0
- knee 355.8
- loin 355.8
- malarial (see also Malaria) 084.6
- mastoid 385.89
- maxilla 352.1
- median thenar 354.1
- metatarsal 355.6
- middle ear 352.1
- migrainous 346.2
- Morton's 355.6
- nerve, cranial — see Disorder, nerve, cranial
- nose 352.0
- occipital 723.8

Neuralgia, neuralgic (see also Neuritis) — continued
- ophthalmic 377.30
  - postherpetic 053.19
- optic 377.30
- penis 607.9
- perineum 355.8
- pleura 511.0
- postherpetic NEC 053.19
  - geniculate ganglion 053.11
  - ophthalmic 053.19
  - trifacial 053.12
  - trigeminal 053.12
- pubic region 355.8
- radial (nerve) 723.4
- rectum 787.99
- sacroiliac joint 724.3
- sciatic (nerve) 724.3
- scrotum 608.9
- seminal vesicle 608.9
- shoulder 354.9
- Sluder's 337.0
- specified nerve NEC — see Disorder, nerve
- spermatic cord 608.9
- sphenopalatine (ganglion) 337.0
- subscapular (nerve) 723.4
- suprascapular (nerve) 723.4
- testis 608.89
- thenar (median) 354.1
- thigh 355.8
- tongue 352.5
- trifacial (nerve) (see also Neuralgia, trigeminal) 350.1
- trigeminal (nerve) 350.1
  - postherpetic 053.12
- tympanic plexus 388.71
- ulnar (nerve) 723.4
- vagus (nerve) 352.3
- wrist 354.9
- writers' 300.89
  - organic 333.84

Neurapraxia — see Injury, nerve, by site

Neurasthenia 300.5
- cardiac 306.2
- gastric 306.4
- heart 306.2
- postfebrile 780.79
- postviral 780.79

Neurilemmoma (M9560/0) — see also Neoplasm, connective tissue, benign
- acoustic (nerve) 225.1
- malignant (M9560/3) — see also Neoplasm, connective tissue, malignant
  - acoustic (nerve) 192.0

Neurilemmosarcoma (M9560/3) — see Neoplasm, connective tissue, malignant

Neurilemoma — see Neurilemmoma

Neurinoma (M9560/0) — see Neurilemmoma

Neurinomatosis (M9560/1) — see also Neoplasm, connective tissue, uncertain behavior
- centralis 759.5

Neuritis (see also Neuralgia) 729.2
- abducens (nerve) 378.54
- accessory (nerve) 352.4
- acoustic (nerve) 388.5
  - syphilitic 094.86
- alcoholic 357.5
  - with psychosis 291.1
- amyloid, any site 277.3 [357.4]
- anterior crural 355.8
- arising during pregnancy 646.4
- arm 723.4
- ascending 355.2
- auditory (nerve) 388.5
- brachial (nerve) NEC 723.4
  - due to displacement, intervertebral disc 722.0
- cervical 723.4
- chest (wall) 353.8
- costal region 353.8
- cranial nerve — see also Disorder, nerve, cranial
  - first or olfactory 352.0
  - second or optic 377.30
  - third or oculomotor 378.52
  - fourth or trochlear 378.53

Neuritis

Neuritis (see also Neuralgia) — continued
  cranial nerve — see also Disorder, nerve, cranial — continued
    fifth or trigeminal (see also Neuralgia, trigeminal) 350.1
    sixth or abducens 378.54
    seventh or facial 351.8
      newborn 767.5
    eighth or acoustic 388.5
    ninth or glossopharyngeal 352.1
    tenth or vagus 352.3
    eleventh or accessory 352.4
    twelfth or hypoglossal 352.5
  Déjérine-Sottas 356.0
  diabetic 250.6 ✓5th [357.2]
  diphtheritic 032.89 [357.4]
  due to
    beriberi 265.0 [357.4]
    displacement, prolapse, protrusion, or rupture of intervertebral disc 722.2
      cervical 722.0
      lumbar, lumbosacral 722.10
      thoracic, thoracolumbar 722.11
    herniation, nucleus pulposus 722.2
      cervical 722.0
      lumbar, lumbosacral 722.10
      thoracic, thoracolumbar 722.11
  endemic 265.0 [357.4]
  facial (nerve) 351.8
    newborn 767.5
  general — see Polyneuropathy
  geniculate ganglion 351.1
    due to herpes 053.11
  glossopharyngeal (nerve) 352.1
  gouty 274.89 [357.4]
  hypoglossal (nerve) 352.5
  ilioinguinal (nerve) 355.8
  in diseases classified elsewhere — see Polyneuropathy, in
  infectious (multiple) 357.0
  intercostal (nerve) 353.8
  interstitial hypertrophic progressive NEC 356.9
  leg 355.8
  lumbosacral NEC 724.4
  median (nerve) 354.1
    thenar 354.1
  multiple (acute) (infective) 356.9
    endemic 265.0 [357.4]
  multiplex endemica 265.0 [357.4]
  nerve root (see also Radiculitis) 729.2
  oculomotor (nerve) 378.52
  olfactory (nerve) 352.0
  optic (nerve) 377.30
    in myelitis 341.0
    meningococcal 036.81
  pelvic 355.8
  peripheral (nerve) — see also Neuropathy, peripheral
    complicating pregnancy or puerperium 646.4 ✓5th
    specified nerve NEC — see Mononeuritis
  pneumogastric (nerve) 352.3
  postchickenpox 052.7
  postherpetic 053.19
  progressive hypertrophic interstitial NEC 356.9
  puerperal, postpartum 646.4 ✓5th
  radial (nerve) 723.4
  retrobulbar 377.32
    syphilitic 094.85
  rheumatic (chronic) 729.2
  sacral region 355.8
  sciatic (nerve) 724.3
    due to displacement of intervertebral disc 722.10
  serum 999.5
  specified nerve NEC — see Disorder, nerve
  spinal (nerve) 355.9
    root (see also Radiculitis) 729.2
  subscapular (nerve) 723.4
  suprascapular (nerve) 723.4
  syphilitic 095.8
  thenar (median) 354.1
  thoracic NEC 724.4
  toxic NEC 357.7
  trochlear (nerve) 378.53
  ulnar (nerve) 723.4
  vagus (nerve) 352.3

Neuroangiomatosis, encephalofacial 759.6
Neuroastrocytoma (M9505/1) — see Neoplasm, by site, uncertain behavior
Neuro-avitaminosis 269.2
Neuroblastoma (M9500/3)
  olfactory (M9522/3) 160.0
  specified site — see Neoplasm, by site, malignant
  unspecified site 194.0
Neurochorioretinitis (see also Chorioretinitis) 363.20
Neurocirculatory asthenia 306.2
Neurocytoma (M9506/0) — see Neoplasm, by site, benign
Neurodermatitis (circumscribed) (circumscripta) (local) 698.3
  atopic 691.8
  diffuse (Brocq) 691.8
  disseminated 691.8
  nodulosa 698.3
Neuroencephalomyelopathy, optic 341.0
Neuroepithelioma (M9503/3) — see also Neoplasm, by site, malignant
  olfactory (M9521/3) 160.0
Neurofibroma (M9540/0) — see also Neoplasm, connective tissue, benign
  melanotic (M9541/0) — see Neoplasm, connective tissue, benign
  multiple (M9540/1) 237.70
    type 1 237.71
    type 2 237.72
  plexiform (M9550/0) — see Neoplasm, connective tissue, benign
Neurofibromatosis (multiple) (M9540/1) 237.70
  acoustic 237.72
  malignant (M9540/3) — see Neoplasm, connective tissue, malignant
  type 1 237.71
  type 2 237.72
  von Recklinghausen's 237.71
Neurofibrosarcoma (M9540/3) — see Neoplasm, connective tissue, malignant
Neurogenic — see also condition
  bladder (atonic) (automatic) (autonomic) (flaccid) (hypertonic) (hypotonic) (inertia) (infranuclear) (irritable) (motor) (nonreflex) (nuclear) (paralysis) (reflex) (sensory) (spastic) (supranuclear) (uninhibited) 596.54
    with cauda equina syndrome 344.61
  bowel 564.81
  heart 306.2
Neuroglioma (M9505/1) — see Neoplasm, by site, uncertain behavior
Neurolabyrinthitis (of Dix and Hallpike) 386.12
Neurolathyrism 988.2
Neuroleprosy 030.1
Neuroleptic malignant syndrome 333.92
Neurolipomatosis 272.8
Neuroma (M9570/0) — see also Neoplasm, connective tissue, benign
  acoustic (nerve) (M9560/0) 225.1
  amputation (traumatic) — see also Injury, nerve, by site
    surgical complication (late) 997.61
  appendix 211.3
  auditory nerve 225.1
  digital 355.6
    toe 355.6
  interdigital (toe) 355.6
  intermetatarsal 355.6
  Morton's 355.6
  multiple 237.70
    type 1 237.71
    type 2 237.72
  nonneoplastic 355.9
    arm NEC 354.9
    leg NEC 355.8
    lower extremity NEC 355.8
    specified site NEC — see Mononeuritis, by site
    upper extremity NEC 354.9
  optic (nerve) 225.1
  plantar 355.6

Neuroma — see also Neoplasm, connective tissue, benign — continued
  plexiform (M9550/0) — see Neoplasm, connective tissue, benign
  surgical (nonneoplastic) 355.9
    arm NEC 354.9
    leg NEC 355.8
    lower extremity NEC 355.8
    upper extremity NEC 354.9
  traumatic — see also Injury, nerve, by site
    old — see Neuroma, nonneoplastic
Neuromyalgia 729.1
Neuromyasthenia (epidemic) 049.8
Neuromyelitis 341.8
  ascending 357.0
  optica 341.0
Neuromyopathy NEC 358.9
Neuromyositis 729.1
Neuronevus (M8725/0) — see Neoplasm, skin, benign
Neuronitis 357.0
  ascending (acute) 355.2
  vestibular 386.12
Neuroparalytic — see condition
Neuropathy, neuropathic (see also Disorder, nerve) 355.9
  acute motor 357.82
  alcoholic 357.5
    with psychosis 291.1
  arm NEC 354.9
  autonomic (peripheral) — see Neuropathy, peripheral, autonomic
  axillary nerve 353.0
  brachial plexus 353.0
  cervical plexus 353.2
  chronic
    progressive segmentally demyelinating 357.89
    relapsing demyelinating 357.89
  congenital sensory 356.2
  Déjérine-Sottas 356.0
  diabetic 250.6 ✓5th [357.2]
  entrapment 355.9
    iliohypogastric nerve 355.79
    ilioinguinal nerve 355.79
    lateral cutaneous nerve of thigh 355.1
    median nerve 354.0
    obturator nerve 355.79
    peroneal nerve 355.3
    posterior tibial nerve 355.5
    saphenous nerve 355.79
    ulnar nerve 354.2
  facial nerve 351.9
  hereditary 356.9
    peripheral 356.0
    sensory (radicular) 356.2
  hypertrophic
    Charcôt-Marie-Tooth 356.1
    Déjérine-Sottas 356.0
    interstitial 356.9
    Refsum 356.3
  intercostal nerve 354.8
  ischemic — see Disorder, nerve
  Jamaican (ginger) 357.7
  leg NEC 355.8
  lower extremity NEC 355.8
  lumbar plexus 353.1
  median nerve 354.1
  motor
    acute 357.82
  multiple (acute) (chronic) (see also Polyneuropathy) 356.9
  optic 377.39
    ischemic 377.41
    nutritional 377.33
    toxic 377.34
  peripheral (nerve) (see also Polyneuropathy) 356.9
    arm NEC 354.9
    autonomic 337.9
      amyloid 277.3 [337.1]
      idiopathic 337.0
    in
      amyloidosis 277.3 [337.1]
      diabetes (mellitus) 250.6 ✓5th [337.1]
      diseases classified elsewhere 337.1

Index to Diseases

Neuropathy, neuropathic (see also Disorder, nerve) — continued
  peripheral (see also Polyneuropathy) — continued
    autonomic — continued
      in — continued
        gout 274.89 [337.1]
        hyperthyroidism 242.9 ✓5ᵗʰ [337.1]
      due to
        antitetanus serum 357.6
        arsenic 357.7
        drugs 357.6
        lead 357.7
        organophosphate compounds 357.7
        toxic agent NEC 357.7
      hereditary 356.0
      idiopathic 356.9
        progressive 356.4
        specified type NEC 356.8
      in diseases classified elsewhere — see Polyneuropathy, in
      leg NEC 355.8
      lower extremity NEC 355.8
      upper extremity NEC 354.9
      plantar nerves 355.6
      progressive hypertrophic interstitial 356.9
      radicular NEC 729.2
        brachial 723.4
        cervical NEC 723.4
        hereditary sensory 356.2
        lumbar 724.4
        lumbosacral 724.4
        thoracic NEC 724.4
      sacral plexus 353.1
      sciatic 355.0
      spinal nerve NEC 355.9
        root (see also Radiculitis) 729.2
      toxic 357.7
      trigeminal sensory 350.8
      ulnar nerve 354.2
      upper extremity NEC 354.9
      uremic 585 [357.4]
      vitamin B_{12} 266.2 [357.4]
        with anemia (pernicious) 281.0 [357.4]
          due to dietary deficiency 281.1 [357.4]

Neurophthisis — (see also Disorder, nerve peripheral) 356.9
  diabetic 250.6 ✓5ᵗʰ [357.2]

Neuropraxia — see Injury, nerve

Neuroretinitis 363.05
  syphilitic 094.85

Neurosarcoma (M9540/3) — see Neoplasm, connective tissue, malignant

Neurosclerosis — see Disorder, nerve

Neurosis, neurotic 300.9
  accident 300.16
  anancastic, anankastic 300.3
  anxiety (state) 300.00
    generalized 300.02
    panic type 300.01
  asthenic 300.5
  bladder 306.53
  cardiac (reflex) 306.2
  cardiovascular 306.2
  climacteric, unspecified type 627.2
  colon 306.4
  compensation 300.16
  compulsive, compulsion 300.3
  conversion 300.11
  craft 300.89
  cutaneous 306.3
  depersonalization 300.6
  depressive (reaction) (type) 300.4
  endocrine 306.6
  environmental 300.89
  fatigue 300.5
  functional (see also Disorder, psychosomatic) 306.9
  gastric 306.4
  gastrointestinal 306.4
  genitourinary 306.50
  heart 306.2
  hypochondriacal 300.7
  hysterical 300.10
    conversion type 300.11
    dissociative type 300.15

Neurosis, neurotic — continued
  impulsive 300.3
  incoordination 306.0
    larynx 306.1
    vocal cord 306.1
  intestine 306.4
  larynx 306.1
    hysterical 300.11
    sensory 306.1
  menopause, unspecified type 627.2
  mixed NEC 300.89
  musculoskeletal 306.0
  obsessional 300.3
    phobia 300.3
  obsessive-compulsive 300.3
  occupational 300.89
  ocular 306.7
  oral 307.0
  organ (see also Disorder, psychosomatic) 306.9
  pharynx 306.1
  phobic 300.20
  posttraumatic (acute) (situational) 308.3
    chronic 309.81
  psychasthenic (type) 300.89
  railroad 300.16
  rectum 306.4
  respiratory 306.1
  rumination 306.4
  senile 300.89
  sexual 302.70
  situational 300.89
  specified type NEC 300.89
  state 300.9
    with depersonalization episode 300.6
  stomach 306.4
  vasomotor 306.2
  visceral 306.4
  war 300.16

Neurospongioblastosis diffusa 759.5

Neurosyphilis (arrested) (early) (inactive) (late) (latent) (recurrent) 094.9
  with ataxia (cerebellar) (locomotor) (spastic) (spinal) 094.0
  acute meningitis 094.2
  aneurysm 094.89
  arachnoid (adhesive) 094.2
  arteritis (any artery) 094.89
  asymptomatic 094.3
  congenital 090.40
  dura (mater) 094.89
  general paresis 094.1
  gumma 094.9
  hemorrhagic 094.9
  juvenile (asymptomatic) (meningeal) 090.40
  leptomeninges (aseptic) 094.2
  meningeal 094.2
  meninges (adhesive) 094.2
  meningovascular (diffuse) 094.2
  optic atrophy 094.84
  parenchymatous (degenerative) 094.1
  paresis (see also Paresis, general) 094.1
  paretic (see also Paresis, general) 094.1
  relapse 094.9
  remission in (sustained) 094.9
  serological 094.3
  specified nature or site NEC 094.89
  tabes (dorsalis) 094.0
    juvenile 090.40
  tabetic 094.0
    juvenile 090.40
  taboparesis 094.1
    juvenile 090.40
  thrombosis 094.89
  vascular 094.89

Neurotic (see also Neurosis) 300.9
  excoriation 698.4
    psychogenic 306.3

Neurotmesis — see Injury, nerve, by site

Neurotoxemia — see Toxemia

Neutroclusion 524.2

Neutropenia, neutropenic (chronic) (cyclic) (drug-induced) (genetic) (idiopathic) (immune) (infantile) (malignant) (periodic) (pernicious) (primary) (splenic) (splenomegaly) (toxic) 288.0
  chronic hypoplastic 288.0

Neutropenia, neutropenic — continued
  congenital (nontransient) 288.0
  fever 288.0
  neonatal, transitory (isoimmune) (maternal transfer) 776.7

Neutrophilia, hereditary giant 288.2

Nevocarcinoma (M8720/3) — see Melanoma

Nevus (M8720/0) — see also Neoplasm, skin, benign

> Note — Except where otherwise indicated, varieties of nevus in the list below that are followed by a morphology code number (M----/0) should be coded by site as for "Neoplasm, skin, benign."

  acanthotic 702.8
  achromic (M8730/0)
  amelanotic (M8730/0)
  anemic, anemicus 709.09
  angiomatous (M9120/0) (see also Hemangioma) 228.00
  araneus 448.1
  avasculosus 709.09
  balloon cell (M8722/0)
  bathing trunk (M8761/1) 238.2
  blue (M8780/0)
    cellular (M8790/0)
    giant (M8790/0)
    Jadassohn's (M8780/0)
    malignant (M8780/3) — see Melanoma
  capillary (M9131/0) (see also Hemangioma) 228.00
  cavernous (M9121/0) (see also Hemangioma) 228.00
  cellular (M8720/0)
    blue (M8790/0)
  comedonicus 757.33
  compound (M8760/0)
  conjunctiva (M8720/0) 224.3
  dermal (M8750/0)
    and epidermal (M8760/0)
  epithelioid cell (and spindle cell) (M8770/0)
  flammeus 757.32
    osteohypertrophic 759.89
  hairy (M8720/0)
  halo (M8723/0)
  hemangiomatous (M9120/0) (see also Hemangioma) 228.00
  intradermal (M8750/0)
  intraepidermal (M8740/0)
  involuting (M8724/0)
  Jadassohn's (blue) (M8780/0)
  junction, junctional (M8740/0)
    malignant melanoma in (M8740/3) — see Melanoma
  juvenile (M8770/0)
  lymphatic (M9170/0) 228.1
  magnocellular (M8726/0)
    specified site — see Neoplasm, by site, benign
    unspecified site 224.0
  malignant (M8720/3) — see Melanoma
  meaning hemangioma (M9120/0) (see also Hemangioma) 228.00
  melanotic (pigmented) (M8720/0)
  multiplex 759.5
  nonneoplastic 448.1
  nonpigmented (M8730/0)
  nonvascular (M8720/0)
  oral mucosa, white sponge 750.26
  osteohypertrophic, flammeus 759.89
  papillaris (M8720/0)
  papillomatosus (M8720/0)
  pigmented (M8720/0)
    giant (M8761/1) — see also Neoplasm, skin, uncertain behavior
      malignant melanoma in (M8761/3) — see Melanoma
    systematicus 757.33
  pilosus (M8720/0)
  port wine 757.32
  sanguineous 757.32
  sebaceous (senile) 702.8
  senile 448.1
  spider 448.1
  spindle cell (and epithelioid cell) (M8770/0)

Nevus — see also Neoplasm, skin, benign — continued
- stellar 448.1
- strawberry 757.32
- syringocystadenomatous papilliferous (M8406/0)
- unius lateris 757.33
- Unna's 757.32
- vascular 757.32
- verrucous 757.33
- white sponge (oral mucosa) 750.26

Newborn (infant) (liveborn)
- gestation
  - 24 completed weeks 765.22
  - 25-26 completed weeks 765.23
  - 27-28 completed weeks 765.24
  - 29-30 completed weeks 765.25
  - 31-32 completed weeks 765.26
  - 33-34 completed weeks 765.27
  - 35-36 completed weeks 765.28
  - 37 or more completed weeks 765.29
  - less than 24 completed weeks 765.21
  - unspecified completed weeks 765.20
- multiple NEC
  - born in hospital (without mention of cesarean delivery or section) V37.00
    - with cesarean delivery or section V37.01
  - born outside hospital
    - hospitalized V37.1
    - not hospitalized V37.2
  - mates all liveborn
    - born in hospital (without mention of cesarean delivery or section) V34.00
      - with cesarean delivery or section V34.01
    - born outside hospital
      - hospitalized V34.1
      - not hospitalized V34.2
  - mates all stillborn
    - born in hospital (without mention of cesarean delivery or section) V35.00
      - with cesarean delivery or section V35.01
    - born outside hospital
      - hospitalized V35.1
      - not hospitalized V35.2
  - mates liveborn and stillborn
    - born in hospital (without mention of cesarean delivery or section) V36.00
      - with cesarean delivery or section V36.01
    - born outside hospital
      - hospitalized V36.1
      - not hospitalized V36.2
- single
  - born in hospital (without mention of cesarean delivery or section) V30.00
    - with cesarean delivery or section V30.01
  - born outside hospital
    - hospitalized V30.1
    - not hospitalized V30.2
- twin NEC
  - born in hospital (without mention of cesarean delivery or section) V33.00
    - with cesarean delivery or section V33.01
  - born outside hospital
    - hospitalized V33.1
    - not hospitalized V33.2
  - mate liveborn
    - born in hospital V31.0
    - born outside hospital
      - hospitalized V31.1
      - not hospitalized V31.2
  - mate stillborn
    - born in hospital V32.0
    - born outside hospital
      - hospitalized V32.1
      - not hospitalized V32.2
- unspecified as to single or multiple birth
  - born in hospital (without mention of cesarean delivery or section) V39.00
    - with cesarean delivery or section V39.01
  - born outside hospital
    - hospitalized V39.1
    - not hospitalized V39.2

Newcastle's conjunctivitis or disease 077.8

Nezelof's syndrome (pure alymphocytosis) 279.13
Niacin (amide) deficiency 265.2
Nicolas-Durand-Favre disease (climatic bubo) 099.1
Nicolas-Favre disease (climatic bubo) 099.1
Nicotinic acid (amide) deficiency 265.2
Niemann-Pick disease (lipid histiocytosis) (splenomegaly) 272.7
Night
- blindness (see also Blindness, night) 368.60
  - congenital 368.61
  - vitamin A deficiency 264.5
- cramps 729.82
- sweats 780.8
- terrors, child 307.46

Nightmare 307.47
- REM-sleep type 307.47

Nipple — see condition
Nisbet's chancre 099.0
Nishimoto (-Takeuchi) disease 437.5
Nitritoid crisis or reaction — see Crisis, nitritoid
Nitrogen retention, extrarenal 788.9
Nitrosohemoglobinemia 289.8
Njovera 104.0
No
- diagnosis 799.9
- disease (found) V71.9
- room at the inn V65.0

Nocardiasis — see Nocardiosis
Nocardiosis 039.9
- with pneumonia 039.1
- lung 039.1
- specified type NEC 039.8

Nocturia 788.43
- psychogenic 306.53

Nocturnal — see also condition
- dyspnea (paroxysmal) 786.09
- emissions 608.89
- enuresis 788.36
  - psychogenic 307.6
- frequency (micturition) 788.43
  - psychogenic 306.53

Nodal rhythm disorder 427.89
Nodding of head 781.0
Node(s) — see also Nodule
- Heberden's 715.04
- larynx 478.79
- lymph — see condition
- milkers' 051.1
- Osler's 421.0
- rheumatic 729.89
- Schmorl's 722.30
  - lumbar, lumbosacral 722.32
  - specified region NEC 722.39
  - thoracic, thoracolumbar 722.31
- singers' 478.5
- skin NEC 782.2
- tuberculous — see Tuberculosis, lymph gland
- vocal cords 478.5

Nodosities, Haygarth's 715.04
Nodule(s), nodular
- actinomycotic (see also Actinomycosis) 039.9
- arthritic — see Arthritis, nodosa
- cutaneous 782.2
- Haygarth's 715.04
- inflammatory — see Inflammation
- juxta-articular 102.7
  - syphilitic 095.7
  - yaws 102.7
- larynx 478.79
- lung, solitary 518.89
  - emphysematous 492.8
- milkers' 051.1
- prostate 600.1
- rheumatic 729.89
- rheumatoid — see Arthritis, rheumatoid
- scrotum (inflammatory) 608.4
- singers' 478.5
- skin NEC 782.2
- solitary, lung 518.89
  - emphysematous 492.8
- subcutaneous 782.2

Nodule(s), nodular — continued
- thyroid (gland) (nontoxic) (uninodular) 241.0
  - with
    - hyperthyroidism 242.1
    - thyrotoxicosis 242.1
  - toxic or with hyperthyroidism 242.1
- vocal cords 478.5

Noma (gangrenous) (hospital) (infective) 528.1
- auricle (see also Gangrene) 785.4
- mouth 528.1
- pudendi (see also Vulvitis) 616.10
- vulvae (see also Vulvitis) 616.10

Nomadism V60.0
Non-adherence
- artificial skin graft 996.55
- decellularized allodermis graft 996.55

Non-autoimmune hemolytic anemia NEC 283.10
Nonclosure — see also Imperfect, closure
- ductus
  - arteriosus 747.0
  - Botalli 747.0
- Eustachian valve 746.89
- foramen
  - Botalli 745.5
  - ovale 745.5

Noncompliance with medical treatment V15.81
Nondescent (congenital) — see also Malposition, congenital
- cecum 751.4
- colon 751.4
- testis 752.51

Nondevelopment
- brain 742.1
  - specified part 742.2
- heart 746.89
- organ or site, congenital NEC — see Hypoplasia

Nonengagement
- head NEC 652.5
  - in labor 660.1
    - affecting fetus or newborn 763.1

Nonexanthematous tick fever 066.1
Nonexpansion, lung (newborn) NEC 770.4
Nonfunctioning
- cystic duct (see also Disease, gallbladder) 575.8
- gallbladder (see also Disease, gallbladder) 575.8
- kidney (see also Disease, renal) 593.9
- labyrinth 386.58

Nonhealing
- stump (surgical) 997.69
- wound, surgical 998.83

Nonimplantation of ovum, causing infertility 628.3
Noninsufflation, fallopian tube 628.2
Nonne-Milroy-Meige syndrome (chronic hereditary edema) 757.0
Nonovulation 628.0
Nonpatent fallopian tube 628.2
Nonpneumatization, lung NEC 770.4
Nonreflex bladder 596.54
- with cauda equina 344.61

Nonretention of food — see Vomiting
Nonrotation — see Malrotation
Nonsecretion, urine (see also Anuria) 788.5
- newborn 753.3

Nonunion
- fracture 733.82
- organ or site, congenital NEC — see Imperfect, closure
- symphysis pubis, congenital 755.69
- top sacrum, congenital 756.19

Nonviability 765.0
Nonvisualization, gallbladder 793.3
Nonvitalized tooth 522.9
Normal
- delivery — see category 650
- menses V65.5
- state (feared complaint unfounded) V65.5

Normoblastosis 289.8

Normocytic anemia (infectional) 285.9
  due to blood loss (chronic) 280.0
    acute 285.1
Norrie's disease (congenital) (progressive oculoacousticocerebral degeneration) 743.8
North American blastomycosis 116.0
Norwegian itch 133.0
Nose, nasal — *see* condition
Nosebleed 784.7
Nosomania 298.9
Nosophobia 300.29
Nostalgia 309.89
Notch of iris 743.46
Notched lip, congenital (*see also* Cleft, lip) 749.10
Notching nose, congenital (tip) 748.1
Nothnagel's
  syndrome 378.52
  vasomotor acroparesthesia 443.89
Novy's relapsing fever (American) 087.1
Noxious
  foodstuffs, poisoning by
    fish 988.0
    fungi 988.1
    mushrooms 988.1
    plants (food) 988.2
    shellfish 988.0
    specified type NEC 988.8
    toadstool 988.1
  substances transmitted through placenta or breast milk 760.70
    alcohol 760.71
    anti-infective agents 760.74
    cocaine 760.75
    "crack" 760.75
    diethylstilbestrol (DES) 760.76
    hallucinogenic agents NEC 760.73
    medicinal agents NEC 760.79
    narcotics 760.72
    obstetric anesthetic or analgesic 763.5
    specified agent NEC 760.79
    suspected, affecting management of pregnancy 655.5 ✓5th
Nuchal hitch (arm) 652.8 ✓5th
Nucleus pulposus — *see* condition
Numbness 782.0
Nuns' knee 727.2
Nursemaid's
  elbow 832.0 ✓5th
  shoulder 831.0 ✓5th
Nutmeg liver 573.8
Nutrition, deficient or insufficient (particular kind of food) 269.9
  due to
    insufficient food 994.2
    lack of
      care (child) (infant) 995.52
        adult 995.84
      food 994.2
Nyctalopia (*see also* Blindness, night) 368.60
  vitamin A deficiency 264.5
Nycturia 788.43
  psychogenic 306.53
Nymphomania 302.89
Nystagmus 379.50
  associated with vestibular system disorders 379.54
  benign paroxysmal positional 386.11
  central positional 386.2
  congenital 379.51
  deprivation 379.53
  dissociated 379.55
  latent 379.52
  miners' 300.89
  positional
    benign paroxysmal 386.11
    central 386.2
  specified NEC 379.56
  vestibular 379.54
  visual deprivation 379.53

Index to Diseases

O

Oasthouse urine disease 270.2
Obermeyer's relapsing fever (European) 087.0
Obesity (constitutional) (exogenous) (familial) (nutritional) (simple) 278.00
  adrenal 255.8
  due to hyperalimentation 278.00
  endocrine NEC 259.9
  endogenous 259.9
  Fröhlich's (adiposogenital dystrophy) 253.8
  glandular NEC 259.9
  hypothyroid (*see also* Hypothyroidism) 244.9
  morbid 278.01
  of pregnancy 646.1 ☑5ᵗʰ
  pituitary 253.8
  thyroid (*see also* Hypothyroidism) 244.9
Oblique — *see also* condition
  lie before labor, affecting fetus or newborn 761.7
Obliquity, pelvis 738.6
Obliteration
  abdominal aorta 446.7
  appendix (lumen) 543.9
  artery 447.1
  ascending aorta 446.7
  bile ducts 576.8
    with calculus, choledocholithiasis, or stones — *see* Choledocholithiasis
    congenital 751.61
      jaundice from 751.61 [774.5]
  common duct 576.8
    with calculus, choledocholithiasis, or stones — *see* Choledocholithiasis
    congenital 751.61
  cystic duct 575.8
    with calculus, choledocholithiasis, or stones — *see* Choledocholithiasis
  disease, arteriolar 447.1
  endometrium 621.8
  eye, anterior chamber 360.34
  fallopian tube 628.2
  lymphatic vessel 457.1
    postmastectomy 457.0
  organ or site, congenital NEC — *see* Atresia
  placental blood vessels — *see* Placenta, abnormal
  supra-aortic branches 446.7
  ureter 593.89
  urethra 599.84
  vein 459.9
  vestibule (oral) 525.8
Observation (for) V71.9
  without need for further medical care V71.9
  accident NEC V71.4
    at work V71.3
  criminal V71.6
  deleterious agent ingestion V71.89
  disease V71.9
    cardiovascular V71.7
    heart V71.7
    mental V71.09
    specified condition NEC V71.89
  foreign body ingestion V71.89
  growth and development variations V21.8
  injuries (accidental) V71.4
    inflicted NEC V71.6
      during alleged rape or seduction V71.5
  malignant neoplasm, suspected V71.1
  postpartum
    immediately after delivery V24.0
    routine follow-up V24.2
  pregnancy
    high-risk V23.9
      specified problem NEC V23.8 ☑5ᵗʰ
    normal (without complication) V22.1
      with nonobstetric complication V22.2
      first V22.0
  rape or seduction, alleged V71.5
    injury during V71.5
  suicide attempt, alleged V71.89
  suspected (undiagnosed) (unproven)
    abuse V71.81
    cardiovascular disease V71.7
    child or wife battering victim V71.6
    concussion (cerebral) V71.6

Observation — *continued*
  suspected — *continued*
    condition NEC V71.89
      infant — *see* Observation, suspected, condition, newborn
    newborn V29.9
      cardiovascular disease V29.8
      congenital anomaly V29.8
      genetic V29.3
      infectious V29.0
      ingestion foreign object V29.8
      injury V29.8
      metabolic V29.3
      neoplasm V29.8
      neurological V29.1
      poison, poisoning V29.8
      respiratory V29.2
      specified NEC V29.8
    exposure
      anthrax V71.82
      biologic agent NEC V71.83
    infectious disease not requiring isolation V71.89
    malignant neoplasm V71.1
    mental disorder V71.09
    neglect V71.81
    neoplasm
      benign V71.89
      malignant V71.1
    specified condition NEC V71.89
    tuberculosis V71.2
  tuberculosis, suspected V71.2
Obsession, obsessional 300.3
  ideas and mental images 300.3
  impulses 300.3
  neurosis 300.3
  phobia 300.3
  psychasthenia 300.3
  ruminations 300.3
  state 300.3
  syndrome 300.3
Obsessive-compulsive 300.3
  neurosis 300.3
  reaction 300.3
Obstetrical trauma NEC (complicating delivery) 665.9 ☑5ᵗʰ
  with
    abortion — *see* Abortion, by type, with damage to pelvic organs
    ectopic pregnancy (*see also* categories 633.0-633.9) 639.2
    molar pregnancy (*see also* categories 630-632) 639.2
  affecting fetus or newborn 763.89
  following
    abortion 639.2
    ectopic or molar pregnancy 639.2
Obstipation (*see also* Constipation) 564.00
  psychogenic 306.4
Obstruction, obstructed, obstructive
  airway NEC 519.8
    with
      allergic alveolitis NEC 495.9
      asthma NEC (*see also* Asthma) 493.9 ☑5ᵗʰ
      bronchiectasis 494.0
        with acute exacerbation 494.1
      bronchitis (chronic) (*see also* Bronchitis, with, obstruction) 491.20
      emphysema NEC 492.8
    chronic 496
      with
        allergic alveolitis NEC 495.5
        asthma NEC (*see also* Asthma) 493.2 ☑5ᵗʰ
        bronchiectasis 494.0
          with acute exacerbation 494.1
        bronchitis (chronic) (*see also* Bronchitis, with, obstruction) 491.20
        emphysema NEC 492.8
    due to
      bronchospasm 519.1
      foreign body 934.9
      inhalation of fumes or vapors 506.9
      laryngospasm 478.75

Obstruction, obstructed, obstructive — *continued*
  alimentary canal (*see also* Obstruction, intestine) 560.9
  ampulla of Vater 576.2
    with calculus, cholelithiasis, or stones — *see* Choledocholithiasis
  aortic (heart) (valve) (*see also* Stenosis, aortic) 424.1
    rheumatic (*see also* Stenosis, aortic, rheumatic) 395.0
  aortoiliac 444.0
  aqueduct of Sylvius 331.4
    congenital 742.3
      with spina bifida (*see also* Spina bifida) 741.0 ☑5ᵗʰ
  Arnold-Chiari (*see also* Spina bifida) 741.0 ☑5ᵗʰ
  artery (*see also* Embolism, artery) 444.9
    basilar (complete) (partial) (*see also* Occlusion, artery, basilar) 433.0 ☑5ᵗʰ
    carotid (complete) (partial) (*see also* Occlusion, artery, carotid) 433.1 ☑5ᵗʰ
    precerebral — *see* Occlusion, artery, precerebral NEC
    retinal (central) (*see also* Occlusion, retina) 362.30
    vertebral (complete) (partial) (*see also* Occlusion, artery, vertebral) 433.2 ☑5ᵗʰ
  asthma (chronic) (with obstructive pulmonary disease) 493.2 ☑5ᵗʰ
  band (intestinal) 560.81
  bile duct or passage (*see also* Obstruction, biliary) 576.2
    congenital 751.61
      jaundice from 751.61 [774.5]
  biliary (duct) (tract) 576.2
    with calculus 574.51
      with cholecystitis (chronic) 574.41
        acute 574.31
    congenital 751.61
      jaundice from 751.61 [774.5]
    gallbladder 575.2
      with calculus 574.21
        with cholecystitis (chronic) 574.11
          acute 574.01
  bladder neck (acquired) 596.0
    congenital 753.6
  bowel (*see also* Obstruction, intestine) 560.9
  bronchus 519.1
  canal, ear (*see also* Stricture, ear canal, acquired) 380.50
  cardia 537.89
  caval veins (inferior) (superior) 459.2
  cecum (*see also* Obstruction, intestine) 560.9
  circulatory 459.9
  colon (*see also* Obstruction, intestine) 560.9
    sympathicotonic 560.89
  common duct (*see also* Obstruction, biliary) 576.2
    congenital 751.61
  coronary (artery) (heart) — *see also* Arteriosclerosis, coronary
    acute (*see also* Infarct, myocardium) 410.9 ☑5ᵗʰ
      without myocardial infarction 411.81
  cystic duct (*see also* Obstruction, gallbladder) 575.2
    congenital 751.61
  device, implant, or graft — *see* Complications, due to (presence of) any device, implant, or graft classified to 996.0-996.5 NEC
  due to foreign body accidentally left in operation wound 998.4
  duodenum 537.3
    congenital 751.1
    due to
      compression NEC 537.3
      cyst 537.3
      intrinsic lesion or disease NEC 537.3
      scarring 537.3
      torsion 537.3
      ulcer 532.91
      volvulus 537.3
  ejaculatory duct 608.89
  endocardium 424.90
    arteriosclerotic 424.99
    specified cause, except rheumatic 424.99

Obstruction, obstructed, obstructive

Obstruction, obstructed, obstructive — *continued*
- esophagus 530.3
- eustachian tube (complete) (partial) 381.60
    - cartilaginous
        - extrinsic 381.63
        - intrinsic 381.62
    - due to
        - cholesteatoma 381.61
        - osseous lesion NEC 381.61
        - polyp 381.61
    - osseous 381.61
- fallopian tube (bilateral) 628.2
- fecal 560.39
    - with hernia — *see also* Hernia, by site, with obstruction
        - gangrenous — *see* Hernia, by site, with gangrene
- foramen of Monro (congenital) 742.3
    - with spina bifida (*see also* Spina bifida) 741.0 ✓5th
- foreign body — *see* Foreign body
- gallbladder 575.2
    - with calculus, cholelithiasis, or stones 574.21
        - with cholecystitis (chronic) 574.11
            - acute 574.01
    - congenital 751.69
        - jaundice from 751.69 [774.5]
- gastric outlet 537.0
- gastrointestinal (*see also* Obstruction, intestine) 560.9
- glottis 478.79
- hepatic 573.8
    - duct (*see also* Obstruction, biliary) 576.2
        - congenital 751.61
    - icterus (*see also* Obstruction, biliary) 576.8
        - congenital 751.61
- ileocecal coil (*see also* Obstruction, intestine) 560.9
- ileum (*see also* Obstruction, intestine) 560.9
- iliofemoral (artery) 444.81
- internal anastomosis — *see* Complications, mechanical, graft
- intestine (mechanical) (neurogenic) (paroxysmal) (postinfectional) (reflex) 560.9
    - with
        - adhesions (intestinal) (peritoneal) 560.81
        - hernia — *see also* Hernia, by site, with obstruction
            - gangrenous — *see* Hernia, by site, with gangrene
    - adynamic (*see also* Ileus) 560.1
    - by gallstone 560.31
    - congenital or infantile (small) 751.1
        - large 751.2
    - due to
        - Ascaris lumbricoides 127.0
        - mural thickening 560.89
        - procedure 997.4
            - involving urinary tract 997.5
    - impaction 560.39
    - infantile — *see* Obstruction, intestine, congenital
    - newborn
        - due to
            - fecaliths 777.1
            - inspissated milk 777.2
            - meconium (plug) 777.1
                - in mucoviscidosis 277.01
            - transitory 777.4
        - specified cause NEC 560.89
        - transitory, newborn 777.4
        - volvulus 560.2
- intracardiac ball valve prosthesis 996.02
- jaundice (*see also* Obstruction, biliary) 576.8
    - congenital 751.61
- jejunum (*see also* Obstruction, intestine) 560.9
- kidney 593.89
- labor 660.9 ✓5th
    - affecting fetus or newborn 763.1
    - by
        - bony pelvis (conditions classifiable to 653.0-653.9) 660.1 ✓5th
        - deep transverse arrest 660.3 ✓5th
        - impacted shoulder 660.4 ✓5th

Obstruction, obstructed, obstructive — *continued*
- labor — *continued*
    - by — *continued*
        - locked twins 660.5 ✓5th
        - malposition (fetus) (conditions classifiable to 652.0-652.9) 660.0 ✓5th
            - head during labor 660.3 ✓5th
        - persistent occipitoposterior position 660.3 ✓5th
        - soft tissue, pelvic (conditions classifiable to 654.0-654.9) 660.2 ✓5th
- lacrimal
    - canaliculi 375.53
    - congenital 743.65
    - punctum 375.52
    - sac 375.54
- lacrimonasal duct 375.56
    - congenital 743.65
    - neonatal 375.55
- lacteal, with steatorrhea 579.2
- laryngitis (*see also* Laryngitis) 464.01
- larynx 478.79
    - congenital 748.3
- liver 573.8
    - cirrhotic (*see also* Cirrhosis, liver) 571.5
- lung 518.89
    - with
        - asthma — *see* Asthma
        - bronchitis (chronic) 491.2 ✓5th
        - emphysema NEC 492.8
    - airway, chronic 496
    - chronic NEC 496
        - with
            - asthma (chronic) (obstructive) 493.2 ✓5th
    - disease, chronic 496
        - with
            - asthma (chronic) (obstructive) 493.2 ✓5th
    - emphysematous 492.8
- lymphatic 457.1
- meconium
    - fetus or newborn 777.1
        - in mucoviscidosis 277.01
    - newborn due to fecaliths 777.1
- mediastinum 519.3
- mitral (rheumatic) — *see* Stenosis, mitral
- nasal 478.1
    - duct 375.56
        - neonatal 375.55
    - sinus — *see* Sinusitis
- nasolacrimal duct 375.56
    - congenital 743.65
    - neonatal 375.55
- nasopharynx 478.29
- nose 478.1
- organ or site, congenital NEC — *see* Atresia
- pancreatic duct 577.8
- parotid gland 527.8
- pelviureteral junction (*see also* Obstruction, ureter) 593.4
- pharynx 478.29
- portal (circulation) (vein) 452
- prostate 600.9
    - valve (urinary) 596.0
- pulmonary
    - valve (heart) (*see also* Endocarditis, pulmonary) 424.3
    - vein, isolated 747.49
- pyemic — *see* Septicemia
- pylorus (acquired) 537.0
    - congenital 750.5
    - infantile 750.5
- rectosigmoid (*see also* Obstruction, intestine) 560.9
- rectum 569.49
- renal 593.89
- respiratory 519.8
    - chronic 496
- retinal (artery) (vein) (central) (*see also* Occlusion, retina) 362.30
- salivary duct (any) 527.8
    - with calculus 527.5
- sigmoid (*see also* Obstruction, intestine) 560.9
- sinus (accessory) (nasal) (*see also* Sinusitis) 473.9

Obstruction, obstructed, obstructive — *continued*
- Stensen's duct 527.8
- stomach 537.89
    - acute 536.1
    - congenital 750.7
- submaxillary gland 527.8
    - with calculus 527.5
- thoracic duct 457.1
- thrombotic — *see* Thrombosis
- tooth eruption 520.6
- trachea 519.1
- tracheostomy airway 519.09
- tricuspid — *see* Endocarditis, tricuspid
- upper respiratory, congenital 748.8
- ureter (functional) 593.4
    - congenital 753.20
    - due to calculus 592.1
- ureteropelvic junction, congenital 753.21
- ureterovesical junction, congenital 753.22
- urethra 599.6
    - congenital 753.6
- urinary (moderate) 599.6
    - organ or tract (lower) 599.6
    - prostatic valve 596.0
- uropathy 599.6
- uterus 621.8
- vagina 623.2
- valvular — *see* Endocarditis
- vascular graft or shunt 996.1
    - atherosclerosis — *see* Arteriosclerosis, coronary
    - embolism 996.74
    - occlusion NEC 996.74
    - thrombus 996.74
- vein, venous 459.2
    - caval (inferior) (superior) 459.2
    - thrombotic — *see* Thrombosis
- vena cava (inferior) (superior) 459.2
- ventricular shunt 996.2
- vesical 596.0
- vesicourethral orifice 596.0
- vessel NEC 459.9

Obturator — *see* condition

Occlusal wear, teeth 521.1

Occlusion
- anus 569.49
    - congenital 751.2
    - infantile 751.2
- aortoiliac (chronic) 444.0
- aqueduct of Sylvius 331.4
    - congenital 742.3
        - with spina bifida (*see also* Spina bifida) 741.0 ✓5th
- arteries of extremities, lower 444.22
    - without thrombus or embolus (*see also* Arteriosclerosis, extremities) 440.20
    - due to stricture or stenosis 447.1
    - upper 444.21
        - without thrombus or embolus (*see also* Arteriosclerosis, extremities) 440.20
        - due to stricture or stenosis 447.1
- artery NEC (*see also* Embolism, artery) 444.9
    - auditory, internal 433.8 ✓5th
    - basilar 433.0 ✓5th
        - with other precerebral artery 433.3 ✓5th
        - bilateral 433.3 ✓5th
    - brain or cerebral (*see also* Infarct, brain) 434.9 ✓5th
    - carotid 433.1 ✓5th
        - with other precerebral artery 433.3 ✓5th
        - bilateral 433.3 ✓5th
    - cerebellar (anterior inferior) (posterior inferior) (superior) 433.8 ✓5th
    - cerebral (*see also* Infarct, brain) 434.9 ✓5th
    - choroidal (anterior) 433.8 ✓5th
    - communicating posterior 433.8 ✓5th
    - coronary (thrombotic) (*see also* Infarct, myocardium) 410.9 ✓5th
        - acute 410.9 ✓5th
            - without myocardial infarction 411.81
        - healed or old 412
    - hypophyseal 433.8 ✓5th
    - iliac 444.81

Occlusion — continued
artery NEC (see also Embolism, artery) — continued
  mesenteric (embolic) (thrombotic) (with gangrene) 557.0
  pontine 433.8 ✓5th
  precerebral NEC 433.9 ✓5th
    late effect — see Late effect(s) (of) cerebrovascular disease
    multiple or bilateral 433.3 ✓5th
    puerperal, postpartum, childbirth 674.0 ✓5th
    specified NEC 433.8 ✓5th
  renal 593.81
  retinal — see Occlusion, retina, artery
  spinal 433.8 ✓5th
  vertebral 433.2 ✓5th
    with other precerebral artery 433.3 ✓5th
    bilateral 433.3 ✓5th
basilar (artery) — see Occlusion, artery, basilar
bile duct (any) (see also Obstruction, biliary) 576.2
bowel (see also Obstruction, intestine) 560.9
brain (artery) (vascular) (see also Infarct, brain) 434.9 ✓5th
breast (duct) 611.8
carotid (artery) (common) (internal) — see Occlusion, artery, carotid
cerebellar (anterior inferior) (artery) (posterior inferior) (superior) 433.8 ✓5th
cerebral (artery) (see also Infarct, brain) 434.9 ✓5th
cerebrovascular (see also Infarct, brain) 434.9 ✓5th
  diffuse 437.0
cervical canal (see also Stricture, cervix) 622.4
  by falciparum malaria 084.0
cervix (uteri) (see also Stricture, cervix) 622.4
choanal 748.0
choroidal (artery) 433.8 ✓5th
colon (see also Obstruction, intestine) 560.9
communicating posterior artery 433.8 ✓5th
coronary (artery) (thrombotic) (see also Infarct, myocardium) 410.9 ✓5th
  acute 410.9 ✓5th
    without myocardial infarction 411.81
  healed or old 412
  without myocardial infarction 411.81
cystic duct (see also Obstruction, gallbladder) 575.2
  congenital 751.69
embolic — see Embolism
fallopian tube 628.2
  congenital 752.19
gallbladder (see also Obstruction, gallbladder) 575.2
  congenital 751.69
    jaundice from 751.69 [774.5]
gingiva, traumatic 523.8
hymen 623.3
  congenital 752.42
hypophyseal (artery) 433.8 ✓5th
iliac artery 444.81
intestine (see also Obstruction, intestine) 560.9
kidney 593.89
lacrimal apparatus — see Stenosis, lacrimal
lung 518.89
lymph or lymphatic channel 457.1
mammary duct 611.8
mesenteric artery (embolic) (thrombotic) (with gangrene) 557.0
nose 478.1
  congenital 748.0
organ or site, congenital NEC — see Atresia
oviduct 628.2
  congenital 752.19
periodontal, traumatic 523.8
peripheral arteries (lower extremity) 444.22
  without thrombus or embolus (see also Arteriosclerosis, extremities) 440.20
  due to stricture or stenosis 447.1
  upper extremity 444.21
    without thrombus or embolus (see also Arteriosclerosis, extremities) 440.20
    due to stricture or stenosis 447.1
pontine (artery) 433.8 ✓5th
posterior lingual, of mandibular teeth 524.2

Occlusion — continued
precerebral artery — see Occlusion, artery, precerebral NEC
puncta lacrimalia 375.52
pupil 364.74
pylorus (see also Stricture, pylorus) 537.0
renal artery 593.81
retina, retinal (vascular) 362.30
  artery, arterial 362.30
    branch 362.32
    central (total) 362.31
    partial 362.33
    transient 362.34
    tributary 362.32
  vein 362.30
    branch 362.36
    central (total) 362.35
    incipient 362.37
    partial 362.37
    tributary 362.36
spinal artery 433.8 ✓5th
stent
  coronary 996.72
teeth (mandibular) (posterior lingual) 524.2
thoracic duct 457.1
tubal 628.2
ureter (complete) (partial) 593.4
  congenital 753.29
urethra (see also Stricture, urethra) 598.9
  congenital 753.6
uterus 621.8
vagina 623.2
vascular NEC 459.9
vein — see Thrombosis
vena cava (inferior) (superior) 453.2
ventricle (brain) NEC 331.4
vertebral (artery) — see Occlusion, artery, vertebral
vessel (blood) NEC 459.9
vulva 624.8

Occlusio pupillae 364.74

Occupational
problems NEC V62.2
therapy V57.21

Ochlophobia 300.29

Ochronosis (alkaptonuric) (congenital) (endogenous) 270.2
with chloasma of eyelid 270.2

Ocular muscle — see also condition
myopathy 359.1
torticollis 781.93

Oculoauriculovertebral dysplasia 756.0

Oculogyric
crisis or disturbance 378.87
psychogenic 306.7

Oculomotor syndrome 378.81

Oddi's sphincter spasm 576.5

Odelberg's disease (juvenile osteochondrosis) 732.1

Odontalgia 525.9

Odontoameloblastoma (M9311/0) 213.1
upper jaw (bone) 213.0

Odontoclasia 521.05

Odontoclasis 873.63
complicated 873.73

Odontodysplasia, regional 520.4

Odontogenesis imperfecta 520.5

Odontoma (M9280/0) 213.1
ameloblastic (M9311/0) 213.1
  upper jaw (bone) 213.0
calcified (M9280/0) 213.1
  upper jaw (bone) 213.0
complex (M9282/0) 213.1
  upper jaw (bone) 213.0
compound (M9281/0) 213.1
  upper jaw (bone) 213.0
fibroameloblastic (M9290/0) 213.1
  upper jaw (bone) 213.0
follicular 526.0
  upper jaw (bone) 213.0

Odontomyelitis (closed) (open) 522.0

Odontonecrosis 521.09

Odontorrhagia 525.8

Odontosarcoma, ameloblastic (M9290/3) 170.1
upper jaw (bone) 170.0

Odynophagia 787.2

Oesophagostomiasis 127.7

Oesophagostomum infestation 127.7

Oestriasis 134.0

Ogilvie's syndrome (sympathicotonic colon obstruction) 560.89

Oguchi's disease (retina) 368.61

Ohara's disease (see also Tularemia) 021.9

Oidiomycosis (see also Candidiasis) 112.9

Oidiomycotic meningitis 112.83

Oidium albicans infection (see also Candidiasis) 112.9

Old age 797
dementia (of) 290.0

Olfactory — see condition

Oligemia 285.9

Oligergasia (see also Retardation, mental) 319

Oligoamnios 658.0 ✓5th
affecting fetus or newborn 761.2

Oligoastrocytoma, mixed (M9382/3)
specified site — see Neoplasm, by site, malignant
unspecified site 191.9

Oligocythemia 285.9

Oligodendroblastoma (M9460/3)
specified site — see Neoplasm, by site, malignant
unspecified site 191.9

Oligodendroglioma (M9450/3)
anaplastic type (M9451/3)
  specified site — see Neoplasm, by site, malignant
  unspecified site 191.9
specified site — see Neoplasm, by site, malignant
unspecified site 191.9

Oligodendroma — see Oligodendroglioma

Oligodontia (see also Anodontia) 520.0

Oligoencephalon 742.1

Oligohydramnios 658.0 ✓5th
affecting fetus or newborn 761.2
due to premature rupture of membranes 658.1 ✓5th
  affecting fetus or newborn 761.2

Oligohydrosis 705.0

Oligomenorrhea 626.1

Oligophrenia (see also Retardation, mental) 319
phenylpyruvic 270.1

Oligospermia 606.1

Oligotrichia 704.09
congenita 757.4

Oliguria 788.5
with
  abortion — see Abortion, by type, with renal failure
  ectopic pregnancy (see also categories 633.0-633.9) 639.3
  molar pregnancy (see also categories 630-632) 639.3
complicating
  abortion 639.3
  ectopic or molar pregnancy 639.3
  pregnancy 646.2 ✓5th
    with hypertension — see Toxemia, of pregnancy
  due to a procedure 997.5
  following labor and delivery 669.3 ✓5th
  heart or cardiac — see Failure, heart
  puerperal, postpartum 669.3 ✓5th
  specified due to a procedure 997.5

Ollier's disease (chondrodysplasia) 756.4

Omentitis (see also Peritonitis) 567.9

Omentocele (see also Hernia, omental) 553.8

Omentum, omental — see condition

Omphalitis (congenital) (newborn) 771.4
not of newborn 686.9
tetanus 771.3

Omphalocele 756.79

Omphalomesenteric duct, persistent 751.0

Omphalorrhagia, newborn 772.3
Omsk hemorrhagic fever 065.1
Onanism 307.9
Onchocerciasis 125.3
   eye 125.3 [360.13]
Onchocercosis 125.3
Oncocytoma (M8290/0) — see Neoplasm, by site, benign
Ondine's curse 348.8
Oneirophrenia (see also Schizophrenia) 295.4
Onychauxis 703.8
   congenital 757.5
Onychia (with lymphangitis) 681.9
   dermatophytic 110.1
   finger 681.02
   toe 681.11
Onychitis (with lymphangitis) 681.9
   finger 681.02
   toe 681.11
Onychocryptosis 703.0
Onychodystrophy 703.8
   congenital 757.5
Onychogryphosis 703.8
Onychogryposis 703.8
Onycholysis 703.8
Onychomadesis 703.8
Onychomalacia 703.8
Onychomycosis 110.1
   finger 110.1
   toe 110.1
Onycho-osteodysplasia 756.89
Onychophagy 307.9
Onychoptosis 703.8
Onychorrhexis 703.8
   congenital 757.5
Onychoschizia 703.8
Onychotrophia (see also Atrophy, nail) 703.8
O'nyong-nyong fever 066.3
Onyxis (finger) (toe) 703.0
Onyxitis (with lymphangitis) 681.9
   finger 681.02
   toe 681.11
Oophoritis (cystic) (infectional) (interstitial) (see also Salpingo-oophoritis) 614.2
   complicating pregnancy 646.6
   fetal (acute) 752.0
   gonococcal (acute) 098.19
      chronic or duration of 2 months or over 098.39
   tuberculous (see also Tuberculosis) 016.6
Opacity, opacities
   cornea 371.00
      central 371.03
      congenital 743.43
         interfering with vision 743.42
      degenerative (see also Degeneration, cornea) 371.40
      hereditary (see also Dystrophy, cornea) 371.50
      inflammatory (see also Keratitis) 370.9
      late effect of trachoma (healed) 139.1
      minor 371.01
      peripheral 371.02
   enamel (fluoride) (nonfluoride) (teeth) 520.3
   lens (see also Cataract) 366.9
   snowball 379.22
   vitreous (humor) 379.24
      congenital 743.51
Opalescent dentin (hereditary) 520.5
Open, opening
   abnormal, organ or site, congenital — see Imperfect, closure
   angle with
      borderline intraocular pressure 365.01
      cupping of discs 365.01
   bite (anterior) (posterior) 524.2
   false — see Imperfect, closure
   wound — see Wound, open, by site

Operation
   causing mutilation of fetus 763.89
   destructive, on live fetus, to facilitate birth 763.89
   for delivery, fetus or newborn 763.89
   maternal, unrelated to current delivery, affecting fetus or newborn 760.6
Operational fatigue 300.89
Operative — see condition
Operculitis (chronic) 523.4
   acute 523.3
Operculum, retina 361.32
   with detachment 361.01
Ophiasis 704.01
Ophthalmia (see also Conjunctivitis) 372.30
   actinic rays 370.24
   allergic (acute) 372.05
      chronic 372.14
   blennorrhagic (neonatorum) 098.40
   catarrhal 372.03
   diphtheritic 032.81
   Egyptian 076.1
   electric, electrica 370.24
   gonococcal (neonatorum) 098.40
   metastatic 360.11
   migraine 346.8
   neonatorum, newborn 771.6
      gonococcal 098.40
   nodosa 360.14
   phlyctenular 370.31
      with ulcer (see also Ulcer, cornea) 370.00
   sympathetic 360.11
Ophthalmitis — see Ophthalmia
Ophthalmocele (congenital) 743.66
Ophthalmoneuromyelitis 341.0
Ophthalmopathy, infiltrative with thyrotoxicosis 242.0
Ophthalmoplegia (see also Strabismus) 378.9
   anterior internuclear 378.86
   ataxia-areflexia syndrome 357.0
   bilateral 378.9
   diabetic 250.5 [378.86]
   exophthalmic 242.0 [376.22]
   external 378.55
      progressive 378.72
      total 378.56
   interna(l) (complete) (total) 367.52
   internuclear 378.86
   migraine 346.8
   painful 378.55
   Parinaud's 378.81
   progressive external 378.72
   supranuclear, progressive 333.0
   total (external) 378.56
      internal 367.52
   unilateral 378.9
Opisthognathism 524.00
Opisthorchiasis (felineus) (tenuicollis) (viverrini) 121.0
Opisthotonos, opisthotonus 781.0
Opitz's disease (congestive splenomegaly) 289.51
Opiumism (see also Dependence) 304.0
Oppenheim's disease 358.8
Oppenheim-Urbach disease or syndrome (necrobiosis lipoidica diabeticorum) 250.8 [709.3]
Opsoclonia 379.59
Optic nerve — see condition
Orbit — see condition
Orchioblastoma (M9071/3) 186.9
Orchitis (nonspecific) (septic) 604.90
   with abscess 604.0
   blennorrhagic (acute) 098.13
      chronic or duration of 2 months or over 098.33
   diphtheritic 032.89 [604.91]
   filarial 125.9 [604.91]
   gangrenous 604.99
   gonococcal (acute) 098.13
      chronic or duration of 2 months or over 098.33
   mumps 072.0
   parotidea 072.0

Orchitis — continued
   suppurative 604.99
   syphilitic 095.8 [604.91]
   tuberculous (see also Tuberculosis) 016.5 [608.81]
Orf 051.2
Organic — see also condition
   heart — see Disease, heart
   insufficiency 799.8
Oriental
   bilharziasis 120.2
   schistosomiasis 120.2
   sore 085.1
Orifice — see condition
Origin, both great vessels from right ventricle 745.11
Ormond's disease or syndrome 593.4
Ornithosis 073.9
   with
      complication 073.8
         specified NEC 073.7
      pneumonia 073.0
      pneumonitis (lobular) 073.0
Orodigitofacial dysostosis 759.89
Oropouche fever 066.3
Orotaciduria, oroticaciduria (congenital) (hereditary) (pyrimidine deficiency) 281.4
Oroya fever 088.0
Orthodontics V58.5
   adjustment V53.4
   aftercare V58.5
   fitting V53.4
Orthopnea 786.02
Orthoptic training V57.4
Os, uterus — see condition
Osgood-Schlatter
   disease 732.4
   osteochondrosis 732.4
Osler's
   disease (M9950/1) (polycythemia vera) 238.4
   nodes 421.0
Osler-Rendu disease (familial hemorrhagic telangiectasia) 448.0
Osler-Vaquez disease (M9950/1) (polycythemia vera) 238.4
Osler-Weber-Rendu syndrome (familial hemorrhagic telangiectasia) 448.0
Osmidrosis 705.89
Osseous — see condition
Ossification
   artery — see Arteriosclerosis
   auricle (ear) 380.39
   bronchus 519.1
   cardiac (see also Degeneration, myocardial) 429.1
   cartilage (senile) 733.99
   coronary (artery) — see Arteriosclerosis, coronary
   diaphragm 728.10
   ear 380.39
      middle (see also Otosclerosis) 387.9
   falx cerebri 349.2
   fascia 728.10
   fontanel
      defective or delayed 756.0
      premature 756.0
   heart (see also Degeneration, myocardial) 429.1
      valve — see Endocarditis
   larynx 478.79
   ligament
      posterior longitudinal 724.8
         cervical 723.7
   meninges (cerebral) 349.2
      spinal 336.8
   multiple, eccentric centers 733.99
   muscle 728.10
      heterotopic, postoperative 728.13
   myocardium, myocardial (see also Degeneration, myocardial) 429.1
   penis 607.81
   periarticular 728.89
   sclera 379.16
   tendon 727.82

Index to Diseases

Ossification — *continued*
   trachea 519.1
   tympanic membrane (*see also*
      Tympanosclerosis) 385.00
   vitreous (humor) 360.44
Osteitis (*see also* Osteomyelitis) 730.2 ✓5ᵗʰ
   acute 730.0 ✓5ᵗʰ
   alveolar 526.5
   chronic 730.1 ✓5ᵗʰ
   condensans (ilii) 733.5
   deformans (Paget's) 731.0
      due to or associated with malignant
         neoplasm (*see also* Neoplasm, bone,
         malignant) 170.9 *[731.1]*
   due to yaws 102.6
   fibrosa NEC 733.29
      cystica (generalisata) 252.0
      disseminata 756.59
      osteoplastica 252.0
   fragilitans 756.51
   Garré's (sclerosing) 730.1 ✓5ᵗʰ
   infectious (acute) (subacute) 730.0 ✓5ᵗʰ
      chronic or old 730.1 ✓5ᵗʰ
   jaw (acute) (chronic) (lower) (neonatal)
      (suppurative) (upper) 526.4
   parathyroid 252.0
   petrous bone (*see also* Petrositis) 383.20
   pubis 733.5
   sclerotic, nonsuppurative 730.1 ✓5ᵗʰ
   syphilitic 095.5
   tuberculosa
      cystica (of Jüngling) 135
      multiplex cystoides 135
Osteoarthritica spondylitis (spine) (*see also*
   Spondylosis) 721.90
Osteoarthritis (*see also* Osteoarthrosis) 715.9 ✓5ᵗʰ
   distal interphalangeal 715.9 ✓5ᵗʰ
   hyperplastic 731.2
   interspinalis (*see also* Spondylosis) 721.90
   spine, spinal NEC (*see also* Spondylosis)
      721.90
Osteoarthropathy (*see also* Osteoarthrosis)
   715.9 ✓5ᵗʰ
   chronic idiopathic hypertrophic 757.39
   familial idiopathic 757.39
   hypertrophic pulmonary 731.2
      secondary 731.2
   idiopathic hypertrophic 757.39
   primary hypertrophic 731.2
   pulmonary hypertrophic 731.2
   secondary hypertrophic 731.2
Osteoarthrosis (degenerative) (hypertrophic)
   (rheumatoid) 715.9 ✓5ᵗʰ

> Note — Use the following fifth-digit
> subclassification with category 715:
>
> 0   site unspecified
> 1   shoulder region
> 2   upper arm
> 3   forearm
> 4   hand
> 5   pelvic region and thigh
> 6   lower leg
> 7   ankle and foot
> 8   other specified sites except spine
> 9   multiple sites

   Deformans alkaptonurica 270.2
   generalized 715.09
   juvenilis (Köhler's) 732.5
   localized 715.3 ✓5ᵗʰ
      idiopathic 715.1 ✓5ᵗʰ
      primary 715.1 ✓5ᵗʰ
      secondary 715.2 ✓5ᵗʰ
   multiple sites, not specified as generalized
      715.89
   polyarticular 715.09
   spine (*see also* Spondylosis) 721.90
   temporomandibular joint 524.69
Osteoblastoma (M9200/0) — *see* Neoplasm,
   bone, benign
Osteochondritis (*see also* Osteochondrosis) 732.9
   dissecans 732.7
      hip 732.7

Osteochondritis (*see also* Osteochondrosis) —
   continued
   ischiopubica 732.1
   multiple 756.59
   syphilitic (congenital) 090.0
Osteochondrodermodysplasia 756.59
Osteochondrodystrophy 277.5
   deformans 277.5
   familial 277.5
   fetalis 756.4
Osteochondrolysis 732.7
Osteochondroma (M9210/0) — *see also*
   Neoplasm, bone, benign
   multiple, congenital 756.4
Osteochondromatosis (M9210/1) 238.0
   synovial 727.82
Osteochondromyxosarcoma (M9180/3) — *see*
   Neoplasm, bone, malignant
Osteochondropathy NEC 732.9
Osteochondrosarcoma (M9180/3) — *see*
   Neoplasm, bone, malignant
Osteochondrosis 732.9
   acetabulum 732.1
   adult spine 732.8
   astragalus 732.5
   Blount's 732.4
   Buchanan's (juvenile osteochondrosis of iliac
      crest) 732.1
   Buchman's (juvenile osteochondrosis) 732.1
   Burns' 732.3
   calcaneus 732.5
   capitular epiphysis (femur) 732.1
   carpal
      lunate (wrist) 732.3
      scaphoid 732.3
   coxae juvenilis 732.1
   deformans juvenilis (coxae) (hip) 732.1
      Scheuermann's 732.0
      spine 732.0
      tibia 732.4
      vertebra 732.0
   Diaz's (astragalus) 732.5
   dissecans (knee) (shoulder) 732.7
   femoral capital epiphysis 732.1
   femur (head) (juvenile) 732.1
   foot (juvenile) 732.5
   Freiberg's (disease) (second metatarsal) 732.5
   Haas' 732.3
   Haglund's (os tibiale externum) 732.5
   hand (juvenile) 732.3
   head of
      femur 732.1
      humerus (juvenile) 732.3
   hip (juvenile) 732.1
   humerus (juvenile) 732.3
   iliac crest (juvenile) 732.1
   ilium (juvenile) 732.1
   ischiopubic synchondrosis 732.1
   Iselin's (osteochondrosis fifth metatarsal) 732.5
   juvenile, juvenilis 732.6
      arm 732.3
      capital femoral epiphysis 732.1
      capitellum humeri 732.3
      capitular epiphysis 732.1
      carpal scaphoid 732.3
      clavicle, sternal epiphysis 732.6
      coxae 732.1
      deformans 732.1
      foot 732.5
      hand 732.3
      hip and pelvis 732.1
      lower extremity, except foot 732.4
      lunate, wrist 732.3
      medial cuneiform bone 732.5
      metatarsal (head) 732.5
      metatarsophalangeal 732.5
      navicular, ankle 732.5
      patella 732.4
      primary patellar center (of Köhler) 732.4
      specified site NEC 732.6
      spine 732.0
      tarsal scaphoid 732.5
      tibia (epiphysis) (tuberosity) 732.4
      upper extremity 732.3
      vertebra (body) (Calvé) 732.0
         epiphyseal plates (of Scheuermann) 732.0

Osteochondrosis — *continued*
   Kienböck's (disease) 732.3
   Köhler's (disease) (navicular, ankle) 732.5
      patellar 732.4
      tarsal navicular 732.5
   Legg-Calvé-Perthes (disease) 732.1
   lower extremity (juvenile) 732.4
   lunate bone 732.3
   Mauclaire's 732.3
   metacarpal heads (of Mauclaire) 732.3
   metatarsal (fifth) (head) (second) 732.5
   navicular, ankle 732.5
   os calcis 732.5
   Osgood-Schlatter 732.4
   os tibiale externum 732.5
   Panner's 732.3
   patella (juvenile) 732.4
   patellar center
      primary (of Köhler) 732.4
      secondary (of Sinding-Larsen) 732.4
   pelvis (juvenile) 732.1
   Pierson's 732.1
   radial head (juvenile) 732.3
   Scheuermann's 732.0
   Sever's (calcaneum) 732.5
   Sinding-Larsen (secondary patellar center)
      732.4
   spine (juvenile) 732.0
      adult 732.8
   symphysis pubis (of Pierson) (juvenile) 732.1
   syphilitic (congenital) 090.0
   tarsal (navicular) (scaphoid) 732.5
   tibia (proximal) (tubercle) 732.4
   tuberculous — *see* Tuberculosis, bone
   ulna 732.3
   upper extremity (juvenile) 732.3
   van Neck's (juvenile osteochondrosis) 732.1
   vertebral (juvenile) 732.0
      adult 732.8
Osteoclastoma (M9250/1) 238.0
   malignant (M9250/3) — *see* Neoplasm, bone,
      malignant
Osteocopic pain 733.90
Osteodynia 733.90
Osteodystrophy
   azotemic 588.0
   chronica deformans hypertrophica 731.0
   congenital 756.50
      specified type NEC 756.59
   deformans 731.0
   fibrosa localisata 731.0
   parathyroid 252.0
   renal 588.0
Osteofibroma (M9262/0) — *see* Neoplasm, bone,
   benign
Osteofibrosarcoma (M9182/3) — *see* Neoplasm,
   bone, malignant
Osteogenesis imperfecta 756.51
Osteogenic — *see* condition
Osteoma (M9180/0) — *see also* Neoplasm, bone,
   benign
   osteoid (M9191/0) — *see also* Neoplasm, bone,
      benign
      giant (M9200/0) — *see* Neoplasm, bone,
         benign
Osteomalacia 268.2
   chronica deformans hypertrophica 731.0
   due to vitamin D deficiency 268.2
   infantile (*see also* Rickets) 268.0
   juvenile (*see also* Rickets) 268.0
   pelvis 268.2
   vitamin D-resistant 275.3
Osteomalacic bone 268.2
Osteomalacosis 268.2

Osteomyelitis

Osteomyelitis (general) (infective) (localized) (neonatal) (purulent) (pyogenic) (septic) (staphylococcal) (streptococcal) (suppurative) (with periostitis) 730.2

> Note — Use the following fifth-digit subclassification with category 730:
>
> 0   site unspecified
> 1   shoulder region
> 2   upper arm
> 3   forearm
> 4   hand
> 5   pelvic region and thigh
> 6   lower leg
> 7   ankle and foot
> 8   other specified sites
> 9   multiple sites

  acute or subacute 730.0
  chronic or old 730.1
  due to or associated with
    diabetes mellitus 250.8 [731.8]
    tuberculosis (see also Tuberculosis, bone)
      015.9 [730.8]
      limb bones 015.5 [730.8]
      specified bones NEC
        015.7 [730.8]
      spine 015.0 [730.8]
    typhoid 002.0 [730.8]
  Garré's 730.1
  jaw (acute) (chronic) (lower) (neonatal) (suppurative) (upper) 526.4
  nonsuppurating 730.1
  orbital 376.03
  petrous bone (see also Petrositis) 383.20
  Salmonella 003.24
  sclerosing, nonsuppurative 730.1
  sicca 730.1
  syphilitic 095.5
    congenital 090.0 [730.8]
  tuberculous — see Tuberculosis, bone
  typhoid 002.0 [730.8]
Osteomyelofibrosis 289.8
Osteomyelosclerosis 289.8
Osteonecrosis 733.40
  meaning osteomyelitis 730.1
Osteo-onycho-arthro dysplasia 756.89
Osteo-onychodysplasia, hereditary 756.89
Osteopathia
  condensans disseminata 756.53
  hyperostotica multiplex infantilis 756.59
  hypertrophica toxica 731.2
  striata 756.4
Osteopathy resulting from poliomyelitis (see also Poliomyelitis) 045.9 [730.7]
  familial dysplastic 731.2
Osteopecilia 756.53
Osteopenia 733.90
Osteoperiostitis (see also Osteomyelitis) 730.2
  ossificans toxica 731.2
  toxica ossificans 731.2
Osteopetrosis (familial) 756.52
Osteophyte — see Exostosis
Osteophytosis — see Exostosis
Osteopoikilosis 756.53
Osteoporosis (generalized) 733.00
  circumscripta 731.0
  disuse 733.03
  drug-induced 733.09
  idiopathic 733.02
  postmenopausal 733.01
  posttraumatic 733.7
  screening V82.81
  senile 733.01
  specified type NEC 733.09
Osteoporosis-osteomalacia syndrome 268.2
Osteopsathyrosis 756.51
Osteoradionecrosis, jaw 526.89
Osteosarcoma (M9180/3) — see also Neoplasm, bone, malignant
  chondroblastic (M9181/3) — see Neoplasm, bone, malignant

Osteosarcoma (M9180/3) — see also Neoplasm, bone, malignant — continued
  fibroblastic (M9182/3) — see Neoplasm, bone, malignant
  in Paget's disease of bone (M9184/3) — see Neoplasm, bone, malignant
  juxtacortical (M9190/3) — see Neoplasm, bone, malignant
  parosteal (M9190/3) — see Neoplasm, bone, malignant
  telangiectatic (M9183/3) — see Neoplasm, bone, malignant
Osteosclerosis 756.52
  fragilis (generalisata) 756.52
  myelofibrosis 289.8
Osteosclerotic anemia 289.8
Osteosis
  acromegaloid 757.39
  cutis 709.3
  parathyroid 252.0
  renal fibrocystic 588.0
Österreicher-Turner syndrome 756.89
Ostium
  atrioventriculare commune 745.69
  primum (arteriosum) (defect) (persistent) 745.61
  secundum (arteriosum) (defect) (patent) (persistent) 745.5
Ostrum-Furst syndrome 756.59
Otalgia 388.70
  otogenic 388.71
  referred 388.72
Othematoma 380.31
Otitic hydrocephalus 348.2
Otitis 382.9
  with effusion 381.4
    purulent 382.4
    secretory 381.4
    serous 381.4
    suppurative 382.4
  acute 382.9
  adhesive (see also Adhesions, middle ear) 385.10
  chronic 382.9
    with effusion 381.3
    mucoid, mucous (simple) 381.20
    purulent 382.3
    secretory 381.3
    serous 381.10
    suppurative 382.3
  diffuse parasitic 136.8
  externa (acute) (diffuse) (hemorrhagica) 380.10
    actinic 380.22
    candidal 112.82
    chemical 380.22
    chronic 380.23
      mycotic — see Otitis, externa, mycotic
      specified type NEC 380.23
    circumscribed 380.10
    contact 380.22
    due to
      erysipelas 035 [380.13]
      impetigo 684 [380.13]
      seborrheic dermatitis 690.10 [380.13]
    eczematoid 380.22
    furuncular 680.0 [380.13]
    infective 380.10
      chronic 380.16
    malignant 380.14
    mycotic (chronic) 380.15
      due to
        aspergillosis 117.3 [380.15]
        moniliasis 112.82
        otomycosis 111.8 [380.15]
    reactive 380.22
    specified type NEC 380.22
    tropical 111.8 [380.15]
  insidiosa (see also Otosclerosis) 387.9
  interna (see also Labyrinthitis) 386.30
  media (hemorrhagic) (staphylococcal) (streptococcal) 382.9
    acute 382.9
      with effusion 381.00
      allergic 381.04
        mucoid 381.05
        sanguineous 381.06

Otitis — continued
  media — continued
    acute — continued
      allergic — continued
        serous 381.04
      catarrhal 381.00
      exudative 381.00
      mucoid 381.02
        allergic 381.05
      necrotizing 382.00
        with spontaneous rupture of ear drum 382.01
        in
          influenza 487.8 [382.02]
          measles 055.2
          scarlet fever 034.1 [382.02]
      nonsuppurative 381.00
      purulent 382.00
        with spontaneous rupture of ear drum 382.01
      sanguineous 381.03
        allergic 381.06
      secretory 381.01
      seromucinous 381.02
      serous 381.01
        allergic 381.04
      suppurative 382.00
        with spontaneous rupture of ear drum 382.01
        due to
          influenza 487.8 [382.02]
          scarlet fever 034.1 [382.02]
      transudative 381.00
    adhesive (see also Adhesions, middle ear) 385.10
    allergic 381.4
      acute 381.04
        mucoid 381.05
        sanguineous 381.06
        serous 381.04
      chronic 381.3
    catarrhal 381.4
      acute 381.00
      chronic (simple) 381.10
    chronic 382.9
      with effusion 381.3
      adhesive (see also Adhesions, middle ear) 385.10
      allergic 381.3
      atticoantral, suppurative (with posterior or superior marginal perforation of ear drum) 382.2
      benign suppurative (with anterior perforation of ear drum) 382.1
      catarrhal 381.10
      exudative 381.3
      mucinous 381.20
      mucoid, mucous (simple) 381.20
      mucosanguineous 381.29
      nonsuppurative 381.3
      purulent 382.3
      secretory 381.3
      seromucinous 381.3
      serosanguineous 381.19
      serous (simple) 381.10
      suppurative 382.3
        atticoantral (with posterior or superior marginal perforation of ear drum) 382.2
        benign (with anterior perforation of ear drum) 382.1
      tuberculous (see also Tuberculosis) 017.4
      tubotympanic 382.1
      transudative 381.3
    exudative 381.4
      acute 381.00
      chronic 381.3
    fibrotic (see also Adhesions, middle ear) 385.10
    mucoid, mucous 381.4
      acute 381.02
      chronic (simple) 381.20
    mucosanguineous, chronic 381.29
    nonsuppurative 381.4
      acute 381.00
      chronic 381.3
    postmeasles 055.2

Index to Diseases

Otitis — continued
  media — continued
    purulent 382.4
      acute 382.00
        with spontaneous rupture of ear drum 382.01
      chronic 382.3
    sanguineous, acute 381.03
      allergic 381.06
    secretory 381.4
      acute or subacute 381.01
      chronic 381.3
    seromucinous 381.4
      acute or subacute 381.02
      chronic 381.3
    serosanguineous, chronic 381.19
    serous 381.4
      acute or subacute 381.01
      chronic (simple) 381.10
    subacute — see Otitis, media, acute
    suppurative 382.4
      acute 382.00
        with spontaneous rupture of ear drum 382.01
      chronic 382.3
        atticoantral 382.2
        benign 382.1
        tuberculous (see also Tuberculosis) 017.4 ✓5ᵗʰ
        tubotympanic 382.1
    transudative 381.4
      acute 381.00
      chronic 381.3
    tuberculous (see also Tuberculosis) 017.4 ✓5ᵗʰ
    postmeasles 055.2
Otoconia 386.8
Otolith syndrome 386.19
Otomycosis 111.8 [380.15]
  in
    aspergillosis 117.3 [380.15]
    moniliasis 112.82
Otopathy 388.9
Otoporosis (see also Otosclerosis) 387.9
Otorrhagia 388.69
  traumatic — see nature of injury
Otorrhea 388.60
  blood 388.69
  cerebrospinal (fluid) 388.61
Otosclerosis (general) 387.9
  cochlear (endosteal) 387.2
  involving
    otic capsule 387.2
    oval window
      nonobliterative 387.0
      obliterative 387.1
    round window 387.2
  nonobliterative 387.0
  obliterative 387.1
  specified type NEC 387.8
Otospongiosis (see also Otosclerosis) 387.9
Otto's disease or pelvis 715.35
Outburst, aggressive (see also Disturbance, conduct) 312.0 ✓5ᵗʰ
  in children and adolescents 313.9
Outcome of delivery
  multiple birth NEC V27.9
    all liveborn V27.5
    all stillborn V27.7
    some liveborn V27.6
    unspecified V27.9
  single V27.9
    liveborn V27.0
    stillborn V27.1
  twins V27.9
    both liveborn V27.2
    both stillborn V27.4
    one liveborn, one stillborn V27.3
Outlet — see also condition
  syndrome (thoracic) 353.0
Outstanding ears (bilateral) 744.29
Ovalocytosis (congenital) (hereditary) (see also Elliptocytosis) 282.1

Ovarian — see also condition
  pregnancy — see Pregnancy, ovarian
  remnant syndrome 620.8
  vein syndrome 593.4
Ovaritis (cystic) (see also Salpingo-oophoritis) 614.2
Ovary, ovarian — see condition
Overactive — see also Hyperfunction
  bladder 596.51
  eye muscle (see also Strabismus) 378.9
  hypothalamus 253.8
  thyroid (see also Thyrotoxicosis) 242.9 ✓5ᵗʰ
Overactivity, child 314.01
Overbite (deep) (excessive) (horizontal) (vertical) 524.2
Overbreathing (see also Hyperventilation) 786.01
Overconscientious personality 301.4
Overdevelopment — see also Hypertrophy
  breast (female) (male) 611.1
  nasal bones 738.0
  prostate, congenital 752.8
Overdistention — see Distention
Overdose, overdosage (drug) 977.9
  specified drug or substance — see Table of Drugs and Chemicals
Overeating 783.6
  with obesity 278.0 ✓5ᵗʰ
  nonorganic origin 307.51
Overexertion (effects) (exhaustion) 994.5
Overexposure (effects) 994.9
  exhaustion 994.4
Overfeeding (see also Overeating) 783.6
Overgrowth, bone NEC 733.99
Overheated (effects) (places) — see Heat
Overinhibited child 313.0
Overjet 524.2
Overlaid, overlying (suffocation) 994.7
Overlapping toe (acquired) 735.8
  congenital (fifth toe) 755.66
Overload
  fluid 276.6
  potassium (K) 276.7
  sodium (Na) 276.0
Overnutrition (see also Hyperalimentation) 783.6
Overproduction — see also Hypersecretion
  ACTH 255.3
  cortisol 255.0
  growth hormone 253.0
  thyroid-stimulating hormone (TSH) 242.8 ✓5ᵗʰ
Overriding
  aorta 747.21
  finger (acquired) 736.29
    congenital 755.59
  toe (acquired) 735.8
    congenital 755.66
Oversize
  fetus (weight of 4500 grams or more) 766.0
    affecting management of pregnancy 656.6 ✓5ᵗʰ
    causing disproportion 653.5 ✓5ᵗʰ
      with obstructed labor 660.1 ✓5ᵗʰ
        affecting fetus or newborn 763.1
Overstimulation, ovarian 256.1
Overstrained 780.79
  heart — see Hypertrophy, cardiac
Overweight (see also Obesity) 278.00
Overwork 780.79
Oviduct — see condition
Ovotestis 752.7
Ovulation (cycle)
  failure or lack of 628.0
  pain 625.2
Ovum
  blighted 631
  dropsical 631
  pathologic 631
Owren's disease or syndrome (parahemophilia) (see also Defect, coagulation) 286.3
Oxalosis 271.8
Oxaluria 271.8

Ox heart — see Hypertrophy, cardiac
OX syndrome 758.6
Oxycephaly, oxycephalic 756.0
  syphilitic, congenital 090.0
Oxyuriasis 127.4
Oxyuris vermicularis (infestation) 127.4
Ozena 472.0

P

Pacemaker syndrome 429.4
Pachyderma, pachydermia 701.8
  laryngis 478.5
  laryngitis 478.79
  larynx (verrucosa) 478.79
Pachydermatitis 701.8
Pachydermatocele (congenital) 757.39
  acquired 701.8
Pachydermatosis 701.8
Pachydermoperiostitis
  secondary 731.2
Pachydermoperiostosis
  primary idiopathic 757.39
  secondary 731.2
Pachymeningitis (adhesive) (basal) (brain) (cerebral) (cervical) (chronic) (circumscribed) (external) (fibrous) (hemorrhagic) (hypertrophic) (internal) (purulent) (spinal) (suppurative) (see also Meningitis) 322.9
  gonococcal 098.82
Pachyonychia (congenital) 757.5
  acquired 703.8
Pachyperiosteodermia
  primary or idiopathic 757.39
  secondary 731.2
Pachyperiostitis
  primary or idiopathic 757.39
  secondary 731.2
Pachyperiostosis
  primary or idiopathic 757.39
  secondary 731.2
Pacinian tumor (M9507/0) — see Neoplasm, skin, benign
Pads, knuckle or Garrod's 728.79
Paget's disease (osteitis deformans) 731.0
  with infiltrating duct carcinoma of the breast (M8541/3) — see Neoplasm, breast, malignant
  bone 731.0
    osteosarcoma in (M9184/3) — see Neoplasm, bone, malignant
  breast (M8540/3) 174.0
  extramammary (M8542/3) — see also Neoplasm, skin, malignant
    anus 154.3
    skin 173.5
  malignant (M8540/3)
    breast 174.0
    specified site NEC (M8542/3) — see Neoplasm, skin, malignant
    unspecified site 174.0
  mammary (M8540/3) 174.0
  necrosis of bone 731.0
  nipple (M8540/3) 174.0
  osteitis deformans 731.0
Paget-Schroetter syndrome (intermittent venous claudication) 453.8
Pain(s)
  abdominal 789.0 ✓5ᵗʰ
  adnexa (uteri) 625.9
  alimentary, due to vascular insufficiency 557.9
  anginoid (see also Pain, precordial) 786.51
  anus 569.42
  arch 729.5
  arm 729.5
  back (postural) 724.5
    low 724.2
    psychogenic 307.89
  bile duct 576.9
  bladder 788.9
  bone 733.90
  breast 611.71
    psychogenic 307.89
  broad ligament 625.9
  cartilage NEC 733.90
  cecum 789.0 ✓5ᵗʰ

Pain(s)

Pain(s) — continued
- cervicobrachial 723.3
- chest (central) 786.50
    - atypical 786.59
    - midsternal 786.51
    - musculoskeletal 786.59
    - noncardiac 786.59
    - substernal 786.51
    - wall (anterior) 786.52
- coccyx 724.79
- colon 789.0 ✓5ᵗʰ
- common duct 576.9
- coronary — see Angina
- costochondral 786.52
- diaphragm 786.52
- due to (presence of) any device, implant, or graft classifiable to 996.0-996.5 — see Complications, due to (presence of) any device, implant, or graft classified to 996.0-996.5 NEC
- ear (see also Otalgia) 388.70
- epigastric, epigastrium 789.0 ✓5ᵗʰ
- extremity (lower) (upper) 729.5
- eye 379.91
- face, facial 784.0
    - atypical 350.2
    - nerve 351.8
- false (labor) 644.1 ✓5ᵗʰ
- female genital organ NEC 625.9
    - psychogenic 307.89
- finger 729.5
- flank 789.0 ✓5ᵗʰ
- foot 729.5
- gallbladder 575.9
- gas (intestinal) 787.3
- gastric 536.8
- generalized 780.99 ▲
- genital organ
    - female 625.9
    - male 608.9
    - psychogenic 307.89
- groin 789.0 ✓5ᵗʰ
- growing 781.99
- hand 729.5
- head (see also Headache) 784.0
- heart (see also Pain, precordial) 786.51
- infraorbital (see also Neuralgia, trigeminal) 350.1
- intermenstrual 625.2
- jaw 526.9
- joint 719.40
    - ankle 719.47
    - elbow 719.42
    - foot 719.47
    - hand 719.44
    - hip 719.45
    - knee 719.46
    - multiple sites 719.49
    - pelvic region 719.45
    - psychogenic 307.89
    - shoulder (region) 719.41
    - specified site NEC 719.48
    - wrist 719.43
- kidney 788.0
- labor, false or spurious 644.1 ✓5ᵗʰ
- laryngeal 784.1
- leg 729.5
- limb 729.5
- low back 724.2
- lumbar region 724.2
- mastoid (see also Otalgia) 388.70
- maxilla 526.9
- metacarpophalangeal (joint) 719.44
- metatarsophalangeal (joint) 719.47
- mouth 528.9
- muscle 729.1
    - intercostal 786.59
- nasal 478.1
- nasopharynx 478.29
- neck NEC 723.1
    - psychogenic 307.89
- nerve NEC 729.2
- neuromuscular 729.1
- nose 478.1
- ocular 379.91
- ophthalmic 379.91
- orbital region 379.91
- osteocopic 733.90

Pain(s) — continued
- ovary 625.9
    - psychogenic 307.89
- over heart (see also Pain, precordial) 786.51
- ovulation 625.2
- pelvic (female) 625.9
    - male NEC 789.0 ✓5ᵗʰ
        - psychogenic 307.89
    - psychogenic 307.89
- penis 607.9
    - psychogenic 307.89
- pericardial (see also Pain, precordial) 786.51
- perineum
    - female 625.9
    - male 608.9
- pharynx 478.29
- pleura, pleural, pleuritic 786.52
- post-operative — see Pain, by site
- preauricular 388.70
- precordial (region) 786.51
    - psychogenic 307.89
- psychogenic 307.80
    - cardiovascular system 307.89
    - gastrointestinal system 307.89
    - genitourinary system 307.89
    - heart 307.89
    - musculoskeletal system 307.89
    - respiratory system 307.89
    - skin 306.3
- radicular (spinal) (see also Radiculitis) 729.2
- rectum 569.42
- respiration 786.52
- retrosternal 786.51
- rheumatic NEC 729.0
    - muscular 729.1
- rib 786.50
- root (spinal) (see also Radiculitis) 729.2
- round ligament (stretch) 625.9
- sacroiliac 724.6
- sciatic 724.3
- scrotum 608.9
    - psychogenic 307.89
- seminal vesicle 608.9
- sinus 478.1
- skin 782.0
- spermatic cord 608.9
- spinal root (see also Radiculitis) 729.2
- stomach 536.8
    - psychogenic 307.89
- substernal 786.51
- temporomandibular (joint) 524.62
- temporomaxillary joint 524.62
- testis 608.9
    - psychogenic 307.89
- thoracic spine 724.1
    - with radicular and visceral pain 724.4
- throat 784.1
- tibia 733.90
- toe 729.5
- tongue 529.6
- tooth 525.9
- trigeminal (see also Neuralgia, trigeminal) 350.1
- umbilicus 789.0 ✓5ᵗʰ
- ureter 788.0
- urinary (organ) (system) 788.0
- uterus 625.9
    - psychogenic 307.89
- vagina 625.9
- vertebrogenic (syndrome) 724.5
- vesical 788.9
- vulva 625.9
- xiphoid 733.90

Painful — see also Pain
- arc syndrome 726.19
- coitus
    - female 625.0
    - male 608.89
    - psychogenic 302.76
- ejaculation (semen) 608.89
    - psychogenic 302.79
- erection 607.3
- feet syndrome 266.2
- menstruation 625.3
    - psychogenic 306.52
- micturition 788.1
- ophthalmoplegia 378.55

Painful — see also Pain — continued
- respiration 786.52
- scar NEC 709.2
- urination 788.1
- wire sutures 998.89

Painters' colic 984.9
- specified type of lead — see Table of Drugs and Chemicals

Palate — see condition

Palatoplegia 528.9

Palatoschisis (see also Cleft, palate) 749.00

Palilalia 784.69

Palindromic arthritis (see also Rheumatism, palindromic) 719.3 ✓5ᵗʰ

Palliative care V66.7

Pallor 782.61
- temporal, optic disc 377.15

Palmar — see also condition
- fascia — see condition

Palpable
- cecum 569.89
- kidney 593.89
- liver 573.9
- lymph nodes 785.6
- ovary 620.8
- prostate 602.9
- spleen (see also Splenomegaly) 789.2
- uterus 625.8

Palpitation (heart) 785.1
- psychogenic 306.2

Palsy (see also Paralysis) 344.9
- atrophic diffuse 335.20
- Bell's 351.0
    - newborn 767.5
- birth 767.7
- brachial plexus 353.0
    - fetus or newborn 767.6
- brain — see also Palsy, cerebral
    - noncongenital or noninfantile 344.89
        - due to vascular lesion — see category 438 ✓4ᵗʰ
        - late effect — see Late effect(s) (of) cerebrovascular disease
    - syphilitic 094.89
        - congenital 090.49
- bulbar (chronic) (progressive) 335.22
    - pseudo NEC 335.23
    - supranuclear NEC 344.8 ✓5ᵗʰ
- cerebral (congenital) (infantile) (spastic) 343.9
    - athetoid 333.7
    - diplegic 343.0
        - due to previous vascular lesion — see category 438 ✓4ᵗʰ
        - late effect — see Late effect(s) (of) cerebrovascular disease
    - hemiplegic 343.1
    - monoplegic 343.3
    - noncongenital or noninfantile 437.8
        - due to previous vascular lesion — see category 438 ✓4ᵗʰ
        - late effect — see Late effect(s) (of) cerebrovascular disease
    - paraplegic 343.0
    - quadriplegic 343.2
    - spastic, not congenital or infantile 344.8 ✓5ᵗʰ
    - syphilitic 094.89
        - congenital 090.49
    - tetraplegic 343.2
- cranial nerve — see also Disorder, nerve, cranial
    - multiple 352.6
- creeping 335.21
- divers' 993.3
- Erb's (birth injury) 767.6
- facial 351.0
    - newborn 767.5
- glossopharyngeal 352.2
- Klumpke (-Déjérine) 767.6
- lead 984.9
    - specified type of lead — see Table of Drugs and Chemicals
- median nerve (tardy) 354.0
- peroneal nerve (acute) (tardy) 355.3
- progressive supranuclear 333.0
- pseudobulbar NEC 335.23

Palsy (see also Paralysis) — continued
  radial nerve (acute) 354.3
  seventh nerve 351.0
    newborn 767.5
  shaking (see also Parkinsonism) 332.0
  spastic (cerebral) (spinal) 343.9
    hemiplegic 343.1
  specified nerve NEC — see Disorder, nerve
  supranuclear NEC 356.8
    progressive 333.0
  ulnar nerve (tardy) 354.2
  wasting 335.21
Paltauf-Sternberg disease 201.9 ✓5ᵗʰ
Paludism — see Malaria
Panama fever 084.0
Panaris (with lymphangitis) 681.9
  finger 681.02
  toe 681.11
Panaritium (with lymphangitis) 681.9
  finger 681.02
  toe 681.11
Panarteritis (nodosa) 446.0
  brain or cerebral 437.4
Pancake heart 793.2
  with cor pulmonale (chronic) 416.9
Pancarditis (acute) (chronic) 429.89
  with
    rheumatic
      fever (active) (acute) (chronic) (subacute) 391.8
        inactive or quiescent 398.99
  rheumatic, acute 391.8
    chronic or inactive 398.99
Pancoast's syndrome or tumor (carcinoma, pulmonary apex) (M8010/3) 162.3
Pancoast-Tobias syndrome (M8010/3) (carcinoma, pulmonary apex) 162.3
Pancolitis 556.6
Pancreas, pancreatic — see condition
Pancreatitis 577.0
  acute (edematous) (hemorrhagic) (recurrent) 577.0
  annular 577.0
  apoplectic 577.0
  calcerous 577.0
  chronic (infectious) 577.1
    recurrent 577.1
  cystic 577.2
  fibrous 577.8
  gangrenous 577.0
  hemorrhagic (acute) 577.0
  interstitial (chronic) 577.1
    acute 577.0
  malignant 577.0
  mumps 072.3
  painless 577.1
  recurrent 577.1
  relapsing 577.1
  subacute 577.0
  suppurative 577.0
  syphilitic 095.8
Pancreatolithiasis 577.8
Pancytolysis 289.9
Pancytopenia (acquired) 284.8
  with malformations 284.0
  congenital 284.0
Panencephalitis — see also Encephalitis
  subacute, sclerosing 046.2
Panhematopenia 284.8
  congenital 284.0
  constitutional 284.0
  splenic, primary 289.4
Panhemocytopenia 284.8
  congenital 284.0
  constitutional 284.0
Panhypogonadism 257.2
Panhypopituitarism 253.2
  prepubertal 253.3
Panic (attack) (state) 300.01
  reaction to exceptional stress (transient) 308.0
Panmyelopathy, familial constitutional 284.0
Panmyelophthisis 284.9
  acquired (secondary) 284.8

Panmyelophthisis — continued
  congenital 284.0
  idiopathic 284.9
Panmyelosis (acute) (M9951/1) 238.7
Panner's disease 732.3
  capitellum humeri 732.3
  head of humerus 732.3
  tarsal navicular (bone) (osteochondrosis) 732.5
Panneuritis endemica 265.0 [357.4]
Panniculitis 729.30
  back 724.8
  knee 729.31
  neck 723.6
  nodular, nonsuppurative 729.30
  sacral 724.8
  specified site NEC 729.39
Panniculus adiposus (abdominal) 278.1
Pannus 370.62
  allergic eczematous 370.62
  degenerativus 370.62
  keratic 370.62
  rheumatoid — see Arthritis, rheumatoid
  trachomatosus, trachomatous (active) 076.1 [370.62]
    late effect 139.1
Panophthalmitis 360.02
Panotitis — see Otitis media
Pansinusitis (chronic) (hyperplastic) (nonpurulent) (purulent) 473.8
  acute 461.8
  due to fungus NEC 117.9
  tuberculous (see also Tuberculosis) 012.8 ✓5ᵗʰ
Panuveitis 360.12
  sympathetic 360.11
Panvalvular disease — see Endocarditis, mitral
Papageienkrankheit 073.9
Papanicolaou smear
  cervix (screening test) V76.2
    as part of gynecological examination V72.3
    for suspected malignant neoplasm V76.2
      no disease found V71.1
    nonspecific abnormal finding 795.00 ▲
      atypical squamous cell changes of undetermined significance ●
        favor benign (ASCUS favor benign) 795.01 ●
        favor dysplasia (ASCUS favor dysplasia) 795.02 ●
      nonspecific finding NEC 795.09 ●
      unsatisfactory 795.09 ●
  other specified site — see also Screening, malignant neoplasm
    for suspected malignant neoplasm — see also Screening, malignant neoplasm
      no disease found V71.1
    nonspecific abnormal finding 795.1
  vagina V76.47
    following hysterectomy for malignant condition V67.01
Papilledema 377.00
  associated with
    decreased ocular pressure 377.02
    increased intracranial pressure 377.01
    retinal disorder 377.03
  choked disc 377.00
  infectional 377.00
Papillitis 377.31
  anus 569.49
  chronic lingual 529.4
  necrotizing, kidney 584.7
  optic 377.31
  rectum 569.49
  renal, necrotizing 584.7
  tongue 529.0
Papilloma (M8050/0) — see also Neoplasm, by site, benign

Note — Except where otherwise indicated, the morphological varieties of papilloma in the list below should be coded by site as for "Neoplasm, benign."

  acuminatum (female) (male) 078.1 ✓5ᵗʰ

Papilloma (M8050/0) — see also Neoplasm, by site, benign — continued
  bladder (urinary) (transitional cell) (M8120/1) 236.7
    benign (M8120/0) 223.3
  choroid plexus (M9390/0) 225.0
    anaplastic type (M9390/3) 191.5
    malignant (M9390/3) 191.5
  ductal (M8503/0)
  dyskeratotic (M8052/0)
  epidermoid (M8052/0)
  hyperkeratotic (M8052/0)
  intracystic (M8504/0)
  intraductal (M8503/0)
  inverted (M8053/0)
  keratotic (M8052/0)
  parakeratotic (M8052/0)
  pinta (primary) 103.0
  renal pelvis (transitional cell) (M8120/1) 236.99
    benign (M8120/0) 223.1
  Schneiderian (M8121/0)
    specified site — see Neoplasm, by site, benign
    unspecified site 212.0
  serous surface (M8461/0)
    borderline malignancy (M8461/1)
      specified site — see Neoplasm, by site, uncertain behavior
      unspecified site 236.2
    specified site — see Neoplasm, by site, benign
    unspecified site 220
  squamous (cell) (M8052/0)
  transitional (cell) (M8120/0)
    bladder (urinary) (M8120/1) 236.7
    inverted type (M8121/1) — see Neoplasm, by site, uncertain behavior
    renal pelvis (M8120/1) 236.91
    ureter (M8120/1) 236.91
  ureter (transitional cell) (M8120/1) 236.91
    benign (M8120/0) 223.2
  urothelial (M8120/1) — see Neoplasm, by site, uncertain behavior
  verrucous (M8051/0)
  villous (M8261/1) — see Neoplasm, by site, uncertain behavior
  yaws, plantar or palmar 102.1
Papillomata, multiple, of yaws 102.1
Papillomatosis (M8060/0) — see also Neoplasm, by site, benign
  confluent and reticulate 701.8
  cutaneous 701.8
  ductal, breast 610.1
  Gougerot-Carteaud (confluent reticulate) 701.8
  intraductal (diffuse) (M8505/0) — see Neoplasm, by site, benign
  subareolar duct (M8506/0) 217
Papillon-Léage and Psaume syndrome (orodigitofacial dysostosis) 759.89
Papule 709.8
  carate (primary) 103.0
  fibrous, of nose (M8724/0) 216.3
  pinta (primary) 103.0
Papulosis, malignant 447.8
Papyraceous fetus 779.89 ▲
  complicating pregnancy 646.0 ✓5ᵗʰ
Paracephalus 759.7
Parachute mitral valve 746.5
Paracoccidioidomycosis 116.1
  mucocutaneous-lymphangitic 116.1
  pulmonary 116.1
  visceral 116.1
Paracoccidiomycosis — see Paracoccidioidomycosis
Paracusis 388.40
Paradentosis 523.5
Paradoxical facial movements 374.43
Paraffinoma 999.9
Paraganglioma (M8680/1)
  adrenal (M8700/0) 227.0
    malignant (M8700/3) 194.0
  aortic body (M8691/1) 237.3
    malignant (M8691/3) 194.6
  carotid body (M8692/1) 237.3
    malignant (M8692/3) 194.5

Paraganglioma — *continued*
   chromaffin (M8700/0) — *see also* Neoplasm, by site, benign
      malignant (M8700/3) — *see* Neoplasm, by site, malignant
   extra-adrenal (M8693/1)
      malignant (M8693/3)
         specified site — *see* Neoplasm, by site, malignant
         unspecified site 194.6
      specified site — *see* Neoplasm, by site, uncertain behavior
      unspecified site 237.3
   glomus jugulare (M8690/1) 237.3
      malignant (M8690/3) 194.6
   jugular (M8690/1) 237.3
      malignant (M8680/3)
         specified site — *see* Neoplasm, by site, malignant
         unspecified site 194.6
   nonchromaffin (M8693/1)
      malignant (M8693/3)
         specified site — *see* Neoplasm, by site, malignant
         unspecified site 194.6
      specified site — *see* Neoplasm, by site, uncertain behavior
      unspecified site 237.3
   parasympathetic (M8682/1)
      specified site — *see* Neoplasm, by site, uncertain behavior
      unspecified site 237.3
   specified site — *see* Neoplasm, by site, uncertain behavior
   sympathetic (M8681/1)
      specified site — *see* Neoplasm, by site, uncertain behavior
      unspecified site 237.3
   unspecified site 237.3

Parageusia 781.1
   psychogenic 306.7

Paragonimiasis 121.2

Paragranuloma, Hodgkin's (M9660/3) 201.0 ✓5ᵗʰ

Parahemophilia (*see also* Defect, coagulation) 286.3

Parakeratosis 690.8
   psoriasiformis 696.2
   variegata 696.2

Paralysis, paralytic (complete) (incomplete) 344.9
   with
      broken
         back — *see* Fracture, vertebra, by site, with spinal cord injury
         neck — *see* Fracture, vertebra, cervical, with spinal cord injury
      fracture, vertebra — *see* Fracture, vertebra, by site, with spinal cord injury
      syphilis 094.89
   abdomen and back muscles 355.9
   abdominal muscles 355.9
   abducens (nerve) 378.54
   abductor 355.9
      lower extremity 355.8
      upper extremity 354.9
   accessory nerve 352.4
   accommodation 367.51
      hysterical 300.11
   acoustic nerve 388.5
   agitans 332.0
      arteriosclerotic 332.0
   alternating 344.89
      oculomotor 344.89
   amyotrophic 335.20
   ankle 355.8
   anterior serratus 355.9
   anus (sphincter) 569.49
   apoplectic (current episode) (*see also* Disease, cerebrovascular, acute) 436
      late effect — *see* Late effect(s) (of) cerebrovascular disease
   arm 344.40
      affecting
         dominant side 344.41
         nondominant side 344.42
      both 344.2
      due to old CVA — *see* category 438 ✓4ᵗʰ

Paralysis, paralytic — *continued*
   arm — *continued*
      hysterical 300.11
      late effect — *see* Late effect(s) (of) cerebrovascular disease
      psychogenic 306.0 transient 781.4
         traumatic NEC (*see also* Injury, nerve, upper limb) 955.9
   arteriosclerotic (current episode) 437.0
      late effect — *see* Late effect(s) (of) cerebrovascular disease
   ascending (spinal), acute 357.0
   associated, nuclear 344.89
   asthenic bulbar 358.0
   ataxic NEC 334.9
      general 094.1
   athetoid 333.7
   atrophic 356.9
      infantile, acute (*see also* Poliomyelitis, with paralysis) 045.1 ✓5ᵗʰ
      muscle NEC 355.9
      progressive 335.21
      spinal (acute) (*see also* Poliomyelitis, with paralysis) 045.1 ✓5ᵗʰ
   attack (*see also* Disease, cerebrovascular, acute) 436
   axillary 353.0
   Babinski-Nageotte's 344.89
   Bell's 351.0
      newborn 767.5
   Benedikt's 344.89
   birth (injury) 767.7
      brain 767.0
      intracranial 767.0
      spinal cord 767.4
   bladder (sphincter) 596.53
      neurogenic 596.54
         with cauda equina syndrome 344.61
      puerperal, postpartum, childbirth 665.5 ✓5ᵗʰ
      sensory 344.61
         with cauda equina 344.61
      spastic 344.61
         with cauda equina 344.61
   bowel, colon, or intestine (*see also* Ileus) 560.1
   brachial plexus 353.0
      due to birth injury 767.6
      newborn 767.6
   brain
      congenital — *see* Palsy, cerebral
      current episode 437.8
      diplegia 344.2
      due to previous vascular lesion — *see* category 438 ✓4ᵗʰ
      hemiplegia 342.9
         due to previous vascular lesion — *see* category 438 ✓4ᵗʰ
         late effect — *see* Late effect(s) (of) cerebrovascular disease
      infantile — *see* Palsy, cerebral
      late effect — *see* Late effect(s) (of) cerebrovascular disease
      monoplegia — *see also* Monoplegia
         due to previous vascular lesion — *see* category 438 ✓4ᵗʰ
         late effect — *see* Late effect(s) (of) cerebrovascular disease
      paraplegia 344.1
      quadriplegia — *see* Quadriplegia
      syphilitic, congenital 090.49
      triplegia 344.89
   bronchi 519.1
   Brown-Séquard's 344.89
   bulbar (chronic) (progressive) 335.22
      infantile (*see also* Poliomyelitis, bulbar) 045.0 ✓5ᵗʰ
      poliomyelitic (*see also* Poliomyelitis, bulbar) 045.0 ✓5ᵗʰ
      pseudo 335.23
      supranuclear 344.89
   bulbospinal 358.0
   cardiac (*see also* Failure, heart) 428.9
   cerebral
      current episode 437.8
      spastic, infantile — *see* Palsy, cerebral
   cerebrocerebellar 437.8
      diplegic infantile 343.0

Paralysis, paralytic — *continued*
   cervical
      plexus 353.2
      sympathetic NEC 337.0
   Céstan-Chenais 344.89
   Charcôt-Marie-Tooth type 356.1
   childhood — *see* Palsy, cerebral
   Clark's 343.9
   colon (*see also* Ileus) 560.1
   compressed air 993.3
   compression
      arm NEC 354.9
      cerebral — *see* Paralysis, brain
      leg NEC 355.8
      lower extremity NEC 355.8
      upper extremity NEC 354.9
   congenital (cerebral) (spastic) (spinal) — *see* Palsy, cerebral
   conjugate movement (of eye) 378.81
      cortical (nuclear) (supranuclear) 378.81
   convergence 378.83
   cordis (*see also* Failure, heart) 428.9
   cortical (*see also* Paralysis, brain) 437.8
   cranial or cerebral nerve (*see also* Disorder, nerve, cranial) 352.9
   creeping 335.21
   crossed leg 344.89
   crutch 953.4
   deglutition 784.9
      hysterical 300.11
   dementia 094.1
   descending (spinal) NEC 335.9
   diaphragm (flaccid) 519.4
      due to accidental section of phrenic nerve during procedure 998.2
   digestive organs NEC 564.89
   diplegic — *see* Diplegia
   divergence (nuclear) 378.85
   divers' 993.3
   Duchenne's 335.22
   due to intracranial or spinal birth injury — *see* Palsy, cerebral
   embolic (current episode) (*see also* Embolism, brain) 434.1 ✓5ᵗʰ
      late effect — *see* Late effect(s) (of) cerebrovascular disease
   enteric (*see also* Ileus) 560.1
      with hernia — *see* Hernia, by site, with obstruction
   Erb's syphilitic spastic spinal 094.89
   Erb (-Duchenne) (birth) (newborn) 767.6
   esophagus 530.8 ✓5ᵗʰ
   essential, infancy (*see also* Poliomyelitis) 045.9 ✓5ᵗʰ
   extremity
      lower — *see* Paralysis, leg
      spastic (hereditary) 343.3
         noncongenital or noninfantile 344.1
      transient (cause unknown) 781.4
      upper — *see* Paralysis, arm
   eye muscle (extrinsic) 378.55
      intrinsic 367.51
   facial (nerve) 351.0
      birth injury 767.5
      congenital 767.5
      following operation NEC 998.2
      newborn 767.5
   familial 359.3
      periodic 359.3
      spastic 334.1
   fauces 478.29
   finger NEC 354.9
   foot NEC 355.8
   gait 781.2
   gastric nerve 352.3
   gaze 378.81
   general 094.1
      ataxic 094.1
      insane 094.1
      juvenile 090.40
      progressive 094.1
      tabetic 094.1
   glossopharyngeal (nerve) 352.2
   glottis (*see also* Paralysis, vocal cord) 478.30
   gluteal 353.4
   Gubler (-Millard) 344.89
   hand 354.9
      hysterical 300.11

Paralysis, paralytic — continued
  hand — continued
    psychogenic 306.0
  heart (see also Failure, heart) 428.9
  hemifacial, progressive 349.89
  hemiplegic — see Hemiplegia
  hyperkalemic periodic (familial) 359.3
  hypertensive (current episode) 437.8
  hypoglossal (nerve) 352.5
  hypokalemic periodic 359.3
  Hyrtl's sphincter (rectum) 569.49
  hysterical 300.11
  ileus (see also Ileus) 560.1
  infantile (see also Poliomyelitis) 045.9 ✓5ᵗʰ
    atrophic acute 045.1 ✓5ᵗʰ
    bulbar 045.0 ✓5ᵗʰ
    cerebral — see Palsy, cerebral
    paralytic 045.1 ✓5ᵗʰ
    progressive acute 045.9 ✓5ᵗʰ
    spastic — see Palsy, cerebral
    spinal 045.9 ✓5ᵗʰ
  infective (see also Poliomyelitis) 045.9 ✓5ᵗʰ
  inferior nuclear 344.9
  insane, general or progressive 094.1
  internuclear 378.86
  interosseous 355.9
  intestine (see also Ileus) 560.1
  intracranial (current episode) (see also Paralysis, brain) 437.8
    due to birth injury 767.0
  iris 379.49
    due to diphtheria (toxin) 032.81 [379.49]
  ischemic, Volkmann's (complicating trauma) 958.6
  Jackson's 344.8 ✓5ᵗʰ
  jake 357.7
  Jamaica ginger (jake) 357.7
  juvenile general 090.40
  Klumpke (-Déjérine) (birth) (newborn) 767.6
  labioglossal (laryngeal) (pharyngeal) 335.22
  Landry's 357.0
  laryngeal nerve (recurrent) (superior) (see also Paralysis, vocal cord) 478.30
  larynx (see also Paralysis, vocal cord) 478.30
    due to diphtheria (toxin) 032.3
  late effect
    due to
      birth injury, brain or spinal (cord) — see Palsy, cerebral
      edema, brain or cerebral — see Paralysis, brain
    lesion
      cerebrovascular — see category 438 ✓4ᵗʰ
        late effect — see Late effect(s) (of) cerebrovascular disease
      spinal (cord) — see Paralysis, spinal
  lateral 335.24
  lead 984.9
    specified type of lead — see Table of Drugs and Chemicals
  left side — see Hemiplegia
  leg 344.30
    affecting
      dominant side 344.31
      nondominant side 344.32
    both (see also Paraplegia) 344.1
    crossed 344.89
    hysterical 300.11
    psychogenic 306.0
    transient or transitory 781.4
      traumatic NEC (see also Injury, nerve, lower limb) 956.9
  levator palpebrae superioris 374.31
  limb NEC 344.5
    all four — see Quadriplegia
    quadriplegia — see Quadriplegia
  lip 528.5
  Lissauer's 094.1
  local 355.9
  lower limb — see also Paralysis, leg
    both (see also Paraplegia) 344.1
  lung 518.89
    newborn 770.89
  median nerve 354.1
  medullary (tegmental) 344.89

Paralysis, paralytic — continued
  mesencephalic NEC 344.89
    tegmental 344.89
  middle alternating 344.89
  Millard-Gubler-Foville 344.89
  monoplegic — see Monoplegia
  motor NEC 344.9
    cerebral — see Paralysis, brain
    spinal — see Paralysis, spinal
  multiple
    cerebral — see Paralysis, brain
    spinal — see Paralysis, spinal
  muscle (flaccid) 359.9
    due to nerve lesion NEC 355.9
    eye (extrinsic) 378.55
      intrinsic 367.51
      oblique 378.51
    iris sphincter 364.8
    ischemic (complicating trauma) (Volkmann's) 958.6
    pseudohypertrophic 359.1
  muscular (atrophic) 359.9
    progressive 335.21
  musculocutaneous nerve 354.9
  musculospiral 354.9
  nerve — see also Disorder, nerve
    third or oculomotor (partial) 378.51
      total 378.52
    fourth or trochlear 378.53
    sixth or abducens 378.54
    seventh or facial 351.0
      birth injury 767.5
      due to
        injection NEC 999.9
        operation NEC 997.09
      newborn 767.5
    accessory 352.4
    auditory 388.5
    birth injury 767.7
    cranial or cerebral (see also Disorder, nerve, cranial) 352.9
    facial 351.0
      birth injury 767.5
      newborn 767.5
    laryngeal (see also Paralysis, vocal cord) 478.30
      newborn 767.7
    phrenic 354.8
      newborn 767.7
    radial 354.3
      birth injury 767.6
      newborn 767.6
    syphilitic 094.89
    traumatic NEC (see also Injury, nerve, by site) 957.9
    trigeminal 350.9
    ulnar 354.2
  newborn NEC 767.0
  normokalemic periodic 359.3
  obstetrical, newborn 767.7
  ocular 378.9
  oculofacial, congenital 352.6
  oculomotor (nerve) (partial) 378.51
    alternating 344.89
    external bilateral 378.55
    total 378.52
  olfactory nerve 352.0
  palate 528.9
  palatopharyngolaryngeal 352.6
  paratrigeminal 350.9
  periodic (familial) (hyperkalemic) (hypokalemic) (normokalemic) (secondary) 359.3
  peripheral
    autonomic nervous system — see Neuropathy, peripheral, autonomic
    nerve NEC 355.9
  peroneal (nerve) 355.3
  pharynx 478.29
  phrenic nerve 354.8
  plantar nerves 355.6
  pneumogastric nerve 352.3
  poliomyelitis (current) (see also Poliomyelitis, with paralysis) 045.1 ✓5ᵗʰ
    bulbar 045.0 ✓5ᵗʰ
  popliteal nerve 355.3
  pressure (see also Neuropathy, entrapment) 355.9

Paralysis, paralytic — continued
  progressive 335.21
    atrophic 335.21
    bulbar 335.22
    general 094.1
    hemifacial 349.89
    infantile, acute (see also Poliomyelitis) 045.9 ✓5ᵗʰ
    multiple 335.20
  pseudobulbar 335.23
  pseudohypertrophic 359.1
    muscle 359.1
  psychogenic 306.0
  pupil, pupillary 379.49
  quadriceps 355.8
  quadriplegic (see also Quadriplegia) 344.0
  radial nerve 354.3
    birth injury 767.6
  rectum (sphincter) 569.49
  rectus muscle (eye) 378.55
  recurrent laryngeal nerve (see also Paralysis, vocal cord) 478.30
  respiratory (muscle) (system) (tract) 786.09
    center NEC 344.89
      fetus or newborn 770.89 ▲
    congenital 768.9
    newborn 768.9
  right side — see Hemiplegia
  Saturday night 354.3
  saturnine 984.9
    specified type of lead — see Table of Drugs and Chemicals
  sciatic nerve 355.0
  secondary — see Paralysis, late effect
  seizure (cerebral) (current episode) (see also Disease, cerebrovascular, acute) 436
    late effect — see Late effect(s) (of) cerebrovascular disease
  senile NEC 344.9
  serratus magnus 355.9
  shaking (see also Parkinsonism) 332.0
  shock (see also Disease, cerebrovascular, acute) 436
    late effect — see Late effect(s) (of) cerebrovascular disease
  shoulder 354.9
  soft palate 528.9
  spasmodic — see Paralysis, spastic
  spastic 344.9
    cerebral infantile — see Palsy, cerebral
    congenital (cerebral) — see Palsy, cerebral
    familial 334.1
    hereditary 334.1
    infantile 343.9
    noncongenital or noninfantile, cerebral 344.9
    syphilitic 094.0
      spinal 094.89
  sphincter, bladder (see also Paralysis, bladder) 596.53
  spinal (cord) NEC 344.1
    accessory nerve 352.4
    acute (see also Poliomyelitis) 045.9 ✓5ᵗʰ
    ascending acute 357.0
    atrophic (acute) (see also Poliomyelitis, with paralysis) 045.1 ✓5ᵗʰ
      spastic, syphilitic 094.89
    congenital NEC 343.9
    hemiplegic — see Hemiplegia
    hereditary 336.8
    infantile (see also Poliomyelitis) 045.9 ✓5ᵗʰ
    late effect NEC 344.89
    monoplegic — see Monoplegia
    nerve 355.9
    progressive 335.10
    quadriplegic — see Quadriplegia
    spastic NEC 343.9
    traumatic — see Injury, spinal, by site
  sternomastoid 352.4
  stomach 536.3
    nerve 352.3
  stroke (current episode) (see also Disease, cerebrovascular, acute) 436
    late effect — see Late effect(s) (of) cerebrovascular disease
  subscapularis 354.8
  superior nuclear NEC 334.9

Paralysis, paralytic — *continued*
- supranuclear 356.8
- sympathetic
  - cervical NEC 337.0
  - nerve NEC (*see also* Neuropathy, peripheral, autonomic) 337.9
  - nervous system — *see* Neuropathy, peripheral, autonomic
- syndrome 344.9
  - specified NEC 344.89
- syphilitic spastic spinal (Erb's) 094.89
- tabetic general 094.1
- thigh 355.8
- throat 478.29
  - diphtheritic 032.0
  - muscle 478.29
- thrombotic (current episode) (*see also* Thrombosis, brain) 434.0 ✓5ᵗʰ
  - late effect — *see* Late effect(s) (of) cerebrovascular disease
  - old — *see* category 438 ✓4ᵗʰ
- thumb NEC 354.9
- tick (-bite) 989.5
- Todd's (postepileptic transitory paralysis) 344.89
- toe 355.6
- tongue 529.8
- transient
  - arm or leg NEC 781.4
  - traumatic NEC (*see also* Injury, nerve, by site) 957.9
- trapezius 352.4
- traumatic, transient NEC (*see also* Injury, nerve, by site) 957.9
- trembling (*see also* Parkinsonism) 332.0
- triceps brachii 354.9
- trigeminal nerve 350.9
- trochlear nerve 378.53
- ulnar nerve 354.2
- upper limb — *see also* Paralysis, arm
  - both (*see also* Diplegia) 344.2
- uremic — *see* Uremia
- uveoparotitic 135
- uvula 528.9
  - hysterical 300.11
  - postdiphtheritic 032.0
- vagus nerve 352.3
- vasomotor NEC 337.9
- velum palati 528.9
- vesical (*see also* Paralysis, bladder) 596.53
- vestibular nerve 388.5
- visual field, psychic 368.16
- vocal cord 478.30
  - bilateral (partial) 478.33
    - complete 478.34
  - complete (bilateral) 478.34
  - unilateral (partial) 478.31
    - complete 478.32
- Volkmann's (complicating trauma) 958.6
- wasting 335.21
- Weber's 344.89
- wrist NEC 354.9

Paramedial orifice, urethrovesical 753.8
Paramenia 626.9
Parametritis (chronic) (*see also* Disease, pelvis, inflammatory) 614.4
- acute 614.3
- puerperal, postpartum, childbirth 670 ✓4ᵗʰ

Parametrium, parametric — *see* condition
Paramnesia (*see also* Amnesia) 780.99 ▲
Paramolar 520.1
- causing crowding 524.3

Paramyloidosis 277.3
Paramyoclonus multiplex 333.2
Paramyotonia 359.2
- congenita 359.2

Paraneoplastic syndrome — *see* condition
Parangi (*see also* Yaws) 102.9
Paranoia 297.1
- alcoholic 291.5
- querulans 297.8
- senile 290.20

Paranoid
- dementia (*see also* Schizophrenia) 295.3 ✓5ᵗʰ
  - praecox (acute) 295.3 ✓5ᵗʰ
  - senile 290.20

Paranoid — *continued*
- personality 301.0
- psychosis 297.9
  - alcoholic 291.5
  - climacteric 297.2
  - drug-induced 292.11
  - involutional 297.2
  - menopausal 297.2
  - protracted reactive 298.4
  - psychogenic 298.4
    - acute 298.3
  - senile 290.20
- reaction (chronic) 297.9
  - acute 298.3
- schizophrenia (acute) (*see also* Schizophrenia) 295.3 ✓5ᵗʰ
- state 297.9
  - alcohol-induced 291.5
  - climacteric 297.2
  - drug-induced 292.11
  - due to or associated with
    - arteriosclerosis (cerebrovascular) 290.42
    - presenile brain disease 290.12
    - senile brain disease 290.20
  - involutional 297.2
  - menopausal 297.2
  - senile 290.20
  - simple 297.0
  - specified type NEC 297.8
- tendencies 301.0
- traits 301.0
- trends 301.0
- type, psychopathic personality 301.0

Paraparesis (*see also* Paralysis) 344.9
Paraphasia 784.3
Paraphilia (*see also* Deviation, sexual) 302.9
Paraphimosis (congenital) 605
- chancroidal 099.0

Paraphrenia, paraphrenic (late) 297.2
- climacteric 297.2
- dementia (*see also* Schizophrenia) 295.3 ✓5ᵗʰ
- involutional 297.2
- menopausal 297.2
- schizophrenia (acute) (*see also* Schizophrenia) 295.3 ✓5ᵗʰ

Paraplegia 344.1
- with
  - broken back — *see* Fracture, vertebra, by site, with spinal cord injury
  - fracture, vertebra — *see* Fracture, vertebra, by site, with spinal cord injury
- ataxic — *see* Degeneration, combined, spinal cord
- brain (current episode) (*see also* Paralysis, brain) 437.8
- cerebral (current episode) (*see also* Paralysis, brain) 437.8
- congenital or infantile (cerebral) (spastic) (spinal) 343.0
- cortical — *see* Paralysis, brain
- familial spastic 334.1
- functional (hysterical) 300.11
- hysterical 300.11
- infantile 343.0
- late effect 344.1
- Pott's (*see also* Tuberculosis) 015.0 ✓5ᵗʰ [730.88]
- psychogenic 306.0
- spastic
  - Erb's spinal 094.89
  - hereditary 334.1
  - not infantile or congenital 344.1
- spinal (cord)
  - traumatic NEC — *see* Injury, spinal, by site
- syphilitic (spastic) 094.89
- traumatic NEC — *see* Injury, spinal, by site

Paraproteinemia 273.2
- benign (familial) 273.1
- monoclonal 273.1
- secondary to malignant or inflammatory disease 273.1

Parapsoriasis 696.2
- en plaques 696.2
- guttata 696.2

Parapsoriasis — *continued*
- lichenoides chronica 696.2
- retiformis 696.2
- varioliformis (acuta) 696.2

Parascarlatina 057.8
Parasitic — *see also* condition
- disease NEC (*see also* Infestation, parasitic) 136.9
  - contact V01.89 ▲
  - exposure to V01.89 ▲
  - intestinal NEC 129
  - skin NEC 134.9
- stomatitis 112.0
- sycosis 110.0
  - beard 110.0
  - scalp 110.0
- twin 759.4

Parasitism NEC 136.9
- intestinal NEC 129
- skin NEC 134.9
- specified — *see* Infestation

Parasitophobia 300.29
Parasomnia 780.59
- nonorganic origin 307.47

Paraspadias 752.69
Paraspasm facialis 351.8
Parathyroid gland — *see* condition
Parathyroiditis (autoimmune) 252.1
Parathyroprival tetany 252.1
Paratrachoma 077.0
Paratyphilitis (*see also* Appendicitis) 541
Paratyphoid (fever) — *see* Fever, paratyphoid
Paratyphus — *see* Fever, paratyphoid
Paraurethral duct 753.8
Para-urethritis 597.89
- gonococcal (acute) 098.0
  - chronic or duration of 2 months or over 098.2

Paravaccinia NEC 051.9
- milkers' node 051.1

Paravaginitis (*see also* Vaginitis) 616.10
Parencephalitis (*see also* Encephalitis) 323.9
- late effect — *see* category 326

Parergasia 298.9
Paresis (*see also* Paralysis) 344.9
- accommodation 367.51
- bladder (spastic) (sphincter) (*see also* Paralysis, bladder) 596.53
  - tabetic 094.0
- bowel, colon, or intestine (*see also* Ileus) 560.1
- brain or cerebral — *see* Paralysis, brain
- extrinsic muscle, eye 378.55
- general 094.1
  - arrested 094.1
  - brain 094.1
  - cerebral 094.1
  - insane 094.1
  - juvenile 090.40
    - remission 090.49
  - progressive 094.1
  - remission (sustained) 094.1
  - tabetic 094.1
- heart (*see also* Failure, heart) 428.9
- infantile (*see also* Poliomyelitis) 045.9 ✓5ᵗʰ
- insane 094.1
- juvenile 090.40
- late effect — *see* Paralysis, late effect
- luetic (general) 094.1
- peripheral progressive 356.9
- pseudohypertrophic 359.1
- senile NEC 344.9
- stomach 536.3
- syphilitic (general) 094.1
  - congenital 090.40
- transient, limb 781.4
- vesical (sphincter) NEC 596.53

Paresthesia (*see also* Disturbance, sensation) 782.0
- Berger's (paresthesia of lower limb) 782.0
- Bernhardt 355.1
- Magnan's 782.0

Paretic — *see* condition

Index to Diseases

Parinaud's
  conjunctivitis 372.02
  oculoglandular syndrome 372.02
  ophthalmoplegia 378.81
  syndrome (paralysis of conjugate upward gaze) 378.81
Parkes Weber and Dimitri syndrome (encephalocutaneous angiomatosis) 759.6
Parkinson's disease, syndrome, or tremor — see Parkinsonism
Parkinsonism (arteriosclerotic) (idiopathic) (primary) 332.0
  associated with orthostatic hypotension (idiopathic) (symptomatic) 333.0
  due to drugs 332.1
  secondary 332.1
  syphilitic 094.82
Parodontitis 523.4
Parodontosis 523.5
Paronychia (with lymphangitis) 681.9
  candidal (chronic) 112.3
  chronic 681.9
    candidal 112.3
    finger 681.02
    toe 681.11
  finger 681.02
  toe 681.11
  tuberculous (primary) (see also Tuberculosis) 017.0
Parorexia NEC 307.52
  hysterical 300.11
Parosmia 781.1
  psychogenic 306.7
Parotid gland — see condition
Parotiditis (see also Parotitis) 527.2
  epidemic 072.9
  infectious 072.9
Parotitis 527.2
  allergic 527.2
  chronic 527.2
  epidemic (see also Mumps) 072.9
  infectious (see also Mumps) 072.9
  noninfectious 527.2
  nonspecific toxic 527.2
  not mumps 527.2
  postoperative 527.2
  purulent 527.2
  septic 527.2
  suppurative (acute) 527.2
  surgical 527.2
  toxic 527.2
Paroxysmal — see also condition
  dyspnea (nocturnal) 786.09
Parrot's disease (syphilitic osteochondritis) 090.0
Parrot fever 073.9
Parry's disease or syndrome (exophthalmic goiter) 242.0
Parry-Romberg syndrome 349.89
Parson's disease (exophthalmic goiter) 242.0
Parsonage-Aldren-Turner syndrome 353.5
Parsonage-Turner syndrome 353.5
Pars planitis 363.21
Particolored infant 757.39
Parturition — see Delivery
Passage
  false, urethra 599.4
  of sounds or bougies (see also Attention to artificial opening) V55.9
Passive — see condition
Pasteurella septica 027.2
Pasteurellosis (see also Infection, Pasteurella) 027.2
PAT (paroxysmal atrial tachycardia) 427.0
Patau's syndrome (trisomy D) 758.1
Patch
  herald 696.3
Patches
  mucous (syphilitic) 091.3
    congenital 090.0
  smokers' (mouth) 528.6
Patellar — see condition

Patellofemoral syndrome 719.46
Patent — see also Imperfect closure
  atrioventricular ostium 745.69
  canal of Nuck 752.41
  cervix 622.5
    complicating pregnancy 654.5
      affecting fetus or newborn 761.0
  ductus arteriosus or Botalli 747.0
  Eustachian
    tube 381.7
    valve 746.89
  foramen
    Botalli 745.5
    ovale 745.5
  interauricular septum 745.5
  interventricular septum 745.4
  omphalomesenteric duct 751.0
  os (uteri) — see Patent, cervix
  ostium secundum 745.5
  urachus 753.7
  vitelline duct 751.0
Paternity testing V70.4
Paterson's syndrome (sideropenic dysphagia) 280.8
Paterson (-Brown) (-Kelly) syndrome (sideropenic dysphagia) 280.8
Paterson-Kelly syndrome or web (sideropenic dysphagia) 280.8
Pathologic, pathological — see also condition
  asphyxia 799.0
  drunkenness 291.4
  emotionality 301.3
  liar 301.7
  personality 301.9
  resorption, tooth 521.4
  sexuality (see also Deviation, sexual) 302.9
Pathology (of) — see Disease
Patterned motor discharge, idiopathic (see also Epilepsy) 345.5
Patulous — see also Patent
  anus 569.49
  Eustachian tube 381.7
Pause, sinoatrial 427.81
Pavor nocturnus 307.46
Pavy's disease 593.6
Paxton's disease (white piedra) 111.2
Payr's disease or syndrome (splenic flexure syndrome) 569.89
Pearls
  Elschnig 366.51
  enamel 520.2
Pearl-workers' disease (chronic osteomyelitis) (see also Osteomyelitis) 730.1
Pectenitis 569.49
Pectenosis 569.49
Pectoral — see condition
Pectus
  carinatum (congenital) 754.82
    acquired 738.3
    rachitic (see also Rickets) 268.0
  excavatum (congenital) 754.81
    acquired 738.3
    rachitic (see also Rickets) 268.0
  recurvatum (congenital) 754.81
    acquired 738.3
Pedatrophia 261
Pederosis 302.2
Pediculosis (infestation) 132.9
  capitis (head louse) 132.0
  corporis (body louse) (any site) 132.1
  eyelid 132.0 [373.6]
  mixed (classifiable to more than one category in 132.0-132.2) 132.3
  pubis (pubic louse) (any site) 132.2
  vestimenti 132.1
  vulvae 132.2
Pediculus (infestation) — see Pediculosis
Pedophilia 302.2
Peg-shaped teeth 520.2
Pel's crisis 094.0
Pel-Ebstein disease — see Disease, Hodgkin's
Pelade 704.01

Penetration, pregnant uterus by instrument

Pelger-Huât anomaly or syndrome (hereditary hyposegmentation) 288.2
Peliosis (rheumatica) 287.0
Pelizaeus-Merzbacher
  disease 330.0
  sclerosis, diffuse cerebral 330.0
Pellagra (alcoholic or with alcoholism) 265.2
  with polyneuropathy 265.2 [357.4]
Pellagra-cerebellar-ataxia-renal aminoaciduria syndrome 270.0
Pellegrini's disease (calcification, knee joint) 726.62
Pellegrini (-Stieda) disease or syndrome (calcification, knee joint) 726.62
Pellizzi's syndrome (pineal) 259.8
Pelvic — see also condition
  congestion-fibrosis syndrome 625.5
  kidney 753.3
Pelvioectasis 591
Pelviolithiasis 592.0
Pelviperitonitis
  female (see also Peritonitis, pelvic, female) 614.5
  male (see also Peritonitis) 567.2
Pelvis, pelvic — see also condition or type
  infantile 738.6
  Nägele's 738.6
  obliquity 738.6
  Robert's 755.69
Pemphigoid 694.5
  benign, mucous membrane 694.60
    with ocular involvement 694.61
  bullous 694.5
  cicatricial 694.60
    with ocular involvement 694.61
  juvenile 694.2
Pemphigus 694.4
  benign 694.5
    chronic familial 757.39
  Brazilian 694.4
  circinatus 694.0
  congenital, traumatic 757.39
  conjunctiva 694.61
  contagiosus 684
  erythematodes 694.4
  erythematosus 694.4
  foliaceus 694.4
  frambesiodes 694.4
  gangrenous (see also Gangrene) 785.4
  malignant 694.4
  neonatorum, newborn 684
  ocular 694.61
  papillaris 694.4
  seborrheic 694.4
  South American 694.4
  syphilitic (congenital) 090.0
  vegetans 694.4
  vulgaris 694.4
  wildfire 694.4
Pendred's syndrome (familial goiter with deafmutism) 243
Pendulous
  abdomen 701.9
    in pregnancy or childbirth 654.4
      affecting fetus or newborn 763.89
  breast 611.8
Penetrating wound — see also Wound, open, by site
  with internal injury — see Injury, internal, by site, with open wound
  eyeball 871.7
    with foreign body (nonmagnetic) 871.6
      magnetic 871.5
  ocular (see also Penetrating wound, eyeball) 871.7
    adnexa 870.3
      with foreign body 870.4
    orbit 870.3
      with foreign body 870.4
Penetration, pregnant uterus by instrument
  with
    abortion — see Abortion, by type, with damage to pelvic organs

Penetration, pregnant uterus by instrument — *continued*
  with — *continued*
    ectopic pregnancy (*see also* categories 633.0-633.9) 639.2
    molar pregnancy (*see also* categories 630-632) 639.2
  complication of delivery 665.1 ✓5ᵗʰ
    affecting fetus or newborn 763.89
  following
    abortion 639.2
    ectopic or molar pregnancy 639.2
Penfield's syndrome (*see also* Epilepsy) 345.5 ✓5ᵗʰ
Penicilliosis of lung 117.3
Penis — *see* condition
Penitis 607.2
Penta X syndrome 758.81
Pentalogy (of Fallot) 745.2
Pentosuria (benign) (essential) 271.8
Peptic acid disease 536.8
Peregrinating patient V65.2
Perforated — *see* Perforation
Perforation, perforative (nontraumatic)
  antrum (*see also* Sinusitis, maxillary) 473.0
  appendix 540.0
    with peritoneal abscess 540.1
  atrial septum, multiple 745.5
  attic, ear 384.22
    healed 384.81
  bile duct, except cystic (*see also* Disease, biliary) 576.3
    cystic 575.4
  bladder (urinary) 596.6
    with
      abortion — *see* Abortion, by type, with damage to pelvic organs
      ectopic pregnancy (*see also* categories 633.0-633.9) 639.2
      molar pregnancy (*see also* categories 630-632) 639.2
    following
      abortion 639.2
      ectopic or molar pregnancy 639.2
    obstetrical trauma 665.5 ✓5ᵗʰ
  bowel 569.83
    with
      abortion — *see* Abortion, by type, with damage to pelvic organs
      ectopic pregnancy (*see also* categories 633.0-633.9) 639.2
      molar pregnancy (*see also* categories 630-632) 639.2
    fetus or newborn 777.6
    following
      abortion 639.2
      ectopic or molar pregnancy 639.2
    obstetrical trauma 665.5 ✓5ᵗʰ
  broad ligament
    with
      abortion — *see* Abortion, by type, with damage to pelvic organs
      ectopic pregnancy (*see also* categories 633.0-633.9) 639.2
      molar pregnancy (*see also* categories 630-632) 639.2
    following
      abortion 639.2
      ectopic or molar pregnancy 639.2
    obstetrical trauma 665.6 ✓5ᵗʰ
  by
    device, implant, or graft — *see* Complications, mechanical
    foreign body left accidentally in operation wound 998.4
    instrument (any) during a procedure, accidental 998.2
  cecum 540.0
    with peritoneal abcess 540.1
  cervix (uteri) — *see also* Injury, internal, cervix
    with
      abortion — *see* Abortion, by type, with damage to pelvic organs
      ectopic pregnancy (*see also* categories 633.0-633.9) 639.2

Perforation, perforative — *continued*
  cervix (uteri) — *see also* Injury, internal, cervix — *continued*
    with — *continued*
      molar pregnancy (*see also* categories 630-632) 639.2
    following
      abortion 639.2
      ectopic or molar pregnancy 639.2
    obstetrical trauma 665.3 ✓5ᵗʰ
  colon 569.83
  common duct (bile) 576.3
  cornea (*see also* Ulcer, cornea) 370.00
    due to ulceration 370.06
  cystic duct 575.4
  diverticulum (*see also* Diverticula) 562.10
    small intestine 562.00
  duodenum, duodenal (ulcer) — *see* Ulcer, duodenum, with perforation
  ear drum — *see* Perforation, tympanum
  enteritis — *see* Enteritis
  esophagus 530.4
  ethmoidal sinus (*see also* Sinusitis, ethmoidal) 473.2
  foreign body (external site) — *see also* Wound, open, by site, complicated
    internal site, by ingested object — *see* Foreign body
  frontal sinus (*see also* Sinusitis, frontal) 473.1
  gallbladder or duct (*see also* Disease, gallbladder) 575.4
  gastric (ulcer) — *see* Ulcer, stomach, with perforation
  heart valve — *see* Endocarditis
  ileum (*see also* Perforation, intestine) 569.83
  instrumental
    external — *see* Wound, open, by site
    pregnant uterus, complicating delivery 665.9 ✓5ᵗʰ
    surgical (accidental) (blood vessel) (nerve) (organ) 998.2
  intestine 569.83
    with
      abortion — *see* Abortion, by type, with damage to pelvic organs
      ectopic pregnancy (*see also* categories 633.0-633.9) 639.2
      molar pregnancy (*see also* categories 630-632) 639.2
    fetus or newborn 777.6
    obstetrical trauma 665.5 ✓5ᵗʰ
    ulcerative NEC 569.83
  jejunum, jejunal 569.83
    ulcer — *see* Ulcer, gastrojejunal, with perforation
  mastoid (antrum) (cell) 383.89
  maxillary sinus (*see also* Sinusitis, maxillary) 473.0
  membrana tympani — *see* Perforation, tympanum
  nasal
    septum 478.1
      congenital 748.1
      syphilitic 095.8
    sinus (*see also* Sinusitis) 473.9
      congenital 748.1
  palate (hard) 526.89
    soft 528.9
      syphilitic 095.8
        syphilitic 095.8
  palatine vault 526.89
    syphilitic 095.8
      congenital 090.5
  pelvic
    floor
      with
        abortion — *see* Abortion, by type, with damage to pelvic organs
        ectopic pregnancy (*see also* categories 633.0-633.9) 639.2
        molar pregnancy (*see also* categories 630-632) 639.2
      obstetrical trauma 664.1 ✓5ᵗʰ
    organ
      with
        abortion — *see* Abortion, by type, with damage to pelvic organs

Perforation, perforative — *continued*
  pelvic — *continued*
    organ — *continued*
      with — *continued*
        ectopic pregnancy (*see also* categories 633.0-633.9) 639.2
        molar pregnancy (*see also* categories 630-632) 639.2
      following
        abortion 639.2
        ectopic or molar pregnancy 639.2
      obstetrical trauma 665.5 ✓5ᵗʰ
  perineum — *see* Laceration, perineum
  periurethral tissue
    with
      abortion — *see* Abortion, by type, with damage to pelvic organs
      ectopic pregnancy (*see also* categories 630-632) 639.2
      molar pregnancy (*see also* categories 630-632) 639.2
  pharynx 478.29
  pylorus, pyloric (ulcer) — *see* Ulcer, stomach, with perforation
  rectum 569.49
  sigmoid 569.83
  sinus (accessory) (chronic) (nasal) (*see also* Sinusitis) 473.9
  sphenoidal sinus (*see also* Sinusitis, sphenoidal) 473.3
  stomach (due to ulcer) — *see* Ulcer, stomach, with perforation
  surgical (accidental) (by instrument) (blood vessel) (nerve) (organ) 998.2
  traumatic
    external — *see* Wound, open, by site
    eye (*see also* Penetrating wound, ocular) 871.7
    internal organ — *see* Injury, internal, by site
  tympanum (membrane) (persistent posttraumatic) (postinflammatory) 384.20
    with
      otitis media — *see* Otitis media
    attic 384.22
    central 384.21
    healed 384.81
    marginal NEC 384.23
    multiple 384.24
    pars flaccida 384.22
    total 384.25
    traumatic — *see* Wound, open, ear, drum
  typhoid, gastrointestinal 002.0
  ulcer — *see* Ulcer, by site, with perforation
  ureter 593.89
  urethra
    with
      abortion — *see* Abortion, by type, with damage to pelvic organs
      ectopic pregnancy (*see also* categories 633.0-633.9) 639.2
      molar pregnancy (*see also* categories 630-632) 639.2
    following
      abortion 639.2
      ectopic or molar pregnancy 639.2
    obstetrical trauma 665.5 ✓5ᵗʰ
  uterus — *see also* Injury, internal, uterus
    with
      abortion — *see* Abortion, by type, with damage to pelvic organs
      ectopic pregnancy (*see also* categories 633.0-633.9) 639.2
      molar pregnancy (*see also* categories 630-632) 639.2
    by intrauterine contraceptive device 996.32
    following
      abortion 639.2
      ectopic or molar pregnancy 639.2
    obstetrical trauma — *see* Injury, internal, uterus, obstetrical trauma
  uvula 528.9
    syphilitic 095.8
  vagina — *see* Laceration, vagina
  viscus NEC 799.8
    traumatic 868.00
      with open wound into cavity 868.10
Periadenitis mucosa necrotica recurrens 528.2

Periangiitis 446.0
Periantritis 535.4
Periappendicitis (acute) (see also Appendicitis) 541
Periarteritis (disseminated) (infectious) (necrotizing) (nodosa) 446.0
Periarthritis (joint) 726.90
  Duplay's 726.2
  gonococcal 098.50
  humeroscapularis 726.2
  scapulohumeral 726.2
  shoulder 726.2
  wrist 726.4
Periarthrosis (angioneural) — see Periarthritis
Peribronchitis 491.9
  tuberculous (see also Tuberculosis) 011.3
Pericapsulitis, adhesive (shoulder) 726.0
Pericarditis (granular) (with decompensation) (with effusion) 423.9
  with
    rheumatic fever (conditions classifiable to 390)
      active (see also Pericarditis, rheumatic) 391.0
      inactive or quiescent 393
  actinomycotic 039.8 [420.0]
  acute (nonrheumatic) 420.90
    with chorea (acute) (rheumatic) (Sydenham's) 392.0
    bacterial 420.99
    benign 420.91
    hemorrhagic 420.90
    idiopathic 420.91
    infective 420.90
    nonspecific 420.91
    rheumatic 391.0
      with chorea (acute) (rheumatic) (Sydenham's) 392.0
    sicca 420.90
    viral 420.91
  adhesive or adherent (external) (internal) 423.1
    acute — see Pericarditis, acute
    rheumatic (external) (internal) 393
  amebic 006.8 [420.0]
  bacterial (acute) (subacute) (with serous or seropurulent effusion) 420.99
  calcareous 423.2
  cholesterol (chronic) 423.8
    acute 420.90
  chronic (nonrheumatic) 423.8
    rheumatic 393
  constrictive 423.2
  Coxsackie 074.21
  due to
    actinomycosis 039.8 [420.0]
    amebiasis 006.8 [420.0]
    Coxsackie (virus) 074.21
    histoplasmosis (see also Histoplasmosis) 115.93
    nocardiosis 039.8 [420.0]
    tuberculosis (see also Tuberculosis) 017.9 [420.0]
  fibrinocaseous (see also Tuberculosis) 017.9 [420.0]
  fibrinopurulent 420.99
  fibrinous — see Pericarditis, rheumatic
  fibropurulent 420.99
  fibrous 423.1
  gonococcal 098.83
  hemorrhagic 423.0
  idiopathic (acute) 420.91
  infective (acute) 420.90
  meningococcal 036.41
  neoplastic (chronic) 423.8
    acute 420.90
  nonspecific 420.91
  obliterans, obliterating 423.1
  plastic 423.1
  pneumococcal (acute) 420.99
  postinfarction 411.0
  purulent (acute) 420.99
  rheumatic (active) (acute) (with effusion) (with pneumonia) 391.0
    with chorea (acute) (rheumatic) (Sydenham's) 392.0
    chronic or inactive (with chorea) 393

Pericarditis — continued
  septic (acute) 420.99
  serofibrinous — see Pericarditis, rheumatic
  staphylococcal (acute) 420.99
  streptococcal (acute) 420.99
  suppurative (acute) 420.99
  syphilitic 093.81
  tuberculous (acute) (chronic) (see also Tuberculosis) 017.9 [420.0]
  uremic 585 [420.0]
  viral (acute) 420.91
Pericardium, pericardial — see condition
Pericellulitis (see also Cellulitis) 682.9
Pericementitis 523.4
  acute 523.3
  chronic (suppurative) 523.4
Pericholecystitis (see also Cholecystitis) 575.10
Perichondritis
  auricle 380.00
    acute 380.01
    chronic 380.02
  bronchus 491.9
  ear (external) 380.00
    acute 380.01
    chronic 380.02
  larynx 478.71
    syphilitic 095.8
    typhoid 002.0 [478.71]
  nose 478.1
  pinna 380.00
    acute 380.01
    chronic 380.02
  trachea 478.9
Periclasia 523.5
Pericolitis 569.89
Pericoronitis (chronic) 523.4
  acute 523.3
Pericystitis (see also Cystitis) 595.9
Pericytoma (M9150/1) — see also Neoplasm, connective tissue, uncertain behavior
  benign (M9150/0) — see Neoplasm, connective tissue, benign
  malignant (M9150/3) — see Neoplasm, connective tissue, malignant
Peridacryocystitis, acute 375.32
Peridiverticulitis (see also Diverticulitis) 562.11
Periduodenitis 535.6
Periendocarditis (see also Endocarditis) 424.90
  acute or subacute 421.9
Periepididymitis (see also Epididymitis) 604.90
Perifolliculitis (abscedens) 704.8
  capitis, abscedens et suffodiens 704.8
  dissecting, scalp 704.8
  scalp 704.8
  superficial pustular 704.8
Perigastritis (acute) 535.0
Perigastrojejunitis (acute) 535.0
Perihepatitis (acute) 573.3
  chlamydial 099.56
  gonococcal 098.86
Peri-ileitis (subacute) 569.89
Perilabyrinthitis (acute) — see Labyrinthitis
Perimeningitis — see Meningitis
Perimetritis (see also Endometritis) 615.9
Perimetrosalpingitis (see also Salpingo-oophoritis) 614.2
Perinephric — see condition
Perinephritic — see condition
Perinephritis (see also Infection, kidney) 590.9
  purulent (see also Abscess, kidney) 590.2
Perineum, perineal — see condition
Perineuritis NEC 729.2
Periodic — see also condition
  disease (familial) 277.3
  edema 995.1
    hereditary 277.6
  fever 277.3
  paralysis (familial) 359.3
  peritonitis 277.3
  polyserositis 277.3
  somnolence 347

Periodontal
  cyst 522.8
  pocket 523.8
Periodontitis (chronic) (complex) (compound) (local) (simplex) 523.4
  acute 523.3
  apical 522.6
    acute (pulpal origin) 522.4
Periodontoclasia 523.5
Periodontosis 523.5
Periods — see also Menstruation
  heavy 626.2
  irregular 626.4
Perionychia (with lymphangitis) 681.9
  finger 681.02
  toe 681.11
Perioophoritis (see also Salpingo-oophoritis) 614.2
Periorchitis (see also Orchitis) 604.90
Periosteum, periosteal — see condition
Periostitis (circumscribed) (diffuse) (infective) 730.3

Note — Use the following fifth-digit subclassification with category 730:

  0   site unspecified
  1   shoulder region
  2   upper arm
  3   forearm
  4   hand
  5   pelvic region and thigh
  6   lower leg
  7   ankle and foot
  8   other specified sites
  9   multiple sites

  with osteomyelitis (see also Osteomyelitis) 730.2
    acute or subacute 730.0
    chronic or old 730.1
  albuminosa, albuminosus 730.3
  alveolar 526.5
  alveolodental 526.5
  dental 526.5
  gonorrheal 098.89
  hyperplastica, generalized 731.2
  jaw (lower) (upper) 526.4
  monomelic 733.99
  orbital 376.02
  syphilitic 095.5
    congenital 090.0 [730.8]
    secondary 091.61
  tuberculous (see also Tuberculosis, bone) 015.9 [730.8]
  yaws (early) (hypertrophic) (late) 102.6
Periostosis (see also Periostitis) 730.3
  with osteomyelitis (see also Osteomyelitis) 730.2
    acute or subacute 730.0
    chronic or old 730.1
  hyperplastic 756.59
Periphlebitis (see also Phlebitis) 451.9
  lower extremity 451.2
    deep (vessels) 451.19
    superficial (vessels) 451.0
  portal 572.1
  retina 362.18
  superficial (vessels) 451.0
  tuberculous (see also Tuberculosis) 017.9
    retina 017.3 [362.18]
Peripneumonia — see Pneumonia
Periproctitis 569.49
Periprostatitis (see also Prostatitis) 601.9
Perirectal — see condition
Perirenal — see condition
Perisalpingitis (see also Salpingo-oophoritis) 614.2
Perisigmoiditis 569.89
Perisplenitis (infectional) 289.59
Perispondylitis — see Spondylitis
Peristalsis reversed or visible 787.4

Peritendinitis (see also Tenosynovitis) 726.90
- adhesive (shoulder) 726.0

Perithelioma (M9150/1) — see Pericytoma

Peritoneum, peritoneal — see also condition
- equilibration test V56.32

Peritonitis (acute) (adhesive) (fibrinous) (hemorrhagic) (idiopathic) (localized) (perforative) (primary) (with adhesions) (with effusion) 567.9
- with or following
  - abortion — see Abortion, by type, with sepsis
  - abscess 567.2
  - appendicitis 540.0
    - with peritoneal abcess 540.1
  - ectopic pregnancy (see also categories 633.0-633.9) 639.0
  - molar pregnancy (see also categories 630-632) 639.0
- aseptic 998.7
- bacterial 567.2
- bile, biliary 567.8
- chemical 998.7
- chlamydial 099.56
- chronic proliferative 567.8
- congenital NEC 777.6
- diaphragmatic 567.2
- diffuse NEC 567.2
- diphtheritic 032.83
- disseminated NEC 567.2
- due to
  - bile 567.8
  - foreign
    - body or object accidentally left during a procedure (instrument) (sponge) (swab) 998.4
    - substance accidentally left during a procedure (chemical) (powder) (talc) 998.7
  - talc 998.7
  - urine 567.8
- fibrinopurulent 567.2
- fibrinous 567.2
- fibrocaseous (see also Tuberculosis) 014.0 ✓5ᵗʰ
- fibropurulent 567.2
- general, generalized (acute) 567.2
- gonococcal 098.86
- in infective disease NEC 136.9 [567.0]
- meconium (newborn) 777.6
- pancreatic 577.8
- paroxysmal, benign 277.3
- pelvic
  - female (acute) 614.5
    - chronic NEC 614.7
      - with adhesions 614.6
    - puerperal, postpartum, childbirth 670 ✓4ᵗʰ
  - male (acute) 567.2
- periodic (familial) 277.3
- phlegmonous 567.2
- pneumococcal 567.1
- postabortal 639.0
- proliferative, chronic 567.8
- puerperal, postpartum, childbirth 670 ✓4ᵗʰ
- purulent 567.2
- septic 567.2
- staphylococcal 567.2
- streptococcal 567.2
- subdiaphragmatic 567.2
- subphrenic 567.2
- suppurative 567.2
- syphilitic 095.2
  - congenital 090.0 [567.0]
- talc 998.7
- tuberculous (see also Tuberculosis) 014.0 ✓5ᵗʰ
- urine 567.8

Peritonsillar — see condition

Peritonsillitis 475

Perityphlitis (see also Appendicitis) 541

Periureteritis 593.89

Periurethral — see condition

Periurethritis (gangrenous) 597.89

Periuterine — see condition

Perivaginitis (see also Vaginitis) 616.10

Perivasculitis, retinal 362.18

Perivasitis (chronic) 608.4

Periventricular leukomalacia 779.7

Perivesiculitis (seminal) (see also Vesiculitis) 608.0

Perlèche 686.8
- due to
  - moniliasis 112.0
  - riboflavin deficiency 266.0

Pernicious — see condition

Pernio, perniosis 991.5

Persecution
- delusion 297.9
- social V62.4

Perseveration (tonic) 784.69

Persistence, persistent (congenital) 759.89
- anal membrane 751.2
- arteria stapedia 744.04
- atrioventricular canal 745.69
- bloody ejaculate 792.2
- branchial cleft 744.41
- bulbus cordis in left ventricle 745.8
- canal of Cloquet 743.51
- capsule (opaque) 743.51
- cilioretinal artery or vein 743.51
- cloaca 751.5
- communication — see Fistula, congenital
- convolutions
  - aortic arch 747.21
  - fallopian tube 752.19
  - oviduct 752.19
  - uterine tube 752.19
- double aortic arch 747.21
- ductus
  - arteriosus 747.0
  - Botalli 747.0
- fetal
  - circulation 747.83 ▲
  - form of cervix (uteri) 752.49
  - hemoglobin (hereditary) ("Swiss variety") 282.7
  - pulmonary hypertension 747.83 ▲
- foramen
  - Botalli 745.5
  - ovale 745.5
- Gartner's duct 752.11
- hemoglobin, fetal (hereditary) (HPFH) 282.7
- hyaloid
  - artery (generally incomplete) 743.51
  - system 743.51
- hymen (tag)
  - in pregnancy or childbirth 654.8 ✓5ᵗʰ
    - causing obstructed labor 660.2 ✓5ᵗʰ
- lanugo 757.4
- left
  - posterior cardinal vein 747.49
  - root with right arch of aorta 747.21
  - superior vena cava 747.49
- Meckel's diverticulum 751.0
- mesonephric duct 752.8
  - fallopian tube 752.11
- mucosal disease (middle ear) (with posterior or superior marginal perforation of ear drum) 382.2
- nail(s), anomalous 757.5
- occiput, anterior or posterior 660.3 ✓5ᵗʰ
  - fetus or newborn 763.1
- omphalomesenteric duct 751.0
- organ or site NEC — see Anomaly, specified type NEC
- ostium
  - atrioventriculare commune 745.69
  - primum 745.61
  - secundum 745.5
- ovarian rests in fallopian tube 752.19
- pancreatic tissue in intestinal tract 751.5
- primary (deciduous)
  - teeth 520.6
  - vitreous hyperplasia 743.51
- pulmonary hypertension 747.83 ▲
- pupillary membrane 743.46
  - iris 743.46
- Rhesus (Rh) titer 999.7
- right aortic arch 747.21
- sinus
  - urogenitalis 752.8

Persistence, persistent — continued
- sinus — continued
  - venosus with imperfect incorporation in right auricle 747.49
- thymus (gland) 254.8
  - hyperplasia 254.0
- thyroglossal duct 759.2
- thyrolingual duct 759.2
- truncus arteriosus or communis 745.0
- tunica vasculosa lentis 743.39
- umbilical sinus 753.7
- urachus 753.7
- vegetative state 780.03
- vitelline duct 751.0
- wolffian duct 752.8

Person (with)
- admitted for clinical research, as participant or control subject V70.7
- awaiting admission to adequate facility elsewhere V63.2
  - undergoing social agency investigation V63.8
- concern (normal) about sick person in family V61.49
- consulting on behalf of another V65.1
- feared
  - complaint in whom no diagnosis was made V65.5
  - condition not demonstrated V65.5
- feigning illness V65.2
- healthy, accompanying sick person V65.0
- living (in)
  - alone V60.3
  - boarding school V60.6
  - residence remote from hospital or medical care facility V63.0
  - residential institution V60.6
  - without
    - adequate
      - financial resources V60.2
      - housing (heating) (space) V60.1
    - housing (permanent) (temporary) V60.0
    - material resources V60.2
    - person able to render necessary care V60.4
    - shelter V60.0
- medical services in home not available V63.1
- on waiting list V63.2
  - undergoing social agency investigation V63.8
- sick or handicapped in family V61.49
- "worried well" V65.5

Personality
- affective 301.10
- aggressive 301.3
- amoral 301.7
- anancastic, anankastic 301.4
- antisocial 301.7
- asocial 301.7
- asthenic 301.6
- avoidant 301.82
- borderline 301.83
- change 310.1
- compulsive 301.4
- cycloid 301.13
- cyclothymic 301.13
- dependent 301.6
- depressive (chronic) 301.12
- disorder, disturbance NEC 301.9
  - with
    - antisocial disturbance 301.7
    - pattern disturbance NEC 301.9
    - sociopathic disturbance 301.7
    - trait disturbance 301.9
- dual 300.14
- dyssocial 301.7
- eccentric 301.89
  - "haltlose" type 301.89
- emotionally unstable 301.59
- epileptoid 301.3
- explosive 301.3
- fanatic 301.0
- histrionic 301.50
- hyperthymic 301.11
- hypomanic 301.11
- hypothymic 301.12
- hysterical 301.50
- immature 301.89
- inadequate 301.6

Index to Diseases — Phlebitis

Personality — *continued*
- labile 301.59
- masochistic 301.89
- morally defective 301.7
- multiple 300.14
- narcissistic 301.81
- obsessional 301.4
- obsessive (-compulsive) 301.4
- overconscientious 301.4
- paranoid 301.0
- passive (-dependent) 301.6
- passive-aggressive 301.84
- pathologic NEC 301.9
- pattern defect or disturbance 301.9
- pseudosocial 301.7
- psychoinfantile 301.59
- psychoneurotic NEC 301.89
- psychopathic 301.9
  - with
    - amoral trend 301.7
    - antisocial trend 301.7
    - asocial trend 301.7
    - pathologic sexuality (*see also* Deviation, sexual) 302.9
  - mixed types 301.9
  - schizoid 301.20
    - introverted 301.21
    - schizotypal 301.22
    - with sexual deviation (*see also* Deviation, sexual) 302.9
    - antisocial 301.7
    - dyssocial 301.7
  - type A 301.4
  - unstable (emotional) 301.59

Perthes' disease (capital femoral osteochondrosis) 732.1

Pertussis (*see also* Whooping cough) 033.9
- vaccination, prophylactic (against) V03.6

Peruvian wart 088.0

Perversion, perverted
- appetite 307.52
  - hysterical 300.11
- function
  - pineal gland 259.8
  - pituitary gland 253.9
    - anterior lobe
      - deficient 253.2
      - excessive 253.1
    - posterior lobe 253.6
  - placenta — *see* Placenta, abnormal
- sense of smell or taste 781.1
  - psychogenic 306.7
- sexual (*see also* Deviation, sexual) 302.9

Pervious, congenital — *see also* Imperfect, closure
- ductus arteriosus 747.0

Pes (congenital) (*see also* Talipes) 754.70
- abductus (congenital) 754.60
  - acquired 736.79
- acquired NEC 736.79
  - planus 734
- adductus (congenital) 754.79
  - acquired 736.79
- cavus 754.71
  - acquired 736.73
- planovalgus (congenital) 754.69
  - acquired 736.79
- planus (acquired) (any degree) 734
  - congenital 754.61
  - rachitic 268.1
- valgus (congenital) 754.61
  - acquired 736.79
- varus (congenital) 754.50
  - acquired 736.79

Pest (*see also* Plague) 020.9

Pestis (*see also* Plague) 020.9
- bubonica 020.0
- fulminans 020.0
- minor 020.8
- pneumonica — *see* Plague, pneumonic

Petechia, petechiae 782.7
- fetus or newborn 772.6

Petechial
- fever 036.0
- typhus 081.9

Petges-Cléjat or Petges-Clégat syndrome (poikilodermatomyositis) 710.3

Petit's
- disease (*see also* Hernia, lumbar) 553.8

Petit mal (idiopathic) (*see also* Epilepsy) 345.0
- status 345.2

Petrellidosis 117.6

Petrositis 383.20
- acute 383.21
- chronic 383.22

Peutz-Jeghers disease or syndrome 759.6

Peyronie's disease 607.89

Pfeiffer's disease 075

Phacentocele 379.32
- traumatic 921.3

Phacoanaphylaxis 360.19

Phacocele (old) 379.32
- traumatic 921.3

Phaehyphomycosis 117.8

Phagedena (dry) (moist) (*see also* Gangrene) 785.4
- arteriosclerotic 440.2 [785.4]
- geometric 686.09
- penis 607.89
- senile 440.2 [785.4]
- sloughing 785.4
- tropical (*see also* Ulcer, skin) 707.9
- vulva 616.50

Phagedenic — *see also* condition
- abscess — *see also* Abscess
  - chancroid 099.0
- bubo NEC 099.8
- chancre 099.0
- ulcer (tropical) (*see also* Ulcer, skin) 707.9

Phagomania 307.52

Phakoma 362.89

Phantom limb (syndrome) 353.6

Pharyngeal — *see also* condition
- arch remnant 744.41
- pouch syndrome 279.11

Pharyngitis (acute) (catarrhal) (gangrenous) (infective) (malignant) (membranous) (phlegmonous) (pneumococcal) (pseudomembranous) (simple) (staphylococcal) (subacute) (suppurative) (ulcerative) (viral) 462
- with influenza, flu, or grippe 487.1
- aphthous 074.0
- atrophic 472.1
- chronic 472.1
- chlamydial 099.51
- coxsackie virus 074.0
- diphtheritic (membranous) 032.0
- follicular 472.1
- fusospirochetal 101
- gonococcal 098.6
- granular (chronic) 472.1
- herpetic 054.79
- hypertrophic 472.1
- infectional, chronic 472.1
- influenzal 487.1
- lymphonodular, acute 074.8
- septic 034.0
- streptococcal 034.0
- tuberculous (*see also* Tuberculosis) 012.8
- vesicular 074.0

Pharyngoconjunctival fever 077.2

Pharyngoconjunctivitis, viral 077.2

Pharyngolaryngitis (acute) 465.0
- chronic 478.9
- septic 034.0

Pharyngoplegia 478.29

Pharyngotonsillitis 465.8
- tuberculous 012.8

Pharyngotracheitis (acute) 465.8
- chronic 478.9

Pharynx, pharyngeal — *see* condition

Phase of life problem NEC V62.89

Phenomenon
- Arthus' — *see* Arthus' phenomenon
- flashback (drug) 292.89
- jaw-winking 742.8
- Jod-Basedow 242.8
- L. E. cell 710.0
- lupus erythematosus cell 710.0

Phenomenon — *continued*
- Pelger-Huët (hereditary hyposegmentation) 288.2
- Raynaud's (paroxysmal digital cyanosis) (secondary) 443.0
- Reilly's (*see also* Neuropathy, peripheral, autonomic) 337.9
- vasomotor 780.2
- vasospastic 443.9
- vasovagal 780.2
- Wenckebach's, heart block (second degree) 426.13

Phenylketonuria (PKU) 270.1

Phenylpyruvicaciduria 270.1

Pheochromoblastoma (M8700/3)
- specified site — *see* Neoplasm, by site, malignant
- unspecified site 194.0

Pheochromocytoma (M8700/0)
- malignant (M8700/3)
  - specified site — *see* Neoplasm, by site, malignant
  - unspecified site 194.0
- specified site — *see* Neoplasm, by site, benign
- unspecified site 227.0

Phimosis (congenital) 605
- chancroidal 099.0
- due to infection 605

Phlebectasia (*see also* Varicose, vein) 454.9
- congenital 747.6
- esophagus (*see also* Varix, esophagus) 456.1
  - with hemorrhage (*see also* Varix, esophagus, bleeding) 456.0

Phlebitis (infective) (pyemic) (septic) (suppurative) 451.9
- antecubital vein 451.82
- arm NEC 451.84
  - axillary vein 451.89
  - basilic vey 451.82
  - deep 451.83
  - superficial 451.82
- basilic vein 451.82
- blue 451.19
- brachial vein 451.83
- breast, superficial 451.89
- cavernous (venous) sinus — *see* Phlebitis, intracranial sinus
- cephalic vein 451.82
- cerebral (venous) sinus — *see* Phlebitis, intracranial sinus
- chest wall, superficial 451.89
- complicating pregnancy or puerperium 671.9
  - affecting fetus or newborn 760.3
- cranial (venous) sinus — *see* Phlebitis, intracranial sinus
- deep (vessels) 451.19
  - femoral vein 451.11
  - specified vessel NEC 451.19
- due to implanted device — *see* Complications, due to (presence of) any device, implant or graft classified to 996.0-996.5 NEC
- during or resulting from a procedure 997.2
- femoral vein (deep) 451.11
- femoropopliteal 451.0
- following infusion, perfusion, or transfusion 999.2
- gouty 274.89 [451.9]
- hepatic veins 451.89
- iliac vein 451.81
- iliofemoral 451.11
- intracranial sinus (any) (venous) 325
  - late effect — *see* category 326
  - nonpyogenic 437.6
  - in pregnancy or puerperium 671.5
- jugular vein 451.89
- lateral (venous) sinus — *see* Phlebitis, intracranial sinus
- leg 451.2
  - deep (vessels) 451.19
    - femoral vein 451.11
    - specified vessel NEC 451.19
  - superficial (vessels) 451.0
    - femoral vein 451.11
- longitudinal sinus — *see* Phlebitis, intracranial sinus

Phlebitis — continued
　lower extremity 451.2
　　deep (vessels) 451.19
　　　femoral vein 451.11
　　　specified vessel NEC 451.19
　　superficial (vessels) 451.0
　　　femoral vein 451.11
　migrans, migrating (superficial) 453.1
　pelvic
　　with
　　　abortion — see Abortion, by type, with sepsis
　　　ectopic pregnancy (see also categories 633.0-633.9) 639.0
　　　molar pregnancy (see also categories 630-632) 639.0
　　following
　　　abortion 639.0
　　　ectopic or molar pregnancy 639.0
　　puerperal, postpartum 671.4 ✓5ᵗʰ
　popliteal vein 451.19
　portal (vein) 572.1
　postoperative 997.2
　pregnancy 671.9 ✓5ᵗʰ
　　deep 671.3 ✓5ᵗʰ
　　specified type NEC 671.5 ✓5ᵗʰ
　　superficial 671.2 ✓5ᵗʰ
　puerperal, postpartum, childbirth 671.9 ✓5ᵗʰ
　　deep 671.4 ✓5ᵗʰ
　　lower extremities 671.2 ✓5ᵗʰ
　　pelvis 671.4 ✓5ᵗʰ
　　specified site NEC 671.5 ✓5ᵗʰ
　　superficial 671.2 ✓5ᵗʰ
　radial vein 451.83
　retina 362.18
　saphenous (great) (long) 451.0
　　accessory or small 451.0
　sinus (meninges) — see Phlebitis, intracranial sinus
　specified site NEC 451.89
　subclavian vein 451.89
　syphilitic 093.89
　tibial vein 451.19
　ulcer, ulcerative 451.9
　　leg 451.2
　　　deep (vessels) 451.19
　　　　femoral vein 451.11
　　　　specified vessel NEC 451.19
　　　superficial (vessels) 451.0
　　　　femoral vein 451.11
　　lower extremity 451.2
　　　deep (vessels) 451.19
　　　　femoral vein 451.11
　　　　specified vessel NEC 451.19
　　　superficial (vessels) 451.0
　ulnar vein 451.83
　umbilicus 451.89
　upper extremity — see Phlebitis, arm
　uterus (septic) (see also Endometritis) 615.9
　varicose (leg) (lower extremity) (see also Varicose, vein) 454.1
Phlebofibrosis 459.89
Pheboliths 459.89
Phlebosclerosis 459.89
Phlebothrombosis — see Thrombosis
Phlebotomus fever 066.0
Phlegm, choked on 933.1
Phlegmasia
　alba dolens (deep vessels) 451.19
　　complicating pregnancy 671.3 ✓5ᵗʰ
　　nonpuerperal 451.19
　　puerperal, postpartum, childbirth 671.4 ✓5ᵗʰ
　cerulea dolens 451.19
Phlegmon (see also Abscess) 682.9
　erysipelatous (see also Erysipelas) 035
　iliac 682.2
　　fossa 540.1
　throat 478.29
Phlegmonous — see condition
Phlyctenulosis (allergic) (keratoconjunctivitis) (nontuberculous) 370.31
　cornea 370.31
　　with ulcer (see also Ulcer, cornea) 370.00
　tuberculous (see also Tuberculosis) 017.3 ✓5ᵗʰ [370.31]

Phobia, phobic (reaction) 300.20
　animal 300.29
　isolated NEC 300.29
　obsessional 300.3
　simple NEC 300.29
　social 300.23
　specified NEC 300.29
　state 300.20
Phocas' disease 610.1
Phocomelia 755.4
　lower limb 755.32
　　complete 755.33
　　distal 755.35
　　proximal 755.34
　upper limb 755.22
　　complete 755.23
　　distal 755.25
　　proximal 755.24
Phoria (see also Heterophoria) 378.40
Phosphate-losing tubular disorder 588.0
Phosphatemia 275.3
Phosphaturia 275.3
Photoallergic response 692.72
Photocoproporphyria 277.1
Photodermatitis (sun) 692.72
　light other than sun 692.82
Photokeratitis 370.24
Photo-ophthalmia 370.24
Photophobia 368.13
Photopsia 368.15
Photoretinitis 363.31
Photoretinopathy 363.31
Photosensitiveness (sun) 692.72
　light other than sun 692.82
Photosensitization (sun) skin 692.72
　light other than sun 692.82
Phototoxic response 692.72
Phrenitis 323.9
Phrynoderma 264.8
Phthiriasis (pubis) (any site) 132.2
　with any infestation classifiable to 132.0, 132.1 and 132.3
Phthirus infestation — see Phthiriasis
Phthisis (see also Tuberculosis) 011.9 ✓5ᵗʰ
　bulbi (infectional) 360.41
　colliers' 011.4 ✓5ᵗʰ
　cornea 371.05
　eyeball (due to infection) 360.41
　millstone makers' 011.4 ✓5ᵗʰ
　miners' 011.4 ✓5ᵗʰ
　potters' 011.4 ✓5ᵗʰ
　sandblasters' 011.4 ✓5ᵗʰ
　stonemasons' 011.4 ✓5ᵗʰ
Phycomycosis 117.7
Physalopteriasis 127.7
Physical therapy NEC V57.1
　breathing exercises V57.0
Physiological cup, optic papilla
　borderline, glaucoma suspect 365.00
　enlarged 377.14
　glaucomatous 377.14
Phytobezoar 938
　intestine 936
　stomach 935.2
Pian (see also Yaws) 102.9
Pianoma 102.1
Piarhemia, piarrhemia (see also Hyperlipemia) 272.4
　bilharziasis 120.9
Pica 307.52
　hysterical 300.11
Pick's
　cerebral atrophy 331.1
　　with dementia
　　　with behavioral disturbance 331.1 [294.11]
　　　without behavioral disturbance 331.1 [294.10]

Pick's — continued
　disease
　　brain 331.1
　　　dementia in
　　　　with behavioral disturbance 331.1 [294.11]
　　　　without behavioral disturbance 331.1 [294.10]
　　lipid histiocytosis 272.7
　　liver (pericardial pseudocirrhosis of liver) 423.2
　　pericardium (pericardial pseudocirrhosis of liver) 423.2
　　polyserositis (pericardial pseudocirrhosis of liver) 423.2
　syndrome
　　heart (pericardial pseudocirrhosis of liver) 423.2
　　liver (pericardial pseudocirrhosis of liver) 423.2
　tubular adenoma (M8640/0)
　　specified site — see Neoplasm, by site, benign
　　unspecified site
　　　female 220
　　　male 222.0
Pick-Herxheimer syndrome (diffuse idiopathic cutaneous atrophy) 701.8
Pick-Niemann disease (lipid histiocytosis) 272.7
Pickwickian syndrome (cardiopulmonary obesity) 278.8
Piebaldism, classic 709.09
Piedra 111.2
　beard 111.2
　　black 111.3
　　white 111.2
　black 111.3
　scalp 111.3
　　black 111.3
　　white 111.2
　white 111.2
Pierre Marie's syndrome (pulmonary hypertrophic osteoarthropathy) 731.2
Pierre Marie-Bamberger syndrome (hypertrophic pulmonary osteoarthropathy) 731.2
Pierre Mauriac's syndrome (diabetes-dwarfism-obesity) 258.1
Pierre Robin deformity or syndrome (congenital) 756.0
Pierson's disease or osteochondrosis 732.1
Pigeon
　breast or chest (acquired) 738.3
　　congenital 754.82
　　rachitic (see also Rickets) 268.0
　breeders' disease or lung 495.2
　fanciers' disease or lung 495.2
　toe 735.8
Pigmentation (abnormal) 709.00
　anomaly 709.00
　　congenital 757.33
　　specified NEC 709.09
　conjunctiva 372.55
　cornea 371.10
　　anterior 371.11
　　posterior 371.13
　　stromal 371.12
　lids (congenital) 757.33
　　acquired 374.52
　limbus corneae 371.10
　metals 709.00
　optic papilla, congenital 743.57
　retina (congenital) (grouped) (nevoid) 743.53
　　acquired 362.74
　scrotum, congenital 757.33
Piles — see Hemorrhoids
Pili
　annulati or torti (congenital) 757.4
　incarnati 704.8
Pill roller hand (intrinsic) 736.09
Pilomatrixoma (M8110/0) — see Neoplasm, skin, benign
Pilonidal — see condition
Pimple 709.8
PIN I (prostatic intraepithelial neoplasia I) 602.3

Index to Diseases — Pleurisy

PIN II (prostatic intraepithelial neoplasia II) 602.3
PIN III (prostatic intraepithelial neoplasia III) 233.4
Pinched nerve — see Neuropathy, entrapment
Pineal body or gland — see condition
Pinealoblastoma (M9362/3) 194.4
Pinealoma (M9360/1) 237.1
    malignant (M9360/3) 194.4
Pineoblastoma (M9362/3) 194.4
Pineocytoma (M9361/1) 237.1
Pinguecula 372.51
Pinhole meatus (see also Stricture, urethra) 598.9
Pink
    disease 985.0
    eye 372.03
    puffer 492.8
Pinkus' disease (lichen nitidus) 697.1
Pinpoint
    meatus (see also Stricture, urethra) 598.9
    os uteri (see also Stricture, cervix) 622.4
Pinselhaare (congenital) 757.4
Pinta 103.9
    cardiovascular lesions 103.2
    chancre (primary) 103.0
    erythematous plaques 103.1
    hyperchromic lesions 103.1
    hyperkeratosis 103.1
    lesions 103.9
        cardiovascular 103.2
        hyperchromic 103.1
        intermediate 103.1
        late 103.2
        mixed 103.3
        primary 103.0
        skin (achromic) (cicatricial) (dyschromic) 103.2
            hyperchromic 103.1
            mixed (achromic and hyperchromic) 103.3
    papule (primary) 103.0
    skin lesions (achromic) (cicatricial) (dyschromic) 103.2
        hyperchromic 103.1
        mixed (achromic and hyperchromic) 103.3
    vitiligo 103.2
Pintid 103.0
Pinworms (disease) (infection) (infestation) 127.4
Piry fever 066.8
Pistol wound — see Gunshot wound
Pit, lip (mucus), congenital 750.25
Pitchers' elbow 718.82
Pithecoid pelvis 755.69
    with disproportion (fetopelvic) 653.2 ✓5ᵗʰ
        affecting fetus or newborn 763.1
        causing obstructed labor 660.1 ✓5ᵗʰ
Pithiatism 300.11
Pitted — see also Pitting
    teeth 520.4
Pitting (edema) (see also Edema) 782.3
    lip 782.3
    nail 703.8
        congenital 757.5
Pituitary gland — see condition
Pituitary snuff-takers' disease 495.8
Pityriasis 696.5
    alba 696.5
    capitis 690.11
    circinata (et maculata) 696.3
    Hebra's (exfoliative dermatitis) 695.89
    lichenoides et varioliformis 696.2
    maculata (et circinata) 696.3
    nigra 111.1
    pilaris 757.39
        acquired 701.1
        Hebra's 696.4
    rosea 696.3
    rotunda 696.3
    rubra (Hebra) 695.89
        pilaris 696.4
    sicca 690.18

Pityriasis — continued
    simplex 690.18
    specified type NEC 696.5
    streptogenes 696.5
    versicolor 111.0
        scrotal 111.0
Placenta, placental
    ablatio 641.2 ✓5ᵗʰ
        affecting fetus or newborn 762.1
    abnormal, abnormality 656.7 ✓5ᵗʰ
        with hemorrhage 641.8 ✓5ᵗʰ
            affecting fetus or newborn 762.1
        affecting fetus or newborn 762.2
    abruptio 641.2 ✓5ᵗʰ
        affecting fetus or newborn 762.1
    accessory lobe — see Placenta, abnormal
    accreta (without hemorrhage) 667.0 ✓5ᵗʰ
        with hemorrhage 666.0 ✓5ᵗʰ
    adherent (without hemorrhage) 667.0 ✓5ᵗʰ
        with hemorrhage 666.0 ✓5ᵗʰ
    apoplexy — see Placenta, separation
    battledore — see Placenta, abnormal
    bilobate — see Placenta, abnormal
    bipartita — see Placenta, abnormal
    carneous mole 631
    centralis — see Placenta, previa
    circumvallata — see Placenta, abnormal
    cyst (amniotic) — see Placenta, abnormal
    deficiency — see Placenta, insufficiency
    degeneration — see Placenta, insufficiency
    detachment (partial) (premature) (with hemorrhage) 641.2 ✓5ᵗʰ
        affecting fetus or newborn 762.1
    dimidiata — see Placenta, abnormal
    disease 656.7 ✓5ᵗʰ
        affecting fetus or newborn 762.2
    duplex — see Placenta, abnormal
    dysfunction — see Placenta, insufficiency
    fenestrata — see Placenta, abnormal
    fibrosis — see Placenta, abnormal
    fleshy mole 631
    hematoma — see Placenta, abnormal
    hemorrhage NEC — see Placenta, separation
    hormone disturbance or malfunction — see Placenta, abnormal
    hyperplasia — see Placenta, abnormal
    increta (without hemorrhage) 667.0 ✓5ᵗʰ
        with hemorrhage 666.0 ✓5ᵗʰ
    infarction 656.7 ✓5ᵗʰ
        affecting fetus or newborn 762.2
    insertion, vicious — see Placenta, previa
    insufficiency
        affecting
            fetus or newborn 762.2
            management of pregnancy 656.5 ✓5ᵗʰ
    lateral — see Placenta, previa
    low implantation or insertion — see Placenta, previa
    low-lying — see Placenta, previa
    malformation — see Placenta, abnormal
    malposition — see Placenta, previa
    marginalis, marginata — see Placenta, previa
    marginal sinus (hemorrhage) (rupture) 641.2 ✓5ᵗʰ
        affecting fetus or newborn 762.1
    membranacea — see Placenta, abnormal
    multilobed — see Placenta, abnormal
    multipartita — see Placenta, abnormal
    necrosis — see Placenta, abnormal
    percreta (without hemorrhage) 667.0 ✓5ᵗʰ
        with hemorrhage 666.0 ✓5ᵗʰ
    polyp 674.4 ✓5ᵗʰ
    previa (central) (centralis) (complete) (lateral) (marginal) (marginalis) (partial) (partialis) (total) (with hemorrhage) 641.1 ✓5ᵗʰ
        affecting fetus or newborn 762.0
        noted
            before labor, without hemorrhage (with cesarean delivery) 641.0 ✓5ᵗʰ
            during pregnancy (without hemorrhage) 641.0 ✓5ᵗʰ
        without hemorrhage (before labor and delivery) (during pregnancy) 641.0 ✓5ᵗʰ
    retention (with hemorrhage) 666.0 ✓5ᵗʰ
        fragments, complicating puerperium (delayed hemorrhage) 666.2 ✓5ᵗʰ

Placenta, placental — continued
    retention — continued
        fragments, complicating puerperium — continued
            without hemorrhage 667.1 ✓5ᵗʰ
        postpartum, puerperal 666.2 ✓5ᵗʰ
        without hemorrhage 667.0 ✓5ᵗʰ
    separation (normally implanted) (partial) (premature) (with hemorrhage) 641.2 ✓5ᵗʰ
        affecting fetus or newborn 762.1
    septuplex — see Placenta, abnormal
    small — see Placenta, insufficiency
    softening (premature) — see Placenta, abnormal
    spuria — see Placenta, abnormal
    succenturiata — see Placenta, abnormal
    syphilitic 095.8
    transfusion syndromes 762.3
    transmission of chemical substance — see Absorption, chemical, through placenta
    trapped (with hemorrhage) 666.0 ✓5ᵗʰ
        without hemorrhage 667.0 ✓5ᵗʰ
    trilobate — see Placenta, abnormal
    tripartita — see Placenta, abnormal
    triplex — see Placenta, abnormal
    varicose vessel — see Placenta, abnormal
    vicious insertion — see Placenta, previa
Placentitis
    affecting fetus or newborn 762.7
    complicating pregnancy 658.4 ✓5ᵗʰ
Plagiocephaly (skull) 754.0
Plague 020.9
    abortive 020.8
    ambulatory 020.8
    bubonic 020.0
    cellulocutaneous 020.1
    lymphatic gland 020.0
    pneumonic 020.5
        primary 020.3
        secondary 020.4
    pulmonary — see Plague, pneumonic
    pulmonic — see Plague, pneumonic
    septicemic 020.2
    tonsillar 020.9
        septicemic 020.2
    vaccination, prophylactic (against) V03.3
Planning, family V25.09
    contraception V25.9
    procreation V26.4
Plaque
    artery, arterial — see Arteriosclerosis
    calcareous — see Calcification
    Hollenhorst's (retinal) 362.33
    tongue 528.6
Plasma cell myeloma 203.0 ✓5ᵗʰ
Plasmacytoma, plasmocytoma (solitary) (M9731/1) 238.6
    benign (M9731/0) — see Neoplasm, by site, benign
    malignant (M9731/3) 203.8 ✓5ᵗʰ
Plasmacytosis 288.8
Plaster ulcer (see also Decubitus) 707.0
Platybasia 756.0
Platyonychia (congenital) 757.5
    acquired 703.8
Platypelloid pelvis 738.6
    with disproportion (fetopelvic) 653.2 ✓5ᵗʰ
        affecting fetus or newborn 763.1
        causing obstructed labor 660.1 ✓5ᵗʰ
            affecting fetus or newborn 763.1
    congenital 755.69
Platyspondylia 756.19
Plethora 782.62
    newborn 776.4
Pleura, pleural — see condition
Pleuralgia 786.52
Pleurisy (acute) (adhesive) (chronic) (costal) (diaphragmatic) (double) (dry) (fetid) (fibrinous) (fibrous) (interlobar) (latent) (lung) (old) (plastic) (primary) (residual) (sicca) (sterile) (subacute) (unresolved) (with adherent pleura) 511.0

Pleurisy

Pleurisy — continued
- with
  - effusion (without mention of cause) 511.9
    - bacterial, nontuberculous 511.1
      - nontuberculous NEC 511.9
        - bacterial 511.1
      - pneumococcal 511.1
      - specified type NEC 511.8
      - staphylococcal 511.1
      - streptococcal 511.1
      - tuberculous (see also Tuberculosis, pleura) 012.0 ✓5ᵗʰ
        - primary, progressive 010.1 ✓5ᵗʰ
  - influenza, flu, or grippe 487.1
  - tuberculosis — see Pleurisy, tuberculous
- encysted 511.8
- exudative (see also Pleurisy, with effusion) 511.9
  - bacterial, nontuberculous 511.1
- fibrinopurulent 510.9
  - with fistula 510.0
- fibropurulent 510.9
  - with fistula 510.0
- hemorrhagic 511.8
- influenzal 487.1
- pneumococcal 511.0
  - with effusion 511.1
- purulent 510.9
  - with fistula 510.0
- septic 510.9
  - with fistula 510.0
- serofibrinous (see also Pleurisy, with effusion) 511.9
  - bacterial, nontuberculous 511.1
- seropurulent 510.9
  - with fistula 510.0
- serous (see also Pleurisy, with effusion) 511.9
  - bacterial, nontuberculous 511.1
- staphylococcal 511.0
  - with effusion 511.1
- streptococcal 511.0
  - with effusion 511.1
- suppurative 510.9
  - with fistula 510.0
- traumatic (post) (current) 862.29
  - with open wound into cavity 862.39
- tuberculous (with effusion) (see also Tuberculosis, pleura) 012.0 ✓5ᵗʰ
  - primary, progressive 010.1 ✓5ᵗʰ

Pleuritis sicca — see Pleurisy
Pleurobronchopneumonia (see also Pneumonia, broncho-) 485
Pleurodynia 786.52
- epidemic 074.1
- viral 074.1

Pleurohepatitis 573.8
Pleuropericarditis (see also Pericarditis) 423.9
- acute 420.90

Pleuropneumonia (acute) (bilateral) (double) (septic) (see also Pneumonia) 486
- chronic (see also Fibrosis, lung) 515

Pleurorrhea (see also Hydrothorax) 511.8
Plexitis, brachial 353.0
Plica
- knee 727.83
- polonica 132.0
- tonsil 474.8

Plicae dysphonia ventricularis 784.49
Plicated tongue 529.5
- congenital 750.13

Plug
- bronchus NEC 519.1
- meconium (newborn) NEC 777.1
- mucus — see Mucus, plug

Plumbism 984.9
- specified type of lead — see Table of Drugs and Chemicals

Plummer's disease (toxic nodular goiter) 242.3 ✓5ᵗʰ
Plummer-Vinson syndrome (sideropenic dysphagia) 280.8
Pluricarential syndrome of infancy 260
Pluridefiency syndrome of infancy 260

Plus (and minus) hand (intrinsic) 736.09
PMS 625.4
Pneumathemia — see Air, embolism, by type
Pneumatic drill or hammer disease 994.9
Pneumatocele (lung) 518.89
- intracranial 348.8
- tension 492.0

Pneumatosis
- cystoides intestinalis 569.89
- peritonei 568.89
- pulmonum 492.8

Pneumaturia 599.84
Pneumoblastoma (M8981/3) — see Neoplasm, lung, malignant
Pneumocephalus 348.8
Pneumococcemia 038.2
Pneumococcus, pneumococcal — see condition
Pneumoconiosis (due to) (inhalation of) 505
- aluminum 503
- asbestos 501
- bagasse 495.1
- bauxite 503
- beryllium 503
- carbon electrode makers' 503
- coal
  - miners' (simple) 500
  - workers' (simple) 500
- cotton dust 504
- diatomite fibrosis 502
- dust NEC 504
  - inorganic 503
  - lime 502
  - marble 502
  - organic NEC 504
- fumes or vapors (from silo) 506.9
- graphite 503
- hard metal 503
- mica 502
- moldy hay 495.0
- rheumatoid 714.81
- silica NEC 502
  - and carbon 500
- silicate NEC 502
- talc 502

Pneumocystis carinii pneumonia 136.3
Pneumocystosis 136.3
- with pneumonia 136.3

Pneumoenteritis 025
Pneumohemopericardium (see also Pericarditis) 423.9
Pneumohemothorax (see also Hemothorax) 511.8
- traumatic 860.4
  - with open wound into thorax 860.5

Pneumohydropericardium (see also Pericarditis) 423.9
Pneumohydrothorax (see also Hydrothorax) 511.8
Pneumomediastinum 518.1
- congenital 770.2
- fetus or newborn 770.2

Pneumomycosis 117.9
Pneumonia (acute) (Alpenstich) (benign) (bilateral) (brain) (cerebral) (circumscribed) (congestive) (creeping) (delayed resolution) (double) (epidemic) (fever) (flash) (fulminant) (fungoid) (granulomatous) (hemorrhagic) (incipient) (infantile) (infectious) (infiltration) (insular) (intermittent) (latent) (lobe) (migratory) (newborn) (organized) (overwhelming) (primary) (progressive) (pseudolobar) (purulent) (resolved) (secondary) (senile) (septic) (suppurative) (terminal) (true) (unresolved) (vesicular) 486
- with influenza, flu, or grippe 487.0
- adenoviral 480.0
- adynamic 514
- alba 090.0
- allergic 518.3
- alveolar — see Pneumonia, lobar
- anaerobes 482.81
- anthrax 022.1 [484.5]
- apex, apical — see Pneumonia, lobar
- ascaris 127.0 [484.8]

Index to Diseases

Pneumonia — continued
- aspiration 507.0
  - due to
    - aspiration of microorganisms
      - bacterial 482.9
        - specified type NEC 482.89
      - specified organism NEC 483.8
        - bacterial NEC 482.89
      - viral 480.9
        - specified type NEC 480.8
    - food (regurgitated) 507.0
    - gastric secretions 507.0
    - milk 507.0
    - oils, essences 507.1
    - solids, liquids NEC 507.8
    - vomitus 507.0
  - newborn 770.1
- asthenic 514
- atypical (disseminated, focal) (primary) 486
  - with influenza 487.0
- bacillus 482.9
  - specified type NEC 482.89
- bacterial 482.9
  - specified type NEC 482.89
- Bacteroides (fragilis) (oralis) (melaninogenicus) 482.81
- basal, basic, basilar — see Pneumonia, lobar
- broncho-, bronchial (confluent) (croupous) (diffuse) (disseminated) (hemorrhagic) (involving lobes) (lobar) (terminal) 485
  - with influenza 487.0
  - allergic 518.3
  - aspiration (see also Pneumonia, aspiration) 507.0
  - bacterial 482.9
    - specified type NEC 482.89
  - capillary 466.19
    - with bronchospasm or obstruction 466.19
  - chronic (see also Fibrosis, lung) 515
  - congenital (infective) 770.0
  - diplococcal 481
  - Eaton's agent 483.0
  - Escherichia coli (E. coli) 482.82
  - Friedländer's bacillus 482.0
  - Hemophilus influenzae 482.2
  - hiberno-vernal 083.0 [484.8]
  - hypostatic 514
  - influenzal 487.0
  - inhalation (see also Pneumonia, aspiration) 507.0
    - due to fumes or vapors (chemical) 506.0
  - Klebsiella 482.0
  - lipid 507.1
    - endogenous 516.8
  - Mycoplasma (pneumoniae) 483.0
  - ornithosis 073.0
  - pleuropneumonia-like organisms (PPLO) 483.0
  - pneumococcal 481
  - Proteus 482.83
  - pseudomonas 482.1
  - specified organism NEC 483.8
    - bacterial NEC 482.89
  - staphylococcal 482.40
    - aureus 482.41
    - specified type NEC 482.49
  - streptococcal — see Pneumonia, streptococcal
  - typhoid 002.0 [484.8]
  - viral, virus (see also Pneumonia, viral) 480.9
- butyrivibrio (fibriosolvens) 482.81
- Candida 112.4
- capillary 466.19
  - with bronchospasm or obstruction 466.19
- caseous (see also Tuberculosis) 011.6 ✓5ᵗʰ
- catarrhal — see Pneumonia, broncho-central — see Pneumonia, lobar
- Chlamydia, chlamydial 483.1
  - pneumoniae 483.1
  - psittaci 073.0
  - specified type NEC 483.1
  - trachomatis 483.1
- cholesterol 516.8
- chronic (see also Fibrosis, lung) 515
- Clostridium (haemolyticum) (novyi) NEC 482.81
- confluent — see Pneumonia, broncho-

Index to Diseases

Pneumonia — continued
- congenital (infective) 770.0
  - aspiration 770.1
- croupous — *see* Pneumonia, lobar
- cytomegalic inclusion 078.5 *[484.1]*
- deglutition (*see also* Pneumonia, aspiration) 507.0
- desquamative interstitial 516.8
- diffuse — *see* Pneumonia, broncho-
- diplococcal, diplococcus (broncho-) (lobar) 481
- disseminated (focal) — *see* Pneumonia, broncho-
- due to
  - adenovirus 480.0
  - Bacterium anitratum 482.83
  - Chlamydia, chlamydial 483.1
    - pneumoniae 483.1
    - psittaci 073.0
    - specified type NEC 483.1
    - trachomatis 483.1
  - coccidioidomycosis 114.0
  - Diplococcus (pneumoniae) 481
  - Eaton's agent 483.0
  - Escherichia coli (E. coli) 482.82
  - Friedländer's bacillus 482.0
  - fumes or vapors (chemical) (inhalation) 506.0
  - fungus NEC 117.9 *[484.7]*
    - coccidioidomycosis 114.0
  - Hemophilus influenzae (H. influenzae) 482.2
  - Herellea 482.83
  - influenza 487.0
  - Klebsiella pneumoniae 482.0
  - Mycoplasma (pneumoniae) 483.0
  - parainfluenza virus 480.2
  - pleuropneumonia-like organism (PPLO) 483.0
  - Pneumococcus 481
  - Pneumocystis carinii 136.3
  - Proteus 482.83
  - pseudomonas 482.1
  - respiratory syncytial virus 480.1
  - rickettsia 083.9 *[484.8]*
  - specified
    - bacteria NEC 482.89
    - organism NEC 483.8
    - virus NEC 480.8
  - Staphylococcus 482.40
    - aureus 482.41
    - specified type NEC 482.49
  - Streptococcus — *see* Pneumonia, streptococcal
  - pneumoniae 481
  - virus (*see also* Pneumonia, viral) 480.9
- Eaton's agent 483.0
- embolic, embolism (*see also* Embolism, pulmonary) 415.1 ✓5ᵗʰ
- eosinophilic 518.3
- Escherichia coli (E. coli) 482.82
- Eubacterium 482.81
- fibrinous — *see* Pneumonia, lobar
- fibroid (chronic)(*see also* Fibrosis, lung) 515
- fibrous (*see also* Fibrosis, lung) 515
- Friedländer's bacillus 482.0
- Fusobacterium (nucleatum) 482.81
- gangrenous 513.0
- giant cell (*see also* Pneumonia, viral) 480.9
- gram-negative bacteria NEC 482.83
  - anaerobic 482.81
- grippal 487.0
- Hemophilus influenzae (bronchial) (lobar) 482.2
- hypostatic (broncho-) (lobar) 514
- in
  - actinomycosis 039.1
  - anthrax 022.1 *[484.5]*
  - aspergillosis 117.3 *[484.6]*
  - candidiasis 112.4
  - coccidioidomycosis 114.0
  - cytomegalic inclusion disease 078.5 *[484.1]*
  - histoplasmosis (*see also* Histoplasmosis) 115.95
  - infectious disease NEC 136.9 *[484.8]*
  - measles 055.1
  - mycosis, systemic NEC 117.9 *[484.7]*
  - nocardiasis, nocardiosis 039.1
  - ornithosis 073.0
  - pneumocystosis 136.3

Pneumonia — continued
- in — *continued*
  - psittacosis 073.0
  - Q fever 083.0 *[484.8]*
  - salmonellosis 003.22
  - toxoplasmosis 130.4
  - tularemia 021.2
  - typhoid (fever) 002.0 *[484.8]*
  - varicella 052.1
  - whooping cough (*see also* Whooping cough) 033.9 *[484.3]*
- infective, acquired prenatally 770.0
- influenzal (broncho) (lobar) (virus) 487.0
- inhalation (*see also* Pneumonia, aspiration) 507.0
  - fumes or vapors (chemical) 506.0
- interstitial 516.8
  - with influenzal 487.0
  - acute 136.3
  - chronic (*see also* Fibrosis, lung) 515
  - desquamative 516.8
  - hypostatic 514
  - lipoid 507.1
  - lymphoid 516.8
  - plasma cell 136.3
  - pseudomonas 482.1
- intrauterine (infective) 770.0
  - aspiration 770.1
- Klebsiella pneumoniae 482.0
- Legionnaires' 482.84
- lipid, lipoid (exogenous) (interstitial) 507.1
  - endogenous 516.8
- lobar (diplococcal) (disseminated) (double) (interstitial) (pneumococcal, any type) 481
  - with influenza 487.0
  - bacterial 482.9
    - specified type NEC 482.89
  - chronic (*see also* Fibrosis, lung) 515
  - Escherichia coli (E. coli) 482.82
  - Friedländer's bacillus 482.0
  - Hemophilus influenzae (H. influenzae) 482.2
  - hypostatic 514
  - influenzal 487.0
  - Klebsiella 482.0
  - ornithosis 073.0
  - Proteus 482.83
  - pseudomonas 482.1
  - psittacosis 073.0
  - specified organism NEC 483.8
    - bacterial NEC 482.89
  - staphylococcal 482.40
    - aureus 482.41
    - specified type NEC 482.49
  - streptococcal — *see* Pneumonia, streptococcal
  - viral, virus (*see also* Pneumonia, viral) 480.9
- lobular (confluent) — *see* Pneumonia, broncho-
- Löffler's 518.3
- massive — *see* Pneumonia, lobar
- meconium 770.1
- metastatic NEC 038.8 *[484.8]*
- Mycoplasma (pneumoniae) 483.0
- necrotic 513.0
- nitrogen dioxide 506.9
- orthostatic 514
- parainfluenza virus 480.2
- parenchymatous (*see also* Fibrosis, lung) 515
- passive 514
- patchy — *see* Pneumonia, broncho-
- Peptococcus 482.81
- Peptostreptococcus 482.81
- plasma cell 136.3
- pleurolobar — *see* Pneumonia, lobar
- pleuropneumonia-like organism (PPLO) 483.0
- pneumococcal (broncho) (lobar) 481
- Pneumocystis (carinii) 136.3
- postinfectional NEC 136.9 *[484.8]*
- postmeasles 055.1
- postoperative 997.3
- primary atypical 486
- Proprionibacterium 482.81
- Proteus 482.83
- pseudomonas 482.1
- psittacosis 073.0
- radiation 508.0
- respiratory syncytial virus 480.1
- resulting from a procedure 997.3
- rheumatic 390 *[517.1]*

Pneumonia — continued
- Salmonella 003.22
- segmented, segmental — *see* Pneumonia, broncho-
- Serratia (marcescens) 482.83
- specified
  - bacteria NEC 482.89
  - organism NEC 483.8
  - virus NEC 480.8
- spirochetal 104.8 *[484.8]*
- staphylococcal (broncho) (lobar) 482.40
  - aureus 482.41
  - specified type NEC 482.49
- static, stasis 514
- streptococcal (broncho) (lobar) NEC 482.30
  - Group
    - A 482.31
    - B 482.32
    - specified NEC 482.39
  - pneumoniae 481
  - specified type NEC 482.39
- Streptococcus pneumoniae 481
- traumatic (complication) (early) (secondary) 958.8
- tuberculous (any) (*see also* Tuberculosis) 011.6 ✓5ᵗʰ
- tularemic 021.2
- TWAR agent 483.1
- varicella 052.1
- Veillonella 482.81
- viral, virus (broncho) (interstitial) (lobar) 480.9
  - with influenza, flu, or grippe 487.0
  - adenoviral 480.0
  - parainfluenza 480.2
  - respiratory syncytial 480.1
  - specified type NEC 480.8
- white (congenital) 090.0

Pneumonic — *see* condition

Pneumonitis (acute) (primary) (*see also* Pneumonia) 486
- allergic 495.9
  - specified type NEC 495.8
- aspiration 507.0
  - due to fumes or gases 506.0
  - newborn 770.1
  - obstetric 668.0 ✓5ᵗʰ
- chemical 506.0
  - due to fumes or gases 506.0
- cholesterol 516.8
- chronic (*see also* Fibrosis, lung) 515
- congenital rubella 771.0
- due to
  - fumes or vapors 506.0
  - inhalation
    - food (regurgitated), milk, vomitus 507.0
    - oils, essences 507.1
    - saliva 507.0
    - solids, liquids NEC 507.8
  - toxoplasmosis (acquired) 130.4
    - congenital (active) 771.2 *[484.8]*
- eosinophilic 518.3
- fetal aspiration 770.1
- hypersensitivity 495.9
- interstitial (chronic) (*see also* Fibrosis, lung) 515
- lymphoid 516.8
- lymphoid, interstitial 516.8
- meconium 770.1
- postanesthetic
  - correct substance properly administered 507.0
  - obstetric 668.0 ✓5ᵗʰ
  - overdose or wrong substance given 968.4
    - specified anesthetic — *see* Table of Drugs and Chemicals
- postoperative 997.3
  - obstetric 668.0 ✓5ᵗʰ
- radiation 508.0
- rubella, congenital 771.0
- "ventilation" 495.7
- wood-dust 495.8

Pneumonoconiosis — *see* Pneumoconiosis

Pneumoparotid 527.8

Pneumopathy NEC 518.89
- alveolar 516.9
  - specified NEC 516.8

Pneumopathy NEC — *continued*
 due to dust NEC 504
 parietoalveolar 516.9
  specified condition NEC 516.8
Pneumopericarditis (*see also* Pericarditis) 423.9
 acute 420.90
Pneumopericardium — *see also* Pericarditis
 congenital 770.2
 fetus or newborn 770.2
 traumatic (post) (*see also* Pneumothorax, traumatic) 860.0
  with open wound into thorax 860.1
Pneumoperitoneum 568.89
 fetus or newborn 770.2
Pneumophagia (psychogenic) 306.4
Pneumopleurisy, pneumopleuritis (*see also* Pneumonia) 486
Pneumopyopericardium 420.99
Pneumopyothorax (*see also* Pyopneumothorax) 510.9
 with fistula 510.0
Pneumorrhagia 786.3
 newborn 770.3
 tuberculous (*see also* Tuberculosis, pulmonary) 011.9 ☑5ᵗʰ
Pneumosiderosis (occupational) 503
Pneumothorax (acute) (chronic) 512.8
 congenital 770.2
 due to operative injury of chest wall or lung 512.1
  accidental puncture or laceration 512.1
 fetus or newborn 770.2
 iatrogenic 512.1
 postoperative 512.1
 spontaneous 512.8
  fetus or newborn 770.2
  tension 512.0
 sucking 512.8
  iatrogenic 512.1
  postoperative 512.1
 tense valvular, infectional 512.0
 tension 512.0
  iatrogenic 512.1
  postoperative 512.1
  spontaneous 512.0
 traumatic 860.0
  with
   hemothorax 860.4
    with open wound into thorax 860.5
   open wound into thorax 860.1
 tuberculous (*see also* Tuberculosis) 011.7 ☑5ᵗʰ
Pocket(s)
 endocardial (*see also* Endocarditis) 424.90
 periodontal 523.8
Podagra 274.9
Podencephalus 759.89
Poikilocytosis 790.09
Poikiloderma 709.09
 Civatte's 709.09
 congenital 757.33
 vasculare atrophicans 696.2
Poikilodermatomyositis 710.3
Pointed ear 744.29
Poise imperfect 729.9
Poisoned — *see* Poisoning
Poisoning (acute) — *see also* Table of Drugs and Chemicals
 Bacillus, B.
  aertrycke (*see also* Infection, Salmonella) 003.9
  botulinus 005.1
  cholerae (suis) (*see also* Infection, Salmonella) 003.9
  paratyphosus (*see also* Infection, Salmonella) 003.9
  suipestifer (*see also* Infection, Salmonella) 003.9
 bacterial toxins NEC 005.9
 berries, noxious 988.2
 blood (general) — *see* Septicemia
 botulism 005.1
 bread, moldy, mouldy — *see* Poisoning, food
 damaged meat — *see* Poisoning, food

Poisoning (acute) — *see also* Table of Drugs and Chemicals — *continued*
 death-cap (Amanita phalloides) (Amanita verna) 988.1
 decomposed food — *see* Poisoning, food
 diseased food — *see* Poisoning, food
 drug — *see* Table of Drugs and Chemicals
 epidemic, fish, meat, or other food — *see* Poisoning, food
 fava bean 282.2
 fish (bacterial) — *see also* Poisoning, food
  noxious 988.0
 food (acute) (bacterial) (diseased) (infected) NEC 005.9
  due to
   bacillus
    aertrycke (*see also* Poisoning, food, due to Salmonella) 003.9
    botulinus 005.1
    cereus 005.89
    choleraesuis (*see also* Poisoning, food, due to Salmonella) 003.9
    paratyphosus (*see also* Poisoning, food, due to Salmonella) 003.9
    suipestifer (*see also* Poisoning, food, due to Salmonella) 003.9
   Clostridium 005.3
    botulinum 005.1
    perfringens 005.2
    welchii 005.2
   Salmonella (aertrycke) (callinarum) (choleraesuis) (enteritidis) (paratyphi) (suipestifer) 003.9
    with
     gastroenteritis 003.0
     localized infection(s) (*see also* Infection, Salmonella) 003.20
     septicemia 003.1
     specified manifestation NEC 003.8
   specified bacterium NEC 005.89
   Staphylococcus 005.0
   Streptococcus 005.8 ☑5ᵗʰ
   Vibrio parahaemolyticus 005.4
   Vibrio vulnificus 005.81
  noxious or naturally toxic 988.0
   berries 988.2
   fish 988.0
   mushroom 988.1
   plants NEC 988.2
 ice cream — *see* Poisoning, food
 ichthyotoxism (bacterial) 005.9
 kreotoxism, food 005.9
 malarial — *see* Malaria
 meat — *see* Poisoning, food
 mushroom (noxious) 988.1
 mussel — *see also* Poisoning, food
  noxious 988.0
 noxious foodstuffs (*see also* Poisoning, food, noxious) 988.9
  specified type NEC 988.8
 plants, noxious 988.2
 pork — *see also* Poisoning, food
  specified NEC 988.8
  Trichinosis 124
 ptomaine — *see* Poisoning, food
 putrefaction, food — *see* Poisoning, food
 radiation 508.0
 Salmonella (*see also* Infection, Salmonella) 003.9
 sausage — *see also* Poisoning, food
  Trichinosis 124
 saxitoxin 988.0
 shellfish — *see also* Poisoning, food
  noxious 988.0
 Staphylococcus, food 005.0
 toxic, from disease NEC 799.8
 truffles — *see* Poisoning, food
 uremic — *see* Uremia
 uric acid 274.9
Poison ivy, oak, sumac or other plant dermatitis 692.6
Poker spine 720.0
Policeman's disease 729.2
Polioencephalitis (acute) (bulbar) (*see also* Poliomyelitis, bulbar) 045.0 ☑5ᵗʰ
 inferior 335.22

Polioencephalitis (*see also* Poliomyelitis, bulbar) — *continued*
 influenzal 487.8
 superior hemorrhagic (acute) (Wernicke's) 265.1
 Wernicke's (superior hemorrhagic) 265.1
Polioencephalomyelitis (acute) (anterior) (bulbar) (*see also* Polioencephalitis) 045.0 ☑5ᵗʰ
Polioencephalopathy, superior hemorrhagic 265.1
 with
  beriberi 265.0
  pellagra 265.2
Poliomeningoencephalitis — *see* Meningoencephalitis
Poliomyelitis (acute) (anterior) (epidemic) 045.9 ☑5ᵗʰ

 Note — *Use the following fifth-digit subclassification with category 045:*

 0 poliovirus, unspecified type
 1 poliovirus, type I
 2 poliovirus, type II
 3 poliovirus, type III

 with
  paralysis 045.1 ☑5ᵗʰ
   bulbar 045.0 ☑5ᵗʰ
  abortive 045.2 ☑5ᵗʰ
  ascending 045.9 ☑5ᵗʰ
   progressive 045.9 ☑5ᵗʰ
  bulbar 045.0 ☑5ᵗʰ
  cerebral 045.0 ☑5ᵗʰ
  chronic 335.21
  congenital 771.2
  contact V01.2
  deformities 138
  exposure to V01.2
  late effect 138
  nonepidemic 045.9 ☑5ᵗʰ
  nonparalytic 045.2 ☑5ᵗʰ
  old with deformity 138
  posterior, acute 053.19
  residual 138
  sequelae 138
  spinal, acute 045.9 ☑5ᵗʰ
  syphilitic (chronic) 094.89
  vaccination, prophylactic (against) V04.0
Poliosis (eyebrow) (eyelashes) 704.3
 circumscripta (congenital) 757.4
  acquired 704.3
 congenital 757.4
Pollakiuria 788.4 ☑5ᵗʰ
 psychogenic 306.53
Pollinosis 477.0
Pollitzer's disease (hidradenitis suppurativa) 705.83
Polyadenitis (*see also* Adenitis) 289.3
 malignant 020.0
Polyalgia 729.9
Polyangiitis (essential) 446.0
Polyarteritis (nodosa) (renal) 446.0
Polyarthralgia 719.49
 psychogenic 306.0
Polyarthritis, polyarthropathy NEC 716.59
 due to or associated with other specified conditions — *see* Arthritis, due to or associated with
 endemic (*see also* Disease, Kaschin-Beck) 716.0 ☑5ᵗʰ
 inflammatory 714.9
  specified type NEC 714.89
 juvenile (chronic) 714.30
  acute 714.31
 migratory — *see* Fever, rheumatic
 rheumatic 714.0
  fever (acute) — *see* Fever, rheumatic
Polycarential syndrome of infancy 260
Polychondritis (atrophic) (chronic) (relapsing) 733.99
Polycoria 743.46
Polycystic (congenital) (disease) 759.89
 degeneration, kidney — *see* Polycystic, kidney

Polycystic — *continued*
  kidney (congenital) 753.12
    adult type (APKD) 753.13
      autosomal dominant 753.13
      autosomal recessive 753.14
    childhood type (CPKD) 753.14
    infantile type 753.14
  liver 751.62
  lung 518.89
    congenital 748.4
  ovary, ovaries 256.4
  spleen 759.0
Polycythemia (primary) (rubra) (vera) (M9950/1) 238.4
  acquired 289.0
  benign 289.0
    familial 289.6
  due to
    donor twin 776.4
    fall in plasma volume 289.0
    high altitude 289.0
    maternal-fetal transfusion 776.4
    stress 289.0
  emotional 289.0
  erythropoietin 289.0
  familial (benign) 289.6
  Gaisböck's (hypertonica) 289.0
  high altitude 289.0
  hypertonica 289.0
  hypoxemic 289.0
  neonatorum 776.4
  nephrogenous 289.0
  relative 289.0
  secondary 289.0
  spurious 289.0
  stress 289.0
Polycytosis cryptogenica 289.0
Polydactylism, polydactyly 755.00
  fingers 755.01
  toes 755.02
Polydipsia 783.5
Polydystrophic oligophrenia 277.5
Polyembryoma (M9072/3) — *see* Neoplasm, by site, malignant
Polygalactia 676.6 ✓5ᵗʰ
Polyglandular
  deficiency 258.9
  dyscrasia 258.9
  dysfunction 258.9
  syndrome 258.8
Polyhydramnios (*see also* Hydramnios) 657 ✓5ᵗʰ
Polymastia 757.6
Polymenorrhea 626.2
Polymicrogyria 742.2
Polymyalgia 725
  arteritica 446.5
  rheumatica 725
Polymyositis (acute) (chronic) (hemorrhagic) 710.4
  with involvement of
    lung 710.4 [517.8]
    skin 710.3
  ossificans (generalisata) (progressiva) 728.19
  Wagner's (dermatomyositis) 710.3
Polyneuritis, polyneuritic (*see also* Polyneuropathy) 356.9
  alcoholic 357.5
    with psychosis 291.1
  cranialis 352.6
  diabetic 250.6 ✓5ᵗʰ [357.2]
  demyelinating, chronic inflammatory 357.81▲
  due to lack of vitamin NEC 269.2 [357.4]
  endemic 265.0 [357.4]
  erythredema 985.0
  febrile 357.0
  hereditary ataxic 356.3
  idiopathic, acute 357.0
  infective (acute) 357.0
  nutritional 269.9 [357.4]
  postinfectious 357.0
Polyneuropathy (peripheral) 356.9
  alcoholic 357.5
  amyloid 277.3 [357.4]
  arsenical 357.7
  critical illness 357.82

Polyneuropathy — *continued*
  diabetic 250.6 ✓5ᵗʰ [357.2]
  due to
    antitetanus serum 357.6
    arsenic 357.7
    drug or medicinal substance 357.6
      correct substance properly administered 357.6
      overdose or wrong substance given or taken 977.9
      specified drug — *see* Table of Drugs and Chemicals
    lack of vitamin NEC 269.2 [357.4]
    lead 357.7
    organophosphate compounds 357.7
    pellagra 265.2 [357.4]
    porphyria 277.1 [357.4]
    serum 357.6
    toxic agent NEC 357.7
  hereditary 356.0
  idiopathic 356.9
    progressive 356.4
  in
    amyloidosis 277.3 [357.4]
    avitaminosis 269.2 [357.4]
      specified NEC 269.1 [357.4]
    beriberi 265.0 [357.4]
    collagen vascular disease NEC 710.9 [357.1]
    deficiency
      B-complex NEC 266.2 [357.4]
      vitamin B 266.9 [357.4]
      vitamin B 266.1 [357.4]
    diabetes 250.6 ✓5ᵗʰ [357.2]
    diphtheria (*see also* Diphtheria) 032.89 [357.4]
    disseminated lupus erythematosus 710.0 [357.1]
    herpes zoster 053.13
    hypoglycemia 251.2 [357.4]
    malignant neoplasm (M8000/3) NEC 199.1 [357.3]
    mumps 072.72
    pellagra 265.2 [357.4]
    polyarteritis nodosa 446.0 [357.1]
    porphyria 277.1 [357.4]
    rheumatoid arthritis 714.0 [357.1]
    sarcoidosis 135 [357.4]
    uremia 585 [357.4]
  lead 357.7
  nutritional 269.9 [357.4]
    specified NEC 269.8 [357.4]
  postherpetic 053.13
  progressive 356.4
  sensory (hereditary) 356.2
Polyonychia 757.5
Polyopia 368.2
  refractive 368.15
Polyorchism, polyorchidism (three testes) 752.8
Polyorrhymenitis (peritoneal) (*see also* Polyserositis) 568.82
  pericardial 423.2
Polyostotic fibrous dysplasia 756.54
Polyotia 744.1
Polyp, polypus

> Note — Polyps of organs or sites that do not appear in the list below should be coded to the residual category for diseases of the organ or site concerned.

  accessory sinus 471.8
  adenoid tissue 471.0
  adenomatous (M8210/0) — *see also* Neoplasm, by site, benign
    adenocarcinoma in (M8210/3) — *see* Neoplasm, by site, malignant
    carcinoma in (M8210/3) — *see* Neoplasm, by site, malignant
    multiple (M8221/0) — *see* Neoplasm, by site, benign
  antrum 471.8
  anus, anal (canal) (nonadenomatous) 569.0
    adenomatous 211.4
  Bartholin's gland 624.6
  bladder (M8120/1) 236.7
  broad ligament 620.8

Polyp, polypus — *continued*
  cervix 622.7
    adenomatous 219.0
    in pregnancy or childbirth 654.6 ✓5ᵗʰ
      affecting fetus or newborn 763.89
      causing obstructed labor 660.2 ✓5ᵗʰ
    mucous 622.7
    nonneoplastic 622.7
  choanal 471.0
  cholesterol 575.6
  clitoris 624.6
  colon (M8210/0) (*see also* Polyp, adenomatous) 211.3
  corpus uteri 621.0
  dental 522.0
  ear (middle) 385.30
  endometrium 621.0
  ethmoidal (sinus) 471.8
  fallopian tube 620.8
  female genital organs NEC 624.8
  frontal (sinus) 471.8
  gallbladder 575.6
  gingiva 523.8
  gum 523.8
  labia 624.6
  larynx (mucous) 478.4
  malignant (M8000/3) — *see* Neoplasm, by site, malignant
  maxillary (sinus) 471.8
  middle ear 385.30
  myometrium 621.0
  nares
    anterior 471.9
    posterior 471.0
  nasal (mucous) 471.9
    cavity 471.0
    septum 471.9
  nasopharyngeal 471.0
  neoplastic (M8210/0) — *see* Neoplasm, by site, benign
  nose (mucous) 471.9
  oviduct 620.8
  paratubal 620.8
  pharynx 478.29
    congenital 750.29
  placenta, placental 674.4 ✓5ᵗʰ
  prostate 600.2
  pudenda 624.6
  pulp (dental) 522.0
  rectosigmoid 211.4
  rectum (nonadenomatous) 569.0
    adenomatous 211.4
  septum (nasal) 471.9
  sinus (accessory) (ethmoidal) (frontal) (maxillary) (sphenoidal) 471.8
  sphenoidal (sinus) 471.8
  stomach (M8210/0) 211.1
  tube, fallopian 620.8
  turbinate, mucous membrane 471.8
  ureter 593.89
  urethra 599.3
  uterine
    ligament 620.8
    tube 620.8
  uterus (body) (corpus) (mucous) 621.0
    in pregnancy or childbirth 654.1 ✓5ᵗʰ
      affecting fetus or newborn 763.89
      causing obstructed labor 660.2 ✓5ᵗʰ
  vagina 623.7
  vocal cord (mucous) 478.4
  vulva 624.6
Polyphagia 783.6
Polypoid — *see* condition
Polyposis — *see also* Polyp
  coli (adenomatous) (M8220/0) 211.3
    adenocarcinoma in (M8220/3) 153.9
    carcinoma in (M8220/3) 153.9
  familial (M8220/0) 211.3
  intestinal (adenomatous) (M8220/0) 211.3
  multiple (M8221/0) — *see* Neoplasm, by site, benign
Polyradiculitis (acute) 357.0
Polyradiculoneuropathy (acute) (segmentally demyelinating) 357.0
Polysarcia 278.00

Polyserositis (peritoneal) 568.82
- due to pericarditis 423.2
- paroxysmal (familial) 277.3
- pericardial 423.2
- periodic 277.3
- pleural — see Pleurisy
- recurrent 277.3
- tuberculous (see also Tuberculosis, polyserositis) 018.9

Polysialia 527.7
Polysplenia syndrome 759.0
Polythelia 757.6
Polytrichia (see also Hypertrichosis) 704.1
Polyunguia (congenital) 757.5
- acquired 703.8

Polyuria 788.42
Pompe's disease (glycogenosis II) 271.0
Pompholyx 705.81
Poncet's disease (tuberculous rheumatism) (see also Tuberculosis) 015.9
Pond fracture — see Fracture, skull, vault
Ponos 085.0
Pons, pontine — see condition
Poor
- contractions, labor 661.2
  - affecting fetus or newborn 763.7
- fetal growth NEC 764.9
  - affecting management of pregnancy 656.5
- incorporation
  - artificial skin graft 996.55
  - decellularized allodermis graft 996.55
- obstetrical history V13.49
  - affecting management of current pregnancy V23.49
    - pre-term labor V23.41
  - pre-term labor V13.41
- sucking reflex (newborn) 796.1
- vision NEC 369.9

Poradenitis, nostras 099.1
Porencephaly (congenital) (developmental) (true) 742.4
- acquired 348.0
- nondevelopmental 348.0
- traumatic (post) 310.2

Porocephaliasis 134.1
Porokeratosis 757.39
- disseminated superficial actinic (DSAP) 692.75

Poroma, eccrine (M8402/0) — see Neoplasm, skin, benign
Porphyria (acute) (congenital) (constitutional) (erythropoietic) (familial) (hepatica) (idiopathic) (idiosyncratic) (intermittent) (latent) (mixed hepatic) (photosensitive) (South African genetic) (Swedish) 277.1
- acquired 277.1
- cutaneatarda
  - hereditaria 277.1
  - symptomatica 277.1
- due to drugs
  - correct substance properly administered 277.1
  - overdose or wrong substance given or taken 977.9
    - specified drug — see Table of Drugs and Chemicals
- secondary 277.1
- toxic NEC 277.1
- variegata 277.1

Porphyrinuria (acquired) (congenital) (secondary) 277.1
Porphyruria (acquired) (congenital) 277.1
Portal — see condition
Port wine nevus or mark 757.32
Posadas-Wernicke disease 114.9
Position
- fetus, abnormal (see also Presentation, fetal) 652.9
- teeth, faulty 524.3

Positive
- culture (nonspecific) 795.39 ▲
  - AIDS virus V08
  - blood 790.7
- culture — continued
  - HIV V08
  - human immunodeficiency virus V08
  - nose 795.39 ▲
  - skin lesion NEC 795.39 ▲
  - spinal fluid 792.0
  - sputum 795.39 ▲
  - stool 792.1
  - throat 795.39 ▲
  - urine 791.9
  - wound 795.39 ▲
- findings, anthrax 795.31 ●
- HIV V08
- human immunodeficiency virus (HIV) V08
- PPD 795.5
- serology
  - AIDS virus V08
    - inconclusive 795.71
  - HIV V08
    - inconclusive 795.71
  - human immunodeficiency virus (HIV) V08
    - inconclusive 795.71
  - syphilis 097.1
    - with signs or symptoms — see Syphilis, by site and stage
    - false 795.6
- skin test 795.7
  - tuberculin (without active tuberculosis) 795.5
- VDRL 097.1
  - with signs or symptoms — see Syphilis, by site and stage
  - false 795.6
- Wassermann reaction 097.1
  - false 795.6

Postcardiotomy syndrome 429.4
Postcaval ureter 753.4
Postcholecystectomy syndrome 576.0
Postclimacteric bleeding 627.1
Postcommissurotomy syndrome 429.4
Postconcussional syndrome 310.2
Postcontusional syndrome 310.2
Postcricoid region — see condition
Post-dates (pregnancy) — see Pregnancy
Postencephalitic — see also condition
- syndrome 310.8

Posterior — see condition
Posterolateral sclerosis (spinal cord) — see Degeneration, combined
Postexanthematous — see condition
Postfebrile — see condition
Postgastrectomy dumping syndrome 564.2
Posthemiplegic chorea 344.89
Posthemorrhagic anemia (chronic) 280.0
- acute 285.1
- newborn 776.5

Posthepatitis syndrome 780.79
Postherpetic neuralgia (intercostal) (syndrome) (zoster) 053.19
- geniculate ganglion 053.11
- ophthalmica 053.19
- trigeminal 053.12

Posthitis 607.1
Postimmunization complication or reaction — see Complications, vaccination
Postinfectious — see condition
Postinfluenzal syndrome 780.79
Postlaminectomy syndrome 722.80
- cervical, cervicothoracic 722.81
- kyphosis 737.12
- lumbar, lumbosacral 722.83
- thoracic, thoracolumbar 722.82

Postleukotomy syndrome 310.0
Postlobectomy syndrome 310.0
Postmastectomy lymphedema (syndrome) 457.0
Postmaturity, postmature (fetus or newborn) 766.2
- affecting management of pregnancy
  - post term pregnancy 645.1
  - prolonged pregnancy 645.2
- syndrome 766.2

Postmeasles — see also condition
- complication 055.8
- specified NEC 055.79

Postmenopausal
- endometrium (atrophic) 627.8
  - suppurative (see also Endometritis) 615.9
- hormone replacement V07.4
- status (age related) (natural) V49.81

Postnasal drip — see Sinusitis
Postnatal — see condition
Postoperative — see also condition
- confusion state 293.9
- psychosis 293.9
- status NEC (see also Status (post)) V45.89

Postpancreatectomy hyperglycemia 251.3
Postpartum — see also condition
- observation
  - immediately after delivery V24.0
  - routine follow-up V24.2

Postperfusion syndrome NEC 999.8
- bone marrow 996.85

Postpoliomyelitic — see condition
Postsurgery status NEC (see also Status (post)) V45.89
Post-term (pregnancy) 645.1
- infant (294 days or more gestation) 766.2

Posttraumatic — see condition
Posttraumatic brain syndrome, nonpsychotic 310.2
Post-typhoid abscess 002.0
Postures, hysterical 300.11
Postvaccinal reaction or complication — see Complications, vaccination
Postvagotomy syndrome 564.2
Postvalvulotomy syndrome 429.4
Postvasectomy sperm count V25.8
Potain's disease (pulmonary edema) 514
Potain's syndrome (gastrectasis with dyspepsia) 536.1
Pott's
- curvature (spinal) (see also Tuberculosis) 015.0 [737.43]
- disease or paraplegia (see also Tuberculosis) 015.0 [730.88]
- fracture (closed) 824.4
  - open 824.5
- gangrene 440.24
- osteomyelitis (see also Tuberculosis) 015.0 [730.88]
- spinal curvature (see also Tuberculosis) 015.0 [737.43]
- tumor, puffy (see also Osteomyelitis) 730.2

Potter's
- asthma 502
- disease 753.0
- facies 754.0
- lung 502
- syndrome (with renal agenesis) 753.0

Pouch
- bronchus 748.3
- Douglas' — see condition
- esophagus, esophageal (congenital) 750.4
  - acquired 530.6
- gastric 537.1
- Hartmann's (abnormal sacculation of gallbladder neck) 575.8
- of intestine V44.3
  - attention to V55.3
- pharynx, pharyngeal (congenital) 750.27

Poulet's disease 714.2
Poultrymen's itch 133.8
Poverty V60.2
Prader-Labhart-Willi-Fanconi syndrome (hypogenital dystrophy with diabetic tendency) 759.81
Prader-Willi syndrome (hypogenital dystrophy with diabetic tendency) 759.81
Preachers' voice 784.49
Pre-AIDS — see Human immunodeficiency virus (disease) (illness) (infection)
Preauricular appendage 744.1

Index to Diseases

Prebetalipoproteinemia (acquired) (essential) (familial) (hereditary) (primary) (secondary) 272.1
  with chylomicronemia 272.3
Precipitate labor 661.3 ✓5ᵗʰ
  affecting fetus or newborn 763.6
Preclimacteric bleeding 627.0
  menorrhagia 627.0
Precocious
  adrenarche 259.1
  menarche 259.1
  menstruation 626.8
  pubarche 259.1
  puberty NEC 259.1
  sexual development NEC 259.1
  thelarche 259.1
Precocity, sexual (constitutional) (cryptogenic) (female) (idiopathic) (male) NEC 259.1
  with adrenal hyperplasia 255.2
Precordial pain 786.51
  psychogenic 307.89
Predeciduous teeth 520.2
Prediabetes, prediabetic 790.2
  complicating pregnancy, childbirth, or puerperium 648.8 ✓5ᵗʰ
  fetus or newborn 775.8
Predislocation status of hip, at birth (see also Subluxation, congenital, hip) 754.32
Preeclampsia (mild) 642.4 ✓5ᵗʰ
  with pre-existing hypertension 642.7 ✓5ᵗʰ
  affecting fetus or newborn 760.0
  severe 642.5 ✓5ᵗʰ
  superimposed on pre-existing hypertensive disease 642.7 ✓5ᵗʰ
Preeruptive color change, teeth, tooth 520.8
Preexcitation 426.7
  atrioventricular conduction 426.7
  ventricular 426.7
Preglaucoma 365.00
Pregnancy (single) (uterine) (without sickness) V22.2

> Note — Use the following fifth-digit subclassification with categories 640-648, 651-676:
>
> 0 unspecified as to episode of care
> 1 delivered, with or without mention of antepartum condition
> 2 delivered, with mention of postpartum complication
> 3 antepartum condition or complication
> 4 postpartum condition or complication

  abdominal (ectopic) 633.00 ▲
    with intrauterine pregnancy 633.01 ●
    affecting fetus or newborn 761.4
  abnormal NEC 646.9 ✓5ᵗʰ
  ampullar — see Pregnancy, tubal
  broad ligament — see Pregnancy, cornual
  cervical — see Pregnancy, cornual
  combined (extrauterine and intrauterine) — see Pregnancy, cornual
  complicated (by)
    abnormal, abnormality NEC 646.9 ✓5ᵗʰ
      cervix 654.6 ✓5ᵗʰ
      cord (umbilical) 663.9 ✓5ᵗʰ
      glucose tolerance (conditions classifiable to 790.2) 648.8 ✓5ᵗʰ
      injury 648.9 ✓5ᵗʰ
        obstetrical NEC 665.9 ✓5ᵗʰ
        obstetrical trauma NEC 665.9 ✓5ᵗʰ
      pelvic organs or tissues NEC 654.9 ✓5ᵗʰ
      pelvis (bony) 653.0 ✓5ᵗʰ
      perineum or vulva 654.8 ✓5ᵗʰ
      placenta, placental (vessel) 656.7 ✓5ᵗʰ
      position
        cervix 654.4 ✓5ᵗʰ
        placenta 641.1 ✓5ᵗʰ
          without hemorrhage 641.0 ✓5ᵗʰ
        uterus 654.4 ✓5ᵗʰ

Pregnancy — continued
  complicated (by) — continued
    abnormal, abnormality NEC — continued
      size, fetus 653.5 ✓5ᵗʰ
      uterus (congenital) 654.0 ✓5ᵗʰ
    abscess or cellulitis
      bladder 646.6 ✓5ᵗʰ
      genitourinary tract (conditions classifiable to 590, 595, 597, 599.0, 614-616) 646.6 ✓5ᵗʰ
      kidney 646.6 ✓5ᵗʰ
      urinary tract NEC 646.6 ✓5ᵗʰ
    air embolism 673.0 ✓5ᵗʰ
    albuminuria 646.2 ✓5ᵗʰ
      with hypertension — see Toxemia, of pregnancy
    amnionitis 658.4 ✓5ᵗʰ
    amniotic fluid embolism 673.1 ✓5ᵗʰ
    anemia (conditions classifiable to 280-285) 648.2 ✓5ᵗʰ
    atrophy, yellow (acute) (liver) (subacute) 646.7 ✓5ᵗʰ
    bacilluria, asymptomatic 646.5 ✓5ᵗʰ
    bacteriuria, asymptomatic 646.5 ✓5ᵗʰ
    bicornis or bicornuate uterus 654.0 ✓5ᵗʰ
    bone and joint disorders (conditions classifiable to 720-724 or conditions affecting lower limbs classifiable to 711-719, 725-738) 648.7 ✓5ᵗʰ
    breech presentation 652.2 ✓5ᵗʰ
      with successful version 652.1 ✓5ᵗʰ
    cardiovascular disease (conditions classifiable to 390-398, 410-429) 648.6 ✓5ᵗʰ
      congenital (conditions classifiable to 745-747) 648.5 ✓5ᵗʰ
    cerebrovascular disorders (conditions classifiable to 430-434, 436-437) 674.0 ✓5ᵗʰ
    cervicitis (conditions classifiable to 616.0) 646.6 ✓5ᵗʰ
    chloasma (gravidarum) 646.8 ✓5ᵗʰ
    chorea (gravidarum) — see Eclampsia, pregnancy
    cholelithiasis 646.8 ✓5ᵗʰ ●
    contraction, pelvis (general) 653.1 ✓5ᵗʰ
      inlet 653.2 ✓5ᵗʰ
      outlet 653.3 ✓5ᵗʰ
    convulsions (eclamptic) (uremic) 642.6 ✓5ᵗʰ
      with pre-existing hypertension 642.7 ✓5ᵗʰ
    current disease or condition (nonobstetric)
      abnormal glucose tolerance 648.8 ✓5ᵗʰ
      anemia 648.2 ✓5ᵗʰ
      bone and joint (lower limb) 648.7 ✓5ᵗʰ
      cardiovascular 648.6 ✓5ᵗʰ
        congenital 648.5 ✓5ᵗʰ
      cerebrovascular 674.0 ✓5ᵗʰ
      diabetic 648.0 ✓5ᵗʰ
      drug dependence 648.3 ✓5ᵗʰ
      genital organ or tract 646.6 ✓5ᵗʰ
      gonorrheal 647.1 ✓5ᵗʰ
      hypertensive 642.2 ✓5ᵗʰ
        renal 642.1 ✓5ᵗʰ
      infectious 647.9 ✓5ᵗʰ
        specified type NEC 647.8 ✓5ᵗʰ
      liver 646.7 ✓5ᵗʰ
      malarial 647.4 ✓5ᵗʰ
      nutritional deficiency 648.9 ✓5ᵗʰ
      parasitic NEC 647.8 ✓5ᵗʰ
      renal 646.2 ✓5ᵗʰ
        hypertensive 642.1 ✓5ᵗʰ
      rubella 647.5 ✓5ᵗʰ
      specified condition NEC 648.9 ✓5ᵗʰ
      syphilitic 647.0 ✓5ᵗʰ
      thyroid 648.1 ✓5ᵗʰ
      tuberculous 647.3 ✓5ᵗʰ
      urinary 646.6 ✓5ᵗʰ
      venereal 647.2 ✓5ᵗʰ
      viral NEC 647.6 ✓5ᵗʰ
    cystitis 646.6 ✓5ᵗʰ
    cystocele 654.4 ✓5ᵗʰ
    death of fetus (near term) 656.4 ✓5ᵗʰ
      early pregnancy (before 22 completed weeks gestation) 632
    deciduitis 646.6 ✓5ᵗʰ
    decreased fetal movements 655.7

Pregnancy — continued
  complicated (by) — continued
    diabetes (mellitus) (conditions classifiable to 250) 648.0 ✓5ᵗʰ
    disorders of liver 646.7 ✓5ᵗʰ
    displacement, uterus NEC 654.4 ✓5ᵗʰ
    disproportion — see Disproportion
    double uterus 654.0 ✓5ᵗʰ
    drug dependence (conditions classifiable to 304) 648.3 ✓5ᵗʰ
    dysplasia, cervix 654.6 ✓5ᵗʰ
    early onset of delivery (spontaneous) 644.2 ✓5ᵗʰ
    eclampsia, eclamptic (coma) (convulsions) (delirium) (nephritis) (uremia) 642.6 ✓5ᵗʰ
      with pre-existing hypertension 642.7 ✓5ᵗʰ
    edema 646.1 ✓5ᵗʰ
      with hypertension — see Toxemia, of pregnancy
    effusion, amniotic fluid 658.1 ✓5ᵗʰ
      delayed delivery following 658.2 ✓5ᵗʰ
    embolism
      air 673.0 ✓5ᵗʰ
      amniotic fluid 673.1 ✓5ᵗʰ
      blood-clot 673.2 ✓5ᵗʰ
      cerebral 674.0 ✓5ᵗʰ
      pulmonary NEC 673.2 ✓5ᵗʰ
      pyemic 673.3 ✓5ᵗʰ
      septic 673.3 ✓5ᵗʰ
    emesis (gravidarum) — see Pregnancy, complicated, vomiting
    endometritis (conditions classifiable to 615.0-615.9) 646.6 ✓5ᵗʰ
      decidual 646.6 ✓5ᵗʰ
    excessive weight gain NEC 646.1 ✓5ᵗʰ
    face presentation 652.4 ✓5ᵗʰ
    failure, fetal head to enter pelvic brim 652.5 ✓5ᵗʰ
    false labor (pains) 644.1 ✓5ᵗʰ
    fatigue 646.8 ✓5ᵗʰ
    fatty metamorphosis of liver 646.7 ✓5ᵗʰ
    fetal
      death (near term) 656.4 ✓5ᵗʰ
        early (before 22 completed weeks gestation) 632
      deformity 653.7 ✓5ᵗʰ
      distress 656.8 ✓5ᵗʰ
    fibroid (tumor) (uterus) 654.1 ✓5ᵗʰ
    footling presentation 652.8 ✓5ᵗʰ
      with successful version 652.1 ✓5ᵗʰ
    gallbladder disease 646.8 ✓5ᵗʰ ●
    goiter 648.1 ✓5ᵗʰ
    gonococcal infection (conditions classifiable to 098) 647.1 ✓5ᵗʰ
    gonorrhea (conditions classifiable to 098) 647.1 ✓5ᵗʰ
    hemorrhage 641.9 ✓5ᵗʰ
      accidental 641.2 ✓5ᵗʰ
      before 22 completed weeks gestation NEC 640.9 ✓5ᵗʰ
      cerebrovascular 674.0 ✓5ᵗʰ
      due to
        afibrinogenemia or other coagulation defect (conditions classifiable to 286.0-286.9) 641.3 ✓5ᵗʰ
        leiomyoma, uterine 641.8 ✓5ᵗʰ
        marginal sinus (rupture) 641.2 ✓5ᵗʰ
        premature separation, placenta 641.2 ✓5ᵗʰ
        trauma 641.8 ✓5ᵗʰ
      early (before 22 completed weeks gestation) 640.9 ✓5ᵗʰ
      threatened abortion 640.0 ✓5ᵗʰ
      unavoidable 641.1 ✓5ᵗʰ
    hepatitis (acute) (malignant) (subacute) 646.7 ✓5ᵗʰ
      viral 647.6 ✓5ᵗʰ
    herniation of uterus 654.4 ✓5ᵗʰ
    high head at term 652.5 ✓5ᵗʰ
    hydatidiform mole (delivered) (undelivered) 630
    hydramnios 657 ✓5ᵗʰ
    hydrocephalic fetus 653.6 ✓5ᵗʰ
    hydrops amnii 657 ✓5ᵗʰ
    hydrorrhea 658.1 ✓5ᵗʰ
    hyperemesis (gravidarum) — see Hyperemesis, gravidarum

Pregnancy — *continued*
  complicated (by) — *continued*
    hypertension — *see* Hypertension, complicating pregnancy
    hypertensive
      heart and renal disease 642.2 ✓5
      heart disease 642.2 ✓5
      renal disease 642.2 ✓5
    hyperthyroidism 648.1 ✓5
    hypothyroidism 648.1 ✓5
    hysteralgia 646.8 ✓5
    icterus gravis 646.7 ✓5
    incarceration, uterus 654.3 ✓5
    incompetent cervix (os) 654.5 ✓5
    infection 647.9 ✓5
      amniotic fluid 658.4 ✓5
      bladder 646.6 ✓5
      genital organ (conditions classifiable to 614-616) 646.6 ✓5
      kidney (conditions classifiable to 590.0-590.9) 646.6 ✓5
      urinary (tract) 646.6 ✓5
        asymptomatic 646.5 ✓5
    infective and parasitic diseases NEC 647.8 ✓5
    inflammation
      bladder 646.6 ✓5
      genital organ (conditions classifiable to 614-616) 646.6 ✓5
      urinary tract NEC 646.6 ✓5
    insufficient weight gain 646.8 ✓5
    intrauterine fetal death (near term) NEC 656.4 ✓5
      early (before 22 completed weeks' gestation) 632
    malaria (conditions classifiable to 084) 647.4 ✓5
    malformation, uterus (congenital) 654.0 ✓5
    malnutrition (conditions classifiable to 260-269) 648.9 ✓5
    malposition
      fetus — *see* Pregnancy, complicated, malpresentation
      uterus or cervix 654.4 ✓5
    malpresentation 652.9 ✓5
      with successful version 652.1 ✓5
      in multiple gestation 652.6 ✓5
      specified type NEC 652.8 ✓5
    marginal sinus hemorrhage or rupture 641.2 ✓5
    maternal obesity syndrome 646.1 ✓5
    menstruation 640.8 ✓5
    mental disorders (conditions classifiable to 290-303, 305-316, 317-319) 648.4 ✓5
    mentum presentation 652.4 ✓5
    missed
      abortion 632
      delivery (at or near term) 656.4 ✓5
      labor (at or near term) 656.4 ✓5
    necrosis
      genital organ or tract (conditions classifiable to 614-616) 646.6 ✓5
      liver (conditions classifiable to 570) 646.7 ✓5
      renal, cortical 646.2 ✓5
    nephritis or nephrosis (conditions classifiable to 580-589) 646.2 ✓5
      with hypertension 642.1 ✓5
    nephropathy NEC 646.2 ✓5
    neuritis (peripheral) 646.4 ✓5
    nutritional deficiency (conditions classifiable to 260-269) 648.9 ✓5
    oblique lie or presentation 652.3 ✓5
      with successful version 652.1 ✓5
    obstetrical trauma NEC 665.9 ✓5
    oligohydramnios NEC 658.0 ✓5
    onset of contractions before 37 weeks 644.0 ✓5
    oversize fetus 653.5 ✓5
    papyraceous fetus 646.0 ✓5
    patent cervix 654.5 ✓5
    pelvic inflammatory disease (conditions classifiable to 614-616) 646.6 ✓5
    placenta, placental
      abnormality 656.7 ✓5
        abruptio or ablatio 641.2 ✓5
        detachment 641.2 ✓5

Pregnancy — *continued*
  complicated (by) — *continued*
    placenta, placental — *continued*
      disease 656.7 ✓5
      infarct 656.7 ✓5
      low implantation 641.1 ✓5
        without hemorrhage 641.0 ✓5
      malformation 656.7 ✓5
      malposition 641.1 ✓5
        without hemorrhage 641.0 ✓5
      marginal sinus hemorrhage 641.2 ✓5
      previa 641.1 ✓5
        without hemorrhage 641.0 ✓5
      separation (premature) (undelivered) 641.2 ✓5
    placentitis 658.4 ✓5
    polyhydramnios 657 ✓5
    postmaturity
      post term 645.1 ✓5
      prolonged 645.2 ✓5
    prediabetes 648.8 ✓5
    pre-eclampsia (mild) 642.4 ✓5
      severe 642.5 ✓5
      superimposed on pre-existing hypertensive disease 642.7 ✓5
    premature rupture of membranes 658.1 ✓5
      with delayed delivery 658.2 ✓5
    previous
      infertility V23.0
      nonobstetric condition V23.8 ✓5
      poor obstetrical history V23.49 ▲
      premature delivery V23.41 ▲
      trophoblastic disease (conditions classifiable to 630) V23.1
    prolapse, uterus 654.4 ✓5
    proteinuria (gestational) 646.2 ✓5
      with hypertension — *see* Toxemia, of pregnancy
    pruritus (neurogenic) 646.8 ✓5
    psychosis or psychoneurosis 648.4 ✓5
    ptyalism 646.8 ✓5
    pyelitis (conditions classifiable to 590.0-590.9) 646.6 ✓5
    renal disease or failure NEC 646.2 ✓5
      with secondary hypertension 642.1 ✓5
      hypertensive 642.2 ✓5
    retention, retained dead ovum 631
    retroversion, uterus 654.3 ✓5
    Rh immunization, incompatibility, or sensitization 656.1 ✓5
    rubella (conditions classifiable to 056) 647.5 ✓5
    rupture
      amnion (premature) 658.1 ✓5
        with delayed delivery 658.2 ✓5
      marginal sinus (hemorrhage) 641.2 ✓5
      membranes (premature) 658.1 ✓5
        with delayed delivery 658.2 ✓5
      uterus (before onset of labor) 665.0 ✓5
    salivation (excessive) 646.8 ✓5
    salpingo-oophoritis (conditions classifiable to 614.0-614.2) 646.6 ✓5
    septicemia (conditions classifiable to 038.0-038.9) 647.8 ✓5
      postpartum 670 ✓4
      puerperal 670 ✓4
    spasms, uterus (abnormal) 646.8 ✓5
    specified condition NEC 646.8 ✓5
    spurious labor pains 644.1 ✓5
    superfecundation 651.9 ✓5
    superfetation 651.9 ✓5
    syphilis (conditions classifiable to 090-097) 647.0 ✓5
    threatened
      abortion 640.0 ✓5
      premature delivery 644.2 ✓5
      premature labor 644.0 ✓5
    thrombophlebitis (superficial) 671.2 ✓5
      deep 671.3 ✓5
    thrombosis 671.9 ✓5
      venous (superficial) 671.2 ✓5
        deep 671.3 ✓5
    thyroid dysfunction (conditions classifiable to 240-246) 648.1 ✓5
    thyroiditis 648.1 ✓5
    thyrotoxicosis 648.1 ✓5
    torsion of uterus 654.4 ✓5

Pregnancy — *continued*
  complicated (by) — *continued*
    toxemia — *see* Toxemia, of pregnancy
    transverse lie or presentation 652.3 ✓5
      with successful version 652.1 ✓5
    tuberculosis (conditions classifiable to 010-018) 647.3 ✓5
    tumor
      cervix 654.6 ✓5
      ovary 654.4 ✓5
      pelvic organs or tissue NEC 654.4 ✓5
      uterus (body) 654.1 ✓5
        cervix 654.6 ✓5
      vagina 654.7 ✓5
      vulva 654.8 ✓5
    unstable lie 652.0 ✓5
    uremia — *see* Pregnancy, complicated, renal disease
    urethritis 646.6 ✓5
    vaginitis or vulvitis (conditions classifiable to 616.1) 646.6 ✓5
    varicose
      placental vessels 656.7 ✓5
      veins (legs) 671.0 ✓5
        perineum 671.1 ✓5
        vulva 671.1 ✓5
    varicosity, labia or vulva 671.1 ✓5
    venereal disease NEC (conditions classifiable to 099) 647.2 ✓5
    viral disease NEC (conditions classifiable to 042, 050-055, 057-079) 647.6 ✓5
    vomiting (incoercible) (pernicious) (persistent) (uncontrollable) (vicious) 643.9 ✓5
      due to organic disease or other cause 643.8 ✓5
      early — *see* Hyperemesis, gravidarum
      late (after 22 completed weeks gestation) 643.2 ✓5
    young maternal age 659.8 ✓5
  complications NEC 646.9 ✓5
  cornual 633.80 ▲
    with intrauterine pregnancy 633.81 ●
    affecting fetus or newborn 761.4
  death, maternal NEC 646.9 ✓5
  delivered — *see* Delivery
  ectopic (ruptured) NEC 633.90 ▲
    with intrauterine pregnancy 633.91 ●
    abdominal — *see* Pregnancy, abdominal
    affecting fetus or newborn 761.4
    combined (extrauterine and intrauterine) — *see* Pregnancy, cornual
    ovarian — *see* Pregnancy, ovarian
    specified type NEC 633.80 ▲
      with intrauterine pregnancy 633.81 ●
      affecting fetus or newborn 761.4
    tubal — *see* Pregnancy, tubal
  examination, pregnancy not confirmed V72.4
  extrauterine — *see* Pregnancy, ectopic
  fallopian — *see* Pregnancy, tubal
  false 300.11
    labor (pains) 644.1 ✓5
  fatigue 646.8 ✓5
  illegitimate V61.6
  incidental finding V22.2
  in double uterus 654.0 ✓5
  interstitial — *see* Pregnancy, cornual
  intraligamentous — *see* Pregnancy, cornual
  intramural — *see* Pregnancy, cornual
  intraperitoneal — *see* Pregnancy, abdominal
  isthmian — *see* Pregnancy, tubal
  management affected by
    abnormal, abnormality
      fetus (suspected) 655.9 ✓5
        specified NEC 655.8 ✓5
      placenta 656.7 ✓5
    advanced maternal age NEC 659.6 ✓5
      multigravida 659.6 ✓5
      primigravida 659.5 ✓5
    antibodies (maternal)
      anti-c 656.1 ✓5
      anti-d 656.1 ✓5
      anti-e 656.1 ✓5
      blood group (ABO) 656.2 ✓5
        Rh(esus) 656.1 ✓5
    elderly multigravida 659.6 ✓5
    elderly primigravida 659.5 ✓5

Index to Diseases

Pregnancy — *continued*
  management affected by — *continued*
    fetal (suspected)
      abnormality 655.9 ✓5ᵗʰ
        acid-base balance 656.8 ✓5ᵗʰ
        heart rate or rhythm 659.7 ✓5ᵗʰ
        specified NEC 655.8 ✓5ᵗʰ
      acidemia 656.3 ✓5ᵗʰ
      anencephaly 655.0 ✓5ᵗʰ
      bradycardia 659.7 ✓5ᵗʰ
      central nervous system malformation 655.0 ✓5ᵗʰ
      chromosomal abnormalities (conditions classifiable to 758.0-758.9) 655.1 ✓5ᵗʰ
      damage from
        drugs 655.5 ✓5ᵗʰ
          obstetric, anesthetic, or sedative 655.5 ✓5ᵗʰ
        environmental toxins 655.8 ✓5ᵗʰ
        intrauterine contraceptive device 655.8 ✓5ᵗʰ
        maternal
          alcohol addiction 655.4 ✓5ᵗʰ
          disease NEC 655.4 ✓5ᵗʰ
          drug use 655.5 ✓5ᵗʰ
          listeriosis 655.4 ✓5ᵗʰ
          rubella 655.3 ✓5ᵗʰ
          toxoplasmosis 655.4 ✓5ᵗʰ
          viral infection 655.3 ✓5ᵗʰ
        radiation 655.6 ✓5ᵗʰ
      death (near term) 656.4 ✓5ᵗʰ
        early (before 22 completed weeks' gestation) 632
      distress 656.8 ✓5ᵗʰ
      excessive growth 656.6 ✓5ᵗʰ
      growth retardation 656.5 ✓5ᵗʰ
      hereditary disease 655.2 ✓5ᵗʰ
      hydrocephalus 655.0 ✓5ᵗʰ
      intrauterine death 656.4 ✓5ᵗʰ
      poor growth 656.5 ✓5ᵗʰ
      spina bifida (with myelomeningocele) 655.0 ✓5ᵗʰ
    fetal-maternal hemorrhage 656.0 ✓5ᵗʰ
    hereditary disease in family (possibly) affecting fetus 655.2 ✓5ᵗʰ
    incompatibility, blood groups (ABO) 656.2 ✓5ᵗʰ
      rh(esus) 656.1 ✓5ᵗʰ
    insufficient prenatal care V23.7
    intrauterine death 656.4 ✓5ᵗʰ
    isoimmunization (ABO) 656.2 ✓5ᵗʰ
      rh(esus) 656.1 ✓5ᵗʰ
    large-for-dates fetus 656.6 ✓5ᵗʰ
    light-for-dates fetus 656.5 ✓5ᵗʰ
    meconium in liquor 656.8 ✓5ᵗʰ
    mental disorder (conditions classifiable to 290-303, 305-316, 317-319) 648.4 ✓5ᵗʰ
    multiparity (grand) 659.4 ✓5ᵗʰ
    poor obstetric history V23.49 ▲
      pre-term labor V23.41 ●
    postmaturity
      post term 645.1 ✓5ᵗʰ
      prolonged 645.2 ✓5ᵗʰ
    post term pregnancy 645.1 ✓5ᵗʰ
    previous
      abortion V23.2
        habitual 646.3 ✓5ᵗʰ
      cesarean delivery 654.2 ✓5ᵗʰ
      difficult delivery V23.49 ▲
      forceps delivery V23.49 ▲
      habitual abortions 646.3 ✓5ᵗʰ
      hemorrhage, antepartum or postpartum V23.49 ▲
      hydatidiform mole V23.1
      infertility V23.0
      malignancy NEC V23.8 ✓5ᵗʰ
      nonobstetrical conditions V23.8 ✓5ᵗʰ
      premature delivery V23.41 ▲
      trophoblastic disease (conditions in 630) V23.1
      vesicular mole V23.1
    prolonged pregnancy 645.2 ✓5ᵗʰ
    small-for-dates fetus 656.5 ✓5ᵗʰ
    young maternal age 659.8 ✓5ᵗʰ
  maternal death NEC 646.9 ✓5ᵗʰ

Pregnancy — *continued*
  mesometric (mural) — *see* Pregnancy, cornual
  molar 631
    hydatidiform (*see also* Hydatidiform mole) 630
      previous, affecting management of pregnancy V23.1
    previous, affecting management of pregnancy V23.49 ▲
  multiple NEC 651.9 ✓5ᵗʰ
    with fetal loss and retention of one or more fetus(es) 651.6 ✓5ᵗʰ
    affecting fetus or newborn 761.5
    specified type NEC 651.8 ✓5ᵗʰ
      with fetal loss and retention of one or more fetus(es) 651.6 ✓5ᵗʰ
  mural — *see* Pregnancy, cornual
  observation NEC V22.1
    first pregnancy V22.0
    high-risk V23.9
      specified problem NEC V23.8 ✓5ᵗʰ
  ovarian 633.20 ▲
    with intrauterine pregnancy 633.21 ●
    affecting fetus or newborn 761.4
  postmature
    post term 645.1 ✓5ᵗʰ
    prolonged 645.2 ✓5ᵗʰ
  post term 645.1 ✓5ᵗʰ
  prenatal care only V22.1
    first pregnancy V22.0
    high-risk V23.9
      specified problem NEC V23.8 ✓5ᵗʰ
  prolonged 645.2 ✓5ᵗʰ
  quadruplet NEC 651.2 ✓5ᵗʰ
    with fetal loss and retention of one or more fetus(es) 651.5 ✓5ᵗʰ
    affecting fetus or newborn 761.5
  quintuplet NEC 651.8 ✓5ᵗʰ
    with fetal loss and retention of one or more fetus(es) 651.6 ✓5ᵗʰ
    affecting fetus or newborn 761.5
  sextuplet NEC 651.8 ✓5ᵗʰ
    with fetal loss and retention of one or more fetus(es) 651.6 ✓5ᵗʰ
    affecting fetus or newborn 761.5
  spurious 300.11
  superfecundation NEC 651.9 ✓5ᵗʰ
    with fetal loss and retention of one or more fetus(es) 651.6 ✓5ᵗʰ
  superfetation NEC 651.9 ✓5ᵗʰ
    with fetal loss and retention of one or more fetus(es) 651.6 ✓5ᵗʰ
  supervision (of) (for) — *see also* Pregnancy, management affected by
    elderly
      multigravida V23.82
      primigravida V23.81
    high-risk V23.9
      insufficient prenatal care V23.7
      specified problem NEC V23.8 ✓5ᵗʰ
    multiparity V23.3
    normal NEC V22.1
      first V22.0
    poor
      obstetric history V23.49 ▲
        pre-term labor V23.41 ●
      reproductive history V23.5
    previous
      abortion V23.2
      hydatidiform mole V23.1
      infertility V23.0
      neonatal death V23.5
      stillbirth V23.5
      trophoblastic disease V23.1
      vesicular mole V23.1
    specified problem NEC V23.8 ✓5ᵗʰ
    young
      multigravida V23.84
      primigravida V23.83
  triplet NEC 651.1 ✓5ᵗʰ
    with fetal loss and retention of one or more fetus(es) 651.4 ✓5ᵗʰ
    affecting fetus or newborn 761.5
  tubal (with rupture) 633.10 ▲
    with intrauterine pregnancy 633.11 ●
    affecting fetus or newborn 761.4

Prescription of contraceptives

Pregnancy — *continued*
  twin NEC 651.0 ✓5ᵗʰ
    with fetal loss and retention of one fetus 651.3 ✓5ᵗʰ
    affecting fetus or newborn 761.5
  unconfirmed V72.4
  undelivered (no other diagnosis) V22.2
    with false labor 644.1 ✓5ᵗʰ
    high-risk V23.9
      specified problem NEC V23.8 ✓5ᵗʰ
  unwanted NEC V61.7

Pregnant uterus — *see* condition

Preiser's disease (osteoporosis) 733.09

Prekwashiorkor 260

Preleukemia 238.7

Preluxation of hip, congenital (*see also* Subluxation, congenital, hip) 754.32

Premature — *see also* condition
  beats (nodal) 427.60
    atrial 427.61
    auricular 427.61
    postoperative 997.1
    specified type NEC 427.69
    supraventricular 427.61
    ventricular 427.69
  birth NEC 765.1 ✓5ᵗʰ
  closure
    cranial suture 756.0
    fontanel 756.0
    foramen ovale 745.8
  contractions 427.60
    atrial 427.61
    auricular 427.61
    auriculoventricular 427.61
    heart (extrasystole) 427.60
    junctional 427.60
    nodal 427.60
    postoperative 997.1
    ventricular 427.69
  ejaculation 302.75
  infant NEC 765.1 ✓5ᵗʰ
    excessive 765.0 ✓5ᵗʰ
    light-for-dates — *see* Light-for-dates
  labor 644.2 ✓5ᵗʰ
    threatened 644.0 ✓5ᵗʰ
  lungs 770.4
  menopause 256.31
  puberty 259.1
  rupture of membranes or amnion 658.1 ✓5ᵗʰ
    affecting fetus or newborn 761.1
    delayed delivery following 658.2 ✓5ᵗʰ
  senility (syndrome) 259.8
  separation, placenta (partial) — *see* Placenta, separation
  ventricular systole 427.69

Prematurity NEC 765.1 ✓5ᵗʰ
  extreme 765.0 ✓5ᵗʰ

Premenstrual syndrome 625.4

Premenstrual tension 625.4

Premolarization, cuspids 520.2

Premyeloma 273.1

Prenatal
  care, normal pregnancy V22.1
    first V22.0
  death, cause unknown — *see* Death, fetus
  screening — *see* Antenatal, screening

Prepartum — *see* condition

Preponderance, left or right ventricular 429.3

Prepuce — *see* condition

Presbycardia 797
  hypertensive (*see also* Hypertension, heart) 402.90

Presbycusis 388.01

Presbyesophagus 530.89

Presbyophrenia 310.1

Presbyopia 367.4

Prescription of contraceptives NEC V25.02
  diaphragm V25.02
  oral (pill) V25.01
    repeat V25.41
  repeat V25.40
    oral (pill) V25.41

Presenile

Presenile — see also condition
- aging 259.8
- dementia (see also Dementia, presenile) 290.10

Presenility 259.8

Presentation, fetal
- abnormal 652.9 ✓5th
  - with successful version 652.1 ✓5th
  - before labor, affecting fetus or newborn 761.7
  - causing obstructed labor 660.0 ✓5th
    - affecting fetus or newborn, any, except breech 763.1
  - in multiple gestation (one or more) 652.6 ✓5th
  - specified NEC 652.8 ✓5th
- arm 652.7 ✓5th
  - causing obstructed labor 660.0 ✓5th
- breech (buttocks) (complete) (frank) 652.2 ✓5th
  - with successful version 652.1 ✓5th
    - before labor, affecting fetus or newborn 761.7
  - before labor, affecting fetus or newborn 761.7
- brow 652.4 ✓5th
  - causing obstructed labor 660.0 ✓5th
- buttocks 652.2 ✓5th
- chin 652.4 ✓5th
- complete 652.2 ✓5th
- compound 652.8 ✓5th
- cord 663.0 ✓5th
- extended head 652.4 ✓5th
- face 652.4 ✓5th
  - to pubes 652.8 ✓5th
- footling 652.8 ✓5th
- frank 652.2 ✓5th
- hand, leg, or foot NEC 652.8 ✓5th
- incomplete 652.8 ✓5th
- mentum 652.4 ✓5th
- multiple gestation (one fetus or more) 652.6 ✓5th
- oblique 652.3 ✓5th
  - with successful version 652.1 ✓5th
- shoulder 652.8 ✓5th
  - affecting fetus or newborn 763.1
- transverse 652.3 ✓5th
  - with successful version 652.1 ✓5th
- umbilical cord 663.0 ✓5th
- unstable 652.0 ✓5th

Prespondylolisthesis (congenital) (lumbosacral) 756.11

Pressure
- area, skin ulcer (see also Decubitus) 707.0
- atrophy, spine 733.99
- birth, fetus or newborn NEC 767.9
- brachial plexus 353.0
- brain 348.4
  - injury at birth 767.0
- cerebral — see Pressure, brain
- chest 786.59
- cone, tentorial 348.4
  - injury at birth 767.0
- funis — see Compression, umbilical cord
- hyposystolic (see also Hypotension) 458.9
- increased
  - intracranial 781.99
    - due to
      - benign intracranial hypertension 348.2
      - hydrocephalus — see hydrocephalus
    - injury at birth 767.8
  - intraocular 365.00
- lumbosacral plexus 353.1
- mediastinum 519.3
- necrosis (chronic) (skin) (see also Decubitus) 707.0
- nerve — see Compression, nerve
- paralysis (see also Neuropathy, entrapment) 355.9
- sore (chronic) (see also Decubitus) 707.0
- spinal cord 336.9
- ulcer (chronic) (see also Decubitus) 707.0
- umbilical cord — see Compression, umbilical cord
- venous, increased 459.89

Pre-syncope 780.2

Preterm infant NEC 765.1 ✓5th
- extreme 765.0 ✓5th

Priapism (penis) 607.3

Prickling sensation (see also Disturbance, sensation) 782.0

Prickly heat 705.1

Primary — see condition

Primigravida, elderly
- affecting
  - fetus or newborn 763.89
  - management of pregnancy, labor, and delivery 659.5 ✓5th

Primipara, old
- affecting
  - fetus or newborn 763.89
  - management of pregnancy, labor, and delivery 659.5 ✓5th

Primula dermatitis 692.6

Primus varus (bilateral) (metatarsus) 754.52

P.R.I.N.D. 436

Pringle's disease (tuberous sclerosis) 759.5

Prinzmetal's angina 413.1

Prinzmetal-Massumi syndrome (anterior chest wall) 786.52

Prizefighter ear 738.7

Problem (with) V49.9
- academic V62.3
- acculturation V62.4
- adopted child V61.29
- aged
  - in-law V61.3
  - parent V61.3
  - person NEC V61.8
- alcoholism in family V61.41
- anger reaction (see also Disturbance, conduct) 312.0 ✓5th
- behavior, child 312.9
- behavioral V40.9
  - specified NEC V40.3
- betting V69.3
- cardiorespiratory NEC V47.2
- care of sick or handicapped person in family or household V61.49
- career choice V62.2
- communication V40.1
- conscience regarding medical care V62.6
- delinquency (juvenile) 312.9
- diet, inappropriate V69.1
- digestive NEC V47.3
- ear NEC V41.3
- eating habits, inappropriate V69.1
- economic V60.2
  - affecting care V60.9
  - specified type NEC V60.8
- educational V62.3
- enuresis, child 307.6
- exercise, lack of V69.0
- eye NEC V41.1
- family V61.9
  - specified circumstance NEC V61.8
- fear reaction, child 313.0
- feeding (elderly) (infant) 783.3
  - newborn 779.3
  - nonorganic 307.50
- fetal, affecting management of pregnancy 656.9 ✓5th
  - specified type NEC 656.8 ✓5th
- financial V60.2
- foster child V61.29
  - specified NEC V41.8
- functional V41.9
  - specified type NEC V41.8
- gambling V69.3
- genital NEC V47.5
- head V48.9
  - deficiency V48.0
  - disfigurement V48.6
  - mechanical V48.2
  - motor V48.2
  - movement of V48.2
  - sensory V48.4
  - specified condition NEC V48.8
- hearing V41.2
- high-risk sexual behavior V69.2
- influencing health status NEC V49.89
- internal organ NEC V47.9
  - deficiency V47.0

Problem (with) — continued
- internal organ NEC — continued
  - mechanical or motor V47.1
- interpersonal NEC V62.81
- jealousy, child 313.3
- learning V40.0
- legal V62.5
- life circumstance NEC V62.89
- lifestyle V69.9
  - specified NEC V69.8
- limb V49.9
  - deficiency V49.0
  - disfigurement V49.4
  - mechanical V49.1
  - motor V49.2
  - movement, involving
    - musculoskeletal system V49.1
    - nervous system V49.2
  - sensory V49.3
  - specified condition NEC V49.5
- litigation V62.5
- living alone V60.3
- loneliness NEC V62.89
- marital V61.10
  - involving
    - divorce V61.0
    - estrangement V61.0
    - psychosexual disorder 302.9
    - sexual function V41.7
- mastication V41.6
- medical care, within family V61.49
- mental V40.9
  - specified NEC V40.2
- mental hygiene, adult V40.9
- multiparity V61.5
- nail biting, child 307.9
- neck V48.9
  - deficiency V48.1
  - disfigurement V48.7
  - mechanical V48.3
  - motor V48.3
  - movement V48.3
  - sensory V48.5
  - specified condition NEC V48.8
- neurological NEC 781.99
- none (feared complaint unfounded) V65.5
- occupational V62.2
- parent-child V61.20
- partner V61.10
- personal NEC V62.89
  - interpersonal conflict NEC V62.81
- personality (see also Disorder, personality) 301.9
- phase of life V62.89
- placenta, affecting managment of pregnancy 656.9 ✓5th
  - specified type NEC 656.8 ✓5th
- poverty V60.2
- presence of sick or handicapped person in family or household V61.49
- psychiatric 300.9
- psychosocial V62.9
  - specified type NEC V62.89
- relational NEC V62.81
- relationship, childhood 313.3
- religious or spiritual belief
  - other than medical care V62.89
  - regarding medical care V62.6
- self-damaging behavior V69.8
- sexual
  - behavior, high-risk V69.2
  - function NEC V41.7
- sibling relational V61.8
- sight V41.0
- sleep disorder, child 307.40
- smell V41.5
- speech V40.1
- spite reaction, child (see also Disturbance, conduct) 312.0 ✓5th
- spoiled child reaction (see also Disturbance, conduct) 312.1 ✓5th
- swallowing V41.6
- tantrum, child (see also Disturbance, conduct) 312.1 ✓5th
- taste V41.5
- thumb sucking, child 307.9
- tic, child 307.21

Problem (with) — *continued*
- trunk V48.9
  - deficiency V48.1
  - disfigurement V48.7
  - mechanical V48.3
  - motor V48.3
  - movement V48.3
  - sensory V48.5
  - specified condition NEC V48.8
- unemployment V62.0
- urinary NEC V47.4
- voice production V41.4

Procedure (surgical) not done NEC V64.3
- because of
  - contraindication V64.1
  - patient's decision V64.2
    - for reasons of conscience or religion V62.6
  - specified reason NEC V64.3

Procidentia
- anus (sphincter) 569.1
- rectum (sphincter) 569.1
- stomach 537.89
- uteri 618.1

Proctalgia 569.42
- fugax 564.6
- spasmodic 564.6
  - psychogenic 307.89

Proctitis 569.49
- amebic 006.8
- chlamydial 099.52
- gonococcal 098.7
- granulomatous 555.1
- idiopathic 556.2
  - with ulcerative sigmoiditis 556.3
- tuberculous (*see also* Tuberculosis) 014.8 ✓5
- ulcerative (chronic) (nonspecific) 556.2
  - with ulcerative sigmoiditis 556.3

Proctocele
- female (without uterine prolapse) 618.0
  - with uterine prolapse 618.4
    - complete 618.3
    - incomplete 618.2
- male 569.49

Proctocolitis, idiopathic 556.2
- with ulcerative sigmoiditis 556.3

Proctoptosis 569.1

Proctosigmoiditis 569.89
- ulcerative (chronic) 556.3

Proctospasm 564.6
- psychogenic 306.4

Prodromal-AIDS — *see* Human immunodeficiency virus (disease) (illness) (infection)

Profichet's disease or syndrome 729.9

Progeria (adultorum) (syndrome) 259.8

Prognathism (mandibular) (maxillary) 524.00

Progonoma (melanotic) (M9363/0) — *see* Neoplasm, by site, benign

Progressive — *see* condition

Prolapse, prolapsed
- anus, anal (canal) (sphincter) 569.1
- arm or hand, complicating delivery 652.7 ✓5
  - causing obstructed labor 660.0 ✓5
    - affecting fetus or newborn 763.1
  - fetus or newborn 763.1
- bladder (acquired) (mucosa) (sphincter)
  - congenital (female) (male) 756.71
  - female 618.0
  - male 596.8
- breast implant (prosthetic) 996.54
- cecostomy 569.69
- cecum 569.89
- cervix, cervical (stump) (hypertrophied) 618.1
  - anterior lip, obstructing labor 660.2 ✓5
    - affecting fetus or newborn 763.1
  - congenital 752.49
  - postpartal (old) 618.1
- ciliary body 871.1
- colon (pedunculated) 569.89
- colostomy 569.69
- conjunctiva 372.73
- cord — *see* Prolapse, umbilical cord
- disc (intervertebral) — *see* Displacement, intervertebral disc

Prolapse, prolapsed — *continued*
- duodenum 537.89
- eye implant (orbital) 996.59
  - lens (ocular) 996.53
- fallopian tube 620.4
- fetal extremity, complicating delivery 652.8 ✓5
  - causing obstructed labor 660.0 ✓5
  - fetus or newborn 763.1
- funis — *see* Prolapse, umbilical cord
- gastric (mucosa) 537.89
- genital, female 618.9
  - specified NEC 618.8
- globe 360.81
- ileostomy bud 569.69
- intervertebral disc — *see* Displacement, intervertebral disc
- intestine (small) 569.89
- iris 364.8
  - traumatic 871.1
- kidney (*see also* Disease, renal) 593.0
  - congenital 753.3
- laryngeal muscles or ventricle 478.79
- leg, complicating delivery 652.8 ✓5
  - causing obstructed labor 660.0 ✓5
  - fetus or newborn 763.1
- liver 573.8
- meatus urinarius 599.5
- mitral valve 424.0
- ocular lens implant 996.53
- organ or site, congenital NEC — *see* Malposition, congenital
- ovary 620.4
- pelvic (floor), female 618.8
- perineum, female 618.8
- pregnant uterus 654.4 ✓5
- rectum (mucosa) (sphincter) 569.1
  - due to Trichuris trichiuria 127.3
- spleen 289.59
- stomach 537.89
- umbilical cord
  - affecting fetus or newborn 762.4
  - complicating delivery 663.0 ✓5
- ureter 593.89
  - with obstruction 593.4
- ureterovesical orifice 593.89
- urethra (acquired) (infected) (mucosa) 599.5
  - congenital 753.8
- uterovaginal 618.4
  - complete 618.3
  - incomplete 618.2
  - specified NEC 618.8
- uterus (first degree) (second degree) (third degree) (complete) (without vaginal wall prolapse) 618.1
  - with mention of vaginal wall prolapse — *see* Prolapse, uterovaginal
  - congenital 752.3
  - in pregnancy or childbirth 654.4 ✓5
    - affecting fetus or newborn 763.1
    - causing obstructed labor 660.2 ✓5
      - affecting fetus or newborn 763.1
  - postpartal (old) 618.1
- uveal 871.1
- vagina (anterior) (posterior) (vault) (wall) (without uterine prolapse) 618.0
  - with uterine prolapse 618.4
    - complete 618.3
    - incomplete 618.2
  - posthysterectomy 618.5
- vitreous (humor) 379.26
  - traumatic 871.1
- womb — *see* Prolapse, uterus

Prolapsus, female 618.9

Proliferative — *see* condition

Prolinemia 270.8

Prolinuria 270.8

Prolonged, prolongation
- bleeding time (*see also* Defect, coagulation) 790.92
  - "idiopathic" (in von Willebrand's disease) 286.4
- coagulation time (*see also* Defect, coagulation) 790.92
- gestation syndrome 766.2
- labor 662.1 ✓5
  - affecting fetus or newborn 763.89
  - first stage 662.0 ✓5

Prolonged, prolongation — *continued*
- labor — *continued*
  - second stage 662.2 ✓5
- pregnancy 645.2 ✓5
- PR interval 426.11
- prothrombin time (*see also* Defect, coagulation) 790.92
- rupture of membranes (24 hours or more prior to onset of labor) 658.2 ✓5
- uterine contractions in labor 661.4 ✓5
  - affecting fetus or newborn 763.7

Prominauris 744.29

Prominence
- auricle (ear) (congenital) 744.29
  - acquired 380.32
- ischial spine or sacral promontory
  - with disproportion (fetopelvic) 653.3 ✓5
    - affecting fetus or newborn 763.1
    - causing obstructed labor 660.1 ✓5
      - affecting fetus or newborn 763.1
- nose (congenital) 748.1
  - acquired 738.0

Pronation
- ankle 736.79
- foot 736.79
  - congenital 755.67

Prophylactic
- administration of
  - antibiotics V07.39
  - antitoxin, any V07.2
  - antivenin V07.2
  - chemotherapeutic agent NEC V07.39
    - fluoride V07.31
  - diphtheria antitoxin V07.2
  - gamma globulin V07.2
  - immune sera (gamma globulin) V07.2
  - RhoGAM V07.2
  - tetanus antitoxin V07.2
- chemotherapy NEC V07.39
  - fluoride V07.31
- immunotherapy V07.2
- measure V07.9
  - specified type NEC V07.8
- postmenopausal hormone replacement V07.4
- sterilization V25.2

Proptosis (ocular) (*see also* Exophthalmos) 376.30
- thyroid 242.0 ✓5

Propulsion
- eyeball 360.81

Prosecution, anxiety concerning V62.5

Prostate, prostatic — *see* condition

Prostatism 600.9

Prostatitis (congestive) (suppurative) 601.9
- acute 601.0
- cavitary 601.8
- chlamydial 099.54
- chronic 601.1
- diverticular 601.8
- due to Trichomonas (vaginalis) 131.03
- fibrous 600.9
- gonococcal (acute) 098.12
  - chronic or duration of 2 months or over 098.32
- granulomatous 601.8
- hypertrophic 600.0
- specified type NEC 601.8
- subacute 601.1
- trichomonal 131.03
- tuberculous (*see also* Tuberculosis) 016.5 ✓5 [601.4]

Prostatocystitis 601.3

Prostatorrhea 602.8

Prostatoseminovesiculitis, trichomonal 131.03

Prostration 780.79
- heat 992.5
  - anhydrotic 992.3
  - due to
    - salt (and water) depletion 992.4
    - water depletion 992.3
- nervous 300.5
- newborn 779.89 ▲
- senile 797

Protanomaly 368.51

Protanopia (anomalous trichromat) (complete) (incomplete) 368.51
Protein
  deficiency 260
  malnutrition 260
  sickness (prophylactic) (therapeutic) 999.5
Proteinemia 790.99
Proteinosis
  alveolar, lung or pulmonary 516.0
  lipid 272.8
  lipoid (of Urbach) 272.8
Proteinuria (see also Albuminuria) 791.0
  Bence-Jones NEC 791.0
  gestational 646.2
    with hypertension — see Toxemia, of pregnancy
  orthostatic 593.6
  postural 593.6
Proteolysis, pathologic 286.6
Protocoproporphyria 277.1
Protoporphyria (erythrohepatic) (erythropoietic) 277.1
Protrusio acetabuli 718.65
Protrusion
  acetabulum (into pelvis) 718.65
  device, implant, or graft — see Complications, mechanical
  ear, congenital 744.29
  intervertebral disc — see Displacement, intervertebral disc
  nucleus pulposus — see Displacement, intervertebral disc
Proud flesh 701.5
Prune belly (syndrome) 756.71
Prurigo (ferox) (gravis) (Hebra's) (hebrae) (mitis) (simplex) 698.2
  agria 698.3
  asthma syndrome 691.8
  Besnier's (atopic dermatitis) (infantile eczema) 691.8
  eczematodes allergicum 691.8
  estivalis (Hutchinson's) 692.72
  Hutchinson's 692.72
  nodularis 698.3
  psychogenic 306.3
Pruritus, pruritic 698.9
  ani 698.0
    psychogenic 306.3
  conditions NEC 698.9
    psychogenic 306.3
  due to Onchocerca volvulus 125.3
  ear 698.9
  essential 698.9
  genital organ(s) 698.1
    psychogenic 306.3
  gravidarum 646.8
  hiemalis 698.8
  neurogenic (any site) 306.3
  perianal 698.0
  psychogenic (any site) 306.3
  scrotum 698.1
    psychogenic 306.3
  senile, senilis 698.8
  Trichomonas 131.9
  vulva, vulvae 698.1
    psychogenic 306.3
Psammocarcinoma (M8140/3) — see Neoplasm, by site, malignant
Pseudarthrosis, pseudoarthrosis (bone) 733.82
  joint following fusion V45.4
Pseudoacanthosis
  nigricans 701.8
Pseudoaneurysm — see Aneurysm
Pseudoangina (pectoris) — see Angina
Pseudoangioma 452
Pseudo-Argyll-Robertson pupil 379.45
Pseudoarteriosus 747.89
Pseudoarthrosis — see Pseudarthrosis
Pseudoataxia 799.8
Pseudobursa 727.89
Pseudocholera 025
Pseudochromidrosis 705.89

Pseudocirrhosis, liver, pericardial 423.2
Pseudocoarctation 747.21
Pseudocowpox 051.1
Pseudocoxalgia 732.1
Pseudocroup 478.75
Pseudocyesis 300.11
Pseudocyst
  lung 518.89
  pancreas 577.2
  retina 361.19
Pseudodementia 300.16
Pseudoelephantiasis neuroarthritica 757.0
Pseudoemphysema 518.89
Pseudoencephalitis
  superior (acute) hemorrhagic 265.1
Pseudoerosion cervix, congenital 752.49
Pseudoexfoliation, lens capsule 366.11
Pseudofracture (idiopathic) (multiple) (spontaneous) (symmetrical) 268.2
Pseudoglanders 025
Pseudoglioma 360.44
Pseudogout — see Chondrocalcinosis
Pseudohallucination 780.1
Pseudohemianesthesia 782.0
Pseudohemophilia (Bernuth's) (hereditary) (type B) 286.4
  type A 287.8
  vascular 287.8
Pseudohermaphroditism 752.7
  with chromosomal anomaly — see Anomaly, chromosomal
  adrenal 255.2
  female (without adrenocortical disorder) 752.7
    with adrenocortical disorder 255.2
    adrenal 255.2
  male (without gonadal disorder) 752.7
    with
      adrenocortical disorder 255.2
      cleft scrotum 752.7
      feminizing testis 257.8
      gonadal disorder 257.9
    adrenal 255.2
Pseudohole, macula 362.54
Pseudo-Hurler's disease (mucolipidosis III) 272.7
Pseudohydrocephalus 348.2
Pseudohypertrophic muscular dystrophy (Erb's) 359.1
Pseudohypertrophy, muscle 359.1
Pseudohypoparathyroidism 275.49
Pseudoinfluenza 487.1
Pseudoinsomnia 307.49
Pseudoleukemia 288.8
  infantile 285.8
Pseudomembranous — see condition
Pseudomeningocele (cerebral) (infective) (surgical) 349.2
  spinal 349.2
Pseudomenstruation 626.8
Pseudomucinous
  cyst (ovary) (M8470/0) 220
  peritoneum 568.89
Pseudomyeloma 273.1
Pseudomyxoma peritonei (M8480/6) 197.6
Pseudoneuritis optic (nerve) 377.24
  papilla 377.24
  congenital 743.57
Pseudoneuroma — see Injury, nerve, by site
Pseudo-obstruction
  intestine 564.89
Pseudopapilledema 377.24.
Pseudoparalysis
  arm or leg 781.4
  atonic, congenital 358.8
Pseudopelade 704.09
Pseudophakia V43.1
Pseudopolycythemia 289.0
Pseudopolyposis, colon 556.4
Pseudoporencephaly 348.0

Pseudopseudohypoparathyroidism 275.49
Pseudopsychosis 300.16
Pseudopterygium 372.52
Pseudoptosis (eyelid) 374.34
Pseudorabies 078.89
Pseudoretinitis, pigmentosa 362.65
Pseudorickets 588.0
  senile (Pozzi's) 731.0
Pseudorubella 057.8
Pseudoscarlatina 057.8
Pseudosclerema 778.1
Pseudosclerosis (brain)
  Jakob's 046.1
  of Westphal (-Strümpell) (hepatolenticular degeneration) 275.1
  spastic 046.1
    with dementia
      with behavioral disturbance 046.1 [294.11]
      without behavioral disturbance 046.1 [294.10]
Pseudoseizure 780.39
  non-psychiatric 780.39
  psychiatric 300.11
Pseudotabes 799.8
  diabetic 250.6 [337.1]
Pseudotetanus (see also Convulsions) 780.39
Pseudotetany 781.7
  hysterical 300.11
Pseudothalassemia 285.0
Pseudotrichinosis 710.3
Pseudotruncus arteriosus 747.29
Pseudotuberculosis, pasteurella (infection) 027.2
Pseudotumor
  cerebri 348.2
  orbit (inflammatory) 376.11
Pseudo-Turner's syndrome 759.89
Pseudoxanthoma elasticum 757.39
Psilosis (sprue) (tropical) 579.1
  Monilia 112.89
  nontropical 579.0
  not sprue 704.00
Psittacosis 073.9
Psoitis 728.89
Psora NEC 696.1
Psoriasis 696.1
  any type, except arthropathic 696.1
  arthritic, arthropathic 696.0
  buccal 528.6
  flexural 696.1
  follicularis 696.1
  guttate 696.1
  inverse 696.1
  mouth 528.6
  nummularis 696.1
  psychogenic 316 [696.1]
  punctata 696.1
  pustular 696.1
  rupioides 696.1
  vulgaris 696.1
Psorospermiasis 136.4
Psorospermosis 136.4
  follicularis (vegetans) 757.39
Psychalgia 307.80
Psychasthenia 300.89
  compulsive 300.3
  mixed compulsive states 300.3
  obsession 300.3
Psychiatric disorder or problem NEC 300.9
Psychogenic — see also condition
  factors associated with physical conditions 316
Psychoneurosis, psychoneurotic (see also Neurosis) 300.9
  anxiety (state) 300.00
  climacteric 627.2
  compensation 300.16
  compulsion 300.3
  conversion hysteria 300.11
  depersonalization 300.6
  depressive type 300.4
  dissociative hysteria 300.15

Index to Diseases

Psychoneurosis

Psychoneurosis, psychoneurotic (see also Neurosis) — continued
- hypochondriacal 300.7
- hysteria 300.10
  - conversion type 300.11
  - dissociative type 300.15
- mixed NEC 300.89
- neurasthenic 300.5
- obsessional 300.3
- obsessive-compulsive 300.3
- occupational 300.89
- personality NEC 301.89
- phobia 300.20
- senile NEC 300.89

Psychopathic — see also condition
- constitution, posttraumatic 310.2
  - with psychosis 293.9
- personality 301.9
  - amoral trends 301.7
  - antisocial trends 301.7
  - asocial trends 301.7
  - mixed types 301.7
- state 301.9

Psychopathy, sexual (see also Deviation, sexual) 302.9

Psychophysiologic, psychophysiological condition — see Reaction, psychophysiologic

Psychose passionelle 297.8

Psychosexual identity disorder 302.6
- adult-life 302.85
- childhood 302.6

Psychosis 298.9
- acute hysterical 298.1
- affecting management of pregnancy, childbirth, or puerperium 648.4 ✓5
- affective NEC 296.90

> Note — Use the following fifth-digit subclassification with categories 296.0-296.6:
>
> 0 unspecified
> 1 mild
> 2 moderate
> 3 severe, without mention of psychotic behavior
> 4 severe, specified as with psychotic behavior
> 5 in partial or unspecified remission
> 6 in full remission

- drug-induced 292.84
- due to or associated with physical condition 293.83
- involutional 296.2 ✓5
  - recurrent episode 296.3 ✓5
  - single episode 296.2 ✓5
- manic-depressive 296.80
  - circular (alternating) 296.7
    - currently depressed 296.5 ✓5
    - currently manic 296.4 ✓5
  - depressed type 296.2 ✓5
    - atypical 296.82
    - recurrent episode 296.3 ✓5
    - single episode 296.2 ✓5
  - manic 296.0 ✓5
    - atypical 296.81
    - recurrent episode 296.1 ✓5
    - single episode 296.0 ✓5
  - mixed type NEC 296.89
  - specified type NEC 296.89
- senile 290.21
- specified type NEC 296.99
- alcoholic 291.9
  - with
    - anxiety 291.89
    - delirium tremens 291.0
    - delusions 291.5
    - dementia 291.2
    - hallucinosis 291.3
    - mood disturbance 291.89
    - jealousy 291.5
    - paranoia 291.5
    - persisting amnesia 291.1

Psychosis — continued
- alcoholic — continued
  - with — continued
    - sexual dysfunction 291.89
    - sleep disturbance 291.89
  - amnestic confabulatory 291.1
  - delirium tremens 291.0
  - hallucinosis 291.3
  - Korsakoff's, Korsakov's, Korsakow's 291.1
  - paranoid type 291.5
  - pathological intoxication 291.4
  - polyneuritic 291.1
  - specified type NEC 291.89
- alternating (see also Psychosis, manic-depressive, circular) 296.7
- anergastic (see also Psychosis, organic) 294.9
- arteriosclerotic 290.40
  - with
    - acute confusional state 290.41
    - delirium 290.41
    - delusional features 290.42
    - depressive features 290.43
  - depressed type 290.43
  - paranoid type 290.42
  - simple type 290.40
  - uncomplicated 290.40
- atypical 298.9
  - depressive 296.82
  - manic 296.81
- borderline (schizophrenia) (see also Schizophrenia) 295.5 ✓5
  - of childhood (see also Psychosis, childhood) 299.8 ✓5
  - prepubertal 299.8 ✓5
- brief reactive 298.8
- childhood, with origin specific to 299.9 ✓5

> Note — Use the following fifth-digit subclassification with category 299:
>
> 0 current or active state
> 1 residual state

  - atypical 299.8 ✓5
  - specified type NEC 299.8 ✓5
- circular (see also Psychosis, manic-depressive, circular) 296.7
- climacteric (see also Psychosis, involutional) 298.8
- confusional 298.9
  - acute 293.0
  - reactive 298.2
  - subacute 293.1
- depressive (see also Psychosis, affective) 296.2 ✓5
  - atypical 296.82
  - involutional 296.2 ✓5
    - recurrent episode 296.3 ✓5
    - single episode 296.2 ✓5
  - psychogenic 298.0
  - reactive (emotional stress) (psychological trauma) 298.0
  - recurrent episode 296.3 ✓5
    - with hypomania (bipolar II) 296.89
  - single episode 296.2 ✓5
- disintegrative (childhood) (see also Psychosis, childhood) 299.1 ✓5
- drug 292.9
  - with
    - affective syndrome 292.84
    - amnestic syndrome 292.83
    - anxiety 292.89
    - delirium 292.81
      - withdrawal 292.0
    - delusional syndrome 292.11
    - dementia 292.82
    - depressive state 292.84
    - hallucinosis 292.12
    - mood disturbance 292.84
    - organic personality syndrome NEC 292.89
    - sexual dysfunction 292.89
    - sleep disturbance 292.89
    - withdrawal syndrome (and delirium) 292.0
  - affective syndrome 292.84
  - delusional state 292.11
  - hallucinatory state 292.12

Psychosis — continued
- drug — continued
  - hallucinosis 292.12
  - paranoid state 292.11
  - specified type NEC 292.89
  - withdrawal syndrome (and delirium) 292.0
- due to or associated with physical condition (see also Psychosis, organic) 293.9
- epileptic NEC 294.8
- excitation (psychogenic) (reactive) 298.1
- exhaustive (see also Reaction, stress, acute) 308.9
- hypomanic (see also Psychosis, affective) 296.0 ✓5
  - recurrent episode 296.1 ✓5
  - single episode 296.0 ✓5
- hysterical 298.8
  - acute 298.1
- incipient 298.8
  - schizophrenic (see also Schizophrenia) 295.5 ✓5
- induced 297.3
- infantile (see also Psychosis, childhood) 299.0 ✓5
- infective 293.9
  - acute 293.0
  - subacute 293.1
- in pregnancy, childbirth, or puerperium 648.4 ✓5
- interactional (childhood) (see also Psychosis, childhood) 299.1 ✓5
- involutional 298.8
  - depressive (see also Psychosis, affective) 296.2 ✓5
    - recurrent episode 296.3 ✓5
    - single episode 296.2 ✓5
  - melancholic 296.2 ✓5
    - recurrent episode 296.3 ✓5
    - single episode 296.2 ✓5
  - paranoid state 297.2
  - paraphrenia 297.2
- Korsakoff's, Korakov's, Korsakow's (nonalcoholic) 294.0
  - alcoholic 291.1
- mania (phase) (see also Psychosis, affective) 296.0 ✓5
  - recurrent episode 296.1 ✓5
  - single episode 296.0 ✓5
- manic (see also Psychosis, affective) 296.0 ✓5
  - atypical 296.81
  - recurrent episode 296.1 ✓5
  - single episode 296.0 ✓5
- manic-depressive 296.80
  - circular 296.7
    - currently
      - depressed 296.5 ✓5
      - manic 296.4 ✓5
    - mixed 296.6 ✓5
  - depressive 296.2 ✓5
    - recurrent episode 296.3 ✓5
      - with hypomania (bipolar II) 296.89
    - single episode 296.2 ✓5
  - hypomanic 296.0 ✓5
    - recurrent episode 296.1 ✓5
    - single episode 296.0 ✓5
  - manic 296.0 ✓5
    - atypical 296.81
    - recurrent episode 296.1 ✓5
    - single episode 296.0 ✓5
  - mixed NEC 296.89
  - perplexed 296.89
  - stuporous 296.89
- menopausal (see also Psychosis, involutional) 298.8
- mixed schizophrenic and affective (see also Schizophrenia) 295.7 ✓5
- multi-infarct (cerebrovascular) (see also Psychosis, arteriosclerotic) 290.40
- organic NEC 294.9
  - due to or associated with
    - addiction
      - alcohol (see also Psychosis, alcoholic) 291.9
      - drug (see also Psychosis, drug) 292.9
    - alcohol intoxication, acute (see also Psychosis, alcoholic) 291.9

Psychosis — continued
  organic NEC — continued
    due to or associated with — continued
      alcoholism (see also Psychosis, alcoholic) 291.9
      arteriosclerosis (cerebral) (see also Psychosis, arteriosclerotic) 290.40
      cerebrovascular disease
        acute (psychosis) 293.0
        arteriosclerotic (see also Psychosis, arteriosclerotic) 290.40
      childbirth — see Psychosis, puerperal
      dependence
        alcohol (see also Psychosis, alcoholic) 291.9
        drug 292.9
      disease
        alcoholic liver (see also Psychosis, alcoholic) 291.9
        brain
          arteriosclerotic (see also Psychosis, arteriosclerotic) 290.40
        cerebrovascular
          acute (psychosis) 293.0
          arteriosclerotic (see also Psychosis, arteriosclerotic) 290.40
        endocrine or metabolic 293.9
          acute (psychosis) 293.0
          subacute (psychosis) 293.1
        Jakob-Creutzfeldt
          with behavioral disturbance 046.1 [294.11]
          without behavioral disturbance 046.1 [294.10]
        liver, alcoholic (see also Psychosis, alcoholic) 291.9
      disorder
        cerebrovascular
          acute (psychosis) 293.0
        endocrine or metabolic 293.9
          acute (psychosis) 293.0
          subacute (psychosis) 293.1
      epilepsy
        with behavioral disturbance 345.9 [294.11]
        without behavioral disturbance 345.9 [294.10]
        transient (acute) 293.0
      Huntington's chorea
        with behavioral disturbance 333.4 [294.11]
        without behavioral disturbance 333.4 [294.10]
      infection
        brain 293.9
          acute (psychosis) 293.0
          chronic 294.8
          subacute (psychosis) 293.1
        intracranial NEC 293.9
          acute (psychosis) 293.0
          chronic 294.8
          subacute (psychosis) 293.1
      intoxication
        alcoholic (acute) (see also Psychosis, alcoholic) 291.9
        pathological 291.4
        drug (see also Psychosis, drug) 292.2
      ischemia
        cerebrovascular (generalized) (see also Psychosis, arteriosclerotic) 290.40
      Jakob-Creutzfeldt disease or syndrome
        with behavioral disturbance 046.1 [294.11]
        without behavioral disturbance 046.1 [294.10]
      multiple sclerosis
        with behavioral disturbance 340 [294.11]
        without behavioral disturbance 340 [294.10]
      physical condition NEC 293.9
        with
          delusions 293.81
          hallucinations 293.82

Psychosis — continued
  organic NEC — continued
    due to or associated with — continued
      presenility 290.10
      puerperium — see Psychosis, puerperal
      sclerosis, multiple
        with behavioral disturbance 340 [294.11]
        without behavioral disturbance 340 [294.10]
      senility 290.20
      status epilepticus
        with behavioral disturbance 345.3 [294.11]
        without behavioral disturbance 345.3 [294.10]
      trauma
        brain (birth) (from electrical current) (surgical) 293.9
          acute (psychosis) 293.0
          chronic 294.8
          subacute (psychosis) 293.1
        unspecified physical condition 294.9
      infective 293.9
        acute (psychosis) 293.0
        subacute 293.1
      posttraumatic 293.9
        acute 293.0
        subacute 293.1
      specified type NEC 294.8
      transient 293.9
        with
          anxiety 293.84
          delusions 293.81
          depression 293.83
          hallucinations 293.82
        depressive type 293.83
        hallucinatory type 293.82
        paranoid type 293.81
        specified type NEC 293.89
  paranoic 297.1
  paranoid (chronic) 297.9
    alcoholic 291.5
    chronic 297.1
    climacteric 297.2
    involuntional 297.2
    menopausal 297.2
    protracted reactive 298.4
    psychogenic 298.4
      acute 298.3
    schizophrenic (see also Schizophrenia) 295.3
    senile 290.20
  paroxysmal 298.9
    senile 290.20
  polyneuritic, alcoholic 291.1
  postoperative 293.9
  postpartum — see Psychosis, puerperal
  prepsychotic (see also Schizophrenia) 295.5
  presbyophrenic (type) 290.8
  presenile (see also Dementia, presenile) 290.10
  prison 300.16
  psychogenic 298.8
    depressive 298.0
    paranoid 298.4
      acute 298.3
  puerperal
    specified type — see categories 295-298
    unspecified type 293.89
      acute 293.0
      chronic 293.89
      subacute 293.1
  reactive (emotional stress) (psychological trauma) 298.8
    brief 298.8
    confusion 298.2
    depressive 298.0
    excitation 298.1
  schizo-affective (depressed) (excited) (see also Schizophrenia) 295.7
  schizophrenia, schizophrenic (see also Schizophrenia) 295.9
    borderline type 295.5
      of childhood (see also Psychosis, childhood) 299.8
    catatonic (excited) (withdrawn) 295.2

Psychosis — continued
  schizophrenia, schizophrenic (see also Schizophrenia) — continued
    childhood type (see also Psychosis, childhood) 299.9
    hebephrenic 295.1
    incipient 295.5
    latent 295.5
    paranoid 295.3
    prepsychotic 295.5
    prodromal 295.5
    pseudoneurotic 295.5
    pseudopsychopathic 295.5
    schizophreniform 295.4
    simple 295.0
  schizophreniform 295.4
  senile NEC 290.20
    with
      delusional features 290.20
      depressive features 290.21
    depressed type 290.21
    paranoid type 290.20
    simple deterioration 290.20
    specified type — see categories 295-298
  shared 297.3
  situational (reactive) 298.8
  symbiotic (childhood) (see also Psychosis, childhood) 299.1
  toxic (acute) 293.9

Psychotic (see also condition) 298.9
  episode 298.9
    due to or associated with physical conditions (see also Psychosis, organic) 293.9

Pterygium (eye) 372.40
  central 372.43
  colli 744.5
  double 372.44
  peripheral (stationary) 372.41
    progressive 372.42
  recurrent 372.45

Ptilosis 374.55

Ptomaine (poisoning) (see also Poisoning, food) 005.9

Ptosis (adiposa) 374.30
  breast 611.8
  cecum 569.89
  colon 569.89
  congenital (eyelid) 743.61
    specified site NEC — see Anomaly, specified type NEC
  epicanthus syndrome 270.2
  eyelid 374.30
    congenital 743.61
    mechanical 374.33
    myogenic 374.32
    paralytic 374.31
  gastric 537.5
  intestine 569.89
  kidney (see also Disease, renal) 593.0
    congenital 753.3
  liver 573.8
  renal (see also Disease, renal) 593.0
    congenital 753.3
  splanchnic 569.89
  spleen 289.59
  stomach 537.5
  viscera 569.89

Ptyalism 527.7
  hysterical 300.11
  periodic 527.2
  pregnancy 646.8
  psychogenic 306.4

Ptyalolithiasis 527.5

Pubalgia 848.8

Pubarche, precocious 259.1

Pubertas praecox 259.1

Puberty V21.1
  abnormal 259.9
  bleeding 626.3
  delayed 259.0
  precocious (constitutional) (cryptogenic) (idiopathic) NEC 259.1

Index to Diseases

Puberty — *continued*
  precocious — *continued*
    due to
      adrenal
        cortical hyperfunction 255.2
        hyperplasia 255.2
      cortical hyperfunction 255.2
      ovarian hyperfunction 256.1
        estrogen 256.0
      pineal tumor 259.8
      testicular hyperfunction 257.0
  premature 259.1
    due to
      adrenal cortical hyperfunction 255.2
      pineal tumor 259.8
      pituitary (anterior) hyperfunction 253.1
Puckering, macula 362.56
Pudenda, pudendum — *see* condition
Puente's disease (simple glandular cheilitis) 528.5
Puerperal
  abscess
    areola 675.1 ✓5ᵗʰ
    Bartholin's gland 646.6 ✓5ᵗʰ
    breast 675.1 ✓5ᵗʰ
    cervix (uteri) 670 ✓4ᵗʰ
    fallopian tube 670 ✓4ᵗʰ
    genital organ 670 ✓4ᵗʰ
    kidney 646.6 ✓5ᵗʰ
    mammary 675.1 ✓5ᵗʰ
    mesosalpinx 670 ✓4ᵗʰ
    nabothian 646.6 ✓5ᵗʰ
    nipple 675.0 ✓5ᵗʰ
    ovary, ovarian 670 ✓4ᵗʰ
    oviduct 670 ✓4ᵗʰ
    parametric 670 ✓4ᵗʰ
    para-uterine 670 ✓4ᵗʰ
    pelvic 670 ✓4ᵗʰ
    perimetric 670 ✓4ᵗʰ
    periuterine 670 ✓4ᵗʰ
    retro-uterine 670 ✓4ᵗʰ
    subareolar 675.1 ✓5ᵗʰ
    suprapelvic 670 ✓4ᵗʰ
    tubal (ruptured) 670 ✓4ᵗʰ
    tubo-ovarian 670 ✓4ᵗʰ
    urinary tract NEC 646.6 ✓5ᵗʰ
    uterine, uterus 670 ✓4ᵗʰ
    vagina (wall) 646.6 ✓5ᵗʰ
    vaginorectal 646.6 ✓5ᵗʰ
    vulvovaginal gland 646.6 ✓5ᵗʰ
  accident 674.9 ✓5ᵗʰ
  adnexitis 670 ✓4ᵗʰ
  afibrinogenemia, or other coagulation defect 666.3 ✓5ᵗʰ
  albuminuria (acute) (subacute) 646.2 ✓5ᵗʰ
    pre-eclamptic 642.4 ✓5ᵗʰ
  anemia (conditions classifiable to 280-285) 648.2 ✓5ᵗʰ
  anuria 669.3 ✓5ᵗʰ
  apoplexy 674.0 ✓5ᵗʰ
  asymptomatic bacteriuria 646.5 ✓5ᵗʰ
  atrophy, breast 676.3 ✓5ᵗʰ
  blood dyscrasia 666.3 ✓5ᵗʰ
  caked breast 676.2 ✓5ᵗʰ
  cardiomyopathy 674.8 ✓5ᵗʰ
  cellulitis — *see* Puerperal, abscess
  cerebrovascular disorder (conditions classifiable to 430-434, 436-437) 674.0 ✓5ᵗʰ
  cervicitis (conditions classifiable to 616.0) 646.6 ✓5ᵗʰ
  coagulopathy (any) 666.3 ✓5ᵗʰ
  complications 674.9 ✓5ᵗʰ
    specified type NEC 674.8 ✓5ᵗʰ
  convulsions (eclamptic) (uremic) 642.6 ✓5ᵗʰ
    with pre-existing hypertension 642.7 ✓5ᵗʰ
  cracked nipple 676.1 ✓5ᵗʰ
  cystitis 646.6 ✓5ᵗʰ
  cystopyelitis 646.6 ✓5ᵗʰ
  deciduitis (acute) 670 ✓4ᵗʰ
  delirium NEC 293.9
  diabetes (mellitus) (conditions classifiable to 250) 648.0 ✓5ᵗʰ
  disease 674.9 ✓5ᵗʰ
    breast NEC 676.3 ✓5ᵗʰ
    cerebrovascular (acute) 674.0 ✓5ᵗʰ

Puerperal — *continued*
  disease — *continued*
    nonobstetric NEC (*see also* Pregnancy, complicated, current disease or condition) 648.9 ✓5ᵗʰ
    pelvis inflammatory 670 ✓4ᵗʰ
    renal NEC 646.2 ✓5ᵗʰ
    tubo-ovarian 670 ✓4ᵗʰ
    Valsuani's (progressive pernicious anemia) 648.2 ✓5ᵗʰ
  disorder
    lactation 676.9 ✓5ᵗʰ
      specified type NEC 676.8 ✓5ᵗʰ
    nonobstetric NEC (*see also* Pregnancy, complicated, current disease or condition) 648.9 ✓5ᵗʰ
  disruption
    cesarean wound 674.1 ✓5ᵗʰ
    episiotomy wound 674.2 ✓5ᵗʰ
    perineal laceration wound 674.2 ✓5ᵗʰ
  drug dependence (conditions classifiable to 304) 648.3 ✓5ᵗʰ
  eclampsia 642.6 ✓5ᵗʰ
    with pre-existing hypertension 642.7 ✓5ᵗʰ
  embolism (pulmonary) 673.2 ✓5ᵗʰ
    air 673.0 ✓5ᵗʰ
    amniotic fluid 673.1 ✓5ᵗʰ
    blood-clot 673.2 ✓5ᵗʰ
    brain or cerebral 674.0 ✓5ᵗʰ
    cardiac 674.8 ✓5ᵗʰ
    fat 673.8 ✓5ᵗʰ
    intracranial sinus (venous) 671.5 ✓5ᵗʰ
    pyemic 673.3 ✓5ᵗʰ
    septic 673.3 ✓5ᵗʰ
    spinal cord 671.5 ✓5ᵗʰ
  endometritis (conditions classifiable to 615.0-615.9) 670 ✓4ᵗʰ
  endophlebitis — *see* Puerperal, phlebitis
  endotrachelitis 646.6 ✓5ᵗʰ
  engorgement, breasts 676.2 ✓5ᵗʰ
  erysipelas 670 ✓4ᵗʰ
  failure
    lactation 676.4 ✓5ᵗʰ
    renal, acute 669.3 ✓5ᵗʰ
  fever 670 ✓4ᵗʰ
    meaning pyrexia (of unknown origin) 672 ✓5ᵗʰ
    meaning sepsis 670 ✓4ᵗʰ
  fissure, nipple 676.1 ✓5ᵗʰ
  fistula
    breast 675.1 ✓5ᵗʰ
    mammary gland 675.1 ✓5ᵗʰ
    nipple 675.0 ✓5ᵗʰ
  galactophoritis 675.2 ✓5ᵗʰ
  galactorrhea 676.6 ✓5ᵗʰ
  gangrene
    gas 670 ✓4ᵗʰ
    uterus 670 ✓4ᵗʰ
  gonorrhea (conditions classifiable to 098) 647.1 ✓5ᵗʰ
  hematoma, subdural 674.0 ✓5ᵗʰ
  hematosalpinx, infectional 670 ✓4ᵗʰ
  hemiplegia, cerebral 674.0 ✓5ᵗʰ
  hemorrhage 666.1 ✓5ᵗʰ
    brain 674.0 ✓5ᵗʰ
    bulbar 674.0 ✓5ᵗʰ
    cerebellar 674.0 ✓5ᵗʰ
    cerebral 674.0 ✓5ᵗʰ
    cortical 674.0 ✓5ᵗʰ
    delayed (after 24 hours) (uterine) 666.2 ✓5ᵗʰ
    extradural 674.0 ✓5ᵗʰ
    internal capsule 674.0 ✓5ᵗʰ
    intracranial 674.0 ✓5ᵗʰ
    intrapontine 674.0 ✓5ᵗʰ
    meningeal 674.0 ✓5ᵗʰ
    pontine 674.0 ✓5ᵗʰ
    subarachnoid 674.0 ✓5ᵗʰ
    subcortical 674.0 ✓5ᵗʰ
    subdural 674.0 ✓5ᵗʰ
    uterine, delayed 666.2 ✓5ᵗʰ
    ventricular 674.0 ✓5ᵗʰ
  hemorrhoids 671.8 ✓5ᵗʰ
  hepatorenal syndrome 674.8 ✓5ᵗʰ
  hypertrophy
    breast 676.3 ✓5ᵗʰ
    mammary gland 676.3 ✓5ᵗʰ
  induration breast (fibrous) 676.3 ✓5ᵗʰ

Puerperal — *continued*
  infarction
    lung — *see* Puerperal, embolism
    pulmonary — *see* Puerperal, embolism
  infection
    Bartholin's gland 646.6 ✓5ᵗʰ
    breast 675.2 ✓5ᵗʰ
      with nipple 675.9 ✓5ᵗʰ
        specified type NEC 675.8 ✓5ᵗʰ
    cervix 646.6 ✓5ᵗʰ
    endocervix 646.6 ✓5ᵗʰ
    fallopian tube 670 ✓4ᵗʰ
    generalized 670 ✓4ᵗʰ
    genital tract (major) 670 ✓4ᵗʰ
      minor or localized 646.6 ✓5ᵗʰ
    kidney (bacillus coli) 646.6 ✓5ᵗʰ
    mammary gland 675.2 ✓5ᵗʰ
      with nipple 675.9 ✓5ᵗʰ
        specified type NEC 675.8 ✓5ᵗʰ
    nipple 675.0 ✓5ᵗʰ
      with breast 675.9 ✓5ᵗʰ
        specified type NEC 675.8 ✓5ᵗʰ
    ovary 670 ✓4ᵗʰ
    pelvic 670 ✓4ᵗʰ
    peritoneum 670 ✓4ᵗʰ
    renal 646.6 ✓5ᵗʰ
    tubo-ovarian 670 ✓4ᵗʰ
    urinary (tract) NEC 646.6 ✓5ᵗʰ
      asymptomatic 646.5 ✓5ᵗʰ
    uterus, uterine 670 ✓4ᵗʰ
    vagina 646.6 ✓5ᵗʰ
  inflammation — *see also* Puerperal, infection
    areola 675.1 ✓5ᵗʰ
    Bartholin's gland 646.6 ✓5ᵗʰ
    breast 675.2 ✓5ᵗʰ
    broad ligament 670 ✓4ᵗʰ
    cervix (uteri) 646.6 ✓5ᵗʰ
    fallopian tube 670 ✓4ᵗʰ
    genital organs 670 ✓4ᵗʰ
      localized 646.6 ✓5ᵗʰ
    mammary gland 675.2 ✓5ᵗʰ
    nipple 675.0 ✓5ᵗʰ
    ovary 670 ✓4ᵗʰ
    oviduct 670 ✓4ᵗʰ
    pelvis 670 ✓4ᵗʰ
    periuterine 670 ✓4ᵗʰ
    tubal 670 ✓4ᵗʰ
    vagina 646.6 ✓5ᵗʰ
    vein — *see* Puerperal, phlebitis
  inversion, nipple 676.3 ✓5ᵗʰ
  ischemia, cerebral 674.0 ✓5ᵗʰ
  lymphangitis 670 ✓4ᵗʰ
    breast 675.2 ✓5ᵗʰ
  malaria (conditions classifiable to 084) 647.4 ✓5ᵗʰ
  malnutrition 648.9 ✓5ᵗʰ
  mammillitis 675.0 ✓5ᵗʰ
  mammitis 675.2 ✓5ᵗʰ
  mania 296.0 ✓5ᵗʰ
    recurrent episode 296.1 ✓5ᵗʰ
    single episode 296.0 ✓5ᵗʰ
  mastitis 675.2 ✓5ᵗʰ
    purulent 675.1 ✓5ᵗʰ
    retromammary 675.1 ✓5ᵗʰ
    submammary 675.1 ✓5ᵗʰ
  melancholia 296.2 ✓5ᵗʰ
    recurrent episode 296.3 ✓5ᵗʰ
    single episode 296.2 ✓5ᵗʰ
  mental disorder (conditions classifiable to 290-303, 305-316, 317-319) 648.4 ✓5ᵗʰ
  metritis (septic) (suppurative) 670 ✓4ᵗʰ
  metroperitonitis 670 ✓4ᵗʰ
  metrorrhagia 666.2 ✓5ᵗʰ
  metrosalpingitis 670 ✓4ᵗʰ
  metrovaginitis 670 ✓4ᵗʰ
  milk leg 671.4 ✓5ᵗʰ
  monoplegia, cerebral 674.0 ✓5ᵗʰ
  necrosis
    kidney, tubular 669.3 ✓5ᵗʰ
    liver (acute) (subacute) (conditions classifiable to 570) 674.8 ✓5ᵗʰ
    ovary 670 ✓4ᵗʰ
    renal cortex 669.3 ✓5ᵗʰ
  nephritis or nephrosis (conditions classifiable to 580-589) 646.2 ✓5ᵗʰ
    with hypertension 642.1 ✓5ᵗʰ

Puerperal — continued

Puerperal — *continued*
- nutritional deficiency (conditions classifiable to 260-269) 648.9 ✓5th
- occlusion, precerebral artery 674.0 ✓5th
- oliguria 669.3 ✓5th
- oophoritis 670 ✓4th
- ovaritis 670 ✓4th
- paralysis
  - bladder (sphincter) 665.5 ✓5th
  - cerebral 674.0 ✓5th
- paralytic stroke 674.0 ✓5th
- parametritis 670 ✓4th
- paravaginitis 646.6 ✓5th
- pelviperitonitis 670 ✓4th
- perimetritis 670 ✓4th
- perimetrosalpingitis 670 ✓4th
- perinephritis 646.6 ✓5th
- periooophoritis 670 ✓4th
- periphlebitis — see Puerperal, phlebitis
- perisalpingitis 670 ✓4th
- peritoneal infection 670 ✓4th
- peritonitis (pelvic) 670 ✓4th
- perivaginitis 646.6 ✓5th
- phlebitis 671.9 ✓5th
  - deep 671.4 ✓5th
  - intracranial sinus (venous) 671.5 ✓5th
  - pelvic 671.4 ✓5th
  - specified site NEC 671.5 ✓5th
  - superficial 671.2 ✓5th
- phlegmasia alba dolens 671.4 ✓5th
- placental polyp 674.4 ✓5th
- pneumonia, embolic — see Puerperal, embolism
- prediabetes 648.8 ✓5th
- pre-eclampsia (mild) 642.4 ✓5th
  - with pre-existing hypertension 642.7 ✓5th
  - severe 642.5 ✓5th
- psychosis, unspecified (see also Psychosis, puerperal) 293.89
- pyelitis 646.6 ✓5th
- pyelocystitis 646.6 ✓5th
- pyelohydronephrosis 646.6 ✓5th
- pyelonephritis 646.6 ✓5th
- pyelonephrosis 646.6 ✓5th
- pyemia 670 ✓4th
- pyocystitis 646.6 ✓5th
- pyohemia 670 ✓4th
- pyometra 670 ✓4th
- pyonephritis 646.6 ✓5th
- pyonephrosis 646.6 ✓5th
- pyo-oophoritis 670 ✓4th
- pyosalpingitis 670 ✓4th
- pyosalpinx 670 ✓4th
- pyrexia (of unknown origin) 672 ✓5th
- renal
  - disease NEC 646.2 ✓5th
  - failure, acute 669.3 ✓5th
- retention
  - decidua (fragments) (with delayed hemorrhage) 666.2 ✓5th
    - without hemorrhage 667.1 ✓5th
  - placenta (fragments) (with delayed hemorrhage) 666.2 ✓5th
    - without hemorrhage 667.1 ✓5th
  - secundines (fragments) (with delayed hemorrhage) 666.2 ✓5th
    - without hemorrhage 667.1 ✓5th
- retracted nipple 676.0 ✓5th
- rubella (conditions classifiable to 056) 647.5 ✓5th
- salpingitis 670 ✓4th
- salpingo-oophoritis 670 ✓4th
- salpingo-ovaritis 670 ✓4th
- salpingoperitonitis 670 ✓4th
- sapremia 670 ✓4th
- secondary perineal tear 674.2 ✓5th
- sepsis (pelvic) 670 ✓4th
- septicemia 670 ✓4th
- subinvolution (uterus) 674.8 ✓5th
- sudden death (cause unknown) 674.9 ✓5th
- suppuration — see Puerperal, abscess
- syphilis (conditions classifiable to 090-097) 647.0 ✓5th
- tetanus 670 ✓4th
- thelitis 675.0 ✓5th
- thrombocytopenia 666.3 ✓5th
- thrombophlebitis (superficial) 671.2 ✓5th
  - deep 671.4 ✓5th

Puerperal — *continued*
- thrombophlebitis — *continued*
  - pelvic 671.4 ✓5th
  - specified site NEC 671.5 ✓5th
- thrombosis (venous) — see Thrombosis, puerperal
- thyroid dysfunction (conditions classifiable to 240-246) 648.1 ✓5th
- toxemia (see also Toxemia, of pregnancy) 642.4 ✓5th
  - eclamptic 642.6 ✓5th
    - with pre-existing hypertension 642.7 ✓5th
  - pre-eclamptic (mild) 642.4 ✓5th
    - with
      - convulsions 642.6 ✓5th
      - pre-existing hypertension 642.7 ✓5th
    - severe 642.5 ✓5th
- tuberculosis (conditions classifiable to 010-018) 647.3 ✓5th
- uremia 669.3 ✓5th
- vaginitis (conditions classifiable to 616.1) 646.6 ✓5th
- varicose veins (legs) 671.0 ✓5th
  - vulva or perineum 671.1 ✓5th
- vulvitis (conditions classifiable to 616.1) 646.6 ✓5th
- vulvovaginitis (conditions classifiable to 616.1) 646.6 ✓5th
- white leg 671.4 ✓5th

Pulled muscle — see Sprain, by site

Pulmolithiasis 518.89

Pulmonary — see condition

Pulmonitis (unknown etiology) 486

Pulpitis (acute) (anachoretic) (chronic) (hyperplastic) (putrescent) (suppurative) (ulcerative) 522.0

Pulpless tooth 522.9

Pulse
- alternating 427.89
  - psychogenic 306.2
- bigeminal 427.89
- fast 785.0
- feeble, rapid, due to shock following injury 958.4
- rapid 785.0
- slow 427.89
- strong 785.9
- trigeminal 427.89
- water-hammer (see also Insufficiency, aortic) 424.1
- weak 785.9

Pulseless disease 446.7

Pulsus
- alternans or trigeminy 427.89
  - psychogenic 306.2

Punch drunk 310.2

Puncta lacrimalia occlusion 375.52

Punctiform hymen 752.49

Puncture (traumatic) — see also Wound, open, by site
- accidental, complicating surgery 998.2
- bladder, nontraumatic 596.6
- by
  - device, implant, or graft — see Complications, mechanical
  - foreign body
    - internal organs — see also Injury, internal, by site
    - by ingested object — see Foreign body
  - left accidentally in operation wound 998.4
- instrument (any) during a procedure, accidental 998.2
- internal organs, abdomen, chest, or pelvis — see Injury, internal, by site
- kidney, nontraumatic 593.89

Pupil — see condition

Pupillary membrane 364.74
- persistent 743.46

Pupillotonia 379.46
- pseudotabetic 379.46

Purpura 287.2
- abdominal 287.0
- allergic 287.0

Purpura — *continued*
- anaphylactoid 287.0
- annularis telangiectodes 709.1
- arthritic 287.0
- autoerythrocyte sensitization 287.2
- autoimmune 287.0
- bacterial 287.0
- Bateman's (senile) 287.2
- capillary fragility (hereditary) (idiopathic) 287.8
- cryoglobulinemic 273.2
- devil's pinches 287.2
- fibrinolytic (see also Fibrinolysis) 286.6
- fulminans, fulminous 286.6
- gangrenous 287.0
- hemorrhagic (see also Purpura, thrombocytopenic) 287.3
  - nodular 272.7
  - nonthrombocytopenic 287.0
  - thrombocytopenic 287.3
- Henoch's (purpura nervosa) 287.0
- Henoch-Schönlein (allergic) 287.0
- hypergammaglobulinemic (benign primary) (Waldenström's) 273.0
- idiopathic 287.3
  - nonthrombocytopenic 287.0
  - thrombocytopenic 287.3
- infectious 287.0
- malignant 287.0
- neonatorum 772.6
- nervosa 287.0
- newborn NEC 772.6
- nonthrombocytopenic 287.2
  - hemorrhagic 287.0
  - idiopathic 287.0
- nonthrombopenic 287.2
- peliosis rheumatica 287.0
- pigmentaria, progressiva 709.09
- posttransfusion 287.4
- primary 287.0
- primitive 287.0
- red cell membrane sensitivity 287.2
- rheumatica 287.0
- Schönlein (-Henoch) (allergic) 287.0
- scorbutic 267
- senile 287.2
- simplex 287.2
- symptomatica 287.0
- telangiectasia annularis 709.1
- thrombocytopenic (congenital) (essential) (hereditary) (idiopathic) (primary) (see also Thrombocytopenia) 287.3
  - neonatal, transitory (see also Thrombocytopenia, neonatal transitory) 776.1
  - puerperal, postpartum 666.3 ✓5th
  - thrombotic 446.6
- thrombohemolytic (see also Fibrinolysis) 286.6
- thrombopenic (congenital) (essential) (see also Thrombocytopenia) 287.3
  - thrombotic 446.6
    - thrombocytic 446.6
    - thrombocytopenic 446.6
- toxic 287.0
- variolosa 050.0
- vascular 287.0
- visceral symptoms 287.0
- Werlhof's (see also Purpura, thrombocytopenic) 287.3

Purpuric spots 782.7

Purulent — see condition

Pus
- absorption, general — see Septicemia
- in
  - stool 792.1
  - urine 791.9
- tube (rupture) (see also Salpingo-oophoritis) 614.2

Pustular rash 782.1

Pustule 686.9
- malignant 022.0
- nonmalignant 686.9

Putnam's disease (subacute combined sclerosis with pernicious anemia) 281.0 [336.2]

Putnam-Dana syndrome (subacute combined sclerosis with pernicious anemia) 281.0 [336.2]

Putrefaction, intestinal 569.89

Putrescent pulp (dental) 522.1
Pyarthritis — see Pyarthrosis
Pyarthrosis (see also Arthritis, pyogenic) 711.0
   tuberculous — see Tuberculosis, joint
Pycnoepilepsy, pycnolepsy (idiopathic) (see also Epilepsy) 345.0
Pyelectasia 593.89
Pyelectasis 593.89
Pyelitis (congenital) (uremic) 590.80
  with
    abortion — see Abortion, by type, with specified complication NEC
    contracted kidney 590.00
    ectopic pregnancy (see also categories 633.0-633.9) 639.8
    molar pregnancy (see also categories 630-632) 639.8
  acute 590.10
    with renal medullary necrosis 590.11
  chronic 590.00
    with
      renal medullary necrosis 590.01
    complicating pregnancy, childbirth, or puerperium 646.6
      affecting fetus or newborn 760.1
  cystica 590.3
    following
      abortion 639.8
      ectopic or molar pregnancy 639.8
  gonococcal 098.19
    chronic or duration of 2 months or over 098.39
  tuberculous (see also Tuberculosis) 016.0 [590.81]
Pyelocaliectasis 593.89
Pyelocystitis (see also Pyelitis) 590.80
Pyelohydronephrosis 591
Pyelonephritis (see also Pyelitis) 590.80
  acute 590.10
    with renal medullary necrosis 590.11
  chronic 590.00
  syphilitic (late) 095.4
  tuberculous (see also Tuberculosis) 016.0 [590.81]
Pyelonephrosis (see also Pyelitis) 590.80
  chronic 590.00
Pyelophlebitis 451.89
Pyelo-ureteritis cystica 590.3
Pyemia, pyemic (purulent) (see also Septicemia) 038.9
  abscess — see Abscess
  arthritis (see also Arthritis, pyogenic) 711.0
  Bacillus coli 038.42
  embolism — see Embolism, pyemic
  fever 038.9
  infection 038.9
  joint (see also Arthritis, pyogenic) 711.0
  liver 572.1
  meningococcal 036.2
  newborn 771.81 ▲
  phlebitis — see Phlebitis
  pneumococcal 038.2
  portal 572.1
  postvaccinal 999.3
  specified organism NEC 038.8
  staphylococcal 038.10
    aureus 038.11
    specified organism NEC 038.19
  streptococcal 038.0
  tuberculous — see Tuberculosis, miliary
Pygopagus 759.4
Pykno-epilepsy, pyknolepsy (idiopathic) (see also Epilepsy) 345.0
Pyle (-Cohn) disease (craniometaphyseal dysplasia) 756.89
Pylephlebitis (suppurative) 572.1
Pylethrombophlebitis 572.1
Pylethrombosis 572.1
Pyloritis (see also Gastritis) 535.5
Pylorospasm (reflex) 537.81
  congenital or infantile 750.5
  neurotic 306.4
  newborn 750.5
  psychogenic 306.4
Pylorus, pyloric — see condition
Pyoarthrosis — see Pyarthrosis

Pyocele
  mastoid 383.00
  sinus (accessory) (nasal) (see also Sinusitis) 473.9
  turbinate (bone) 473.9
  urethra (see also Urethritis) 597.0
Pyococcal dermatitis 686.00
Pyococcide, skin 686.00
Pyocolpos (see also Vaginitis) 616.10
Pyocyaneus dermatitis 686.09
Pyocystitis (see also Cystitis) 595.9
Pyoderma, pyodermia 686.00
  gangrenosum 686.01
  specified type NEC 686.09
  vegetans 686.8
Pyodermatitis 686.00
  vegetans 686.8
Pyogenic — see condition
Pyohemia — see Septicemia
Pyohydronephrosis (see also Pyelitis) 590.80
Pyometra 615.9
Pyometritis (see also Endometritis) 615.9
Pyometrium (see also Endometritis) 615.9
Pyomyositis 728.0
  ossificans 728.19
  tropical (bungpagga) 040.81
Pyonephritis (see also Pyelitis) 590.80
  chronic 590.00
Pyonephrosis (congenital) (see also Pyelitis) 590.80
  acute 590.10
Pyo-oophoritis (see also Salpingo-oophoritis) 614.2
Pyo-ovarium (see also Salpingo-oophoritis) 614.2
Pyopericarditis 420.99
Pyopericardium 420.99
Pyophlebitis — see Phlebitis
Pyopneumopericardium 420.99
Pyopneumothorax (infectional) 510.9
  with fistula 510.0
  subdiaphragmatic (see also Peritonitis) 567.2
  subphrenic (see also Peritonitis) 567.2
  tuberculous (see also Tuberculosis, pleura) 012.0
Pyorrhea (alveolar) (alveolaris) 523.4
  degenerative 523.5
Pyosalpingitis (see also Salpingo-oophoritis) 614.2
Pyosalpinx (see also Salpingo-oophoritis) 614.2
Pyosepticemia — see Septicemia
Pyosis
  Corlett's (impetigo) 684
  Manson's (pemphigus contagiosus) 684
Pyothorax 510.9
  with fistula 510.0
  tuberculous (see also Tuberculosis, pleura) 012.0
Pyoureter 593.89
  tuberculous (see also Tuberculosis) 016.2
Pyramidopallidonigral syndrome 332.0
Pyrexia (of unknown origin) (P.U.O.) 780.6
  atmospheric 992.0
  during labor 659.2
  environmentally-induced newborn 778.4
  heat 992.0
  newborn, environmentally-induced 778.4
  puerperal 672
Pyroglobulinemia 273.8
Pyromania 312.33
Pyrosis 787.1
Pyrroloporphyria 277.1
Pyuria (bacterial) 791.9

Q

Q fever 083.0
  with pneumonia 083.0 [484.8]
Quadricuspid aortic valve 746.89
Quadrilateral fever 083.0

Quadriparesis — see Quadriplegia
Quadriplegia 344.00
  with fracture, vertebra (process) — see Fracture, vertebra, cervical, with spinal cord injury
  brain (current episode) 437.8
  C1-C4
    complete 344.01
    incomplete 344.02
  C5-C7
    complete 344.03
    incomplete 344.04
  cerebral (current episode) 437.8
  congenital or infantile (cerebral) (spastic) (spinal) 343.2
  cortical 437.8
  embolic (current episode) (see also Embolism, brain) 434.1
  infantile (cerebral) (spastic) (spinal) 343.2
  newborn NEC 767.0
  specified NEC 344.09
  thrombotic (current episode) (see also Thrombosis, brain) 434.0
  traumatic — see Injury, spinal, cervical
Quadruplet
  affected by maternal complications of pregnancy 761.5
  healthy liveborn — see Newborn, multiple
  pregnancy (complicating delivery) NEC 651.8
    with fetal loss and retention of one or more fetus(es) 651.5
Quarrelsomeness 301.3
Quartan
  fever 084.2
  malaria (fever) 084.2
Queensland fever 083.0
  coastal 083.0
  seven-day 100.89
Quervain's disease 727.04
  thyroid (subacute granulomatous thyroiditis) 245.1
Queyrat's erythroplasia (M8080/2)
  specified site — see Neoplasm, skin, in situ
  unspecified site 233.5
Quincke's disease or edema — see Edema, angioneurotic
Quinquaud's disease (acne decalvans) 704.09
Quinsy (gangrenous) 475
Quintan fever 083.1
Quintuplet
  affected by maternal complications of pregnancy 761.5
  healthy liveborn — see Newborn, multiple
  pregnancy (complicating delivery) NEC 651.2
    with fetal loss and retention of one or more fetus(es) 651.6
Quotidian
  fever 084.0
  malaria (fever) 084.0

R

Rabbia 071
Rabbit fever (see also Tularemia) 021.9
Rabies 071
  contact V01.5
  exposure to V01.5
  inoculation V04.5
    reaction — see Complications, vaccination
  vaccination, prophylactic (against) V04.5
Rachischisis (see also Spina bifida) 741.9
Rachitic — see also condition
  deformities of spine 268.1
  pelvis 268.1
    with disproportion (fetopelvic) 653.2
      affecting fetus or newborn 763.1
      causing obstructed labor 660.1
        affecting fetus or newborn 763.1
Rachitis, rachitism — see also Rickets
  acute 268.0
  fetalis 756.4

Rachitis, rachitism

Rachitis, rachitism — *see also* Rickets — *continued*
  renalis 588.0
  tarda 268.0
Racket nail 757.5
Radial nerve — *see* condition
Radiation effects or sickness — *see also* Effect, adverse, radiation
  cataract 366.46
  dermatitis 692.82
    sunburn (*see also* Sunburn) 692.71
Radiculitis (pressure) (vertebrogenic) 729.2
  accessory nerve 723.4
  anterior crural 724.4
  arm 723.4
  brachial 723.4
  cervical NEC 723.4
  due to displacement of intervertebral disc — *see* Neuritis, due to, displacement intervertebral disc
  leg 724.4
  lumbar NEC 724.4
  lumbosacral 724.4
  rheumatic 729.2
  syphilitic 094.89
  thoracic (with visceral pain) 724.4
Radiculomyelitis 357.0
  toxic, due to
    Clostridium tetani 037
    Corynebacterium diphtheriae 032.89
Radiculopathy (*see also* Radiculitis) 729.2
Radioactive substances, adverse effect — *see* Effect, adverse, radioactive substance
Radiodermal burns (acute) (chronic) (occupational) — *see* Burn, by site
Radiodermatitis 692.82
Radionecrosis — *see* Effect, adverse, radiation
Radiotherapy session V58.0
Radium, adverse effect — *see* Effect, adverse, radioactive substance
Raeder-Harbitz syndrome (pulseless disease) 446.7
Rage (*see also* Disturbance, conduct) 312.0 ✓5ᵗʰ
  meaning rabies 071
Rag sorters' disease 022.1
Raillietiniasis 123.8
Railroad neurosis 300.16
Railway spine 300.16
Raised — *see* Elevation
Raiva 071
Rake teeth, tooth 524.3
Rales 786.7
Ramifying renal pelvis 753.3
Ramsay Hunt syndrome (herpetic geniculate ganglionitis) 053.11
  meaning dyssynergia cerebellaris myoclonica 334.2
Ranke's primary infiltration (*see also* Tuberculosis) 010.0 ✓5ᵗʰ
Ranula 527.6
  congenital 750.26
Rape — *see* Injury, by site
  alleged, observation or examination V71.5
Rapid
  feeble pulse, due to shock, following injury 958.4
  heart (beat) 785.0
    psychogenic 306.2
  respiration 786.06
    psychogenic 306.1
  second stage (delivery) 661.3 ✓5ᵗʰ
    affecting fetus or newborn 763.6
  time-zone change syndrome 307.45
Rarefaction, bone 733.99
Rash 782.1
  canker 034.1
  diaper 691.0
  drug (internal use) 693.0
    contact 692.3
  ECHO 9 virus 078.89
  enema 692.89

Rash — *continued*
  food (*see also* Allergy, food) 693.1
  heat 705.1
  napkin 691.0
  nettle 708.8
  pustular 782.1
  rose 782.1
    epidemic 056.9
    of infants 057.8
  scarlet 034.1
  serum (prophylactic) (therapeutic) 999.5
  toxic 782.1
  wandering tongue 529.1
Rasmussen's aneurysm (*see also* Tuberculosis) 011.2 ✓5ᵗʰ
Rat-bite fever 026.9
  due to Streptobacillus moniliformis 026.1 ✓5ᵗʰ
  spirochetal (morsus muris) 026.0 ✓5ᵗʰ
Rathke's pouch tumor (M9350/1) 237.0
Raymond (-Céstan) syndrome 433.8 ✓5ᵗʰ
Raynaud's
  disease or syndrome (paroxysmal digital cyanosis) 443.0
  gangrene (symmetric) 443.0 [785.4]
  phenomenon (paroxysmal digital cyanosis) (secondary) 443.0
RDS 769
Reaction
  acute situational maladjustment (*see also* Reaction, adjustment) 309.9
  adaptation (*see also* Reaction, adjustment) 309.9
  adjustment 309.9
    with
      anxious mood 309.24
        with depressed mood 309.28
      conduct disturbance 309.3
        combined with disturbance of emotions 309.4
      depressed mood 309.0
        brief 309.0
          with anxious mood 309.28
        prolonged 309.1
      elective mutism 309.83
      mixed emotions and conduct 309.4
      mutism, elective 309.83
      physical symptoms 309.82
      predominant disturbance (of)
        conduct 309.3
        emotions NEC 309.29
          mixed 309.28
        mixed, emotions and conduct 309.4
        specified type NEC 309.89
      specific academic or work inhibition 309.23
      withdrawal 309.83
        depressive 309.0
          with conduct disturbance 309.4
          brief 309.0
          prolonged 309.1
    specified type NEC 309.89
  adverse food NEC 995.7
  affective (*see also* Psychosis, affective) 296.90
    specified type NEC 296.99
  aggressive 301.3
    unsocialized (*see also* Disturbance, conduct) 312.0 ✓5ᵗʰ
  allergic (*see also* Allergy) 995.3
    drug, medicinal substance, and biological — *see* Allergy, drug
    food — *see* Allergy, food
    serum 999.5
  anaphylactic — *see* Shock, anaphylactic
  anesthesia — *see* Anesthesia, complication
  anger 312.0 ✓5ᵗʰ
  antisocial 301.7
  antitoxin (prophylactic) (therapeutic) — *see* Complications, vaccination
  anxiety 300.00
  asthenic 300.5
  compulsive 300.3
  conversion (anesthetic) (autonomic) (hyperkinetic) (mixed paralytic) (paresthetic) 300.11
  deoxyribonuclease (DNA) (DNase)
    hypersensitivity NEC 287.2

Reaction — *continued*
  depressive 300.4
    acute 309.0
    affective (*see also* Psychosis, affective) 296.2 ✓5ᵗʰ
      recurrent episode 296.3 ✓5ᵗʰ
      single episode 296.2 ✓5ᵗʰ
    brief 309.0
    manic (*see also* Psychosis, affective) 296.80
    neurotic 300.4
    psychoneurotic 300.4
    psychotic 298.0
  dissociative 300.15
  drug NEC (*see also* Table of Drugs and Chemicals) 995.2
    allergic — *see* Allergy, drug
    correct substance properly administered 995.2
    obstetric anesthetic or analgesic NEC 668.9 ✓5ᵗʰ
      affecting fetus or newborn 763.5
      specified drug — *see* Table of Drugs and Chemicals
    overdose or poisoning 977.9
      specified drug — *see* Table of Drugs and Chemicals
    specific to newborn 779.4
    transmitted via placenta or breast milk — *see* Absorption, drug, through placenta
    withdrawal NEC 292.0
      infant of dependent mother 779.5
    wrong substance given or taken in error 977.9
      specified drug — *see* Table of Drugs and Chemicals
  dyssocial 301.7
  erysipeloid 027.1
  fear 300.20
    child 313.0
  fluid loss, cerebrospinal 349.0
  food — *see also* Allergy, food
    adverse NEC 995.7
    anaphylactic shock — *see* Anaphylactic shock, due to, food
  foreign
    body NEC 728.82
      in operative wound (inadvertently left) 998.4
        due to surgical material intentionally left — *see* Complications, due to (presence of) any device, implant, or graft classified to 996.0-996.5 NEC
    substance accidentally left during a procedure (chemical) (powder) (talc) 998.7
    body or object (instrument) (sponge) (swab) 998.4
  graft-versus-host (GVH) 996.85
  grief (acute) (brief) 309.0
    prolonged 309.1
  gross stress (*see also* Reaction, stress, acute) 308.9
  group delinquent (*see also* Disturbance, conduct) 312.2 ✓5ᵗʰ
  Herxheimer's 995.0
  hyperkinetic (*see also* Hyperkinesia) 314.9
  hypochondriacal 300.7
  hypoglycemic, due to insulin 251.0
    therapeutic misadventure 962.3
  hypomanic (*see also* Psychosis, affective) 296.0 ✓5ᵗʰ
    recurrent episode 296.1 ✓5ᵗʰ
    single episode 296.0 ✓5ᵗʰ
  hysterical 300.10
    conversion type 300.11
    dissociative 300.15
  id (bacterial cause) 692.89
  immaturity NEC 301.89
    aggressive 301.3
    emotional instability 301.59
  immunization — *see* Complications, vaccination
  incompatibility
    blood group (ABO) (infusion) (transfusion) 999.6

Index to Diseases

Reaction — *continued*
  incompatibility — *continued*
    Rh (factor) (infusion) (transfusion) 999.7
  inflammatory — *see* Infection
  infusion — *see* Complications, infusion
  inoculation (immune serum) — *see*
    Complications, vaccination
  insulin 995.2
  involutional
    paranoid 297.2
    psychotic (*see also* Psychosis, affective,
      depressive) 296.2 ✓5ᵗʰ
  leukemoid (lymphocytic) (monocytic)
    (myelocytic) 288.8
  LSD (*see also* Abuse, drugs, nondependent)
    305.3 ✓5ᵗʰ
  lumbar puncture 349.0
  manic-depressive (*see also* Psychosis, affective)
    296.80
    depressed 296.2 ✓5ᵗʰ
      recurrent episode 296.3 ✓5ᵗʰ
      single episode 296.2 ✓5ᵗʰ
    hypomanic 296.0 ✓5ᵗʰ
  neurasthenic 300.5
  neurogenic (*see also* Neurosis) 300.9
  neurotic NEC 300.9
  neurotic-depressive 300.4
  nitritoid — *see* Crisis, nitritoid
  obsessive (-compulsive) 300.3
  organic 293.9
    acute 293.0
    subacute 293.1
  overanxious, child or adolescent 313.0
  paranoid (chronic) 297.9
    acute 298.3
    climacteric 297.2
    involutional 297.2
    menopausal 297.2
    senile 290.20
    simple 297.0
  passive
    aggressive 301.84
    dependency 301.6
  personality (*see also* Disorder, personality)
    301.9
  phobic 300.20
  postradiation — *see* Effect, adverse, radiation
  psychogenic NEC 300.9
  psychoneurotic (*see also* Neurosis) 300.9
    anxiety 300.00
    compulsive 300.3
    conversion 300.11
    depersonalization 300.6
    depressive 300.4
    dissociative 300.15
    hypochondriacal 300.7
    hysterical 300.10
      conversion type 300.11
      dissociative type 300.15
    neurasthenic 300.5
    obsessive 300.3
    obsessive-compulsive 300.3
    phobic 300.20
    tension state 300.9
  psychophysiologic NEC (*see also* Disorder,
    psychosomatic) 306.9
    cardiovascular 306.2
    digestive 306.4
    endocrine 306.6
    gastrointestinal 306.4
    genitourinary 306.50
    heart 306.2
    hemic 306.8
    intestinal (large) (small) 306.4
    laryngeal 306.1
    lymphatic 306.8
    musculoskeletal 306.0
    pharyngeal 306.1
    respiratory 306.1
    skin 306.3
    special sense organs 306.7
  psychosomatic (*see also* Disorder,
    psychosomatic) 306.9
  psychotic (*see also* Psychosis) 298.9
    depressive 298.0
    due to or associated with physical condition
      (*see also* Psychosis, organic) 293.9

Reaction — *continued*
  psychotic (*see also* Psychosis) — *continued*
    involutional (*see also* Psychosis, affective)
      296.2 ✓5ᵗʰ
      recurrent episode 296.3 ✓5ᵗʰ
      single episode 296.2 ✓5ᵗʰ
  pupillary (myotonic) (tonic) 379.46
  radiation — *see* Effect, adverse, radiation
  runaway — *see also* Disturbance, conduct
    socialized 312.2 ✓5ᵗʰ
    undersocialized, unsocialized 312.1 ✓5ᵗʰ
  scarlet fever toxin — *see* Complications,
    vaccination
  schizophrenic (*see also* Schizophrenia)
    295.9 ✓5ᵗʰ
    latent 295.5 ✓5ᵗʰ
  serological for syphilis — *see* Serology for
    syphilis
  serum (prophylactic) (therapeutic) 999.5
    immediate 999.4
  situational (*see also* Reaction, adjustment)
    309.9
    acute, to stress 308.3
    adjustment (*see also* Reaction, adjustment)
      309.9
  somatization (*see also* Disorder, psychosomatic)
    306.9
  spinal puncture 349.0
  spite, child (*see also* Disturbance, conduct)
    312.0 ✓5ᵗʰ
  stress, acute 308.9
    with predominant disturbance (of)
      consciousness 308.1
      emotions 308.0
      mixed 308.4
      psychomotor 308.2
      specified type NEC 308.3
  bone or cartilage — *see* Fracture, stress
  surgical procedure — *see* Complications,
    surgical procedure
  tetanus antitoxin — *see* Complications,
    vaccination
  toxin-antitoxin — *see* Complications,
    vaccination
  transfusion (blood) (bone marrow)
    (lymphocytes) (allergic) — *see*
    Complications, transfusion
  tuberculin skin test, nonspecific (without active
    tuberculosis) 795.5
    positive (without active tuberculosis) 795.5
  ultraviolet — *see* Effect, adverse, ultraviolet
  undersocialized, unsocialized — *see also*
    Disturbance, conduct
    aggressive (type) 312.0 ✓5ᵗʰ
    unaggressive (type) 312.1 ✓5ᵗʰ
  vaccination (any) — *see* Complications,
    vaccination
  white graft (skin) 996.52
  withdrawing, child or adolescent 313.22
  x-ray — *see* Effect, adverse, x-rays
Reactive depression (*see also* Reaction,
  depressive) 300.4
  neurotic 300.4
  psychoneurotic 300.4
  psychotic 298.0
Rebound tenderness 789.6 ✓5ᵗʰ
Recalcitrant patient V15.81
Recanalization, thrombus — *see* Thrombosis
Recession, receding
  chamber angle (eye) 364.77
  chin 524.06
  gingival (generalized) (localized) (postinfective)
    (postoperative) 523.2
Recklinghausen's disease (M9540/1) 237.71
  bones (osteitis fibrosa cystica) 252.0
Recklinghausen-Applebaum disease
  (hemochromatosis) 275.0
Reclus' disease (cystic) 610.1
Recrudescent typhus (fever) 081.1
Recruitment, auditory 388.44
Rectalgia 569.42
Rectitis 569.49

Rectocele
  female (without uterine prolapse) 618.0
    with uterine prolapse 618.4
      complete 618.3
      incomplete 618.2
  in pregnancy or childbirth 654.4 ✓5ᵗʰ
    causing obstructed labor 660.2 ✓5ᵗʰ
      affecting fetus or newborn 763.1
  male 569.49
  vagina, vaginal (outlet) 618.0
Rectosigmoiditis 569.89
  ulcerative (chronic) 556.3
Rectosigmoid junction — *see* condition
Rectourethral — *see* condition
Rectovaginal — *see* condition
Rectovesical — *see* condition
Rectum, rectal — *see* condition
Recurrent — *see* condition
Red bugs 133.8
Red cedar asthma 495.8
Redness
  conjunctiva 379.93
  eye 379.93
  nose 478.1
Reduced ventilatory or vital capacity 794.2
Reduction
  function
    kidney (*see also* Disease, renal) 593.9
    liver 573.8
  ventilatory capacity 794.2
  vital capacity 794.2
Redundant, redundancy
  abdomen 701.9
  anus 751.5
  cardia 537.89
  clitoris 624.2
  colon (congenital) 751.5
  foreskin (congenital) 605
  intestine 751.5
  labia 624.3
  organ or site, congenital NEC — *see* Accessory
  panniculus (abdominal) 278.1
  prepuce (congenital) 605
  pylorus 537.89
  rectum 751.5
  scrotum 608.89
  sigmoid 751.5
  skin (of face) 701.9
    eyelids 374.30
  stomach 537.89
  uvula 528.9
  vagina 623.8
Reduplication — *see* Duplication
Referral
  adoption (agency) V68.89
  nursing care V63.8
  patient without examination or treatment
    V68.81
  social services V63.8
Reflex — *see also* condition
  blink, deficient 374.45
  hyperactive gag 478.29
  neurogenic bladder NEC 596.54
    atonic 596.54
      with cauda equina syndrome 344.61
  vasoconstriction 443.9
  vasovagal 780.2
Reflux
  esophageal 530.81
  esophagitis 530.11
  gastroesophageal 530.81
  mitral — *see* Insufficiency, mitral
  ureteral — *see* Reflux, vesicoureteral
  vesicoureteral 593.70
    with
      reflux nephropathy 593.73
        bilateral 593.72
        unilateral 593.71
Reformed gallbladder 576.0
Reforming, artificial openings (*see also*
  Attention to, artificial, opening) V55.9
Refractive error (*see also* Error, refractive) 367.9

Refsum's disease or syndrome

Refsum's disease or syndrome (heredopathia atactica polyneuritiformis) 356.3
Refusal of
   food 307.59
      hysterical 300.11
   treatment because of, due to
      patient's decision NEC V64.2
      reason of conscience or religion V62.6
Regaud
   tumor (M8082/3) — see Neoplasm, nasopharynx, malignant
   type carcinoma (M8082/3) — see Neoplasm, nasopharynx, malignant
Regional — see condition
Regulation feeding (elderly) (infant) 783.3
   newborn 779.3
Regurgitated
   food, choked on 933.1
   stomach contents, choked on 933.1
Regurgitation
   aortic (valve) (see also Insufficiency, aortic) 424.1
      congenital 746.4
      syphilitic 093.22
   food — see also Vomiting
      with reswallowing — see Rumination
      newborn 779.3
   gastric contents — see Vomiting
   heart — see Endocarditis
   mitral (valve) — see also Insufficiency, mitral
      congenital 746.6
   myocardial — see Endocarditis
   pulmonary (heart) (valve) (see also Endocarditis, pulmonary) 424.3
   stomach — see Vomiting
   tricuspid — see Endocarditis, tricuspid
   valve, valvular — see Endocarditis
   vesicoureteral — see Reflux, vesicoureteral
Rehabilitation V57.9
   multiple types V57.89
   occupational V57.21
   specified type NEC V57.89
   speech V57.3
   vocational V57.22
Reichmann's disease or syndrome (gastrosuccorrhea) 536.8
Reifenstein's syndrome (hereditary familial hypogonadism, male) 257.2
Reilly's syndrome or phenomenon (see also Neuropathy, peripheral, autonomic) 337.9
Reimann's periodic disease 277.3
Reinsertion, contraceptive device V25.42
Reiter's disease, syndrome, or urethritis 099.3 [711.1]
Rejection
   food, hysterical 300.11
   transplant 996.80
      bone marrow 996.85
      corneal 996.51
      organ (immune or nonimmune cause) 996.80
         bone marrow 996.85
         heart 996.83
         intestines 996.87
         kidney 996.81
         liver 996.82
         lung 996.84
         pancreas 996.86
         specified NEC 996.89
      skin 996.52
         artificial 996.55
         decellularized allodermis 996.55
Relapsing fever 087.9
   Carter's (Asiatic) 087.0
   Dutton's (West African) 087.1
   Koch's 087.9
   louse-borne (epidemic) 087.0
   Novy's (American) 087.1
   Obermeyer's (European) 087.0
   Spirillum 087.9
   tick-borne (endemic) 087.1
Relaxation
   anus (sphincter) 569.49
      due to hysteria 300.11

Relaxation — continued
   arch (foot) 734
      congenital 754.61
   back ligaments 728.4
   bladder (sphincter) 596.59
   cardio-esophageal 530.89
   cervix (see also Incompetency, cervix) 622.5
   diaphragm 519.4
   inguinal rings — see Hernia, inguinal
   joint (capsule) (ligament) (paralytic) (see also Derangement, joint) 718.90
      congenital 755.8
   lumbosacral joint 724.6
   pelvic floor 618.8
   pelvis 618.8
   perineum 618.8
   posture 729.9
   rectum (sphincter) 569.49
   sacroiliac (joint) 724.6
   scrotum 608.89
   urethra (sphincter) 599.84
   uterus (outlet) 618.8
   vagina (outlet) 618.8
   vesical 596.59
Remains
   canal of Cloquet 743.51
   capsule (opaque) 743.51
Remittent fever (malarial) 084.6
Remnant
   canal of Cloquet 743.51
   capsule (opaque) 743.51
   cervix, cervical stump (acquired) (postoperative) 622.8
   cystic duct, postcholecystectomy 576.0
   fingernail 703.8
      congenital 757.5
   meniscus, knee 717.5
   thyroglossal duct 759.2
   tonsil 474.8
      infected 474.00
   urachus 753.7
Remote effect of cancer — see condition
Removal (of)
   catheter (urinary) (indwelling) V53.6
      from artificial opening — see Attention to, artificial, opening
      non-vascular V58.82
      vascular V58.81
   cerebral ventricle (communicating) shunt V53.01
   device — see also Fitting (of)
      contraceptive V25.42
      fixation
         external V54.89 ▲
         internal V54.0
      traction V54.89 ▲
   dressing V58.3
   ileostomy V55.2
   Kirschner wire V54.89 ▲
   nonvascular catheter V58.82
   pin V54.0
   plaster cast V54.89 ▲
   plate (fracture) V54.0
   rod V54.0
   screw V54.0
   splint, external V54.89 ▲
   subdermal implantable contraceptive V25.43
   suture V58.3
   traction device, external V54.89 ▲
   vascular catheter V58.81
Ren
   arcuatus 753.3
   mobile, mobilis (see also Disease, renal) 593.0
      congenital 753.3
   unguliformis 753.3
Renal — see also condition
   glomerulohyalinosis-diabetic syndrome 250.4 [581.81]
Rendu-Osler-Weber disease or syndrome (familial hemorrhagic telangiectasia) 448.0
Reninoma (M8361/1) 236.91
Rénon-Delille syndrome 253.8

Repair
   pelvic floor, previous, in pregnancy or childbirth 654.4
      affecting fetus or newborn 763.89
   scarred tissue V51
Replacement by artificial or mechanical device or prosthesis of (see also Fitting (of))
   artificial skin V43.83
   bladder V43.5
   blood vessel V43.4
   breast V43.82
   eye globe V43.0
   heart V43.2
      valve V43.3
   intestine V43.89
   joint V43.60
      ankle V43.66
      elbow V43.62
      finger V43.69
      hip (partial) (total) V43.64
      knee V43.65
      shoulder V43.61
      specified NEC V43.69
      wrist V43.63
   kidney V43.89
   larynx V43.81
   lens V43.1
   limb(s) V43.7
   liver V43.89
   lung V43.89
   organ NEC V43.89
   pancreas V43.89
   skin (artificial) V43.83
   tissue NEC V43.89
Reprogramming
   cardiac pacemaker V53.31
Request for expert evidence V68.2
Reserve, decreased or low
   cardiac — see Disease, heart
   kidney (see also Disease, renal) 593.9
Residual — see also condition
   bladder 596.8
   foreign body — see Retention, foreign body
   state, schizophrenic (see also Schizophrenia) 295.6
   urine 788.69
Resistance, resistant (to)

> Note — use the following subclassification for categories V09.5, V09.7, V09.8, V09.9:
>
> 0   without mention of resistance to multiple drugs
> 1   with resistance to multiple drugs
>   V09.5   quinolones and fluoroquinolones
>   V09.7   antimycobacterial agents
>   V09.8   specified drugs NEC
>   V09.9   unspecified drugs
> 9   multiple sites

   drugs by microorganisms V09.9
      Amikacin V09.4
      aminoglycosides V09.4
      Amodiaquine V09.5
      Amoxicillin V09.0
      Ampicillin V09.0
      antimycobacterial agents V09.7 ●
      Azithromycin V09.2
      Azlocillin V09.0
      Aztreonam V09.1
      B-lactam antibiotics V09.1
      bacampicillin V09.0
      Bacitracin V09.8
      Benznidazole V09.8
      Capreomycin V09.7
      Carbenicillin V09.0
      Cefaclor V09.1
      Cefadroxil V09.1
      Cefamandole V09.1
      Cefatetan V09.1
      Cefazolin V09.1
      Cefixime V09.1
      Cefonicid V09.1
      Cefoperazone V09.1
      Ceforanide V09.1

Index to Diseases

Resistance, resistant (to) — continued
  drugs by microorganisms — continued
    Cefotaxime V09.1
    Cefoxitin V09.1
    Ceftazidime V09.1
    Ceftizoxime V09.1
    Ceftriaxone V09.1
    Cefuroxime V09.1
    Cephalexin V09.1
    Cephaloglycin V09.1
    Cephaloridine V09.1
    Cephalosporins V09.1
    Cephalothin V09.1
    Cephapirin V09.1
    Cephradine V09.1
    Chloramphenicol V09.8 ✓5ᵗʰ
    Chloraquine V09.5 ✓5ᵗʰ
    Chlorguanide V09.8 ✓5ᵗʰ
    Chlorproguanil V09.8 ✓5ᵗʰ
    Chlortetracyline V09.3
    Cinoxacin V09.5 ✓5ᵗʰ
    Ciprofloxacin V09.5 ✓5ᵗʰ
    Clarithromycin V09.2
    Clindamycin V09.8 ✓5ᵗʰ
    Clioquinol V09.5 ✓5ᵗʰ
    Clofazimine V09.7 ✓5ᵗʰ
    Cloxacillin V09.0
    Cyclacillin V09.0
    Cycloserine V09.7 ✓5ᵗʰ
    Dapsone [DZ] V09.7 ✓5ᵗʰ
    Demeclocycline V09.3
    Dicloxacillin V09.0
    Doxycycline V09.3
    Enoxacin V09.5 ✓5ᵗʰ
    Erythromycin V09.2
    Ethambutol [EMB] V09.7 ✓5ᵗʰ
    Ethionamide [ETA] V09.7 ✓5ᵗʰ
    fluoroquinolones V09.5 ✓5ᵗʰ
    Gentamicin V09.4
    Halofantrine V09.8 ✓5ᵗʰ
    Imipenem V09.1
    Iodoquinol V09.5 ✓5ᵗʰ
    Isoniazid [INH] V09.7 ✓5ᵗʰ
    Kanamycin V09.4
    macrolides V09.2
    Mafenide V09.6
    Mefloquine V09.8 ✓5ᵗʰ
    Melasoprol V09.8 ✓5ᵗʰ
    Methacycline V09.3
    Methenamine V09.8 ✓5ᵗʰ
    Methicillin V09.0
    Metronidazole V09.8 ✓5ᵗʰ
    Mezlocillin V09.0
    Minocycline V09.3
    Nafcillin V09.0
    Nalidixic acid V09.5 ✓5ᵗʰ
    Natamycin V09.2
    Neomycin V09.4
    Netilmicin V09.4
    Nifurtimox V09.8 ✓5ᵗʰ
    Nimorazole V09.8 ✓5ᵗʰ
    Nitrofurantoin V09.8 ✓5ᵗʰ
    Norfloxacin V09.5 ✓5ᵗʰ
    Nystatin V09.2
    Ofloxacin V09.5 ✓5ᵗʰ
    Oleandomycin V09.2
    Oxacillin V09.0
    Oxytetracycline V09.3
    Para-amino salicylic acid [PAS] V09.7 ✓5ᵗʰ
    Paromomycin V09.4
    Penicillin (G) (V) (VK) V09.0
    penicillins V09.0
    Pentamidine V09.8 ✓5ᵗʰ
    Piperacillin V09.0
    Primaquine V09.5 ✓5ᵗʰ
    Proguanil V09.8 ✓5ᵗʰ
    Pyrazinamide [PZA] V09.7 ✓5ᵗʰ
    Pyrimethamine/sulfalene V09.8 ✓5ᵗʰ
    Pyrimethamine/sulfodoxine V09.8 ✓5ᵗʰ
    Quinacrine V09.5 ✓5ᵗʰ
    Quinidine V09.8 ✓5ᵗʰ
    Quinine V09.8 ✓5ᵗʰ
    quinolones V09.5 ✓5ᵗʰ
    Rifabutin V09.7 ✓5ᵗʰ
    Rifampin [RIF] V09.7 ✓5ᵗʰ
    Rifamycin V09.7 ✓5ᵗʰ
    Rolitetracycline V09.3

Resistance, resistant (to) — continued
  drugs by microorganisms — continued
    Specified drugs NEC V09.8 ✓5ᵗʰ
    Spectinomycin V09.8 ✓5ᵗʰ
    Spiramycin V09.2
    Streptomycin [SM] V09.4
    Sulfacetamide V09.6
    Sulfacytine V09.6
    Sulfadiazine V09.6
    Sulfadoxine V09.6
    Sulfamethoxazole V09.6
    Sulfapyridine V09.6
    Sulfasalizine V09.6
    Sulfasoxazone V09.6
    sulfonamides V09.6
    Sulfoxone V09.7 ✓5ᵗʰ
    tetracycline V09.3
    tetracyclines V09.3
    Thiamphenicol V09.8 ✓5ᵗʰ
    Ticarcillin V09.0
    Tinidazole V09.8 ✓5ᵗʰ
    Tobramycin V09.4
    Triamphenicol V09.8 ✓5ᵗʰ
    Trimethoprim V09.8 ✓5ᵗʰ
    Vancomycin V09.8 ✓5ᵗʰ
Resorption
  biliary 576.8
    purulent or putrid (see also Cholecystitis) 576.8
  dental (roots) 521.4
    alveoli 525.8
  septic — see Septicemia
  teeth (external) (internal) (pathological) (roots) 521.4
Respiration
  asymmetrical 786.09
  bronchial 786.09
  Cheyne-Stokes (periodic respiration) 786.04
  decreased, due to shock following injury 958.4
  disorder of 786.00
    psychogenic 306.1
    specified NEC 786.09
  failure 518.81
    acute 518.81
    acute and chronic 518.84
    chronic 518.83
    newborn 770.84 ▲
  insufficiency 786.09
    acute 518.82
    newborn NEC 770.89 ▲
  Kussmaul (air hunger) 786.09
  painful 786.52
  periodic 786.09
  poor 786.09
    newborn NEC 770.89 ▲
  sighing 786.7
    psychogenic 306.1
  wheezing 786.07
Respiratory — see also condition
  distress 786.09
    acute 518.82
    fetus or newborn NEC 770.89 ▲
    syndrome (newborn) 769
      adult (following shock, surgery, or trauma) 518.5
      specified NEC 518.82
  failure 518.81
    acute 518.81
    acute and chronic 518.8
    chronic 518.83
Respiratory syncytial virus (RSV) 079.6
  bronchiolitis 466.11
  pneumonia 480.1
Response
  photoallergic 692.72
  phototoxic 692.72
Rest, rests
  mesonephric duct 752.8
    fallopian tube 752.11
  ovarian, in fallopian tubes 752.19
  wolffian duct 752.8
Restless leg (syndrome) 333.99
Restlessness 799.2
Restoration of organ continuity from previous sterilization (tuboplasty) (vasoplasty) V26.0

Restriction of housing space V60.1
Restzustand, schizophrenic (see also Schizophrenia) 295.6 ✓5ᵗʰ
Retained — see Retention
Retardation
  development, developmental, specific (see also Disorder, development, specific) 315.9
    learning, specific 315.2
      arithmetical 315.1
      language (skills) 315.31
        expressive 315.31
        mixed receptive-expressive 315.32
      mathematics 315.1
      reading 315.00
        phonological 315.39
      written expression 315.2
    motor 315.4
  endochondral bone growth 733.91
  growth (physical) in childhood 783.43
    due to malnutrition 263.2
  fetal (intrauterine) 764.9 ✓5ᵗʰ
    affecting management of pregnancy 656.5 ✓5ᵗʰ
  intrauterine growth 764.9 ✓5ᵗʰ
    affecting management of pregnancy 656.5 ✓5ᵗʰ
  mental 319
    borderline V62.89
    mild, IQ 50-70 317
    moderate, IQ 35-49 318.0
    profound, IQ under 20 318.2
    severe, IQ 20-34 318.1
  motor, specific 315.4
  physical 783.43
    child 783.43
    due to malnutrition 263.2
    fetus (intrauterine) 764.9 ✓5ᵗʰ
      affecting management of pregnancy 656.5 ✓5ᵗʰ
  psychomotor NEC 307.9
  reading 315.00
Retching — see Vomiting
Retention, retained
  bladder NEC (see also Retention, urine) 788.20
    psychogenic 306.53
  carbon dioxide 276.2
  cyst — see Cyst
  dead
    fetus (after 22 completed weeks gestation) 656.4 ✓5ᵗʰ
      early fetal death (before 22 completed weeks gestation) 632
    ovum 631
  decidua (following delivery) (fragments) (with hemorrhage) 666.2 ✓5ᵗʰ
    without hemorrhage 667.1 ✓5ᵗʰ
  deciduous tooth 520.6
  dental root 525.3
  fecal (see also Constipation) 564.00
  fluid 276.6
  foreign body — see also Foreign body, retained
    bone 733.99
    current trauma — see Foreign body, by site or type
    middle ear 385.83
    muscle 729.6
    soft tissue NEC 729.6
  gastric 536.8
  membranes (following delivery) (with hemorrhage) 666.2 ✓5ᵗʰ
    with abortion — see Abortion, by type
    without hemorrhage 667.1 ✓5ᵗʰ
  menses 626.8
  milk (puerperal) 676.2 ✓5ᵗʰ
  nitrogen, extrarenal 788.9
  placenta (total) (with hemorrhage) 666.0 ✓5ᵗʰ
    with abortion — see Abortion, by type
    portions or fragments 666.2 ✓5ᵗʰ
      without hemorrhage 667.1 ✓5ᵗʰ
    without hemorrhage 667.0 ✓5ᵗʰ
  products of conception
    early pregnancy (fetal death before 22 completed weeks gestation) 632
    following
      abortion — see Abortion, by type

Retention, retained — continued
 products of conception — continued
  following — continued
   delivery 666.2 ✓5ᵗʰ
    with hemorrhage 666.2 ✓5ᵗʰ
    without hemorrhage 667.1 ✓5ᵗʰ
  secundines (following delivery) (with hemorrhage) 666.2 ✓5ᵗʰ
  with abortion — see Abortion, by type
  complicating puerperium (delayed hemorrhage) 666.2 ✓5ᵗʰ
   without hemorrhage 667.1 ✓5ᵗʰ
 smegma, clitoris 624.8
 urine NEC 788.20
  bladder, incomplete emptying 788.21
  psychogenic 306.53
  specified NEC 788.29
 water (in tissue) (see also Edema) 782.3
Reticulation, dust (occupational) 504
Reticulocytosis NEC 790.99
Reticuloendotheliosis
 acute infantile (M9722/3) 202.5 ✓5ᵗʰ
 leukemic (M9940/3) 202.4 ✓5ᵗʰ
 malignant (M9720/3) 202.3 ✓5ᵗʰ
 nonlipid (M9722/3) 202.5 ✓5ᵗʰ
Reticulohistiocytoma (giant cell) 277.8
Reticulohistiocytosis, multicentric 272.8
Reticulolymphosarcoma (diffuse) (M9613/3) 200.8 ✓5ᵗʰ
 follicular (M9691/3) 202.0 ✓5ᵗʰ
 nodular (M9691/3) 202.0 ✓5ᵗʰ
Reticulosarcoma (M9640/3) 200.0 ✓5ᵗʰ
 nodular (M9642/3) 200.0 ✓5ᵗʰ
 pleomorphic cell type (M9641/3) 200.0 ✓5ᵗʰ
Reticulosis (skin)
 acute of infancy (M9722/3) 202.5 ✓5ᵗʰ
 histiocytic medullary (M9721/3) 202.3 ✓5ᵗʰ
 lipomelanotic 695.89
 malignant (M9720/3) 202.3 ✓5ᵗʰ
 Sézary's (M9701/3) 202.2 ✓5ᵗʰ
Retina, retinal — see condition
Retinitis (see also Chorioretinitis) 363.20
 albuminurica 585 [363.10]
 arteriosclerotic 440.8 [362.13]
 central angiospastic 362.41
 Coat's 362.12
 diabetic 250.5 ✓5ᵗʰ [362.01]
 disciformis 362.52
 disseminated 363.10
  metastatic 363.14
  neurosyphilitic 094.83
  pigment epitheliopathy 363.15
 exudative 362.12
 focal 363.00
  in histoplasmosis 115.92
   capsulatum 115.02
   duboisii 115.12
  juxtapapillary 363.05
  macular 363.06
  paramacular 363.06
  peripheral 363.08
  posterior pole NEC 363.07
 gravidarum 646.8 ✓5ᵗʰ
 hemorrhagica externa 362.12
 juxtapapillary (Jensen's) 363.05
 luetic — see Retinitis, syphilitic
 metastatic 363.14
 pigmentosa 362.74
 proliferans 362.29
 proliferating 362.29
 punctata albescens 362.76
 renal 585 [363.13]
 syphilitic (secondary) 091.51
  congenital 090.0 [363.13]
  early 091.51
  late 095.8 [363.13]
 syphilitica, central, recurrent 095.8 [363.13]
 tuberculous (see also Tuberculous) 017.3 ✓5ᵗʰ [363.13]
Retinoblastoma (M9510/3) 190.5
 differentiated type (M9511/3) 190.5
 undifferentiated type (M9512/3) 190.5

Retinochoroiditis (see also Chorioretinitis) 363.20
 central angiospastic 362.41
 disseminated 363.10
  metastatic 363.14
  neurosyphilitic 094.83
  pigment epitheliopathy 363.15
  syphilitic 094.83
 due to toxoplasmosis (acquired) (focal) 130.2
 focal 363.00
  in histoplasmosis 115.92
   capsulatum 115.02
   duboisii 115.12
  juxtapapillary (Jensen's) 363.05
  macular 363.06
  paramacular 363.06
  peripheral 363.08
  posterior pole NEC 363.07
 juxtapapillaris 363.05
 syphilitic (disseminated) 094.83
Retinopathy (background) 362.10
 arteriosclerotic 440.8 [362.13]
 atherosclerotic 440.8 [362.13]
 central serous 362.41
 circinate 362.10
 Coat's 362.12
 diabetic 250.5 ✓5ᵗʰ [362.01]
  proliferative 250.5 ✓5ᵗʰ [362.02]
 exudative 362.12
 hypertensive 362.11
 of prematurity 362.21
 pigmentary, congenital 362.74
 proliferative 362.29
  diabetic 250.5 [362.02]
  sickle-cell 282.60 [362.29]
 solar 363.31
Retinoschisis 361.10
 bullous 361.12
 congenital 743.56
 flat 361.11
 juvenile 362.73
Retractile testis 752.52
Retraction
 cervix (see also Retroversion, uterus) 621.6
 drum (membrane) 384.82
 eyelid 374.41
 finger 736.29
 head 781.0
 lid 374.41
 lung 518.89
 mediastinum 519.3
 nipple 611.79
  congenital 757.6
  puerperal, postpartum 676.0 ✓5ᵗʰ
 palmar fascia 728.6
 pleura (see also Pleurisy) 511.0
 ring, uterus (Bandl's) (pathological) 661.4 ✓5ᵗʰ
  affecting fetus or newborn 763.7
 sternum (congenital) 756.3
  acquired 738.3
  during respiration 786.9
 substernal 738.3
 supraclavicular 738.8
 syndrome (Duane's) 378.71
 uterus (see also Retroversion, uterus) 621.6
 valve (heart) — see Endocarditis
Retrobulbar — see condition
Retrocaval ureter 753.4
Retrocecal — see also condition
 appendix (congenital) 751.5
Retrocession — see Retroversion
Retrodisplacement — see Retroversion
Retroflection, retroflexion — see Retroversion
Retrognathia, retrognathism (mandibular) (maxillary) 524.06
Retrograde
 ejaculation 608.87
 menstruation 626.8
Retroiliac ureter 753.4
Retroperineal — see condition
Retroperitoneal — see condition
Retroperitonitis (see also Peritonitis) 567.9
Retropharyngeal — see condition
Retroplacental — see condition

Retroposition — see Retroversion
Retrosternal thyroid (congenital) 759.2
Retroversion, retroverted
 cervix (see also Retroversion, uterus) 621.6
 female NEC (see also Retroversion, uterus) 621.6
 iris 364.70
 testis (congenital) 752.51
 uterus, uterine (acquired) (acute) (adherent) (any degree) (asymptomatic) (cervix) (postinfectional) (postpartal, old) 621.6
  congenital 752.3
  in pregnancy or childbirth 654.3 ✓5ᵗʰ
   affecting fetus or newborn 763.89
   causing obstructed labor 660.2 ✓5ᵗʰ
    affecting fetus or newborn 763.1
Retrusion, premaxilla (developmental) 524.04
Rett's syndrome 330.8
Reverse, reversed
 peristalsis 787.4
Reye's syndrome 331.81
Reye-Sheehan syndrome (postpartum pituitary necrosis) 253.2
Rh (factor)
 hemolytic disease 773.0
 incompatibility, immunization, or sensitization
  affecting management of pregnancy 656.1 ✓5ᵗʰ
  fetus or newborn 773.0
  transfusion reaction 999.7
 negative mother, affecting fetus or newborn 773.0
 titer elevated 999.7
 transfusion reaction 999.7
Rhabdomyolysis (idiopathic) 728.89
Rhabdomyoma (M8900/0) — see also Neoplasm, connective tissue, benign
 adult (M8904/0) — see Neoplasm, connective tissue, benign
 fetal (M8903/0) — see Neoplasm, connective tissue, benign
 glycogenic (M8904/0) — see Neoplasm, connective tissue, benign
Rhabdomyosarcoma (M8900/3) — see also Neoplasm, connective tissue, malignant
 alveolar (M8920/3) — see Neoplasm, connective tissue, malignant
 embryonal (M8910/3) — see Neoplasm, connective tissue, malignant
 mixed type (M8902/3) — see Neoplasm, connective tissue, malignant
 pleomorphic (M8901/3) — see Neoplasm, connective tissue, malignant
Rhabdosarcoma (M8900/3) — see Rhabdomyosarcoma
Rhesus (factor) (Rh) incompatibility — see Rh, incompatibility
Rheumaticosis — see Rheumatism
Rheumatism, rheumatic (acute NEC) 729.0
 adherent pericardium 393
 arthritis
  acute or subacute — see Fever, rheumatic
  chronic 714.0
   spine 720.0
  articular (chronic) NEC (see also Arthritis) 716.9 ✓5ᵗʰ
   acute or subacute — see Fever, rheumatic
 back 724.9
 blennorrhagic 098.59
 carditis — see Disease, heart, rheumatic
 cerebral — see Fever, rheumatic
 chorea (acute) — see Chorea, rheumatic
 chronic NEC 729.0
 coronary arteritis 391.9
  chronic 398.99
 degeneration, myocardium (see also Degeneration, myocardium, with rheumatic fever) 398.0
 desert 114.0
 febrile — see Fever, rheumatic
 fever — see Fever, rheumatic
 gonococcal 098.59
 gout 274.0

Index to Diseases

Rheumatism, rheumatic — *continued*
  heart
    disease (*see also* Disease, heart, rheumatic) 398.90
    failure (chronic) (congestive) (inactive) 398.91
  hemopericardium — *see* Rheumatic, pericarditis
  hydropericardium — *see* Rheumatic, pericarditis
  inflammatory (acute) (chronic) (subacute) — *see* Fever, rheumatic
  intercostal 729.0
    meaning Tietze's disease 733.6
  joint (chronic) NEC (*see also* Arthritis) 716.9
    acute — *see* Fever, rheumatic
  mediastinopericarditis — *see* Rheumatic, pericarditis
  muscular 729.0
  myocardial degeneration (*see also* Degeneration, myocardium, with rheumatic fever) 398.0
  myocarditis (chronic) (inactive) (with chorea) 398.0
    active or acute 391.2
      with chorea (acute) (rheumatic) (Sydenham's) 392.0
  myositis 729.1
  neck 724.9
  neuralgic 729.0
  neuritis (acute) (chronic) 729.2
  neuromuscular 729.0
  nodose — *see* Arthritis, nodosa
  nonarticular 729.0
  palindromic 719.30
    ankle 719.37
    elbow 719.32
    foot 719.37
    hand 719.34
    hip 719.35
    knee 719.36
    multiple sites 719.39
    pelvic region 719.35
    shoulder (region) 719.31
    specified site NEC 719.38
    wrist 719.33
  pancarditis, acute 391.8
    with chorea (acute) (rheumatic) (Sydenham's) 392.0
    chronic or inactive 398.99
  pericarditis (active) (acute) (with effusion) (with pneumonia) 391.0
    with chorea (acute) (rheumatic) (Sydenham's) 392.0
    chronic or inactive 393
  pericardium — *see* Rheumatic, pericarditis
  pleuropericarditis — *see* Rheumatic, pericarditis
  pneumonia 390 [517.1]
  pneumonitis 390 [517.1]
  pneumopericarditis — *see* Rheumatic, pericarditis
  polyarthritis
    acute or subacute — *see* Fever, rheumatic
    chronic 714.0
  polyarticular NEC (*see also* Arthritis) 716.9
  psychogenic 306.0
  radiculitis 729.2
  sciatic 724.3
  septic — *see* Fever, rheumatic
  spine 724.9
  subacute NEC 729.0
  torticollis 723.5
  tuberculous NEC (*see also* Tuberculosis) 015.9
  typhoid fever 002.0
Rheumatoid — *see also* condition
  lungs 714.81
Rhinitis (atrophic) (catarrhal) (chronic) (croupous) (fibrinous) (hyperplastic) (hypertrophic) (membranous) (purulent) (suppurative) (ulcerative) 472.0
  with
    hay fever (*see also* Fever, hay) 477.9
      with asthma (bronchial) 493.0
    sore throat — *see* Nasopharyngitis

Rhinitis — *continued*
  acute 460
  allergic (nonseasonal) (seasonal) (*see also* Fever, hay) 477.9
    with asthma (*see also* Asthma) 493.0
    due to food 477.1
  granulomatous 472.0
  infective 460
  obstructive 472.0
  pneumococcal 460
  syphilitic 095.8
    congenital 090.0
  tuberculous (*see also* Tuberculosis) 012.8
  vasomotor (*see also* Fever, hay) 477.9
Rhinoantritis (chronic) 473.0
  acute 461.0
Rhinodacryolith 375.57
Rhinolalia (aperta) (clausa) (open) 784.49
Rhinolith 478.1
  nasal sinus (*see also* Sinusitis) 473.9
Rhinomegaly 478.1
Rhinopharyngitis (acute) (subacute) (*see also* Nasopharyngitis) 460
  chronic 472.2
  destructive ulcerating 102.5
  mutilans 102.5
Rhinophyma 695.3
Rhinorrhea 478.1
  cerebrospinal (fluid) 349.81
  paroxysmal (*see also* Fever, hay) 477.9
  spasmodic (*see also* Fever, hay) 477.9
Rhinosalpingitis 381.50
  acute 381.51
  chronic 381.52
Rhinoscleroma 040.1
Rhinosporidiosis 117.0
Rhinovirus infection 079.3
Rhizomelique, pseudopolyarthritic 446.5
Rhoads and Bomford anemia (refractory) 284.9
Rhus
  diversiloba dermatitis 692.6
  radicans dermatitis 692.6
  toxicodendron dermatitis 692.6
  venenata dermatitis 692.6
  verniciflua dermatitis 692.6
Rhythm
  atrioventricular nodal 427.89
  disorder 427.9
    coronary sinus 427.89
    ectopic 427.89
    nodal 427.89
  escape 427.89
  heart, abnormal 427.9
    fetus or newborn — *see* Abnormal, heart rate
  idioventricular 426.89
    accelerated 427.89
  nodal 427.89
  sleep, inversion 780.55
    nonorganic origin 307.45
Rhytidosis facialis 701.8
Rib — *see also* condition
  cervical 756.2
Riboflavin deficiency 266.0
Rice bodies (*see also* Loose, body, joint) 718.1
  knee 717.6
Richter's hernia — *see* Hernia, Richter's
Ricinism 988.2
Rickets (active) (acute) (adolescent) (adult) (chest wall) (congenital) (current) (infantile) (intestinal) 268.0
  celiac 579.0
  fetal 756.4
  hemorrhagic 267
  hypophosphatemic with nephroticglycosuric dwarfism 270.0
  kidney 588.0
  late effect 268.1
  renal 588.0
  scurvy 267
  vitamin D-resistant 275.3

Rickettsial disease 083.9
  specified type NEC 083.8
Rickettsialpox 083.2
Rickettsiosis NEC 083.9
  specified type NEC 083.8
  tick-borne 082.9
    specified type NEC 082.8
  vesicular 083.2
Ricord's chancre 091.0
Riddoch's syndrome (visual disorientation) 368.16
Rider's
  bone 733.99
  chancre 091.0
Ridge, alveolus — *see also* condition
  flabby 525.2
Ridged ear 744.29
Riedel's
  disease (ligneous thyroiditis) 245.3
  lobe, liver 751.69
  struma (ligneous thyroiditis) 245.3
  thyroiditis (ligneous) 245.3
Rieger's anomaly or syndrome (mesodermal dysgenesis, anterior ocular segment) 743.44
Riehl's melanosis 709.09
Rietti-Greppi-Micheli anemia or syndrome 282.4
Rieux's hernia — *see* Hernia, Rieux's
Rift Valley fever 066.3
Riga's disease (cachectic aphthae) 529.0
Riga-Fede disease (cachectic aphthae) 529.0
Riggs' disease (compound periodontitis) 523.4
Right middle lobe syndrome 518.0
Rigid, rigidity — *see also* condition
  abdominal 789.4
  articular, multiple congenital 754.89
  back 724.8
  cervix uteri
    in pregnancy or childbirth 654.6
      affecting fetus or newborn 763.89
      causing obstructed labor 660.2
        affecting fetus or newborn 763.1
  hymen (acquired) (congenital) 623.3
  nuchal 781.6
  pelvic floor
    in pregnancy or childbirth 654.4
      affecting fetus or newborn 763.89
      causing obstructed labor 660.2
        affecting fetus or newborn 763.1
  perineum or vulva
    in pregnancy or childbirth 654.8
      affecting fetus or newborn 763.89
      causing obstructed labor 660.2
        affecting fetus or newborn 763.1
  spine 724.8
  vagina
    in pregnancy or childbirth 654.7
      affecting fetus or newborn 763.89
      causing obstructed labor 660.2
        affecting fetus or newborn 763.1
Rigors 780.99
Riley-Day syndrome (familial dysautonomia) 742.8
Ring(s)
  aorta 747.21
  Bandl's, complicating delivery 661.4
    affecting fetus or newborn 763.7
  contraction, complicating delivery 661.4
    affecting fetus or newborn 763.7
  esophageal (congenital) 750.3
  Fleischer (-Kayser) (cornea) 275.1 [371.14]
  hymenal, tight (acquired) (congenital) 623.3
  Kayser-Fleischer (cornea) 275.1 [371.14]
  retraction, uterus, pathological 661.4
    affecting fetus or newborn 763.7
  Schatzki's (esophagus) (congenital) (lower) 750.3
    acquired 530.3
  Soemmering's 366.51
  trachea, abnormal 748.3
  vascular (congenital) 747.21
  Vossius' 921.3
    late effect 366.21

Ringed hair

Ringed hair (congenital) 757.4
Ringing in the ear (see also Tinnitus) 388.30
Ringworm 110.9
  beard 110.0
  body 110.5
  Burmese 110.9
  corporeal 110.5
  foot 110.4
  groin 110.3
  hand 110.2
  honeycomb 110.0
  nails 110.1
  perianal (area) 110.3
  scalp 110.0
  specified site NEC 110.8
  Tokelau 110.5
Rise, venous pressure 459.89
Risk
  factor — see Problem
  suicidal 300.9
Ritter's disease (dermatitis exfoliativa neonatorum) 695.81
Rivalry, sibling 313.3
Rivalta's disease (cervicofacial actinomycosis) 039.3
River blindness 125.3 [360.13]
Robert's pelvis 755.69
  with disproportion (fetopelvic) 653.0 ✓5ᵗʰ
    affecting fetus or newborn 763.1
  causing obstructed labor 660.1 ✓5ᵗʰ
    affecting fetus or newborn 763.1
Robin's syndrome 756.0
Robinson's (hidrotic) ectodermal dysplasia 757.31
Robles' disease (onchocerciasis) 125.3 [360.13]
Rochalimea — see Rickettsial disease
Rocky Mountain fever (spotted) 082.0
Rodent ulcer (M8090/3) — see also Neoplasm, skin, malignant
  cornea 370.07
Roentgen ray, adverse effect — see Effect, adverse, x-ray
Roetheln 056.9
Roger's disease (congenital interventricular septal defect) 745.4
Rokitansky's
  disease (see also Necrosis, liver) 570
  tumor 620.2
Rokitansky-Aschoff sinuses (mucosal outpouching of gallbladder) (see also Disease, gallbladder) 575.8
Rokitansky-Kuster-Hauser syndrome (congenital absence vagina) 752.49
Rollet's chancre (syphilitic) 091.0
Rolling of head 781.0
Romano-Ward syndrome (prolonged Q-T interval) 794.31
Romanus lesion 720.1
Romberg's disease or syndrome 349.89
Roof, mouth — see condition
Rosacea 695.3
  acne 695.3
  keratitis 695.3 [370.49]
Rosary, rachitic 268.0
Rose
  cold 477.0
  fever 477.0
  rash 782.1
    epidemic 056.9
    of infants 057.8
Rosen-Castleman-Liebow syndrome (pulmonary proteinosis) 516.0
Rosenbach's erysipelatoid or erysipeloid 027.1
Rosenthal's disease (factor XI deficiency) 286.2
Roseola 057.8
  infantum, infantilis 057.8
Rossbach's disease (hyperchlorhydria) 536.8
  psychogenic 306.4
Rössle-Urbach-Wiethe lipoproteinosis 272.8
Ross river fever 066.3

Rostan's asthma (cardiac) (see also Failure, ventricular, left) 428.1
Rot
  Barcoo (see also Ulcer, skin) 707.9
  knife-grinders' (see also Tuberculosis) 011.4 ✓5ᵗʰ
Rot-Bernhardt disease 355.1
Rotation
  anomalous, incomplete or insufficient — see Malrotation
  cecum (congenital) 751.4
  colon (congenital) 751.4
  manual, affecting fetus or newborn 763.89
  spine, incomplete or insufficient 737.8
  tooth, teeth 524.3
  vertebra, incomplete or insufficient 737.8
Röteln 056.9
Roth's disease or meralgia 355.1
Roth-Bernhardt disease or syndrome 355.1
Rothmund (-Thomson) syndrome 757.33
Rotor's disease or syndrome (idiopathic hyperbilirubinemia) 277.4
Rotundum ulcus — see Ulcer, stomach
Round
  back (with wedging of vertebrae) 737.10
    late effect of rickets 268.1
  hole, retina 361.31
    with detachment 361.01
  ulcer (stomach) — see Ulcer, stomach
  worms (infestation) (large) NEC 127.0
Roussy-Lévy syndrome 334.3
Routine postpartum follow-up V24.2
Roy (-Jutras) syndrome (acropachyderma) 757.39
Rubella (German measles) 056.9
  complicating pregnancy, childbirth, or puerperium 647.5 ✓5ᵗʰ
  complication 056.8
    neurological 056.00
      encephalomyelitis 056.01
      specified type NEC 056.09
    specified type NEC 056.79
  congenital 771.0
  contact V01.4
  exposure to V01.4
  maternal
    with suspected fetal damage affecting management of pregnancy 655.3 ✓5ᵗʰ
      affecting fetus or newborn 760.2
      manifest rubella in infant 771.0
  specified complications NEC 056.79
  vaccination, prophylactic (against) V04.3
Rubeola (measles) (see also Measles) 055.9
  complicated 055.8
  meaning rubella (see also Rubella) 056.9
  scarlatinosis 057.8
Rubeosis iridis 364.42
  diabetica 250.5 ✓5ᵗʰ [364.42]
Rubinstein-Taybi's syndrome (brachydactylia, short stature, and mental retardation) 759.89
Rud's syndrome (mental deficiency, epilepsy, and infantilism) 759.89
Rudimentery (congenital) — see also Agenesis
  arm 755.22
  bone 756.9
  cervix uteri 752.49
  eye (see also Microphthalmos) 743.10
  fallopian tube 752.19
  leg 755.32
  lobule of ear 744.21
  patella 755.64
  respiratory organs in thoracopagus 759.4
  tracheal bronchus 748.3
  uterine horn 752.3
  uterus 752.3
    in male 752.7
    solid or with cavity 752.3
  vagina 752.49
Ruiter-Pompen (-Wyers) syndrome (angiokeratoma corporis diffusum) 272.7
Ruled out condition (see also Observation, suspected) V71.9

Rumination — see also Vomiting
  neurotic 300.3
  obsessional 300.3
  psychogenic 307.53
Runaway reaction — see also Disturbance, conduct
  socialized 312.2 ✓5ᵗʰ
  undersocialized, unsocialized 312.1 ✓5ᵗʰ
Runeberg's disease (progressive pernicious anemia) 281.0
Runge's syndrome (postmaturity) 766.2
Rupia 091.3
  congenital 090.0
  tertiary 095.9
Rupture, ruptured 553.9
  abdominal viscera NEC 799.8
    obstetrical trauma 665.5 ✓5ᵗʰ
  abscess (spontaneous) — see Abscess, by site
  amnion — see Rupture, membranes
  aneurysm — see Aneurysm
  anus (sphincter) — see Laceration, anus
  aorta, aortic 441.5
    abdominal 441.3
    arch 441.1
    ascending 441.1
    descending 441.5
      abdominal 441.3
      thoracic 441.1
    syphilitic 093.0
    thoracoabdominal 441.6
    thorax, thoracic 441.1
    transverse 441.1
    traumatic (thoracic) 901.0
      abdominal 902.0
    valve or cusp (see also Endocarditis, aortic) 424.1
  appendix (with peritonitis) 540.0
    with peritoneal abscess 540.1
    traumatic — see Injury, internal, gastrointestinal tract
  arteriovenous fistula, brain (congenital) 430
  artery 447.2
    brain (see also Hemorrhage, brain) 431
    coronary (see also Infarct, myocardium) 410.9 ✓5ᵗʰ
    heart (see also Infarct, myocardium) 410.9 ✓5ᵗʰ
    pulmonary 417.8
    traumatic (complication) (see also Injury, blood vessel, by site) 904.9
  bile duct, except cystic (see also Disease, biliary) 576.3
    cystic 575.4
    traumatic — see Injury, internal, intra-abdominal
  bladder (sphincter) 596.6
    with
      abortion — see Abortion, by type, with damage to pelvic organs
      ectopic pregnancy (see also categories 633.0-633.9) 639.2
      molar pregnancy (see also categories 630-632) 639.2
    following
      abortion 639.2
      ectopic or molar pregnancy 639.2
    nontraumatic 596.6
    obstetrical trauma 665.5 ✓5ᵗʰ
    spontaneous 596.6
    traumatic — see Injury, internal, bladder
  blood vessel (see also Hemorrhage) 459.0
    brain (see also Hemorrhage, brain) 431
    heart (see also Infarct, myocardium) 410.9 ✓5ᵗʰ
    traumatic (complication) (see also Injury, blood vessel, by site) 904.9
  bone — see Fracture, by site
  bowel 569.89
    traumatic — see Injury, internal, intestine
  Bowman's membrane 371.31
  brain
    aneurysm (congenital) (see also Hemorrhage, subarachnoid) 430
      late effect — see Late effect(s) (of) cerebrovascular disease
    syphilitic 094.87

Index to Diseases

Rupture, ruptured — *continued*
  brain — *continued*
    hemorrhagic (*see also* Hemorrhage, brain) 431
    injury at birth 767.0
    syphilitic 094.89
  capillaries 448.9
  cardiac (*see also* Infarct, myocardium) 410.9 ✓5ᵗʰ
  cartilage (articular) (current) — *see also* Sprain, by site
    knee — *see* Tear, meniscus
    semilunar — *see* Tear, meniscus
  cecum (with peritonitis) 540.0
    with peritoneal abscess 540.1
    traumatic 863.89
      with open wound into cavity 863.99
  cerebral aneurysm (congenital) (*see also* Hemorrhage, subarachnoid) 430
    late effect — *see* Late effect(s) (of) cerebrovascular disease
  cervix (uteri)
    with
      abortion — *see* Abortion, by type, with damage to pelvic organs
      ectopic pregnancy (*see also* categories 633.0-633.9) 639.2
      molar pregnancy (*see also* categories 630-632) 639.2
    following
      abortion 639.2
      ectopic or molar pregnancy 639.2
    obstetrical trauma 665.3 ✓5ᵗʰ
    traumatic — *see* Injury, internal, cervix
  chordae tendineae 429.5
  choroid (direct) (indirect) (traumatic) 363.63
  circle of Willis (*see also* Hemorrhage, subarachnoid) 430
    late effect — *see* Late effect(s) (of) cerebrovascular disease
  colon 569.89
    traumatic — *see* Injury, internal, colon
  cornea (traumatic) — *see also* Rupture, eye
    due to ulcer 370.00
  coronary (artery) (thrombotic) (*see also* Infarct, myocardium) 410.9 ✓5ᵗʰ
  corpus luteum (infected) (ovary) 620.1
  cyst — *see* Cyst
  cystic duct (*see also* Disease, gallbladder) 575.4
  Descemet's membrane 371.33
    traumatic — *see* Rupture, eye
  diaphragm — *see also* Hernia, diaphragm
    traumatic — *see* Injury, internal, diaphragm
  diverticulum
    bladder 596.3
    intestine (large) (*see also* Diverticula) 562.10
      small 562.00
  duodenal stump 537.89
  duodenum (ulcer) — *see* Ulcer, duodenum, with perforation
  ear drum (*see also* Perforation, tympanum) 384.20
    with otitis media — *see* Otitis media
    traumatic — *see* Wound, open, ear
  esophagus 530.4
    traumatic 862.22
      with open wound into cavity 862.32
      cervical region — *see* Wound, open, esophagus
  eye (without prolapse of intraocular tissue) 871.0
    with
      exposure of intraocular tissue 871.1
      partial loss of intraocular tissue 871.2
      prolapse of intraocular tissue 871.1
    due to burn 940.5
  fallopian tube 620.8
    due to pregnancy — *see* Pregnancy, tubal
    traumatic — *see* Injury, internal, fallopian tube
  fontanel 767.3
  free wall (ventricle) (*see also* Infarct, myocardium) 410.9 ✓5ᵗʰ
  gallbladder or duct (*see also* Disease, gallbladder) 575.4
    traumatic — *see* Injury, internal, gallbladder

Rupture, ruptured — *continued*
  gastric (*see also* Rupture, stomach) 537.89
    vessel 459.0
  globe (eye) (traumatic) — *see* Rupture, eye
  graafian follicle (hematoma) 620.0
  heart (auricle) (ventricle) (*see also* Infarct, myocardium) 410.9 ✓5ᵗʰ
    infectional 422.90
    traumatic — *see* Rupture, myocardium, traumatic
  hymen 623.8
  internal
    organ, traumatic — *see also* Injury, internal, by site
      heart — *see* Rupture, myocardium, traumatic
      kidney — *see* Rupture, kidney
      liver — *see* Rupture, liver
      spleen — *see* Rupture, spleen, traumatic
    semilunar cartilage — *see* Tear, meniscus
  intervertebral disc — *see* Displacement, intervertebral disc
    traumatic (current) — *see* Dislocation, vertebra
  intestine 569.89
    traumatic — *see* Injury, internal, intestine
  intracranial, birth injury 767.0
  iris 364.76
    traumatic — *see* Rupture, eye
  joint capsule — *see* Sprain, by site
  kidney (traumatic) 866.03
    with open wound into cavity 866.13
    due to birth injury 767.8
    nontraumatic 593.89
  lacrimal apparatus (traumatic) 870.2
  lens (traumatic) 366.20
  ligament — *see also* Sprain, by site
    with open wound — *see* Wound, open, by site
    old (*see also* Disorder, cartilage, articular) 718.0 ✓5ᵗʰ
  liver (traumatic) 864.04
    with open wound into cavity 864.14
    due to birth injury 767.8
    nontraumatic 573.8
  lymphatic (node) (vessel) 457.8
  marginal sinus (placental) (with hemorrhage) 641.2 ✓5ᵗʰ
    affecting fetus or newborn 762.1
  meaning hernia — *see* Hernia
  membrana tympani (*see also* Perforation, tympanum) 384.20
    with otitis media — *see* Otitis media
    traumatic — *see* Wound, open, ear
  membranes (spontaneous)
    artificial
      delayed delivery following 658.3 ✓5ᵗʰ
        affecting fetus or newborn 761.1
    fetus or newborn 761.1
    delayed delivery following 658.2 ✓5ᵗʰ
      affecting fetus or newborn 761.1
    premature (less than 24 hours prior to onset of labor) 658.1 ✓5ᵗʰ
      affecting fetus or newborn 761.1
      delayed delivery following 658.2 ✓5ᵗʰ
        affecting fetus or newborn 761.1
  meningeal artery (*see also* Hemorrhage, subarachnoid) 430
    late effect — *see* Late effect(s) (of) cerebrovascular diseas
  meniscus (knee) — *see also* Tear, meniscus
    old (*see also* Derangement, meniscus) 717.5
      site other than knee — *see* Disorder, cartilage, articular
    site other than knee — *see* Sprain, by site
  mesentery 568.89
    traumatic — *see* Injury, internal, mesentery
  mitral — *see* Insufficiency, mitral
  muscle (traumatic) NEC — *see also* Sprain, by site
    with open wound — *see* Wound, open, by site
    nontraumatic 728.83
  musculotendinous cuff (nontraumatic) (shoulder) 840.4

Rupture, ruptured — *continued*
  mycotic aneurysm, causing cerebral hemorrhage (*see also* Hemorrhage, subarachnoid) 430
    late effect — *see* Late effect(s) (of) cerebrovascular disease
  myocardium, myocardial (*see also* Infarct, myocardium) 410.9 ✓5ᵗʰ
    traumatic 861.03
      with open wound into thorax 861.13
  nontraumatic (meaning hernia) (*see also* Hernia, by site) 553.9
  obstructed (*see also* Hernia, by site, with obstruction) 552.9
    gangrenous (*see also* Hernia, by site, with gangrene) 551.9
  operation wound 998.32 ▲
    internal 998.31 ●
  ovary, ovarian 620.8
    corpus luteum 620.1
    follicle (graafian) 620.0
  oviduct 620.8
    due to pregnancy — *see* Pregnancy, tubal
  pancreas 577.8
    traumatic — *see* Injury, internal, pancreas
  papillary muscle (ventricular) 429.6
  pelvic
    floor, complicating delivery 664.1 ✓5ᵗʰ
    organ NEC — *see* Injury, pelvic, organs
  penis (traumatic) — *see* Wound, open, penis
  perineum 624.8
    during delivery (*see also* Laceration, perineum, complicating delivery) 664.4 ✓5ᵗʰ
  pharynx (nontraumatic) (spontaneous) 478.29
  pregnant uterus (before onset of labor) 665.0 ✓5ᵗʰ
  prostate (traumatic) — *see* Injury, internal, prostate
  pulmonary
    artery 417.8
    valve (heart) (*see also* Endocarditis, pulmonary) 424.3
    vein 417.8
    vessel 417.8
  pupil, sphincter 364.75
  pus tube (*see also* Salpingo-oophoritis) 614.2
  pyosalpinx (*see also* Salpingo-oophoritis) 614.2
  rectum 569.49
    traumatic — *see* Injury, internal, rectum
  retina, retinal (traumatic) (without detachment) 361.30
    with detachment (*see also* Detachment, retina, with retinal defect) 361.00
  rotator cuff (capsule) (traumatic) 840.4
    nontraumatic, complete 727.61
  sclera 871.0
  semilunar cartilage, knee (*see also* Tear, meniscus) 836.2
    old (*see also* Derangement, meniscus) 717.5
  septum (cardiac) 410.8 ✓5ᵗʰ
  sigmoid 569.89
    traumatic — *see* Injury, internal, colon, sigmoid
  sinus of Valsalva 747.29
  spinal cord — *see also* Injury, spinal, by site
    due to injury at birth 767.4
    fetus or newborn 767.4
    syphilitic 094.89
    traumatic — *see also* Injury, spinal, by site
      with fracture — *see* Fracture, vertebra, by site, with spinal cord injury
  spleen 289.59
    congenital 767.8
    due to injury at birth 767.8
    malarial 084.9
    nontraumatic 289.59
    spontaneous 289.59
    traumatic 865.04
      with open wound into cavity 865.14
  splenic vein 459.0
  stomach 537.89
    due to injury at birth 767.8
    traumatic — *see* Injury, internal, stomach
    ulcer — *see* Ulcer, stomach, with perforation
  synovium 727.50
    specified site NEC 727.59

Rupture, ruptured — *continued*
- tendon (traumatic) — *see also* Sprain, by site
  - with open wound — *see* Wound, open, by site
  - Achilles 845.09
    - nontraumatic 727.67
  - ankle 845.09
    - nontraumatic 727.68
  - biceps (long head) 840.8
    - nontraumatic 727.62
  - foot 845.10
    - interphalangeal (joint) 845.13
    - metatarsophalangeal (joint) 845.12
    - nontraumatic 727.68
    - specified site NEC 845.19
    - tarsometatarsal (joint) 845.11
  - hand 842.10
    - carpometacarpal (joint) 842.11
    - interphalangeal (joint) 842.13
    - metacarpophalangeal (joint) 842.12
    - nontraumatic 727.63
      - extensors 727.63
      - flexors 727.64
    - specified site NEC 842.19
  - nontraumatic 727.60
    - specified site NEC 727.69
  - patellar 844.8
    - nontraumatic 727.66
  - quadriceps 844.8
    - nontraumatic 727.65
  - rotator cuff (capsule) 840.4
    - nontraumatic, complete 727.61
  - wrist 842.00
    - carpal (joint) 842.01
    - nontraumatic 727.63
      - extensors 727.63
      - flexors 727.64
    - radiocarpal (joint) (ligament) 842.02
    - radioulnar (joint), distal 842.09
    - specified site NEC 842.09
- testis (traumatic) 878.2
  - complicated 878.3
  - due to syphilis 095.8
- thoracic duct 457.8
- tonsil 474.8
- traumatic
  - with open wound — *see* Wound, open, by site
  - aorta — *see* Rupture, aorta, traumatic
  - ear drum — *see* Wound, open, ear, drum
  - external site — *see* Wound, open, by site
  - eye 871.2
  - globe (eye) — *see* Wound, open, eyeball
  - internal organ (abdomen, chest, or pelvis) — *see also* Injury, internal, by site
    - heart — *see* Rupture, myocardium, traumatic
    - kidney — *see* Rupture, kidney
    - liver — *see* Rupture, liver
    - spleen — *see* Rupture, spleen, traumatic
  - ligament, muscle, or tendon — *see also* Sprain, by site
    - with open wound — *see* Wound, open, by site
  - meaning hernia — *see* Hernia
  - tricuspid (heart) (valve) — *see* Endocarditis, tricuspid
- tube, tubal 620.8
  - abscess (*see also* Salpingo-oophoritis) 614.2
  - due to pregnancy — *see* Pregnancy, tubal
- tympanum, tympanic (membrane) (*see also* Perforation, tympanum) 384.20
  - with otitis media — *see* Otitis media
  - traumatic — *see* Wound, open, ear, drum
- umbilical cord 663.8 ✓5ᵗʰ
  - fetus or newborn 772.0
- ureter (traumatic) (*see also* Injury, internal, ureter) 867.2
  - nontraumatic 593.89
- urethra 599.84
  - with
    - abortion — *see* Abortion, by type, with damage to pelvic organs
    - ectopic pregnancy (*see also* categories 633.0-633.9) 639.2
    - molar pregnancy (*see also* categories 630-632) 639.2

Rupture, ruptured — *continued*
- urethra — *continued*
  - following
    - abortion 639.2
    - ectopic or molar pregnancy 639.2
  - obstetrical trauma 665.5 ✓5ᵗʰ
  - traumatic — *see* Injury, internal urethra
- uterosacral ligament 620.8
- uterus (traumatic) — *see also* Injury, internal uterus
  - affecting fetus or newborn 763.89
  - during labor 665.1 ✓5ᵗʰ
  - nonpuerperal, nontraumatic 621.8
  - nontraumatic 621.8
  - pregnant (during labor) 665.1 ✓5ᵗʰ
    - before labor 665.0 ✓5ᵗʰ
- vagina 878.6
  - complicated 878.7
  - complicating delivery — *see* Laceration, vagina, complicating delivery
- valve, valvular (heart) — *see* Endocarditis
- varicose vein — *see* Varicose, vein
- varix — *see* Varix
- vena cava 459.0
- ventricle (free wall) (left) (*see also* Infarct, myocardium) 410.9 ✓5ᵗʰ
- vesical (urinary) 596.6
  - traumatic — *see* Injury, internal, bladder
- vessel (blood) 459.0
  - pulmonary 417.8
- viscus 799.8
- vulva 878.4
  - complicated 878.5
  - complicating delivery 664.0 ✓5ᵗʰ

Russell's dwarf (uterine dwarfism and craniofacial dysostosis) 759.89

Russell's dysentery 004.8

Russell (-Silver) syndrome (congenital hemihypertrophy and short stature) 759.89

Russian spring-summer type encephalitis 063.0

Rust's disease (tuberculous spondylitis) 015.0 ✓5ᵗʰ [720.81]

Rustitskii's disease (multiple myeloma) (M9730/3) 203.0 ✓5ᵗʰ

Ruysch's disease (Hirschsprung's disease) 751.3

Rytand-Lipsitch syndrome (complete atrioventricular bloc) 426.0

Index to Diseases

S

Saber
   shin 090.5
   tibia 090.5
Sac, lacrimal — see condition
Saccharomyces infection (see also Candidiasis) 112.9
Saccharopinuria 270.7
Saccular — see condition
Sacculation
   aorta (nonsyphilitic) (see also Aneurysm, aorta) 441.9
      ruptured 441.5
      syphilitic 093.0
   bladder 596.3
   colon 569.89
   intralaryngeal (congenital) (ventricular) 748.3
   larynx (congenital) (ventricular) 748.3
   organ or site, congenital — see Distortion
   pregnant uterus, complicating delivery 654.4 ✓5ᵗʰ
      affecting fetus or newborn 763.1
      causing obstructed labor 660.2 ✓5ᵗʰ
         affecting fetus or newborn 763.1
   rectosigmoid 569.89
   sigmoid 569.89
   ureter 593.89
   urethra 599.2
   vesical 596.3
Sachs (-Tay) disease (amaurotic familial idiocy) 330.1
Sacks-Libman disease 710.0 [424.91]
Sacralgia 724.6
Sacralization
   fifth lumbar vertebra 756.15
   incomplete (vertebra) 756.15
Sacrodynia 724.6
Sacroiliac joint — see condition
Sacroiliitis NEC 720.2
Sacrum — see condition
Saddle
   back 737.8
   embolus, aorta 444.0
   nose 738.0
      congenital 754.0
      due to syphilis 090.5
Sadism (sexual) 302.84
Saemisch's ulcer 370.04
Saenger's syndrome 379.46
Sago spleen 277.3
Sailors' skin 692.74
Saint
   Anthony's fire (see also Erysipelas) 035
   Guy's dance — see Chorea
   Louis-type encephalitis 062.3
   triad (see also Hernia, diaphragm) 553.3
   Vitus' dance — see Chorea
Salicylism
   correct substance properly administered 535.4 ✓5ᵗʰ
   overdose or wrong substance given or taken 965.1
Salivary duct or gland — see also condition
   virus disease 078.5
Salivation (excessive) (see also Ptyalism) 527.7
Salmonella (aertrycke) (choleraesuis) (enteritidis) (gallinarum) (suipestifer) (typhimurium) (see also Infection, Salmonella) 003.9
   arthritis 003.23
   carrier (suspected) of V02.3
   meningitis 003.21
   osteomyelitis 003.24
   pneumonia 003.22
   septicemia 003.1
   typhosa 002.0
      carrier (suspected) of V02.1
Salmonellosis 003.0
   with pneumonia 003.22

Salpingitis (catarrhal) (fallopian tube) (nodular) (pseudofollicular) (purulent) (septic) (see also Salpingo-oophoritis) 614.2
   ear 381.50
      acute 381.51
      chronic 381.52
Salpingitis
   Eustachian (tube) 381.50
      acute 381.51
      chronic 381.52
   follicularis 614.1
   gonococcal (chronic) 098.37
      acute 098.17
   interstitial, chronic 614.1
   isthmica nodosa 614.1
   old — see Salpingo-oophoritis, chronic
   puerperal, postpartum, childbirth 670 ✓5ᵗʰ
   specific (chronic) 098.37
      acute 098.17
   tuberculous (acute) (chronic) (see also Tuberculosis) 016.6 ✓5ᵗʰ
   venereal (chronic) 098.37
      acute 098.17
Salpingocele 620.4
Salpingo-oophoritis (catarrhal) (purulent) (ruptured) (septic) (suppurative) 614.2
   acute 614.0
      with
         abortion — see Abortion, by type, with sepsis
         ectopic pregnancy (see also categories 633.0-633.9) 639.0
         molar pregnancy (see also categories 630-632) 639.0
      following
         abortion 639.0
         ectopic or molar pregnancy 639.0
      gonococcal 098.17
      puerperal, postpartum, childbirth 670 ✓4ᵗʰ
      tuberculous (see also Tuberculosis) 016.6 ✓5ᵗʰ
   chronic 614.1
      gonococcal 098.37
      tuberculous (see also Tuberculosis) 016.6 ✓5ᵗʰ
   complicating pregnancy 646.6 ✓5ᵗʰ
      affecting fetus or newborn 760.8
   gonococcal (chronic) 098.37
      acute 098.17
   old — see Salpingo-oophoritis, chronic
   puerperal 670 ✓4ᵗʰ
   specific — see Salpingo-oophoritis, gonococcal
   subacute (see also Salpingo-oophoritis, acute) 614.0
   tuberculous (acute) (chronic) (see also Tuberculosis) 016.6 ✓5ᵗʰ
   venereal — see Salpingo-oophoritis, gonococcal
Salpingo-ovaritis (see also Salpingooophoritis) 614.2
Salpingoperitonitis (see also Salpingo-oophoritis) 614.2
Salt-losing
   nephritis (see also Disease, renal) 593.9
   syndrome (see also Disease, renal) 593.9
Salt-rheum (see also Eczema) 692.9
Salzmann's nodular dystrophy 371.46
Sampson's cyst or tumor 617.1
Sandblasters'
   asthma 502
   lung 502
Sander's disease (paranoia) 297.1
Sandfly fever 066.0
Sandhoff's disease 330.1
Sanfilippo's syndrome (mucopolysaccharidosis III) 277.5
Sanger-Brown's ataxia 334.2
San Joaquin Valley fever 114.0
Sao Paulo fever or typhus 082.0
Saponification, mesenteric 567.8
Sapremia — see Septicemia
Sarcocele (benign)
   syphilitic 095.8
      congenital 090.5

Sarcoepiplocele (see also Hernia) 553.9
Sarcoepiplomphalocele (see also Hernia, umbilicus) 553.1
Sarcoid (any site) 135
   with lung involvement 135 [517.8]
   Boeck's 135
   Darier-Roussy 135
   Spiegler-Fendt 686.8
Sarcoidosis 135
   cardiac 135 [425.8]
   lung 135 [517.8]
Sarcoma (M8800/3) — see also Neoplasm, connective tissue, malignant
   alveolar soft part (M9581/3) — see Neoplasm, connective tissue, malignant
   ameloblastic (M9330/3) 170.1
      upper jaw (bone) 170.0
   botryoid (M8910/3) — see Neoplasm, connective tissue, malignant
   botryoides (M8910/3) — see Neoplasm, connective tissue, malignant
   cerebellar (M9480/3) 191.6
      circumscribed (arachnoidal) (M9471/3) 191.6
   circumscribed (arachnoidal) cerebellar (M9471/3) 191.6
   clear cell, of tendons and aponeuroses (M9044/3) — see Neoplasm, connective tissue, malignant
   embryonal (M8991/3) — see Neoplasm, connective tissue, malignant
   endometrial (stromal) (M8930/3) 182.0
      isthmus 182.1
   endothelial (M9130/3) — see also Neoplasm, connective tissue, malignant
      bone (M9260/3) — see Neoplasm, bone, malignant
   epithelioid cell (M8804/3) — see Neoplasm, connective tissue, malignant
   Ewing's (M9260/3) — see Neoplasm, bone, malignant
   germinoblastic (diffuse) (M9632/3) 202.8 ✓5ᵗʰ
      follicular (M9697/3) 202.0 ✓5ᵗʰ
   giant cell (M8802/3) — see also Neoplasm, connective tissue, malignant
      bone (M9250/3) — see Neoplasm, bone, malignant
   glomoid (M8710/3) — see Neoplasm, connective tissue, malignant
   granulocytic (M9930/3) 205.3 ✓5ᵗʰ
   hemangioendothelial (M9130/3) — see Neoplasm, connective tissue, malignant
   hemorrhagic, multiple (M9140/3) — see Kaposi's, sarcoma
   Hodgkin's (M9662/3) 201.2 ✓5ᵗʰ
   immunoblastic (M9612/3) 200.8 ✓5ᵗʰ
   Kaposi's (M9140/3) — see Kaposi's, sarcoma
   Kupffer cell (M9124/3) 155.0
   leptomeningeal (M9530/3) — see Neoplasm, meninges, malignant
   lymphangioendothelial (M9170/3) — see Neoplasm, connective tissue, malignant
   lymphoblastic (M9630/3) 200.1 ✓5ᵗʰ
   lymphocytic (M9620/3) 200.1 ✓5ᵗʰ
   mast cell (M9740/3) 202.6 ✓5ᵗʰ
   melanotic (M8720/3) — see Melanoma
   meningeal (M9530/3) — see Neoplasm, meninges, malignant
   meningothelial (M9530/3) — see Neoplasm, meninges, malignant
   mesenchymal (M8800/3) — see also Neoplasm, connective tissue, malignant
      mixed (M8990/3) — see Neoplasm, connective tissue, malignant
   mesothelial (M9050/3) — see Neoplasm, by site, malignant
   monstrocellular (M9481/3)
      specified site — see Neoplasm, by site, malignant
      unspecified site 191.9
   myeloid (M9930/3) 205.3 ✓5ᵗʰ
   neurogenic (M9540/3) — see Neoplasm, connective tissue, malignant
   odontogenic (M9270/3) 170.1
      upper jaw (bone) 170.0
   osteoblastic (M9180/3) — see Neoplasm, bone, malignant

Sarcoma — see also Neoplasm, connective tissue, malignant — continued
- osteogenic (M9180/3) — see also Neoplasm, bone, malignant
  - juxtacortical (M9190/3) — see Neoplasm, bone, malignant
  - periosteal (M9190/3) — see Neoplasm, bone, malignant
- periosteal (M8812/3) — see also Neoplasm, bone, malignant
  - osteogenic (M9190/3) — see Neoplasm, bone, malignant
- plasma cell (M9731/3) 203.8 ✓5th
- pleomorphic cell (M8802/3) — see Neoplasm, connective tissue, malignant
- reticuloendothelial (M9720/3) 202.3 ✓5th
- reticulum cell (M9640/3) 200.0 ✓5th
  - nodular (M9642/3) 200.0 ✓5th
  - pleomorphic cell type (M9641/3) 200.0 ✓5th
- round cell (M8803/3) — see Neoplasm, connective tissue, malignant
- small cell (M8803/3) — see Neoplasm, connective tissue, malignant
- spindle cell (M8801/3) — see Neoplasm, connective tissue, malignant
- stromal (endometrial) (M8930/3) 182.0
  - isthmus 182.1
- synovial (M9040/3) — see also Neoplasm, connective tissue, malignant
  - biphasic type (M9043/3) — see Neoplasm, connective tissue, malignant
  - epithelioid cell type (M9042/3) — see Neoplasm, connective tissue, malignant
  - spindle cell type (M9041/3) — see Neoplasm, connective tissue, malignant

Sarcomatosis
- meningeal (M9539/3) — see Neoplasm, meninges, malignant
- specified site NEC (M8800/3) — see Neoplasm, connective tissue, malignant
- unspecified site (M8800/6) 171.9

Sarcosinemia 270.8
Sarcosporidiosis 136.5
Saturnine — see condition
Saturnism 984.9
- specified type of lead — see Table of Drugs and Chemicals

Satyriasis 302.89
Sauriasis — see Ichthyosis
Sauriderma 757.39
Sauriosis — see Ichthyosis
Savill's disease (epidemic exfoliative dermatitis) 695.89
SBE (subacute bacterial endocarditis) 421.0
Scabies (any site) 133.0
Scabs 782.8
Scaglietti-Dagnini syndrome (acromegalic macrospondylitis) 253.0
Scald, scalded — see also Burn, by site
- skin syndrome 695.1

Scalenus anticus (anterior) syndrome 353.0
Scales 782.8
Scalp — see condition
Scaphocephaly 756.0
Scaphoiditis, tarsal 732.5
Scapulalgia 733.90
Scapulohumeral myopathy 359.1
Scar, scarring (see also Cicatrix) 709.2
- adherent 709.2
- atrophic 709.2
- cervix
  - in pregnancy or childbirth 654.6 ✓5th
    - affecting fetus or newborn 763.89
    - causing obstructed labor 660.2 ✓5th
      - affecting fetus or newborn 763.1
- cheloid 701.4
- chorioretinal 363.30
  - disseminated 363.35
  - macular 363.32
  - peripheral 363.34

Scar, scarring (see also Cicatrix) — continued
- chorioretinal — continued
  - posterior pole NEC 363.33
- choroid (see also Scar, chorioretinal) 363.30
- compression, pericardial 423.9
- congenital 757.39
- conjunctiva 372.64
- cornea 371.00
  - xerophthalmic 264.6
- due to previous cesarean delivery, complicating pregnancy or childbirth 654.2 ✓5th
  - affecting fetus or newborn 763.89
- duodenal (bulb) (cap) 537.3
- hypertrophic 701.4
- keloid 701.4
- labia 624.4
- lung (base) 518.89
- macula 363.32
  - disseminated 363.35
  - peripheral 363.34
- muscle 728.89
- myocardium, myocardial 412
- painful 709.2
- papillary muscle 429.81
- posterior pole NEC 363.33
  - macular — see Scar, macula
- postnecrotic (hepatic) (liver) 571.9
- psychic V15.49
- retina (see also Scar, chorioretinal) 363.30
- trachea 478.9
- uterus 621.8
  - in pregnancy or childbirth NEC 654.9 ✓5th
    - affecting fetus or newborn 763.89
    - due to previous cesarean delivery 654.2 ✓5th
- vulva 624.4

Scarabiasis 134.1
Scarlatina 034.1
- anginosa 034.1
- maligna 034.1
- myocarditis, acute 034.1 [422.0]
- old (see also Myocarditis) 429.0
- otitis media 034.1 [382.02]
- ulcerosa 034.1

Scarlatinella 057.8
Scarlet fever (albuminuria) (angina) (convulsions) (lesions of lid) (rash) 034.1
Schamberg's disease, dermatitis, or dermatosis (progressive pigmentary dermatosis) 709.09
Schatzki's ring (esophagus) (lower) (congenital) 750.3
- acquired 530.3

Schaufenster krankheit 413.9
Schaumann's
- benign lymphogranulomatosis 135
- disease (sarcoidosis) 135
- syndrome (sarcoidosis) 135

Scheie's syndrome (mucopolysaccharidosis IS) 277.5
Schenck's disease (sporotrichosis) 117.1
Scheuermann's disease or osteochondrosis 732.0
Scheuthauer-Marie-Sainton syndrome (cleidocranialis dysostosis) 755.59
Schilder (-Flatau) disease 341.1
Schilling-type monocytic leukemia (M9890/3) 206.9 ✓5th
Schimmelbusch's disease, cystic mastitis, or hyperplasia 610.1
Schirmer's syndrome (encephalocutaneous angiomatosis) 759.6
Schistocelia 756.79
Schistoglossia 750.13
Schistosoma infestation — see Infestation, Schistosoma
Schistosomiasis 120.9
- Asiatic 120.2
- bladder 120.0
- chestermani 120.8
- colon 120.1
- cutaneous 120.3
- due to
  - S. hematobium 120.0
  - S. japonicum 120.2

Schistosomiasis — continued
- due to — continued
  - S. mansoni 120.1
  - S. mattheii 120.8
- eastern 120.2
- genitourinary tract 120.0
- intestinal 120.1
- lung 120.2
- Manson's (intestinal) 120.1
- Oriental 120.2
- pulmonary 120.2
- specified type NEC 120.8
- vesical 120.0

Schizencephaly 742.4
Schizo-affective psychosis (see also Schizophrenia) 295.7 ✓5th
Schizodontia 520.2
Schizoid personality 301.20
- introverted 301.21
- schizotypal 301.22

Schizophrenia, schizophrenic (reaction) 295.9 ✓5th

> Note — Use the following fifth-digit subclassification with category 295:
> 0 unspecified
> 1 subchronic
> 2 chronic
> 3 subchronic with acute exacerbation
> 4 chronic with acute exacerbation
> 5 in remission

- acute (attack) NEC 295.8 ✓5th
  - episode 295.4 ✓5th
- atypical form 295.8 ✓5th
- borderline 295.5 ✓5th
- catalepsy 295.2 ✓5th
- catatonic (type) (acute) (excited) (withdrawn) 295.2 ✓5th
- childhood (type) (see also Psychosis, childhood) 299.9 ✓5th
- chronic NEC 295.6 ✓5th
- coenesthesiopathic 295.8 ✓5th
- cyclic (type) 295.7 ✓5th
- disorganized (type) 295.1 ✓5th
- flexibilitas cerea 295.2 ✓5th
- hebephrenic (type) (acute) 295.1 ✓5th
- incipient 295.5 ✓5th
- latent 295.5 ✓5th
- paranoid (type) (acute) 295.3 ✓5th
- paraphrenic (acute) 295.3 ✓5th
- prepsychotic 295.5 ✓5th
- primary (acute) 295.0 ✓5th
- prodromal 295.5 ✓5th
- pseudoneurotic 295.5 ✓5th
- pseudopsychopathic 295.5 ✓5th
- reaction 295.9 ✓5th
- residual (state) (type) 295.6 ✓5th
- restzustand 295.6 ✓5th
- schizo-affective (type) (depressed) (excited) 295.7 ✓5th
- schizophreniform type 295.4 ✓5th
- simple (type) (acute) 295.0 ✓5th
- simplex (acute) 295.0 ✓5th
- specified type NEC 295.8 ✓5th
- syndrome of childhood NEC (see also Psychosis, childhood) 299.9 ✓5th
- undifferentiated 295.9 ✓5th
  - acute 295.8 ✓5th
  - chronic 295.6 ✓5th

Schizothymia 301.20
- introverted 301.21
- schizotypal 301.22

Schlafkrankheit 086.5
Schlatter's tibia (osteochondrosis) 732.4
Schlatter-Osgood disease (osteochondrosis, tibial tubercle) 732.4
Schloffer's tumor (see also Peritonitis) 567.2
Schmidt's syndrome
- sphallo-pharyngo-laryngeal hemiplegia 352.6
- thyroid-adrenocortical insufficiency 258.1
- vagoaccessory 352.6

Index to Diseases — Sclerosis, sclerotic

Schmincke
  carcinoma (M8082/3) — *see* Neoplasm, nasopharynx, malignant
  tumor (M8082/3) — *see* Neoplasm, nasopharynx, malignant
Schmitz (-Stutzer) dysentery 004.0
Schmorl's disease or nodes 722.30
  lumbar, lumbosacral 722.32
  specified region NEC 722.39
  thoracic, thoracolumbar 722.31
Schneider's syndrome 047.9
Schneiderian
  carcinoma (M8121/3)
    specified site — *see* Neoplasm, by site, malignant
    unspecified site 160.0
  papilloma (M8121/0)
    specified site — *see* Neoplasm, by site, benign
    unspecified site 212.0
Schoffer's tumor (*see also* Peritonitis) 567.2
Scholte's syndrome (malignant carcinoid) 259.2
Scholz's disease 330.0
Scholz (-Bielschowsky-Henneberg) syndrome 330.0
Schönlein (-Henoch) disease (primary) (purpura) (rheumatic) 287.0
School examination V70.3
Schottmüller's disease (*see also* Fever, paratyphoid) 002.9
Schroeder's syndrome (endocrine-hypertensive) 255.3
Schüller-Christian disease or syndrome (chronic histiocytosis X) 277.8
Schultz's disease or syndrome (agranulocytosis) 288.0
Schultze's acroparesthesia, simple 443.89
Schwalbe-Ziehen-Oppenheimer disease 333.6
Schwannoma (M9560/0) — *see also* Neoplasm, connective tissue, benign
  malignant (M9560/3) — *see* Neoplasm, connective tissue, malignant
Schwartz (-Jampel) syndrome 756.89
Schwartz-Bartter syndrome (inappropriate secretion of antidiuretic hormone) 253.6
Schweninger-Buzzi disease (macular atrophy) 701.3
Sciatic — *see* condition
Sciatica (infectional) 724.3
  due to
    displacement of intervertebral disc 722.10
    herniation, nucleus pulposus 722.10
Scimitar syndrome (anomalous venous drainage, right lung to inferior vena cava) 747.49
Sclera — *see* condition
Sclerectasia 379.11
Scleredema
  adultorum 710.1
  Buschke's 710.1
  newborn 778.1
Sclerema
  adiposum (newborn) 778.1
  adultorum 710.1
  edematosum (newborn) 778.1
  neonatorum 778.1
  newborn 778.1
Scleriasis — *see* Scleroderma
Scleritis 379.00
  with corneal involvement 379.05
  anterior (annular) (localized) 379.03
  brawny 379.06
  granulomatous 379.09
  posterior 379.07
  specified NEC 379.09
  suppurative 379.09
  syphilitic 095.0
  tuberculous (nodular) (*see also* Tuberculosis) 017.3 [379.09]
Sclerochoroiditis (*see also* Scleritis) 379.00
Scleroconjunctivitis (*see also* Scleritis) 379.00
Sclerocystic ovary (syndrome) 256.4
Sclerodactylia 701.0
Scleroderma, sclerodermia (acrosclerotic) (diffuse) (generalized) (progressive) (pulmonary) 710.1
  circumscribed 701.0
  linear 701.0
  localized (linear) 701.0
  newborn 778.1
Sclerokeratitis 379.05
  meaning sclerosing keratitis 370.54
  tuberculous (*see also* Tuberculosis) 017.3 [379.09]
Scleroma, trachea 040.1
Scleromalacia
  multiple 731.0
  perforans 379.04
Scleromyxedema 701.8
Scleroperikeratitis 379.05
Sclerose en plaques 340
Sclerosis, sclerotic
  adrenal (gland) 255.8
  Alzheimer's 331.0
    with dementia — *see* Alzheimer's, dementia
  amyotrophic (lateral) 335.20
  annularis fibrosi
    aortic 424.1
    mitral 424.0
  aorta, aortic 440.0
    valve (*see also* Endocarditis, aortic) 424.1
  artery, arterial, arteriolar, arteriovascular — *see* Arteriosclerosis
  ascending multiple 340
  Baló's (concentric) 341.1
  basilar — *see* Sclerosis, brain
  bone (localized) NEC 733.99
  brain (general) (lobular) 341.9
    Alzheimer's — *see* Alzheimer's, dementia
    artery, arterial 437.0
    atrophic lobar 331.0
      with dementia
        with behavioral disturbance 331.0 [294.11]
        without behavioral disturbance 331.0 [294.10]
    diffuse 341.1
      familial (chronic) (infantile) 330.0
      infantile (chronic) (familial) 330.0
      Pelizaeus-Merzbacher type 330.0
    disseminated 340
    hereditary 334.2
    infantile, (degenerative) (diffuse) 330.0
    insular 340
    Krabbe's 330.0
    miliary 340
    multiple 340
    Pelizaeus-Merzbacher 330.0
    progressive familial 330.0
    senile 437.0
    tuberous 759.5
  bulbar, progressive 340
  bundle of His 426.50
    left 426.3
    right 426.4
  cardiac — *see* Arteriosclerosis, coronary
  cardiorenal (*see also* Hypertension, cardiorenal) 404.90
  cardiovascular (*see also* Disease, cardiovascular) 429.2
    renal (*see also* Hypertension, cardiorenal) 404.90
  centrolobar, familial 330.0
  cerebellar — *see* Sclerosis, brain
  cerebral — *see* Sclerosis, brain
  cerebrospinal 340
    disseminated 340
    multiple 340
  cerebrovascular 437.0
  choroid 363.40
    diffuse 363.56
  combined (spinal cord) — *see also* Degeneration, combined
    multiple 340
  concentric, Baló's 341.1
  cornea 370.54
  coronary (artery) — *see* Arteriosclerosis, coronary
Sclerosis, sclerotic — *continued*
  corpus cavernosum
    female 624.8
    male 607.89
  Dewitzky's
    aortic 424.1
    mitral 424.0
  diffuse NEC 341.1
  disease, heart — *see* Arteriosclerosis, coronary
  disseminated 340
  dorsal 340
  dorsolateral (spinal cord) — *see* Degeneration, combined
  endometrium 621.8
  extrapyramidal 333.90
  eye, nuclear (senile) 366.16
  Friedreich's (spinal cord) 334.0
  funicular (spermatic cord) 608.89
  gastritis 535.4
  general (vascular) — *see* Arteriosclerosis
  gland (lymphatic) 457.8
  hepatic 571.9
  hereditary
    cerebellar 334.2
    spinal 334.0
  idiopathic cortical (Garré's) (*see also* Osteomyelitis) 730.1
  ilium, piriform 733.5
  insular 340
    pancreas 251.8
  Islands of Langerhans 251.8
  kidney — *see* Sclerosis, renal
  larynx 478.79
  lateral 335.24
    amyotrophic 335.20
    descending 335.24
    primary 335.24
    spinal 335.24
  liver 571.9
  lobar, atrophic (of brain) 331.0
    with dementia
      with behavioral disturbance 331.0 [294.11]
      without behavioral disturbance 331.0 [294.10]
  lung (*see also* Fibrosis, lung) 515
  mastoid 383.1
  mitral — *see* Endocarditis, mitral
  Mönckeberg's (medial) (*see also* Arteriosclerosis, extremities) 440.20
  multiple (brain stem) (cerebral) (generalized) (spinal cord) 340
  myocardium, myocardial — *see* Arteriosclerosis, coronary
  nuclear (senile), eye 366.16
  ovary 620.8
  pancreas 577.8
  penis 607.89
  peripheral arteries NEC (*see also* Arteriosclerosis, extremities) 440.20
  plaques 340
  pluriglandular 258.8
  polyglandular 258.8
  posterior (spinal cord) (syphilitic) 094.0
  posterolateral (spinal cord) — *see* Degeneration, combined
  prepuce 607.89
  primary lateral 335.24
  progressive systemic 710.1
  pulmonary (*see also* Fibrosis, lung) 515
    artery 416.0
    valve (heart) (*see also* Endocarditis, pulmonary) 424.3
  renal 587
    with
      cystine storage disease 270.0
      hypertension (*see also* Hypertension, kidney) 403.90
      hypertensive heart disease (conditions classifiable to 402) (*see also* Hypertension, cardiorenal) 404.90
      arteriolar (hyaline) (*see also* Hypertension, kidney) 403.90
      hyperplastic (*see also* Hypertension, kidney) 403.90
  retina (senile) (vascular) 362.17
  rheumatic
    aortic valve 395.9

Sclerosis, sclerotic

Sclerosis, sclerotic — continued
- rheumatic — continued
  - mitral valve 394.9
- Schilder's 341.1
- senile — see Arteriosclerosis
- spinal (cord) (general) (progressive) (transverse) 336.8
  - ascending 357.0
  - combined — see also Degeneration, combined
    - multiple 340
    - syphilitic 094.89
  - disseminated 340
  - dorsolateral — see Degeneration, combined
  - hereditary (Friedreich's) (mixed form) 334.0
  - lateral (amyotrophic) 335.24
  - multiple 340
  - posterior (syphilitic) 094.0
- stomach 537.89
- subendocardial, congenital 425.3
- systemic (progressive) 710.1
  - with lung involvement 710.1 [517.2]
- tricuspid (heart) (valve) — see Endocarditis, tricuspid
- tuberous (brain) 759.5
- tympanic membrane (see also Tympanosclerosis) 385.00
- valve, valvular (heart) — see Endocarditis
- vascular — see Arteriosclerosis
- vein 459.89

Sclerotenonitis 379.07

Sclerotitis (see also Scleritis) 379.00
- syphilitic 095.0
- tuberculous (see also Tuberculosis) 017.3 [379.09]

Scoliosis (acquired) (postural) 737.30
- congenital 754.2
- due to or associated with
  - Charcôt-Marie-Tooth disease 356.1 [737.43]
  - mucopolysaccharidosis 277.5 [737.43]
  - neurofibromatosis 237.71 [737.43]
  - osteitis
    - deformans 731.0 [737.43]
    - fibrosa cystica 252.0 [737.43]
  - osteoporosis (see also Osteoporosis) 733.00 [737.43]
  - poliomyelitis 138 [737.43]
  - radiation 737.33
  - tuberculosis (see also Tuberculosis) 015.0 [737.43]
- idiopathic 737.30
  - infantile
    - progressive 737.32
    - resolving 737.31
- paralytic 737.39
- rachitic 268.1
- sciatic 724.3
- specified NEC 737.39
- thoracogenic 737.34
- tuberculous (see also Tuberculosis) 015.0 [737.43]

Scoliotic pelvis 738.6
- with disproportion (fetopelvic) 653.0
  - affecting fetus or newborn 763.1
  - causing obstructed labor 660.1
    - affecting fetus or newborn 763.1

Scorbutus, scorbutic 267
- anemia 281.8

Scotoma (ring) 368.44
- arcuate 368.43
- Bjerrum 368.43
- blind spot area 368.42
- central 368.41
- centrocecal 368.41
- paracecal 368.42
- paracentral 368.41
- scintillating 368.12
- Seidel 368.43

Scratch — see Injury, superficial, by site

Screening (for) V82.9
- alcoholism V79.1
- anemia, deficiency NEC V78.1
  - iron V78.0
- anomaly, congenital V82.89
- antenatal V28.9
  - alphafetoprotein levels, raised V28.1

Screening (for) — continued
- antenatal — continued
  - based on amniocentesis V28.2
    - chromosomal anomalies V28.0
    - raised alphafetoprotein levels V28.1
  - fetal growth retardation using ultrasonics V28.4
  - isoimmunization V28.5
  - malformations using ultrasonics V28.3
  - raised alphafetoprotein levels V28.1
  - specified condition NEC V28.8
  - Streptococcus B V28.6
- arterial hypertension V81.1
- arthropod-borne viral disease NEC V73.5
- asymptomatic bacteriuria V81.5
- bacterial
  - conjunctivitis V74.4
  - disease V74.9
    - specified condition NEC V74.8
- bacteriuria, asymptomatic V81.5
- blood disorder NEC V78.9
  - specified type NEC V78.8
- bronchitis, chronic V81.3
- brucellosis V74.8
- cancer — see Screening, malignant neoplasm
- cardiovascular disease NEC V81.2
- cataract V80.2
- Chagas' disease V75.3
- chemical poisoning V82.5
- cholera V74.0
- cholesterol level V77.91
- chromosomal
  - anomalies
    - by amniocentesis, antenatal V28.0
    - maternal postnatal V82.4
  - athletes V70.3
- condition
  - cardiovascular NEC V81.2
  - eye NEC V80.2
  - genitourinary NEC V81.6
  - neurological V80.0
  - respiratory NEC V81.4
  - skin V82.0
  - specified NEC V82.89
- congenital
  - anomaly V82.89
    - eye V80.2
  - dislocation of hip V82.3
  - eye condition or disease V80.2
- conjunctivitis, bacterial V74.4
- contamination NEC (see also Poisoning) V82.5
- coronary artery disease V81.0
- cystic fibrosis V77.6
- deficiency anemia NEC V78.1
  - iron V78.0
- dengue fever V73.5
- depression V79.0
- developmental handicap V79.9
  - in early childhood V79.3
  - specified type NEC V79.8
- diabetes mellitus V77.1
- diphtheria V74.3
- disease or disorder V82.9
  - bacterial V74.9
    - specified NEC V74.8
  - blood V78.9
    - specified type NEC V78.8
  - blood-forming organ V78.9
    - specified type NEC V78.8
  - cardiovascular NEC V81.2
    - hypertensive V81.1
    - ischemic V81.0
  - Chagas' V75.3
  - chlamydial V73.98
    - specified NEC V73.88
  - ear NEC V80.3
  - endocrine NEC V77.99
  - eye NEC V80.2
  - genitourinary NEC V81.6
  - heart NEC V81.2
    - hypertensive V81.1
    - ischemic V81.0
  - immunity NEC V77.99
  - infectious NEC V75.9
  - lipoid NEC V77.91
  - mental V79.9
    - specified type NEC V79.8

Screening (for) — continued
- disease or disorder — continued
  - metabolic NEC V77.99
    - inborn NEC V77.7
  - neurological V80.0
  - nutritional NEC V77.99
  - rheumatic NEC V82.2
  - rickettsial V75.0
  - sickle-cell V78.2
    - trait V78.2
  - specified type NEC V82.89
  - thyroid V77.0
  - vascular NEC V81.2
    - ischemic V81.0
  - venereal V74.5
  - viral V73.99
    - arthropod-borne NEC V73.5
    - specified type NEC V73.89
- dislocation of hip, congenital V82.3
- drugs in athletes V70.3
- emphysema (chronic) V81.3
- encephalitis, viral (mosquito or tick borne) V73.5
- endocrine disorder NEC V77.99
- eye disorder NEC V80.2
  - congenital V80.2
- fever
  - dengue V73.5
  - hemorrhagic V73.5
  - yellow V73.4
- filariasis V75.6
- galactosemia V77.4
- genitourinary condition NEC V81.6
- glaucoma V80.1
- gonorrhea V74.5
- gout V77.5
- Hansen's disease V74.2
- heart disease NEC V81.2
  - hypertensive V81.1
  - ischemic V81.0
- heavy metal poisoning V82.5
- helminthiasis, intestinal V75.7
- hematopoietic malignancy V76.89
- hemoglobinopathies NEC V78.3
- hemorrhagic fever V73.5
- Hodgkin's disease V76.89
- hormones in athletes V70.3
- hypercholesterolemia V77.91
- hyperlipidemia V77.91
- hypertension V81.1
- immunity disorder NEC V77.99
- inborn errors of metabolism NEC V77.7
- infection
  - bacterial V74.9
    - specified type NEC V74.8
  - mycotic V75.4
  - parasitic NEC V75.8
- infectious disease V75.9
  - specified type NEC V75.8
- ingestion of radioactive substance V82.5
- intestinal helminthiasis V75.7
- iron deficiency anemia V78.0
- ischemic heart disease V81.0
- lead poisoning V82.5
- leishmaniasis V75.2
- leprosy V74.2
- leptospirosis V74.8
- leukemia V76.89
- lipoid disorder NEC V77.91
- lymphoma V76.89
- malaria V75.1
- malignant neoplasm (of) V76.9
  - bladder V76.3
  - blood V76.89
  - breast V76.10
    - mammogram NEC V76.12
      - for high-risk patient V76.11
    - specified type NEC V76.19
  - cervix V76.2
  - colon V76.51
  - colorectal V76.51
  - hematopoietic system V76.89
  - intestine V76.50
    - colon V76.51
    - small V76.52
  - lymph (glands) V76.89
  - nervous system V76.81

Index to Diseases

Screening (for) — *continued*
  malignant neoplasm (of) — *continued*
    oral cavity V76.42
    other specified neoplasm NEC V76.89
    ovary V76.46
    prostate V76.44
    rectum V76.41
    respiratory organs V76.0
    skin V76.43
    specified sites NEC V76.49
    testis V76.45
    vagina V76.47
      following hysterectomy for malignant condition V67.01
  maternal postnatal chromosomal anomalies V82.4
  malnutrition V77.2
  mammogram NEC V76.12
    for high-risk patient V76.11
  measles V73.2
  mental
    disorder V79.9
      specified type NEC V79.8
    retardation V79.2
  metabolic disorder NEC V77.99
  metabolic errors, inborn V77.7
  mucoviscidosis V77.6
  multiphasic V82.6
  mycosis V75.4
  mycotic infection V75.4
  nephropathy V81.5
  neurological condition V80.0
  nutritional disorder V77.99
  obesity V77.8
  osteoporosis V82.81
  parasitic infection NEC V75.8
  phenylketonuria V77.3
  plague V74.8
  poisoning
    chemical NEC V82.5
      contaminated water supply V82.5
        heavy metal V82.5
  poliomyelitis V73.0
  postnatal chromosomal anomalies, maternal V82.4
  prenatal — *see* Screening, antenatal
  pulmonary tuberculosis V74.1
  radiation exposure V82.5
  renal disease V81.5
  respiratory condition NEC V81.4
  rheumatic disorder NEC V82.2
  rheumatoid arthritis V82.1
  rickettsial disease V75.0
  rubella V73.3
  schistosomiasis V75.5
  senile macular lesions of eye V80.2
  sickle-cell anemia, disease, or trait V78.2
  skin condition V82.0
  sleeping sickness V75.3
  smallpox V73.1
  special V82.9
    specified condition NEC V82.89
  specified type NEC V82.89
  spirochetal disease V74.9
    specified type NEC V74.8
  stimulants in athletes V70.3
  syphilis V74.5
  tetanus V74.8
  thyroid disorder V77.0
  trachoma V73.6
  trypanosomiasis V75.3
  tuberculosis, pulmonary V74.1
  venereal disease V74.5
  viral encephalitis
    mosquito-borne V73.5
    tick-borne V73.5
  whooping cough V74.8
  worms, intestinal V75.7
  yaws V74.6
  yellow fever V73.4
Scrofula (*see also* Tuberculosis) 017.2
Scrofulide (primary) (*see also* Tuberculosis) 017.0
Scrofuloderma, scrofulodermia (any site) (primary) (*see also* Tuberculosis) 017.0
Scrofulosis (universal) (*see also* Tuberculosis) 017.2

Scrofulosis lichen (primary) (*see also* Tuberculosis) 017.0
Scrofulous — *see* condition
Scrotal tongue 529.5
  congenital 750.13
Scrotum — *see* condition
Scurvy (gum) (infantile) (rickets) (scorbutic) 267
Sea-blue histiocyte syndrome 272.7
Seabright-Bantam syndrome (pseudohypoparathyroidism) 275.49
Seasickness 994.6
Seatworm 127.4
Sebaceous
  cyst (*see also* Cyst, sebaceous) 706.2
  gland disease NEC 706.9
Sebocystomatosis 706.2
Seborrhea, seborrheic 706.3
  adiposa 706.3
  capitis 690.11
  congestiva 695.4
  corporis 706.3
  dermatitis 690.10
    infantile 690.12
  diathesis in infants 695.89
  eczema 690.18
    infantile 691.12
  keratosis 702.19
    inflamed 702.11
  nigricans 705.89
  sicca 690.18
  wart 702.19
    inflamed 702.11
Seckel's syndrome 759.89
Seclusion pupil 364.74
Seclusiveness, child 313.22
Secondary — *see also* condition
  neoplasm — *see* Neoplasm, by site, malignant, secondary
Secretan's disease or syndrome (posttraumatic edema) 782.3
Secretion
  antidiuretic hormone, inappropriate (syndrome) 253.6
  catecholamine, by pheochromocytoma 255.6
  hormone
    antidiuretic, inappropriate (syndrome) 253.6
    by
      carcinoid tumor 259.2
      pheochromocytoma 255.6
    ectopic NEC 259.3
  urinary
    excessive 788.42
    suppression 788.5
Section
  cesarean
    affecting fetus or newborn 763.4
    post mortem, affecting fetus or newborn 761.6
    previous, in pregnancy or childbirth 654.2
      affecting fetus or newborn 763.89
  nerve, traumatic — *see* Injury, nerve, by site
Seeligmann's syndrome (ichthyosis congenita) 757.1
Segmentation, incomplete (congenital) — *see also* Fusion
  bone NEC 756.9
  lumbosacral (joint) 756.15
  vertebra 756.15
    lumbosacral 756.15
Seizure 780.39
  akinetic (idiopathic) (*see also* Epilepsy) 345.0
    psychomotor 345.4
  apoplexy, apoplectic (*see also* Disease, cerebrovascular, acute) 436
  atonic (*see also* Epilepsy) 345.0
  autonomic 300.11
  brain or cerebral (*see also* Disease, cerebrovascular, acute) 436
  convulsive (*see also* Convulsions) 780.39
  cortical (focal) (motor) (*see also* Epilepsy) 345.5

Seizure — *continued*
  epilepsy, epileptic (cryptogenic) (*see also* Epilepsy) 345.9
  epileptiform, epileptoid 780.39
    focal (*see also* Epilepsy) 345.5
  febrile 780.31
  heart — *see* Disease, heart
  hysterical 300.11
  Jacksonian (focal) (*see also* Epilepsy) 345.5
    motor type 345.5
    sensory type 345.5
  newborn 779.0
  paralysis (*see also* Disease, cerebrovascular, acute) 436
  recurrent 780.39
    epileptic — *see* Epilepsy
  repetitive 780.39
    epileptic — *see* Epilepsy
  salaam (*see also* Epilepsy) 345.6
  uncinate (*see also* Epilepsy) 345.4
Self-mutilation 300.9
Semicoma 780.09
Semiconsciousness 780.09
Seminal
  vesicle — *see* condition
  vesiculitis (*see also* Vesiculitis) 608.0
Seminoma (M9061/3)
  anaplastic type (M9062/3)
    specified site — *see* Neoplasm, by site, malignant
    unspecified site 186.9
  specified site — *see* Neoplasm, by site, malignant
  spermatocytic (M9063/3)
    specified site — *see* Neoplasm, by site, malignant
    unspecified site 186.9
  unspecified site 186.9
Semliki Forest encephalitis 062.8
Senear-Usher disease or syndrome (pemphigus erythematosus) 694.4
Senecio jacobae dermatitis 692.6
Senectus 797
Senescence 797
Senile (*see also* condition) 797
  cervix (atrophic) 622.8
  degenerative atrophy, skin 701.3
  endometrium (atrophic) 621.8
  fallopian tube (atrophic) 620.3
  heart (failure) 797
  lung 492.8
  ovary (atrophic) 620.3
  syndrome 259.8
  vagina, vaginitis (atrophic) 627.3
  wart 702.0
Senility 797
  with
    acute confusional state 290.3
    delirium 290.3
    mental changes 290.9
    psychosis NEC (*see also* Psychosis, senile) 290.20
  premature (syndrome) 259.8
Sensation
  burning (*see also* Disturbance, sensation) 782.0
    tongue 529.6
  choking 784.9
  loss of (*see also* Disturbance, sensation) 782.0
  prickling (*see also* Disturbance, sensation) 782.0
  tingling (*see also* Disturbance, sensation) 782.0
Sense loss (touch) (*see also* Disturbance, sensation) 782.0
  smell 781.1
  taste 781.1
Sensibility disturbance NEC (cortical) (deep) (vibratory) (*see also* Disturbance, sensation) 782.0
Sensitive dentine 521.8
Sensitiver Beziehungswahn 297.8
Sensitivity, sensitization — *see also* Allergy
  autoerythrocyte 287.2
  carotid sinus 337.0

Sensitivity, sensitization — see also Allergy — continued
- child (excessive) 313.21
- cold, autoimmune 283.0
- methemoglobin 289.7
- suxamethonium 289.8
- tuberculin, without clinical or radiological symptoms 795.5

Sensory
- extinction 781.8
- neglect 781.8

Separation
- acromioclavicular — see Dislocation, acromioclavicular
- anxiety, abnormal 309.21
- apophysis, traumatic — see Fracture, by site
- choroid 363.70
  - hemorrhagic 363.72
  - serous 363.71
- costochondral (simple) (traumatic) — see Dislocation, costochondral
- epiphysis, epiphyseal
  - nontraumatic 732.9
    - upper femoral 732.2
  - traumatic — see Fracture, by site
- fracture — see Fracture, by site
- infundibulum cardiac from right ventricle by a partition 746.83
- joint (current) (traumatic) — see Dislocation, by site
- placenta (normally implanted) — see Placenta, separation
- pubic bone, obstetrical trauma 665.6 ✓5ᵗʰ
- retina, retinal (see also Detachment, retina) 361.9
  - layers 362.40
    - sensory (see also Retinoschisis) 361.10
    - pigment epithelium (exudative) 362.42
      - hemorrhagic 362.43
- sternoclavicular (traumatic) — see Dislocation, sternoclavicular
- symphysis pubis, obstetrical trauma 665.6 ✓5ᵗʰ
- tracheal ring, incomplete (congenital) 748.3

Sepsis (generalized) (see also Septicemia) 038.9
- with
  - abortion — see Abortion, by type, with sepsis
  - ectopic pregnancy (see also categories 633.0-633.9) 639.0
  - molar pregnancy (see also categories 630-632) 639.0
- buccal 528.3
- complicating labor 659.3 ✓5ᵗʰ
- dental (pulpal origin) 522.4
- female genital organ NEC 614.9
- fetus (intrauterine) 771.81 ▲
- following
  - abortion 639.0
  - ectopic or molar pregnancy 639.0
  - infusion, perfusion, or transfusion 999.3
- Friedländer's 038.49
- intraocular 360.00
- localized
  - in operation wound 998.59
  - skin (see also Abscess) 682.9
- malleus 024
- nadir 038.9
- newborn (organism unspecified) NEC 771.81 ▲
- oral 528.3
- puerperal, postpartum, childbirth (pelvic) 670 ✓4ᵗʰ
- resulting from infusion, injection, transfusion, or vaccination 999.3
- severe 995.92 ●
- skin, localized (see also Abscess) 682.9
- umbilical (newborn) (organism unspecified) 771.89 ▲
  - tetanus 771.3
- urinary 599.0

Septate — see also Septum

Septic — see also condition
- adenoids 474.01
  - and tonsils 474.02
- arm (with lymphangitis) 682.3
- embolus — see Embolism

Septic — see also condition — continued
- finger (with lymphangitis) 681.00
- foot (with lymphangitis) 682.7
- gallbladder (see also Cholecystitis) 575.8
- hand (with lymphangitis) 682.4
- joint (see also Arthritis, septic) 711.0 ✓5ᵗʰ
- kidney (see also Infection, kidney) 590.9
- leg (with lymphangitis) 682.6
- mouth 528.3
- nail 681.9
  - finger 681.02
  - toe 681.11
- shock (endotoxic) 785.59
- sore (see also Abscess) 682.9
  - throat 034.0
    - milk-borne 034.0
    - streptococcal 034.0
- spleen (acute) 289.59
- teeth (pulpal origin) 522.4
- throat 034.0
- thrombus — see Thrombosis
- toe (with lymphangitis) 681.0 ✓5ᵗʰ
- tonsils 474.00
  - and adenoids 474.02
- umbilical cord (newborn) (organism unspecified) 771.89 ▲
- uterus (see also Endometritis) 615.9

Septicemia, septicemic (generalized) (suppurative) 038.9
- with
  - abortion — see Abortion, by type, with sepsis
  - ectopic pregnancy (see also categories 633.0-633.9) 639.0
  - molar pregnancy (see also categories 630-632) 639.0
- Aerobacter aerogenes 038.49
- anaerobic 038.3
- anthrax 022.3
- Bacillus coli 038.42
- Bacteroides 038.3
- Clostridium 038.3
- complicating labor 659.3 ✓5ᵗʰ
- cryptogenic 038.9
- enteric gram-negative bacilli 038.40
- Enterobacter aerogenes 038.49
- Erysipelothrix (insidiosa) (rhusiopathiae) 027.1
- Escherichia coli 038.42
- following
  - abortion 639.0
  - ectopic or molar pregnancy 639.0
  - infusion, injection, transfusion, or vaccination 999.3
- Friedländer's (bacillus) 038.49
- gangrenous 038.9
- gonococcal 098.89
- gram-negative (organism) 038.40
  - anaerobic 038.3
- Hemophilus influenzae 038.41
- herpes (simplex) 054.5
- herpetic 054.5
- Listeria monocytogenes 027.0
- meningeal — see Meningitis
- meningococcal (chronic) (fulminating) 036.2
- navel, newborn (organism unspecified) 771.89 ▲
- newborn (organism unspecified) 771.81 ▲
- plague 020.2
- pneumococcal 038.2
- postabortal 639.0
- postoperative 998.59
- Proteus vulgaris 038.49
- Pseudomonas (aeruginosa) 038.43
- puerperal, postpartum 670 ✓4ᵗʰ
- Salmonella (aertrycke) (callinarum) (choleraesuis) (enteritidis) (suipestifer) 003.1
- Serratia 038.44
- Shigella (see also Dysentery, bacillary) 004.9
- specified organism NEC 038.8
- staphylococcal 038.10
  - aureus 038.11
  - specified organism NEC 038.19
- streptococcal (anaerobic) 038.0
- suipestifer 003.1

Septicemia, septicemic — continued
- umbilicus, newborn (organism unspecified) 771.89 ▲
- viral 079.99
- Yersinia enterocolitica 038.49

Septum, septate (congenital) — see also Anomaly, specified type NEC
- anal 751.2
- aqueduct of Sylvius 742.3
  - with spina bifida (see also Spina bifida) 741.0 ✓5ᵗʰ
- hymen 752.49
- uterus (see also Double, uterus) 752.2
- vagina 752.49
  - in pregnancy or childbirth 654.7 ✓5ᵗʰ
    - affecting fetus or newborn 763.89
    - causing obstructed labor 660.2 ✓5ᵗʰ
      - affecting fetus or newborn 763.1

Sequestration
- lung (congenital) (extralobar) (intralobar) 748.5
- orbit 376.10
- pulmonary artery (congenital) 747.3

Sequestrum
- bone (see also Osteomyelitis) 730.1 ✓5ᵗʰ
  - jaw 526.4
- dental 525.8
- jaw bone 526.4
- sinus (accessory) (nasal) (see also Sinusitis) 473.9
  - maxillary 473.0

Sequoiosis asthma 495.8

Serology for syphilis
- doubtful
  - with signs or symptoms — see Syphilis, by site and stage
  - follow-up of latent syphilis — see Syphilis, latent
- false positive 795.6
- negative, with signs or symptoms — see Syphilis, by site and stage
- positive 097.1
  - with signs or symptoms — see Syphilis, by site and stage
  - false 795.6
  - follow-up of latent syphilis — see Syphilis, latent
  - only finding — see Syphilis, latent
- reactivated 097.1

Seroma (postoperative) (non-infected) 998.13
- infected 998.51

Seropurulent — see condition

Serositis, multiple 569.89
- pericardial 423.2
- peritoneal 568.82
- pleural — see Pleurisy

Serotonin syndrome 333.99

Serous — see condition

Sertoli cell
- adenoma (M8640/0)
  - specified site — see Neoplasm, by site, benign
  - unspecified site
    - female 220
    - male 222.0
- carcinoma (M8640/3)
  - specified site — see Neoplasm, by site, malignant
  - unspecified site 186.9
- syndrome (germinal aplasia) 606.0
- tumor (M8640/0)
  - with lipid storage (M8641/0)
    - specified site — see Neoplasm, by site, benign
    - unspecified site
      - female 220
      - male 222.0
  - specified site — see Neoplasm, by site, benign
  - unspecified site
    - female 220
    - male 222.0

Sertoli-Leydig cell tumor (M8631/0)
- specified site — see Neoplasm, by site, benign
- unspecified site
  - female 220
  - male 222.0

Index to Diseases

Serum
  allergy, allergic reaction 999.5
    shock 999.4
  arthritis 999.5 [713.6]
  complication or reaction NEC 999.5
  disease NEC 999.5
  hepatitis 070.3 ✓5ᵗʰ
  intoxication 999.5
  jaundice (homologous) — see Hepatitis, viral
  neuritis 999.5
  poisoning NEC 999.5
  rash NEC 999.5
  reaction NEC 999.5
  sickness NEC 999.5
Sesamoiditis 733.99
Seven-day fever 061
  of
    Japan 100.89
    Queensland 100.89
Sever's disease or osteochondrosis (calcaneum) 732.5
Sex chromosome mosaics 758.81
Sextuplet
  affected by maternal complications of pregnancy 761.5
  healthy liveborn — see Newborn, multiple
  pregnancy (complicating delivery) NEC 651.8 ✓5ᵗʰ
    with fetal loss and retention of one or more fetus(es) 651.6 ✓5ᵗʰ
Sexual
  anesthesia 302.72
  deviation (see also Deviation, sexual) 302.9
  disorder (see also Deviation, sexual) 302.9
  frigidity (female) 302.72
  function, disorder of (psychogenic) 302.70
    specified type NEC 302.79
  immaturity (female) (male) 259.0
  impotence (psychogenic) 302.72
    organic origin NEC 607.84
  precocity (constitutional) (cryptogenic) (female) (idiopathic) (male) NEC 259.1
    with adrenal hyperplasia 255.2
  sadism 302.84
Sexuality, pathological (see also Deviation, sexual) 302.9
Sézary's disease, reticulosis, or syndrome (M9701/3) 202.2 ✓5ᵗʰ
Shadow, lung 793.1
Shaken infant syndrome 995.55
Shaking
  head (tremor) 781.0
  palsy or paralysis (see also Parkinsonism) 332.0
Shallowness, acetabulum 736.39
Shaver's disease or syndrome (bauxite pneumoconiosis) 503
Shearing
  artificial skin graft 996.55
  decellularized allodermis graft 996.55
Sheath (tendon) — see condition
Shedding
  nail 703.8
  teeth, premature, primary (deciduous) 520.6
Sheehan's disease or syndrome (postpartum pituitary necrosis) 253.2
Shelf, rectal 569.49
Shell
  shock (current) (see also Reaction, stress, acute) 308.9
    lasting state 300.16
  teeth 520.5
Shield kidney 753.3
Shift, mediastinal 793.2
Shifting
  pacemaker 427.89
  sleep-work schedule (affecting sleep) 307.45
Shiga's
  bacillus 004.0
  dysentery 004.0
Shigella (dysentery) (see also Dysentery, bacillary) 004.9
  carrier (suspected) of V02.3

Shigellosis (see also Dysentery, bacillary) 004.9
Shingles (see also Herpes, zoster) 053.9
  eye NEC 053.29
Shin splints 844.9
Shipyard eye or disease 077.1
Shirodkar suture, in pregnancy 654.5 ✓5ᵗʰ
Shock 785.50
  with
    abortion — see Abortion, by type, with shock
    ectopic pregnancy (see also categories 633.0-633.9) 639.5
    molar pregnancy (see also categories 630-632) 639.5
  allergic — see Shock, anaphylactic
  anaclitic 309.21
  anaphylactic 995.0
    chemical — see Table of Drugs and Chemicals
    correct medicinal substance properly administered 995.0
    drug or medicinal substance
      correct substance properly administered 995.0
      overdose or wrong substance given or taken 977.9
        specified drug — see Table of Drugs and Chemicals
    following sting(s) 989.5
    food — see Anaphylactic shock, due to, food
    immunization 999.4
    serum 999.4
  anaphylactoid — see Shock, anaphylactic
  anesthetic
    correct substance properly administered 995.4
    overdose or wrong substance given 968.4
      specified anesthetic — see Table of Drugs and Chemicals
  birth, fetus or newborn NEC 779.89 ▶◀
  cardiogenic 785.51
  chemical substance — see Table of Drugs and Chemicals
  circulatory 785.59
  complicating
    abortion — see Abortion, by type, with shock
    ectopic pregnancy (see also categories 633.0-633.9) 639.5
    labor and delivery 669.1 ✓5ᵗʰ
    molar pregnancy (see also categories 630-632) 639.5
  culture 309.29
  due to
    drug 995.0
      correct substance properly administered 995.0
      overdose or wrong substance given or taken 977.9
        specified drug — see Table of Drugs and Chemicals
    food — see Anaphylactic shock, due to, food
  during labor and delivery 669.1 ✓5ᵗʰ
  electric 994.8
  endotoxic 785.59
    due to surgical procedure 998.0
  following
    abortion 639.5
    ectopic or molar pregnancy 639.5
    injury (immediate) (delayed) 958.4
    labor and delivery 669.1 ✓5ᵗʰ
  gram-negative 785.59
  hematogenic 785.59
  hemorrhagic
    due to
      disease 785.59
      surgery (intraoperative) (postoperative) 998.0
      trauma 958.4
  hypovolemic NEC 785.59
    surgical 998.0
    traumatic 958.4
  insulin 251.0
    therapeutic misadventure 962.3
  kidney 584.5
    traumatic (following crushing) 958.5

Shock — continued
  lightning 994.0
  lung 518.5
  nervous (see also Reaction, stress, acute) 308.9
  obstetric 669.1 ✓5ᵗʰ
    with
      abortion — see Abortion, by type, with shock
      ectopic pregnancy (see also categories 633.0-633.9) 639.5
      molar pregnancy (see also categories 630-632) 639.5
    following
      abortion 639.5
      ectopic or molar pregnancy 639.5
  paralysis, paralytic (see also Disease, cerebrovascular, acute) 436
    late effect — see Late effect(s) (of) cerebrovascular disease
  pleural (surgical) 998.0
    due to trauma 958.4
  postoperative 998.0
    with
      abortion — see Abortion, by type, with shock
      ectopic pregnancy (see also categories 633.0-633.9) 639.5
      molar pregnancy (see also categories 630-632) 639.5
    following
      abortion 639.5
      ectopic or molar pregnancy 639.5
  psychic (see also Reaction, stress, acute) 308.9
    past history (of) V15.49
  psychogenic (see also Reaction, stress, acute) 308.9
  septic 785.59
    with
      abortion — see Abortion, by type, with shock
      ectopic pregnancy (categories 633.0-633.9) 639.5
      molar pregnancy (see also categories 630-632) 639.5
    due to
      surgical procedure 998.0
      transfusion NEC 999.8
        bone marrow 996.85
    following
      abortion 639.5
      ectopic or molar pregnancy 639.5
      surgical procedure 998.0
      transfusion NEC 999.8
        bone marrow 996.85
  spinal — see also Injury, spinal, by site
    with spinal bone injury — see Fracture, vertebra, by site, with spinal cord injury
  surgical 998.0
  therapeutic misadventure NEC (see also Complications) 998.89
  thyroxin 962.7
  toxic 040.82 ▲
  transfusion — see Complications, transfusion
  traumatic (immediate) (delayed) 958.4
Shoemakers' chest 738.3
Short, shortening, shortness
  Achilles tendon (acquired) 727.81
  arm 736.89
    congenital 755.20
  back 737.9
  bowel syndrome 579.3
  breath 786.05
  common bile duct, congenital 751.69
  cord (umbilical) 663.4 ✓5ᵗʰ
    affecting fetus or newborn 762.6
  cystic duct, congenital 751.69
  esophagus (congenital) 750.4
  femur (acquired) 736.81
    congenital 755.34
  frenulum linguae 750.0
  frenum, lingual 750.0
  hamstrings 727.81
  hip (acquired) 736.39
    congenital 755.63
  leg (acquired) 736.81
    congenital 755.30

Short, shortening, shortness — *continued*
- metatarsus (congenital) 754.79
  - acquired 736.79
- organ or site, congenital NEC — *see* Distortion
- palate (congenital) 750.26
- P-R interval syndrome 426.81
- radius (acquired) 736.09
  - congenital 755.26
- round ligament 629.8
- sleeper 307.49
- stature, constitutional (hereditary) 783.43
- tendon 727.81
  - Achilles (acquired) 727.81
    - congenital 754.79
  - congenital 756.89
- thigh (acquired) 736.81
  - congenital 755.34
- tibialis anticus 727.81
- umbilical cord 663.4 ✓5th
  - affecting fetus or newborn 762.6
- urethra 599.84
- uvula (congenital) 750.26
- vagina 623.8

Shortsightedness 367.1

Shoshin (acute fulminating beriberi) 265.0

Shoulder — *see* condition

Shovel-shaped incisors 520.2

Shower, thromboembolic — *see* Embolism

Shunt (status)
- aortocoronary bypass V45.81
- arterial-venous (dialysis) V45.1
- arteriovenous, pulmonary (acquired) 417.0
  - congenital 747.3
  - traumatic (complication) 901.40
- cerebral ventricle (communicating) in situ V45.2
- coronary artery bypass V45.81
- surgical, prosthetic, with complications — *see* Complications, shunt
- vascular NEC V45.89

Shutdown
- renal 586
  - with
    - abortion — *see* Abortion, by type, with renal failure
    - ectopic pregnancy (*see also* categories 633.0-633.9) 639.3
    - molar pregnancy (*see also* categories 630-632) 639.3
  - complicating
    - abortion 639.3
    - ectopic or molar pregnancy 639.3
  - following labor and delivery 669.3 ✓5th

Shwachman's syndrome 288.0

Shy-Drager syndrome (orthostatic hypotension with multisystem degeneration) 333.0

Sialadenitis (any gland) (chronic) (suppurative) 527.2
- epidemic — *see* Mumps

Sialadenosis, periodic 527.2

Sialaporia 527.7

Sialectasia 527.8

Sialitis 527.2

Sialoadenitis (*see also* Sialadenitis) 527.2

Sioloangitis 527.2

Sialodochitis (fibrinosa) 527.2

Sialodocholithiasis 527.5

Sialolithiasis 527.5

Sialorrhea (*see also* Ptyalism) 527.7
- periodic 527.2

Sialosis 527.8
- rheumatic 710.2

Siamese twin 759.4

Sicard's syndrome 352.6

Sicca syndrome (keratoconjunctivitis) 710.2

Sick 799.9
- cilia syndrome 759.89
- or handicapped person in family V61.49

Sickle-cell
- anemia (*see also* Disease, sickle-cell) 282.60
- disease (*see also* Disease, sickle-cell) 282.60

Sickle-cell — *continued*
- hemoglobin
  - C disease 282.63
  - D disease 282.69
  - E disease 282.69
- thalassemia 282.4
- trait 282.5

Sicklemia (*see also* Disease, sickle-cell) 282.60
- trait 282.5

Sickness
- air (travel) 994.6
- airplane 994.6
- alpine 993.2
- altitude 993.2
- Andes 993.2
- aviators' 993.2
- balloon 993.2
- car 994.6
- compressed air 993.3
- decompression 993.3
- green 280.9
- harvest 100.89
- milk 988.8
- morning 643.0 ✓5th
- motion 994.6
- mountain 993.2
  - acute 289.0
- protein (*see also* Complications, vaccination) 999.5
- radiation NEC 990
- roundabout (motion) 994.6
- sea 994.6
- serum NEC 999.5
- sleeping (African) 086.5
  - by Trypanosoma 086.5
    - gambiense 086.3
    - rhodesiense 086.4
  - Gambian 086.3
  - late effect 139.8
  - Rhodesian 086.4
- sweating 078.2
- swing (motion) 994.6
- train (railway) (travel) 994.6
- travel (any vehicle) 994.6

Sick sinus syndrome 427.81

Sideropenia (*see also* Anemia, iron deficiency) 280.9

Siderosis (lung) (occupational) 503
- cornea 371.15
- eye (bulbi) (vitreous) 360.23
- lens 360.23

Siegal-Cattan-Mamou disease (periodic) 277.3

Siemens' syndrome
- ectodermal dysplasia 757.31
- keratosis follicularis spinulosa (decalvans) 757.39

Sighing respiration 786.7

Sigmoid
- flexure — *see* condition
- kidney 753.3

Sigmoiditis — *see* Enteritis

Silfverskiöld's syndrome 756.5 ✓5th

Silicosis, silicotic (complicated) (occupational) (simple) 502
- fibrosis, lung (confluent) (massive) (occupational) 502
- non-nodular 503
- pulmonum 502

Silicotuberculosis (*see also* Tuberculosis) 011.4 ✓5th

Silo fillers' disease 506.9

Silver's syndrome (congenital hemihypertrophy and short stature) 759.89

Silver wire arteries, retina 362.13

Silvestroni-Bianco syndrome (thalassemia minima) 282.4

Simian crease 757.2

Simmonds' cachexia or disease (pituitary cachexia) 253.2

Simons' disease or syndrome (progressive lipodystrophy) 272.6

Simple, simplex — *see* condition

Sinding-Larsen disease (juvenile osteopathia patellae) 732.4

Singapore hemorrhagic fever 065.4

Singers' node or nodule 478.5

Single
- atrium 745.69
- coronary artery 746.85
- umbilical artery 747.5
- ventricle 745.3

Singultus 786.8
- epidemicus 078.89

Sinus — *see also* Fistula
- abdominal 569.81
- arrest 426.6
- arrhythmia 427.89
- bradycardia 427.89
  - chronic 427.81
- branchial cleft (external) (internal) 744.41
- coccygeal (infected) 685.1
  - with abscess 685.0
- dental 522.7
- dermal (congenital) 685.1
  - with abscess 685.0
- draining — *see* Fistula
- infected, skin NEC 686.9
- marginal, ruptured or bleeding 641.2 ✓5th
  - affecting fetus or newborn 762.1
- pause 426.6
- pericranii 742.0
- pilonidal (infected) (rectum) 685.1
  - with abscess 685.0
- preauricular 744.46
- rectovaginal 619.1
- sacrococcygeal (dermoid) (infected) 685.1
  - with abscess 685.0
- skin
  - infected NEC 686.9
  - noninfected — *see* Ulcer, skin
- tachycardia 427.89
- tarsi syndrome 726.79
- testis 608.89
- tract (postinfectional) — *see* Fistula
- urachus 753.7

Sinuses, Rokitansky-Aschoff (*see also* Disease, gallbladder) 575.8

Sinusitis (accessory) (nasal) (hyperplastic) (nonpurulent) (purulent) (chronic) 473.9
- with influenza, flu, or grippe 487.1
- acute 461.9
  - ethmoidal 461.2
  - frontal 461.1
  - maxillary 461.0
  - specified type NEC 461.8
  - sphenoidal 461.3
- allergic (*see also* Fever, hay) 477.9
- antrum — *see* Sinusitis, maxillary
- due to
  - fungus, any sinus 117.9
  - high altitude 993.1
- ethmoidal 473.2
  - acute 461.2
- frontal 473.1
  - acute 461.1
- influenzal 478.1
- maxillary 473.0
  - acute 461.0
- specified site NEC 473.8
- sphenoidal 473.3
  - acute 461.3
- syphilitic, any sinus 095.8
- tuberculous, any sinus (*see also* Tuberculosis) 012.8 ✓5th

Sinusitis-bronchiectasis-situs inversus (syndrome) (triad) 759.3

Sipple's syndrome (medullary thyroid carcinoma-pheochromocytoma) 193

Sirenomelia 759.89

Siriasis 992.0

Sirkari's disease 085.0

SIRS (systemic inflammatory response syndrome) 995.90
- due to
  - infectious process 995.91
    - with organ dysfunction 995.92
  - non-infectious process 995.93
    - with organ dysfunction 995.94

Index to Diseases

Siti 104.0
Sitophobia 300.29
Situation, psychiatric 300.9
Situational
　disturbance (transient) (*see also* Reaction, adjustment) 309.9
　　acute 308.3
　maladjustment, acute (*see also* Reaction, adjustment) 309.9
　reaction (*see also* Reaction, adjustment) 309.9
　　acute 308.3
Situs inversus or transversus 759.3
　abdominalis 759.3
　thoracis 759.3
Sixth disease 057.8
Sjögren (-Gougerot) syndrome or disease (keratoconjunctivitis sicca) 710.2
　with lung involvement 710.2 [517.8]
Sjögren-Larsson syndrome (ichthyosis congenita) 757.1
Skeletal — *see* condition
Skene's gland — *see* condition
Skenitis (*see also* Urethritis) 597.89
　gonorrheal (acute) 098.0
　　chronic or duration of 2 months or over 098.2
Skerljevo 104.0
Skevas-Zerfus disease 989.5
Skin — *see also* condition
　donor V59.1
　hidebound 710.9
SLAP lesion (superior glenoid labrum) 840.7
Slate-dressers' lung 502
Slate-miners' lung 502
Sleep
　disorder 780.50
　　with apnea — *see* Apnea, sleep
　　child 307.40
　　nonorganic origin 307.40
　　　specified type NEC 307.49
　disturbance 780.50
　　with apnea — *see* Apnea, sleep
　　nonorganic origin 307.40
　　　specified type NEC 307.49
　drunkenness 307.47
　paroxysmal 347
　rhythm inversion 780.55
　　nonorganic origin 307.45
　walking 307.46
　　hysterical 300.13
Sleeping sickness 086.5
　late effect 139.8
Sleeplessness (*see also* Insomnia) 780.52
　menopausal 627.2
　nonorganic origin 307.41
Slipped, slipping
　epiphysis (postinfectional) 732.9
　　traumatic (old) 732.9
　　　current — *see* Fracture, by site
　　upper femoral (nontraumatic) 732.2
　intervertebral disc — *see* Displacement, intervertebral disc
　ligature, umbilical 772.3
　patella 717.89
　rib 733.99
　sacroiliac joint 724.6
　tendon 727.9
　ulnar nerve, nontraumatic 354.2
　vertebra NEC (*see also* Spondylolisthesis) 756.12
Slocumb's syndrome 255.3
Sloughing (multiple) (skin) 686.9
　abscess — *see* Abscess, by site
　appendix 543.9
　bladder 596.8
　fascia 728.9
　graft — *see* Complications, graft
　phagedena (*see also* Gangrene) 785.4
　reattached extremity (*see also* Complications, reattached extremity) 996.90
　rectum 569.49
　scrotum 608.89
　tendon 727.9

Sloughing — *continued*
　transplanted organ (*see also* Rejection, transplant, organ, by site) 996.80
　ulcer (*see also* Ulcer, skin) 707.9
Slow
　feeding newborn 779.3
　fetal, growth NEC 764.9 ✓5ᵗʰ
　　affecting management of pregnancy 656.5 ✓5ᵗʰ
Slowing
　heart 427.89
　urinary stream 788.62
Sluder's neuralgia or syndrome 337.0
Slurred, slurring, speech 784.5
Small, smallness
　cardiac reserve — *see* Disease, heart
　for dates
　　fetus or newborn 764.0 ✓5ᵗʰ
　　　with malnutrition 764.1 ✓5ᵗʰ
　　　affecting management of pregnancy 656.5 ✓5ᵗʰ
　　infant, term 764.0 ✓5ᵗʰ
　　　with malnutrition 764.1 ✓5ᵗʰ
　　　affecting management of pregnancy 656.5 ✓5ᵗʰ
　introitus, vagina 623.3
　kidney, unknown cause 589.9
　　bilateral 589.1
　　unilateral 589.0
　ovary 620.8
　pelvis
　　with disproportion (fetopelvic) 653.1 ✓5ᵗʰ
　　　affecting fetus or newborn 763.1
　　causing obstructed labor 660.1 ✓5ᵗʰ
　　　affecting fetus or newborn 763.1
　placenta — *see* Placenta, insufficiency
　uterus 621.8
　white kidney 582.9
Small-for-dates (*see also* Light-for-dates) 764.0 ✓5ᵗʰ
　affecting management of pregnancy 656.5 ✓5ᵗʰ
Smallpox 050.9
　contact V01.3
　exposure to V01.3
　hemorrhagic (pustular) 050.0
　malignant 050.0
　modified 050.2
　vaccination
　　complications — *see* Complications, vaccination
　　prophylactic (against) V04.1
Smith's fracture (separation) (closed) 813.41
　open 813.51
Smith-Lemli Opitz syndrome (cerebrohepatorenal syndrome) 759.89
Smith-Strang disease (oasthouse urine) 270.2
Smokers'
　bronchitis 491.0
　cough 491.0
　syndrome (*see also* Abuse, drugs, nondependent) 305.1
　throat 472.1
　tongue 528.6
Smothering spells 786.09
Snaggle teeth, tooth 524.3
Snapping
　finger 727.05
　hip 719.65
　jaw 524.69
　knee 717.9
　thumb 727.05
Sneddon-Wilkinson disease or syndrome (subcorneal pustular dermatosis) 694.1
Sneezing 784.9
　intractable 478.1
Sniffing
　cocaine (*see also* Dependence) 304.2 ✓5ᵗʰ
　ether (*see also* Dependence) 304.6 ✓5ᵗʰ
　glue (airplane) (*see also* Dependence) 304.6 ✓5ᵗʰ
Snoring 786.09
Snow blindness 370.24
Snuffles (nonsyphilitic) 460
　syphilitic (infant) 090.0

Social migrant V60.0
Sodoku 026.0
Soemmering's ring 366.51
Soft — *see also* condition
　enlarged prostate 600.0
　nails 703.8
Softening
　bone 268.2
　brain (necrotic) (progressive) 434.9 ✓5ᵗʰ
　　arteriosclerotic 437.0
　　congenital 742.4
　　embolic (*see also* Embolism, brain) 434.1 ✓5ᵗʰ
　　hemorrhagic (*see also* Hemorrhage, brain) 431
　　occlusive 434.9 ✓5ᵗʰ
　　thrombotic (*see also* Thrombosis, brain) 434.0 ✓5ᵗʰ
　cartilage 733.92
　cerebellar — *see* Softening, brain
　cerebral — *see* Softening, brain
　cerebrospinal — *see* Softening, brain
　myocardial, heart (*see also* Degeneration, myocardial) 429.1
　nails 703.8
　spinal cord 336.8
　stomach 537.89
Solar fever 061
Soldier's
　heart 306.2
　patches 423.1
Solitary
　cyst
　　bone 733.21
　　kidney 593.2
　kidney (congenital) 753.0
　tubercle, brain (*see also* Tuberculosis, brain) 013.2 ✓5ᵗʰ
　ulcer, bladder 596.8
Somatization reaction, somatic reaction (*see also* Disorder, psychosomatic) 306.9
　disorder 300.81
Somatoform disorder 300.82
　atypical 300.82
　severe 300.81
　undifferentiated 300.82
Somnambulism 307.46
　hysterical 300.13
Somnolence 780.09
　nonorganic origin 307.43
　periodic 349.89
Sonne dysentery 004.3
Soor 112.0
Sore
　Delhi 085.1
　desert (*see also* Ulcer, skin) 707.9
　eye 379.99
　Lahore 085.1
　mouth 528.9
　　canker 528.2
　　due to dentures 528.9
　muscle 729.1
　Naga (*see also* Ulcer, skin) 707.9
　oriental 085.1
　pressure 707.0
　　with gangrene 707.0 [785.4]
　skin NEC 709.9
　soft 099.0
　throat 462
　　with influenza, flu, or grippe 487.1
　　acute 462
　　chronic 472.1
　　clergyman's 784.49
　　coxsackie (virus) 074.0
　　diphtheritic 032.0
　　epidemic 034.0
　　gangrenous 462
　　herpetic 054.79
　　influenzal 487.1
　　malignant 462
　　purulent 462
　　putrid 462
　　septic 034.0
　　streptococcal (ulcerative) 034.0
　　ulcerated 462

Sore

Sore — continued
- throat — continued
  - viral NEC 462
    - Coxsackie 074.0
  - tropical (see also Ulcer, skin) 707.9
  - veldt (see also Ulcer, skin) 707.9
- **Sotos' syndrome** (cerebral gigantism) 253.0
- **Sounds**
  - friction, pleural 786.7
  - succussion, chest 786.7
- **South African cardiomyopathy syndrome** 425.2
- **South American**
  - blastomycosis 116.1
  - trypanosomiasis — see Trypanosomiasis
- **Southeast Asian hemorrhagic fever** 065.4
- **Spacing, teeth, abnormal** 524.3
- **Spade-like hand** (congenital) 754.89
- **Spading nail** 703.8
  - congenital 757.5
- **Spanemia** 285.9
- **Spanish collar** 605
- **Sparganosis** 123.5
- **Spasm, spastic, spasticity** (see also condition) 781.0
  - accommodation 367.53
  - ampulla of Vater (see also Disease, gallbladder) 576.8
  - anus, ani (sphincter) (reflex) 564.6
    - psychogenic 306.4
  - artery NEC 443.9
    - basilar 435.0
    - carotid 435.8
    - cerebral 435.9
      - specified artery NEC 435.8
    - retinal (see also Occlusion, retinal, artery) 362.30
    - vertebral 435.1
    - vertebrobasilar 435.3
  - Bell's 351.0
  - bladder (sphincter, external or internal) 596.8
  - bowel 564.9
    - psychogenic 306.4
  - bronchus, bronchiole 519.1
  - cardia 530.0
  - cardiac — see Angina
  - carpopedal (see also Tetany) 781.7
  - cecum 564.9
    - psychogenic 306.4
  - cerebral (arteries) (vascular) 435.9
    - specified artery NEC 435.8
  - cerebrovascular 435.9
  - cervix, complicating delivery 661.4 ✓5ᵗʰ
    - affecting fetus or newborn 763.7
  - ciliary body (of accommodation) 367.53
  - colon 564.1
    - psychogenic 306.4
  - common duct (see also Disease, biliary) 576.8
  - compulsive 307.22
  - conjugate 378.82
  - convergence 378.84
  - coronary (artery) — see Angina
  - diaphragm (reflex) 786.8
    - psychogenic 306.1
  - duodenum, duodenal (bulb) 564.89
  - esophagus (diffuse) 530.5
    - psychogenic 306.4
  - facial 351.8
  - fallopian tube 620.8
  - gait 781.2
  - gastrointestinal (tract) 536.8
    - psychogenic 306.4
  - glottis 478.75
    - hysterical 300.11
    - psychogenic 306.1
      - specified as conversion reaction 300.11
    - reflex through recurrent laryngeal nerve 478.75
  - habit 307.20
    - chronic 307.22
    - transient of childhood 307.21
  - heart — see Angina
  - hourglass — see Contraction, hourglass
  - hysterical 300.11
  - infantile (see also Epilepsy) 345.6 ✓5ᵗʰ
  - internal oblique, eye 378.51

Spasm, spastic, spasticity (see also condition) — continued
- intestinal 564.9
  - psychogenic 306.4
- larynx, laryngeal 478.75
  - hysterical 300.11
  - psychogenic 306.1
    - specified as conversion reaction 300.11
- levator palpebrae superioris 333.81
- lightning (see also Epilepsy) 345.6 ✓5ᵗʰ
- mobile 781.0
- muscle 728.85
  - back 724.8
  - psychogenic 306.0
- nerve, trigeminal 350.1
- nervous 306.0
- nodding 307.3
  - infantile (see also Epilepsy) 345.6 ✓5ᵗʰ
- occupational 300.89
- oculogyric 378.87
- ophthalmic artery 362.30
- orbicularis 781.0
- perineal 625.8
- peroneo-extensor (see also Flat, foot) 734
- pharynx (reflex) 478.29
  - hysterical 300.11
  - psychogenic 306.1
    - specified as conversion reaction 300.11
- pregnant uterus, complicating delivery 661.4 ✓5ᵗʰ
- psychogenic 306.0
- pylorus 537.81
  - adult hypertrophic 537.0
  - congenital or infantile 750.5
  - psychogenic 306.4
- rectum (sphincter) 564.6
  - psychogenic 306.4
- retinal artery NEC (see also Occlusion, retina, artery) 362.30
- sacroiliac 724.6
- salaam (infantile) (see also Epilepsy) 345.6 ✓5ᵗʰ
- saltatory 781.0
- sigmoid 564.9
  - psychogenic 306.4
- sphincter of Oddi (see also Disease, gallbladder) 576.5
- stomach 536.8
  - neurotic 306.4
- throat 478.29
  - hysterical 300.11
  - psychogenic 306.1
    - specified as conversion reaction 300.11
- tic 307.20
  - chronic 307.22
  - transient of childhood 307.21
- tongue 529.8
- torsion 333.6
- trigeminal nerve 350.1
  - postherpetic 053.12
- ureter 593.89
- urethra (sphincter) 599.84
- uterus 625.8
  - complicating labor 661.4 ✓5ᵗʰ
    - affecting fetus or newborn 763.7
- vagina 625.1
  - psychogenic 306.51
- vascular NEC 443.9
- vasomotor NEC 443.9
- vein NEC 459.89
- vesical (sphincter, external or internal) 596.8
- viscera 789.0 ✓5ᵗʰ

Spasmodic — see condition
Spasmophilia (see also Tetany) 781.7
Spasmus nutans 307.3
Spastic — see also Spasm
- child 343.9

Spasticity — see also Spasm
- cerebral, child 343.9

Speakers' throat 784.49
Specific, specified — see condition
Speech
- defect, disorder, disturbance, impediment NEC 784.5
  - psychogenic 307.9
- therapy V57.3

Spells 780.39
- breath-holding 786.9
Spencer's disease (epidemic vomiting) 078.82
Spens' syndrome (syncope with heart block) 426.9
Spermatic cord — see condition
Spermatocele 608.1
- congenital 752.8
Spermatocystitis 608.4
Spermatocytoma (M9063/3)
- specified site — see Neoplasm, by site, malignant
- unspecified site 186.9
Spermatorrhea 608.89
Sperm counts
- fertility testing V26.21
- following sterilization reversal V26.22
- postvasectomy V25.8
Sphacelus (see also Gangrene) 785.4
Sphenoidal — see condition
Sphenoiditis (chronic) (see also Sinusitis, sphenoidal) 473.3
Sphenopalatine ganglion neuralgia 337.0
Sphericity, increased, lens 743.36
Spherocytosis (congenital) (familial) (hereditary) 282.0
- hemoglobin disease 282.7
- sickle-cell (disease) 282.60
Spherophakia 743.36
Sphincter — see condition
Sphincteritis, sphincter of Oddi (see also Cholecystitis) 576.8
Sphingolipidosis 272.7
Sphingolipodystrophy 272.7
Sphingomyelinosis 272.7
Spicule tooth 520.2
Spider
- finger 755.59
- nevus 448.1
- vascular 448.1
Spiegler-Fendt sarcoid 686.8
Spielmeyer-Stock disease 330.1
Spielmeyer-Vogt disease 330.1
Spina bifida (aperta) 741.9 ✓5ᵗʰ

> Note — Use the following fifth-digit subclassification with category 741:
>
> 0   unspecified region
> 1   cervical region
> 2   dorsal [thoracic] region
> 3   lumbar region

- with hydrocephalus 741.0 ✓5ᵗʰ
- fetal (suspected), affecting management of pregnancy 655.0 ✓5ᵗʰ
- occulta 756.17
Spindle, Krukenberg's 371.13
Spine, spinal — see condition
Spiradenoma (eccrine) (M8403/0) — see Neoplasm, skin, benign
Spirillosis NEC (see also Fever, relapsing) 087.9
Spirillum minus 026.0
Spirillum obermeieri infection 087.0
Spirochetal — see condition
Spirochetosis 104.9
- arthritic, arthritica 104.9 [711.8] ✓5ᵗʰ
- bronchopulmonary 104.8
- icterohemorrhagica 100.0
- lung 104.8
Spitting blood (see also Hemoptysis) 786.3
Splanchnomegaly 569.89
Splanchnoptosis 569.89
Spleen, splenic — see also condition
- agenesis 759.0
- flexure syndrome 569.89
- neutropenia syndrome 288.0
- sequestration syndrome 282.60
Splenectasis (see also Splenomegaly) 789.2

Index to Diseases

Splenitis (interstitial) (malignant) (nonspecific) 289.59
  malarial (see also Malaria) 084.6
  tuberculous (see also Tuberculosis) 017.7 ✓5ᵗʰ
Splenocele 289.59
Splenomegalia — see Splenomegaly
Splenomegalic — see condition
Splenomegaly 789.2
  Bengal 789.2
  cirrhotic 289.51
  congenital 759.0
  congestive, chronic 289.51
  cryptogenic 789.2
  Egyptian 120.1
  Gaucher's (cerebroside lipidosis) 272.7
  idiopathic 789.2
  malarial (see also Malaria) 084.6
  neutropenic 288.0
  Niemann-Pick (lipid histiocytosis) 272.7
  siderotic 289.51
  syphilitic 095.8
    congenital 090.0
  tropical (Bengal) (idiopathic) 789.2
Splenopathy 289.50
Splenopneumonia — see Pneumonia
Splenoptosis 289.59
Splinter — see Injury, superficial, by site
Split, splitting
  heart sounds 427.89
  lip, congenital (see also Cleft, lip) 749.10
  nails 703.8
  urinary stream 788.61
Spoiled child reaction (see also Disturbance, conduct) 312.1 ✓5ᵗʰ
Spondylarthritis (see also Spondylosis) 721.90
Spondylarthrosis (see also Spondylosis) 721.90
Spondylitis 720.9
  ankylopoietica 720.0
  ankylosing (chronic) 720.0
  atrophic 720.9
    ligamentous 720.9
  chronic (traumatic) (see also Spondylosis) 721.90
  deformans (chronic) (see also Spondylosis) 721.90
  gonococcal 098.53
  gouty 274.0
  hypertrophic (see also Spondylosis) 721.90
  infectious NEC 720.9
  juvenile (adolescent) 720.0
  Kümmell's 721.7
  Marie-Strümpell (ankylosing) 720.0
  muscularis 720.9
  ossificans ligamentosa 721.6
  osteoarthritica (see also Spondylosis) 721.90
  posttraumatic 721.7
  proliferative 720.0
  rheumatoid 720.0
  rhizomelica 720.0
  sacroiliac NEC 720.2
  senescent (see also Spondylosis) 721.90
  senile (see also Spondylosis) 721.90
  static (see also Spondylosis) 721.90
  traumatic (chronic) (see also Spondylosis) 721.90
  tuberculous (see also Tuberculosis) 015.0 ✓5ᵗʰ [720.81]
  typhosa 002.0 [720.81]
Spondyloarthrosis (see also Spondylosis) 721.90
Spondylolisthesis (congenital) (lumbosacral) 756.12
  with disproportion (fetopelvic) 653.3 ✓5ᵗʰ
    affecting fetus or newborn 763.1
    causing obstructed labor 660.1 ✓5ᵗʰ
      affecting fetus or newborn 763.1
  acquired 738.4
  degenerative 738.4
  traumatic 738.4
    acute (lumbar) — see Fracture, vertebra, lumbar
      site other than lumbosacral — see Fracture, vertebra, by site
Spondylolysis (congenital) 756.11
  acquired 738.4
  cervical 756.19

Spondylolysis — continued
  lumbosacral region 756.11
    with disproportion (fetopelvic) 653.3 ✓5ᵗʰ
      affecting fetus or newborn 763.1
      causing obstructed labor 660.1 ✓5ᵗʰ
        affecting fetus or newborn 763.1
Spondylopathy
  inflammatory 720.9
    specified type NEC 720.89
  traumatic 721.7
Spondylose rhizomelique 720.0
Spondylosis 721.90
  with
    disproportion 653.3 ✓5ᵗʰ
      affecting fetus or newborn 763.1
      causing obstructed labor 660.1 ✓5ᵗʰ
        affecting fetus or newborn 763.1
    myelopathy NEC 721.91
  cervical, cervicodorsal 721.0
    with myelopathy 721.1
  inflammatory 720.9
  lumbar, lumbosacral 721.3
    with myelopathy 721.42
  sacral 721.3
    with myelopathy 721.42
  thoracic 721.2
    with myelopathy 721.41
  traumatic 721.7
Sponge
  divers' disease 989.5
  inadvertently left in operation wound 998.4
  kidney (medullary) 753.17
Spongioblastoma (M9422/3)
  multiforme (M9440/3)
    specified site — see Neoplasm, by site, malignant
    unspecified site 191.9
  polare (M9423/3)
    specified site — see Neoplasm, by site, malignant
    unspecified site 191.9
  primitive polar (M9443/3)
    specified site — see Neoplasm, by site, malignant
    unspecified site 191.9
  specified site — see Neoplasm, by site, malignant
  unspecified site 191.9
Spongiocytoma (M9400/3)
  specified site — see Neoplasm, by site, malignant
  unspecified site 191.9
Spongioneuroblastoma (M9504/3) — see Neoplasm, by site, malignant
Spontaneous — see also condition
  fracture — see Fracture, pathologic
Spoon nail 703.8
  congenital 757.5
Sporadic — see condition
Sporotrichosis (bones) (cutaneous) (disseminated) (epidermal) (lymphatic) (lymphocutaneous) (mucous membranes) (pulmonary) (skeletal) (visceral) 117.1
Sporotrichum schenckii infection 117.1
Spots, spotting
  atrophic (skin) 701.3
  Bitôt's (in the young child) 264.1
  café au lait 709.09
  cayenne pepper 448.1
  cotton wool (retina) 362.83
  de Morgan's (senile angiomas) 448.1
  Fúchs' black (myopic) 360.21
  intermenstrual
    irregular 626.6
    regular 626.5
  interpalpebral 372.53
  Koplik's 055.9
  liver 709.09
  Mongolian (pigmented) 757.33
  of pregnancy 641.9 ✓5ᵗʰ
  purpuric 782.7
  ruby 448.1
Spotted fever — see Fever, spotted

Sprain, strain (joint) (ligament) (muscle) (tendon) 848.9
  abdominal wall (muscle) 848.8
  Achilles tendon 845.09
  acromioclavicular 840.0
  ankle 845.00
    and foot 845.00
  anterior longitudinal, cervical 847.0
  arm 840.9
    upper 840.9
      and shoulder 840.9
  astragalus 845.00
  atlanto-axial 847.0
  atlanto-occipital 847.0
  atlas 847.0
  axis 847.0
  back (see also Sprain, spine) 847.9
  breast bone 848.40
  broad ligament — see Injury, internal, broad ligament
  calcaneofibular 845.02
  carpal 842.01
  carpometacarpal 842.11
  cartilage
    costal, without mention of injury to sternum 848.3
      involving sternum 848.42
    ear 848.8
    knee 844.9
      with current tear (see also Tear, meniscus) 836.2
    semilunar (knee) 844.8
      with current tear (see also Tear, meniscus) 836.2
    septal, nose 848.0
    thyroid region 848.2
    xiphoid 848.49
  cervical, cervicodorsal, cervicothoracic 847.0
  chondrocostal, without mention of injury to sternum 848.3
    involving sternum 848.42
  chondrosternal 848.42
  chronic (joint) — see Derangement, joint
  clavicle 840.9
  coccyx 847.4
  collar bone 840.9
  collateral, knee (medial) (tibial) 844.1
    lateral (fibular) 844.0
    recurrent or old 717.89
      lateral 717.81
      medial 717.82
  coracoacromial 840.8
  coracoclavicular 840.1
  coracohumeral 840.2
  coracoid (process) 840.9
  coronary, knee 844.8
  costal cartilage, without mention of injury to sternum 848.3
    involving sternum 848.42
  cricoarytenoid articulation 848.2
  cricothyroid articulation 848.2
  cruciate
    knee 844.2
    old 717.89
      anterior 717.83
      posterior 717.84
  deltoid
    ankle 845.01
    shoulder 840.8
  dorsal (spine) 847.1
  ear cartilage 848.8
  elbow 841.9
    and forearm 841.9
    specified site NEC 841.8
  femur (proximal end) 843.9
    distal end 844.9
  fibula (proximal end) 844.9
    distal end 845.00
  fibulocalcaneal 845.02
  finger(s) 842.10
  foot 845.10
    and ankle 845.00
  forearm 841.9
    and elbow 841.9
    specified site NEC 841.8
  glenoid (shoulder) (see also SLAP lesion) 840.8
  hand 842.10

Sprain, strain — continued

hip 843.9
  and thigh 843.9
humerus (proximal end) 840.9
  distal end 841.9
iliofemoral 843.0
infraspinatus 840.3
innominate
  acetabulum 843.9
  pubic junction 848.5
  sacral junction 846.1
internal
  collateral, ankle 845.01
  semilunar cartilage 844.8
    with current tear (see also Tear, meniscus) 836.2
    old 717.5
interphalangeal
  finger 842.13
  toe 845.13
ischiocapsular 843.1
jaw (cartilage) (meniscus) 848.1
  old 524.69
knee 844.9
  and leg 844.9
  old 717.5
    collateral
      lateral 717.81
      medial 717.82
    cruciate
      anterior 717.83
      posterior 717.84
late effect — see Late, effects (of), sprain
lateral collateral, knee 844.0
  old 717.81
leg 844.9
  and knee 844.9
ligamentum teres femoris 843.8
low back 846.9
lumbar (spine) 847.2
lumbosacral 846.0
  chronic or old 724.6
mandible 848.1
  old 524.69
maxilla 848.1
medial collateral, knee 844.1
  old 717.82
meniscus
  jaw 848.1
    old 524.69
  knee 844.8
    with current tear (see also Tear, meniscus) 836.2
    old 717.5
  mandible 848.1
    old 524.69
  specified site NEC 848.8
metacarpal 842.10
  distal 842.12
  proximal 842.11
metacarpophalangeal 842.12
metatarsal 845.10
metatarsophalangeal 845.12
midcarpal 842.19
midtarsal 845.19
multiple sites, except fingers alone or toes alone 848.8
neck 847.0
nose (septal cartilage) 848.0
occiput from atlas 847.0
old — see Derangement, joint
orbicular, hip 843.8
patella(r) 844.8
  old 717.89
pelvis 848.5
phalanx
  finger 842.10
  toe 845.10
radiocarpal 842.02
radiohumeral 841.2
radioulnar 841.9
  distal 842.09
radius, radial (proximal end) 841.9
  and ulna 841.9
    distal 842.09
  collateral 841.0
  distal end 842.00

Sprain, strain — continued

recurrent — see Sprain, by site
rib (cage), without mention of injury to sternum 848.3
  involving sternum 848.42
rotator cuff (capsule) 840.4
round ligament — see also Injury, internal, round ligament
  femur 843.8
sacral (spine) 847.3
sacrococcygeal 847.3
sacroiliac (region) 846.9
  chronic or old 724.6
  ligament 846.1
  specified site NEC 846.8
sacrospinatus 846.2
sacrospinous 846.2
sacrotuberous 846.3
scaphoid bone, ankle 845.00
scapula(r) 840.9
semilunar cartilage (knee) 844.8
  with current tear (see also Tear, meniscus) 836.2
  old 717.5
septal cartilage (nose) 848.0
shoulder 840.9
  and arm, upper 840.9
  blade 840.9
specified site NEC 848.8
spine 847.9
  cervical 847.0
  coccyx 847.4
  dorsal 847.1
  lumbar 847.2
  lumbosacral 846.0
    chronic or old 724.6
  sacral 847.3
  sacroiliac (see also Sprain, sacroiliac) 846.9
    chronic or old 724.6
  thoracic 847.1
sternoclavicular 848.41
sternum 848.40
subglenoid (see also SLAP lesion) 840.8
subscapularis 840.5
supraspinatus 840.6
symphysis
  jaw 848.1
    old 524.69
  mandibular 848.1
    old 524.69
  pubis 848.5
talofibular 845.09
tarsal 845.10
tarsometatarsal 845.11
temporomandibular 848.1
  old 524.69
teres
  ligamentum femoris 843.8
  major or minor 840.8
thigh (proximal end) 843.9
  and hip 843.9
  distal end 844.9
thoracic (spine) 847.1
thorax 848.8
thumb 842.10
thyroid cartilage or region 848.2
tibia (proximal end) 844.9
  distal end 845.00
tibiofibular
  distal 845.03
  superior 844.3
toe(s) 845.10
trachea 848.8
trapezoid 840.8
ulna, ulnar (proximal end) 841.9
  collateral 841.1
  distal end 842.00
ulnohumeral 841.3
vertebrae (see also Sprain, spine) 847.9
  cervical, cervicodorsal, cervicothoracic 847.0
wrist (cuneiform) (scaphoid) (semilunar) 842.00
xiphoid cartilage 848.49

Sprengel's deformity (congenital) 755.52
Spring fever 309.23
Sprue 579.1
  celiac 579.0
  idiopathic 579.0

Sprue — continued

  meaning thrush 112.0
  nontropical 579.0
  tropical 579.1
Spur — see also Exostosis
  bone 726.91
    calcaneal 726.73
  calcaneal 726.73
  iliac crest 726.5
  nose (septum) 478.1
    bone 726.91
  septal 478.1
Spuria placenta — see Placenta, abnormal
Spurway's syndrome (brittle bones and blue sclera) 756.51
Sputum, abnormal (amount) (color) (excessive) (odor) (purulent) 786.4
  bloody 786.3
Squamous — see also condition
  cell metaplasia
    bladder 596.8
    cervix — see condition
  epithelium in
    cervical canal (congenital) 752.49
    uterine mucosa (congenital) 752.3
  metaplasia
    bladder 596.8
    cervix — see condition
Squashed nose 738.0
  congenital 754.0
Squeeze, divers' 993.3
Squint (see also Strabismus) 378.9
  accommodative (see also Esotropia) 378.00
  concomitant (see also Heterotropia) 378.30
Stab — see also Wound, open, by site
  internal organs — see Injury, internal, by site, with open wound
Staggering gait 781.2
  hysterical 300.11
Staghorn calculus 592.0
Stälh's
  ear 744.29
  pigment line (cornea) 371.11
Stälhi's pigment lines (cornea) 371.11
Stain
  port wine 757.32
  tooth, teeth (hard tissues) 521.7
    due to
      accretions 523.6
      deposits (betel) (black) (green) (materia alba) (orange) (tobacco) 523.6
      metals (copper) (silver) 521.7
      nicotine 523.6
      pulpal bleeding 521.7
      tobacco 523.6
Stammering 307.0
Standstill
  atrial 426.6
  auricular 426.6
  cardiac (see also Arrest, cardiac) 427.5
  sinoatrial 429.6
  sinus 426.6
  ventricular (see also Arrest, cardiac) 427.5
Stannosis 503
Stanton's disease (melioidosis) 025
Staphylitis (acute) (catarrhal) (chronic) (gangrenous) (membranous) (suppurative) (ulcerative) 528.3
Staphylococcemia 038.10
  aureus 038.11
  specified organism NEC 038.19
Staphylococcus, staphylococcal — see condition
Staphyloderma (skin) 686.00
Staphyloma 379.11
  anterior, localized 379.14
  ciliary 379.11
  cornea 371.73
  equatorial 379.13
  posterior 379.12
  posticum 379.12
  ring 379.15
  sclera NEC 379.11
Starch eating 307.52

Index to Diseases

Stargardt's disease 362.75
Starvation (inanition) (due to lack of food) 994.2
   edema 262
   voluntary NEC 307.1
Stasis
   bile (duct) (see also Disease, biliary) 576.8
   bronchus (see also Bronchitis) 490
   cardiac (see also Failure, heart) 428.0
   cecum 564.89
   colon 564.89
   dermatitis (see also Varix, with stasis
      dermatitis) 454.1
   duodenal 536.8
   eczema (see also Varix, with stasis dermatitis)
      454.1
   edema (see also Hypertension, venous)
      459.30
   foot 991.4
   gastric 536.3
   ileocecal coil 564.89
   ileum 564.89
   intestinal 564.89
   jejunum 564.89
   kidney 586
   liver 571.9
      cirrhotic — see Cirrhosis, liver
   lymphatic 457.8
   pneumonia 514
   portal 571.9
   pulmonary 514
   rectal 564.89
   renal 586
      tubular 584.5
   stomach 536.3
   ulcer
      with varicose veins 454.0
      without varicose veins 459.81
   urine NEC (see also Retention, urine) 788.20
   venous 459.81
State
   affective and paranoid, mixed, organic
      psychotic 294.8
   agitated 307.9
      acute reaction to stress 308.2
   anxiety (neurotic) (see also Anxiety) 300.00
      specified type NEC 300.09
   apprehension (see also Anxiety) 300.00
      specified type NEC 300.09
   climacteric, female 627.2
      following induced menopause 627.4
   clouded
      epileptic (see also Epilepsy) 345.9 ✓5ᵗʰ
      paroxysmal (idiopathic) (see also Epilepsy)
         345.9 ✓5ᵗʰ
   compulsive (mixed) (with obsession) 300.3
   confusional 298.9
      acute 293.0
         with
            arteriosclerotic dementia 290.41
            presenile brain disease 290.11
            senility 290.3
      alcoholic 291.0
      drug-induced 292.81
      epileptic 293.0
      postoperative 293.9
      reactive (emotional stress) (psychological
         trauma) 298.2
      subacute 293.1
   constitutional psychopathic 301.9
   convulsive (see also Convulsions) 780.39
   depressive NEC 311
      induced by drug 292.84
      neurotic 300.4
   dissociative 300.15
   hallucinatory 780.1
      induced by drug 292.12
   hyperdynamic beta-adrenergic circulatory
      429.82
   locked-in 344.81
   menopausal 627.2
      artificial 627.4
      following induced menopause 627.4
   neurotic NEC 300.9
      with depersonalization episode 300.6
   obsessional 300.3
   oneiroid (see also Schizophrenia) 295.4 ✓5ᵗʰ
   panic 300.01

State — continued
   paranoid 297.9
      alcohol-induced 291.5
      arteriosclerotic 290.42
      climacteric 297.2
      drug-induced 292.11
      in
         presenile brain disease 290.12
         senile brain disease 290.20
      involutional 297.2
      menopausal 297.2
      senile 290.20
      simple 297.0
   postleukotomy 310.0
   pregnant (see also Pregnancy) V22.2
   psychogenic, twilight 298.2
   psychotic, organic (see also Psychosis, organic)
      294.9
      mixed paranoid and affective 294.8
      senile or presenile NEC 290.9
      transient NEC 293.9
         with
            anxiety 293.84
            delusions 293.81
            depression 293.83
            hallucinations 293.82
   residual schizophrenic (see also Schizophrenia)
      295.6 ✓5ᵗʰ
   tension (see also Anxiety) 300.9
   transient organic psychotic 293.9
      anxiety type 293.84
      depressive type 293.83
      hallucinatory type 293.83
      paranoid type 293.81
      specified type NEC 293.89
   twilight
      epileptic 293.0
      psychogenic 298.2
   vegetative (persistent) 780.03
Status (post)
   absence
      epileptic (see also Epilepsy) 345.2
      of organ, acquired (postsurgical) — see
         Absence, by site, acquired
   anastomosis of intestine (for bypass) V45.3
   angioplasty, percutaneous transluminal
      coronary V45.82
   anginosus 413.9
   ankle prosthesis V43.66
   aortocoronary bypass or shunt V45.81
   arthrodesis V45.4
   artificially induced condition NEC V45.89
   artificial opening (of) V44.9
      gastrointestinal tract NEC V44.4
      specified site NEC V44.8
      urinary tract NEC V44.6
      vagina V44.7
   aspirator V46.0
   asthmaticus (see also Asthma) 493.9 ✓5ᵗʰ
   breast implant removal V45.83
   cardiac
      device (in situ) V45.00
         carotid sinus V45.09
            fitting or adjustment V53.39
         defibrillator, automatic implantable
            V45.02
         pacemaker V45.01
            fitting or adjustmanet V53.31
   carotid sinus stimulator V45.09
   cataract extraction V45.61
   chemotherapy V66.2
      current V58.69
   colostomy V44.3
   contraceptive device V45.59
      intrauterine V45.51
      subdermal V45.52
   convulsivus idiopathicus (see also Epilepsy)
      345.3
   coronary artery bypass or shunt V45.81
   cystostomy V44.50
      appendico-vesicostomy V44.52
      cutaneous-vesicostomy V44.51
      specified type NEC V44.59
   defibrillator, automatic implant-able cardiac
      V45.02
   dental crowns V45.84
   dental fillings V45.84

Status — continued
   dental restoration V45.84
   dental sealant V49.82
   dialysis V45.1
   donor V59.9
   drug therapy or regimen V67.59
      high-risk medication NEC V67.51
   elbow prosthesis V43.62
   enterostomy V44.4
   epileptic, epilepticus (absence) (grand mal) (see
      also Epilepsy) 345.3
      focal motor 345.7 ✓5ᵗʰ
      partial 345.7 ✓5ᵗʰ
      petit mal 345.2
      psychomotor 345.7 ✓5ᵗʰ
      temporal lobe 345.7 ✓5ᵗʰ
   eye (adnexa) surgery V45.69
   filtering bleb (eye) (postglaucoma) V45.69
      with rupture or complication 997.99
      pastcataract extraction (complication)
         997.99
   finger joint prosthesis V43.69
   gastrostomy V44.1
   grand mal 345.3
   heart valve prosthesis V43.3
   hip prosthesis (joint) (partial) (total) V43.64
   ileostomy V44.2
   intestinal bypass V45.3
   intrauterine contraceptive device V45.51
   jejunostomy V44.4
   knee joint prosthesis V43.65
   lacunaris 437.8
   lacunosis 437.8
   low birth weight V21.30
      less than 500 grams V21.31
      500-999 grams V21.32
      1000-1499 grams V21.33
      1500-1999 grams V21.34
      2000-2500 grams V21.35
   lymphaticus 254.8
   malignant neoplasm, ablated or excised — see
      History, malignant neoplasm
   marmoratus 333.7
   nephrostomy V44.6
   neuropacemaker NEC V45.89
      brain V45.89
      carotid sinus V45.09
      neurologic NEC V45.89
   organ replacement
      by artificial or mechanical device or
         prosthesis of
            artery V43.4
            artificial skin V43.83
            bladder V43.5
            blood vessel V43.4
            breast V43.82
            eye globe V43.0
            heart V43.2
               valve V43.3
            intestine V43.89
            joint V43.60
               ankle V43.66
               elbow V43.62
               finger V43.69
               hip (partial) (total) V43.64
               knee V43.65
               shoulder V43.61
               specified NEC V43.69
               wrist V43.63
            kidney V43.89
            larynx V43.81
            lens V43.1
            limb(s) V43.7
            liver V43.89
            lung V43.89
            organ NEC V43.89
            pancreas V43.89
            skin (artificial) V43.83
            tissue NEC V43.89
            vein V43.4
      by organ transplant (heterologous)
         (homologous) — see Status, transplant
   pacemaker
      brain V45.89
      cardiac V45.01
      carotid sinus V45.09
      neurologic NEC V45.89

Status — *continued*
  pacemaker — *continued*
    specified site NEC V45.89
  percutaneous transluminal coronary
      angioplasty V45.82
  petit mal 345.2
  postcommotio cerebri 310.2
  postmenopausal (age related) (natural) V49.81
  postoperative NEC V45.89
  postpartum NEC V24.2
    care immediately following delivery V24.0
    routine follow-up V24.2
  postsurgical NEC V45.89
  renal dialysis V45.1
  respirator V46.1
  reversed jejunal transposition (for bypass) V45.3
  shoulder prosthesis V43.61
  shunt
    aortocoronary bypass V45.81
    arteriovenous (for dialysis) V45.1
    cerebrospinal fluid V45.2
    vascular NEC V45.89
      aortocoronary (bypass) V45.81
    ventricular (communicating) (for drainage) V45.2
  sterilization
    tubal ligation V26.51
    vasectomy V26.52
  subdermal contraceptive device V45.52
  thymicolymphaticus 254.8
  thymicus 254.8
  thymolymphaticus 254.8
  tooth extraction 525.10
  tracheostomy V44.0
  transplant
    blood vessel V42.89
    bone V42.4
      marrow V42.81
    cornea V42.5
    heart V42.1
      valve V42.2
    intestine V42.84
    kidney V42.0
    liver V42.7
    lung V42.6
    organ V42.9
      specified site NEC V42.89
    pancreas V42.83
    peripheral stem cells V42.82
    skin V42.3
    stem cells, peripheral V42.82
    tissue V42.9
      specified type NEC V42.89
    vessel, blood V42.89
  tubal ligation V26.51
  ureterostomy V44.6
  urethrostomy V44.6
  vagina, artificial V44.7
  vascular shunt NEC V45.89
    aortocoronary (bypass) V45.81
  vasectomy V26.52
  ventilator V46.1
  wrist prosthesis V43.63
Stave fracture — *see* Fracture, metacarpus, metacarpal bone(s)
Steal
  subclavian artery 435.2
  vertebral artery 435.1
Stealing, solitary, child problem (*see also* Disturbance, conduct) 312.1 ✓5ᵗʰ
Steam burn — *see* Burn, by site
Steatocystoma multiplex 706.2
Steatoma (infected) 706.2
  eyelid (cystic) 374.84
    infected 373.13
Steatorrhea (chronic) 579.8
  with lacteal obstruction 579.2
  idiopathic 579.0
    adult 579.0
    infantile 579.0
  pancreatic 579.4
  primary 579.0
  secondary 579.8
  specified cause NEC 579.8
  tropical 579.1

Steatosis 272.8
  heart (*see also* Degeneration, myocardial) 429.1
  kidney 593.89
  liver 571.8
Steele-Richardson (-Olszewski) Syndrome 333.0
Stein's syndrome (polycystic ovary) 256.4
Stein-Leventhal syndrome (polycystic ovary) 256.4
Steinbrocker's syndrome (*see also* Neuropathy, peripheral, autonomic) 337.9
Steinert's disease 359.2
Stenocardia (*see also* Angina) 413.9
Stenocephaly 756.0
Stenosis (cicatricial) — *see also* Stricture
  ampulla of Vater 576.2
    with calculus, cholelithiasis, or stones — *see* Choledocholithiasis
  anus, anal (canal) (sphincter) 569.2
    congenital 751.2
  aorta (ascending) 747.22
    arch 747.10
    arteriosclerotic 440.0
    calcified 440.0
  aortic (valve) 424.1
    with
      mitral (valve)
        insufficiency or incompetence 396.2
        stenosis or obstruction 396.0
    atypical 396.0
    congenital 746.3
    rheumatic 395.0
      with
        insufficiency, incompetency or regurgitation 395.2
          with mitral (valve) disease 396.8
        mitral (valve)
          disease (stenosis) 396.0
          insufficiency or incompetence 396.2
          stenosis or obstruction 396.0
    specified cause, except rheumatic 424.1
    syphilitic 093.22
  aqueduct of Sylvius (congenital) 742.3
    with spina bifida (*see also* Spina bifida) 741.0 ✓5ᵗʰ
    acquired 331.4
  artery NEC 447.1
    basilar — *see* Narrowing, artery, basilar
    carotid (common) (internal) — *see* Narrowing, artery, carotid
    celiac 447.4
    cerebral 437.0
      due to
        embolism (*see also* Embolism, brain) 434.1 ✓5ᵗʰ
        thrombus (*see also* Thrombosis, brain) 434.0 ✓5ᵗʰ
    precerebral — *see* Narrowing, artery, precerebral
    pulmonary (congenital) 747.3
      acquired 417.8
    renal 440.1
    vertebral — *see* Narrowing, artery, vertebral
  bile duct or biliary passage (*see also* Obstruction, biliary) 576.2
    congenital 751.61
  bladder neck (acquired) 596.0
    congenital 753.6
  brain 348.8
  bronchus 519.1
    syphilitic 095.8
  cardia (stomach) 537.89
    congenital 750.7
  cardiovascular (*see also* Disease, cardiovascular) 429.2
  carotid artery — *see* Narrowing, artery, carotid
  cervix, cervical (canal) 622.4
    congenital 752.49
    in pregnancy or childbirth 654.6 ✓5ᵗʰ
      affecting fetus or newborn 763.89
      causing obstructed labor 660.2 ✓5ᵗʰ
        affecting fetus or newborn 763.1
  colon (*see also* Obstruction, intestine) 560.9
    congenital 751.2
  colostomy 569.62
  common bile duct (*see also* Obstruction, biliary) 576.2
    congenital 751.61

Stenosis — *see also* Stricture — *continued*
  coronary (artery) — *see* Arteriosclerosis, coronary
  cystic duct (*see also* Obstruction, gallbladder) 575.2
    congenital 751.61
  due to (presence of) any device, implant, or graft classifiable to 996.0-996.5 — *see* Complications, due to (presence of) any device, implant, or graft classified to 996.0-996.5 NEC
  duodenum 537.3
    congenital 751.1
  ejaculatory duct NEC 608.89
  endocervical os — *see* Stenosis, cervix
  enterostomy 569.62
  esophagus 530.3
    congenital 750.3
    syphilitic 095.8
      congenital 090.5
  external ear canal 380.50
    secondary to
      inflammation 380.53
      surgery 380.52
      trauma 380.51
  gallbladder (*see also* Obstruction, gallbladder) 575.2
  glottis 478.74
  heart valve (acquired) — *see also* Endocarditis
    congenital NEC 746.89
      aortic 746.3
      mitral 746.5
      pulmonary 746.02
      tricuspid 746.1
  hepatic duct (*see also* Obstruction, biliary) 576.2
  hymen 623.3
  hypertrophic subaortic (idiopathic) 425.1
  infundibulum cardiac 746.83
  intestine (*see also* Obstruction, intestine) 560.9
    congenital (small) 751.1
      large 751.2
  lacrimal
    canaliculi 375.53
    duct 375.56
      congenital 743.65
    punctum 375.52
      congenital 743.65
    sac 375.54
      congenital 743.65
  lacrimonasal duct 375.56
    congenital 743.65
    neonatal 375.55
  larynx 478.74
    congenital 748.3
    syphilitic 095.8
      congenital 090.5
  mitral (valve) (chronic) (inactive) 394.0
    with
      aortic (valve)
        disease (insufficiency) 396.1
        insufficiency or incompetence 396.1
        stenosis or obstruction 396.0
      incompetency, insufficiency or regurgitation 394.2
        with aortic valve disease 396.8
      active or acute 391.1
        with chorea (acute) (rheumatic) (Sydenham's) 392.0
      congenital 746.5
      specified cause, except rheumatic 424.0
      syphilitic 093.21
  myocardium, myocardial (*see also* Degeneration, myocardial) 429.1
    hypertrophic subaortic (idiopathic) 425.1
  nares (anterior) (posterior) 478.1
    congenital 748.0
  nasal duct 375.56
    congenital 743.65
  nasolacrimal duct 375.56
    congenital 743.65
    neonatal 375.55
  organ or site, congenital NEC — *see* Atresia
  papilla of Vater 576.2
    with calculus, cholelithiasis, or stones — *see* Choledocholithiasis

Stenosis — *see also* Stricture — *continued*
  pulmonary (artery) (congenital) 747.3
    with ventricular septal defect, dextraposition of aorta and hypertrophy of right ventricle 745.2
    acquired 417.8
    infundibular 746.83
    in tetralogy of Fallot 745.2
    subvalvular 746.83
    valve (*see also* Endocarditis, pulmonary) 424.3
      congenital 746.02
    vein 747.49
      acquired 417.8
    vessel NEC 417.8
  pulmonic (congenital) 746.02
    infundibular 746.83
    subvalvular 746.83
  pylorus (hypertrophic) 537.0
    adult 537.0
    congenital 750.5
    infantile 750.5
  rectum (sphincter) (*see also* Stricture, rectum) 569.2
  renal artery 440.1
  salivary duct (any) 527.8
  sphincter of Oddi (*see also* Obstruction, biliary) 576.2
  spinal 724.00
    cervical 723.0
    lumbar, lumbosacral 724.02
    nerve (root) NEC 724.9
    specified region NEC 724.09
    thoracic, thoracolumbar 724.01
  stomach, hourglass 537.6
  subaortic 746.81
    hypertrophic (idiopathic) 425.1
  supra (valvular)-aortic 747.22
  trachea 519.1
    congenital 748.3
    syphilitic 095.8
    tuberculous (*see also* Tuberculosis) 012.8
  tracheostomy 519.02
  tricuspid (valve) (*see also* Endocarditis, tricuspid) 397.0
    congenital 746.1
    nonrheumatic 424.2
  tubal 628.2
  ureter (*see also* Stricture, ureter) 593.3
    congenital 753.29
  urethra (*see also* Stricture, urethra) 598.9
  vagina 623.2
    congenital 752.49
    in pregnancy or childbirth 654.7
      affecting fetus or newborn 763.89
      causing obstructed labor 660.2
        affecting fetus or newborn 763.1
  valve (cardiac) (heart) (*see also* Endocarditis) 424.90
    congenital NEC 746.89
      aortic 746.3
      mitral 746.5
      pulmonary 746.02
      tricuspid 746.1
      urethra 753.6
  valvular (*see also* Endocarditis) 424.90
    congenital NEC 746.89
      urethra 753.6
  vascular graft or shunt 996.1
    atherosclerosis — *see* Arteriosclerosis, extremities
    embolism 996.74
    occlusion NEC 996.74
    thrombus 996.74
  vena cava (inferior) (superior) 459.2
    congenital 747.49
  ventricular shunt 996.2
  vulva 624.8
Stercolith (*see also* Fecalith) 560.39
  appendix 543.9
Stercoraceous, stercoral ulcer 569.82
  anus or rectum 569.41
Stereopsis, defective
  with fusion 368.33
  without fusion 368.32
Stereotypes NEC 307.3

Sterility
  female — *see* Infertility, female
  male (*see also* Infertility, male) 606.9
Sterilization, admission for V25.2
  status
    tubal ligation V26.51
    vasectomy V26.52
Sternalgia (*see also* Angina) 413.9
Sternopagus 759.4
Sternum bifidum 756.3
Sternutation 784.9
Steroid
  effects (adverse) (iatrogenic)
    cushingoid
      correct substance properly administered 255.0
      overdose or wrong substance given or taken 962.0
    diabetes
      correct substance properly administered 251.8
      overdose or wrong substance given or taken 962.0
    due to
      correct substance properly administered 255.8
      overdose or wrong substance given or taken 962.0
    fever
      correct substance properly administered 780.6
      overdose or wrong substance given or taken 962.0
    withdrawal
      correct substance properly administered 255.4
      overdose or wrong substance given or taken 962.0
  responder 365.03
Stevens-Johnson disease or syndrome (erythema multiforme exudativum) 695.1
Stewart-Morel syndrome (hyperostosis frontalis interna) 733.3
Sticker's disease (erythema infectiosum) 057.0
Sticky eye 372.03
Stieda's disease (calcification, knee joint) 726.62
Stiff
  back 724.8
  neck (*see also* Torticollis) 723.5
Stiff-man syndrome 333.91
Stiffness, joint NEC 719.50
  ankle 719.57
  back 724.8
  elbow 719.52
  finger 719.54
  hip 719.55
  knee 719.56
  multiple sites 719.59
  sacroiliac 724.6
  shoulder 719.51
  specified site NEC 719.58
  spine 724.9
  surgical fusion V45.4
  wrist 719.53
Stigmata, congenital syphilis 090.5
Still's disease or syndrome 714.30
Still-Felty syndrome (rheumatoid arthritis with splenomegaly and leukopenia) 714.1
Stillbirth, stillborn NEC 779.9
Stiller's disease (asthenia) 780.79
Stilling-Türk-Duane syndrome (ocular retraction syndrome) 378.71
Stimulation, ovary 256.1
Sting (animal) (bee) (fish) (insect) (jellyfish) (Portuguese man-o-war) (wasp) (venomous) 989.5
  anaphylactic shock or reaction 989.5
  plant 692.6
Stippled epiphyses 756.59

Stitch
  abscess 998.59
  burst (in ►external◄ operation wound) 998.32
    internal 998.31
  in back 724.5
Stojano's (subcostal) syndrome 098.86
Stokes' disease (exophthalmic goiter) 242.0
Stokes-Adams syndrome (syncope with heart block) 426.9
Stokvis' (-Talma) disease (enterogenous cyanosis) 289.7
Stomach — *see* condition
Stoma malfunction
  colostomy 569.62
  cystostomy 997.5
  enterostomy 569.62
  gastrostomy 536.42
  ileostomy 569.62
  nephrostomy 997.5
  tracheostomy 519.02
  ureterostomy 997.5
Stomatitis 528.0
  angular 528.5
    due to dietary or vitamin deficiency 266.0
  aphthous 528.2
  candidal 112.0
  catarrhal 528.0
  denture 528.9
  diphtheritic (membranous) 032.0
  due to
    dietary deficiency 266.0
    thrush 112.0
    vitamin deficiency 266.0
  epidemic 078.4
  epizootic 078.4
  follicular 528.0
  gangrenous 528.1
  herpetic 054.2
  herpetiformis 528.2
  malignant 528.0
  membranous acute 528.0
  monilial 112.0
  mycotic 112.0
  necrotic 528.1
    ulcerative 101
  necrotizing ulcerative 101
  parasitic 112.0
  septic 528.0
  spirochetal 101
  suppurative (acute) 528.0
  ulcerative 528.0
    necrotizing 101
  ulceromembranous 101
  vesicular 528.0
    with exanthem 074.3
  Vincent's 101
Stomatocytosis 282.8
Stomatomycosis 112.0
Stomatorrhagia 528.9
Stone(s) — *see also* Calculus
  bladder 594.1
    diverticulum 594.0
  cystine 270.0
  heart syndrome (*see also* Failure, ventricular, left) 428.1
  kidney 592.0
  prostate 602.0
  pulp (dental) 522.2
  renal 592.0
  salivary duct or gland (any) 527.5
  ureter 592.1
  urethra (impacted) 594.2
  urinary (duct) (impacted) (passage) 592.9
    bladder 594.1
      diverticulum 594.0
    lower tract NEC 594.9
    specified site 594.8
  xanthine 277.2
Stonecutters' lung 502
  tuberculous (*see also* Tuberculosis) 011.4
Stonemasons'
  asthma, disease, or lung 502
  tuberculous (*see also* Tuberculosis) 011.4

Stonemasons' — *continued*
  phthisis (*see also* Tuberculosis) 011.4
Stoppage
  bowel (*see also* Obstruction, intestine) 560.9
  heart (*see also* Arrest, cardiac) 427.5
  intestine (*see also* Obstruction, intestine) 560.9
  urine NEC (*see also* Retention, urine) 788.20
Storm, thyroid (apathetic) (*see also* Thyrotoxicosis) 242.9
Strabismus (alternating) (congenital) (nonparalytic) 378.9
  concomitant (*see also* Heterotropia) 378.30
    convergent (*see also* Esotropia) 378.00
    divergent (*see also* Exotropia) 378.10
  convergent (*see also* Esotropia) 378.00
  divergent (*see also* Exotropia) 378.10
  due to adhesions, scars — *see* Strabismus, mechanical
  in neuromuscular disorder NEC 378.73
    intermittent 378.20
      vertical 378.31
    latent 378.40
      convergent (esophoria) 378.41
      divergent (exophoria) 378.42
      vertical 378.43
    mechanical 378.60
      due to
        Brown's tendon sheath syndrome 378.61
        specified musculofascial disorder NEC 378.62
    paralytic 378.50
      third or oculomotor nerve (partial) 378.51
        total 378.52
      fourth or trochlear nerve 378.53
      sixth or abducens nerve 378.54
    specified type NEC 378.73
    vertical (hypertropia) 378.31
Strain — *see also* Sprain, by site
  eye NEC 368.13
  heart — *see* Disease, heart
  meaning gonorrhea — *see* Gonorrhea
  physical NEC V62.89
  postural 729.9
  psychological NEC V62.89
Strands
  conjunctiva 372.62
  vitreous humor 379.25
Strangulation, strangulated 994.7
  appendix 543.9
  asphyxiation or suffocation by 994.7
  bladder neck 596.0
  bowel — *see* Strangulation, intestine
  colon — *see* Strangulation, intestine
  cord (umbilical) — *see* Compression, umbilical cord
  due to birth injury 767.8
  food or foreign body (*see also* Asphyxia, food) 933.1
  hemorrhoids 455.8
    external 455.5
    internal 455.2
  hernia — *see also* Hernia, by site, with obstruction
    gangrenous — *see* Hernia, by site, with gangrene
  intestine (large) (small) 560.2
    with hernia — *see also* Hernia, by site, with obstruction
      gangrenous — *see* Hernia, by site, with gangrene
    congenital (small) 751.1
      large 751.2
  mesentery 560.2
  mucus (*see also* Asphyxia, mucus) 933.1
    newborn 770.1
  omentum 560.2
  organ or site, congenital NEC — *see* Atresia
  ovary 620.8
    due to hernia 620.4
  penis 607.89
    foreign body 939.3
  rupture (*see also* Hernia, by site, with obstruction) 552.9
    gangrenous (*see also* Hernia, by site, with gangrene) 551.9

Strangulation, strangulated — *continued*
  stomach, due to hernia (*see also* Hernia, by site, with obstruction) 552.9
    with gangrene (*see also* Hernia, by site, with gangrene) 551.9
  umbilical cord — *see* Compression, umbilical cord
  vesicourethral orifice 596.0
Strangury 788.1
Strawberry
  gallbladder (*see also* Disease, gallbladder) 575.6
  mark 757.32
  tongue (red) (white) 529.3
Straw itch 133.8
Streak, ovarian 752.0
Strephosymbolia 315.01
  secondary to organic lesion 784.69
Streptobacillary fever 026.1
Streptobacillus moniliformis 026.1
Streptococcemia 038.0
Streptococcicosis — *see* Infection, streptococcal
Streptococcus, streptococcal — *see* condition
Streptoderma 686.00
Streptomycosis — *see* Actinomycosis
Streptothricosis — *see* Actinomycosis
Streptothrix — *see* Actinomycosis
Streptotrichosis — *see* Actinomycosis
Stress
  fracture — *see* Fracture, stress
  polycythemia 289.0
  reaction (gross) (*see also* Reaction, stress, acute) 308.9
Stretching, nerve — *see* Injury, nerve, by site
Striae (albicantes) (atrophicae) (cutis distensae) (distensae) 701.3
Striations of nails 703.8
Stricture (*see also* Stenosis) 799.8
  ampulla of Vater 576.2
    with calculus, cholelithiasis, or stones — *see* Choledocholithiasis
  anus (sphincter) 569.2
    congenital 751.2
    infantile 751.2
  aorta (ascending) 747.22
    arch 747.10
    arteriosclerotic 440.0
    calcified 440.0
  aortic (valve) (*see also* Stenosis, aortic) 424.1
    congenital 746.3
  aqueduct of Sylvius (congenital) 742.3
    with spina bifida (*see also* Spina bifida) 741.0
    acquired 331.4
  artery 447.1
    basilar — *see* Narrowing, artery, basilar
    carotid (common) (internal) — *see* Narrowing, artery, carotid
    celiac 447.4
    cerebral 437.0
      congenital 747.81
      due to
        embolism (*see also* Embolism, brain) 434.1
        thrombus (*see also* Thrombosis, brain) 434.0
    congenital (peripheral) 747.60
      cerebral 747.81
      coronary 746.85
      gastrointestinal 747.61
      lower limb 747.64
      renal 747.62
      retinal 743.58
      specified NEC 747.69
      spinal 747.82
      umbilical 747.5
      upper limb 747.63
    coronary — *see* Arteriosclerosis, coronary
      congenital 746.85
    precerebral — *see* Narrowing, artery, precerebral NEC
    pulmonary (congenital) 747.3
      acquired 417.8

Stricture (*see also* Stenosis) — *continued*
  artery — *continued*
    renal 440.1
    vertebral — *see* Narrowing, artery, vertebral
  auditory canal (congenital) (external) 744.02
    acquired (*see also* Stricture, ear canal, acquired) 380.50
  bile duct or passage (any) (postoperative) (*see also* Obstruction, biliary) 576.2
    congenital 751.61
  bladder 596.8
    congenital 753.6
    neck 596.0
      congenital 753.6
  bowel (*see also* Obstruction, intestine) 560.9
  brain 348.8
  bronchus 519.1
    syphilitic 095.8
  cardia (stomach) 537.89
    congenital 750.7
  cardiac — *see* Disease, heart
    orifice (stomach) 537.89
  cardiovascular (*see also* Disease, cardiovascular) 429.2
  carotid artery — *see* Narrowing, artery, carotid
  cecum (*see also* Obstruction, intestine) 560.9
  cervix, cervical (canal) 622.4
    congenital 752.49
    in pregnancy or childbirth 654.6
      affecting fetus or newborn 763.89
      causing obstructed labor 660.2
        affecting fetus or newborn 763.1
  colon (*see also* Obstruction, intestine) 560.9
    congenital 751.2
  colostomy 569.62
  common bile duct (*see also* Obstruction, biliary) 576.2
    congenital 751.61
  coronary (artery) — *see* Arteriosclerosis, coronary
    congenital 746.85
  cystic duct (*see also* Obstruction, gallbladder) 575.2
    congenital 751.61
  cystostomy 997.5
  digestive organs NEC, congenital 751.8
  duodenum 537.3
    congenital 751.1
  ear canal (external) (congenital) 744.02
    acquired 380.50
      secondary to
        inflammation 380.53
        surgery 380.52
        trauma 380.51
  ejaculatory duct 608.85
  enterostomy 569.62
  esophagus (corrosive) (peptic) 530.3
    congenital 750.3
    syphilitic 095.8
      congenital 090.5
  eustachian tube (*see also* Obstruction, Eustachian tube) 381.60
    congenital 744.24
  fallopian tube 628.2
    gonococcal (chronic) 098.37
      acute 098.17
    tuberculous (*see also* Tuberculosis) 016.6
  gallbladder (*see also* Obstruction, gallbladder) 575.2
    congenital 751.69
  glottis 478.74
  heart — *see also* Disease, heart
    congenital NEC 746.89
    valve — *see also* Endocarditis
      congenital NEC 746.89
        aortic 746.3
        mitral 746.5
        pulmonary 746.02
        tricuspid 746.1
  hepatic duct (*see also* Obstruction, biliary) 576.2
  hourglass, of stomach 537.6
  hymen 623.3
  hypopharynx 478.29

Index to Diseases

Stricture (see also Stenosis) — continued
  intestine (see also Obstruction, intestine) 560.9
    congenital (small) 751.1
      large 751.2
    ischemic 557.1
  lacrimal
    canaliculi 375.53
      congenital 743.65
    punctum 375.52
      congenital 743.65
    sac 375.54
      congenital 743.65
  lacrimonasal duct 375.56
    congenital 743.65
    neonatal 375.55
  larynx 478.79
    congenital 748.3
    syphilitic 095.8
      congenital 090.5
  lung 518.89
  meatus
    ear (congenital) 744.02
      acquired (see also Stricture, ear canal, acquired) 380.50
      osseous (congenital) (ear) 744.03
        acquired (see also Stricture, ear canal, acquired) 380.50
    urinarius (see also Stricture, urethra) 598.9
      congenital 753.6
  mitral (valve) (see also Stenosis, mitral) 394.0
    congenital 746.5
    specified cause, except rheumatic 424.0
  myocardium, myocardial (see also Degeneration, myocardial) 429.1
    hypertrophic subaortic (idiopathic) 425.1
  nares (anterior) (posterior) 478.1
    congenital 748.0
  nasal duct 375.56
    congenital 743.65
    neonatal 375.55
  nasolacrimal duct 375.56
    congenital 743.65
    neonatal 375.55
  nasopharynx 478.29
    syphilitic 095.8
  nephrostomy 997.5
  nose 478.1
    congenital 748.0
  nostril (anterior) (posterior) 478.1
    congenital 748.0
  organ or site, congenital NEC — see Atresia
  osseous meatus (congenital) (ear) 744.03
    acquired (see also Stricture, ear canal, acquired) 380.50
  os uteri (see also Stricture, cervix) 622.4
  oviduct — see Stricture, fallopian tube
  pelviureteric junction 593.3
  pharynx (dilation) 478.29
  prostate 602.8
  pulmonary, pulmonic
    artery (congenital) 747.3
      acquired 417.8
      noncongenital 417.8
    infundibulum (congenital) 746.83
    valve (see also Endocarditis, pulmonary) 424.3
      congenital 746.02
    vein (congenital) 747.49
      acquired 417.8
    vessel NEC 417.8
  punctum lacrimale 375.52
    congenital 743.65
  pylorus (hypertrophic) 537.0
    adult 537.0
    congenital 750.5
    infantile 750.5
  rectosigmoid 569.89
  rectum (sphincter) 569.2
    congenital 751.2
    due to
      chemical burn 947.3
      irradiation 569.2
      lymphogranuloma venereum 099.1
    gonococcal 098.7
    inflammatory 099.1
    syphilitic 095.8

Stricture (see also Stenosis) — continued
  rectum — continued
    tuberculous (see also Tuberculosis) 014.8
  renal artery 440.1
  salivary duct or gland (any) 527.8
  sigmoid (flexure) (see also Obstruction, intestine) 560.9
  spermatic cord 608.85
  stoma (following) (of)
    colostomy 569.62
    cystostomy 997.5
    enterostomy 569.62
    gastrostomy 536.42
    ileostomy 569.62
    nephrostomy 997.5
    tracheostomy 519.02
    ureterostomy 997.5
  stomach 537.89
    congenital 750.7
    hourglass 537.6
  subaortic 746.81
    hypertrophic (acquired) (idiopathic) 425.1
  subglottic 478.74
  syphilitic NEC 095.8
  tendon (sheath) 727.81
  trachea 519.1
    congenital 748.3
    syphilitic 095.8
    tuberculous (see also Tuberculosis) 012.8
  tracheostomy 519.02
  tricuspid (valve) (see also Endocarditis, tricuspid) 397.0
    congenital 746.1
    nonrheumatic 424.2
  tunica vaginalis 608.85
  ureter (postoperative) 593.3
    congenital 753.29
    tuberculous (see also Tuberculosis) 016.2
  ureteropelvic junction 593.3
    congenital 753.21
  ureterovesical orifice 593.3
    congenital 753.22
  urethra (anterior) (meatal) (organic) (posterior) (spasmodic) 598.9
    associated with schistosomiasis (see also Schistosomiasis) 120.9 [598.01]
    congenital (valvular) 753.6
    due to
      infection 598.00
        syphilis 095.8 [598.01]
      trauma 598.1
    gonococcal 098.2 [598.01]
    gonorrheal 098.2 [598.01]
    infective 598.00
    late effect of injury 598.1
    postcatheterization 598.2
    postobstetric 598.1
    postoperative 598.2
    specified cause NEC 598.8
    syphilitic 095.8 [598.01]
    traumatic 598.1
    valvular, congenital 753.6
  urinary meatus (see also Stricture, urethra) 598.9
    congenital 753.6
  uterus, uterine 621.5
    os (external) (internal) — see Stricture, cervix
  vagina (outlet) 623.2
    congenital 752.49
  valve (cardiac) (heart) (see also Endocarditis) 424.90
    congenital (cardiac) (heart) NEC 746.89
      aortic 746.3
      mitral 746.5
      pulmonary 746.02
      tricuspid 746.1
      urethra 753.6
  valvular (see also Endocarditis) 424.90
  vascular graft or shunt 996.1
    atherosclerosis — see Arteriosclersis, extremities
    embolism 996.74
    occlusion NEC 996.74
    thrombus 996.74

Stricture (see also Stenosis) — continued
  vas deferens 608.85
    congenital 752.8
  vein 459.2
  vena cava (inferior) (superior) NEC 459.2
    congenital 747.49
  ventricular shunt 996.2
  vesicourethral orifice 596.0
    congenital 753.6
  vulva (acquired) 624.8

Stridor 786.1
  congenital (larynx) 748.3

Stridulous — see condition

Strippling of nails 703.8

Stroke (see also Disease, cerebrovascular, acute) 436
  apoplectic (see also Disease, cerebrovascular, acute) 436
  brain (see also Disease, cerebrovascular, acute) 436
  epileptic — see Epilepsy
  healed or old V12.59
  heart — see Disease, heart
  heat 992.0
  iatrogenic 997.02
  in evolution 435.9
  late effect — see Late effect(s) (of) cerebrovascular disease
  lightning 994.0
  paralytic (see also Disease, cerebrovascular, acute) 436
  postoperative 997.02
  progressive 435.9

Stromatosis, endometrial (M8931/1) 236.0

Strong pulse 785.9

Strongyloides stercoralis infestation 127.2

Strongyloidiasis 127.2

Strongyloidosis 127.2

Strongylus (gibsoni) infestation 127.7

Strophulus (newborn) 779.89 ▲
  pruriginosus 698.2

Struck by lightning 994.0

Struma (see also Goiter) 240.9
  fibrosa 245.3
  Hashimoto (struma lymphomatosa) 245.2
  lymphomatosa 245.2
  nodosa (simplex) 241.9
    endemic 241.9
    multinodular 241.1
    sporadic 241.9
    toxic or with hyperthyroidism 242.3
      multinodular 242.2
      uninodular 242.1
    toxicosa 242.3
      multinodular 242.2
      uninodular 242.1
    uninodular 241.0
  ovarii (M9090/0) 220
    and carcinoid (M9091/1) 236.2
    malignant (M9090/3) 183.0
  Riedel's (ligneous thyroiditis) 245.3
  scrofulous (see also Tuberculosis) 017.2
  tuberculous (see also Tuberculosis) 017.2
    abscess 017.2
    adenitis 017.2
    lymphangitis 017.2
    ulcer 017.2

Strumipriva cachexia (see also Hypothyroidism) 244.9

Strümpell-Marie disease or spine (ankylosing spondylitis) 720.0

Strümpell-Westphal pseudosclerosis (hepatolenticular degeneration) 275.1

Stuart's disease (congenital factor X deficiency) (see also Defect, coagulation) 286.3

Stuart-Prower factor deficiency (congenital factor X deficiency) (see also Defect, coagulation) 286.3

Students' elbow 727.2

Stuffy nose 478.1

Stump — see also Amputation
  cervix, cervical (healed) 622.8

Stupor 780.09
- catatonic (see also Schizophrenia) 295.2
- circular (see also Psychosis, manic-depressive, circular) 296.7
- manic 296.89
- manic-depressive (see also Psychosis, affective) 296.89
- mental (anergic) (delusional) 298.9
- psychogenic 298.8
- reaction to exceptional stress (transient) 308.2
- traumatic NEC — see also Injury, intracranial
  - with spinal (cord)
    - lesion — see Injury, spinal, by site
    - shock — see Injury, spinal, by site

Sturge (-Weber) (-Dimitri) disease or syndrome (encephalocutan-eous angiomatosis) 759.6

Sturge-Kalischer-Weber syndrome (encephalocutaneous angiomatosis) 759.6

Stuttering 307.0

Sty, stye 373.11
- external 373.11
- internal 373.12
- meibomian 373.12

Subacidity, gastric 536.8
- psychogenic 306.4

Subacute — see condition

Subarachnoid — see condition

Subclavian steal syndrome 435.2

Subcortical — see condition

Subcostal syndrome 098.86
- nerve compression 354.8

Subcutaneous, subcuticular — see condition

Subdelirium 293.1

Subdural — see condition

Subendocardium — see condition

Subependymoma (M9383/1) 237.5

Suberosis 495.3

Subglossitis — see Glossitis

Subhemophilia 286.0

Subinvolution (uterus) 621.1
- breast (postlactational) (postpartum) 611.8
- chronic 621.1
- puerperal, postpartum 674.8

Sublingual — see condition

Sublinguitis 527.2

Subluxation — see also Dislocation, by site
- congenital NEC — see also Malposition, congenital
  - hip (unilateral) 754.32
    - with dislocation of other hip 754.35
    - bilateral 754.33
  - joint
    - lower limb 755.69
    - shoulder 755.59
    - upper limb 755.59
  - lower limb (joint) 755.69
  - shoulder (joint) 755.59
  - upper limb (joint) 755.59
- lens 379.32
  - anterior 379.33
  - posterior 379.34
- rotary, cervical region of spine — see Fracture, vertebra, cervical

Submaxillary — see condition

Submersion (fatal) (nonfatal) 994.1

Submissiveness (undue), in child 313.0

Submucous — see condition

Subnormal, subnormality
- accommodation (see also Disorder, accommodation) 367.9
- mental (see also Retardation, mental) 319
  - mild 317
  - moderate 318.0
  - profound 318.2
  - severe 318.1
- temperature (accidental) 991.6
  - not associated with low environmental temperature 780.99 ▲

Subphrenic — see condition

Subscapular nerve — see condition

Subseptus uterus 752.3

Subsiding appendicitis 542

Substernal thyroid (see also Goiter) 240.9
- congenital 759.2

Substitution disorder 300.11

Subtentorial — see condition

Subtertian
- fever 084.0
- malaria (fever) 084.0

Subthyroidism (acquired) (see also Hypothyroidism) 244.9
- congenital 243

Succenturiata placenta — see Placenta, abnormal

Succussion sounds, chest 786.7

Sucking thumb, child 307.9

Sudamen 705.1

Sudamina 705.1

Sudanese kala-azar 085.0

Sudden
- death, cause unknown (less than 24 hours) 798.1
  - during childbirth 669.9
  - infant 798.0
  - puerperal, postpartum 674.9
- hearing loss NEC 388.2
- heart failure (see also Failure, heart) 428.9
- infant death syndrome 798.0

Sudeck's atrophy, disease, or syndrome 733.7

SUDS (Sudden unexplained death) 798.2

Suffocation (see also Asphyxia) 799.0
- by
  - bed clothes 994.7
  - bunny bag 994.7
  - cave-in 994.7
  - constriction 994.7
  - drowning 994.1
  - inhalation
    - food or foreign body (see also Asphyxia, food or foreign body) 933.1
    - oil or gasoline (see also Asphyxia, food or foreign body) 933.1
  - overlying 994.7
  - plastic bag 994.7
  - pressure 994.7
  - strangulation 994.7
- during birth 768.1
- mechanical 994.7

Sugar
- blood
  - high 790.2
  - low 251.2
- in urine 791.5

Suicide, suicidal (attempted)
- by poisoning — see Table of Drugs and Chemicals
- risk 300.9
- tendencies 300.9
- trauma NEC (see also nature and site of injury) 959.9

Suipestifer infection (see also Infection, Salmonella) 003.9

Sulfatidosis 330.0

Sulfhemoglobinemia, sulphemoglobinemia (acquired) (congenital) 289.7

Sumatran mite fever 081.2

Summer — see condition

Sunburn 692.71
- dermatitis 692.71
- due to
  - other ultraviolet radiation 692.82
  - tanning bed 692.82
- first degree 692.71
- second degree 692.76
- third degree 692.77

Sunken
- acetabulum 718.85
- fontanels 756.0

Sunstroke 992.0

Superfecundation 651.9
- with fetal loss and retention of one or more fetus(es) 651.6

Superfetation 651.9
- with fetal loss and retention of one or more fetus(es) 651.6

Superinvolution uterus 621.8

Supernumerary (congenital)
- aortic cusps 746.89
- auditory ossicles 744.04
- bone 756.9
- breast 757.6
- carpal bones 755.56
- cusps, heart valve NEC 746.89
  - mitral 746.5
  - pulmonary 746.09
- digit(s) 755.00
  - finger 755.01
  - toe 755.02
- ear (lobule) 744.1
- fallopian tube 752.19
- finger 755.01
- hymen 752.49
- kidney 753.3
- lacrimal glands 743.64
- lacrimonasal duct 743.65
- lobule (ear) 744.1
- mitral cusps 746.5
- muscle 756.82
- nipples 757.6
- organ or site NEC — see Accessory
- ossicles, auditory 744.04
- ovary 752.0
- oviduct 752.19
- pulmonic cusps 746.09
- rib 756.3
  - cervical or first 756.2
  - syndrome 756.2
- roots (of teeth) 520.2
- spinal vertebra 756.19
- spleen 759.0
- tarsal bones 755.67
- teeth 520.1
  - causing crowding 524.3
- testis 752.8
- thumb 755.01
- toe 755.02
- uterus 752.2
- vagina 752.49
- vertebra 756.19

Supervision (of)
- contraceptive method previously prescribed V25.40
  - intrauterine device V25.42
  - oral contraceptive (pill) V25.41
  - specified type NEC V25.49
  - subdermal implantable contraceptive V25.43
- dietary (for) V65.3
  - allergy (food) V65.3
  - colitis V65.3
  - diabetes mellitus V65.3
  - food allergy intolerance V65.3
  - gastritis V65.3
  - hypercholesterolemia V65.3
  - hypoglycemia V65.3
  - intolerance (food) V65.3
  - obesity V65.3
  - specified NEC V65.3
- lactation V24.1
- pregnancy — see Pregnancy, supervision of

Supplemental teeth 520.1
- causing crowding 524.3

Suppression
- binocular vision 368.31
- lactation 676.5
- menstruation 626.8
- ovarian secretion 256.39
- renal 586
- urinary secretion 788.5
- urine 788.5

Suppuration, suppurative — see also condition
- accessory sinus (chronic) (see also Sinusitis) 473.9
- adrenal gland 255.8
- antrum (chronic) (see also Sinusitis, maxillary) 473.0
- bladder (see also Cystitis) 595.89
- bowel 569.89
- brain 324.0
  - late effect 326
- breast 611.0
  - puerperal, postpartum 675.1
- dental periosteum 526.5

Suppuration, suppurative — see also condition — continued
  diffuse (skin) 686.00
  ear (middle) (see also Otitis media) 382.4
    external (see also Otitis, externa) 380.10
    internal 386.33
  ethmoidal (sinus) (chronic) (see also Sinusitis, ethmoidal) 473.2
  fallopian tube (see also Salpingo-oophoritis) 614.2
  frontal (sinus) (chronic) (see also Sinusitis, frontal) 473.1
  gallbladder (see also Cholecystitis, acute) 575.0
  gum 523.3
  hernial sac — see Hernia, by site
  intestine 569.89
  joint (see also Arthritis, suppurative) 711.0 ✓5ᵗʰ
  labyrinthine 386.33
  lung 513.0
  mammary gland 611.0
    puerperal, postpartum 675.1 ✓5ᵗʰ
  maxilla, maxillary 526.4
    sinus (chronic) (see also Sinusitis, maxillary) 473.0
  muscle 728.0
  nasal sinus (chronic) (see also Sinusitis) 473.9
  pancreas 577.0
  parotid gland 527.2
  pelvis, pelvic
    female (see also Disease, pelvis, inflammatory) 614.4
      acute 614.3
    male (see also Peritonitis) 567.2
  pericranial (see also Osteomyelitis) 730.2 ✓5ᵗʰ
  salivary duct or gland (any) 527.2
  sinus (nasal) (see also Sinusitis) 473.9
  sphenoidal (sinus) (chronic) (see also Sinusitis, sphenoidal) 473.3
  thymus (gland) 254.1
  thyroid (gland) 245.0
  tonsil 474.8
  uterus (see also Endometritis) 615.9
  vagina 616.10
  wound — see also Wound, open, by site, complicated
    dislocation — see Dislocation, by site, compound
    fracture — see Fracture, by site, open
    scratch or other superficial injury — see Injury, superficial, by site

Supraglottitis 464.50
  with obstruction 464.51
Suprapubic drainage 596.8
Suprarenal (gland) — see condition
Suprascapular nerve — see condition
Suprasellar — see condition
Supraspinatus syndrome 726.10
Surfer knots 919.8
  infected 919.9
Surgery
  cosmetic NEC V50.1
    following healed injury or operation V51
    hair transplant V50.0
  elective V50.9
    breast augmentation or reduction V50.1
    circumcision, ritual or routine (in absence of medical indication) V50.2
    cosmetic NEC V50.1
    ear piercing V50.3
    face-lift V50.1
    following healed injury or operation V51
    hair transplant V50.0
  not done because of
    contraindication V64.1
    patient's decision V64.2
    specified reason NEC V64.3
  plastic
    breast augmentation or reduction V50.1
    cosmetic V50.1
    face-lift V50.1
    following healed injury or operation V51
    repair of scarred tissue (following healed injury or operation) V51
    specified type NEC V50.8

Surgery — continued
  previous, in pregnancy or childbirth
    cervix 654.6 ✓5ᵗʰ
      affecting fetus or newborn 763.89
      causing obstructed labor 660.2 ✓5ᵗʰ
        affecting fetus or newborn 763.1
    pelvic soft tissues NEC 654.9 ✓5ᵗʰ
      affecting fetus or newborn 763.89
      causing obstructed labor 660.2 ✓5ᵗʰ
        affecting fetus or newborn 763.1
    perineum or vulva 654.8 ✓5ᵗʰ
    uterus NEC 654.9 ✓5ᵗʰ
      affecting fetus or newborn 763.89
      causing obstructed labor 660.2 ✓5ᵗʰ
        affecting fetus or newborn 763.1
      due to previous cesarean delivery 654.2 ✓5ᵗʰ
    vagina 654.7 ✓5ᵗʰ
Surgical
  abortion — see Abortion, legal
  emphysema 998.81
  kidney (see also Pyelitis) 590.80
  operation NEC 799.9
  procedures, complication or misadventure — see Complications, surgical procedure
  shock 998.0
Suspected condition, ruled out (see also Observation, suspected) V71.9
  specified condition NEC V71.89
Suspended uterus, in pregnancy or childbirth 654.4 ✓5ᵗʰ
  affecting fetus or newborn 763.89
  causing obstructed labor 660.2 ✓5ᵗʰ
    affecting fetus or newborn 763.1
Sutton's disease 709.09
Sutton and Gull's disease (arteriolar nephrosclerosis) (see also Hypertension, kidney) 403.90
Suture
  burst (in ►external◄ operation wound) 998.32 ▲
    internal 998.31 ●
  inadvertently left in operation wound 998.4
  removal V58.3
  Shirodkar, in pregnancy (with or without cervical incompetence) 654.5 ✓5ᵗʰ
Swab inadvertently left in operation wound 998.4
Swallowed, swallowing
  difficulty (see also Dysphagia) 787.2
  foreign body NEC (see also Foreign body) 938
Swamp fever 100.89
Swan neck hand (intrinsic) 736.09
Sweat(s), sweating
  disease or sickness 078.2
  excessive 780.8
  fetid 705.89
  fever 078.2
  gland disease 705.9
    specified type NEC 705.89
  miliary 078.2
  night 780.8
Sweeley-Klionsky disease (angiokeratoma corporis diffusum) 272.7
Sweet's syndrome (acute febrile neutrophilic dermatosis) 695.89
Swelling
  abdominal (not referable to specific organ) 789.3 ✓5ᵗʰ
  adrenal gland, cloudy 255.8
  ankle 719.07
  anus 787.99
  arm 729.81
  breast 611.72
  Calabar 125.2
  cervical gland 785.6
  cheek 784.2
  chest 786.6
  ear 388.8
  epigastric 789.3 ✓5ᵗʰ
  extremity (lower) (upper) 729.81
  eye 379.92
  female genital organ 625.8
  finger 729.81
  foot 729.81

Swelling — continued
  glands 785.6
  gum 784.2
  hand 729.81
  head 784.2
  inflammatory — see Inflammation
  joint (see also Effusion, joint) 719.0 ✓5ᵗʰ
    tuberculous — see Tuberculosis, joint
  kidney, cloudy 593.89
  leg 729.81
  limb 729.81
  liver 573.8
  lung 786.6
  lymph nodes 785.6
  mediastinal 786.6
  mouth 784.2
  muscle (limb) 729.81
  neck 784.2
  nose or sinus 784.2
  palate 784.2
  pelvis 789.3 ✓5ᵗʰ
  penis 607.83
  perineum 625.8
  rectum 787.99
  scrotum 608.86
  skin 782.2
  splenic (see also Splenomegaly) 789.2
  substernal 786.6
  superficial, localized (skin) 782.2
  testicle 608.86
  throat 784.2
  toe 729.81
  tongue 784.2
  tubular (see also Disease, renal) 593.9
  umbilicus 789.3 ✓5ᵗʰ
  uterus 625.8
  vagina 625.8
  vulva 625.8
  wandering, due to Gnathostoma (spinigerum) 128.1
  white — see Tuberculosis, arthritis
Swift's disease 985.0
Swimmers'
  ear (acute) 380.12
  itch 120.3
Swimming in the head 780.4
Swollen — see also Swelling
  glands 785.6
Swyer-James syndrome (unilateral hyperlucent lung) 492.8
Swyer's syndrome (XY pure gonadal dysgenesis) 752.7
Sycosis 704.8
  barbae (not parasitic) 704.8
  contagiosa 110.0
  lupoid 704.8
  mycotic 110.0
  parasitic 110.0
  vulgaris 704.8
Sydenham's chorea — see Chorea, Sydenham's
Sylvatic yellow fever 060.0
Sylvest's disease (epidemic pleurodynia) 074.1
Symblepharon 372.63
  congenital 743.62
Symonds' syndrome 348.2
Sympathetic — see condition
Sympatheticotonia (see also Neuropathy, peripheral, autonomic) 337.9
Sympathicoblastoma (M9500/3)
  specified site — see Neoplasm, by site, malignant
  unspecified site 194.0
Sympathicogonioma (M9500/3) — see Sympathicoblastoma
Sympathoblastoma (M9500/3) — see Sympathicoblastoma
Sympathogonioma (M9500/3) — see Sympathicoblastoma
Symphalangy (see also Syndactylism) 755.10
Symptoms, specified (general) NEC 780.99 ▲
  abdomen NEC 789.9
  bone NEC 733.90
  breast NEC 611.79
  cardiac NEC 785.9

Symptoms, specified

Symptoms, specified NEC — *continued*
- cardiovascular NEC 785.9
- chest NEC 786.9
- development NEC 783.9
- digestive system NEC 787.99
- eye NEC 379.99
- gastrointestinal tract NEC 787.99
- genital organs NEC
  - female 625.9
  - male 608.9
- head and neck NEC 784.9
- heart NEC 785.9
- joint NEC 719.60
  - ankle 719.67
  - elbow 719.62
  - foot 719.67
  - hand 719.64
  - hip 719.65
  - knee 719.66
  - multiple sites 719.69
  - pelvic region 719.65
  - shoulder (region) 719.61
  - specified site NEC 719.68
  - wrist 719.63
- larynx NEC 784.9
- limbs NEC 729.89
- lymphatic system NEC 785.9
- menopausal 627.2
- metabolism NEC 783.9
- mouth NEC 528.9
- muscle NEC 728.9
- musculoskeletal NEC 781.99
  - limbs NEC 729.89
- nervous system NEC 781.99
- neurotic NEC 300.9
- nutrition, metabolism, and development NEC 783.9
- pelvis NEC 789.9
  - female 625.9
- peritoneum NEC 789.9
- respiratory system NEC 786.9
- skin and integument NEC 782.9
- subcutaneous tissue NEC 782.9
- throat NEC 784.9
- tonsil NEC 784.9
- urinary system NEC 788.9
- vascular NEC 785.9

Sympus 759.89
Synarthrosis 719.80
- ankle 719.87
- elbow 719.82
- foot 719.87
- hand 719.84
- hip 719.85
- knee 719.86
- multiple sites 719.89
- pelvic region 719.85
- shoulder (region) 719.81
- specified site NEC 719.88
- wrist 719.83

Syncephalus 759.4
Synchondrosis 756.9
- abnormal (congenital) 756.9
- ischiopubic (van Neck's) 732.1

Synchysis (senile) (vitreous humor) 379.21
- scintillans 379.22

Syncope (near) (pre-) 780.2
- anginosa 413.9
- bradycardia 427.89
- cardiac 780.2
- carotid sinus 337.0
- complicating delivery 669.2 ✓5ᵗʰ
- due to lumbar puncture 349.0
- fatal 798.1
- heart 780.2
- heat 992.1
- laryngeal 786.2
- tussive 786.2
- vasoconstriction 780.2
- vasodepressor 780.2
- vasomotor 780.2
- vasovagal 780.2

Syncytial infarct — *see* Placenta, abnormal
Syndactylism, syndactyly (multiple sites) 755.10
- fingers (without fusion of bone) 755.11
  - with fusion of bone 755.12

Syndactylism, syndactyly — *continued*
- toes (without fusion of bone) 755.13
  - with fusion of bone 755.14

Syndrome — *see also* Disease
- abdominal
  - acute 789.0 ✓5ᵗʰ
  - migraine 346.2 ✓5ᵗʰ
  - muscle deficiency 756.79
- Abercrombie's (amyloid degeneration) 277.3
- abnormal innervation 374.43
- abstinence
  - alcohol 291.81
  - drug 292.0
- Abt-Letterer-Siwe (acute histiocytosis X) (M9722/3) 202.5 ✓5ᵗʰ
- Achard-Thiers (adrenogenital) 255.2
- acid pulmonary aspiration 997.3
  - obstetric (Mendelson's) 668.0 ✓5ᵗʰ
- acquired immune deficiency 042
- acquired immunodeficiency 042
- acrocephalosyndactylism 755.55
- acute abdominal 789.0 ✓5ᵗʰ
- acute chest 282.62 ●
- acute coronary 411.1 ●
- Adair-Dighton (brittle bones and blue sclera, deafness) 756.51
- Adams-Stokes (-Morgagni) (syncope with heart block) 426.9
- addisonian 255.4
- Adie (-Holmes) (pupil) 379.46
- adiposogenital 253.8
- adrenal
  - hemorrhage 036.3
  - meningococcic 036.3
- adrenocortical 255.3
- adrenogenital (acquired) (congenital) 255.2
  - feminizing 255.2
  - iatrogenic 760.79
  - virilism (acquired) (congenital) 255.2
- affective organic NEC 293.89
  - drug-induced 292.84
- afferent loop NEC 537.89
- African macroglobulinemia 273.3
- Ahumada-Del Castillo (nonpuerperal galactorrhea and amenorrhea) 253.1
- air blast concussion — *see* Injury, internal, by site
- Albright (-Martin) (pseudohypoparathyroidism) 275.49
- Albright-McCune-Sternberg (osteitis fibrosa disseminata) 756.59
- alcohol withdrawal 291.81
- Alder's (leukocyte granulation anomaly) 288.2
- Aldrich (-Wiskott) (eczema-thrombocytopenia) 279.12
- Alibert-Bazin (mycosis fungoides) (M9700/3) 202.1 ✓5ᵗʰ
- Alice in Wonderland 293.89
- Allen-Masters 620.6
- Alligator baby (ichthyosis congenita) 757.1
- Alport's (hereditary hematuria-nephropathy-deafness) 759.89
- Alvarez (transient cerebral ischemia) 435.9
- alveolar capillary block 516.3
- Alzheimer's 331.0
  - with dementia — *see* Alzheimer's, dementia
- amnestic (confabulatory) 294.0
  - alcoholic 291.1
  - drug-induced 292.83
  - posttraumatic 294.0
- amotivational 292.89
- amyostatic 275.1
- amyotrophic lateral sclerosis 335.20
- angina (*see also* Angina) 413.9
- ankyloglossia superior 750.0
- anterior
  - chest wall 786.52
  - compartment (tibial) 958.8
  - spinal artery 433.8 ✓5ᵗʰ
    - compression 721.1
  - tibial (compartment) 958.8
- antibody deficiency 279.00
  - agammaglobulinemic 279.00
  - congenital 279.04
  - hypogammaglobulinemic 279.00
- anticardiolipin antibody 795.79
- antimongolism 758.3

Syndrome — *see also* Disease — *continued*
- antiphospholipid antibody 795.79
- Anton (-Babinski) (hemiasomatognosia) 307.9
- anxiety (*see also* Anxiety) 300.00
  - organic 293.84
- aortic
  - arch 446.7
  - bifurcation (occlusion) 444.0
  - ring 747.21
- Apert's (acrocephalosyndactyly) 755.55
- Apert-Gallais (adrenogenital) 255.2
- aphasia-apraxia-alexia 784.69
- "approximate answers" 300.16
- arcuate ligament (-celiac axis) 447.4
- arcus aortae 446.7
- arc-welders' 370.24
- argentaffin, argintaffinoma 259.2
- Argonz-Del Castillo (nonpuerperal galactorrhea and amenorrhea) 253.1
- Argyll Robertson's (syphilitic) 094.89
  - nonsyphilitic 379.45
- arm-shoulder (*see also* Neuropathy, peripheral, autonomic) 337.9
- Arnold-Chiari (*see also* Spina bifida) 741.0 ✓5ᵗʰ
  - type I 348.4
  - type II 741.0 ✓5ᵗʰ
  - type III 742.0
  - type IV 742.2
- Arrillaga-Ayerza (pulmonary artery sclerosis with pulmonary hypertension) 416.0
- arteriomesenteric duodenum occlusion 537.89
- arteriovenous steal 996.73
- arteritis, young female (obliterative brachiocephalic) 446.7
- aseptic meningitis — *see* Meningitis, aseptic
- Asherman's 621.5
- asphyctic (*see also* Anxiety) 300.00
- aspiration, of newborn, massive or meconium 770.1
- ataxia-telangiectasia 334.8
- Audry's (acropachyderma) 757.39
- auriculotemporal 350.8
- autosomal — *see also* Abnormal, autosomes NEC
  - deletion 758.3
- Avellis' 344.89
- Axenfeld's 743.44
- Ayerza (-Arrillaga) (pulmonary artery sclerosis with pulmonary hypertension) 416.0
- Baader's (erythema multiforme exudativum) 695.1
- Baastrup's 721.5
- Babinski (-Vaquez) (cardiovascular syphilis) 093.89
- Babinski-Fröhlich (adiposogenital dystrophy) 253.8
- Babinski-Nageotte 344.89
- Bagratuni's (temporal arteritis) 446.5
- Bakwin-Krida (craniometaphyseal dysplasia) 756.89
- Balint's (psychic paralysis of visual disorientation) 368.16
- Ballantyne (-Runge) (postmaturity) 766.2
- ballooning posterior leaflet 424.0
- Banti's — *see* Cirrhosis, liver
- Bard-Pic's (carcinoma, head of pancreas) 157.0
- Bardet-Biedl (obesity, polydactyly, and mental retardation) 759.89
- Barlow's (mitral valve prolapse) 424.0
- Barlow (-Möller) (infantile scurvy) 267
- Baron Munchausen's 301.51
- Barré-Guillain 357.0
- Barré-Liéou (posterior cervical sympathetic) 723.2
- Barrett's (chronic peptic ulcer of esophagus) 530.2
- Bársony-Polgár (corkscrew esophagus) 530.5
- Bársony-Teschendorf (corkscrew esophagus) 530.5
- Bartter's (secondary hyperaldosteronism with juxtaglomerular hyperplasia) 255.1
- Basedow's (exophthalmic goiter) 242.0 ✓5ᵗʰ
- basilar artery 435.0
- basofrontal 377.04
- Bassen-Kornzweig (abetalipoproteinemia) 272.5
- Batten-Steinert 359.2
- battered
  - adult 995.81

Index to Diseases

Syndrome — see also Disease — continued
  battered — continued
    baby or child 995.54
      spouse 995.81
  Baumgarten-Cruveilhier (cirrhosis of liver) 571.5
  Bearn-Kunkel (-Slater) (lupoid hepatitis) 571.49
  Beau's (see also Degeneration, myocardial) 429.1
  Bechterew-Strümpell-Marie (ankylosing spondylitis) 720.0
  Beck's (anterior spinal artery occlusion) 433.8 ✓5
  Beckwith (-Wiedemann) 759.89
  Behçet's 136.1
  Bekhterev-Strümpell-Marie (ankylosing spondylitis) 720.0
  Benedikt's 344.89
  Béquez César (-Steinbrinck-Chédiak- Higashi) (congenital gigantism of peroxidase granules) 288.2
  Bernard-Horner (see also Neuropathy, peripheral, autonomic) 337.9
  Bernard-Sergent (acute adrenocortical insufficiency) 255.4
  Bernhardt-Roth 355.1
  Bernheim's (see also Failure, heart) 428.0
  Bertolotti's (sacralization of fifth lumbar vertebra) 756.15
  Besnier-Boeck-Schaumann (sarcoidosis) 135
  Bianchi's (aphasia-apraxia-alexia syndrome) 784.69
  Biedl-Bardet (obesity, polydactyly, and mental retardation) 759.89
  Biemond's (obesity, polydactyly, and mental retardation) 759.89
  big spleen 289.4
  bilateral polycystic ovarian 256.4
  Bing-Horton's 346.2 ✓5
  Biörck (-Thorson) (malignant carcinoid) 259.2
  Blackfan-Diamond (congenital hypoplastic anemia) 284.0
  black lung 500
  black widow spider bite 989.5
  bladder neck (see also Incontinence, urine) 788.30
  blast (concussion) — see Blast, injury
  blind loop (postoperative) 579.2
  Bloch-Siemens (incontinentia pigmenti) 757.33
  Bloch-Sulzberger (incontinentia pigmenti) 757.33
  Bloom (-Machacek) (-Torre) 757.39
  Blount-Barber (tibia vara) 732.4
  blue
    bloater 491.2 ✓5
    diaper 270.0
    drum 381.02
    sclera 756.51
    toe — see Atherosclerosis
  Boder-Sedgwick (ataxia-telangiectasia) 334.8
  Boerhaave's (spontaneous esophageal rupture) 530.4
  Bonnevie-Ullrich 758.6
  Bonnier's 386.19
  Bouillaud's (rheumatic heart disease) 391.9
  Bourneville (-Pringle) (tuberous sclerosis) 759.5
  Bouveret (-Hoffmann) (paroxysmal tachycardia) 427.2
  brachial plexus 353.0
  Brachman-de Lange (Amsterdam dwarf, mental retardation, and brachycephaly) 759.89
  bradycardia-tachycardia 427.81
  Brailsford-Morquio (dystrophy) (mucopolysaccharidosis IV) 277.5
  brain (acute) (chronic) (nonpsychotic) (organic) (with behavioral reaction) (with neurotic reaction) 310.9
    with
      presenile brain disease (see also Dementia, presenile) 290.10
      psychosis, psychotic reaction (see also Psychosis, organic) 294.9
    chronic alcoholic 291.2
    congenital (see also Retardation, mental) 319
    postcontusional 310.2
    posttraumatic
      nonpsychotic 310.2

Syndrome — see also Disease — continued
  brain — continued
    posttraumatic — continued
      psychotic 293.9
        acute 293.0
        chronic (see also Psychosis, organic) 294.8
        subacute 293.1
    psycho-organic (see also Syndrome, psycho-organic) 310.9
    psychotic (see also Psychosis, organic) 294.9
    senile (see also Dementia, senile) 290.0
  branchial arch 744.41
  Brandt's (acrodermatitis enteropathica) 686.8
  Brennemann's 289.2
  Briquet's 300.81
  Brissaud-Meige (infantile myxedema) 244.9
  broad ligament laceration 620.6
  Brock's (atelectasis due to enlarged lymph nodes) 518.0
  Brown's tendon sheath 378.61
  Brown-Séquard 344.89
  brown spot 756.59
  Brugada 746.89
  Brugsch's (acropachyderma) 757.39
  bubbly lung 770.7
  Buchem's (hyperostosis corticalis) 733.3
  Budd-Chiari (hepatic vein thrombosis) 453.0
  Büdinger-Ludloff-Läwen 717.89
  bulbar 335.22
    lateral (see also Disease, cerebrovascular, acute) 436
  Bullis fever 082.8
  bundle of Kent (anomalous atrioventricular excitation) 426.7
  Bürger-Grütz (essential familial hyperlipemia) 272.3
  Burke's (pancreatic insufficiency and chronic neutropenia) 577.8
  Burnett's (milk-alkali) 999.9
  Burnier's (hypophyseal dwarfism) 253.3
  burning feet 266.2
  Bywaters' 958.5
  Caffey's (infantile cortical hyperostosis) 756.59
  Calvé-Legg-Perthes (osteochondrosis, femoral capital) 732.1
  Caplan (-Colinet) syndrome 714.81
  capsular thrombosis (see also Thrombosis, brain) 434.0 ✓5
  carcinogenic thrombophlebitis 453.1
  carcinoid 259.2
  cardiac asthma (see also Failure, ventricular, left) 428.1
  cardiacos negros 416.0
  cardiopulmonary obesity 278.8
  cardiorenal (see also Hypertension, cardiorenal) 404.90
  cardiorespiratory distress (idiopathic), newborn 769
  cardiovascular renal (see also Hypertension, cardiorenal) 404.90
  cardiovasorenal 272.7
  Carini's (ichthyosis congenita) 757.1
  carotid
    artery (internal) 435.8
    body or sinus 337.0
  carpal tunnel 354.0
  Carpenter's 759.89
  Cassidy (-Scholte) (malignant carcinoid) 259.2
  cat-cry 758.3
  cauda equina 344.60
  causalgia 355.9
    lower limb 355.71
    upper limb 354.4
  cavernous sinus 437.6
  celiac 579.1
    artery compression 447.4
    axis 447.4
  cerebellomedullary malformation (see also Spina bifida) 741.0 ✓5
  cerebral gigantism 253.0
  cerebrohepatorenal 759.89
  cervical (root) (spine) NEC 723.8
    disc 722.71
    posterior, sympathetic 723.2
    rib 353.0
    sympathetic paralysis 337.0
    traumatic (acute) NEC 847.0

Syndrome — see also Disease — continued
  cervicobrachial (diffuse) 723.3
  cervicocranial 723.2
  cervicodorsal outlet 353.2
  Céstan's 344.89
  Céstan (-Raymond) 433.8 ✓5
  Céstan-Chenais 344.89
  chancriform 114.1
  Charcôt's (intermittent claudication) 443.9
    angina cruris 443.9
    due to atherosclerosis 440.21
  Charcôt-Marie-Tooth 356.1
  Charcôt-Weiss-Baker 337.0
  Cheadle (-Möller) (-Barlow) (infantile scurvy) 267
  Chédiak-Higashi (-Steinbrinck) (congenital gigantism of peroxidase granules) 288.2
  chest wall 786.52
  Chiari's (hepatic vein thrombosis) 453.0
  Chiari-Frommel 676.6 ✓5
  chiasmatic 368.41
  Chilaiditi's (subphrenic displacement, colon) 751.4
  chondroectodermal dysplasia 756.55
  chorea-athetosis-agitans 275.1
  Christian's (chronic histiocytosis X) 277.8
  chromosome 4 short arm deletion 758.3
  Churg-Strauss 446.4
  Clarke-Hadfield (pancreatic infantilism) 577.8
  Claude's 352.6
  Claude Bernard-Horner (see also Neuropathy, peripheral, autonomic) 337.9
  Clérambault's
    automatism 348.8
    erotomania 297.8
  Clifford's (postmaturity) 766.2
  climacteric 627.2
  Clouston's (hidrotic ectodermal dysplasia) 757.31
  clumsiness 315.4
  Cockayne's (microencephaly and dwarfism) 759.89
  Cockayne-Weber (epidermolysis bullosa) 757.39
  Cogan's (nonsyphilitic interstitial keratitis) 370.52
  cold injury (newborn) 778.2
  Collet (-Sicard) 352.6
  combined immunity deficiency 279.2
  compartment(al) (anterior) (deep) (posterior) (tibial) 958.8
    nontraumatic 729.9
  compression 958.5
    cauda equina 344.60
      with neurogenic bladder 344.61
  concussion 310.2
  congenital
    affecting more than one system 759.7
      specified type NEC 759.89
    facial diplegia 352.6
    muscular hypertrophy-cerebral 759.89
  congestion-fibrosis (pelvic) 625.5
  conjunctivourethrosynovial 099.3
  Conn (-Louis) (primary aldosteronism) 255.1
  Conradi (-Hünermann) (chondrodysplasia calcificans congenita) 756.59
  conus medullaris 336.8
  Cooke-Apert-Gallais (adrenogenital) 255.2
  Cornelia de Lange's (Amsterdam dwarf, mental retardation, and brachycephaly) 759.8 ✓5
  coronary insufficiency or intermediate 411.1
  cor pulmonale 416.9
  corticosexual 255.2
  Costen's (complex) 524.60
  costochondral junction 733.6
  costoclavicular 353.0
  costovertebral 253.0
  Cotard's (paranoia) 297.1
  craniovertebral 723.2
  Creutzfeldt-Jakob 046.1
    with dementia
      with behavioral disturbance 046.1 [294.11]
      without behavioral disturbance 046.1 [294.10]
  crib death 798.0
  cricopharyngeal 787.2
  cri-du-chat 758.3

Syndrome — see also Disease — continued
- Crigler-Najjar (congenital hyperbilirubinemia) 277.4
- crocodile tears 351.8
- Cronkhite-Canada 211.3
- croup 464.4
- CRST (cutaneous systemic sclerosis) 710.1
- crush 958.5
- crushed lung (see also Injury, internal, lung) 861.20
- Cruveilhier-Baumgarten (cirrhosis of liver) 571.5
- cubital tunnel 354.2
- Cuiffini-Pancoast (M8010/3) (carcinoma, pulmonary apex) 162.3
- Curschmann (-Batten) (-Steinert) 359.2
- Cushing's (iatrogenic) (idiopathic) (pituitary basophilism) (pituitary-dependent) 255.0
  - overdose or wrong substance given or taken 962.0
- Cyriax's (slipping rib) 733.99
- cystic duct stump 576.0
- Da Costa's (neurocirculatory asthenia) 306.2
- Dameshek's (erythroblastic anemia) 282.4
- Dana-Putnam (subacute combined sclerosis with pernicious anemia) 281.0 [336.2]
- Danbolt (-Closs) (acrodermatitis enteropathica) 686.8
- Dandy-Walker (atresia, foramen of Magendie) 742.3
  - with spina bifida (see also Spina bifida) 741.0 ✓5ᵗʰ
- Danlos' 756.83
- Davies-Colley (slipping rib) 733.99
- dead fetus 641.3 ✓5ᵗʰ
- defeminization 255.2
- defibrination (see also Fibrinolysis) 286.6
- Degos' 447.8
- Deiters' nucleus 386.19
- Déjérine-Roussy 348.8
- Déjérine-Thomas 333.0
- de Lange's (Amsterdam dwarf, mental retardation, and brachycephaly) (Cornelia) 759.89
- Del Castillo's (germinal aplasia) 606.0
- deletion chromosomes 758.3
- delusional
  - induced by drug 292.11
- dementia-aphonia, of childhood (see also Psychosis, childhood) 299.1 ✓5ᵗʰ
- demyelinating NEC 341.9
- denial visual hallucination 307.9
- depersonalization 300.6
- Dercum's (adiposis dolorosa) 272.8
- de Toni-Fanconi (-Debré) (cystinosis) 270.0
- diabetes-dwarfism-obesity (juvenile) 258.1
- diabetes mellitus-hypertension-nephrosis 250.4 ✓5ᵗʰ [581.81]
- diabetes mellitus in newborn infant 775.1
- diabetes-nephrosis 250.4 ✓5ᵗʰ [581.81]
- diabetic amyotrophy 250.6 ✓5ᵗʰ [358.1]
- Diamond-Blackfan (congenital hypoplastic anemia) 284.0
- Diamond-Gardener (autoerythrocyte sensitization) 287.2
- DIC (diffuse or disseminated intravascular coagulopathy) (see also Fibrinolysis) 286.6
- diencephalohypophyseal NEC 253.8
- diffuse cervicobrachial 723.3
- diffuse obstructive pulmonary 496
- DiGeorge's (thymic hypoplasia) 279.11
- Dighton's 756.51
- Di Guglielmo's (erythremic myelosis) (M9841/3) 207.0 ✓5ᵗʰ
- disc — see Displacement, intervertebral disc
- discogenic — see Displacement, intervertebral disc
- disequilibrium 276.9
- disseminated platelet thrombosis 446.6
- Ditthomska 307.81
- Doan-Wiseman (primary splenic neutropenia) 288.0
- Döhle body-panmyelopathic 288.2
- Donohue's (leprechaunism) 259.8
- dorsolateral medullary (see also Disease, cerebrovascular, acute) 436
- double whammy 360.81

Syndrome — see also Disease — continued
- Down's (mongolism) 758.0
- Dresbach's (elliptocytosis) 282.1
- Dressler's (postmyocardial infarction) 411.0
  - hemoglobinuria 283.2
- drug withdrawal, infant, of dependent mother 779.5
- dry skin 701.1
  - eye 375.15
- DSAP (disseminated superficial actinic porokeratosis) 692.75
- Duane's (retraction) 378.71
- Duane-Stilling-Türk (ocular retraction syndrome) 378.71
- Dubin-Johnson (constitutional hyperbilirubinemia) 277.4
- Dubin-Sprinz (constitutional hyperbilirubinemia) 277.4
- Duchenne's 335.22
- due to abnormality
  - autosomal NEC (see also Abnormal, autosomes NEC) 758.5
    - 13 758.1
    - 18 758.2
    - 21 or 22 758.0
    - D 758.1
    - E 758.2
    - G 758.0
  - chromosomal 758.89
  - sex 758.81
- dumping 564.2
  - nonsurgical 536.8
- Duplay's 726.2
- Dupré's (meningism) 781.6
- Dyke-Young (acquired macrocytic hemolytic anemia) 283.9
- dyspraxia 315.4
- dystocia, dystrophia 654.9 ✓5ᵗʰ
- Eagle-Barret 756.71
- Eales' 362.18
- Eaton-Lambert (see also Neoplasm, by site, malignant) 199.1 [358.1]
- Ebstein's (downward displacement, tricuspid valve into right ventricle) 746.2
- ectopic ACTH secretion 255.0
- eczema-thrombocytopenia 279.12
- Eddowes' (brittle bones and blue sclera) 756.51
- Edwards' 758.2
- efferent loop 537.89
- effort (aviators') (psychogenic) 306.2
- Ehlers-Danlos 756.83
- Eisenmenger's (ventricular septal defect) 745.4
- Ekbom's (restless legs) 333.99
- Ekman's (brittle bones and blue sclera) 756.51
- electric feet 266.2
- Elephant man 237.71
- Ellison-Zollinger (gastric hypersecretion with pancreatic islet cell tumor) 251.5
- Ellis-van Creveld (chondroectodermal dysplasia) 756.55
- embryonic fixation 270.2
- empty sella (turcica) 253.8
- endocrine-hypertensive 255.3
- Engel-von Recklinghausen (osteitis fibrosa cystica) 252.0
- enteroarticular 099.3
- entrapment — see Neuropathy, entrapment
- eosinophilia myalgia 710.5
- epidemic vomiting 078.82
- Epstein's — see Nephrosis
- Erb (-Oppenheim) — Goldflam 358.0
- Erdheim's (acromegalic macrospondylitis) 253.0
- Erlacher-Blount (tibia vara) 732.4
- erythrocyte fragmentation 283.19
- euthyroid sick 790.94
- Evans' (thrombocytopenic purpura) 287.3
- excess cortisol, iatrogenic 255.0
- exhaustion 300.5
- extrapyramidal 333.90
- eyelid-malar-mandible 756.0
- eye retraction 378.71
- Faber's (achlorhydric anemia) 280.9
- Fabry (-Anderson) (angiokeratoma corporis diffusum) 272.7
- facet 724.8
- Fallot's 745.2
- falx (see also Hemorrhage, brain) 431
- familial eczema-thrombocytopenia 279.12

Syndrome — see also Disease — continued
- Fanconi's (anemia) (congenital pancytopenia) 284.0
- Fanconi (-de Toni) (-Debré) (cystinosis) 270.0
- Farber (-Uzman) (disseminated lipogranulomatosis) 272.8
- fatigue NEC 300.5
  - chronic 780.71
- faulty bowel habit (idiopathic megacolon) 564.7
- FDH (focal dermal hypoplasia) 757.39
- fecal reservoir 560.39
- Feil-Klippel (brevicollis) 756.16
- Felty's (rheumatoid arthritis with splenomegaly and leukopenia) 714.1
- fertile eunuch 257.2
- fetal alcohol 760.71
  - late effect 760.71
- fibrillation-flutter 427.32
- fibrositis (periarticular) 729.0
- Fiedler's (acute isolated myocarditis) 422.91
- Fiessinger-Leroy (-Reiter) 099.3
- Fiessinger-Rendu (erythema multiforme exudativum) 695.1
- first arch 756.0
- Fisher's 357.0
- Fitz's (acute hemorrhagic pancreatitis) 577.0
- Fitz-Hugh and Curtis (gonococcal peritonitis) 098.86
- Flajani (-Basedow) (exophthalmic goiter) 242.0 ✓5ᵗʰ
- floppy
  - infant 781.99
  - valve (mitral) 424.0
- flush 259.2
- Foix-Alajouanine 336.1
- Fong's (hereditary osteo-onychodysplasia) 756.89
- foramen magnum 348.4
- Forbes-Albright (nonpuerperal amenorrhea and lactation associated with pituitary tumor) 253.1
- Foster-Kennedy 377.04
- Foville's (peduncular) 344.89
- fragile X 759.83
- Franceschetti's (mandibulofacial dysostosis) 756.0
- Fraser's 759.89
- Freeman-Sheldon 759.89
- Frey's (auriculotemporal) 350.8
- Friderichsen-Waterhouse 036.3
- Friedrich-Erb-Arnold (acropachyderma) 757.39
- Fröhlich's (adiposogenital dystrophy) 253.8
- Froin's 336.8
- Frommel-Chiari 676.6 ✓5ᵗʰ
- frontal lobe 310.0
- Fuller Albright's (osteitis fibrosa disseminata) 756.59
- functional
  - bowel 564.9
  - prepubertal castrate 752.8
- Gaisböck's (polycythemia hypertonica) 289.0
- ganglion (basal, brain) 333.90
  - geniculi 351.1
- Ganser's, hysterical 300.16
- Gardner-Diamond (autoerythrocyte sensitization) 287.2
- gastroesophageal junction 530.0
- gastroesophageal laceration-hemorrhage 530.7
- gastrojejunal loop obstruction 537.89
- Gayet-Wernicke's (superior hemorrhagic polioencephalitis) 265.1
- Gee-Herter-Heubner (nontropical sprue) 579.0
- Gélineau's 347
- genito-anorectal 099.1
- Gerhardt's (vocal cord paralysis) 478.30
- Gerstmann's (finger agnosia) 784.69
- Gilbert's 277.4
- Gilford (-Hutchinson) (progeria) 259.8
- Gilles de la Tourette's 307.23
- Gillespie's (dysplasia oculodentodigitalis) 759.89
- Glénard's (enteroptosis) 569.89
- Glinski-Simmonds (pituitary cachexia) 253.2
- glucuronyl transferase 277.4
- glue ear 381.20
- Goldberg (-Maxwell) (-Morris) (testicular feminization) 257.8

Index to Diseases

Syndrome — see also Disease — continued
- Goldenhar's (oculoauriculovertebral dysplasia) 756.0
- Goldflam-Erb 358.0
- Goltz-Gorlin (dermal hypoplasia) 757.39
- Goodpasture's (pneumorenal) 446.21
- Gopalan's (burning feet) 266.2
- Gorlin-Chaudhry-Moss 759.89
- Gougerot (-Houwer) — Sjögren (keratoconjunctivitis sicca) 710.2
- Gougerot-Blum (pigmented purpuric lichenoid dermatitis) 709.1
- Gougerot-Carteaud (confluent reticulate papillomatosis) 701.8
- Gouley's (constrictive pericarditis) 423.2
- Gowers' (vasovagal attack) 780.2
- Gowers-Paton-Kennedy 377.04
- Gradenigo's 383.02
- gray or grey (chloramphenicol) (newborn) 779.4
- Greig's (hypertelorism) 756.0
- Gubler-Millard 344.89
- Guérin-Stern (arthrogryposis multiplex congenita) 754.89
- Guillain-Barré (-Strohl) 357.0
- Gunn's (jaw-winking syndrome) 742.8
- Günther's (congenital erythropoietic porphyria) 277.1
- gustatory sweating 350.8
- H_3O 759.81
- Hadfield-Clarke (pancreatic infantilism) 577.8
- Haglund-Läwen-Fründ 717.89
- hairless women 257.8
- Hallermann-Streiff 756.0
- Hallervorden-Spatz 333.0
- Hamman's (spontaneous mediastinal emphysema) 518.1
- Hamman-Rich (diffuse interstitial pulmonary fibrosis) 516.3
- Hand-Schüller-Christian (chronic histiocytosis X) 277.8
- hand-foot 282.61
- Hanot-Chauffard (-Troisier) (bronze diabetes) 275.0
- Harada's 363.22
- Hare's (M8010/3) (carcinoma, pulmonary apex) 162.3
- Harkavy's 446.0
- harlequin color change 779.89 ▲
- Harris' (organic hyperinsulinism) 251.1
- Hart's (pellagra-cerebellar ataxia-renal aminoaciduria) 270.0
- Hayem-Faber (achlorhydric anemia) 280.9
- Hayem-Widal (acquired hemolytic jaundice) 283.9
- Heberden's (angina pectoris) 413.9
- Hedinger's (malignant carcinoid) 259.2
- Hegglin's 288.2
- Heller's (infantile psychosis) (see also Psychosis, childhood) 299.1 ✓5ᵗʰ
- H.E.L.L.P 642.5 ✓5ᵗʰ
- hemolytic-uremic (adult) (child) 283.11
- Hench-Rosenberg (palindromic arthritis) (see also Rheumatism, palindromic) 719.3 ✓5ᵗʰ
- Henoch-Schönlein (allergic purpura) 287.0
- hepatic flexure 569.89
- hepatorenal 572.4
  - due to a procedure 997.4
  - following delivery 674.8 ✓5ᵗʰ
- hepatourologic 572.4
- Herrick's (hemoglobin S disease) 282.61
- Herter (-Gee) (nontropical sprue) 579.0
- Heubner-Herter (nontropical sprue) 579.0
- Heyd's (hepatorenal) 572.4
- HHHO 759.81
- Hilger's 337.0
- Hoffa (-Kastert) (liposynovitis prepatellaris) 272.8
- Hoffmann's 244.9 [359.5]
- Hoffmann-Bouveret (paroxysmal tachycardia) 427.2
- Hoffmann-Werdnig 335.0
- Holländer-Simons (progressive lipodystrophy) 272.6
- Holmes' (visual disorientation) 368.16
- Holmes-Adie 379.46
- Hoppe-Goldflam 358.0

Syndrome — see also Disease — continued
- Horner's (see also Neuropathy, peripheral, autonomic) 337.9
  - traumatic — see Injury, nerve, cervical sympathetic
- hospital addiction 301.51
- Hunt's (herpetic geniculate ganglionitis) 053.11
  - dyssynergia cerebellaris myoclonica 334.2
- Hunter (-Hurler) (mucopolysaccharidosis II) 277.5
- hunterian glossitis 529.4
- Hurler (-Hunter) (mucopolysaccharidosis II) 277.5
- Hutchinson's incisors or teeth 090.5
- Hutchinson-Boeck (sarcoidosis) 135
- Hutchinson-Gilford (progeria) 259.8
- hydralazine
  - correct substance properly administered 695.4
  - overdose or wrong substance given or taken 972.6
- hydraulic concussion (abdomen) (see also Injury, internal, abdomen) 868.00
- hyperabduction 447.8
- hyperactive bowel 564.9
- hyperaldosteronism with hypokalemic alkalosis (Bartter's) 255.1
- hypercalcemic 275.42
- hypercoagulation NEC 289.8
- hypereosinophilic (idiopathic) 288.3
- hyperkalemic 276.7
- hyperkinetic — see also Hyperkinesia
  - heart 429.82
- hyperlipemia-hemolytic anemia-icterus 571.1
- hypermobility 728.5
- hypernatremia 276.0
- hyperosmolarity 276.0
- hypersomnia-bulimia 349.89
- hypersplenic 289.4
- hypersympathetic (see also Neuropathy, peripheral, autonomic) 337.9
- hypertransfusion, newborn 776.4
- hyperventilation, psychogenic 306.1
- hyperviscosity (of serum) NEC 273.3
  - polycythemic 289.0
  - sclerothymic 282.8
- hypoglycemic (familial) (neonatal) 251.2
  - functional 251.1
- hypokalemic 276.8
- hypophyseal 253.8
- hypophyseothalamic 253.8
- hypopituitarism 253.2
- hypoplastic left heart 746.7
- hypopotassemia 276.8
- hyposmolality 276.1
- hypotension, maternal 669.2 ✓5ᵗʰ
- hypotonia-hypomentia-hypogonadism-obesity 759.81
- ICF (intravascular coagulation-fibrinolysis) (see also Fibrinolysis) 286.6
- idiopathic cardiorespiratory distress, newborn 769
- idiopathic nephrotic (infantile) 581.9
- Imerslund (-Gräsbeck) (anemia due to familial selective vitamin B_{12} malabsorption) 281.1
- immobility (paraplegic) 728.3
- immunity deficiency, combined 279.2
- impending coronary 411.1
- impingement
  - shoulder 726.2
  - vertebral bodies 724.4
- inappropriate secretion of antidiuretic hormone (ADH) 253.6
- incomplete
  - mandibulofacial 756.0
- infant
  - death, sudden (SIDS) 798.0
  - Hercules 255.2
  - of diabetic mother 775.0
  - shaken 995.55
- infantilism 253.3
- inferior vena cava 459.2
- influenza-like 487.1
- inspissated bile, newborn 774.4
- intermediate coronary (artery) 411.1
- internal carotid artery (see also Occlusion, artery, carotid) 433.1 ✓5ᵗʰ

Syndrome — see also Disease — continued
- interspinous ligament 724.8
- intestinal
  - carcinoid 259.2
  - gas 787.3
  - knot 560.2
- intravascular
  - coagulation-fibrinolysis (ICF) (see also Fibrinolysis) 286.6
  - coagulopathy (see also Fibrinolysis) 286.6
- inverted Marfan's 759.89
- IRDS (idiopathic respiratory distress, newborn) 769
- irritable
  - bowel 564.1
  - heart 306.2
  - weakness 300.5
- ischemic bowel (transient) 557.9
  - chronic 557.1
  - due to mesenteric artery insufficiency 557.1
- Itsenko-Cushing (pituitary basophilism) 255.0
- IVC (intravascular coagulopathy) (see also Fibrinolysis) 286.6
- Ivemark's (asplenia with congenital heart disease) 759.0
- Jaccoud's 714.4
- Jackson's 344.89
- Jadassohn-Lewandowski (pachyonchia congenita) 757.5
- Jaffe-Lichtenstein (-Uehlinger) 252.0
- Jahnke's (encephalocutaneous angiomatosis) 759.6
- Jakob-Creutzfeldt 046.1
  - with dementia
    - with behavioral disturbance 046.1 [294.11]
    - without behavioral disturbance 046.1 [294.10]
- Jaksch's (pseudoleukemia infantum) 285.8
- Jaksch-Hayem (-Luzet) (pseudoleukemia infantum) 285.8
- jaw-winking 742.8
- jejunal 564.2
- jet lag 307.45
- Jeune's (asphyxiating thoracic dystrophy of newborn) 756.4
- Job's (chronic granulomatous disease) 288.1
- Jordan's 288.2
- Joseph-Diamond-Blackfan (congenital hypoplastic anemia) 284.0
- Joubert 759.89
- jugular foramen 352.6
- Kahler's (multiple myeloma) (M9730/3) 203.0 ✓5ᵗʰ
- Kalischer's (encephalocutaneous angiomatosis) 759.6
- Kallmann's (hypogonadotropic hypogonadism with anosmia) 253.4
- Kanner's (autism) (see also Psychosis, childhood) 299.0 ✓5ᵗʰ
- Kartagener's (sinusitis, bronchiectasis, situs inversus) 759.3
- Kasabach-Merritt (capillary hemangioma associated with thrombocytopenic purpura) 287.3
- Kast's (dyschondroplasia with hemangiomas) 756.4
- Kaznelson's (congenital hypoplastic anemia) 284.0
- Kelly's (sideropenic dysphagia) 280.8
- Kimmelstiel-Wilson (intercapillary glomerulosclerosis) 250.4 ✓5ᵗʰ [581.81]
- Klauder's (erythema multiforme exudativum) 695.1
- Klein-Waardenburg (ptosis-epicanthus) 270.2
- Kleine-Levin 349.89
- Klinefelter's 758.7
- Klippel-Feil (brevicollis) 756.16
- Klippel-Trenaunay 759.89
- Klumpke (-Déjérine) (injury to brachial plexus at birth) 767.6
- Klüver-Bucy (-Terzian) 310.0
- Köhler-Pellegrini-Stieda (calcification, knee joint) 726.62
- König's 564.89
- Korsakoff's (nonalcoholic) 294.0
  - alcoholic 291.1

Syndrome — see also Disease — continued
  Korsakoff (-Wernicke) (nonalcoholic) 294.0
    alcoholic 291.1
  Kostmann's (infantile genetic agranulocytosis) 288.0
  Krabbe's
    congenital muscle hypoplasia 756.89
    cutaneocerebral angioma 759.6
  Kunkel (lupoid hepatitis) 571.49
  labyrinthine 386.6
  laceration, broad ligament 620.6
  Langdon Down (mongolism) 758.0
  Larsen's (flattened facies and multiple congenital dislocations) 755.8
  lateral
    cutaneous nerve of thigh 355.1
    medullary (see also Disease, cerebrovascular acute) 436
  Launois' (pituitary gigantism) 253.0
  Launois-Cléret (adiposogenital dystrophy) 253.8
  Laurence-Moon (-Bardet) — Biedl (obesity, polydactyly, and mental retardation) 759.89
  Lawford's (encephalocutaneous angiomatosis) 759.6
  lazy
    leukocyte 288.0
    posture 728.3
  Lederer-Brill (acquired infectious hemolytic anemia) 283.19
  Legg-Calvé-Perthes (osteochondrosis capital femoral) 732.1
  Lennox's (see also Epilepsy) 345.0 ✓5ᵗʰ
  lenticular 275.1
  Léopold-Lévi's (paroxysmal thyroid instability) 242.9 ✓5ᵗʰ
  Lepore hemoglobin 282.4
  Léri-Weill 756.59
  Leriche's (aortic bifurcation occlusion) 444.0
  Lermoyez's (see also Disease, Ménière's) 386.00
  Lesch-Nyhan (hypoxanthine-guanine-phosphoribosyltransferase deficiency) 277.2
  Lev's (acquired complete heart block) 426.0
  Levi's (pituitary dwarfism) 253.3
  Lévy-Roussy 334.3
  Lichtheim's (subacute combined sclerosis with pernicious anemia) 281.0 [336.2]
  Li-Fraumeni 758.3
  Lightwood's (renal tubular acidosis) 588.8
  Lignac (-de Toni) (-Fanconi) (-Debré) (cystinosis) 270.0
  Likoff's (angina in menopausal women) 413.9
  liver-kidney 572.4
  Lloyd's 258.1
  lobotomy 310.0
  Löffler's (eosinophilic pneumonitis) 518.3
  Löfgren's (sarcoidosis) 135
  long arm 18 or 21 deletion 758.3
  Looser (-Debray) — Milkman (osteomalacia with pseudofractures) 268.2
  Lorain-Levi (pituitary dwarfism) 253.3
  Louis-Bar (ataxia-telangiectasia) 334.8
  low
    atmospheric pressure 993.2
    back 724.2
      psychogenic 306.0
    output (cardiac) (see also Failure, heart) 428.9
  Lowe's (oculocerebrorenal dystrophy) 270.8
  Lowe-Terrey-MacLachlan (oculocerebrorenal dystrophy) 270.8
  lower radicular, newborn 767.4
  Lown (-Ganong)-Levine (short P-R interval, normal QRS complex, and supraventricular tachycardia) 426.81
  Lucey-Driscoll (jaundice due to delayed conjugation) 774.30
  Luetscher's (dehydration) 276.5
  lumbar vertebral 724.4
  Lutembacher's (atrial septal defect with mitral stenosis) 745.5
  Lyell's (toxic epidermal necrolysis) 695.1
    due to drug
      correct substance properly administered 695.1
      overdose or wrong substance given or taken 977.9

Syndrome — see also Disease — continued
  Lyell's — continued
    due to drug — continued
      overdose or wrong substance given or taken — continued
        specified drug — see Table of Drugs and Chemicals
  MacLeod's 492.8
  macrogenitosomia praecox 259.8
  macroglobulinemia 273.3
  Maffucci's (dyschondroplasia with hemangiomas) 756.4
  Magenblase 306.4
  magnesium-deficiency 781.7
  malabsorption 579.9
    postsurgical 579.3
    spinal fluid 331.3
  malignant carcinoid 259.2
  Mallory-Weiss 530.7
  mandibulofacial dysostosis 756.0
  manic-depressive (see also Psychosis, affective) 296.80
  Mankowsky's (familial dysplastic osteopathy) 731.2
  maple syrup (urine) 270.3
  Marable's (celiac artery compression) 447.4
  Marchesani (-Weill) (brachymorphism and ectopia lentis) 759.89
  Marchiafava-Bignami 341.8
  Marchiafava-Micheli (paroxysmal nocturnal hemoglobinuria) 283.2
  Marcus Gunn's (jaw-winking syndrome) 742.8
  Marfan's (arachnodactyly) 759.82
    meaning congenital syphilis 090.49
      with luxation of lens 090.49 [379.32]
  Marie's (acromegaly) 253.0
    primary or idiopathic (acropachyderma) 757.39
    secondary (hypertrophic pulmonary osteoarthropathy) 731.2
  Markus-Adie 379.46
  Maroteaux-Lamy (mucopolysaccharidosis VI) 277.5
  Martin's 715.27
  Martin-Albright (pseudohypoparathyroidism) 275.49
  Martorell-Fabré (pulseless disease) 446.7
  massive aspiration of newborn 770.1
  Masters-Allen 620.6
  mastocytosis 757.33
  maternal hypotension 669.2 ✓5ᵗʰ
  maternal obesity 646.1 ✓5ᵗʰ
  May (-Hegglin) 288.2
  McArdle (-Schmid) (-Pearson) (glycogenosis V) 271.0
  McCune-Albright (osteitis fibrosa disseminata) 756.59
  McQuarrie's (idiopathic familial hypoglycemia) 251.2
  meconium
    aspiration 770.1
    plug (newborn) NEC 777.1
  median arcuate ligament 447.4
  mediastinal fibrosis 519.3
  Meekeren-Ehlers-Danlos 756.83
  Meige (blepharospasm-oromandibular dystonia) 333.82
    -Milroy (chronic hereditary edema) 757.0
  MELAS 758.89
  Melkersson (-Rosenthal) 351.8
  Mende's (ptosis-epicanthus) 270.2
  Mendelson's (resulting from a procedure) 997.3
    during labor 668.0 ✓5ᵗʰ
    obstetric 668.0 ✓5ᵗʰ
  Ménétrier's (hypertrophic gastritis) 535.2 ✓5ᵗʰ
  Ménière's (see also Disease, Ménière's) 386.00
  meningo-eruptive 047.1
  Menkes' 759.89
    glutamic acid 759.89
    maple syrup (urine) disease 270.3
  menopause 627.2
    postartificial 627.4
  menstruation 625.4
  MERFF 758.89
  mesenteric
    artery, superior 557.1
    vascular insufficiency (with gangrene) 557.1
  metastatic carcinoid 259.2

Syndrome — see also Disease — continued
  Meyenburg-Altherr-Uehlinger 733.99
  Meyer-Schwickerath and Weyers (dysplasia oculodentodigitalis) 759.89
  Micheli-Rietti (thalassemia minor) 282.4
  Michotte's 721.5
  micrognathia-glossoptosis 756.0
  microphthalmos (congenital) 759.89
  midbrain 348.8
  middle
    lobe (lung) (right) 518.0
    radicular 353.0
  Miescher's
    familial acanthosis nigricans 701.2
    granulomatosis disciformis 709.3
  Mieten's 759.89
  migraine 346.0 ✓5ᵗʰ
  Mikity-Wilson (pulmonary dysmaturity) 770.7
  Mikulicz's (dryness of mouth, absent or decreased lacrimation) 527.1
  milk alkali (milk drinkers') 999.9
  Milkman (-Looser) (osteomalacia with pseudofractures) 268.2
  Millard-Gubler 344.89
  Miller Fisher's 357.0
  Milles' (encephalocutaneous angiomatosis) 759.6
  Minkowski-Chauffard (see also Spherocytosis) 282.0
  Mirizzi's (hepatic duct stenosis) 576.2
    with calculus, cholelithiasis, or stones — see Choledocholithiasis
  mitral
    click (-murmur) 785.2
    valve prolapse 424.0
  Möbius'
    congenital oculofacial paralysis 352.6
    ophthalmoplegic migraine 346.8 ✓5ᵗʰ
  Mohr's (types I and II) 759.89
  monofixation 378.34
  Moore's (see also Epilepsy) 345.5 ✓5ᵗʰ
  Morel-Moore (hyperostosis frontalis interna) 733.3
  Morel-Morgagni (hyperostosis frontalis interna) 733.3
  Morgagni (-Stewart-Morel) (hyperostosis frontalis interna) 733.3
  Morgagni-Adams-Stokes (syncope with heart block) 426.9
  Morquio (-Brailsford) (-Ullrich) (mucopolysaccharidosis IV) 277.5
  Morris (testicular feminization) 257.8
  Morton's (foot) (metatarsalgia) (metatarsal neuralgia) (neuralgia) (neuroma) (toe) 355.6
  Moschcowitz (-Singer-Symmers) (thrombotic thrombocytopenic purpura) 446.6
  Mounier-Kuhn 494.0
    with acute exacerbation 494.1
  Mucha-Haberman (acute parapsoriasis varioliformis) 696.2
  mucocutaneous lymph node (acute) (febrile) (infantile) (MCLS) 446.1
  multiple
    deficiency 260
    operations 301.51
  Munchausen's 301.51
  Münchmeyer's (exostosis luxurians) 728.11
  Murchison-Sanderson — see Disease, Hodgkin's
  myasthenic — see Myasthenia, syndrome
  myelodysplastic 238.7
  myeloproliferative (chronic) (M9960/1) 238.7
  myofascial pain NEC 729.1
  Naffziger's 353.0
  Nager-de Reynier (dysostosis mandibularis) 756.0
  nail-patella (hereditary osteo-onychodysplasia) 756.89
  Nebécourt's 253.3
  Neill-Dingwall (microencephaly and dwarfism) 759.89
  nephrotic (see also Nephrosis) 581.9
    diabetic 250.4 ✓5ᵗʰ [581.81]
  Netherton's (ichthyosiform erythroderma) 757.1
  neurocutaneous 759.6
  neuroleptic malignant 333.92
  Nezelof's (pure alymphocytosis) 279.13

Index to Diseases

Syndrome — see also Disease — continued
  Niemann-Pick (lipid histiocytosis) 272.7
  Nonne-Milroy-Meige (chronic hereditary edema) 757.0
  nonsense 300.16
  Noonan's 759.89
  Nothnagel's
    ophthalmoplegia-cerebellar ataxia 378.52
    vasomotor acroparesthesia 443.89
  nucleus ambiguus-hypoglossal 352.6
  OAV (oculoauriculovertebral dysplasia) 756.0
  obsessional 300.3
  oculocutaneous 364.24
  oculomotor 378.81
  oculourethroarticular 099.3
  Ogilvie's (sympathicotonic colon obstruction) 560.89
  ophthalmoplegia-cerebellar ataxia 378.52
  Oppenheim-Urbach (necrobiosis lipoidica diabeticorum) 250.8 ✓5ᵗʰ [709.3]
  oral-facial-digital 759.89
  organic
    affective NEC 293.83
      drug-induced 292.84
    anxiety 293.84
    delusional 293.81
      alcohol-induced 291.5
      drug-induced 292.11
      due to or associated with
        arteriosclerosis 290.42
        presenile brain disease 290.12
        senility 290.20
    depressive 293.83
      drug-induced 292.84
      due to or associated with
        arteriosclerosis 290.43
        presenile brain disease 290.13
        senile brain disease 290.21
    hallucinosis 293.82
      drug-induced 292.84
  organic affective 293.83
    induced by drug 292.84
  organic personality 310.1
    induced by drug 292.89
  Ormond's 593.4
  orodigitofacial 759.89
  orthostatic hypotensive-dysautonomic dyskinetic 333.0
  Osler-Weber-Rendu (familial hemorrhagic telangiectasia) 448.0
  osteodermopathic hyperostosis 757.39
  osteoporosis-osteomalacia 268.2
  Österreicher-Turner (hereditary osteo-onychodysplasia) 756.89
  Ostrum-Furst 756.59
  otolith 386.19
  otopalatodigital 759.89
  outlet (thoracic) 353.0
  ovarian remant 620.8
  ovarian vein 593.4
  Owren's (see also Defect, coagulation) 286.3
  OX 758.6
  pacemaker 429.4
  Paget-Schroetter (intermittent venous claudication) 453.8
  pain — see Pain
  painful
    apicocostal vertebral (M8010/3) 162.3
    arc 726.19
    bruising 287.2
    feet 266.2
  Pancoast's (carcinoma, pulmonary apex) (M8010/3) 162.3
  panhypopituitary (postpartum) 253.2
  papillary muscle 429.81
    with myocardial infarction 410.8 ✓5ᵗʰ
  Papillon-Léage and Psaume (orodigitofacial dysostosis) 759.89
  parabiotic (transfusion)
    donor (twin) 772.0
    recipient (twin) 776.4
  paralysis agitans 332.0
  paralytic 344.9
    specified type NEC 344.89
  paraneoplastic — see condition
  Parinaud's (paralysis of conjugate upward gaze) 378.81

Syndrome — see also Disease — continued
  Parinaud's — continued
    oculoglandular 372.02
  Parkes Weber and Dimitri (encephalocutaneous angiomatosis) 759.6
  Parkinson's (see also Parkinsonism) 332.0
  parkinsonian (see also Parkinsonism) 332.0
  Parry's (exophthalmic goiter) 242.0 ✓5ᵗʰ
  Parry-Romberg 349.89
  Parsonage-Aldren-Turner 353.5
  Parsonage-Turner 353.5
  Patau's (trisomy D) 758.1
  patellofemoral 719.46
  Paterson (-Brown) (-Kelly) (sideropenic dysphagia) 280.8
  Payr's (splenic flexure syndrome) 569.89
  pectoral girdle 447.8
  pectoralis minor 447.8
  Pelger-Huët (hereditary hyposegmentation) 288.2
  pellagra-cerebellar ataxia-renal aminoaciduria 270.0
  Pellegrini-Stieda 726.62
  pellagroid 265.2
  Pellizzi's (pineal) 259.8
  pelvic congestion (-fibrosis) 625.5
  Pendred's (familial goiter with deaf-mutism) 243
  Penfield's (see also Epilepsy) 345.5 ✓5ᵗʰ
  Penta X 758.81
  peptic ulcer — see Ulcer, peptic 533.9 ✓5ᵗʰ
  perabduction 447.8
  periodic 277.3
  periurethral fibrosis 593.4
  persistent fetal circulation 747.83 ▲
  Petges-Cléjat (poikilodermatomyositis) 710.3
  Peutz-Jeghers 759.6
  Pfeiffer (acrocephalosyndactyly) 755.55
  phantom limb 353.6
  pharyngeal pouch 279.11
  Pick's (pericardial pseudocirrhosis of liver) 423.2
    heart 423.2
    liver 423.2
  Pick-Herxheimer (diffuse idiopathic cutaneous atrophy) 701.8
  Pickwickian (cardiopulmonary obesity) 278.8
  PIE (pulmonary infiltration with eosinophilia) 518.3
  Pierre Marie-Bamberger (hypertrophic pulmonary osteoarthropathy) 731.2
  Pierre Mauriac's (diabetes-dwarfism-obesity) 258.1
  Pierre Robin 756.0
  pigment dispersion, iris 364.53
  pineal 259.8
  pink puffer 492.8
  pituitary 253.0
  placental
    dysfunction 762.2
    insufficiency 762.2
    transfusion 762.3
  plantar fascia 728.71
  plica knee 727.83
  Plummer-Vinson (sideropenic dysphagia) 280.8
  pluricarential of infancy 260
  plurideficiency of infancy 260
  pluriglandular (compensatory) 258.8
  polycarential of infancy 260
  polyglandular 258.8
  polysplenia 759.0
  pontine 433.8 ✓5ᵗʰ
  popliteal
    artery entrapment 447.8
    web 756.89
  postartificial menopause 627.4
  postcardiotomy 429.4
  postcholecystectomy 576.0
  postcommissurotomy 429.4
  postconcussional 310.2
  postcontusional 310.2
  postencephalitic 310.8
  posterior
    cervical sympathetic 723.2
    fossa compression 348.4
    inferior cerebellar artery (see also Disease, cerebrovascular, acute) 436
  postgastrectomy (dumping) 564.2

Syndrome — see also Disease — continued
  post-gastric surgery 564.2
  posthepatitis 780.79
  postherpetic (neuralgia) (zoster) 053.19
    geniculate ganglion 053.11
    ophthalmica 053.19
  postimmunization — see Complications, vaccination
  postinfarction 411.0
  postinfluenza (asthenia) 780.79
  postirradiation 990
  postlaminectomy 722.80
    cervical, cervicothoracic 722.81
    lumbar, lumbosacral 722.83
    thoracic, thoracolumbar 722.82
  postleukotomy 310.0
  postlobotomy 310.0
  postmastectomy lymphedema 457.0
  postmature (of newborn) 766.2
  postmyocardial infarction 411.0
  postoperative NEC 998.9
    blind loop 579.2
  postpartum panhypopituitary 253.2
  postperfusion NEC 999.8
    bone marrow 996.85
  postpericardiotomy 429.4
  postphlebitic ▶(asymptomatic)◀ 459.10 ▲
    with
      complications NEC 459.19   •
      inflammation 459.12   •
        and ulcer 459.13   •
      stasis dermatitis 459.12   •
        with ulcer 459.13   •
      ulcer 459.11   •
        with inflammation 459.13   •
  postpolio (myelitis) 138
  postvagotomy 564.2
  postvalvulotomy 429.4
  postviral (asthenia) NEC 780.79
  Potain's (gastrectasis with dyspepsia) 536.1
  potassium intoxication 276.7
  Potter's 753.0
  Prader (-Labhart) -Willi (-Fanconi) 759.81
  preinfarction 411.1
  preleukemic 238.7
  premature senility 259.8
  premenstrual 625.4
  premenstrual tension 625.4
  pre ulcer 536.9
  Prinzmetal-Massumi (anterior chest wall syndrome) 786.52
  Profichet's 729.9
  progeria 259.8
  progressive pallidal degeneration 333.0
  prolonged gestation 766.2
  Proteus (dermal hypoplasia) 757.39
  prune belly 756.71
  prurigo-asthma 691.8
  pseudocarpal tunnel (sublimis) 354.0
  pseudohermaphroditism-virilism-hirsutism 255.2
  pseudoparalytica 358.0
  pseudo-Turner's 759.89
  psycho-organic 293.9
    acute 293.0
    anxiety type 293.84
    depressive type 293.83
    hallucinatory type 293.82
    nonpsychotic severity 310.1
      specified focal (partial) NEC 310.8
    paranoid type 293.81
    specified type NEC 293.89
    subacute 293.1
  pterygolymphangiectasia 758.6
  ptosis-epicanthus 270.2
  pulmonary 660.1 ✓5ᵗʰ
    arteriosclerosis 416.0
    hypoperfusion (idiopathic) 769
    renal (hemorrhagic) 446.21
  pulseless 446.7
  Putnam-Dana (subacute combined sclerosis with pernicious anemia) 281.0 [336.2]
  pyloroduodenal 537.89
  pyramidopallidonigral 332.0
  pyriformis 355.0
  Q-T interval prolongation 794.31
  radicular NEC 729.2
    lower limbs 724.4

Syndrome — see also Disease — continued
  radicular NEC — continued
    upper limbs 723.4
      newborn 767.4
  Raeder-Harbitz (pulseless disease) 446.7
  Ramsay Hunt's
    dyssynergia cerebellaris myoclonica 334.2
    herpetic geniculate ganglionitis 053.11
  rapid time-zone change 307.45
  Raymond (-Céstan) 433.8 ✓5ᵗʰ
  Raynaud's (paroxysmal digital cyanosis) 443.0
  RDS (respiratory distress syndrome, newborn) 769
  Refsum's (heredopathia atactica polyneuritiformis) 356.3
  Reichmann's (gastrosuccorrhea) 536.8
  Reifenstein's (hereditary familial hypogonadism, male) 257.2
  Reilly's (see also Neuropathy, peripheral, autonomic) 337.9
  Reiter's 099.3
  renal glomerulohyalinosis-diabetic 250.4 ✓5ᵗʰ [581.81]
  Rendu-Osler-Weber (familial hemorrhagic telangiectasia) 448.0
  renofacial (congenital biliary fibroangiomatosis) 753.0
  Rénon-Delille 253.8
  respiratory distress (idiopathic) (newborn) 769
    adult (following shock, surgery, or trauma) 518.5
    specified NEC 518.82
  restless leg 333.99
  retraction (Duane's) 378.71
  retroperitoneal fibrosis 593.4
  Rett's 330.8
  Reye's 331.81
  Reye-Sheehan (postpartum pituitary necrosis) 253.2
  Riddoch's (visual disorientation) 368.16
  Ridley's (see also Failure, ventricular, left) 428.1
  Rieger's (mesodermal dysgenesis, anterior ocular segment) 743.44
  Rietti-Greppi-Micheli (thalassemia minor) 282.4
  right ventricular obstruction — see Failure, heart
  Riley-Day (familial dysautonomia) 742.8
  Robin's 756.0
  Rokitansky-Kuster-Hauser (congenital absence, vagina) 752.49
  Romano-Ward (prolonged Q-T interval) 794.31
  Romberg's 349.89
  Rosen-Castleman-Liebow (pulmonary proteinosis) 516.0
  rotator cuff, shoulder 726.10
  Roth's 355.1
  Rothmund's (congenital poikiloderma) 757.33
  Rotor's (idiopathic hyperbilirubinemia) 277.4
  Roussy-Lévy 334.3
  Roy (-Jutras) (acropachyderma) 757.39
  rubella (congenital) 771.0
  Rubinstein-Taybi's (brachydactylia, short stature, and mental retardation) 759.89
  Rud's (mental deficiency, epilepsy, and infantilism) 759.89
  Ruiter-Pompen (-Wyers) (angiokeratoma corporis diffusum) 272.7
  Runge's (postmaturity) 766.2
  Russell (-Silver) (congenital hemihypertrophy and short stature) 759.89
  Rytand-Lipsitch (complete atrioventricular block) 426.0
  sacralization-scoliosis-sciatica 756.15
  sacroiliac 724.6
  Saenger's 379.46
  salt
    depletion (see also Disease, renal) 593.9
      due to heat NEC 992.8
        causing heat exhaustion or prostration 992.4
    low (see also Disease, renal) 593.9
  salt-losing (see also Disease, renal) 593.9
  Sanfilippo's (mucopolysaccharidosis III) 277.5
  Scaglietti-Dagnini (acromegalic macrospondylitis) 253.0
  scalded skin 695.1
  scalenus anticus (anterior) 353.0

Syndrome — see also Disease — continued
  scapulocostal 354.8
  scapuloperoneal 359.1
  scapulovertebral 723.4
  Schaumann's (sarcoidosis) 135
  Scheie's (mucopolysaccharidosis IS) 277.5
  Scheuthauer-Marie-Sainton (cleidocranialis dysostosis) 755.59
  Schirmer's (encephalocutaneous angiomatosis) 759.6
  schizophrenic, of childhood NEC (see also Psychosis, childhood) 299.9 ✓5ᵗʰ
  Schmidt's
    sphallo-pharyngo-laryngeal hemiplegia 352.6
    thyroid-adrenocortical insufficiency 258.1
    vagoaccessory 352.6
  Schneider's 047.9
  Scholte's (malignant carcinoid) 259.2
  Scholz (-Bielschowsky-Henneberg) 330.0
  Schroeder's (endocrine-hypertensive) 255.3
  Schüller-Christian (chronic histiocytosis X) 277.8
  Schultz's (agranulocytosis) 288.0
  Schwartz (-Jampel) 756.89
  Schwartz-Bartter (inappropriate secretion of antidiuretic hormone) 253.6
  Scimitar (anomalous venous drainage, right lung to inferior vena cava) 747.49
  sclerocystic ovary 256.4
  sea-blue histiocyte 272.7
  Seabright-Bantam (pseudohypoparathyroidism) 275.49
  Seckel's 759.89
  Secretan's (posttraumatic edema) 782.3
  secretoinhibitor (keratoconjunctivitis sicca) 710.2
  Seeligmann's (ichthyosis congenita) 757.1
  Senear-Usher (pemphigus erythematosus) 694.4
  senilism 259.8
  serotonin 333.99
  serous meningitis 348.2
  Sertoli cell (germinal aplasia) 606.0
  sex chromosome mosaic 758.81
  Sézary's (reticulosis) (M9701/3) 202.2 ✓5ᵗʰ
  shaken infant 995.55
  Shaver's (bauxite pneumoconiosis) 503
  Sheehan's (postpartum pituitary necrosis) 253.2
  shock (traumatic) 958.4
    kidney 584.5
      following crush injury 958.5
    lung 518.5
    neurogenic 308.9
    psychic 308.9
  short
    bowel 579.3
    P-R interval 426.81
  shoulder-arm (see also Neuropathy, peripheral, autonomic) 337.9
  shoulder-girdle 723.4
  shoulder-hand (see also Neuropathy, peripheral, autonomic) 337.9
  Shwachman's 288.0
  Shy-Drager (orthostatic hypotension with multisystem degeneration) 333.0
  Sicard's 352.6
  sicca (keratoconjunctivitis) 710.2
  sick
    cell 276.1
    cilia 759.89
    sinus 427.81
  sideropenic 280.8
  Siemens'
    ectodermal dysplasia 757.31
    keratosis follicularis spinulosa (decalvans) 757.39
  Silfverskiöld's (osteochondrodysplasia, extremities) 756.50
  Silver's (congenital hemihypertrophy and short stature) 759.89
  Silvestroni-Bianco (thalassemia minima) 282.4
  Simons' (progressive lipodystrophy) 272.6
  sinus 726.79
  sinusitis-bronchiectasis-situs inversus 759.3
  Sipple's (medullary thyroid carcinoma-pheochromocytoma) 193

Syndrome — see also Disease — continued
  Sjögren (-Gougerot) (keratoconjunctivitis sicca) 710.2
    with lung involvement 710.2 [517.8]
  Sjögren-Larsson (ichthyosis congenita) 757.1
  Slocumb's 255.3
  Sluder's 337.0
  Smith-Lemli-Opitz (cerebrohepatorenal syndrome) 759.89
  smokers' 305.1
  Sneddon-Wilkinson (subcorneal pustular dermatosis) 694.1
  Sotos' (cerebral gigantism) 253.0
  South African cardiomyopathy 425.2
  spasmodic
    upward movement, eye(s) 378.82
    winking 307.20
  Spens' (syncope with heart block) 426.9
  spherophakia-brachymorphia 759.89
  spinal cord injury — see also Injury, spinal, by site
    with fracture, vertebra — see Fracture, vertebra, by site, with spinal cord injury
    cervical — see Injury, spinal, cervical
    fluid malabsorption (acquired) 331.3
  splenic
    agenesis 759.0
    flexure 569.89
    neutropenia 288.0
    sequestration 282.60
  Spurway's (brittle bones and blue sclera) 756.51
  staphylococcal scalded skin 695.1
  Stein's (polycystic ovary) 256.4
  Stein-Leventhal (polycystic ovary) 256.4
  Steinbrocker's (see also Neuropathy, peripheral, autonomic) 337.9
  Stevens-Johnson (erythema multiforme exudativum) 695.1
  Stewart-Morel (hyperostosis frontalis interna) 733.3
  stiff-man 333.91
  Still's (juvenile rheumatoid arthritis) 714.30
  Still-Felty (rheumatoid arthritis with splenomegaly and leukopenia) 714.1
  Stilling-Türk-Duane (ocular retraction syndrome) 378.71
  Stojano's (subcostal) 098.86
  Stokes (-Adams) (syncope with heart block) 426.9
  Stokvis-Talma (enterogenous cyanosis) 289.7
  stone heart (see also Failure, ventricular, left) 428.1
  straight-back 756.19
  stroke (see also Disease, cerebrovascular, acute) 436
    little 435.9
  Sturge-Kalischer-Weber (encephalotrigeminal angiomatosis) 759.6
  Sturge-Weber (-Dimitri) (encephalocutaneous angiomatosis) 759.6
  subclavian-carotid obstruction (chronic) 446.7
  subclavian steal 435.2
  subcoracoid-pectoralis minor 447.8
  subcostal 098.86
    nerve compression 354.8
  subperiosteal hematoma 267
  subphrenic interposition 751.4
  sudden infant death (SIDS) 798.0
  Sudeck's 733.7
  Sudeck-Leriche 733.7
  superior
    cerebellar artery (see also Disease, cerebrovascular, acute) 436
    mesenteric artery 557.1
    pulmonary sulcus (tumor) (M8010/3) 162.3
    vena cava 459.2
  suprarenal cortical 255.3
  supraspinatus 726.10
  swallowed blood 777.3
  sweat retention 705.1
  Sweet's (acute febrile neutrophilic dermatosis) 695.89
  Swyer-James (unilateral hyperlucent lung) 492.8
  Swyer's (XY pure gonadal dysgenesis) 752.7
  Symonds' 348.2

Syndrome — see also Disease — continued
  sympathetic
    cervical paralysis 337.0
    pelvic 625.5
  syndactylic oxycephaly 755.55
  syphilitic-cardiovascular 093.89
  systemic
    fibrosclerosing 710.8
    inflammatory response (SIRS) 995.90
      due to
        infectious process 995.91
          with organ dysfunction 995.92
        non-infectious process 995.93
          with organ dysfunction 995.94
  systolic click (-murmur) 785.2
  Tabagism 305.1
  tachycardia-bradycardia 427.81
  Takayasu (-Onishi) (pulseless disease) 446.7
  Tapia's 352.6
  tarsal tunnel 355.5
  Taussig-Bing (transposition, aorta and overriding pulmonary artery) 745.11
  Taybi's (otopalatodigital) 759.89
  Taylor's 625.5
  teething 520.7
  tegmental 344.89
  telangiectasis-pigmentation-cataract 757.33
  temporal 383.02
    lobectomy behavior 310.0
  temporomandibular joint-pain-dysfunction [TMJ] NEC 524.60
    specified NEC 524.69
  Terry's 362.21
  testicular feminization 257.8
  testis, nonvirilizing 257.8
  tethered (spinal) cord 742.59
  thalamic 348.8
  Thibierge-Weissenbach (cutaneous systemic sclerosis) 710.1
  Thiele 724.6
  thoracic outlet (compression) 353.0
  thoracogenous rheumatic (hypertrophic pulmonary osteoarthropathy) 731.2
  Thorn's (see also Disease, renal) 593.9
  Thorson-Biörck (malignant carcinoid) 259.2
  thrombopenia-hemangioma 287.3
  thyroid-adrenocortical insufficiency 258.1
  Tietze's 733.6
  time-zone (rapid) 307.45
  Tobias' (carcinoma, pulmonary apex) (M8010/3) 162.3
  toilet seat 926.0
  Tolosa-Hunt 378.55
  Toni-Fanconi (cystinosis) 270.0
  Touraine's (hereditary osteo-onychodysplasia) 756.89
  Touraine-Solente-Golé (acropachyderma) 757.39
  toxic
    oil 710.5
    shock 040.82
  transfusion
    fetal-maternal 772.0
    twin
      donor (infant) 772.0
      recipient (infant) 776.4
  Treacher Collins' (incomplete mandibulofacial dysostosis) 756.0
  trigeminal plate 259.8
  triple X female 758.81
  trisomy NEC 758.5
    13 or D₁ 758.1
    16-18 or E 758.2
    18 or E₃ 758.2
    20 758.5
    21 or G (mongolism) 758.0
    22 or G (mongolism) 758.0
    G 758.0
  Troisier-Hanot-Chauffard (bronze diabetes) 275.0
  tropical wet feet 991.4
  Trousseau's (thrombophlebitis migrans visceral cancer) 453.1
  Türk's (ocular retraction syndrome) 378.71
  Turner's 758.6

Syndrome — see also Disease — continued
  Turner-Varny 758.6
  twin-to-twin transfusion 762.3
    recipient twin 776.4
  Uehlinger's (acropachyderma) 757.39
  Ullrich (-Bonnevie) (-Turner) 758.6
  Ullrich-Feichtiger 759.89
  underwater blast injury (abdominal) (see also Injury, internal, abdomen) 868.00
  universal joint, cervix 620.6
  Unverricht (-Lundborg) 333.2
  Unverricht-Wagner (dermatomyositis) 710.3
  upward gaze 378.81
  Urbach-Oppenheim (necrobiosis lipoidica diabeticorum) 250.8 [709.3]
  Urbach-Wiethe (lipoid proteinosis) 272.8
  uremia, chronic 585
  urethral 597.81
  urethro-oculoarticular 099.3
  urethro-oculosynovial 099.3
  urohepatic 572.4
  uveocutaneous 364.24
  uveomeningeal, uveomeningitis 363.22
  vagohypoglossal 352.6
  vagovagal 780.2
  van Buchem's (hyperostosis corticalis) 733.3
  van der Hoeve's (brittle bones and blue sclera, deafness) 756.51
  van der Hoeve-Halbertsma-Waardenburg (ptosis-epicanthus) 270.2
  van der Hoeve-Waardenburg-Gualdi (ptosis-epicanthus) 270.2
  van Neck-Odelberg (juvenile osteochondrosis) 732.1
  vanishing twin 651.33
  vascular splanchnic 557.0
  vasomotor 443.9
  vasovagal 780.2
  VATER 759.89
  Velo-cardio-facial 759.89
    with chromosomal deletion 758.5
  vena cava (inferior) (superior) (obstruction) 459.2
  Verbiest's (claudicatio intermittens spinalis) 435.1
  Vernet's 352.6
  vertebral
    artery 435.1
      compression 721.1
    lumbar 724.4
    steal 435.1
  vertebrogenic (pain) 724.5
  vertiginous NEC 386.9
  video display tube 723.8
  Villaret's 352.6
  Vinson-Plummer (sideropenic dysphagia) 280.8
  virilizing adrenocortical hyperplasia, congenital 255.2
  virus, viral 079.99
  visceral larval migrans 128.0
  visual disorientation 368.16
  vitamin B₆ deficiency 266.1
  vitreous touch 997.99
  Vogt's (corpus striatum) 333.7
  Vogt-Koyanagi 364.24
  Volkmann's 958.6
  von Bechterew-Strümpell (ankylosing spondylitis) 720.0
  von Graefe's 378.72
  von Hippel-Lindau (angiomatosis retinocerebellosa) 759.6
  von Schroetter's (intermittent venous claudication) 453.8
  von Willebrand (-Jürgens) (angiohemophilia) 286.4
  Waardenburg-Klein (ptosis epicanthus) 270.2
  Wagner (-Unverricht) (dermatomyositis) 710.3
  Waldenström's (macroglobulinemia) 273.3
  Waldenström-Kjellberg (sideropenic dysphagia) 280.8
  Wallenberg's (posterior inferior cerebellar artery) (see also Disease, cerebrovascular, acute) 436
  Waterhouse (-Friderichsen) 036.3
  water retention 276.6
  Weber's 344.89
  Weber-Christian (nodular nonsuppurative panniculitis) 729.30

Syndrome — see also Disease — continued
  Weber-Cockayne (epidermolysis bullosa) 757.39
  Weber-Dimitri (encephalocutaneous angiomatosis) 759.6
  Weber-Gubler 344.89
  Weber-Leyden 344.89
  Weber-Osler (familial hemorrhagic telangiectasia) 448.0
  Wegener's (necrotizing respiratory granulomatosis) 446.4
  Weill-Marchesani (brachymorphism and ectopia lentis) 759.89
  Weingarten's (tropical eosinophilia) 518.3
  Weiss-Baker (carotid sinus syncope) 337.0
  Weissenbach-Thibierge (cutaneous systemic sclerosis) 710.1
  Werdnig-Hoffmann 335.0
  Werlhof-Wichmann (see also Purpura, thrombocytopenic) 287.3
  Wermer's (polyendocrine adenomatosis) 258.0
  Werner's (progeria adultorum) 259.8
  Wernicke's (nonalcoholic) (superior hemorrhagic polioencephalitis) 265.1
  Wernicke-Korsakoff (nonalcoholic) 294.0
    alcoholic 291.1
  Westphal-Strümpell (hepatolenticular degeneration) 275.1
  wet
    brain (alcoholic) 303.9
    feet (maceration) (tropical) 991.4
    lung
      adult 518.5
      newborn 770.6
  whiplash 847.0
  Whipple's (intestinal lipodystrophy) 040.2
  "whistling face" (craniocarpotarsal dystrophy) 759.89
  Widal (-Abrami) (acquired hemolytic jaundice) 283.9
  Wilkie's 557.1
  Wilkinson-Sneddon (subcorneal pustular dermatosis) 694.1
  Willan-Plumbe (psoriasis) 696.1
  Willebrand (-Jürgens) (angiohemophilia) 286.4
  Willi-Prader (hypogenital dystrophy with diabetic tendency) 759.81
  Wilson's (hepatolenticular degeneration) 275.1
  Wilson-Mikity 770.7
  Wiskott-Aldrich (eczema-thrombocytopenia) 279.12
  withdrawal
    alcohol 291.81
    drug 292.0
      infant of dependent mother 779.5
  Woakes' (ethmoiditis) 471.1
  Wolff-Parkinson-White (anomalous atrioventricular excitation) 426.7
  Wright's (hyperabduction) 447.8
  X
    cardiac 413.9
    dysmetabolic 277.7
  xiphoidalgia 733.99
  XO 758.6
  XXX 758.81
  XXXXY 758.81
  XXY 758.7
  yellow vernix (placental dysfunction) 762.2
  Zahorsky's 074.0
  Zieve's (jaundice, hyperlipemia and hemolytic anemia) 571.1
  Zollinger-Ellison (gastric hypersecretion with pancreatic islet cell tumor) 251.5
  Zuelzer-Ogden (nutritional megaloblastic anemia) 281.2
Synechia (iris) (pupil) 364.70
  anterior 364.72
    peripheral 364.73
  intrauterine (traumatic) 621.5
  posterior 364.71
  vulvae, congenital 752.49
Synesthesia (see also Disturbance, sensation) 782.0
Synodontia 520.2
Synophthalmus 759.89
Synorchidism 752.8
Synorchism 752.8

Synostosis (congenital) 756.59
  astragaloscaphoid 755.67
  radioulnar 755.53
  talonavicular (bar) 755.67
  tarsal 755.67
Synovial — see condition
Synovioma (M9040/3) — see also Neoplasm, connective tissue, malignant
  benign (M9040/0) — see Neoplasm, connective tissue, benign
Synoviosarcoma (M9040/3) — see Neoplasm, connective tissue, malignant
Synovitis 727.00
  chronic crepitant, wrist 727.2
  due to crystals — see Arthritis, due to crystals
  gonococcal 098.51
  gouty 274.0
  syphilitic 095.7
    congenital 090.0
  traumatic, current — see Sprain, by site
  tuberculous — see Tuberculosis, synovitis
  villonodular 719.20
    ankle 719.27
    elbow 719.22
    foot 719.27
    hand 719.24
    hip 719.25
    knee 719.26
    multiple sites 719.29
    pelvic region 719.25
    shoulder (region) 719.21
    specified site NEC 719.28
    wrist 719.23
Syphilide 091.3
  congenital 090.0
  newborn 090.0
  tubercular 095.8
    congenital 090.0
Syphilis, syphilitic (acquired) 097.9
  with lung involvement 095.1
  abdomen (late) 095.2
  acoustic nerve 094.86
  adenopathy (secondary) 091.4
  adrenal (gland) 095.8
    with cortical hypofunction 095.8
  age under 2 years NEC (see also Syphilis, congenital) 090.9
    acquired 097.9
  alopecia (secondary) 091.82
  anemia 095.8
  aneurysm (artery) (ruptured) 093.89
    aorta 093.0
    central nervous system 094.89
    congenital 090.5
  anus 095.8
    primary 091.1
    secondary 091.3
  aorta, aortic (arch) (abdominal) (insufficiency) (pulmonary) (regurgitation) (stenosis) (thoracic) 093.89
    aneurysm 093.0
  arachnoid (adhesive) 094.2
  artery 093.89
    cerebral 094.89
    spinal 094.89
  arthropathy (neurogenic) (tabetic) 094.0 [713.5]
  asymptomatic — see Syphilis, latent
  ataxia, locomotor (progressive) 094.0
  atrophoderma maculatum 091.3
  auricular fibrillation 093.89
  Bell's palsy 094.89
  bladder 095.8
  bone 095.5
    secondary 091.61
  brain 094.89
  breast 095.8
  bronchus 095.8
  bubo 091.0
  bulbar palsy 094.89
  bursa (late) 095.7
  cardiac decompensation 093.89
  cardiovascular (early) (late) (primary) (secondary) (tertiary) 093.89
    specified type and site NEC 093.89
  causing death under 2 years of age (see also Syphilis, congenital) 090.9
    stated to be acquired NEC 097.9

Syphilis, syphilitic — continued
  central nervous system (any site) (early) (late) (latent) (primary) (recurrent) (relapse) (secondary) (tertiary) 094.9
    with
      ataxia 094.0
      paralysis, general 094.1
        juvenile 090.40
      paresis (general) 094.1
        juvenile 090.40
      tabes (dorsalis) 094.0
        juvenile 090.40
      taboparesis 094.1
        juvenile 090.40
    aneurysm (ruptured) 094.87
    congenital 090.40
    juvenile 090.40
    remission in (sustained) 094.9
    serology doubtful, negative, or positive 094.9
    specified nature or site NEC 094.89
    vascular 094.89
  cerebral 094.89
    meningovascular 094.2
    nerves 094.89
    sclerosis 094.89
    thrombosis 094.89
  cerebrospinal 094.89
    tabetic 094.0
  cerebrovascular 094.89
  cervix 095.8
  chancre (multiple) 091.0
    extragenital 091.2
    Rollet's 091.0
  Charcôt's joint 094.0 [713.5]
  choked disc 094.89 [377.00]
  chorioretinitis 091.51
    congenital 090.0 [363.13]
    late 094.83
  choroiditis 091.51
    congenital 090.0 [363.13]
    late 094.83
    prenatal 090.0 [363.13]
  choroidoretinitis (secondary) 091.51
    congenital 090.0 [363.13]
    late 094.83
  ciliary body (secondary) 091.52
    late 095.8 [364.11]
  colon (late) 095.8
  combined sclerosis 094.89
  complicating pregnancy, childbirth or puerperium 647.0
    affecting fetus or newborn 760.2
  condyloma (latum) 091.3
  congenital 090.9
    with
      encephalitis 090.41
      paresis (general) 090.40
      tabes (dorsalis) 090.40
      taboparesis 090.40
    chorioretinitis, choroiditis 090.0 [363.13]
    early or less than 2 years after birth NEC 090.2
      with manifestations 090.0
      latent (without manifestations) 090.1
        negative spinal fluid test 090.1
        serology, positive 090.1
      symptomatic 090.0
    interstitial keratitis 090.3
    juvenile neurosyphilis 090.40
    late or 2 years or more after birth NEC 090.7
      chorioretinitis, choroiditis 090.5 [363.13]
      interstitial keratitis 090.3
      juvenile neurosyphilis NEC 090.40
      latent (without manifestations) 090.6
        negative spinal fluid test 090.6
        serology, positive 090.6
      symptomatic or with manifestations NEC 090.5
      interstitial keratitis 090.3
  conjugal 097.9
    tabes 094.0
  conjunctiva 095.8 [372.10]
  contact V01.6
  cord, bladder 094.0
  cornea, late 095.8 [370.59]
  coronary (artery) 093.89
    sclerosis 093.89

Syphilis, syphilitic — continued
  coryza 095.8
    congenital 090.0
  cranial nerve 094.89
  cutaneous — see Syphilis, skin
  dacryocystitis 095.8
  degeneration, spinal cord 094.89
  d'emblée 095.8
  dementia 094.1
    paralytica 094.1
      juvenilis 090.40
  destruction of bone 095.5
  dilatation, aorta 093.0
  due to blood transfusion 097.9
  dura mater 094.89
  ear 095.8
    inner 095.8
      nerve (eighth) 094.86
      neurorecurrence 094.86
  early NEC 091.0
    cardiovascular 093.9
    central nervous system 094.9
      paresis 094.1
      tabes 094.0
    latent (without manifestations) (less than 2 years after infection) 092.9
      negative spinal fluid test 092.9
      serological relapse following treatment 092.0
      serology positive 092.9
    paresis 094.1
    relapse (treated, untreated) 091.7
    skin 091.3
    symptomatic NEC 091.89
      extragenital chancre 091.2
      primary, except extragenital chancre 091.0
      secondary (see also Syphilis, secondary) 091.3
        relapse (treated, untreated) 091.7
    tabes 094.0
    ulcer 091.3
  eighth nerve 094.86
  endemic, nonvenereal 104.0
  endocarditis 093.20
    aortic 093.22
    mitral 093.21
    pulmonary 093.24
    tricuspid 093.23
  epididymis (late) 095.8
  epiglottis 095.8
  epiphysitis (congenital) 090.0
  esophagus 095.8
  Eustachian tube 095.8
  exposure to V01.6
  eye 095.8 [363.13]
    neuromuscular mechanism 094.85
  eyelid 095.8 [373.5]
    with gumma 095.8 [373.5]
    ptosis 094.89
  fallopian tube 095.8
  fracture 095.5
  gallbladder (late) 095.8
  gastric 095.8
    crisis 094.0
    polyposis 095.8
  general 097.9
    paralysis 094.1
      juvenile 090.40
  genital (primary) 091.0
  glaucoma 095.8
  gumma (late) NEC 095.9
    cardiovascular system 093.9
    central nervous system 094.9
    congenital 090.5
    heart or artery 093.89
  heart 093.89
    block 093.89
    decompensation 093.89
    disease 093.89
    failure 093.89
    valve (see also Syphilis, endocarditis) 093.20
  hemianesthesia 094.89
  hemianopsia 095.8
  hemiparesis 094.89
  hemiplegia 094.89
  hepatic artery 093.89

Index to Diseases

Syphilis, syphilitic — continued
- hepatitis 095.3
- hepatomegaly 095.3
  - congenital 090.0
- hereditaria tarda (see also Syphilis, congenital, late) 090.7 ✓5th
- hereditary (see also Syphilis, congenital) 090.9 ✓5th
  - interstitial keratitis 090.3
- Hutchinson's teeth 090.5
- hyalitis 095.8
- inactive — see Syphilis, latent
- infantum NEC (see also Syphilis, congenital) 090.9 ✓5th
- inherited — see Syphilis, congenital
- internal ear 095.8
- intestine (late) 095.8
- iris, iritis (secondary) 091.52
  - late 095.8 [364.11]
- joint (late) 095.8
- keratitis (congenital) (early) (interstitial) (late) (parenchymatous) (punctata profunda) 090.3
- kidney 095.4
- lacrimal apparatus 095.8
- laryngeal paralysis 095.8
- larynx 095.8
- late 097.0
  - cardiovascular 093.9
  - central nervous system 094.9
  - latent or 2 years or more after infection (without manifestations) 096
    - negative spinal fluid test 096
    - serology positive 096
  - paresis 094.1
  - specified site NEC 095.8
  - symptomatic or with symptoms 095.9
  - tabes 094.0
- latent 097.1
  - central nervous system 094.9
  - date of infection unspecified 097.1
  - early or less than 2 years after infection 092.9
  - late or 2 years or more after infection 096
  - serology
    - doubtful
      - follow-up of latent syphilis 097.1
        - central nervous system 094 ✓4th
        - date of infection unspecified 097.1
        - early or less than 2 years after infection 092 ✓4th
        - late or 2 years or more after infection 096
    - positive, only finding 097.1
      - date of infection unspecified 097.1
      - early or less than 2 years after infection 097.1
      - late or 2 years or more after infection 097.1
- lens 095.8
- leukoderma 091.3
  - late 095.8
- lienis 095.8
- lip 091.3
  - chancre 091.2
  - late 095.8
  - primary 091.2
- Lissauer's paralysis 094.1
- liver 095.3
  - secondary 091.62
- locomotor ataxia 094.0
- lung 095.1
- lymphadenitis (secondary) 091.4
- lymph gland (early) (secondary) 091.4
  - late 095.8
- macular atrophy of skin 091.3
  - striated 095.8
- maternal, affecting fetus or newborn 760.2
  - manifest syphilis in newborn — see Syphilis, congenital
- mediastinum (late) 095.8
- meninges (adhesive) (basilar) (brain) (spinal cord) 094.2
- meningitis 094.2
  - acute 091.81
  - congenital 090.42
- meningoencephalitis 094.2

Syphilis, syphilitic — continued
- meningovascular 094.2
  - congenital 090.49
- mesarteritis 093.89
  - brain 094.89
  - spine 094.89
- middle ear 095.8
- mitral stenosis 093.21
- monoplegia 094.89
- mouth (secondary) 091.3
  - late 095.8
- mucocutaneous 091.3
  - late 095.8
- mucous
  - membrane 091.3
    - late 095.8
  - patches 091.3
    - congenital 090.0
- mulberry molars 090.5
- muscle 095.6
- myocardium 093.82
- myositis 095.6
- nasal sinus 095.8
- neonatorum NEC (see also Syphilis, congenital) 090.9 ✓5th
- nerve palsy (any cranial nerve) 094.89
- nervous system, central 094.9
- neuritis 095.8
  - acoustic nerve 094.86
- neurorecidive of retina 094.83
- neuroretinitis 094.85
- newborn (see also Syphilis, congenital) 090.9 ✓5th
- nodular superficial 095.8
- nonvenereal, endemic 104.0
- nose 095.8
  - saddle back deformity 090.5
  - septum 095.8
    - perforated 095.8
- occlusive arterial disease 093.89
- ophthalmic 095.8 [363.13]
- ophthalmoplegia 094.89
- optic nerve (atrophy) (neuritis) (papilla) 094.84
- orbit (late) 095.8
- orchitis 095.8
- organic 097.9
- osseous (late) 095.5
- osteochondritis (congenital) 090.0
- osteoporosis 095.5
- ovary 095.8
- oviduct 095.8
- palate 095.8
  - gumma 095.8
  - perforated 090.5
- pancreas (late) 095.8
- pancreatitis 095.8
- paralysis 094.89
  - general 094.1
  - juvenile 090.40
- paraplegia 094.89
- paresis (general) 094.1
  - juvenile 090.40
- paresthesia 094.89
- Parkinson's disease or syndrome 094.82
- paroxysmal tachycardia 093.89
- pemphigus (congenital) 090.0
- penis 091.0
  - chancre 091.0
  - late 095.8
- pericardium 093.81
- perichondritis, larynx 095.8
- periosteum 095.5
  - congenital 090.0
  - early 091.61
  - secondary 091.61
- peripheral nerve 095.8
- petrous bone (late) 095.5
- pharynx 095.8
  - secondary 091.3
- pituitary (gland) 095.8
- placenta 095.8
- pleura (late) 095.8
- pneumonia, white 090.0
- pontine (lesion) 094.89
- portal vein 093.89
- primary NEC 091.2
  - anal 091.1

Syphilis, syphilitic — continued
- primary NEC — continued
  - and secondary (see also Syphilis, secondary) 091.9
  - cardiovascular 093.9
  - central nervous system 094.9
  - extragenital chancre NEC 091.2
  - fingers 091.2
  - genital 091.0
  - lip 091.2
  - specified site NEC 091.2
  - tonsils 091.2
- prostate 095.8
- psychosis (intracranial gumma) 094.89
- ptosis (eyelid) 094.89
- pulmonary (late) 095.1
  - artery 093.89
- pulmonum 095.1
- pyelonephritis 095.4
- recently acquired, symptomatic NEC 091.89
- rectum 095.8
- respiratory tract 095.8
- retina
  - late 094.83
  - neurorecidive 094.83
- retrobulbar neuritis 094.85
- salpingitis 095.8
- sclera (late) 095.0
- sclerosis
  - cerebral 094.89
  - coronary 093.89
  - multiple 094.89
  - subacute 094.89
- scotoma (central) 095.8
- scrotum 095.8
- secondary (and primary) 091.9
  - adenopathy 091.4
  - anus 091.3
  - bone 091.61
  - cardiovascular 093.9
  - central nervous system 094.9
  - chorioretinitis, choroiditis 091.51
  - hepatitis 091.62
  - liver 091.62
  - lymphadenitis 091.4
  - meningitis, acute 091.81
  - mouth 091.3
  - mucous membranes 091.3
  - periosteum 091.61
  - periostitis 091.61
  - pharynx 091.3
  - relapse (treated) (untreated) 091.7
  - skin 091.3
  - specified form NEC 091.89
  - tonsil 091.3
  - ulcer 091.3
  - viscera 091.69
  - vulva 091.3
- seminal vesicle (late) 095.8
- seronegative
  - with signs or symptoms — see Syphilis, by site and stage
- seropositive
  - with signs or symptoms — see Syphilis, by site and stage
  - follow-up of latent syphilis — see Syphilis, latent
  - only finding — see Syphilis, latent
- seventh nerve (paralysis) 094.89
- sinus 095.8
- sinusitis 095.8
- skeletal system 095.5
- skin (early) (secondary) (with ulceration) 091.3
  - late or tertiary 095.8
- small intestine 095.8
- spastic spinal paralysis 094.0
- spermatic cord (late) 095.8
- spinal (cord) 094.89
  - with
    - paresis 094.1
    - tabes 094.0
- spleen 095.8
- splenomegaly 095.8
- spondylitis 095.5
- staphyloma 095.8
- stigmata (congenital) 090.5
- stomach 095.8
- synovium (late) 095.7

Syphilis, syphilitic

Syphilis, syphilitic — *continued*
  tabes dorsalis (early) (late) 094.0
    juvenile 090.40
  tabetic type 094.0
    juvenile 090.40
  taboparesis 094.1
    juvenile 090.40
  tachycardia 093.89
  tendon (late) 095.7
  tertiary 097.0
    with symptoms 095.8
    cardiovascular 093.9
    central nervous system 094.9
    multiple NEC 095.8
    specified site NEC 095.8
  testis 095.8
  thorax 095.8
  throat 095.8
  thymus (gland) 095.8
  thyroid (late) 095.8
  tongue 095.8
  tonsil (lingual) 095.8
    primary 091.2
    secondary 091.3
  trachea 095.8
  tricuspid valve 093.23
  tumor, brain 094.89
  tunica vaginalis (late) 095.8
  ulcer (any site) (early) (secondary) 091.3
    late 095.9
    perforating 095.9
      foot 094.0
  urethra (stricture) 095.8
  urogenital 095.8
  uterus 095.8
  uveal tract (secondary) 091.50
    late 095.8 [363.13]
  uveitis (secondary) 091.50
    late 095.8 [363.13]
  uvula (late) 095.8
    perforated 095.8
  vagina 091.0
    late 095.8
  valvulitis NEC 093.20
  vascular 093.89
    brain or cerebral 094.89
  vein 093.89
    cerebral 094.89
  ventriculi 095.8
  vesicae urinariae 095.8
  viscera (abdominal) 095.2
    secondary 091.69
  vitreous (hemorrhage) (opacities) 095.8
  vulva 091.0
    late 095.8
    secondary 091.3
Syphiloma 095.9
  cardiovascular system 093.9
  central nervous system 094.9
  circulatory system 093.9
  congenital 090.5
Syphilophobia 300.29
Syringadenoma (M8400/0) — *see also* Neoplasm, skin, benign
  papillary (M8406/0) — *see* Neoplasm, skin, benign
Syringobulbia 336.0
Syringocarcinoma (M8400/3) — *see* Neoplasm, skin, malignant
Syringocystadenoma (M8400/0) — *see also* Neoplasm, skin, benign
  papillary (M8406/0) — *see* Neoplasm, skin, benign
Syringocystoma (M8407/0) — *see* Neoplasm, skin, benign
Syringoma (M8407/0) — *see also* Neoplasm, skin, benign
  chondroid (M8940/0) — *see* Neoplasm, by site, benign
Syringomyelia 336.0
Syringomyelitis 323.9
  late effect — *see* category 326
Syringomyelocele (*see also* Spina bifida) 741.9
Syringopontia 336.0

System, systemic — *see also* condition
  disease, combined — *see* Degeneration, combined
  fibrosclerosing syndrome 710.8
  inflammatory response syndrome (SIRS) 995.90
    due to
      infectious process 995.91
        with organ dsfunction 995.92
      non-infectious process 995.93
        with organ dysfunction 995.94
  lupus erythematosus 710.0
    inhibitor 286.5

T

Tab — *see* Tag
Tabacism 989.8
Tabacosis 989.8
Tabardillo 080
  flea-borne 081.0
  louse-borne 080
Tabes, tabetic
  with
    central nervous system syphilis 094.0
    Charcôt's joint 094.0 [713.5]
    cord bladder 094.0
    crisis, viscera (any) 094.0
    paralysis, general 094.1
    paresis (general) 094.1
    perforating ulcer 094.0
  arthropathy 094.0 [713.5]
  bladder 094.0
  bone 094.0
  cerebrospinal 094.0
  congenital 090.40
  conjugal 094.0
  dorsalis 094.0
    neurosyphilis 094.0
  early 094.0
  juvenile 090.40
  latent 094.0
  mesenterica (*see also* Tuberculosis) 014.8
  paralysis insane, general 094.1
  peripheral (nonsyphilitic) 799.8
  spasmodic 094.0
    not dorsal or dorsalis 343.9
  syphilis (cerebrospinal) 094.0
Taboparalysis 094.1
Taboparesis (remission) 094.1
  with
    Charcôt's joint 094.1 [713.5]
    cord bladder 094.1
    perforating ulcer 094.1
  juvenile 090.40
Tachyalimentation 579.3
Tachyarrhythmia, tachyrhythmia — *see also* Tachycardia
  paroxysmal with sinus bradycardia 427.81
Tachycardia 785.0
  atrial 427.89
  auricular 427.89
  newborn 779.82
  nodal 427.89
    nonparoxysmal atrioventricular 426.89
    nonparoxysmal atrioventricular (nodal) 426.89
  paroxysmal 427.2
    with sinus bradycardia 427.81
    atrial (PAT) 427.0
      psychogenic 316 [427.0]
    atrioventricular (AV) 427.0
      psychogenic 316 [427.0]
    essential 427.2
    junctional 427.0
    nodal 427.0
    psychogenic 316 [427.2]
      atrial 316 [427.0]
      supraventricular 316 [427.0]
      ventricular 316 [427.1]
    supraventricular 427.0
      psychogenic 316 [427.0]
    ventricular 427.1
      psychogenic 316 [427.1]
  postoperative 997.1
  psychogenic 306.2
  sick sinus 427.81

Tachycardia — *continued*
  sinoauricular 427.89
  sinus 427.89
  supraventricular 427.89
  ventricular (paroxysmal) 427.1
    psychogenic 316 [427.1]
Tachypnea 786.06
  hysterical 300.11
  newborn (idiopathic) (transitory) 770.6
  psychogenic 306.1
  transitory, of newborn 770.6
Taenia (infection) (infestation) (*see also* Infestation, taenia) 123.3
  diminuta 123.6
  echinococcal infestation (*see also* Echinococcus) 122.9
  nana 123.6
  saginata infestation 123.2
  solium (intestinal form) 123.0
    larval form 123.1
Taeniasis (intestine) (*see also* Infestation, Taenia) 123.3
  saginata 123.2
  solium 123.0
Taenzer's disease 757.4
Tag (hypertrophied skin) (infected) 701.9
  adenoid 474.8
  anus 455.9
  endocardial (*see also* Endocarditis) 424.90
  hemorrhoidal 455.9
  hymen 623.8
  perineal 624.8
  preauricular 744.1
  rectum 455.9
  sentinel 455.9
  skin 701.9
    accessory 757.39
    anus 455.9
    congenital 757.39
    preauricular 744.1
    rectum 455.9
  tonsil 474.8
  urethra, urethral 599.84
  vulva 624.8
Tahyna fever 062.5
Takayasu (-Onishi) disease or syndrome (pulseless disease) 446.7
Talc granuloma 728.82
Talcosis 502
Talipes (congenital) 754.70
  acquired NEC 736.79
    planus 734
  asymmetric 754.79
    acquired 736.79
  calcaneovalgus 754.62
    acquired 736.76
  calcaneovarus 754.59
    acquired 736.76
  calcaneus 754.79
    acquired 736.76
  cavovarus 754.59
    acquired 736.75
  cavus 754.71
    acquired 736.73
  equinovalgus 754.69
    acquired 736.72
  equinovarus 754.51
    acquired 736.71
  equinus 754.79
    acquired, NEC 736.72
  percavus 754.71
    acquired 736.73
  planovalgus 754.69
    acquired 736.79
  planus (acquired) (any degree) 734
    congenital 754.61
    due to rickets 268.1
  valgus 754.60
    acquired 736.79
  varus 754.50
    acquired 736.79
Talma's disease 728.85
Tamponade heart (Rose's) (*see also* Pericarditis) 423.9
Tanapox 078.89

Index to Diseases

Tangier disease (familial high-density lipoprotein deficiency) 272.5
Tank ear 380.12
Tantrum (childhood) (*see also* Disturbance, conduct) 312.1 ✓5ᵗʰ
Tapeworm (infection) (infestation) (*see also* Infestation, tapeworm) 123.9
Tapia's syndrome 352.6
Tarantism 297.8
Target-oval cell anemia 282.4
Tarlov's cyst 355.9
Tarral-Besnier disease (pityriasis rubra pilaris) 696.4
Tarsalgia 729.2
Tarsal tunnel syndrome 355.5
Tarsitis (eyelid) 373.00
  syphilitic 095.8 [373.00]
  tuberculous (*see also* Tuberculosis) 017.0 ✓5ᵗʰ [373.4]
Tartar (teeth) 523.6
Tattoo (mark) 709.09
Taurodontism 520.2
Taussig-Bing defect, heart, or syndrome (transposition, aorta and overriding pulmonary artery) 745.11
Tay's choroiditis 363.41
Tay-Sachs
  amaurotic familial idiocy 330.1
  disease 330.1
Taybi's syndrome (otopalatodigital) 759.89
Taylor's
  disease (diffuse idiopathic cutaneous atrophy) 701.8
  syndrome 625.5
Tear, torn (traumatic) — *see also* Wound, open, by site
  anus, anal (sphincter) 863.89
    with open wound in cavity 863.99
    complicating delivery 664.2 ✓5ᵗʰ
      with mucosa 664.3 ✓5ᵗʰ
    nontraumatic, nonpuerperal 565.0
  articular cartilage, old (*see also* Disorder, cartilage, articular) 718.0 ✓5ᵗʰ
  bladder
    with
      abortion — *see* Abortion, by type, with damage to pelvic organs
      ectopic pregnancy (*see also* categories 633.0-633.9) 639.2
      molar pregnancy (*see also* categories 630-632) 639.2
    following
      abortion 639.2
      ectopic or molar pregnancy 639.2
    obstetrical trauma 665.5 ✓5ᵗʰ
  bowel
    with
      abortion — *see* Abortion, by type, with damage to pelvic organs
      ectopic pregnancy (*see also* categories 633.0-633.9) 639.2
      molar pregnancy (*see also* categories 630-632) 639.2
    following
      abortion 639.2
      ectopic or molar pregnancy 639.2
    obstetrical trauma 665.5 ✓5ᵗʰ
  broad ligament
    with
      abortion — *see* Abortion, by type, with damage to pelvic organs
      ectopic pregnancy (*see also* categories 633.0-633.9) 639.2
      molar pregnancy (*see also* categories 630-632) 639.2
    following
      abortion 639.2
      ectopic or molar pregnancy 639.2
    obstetrical trauma 665.6 ✓5ᵗʰ
  bucket handle (knee) (meniscus) — *see* Tear, meniscus

Tear, torn — *see also* Wound, open, by site — *continued*
  capsule
    joint — *see* Sprain, by site
    spleen — *see* Laceration, spleen, capsule
  cartilage — *see also* Sprain, by site
    articular, old (*see also* Disorder, cartilage, articular) 718.0 ✓5ᵗʰ
    knee — *see* Tear, meniscus
    semilunar (knee) (current injury) — *see* Tear, meniscus
  cervix
    with
      abortion — *see* Abortion, by type, with damage to pelvic organs
      ectopic pregnancy (*see also* categories 633.0-633.9) 639.2
      molar pregnancy (*see also* categories 630-632) 639.2
    following
      abortion 639.2
      ectopic or molar pregnancy 639.2
    obstetrical trauma (current) 665.3 ✓5ᵗʰ
    old 622.3
  internal organ (abdomen, chest, or pelvis) — *see* Injury, internal, by site
  ligament — *see also* Sprain, by site
    with open wound — *see* Wound, open by site
  meniscus (knee) (current injury) 836.2
    bucket handle 836.0
      old 717.0
    lateral 836.1
      anterior horn 836.1
        old 717.42
      bucket handle 836.1
        old 717.41
      old 717.40
      posterior horn 836.1
        old 717.43
      specified site NEC 836.1
        old 717.49
    medial 836.0
      anterior horn 836.0
        old 717.1
      bucket handle 836.0
        old 717.0
      old 717.3
      posterior horn 836.0
        old 717.2
    old NEC 717.5
    site other than knee — *see* Sprain, by site
  muscle — *see also* Sprain, by site
    with open wound — *see* Wound, open by site
  pelvic
    floor, complicating delivery 664.1 ✓5ᵗʰ
    organ NEC
      with
        abortion — *see* Abortion, by type, with damage to pelvic organs
        ectopic pregnancy (*see also* categories 633.0-633.9) 639.2
        molar pregnancy (*see also* categories 630-632) 639.2
      following
        abortion 639.2
        ectopic or molar pregnancy 639.2
      obstetrical trauma 665.5 ✓5ᵗʰ
  perineum — *see also* Laceration, perineum
    obstetrical trauma 665.5 ✓5ᵗʰ
  periurethral tissue
    with
      abortion — *see* Abortion, by type, with damage to pelvic organs
      ectopic pregnancy (*see also* categories 633.0-633.9) 639.2
      molar pregnancy (*see also* categories 630-632) 639.2
    following
      abortion 639.2
      ectopic or molar pregnancy 639.2
    obstetrical trauma 665.5 ✓5ᵗʰ
  rectovaginal septum — *see* Laceration, rectovaginal septum
  retina, retinal (recent) (with detachment) 361.00

Tear, torn — *see also* Wound, open, by site — *continued*
  retina, retinal — *continued*
    without detachment 361.30
    dialysis (juvenile) (with detachment) 361.04
    giant (with detachment) 361.03
    horseshoe (without detachment) 361.32
    multiple (with detachment) 361.02
      without detachment 361.33
    old
      delimited (partial) 361.06
      partial 361.06
      total or subtotal 361.07
    partial (without detachment)
      giant 361.03
      multiple defects 361.02
      old (delimited) 361.06
      single defect 361.01
    round hole (without detachment) 361.31
    single defect (with detachment) 361.01
    total or subtotal (recent) 361.05
      old 361.07
  rotator cuff (traumatic) 840.4
    current injury 840.4
    degenerative 726.10
    nontraumatic 727.61
  semilunar cartilage, knee (*see also* Tear, meniscus) 836.2
    old 717.5
  tendon — *see also* Sprain, by site
    with open wound — *see* Wound, open by site
  tentorial, at birth 767.0
  umbilical cord
    affecting fetus or newborn 772.0
    complicating delivery 663.8 ✓5ᵗʰ
  urethra
    with
      abortion — *see* Abortion, by type, with damage to pelvic organs
      ectopic pregnancy (*see also* categories 633.0-633.9) 639.2
      molar pregnancy (*see also* categories 630-632) 639.2
    following
      abortion 639.2
      ectopic or molar pregnancy 639.2
    obstetrical trauma 665.5 ✓5ᵗʰ
  uterus — *see* Injury, internal, uterus
  vagina — *see* Laceration, vagina
  vessel, from catheter 998.2
  vulva, complicating delivery 664.0 ✓5ᵗʰ
Tear stone 375.57
Teeth, tooth — *see also* condition
  grinding 306.8
Teething 520.7
  syndrome 520.7
Tegmental syndrome 344.89
Telangiectasia, telangiectasis (verrucous) 448.9
  ataxic (cerebellar) 334.8
  familial 448.0
  hemorrhagic, hereditary (congenital) (senile) 448.0
  hereditary hemorrhagic 448.0
  retina 362.15
  spider 448.1
Telecanthus (congenital) 743.63
Telescoped bowel or intestine (*see also* Intussusception) 560.0
Teletherapy, adverse effect NEC 990
Telogen effluvium 704.02
Temperature
  body, high (of unknown origin) (*see also* Pyrexia) 780.6
  cold, trauma from 991.9
    newborn 778.2
    specified effect NEC 991.8
  high
    body (of unknown origin) (*see also* Pyrexia) 780.6
    trauma from — *see* Heat
Temper tantrum (childhood) (*see also* Disturbance, conduct) 312.1 ✓5ᵗʰ
Temple — *see* condition

Temporal — see also condition
  lobe syndrome 310.0
Temporomandibular joint-pain-dysfunction syndrome 524.60
Temporosphenoidal — see condition
Tendency
  bleeding (see also Defect, coagulation) 286.9
  homosexual, ego-dystonic 302.0
  paranoid 301.0
  suicide 300.9
Tenderness
  abdominal (generalized) (localized) 789.6 ✓5
  rebound 789.6 ✓5
  skin 782.0
Tendinitis, tendonitis (see also Tenosynovitis) 726.90
  Achilles 726.71
  adhesive 726.90
    shoulder 726.0
  calcific 727.82
    shoulder 726.11
  gluteal 726.5
  patellar 726.64
  peroneal 726.79
  pes anserinus 726.61
  psoas 726.5
  tibialis (anterior) (posterior) 726.72
  trochanteric 726.5
Tendon — see condition
Tendosynovitis — see Tenosynovitis
Tendovaginitis — see Tenosynovitis
Tenesmus 787.99
  rectal 787.99
  vesical 788.9
Tenia — see Taenia
Teniasis — see Taeniasis
Tennis elbow 726.32
Tenonitis — see also Tenosynovitis
  eye (capsule) 376.04
Tenontosynovitis — see Tenosynovitis
Tenontothecitis — see Tenosynovitis
Tenophyte 727.9
Tenosynovitis 727.00
  adhesive 726.90
    shoulder 726.0
  ankle 727.06
  bicipital (calcifying) 726.12
  buttock 727.09
  due to crystals — see Arthritis, due to crystals
  elbow 727.09
  finger 727.05
  foot 727.06
  gonococcal 098.51
  hand 727.05
  hip 727.09
  knee 727.09
  radial styloid 727.04
  shoulder 726.10
    adhesive 726.0
  spine 720.1
  supraspinatus 726.10
  toe 727.06
  tuberculous — see Tuberculosis, tenosynovitis
  wrist 727.05
Tenovaginitis — see Tenosynovitis
Tension
  arterial, high (see also Hypertension) 401.9
    without diagnosis of hypertension 796.2
  headache 307.81
  intraocular (elevated) 365.00
  nervous 799.2
  ocular (elevated) 365.00
  pneumothorax 512.0
    iatrogenic 512.1
    postoperative 512.1
    spontaneous 512.0
  premenstrual 625.4
  state 300.9
Tentorium — see condition
Teratencephalus 759.89
Teratism 759.7
Teratoblastoma (malignant) (M9080/3) — see Neoplasm, by site, malignant

Teratocarcinoma (M9081/3) — see also Neoplasm, by site, malignant
  liver 155.0
Teratoma (solid) (M9080/1) — see also Neoplasm, by site, uncertain behavior
  adult (cystic) (M9080/0) — see Neoplasm, by site, benign
  and embryonal carcinoma, mixed (M9081/3) — see Neoplasm, by site, malignant
  benign (M9080/0) — see Neoplasm, by site, benign
  combined with choriocarcinoma (M9101/3) — see Neoplasm, by site, malignant
  cystic (adult) (M9080/0) — see Neoplasm, by site, benign
  differentiated type (M9080/0) — see Neoplasm, by site, benign
  embryonal (M9080/3) — see also Neoplasm, by site, malignant
    liver 155.0
  fetal
    sacral, causing fetopelvic disproportion 653.7 ✓5
  immature (M9080/3) — see Neoplasm, by site, malignant
  liver (M9080/3) 155.0
    adult, benign, cystic, differentiated type or mature (M9080/0) 211.5
  malignant (M9080/3) — see also Neoplasm, by site, malignant
    anaplastic type (M9082/3) — see Neoplasm, by site, malignant
    intermediate type (M9083/3) — see Neoplasm, by site, malignant
    liver (M9080/3) 155.0
    trophoblastic (M9102/3)
      specified site — see Neoplasm, by site, malignant
      unspecified site 186.9
    undifferentiated type (M9082/3) — see Neoplasm, by site, malignant
  mature (M9080/0) — see Neoplasm, by site, benign
  ovary (M9080/0) 220
    embryonal, immature, or malignant (M9080/3) 183.0
  suprasellar (M9080/3) — see Neoplasm, by site, malignant
  testis (M9080/3) 186.9
    adult, benign, cystic, differentiated type or mature (M9080/0) 222.0
  undescended 186.0
Terminal care V66.7
Termination
  anomalous — see also Malposition, congenital
    portal vein 747.49
    right pulmonary vein 747.42
  pregnancy (legal) (therapeutic) (see Abortion, legal) 635.9 ✓5
    fetus NEC 779.6
  illegal (see also Abortion, illegal) 636.9 ✓5
Ternidens diminutus infestation 127.7
Terrors, night (child) 307.46
Terry's syndrome 362.21
Tertiary — see condition
Tessellated fundus, retina (tigroid) 362.89
Test(s)
  AIDS virus V72.6
  adequacy
    hemodialysis V56.31
    peritoneal dialysis V56.32
  allergen V72.7
  bacterial disease NEC (see also Screening, by name of disease) V74.9
  basal metabolic rate V72.6
  blood-alcohol V70.4
  blood-drug V70.4
    for therapeutic drug monitoring V58.83
  developmental, infant or child V20.2
  Dick V74.8
  fertility V26.21
  genetic V26.3
  hearing V72.1
  HIV V72.6
  human immunodeficiency virus V72.6
  Kveim V82.89

Test(s) — continued
  laboratory V72.6
    for medicolegal reason V70.4
  Mantoux (for tuberculosis) V74.1
  mycotic organism V75.4
  parasitic agent NEC V75.8
  paternity V70.4
  peritoneal equilibration V56.32
  pregnancy
    positive V22.1
      first pregnancy V22.0
    unconfirmed V72.4
  preoperative V72.84
    cardiovascular V72.81
    respiratory V72.82
    specified NEC V72.83
  procreative management NEC V26.29
  sarcoidosis V82.89
  Schick V74.3
  Schultz-Charlton V74.8
  skin, diagnostic
    allergy V72.7
    bacterial agent NEC (see also Screening, by name of disease) V74.9
    Dick V74.8
    hypersensitivity V72.7
    Kveim V82.89
    Mantoux V74.1
    mycotic organism V75.4
    parasitic agent NEC V75.8
    sarcoidosis V82.89
    Schick V74.3
    Schultz-Charlton V74.8
    tuberculin V74.1
  specified type NEC V72.8 ✓5
  tuberculin V74.1
  vision V72.0
  Wassermann
    positive (see also Serology for syphilis, positive) 097.1
      false 795.6
Testicle, testicular, testis — see also condition
  feminization (syndrome) 257.8
Tetanus, tetanic (cephalic) (convulsions) 037
  with
    abortion — see Abortion, by type, with sepsis
    ectopic pregnancy (see also categories 633.0-633.9) 639.0
    molar pregnancy (see categories 630-632) 639.0
  following
    abortion 639.0
    ectopic or molar pregnancy 639.0
  inoculation V03.7
    reaction (due to serum) — see Complications, vaccination
  neonatorum 771.3
  puerperal, postpartum, childbirth 670 ✓4
Tetany, tetanic 781.7
  alkalosis 276.3
  associated with rickets 268.0
  convulsions 781.7
    hysterical 300.11
  functional (hysterical) 300.11
  hyperkinetic 781.7
    hysterical 300.11
  hyperpnea 786.01
    hysterical 300.11
    psychogenic 306.1
  hyperventilation 786.01
    hysterical 300.11
    psychogenic 306.1
  hypocalcemic, neonatal 775.4
  hysterical 300.11
  neonatal 775.4
  parathyroid (gland) 252.1
  parathyroprival 252.1
  postoperative 252.1
  postthyroidectomy 252.1
  pseudotetany 781.7
    hysterical 300.11
  psychogenic 306.1
    specified as conversion reaction 300.11
Tetralogy of Fallot 745.2
Tetraplegia — see Quadriplegia

Index to Diseases

Thailand hemorrhagic fever 065.4
Thalassanemia 282.4
Thalassemia (alpha) (beta) (disease) (Hb-C) (Hb-D) (Hb-E) (Hb-H) (Hb-I) (Hb-S) (high fetal gene) (high fetal hemoglobin) (intermedia) (major) (minima) (minor) (mixed) (sickle-cell) (trait) (with other hemoglobinopathy) 282.4
Thalassemic variants 282.4
Thaysen-Gee disease (nontropical sprue) 579.0
Thecoma (M8600/0) 220
   malignant (M8600/3) 183.0
Thelarche, precocious 259.1
Thelitis 611.0
   puerperal, postpartum 675.0 ✓5th
Therapeutic — see condition
Therapy V57.9
   blood transfusion, without reported diagnosis V58.2
   breathing V57.0
   chemotherapy V58.1
      fluoride V07.31
      prophylactic NEC V07.39
   dialysis (intermittent) (treatment)
      extracorporeal V56.0
      peritoneal V56.8
      renal V56.0
      specified type NEC V56.8
   exercise NEC V57.1
      breathing V57.0
   extracorporeal dialysis (renal) V56.0
   fluoride prophylaxis V07.31
   hemodialysis V56.0
   long term oxygen therapy V46.2
   occupational V57.21
   orthoptic V57.4
   orthotic V57.81
   peritoneal dialysis V56.8
   physical NEC V57.1
   postmenopausal hormone replacement V07.4
   radiation V58.0
   speech V57.3
   vocational V57.22
Thermalgesia 782.0
Thermalgia 782.0
Thermanalgesia 782.0
Thermanesthesia 782.0
Thermic — see condition
Thermography (abnormal) 793.9
   breast 793.89
Thermoplegia 992.0
Thesaurismosis
   amyloid 277.3
   bilirubin 277.4
   calcium 275.40
   cystine 270.0
   glycogen (see also Disease, glycogen storage) 271.0
   kerasin 272.7
   lipoid 272.7
   melanin 255.4
   phosphatide 272.7
   urate 274.9
Thiaminic deficiency 265.1
   with beriberi 265.0
Thibierge-Weissenbach syndrome (cutaneous systemic sclerosis) 710.1
Thickened endometrium 793.5
Thickening
   bone 733.99
      extremity 733.99
   breast 611.79
   hymen 623.3
   larynx 478.79
   nail 703.8
      congenital 757.5
   periosteal 733.99
   pluera (see also Pleurisy) 511.0
   skin 782.8
   subepiglottic 478.79
   tongue 529.8
   valve, heart — see Endocarditis
Thiele syndrome 724.6
Thigh — see condition

Thinning vertebra (see also Osteoporosis) 733.00
Thirst, excessive 783.5
   due to deprivation of water 994.3
Thomsen's disease 359.2
Thomson's disease (congenital poikiloderma) 757.33
Thoracic — see also condition
   kidney 753.3
   outlet syndrome 353.0
   stomach — see Hernia, diaphragm
Thoracogastroschisis (congenital) 759.89
Thoracopagus 759.4
Thoracoschisis 756.3
Thorax — see condition
Thorn's syndrome (see also Disease, renal) 593.9
Thornwaldt's, Tornwaldt's
   bursitis (pharyngeal) 478.29
   cyst 478.26
   disease (pharyngeal bursitis) 478.29
Thorson-Biörck syndrome (malignant carcinoid) 259.2
Threadworm (infection) (infestation) 127.4
Threatened
   abortion or miscarriage 640.0 ✓5th
      with subsequent abortion (see also Abortion, spontaneous) 634.9 ✓5th
      affecting fetus 762.1
   labor 644.1 ✓5th
      affecting fetus or newborn 761.8
      premature 644.0 ✓5th
   miscarriage 640.0 ✓5th
      affecting fetus 762.1
   premature
      delivery 644.2 ✓5th
         affecting fetus or newborn 761.8
      labor 644.0 ✓5th
         before 22 completed weeks gestation 640.0 ✓5th
Three-day fever 066.0
Threshers' lung 495.0
Thrix annulata (congenital) 757.4
Throat — see condition
Thrombasthenia (Glanzmann's) (hemorrhagic) (hereditary) 287.1
Thromboangiitis 443.1
   obliterans (general) 443.1
      cerebral 437.1
      vessels
         brain 437.1
         spinal cord 437.1
Thromboarteritis — see Arteritis
Thromboasthenia (Glanzmann's) (hemorrhagic) (hereditary) 287.1
Thrombocytasthenia (Glanzmann's) 287.1
Thrombocythemia (essential) (hemorrhagic) (primary) (M9962/1) 238.7
   idiopathic (M9962/1) 238.7
Thrombocytopathy (dystrophic) (granulopenic) 287.1
Thrombocytopenia, thrombocytopenic 287.5
   with giant hemangioma 287.3
   amegakaryocytic, congenital 287.3
   congenital 287.3
   cyclic 287.3
   dilutional 287.4
   due to
      drugs 287.4
      extracorporeal circulation of blood 287.4
      massive blood transfusion 287.4
      platelet alloimmunization 287.4
   essential 287.3
   hereditary 287.3
   Kasabach-Merritt 287.3
   neonatal, transitory 776.1
      due to
         exchange transfusion 776.1
         idiopathic maternal thrombocytopenia 776.1
         isoimmunization 776.1
   primary 287.3
   puerperal, postpartum 666.3 ✓5th

Thrombocytopenia, thrombocytopenic — continued
   purpura (see also Purpura, thrombocytopenic) 287.3
      thrombotic 446.6
   secondary 287.4
   sex-linked 287.3
Thrombocytosis, essential 289.9
Thromboembolism — see Embolism
Thrombopathy (Bernard-Soulier) 287.1
   constitutional 286.4
   Willebrand-Jürgens (angiohemophilia) 286.4
Thrombopenia (see also Thrombocytopenia) 287.5
Thrombophlebitis 451.9
   antecubital vein 451.82
   antepartum (superficial) 671.2 ✓5th
      affecting fetus or newborn 760.3
      deep 671.3 ✓5th
   arm 451.89
      deep 451.83
      superficial 451.82
   breast, superficial 451.89
   cavernous (venous) sinus — see Thrombophlebitis, intracranial venous sinus
   cephalic vein 451.82
   cerebral (sinus) (vein) 325
      late effect — see category 326
      nonpyogenic 437.6
         in pregnancy or puerperium 671.5 ✓5th
         late effect — see Late effect(s) (of) cerebrovascular disease
   due to implanted device — see Complications, due to (presence of) any device, implant or graft classified to 996.0-996.5 NEC
   during or resulting from a procedure NEC 997.2
   femoral 451.11
   femoropopliteal 451.19
   following infusion, perfusion, or transfusion 999.2
   hepatic (vein) 451.89
   idiopathic, recurrent 453.1
   iliac vein 451.81
   iliofemoral 451.11
   intracranial venous sinus (any) 325
      late effect — see category 326
      nonpyogenic 437.6
         in pregnancy or puerperium 671.5 ✓5th
         late effect — see Late effect(s) (of) cerebrovascular disease
   jugular vein 451.89
   lateral (venous) sinus — see Thrombophlebitis, intracranial venous sinus
   leg 451.2
      deep (vessels) 451.19
         femoral vein 451.11
         specified vessel NEC 451.19
      superficial (vessels) 451.0
         femoral vein 451.11
   longitudinal (venous) sinus — see Thrombophlebitis, intracranial venous sinus
   lower extremity 451.2
      deep (vessels) 451.19
         femoral vein 451.11
         specified vessel NEC 451.19
      superficial (vessels) 451.0
   migrans, migrating 453.1
   pelvic
      with
         abortion — see Abortion, by type, with sepsis
         ectopic pregnancy — (see also categories 633.0-633.9) 639.0
         molar pregnancy — (see also categories 630-632) 639.0
      following
         abortion 639.0
         ectopic or molar pregnancy 639.0
      puerperal 671.4 ✓5th
   popliteal vein 451.19
   portal (vein) 572.1
   postoperative 997.2
   pregnancy (superficial) 671.2 ✓5th
      affecting fetus or newborn 760.3

Thrombophlebitis — continued
pregnancy — continued
 deep 671.3 ✓5
 puerperal, postpartum, childbirth (extremities) (superficial) 671.2 ✓5
  deep 671.4 ✓5
  pelvic 671.4 ✓5
  specified site NEC 671.5 ✓5
radial vein 451.83
saphenous (greater) (lesser) 451.0
sinus (intracranial) — see Thrombophlebitis, intracranial venous sinus
specified site NEC 451.89
tibial vein 451.19

Thrombosis, thrombotic (marantic) (multiple) (progressive) (septic) (vein) (vessel) 453.9
with childbirth or during the puerperium — see Thrombosis, puerperal, postpartum
antepartum — see Thrombosis, pregnancy
aorta, aortic 444.1
 abdominal 444.0
 bifurcation 444.0
 saddle 444.0
 terminal 444.0
 thoracic 444.1
 valve — see Endocarditis, aortic
apoplexy (see also Thrombosis, brain) 434.0 ✓5
 late effect — see Late effect(s) (of) cerebrovascular disease
appendix, septic — see Appendicitis, acute
arteriolar-capillary platelet, disseminated 446.6
artery, arteries (postinfectional) 444.9
 auditory, internal 433.8 ✓5
 basilar (see also Occlusion, artery, basilar) 433.0 ✓5
 carotid (common) (internal) (see also Occlusion, artery, carotid) 433.1 ✓5
  with other precerebral artery 433.3 ✓5
 cerebellar (anterior inferior) (posterior inferior) (superior) 433.8 ✓5
 cerebral (see also Thrombosis, brain) 434.0 ✓5
 choroidal (anterior) 433.8 ✓5
 communicating posterior 433.8 ✓5
 coronary (see also Infarct, myocardium) 410.9 ✓5
  without myocardial infarction 411.81
  due to syphilis 093.89
  healed or specified as old 412
 extremities 444.22
  lower 444.22
  upper 444.21
 femoral 444.22
 hepatic 444.89
 hypophyseal 433.8 ✓5
 meningeal, anterior or posterior 433.8 ✓5
 mesenteric (with gangrene) 557.0
 ophthalmic (see also Occlusion, retina) 362.30
 pontine 433.8 ✓5
 popliteal 444.22
 precerebral — see Occlusion, artery, precerebral NEC
 pulmonary 415.19
  iatrogenic 415.11
  postoperative 415.11
 renal 593.81
 retinal (see also Occlusion, retina) 362.30
 specified site NEC 444.89
 spinal, anterior or posterior 433.8 ✓5
  traumatic (complication) (early) (see also Injury, blood vessel, by site) 904.9
 vertebral (see also Occlusion, artery, vertebral) 433.2 ✓5
  with other precerebral artery 433.3 ✓5
atrial (endocardial) 424.90
 due to syphilis 093.89
auricular (see also Infarct, myocardium) 410.9 ✓5
axillary (vein) 453.8
basilar (artery) (see also Occlusion, artery, basilar) 433.0 ✓5
bland NEC 453.9
brain (artery) (stem) 434.0 ✓5
 due to syphilis 094.89
 iatrogenic 997.02

Thrombosis, thrombotic — continued
brain — continued
 late effect — see Late effect(s) (of) cerebrovascular disease
 postoperative 997.02
 puerperal, postpartum, childbirth 674.0 ✓5
 sinus (see also Thrombosis, intracranial venous sinus) 325
capillary 448.9
 arteriolar, generalized 446.6
cardiac (see also Infarct, myocardium) 410.9 ✓5
 due to syphilis 093.89
 healed or specified as old 412
 valve — see Endocarditis
carotid (artery) (common) (internal) (see also Occlusion, artery, carotid) 433.1 ✓5
 with other precerebral artery 433.3 ✓5
cavernous sinus (venous) — see Thrombosis, intracranial venous sinus
cerebellar artery (anterior inferior) (posterior inferior) (superior) 433.8 ✓5
 late effect — see Late effect(s) (of) cerebrovascular disease
cerebral (arteries) (see also Thrombosis, brain) 434.0 ✓5
 late effect — see Late effect(s) (of) cerebrovascular disese
coronary (artery) (see also Infarct, myocardium) 410.9 ✓5
 without myocardial infarction 411.81
 due to syphilis 093.89
 healed or specified as old 412
corpus cavernosum 607.82
cortical (see also Thrombosis, brain) 434.0 ✓5
due to (presence of) any device, implant, or graft classifiable to 996.0-996.5 — see Complications, due to (presence of) any device, implant, or graft classified to 996.0-996.5 NEC
effort 453.8
endocardial — see Infarct, myocardium
eye (see also Occlusion, retina) 362.30
femoral (vein) (deep) 453.8
 with inflammation or phlebitis 451.11
 artery 444.22
genital organ, male 608.83
heart (chamber) (see also Infarct, myocardium) 410.9 ✓5
hepatic (vein) 453.0
 artery 444.89
 infectional or septic 572.1
iliac (vein) 453.8
 with inflammation or phlebitis 451.81
 artery (common) (external) (internal) 444.81
inflammation, vein — see Thrombophlebitis
internal carotid artery (see also Occlusion, artery, carotid) 433.1 ✓5
 with other precerebral artery 433.3 ✓5
intestine (with gangrene) 557.0
intracranial (see also Thrombosis, brain) 434.0 ✓5
 venous sinus (any) 325
  nonpyogenic origin 437.6
  in pregnancy or puerperium 671.5 ✓5
intramural (see also Infarct, myocardium) 410.9 ✓5
 without
  cardiac condition 429.89
  coronary artery disease 429.89
  myocardial infarction 429.89
 healed or specified as old 412
jugular (bulb) 453.8
kidney 593.81
 artery 593.81
lateral sinus (venous) — see Thrombosis, intracranial venous sinus
leg 453.8
 with inflammation or phlebitis — see Thrombophlebitis
 deep (vessels) 453.8
 superficial (vessels) 453.8
liver (venous) 453.0
 artery 444.89
 infectional or septic 572.1
 portal vein 452
longitudinal sinus (venous) — see Thrombosis, intracranial venous sinus

Thrombosis, thrombotic — continued
lower extremity — see Thrombosis, leg
lung 415.19
 iatrogenic 415.11
 postoperative 415.11
marantic, dural sinus 437.6
meninges (brain) (see also Thrombosis, brain) 434.0 ✓5
mesenteric (artery) (with gangrene) 557.0
 vein (inferior) (superior) 557.0
mitral — see Insufficiency, mitral
mural (heart chamber) (see also Infarct, myocardium) 410.9 ✓5
 without
  cardiac condition 429.89
  coronary artery disease 429.89
  myocardial infarction 429.89
 due to syphilis 093.89
 following myocardial infarction 429.79
 healed or specified as old 412
omentum (with gangrene) 557.0
ophthalmic (artery) (see also Occlusion, retina) 362.30
pampiniform plexus (male) 608.83
 female 620.8
parietal (see also Infarct, myocardium) 410.9 ✓5
penis, penile 607.82
peripheral arteries 444.22
 lower 444.22
 upper 444.21
platelet 446.6
portal 452
 due to syphilis 093.89
 infectional or septic 572.1
precerebral artery — see also Occlusion, artery, precerebral NEC
pregnancy 671.9 ✓5
 deep (vein) 671.3 ✓5
 superficial (vein) 671.2 ✓5
puerperal, postpartum, childbirth 671.9 ✓5
 brain (artery) 674.0 ✓5
  venous 671.5 ✓5
 cardiac 674.8 ✓5
 cerebral (artery) 674.0 ✓5
  venous 671.5 ✓5
 deep (vein) 671.4 ✓5
 intracranial sinus (nonpyogenic) (venous) 671.5 ✓5
 pelvic 671.4 ✓5
 pulmonary (artery) 673.2 ✓5
 specified site NEC 671.5 ✓5
 superficial 671.2 ✓5
pulmonary (artery) (vein) 415.19
 iatrogenic 415.11
 postoperative 415.11
renal (artery) 593.81
 vein 453.3
resulting from presence of shunt or other internal prosthetic device — see Complications, due to (presence of) any device, implant, or graft classified to 996.0-996.5 NEC
retina, retinal (artery) 362.30
 arterial branch 362.32
 central 362.31
 partial 362.33
 vein
  central 362.35
  tributary (branch) 362.36
scrotum 608.83
seminal vesicle 608.83
sigmoid (venous) sinus (see Thrombosis, intracranial venous sinus) 325
silent NEC 453.9
sinus, intracranial (venous) (any) (see also Thrombosis, intracranial venous sinus) 325
softening, brain (see also Thrombosis, brain) 434.0 ✓5
specified site NEC 453.8
spermatic cord 608.83
spinal cord 336.1
 due to syphilis 094.89
 in pregnancy or puerperium 671.5 ✓5
 pyogenic origin 324.1
  late effect — see category 326

Index to Diseases

Thrombosis, thrombotic — *continued*
  spleen, splenic 289.59
    artery 444.89
  testis 608.83
  traumatic (complication) (early) (*see also* Injury, blood vessel, by site) 904.9
  tricuspid — *see* Endocarditis, tricuspid
  tunica vaginalis 608.83
  umbilical cord (vessels) 663.6 ✓5th
    affecting fetus or newborn 762.6
  vas deferens 608.83
  vena cava (inferior) (superior) 453.2
Thrombus — *see* Thrombosis
Thrush 112.0
  newborn 771.7
Thumb — *see also* condition
  gamekeeper's 842.12
  sucking (child problem) 307.9
Thygeson's superficial punctate keratitis 370.21
Thymergasia (*see also* Psychosis, affective) 296.80
Thymitis 254.8
Thymoma (benign) (M8580/0) 212.6
  malignant (M8580/3) 164.0
Thymus, thymic (gland) — *see* condition
Thyrocele (*see also* Goiter) 240.9
Thyroglossal — *see also* condition
  cyst 759.2
  duct, persistent 759.2
Thyroid (body) (gland) — *see also* condition
  lingual 759.2
Thyroiditis 245.9
  acute (pyogenic) (suppurative) 245.0
    nonsuppurative 245.0
  autoimmune 245.2
  chronic (nonspecific) (sclerosing) 245.8
    fibrous 245.3
    lymphadenoid 245.2
    lymphocytic 245.2
    lymphoid 245.2
  complicating pregnancy, childbirth, or puerperium 648.1 ✓5th
  de Quervain's (subacute granulomatous) 245.1
  fibrous (chronic) 245.3
  giant (cell) (follicular) 245.1
  granulomatous (de Quervain's) (subacute) 245.1
  Hashimoto's (struma lymphomatosa) 245.2
  iatrogenic 245.4
  invasive (fibrous) 245.3
  ligneous 245.3
  lymphocytic (chronic) 245.2
  lymphoid 245.2
  lymphomatous 245.2
  pseudotuberculous 245.1
  pyogenic 245.0
  radiation 245.4
  Riedel's (ligneous) 245.3
  subacute 245.1
  suppurative 245.0
  tuberculous (*see also* Tuberculosis) 017.5 ✓5th
  viral 245.1
  woody 245.3
Thyrolingual duct, persistent 759.2
Thyromegaly 240.9
Thyrotoxic
  crisis or storm (*see also* Thyrotoxicosis) 242.9 ✓5th
  heart failure (*see also* Thyrotoxicosis) 242.9 ✓5th [425.7]
Thyrotoxicosis 242.9 ✓5th

> *Note* — *Use the following fifth-digit subclassification with category 242:*
> 0 *without mention of thyrotoxic crisis or storm*
> 1 *with mention of thyrotoxic crisis or storm*

  with
    goiter (diffuse) 242.0 ✓5th
      adenomatous 242.3 ✓5th
        multinodular 242.2 ✓5th

Thyrotoxicosis — *continued*
  with — *continued*
    goiter — *continued*
      adenomatous — *continued*
        uninodular 242.1 ✓5th
        nodular 242.3 ✓5th
          multinodular 242.2 ✓5th
          uninodular 242.1 ✓5th
      infiltrative
        dermopathy 242.0 ✓5th
        ophthalmopathy 242.0 ✓5th
      thyroid acropachy 242.0 ✓5th
    complicating pregnancy, childbirth, or puerperium 648.1 ✓5th
    due to
      ectopic thyroid nodule 242.4 ✓5th
      ingestion of (excessive) thyroid material 242.8 ✓5th
      specified cause NEC 242.8 ✓5th
    factitia 242.8 ✓5th
    heart 242.9 ✓5th [425.7]
    neonatal (transient) 775.3
TIA (transient ischemic attack) 435.9
  with transient neurologic deficit 435.9
  late effect — *see* Late effect(s) (of) cerebrovascular disease
Tibia vara 732.4
Tic 307.20
  breathing 307.20
  child problem 307.21
  compulsive 307.22
  convulsive 307.20
  degenerative (generalized) (localized) 333.3
    facial 351.8
  douloureux (*see also* Neuralgia, trigeminal) 350.1
    atypical 350.2
  habit 307.20
    chronic (motor or vocal) 307.22
    transient of childhood 307.21
  lid 307.20
    transient of childhood 307.21
  motor-verbal 307.23
  occupational 300.89
  orbicularis 307.20
    transient of childhood 307.21
  organic origin 333.3
  postchoreic — *see* Chorea
  psychogenic 307.20
    compulsive 307.22
  salaam 781.0
  spasm 307.20
    chronic (motor or vocal) 307.22
    transient of childhood 307.21
Tick (-borne) fever NEC 066.1
  American mountain 066.1
  Colorado 066.1
  hemorrhagic NEC 065.3
    Crimean 065.0
    Kyasanur Forest 065.2
    Omsk 065.1
  mountain 066.1
  nonexanthematous 066.1
Tick-bite fever NEC 066.1
  African 087.1
  Colorado (virus) 066.1
  Rocky Mountain 082.0
Tick paralysis 989.5
Tics and spasms, compulsive 307.22
Tietze's disease or syndrome 733.6
Tight, tightness
  anus 564.89
  chest 786.59
  fascia (lata) 728.9
  foreskin (congenital) 605
  hymen 623.3
  introitus (acquired) (congenital) 623.3
  rectal sphincter 564.89
  tendon 727.81
    Achilles (heel) 727.81
  urethral sphincter 598.9
Tilting vertebra 737.9
Timidity, child 313.21
Tinea (intersecta) (tarsi) 110.9
  amiantacea 110.0

Tinea — *continued*
  asbestina 110.0
  barbae 110.0
  beard 110.0
  black dot 110.0
  blanca 111.2
  capitis 110.0
  corporis 110.5
  cruris 110.3
  decalvans 704.09
  flava 111.0
  foot 110.4
  furfuracea 111.0
  imbricata (Tokelau) 110.5
  lepothrix 039.0
  manuum 110.2
  microsporic (*see also* Dermatophytosis) 110.9
  nigra 111.1
  nodosa 111.2
  pedis 110.4
  scalp 110.0
  specified site NEC 110.8
  sycosis 110.0
  tonsurans 110.0
  trichophytic (*see also* Dermatophytosis) 110.9
  unguium 110.1
  versicolor 111.0
Tingling sensation (*see also* Disturbance, sensation) 782.0
Tin-miners' lung 503
Tinnitus (aurium) 388.30
  audible 388.32
  objective 388.32
  subjective 388.31
Tipping pelvis 738.6
  with disproportion (fetopelvic) 653.0 ✓5th
    affecting fetus or newborn 763.1
    causing obstructed labor 660.1 ✓5th
      affecting fetus or newborn 763.1
Tiredness 780.79
Tissue — *see* condition
Tobacco
  abuse (affecting health) NEC (*see also* Abuse, drugs, nondependent) 305.1
  heart 989.8 ✓5th
Tobias' syndrome (carcinoma, pulmonary apex) (M8010/3) 162.3
Tocopherol deficiency 269.1
Todd's
  cirrhosis — *see* Cirrhosis, biliary
  paralysis (postepileptic transitory paralysis) 344.8 ✓5th
Toe — *see* condition
Toilet, artificial opening (*see also* Attention to, artificial, opening) V55.9
Tokelau ringworm 110.5
Tollwut 071
Tolosa-Hunt syndrome 378.55
Tommaselli's disease
  correct substance properly administered 599.7
  overdose or wrong substance given or taken 961.4
Tongue — *see also* condition
  worms 134.1
Tongue tie 750.0
Toni-Fanconi syndrome (cystinosis) 270.0
Tonic pupil 379.46
Tonsil — *see* condition
Tonsillitis (acute) (catarrhal) (croupous) (follicular) (gangrenous) (infective) (lacunar) (lingual) (malignant) (membranous) (phlegmonous) (pneumococcal) (pseudomembranous) (purulent) (septic) (staphylococcal) (subacute) (suppurative) (toxic) (ulcerative) (vesicular) (viral) 463
  with influenza, flu, or grippe 487.1
  chronic 474.00
  diphtheritic (membranous) 032.0
  hypertrophic 474.00
  influenzal 487.1
  parenchymatous 475
  streptococcal 034.0
  tuberculous (*see also* Tuberculosis) 012.8 ✓5th

Tonsillitis

Tonsillitis — *continued*
    Vincent's 101
Tonsillopharyngitis 465.8
Tooth, teeth — *see* condition
Toothache 525.9
Topagnosis 782.0
Tophi (gouty) 274.0
    ear 274.81
    heart 274.82
    specified site NEC 274.82
Torn — *see* Tear, torn
Tornwaldt's bursitis (disease) (pharyngeal bursitis) 478.29
    cyst 478.26
Torpid liver 573.9
Torsion
    accessory tube 620.5
    adnexa (female) 620.5
    aorta (congenital) 747.29
        acquired 447.1
    appendix epididymis 608.2
    bile duct 576.8
        with calculus, choledocholithiasis or stones — *see* Choledocholithiasis
        congenital 751.69
    bowel, colon, or intestine 560.2
    cervix (*see also* Malposition, uterus) 621.6
    duodenum 537.3
    dystonia — *see* Dystonia, torsion
    epididymis 608.2
        appendix 608.2
    fallopian tube 620.5
    gallbladder (*see also* Disease, gallbladder) 575.8
        congenital 751.69
    gastric 537.89
    hydatid of Morgagni (female) 620.5
    kidney (pedicle) 593.89
    Meckel's diverticulum (congenital) 751.0
    mesentery 560.2
    omentum 560.2
    organ or site, congenital NEC — *see* Anomaly, specified type NEC
    ovary (pedicle) 620.5
        congenital 752.0
    oviduct 620.5
    penis 607.89
        congenital 752.69
    renal 593.89
    spasm — *see* Dystonia, torsion
    spermatic cord 608.2
    spleen 289.59
    testicle, testis 608.2
    tibia 736.89
    umbilical cord — *see* Compression, umbilical cord
    uterus (*see also* Malposition, uterus) 621.6
Torticollis (intermittent) (spastic) 723.5
    congenital 754.1
        sternomastoid 754.1
    due to birth injury 767.8
    hysterical 300.11
    ocular 781.93
    psychogenic 306.0
        specified as conversion reaction 300.11
    rheumatic 723.5
    rheumatoid 714.0
    spasmodic 333.83
    traumatic, current NEC 847.0
Tortuous
    artery 447.1
    fallopian tube 752.19
    organ or site, congenital NEC — *see* Distortion
    renal vessel, congenital 747.62
    retina vessel (congenital) 743.58
        acquired 362.17
    ureter 593.4
    urethra 599.84
    vein — *see* Varicose, vein
Torula, torular (infection) 117.5
    histolytica 117.5
    lung 117.5
Torulosis 117.5

Torus
    fracture
        fibula 823.41
            with tibia 823.42
        radius 813.45
        tibia 823.40
            with fibula 823.42
    mandibularis 526.81
    palatinus 526.81
Touch, vitreous 997.99
Touraine's syndrome (hereditary osteo-onychodysplasia) 756.89
Touraine-Solente-Golé syndrome (acropachyderma) 757.39
Tourette's disease (motor-verbal tic) 307.23
Tower skull 756.0
    with exophthalmos 756.0
Toxemia 799.8
    with
        abortion — *see* Abortion, by type, with toxemia
    bacterial — *see* Septicemia
    biliary (*see also* Disease, biliary) 576.8
    burn — *see* Burn, by site
    congenital NEC 779.89
    eclamptic 642.6
        with pre-existing hypertension 642.7
    erysipelatous (*see also* Erysipelas) 035
    fatigue 799.8
    fetus or newborn NEC 779.89
    food (*see also* Poisoning, food) 005.9
    gastric 537.89
    gastrointestinal 558.2
    intestinal 558.2
    kidney (*see also* Disease, renal) 593.9
    lung 518.89
    malarial NEC (*see also* Malaria) 084.6
    maternal (of pregnancy), affecting fetus or newborn 760.0
    myocardial — *see* Myocarditis, toxic
    of pregnancy (mild) (pre-eclamptic) 642.4
        with
            convulsions 642.6
            pre-existing hypertension 642.7
        affecting fetus or newborn 760.0
        severe 642.5
    pre-eclamptic — *see* Toxemia, of pregnancy
    puerperal, postpartum — *see* Toxemia, of pregnancy
    pulmonary 518.89
    renal (*see also* Disease, renal) 593.9
    septic (*see also* Septicemia) 038.9
    small intestine 558.2
    staphylococcal 038.10
        aureus 038.11
        due to food 005.0
        specified organism NEC 038.19
    stasis 799.8
    stomach 537.89
    uremic (*see also* Uremia) 586
    urinary 586
Toxemica cerebropathia psychica (nonalcoholic) 294.0
    alcoholic 291.1
Toxic (poisoning) — *see also* condition
    from drug or poison — *see* Table of Drugs and Chemicals
    oil syndrome 710.5
    shock syndrome 040.82
    thyroid (gland) (*see also* Thyrotoxicosis) 242.9
Toxicemia — *see* Toxemia
Toxicity
    dilantin
        asymptomatic 796.0
        symptomatic — *see* Table of Drugs and Chemicals
    drug
        asymptomatic 796.0
        symptomatic — *see* Table of Drugs and Chemicals
    fava bean 282.2
    from drug or poison
        asymptomatic 796.0
        symptomatic — *see* Table of Drugs and Chemicals

Toxicosis (*see also* Toxemia) 799.8
    capillary, hemorrhagic 287.0
Toxinfection 799.8
    gastrointestinal 558.2
Toxocariasis 128.0
Toxoplasma infection, generalized 130.9
Toxoplasmosis (acquired) 130.9
    with pneumonia 130.4
    congenital, active 771.2
    disseminated (multisystemic) 130.8
    maternal
        with suspected damage to fetus affecting management of pregnancy 655.4
        affecting fetus or newborn 760.2
            manifest toxoplasmosis in fetus or newborn 771.2
    multiple sites 130.8
    multisystemic disseminated 130.8
    specified site NEC 130.7
Trabeculation, bladder 596.8
Trachea — *see* condition
Tracheitis (acute) (catarrhal) (infantile) (membranous) (plastic) (pneumococcal) (septic) (suppurative) (viral) 464.10
    with
        bronchitis 490
            acute or subacute 466.0
            chronic 491.8
            tuberculosis — *see* Tuberculosis, pulmonary
        laryngitis (acute) 464.20
            with obstruction 464.21
            chronic 476.1
            tuberculous (*see also* Tuberculosis, larynx) 012.3
        obstruction 464.11
    chronic 491.8
        with
            bronchitis (chronic) 491.8
            laryngitis (chronic) 476.1
            due to external agent — *see* Condition, respiratory, chronic, due to
    diphtheritic (membranous) 032.3
        due to external agent — *see* Inflammation, respiratory, upper, due to
    edematous 464.11
    influenzal 487.1
    streptococcal 034.0
    syphilitic 095.8
    tuberculous (*see also* Tuberculosis) 012.8
Trachelitis (nonvenereal) (*see also* Cervicitis) 616.0
    trichomonal 131.09
Tracheobronchial — *see* condition
Tracheobronchitis (*see also* Bronchitis) 490
    acute or subacute 466.0
        with bronchospasm or obstruction 466.0
    chronic 491.8
    influenzal 487.1
    senile 491.8
Tracheobronchomegaly (congenital) 748.3
Tracheobronchopneumonitis — *see* Pneumonia, broncho
Tracheocele (external) (internal) 519.1
    congenital 748.3
Tracheomalacia 519.1
    congenital 748.3
Tracheopharyngitis (acute) 465.8
    chronic 478.9
    due to external agent — *see* Condition, respiratory, chronic, due to
    due to external agent — *see* Inflammation, respiratory, upper, due to
Tracheostenosis 519.1
    congenital 748.3
Tracheostomy
    attention to V55.0
    complication 519.00
    hemorrhage 519.09
    infection 519.01
    malfunctioning 519.02
    obstruction 519.09
    sepsis 519.01
    status V44.0

Tracheostomy — continued
  stenosis 519.02
Trachoma, trachomatous 076.9
  active (stage) 076.1
  contraction of conjunctiva 076.1
  dubium 076.0
  healed or late effect 139.1
  initial (stage) 076.0
  Türck's (chronic catarrhal laryngitis) 476.0
Trachyphonia 784.49
Training
  orthoptic V57.4
  orthotic V57.81
Train sickness 994.6
Trait
  hemoglobin
    abnormal NEC 282.7
      with thalassemia 282.4
    C (see also Disease, hemoglobin, C) 282.7
      with elliptocytosis 282.7
    S (Hb-S) 282.5
  Lepore 282.4
    with other abnormal hemoglobin NEC 282.4
  paranoid 301.0
  sickle-cell 282.5
    with
      elliptocytosis 282.5
      spherocytosis 282.5
Traits, paranoid 301.0
Tramp V60.0
Trance 780.09
  hysterical 300.13
Transaminasemia 790.4
Transfusion, blood
  donor V59.01
    stem cells V59.02
  incompatible 999.6
  reaction or complication — see Complications, transfusion
  syndrome
    fetomaternal 772.0
    twin-to-twin
      blood loss (donor twin) 772.0
      recipient twin 776.4
  without reported diagnosis V58.2
Transient — see also condition
  alteration of awareness 780.02
  blindness 368.12
  deafness (ischemic) 388.02
  global amnesia 437.7
  person (homeless) NEC V60.0
Transitional, lumbosacral joint of vertebra 756.19
Translocation
  autosomes NEC 758.5
    13-15 758.1
    16-18 758.2
    21 or 22 758.0
    balanced in normal individual 758.4
    D$_1$ 758.1
    E$_3$ 758.2
    G 758.0
  balanced autosomal in normal individual 758.4
  chromosomes NEC 758.89
  Down's syndrome 758.0
Translucency, iris 364.53
Transmission of chemical substances through the placenta (affecting fetus or newborn) 760.70
  alcohol 760.71
  anti-infective agents 760.74
  cocaine 760.75
  "crack" 760.75
  diethylstilbestrol [DES] 760.76
  hallucinogenic agents 760.73
  medicinal agents NEC 760.79
  narcotics 760.72
  obstetric anesthetic or analgesic drug 763.5
  specified agent NEC 760.79
  suspected, affecting management of pregnancy 655.5
Transplant(ed)
  bone V42.4
    marrow V42.81

Transplant(ed) — continued
  complication — see also Complications, due to (presence of) any device, implant, or graft classified to 996.0-996.5 NEC
    bone marrow 996.85
    corneal graft NEC 996.79
      infection or inflammation 996.69
      reaction 996.51
      rejection 996.51
    organ (failure) (immune or nonimmune cause) (infection) (rejection) 996.87
      bone marrow 996.85
      heart 996.83
      intestines 996.87
      kidney 996.81
      liver 996.82
      lung 996.84
      pancreas 996.86
      specified NEC 996.89
    skin NEC 996.79
      infection or inflammation 996.69
      rejection 996.52
        artificial 996.55
        decellularized allodermis 996.55
  cornea V42.5
  hair V50.0
  heart V42.1
    valve V42.2
  intestine V42.84
  kidney V42.0
  liver V42.7
  lung V42.6
  organ V42.9
    specified NEC V42.89
  pancreas V42.83
  peripheral stem cells V42.82
  skin V42.3
  stem cells, peripheral V42.82
  tissue V42.9
    specified NEC V42.89
Transplants, ovarian, endometrial 617.1
Transposed — see Transposition
Transposition (congenital) — see also Malposition, congenital
  abdominal viscera 759.3
  aorta (dextra) 745.11
  appendix 751.5
  arterial trunk 745.10
  colon 751.5
  great vessels (complete) 745.10
    both originating from right ventricle 745.11
    corrected 745.12
    double outlet right ventricle 745.11
    incomplete 745.11
    partial 745.11
    specified type NEC 745.19
  heart 746.87
    with complete transposition of viscera 759.3
  intestine (large) (small) 751.5
  pulmonary veins 747.49
  reversed jejunal (for bypass) (status) V45.3
  stomach 750.7
    with general transposition of viscera 759.3
  teeth, tooth 524.3
  vessels (complete) 745.10
    partial 745.11
  viscera (abdominal) (thoracic) 759.3
Trans-sexualism 302.50
  with
    asexual history 302.51
    heterosexual history 302.53
    homosexual history 302.52
Transverse — see also condition
  arrest (deep), in labor 660.3
    affecting fetus or newborn 763.1
  lie 652.3
    before labor, affecting fetus or newborn 761.7
    causing obstructed labor 660.0
      affecting fetus or newborn 763.1
    during labor, affecting fetus or newborn 763.1
Transvestism, transvestitism (transvestic fetishism) 302.3
Trapped placenta (with hemorrhage) 666.0
  without hemorrhage 667.0

Trauma, traumatism (see also Injury, by site) 959.9
  birth — see Birth, injury NEC
  causing hemorrhage of pregnancy or delivery 641.8
  complicating
    abortion — see Abortion, by type, with damage to pelvic organs
    ectopic pregnancy (see also categories 633.0-633.9) 639.2
    molar pregnancy (see also categories 630-632) 639.2
  during delivery NEC 665.9
  following
    abortion 639.2
    ectopic or molar pregnancy 639.2
  maternal, during pregnancy, affecting fetus or newborn 760.5
  neuroma — see Injury, nerve, by site
  previous major, affecting management of pregnancy, childbirth, or puerperium V23.8
  psychic (current) — see also Reaction, adjustment
    previous (history) V15.49
  psychologic, previous (affecting health) V15.49
  transient paralysis — see Injury, nerve, by site
Traumatic — see condition
Treacher Collins' syndrome (incomplete facial dysostosis) 756.0
Treitz's hernia — see Hernia, Treitz's
Trematode infestation NEC 121.9
Trematodiasis NEC 121.9
Trembles 988.8
Trembling paralysis (see also Parkinsonism) 332.0
Tremor 781.0
  essential (benign) 333.1
  familial 333.1
  flapping (liver) 572.8
  hereditary 333.1
  hysterical 300.11
  intention 333.1
  mercurial 985.0
  muscle 728.85
  Parkinson's (see also Parkinsonism) 332.0
  psychogenic 306.0
    specified as conversion reaction 300.11
  senilis 797
  specified type NEC 333.1
Trench
  fever 083.1
  foot 991.4
  mouth 101
  nephritis — see Nephritis, acute
Treponema pallidum infection (see also Syphilis) 097.9
Treponematosis 102.9
  due to
    T. pallidum — see Syphilis
    T. pertenue (yaws) (see also Yaws) 102.9
Triad
  Kartagener's 759.3
  Reiter's (complete) (incomplete) 099.3
  Saint's (see also Hernia, diaphragm) 553.3
Trichiasis 704.2
  cicatricial 704.2
  eyelid 374.05
    with entropion (see also Entropion) 374.00
Trichinella spiralis (infection) (infestation) 124
Trichinelliasis 124
Trichinellosis 124
Trichiniasis 124
Trichinosis 124
Trichobezoar 938
  intestine 936
  stomach 935.2
Trichocephaliasis 127.3
Trichocephalosis 127.3
Trichocephalus infestation 127.3
Trichoclasis 704.2

Trichoepithelioma

Trichoepithelioma (M8100/0) — see also Neoplasm, skin, benign
- breast 217
- genital organ NEC — see Neoplasm, by site, benign
- malignant (M8100/3) — see Neoplasm, skin, malignant

Trichofolliculoma (M8101/0) — see Neoplasm, skin, benign

Tricholemmoma (M8102/0) — see Neoplasm, skin, benign

Trichomatosis 704.2

Trichomoniasis 131.9
- bladder 131.09
- cervix 131.09
- intestinal 007.3
- prostate 131.03
- seminal vesicle 131.09
- specified site NEC 131.8
- urethra 131.02
- urogenitalis 131.00
- vagina 131.01
- vulva 131.01
- vulvovaginal 131.01

Trichomycosis 039.0
- axillaris 039.0
- nodosa 111.2
- nodularis 111.2
- rubra 039.0

Trichonocardiosis (axillaris) (palmellina) 039.0

Trichonodosis 704.2

Trichophytid, trichophyton infection (see also Dermatophytosis) 110.9

Trichophytide — see Dermatophytosis

Trichophytobezoar 938
- intestine 936
- stomach 935.2

Trichophytosis — see Dermatophytosis

Trichoptilosis 704.2

Trichorrhexis (nodosa) 704.2

Trichosporosis nodosa 111.2

Trichostasis spinulosa (congenital) 757.4

Trichostrongyliasis (small intestine) 127.6

Trichostrongylosis 127.6

Trichostrongylus (instabilis) infection 127.6

Trichotillomania 312.39

Trichromat, anomalous (congenital) 368.59

Trichromatopsia, anomalous (congenital) 368.59

Trichuriasis 127.3

Trichuris trichiuria (any site) (infection) (infestation) 127.3

Tricuspid (valve) — see condition

Trifid — see also Accessory
- kidney (pelvis) 753.3
- tongue 750.13

Trigeminal neuralgia (see also Neuralgia, trigeminal) 350.1

Trigeminoencephaloangiomatosis 759.6

Trigeminy 427.89
- postoperative 997.1

Trigger finger (acquired) 727.03
- congenital 756.89

Trigonitis (bladder) (chronic) (pseudomembranous) 595.3
- tuberculous (see also Tuberculosis) 016.1

Trigonocephaly 756.0

Trihexosidosis 272.7

Trilobate placenta — see Placenta, abnormal

Trilocular heart 745.8

Tripartita placenta — see Placenta, abnormal

Triple — see also Accessory
- kidneys 753.3
- uteri 752.2
- X female 758.81

Triplegia 344.89
- congenital or infantile 343.8

Triplet
- affected by maternal complications of pregnancy 761.5
- healthy liveborn — see Newborn, multiple

Triplet — continued
- pregnancy (complicating delivery) NEC 651.1
  - with fetal loss and retention of one or more fetus(es) 651.4

Triplex placenta — see Placenta, abnormal

Triplication — see Accessory

Trismus 781.0
- neonatorum 771.3
- newborn 771.3

Trisomy (syndrome) NEC 758.5
- 13 (partial) 758.1
- 16-18 758.2
- 18 (partial) 758.2
- 21 (partial) 758.0
- 22 758.0
- autosomes NEC 758.5
- D₁ 758.1
- E₃ 758.2
- G (group) 758.0
- group D₁ 758.1
- group E 758.2
- group G 758.0

Tritanomaly 368.53

Tritanopia 368.53

Troisier-Hanot-Chauffard syndrome (bronze diabetes) 275.0

Trombidiosis 133.8

Trophedema (hereditary) 757.0
- congenital 757.0

Trophoblastic disease (see also Hydatidiform mole) 630
- previous, affecting management of pregnancy V23.1

Tropholymphedema 757.0

Trophoneurosis NEC 356.9
- arm NEC 354.9
- disseminated 710.1
- facial 349.89
- leg NEC 355.8
- lower extremity NEC 355.8
- upper extremity NEC 354.9

Tropical — see also condition
- maceration feet (syndrome) 991.4
- wet foot (syndrome) 991.4

Trouble — see also Disease
- bowel 569.9
- heart — see Disease, heart
- intestine 569.9
- kidney (see also Disease, renal) 593.9
- nervous 799.2
- sinus (see also Sinusitis) 473.9

Trousseau's syndrome (thrombophlebitis migrans) 453.1

Truancy, childhood — see also Disturbance, conduct
- socialized 312.2
- undersocialized, unsocialized 312.1

Truncus
- arteriosus (persistent) 745.0
- common 745.0
- communis 745.0

Trunk — see condition

Trychophytide — see Dermatophytosis

Trypanosoma infestation — see Trypanosomiasis

Trypanosomiasis 086.9
- with meningoencephalitis 086.9 [323.2]
- African 086.5
  - due to Trypanosoma 086.5
    - gambiense 086.3
    - rhodesiense 086.4
- American 086.2
  - with
    - heart involvement 086.0
    - other organ involvement 086.1
  - without mention of organ involvement 086.2
- Brazilian — see Trypanosomiasis, American
- Chagas' — see Trypanosomiasis, American
- due to Trypanosoma
  - cruzi — see Trypanosomiasis, American
  - gambiense 086.3
  - rhodesiense 086.4

Trypanosomiasis — continued
- gambiensis, Gambian 086.3
- North American — see Trypanosomiasis, American
- rhodesiensis, Rhodesian 086.4
- South American — see Trypanosomiasis, American

T-shaped incisors 520.2

Tsutsugamushi fever 081.2

Tube, tubal, tubular — see also condition
- ligation, admission for V25.2

Tubercle — see also Tuberculosis
- brain, solitary 013.2
- Darwin's 744.29
- epithelioid noncaseating 135
- Ghon, primary infection 010.0

Tuberculid, tuberculide (indurating) (lichenoid) (miliary) (papulonecrotic) (primary) (skin) (subcutaneous) (see also Tuberculosis) 017.0

Tuberculoma — see also Tuberculosis
- brain (any part) 013.2
- meninges (cerebral) (spinal) 013.1
- spinal cord 013.4

Tuberculosis, tubercular, tuberculous (calcification) (calcified) (caseous) (chromogenic acid-fast bacilli) (congenital) (degeneration) (disease) (fibrocaseous) (fistula) (gangrene) (interstitial) (isolated circumscribed lesions) (necrosis) (parenchymatous) (ulcerative) 011.9

> Note — Use the following fifth-digit subclassification with categories 010-018:
>
> 0   unspecified
>
> 1   bacteriological or histological examination not done
>
> 2   bacteriological or histological examination unknown (at present)
>
> 3   tubercle bacilli found (in sputum) by microscopy
>
> 4   tubercle bacilli not found (in sputum) by microscopy, but found by bacterial culture
>
> 5   tubercle bacilli not found by bacteriological exam-ination, but tuberculosis confirmed histologically
>
> 6   tubercle bacilli not found by bacteriological or histological examination, but tuberculosis confirmed by other methods [inoculation of animals]
>
> For tuberculous conditions specified as late effects or sequelae, see category 137.

- abdomen 014.8
- lymph gland 014.8
- abscess 011.9
  - arm 017.9
  - bone (see also Osteomyelitis, due to, tuberculosis) 015.9 [730.8]
    - hip 015.1 [730.85]
    - knee 015.2 [730.96]
    - sacrum 015.0 [730.88]
    - specified site NEC 015.7 [730.88]
    - spinal 015.0 [730.88]
    - vertebra 015.0 [730.88]
  - brain 013.3
  - breast 017.9
  - Cowper's gland 016.5
  - dura (mater) 013.8
    - brain 013.3
    - spinal cord 013.5
  - epidural 013.8
    - brain 013.3
    - spinal cord 013.5
  - frontal sinus — see Tuberculosis, sinus
  - genital organs NEC 016.9
    - female 016.7
    - male 016.5
  - genitourinary NEC 016.9
  - gland (lymphatic) — see Tuberculosis, lymph gland
  - hip 015.1

Index to Diseases

Tuberculosis, tubercular, tuberculous — *continued*
- abscess — *continued*
  - iliopsoas 015.0 ✓5 [730.88]
  - intestine 014.8 ✓5
  - ischiorectal 014.8 ✓5
  - joint 015.9 ✓5
    - hip 015.1 ✓5
    - knee 015.2 ✓5
    - specified joint NEC 015.8 ✓5
    - vertebral 015.0 ✓5 [730.88]
  - kidney 016.0 ✓5 [590.81]
  - knee 015.2 ✓5
  - lumbar 015.0 ✓5 [730.88]
  - lung 011.2 ✓5
    - primary, progressive 010.8 ✓5
  - meninges (cerebral) (spinal) 013.0 ✓5
  - pelvic 016.9 ✓5
    - female 016.7 ✓5
    - male 016.5 ✓5
  - perianal 014.8 ✓5
    - fistula 014.8 ✓5
  - perinephritic 016.0 ✓5 [590.81]
  - perineum 017.9 ✓5
  - perirectal 014.8 ✓5
  - psoas 015.0 ✓5 [730.88]
  - rectum 014.8 ✓5
  - retropharyngeal 012.8 ✓5
  - sacrum 015.0 ✓5 [730.88]
  - scrofulous 017.2 ✓5
  - scrotum 016.5 ✓5
  - skin 017.0 ✓5
    - primary 017.0 ✓5
  - spinal cord 013.5 ✓5
  - spine or vertebra (column) 015.0 ✓5 [730.88]
  - strumous 017.2 ✓5
  - subdiaphragmatic 014.8 ✓5
  - testis 016.5 ✓5
  - thigh 017.9 ✓5
  - urinary 016.3 ✓5
    - kidney 016.0 ✓5 [590.81]
  - uterus 016.7 ✓5
- accessory sinus — *see* Tuberculosis, sinus
- Addison's disease 017.6 ✓5
- adenitis (*see also* Tuberculosis, lymph gland) 017.2 ✓5
- adenoids 012.8 ✓5
- adenopathy (*see also* Tuberculosis, lymph gland) 017.2 ✓5
  - tracheobronchial 012.1 ✓5
    - primary progressive 010.8 ✓5
- adherent pericardium 017.9 ✓5 [420.0]
- adnexa (uteri) 016.7 ✓5
- adrenal (capsule) (gland) 017.6 ✓5
- air passage NEC 012.8 ✓5
- alimentary canal 014.8 ✓5
- anemia 017.9 ✓5
- ankle (joint) 015.8 ✓5
  - bone 015.5 ✓5 [730.87]
- anus 014.8 ✓5
- apex (*see also* Tuberculosis, pulmonary) 011.9 ✓5
- apical (*see also* Tuberculosis, pulmonary) 011.9 ✓5
- appendicitis 014.8 ✓5
- appendix 014.8 ✓5
- arachnoid 013.0 ✓5
- artery 017.9 ✓5
- arthritis (chronic) (synovial) 015.9 ✓5 [711.40]
  - ankle 015.8 ✓5 [730.87]
  - hip 015.1 ✓5 [711.45]
  - knee 015.2 ✓5 [711.46]
  - specified site NEC 015.8 ✓5 [711.48]
  - spine or vertebra (column) 015.0 ✓5 [720.81]
  - wrist 015.8 ✓5 [730.83]
- articular — *see* Tuberculosis, joint
- ascites 014.0 ✓5
- asthma (*see also* Tuberculosis, pulmonary) 011.9 ✓5
- axilla, axillary 017.2 ✓5
  - gland 017.2 ✓5
- bilateral (*see also* Tuberculosis, pulmonary) 011.9 ✓5
- bladder 016.1 ✓5

Tuberculosis, tubercular, tuberculous — *continued*
- bone (*see also* Osteomyelitis, due to, tuberculosis) 015.9 ✓5 [730.8] ✓5
  - hip 015.1 ✓5 [730.85]
  - knee 015.2 ✓5 [730.86]
  - limb NEC 015.5 ✓5 [730.88]
  - sacrum 015.0 ✓5 [730.88]
  - specified site NEC 015.7 ✓5 [730.88]
  - spinal or vertebral column 015.0 ✓5 [730.88]
- bowel 014.8 ✓5
  - miliary 018.9 ✓5
- brain 013.2 ✓5
- breast 017.9 ✓5
- broad ligament 016.7 ✓5
- bronchi, bronchial, bronchus 011.3 ✓5
  - ectasia, ectasis 011.5 ✓5
  - fistula 011.3 ✓5
    - primary, progressive 010.8 ✓5
  - gland 012.1 ✓5
    - primary, progressive 010.8 ✓5
    - isolated 012.2 ✓5
  - lymph gland or node 012.1 ✓5
    - primary, progressive 010.8 ✓5
- bronchiectasis 011.5 ✓5
- bronchitis 011.3 ✓5
- bronchopleural 012.0 ✓5
- bronchopneumonia, bronchopneumonic 011.6 ✓5
- bronchorrhagia 011.3 ✓5
- bronchotracheal 011.3 ✓5
  - isolated 012.2 ✓5
- bronchus — *see* Tuberculosis, bronchi
- bronze disease (Addison's) 017.6 ✓5
- buccal cavity 017.9 ✓5
- bulbourethral gland 016.5 ✓5
- bursa (*see also* Tuberculosis, joint) 015.9 ✓5
- cachexia NEC (*see also* Tuberculosis, pulmonary) 011.9 ✓5
- cardiomyopathy 017.9 ✓5 [425.8]
- caries (*see also* Tuberculosis, bone) 015.9 ✓5 [730.8] ✓5
- cartilage (*see also* Tuberculosis, bone) 015.9 ✓5 [730.8] ✓5
  - intervertebral 015.0 ✓5 [730.88]
- catarrhal (*see also* Tuberculosis, pulmonary) 011.9 ✓5
- cecum 014.8 ✓5
- cellular tissue (primary) 017.0 ✓5
- cellulitis (primary) 017.0 ✓5
- central nervous system 013.9 ✓5
  - specified site NEC 013.8 ✓5
- cerebellum (current) 013.2 ✓5
- cerebral (current) 013.2 ✓5
  - meninges 013.0 ✓5
- cerebrospinal 013.6 ✓5
  - meninges 013.0 ✓5
- cerebrum (current) 013.2 ✓5
- cervical 017.2 ✓5
  - gland 017.2 ✓5
  - lymph nodes 017.2 ✓5
- cervicitis (uteri) 016.7 ✓5
- cervix 016.7 ✓5
- chest (*see also* Tuberculosis, pulmonary) 011.9 ✓5
- childhood type or first infection 010.0 ✓5
- choroid 017.3 ✓5 [363.13]
- choroiditis 017.3 ✓5 [363.13]
- ciliary body 017.3 ✓5 [364.11]
- colitis 014.8 ✓5
- colliers' 011.4 ✓5
- colliquativa (primary) 017.0 ✓5
- colon 014.8 ✓5
  - ulceration 014.8 ✓5
- complex, primary 010.0 ✓5
- complicating pregnancy, childbirth, or puerperium 647.3 ✓5
  - affecting fetus or newborn 760.2
- congenital 771.2
- conjunctiva 017.3 ✓5 [370.31]
- connective tissue 017.9 ✓5
  - bone — *see* Tuberculosis, bone
- contact V01.1
- converter (tuberculin test) (without disease) 795.5
- cornea (ulcer) 017.3 ✓5 [370.31]
- Cowper's gland 016.5 ✓5

Tuberculosis, tubercular, tuberculous — *continued*
- coxae 015.1 ✓5 [730.85]
- coxalgia 015.1 ✓5 [730.85]
- cul-de-sac of Douglas 014.8 ✓5
- curvature, spine 015.0 ✓5 [737.40]
- cutis (colliquativa) (primary) 017.0 ✓5
- cyst, ovary 016.6 ✓5
- cystitis 016.1 ✓5
- dacryocystitis 017.3 ✓5 [375.32]
- dactylitis 015.5 ✓5
- diarrhea 014.8 ✓5
- diffuse (*see also* Tuberculosis, miliary) 018.9 ✓5
  - lung — *see* Tuberculosis, pulmonary
  - meninges 013.0 ✓5
- digestive tract 014.8 ✓5
- disseminated (*see also* Tuberculosis, miliary) 018.9 ✓5
  - meninges 013.0 ✓5
- duodenum 014.8 ✓5
- dura (mater) 013.9 ✓5
  - abscess 013.8 ✓5
    - cerebral 013.3 ✓5
    - spinal 013.5 ✓5
- dysentery 014.8 ✓5
- ear (inner) (middle) 017.4 ✓5
  - bone 015.6 ✓5
  - external (primary) 017.0 ✓5
  - skin (primary) 017.0 ✓5
- elbow 015.8 ✓5
- emphysema — *see* Tuberculosis, pulmonary
- empyema 012.0 ✓5
- encephalitis 013.6 ✓5
- endarteritis 017.9 ✓5
- endocarditis (any valve) 017.9 ✓5 [424.91]
- endocardium (any valve) 017.9 ✓5 [424.91]
- endocrine glands NEC 017.9 ✓5
- endometrium 016.7 ✓5
- enteric, enterica 014.8 ✓5
- enteritis 014.8 ✓5
- enterocolitis 014.8 ✓5
- epididymis 016.4 ✓5
- epididymitis 016.4 ✓5
- epidural abscess 013.8 ✓5
  - brain 013.3 ✓5
  - spinal cord 013.5 ✓5
- epiglottis 012.3 ✓5
- episcleritis 017.3 ✓5 [379.00]
- erythema (induratum) (nodosum) (primary) 017.1 ✓5
- esophagus 017.8 ✓5
- Eustachian tube 017.4 ✓5
- exposure to V01.1
- exudative 012.0 ✓5
  - primary, progressive 010.1 ✓5
- eye 017.3 ✓5
  - glaucoma 017.3 ✓5 [365.62]
- eyelid (primary) 017.0 ✓5
  - lupus 017.0 ✓5 [373.4]
- fallopian tube 016.6 ✓5
- fascia 017.9 ✓5
- fauces 012.8 ✓5
- finger 017.9 ✓5
- first infection 010.0 ✓5
- fistula, perirectal 014.8 ✓5
- Florida 011.6 ✓5
- foot 017.9 ✓5
- funnel pelvis 137.3
- gallbladder 017.9 ✓5
- galloping (*see also* Tuberculosis, pulmonary) 011.9 ✓5
- ganglionic 015.9 ✓5
- gastritis 017.9 ✓5
- gastrocolic fistula 014.8 ✓5
- gastroenteritis 014.8 ✓5
- gastrointestinal tract 014.8 ✓5
- general, generalized 018.9 ✓5
  - acute 018.0 ✓5
  - chronic 018.8 ✓5
- genital organs NEC 016.9 ✓5
  - female 016.7 ✓5
  - male 016.5 ✓5
- genitourinary NEC 016.9 ✓5
- genu 015.2 ✓5
- glandulae suprarenalis 017.6 ✓5
- glandular, general 017.2 ✓5
- glottis 012.3 ✓5

Tuberculosis, tubercular, tuberculous — continued
- grinders' 011.4 ✓5th
- groin 017.2 ✓5th
- gum 017.9 ✓5th
- hand 017.9 ✓5th
- heart 017.9 ✓5th [425.8]
- hematogenous — see Tuberculosis, miliary
- hemoptysis (see also Tuberculosis, pulmonary) 011.9 ✓5th
- hemorrhage NEC (see also Tuberculosis, pulmonary) 011.9 ✓5th
- hemothorax 012.0 ✓5th
- hepatitis 017.9 ✓5th
- hilar lymph nodes 012.1 ✓5th
  - primary, progressive 010.8 ✓5th
- hip (disease) (joint) 015.1 ✓5th
  - bone 015.1 ✓5th [730.85]
- hydrocephalus 013.8 ✓5th
- hydropneumothorax 012.0 ✓5th
- hydrothorax 012.0 ✓5th
- hypoadrenalism 017.6 ✓5th
- hypopharynx 012.8 ✓5th
- ileocecal (hyperplastic) 014.8 ✓5th
- ileocolitis 014.8 ✓5th
- ileum 014.8 ✓5th
- iliac spine (superior) 015.0 ✓5th [730.88]
- incipient NEC (see also Tuberculosis, pulmonary) 011.9 ✓5th
- indurativa (primary) 017.1 ✓5th
- infantile 010.0 ✓5th
- infection NEC 011.9 ✓5th
  - without clinical manifestation 010.0 ✓5th
- infraclavicular gland 017.2 ✓5th
- inguinal gland 017.2 ✓5th
- inguinalis 017.2 ✓5th
- intestine (any part) 014.8 ✓5th
- iris 017.3 ✓5th [364.11]
- iritis 017.3 ✓5th [364.11]
- ischiorectal 014.8 ✓5th
- jaw 015.7 ✓5th [730.88]
- jejunum 014.8 ✓5th
- joint 015.9 ✓5th
  - hip 015.1 ✓5th
  - knee 015.2 ✓5th
  - specified site NEC 015.8 ✓5th
  - vertebral 015.0 ✓5th [730.88]
- keratitis 017.3 ✓5th [370.31]
  - interstitial 017.3 ✓5th [370.59]
- keratoconjunctivitis 017.3 ✓5th [370.31]
- kidney 016.0 ✓5th
- knee (joint) 015.2 ✓5th
- kyphoscoliosis 015.0 ✓5th [737.43]
- kyphosis 015.0 ✓5th [737.41]
- lacrimal apparatus, gland 017.3 ✓5th
- laryngitis 012.3 ✓5th
- larynx 012.3 ✓5th
- leptomeninges, leptomeningitis (cerebral) (spinal) 013.0 ✓5th
- lichenoides (primary) 017.0 ✓5th
- linguae 017.9 ✓5th
- lip 017.9 ✓5th
- liver 017.9 ✓5th
- lordosis 015.0 ✓5th [737.42]
- lung — see Tuberculosis, pulmonary
- luposa 017.0 ✓5th
  - eyelid 017.0 ✓5th [373.4]
- lymphadenitis — see Tuberculosis, lymph gland
- lymphangitis — see Tuberculosis, lymph gland
- lymphatic (gland) (vessel) — see Tuberculosis, lymph gland
- lymph gland or node (peripheral) 017.2 ✓5th
  - abdomen 014.8 ✓5th
  - bronchial 012.1 ✓5th
    - primary, progressive 010.8 ✓5th
  - cervical 017.2 ✓5th
  - hilar 012.1 ✓5th
    - primary, progressive 010.8 ✓5th
  - intrathoracic 012.1 ✓5th
    - primary, progressive 010.8 ✓5th
  - mediastinal 012.1 ✓5th
    - primary, progressive 010.8 ✓5th
  - mesenteric 014.8 ✓5th
  - peripheral 017.2 ✓5th
  - retroperitoneal 014.8 ✓5th
  - tracheobronchial 012.1 ✓5th
    - primary, progressive 010.8 ✓5th

Tuberculosis, tubercular, tuberculous — continued
- malignant NEC (see also Tuberculosis, pulmonary) 011.9 ✓5th
- mammary gland 017.9 ✓5th
- marasmus NEC (see also Tuberculosis, pulmonary) 011.9 ✓5th
- mastoiditis 015.6 ✓5th
- maternal, affecting fetus or newborn 760.2
- mediastinal (lymph) gland or node 012.1 ✓5th
  - primary, progressive 010.8 ✓5th
- mediastinitis 012.8 ✓5th
  - primary, progressive 010.8 ✓5th
- mediastinopericarditis 017.9 ✓5th [420.0]
- mediastinum 012.8 ✓5th
  - primary, progressive 010.8 ✓5th
- medulla 013.9 ✓5th
  - brain 013.2 ✓5th
  - spinal cord 013.4 ✓5th
- melanosis, Addisonian 017.6 ✓5th
- membrane, brain 013.0 ✓5th
- meninges (cerebral) (spinal) 013.0 ✓5th
- meningitis (basilar) (brain) (cerebral) (cerebrospinal) (spinal) 013.0 ✓5th
- meningoencephalitis 013.0 ✓5th
- mesentery, mesenteric 014.8 ✓5th
  - lymph gland or node 014.8 ✓5th
- miliary (any site) 018.9 ✓5th
  - acute 018.0 ✓5th
  - chronic 018.8 ✓5th
  - specified type NEC 018.8 ✓5th
- millstone makers' 011.4 ✓5th
- miners' 011.4 ✓5th
- moulders' 011.4 ✓5th
- mouth 017.9 ✓5th
- multiple 018.9 ✓5th
  - acute 018.0 ✓5th
  - chronic 018.8 ✓5th
- muscle 017.9 ✓5th
- myelitis 013.6 ✓5th
- myocarditis 017.9 ✓5th [422.0]
- myocardium 017.9 ✓5th [422.0]
- nasal (passage) (sinus) 012.8 ✓5th
- nasopharynx 012.8 ✓5th
- neck gland 017.2 ✓5th
- nephritis 016.0 ✓5th [583.81] ✓5th
- nerve 017.9 ✓5th
- nose (septum) 012.8 ✓5th
- ocular 017.3 ✓5th
- old NEC 137.0
  - without residuals V12.01
- omentum 014.8 ✓5th
- oophoritis (acute) (chronic) 016.6 ✓5th
- optic 017.3 ✓5th [377.39]
  - nerve trunk 017.3 ✓5th [377.39]
  - papilla, papillae 017.3 ✓5th [377.39]
- orbit 017.3 ✓5th
- orchitis 016.5 ✓5th [608.81]
- organ, specified NEC 017.9 ✓5th
- orificialis (primary) 017.0 ✓5th
- osseous (see also Tuberculosis, bone) 015.9 ✓5th [730.8] ✓5th
- osteitis (see also Tuberculosis, bone) 015.9 ✓5th [730.8] ✓5th
- osteomyelitis (see also Tuberculosis, bone) 015.9 ✓5th [730.8] ✓5th
- otitis (media) 017.4 ✓5th
- ovaritis (acute) (chronic) 016.6 ✓5th
- ovary (acute) (chronic) 016.6 ✓5th
- oviducts (acute) (chronic) 016.6 ✓5th
- pachymeningitis 013.0 ✓5th
- palate (soft) 017.9 ✓5th
- pancreas 017.9 ✓5th
- papulonecrotic (primary) 017.0 ✓5th
- parathyroid glands 017.9 ✓5th
- paronychia (primary) 017.0 ✓5th
- parotid gland or region 017.9 ✓5th
- pelvic organ NEC 016.9 ✓5th
  - female 016.7 ✓5th
  - male 016.5 ✓5th
- pelvis (bony) 015.7 ✓5th [730.85]
- penis 016.5 ✓5th
- peribronchitis 011.3 ✓5th
- pericarditis 017.9 ✓5th [420.0]
- pericardium 017.9 ✓5th [420.0]
- perichondritis, larynx 012.3 ✓5th
- perineum 017.9 ✓5th

Tuberculosis, tubercular, tuberculous — continued
- periostitis (see also Tuberculosis, bone) 015.9 ✓5th [730.8]
- periphlebitis 017.9 ✓5th
  - eye vessel 017.3 ✓5th [362.18]
  - retina 017.3 ✓5th [362.18]
- perirectal fistula 014.8 ✓5th
- peritoneal gland 014.8 ✓5th
- peritoneum 014.0 ✓5th
- peritonitis 014.0 ✓5th
- pernicious NEC (see also Tuberculosis, pulmonary) 011.9 ✓5th
- pharyngitis 012.8 ✓5th
- pharynx 012.8 ✓5th
- phlyctenulosis (conjunctiva) 017.3 ✓5th [370.31]
- phthisis NEC (see also Tuberculosis, pulmonary) 011.9 ✓5th
- pituitary gland 017.9 ✓5th
- placenta 016.7 ✓5th
- pleura, pleural, pleurisy, pleuritis (fibrinous) (obliterative) (purulent) (simple plastic) (with effusion) 012.0 ✓5th
  - primary, progressive 010.1 ✓5th
- pneumonia, pneumonic 011.6 ✓5th
- pneumothorax 011.7 ✓5th
- polyserositis 018.9 ✓5th
  - acute 018.0 ✓5th
  - chronic 018.8 ✓5th
- potters' 011.4 ✓5th
- prepuce 016.5 ✓5th
- primary 010.9 ✓5th
  - complex 010.0 ✓5th
  - complicated 010.8 ✓5th
    - with pleurisy or effusion 010.1 ✓5th
  - progressive 010.8 ✓5th
    - with pleurisy or effusion 010.1 ✓5th
  - skin 017.0 ✓5th
- proctitis 014.8 ✓5th
- prostate 016.5 ✓5th [601.4]
- prostatitis 016.5 ✓5th [601.4]
- pulmonaris (see also Tuberculosis, pulmonary) 011.9 ✓5th
- pulmonary (artery) (incipient) (malignant) (multiple round foci) (pernicious) (reinfection stage) 011.9 ✓5th
  - cavitated or with cavitation 011.2 ✓5th
    - primary, progressive 010.8 ✓5th
  - childhood type or first infection 010.0 ✓5th
  - chromogenic acid-fast bacilli 795.39 ▲
  - fibrosis or fibrotic 011.4 ✓5th
  - infiltrative 011.0 ✓5th
    - primary, progressive 010.9 ✓5th
  - nodular 011.1 ✓5th
  - specified NEC 011.8 ✓5th
  - sputum positive only 795.39 ▲
  - status following surgical collapse of lung NEC 011.9 ✓5th
- pyelitis 016.0 ✓5th [590.81]
- pyelonephritis 016.0 ✓5th [590.81]
- pyemia — see Tuberculosis, miliary
- pyonephrosis 016.0 ✓5th
- pyopneumothorax 012.0 ✓5th
- pyothorax 012.0 ✓5th
- rectum (with abscess) 014.8 ✓5th
  - fistula 014.8 ✓5th
- reinfection stage (see also Tuberculosis, pulmonary) 011.9 ✓5th
- renal 016.0 ✓5th
- renis 016.0 ✓5th
- reproductive organ 016.7 ✓5th
- respiratory NEC (see also Tuberculosis, pulmonary) 011.9 ✓5th
  - specified site NEC 012.8 ✓5th
- retina 017.3 ✓5th [363.13]
- retroperitoneal (lymph gland or node) 014.8 ✓5th
  - gland 014.8 ✓5th
- retropharyngeal abscess 012.8 ✓5th
- rheumatism 015.9 ✓5th
- rhinitis 012.8 ✓5th
- sacroiliac (joint) 015.8 ✓5th
- sacrum 015.0 ✓5th [730.88]
- salivary gland 017.9 ✓5th
- salpingitis (acute) (chronic) 016.6 ✓5th
- sandblasters' 011.4 ✓5th
- sclera 017.3 ✓5th [379.09]
- scoliosis 015.0 ✓5th [737.43]
- scrofulous 017.2 ✓5th

Index to Diseases

Tuberculosis, tubercular, tuberculous — *continued*
- scrotum 016.5
- seminal tract or vesicle 016.5 [608.81]
- senile NEC (*see also* Tuberculosis, pulmonary) 011.9
- septic NEC (*see also* Tuberculosis, miliary) 018.9
- shoulder 015.8
  - blade 015.7 [730.8]
- sigmoid 014.8
- sinus (accessory) (nasal) 012.8
  - bone 015.7 [730.88]
  - epididymis 016.4
- skeletal NEC (*see also* Osteomyelitis, due to tuberculosis) 015.9 [730.8]
- skin (any site) (primary) 017.0
- small intestine 014.8
- soft palate 017.9
- spermatic cord 016.5
- spinal
  - column 015.0 [730.88]
  - cord 013.4
  - disease 015.0 [730.88]
  - medulla 013.4
  - membrane 013.0
  - meninges 013.0
- spine 015.0 [730.88]
- spleen 017.7
- splenitis 017.7
- spondylitis 015.0 [720.81]
- spontaneous pneumothorax — *see* Tuberculosis, pulmonary
- sternoclavicular joint 015.8
- stomach 017.9
- stonemasons' 011.4
- struma 017.2
- subcutaneous tissue (cellular) (primary) 017.0
- subcutis (primary) 017.0
- subdeltoid bursa 017.9
- submaxillary 017.9
  - region 017.9
- supraclavicular gland 017.2
- suprarenal (capsule) (gland) 017.6
- swelling, joint (*see also* Tuberculosis, joint) 015.9
- symphysis pubis 015.7 [730.88]
- synovitis 015.9 [727.01]
  - hip 015.1 [727.01]
  - knee 015.2 [727.01]
  - specified site NEC 015.8 [727.01]
  - spine or vertebra 015.0 [727.01]
- systemic — *see* Tuberculosis, miliary
- tarsitis (eyelid) 017.0 [373.4]
  - ankle (bone) 015.5 [730.87]
- tendon (sheath) — *see* Tuberculosis, tenosynovitis
- tenosynovitis 015.9 [727.01]
  - hip 015.1 [727.01]
  - knee 015.2 [727.01]
  - specified site NEC 015.8 [727.01]
  - spine or vertebra 015.0 [727.01]
- testis 016.5 [608.81]
- throat 012.8
- thymus gland 017.9
- thyroid gland 017.5
- toe 017.9
- tongue 017.9
- tonsil (lingual) 012.8
- tonsillitis 012.8
- trachea, tracheal 012.8
  - gland 012.1
    - primary, progressive 010.8
    - isolated 012.2
- tracheobronchial 011.3
  - glandular 012.1
    - primary, progressive 010.8
    - isolated 012.2
  - lymph gland or node 012.1
    - primary, progressive 010.8
- tubal 016.6
- tunica vaginalis 016.5
- typhlitis 014.8
- ulcer (primary) (skin) 017.0
  - bowel or intestine 014.8
  - specified site NEC — *see* Tuberculosis, by site

Tuberculosis, tubercular, tuberculous — *continued*
- unspecified site — *see* Tuberculosis, pulmonary
- ureter 016.2
- urethra, urethral 016.3
- urinary organ or tract 016.3
  - kidney 016.0
- uterus 016.7
- uveal tract 017.3 [363.13]
- uvula 017.9
- vaccination, prophylactic (against) V03.2
- vagina 016.7
- vas deferens 016.5
- vein 017.9
- verruca (primary) 017.0
- verrucosa (cutis) (primary) 017.0
- vertebra (column) 015.0 [730.88]
- vesiculitis 016.5 [608.81]
- viscera NEC 014.8
- vulva 016.7 [616.51]
- wrist (joint) 015.8
  - bone 015.5 [730.83]

Tuberculum
- auriculae 744.29
- occlusal 520.2
- paramolare 520.2

Tuberous sclerosis (brain) 759.5

Tubo-ovarian — *see* condition

Tuboplasty, after previous sterilization V26.0

Tubotympanitis 381.10

Tularemia 021.9
- with
  - conjunctivitis 021.3
  - pneumonia 021.2
- bronchopneumonic 021.2
- conjunctivitis 021.3
- cryptogenic 021.1
- disseminated 021.8
- enteric 021.1
- generalized 021.8
- glandular 021.8
- intestinal 021.1
- oculoglandular 021.3
- ophthalmic 021.3
- pneumonia 021.2
- pulmonary 021.2
- specified NEC 021.8
- typhoidal 021.1
- ulceroglandular 021.0
- vaccination, prophylactic (against) V03.4

Tularensis conjunctivitis 021.3

Tumefaction — *see also* Swelling
- liver (*see also* Hypertrophy, liver) 789.1

Tumor (M8000/1) — *see also* Neoplasm, by site, unspecified nature
- Abrikossov's (M9580/0) — *see also* Neoplasm, connective tissue, benign
  - malignant (M9580/3) — *see* Neoplasm, connective tissue, malignant
- acinar cell (M8550/1) — *see* Neoplasm, by site, uncertain behavior
- acinic cell (M8550/1) — *see* Neoplasm, by site, uncertain behavior
- adenomatoid (M9054/0) — *see also* Neoplasm, by site, benign
  - odontogenic (M9300/0) 213.1
    - upper jaw (bone) 213.0
- adnexal (skin) (M8390/0) — *see* Neoplasm, skin, benign
- adrenal
  - cortical (benign) (M8370/0) 227.0
    - malignant (M8370/3) 194.0
  - rest (M8671/0) — *see* Neoplasm, by site, benign
- alpha cell (M8152/0)
  - malignant (M8152/3)
    - pancreas 157.4
    - specified site NEC — *see* Neoplasm, by site, malignant
    - unspecified site 157.4
  - pancreas 211.7
  - specified site NEC — *see* Neoplasm, by site, benign
  - unspecified site 211.7
- aneurysmal (*see also* Aneurysm) 442.9

Tumor — *see also* Neoplasm, by site, unspecified nature — *continued*
- aortic body (M8691/1) 237.3
  - malignant (M8691/3) 194.6
- argentaffin (M8241/1) — *see* Neoplasm, by site, uncertain behavior
- basal cell (M8090/1) — *see also* Neoplasm, skin, uncertain behavior
- benign (M8000/0) — *see* Neoplasm, by site, benign
- beta cell (M8151/0)
  - malignant (M8151/3)
    - pancreas 157.4
    - specified site — *see* Neoplasm, by site, malignant
    - unspecified site 157.4
  - pancreas 211.7
  - specified site NEC — *see* Neoplasm, by site, benign
  - unspecified site 211.7
- blood — *see* Hematoma
- Brenner (M9000/0) 220
  - borderline malignancy (M9000/1) 236.2
  - malignant (M9000/3) 183.0
  - proliferating (M9000/1) 236.2
- Brooke's (M8100/0) — *see* Neoplasm, skin, benign
- brown fat (M8880/0) — *see* Lipoma, by site
- Burkitt's (M9750/3) 200.2
- calcifying epithelial odontogenic (M9340/0) 213.1
  - upper jaw (bone) 213.0
- carcinoid (M8240/1) — *see* Carcinoid
- carotid body (M8692/1) 237.3
  - malignant (M8692/3) 194.5
- Castleman's (mediastinal lymph node hyperplasia) 785.6
- cells (M8001/1) — *see also* Neoplasm, by site, unspecified nature
  - benign (M8001/0) — *see* Neoplasm, by site, benign
  - malignant (M8001/3) — *see* Neoplasm, by site, malignant
  - uncertain whether benign or malignant (M8001/1) — *see* Neoplasm, by site, uncertain nature
- cervix
  - in pregnancy or childbirth 654.6
    - affecting fetus or newborn 763.89
    - causing obstructed labor 660.2
      - affecting fetus or newborn 763.1
- chondromatous giant cell (M9230/0) — *see* Neoplasm, bone, benign
- chromaffin (M8700/0) — *see also* Neoplasm, by site, benign
  - malignant (M8700/3) — *see* Neoplasm, by site, malignant
- Cock's peculiar 706.2
- Codman's (benign chondroblastoma) (M9230/0) — *see* Neoplasm, bone, benign
- dentigerous, mixed (M9282/0) 213.1
  - upper jaw (bone) 213.0
- dermoid (M9084/0) — *see* Neoplasm, by site, benign
  - with malignant transformation (M9084/3) 183.0
- desmoid (extra-abdominal) (M8821/1) — *see also* Neoplasm, connective tissue, uncertain behavior
  - abdominal (M8822/1) — *see* Neoplasm, connective tissue, uncertain behavior
- embryonal (mixed) (M9080/1) — *see also* Neoplasm, by site, uncertain behavior
  - liver (M9080/3) 155.0
- endodermal sinus (M9071/3)
  - specified site — *see* Neoplasm, by site, malignant
  - unspecified site
    - female 183.0
    - male 186.9
- epithelial
  - benign (M8010/0) — *see* Neoplasm, by site, benign
  - malignant (M8010/3) — *see* Neoplasm, by site, malignant
- Ewing's (M9260/3) — *see* Neoplasm, bone, malignant

Tumor — see also Neoplasm, by site, unspecified nature — continued
- fatty — see Lipoma
- fetal, causing disproportion 653.7 ✓5
  - causing obstructed labor 660.1 ✓5
- fibroid (M8890/0) — see Leiomyoma
- G cell (M8153/1)
  - malignant (M8153/3)
    - pancreas 157.4
    - specified site NEC — see Neoplasm, by site, malignant
    - unspecified site 157.4
  - specified site — see Neoplasm, by site, uncertain behavior
  - unspecified site 235.5
- giant cell (type) (M8003/1) — see also Neoplasm, by site, unspecified nature
  - bone (M9250/1) 238.0
    - malignant (M9250/3) — see Neoplasm, bone, malignant
  - chondromatous (M9230/0) — see Neoplasm, bone, benign
  - malignant (M8003/3) — see Neoplasm, by site, malignant
  - peripheral (gingiva) 523.8
  - soft parts (M9251/1) — see also Neoplasm, connective tissue, uncertain behavior
    - malignant (M9251/3) — see Neoplasm, connective tissue, malignant
  - tendon sheath 727.02
- glomus (M8711/0) — see also Hemangioma, by site
  - jugulare (M8690/1) 237.3
  - malignant (M8690/3) 194.6
- gonadal stromal (M8590/1) — see Neoplasm, by site, uncertain behavior
- granular cell (M9580/0) — see also Neoplasm, connective tissue, benign
  - malignant (M9580/3) — see Neoplasm, connective tissue, malignant
- granulosa cell (M8620/1) 236.2
  - malignant (M8620/3) 183.0
- granulosa cell-theca cell (M8621/1) 236.2
  - malignant (M8621/3) 183.0
- Grawitz's (hypernephroma) (M8312/3) 189.0
- hazard-crile (M8350/3) 193
- hemorrhoidal — see Hemorrhoids
- hilar cell (M8660/0) 220
- Hürthle cell (benign) (M8290/0) 226
  - malignant (M8290/3) 193
- hydatid (see also Echinococcus) 122.9
- hypernephroid (M8311/1) — see also Neoplasm, by site, uncertain behavior
- interstitial cell (M8650/1) — see also Neoplasm, by site, uncertain behavior
  - benign (M8650/0) — see Neoplasm, by site, benign
  - malignant (M8650/3) — see Neoplasm, by site, malignant
- islet cell (M8150/0)
  - malignant (M8150/3)
    - pancreas 157.4
    - specified site — see Neoplasm, by site, malignant
    - unspecified site 157.4
  - pancreas 211.7
  - specified site NEC — see Neoplasm, by site, benign
  - unspecified site 211.7
- juxtaglomerular (M8361/1) 236.91
- Krukenberg's (M8490/6) 198.6
- Leydig cell (M8650/1)
  - benign (M8650/0)
    - specified site — see Neoplasm, by site, benign
    - unspecified site
      - female 220
      - male 222.0
  - malignant (M8650/3)
    - specified site — see Neoplasm, by site, malignant
    - unspecified site
      - female 183.0
      - male 186.9
  - specified site — see Neoplasm, by site, uncertain behavior

Tumor — see also Neoplasm, by site, unspecified nature — continued
- Leydig cell — continued
  - unspecified site
    - female 236.2
    - male 236.4
- lipid cell, ovary (M8670/0) 220
- lipoid cell, ovary (M8670/0) 220
- lymphomatous, benign (M9590/0) — see also Neoplasm, by site, benign
- Malherbe's (M8110/0) — see Neoplasm, skin, benign
- malignant (M8000/3) — see also Neoplasm, by site, malignant
  - fusiform cell (type) (M8004/3) — see Neoplasm, by site, malignant
  - giant cell (type) (M8003/3) — see Neoplasm, by site, malignant
  - mixed NEC (M8940/3) — see Neoplasm, by site, malignant
  - small cell (type) (M8002/3) — see Neoplasm, by site, malignant
  - spindle cell (type) (M8004/3) — see Neoplasm, by site, malignant
- mast cell (M9740/1) 238.5
  - malignant (M9740/3) 202.6 ✓5
- melanotic, neuroectodermal (M9363/0) — see Neoplasm, by site, benign
- Merkel cell — see Neoplasm, by site, malignant
- mesenchymal
  - malignant (M8800/3) — see Neoplasm, connective tissue, malignant
  - mixed (M8990/1) — see Neoplasm, connective tissue, uncertain behavior
- mesodermal, mixed (M8951/3) — see also Neoplasm, by site, malignant
  - liver 155.0
- mesonephric (M9110/1) — see also Neoplasm, by site, uncertain behavior
  - malignant (M9110/3) — see Neoplasm, by site, malignant
- metastatic
  - from specified site (M8000/3) — see Neoplasm, by site, malignant
  - to specified site (M8000/6) — see Neoplasm, by site, secondary
- mixed NEC (M8940/0) — see Neoplasm, by site, benign
  - malignant (M8940/3) — see Neoplasm, by site, malignant
- mucocarcinoid, malignant (M8243/3) — see Neoplasm, by site, malignant
- mucoepidermoid (M8430/1) — see Neoplasm, by site, uncertain behavior
- Mullerian, mixed (M8950/3) — see Neoplasm, by site, malignant
- myoepithelial (M8982/0) — see Neoplasm, by site, benign
- neurogenic olfactory (M9520/3) 160.0
- nonencapsulated sclerosing (M8350/3) 193
- odontogenic (M9270/1) 238.0
  - adenomatoid (M9300/0) 213.1
    - upper jaw (bone) 213.0
  - benign (M9270/0) 213.1
    - upper jaw (bone) 213.0
  - calcifying epithelial (M9340/0) 213.1
    - upper jaw (bone) 213.0
  - malignant (M9270/3) 170.1
    - upper jaw (bone) 170.0
  - squamous (M9312/0) 213.1
    - upper jaw (bone) 213.0
- ovarian stromal (M8590/1) 236.2
- ovary
  - in pregnancy or childbirth 654.4 ✓5
    - affecting fetus or newborn 763.89
  - causing obstructed labor 660.2 ✓5
    - affecting fetus or newborn 763.1
- pacinian (M9507/0) — see Neoplasm, skin, benign
- Pancoast's (M8010/3) 162.3
- papillary — see Papilloma
- pelvic, in pregnancy or childbirth 654.9 ✓5
  - affecting fetus or newborn 763.89
  - causing obstructed labor 660.2 ✓5
    - affecting fetus or newborn 763.1
- phantom 300.11

Tumor — see also Neoplasm, by site, unspecified nature — continued
- plasma cell (M9731/1) 238.6
  - benign (M9731/0) — see Neoplasm, by site, benign
  - malignant (M9731/3) 203.8 ✓5
- polyvesicular vitelline (M9071/3)
  - specified site — see Neoplasm, by site, malignant
  - unspecified site
    - female 183.0
    - male 186.9
- Pott's puffy (see also Osteomyelitis) 730.2 ✓5
- Rathke's pouch (M9350/1) 237.0
- regaud's (M8082/3) — see Neoplasm, nasopharynx, malignant
- rete cell (M8140/0) 222.0
- retinal anlage (M9363/0) — see Neoplasm, by site, benign
- Rokitansky's 620.2
- salivary gland type, mixed (M8940/0) — see also Neoplasm, by site, benign
  - malignant (M8940/3) — see Neoplasm, by site, malignant
- Sampson's 617.1
- Schloffer's (see also Peritonitis) 567.2
- Schmincke (M8082/3) — see Neoplasm, nasopharynx, malignant
- sebaceous (see also Cyst, sebaceous) 706.2
- secondary (M8000/6) — see Neoplasm, by site, secondary
- Sertoli cell (M8640/0)
  - with lipid storage (M8641/0)
    - specified site — see Neoplasm, by site, benign
    - unspecified site
      - female 220
      - male 222.0
  - specified site — see Neoplasm, by site, benign
  - unspecified site
    - female 220
    - male 222.0
- Sertoli-Leydig cell (M8631/0)
  - specified site, — see Neoplasm, by site, benign
  - unspecified site
    - female 220
    - male 222.0
- sex cord (-stromal) (M8590/1) — see Neoplasm, by site, uncertain behavior
- skin appendage (M8390/0) — see Neoplasm, skin, benign
- soft tissue
  - benign (M8800/0) — see Neoplasm, connective tissue, benign
  - malignant (M8800/3) — see Neoplasm, connective tissue, malignant
- sternomastoid 754.1
- superior sulcus (lung) (pulmonary) (syndrome) (M8010/3) 162.3
- suprasulcus (M8010/3) 162.3
- sweat gland (M8400/1) — see also Neoplasm, skin, uncertain behavior
  - benign (M8400/0) — see Neoplasm, skin, benign
  - malignant (M8400/3) — see Neoplasm, skin, malignant
- syphilitic brain 094.89
  - congenital 090.49
- testicular stromal (M8590/1) 236.4
- theca cell (M8600/0) 220
- theca cell-granulosa cell (M8621/1) 236.2
- theca-lutein (M8610/0) 220
- turban (M8200/0) 216.4
- uterus
  - in pregnancy or childbirth 654.1 ✓5
    - affecting fetus or newborn 763.89
    - causing obstructed labor 660.2 ✓5
      - affecting fetus or newborn 763.1
- vagina
  - in pregnancy or childbirth 654.7 ✓5
    - affecting fetus or newborn 763.89
    - causing obstructed labor 660.2 ✓5
      - affecting fetus or newborn 763.1
- varicose (see also Varicose, vein) 454.9
- von Recklinghausen's (M9540/1) 237.71

Index to Diseases

Tumor — see also Neoplasm, by site, unspecified
  nature — continued
  vulva
    in pregnancy or childbirth 654.8 ✓5ᵗʰ
      affecting fetus or newborn 763.89
      causing obstructed labor 660.2 ✓5ᵗʰ
        affecting fetus or newborn 763.1
  Warthin's (salivary gland) (M8561/0) 210.2
  white — see also Tuberculosis, arthritis
  White-Darier 757.39
  Wilms' (nephroblastoma) (M8960/3) 189.0
  yolk sac (M9071/3)
    specified site — see Neoplasm, by site, malignant
    unspecified site
      female 183.0
      male 186.9

Tumorlet (M8040/1) — see Neoplasm, by site, uncertain behavior
Tungiasis 134.1
Tunica vasculosa lentis 743.39
Tunnel vision 368.45
Turban tumor (M8200/0) 216.4
Türck's trachoma (chronic catarrhal laryngitis) 476.0
Türk's syndrome (ocular retraction syndrome) 378.71
Turner's
  hypoplasia (tooth) 520.4
  syndrome 758.6
  tooth 520.4
Turner-Kieser syndrome (hereditary osteo-onychodysplasia) 756.89
Turner-Varny syndrome 758.6
Turricephaly 756.0
Tussis convulsiva (see also Whooping cough) 033.9
Twin
  affected by maternal complications of pregnancy 761.5
  conjoined 759.4
  healthy liveborn — see Newborn, twin
  pregnancy (complicating delivery) NEC 651.0 ✓5ᵗʰ
    with fetal loss and retention of one fetus 651.3 ✓5ᵗʰ
Twinning, teeth 520.2
Twist, twisted
  bowel, colon, or intestine 560.2
  hair (congenital) 757.4
  mesentery 560.2
  omentum 560.2
  organ or site, congenital NEC — see Anomaly, specified type NEC
  ovarian pedicle 620.5
    congenital 752.0
  umbilical cord — see Compression, umbilical cord
Twitch 781.0
Tylosis 700
  buccalis 528.6
  gingiva 523.8
  linguae 528.6
  palmaris et plantaris 757.39
Tympanism 787.3
Tympanites (abdominal) (intestine) 787.3
Tympanitis — see Myringitis
Tympanosclerosis 385.00
  involving
    combined sites NEC 385.09
      with tympanic membrane 385.03
    tympanic membrane 385.01
      with ossicles 385.02
      and middle ear 385.03
Tympanum — see condition
Tympany
  abdomen 787.3
  chest 786.7
Typhlitis (see also Appendicitis) 541
Typhoenteritis 002.0
Typhogastric fever 002.0

Typhoid (abortive) (ambulant) (any site) (fever) (hemorrhagic) (infection) (intermittent) (malignant) (rheumatic) 002.0
  with pneumonia 002.0 [484.8]
  abdominal 002.0
  carrier (suspected) of V02.1
  cholecystitis (current) 002.0
  clinical (Widal and blood test negative) 002.0
  endocarditis 002.0 [421.1]
  inoculation reaction — see Complications, vaccination
  meningitis 002.0 [320.7]
  mesenteric lymph nodes 002.0
  myocarditis 002.0 [422.0]
  osteomyelitis (see also Osteomyelitis, due to, typhoid) 002.0 [730.8] ✓5ᵗʰ
  perichondritis, larynx 002.0 [478.71]
  pneumonia 002.0 [484.8]
  spine 002.0 [720.81]
  ulcer (perforating) 002.0
  vaccination, prophylactic (against) V03.1
  Widal negative 002.0
Typhomalaria (fever) (see also Malaria) 084.6
Typhomania 002.0
Typhoperitonitis 002.0
Typhus (fever) 081.9
  abdominal, abdominalis 002.0
  African tick 082.1
  amarillic (see also Fever, Yellow) 060.9
  brain 081.9
  cerebral 081.9
  classical 080
  endemic (flea-borne) 081.0
  epidemic (louse-borne) 080
  exanthematic NEC 080
  exanthematicus SAI 080
    brillii SAI 081.1
    Mexicanus SAI 081.0
    pediculo vestimenti causa 080
    typhus murinus 081.0
  flea-borne 081.0
  Indian tick 082.1
  Kenya tick 082.1
  louse-borne 080
  Mexican 081.0
    flea-borne 081.0
    louse-borne 080
    tabardillo 080
  mite-borne 081.2
  murine 081.0
  North Asian tick-borne 082.2
  petechial 081.9
  Queensland tick 082.3
  rat 081.0
  recrudescent 081.1
  recurrent (see also Fever, relapsing) 087.9
  São Paulo 082.0
  scrub (China) (India) (Malaya) (New Guinea) 081.2
  shop (of Malaya) 081.0
  Siberian tick 082.2
  tick-borne NEC 082.9
  tropical 081.2
  vaccination, prophylactic (against) V05.8
Tyrosinemia 270.2
  neonatal 775.8
Tyrosinosis (Medes) (Sakai) 270.2
Tyrosinuria 270.2
Tyrosyluria 270.2

U

Uehlinger's syndrome (acropachyderma) 757.39
Uhl's anomaly or disease (hypoplasia of myocardium, right ventricle) 746.84
Ulcer, ulcerated, ulcerating, ulceration, ulcerative 707.9
  with gangrene 707.9 [785.4]
  abdomen (wall) (see also Ulcer, skin) 707.8
  ala, nose 478.1
  alveolar process 526.5
  amebic (intestine) 006.9
    skin 006.6
  anastomotic — see Ulcer, gastrojejunal
  anorectal 569.41

Ulcer, ulcerated, ulcerating, ulceration, ulcerative — continued
  antral — see Ulcer, stomach
  anus (sphincter) (solitary) 569.41
    varicose — see Varicose, ulcer, anus
  aphthous (oral) (recurrent) 528.2
    genital organ(s)
      female 616.8
      male 608.89
    mouth 528.2
  arm (see also Ulcer, skin) 707.8
  arteriosclerotic plaque — see Arteriosclerosis, by site
  artery NEC 447.2
    without rupture 447.8
  atrophic NEC — see Ulcer, skin
  Barrett's (chronic peptic ulcer of esophagus) 530.2
  bile duct 576.8
  bladder (solitary) (sphincter) 596.8
    bilharzial (see also Schistosomiasis) 120.9 [595.4]
    submucosal (see also Cystitis) 595.1
    tuberculous (see also Tuberculosis) 016.1 ✓5ᵗʰ
  bleeding NEC — see Ulcer, peptic, with hemorrhage
  bone 730.9 ✓5ᵗʰ
  bowel (see also Ulcer, intestine) 569.82
  breast 611.0
  bronchitis 491.8
  bronchus 519.1
  buccal (cavity) (traumatic) 528.9
  burn (acute) — see Ulcer, duodenum
  Buruli 031.1
  buttock (see also Ulcer, skin) 707.8
    decubitus (see also Ulcer, decubitus) 707.0
  cancerous (M8000/3) — see Neoplasm, by site, malignant
  cardia — see Ulcer, stomach
  cardio-esophageal (peptic) 530.2
  cecum (see also Ulcer, intestine) 569.82
  cervix (uteri) (trophic) 622.0
    with mention of cervicitis 616.0
  chancroidal 099.0
  chest (wall) (see also Ulcer, skin) 707.8
  Chiclero 085.4
  chin (pyogenic) (see also Ulcer, skin) 707.8
  chronic (cause unknown) — see also Ulcer, skin
    penis 607.89
  Cochin-China 085.1
  colitis — see Colitis, ulcerative
  colon (see also Ulcer, intestine) 569.82
  conjunctiva (acute) (postinfectional) 372.00
  cornea (infectional) 370.00
    with perforation 370.06
    annular 370.02
    catarrhal 370.01
    central 370.03
    dendritic 054.42
    marginal 370.01
    mycotic 370.05
    phlyctenular, tuberculous (see also Tuberculosis) 017.3 ✓5ᵗʰ [370.31]
    ring 370.02
    rodent 370.07
    serpent, serpiginous 370.04
    superficial marginal 370.01
    tuberculous (see also Tuberculosis) 017.3 ✓5ᵗʰ [370.31]
  corpus cavernosum (chronic) 607.89
  crural — see Ulcer, lower extremity
  Curling's — see Ulcer, duodenum
  Cushing's — see Ulcer, peptic
  cystitis (interstitial) 595.1
  decubitus (any site) 707.0
    with gangrene 707.0 [785.4]
  dendritic 054.42
  diabetes, diabetic (mellitus) 250.8 ✓5ᵗʰ [707.9]
    lower limb 250.8 ✓5ᵗʰ [707.10]
    ankle 250.8 ✓5ᵗʰ [707.13]
    calf 250.8 ✓5ᵗʰ [707.12]
    foot 250.8 ✓5ᵗʰ [707.15]
    heel 250.8 ✓5ᵗʰ [707.14]
    knee 250.8 ✓5ᵗʰ [707.19]
    specified site NEC 250.8 ✓5ᵗʰ [707.19]

Ulcer, ulcerated, ulcerating, ulceration, ulcerative — *continued*
  diabetes, diabetic — *continued*
    lower limb — *continued*
      thigh 250.8 ✓5ᵗʰ [707.11]
      toes 250.8 ✓5ᵗʰ [707.15]
      specified site NEC 250.8 ✓5ᵗʰ [707.8]
  Dieulafoy — *see* ▶Lesion, Dieulafoy◀
  due to
    infection NEC — *see* Ulcer, skin
    radiation, radium — *see* Ulcer, by site
    trophic disturbance (any region) — *see* Ulcer, skin
    x-ray — *see* Ulcer, by site
  duodenum, duodenal (eroded) (peptic) 532.9 ✓5ᵗʰ

Note — *Use the following fifth-digit subclassification with categories 531-534:*
  0 *without mention of obstruction*
  1 *with obstruction*

    with
      hemorrhage (chronic) 532.4 ✓5ᵗʰ
        and perforation 532.6 ✓5ᵗʰ
      perforation (chronic) 532.5 ✓5ᵗʰ
        and hemorrhage 532.6 ✓5ᵗʰ
    acute 532.3 ✓5ᵗʰ
      with
        hemorrhage 532.0 ✓5ᵗʰ
          and perforation 532.2 ✓5ᵗʰ
        perforation 532.1 ✓5ᵗʰ
          and hemorrhage 532.2 ✓5ᵗʰ
    bleeding (recurrent) — *see* Ulcer, duodenum, with hemorrhage
    chronic 532.7 ✓5ᵗʰ
      with
        hemorrhage 532.4 ✓5ᵗʰ
          and perforation 532.6 ✓5ᵗʰ
        perforation 532.5 ✓5ᵗʰ
          and hemorrhage 532.6 ✓5ᵗʰ
    penetrating — *see* Ulcer, duodenum, with perforation
    perforating — *see* Ulcer, duodenum, with perforation
  dysenteric NEC 009.0
  elusive 595.1
  endocarditis (any valve) (acute) (chronic) (subacute) 421.0
  enteritis — *see* Colitis, ulcerative
  enterocolitis 556.0
  epiglottis 478.79
  esophagus (peptic) 530.2
    due to ingestion
      aspirin 530.2
      chemicals 530.2
      medicinal agents 530.2
    fungal 530.2
    infectional 530.2
    varicose (*see also* Varix, esophagus) 456.1
      bleeding (*see also* Varix, esophagus, bleeding) 456.0
  eye NEC 360.00
    dendritic 054.42
  eyelid (region) 373.01
  face (*see also* Ulcer, skin) 707.8
  fauces 478.29
  Fenwick (-Hunner) (solitary) (*see also* Cystitis) 595.1
  fistulous NEC — *see* Ulcer, skin
  foot (indolent) (*see also* Ulcer, lower extremity) 707.15
    perforating 707.15
      leprous 030.1
      syphilitic 094.0
    trophic 707.15
    varicose 454.0
      inflamed or infected 454.2
  frambesial, initial or primary 102.0
  gallbladder or duct 575.8
  gall duct 576.2
  gangrenous (*see also* Gangrene) 785.4
  gastric — *see* Ulcer, stomach
  gastrocolic — *see* Ulcer, gastrojejunal
  gastroduodenal — *see* Ulcer, peptic
  gastroesophageal — *see* Ulcer, stomach
  gastrohepatic — *see* Ulcer, stomach

Ulcer, ulcerated, ulcerating, ulceration, ulcerative — *continued*
  gastrointestinal — *see* Ulcer, gastrojejunal
  gastrojejunal (eroded) (peptic) 534.9

Note — *Use the following fifth-digit subclassification with categories 531-534:*
  0 *without mention of obstruction*
  1 *with obstruction*

    with
      hemorrhage (chronic) 534.4 ✓5ᵗʰ
        and perforation 534.6 ✓5ᵗʰ
      perforation 534.5 ✓5ᵗʰ
        and hemorrhage 534.6 ✓5ᵗʰ
    acute 534.3 ✓5ᵗʰ
      with
        hemorrhage 534.0 ✓5ᵗʰ
          and perforation 534.2 ✓5ᵗʰ
        perforation 534.1 ✓5ᵗʰ
          and hemorrhage 534.2 ✓5ᵗʰ
    bleeding (recurrent) — *see* Ulcer, gastrojejunal, with hemorrhage
    chronic 534.7 ✓5ᵗʰ
      with
        hemorrhage 534.4 ✓5ᵗʰ
          and perforation 534.6 ✓5ᵗʰ
        perforation 534.5 ✓5ᵗʰ
          and hemorrhage 534.6 ✓5ᵗʰ
    penetrating — *see* Ulcer, gastrojejunal, with perforation
    perforating — *see* Ulcer, gastrojejunal, with perforation
  gastrojejunocolic — *see* Ulcer, gastrojejunal
  genital organ
    female 629.8
    male 608.89
  gingiva 523.8
  gingivitis 523.1
  glottis 478.79
  granuloma of pudenda 099.2
  groin (*see also* Ulcer, skin) 707.8
  gum 523.8
  gumma, due to yaws 102.4
  hand (*see also* Ulcer, skin) 707.8
  hard palate 528.9
  heel (*see also* Ulcer, lower extremity) 707.14
    decubitus (*see also* Ulcer, decubitus) 707.0
  hemorrhoids 455.8
    external 455.5
    internal 455.2
  hip (*see also* Ulcer, skin) 707.8
    decubitus (*see also* Ulcer, decubitus) 707.0
  Hunner's 595.1
  hypopharynx 478.29
  hypopyon (chronic) (subacute) 370.04
  hypostaticum — *see* Ulcer, varicose
  ileocolitis 556.1
  ileum (*see also* Ulcer, intestine) 569.82
  intestine, intestinal 569.82
    with perforation 569.83
    amebic 006.9
    duodenal — *see* Ulcer, duodenum
    granulocytopenic (with hemorrhage) 288.0
    marginal 569.82
    perforating 569.83
    small, primary 569.82
    stercoraceous 569.82
    stercoral 569.82
    tuberculous (*see also* Tuberculosis) 014.8 ✓5ᵗʰ
    typhoid (fever) 002.0
    varicose 456.8
  ischemic 707.9
    lower extremity (*see also* Ulcer, lower extremity) 707.10
      ankle 707.13
      calf 707.12
      foot 707.15
      heel 707.14
      knee 707.19
      specified site NEC 707.19
      thigh 707.11
      toes 707.15
  jejunum, jejunal — *see* Ulcer, gastrojejunal
  keratitis (*see also* Ulcer, cornea) 370.00
  knee — *see* Ulcer, lower extremity

Ulcer, ulcerated, ulcerating, ulceration, ulcerative — *continued*
  labium (majus) (minus) 616.50
  laryngitis (*see also* Laryngitis) 464.00
    with obstruction 464.01
  larynx (aphthous) (contact) 478.79
    diphtheritic 032.3
  leg — *see* Ulcer, lower extremity
  lip 528.5
  Lipschütz's 616.50
  lower extremity (atrophic) (chronic) (neurogenic) (perforating) (pyogenic) (trophic) (tropical) 707.10
    with gangrene (*see also* Ulcer, lower extremity) 707.10 [785.4]
      arteriosclerotic 440.24
    ankle 707.13
    arteriosclerotic 440.23
      with gangrene 440.24
    calf 707.12
    decubitus 707.0
      with gangrene 707.0 [785.4]
    foot 707.15
    heel 707.14
    knee 707.19
    specified site NEC 707.19
    thigh 707.11
    toes 707.15
    varicose 454.0
      inflamed or infected 454.2
  luetic — *see* Ulcer, syphilitic
  lung 518.89
    tuberculous (*see also* Tuberculosis) 011.2 ✓5ᵗʰ
  malignant (M8000/3) — *see* Neoplasm, by site, malignant
  marginal NEC — *see* Ulcer, gastrojejunal
  meatus (urinarius) 597.89
  Meckel's diverticulum 751.0
  Meleney's (chronic undermining) 686.09
  Mooren's (cornea) 370.07
  mouth (traumatic) 528.9
  mycobacterial (skin) 031.1
  nasopharynx 478.29
  navel cord (newborn) 771.4
  neck (*see also* Ulcer, skin) 707.8
    uterus 622.0
  neurogenic NEC — *see* Ulcer, skin
  nose, nasal (infectional) (passage) 478.1
    septum 478.1
      varicose 456.8
    skin — *see* Ulcer, skin
    spirochetal NEC 104.8
  oral mucosa (traumatic) 528.9
  palate (soft) 528.9
  penetrating NEC — *see* Ulcer, peptic, with perforation
  penis (chronic) 607.89
  peptic (site unspecified) 533.9

Note — *Use the following fifth-digit subclassification with categories 531-534:*
  0 *without mention of obstruction*
  1 *with obstruction*

    with
      hemorrhage 533.4 ✓5ᵗʰ
        and perforation 533.6 ✓5ᵗʰ
      perforation (chronic) 533.5 ✓5ᵗʰ
        and hemorrhage 533.6 ✓5ᵗʰ
    acute 533.3 ✓5ᵗʰ
      with
        hemorrhage 533.0 ✓5ᵗʰ
          and perforation 533.2 ✓5ᵗʰ
        perforation 533.1 ✓5ᵗʰ
          and hemorrhage 533.2 ✓5ᵗʰ
    bleeding (recurrent) — *see* Ulcer, peptic, with hemorrhage
    chronic 533.7 ✓5ᵗʰ
      with
        hemorrhage 533.4 ✓5ᵗʰ
          and perforation 533.6 ✓5ᵗʰ
        perforation 533.5 ✓5ᵗʰ
          and hemorrhage 533.6 ✓5ᵗʰ
    penetrating — *see* Ulcer, peptic, with perforation

Index to Diseases

Ulcer, ulcerated, ulcerating, ulceration, ulcerative — *continued*
- perforating NEC (*see also* Ulcer, peptic, with perforation) 533.5 ✓5ᵗʰ
  - skin 707.9
- perineum (*see also* Ulcer, skin) 707.8
- peritonsillar 474.8
- phagedenic (tropical) NEC — *see* Ulcer, skin
- pharynx 478.29
- phlebitis — *see* Phlebitis
- plaster (*see also* Ulcer, decubitus) 707.0
- popliteal space — *see* Ulcer, lower extremity
- postpyloric — *see* Ulcer, duodenum
- prepuce 607.89
- prepyloric — *see* Ulcer, stomach
- pressure (*see also* Ulcer, decubitus) 707.0
- primary of intestine 569.82
  - with perforation 569.83
- proctitis 556.2
  - with ulcerative sigmoiditis 556.3
- prostate 601.8
- pseudopeptic — *see* Ulcer, peptic
- pyloric — *see* Ulcer, stomach
- rectosigmoid 569.82
  - with perforation 569.83
- rectum (sphincter) (solitary) 569.41
  - stercoraceous, stercoral 569.41
  - varicose — *see* Varicose, ulcer, anus
- retina (*see also* Chorioretinitis) 363.20
- rodent (M8090/3) — *see also* Neoplasm, skin, malignant
  - cornea 370.07
- round — *see* Ulcer, stomach
- sacrum (region) (*see also* Ulcer, skin) 707.8
- Saemisch's 370.04
- scalp (*see also* Ulcer, skin) 707.8
- sclera 379.09
- scrofulous (*see also* Tuberculosis) 017.2 ✓5ᵗʰ
- scrotum 608.89
  - tuberculous (*see also* Tuberculosis) 016.5 ✓5ᵗʰ
  - varicose 456.4
- seminal vesicle 608.89
- sigmoid 569.82
  - with perforation 569.83
- skin (atrophic) (chronic) (neurogenic) (non-healing) (perforating) (pyogenic) (trophic) 707.9
  - with gangrene 707.9 [785.4]
  - amebic 006.6
  - decubitus 707.0
    - with gangrene 707.0 [785.4]
  - in granulocytopenia 288.0
  - lower extremity (*see also* Ulcer, lower extremity) 707.10
    - with gangrene 707.10 [785.4]
      - arteriosclerotic 440.24
    - ankle 707.13
    - arteriosclerotic 440.23
      - with gangrene 440.24
    - calf 707.12
    - foot 707.15
    - heel 707.14
    - knee 707.19
    - specified site NEC 707.19
    - thigh 707.11
    - toes 707.15
  - mycobacterial 031.1
  - syphilitic (early) (secondary) 091.3
  - tuberculous (primary) (*see also* Tuberculosis) 017.0 ✓5ᵗʰ
  - varicose — *see* Ulcer, varicose
- sloughing NEC — *see* Ulcer, skin
- soft palate 528.9
- solitary, anus or rectum (sphincter) 569.41
- sore throat 462
  - streptococcal 034.0
- spermatic cord 608.89
- spine (tuberculous) 015.0 ✓5ᵗʰ [730.88]
- stasis (leg) (venous) 454.0
  - inflamed or infected 454.2
  - without varicose veins 459.81
- stercoral, stercoraceous 569.82
  - with perforation 569.83
  - anus or rectum 569.41
- stoma, stomal — *see* Ulcer, gastrojejunal

Ulcer, ulcerated, ulcerating, ulceration, ulcerative — *continued*
- stomach (eroded) (peptic) (round) 531.9

> Note — Use the following fifth-digit subclassification with categories 531-534:
> 0 without mention of obstruction
> 1 with obstruction

  - with
    - hemorrhage 531.4 ✓5ᵗʰ
      - and perforation 531.6 ✓5ᵗʰ
    - perforation (chronic) 531.5 ✓5ᵗʰ
      - and hemorrhage 531.6 ✓5ᵗʰ
  - acute 531.3 ✓5ᵗʰ
    - with
      - hemorrhage 531.0 ✓5ᵗʰ
        - and perforation 531.2 ✓5ᵗʰ
      - perforation 531.1 ✓5ᵗʰ
        - and hemorrhage 531.2 ✓5ᵗʰ
  - bleeding (recurrent) — *see* Ulcer, stomach, with hemorrhage
  - chronic 531.7 ✓5ᵗʰ
    - with
      - hemorrhage 531.4 ✓5ᵗʰ
        - and perforation 531.6 ✓5ᵗʰ
      - perforation 531.5 ✓5ᵗʰ
        - and hemorrhage 531.6 ✓5ᵗʰ
  - penetrating — *see* Ulcer, stomach, with perforation
  - perforating — *see* Ulcer, stomach, with perforation
- stomatitis 528.0
- stress — *see* Ulcer, peptic
- strumous (tuberculous) (*see also* Tuberculosis) 017.2 ✓5ᵗʰ
- submental (*see also* Ulcer, skin) 707.8
- submucosal, bladder 595.1
- syphilitic (any site) (early) (secondary) 091.3
  - late 095.9
  - perforating 095.9
  - foot 094.0
- testis 608.89
- thigh — *see* Ulcer, lower extremity
- throat 478.29
  - diphtheritic 032.0
- toe — *see* Ulcer, lower extremity
- tongue (traumatic) 529.0
- tonsil 474.8
  - diphtheritic 032.0
- trachea 519.1
- trophic — *see* Ulcer, skin
- tropical NEC (*see also* Ulcer, skin) 707.9
- tuberculous — *see* Tuberculosis, ulcer
- tunica vaginalis 608.89
- turbinate 730.9 ✓5ᵗʰ
- typhoid (fever) 002.0
  - perforating 002.0
- umbilicus (newborn) 771.4
- unspecified site NEC — *see* Ulcer, skin
- urethra (meatus) (*see also* Urethritis) 597.89
- uterus 621.8
  - cervix 622.0
    - with mention of cervicitis 616.0
  - neck 622.0
    - with mention of cervicitis 616.0
- vagina 616.8
- valve, heart 421.0
- varicose (lower extremity, any part) 454.0
  - anus — *see* Varicose, ulcer, anus
  - broad ligament 456.5
  - esophagus (*see also* Varix, esophagus) 456.1
    - bleeding (*see also* Varix, esophagus, bleeding) 456.0
  - inflamed or infected 454.2
  - nasal septum 456.8
  - perineum 456.6
  - rectum — *see* Varicose, ulcer, anus
  - scrotum 456.4
  - specified site NEC 456.8
  - sublingual 456.3
  - vulva 456.6
- vas deferens 608.89
- vesical (*see also* Ulcer, bladder) 596.8
- vulva (acute) (infectional) 616.50
  - Behçet's syndrome 136.1 [616.51]

Ulcer, ulcerated, ulcerating, ulceration, ulcerative — *continued*
- vulva — *continued*
  - herpetic 054.12
  - tuberculous 016.7 ✓5ᵗʰ [616.51]
  - vulvobuccal, recurring 616.50
  - x-ray — *see* Ulcer, by site
  - yaws 102.4

Ulcerosa scarlatina 034.1

Ulcus — *see also* Ulcer
- cutis tuberculosum (*see also* Tuberculosis) 017.0 ✓5ᵗʰ
- duodeni — *see* Ulcer, duodenum
- durum 091.0
  - extragenital 091.2
- gastrojejunale — *see* Ulcer, gastrojejunal
- hypostaticum — *see* Ulcer, varicose
- molle (cutis) (skin) 099.0
- serpens corneae (pneumococcal) 370.04
- ventriculi — *see* Ulcer, stomach

Ulegyria 742.4

Ulerythema
- acneiforma 701.8
- centrifugum 695.4
- ophryogenes 757.4

Ullrich (-Bonnevie) (-Turner) syndrome 758.6

Ullrich-Feichtiger syndrome 759.89

Ulnar — *see* condition

Ulorrhagia 523.8

Ulorrhea 523.8

Umbilicus, umbilical — *see also* condition
- cord necrosis, affecting fetus or newborn 762.6

Unavailability of medical facilities (at) V63.9
- due to
  - investigation by social service agency V63.8
  - lack of services at home V63.1
  - remoteness from facility V63.0
  - waiting list V63.2
- home V63.1
- outpatient clinic V63.0
- specified reason NEC V63.8

Uncinaria americana infestion 126.1

Uncinariasis (*see also* Ancylostomiasis) 126.9

Unconscious, unconsciousness 780.09

Underdevelopment — *see also* Undeveloped
- sexual 259.0

Undernourishment 269.9

Undernutrition 269.9

Under observation — *see* Observation

Underweight 783.22
- for gestational age — *see* Light-for-dates

Underwood's disease (sclerema neonatorum) 778.1

Undescended — *see also* Malposition, congenital
- cecum 751.4
- colon 751.4
- testis 752.51

Undetermined diagnosis or cause 799.9

Undeveloped, undevelopment — *see also* Hypoplasia
- brain (congenital) 742.1
- cerebral (congenital) 742.1
- fetus or newborn 764.9 ✓5ᵗʰ
- heart 746.89
- lung 748.5
- testis 257.2
- uterus 259.0

Undiagnosed (disease) 799.9

Undulant fever (*see also* Brucellosis) 023.9

Unemployment, anxiety concerning V62.0

Unequal leg (acquired) (length) 736.81
- congenital 755.30

Unerupted teeth, tooth 520.6

Unextracted dental root 525.3

Unguis incarnatus 703.0

Unicornis uterus 752.3

Unicorporeus uterus 752.3

Uniformis uterus 752.3

Unilateral — *see also* condition
- development, breast 611.8
- organ or site, congenital NEC — *see* Agenesis

Unilateral — see also condition — continued
  vagina 752.49
Unilateralis uterus 752.3
Unilocular heart 745.8
Uninhibited bladder 596.54
  with cauda equina syndrome 344.61
  neurogenic — see Neurogenic, bladder 596.54
Union, abnormal — see also Fusion
  divided tendon 727.89
  larynx and trachea 748.3
Universal
  joint, cervix 620.6
  mesentery 751.4
Unknown
  cause of death 799.9
  diagnosis 799.9
Unna's disease (seborrheic dermatitis) 690.10
Unresponsiveness, adrenocorticotropin (ACTH) 255.4
Unsoundness of mind (see also Psychosis) 298.9
Unspecified cause of death 799.9
Unstable
  back NEC 724.9
  colon 569.89
  joint — see Instability, joint
  lie 652.0
    affecting fetus or newborn (before labor) 761.7
    causing obstructed labor 660.0
      affecting fetus or newborn 763.1
  lumbosacral joint (congenital) 756.19
    acquired 724.6
  sacroiliac 724.6
  spine NEC 724.9
Untruthfulness, child problem (see also Disturbance, conduct) 312.0
Unverricht (-Lundborg) disease, syndrome, or epilepsy 333.2
Unverricht-Wagner syndrome (dermatomyositis) 710.3
Upper respiratory — see condition
Upset
  gastric 536.8
    psychogenic 306.4
  gastrointestinal 536.8
    psychogenic 306.4
    virus (see also Enteritis, viral) 008.8
  intestinal (large) (small) 564.9
    psychogenic 306.4
  menstruation 626.9
  mental 300.9
  stomach 536.8
    psychogenic 306.4
Urachus — see also condition
  patent 753.7
  persistent 753.7
Uratic arthritis 274.0
Urbach's lipoid proteinosis 272.8
Urbach-Oppenheim disease or syndrome (necrobiosis lipoidica diabeticorum) 250.8 [709.3]
Urbach-Wiethe disease or syndrome (lipoid proteinosis) 272.8
Urban yellow fever 060.1
Urea, blood, high — see Uremia
Uremia, uremic (absorption) (amaurosis) (amblyopia) (aphasia) (apoplexy) (coma) (delirium) (dementia) (dropsy) (dyspnea) (fever) (intoxication) (mania) (paralysis) (poisoning) (toxemia) (vomiting) 586
  with
    abortion — see Abortion, by type, with renal failure
    ectopic pregnancy (see also categories 633.0-633.9) 639.3
    hypertension (see also Hypertension, kidney) 403.91
    molar pregnancy (see also categories 630-632) 639.3
  chronic 585
  complicating
    abortion 639.3
    ectopic or molar pregnancy 639.3

Uremia, uremic — continued
  complicating — continued
    hypertension (see also Hypertension, kidney) 403.91
    labor and delivery 669.3
  congenital 779.89
  extrarenal 788.9
  hypertensive (chronic) (see also Hypertension, kidney) 403.91
  maternal NEC, affecting fetus or newborn 760.1
  neuropathy 585 [357.4]
  pericarditis 585 [420.0]
  prerenal 788.9
  pyelitic (see also Pyelitis) 590.80
Ureter, ureteral — see condition
Ureteralgia 788.0
Ureterectasis 593.89
Ureteritis 593.89
  cystica 590.3
  due to calculus 592.1
  gonococcal (acute) 098.19
    chronic or duration of 2 months or over 098.39
  nonspecific 593.89
Ureterocele (acquired) 593.89
  congenital 753.23
Ureterolith 592.1
Ureterolithiasis 592.1
Ureterostomy status V44.6
  with complication 997.5
Urethra, urethral — see condition
Urethralgia 788.9
Urethritis (abacterial) (acute) (allergic) (anterior) (chronic) (nonvenereal) (posterior) (recurrent) (simple) (subacute) (ulcerative) (undifferentiated) 597.80
  diplococcal (acute) 098.0
    chronic or duration of 2 months or over 098.2
  due to Trichomonas (vaginalis) 131.02
  gonococcal (acute) 098.0
    chronic or duration of 2 months or over 098.2
  nongonococcal (sexually transmitted) 099.40
    Chlamydia trachomatis 099.41
    Reiter's 099.3
    specified organism NEC 099.49
  nonspecific (sexually transmitted) (see also Urethritis, nongonococcal) 099.40
  not sexually transmitted 597.80
  Reiter's 099.3
  trichomonal or due to Trichomonas (vaginalis) 131.02
  tuberculous (see also Tuberculosis) 016.3
  venereal NEC (see also Urethritis, nongonococcal) 099.40
Urethrocele
  female 618.0
    with uterine prolapse 618.4
      complete 618.3
      incomplete 618.2
  male 599.5
Urethrolithiasis 594.2
Urethro-oculoarticular syndrome 099.3
Urethro-oculosynovial syndrome 099.3
Urethrorectal — see condition
Urethrorrhagia 599.84
Urethrorrhea 788.7
Urethrostomy status V44.6
  with complication 997.5
Urethrotrigonitis 595.3
Urethrovaginal — see condition
Urhidrosis, uridrosis 705.89
Uric acid
  diathesis 274.9
  in blood 790.6
Uricacidemia 790.6
Uricemia 790.6
Uricosuria 791.9

Urination
  frequent 788.41
  painful 788.1
Urine, urinary — see also condition
  abnormality NEC 788.69
  blood in (see also Hematuria) 599.7
  discharge, excessive 788.42
  enuresis 788.30
    nonorganic origin 307.6
  extravasation 788.8
  frequency 788.41
  incontinence 788.30
    active 788.30
    female 788.30
      stress 625.6
        and urge 788.33
    male 788.30
      stress 788.32
        and urge 788.33
    mixed (stress and urge) 788.33
    neurogenic 788.39
    nonorganic origin 307.6
    stress (female) 625.6
      male NEC 788.32
  intermittent stream 788.61
  pus in 791.9
  retention or stasis NEC 788.20
    bladder, incomplete emptying 788.21
    psychogenic 306.53
    specified NEC 788.29
  secretion
    deficient 788.5
    excessive 788.42
    frequency 788.41
  stream
    intermittent 788.61
    slowing 788.62
    splitting 788.61
    weak 788.62
Urinemia — see Uremia
Urinoma NEC 599.9
  bladder 596.8
  kidney 593.89
  renal 593.89
  ureter 593.89
  urethra 599.84
Uroarthritis, infectious 099.3
Urodialysis 788.5
Urolithiasis 592.9
Uronephrosis 593.89
Uropathy 599.9
  obstructive 599.6
Urosepsis 599.0
  meaning sepsis 038.9
  meaning urinary tract infection 599.0
Urticaria 708.9
  with angioneurotic edema 995.1
    hereditary 277.6
  allergic 708.0
  cholinergic 708.5
  chronic 708.8
  cold, familial 708.2
  dermatographic 708.3
  due to
    cold or heat 708.2
    drugs 708.0
    food 708.0
    inhalants 708.0
    plants 708.8
    serum 999.5
  factitial 708.3
  giant 995.1
    hereditary 277.6
  gigantea 995.1
    hereditary 277.6
  idiopathic 708.1
  larynx 995.1
    hereditary 277.6
  neonatorum 778.8
  nonallergic 708.1
  papulosa (Hebra) 698.2
  perstans hemorrhagica 757.39
  pigmentosa 757.33
  recurrent periodic 708.8
  serum 999.5
  solare 692.72

Index to Diseases

Urticaria — *continued*
  specified type NEC 708.8
  thermal (cold) (heat) 708.2
  vibratory 708.4
Urticarioides acarodermatitis 133.9
Use of
  nonprescribed drugs (*see also* Abuse, drugs,
      nondependent) 305.9 ✓5ᵗʰ
  patent medicines (*see also* Abuse, drugs,
      nondependent) 305.9 ✓5ᵗʰ
Usher-Senear disease (pemphigus erythematosus)
    694.4
Uta 085.5
Uterine size-date discrepancy 646.8 ✓5ᵗʰ
Uteromegaly 621.2
Uterovaginal — *see* condition
Uterovesical — *see* condition
Uterus — *see* condition
Utriculitis (utriculus prostaticus) 597.89
Uveal — *see* condition
Uveitis (anterior) (*see also* Iridocyclitis) 364.3
  acute or subacute 364.00
    due to or associated with
      gonococcal infection 098.41
      herpes (simplex) 054.44
        zoster 053.22
    primary 364.01
    recurrent 364.02
    secondary (noninfectious) 364.04
      infectious 364.03
  allergic 360.11
  chronic 364.10
    due to or associated with
      sarcoidosis 135 [364.11]
      tuberculosis (*see also* Tuberculosis)
        017.3 ✓5ᵗʰ [364.11]
  due to
    operation 360.11
    toxoplasmosis (acquired) 130.2
      congenital (active) 771.2
  granulomatous 364.10
  heterochromic 364.21
  lens-induced 364.23
  nongranulomatous 364.00
  posterior 363.20
    disseminated — *see* Chorioretinitis,
        disseminated
    focal — *see* Chorioretinitis, focal
  recurrent 364.02
  sympathetic 360.11
  syphilitic (secondary) 091.50
    congenital 090.0 [363.13]
    late 095.8 [363.13]
  tuberculous (*see also* Tuberculosis)
    017.3 ✓5ᵗʰ [364.11]
Uveoencephalitis 363.22
Uveokeratitis (*see also* Iridocyclitis) 364.3
Uveoparotid fever 135
Uveoparotitis 135
Uvula — *see* condition
Uvulitis (acute) (catarrhal) (chronic) (gangrenous)
    (membranous) (suppurative) (ulcerative)
    528.3

Index to Diseases

V

Vaccination
 complication or reaction — *see* Complications, vaccination
 not done (contraindicated) V64.0
  because of patient's decision V64.2
 prophylactic (against) V05.9
  arthropod-borne viral
   disease NEC V05.1
   encephalitis V05.0
  chickenpox V05.4
  cholera (alone) V03.0
   with typhoid-paratyphoid (cholera + TAB) V06.0
  common cold V04.7
  diphtheria (alone) V03.5
   with
    poliomyelitis (DTP+ polio) V06.3
    tetanus V06.5
     pertussis combined (DTP) V06.1
    typhoid-paratyphoid (DTP + TAB) V06.2
  disease (single) NEC V05.9
   bacterial NEC V03.9
    specified type NEC V03.89
   combinations NEC V06.9
    specified type NEC V06.8
   specified type NEC V05.8
  encephalitis, viral, arthropod-borne V05.0
  Hemophilus influenzae, type B [Hib] V03.81
  hepatitis, viral V05.3
  influenza V04.8
   with
    Streptococcus pneumoniae [pneumococcus] V06.6
  lileieshmaniasis V05.2
  measles (alone) V04.2
   with mumps-rubella (MMR) V06.4
  mumps (alone) V04.6
   with measles and rubella (MMR) V06.4
  pertussis alone V03.6
  plague V03.3
  poliomyelitis V04.0
   with diphtheria-tetanus-pertussis (DTP + polio) V06.3
  rabies V04.5
  rubella (alone) V04.3
   with measles and mumps (MMR) V06.4
  smallpox V04.1
  Streptococcus pneumoniae [pneumococcus] V03.82
   with
    influenza V06.6
  tetanus toxoid (alone) V03.7
   with diphtheria [Td] V06.5
    with
     pertussis (DTP) V06.1
      with poliomyelitis (DTP+polio) V06.3
  tuberculosis (BCG) V03.2
  tularemia V03.4
  typhoid-paratyphoid (TAB) (alone) V03.1
   with diphtheria-tetanus-pertussis (TAB + DTP) V06.2
  varicella V05.4
  viral
   encephalitis, arthropod-borne V05.0
   hepatitis V05.3
  yellow fever V04.4

Vaccinia (generalized) 999.0
 congenital 771.2
 conjunctiva 999.3
 eyelids 999.0 [373.5]
 localized 999.3
 nose 999.3
 not from vaccination 051.0
  eyelid 051.0 [373.5]
 sine vaccinatione 051.0
 without vaccination 051.0

Vacuum
 extraction of fetus or newborn 763.3
 in sinus (accessory) (nasal) (*see also* Sinusitis) 473.9

Vagabond V60.0
Vagabondage V60.0
Vagabonds' disease 132.1
Vagina, vaginal — *see* condition
Vaginalitis (tunica) 608.4
Vaginismus (reflex) 625.1
 functional 306.51
 hysterical 300.11
 psychogenic 306.51
Vaginitis (acute) (chronic) (circumscribed) (diffuse) (emphysematous) (Hemophilus vaginalis) (nonspecific) (nonvenereal) (ulcerative) 616.10
 with
  abortion — *see* Abortion, by type, with sepsis
  ectopic pregnancy (*see also* categories 633.0-633.9) 639.0
  molar pregnancy (*see also* categories 630-632) 639.0
 adhesive, congenital 752.49
 atrophic, postmenopausal 627.3
 bacterial 616.10
 blennorrhagic (acute) 098.0
  chronic or duration of 2 months or over 098.2
 candidal 112.1
 chlamydial 099.53
 complicating pregnancy or puerperium 646.6 ✓5ᵗʰ
  affecting fetus or newborn 760.8
 congenital (adhesive) 752.49
 due to
  C. albicans 112.1
  Trichomonas (vaginalis) 131.01
 following
  abortion 639.0
  ectopic or molar pregnancy 639.0
 gonococcal (acute) 098.0
  chronic or duration of 2 months or over 098.2
 granuloma 099.2
 Monilia 112.1
 mycotic 112.1
 pinworm 127.4 [616.11]
 postirradiation 616.10
 postmenopausal atrophic 627.3
 senile (atrophic) 627.3
 syphilitic (early) 091.0
  late 095.8
 trichomonal 131.01
 tuberculous (*see also* Tuberculosis) 016.7 ✓5ᵗʰ
 venereal NEC 099.8
Vaginosis — *see* Vaginitis
Vagotonia 352.3
Vagrancy V60.0
Vallecula — *see* condition
Valley fever 114.0
Valsuani's disease (progressive pernicious anemia, puerperal) 648.2 ✓5ᵗʰ
Valve, valvular (formation) — *see also* condition
 cerebral ventricle (communicating) in situ V45.2
 cervix, internal os 752.49
 colon 751.5
 congenital NEC — *see* Atresia
 formation, congenital NEC — *see* Atresia
 heart defect — *see* Anomaly, heart, valve
 ureter 753.29
  pelvic junction 753.21
  vesical orifice 753.22
 urethra 753.6
Valvulitis (chronic) (*see also* Endocarditis) 424.90
 rheumatic (chronic) (inactive) (with chorea) 397.9
  active or acute (aortic) (mitral) (pulmonary) (tricuspid) 391.1
 syphilitic NEC 093.20
  aortic 093.22
  mitral 093.21
  pulmonary 093.24
  tricuspid 093.23
Valvulopathy — *see* Endocarditis
van Bogaert's leukoencephalitis (sclerosing) (subacute) 046.2
van Bogaert-Nijssen (-Peiffer) disease 330.0

van Buchem's syndrome (hyperostosis corticalis) 733.3
van Creveld-von Gierke disease (glycogenosis I) 271.0
van den Bergh's disease (enterogenous cyanosis) 289.7
van der Hoeve's syndrome (brittle bones and blue sclera, deafness) 756.51
van der Hoeve-Halbertsma-Waardenburg syndrome (ptosis-epicanthus) 270.2
van der Hoeve-Waardenburg-Gualdi syndrome (ptosis epicanthus) 270.2
Vanillism 692.89
Vanishing lung 492.0
van Neck (-Odelberg) disease or syndrome (juvenile osteochondrosis) 732.1
Vanishing twin 651.33
Vapor asphyxia or suffocation NEC 987.9
 specified agent — *see* Table of Drugs and Chemicals
Vaquez's disease (M9950/1) 238.4
Vaquez-Osler disease (polycythemia vera) (M9950/1) 238.4
Variance, lethal ball, prosthetic heart valve 996.02
Variants, thalassemic 282.4
Variations in hair color 704.3
Varicella 052.9
 with
  complication 052.8
   specified NEC 052.7
  pneumonia 052.1
  vaccination and inoculation (prophylactic) V05.4
Varices — *see* Varix
Varicocele (scrotum) (thrombosed) 456.4
 ovary 456.5
 perineum 456.6
 spermatic cord (ulcerated) 456.4
Varicose
 aneurysm (ruptured) (*see also* Aneurysm) 442.9
 dermatitis (lower extremity) — *see* Varicose, vein, inflamed or infected
 eczema — *see* Varicose, vein
 phlebitis — *see* Varicose, vein, inflamed or infected
 placental vessel — *see* Placenta, abnormal
 tumor — *see* Varicose, vein
 ulcer (lower extremity, any part) 454.0
  anus 455.8
   external 455.5
   internal 455.2
  esophagus (*see also* Varix, esophagus) 456.1
   bleeding (*see also* Varix, esophagus, bleeding) 456.0
  inflamed or infected 454.2
  nasal septum 456.8
  perineum 456.6
  rectum — *see* Varicose, ulcer, anus
  scrotum 456.4
  specified site NEC 456.8
 vein (lower extremity) (ruptured) (*see also* Varix) 454.9
  with
   complications NEC 454.8 ●
   edema 454.8 ●
   inflammation or infection 454.1
    ulcerated 454.2
   pain 454.8 ●
   stasis dermatitis 454.1
    with ulcer 454.2
   swelling 454.8 ●
   ulcer 454.0
    inflamed or infected 454.2
  anus — *see* Hemorrhoids
  broad ligament 456.5
  congenital (peripheral) NEC 747.60
   gastrointestinal 747.61
   lower limb 747.64
   renal 747.62
   specified NEC 747.69
   upper limb 747.63

Varicose | Index to Diseases

Varicose — *continued*
  vein (*see also* Varix) — *continued*
    esophagus (ulcerated) (*see also* Varix, esophagus) 456.1
      bleeding (*see also* Varix, esophagus, bleeding) 456.0
      inflamed or infected 454.1
        with ulcer 454.2
      in pregnancy or puerperium 671.0 ✓5ᵗʰ
        vulva or perineum 671.1 ✓5ᵗʰ
      nasal septum (with ulcer) 456.8
      pelvis 456.5
      perineum 456.6
        in pregnancy, childbirth, or puerperium 671.1 ✓5ᵗʰ
      rectum — *see* Hemorrhoids
      scrotum (ulcerated) 456.4
      specified site NEC 456.8
      sublingual 456.3
      ulcerated 454.0
        inflamed or infected 454.2
      umbilical cord, affecting fetus or newborn 762.6
      urethra 456.8
      vulva 456.6
        in pregnancy, childbirth, or puerperium 671.1 ✓5ᵗʰ
    vessel — *see also* Varix
      placenta — *see* Placenta, abnormal
Varicosis, varicosities, varicosity (*see also* Varix) 454.9
Variola 050.9
  hemorrhagic (pustular) 050.0
  major 050.0
  minor 050.1
  modified 050.2
Varioloid 050.2
Variolosa, purpura 050.0
Varix (lower extremity) (ruptured) 454.9
  with
    complications NEC 454.8 ●
    edema 454.8 ●
    inflammation or infection 454.1
      with ulcer 454.2
    pain 454.8 ●
    stasis dermatitis 454.1
      with ulcer 454.2
    swelling 454.8 ●
    ulcer 454.0
      with inflammation or infection 454.2
  aneurysmal (*see also* Aneurysm) 442.9
  anus — *see* Hemorrhoids
  arteriovenous (congenital) (peripheral) NEC 747.60
    gastrointestinal 747.61
    lower limb 747.64
    renal 747.62
    specified NEC 747.69
    spinal 747.82
    upper limb 747.63
  bladder 456.5
  broad ligament 456.5
  congenital (peripheral) NEC 747.60
  esophagus (ulcerated) 456.1
    bleeding 456.0
      in
        cirrhosis of liver 571.5 [456.20]
        portal hypertension 572.3 [456.20]
    congenital 747.69
      in
        cirrhosis of liver 571.5 [456.21]
          with bleeding 571.5 [456.20]
        portal hypertension 572.3 [456.21]
          with bleeding 572.3 [456.20]
  gastric 456.8
  inflamed or infected 454.1
    ulcerated 454.2
  in pregnancy or puerperium 671.0 ✓5ᵗʰ
    perineum 671.1 ✓5ᵗʰ
    vulva 671.1 ✓5ᵗʰ
  labia (majora) 456.6
  orbit 456.8
    congenital 747.69
  ovary 456.5
  papillary 448.1
  pelvis 456.5

Varix — *continued*
  perineum 456.6
    in pregnancy or puerperium 671.1 ✓5ᵗʰ
  pharynx 456.8
  placenta — *see* Placenta, abnormal
  prostate 456.8
  rectum — *see* Hemorrhoids
  renal papilla 456.8
  retina 362.17
  scrotum (ulcerated) 456.4
  sigmoid colon 456.8
  specified site NEC 456.8
  spinal (cord) (vessels) 456.8
  spleen, splenic (vein) (with phlebolith) 456.8
  sublingual 456.3
  ulcerated 454.0
    inflamed or infected 454.2
  umbilical cord, affecting fetus or newborn 762.6
  uterine ligament 456.5
  vocal cord 456.8
  vulva 456.6
    in pregnancy, childbirth, or puerperium 671.1 ✓5ᵗʰ
Vasa previa 663.5 ✓5ᵗʰ
  affecting fetus or newborn 762.6
  hemorrhage from, affecting fetus or newborn 772.0
Vascular — *see also* condition
  loop on papilla (optic) 743.57
  sheathing, retina 362.13
  spasm 443.9
  spider 448.1
Vascularity, pulmonary, congenital 747.3
Vascularization
  choroid 362.16
  cornea 370.60
    deep 370.63
    localized 370.61
  retina 362.16
  subretinal 362.16
Vasculitis 447.6
  allergic 287.0
  cryoglobulinemic 273.2
  disseminated 447.6
  kidney 447.8
  leukocytoclastic 446.29
  nodular 695.2
  retinal 362.18
  rheumatic — *see* Fever, rheumatic
Vas deferens — *see* condition
Vas deferentitis 608.4
Vasectomy, admission for V25.2
Vasitis 608.4
  nodosa 608.4
  scrotum 608.4
  spermatic cord 608.4
  testis 608.4
  tuberculous (*see also* Tuberculosis) 016.5 ✓5ᵗʰ
  tunica vaginalis 608.4
  vas deferens 608.4
Vasodilation 443.9
Vasomotor — *see* condition
Vasoplasty, after previous sterilization V26.0
Vasoplegia, splanchnic (*see also* Neuropathy, peripheral, autonomic) 337.9
Vasospasm 443.9
  cerebral (artery) 435.9
    with transient neurologic deficit 435.9
  nerve
    arm NEC 354.9
    autonomic 337.9
    brachial plexus 353.0
    cervical plexus 353.2
    leg NEC 355.8
    lower extremity NEC 355.8
    peripheral NEC 355.9
    spinal NEC 355.9
    sympathetic 337.9
    upper extremity NEC 354.9
  peripheral NEC 443.9
  retina (artery) (*see also* Occlusion, retinal, artery) 362.30
Vasospastic — *see* condition

Vasovagal attack (paroxysmal) 780.2
  psychogenic 306.2
Vater's ampulla — *see* condition
VATER syndrome 759.89
Vegetation, vegetative
  adenoid (nasal fossa) 474.2
  consciousness (persistent) 780.03
  endocarditis (acute) (any valve) (chronic) (subacute) 421.0
  heart (mycotic) (valve) 421.0
  state (persistent) 780.03
Veil
  Jackson's 751.4
  over face (causing asphyxia) 768.9
Vein, venous — *see* condition
Veldt sore (*see also* Ulcer, skin) 707.9
Velpeau's hernia — *see* Hernia, femoral
Venereal
  balanitis NEC 099.8
  bubo 099.1
  disease 099.9
    specified nature or type NEC 099.8
  granuloma inguinale 099.2
  lymphogranuloma (Durand-Nicolas-Favre), any site 099.1
  salpingitis 098.37
  urethritis (*see also* Urethritis, nongonococcal) 099.40
  vaginitis NEC 099.8
  warts 078.19
Vengefulness, in child (*see also* Disturbance, conduct) 312.0 ✓5ᵗʰ
Venofibrosis 459.89
Venom, venomous
  bite or sting (animal or insect) 989.5
  poisoning 989.5
Venous — *see* condition
Ventouse delivery NEC 669.5 ✓5ᵗʰ
  affecting fetus or newborn 763.3
Ventral — *see* condition
Ventricle, ventricular — *see also* condition
  escape 427.69
  standstill (*see also* Arrest, cardiac) 427.5
Ventriculitis, cerebral (*see also* Meningitis) 322.9
Ventriculostomy status V45.2
Verbiest's syndrome (claudicatio intermittens spinalis) 435.1
Vernet's syndrome 352.6
Verneuil's disease (syphilitic bursitis) 095.7
Verruca (filiformis) 078.10
  acuminata (any site) 078.11
  necrogenica (primary) (*see also* Tuberculosis) 017.0 ✓5ᵗʰ
  plana (juvenilis) 078.19
  peruana 088.0
  peruviana 088.0
  plantaris 078.19
  seborrheica 702.19
    inflamed 702.11
  senilis 702.0
  tuberculosa (primary) (*see also* Tuberculosis) 017.0 ✓5ᵗʰ
  venereal 078.19
  viral NEC 078.10
Verrucosities (*see also* Verruca) 078.10
Verrucous endocarditis (acute) (any valve) (chronic) (subacute) 710.0 [424.91]
  nonbacterial 710.0 [424.91]
Verruga
  peruana 088.0
  peruviana 088.0
Verse's disease (calcinosis intervertebralis) 275.49 [722.90]
Version
  before labor, affecting fetus or newborn 761.7
  cephalic (correcting previous malposition) 652.1 ✓5ᵗʰ
    affecting fetus or newborn 763.1
  cervix (*see also* Malposition, uterus) 621.6
  uterus (postinfectional) (postpartal, old) (*see also* Malposition, uterus) 621.6
    forward — *see* Anteversion, uterus
    lateral — *see* Lateroversion, uterus

Vertebra, vertebral — see condition
Vertigo 780.4
  auditory 386.19
  aural 386.19
  benign paroxysmal positional 386.11
  central origin 386.2
  cerebral 386.2
  Dix and Hallpike (epidemic) 386.12
  endemic paralytic 078.81
  epidemic 078.81
    Dix and Hallpike 386.12
    Gerlier's 078.81
    Pedersen's 386.12
    vestibular neuronitis 386.12
  epileptic — see Epilepsy
  Gerlier's (epidemic) 078.81
  hysterical 300.11
  labyrinthine 386.10
  laryngeal 786.2
  malignant positional 386.2
  Ménière's (see also Disease, Ménière's) 386.00
  menopausal 627.2
  otogenic 386.19
  paralytic 078.81
  paroxysmal positional, benign 386.11
  Pedersen's (epidemic) 386.12
  peripheral 386.10
    specified type NEC 386.19
  positional
    benign paroxysmal 386.11
    malignant 386.2
Verumontanitis (chronic) (see also Urethritis) 597.89
Vesania (see also Psychosis) 298.9
Vesical — see condition
Vesicle
  cutaneous 709.8
  seminal — see condition
  skin 709.8
Vesicocolic — see condition
Vesicoperineal — see condition
Vesicorectal — see condition
Vesicourethrorectal — see condition
Vesicovaginal — see condition
Vesicular — see condition
Vesiculitis (seminal) 608.0
  amebic 006.8
  gonorrheal (acute) 098.14
    chronic or duration of 2 months or over 098.34
  trichomonal 131.09
  tuberculous (see also Tuberculosis) 016.5 [608.81]
Vestibulitis (ear) (see also Labyrinthitis) 386.30
  nose (external) 478.1
  vulvar 616.10
Vestibulopathy, acute peripheral (recurrent) 386.12
Vestige, vestigial — see also Persistence
  branchial 744.41
  structures in vitreous 743.51
Vibriosis NEC 027.9
Vidal's disease (lichen simplex chronicus) 698.3
Video display tube syndrome 723.8
Vienna type encephalitis 049.8
Villaret's syndrome 352.6
Villous — see condition
VIN I (vulvar intraepithelial neoplasia I) 624.8
VIN II (vulvar intraepithelial neoplasia II) 624.8
VIN III (vulvar intraepithelial neoplasia III) 233.3
Vincent's
  angina 101
  bronchitis 101
  disease 101
  gingivitis 101
  infection (any site) 101
  laryngitis 101
  stomatitis 101
  tonsillitis 101
Vinson-Plummer syndrome (sideropenic dysphagia) 280.8

Viosterol deficiency (see also Deficiency, calciferol) 268.9
Virchow's disease 733.99
Viremia 790.8
Virilism (adrenal) (female) NEC 255.2
  with
    3-beta-hydroxysteroid dehydrogenase defect 255.2
    11-hydroxylase defect 255.2
    21-hydroxylase defect 255.2
  adrenal
    hyperplasia 255.2
    insufficiency (congenital) 255.2
  cortical hyperfunction 255.2
Virilization (female) (suprarenal) (see also Virilism) 255.2
  isosexual 256.4
Virulent bubo 099.0
Virus, viral — see also condition
  infection NEC (see also Infection, viral) 079.99
  septicemia 079.99
Viscera, visceral — see condition
Visceroptosis 569.89
Visible peristalsis 787.4
Vision, visual
  binocular, suppression 368.31
  blurred, blurring 368.8
    hysterical 300.11
  defect, defective (see also Impaired, vision) 369.9
  disorientation (syndrome) 368.16
  disturbance NEC (see also Disturbance, vision) 368.9
    hysterical 300.11
  examination V72.0
  field, limitation 368.40
  fusion, with defective steropsis 368.33
  hallucinations 368.16
  halos 368.16
  loss 369.9
    both eyes (see also Blindness, both eyes) 369.3
    complete (see also Blindness, both eyes) 369.00
    one eye 369.8
    sudden 368.16
  low (both eyes) 369.20
    one eye (other eye normal) (see also Impaired, vision) 369.70
      blindness, other eye 369.10
  perception, simultaneous without fusion 368.32
  tunnel 368.45
Vitality, lack or want of 780.79
  newborn 779.89
Vitamin deficiency NEC (see also Deficiency, vitamin) 269.2
Vitelline duct, persistent 751.0
Vitiligo 709.01
  due to pinta (carate) 103.2
  eyelid 374.53
  vulva 624.8
Vitium cordis — see Disease, heart
Vitreous — see also condition
  touch syndrome 997.99
Vocal cord — see condition
Vocational rehabilitation V57.22
Vogt's (Cecile) disease or syndrome 333.7
Vogt-Koyanagi syndrome 364.24
Vogt-Spielmeyer disease (amaurotic familial idiocy) 330.1
Voice
  change (see also Dysphonia) 784.49
  loss (see also Aphonia) 784.41
Volhard-Fahr disease (malignant nephrosclerosis) 403.00
Volhynian fever 083.1
Volkmann's ischemic contracture or paralysis (complicating trauma) 958.6
Voluntary starvation 307.1

Volvulus (bowel) (colon) (intestine) 560.2
  with
    hernia — see also Hernia, by site, with obstruction
      gangrenous — see Hernia, by site, with gangrene
    perforation 560.2
  congenital 751.5
  duodenum 537.3
  fallopian tube 620.5
  oviduct 620.5
  stomach (due to absence of gastrocolic ligament) 537.89
Vomiting 787.03
  with nausea 787.01
  allergic 535.4
  asphyxia 933.1
  bilious (cause unknown) 787.0
    following gastrointestinal surgery 564.3
  blood (see also Hematemesis) 578.0
  causing asphyxia, choking, or suffocation (see also Asphyxia, food) 933.1
  cyclical 536.2
    psychogenic 306.4
  epidemic 078.82
  fecal matter 569.89
  following gastrointestinal surgery 564.3
  functional 536.8
    psychogenic 306.4
  habit 536.2
  hysterical 300.11
  nervous 306.4
  neurotic 306.4
  newborn 779.3
  of or complicating pregnancy 643.9
    due to
      organic disease 643.8
      specific cause NEC 643.8
    early — see Hyperemesis, gravidarum
    late (after 22 completed weeks of gestation) 643.2
  pernicious or persistent 536.2
    complicating pregnancy — see Hyperemesis, gravidarum
    psychogenic 306.4
  physiological 787.0
  psychic 306.4
  psychogenic 307.54
  stercoral 569.89
  uncontrollable 536.2
    psychogenic 306.4
  uremic — see Uremia
  winter 078.82
von Bechterew (-Strumpell) disease or syndrome (ankylosing spondylitis) 720.0
von Bezold's abscess 383.01
von Economo's disease (encephalitis lethargica) 049.8
von Eulenburg's disease (congenital paramyotonia) 359.2
von Gierke's disease (glycogenosis I) 271.0
von Gies' joint 095.8
von Graefe's disease or syndrome 378.72
von Hippel (-Lindau) disease or syndrome (retinocerebral angiomatosis) 759.6
von Jaksch's anemia or disease (pseudoleukemia infantum) 285.8
von Recklinghausen's
  disease or syndrome (nerves) (skin) (M9540/1) 237.71
    bones (osteitis fibrosa cystica) 252.0
  tumor (M9540/1) 237.71
von Recklinghausen-Applebaum disease (hemochromatosis) 275.0
von Schroetter's syndrome (intermittent venous claudication) 453.8
von Willebrand (-Jürgens) (-Minot) disease or syndrome (angiohemophilia) 286.4
von Zambusch's disease (lichen sclerosus et atrophicus) 701.0
Voorhoeve's disease or dyschondroplasia 756.4
Vossius' ring 921.3
  late effect 366.21
Voyeurism 302.82

Vrolik's disease (osteogenesis imperfecta) 756.51
Vulva — see condition
Vulvismus 625.1
Vulvitis (acute) (allergic) (aphthous) (chronic) (gangrenous) (hypertrophic) (intertriginous) 616.10
  with
    abortion — see Abortion, by type, with sepsis
    ectopic pregnancy (see also categories 633.0-633.9) 639.0
    molar pregnancy (see also categories 630-632) 639.0
  adhesive, congenital 752.49
  blennorhagic (acute) 098.0
    chronic or duration of 2 months or over 098.2
  chlamydial 099.53
  complicating pregnancy or puerperium 646.6 ✓5ᵗʰ
  due to Ducrey's bacillus 099.0
  following
    abortion 639.0
    ectopic or molar pregnancy 639.0
  gonococcal (acute) 098.0
    chronic or duration of 2 months or over 098.2
  herpetic 054.11
  leukoplakic 624.0
  monilial 112.1
  puerperal, postpartum, childbirth 646.6 ✓5ᵗʰ
  syphilitic (early) 091.0
    late 095.8
  trichomonal 131.01
Vulvodynia 625.9
Vulvorectal — see condition
Vulvovaginitis (see also Vulvitis) 616.10
  amebic 006.8
  chlamydial 099.53
  gonococcal (acute) 098.0
    chronic or duration of 2 months or over 098.2
  herpetic 054.11
  monilial 112.1
  trichomonal (Trichomonas vaginalis) 131.01

W

Waardenburg's syndrome 756.89
  meaning ptosis-epicanthus 270.2
Waardenburg-Klein syndrome (ptosis-epicanthus) 270.2
Wagner's disease (colloid milium) 709.3
Wagner (-Unverricht) syndrome (dermatomyositis) 710.3
Waiting list, person on V63.2
  undergoing social agency investigation V63.8
Wakefulness disorder (see also Hypersomnia) 780.54
  nonorganic origin 307.43
Waldenström's
  disease (osteochondrosis, capital femoral) 732.1
  hepatitis (lupoid hepatitis) 571.49
  hypergammaglobulinemia 273.0
  macroglobulinemia 273.3
  purpura, hypergammaglobulinemic 273.0
  syndrome (macroglobulinemia) 273.3
Waldenström-Kjellberg syndrome (sideropenic dysphagia) 280.8
Walking
  difficulty 719.7 ✓5ᵗʰ
    psychogenic 307.9
  sleep 307.46
    hysterical 300.13
Wall, abdominal — see condition
Wallenberg's syndrome (posterior inferior cerebellar artery) (see also Disease, cerebrovascular, acute) 436
Wallgren's
  disease (obstruction of splenic vein with collateral circulation) 459.89
  meningitis (see also Meningitis, aseptic) 047.9

Wandering
  acetabulum 736.39
  gallbladder 751.69
  kidney, congenital 753.3
  organ or site, congenital NEC — see Malposition, congenital
  pacemaker (atrial) (heart) 427.89
  spleen 289.59
Wardrop's disease (with lymphangitis) 681.9
  finger 681.02
  toe 681.11
War neurosis 300.16
Wart (common) (digitate) (filiform) (infectious) (juvenile) (plantar) (viral) 078.10
  external genital organs (venereal) 078.19
  fig 078.19
  Hassall-Henle's (of cornea) 371.41
  Henle's (of cornea) 371.41
  juvenile 078.19
  moist 078.10
  Peruvian 088.0
  plantar 078.19
  prosector (see also Tuberculosis) 017.0 ✓5ᵗʰ
  seborrheic 702.19
    inflamed 702.11
  senile 702.0
  specified NEC 078.19
  syphilitic 091.3
  tuberculous (see also Tuberculosis) 017.0 ✓5ᵗʰ
  venereal (female) (male) 078.19
Warthin's tumor (salivary gland) (M8561/0) 210.2
Washerwoman's itch 692.4
Wassilieff's disease (leptospiral jaundice) 100.0
Wasting
  disease 799.4
    due to malnutrition 261
  extreme (due to malnutrition) 261
  muscular NEC 728.2
  palsy, paralysis 335.21
Water
  clefts 366.12
  deprivation of 994.3
  in joint (see also Effusion, joint) 719.0 ✓5ᵗʰ
  intoxication 276.6
  itch 120.3
  lack of 994.3
  loading 276.6
  on
    brain — see Hydrocephalus
    chest 511.8
  poisoning 276.6
Waterbrash 787.1
Water-hammer pulse (see also Insufficiency, aortic) 424.1
Waterhouse (-Friderichsen) disease or syndrome 036.3
Water-losing nephritis 588.8
Wax in ear 380.4
Waxy
  degeneration, any site 277.3
  disease 277.3
  kidney 277.3 [583.81]
  liver (large) 277.3
  spleen 277.3
Weak, weakness (generalized) 780.79
  arches (acquired) 734
    congenital 754.61
  bladder sphincter 596.59
  congenital 779.89 ▲
  eye muscle — see Strabismus
  foot (double) — see Weak, arches
  heart, cardiac (see also Failure, heart) 428.9
    congenital 746.9
  mind 317
  muscle 728.9
  myocardium (see also Failure, heart) 428.9
  newborn 779.89 ▲
  pelvic fundus 618.8
  pulse 785.9
  senile 797
  valvular — see Endocarditis
Wear, worn, tooth, teeth (approximal) (hard tissues) (interproximal) (occlusal) 521.1

Weather, weathered
  effects of
    cold NEC 991.9
      specified effect NEC 991.8
    hot (see also Heat) 992.9
  skin 692.74
Web, webbed (congenital) — see also Anomaly, specified type NEC
  canthus 743.63
  digits (see also Syndactylism) 755.10
  esophagus 750.3
  fingers (see also Syndactylism, fingers) 755.11
  larynx (glottic) (subglottic) 748.2
  neck (pterygium colli) 744.5
  Paterson-Kelly (sideropenic dysphagia) 280.8
  popliteal syndrome 756.89
  toes (see also Syndactylism, toes) 755.13
Weber's paralysis or syndrome 344.89
Weber-Christian disease or syndrome (nodular nonsuppurative panniculitis) 729.30
Weber-Cockayne syndrome (epidermolysis bullosa) 757.39
Weber-Dimitri syndrome 759.6
Weber-Gubler syndrome 344.89
Weber-Leyden syndrome 344.89
Weber-Osler syndrome (familial hemorrhagic telangiectasia) 448.0
Wedge-shaped or wedging vertebra (see also Osteoporosis) 733.00
Wegener's granulomatosis or syndrome 446.4
Wegner's disease (syphilitic osteochondritis) 090.0
Weight
  gain (abnormal) (excessive) 783.1
    during pregnancy 646.1 ✓5ᵗʰ
      insufficient 646.8 ✓5ᵗʰ
  less than 1000 grams at birth 765.0 ✓5ᵗʰ
  loss (cause unknown) 783.21
Weightlessness 994.9
Weil's disease (leptospiral jaundice) 100.0
Weill-Marchesani syndrome (brachymorphism and ectopia lentis) 759.89
Weingarten's syndrome (tropical eosinophilia) 518.3
Weir Mitchell's disease (erythromelalgia) 443.89
Weiss-Baker syndrome (carotid sinus syncope) 337.0
Weissenbach-Thibierge syndrome (cutaneous systemic sclerosis) 710.1
Wen (see also Cyst, sebaceous) 706.2
Wenckebach's phenomenon, heart block (second degree) 426.13
Werdnig-Hoffmann syndrome (muscular atrophy) 335.0
Werlhof's disease (see also Purpura, thrombocytopenic) 287.3
Werlhof-Wichmann syndrome (see also Purpura, thrombocytopenic) 287.3
Wermer's syndrome or disease (polyendocrine adenomatosis) 258.0
Werner's disease or syndrome (progeria adultorum) 259.8
Werner-His disease (trench fever) 083.1
Werner-Schultz disease (agranulocytosis) 288.0
Wernicke's encephalopathy, disease, or syndrome (superior hemorrhagic polioencephalitis) 265.1
Wernicke-Korsakoff syndrome or psychosis (nonalcoholic) 294.0
  alcoholic 291.1
Wernicke-Posadas disease (see also Coccidioidomycosis) 114.9
Wesselsbron fever 066.3
West African fever 084.8
West Nile fever 066.4 ▲
West Nile virus 066.4 ●
Westphal-Strümpell syndrome (hepatolenticular degeneration) 275.1
Wet
  brain (alcoholic) (see also Alcoholism) 303.9 ✓5ᵗʰ

Index to Diseases

Wet — *continued*
  feet, tropical (syndrome) (maceration) 991.4
  lung (syndrome)
    adult 518.5
    newborn 770.6
Wharton's duct — *see* condition
Wheal 709.8
Wheezing 786.07
Whiplash injury or syndrome 847.0
Whipple's disease or syndrome (intestinal lipodystrophy) 040.2
Whipworm 127.3
"Whistling face" syndrome (craniocarpotarsal dystrophy) 759.89
White — *see also* condition
  kidney
    large — *see* Nephrosis
    small 582.9
  leg, puerperal, postpartum, childbirth 671.4 ✓5ᵗʰ
    nonpuerperal 451.19
  mouth 112.0
  patches of mouth 528.6
  sponge nevus of oral mucosa 750.26
  spot lesions, teeth 521.01
White's disease (congenital) (keratosis follicularis) 757.39
Whitehead 706.2
Whitlow (with lymphangitis) 681.01
  herpetic 054.6
Whitmore's disease or fever (melioidosis) 025
Whooping cough 033.9
  with pneumonia 033.9 [484.3]
  due to
    Bordetella
      bronchoseptica 033.8
        with pneumonia 033.8 [484.3]
      parapertussis 033.1
        with pneumonia 033.1 [484.3]
      pertussis 033.0
        with pneumonia 033.0 [484.3]
    specified organism NEC 033.8
      with pneumonia 033.8 [484.3]
  vaccination, prophylactic (against) V03.6
Wichmann's asthma (laryngismus stridulus) 478.75
Widal (-Abrami) syndrome (acquired hemolytic jaundice) 283.9
Widening aorta (*see also* Aneurysm, aorta) 441.9
  ruptured 441.5
Wilkie's disease or syndrome 557.1
Wilkinson-Sneddon disease or syndrome (subcorneal pustular dermatosis) 694.1
Willan's lepra 696.1
Willan-Plumbe syndrome (psoriasis) 696.1
Willebrand (-Jürgens) syndrome or thrombopathy (angiohemophilia) 286.4
Willi-Prader syndrome (hypogenital dystrophy with diabetic tendency) 759.81
Willis' disease (diabetes mellitus) (*see also* Diabetes) 250.0 ✓5ᵗʰ
Wilms' tumor or neoplasm (nephroblastoma) (M8960/3) 189.0
Wilson's
  disease or syndrome (hepatolenticular degeneration) 275.1
  hepatolenticular degeneration 275.1
  lichen ruber 697.0
Wilson-Brocq disease (dermatitis exfoliativa) 695.89
Wilson-Mikity syndrome 770.7
Window — *see also* Imperfect, closure
  aorticopulmonary 745.0
Winged scapula 736.89
Winter — *see also* condition
  vomiting disease 078.82
Wise's disease 696.2
Wiskott-Aldrich syndrome (eczema-thrombocytopenia) 279.12

Withdrawal symptoms, syndrome
  alcohol 291.81
    delirium (acute) 291.0
      chronic 291.1
      newborn 760.71
  drug or narcotic 292.0
  newborn, infant of dependent mother 779.5
  steroid NEC
    correct substance properly administered 255.4
    overdose or wrong substance given or taken 962.0
Withdrawing reaction, child or adolescent 313.22
Witts' anemia (achlorhydric anemia) 280.9
Witzelsucht 301.9
Woakes' syndrome (ethmoiditis) 471.1
Wohlfart-Kugelberg-Welander disease 335.11
Woillez's disease (acute idiopathic pulmonary congestion) 518.5
Wolff-Parkinson-White syndrome (anomalous atrioventricular excitation) 426.7
Wolhynian fever 083.1
Wolman's disease (primary familial xanthomatosis) 272.7
Wood asthma 495.8
Woolly, wooly hair (congenital) (nevus) 757.4
Wool-sorters' disease 022.1
Word
  blindness (congenital) (developmental) 315.01
    secondary to organic lesion 784.61
  deafness (secondary to organic lesion) 784.69
    developmental 315.31
Worm(s) (colic) (fever) (infection) (infestation) (*see also* Infestation) 128.9
  guinea 125.7
  in intestine NEC 127.9
Worm-eaten soles 102.3
Worn out (*see also* Exhaustion) 780.79
"Worried well" V65.5
Wound, open (by cutting or piercing instrument) (by firearms) (cut) (dissection) (incised) (laceration) (penetration) (perforating) (puncture) (with initial hemorrhage, not internal) 879.8

> *Note* — For fracture with open wound, see Fracture.
>
> For laceration, traumatic rupture, tear or penetrating wound of internal organs, such as heart, lung, liver, kidney, pelvic organs, etc., whether or not accompanied by open wound or fracture in the same region, see Injury, internal.
>
> For contused wound, see Contusion. For crush injury, see Crush. For abrasion, insect bite (nonvenomous), blister, or scratch, see Injury, superficial.
>
> Complicated includes wounds with:
>   delayed healing
>   delayed treatment
>   foreign body
>   primary infection
>
> For late effect of open wound, see Late, effect, wound, open, by site.

  abdomen, abdominal (external) (muscle) 879.2
    complicated 879.3
    wall (anterior) 879.2
      complicated 879.3
      lateral 879.4
        complicated 879.5
  alveolar (process) 873.62
    complicated 873.72
  ankle 891.0
    with tendon involvement 891.2
    complicated 891.1
  anterior chamber, eye (*see also* Wound, open, intraocular) 871.9
  anus 879.6
    complicated 879.7
  arm 884.0
    with tendon involvement 884.2

Wound, open — *continued*
  arm — *continued*
    complicated 884.1
    forearm 881.00
      with tendon involvement 881.20
      complicated 881.10
    multiple sites — *see* Wound, open, multiple, upper limb
    upper 880.03
      with tendon involvement 880.23
      complicated 880.13
      multiple sites (with axillary or shoulder regions) 880.09
        with tendon involvement 880.29
        complicated 880.19
  artery — *see* Injury, blood vessel, by site
  auditory
    canal (external) (meatus) 872.02
      complicated 872.12
    ossicles (incus) (malleus) (stapes) 872.62
      complicated 872.72
  auricle, ear 872.01
    complicated 872.11
  axilla 880.02
    with tendon involvement 880.22
    complicated 880.12
      with tendon involvement 880.29
    involving other sites of upper arm 880.09
      complicated 880.19
  back 876.0
    complicated 876.1
  bladder — *see* Injury, internal, bladder
  blood vessel — *see* Injury, blood vessel, by site
  brain — *see* Injury, intracranial, with open intracranial wound
  breast 879.0
    complicated 879.1
  brow 873.42
    complicated 873.52
  buccal mucosa 873.61
    complicated 873.71
  buttock 877.0
    complicated 877.1
  calf 891.0
    with tendon involvement 891.2
    complicated 891.1
  canaliculus lacrimalis 870.8
    with laceration of eyelid 870.2
  canthus, eye 870.8
    laceration — *see* Laceration, eyelid
  cavernous sinus — *see* Injury, intracranial
  cerebellum — *see* Injury, intracranial
  cervical esophagus 874.4
    complicated 874.5
  cervix — *see* Injury, internal, cervix
  cheek(s) (external) 873.41
    complicated 873.51
    internal 873.61
      complicated 873.71
  chest (wall) (external) 875.0
    complicated 875.1
  chin 873.44
    complicated 873.54
  choroid 363.63
  ciliary body (eye) (*see also* Wound, open, intraocular) 871.9
  clitoris 878.8
    complicated 878.9
  cochlea 872.64
    complicated 872.74
  complicated 879.9
  conjunctiva — *see* Wound, open, intraocular
  cornea (nonpenetrating) (*see also* Wound, open, intraocular) 871.9
  costal region 875.0
    complicated 875.1
  Descemet's membrane (*see also* Wound, open, intraocular) 871.9
  digit(s)
    foot 893.0
      with tendon involvement 893.2
      complicated 893.1
    hand 883.0
      with tendon involvement 883.2
      complicated 883.1
  drumhead, ear 872.61
    complicated 872.71

Wound, open

Wound, open — *continued*
  ear 872.8
    canal 872.02
      complicated 872.12
    complicated 872.9
    drum 872.61
      complicated 872.71
    external 872.00
      complicated 872.10
    multiple sites 872.69
      complicated 872.79
    ossicles (incus) (malleus) (stapes) 872.62
      complicated 872.72
    specified part NEC 872.69
      complicated 872.79
  elbow 881.01
    with tendon involvement 881.21
    complicated 881.11
  epididymis 878.2
    complicated 878.3
  epigastric region 879.2
    complicated 879.3
  epiglottis 874.01
    complicated 874.11
  esophagus (cervical) 874.4
    complicated 874.5
    thoracic — *see* Injury, internal, esophagus
  Eustachian tube 872.63
    complicated 872.73
  extremity
    lower (multiple) NEC 894.0
      with tendon involvement 894.2
      complicated 894.1
    upper (multiple) NEC 884.0
      with tendon involvement 884.2
      complicated 884.1
  eye(s) (globe) — *see* Wound, open, intraocular
  eyeball NEC 871.9
    laceration (*see also* Laceration, eyeball) 871.4
    penetrating (*see also* Penetrating wound, eyeball) 871.7
  eyebrow 873.42
    complicated 873.52
  eyelid NEC 870.8
    laceration — *see* Laceration, eyelid
  face 873.40
    complicated 873.50
    multiple sites 873.49
      complicated 873.59
    specified part NEC 873.49
      complicated 873.59
  fallopian tube — *see* Injury, internal, fallopian tube
  finger(s) (nail) (subungual) 883.0
    with tendon involvement 883.2
    complicated 883.1
  flank 879.4
    complicated 879.5
  foot (any part except toe(s) alone) 892.0
    with tendon involvement 892.2
    complicated 892.1
  forearm 881.00
    with tendon involvement 881.20
    complicated 881.10
  forehead 873.42
    complicated 873.52
  genital organs (external) NEC 878.8
    complicated 878.9
    internal — *see* Injury, internal, by site
  globe (eye) (*see also* Wound, open, eyeball) 871.9
  groin 879.4
    complicated 879.5
  gum(s) 873.62
    complicated 873.72
  hand (except finger(s) alone) 882.0
    with tendon involvement 882.2
    complicated 882.1
  head NEC 873.8
    with intracranial injury — *see* Injury, intracranial
      due to or associated with skull fracture — *see* Fracture, skull
    complicated 873.9
    scalp — *see* Wound, open, scalp

Wound, open — *continued*
  heel 892.0
    with tendon involvement 892.2
    complicated 892.1
  high-velocity (grease gun) — *see* Wound, open, complicated, by site
  hip 890.0
    with tendon involvement 890.2
    complicated 890.1
  hymen 878.6
    complicated 878.7
  hypochondrium 879.4
    complicated 879.5
  hypogastric region 879.2
    complicated 879.3
  iliac (region) 879.4
    complicated 879.5
  incidental to
    dislocation — *see* Dislocation, open, by site
    fracture — *see* Fracture, open, by site
    intracranial injury — *see* Injury, intracranial, with open intracranial wound
    nerve injury — *see* Injury, nerve, by site
  inguinal region 879.4
    complicated 879.5
  instep 892.0
    with tendon involvement 892.2
    complicated 892.1
  interscapular region 876.0
    complicated 876.1
  intracranial — *see* Injury, intracranial, with open intracranial wound
  intraocular 871.9
    with
      partial loss (of intraocular tissue) 871.2
      prolapse or exposure (of intraocular tissue) 871.1
    aceration (*see also* Laceration, eyeball) 871.4
    penetrating 871.7
      with foreign body (nonmagnetic) 871.6
        magnetic 871.5
    without prolapse (of intraocular tissue) 871.0
  iris (*see also* Wound, open, eyeball) 871.9
  jaw (fracture not involved) 873.44
    with fracture — *see* Fracture, jaw
    complicated 873.54
  knee 891.0
    with tendon involvement 891.2
    complicated 891.1
  labium (majus) (minus) 878.4
    complicated 878.5
  lacrimal apparatus, gland, or sac 870.8
    with laceration of eyelid 870.2
  larynx 874.01
    with trachea 874.00
      complicated 874.10
    complicated 874.11
  leg (multiple) 891.0
    with tendon involvement 891.2
    complicated 891.1
    lower 891.0
      with tendon involvement 891.2
      complicated 891.1
    thigh 890.0
      with tendon involvement 890.2
      complicated 890.1
    upper 890.0
      with tendon involvement 890.2
      complicated 890.1
  lens (eye) (alone) (*see also* Cataract, traumatic) 366.20
    with involvement of other eye structures — *see* Wound, open, eyeball
  limb
    lower (multiple) NEC 894.0
      with tendon involvement 894.2
      complicated 894.1
    upper (multiple) NEC 884.0
      with tendon involvement 884.2
      complicated 884.1
  lip 873.43
    complicated 873.53
  loin 876.0
    complicated 876.1

Wound, open — *continued*
  lumbar region 876.0
    complicated 876.1
  malar region 873.41
    complicated 873.51
  mastoid region 873.49
    complicated 873.59
  mediastinum — *see* Injury, internal, mediastinum
  midthoracic region 875.0
    complicated 875.1
  mouth 873.60
    complicated 873.70
    floor 873.64
      complicated 873.74
    multiple sites 873.69
      complicated 873.79
    specified site NEC 873.69
      complicated 873.79
  multiple, unspecified site(s) 879.8

> *Note* — Multiple open wounds of sites classifiable to the same four-digit category should be classified to that category unless they are in different limbs.
>
> Multiple open wounds of sites classifiable to different four-digit categories, or to different limbs, should be coded separately.

    complicated 879.9
    lower limb(s) (one or both) (sites classifiable to more than one three-digit category in 890 to 893) 894.0
      with tendon involvement 894.2
      complicated 894.1
    upper limb(s) (one or both) (sites classifiable to more than one three-digit category in 880 to 883) 884.0
      with tendon involvement 884.2
      complicated 884.1
  muscle — *see* Sprain, by site
  nail
    finger(s) 883.0
      complicated 883.1
    thumb 883.0
      complicated 883.1
    toe(s) 893.0
      complicated 893.1
  nape (neck) 874.8
    complicated 874.9
    specified part NEC 874.8
      complicated 874.9
  nasal — *see also* Wound, open, nose
    cavity 873.22
      complicated 873.32
    septum 873.21
      complicated 873.31
    sinuses 873.23
      complicated 873.33
  nasopharynx 873.22
    complicated 873.32
  neck 874.8
    complicated 874.9
    nape 874.8
      complicated 874.9
    specified part NEC 874.8
      complicated 874.9
  nerve — *see* Injury, nerve, by site
  non-healing surgical 998.83
  nose 873.20
    complicated 873.30
    multiple sites 873.29
      complicated 873.39
    septum 873.21
      complicated 873.31
    sinuses 873.23
      complicated 873.33
  occipital region — *see* Wound, open, scalp
  ocular NEC 871.9
    adnexa 870.9
      specified region NEC 870.8
    laceration (*see also* Laceration, ocular) 871.4
    muscle (extraocular) 870.3
      with foreign body 870.4
      eyelid 870.1
      intraocular — *see* Wound, open, eyeball

Wound, open — *continued*
  ocular NEC — *continued*
    penetrating (*see also* Penetrating wound, ocular) 871.7
    orbit 870.8
      penetrating 870.3
        with foreign body 870.4
    orbital region 870.9
  ovary — *see* Injury, internal, pelvic organs
  palate 873.65
    complicated 873.75
  palm 882.0
    with tendon involvement 882.2
    complicated 882.1
  parathyroid (gland) 874.2
    complicated 874.3
  parietal region — *see* Wound, open, scalp
  pelvic floor or region 879.6
    complicated 879.7
  penis 878.0
    complicated 878.1
  perineum 879.6
    complicated 879.7
  periocular area 870.8
    laceration of skin 870.0
  pharynx 874.4
    complicated 874.5
  pinna 872.01
    complicated 872.11
  popliteal space 891.0
    with tendon involvement 891.2
    complicated 891.1
  prepuce 878.0
    complicated 878.1
  pubic region 879.2
    complicated 879.3
  pudenda 878.8
    complicated 878.9
  rectovaginal septum 878.8
    complicated 878.9
  sacral region 877.0
    complicated 877.1
  sacroiliac region 877.0
    complicated 877.1
  salivary (ducts) (glands) 873.69
    complicated 873.79
  scalp 873.0
    complicated 873.1
  scalpel, fetus or newborn 767.8
  scapular region 880.01
    with tendon involvement 880.21
    complicated 880.11
    involving other sites of upper arm 880.09
      with tendon involvement 880.29
      complicated 880.19
  sclera — (*see also* Wound, open, intraocular) 871.9
  scrotum 878.2
    complicated 878.3
  seminal vesicle — *see* Injury, internal, pelvic organs
  shin 891.0
    with tendon involvement 891.2
    complicated 891.1
  shoulder 880.00
    with tendon involvement 880.20
    complicated 880.10
    involving other sites of upper arm 880.09
      with tendon involvement 880.29
      complicated 880.19
  skin NEC 879.8
    complicated 879.9
  skull — *see also* Injury, intracranial, with open intracranial wound
    with skull fracture — *see* Fracture, skull
  spermatic cord (scrotal) 878.2
    complicated 878.3
    pelvic region — *see* Injury, internal, spermatic cord
  spinal cord — *see* Injury, spinal
  sternal region 875.0
    complicated 875.1
  subconjunctival — *see* Wound, open, intraocular
  subcutaneous NEC 879.8
    complicated 879.9
  submaxillary region 873.44
    complicated 873.54

Wound, open — *continued*
  submental region 873.44
    complicated 873.54
  subungual
    finger(s) (thumb) — *see* Wound, open, finger
    toe(s) — *see* Wound, open, toe
  supraclavicular region 874.8
    complicated 874.9
  supraorbital 873.42
    complicated 873.52
  surgical, non-healing 998.83
  temple 873.49
    complicated 873.59
  temporal region 873.49
    complicated 873.59
  testis 878.2
    complicated 878.3
  thigh 890.0
    with tendon involvement 890.2
    complicated 890.1
  thorax, thoracic (external) 875.0
    complicated 875.1
  throat 874.8
    complicated 874.9
  thumb (nail) (subungual) 883.0
    with tendon involvement 883.2
    complicated 883.1
  thyroid (gland) 874.2
    complicated 874.3
  toe(s) (nail) (subungual) 893.0
    with tendon involvement 893.2
    complicated 893.1
  tongue 873.64
    complicated 873.74
  tonsil — *see* Wound, open, neck
  trachea (cervical region) 874.02
    with larynx 874.00
      complicated 874.10
    complicated 874.12
    intrathoracic — *see* Injury, internal, trachea
  trunk (multiple) NEC 879.6
    complicated 879.7
    specified site NEC 879.6
      complicated 879.7
  tunica vaginalis 878.2
    complicated 878.3
  tympanic membrane 872.61
    complicated 872.71
  tympanum 872.61
    complicated 872.71
  umbilical region 879.2
    complicated 879.3
  ureter — *see* Injury, internal, ureter
  urethra — *see* Injury, internal, urethra
  uterus — *see* Injury, internal, uterus
  uvula 873.69
    complicated 873.79
  vagina 878.6
    complicated 878.7
  vas deferens — *see* Injury, internal, vas deferens
  vitreous (humor) 871.2
  vulva 878.4
    complicated 878.5
  wrist 881.02
    with tendon involvement 881.22
    complicated 881.12

Wright's syndrome (hyperabduction) 447.8
  pneumonia 390 [517.1]

Wringer injury — *see* Crush injury, by site

Wrinkling of skin 701.8

Wrist — *see also* condition
  drop (acquired) 736.05

Wrong drug (given in error) NEC 977.9
  specified drug or substance — *see* Table of Drugs and Chemicals

Wry neck — *see also* Torticollis
  congenital 754.1

Wuchereria infestation 125.0
  bancrofti 125.0
  Brugia malayi 125.1
  malayi 125.1

Wuchereriasis 125.0

Wuchereriosis 125.0

Wuchernde struma langhans (M8332/3) 193

X

Xanthelasma 272.2
  eyelid 272.2 [374.51]
  palpebrarum 272.2 [374.51]
Xanthelasmatosis (essential) 272.2
Xanthelasmoidea 757.33
Xanthine stones 277.2
Xanthinuria 277.2
Xanthofibroma (M8831/0) — *see* Neoplasm, connective tissue, benign
Xanthoma(s), xanthomatosis 272.2
  with
    hyperlipoproteinemia
      type I 272.3
      type III 272.2
      type IV 272.1
      type V 272.3
  bone 272.7
  craniohypophyseal 277.8
  cutaneotendinous 272.7
  diabeticorum 250.8 [272.2]
  disseminatum 272.7
  eruptive 272.2
  eyelid 272.2 [374.51]
  familial 272.7
  hereditary 272.7
  hypercholesterinemic 272.0
  hypercholesterolemic 272.0
  hyperlipemic 272.4
  hyperlipidemic 272.4
  infantile 272.7
  joint 272.7
  juvenile 272.7
  multiple 272.7
  multiplex 272.7
  primary familial 272.7
  tendon (sheath) 272.7
  tuberosum 272.2
  tuberous 272.2
  tubo-eruptive 272.2
Xanthosis 709.09
  surgical 998.81
Xenophobia 300.29
Xeroderma (congenital) 757.39
  acquired 701.1
    eyelid 373.33
  eyelid 373.33
  pigmentosum 757.33
  vitamin A deficiency 264.8
Xerophthalmia 372.53
  vitamin A deficiency 264.7
Xerosis
  conjunctiva 372.53
    with Bitôt's spot 372.53
      vitamin A deficiency 264.1
    vitamin A deficiency 264.0
  cornea 371.40
    with corneal ulceration 370.00
      vitamin A deficiency 264.3
    vitamin A deficiency 264.2
  cutis 706.8
  skin 706.8
Xerostomia 527.7
Xiphodynia 733.90
Xiphoidalgia 733.90
Xiphoiditis 733.99
Xiphopagus 759.4
XO syndrome 758.6
X-ray
  effects, adverse, NEC 990
  of chest
    for suspected tuberculosis V71.2
    routine V72.5
XXX syndrome 758.81
XXXXY syndrome 758.81
XXY syndrome 758.7
Xyloketosuria 271.8
Xylosuria 271.8
Xylulosuria 271.8
XYY syndrome 758.81

Y

Yawning 786.09
- psychogenic 306.1

Yaws 102.9
- bone or joint lesions 102.6
- butter 102.1
- chancre 102.0
- cutaneous, less than five years after infection 102.2
- early (cutaneous) (macular) (maculopapular) (micropapular) (papular) 102.2
  - frambeside 102.2
  - skin lesions NEC 102.2
- eyelid 102.9 [373.4]
- ganglion 102.6
- gangosis, gangosa 102.5
- gumma, gummata 102.4
  - bone 102.6
- gummatous
  - frambeside 102.4
  - osteitis 102.6
  - periostitis 102.6
- hydrarthrosis 102.6
- hyperkeratosis (early) (late) (palmar) (plantar) 102.3
- initial lesions 102.0
- joint lesions 102.6
- juxta-articular nodules 102.7
- late nodular (ulcerated) 102.4
- latent (without clinical manifestations) (with positive serology) 102.8
- mother 102.0
- mucosal 102.7
- multiple papillomata 102.1
- nodular, late (ulcerated) 102.4
- osteitis 102.6
- papilloma, papillomata (palmar) (plantar) 102.1
- periostitis (hypertrophic) 102.6
- ulcers 102.4
- wet crab 102.1

Yeast infection (see also Candidiasis) 112.9

Yellow
- atrophy (liver) 570
  - chronic 571.8
  - resulting from administration of blood, plasma, serum, or other biological substance (within 8 months of administration) — see Hepatitis, viral
- fever — see Fever, yellow
- jack (see also Fever, yellow) 060.9
- jaundice (see also Jaundice) 782.4

Yersinia septica 027.8

Z

Zagari's disease (xerostomia) 527.7

Zahorsky's disease (exanthema subitum) 057.8
- syndrome (herpangina) 074.0

Zenker's diverticulum (esophagus) 530.6

Ziehen-Oppenheim disease 333.6

Zieve's syndrome (jaundice, hyperlipemia, and hemolytic anemia) 571.1

Zika fever 066.3

Zollinger-Ellison syndrome (gastric hypersecretion with pancreatic islet cell tumor) 251.5

Zona (see also Herpes, zoster) 053.9

Zoophilia (erotica) 302.1

Zoophobia 300.29

Zoster (herpes) (see also Herpes, zoster) 053.9

Zuelzer (-Ogden) anemia or syndrome (nutritional megaloblastic anemia) 281.2

Zygodactyly (see also Syndactylism) 755.10

Zygomycosis 117.7

Zymotic — see condition

SECTION 2

Alphabetic Index to Poisoning and External Causes of Adverse Effects of Drugs and Other Chemical Substances

TABLE OF DRUGS AND CHEMICALS

This table contains a classification of drugs and other chemical substances to identify poisoning states and external causes of adverse effects.

Each of the listed substances in the table is assigned a code according to the poisoning classification (960-989). These codes are used when there is a statement of poisoning, overdose, wrong substance given or taken, or intoxication.

The table also contains a listing of external causes of adverse effects. An adverse effect is a pathologic manifestation due to ingestion or exposure to drugs or other chemical substances (e.g., dermatitis, hypersensitivity reaction, aspirin gastritis). The adverse effect is to be identified by the appropriate code found in Section 1, Index to Diseases and Injuries. An external cause code can then be used to identify the circumstances involved. The table headings pertaining to external causes are defined below:

> **Accidental poisoning (E850-E869)** — accidental overdose of drug, wrong substance given or taken, drug taken inadvertently, accidents in the usage of drugs and biologicals in medical and surgical procedures, and to show external causes of poisonings classifiable to 980-989.
>
> **Therapeutic use (E930-E949)** — a correct substance properly administered in therapeutic or prophylactic dosage as the external cause of adverse effects.
>
> **Suicide attempt (E950-E952)** — instances in which self-inflicted injuries or poisonings are involved.
>
> **Assault (E961-E962)** — injury or poisoning inflicted by another person with the intent to injure or kill.
>
> **Undetermined (E980-E982)** — to be used when the intent of the poisoning or injury cannot be determined whether it was intentional or accidental.

The American Hospital Formulary Service list numbers are included in the table to help classify new drugs not identified in the table by name. The AHFS list numbers are keyed to the continually revised American Hospital Formulary Service (AHFS).* These listings are found in the table under the main term **Drug.**

Excluded from the table are radium and other radioactive substances. The classification of adverse effects and complications pertaining to these substances will be found in Section 1, Index to Diseases and Injuries, and Section 3, Index to External Causes of Injuries.

Although certain substances are indexed with one or more subentries, the majority are listed according to one use or state. It is recognized that many substances may be used in various ways, in medicine and in industry, and may cause adverse effects whatever the state of the agent (solid, liquid, or fumes arising from a liquid). In cases in which the reported data indicates a use or state not in the table, or which is clearly different from the one listed, an attempt should be made to classify the substance in the form which most nearly expresses the reported facts.

*American Hospital Formulary Service, 2 vol. (Washington, D.C.: American Society of Hospital Pharmacists, 1959-)

Table of Drugs and Chemicals

		External Cause (E-Code)				
	Poisoning	Accident	Therapeutic Use	Suicide Attempt	Assault	Undetermined
1-propanol	980.3	E860.4	—	E950.9	E962.1	E980.9
2-propanol	980.2	E860.3	—	E950.9	E962.1	E980.9
2, 4-D (dichlorophenoxyacetic acid)	989.4	E863.5	—	E950.6	E962.1	E980.7
2, 4-toluene diisocyanate	983.0	E864.0	—	E950.7	E962.1	E980.6
2, 4, 5-T (trichlorophenoxyacetic acid)	989.2	E863.5	—	E950.6	E962.1	E980.7
14-hydroxydihydromorphinone	965.09	E850.2	E935.2	E950.0	E962.0	E980.0
ABOB	961.7	E857	E931.7	E950.4	E962.0	E980.4
Abrus (seed)	988.2	E865.3	—	E950.9	E962.1	E980.9
Absinthe	980.0	E860.1	—	E950.9	E962.1	E980.9
beverage	980.0	E860.0	—	E950.9	E962.1	E980.9
Acenocoumarin, acenocoumarol	964.2	E858.2	E934.2	E950.4	E962.0	E980.4
Acepromazine	969.1	E853.0	E939.1	E950.3	E962.0	E980.3
Acetal	982.8	E862.4	—	E950.9	E962.1	E980.9
Acetaldehyde (vapor)	987.8	E869.8	—	E952.8	E962.2	E982.8
liquid	989.89	E866.8	—	E950.9	E962.1	E980.9
Acetaminophen	965.4	E850.4	E935.4	E950.0	E962.0	E980.0
Acetaminosalol	965.1	E850.3	E935.3	E950.0	E962.0	E980.0
Acetanilid(e)	965.4	E850.4	E935.4	E950.0	E962.0	E980.0
Acetarsol, acetarsone	961.1	E857	E931.1	E950.4	E962.0	E980.4
Acetazolamide	974.2	E858.5	E944.2	E950.4	E962.0	E980.4
Acetic						
acid	983.1	E864.1	—	E950.7	E962.1	E980.6
with sodium acetate (ointment)	976.3	E858.7	E946.3	E950.4	E962.0	E980.4
irrigating solution	974.5	E858.5	E944.5	E950.4	E962.0	E980.4
lotion	976.2	E858.7	E946.2	E950.4	E962.0	E980.4
anhydride	983.1	E864.1	—	E950.7	E962.1	E980.6
ether (vapor)	982.8	E862.4	—	E950.9	E962.1	E980.9
Acetohexamide	962.3	E858.0	E932.3	E950.4	E962.0	E980.4
Acetomenaphthone	964.3	E858.2	E934.3	E950.4	E962.0	E980.4
Acetomorphine	965.01	E850.0	E935.0	E950.0	E962.0	E980.0
Acetone (oils) (vapor)	982.8	E862.4	—	E950.9	E962.1	E980.9
Acetophenazine (maleate)	969.1	E853.0	E939.1	E950.3	E962.0	E980.3
Acetophenetidin	965.4	E850.4	E935.4	E950.0	E962.0	E980.0
Acetophenone	982.0	E862.4	—	E950.9	E962.1	E980.9
Acetorphine	965.09	E850.2	E935.2	E950.0	E962.0	E980.0
Acetosulfone (sodium)	961.8	E857	E931.8	E950.4	E962.0	E980.4
Acetrizoate (sodium)	977.8	E858.8	E947.8	E950.4	E962.0	E980.4
Acetylcarbromal	967.3	E852.2	E937.3	E950.2	E962.0	E980.2
Acetylcholine (chloride)	971.0	E855.3	E941.0	E950.4	E962.0	E980.4
Acetylcysteine	975.5	E858.6	E945.5	E950.4	E962.0	E980.4
Acetyldigitoxin	972.1	E858.3	E942.1	E950.4	E962.0	E980.4
Acetyldihydrocodeine	965.09	E850.2	E935.2	E950.0	E962.0	E980.0
Acetyldihydrocodeinone	965.09	E850.2	E935.2	E950.0	E962.0	E980.0
Acetylene (gas) (industrial)	987.1	E868.1	—	E951.8	E962.2	E981.8
incomplete combustion of — see Carbon monoxide, fuel, utility						
tetrachloride (vapor)	982.3	E862.4	—	E950.9	E962.1	E980.9
Acetyliodosalicylic acid	965.1	E850.3	E935.3	E950.0	E962.0	E980.0
Acetylphenylhydrazine	965.8	E850.8	E935.8	E950.0	E962.0	E980.0
Acetylsalicylic acid	965.1	E850.3	E935.3	E950.0	E962.0	E980.0
Achromycin	960.4	E856	E930.4	E950.4	E962.0	E980.4
ophthalmic preparation	976.5	E858.7	E946.5	E950.4	E962.0	E980.4
topical NEC	976.0	E858.7	E946.0	E950.4	E962.0	E980.4
Acidifying agents	963.2	E858.1	E933.2	E950.4	E962.0	E980.4
Acids (corrosive) NEC	983.1	E864.1	—	E950.7	E962.1	E980.6
Aconite (wild)	988.2	E865.4	—	E950.9	E962.1	E980.9
Aconitine (liniment)	976.8	E858.7	E946.8	E950.4	E962.0	E980.4
Aconitum ferox	988.2	E865.4	—	E950.9	E962.1	E980.9
Acridine	983.0	E864.0	—	E950.7	E962.1	E980.6
vapor	987.8	E869.8	—	E952.8	E962.2	E982.8
Acriflavine	961.9	E857	E931.9	E950.4	E962.0	E980.4
Acrisorcin	976.0	E858.7	E946.0	E950.4	E962.0	E980.4
Acrolein (gas)	987.8	E869.8	—	E952.8	E962.2	E982.8
liquid	989.89	E866.8	—	E950.9	E962.1	E980.9
Actaea spicata	988.2	E865.4	—	E950.9	E962.1	E980.9
Acterol	961.5	E857	E931.5	E950.4	E962.0	E980.4
ACTH	962.4	E858.0	E932.4	E950.4	E962.0	E980.4
Acthar	962.4	E858.0	E932.4	E950.4	E962.0	E980.4
Actinomycin (C)(D)	960.7	E856	E930.7	E950.4	E962.0	E980.4
Adalin (acetyl)	967.3	E852.2	E937.3	E950.2	E962.0	E980.2
Adenosine (phosphate)	977.8	E858.8	E947.8	E950.4	E962.0	E980.4
Adhesives	989.89	E866.6	—	E950.9	E962.1	E980.9
ADH	962.5	E858.0	E932.5	E950.4	E962.0	E980.4
Adicillin	960.0	E856	E930.0	E950.4	E962.0	E980.4
Adiphenine	975.1	E855.6	E945.1	E950.4	E962.0	E980.4
Adjunct, pharmaceutical	977.4	E858.8	E947.4	E950.4	E962.0	E980.4
Adrenal (extract, cortex or medulla) (glucocorticoids) (hormones) (mineralocorticoids)	962.0	E858.0	E932.0	E950.4	E962.0	E980.4
ENT agent	976.6	E858.7	E946.6	E950.4	E962.0	E980.4
ophthalmic preparation	976.5	E858.7	E946.5	E950.4	E962.0	E980.4
topical NEC	976.0	E858.7	E946.0	E950.4	E962.0	E980.4
Adrenalin	971.2	E855.5	E941.2	E950.4	E962.0	E980.4

Table of Drugs and Chemicals

		External Cause (E-Code)				
	Poisoning	Accident	Therapeutic Use	Suicide Attempt	Assault	Undetermined
Adrenergic blocking agents	971.3	E855.6	E941.3	E950.4	E962.0	E980.4
Adrenergics	971.2	E855.5	E941.2	E950.4	E962.0	E980.4
Adrenochrome (derivatives)	972.8	E858.3	E942.8	E950.4	E962.0	E980.4
Adrenocorticotropic hormone	962.4	E858.0	E932.4	E950.4	E962.0	E980.4
Adrenocorticotropin	962.4	E858.0	E932.4	E950.4	E962.0	E980.4
Adriamycin	960.7	E856	E930.7	E950.4	E962.0	E980.4
Aerosol spray — see Sprays						
Aerosporin	960.8	E856	E930.8	E950.4	E962.0	E980.4
ENT agent	976.6	E858.7	E946.6	E950.4	E962.0	E980.4
ophthalmic preparation	976.5	E858.7	E946.5	E950.4	E962.0	E980.4
topical NEC	976.0	E858.7	E946.0	E950.4	E962.0	E980.4
Aethusa cynapium	988.2	E865.4	—	E950.9	E962.1	E980.9
Afghanistan black	969.6	E854.1	E939.6	E950.3	E962.0	E980.3
Aflatoxin	989.7	E865.9	—	E950.9	E962.1	E980.9
African boxwood	988.2	E865.4	—	E950.9	E962.1	E980.9
Agar (-agar)	973.3	E858.4	E943.3	E950.4	E962.0	E980.4
Agricultural agent NEC	989.89	E863.9	—	E950.6	E962.1	E980.7
Agrypnal	967.0	E851	E937.0	E950.1	E962.0	E980.1
Air contaminant(s), source or type not specified	987.9	E869.9	—	E952.9	E962.2	E982.9
specified type — see specific substance						
Akee	988.2	E865.4	—	E950.9	E962.1	E980.9
Akrinol	976.0	E858.7	E946.0	E950.4	E962.0	E980.4
Alantolactone	961.6	E857	E931.6	E950.4	E962.0	E980.4
Albamycin	960.8	E856	E930.8	E950.4	E962.0	E980.4
Albumin (normal human serum)	964.7	E858.2	E934.7	E950.4	E962.0	E980.4
Albuterol ●	975.7	E858.6	E945.7	E950.4	E962.0	E980.4
Alcohol	980.9	E860.9	—	E950.9	E962.1	E980.9
absolute	980.0	E860.1	—	E950.9	E962.1	E980.9
beverage	980.0	E860.0	E947.8	E950.9	E962.1	E980.9
amyl	980.3	E860.4	—	E950.9	E962.1	E980.9
antifreeze	980.1	E860.2	—	E950.9	E962.1	E980.9
butyl	980.3	E860.4	—	E950.9	E962.1	E980.9
dehydrated	980.0	E860.1	—	E950.9	E862.1	E980.9
beverage	980.0	E860.0	E947.8	E950.9	E962.1	E980.9
denatured	980.0	E860.1	—	E950.9	E962.1	E980.9
deterrents	977.3	E858.8	E947.3	E950.4	E962.0	E980.4
diagnostic (gastric function)	977.8	E858.8	E947.8	E950.4	E962.0	E980.4
ethyl	980.0	E860.1	—	E950.9	E962.1	E980.9
beverage	980.0	E860.0	E947.8	E950.9	E962.1	E980.9
grain	980.0	E860.1	—	E950.9	E962.1	E980.9
beverage	980.0	E860.0	E947.8	E950.9	E962.1	E980.9
industrial	980.9	E860.9	—	E950.9	E962.1	E980.9
isopropyl	980.2	E860.3	—	E950.9	E962.1	E980.9
methyl	980.1	E860.2	—	E950.9	E962.1	E980.9
preparation for consumption	980.0	E860.0	E947.8	E950.9	E962.1	E980.9
propyl	980.3	E860.4	—	E950.9	E962.1	E980.9
secondary	980.2	E860.3	—	E950.9	E962.1	E980.9
radiator	980.1	E860.2	—	E950.9	E962.1	E980.9
rubbing	980.2	E860.3	—	E950.9	E962.1	E980.9
specified type NEC	980.8	E860.8	—	E950.9	E962.1	E980.9
surgical	980.9	E860.9	—	E950.9	E962.1	E980.9
vapor (from any type of alcohol)	987.8	E869.8	—	E952.8	E962.2	E982.8
wood	980.1	E860.2	—	E950.9	E962.1	E980.9
Alcuronium chloride	975.2	E858.6	E945.2	E950.4	E962.0	E980.4
Aldactone	974.4	E858.5	E944.4	E950.4	E962.0	E980.4
Aldicarb	989.3	E863.2	—	E950.6	E962.1	E980.7
Aldomet	972.6	E858.3	E942.6	E950.4	E962.0	E980.4
Aldosterone	962.0	E858.0	E932.0	E950.4	E962.0	E980.4
Aldrin (dust)	989.2	E863.0	—	E950.6	E962.1	E980.7
Algeldrate	973.0	E858.4	E943.0	E950.4	E962.0	E980.4
Alidase	963.4	E858.1	E933.4	E950.4	E962.0	E980.4
Aliphatic thiocyanates	989.0	E866.8	—	E950.9	E962.1	E980.9
Alkaline antiseptic solution (aromatic)	976.6	E858.7	E946.6	E950.4	E962.0	E980.4
Alkalinizing agents (medicinal)	963.3	E858.1	E933.3	E950.4	E962.0	E980.4
Alkalis, caustic	983.2	E864.2	—	E950.7	E962.1	E980.6
Alkalizing agents (medicinal)	963.3	E858.1	E933.3	E950.4	E962.0	E980.4
Alka-seltzer	965.1	E850.3	E935.3	E950	E962.0	E980
Alkavervir	972.6	E858.3	E942.6	E950.4	E962.0	E980.4
Allegron	969.0	E854.0	E939.0	E950.3	E962.0	E980.3
Alleve — see Naproxen						
Allobarbital, allobarbitone	967.0	E851	E937.0	E950.1	E962.0	E980.1
Allopurinol	974.7	E858.5	E944.7	E950.4	E962.0	E980.4
Allylestrenol	962.2	E858.0	E932.2	E950.4	E962.0	E980.4
Allylisopropylacetylurea	967.8	E852.8	E937.8	E950.2	E962.0	E980.2
Allylisopropylmalonylurea	967.0	E851	E937.0	E950.1	E962.0	E980.1
Allyltribromide	967.3	E852.2	E937.3	E950.2	E962.0	E980.2
Aloe, aloes, aloin	973.1	E858.4	E943.1	E950.4	E962.0	E980.4
Alosetron	973.8	E858.4	E943.8	E950.4	E962.0	E980.4
Aloxidone	966.0	E855.0	E936.0	E950.4	E962.0	E980.4
Aloxiprin	965.1	E850.3	E935.3	E950.0	E962.0	E980.0
Alpha amylase	963.4	E858.1	E933.4	E950.4	E962.0	E980.4

Table of Drugs and Chemicals

		External Cause (E-Code)				
	Poisoning	Accident	Therapeutic Use	Suicide Attempt	Assault	Undetermined
Alphaprodine (hydrochloride)	965.09	E850.2	E935.2	E950.0	E962.0	E980.0
Alpha tocopherol	963.5	E858.1	E933.5	E950.4	E962.0	E980.4
Alseroxylon	972.6	E858.3	E942.6	E950.4	E962.0	E980.4
Alum (ammonium) (potassium)	983.2	E864.2	—	E950.7	E962.1	E980.6
medicinal (astringent) NEC	976.2	E858.7	E946.2	E950.4	E962.0	E980.4
Aluminium, aluminum (gel) (hydroxide)	973.0	E858.4	E943.0	E950.4	E962.0	E980.4
acetate solution	976.2	E858.7	E946.2	E950.4	E962.0	E980.4
aspirin	965.1	E850.3	E935.3	E950.0	E962.0	E980.0
carbonate	973.0	E858.4	E943.0	E950.4	E962.0	E980.4
glycinate	973.0	E858.4	E943.0	E950.4	E962.0	E980.4
nicotinate	972.2	E858.3	E942.2	E950.4	E962.0	E980.4
ointment (surgical) (topical)	976.3	E858.7	E946.3	E950.4	E962.0	E980.4
phosphate	973.0	E858.4	E943.0	E950.4	E962.0	E980.4
subacetate	976.2	E858.7	E946.2	E950.4	E962.0	E980.4
topical NEC	976.3	E858.7	E946.3	E950.4	E962.0	E980.4
Alurate	967.0	E851	E937.0	E950.1	E962.0	E980.1
Alverine (citrate)	975.1	E858.6	E945.1	E950.4	E962.0	E980.4
Alvodine	965.09	E850.2	E935.2	E950.0	E962.0	E980.0
Amanita phalloides	988.1	E865.5	—	E950.9	E962.1	E980.9
Amantadine (hydrochloride)	966.4	E855.0	E936.4	E950.4	E962.0	E980.4
Ambazone	961.9	E857	E931.9	E950.4	E962.0	E980.4
Ambenonium	971.0	E855.3	E941.0	E950.4	E962.0	E980.4
Ambutonium bromide	971.1	E855.4	E941.1	E950.4	E962.0	E980.4
Ametazole	977.8	E858.8	E947.8	E950.4	E962.0	E980.4
Amethocaine (infiltration) (topical)	968.5	E855.2	E938.5	E950.4	E962.0	E980.4
nerve block (peripheral) (plexus)	968.6	E855.2	E938.6	E950.4	E962.0	E980.4
spinal	968.7	E855.2	E938.7	E950.4	E962.0	E980.4
Amethopterin	963.1	E858.1	E933.1	E950.4	E962.0	E980.4
Amfepramone	977.0	E858.8	E947.0	E950.4	E962.0	E980.4
Amidon	965.02	E850.1	E935.1	E950.0	E962.0	E980.0
Amidopyrine	965.5	E850.5	E935.5	E950.0	E962.0	E980.0
Aminacrine	976.0	E858.7	E946.0	E950.4	E962.0	E980.4
Aminitrozole	961.5	E857	E931.5	E950.4	E962.0	E980.4
Aminoacetic acid	974.5	E858.5	E944.5	E950.4	E962.0	E980.4
Amino acids	974.5	E858.5	E944.5	E950.4	E962.0	E980.4
Aminocaproic acid	964.4	E858.2	E934.4	E950.4	E962.0	E980.4
Aminoethylisothiourium	963.8	E858.1	E933.8	E950.4	E962.0	E980.4
Aminoglutethimide	966.3	E855.0	E936.3	E950.4	E962.0	E980.4
Aminometradine	974.3	E858.5	E944.3	E950.4	E962.0	E980.4
Aminopentamide	971.1	E855.4	E941.1	E950.4	E962.0	E980.4
Aminophenazone	965.5	E850.5	E935.5	E950.0	E962.0	E980.0
Aminophenol	983.0	E864.0	—	E950.7	E962.1	E980.6
Aminophenylpyridone	969.5	E853.8	E939.5	E950.3	E962.0	E980.3
Aminophyllin	975.7	E858.6	E945.7	E950.4	E962.0	E980.4
Aminopterin	963.1	E858.1	E933.1	E950.4	E962.0	E980.4
Aminopyrine	965.5	E850.5	E935.5	E950.0	E962.0	E980.0
Aminosalicylic acid	961.8	E857	E931.8	E950.4	E962.0	E980.4
Amiphenazole	970.1	E854.3	E940.1	E950.4	E962.0	E980.4
Amiquinsin	972.6	E858.3	E942.6	E950.4	E962.0	E980.4
Amisometradine	974.3	E858.5	E944.3	E950.4	E962.0	E980.4
Amitriptyline	969.0	E854.0	E939.0	E950.3	E962.0	E980.3
Ammonia (fumes) (gas) (vapor)	987.8	E869.8	—	E952.8	E962.2	E982.8
liquid (household) NEC	983.2	E861.4	—	E950.7	E962.1	E980.6
spirit, aromatic	970.8	E854.3	E940.8	E950.4	E962.0	E980.4
Ammoniated mercury	976.0	E858.7	E946.0	E950.4	E962.0	E980.4
Ammonium						
carbonate	983.2	E864.2	—	E950.7	E962.1	E980.6
chloride (acidifying agent)	963.2	E858.1	E933.2	E950.4	E962.0	E980.4
expectorant	975.5	E858.6	E945.5	E950.4	E962.0	E980.4
compounds (household) NEC	983.2	E861.4	—	E950.7	E962.1	E980.6
fumes (any usage)	987.8	E869.8	—	E952.8	E962.2	E982.8
industrial	983.2	E864.2	—	E950.7	E962.1	E980.6
ichthyosulfonate	976.4	E858.7	E946.4	E950.4	E962.0	E980.4
mandelate	961.9	E857	E931.9	E950.4	E962.0	E980.4
Amobarbital	967.0	E851	E937.0	E950.1	E962.0	E980.1
Amodiaquin(e)	961.4	E857	E931.4	E950.4	E962.0	E980.4
Amopyroquin(e)	961.4	E857	E931.4	E950.4	E962.0	E980.4
Amphenidone	969.5	E853.8	E939.5	E950.3	E962.0	E980.3
Amphetamine	969.7	E854.2	E939.7	E950.3	E962.0	E980.3
Amphomycin	960.8	E856	E930.8	E950.4	E962.0	E980.4
Amphotericin B	960.1	E856	E930.1	E950.4	E962.0	E980.4
topical	976.0	E858.7	E946.0	E950.4	E962.0	E980.4
Ampicillin	960.0	E856	E930.0	E950.4	E962.0	E980.4
Amprotropine	971.1	E855.4	E941.1	E950.4	E962.0	E980.4
Amygdalin	977.8	E858.8	E947.8	E950.4	E962.0	E980.4
Amyl						
acetate (vapor)	982.8	E862.4	—	E950.9	E962.1	E980.9
alcohol	980.3	E860.4	—	E950.9	E962.1	E980.9
nitrite (medicinal)	972.4	E858.3	E942.4	E950.4	E962.0	E980.4
Amylase (alpha)	963.4	E858.1	E933.4	E950.4	E962.0	E980.4
Amylene hydrate	980.8	E860.8	—	E950.9	E962.1	E980.9

Table of Drugs and Chemicals — Antifertility pills

		External Cause (E-Code)				
	Poisoning	Accident	Therapeutic Use	Suicide Attempt	Assault	Undetermined
Amylobarbitone	967.0	E851	E937.0	E950.1	E962.0	E980.1
Amylocaine	968.9	E855.2	E938.9	E950.4	E962.0	E980.4
infiltration (subcutaneous)	968.5	E855.2	E938.5	E950.4	E962.0	E980.4
nerve block (peripheral) (plexus)	968.6	E855.2	E938.6	E950.4	E962.0	E980.4
spinal	968.7	E855.2	E938.7	E950.4	E962.0	E980.4
topical (surface)	968.5	E855.2	E938.5	E950.4	E962.0	E980.4
Amytal (sodium)	967.0	E851	E937.0	E950.1	E962.0	E980.1
Analeptics	970.0	E854.3	E940.0	E950.4	E962.0	E980.4
Analgesics	965.9	E850.9	E935.9	E950.0	E962.0	E980.0
aromatic NEC	965.4	E850.4	E935.4	E950.0	E962.0	E980.0
non-narcotic NEC	965.7	E850.7	E935.7	E950.0	E962.0	E980.0
specified NEC	965.8	E850.8	E935.8	E950.0	E962.0	E980.0
Anamirta cocculus	988.2	E865.3	—	E950.9	E962.1	E980.9
Ancillin	960.0	E856	E930.0	E950.4	E962.0	E980.4
Androgens (anabolic congeners)	962.1	E858.0	E932.1	E950.4	E962.0	E980.4
Androstalone	962.1	E858.0	E932.1	E950.4	E962.0	E980.4
Androsterone	962.1	E858.0	E932.1	E950.4	E962.0	E980.4
Anemone pulsatilla	988.2	E865.4	—	E950.9	E962.1	E980.9
Anesthesia, anesthetic (general) NEC	968.4	E855.1	E938.4	E950.4	E962.0	E980.4
block (nerve) (plexus)	968.6	E855.2	E938.6	E950.4	E962.0	E980.4
gaseous NEC	968.2	E855.1	E938.2	E950.4	E962.0	E980.4
halogenated hydrocarbon derivatives NEC	968.2	E855.1	E938.2	E950.4	E962.0	E980.4
infiltration (intradermal) (subcutaneous) (submucosal)	968.5	E855.2	E938.5	E950.4	E962.0	E980.4
intravenous	968.3	E855.1	E938.3	E950.4	E962.0	E980.4
local NEC	968.9	E855.2	E938.9	E950.4	E962.0	E980.4
nerve blocking (peripheral) (plexus)	968.6	E855.2	E938.6	E950.4	E962.0	E980.4
rectal NEC	968.3	E855.1	E938.3	E950.4	E962.0	E980.4
spinal	968.7	E855.2	E938.7	E950.4	E962.0	E980.4
surface	968.5	E855.2	E938.5	E950.4	E962.0	E980.4
topical	968.5	E855.2	E938.5	E950.4	E962.0	E980.4
Aneurine	963.5	E858.1	E933.5	E950.4	E962.0	E980.4
Angio-Conray	977.8	E858.8	E947.8	E950.4	E962.0	E980.4
Angiotensin	971.2	E855.5	E941.2	E950.4	E962.0	E980.4
Anhydrohydroxyprogesterone	962.2	E858.0	E932.2	E950.4	E962.0	E980.4
Anhydron	974.3	E858.5	E944.3	E950.4	E962.0	E980.4
Anileridine	965.09	E850.2	E935.2	E950.0	E962.0	E980.0
Aniline (dye) (liquid)	983.0	E864.0	—	E950.7	E962.1	E980.6
analgesic	965.4	E850.4	E935.4	E950.0	E962.0	E980.0
derivatives, therapeutic NEC	965.4	E850.4	E935.4	E950.0	E962.0	E980.0
vapor	987.8	E869.8	—	E952.8	E962.2	E982.8
Anisindione	964.2	E858.2	E934.2	E950.4	E962.0	E980.4
Aniscoropine	971.1	E855.4	E941.1	E950.4	E962.0	E980.4
Anorexic agents	977.0	E858.8	E947.0	E950.4	E962.0	E980.4
Ant (bite) (sting)	989.5	E905.5	—	E950.9	E962.1	E980.9
Antabuse	977.3	E858.8	E947.3	E950.4	E962.0	E980.4
Antacids	973.0	E858.4	E943.0	E950.4	E962.0	E980.4
Antazoline	963.0	E858.1	E933.0	E950.4	E962.0	E980.4
Anthelmintics	961.6	E857	E931.6	E950.4	E962.0	E980.4
Anthralin	976.4	E858.7	E946.4	E950.4	E962.0	E980.4
Anthramycin	960.7	E856	E930.7	E950.4	E962.0	E980.4
Antiadrenergics	971.3	E855.6	E941.3	E950.4	E962.0	E980.4
Antiallergic agents	963.0	E858.1	E933.0	E950.4	E962.0	E980.4
Antianemic agents NEC	964.1	E858.2	E934.1	E950.4	E962.0	E980.4
Antiaris toxicaria	988.2	E865.4	—	E950.9	E962.1	E980.9
Antiarteriosclerotic agents	972.2	E858.3	E942.2	E950.4	E962.0	E980.4
Antiasthmatics	975.7	E858.6	E945.7	E950.4	E962.0	E980.4
Antibiotics	960.9	E856	E930.9	E950.4	E962.0	E980.4
antifungal	960.1	E856	E930.1	E950.4	E962.0	E980.4
antimycobacterial	960.6	E856	E930.6	E950.4	E962.0	E980.4
antineoplastic	960.7	E856	E930.7	E950.4	E962.0	E980.4
cephalosporin (group)	960.5	E856	E930.5	E950.4	E962.0	E980.4
chloramphenicol (group)	960.2	E856	E930.2	E950.4	E962.0	E980.4
macrolides	960.3	E856	E930.3	E950.4	E962.0	E980.4
specified NEC	960.8	E856	E930.8	E950.4	E962.0	E980.4
tetracycline (group)	960.4	E856	E930.4	E950.4	E962.0	E980.4
Anticancer agents NEC	963.1	E858.1	E933.1	E950.4	E962.0	E980.4
antibiotics	960.7	E856	E930.7	E950.4	E962.0	E980.4
Anticholinergics	971.1	E855.4	E941.1	E950.4	E962.0	E980.4
Anticholinesterase (organophosphorus) (reversible)	971.0	E855.3	E941.0	E950.4	E962.0	E980.4
Anticoagulants	964.2	E858.2	E934.2	E950.4	E962.0	E980.4
antagonists	964.5	E858.2	E934.5	E950.4	E962.0	E980.4
Anti-common cold agents NEC	975.6	E858.6	E945.6	E950.4	E962.0	E980.4
Anticonvulsants NEC	966.3	E855.0	E936.3	E950.4	E962.0	E980.4
Antidepressants	969.0	E854.0	E939.0	E950.3	E962.0	E980.3
Antidiabetic agents	962.3	E858.0	E932.3	E950.4	E962.0	E980.4
Antidiarrheal agents	973.5	E858.4	E943.5	E950.4	E962.0	E980.4
Antidiuretic hormone	962.5	E858.0	E932.5	E950.4	E962.0	E980.4
Antidotes NEC	977.2	E858.8	E947.2	E950.4	E962.0	E980.4
Antiemetic agents	963.0	E858.1	E933.0	E950.4	E962.0	E980.4
Antiepilepsy agent NEC	966.3	E855.0	E936.3	E950.4	E962.0	E980.4
Antifertility pills	962.2	E858.0	E932.2	E950.4	E962.0	E980.4

Antiflatulents

Table of Drugs and Chemicals

		External Cause (E-Code)				
	Poisoning	Accident	Therapeutic Use	Suicide Attempt	Assault	Undetermined
Antiflatulents	973.8	E858.4	E943.8	E950.4	E962.0	E980.4
Antifreeze	989.89	E866.8	—	E950.9	E962.1	E980.9
alcohol	980.1	E860.2	—	E950.9	E962.1	E980.9
ethylene glycol	982.8	E862.4	—	E950.9	E962.1	E980.9
Antifungals (nonmedicinal) (sprays)	989.4	E863.6	—	E950.6	E962.1	E980.7
medicinal NEC	961.9	E857	E931.9	E950.4	E962.0	E980.4
antibiotic	960.1	E856	E930.1	E950.4	E962.0	E980.4
topical	976.0	E858.7	E946.0	E950.4	E962.0	E980.4
Antigastric secretion agents	973.0	E858.4	E943.0	E950.4	E962.0	E980.4
Anthelmintics	961.6	E857	E931.6	E950.4	E962.0	E980.4
Antihemophilic factor (human)	964.7	E858.2	E934.7	E950.4	E962.0	E980.4
Antihistamine	963.0	E858.1	E933.0	E950.4	E962.0	E980.4
Antihypertensive agents NEC	972.6	E858.3	E942.6	E950.4	E962.0	E980.4
Anti-infectives NEC	961.9	E857	E931.9	E950.4	E962.0	E980.4
antibiotics	960.9	E856	E930.9	E950.4	E962.0	E980.4
specified NEC	960.8	E856	E930.8	E950.4	E962.0	E980.4
anthelmintic	961.6	E857	E931.6	E950.4	E962.0	E980.4
antimalarial	961.4	E857	E931.4	E950.4	E962.0	E980.4
antimycobacterial NEC	961.8	E857	E931.8	E950.4	E962.0	E980.4
antibiotics	960.6	E856	E930.6	E950.4	E962.0	E980.4
antiprotozoal NEC	961.5	E857	E931.5	E950.4	E962.0	E980.4
blood	961.4	E857	E931.4	E950.4	E962.0	E980.4
antiviral	961.7	E857	E931.7	E950.4	E962.0	E980.4
arsenical	961.1	E857	E931.1	E950.4	E962.0	E980.4
ENT agents	976.6	E858.7	E946.6	E950.4	E962.0	E980.4
heavy metals NEC	961.2	E857	E931.2	E950.4	E962.0	E980.4
local	976.0	E858.7	E946.0	E950.4	E962.0	E980.4
ophthalmic preparation	976.5	E858.7	E946.5	E950.4	E962.0	E980.4
topical NEC	976.0	E858.7	E946.0	E950.4	E962.0	E980.4
Anti-inflammatory agents (topical)	976.0	E858.7	E946.0	E950.4	E962.0	E980.4
Antiknock (tetraethyl lead)	984.1	E862.1	—	E950.9	E962.1	E980.9
Antilipemics	972.2	E858.3	E942.2	E950.4	E962.0	E980.4
Antimalarials	961.4	E857	E931.4	E950.4	E962.0	E980.4
Antimony (compounds) (vapor) NEC	985.4	E866.2	—	E950.9	E962.1	E980.9
anti-infectives	961.2	E857	E931.2	E950.4	E962.0	E980.4
pesticides (vapor)	985.4	E863.4	—	E950.6	E962.2	E980.7
potassium tartrate	961.2	E857	E931.2	E950.4	E962.0	E980.4
tartrated	961.2	E857	E931.2	E950.4	E962.0	E980.4
Antimuscarinic agents	971.1	E855.4	E941.1	E950.4	E962.0	E980.4
Antimycobacterials NEC	961.8	E857	E931.8	E950.4	E962.0	E980.4
antibiotics	960.6	E856	E930.6	E950.4	E962.0	E980.4
Antineoplastic agents	963.1	E858.1	E933.1	E950.4	E962.0	E980.4
antibiotics	960.7	E856	E930.7	E950.4	E962.0	E980.4
Anti-Parkinsonism agents	966.4	E855.0	E936.4	E950.4	E962.0	E980.4
Antiphlogistics	965.69	E850.6	E935.6	E950.0	E962.0	E980.0
Antiprotozoals NEC	961.5	E857	E931.5	E950.4	E962.0	E980.4
blood	961.4	E857	E931.4	E950.4	E962.0	E980.4
Antipruritics (local)	976.1	E858.7	E946.1	E950.4	E962.0	E980.4
Antipsychotic agents NEC	969.3	E853.8	E939.3	E950.3	E962.0	E980.3
Antipyretics	965.9	E850.9	E935.9	E950.0	E962.0	E980.0
specified NEC	965.8	E850.8	E935.8	E950.0	E962.0	E980.0
Antipyrine	965.5	E850.5	E935.5	E950.0	E962.0	E980.0
Antirabies serum (equine)	979.9	E858.8	E949.9	E950.4	E962.0	E980.4
Antirheumatics	965.69	E850.6	E935.6	E950.0	E962.0	E980.0
Antiseborrheics	976.4	E858.7	E946.4	E950.4	E962.0	E980.4
Antiseptics (external) (medicinal)	976.0	E858.7	E946.0	E950.4	E962.0	E980.4
Antistine	963.0	E858.1	E933.0	E950.4	E962.0	E980.4
Antithyroid agents	962.8	E858.0	E932.8	E950.4	E962.0	E980.4
Antitoxin, any	979.9	E858.8	E949.9	E950.4	E962.0	E980.4
Antituberculars	961.8	E857	E931.8	E950.4	E962.0	E980.4
antibiotics	960.6	E856	E930.6	E950.4	E962.0	E980.4
Antitussives	975.4	E858.6	E945.4	E950.4	E962.0	E980.4
Antivaricose agents (sclerosing)	972.7	E858.3	E942.7	E950.4	E962.0	E980.4
Antivenin (crotaline) (spider-bite)	979.9	E858.8	E949.9	E950.4	E962.0	E980.4
Antivert	963.0	E858.1	E933.0	E950.4	E962.0	E980.4
Antivirals NEC	961.7	E857	E931.7	E950.4	E962.0	E980.4
Ant poisons — see Pesticides						
Antrol	989.4	E863.4	—	E950.6	E962.1	E980.7
fungicide	989.4	E863.6	—	E950.6	E962.1	E980.7
Apomorphine hydrochloride (emetic)	973.6	E858.4	E943.6	E950.4	E962.0	E980.4
Appetite depressants, central	977.0	E858.8	E947.0	E950.4	E962.0	E980.4
Apresoline	972.6	E858.3	E942.6	E950.4	E962.0	E980.4
Aprobarbital, aprobarbitone	967.0	E851	E937.0	E950.1	E962.0	E980.1
Apronalide	967.8	E852.8	E937.8	E950.2	E962.0	E980.2
Aqua fortis	983.1	E864.1	—	E950.7	E962.1	E980.6
Arachis oil (topical)	976.3	E858.7	E946.3	E950.4	E962.0	E980.4
cathartic	973.2	E858.4	E943.2	E950.4	E962.0	E980.4
Aralen	961.4	E857	E931.4	E950.4	E962.0	E980.4
Arginine salts	974.5	E858.5	E944.5	E950.4	E962.0	E980.4
Argyrol	976.0	E858.7	E946.0	E950.4	E962.0	E980.4
ENT agent	976.6	E858.7	E946.6	E950.4	E962.0	E980.4

Table of Drugs and Chemicals — Benadryl

		External Cause (E-Code)				
	Poisoning	Accident	Therapeutic Use	Suicide Attempt	Assault	Undetermined
Argyrol — *continued*						
ophthalmic preparation	976.5	E858.7	E946.5	E950.4	E962.0	E980.4
Aristocort	962.0	E858.0	E932.0	E950.4	E962.0	E980.4
ENT agent	976.6	E858.7	E946.6	E950.4	E962.0	E980.4
ophthalmic preparation	976.5	E858.7	E946.5	E950.4	E962.0	E980.4
topical NEC	976.0	E858.7	E946.0	E950.4	E962.0	E980.4
Aromatics, corrosive	983.0	E864.0	—	E950.7	E962.1	E980.6
disinfectants	983.0	E861.4	—	E950.7	E962.1	E980.6
Arsenate of lead (insecticide)	985.1	E863.4	—	E950.8	E962.1	E980.8
herbicide	985.1	E863.5	—	E950.8	E962.1	E980.8
Arsenic, arsenicals (compounds) (dust) (fumes) (vapor) NEC	985.1	E866.3	—	E950.8	E962.1	E980.8
anti-infectives	961.1	E857	E931.1	E950.4	E962.0	E980.4
pesticide (dust) (fumes)	985.1	E863.4	—	E950.8	E962.1	E980.8
Arsine (gas)	985.1	E866.3	—	E950.8	E962.1	E980.8
Arsphenamine (silver)	961.1	E857	E931.1	E950.4	E962.0	E980.4
Arsthinol	961.1	E857	E931.1	E950.4	E962.0	E980.4
Artane	971.1	E855.4	E941.1	E950.4	E962.0	E980.4
Arthropod (venomous) NEC	989.5	E905.5	—	E950.9	E962.1	E980.9
Asbestos	989.81	E866.8	—	E950.9	E962.1	E980.9
Ascaridole	961.6	E857	E931.6	E950.4	E962.0	E980.4
Ascorbic acid	963.5	E858.1	E933.5	E950.4	E962.0	E980.4
Asiaticoside	976.0	E858.7	E946.0	E950.4	E962.0	E980.4
Aspidium (oleoresin)	961.6	E857	E931.6	E950.4	E962.0	E980.4
Aspirin	965.1	E850.3	E935.3	E950.0	E962.0	E980.0
Astringents (local)	976.2	E858.7	E946.2	E950.4	E962.0	E980.4
Atabrine	961.3	E857	E931.3	E950.4	E962.0	E980.4
Ataractics	969.5	E853.8	E939.5	E950.3	E962.0	E980.3
Atonia drug, intestinal	973.3	E858.4	E943.3	E950.4	E962.0	E980.4
Atophan	974.7	E858.5	E944.7	E950.4	E962.0	E980.4
Atropine	971.1	E855.4	E941.1	E950.4	E962.0	E980.4
Attapulgite	973.5	E858.4	E943.5	E950.4	E962.0	E980.4
Attenuvax	979.4	E858.8	E949.4	E950.4	E962.0	E980.4
Aureomycin	960.4	E856	E930.4	E950.4	E962.0	E980.4
ophthalmic preparation	976.5	E858.7	E946.5	E950.4	E962.0	E980.4
topical NEC	976.0	E858.7	E946.0	E950.4	E962.0	E980.4
Aurothioglucose	965.69	E850.6	E935.6	E950.0	E962.0	E980.0
Aurothioglycanide	965.69	E850.6	E935.6	E950.0	E962.0	E980.0
Aurothiomalate	965.69	E850.6	E935.6	E950.0	E962.0	E980.0
Automobile fuel	981	E862.1	—	E950.9	E962.1	E980.9
Autonomic nervous system agents NEC	971.9	E855.9	E941.9	E950.4	E962.0	E980.4
Avlosulfon	961.8	E857	E931.8	E950.4	E962.0	E980.4
Avomine	967.8	E852.8	E937.8	E950.2	E962.0	E980.2
Azacyclonol	969.5	E853.8	E939.5	E950.3	E962.0	E980.3
Azapetine	971.3	E855.6	E941.3	E950.4	E962.0	E980.4
Azaribine	963.1	E858.1	E933.1	E950.4	E962.0	E980.4
Azaserine	960.7	E856	E930.7	E950.4	E962.0	E980.4
Azathioprine	963.1	E858.1	E933.1	E950.4	E962.0	E980.4
Azosulfamide	961.0	E857	E931.0	E950.4	E962.0	E980.4
Azulfidine	961.0	E857	E931.0	E950.4	E962.0	E980.4
Azuresin	977.8	E858.8	E947.8	E950.4	E962.0	E980.4
Bacimycin	976.0	E858.7	E946.0	E950.4	E962.0	E980.4
ophthalmic preparation	976.5	E858.7	E946.5	E950.4	E962.0	E980.4
Bacitracin	960.8	E856	E930.8	E950.4	E962.0	E980.4
ENT agent	976.6	E858.7	E946.6	E950.4	E962.0	E980.4
ophthalmic preparation	976.5	E858.7	E946.5	E950.4	E962.0	E980.4
topical NEC	976.0	E858.7	E946.0	E950.4	E962.0	E980.4
Baking soda	963.3	E858.1	E933.3	E950.4	E962.0	E980.4
BAL	963.8	E858.1	E933.8	E950.4	E962.0	E980.4
Bamethan (sulfate)	972.5	E858.3	E942.5	E950.4	E962.0	E980.4
Bamipine	963.0	E858.1	E933.0	E950.4	E962.0	E980.4
Baneberry	988.2	E865.4	—	E950.9	E962.1	E980.9
Banewort	988.2	E865.4	—	E950.9	E962.1	E980.9
Barbenyl	967.0	E851	E937.0	E950.1	E962.0	E980.1
Barbital, barbitone	967.0	E851	E937.0	E950.1	E962.0	E980.1
Barbiturates, barbituric acid	967.0	E851	E937.0	E950.1	E962.0	E980.1
anesthetic (intravenous)	968.3	E855.1	E938.3	E950.4	E962.0	E980.4
Barium (carbonate) (chloride) (sulfate)	985.8	E866.4	—	E950.9	E962.1	E980.9
diagnostic agent	977.8	E858.8	E947.8	E950.4	E962.0	E980.4
pesticide	985.8	E863.4	—	E950.6	E962.1	E980.7
rodenticide	985.8	E863.7	—	E950.6	E962.1	E980.7
Barrier cream	976.3	E858.7	E946.3	E950.4	E962.0	E980.4
Battery acid or fluid	983.1	E864.1	—	E950.7	E962.1	E980.6
Bay rum	980.8	E860.8	—	E950.9	E962.1	E980.9
BCG vaccine	978.0	E858.8	E948.0	E950.4	E962.0	E980.4
Bearsfoot	988.2	E865.4	—	E950.9	E962.1	E980.9
Beclamide	966.3	E855.0	E936.3	E950.4	E962.0	E980.4
Bee (sting) (venom)	989.5	E905.3	—	E950.9	E962.1	E980.9
Belladonna (alkaloids)	971.1	E855.4	E941.1	E950.4	E962.0	E980.4
Bemegride	970.0	E854.3	E940.0	E950.4	E962.0	E980.4
Benactyzine	969.8	E855.8	E939.8	E950.3	E962.0	E980.3
Benadryl	963.0	E858.1	E933.0	E950.4	E962.0	E980.4

Bendrofluazide — Table of Drugs and Chemicals

		External Cause (E-Code)				
	Poisoning	Accident	Therapeutic Use	Suicide Attempt	Assault	Undetermined
Bendrofluazide	974.3	E858.5	E944.3	E950.4	E962.0	E980.4
Bendroflumethiazide	974.3	E858.5	E944.3	E950.4	E962.0	E980.4
Benemid	974.7	E858.5	E944.7	E950.4	E962.0	E980.4
Benethamine penicillin G	960.0	E856	E930.0	E950.4	E962.0	E980.4
Benisone	976.0	E858.7	E946.0	E950.4	E962.0	E980.4
Benoquin	976.8	E858.7	E946.8	E950.4	E962.0	E980.4
Benoxinate	968.5	E855.2	E938.5	E950.4	E962.0	E980.4
Bentonite	976.3	E858.7	E946.3	E950.4	E962.0	E980.4
Benzalkonium (chloride)	976.0	E858.7	E946.0	E950.4	E962.0	E980.4
ophthalmic preparation	976.5	E858.7	E946.5	E950.4	E962.0	E980.4
Benzamidosalicylate (calcium)	961.8	E857	E931.8	E950.4	E962.0	E980.4
Benzathine penicillin	960.0	E856	E930.0	E950.4	E962.0	E980.4
Benzcarbimine	963.1	E858.1	E933.1	E950.4	E962.0	E980.4
Benzedrex	971.2	E855.5	E941.2	E950.4	E962.0	E980.4
Benzedrine (amphetamine)	969.7	E854.2	E939.7	E950.3	E962.0	E980.3
Benzene (acetyl) (dimethyl) (methyl) (solvent) (vapor)	982.0	E862.4	—	E950.9	E962.1	E980.9
hexachloride (gamma) (insecticide) (vapor)	989.2	E863.0	—	E950.6	E962.1	E980.7
Benzethonium	976.0	E858.7	E946.0	E950.4	E962.0	E980.4
Benzhexol (chloride)	966.4	E855.0	E936.4	E950.4	E962.0	E980.4
Benzilonium	971.1	E855.4	E941.1	E950.4	E962.0	E980.4
Benzin(e) — see Ligroin						
Benziodarone	972.4	E858.3	E942.4	E950.4	E962.0	E980.4
Benzocaine	968.5	E855.2	E938.5	E950.4	E962.0	E980.4
Benzodiapin	969.4	E853.2	E939.4	E950.3	E962.0	E980.3
Benzodiazepines (tranquilizers) NEC	969.4	E853.2	E939.4	E950.3	E962.0	E980.3
Benzoic acid (with salicylic acid) (anti-infective)	976.0	E858.7	E946.0	E950.4	E962.0	E980.4
Benzoin	976.3	E858.7	E946.3	E950.4	E962.0	E980.4
Benzol (vapor)	982.0	E862.4	—	E950.9	E962.1	E980.9
Benzomorphan	965.09	E850.2	E935.2	E950.0	E962.0	E980.0
Benzonatate	975.4	E858.6	E945.4	E950.4	E962.0	E980.4
Benzothiadiazides	974.3	E858.5	E944.3	E950.4	E962.0	E980.4
Benzoylpas	961.8	E857	E931.8	E950.4	E962.0	E980.4
Benzperidol	969.5	E853.8	E939.5	E950.3	E962.0	E980.3
Benzphetamine	977.0	E858.8	E947.0	E950.4	E962.0	E980.4
Benzpyrinium	971.0	E855.3	E941.0	E950.4	E962.0	E980.4
Benzquinamide	963.0	E858.1	E933.0	E950.4	E962.0	E980.4
Benzthiazide	974.3	E858.5	E944.3	E950.4	E962.0	E980.4
Benztropine	971.1	E855.4	E941.1	E950.4	E962.0	E980.4
Benzyl						
acetate	982.8	E862.4	—	E950.9	E962.1	E980.9
benzoate (anti-infective)	976.0	E858.7	E946.0	E950.4	E962.0	E980.4
morphine	965.09	E850.2	E935.2	E950.0	E962.0	E980.0
penicillin	960.0	E856	E930.0	E950.4	E962.0	E980.4
Bephenium hydroxynapthoate	961.6	E857	E931.6	E950.4	E962.0	E980.4
Bergamot oil	989.89	E866.8	—	E950.9	E962.1	E980.9
Berries, poisonous	988.2	E865.3	—	E950.9	E962.1	E980.9
Beryllium (compounds) (fumes)	985.3	E866.4	—	E950.9	E962.1	E980.9
Beta-carotene	976.3	E858.7	E946.3	E950.4	E962.0	E980.4
Beta-Chlor	967.1	E852.0	E937.1	E950.2	E962.0	E980.2
Betamethasone	962.0	E858.0	E932.0	E950.4	E962.0	E980.4
topical	976.0	E858.7	E946.0	E950.4	E962.0	E980.4
Betazole	977.8	E858.8	E947.8	E950.4	E962.0	E980.4
Bethanechol	971.0	E855.3	E941.0	E950.4	E962.0	E980.4
Bethanidine	972.6	E858.3	E942.6	E950.4	E962.0	E980.4
Betula oil	976.3	E858.7	E946.3	E950.4	E962.0	E980.4
Bhang	969.6	E854.1	E939.6	E950.3	E962.0	E980.3
Bialamicol	961.5	E857	E931.5	E950.4	E962.0	E980.4
Bichloride of mercury — see Mercury, chloride						
Bichromates (calcium) (crystals) (potassium) (sodium)	983.9	E864.3	—	E950.7	E962.1	E980.6
fumes	987.8	E869.8	—	E952.8	E962.2	E982.8
Biguanide derivatives, oral	962.3	E858.0	E932.3	E950.4	E962.0	E980.4
Biligrafin	977.8	E858.8	E947.8	E950.4	E962.0	E980.4
Bilopaque	977.8	E858.8	E947.8	E950.4	E962.0	E980.4
Bioflavonoids	972.8	E858.3	E942.8	E950.4	E962.0	E980.4
Biological substance NEC	979.9	E858.8	E949.9	E950.4	E962.0	E980.4
Biperiden	966.4	E855.0	E936.4	E950.4	E962.0	E980.4
Bisacodyl	973.1	E858.4	E943.1	E950.4	E962.0	E980.4
Bishydroxycoumarin	964.2	E858.2	E934.2	E950.4	E962.0	E980.4
Bismarsen	961.1	E857	E931.1	E950.4	E962.0	E980.4
Bismuth (compounds) NEC	985.8	E866.4	—	E950.9	E962.1	E980.9
anti-infectives	961.2	E857	E931.2	E950.4	E962.0	E980.4
subcarbonate	973.5	E858.4	E943.5	E950.4	E962.0	E980.4
sulfarsphenamine	961.1	E857	E931.1	E950.4	E962.0	E980.4
Bithionol	961.6	E857	E931.6	E950.4	E962.0	E980.4
Bitter almond oil	989.0	E866.8	—	E950.9	E962.1	E980.9
Bittersweet	988.2	E865.4	—	E950.9	E962.1	E930.9
Black						
flag	989.4	E863.4	—	E950.6	E962.1	E980.7
henbane	988.2	E865.4	—	E950.9	E962.1	E980.9
leaf (40)	989.4	E863.4	—	E950.6	E962.1	E980.7
widow spider (bite)	989.5	E905.1	—	E950.9	E962.1	E980.9

✓4ᵗʰ Fourth-digit Required   ✓5ᵗʰ Fifth-digit Required   ▶◀ Revised Text   ● New Line   ▲ Revised Code

Table of Drugs and Chemicals

		External Cause (E-Code)				
	Poisoning	Accident	Therapeutic Use	Suicide Attempt	Assault	Undetermined
Black — *continued*						
widow spider — *continued*						
antivenin	979.9	E858.8	E949.9	E950.4	E962.0	E980.4
Blast furnace gas (carbon monoxide from)	986	E868.8	—	E952.1	E962.2	E982.1
Bleach NEC	983.9	E864.3	—	E950.7	E962.1	E980.6
Bleaching solutions	983.9	E864.3	—	E950.7	E962.1	E980.6
Bleomycin (sulfate)	960.7	E856	E930.7	E950.4	E962.0	E980.4
Blockain	968.9	E855.2	E938.9	E950.4	E962.0	E980.4
infiltration (subcutaneous)	968.5	E855.2	E938.5	E950.4	E962.0	E980.4
nerve block (peripheral) (plexus)	968.6	E855.2	E938.6	E950.4	E962.0	E980.4
topical (surface)	968.5	E855.2	E938.5	E950.4	E962.0	E980.4
Blood (derivatives) (natural) (plasma) (whole)	964.7	E858.2	E934.7	E950.4	E962.0	E980.4
affecting agent	964.9	E858.2	E934.9	E950.4	E962.0	E980.4
specified NEC	964.8	E858.2	E934.8	E950.4	E962.0	E980.4
substitute (macromolecular)	964.8	E858.2	E934.8	E950.4	E962.0	E980.4
Blue velvet	965.09	E850.2	E935.2	E950.0	E962.0	E980.0
Bone meal	989.89	E866.5	—	E950.9	E962.1	E980.9
Bonine	963.0	E858.1	E933.0	E950.4	E962.0	E980.4
Boracic acid	976.0	E858.7	E946.0	E950.4	E962.0	E980.4
ENT agent	976.6	E858.7	E946.6	E950.4	E962.0	E980.4
ophthalmic preparation	976.5	E858.7	E946.5	E950.4	E962.0	E980.4
Borate (cleanser) (sodium)	989.6	E861.3	—	E950.9	E962.1	E980.9
Borax (cleanser)	989.6	E861.3	—	E950.9	E962.1	E980.9
Boric acid	976.0	E858.7	E946.0	E950.4	E962.0	E980.4
ENT agent	976.6	E858.7	E946.6	E950.4	E962.0	E980.4
ophthalmic preparation	976.5	E858.7	E946.5	E950.4	E962.0	E980.4
Boron hydride NEC	989.89	E866.8	—	E950.9	E962.1	E980.9
fumes or gas	987.8	E869.8	—	E952.8	E962.2	E982.8
Brake fluid vapor	987.8	E869.8	—	E952.8	E962.2	E982.8
Brass (compounds) (fumes)	985.8	E866.4	—	E950.9	E962.1	E980.9
Brasso	981	E861.3	—	E950.9	E962.1	E980.9
Bretylium (tosylate)	972.6	E858.3	E942.6	E950.4	E962.0	E980.4
Brevital (sodium)	968.3	E855.1	E938.3	E950.4	E962.0	E980.4
British antilewisite	963.8	E858.1	E933.8	E950.4	E962.0	E980.4
Bromal (hydrate)	967.3	E852.2	E937.3	E950.2	E962.0	E980.2
Bromelains	963.4	E858.1	E933.4	E950.4	E962.0	E980.4
Bromides NEC	967.3	E852.2	E937.3	E950.2	E962.0	E980.2
Bromine (vapor)	987.8	E869.8	—	E952.8	E962.2	E982.8
compounds (medicinal)	967.3	E852.2	E937.3	E950.2	E962.0	E980.2
Bromisovalum	967.3	E852.2	E937.3	E950.2	E962.0	E980.2
Bromobenzyl cyanide	987.5	E869.3	—	E952.8	E962.2	E982.8
Bromodiphenhydramine	963.0	E858.1	E933.0	E950.4	E962.0	E980.4
Bromoform	967.3	E852.2	E937.3	E950.2	E962.0	E980.2
Bromophenol blue reagent	977.8	E858.8	E947.8	E950.4	E962.0	E980.4
Bromosalicylhydroxamic acid	961.8	E857	E931.8	E950.4	E962.0	E980.4
Bromo-seltzer	965.4	E850.4	E935.4	E950.0	E962.0	E980.0
Brompheniramine	963.0	E858.1	E933.0	E950.4	E962.0	E980.4
Bromural	967.3	E852.2	E937.3	E950.2	E962.0	E980.2
Brown spider (bite) (venom)	989.5	E905.1	—	E950.9	E962.1	E980.9
Brucia	988.2	E865.3	—	E950.9	E962.1	E980.9
Brucine	989.1	E863.7	—	E950.6	E962.1	E980.7
Brunswick green — *see* Copper						
Bruten — *see* Ibuprofen						
Bryonia (alba) (dioica)	988.2	E865.4	—	E950.9	E962.1	E980.9
Buclizine	969.5	E853.8	E939.5	E950.3	E962.0	E980.3
Bufferin	965.1	E850.3	E935.3	E950.0	E962.0	E980.0
Bufotenine	969.6	E854.1	E939.6	E950.3	E962.0	E980.3
Buphenine	971.2	E855.5	E941.2	E950.4	E962.0	E980.4
Bupivacaine	968.9	E855.2	E938.9	E950.4	E962.0	E980.4
infiltration (subcutaneous)	968.5	E855.2	E938.5	E950.4	E962.0	E980.4
nerve block (peripheral) (plexus)	968.6	E855.2	E938.6	E950.4	E962.0	E980.4
Busulfan	963.1	E858.1	E933.1	E950.4	E962.0	E980.4
Butabarbital (sodium)	967.0	E851	E937.0	E950.1	E962.0	E980.1
Butabarbitone	967.0	E851	E937.0	E950.1	E962.0	E980.1
Butabarpal	967.0	E851	E937.0	E950.1	E962.0	E980.1
Butacaine	968.5	E855.2	E938.5	E950.4	E962.0	E980.4
Butallylonal	967.0	E851	E937.0	E950.1	E962.0	E980.1
Butane (distributed in mobile container)	987.0	E868.0	—	E951.1	E962.2	E981.1
distributed through pipes	987.0	E867	—	E951.0	E962.2	E981.0
incomplete combustion of — *see* Carbon monoxide, butane						
Butanol	980.3	E860.4	—	E950.9	E962.1	E980.9
Butanone	982.8	E862.4	—	E950.9	E962.1	E980.9
Butaperazine	969.1	E853.0	E939.1	E950.3	E962.0	E980.3
Butazolidin	965.5	E850.5	E935.5	E950.0	E962.0	E980.0
Butethal	967.0	E851	E937.0	E950.1	E962.0	E980.1
Butethamate	971.1	E855.4	E941.1	E950.4	E962.0	E980.4
Buthalitone (sodium)	968.3	E855.1	E938.3	E950.4	E962.0	E980.4
Butisol (sodium)	967.0	E851	E937.0	E950.1	E962.0	E980.1
Butobarbital, butobarbitone	967.0	E851	E937.0	E950.1	E962.0	E980.1
Butriptyline	969.0	E854.0	E939.0	E950.3	E962.0	E980.3
Buttercups	988.2	E865.4	—	E950.9	E962.1	E980.9

Table of Drugs and Chemicals

Butter of antimony — Carbon

	Poisoning	External Cause (E-Code)				
		Accident	Therapeutic Use	Suicide Attempt	Assault	Undetermined
Butter of antimony — see Antimony						
Butyl						
acetate (secondary)	982.8	E862.4	—	E950.9	E962.1	E980.9
alcohol	980.3	E860.4	—	E950.9	E962.1	E980.9
carbinol	980.8	E860.8	—	E950.9	E962.1	E980.9
carbitol	982.8	E862.4	—	E950.9	E962.1	E980.9
cellosolve	982.8	E862.4	—	E950.9	E962.1	E980.9
chloral (hydrate)	967.1	E852.0	E937.1	E950.2	E962.0	E980.2
formate	982.8	E862.4	—	E950.9	E962.1	E980.9
scopolammonium bromide	971.1	E855.4	E941.1	E950.4	E962.0	E980.4
Butyn	968.5	E855.2	E938.5	E950.4	E962.0	E980.4
Butyrophenone (-based tranquilizers)	969.2	E853.1	E939.2	E950.3	E962.0	E980.3
Cacodyl, cacodylic acid — see Arsenic						
Cactinomycin	960.7	E856	E930.7	E950.4	E962.0	E980.4
Cade oil	976.4	E858.7	E946.4	E950.4	E962.0	E980.4
Cadmium (chloride) (compounds) (dust) (fumes) (oxide)	985.5	E866.4	—	E950.9	E962.1	E980.9
sulfide (medicinal) NEC	976.4	E858.7	E946.4	E950.4	E962.0	E980.4
Caffeine	969.7	E854.2	E939.7	E950.3	E962.0	E980.3
Calabar bean	988.2	E865.4	—	E950.9	E962.1	E980.9
Caladium seguinium	988.2	E865.4	—	E950.9	E962.1	E980.9
Calamine (liniment) (lotion)	976.3	E858.7	E946.3	E950.4	E962.0	E980.4
Calciferol	963.5	E858.1	E933.5	E950.4	E962.0	E980.4
Calcium (salts) NEC	974.5	E858.5	E944.5	E950.4	E962.0	E980.4
acetylsalicylate	965.1	E850.3	E935.3	E950.0	E962.0	E980.0
benzamidosalicylate	961.8	E857	E931.8	E950.4	E962.0	E980.4
carbaspirin	965.1	E850.3	E935.3	E950.0	E962.0	E980.0
carbimide (citrated)	977.3	E858.8	E947.3	E950.4	E962.0	E980.4
carbonate (antacid)	973.0	E858.4	E943.0	E950.4	E962.0	E980.4
cyanide (citrated)	977.3	E858.8	E947.3	E950.4	E962.0	E980.4
dioctyl sulfosuccinate	973.2	E858.4	E943.2	E950.4	E962.0	E980.4
disodium edathamil	963.8	E858.1	E933.8	E950.4	E962.0	E980.4
disodium edetate	963.8	E858.1	E933.8	E950.4	E962.0	E980.4
EDTA	963.8	E858.1	E933.8	E950.4	E962.0	E980.4
hydrate, hydroxide	983.2	E864.2	—	E950.7	E962.1	E980.6
mandelate	961.9	E857	E931.9	E950.4	E962.0	E980.4
oxide	983.2	E864.2	—	E950.7	E962.1	E980.6
Calomel — see Mercury, chloride						
Caloric agents NEC	974.5	E858.5	E944.5	E950.4	E962.0	E980.4
Calusterone	963.1	E858.1	E933.1	E950.4	E962.0	E980.4
Camoquin	961.4	E857	E931.4	E950.4	E962.0	E980.4
Camphor (oil)	976.1	E858.7	E946.1	E950.4	E962.0	E980.4
Candeptin	976.0	E858.7	E946.0	E950.4	E962.0	E980.4
Candicidin	976.0	E858.7	E946.0	E950.4	E962.0	E980.4
Cannabinols	969.6	E854.1	E939.6	E950.3	E962.0	E980.3
Cannabis (derivatives) (indica) (sativa)	969.6	E854.1	E939.6	E950.3	E962.0	E980.3
Canned heat	980.1	E860.2	—	E950.9	E962.1	E980.9
Cantharides, cantharidin, cantharis	976.8	E858.7	E946.8	E950.4	E962.0	E980.4
Capillary agents	972.8	E858.3	E942.8	E950.4	E962.0	E980.4
Capreomycin	960.6	E856	E930.6	E950.4	E962.0	E980.4
Captodiame, captodiamine	969.5	E853.8	E939.5	E950.3	E962.0	E980.3
Caramiphen (hydrochloride)	971.1	E855.4	E941.1	E950.4	E962.0	E980.4
Carbachol	971.0	E855.3	E941.0	E950.4	E962.0	E980.4
Carbacrylamine resins	974.5	E858.5	E944.5	E950.4	E962.0	E980.4
Carbamate (sedative)	967.8	E852.8	E937.8	E950.2	E962.0	E980.2
herbicide	989.3	E863.5	—	E950.6	E962.1	E980.7
insecticide	989.3	E863.2	—	E950.6	E962.1	E980.7
Carbamazepine	966.3	E855.0	E936.3	E950.4	E962.0	E980.4
Carbamic esters	967.8	E852.8	E937.8	E950.2	E962.0	E980.2
Carbamide	974.4	E858.5	E944.4	E950.4	E962.0	E980.4
topical	976.8	E858.7	E946.8	E950.4	E962.0	E980.4
Carbamylcholine chloride	971.0	E855.3	E941.0	E950.4	E962.0	E980.4
Carbarsone	961.1	E857	E931.1	E950.4	E962.0	E980.4
Carbaryl	989.3	E863.2	—	E950.6	E962.1	E980.7
Carbaspirin	965.1	E850.3	E935.3	E950.0	E962.0	E980.0
Carbazochrome	972.8	E858.3	E942.8	E950.4	E962.0	E980.4
Carbenicillin	960.0	E856	E930.0	E950.4	E962.0	E980.4
Carbenoxolone	973.8	E858.4	E943.8	E950.4	E962.0	E980.4
Carbetapentane	975.4	E858.6	E945.4	E950.4	E962.0	E980.4
Carbimazole	962.8	E858.0	E932.8	E950.4	E962.0	E980.4
Carbinol	980.1	E860.2	—	E950.9	E962.1	E980.9
Carbinoxamine	963.0	E858.1	E933.0	E950.4	E962.0	E980.4
Carbitol	982.8	E862.4	—	E950.9	E962.1	E980.9
Carbocaine	968.9	E855.2	E938.9	E950.4	E962.0	E980.4
infiltration (subcutaneous)	968.5	E855.2	E938.5	E950.4	E962.0	E980.4
nerve block (peripheral) (plexus)	968.6	E855.2	E938.6	E950.4	E962.0	E980.4
topical (surface)	968.5	E855.2	E938.5	E950.4	E962.0	E980.4
Carbol-fuchsin solution	976.0	E858.7	E946.0	E950.4	E962.0	E980.4
Carbolic acid (see also Phenol)	983.0	E864.0	—	E950.7	E962.1	E980.6
Carbomycin	960.8	E856	E930.8	E950.4	E962.0	E980.4
Carbon						
bisulfide (liquid) (vapor)	982.2	E862.4	—	E950.9	E962.1	E980.9

Table of Drugs and Chemicals — Caustic(s)

	Poisoning	External Cause (E-Code)				
		Accident	Therapeutic Use	Suicide Attempt	Assault	Undetermined
Carbon — *continued*						
dioxide (gas)	987.8	E869.8	—	E952.8	E962.2	E982.8
disulfide (liquid) (vapor)	982.2	E862.4	—	E950.9	E962.1	E980.9
monoxide (from incomplete combustion of) (in) NEC	986	E868.9	—	E952.1	E962.2	E982.1
blast furnace gas	986	E868.8	—	E952.1	E962.2	E982.1
butane (distributed in mobile container)	986	E868.0	—	E951.1	E962.2	E981.1
distributed through pipes	986	E867	—	E951.0	E962.2	E981.0
charcoal fumes	986	E868.3	—	E952.1	E962.2	E982.1
coal						
gas (piped)	986	E867	—	E951.0	E962.2	E981.0
solid (in domestic stoves, fireplaces)	986	E868.3	—	E952.1	E962.2	E982.1
coke (in domestic stoves, fireplaces)	986	E868.3	—	E952.1	E962.2	E982.1
exhaust gas (motor) not in transit	986	E868.2	—	E952.0	E962.2	E982.0
combustion engine, any not in watercraft	986	E868.2	—	E952.0	E962.2	E982.0
farm tractor, not in transit	986	E868.2	—	E952.0	E962.2	E982.0
gas engine	986	E868.2	—	E952.0	E962.2	E982.0
motor pump	986	E868.2	—	E952.0	E962.2	E982.0
motor vehicle, not in transit	986	E868.2	—	E952.0	E962.2	E982.0
fuel (in domestic use)	986	E868.3	—	E952.1	E962.2	E982.1
gas (piped)	986	E867	—	E951.0	E962.2	E981.0
in mobile container	986	E868.0	—	E951.1	E962.2	E981.1
utility	986	E868.1	—	E951.8	E962.2	E981.1
in mobile container	986	E868.0	—	E951.1	E962.2	E981.1
piped (natural)	986	E867	—	E951.0	E962.2	E981.0
illuminating gas	986	E868.1	—	E951.8	E962.2	E981.8
industrial fuels or gases, any	986	E868.8	—	E952.1	E962.2	E982.1
kerosene (in domestic stoves, fireplaces)	986	E868.3	—	E952.1	E962.2	E982.1
kiln gas or vapor	986	E868.8	—	E952.1	E962.2	E982.1
motor exhaust gas, not in transit	986	E868.2	—	E952.0	E962.2	E982.0
piped gas (manufactured) (natural)	986	E867	—	E951.0	E962.2	E981.0
producer gas	986	E868.8	—	E952.1	E962.2	E982.1
propane (distributed in mobile container)	986	E868.0	—	E951.1	E962.2	E981.1
distributed through pipes	986	E867	—	E951.0	E962.2	E981.0
specified source NEC	986	E868.8	—	E952.1	E962.2	E982.1
stove gas	986	E868.1	—	E951.8	E962.2	E981.8
piped	986	E867	—	E951.0	E962.2	E981.0
utility gas	986	E868.1	—	E951.8	E962.2	E981.8
piped	986	E867	—	E951.0	E962.2	E981.0
water gas	986	E868.1	—	E951.8	E962.2	E981.8
wood (in domestic stoves, fireplaces)	986	E868.3	—	E952.1	E962.2	E982.1
tetrachloride (vapor) NEC	987.8	E869.8	—	E952.8	E962.2	E982.8
liquid (cleansing agent) NEC	982.1	E861.3	—	E950.9	E962.1	E980.9
solvent	982.1	E862.4	—	E950.9	E962.1	E980.9
Carbonic acid (gas)	987.8	E869.8	—	E952.8	E962.2	E982.8
anhydrase inhibitors	974.2	E858.5	E944.2	E950.4	E962.0	E980.4
Carbowax	976.3	E858.7	E946.3	E950.4	E962.0	E980.4
Carbrital	967.0	E851	E937.0	E950.1	E962.0	E980.1
Carbromal (derivatives)	967.3	E852.2	E937.3	E950.2	E962.0	E980.2
Cardiac						
depressants	972.0	E858.3	E942.0	E950.4	E962.0	E980.4
rhythm regulators	972.0	E858.3	E942.0	E950.4	E962.0	E980.4
Cardiografin	977.8	E858.8	E947.8	E950.4	E962.0	E980.4
Cardio-green	977.8	E858.8	E947.8	E950.4	E962.0	E980.4
Cardiotonic glycosides	972.1	E858.3	E942.1	E950.4	E962.0	E980.4
Cardiovascular agents NEC	972.9	E858.3	E942.9	E950.4	E962.0	E980.4
Cardrase	974.2	E858.5	E944.2	E950.4	E962.0	E980.4
Carfusin	976.0	E858.7	E946.0	E950.4	E962.0	E980.4
Carisoprodol	968.0	E855.1	E938.0	E950.4	E962.0	E980.4
Carmustine	963.1	E858.1	E933.1	E950.4	E962.0	E980.4
Carotene	963.5	E858.1	E933.5	E950.4	E962.0	E980.4
Carphenazine (maleate)	969.1	E853.0	E939.1	E950.3	E962.0	E980.3
Carter's Little Pills	973.1	E858.4	E943.1	E950.4	E962.0	E980.4
Cascara (sagrada)	973.1	E858.4	E943.1	E950.4	E962.0	E980.4
Cassava	988.2	E865.4	—	E950.9	E962.1	E980.9
Castellani's paint	976.0	E858.7	E946.0	E950.4	E962.0	E980.4
Castor						
bean	988.2	E865.3	—	E950.9	E962.1	E980.9
oil	973.1	E858.4	E943.1	E950.4	E962.0	E980.4
Caterpillar (sting)	989.5	E905.5	—	E950.9	E962.1	E980.9
Catha (edulis)	970.8	E854.3	E940.8	E950.4	E962.0	E980.4
Cathartics NEC	973.3	E858.4	E943.3	E950.4	E962.0	E980.4
contact	973.1	E858.4	E943.1	E950.4	E962.0	E980.4
emollient	973.2	E858.4	E943.2	E950.4	E962.0	E980.4
intestinal irritants	973.1	E858.4	E943.1	E950.4	E962.0	E980.4
saline	973.3	E858.4	E943.3	E950.4	E962.0	E980.4
Cathomycin	960.8	E856	E930.8	E950.4	E962.0	E980.4
Caustic(s)	983.9	E864.4	—	E950.7	E962.1	E980.6
alkali	983.2	E864.2	—	E950.7	E962.1	E980.6
hydroxide	983.2	E864.2	—	E950.7	E962.1	E980.6

Caustic(s) — Table of Drugs and Chemicals

	Poisoning	External Cause (E-Code)				
		Accident	Therapeutic Use	Suicide Attempt	Assault	Undetermined
Caustic(s) — *continued*						
potash	983.2	E864.2	—	E950.7	E962.1	E980.6
soda	983.2	E864.2	—	E950.7	E962.1	E980.6
specified NEC	983.9	E864.3	—	E950.7	E962.1	E980.6
Ceepryn	976.0	E858.7	E946.0	E950.4	E962.0	E980.4
ENT agent	976.6	E858.7	E946.6	E950.4	E962.0	E980.4
lozenges	976.6	E858.7	E946.6	E950.4	E962.0	E980.4
Celestone	962.0	E858.0	E932.0	E950.4	E962.0	E980.4
topical	976.0	E858.7	E946.0	E950.4	E962.0	E980.4
Cellosolve	982.8	E862.4	—	E950.9	E962.1	E980.9
Cell stimulants and proliferants	976.8	E858.7	E946.8	E950.4	E962.0	E980.4
Cellulose derivatives, cathartic	973.3	E858.4	E943.3	E950.4	E962.0	E980.4
nitrates (topical)	976.3	E858.7	E946.3	E950.4	E962.0	E980.4
Centipede (bite)	989.5	E905.4	—	E950.9	E962.1	E980.9
Central nervous system						
depressants	968.4	E855.1	E938.4	E950.4	E962.0	E980.4
anesthetic (general) NEC	968.4	E855.1	E938.4	E950.4	E962.0	E980.4
gases NEC	968.2	E855.1	E938.2	E950.4	E962.0	E980.4
intravenous	968.3	E855.1	E938.3	E950.4	E962.0	E980.4
barbiturates	967.0	E851	E937.0	E950.1	E962.0	E980.1
bromides	967.3	E852.2	E937.3	E950.2	E962.0	E980.2
cannabis sativa	969.6	E854.1	E939.6	E950.3	E962.0	E980.3
chloral hydrate	967.1	E852.0	E937.1	E950.2	E962.0	E980.2
hallucinogenics	969.6	E854.1	E939.6	E950.3	E962.0	E980.3
hypnotics	967.9	E852.9	E937.9	E950.2	E962.0	E980.2
specified NEC	967.8	E852.8	E937.8	E950.2	E962.0	E980.2
muscle relaxants	968.0	E855.1	E938.0	E950.4	E962.0	E980.4
paraldehyde	967.2	E852.1	E937.2	E950.2	E962.0	E980.2
sedatives	967.9	E852.9	E937.9	E950.2	E962.0	E980.2
mixed NEC	967.6	E852.5	E937.6	E950.2	E962.0	E980.2
specified NEC	967.8	E852.8	E937.8	E950.2	E962.0	E980.2
muscle-tone depressants	968.0	E855.1	E938.0	E950.4	E962.0	E980.4
stimulants	970.9	E854.3	E940.9	E950.4	E962.0	E980.4
amphetamines	969.7	E854.2	E939.7	E950.3	E962.0	E980.3
analeptics	970.0	E854.3	E940.0	E950.4	E962.0	E980.4
antidepressants	969.0	E854.0	E939.0	E950.3	E962.0	E980.3
opiate antagonists	970.1	E854.3	E940.1	E950.4	E962.0	E980.4
specified NEC	970.8	E854.3	E940.8	E950.4	E962.0	E980.4
Cephalexin	960.5	E856	E930.5	E950.4	E962.0	E980.4
Cephaloglycin	960.5	E856	E930.5	E950.4	E962.0	E980.4
Cephaloridine	960.5	E856	E930.5	E950.4	E962.0	E980.4
Cephalosporins NEC	960.5	E856	E930.5	E950.4	E962.0	E980.4
N (adicillin)	960.0	E856	E930.0	E950.4	E962.0	E980.4
Cephalothin (sodium)	960.5	E856	E930.5	E950.4	E962.0	E980.4
Cerbera (odallam)	988.2	E865.4	—	E950.9	E962.1	E980.9
Cerberin	972.1	E858.3	E942.1	E950.4	E962.0	E980.4
Cerebral stimulants	970.9	E854.3	E940.9	E950.4	E962.0	E980.4
psychotherapeutic	969.7	E854.2	E939.7	E950.3	E962.0	E980.3
specified NEC	970.8	E854.3	E940.8	E950.4	E962.0	E980.4
Cetalkonium (chloride)	976.0	E858.7	E946.0	E950.4	E962.0	E980.4
Cetoxime	963.0	E858.1	E933.0	E950.4	E962.0	E980.4
Cetrimide	976.2	E858.7	E946.2	E950.4	E962.0	E980.4
Cetylpyridinium	976.0	E858.7	E946.0	E950.4	E962.0	E980.4
ENT agent	976.6	E858.7	E946.6	E950.4	E962.0	E980.4
lozenges	976.6	E858.7	E946.6	E950.4	E962.0	E980.4
Cevadilla — *see* Sabadilla						
Cevitamic acid	963.5	E858.1	E933.5	E950.4	E962.0	E980.4
Chalk, precipitated	973.0	E858.4	E943.0	E950.4	E962.0	E980.4
Charcoal						
fumes (carbon monoxide)	986	E868.3	—	E952.1	E962.2	E982.1
industrial	986	E868.8	—	E952.1	E962.2	E982.1
medicinal (activated)	973.0	E858.4	E943.0	E950.4	E962.0	E980.4
Chelating agents NEC	977.2	E858.8	E947.2	E950.4	E962.0	E980.4
Chelidonium majus	988.2	E865.4	—	E950.9	E962.1	E980.9
Chemical substance	989.9	E866.9	—	E950.9	E962.1	E980.9
specified NEC	989.89	E866.8	—	E950.9	E962.1	E980.9
Chemotherapy, antineoplastic	963.1	E858.1	E933.1	E950.4	E962.0	E980.4
Chenopodium (oil)	961.6	E857	E931.6	E950.4	E962.0	E980.4
Cherry laurel	988.2	E865.4	—	E950.9	E962.1	E980.9
Chiniofon	961.3	E857	E931.3	E950.4	E962.0	E980.4
Chlophedianol	975.4	E858.6	E945.4	E950.4	E962.0	E980.4
Chloral (betaine) (formamide) (hydrate)	967.1	E852.0	E937.1	E950.2	E962.0	E980.2
Chloralamide	967.1	E852.0	E937.1	E950.2	E962.0	E980.2
Chlorambucil	963.1	E858.1	E933.1	E950.4	E962.0	E980.4
Chloramphenicol	960.2	E856	E930.2	E950.4	E962.0	E980.4
ENT agent	976.6	E858.7	E946.6	E950.4	E962.0	E980.4
ophthalmic preparation	976.5	E858.7	E946.5	E950.4	E962.0	E980.4
topical NEC	976.0	E858.7	E946.0	E950.4	E962.0	E980.4
Chlorate(s) (potassium) (sodium) NEC	983.9	E864.3	—	E950.7	E962.1	E980.6
herbicides	989.4	E863.5	—	E950.6	E962.1	E980.7

Table of Drugs and Chemicals

	Poisoning	External Cause (E-Code)				
		Accident	Therapeutic Use	Suicide Attempt	Assault	Undetermined
Chlorcylizine	963.0	E858.1	E933.0	E950.4	E962.0	E980.4
Chlordan(e) (dust)	989.2	E863.0	—	E950.6	E962.1	E980.7
Chlordantoin	976.0	E858.7	E946.0	E950.4	E962.0	E980.4
Chlordiazepoxide	969.4	E853.2	E939.4	E950.3	E962.0	E980.3
Chloresium	976.8	E858.7	E946.8	E950.4	E962.0	E980.4
Chlorethiazol	967.1	E852.0	E937.1	E950.2	E962.0	E980.2
Chlorethyl — see Ethyl, chloride						
Chloretone	967.1	E852.0	E937.1	E950.2	E962.0	E980.2
Chlorex	982.3	E862.4	—	E950.9	E962.1	E980.9
Chlorhexadol	967.1	E852.0	E937.1	E950.2	E962.0	E980.2
Chlorhexidine (hydrochloride)	976.0	E858.7	E946.0	E950.4	E962.0	E980.4
Chlorhydroxyquinolin	976.0	E858.7	E946.0	E950.4	E962.0	E980.4
Chloride of lime (bleach)	983.9	E864.3	—	E950.7	E962.1	E980.6
Chlorinated						
camphene	989.2	E863.0	—	E950.6	E962.1	E980.7
diphenyl	989.89	E866.8	—	E950.9	E962.1	E980.9
hydrocarbons NEC	989.2	E863.0	—	E950.6	E962.1	E980.7
solvent	982.3	E862.4	—	E950.9	E962.1	E980.9
lime (bleach)	983.9	E864.3	—	E950.7	E962.1	E980.6
naphthalene — see Naphthalene						
pesticides NEC	989.2	E863.0	—	E950.6	E962.1	E980.7
soda — see Sodium, hypochlorite						
Chlorine (fumes) (gas)	987.6	E869.8	—	E952.8	E962.2	E982.8
bleach	983.9	E864.3	—	E950.7	E962.1	E980.6
compounds NEC	983.9	E864.3	—	E950.7	E962.1	E980.6
disinfectant	983.9	E861.4	—	E950.7	E962.1	E980.6
releasing agents NEC	983.9	E864.3	—	E950.7	E962.1	E980.6
Chlorisondamine	972.3	E858.3	E942.3	E950.4	E962.0	E980.4
Chlormadinone	962.2	E858.0	E932.2	E950.4	E962.0	E980.4
Chlormerodrin	974.0	E858.5	E944.0	E950.4	E962.0	E980.4
Chlormethiazole	967.1	E852.0	E937.1	E950.2	E962.0	E980.2
Chlormethylenecycline	960.4	E856	E930.4	E950.4	E962.0	E980.4
Chlormezanone	969.5	E853.8	E939.5	E950.3	E962.0	E980.3
Chloroacetophenone	987.5	E869.3	—	E952.8	E962.2	E982.8
Chloroaniline	983.0	E864.0	—	E950.7	E962.1	E980.6
Chlorobenzene, chlorobenzol	982.0	E862.4	—	E950.9	E962.1	E980.9
Chlorobutanol	967.1	E852.0	E937.1	E950.2	E962.0	E980.2
Chlorodinitrobenzene	983.0	E864.0	—	E950.7	E962.1	E980.6
dust or vapor	987.8	E869.8	—	E952.8	E962.2	E982.8
Chloroethane — see Ethyl, chloride						
Chloroform (fumes) (vapor)	987.8	E869.8	—	E952.8	E962.2	E982.8
anesthetic (gas)	968.2	E855.1	E938.2	E950.4	E962.0	E980.4
liquid NEC	968.4	E855.1	E938.4	E950.4	E962.0	E980.4
solvent	982.3	E862.4	—	E950.9	E962.1	E980.9
Chloroguanide	961.4	E857	E931.4	E950.4	E962.0	E980.4
Chloromycetin	960.2	E856	E930.2	E950.4	E962.0	E980.4
ENT agent	976.6	E858.7	E946.6	E950.4	E962.0	E980.4
ophthalmic preparation	976.5	E858.7	E946.5	E950.4	E962.0	E980.4
otic solution	976.6	E858.7	E946.6	E950.4	E962.0	E980.4
topical NEC	976.0	E858.7	E946.0	E950.4	E962.0	E980.4
Chloronitrobenzene	983.0	E864.0	—	E950.7	E962.1	E980.6
dust or vapor	987.8	E869.8	—	E952.8	E962.2	E982.8
Chlorophenol	983.0	E864.0	—	E950.7	E962.1	E980.6
Chlorophenothane	989.2	E863.0	—	E950.6	E962.1	E980.7
Chlorophyll (derivatives)	976.8	E858.7	E946.8	E950.4	E962.0	E980.4
Chloropicrin (fumes)	987.8	E869.8	—	E952.8	E962.2	E982.8
fumigant	989.4	E863.8	—	E950.6	E962.1	E980.7
fungicide	989.4	E863.6	—	E950.6	E962.1	E980.7
pesticide (fumes)	989.4	E863.4	—	E950.6	E962.1	E980.7
Chloroprocaine	968.9	E855.2	E938.9	E950.4	E962.0	E980.4
infiltration (subcutaneous)	968.5	E855.2	E938.5	E950.4	E962.0	E980.4
nerve block (peripheral) (plexus)	968.6	E855.2	E938.6	E950.4	E962.0	E980.4
Chloroptic	976.5	E858.7	E946.5	E950.4	E962.0	E980.4
Chloropurine	963.1	E858.1	E933.1	E950.4	E962.0	E980.4
Chloroquine (hydrochloride) (phosphate)	961.4	E857	E931.4	E950.4	E962.0	E980.4
Chlorothen	963.0	E858.1	E933.0	E950.4	E962.0	E980.4
Chlorothiazide	974.3	E858.5	E944.3	E950.4	E962.0	E980.4
Chlorotrianisene	962.2	E858.0	E932.2	E950.4	E962.0	E980.4
Chlorovinyldichloroarsine	985.1	E866.3	—	E950.8	E962.1	E980.8
Chloroxylenol	976.0	E858.7	E946.0	E950.4	E962.0	E980.4
Chlorphenesin (carbamate)	968.0	E855.1	E938.0	E950.4	E962.0	E980.4
topical (antifungal)	976.0	E858.7	E946.0	E950.4	E962.0	E980.4
Chlorpheniramine	963.0	E858.1	E933.0	E950.4	E962.0	E980.4
Chlorphenoxamine	966.4	E855.0	E936.4	E950.4	E962.0	E980.4
Chlorphentermine	977.0	E858.8	E947.0	E950.4	E962.0	E980.4
Chlorproguanil	961.4	E857	E931.4	E950.4	E962.0	E980.4
Chlorpromazine	969.1	E853.0	E939.1	E950.3	E962.0	E980.3
Chlorpropamide	962.3	E858.0	E932.3	E950.4	E962.0	E980.4
Chlorprothixene	969.3	E853.8	E939.3	E950.3	E962.0	E980.3
Chlorquinaldol	976.0	E858.7	E946.0	E950.4	E962.0	E980.4

Chlortetracycline — Table of Drugs and Chemicals

		External Cause (E-Code)				
	Poisoning	Accident	Therapeutic Use	Suicide Attempt	Assault	Undetermined
Chlortetracycline	960.4	E856	E930.4	E950.4	E962.0	E980.4
Chlorthalidone	974.4	E858.5	E944.4	E950.4	E962.0	E980.4
Chlortrianisene	962.2	E858.0	E932.2	E950.4	E962.0	E980.4
Chlor-Trimeton	963.0	E858.1	E933.0	E950.4	E962.0	E980.4
Chlorzoxazone	968.0	E855.1	E938.0	E950.4	E962.0	E980.4
Choke damp	987.8	E869.8	—	E952.8	E962.2	E982.8
Cholebrine	977.8	E858.8	E947.8	E950.4	E962.0	E980.4
Cholera vaccine	978.2	E858.8	E948.2	E950.4	E962.0	E980.4
Cholesterol-lowering agents	972.2	E858.3	E942.2	E950.4	E962.0	E980.4
Cholestyramine (resin)	972.2	E858.3	E942.2	E950.4	E962.0	E980.4
Cholic acid	973.4	E858.4	E943.4	E950.4	E962.0	E980.4
Choline						
dihydrogen citrate	977.1	E858.8	E947.1	E950.4	E962.0	E980.4
salicylate	965.1	E850.3	E935.3	E950.0	E962.0	E980.0
theophyllinate	974.1	E858.5	E944.1	E950.4	E962.0	E980.4
Cholinergics	971.0	E855.3	E941.0	E950.4	E962.0	E980.4
Cholografin	977.8	E858.8	E947.8	E950.4	E962.0	E980.4
Chorionic gonadotropin	962.4	E858.0	E932.4	E950.4	E962.0	E980.4
Chromates	983.9	E864.3	—	E950.7	E962.1	E980.6
dust or mist	987.8	E869.8	—	E952.8	E962.2	E982.8
lead	984.0	E866.0	—	E950.9	E962.1	E980.9
paint	984.0	E861.5	—	E950.9	E962.1	E980.9
Chromic acid	983.9	E864.3	—	E950.7	E962.1	E980.6
dust or mist	987.8	E869.8	—	E952.8	E962.2	E982.8
Chromium	985.6	E866.4	—	E950.9	E962.1	E980.9
compounds — see Chromates						
Chromonar	972.4	E858.3	E942.4	E950.4	E962.0	E980.4
Chromyl chloride	983.9	E864.3	—	E950.7	E962.1	E980.6
Chrysarobin (ointment)	976.4	E858.7	E946.4	E950.4	E962.0	E980.4
Chrysazin	973.1	E858.4	E943.1	E950.4	E962.0	E980.4
Chymar	963.4	E858.1	E933.4	E950.4	E962.0	E980.4
ophthalmic preparation	976.5	E858.7	E946.5	E950.4	E962.0	E980.4
Chymotrypsin	963.4	E858.1	E933.4	E950.4	E962.0	E980.4
ophthalmic preparation	976.5	E858.7	E946.5	E950.4	E962.0	E980.4
Cicuta maculata or virosa	988.2	E865.4	—	E950.9	E962.1	E980.9
Cigarette lighter fluid	981	E862.1	—	E950.9	E962.1	E980.9
Cinchocaine (spinal)	968.7	E855.2	E938.7	E950.4	E962.0	E980.4
topical (surface)	968.5	E855.2	E938.5	E950.4	E962.0	E980.4
Cinchona	961.4	E857	E931.4	E950.4	E962.0	E980.4
Cinchonine alkaloids	961.4	E857	E931.4	E950.4	E962.0	E980.4
Cinchophen	974.7	E858.5	E944.7	E950.4	E962.0	E980.4
Cinnarizine	963.0	E858.1	E933.0	E950.4	E962.0	E980.4
Citanest	968.9	E855.2	E938.9	E950.4	E962.0	E980.4
infiltration (subcutaneous)	968.5	E855.2	E938.5	E950.4	E962.0	E980.4
nerve block (peripheral) (plexus)	968.6	E855.2	E938.6	E950.4	E962.0	E980.4
Citric acid	989.89	E866.8	—	E950.9	E962.1	E980.9
Citrovorum factor	964.1	E858.2	E934.1	E950.4	E962.0	E980.4
Claviceps purpurea	988.2	E865.4	—	E950.9	E962.1	E980.9
Cleaner, cleansing agent NEC	989.89	E861.3	—	E950.9	E962.1	E980.9
of paint or varnish	982.8	E862.9	—	E950.9	E962.1	E980.9
Clematis vitalba	988.2	E865.4	—	E950.9	E962.1	E980.9
Clemizole	963.0	E858.1	E933.0	E950.4	E962.0	E980.4
penicillin	960.0	E856	E930.0	E950.4	E962.0	E980.4
Clidinium	971.1	E855.4	E941.1	E950.4	E962.0	E980.4
Clindamycin	960.8	E856	E930.8	E950.4	E962.0	E980.4
Cliradon	965.09	E850.2	E935.2	E950.0	E962.0	E980.0
Clocortolone	962.0	E858.0	E932.0	E950.4	E962.0	E980.4
Clofedanol	975.4	E858.6	E945.4	E950.4	E962.0	E980.4
Clofibrate	972.2	E858.3	E942.2	E950.4	E962.0	E980.4
Clomethiazole	967.1	E852.2	E937.1	E950.2	E962.0	E980.2
Clomiphene	977.8	E858.8	E947.8	E950.4	E962.0	E980.4
Clonazepam	969.4	E853.2	E939.4	E950.3	E962.0	E980.3
Clonidine	972.6	E858.3	E942.6	E950.4	E962.0	E980.4
Clopamide	974.3	E858.5	E944.3	E950.4	E962.0	E980.4
Clorazepate	969.4	E853.2	E939.4	E950.3	E962.0	E980.3
Clorexolone	974.4	E858.5	E944.4	E950.4	E962.0	E980.4
Clorox (bleach)	983.9	E864.3	—	E950.7	E962.1	E980.6
Clortermine	977.0	E858.8	E947.0	E950.4	E962.0	E980.4
Clotrimazole	976.0	E858.7	E946.0	E950.4	E962.0	E980.4
Cloxacillin	960.0	E856	E930.0	E950.4	E962.0	E980.4
Coagulants NEC	964.5	E858.2	E934.5	E950.4	E962.0	E980.4
Coal (carbon monoxide from) — see also Carbon, monoxide, coal						
oil — see Kerosene						
tar NEC	983.0	E864.0	—	E950.7	E962.1	E980.6
fumes	987.8	E869.8	—	E952.8	E962.2	E982.8
medicinal (ointment)	976.4	E858.7	E946.4	E950.4	E962.0	E980.4
analgesics NEC	965.5	E850.5	E935.5	E950.0	E962.0	E980.0
naphtha (solvent)	981	E862.0	—	E950.9	E962.1	E980.9
Cobalt (fumes) (industrial)	985.8	E866.4	—	E950.9	E962.1	E980.9
Cobra (venom)	989.5	E905.0	—	E950.9	E962.1	E980.9

Table of Drugs and Chemicals

		External Cause (E-Code)				
	Poisoning	Accident	Therapeutic Use	Suicide Attempt	Assault	Undetermined
Coca (leaf)	970.8	E854.3	E940.8	E950.4	E962.0	E980.4
Cocaine (hydrochloride) (salt)	970.8 ▲	E854.3 ▲	E940.8 ▲	E950.4	E962.0	E980.4
topical anesthetic ●	968.5	E855.2	E938.5	E950.4	E962.0	E980.4
Coccidioidin	977.8	E858.8	E947.8	E950.4	E962.0	E980.4
Cocculus indicus	988.2	E865.3	—	E950.9	E962.1	E980.9
Cochineal	989.89	E866.8	—	E950.9	E962.1	E980.9
medicinal products	977.4	E858.8	E947.4	E950.4	E962.0	E980.4
Codeine	965.09	E850.2	E935.2	E950.0	E962.0	E980.0
Coffee	989.89	E866.8	—	E950.9	E962.1	E980.9
Cogentin	971.1	E855.4	E941.1	E950.4	E962.0	E980.4
Coke fumes or gas (carbon monoxide)	986	E868.3	—	E952.1	E962.2	E982.1
industrial use	986	E868.8	—	E952.1	E962.2	E982.1
Colace	973.2	E858.4	E943.2	E950.4	E962.0	E980.4
Colchicine	974.7	E858.5	E944.7	E950.4	E962.0	E980.4
Colchicum	988.2	E865.3	—	E950.9	E962.1	E980.9
Cold cream	976.3	E858.7	E946.3	E950.4	E962.0	E980.4
Colestipol	972.2	E858.3	E942.2	E950.4	E962.0	E980.4
Colistimethate	960.8	E856	E930.8	E950.4	E962.0	E980.4
Colistin	960.8	E856	E930.8	E950.4	E962.0	E980.4
Collagenase	976.8	E858.7	E946.8	E950.4	E962.0	E980.4
Collagen	977.8	E866.8	E947.8	E950.9	E962.1	E980.9
Collodion (flexible)	976.3	E858.7	E946.3	E950.4	E962.0	E980.4
Colocynth	973.1	E858.4	E943.1	E950.4	E962.0	E980.4
Coloring matter — see Dye(s)						
Combustion gas — see Carbon, monoxide						
Compazine	969.1	E853.0	E939.1	E950.3	E962.0	E980.3
Compound						
42 (warfarin)	989.4	E863.7	—	E950.6	E962.1	E980.7
269 (endrin)	989.2	E863.0	—	E950.6	E962.1	E980.7
497 (dieldrin)	989.2	E863.0	—	E950.6	E962.1	E980.7
1080 (sodium fluoroacetate)	989.4	E863.7	—	E950.6	E962.1	E980.7
3422 (parathion)	989.3	E863.1	—	E950.6	E962.1	E980.7
3911 (phorate)	989.3	E863.1	—	E950.6	E962.1	E980.7
3956 (toxaphene)	989.2	E863.0	—	E950.6	E962.1	E980.7
4049 (malathion)	989.3	E863.1	—	E950.6	E962.1	E980.7
4124 (dicapthon)	989.4	E863.4	—	E950.6	E962.1	E980.7
E (cortisone)	962.0	E858.0	E932.0	E950.4	E962.0	E980.4
F (hydrocortisone)	962.0	E858.0	E932.0	E950.4	E962.0	E980.4
Congo red	977.8	E858.8	E947.8	E950.4	E962.0	E980.4
Coniine, conine	965.7	E850.7	E935.7	E950.0	E962.0	E980.0
Conium (maculatum)	988.2	E865.4	—	E950.9	E962.1	E980.9
Conjugated estrogens (equine)	962.2	E858.0	E932.2	E950.4	E962.0	E980.4
Contac	975.6	E858.6	E945.6	E950.4	E962.0	E980.4
Contact lens solution	976.5	E858.7	E946.5	E950.4	E962.0	E980.4
Contraceptives (oral)	962.2	E858.0	E932.2	E950.4	E962.0	E980.4
vaginal	976.8	E858.7	E946.8	E950.4	E962.0	E980.4
Contrast media (roentgenographic)	977.8	E858.8	E947.8	E950.4	E962.0	E980.4
Convallaria majalis	988.2	E865.4	—	E950.9	E962.1	E980.9
Copper (dust) (fumes) (salts) NEC	985.8	E866.4	—	E950.9	E962.1	E980.9
arsenate, arsenite	985.1	E866.3	—	E950.8	E962.1	E980.8
insecticide	985.1	E863.4	—	E950.8	E962.1	E980.8
emetic	973.6	E858.4	E943.6	E950.4	E962.0	E980.4
fungicide	985.8	E863.6	—	E950.6	E962.1	E980.7
insecticide	985.8	E863.4	—	E950.6	E962.1	E980.7
oleate	976.0	E858.7	E946.0	E950.4	E962.0	E980.4
sulfate	983.9	E864.3	—	E950.7	E962.1	E980.6
fungicide	983.9	E863.6	—	E950.7	E962.1	E980.6
cupric	973.6	E858.4	E943.6	E950.4	E962.0	E980.4
cuprous	983.9	E864.3	—	E950.7	E962.1	E980.6
Copperhead snake (bite) (venom)	989.5	E905.0	—	E950.9	E962.1	E980.9
Coral (sting)	989.5	E905.6	—	E950.9	E962.1	E980.9
snake (bite) (venom)	989.5	E905.0	—	E950.9	E962.1	E980.9
Cordran	976.0	E858.7	E946.0	E950.4	E962.0	E980.4
Corn cures	976.4	E858.7	E946.4	E950.4	E962.0	E980.4
Cornhusker's lotion	976.3	E858.7	E946.3	E950.4	E962.0	E980.4
Corn starch	976.3	E858.7	E946.3	E950.4	E962.0	E980.4
Corrosive	983.9	E864.4	—	E950.7	E962.1	E980.6
acids NEC	983.1	E864.1	—	E950.7	E962.1	E980.6
aromatics	983.0	E864.0	—	E950.7	E962.1	E980.6
disinfectant	983.0	E861.4	—	E950.7	E962.1	E980.6
fumes NEC	987.9	E869.9	—	E952.9	E962.2	E982.9
specified NEC	983.9	E864.3	—	E950.7	E962.1	E980.6
sublimate — see Mercury, chloride						
Cortate	962.0	E858.0	E932.0	E950.4	E962.0	E980.4
Cort-Dome	962.0	E858.0	E932.0	E950.4	E962.0	E980.4
ENT agent	976.6	E858.7	E946.6	E950.4	E962.0	E980.4
ophthalmic preparation	976.5	E858.7	E946.5	E950.4	E962.0	E980.4
topical NEC	976.0	E858.7	E946.0	E950.4	E962.0	E980.4
Cortef	962.0	E858.0	E932.0	E950.4	E962.0	E980.4
ENT agent	976.6	E858.7	E946.6	E950.4	E962.0	E980.4
ophthalmic preparation	976.5	E858.7	E946.5	E950.4	E962.0	E980.4

Table of Drugs and Chemicals

	Poisoning	External Cause (E-Code)				
		Accident	Therapeutic Use	Suicide Attempt	Assault	Undetermined
Cortef — *continued*						
topical NEC	976.0	E858.7	E946.0	E950.4	E962.0	E980.4
Corticosteroids (fluorinated)	962.0	E858.0	E932.0	E950.4	E962.0	E980.4
ENT agent	976.6	E858.7	E946.6	E950.4	E962.0	E980.4
ophthalmic preparation	976.5	E858.7	E946.5	E950.4	E962.0	E980.4
topical NEC	976.0	E858.7	E946.0	E950.4	E962.0	E980.4
Corticotropin	962.4	E858.0	E932.4	E950.4	E962.0	E980.4
Cortisol	962.0	E858.0	E932.0	E950.4	E962.0	E980.4
ENT agent	976.6	E858.7	E946.6	E950.4	E962.0	E980.4
ophthalmic preparation	976.5	E858.7	E946.5	E950.4	E962.0	E980.4
topical NEC	976.0	E858.7	E946.0	E950.4	E962.0	E980.4
Cortisone derivatives (acetate)	962.0	E858.0	E932.0	E950.4	E962.0	E980.4
ENT agent	976.6	E858.7	E946.6	E950.4	E962.0	E980.4
ophthalmic preparation	976.5	E858.7	E946.5	E950.4	E962.0	E980.4
topical NEC	976.0	E858.7	E946.0	E950.4	E962.0	E980.4
Cortogen	962.0	E858.0	E932.0	E950.4	E962.0	E980.4
ENT agent	976.6	E858.7	E946.6	E950.4	E962.0	E980.4
ophthalmic preparation	976.5	E858.7	E946.5	E950.4	E962.0	E980.4
Cortone	962.0	E858.0	E932.0	E950.4	E962.0	E980.4
ENT agent	976.6	E858.7	E946.6	E950.4	E962.0	E980.4
ophthalmic preparation	976.5	E858.7	E946.5	E950.4	E962.0	E980.4
Cortril	962.0	E858.0	E932.0	E950.4	E962.0	E980.4
ENT agent	976.6	E858.7	E946.6	E950.4	E962.0	E980.4
ophthalmic preparation	976.5	E858.7	E946.5	E950.4	E962.0	E980.4
topical NEC	976.0	E858.7	E946.0	E950.4	E962.0	E980.4
Cosmetics	989.89	E866.7	—	E950.9	E962.1	E980.9
Cosyntropin	977.8	E858.8	E947.8	E950.4	E962.0	E980.4
Cotarnine	964.5	E858.2	E934.5	E950.4	E962.0	E980.4
Cottonseed oil	976.3	E858.7	E946.3	E950.4	E962.0	E980.4
Cough mixtures (antitussives)	975.4	E858.6	E945.4	E950.4	E962.0	E980.4
containing opiates	965.09	E850.2	E935.2	E950.0	E962.0	E980.0
expectorants	975.5	E858.6	E945.5	E950.4	E962.0	E980.4
Coumadin	964.2	E858.2	E934.2	E950.4	E962.0	E980.4
rodenticide	989.4	E863.7	—	E950.6	E962.1	E980.7
Coumarin	964.2	E858.2	E934.2	E950.4	E962.0	E980.4
Coumetarol	964.2	E858.2	E934.2	E950.4	E962.0	E980.4
Cowbane	988.2	E865.4	—	E950.9	E962.1	E980.9
Cozyme	963.5	E858.1	E933.5	E950.4	E962.0	E980.4
Crack ●	970.8	E854.3	E940.8	E950.4	E962.0	E980.4
Creolin	983.0	E864.0	—	E950.7	E962.1	E980.6
disinfectant	983.0	E861.4	—	E950.7	E962.1	E980.6
Creosol (compound)	983.0	E864.0	—	E950.7	E962.1	E980.6
Creosote (beechwood) (coal tar)	983.0	E864.0	—	E950.7	E962.1	E980.6
medicinal (expectorant)	975.5	E858.6	E945.5	E950.4	E962.0	E980.4
syrup	975.5	E858.6	E945.5	E950.4	E962.0	E980.4
Cresol	983.0	E864.0	—	E950.7	E962.1	E980.6
disinfectant	983.0	E861.4	—	E950.7	E962.1	E980.6
Cresylic acid	983.0	E864.0	—	E950.7	E962.1	E980.6
Cropropamide	965.7	E850.7	E935.7	E950.0	E962.0	E980.0
with crotethamide	970.0	E854.3	E940.0	E950.4	E962.0	E980.4
Crotamiton	976.0	E858.7	E946.0	E950.4	E962.0	E980.4
Crotethamide	965.7	E850.7	E935.7	E950.0	E962.0	E980.0
with cropropamide	970.0	E854.3	E940.0	E950.4	E962.0	E980.4
Croton (oil)	973.1	E858.4	E943.1	E950.4	E962.0	E980.4
chloral	967.1	E852.0	E937.1	E950.2	E962.0	E980.2
Crude oil	981	E862.1	—	E950.9	E962.1	E980.9
Cryogenine	965.8	E850.8	E935.8	E950.0	E962.0	E980.0
Cryolite (pesticide)	989.4	E863.4	—	E950.6	E962.1	E980.7
Cryptenamine	972.6	E858.3	E942.6	E950.4	E962.0	E980.4
Crystal violet	976.0	E858.7	E946.0	E950.4	E962.0	E980.4
Cuckoopint	988.2	E865.4	—	E950.9	E962.1	E980.9
Cumetharol	964.2	E858.2	E934.2	E950.4	E962.0	E980.4
Cupric sulfate	973.6	E858.4	E943.6	E950.4	E962.0	E980.4
Cuprous sulfate	983.9	E864.3	—	E950.7	E962.1	E980.6
Curare, curarine	975.2	E858.6	E945.2	E950.4	E962.0	E980.4
Cyanic acid — *see* Cyanide(s)						
Cyanide(s) (compounds) (hydrogen) (potassium) (sodium) NEC	989.0	E866.8	—	E950.9	E962.1	E980.9
dust or gas (inhalation) NEC	987.7	E869.8	—	E952.8	E962.2	E982.8
fumigant	989.0	E863.8	—	E950.6	E962.1	E980.7
mercuric — *see* Mercury						
pesticide (dust) (fumes)	989.0	E863.4	—	E950.6	E962.1	E980.7
Cyanocobalamin	964.1	E858.2	E934.1	E950.4	E962.0	E980.4
Cyanogen (chloride) (gas) NEC	987.8	E869.8	—	E952.8	E962.2	E982.8
Cyclaine	968.5	E855.2	E938.5	E950.4	E962.0	E980.4
Cyclamen europaeum	988.2	E865.4	—	E950.9	E962.1	E980.9
Cyclandelate	972.5	E858.3	E942.5	E950.4	E962.0	E980.4
Cyclazocine	965.09	E850.2	E935.2	E950.0	E962.0	E980.0
Cyclizine	963.0	E858.1	E933.0	E950.4	E962.0	E980.4
Cyclobarbital, cyclobarbitone	967.0	E851	E937.0	E950.1	E962.0	E980.1
Cycloguanil	961.4	E857	E931.4	E950.4	E962.0	E980.4
Cyclohexane	982.0	E862.4	—	E950.9	E962.1	E980.9

Table of Drugs and Chemicals

		External Cause (E-Code)				
	Poisoning	Accident	Therapeutic Use	Suicide Attempt	Assault	Undetermined
Cyclohexanol	980.8	E860.8	—	E950.9	E962.1	E980.9
Cyclohexanone	982.8	E862.4	—	E950.9	E962.1	E980.9
Cyclomethycaine	968.5	E855.2	E938.5	E950.4	E962.0	E980.4
Cyclopentamine	971.2	E855.5	E941.2	E950.4	E962.0	E980.4
Cyclopenthiazide	974.3	E858.5	E944.3	E950.4	E962.0	E980.4
Cyclopentolate	971.1	E855.4	E941.1	E950.4	E962.0	E980.4
Cyclophosphamide	963.1	E858.1	E933.1	E950.4	E962.0	E980.4
Cyclopropane	968.2	E855.1	E938.2	E950.4	E962.0	E980.4
Cycloserine	960.6	E856	E930.6	E950.4	E962.0	E980.4
Cyclothiazide	974.3	E858.5	E944.3	E950.4	E962.0	E980.4
Cycrimine	966.4	E855.0	E936.4	E950.4	E962.0	E980.4
Cymarin	972.1	E858.3	E942.1	E950.4	E962.0	E980.4
Cyproheptadine	963.0	E858.1	E933.0	E950.4	E962.0	E980.4
Cyprolidol	969.0	E854.0	E939.0	E950.3	E962.0	E980.3
Cytarabine	963.1	E858.1	E933.1	E950.4	E962.0	E980.4
Cytisus						
laburnum	988.2	E865.4	—	E950.9	E962.1	E980.9
scoparius	988.2	E865.4	—	E950.9	E962.1	E980.9
Cytomel	962.7	E858.0	E932.7	E950.4	E962.0	E980.4
Cytosine (antineoplastic)	963.1	E858.1	E933.1	E950.4	E962.0	E980.4
Cytoxan	963.1	E858.1	E933.1	E950.4	E962.0	E980.4
Dacarbazine	963.1	E858.1	E933.1	E950.4	E962.0	E980.4
Dactinomycin	960.7	E856	E930.7	E950.4	E962.0	E980.4
DADPS	961.8	E857	E931.8	E950.4	E962.0	E980.4
Dakin's solution (external)	976.0	E858.7	E946.0	E950.4	E962.0	E980.4
Dalmane	969.4	E853.2	E939.4	E950.3	E962.0	E980.3
DAM	977.2	E858.8	E947.2	E950.4	E962.0	E980.4
Danilone	964.2	E858.2	E934.2	E950.4	E962.0	E980.4
Danthron	973.1	E858.4	E943.1	E950.4	E962.0	E980.4
Dantrolene	975.2	E858.6	E945.2	E950.4	E962.0	E980.4
Daphne (gnidium) (mezereum)	988.2	E865.4	—	E950.9	E962.1	E980.9
berry	988.2	E865.3	—	E950.9	E962.1	E980.9
Dapsone	961.8	E857	E931.8	E950.4	E962.0	E980.4
Daraprim	961.4	E857	E931.4	E950.4	E962.0	E980.4
Darnel	988.2	E865.3	—	E950.9	E962.1	E980.9
Darvon	965.8	E850.8	E935.8	E950.0	E962.0	E980.0
Daunorubicin	960.7	E856	E930.7	E950.4	E962.0	E980.4
DBI	962.3	E858.0	E932.3	E950.4	E962.0	E980.4
D-Con (rodenticide)	989.4	E863.7	—	E950.6	E962.1	E980.7
DDS	961.8	E857	E931.8	E950.4	E962.0	E980.4
DDT	989.2	E863.0	—	E950.6	E962.1	E980.7
Deadly nightshade	988.2	E865.4	—	E950.9	E962.1	E980.9
berry	988.2	E865.3	—	E950.9	E962.1	E980.9
Deanol	969.7	E854.2	E939.7	E950.3	E962.0	E980.3
Debrisoquine	972.6	E858.3	E942.6	E950.4	E962.0	E980.4
Decaborane	989.89	E866.8	—	E950.9	E962.1	E980.9
fumes	987.8	E869.8	—	E952.8	E962.2	E982.8
Decadron	962.0	E858.0	E932.0	E950.4	E962.0	E980.4
ENT agent	976.6	E858.7	E946.6	E950.4	E962.0	E980.4
ophthalmic preparation	976.5	E858.7	E946.5	E950.4	E962.0	E980.4
topical NEC	976.0	E858.7	E946.0	E950.4	E962.0	E980.4
Decahydronaphthalene	982.0	E862.4	—	E950.9	E962.1	E980.9
Decalin	982.0	E862.4	—	E950.9	E962.1	E980.9
Decamethonium	975.2	E858.6	E945.2	E950.4	E962.0	E980.4
Decholin	973.4	E858.4	E943.4	E950.4	E962.0	E980.4
sodium (diagnostic)	977.8	E858.8	E947.8	E950.4	E962.0	E980.4
Declomycin	960.4	E856	E930.4	E950.4	E962.0	E980.4
Deferoxamine	963.8	E858.1	E933.8	E950.4	E962.0	E980.4
Dehydrocholic acid	973.4	E858.4	E943.4	E950.4	E962.0	E980.4
DeKalin	982.0	E862.4	—	E950.9	E962.1	E980.9
Delalutin	962.2	E858.0	E932.2	E950.4	E962.0	E980.4
Delphinium	988.2	E865.3	—	E950.9	E962.1	E980.9
Deltasone	962.0	E858.0	E932.0	E950.4	E962.0	E980.4
Delta	962.0	E858.0	E932.0	E950.4	E962.0	E980.4
Delvinal	967.0	E851	E937.0	E950.1	E962.0	E980.1
Demecarium (bromide)	971.0	E855.3	E941.0	E950.4	E962.0	E980.4
Demeclocycline	960.4	E856	E930.4	E950.4	E962.0	E980.4
Demecolcine	963.1	E858.1	E933.1	E950.4	E962.0	E980.4
Demelanizing agents	976.8	E858.7	E946.8	E950.4	E962.0	E980.4
Demerol	965.09	E850.2	E935.2	E950.0	E962.0	E980.0
Demethylchlortetracycline	960.4	E856	E930.4	E950.4	E962.0	E980.4
Demethyltetracycline	960.4	E856	E930.4	E950.4	E962.0	E980.4
Demeton	989.3	E863.1	—	E950.6	E962.1	E980.7
Demulcents	976.3	E858.7	E946.3	E950.4	E962.0	E980.4
Demulen	962.2	E858.0	E932.2	E950.4	E962.0	E980.4
Denatured alcohol	980.0	E860.1	—	E950.9	E962.1	E980.9
Dendrid	976.5	E858.7	E946.5	E950.4	E962.0	E980.4
Dental agents, topical	976.7	E858.7	E946.7	E950.4	E962.0	E980.4
Deodorant spray (feminine hygiene)	976.8	E858.7	E946.8	E950.4	E962.0	E980.4
Deoxyribonuclease	963.4	E858.1	E933.4	E950.4	E962.0	E980.4

Table of Drugs and Chemicals

Depressants — Dichlorvos

	Poisoning	External Cause (E-Code)				
		Accident	Therapeutic Use	Suicide Attempt	Assault	Undetermined
Depressants	977.0	E858.8	E947.0	E950.4	E962.0	E980.4
appetite, central	972.0	E858.3	E942.0	E950.4	E962.0	E980.4
cardiac	968.4	E855.1	E938.4	E950.4	E962.0	E980.4
central nervous system (anesthetic)	969.5	E853.9	E939.5	E950.3	E962.0	E980.3
psychotherapeutic	976.0	E858.7	E946.0	E950.4	E962.0	E980.4
Dequalinium	976.2	E858.7	E946.2	E950.4	E962.0	E980.4
Dermolate	962.2	E858.0	E932.2	E950.4	E962.0	E980.4
DES	976.0	E858.7	E946.0	E950.4	E962.0	E980.4
Desenex	972.6	E858.3	E942.6	E950.4	E962.0	E980.4
Deserpidine	969.0	E854.0	E939.0	E950.3	E962.0	E980.3
Desipramine	972.1	E858.3	E942.1	E950.4	E962.0	E980.4
Deslanoside	965.09	E850.2	E935.2	E950.0	E962.0	E980.0
Desocodeine	965.09	E850.2	E935.2	E950.0	E962.0	E980.0
Desomorphine	976.0	E858.7	E946.0	E950.4	E962.0	E980.4
Desonide	962.0	E858.0	E932.0	E950.4	E962.0	E980.4
Desoxycorticosterone derivatives	969.7	E854.2	E939.7	E950.3	E962.0	E980.3
Desoxyephedrine	969.6	E854.1	E939.6	E950.3	E962.0	E980.3
DET	989.6	E861.0	—	E950.9	E962.1	E980.9
Detergents (ingested) (synthetic)	976.2	E858.7	E946.2	E950.4	E962.0	E980.4
external medication	977.3	E858.8	E947.3	E950.4	E962.0	E980.4
Deterrent, alcohol	962.7	E858.0	E932.7	E950.4	E962.0	E980.4
Detrothyronine	976.0	E858.7	E946.0	E950.4	E962.0	E980.4
Dettol (external medication)	962.0	E858.0	E932.0	E950.4	E962.0	E980.4
Dexamethasone	976.6	E858.7	E946.6	E950.4	E962.0	E980.4
ENT agent	976.5	E858.7	E946.5	E950.4	E962.0	E980.4
ophthalmic preparation	976.0	E858.7	E946.0	E950.4	E962.0	E980.4
topical NEC	969.7	E854.2	E939.7	E950.3	E962.0	E980.3
Dexamphetamine	969.7	E854.2	E939.7	E950.3	E962.0	E980.3
Dexedrine	963.5	E858.1	E933.5	E950.4	E962.0	E980.4
Dexpanthenol	964.8	E858.2	E934.8	E950.4	E962.0	E980.4
Dextran	964.0	E858.2	E934.0	E950.4	E962.0	E980.4
Dextriferron	969.7	E854.2	E939.7	E950.3	E962.0	E980.3
Dextroamphetamine	963.5	E858.1	E933.5	E950.4	E962.0	E980.4
Dextro calcium pantothenate	975.4	E858.6	E945.4	E950.4	E962.0	E980.4
Dextromethorphan	965.09	E850.2	E935.2	E950.0	E962.0	E980.0
Dextromoramide	963.5	E858.1	E933.5	E950.4	E962.0	E980.4
Dextro pantothenyl alcohol	976.8	E858.7	E946.8	E950.4	E962.0	E980.4
topical	965.8	E850.8	E935.8	E950.0	E962.0	E980.0
Dextropropoxyphene (hydrochloride)	965.09	E850.2	E935.2	E950.0	E962.0	E980.0
Dextrorphan	974.5	E858.5	E944.5	E950.4	E962.0	E980.4
Dextrose NEC	962.7	E858.0	E932.7	E950.4	E962.0	E980.4
Dextrothyroxin	971.0	E855.3	E941.0	E950.4	E962.0	E980.4
DFP	972.9	E858.3	E942.9	E950.4	E962.0	E980.4
DHE-45	962.3	E858.0	E932.3	E950.4	E962.0	E980.4
Diabinese	977.2	E858.8	E947.2	E950.4	E962.0	E980.4
Diacetyl monoxime	965.01	E850.0	E935.0	E950.0	E962.0	E980.0
Diacetylmorphine	977.8	E858.8	E947.8	E950.4	E962.0	E980.4
Diagnostic agents	976.2	E858.7	E946.2	E950.4	E962.0	E980.4
Dial (soap)	967.0	E851	E937.0	E950.1	E962.0	E980.1
sedative	967.0	E851	E937.0	E950.1	E962.0	E980.1
Diallylbarbituric acid	961.8	E857	E931.8	E950.4	E962.0	E980.4
Diaminodiphenylsulfone	965.01	E850.0	E935.0	E950.0	E962.0	E980.0
Diamorphine	974.2	E858.5	E944.2	E950.4	E962.0	E980.4
Diamox	976.0	E858.7	E946.0	E950.4	E962.0	E980.4
Diamthazole	961.8	E857	E931.8	E950.4	E962.0	E980.4
Diaphenylsulfone	961.8	E857	E931.8	E950.4	E962.0	E980.4
Diasone (sodium)	969.4	E853.2	E939.4	E950.3	E962.0	E980.3
Diazepam	989.3	E863.1	—	E950.6	E962.1	E980.7
Diazinon	987.8	E869.8	—	E952.8	E962.2	E982.8
Diazomethane (gas)	972.5	E858.3	E942.5	E950.4	E962.0	E980.4
Diazoxide	971.3	E855.6	E941.3	E950.4	E962.0	E980.4
Dibenamine	963.0	E858.1	E933.0	E950.4	E962.0	E980.4
Dibenzheptropine	971.3	E855.6	E941.3	E950.4	E962.0	E980.4
Dibenzyline	987.8	E869.8	—	E952.8	E962.2	E982.8
Diborane (gas)	963.1	E858.1	E933.1	E950.4	E962.0	E980.4
Dibromomannitol	968.7	E855.2	E938.7	E950.4	E962.0	E980.4
Dibucaine (spinal)	968.5	E855.2	E938.5	E950.4	E962.0	E980.4
topical (surface)	975.4	E858.6	E945.4	E950.4	E962.0	E980.4
Dibunate sodium	971.1	E855.4	E941.1	E950.4	E962.0	E980.4
Dibutoline	989.4	E863.4	—	E950.6	E962.1	E980.7
Dicapthon	967.1	E852.0	E937.1	E950.2	E962.0	E980.2
Dichloralphenazone	987.4	E869.2	—	E952.8	E962.2	E982.8
Dichlorodifluoromethane	982.3	E862.4	—	E950.9	E962.1	E980.9
Dichloroethane	982.3	E862.4	—	E950.9	E962.1	E980.9
Dichloroethylene	987.8	E869.8	—	E952.8	E962.2	E982.8
Dichloroethyl sulfide	982.3	E862.4	—	E950.9	E962.1	E980.9
Dichlorohydrin	982.3	E862.4	—	E950.9	E962.1	E980.9
Dichloromethane (solvent) (vapor)	961.6	E857	E931.6	E950.4	E962.0	E980.4
Dichlorophen(e)	974.2	E858.5	E944.2	E950.4	E962.0	E980.4
Dichlorphenamide	989.3	E863.1	—	E950.6	E962.1	E980.7
Dichlorvos						

Table of Drugs and Chemicals

	Poisoning	External Cause (E-Code)				
		Accident	Therapeutic Use	Suicide Attempt	Assault	Undetermined
Diclofenac sodium	965.69	E850.6	E935.6	E950.0	E962.0	E980.0
Dicoumarin, dicumarol	964.2	E858.2	E934.2	E950.4	E962.0	E980.4
Dicyanogen (gas)	987.8	E869.8	—	E952.8	E962.2	E982.8
Dicyclomine	971.1	E855.4	E941.1	E950.4	E962.0	E980.4
Dieldrin (vapor)	989.2	E863.0	—	E950.6	E962.1	E980.7
Dienestrol	962.2	E858.0	E932.2	E950.4	E962.0	E980.4
Dietetics	977.0	E858.8	E947.0	E950.4	E962.0	E980.4
Diethazine	966.4	E855.0	E936.4	E950.4	E962.0	E980.4
Diethyl						
barbituric acid	967.0	E851	E937.0	E950.1	E962.0	E980.1
carbamazine	961.6	E857	E931.6	E950.4	E962.0	E980.4
carbinol	980.8	E860.8	—	E950.9	E962.1	E980.9
carbonate	982.8	E862.4	—	E950.9	E962.1	E980.9
ether (vapor) — see Ether(s)						
propion	977.0	E858.8	E947.0	E950.4	E962.0	E980.4
stilbestrol	962.2	E858.0	E932.2	E950.4	E962.0	E980.4
Diethylene						
dioxide	982.8	E862.4	—	E950.9	E962.1	E980.9
glycol (monoacetate) (monoethyl ether)	982.8	E862.4	—	E950.9	E962.1	E980.9
Diethylsulfone-diethylmethane	967.8	E852.8	E937.8	E950.2	E962.0	E980.2
Difencloxazine	965.09	E850.2	E935.2	E950.0	E962.0	E980.0
Diffusin	963.4	E858.1	E933.4	E950.4	E962.0	E980.4
Diflos	971.0	E855.3	E941.0	E950.4	E962.0	E980.4
Digestants	973.4	E858.4	E943.4	E950.4	E962.0	E980.4
Digitalin(e)	972.1	E858.3	E942.1	E950.4	E962.0	E980.4
Digitalis glycosides	972.1	E858.3	E942.1	E950.4	E962.0	E980.4
Digitoxin	972.1	E858.3	E942.1	E950.4	E962.0	E980.4
Digoxin	972.1	E858.3	E942.1	E950.4	E962.0	E980.4
Dihydrocodeine	965.09	E850.2	E935.2	E950.0	E962.0	E980.0
Dihydrocodeinone	965.09	E850.2	E935.2	E950.0	E962.0	E980.0
Dihydroergocristine	972.9	E858.3	E942.9	E950.4	E962.0	E980.4
Dihydroergotamine	972.9	E858.3	E942.9	E950.4	E962.0	E980.4
Dihydroergotoxine	972.9	E858.3	E942.9	E950.4	E962.0	E980.4
Dihydrohydroxycodeinone	965.09	E850.2	E935.2	E950.0	E962.0	E980.0
Dihydrohydroxymorphinone	965.09	E850.2	E935.2	E950.0	E962.0	E980.0
Dihydroisocodeine	965.09	E850.2	E935.2	E950.0	E962.0	E980.0
Dihydromorphine	965.09	E850.2	E935.2	E950.0	E962.0	E980.0
Dihydromorphinone	965.09	E850.2	E935.2	E950.0	E962.0	E980.0
Dihydrostreptomycin	960.6	E856	E930.6	E950.4	E962.0	E980.4
Dihydrotachysterol	962.6	E858.0	E932.6	E950.4	E962.0	E980.4
Dihydroxyanthraquinone	973.1	E858.4	E943.1	E950.4	E962.0	E980.4
Dihydroxycodeinone	965.09	E850.2	E935.2	E950.0	E962.0	E980.0
Diiodohydroxyquin	961.3	E857	E931.3	E950.4	E962.0	E980.4
topical	976.0	E858.7	E946.0	E950.4	E962.0	E980.4
Diiodohydroxyquinoline	961.3	E857	E931.3	E950.4	E962.0	E980.4
Dilantin	966.1	E855.0	E936.1	E950.4	E962.0	E980.4
Dilaudid	965.09	E850.2	E935.2	E950.0	E962.0	E980.0
Diloxanide	961.5	E857	E931.5	E950.4	E962.0	E980.4
Dimefline	970.0	E854.3	E940.0	E950.4	E962.0	E980.4
Dimenhydrinate	963.0	E858.1	E933.0	E950.4	E962.0	E980.4
Dimercaprol	963.8	E858.1	E933.8	E950.4	E962.0	E980.4
Dimercaptopropanol	963.8	E858.1	E933.8	E950.4	E962.0	E980.4
Dimetane	963.0	E858.1	E933.0	E950.4	E962.0	E980.4
Dimethicone	976.3	E858.7	E946.3	E950.4	E962.0	E980.4
Dimethindene	963.0	E858.1	E933.0	E950.4	E962.0	E980.4
Dimethisoquin	968.5	E855.2	E938.5	E950.4	E962.0	E980.4
Dimethisterone	962.2	E858.0	E932.2	E950.4	E962.0	E980.4
Dimethoxanate	975.4	E858.6	E945.4	E950.4	E962.0	E980.4
Dimethyl						
arsine, arsinic acid — see Arsenic						
carbinol	980.2	E860.3	—	E950.9	E962.1	E980.9
diguanide	962.3	E858.0	E932.3	E950.4	E962.0	E980.4
ketone	982.8	E862.4	—	E950.9	E962.1	E980.9
vapor	987.8	E869.8	—	E952.8	E962.2	E982.8
meperidine	965.09	E850.2	E935.2	E950.0	E962.0	E980.0
parathion	989.3	E863.1	—	E950.6	E962.1	E980.7
polysiloxane	973.8	E858.4	E943.8	E950.4	E962.0	E980.4
sulfate (fumes)	987.8	E869.8	—	E952.8	E962.2	E982.8
liquid	983.9	E864.3	—	E950.7	E962.1	E980.6
sulfoxide NEC	982.8	E862.4	—	E950.9	E962.1	E980.9
medicinal	976.4	E858.7	E946.4	E950.4	E962.0	E980.4
triptamine	969.6	E854.1	E939.6	E950.3	E962.0	E980.3
tubocurarine	975.2	E858.6	E945.2	E950.4	E962.0	E980.4
Dindevan	964.2	E858.2	E934.2	E950.4	E962.0	E980.4
Dinitro (-ortho-) cresol (herbicide) (spray)	989.4	E863.5	—	E950.6	E962.1	E980.7
insecticide	989.4	E863.4	—	E950.6	E962.1	E980.7
Dinitrobenzene	983.0	E864.0	—	E950.7	E962.1	E980.6
vapor	987.8	E869.8	—	E952.8	E962.2	E982.8
Dinitro-orthocresol (herbicide)	989.4	E863.5	—	E950.6	E962.1	E980.7
insecticide	989.4	E863.4	—	E950.6	E962.1	E980.7

Dinitrophenol — Droperidol

Table of Drugs and Chemicals

	Poisoning	Accident	Therapeutic Use	Suicide Attempt	Assault	Undetermined
			External Cause (E-Code)			
Dinitrophenol (herbicide) (spray)	989.4	E863.5	—	E950.6	E962.1	E980.7
insecticide	989.4	E863.4	—	E950.6	E962.1	E980.7
Dinoprost	975.0	E858.6	E945.0	E950.4	E962.0	E980.4
Dioctyl sulfosuccinate (calcium) (sodium)	973.2	E858.4	E943.2	E950.4	E962.0	E980.4
Diodoquin	961.3	E857	E931.3	E950.4	E962.0	E980.4
Dione derivatives NEC	966.3	E855.0	E936.3	E950.4	E962.0	E980.4
Dionin	965.09	E850.2	E935.2	E950.0	E962.0	E980.0
Dioxane	982.8	E862.4	—	E950.9	E962.1	E980.9
Dioxin — see Herbicide						
Dioxyline	972.5	E858.3	E942.5	E950.4	E962.0	E980.4
Dipentene	982.8	E862.4	—	E950.9	E962.1	E980.9
Diphemanil	971.1	E855.4	E941.1	E950.4	E962.0	E980.4
Diphenadione	964.2	E858.2	E934.2	E950.4	E962.0	E980.4
Diphenhydramine	963.0	E858.1	E933.0	E950.4	E962.0	E980.4
Diphenidol	963.0	E858.1	E933.0	E950.4	E962.0	E980.4
Diphenoxylate	973.5	E858.4	E943.5	E950.4	E962.0	E980.4
Diphenylchloroarsine	985.1	E866.3	—	E950.8	E962.1	E980.8
Diphenylhydantoin (sodium)	966.1	E855.0	E936.1	E950.4	E962.0	E980.4
Diphenylpyraline	963.0	E858.1	E933.0	E950.4	E962.0	E980.4
Diphtheria						
antitoxin	979.9	E858.8	E949.9	E950.4	E962.0	E980.4
toxoid	978.5	E858.8	E948.5	E950.4	E962.0	E980.4
with tetanus toxoid	978.9	E858.8	E948.9	E950.4	E962.0	E980.4
with pertussis component	978.6	E858.8	E948.6	E950.4	E962.0	E980.4
vaccine	978.5	E858.8	E948.5	E950.4	E962.0	E980.4
Dipipanone	965.09	E850.2	E935.2	E950.0	E962.0	E980.0
Diplovax	979.5	E858.8	E949.5	E950.4	E962.0	E980.4
Diprophylline	975.1	E858.6	E945.1	E950.4	E962.0	E980.4
Dipyridamole	972.4	E858.3	E942.4	E950.4	E962.0	E980.4
Dipyrone	965.5	E850.5	E935.5	E950.0	E962.0	E980.0
Diquat	989.4	E863.5	—	E950.6	E962.1	E980.7
Disinfectant NEC	983.9	E861.4	—	E950.7	E962.1	E980.6
alkaline	983.2	E861.4	—	E950.7	E962.1	E980.6
aromatic	983.0	E861.4	—	E950.7	E962.1	E980.6
Disipal	966.4	E855.0	E936.4	E950.4	E962.0	E980.4
Disodium edetate	963.8	E858.1	E933.8	E950.4	E962.0	E980.4
Disulfamide	974.4	E858.5	E944.4	E950.4	E962.0	E980.4
Disulfanilamide	961.0	E857	E931.0	E950.4	E962.0	E980.4
Disulfiram	977.3	E858.8	E947.3	E950.4	E962.0	E980.4
Dithiazanine	961.6	E857	E931.6	E950.4	E962.0	E980.4
Dithioglycerol	963.8	E858.1	E933.8	E950.4	E962.0	E980.4
Dithranol	976.4	E858.7	E946.4	E950.4	E962.0	E980.4
Diucardin	974.3	E858.5	E944.3	E950.4	E962.0	E980.4
Diupres	974.3	E858.5	E944.3	E950.4	E962.0	E980.4
Diuretics NEC	974.4	E858.5	E944.4	E950.4	E962.0	E980.4
carbonic acid anhydrase inhibitors	974.2	E858.5	E944.2	E950.4	E962.0	E980.4
mercurial	974.0	E858.5	E944.0	E950.4	E962.0	E980.4
osmotic	974.4	E858.5	E944.4	E950.4	E962.0	E980.4
purine derivatives	974.1	E858.5	E944.1	E950.4	E962.0	E980.4
saluretic	974.3	E858.5	E944.3	E950.4	E962.0	E980.4
Diuril	974.3	E858.5	E944.3	E950.4	E962.0	E980.4
Divinyl ether	968.2	E855.1	E938.2	E950.4	E962.0	E980.4
D-lysergic acid diethylamide	969.6	E854.1	E939.6	E950.3	E962.0	E980.3
DMCT	960.4	E856	E930.4	E950.4	E962.0	E980.4
DMSO	982.8	E862.4	—	E950.9	E962.1	E980.9
DMT	969.6	E854.1	E939.6	E950.3	E962.0	E980.3
DNOC	989.4	E863.5	—	E950.6	E962.1	E980.7
DOCA	962.0	E858.0	E932.0	E950.4	E962.0	E980.4
Dolophine	965.02	E850.1	E935.1	E950.0	E962.0	E980.0
Doloxene	965.8	E850.8	E935.8	E950.0	E962.0	E980.0
DOM	969.6	E854.1	E939.6	E950.3	E962.0	E980.3
Domestic gas — see Gas, utility						
Domiphen (bromide) (lozenges)	976.6	E858.7	E946.6	E950.4	E962.0	E980.4
Dopa (levo)	966.4	E855.0	E936.4	E950.4	E962.0	E980.4
Dopamine	971.2	E855.5	E941.2	E950.4	E962.0	E980.4
Doriden	967.5	E852.4	E937.5	E950.2	E962.0	E980.2
Dormiral	967.0	E851	E937.0	E950.1	E962.0	E980.1
Dormison	967.8	E852.8	E937.8	E950.2	E962.0	E980.2
Dornase	963.4	E858.1	E933.4	E950.4	E962.0	E980.4
Dorsacaine	968.5	E855.2	E938.5	E950.4	E962.0	E980.4
Dothiepin hydrochloride	969.0	E854.0	E939.0	E950.3	E962.0	E980.3
Doxapram	970.0	E854.3	E940.0	E950.4	E962.0	E980.4
Doxepin	969.0	E854.0	E939.0	E950.3	E962.0	E980.3
Doxorubicin	960.7	E856	E930.7	E950.4	E962.0	E980.4
Doxycycline	960.4	E856	E930.4	E950.4	E962.0	E980.4
Doxylamine	963.0	E858.1	E933.0	E950.4	E962.0	E980.4
Dramamine	963.0	E858.1	E933.0	E950.4	E962.0	E980.4
Drano (drain cleaner)	983.2	E864.2	—	E950.7	E962.1	E980.6
Dromoran	965.09	E850.2	E935.2	E950.0	E962.0	E980.0
Dromostanolone	962.1	E858.0	E932.1	E950.4	E962.0	E980.4
Droperidol	969.2	E853.1	E939.2	E950.3	E962.0	E980.3

Table of Drugs and Chemicals

		External Cause (E-Code)				
	Poisoning	Accident	Therapeutic Use	Suicide Attempt	Assault	Undetermined
Drug	977.9	E858.9	E947.9	E950.5	E962.0	E980.5
specified NEC	977.8	E858.8	E947.8	E950.4	E962.0	E980.4
AHFS List						
4:00 antihistamine drugs	963.0	E858.1	E933.0	E950.4	E962.0	E980.4
8:04 amebacides	961.5	E857	E931.5	E950.4	E962.0	E980.4
arsenical anti-infectives	961.1	E857	E931.1	E950.4	E962.0	E980.4
quinoline derivatives	961.3	E857	E931.3	E950.4	E962.0	E980.4
8:08 anthelmintics	961.6	E857	E931.6	E950.4	E962.0	E980.4
quinoline derivatives	961.3	E857	E931.3	E950.4	E962.0	E980.4
8:12.04 antifungal antibiotics	960.1	E856	E930.1	E950.4	E962.0	E980.4
8:12.06 cephalosporins	960.5	E856	E930.5	E950.4	E962.0	E980.4
8:12.08 chloramphenicol	960.2	E856	E930.2	E950.4	E962.0	E980.4
8:12.12 erythromycins	960.3	E856	E930.3	E950.4	E962.0	E980.4
8:12.16 penicillins	960.0	E856	E930.0	E950.4	E962.0	E980.4
8:12.20 streptomycins	960.6	E856	E930.6	E950.4	E962.0	E980.4
8:12.24 tetracyclines	960.4	E856	E930.4	E950.4	E962.0	E980.4
8:12.28 other antibiotics	960.8	E856	E930.8	E950.4	E962.0	E980.4
antimycobacterial	960.6	E856	E930.6	E950.4	E962.0	E980.4
macrolides	960.3	E856	E930.3	E950.4	E962.0	E980.4
8:16 antituberculars	961.8	E857	E931.8	E950.4	E962.0	E980.4
antibiotics	960.6	E856	E930.6	E950.4	E962.0	E980.4
8:18 antivirals	961.7	E857	E931.7	E950.4	E962.0	E980.4
8:20 plasmodicides (antimalarials)	961.4	E857	E931.4	E950.4	E962.0	E980.4
8:24 sulfonamides	961.0	E857	E931.0	E950.4	E962.0	E980.4
8:26 sulfones	961.8	E857	E931.8	E950.4	E962.0	E980.4
8:28 treponemicides	961.2	E857	E931.2	E950.4	E962.0	E980.4
8:32 trichomonacides	961.5	E857	E931.5	E950.4	E962.0	E980.4
quinoline derivatives	961.3	E857	E931.3	E950.4	E962.0	E980.4
nitrofuran derivatives	961.9	E857	E931.9	E950.4	E962.0	E980.4
8:36 urinary germicides	961.9	E857	E931.9	E950.4	E962.0	E980.4
quinoline derivatives	961.3	E857	E931.3	E950.4	E962.0	E980.4
8:40 other anti-infectives	961.9	E857	E931.9	E950.4	E962.0	E980.4
10:00 antineoplastic agents	963.1	E858.1	E933.1	E950.4	E962.0	E980.4
antibiotics	960.7	E856	E930.7	E950.4	E962.0	E980.4
progestogens	962.2	E858.0	E932.2	E950.4	E962.0	E980.4
12:04 parasympathomimetic (cholinergic) agents	971.0	E855.3	E941.0	E950.4	E962.0	E980.4
12:08 parasympatholytic (cholinergic-blocking) agents	971.1	E855.4	E941.1	E950.4	E962.0	E980.4
12:12 Sympathomimetic (adrenergic) agents	971.2	E855.5	E941.2	E950.4	E962.0	E980.4
12:16 sympatholytic (adrenergic-blocking) agents	971.3	E855.6	E941.3	E950.4	E962.0	E980.4
12:20 skeletal muscle relaxants						
central nervous system muscle-tone depressants	968.0	E855.1	E938.0	E950.4	E962.0	E980.4
myoneural blocking agents	975.2	E858.6	E945.2	E950.4	E962.0	E980.4
16:00 blood derivatives	964.7	E858.2	E934.7	E950.4	E962.0	E980.4
20:04 antianemia drugs	964.1	E858.2	E934.1	E950.4	E962.0	E980.4
20:04.04 iron preparations	964.0	E858.2	E934.0	E950.4	E962.0	E980.4
20:04.08 liver and stomach preparations	964.1	E858.2	E934.1	E950.4	E962.0	E980.4
20:12.04 anticoagulants	964.2	E858.2	E934.2	E950.4	E962.0	E980.4
20:12.08 antiheparin agents	964.5	E858.2	E934.5	E950.4	E962.0	E980.4
20:12.12 coagulants	964.5	E858.2	E934.5	E950.4	E962.0	E980.4
20:12.16 hemostatics NEC	964.5	E858.2	E934.5	E950.4	E962.0	E980.4
capillary active drugs	972.8	E858.3	E942.8	E950.4	E962.0	E980.4
24:04 cardiac drugs	972.9	E858.3	E942.9	E950.4	E962.0	E980.4
cardiotonic agents	972.1	E858.3	E942.1	E950.4	E962.0	E980.4
rhythm regulators	972.0	E858.3	E942.0	E950.4	E962.0	E980.4
24:06 antilipemic agents	972.2	E858.3	E942.2	E950.4	E962.0	E980.4
thyroid derivatives	962.7	E858.0	E932.7	E950.4	E962.0	E980.4
24:08 hypotensive agents	972.6	E858.3	E942.6	E950.4	E962.0	E980.4
adrenergic blocking agents	971.3	E855.6	E941.3	E950.4	E962.0	E980.4
ganglion blocking agents	972.3	E858.3	E942.3	E950.4	E962.0	E980.4
vasodilators	972.5	E858.3	E942.5	E950.4	E962.0	E980.4
24:12 vasodilating agents NEC	972.5	E858.3	E942.5	E950.4	E962.0	E980.4
coronary	972.4	E858.3	E942.4	E950.4	E962.0	E980.4
nicotinic acid derivatives	972.2	E858.3	E942.2	E950.4	E962.0	E980.4
24:16 sclerosing agents	972.7	E858.3	E942.7	E950.4	E962.0	E980.4
28:04 general anesthetics	968.4	E855.1	E938.4	E950.4	E962.0	E980.4
gaseous anesthetics	968.2	E855.1	E938.2	E950.4	E962.0	E980.4
halothane	968.1	E855.1	E938.1	E950.4	E962.0	E980.4
intravenous anesthetics	968.3	E855.1	E938.3	E950.4	E962.0	E980.4
28:08 analgesics and antipyretics	965.9	E850.9	E935.9	E950.0	E962.0	E980.0
antirheumatics	965.69	E850.6	E935.6	E950.0	E962.0	E980.0
aromatic analgesics	965.4	E850.4	E935.4	E950.0	E962.0	E980.0
non-narcotic NEC	965.7	E850.7	E935.7	E950.0	E962.0	E980.0
opium alkaloids	965.00	E850.2	E935.2	E950.0	E962.0	E980.0
heroin	965.01	E850.0	E935.0	E950.0	E962.0	E980.0
methadone	965.02	E850.1	E935.1	E950.0	E962.0	E980.0
specified type NEC	965.09	E850.2	E935.2	E950.0	E962.0	E980.0
pyrazole derivatives	965.5	E850.5	E935.5	E950.0	E962.0	E980.0
salicylates	965.1	E850.3	E935.3	E950.0	E962.0	E980.0
specified NEC	965.8	E850.8	E935.8	E950.0	E962.0	E980.0
28:10 narcotic antagonists	970.1	E854.3	E940.1	E950.4	E962.0	E980.4

Drug

Table of Drugs and Chemicals

		External Cause (E-Code)				
	Poisoning	Accident	Therapeutic Use	Suicide Attempt	Assault	Undetermined
Drug — *continued*						
28:12 anticonvulsants	966.3	E855.0	E936.3	E950.4	E962.0	E980.4
barbiturates	967.0	E851	E937.0	E950.1	E962.0	E980.1
benzodiazepine-based tranquilizers	969.4	E853.2	E939.4	E950.3	E962.0	E980.3
bromides	967.3	E852.2	E937.3	E950.2	E962.0	E980.2
hydantoin derivatives	966.1	E855.0	E936.1	E950.4	E962.0	E980.4
oxazolidine (derivatives)	966.0	E855.0	E936.0	E950.4	E962.0	E980.4
succinimides	966.2	E855.0	E936.2	E950.4	E962.0	E980.4
28:16.04 antidepressants	969.0	E854.0	E939.0	E950.3	E962.0	E980.3
28:16.08 tranquilizers	969.5	E853.9	E939.5	E950.3	E962.0	E980.3
benzodiazepine-based	969.4	E853.2	E939.4	E950.3	E962.0	E980.3
butyrophenone-based	969.2	E853.1	E939.2	E950.3	E962.0	E980.3
major NEC	969.3	E853.8	E939.3	E950.3	E962.0	E980.3
phenothiazine-based	969.1	E853.0	E939.1	E950.3	E962.0	E980.3
28:16.12 other psychotherapeutic agents	969.8	E855.8	E939.8	E950.3	E962.0	E980.3
28:20 respiratory and cerebral stimulants	970.9	E854.3	E940.9	E950.4	E962.0	E980.4
analeptics	970.0	E854.3	E940.0	E950.4	E962.0	E980.4
anorexigenic agents	977.0	E858.8	E947.0	E950.4	E962.0	E980.4
psychostimulants	969.7	E854.2	E939.7	E950.3	E962.0	E980.3
specified NEC	970.8	E854.3	E940.8	E950.4	E962.0	E980.4
28:24 sedatives and hypnotics	967.9	E852.9	E937.9	E950.2	E962.0	E980.2
barbiturates	967.0	E851	E937.0	E950.1	E962.0	E980.1
benzodiazepine-based tranquilizers	969.4	E853.2	E939.4	E950.3	E962.0	E980.3
chloral hydrate (group)	967.1	E852.0	E937.1	E950.2	E962.0	E980.2
glutethamide group	967.5	E852.4	E937.5	E950.2	E962.0	E980.2
intravenous anesthetics	968.3	E855.1	E938.3	E950.4	E962.0	E980.4
methaqualone (compounds)	967.4	E852.3	E937.4	E950.2	E962.0	E980.2
paraldehyde	967.2	E852.1	E937.2	E950.2	E962.0	E980.2
phenothiazine-based tranquilizers	969.1	E853.0	E939.1	E950.3	E962.0	E980.3
specified NEC	967.8	E852.8	E937.8	E950.2	E962.0	E980.2
thiobarbiturates	968.3	E855.1	E938.3	E950.4	E962.0	E980.4
tranquilizer NEC	969.5	E853.9	E939.5	E950.3	E962.0	E980.3
36:04 to 36:88 diagnostic agents	977.8	E858.8	E947.8	E950.4	E962.0	E980.4
40:00 electrolyte, caloric, and water balance agents NEC	974.5	E858.5	E944.5	E950.4	E962.0	E980.4
40:04 acidifying agents	963.2	E858.1	E933.2	E950.4	E962.0	E980.4
40:08 alkalinizing agents	963.3	E858.1	E933.3	E950.4	E962.0	E980.4
40:10 ammonia detoxicants	974.5	E858.5	E944.5	E950.4	E962.0	E980.4
40:12 replacement solutions	974.5	E858.5	E944.5	E950.4	E962.0	E980.4
plasma expanders	964.8	E858.2	E934.8	E950.4	E962.0	E980.4
40:16 sodium-removing resins	974.5	E858.5	E944.5	E950.4	E962.0	E980.4
40:18 potassium-removing resins	974.5	E858.5	E944.5	E950.4	E962.0	E980.4
40:20 caloric agents	974.5	E858.5	E944.5	E950.4	E962.0	E980.4
40:24 salt and sugar substitutes	974.5	E858.5	E944.5	E950.4	E962.0	E980.4
40:28 diuretics NEC	974.4	E858.5	E944.4	E950.4	E962.0	E980.4
carbonic acid anhydrase inhibitors	974.2	E858.5	E944.2	E950.4	E962.0	E980.4
mercurials	974.0	E858.5	E944.0	E950.4	E962.0	E980.4
purine derivatives	974.1	E858.5	E944.1	E950.4	E962.0	E980.4
saluretics	974.3	E858.5	E944.3	E950.4	E962.0	E980.4
thiazides	974.3	E858.5	E944.3	E950.4	E962.0	E980.4
40:36 irrigating solutions	974.5	E858.5	E944.5	E950.4	E962.0	E980.4
40:40 uricosuric agents	974.7	E858.5	E944.7	E950.4	E962.0	E980.4
44:00 enzymes	963.4	E858.1	E933.4	E950.4	E962.0	E980.4
fibrinolysis-affecting agents	964.4	E858.2	E934.4	E950.4	E962.0	E980.4
gastric agents	973.4	E858.4	E943.4	E950.4	E962.0	E980.4
48:00 expectorants and cough preparations						
antihistamine agents	963.0	E858.1	E933.0	E950.4	E962.0	E980.4
antitussives	975.4	E858.6	E945.4	E950.4	E962.0	E980.4
codeine derivatives	965.09	E850.2	E935.2	E950.0	E962.0	E980.0
expectorants	975.5	E858.6	E945.5	E950.4	E962.0	E980.4
narcotic agents NEC	965.09	E850.2	E935.2	E950.0	E962.0	E980.0
52:04 anti-infectives (EENT)						
ENT agent	976.6	E858.7	E946.6	E950.4	E962.0	E980.4
ophthalmic preparation	976.5	E858.7	E946.5	E950.4	E962.0	E980.4
52:04.04 antibiotics (EENT)						
ENT agent	976.6	E858.7	E946.6	E950.4	E962.0	E980.4
ophthalmic preparation	976.5	E858.7	E946.5	E950.4	E962.0	E980.4
52:04.06 antivirals (EENT)						
ENT agent	976.6	E858.7	E946.6	E950.4	E962.0	E980.4
ophthalmic preparation	976.5	E858.7	E946.5	E950.4	E962.0	E980.4
52:04.08 sulfonamides (EENT)						
ENT agent	976.6	E858.7	E946.6	E950.4	E962.0	E980.4
ophthalmic preparation	976.5	E858.7	E946.5	E950.4	E962.0	E980.4
52:04.12 miscellaneous anti-infectives (EENT)						
ENT agent	976.6	E858.7	E946.6	E950.4	E962.0	E980.4
ophthalmic preparation	976.5	E858.7	E946.5	E950.4	E962.0	E980.4
52:08 anti-inflammatory agents (EENT)						
ENT agent	976.6	E858.7	E946.6	E950.4	E962.0	E980.4
ophthalmic preparation	976.5	E858.7	E946.5	E950.4	E962.0	E980.4
52:10 carbonic anhydrase inhibitors	974.2	E858.5	E944.2	E950.4	E962.0	E980.4
52:12 contact lens solutions	976.5	E858.7	E946.5	E950.4	E962.0	E980.4

Table of Drugs and Chemicals

		External Cause (E-Code)				
	Poisoning	Accident	Therapeutic Use	Suicide Attempt	Assault	Undetermined
Drug — continued						
52:16 local anesthetics (EENT)	968.5	E855.2	E938.5	E950.4	E962.0	E980.4
52:20 miotics	971.0	E855.3	E941.0	E950.4	E962.0	E980.4
52:24 mydriatics						
adrenergics	971.2	E855.5	E941.2	E950.4	E962.0	E980.4
anticholinergics	971.1	E855.4	E941.1	E950.4	E962.0	E980.4
antimuscarinics	971.1	E855.4	E941.1	E950.4	E962.0	E980.4
parasympatholytics	971.1	E855.4	E941.1	E950.4	E962.0	E980.4
spasmolytics	971.1	E855.4	E941.1	E950.4	E962.0	E980.4
sympathomimetics	971.2	E855.5	E941.2	E950.4	E962.0	E980.4
52:28 mouth washes and gargles	976.6	E858.7	E946.6	E950.4	E962.0	E980.4
52:32 vasoconstrictors (EENT)	971.2	E855.5	E941.2	E950.4	E962.0	E980.4
52:36 unclassified agents (EENT)						
ENT agent	976.6	E858.7	E946.6	E950.4	E962.0	E980.4
ophthalmic preparation	976.5	E858.7	E946.5	E950.4	E962.0	E980.4
56:04 antacids and adsorbents	973.0	E858.4	E943.0	E950.4	E962.0	E980.4
56:08 antidiarrhea agents	973.5	E858.4	E943.5	E950.4	E962.0	E980.4
56:10 antiflatulents	973.8	E858.4	E943.8	E950.4	E962.0	E980.4
56:12 cathartics NEC	973.3	E858.4	E943.3	E950.4	E962.0	E980.4
emollients	973.2	E858.4	E943.2	E950.4	E962.0	E980.4
irritants	973.1	E858.4	E943.1	E950.4	E962.0	E980.4
56:16 digestants	973.4	E858.4	E943.4	E950.4	E962.0	E980.4
56:20 emetics and antiemetics						
antiemetics	963.0	E858.1	E933.0	E950.4	E962.0	E980.4
emetics	973.6	E858.4	E943.6	E950.4	E962.0	E980.4
56:24 lipotropic agents	977.1	E858.8	E947.1	E950.4	E962.0	E980.4
56:40 miscellaneous G.I. drugs	973.8	E858.4	E943.8	E950.4	E962.0	E980.4
60:00 gold compounds	965.69	E850.6	E935.6	E950.0	E962.0	E980.0
64:00 heavy metal antagonists	963.8	E858.1	E933.8	E950.4	E962.0	E980.4
68:04 adrenals	962.0	E858.0	E932.0	E950.4	E962.0	E980.4
68:08 androgens	962.1	E858.0	E932.1	E950.4	E962.0	E980.4
68:12 contraceptives, oral	962.2	E858.0	E932.2	E950.4	E962.0	E980.4
68:16 estrogens	962.2	E858.0	E932.2	E950.4	E962.0	E980.4
68:18 gonadotropins	962.4	E858.0	E932.4	E950.4	E962.0	E980.4
68:20 insulins and antidiabetic agents	962.3	E858.0	E932.3	E950.4	E962.0	E980.4
68:20.08 insulins	962.3	E858.0	E932.3	E950.4	E962.0	E980.4
68:24 parathyroid	962.6	E858.0	E932.6	E950.4	E962.0	E980.4
68:28 pituitary (posterior)	962.5	E858.0	E932.5	E950.4	E962.0	E980.4
anterior	962.4	E858.0	E932.4	E950.4	E962.0	E980.4
68:32 progestogens	962.2	E858.0	E932.2	E950.4	E962.0	E980.4
68:34 other corpus luteum						
hormones NEC	962.2	E858.0	E932.2	E950.4	E962.0	E980.4
68:36 thyroid and antithyroid						
antithyroid	962.8	E858.0	E932.8	E950.4	E962.0	E980.4
thyroid (derivatives)	962.7	E858.0	E932.7	E950.4	E962.0	E980.4
72:00 local anesthetics NEC	968.9	E855.2	E938.9	E950.4	E962.0	E980.4
topical (surface)	968.5	E855.2	E938.5	E950.4	E962.0	E980.4
infiltration (intradermal) (subcutaneous) (submucosal)	968.5	E855.2	E938.5	E950.4	E962.0	E980.4
nerve blocking (peripheral) (plexus) (regional)	968.6	E855.2	E938.6	E950.4	E962.0	E980.4
spinal	968.7	E855.2	E938.7	E950.4	E962.0	E980.4
76:00 oxytocics	975.0	E858.6	E945.0	E950.4	E962.0	E980.4
78:00 radioactive agents	990	—	—	—	—	—
80:04 serums NEC	979.9	E858.8	E949.9	E950.4	E962.0	E980.4
immune gamma globulin (human)	964.6	E858.2	E934.6	E950.4	E962.0	E980.4
80:08 toxoids NEC	978.8	E858.8	E948.8	E950.4	E962.0	E980.4
diphtheria	978.5	E858.8	E948.5	E950.4	E962.0	E980.4
and tetanus	978.9	E858.8	E948.9	E950.4	E962.0	E980.4
with pertussis component	978.6	E858.8	E948.6	E950.4	E962.0	E980.4
tetanus	978.4	E858.8	E948.4	E950.4	E962.0	E980.4
and diphtheria	978.9	E858.8	E948.9	E950.4	E962.0	E980.4
with pertussis component	978.6	E858.8	E948.6	E950.4	E962.0	E980.4
80:12 vaccines	979.9	E858.8	E949.9	E950.4	E962.0	E980.4
bacterial NEC	978.8	E858.8	E948.8	E950.4	E962.0	E980.4
with						
other bacterial components	978.9	E858.8	E948.9	E950.4	E962.0	E980.4
pertussis component	978.6	E858.8	E948.6	E950.4	E962.0	E980.4
viral and rickettsial components	979.7	E858.8	E949.7	E950.4	E962.0	E980.4
rickettsial NEC	979.6	E858.8	E949.6	E950.4	E962.0	E980.4
with						
bacterial component	979.7	E858.8	E949.7	E950.4	E962.0	E980.4
pertussis component	978.6	E858.8	E948.6	E950.4	E962.0	E980.4
viral component	979.7	E858.8	E949.7	E950.4	E962.0	E980.4
viral NEC	979.6	E858.8	E949.6	E950.4	E962.0	E980.4
with						
bacterial component	979.7	E858.8	E949.7	E950.4	E962.0	E980.4
pertussis component	978.6	E858.8	E948.6	E950.4	E962.0	E980.4
rickettsial component	979.7	E858.8	E949.7	E950.4	E962.0	E980.4
84:04.04 antibiotics (skin and mucous membrane)	976.0	E858.7	E946.0	E950.4	E962.0	E980.4
84:04.08 fungicides (skin and mucous membrane)	976.0	E858.7	E946.0	E950.4	E962.0	E980.4
84:04.12 scabicides and pediculicides (skin and mucous membrane)	976.0	E858.7	E946.0	E950.4	E962.0	E980.4

Table of Drugs and Chemicals

		External Cause (E-Code)				
	Poisoning	Accident	Therapeutic Use	Suicide Attempt	Assault	Undetermined
Drug — *continued*						
84:04.16 miscellaneous local anti-infectives (skin and mucous membrane)	976.0	E858.7	E946.0	E950.4	E962.0	E980.4
84:06 anti-inflammatory agents (skin and mucous membrane)	976.0	E858.7	E946.0	E950.4	E962.0	E980.4
84:08 antipruritics and local anesthetics						
antipruritics	976.1	E858.7	E946.1	E950.4	E962.0	E980.4
local anesthetics	968.5	E855.2	E938.5	E950.4	E962.0	E980.4
84:12 astringents	976.2	E858.7	E946.2	E950.4	E962.0	E980.4
84:16 cell stimulants and proliferants	976.8	E858.7	E946.8	E950.4	E962.0	E980.4
84:20 detergents	976.2	E858.7	E946.2	E950.4	E962.0	E980.4
84:24 emollients, demulcents, and protectants	976.3	E858.7	E946.3	E950.4	E962.0	E980.4
84:28 keratolytic agents	976.4	E858.7	E946.4	E950.4	E962.0	E980.4
84:32 keratoplastic agents	976.4	E858.7	E946.4	E950.4	E962.0	E980.4
84:36 miscellaneous agents (skin and mucous membrane)	976.8	E858.7	E946.8	E950.4	E962.0	E980.4
86:00 spasmolytic agents	975.1	E858.6	E945.1	E950.4	E962.0	E980.4
antiasthmatics	975.7	E858.6	E945.7	E950.4	E962.0	E980.4
papaverine	972.5	E858.3	E942.5	E950.4	E962.0	E980.4
theophylline	974.1	E858.5	E944.1	E950.4	E962.0	E980.4
88:04 vitamin A	963.5	E858.1	E933.5	E950.4	E962.0	E980.4
88:08 vitamin B complex	963.5	E858.1	E933.5	E950.4	E962.0	E980.4
hematopoietic vitamin	964.1	E858.2	E934.1	E950.4	E962.0	E980.4
nicotinic acid derivatives	972.2	E858.3	E942.2	E950.4	E962.0	E980.4
88:12 vitamin C	963.5	E858.1	E933.5	E950.4	E962.0	E980.4
88:16 vitamin D	963.5	E858.1	E933.5	E950.4	E962.0	E980.4
88:20 vitamin E	963.5	E858.1	E933.5	E950.4	E962.0	E980.4
88:24 vitamin K activity	964.3	E858.2	E934.3	E950.4	E962.0	E980.4
88:28 multivitamin preparations	963.5	E858.1	E933.5	E950.4	E962.0	E980.4
92:00 unclassified therapeutic agents	977.8	E858.8	E947.8	E950.4	E962.0	E980.4
Duboisine	971.1	E855.4	E941.1	E950.4	E962.0	E980.4
Dulcolax	973.1	E858.4	E943.1	E950.4	E962.0	E980.4
Duponol (C) (EP)	976.2	E858.7	E946.2	E950.4	E962.0	E980.4
Durabolin	962.1	E858.0	E932.1	E950.4	E962.0	E980.4
Dyclone	968.5	E855.2	E938.5	E950.4	E962.0	E980.4
Dyclonine	968.5	E855.2	E938.5	E950.4	E962.0	E980.4
Dydrogesterone	962.2	E858.0	E932.2	E950.4	E962.0	E980.4
Dyes NEC	989.89	E866.8	—	E950.9	E962.1	E980.9
diagnostic agents	977.8	E858.8	E947.8	E950.4	E962.0	E980.4
pharmaceutical NEC	977.4	E858.8	E947.4	E950.4	E962.0	E980.4
Dyfols	971.0	E855.3	E941.0	E950.4	E962.0	E980.4
Dymelor	962.3	E858.0	E932.3	E950.4	E962.0	E980.4
Dynamite	989.89	E866.8	—	E950.9	E962.1	E980.9
fumes	987.8	E869.8	—	E952.8	E962.2	E982.8
Dyphylline	975.1	E858.6	E945.1	E950.4	E962.0	E980.4
Ear preparations	976.6	E858.7	E946.6	E950.4	E962.0	E980.4
Echothiopate, ecothiopate	971.0	E855.3	E941.0	E950.4	E962.0	E980.4
Ectylurea	967.8	E852.8	E937.8	E950.2	E962.0	E980.2
Edathamil disodium	963.8	E858.1	E933.8	E950.4	E962.0	E980.4
Edecrin	974.4	E858.5	E944.4	E950.4	E962.0	E980.4
Edetate, disodium (calcium)	963.8	E858.1	E933.8	E950.4	E962.0	E980.4
Edrophonium	971.0	E855.3	E941.0	E950.4	E962.0	E980.4
Elase	976.8	E858.7	E946.8	E950.4	E962.0	E980.4
Elaterium	973.1	E858.4	E943.1	E950.4	E962.0	E980.4
Elder	988.2	E865.4	—	E950.9	E962.1	E980.9
berry (unripe)	988.2	E865.3	—	E950.9	E962.1	E980.9
Electrolytes NEC	974.5	E858.5	E944.5	E950.4	E962.0	E980.4
Electrolytic agent NEC	974.5	E858.5	E944.5	E950.4	E962.0	E980.4
Embramine	963.0	E858.1	E933.0	E950.4	E962.0	E980.4
Emetics	973.6	E858.4	E943.6	E950.4	E962.0	E980.4
Emetine (hydrochloride)	961.5	E857	E931.5	E950.4	E962.0	E980.4
Emollients	976.3	E858.7	E946.3	E950.4	E962.0	E980.4
Emylcamate	969.5	E853.8	E939.5	E950.3	E962.0	E980.3
Encyprate	969.0	E854.0	E939.0	E950.3	E962.0	E980.3
Endocaine	968.5	E855.2	E938.5	E950.4	E962.0	E980.4
Endrin	989.2	E863.0	—	E950.6	E962.1	E980.7
Enflurane	968.2	E855.1	E938.2	E950.4	E962.0	E980.4
Enovid	962.2	E858.0	E932.2	E950.4	E962.0	E980.4
ENT preparations (anti-infectives)	976.6	E858.7	E946.6	E950.4	E962.0	E980.4
Enzodase	963.4	E858.1	E933.4	E950.4	E962.0	E980.4
Enzymes NEC	963.4	E858.1	E933.4	E950.4	E962.0	E980.4
Epanutin	966.1	E855.0	E936.1	E950.4	E962.0	E980.4
Ephedra (tincture)	971.2	E855.5	E941.2	E950.4	E962.0	E980.4
Ephedrine	971.2	E855.5	E941.2	E950.4	E962.0	E980.4
Epiestriol	962.2	E858.0	E932.2	E950.4	E962.0	E980.4
Epilim — *see* Sodium Valproate						
Epinephrine	971.2	E855.5	E941.2	E950.4	E962.0	E980.4
Epsom salt	973.3	E858.4	E943.3	E950.4	E962.0	E980.4
Equanil	969.5	E853.8	E939.5	E950.3	E962.0	E980.3
Equisetum (diuretic)	974.4	E858.5	E944.4	E950.4	E962.0	E980.4
Ergometrine	975.0	E858.6	E945.0	E950.4	E962.0	E980.4
Ergonovine	975.0	E858.6	E945.0	E950.4	E962.0	E980.4

Table of Drugs and Chemicals

	Poisoning	External Cause (E-Code)				
		Accident	Therapeutic Use	Suicide Attempt	Assault	Undetermined
Ergot NEC	988.2	E865.4	—	E950.9	E962.1	E980.9
medicinal (alkaloids)	975.0	E858.6	E945.0	E950.4	E962.0	E980.4
Ergotamine (tartrate) (for migraine) NEC	972.9	E858.3	E942.9	E950.4	E962.0	E980.4
Ergotrate	975.0	E858.6	E945.0	E950.4	E962.0	E980.4
Erythrityl tetranitrate	972.4	E858.3	E942.4	E950.4	E962.0	E980.4
Erythrol tetranitrate	972.4	E858.3	E942.4	E950.4	E962.0	E980.4
Erythromycin	960.3	E856	E930.3	E950.4	E962.0	E980.4
ophthalmic preparation	976.5	E858.7	E946.5	E950.4	E962.0	E980.4
topical NEC	976.0	E858.7	E946.0	E950.4	E962.0	E980.4
Eserine	971.0	E855.3	E941.0	E950.4	E962.0	E980.4
Eskabarb	967.0	E851	E937.0	E950.1	E962.0	E980.1
Eskalith	969.8	E855.8	E939.8	E950.3	E962.0	E980.3
Estradiol (cypionate) (dipropionate) (valerate)	962.2	E858.0	E932.2	E950.4	E962.0	E980.4
Estriol	962.2	E858.0	E932.2	E950.4	E962.0	E980.4
Estrogens (with progestogens)	962.2	E858.0	E932.2	E950.4	E962.0	E980.4
Estrone	962.2	E858.0	E932.2	E950.4	E962.0	E980.4
Etafedrine	971.2	E855.5	E941.2	E950.4	E962.0	E980.4
Ethacrynate sodium	974.4	E858.5	E944.4	E950.4	E962.0	E980.4
Ethacrynic acid	974.4	E858.5	E944.4	E950.4	E962.0	E980.4
Ethambutol	961.8	E857	E931.8	E950.4	E962.0	E980.4
Ethamide	974.2	E858.5	E944.2	E950.4	E962.0	E980.4
Ethamivan	970.0	E854.3	E940.0	E950.4	E962.0	E980.4
Ethamsylate	964.5	E858.2	E934.5	E950.4	E962.0	E980.4
Ethanol	980.0	E860.1	—	E950.9	E962.1	E980.9
beverage	980.0	E860.0	—	E950.9	E962.1	E980.9
Ethchlorvynol	967.8	E852.8	E937.8	E950.2	E962.0	E980.2
Ethebenecid	974.7	E858.5	E944.7	E950.4	E962.0	E980.4
Ether(s) (diethyl) (ethyl) (vapor)	987.8	E869.8	—	E952.8	E962.2	E982.8
anesthetic	968.2	E855.1	E938.2	E950.4	E962.0	E980.4
petroleum — see Ligroin						
solvent	982.8	E862.4	—	E950.9	E962.1	E980.9
Ethidine chloride (vapor)	987.8	E869.8	—	E952.8	E962.2	E982.8
liquid (solvent)	982.3	E862.4	—	E950.9	E962.1	E980.9
Ethinamate	967.8	E852.8	E937.8	E950.2	E962.0	E980.2
Ethinylestradiol	962.2	E858.0	E932.2	E950.4	E962.0	E980.4
Ethionamide	961.8	E857	E931.8	E950.4	E962.0	E980.4
Ethisterone	962.2	E858.0	E932.2	E950.4	E962.0	E980.4
Ethobral	967.0	E851	E937.0	E950.1	E962.0	E980.1
Ethocaine (infiltration) (topical)	968.5	E855.2	E938.5	E950.4	E962.0	E980.4
nerve block (peripheral) (plexus)	968.6	E855.2	E938.6	E950.4	E962.0	E980.4
spinal	968.7	E855.2	E938.7	E950.4	E962.0	E980.4
Ethoheptazine (citrate)	965.7	E850.7	E935.7	E950.0	E962.0	E980.0
Ethopropazine	966.4	E855.0	E936.4	E950.4	E962.0	E980.4
Ethosuximide	966.2	E855.0	E936.2	E950.4	E962.0	E980.4
Ethotoin	966.1	E855.0	E936.1	E950.4	E962.0	E980.4
Ethoxazene	961.9	E857	E931.9	E950.4	E962.0	E980.4
Ethoxzolamide	974.2	E858.5	E944.2	E950.4	E962.0	E980.4
Ethyl						
acetate (vapor)	982.8	E862.4	—	E950.9	E962.1	E980.9
alcohol	980.0	E860.1	—	E950.9	E962.1	E980.9
beverage	980.0	E860.0	—	E950.9	E962.1	E980.9
aldehyde (vapor)	987.8	E869.8	—	E952.8	E962.2	E982.8
liquid	989.89	E866.8	—	E950.9	E962.1	E980.9
aminobenzoate	968.5	E855.2	E938.5	E950.4	E962.0	E980.4
biscoumacetate	964.2	E858.2	E934.2	E950.4	E962.0	E980.4
bromide (anesthetic)	968.2	E855.1	E938.2	E950.4	E962.0	E980.4
carbamate (antineoplastic)	963.1	E858.1	E933.1	E950.4	E962.0	E980.4
carbinol	980.3	E860.4	—	E950.9	E962.1	E980.9
chaulmoograte	961.8	E857	E931.8	E950.4	E962.0	E980.4
chloride (vapor)	987.8	E869.8	—	E952.8	E962.2	E982.8
anesthetic (local)	968.5	E855.2	E938.5	E950.4	E962.0	E980.4
inhaled	968.2	E855.1	E938.2	E950.4	E962.0	E980.4
solvent	982.3	E862.4	—	E950.9	E962.1	E980.9
estranol	962.1	E858.0	E932.1	E950.4	E962.0	E980.4
ether — see Ether(s)						
formate (solvent) NEC	982.8	E862.4	—	E950.9	E962.1	E980.9
iodoacetate	987.5	E869.3	—	E952.8	E962.2	E982.8
lactate (solvent) NEC	982.8	E862.4	—	E950.9	E962.1	E980.9
methylcarbinol	980.8	E860.8	—	E950.9	E962.1	E980.9
morphine	965.09	E850.2	E935.2	E950.0	E962.0	E980.0
Ethylene (gas)	987.1	E869.8	—	E952.8	E962.2	E982.8
anesthetic (general)	968.2	E855.1	E938.2	E950.4	E962.0	E980.4
chlorohydrin (vapor)	982.3	E862.4	—	E950.9	E962.1	E980.9
dichloride (vapor)	982.3	E862.4	—	E950.9	E962.1	E980.9
glycol(s) (any) (vapor)	982.8	E862.4	—	E950.9	E962.1	E980.9
Ethylidene						
chloride NEC	982.3	E862.4	—	E950.9	E962.1	E980.9
diethyl ether	982.8	E862.4	—	E950.9	E962.1	E980.9
Ethynodiol	962.2	E858.0	E932.2	E950.4	E962.0	E980.4
Etidocaine	968.9	E855.2	E938.9	E950.4	E962.0	E980.4
infiltration (subcutaneous)	968.5	E855.2	E938.5	E950.4	E962.0	E980.4

Table of Drugs and Chemicals

	Poisoning	External Cause (E-Code)				
		Accident	Therapeutic Use	Suicide Attempt	Assault	Undetermined
Etidocaine — *continued*						
nerve (peripheral) (plexus)	968.6	E855.2	E938.6	E950.4	E962.0	E980.4
Etilfen	967.0	E851	E937.0	E950.1	E962.0	E980.1
Etomide	965.7	E850.7	E935.7	E950.0	E962.0	E980.0
Etorphine	965.09	E850.2	E935.2	E950.0	E962.0	E980.0
Etoval	967.0	E851	E937.0	E950.1	E962.0	E980.1
Etryptamine	969.0	E854.0	E939.0	E950.3	E962.0	E980.3
Eucaine	968.5	E855.2	E938.5	E950.4	E962.0	E980.4
Eucalyptus (oil) NEC	975.5	E858.6	E945.5	E950.4	E962.0	E980.4
Eucatropine	971.1	E855.4	E941.1	E950.4	E962.0	E980.4
Eucodal	965.09	E850.2	E935.2	E950.0	E962.0	E980.0
Euneryl	967.0	E851	E937.0	E950.1	E962.0	E980.1
Euphthalmine	971.1	E855.4	E941.1	E950.4	E962.0	E980.4
Eurax	976.0	E858.7	E946.0	E950.4	E962.0	E980.4
Euresol	976.4	E858.7	E946.4	E950.4	E962.0	E980.4
Euthroid	962.7	E858.0	E932.7	E950.4	E962.0	E980.4
Evans blue	977.8	E858.8	E947.8	E950.4	E962.0	E980.4
Evipal	967.0	E851	E937.0	E950.1	E962.0	E980.1
sodium	968.3	E855.1	E938.3	E950.4	E962.0	E980.4
Evipan	967.0	E851	E937.0	E950.1	E962.0	E980.1
sodium	968.3	E855.1	E938.3	E950.4	E962.0	E980.4
Exalgin	965.4	E850.4	E935.4	E950.0	E962.0	E980.0
Excipients, pharmaceutical	977.4	E858.8	E947.4	E950.4	E962.0	E980.4
Exhaust gas — *see* Carbon, monoxide						
Ex-Lax (phenolphthalein)	973.1	E858.4	E943.1	E950.4	E962.0	E980.4
Expectorants	975.5	E858.6	E945.5	E950.4	E962.0	E980.4
External medications (skin) (mucous membrane)	976.9	E858.7	E946.9	E950.4	E962.0	E980.4
dental agent	976.7	E858.7	E946.7	E950.4	E962.0	E980.4
ENT agent	976.6	E858.7	E946.6	E950.4	E962.0	E980.4
ophthalmic preparation	976.5	E858.7	E946.5	E950.4	E962.0	E980.4
specified NEC	976.8	E858.7	E946.8	E950.4	E962.0	E980.4
Eye agents (anti-infective)	976.5	E858.7	E946.5	E950.4	E962.0	E980.4
Factor IX complex (human)	964.5	E858.2	E934.5	E950.4	E962.0	E980.4
Fecal softeners	973.2	E858.4	E943.2	E950.4	E962.0	E980.4
Fenbutrazate	977.0	E858.8	E947.0	E950.4	E962.0	E980.4
Fencamfamin	970.8	E854.3	E940.8	E950.4	E962.0	E980.4
Fenfluramine	977.0	E858.8	E947.0	E950.4	E962.0	E980.4
Fenoprofen	965.61	E850.6	E935.6	E950.0	E962.0	E980.0
Fentanyl	965.09	E850.2	E935.2	E950.0	E962.0	E980.0
Fentazin	969.1	E853.0	E939.1	E950.3	E962.0	E980.3
Fenticlor, fentichlor	976.0	E858.7	E946.0	E950.4	E962.0	E980.4
Fer de lance (bite) (venom)	989.5	E905.0	—	E950.9	E962.1	E980.9
Ferric — *see* Iron						
Ferrocholinate	964.0	E858.2	E934.0	E950.4	E962.0	E980.4
Ferrous fumerate, gluconate, lactate, salt NEC, sulfate (medicinal)	964.0	E858.2	E934.0	E950.4	E962.0	E980.4
Ferrum — *see* Iron						
Fertilizers NEC	989.89	E866.5	—	E950.9	E962.1	E980.4
with herbicide mixture	989.4	E863.5	—	E950.6	E962.1	E980.7
Fibrinogen (human)	964.7	E858.2	E934.7	E950.4	E962.0	E980.4
Fibrinolysin	964.4	E858.2	E934.4	E950.4	E962.0	E980.4
Fibrinolysis-affecting agents	964.4	E858.2	E934.4	E950.4	E962.0	E980.4
Filix mas	961.6	E857	E931.6	E950.4	E962.0	E980.4
Fiorinal	965.1	E850.3	E935.3	E950.0	E962.0	E980.0
Fire damp	987.1	E869.8	—	E952.8	E962.2	E982.8
Fish, nonbacterial or noxious	988.0	E865.2	—	E950.9	E962.1	E980.9
shell	988.0	E865.1	—	E950.9	E962.1	E980.9
Flagyl	961.5	E857	E931.5	E950.4	E962.0	E980.4
Flavoxate	975.1	E858.6	E945.1	E950.4	E962.0	E980.4
Flaxedil	975.2	E858.6	E945.2	E950.4	E962.0	E980.4
Flaxseed (medicinal)	976.3	E858.7	E946.3	E950.4	E962.0	E980.4
Florantyrone	973.4	E858.4	E943.4	E950.4	E962.0	E980.4
Floraquin	961.3	E857	E931.3	E950.4	E962.0	E980.4
Florinef	962.0	E858.0	E932.0	E950.4	E962.0	E980.4
ENT agent	976.6	E858.7	E946.6	E950.4	E962.0	E980.4
ophthalmic preparation	976.5	E858.7	E946.5	E950.4	E962.0	E980.4
topical NEC	976.0	E858.7	E946.0	E950.4	E962.0	E980.4
Flowers of sulfur	976.4	E858.7	E946.4	E950.4	E962.0	E980.4
Floxuridine	963.1	E858.1	E933.1	E950.4	E962.0	E980.4
Flucytosine	961.9	E857	E931.9	E950.4	E962.0	E980.4
Fludrocortisone	962.0	E858.0	E932.0	E950.4	E962.0	E980.4
ENT agent	976.6	E858.7	E946.6	E950.4	E962.0	E980.4
ophthalmic preparation	976.5	E858.7	E946.5	E950.4	E962.0	E980.4
topical NEC	976.0	E858.7	E946.0	E950.4	E962.0	E980.4
Flumethasone	976.0	E858.7	E946.0	E950.4	E962.0	E980.4
Flumethiazide	974.3	E858.5	E944.3	E950.4	E962.0	E980.4
Flumidin	961.7	E857	E931.7	E950.4	E962.0	E980.4
Flunitrazepam	969.4	E853.2	E939.4	E950.3	E962.0	E980.3 ▲
Fluocinolone	976.0	E858.7	E946.0	E950.4	E962.0	E980.4
Fluocortolone	962.0	E858.0	E932.0	E950.4	E962.0	E980.4
Fluohydrocortisone	962.0	E858.0	E932.0	E950.4	E962.0	E980.4
ENT agent	976.6	E858.7	E946.6	E950.4	E962.0	E980.4

Table of Drugs and Chemicals

		External Cause (E-Code)				
	Poisoning	Accident	Therapeutic Use	Suicide Attempt	Assault	Undetermined
Fluohydrocortisone — *continued*						
ophthalmic preparation	976.5	E858.7	E946.5	E950.4	E962.0	E980.4
topical NEC	976.0	E858.7	E946.0	E950.4	E962.0	E980.4
Fluonid	976.0	E858.7	E946.0	E950.4	E962.0	E980.4
Fluopromazine	969.1	E853.0	E939.1	E950.3	E962.0	E980.3
Fluoracetate	989.4	E863.7	—	E950.6	E962.1	E980.7
Fluorescein (sodium)	977.8	E858.8	E947.8	E950.4	E962.0	E980.4
Fluoride(s) (pesticides) (sodium) NEC	989.4	E863.4	—	E950.6	E962.1	E980.7
hydrogen — *see* Hydrofluoric acid						
medicinal	976.7	E858.7	E946.7	E950.4	E962.0	E980.4
not pesticide NEC	983.9	E864.4	—	E950.7	E962.1	E980.6
stannous	976.7	E858.7	E946.7	E950.4	E962.0	E980.4
Fluorinated corticosteroids	962.0	E858.0	E932.0	E950.4	E962.0	E980.4
Fluorine (compounds) (gas)	987.8	E869.8	—	E952.8	E962.2	E982.8
salt — *see* Fluoride(s)						
Fluoristan	976.7	E858.7	E946.7	E950.4	E962.0	E980.4
Fluoroacetate	989.4	E863.7	—	E950.6	E962.1	E980.7
Fluorodeoxyuridine	963.1	E858.1	E933.1	E950.4	E962.0	E980.4
Fluorometholone (topical) NEC	976.0	E858.7	E946.0	E950.4	E962.0	E980.4
ophthalmic preparation	976.5	E858.7	E946.5	E950.4	E962.0	E980.4
Fluorouracil	963.1	E858.1	E933.1	E950.4	E962.0	E980.4
Fluothane	968.1	E855.1	E938.1	E950.4	E962.0	E980.4
Fluoxetine hydrochloride	969.0	E854.0	E939.0	E950.3	E962.0	E980.3
Fluoxymesterone	962.1	E858.0	E932.1	E950.4	E962.0	E980.4
Fluphenazine	969.1	E853.0	E939.1	E950.3	E962.0	E980.3
Fluprednisolone	962.0	E858.0	E932.0	E950.4	E962.0	E980.4
Flurandrenolide	976.0	E858.7	E946.0	E950.4	E962.0	E980.4
Flurazepam (hydrochloride)	969.4	E853.2	E939.4	E950.3	E962.0	E980.3
Flurbiprofen	965.61	E850.6	E935.6	E950.0	E962.0	E980.0
Flurobate	976.0	E858.7	E946.0	E950.4	E962.0	E980.4
Flurothyl	969.8	E855.8	E939.8	E950.3	E962.0	E980.3
Fluroxene	968.2	E855.1	E938.2	E950.4	E962.0	E980.4
Folacin	964.1	E858.2	E934.1	E950.4	E962.0	E980.4
Folic acid	964.1	E858.2	E934.1	E950.4	E962.0	E980.4
Follicle stimulating hormone	962.4	E858.0	E932.4	E950.4	E962.0	E980.4
Food, foodstuffs, nonbacterial or noxious	988.9	E865.9	—	E950.9	E962.1	E980.9
berries, seeds	988.2	E865.3	—	E950.9	E962.1	E980.9
fish	988.0	E865.2	—	E950.9	E962.1	E980.9
mushrooms	988.1	E865.5	—	E950.9	E962.1	E980.9
plants	988.2	E865.9	—	E950.9	E962.1	E980.9
specified type NEC	988.2	E865.4	—	E950.9	E962.1	E980.9
shellfish	988.0	E865.1	—	E950.9	E962.1	E980.9
specified NEC	988.8	E865.8	—	E950.9	E962.1	E980.9
Fool's parsley	988.2	E865.4	—	E950.9	E962.1	E980.9
Formaldehyde (solution)	989.89	E861.4	—	E950.9	E962.1	E980.9
fungicide	989.4	E863.6	—	E950.6	E962.1	E980.7
gas or vapor	987.8	E869.8	—	E952.8	E962.2	E982.8
Formalin	989.89	E861.4	—	E950.9	E962.1	E980.9
fungicide	989.4	E863.6	—	E950.6	E962.1	E980.7
vapor	987.8	E869.8	—	E952.8	E962.2	E982.8
Formic acid	983.1	E864.1	—	E950.7	E962.1	E980.6
vapor	987.8	E869.8	—	E952.8	E962.2	E982.8
Fowler's solution	985.1	E866.3	—	E950.8	E962.1	E980.8
Foxglove	988.2	E865.4	—	E950.9	E962.1	E980.9
Fox green	977.8	E858.8	E947.8	E950.4	E962.0	E980.4
Framycetin	960.8	E856	E930.8	E950.4	E962.0	E980.4
Frangula (extract)	973.1	E858.4	E943.1	E950.4	E962.0	E980.4
Frei antigen	977.8	E858.8	E947.8	E950.4	E962.0	E980.4
Freons	987.4	E869.2	—	E952.8	E962.2	E982.8
Fructose	974.5	E858.5	E944.5	E950.4	E962.0	E980.4
Frusemide	974.4	E858.5	E944.4	E950.4	E962.0	E980.4
FSH	962.4	E858.0	E932.4	E950.4	E962.0	E980.4
Fuel						
automobile	981	E862.1	—	E950.9	E962.1	E980.9
exhaust gas, not in transit	986	E868.2	—	E952.0	E962.2	E982.0
vapor NEC	987.1	E869.8	—	E952.8	E962.2	E982.8
gas (domestic use) — *see also* Carbon, monoxide, fuel						
utility	987.1	E868.1	—	E951.8	E962.2	E981.8
incomplete combustion of — *see* Carbon, monoxide, fuel, utility						
in mobile container	987.0	E868.0	—	E951.1	E962.2	E981.1
piped (natural)	987.1	E867	—	E951.0	E962.2	E981.0
industrial, incomplete combustion	986	E868.3	—	E952.1	E962.2	E982.1
Fugillin	960.8	E856	E930.8	E950.4	E962.0	E980.4
Fulminate of mercury	985.0	E866.1	—	E950.9	E962.1	E980.9
Fulvicin	960.1	E856	E930.1	E950.4	E962.0	E980.4
Fumadil	960.8	E856	E930.8	E950.4	E962.0	E980.4
Fumagillin	960.8	E856	E930.8	E950.4	E962.0	E980.4
Fumes (from)	987.9	E869.9	—	E952.9	E962.2	E982.9
carbon monoxide — *see* Carbon, monoxide						
charcoal (domestic use)	986	E868.3	—	E952.1	E962.2	E982.1

Fumes

Table of Drugs and Chemicals

	Poisoning	External Cause (E-Code)				
		Accident	Therapeutic Use	Suicide Attempt	Assault	Undetermined
Fumes — continued						
chloroform — see Chloroform						
coke (in domestic stoves, fireplaces)	986	E868.3	—	E952.1	E962.2	E982.1
corrosive NEC	987.8	E869.8	—	E952.8	E962.2	E982.8
ether — see Ether(s)						
freons	987.4	E869.2	—	E952.8	E962.2	E982.8
hydrocarbons	987.1	E869.8	—	E952.8	E962.2	E982.8
petroleum (liquefied)	987.0	E868.0	—	E951.1	E962.2	E981.1
distributed through pipes (pure or mixed with air)	987.0	E867	—	E951.0	E962.2	E981.0
lead — see Lead						
metals — see specified metal						
nitrogen dioxide	987.2	E869.0	—	E952.8	E962.2	E982.8
pesticides — see Pesticides						
petroleum (liquefied)	987.0	E868.0	—	E951.1	E962.2	E981.1
distributed through pipes (pure or mixed with air)	987.0	E867	—	E951.0	E962.2	E981.0
polyester	987.8	E869.8	—	E952.8	E962.2	E982.8
specified source other (see also substance specified)	987.8	E869.8	—	E952.8	E962.2	E982.8
sulfur dioxide	987.3	E869.1	—	E952.8	E962.2	E982.8
Fumigants	989.4	E863.8	—	E950.6	E962.1	E980.7
Fungi, noxious, used as food	988.1	E865.5	—	E950.9	E962.1	E980.9
Fungicides (see also Antifungals)	989.4	E863.6	—	E950.6	E962.1	E980.7
Fungizone	960.1	E856	E930.1	E950.4	E962.0	E980.4
topical	976.0	E858.7	E946.0	E950.4	E962.0	E980.4
Furacin	976.0	E858.7	E946.0	E950.4	E962.0	E980.4
Furadantin	961.9	E857	E931.9	E950.4	E962.0	E980.4
Furazolidone	961.9	E857	E931.9	E950.4	E962.0	E980.4
Furnace (coal burning) (domestic), gas from	986	E868.3	—	E952.1	E962.2	E982.1
industrial	986	E868.8	—	E952.1	E962.2	E982.1
Furniture polish	989.89	E861.2	—	E950.9	E962.1	E980.9
Furosemide	974.4	E858.5	E944.4	E950.4	E962.0	E980.4
Furoxone	961.9	E857	E931.9	E950.4	E962.0	E980.4
Fusel oil (amyl) (butyl) (propyl)	980.3	E860.4	—	E950.9	E962.1	E980.9
Fusidic acid	960.8	E856	E930.8	E950.4	E962.0	E980.4
Gallamine	975.2	E858.6	E945.2	E950.4	E962.0	E980.4
Gallotannic acid	976.2	E858.7	E946.2	E950.4	E962.0	E980.4
Gamboge	973.1	E858.4	E943.1	E950.4	E962.0	E980.4
Gamimune	964.6	E858.2	E934.6	E950.4	E962.0	E980.4
Gamma-benzene hexachloride (vapor)	989.2	E863.0	—	E950.6	E962.1	E980.7
Gamma globulin	964.6	E858.2	E934.6	E950.4	E962.0	E980.4
Gamma Hydroxy Butyrate (GHB)	968.4	E855.1	E938.4	E950.4	E962.0	E980.4
Gamulin	964.6	E858.2	E934.6	E950.4	E962.0	E980.4
Ganglionic blocking agents	972.3	E858.3	E942.3	E950.4	E962.0	E980.4
Ganja	969.6	E854.1	E939.6	E950.3	E962.0	E980.3
Garamycin	960.8	E856	E930.8	E950.4	E962.0	E980.4
ophthalmic preparation	976.5	E858.7	E946.5	E950.4	E962.0	E980.4
topical NEC	976.0	E858.7	E946.0	E950.4	E962.0	E980.4
Gardenal	967.0	E851	E937.0	E950.1	E962.0	E980.1
Gardepanyl	967.0	E851	E937.0	E950.1	E962.0	E980.1
Gas	987.9	E869.9	—	E952.9	E962.2	E982.9
acetylene	987.1	E868.1	—	E951.8	E962.2	E981.8
incomplete combustion of — see Carbon, monoxide, fuel, utility						
air contaminants, source or type not specified	987.9	E869.9	—	E952.9	E962.2	E982.9
anesthetic (general) NEC	968.2	E855.1	E938.2	E950.4	E962.0	E980.4
blast furnace	986	E868.8	—	E952.1	E962.2	E982.1
butane — see Butane						
carbon monoxide — see Carbon, monoxide						
chlorine	987.6	E869.8	—	E952.8	E962.2	E982.8
coal — see Carbon, monoxide, coal						
cyanide	987.7	E869.8	—	E952.8	E962.2	E982.8
dicyanogen	987.8	E869.8	—	E952.8	E962.2	E982.8
domestic — see Gas, utility						
exhaust — see Carbon, monoxide, exhaust gas						
from wood- or coal-burning stove or fireplace	986	E868.3	—	E952.1	E962.2	E982.1
fuel (domestic use) — see also Carbon, monoxide, fuel						
industrial use	986	E868.8	—	E952.1	E962.2	E982.1
utility	987.1	E868.1	—	E951.8	E962.2	E981.8
incomplete combustion of — see Carbon, monoxide, fuel, utility						
in mobile container	987.0	E868.0	—	E951.1	E962.2	E981.1
piped (natural)	987.1	E867	—	E951.0	E962.2	E981.0
garage	986	E868.2	—	E952.0	E962.2	E982.0
hydrocarbon NEC	987.1	E869.8	—	E952.8	E962.2	E982.8
incomplete combustion of — see Carbon, monoxide, fuel, utility						
liquefied (mobile container)	987.0	E868.0	—	E951.1	E962.2	E981.1
piped	987.0	E867	—	E951.0	E962.2	E981.0
hydrocyanic acid	987.7	E869.8	—	E952.8	E962.2	E982.8
illuminating — see Gas, utility						
incomplete combustion, any — see Carbon, monoxide						
kiln	986	E868.8	—	E952.1	E962.2	E982.1
lacrimogenic	987.5	E869.3	—	E952.8	E962.2	E982.8
marsh	987.1	E869.8	—	E952.8	E962.2	E982.8

Table of Drugs and Chemicals

		External Cause (E-Code)				
	Poisoning	Accident	Therapeutic Use	Suicide Attempt	Assault	Undetermined
Gas — *continued*						
motor exhaust, not in transit	986	E868.8	—	E952.1	E962.2	E982.1
mustard — *see* Mustard, gas						
natural	987.1	E867	—	E951.0	E962.2	E981.0
nerve (war)	987.9	E869.9	—	E952.9	E962.2	E982.9
oils	981	E862.1	—	E950.9	E962.1	E980.9
petroleum (liquefied) (distributed in mobile containers)	987.0	E868.0	—	E951.1	E962.2	E981.1
piped (pure or mixed with air)	987.0	E867	—	E951.1	E962.2	E981.1
piped (manufactured) (natural) NEC	987.1	E867	—	E951.0	E962.2	E981.0
producer	986	E868.8	—	E952.1	E962.2	E982.1
propane — *see* Propane						
refrigerant (freon)	987.4	E869.2	—	E952.8	E962.2	E982.8
not freon	987.9	E869.9	—	E952.9	E962.2	E982.9
sewer	987.8	E869.8	—	E952.8	E962.2	E982.8
specified source NEC (*see also* substance specified)	987.8	E869.8	—	E952.8	E962.2	E982.8
stove — *see* Gas, utility						
tear	987.5	E869.3	—	E952.8	E962.2	E982.8
utility (for cooking, heating, or lighting) (piped) NEC	987.1	E868.1	—	E951.8	E962.2	E981.8
incomplete combustion of — *see* Carbon, monoxide, fuel, utilty						
in mobile container	987.0	E868.0	—	E951.1	E962.2	E981.1
piped (natural)	987.1	E867	—	E951.0	E962.2	E981.0
water	987.1	E868.1	—	E951.8	E962.2	E981.8
incomplete combustion of — *see* Carbon, monoxide, fuel, utility						
Gaseous substance — *see* Gas						
Gasoline, gasolene	981	E862.1	—	E950.9	E962.1	E980.9
vapor	987.1	E869.8	—	E952.8	E962.2	E982.8
Gastric enzymes	973.4	E858.4	E943.4	E950.4	E962.0	E980.4
Gastrografin	977.8	E858.8	E947.8	E950.4	E962.0	E980.4
Gastrointestinal agents	973.9	E858.4	E943.9	E950.4	E962.0	E980.4
specified NEC	973.8	E858.4	E943.8	E950.4	E962.0	E980.4
Gaultheria procumbens	988.2	E865.4	—	E950.9	E962.1	E980.9
Gelatin (intravenous)	964.8	E858.2	E934.8	E950.4	E962.0	E980.4
absorbable (sponge)	964.5	E858.2	E934.5	E950.4	E962.0	E980.4
Gelfilm	976.8	E858.7	E946.8	E950.4	E962.0	E980.4
Gelfoam	964.5	E858.2	E934.5	E950.4	E962.0	E980.4
Gelsemine	970.8	E854.3	E940.8	E950.4	E962.0	E980.4
Gelsemium (sempervirens)	988.2	E865.4	—	E950.9	E962.1	E980.9
Gemonil	967.0	E851	E937.0	E950.1	E962.0	E980.1
Gentamicin	960.8	E856	E930.8	E950.4	E962.0	E980.4
ophthalmic preparation	976.5	E858.7	E946.5	E950.4	E962.0	E980.4
topical NEC	976.0	E858.7	E946.0	E950.4	E962.0	E980.4
Gentian violet	976.0	E858.7	E946.0	E950.4	E962.0	E980.4
Gexane	976.0	E858.7	E946.0	E950.4	E962.0	E980.4
Gila monster (venom)	989.5	E905.0	—	E950.9	E962.1	E980.9
Ginger, Jamaica	989.89	E866.8	—	E950.9	E962.1	E980.9
Gitalin	972.1	E858.3	E942.1	E950.4	E962.0	E980.4
Gitoxin	972.1	E858.3	E942.1	E950.4	E962.0	E980.4
Glandular extract (medicinal) NEC	977.9	E858.9	E947.9	E950.5	E962.0	E980.5
Glaucarubin	961.5	E857	E931.5	E950.4	E962.0	E980.4
Globin zinc insulin	962.3	E858.0	E932.3	E950.4	E962.0	E980.4
Glucagon	962.3	E858.0	E932.3	E950.4	E962.0	E980.4
Glucochloral	967.1	E852.0	E937.1	E950.2	E962.0	E980.2
Glucocorticoids	962.0	E858.0	E932.0	E950.4	E962.0	E980.4
Glucose	974.5	E858.5	E944.5	E950.4	E962.0	E980.4
oxidase reagent	977.8	E858.8	E947.8	E950.4	E962.0	E980.4
Glucosulfone sodium	961.8	E857	E931.8	E950.4	E962.0	E980.4
Glue(s)	989.89	E866.6	—	E950.9	E962.1	E980.9
Glutamic acid (hydrochloride)	973.4	E858.4	E943.4	E950.4	E962.0	E980.4
Glutathione	963.8	E858.1	E933.8	E950.4	E962.0	E980.4
Glutethimide (group)	967.5	E852.4	E937.5	E950.2	E962.0	E980.2
Glycerin (lotion)	976.3	E858.7	E946.3	E950.4	E962.0	E980.4
Glycerol (topical)	976.3	E858.7	E946.3	E950.4	E962.0	E980.4
Glyceryl						
guaiacolate	975.5	E858.6	E945.5	E950.4	E962.0	E980.4
triacetate (topical)	976.0	E858.7	E946.0	E950.4	E962.0	E980.4
trinitrate	972.4	E858.3	E942.4	E950.4	E962.0	E980.4
Glycine	974.5	E858.5	E944.5	E950.4	E962.0	E980.4
Glycobiarsol	961.1	E857	E931.1	E950.4	E962.0	E980.4
Glycols (ether)	982.8	E862.4	—	E950.9	E962.1	E980.9
Glycopyrrolate	971.1	E855.4	E941.1	E950.4	E962.0	E980.4
Glymidine	962.3	E858.0	E932.3	E950.4	E962.0	E980.4
Gold (compounds) (salts)	965.69	E850.6	E935.6	E950.0	E962.0	E980.0
Golden sulfide of antimony	985.4	E866.2	—	E950.9	E962.1	E980.9
Goldylocks	988.2	E865.4	—	E950.9	E962.1	E980.9
Gonadal tissue extract	962.9	E858.0	E932.9	E950.4	E962.0	E980.4
female	962.2	E858.0	E932.2	E950.4	E962.0	E980.4
male	962.1	E858.0	E932.1	E950.4	E962.0	E980.4
Gonadotropin	962.4	E858.0	E932.4	E950.4	E962.0	E980.4
Grain alcohol	980.0	E860.1	—	E950.9	E962.1	E980.9
beverage	980.0	E860.0	—	E950.9	E962.1	E980.9
Gramicidin	960.8	E856	E930.8	E950.4	E962.0	E980.4

Table of Drugs and Chemicals

Gratiola officinalis — Homatropine

		External Cause (E-Code)				
	Poisoning	Accident	Therapeutic Use	Suicide Attempt	Assault	Undetermined
Gratiola officinalis	988.2	E865.4	—	E950.9	E962.1	E980.9
Grease	989.89	E866.8	—	E950.9	E962.1	E980.9
Green hellebore	988.2	E865.4	—	E950.9	E962.1	E980.9
Green soap	976.2	E858.7	E946.2	E950.4	E962.0	E980.4
Grifulvin	960.1	E856	E930.1	E950.4	E962.0	E980.4
Griseofulvin	960.1	E856	E930.1	E950.4	E962.0	E980.4
Growth hormone	962.4	E858.0	E932.4	E950.4	E962.0	E980.4
Guaiacol	975.5	E858.6	E945.5	E950.4	E962.0	E980.4
Guaiac reagent	977.8	E858.8	E947.8	E950.4	E962.0	E980.4
Guaifenesin	975.5	E858.6	E945.5	E950.4	E962.0	E980.4
Guaiphenesin	975.5	E858.6	E945.5	E950.4	E962.0	E980.4
Guanatol	961.4	E857	E931.4	E950.4	E962.0	E980.4
Guanethidine	972.6	E858.3	E942.6	E950.4	E962.0	E980.4
Guano	989.89	E866.5	—	E950.9	E962.1	E980.9
Guanochlor	972.6	E858.3	E942.6	E950.4	E962.0	E980.4
Guanoctine	972.6	E858.3	E942.6	E950.4	E962.0	E980.4
Guanoxan	972.6	E858.3	E942.6	E950.4	E962.0	E980.4
Hair treatment agent NEC	976.4	E858.7	E946.4	E950.4	E962.0	E980.4
Halcinonide	976.0	E858.7	E946.0	E950.4	E962.0	E980.4
Halethazole	976.0	E858.7	E946.0	E950.4	E962.0	E980.4
Hallucinogens	969.6	E854.1	E939.6	E950.3	E962.0	E980.3
Haloperidol	969.2	E853.1	E939.2	E950.3	E962.0	E980.3
Haloprogin	976.0	E858.7	E946.0	E950.4	E962.0	E980.4
Halotex	976.0	E858.7	E946.0	E950.4	E962.0	E980.4
Halothane	968.1	E855.1	E938.1	E950.4	E962.0	E980.4
Halquinols	976.0	E858.7	E946.0	E950.4	E962.0	E980.4
Harmonyl	972.6	E858.3	E942.6	E950.4	E962.0	E980.4
Hartmann's solution	974.5	E858.5	E944.5	E950.4	E962.0	E980.4
Hashish	969.6	E854.1	E939.6	E950.3	E962.0	E980.3
Hawaiian wood rose seeds	969.6	E854.1	E939.6	E950.3	E962.0	E980.3
Headache cures, drugs, powders NEC	977.9	E858.9	E947.9	E950.5	E962.0	E980.9
Heavenly Blue (morning glory)	969.6	E854.1	E939.6	E950.3	E962.0	E980.3
Heavy metal antagonists	963.8	E858.1	E933.8	E950.4	E962.0	E980.4
anti-infectives	961.2	E857	E931.2	E950.4	E962.0	E980.4
Hedaquinium	976.0	E858.7	E946.0	E950.4	E962.0	E980.4
Hedge hyssop	988.2	E865.4	—	E950.9	E962.1	E980.9
Heet	976.8	E858.7	E946.8	E950.4	E962.0	E980.4
Helenin	961.6	E857	E931.6	E950.4	E962.0	E980.4
Hellebore (black) (green) (white)	988.2	E865.4	—	E950.9	E962.1	E980.9
Hemlock	988.2	E865.4	—	E950.9	E962.1	E980.9
Hemostatics	964.5	E858.2	E934.5	E950.4	E962.0	E980.4
capillary active drugs	972.8	E858.3	E942.8	E950.4	E962.0	E980.4
Henbane	988.2	E865.4	—	E950.9	E962.1	E980.9
Heparin (sodium)	964.2	E858.2	E934.2	E950.4	E962.0	E980.4
Heptabarbital, heptabarbitone	967.0	E851	E937.0	E950.1	E962.0	E980.1
Heptachlor	989.2	E863.0	—	E950.6	E962.1	E980.7
Heptalgin	965.09	E850.2	E935.2	E950.0	E962.0	E980.0
Herbicides	989.4	E863.5	—	E950.6	E962.1	E980.7
Heroin	965.01	E850.0	E935.0	E950.0	E962.0	E980.0
Herplex	976.5	E858.7	E946.5	E950.4	E962.0	E980.4
HES	964.8	E858.2	E934.8	E950.4	E962.0	E980.4
Hetastarch	964.8	E858.2	E934.8	E950.4	E962.0	E980.4
Hexachlorocyclohexane	989.2	E863.0	—	E950.6	E962.1	E980.7
Hexachlorophene	976.2	E858.7	E946.2	E950.4	E962.0	E980.4
Hexadimethrine (bromide)	964.5	E858.2	E934.5	E950.4	E962.0	E980.4
Hexafluorenium	975.2	E858.6	E945.2	E950.4	E962.0	E980.4
Hexa-germ	976.2	E858.7	E946.2	E950.4	E962.0	E980.4
Hexahydrophenol	980.8	E860.8	—	E950.9	E962.1	E980.9
Hexalin	980.8	E860.8	—	E950.9	E962.1	E980.9
Hexamethonium	972.3	E858.3	E942.3	E950.4	E962.0	E980.4
Hexamethyleneamine	961.9	E857	E931.9	E950.4	E962.0	E980.4
Hexamine	961.9	E857	E931.9	E950.4	E962.0	E980.4
Hexanone	982.8	E862.4	—	E950.9	E962.1	E980.9
Hexapropymate	967.8	E852.8	E937.8	E950.2	E962.0	E980.2
Hexestrol	962.2	E858.0	E932.2	E950.4	E962.0	E980.4
Hexethal (sodium)	967.0	E851	E937.0	E950.1	E962.0	E980.1
Hexetidine	976.0	E858.7	E946.0	E950.4	E962.0	E980.4
Hexobarbital, hexobarbitone	967.0	E851	E937.0	E950.1	E962.0	E980.1
sodium (anesthetic)	968.3	E855.1	E938.3	E950.4	E962.0	E980.4
soluble	968.3	E855.1	E938.3	E950.4	E962.0	E980.4
Hexocyclium	971.1	E855.4	E941.1	E950.4	E962.0	E980.4
Hexoestrol	962.2	E858.0	E932.2	E950.4	E962.0	E980.4
Hexone	982.8	E862.4	—	E950.9	E962.1	E980.9
Hexylcaine	968.5	E855.2	E938.5	E950.4	E962.0	E980.4
Hexylresorcinol	961.6	E857	E931.6	E950.4	E962.0	E980.4
Hinkle's pills	973.1	E858.4	E943.1	E950.4	E962.0	E980.4
Histalog	977.8	E858.8	E947.8	E950.4	E962.0	E980.4
Histamine (phosphate)	972.5	E858.3	E942.5	E950.4	E962.0	E980.4
Histoplasmin	977.8	E858.8	E947.8	E950.4	E962.0	E980.4
Holly berries	988.2	E865.3	—	E950.9	E962.1	E980.9
Homatropine	971.1	E855.4	E941.1	E950.4	E962.0	E980.4

Table of Drugs and Chemicals

		External Cause (E-Code)				
	Poisoning	Accident	Therapeutic Use	Suicide Attempt	Assault	Undetermined
Homo-tet	964.6	E858.2	E934.6	E950.4	E962.0	E980.4
Hormones (synthetic substitute) NEC	962.9	E858.0	E932.9	E950.4	E962.0	E980.4
adrenal cortical steroids	962.0	E858.0	E932.0	E950.4	E962.0	E980.4
antidiabetic agents	962.3	E858.0	E932.3	E950.4	E962.0	E980.4
follicle stimulating	962.4	E858.0	E932.4	E950.4	E962.0	E980.4
gonadotropic	962.4	E858.0	E932.4	E950.4	E962.0	E980.4
growth	962.4	E858.0	E932.4	E950.4	E962.0	E980.4
ovarian (substitutes)	962.2	E858.0	E932.2	E950.4	E962.0	E980.4
parathyroid (derivatives)	962.6	E858.0	E932.6	E950.4	E962.0	E980.4
pituitary (posterior)	962.5	E858.0	E932.5	E950.4	E962.0	E980.4
anterior	962.4	E858.0	E932.4	E950.4	E962.0	E980.4
thyroid (derivative)	962.7	E858.0	E932.7	E950.4	E962.0	E980.4
Hornet (sting)	989.5	E905.3	—	E950.9	E962.1	E980.9
Horticulture agent NEC	989.4	E863.9		E950.6	E962.1	E980.7
Hyaluronidase	963.4	E858.1	E933.4	E950.4	E962.0	E980.4
Hyazyme	963.4	E858.1	E933.4	E950.4	E962.0	E980.4
Hycodan	965.09	E850.2	E935.2	E950.0	E962.0	E980.0
Hydantoin derivatives	966.1	E855.0	E936.1	E950.4	E962.0	E980.4
Hydeltra	962.0	E858.0	E932.0	E950.4	E962.0	E980.4
Hydergine	971.3	E855.6	E941.3	E950.4	E962.0	E980.4
Hydrabamine penicillin	960.0	E856	E930.0	E950.4	E962.0	E980.4
Hydralazine, hydrallazine	972.6	E858.3	E942.6	E950.4	E962.0	E980.4
Hydrargaphen	976.0	E858.7	E946.0	E950.4	E962.0	E980.4
Hydrazine	983.9	E864.3	—	E950.7	E962.1	E980.6
Hydriodic acid	975.5	E858.6	E945.5	E950.4	E962.0	E980.4
Hydrocarbon gas	987.1	E869.8	—	E952.8	E962.2	E982.8
incomplete combustion of — see Carbon, monoxide, fuel, utility						
liquefied (mobile container)	987.0	E868.0	—	E951.1	E962.2	E981.1
piped (natural)	987.0	E867	—	E951.0	E962.2	E981.0
Hydrochloric acid (liquid)	983.1	E864.1	—	E950.7	E962.1	E980.6
medicinal	973.4	E858.4	E943.4	E950.4	E962.0	E980.4
vapor	987.8	E869.8	—	E952.8	E962.2	E982.8
Hydrochlorothiazide	974.3	E858.5	E944.3	E950.4	E962.0	E980.4
Hydrocodone	965.09	E850.2	E935.2	E950.0	E962.0	E980.0
Hydrocortisone	962.0	E858.0	E932.0	E950.4	E962.0	E980.4
ENT agent	976.6	E858.7	E946.6	E950.4	E962.0	E980.4
ophthalmic preparation	976.5	E858.7	E946.5	E950.4	E962.0	E980.4
topical NEC	976.0	E858.7	E946.0	E950.4	E962.0	E980.4
Hydrocortone	962.0	E858.0	E932.0	E950.4	E962.0	E980.4
ENT agent	976.6	E858.7	E946.6	E950.4	E962.0	E980.4
ophthalmic preparation	976.5	E858.7	E946.5	E950.4	E962.0	E980.4
topical NEC	976.0	E858.7	E946.0	E950.4	E962.0	E980.4
Hydrocyanic acid — see Cyanide(s)						
Hydroflumethiazide	974.3	E858.5	E944.3	E950.4	E962.0	E980.4
Hydrofluoric acid (liquid)	983.1	E864.1	—	E950.7	E962.1	E980.6
vapor	987.8	E869.8	—	E952.8	E962.2	E982.8
Hydrogen	987.8	E869.8	—	E952.8	E962.2	E982.8
arsenide	985.1	E866.3	—	E950.8	E962.1	E980.8
arseniureted	985.1	E866.3	—	E950.8	E962.1	E980.8
cyanide (salts)	989.0	E866.8	—	E950.9	E962.1	E980.9
gas	987.7	E869.8	—	E952.8	E962.2	E982.8
fluoride (liquid)	983.1	E864.1	—	E950.7	E962.1	E980.6
vapor	987.8	E869.8	—	E952.8	E962.2	E982.8
peroxide (solution)	976.6	E858.7	E946.6	E950.4	E962.0	E980.4
phosphureted	987.8	E869.8	—	E952.8	E962.2	E982.8
sulfide (gas)	987.8	E869.8	—	E952.8	E962.2	E982.8
arseniureted	985.1	E866.3	—	E950.8	E962.1	E980.8
sulfureted	987.8	E869.8	—	E952.8	E962.2	E982.8
Hydromorphinol	965.09	E850.2	E935.2	E950.0	E962.0	E980.0
Hydromorphinone	965.09	E850.2	E935.2	E950.0	E962.0	E980.0
Hydromorphone	965.09	E850.2	E935.2	E950.0	E962.0	E980.0
Hydromox	974.3	E858.5	E944.3	E950.4	E962.0	E980.4
Hydrophilic lotion	976.3	E858.7	E946.3	E950.4	E962.0	E980.4
Hydroquinone	983.0	E864.0	—	E950.7	E962.1	E980.6
vapor	987.8	E869.8	—	E952.8	E962.2	E982.8
Hydrosulfuric acid (gas)	987.8	E869.8	—	E952.8	E962.2	E982.8
Hydrous wool fat (lotion)	976.3	E858.7	E946.3	E950.4	E962.0	E980.4
Hydroxide, caustic	983.2	E864.2	—	E950.7	E962.1	E980.6
Hydroxocobalamin	964.1	E858.2	E934.1	E950.4	E962.0	E980.4
Hydroxyamphetamine	971.2	E855.5	E941.2	E950.4	E962.0	E980.4
Hydroxychloroquine	961.4	E857	E931.4	E950.4	E962.0	E980.4
Hydroxydihydrocodeinone	965.09	E850.2	E935.2	E950.0	E962.0	E980.0
Hydroxyethyl starch	964.8	E858.2	E934.8	E950.4	E962.0	E980.4
Hydroxyphenamate	969.5	E853.8	E939.5	E950.3	E962.0	E980.3
Hydroxyphenylbutazone	965.5	E850.5	E935.5	E950.0	E962.0	E980.0
Hydroxyprogesterone	962.2	E858.0	E932.2	E950.4	E962.0	E980.4
Hydroxyquinoline derivatives	961.3	E857	E931.3	E950.4	E962.0	E980.4
Hydroxystilbamidine	961.5	E857	E931.5	E950.4	E962.0	E980.4
Hydroxyurea	963.1	E858.1	E933.1	E950.4	E962.0	E980.4
Hydroxyzine	969.5	E853.8	E939.5	E950.3	E962.0	E980.3
Hyoscine (hydrobromide)	971.1	E855.4	E941.1	E950.4	E962.0	E980.4

Table of Drugs and Chemicals

	Poisoning	External Cause (E-Code)				
		Accident	Therapeutic Use	Suicide Attempt	Assault	Undetermined
Hyoscyamine	971.1	E855.4	E941.1	E950.4	E962.0	E980.4
Hyoscyamus (albus) (niger)	988.2	E865.4	—	E950.9	E962.1	E980.9
Hypaque	977.8	E858.8	E947.8	E950.4	E962.0	E980.4
Hypertussis	964.6	E858.2	E934.6	E950.4	E962.0	E980.4
Hypnotics NEC	967.9	E852.9	E937.9	E950.2	E962.0	E980.2
Hypochlorites — see Sodium, hypochlorite						
Hypotensive agents NEC	972.6	E858.3	E942.6	E950.4	E962.0	E980.4
Ibufenac	965.69	E850.6	E935.6	E950.0	E962.0	E980.0
Ibuprofen	965.61	E850.6	E935.6	E950.0	E962.0	E980.0
ICG	977.8	E858.8	E947.8	E950.4	E962.0	E980.4
Ichthammol	976.4	E858.7	E946.4	E950.4	E962.0	E980.4
Ichthyol	976.4	E858.7	E946.4	E950.4	E962.0	E980.4
Idoxuridine	976.5	E858.7	E946.5	E950.4	E962.0	E980.4
IDU	976.5	E858.7	E946.5	E950.4	E962.0	E980.4
Iletin	962.3	E858.0	E932.3	E950.4	E962.0	E980.4
Ilex	988.2	E865.4	—	E950.9	E962.1	E980.9
Illuminating gas — see Gas, utility						
Ilopan	963.5	E858.1	E933.5	E950.4	E962.0	E980.4
Ilotycin	960.3	E856	E930.3	E950.4	E962.0	E980.4
ophthalmic preparation	976.5	E858.7	E946.5	E950.4	E962.0	E980.4
topical NEC	976.0	E858.7	E946.0	E950.4	E962.0	E980.4
Imipramine	969.0	E854.0	E939.0	E950.3	E962.0	E980.3
Immu-G	964.6	E858.2	E934.6	E950.4	E962.0	E980.4
Immuglobin	964.6	E858.2	E934.6	E950.4	E962.0	E980.4
Immune serum globulin	964.6	E858.2	E934.6	E950.4	E962.0	E980.4
Immunosuppressive agents	963.1	E858.1	E933.1	E950.4	E962.0	E980.4
Immu-tetanus	964.6	E858.2	E934.6	E950.4	E962.0	E980.4
Indandione (derivatives)	964.2	E858.2	E934.2	E950.4	E962.0	E980.4
Inderal	972.0	E858.3	E942.0	E950.4	E962.0	E980.4
Indian						
hemp	969.6	E854.1	E939.6	E950.3	E962.0	E980.3
tobacco	988.2	E865.4	—	E950.9	E962.1	E980.9
Indigo carmine	977.8	E858.8	E947.8	E950.4	E962.0	E980.4
Indocin	965.69	E850.6	E935.6	E950.0	E962.0	E980.0
Indocyanine green	977.8	E858.8	E947.8	E950.4	E962.0	E980.4
Indomethacin	965.69	E850.6	E935.6	E950.0	E962.0	E980.0
Industrial						
alcohol	980.9	E860.9	—	E950.9	E962.1	E980.9
fumes	987.8	E869.8	—	E952.8	E962.2	E982.8
solvents (fumes) (vapors)	982.8	E862.9	—	E950.9	E962.1	E980.9
Influenza vaccine	979.6	E858.8	E949.6	E950.4	E962.0	E982.8
Ingested substances NEC	989.9	E866.9	—	E950.9	E962.1	E980.9
INH (isoniazid)	961.8	E857	E931.8	E950.4	E962.0	E980.4
Inhalation, gas (noxious) — see Gas						
Ink	989.89	E866.8	—	E950.9	E962.1	E980.9
Innovar	967.6	E852.5	E937.6	E950.2	E962.0	E980.2
Inositol niacinate	972.2	E858.3	E942.2	E950.4	E962.0	E980.4
Inproquone	963.1	E858.1	E933.1	E950.4	E962.0	E980.4
Insect (sting), venomous	989.5	E905.5	—	E950.9	E962.1	E980.9
Insecticides (see also Pesticides)	989.4	E863.4	—	E950.6	E962.1	E980.7
chlorinated	989.2	E863.0	—	E950.6	E962.1	E980.7
mixtures	989.4	E863.3	—	E950.6	E962.1	E980.7
organochlorine (compounds)	989.2	E863.0	—	E950.6	E962.1	E980.7
organophosphorus (compounds)	989.3	E863.1	—	E950.6	E962.1	E980.7
Insular tissue extract	962.3	E858.0	E932.3	E950.4	E962.0	E980.4
Insulin (amorphous) (globin) (isophane) (Lente) (NPH) (protamine) (Semilente) (Ultralente) (zinc)	962.3	E858.0	E932.3	E950.4	E962.0	E980.4
Intranarcon	968.3	E855.1	E938.3	E950.4	E962.0	E980.4
Inulin	977.8	E858.8	E947.8	E950.4	E962.0	E980.4
Invert sugar	974.5	E858.5	E944.5	E950.4	E962.0	E980.4
Iodide NEC (see also Iodine)	976.0	E858.7	E946.0	E950.4	E962.0	E980.4
mercury (ointment)	976.0	E858.7	E946.0	E950.4	E962.0	E980.4
methylate	976.0	E858.7	E946.0	E950.4	E962.0	E980.4
potassium (expectorant) NEC	975.5	E858.6	E945.5	E950.4	E962.0	E980.4
Iodinated glycerol	975.5	E858.6	E945.5	E950.4	E962.0	E980.4
Iodine (antiseptic, external) (tincture) NEC	976.0	E858.7	E946.0	E950.4	E962.0	E980.4
diagnostic	977.8	E858.8	E947.8	E950.4	E962.0	E980.4
for thyroid conditions (antithyroid)	962.8	E858.0	E932.8	E950.4	E962.0	E980.4
vapor	987.8	E869.8	—	E952.8	E962.2	E982.8
Iodized oil	977.8	E858.8	E947.8	E950.4	E962.0	E980.4
Iodobismitol	961.2	E857	E931.2	E950.4	E962.0	E980.4
Iodochlorhydroxyquin	961.3	E857	E931.3	E950.4	E962.0	E980.4
topical	976.0	E858.7	E946.0	E950.4	E962.0	E980.4
Iodoform	976.0	E858.7	E946.0	E950.4	E962.0	E980.4
Iodopanoic acid	977.8	E858.8	E947.8	E950.4	E962.0	E980.4
Iodophthalein	977.8	E858.8	E947.8	E950.4	E962.0	E980.4
Ion exchange resins	974.5	E858.5	E944.5	E950.4	E962.0	E980.4
Iopanoic acid	977.8	E858.8	E947.8	E950.4	E962.0	E980.4
Iophendylate	977.8	E858.8	E947.8	E950.4	E962.0	E980.4
Iothiouracil	962.8	E858.0	E932.8	E950.4	E962.0	E980.4
Ipecac	973.6	E858.4	E943.6	E950.4	E962.0	E980.4

Table of Drugs and Chemicals

	Poisoning	External Cause (E-Code)				
		Accident	Therapeutic Use	Suicide Attempt	Assault	Undetermined
Ipecacuanha	973.6	E858.4	E943.6	E950.4	E962.0	E980.4
Ipodate	977.8	E858.8	E947.8	E950.4	E962.0	E980.4
Ipral	967.0	E851	E937.0	E950.1	E962.0	E980.1
Ipratropium ●	975.1	E858.6	E945.1	E950.4	E962.0	E980.4
Iproniazid	969.0	E854.0	E939.0	E950.3	E962.0	E980.3
Iron (compounds) (medicinal) (preparations)	964.0	E858.2	E934.0	E950.4	E962.0	E980.4
dextran	964.0	E858.2	E934.0	E950.4	E962.0	E980.4
nonmedicinal (dust) (fumes) NEC	985.8	E866.4	—	E950.9	E962.1	E980.9
Irritant drug	977.9	E858.9	E947.9	E950.5	E962.0	E980.5
Ismelin	972.6	E858.3	E942.6	E950.4	E962.0	E980.4
Isoamyl nitrite	972.4	E858.3	E942.4	E950.4	E962.0	E980.4
Isobutyl acetate	982.8	E862.4	—	E950.9	E962.1	E980.9
Isocarboxazid	969.0	E854.0	E939.0	E950.3	E962.0	E980.3
Isoephedrine	971.2	E855.5	E941.2	E950.4	E962.0	E980.4
Isoetharine	971.2	E855.5	E941.2	E950.4	E962.0	E980.4
Isofluorophate	971.0	E855.3	E941.0	E950.4	E962.0	E980.4
Isoniazid (INH)	961.8	E857	E931.8	E950.4	E962.0	E980.4
Isopentaquine	961.4	E857	E931.4	E950.4	E962.0	E980.4
Isophane insulin	962.3	E858.0	E932.3	E950.4	E962.0	E980.4
Isopregnenone	962.2	E858.0	E932.2	E950.4	E962.0	E980.4
Isoprenaline	971.2	E855.5	E941.2	E950.4	E962.0	E980.4
Isopropamide	971.1	E855.4	E941.1	E950.4	E962.0	E980.4
Isopropanol	980.2	E860.3	—	E950.9	E962.1	E980.9
topical (germicide)	976.0	E858.7	E946.0	E950.4	E962.0	E980.4
Isopropyl						
acetate	982.8	E862.4	—	E950.9	E962.1	E980.9
alcohol	980.2	E860.3	—	E950.9	E962.1	E980.9
topical (germicide)	976.0	E858.7	E946.0	E950.4	E962.0	E980.4
ether	982.8	E862.4	—	E950.9	E962.1	E980.9
Isoproterenol	971.2	E855.5	E941.2	E950.4	E962.0	E980.4
Isosorbide dinitrate	972.4	E858.3	E942.4	E950.4	E962.0	E980.4
Isothipendyl	963.0	E858.1	E933.0	E950.4	E962.0	E980.4
Isoxazolyl penicillin	960.0	E856	E930.0	E950.4	E962.0	E980.4
Isoxsuprine hydrochloride	972.5	E858.3	E942.5	E950.4	E962.0	E980.4
l-thyroxine sodium	962.7	E858.0	E932.7	E950.4	E962.0	E980.4
Jaborandi (pilocarpus) (extract)	971.0	E855.3	E941.0	E950.4	E962.0	E980.4
Jalap	973.1	E858.4	E943.1	E950.4	E962.0	E980.4
Jamaica						
dogwood (bark)	965.7	E850.7	E935.7	E950.0	E962.0	E980.0
ginger	989.89	E866.8	—	E950.9	E962.1	E980.9
Jatropha	988.2	E865.4	—	E950.9	E962.1	E980.9
curcas	988.2	E865.3	—	E950.9	E962.1	E980.9
Jectofer	964.0	E858.2	E934.0	E950.4	E962.0	E980.4
Jellyfish (sting)	989.5	E905.6	—	E950.9	E962.1	E980.9
Jequirity (bean)	988.2	E865.3	—	E950.9	E962.1	E980.9
Jimson weed	988.2	E865.4	—	E950.9	E962.1	E980.9
seeds	988.2	E865.3	—	E950.9	E962.1	E980.9
Juniper tar (oil) (ointment)	976.4	E858.7	E946.4	E950.4	E962.0	E980.4
Kallikrein	972.5	E858.3	E942.5	E950.4	E962.0	E980.4
Kanamycin	960.6	E856	E930.6	E950.4	E962.0	E980.4
Kantrex	960.6	E856	E930.6	E950.4	E962.0	E980.4
Kaolin	973.5	E858.4	E943.5	E950.4	E962.0	E980.4
Karaya (gum)	973.3	E858.4	E943.3	E950.4	E962.0	E980.4
Kemithal	968.3	E855.1	E938.3	E950.4	E962.0	E980.4
Kenacort	962.0	E858.0	E932.0	E950.4	E962.0	E980.4
Keratolytics	976.4	E858.7	E946.4	E950.4	E962.0	E980.4
Keratoplastics	976.4	E858.7	E946.4	E950.4	E962.0	E980.4
Kerosene, kerosine (fuel) (solvent) NEC	981	E862.1	—	E950.9	E962.1	E980.9
insecticide	981	E863.4	—	E950.6	E962.1	E980.7
vapor	987.1	E869.8	—	E952.8	E962.2	E982.8
Ketamine	968.3	E855.1	E938.3	E950.4	E962.0	E980.4
Ketobemidone	965.09	E850.2	E935.2	E950.0	E962.0	E980.0
Ketols	982.8	E862.4	—	E950.9	E962.1	E980.9
Ketone oils	982.8	E862.4	—	E950.9	E962.1	E980.9
Ketoprofen	965.61	E850.6	E935.6	E950.0	E962.0	E980.0
Kiln gas or vapor (carbon monoxide)	986	E868.8	—	E952.1	E962.2	E982.1
Konsyl	973.3	E858.4	E943.3	E950.4	E962.0	E980.4
Kosam seed	988.2	E865.3	—	E950.9	E962.1	E980.9
Krait (venom)	989.5	E905.0	—	E950.9	E962.1	E980.9
Kwell (insecticide)	989.2	E863.0	—	E950.6	E962.1	E980.7
anti-infective (topical)	976.0	E858.7	E946.0	E950.4	E962.0	E980.4
Laburnum (flowers) (seeds)	988.2	E865.3	—	E950.9	E962.1	E980.9
leaves	988.2	E865.4	—	E950.9	E962.1	E980.9
Lacquers	989.89	E861.6	—	E950.9	E962.1	E980.9
Lacrimogenic gas	987.5	E869.3	—	E952.8	E962.2	E982.8
Lactic acid	983.1	E864.1	—	E950.7	E962.1	E980.6
Lactobacillus acidophilus	973.5	E858.4	E943.5	E950.4	E962.0	E980.4
Lactoflavin	963.5	E858.1	E933.5	E950.4	E962.0	E980.4
Lactuca (virosa) (extract)	967.8	E852.8	E937.8	E950.2	E962.0	E980.2
Lactucarium	967.8	E852.8	E937.8	E950.2	E962.0	E980.2
Laevulose	974.5	E858.5	E944.5	E950.4	E962.0	E980.4

Lanatoside (C) — Lincomycin

Table of Drugs and Chemicals

	Poisoning	External Cause (E-Code)				
		Accident	Therapeutic Use	Suicide Attempt	Assault	Undetermined
Lanatoside (C)	972.1	E858.3	E942.1	E950.4	E962.0	E980.4
Lanolin (lotion)	976.3	E858.7	E946.3	E950.4	E962.0	E980.4
Largactil	969.1	E853.0	E939.1	E950.3	E962.0	E980.3
Larkspur	988.2	E865.3	—	E950.9	E962.1	E980.9
Laroxyl	969.0	E854.0	E939.0	E950.3	E962.0	E980.3
Lasix	974.4	E858.5	E944.4	E950.4	E962.0	E980.4
Latex	989.82	E866.8	—	E950.9	E962.1	E980.9
Lathyrus (seed)	988.2	E865.3	—	E950.9	E962.1	E980.9
Laudanum	965.09	E850.2	E935.2	E950.0	E962.0	E980.0
Laudexium	975.2	E858.6	E945.2	E950.4	E962.0	E980.4
Laurel, black or cherry	988.2	E865.4	—	E950.9	E962.1	E980.9
Laurolinium	976.0	E858.7	E946.0	E950.4	E962.0	E980.4
Lauryl sulfoacetate	976.2	E858.7	E946.2	E950.4	E962.0	E980.4
Laxatives NEC	973.3	E858.4	E943.3	E950.4	E962.0	E980.4
emollient	973.2	E858.4	E943.2	E950.4	E962.0	E980.4
L-dopa	966.4	E855.0	E936.4	E950.4	E962.0	E980.4
Lead (dust) (fumes) (vapor) NEC	984.9	E866.0	—	E950.9	E962.1	E980.9
acetate (dust)	984.1	E866.0	—	E950.9	E962.1	E980.9
anti-infectives	961.2	E857	E931.2	E950.4	E962.0	E980.4
antiknock compound (tetraethyl)	984.1	E862.1	—	E950.9	E962.1	E980.9
arsenate, arsenite (dust) (insecticide) (vapor)	985.1	E863.4	—	E950.8	E962.1	E980.8
herbicide	985.1	E863.5	—	E950.8	E962.1	E980.8
carbonate	984.0	E866.0	—	E950.9	E962.1	E980.9
paint	984.0	E861.5	—	E950.9	E962.1	E980.9
chromate	984.0	E866.0	—	E950.9	E962.1	E980.9
paint	984.0	E861.5	—	E950.9	E962.1	E980.9
dioxide	984.0	E866.0	—	E950.9	E962.1	E980.9
inorganic (compound)	984.0	E866.0	—	E950.9	E962.1	E980.9
paint	984.0	E861.5	—	E950.9	E962.1	E980.9
iodide	984.0	E866.0	—	E950.9	E962.1	E980.9
pigment (paint)	984.0	E861.5	—	E950.9	E962.1	E980.9
monoxide (dust)	984.0	E866.0	—	E950.9	E962.1	E980.9
paint	984.0	E861.5	—	E950.9	E962.1	E980.9
organic	984.1	E866.0	—	E950.9	E962.1	E980.9
oxide	984.0	E866.0	—	E950.9	E962.1	E980.9
paint	984.0	E861.5	—	E950.9	E962.1	E980.9
paint	984.0	E861.5	—	E950.9	E962.1	E980.9
salts	984.0	E866.0	—	E950.9	E962.1	E980.9
specified compound NEC	984.8	E866.0	—	E950.9	E962.1	E980.9
tetra-ethyl	984.1	E862.1	—	E950.9	E962.1	E980.9
Lebanese red	969.6	E854.1	E939.6	E950.3	E962.0	E980.3
Lente Iletin (insulin)	962.3	E858.0	E932.3	E950.4	E962.0	E980.4
Leptazol	970.0	E854.3	E940.0	E950.4	E962.0	E980.4
Leritine	965.09	E850.2	E935.2	E950.0	E962.0	E980.0
Letter	962.7	E858.0	E932.7	E950.4	E962.0	E980.4
Lettuce opium	967.8	E852.8	E937.8	E950.2	E962.0	E980.2
Leucovorin (factor)	964.1	E858.2	E934.1	E950.4	E962.0	E980.4
Leukeran	963.1	E858.1	E933.1	E950.4	E962.0	E980.4
Levalbuterol ●	975.7	E858.6	E945.7	E950.4	E962.0	E980.4
Levallorphan	970.1	E854.3	E940.1	E950.4	E962.0	E980.4
Levanil	967.8	E852.8	E937.8	E950.2	E962.0	E980.2
Levarterenol	971.2	E855.5	E941.2	E950.4	E962.0	E980.4
Levodopa	966.4	E855.0	E936.4	E950.4	E962.0	E980.4
Levo-dromoran	965.09	E850.2	E935.2	E950.0	E962.0	E980.0
Levoid	962.7	E858.0	E932.7	E950.4	E962.0	E980.4
Levo-iso-methadone	965.02	E850.1	E935.1	E950.0	E962.0	E980.0
Levomepromazine	967.8	E852.8	E937.8	E950.2	E962.0	E980.2
Levoprome	967.8	E852.8	E937.8	E950.2	E962.0	E980.2
Levopropoxyphene	975.4	E858.6	E945.4	E950.4	E962.0	E980.4
Levorphan, levophanol	965.09	E850.2	E935.2	E950.0	E962.0	E980.0
Levothyroxine (sodium)	962.7	E858.0	E932.7	E950.4	E962.0	E980.4
Levsin	971.1	E855.4	E941.1	E950.4	E962.0	E980.4
Levulose	974.5	E858.5	E944.5	E950.4	E962.0	E980.4
Lewisite (gas)	985.1	E866.3	—	E950.8	E962.1	E980.8
Librium	969.4	E853.2	E939.4	E950.3	E962.0	E980.3
Lidex	976.0	E858.7	E946.0	E950.4	E962.0	E980.4
Lidocaine (infiltration) (topical)	968.5	E855.2	E938.5	E950.4	E962.0	E980.4
nerve block (peripheral) (plexus)	968.6	E855.2	E938.6	E950.4	E962.0	E980.4
spinal	968.7	E855.2	E938.7	E950.4	E962.0	E980.4
Lighter fluid	981	E862.1	—	E950.9	E962.1	E980.9
Lignocaine (infiltration) (topical)	968.5	E855.2	E938.5	E950.4	E962.0	E980.4
nerve block (peripheral) (plexus)	968.6	E855.2	E938.6	E950.4	E962.0	E980.4
spinal	968.7	E855.2	E938.7	E950.4	E962.0	E980.4
Ligroin(e) (solvent)	981	E862.0	—	E950.9	E962.1	E980.9
vapor	987.1	E869.8	—	E952.8	E962.2	E982.8
Ligustrum vulgare	988.2	E865.3	—	E950.9	E962.1	E980.9
Lily of the valley	988.2	E865.4	—	E950.9	E962.1	E980.9
Lime (chloride)	983.2	E864.2	—	E950.7	E962.1	E980.6
solution, sulferated	976.4	E858.7	E946.4	E950.4	E962.0	E980.4
Limonene	982.8	E862.4	—	E950.9	E962.1	E980.9
Lincomycin	960.8	E856	E930.8	E950.4	E962.0	E980.4

Table of Drugs and Chemicals

		External Cause (E-Code)				
	Poisoning	Accident	Therapeutic Use	Suicide Attempt	Assault	Undetermined
Lindane (insecticide) (vapor)	989.2	E863.0	—	E950.6	E962.1	E980.7
anti-infective (topical)	976.0	E858.7	E946.0	E950.4	E962.0	E980.4
Liniments NEC	976.9	E858.7	E946.9	E950.4	E962.0	E980.4
Linoleic acid	972.2	E858.3	E942.2	E950.4	E962.0	E980.4
Liothyronine	962.7	E858.0	E932.7	E950.4	E962.0	E980.4
Liotrix	962.7	E858.0	E932.7	E950.4	E962.0	E980.4
Lipancreatin	973.4	E858.4	E943.4	E950.4	E962.0	E980.4
Lipo-Lutin	962.2	E858.0	E932.2	E950.4	E962.0	E980.4
Lipotropic agents	977.1	E858.8	E947.1	E950.4	E962.0	E980.4
Liquefied petroleum gases	987.0	E868.0	—	E951.1	E962.2	E981.1
piped (pure or mixed with air)	987.0	E867	—	E951.0	E962.2	E981.0
Liquid petrolatum	973.2	E858.4	E943.2	E950.4	E962.0	E980.4
substance	989.9	E866.9	—	E950.9	E962.1	E980.9
specified NEC	989.89	E866.8	—	E950.9	E962.1	E980.9
Lirugen	979.4	E858.8	E949.4	E950.4	E962.0	E980.4
Lithane	969.8	E855.8	E939.8	E950.3	E962.0	E980.3
Lithium	985.8	E866.4	—	E950.9	E962.1	E980.9
carbonate	969.8	E855.8	E939.8	E950.3	E962.0	E980.3
Lithonate	969.8	E855.8	E939.8	E950.3	E962.0	E980.3
Liver (extract) (injection) (preparations)	964.1	E858.2	E934.1	E950.4	E962.0	E980.4
Lizard (bite) (venom)	989.5	E905.0	—	E950.9	E962.1	E980.9
LMD	964.8	E858.2	E934.8	E950.4	E962.0	E980.4
Lobelia	988.2	E865.4	—	E950.9	E962.1	E980.9
Lobeline	970.0	E854.3	E940.0	E950.4	E962.0	E980.4
Locorten	976.0	E858.7	E946.0	E950.4	E962.0	E980.4
Lolium temulentum	988.2	E865.3	—	E950.9	E962.1	E980.9
Lomotil	973.5	E858.4	E943.5	E950.4	E962.0	E980.4
Lomustine	963.1	E858.1	E933.1	E950.4	E962.0	E980.4
Lophophora williamsii	969.6	E854.1	E939.6	E950.3	E962.0	E980.3
Lorazepam	969.4	E853.2	E939.4	E950.3	E962.0	E980.3
Lotions NEC	976.9	E858.7	E946.9	E950.4	E962.0	E980.4
Lotronex	973.8	E858.4	E943.8	E950.4	E962.0	E980.4
Lotusate	967.0	E851	E937.0	E950.1	E962.0	E980.1
Lowila	976.2	E858.7	E946.2	E950.4	E962.0	E980.4
Loxapine	969.3	E853.8	E939.3	E950.3	E962.0	E980.3
Lozenges (throat)	976.6	E858.7	E946.6	E950.4	E962.0	E980.4
LSD (25)	969.6	E854.1	E939.6	E950.3	E962.0	E980.3
Lubricating oil NEC	981	E862.2	—	E950.9	E962.1	E980.9
Lucanthone	961.6	E857	E931.6	E950.4	E962.0	E980.4
Luminal	967.0	E851	E937.0	E950.1	E962.0	E980.1
Lung irritant (gas) NEC	987.9	E869.9	—	E952.9	E962.2	E982.9
Lutocylol	962.2	E858.0	E932.2	E950.4	E962.0	E980.4
Lutromone	962.2	E858.0	E932.2	E950.4	E962.0	E980.4
Lututrin	975.0	E858.6	E945.0	E950.4	E962.0	E980.4
Lye (concentrated)	983.2	E864.2	—	E950.7	E962.1	E980.6
Lygranum (skin test)	977.8	E858.8	E947.8	E950.4	E962.0	E980.4
Lymecycline	960.4	E856	E930.4	E950.4	E962.0	E980.4
Lymphogranuloma venereum antigen	977.8	E858.8	E947.8	E950.4	E962.0	E980.4
Lynestrenol	962.2	E858.0	E932.2	E950.4	E962.0	E980.4
Lyovac Sodium Edecrin	974.4	E858.5	E944.4	E950.4	E962.0	E980.4
Lypressin	962.5	E858.0	E932.5	E950.4	E962.0	E980.4
Lysergic acid (amide) (diethylamide)	969.6	E854.1	E939.6	E950.3	E962.0	E980.3
Lysergide	969.6	E854.1	E939.6	E950.3	E962.0	E980.3
Lysine vasopressin	962.5	E858.0	E932.5	E950.4	E962.0	E980.4
Lysol	983.0	E864.0	—	E950.7	E962.1	E980.6
Lytta (vitatta)	976.8	E858.7	E946.8	E950.4	E962.0	E980.4
Mace	987.5	E869.3	—	E952.8	E962.2	E982.8
Macrolides (antibiotics)	960.3	E856	E930.3	E950.4	E962.0	E980.4
Mafenide	976.0	E858.7	E946.0	E950.4	E962.0	E980.4
Magaldrate	973.0	E858.4	E943.0	E950.4	E962.0	E980.4
Magic mushroom	969.6	E854.1	E939.6	E950.3	E962.0	E980.3
Magnamycin	960.8	E856	E930.8	E950.4	E962.0	E980.4
Magnesia magma	973.0	E858.4	E943.0	E950.4	E962.0	E980.4
Magnesium (compounds) (fumes) NEC	985.8	E866.4	—	E950.9	E962.1	E980.9
antacid	973.0	E858.4	E943.0	E950.4	E962.0	E980.4
carbonate	973.0	E858.4	E943.0	E950.4	E962.0	E980.4
cathartic	973.3	E858.4	E943.3	E950.4	E962.0	E980.4
citrate	973.3	E858.4	E943.3	E950.4	E962.0	E980.4
hydroxide	973.0	E858.4	E943.0	E950.4	E962.0	E980.4
oxide	973.0	E858.4	E943.0	E950.4	E962.0	E980.4
sulfate (oral)	973.3	E858.4	E943.3	E950.4	E962.0	E980.4
intravenous	966.3	E855.0	E936.3	E950.4	E962.0	E980.4
trisilicate	973.0	E858.4	E943.0	E950.4	E962.0	E980.4
Malathion (insecticide)	989.3	E863.1	—	E950.6	E962.1	E980.7
Male fern (oleoresin)	961.6	E857	E931.6	E950.4	E962.0	E980.4
Mandelic acid	961.9	E857	E931.9	E950.4	E962.0	E980.4
Manganese compounds (fumes) NEC	985.2	E866.4	—	E950.9	E962.1	E980.9
Mannitol (diuretic) (medicinal) NEC	974.4	E858.5	E944.4	E950.4	E962.0	E980.4
hexanitrate	972.4	E858.3	E942.4	E950.4	E962.0	E980.4
mustard	963.1	E858.1	E933.1	E950.4	E962.0	E980.4

Table of Drugs and Chemicals

			External Cause (E-Code)			
	Poisoning	Accident	Therapeutic Use	Suicide Attempt	Assault	Undetermined
Mannomustine	963.1	E858.1	E933.1	E950.4	E962.0	E980.4
MAO inhibitors	969.0	E854.0	E939.0	E950.3	E962.0	E980.3
Mapharsen	961.1	E857	E931.1	E950.4	E962.0	E980.4
Marcaine	968.9	E855.2	E938.9	E950.4	E962.0	E980.4
infiltration (subcutaneous)	968.5	E855.2	E938.5	E950.4	E962.0	E980.4
nerve block (peripheral) (plexus)	968.6	E855.2	E938.6	E950.4	E962.0	E980.4
Marezine	963.0	E858.1	E933.0	E950.4	E962.0	E980.4
Marihuana, marijuana (derivatives)	969.6	E854.1	E939.6	E950.3	E962.0	E980.3
Marine animals or plants (sting)	989.5	E905.6	—	E950.9	E962.1	E980.9
Marplan	969.0	E854.0	E939.0	E950.3	E962.0	E980.3
Marsh gas	987.1	E869.8	—	E952.8	E962.2	E982.8
Marsilid	969.0	E854.0	E939.0	E950.3	E962.0	E980.3
Matulane	963.1	E858.1	E933.1	E950.4	E962.0	E980.4
Mazindol	977.0	E858.8	E947.0	E950.4	E962.0	E980.4
Meadow saffron	988.2	E865.3	—	E950.9	E962.1	E980.9
Measles vaccine	979.4	E858.8	E949.4	E950.4	E962.0	E980.4
Meat, noxious or nonbacterial	988.8	E865.0	—	E950.9	E962.1	E980.9
Mebanazine	969.0	E854.0	E939.0	E950.3	E962.0	E980.3
Mebaral	967.0	E851	E937.0	E950.1	E962.0	E980.1
Mebendazole	961.6	E857	E931.6	E950.4	E962.0	E980.4
Mebeverine	975.1	E858.6	E945.1	E950.4	E962.0	E980.4
Mebhydroline	963.0	E858.1	E933.0	E950.4	E962.0	E980.4
Mebrophenhydramine	963.0	E858.1	E933.0	E950.4	E962.0	E980.4
Mebutamate	969.5	E853.8	E939.5	E950.3	E962.0	E980.3
Mecamylamine (chloride)	972.3	E858.3	E942.3	E950.4	E962.0	E980.4
Mechlorethamine hydrochloride	963.1	E858.1	E933.1	E950.4	E962.0	E980.4
Meclizene (hydrochloride)	963.0	E858.1	E933.0	E950.4	E962.0	E980.4
Meclofenoxate	970.0	E854.3	E940.0	E950.4	E962.0	E980.4
Meclozine (hydrochloride)	963.0	E858.1	E933.0	E950.4	E962.0	E980.4
Medazepam	969.4	E853.2	E939.4	E950.3	E962.0	E980.3
Medicine, medicinal substance	977.9	E858.9	E947.9	E950.5	E962.0	E980.5
specified NEC	977.8	E858.8	E947.8	E950.4	E962.0	E980.4
Medinal	967.0	E851	E937.0	E950.1	E962.0	E980.1
Medomin	967.0	E851	E937.0	E950.1	E962.0	E980.1
Medroxyprogesterone	962.2	E858.0	E932.2	E950.4	E962.0	E980.4
Medrysone	976.5	E858.7	E946.5	E950.4	E962.0	E980.4
Mefenamic acid	965.7	E850.7	E935.7	E950.0	E962.0	E980.0
Megahallucinogen	969.6	E854.1	E939.6	E950.3	E962.0	E980.3
Megestrol	962.2	E858.0	E932.2	E950.4	E962.0	E980.4
Meglumine	977.8	E858.8	E947.8	E950.4	E962.0	E980.4
Meladinin	976.3	E858.7	E946.3	E950.4	E962.0	E980.4
Melanizing agents	976.3	E858.7	E946.3	E950.4	E962.0	E980.4
Melarsoprol	961.1	E857	E931.1	E950.4	E962.0	E980.4
Melia azedarach	988.2	E865.3	—	E950.9	E962.1	E980.9
Mellaril	969.1	E853.0	E939.1	E950.3	E962.0	E980.3
Meloxine	976.3	E858.7	E946.3	E950.4	E962.0	E980.4
Melphalan	963.1	E858.1	E933.1	E950.4	E962.0	E980.4
Menadiol sodium diphosphate	964.3	E858.2	E934.3	E950.4	E962.0	E980.4
Menadione (sodium bisulfite)	964.3	E858.2	E934.3	E950.4	E962.0	E980.4
Menaphthone	964.3	E858.2	E934.3	E950.4	E962.0	E980.4
Meningococcal vaccine	978.8	E858.8	E948.8	E950.4	E962.0	E980.4
Menningovax-C	978.8	E858.8	E948.8	E950.4	E962.0	E980.4
Menotropins	962.4	E858.0	E932.4	E950.4	E962.0	E980.4
Menthol NEC	976.1	E858.7	E946.1	E950.4	E962.0	E980.4
Mepacrine	961.3	E857	E931.3	E950.4	E962.0	E980.4
Meparfynol	967.8	E852.8	E937.8	E950.2	E962.0	E980.2
Mepazine	969.1	E853.0	E939.1	E950.3	E962.0	E980.3
Mepenzolate	971.1	E855.4	E941.1	E950.4	E962.0	E980.4
Meperidine	965.09	E850.2	E935.2	E950.0	E962.0	E980.0
Mephenamin(e)	966.4	E855.0	E936.4	E950.4	E962.0	E980.4
Mephenesin (carbamate)	968.0	E855.1	E938.0	E950.4	E962.0	E980.4
Mephenoxalone	969.5	E853.8	E939.5	E950.3	E962.0	E980.3
Mephentermine	971.2	E855.5	E941.2	E950.4	E962.0	E980.4
Mephenytoin	966.1	E855.0	E936.1	E950.4	E962.0	E980.4
Mephobarbital	967.0	E851	E937.0	E950.1	E962.0	E980.1
Mepiperphenidol	971.1	E855.4	E941.1	E950.4	E962.0	E980.4
Mepivacaine	968.9	E855.2	E938.9	E950.4	E962.0	E980.4
infiltration (subcutaneous)	968.5	E855.2	E938.5	E950.4	E962.0	E980.4
nerve block (peripheral) (plexus)	968.6	E855.2	E938.6	E950.4	E962.0	E980.4
topical (surface)	968.5	E855.2	E938.5	E950.4	E962.0	E980.4
Meprednisone	962.0	E858.0	E932.0	E950.4	E962.0	E980.4
Meprobam	969.5	E853.8	E939.5	E950.3	E962.0	E980.3
Meprobamate	969.5	E853.8	E939.5	E950.3	E962.0	E980.3
Mepyramine (maleate)	963.0	E858.1	E933.0	E950.4	E962.0	E980.4
Meralluride	974.0	E858.5	E944.0	E950.4	E962.0	E980.4
Merbaphen	974.0	E858.5	E944.0	E950.4	E962.0	E980.4
Merbromin	976.0	E858.7	E946.0	E950.4	E962.0	E980.4
Mercaptomerin	974.0	E858.5	E944.0	E950.4	E962.0	E980.4
Mercaptopurine	963.1	E858.1	E933.1	E950.4	E962.0	E980.4
Mercumatilin	974.0	E858.5	E944.0	E950.4	E962.0	E980.4
Mercuramide	974.0	E858.5	E944.0	E950.4	E962.0	E980.4

Table of Drugs and Chemicals — Methoxypsoralen

	Poisoning	External Cause (E-Code)				
		Accident	Therapeutic Use	Suicide Attempt	Assault	Undetermined
Mercuranin	976.0	E858.7	E946.0	E950.4	E962.0	E980.4
Mercurochrome	976.0	E858.7	E946.0	E950.4	E962.0	E980.4
Mercury, mercuric, mercurous (compounds) (cyanide) (fumes)						
(nonmedicinal) (vapor) NEC	985.0	E866.1	—	E950.9	E962.1	E980.9
ammoniated	976.0	E858.7	E946.0	E950.4	E962.0	E980.4
anti-infective	961.2	E857	E931.2	E950.4	E962.0	E980.4
topical	976.0	E858.7	E946.0	E950.4	E962.0	E980.4
chloride (antiseptic) NEC	976.0	E858.7	E946.0	E950.4	E962.0	E980.4
fungicide	985.0	E863.6	—	E950.6	E962.1	E980.7
diuretic compounds	974.0	E858.5	E944.0	E950.4	E962.0	E980.4
fungicide	985.0	E863.6	—	E950.6	E962.1	E980.7
organic (fungicide)	985.0	E863.6	—	E950.6	E962.1	E980.7
Merethoxylline	974.0	E858.5	E944.0	E950.4	E962.0	E980.4
Mersalyl	974.0	E858.5	E944.0	E950.4	E962.0	E980.4
Merthiolate (topical)	976.0	E858.7	E946.0	E950.4	E962.0	E980.4
ophthalmic preparation	976.5	E858.7	E946.5	E950.4	E962.0	E980.4
Meruvax	979.4	E858.8	E949.4	E950.4	E962.0	E980.4
Mescal buttons	969.6	E854.1	E939.6	E950.3	E962.0	E980.3
Mescaline (salts)	969.6	E854.1	E939.6	E950.3	E962.0	E980.3
Mesoridazine besylate	969.1	E853.0	E939.1	E950.3	E962.0	E980.3
Mestanolone	962.1	E858.0	E932.1	E950.4	E962.0	E980.4
Mestranol	962.2	E858.0	E932.2	E950.4	E962.0	E980.4
Metacresylacetate	976.0	E858.7	E946.0	E950.4	E962.0	E980.4
Metaldehyde (snail killer) NEC	989.4	E863.4	—	E950.6	E962.1	E980.7
Metals (heavy) (nonmedicinal) NEC	985.9	E866.4	—	E950.9	E962.1	E980.9
dust, fumes, or vapor NEC	985.9	E866.4	—	E950.9	E962.1	E980.9
light NEC	985.9	E866.4	—	E950.9	E962.1	E980.9
dust, fumes, or vapor NEC	985.9	E866.4	—	E950.9	E962.1	E980.9
pesticides (dust) (vapor)	985.9	E863.4	—	E950.6	E962.1	E980.7
Metamucil	973.3	E858.4	E943.3	E950.4	E962.0	E980.4
Metaphen	976.0	E858.7	E946.0	E950.4	E962.0	E980.4
Metaproterenol	975.1	E858.6	E945.1	E950.4	E962.0	E980.4
Metaraminol	972.8	E858.3	E942.8	E950.4	E962.0	E980.4
Metaxalone	968.0	E855.1	E938.0	E950.4	E962.0	E980.4
Metformin	962.3	E858.0	E932.3	E950.4	E962.0	E980.4
Methacycline	960.4	E856	E930.4	E950.4	E962.0	E980.4
Methadone	965.02	E850.1	E935.1	E950.0	E962.0	E980.0
Methallenestril	962.2	E858.0	E932.2	E950.4	E962.0	E980.4
Methamphetamine	969.7	E854.2	E939.7	E950.3	E962.0	E980.3
Methandienone	962.1	E858.0	E932.1	E950.4	E962.0	E980.4
Methandriol	962.1	E858.0	E932.1	E950.4	E962.0	E980.4
Methandrostenolone	962.1	E858.0	E932.1	E950.4	E962.0	E980.4
Methane gas	987.1	E869.8	—	E952.8	E962.2	E982.8
Methanol	980.1	E860.2	—	E950.9	E962.1	E980.9
vapor	987.8	E869.8	—	E952.8	E962.2	E982.8
Methantheline	971.1	E855.4	E941.1	E950.4	E962.0	E980.4
Methaphenilene	963.0	E858.1	E933.0	E950.4	E962.0	E980.4
Methapyrilene	963.0	E858.1	E933.0	E950.4	E962.0	E980.4
Methaqualone (compounds)	967.4	E852.3	E937.4	E950.2	E962.0	E980.2
Metharbital, metharbitone	967.0	E851	E937.0	E950.1	E962.0	E980.1
Methazolamide	974.2	E858.5	E944.2	E950.4	E962.0	E980.4
Methdilazine	963.0	E858.1	E933.0	E950.4	E962.0	E980.4
Methedrine	969.7	E854.2	E939.7	E950.3	E962.0	E980.3
Methenamine (mandelate)	961.9	E857	E931.9	E950.4	E962.0	E980.4
Methenolone	962.1	E858.0	E932.1	E950.4	E962.0	E980.4
Methergine	975.0	E858.6	E945.0	E950.4	E962.0	E980.4
Methiacil	962.8	E858.0	E932.8	E950.4	E962.0	E980.4
Methicillin (sodium)	960.0	E856	E930.0	E950.4	E962.0	E980.4
Methimazole	962.8	E858.0	E932.8	E950.4	E962.0	E980.4
Methionine	977.1	E858.8	E947.1	E950.4	E962.0	E980.4
Methisazone	961.7	E857	E931.7	E950.4	E962.0	E980.4
Methitural	967.0	E851	E937.0	E950.1	E962.0	E980.1
Methixene	971.1	E855.4	E941.1	E950.4	E962.0	E980.4
Methobarbital, methobarbitone	967.0	E851	E937.0	E950.1	E962.0	E980.1
Methocarbamol	968.0	E855.1	E938.0	E950.4	E962.0	E980.4
Methohexital, methohexitone (sodium)	968.3	E855.1	E938.3	E950.4	E962.0	E980.4
Methoin	966.1	E855.0	E936.1	E950.4	E962.0	E980.4
Methopholine	965.7	E850.7	E935.7	E950.0	E962.0	E980.0
Methorate	975.4	E858.6	E945.4	E950.4	E962.0	E980.4
Methoserpidine	972.6	E858.3	E942.6	E950.4	E962.0	E980.4
Methotrexate	963.1	E858.1	E933.1	E950.4	E962.0	E980.4
Methotrimeprazine	967.8	E852.8	E937.8	E950.2	E962.0	E980.2
Methoxa-Dome	976.3	E858.7	E946.3	E950.4	E962.0	E980.4
Methoxamine	971.2	E855.5	E941.2	E950.4	E962.0	E980.4
Methoxsalen	976.3	E858.7	E946.3	E950.4	E962.0	E980.4
Methoxybenzyl penicillin	960.0	E856	E930.0	E950.4	E962.0	E980.4
Methoxychlor	989.2	E863.0	—	E950.6	E962.1	E980.7
Methoxyflurane	968.2	E855.1	E938.2	E950.4	E962.0	E980.4
Methoxyphenamine	971.2	E855.5	E941.2	E950.4	E962.0	E980.4
Methoxypromazine	969.1	E853.0	E939.1	E950.3	E962.0	E980.3
Methoxypsoralen	976.3	E858.7	E946.3	E950.4	E962.0	E980.4

Table of Drugs and Chemicals

		External Cause (E-Code)				
	Poisoning	Accident	Therapeutic Use	Suicide Attempt	Assault	Undetermined
Methscopolamine (bromide)	971.1	E855.4	E941.1	E950.4	E962.0	E980.4
Methsuximide	966.2	E855.0	E936.2	E950.4	E962.0	E980.4
Methyclothiazide	974.3	E858.5	E944.3	E950.4	E962.0	E980.4
Methyl						
acetate	982.8	E862.4	—	E950.9	E962.1	E980.9
acetone	982.8	E862.4	—	E950.9	E962.1	E980.9
alcohol	980.1	E860.2	—	E950.9	E962.1	E980.9
amphetamine	969.7	E854.2	E939.7	E950.3	E962.0	E980.3
androstanolone	962.1	E858.0	E932.1	E950.4	E962.0	E980.4
atropine	971.1	E855.4	E941.1	E950.4	E962.0	E980.4
benzene	982.0	E862.4	—	E950.9	E962.1	E980.9
bromide (gas)	987.8	E869.8	—	E952.8	E962.2	E982.8
fumigant	987.8	E863.8	—	E950.6	E962.2	E980.7
butanol	980.8	E860.8	—	E950.9	E962.1	E980.9
carbinol	980.1	E860.2	—	E950.9	E962.1	E980.9
cellosolve	982.8	E862.4	—	E950.9	E962.1	E980.9
cellulose	973.3	E858.4	E943.3	E950.4	E962.0	E980.4
chloride (gas)	987.8	E869.8	—	E952.8	E962.2	E982.8
cyclohexane	982.8	E862.4	—	E950.9	E962.1	E980.9
cyclohexanone	982.8	E862.4	—	E950.9	E962.1	E980.9
dihydromorphinone	965.09	E850.2	E935.2	E950.0	E962.0	E980.0
ergometrine	975.0	E858.6	E945.0	E950.4	E962.0	E980.4
ergonovine	975.0	E858.6	E945.0	E950.4	E962.0	E980.4
ethyl ketone	982.8	E862.4	—	E950.9	E962.1	E980.9
hydrazine	983.9	E864.3	—	E950.7	E962.1	E980.6
isobutyl ketone	982.8	E862.4	—	E950.9	E962.1	E980.9
morphine NEC	965.09	E850.2	E935.2	E950.0	E962.0	E980.0
parafynol	967.8	E852.8	E937.8	E950.2	E962.0	E980.2
parathion	989.3	E863.1	—	E950.6	E962.1	E980.7
pentynol NEC	967.8	E852.8	E937.8	E950.2	E962.0	E980.2
peridol	969.2	E853.1	E939.2	E950.3	E962.0	E980.3
phenidate	969.7	E854.2	E939.7	E950.3	E962.0	E980.3
prednisolone	962.0	E858.0	E932.0	E950.4	E962.0	E980.4
ENT agent	976.6	E858.7	E946.6	E950.4	E962.0	E980.4
ophthalmic preparation	976.5	E858.7	E946.5	E950.4	E962.0	E980.4
topical NEC	976.0	E858.7	E946.0	E950.4	E962.0	E980.4
propylcarbinol	980.8	E860.8	—	E950.9	E962.1	E980.9
rosaniline NEC	976.0	E858.7	E946.0	E950.4	E962.0	E980.4
salicylate NEC	976.3	E858.7	E946.3	E950.4	E962.0	E980.4
sulfate (fumes)	987.8	E869.8	—	E952.8	E962.2	E982.8
liquid	983.9	E864.3	—	E950.7	E962.1	E980.6
sulfonal	967.8	E852.8	E937.8	E950.2	E962.0	E980.2
testosterone	962.1	E858.0	E932.1	E950.4	E962.0	E980.4
thiouracil	962.8	E858.0	E932.8	E950.4	E962.0	E980.4
Methylated spirit	980.0	E860.1	—	E950.9	E962.1	E980.9
Methyldopa	972.6	E858.3	E942.6	E950.4	E962.0	E980.4
Methylene						
blue	961.9	E857	E931.9	E950.4	E962.0	E980.4
chloride or dichloride (solvent) NEC	982.3	E862.4	—	E950.9	E962.1	E980.9
Methylhexabital	967.0	E851	E937.0	E950.1	E962.0	E980.1
Methylparaben (ophthalmic)	976.5	E858.7	E946.5	E950.4	E962.0	E980.4
Methyprylon	967.5	E852.4	E937.5	E950.2	E962.0	E980.2
Methysergide	971.3	E855.6	E941.3	E950.4	E962.0	E980.4
Metoclopramide	963.0	E858.1	E933.0	E950.4	E962.0	E980.4
Metofoline	965.7	E850.7	E935.7	E950.0	E962.0	E980.0
Metopon	965.09	E850.2	E935.2	E950.0	E962.0	E980.0
Metronidazole	961.5	E857	E931.5	E950.4	E962.0	E980.4
Metycaine	968.9	E855.2	E938.9	E950.4	E962.0	E980.4
infiltration (subcutaneous)	968.5	E855.2	E938.5	E950.4	E962.0	E980.4
nerve block (peripheral) (plexus)	968.6	E855.2	E938.6	E950.4	E962.0	E980.4
topical (surface)	968.5	E855.2	E938.5	E950.4	E962.0	E980.4
Metyrapone	977.8	E858.8	E947.8	E950.4	E962.0	E980.4
Mevinphos	989.3	E863.1	—	E950.6	E962.1	E980.7
Mezereon (berries)	988.2	E865.3	—	E950.9	E962.1	E980.9
Micatin	976.0	E858.7	E946.0	E950.4	E962.0	E980.4
Miconazole	976.0	E858.7	E946.0	E950.4	E962.0	E980.4
Midol	965.1	E850.3	E935.3	E950.0	E962.0	E980.0
Mifepristone	962.9	E858.0	E932.9	E950.4	E962.0	E980.4
Milk of magnesia	973.0	E858.4	E943.0	E950.4	E962.0	E980.4
Millipede (tropical) (venomous)	989.5	E905.4	—	E950.9	E962.1	E980.9
Miltown	969.5	E853.8	E939.5	E950.3	E962.0	E980.3
Mineral						
oil (medicinal)	973.2	E858.4	E943.2	E950.4	E962.0	E980.4
nonmedicinal	981	E862.1	—	E950.9	E962.1	E980.9
topical	976.3	E858.7	E946.3	E950.4	E962.0	E980.4
salts NEC	974.6	E858.5	E944.6	E950.4	E962.0	E980.4
spirits	981	E862.0	—	E950.9	E962.1	E980.9
Minocycline	960.4	E856	E930.4	E950.4	E962.0	E980.4
Mithramycin (antineoplastic)	960.7	E856	E930.7	E950.4	E962.0	E980.4
Mitobronitol	963.1	E858.1	E933.1	E950.4	E962.0	E980.4
Mitomycin (antineoplastic)	960.7	E856	E930.7	E950.4	E962.0	E980.4

Table of Drugs and Chemicals

		External Cause (E-Code)				
	Poisoning	Accident	Therapeutic Use	Suicide Attempt	Assault	Undetermined
Mitotane	963.1	E858.1	E933.1	E950.4	E962.0	E980.4
Moderil	972.6	E858.3	E942.6	E950.4	E962.0	E980.4
Mogadon — see Nitrazepam						
Molindone	969.3	E853.8	E939.3	E950.3	E962.0	E980.3
Monistat	976.0	E858.7	E946.0	E950.4	E962.0	E980.4
Monkshood	988.2	E865.4	—	E950.9	E962.1	E980.9
Monoamine oxidase inhibitors	969.0	E854.0	E939.0	E950.3	E962.0	E980.3
Monochlorobenzene	982.0	E862.4	—	E950.9	E962.1	E980.9
Monosodium glutamate	989.89	E866.8	—	E950.9	E962.1	E980.9
Monoxide, carbon — see Carbon, monoxide						
Moperone	969.2	E853.1	E939.2	E950.3	E962.0	E980.3
Morning glory seeds	969.6	E854.1	E939.6	E950.3	E962.0	E980.3
Moroxydine (hydrochloride)	961.7	E857	E931.7	E950.4	E962.0	E980.4
Morphazinamide	961.8	E857	E931.8	E950.4	E962.0	E980.4
Morphinans	965.09	E850.2	E935.2	E950.0	E962.0	E980.0
Morphine NEC	965.09	E850.2	E935.2	E950.0	E962.0	E980.0
antagonists	970.1	E854.3	E940.1	E950.4	E962.0	E980.4
Morpholinylethylmorphine	965.09	E850.2	E935.2	E950.0	E962.0	E980.0
Morrhuate sodium	972.7	E858.3	E942.7	E950.4	E962.0	E980.4
Moth balls (see also Pesticides)	989.4	E863.4	—	E950.6	E962.1	E980.7
naphthalene	983.0	E863.4	—	E950.7	E962.1	E980.6
Motor exhaust gas — see Carbon, monoxide, exhaust gas						
Mouth wash	976.6	E858.7	E946.6	E950.4	E962.0	E980.4
Mucolytic agent	975.5	E858.6	E945.5	E950.4	E962.0	E980.4
Mucomyst	975.5	E858.6	E945.5	E950.4	E962.0	E980.4
Mucous membrane agents (external)	976.9	E858.7	E946.9	E950.4	E962.0	E980.4
specified NEC	976.8	E858.7	E946.8	E950.4	E962.0	E980.4
Mumps						
immune globulin (human)	964.6	E858.2	E934.6	E950.4	E962.0	E980.4
skin test antigen	977.8	E858.8	E947.8	E950.4	E962.0	E980.4
vaccine	979.6	E858.8	E949.6	E950.4	E962.0	E980.4
Mumpsvax	979.6	E858.8	E949.6	E950.4	E962.0	E980.4
Muriatic acid — see Hydrochloric acid						
Muscarine	971.0	E855.3	E941.0	E950.4	E962.0	E980.4
Muscle affecting agents NEC	975.3	E858.6	E945.3	E950.4	E962.0	E980.4
oxytocic	975.0	E858.6	E945.0	E950.4	E962.0	E980.4
relaxants	975.3	E858.6	E945.3	E950.4	E962.0	E980.4
central nervous system	968.0	E855.1	E938.0	E950.4	E962.0	E980.4
skeletal	975.2	E858.6	E945.2	E950.4	E962.0	E980.4
smooth	975.1	E858.6	E945.1	E950.4	E962.0	E980.4
Mushrooms, noxious	988.1	E865.5	—	E950.9	E962.1	E980.9
Mussel, noxious	988.0	E865.1	—	E950.9	E962.1	E980.9
Mustard (emetic)	973.6	E858.4	E943.6	E950.4	E962.0	E980.4
gas	987.8	E869.8	—	E952.8	E962.2	E982.8
nitrogen	963.1	E858.1	E933.1	E950.4	E962.0	E980.4
Mustine	963.1	E858.1	E933.1	E950.4	E962.0	E980.4
M-vac	979.4	E858.8	E949.4	E950.4	E962.0	E980.4
Mycifradin	960.8	E856	E930.8	E950.4	E962.0	E980.4
topical	976.0	E858.7	E946.0	E950.4	E962.0	E980.4
Mycitracin	960.8	E856	E930.8	E950.4	E962.0	E980.4
ophthalmic preparation	976.5	E858.7	E946.5	E950.4	E962.0	E980.4
Mycostatin	960.1	E856	E930.1	E950.4	E962.0	E980.4
topical	976.0	E858.7	E946.0	E950.4	E962.0	E980.4
Mydriacyl	971.1	E855.4	E941.1	E950.4	E962.0	E980.4
Myelobromal	963.1	E858.1	E933.1	E950.4	E962.0	E980.4
Myleran	963.1	E858.1	E933.1	E950.4	E962.0	E980.4
Myochrysin(e)	965.69	E850.6	E935.6	E950.0	E962.0	E980.0
Myoneural blocking agents	975.2	E858.6	E945.2	E950.4	E962.0	E980.4
Myristica fragrans	988.2	E865.3	—	E950.9	E962.1	E980.9
Myristicin	988.2	E865.3	—	E950.9	E962.1	E980.9
Mysoline	966.3	E855.0	E936.3	E950.4	E962.0	E980.4
Nafcillin (sodium)	960.0	E856	E930.0	E950.4	E962.0	E980.4
Nail polish remover	982.8	E862.4	—	E950.9	E962.1	E908.9
Nalidixic acid	961.9	E857	E931.9	E950.4	E962.0	E980.4
Nalorphine	970.1	E854.3	E940.1	E950.4	E962.0	E980.4
Naloxone	970.1	E854.3	E940.1	E950.4	E962.0	E980.4
Nandrolone (decanoate) (phenproprioate)	962.1	E858.0	E932.1	E950.4	E962.0	E980.4
Naphazoline	971.2	E855.5	E941.2	E950.4	E962.0	E980.4
Naphtha (painter's) (petroleum)	981	E862.0	—	E950.9	E962.1	E980.9
solvent	981	E862.0	—	E950.9	E962.1	E980.9
vapor	987.1	E869.8	—	E952.8	E962.2	E982.8
Naphthalene (chlorinated)	983.0	E864.0	—	E950.7	E962.1	E980.6
insecticide or moth repellent	983.0	E863.4	—	E950.7	E962.1	E980.6
vapor	987.8	E869.8	—	E952.8	E962.2	E982.8
Naphthol	983.0	E864.0	—	E950.7	E962.1	E980.6
Naphthylamine	983.0	E864.0	—	E950.7	E962.1	E980.6
Naprosyn — see Naproxen						
Naproxen	965.61	E850.6	E935.6	E950.0	E962.0	E980.0
Narcotic (drug)	967.9	E852.9	E937.9	E950.2	E962.0	E980.2
analgesic NEC	965.8	E850.8	E935.8	E950.0	E962.0	E980.0
antagonist	970.1	E854.3	E940.1	E950.4	E962.0	E980.4

Narcotic

Table of Drugs and Chemicals

	Poisoning	External Cause (E-Code)				
		Accident	Therapeutic Use	Suicide Attempt	Assault	Undetermined
Narcotic — *continued*						
specified NEC	967.8	E852.8	E937.8	E950.2	E962.0	E980.2
Narcotine	975.4	E858.6	E945.4	E950.4	E962.0	E980.4
Nardil	969.0	E854.0	E939.0	E950.3	E962.0	E980.3
Natrium cyanide — *see* Cyanide(s)						
Natural						
blood (product)	964.7	E858.2	E934.7	E950.4	E962.0	E980.4
gas (piped)	987.1	E867	—	E951.0	E962.2	E981.0
incomplete combustion	986	E867	—	E951.0	E962.2	E981.0
Nealbarbital, nealbarbitone	967.0	E851	E937.0	E950.1	E962.0	E980.1
Nectadon	975.4	E858.6	E945.4	E950.4	E962.0	E980.4
Nematocyst (sting)	989.5	E905.6	—	E950.9	E962.1	E980.9
Nembutal	967.0	E851	E937.0	E950.1	E962.0	E980.1
Neoarsphenamine	961.1	E857	E931.1	E950.4	E962.0	E980.4
Neocinchophen	974.7	E858.5	E944.7	E950.4	E962.0	E980.4
Neomycin	960.8	E856	E930.8	E950.4	E962.0	E980.4
ENT agent	976.6	E858.7	E946.6	E950.4	E962.0	E980.4
ophthalmic preparation	976.5	E858.7	E946.5	E950.4	E962.0	E980.4
topical NEC	976.0	E858.7	E946.0	E950.4	E962.0	E980.4
Neonal	967.0	E851	E937.0	E950.1	E962.0	E980.1
Neoprontosil	961.0	E857	E931.0	E950.4	E962.0	E980.4
Neosalvarsan	961.1	E857	E931.1	E950.4	E962.0	E980.4
Neosilversalvarsan	961.1	E857	E931.1	E950.4	E962.0	E980.4
Neosporin	960.8	E856	E930.8	E950.4	E962.0	E980.4
ENT agent	976.6	E858.7	E946.6	E950.4	E962.0	E980.4
opthalmic preparation	976.5	E858.7	E946.5	E950.4	E962.0	E980.4
topical NEC	976.0	E858.7	E946.0	E950.4	E962.0	E980.4
Neostigmine	971.0	E855.3	E941.0	E950.4	E962.0	E980.4
Neraval	967.0	E851	E937.0	E950.1	E962.0	E980.1
Neravan	967.0	E851	E937.0	E950.1	E962.0	E980.1
Nerium oleander	988.2	E865.4	—	E950.9	E962.1	E980.9
Nerve gases (war)	987.9	E869.9	—	E952.9	E962.2	E982.9
Nesacaine	968.9	E855.2	E938.9	E950.4	E962.0	E980.4
infiltration (subcutaneous)	968.5	E855.2	E938.5	E950.4	E962.0	E980.4
nerve block (peripheral) (plexus)	968.6	E855.2	E938.6	E950.4	E962.0	E980.4
Neurobarb	967.0	E851	E937.0	E950.1	E962.0	E980.1
Neuroleptics NEC	969.3	E853.8	E939.3	E950.3	E962.0	E980.3
Neuroprotective agent	977.8	E858.8	E947.8	E950.4	E962.0	E980.4
Neutral spirits	980.0	E860.1	—	E950.9	E962.1	E980.9
beverage	980.0	E860.0	—	E950.9	E962.1	E980.9
Niacin, niacinamide	972.2	E858.3	E942.2	E950.4	E962.0	E980.4
Nialamide	969.0	E854.0	E939.0	E950.3	E962.0	E980.3
Nickle (carbonyl) (compounds) (fumes) (tetracarbonyl) (vapor)	985.8	E866.4	—	E950.9	E962.1	E980.9
Niclosamide	961.6	E857	E931.6	E950.4	E962.0	E980.4
Nicomorphine	965.09	E850.2	E935.2	E950.0	E962.0	E980.0
Nicotinamide	972.2	E858.3	E942.2	E950.4	E962.0	E980.4
Nicotine (insecticide) (spray) (sulfate) NEC	989.4	E863.4	—	E950.6	E962.1	E980.7
not insecticide	989.89	E866.8	—	E950.9	E962.1	E980.9
Nicotinic acid (derivatives)	972.2	E858.3	E942.2	E950.4	E962.0	E980.4
Nicotinyl alcohol	972.2	E858.3	E942.2	E950.4	E962.0	E980.4
Nicoumalone	964.2	E858.2	E934.2	E950.4	E962.0	E980.4
Nifenazone	965.5	E850.5	E935.5	E950.0	E962.0	E980.0
Nifuraldezone	961.9	E857	E931.9	E950.4	E962.0	E980.4
Nightshade (deadly)	988.2	E865.4	—	E950.9	E962.1	E980.9
Nikethamide	970.0	E854.3	E940.0	E950.4	E962.0	E980.4
Nilstat	960.1	E856	E930.1	E950.4	E962.0	E980.4
topical	976.0	E858.7	E946.0	E950.4	E962.0	E980.4
Nimodipine	977.8	E858.8	E947.8	E950.4	E962.0	E980.4
Niridazole	961.6	E857	E931.6	E950.4	E962.0	E980.4
Nisentil	965.09	E850.2	E935.2	E950.0	E962.0	E980.0
Nitrates	972.4	E858.3	E942.4	E950.4	E962.0	E980.4
Nitrazepam	969.4	E853.2	E939.4	E950.3	E962.0	E980.3
Nitric						
acid (liquid)	983.1	E864.1	—	E950.7	E962.1	E980.6
vapor	987.8	E869.8	—	E952.8	E962.2	E982.8
oxide (gas)	987.2	E869.0	—	E952.8	E962.2	E982.8
Nitrite, amyl (medicinal) (vapor)	972.4	E858.3	E942.4	E950.4	E962.0	E980.4
Nitroaniline	983.0	E864.0	—	E950.7	E962.1	E980.6
vapor	987.8	E869.8	—	E952.8	E962.2	E982.8
Nitrobenzene, nitrobenzol	983.0	E864.0	—	E950.7	E962.1	E980.6
vapor	987.8	E869.8	—	E952.8	E962.2	E982.8
Nitrocellulose	976.3	E858.7	E946.3	E950.4	E962.0	E980.4
Nitrofuran derivatives	961.9	E857	E931.9	E950.4	E962.0	E980.4
Nitrofurantoin	961.9	E857	E931.9	E950.4	E962.0	E980.4
Nitrofurazone	976.0	E858.7	E946.0	E950.4	E962.0	E980.4
Nitrogen (dioxide) (gas) (oxide)	987.2	E869.0	—	E952.8	E962.2	E982.8
mustard (antineoplastic)	963.1	E858.1	E933.1	E950.4	E962.0	E980.4
Nitroglycerin, nitroglycerol (medicinal)	972.4	E858.3	E942.4	E950.4	E962.0	E980.4
nonmedicinal	989.89	E866.8	—	E950.9	E962.1	E980.9
fumes	987.8	E869.8	—	E952.8	E962.2	E982.8
Nitrohydrochloric acid	983.1	E864.1	—	E950.7	E962.1	E980.6

Table of Drugs and Chemicals — Orphenadrine

	Poisoning	External Cause (E-Code)				
		Accident	Therapeutic Use	Suicide Attempt	Assault	Undetermined
Nitromersol	976.0	E858.7	E946.0	E950.4	E962.0	E980.4
Nitronaphthalene	983.0	E864.0	—	E950.7	E962.2	E980.6
Nitrophenol	983.0	E864.0	—	E950.7	E962.2	E980.6
Nitrothiazol	961.6	E857	E931.6	E950.4	E962.0	E980.4
Nitrotoluene, nitrotoluol	983.0	E864.0	—	E950.7	E962.1	E980.6
vapor	987.8	E869.8	—	E952.8	E962.2	E982.8
Nitrous	968.2	E855.1	E938.2	E950.4	E962.0	E980.4
acid (liquid)	983.1	E864.1	—	E950.7	E962.1	E980.6
fumes	987.2	E869.0	—	E952.8	E962.2	E982.8
oxide (anesthetic) NEC	968.2	E855.1	E938.2	E950.4	E962.0	E980.4
Nitrozone	976.0	E858.7	E946.0	E950.4	E962.0	E980.4
Noctec	967.1	E852.0	E937.1	E950.2	E962.0	E980.2
Noludar	967.5	E852.4	E937.5	E950.2	E962.0	E980.2
Noptil	967.0	E851	E937.0	E950.1	E962.0	E980.1
Noradrenalin	971.2	E855.5	E941.2	E950.4	E962.0	E980.4
Noramidopyrine	965.5	E850.5	E935.5	E950.0	E962.0	E980.0
Norepinephrine	971.2	E855.5	E941.2	E950.4	E962.0	E980.4
Norethandrolone	962.1	E858.0	E932.1	E950.4	E962.0	E980.4
Norethindrone	962.2	E858.0	E932.2	E950.4	E962.0	E980.4
Norethisterone	962.2	E858.0	E932.2	E950.4	E962.0	E980.4
Norethynodrel	962.2	E858.0	E932.2	E950.4	E962.0	E980.4
Norlestrin	962.2	E858.0	E932.2	E950.4	E962.0	E980.4
Norlutin	962.2	E858.0	E932.2	E950.4	E962.0	E980.4
Normison — see Benzodiazepines						
Normorphine	965.09	E850.2	E935.2	E950.0	E962.0	E980.0
Nortriptyline	969.0	E854.0	E939.0	E950.3	E962.0	E980.3
Noscapine	975.4	E858.6	E945.4	E950.4	E962.0	E980.4
Nose preparations	976.6	E858.7	E946.6	E950.4	E962.0	E980.4
Novobiocin	960.8	E856	E930.8	E950.4	E962.0	E980.4
Novocain (infiltration) (topical)	968.5	E855.2	E938.5	E950.4	E962.0	E980.4
nerve block (peripheral) (plexus)	968.6	E855.2	E938.6	E950.4	E962.0	E980.4
spinal	968.7	E855.2	E938.7	E950.4	E962.0	E980.4
Noxythiolin	961.9	E857	E931.9	E950.4	E962.0	E980.4
NPH Iletin (insulin)	962.3	E858.0	E932.3	E950.4	E962.0	E980.4
Numorphan	965.09	E850.2	E935.2	E950.0	E962.0	E980.0
Nunol	967.0	E851	E937.0	E950.1	E962.0	E980.1
Nupercaine (spinal anesthetic)	968.7	E855.2	E938.7	E950.4	E962.0	E980.4
topical (surface)	968.5	E855.2	E938.5	E950.4	E962.0	E980.4
Nutmeg oil (liniment)	976.3	E858.7	E946.3	E950.4	E962.0	E980.4
Nux vomica	989.1	E863.7	—	E950.6	E962.1	E980.7
Nydrazid	961.8	E857	E931.8	E950.4	E962.0	E980.4
Nylidrin	971.2	E855.5	E941.2	E950.4	E962.0	E980.4
Nystatin	960.1	E856	E930.1	E950.4	E962.0	E980.4
topical	976.0	E858.7	E946.0	E950.4	E962.0	E980.4
Nytol	963.0	E858.2	E934.2	E950.4	E962.0	E980.4
Oblivion	967.8	E852.8	E937.8	E950.2	E962.0	E980.2
Octyl nitrite	972.4	E858.3	E942.4	E950.4	E962.0	E980.4
Oestradiol (cypionate) (dipropionate) (valerate)	962.2	E858.0	E932.2	E950.4	E962.0	E980.4
Oestriol	962.2	E858.0	E932.2	E950.4	E962.0	E980.4
Oestrone	962.2	E858.0	E932.2	E950.4	E962.0	E980.4
Oil (of) NEC	989.89	E866.8	—	E950.9	E962.1	E980.9
bitter almond	989.0	E866.8	—	E950.9	E962.1	E980.9
camphor	976.1	E858.7	E946.1	E950.4	E962.0	E980.4
colors	989.89	E861.6	—	E950.9	E962.1	E980.9
fumes	987.8	E869.8	—	E952.8	E962.2	E982.8
lubricating	981	E862.2	—	E950.9	E962.1	E980.9
specified source, other — see substance specified						
vitriol (liquid)	983.1	E864.1	—	E950.7	E962.1	E980.6
fumes	987.8	E869.8	—	E952.8	E962.2	E982.8
wintergreen (bitter) NEC	976.3	E858.7	E946.3	E950.4	E962.0	E980.4
Ointments NEC	976.9	E858.7	E946.9	E950.4	E962.0	E980.4
Oleander	988.2	E865.4	—	E950.9	E962.1	E980.9
Oleandomycin	960.3	E856	E930.3	E950.4	E962.0	E980.4
Oleovitamin A	963.5	E858.1	E933.5	E950.4	E962.0	E980.4
Oleum ricini	973.1	E858.4	E943.1	E950.4	E962.0	E980.4
Olive oil (medicinal) NEC	973.2	E858.4	E943.2	E950.4	E962.0	E980.4
OMPA	989.3	E863.1	—	E950.6	E962.1	E980.7
Oncovin	963.1	E858.1	E933.1	E950.4	E962.0	E980.4
Ophthaine	968.5	E855.2	E938.5	E950.4	E962.0	E980.4
Ophthetic	968.5	E855.2	E938.5	E950.4	E962.0	E980.4
Opiates, opioids, opium NEC	965.00	E850.2	E935.2	E950.0	E962.0	E980.0
antagonists	970.1	E854.3	E940.1	E950.4	E962.0	E980.4
Oracon	962.2	E858.0	E932.2	E950.4	E962.0	E980.4
Oragrafin	977.8	E858.8	E947.8	E950.4	E962.0	E980.4
Oral contraceptives	962.2	E858.0	E932.2	E950.4	E962.0	E980.4
Orciprenaline	975.1	E858.6	E945.1	E950.4	E962.0	E980.4
Organidin	975.5	E858.6	E945.5	E950.4	E962.0	E980.4
Organophosphates	989.3	E863.1	—	E950.6	E962.1	E980.7
Orimune	979.5	E858.8	E949.5	E950.4	E962.0	E980.4
Orinase	962.3	E858.0	E932.3	E950.4	E962.0	E980.4
Orphenadrine	966.4	E855.0	E936.4	E950.4	E962.0	E980.4

		External Cause (E-Code)				
	Poisoning	Accident	Therapeutic Use	Suicide Attempt	Assault	Undetermined
Ortal (sodium)	967.0	E851	E937.0	E950.1	E962.0	E980.1
Orthoboric acid	976.0	E858.7	E946.0	E950.4	E962.0	E980.4
ENT agent	976.6	E858.7	E946.6	E950.4	E962.0	E980.4
ophthalmic preparation	976.5	E858.7	E946.5	E950.4	E962.0	E980.4
Orthocaine	968.5	E855.2	E938.5	E950.4	E962.0	E980.4
Ortho-Novum	962.2	E858.0	E932.2	E950.4	E962.0	E980.4
Orthotolidine (reagent)	977.8	E858.8	E947.8	E950.4	E962.0	E980.4
Osmic acid (liquid)	983.1	E864.1	—	E950.7	E962.1	E980.6
fumes	987.8	E869.8	—	E952.8	E962.2	E982.8
Osmotic diuretics	974.4	E858.5	E944.4	E950.4	E962.0	E980.4
Ouabain	972.1	E858.3	E942.1	E950.4	E962.0	E980.4
Ovarian hormones (synthetic substitutes)	962.2	E858.0	E932.2	E950.4	E962.0	E980.4
Ovral	962.2	E858.0	E932.2	E950.4	E962.0	E980.4
Ovulation suppressants	962.2	E858.0	E932.2	E950.4	E962.0	E980.4
Ovulen	962.2	E858.0	E932.2	E950.4	E962.0	E980.4
Oxacillin (sodium)	960.0	E856	E930.0	E950.4	E962.0	E980.4
Oxalic acid	983.1	E864.1	—	E950.7	E962.1	E980.6
Oxanamide	969.5	E853.8	E939.5	E950.3	E962.0	E980.3
Oxandrolone	962.1	E858.0	E932.1	E950.4	E962.0	E980.4
Oxaprozin	965.61	E850.6	E935.6	E950.0	E962.0	E980.0
Oxazepam	969.4	E853.2	E939.4	E950.3	E962.0	E980.3
Oxazolidine derivatives	966.0	E855.0	E936.0	E950.4	E962.0	E980.4
Ox bile extract	973.4	E858.4	E943.4	E950.4	E962.0	E980.4
Oxedrine	971.2	E855.5	E941.2	E950.4	E962.0	E980.4
Oxeladin	975.4	E858.6	E945.4	E950.4	E962.0	E980.4
Oxethazaine NEC	968.5	E855.2	E938.5	E950.4	E962.0	E980.4
Oxidizing agents NEC	983.9	E864.3	—	E950.7	E962.1	E980.6
Oxolinic acid	961.3	E857	E931.3	E950.4	E962.0	E980.4
Oxophenarsine	961.1	E857	E931.1	E950.4	E962.0	E980.4
Oxsoralen	976.3	E858.7	E946.3	E950.4	E962.0	E980.4
Oxtriphylline	975.7	E858.6	E945.7	E950.4	E962.0	E980.4
Oxybuprocaine	968.5	E855.2	E938.5	E950.4	E962.0	E980.4
Oxybutynin	975.1	E858.6	E945.1	E950.4	E962.0	E980.4
Oxycodone	965.09	E850.2	E935.2	E950.0	E962.0	E980.0
Oxygen	987.8	E869.8	—	E952.8	E962.2	E982.8
Oxylone	976.0	E858.7	E946.0	E950.4	E962.0	E980.4
ophthalmic preparation	976.5	E858.7	E946.5	E950.4	E962.0	E980.4
Oxymesterone	962.1	E858.0	E932.1	E950.4	E962.0	E980.4
Oxymetazoline	971.2	E855.5	E941.2	E950.4	E962.0	E980.4
Oxymetholone	962.1	E858.0	E932.1	E950.4	E962.0	E980.4
Oxymorphone	965.09	E850.2	E935.2	E950.0	E962.0	E980.0
Oxypertine	969.0	E854.0	E939.0	E950.3	E962.0	E980.3
Oxyphenbutazone	965.5	E850.5	E935.5	E950.0	E962.0	E980.0
Oxyphencyclimine	971.1	E855.4	E941.1	E950.4	E962.0	E980.4
Oxyphenisatin	973.1	E858.4	E943.1	E950.4	E962.0	E980.4
Oxyphenonium	971.1	E855.4	E941.1	E950.4	E962.0	E980.4
Oxyquinoline	961.3	E857	E931.3	E950.4	E962.0	E980.4
Oxytetracycline	960.4	E856	E930.4	E950.4	E962.0	E980.4
Oxytocics	975.0	E858.6	E945.0	E950.4	E962.0	E980.4
Oxytocin	975.0	E858.6	E945.0	E950.4	E962.0	E980.4
Ozone	987.8	E869.8	—	E952.8	E962.2	E982.8
PABA	976.3	E858.7	E946.3	E950.4	E962.0	E980.4
Packed red cells	964.7	E858.2	E934.7	E950.4	E962.0	E980.4
Paint NEC	989.89	E861.6	—	E950.9	E962.1	E980.9
cleaner	982.8	E862.9	—	E950.9	E962.1	E980.9
fumes NEC	987.8	E869.8	—	E952.8	E962.1	E982.8
lead (fumes)	984.0	E861.5	—	E950.9	E962.1	E980.9
solvent NEC	982.8	E862.9	—	E950.9	E962.1	E980.9
stripper	982.8	E862.9	—	E950.9	E962.1	E980.9
Palfium	965.09	E850.2	E935.2	E950.0	E962.0	E980.0
Palivizumab	979.9	E858.8	E949.6	E950.4	E962.0	E980.4
Paludrine	961.4	E857	E931.4	E950.4	E962.0	E980.4
PAM	977.2	E855.8	E947.2	E950.4	E962.0	E980.4
Pamaquine (naphthoate)	961.4	E857	E931.4	E950.4	E962.0	E980.4
Pamprin	965.1	E850.3	E935.3	E950.0	E962.0	E980.0
Panadol	965.4	E850.4	E935.4	E950.0	E962.0	E980.0
Pancreatic dornase (mucolytic)	963.4	E858.1	E933.4	E950.4	E962.0	E980.4
Pancreatin	973.4	E858.4	E943.4	E950.4	E962.0	E980.4
Pancrelipase	973.4	E858.4	E943.4	E950.4	E962.0	E980.4
Pangamic acid	963.5	E858.1	E933.5	E950.4	E962.0	E980.4
Panthenol	963.5	E858.1	E933.5	E950.4	E962.0	E980.4
topical	976.8	E858.7	E946.8	E950.4	E962.0	E980.4
Pantopaque	977.8	E858.8	E947.8	E950.4	E962.0	E980.4
Pantopon	965.00	E850.2	E935.2	E950.0	E962.0	E980.0
Pantothenic acid	963.5	E858.1	E933.5	E950.4	E962.0	E980.4
Panwarfin	964.2	E858.2	E934.2	E950.4	E962.0	E980.4
Papain	973.4	E858.4	E943.4	E950.4	E962.0	E980.4
Papaverine	972.5	E858.3	E942.5	E950.4	E962.0	E980.4
Para-aminobenzoic acid	976.3	E858.7	E946.3	E950.4	E962.0	E980.4
Para-aminophenol derivatives	965.4	E850.4	E935.4	E950.0	E962.0	E980.0
Para-aminosalicylic acid (derivatives)	961.8	E857	E931.8	E950.4	E962.0	E980.4

Table of Drugs and Chemicals

		External Cause (E-Code)				
	Poisoning	Accident	Therapeutic Use	Suicide Attempt	Assault	Undetermined
Paracetaldehyde (medicinal)	967.2	E852.1	E937.2	E950.2	E962.0	E980.2
Paracetamol	965.4	E850.4	E935.4	E950.0	E962.0	E980.0
Paracodin	965.09	E850.2	E935.2	E950.0	E962.0	E980.0
Paradione	966.0	E855.0	E936.0	E950.4	E962.0	E980.4
Paraffin(s) (wax)	981	E862.3	—	E950.9	E962.1	E980.9
liquid (medicinal)	973.2	E858.4	E943.2	E950.4	E962.0	E980.4
nonmedicinal (oil)	981	E862.1	—	E950.9	E962.1	E980.9
Paraldehyde (medicinal)	967.2	E852.1	E937.2	E950.2	E962.0	E980.2
Paramethadione	966.0	E855.0	E936.0	E950.4	E962.0	E980.4
Paramethasone	962.0	E858.0	E932.0	E950.4	E962.0	E980.4
Paraquat	989.4	E863.5	—	E950.6	E962.1	E980.7
Parasympatholytics	971.1	E855.4	E941.1	E950.4	E962.0	E980.4
Parasympathomimetics	971.0	E855.3	E941.0	E950.4	E962.0	E980.4
Parathion	989.3	E863.1	—	E950.6	E962.1	E980.7
Parathormone	962.6	E858.0	E932.6	E950.4	E962.0	E980.4
Parathyroid (derivatives)	962.6	E858.0	E932.6	E950.4	E962.0	E980.4
Paratyphoid vaccine	978.1	E858.8	E948.1	E950.4	E962.0	E980.4
Paredrine	971.2	E855.5	E941.2	E950.4	E962.0	E980.4
Paregoric	965.00	E850.2	E935.2	E950.0	E962.0	E980.0
Pargyline	972.3	E858.3	E942.3	E950.4	E962.0	E980.4
Paris green	985.1	E866.3	—	E950.8	E962.1	E980.8
insecticide	985.1	E863.4	—	E950.8	E962.1	E980.8
Parnate	969.0	E854.0	E939.0	E950.3	E962.0	E980.3
Paromomycin	960.8	E856	E930.8	E950.4	E962.0	E980.4
Paroxypropione	963.1	E858.1	E933.1	E950.4	E962.0	E980.4
Parzone	965.09	E850.2	E935.2	E950.0	E962.0	E980.0
PAS	961.8	E857	E931.8	E950.4	E962.0	E980.4
PCBs	981	E862.3	—	E950.9	E962.1	E980.9
PCP (pentachlorophenol)	989.4	E863.6	—	E950.6	E962.1	E980.7
herbicide	989.4	E863.5	—	E950.6	E962.1	E980.7
insecticide	989.4	E863.4	—	E950.6	E962.1	E980.7
phencyclidine	968.3	E855.1	E938.3	E950.4	E962.0	E980.4
Peach kernel oil (emulsion)	973.2	E858.4	E943.2	E950.4	E962.0	E980.4
Peanut oil (emulsion) NEC	973.2	E858.4	E943.2	E950.4	E962.0	E980.4
topical	976.3	E858.7	E946.3	E950.4	E962.0	E980.4
Pearly Gates (morning glory seeds)	969.6	E854.1	E939.6	E950.3	E962.0	E980.3
Pecazine	969.1	E853.0	E939.1	E950.3	E962.0	E980.3
Pecilocin	960.1	E856	E930.1	E950.4	E962.0	E980.4
Pectin (with kaolin) NEC	973.5	E858.4	E943.5	E950.4	E962.0	E980.4
Pelletierine tannate	961.6	E857	E931.6	E950.4	E962.0	E980.4
Pemoline	969.7	E854.2	E939.7	E950.3	E962.0	E980.3
Pempidine	972.3	E858.3	E942.3	E950.4	E962.0	E980.4
Penamecillin	960.0	E856	E930.0	E950.4	E962.0	E980.4
Penethamate hydriodide	960.0	E856	E930.0	E950.4	E962.0	E980.4
Penicillamine	963.8	E858.1	E933.8	E950.4	E962.0	E980.4
Penicillin (any type)	960.0	E856	E930.0	E950.4	E962.0	E980.4
Penicillinase	963.4	E858.1	E933.4	E950.4	E962.0	E980.4
Pentachlorophenol (fungicide)	989.4	E863.6	—	E950.6	E962.1	E980.7
herbicide	989.4	E863.5	—	E950.6	E962.1	E980.7
insecticide	989.4	E863.4	—	E950.6	E962.1	E980.7
Pentaerythritol	972.4	E858.3	E942.4	E950.4	E962.0	E980.4
chloral	967.1	E852.0	E937.1	E950.2	E962.0	E980.2
tetranitrate NEC	972.4	E858.3	E942.4	E950.4	E962.0	E980.4
Pentagastrin	977.8	E858.8	E947.8	E950.4	E962.0	E980.4
Pentalin	982.3	E862.4	—	E950.9	E962.1	E980.9
Pentamethonium (bromide)	972.3	E858.3	E942.3	E950.4	E962.0	E980.4
Pentamidine	961.5	E857	E931.5	E950.4	E962.0	E980.4
Pentanol	980.8	E860.8	—	E950.9	E962.1	E980.9
Pentaquine	961.4	E857	E931.4	E950.4	E962.0	E980.4
Pentazocine	965.8	E850.8	E935.8	E950.0	E962.0	E980.0
Penthienate	971.1	E855.4	E941.1	E950.4	E962.0	E980.4
Pentobarbital, pentobarbitone (sodium)	967.0	E851	E937.0	E950.1	E962.0	E980.1
Pentolinium (tartrate)	972.3	E858.3	E942.3	E950.4	E962.0	E980.4
Pentothal	968.3	E855.1	E938.3	E950.4	E962.0	E980.4
Pentylenetetrazol	970	E854.3	E940.0	E950.4	E962.0	E980.4
Pentylsalicylamide	961.8	E857	E931.8	E950.4	E962.0	E980.4
Pepsin	973.4	E858.4	E943.4	E950.4	E962.0	E980.4
Peptavlon	977.8	E858.8	E947.8	E950.4	E962.0	E980.4
Percaine (spinal)	968.7	E855.2	E938.7	E950.4	E962.0	E980.4
topical (surface)	968.5	E855.2	E938.5	E950.4	E962.0	E980.4
Perchloroethylene (vapor)	982.3	E862.4	—	E950.9	E962.1	E980.9
medicinal	961.6	E857	E931.6	E950.4	E962.0	E980.4
Percodan	965.09	E850.2	E935.2	E950.0	E962.0	E980.0
Percogesic	965.09	E850.2	E935.2	E950.0	E962.0	E980.0
Percorten	962.0	E858.0	E932.0	E950.4	E962.0	E980.4
Pergonal	962.4	E858.0	E932.4	E950.4	E962.0	E980.4
Perhexiline	972.4	E858.3	E942.4	E950.4	E962.0	E980.4
Periactin	963.0	E858.1	E933.0	E950.4	E962.0	E980.4
Periclor	967.1	E852.0	E937.1	E950.2	E962.0	E980.2
Pericyazine	969.1	E853.0	E939.1	E950.3	E962.0	E980.3
Peritrate	972.4	E858.3	E942.4	E950.4	E962.0	E980.4

Table of Drugs and Chemicals

		External Cause (E-Code)				
	Poisoning	Accident	Therapeutic Use	Suicide Attempt	Assault	Undetermined
Permanganates NEC	983.9	E864.3	—	E950.7	E962.1	E980.6
potassium (topical)	976.0	E858.7	E946.0	E950.4	E962.0	E980.4
Pernocton	967.0	E851	E937.0	E950.1	E962.0	E980.1
Pernoston	967.0	E851	E937.0	E950.1	E962.0	E980.1
Peronin(e)	965.09	E850.2	E935.2	E950.0	E962.0	E980.0
Perphenazine	969.1	E853.0	E939.1	E950.3	E962.0	E980.3
Pertofrane	969.0	E854 ⚠4	E939.0	E950.3	E962.0	E980.3
Pertussis						
immune serum (human)	964.6	E858.2	E934.6	E950.4	E962.0	E980.4
vaccine (with diphtheria toxoid) (with tetanus toxoid)	978.6	E858.8	E948.6	E950.4	E962.0	E980.4
Peruvian balsam	976.8	E858.7	E946.8	E950.4	E962.0	E980.4
Pesticides (dust) (fumes) (vapor)	989.4	E863.4	—	E950.6	E962.1	E980.7
arsenic	985.1	E863.4	—	E950.8	E962.1	E980.8
chlorinated	989.2	E863.0	—	E950.6	E962.1	E980.7
cyanide	989.0	E863.4	—	E950.6	E962.1	E980.7
kerosene	981	E863.4	—	E950.6	E962.1	E980.7
mixture (of compounds)	989.4	E863.3	—	E950.6	E962.1	E980.7
naphthalene	983.0	E863.4	—	E950.7	E962.1	E980.6
organochlorine (compounds)	989.2	E863.0	—	E950.6	E962.1	E980.7
petroleum (distillate) (products) NEC	981	E863.4	—	E950.6	E962.1	E980.7
specified ingredient NEC	989.4	E863.4	—	E950.6	E962.1	E980.7
strychnine	989.1	E863.4	—	E950.6	E962.1	E980.7
thallium	985.8	E863.7	—	E950.6	E962.1	E980.7
Pethidine (hydrochloride)	965.09	E850.2	E935.2	E950.0	E962.0	E980.0
Petrichloral	967.1	E852.0	E937.1	E950.2	E962.0	E980.2
Petrol	981	E862.1	—	E950.9	E962.1	E980.9
vapor	987.1	E869.8	—	E952.8	E962.2	E982.8
Petrolatum (jelly) (ointment)	976.3	E858.7	E946.3	E950.4	E962.0	E980.4
hydrophilic	976.3	E858.7	E946.3	E950.4	E962.0	E980.4
liquid	973.2	E858.4	E943.2	E950.4	E962.0	E980.4
topical	976.3	E858.7	E946.3	E950.4	E962.0	E980.4
nonmedicinal	981	E862.1	—	E950.9	E962.1	E980.9
Petroleum (cleaners) (fuels) (products) NEC	981	E862.1	—	E950.9	E962.1	E980.9
benzin(e) — see Ligroin						
ether — see Ligroin						
jelly — see Petrolatum						
naphtha — see Ligroin						
pesticide	981	E863.4	—	E950.6	E962.1	E980.7
solids	981	E862.3	—	E950.9	E962.1	E980.9
solvents	981	E862.0	—	E950.9	E962.1	E980.9
vapor	987.1	E869.8	—	E952.8	E962.2	E982.8
Peyote	969.6	E854.1	E939.6	E950.3	E962.0	E980.3
Phanodorm, phanodorn	967.0	E851	E937.0	E950.1	E962.0	E980.1
Phanquinone, phanquone	961.5	E857	E931.5	E950.4	E962.0	E980.4
Pharmaceutical excipient or adjunct	977.4	E858.8	E947.4	E950.4	E962.0	E980.4
Phenacemide	966.3	E855.0	E936.3	E950.4	E962.0	E980.4
Phenacetin	965.4	E850.4	E935.4	E950.0	E962.0	E980.0
Phenadoxone	965.09	E850.2	E935.2	E950.0	E962.0	E980.0
Phenaglycodol	969.5	E853.8	E939.5	E950.3	E962.0	E980.3
Phenantoin	966.1	E855.0	E936.1	E950.4	E962.0	E980.4
Phenaphthazine reagent	977.8	E858.8	E947.8	E950.4	E962.0	E980.4
Phenazocine	965.09	E850.2	E935.2	E950.0	E962.0	E980.0
Phenazone	965.5	E850.5	E935.5	E950.0	E962.0	E980.0
Phenazopyridine	976.1	E858.7	E946.1	E950.4	E962.0	E980.4
Phenbenicillin	960.0	E856	E930.0	E950.4	E962.0	E980.4
Phenbutrazate	977.0	E858.8	E947.0	E950.4	E962.0	E980.4
Phencyclidine	968.3	E855.1	E938.3	E950.4	E962.0	E980.4
Phendimetrazine	977.0	E858.8	E947.0	E950.4	E962.0	E980.4
Phenelzine	969.0	E854.0	E939.0	E950.3	E962.0	E980.3
Phenergan	967.8	E852.8	E937.8	E950.2	E962.0	E980.2
Phenethicillin (potassium)	960.0	E856	E930.0	E950.4	E962.0	E980.4
Phenetsal	965.1	E850.3	E935.3	E950.0	E962.0	E980.0
Pheneturide	966.3	E855.0	E936.3	E950.4	E962.0	E980.4
Phenformin	962.3	E858.0	E932.3	E950.4	E962.0	E980.4
Phenglutarimide	971.1	E855.4	E941.1	E950.4	E962.0	E980.4
Phenicarbazide	965.8	E850.8	E935.8	E950.0	E962.0	E980.0
Phenindamine (tartrate)	963.0	E858.1	E933.0	E950.4	E962.0	E980.4
Phenindione	964.2	E858.2	E934.2	E950.4	E962.0	E980.4
Pheniprazine	969.0	E854.0	E939.0	E950.3	E962.0	E980.3
Pheniramine (maleate)	963.0	E858.1	E933.0	E950.4	E962.0	E980.4
Phenmetrazine	977.0	E858.8	E947.0	E950.4	E962.0	E980.4
Phenobal	967.0	E851	E937.0	E950.1	E962.0	E980.1
Phenobarbital	967.0	E851	E937.0	E950.1	E962.0	E980.1
Phenobarbitone	967.0	E851	E937.0	E950.1	E962.0	E980.1
Phenoctide	976.0	E858.7	E946.0	E950.4	E962.0	E980.4
Phenol (derivatives) NEC	983.0	E864.0	—	E950.7	E962.1	E980.6
disinfectant	983.0	E864.0	—	E950.7	E962.1	E980.6
pesticide	989.4	E863.4	—	E950.6	E962.1	E980.7
red	977.8	E858.8	E947.8	E950.4	E962.0	E980.4
Phenolphthalein	973.1	E858.4	E943.1	E950.4	E962.0	E980.4
Phenolsulfonphthalein	977.8	E858.8	E947.8	E950.4	E962.0	E980.4

Table of Drugs and Chemicals — Placental extract

	Poisoning	External Cause (E-Code)				
		Accident	Therapeutic Use	Suicide Attempt	Assault	Undetermined
Phenomorphan	965.09	E850.2	E935.2	E950.0	E962.0	E980.0
Phenonyl	967.0	E851	E937.0	E950.1	E962.0	E980.1
Phenoperidine	965.09	E850.2	E935.2	E950.0	E962.0	E980.0
Phenoquin	974.7	E858.5	E944.7	E950.4	E962.0	E980.4
Phenothiazines (tranquilizers) NEC	969.1	E853.0	E939.1	E950.3	E962.0	E980.3
insecticide	989.3	E863.4	—	E950.6	E962.1	E980.7
Phenoxybenzamine	971.3	E855.6	E941.3	E950.4	E962.0	E980.4
Phenoxymethyl penicillin	960.0	E856	E930.0	E950.4	E962.0	E980.4
Phenprocoumon	964.2	E858.2	E934.2	E950.4	E962.0	E980.4
Phensuximide	966.2	E855.0	E936.2	E950.4	E962.0	E980.4
Phentermine	977.0	E858.8	E947.0	E950.4	E962.0	E980.4
Phentolamine	971.3	E855.6	E941.3	E950.4	E962.0	E980.4
Phenyl						
butazone	965.5	E850.5	E935.5	E950.0	E962.0	E980.0
enediamine	983.0	E864.0	—	E950.7	E962.1	E980.6
hydrazine	983.0	E864.0	—	E950.7	E962.1	E980.6
antineoplastic	963.1	E858.1	E933.1	E950.4	E962.0	E980.4
mercuric compounds — see Mercury						
salicylate	976.3	E858.7	E946.3	E950.4	E962.0	E980.4
Phenylephrin	971.2	E855.5	E941.2	E950.4	E962.0	E980.4
Phenylethylbiguanide	962.3	E858.0	E932.3	E950.4	E962.0	E980.4
Phenylpropanolamine	971.2	E855.5	E941.2	E950.4	E962.0	E980.4
Phenylsulfthion	989.3	E863.1	—	E950.6	E962.1	E980.7
Phenyramidol, phenyramidon	965.7	E850.7	E935.7	E950.0	E962.0	E980.0
Phenytoin	966.1	E855.0	E936.1	E950.4	E962.0	E980.4
pHisoHex	976.2	E858.7	E946.2	E950.4	E962.0	E980.4
Pholcodine	965.09	E850.2	E935.2	E950.0	E962.0	E980.0
Phorate	989.3	E863.1	—	E950.6	E962.1	E980.7
Phosdrin	989.3	E863.1	—	E950.6	E962.1	E980.7
Phosgene (gas)	987.8	E869.8	—	E952.8	E962.2	E982.8
Phosphate (tricresyl)	989.89	E866.8	—	E950.9	E962.1	E980.9
organic	989.3	E863.1	—	E950.6	E962.1	E980.7
solvent	982.8	E862.4	—	E950.9	E926.1	E980.9
Phosphine	987.8	E869.8	—	E952.8	E962.2	E982.8
fumigant	987.8	E863.8	—	E950.6	E962.2	E980.7
Phospholine	971.0	E855.3	E941.0	E950.4	E962.0	E980.4
Phosphoric acid	983.1	E864.1	—	E950.7	E962.1	E980.6
Phosphorus (compounds) NEC	983.9	E864.3	—	E950.7	E962.1	E980.6
rodenticide	983.9	E863.7	—	E950.7	E962.1	E980.6
Phthalimidoglutarimide	967.8	E852.8	E937.8	E950.2	E962.0	E980.2
Phthalylsulfathiazole	961.1	E857	E931.0	E950.4	E962.0	E980.4
Phylloquinone	964.3	E858.2	E934.3	E950.4	E962.0	E980.4
Physeptone	965.02	E850.1	E935.1	E950.0	E962.0	E980.0
Physostigma venenosum	988.2	E865.4	—	E950.9	E962.1	E980.9
Physostigmine	971.0	E855.3	E941.0	E950.4	E962.0	E980.4
Phytolacca decandra	988.2	E865.4	—	E950.9	E962.1	E980.9
Phytomenadione	964.3	E858.2	E934.3	E950.4	E962.0	E980.4
Phytonadione	964.3	E858.2	E934.3	E950.4	E962.0	E980.4
Picric (acid)	983.0	E864.0	—	E950.7	E962.1	E980.6
Picrotoxin	970.0	E854.3	E940.0	E950.4	E962.0	E980.4
Pilocarpine	971.0	E855.3	E941.0	E950.4	E962.0	E980.4
Pilocarpus (jaborandi) extract	971.0	E855.3	E941.0	E950.4	E962.0	E980.4
Pimaricin	960.1	E856	E930.1	E950.4	E962.0	E980.4
Piminodine	965.09	E850.2	E935.2	E950.0	E962.0	E980.0
Pine oil, pinesol (disinfectant)	983.9	E861.4	—	E950.7	E962.1	E980.6
Pinkroot	961.6	E857	E931.6	E950.4	E962.0	E980.4
Pipadone	965.09	E850.2	E935.2	E950.0	E962.0	E980.0
Pipamazine	963.0	E858.1	E933.0	E950.4	E962.0	E980.4
Pipazethate	975.4	E858.6	E945.4	E950.4	E962.0	E980.4
Pipenzolate	971.1	E855.4	E941.1	E950.4	E962.0	E980.4
Piperacetazine	969.1	E853.0	E939.1	E950.3	E962.0	E980.3
Piperazine NEC	961.6	E857	E931.6	E950.4	E962.0	E980.4
estrone sulfate	962.2	E858.0	E932.2	E950.4	E962.0	E980.4
Piper cubeba	988.2	E865.4	—	E950.9	E962.1	E980.9
Piperidione	975.4	E858.6	E945.4	E950.4	E962.0	E980.4
Piperidolate	971.1	E855.4	E941.1	E950.4	E962.0	E980.4
Piperocaine	968.9	E855.2	E938.9	E950.4	E962.0	E980.4
infiltration (subcutaneous)	968.5	E855.2	E938.5	E950.4	E962.0	E980.4
nerve block (peripheral) (plexus)	968.6	E855.2	E938.6	E950.4	E962.0	E980.4
topical (surface)	968.5	E855.2	E938.5	E950.4	E962.0	E980.4
Pipobroman	963.1	E858.1	E933.1	E950.4	E962.0	E980.4
Pipradrol	970.8	E854.3	E940.8	E950.4	E962.0	E980.4
Piscidia (bark) (erythrina)	965.7	E850.7	E935.7	E950.0	E962.0	E980.0
Pitch	983.0	E864.0	—	E950.7	E962.1	E980.6
Pitkin's solution	968.7	E855.2	E938.7	E950.4	E962.0	E980.4
Pitocin	975.0	E858.6	E945.0	E950.4	E962.0	E980.4
Pitressin (tannate)	962.5	E858.0	E932.5	E950.4	E962.0	E980.4
Pituitary extracts (posterior)	962.5	E858.0	E932.5	E950.4	E962.0	E980.4
anterior	962.4	E858.0	E932.4	E950.4	E962.0	E980.4
Pituitrin	962.5	E858.0	E932.5	E950.4	E962.0	E980.4
Placental extract	962.9	E858.0	E932.9	E950.4	E962.0	E980.4

Placidyl

Table of Drugs and Chemicals

		External Cause (E-Code)				
	Poisoning	Accident	Therapeutic Use	Suicide Attempt	Assault	Undetermined
Placidyl	967.8	E852.8	E937.8	E950.2	E962.0	E980.2
Plague vaccine	978.3	E858.8	E948.3	E950.4	E962.0	E980.4
Plant foods or fertilizers NEC	989.89	E866.5	—	E950.9	E962.1	E980.9
mixed with herbicides	989.4	E863.5	—	E950.6	E962.1	E980.7
Plants, noxious, used as food	988.2	E865.9	—	E950.9	E962.1	E980.9
berries and seeds	988.2	E865.3	—	E950.9	E962.1	E980.9
specified type NEC	988.2	E865.4	—	E950.9	E962.1	E980.9
Plasma (blood)	964.7	E858.2	E934.7	E950.4	E962.0	E980.4
expanders	964.8	E858.2	E934.8	E950.4	E962.0	E980.4
Plasmanate	964.7	E858.2	E934.7	E950.4	E962.0	E980.4
Plegicil	969.1	E853.0	E939.1	E950.3	E962.0	E980.3
Podophyllin	976.4	E858.7	E946.4	E950.4	E962.0	E980.4
Podophyllum resin	976.4	E858.7	E946.4	E950.4	E962.0	E980.4
Poison NEC	989.9	E866.9	—	E950.9	E962.1	E980.9
Poisonous berries	988.2	E865.3	—	E950.9	E962.1	E980.9
Pokeweed (any part)	988.2	E865.4	—	E950.9	E962.1	E980.9
Poldine	971.1	E855.4	E941.1	E950.4	E962.0	E980.4
Poliomyelitis vaccine	979.5	E858.8	E949.5	E950.4	E962.0	E980.4
Poliovirus vaccine	979.5	E858.8	E949.5	E950.4	E962.0	E980.4
Polish (car) (floor) (furniture) (metal) (silver)	989.89	E861.2	—	E950.9	E962.1	E980.9
abrasive	989.89	E861.3	—	E950.9	E962.1	E980.9
porcelain	989.89	E861.3	—	E950.9	E962.1	E980.9
Poloxalkol	973.2	E858.4	E943.2	E950.4	E962.0	E980.4
Polyaminostyrene resins	974.5	E858.5	E944.5	E950.4	E962.0	E980.4
Polychlorinated biphenyl — see PCBs						
Polycycline	960.4	E856	E930.4	E950.4	E962.0	E980.4
Polyester resin hardener	982.8	E862.4	—	E950.9	E962.1	E980.9
fumes	987.8	E869.8	—	E952.8	E962.2	E982.8
Polyestradiol (phosphate)	962.2	E858.0	E932.2	E950.4	E962.0	E980.4
Polyethanolamine alkyl sulfate	976.2	E858.7	E946.2	E950.4	E962.0	E980.4
Polyethylene glycol	976.3	E858.7	E946.3	E950.4	E962.0	E980.4
Polyferose	964.0	E858.2	E934.0	E950.4	E962.0	E980.4
Polymyxin B	960.8	E856	E930.8	E950.4	E962.0	E980.4
ENT agent	976.6	E858.7	E946.6	E950.4	E962.0	E980.4
ophthalmic preparation	976.5	E858.7	E946.5	E950.4	E962.0	E980.4
topical NEC	976.0	E858.7	E946.0	E950.4	E962.0	E980.4
Polynoxylin(e)	976.0	E858.7	E946.0	E950.4	E962.0	E980.4
Polyoxymethyleneurea	976.0	E858.7	E946.0	E950.4	E962.0	E980.4
Polytetrafluoroethylene (inhaled)	987.8	E869.8	—	E952.8	E962.2	E982.8
Polythiazide	974.3	E858.5	E944.3	E950.4	E962.0	E980.4
Polyvinylpyrrolidone	964.8	E858.2	E934.8	E950.4	E962.0	E980.4
Pontocaine (hydrochloride) (infiltration) (topical)	968.5	E855.2	E938.5	E950.4	E962.0	E980.4
nerve block (peripheral) (plexus)	968.6	E855.2	E938.6	E950.4	E962.0	E980.4
spinal	968.7	E855.2	E938.7	E950.4	E962.0	E980.4
Pot	969.6	E854.1	E939.6	E950.3	E962.0	E980.3
Potash (caustic)	983.2	E864.2	—	E950.7	E962.1	E980.6
Potassic saline injection (lactated)	974.5	E858.5	E944.5	E950.4	E962.0	E980.4
Potassium (salts) NEC	974.5	E858.5	E944.5	E950.4	E962.0	E980.4
aminosalicylate	961.8	E857	E931.8	E950.4	E962.0	E980.4
arsenite (solution)	985.1	E866.3	—	E950.8	E962.1	E980.8
bichromate	983.9	E864.3	—	E950.7	E962.1	E980.6
bisulfate	983.9	E864.3	—	E950.7	E962.1	E980.6
bromide (medicinal) NEC	967.3	E852.2	E937.3	E950.2	E962.0	E980.2
carbonate	983.2	E864.2	—	E950.7	E962.1	E980.6
chlorate NEC	983.9	E864.3	—	E950.7	E962.1	E980.6
cyanide — see Cyanide						
hydroxide	983.2	E864.2	—	E950.7	E962.1	E980.6
iodide (expectorant) NEC	975.5	E858.6	E945.5	E950.4	E962.0	E980.4
nitrate	989.89	E866.8	—	E950.9	E962.1	E980.9
oxalate	983.9	E864.3	—	E950.7	E962.1	E980.6
perchlorate NEC	977.8	E858.8	E947.8	E950.4	E962.0	E980.4
antithyroid	962.8	E858.0	E932.8	E950.4	E962.0	E980.4
permanganate	976.0	E858.7	E946.0	E950.4	E962.0	E980.4
nonmedicinal	983.9	E864.3	—	E950.7	E962.1	E980.6
Povidone-iodine (anti-infective) NEC	976.0	E858.7	E946.0	E950.4	E962.0	E980.4
Practolol	972.0	E858.3	E942.0	E950.4	E962.0	E980.4
Pralidoxime (chloride)	977.2	E858.8	E947.2	E950.4	E962.0	E980.4
Pramoxine	968.5	E855.2	E938.5	E950.4	E962.0	E980.4
Prazosin	972.6	E858.3	E942.6	E950.4	E962.0	E980.4
Prednisolone	962.0	E858.0	E932.0	E950.4	E962.0	E980.4
ENT agent	976.6	E858.7	E946.6	E950.4	E962.0	E980.4
ophthalmic preparation	976.5	E858.7	E946.5	E950.4	E962.0	E980.4
topical NEC	976.0	E858.7	E946.0	E950.4	E962.0	E980.4
Prednisone	962.0	E858.0	E932.0	E950.4	E962.0	E980.4
Pregnanediol	962.2	E858.0	E932.2	E950.4	E962.0	E980.4
Pregneninolone	962.2	E858.0	E932.2	E950.4	E962.0	E980.4
Preludin	977.0	E858.8	E947.0	E950.4	E962.0	E980.4
Premarin	962.2	E858.0	E932.2	E950.4	E962.0	E980.4
Prenylamine	972.4	E858.3	E942.4	E950.4	E962.0	E980.4
Preparation H	976.8	E858.7	E946.8	E950.4	E962.0	E980.4
Preservatives	989.89	E866.8	—	E950.9	E962.1	E980.9

Table of Drugs and Chemicals

		External Cause (E-Code)				
	Poisoning	Accident	Therapeutic Use	Suicide Attempt	Assault	Undetermined
Pride of China	988.2	E865.3	—	E950.9	E962.1	E980.9
Prilocaine	968.9	E855.2	E938.9	E950.4	E962.0	E980.4
infiltration (subcutaneous)	968.5	E855.2	E938.5	E950.4	E962.0	E980.4
nerve block (peripheral) (plexus)	968.6	E855.2	E938.6	E950.4	E962.0	E980.4
Primaquine	961.4	E857	E931.4	E950.4	E962.0	E980.4
Primidone	966.3	E855.0	E936.3	E950.4	E962.0	E980.4
Primula (veris)	988.2	E865.4	—	E950.9	E962.1	E980.9
Prinadol	965.09	E850.2	E935.2	E950.0	E962.0	E980.0
Priscol, Priscoline	971.3	E855.6	E941.3	E950.4	E962.0	E980.4
Privet	988.2	E865.4	—	E950.9	E962.1	E980.9
Privine	971.2	E855.5	E941.2	E950.4	E962.0	E980.4
Pro-Banthine	971.1	E855.4	E941.1	E950.4	E962.0	E980.4
Probarbitol	967.0	E851	E937.0	E950.1	E962.0	E980.1
Probenecid	974.7	E858.5	E944.7	E950.4	E962.0	E980.4
Procainamide (hydrochloride)	972.0	E858.3	E942.0	E950.4	E962.0	E980.4
Procaine (hydrochloride) (infiltration) (topical)	968.5	E855.2	E938.5	E950.4	E962.0	E980.4
nerve block (peripheral) (plexus)	968.6	E855.2	E938.6	E950.4	E962.0	E980.4
penicillin G	960.0	E856	E930.0	E950.4	E962.0	E980.4
spinal	968.7	E855.2	E938.7	E950.4	E962.0	E980.4
Procalmidol	969.5	E853.8	E939.5	E950.3	E962.0	E980.3
Procarbazine	963.1	E858.1	E933.1	E950.4	E962.0	E980.4
Prochlorperazine	969.1	E853.0	E939.1	E950.3	E962.0	E980.3
Procyclidine	966.4	E855.0	E936.4	E950.4	E962.0	E980.4
Producer gas	986	E868.8	—	E952.1	E962.2	E982.1
Profenamine	966.4	E855.0	E936.4	E950.4	E962.0	E980.4
Profenil	975.1	E858.6	E945.1	E950.4	E962.0	E980.4
Progesterones	962.2	E858.0	E932.2	E950.4	E962.0	E980.4
Progestin	962.2	E858.0	E932.2	E950.4	E962.0	E980.4
Progestogens (with estrogens)	962.2	E858.0	E932.2	E950.4	E962.0	E980.4
Progestone	962.2	E858.0	E932.2	E950.4	E962.0	E980.4
Proguanil	961.4	E857	E931.4	E950.4	E962.0	E980.4
Prolactin	962.4	E858.0	E932.4	E950.4	E962.0	E980.4
Proloid	962.7	E858.0	E932.7	E950.4	E962.0	E980.4
Proluton	962.2	E858.0	E932.2	E950.4	E962.0	E980.4
Promacetin	961.8	E857	E931.8	E950.4	E962.0	E980.4
Promazine	969.1	E853.0	E939.1	E950.3	E962.0	E980.3
Promedol	965.09	E850.2	E935.2	E950.0	E962.0	E980.0
Promethazine	967.8	E852.8	E937.8	E950.2	E962.0	E980.2
Promin	961.8	E857	E931.8	E950.4	E962.0	E980.4
Pronestyl (hydrochloride)	972.0	E858.3	E942.0	E950.4	E962.0	E980.4
Pronetalol, pronethalol	972.0	E858.3	E942.0	E950.4	E962.0	E980.4
Prontosil	961.0	E857	E931.0	E950.4	E962.0	E980.4
Propamidine isethionate	961.5	E857	E931.5	E950.4	E962.0	E980.4
Propanal (medicinal)	967.8	E852.8	E937.8	E950.2	E962.0	E980.2
Propane (gas) (distributed in mobile container)	987.0	E868.0	—	E951.1	E962.2	E981.1
distributed through pipes	987.0	E867	—	E951.0	E962.2	E981.0
incomplete combustion of — see Carbon monoxide, Propane						
Propanidid	968.3	E855.1	E938.3	E950.4	E962.0	E980.4
Propanol	980.3	E860.4	—	E950.9	E962.1	E980.9
Propantheline	971.1	E855.4	E941.1	E950.4	E962.0	E980.4
Proparacaine	968.5	E855.2	E938.5	E950.4	E962.0	E980.4
Propatyl nitrate	972.4	E858.3	E942.4	E950.4	E962.0	E980.4
Propicillin	960.0	E856	E930.0	E950.4	E962.0	E980.4
Propiolactone (vapor)	987.8	E869.8	—	E952.8	E962.2	E982.8
Propiomazine	967.8	E852.8	E937.8	E950.2	E962.0	E980.2
Propionaldehyde (medicinal)	967.8	E852.8	E937.8	E950.2	E962.0	E980.2
Propionate compound	976.0	E858.7	E946.0	E950.4	E962.0	E980.4
Propion gel	976.0	E858.7	E946.0	E950.4	E962.0	E980.4
Propitocaine	968.9	E855.2	E938.9	E950.4	E962.0	E980.4
infiltration (subcutaneous)	968.5	E855.2	E938.5	E950.4	E962.0	E980.4
nerve block (peripheral) (plexus)	968.6	E855.2	E938.6	E950.4	E962.0	E980.4
Propoxur	989.3	E863.2	—	E950.6	E962.1	E980.7
Propoxycaine	968.9	E855.2	E938.9	E950.4	E962.0	E980.4
infiltration (subcutaneous)	968.5	E855.2	E938.5	E950.4	E962.0	E980.4
nerve block (peripheral) (plexus)	968.6	E855.2	E938.6	E950.4	E962.0	E980.4
topical (surface)	968.5	E855.2	E938.5	E950.4	E962.0	E980.4
Propoxyphene (hydrochloride)	965.8	E850.8	E935.8	E950.0	E962.0	E980.0
Propranolol	972.0	E858.3	E942.0	E950.4	E962.0	E980.4
Propyl						
alcohol	980.3	E860.4	—	E950.9	E962.1	E980.9
carbinol	980.3	E860.4	—	E950.9	E962.1	E980.9
hexadrine	971.2	E855.5	E941.2	E950.4	E962.0	E980.4
iodone	977.8	E858.8	E947.8	E950.4	E962.0	E980.4
thiouracil	962.8	E858.0	E932.8	E950.4	E962.0	E980.4
Propylene	987.1	E869.8	—	E952.8	E962.2	E982.8
Propylparaben (ophthalmic)	976.5	E858.7	E946.5	E950.4	E962.0	E980.4
Proscillaridin	972.1	E858.3	E942.1	E950.4	E962.0	E980.4
Prostaglandins	975.0	E858.6	E945.0	E950.4	E962.0	E980.4
Prostigmin	971	E855.3	E941.0	E950.4	E962.0	E980.4
Protamine (sulfate)	964.5	E858.2	E934.5	E950.4	E962.0	E980.4
zinc insulin	962.3	E858.0	E932.3	E950.4	E962.0	E980.4

Protectants

Table of Drugs and Chemicals

	Poisoning	External Cause (E-Code)				
		Accident	Therapeutic Use	Suicide Attempt	Assault	Undetermined
Protectants (topical)	976.3	E858.7	E946.3	E950.4	E962.0	E980.4
Protein hydrolysate	974.5	E858.5	E944.5	E950.4	E962.0	E980.4
Prothiaden — see Dothiepin hydrochloride						
Prothionamide	961.8	E857	E931.8	E950.4	E962.0	E980.4
Prothipendyl	969.5	E853.8	E939.5	E950.3	E962.0	E980.3
Protokylol	971.2	E855.5	E941.2	E950.4	E962.0	E980.4
Protopam	977.2	E858.8	E947.2	E950.4	E962.0	E980.4
Protoveratrine(s) (A) (B)	972.6	E858.3	E942.6	E950.4	E962.0	E980.4
Protriptyline	969.0	E854.0	E939.0	E950.3	E962.0	E980.3
Provera	962.2	E858.0	E932.2	E950.4	E962.0	E980.4
Provitamin A	963.5	E858.1	E933.5	E950.4	E962.0	E980.4
Proxymetacaine	968.5	E855.2	E938.5	E950.4	E962.0	E980.4
Proxyphylline	975.1	E858.6	E945.1	E950.4	E962.0	E980.4
Prozac — see Fluoxetine hydrochloride						
Prunus						
laurocerasus	988.2	E865.4	—	E950.9	E962.1	E980.9
virginiana	988.2	E865.4	—	E950.9	E962.1	E980.9
Prussic acid	989.0	E866.8	—	E950.9	E962.1	E980.9
vapor	987.7	E869.8	—	E952.8	E962.2	E982.8
Pseudoephedrine	971.2	E855.5	E941.2	E950.4	E962.0	E980.4
Psilocin	969.6	E854.1	E939.6	E950.3	E962.0	E980.3
Psilocybin	969.6	E854.1	E939.6	E950.3	E962.0	E980.3
PSP	977.8	E858.8	E947.8	E950.4	E962.0	E980.4
Psychedelic agents	969.6	E854.1	E939.6	E950.3	E962.0	E980.3
Psychodysleptics	969.6	E854.1	E939.6	E950.3	E962.0	E980.3
Psychostimulants	969.7	E854.2	E939.7	E950.3	E962.0	E980.3
Psychotherapeutic agents	969.9	E855.9	E939.9	E950.3	E962.0	E980.3
antidepressants	969.0	E854.0	E939.0	E950.3	E962.0	E980.3
specified NEC	969.8	E855.8	E939.8	E950.3	E962.0	E980.3
tranquilizers NEC	969.5	E853.9	E939.5	E950.3	E962.0	E980.3
Psychotomimetic agents	969.6	E854.1	E939.6	E950.3	E962.0	E980.3
Psychotropic agents	969.9	E854.8	E939.3	E950.3	E962.0	E980.3
specified NEC	969.8	E854.8	E939.8	E950.3	E962.0	E980.3
Psyllium	973.3	E858.4	E943.3	E950.4	E962.0	E980.4
Pteroylglutamic acid	964.1	E858.2	E934.1	E950.4	E962.0	E980.4
Pteroyltriglutamate	963.1	E858.1	E933.1	E950.4	E962.0	E980.4
PTFE	987.8	E869.8	—	E952.8	E962.2	E982.8
Pulsatilla	988.2	E865.4	—	E950.9	E962.1	E980.9
Purex (bleach)	983.9	E864.3	—	E950.7	E962.1	E980.6
Purine diuretics	974.1	E858.5	E944.1	E950.4	E962.0	E980.4
Purinethol	963.1	E858.1	E933.1	E950.4	E962.0	E980.4
PVP	964.8	E858.2	E934.8	E950.4	E962.0	E980.4
Pyrabital	965.7	E850.7	E935.7	E950.0	E962.0	E980.0
Pyramidon	965.5	E850.5	E935.5	E950.0	E962.0	E980.0
Pyrantel (pamoate)	961.6	E857	E931.6	E950.4	E962.0	E980.4
Pyrathiazine	963.0	E858.1	E933.0	E950.4	E962.0	E980.4
Pyrazinamide	961.8	E857	E931.8	E950.4	E962.0	E980.4
Pyrazinoic acid (amide)	961.8	E857	E931.8	E950.4	E962.0	E980.4
Pyrazole (derivatives)	965.5	E850.5	E935.5	E950.0	E962.0	E980.0
Pyrazolone (analgesics)	965.5	E850.5	E935.5	E950.0	E962.0	E980.0
Pyrethrins, pyrethrum	989.4	E863.4	—	E950.6	E962.1	E980.7
Pyribenzamine	963.0	E858.1	E933.0	E950.4	E962.0	E980.4
Pyridine (liquid) (vapor)	982.0	E862.4	—	E950.9	E962.1	E980.9
aldoxime chloride	977.2	E858.8	E947.2	E950.4	E962.0	E980.4
Pyridium	976.1	E858.7	E946.1	E950.4	E962.0	E980.4
Pyridostigmine	971.0	E855.3	E941.0	E950.4	E962.0	E980.4
Pyridoxine	963.5	E858.1	E933.5	E950.4	E962.0	E980.4
Pyrilamine	963.0	E858.1	E933.0	E950.4	E962.0	E980.4
Pyrimethamine	961.4	E857	E931.4	E950.4	E962.0	E980.4
Pyrogallic acid	983.0	E864.0	—	E950.7	E962.1	E980.6
Pyroxylin	976.3	E858.7	E946.3	E950.4	E962.0	E980.4
Pyrrobutamine	963.0	E858.1	E933.0	E950.4	E962.0	E980.4
Pyrrocitine	968.5	E855.2	E938.5	E950.4	E962.0	E980.4
Pyrvinium (pamoate)	961.6	E857	E931.6	E950.4	E962.0	E980.4
PZI	962.3	E858.0	E932.3	E950.4	E962.0	E980.4
Quaalude	967.4	E852.3	E937.4	E950.2	E962.0	E980.2
Quaternary ammonium derivatives	971.1	E855.4	E941.1	E950.4	E962.0	E980.4
Quicklime	983.2	E864.2	—	E950.7	E962.1	E980.6
Quinacrine	961.3	E857	E931.3	E950.4	E962.0	E980.4
Quinaglute	972.0	E858.3	E942.0	E950.4	E962.0	E980.4
Quinalbarbitone	967.0	E851	E937.0	E950.1	E962.0	E980.1
Quinestradiol	962.2	E858.0	E932.2	E950.4	E962.0	E980.4
Quinethazone	974.3	E858.5	E944.3	E950.4	E962.0	E980.4
Quinidine (gluconate) (polygalacturonate) (salts) (sulfate)	972.0	E858.3	E942.0	E950.4	E962.0	E980.4
Quinine	961.4	E857	E931.4	E950.4	E962.0	E980.4
Quiniobine	961.3	E857	E931.3	E950.4	E962.0	E980.4
Quinolines	961.3	E857	E931.3	E950.4	E962.0	E980.4
Quotane	968.5	E855.2	E938.5	E950.4	E962.0	E980.4
Rabies						
immune globulin (human)	964.6	E858.2	E934.6	E950.4	E962.0	E980.4
vaccine	979.1	E858.8	E949.1	E950.4	E962.0	E980.4

Table of Drugs and Chemicals — Salicylic acid

	Poisoning	External Cause (E-Code)				
		Accident	Therapeutic Use	Suicide Attempt	Assault	Undetermined
Racemoramide	965.09	E850.2	E935.2	E950.0	E962.0	E980.0
Racemorphan	965.09	E850.2	E935.2	E950.0	E962.0	E980.0
Radiator alcohol	980.1	E860.2	—	E950.9	E962.1	E980.9
Radio-opaque (drugs) (materials)	977.8	E858.8	E947.8	E950.4	E962.0	E980.4
Ranunculus	988.2	E865.4	—	E950.9	E962.1	E980.9
Rat poison	989.4	E863.7	—	E950.6	E962.1	E980.7
Rattlesnake (venom)	989.5	E905.0	—	E950.9	E962.1	E980.9
Raudixin	972.6	E858.3	E942.6	E950.4	E962.0	E980.4
Rautensin	972.6	E858.3	E942.6	E950.4	E962.0	E980.4
Rautina	972.6	E858.3	E942.6	E950.4	E962.0	E980.4
Rautotal	972.6	E858.3	E942.6	E950.4	E962.0	E980.4
Rauwiloid	972.6	E858.3	E942.6	E950.4	E962.0	E980.4
Rauwoldin	972.6	E858.3	E942.6	E950.4	E962.0	E980.4
Rauwolfia (alkaloids)	972.6	E858.3	E942.6	E950.4	E962.0	E980.4
Realgar	985.1	E866.3	—	E950.8	E962.1	E980.8
Red cells, packed	964.7	E858.2	E934.7	E950.4	E962.0	E980.4
Reducing agents, industrial NEC	983.9	E864.3	—	E950.7	E962.1	E980.6
Refrigerant gas (freon)	987.4	E869.2	—	E952.8	E962.2	E982.8
not freon	987.9	E869.9	—	E952.9	E962.2	E982.9
Regroton	974.4	E858.5	E944.4	E950.4	E962.0	E980.4
Rela	968.0	E855.1	E938.0	E950.4	E962.0	E980.4
Relaxants, skeletal muscle (autonomic)	975.2	E858.6	E945.2	E950.4	E962.0	E980.4
central nervous system	968.0	E855.1	E938.0	E950.4	E962.0	E980.4
Renese	974.3	E858.5	E944.3	E950.4	E962.0	E980.4
Renografin	977.8	E858.8	E947.8	E950.4	E962.0	E980.4
Replacement solutions	974.5	E858.5	E944.5	E950.4	E962.0	E980.4
Rescinnamine	972.6	E858.3	E942.6	E950.4	E962.0	E980.4
Reserpine	972.6	E858.3	E942.6	E950.4	E962.0	E980.4
Resorcin, resorcinol	976.4	E858.7	E946.4	E950.4	E962.0	E980.4
Respaire	975.5	E858.6	E945.5	E950.4	E962.0	E980.4
Respiratory agents NEC	975.8	E858.6	E945.8	E950.4	E962.0	E980.4
Retinoic acid	976.8	E858.7	E946.8	E950.4	E962.0	E980.4
Retinol	963.5	E858.1	E933.5	E950.4	E962.0	E980.4
Rh (D) immune globulin (human)	964.6	E858.2	E934.6	E950.4	E962.0	E980.4
Rhodine	965.1	E850.3	E935.3	E950.0	E962.0	E980.0
RhoGAM	964.6	E858.2	E934.6	E950.4	E962.0	E980.4
Riboflavin	963.5	E858.1	E933.5	E950.4	E962.0	E980.4
Ricin	989.89	E866.8	—	E950.9	E962.1	E980.9
Ricinus communis	988.2	E865.3	—	E950.9	E962.1	E980.9
Rickettsial vaccine NEC	979.6	E858.8	E949.6	E950.4	E962.0	E980.4
with viral and bacterial vaccine	979.7	E858.8	E949.7	E950.4	E962.0	E980.4
Rifampin	960.6	E856	E930.6	E950.4	E962.0	E980.4
Rimifon	961.8	E857	E931.8	E950.4	E962.0	E980.4
Ringer's injection (lactated)	974.5	E858.5	E944.5	E950.4	E962.0	E980.4
Ristocetin	960.8	E856	E930.8	E950.4	E962.0	E980.4
Ritalin	969.7	E854.2	E939.7	E950.3	E962.0	E980.3
Roach killers — see Pesticides						
Rocky Mountain spotted fever vaccine	979.6	E858.8	E949.6	E950.4	E962.0	E980.4
Rodenticides	989.4	E863.7	—	E950.6	E962.1	E980.7
Rohypnol	969.4	E853.2	E939.4	E950.3	E962.0	E980.3 ▲
Rolaids	973.0	E858.4	E943.0	E950.4	E962.0	E980.4
Rolitetracycline	960.4	E856	E930.4	E950.4	E962.0	E980.4
Romilar	975.4	E858.6	E945.4	E950.4	E962.0	E980.4
Rose water ointment	976.3	E858.7	E946.3	E950.4	E962.0	E980.4
Rotenone	989.4	E863.7	—	E950.6	E962.1	E980.7
Rotoxamine	963.0	E858.1	E933.0	E950.4	E962.0	E980.4
Rough-on-rats	989.4	E863.7	—	E950.6	E962.1	E980.7
RU486	962.9	E858.0	E932.9	E950.4	E962.0	E980.4
Rubbing alcohol	980.2	E860.3	—	E950.9	E962.1	E980.9
Rubella virus vaccine	979.4	E858.8	E949.4	E950.4	E962.0	E980.4
Rubelogen	979.4	E858.8	E949.4	E950.4	E962.0	E980.4
Rubeovax	979.4	E858.8	E949.4	E950.4	E962.0	E980.4
Rubidomycin	960.7	E856	E930.7	E950.4	E962.0	E980.4
Rue	988.2	E865.4	—	E950.9	E962.1	E980.9
Ruta	988.2	E865.4	—	E950.9	E962.1	E980.9
Sabadilla (medicinal)	976.0	E858.7	E946.0	E950.4	E962.0	E980.4
pesticide	989.4	E863.4	—	E950.6	E962.1	E980.7
Sabin oral vaccine	979.5	E858.8	E949.5	E950.4	E962.0	E980.4
Saccharated iron oxide	964.0	E858.2	E934.0	E950.4	E962.0	E980.4
Saccharin	974.5	E858.5	E944.5	E950.4	E962.0	E980.4
Safflower oil	972.2	E858.3	E942.2	E950.4	E962.0	E980.4
Salbutamol sulfate	975.7	E858.6	E945.7	E950.4	E962.0	E980.4
Salicylamide	965.1	E850.3	E935.3	E950.0	E962.0	E980.0
Salicylate(s)	965.1	E850.3	E935.3	E950.0	E962.0	E980.0
methyl	976.3	E858.7	E946.3	E950.4	E962.0	E980.4
theobromine calcium	974.1	E858.5	E944.1	E950.4	E962.0	E980.4
Salicylazosulfapyridine	961.0	E857	E931.0	E950.4	E962.0	E980.4
Salicylhydroxamic acid	976.0	E858.7	E946.0	E950.4	E962.0	E980.4
Salicylic acid (keratolytic) NEC	976.4	E858.7	E946.4	E950.4	E962.0	E980.4
congeners	965.1	E850.3	E935.3	E950.0	E962.0	E980.0
salts	965.1	E850.3	E935.3	E950.0	E962.0	E980.0

Table of Drugs and Chemicals

		External Cause (E-Code)				
	Poisoning	Accident	Therapeutic Use	Suicide Attempt	Assault	Undetermined
Saliniazid	961.8	E857	E931.8	E950.4	E962.0	E980.4
Salol	976.3	E858.7	E946.3	E950.4	E962.0	E980.4
Salt (substitute) NEC	974.5	E858.5	E944.5	E950.4	E962.0	E980.4
Saluretics	974.3	E858.5	E944.3	E950.4	E962.0	E980.4
Saluron	974.3	E858.5	E944.3	E950.4	E962.0	E980.4
Salvarsan 606 (neosilver) (silver)	961.1	E857	E931.1	E950.4	E962.0	E980.4
Sambucus canadensis	988.2	E865.4	—	E950.9	E962.1	E980.9
berry	988.2	E865.3	—	E950.9	E962.1	E980.9
Sandril	972.6	E858.3	E942.6	E950.4	E962.0	E980.4
Sanguinaria canadensis	988.2	E865.4	—	E950.9	E962.1	E980.9
Saniflush (cleaner)	983.9	E861.3	—	E950.7	E962.1	E980.6
Santonin	961.6	E857	E931.6	E950.4	E962.0	E980.4
Santyl	976.8	E858.7	E946.8	E950.4	E962.0	E980.4
Sarkomycin	960.7	E856	E930.7	E950.4	E962.0	E980.4
Saroten	969.0	E854.0	E939.0	E950.3	E962.0	E980.3
Saturnine — see Lead						
Savin (oil)	976.4	E858.7	E946.4	E950.4	E962.0	E980.4
Scammony	973.1	E858.4	E943.1	E950.4	E962.0	E980.4
Scarlet red	976.8	E858.7	E946.8	E950.4	E962.0	E980.4
Scheele's green	985.1	E866.3	—	E950.8	E962.1	E980.8
insecticide	985.1	E863.4	—	E950.8	E962.1	E980.8
Schradan	989.3	E863.1	—	E950.6	E962.1	E980.7
Schweinfurt(h) green	985.1	E866.3	—	E950.8	E962.1	E980.8
insecticide	985.1	E863.4	—	E950.8	E962.1	E980.8
Scilla — see Squill						
Sclerosing agents	972.7	E858.3	E942.7	E950.4	E962.0	E980.4
Scopolamine	971.1	E855.4	E941.1	E950.4	E962.0	E980.4
Scouring powder	989.89	E861.3	—	E950.9	E962.1	E980.9
Sea						
anemone (sting)	989.5	E905.6	—	E950.9	E962.1	E980.9
cucumber (sting)	989.5	E905.6	—	E950.9	E962.1	E980.9
snake (bite) (venom)	989.5	E905.0	—	E950.9	E962.1	E980.9
urchin spine (puncture)	989.5	E905.6	—	E950.9	E962.1	E980.9
Secbutabarbital	967.0	E851	E937.0	E950.1	E962.0	E980.1
Secbutabarbitone	967.0	E851	E937.0	E950.1	E962.0	E980.1
Secobarbital	967.0	E851	E937.0	E950.1	E962.0	E980.1
Seconal	967.0	E851	E937.0	E950.1	E962.0	E980.1
Secretin	977.8	E858.8	E947.8	E950.4	E962.0	E980.4
Sedatives, nonbarbiturate	967.9	E852.9	E937.9	E950.2	E962.0	E980.2
specified NEC	967.8	E852.8	E937.8	E950.2	E962.0	E980.2
Sedormid	967.8	E852.8	E937.8	E950.2	E962.0	E980.2
Seed (plant)	988.2	E865.3	—	E950.9	E962.1	E980.9
disinfectant or dressing	989.89	E866.5	—	E950.9	E962.1	E980.9
Selenium (fumes) NEC	985.8	E866.4	—	E950.9	E962.1	E980.9
disulfide or sulfide	976.4	E858.7	E946.4	E950.4	E962.0	E980.4
Selsun	976.4	E858.7	E946.4	E950.4	E962.0	E980.4
Senna	973.1	E858.4	E943.1	E950.4	E962.0	E980.4
Septisol	976.2	E858.7	E946.2	E950.4	E962.0	E980.4
Serax	969.4	E853.2	E939.4	E950.3	E962.0	E980.3
Serenesil	967.8	E852.8	E937.8	E950.2	E962.0	E980.2
Serenium (hydrochloride)	961.9	E857	E931.9	E950.4	E962.0	E980.4
Sernyl	968.3	E855.1	E938.3	E950.4	E962.0	E980.4
Serotonin	977.8	E858.8	E947.8	E950.4	E962.0	E980.4
Serpasil	972.6	E858.3	E942.6	E950.4	E962.0	E980.4
Sewer gas	987.8	E869.8	—	E952.8	E962.2	E982.8
Shampoo	989.6	E861.0	—	E950.9	E962.1	E980.9
Shellfish, nonbacterial or noxious	988.0	E865.1	—	E950.9	E962.1	E980.9
Silicones NEC	989.83	E866.8	E947.8	E950.9	E962.1	E980.9
Silvadene	976.0	E858.7	E946.0	E950.4	E962.0	E980.4
Silver (compound) (medicinal) NEC	976.0	E858.7	E946.0	E950.4	E962.0	E980.4
anti-infectives	976.0	E858.7	E946.0	E950.4	E962.0	E980.4
arsphenamine	961.1	E857	E931.1	E950.4	E962.0	E980.4
nitrate	976.0	E858.7	E946.0	E950.4	E962.0	E980.4
ophthalmic preparation	976.5	E858.7	E946.5	E950.4	E962.0	E980.4
toughened (keratolytic)	976.4	E858.7	E946.4	E950.4	E962.0	E980.4
nonmedicinal (dust)	985.8	E866.4	—	E950.9	E962.1	E980.9
protein (mild) (strong)	976.0	E858.7	E946.0	E950.4	E962.0	E980.4
salvarsan	961.1	E857	E931.1	E950.4	E962.0	E980.4
Simethicone	973.8	E858.4	E943.8	E950.4	E962.0	E980.4
Sinequan	969.0	E854.0	E939.0	E950.3	E962.0	E980.3
Singoserp	972.6	E858.3	E942.6	E950.4	E962.0	E980.4
Sintrom	964.2	E858.2	E934.2	E950.4	E962.0	E980.4
Sitosterols	972.2	E858.3	E942.2	E950.4	E962.0	E980.4
Skeletal muscle relaxants	975.2	E858.6	E945.2	E950.4	E962.0	E980.4
Skin						
agents (external)	976.9	E858.7	E946.9	E950.4	E962.0	E980.4
specified NEC	976.8	E858.7	E946.8	E950.4	E962.0	E980.4
test antigen	977.8	E858.8	E947.8	E950.4	E962.0	E980.4
Sleep-eze	963.0	E858.1	E933.0	E950.4	E962.0	E980.4
Sleeping draught (drug) (pill) (tablet)	967.9	E852.9	E937.9	E950.2	E962.0	E980.2
Smallpox vaccine	979.0	E858.8	E949.0	E950.4	E962.0	E980.4

Table of Drugs and Chemicals — Sodium

	Poisoning	External Cause (E-Code)				
		Accident	Therapeutic Use	Suicide Attempt	Assault	Undetermined
Smelter fumes NEC	985.9	E866.4	—	E950.9	E962.1	E980.9
Smog	987.3	E869.1	—	E952.8	E962.2	E982.8
Smoke NEC	987.9	E869.9	—	E952.9	E962.2	E982.9
Smooth muscle relaxant	975.1	E858.6	E945.1	E950.4	E962.0	E980.4
Snail killer	989.4	E863.4	—	E950.6	E962.1	E980.7
Snake (bite) (venom)	989.5	E905.0	—	E950.9	E962.1	E980.9
Snuff	989.89	E866.8	—	E950.9	E962.1	E980.9
Soap (powder) (product)	989.6	E861.1	—	E950.9	E962.1	E980.9
medicinal, soft	976.2	E858.7	E946.2	E950.4	E962.0	E980.4
Soda (caustic)	983.2	E864.2	—	E950.7	E962.1	E980.6
bicarb	963.3	E858.1	E933.3	E950.4	E962.0	E980.4
chlorinated — see Sodium, hypochlorite						
Sodium						
acetosulfone	961.8	E857	E931.8	E950.4	E962.0	E980.4
acetrizoate	977.8	E858.8	E947.8	E950.4	E962.0	E980.4
amytal	967.0	E851	E937.0	E950.1	E962.0	E980.1
arsenate — see Arsenic						
bicarbonate	963.3	E858.1	E933.3	E950.4	E962.0	E980.4
bichromate	983.9	E864.3	—	E950.7	E962.1	E980.6
biphosphate	963.2	E858.1	E933.2	E950.4	E962.0	E980.4
bisulfate	983.9	E864.3	—	E950.7	E962.1	E980.6
borate (cleanser)	989.6	E861.3	—	E950.9	E962.1	E980.9
bromide NEC	967.3	E852.2	E937.3	E950.2	E962.0	E980.2
cacodylate (nonmedicinal) NEC	978.8	E858.8	E948.8	E950.4	E962.0	E980.4
anti-infective	961.1	E857	E931.1	E950.4	E962.0	E980.4
herbicide	989.4	E863.5	—	E950.6	E962.1	E980.7
calcium edetate	963.8	E858.1	E933.8	E950.4	E962.0	E980.4
carbonate NEC	983.2	E864.2	—	E950.7	E962.1	E980.6
chlorate NEC	983.9	E864.3	—	E950.7	E962.1	E980.6
herbicide	983.9	E863.5	—	E950.7	E962.1	E980.6
chloride NEC	974.5	E858.5	E944.5	E950.4	E962.0	E980.4
chromate	983.9	E864.3	—	E950.7	E962.1	E980.6
citrate	963.3	E858.1	E933.3	E950.4	E962.0	E980.4
cyanide — see Cyanide(s)						
cyclamate	974.5	E858.5	E944.5	E950.4	E962.0	E980.4
diatrizoate	977.8	E858.8	E947.8	E950.4	E962.0	E980.4
dibunate	975.4	E858.6	E945.4	E950.4	E962.0	E980.4
dioctyl sulfosuccinate	973.2	E858.4	E943.2	E950.4	E962.0	E980.4
edetate	963.8	E858.1	E933.8	E950.4	E962.0	E980.4
ethacrynate	974.4	E858.5	E944.4	E950.4	E962.0	E980.4
fluoracetate (dust) (rodenticide)	989.4	E863.7	—	E950.6	E962.1	E980.7
fluoride — see Fluoride(s)						
free salt	974.5	E858.5	E944.5	E950.4	E962.0	E980.4
glucosulfone	961.8	E857	E931.8	E950.4	E962.0	E980.4
hydroxide	983.2	E864.2	—	E950.7	E962.1	E980.6
hypochlorite (bleach) NEC	983.9	E864.3	—	E950.7	E962.1	E980.6
disinfectant	983.9	E861.4	—	E950.7	E962.1	E980.6
medicinal (anti-infective) (external)	976.0	E858.7	E946.0	E950.4	E962.0	E980.4
vapor	987.8	E869.8	—	E952.8	E962.2	E982.8
hyposulfite	976.0	E858.7	E946.0	E950.4	E962.0	E980.4
indigotindisulfonate	977.8	E858.8	E947.8	E950.4	E962.0	E980.4
iodide	977.8	E858.8	E947.8	E950.4	E962.0	E980.4
iothalamate	977.8	E858.8	E947.8	E950.4	E962.0	E980.4
iron edetate	964.0	E858.2	E934.0	E950.4	E962.0	E980.4
lactate	963.3	E858.1	E933.3	E950.4	E962.0	E980.4
lauryl sulfate	976.2	E858.7	E946.2	E950.4	E962.0	E980.4
L-triiodothyronine	962.7	E858.0	E932.7	E950.4	E962.0	E980.4
metrizoate	977.8	E858.8	E947.8	E950.4	E962.0	E980.4
monofluoracetate (dust) (rodenticide)	989.4	E863.7	—	E950.6	E962.1	E980.7
morrhuate	972.7	E858.3	E942.7	E950.4	E962.0	E980.4
nafcillin	960.0	E856	E930.0	E950.4	E962.0	E980.4
nitrate (oxidizing agent)	983.9	E864.3	—	E950.7	E962.1	E980.6
nitrite (medicinal)	972.4	E858.3	E942.4	E950.4	E962.0	E980.4
nitroferricyanide	972.6	E858.3	E942.6	E950.4	E962.0	E980.4
nitroprusside	972.6	E858.3	E942.6	E950.4	E962.0	E980.4
para-aminohippurate	977.8	E858.8	E947.8	E950.4	E962.0	E980.4
perborate (nonmedicinal) NEC	989.89	E866.8	—	E950.9	E962.1	E980.9
medicinal	976.6	E858.7	E946.6	E950.4	E962.0	E980.4
soap	989.6	E861.1	—	E950.9	E962.1	E980.9
percarbonate — see Sodium, perborate						
phosphate	973.3	E858.4	E943.3	E950.4	E962.0	E980.4
polystyrene sulfonate	974.5	E858.5	E944.5	E950.4	E962.0	E980.4
propionate	976.0	E858.7	E946.0	E950.4	E962.0	E980.4
psylliate	972.7	E858.3	E942.7	E950.4	E962.0	E980.4
removing resins	974.5	E858.5	E944.5	E950.4	E962.0	E980.4
salicylate	965.1	E850.3	E935.3	E950	E962.0	E980.0
sulfate	973.3	E858.4	E943.3	E950.4	E962.0	E980.4
sulfoxone	961.8	E857	E931.8	E950.4	E962.0	E980.4
tetradecyl sulfate	972.7	E858.3	E942.7	E950.4	E962.0	E980.4
thiopental	968.3	E855.1	E938.3	E950.4	E962.0	E980.4
thiosalicylate	965.1	E850.3	E935.3	E950.0	E962.0	E980.0

☑4ᵗʰ Fourth-digit Required   ☑5ᵗʰ Fifth-digit Required   ▶◀ Revised Text   ● New Line   ▲ Revised Code

Sodium

Table of Drugs and Chemicals

		External Cause (E-Code)				
	Poisoning	Accident	Therapeutic Use	Suicide Attempt	Assault	Undetermined
Sodium — *continued*						
thiosulfate	976.0	E858.7	E946.0	E950.4	E962.0	E980.4
tolbutamide	977.8	E858.8	E947.8	E950.4	E962.0	E980.4
tyropanoate	977.8	E858.8	E947.8	E950.4	E962.0	E980.4
valproate	966.3	E855.0	E936.3	E950.4	E962.0	E980.4
Solanine	977.8	E858.8	E947.8	E950.4	E962.0	E980.4
Solanum dulcamara	988.2	E865.4	—	E950.9	E962.1	E980.9
Solapsone	961.8	E857	E931.8	E950.4	E962.0	E980.4
Solasulfone	961.8	E857	E931.8	E950.4	E962.0	E980.4
Soldering fluid	983.1	E864.1	—	E950.7	E962.1	E980.6
Solid substance	989.9	E866.9	—	E950.9	E962.1	E980.9
specified NEC	989.9	E866.8	—	E950.9	E962.1	E980.9
Solvents, industrial	982.8	E862.9	—	E950.9	E962.1	E980.9
naphtha	981	E862.0	—	E950.9	E962.1	E980.9
petroleum	981	E862.0	—	E950.9	E962.1	E980.9
specified NEC	982.8	E862.4	—	E950.9	E962.1	E980.9
Soma	968.0	E855.1	E938.0	E950.4	E962.0	E980.4
Somatotropin	962.4	E858.0	E932.4	E950.4	E962.0	E980.4
Sominex	963.0	E858.1	E933.0	E950.4	E962.0	E980.4
Somnos	967.1	E852.0	E937.1	E950.2	E962.0	E980.2
Somonal	967.0	E851	E937.0	E950.1	E962.0	E980.1
Soneryl	967.0	E851	E937.0	E950.1	E962.0	E980.1
Soothing syrup	977.9	E858.9	E947.9	E950.5	E962.0	E980.5
Sopor	967.4	E852.3	E937.4	E950.2	E962.0	E980.2
Soporific drug	967.9	E852.9	E937.9	E950.2	E962.0	E980.2
specified type NEC	967.8	E852.8	E937.8	E950.2	E962.0	E980.2
Sorbitol NEC	977.4	E858.8	E947.4	E950.4	E962.0	E980.4
Sotradecol	972.7	E858.3	E942.7	E950.4	E962.0	E980.4
Spacoline	975.1	E858.6	E945.1	E950.4	E962.0	E980.4
Spanish fly	976.8	E858.7	E946.8	E950.4	E962.0	E980.4
Sparine	969.1	E853.0	E939.1	E950.3	E962.0	E980.3
Sparteine	975.0	E858.6	E945.0	E950.4	E962.0	E980.4
Spasmolytics	975.1	E858.6	E945.1	E950.4	E962.0	E980.4
anticholinergics	971.1	E855.4	E941.1	E950.4	E962.0	E980.4
Spectinomycin	960.8	E856	E930.8	E950.4	E962.0	E980.4
Speed	969.7	E854.2	E939.7	E950.3	E962.0	E980.3
Spermicides	976.8	E858.7	E946.8	E950.4	E962.0	E980.4
Spider (bite) (venom)	989.5	E905.1	—	E950.9	E962.1	E980.9
antivenin	979.9	E858.8	E949.9	E950.4	E962.0	E980.4
Spigelia (root)	961.6	E857	E931.6	E950.4	E962.0	E980.4
Spiperone	969.2	E853.1	E939.2	E950.3	E962.0	E980.3
Spiramycin	960.3	E856	E930.3	E950.4	E962.0	E980.4
Spirilene	969.5	E853.8	E939.5	E950.3	E962.0	E980.3
Spirit(s) (neutral) NEC	980.0	E860.1	—	E950.9	E962.1	E980.9
beverage	980.0	E860.0	—	E950.9	E962.1	E980.9
industrial	980.9	E860.9	—	E950.9	E962.1	E980.9
mineral	981	E862.0	—	E950.9	E962.1	E980.9
of salt — *see* Hydrochloric acid						
surgical	980.9	E860.9	—	E950.9	E962.1	E980.9
Spironolactone	974.4	E858.5	E944.4	E950.4	E962.0	E980.4
Sponge, absorbable (gelatin)	964.5	E858.2	E934.5	E950.4	E962.0	E980.4
Sporostacin	976.0	E858.7	E946.0	E950.4	E962.0	E980.4
Sprays (aerosol)	989.89	E866.8	—	E950.9	E962.1	E980.9
cosmetic	989.89	E866.7	—	E950.9	E962.1	E980.9
medicinal NEC	977.9	E858.9	E947.9	E950.5	E962.0	E980.5
pesticides — *see* Pesticides						
specified content — *see* substance specified						
Spurge flax	988.2	E865.4	—	E950.9	E962.1	E980.9
Spurges	988.2	E865.4	—	E950.9	E962.1	E980.9
Squill (expectorant) NEC	975.5	E858.6	E945.5	E950.4	E962.0	E980.4
rat poison	989.4	E863.7	—	E950.6	E962.1	E980.7
Squirting cucumber (cathartic)	973.1	E858.4	E943.1	E950.4	E962.0	E980.4
Stains	989.89	E866.8	—	E950.9	E962.1	E980.9
Stannous — *see also* Tin						
fluoride	976.7	E858.7	E946.7	E950.4	E962.0	E980.4
Stanolone	962.1	E858.0	E932.1	E950.4	E962.0	E980.4
Stanozolol	962.1	E858.0	E932.1	E950.4	E962.0	E980.4
Staphisagria or stavesacre (pediculicide)	976.0	E858.7	E946.0	E950.4	E962.0	E980.4
Stelazine	969.1	E853.0	E939.1	E950.3	E962.0	E980.3
Stemetil	969.1	E853.0	E939.1	E950.3	E962.0	E980.3
Sterculia (cathartic) (gum)	973.3	E858.4	E943.3	E950.4	E962.0	E980.4
Sternutator gas	987.8	E869.8	—	E952.8	E962.2	E982.8
Steroids NEC	962.0	E858.0	E932.0	E950.4	E962.0	E980.4
ENT agent	976.6	E858.7	E946.6	E950.4	E962.0	E980.4
ophthalmic preparation	976.5	E858.7	E946.5	E950.4	E962.0	E980.4
topical NEC	976.0	E858.7	E946.0	E950.4	E962.0	E980.4
Stibine	985.8	E866.4	—	E950.9	E962.1	E980.9
Stibophen	961.2	E857	E931.2	E950.4	E962.0	E980.4
Stilbamide, stilbamidine	961.5	E857	E931.5	E950.4	E962.0	E980.4
Stilbestrol	962.2	E858.0	E932.2	E950.4	E962.0	E980.4

Table of Drugs and Chemicals

Sulfur, sulfureted, sulfuric, sulfurous, sulfuryl

	Poisoning	External Cause (E-Code)				
		Accident	Therapeutic Use	Suicide Attempt	Assault	Undetermined
Stimulants (central nervous system)	970.9	E854.3	E940.9	E950.4	E962.0	E980.4
analeptics	970.0	E854.3	E940.0	E950.4	E962.0	E980.4
opiate antagonist	970.1	E854.3	E940.1	E950.4	E962.0	E980.4
psychotherapeutic NEC	969.0	E854.0	E939.0	E950.3	E962.0	E980.3
specified NEC	970.8	E854.3	E940.8	E950.4	E962.0	E980.4
Storage batteries (acid) (cells)	983.1	E864.1	—	E950.7	E962.1	E980.6
Stovaine	968.9	E855.2	E938.9	E950.4	E962.0	E980.4
infiltration (subcutaneous)	968.5	E855.2	E938.5	E950.4	E962.0	E980.4
nerve block (peripheral) (plexus)	968.6	E855.2	E938.6	E950.4	E962.0	E980.4
spinal	968.7	E855.2	E938.7	E950.4	E962.0	E980.4
topical (surface)	968.5	E855.2	E938.5	E950.4	E962.0	E980.4
Stovarsal	961.1	E857	E931.1	E950.4	E962.0	E980.4
Stove gas — *see* Gas, utility						
Stoxil	976.5	E858.7	E946.5	E950.4	E962.0	E980.4
STP	969.6	E854.1	E939.6	E950.3	E962.0	E980.3
Stramonium (medicinal) NEC	971.1	E855.4	E941.1	E950.4	E962.0	E980.4
natural state	988.2	E865.4	—	E950.9	E962.1	E980.9
Streptodornase	964.4	E858.2	E934.4	E950.4	E962.0	E980.4
Streptoduocin	960.6	E856	E930.6	E950.4	E962.0	E980.4
Streptokinase	964.4	E858.2	E934.4	E950.4	E962.0	E980.4
Streptomycin	960.6	E856	E930.6	E950.4	E962.0	E980.4
Streptozocin	960.7	E856	E930.7	E950.4	E962.0	E980.4
Stripper (paint) (solvent)	982.8	E862.9	—	E950.9	E962.1	E980.9
Strobane	989.2	E863.0	—	E950.6	E962.1	E980.7
Strophanthin	972.1	E858.3	E942.1	E950.4	E962.0	E980.4
Strophanthus hispidus or kombe	988.2	E865.4	—	E950.9	E962.1	E980.9
Strychnine (rodenticide) (salts)	989.1	E863.7	—	E950.6	E962.1	E980.7
medicinal NEC	970.8	E854.3	E940.8	E950.4	E962.0	E980.4
Strychnos (ignatii) — *see* Strychnine						
Styramate	968.0	E855.1	E938.0	E950.4	E962.0	E980.4
Styrene	983.0	E864.0	—	E950.7	E962.1	E980.6
Succinimide (anticonvulsant)	966.2	E855.0	E936.2	E950.4	E962.0	E980.4
mercuric — *see* Mercury						
Succinylcholine	975.2	E858.6	E945.2	E950.4	E962.0	E980.4
Succinylsulfathiazole	961.0	E857	E931.0	E950.4	E962.0	E980.4
Sucrose	974.5	E858.5	E944.5	E950.4	E962.0	E980.4
Sulfacetamide	961.0	E857	E931.0	E950.4	E962.0	E980.4
ophthalmic preparation	976.5	E858.7	E946.5	E950.4	E962.0	E980.4
Sulfachlorpyridazine	961.0	E857	E931.0	E950.4	E962.0	E980.4
Sulfacytine	961.0	E857	E931.0	E950.4	E962.0	E980.4
Sulfadiazine	961.0	E857	E931.0	E950.4	E962.0	E980.4
silver (topical)	976.0	E858.7	E946.0	E950.4	E962.0	E980.4
Sulfadimethoxine	961.0	E857	E931.0	E950.4	E962.0	E980.4
Sulfadimidine	961.0	E857	E931.0	E950.4	E962.0	E980.4
Sulfaethidole	961.0	E857	E931.0	E950.4	E962.0	E980.4
Sulfafurazole	961.0	E857	E931.0	E950.4	E962.0	E980.4
Sulfaguanidine	961.0	E857	E931.0	E950.4	E962.0	E980.4
Sulfamerazine	961.0	E857	E931.0	E950.4	E962.0	E980.4
Sulfameter	961.0	E857	E931.0	E950.4	E962.0	E980.4
Sulfamethizole	961.0	E857	E931.0	E950.4	E962.0	E980.4
Sulfamethoxazole	961.0	E857	E931.0	E950.4	E962.0	E980.4
Sulfamethoxydiazine	961.0	E857	E931.0	E950.4	E962.0	E980.4
Sulfamethoxypyridazine	961.0	E857	E931.0	E950.4	E962.0	E980.4
Sulfamethylthiazole	961.0	E857	E931.0	E950.4	E962.0	E980.4
Sulfamylon	976.0	E858.7	E946.0	E950.4	E962.0	E980.4
Sulfan blue (diagnostic dye)	977.8	E858.8	E947.8	E950.4	E962.0	E980.4
Sulfanilamide	961.0	E857	E931.0	E950.4	E962.0	E980.4
Sulfanilylguanidine	961.0	E857	E931.0	E950.4	E962.0	E980.4
Sulfaphenazole	961.0	E857	E931.0	E950.4	E962.0	E980.4
Sulfaphenylthiazole	961.0	E857	E931.0	E950.4	E962.0	E980.4
Sulfaproxyline	961.0	E857	E931.0	E950.4	E962.0	E980.4
Sulfapyridine	961.0	E857	E931.0	E950.4	E962.0	E980.4
Sulfapyrimidine	961.0	E857	E931.0	E950.4	E962.0	E980.4
Sulfarsphenamine	961.1	E857	E931.1	E950.4	E962.0	E980.4
Sulfasalazine	961.0	E857	E931.0	E950.4	E962.0	E980.4
Sulfasomizole	961.0	E857	E931.0	E950.4	E962.0	E980.4
Sulfasuxidine	961.0	E857	E931.0	E950.4	E962.0	E980.4
Sulfinpyrazone	974.7	E858.5	E944.7	E950.4	E962.0	E980.4
Sulfisoxazole	961.0	E857	E931.0	E950.4	E962.0	E980.4
ophthalmic preparation	976.5	E858.7	E946.5	E950.4	E962.0	E980.4
Sulfomyxin	960.8	E856	E930.8	E950.4	E962.0	E980.4
Sulfonal	967.8	E852.8	E937.8	E950.2	E962.0	E980.2
Sulfonamides (mixtures)	961.0	E857	E931.0	E950.4	E962.0	E980.4
Sulfones	961.8	E857	E931.8	E950.4	E962.0	E980.4
Sulfonethylmethane	967.8	E852.8	E937.8	E950.2	E962.0	E980.2
Sulfonmethane	967.8	E852.8	E937.8	E950.2	E962.0	E980.2
Sulfonphthal, sulfonphthol	977.8	E858.8	E947.8	E950.4	E962.0	E980.4
Sulfonylurea derivatives, oral	962.3	E858.0	E932.3	E950.4	E962.0	E980.4
Sulfoxone	961.8	E857	E931.8	E950.4	E962.0	E980.4
Sulfur, sulfureted, sulfuric, sulfurous, sulfuryl (compounds) NEC	989.89	E866.8	—	E950.9	E962.1	E980.9
acid	983.1	E864.1	—	E950.7	E962.1	E980.6

Sulfur, sulfureted, sulfuric, sulfurous, sulfuryl NEC — Table of Drugs and Chemicals

		External Cause (E-Code)				
	Poisoning	Accident	Therapeutic Use	Suicide Attempt	Assault	Undetermined
Sulfur, sulfureted, sulfuric, sulfurous, sulfuryl NEC — *continued*						
dioxide	987.3	E869.1	—	E952.8	E962.2	E982.8
ether — *see* Ether(s)						
hydrogen	987.8	E869.8	—	E952.8	E962.2	E982.8
medicinal (keratolytic) (ointment) NEC	976.4	E858.7	E946.4	E950.4	E962.0	E980.4
pesticide (vapor)	989.4	E863.4	—	E950.6	E962.1	E980.7
vapor NEC	987.8	E869.8	—	E952.8	E962.2	E982.8
Sulkowitch's reagent	977.8	E858.8	E947.8	E950.4	E962.0	E980.4
Sulph — *see also* Sulf-						
Sulphadione	961.8	E857	E931.8	E950.4	E962.0	E980.4
Sulthiame, sultiame	966.3	E855.0	E936.3	E950.4	E962.0	E980.4
Superinone	975.5	E858.6	E945.5	E950.4	E962.0	E980.4
Suramin	961.5	E857	E931.5	E950.4	E962.0	E980.4
Surfacaine	968.5	E855.2	E938.5	E950.4	E962.0	E980.4
Surital	968.3	E855.1	E938.3	E950.4	E962.0	E980.4
Sutilains	976.8	E858.7	E946.8	E950.4	E962.0	E980.4
Suxamethonium (bromide) (chloride) (iodide)	975.2	E858.6	E945.2	E950.4	E962.0	E980.4
Suxethonium (bromide)	975.2	E858.6	E945.2	E950.4	E962.0	E980.4
Sweet oil (birch)	976.3	E858.7	E946.3	E950.4	E962.0	E980.4
Sym-dichloroethyl ether	982.3	E862.4	—	E950.9	E962.1	E980.9
Sympatholytics	971.3	E855.6	E941.3	E950.4	E962.0	E980.4
Sympathomimetics	971.2	E855.5	E941.2	E950.4	E962.0	E980.4
Synagis	979.6 ▲	E858.8	E949.6	E950.4	E962.0	E980.4
Synalar	976.0	E858.7	E946.0	E950.4	E962.0	E980.4
Synthroid	962.7	E858.0	E932.7	E950.4	E962.0	E980.4
Syntocinon	975.0	E858.6	E945.0	E950.4	E962.0	E950.4
Syrosingopine	972.6	E858.3	E942.6	E950.4	E962.0	E980.4
Systemic agents (primarily)	963.9	E858.1	E933.9	E950.4	E962.0	E980.4
specified NEC	963.8	E858.1	E933.8	E950.4	E962.0	E980.4
Tablets (*see also* specified substance)	977.9	E858.9	E947.9	E950.5	E962.0	E980.5
Tace	962.2	E858.0	E932.2	E950.4	E962.0	E980.4
Tacrine	971.0	E855.3	E941.0	E950.4	E962.0	E980.4
Talbutal	967.0	E851	E937.0	E950.1	E962.0	E980.1
Talc	976.3	E858.7	E946.3	E950.4	E962.0	E980.4
Talcum	976.3	E858.7	E946.3	E950.4	E962.0	E980.4
Tandearil, tanderil	965.5	E850.5	E935.5	E950.0	E962.0	E980.0
Tannic acid	983.1	E864.1	—	E950.7	E962.1	E980.6
medicinal (astringent)	976.2	E858.7	E946.2	E950.4	E962.0	E980.4
Tannin — *see* Tannic acid						
Tansy	988.2	E865.4	—	E950.9	E962.1	E980.9
TAO	960.3	E856	E930.3	E950.4	E962.0	E980.4
Tapazole	962.8	E858.0	E932.8	E950.4	E962.0	E980.4
Tar NEC	983.0	E864.0	—	E950.7	E962.1	E980.6
camphor — *see* Naphthalene						
fumes	987.8	E869.8	—	E952.8	E962.2	E982.8
Taractan	969.3	E853.8	E939.3	E950.3	E962.0	E980.3
Tarantula (venomous)	989.5	E905.1	—	E950.9	E962.1	E980.9
Tartar emetic (anti-infective)	961.2	E857	E931.2	E950.4	E962.0	E980.4
Tartaric acid	983.1	E864.1	—	E950.7	E962.1	E980.6
Tartrated antimony (anti-infective)	961.2	E857	E931.2	E950.4	E962.0	E980.4
TCA — *see* Trichloroacetic acid						
TDI	983.0	E864.0	—	E950.7	E962.1	E980.6
vapor	987.8	E869.8	—	E952.8	E962.2	E982.8
Tear gas	987.5	E869.3	—	E952.8	E962.2	E982.8
Teclothiazide	974.3	E858.5	E944.3	E950.4	E962.0	E980.4
Tegretol	966.3	E855.0	E936.3	E950.4	E962.0	E980.4
Telepaque	977.8	E858.8	E947.8	E950.4	E962.0	E980.4
Tellurium	985.8	E866.4	—	E950.9	E962.1	E980.9
fumes	985.8	E866.4	—	E950.9	E962.1	E980.9
TEM	963.1	E858.1	E933.1	E950.4	E962.0	E980.4
Temazepan — *see* Benzodiazepines						
TEPA	963.1	E858.1	E933.1	E950.4	E962.0	E980.4
TEPP	989.3	E863.1	—	E950.6	E962.1	E980.7
Terbutaline	971.2	E855.5	E941.2	E950.4	E962.0	E980.4
Teroxalene	961.6	E857	E931.6	E950.4	E962.0	E980.4
Terpin hydrate	975.5	E858.6	E945.5	E950.4	E962.0	E980.4
Terramycin	960.4	E856	E930.4	E950.4	E962.0	E980.4
Tessalon	975.4	E858.6	E945.4	E950.4	E962.0	E980.4
Testosterone	962.1	E858.0	E932.1	E950.4	E962.0	E980.4
Tetanus (vaccine)	978.4	E858.8	E948.4	E950.4	E962.0	E980.4
antitoxin	979.9	E858.8	E949.9	E950.4	E962.0	E980.4
immune globulin (human)	964.6	E858.2	E934.6	E950.4	E962.0	E980.4
toxoid	978.4	E858.8	E948.4	E950.4	E962.0	E980.4
with diphtheria toxoid	978.9	E858.8	E948.9	E950.4	E962.0	E980.4
with pertussis	978.6	E858.8	E948.6	E950.4	E962.0	E980.4
Tetrabenazine	969.5	E853.8	E939.5	E950.3	E962.0	E980.3
Tetracaine (infiltration) (topical)	968.5	E855.2	E938.5	E950.4	E962.0	E980.4
nerve block (peripheral) (plexus)	968.6 ▶	E855.2	E938.6	E950.4	E962.0	E980.4
spinal	968.7	E855.2	E938.7	E950.4	E962.0	E980.4
Tetrachlorethylene — *see* Tetrachloroethylene						
Tetrachlormethiazide	974.3	E858.5	E944.3	E950.4	E962.0	E980.4

Table of Drugs and Chemicals

		External Cause (E-Code)				
	Poisoning	Accident	Therapeutic Use	Suicide Attempt	Assault	Undetermined
Tetrachloroethane (liquid) (vapor)	982.3	E862.4	—	E950.9	E962.1	E980.9
paint or varnish	982.3	E861.6	—	E950.9	E962.1	E980.9
Tetrachloroethylene (liquid) (vapor)	982.3	E862.4	—	E950.9	E962.1	E980.9
medicinal	961.6	E857	E931.6	E950.4	E962.0	E980.4
Tetrachloromethane — see Carbon, tetrachloride						
Tetracycline	960.4	E856	E930.4	E950.4	E962.0	E980.4
ophthalmic preparation	976.5	E858.7	E946.5	E950.4	E962.0	E980.4
topical NEC	976.0	E858.7	E946.0	E950.4	E962.0	E980.4
Tetraethylammonium chloride	972.3	E858.3	E942.3	E950.4	E962.0	E980.4
Tetraethyl lead (antiknock compound)	984.1	E862.1	—	E950.9	E962.1	E980.9
Tetraethyl pyrophosphate	989.3	E863.1	—	E950.6	E962.1	E980.7
Tetraethylthiuram disulfide	977.3	E858.8	E947.3	E950.4	E962.0	E980.4
Tetrahydroaminoacridine	971.0	E855.3	E941.0	E950.4	E962.0	E980.4
Tetrahydrocannabinol	969.6	E854.1	E939.6	E950.3	E962.0	E980.3
Tetrahydronaphthalene	982.0	E862.4	—	E950.9	E962.1	E980.9
Tetrahydrozoline	971.2	E855.5	E941.2	E950.4	E962.0	E980.4
Tetralin	982.0	E862.4	—	E950.9	E962.1	E980.9
Tetramethylthiuram (disulfide) NEC	989.4	E863.6	—	E950.6	E962.1	E980.7
medicinal	976.2	E858.7	E946.2	E950.4	E962.0	E980.4
Tetronal	967.8	E852.8	E937.8	E950.2	E962.0	E980.2
Tetryl	983.0	E864.0	—	E950.7	E962.1	E980.6
Thalidomide	967.8	E852.8	E937.8	E950.2	E962.0	E980.2
Thallium (compounds) (dust) NEC	985.8	E866.4	—	E950.9	E962.1	E980.9
pesticide (rodenticide)	985.8	E863.7	—	E950.6	E962.1	E980.7
THC	969.6	E854.1	E939.6	E950.3	E962.0	E980.3
Thebacon	965.09	E850.2	E935.2	E950.0	E962.0	E980.0
Thebaine	965.09	E850.2	E935.2	E950.0	E962.0	E980.0
Theobromine (calcium salicylate)	974.1	E858.5	E944.1	E950.4	E962.0	E980.4
Theophylline (diuretic)	974.1	E858.5	E944.1	E950.4	E962.0	E980.4
ethylenediamine	975.7	E858.6	E945.7	E950.4	E962.0	E980.4
Thiabendazole	961.6	E857	E931.6	E950.4	E962.0	E980.4
Thialbarbital, thialbarbitone	968.3	E855.1	E938.3	E950.4	E962.0	E980.4
Thiamine	963.5	E858.1	E933.5	E950.4	E962.0	E980.4
Thiamylal (sodium)	968.3	E855.1	E938.3	E950.4	E962.0	E980.4
Thiazesim	969.0	E854.0	E939.0	E950.3	E962.0	E980.3
Thiazides (diuretics)	974.3	E858.5	E944.3	E950.4	E962.0	E980.4
Thiethylperazine	963.0	E858.1	E933.0	E950.4	E962.0	E980.4
Thimerosal (topical)	976.0	E858.7	E946.0	E950.4	E962.0	E980.4
ophthalmic preparation	976.5	E858.7	E946.5	E950.4	E962.0	E980.4
Thioacetazone	961.8	E857	E931.8	E950.4	E962.0	E980.4
Thiobarbiturates	968.3	E855.1	E938.3	E950.4	E962.0	E980.4
Thiobismol	961.2	E857	E931.2	E950.4	E962.0	E980.4
Thiocarbamide	962.8	E858.0	E932.8	E950.4	E962.0	E980.4
Thiocarbarsone	961.1	E857	E931.1	E950.4	E962.0	E980.4
Thiocarlide	961.8	E857	E931.8	E950.4	E962.0	E980.4
Thioguanine	963.1	E858.1	E933.1	E950.4	E962.0	E980.4
Thiomercaptomerin	974.0	E858.5	E944.0	E950.4	E962.0	E980.4
Thiomerin	974.0	E858.5	E944.0	E950.4	E962.0	E980.4
Thiopental, thiopentone (sodium)	968.3	E855.1	E938.3	E950.4	E962.0	E980.4
Thiopropazate	969.1	E853.0	E939.1	E950.3	E962.0	E980.3
Thioproperazine	969.1	E853.0	E939.1	E950.3	E962.0	E980.3
Thioridazine	969.1	E853.0	E939.1	E950.3	E962.0	E980.3
Thio-TEPA, thiotepa	963.1	E858.1	E933.1	E950.4	E962.0	E980.4
Thiothixene	969.3	E853.8	E939.3	E950.3	E962.0	E980.3
Thiouracil	962.8	E858.0	E932.8	E950.4	E962.0	E980.4
Thiourea	962.8	E858.0	E932.8	E950.4	E962.0	E980.4
Thiphenamil	971.1	E855.4	E941.1	E950.4	E962.0	E980.4
Thiram NEC	989.4	E863.6	—	E950.6	E962.1	E980.7
medicinal	976.2	E858.7	E946.2	E950.4	E962.0	E980.4
Thonzylamine	963.0	E858.1	E933.0	E950.4	E962.0	E980.4
Thorazine	969.1	E853.0	E939.1	E950.3	E962.0	E980.3
Thornapple	988.2	E865.4	—	E950.9	E962.1	E980.9
Throat preparation (lozenges) NEC	976.6	E858.7	E946.6	E950.4	E962.0	E980.4
Thrombin	964.5	E858.2	E934.5	E950.4	E962.0	E980.4
Thrombolysin	964.4	E858.2	E934.4	E950.4	E962.0	E980.4
Thymol	983.0	E864.0	—	E950.7	E962.1	E980.6
Thymus extract	962.9	E858.0	E932.9	E950.4	E962.0	E980.4
Thyroglobulin	962.7	E858.0	E932.7	E950.4	E962.0	E980.4
Thyroid (derivatives) (extract)	962.7	E858.0	E932.7	E950.4	E962.0	E980.4
Thyrolar	962.7	E858.0	E932.7	E950.4	E962.0	E980.4
Thyrothrophin, thyrotropin	977.8	E858.8	E947.8	E950.4	E962.0	E980.4
Thyroxin(e)	962.7	E858.0	E932.7	E950.4	E962.0	E980.4
Tigan	963.0	E858.1	E933.0	E950.4	E962.0	E980.4
Tigloidine	968.0	E855.1	E938.0	E950.4	E962.0	E980.4
Tin (chloride) (dust) (oxide) NEC	985.8	E866.4	—	E950.9	E962.1	E980.9
anti-infectives	961.2	E857	E931.2	E950.4	E962.0	E980.4
Tinactin	976.0	E858.7	E946.0	E950.4	E962.0	E980.4
Tincture, iodine — see Iodine						
Tindal	969.1	E853.0	E939.1	E950.3	E962.0	E980.3
Titanium (compounds) (vapor)	985.8	E866.4	—	E950.9	E962.1	E980.9
ointment	976.3	E858.7	E946.3	E950.4	E962.0	E980.4

Table of Drugs and Chemicals

	Poisoning	External Cause (E-Code)				
		Accident	Therapeutic Use	Suicide Attempt	Assault	Undetermined
Titroid	962.7	E858.0	E932.7	E950.4	E962.0	E980.4
TMTD — *see* Tetramethylthiuram disulfide						
TNT	989.89	E866.8	—	E950.9	E962.1	E980.9
fumes	987.8	E869.8	—	E952.8	E962.2	E982.8
Toadstool	988.1	E865.5	—	E950.9	E962.1	E980.9
Tobacco NEC	989.84	E866.8	—	E950.9	E962.1	E980.9
Indian	988.2	E865.4	—	E950.9	E962.1	E980.9
smoke, second-hand	987.8	E869.4	—	—	—	—
Tocopherol	963.5	E858.1	E933.5	E950.4	E962.0	E980.4
Tocosamine	975.0	E858.6	E945.0	E950.4	E962.0	E980.4
Tofranil	969.0	E854.0	E939.0	E950.3	E962.0	E980.3
Toilet deodorizer	989.89	E866.8	—	E950.9	E962.1	E980.9
Tolazamide	962.3	E858.0	E932.3	E950.4	E962.0	E980.4
Tolazoline	971.3	E855.6	E941.3	E950.4	E962.0	E980.4
Tolbutamide	962.3	E858.0	E932.3	E950.4	E962.0	E980.4
sodium	977.8	E858.8	E947.8	E950.4	E962.0	E980.4
Tolmetin	965.69	E850.6	E935.6	E950.0	E962.0	E980.0
Tolnaftate	976.0	E858.7	E946.0	E950.4	E962.0	E980.4
Tolpropamine	976.1	E858.7	E946.1	E950.4	E962.0	E980.4
Tolserol	968	E855.1	E938.0	E950.4	E962.0	E980.4
Toluene (liquid) (vapor)	982.0	E862.4	—	E950.9	E962.1	E980.9
diisocyanate	983.0	E864.0	—	E950.7	E962.1	E980.6
Toluidine	983.0	E864.0	—	E950.7	E962.1	E980.6
vapor	987.8	E869.8	—	E952.8	E962.2	E982.8
Toluol (liquid) (vapor)	982.0	E862.4	—	E950.9	E962.1	E980.9
Tolylene-2, 4-diisocyanate	983.0	E864.0	—	E950.7	E962.1	E980.6
Tonics, cardiac	972.1	E858.3	E942.1	E950.4	E962.0	E980.4
Toxaphene (dust) (spray)	989.2	E863.0	—	E950.6	E962.1	E980.7
Toxoids NEC	978.8	E858.8	E948.8	E950.4	E962.0	E980.4
Tractor fuel NEC	981	E862.1	—	E950.9	E962.1	E980.9
Tragacanth	973.3	E858.4	E943.3	E950.4	E962.0	E980.4
Tramazoline	971.2	E855.5	E941.2	E950.4	E962.0	E980.4
Tranquilizers	969.5	E853.9	E939.5	E950.3	E962.0	E980.3
benzodiazepine-based	969.4	E853.2	E939.4	E950.3	E962.0	E980.3
butyrophenone-based	969.2	E853.1	E939.2	E950.3	E962.0	E980.3
major NEC	969.3	E853.8	E939.3	E950.3	E962.0	E980.3
phenothiazine-based	969.1	E853.0	E939.1	E950.3	E962.0	E980.3
specified NEC	969.5	E853.8	E939.5	E950.3	E962.0	E980.3
Trantoin	961.9	E857	E931.9	E950.4	E962.0	E980.4
Tranxene	969.4	E853.2	E939.4	E950.3	E962.0	E980.3
Tranylcypromine (sulfate)	969.0	E854.0	E939.0	E950.3	E962.0	E980.3
Trasentine	975.1	E858.6	E945.1	E950.4	E962.0	E980.4
Travert	974.5	E858.5	E944.5	E950.4	E962.0	E980.4
Trecator	961.8	E857	E931.8	E950.4	E962.0	E980.4
Tretinoin	976.8	E858.7	E946.8	E950.4	E962.0	E980.4
Triacetin	976.0	E858.7	E946.0	E950.4	E962.0	E980.4
Triacetyloleandomycin	960.3	E856	E930.3	E950.4	E962.0	E980.4
Triamcinolone	962.0	E858.0	E932.0	E950.4	E962.0	E980.4
ENT agent	976.6	E858.7	E946.6	E950.4	E962.0	E980.4
ophthalmic preparation	976.5	E858.7	E946.5	E950.4	E962.0	E980.4
topical NEC	976.0	E858.7	E946.0	E950.4	E962.0	E980.4
Triamterene	974.4	E858.5	E944.4	E950.4	E962.0	E980.4
Triaziquone	963.1	E858.1	E933.1	E950.4	E962.0	E980.4
Tribromacetaldehyde	967.3	E852.2	E937.3	E950.2	E962.0	E980.2
Tribromoethanol	968.2	E855.1	E938.2	E950.4	E962.0	E980.4
Tribromomethane	967.3	E852.2	E937.3	E950.2	E962.0	E980.2
Trichlorethane	982.3	E862.4	—	E950.9	E962.1	E980.9
Trichlormethiazide	974.3	E858.5	E944.3	E950.4	E962.0	E980.4
Trichloroacetic acid	983.1	E864.1	—	E950.7	E962.1	E980.6
medicinal (keratolytic)	976.4	E858.7	E946.4	E950.4	E962.0	E980.4
Trichloroethanol	967.1	E852.0	E937.1	E950.2	E962.0	E980.2
Trichloroethylene (liquid) (vapor)	982.3	E862.4	—	E950.9	E962.1	E980.9
anesthetic (gas)	968.2	E855.1	E938.2	E950.4	E962.0	E980.4
Trichloroethyl phosphate	967.1	E852.0	E937.1	E950.2	E962.0	E980.2
Trichlorofluoromethane NEC	987.4	E869.2	—	E952.8	E962.2	E982.8
Trichlorotriethylamine	963.1	E858.1	E933.1	E950.4	E962.0	E980.4
Trichomonacides NEC	961.5	E857	E931.5	E950.4	E962.0	E980.4
Trichomycin	960.1	E856	E930.1	E950.4	E962.0	E980.4
Triclofos	967.1	E852.0	E937.1	E950.2	E962.0	E980.2
Tricresyl phosphate	989.89	E866.8	—	E950.9	E962.1	E980.9
solvent	982.8	E862.4	—	E950.9	E962.1	E980.9
Tricyclamol	966.4	E855.0	E936.4	E950.4	E962.0	E980.4
Tridesilon	976.0	E858.7	E946.0	E950.4	E962.0	E980.4
Tridihexethyl	971.1	E855.4	E941.1	E950.4	E962.0	E980.4
Tridione	966	E855.0	E936.0	E950.4	E962.0	E980.4
Triethanolamine NEC	983.2	E864.2	—	E950.7	E962.1	E980.6
detergent	983.2	E861.0	—	E950.7	E962.1	E980.6
trinitrate	972.4	E858.3	E942.4	E950.4	E962.0	E980.4
Triethanomelamine	963.1	E858.1	E933.1	E950.4	E962.0	E980.4
Triethylene melamine	963.1	E858.1	E933.1	E950.4	E962.0	E980.4
Triethylenephosphoramide	963.1	E858.1	E933.1	E950.4	E962.0	E980.4

Table of Drugs and Chemicals

		External Cause (E-Code)				
	Poisoning	Accident	Therapeutic Use	Suicide Attempt	Assault	Undetermined
Triethylenethiophosphoramide	963.1	E858.1	E933.1	E950.4	E962.0	E980.4
Trifluoperazine	969.1	E853.0	E939.1	E950.3	E962.0	E980.3
Trifluperidol	969.2	E853.1	E939.2	E950.3	E962.0	E980.3
Triflupromazine	969.1	E853.0	E939.1	E950.3	E962.0	E980.3
Trihexyphenidyl	971.1	E855.4	E941.1	E950.4	E962.0	E980.4
Triiodothyronine	962.7	E858.0	E932.7	E950.4	E962.0	E980.4
Trilene	968.2	E855.1	E938.2	E950.4	E962.0	E980.4
Trimeprazine	963.0	E858.1	E933.0	E950.4	E962.0	E980.4
Trimetazidine	972.4	E858.3	E942.4	E950.4	E962.0	E980.4
Trimethadione	966.0	E855.0	E936.0	E950.4	E962.0	E980.4
Trimethaphan	972.3	E858.3	E942.3	E950.4	E962.0	E980.4
Trimethidinium	972.3	E858.3	E942.3	E950.4	E962.0	E980.4
Trimethobenzamide	963.0	E858.1	E933.0	E950.4	E962.0	E980.4
Trimethylcarbinol	980.8	E860.8	—	E950.9	E962.1	E980.9
Trimethylpsoralen	976.3	E858.7	E946.3	E950.4	E962.0	E980.4
Trimeton	963.0	E858.1	E933.0	E950.4	E962.0	E980.4
Trimipramine	969.0	E854.0	E939.0	E950.3	E962.0	E980.3
Trimustine	963.1	E858.1	E933.1	E950.4	E962.0	E980.4
Trinitrin	972.4	E858.3	E942.4	E950.4	E962.0	E980.4
Trinitrophenol	983.0	E864.0	—	E950.7	E962.1	E980.6
Trinitrotoluene	989.89	E866.8	—	E950.9	E962.1	E980.9
fumes	987.8	E869.8	—	E952.8	E962.2	E982.8
Trional	967.8	E852.8	E937.8	E950.2	E962.0	E980.2
Trioxide of arsenic — see Arsenic						
Trioxsalen	976.3	E858.7	E946.3	E950.4	E962.0	E980.4
Tripelennamine	963.0	E858.1	E933.0	E950.4	E962.0	E980.4
Triperidol	969.2	E853.1	E939.2	E950.3	E962.0	E980.3
Triprolidine	963.0	E858.1	E933.0	E950.4	E962.0	E980.4
Trisoralen	976.3	E858.7	E946.3	E950.4	E962.0	E980.4
Troleandomycin	960.3	E856	E930.3	E950.4	E962.0	E980.4
Trolnitrate (phosphate)	972.4	E858.3	E942.4	E950.4	E962.0	E980.4
Trometamol	963.3	E858.1	E933.3	E950.4	E962.0	E980.4
Tromethamine	963.3	E858.1	E933.3	E950.4	E962.0	E980.4
Tronothane	968.5	E855.2	E938.5	E950.4	E962.0	E980.4
Tropicamide	971.1	E855.4	E941.1	E950.4	E962.0	E980.4
Troxidone	966.0	E855.0	E936.0	E950.4	E962.0	E980.4
Tryparsamide	961.1	E857	E931.1	E950.4	E962.0	E980.4
Trypsin	963.4	E858.1	E933.4	E950.4	E962.0	E980.4
Tryptizol	969.0	E854.0	E939.0	E950.3	E962.0	E980.3
Tuaminoheptane	971.2	E855.5	E941.2	E950.4	E962.0	E980.4
Tuberculin (old)	977.8	E858.8	E947.8	E950.4	E962.0	E980.4
Tubocurare	975.2	E858.6	E945.2	E950.4	E962.0	E980.4
Tubocurarine	975.2	E858.6	E945.2	E950.4	E962.0	E980.4
Turkish green	969.6	E854.1	E939.6	E950.3	E962.0	E980.3
Turpentine (spirits of) (liquid) (vapor)	982.8	E862.4	—	E950.9	E962.1	E980.9
Tybamate	969.5	E853.8	E939.5	E950.3	E962.0	E980.3
Tyloxapol	975.5	E858.6	E945.5	E950.4	E962.0	E980.4
Tymazoline	971.2	E855.5	E941.2	E950.4	E962.0	E980.4
Typhoid vaccine	978.1	E858.8	E948.1	E950.4	E962.0	E980.4
Typhus vaccine	979.2	E858.8	E949.2	E950.4	E962.0	E980.4
Tyrothricin	976.0	E858.7	E946.0	E950.4	E962.0	E980.4
ENT agent	976.6	E858.7	E946.6	E950.4	E962.0	E980.4
ophthalmic preparation	976.5	E858.7	E946.5	E950.4	E962.0	E980.4
Undecenoic acid	976.0	E858.7	E946.0	E950.4	E962.0	E980.4
Undecylenic acid	976.0	E858.7	E946.0	E950.4	E962.0	E980.4
Unna's boot	976.3	E858.7	E946.3	E950.4	E962.0	E980.4
Uracil mustard	963.1	E858.1	E933.1	E950.4	E962.0	E980.4
Uramustine	963.1	E858.1	E933.1	E950.4	E962.0	E980.4
Urari	975.2	E858.6	E945.2	E950.4	E962.0	E980.4
Urea	974.4	E858.5	E944.4	E950.4	E962.0	E980.4
topical	976.8	E858.7	E946.8	E950.4	E962.0	E980.4
Urethan(e) (antineoplastic)	963.1	E858.1	E933.1	E950.4	E962.0	E980.4
Urginea (maritima) (scilla) — see Squill						
Uric acid metabolism agents NEC	974.7	E858.5	E944.7	E950.4	E962.0	E980.4
Urokinase	964.4	E858.2	E934.4	E950.4	E962.0	E980.4
Urokon	977.8	E858.8	E947.8	E950.4	E962.0	E980.4
Urotropin	961.9	E857	E931.9	E950.4	E962.0	E980.4
Urtica	988.2	E865.4	—	E950.9	E962.1	E980.9
Utility gas — see Gas, utility						
Vaccine NEC	979.9	E858.8	E949.9	E950.4	E962.0	E980.4
bacterial NEC	978.8	E858.8	E948.8	E950.4	E962.0	E980.4
with						
other bacterial component	978.9	E858.8	E948.9	E950.4	E962.0	E980.4
pertussis component	978.6	E858.8	E948.6	E950.4	E962.0	E980.4
viral-rickettsial component	979.7	E858.8	E949.7	E950.4	E962.0	E980.4
mixed NEC	978.9	E858.8	E948.9	E950.4	E962.0	E980.4
BCG	978.0	E858.8	E948.0	E950.4	E962.0	E980.4
cholera	978.2	E858.8	E948.2	E950.4	E962.0	E980.4
diphtheria	978.5	E858.8	E948.5	E950.4	E962.0	E980.4
influenza	979.6	E858.8	E949.6	E950.4	E962.0	E980.4
measles	979.4	E858.8	E949.4	E950.4	E962.0	E980.4

Vaccine NEC — Table of Drugs and Chemicals

	Poisoning	External Cause (E-Code)				
		Accident	Therapeutic Use	Suicide Attempt	Assault	Undetermined
Vaccine NEC — *continued*						
meningococcal	978.8	E858.8	E948.8	E950.4	E962.0	E980.4
mumps	979.6	E858.8	E949.6	E950.4	E962.0	E980.4
paratyphoid	978.1	E858.8	E948.1	E950.4	E962.0	E980.4
pertussis (with diphtheria toxoid) (with tetanus toxoid)	978.6	E858.8	E948.6	E950.4	E962.0	E980.4
plague	978.3	E858.8	E948.3	E950.4	E962.0	E980.4
poliomyelitis	979.5	E858.8	E949.5	E950.4	E962.0	E980.4
poliovirus	979.5	E858.8	E949.5	E950.4	E962.0	E980.4
rabies	979.1	E858.8	E949.1	E950.4	E962.0	E980.4
respiratory syncytial virus	979.6 ▲	E858.8	E949.6	E950.4	E962.0	E980.4
rickettsial NEC	979.6	E858.8	E949.6	E950.4	E962.0	E980.4
with						
bacterial component	979.7	E858.8	E949.7	E950.4	E962.0	E980.4
pertussis component	978.6	E858.8	E948.6	E950.4	E962.0	E980.4
viral component	979.7	E858.8	E949.7	E950.4	E962.0	E980.4
Rocky mountain spotted fever	979.6	E858.8	E949.6	E950.4	E962.0	E980.4
rotavirus	979.6	E858.8	E949.6	E950.4	E962.0	E980.4
rubella virus	979.4	E858.8	E949.4	E950.4	E962.0	E980.4
sabin oral	979.5	E858.8	E949.5	E950.4	E962.0	E980.4
smallpox	979.0	E858.8	E949.0	E950.4	E962.0	E980.4
tetanus	978.4	E858.8	E948.4	E950.4	E962.0	E980.4
typhoid	978.1	E858.8	E948.1	E950.4	E962.0	E980.4
typhus	979.2	E858.8	E949.2	E950.4	E962.0	E980.4
viral NEC	979.6	E858.8	E949.6	E950.4	E962.0	E980.4
with						
bacterial component	979.7	E858.8	E949.7	E950.4	E962.0	E980.4
pertussis component	978.6	E858.8	E948.6	E950.4	E962.0	E980.4
rickettsial component	979.7	E858.8	E949.7	E950.4	E962.0	E980.4
yellow fever	979.3	E858.8	E949.3	E950.4	E962.0	E980.4
Vaccinia immune globulin (human)	964.6	E858.2	E934.6	E950.4	E962.0	E980.4
Vaginal contraceptives	976.8	E858.7	E946.8	E950.4	E962.0	E980.4
Valethamate	971.1	E855.4	E941.1	E950.4	E962.0	E980.4
Valisone	976.0	E858.7	E946.0	E950.4	E962.0	E980.4
Valium	969.4	E853.2	E939.4	E950.3	E962.0	E980.3
Valmid	967.8	E852.8	E937.8	E950.2	E962.0	E980.2
Vanadium	985.8	E866.4	—	E950.9	E962.1	E980.9
Vancomycin	960.8	E856	E930.8	E950.4	E962.0	E980.4
Vapor (*see also* Gas)	987.9	E869.9	—	E952.9	E962.2	E982.9
kiln (carbon monoxide)	986	E868.8	—	E952.1	E962.2	E982.1
lead — *see* Lead						
specified source NEC (*see also* specific substance)	987.8	E869.8	—	E952.8	E962.2	E982.8
Varidase	964.4	E858.2	E934.4	E950.4	E962.0	E980.4
Varnish	989.89	E861.6	—	E950.9	E962.1	E980.9
cleaner	982.8	E862.9	—	E950.9	E962.1	E980.9
Vaseline	976.3	E858.7	E946.3	E950.4	E962.0	E980.4
Vasodilan	972.5	E858.3	E942.5	E950.4	E962.0	E980.4
Vasodilators NEC	972.5	E858.3	E942.5	E950.4	E962.0	E980.4
coronary	972.4	E858.3	E942.4	E950.4	E962.0	E980.4
Vasopressin	962.5	E858.0	E932.5	E950.4	E962.0	E980.4
Vasopressor drugs	962.5	E858.0	E932.5	E950.4	E962.0	E980.4
Venom, venomous (bite) (sting)	989.5	E905.9	—	E950.9	E962.1	E980.9
arthropod NEC	989.5	E905.5	—	E950.9	E962.1	E980.9
bee	989.5	E905.3	—	E950.9	E962.1	E980.9
centipede	989.5	E905.4	—	E950.9	E962.1	E980.9
hornet	989.5	E905.3	—	E950.9	E962.1	E980.9
lizard	989.5	E905.0	—	E950.9	E962.1	E980.9
marine animals or plants	989.5	E905.6	—	E950.9	E962.1	E980.9
millipede (tropical)	989.5	E905.4	—	E950.9	E962.1	E980.9
plant NEC	989.5	E905.7	—	E950.9	E962.1	E980.9
marine	989.5	E905.6	—	E950.9	E962.1	E980.9
scorpion	989.5	E905.2	—	E950.9	E962.1	E980.9
snake	989.5	E905.0	—	E950.9	E962.1	E980.9
specified NEC	989.5	E905.8	—	E950.9	E962.1	E980.9
spider	989.5	E905.1	—	E950.9	E962.1	E980.9
wasp	989.5	E905.3	—	E950.9	E962.1	E980.9
Veramon	967.0	E851	E937.0	E950.1	E962.0	E980.1
Veratrum						
album	988.2	E865.4	—	E950.9	E962.1	E980.9
alkaloids	972.6	E858.3	E942.6	E950.4	E962.0	E980.4
viride	988.2	E865.4	—	E950.9	E962.1	E980.9
Verdigris (*see also* Copper)	985.8	E866.4	—	E950.9	E962.1	E980.9
Veronal	967.0	E851	E937.0	E950.1	E962.0	E980.1
Veroxil	961.6	E857	E931.6	E950.4	E962.0	E980.4
Versidyne	965.7	E850.7	E935.7	E950.0	E962.0	E980.0
Viagra	972.5	E858.3	E942.5	E950.4	E962.0	E980.4
Vienna						
green	985.1	E866.3	—	E950.8	E962.1	E980.8
insecticide	985.1	E863.4	—	E950.6	E962.1	E980.7
red	989.89	E866.8	—	E950.9	E962.1	E980.9
pharmaceutical dye	977.4	E858.8	E947.4	E950.4	E962.0	E980.4
Vinbarbital, vinbarbitone	967.0	E851	E937.0	E950.1	E962.0	E980.1

Table of Drugs and Chemicals

		External Cause (E-Code)				
	Poisoning	Accident	Therapeutic Use	Suicide Attempt	Assault	Undetermined
Vinblastine	963.1	E858.1	E933.1	E950.4	E962.0	E980.4
Vincristine	963.1	E858.1	E933.1	E950.4	E962.0	E980.4
Vinesthene, vinethene	968.2	E855.1	E938.2	E950.4	E962.0	E980.4
Vinyl						
bital	967.0	E851	E937.0	E950.1	E962.0	E980.1
ether	968.2	E855.1	E938.2	E950.4	E962.0	E980.4
Vioform	961.3	E857	E931.3	E950.4	E962.0	E980.4
topical	976.0	E858.7	E946.0	E930.4	E962.0	E980.4
Viomycin	960.6	E856	E930.6	E950.4	E962.0	E980.4
Viosterol	963.5	E858.1	E933.5	E950.4	E962.0	E980.4
Viper (venom)	989.5	E905.0	—	E950.9	E962.1	E980.9
Viprynium (embonate)	961.6	E857	E931.6	E950.4	E962.0	E980.4
Virugon	961.7	E857	E931.7	E950.4	E962.0	E980.4
Visine	976.5	E858.7	E946.5	E950.4	E962.0	E980.4
Vitamins NEC	963.5	E858.1	E933.5	E950.4	E962.0	E980.4
B_{12}	964.1	E858.2	E934.1	E950.4	E962.0	E980.4
hematopoietic	964.1	E858.2	E934.1	E950.4	E962.0	E980.4
K	964.3	E858.2	E934.3	E950.4	E962.0	E980.4
Vleminckx's solution	976.4	E858.7	E946.4	E950.4	E962.0	E980.4
Voltaren — *see* Diclofenac sodium						
Ventolin — *see* Salbutamol sulfate						
Warfarin (potassium) (sodium)	964.2	E858.2	E934.2	E950.4	E962.0	E980.4
rodenticide	989.4	E863.7	—	E950.6	E962.1	E980.7
Wasp (sting)	989.5	E905.3	—	E950.9	E962.1	E980.9
Water						
balance agents NEC	974.5	E858.5	E944.5	E950.4	E962.0	E980.4
gas	987.1	E868.1	—	E951.8	E962.2	E981.8
incomplete combustion of — *see* Carbon, monoxide, fuel, utility						
hemlock	988.2	E865.4	—	E950.9	E962.1	E980.9
moccasin (venom)	989.5	E905.0	—	E950.9	E962.1	E980.9
Wax (paraffin) (petroleum)	981	E862.3	—	E950.9	E962.1	E980.9
automobile	989.89	E861.2	—	E950.9	E962.1	E980.9
floor	981	E862.0	—	E950.9	E962.1	E980.9
Weed killers NEC	989.4	E863.5	—	E950.6	E962.1	E980.7
Welldorm	967.1	E852.0	E937.1	E950.2	E962.0	E980.2
White						
arsenic — *see* Arsenic						
hellebore	988.2	E865.4	—	E950.9	E962.1	E980.9
lotion (keratolytic)	976.4	E858.7	E946.4	E950.4	E962.0	E980.4
spirit	981	E862.0	—	E950.9	E962.1	E980.9
Whitewashes	989.89	E861.6	—	E950.9	E962.1	E980.9
Whole blood	964.7	E858.2	E934.7	E950.4	E962.0	E980.4
Wild						
black cherry	988.2	E865.4	—	E950.9	E962.1	E980.9
poisonous plants NEC	988.2	E865.4	—	E950.9	E962.1	E980.9
Window cleaning fluid	989.89	E861.3	—	E950.9	E962.1	E980.9
Wintergreen (oil)	976.3	E858.7	E946.3	E950.4	E962.0	E980.4
Witch hazel	976.2	E858.7	E946.2	E950.4	E962.0	E980.4
Wood						
alcohol	980.1	E860.2	—	E950.9	E962.1	E980.9
spirit	980.1	E860.2	—	E950.9	E962.1	E980.9
Woorali	975.2	E858.6	E945.2	E950.4	E962.0	E980.4
Wormseed, American	961.6	E857	E931.6	E950.4	E962.0	E980.4
Xanthine diuretics	974.1	E858.5	E944.1	E950.4	E962.0	E980.4
Xanthocillin	960.0	E856	E930.0	E950.4	E962.0	E980.4
Xanthotoxin	976.3	E858.7	E946.3	E950.4	E962.0	E980.4
Xylene (liquid) (vapor)	982.0	E862.4	—	E950.9	E962.1	E980.9
Xylocaine (infiltration) (topical)	968.5	E855.2	E938.5	E950.4	E962.0	E980.4
nerve block (peripheral) (plexus)	968.6	E855.2	E938.6	E950.4	E962.0	E980.4
spinal	968.7	E855.2	E938.7	E950.4	E962.0	E980.4
Xylol (liquid) (vapor)	982.0	E862.4	—	E950.9	E962.1	E980.9
Xylometazoline	971.2	E855.5	E941.2	E950.4	E962.0	E980.4
Yellow						
fever vaccine	979.3	E858.8	E949.3	E950.4	E962.0	E980.4
jasmine	988.2	E865.4	—	E950.9	E962.1	E980.9
Yew	988.2	E865.4	—	E950.9	E962.1	E980.9
Zactane	965.7	E850.7	E935.7	E950.0	E962.0	E980.0
Zaroxolyn	974.3	E858.5	E944.3	E950.4	E962.0	E980.4
Zephiran (topical)	976.0	E858.7	E946.0	E950.4	E962.0	E980.4
ophthalmic preparation	976.5	E858.7	E946.5	E950.4	E962.0	E980.4
Zerone	980.1	E860.2	—	E950.9	E962.1	E980.9
Zinc (compounds) (fumes) (salts) (vapor) NEC	985.8	E866.4	—	E950.9	E962.1	E980.9
anti-infectives	976.0	E858.7	E946.0	E950.4	E962.0	E980.4
antivaricose	972.7	E858.3	E942.7	E950.4	E962.0	E980.4
bacitracin	976.0	E858.7	E946.0	E950.4	E962.0	E980.4
chloride	976.2	E858.7	E946.2	E950.4	E962.0	E980.4
gelatin	976.3	E858.7	E946.3	E950.4	E962.0	E980.4
oxide	976.3	E858.7	E946.3	E950.4	E962.0	E980.4
peroxide	976.0	E858.7	E946.0	E950.4	E962.0	E980.4
pesticides	985.8	E863.4	—	E950.6	E962.1	E980.7
phosphide (rodenticide)	985.8	E863.7	—	E950.6	E962.1	E980.7

Zinc NEC — Table of Drugs and Chemicals

	Poisoning	External Cause (E-Code)				
		Accident	Therapeutic Use	Suicide Attempt	Assault	Undetermined
Zinc NEC — *continued*						
stearate	976.3	E858.7	E946.3	E950.4	E962.0	E980.4
sulfate (antivaricose)	972.7	E858.3	E942.7	E950.4	E962.0	E980.4
ENT agent	976.6	E858.7	E946.6	E950.4	E962.0	E980.4
ophthalmic solution	976.5	E858.7	E946.5	E950.4	E962.0	E980.4
topical NEC	976.0	E858.7	E946.0	E950.4	E962.0	E980.4
undecylenate	976.0	E858.7	E946.0	E950.4	E962.0	E980.4
Zoxazolamine	968.0	E855.1	E938.0	E950.4	E962.0	E980.4
Zygadenus (venenosus)	988.2	E865.4	—	E950.9	E962.1	E980.9

SECTION 3
Alphabetic Index to External Causes of Injury and Poisoning (E Code)

This section contains the index to the codes which classify environmental events, circumstances, and other conditions as the cause of injury and other adverse effects. Where a code from the section Supplementary Classification of External Causes of Injury and Poisoning (E800-E998) is applicable, it is intended that the E code shall be used in addition to a code from the main body of the classification, Chapters 1 to 17.

The alphabetic index to the E codes is organized by main terms which describe the *accident, circumstance, event,* or *specific agent* which caused the injury or other adverse effect.

Note — Transport accidents (E800-E848) include accidents involving:
      aircraft and spacecraft (E840-E845)
      watercraft (E830-E838)
      motor vehicle (E810-E825)
      railway (E800-E807)
      other road vehicles (E826-E829)

For definitions and examples related to transport accidents — see Volume 1 code categories E800-E848.

The fourth-digit subdivisions for use with categories E800-E848 to identify the injured person are found at the end of this section.

For identifying the place in which an accident or poisoning occurred (circumstances classifiable to categories E850-E869 and E880-E928) — see the listing in this section under "Accident, occurring."

See the Table of Drugs and Chemicals (Section 2 of this volume) for identifying the specific agent involved in drug overdose or a wrong substance given or taken in error, and for intoxication or poisoning by a drug or other chemical substance.

The specific adverse effect, reaction, or localized toxic effect to a correct drug or substance properly administered in therapeutic or prophylactic dosage should be classified according to the nature of the adverse effect (e.g., allergy, dermatitis, tachycardia) listed in Section 1 of this volume.

Index to External Causes

Index to External Causes

A

Abandonment
  causing exposure to weather conditions — see Exposure
  child, with intent to injure or kill E968.4
  helpless person, infant, newborn E904.0
    with intent to injure or kill E968.4
Abortion, criminal, injury to child E968.8
Abuse (alleged) (suspected)
  adult
    by
      child E967.4
      ex-partner E967.3
      ex-spouse E967.3
      father E967.0
      grandchild E967.7
      grandparent E967.6
      mother E967.2
      non-related caregiver E967.8
      other relative E967.7
      other specified person E967.1
      partner E967.3
      sibling E967.5
      spouse E967.3
      stepfather E967.0
      stepmother E967.2
      unspecified person E967.9
  child
    by
      boyfriend of parent or guardian E967.0
      child E967.4
      father E967.0
      female partner of parent or guardian E967.2
      girlfriend of parent or guardian E967.2
      grandchild E967.7
      grandparent E967.6
      male partner of parent or guardian E967.2
      mother E967.2
      non-related caregiver E967.8
      other relative E967.7
      other specified person(s) E967.1
      sibling E967.5
      stepfather E967.0
      stepmother E967.2
      unspecified person E967.9
Accident (to) E928.9
  aircraft (in transit) (powered) E841 ✓4ᵗʰ
    at landing, take-off E840 ✓4ᵗʰ
    due to, caused by cataclysm — see categories E908 ✓4ᵗʰ, E909 ✓4ᵗʰ
    late effect of E929.1
    unpowered (see also Collision, aircraft, unpowered) E842 ✓4ᵗʰ
    while alighting, boarding E843 ✓4ᵗʰ
  amphibious vehicle
    on
      land — see Accident, motor vehicle
      water — see Accident, watercraft
  animal, ridden NEC E828 ✓4ᵗʰ
  animal-drawn vehicle NEC E827 ✓4ᵗʰ
  balloon (see also Collision, aircraft, unpowered) E842 ✓4ᵗʰ
  caused by, due to
    abrasive wheel (metalworking) E919.3
    animal NEC E906.9
      being ridden (in sport or transport) E828 ✓4ᵗʰ
    avalanche NEC E909.2
    band saw E919.4
    bench saw E919.4
    bore, earth-drilling or mining (land) (seabed) E919.1
    bulldozer E919.7
    cataclysmic
      earth surface movement or eruption E909.9
      storm E908.9
    chain
      hoist E919.2
        agricultural operations E919.0
        mining operations E919.1
      saw E920.1
    circular saw E919.4

Accident (to) — continued
  caused by, due to — continued
    cold (excessive) (see also Cold, exposure to) E901.9
    combine E919.0
    conflagration — see Conflagration
    corrosive liquid, substance NEC E924.1
    cotton gin E919.8
    crane E919.2
      agricultural operations E919.0
      mining operations E919.1
    cutting or piercing instrument (see also Cut) E920.9
    dairy equipment E919.8
    derrick E919.2
      agricultural operations E919.0
      mining operations E919.1
    drill E920.1
      earth (land) (seabed) E919.1
      hand (powered) E920.1
        not powered E920.4
      metalworking E919.3
      woodworking E919.4
    earth(-)
      drilling machine E919.1
      moving machine E919.7
      scraping machine E919.7
    electric
      current (see also Electric shock) E925.9
      motor — see also Accident, machine, by type of machine
        current (of) — see Electric shock
    elevator (building) (grain) E919.2
      agricultural operations E919.0
      mining operations E919.1
    environmental factors NEC E928.9
    excavating machine E919.7
    explosive material (see also Explosion) E923.9
    farm machine E919.0
    fire, flames — see also Fire
      conflagration — see Conflagration
    firearm missile — see Shooting
    forging (metalworking) machine E919.3
    forklift (truck) E919.2
      agricultural operations E919.0
      mining operations E919.1
    gas turbine E919.5
    harvester E919.0
    hay derrick, mower, or rake E919.0
    heat (excessive) (see also Heat) E900.9
    hoist (see also Accident, caused by, due to, lift) E919.2
      chain — see Accident, caused by, due to, chain
      shaft E919.1
    hot
      liquid E924.0
        caustic or corrosive E924.1
      object (not producing fire or flames) E924.8
      substance E924.9
        caustic or corrosive E924.1
        liquid (metal) NEC E924.0
        specified type NEC E924.8
    human bite E928.3
    ignition — see Ignition
    internal combustion engine E919.5
    landslide NEC E909.2
    lathe (metalworking) E919.3
      turnings E920.8
      woodworking E919.4
    lift, lifting (appliances) E919.2
      agricultural operations E919.0
      mining operations E919.1
      shaft E919.1
    lightning NEC E907
    machine, machinery — see also Accident, machine
      drilling, metal E919.3
      manufacturing, for manufacture of
        beverages E919.8
        clothing E919.8
        foodstuffs E919.8
        paper E919.8
        textiles E919.8

Accident (to) — continued
  caused by, due to — continued
    machine, machinery — see also Accident, machine — continued
      milling, metal E919.3
      moulding E919.4
      power press, metal E919.3
      printing E919.8
      rolling mill, metal E919.3
      sawing, metal E919.3
      specified type NEC E919.8
      spinning E919.8
      weaving E919.8
    natural factor NEC E928.9
    overhead plane E919.4
    plane E920.4
      overhead E919.4
    powered
      hand tool NEC E920.1
      saw E919.4
        hand E920.1
    printing machine E919.8
    pulley (block) E919.2
      agricultural operations E919.0
      mining operations E919.1
      transmission E919.6
    radial saw E919.4
    radiation — see Radiation
    reaper E919.0
    road scraper E919.7
      when in transport under its own power — see categories E810-E825 ✓4ᵗʰ
    roller coaster E919.8
    sander E919.4
    saw E920.4
      band E919.4
      bench E919.4
      chain E920.1
      circular E919.4
      hand E920.4
        powered E920.1
      powered, except hand E919.4
      radial E919.4
    sawing machine, metal E919.3
    shaft
      hoist E919.1
      lift E919.1
      transmission E919.6
    shears E920.4
      hand E920.4
        powered E920.1
      mechanical E919.3
    shovel E920.4
      steam E919.7
    spinning machine E919.8
    steam — see also Burning, steam
      engine E919.5
      shovel E919.7
    thresher E919.0
    thunderbolt NEC E907
    tractor E919.0
      when in transport under its own power — see categories E810-E825 ✓4ᵗʰ
    transmission belt, cable, chain, gear, pinion, pulley, shaft E919.6
    turbine (gas) (water driven) E919.5
    under-cutter E919.1
    weaving machine E919.8
    winch E919.2
      agricultural operations E919.0
      mining operations E919.1
  diving E883.9
    with insufficient air supply E913.2
  glider (hang) (see also Collision, aircraft, unpowered) E842 ✓4ᵗʰ
  hovercraft
    on
      land — see Accident, motor vehicle
      water — see Accident, watercraft
  ice yacht (see also Accident, vehicle NEC) E848
  in
    medical, surgical procedure
      as, or due to misadventure — see Misadventure

Accident (to) — Andes disease

Accident (to)

Accident (to) — continued
  in — continued
    medical, surgical procedure — continued
      causing an abnormal reaction or later complication without mention of misadventure — see Reaction, abnormal
    kite carrying a person (see also Collision, aircraft, unpowered) E842 ✓4ᵗʰ
    land yacht (see also Accident, vehicle NEC) E848
    late effect of — see Late effect
    launching pad E845 ✓4ᵗʰ
    machine, machinery (see also Accident, caused by, due to, by specific type of machine) E919.9
      agricultural including animal-powered E919.0
      earth-drilling E919.1
      earth moving or scraping E919.7
      excavating E919.7
      involving transport under own power on highway or transport vehicle — see categories E810-E825 ✓4ᵗʰ, E840-E845 ✓4ᵗʰ
      lifting (appliances) E919.2
      metalworking E919.3
      mining E919.1
      prime movers, except electric motors E919.5
        electric motors — see Accident, machine, by specific type of machine
      recreational E919.8
      specified type NEC E919.8
      transmission E919.6
      watercraft (deck) (engine room) (galley) (laundry) (loading) E836 ✓4ᵗʰ
      woodworking or forming E919.4
    motor vehicle (on public highway) (traffic) E819 ✓4ᵗʰ
      due to cataclysm — see categories E908 ✓4ᵗʰ, E909 ✓4ᵗʰ
      involving
        collision (see also Collision, motor vehicle) E812 ✓4ᵗʰ
      nontraffic, not on public highway — see categories E820-E825 ✓4ᵗʰ
      not involving collision — see categories E816-E819 ✓4ᵗʰ
    nonmotor vehicle NEC E829 ✓4ᵗʰ
      nonroad — see Accident, vehicle NEC
      road, except pedal cycle, animal-drawn vehicle, or animal being ridden E829 ✓4ᵗʰ
    nonroad vehicle NEC — see Accident, vehicle NEC
    not elsewhere classifiable involving
      cable car (not on rails) E847
        on rails E829 ✓4ᵗʰ
      coal car in mine E846
      hand truck — see Accident, vehicle NEC
      logging car E846
      sled(ge), meaning snow or ice vehicle E848
      tram, mine or quarry E846
      truck
        mine or quarry E846
        self-propelled, industrial E846
        station baggage E846
      tub, mine or quarry E846
      vehicle NEC E848
        snow and ice E848
        used only on industrial premises E846
      wheelbarrow E848
    occurring (at) (in)
      apartment E849.0
      baseball field, diamond E849.4
      construction site, any E849.3
      dock E849.8
        yard E849.3
      dormitory E849.7
      factory (building) (premises) E849.3
      farm E849.1
        buildings E849.1
        house E849.0
      football field E849.4
      forest E849.8
      garage (place of work) E849.3
        private (home) E849.0

Accident (to) — continued
  occurring (at) (in) — continued
    gravel pit E849.2
    gymnasium E849.4
    highway E849.5
    home (private) (residential) E849.0
      institutional E849.7
    hospital E849.7
    hotel E849.6
    house (private) (residential) E849.0
      movie E849.6
      public E849.6
    institution, residential E849.7
    jail E849.7
    mine E849.2
    motel E849.6
    movie house E849.6
    office (building) E849.6
    orphanage E849.7
    park (public) E849.4
      mobile home E849.8
      trailer E849.8
    parking lot or place E849.8
    place
      industrial NEC E849.3
      parking E849.8
      public E849.8
        specified place NEC E849.5
      recreational NEC E849.4
      sport NEC E849.4
    playground (park) (school) E849.4
    prison E849.6
    public building NEC E849.6
    quarry E849.2
    railway
      line NEC E849.8
      yard E849.3
    residence
      home (private) E849.0
    resort (beach) (lake) (mountain) (seashore) (vacation) E849.4
    restaurant E849.6
    sand pit E849.2
    school (building) (private) (public) (state) E849.6
      reform E849.7
      riding E849.4
    seashore E849.8
      resort E849.4
    shop (place of work) E849.3
      commercial E849.6
    skating rink E849.4
    sports palace E849.4
    stadium E849.4
    store E849.6
    street E849.5
    swimming pool (public) E849.4
      private home or garden E849.0
    tennis court E849.4
    theatre, theater E849.6
    trailer court E849.8
    tunnel E849.8
      under construction E849.2
    warehouse E849.3
    yard
      dock E849.3
      industrial E849.3
      private (home) E849.0
      railway E849.3
  off-road type motor vehicle (not on public highway) NEC E821 ✓4ᵗʰ
    on public highway — see catagories E810-E819 ✓4ᵗʰ
  pedal cycle E826 ✓4ᵗʰ
  railway E807 ✓4ᵗʰ
    due to cataclysm — see categories E908 ✓4ᵗʰ, E909 ✓4ᵗʰ
    involving
      avalanche E909.2
      burning by engine, locomotive, train (see also Explosion, railway engine) E803 ✓4ᵗʰ
      collision (see also Collision, railway) E800 ✓4ᵗʰ
      derailment (see also Derailment, railway) E802 ✓4ᵗʰ

Accident (to) — continued
  railway — continued
    involving — continued
      explosion (see also Explosion, railway engine) E803 ✓4ᵗʰ
      fall (see also Fall, from, railway rolling stock) E804 ✓4ᵗʰ
      fire (see also Explosion, railway engine) E803 ✓4ᵗʰ
      hitting by, being struck by
        object falling in, on, from, rolling stock, train, vehicle E806 ✓4ᵗʰ
        rolling stock, train, vehicle E805 ✓4ᵗʰ
      overturning, railway rolling stock, train, vehicle (see also Derailment, railway) E802 ✓4ᵗʰ
      running off rails, railway (see also Derailment, railway) E802 ✓4ᵗʰ
      specified circumstances NEC E806 ✓4ᵗʰ
      train or vehicle hit by
        avalanche E909 ✓4ᵗʰ
        falling object (earth, rock, tree) E806 ✓4ᵗʰ
          due to cataclysm — see categories E908 ✓4ᵗʰ, E909 ✓4ᵗʰ
        landslide E909 ✓4ᵗʰ
  roller skate E885.1
  scooter (nonmotorized) E885.0 ●
  skateboard E885.2
  ski(ing) E885.3
    jump E884.9
    lift or tow (with chair or gondola) E847
  snow vehicle, motor driven (not on public highway) E820 ✓4ᵗʰ
    on public highway — see catagories E810-E819 ✓4ᵗʰ
  snowboard E885.4
  spacecraft E845 ✓4ᵗʰ
  specified cause NEC E928.8
  street car E829 ✓4ᵗʰ
  traffic NEC E819 ✓4ᵗʰ
  vehicle NEC (with pedestrian) E848
    battery powered
      airport passenger vehicle E846
      truck (baggage) (mail) E846
    powered commercial or industrial (with other vehicle or object within commercial or industrial premises) E846
  watercraft E838 ✓4ᵗʰ
    with
      drowning or submersion resulting from accident other than to watercraft E832 ✓4ᵗʰ
      accident to watercraft E830 ✓4ᵗʰ
      injury, except drowning or submersion, resulting from
        accident other than to watercraft — see categories E833-E838 ✓4ᵗʰ
        accident to watercraft E831 ✓4ᵗʰ
    due to, caused by cataclysm — see categories E908 ✓4ᵗʰ, E909 ✓4ᵗʰ
    machinery E836 ✓4ᵗʰ

Acid throwing E961
Acosta syndrome E902.0
Aeroneurosis E902.1
Aero-otitis media — see Effects of, air pressure
Aerosinusitis — see Effects of, air pressure
After-effect, late — see Late effect
Air
  blast
    in
      terrorism E979.2 ●
      war operations E993
  embolism (traumatic) NEC E928.9
    in
      infusion or transfusion E874.1
      perfusion E874.2
  sickness E903
Alpine sickness E902.0
Altitude sickness — see Effects of, air pressure
Anaphylactic shock, anaphylaxis (see also Table of Drugs and Chemicals) E947.9
  due to bite or sting (venomous) — see Bite, venomous
Andes disease E902.0

Index to External Causes

Apoplexy
   heat — *see* Heat
Arachnidism E905.1
Arson E968.0
Asphyxia, asphyxiation
  by
    chemical
      in
        terrorism E979.7
        war operations E997.2
    explosion — *see* Explosion
    food (bone) (regurgitated food) (seed) E911
    foreign object, exccpt food E912
    fumes
      in
        terrorism (chemical weapons) E979.7
        war operations E997.2
    gas — *see also* Table of Drugs and Chemicals
      in
        terrorism E979.7
        war operations E997.2
      legal
        execution E978
        intervention (tear) E972
      tear E972
    mechanical means (*see also* Suffocation) E913.9
  from
    conflagration — *see* Conflagration
    fire — *see also* Fire E899
      in
        terrorism E979.3
        war operations E990.9
    ignition — *see* Ignition
Aspiration
  foreign body — *see* Foreign body, aspiration
  mucus, not of newborn (with asphyxia, obstruction respiratory passage, suffocation) E912
  phlegm (with asphyxia, obstruction respiratory passage, suffocation) E912
  vomitus (with asphyxia, obstruction respiratory passage, suffocation) (*see also* Foreign body, aspiration, food) E911
Assassination (attempt) (*see also* Assault) E968.9
Assault (homicidal) (by) (in) E968.9
  acid E961
    swallowed E962.1
  air gun E968.6
  BB gun E968.6
  bite NEC E968.8
    of human being E968.7
  bomb ((placed in) car or house) E965.8
    antipersonnel E965.5
    letter E965.7
    petrol E965.7
  brawl (hand) (fists) (foot) E960.0
  burning, burns (by fire) E968.0
    acid E961
      swallowed E962.1
    caustic, corrosive substance E961
      swallowed E962.1
    chemical from swallowing caustic, corrosive substance NEC E962.1
    hot liquid E968.3
    scalding E968.3
    vitriol E961
      swallowed E962.1
  caustic, corrosive substance E961
    swallowed E962.1
  cut, any part of body E966
  dagger E966
  drowning E964
  explosive(s) E965.9
    bomb (*see also* Assault, bomb) E965.8
    dynamite E965.8
  fight (hand) (fists) (foot) E960.0
    with weapon E968.9
      blunt or thrown E968.2
      cutting or piercing E966
      firearm — *see* Shooting, homicide
  fire E968.0
  firearm(s) — *see* Shooting, homicide

Assault — *continued*
  garrotting E963
  gunshot (wound) — *see* Shooting, homicide
  hanging E963
  injury NEC E968.9
  knife E966
  late effect of E969
  ligature E963
  poisoning E962.9
    drugs or medicinals E962.0
    gas(es) or vapors, except drugs and medicinals E962.2
    solid or liquid substances, except drugs and medicinals E962.1
  puncture, any part of body E966
  pushing
    before moving object, train, vehicle E968.5
    from high place E968.1
  rape E960.1
  scalding E968.3
  shooting — *see* Shooting, homicide
  sodomy E960.1
  stab, any part of body E966
  strangulation E963
  submersion E964
  suffocation E963
  transport vehicle E968.5
  violence NEC E968.9
  vitriol E961
    swallowed E962.1
  weapon E968.9
    blunt or thrown E968.2
    cutting or piercing E966
    firearm — *see* Shooting, homicide
  wound E968.9
    cutting E966
    gunshot — *see* Shooting, homicide
    knife E966
    piercing E966
    puncture E966
    stab E966
Attack by animal NEC E906.9
Avalanche E909.2
  falling on or hitting
    motor vehicle (in motion) (on public highway) E909.2
    railway train E909.2
Aviators' disease E902.1

B

Barotitis, barodontalgia, barosinusitis, barotrauma (otitic) (sinus) — *see* Effects of, air pressure
Battered
  baby or child (syndrome) — *see* Abuse, child; category E967
  person other than baby or child — *see* Assault
Bayonet wound (*see also* Cut, by bayonet) E920.3
  in
    legal intervention E974
    terrorism E979.8
    war operations E995
Bean in nose E912
Bed set on fire NEC E898.0
Beheading (by guillotine)
  homicide E966
  legal execution E978
Bending, injury in E927
Bends E902.0
Bite
  animal (nonvenomous) NEC E906.5
    other specified (except arthropod) E906.3
    venomous NEC E905.9
  arthropod (nonvenomous) NEC E906.4
    venomous — *see* Sting
  black widow spider E905.1
  cat E906.3
  centipede E905.4
  cobra E905.0
  copperhead snake E905.0
  coral snake E905.0
  dog E906.0
  fer de lance E905.0
  gila monster E905.0

Bite — *continued*
  human being
    accidental E928.3
    assault E968.7
  insect (nonvenomous) E906.4
    venomous — *see* Sting
  krait E905.0
  late effect of — *see* Late effect
  lizard E906.2
    venomous E905.0
  mamba E905.0
  marine animal
    nonvenomous E906.3
      snake E906.2
    venomous E905.6
      snake E905.0
  millipede E906.4
    venomous E905.4
  moray eel E906.3
  rat E906.1
  rattlesnake E905.0
  rodent, except rat E906.3
  serpent — *see* Bite, snake
  shark E906.3
  snake (venomous) E905.0
    nonvenomous E906.2
    sea E905.0
  spider E905.1
    nonvenomous E906.4
  tarantula (venomous) E905.1
  venomous NEC E905.9
    by specific animal — *see category* E905
  viper E905.0
  water moccasin E905.0
Blast (air)
  from nuclear explosion E996
  in
    terrorism E979.2
      from nuclear explosion E979.5
      underwater E979.0
    war operations E993
      from nuclear explosion E996
      underwater E992
  underwater E992
Blizzard E908.3
Blow E928.9
  by law-enforcing agent, police (on duty) E975
    with blunt object (baton) (nightstick) (stave) (truncheon) E973
Blowing up (*see also* Explosion) E923.9
Brawl (hand) (fists) (foot) E960.0
Breakage (accidental)
  cable of cable car not on rails E847
  ladder (causing fall) E881.0
  part (any) of
    animal-drawn vehicle E827
    ladder (causing fall) E881.0
    motor vehicle
      in motion (on public highway) E818
      not on public highway E825
    nonmotor road vehicle, except animal-drawn vehicle or pedal cycle E829
    off-road type motor vehicle (not on public highway) NEC E821
      on public highway E818
    pedal cycle E826
    scaffolding (causing fall) E881.1
    snow vehicle, motor-driven (not on public highway) E820
      on public highway E818
    vehicle NEC — *see* Accident, vehicle
Broken
  glass
    fall on E888.0
    injury by E920.8
  power line (causing electric shock) E925.1
Bumping against, into (accidentally)
  object (moving) E917.9
    caused by crowd E917.1
      with subsequent fall E917.6
    furniture E917.3
      with subsequent fall E917.7
    in
      running water E917.2
      sports E917.0
        with subsequent fall E917.5

Bumping against, into — *continued*
  object — *continued*
    stationary E917.4
      with subsequent fall E917.8
  person(s) E917.9
    with fall E886.9
      in sports E886.0
    as, or caused by, a crowd E917.1
      with subsequent fall E917.6
    in sports E917.0
      with fall E886.0
Burning, burns (accidental) (by) (from) (on) E899
  acid (any kind) E924.1
    swallowed — *see* Table of Drugs and Chemicals
  bedclothes (*see also* Fire, specified NEC) E898.0
  blowlamp (*see also* Fire, specified NEC) E898.1
  blowtorch (*see also* Fire, specified NEC) E898.1
  boat, ship, watercraft — *see* categories E830 ✓4ᵗʰ, E831 ✓4ᵗʰ, E837 ✓4ᵗʰ
  bonfire (controlled) E897
    uncontrolled E892
  candle (*see also* Fire, specified NEC) E898.1
  caustic liquid, substance E924.1
    swallowed — *see* Table of Drugs and Chemicals
  chemical E924.1
    from swallowing caustic, corrosive substance — *see* Table of Drugs and Chemicals
    in
      terrorism E979.7 •
      war operations E997.2
  cigar(s) or cigarette(s) (*see also* Fire, specified NEC) E898.1
  clothes, clothing, nightdress — *see* Ignition, clothes
    with conflagration — *see* Conflagration
  conflagration — *see* Conflagration
  corrosive liquid, substance E924.1
    swallowed — *see* Table of Drugs and Chemicals
  electric current (*see also* Electric shock) E925.9
  fire, flames (*see also* Fire) E899
  flare, Verey pistol E922.8
  heat
    from appliance (electrical) E924.8
    in local application, or packing during medical or surgical procedure E873.5
  homicide (attempt) (*see also* Assault, burning) E968.0
  hot
    liquid E924.0
      caustic or corrosive E924.1
    object (not producing fire or flames) E924.8
    substance E924.9
      caustic or corrosive E924.1
      liquid (metal) NEC E924.0
      specified type NEC E924.8
    tap water E924.2
  ignition — *see also* Ignition
    clothes, clothing, nightdress — *see also* Ignition, clothes
      with conflagration — *see* Conflagration
    highly inflammable material (benzine) (fat) (gasoline) (kerosene) (paraffin) (petrol) E894
  inflicted by other person
    stated as
      homicidal, intentional (*see also* Assault, burning) E968.0
      undetermined whether accidental or intentional (*see also* Burn, stated as undetermined whether accidental or intentional) E988.1
  internal, from swallowed caustic, corrosive liquid, substance — *see* Table of Drugs and Chemicals
  in
    terrorism E979.3 •
      from nuclear explosion E979.5 •
      petrol bomb E979.3 •

Burning, burns — *continued*
  in — *continued*
    war operations (from fire-producing device or conventional weapon) E990.9 •
      from nuclear explosion E996 •
      petrol bomb E990.0 •
  lamp (*see also* Fire, specified NEC) E898.1
  late effect of NEC E929.4
  lighter (cigar) (cigarette) (*see also* Fire, specified NEC) E898.1
  lightning E907
  liquid (boiling) (hot) (molten) E924.0
    caustic, corrosive (external) E924.1
      swallowed — *see* Table of Drugs and Chemicals
  local application of externally applied substance in medical or surgical care E873.5
  machinery — *see* Accident, machine
  matches (*see also* Fire, specified NEC) E898.1
  medicament, externally applied E873.5
  metal, molten E924.0
  object (hot) E924.8
    producing fire or flames — *see* Fire
  oven (electric) (gas) E924.8
  pipe (smoking) (*see also* Fire, specified NEC) E898.1
  radiation — *see* Radiation
  railway engine, locomotive, train (*see also* Explosion, railway engine) E803 ✓4ᵗʰ
  self-inflicted (unspecified whether accidental or intentional) E988.1
    caustic or corrosive substance NEC E988.7
    stated as intentional, purposeful E958.1
      caustic or corrosive substance NEC E958.7
  stated as undetermined whether accidental or intentional E988.1
    caustic or corrosive substance NEC E988.7
  steam E924.0
    pipe E924.8
  substance (hot) E924.9
    boiling or molten E924.0
    caustic, corrosive (external) E924.1
      swallowed — *see* Table of Drugs and Chemicals
  suicidal (attempt) NEC E958.1
    caustic substance E958.7
    late effect of E959
  tanning bed E926.2
  therapeutic misadventure
    overdose of radiation E873.2
  torch, welding (*see also* Fire, specified NEC) E898.1
  trash fire (*see also* Burning, bonfire) E897
  vapor E924.0
  vitriol E924.1
  x-rays E926.3
    in medical, surgical procedure — *see* Misadventure, failure, in dosage, radiation
Butted by animal E906.8

C

Cachexia, lead or saturnine E866.0
  from pesticide NEC (*see also* Table of Drugs and Chemicals) E863.4
Caisson disease E902.2
Capital punishment (any means) E978
Car sickness E903
Casualty (not due to war) NEC E928.9
  terrorism E979.8 •
  war (*see also* War operations) E995
Cat
  bite E906.3
  scratch E906.8
Cataclysmic (any injury)
  earth surface movement or eruption E909.9
    specified type NEC E909.8
  storm or flood resulting from storm E908.9
    specified type NEC E909.8
Catching fire — *see* Ignition

Caught
  between
    objects (moving) (stationary and moving) E918
      and machinery — *see* Accident, machine
  by cable car, not on rails E847
  in
    machinery (moving parts of) — *see*, Accident, machine
    object E918
Cave-in (causing asphyxia, suffocation (by pressure)) (*see also* Suffocation, due to, cave-in) E913.3
  with injury other than asphyxia or suffocation E916
    with asphyxia or suffocation (*see also* Suffocation, due to, cave-in) E913.3
  struck or crushed by E916
    with asphyxia or suffocation (*see also* Suffocation, due to, cave-in) E913.3
Change(s) in air pressure — *see also* Effects of, air pressure
  sudden, in aircraft (ascent) (descent) (causing aeroneurosis or aviators' disease) E902.1
Chilblains E901.0
  due to manmade conditions E901.1
Choking (on) (any object except food or vomitus) E912
  apple E911
  bone E911
  food, any type (regurgitated) E911
  mucus or phlegm E912
  seed E911
Civil insurrection — *see* War operations
Cloudburst E908.8
Cold, exposure to (accidental) (excessive) (extreme) (place) E901.9
  causing chilblains or immersion foot E901.0
  due to
    manmade conditions E901.1
    specified cause NEC E901.8
    weather (conditions) E901.0
  late effect of NEC E929.5
  self-inflicted (undetermined whether accidental or intentional) E988.3
  suicidal E958.3
  suicide E958.3
Colic, lead, painter's, or saturnine — *see* category E866 ✓4ᵗʰ
Collapse
  building (moveable) E916
    burning ▶(uncontrolled fire)◀ E891.8
      in terrorism E979.3 •
      private E890.8
  dam E909.3
  due to heat — *see* Heat
  machinery — *see* Accident, machine
  man-made structure E909.3
  postoperative NEC E878.9
  structure, burning NEC E891.8
    burning (uncontrolled fire) •
      in terrorism E979.3 •

Index to External Causes

Collision (accidental)

Note — In the case of collisions between different types of vehicles, persons and objects, priority in classification is in the following order:

> *Aircraft*
> *Watercraft*
> *Motor vehicle*
> *Railway vehicle*
> *Pedal cycle*
> *Animal-drawn vehicle*
> *Animal being ridden*
> *Streetcar or other nonmotor road vehicle*
> *Other vehicle*
> *Pedestrian or person using pedestrian conveyance*
> *Object (except where falling from or set in motion by vehicle etc. listed above)*

In the listing below, the combinations are listed only under the vehicle etc. having priority. For definitions, see Volume 1, page 247.

    aircraft (with object or vehicle) (fixed) (movable) (moving) E841 ✓4th
      with
        person (while landing, taking off) (without accident to aircraft) E844 ✓4th
        powered (in transit) (with unpowered aircraft) E841 ✓4th
          while landing, taking off E840 ✓4th
        unpowered E842 ✓4th
          while landing, taking off E840 ✓4th
    animal being ridden (in sport or transport) E828 ✓4th
      and
        animal (being ridden) (herded) (unattended) E828 ✓4th
        nonmotor road vehicle, except pedal cycle or animal-drawn vehicle E828 ✓4th
        object (fallen) (fixed) (movable) (moving) not falling from or set in motion by vehicle of higher priority E828 ✓4th
        pedestrian (conveyance or vehicle) E828 ✓4th
    animal-drawn vehicle E827 ✓4th
      and
        animal (being ridden) (herded) (unattended) E827 ✓4th
        nonmotor road vehicle, except pedal cycle E827 ✓4th
        object (fallen) (fixed) (movable) (moving) not falling from or set in motion by vehicle of higher priority E827 ✓4th
        pedestrian (conveyance or vehicle) E827 ✓4th
        streetcar E827 ✓4th
    motor vehicle (on public highway) (traffic accident) E812 ✓4th
      after leaving, running off, public highway (without antecedent collision) (without re-entry) E816 ✓4th
      with antecedent collision on public highway — see categories E810-E815 ✓4th
      with re-entrance collision with another motor vehicle E811 ✓4th
      and
        abutment (bridge) (overpass) E815 ✓4th
        animal (herded) (unattended) E815 ✓4th
          carrying person, property E813 ✓4th
        animal-drawn vehicle E813 ✓4th
        another motor vehicle (abandoned) (disabled) (parked) (stalled) (stopped) E812 ✓4th

Collision — *continued*
    motor vehicle — *continued*
      and — *continued*
        another motor vehicle — *continued*
          with, involving re-entrance (on same roadway) (across median strip) E811 ✓4th
        any object, person, or vehicle off the public highway resulting from a noncollision motor vehicle nontraffic accident E816 ✓4th
        avalanche, fallen or not moving E815 ✓4th
          falling E909 ✓4th
        boundary fence E815 ✓4th
        culvert E815 ✓4th
        fallen
          stone E815 ✓4th
          tree E815 ✓4th
        falling E909.2
        guard post or guard rail E815 ✓4th
        inter-highway divider E815 ✓4th
        landslide, fallen or not moving E815 ✓4th
          moving E909
        machinery (road) E815 ✓4th
        moving E909.2
        nonmotor road vehicle NEC E813 ✓4th
        object (any object, person, or vehicle off the public highway resulting from a noncollision motor vehicle nontraffic accident) E815 ✓4th
          off, normally not on, public highway resulting from a noncollision motor vehicle traffic accident E816 ✓4th
        pedal cycle E813 ✓4th
        pedestrian (conveyance) E814 ✓4th
        person (using pedestrian conveyance) E814 ✓4th
        post or pole (lamp) (light) (signal) (telephone) (utility) E815 ✓4th
        railway rolling stock, train, vehicle E810 ✓4th
        safety island E815 ✓4th
        street car E813 ✓4th
        traffic signal, sign, or marker (temporary) E815 ✓4th
        tree E815 ✓4th
        tricycle E813 ✓4th
        wall of cut made for road E815 ✓4th
      due to cataclysm — see categories E908 ✓4th, E909
      not on public highway, nontraffic accident E822 ✓4th
      and
        animal (carrying person, property) (herded) (unattended) E822 ✓4th
        animal-drawn vehicle E822 ✓4th
        another motor vehicle (moving), except off-road motor vehicle E822 ✓4th
          stationary E823 ✓4th
        avalanche, fallen, not moving E823 ✓4th
          moving E909 ✓4th
        landslide, fallen, not moving E823 ✓4th
          moving E909 ✓4th
        nonmotor vehicle (moving) E822 ✓4th
          stationary E823 ✓4th
        object (fallen) (normally) (fixed) (movable but not in motion) (stationary) E823 ✓4th
          moving, except when falling from, set in motion by, aircraft or cataclysm E822 ✓4th
        pedal cycle (moving) E822 ✓4th
          stationary E823 ✓4th
        pedestrian (conveyance) E822 ✓4th
        person (using pedestrian conveyance) E822 ✓4th
        railway rolling stock, train, vehicle (moving) E822 ✓4th
          stationary E823 ✓4th
        road vehicle (any) (moving) E822 ✓4th
          stationary E823 ✓4th
        tricycle (moving) E822 ✓4th
          stationary E823 ✓4th
      moving E909.2

Collision — *continued*
    off-road type motor vehicle (not on public highway) E821 ✓4th
      and
        animal (being ridden) (-drawn vehicle) E821 ✓4th
        another off-road motor vehicle, except snow vehicle E821 ✓4th
        other motor vehicle, not on public highway E821 ✓4th
        other object or vehicle NEC, fixed or movable, not set in motion by aircraft, motor vehicle on highway, or snow vehicle, motor driven E821 ✓4th
        pedal cycle E821 ✓4th
        pedestrian (conveyance) E821 ✓4th
        railway train E821 ✓4th
      on public highway — *see* Collision, motor vehicle
    pedal cycle E826 ✓4th
      and
        animal (carrying person, property) (herded) (unherded) E826 ✓4th
        animal-drawn vehicle E826 ✓4th
        another pedal cycle E826 ✓4th
        nonmotor road vehicle E826 ✓4th
        object (fallen) (fixed) (movable) (moving) not falling from or set in motion by aircraft, motor vehicle, or railway train NEC E826 ✓4th
        pedestrian (conveyance) E826 ✓4th
        person (using pedestrian conveyance) E826 ✓4th
        street car E826 ✓4th
    pedestrian(s) (conveyance) E917.9
      with fall E886.9
        in sports E886.0
      and
        crowd, human stampede E917.1
          with subsequent fall E917.6
        furniture E917.3
          with subsequent fall E917.7
        machinery — *see* Accident, machine
        object (fallen) (moving) not falling from NEC, fixed or set in motion by any vehicle classifiable to E800-E848 E917.9
          with subsequent fall E917.6
          caused by a crowd E917.1
            with subsequent fall E917.6
          furniture E917.3
            with subsequent fall E917.7
          in
            running water E917.2
              with drowning or submersion — *see* Submersion
            sports E917.0
              with subsequent fall E917.5
            stationary E917.4
              with subsequent fall E917.8
        vehicle, nonmotor, nonroad E848
      in
        running water E917.2
          with drowning or submersion — *see* Submersion
        sports E917.0
          with fall E886.0
    person(s) (using pedestrian conveyance) (*see also* Collision, pedestrian) E917.9
    railway (rolling stock) (train) (vehicle) (with subsequent) derailment, explosion, fall or fire) E800 ✓4th
      with antecedent derailment E802 ✓4th
      and
        animal (carrying person) (herded) (unattended) E801 ✓4th
        another railway train or vehicle E800 ✓4th
        buffers E801 ✓4th
        fallen tree on railway E801 ✓4th
        farm machinery, nonmotor (in transport) (stationary) E801 ✓4th
        gates E801 ✓4th
        nonmotor vehicle E801 ✓4th

Collision

Collision — *continued*
  railway — *continued*
    and — *continued*
      object (fallen) (fixed) (movable) (moving)
        not falling from, set in motion by, aircraft or motor vehicle NEC E801 ✓4th
      pedal cycle E801 ✓4th
      pedestrian (conveyance) E805 ✓4th
      person (using pedestrian conveyance) E805 ✓4th
      platform E801 ✓4th
      rock on railway E801 ✓4th
      street car E801 ✓4th
  snow vehicle, motor-driven (not on public highway) E820 ✓4th
    and
      animal (being ridden) (-drawn vehicle) E820 ✓4th
      another off-road motor vehicle E820 ✓4th
      other motor vehicle, not on public highway E820 ✓4th
      other object or vehicle NEC, fixed or movable, not set in motion by aircraft or motor vehicle on highway E820 ✓4th
      pedal cycle E820 ✓4th
      pedestrian (conveyance) E820 ✓4th
      railway train E820 ✓4th
    on public highway — *see* Collision, motor vehicle
  street car(s) E829 ✓4th
    and
      animal, herded, not being ridden, unattended E829 ✓4th
      nonmotor road vehicle NEC E829 ✓4th
      object (fallen) (fixed) (movable) (moving) not falling from or set in motion by aircraft, animal-drawn vehicle, animal being ridden, motor vehicle, pedal cycle, or railway train E829 ✓4th
      pedestrian (conveyance) E829 ✓4th
      person (using pedestrian conveyance) E829 ✓4th
  vehicle
    animal-drawn — *see* Collision, animal-drawn vehicle
    motor — *see* Collision, motor vehicle
    nonmotor
      nonroad E848
        and
          another nonmotor, nonroad vehicle E848
          object (fallen) (fixed) (movable) (moving) not falling from or set in motion by aircraft, animal-drawn vehicle, animal being ridden, motor vehicle, nonmotor road vehicle, pedal cycle, railway train, or streetcar E848
      road, except animal being ridden, animal-drawn vehicle, or pedal cycle E829 ✓4th
        and
          animal, herded, not being ridden, unattended E829 ✓4th
          another nonmotor road vehicle, except animal being ridden, animal-drawn vehicle, or pedal cycle E829 ✓4th
          object (fallen) (fixed) (movable) (moving) not falling from or set in motion by, aircraft, animal-drawn vehicle, animal being ridden, motor vehicle, pedal cycle, or railway train E829 ✓4th
          pedestrian (conveyance) E829 ✓4th
          person (using pedestrian conveyance) E829 ✓4th
          vehicle, nonmotor, nonroad E829 ✓4th

Collision — *continued*
  watercraft E838 ✓4th
    and
      person swimming or water skiing E838 ✓4th
    causing
      drowning, submersion E830 ✓4th
      injury except drowning, submersion E831 ✓4th

Combustion, spontaneous — *see* Ignition

Complication of medical or surgical procedure or treatment
  as an abnormal reaction — *see* Reaction, abnormal
  delayed, without mention of misadventure — *see* Reaction, abnormal
  due to misadventure — *see* Misadventure

Compression
  divers' squeeze E902.2
  trachea by
    food E911
    foreign body, except food E912

Conflagration
  building or structure, except private dwelling (barn) (church) (convalescent or residential home) (factory) (farm outbuilding) (hospital) (hotel) (institution (educational) (domitory) (residential)) (school) (shop) (store) (theatre) E891.9
    with or causing (injury due to)
      accident or injury NEC E891.9
        specified circumstance NEC E891.8
      burns, burning E891.3
      carbon monoxide E891.2
      fumes E891.2
        polyvinylchloride (PVC) or similar material E891.1
      smoke E891.2
    causing explosion E891.0
    in terrorism E979.3 ●
  not in building or structure E892
  private dwelling (apartment) (boarding house) (camping place) (caravan) (farmhouse) (home (private)) (house) (lodging house) (private garage) (rooming house) (tenement) E890.9
    with or causing (injury due to)
      accident or injury NEC E890.9
        specified circumstance NEC E890.8
      burns, burning E890.3
      carbon monoxide E890.2
      fumes E890.2
        polyvinylchloride (PVC) or similar material E890.1
      smoke E890.2
    causing explosion E890.0

Contact with
  dry ice E901.1
  liquid air, hydrogen, nitrogen E901.1

Cramp(s)
  Heat — *see* Heat
  swimmers (*see also* category E910 ✓4th) E910.2
    not in recreation or sport E910.3

Cranking (car) (truck) (bus) (engine), injury by E917.9

Crash
  aircraft (in transit) (powered) E841 ✓4th
    at landing, take-off E840 ✓4th
    in
      terrorism E979.1 ●
      war operations E994
    on runway NEC E840 ✓4th
    stated as
      homicidal E968.8
      suicidal E958.6
      undetermined whether accidental or intentional E988.6
    unpowered E842 ✓4th
  glider E842 ✓4th
  motor vehicle — *see also* Accident, motor vehicle
    homicidal E968.5
    suicidal E958.5
    undetermined whether accidental or intentional E988.5

Crushed (accidentally) E928.9
  between
    boat(s), ship(s), watercraft (and dock or pier) (without accident to watercraft) E838 ✓4th
      after accident to, or collision, watercraft E831 ✓4th
    objects (moving) (stationary and moving) E918
  by
    avalanche NEC E909.2
    boat, ship, watercraft after accident to, collision, watercraft E831 ✓4th
    cave-in E916
      with asphyxiation or suffocation (*see also* Suffocation, due to, cave-in) E913.3
    crowd, human stampede E917.1
    falling
      aircraft (*see also* Accident, aircraft) E841 ✓4th
        in
          terrorism E979.1 ●
          war operations E994
      earth, material E916
        with asphyxiation or suffocation (*see also* Suffocation, due to, cave-in) E913.3
      object E916
        on ship, watercraft E838 ✓4th
        while loading, unloading watercraft E838 ✓4th
    landslide NEC E909.2
    lifeboat after abandoning ship E831 ✓4th
    machinery — *see* Accident, machine
    railway rolling stock, train, vehicle (part of) E805 ✓4th
    street car E829 ✓4th
    vehicle NEC — *see* Accident, vehicle NEC
  in
    machinery — *see* Accident, machine
    object E918
    transport accident — *see* categories E800-E848 ✓4th
  late effect of NEC E929.9

Cut, cutting (any part of body) (accidental) E920.9
  by
    arrow E920.8
    axe E920.4
    bayonet (*see also* Bayonet wound) E920.3
    blender E920.2
    broken glass E920.8
      following fall E888.0
    can opener E920.4
      powered E920.2
    chisel E920.4
    circular saw E919.4
    cutting or piercing instrument — *see also* category E920 ✓4th
      following fall E888.0
      late effect of E929.8
    dagger E920.3
    dart E920.8
    drill — *see* Accident, caused by drill
    edge of stiff paper E920.8
    electric
      beater E920.2
      fan E920.2
      knife E920.2
      mixer E920.2
    fork E920.4
    garden fork E920.4
    hand saw or tool (not powered) E920.4
      powered E920.1
    hedge clipper E920.4
      powered E920.1
    hoe E920.4
    ice pick E920.4
    knife E920.3
      electric E920.2
    lathe turnings E920.8
    lawn mower E920.4
      powered E920.0
      riding E919.8
    machine — *see* Accident, machine
    meat
      grinder E919.8

Index to External Causes

Cut, cutting — continued
  by — continued
   meat — continued
    slicer E919.8
   nails E920.8
   needle E920.4
    hypodermic E920.5
   object, edged, pointed, sharp — see category E920 ✓4ᵗʰ
    following fall E888.0
   paper cutter E920.4
   piercing instrument — see also category E920 ✓4ᵗʰ
    late effect of E929.8
   pitchfork E920.4
   powered
    can opener E920.2
    garden cultivator E920.1
     riding E919.8
    hand saw E920.1
    hand tool NEC E920.1
    hedge clipper E920.1
    household appliance or implement E920.2
    lawn mower (hand) E920.0
     riding E919.8
    rivet gun E920.1
    staple gun E920.1
   rake E920.4
   saw
    circular E919.4
    hand E920.4
   scissors E920.4
   screwdriver E920.4
   sewing machine (electric) (powered) E920.2
    not powered E920.4
   shears E920.4
   shovel E920.4
   spade E920.4
   splinters E920.8
   sword E920.3
   tin can lid E920.8
   wood slivers E920.8
  homicide (attempt) E966
  inflicted by other person
   stated as
    intentional, homicidal E966
    undetermined whether accidental or intentional E986
  late effect of NEC E929.8
  legal
   execution E978
   intervention E974
  self-inflicted (unspecified whether accidental or intentional) E986
   stated as intentional, purposeful E956
   stated as undetermined whether accidental or intentional E986
  suicidal (attempt) E956
  terrorism E979.8 ●
  war operations E995
Cyclone E908.1

D

Death due to injury occurring one year or more previous — see Late effect
Decapitation (accidental circumstances) NEC E928.9
  homicidal E966
  legal execution (by guillotine) E978
Deprivation — see also Privation
  homicidal intent E968.4
Derailment (accidental)
  railway (rolling stock) (train) (vehicle) (with subsequent collision) E802 ✓4ᵗʰ
   with
    collision (antecedent) (see also Collision, railway) E800 ✓4ᵗʰ
    explosion (subsequent) (without antecedent collision) E802 ✓4ᵗʰ
     antecedent collision E803 ✓4ᵗʰ
    fall (without collision (antecedent)) E802 ✓4ᵗʰ

Derailment — continued
  railway — continued
   with — continued
    fire (without collision (antecedent)) E802 ✓4ᵗʰ
   street car E829 ✓4ᵗʰ
Descent
  parachute (voluntary) (without accident to aircraft) E844 ✓4ᵗʰ
   due to accident to aircraft — see categories E840-E842 ✓4ᵗʰ
Desertion
  child, with intent to injure or kill E968.4
  helpless person, infant, newborn E904.0
   with intent to injure or kill E968.4
Destitution — see Privation
Disability, late effect or sequela of injury — see Late effect
Disease
  Andes E902.0
  aviators' E902.1
  caisson E902.2
  range E902.0
Divers' disease, palsy, paralysis, squeeze E902.2
Dog bite E906.0
Dragged by
  cable car (not on rails) E847
   on rails E829 ✓4ᵗʰ
  motor vehicle (on highway) E814 ✓4ᵗʰ
   not on highway, nontraffic accident E825 ✓4ᵗʰ
  street car E829 ✓4ᵗʰ
Drinking poison (accidental) — see Table of Drugs and Chemicals
Drowning — see Submersion
Dust in eye E914

E

Earth falling (on) (with asphyxia or suffocation (by pressure)) (see also Suffocation, due to, cave-in) E913.3
  as, or due to, a cataclysm (involving any transport vehicle) — see categories E908 ✓4ᵗʰ, E909 ✓4ᵗʰ
  not due to cataclysmic action E913.3
   motor vehicle (in motion) (on public highway) E810 ✓4ᵗʰ
    not on public highway E825 ✓4ᵗʰ
   nonmotor road vehicle NEC E829 ✓4ᵗʰ
   pedal cycle E826 ✓4ᵗʰ
   railway rolling stock, train, vehicle E806 ✓4ᵗʰ
   street car E829 ✓4ᵗʰ
   struck or crushed by E916
    with asphyxiation or suffocation E913.3
    with injury other than asphyxia, suffocation E916
Earthquake (any injury) E909.0
Effect(s) (adverse) of
  air pressure E902.9
   at high altitude E902.9
    in aircraft E902.1
     residence or prolonged visit (causing conditions classifiable to E902.0) E902.0
    due to
     diving E902.2
     specified cause NEC E902.8
    in aircraft E902.1
  cold, excessive (exposure to) (see also Cold, exposure to) E901.9
  heat (excessive) (see also Heat) E900.9
  hot
   place — see Heat
   weather E900.0
  insulation — see Heat
  late — see Late effect of
  motion E903
  nuclear explosion or weapon
   in
    terrorism E979.5 ●
    war operations (blast) (fireball) (heat) (radiation) (direct) (secondary) E996

Explosion

Effect(s) (adverse) of — continued
  radiation — see Radiation
  terrorism, secondary E979.9 ●
  travel E903
Electric shock, electrocution (accidental) (from exposed wire, faulty appliance, high voltage cable, live rail, open socket) (by) (in) E925.9
  appliance or wiring
   domestic E925.0
   factory E925.2
   farm (building) E925.8
    house E925.0
   home E925.0
   industrial (conductor) (control apparatus) (transformer) E925.2
   outdoors E925.8
   public building E925.8
   residential institution E925.8
   school E925.8
   specified place NEC E925.8
  caused by other person
   stated as
    intentional, homicidal E968.8
    undetermined whether accidental or intentional E988.4
  electric power generating plant, distribution station E925.1
  homicidal (attempt) E968.8
  legal execution E978
  lightning E907
  machinery E925.9
   domestic E925.0
   factory E925.2
   farm E925.8
   home E925.0
  misadventure in medical or surgical procedure in electroshock therapy E873.4
  self-inflicted (undetermined whether accidental or intentional) E988.4
   stated as intentional E958.4
   stated as undetermined whether accidental or intentional E988.4
  suicidal (attempt) E958.4
  transmission line E925.1
Electrocution — see Electric shock
Embolism
  air (traumatic) NEC — see Air, embolism
Encephalitis
  lead or saturnine E866.0
   from pesticide NEC E863.4
Entanglement
  in
   bedclothes, causing suffocation E913.0
   wheel of pedal cycle E826 ✓4ᵗʰ
Entry of foreign body, material, any — see Foreign body
Execution, legal (any method) E978
Exhaustion
  cold — see Cold, exposure to
  due to excessive exertion E927
  heat — see Heat
Explosion (accidental) (in) (of) (on) E923.9
  acetylene E923.2
  aerosol can E921.8
  aircraft (in transit) (powered) E841 ✓4ᵗʰ
   at landing, take-off E840 ✓4ᵗʰ
   in
    terrorism E979.1 ●
    war operations E994
   unpowered E842 ✓4ᵗʰ
  air tank (compressed) (in machinery) E921.1
  anesthetic gas in operating theatre E923.2
  automobile tire NEC E921.8
   causing transport accident — see categories E810-E825 ✓4ᵗʰ
  blasting (cap) (materials) E923.1
  boiler (machinery), not on transport vehicle E921.0
   steamship — see Explosion, watercraft
  bomb E923.8
   in
    terrorism E979.2 ●
    war operations E993
     after cessation of hostilities E998
      atom, hydrogen or nuclear E996

Explosion

Explosion — continued
  bomb — continued
    in — continued
      war operations — continued
        injury by fragments from E991.9
          antipersonnel bomb E991.3
  butane E923.2
  caused by
    other person
      stated as
        intentional, homicidal — see Assault, explosive
        undetermined whether accidental or homicidal E985.5
  coal gas E923.2
  detonator E923.1
  dyamite E923.1
  explosive (material) NEC E923.9
    gas(es) E923.2
    missile E923.8
      in
        terrorism E979.2
        war operations E993
          injury by fragments from E991.9
            antipersonnel bomb E991.3
    used in blasting operations E923.1
  fire-damp E923.2
  fireworks E923.0
  gas E923.2
    cylinder (in machinery) E921.1
    pressure tank (in machinery) E921.1
  gasoline (fumes) (tank) not in moving motor vehicle E923.2
  grain store (military) (munitions) E923.8
  grenade E923.8
    in
      terrorism E979.2
      war operations E993
        injury by fragments from E991.9
  homicide (attempt) — see Assault, explosive
  hot water heater, tank (in machinery) E921.0
  in mine (of explosive gases) NEC E923.2
  late effect of NEC E929.8
  machinery — see also Accident, machine
    pressure vessel — see Explosion, pressure vessel
  methane E923.2
  missile E923.8
    in
      terrorism E979.2
      war operations E993
        injury by fragments from E991.9
  motor vehicle (part of)
    in motion (on public highway) E818 ☑4th
    not on public highway E825 ☑4th
  munitions (dump) (factory) E923.8
    in
      terrorism E979.2
      war operations E993
  of mine E923.8
    in
      terrorism
        at sea or in harbor E979.0
        land E979.2
        marine E979.0
      war operations
        after cessation of hostilities E998
        at sea or in harbor E992
        land E993
          after cessation of hostilities E998
          injury by fragments from E991.9
        marine E992
  own weapons
    in
      terrorism (see also Suicide) E979.2
      war operations E993
        injury by fragments from E991.9
          antipersonnel bomb E991.3
      injury by fragments from E991.9
        antipersonnel bomb E991.3
  pressure
    cooker E921.8
    gas tank (in machinery) E921.1
    vessel (in machinery) E921.9
      on transport vehicle — see categories E800-E848 ☑4th
      specified type NEC E921.8

Explosion — continued
  propane E923.2
  railway engine, locomotive, train (boiler) (with subsequent collision, derailment, fall) E803 ☑4th
    with
      collision (antecedent) (see also Collision, railway) E800 ☑4th
      derailment (antecedent) E802 ☑4th
      fire (without antecedent collision or derailment) E803 ☑4th
  secondary fire resulting from — see Fire
  self-inflicted (unspecified whether accidental or intentional) E985.5
    stated as intentional, purposeful E955.5
  shell (artillery) E923.8
    in
      terrorism E979.2 •
      war operations E993
        injury by fragments from E991.9
  stated as undetermined whether caused accidentally or purposely inflicted E985.5
  steam or water lines (in machinery) E921.0
  suicide (attempted) E955.5
  terrorism — see Terrorism, explosion •
  torpedo E923.8
    in
      terrorism E979.0 •
      war operations E992
  transport accident — see categories E800-E848 ☑4th
  war operations — see War operations, explosion
  watercraft (boiler) E837 ☑4th
    causing drowning, submersion (after jumping from watercraft) E830 ☑4th

Exposure (weather) (conditions) (rain) (wind) E904.3
  with homicidal intent E968.4
  excessive E904.3
    cold (see also Cold, exposure to) E901.9
      self-inflicted — see Cold, exposure to, self-inflicted
    heat (see also Heat) E900.9
  fire — see Fire •
  helpless person, infant, newborn due to abandonment or neglect E904.0
  noise E928.1
  prolonged in deep-freeze unit or refrigerator E901.1
  radiation — see Radiation
  resulting from transport accident — see categories E800-E848 ☑4th
  smoke from, due to
    fire — see Fire
    tobacco, second-hand E869.4
  vibration E928.2

F

Fall, falling (accidental) E888.9
  building E916
    burning E891.8
      private E890.8
  down
    escalator E880.0
    ladder E881.0
      in boat, ship, watercraft E833 ☑4th
    staircase E880.9
    stairs, steps — see Fall, from, stairs
  earth (with asphyxia or suffocation (by pressure)) (see also Earth, falling) E913.3
  from, off
    aircraft (at landing, take-off) (in-transit) (while alighting, boarding) E843 ☑4th
      resulting from accident to aircraft — see categories E840-E842 ☑4th
    animal (in sport or transport) E828 ☑4th
    animal-drawn vehicle E827 ☑4th
    balcony E882
    bed E884.4
    bicycle E826 ☑4th
    boat, ship, watercraft (into water) E832 ☑4th
      after accident to, collision, fire on E830 ☑4th
      and subsequently struck by (part of) boat E831 ☑4th

Fall, falling — continued
  from, off — continued
    boat, ship, watercraft — continued
      and subsequently struck by (part of) boat E831 ☑4th
      burning, crushed, sinking E830 ☑4th
        and subsequently struck by (part of) boat E831 ☑4th
    bridge E882
    building E882
      burning ▶(uncontrolled fire)◀ E891.8
        in terrorism E979.3 •
      private E890.8
    bunk in boat, ship, watercraft E834 ☑4th
      due to accident to watercraft E831 ☑4th
    cable car (not on rails) E847
      on rails E829 ☑4th
    car — see Fall from motor vehicle
    chair E884.2
    cliff E884.1
    commode E884.6
    curb (sidewalk) E880.1
    elevation aboard ship E834 ☑4th
      due to accident to ship E831 ☑4th
    embankment E884.9
    escalator E880.0
    fire escape E882
    flagpole E882
    furniture NEC E884.5
    gangplank (into water) (see also Fall, from, boat) E832 ☑4th
      to deck, dock E834 ☑4th
    hammock on ship E834 ☑4th
      due to accident to watercraft E831 ☑4th
    haystack E884.9
    high place NEC E884.9
      stated as undetermined whether accidental or intentional — see Jumping, from, high place
    horse (in sport or transport) E828 ☑4th
    in-line skates E885.1
    ladder E881.0
      in boat, ship, watercraft E833 ☑4th
      due to accident to watercraft E831 ☑4th
    machinery — see also Accident, machine
      not in operation E884.9
    motor vehicle (in motion) (on public highway) E818 ☑4th
      not on public highway E825 ☑4th
        stationary, except while alighting, boarding, entering, leaving E884.9
        while alighting, boarding, entering, leaving E824 ☑4th
      stationary, except while alighting, boarding, entering, leaving E884.9
      while alighting, boarding, entering, leaving, except off-road type motor vehicle E817 ☑4th
      off-road type — see Fall, from, off-road type motor vehicle
    nonmotor road vehicle (while alighting, boarding) NEC E829 ☑4th
      stationary, except while alighting, boarding, entering, leaving E884.9
    off road type motor vehicle (not on public highway) NEC E821 ☑4th
      on public highway E818 ☑4th
        while alighting, boarding, entering, leaving E817 ☑4th
    snow vehicle — see Fall from snow vehicle, motor-driven
    one
      deck to another on ship E834 ☑4th
        due to accident to ship E831 ☑4th
      level to another NEC E884.9
        boat, ship, or watercraft E834 ☑4th
        due to accident to watercraft E831 ☑4th
    pedal cycle E826 ☑4th
    playground equipment E884.0
    railway rolling stock, train, vehicle, (while alighting, boarding) E804 ☑4th
      with
        collision (see also Collision, railway) E800 ☑4th

☑4th Fourth-digit Required   ▶◀ Revised Text   • New Line   ▲ Revised Code

Index to External Causes

Fall, falling — *continued*
  from, off — *continued*
    railway rolling stock, train, vehicle — *continued*
      with — *continued*
        derailment (*see also* Derailment, railway) E802 ✓4th
        explosion (*see also* Explosion, railway engine) E803 ✓4th
    rigging (aboard ship) E834 ✓4th
      due to accident to watercraft E831 ✓4th
    roller skates E885.1
    scaffolding E881.1
    scooter (nonmotorized) E885.0
    sidewalk (curb) E880.1
      moving E885.9
    skateboard E885.2
    skis E885.3
    snow vehicle, motor-driven (not on public highway) E820 ✓4th
      on public highway E818 ✓4th
        while alighting, boarding, entering, leaving E817 ✓4th
    snowboard E885.4
    stairs, step E880.9
      boat, ship, watercraft E833 ✓4th
        due to accident to watercraft E831 ✓4th
      motor bus, motor vehicle — *see* Fall, from, motor vehicle, while alighting, boarding
      street car E829 ✓4th
    stationary vehicle NEC E884.9
    stepladder E881.0
    street car (while boarding, alighting) E829 ✓4th
      stationary, except while boarding or alighting F884.9 ✓4th
    structure NEC E882
      burning ▶(uncontrolled fire)◀ E891.8
      in terrorism E979.3
    table E884.9
    toilet E884.6
    tower E882
    tree E884.9
    turret E882
    vehicle NEC — *see also* Accident, vehicle NEC
      stationary E884.9
    viaduct E882
    wall E882
    wheelchair E884.3
    window E882
  in, on
    aircraft (at landing, take-off) (in-transit) E843 ✓4th
      resulting from accident to aircraft — *see* categories E840-E842 ✓4th
    boat, ship, watercraft E835 ✓4th
      due to accident to watercraft E831 ✓4th
      one level to another NEC E834 ✓4th
      on ladder, stairs E833 ✓4th
    cutting or piercing instrument or machine E888.0
    deck (of boat, ship, watercraft) E835 ✓4th
      due to accident to watercraft E831 ✓4th
    escalator E880.0
    gangplank E835 ✓4th
    glass, broken E888.0
    knife E888.0
    ladder E881.0
      in boat, ship, watercraft E833 ✓4th
        due to accident to watercraft E831 ✓4th
    object
      edged, pointed or sharp E888.0
      other E888.1
    pitchfork E888.0
    railway rolling stock, train, vehicle (while alighting, boarding) E804 ✓4th
      with
        collision (*see also* Collision, railway) E800 ✓4th
        derailment (*see also* Derailment, railway) E802 ✓4th
        explosion (*see also* Explosion, railway engine) E803 ✓4th
    scaffolding E881.1
    scissors E888.0

Fall, falling — *continued*
  in, on — *continued*
    staircase, stairs, steps (*see also* Fall, from, stairs) E880.9
    street car E829 ✓4th
    water transport (*see also* Fall, in, boat) E835 ✓4th
  into
    cavity E883.9
    dock E883.9
      from boat, ship, watercraft (*see also* Fall, from, boat) E832 ✓4th
    hold (of ship) E834 ✓4th
      due to accident to watercraft E831 ✓4th
    hole E883.9
    manhole E883.2
    moving part of machinery — *see* Accident, machine
    opening in surface NEC E883.9
    pit E883.9
    quarry E883.9
    shaft E883.9
    storm drain E883.2
    tank E883.9
    water (with drowning or submersion) E910.9
    well E883.1
  late effect of NEC E929.3
  object (*see also* Hit by, object, falling) E916
  other E888.8
  over
    animal E885.9
    cliff E884.1
    embankment E884.9
    small object E885
  overboard (*see also* Fall, from, boat) E832 ✓4th
  resulting in striking against object E888.1
    sharp E888.0
  rock E916
  same level NEC E888.9
    aircraft (any kind) E843 ✓4th
      resulting from accident to aircraft — *see* categories E840-E842 ✓4th
    boat, ship, watercraft E835 ✓4th
      due to accident to, collision, watercraft E831 ✓4th
    from
      collision, pushing, shoving, by or with other person(s) E886.9
        as, or caused by, a crowd E917.6
        in sports E886.0
      scooter (nonmotorized) E885.0
      slipping stumbling, tripping E885
  snowslide E916
    as avalanche E909.2
  stone E916
  through
    hatch (on ship) E834 ✓4th
      due to accident to watercraft E831 ✓4th
    roof E882
    window E882
  timber E916
  while alighting from, boarding, entering, leaving
    aircraft (any kind) E843 ✓4th
    motor bus, motor vehicle — *see* Fall, from, motor vehicle, while alighting, boarding
    nonmotor road vehicle NEC E829 ✓4th
    railway train E804 ✓4th
    street car E829 ✓4th

Fallen on by
  animal (horse) (not being ridden) E906.8
    being ridden (in sport or transport) E828 ✓4th

Fell or jumped from high place, so stated — *see* Jumping, from, high place

Felo-de-se (*see also* Suicide) E958.9

Fever
  heat — *see* Heat
  thermic — *see* Heat

Fight (hand) (fist) (foot) (*see also* Assault, fight) E960.9

Fire (accidental) (caused by great heat from appliance (electrical), hot object or hot substance) (secondary, resulting from explosion) E899
  conflagration — *see* Conflagration

Fire — *continued*
  controlled, normal (in brazier, fireplace, furnace, or stove) (charcoal) (coal) (coke) (electric) (gas) (wood)
    bonfire E897
    brazier, not in building or structure E897
    in building or structure, except private dwelling (barn) (church) (convalescent or residential home) (factory) (farm outbuilding) (hospital) (hotel) (institution (educational) (dormitory) (residential)) (private garage) (school) (shop) (store) (theatre) E896
    in private dwelling (apartment) (boarding house) (camping place) (caravan) (farmhouse) (home (private)) (house) (lodging house) (rooming house) (tenement) E895
    not in building or structure E897
    trash E897
  forest (uncontrolled) E892
  grass (uncontrolled) E892
  hay (uncontrolled) E892
  homicide (attempt) E968.0
    late effect of E969
  in, of, on, starting in E892
    aircraft (in transit) (powered) E841 ✓4th
      at landing, take-off E840 ✓4th
      stationary E892
      unpowered (balloon) (glider) E842 ✓4th
    balloon E842 ✓4th
    boat, ship, watercraft — *see* categories E830 ✓4th, E831 ✓4th, E837 ✓4th
    building or structure, except private dwelling (barn) (church) (convalescent or residential home) (factory) (farm outbuilding) (hospital) (hotel) (institution (educational) (dormitory) (residential)) (school) (shop) (store) (theatre) (*see also* Conflagration, building or structure, except private dwelling) E891.9
    forest (uncontrolled) E892
    glider E842 ✓4th
    grass (uncontrolled) E892
    hay (uncontrolled) E892
    lumber (uncontrolled) E892
    machinery — *see* Accident, machine
    mine (uncontrolled) E892
    motor vehicle (in motion) (on public highway) E818 ✓4th
      not on public highway E825 ✓4th
      stationary E892
    prairie (uncontrolled) E892
    private dwelling (apartment) (boarding house) (camping place) (caravan) (farmhouse) (home (private)) (house) (lodging house) (private garage) (rooming house) (tenement) (*see also* Conflagration, private dwelling) E890.9
    railway rolling stock, train, vehicle (*see also* Explosion, railway engine) E803 ✓4th
      stationary E892
    room NEC E898.1
    street car (in motion) E829 ✓4th
      stationary E892
    terrorism (by fire-producing device) E979.3
      fittings or furniture (burning building) (uncontrolled fire) E979.3
      from nuclear explosion E979.5
    transport vehicle, stationary NEC E892
    tunnel (uncontrolled) E892
    war operations (by fire-producing device or conventional weapon) E990.9
      from nuclear explosion E996
      petrol bomb E990.0
  late effect of NEC E929.4
  lumber (uncontrolled) E892
  mine (uncontrolled) E892
  prairie (uncontrolled) E892
  self-inflicted (unspecified whether accidental or intentional) E988.1
    stated as intentional, purposeful E958.1
  specified NEC E898.1
    with
      conflagration — *see* Conflagration

Fire

Fire — continued
  specified — continued
    with — continued
      ignition (of)
        clothing — see Ignition, clothes
        highly inflammable material (benzine)
          (fat) (gasoline) (kerosene)
          (paraffin) (petrol) E894
  started by other person
    stated as
      with intent to injure or kill E968.0
      undetermined whether or not with intent
        to injure or kill E988.1
  suicide (attempted) E958.1
  late effect of E959
  tunnel (uncontrolled) E892

Fireball effects from nuclear explosion
  in
    terrorism E979.5
    war operations E996

Fireworks (explosion) E923.0

Flash burns from explosion (see also Explosion) E923.9

Flood (any injury) (resulting from storm) E908.2
  caused by collapse of dam or manmade structure E909.3

Forced landing (aircraft) E840 ✓4ᵗʰ

Foreign body, object or material (entrance into (accidental))
  air passage (causing injury) E915
    with asphyxia, obstruction, suffocation E912
      food or vomitus E911
    nose (with asphyxia, obstruction, suffocation) E912
    causing injury without asphyxia, obstruction, suffocation E915
  alimentary canal (causing injury) (with obstruction) E915
    with asphyxia, obstruction respiratory passage, suffocation E912
      food E911
    mouth E915
      with asphyxia, obstruction, suffocation E912
        food E911
    pharynx E915
      with asphyxia, obstruction, suffocation E912
        food E911
  aspiration (with asphyxia, obstruction respiratory passage, suffocation) E912
    causing injury without asphyxia, obstruction respiratory passage, suffocation E915
    food (regurgitated) (vomited) E911
      causing injury without asphyxia, obstruction respiratory passage, suffocation E915
    mucus (not of newborn) E912
    phlegm E912
  bladder (causing injury or obstruction) E915
  bronchus, bronchi — see Foreign body, air passages
  conjunctival sac E914
  digestive system — see Foreign body, alimentary canal
  ear (causing injury or obstruction) E915
  esophagus (causing injury or obstruction) (see also Foreign body, alimentary canal) E915
  eye (any part) E914
  eyelid E914
  hairball (stomach) (with obstruction) E915
  ingestion — see Foreign body, alimentary canal
  inhalation — see Foreign body, aspiration
  intestine (causing injury or obstruction) E915
  iris E914
  lacrimal apparatus E914
  larynx — see Foreign body, air passage
  late effect of NEC E929.8
  lung — see Foreign body, air passage
  mouth — see Foreign body, alimentary canal, mouth
  nasal passage — see Foreign body, air passage, nose
  nose — see Foreign body, air passage, nose
  ocular muscle E914

Foreign body, object or material — continued
  operation wound (left in) — see Misadventure, foreign object
  orbit E914
  pharynx — see Foreign body, alimentary canal, pharynx
  rectum (causing injury or obstruction) E915
  stomach (hairball) (causing injury or obstruction) E915
  tear ducts or glands E914
  trachea — see Foreign body, air passage
  urethra (causing injury or obstruction) E915
  vagina (causing injury or obstruction) E915

Found dead, injured
  from exposure (to) — see Exposure
  on
    public highway E819 ✓4ᵗʰ
    railway right of way E807 ✓4ᵗʰ

Fracture (circumstances unknown or unspecified) E887
  due to specified external means — see manner of accident
  late effect of NEC E929.3
  occuring in water transport NEC E835 ✓4ᵗʰ

Freezing — see Cold, exposure to

Frostbite E901.0
  due to manmade conditions E901.1

Frozen — see Cold, exposure to

G

Garrotting, homicidal (attempted) E963

Gored E906.8

Gunshot wound (see also Shooting) E922.9

H

Hailstones, injury by E904.3

Hairball (stomach) (with obstruction) E915

Hanged himself (see also Hanging, self-inflicted) E983.0

Hang gliding E842 ✓4ᵗʰ

Hanging (accidental) E913.8
  caused by other person
    in accidental circumstances E913.8
    stated as
      intentional, homicidal E963
      undetermined whether accidental or intentional E983.0
  homicide (attempt) E963
  in bed or cradle E913.0
  legal execution E978
  self-inflicted (unspecified whether accidental or intentional) E983.0
    in accidental circumstances E913.8
    stated as intentional, purposeful E953.0
    stated as undetermined whether accidental or intentional E983.0
  suicidal (attempt) E953.0

Heat (apoplexy) (collapse) (cramps) (effects of) (excessive) (exhaustion) (fever) (prostration) (stroke) E900.9
  due to
    manmade conditions (as listed in E900.1, except boat, ship, watercraft) E900.1
    weather (conditions) E900.0
  from
    electric heating appartus causing burning E924.8
    nuclear explosion
      in
        terrorism E979.5
        war operations E996
  generated in, boiler, engine, evaporator, fire room of boat, ship, watercraft E838 ✓4ᵗʰ
  inappropriate in local application or packing in medical or surgical procedure E873.5
  late effect of NEC E989

Hemorrhage
  delayed following medical or surgical treatment without mention of misadventure — see Reaction, abnormal
  during medical or surgical treatment as misadventure — see Misadventure, cut

Index to External Causes

High
  altitude, effects E902.9
  level of radioactivity, effects — see Radiation
  pressure effects — see also Effects of, air pressure
    from rapid descent in water (causing caisson or divers' disease, palsy, or paralysis) E902.2
  temperature, effects — see Heat

Hit, hitting (accidental) by
  aircraft (propeller) (without accident to aircraft) E844 ✓4ᵗʰ
    unpowered E842 ✓4ᵗʰ
  avalanche E909.2
  being thrown against object in or part of
    motor vehicle (in motion) (on public highway) E818 ✓4ᵗʰ
      not on public highway E825 ✓4ᵗʰ
    nonmotor road vehicle NEC E829 ✓4ᵗʰ
    street car E829 ✓4ᵗʰ
  boat, ship, watercraft
    after fall from watercraft E838 ✓4ᵗʰ
    damaged, involved in accident E831 ✓4ᵗʰ
    while swimming, water skiing E838 ✓4ᵗʰ
  bullet (see also Shooting) E922.9
    from air gun E922.4
    in
      terrorism E979.4
      war operations E991.2
        rubber E991.0
  flare, Verey pistol (see also Shooting) E922.8
  hailstones E904.3
  landslide E909.2
  law-enforcing agent (on duty) E975
    with blunt object (baton) (night stick) (stave) (truncheon) E973
  machine — see Accident, machine
  missile
    firearm (see also Shooting) E922.9
    in
      terrorism — see Terrorism, mission
      war operations — see War operations, missile
  motor vehicle (on public highway) (traffic accident) E814 ✓4ᵗʰ
    not on public highway, nontraffic accident E822 ✓4ᵗʰ
  nonmotor road vehicle NEC E829 ✓4ᵗʰ
  object
    falling E916
      from, in, on
        aircraft E844 ✓4ᵗʰ
          due to accident to aircraft — see categories E840-E842 ✓4ᵗʰ
          unpowered E842 ✓4ᵗʰ
        boat, ship, watercraft E838 ✓4ᵗʰ
          due to accident to watercraft E831 ✓4ᵗʰ
        building E916
          burning (uncontrolled fire)
            E891.8
            in terrorism E979.3
            private E890.8
        cataclysmic
          earth surface movement or eruption E909.9
          storm E908.9
        cave-in E916
          with asphyxiation or suffocation (see also Suffocation, due to, cave-in) E913.3
        earthquake E909.0
        motor vehicle (in motion) (on public highway) E818 ✓4ᵗʰ
          not on public highway E825 ✓4ᵗʰ
          stationary E916
        nonmotor road vehicle NEC E829 ✓4ᵗʰ
        pedal cycle E826 ✓4ᵗʰ
        railway rolling stock, train, vehicle E806 ✓4ᵗʰ
        street car E829 ✓4ᵗʰ
        structure, burning NEC E891.8
        vehicle, stationary E916
    moving NEC — see Striking against, object
    projected NEC — see Striking against, object

Index to External Causes

Hit, hitting — *continued*
  object — *continued*
    set in motion by
      compressed air or gas, spring, striking, throwing — *see* Striking against, object
      explosion — *see* Explosion
    thrown into, on, or towards
      motor vehicle (in motion) (on public highway) E818 ✓4th
        not on public highway E825 ✓4th
      nonmotor road vehicle NEC E829 ✓4th
      pedal cycle E826 ✓4th
      street car E829 ✓4th
    off-road type motor vehicle (not on public highway) E821 ✓4th
    on public highway E814 ✓4th
  other person(s) E917.9
    with blunt or thrown object E917.9
      in sports E917.0
        with subsequent fall E917.5
      intentionally, homicidal E968.2
    as, or caused by, a crowd E917.1
      with subsequent fall E917.6
    in sports E917.0
  pedal cycle E826 ✓4th
  police (on duty) E975
    with blunt object (baton) (nightstick) (stave) (truncheon) E973
  railway, rolling stock, train, vehicle (part of) E805 ✓4th
  shot — *see* Shooting
  snow vehicle, motor-driven (not on public highway) E820 ✓4th
    on public highway E814 ✓4th
  street car E829 ✓4th
  vehicle NEC — *see* Accident, vehicle NEC

Homicide, homicidal (attempt) (justifiable) (*see also* Assault) E968.9

Hot
  liquid, object, substance, accident caused by — *see also* Accident, caused by, hot, by type of substance
    late effect of E929.8
  place, effects — *see* Heat
  weather, effects E900.0

Humidity, causing problem E904.3

Hunger E904.1
  resulting from
    abandonment or neglect E904.0
    transport accident — *see* categories E800-E848 ✓4th

Hurricane (any injury) E908.0

Hypobarism, hypobaropathy — *see* Effects of, air pressure

Hypothermia — *see* Cold, exposure to

I

Ictus
  caloris — *see* Heat
  solaris E900.0

Ignition (accidental)
  anesthetic gas in operating theatre E923.2
  bedclothes
    with
      conflagration — *see* Conflagration
      ignition (of)
        clothing — *see* Ignition, clothes
        highly inflammable material (benzine) (fat) (gasoline) (kerosene) (paraffin) (petrol) E894
  benzine E894
  clothes, clothing (from controlled fire) (in building) E893.9
    with conflagration — *see* Conflagration
    from
      bonfire E893.2
      highly inflammable material E894
      sources or material as listed in E893.8
      trash fire E893.2
      uncontrolled fire — *see* Conflagration

Ignition — *continued*
  clothes, clothing — *continued*
    in
      private dwelling E893.0
      specified building or structure, except private dwelling E893.1
      not in building or structure E893.2
  explosive material — *see* Explosion
  fat E894
  gasoline E894
  kerosene E894
  material
    explosive — *see* Explosion
    highly inflammable E894
      with conflagration — *see* Conflagration
      with explosion E923.2
  nightdress — *see* Ignition, clothes
  paraffin E894
  petrol E894

Immersion — *see* Submersion

Implantation of quills of porcupine E906.8

Inanition (from) E904.9
  hunger — *see* Lack of, food
  resulting from homicidal intent E968.4
  thirst — *see* Lack of, water

Inattention after, at birth E904.0
  homicidal, infanticidal intent E968.4

Infanticide (*see also* Assault)

Ingestion
  foreign body (causing injury) (with obstruction) — *see* Foreign body, alimentary canal
  poisonous substance NEC — *see* Table of Drugs and Chemicals

Inhalation
  excessively cold substance, manmade E901.1
  foreign body — *see* Foreign body, aspiration
  liquid air, hydrogen, nitrogen E901.1
  mucus, not of newborn (with asphyxia, obstruction respiratory passage, suffocation) E912
  phlegm (with asphyxia, obstruction respiratory passage, suffocation) E912
  poisonous gas — *see* Table of Drugs and Chemicals
  smoke from, due to
    fire — *see* Fire
    tobacco, second-hand E869.4
  vomitus (with asphyxia, obstruction respiratory passage, suffocation) E911

Injury, injured (accidental(ly)) NEC E928.9
  by, caused by, from
    air rifle (BB gun) E922.4
    animal (not being ridden) NEC E906.9
      being ridden (in sport or transport) E828 ✓4th
    assault (*see also* Assault) E968.9
    avalanche E909.2
    bayonet (*see also* Bayonet wound) E920.3
    being thrown against some part of, or object in
      motor vehicle (in motion) (on public highway) E818 ✓4th
        not on public highway E825 ✓4th
      nonmotor road vehicle NEC E829 ✓4th
      off-road motor vehicle NEC E821 ✓4th
      railway train E806 ✓4th
      snow vehicle, motor-driven E820 ✓4th
      street car E829 ✓4th
    bending E927
    broken glass E920.8
    bullet — *see* Shooting
    cave-in (*see also* Suffocation, due to, cave-in) E913.3
      earth surface movement or eruption E909.9
      earthquake E909.0
      flood E908.2
      hurricane E908.0
      landslide E909.2
      storm E908.9
      without asphyxiation or suffocation E916
    cloudburst E908.8
    cutting or piercing instrument (*see also* Cut) E920.9
    cyclone E908.1
    earth surface movement or eruption E909.9

Injury, injured — *continued*
  by, caused by, from — *continued*
    earthquake E909.0
    electric current (*see also* Electric shock) E925.9
    explosion (*see also* Explosion) E923.9
    fire — *see* Fire
    flare, Verey pistol E922.8
    flood E908
    foreign body — *see* Foreign body
    hailstones E904.3
    hurricane E908
    landslide E909 ✓4th
    law-enforcing agent, police, in course of legal intervention — *see* Legal intervention
    lightning E907
    live rail or live wire — *see* Electric shock
    machinery — *see also* Accident, machine
      aircraft, without accident to aircraft E844 ✓4th
      boat, ship, watercraft (deck) (engine room) (galley) (laundry) (loading) E836 ✓4th
    missile
      explosive E923.8
      firearm — *see* Shooting
      in
        terrorism — *see* Terrorism, missile ●
        war operations — *see* War operations, missile
    moving part of motor vehicle (in motion) (on public highway) E818 ✓4th
      not on public highway, nontraffic accident E825 ✓4th
      while alighting, boarding, entering, leaving — *see* Fall, from, motor vehicle, while alighting, boarding
    nail E920.8
    needle (sewing) E920.4
      hypodermic E920.5
    noise E928.1
    object
      fallen on
        motor vehicle (in motion) (on public highway) E818 ✓4th
          not on public highway E825 ✓4th
      falling — *see* Hit by, object, falling
    paintball gun E922.5 ●
    radiation — *see* Radiation
    railway rolling stock, train, vehicle (part of) E805 ✓4th
      door or window E806 ✓4th
    rotating propeller, aircraft E844 ✓4th
    rough landing of off-road type motor vehicle (after leaving ground or rough terrain) E821 ✓4th
    snow vehicle E820 ✓4th
    saber (*see also* Wound, saber) E920.3
    shot — *see* Shooting
    sound waves E928.1
    splinter or sliver, wood E920.8
    straining E927
    street car (door) E829 ✓4th
    suicide (attempt) E958.9
    sword E920.3
    terrorism — *see* Terrorism ●
    third rail — *see* Electric shock
    thunderbolt E907
    tidal wave E909.4
      caused by storm E908.0
    tornado E908.1
    torrential rain E908.2
    twisting E927
    vehicle NEC — *see* Accident, vehicle NEC
    vibration E928.2
    volcanic eruption E909.1
    weapon burst, in war operations E993
    weightlessness (in spacecraft, real or simulated) E928.0
    wood splinter or sliver E920.8
  due to
    civil insurrection — *see* War operations
      occurring after cessation of hostilities E998
    terrorism — *see* Terrorism ●

Injury, injured

Injury, injured — *continued*
  due to — *continued*
    war operations — *see* War operations
      occurring after cessation of hostilities E998
    homicidal (*see also* Assault) E968.9
    in, on
      civil insurrection — *see* War operations
      fight E960.0
      parachute descent (voluntary) (without accident to aircraft) E844 ✓4ᵗʰ
        with accident to aircraft — *see* categories E840-E842 ✓4ᵗʰ
      public highway E819 ✓4ᵗʰ
      railway right of way E807 ✓4ᵗʰ
      terrorism — *see* Terrorism ●
      war operations — *see* War operations
    inflicted (by)
      in course of arrest (attempted), suppression of disturbance, maintenance of order, by law enforcing agents — *see* Legal intervention
      law-enforcing agent (on duty) — *see* Legal intervention
      other person
        stated as
          accidental E928.9
          homicidal, intentional — *see* Assault
          undetermined whether accidental or intentional — *see* Injury, stated as undetermined
      police (on duty) — *see* Legal intervention
  late effect of E929.9
  purposely (inflicted) by other person(s) — *see* Assault
  self-inflicted (unspecified whether accidental or intentional) E988.9
    stated as
      accidental E928.9
      intentionally, purposely E958.9
  specified cause NEC E928.8
  stated as
    undetermined whether accidentally or purposely inflicted (by) E988.9
      cut (any part of body) E986
      cutting or piercing instrument (classifiable to E920) E986
      drowning E984
      explosive(s) (missile) E985.5
      falling from high place E987.9
        manmade structure, except residential E987.1
        natural site E987.2
        residential premises E987.0
      hanging E983.0
      knife E986
      late effect of E989
      puncture (any part of body) E986
      shooting — *see* Shooting, stated as undetermined whether accidental or intentional
      specified means NEC E988.8
      stab (any part of body) E986
      strangulation — *see* Suffocation, stated as undetermined whether accidental or intentional
      submersion E984
      suffocation — *see* Suffocation, stated as undetermined whether accidental or intentional
  to child due to criminal abortion E968.8

Insufficient nourishment — *see also* Lack of, food
  homicidal intent E968.4

Insulation, effects — *see* Heat

Interruption of respiration by
  food lodged in esophagus E911
  foreign body, except food, in esophagus E912

Intervention, legal — *see* Legal intervention

Intoxication, drug or poison — *see* Table of Drugs and Chemicals

Irradiation — *see* Radiation

J

Jammed (accidentally)
  between objects (moving) (stationary and moving) E918
  in object E918

Jumped or fell from high place, so stated — *see* Jumping, from, high place, stated as in undetermined circumstances

Jumping
  before train, vehicle or other moving object (unspecified whether accidental or intentional) E988.0
    stated as
      intentional, purposeful E958.0
      suicidal (attempt) E958.0
  from
    aircraft
      by parachute (voluntarily) (without accident to aircraft) E844 ✓4ᵗʰ
      due to accident to aircraft — *see* categories E840-E842 ✓4ᵗʰ
    boat, ship, watercraft (into water)
      after accident to, fire on, watercraft E830 ✓4ᵗʰ
        and subsequently struck by (part of) boat E831 ✓4ᵗʰ
      burning, crushed, sinking E830 ✓4ᵗʰ
        and subsequently struck by (part of) boat E831 ✓4ᵗʰ
      voluntarily, without accident (to boat)
        with injury other than drowning or submersion E883.0
    building ▶— *see also* Jumping, from, high place◀
      burning ▶(uncontrolled fire)◀ E891.8
        in terrorism E979.3 ●
        private E890.8
    cable car (not on rails) E847
      on rails E829 ✓4ᵗʰ
    high place
      in accidental circumstances or in sport — *see* categories E880-E884 ✓4ᵗʰ
      stated as
        with intent to injure self E957.9
          man-made structures NEC E957.1
          natural sites E957.2
          residential premises E957.0
        in undetermined circumstances E987.9
          man-made structures NEC E987.1
          natural sites E987.2
          residential premises E987.0
        suicidal (attempt) E957.9
          man-made structures NEC E957.1
          natural sites E957.1
          residential premises E957.0
    motor vehicle (in motion) (on public highway) — *see* Fall, from, motor vehicle
    nonmotor road vehicle NEC E829 ✓4ᵗʰ
    street car E829 ✓4ᵗʰ
    structure ▶— *see also* Jumping, from, high place◀
      burning NEC (uncontrolled fire) E891.8 ●
        in terrorism E979.3 ●
  into water
    with injury other than drowning or submersion E883.0
    drowning or submersion — *see* Submersion
    from, off, watercraft — *see* Jumping, from, boat

Justifiable homicide — *see* Assault

K

Kicked by
  animal E906.8
  person(s) (accidentally) E917.9
    with intent to injure or kill E960.0
    as, or caused by a crowd E917.1
      with subsequent fall E917.6
    in fight E960.0

Kicked by — *continued*
  person(s) — *continued*
    in sports E917.9
      with subsequent fall E917.5

Kicking against
  object (moving) E917.9
    in sports E917.0
      with subsequent fall E917.5
    stationary E917.4
      with subsequent fall E917.8
  person — *see* Striking against, person

Killed, killing (accidentally) NEC (*see also* Injury) E928.9
  in
    action — *see* War operations
    brawl, fight (hand) (fists) (foot) E960.0
      by weapon — *see also* Assault
        cutting, piercing E966
        firearm — *see* Shooting, homicide
  self
    stated as
      accident E928.9
      suicide — *see* Suicide
    unspecified whether accidental or suicidal E988.9

Knocked down (accidentally) (by) NEC E928.9
  animal (not being ridden) E906.8
    being ridden (in sport or transport) E828 ✓4ᵗʰ
  blast from explosion (*see also* Explosion) E923.9
  crowd, human stampede E917.6
  late effect of — *see* Late effect
  person (accidentally) E917.9
    in brawl, fight E960.0
    in sports E917.5
  transport vehicle — *see* vehicle involved under Hit by
  while boxing E917.5

L

Laceration NEC E928.9

Lack of
  air (refrigerator or closed place), suffocation by E913.2
  care (helpless person) (infant) (newborn) E904.0
    homicidal intent E968.4
  food except as result of transport accident E904.1
    helpless person, infant, newborn due to abandonment or neglect E904.0
  water except as result of transport accident E904.2
    helpless person, infant, newborn due to abandonment or neglect E904.0

Landslide E909.2
  falling on, hitting
    motor vehicle (any) (in motion) (on or off public highway) E909.2
    railway rolling stock, train, vehicle E909.2

Late effect of
  accident NEC (accident classifiable to E928.9) E929.9
    specified NEC (accident classifiable to E910-E928.8) E929.8
  assault E969
  fall, accidental (accident classifiable to E880-E888) E929.3
  fire, accident caused by (accident classifiable to E890-E899) E929.4
  homicide, attempt (any means) E969
  injury due to terrorism E999.1 ●
  injury undetermined whether accidentally or purposely inflicted (injury classifiable to E980-E988) E989
  legal intervention (injury classifiable to E970-E976) E977
  medical or surgical procedure, test or therapy
    as, or resulting in, or from
      abnormal or delayed reaction or complication — *see* Reaction, abnormal
      misadventure — *see* Misadventure
  motor vehicle accident (accident classifiable to E810-E825) E929.0

Index to External Causes

Late effect of — *continued*
  natural or environmental factor, accident due to (accident classifiable to E900-E909) E929.5
  poisoning, accidental (accident classifiable to E850-E858, E860-E869) E929.2
  suicide, attempt (any means) E959
  transport accident NEC (accident classifiable to E800-E807, E826-E838, E840-E848) E929.1
  war operations, injury due to (injury classifiable to E990-E998) E999.0 ▲

Launching pad accident E845 ☑4ᵗʰ

Legal
  execution, any method E978
  intervention (by) (injury from) E976
    baton E973
    bayonet E974
    blow E975
    blunt object (baton) (nightstick) (stave) (truncheon) E973
    cutting or piercing instrument E974
    dynamite E971
    execution, any method E973
    explosive(s) (shell) E971
    firearm(s) E970
    gas (asphyxiation) (poisoning) (tear) E972
    grenade E971
    late effect of E977
    machine gun E970
    manhandling E975
    mortar bomb E971
    nightstick E973
    revolver E970
    rifle E970
    specified means NEC E975
    stabbing E974
    stave E973
    truncheon E973

Lifting, injury in E927

Lightning (shock) (stroke) (struck by) E907

Liquid (noncorrosive) in eye E914
  corrosive E924.1

Loss of control
  motor vehicle (on public highway) (without antecedent collision) E816 ☑4ᵗʰ
    with
      antecedent collision on public highway — *see* Collision, motor vehicle
      involving any object, person or vehicle not on public highway E816 ☑4ᵗʰ
    on public highway — *see* Collision, motor vehicle
    not on public highway, nontraffic accident E825 ☑4ᵗʰ
      with antecedent collision — *see* Collision, motor vehicle, not on public highway
  off-road type motor vehicle (not on public highway) E821 ☑4ᵗʰ
    on public highway — *see* Loss of control, motor vehicle
  snow vehicle, motor-driven (not on public highway) E820 ☑4ᵗʰ
    on public highway — *see* Loss of control, motor vehicle

Lost at sea E832 ☑4ᵗʰ
  with accident to watercraft E830 ☑4ᵗʰ
  in war operations E995

Low
  pressure, effects — *see* Effects of, air pressure
  temperature, effects — *see* Cold, exposure to

Lying before train, vehicle or other moving object (unspecified whether accidental or intentional) E988.0
  stated as intentional, purposeful, suicidal (attempt) E958.0

Lynching (*see also* Assault) E968.9

M

Malfunction, atomic power plant in water transport E838 ☑4ᵗʰ

Mangled (accidentally) NEC E928.9

Manhandling (in brawl, fight) E960.0
  legal intervention E975

Manslaughter (nonaccidental) — *see* Assault

Marble in nose E912

Mauled by animal E906.8

Medical procedure, complication of
  delayed or as an abnormal reaction without mention of misadventure — *see* Reaction, abnormal
  due to or as a result of misadventure — *see* Misadventure

Melting of fittings and furniture in burning ●
  in terrorism E979.3 ●

Minamata disease E865.2

Misadventure(s) to patient(s) during surgical or medical care E876.9
  contaminated blood, fluid, drug or biological substance (presence of agents and toxins as listed in E875) E875.9
    administered (by) NEC E875.9
      infusion E875.0
      injection E875.1
      specified means NEC E875.2
      transfusion E875.0
      vaccination E875.1
  cut, cutting, puncture, perforation or hemorrhage (accidental) (inadvertent) (inappropriate) (during) E870.9
    aspiration of fluid or tissue (by puncture or catheterization, except heart) E870.5
      biopsy E870.8
      needle (aspirating) E870.5
    blood sampling E870.5
    catheterization E870.5
      heart E870.6
    dialysis (kidney) E870.2
    endoscopic examination E870.4
    enema E870.7
    infusion E870.1
    injection E870.3
    lumbar puncture E870.5
    needle biopsy E870.5
    paracentesis, abdominal E870.5
    perfusion E870.2
    specified procedure NEC E870.8
    surgical operation E870.0
    thoracentesis E870.5
    transfusion E870.1
    vaccination E870.3
  excessive amount of blood or other fluid during transfusion or infusion E873.0
  failure
    in dosage E873.9
      electroshock therapy E873.4
      inappropriate temperature (too hot or too cold) in local application and packing E873.5
      infusion
        excessive amount of fluid E873.0
        incorrect dilution of fluid E873.1
      insulin-shock therapy E873.4
      nonadministration of necessary drug or medicinal E873.6
      overdose — *see also* Overdose
        radiation, in therapy E873.2
      radiation
        inadvertent exposure of patient (receiving radiation for test or therapy) E873.3
        not receiving radiation for test or therapy — *see* Radiation
        overdose E873.2
      specified procedure NEC E873.8
      transfusion
        excessive amount of blood E873.0
    mechanical, of instrument or apparatus (during procedure) E874.9
      aspiration of fluid or tissue (by puncture or catheterization, except of heart) E874.4
      biopsy E874.8
        needle (aspirating) E874.4
      blood sampling E874.4
      catheterization E874.4
        heart E874.5

Misadventure(s) to patient(s) during surgical or medical care — *continued*
  failure — *continued*
    mechanical, of instrument or apparatus — *continued*
      dialysis (kidney) E874.2
      endoscopic examination E874.3
      enema E874.8
      infusion E874.1
      injection E874.8
      lumbar puncture E874.4
      needle biopsy E874.4
      paracentesis, abdominal E874.4
      perfusion E874.2
      specified procedure NEC E874.8
      surgical operation E874.0
      thoracentesis E874.4
      transfusion E874.1
      vaccination E874.8
    sterile precautions (during procedure) E872.9
      aspiration of fluid or tissue (by puncture or catheterization, except heart) E872.5
      biopsy E872.8
        needle (aspirating) E872.5
      blood sampling E872.5
      catheterization E872.5
        heart E872.6
      dialysis (kidney) E872.2
      endoscopic examination E872.4
      enema E872.8
      infusion E872.1
      injection E872.3
      lumbar puncture E872.5
      needle biopsy E872.5
      paracentesis, abdominal E872.5
      perfusion E872.2
      removal of catheter or packing E872.8
      specified procedure NEC E872.8
      surgical operation E872.0
      thoracentesis E872.5
      transfusion E872.1
      vaccination E872.3
    suture or ligature during surgical procedure E876.2
    to introduce or to remove tube or instrument E876.4
      foreign object left in body — *see* Misadventure, foreign object
  foreign object left in body (during procedure) E871.9
    aspiration of fluid or tissue (by puncture or catheterization, except heart) E871.5
    biopsy E871.8
      needle (aspirating) E871.5
    blood sampling E871.5
    catheterization E871.5
      heart E871.6
    dialysis (kidney) E871.2
    endoscopic examination E871.4
    enema E871.8
    infusion E871.1
    injection E871.3
    lumbar puncture E871.5
    needle biopsy E871.5
    paracentesis, abdominal E871.5
    perfusion E871.2
    removal of catheter or packing E871.7
    specified procedure NEC E871.8
    surgical operation E871.0
    thoracentesis E871.5
    transfusion E871.1
    vaccination E871.3
  hemorrhage — *see* Misadventure, cut
  inadvertent exposure of patient to radiation (being received for test or therapy) E873.3
  inappropriate
    operation performed E876.5
    temperature (too hot or too cold) in local application or packing E873.5
  infusion — *see also* Misadventure, by specific type, infusion
    excessive amount of fluid E873.0
    incorrect dilution of fluid E873.1
    wrong fluid E876.1
  mismatched blood in transfusion E876.0

Misadventure(s) to patient(s) during surgical or medical care — continued
  nonadministration of necessary drug or medicinal E873.6
  overdose — see also Overdose
  radiation, in therapy E873.2
  perforation — see Misadventure, cut
  performance of inappropriate operation E876.5
  puncture — see Misadventure, cut
  specified type NEC E876.8
  failure
    suture or ligature during surgical operation E876.2
    to introduce or to remove tube or instrument E876.4
    foreign object left in body E871.9
  infusion of wrong fluid E876.1
  performance of inappropriate operation E876.5
  transfusion of mismatched blood E876.0
  wrong
    fluid in infusion E876.1
    placement of endotracheal tube during anesthetic procedure E876.3
  transfusion — see also Misadventure, by specific type, transfusion
    excessive amount of blood E873.0
    mismatched blood E876.0
  wrong
    drug given in error — see Table of Drugs and Chemicals
    fluid in infusion E876.1
    placement of endotracheal tube during anesthetic procedure E876.3

Motion (effects) E903
  sickness E903
Mountain sickness E902.0
Mucus aspiration or inhalation, not of newborn (with asphyxia, obstruction respiratory passage, suffocation) E912
Mudslide of cataclysmic nature E909.2
Murder (attempt) (see also Assault) E968.9

N

Nail, injury by E920.8
Needlestick (sewing needle) E920.4
  hypodermic E920.5
Neglect — see also Privation
  criminal E968.4
  homicidal intent E968.4
Noise (causing injury) (pollution) E928.1

O

Object
  falling
    from, in, on, hitting
      aircraft E844 ✓4ᵗʰ
        due to accident to aircraft — see categories E840-E842 ✓4ᵗʰ
      machinery — see also Accident, machine
        not in operation E916
      motor vehicle (in motion) (on public highway) E818 ✓4ᵗʰ
        not on public highway E825 ✓4ᵗʰ
        stationary E916
      nonmotor road vehicle NEC E829 ✓4ᵗʰ
      pedal cycle E826 ✓4ᵗʰ
      person E916
      railway rolling stock, train, vehicle E806 ✓4ᵗʰ
      street car E829 ✓4ᵗʰ
      watercraft E838 ✓4ᵗʰ
        due to accident to watercraft E831 ✓4ᵗʰ
  set in motion by
    accidental explosion of pressure vessel — see category E921 ✓4ᵗʰ
    firearm — see category E922 ✓4ᵗʰ
    machine(ry) — see Accident, machine
    transport vehicle — see categories E800-E848 ✓4ᵗʰ

Object — continued
  thrown from, in, on, towards
    aircraft E844 ✓4ᵗʰ
    cable car (not on rails) E847
      on rails E829 ✓4ᵗʰ
    motor vehicle (in motion) (on public highway) E818 ✓4ᵗʰ
      not on public highway E825 ✓4ᵗʰ
    nonmotor road vehicle NEC E829 ✓4ᵗʰ
    pedal cycle E826 ✓4ᵗʰ
    street car E829 ✓4ᵗʰ
    vehicle NEC — see Accident, vehicle NEC
Obstruction
  air passages, larynx, respiratory passages by
    external means NEC — see Suffocation
    food, any type (regurgitated) (vomited) E911
    material or object, except food E912
    mucus E912
    phlegm E912
    vomitus E911
  digestive tract, except mouth or pharynx by
    food, any type E915
    foreign body (any) E915
  esophagus
    food E911
    foreign body, except food E912
    without asphyxia or obstruction of respiratory passage E915
  mouth or pharynx by
    food, any type E911
    material or object, except food E912
  respiration — see Obstruction, air passages
Oil in eye E914
Overdose
  anesthetic (drug) — see Table of Drugs and Chemicals
  drug — see Table of Drugs and Chemicals
Overexertion (lifting) (pulling) (pushing) E927
Overexposure (accidental) (to)
  cold (see also Cold, exposure to) E901.9
    due to manmade conditions E901.1
  heat (see also Heat) E900.9
  radiation — see Radiation
  radioactivity — see Radiation
  sun, except sunburn E900.0
  weather — see Exposure
  wind — see Exposure
Overheated (see also Heat) E900.9
Overlaid E913.0
Overturning (accidental)
  animal-drawn vehicle E827 ✓4ᵗʰ
  boat, ship, watercraft
    causing
      drowning, submersion E830 ✓4ᵗʰ
      injury except drowning, submersion E831 ✓4ᵗʰ
  machinery — see Accident, machine
  motor vehicle (see also Loss of control, motor vehicle) E816 ✓4ᵗʰ
    with antecedent collision on public highway — see Collision, motor vehicle
    not on public highway, nontraffic accident E825 ✓4ᵗʰ
      with antecedent collision — see Collision, motor vehicle, not on public highway
  nonmotor road vehicle NEC E829 ✓4ᵗʰ
  off-road type motor vehicle — see Loss of control, off-road type motor vehicle
  pedal cycle E826 ✓4ᵗʰ
  railway rolling stock, train, vehicle (see also Derailment, railway) E802 ✓4ᵗʰ
  street car E829 ✓4ᵗʰ
  vehicle NEC — see Accident, vehicle NEC

P

Palsy, divers' E902.2
Parachuting (voluntary) (without accident to aircraft) E844 ✓4ᵗʰ

Parachuting — continued
  due to accident to aircraft — see categories E840-E842 ✓4ᵗʰ
Paralysis
  divers' E902.2
  lead or saturnine E866.0
    from pesticide NEC E863.4
Pecked by bird E906.8
Phlegm aspiration or inhalation (with asphyxia, obstruction respiratory passage, suffocation) E912
Piercing (see also Cut) E920.9
Pinched
  between objects (moving) (stationary and moving) E918
  in object E918
Pinned under
  machine(ry) — see Accident, machine
Place of occurrence of accident — see Accident (to), occurring (at) (in)
Plumbism E866.0
  from insecticide NEC E863.4
Poisoning (accidental) (by) — see also Table of Drugs and Chemicals
  carbon monoxide
    generated by
      aircraft in transit E844 ✓4ᵗʰ
      motor vehicle
        in motion (on public highway) E818 ✓4ᵗʰ
        not on public highway E825 ✓4ᵗʰ
      watercraft (in transit) (not in transit) E838 ✓4ᵗʰ
  caused by injection of poisons or toxins into or through skin by plant thorns, spines, or other mechanism E905.7
    marine or sea plants E905.6
  fumes or smoke due to
    conflagration — see Conflagration
    explosion or fire — see Fire
    ignition — see Ignition
  gas
    in legal intervention E972
    legal execution, by E978
    on watercraft E838 ✓4ᵗʰ
    used as anesthetic — see Table of Drugs and Chemicals
  in
    terrorism (chemical weapons) E979.7 ●
    war operations E997.2
  late effect of — see Late effect
  legal
    execution E978
    intervention
      by gas E972
Pressure, external, causing asphyxia, suffocation (see also Suffocation) E913.9
Privation E904.9
  food (see also Lack of, food) E904.1
  helpless person, infant, newborn due to abandonment or neglect E904.0
  late effect of NEC E929.5
  resulting from transport accident — see categories E800-E848 ✓4ᵗʰ
  water (see also Lack of, water) E904.2
Projected objects, striking against or struck by — see Striking against, object
Prolonged stay in
  high altitude (causing conditions as listed in E902.0) E902.0
  weightless environment E928.0
Prostration
  heat — see Heat
Pulling, injury in E927
Puncture, puncturing (see also Cut) E920.9
  by
    plant thorns or spines E920.8
      toxic reaction E905.7
        marine or sea plants E905.6
    sea-urchin spine E905.6

Index to External Causes

Pushing (injury in) (overexertion) E927
  by other person(s) (accidental) E917.9
    as, or caused by, a crowd, human stampede E917.1
      with subsequent fall E917.6
    before moving vehicle or object
      stated as
        intentional, homicidal E968.5
        undetemined whether accidental or intentional E988.8
    from
      high place
        in accidental circum-stances — see categories E880-E884
        stated as
          intentional, homicidal E968.1
          undetermined whether accidental or intentional E987.9
        man-made structure, except residential E987.1
        natural site E987.2
        residential E987.0
      motor vehicle (see also Fall, from, motor vehicle) E818
        stated as
          intentional, homicidal E968.5
          undetermined whether accidental or intentional E988.8
    in sports E917.0
      with fall E886.0
    with fall E886.9
      in sports E886.0

R

Radiation (exposure to) E926.9
  abnormal reaction to medical test or therapy E879.2
  arc lamps E926.2
  atomic power plant (malfunction) NEC E926.9
    in water transport E838
  electromagnetic, ionizing E926.3
  gamma rays E926.3
    in
      terrorism (from or following nuclear explosion) (direct) (secondary) E979.5
        laser E979.8
      war operations (from or following nuclear explosion) (direct) (secondary) E996
        laser(s) E997.0
      water transport E838
  inadvertent exposure of patient (receiving test or therapy) E873.3
  infrared (heaters and lamps) E926.1
    excessive heat E900.1
  ionized, ionizing (particles, artificially accelerated) E926.8
    electromagnetic E926.3
  isotopes, radioactive — see Radiation, radioactive isotopes
  laser(s) E926.4
    in
      terrorism E979.8
      war operations E997.0
    misadventure in medical care — see Misadventure, failure, in dosage, radiation
  late effect of NEC E929.8
    excessive heat from — see Heat
  light sources (visible) (ultraviolet) E926.2
  misadventure in medical or surgical procedure — see Misadventure, failure, in dosage, radiation
  overdose (in medical or surgical procedure) E873.2
  radar E926.0
  radioactive isotopes E926.5
    atomic power plant malfunction E926.5
      in water transport E838
    misadventure in medical or surgical treatment — see Misadventure, failure, in dosage, radiation
  radiobiologicals — see Radiation, radioactive isotopes
  radiofrequency E926.0

Radiation — continued
  radiopharmaceuticals — see Radiation, radioactive isotopes
  radium NEC E926.9
  sun E926.2
    excessive heat from E900.0
  tanning bed E926.2
  welding arc or torch E926.2
    excessive heat from E900.1
  x-rays (hard) (soft) E926.3
    misadventure in medical or surgical treatment — see Misadventure, failure, in dosage, radiation

Rape E960.1

Reaction, abnormal to or following (medical or surgical procedure) E879.9
  amputation (of limbs) E878.5
  anastomosis (arteriovenous) (blood vessel) (gastrojejunal) (skin) (tendon) (natural, artificial material, tissue) E878.2
    external stoma, creation of E878.3
  aspiration (of fluid) E879.4
    tissue E879.8
  biopsy E879.8
  blood
    sampling E879.7
    transfusion
      procedure E879.8
  bypass — see Reaction, abnormal, anastomosis
  catheterization
    cardiac E879.0
    urinary E879.6
  colostomy E878.3
  cystostomy E878.3
  dialysis (kidney) E879.1
  drugs or biologicals — see Table of Drugs and Chemicals
  duodenostomy E878.3
  electroshock therapy E879.3
  formation of external stoma E878.3
  gastrostomy E878.3
  graft — see Reaction, abnormal, anastomosis
  hypothermia E879.8
  implant, implantation (of)
    artificial
      internal device (cardiac pacemaker) (electrodes in brain) (heart valve prosthesis) (orthopedic) E878.1
      material or tissue (for anastomosis or bypass) E878.2
        with creation of external stoma E878.3
    natural tissues (for anastomosis or bypass) E878.2
      as transplantation — see Reaction, abnormal, transplant
      with creation of external stoma E878.3
  infusion
    procedure E879.8
  injection
    procedure E879.8
  insertion of gastric or duodenal sound E879.5
  insulin-shock therapy E879.3
  lumbar puncture E879.4
  perfusion E879.1
  procedures other than surgical operation (see also Reaction, abnormal, by specific type of procedure) E879.9
    specified procedure NEC E879.8
  radiological procedure or therapy E879.2
  removal of organ (partial) (total) NEC E878.6
    with
      anastomosis, bypass or graft E878.2
      formation of external stoma E878.3
      implant of artificial internal device E878.1
      transplant(ation)
        partial organ E878.4
        whole organ E878.0
  sampling
    blood E879.7
    fluid NEC E879.4
    tissue E879.8
  shock therapy E879.3
  surgical operation (see also Reaction, abnormal, by specified type of operation) E878.9

Reaction, abnormal to or following — continued
  surgical operation (see also Reaction, abnormal, by specified type of operation) — continued
    restorative NEC E878.4
      with
        anastomosis, bypass or graft E878.2
        fomation of external stoma E878.3
        implant(ation) — see Reaction, abnormal, implant
        transplant(ation) — see Reaction, abnormal, transplant
    specified operation NEC E878.8
  thoracentesis E879.4
  transfusion
    procedure E879.8
  transplant, transplantation (heart) (kidney) (liver) E878.0
    partial organ E878.4
  ureterostomy E878.3
  vaccination E879.8

Reduction in
  atmospheric pressure — see also Effects of, air pressure
    while surfacing from
      deep water diving causing caisson or divers' disease, palsy or paralysis E902.2
      underground E902.8

Residual (effect) — see Late effect

Rock falling on or hitting (accidentally)
  motor vehicle (in motion) (on public highway) E818
    not on public highway E825
  nonmotor road vehicle NEC E829
  pedal cycle E826
  person E916
  railway rolling stock, train, vehicle E806

Running off, away
  animal (being ridden) (in sport or transport) E829
    not being ridden E906.8
  animal-drawn vehicle E827
  rails, railway (see also Derailment) E802
  roadway
    motor vehicle (without antecedent collision) E816
      nontraffic accident E825
        with antecedent collision — see Collision, motor vehicle, not on public highway
      with
        antecedent collision — see Collision motor vehicle
        subsequent collision
          involving any object, person or vehicle not on public highway E816
          on public highway E811
    nonmotor road vehicle NEC E829
    pedal cycle E826

Run over (accidentally) (by)
  animal (not being ridden) E906.8
    being ridden (in sport or transport) E828
  animal-drawn vehicle E827
  machinery — see Accident, machine
  motor vehicle (on public highway) — see Hit by, motor vehicle
  nonmotor road vehicle NEC E829
  railway train E805
  street car E829
  vehicle NEC E848

S

Saturnism E866.0
  from insecticide NEC E863.4

Scald, scalding (accidental) (by) (from) (in) E924.0
  acid — see Scald, caustic
  boiling tap water E924.2
  caustic or corrosive liquid, substance E924.1
    swallowed — see Table of Drugs and Chemicals
  homicide (attempt) — see Assault, burning

Scald, scalding

Scald, scalding — *continued*
  inflicted by other person
    stated as
      intentional or homicidal E968.3
      undetermined whether accidental or intentional E988.2
  late effect of NEC E929.8
  liquid (boiling) (hot) E924.0
  local application of externally applied substance in medical or surgical care E873.5
  molten metal E924.0
  self-inflicted (unspecified whether accidental or intentional) E988.2
    stated as intentional, purposeful E958.2
    stated as undetermined whether accidental or intentional E988.2
  steam E924.0
  tap water (boiling) E924.2
  transport accident — *see* catagories E800-E848
  vapor E924.0

Scratch, cat E906.8

Sea
  sickness E903

Self-mutilation — *see* Suicide

Sequelae (of)
  in
    terrorism E999.1
    war operations E999.0

Shock
  anaphylactic (*see also* Table of Drugs and Chemicals) E947.9
    due to
      bite (venomous) — *see* Bite, venomous NEC
      sting — *see* Sting
  electric (*see also* Electric shock) E925.9
  from electric appliance or current (*see also* Electric shock) E925.9

Shooting, shot (accidental(ly)) E922.9
  air gun E922.4
  BB gun E922.4
  hand gun (pistol) (revolver) E922.0
  himself (*see also* Shooting, self-inflicted) E985.4
    hand gun (pistol) (revolver) E985.0
    military firearm, except hand gun E985.3
      hand gun (pistol) (revolver) E985.0
    rifle (hunting) E985.2
      military E985.3
    shotgun (automatic) E985.1
    specified firearm NEC E985.4
    Verey pistol E985.4
  homicide (attempt) E965.4
    air gun E968.6
    BB gun E968.6
    hand gun (pistol) (revolver) E965.0
    military firearm, except hand gun E965.3
      hand gun (pistol) (revolver) E965.0
    paintball gun E965.4
    rifle (hunting) E965.2
      military E965.3
    shotgun (automatic) E965.1
    specified firearm NEC E965.4
    Verey pistol E965.4
  inflicted by other person
    in accidental circumstances E922.9
      hand gun (pistol) (revolver) E922.0
      military firearm, except hand gun E922.3
        hand gun (pistol) (revolver) E922.0
      rifle (hunting) E922.2
        military E922.3
      shotgun (automatic) E922.1
      specified firearm NEC E922.8
      Verey pistol E922.8
    stated as
      intentional, homicidal E965.4
        hand gun (pistol) (revolver) E965.0
        military firearm, except hand gun E965.3
          hand gun (pistol) (revolver) E965.0
        paintball gun E965.4
        rifle (hunting) E965.2
          military E965.3
        shotgun (automatic) E965.1
        specified firearm E965.4

Shooting, shot — *continued*
  inflicted by other person — *continued*
    stated as — *continued*
      intentional, homicidal — *continued*
        Verey pistol E965.4
      undetermined whether accidental or intentional E985.4
        air gun E985.6
        BB gun E985.6
        hand gun (pistol) (revolver) E985.0
        military firearm, except hand gun E985.3
          hand gun (pistol) (revolver) E985.0
        paintball gun E985.7
        rifle (hunting) E985.2
        shotgun (automatic) E985.1
        specified firearm NEC E985.4
        Verey pistol E985.4
  in
    terrorism — *see* Terrorism, shooting
    war operations — *see* War operations, shooting
  legal
    execution E978
    intervention E970
  military firearm, except hand gun E922.3
    hand gun (pistol) (revolver) E922.0
  paintball gun E922.5
  rifle (hunting) E922.2
    military E922.3
  self-inflicted (unspecified whether accidental or intentional) E985.4
    air gun E985.6
    BB gun E985.6
    hand gun (pistol) (revolver) E985.0
    military firearm, except hand gun E985.3
      hand gun (pistol) (revolver) E985.0
    paintball gun E985.7
    rifle (hunting) E985.2
      military E985.3
    shotgun (automatic) E985.1
    specified firearm NEC E985.4
    stated as
      accidental E922.9
        hand gun (pistol) (revolver) E922.0
        military firearm, except hand gun E922.3
          hand gun (pistol) (revolver) E922.0
        paintball gun E922.5
        rifle (hunting) E922.2
          military E922.3
        shotgun (automatic) E922.1
        specified firearm NEC E922.8
        Verey pistol E922.8
      intentional, purposeful E955.4
        hand gun (pistol) (revolver) E955.0
        military firearm, except hand gun E955.3
          hand gun (pistol) (revolver) E955.0
        paintball gun E955.7
        rifle (hunting) E955.2
          military E955.3
        shotgun (automatic) E955.1
        specified firearm NEC E955.4
        Verey pistol E955.4
  shotgun (automatic) E922.1
  specified firearm NEC E922.8
  stated as undetermined whether accidental or intentional E985.4
    hand gun (pistol) (revolver) E985.0
    military firearm, except hand gun E985.3
      hand gun (pistol) (revolver) E985.0
    paintball gun E985.7
    rifle (hunting) E985.2
      military E985.3
    shotgun (automatic) E985.1
    specified firearm NEC E985.4
    Verey pistol E985.4
  suicidal (attempt) E955.4
    air gun E955.6
    BB gun E955.6
    hand gun (pistol) (revolver) E955.0
    military firearm, except hand gun E955.3
      hand gun (pistol) (revolver) E955.0
    paintball gun E955.7
    rifle (hunting) E955.2
      military E955.3

Shooting, shot — *continued*
  suicidal — *continued*
    shotgun (automatic) E955.1
    specified firearm NEC E955.4
    Verey pistol E955.4
  Verey pistol E922.8

Shoving (accidentally) by other person (*see also* Pushing by other person) E917.9

Sickness
  air E903
  alpine E902.0
  car E903
  motion E903
  mountain E902.0
  sea E903
  travel E903

Sinking (accidental)
  boat, ship, watercraft (causing drowning, submersion) E830 ◢4ᵗʰ
    causing injury except drowning, submersion E831 ◢4ᵗʰ

Siriasis E900.0

Skydiving E844 ◢4ᵗʰ

Slashed wrists (*see also* Cut, self-inflicted) E986

Slipping (accidental)
  on
    deck (of boat, ship, watercraft) (icy) (oily) (wet) E835 ◢4ᵗʰ
    ice E885
    ladder of ship E833 ◢4ᵗʰ
      due to accident to watercraft E831 ◢4ᵗʰ
    mud E885
    oil E885
    snow E885
    stairs of ship E833 ◢4ᵗʰ
      due to accident to watercraft E831 ◢4ᵗʰ
    surface
      slippery E885
      wet E885

Sliver, wood, injury by E920.8

Smouldering building or structure in terrorism E979.3

Smothering, smothered (*see also* Suffocation) E913.9

Sodomy (assault) E960.1

Solid substance in eye (any part) or adnexa E914

Sound waves (causing injury) E928.1

Splinter, injury by E920.8

Stab, stabbing E966
  accidental — *see* Cut

Starvation E904.1
  helpless person, infant, newborn — *see* Lack of food
  homicidal intent E968.4
  late effect of NEC E929.5
  resulting from accident connected with transport — *see* catagories E800-E848

Stepped on
  by
    animal (not being ridden) E906.8
      being ridden (in sport or transport) E828 ◢4ᵗʰ
    crowd E917.1
    person E917.9
      in sports E917.0
  in sports E917.0

Stepping on
  object (moving) E917.9
    in sports E917.0
      with subsequent fall E917.5
    stationary E917.4
      with subsequent fall E917.8
  person E917.9
    as, or caused by a crowd E917.1
      with subsequent fall E917.6
    in sports E917.0

Sting E905.9
  ant E905.5
  bee E905.3
  caterpillar E905.5
  coral E905.6
  hornet E905.3
  insect NEC E905.5
  jellyfish E905.6

Index to External Causes

Sting — *continued*
  marine animal or plant E905.6
  nematocysts E905.6
  scorpion E905.2
  sea anemone E905.6
  sea cucumber E905.6
  wasp E905.3
  yellow jacket E905.3
Storm E908.9
  specified type NEC E908.8
Straining, injury in E927
Strangling — *see* Suffocation
Strangulation — *see* Suffocation
Strenuous movements (in recreational or other activities) E927
Striking against
  bottom (when jumping or diving into water) E883.0
  object (moving) E917.9
    caused by crowd E917.1
      with subsequent fall E917.6
    furniture E917.3
      with subsequent fall E917.7
    in
      running water E917.2
        with drowning or submersion — *see* Submersion
      sports E917.0
        with subsequent fall E917.5
    stationary E917.4
      with subsequent fall E917.8
  person(s) E917.9
    with fall E886.9
      in sports E886.0
    as, or caused by, a crowd E917.1
      with subsequent fall E917.6
    in sports E917.0
      with fall E886.0
Stroke
  heat — *see* Heat
  lightning E907
Struck by — *see also* Hit by
  bullet
    in
      terrorism E979.4
      war operations E991.2
        rubber E991.0
  lightning E907
  missile
    in terrorism — *see* Terrorism, missile
  object
    falling
      from, in, on
        building
          burning (uncontrolled fire)
            in terrorism E979.3
  thunderbolt E907
Stumbling over animal, carpet, curb, rug or (small) object (with fall) E885
  without fall — *see* Striking against, object
Submersion (accidental) E910.8
  boat, ship, watercraft (causing drowning, submersion) E830 ✓4ᵗʰ
    causing injury except drowning, submersion E831 ✓4ᵗʰ
  by other person
    in accidental circumstances — *see* category E910 ✓4ᵗʰ
    intentional, homicidal E964
    stated as undetermined whether due to accidental or intentional E984
  due to
    accident
      machinery — *see* Accident, machine
      to boat, ship, watercraft E830 ✓4ᵗʰ
      transport — *see* categories E800-E848 ✓4ᵗʰ
    avalanche E909.2
    cataclysmic
      earth surface movement or eruption E909.9
      storm E908.9
    cloudburst E908.8
    cyclone E908.1

Submersion — *continued*
  due to — *continued*
    fall
      from
        boat, ship, watercraft (not involved in accident) E832 ✓4ᵗʰ
          burning, crushed E830 ✓4ᵗʰ
          involved in accident, collision E830 ✓4ᵗʰ
        gangplank (into water) E832 ✓4ᵗʰ
      overboard NEC E832 ✓4ᵗʰ
    flood E908.2
    hurricane E908.0
    jumping into water E910.8
      from boat, ship, watercraft
        burning, crushed, sinking E830 ✓4ᵗʰ
        involved in accident, collision E830 ✓4ᵗʰ
        not involved in accident, for swim E910.2
      in recreational activity (without diving equipment) E910.2
        with or using diving equipment E910.1
      to rescue another person E910.3
  homicide (attempt) E964
  in
    bathtub E910.4
    specified activity, not sport, transport or recreational E910.3
    sport or recreational activity (without diving equipment) E910.2
      with or using diving equipment E910.1
      water skiing E910.0
    swimming pool NEC E910.8
    terrorism E979.8
    war operations E995
    water transport E832 ✓4ᵗʰ
      due to accident to boat, ship, watercraft E830 ✓4ᵗʰ
  landslide E909.2
  overturning boat, ship, watercraft E909.2
  sinking boat, ship, watercraft E909.2
  submersion boat, ship, watercraft E909.2
  tidal wave E909.4
    caused by storm E908.0
  torrential rain E908.2
  late effect of NEC E929.8
  quenching tank E910.8
  self-inflicted (unspecified whether accidental or intentional) E984
    in accidental circumstances — *see* category E910 ✓4ᵗʰ
    stated as intentional, purposeful E954
  stated as undetermined whether accidental or intentional E984
  suicidal (attempted) E954
  while
    attempting rescue of another person E910.3
    engaged in
      marine salvage E910.3
      underwater construction or repairs E910.3
    fishing, not from boat E910.2
    hunting, not from boat E910.2
    ice skating E910.2
    pearl diving E910.3
    placing fishing nets E910.3
    playing in water E910.2
    scuba diving E910.1
      nonrecreational E910.3
    skin diving E910.1
    snorkel diving E910.2
    spear fishing underwater E910.1
    surfboarding E910.2
    swimming (swimming pool) E910.2
    wading (in water) E910.2
    water skiing E910.0
Sucked
  into
    jet (aircraft) E844 ✓4ᵗʰ
Suffocation (accidental) (by external means) (by pressure) (mechanical) E913.9
  caused by other person
    in accidental circumstances — *see* category E913 ✓4ᵗʰ

Suffocation — *continued*
  caused by other person — *continued*
    stated as
      intentional, homicidal E963
      undetermined whether accidental or intentional E983.9
        by, in
          hanging E983.0
          plastic bag E983.1
          specified means NEC E983.8
  due to, by
    avalanche E909.2
    bedclothes E913.0
    bib E913.0
    blanket E913.0
    cave-in E913.3
      caused by cataclysmic earth surface movement or eruption E909.9
    conflagration — *see* Conflagration
    explosion — *see* Explosion
    falling earth, other substance E913.3
    fire — *see* Fire
    food, any type (ingestion) (inhalation) (regurgitated) (vomited) E911
    foreign body, except food (ingestion) (inhalation) E912
    ignition — *see* Ignition
    landslide E909.2
    machine(ry) — *see* Accident, machine
    material, object except food entering by nose or mouth, ingested, inhaled E912
    mucus (aspiration) (inhalation), not of newborn E912
    phlegm (aspiration) (inhalation) E912
    pillow E913.0
    plastic bag — *see* Suffocation, in, plastic bag
    sheet (plastic) E913.0
    specified means NEC E913.8
    vomitus (aspiration) (inhalation) E911
  homicidal (attempt) E963
  in
    airtight enclosed place E913.2
    baby carriage E913.0
    bed E913.0
    closed place E913.2
    cot, cradle E913.0
    perambulator E913.0
    plastic bag (in accidental circumstances) E913.1
      homicidal, purposely inflicted by other person E963
      self-inflicted (unspecified whether accidental or intentional) E983.1
        in accidental circumstances E913.1
        intentional, suicidal E953.1
      stated as undetermined whether accidentally or purposely inflicted E983.1
      suicidal, purposely self-inflicted E953.1
    refrigerator E913.2
  self-inflicted — *see also* Suffocation, stated as undetermined whether accidental or intentional E953.9
    in accidental circumstances — *see* category E913 ✓4ᵗʰ
    stated as intentional, purposeful — *see* Suicide, suffocation
  stated as undetermined whether accidental or intentional E983.9
    by, in
      hanging E983.0
      plastic bag E983.1
      specified means NEC E983.8
  suicidal — *see* Suicide, suffocation
Suicide, suicidal (attempted) (by) E958.9
  burning, burns E958.1
  caustic substance E958.7
    poisoning E950.7
    swallowed E950.7
  cold, extreme E958.3
  cut (any part of body) E956
  cutting or piercing instrument (classifiable to E920) E956
  drowning E954
  electrocution E958.4
  explosive(s) (classifiable to E923) E955.5
  fire E958.1

Suicide, suicidal

Suicide, suicidal — *continued*
  firearm (classifiable to E922) — *see* Shooting, suicidal
  hanging E953.0
  jumping
    before moving object, train, vehicle E958.0
    from high place — *see* Jumping, from, high place, stated as, suicidal
  knife E956
  late effect of E959
  motor vehicle, crashing of E958.5
  poisoning — *see* Table of Drugs and Chemicals
  puncture (any part of body) E956
  scald E958.2
  shooting — *see* Shooting, suicidal
  specified means NEC E958.8
  stab (any part of body) E956
  strangulation — *see* Suicide, suffocation
  submersion E954
  suffocation E953.9
    by, in
      hanging E953.0
      plastic bag E953.1
      specified means NEC E953.8
  wound NEC E958.9
Sunburn E926.2
Sunstroke E900.0
Supersonic waves (causing injury) E928.1
Surgical procedure, complication of
  delayed or as an abnormal reaction without mention of misadventure — *see* Reaction, abnormal
  due to or as a result of misadventure — *see* Misadventure
Swallowed, swallowing
  foreign body — *see* Foreign body, alimentary canal
  poison — *see* Table of Drugs and Chemicals
  substance
    caustic — *see* Table of Drugs and Chemicals
    corrosive — *see* Table or drugs and chemicals
    poisonous — *see* Table of Drugs and Chemicals
Swimmers cramp (*see also* category E910 ☑4ᵗʰ) E910.2
  not in recreation or sport E910.3
Syndrome, battered
  baby or child — *see* Abuse, child
  wife — *see* Assault

T

Tackle in sport E886.0
Terrorism (injury) (by) (in) E979.8 ●
  air blast E979.2 ●
  aircraft burned, destroyed, exploded, shot down E979.1 ●
    used as a weapon E979.1 ●
  anthrax E979.6 ●
  asphyxia from
    chemical (weapons) E979.7 ●
    fire, conflagration (caused by fire-producing device) E979.3 ●
    from nuclear explosion E979.5 ●
    gas or fumes E979.7 ●
  bayonet E979.8 ●
  biological agents E979.6 ●
  blast (air) (effects) E979.2 ●
    from nuclear explosion E979.5 ●
    underwater E979.0 ●
  bomb (antipersonnel) (mortar) (explosion) (fragments) E979.2 ●
  bullet(s) (from carbine, machine gun, pistol, rifle, shotgun) E979.4 ●
  burn from
    chemical E979.7 ●
    fire, conflagration (caused by fire-producing device) E979.3 ●
    from nuclear explosion E979.5 ●
    gas E979.7 ●
  burning aircraft E979.1 ●
  chemical E9797.7 ●
  cholera E979.6 ●
  conflagration E9779.3 ●
  crushed by falling aircraft E979.1 ●

Terrorism — *continued*
  depth-charge E979.0 ●
  destruction of aircraft E979.1 ●
  disability, as sequelae one year or more after injury E999.1 ●
  drowning E979.8 ●
  effect
    of nuclear weapon (direct) (secondary) E979.5 ●
    secondary NEC E979.9 ●
    sequelae E999.1 ●
  explosion (artillery shell) (breech-block) (cannon block) E979 2 ●
    aircraft E979.1 ●
    bomb (antipersonnel) (mortar) E979.2 ●
      nuclear (atom) (hydrogen) E979.5 ●
    depth-charge E979.0 ●
    grenade E979.2 ●
    injury by fragments from E979.2 ●
    land-mine E979.2 ●
    marine weapon E979.0 ●
    mine (land) E979.2 ●
      at sea or in harbor E979.0 ●
      marine E979.0 ●
    missile (explosive) NEC E979.2 ●
    munitions (dump) (factory) E979.2 ●
    nuclear (weapon) E979.5 ●
      other direct and secondary effects of E979.5 ●
    sea-based artillery shell E979.0 ●
    torpedo E979.0 ●
  exposure to ionizing radiation from nuclear explosion E979.5 ●
  falling aircraft E979.1 ●
  fire or fire-producing device E979.3 ●
  firearms E979.4 ●
  fireball effects from nuclear explosion E979.5 ●
  fragments from artillery shell, bomb NEC, grenade, guided missile, land-mine, rocket, shell, shrapnel E979.2 ●
  gas or fumes E979.7 ●
  grenade (explosion) (fragments) E979.2 ●
  guided missile (explosion) (fragments) E979.2 ●
    nuclear E979.5 ●
  heat from nuclear explosion E979.5 ●
  hot substances E979.3 ●
  hydrogen cyanide E979.7 ●
  land-mine (explosion) (fragments) E979.2 ●
  laser(s) E979.8 ●
  late effect of E999.1 ●
  lewisite E979.7 ●
  lung irritant (chemical) (fumes) (gas) E979.7 ●
  marine mine E979.0 ●
  mine E979.2 ●
    at sea E979.0 ●
    in harbor E979.0 ●
    land (explosion) (fragments) E979.2 ●
    marine E979.0 ●
  missile (explosion) (fragments) (guided) E979.2 ●
    marine E979.0 ●
    nuclear E979.5 ●
  mortar bomb (explosion) (fragments) E979.2 ●
  mustard gas E979.7 ●
  nerve gas E979.7 ●
  nuclear weapons E979.5 ●
  pellets (shotgun) E979.4 ●
  petrol bomb E979.3 ●
  piercing object E979.8 ●
  phosgene E979.7 ●
  poisoning (chemical) (fumes) (gas) E979.7 ●
  radiation, ioninizing from nuclear explosion E979.5 ●
  rocket (explosion) (fragments) E979.2 ●
  saber, sabre E979.8 ●
  sarin E979.7 ●
  screening smoke E979.7 ●
  sequelae effect (of) E999.1 ●
  shell (aircraft) (artillery) (cannon) (land-based) (explosion) (fragments) E979.2 ●
    sea-based E979.0 ●
  shooting E979.4 ●
    bullet(s) E979.4 ●
    pellet(s) (rifle) (shotgun) E979.4 ●
  shrapnel E979.2 ●

Terrorism — *continued*
  smallpox E979.7 ●
  stabbing object(s) E979.8 ●
  submersion E979.8 ●
  torpedo E979.0 ●
  underwater blast E979.0 ●
  vesicant (chemical) (fumes) (gas) E979.7 ●
  weapon burst E979.2 ●
Thermic fever E900.9
Thermoplegia E900.9
Thirst — *see also* Lack of water
  resulting from accident connected with transport — *see* categories E800-E848 ☑4ᵗʰ
Thrown (accidentally)
  against object in or part of vehicle
    by motion of vehicle
      aircraft E844 ☑4ᵗʰ
      boat, ship, watercraft E838 ☑4ᵗʰ
      motor vehicle (on public highway) E818 ☑4ᵗʰ
        not on public highway E825 ☑4ᵗʰ
        off-road type (not on public highway) E821 ☑4ᵗʰ
        on public highway E818 ☑4ᵗʰ
        snow vehicle E820 ☑4ᵗʰ
          on public high-way E818 ☑4ᵗʰ
      nonmotor road vehicle NEC E829 ☑4ᵗʰ
      railway rolling stock, train, vehicle E806 ☑4ᵗʰ
      street car E829 ☑4ᵗʰ
  from
    animal (being ridden) (in sport or transport) E828 ☑4ᵗʰ
    high place, homicide (attempt) E968.1
    machinery — *see* Accident, machine
    vehicle NEC — *see* Accident, vehicle NEC
  off — *see* Thrown, from
  overboard (by motion of boat, ship, watercraft) E832 ☑4ᵗʰ
    by accident to boat, ship, watercraft E830 ☑4ᵗʰ
Thunderbolt NEC E907
Tidal wave (any injury) E909.4
  caused by storm E908.0
Took
  overdose of drug — *see* Table of Drugs and Chemicals
  poison — *see* Table of Drugs and Chemicals
Tornado (any injury) E908.1
Torrential rain (any injury) E908.2
Traffic accident NEC E819 ☑4ᵗʰ
Trampled by animal E906.8
  being ridden (in sport or transport) E828 ☑4ᵗʰ
Trapped (accidentally)
  between
    objects (moving) (stationary and moving) E918
  by
    door of
      elevator E918
      motor vehicle (on public highway) (while alighting, boarding) — *see* Fall, from, motor vehicle, while alighting
      railway train (underground) E806 ☑4ᵗʰ
      street car E829 ☑4ᵗʰ
      subway train E806 ☑4ᵗʰ
  in object E918
Travel (effects) E903
  sickness E903
Tree
  falling on or hitting E916
    motor vehicle (in motion) (on public highway) E818 ☑4ᵗʰ
      not on public highway E825 ☑4ᵗʰ
    nonmotor road vehicle NEC E829 ☑4ᵗʰ
    pedal cycle E826 ☑4ᵗʰ
    person E916
    railway rolling stock, train, vehicle E806 ☑4ᵗʰ
    street car E829 ☑4ᵗʰ
Trench foot E901.0
Tripping over animal, carpet, curb, rug, or small object (with fall) E885
  without fall — *see* Striking against, object

Index to External Causes

Tsunami E909.4
Twisting, injury in E927

V

Violence, nonaccidental (see also Assault) E968.9
Volcanic eruption (any injury) E909.1
Vomitus in air passages (with asphyxia, obstruction or suffocation) E911

W

War operations (during hostilities) (injury) (by) (in) E995
  after cessation of hostilities, injury due to E998
  air blast E993
  aircraft burned, destroyed, exploded, shot down E994
  asphyxia from
    chemical E997.2
    fire, conflagration (caused by fire producing device or conventional weapon) E990.9
      from nuclear explosion E996
      petrol bomb E990.0
    fumes E997.2
    gas E997.2
  battle wound NEC E995
  bayonet E995
  biological warfare agents E997.1
  blast (air) (effects) E993
    from nuclear explosion E996
    underwater E992
  bomb (mortar) (explosion) E993
    after cessation of hostilities E998
    fragments, injury by E991.9
      antipersonnel E991.3
  bullet(s) (from carbine, machine gun, pistol, rifle, shotgun) E991.2
    rubber E991.0
  burn from
    chemical E997.2
    fire, conflagration (caused by fire-producing device or conventional weapon) E990.9
      from nuclear explosion E996
      petrol bomb E990.0
    gas E997.2
  burning aircraft E994
  chemical E997.2
  chlorine E997.2
  conventional warfare, specified from NEC E995
  crushing by falling aircraft E994
  depth charge E992
  destruction of aircraft E994
  disability as sequela one year or more after injury E999.0 ▲
  drowning E995
  effect (direct) (secondary) nuclear weapon E996
  explosion (artillery shell) (breech block) (cannon shell) E993
    after cessation of hostilities of bomb, mine placed in war E998
    aircraft E994
    bomb (mortar) E993
      atom E996
      hydrogen E996
      injury by fragments from E991.9
        antipersonnel E991.3
        nuclear E996
    depth charge E992
    injury by fragments from E991.9
      antipersonnel E991.3
    marine weapon E992
    mine
      at sea or in harbor E992
      land E993
        injury by fragments from E991.9
        marine E992
    munitions (accidental) (being used in war) (dump) (factory) E993
    nuclear (weapon) E996
    own weapons (accidental) E993
      injury by fragments from E991.9
        antipersonnel E991.3
    sea-based artillery shell E992
    torpedo E992

War operations — continued
  exposure to ionizing radiation from nuclear explosion E996
  falling aircraft E994
  fire or fire-producing device E990.9
    petrol bomb E990.0
  fireball effects from nuclear explosion E996
  fragments from
    antipersonnel bomb E991.3
    artillery shell, bomb NEC, grenade, guided missile, land mine, rocket, shell, shrapnel E991.9
  fumes E997.2
  gas E997.2
  grenade (explosion) E993
    fragments, injury by E991.9
  guided missile (explosion) E993
    fragments, injury by E991.9
    nuclear E996
  heat from nuclear explosion E996
  injury due to, but occurring after cessation of hostilities E998
  lacrimator (gas) (chemical) E997.2
  land mine (explosion) E993
    after cessation of hostilities E998
    fragments, injury by E991.9
  laser(s) E997.0
  late effect of E999.0 ▲
  lewisite E997.2
  lung irritant (chemical) (fumes) (gas) E997.2
  marine mine E992
  mine
    after cessation of hostilities E998
    at sea E992
    in harbor E992
    land (explosion) E993
      fragments, injury by E991.9
    marine E992
  missile (guided) (explosion) E993
    fragments, injury by E991.9
    marine E992
    nuclear E996
  mortar bomb (explosion) E993
    fragments, injury by E991.9
  mustard gas E997.2
  nerve gas E997.2
  phosgene E997.2
  poisoning (chemical) (fumes) (gas) E997.2
  radiation, ionizing from nuclear explosion E996
  rocket (explosion) E993
    fragments, injury by E991.9
  saber, sabre E995
  screening smoke E997.8
  shell (aircraft) (artillery) (cannon) (land based) (explosion) E993
    fragments, injury by E991.9
    sea-based E992
  shooting E991.2
    after cessation of hostilities E998
    bullet(s) E991.2
      rubber E991.0
    pellet(s) (rifle) E991.1
    shrapnel E991.9
    submersion E995
    torpedo E992
  unconventional warfare, except by nuclear weapon E997.9
    biological (warfare) E997.1
    gas, fumes, chemicals E997.2
    laser(s) E997.0
    specified type NEC E997.8
  underwater blast E992
  vesicant (chemical) (fumes) (gas) E997.2
  weapon burst E993
Washed
  away by flood — see Flood
  away by tidal wave — see Tidal wave
  off road by storm (transport vehicle) E908.9
  overboard E832
Weather exposure — see also Exposure
  cold E901.0
  hot E900.0
Weightlessness (causing injury) (effects of) (in spacecraft, real or simulated) E928.0

Wound (accidental) NEC (see also Injury) E928.9
  battle (see also War operations) E995
  bayonet E920.3
    in
      legal intervention E974
      war operations E995
  gunshot — see Shooting
  incised — see Cut
  saber, sabre E920.3
    in war operations E995

Railway Accidents (E800-E807)

The following fourth-digit subdivisions are for use with categories E800-E807 to identify the injured person:

.0 **Railway employee**
Any person who by virtue of his employment in connection with a railway, whether by the railway company or not, is at increased risk of involvement in a railway accident, such as:

    catering staff on train
    postal staff on train
    driver
    railway fireman
    guard
    shunter
    porter

    sleeping car attendant

.1 **Passenger on railway**
Any authorized person traveling on a train, except a railway employee
EXCLUDES intending passenger waiting at station (.8)
unauthorized rider on railway vehicle (.8)

.2 **Pedestrian**
See definition (r), Vol. 1, page 248

.3 **Pedal cyclist**
See definition (p), Vol. 1, page 248

.8 **Other specified person**
Intending passenger waiting at station
Unauthorized rider on railway vehicle

.9 **Unspecified person**

Motor Vehicle Traffic and Nontraffic Accidents (E810-E825)

The following fourth-digit subdivisions are for use with categories E810-E819 and E820-E825 to identify the injured person:

.0 **Driver of motor vehicle other than motorcycle**
See definition (1), Vol. 1, page 248

.1 **Passenger in motor vehicle other than motorcycle**
See definition (1), Vol. 1, page 248

.2 **Motorcyclist**
See definition (1), Vol. 1, page 248

.3 **Passenger on motorcycle**
See definition (1), Vol. 1, page 248

.4 **Occupant of streetcar**

.5 **Rider of animal; occupant of animal-drawn vehicle**

.6 **Pedal cyclist**
See definition (p), Vol. 1, page 248

.7 **Pedestrian**
See definition (r), Vol. 1, page 248

.8 **Other specified person**
Occupant of vehicle other than above
Person in railway train involved in accident
Unauthorized rider of motor vehicle

.9 **Unspecified person**

Index to External Causes

Other Road Vehicle Accidents (E826-E829)

(animal-drawn vehicle, streetcar, pedal cycle, and other nonmotor road vehicle accidents)

The following fourth-digit subdivisions are for use with categories E826-E829 to identify the injured person:

.0 **Pedestrian**
See definition (r), Vol. 1, page 248

.1 **Pedal cyclist** (does not apply to codes E827, E828, E829)
See definition (p), Vol. 1, page 248

.2 **Rider of animal** (does not apply to code E829)

.3 **Occupant of animal-drawn vehicle** (does not apply to codes E828, E829)

.4 **Occupant of streetcar**

.8 **Other specified person**

.9 **Unspecified person**

Water Transport Accidents (E830-E838)

The following fourth-digit subdivisions are for use with categories E830-E838 to identify the injured person:

.0 **Occupant of small boat, unpowered**

.1 **Occupant of small boat, powered**
See definition (t), Vol. 1, page 248

   EXCLUDES water skier (.4)

.2 **Occupant of other watercraft — crew**
Persons:

   engaged in operation of watercraft

   providing passenger services [cabin attendants, ship's physician, catering personnel]

   working on ship during voyage in other capacity [musician in band, operators of shops and beauty parlors]

.3 **Occupant of other watercraft — other than crew**
Passenger
Occupant of lifeboat, other than crew, after abandoning ship

.4 **Water skier**

.5 **Swimmer**

.6 **Dockers, stevedores**
Longshoreman employed on the dock in loading and unloading ships

.8 **Other specified person**
Immigration and custom officials on board ship
Persons:

   accompanying passenger or member of crew visiting boat

   Pilot (guiding ship into port)

.9 **Unspecified person**

Air and Space Transport Accidents (E840-E845)

The following fourth-digit subdivisions are for use with categories E840-E845 to identify the injured person:

.0 **Occupant of spacecraft**

.1 **Occupant of military aircraft, any**

> Crew
> Passenger (civilian) (military)
> Troops
> } in military aircraft [air force] [army] [national guard] [navy]

>> **EXCLUDES** occupants of aircraft operated under jurisdiction of police departments (.5)
>> parachutist (.7)

.2 **Crew of commercial aircraft (powered) in surface to surface transport**

.3 **Other occupant of commercial aircraft (powered) in surface to surface transport**

> Flight personnel:
>   not part of crew
>   on familiarization flight

> Passenger on aircraft

.4 **Occupant of commercial aircraft (powered) in surface to air transport**

> Occupant [crew] [passenger] of aircraft (powered) engaged in activities, such as:

>> air drops of emergency supplies
>> air drops of parachutists, except from military craft
>> crop dusting
>> lowering of construction material [bridge or telephone pole]
>> sky writing

.5 **Occupant of other powered aircraft**

> Occupant [crew] [passenger] of aircraft (powered) engaged in activities, such as:

>> aerial spraying (crops) (fire retardants)
>> aerobatic flying
>> aircraft racing
>> rescue operation
>> storm surveillance
>> traffic surveillance

> Occupant of private plane NOS

.6 **Occupant of unpowered aircraft, except parachutist**
> Occupant of aircraft classifiable to E842

.7 **Parachutist (military) (other)**
> Person making voluntary descent

>> **EXCLUDES** person making descent after accident to aircraft (.1-.6)

.8 **Ground crew, airline employee**
> Persons employed at airfields (civil) (military) or launching pads, not occupants of aircraft

.9 **Other person**

INFECTIOUS AND PARASITIC DISEASES

1. INFECTIOUS AND PARASITIC DISEASES (001-139)

Note: Categories for "late effects" of infectious and parasitic diseases are to be found at 137-139.

INCLUDES diseases generally recognized as communicable or transmissible as well as a few diseases of unknown but possibly infectious origin

EXCLUDES acute respiratory infections (460-466)
carrier or suspected carrier of infectious organism (V02.0-V02.9)
certain localized infections
influenza (487.0-487.8)

INTESTINAL INFECTIOUS DISEASES (001-009)

EXCLUDES helminthiases (120.0-129)

✓4th **001 Cholera**

DEF: An acute infectious enteritis caused by a potent enterotoxin elaborated by *Vibrio cholerae*; the vibrio produces a toxin in the intestinal tract that changes the permeability of the mucosa leading to diarrhea and dehydration.

- 001.0 Due to Vibrio cholerae
- 001.1 Due to Vibrio cholerae el tor
- 001.9 Cholera, unspecified

✓4th **002 Typhoid and paratyphoid fevers**

DEF: Typhoid fever: an acute generalized illness caused by *Salmonella typhi*; notable clinical features are fever, headache, abdominal pain, cough, toxemia, leukopenia, abnormal pulse, rose spots on the skin, bacteremia, hyperplasia of intestinal lymph nodes, mesenteric lymphadenopathy, and Peyer's patches in the intestines.

DEF: Paratyphoid fever: a prolonged febrile illness, much like typhoid but usually less severe; caused by salmonella serotypes other than *S. typhi*, especially *S. enteritidis* serotypes paratyphi A and B and *S. choleraesuis*.

- 002.0 Typhoid fever
    Typhoid (fever) (infection) [any site]
- 002.1 Paratyphoid fever A
- 002.2 Paratyphoid fever B
- 002.3 Paratyphoid fever C
- 002.9 Paratyphoid fever, unspecified

✓4th **003 Other salmonella infections**

INCLUDES infection or food poisoning by Salmonella [any serotype]

DEF: Infections caused by a genus of gram-negative, anaerobic bacteria of the family *Enterobacteriaceae*; affecting warm-blooded animals, like humans; major symptoms are enteric fevers, acute gastroenteritis and septicemia.

- 003.0 Salmonella gastroenteritis
    Salmonellosis
- 003.1 Salmonella septicemia [HIV]
- ✓5th 003.2 Localized salmonella infections
    - 003.20 **Localized salmonella infection, unspecified** [HIV]
    - 003.21 Salmonella meningitis [HIV]
    - 003.22 Salmonella pneumonia [HIV]
    - 003.23 Salmonella arthritis [HIV]
    - 003.24 Salmonella osteomyelitis [HIV]
    - 003.29 Other [HIV]
- 003.8 Other specified salmonella infections [HIV]
- 003.9 Salmonella infection, unspecified [HIV]

✓4th **004 Shigellosis**

INCLUDES bacillary dysentery

DEF: Acute infectious dysentery caused by the genus *Shigella*, of the family *Enterobacteriaceae*; affecting the colon causing the release of blood-stained stools with accompanying tenesmus, abdominal cramps and fever.

- 004.0 Shigella dysenteriae
    Infection by group A Shigella (Schmitz) (Shiga)
- 004.1 Shigella flexneri
    Infection by group B Shigella
- 004.2 Shigella boydii
    Infection by group C Shigella
- 004.3 Shigella sonnei
    Infection by group D Shigella
- 004.8 Other specified Shigella infections
- 004.9 Shigellosis, unspecified

✓4th **005 Other food poisoning (bacterial)**

EXCLUDES salmonella infections (003.0-003.9)
toxic effect of:
    food contaminants (989.7)
    noxious foodstuffs (988.0-988.9)

DEF: Enteritis caused by ingesting contaminated foods and characterized by diarrhea, abdominal pain, vomiting; symptoms may be mild or life threatening.

- 005.0 Staphylococcal food poisoning
    Staphylococcal toxemia specified as due to food
- 005.1 Botulism
    Food poisoning due to Clostridium botulinum
- 005.2 Food poisoning due to Clostridium perfringens [C. welchii]
    Enteritis necroticans
- 005.3 Food poisoning due to other Clostridia
- 005.4 Food poisoning due to Vibrio parahaemolyticus
- ✓5th 005.8 Other bacterial food poisoning
    EXCLUDES salmonella food poisoning (003.0-003.9)
    - 005.81 Food poisoning due to Vibrio vulnificus
    - 005.89 Other bacterial food poisoning
        Food poisoning due to Bacillus cereus
- 005.9 Food poisoning, unspecified

✓4th **006 Amebiasis**

INCLUDES infection due to Entamoeba histolytica
EXCLUDES amebiasis due to organisms other than Entamoeba histolytica (007.8)

DEF: Infection of the large intestine caused by *Entamoeba histolytica*; usually asymptomatic but symptoms may range from mild diarrhea to profound life-threatening dysentery. Extraintestinal complications include hepatic abscess, which may rupture into the lung, pericardium or abdomen, causing life-threatening infections.

- 006.0 Acute amebic dysentery without mention of abscess
    Acute amebiasis
    DEF: Sudden, severe *Entamoeba histolytica* infection causing bloody stools.
- 006.1 Chronic intestinal amebiasis without mention of abscess
    Chronic:
        amebiasis
        amebic dysentery
- 006.2 Amebic nondysenteric colitis
    DEF: *Entamoeba histolytica* infection with inflamed colon but no dysentery.
- 006.3 Amebic liver abscess
    Hepatic amebiasis
- 006.4 Amebic lung abscess
    Amebic abscess of lung (and liver)
- 006.5 Amebic brain abscess
    Amebic abscess of brain (and liver) (and lung)
- 006.6 Amebic skin ulceration
    Cutaneous amebiasis
- 006.8 Amebic infection of other sites
    Amebic: Ameboma
        appendicitis
        balanitis
    EXCLUDES specific infections by free-living amebae (136.2)
- 006.9 Amebiasis, unspecified
    Amebiasis NOS

INFECTIOUS AND PARASITIC DISEASES

007 Other protozoal intestinal diseases
INCLUDES protozoal:
- colitis
- diarrhea
- dysentery

007.0 Balantidiasis
Infection by Balantidium coli

007.1 Giardiasis
Infection by Giardia lamblia   Lambliasis

007.2 Coccidiosis
Infection by Isospora belli and Isospora hominis
Isosporiasis

007.3 Intestinal trichomoniasis
DEF: Colitis, diarrhea, or dysentery caused by the protozoa *Trichomonas*.

007.4 Cryptosporidiosis
AHA: 4Q, '97, 30

DEF: An intestinal infection by protozoan parasites causing intractable diarrhea in patients with AIDS and other immunosuppressed individuals.

007.5 Cyclosporiasis
AHA: 4Q, '00, 38

DEF: An infection of the small intestine by the protozoal organism, *Cyclospora caytenanesis*, spread to humans though ingestion of contaminated water or food. Symptoms include watery diarrhea with frequent explosive bowel movements, loss of appetite, loss of weight, bloating, increased gas, stomach cramps, nausea, vomiting, muscle aches, low grade fever, and fatigue.

007.8 Other specified protozoal intestinal diseases
Amebiasis due to organisms other than Entamoeba histolytica

007.9 Unspecified protozoal intestinal disease
Flagellate diarrhea   Protozoal dysentery NOS

008 Intestinal infections due to other organisms
INCLUDES any condition classifiable to 009.0-009.3 with mention of the responsible organisms
EXCLUDES food poisoning by these organisms (005.0-005.9)

008.0 Escherichia coli [E. coli]
AHA: 4Q, '92, 17

008.00 E. coli, unspecified
E. coli enteritis NOS

008.01 Enteropathogenic E. coli
DEF: *E. coli* causing inflammation of intestines.

008.02 Enterotoxigenic E. coli
DEF: A toxic reaction to *E. coli* of the intestinal mucosa, causing voluminous watery secretions.

008.03 Enteroinvasive E. coli
DEF: *E. coli* infection penetrating intestinal mucosa.

008.04 Enterohemorrhagic E. coli
DEF: *E. coli* infection penetrating the intestinal mucosa, producing microscopic ulceration and bleeding.

008.09 Other intestinal E. coli infections

008.1 Arizona group of paracolon bacilli
008.2 Aerobacter aerogenes
Enterobacter aeogenes
008.3 Proteus (mirabilis) (morganii)
008.4 Other specified bacteria
AHA: 4Q, '92, 18

008.41 Staphylococcus
Staphylococcal enterocolitis

CC Excl: 001.1, 002.0, 002.9, 003.0, 004.9, 005.0-005.2, 006.0-006.2, 006.9, 007.1-007.9, 008.00-008.49, 008.5, 008.61-008.69, 008.8, 009.0, 014.80-014.86, 112.85, 129, 487.8, 536.3, 536.8, 555.0-555.9, 556.0-556.9, 557.0-557.9, 558.2, 558.3, 558.9, 564.1, 775.0-775.9, 777.5, 777.8

008.42 Pseudomonas
CC Excl: See code 008.41
AHA: 2Q, '89, 10

008.43 Campylobacter
CC Excl: See code 008.41

008.44 Yersinia enterocolitica
CC Excl: See code 008.41

008.45 Clostridium difficile
Pseudomembranous colitis
CC Excl: See code 008.41

DEF: An overgrowth of a species of bacterium that is a part of the normal colon flora in human infants and sometimes in adults; produces a toxin that causes pseudomembranous enterocolitis.; typically is seen in patients undergoing antibiotic therapy.

008.46 Other anaerobes
Anaerobic enteritis NOS
Bacteroides (fragilis)
Gram-negative anaerobes
CC Excl: See code 008.41

008.47 Other gram-negative bacteria
Gram-negative enteritis NOS
EXCLUDES gram-negative anaerobes (008.46)
CC Excl: See code 008.41

008.49 Other
CC Excl: See code 008.41
AHA: 2Q, '89, 10; 1Q, '88, 6

008.5 Bacterial enteritis, unspecified
008.6 Enteritis due to specified virus
AHA: 4Q, '92, 18

008.61 Rotavirus
008.62 Adenovirus
008.63 Norwalk virus
Norwalk-like agent
008.64 Other small round viruses [SRVs]
Small round virus NOS
008.65 Calicivirus
DEF: Enteritis due to a subgroup of *Picornaviruses*.
008.66 Astrovirus
008.67 Enterovirus NEC
Coxsackie virus   Echovirus
EXCLUDES poliovirus (045.0-045.9)
008.69 Other viral enteritis
Torovirus

008.8 Other organism, not elsewhere classified
Viral: Viral:
 enteritis NOS   gastroenteritis
EXCLUDES influenza with involvement of gastrointestinal tract (487.8)

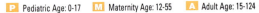

Tabular List — **INFECTIOUS AND PARASITIC DISEASES** — 009–011.9

√4th **009 Ill-defined intestinal infections**
> EXCLUDES diarrheal disease or intestinal infection due to specified organism (001.0-008.8)
> diarrhea following gastrointestinal surgery (564.4)
> intestinal malabsorption (579.0-579.9)
> ischemic enteritis (557.0-557.9)
> other noninfectious gastroenteritis and colitis (558.1-558.9)
> regional enteritis (555.0-555.9)
> ulcerative colitis (556)

009.0 Infectious colitis, enteritis, and gastroenteritis
Colitis
Enteritis } septic
Gastroenteritis

Dysentery: Dysentery:
  NOS   hemorrhagic
  catarrhal

AHA: 3Q, '99, 4

DEF: Colitis: An inflammation of mucous membranes of the colon Enteritis: An inflammation of mucous membranes of the small intestine. Gastroenteritis: An inflammation of mucous membranes of stomach and intestines.

009.1 Colitis, enteritis, and gastroenteritis of presumed infectious origin
> EXCLUDES colitis NOS (558.9)
> enteritis NOS (558.9)
> gastroenteritis NOS (558.9)

AHA: 3Q, '99, 6

009.2 Infectious diarrhea
Diarrhea:
  dysenteric
  epidemic
Infectious diarrheal disease NOS

009.3 Diarrhea of presumed infectious origin
> EXCLUDES diarrhea NOS (787.91)

AHA: N-D, '87, 7

TUBERCULOSIS (010-018)

> INCLUDES infection by Mycobacterium tuberculosis (human) (bovine)
> EXCLUDES congenital tuberculosis (771.2)
> late effects of tuberculosis (137.0-137.4)

The following fifth-digit subclassification is for use with categories 010-018:
0 unspecified
1 bacteriological or histological examination not done
2 bacteriological or histological examination unknown (at present)
3 tubercle bacilli found (in sputum) by microscopy
4 tubercle bacilli not found (in sputum) by microscopy, but found by bacterial culture
5 tubercle bacilli not found by bacteriological examination, but tuberculosis confirmed histologically
6 tubercle bacilli not found by bacteriological or histological examination but tuberculosis confirmed by other methods [inoculation of animals]

DEF: An infection by *Mycobacterium tuberculosis* causing the formation of small, rounded nodules, called tubercles, that can disseminate throughout the body via lymph and blood vessels. Localized tuberculosis is most often seen in the lungs.

√4th **010 Primary tuberculous infection**
DEF: Tuberculosis of the lungs occurring when the patient is first infected.

§ √5th **010.0 Primary tuberculous infection** [HIV]
> EXCLUDES nonspecific reaction to tuberculin skin test without active tuberculosis (795.5)
> positive PPD (795.5)
> positive tuberculin skin test without active tuberculosis (795.5)

DEF: Hilar or paratracheal lymph node enlargement in pulmonary tuberculosis.

§ √5th **010.1 Tuberculous pleurisy in primary progressive tuberculosis** [HIV]
DEF: Inflammation and exudation in the lining of the tubercular lung.

§ √5th **010.8 Other primary progressive tuberculosis** [HIV]
> EXCLUDES tuberculous erythema nodosum (017.1)

§ √5th **010.9 Primary tuberculous infection, unspecified** [HIV]

√4th **011 Pulmonary tuberculosis** [HIV]
Use additional code to identify any associated silicosis (502)

§ √5th **011.0 Tuberculosis of lung, infiltrative** [CC] [HIV]
CC Excl: 011.00-011.96, 012.00-012.86, 017.90-017.96, 018.00-018.96, 031.0, 031.2, 031.8-031.9, 041.81-041.89, 041.9, 137.0, 139.8, 480.0-487.1, 494.0-494.1, 495.0-495.9, 496, 500-505, 506.0-506.9, 507.0-507.8, 508.0-508.9, 517.1, 518.89

§ √5th **011.1 Tuberculosis of lung, nodular** [CC] [HIV]
CC Excl: See code 011.0

§ √5th **011.2 Tuberculosis of lung with cavitation** [CC] [HIV]
CC Excl: See code 011.0

§ √5th **011.3 Tuberculosis of bronchus** [CC] [HIV]
> EXCLUDES isolated bronchial tuberculosis (012.2)

CC Excl: See code 011.0

§ √5th **011.4 Tuberculous fibrosis of lung** [CC] [HIV]
CC Excl: See code 011.0

§ √5th **011.5 Tuberculous bronchiectasis** [CC] [HIV]
CC Excl: See code 011.0

§ √5th **011.6 Tuberculous pneumonia [any form]** [CC] [HIV]
CC Excl: For codes 011.60-011.65: See code 011.0

CC Excl: For code 011.66: 011.66, 139.8, 480.0-487.1, 494.0-494.1, 495.0-495.9, 496, 500-505, 506.0-506.9, 507.0-507.8, 508.0-508.9, 517.1, 518.89

DEF: Inflammatory pulmonary reaction to tuberculous cells.

§ √5th **011.7 Tuberculous pneumothorax** [CC] [HIV]
CC Excl: See code 011.0

DEF: Spontaneous rupture of damaged tuberculous pulmonary tissue.

§ √5th **011.8 Other specified pulmonary tuberculosis** [CC] [HIV]
CC Excl: See code 011.0

§ √5th **011.9 Pulmonary tuberculosis, unspecified** [CC] [HIV]
Respiratory tuberculosis NOS
Tuberculosis of lung NOS
CC Excl: See code 011.0

§ Requires fifth-digit. See beginning of section 010-018 for codes and definitions.

INFECTIOUS AND PARASITIC DISEASES

√4th 012 Other respiratory tuberculosis
EXCLUDES respiratory tuberculosis, unspecified (011.9)

§ √5th 012.0 Tuberculous pleurisy
Tuberculosis of pleura
Tuberculous empyema
Tuberculous hydrothorax
EXCLUDES pleurisy with effusion without mention of cause (511.9)
tuberculous pleurisy in primary progressive tuberculosis (010.1)

CC Excl: See code 011.0

DEF: Inflammation and exudation in the lining of the tubercular lung.

§ √5th 012.1 Tuberculosis of intrathoracic lymph nodes
Tuberculosis of lymph nodes:
  hilar
  mediastinal
  tracheobronchial
Tuberculous tracheobronchial adenopathy
EXCLUDES that specified as primary (010.0-010.9)

CC Excl: See code 011.0

§ √5th 012.2 Isolated tracheal or bronchial tuberculosis
§ √5th 012.3 Tuberculous laryngitis
Tuberculosis of glottis
§ √5th 012.8 Other specified respiratory tuberculosis
Tuberculosis of: Tuberculosis of:
  mediastinum   nose (septum)
  nasopharynx   sinus (any nasal)

√4th 013 Tuberculosis of meninges and central nervous system

§ √5th 013.0 Tuberculous meningitis
Tuberculosis of meninges (cerebral) (spinal)
Tuberculous:
  leptomeningitis
  meningoencephalitis
EXCLUDES tuberculoma of meninges (013.1)

CC Excl: 003.21, 013.00-013.16, 013.40-013.56, 013.80-013.96, 017.90-017.96, 031.2, 031.8-031.9, 036.0, 041.81-041.89, 041.9, 047.0-047.9, 049.0-049.1, 053.0, 054.72, 072.1, 090.42, 091.81, 094.2, 098.89, 100.81, 112.83, 114.2, 115.01, 115.11, 115.91, 130.0, 137.1, 139.8, 320.0-320.9, 321.0-321.8, 322.0-322.9, 349.89, 349.9, 357.0

§ √5th 013.1 Tuberculoma of meninges
CC Excl: See code 013.0

§ √5th 013.2 Tuberculoma of brain
Tuberculosis of brain (current disease)
CC Excl: 013.20-013.36, 013.60-013.96, 017.90-017.96, 031.2, 031.8-031.9, 041.81-041.89, 041.9, 137.1, 139.8

§ √5th 013.3 Tuberculous abscess of brain
CC Excl: See code 013.2

§ √5th 013.4 Tuberculoma of spinal cord
CC Excl: 013.00-013.16, 013.40-013.56, 013.80-013.96, 017.90-017.96, 031.2, 031.8-031.9, 041.81-041.89, 041.9, 137.1, 139.8

§ √5th 013.5 Tuberculous abscess of spinal cord
CC Excl: See code 013.4

§ √5th 013.6 Tuberculous encephalitis or myelitis
CC Excl: 013.20-013.36, 013.60-013.96, 017.90-017.96, 031.2, 031.8-031.9, 041.81-041.89, 041.9, 137.1, 139.8

§ √5th 013.8 Other specified tuberculosis of central nervous system
CC Excl: 013.80-013.96, 017.90-017.96, 031.2, 031.8-031.9, 041.81-041.89, 041.9, 137.1, 139.8

§ √5th 013.9 Unspecified tuberculosis of central nervous system
Tuberculosis of central nervous system NOS
CC Excl: See code 013.8

√4th 014 Tuberculosis of intestines, peritoneum, and mesenteric glands

§ √5th 014.0 Tuberculous peritonitis
Tuberculous ascites
CC Excl: 014.00-014.86, 017.90-017.96, 031.2, 031.8-031.9, 041.81-041.89, 041.9, 139.8

DEF: Tuberculous inflammation of the membrane lining the abdomen.

§ √5th 014.8 Other
Tuberculosis (of):
  anus
  intestine (large) (small)
  mesenteric glands
  rectum
  retroperitoneal (lymph nodes)
Tuberculous enteritis

CC Excl: For code 014.80: See code 014.0

CC Excl: For code 014.81: 014.81, 139.8

CC Excl: For code 014.82: 014.00-014.86, 017.90-017.96, 031.2, 031.8-031.9, 041.81-041.89, 041.9, 139.8

CC Excl: For code 014.83-014.86: See code 014.82

√4th 015 Tuberculosis of bones and joints
Use additional code to identify manifestation, as:
tuberculous:
  arthropathy (711.4)
  necrosis of bone (730.8)
  osteitis (730.8)
  osteomyelitis (730.8)
  synovitis (727.01)
  tenosynovitis (727.01)

§ √5th 015.0 Vertebral column
Pott's disease
Use additional code to identify manifestation, as:
  curvature of spine [Pott's] (737.4)
  kyphosis (737.4)
  spondylitis (720.81)

§ √5th 015.1 Hip
§ √5th 015.2 Knee
§ √5th 015.5 Limb bones
Tuberculous dactylitis
§ √5th 015.6 Mastoid
Tuberculous mastoiditis
§ √5th 015.7 Other specified bone
§ √5th 015.8 Other specified joint
§ √5th 015.9 Tuberculosis of unspecified bones and joints

√4th 016 Tuberculosis of genitourinary system

§ √5th 016.0 Kidney
Renal tuberculosis
Use additional code to identify manifestation, as:
tuberculous:
  nephropathy (583.81)
  pyelitis (590.81)
  pyelonephritis (590.81)
CC Excl: 016.00-016.36, 016.90-016.96, 017.90-017.96, 031.2, 031.8-031.9, 041.81-041.89, 041.9, 137.2, 139.8

§ √5th 016.1 Bladder
CC Excl: See code 016.0

§ √5th 016.2 Ureter
CC Excl: See code 016.0

§ √5th 016.3 Other urinary organs
CC Excl: See code 016.0

---

§ Requires fifth-digit. See beginning of section 010-018 for codes and definitions.

INFECTIOUS AND PARASITIC DISEASES   016.4–020.9

§ ✓5th 016.4   Epididymis   CC HIV ♂
   CC Excl: 016.40-016.56, 016.90-016.96, 017.90-017.96, 031.2, 031.8-031.9, 041.81-041.89, 041.9, 137.2, 139.8

§ ✓5th 016.5   Other male genital organs   CC HIV ♂
   Use additional code to identify manifestation, as:
      tuberculosis of:
         prostate (601.4)
         seminal vesicle (608.81)
         testis (608.81)
   CC Excl: See code 016.4

§ ✓5th 016.6   Tuberculous oophoritis and salpingitis   CC HIV ♀
   CC Excl: 016.60-016.96, 017.90-017.96, 031.2, 031.8-031.9, 041.81-041.89, 041.9, 137.2, 139.8

§ ✓5th 016.7   Other female genital organs   CC HIV ♀
   Tuberculous:
      cervicitis
      endometritis
   CC Excl: See code 016.6

§ ✓5th 016.9   Genitourinary tuberculosis, unspecified   CC HIV
   CC Excl: 016.90-016.96, 017.90-017.96, 031.2, 031.8-031.9, 041.81-041.89, 041.9, 137.2, 139.8

✓4th 017   Tuberculosis of other organs

§ ✓5th 017.0   Skin and subcutaneous cellular tissue   HIV
   Lupus: Tuberculosis:
      exedens   cutis
      vulgaris   lichenoides
   Scrofuloderma   papulonecrotica
   Tuberculosis: verrucosa cutis
      colliquativa
   EXCLUDES   lupus erythematosus (695.4)
                  disseminated (710.0)
                  lupus NOS (710.0)
                  nonspecific reaction to tuberculin skin
                     test without active tuberculosis
                     (795.5)
                  positive PPD (795.5)
                  positive tuberculin skin test without
                     active tuberculosis (795.5)

§ ✓5th 017.1   Erythema nodosum with hypersensitivity   HIV
   reaction in tuberculosis
      Bazin's disease   Erythema:
      Erythema: nodosum, tuberculous
         induratum   Tuberculosis indurativa
   EXCLUDES   erythema nodosum NOS (695.2)
   DEF: Tender, inflammatory, bilateral nodules appearing on the shins and thought to be an allergic reaction to tuberculotoxin.

§ ✓5th 017.2   Peripheral lymph nodes   CC HIV
      Scrofula   Tuberculous adenitis
      Scrofulous abscess
   EXCLUDES   tuberculosis of lymph nodes:
                  bronchial and mediastinal (012.1)
                  mesenteric and retroperitoneal
                     (014.8)
                  tuberculous tracheobronchial
                     adenopathy (012.1)
   CC Excl: 017.20-017.26, 017.90-017.96, 031.2, 031.8-031.9, 041.81-041.89, 041.9, 139.8
   DEF: Scrofula: Old name for tuberculous cervical lymphadenitis.

§ ✓5th 017.3   Eye   CC HIV
   Use additional code to identify manifestation, as:
      tuberculous:
         chorioretinitis, disseminated (363.13)
         episcleritis (379.09)
         interstitial keratitis (370.59)
         iridocyclitis, chronic (364.11)
         keratoconjunctivitis (phlyctenular) (370.31)
   CC Excl: 017.30-017.36, 017.90-017.96, 031.2, 031.8-031.9, 041.81-041.89, 041.9, 139.8

§ ✓5th 017.4   Ear   CC HIV
   Tuberculosis of ear
   Tuberculous otitis media
   EXCLUDES   tuberculous mastoiditis (015.6)
   CC Excl: 017.40-017.46, 017.90-017.96, 031.2, 031.8-031.9, 041.81-041.89, 041.9, 139.8

§ ✓5th 017.5   Thyroid gland   CC HIV
   CC Excl: 017.50-017.56, 017.90-017.96, 031.2, 031.8-031.9, 041.81-041.89, 041.9, 139.8

§ ✓5th 017.6   Adrenal glands   CC HIV
   Addison's disease, tuberculous
   CC Excl: 017.60-017.66, 017.90-017.96, 031.2, 031.8-031.9, 041.81-041.89, 041.9, 139.8

§ ✓5th 017.7   Spleen   CC HIV
   CC Excl: 017.70-017.76, 017.90-017.96, 031.2, 031.8-031.9, 041.81-041.89, 041.9, 139.8

§ ✓5th 017.8   Esophagus   CC HIV
   CC Excl: 017.80-017.96, 031.2, 031.8-031.9, 041.81-041.89, 041.9, 139.8

§ ✓5th 017.9   Other specified organs   CC HIV
   Use additional code to identify manifestation, as:
      tuberculosis of:
         endocardium [any valve] (424.91)
         myocardium (422.0)
         pericardium (420.0)
   CC Excl: 017.90-017.96, 031.2, 031.8-031.9, 041.81-041.89, 041.9, 139.8

✓4th 018   Miliary tuberculosis
   INCLUDES   tuberculosis:
                  disseminated
                  generalized
                  miliary, whether of a single specified site,
                     multiple sites, or unspecified site
                  polyserositis
   DEF: A form of tuberculosis caused by caseous material carried through the bloodstream planting seedlike tubercles in various body organs.

§ ✓5th 018.0   Acute miliary tuberculosis   CC HIV
   CC Excl: 017.90-017.96, 018.00-018.96, 031.2, 031.8-031.9, 041.81-041.89, 041.9, 139.8

§ ✓5th 018.8   Other specified miliary tuberculosis   CC HIV
   CC Excl: See code 018.0

§ ✓5th 018.9   Miliary tuberculosis, unspecified   CC HIV
   CC Excl: See code 018.0

ZOONOTIC BACTERIAL DISEASES (020-027)

✓4th 020   Plague
   INCLUDES   infection by Yersinia [Pasteurella] pestis

   020.0   Bubonic
      DEF: Most common acute and severe form of plague characterized by lymphadenopathy (buboes), chills, fever and headache.

   020.1   Cellulocutaneous
      DEF: Plague characterized by inflammation and necrosis of skin.

   020.2   Septicemic
      DEF: Plague characterized by massive infection in the bloodstream.

   020.3   Primary pneumonic
      DEF: Plague characterized by massive pulmonary infection.

   020.4   Secondary pneumonic
      DEF: Lung infection as a secondary complication of plague.

   020.5   Pneumonic, unspecified

   020.8   Other specified types of plague
      Abortive plague   Pestis minor
      Ambulatory plague

   020.9   Plague, unspecified

§ Requires fifth-digit. See beginning of section 010-018 for codes and definitions.

 Additional Digit Required   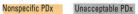 Nonspecific PDx   Unacceptable PDx   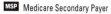 Manifestation Code   MSP Medicare Secondary Payer   ▶◀ Revised Text   ● New Code   ▲ Revised Code Title

2002 Ingenix, Inc.   Volume 1 — 5

INFECTIOUS AND PARASITIC DISEASES

✓4th 021 Tularemia
INCLUDES deerfly fever
infection by Francisella [Pasteurella] tularensis
rabbit fever

DEF: A febrile disease transmitted by the bites of deer flies, fleas and ticks, by inhalations of aerosolized *F. tularensis* or by ingestion of contaminated food or water; patients quickly develop fever, chills, weakness, headache, backache and malaise.

021.0 Ulceroglandular tularemia
DEF: Lesions occur at the site *Francisella tularensis* organism enters body, usually the fingers or hands.

021.1 Enteric tularemia
Tularemia: Tularemia:
cryptogenic   typhoidal
intestinal

021.2 Pulmonary tularemia
Bronchopneumonic tularemia

021.3 Oculoglandular tularemia
DEF: Painful conjunctival infection by *Francisella tularensis* organism with possible corneal, preauricular lymph, or lacrimal involvement.

021.8 Other specified tularemia
Tularemia: Tularemia:
generalized or disseminated   glandular

021.9 Unspecified tularemia

✓4th 022 Anthrax
DEF: An infectious bacterial disease usually transmitted by contact with infected animals or their discharges or products; it is classified by primary routes of inoculation as cutaneous, gastrointestinal and by inhalation.

022.0 Cutaneous anthrax
Malignant pustule

022.1 Pulmonary anthrax
Respiratory anthrax
Wool-sorters' disease

022.2 Gastrointestinal anthrax
022.3 Anthrax septicemia
022.8 Other specified manifestations of anthrax
022.9 Anthrax, unspecified

✓4th 023 Brucellosis
INCLUDES fever:
Malta
Mediterranean
undulant

DEF: An infectious disease caused by gram-negative, aerobic coccobacilli organisms; it is transmitted to humans through contact with infected tissue or dairy products; fever, sweating, weakness and aching are symptoms.

023.0 Brucella melitensis
DEF: Infection from direct or indirect contact with infected sheep or goats.

023.1 Brucella abortus
DEF: Infection from direct or indirect contact with infected cattle.

023.2 Brucella suis
DEF: Infection from direct or indirect contact with infected swine.

023.3 Brucella canis
DEF: Infection from direct or indirect contact with infected dogs.

023.8 Other brucellosis
Infection by more than one organism

023.9 Brucellosis, unspecified

024 Glanders
Infection by:
Actinobacillus mallei   Farcy
Malleomyces mallei   Malleus
Pseudomonas mallei

DEF: Equine infection causing mucosal inflammation and skin ulcers in humans.

025 Melioidosis
Infection by: Infection by:
Malleomyces pseudomallei   Pseudoglanders
Pseudomonas pseudomallei   Whitmore's bacillus

DEF: Rare infection caused by *Pseudomonas pseudomallei*; clinical symptoms range from localized infection to fatal septicemia.

✓4th 026 Rat-bite fever
026.0 Spirillary fever
Rat-bite fever due to Spirillum minor [S. minus]
Sodoku

026.1 Streptobacillary fever
Epidemic arthritic erythema
Haverhill fever
Rat-bite fever due to Streptobacillus moniliformis

026.9 Unspecified rat-bite fever

✓4th 027 Other zoonotic bacterial diseases
027.0 Listeriosis
Infection } by Listeria monocytogenes
Septicemia

Use additional code to identify manifestation, as meningitis (320.7)

EXCLUDES congenital listeriosis (771.2)

027.1 Erysipelothrix infection
Erysipeloid (of Rosenbach)
Infection } by Erysipelothrix insidiosa
Septicemia   [E. rhusiopathiae]

DEF: Usually associated with handling of fish, meat, or poultry; symptoms range from localized inflammation to septicemia.

027.2 Pasteurellosis
Pasteurella pseudotuberculosis infection
Mesenteric adenitis
Septic infection (cat } by Pasteurella multocida
bite) (dog bite)   [P. septica]

EXCLUDES infection by:
Francisella [Pasteurella] tularensis (021.0-021.9)
Yersinia [Pasteurella] pestis (020.0-020.9)

DEF: Swelling, abscesses, or septicemia from *Pasteurella multocida*, commonly transmitted to humans by a dog or cat scratch.

027.8 Other specified zoonotic bacterial diseases
027.9 Unspecified zoonotic bacterial disease

OTHER BACTERIAL DISEASES (030-041)
EXCLUDES bacterial venereal diseases (098.0-099.9)
bartonellosis (088.0)

✓4th 030 Leprosy
INCLUDES Hansen's disease
infection by Mycobacterium leprae

030.0 Lepromatous [type L]
Lepromatous leprosy (macular) (diffuse) (infiltrated) (nodular) (neuritic)

DEF: Infectious, disseminated leprosy bacilli with lesions and deformities.

030.1 Tuberculoid [type T]
Tuberculoid leprosy (macular) (maculoanesthetic) (major) (minor) (neuritic)

DEF: Relatively benign, self-limiting leprosy with neuralgia and scales.

030.2 Indeterminate [group I]
Indeterminate [uncharacteristic] leprosy (macular) (neuritic)

DEF: Uncharacteristic leprosy, frequently an early manifestation.

030.3 Borderline [group B]
Borderline or dimorphous leprosy (infiltrated) (neuritic)

DEF: Transitional form of leprosy, neither lepromatous nor tuberculoid.

INFECTIOUS AND PARASITIC DISEASES

- 030.8 Other specified leprosy
- 030.9 Leprosy, unspecified
- ✓4th **031 Diseases due to other mycobacteria**
  - **031.0 Pulmonary** [CC]
    - Battey disease
    - Infection by Mycobacterium:
      - avium
      - intracellulare [Battey bacillus]
      - kansasii
    - **CC Excl:** 011.00-011.96, 012.00-012.86, 017.90-017.96, 031.0, 031.2, 031.8-031.9, 041.81-041.89, 041.9, 137.0, 139.8, 480.0-480.9, 481, 482.0-482.9, 483.0, 483.1, 483.8, 484.1-484.8, 485-486, 487.0-487.1, 494.0-494.1, 495.0-495.9, 496, 500-505, 506.0-506.9, 507.0-507.8, 508.0-508.9, 517.1, 518.89
  - **031.1 Cutaneous**
    - Buruli ulcer
    - Infection by Mycobacterium:
      - marinum [M. balnei]
      - ulcerans
  - **031.2 Disseminated** [HIV]
    - Disseminated mycobacterium avium-intracellulare complex (DMAC)
    - Mycobacterium avium-intracellulare complex (MAC) bacteremia
    - **AHA:** 4Q, '97, 31
    - **DEF:** Disseminated mycobacterium avium-intracellulare complex (DMAC): A serious systemic form of MAC commonly observed in patients in the late course of AIDS.
    - **DEF:** Mycobacterium avium-intracellulare complex (MAC) bacterium: Human pulmonary disease, lymphadenitis in children and systemic disease in immunocompromised individuals caused by a slow growing, gram-positive, aerobic organism.
  - **031.8 Other specified mycobacterial diseases** [HIV]
  - **031.9 Unspecified diseases due to mycobacteria** [HIV]
    - Atypical mycobacterium infection NOS
- ✓4th **032 Diphtheria**
  - **INCLUDES** infection by Corynebacterium diphtheriae
  - **032.0 Faucial diphtheria**
    - Membranous angina, diphtheritic
    - **DEF:** Diphtheria of the throat.
  - **032.1 Nasopharyngeal diphtheria**
  - **032.2 Anterior nasal diphtheria**
  - **032.3 Laryngeal diphtheria**
    - Laryngotracheitis, diphtheritic
  - ✓5th **032.8 Other specified diphtheria**
    - **032.81 Conjunctival diphtheria**
      - Pseudomembranous diphtheritic conjunctivitis
    - **032.82 Diphtheritic myocarditis**
    - **032.83 Diphtheritic peritonitis**
    - **032.84 Diphtheritic cystitis**
    - **032.85 Cutaneous diphtheria**
    - **032.89 Other**
  - **032.9 Diphtheria, unspecified**
- ✓4th **033 Whooping cough**
  - **INCLUDES** pertussis
  - Use additional code to identify any associated pneumonia (484.3)
  - **DEF:** An acute, highly contagious respiratory tract infection caused by *Bordetella pertussis* and *B. bronchiseptica*; characteristic paroxysmal cough.
  - **033.0 Bordetella pertussis [B. pertussis]**
  - **033.1 Bordetella parapertussis [B. parapertussis]**
  - **033.8 Whooping cough due to other specified organism**
    - Bordetella bronchiseptica [B. bronchiseptica]
  - **033.9 Whooping cough, unspecified organism**

- ✓4th **034 Streptococcal sore throat and scarlet fever**
  - **034.0 Streptococcal sore throat**
    - Septic:
      - angina
      - sore throat
    - Streptococcal:
      - angina
    - Streptococcal:
      - laryngitis
      - pharyngitis
      - tonsillitis
  - **034.1 Scarlet fever**
    - Scarlatina
    - **EXCLUDES** parascarlatina (057.8)
    - **DEF:** Streptococcal infection and fever with red rash spreading from trunk.
- **035 Erysipelas**
  - **EXCLUDES** postpartum or puerperal erysipelas (670)
  - **DEF:** An acute superficial cellulitis involving the dermal lymphatics; it is often caused by group A streptococci.
- ✓4th **036 Meningococcal infection**
  - **036.0 Meningococcal meningitis** [CC]
    - Cerebrospinal fever (meningococcal)
    - Meningitis:
      - cerebrospinal
      - epidemic
    - **CC Excl:** 003.21, 013.00-013.16, 036.0, 036.89, 036.9, 041.81-041.89, 041.9, 047.0-047.9, 049.0-049.1, 053.0, 054.72, 072.1, 090.42, 091.81, 094.2, 098.89, 100.81, 112.83, 114.2, 115.01, 115.11, 115.91, 130.0, 139.8, 320.0-320.9, 321.0-321.8, 322.0-322.9, 349.89, 349.9, 357.0
  - **036.1 Meningococcal encephalitis** [CC]
    - **CC Excl:** 036.1, 036.89, 036.9, 041.81-041.89, 041.9, 139.8
  - **036.2 Meningococcemia** [CC]
    - Meningococcal septicemia
    - **CC Excl:** 003.1, 020.2, 036.2, 036.89, 036.9, 038.0, 038.10-038.11, 038.19, 038.2-038.9, 041.81-041.89, 041.9, 054.5, 139.8, ▶995.90-995.94◀
  - **036.3 Waterhouse-Friderichsen syndrome, meningococcal** [CC]
    - Meningococcal hemorrhagic adrenalitis
    - Meningoccic adrenal syndrome
    - Waterhouse-Friderichsen syndrome NOS
    - **CC Excl:** 036.3, 036.89, 036.9, 041.81-041.89, 041.9, 139.8
  - ✓5th **036.4 Meningococcal carditis**
    - **036.40 Meningococcal carditis, unspecified** [CC]
      - **CC Excl:** 036.40, 036.89, 036.9, 041.81-041.89, 041.9, 139.8
    - **036.41 Meningococcal pericarditis** [CC]
      - **CC Excl:** 036.41, 036.89, 036.9, 041.81-041.89, 041.9, 139.8
      - **DEF:** Meningococcal infection of the outer membrane of the heart.
    - **036.42 Meningococcal endocarditis** [CC]
      - **CC Excl:** 036.42, 036.89, 036.9, 041.81-041.89, 041.9, 139.8
      - **DEF:** Meningococcal infection of the membranes lining the cavities of the heart.
    - **036.43 Meningococcal myocarditis** [CC]
      - **CC Excl:** 036.43, 041.81-041.89, 041.9, 139.8
      - **DEF:** Meningococcal infection of the muscle of the heart.
  - ✓5th **036.8 Other specified meningococcal infections**
    - **036.81 Meningococcal optic neuritis** [CC]
      - **CC Excl:** 036.81, 036.89, 036.9, 041.81-041.89, 041.9, 139.8
    - **036.82 Meningococcal arthropathy** [CC]
      - **CC Excl:** 036.82, 036.89, 036.9, 041.81-041.89, 041.9, 139.8
    - **036.89 Other** [CC]
      - **CC Excl:** 036.89, 036.9, 041.81-041.89, 041.9, 139.8
  - **036.9 Meningococcal infection, unspecified** [CC]
    - Meningococcal infection NOS
    - **CC Excl:** See code 036.89

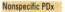 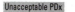 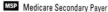

Additional Digit Required | Nonspecific PDx | Unacceptable PDx | Manifestation Code | MSP Medicare Secondary Payer | ▶◀ Revised Text | ● New Code | ▲ Revised Code Title

INFECTIOUS AND PARASITIC DISEASES

037 Tetanus `CC`
 EXCLUDES tetanus:
   complicating:
     abortion (634-638 with .0, 639.0)
     ectopic or molar pregnancy (639.0)
   neonatorum (771.3)
   puerperal (670)

 CC Excl: 037, 139.8

 DEF: An acute, often fatal, infectious disease caused by the anaerobic, spore-forming bacillus *Clostridium tetani*; the bacillus most often enters the body through a contaminated wound, burns, surgical wounds, or cutaneous ulcers. Symptoms include lockjaw, spasms, seizures, and paralysis.

√4th **038 Septicemias**
 EXCLUDES bacteremia (790.7)
   during labor (659.3)
   following ectopic or molar pregnancy (639.0)
   following infusion, injection, transfusion, or vaccination (999.3)
   postpartum, puerperal (670)
   ▶septicemia (sepsis) of newborn (771.81)◀
   that complicating abortion (634-638 with .0, 639.0)

 AHA: 4Q, '88, 10; 3Q, '88, 12

 DEF: A systemic disease associated with the presence and persistence of pathogenic microorganisms or their toxins in the blood.

 038.0 Streptococcal septicemia `CC` `HIV`
  CC Excl: 003.1, 020.2, 036.2, 038.0-038.9, 040.82, 040.89, 041.00-041.05, 041.09-041.11, 041.19, 041.2-041.7, 041.81-041.86, 041.89, 041.9, 054.5, 139.8, V09.0-V09.91, ▶995.90-995.94◀

  AHA: 2Q, '96. 5

 √5th **038.1 Staphylococcal septicemia**
  AHA: 4Q, '97, 32

  038.10 Staphylococcal septicemia, unspecified `CC` `HIV`
   CC Excl: See code 038.0

  038.11 Staphylococcus aureus septicemia `CC` `HIV`
   CC Excl: See code 038.0
   AHA: 2Q, '00, 5; 4Q, '98, 42

  038.19 Other staphylococcal septicemia `CC` `HIV`
   CC Excl: See code 038.0
   AHA: 2Q, '00, 5

 038.2 Pneumococcal septicemia [Streptococcus pneumoniae septicemia] `CC` `HIV`
  CC Excl: See code 038.0
  AHA: 2Q, '96, 5; 1Q, '91, 13

 038.3 Septicemia due to anaerobes `CC` `HIV`
  Septicemia due to bacteroides
  EXCLUDES gas gangrene (040.0)
    that due to anaerobic streptococci (038.0)
  CC Excl: See code 038.0
  DEF: Infection of blood by microorganisms that thrive without oxygen.

 √5th **038.4 Septicemia due to other gram-negative organisms**
  DEF: Infection of blood by microorganisms categorized as gram-negative by Gram's method of staining for identification of bacteria.

  038.40 Gram-negative organism, unspecified `CC` `HIV`
   Gram-negative septicemia NOS
   CC Excl: See code 038.0

  038.41 Hemophilus influenzae [H. influenzae] `CC` `HIV`
   CC Excl: See code 038.0

  038.42 Escherichia coli [E. coli] `CC` `HIV`
   CC Excl: See code 038.0
   DRG 416

  038.43 Pseudomonas `CC` `HIV`
   CC Excl: See code 038.0

  038.44 Serratia `CC` `HIV`
   CC Excl: See code 038.0

  038.49 Other `CC` `HIV`
   CC Excl: See code 038.0
   DRG 416

 038.8 Other specified septicemias `CC` `HIV`
  EXCLUDES septicemia (due to):
    anthrax (022.3)
    gonococcal (098.89)
    herpetic (054.5)
    meningococcal (036.2)
    septicemic plague (020.2)
  CC Excl: See code 038.0

 038.9 Unspecified septicemia `CC` `HIV`
  Septicemia NOS
  EXCLUDES bacteremia NOS (790.7)
  CC Excl: See code 038.0
  AHA: 2Q, '00, 3; 3Q, '99. 5. 9; 1Q, '98, 5; 3Q, '96, 16; 2Q, '96, 6
  DRG 416

√4th **039 Actinomycotic infections**
 INCLUDES actinomycotic mycetoma
   infection by Actinomycetales, such as species of Actinomyces, Actinomadura, Nocardia, Streptomyces
   maduromycosis (actinomycotic)
   schizomycetoma (actinomycotic)

 DEF: Inflammatory lesions and abscesses at site of infection by *Actinomyces israeli*.

 039.0 Cutaneous `HIV`
   Erythrasma   Trichomycosis axillaris
 039.1 Pulmonary `HIV`
   Thoracic actinomycosis
 039.2 Abdominal `HIV`
 039.3 Cervicofacial
 039.4 Madura foot `HIV`
   EXCLUDES madura foot due to mycotic infection (117.4)
 039.8 Of other specified sites `HIV`
 039.9 Of unspecified site `HIV`
   Actinomycosis NOS   Nocardiosis NOS
   Maduromycosis NOS

√4th **040 Other bacterial diseases**
 EXCLUDES bacteremia NOS (790.7)
   bacterial infection NOS (041.9)

 040.0 Gas gangrene `CC`
   Gas bacillus infection or gangrene
   Infection by Clostridium:
     histolyticum
     oedematiens
     perfringens [welchii]
     septicum
     sordellii
   Malignant edema
   Myonecrosis, clostridial
   Myositis, clostridial
   CC Excl: 040.0, 139.8
   AHA: 1Q, '95, 11

 040.1 Rhinoscleroma
   DEF: Growths on the nose and nasopharynx caused by *Klebsiella rhinoscleromatis*.

Tabular List — INFECTIOUS AND PARASITIC DISEASES — 040.2–046.1

040.2 Whipple's disease
Intestinal lipodystrophy

040.3 Necrobacillosis
DEF: Infection with *Fusobacterium necrophorum* causing abscess or necrosis.

√5th **040.8 Other specified bacterial diseases**
  040.81 Tropical pyomyositis
  040.82 Toxic shock syndrome CC
    Use additional code to identify the organism
    CC Excl: 040.82, 780.91-780.99, 785.50-785.59, 785.9, 799.8
  040.89 Other
    AHA: N-D, '86, 7

√4th **041 Bacterial infection in conditions classified elsewhere and of unspecified site**
  Note: This category is provided to be used as an additional code to identify the bacterial agent in diseases classified elsewhere. This category will also be used to classify bacterial infections of unspecified nature or site.
  EXCLUDES bacteremia NOS (790.7)
           septicemia (038.0-038.9)
  AHA: 2Q, '01, 12; J-A, '84, 19

√5th **041.0 Streptococcus**
  041.00 Streptococcus, unspecified
  041.01 Group A
    AHA: ▶1Q, '02, 3◀
  041.02 Group B
  041.03 Group C
  041.04 Group D [Enterococcus]
  041.05 Group G
  041.09 Other Streptococcus

√5th **041.1 Staphylococcus**
  041.10 Staphylococcus, unspecified
  041.11 Staphylococcus aureus
    AHA: 2Q, '01, 11; 4Q, '98, 42, 54; 4Q, '97, 32
  041.19 Other Staphylococcus

041.2 Pneumococcus
041.3 Friedländer's bacillus
  Infection by Klebsiella pneumoniae
041.4 Escherichia coli [E. coli]
041.5 Hemophilus influenzae [H. influenzae]
041.6 Proteus (mirabilis) (morganii)
041.7 Pseudomonas

√5th **041.8 Other specified bacterial infections**
  041.81 Mycoplasma
    Eaton's agent
    Pleuropneumonia-like organisms [PPLO]
  041.82 Bacillus fragilis
  041.83 Clostridium perfringens
  041.84 Other anaerobes
    Bacteroides (fragilis)
    Gram-negative anaerobes
    EXCLUDES Helicobacter pylori (041.86)
  041.85 Other gram-negative organisms
    Aerobacter aerogenes
    Gram-negative bacteria NOS
    Mima polymorpha
    Serratia
    EXCLUDES gram-negative anaerobes (041.84)
    AHA: 1Q, 95, 18
  041.86 Helicobacter pylori (H. pylori)
    AHA: 4Q, '95, 60
  041.89 Other specified bacteria

041.9 Bacterial infection, unspecified
  AHA: 2Q, '91, 9

HUMAN IMMUNODEFICIENCY VIRUS (HIV) INFECTION (042)

042 Human immunodeficiency virus [HIV] disease CC
  Acquired immune deficiency syndrome
  Acquired immunodeficiency syndrome
  AIDS
  AIDS-like syndrome
  AIDS-related complex
  ARC
  HIV infection, symptomatic
  Use additional code(s) to identify all manifestations of HIV
  Use additional code to identify HIV-2 infection (079.53)
  EXCLUDES asymptomatic HIV infection status (V08)
           exposure to HIV virus (V01.7)
           nonspecific serologic evidence of HIV (795.71)
  CC Excl: 042, 139.8
  AHA: 1Q, '99, 14, 4Q, '97, 30, 31; 1Q, '93, 21; 2Q, '92, 11; 3Q, '90, 17; J-A, '87, 8

POLIOMYELITIS AND OTHER NON-ARTHROPOD-BORNE VIRAL DISEASES OF CENTRAL NERVOUS SYSTEM (045-049)

√4th **045 Acute poliomyelitis**
  EXCLUDES late effects of acute poliomyelitis (138)
  The following fifth-digit subclassification is for use with category 045:
  0 poliovirus, unspecified type
  1 poliovirus type I
  2 poliovirus type II
  3 poliovirus type III

√5th **045.0 Acute paralytic poliomyelitis specified as bulbar**
  Infantile paralysis (acute)   } specified as bulbar
  Poliomyelitis (acute) (anterior)
  Polioencephalitis (acute) (bulbar)
  Polioencephalomyelitis (acute) (anterior) (bulbar)
  DEF: Acute paralytic infection occurring where the brain merges with the spinal cord; affecting breathing, swallowing, and heart rate.

√5th **045.1 Acute poliomyelitis with other paralysis**
  Paralysis: acute atrophic, spinal
  Paralysis: infantile, paralytic
  Poliomyelitis (acute) anterior epidemic } with paralysis except bulbar
  DEF: Paralytic infection affecting peripheral or spinal nerves.

√5th **045.2 Acute nonparalytic poliomyelitis**
  Poliomyelitis (acute) anterior epidemic } specified as nonparalytic
  DEF: Nonparalytic infection causing pain, stiffness, and paresthesias.

√5th **045.9 Acute poliomyelitis, unspecified**
  Infantile paralysis
  Poliomyelitis (acute) anterior epidemic } unspecified whether paralytic or nonparalytic

√4th **046 Slow virus infection of central nervous system**
  046.0 Kuru
    DEF: A chronic, progressive, fatal nervous system disorder; clinical symptoms include cerebellar ataxia, trembling, spasticity and progressive dementia.
  046.1 Jakob-Creutzfeldt disease
    Subacute spongiform encephalopathy
    DEF: Communicable, progressive spongiform encephalopathy thought to be caused by an infectious particle known as a "prion" (proteinaceous infection particle). This is a progressive, fatal disease manifested principally by mental deterioration.

INFECTIOUS AND PARASITIC DISEASES

046.2 Subacute sclerosing panencephalitis [CC]
Dawson's inclusion body encephalitis
Van Bogaert's sclerosing leukoencephalitis
CC Excl: 046.2, 139.8

DEF: Progressive viral infection causing cerebral dysfunction, blindness, dementia, and death (SSPE).

046.3 Progressive multifocal leukoencephalopathy [HIV]
Multifocal leukoencephalopathy NOS

DEF: Infection affecting cerebral cortex in patients with weakened immune systems.

046.8 Other specified slow virus infection of central nervous system [HIV]

046.9 Unspecified slow virus infection of central nervous system [HIV]

√4th 047 Meningitis due to enterovirus
INCLUDES   meningitis: meningitis:
           abacterial   viral
           aseptic

EXCLUDES   meningitis due to:
           adenovirus (049.1)
           arthropod-borne virus (060.0-066.9)
           leptospira (100.81)
           virus of:
               herpes simplex (054.72)
               herpes zoster (053.0)
               lymphocytic choriomeningitis (049.0)
               mumps (072.1)
               poliomyelitis (045.0-045.9)
           any other infection specifically classified
               elsewhere

AHA: J-F, '87, 6

047.0 Coxsackie virus
047.1 ECHO virus
Meningo-eruptive syndrome
047.8 Other specified viral meningitis
047.9 Unspecified viral meningitis
Viral meningitis NOS

048 Other enterovirus diseases of central nervous system
Boston exanthem

√4th 049 Other non-arthropod-borne viral diseases of central nervous system
EXCLUDES   late effects of viral encephalitis (139.0)

049.0 Lymphocytic choriomeningitis
Lymphocytic:
    meningitis (serous) (benign)
    meningoencephalitis (serous) (benign)

049.1 Meningitis due to adenovirus
DEF: Inflammation of lining of brain caused by Arenaviruses and usually occurring in adults in fall and winter months.

049.8 Other specified non-arthropod-borne viral diseases of central nervous system
Encephalitis: Encephalitis:
    acute: lethargica
        inclusion body   Rio Bravo
        necrotizing   von Economo's disease
        epidemic

049.9 Unspecified non-arthropod-borne viral diseases of central nervous system
Viral encephalitis NOS

VIRAL DISEASES ACCOMPANIED BY EXANTHEM (050-057)
EXCLUDES   arthropod-borne viral diseases (060.0-066.9)
           Boston exanthem (048)

√4th 050 Smallpox
050.0 Variola major
Hemorrhagic (pustular) smallpox
Malignant smallpox
Purpura variolosa

DEF: Form of smallpox known for its high mortality; exists only in laboratories.

050.1 Alastrim
Variola minor
DEF: Mild form of smallpox known for its low mortality rate.

050.2 Modified smallpox
Varioloid
DEF: Mild form occurring in patients with history of infection or vaccination.

050.9 Smallpox, unspecified

√4th 051 Cowpox and paravaccinia
051.0 Cowpox
Vaccinia not from vaccination
EXCLUDES   vaccinia (generalized) (from vaccination) (999.0)

DEF: A disease contracted by milking infected cows; vesicles usually appear on the fingers, may spread to hands and adjacent areas and usually disappear without scarring; other associated features of the disease may include local edema, lymphangitis and regional lymphadenitis with or without fever.

051.1 Pseudocowpox
Milkers' node
DEF: Hand lesions and mild fever in dairy workers caused by exposure to paravaccinia.

051.2 Contagious pustular dermatitis
Ecthyma contagiosum
Orf
DEF: Skin eruptions caused by exposure to poxvirus-infected sheep or goats.

051.9 Paravaccinia, unspecified

√4th 052 Chickenpox
DEF: Contagious infection by *Varicella-zoster* virus causing rash with pustules and fever.

052.0 Postvaricella encephalitis [CC]
Postchickenpox encephalitis
CC Excl: 051.9, 052.0, 052.7-052.9, 078.88-078.89, 079.81, 079.88-079.89, 079.98-079.99, 139.8

052.1 Varicella (hemorrhagic) pneumonitis [CC]
CC Excl: 051.9, 052.1, 052.7-052.9, 078.88-078.89, 079.81, 079.88-079.89, 079.98-079.99, 139.8

052.7 With other specified complications [CC]
CC Excl: 051.9, 052.7-052.9, 078.88-078.89, 079.81, 079.88-079.89, 079.98-079.99, 139.8
AHA: ▶1Q, '02, 3◀

052.8 With unspecified complication [CC]
CC Excl: See code 052.7

052.9 Varicella without mention of complication [CC]
Chickenpox NOS   Varicella NOS
CC Excl: See code 052.7

√4th 053 Herpes zoster
INCLUDES   shingles
           zona

DEF: Self-limiting infection by *varicella-zoster* virus causing unilateral eruptions and neuralgia along affected nerves.

053.0 With meningitis [CC] [HIV]
CC Excl: 003.21, 013.00-013.16, 036.0, 047.0-047.9, 049.0-049.1, 053.0-053.19, 053.79, 053.8-053.9, 054.72, 054.79, 054.8-054.9, 072.1, 078.88-078.89, 079.81, 079.88-079.89, 079.98-079.99, 090.42, 091.81, 094.2, 098.89, 100.81, 112.83, 114.2, 115.01, 115.11, 115.91, 130.0, 139.8, 320.0-320.9, 321.0-321.8, 322.0-322.9, 349.89, 349.9, 357.0

DEF: *Varicella-zoster* virus infection causing inflammation of the lining of the brain and/or spinal cord.

√5th 053.1 With other nervous system complications
053.10 With unspecified nervous system complication [CC] [HIV]
CC Excl: 053.0-053.19, 053.79, 053.8-053.9, 054.72, 054.79, 054.8-054.9, 078.88-078.89, 079.81, 079.88-079.89, 079.98-079.99, 139.8

INFECTIOUS AND PARASITIC DISEASES

053.11 Geniculate herpes zoster `CC` `HIV`
Herpetic geniculate ganglionitis
CC Excl: See code 053.10

DEF: Unilateral eruptions and neuralgia along the facial nerve geniculum affecting face and outer and middle ear.

053.12 Postherpetic trigeminal neuralgia `CC` `HIV`
CC Excl: See code 053.10

DEF: Severe oral or nasal pain following a herpes zoster infection.

053.13 Postherpetic polyneuropathy `CC` `HIV`
CC Excl: See code 053.10

DEF: Multiple areas of pain following a herpes zoster infection.

053.19 Other `CC` `HIV`
CC Excl: See code 053.10

√5th **053.2 With ophthalmic complications**
053.20 Herpes zoster dermatitis of eyelid `HIV`
Herpes zoster ophthalmicus
053.21 Herpes zoster keratoconjunctivitis `HIV`
053.22 Herpes zoster iridocyclitis `HIV`
053.29 Other `HIV`

√5th **053.7 With other specified complications**
053.71 Otitis externa due to herpes zoster `HIV`
053.79 Other `CC` `HIV`
CC Excl: 053.0-053.9, 054.0-054.71, 054.73, 054.79, 054.8-054.9, 078.88-078.89, 079.81, 079.88-079.89, 079.98-079.99, 139.8

053.8 With unspecified complication `CC` `HIV`
CC Excl: See code 053.79

053.9 Herpes zoster without mention of complication `HIV`
Herpes zoster NOS

√4th **054 Herpes simplex**
EXCLUDES   congenital herpes simplex (771.2)

054.0 Eczema herpeticum `HIV`
Kaposi's varicelliform eruption
DEF: Herpes simplex virus invading site of preexisting skin inflammation.

√5th **054.1 Genital herpes**
AHA: J-F, '87, 15, 16

054.10 Genital herpes, unspecified `HIV`
Herpes progenitalis
054.11 Herpetic vulvovaginitis `HIV` ♀
054.12 Herpetic ulceration of vulva `HIV` ♀
054.13 Herpetic infection of penis `HIV` ♂
054.19 Other `HIV`

054.2 Herpetic gingivostomatitis `HIV`
054.3 Herpetic meningoencephalitis `CC` `HIV`
Herpes encephalitis   Simian B disease
CC Excl: 054.3, 054.79, 054.8-054.9, 139.8

DEF: Inflammation of the brain and its lining, caused by infection of herpes simplex 1 in adults and simplex 2 in newborns.

√5th **054.4 With ophthalmic complications**
054.40 With unspecified ophthalmic complication `HIV`
054.41 Herpes simplex dermatitis of eyelid `HIV`
054.42 Dendritic keratitis `HIV`
054.43 Herpes simplex disciform keratitis `HIV`
054.44 Herpes simplex iridocyclitis `HIV`
054.49 Other `HIV`

054.5 Herpetic septicemia `CC` `HIV`
CC Excl: 003.1, 020.2, 036.2, 038.0, 038.10-038.11, 038.19, 038.2-038.9, 054.5, 054.79, 054.8-054.9, 139.8, ▶995.90-995.94◀
AHA: 2Q, '00, 5

054.6 Herpetic whitlow `HIV`
Herpetic felon
DEF: A primary infection of the terminal segment of a finger by herpes simplex; intense itching and pain start the disease, vesicles form, and tissue ultimately is destroyed.

√5th **054.7 With other specified complications**
054.71 Visceral herpes simplex `CC` `HIV`
CC Excl: 054.71, 054.72, 054.79, 054.8-054.9, 139.8
054.72 Herpes simplex meningitis `CC` `HIV`
CC Excl: 003.21, 013.00-013.16, 036.0, 047.0-047.9, 049.0-049.1, 053.0, 054.72, 054.79, 054.8-054.9, 072.1, 090.42, 091.81, 094.2, 098.89, 100.81, 112.83, 114.2, 115.01, 115.11, 115.91, 130.0, 139.8, 320.0-320.9, 321.0-321.8, 322.0-322.9, 349.89, 349.9, 357.0
054.73 Herpes simplex otitis externa `HIV`
054.79 Other `CC` `HIV`
CC Excl: 054.79, 054.8-054.9, 078.88-078.89, 079.81, 079.88-079.89, 079.98-079.99, 139.8

054.8 With unspecified complication `CC` `HIV`
CC Excl: See code 054.79

054.9 Herpes simplex without mention of complication `HIV`

√4th **055 Measles**
INCLUDES   morbilli   rubeola

055.0 Postmeasles encephalitis `CC`
CC Excl: 055.0, 055.79, 055.8-055.9, 078.88-078.89, 079.81, 079.88-079.89, 079.98-079.99, 139

055.1 Postmeasles pneumonia `CC`
CC Excl: 055.1, 055.79, 055.8-055.9, 078.88-078.89, 079.81, 079.88-079.89, 079.98-079.99, 139.8

055.2 Postmeasles otitis media `CC`
CC Excl: 055.2, 055.79, 055.8-055.9, 078.88-078.89, 079.81, 079.88-079.89, 079.98-079.99, 139.8

√5th **055.7 With other specified complications**
055.71 Measles keratoconjunctivitis `CC`
Measles keratitis
CC Excl: 055.71, 055.79, 055.8-055.9, 078.88-078.89, 079.81, 079.88-079.89, 079.98-079.99, 139.8

055.79 Other `CC`
CC Excl: 055.79, 055.8-055.9, 078.88-078.89, 079.81, 079.88-079.89, 079.98-079.99, 139.8

055.8 With unspecified complication `CC`
CC Excl: 055.79, 055.8-055.9, 056.09, 078.88-078.89, 079.81, 079.88-079.89, 079.98-079.99, 139.8

055.9 Measles without mention of complication

√4th **056 Rubella**
INCLUDES   German measles
EXCLUDES   congenital rubella (771.0)

DEF: Acute but usually benign togavirus infection causing fever, sore throat, and rash; associated with complications to fetus as a result of maternal infection.

√5th **056.0 With neurological complications**
056.00 With unspecified neurological complication `CC`
CC Excl: 056.00-056.09, 056.79, 056.8-056.9, 078.88-078.89, 079.81, 079.88-079.89, 079.98-079.99, 139.8

056.01 Encephalomyelitis due to rubella `CC`
Encephalitis } due to rubella
Meningoencephalitis
CC Excl: See code 056.00

056.09 Other `CC`
CC Excl: See code 056.00

INFECTIOUS AND PARASITIC DISEASES

√5ᵗʰ 056.7 With other specified complications
    056.71 Arthritis due to rubella [CC]
        CC Excl: 056.71-056.9, 078.88-078.89, 079.81,
        079.88-079.89, 079.98-079.99, 139.8

    056.79 Other [CC]
        CC Excl: See code 056.00

056.8 With unspecified complications [CC]
    CC Excl: 056., 056.01, 056.79, 056.8-056.9, 078.88-078.89,
    079.81, 079.88-079.89, 079.98-079.99, 139.8

056.9 Rubella without mention of complication

√4ᵗʰ 057 Other viral exanthemata
    DEF: Skin eruptions or rashes and fever caused by viruses, including poxviruses.

    057.0 Erythema infectiosum [fifth disease]
        DEF: A moderately contagious, benign, epidemic disease, usually seen in children, and of probable viral etiology; a red macular rash appears on the face and may spread to the limbs and trunk.

    057.8 Other specified viral exanthemata
        Dukes (-Filatow) disease
        Exanthema subitum [sixth disease]
        Fourth disease
        Parascarlatina
        Pseudoscarlatina
        Roseola infantum

    057.9 Viral exanthem, unspecified

ARTHROPOD-BORNE VIRAL DISEASES (060-066)
    Use additional code to identify any associated meningitis (321.2)
    EXCLUDES *late effects of viral encephalitis (139.0)*

√4ᵗʰ 060 Yellow fever
    DEF: Fever and jaundice from infection by mosquito-borne virus of genus *Flavivirus*.

    060.0 Sylvatic
        Yellow fever: Yellow fever:
          jungle   sylvan
        DEF: Yellow fever transmitted from animal to man, via mosquito.

    060.1 Urban
        DEF: Yellow fever transmitted from man to man, via mosquito.

    060.9 Yellow fever, unspecified

061 Dengue
    Breakbone fever
    EXCLUDES *hemorrhagic fever caused by dengue virus (065.4)*
    DEF: Acute, self-limiting infection by mosquito-borne virus characterized by fever and generalized aches.

√4ᵗʰ 062 Mosquito-borne viral encephalitis
    062.0 Japanese encephalitis
        Japanese B encephalitis
        DEF: Flavivirus causing inflammation of the brain, and Russia, with a wide range of clinical manifestations.

    062.1 Western equine encephalitis
        DEF: Alphavirus WEE infection causing inflammation of the brain, found in areas west of the Mississippi; transmitted horse to mosquito to man.

    062.2 Eastern equine encephalitis
        EXCLUDES *Venezuelan equine encephalitis (066.2)*
        DEF: Alphavirus EEE causing inflammation of the brain and spinal cord, found as far north as Canada and south into South America and Mexico; transmitted horse to mosquito to man.

    062.3 St. Louis encephalitis
        DEF: Epidemic form caused by Flavivirus and transmitted by mosquito, and characterized by fever, difficulty in speech, and headache.

    062.4 Australian encephalitis
        Australian arboencephalitis   Murray Valley
        Australian X disease   encephalitis
        DEF: Flavivirus causing inflammation of the brain, occurring in Australia and New Guinea.

    062.5 California virus encephalitis
        Encephalitis: Tahyna fever
          California
          La Crosse
        DEF: Bunyamwere causing inflammation of the brain.

    062.8 Other specified mosquito-borne viral encephalitis
        Encephalitis by Ilheus virus
        EXCLUDES ▶*West Nile virus (066.4)*◀

    062.9 Mosquito-borne viral encephalitis, unspecified

√4ᵗʰ 063 Tick-borne viral encephalitis
    INCLUDES diphasic meningoencephalitis

    063.0 Russian spring-summer [taiga] encephalitis
    063.1 Louping ill
        DEF: Inflammation of brain caused by virus transmitted sheep to tick to man; incidence usually limited to British Isles.

    063.2 Central European encephalitis
        DEF: Inflammation of brain caused by virus transmitted by tick; limited to central Europe and presenting with two distinct phases.

    063.8 Other specified tick-borne viral encephalitis
        Langat encephalitis
        Powassan encephalitis

    063.9 Tick-borne viral encephalitis, unspecified

064 Viral encephalitis transmitted by other and unspecified arthropods
    Arthropod-borne viral encephalitis, vector unknown
    Negishi virus encephalitis
    EXCLUDES *viral encephalitis NOS (049.9)*

√4ᵗʰ 065 Arthropod-borne hemorrhagic fever
    065.0 Crimean hemorrhagic fever [CHF Congo virus]
        Central Asian hemorrhagic fever
    065.1 Omsk hemorrhagic fever
    065.2 Kyasanur Forest disease
    065.3 Other tick-borne hemorrhagic fever
    065.4 Mosquito-borne hemorrhagic fever
        Chikungunya hemorrhagic fever
        Dengue hemorrhagic fever
        EXCLUDES *Chikungunya fever (066.3)*
                            dengue (061)
                            yellow fever (060.0-060.9)

    065.8 Other specified arthropod-borne hemorrhagic fever
        Mite-borne hemorrhagic fever

    065.9 Arthropod-borne hemorrhagic fever, unspecified
        Arbovirus hemorrhagic fever NOS

√4ᵗʰ 066 Other arthropod-borne viral diseases
    066.0 Phlebotomus fever
        Changuinola fever
        Sandfly fever
        DEF: Sandfly-borne viral infection occurring in Asia, Mideast and South America.

    066.1 Tick-borne fever
        Nairobi sheep disease
        Tick fever:
          American mountain
          Colorado
          Kemerovo
          Quaranfil

    066.2 Venezuelan equine fever
        Venezuelan equine encephalitis
        DEF: Alphavirus VEE infection causing inflammation of the brain, usually limited to South America, Mexico, and Florida; transmitted horse to mosquito to man

INFECTIOUS AND PARASITIC DISEASES

066.3 Other mosquito-borne fever
Fever (viral):
- Bunyamwera
- Bwamba
- Chikungunya
- Guama
- Mayaro
- Mucambo
- O'Nyong-Nyong

Fever (viral):
- Oropouche
- Pixuna
- Rift valley
- Ross river
- Wesselsbron
- Zika

EXCLUDES: dengue (061)
yellow fever (060.0-060.9)

066.4 West Nile fever
West Nile encephalitis
West Nile encephalomyelitis
West Nile virus

066.8 Other specified arthropod-borne viral diseases
Chandipura fever   Piry fever

066.9 Arthropod-borne viral disease, unspecified
Arbovirus infection NOS

OTHER DISEASES DUE TO VIRUSES AND CHLAMYDIAE (070-079)

070 Viral hepatitis
INCLUDES: viral hepatitis (acute) (chronic)
EXCLUDES: cytomegalic inclusion virus hepatitis (078.5)

DEF: Hepatitis A: HAV infection is self-limiting with flulike symptoms; transmission, fecal-oral.

DEF: Hepatitis B: HBV infection can be chronic and systemic; transmission, bodily fluids.

DEF: Hepatitis C: HCV infection can be chronic and systemic; transmission, blood transfusion and unidentified agents.

DEF: Hepatitis D (delta): HDV occurs only in the presence of hepatitis B virus.

DEF: Hepatitis E: HEV is epidemic form; transmission and nature under investigation.

070.0 Viral hepatitis A with hepatic coma

070.1 Viral hepatitis A without mention of hepatic coma
Infectious hepatitis

The following fifth-digit subclassification is for use with categories 070.2 and 070.3:
- 0 acute or unspecified, without mention of hepatitis delta
- 1 acute or unspecified, with hepatitis delta
- 2 chronic, without mention of hepatitis delta
- 3 chronic, with hepatitis delta

070.2 Viral hepatitis B with hepatic coma
CC Excl: 070.0-070.9, 078.88-078.89, 079.81, 079.88-079.89, 079.98-079.99, 139.8
AHA: 4Q, '91, 28

070.3 Viral hepatitis B without mention of hepatic coma
Serum hepatitis
CC Excl: See code 070.2
AHA: 1Q, '93, 28; 4Q, '91, 28

070.4 Other specified viral hepatitis with hepatic coma
AHA: 4Q, '91, 28

070.41 Acute or unspecified hepatitis C with hepatic coma
CC Excl: See code 070.2

070.42 Hepatitis delta without mention of active hepatitis B disease with hepatic coma
Hepatitis delta with hepatitis B carrier state
CC Excl: See code 070.2

070.43 Hepatitis E with hepatic coma
CC Excl: See code 070.2

070.44 Chronic hepatitis C with hepatic coma
CC Excl: See code 070.2

070.49 Other specified viral hepatitis with hepatic coma
CC Excl: See code 070.2

070.5 Other specified viral hepatitis without mention of hepatic coma
AHA: 4Q, '91, 28

070.51 Acute or unspecified hepatitis C without mention of hepatic coma
CC Excl: See code 070.2

070.52 Hepatitis delta without mention of active hepatititis B disease or hepatic coma
CC Excl: See code 070.2

070.53 Hepatitis E without mention of hepatic coma
CC Excl: See code 070.2

070.54 Chronic hepatitis C without mention of hepatic coma
CC Excl: See code 070.2

070.59 Other specified viral hepatitis without mention of hepatic coma
CC Excl: See code 070.2

070.6 Unspecified viral hepatitis with hepatic coma
CC Excl: See code 070.2

070.9 Unspecified viral hepatitis without mention of hepatic coma
Viral hepatitis NOS
CC Excl: See code 070.2

071 Rabies
Hydrophobia
Lyssa

DEF: Acute infectious disease of the CNS caused by a rhabdovirus; usually spread by virus-laden saliva from bites by infected animals; it progresses from fever, restlessness, and extreme excitability, to hydrophobia, seizures, confusion and death.

072 Mumps
DEF: Acute infectious disease caused by paramyxovirus; usually seen in children less than 15 years of age; salivary glands are typically enlarged, and other organs, such as testes, pancreas and meninges, are often involved.

072.0 Mumps orchitis
CC Excl: 072.0, 072.79, 072.8-072.9, 078.88-078.89, 079.81, 079.88-079.89, 079.98-079.99, 139.8

072.1 Mumps meningitis
CC Excl: 003.21, 013.00-013.16, 036.0, 047.0-047.9, 049.0-049.1, 053.0, 054.72, 072.1, 072.79, 072.8-072.9, 078.88-078.89, 079.81, 079.98-079.99, 090.42, 091.81, 094.2, 098.89, 100.81, 112.83, 114.2, 115.01, 115.11, 115.91, 130.0, 139.8, 320.0-320.9, 321.0-321.8, 322.0-322.9, 349.89, 349.9, 357.0

072.2 Mumps encephalitis
Mumps meningoencephalitis
CC Excl: 072.2, 072.79, 072.8-072.9, 078.88-078.89, 079.81, 079.88-079.89, 079.98-079.99, 139.8

072.3 Mumps pancreatitis
CC Excl: 072.3, 072.79, 072.8-072.9, 078.88-078.89, 079.81, 079.88-079.89, 079.98-079.99, 139.8

072.7 Mumps with other specified complications

072.71 Mumps hepatitis
CC Excl: 072.71, 072.79, 072.8-072.9, 078.88-078.89, 079.81, 079.88-079.89, 079.98-079.99, 139.8

072.72 Mumps polyneuropathy
CC Excl: 072.72, 072.79, 072.8-072.9, 078.88-078.89, 079.81, 079.88-079.89, 079.98-079.99, 139.8

072.79 Other
CC Excl: 072.79, 072.8-072.9, 078.88-078.89, 079.81, 079.88-079.89, 079.98-079.99, 139.8

072.8–078.3 INFECTIOUS AND PARASITIC DISEASES

072.8 Mumps with unspecified complication [CC]
CC Excl: 072.79, 072.8-072.9, 078.88-078.89, 079.81, 079.88-079.89, 079.98-079.99

072.9 Mumps without mention of complication
Epidemic parotitis Infectious parotitis

√4th 073 Ornithosis
INCLUDES parrot fever
psittacosis
DEF: *Chlamydia psittaci* infection often transmitted from birds to humans.

073.0 With pneumonia
Lobular pneumonitis due to ornithosis

073.7 With other specified complications

073.8 With unspecified complication

073.9 Ornithosis, unspecified

√4th 074 Specific diseases due to Coxsackie virus
EXCLUDES Coxsackie virus:
  infection NOS (079.2)
  meningitis (047.0)

074.0 Herpangina
Vesicular pharyngitis
DEF: Acute infectious coxsackie virus infection causing throat lesions, fever, and vomiting; generally affects children in summer.

074.1 Epidemic pleurodynia
Bornholm disease   Epidemic:
Devil's grip   myalgia
                      myositis
DEF: Paroxysmal pain in chest, accompanied by fever and usually limited to children and young adults; caused by coxsackie virus.

√5th 074.2 Coxsackie carditis
074.20 Coxsackie carditis, unspecified
074.21 Coxsackie pericarditis
DEF: Coxsackie infection of the outer lining of the heart.
074.22 Coxsackie endocarditis
DEF: Coxsackie infection within the heart's cavities.
074.23 Coxsackie myocarditis
Aseptic myocarditis of newborn
DEF: Coxsackie infection of the muscle of the heart.

074.3 Hand, foot, and mouth disease
Vesicular stomatitis and exanthem
DEF: Mild coxsackie infection causing lesions on hands, feet and oral mucosa, and most commonly seen in preschool children.

074.8 Other specified diseases due to Coxsackie virus
Acute lymphonodular pharyngitis

075 Infectious mononucleosis
Glandular fever   Pfeiffer's disease
Monocytic angina
AHA: ▶3Q, '01, 13;◀ M-A, '87, 8
DEF: Acute infection by Epstein-Barr virus causing fever, sore throat, enlarged lymph glands and spleen, and fatigue; usually seen in teens and young adults.

√4th 076 Trachoma
EXCLUDES late effect of trachoma (139.1)
DEF: A chronic infectious disease of the cornea and conjunctiva caused by a strain of the bacteria *Chlamydia trachomatis*; the infection can cause photophobia, pain, excessive tearing and sometimes blindness.

076.0 Initial stage
Trachoma dubium

076.1 Active stage
Granular conjunctivitis (trachomatous)
Trachomatous:
  follicular conjunctivitis
  pannus

076.9 Trachoma, unspecified
Trachoma NOS

√4th 077 Other diseases of conjunctiva due to viruses and Chlamydiae
EXCLUDES ophthalmic complications of viral diseases classified elsewhere

077.0 Inclusion conjunctivitis
Paratrachoma   Swimming pool conjunctivitis
EXCLUDES inclusion blennorrhea (neonatal) (771.6)
DEF: Pus in conjunctiva caused by *Chlamydiae trachomatis*.

077.1 Epidemic keratoconjunctivitis
Shipyard eye
DEF: Highly contagious corneal or conjunctival infection caused by adenovirus type 8; symptoms include inflammation and corneal infiltrates.

077.2 Pharyngoconjunctival fever
Viral pharyngoconjunctivitis

077.3 Other adenoviral conjunctivitis
Acute adenoviral follicular conjunctivitis

077.4 Epidemic hemorrhagic conjunctivitis
Apollo:
  conjunctivitis
  disease
Conjunctivitis due to enterovirus type 70
Hemorrhagic conjunctivitis (acute) (epidemic)

077.8 Other viral conjunctivitis
Newcastle conjunctivitis

√5th 077.9 Unspecified diseases of conjunctiva due to viruses and Chlamydiae
DEF: A genus of the family Chlamydiaceae; *C. psittaci* causes psittacosis in man and ornithosis in birds, and *C. trachomatis* causes trachoma, conjunctivitis, lymphogranuloma venereum, pneumonitis and pneumonia.

077.98 Due to Chlamydiae
077.99 Due to viruses
Viral conjunctivitis NOS

√4th 078 Other diseases due to viruses and Chlamydiae
EXCLUDES viral infection NOS (079.0-079.9)
viremia NOS (790.8)

078.0 Molluscum contagiosum
DEF: Benign poxvirus infection causing small bumps on the skin or conjunctiva; transmitted by close contact.

√5th 078.1 Viral warts
Viral warts due to human papilloma virus
AHA: 2Q, '97, 9; 4Q, '93, 22
DEF: A keratotic papilloma of the epidermis caused by the human papilloma virus; the superficial vegetative lesions last for varying durations and eventually regress spontaneously.

078.10 Viral warts, unspecified
Condyloma NOS   Verruca:
Verruca: Vulgaris
  NOS   Warts (infectious)

078.11 Condyloma acuminatum
DEF: Clusters of mucosa or epidermal lesions on external genitalia; viral infection is sexually transmitted.

078.19 Other specified viral warts
Genital warts NOS   Verruca:
Verruca: plantaris
  plana

078.2 Sweating fever
Miliary fever   Sweating disease
DEF: A viral infection characterized by profuse sweating; various papular, vesicular and other eruptions cause the blockage of sweat glands.

078.3 Cat-scratch disease
Benign lymphoreticulosis (of inoculation)
Cat-scratch fever

INFECTIOUS AND PARASITIC DISEASES 078.4–082.0

078.4 Foot and mouth disease
Aphthous fever
Epizootic:
  Epizootic: stomatitis
  aphthae
DEF: Ulcers on oral mucosa, legs, and feet after exposure to infected animal.

078.5 Cytomegaloviral disease [HIV]
Cytomegalic inclusion disease
Salivary gland virus disease
Use additional code to identify manifestation, as:
  cytomegalic inclusion virus:
    hepatitis (573.1)
    pneumonia (484.1)
EXCLUDES congenital cytomegalovirus infection (771.1)
AHA: 3Q, '98, 4; 2Q, '93, 11; 1Q, '89, 9

DEF: A herpes virus inclusion associated with serious disease morbidity including fever, leukopenia, pneumonia, retinitis, hepatitis and organ transplant; often leads to syndromes such as hepatomegaly, splenomegaly and thrombocytopenia; a common post-transplant complication for organ transplant recipients.

078.6 Hemorrhagic nephrosonephritis
Hemorrhagic fever: Hemorrhagic fever:
  epidemic   Russian
  Korean   with renal syndrome
DEF: Viral infection causing kidney dysfunction and bleeding disorders.

078.7 Arenaviral hemorrhagic fever
Hemorrhagic fever: Hemorrhagic fever:
  Argentine   Junin virus
  Bolivian   Machupo virus

078.8 Other specified diseases due to viruses and Chlamydiae
EXCLUDES epidemic diarrhea (009.2)
          lymphogranuloma venereum (099.1)
  078.81 Epidemic vertigo
  078.82 Epidemic vomiting syndrome
    Winter vomiting disease
  078.88 Other specified diseases due to Chlamydiae
    AHA: 4Q, '96, 22
  078.89 Other specified diseases due to viruses
    Epidemic cervical myalgia
    Marburg disease
    Tanapox

079 Viral and chlamydial infection in conditions classified elsewhere and of unspecified site
Note: This category is provided to be used as an additional code to identify the viral agent in diseases classifiable elsewhere. This category will also be used to classify virus infection of unspecified nature or site.

079.0 Adenovirus
079.1 ECHO virus
DEF: An "orphan" enteric RNA virus, certain serotypes of which are associated with human disease, especially aseptic meningitis.

079.2 Coxsackie virus
DEF: A heterogenous group of viruses associated with aseptic meningitis, myocarditis, pericarditis, and acute onset juvenile diabetes.

079.3 Rhinovirus
DEF: Rhinoviruses affect primarily the upper respiratory tract. Over 100 distinct types infect humans.

079.4 Human papillomavirus
AHA: 2Q, '97, 9; 4Q, '93, 22
DEF: Viral infection caused by the genus *Papillomavirus* causing cutaneous and genital warts, including verruca vulgaris and condyloma acuminatum; certain types are associated with cervical dysplasia, cancer and other genital malignancies.

079.5 Retrovirus
EXCLUDES human immunodeficiency virus, type 1 [HIV-1] (042)
          human T-cell lymphotrophic virus, type III [HTLV-III] (042)
          lymphadenopathy-associated virus [LAV] (042)
AHA: 4Q, '93, 22, 23
DEF: A large group of RNA viruses that carry reverse transcriptase and include the leukoviruses and lentiviruses.

  079.50 Retrovirus, unspecified
  079.51 Human T-cell lymphotrophic virus, type I [HTLV-I]
  079.52 Human T-cell lymphotrophic virus, type II [HTLV-II]
  079.53 Human immunodeficiency virus, type 2 [HIV-2]
  079.59 Other specified retrovirus

079.6 Respiratory syncytial virus (RSV)
AHA: 4Q, '96, 27, 28
DEF: The major respiratory pathogen of young children, causing severe bronchitis and bronchopneumonia, and minor infection in adults.

079.8 Other specified viral and chlamydial infections
AHA: 1Q, '88, 12
  079.81 Hantavirus
    AHA: 4Q, '95, 60
    DEF: An infection caused by the Muerto Canyon virus whose primary rodent reservoir is the deer mouse *Peromyscus maniculatus*; commonly characterized by fever, myalgias, headache, cough and rapid decline.
  079.88 Other specified chlamydial infection
  079.89 Other specified viral infection

079.9 Unspecified viral and chlamydial infections
EXCLUDES viremia NOS (790.8)
AHA: 2Q, '91, 8
  079.98 Unspecified chlamydial infection
    Chlamydial infections NOS
  079.99 Unspecified viral infection
    Viral infections NOS

RICKETTSIOSES AND OTHER ARTHROPOD-BORNE DISEASES (080-088)
EXCLUDES arthropod-borne viral diseases (060.0-066.9)

080 Louse-borne [epidemic] typhus
Typhus (fever):   Typhus (fever):
  classical   exanthematic NOS
  epidemic   louse-borne
DEF: *Rickettsia prowazekii*; causes severe headache, rash, high fever.

081 Other typhus
  081.0 Murine [endemic] typhus
    Typhus (fever):   Typhus (fever):
      endemic   flea-borne
    DEF: Milder typhus caused by *Rickettsia typhi (mooseri)*; transmitted by rat flea.
  081.1 Brill's disease
    Brill-Zinsser disease
    Recrudescent typhus (fever)
  081.2 Scrub typhus
    Japanese river fever   Mite-borne typhus
    Kedani fever   Tsutsugamushi
  081.9 Typhus, unspecified
    Typhus (fever) NOS

082 Tick-borne rickettsioses
  082.0 Spotted fevers
    Rocky mountain spotted fever
    Sao Paulo fever

INFECTIOUS AND PARASITIC DISEASES

082.1 **Boutonneuse fever**
African tick typhus Marseilles fever
India tick typhus Mediterranean tick fever
Kenya tick typhus

082.2 **North Asian tick fever**
Siberian tick typhus

082.3 **Queensland tick typhus**

√5th **082.4** **Ehrlichiosis**
AHA: 4Q, '00, 38

  082.40 **Ehrlichiosis, unspecified**
  082.41 **Ehrlichiosis chaffeensis [E. chaffeensis]**
  DEF: A febrile illness caused by bacterial infection, also called human monocytic ehrlichiosis (HME). Causal organism is *Ehrlichia chaffeensis*, transmitted by the Lone Star tick, *Amblyomma americanum*. Symptoms include fever, chills, myalgia, nausea, vomiting, diarrhea, confusion, and severe headache occurring one week after a tick bite. Clinical findings are lymphadenopathy, rash, thrombocytopenia, leukopenia, and abnormal liver function tests.

  082.49 **Other ehrlichiosis**

082.8 **Other specified tick-borne rickettsioses**
Lone star fever
AHA: 4Q, '99, 19

082.9 **Tick-borne rickettsiosis, unspecified**
Tick-borne typhus NOS

√4th **083** **Other rickettsioses**

083.0 **Q fever**
DEF: Infection of *Coxiella burnettii* usually acquired through airborne organisms.

083.1 **Trench fever**
Quintan fever Wolhynian fever

083.2 **Rickettsialpox**
Vesicular rickettsiosis
DEF: Infection of *Rickettsia akari* usually acquired through a mite bite.

083.8 **Other specified rickettsioses**

083.9 **Rickettsiosis, unspecified**

√4th **084** **Malaria**
Note: Subcategories 084.0-084.6 exclude the listed conditions with mention of pernicious complications (084.8-084.9).
  EXCLUDES congenital malaria (771.2)
DEF: Mosquito-borne disease causing high fever and prostration and cataloged by species of *Plasmodium: P. falciparum, P. malariae, P. ovale,* and *P. vivax*.

084.0 **Falciparum malaria [malignant tertian]**
Malaria (fever):
  by Plasmodium falciparum
  subtertian

084.1 **Vivax malaria [benign tertian]**
Malaria (fever) by Plasmodium vivax

084.2 **Quartan malaria**
Malaria (fever) by Plasmodium malariae
Malariae malaria

084.3 **Ovale malaria**
Malaria (fever) by Plasmodium ovale

084.4 **Other malaria**
Monkey malaria

084.5 **Mixed malaria**
Malaria (fever) by more than one parasite

084.6 **Malaria, unspecified**
Malaria (fever) NOS

084.7 **Induced malaria**
Therapeutically induced malaria
  EXCLUDES accidental infection from syringe, blood transfusion, etc. (084.0-084.6, above, according to parasite species)
  transmission from mother to child during delivery (771.2)

084.8 **Blackwater fever**
Hemoglobinuric: Malarial hemoglobinuria
  fever (bilious)
  malaria
DEF: Severe hemic and renal complication of *Plasmodium falciparum* infection.

084.9 **Other pernicious complications of malaria**
Algid malaria
Cerebral malaria
Use additional code to identify complication, as:
  malarial:
    hepatitis (573.2)
    nephrosis (581.81)

√4th **085** **Leishmaniasis**

085.0 **Visceral [kala-azar]**
Dumdum fever Leishmaniasis:
Infection by Leishmania: dermal, post-kala-azar
  donovani Mediterranean
  infantum visceral (Indian)

085.1 **Cutaneous, urban**
Aleppo boil Leishmaniasis, cutaneous:
Baghdad boil dry form
Delhi boil late
Infection by Leishmania recurrent
  tropica (minor) ulcerating
  Oriental sore

085.2 **Cutaneous, Asian desert**
Infection by Leishmania tropica major
Leishmaniasis, cutaneous:
  acute necrotizing
  rural
  wet form
  zoonotic form

085.3 **Cutaneous, Ethiopian**
Infection by Leishmania ethiopica
Leishmaniasis, cutaneous:
  diffuse
  lepromatous

085.4 **Cutaneous, American**
Chiclero ulcer
Infection by Leishmania mexicana
Leishmaniasis tegumentaria diffusa

085.5 **Mucocutaneous (American)**
Espundia
Infection by Leishmania braziliensis
Uta

085.9 **Leishmaniasis, unspecified**

√4th **086** **Trypanosomiasis**
Use additional code to identify manifestations, as:
  trypanosomiasis:
    encephalitis (323.2)
    meningitis (321.3)

086.0 **Chagas' disease with heart involvement** CC
American trypanosomiasis } with heart
Infection by Trypanosoma } involvement
  cruzi

Any condition classifiable to 086.2 with heart involvement

CC Excl: 086.0, 139.8

INFECTIOUS AND PARASITIC DISEASES

086.1 **Chagas' disease with other organ involvement**
American trypanosomiasis } with heart
Infection by Trypanosoma } involvement
    cruzi
Any condition classifiable to 086.2 with heart involvement

086.2 **Chagas' disease without mention of organ involvement**
American trypanosomiasis
Infection by Trypanosoma cruzi

086.3 **Gambian trypanosomiasis**
Gambian sleeping sickness
Infection by Trypanosoma gambiense

086.4 **Rhodesian trypanosomiasis**
Infection by Trypanosoma rhodesiense
Rhodesian sleeping sickness

086.5 **African trypanosomiasis, unspecified**
Sleeping sickness NOS

086.9 **Trypanosomiasis, unspecified**

✓4ᵗʰ 087 Relapsing fever
INCLUDES recurrent fever

DEF: Infection of *Borrelia*; symptoms are episodic and include fever and arthralgia.

087.0 Louse-borne
087.1 Tick-borne
087.9 Relapsing fever, unspecified

✓4ᵗʰ 088 Other arthropod-borne diseases

088.0 **Bartonellosis**
Carrión's disease   Verruga peruana
Oroya fever

✓5ᵗʰ 088.8 Other specified arthropod-borne diseases

088.81 Lyme disease
Erythema chronicum migrans
AHA: 4Q, '91, 15; 3Q, '90, 14; 2Q, '89, 10

DEF: A recurrent multisystem disorder caused by the spirochete *Borrelia burgdorferi* with the carrier being the tick *Ixodes dammini*; the disease begins with lesions of erythema chronicum migrans; it is followed by arthritis of the large joints, myalgia, malaise, and neurological and cardiac manifestations.

088.82 Babesiosis
Babesiasis
AHA: 4Q, '93, 23

DEF: A tick-borne disease caused by infection of *Babesia*, characterized by fever, malaise, listlessness, severe anemia and hemoglobinuria.

088.89 Other
088.9 Arthropod-borne disease, unspecified

SYPHILIS AND OTHER VENEREAL DISEASES (090-099)

EXCLUDES nonvenereal endemic syphilis (104.0)
    urogenital trichomoniasis (131.0)

✓4ᵗʰ 090 Congenital syphilis

DEF: Infection by spirochete *Treponema pallidum* acquired in utero from the infected mother.

090.0 **Early congenital syphilis, symptomatic**
Congenital syphilitic: Congenital syphilitic:
  choroiditis   splenomegaly
  coryza (chronic) Syphilitic (congenital):
  hepatomegaly   epiphysitis
  mucous patches   osteochondritis
  periostitis   pemphigus
Any congenital syphilitic condition specified as early or manifest less than two years after birth

090.1 **Early congenital syphilis, latent**
Congenital syphilis without clinical manifestations, with positive serological reaction and negative spinal fluid test, less than two years after birth

090.2 **Early congenital syphilis, unspecified**
Congenital syphilis NOS, less than two years after birth

090.3 **Syphilitic interstitial keratitis**
Syphilitic keratitis: Syphilitic keratitis:
  parenchymatous   punctata profunda
EXCLUDES interstitial keratitis NOS (370.50)

✓5ᵗʰ 090.4 Juvenile neurosyphilis
Use additional code to identify any associated mental disorder

DEF: *Treponema pallidum* infection involving the nervous system.

090.40 Juvenile neurosyphilis, unspecified CC
Congenital neurosyphilis
Dementia paralytica juvenilis
Juvenile:
  general paresis
  tabes
  taboparesis
CC Excl: 090.0-090.9, 091.0-091.9, 092.0, 092.9, 093.0-093.9, 094.0-094.9, 095.0-095.9, 096, 097.0-097.9, 099.40-099.59, 099.8, 099.9, 139.8

090.41 Congenital syphilitic encephalitis CC
CC Excl: See code 090.40

DEF: Congenital *Treponema pallidum* infection involving the brain.

090.42 Congenital syphilitic meningitis CC
CC Excl: 003.21, 013.00-013.16, 036.0, 047.0-047.9, 049.0-049.1, 053.0, 054.72, 072.1, 090.0-090.9, 091.0-091.9, 092.0, 092.9, 093.0-093.9, 094.0-094.9, 095.0-095.9, 096, 097.0-097.9, 098.89, 099.40-099.59, 099.8, 099.9, 100.81, 112.83, 114.2, 115.01, 115.11, 115.91, 130.0, 139.8, 320.0-320.9, 321.0-321.8, 322.0-322.9, 349.89, 349.9, 357.0

DEF: Congenital *Treponema pallidum* infection involving the lining of the brain and/or spinal cord.

090.49 Other CC
CC Excl: See code 090.40

090.5 **Other late congenital syphilis, symptomatic**
Gumma due to congenital syphilis
Hutchinson's teeth
Syphilitic saddle nose
Any congenital syphilitic condition specified as late or manifest two years or more after birth

090.6 **Late congenital syphilis, latent**
Congenital syphilis without clinical manifestations, with positive serological reaction and negative spinal fluid test, two years or more after birth

090.7 **Late congenital syphilis, unspecified**
Congenital syphilis NOS, two years or more after birth

090.9 **Congenital syphilis, unspecified**

✓4ᵗʰ 091 Early syphilis, symptomatic
EXCLUDES early cardiovascular syphilis (093.0-093.9)
    early neurosyphilis (094.0-094.9)

091.0 **Genital syphilis (primary)**
Genital chancre

DEF: Genital lesion at the site of initial infection by *Treponema pallidum*.

091.1 **Primary anal syphilis**

DEF: Anal lesion at the site of initial infection by *Treponema pallidum*.

091.2 **Other primary syphilis**
Primary syphilis of: Primary syphilis of:
  breast   lip
  fingers   tonsils

DEF: Lesion at the site of initial infection by *Treponema pallidum*.

INFECTIOUS AND PARASITIC DISEASES

091.3 **Secondary syphilis of skin or mucous membranes**
Condyloma latum
Secondary syphilis of:
  anus
  mouth
  pharynx
Secondary syphilis of:
  skin
  tonsils
  vulva

DEF: Transitory or chronic lesions following initial syphillis infection.

091.4 **Adenopathy due to secondary syphilis**
Syphilitic adenopathy (secondary)
Syphilitic lymphadenitis (secondary)

√5ᵗʰ **091.5** **Uveitis due to secondary syphilis**
  091.50 Syphilitic uveitis, unspecified
  091.51 Syphilitic chorioretinitis (secondary)
    DEF: Inflammation of choroid and retina as a secondary infection.
  091.52 Syphilitic iridocyclitis (secondary)
    DEF: Inflammation of iris and ciliary body as a secondary infection.

√5ᵗʰ **091.6** **Secondary syphilis of viscera and bone**
  091.61 Secondary syphilitic periostitis
    DEF: Inflammation of outer layers of bone as a secondary infection.
  091.62 Secondary syphilitic hepatitis
    Secondary syphilis of liver
  091.69 Other viscera

091.7 **Secondary syphilis, relapse**
Secondary syphilis, relapse (treated) (untreated)
DEF: Return of symptoms of syphillis following asymptomatic period.

√5ᵗʰ **091.8** **Other forms of secondary syphilis**
  091.81 Acute syphilitic meningitis (secondary)
    DEF: Sudden, severe inflammation of the lining of the brain and/or spinal cord as a secondary infection.
  091.82 Syphilitic alopecia
    DEF: Hair loss following initial syphillis infection.
  091.89 Other

091.9 **Unspecified secondary syphilis**

√4ᵗʰ **092** **Early syphilis, latent**
INCLUDES syphilis (acquired) without clinical manifestations, with positive serological reaction and negative spinal fluid test, less than two years after infection

  092.0 Early syphilis, latent, serological relapse after treatment
  092.9 Early syphilis, latent, unspecified

√4ᵗʰ **093** **Cardiovascular syphilis**
  093.0 Aneurysm of aorta, specified as syphilitic CC
    Dilatation of aorta, specified as syphilitic
    CC Excl: See code 090.40

  093.1 Syphilitic aortitis CC
    CC Excl: See code 090.40
    DEF: Inflammation of the aorta – the main artery leading from the heart.

√5ᵗʰ **093.2** Syphilitic endocarditis
    DEF: Inflammation of the tissues lining the cavities of the heart.
  093.20 Valve, unspecified CC
    Syphilitic ostial coronary disease
    CC Excl: See code 090.40
  093.21 Mitral valve CC
    CC Excl: See code 090.40
  093.22 Aortic valve CC
    Syphilitic aortic incompetence or stenosis
    CC Excl: See code 090.40
  093.23 Tricuspid valve CC
    CC Excl: See code 090.40
  093.24 Pulmonary valve CC
    CC Excl: See code 090.40

√5ᵗʰ **093.8** **Other specified cardiovascular syphilis**
  093.81 Syphilitic pericarditis CC
    CC Excl: See code 090.40
    DEF: Inflammation of the outer lining of the heart.
  093.82 Syphilitic myocarditis CC
    CC Excl: See code 090.40
    DEF: Inflammation of the muscle of the heart.
  093.89 Other CC
    CC Excl: See code 090.40

093.9 **Cardiovascular syphilis, unspecified** CC
  CC Excl: See code 090.40

√4ᵗʰ **094** **Neurosyphilis**
Use additional code to identify any associated mental disorder

  094.0 Tabes dorsalis CC
    Locomotor ataxia (progressive)
    Posterior spinal sclerosis (syphilitic)
    Tabetic neurosyphilis
    Use additional code to identify manifestation, as: neurogenic arthropathy [Charcot's joint disease] (713.5)
    CC Excl: See code 090.40
    DEF: Progressive degeneration of nerves associated with long-term syphillis; causing pain, wasting away, incontinence, and ataxia.

  094.1 General paresis CC
    Dementia paralytica
    General paralysis (of the insane) (progressive)
    Paretic neurosyphilis
    Taboparesis
    CC Excl: See code 090.40
    DEF: Degeneration of brain associated with long-term syphillis, causing loss of brain function, progressive dementia, and paralysis.

  094.2 Syphilitic meningitis CC
    Meningovascular syphilis
    EXCLUDES acute syphilitic meningitis (secondary) (091.81)
    CC Excl: 003.21, 013.00-013.16, 036.0, 047.0-047.9, 049.0-049.1, 053.0, 054.72, 072.1, 090.0-090.9, 091.0-091.9, 092.0, 092.9, 093.0-093.9, 094.0-094.9, 095.0-095.9, 096, 097.0-097.9, 098.89, 099.40-099.59, 099.8, 099.9, 100.81, 112.83, 114.2, 115.01, 115.11, 115.91, 130.0, 139.8, 320.0-320.9, 321.0-321.8, 322.0-322.9, 349.89, 349.9, 357.0
    DEF: Inflammation of the lining of the brain and/or spinal cord.

  094.3 Asymptomatic neurosyphilis CC
    CC Excl: See code 090.40

√5ᵗʰ **094.8** **Other specified neurosyphilis**
  094.81 Syphilitic encephalitis CC
    CC Excl: See code 090.40
  094.82 Syphilitic Parkinsonism
    DEF: Decreased motor function, tremors, and muscular rigidity.
  094.83 Syphilitic disseminated retinochoroiditis
    DEF: Inflammation of retina and choroid due to neurosyphillis.
  094.84 Syphilitic optic atrophy
    DEF: Degeneration of the eye and its nerves due to neurosyphillis.

INFECTIOUS AND PARASITIC DISEASES

094.85 Syphilitic retrobulbar neuritis
DEF: Inflammation of the posterior optic nerve to neurosyphillis.

094.86 Syphilitic acoustic neuritis
DEF: Inflammation of acoustic nerve due to neurosyphillis.

094.87 Syphilitic ruptured cerebral aneurysm CC
CC Excl: See code 090.40

094.89 Other CC
CC Excl: See code 090.40

094.9 Neurosyphilis, unspecified CC
Gumma (syphilitic)
Syphilis (early) (late) } of central nervous system NOS
Syphiloma

CC Excl: See code 090.40

√4th **095 Other forms of late syphilis, with symptoms**
INCLUDES: gumma (syphilitic)
syphilis, late, tertiary, or unspecified stage

095.0 Syphilitic episcleritis
095.1 Syphilis of lung
095.2 Syphilitic peritonitis
095.3 Syphilis of liver
095.4 Syphilis of kidney
095.5 Syphilis of bone
095.6 Syphilis of muscle
Syphilitic myositis
095.7 Syphilis of synovium, tendon, and bursa
Syphilitic: Syphilitic:
  bursitis   synovitis
095.8 Other specified forms of late symptomatic syphilis
EXCLUDES: cardiovascular syphilis (093.0-093.9)
neurosyphilis (094.0-094.9)
095.9 Late symptomatic syphilis, unspecified

096 Late syphilis, latent
Syphilis (acquired) without clinical manifestations, with positive serological reaction and negative spinal fluid test, two years or more after infection

√4th **097 Other and unspecified syphilis**
097.0 Late syphilis, unspecified
097.1 Latent syphilis, unspecified
Positive serological reaction for syphilis
097.9 Syphilis, unspecified
Syphilis (acquired) NOS
EXCLUDES: syphilis NOS causing death under two years of age (090.9)

√4th **098 Gonococcal infections**
DEF: *Neisseria gonorrhoeae* infection generally acquired in utero or in sexual congress.

098.0 Acute, of lower genitourinary tract CC
Gonococcal: Gonorrhea (acute):
  Bartholinitis (acute)   NOS
  urethritis (acute)   genitourinary (tract) NOS
  vulvovaginitis (acute)

CC Excl: 098.0-098.39, 098.89, 099.40-099.59, 099.8, 099.9, 139.8

√5th **098.1 Acute, of upper genitourinary tract**
098.10 Gonococcal infection (acute) of upper genitourinary tract, site unspecified CC
CC Excl: See code 098.0

098.11 Gonococcal cystitis (acute) CC
Gonorrhea (acute) of bladder
CC Excl: See code 098.0

098.12 Gonococcal prostatitis (acute) CC ♂
CC Excl: See code 098.0

098.13 Gonococcal epididymo-orchitis (acute) CC ♂
Gonococcal orchitis (acute)
CC Excl: See code 098.0
DEF: Acute inflammation of the testes.

098.14 Gonococcal seminal vesiculitis (acute) CC ♂
Gonorrhea (acute) of seminal vesicle
CC Excl: See code 098.0

098.15 Gonococcal cervicitis (acute) CC ♀
Gonorrhea (acute) of cervix
CC Excl: See code 098.0

098.16 Gonococcal endometritis (acute) CC ♀
Gonorrhea (acute) of uterus
CC Excl: See code 098.0

098.17 Gonococcal salpingitis, specified as acute CC ♀
CC Excl: See code 098.0
DEF: Acute inflammation of the fallopian tubes.

098.19 Other CC
CC Excl: See code 098.0

098.2 Chronic, of lower genitourinary tract
Gonococcal:
  Bartholinitis
  urethritis   } specified as chronic
  vulvovaginitis   or with duration of
Gonorrhea: two months
  NOS   or more
  genitourinary (tract)

Any condition classifiable to 098.0 specified as chronic or with duration of two months or more

√5th **098.3 Chronic, of upper genitourinary tract**
INCLUDES: any condition classifiable to 098.1 stated as chronic or with a duration of two months or more

098.30 Chronic gonococcal infection of upper genitourinary tract, site unspecified

098.31 Gonococcal cystitis, chronic
Any condition classifiable to 098.11, specified as chronic
Gonorrhea of bladder, chronic

098.32 Gonococcal prostatitis, chronic ♂
Any condition classifiable to 098.12, specified as chronic

098.33 Gonococcal epididymo-orchitis, chronic ♂
Any condition classifiable to 098.13, specified as chronic
Chronic gonococcal orchitis
DEF: Chronic inflammation of the testes.

098.34 Gonococcal seminal vesiculitis, chronic ♂
Any condition classifiable to 098.14, specified as chronic
Gonorrhea of seminal vesicle, chronic

098.35 Gonococcal cervicitis, chronic ♀
Any condition classifiable to 098.15, specified as chronic
Gonorrhea of cervix, chronic

098.36 Gonococcal endometritis, chronic ♀
Any condition classifiable to 098.16, specified as chronic
DEF: Chronic inflammation of the uterus.

098.37 Gonococcal salpingitis (chronic) ♀
DEF: Chronic inflammation of the fallopian tubes.

098.39 Other

INFECTIOUS AND PARASITIC DISEASES

098.4 Gonococcal infection of eye
- **098.40** Gonococcal conjunctivitis (neonatorum)
  Gonococcal ophthalmia (neonatorum)
  DEF: Infection of conjunctiva present at birth.
- **098.41** Gonococcal iridocyclitis
  DEF: Inflammation and infection of iris and ciliary body.
- **098.42** Gonococcal endophthalmia
  DEF: Inflammation and infection of contents of eyeball.
- **098.43** Gonococcal keratitis
  DEF: Inflammation and infection of the cornea.
- **098.49** Other

098.5 Gonococcal infection of joint
- **098.50** Gonococcal arthritis
  Gonococcal infection of joint NOS
- **098.51** Gonococcal synovitis and tenosynovitis
- **098.52** Gonococcal bursitis
  DEF: Inflammation of the sac-like cavities in a joint.
- **098.53** Gonococcal spondylitis
- **098.59** Other
  Gonococcal rheumatism

098.6 Gonococcal infection of pharynx

098.7 Gonococcal infection of anus and rectum
  Gonococcal proctitis

098.8 Gonococcal infection of other specified sites
- **098.81** Gonococcal keratosis (blennorrhagica)
  DEF: Pustular skin lesions caused by *Neisseria gonorrhoeae*.
- **098.82** Gonococcal meningitis
  DEF: Inflammation of lining of brain and/or spinal cord.
- **098.83** Gonococcal pericarditis
  DEF: Inflammation of the outer lining of the heart.
- **098.84** Gonococcal endocarditis
  DEF: Inflammation of tissues lining the cavities of heart.
- **098.85** Other gonococcal heart disease
- **098.86** Gonococcal peritonitis
  DEF: Inflammation of the membrane lining the abdomen.
- **098.89** Other
  Gonococcemia

099 Other venereal diseases
- **099.0** Chancroid
  Bubo (inguinal):
    chancroidal
    due to Hemophilus
    ducreyi
  Chancre:
    Ducrey's
    simple
    soft
  Ulcus molle (cutis) (skin)
  DEF: A sexually transmitted disease caused by *Haemophilus ducreyi*; it is identified by a painful primary ulcer at the site of inoculation (usually external genitalia) with related lymphadenitis.

- **099.1** Lymphogranuloma venereum
  Climatic or tropical bubo
  (Durand-) Nicolas-Favre disease
  Esthiomene
  Lymphogranuloma inguinale
  DEF: Sexually transmitted infection of *Chlamydia trachomatis* causing skin lesions.

- **099.2** Granuloma inguinale
  Donovanosis
  Granuloma pudendi (ulcerating)
  Granuloma venereum
  Pudendal ulcer
  DEF: Chronic, sexually transmitted infection of *Calymmatobacterium granulomatis* causing progressive, anogenital skin ulcers.

- **099.3** Reiter's disease
  Reiter's syndrome
  Use additional code for associated:
    arthropathy (711.1)
    conjunctivitis (372.33)
  DEF: A symptom complex of unknown etiology consisting of urethritis, conjunctivitis, arthritis and myocutaneous lesions. It occurs most commonly in young men and patients with HIV and may precede or follow AIDS. Also a form of reactive arthritis.

- **099.4** Other nongonococcal urethritis [NGU]
  - **099.40** Unspecified
    Nonspecific urethritis
  - **099.41** Chlamydia trachomatis
  - **099.49** Other specified organism

- **099.5** Other venereal diseases due to Chlamydia trachomatis
  EXCLUDES *Chlamydia trachomatis* infection of conjunctiva (076.0-076.9, 077.0, 077.9)
    Lymphogranuloma venereum (099.1)
  DEF: Venereal diseases caused by *Chlamydia trachomatis* at other sites besides the urethra (e.g., pharynx, anus and rectum, conjunctiva and peritoneum).
  - **099.50** Unspecified site
  - **099.51** Pharynx
  - **099.52** Anus and rectum
  - **099.53** Lower genitourinary sites
    EXCLUDES urethra (099.41)
    Use additional code to specify site of infection, such as:
      bladder (595.4)
      cervix (616.0)
      vagina and vulva (616.11)
  - **099.54** Other genitourinary sites
    Use additional code to specify site of infection, such as:
      pelvic inflammatory disease NOS (614.9)
      testis and epididymis (604.91)
  - **099.55** Unspecified genitourinary site
  - **099.56** Peritoneum
    Perihepatitis
  - **099.59** Other specified site

- **099.8** Other specified venereal diseases
- **099.9** Venereal disease, unspecified

OTHER SPIROCHETAL DISEASES (100-104)

100 Leptospirosis
DEF: An infection of any spirochete of the genus Leptospire in blood. This zoonosis is transmitted to humans most often by exposure with contaminated animal tissues or water and less often by contact with urine. Patients present with flulike symptoms, the most common being muscle aches involving the thighs and low back. Treatment is with hydration and antibiotics.

- **100.0** Leptospirosis icterohemorrhagica
  Leptospiral or spirochetal jaundice (hemorrhagic)
  Weil's disease

- **100.8** Other specified leptospiral infections
  - **100.81** Leptospiral meningitis (aseptic)
  - **100.89** Other
    Fever:
      Fort Bragg
      pretibial
      swamp
    Infection by Leptospira:
      australis
      bataviae
      pyrogenes

- **100.9** Leptospirosis, unspecified

INFECTIOUS AND PARASITIC DISEASES

101 Vincent's angina
Acute necrotizing ulcerative: Trench mouth
  gingivitis   Vincent's:
  stomatitis   gingivitis
Fusospirochetal pharyngitis   infection [any site]
Spirochetal stomatitis

DEF: Painful ulceration with edema and hypermic patches of the oropharyngeal and throat membranes; it is caused by spreading of acute ulcerative gingivitis.

✓4th 102 Yaws
INCLUDES   frambesia
           pian

DEF: An infectious, endemic, tropical disease caused by *Treponema pertenue*; it usually affects persons 15 years old or younger; a primary cutaneous lesion develops, then a granulomatous skin eruption, and occasionally lesions that destroy skin and bone.

102.0 Initial lesions
Chancre of yaws
Frambesia, initial or primary
Initial frambesial ulcer
Mother yaw

102.1 Multiple papillomata and wet crab yaws
Butter yaws   Plantar or palmar
Frambesioma   papilloma of yaws
Pianoma

102.2 Other early skin lesions
Cutaneous yaws, less than five years after infection
Early yaws (cutaneous) (macular) (papular)
  (maculopapular) (micropapular)
Frambeside of early yaws

102.3 Hyperkeratosis
Ghoul hand
Hyperkeratosis, palmar or plantar (early) (late) due
  to yaws
Worm-eaten soles

DEF: Overgrowth of skin of palm of bottoms of feet, due to yaws.

102.4 Gummata and ulcers
Gummatous frambeside
Nodular late yaws (ulcerated)

DEF: Rubbery lesions and areas of dead skin caused by yaws.

102.5 Gangosa
Rhinopharyngitis mutilans

DEF: Massive, mutilating lesions of the nose and oral cavity caused by yaws.

102.6 Bone and joint lesions
Goundou
Gumma, bone
Gummatous osteitis or   } of yaws (late)
  periostitis

Hydrarthrosis
Osteitis   } of yaws (early) (late)
Periostitis (hypertrophic)

102.7 Other manifestations
Juxta-articular nodules of yaws
Mucosal yaws

102.8 Latent yaws
Yaws without clinical manifestations, with positive serology

102.9 Yaws, unspecified

✓4th 103 Pinta
DEF: A chronic form of treponema-tosis, endemic in areas of tropical America; it is identified by the presence of red, violet, blue, coffee-colored or white spots on the skin.

103.0 Primary lesions
Chancre (primary)
Papule (primary)   } of pinta [carate]
Pintid

103.1 Intermediate lesions
Erythematous plaques
Hyperchromic lesions   } of pinta [carate]
Hyperkeratosis

103.2 Late lesions
Cardiovascular lesions
Skin lesions:
  achromic
  cicatricial   } of pinta [carate]
  dyschromic
Vitiligo

103.3 Mixed lesions
Achromic and hyperchromic skin lesions of pinta [carate]

103.9 Pinta, unspecified

✓4th 104 Other spirochetal infection
104.0 Nonvenereal endemic syphilis
Bejel   Njovera

DEF: *Treponema pallidum*, *T. pertenue*, or *T. caroteum* infection transmitted non-sexually, causing lesions on mucosa and skin.

104.8 Other specified spirochetal infections
EXCLUDES relapsing fever (087.0-087.9)
          syphilis (090.0-097.9)

104.9 Spirochetal infection, unspecified

MYCOSES (110-118)
Use additional code to identify manifestation as:
  arthropathy (711.6)
  meningitis (321.0-321.1)
  otitis externa (380.15)

EXCLUDES infection by Actinomycetales, such as species of Actinomyces, Actinomadura, Nocardia, Streptomyces (039.0-039.9)

✓4th 110 Dermatophytosis
INCLUDES infection by species of Epidermophyton, Microsporum, and Trichophyton
          tinea, any type except those in 111

DEF: Superficial infection of the skin caused by a parasitic fungus.

110.0 Of scalp and beard
Kerion   Trichophytic tinea
Sycosis, mycotic   [black dot tinea], scalp

110.1 Of nail
Dermatophytic onychia   Tinea unguium
Onychomycosis

110.2 Of hand
Tinea manuum

110.3 Of groin and perianal area
Dhobie itch   Tinea cruris
Eczema marginatum

110.4 Of foot
Athlete's foot   Tinea pedis

110.5 Of the body
Herpes circinatus   Tinea imbricata [Tokelau]

110.6 Deep seated dermatophytosis
Granuloma trichophyticum
Majocchi's granuloma

110.8 Of other specified sites

110.9 Of unspecified site
Favus NOS   Ringworm NOS
Microsporic tinea NOS

✓4th 111 Dermatomycosis, other and unspecified
111.0 Pityriasis versicolor
Infection by Malassezia [Pityrosporum] furfur
Tinea flava
Tinea versicolor

INFECTIOUS AND PARASITIC DISEASES

111.1 Tinea nigra
   Infection by Cladosporium species
   Keratomycosis nigricans
   Microsporosis nigra
   Pityriasis nigra
   Tinea palmaris nigra

111.2 Tinea blanca
   Infection by Trichosporon (beigelii) cutaneum
   White piedra

111.3 Black piedra
   Infection by Piedraia hortai

111.8 Other specified dermatomycoses

111.9 Dermatomycosis, unspecified

✓4th 112 Candidiasis
   INCLUDES: infection by Candida species
   moniliasis
   EXCLUDES: neonatal monilial infection (771.7)

   DEF: Fungal infection caused by Candida; usually seen in mucous membranes or skin.

112.0 Of mouth [CC] [HIV]
   Thrush (oral)
   CC Excl: 112.0-112.9, 117.9, 139.8

112.1 Of vulva and vagina ♀
   Candidal vulvovaginitis   Monilial vulvovaginitis

112.2 Of other urogenital sites
   Candidal balanitis
   AHA: 4Q, '96, 33

112.3 Of skin and nails [HIV]
   Candidal intertrigo
   Candidal onychia
   Candidal perionyxis [paronychia]

112.4 Of lung [CC] [HIV]
   Candidal pneumonia
   CC Excl: See code 112.0
   AHA: 2Q, '98, 7

112.5 Disseminated [CC] [HIV]
   Systemic candidiasis
   CC Excl: See code 112.0
   AHA: 2Q, '00, 5; 2Q, '89, 10

✓5th 112.8 Of other specified sites

   112.81 Candidal endocarditis [CC] [HIV]
   CC Excl: See code 112.0

   112.82 Candidal otitis externa [CC] [HIV]
   Otomycosis in moniliasis
   CC Excl: See code 112.0

   112.83 Candidal meningitis [CC] [HIV]
   CC Excl: 003.21, 013.00-013.16, 036.0, 047.0-047.9, 049.0-049.1, 053.0, 054.72, 072.1, 090.42, 091.81, 094.2, 098.89, 100.81, 112.0-112.9, 114.2, 115.01, 115.11, 115.91, 117.9, 130.0, 139.8, 320.0-320.9, 321.0-321.8, 322.0-322.9, 349.89, 349.9, 357.0

   112.84 Candidal esophagitis [CC] [HIV]
   CC Excl: See code 112.0
   AHA: 4Q, '92, 19

   112.85 Candidal enteritis [CC] [HIV]
   CC Excl: See code 112.0
   AHA: 4Q, '92, 19

   112.89 Other
   AHA: 1Q, '92, 17; 3Q, '91, 20

112.9 Of unspecified site [HIV]

✓4th 114 Coccidioidomycosis
   INCLUDES: infection by Coccidioides (immitis)
   Posada-Wernicke disease
   AHA: 4Q, '93, 23

   DEF: A fungal disease caused by inhalation of dust particles containing arthrospores of *Coccidioides immitis*; a self-limited respiratory infection; the primary form is known as San Joaquin fever, desert fever or valley fever.

114.0 Primary coccidioidomycosis (pulmonary) [CC] [HIV]
   Acute pulmonary coccidioidomycosis
   Coccidioidomycotic pneumonitis
   Desert rheumatism
   Pulmonary coccidioidomycosis
   San Joaquin Valley fever
   CC Excl: 114.0, 114.3, 114.4-114.5, 114.9, 117.9, 139.8
   DEF: Acute, self-limiting *Coccidioides immitis* infection of the lung.

114.1 Primary extrapulmonary coccidioidomycosis [HIV]
   Chancriform syndrome
   Primary cutaneous coccidioidomycosis
   DEF: Acute, self-limiting *Coccidioides immitis* infection in nonpulmonary site.

114.2 Coccidioidal meningitis [CC] [HIV]
   CC Excl: 003.21, 013.00-013.16, 036.0, 047.0-047.9, 049.0-049.1, 053.0, 054.72, 072.1, 090.42, 091.81, 094.2, 098.89, 100.81, 112.83, 114.2-114.9, 115.01, 115.11, 115.91, 117.9, 130.0, 139.8, 320.0-320.9, 321.0-321.8, 322.0-322.9, 349.89, 349.9, 357.0
   DEF: *Coccidioides immitis* infection of the lining of the brain and/or spinal cord.

114.3 Other forms of progressive coccidioidomycosis [CC] [HIV]
   Coccidioidal granuloma
   Disseminated coccidioidomycosis
   CC Excl: 114.3, 114.9, 117.9, 139.8

114.4 Chronic pulmonary coccidioidomycosis [HIV]

114.5 Pulmonary coccidioidomycosis, unspecified [HIV]

114.9 Coccidioidomycosis, unspecified [CC] [HIV]
   CC Excl: See code 114.3

✓4th 115 Histoplasmosis
   The following fifth-digit subclassification is for use with category 115:
   0 without mention of manifestation
   1 meningitis
   2 retinitis
   3 pericarditis
   4 endocarditis
   5 pneumonia
   9 other

✓5th 115.0 Infection by Histoplasma capsulatum [CC 0-5] [HIV]
   American histoplasmosis
   Darling's disease
   Reticuloendothelial cytomycosis
   Small form histoplasmosis
   CC Excl: For code 115.00: 115.00, 115.09, 115.90, 115.99, 117.9, 139.8; CC Excl: For code 115.01: 003.21, 013.00-013.16, 036.0, 047.0-047.9, 049.0-049.1, 053.0, 054.72, 072.1, 090.42, 091.81, 094.2, 098.89, 100.81, 112.83, 114.2, 115.00-115.01, 115.09, 115.11, 115.90-115.91, 115.99, 117.9, 130.0, 139.8, 320.0-320.9, 321.0-321.8, 322.0-322.9, 349.89, 349.9, 357.0; CC Excl: For code 115.02: 115.00, 115.02, 115.09, 115.90, 115.92, 115.99, 117.9, 139.8; CC Excl: For code 115.03: 115.00, 115.03, 115.09, 115.90, 115.93, 115.99, 117.9, 139.8; CC Excl: For code 115.04: 115.00, 115.04, 115.09, 115.90, 115.94, 115.99, 117.9, 139.8; CC Excl: For code 115.05: 115.00, 115.05, 115.09, 115.90, 115.95, 115.99, 117.9, 139.8, 480.0-480.9, 481, 482.0-482.7, 482.81-482.84, 482.89, 482.9, 483.0, 483.1, 483.8, 484.1-484.8, 485-486, 487.0-487.1, 494.0-494.1, 495.0-495.9, 496, 500-505, 506.0-506.9, 507.0-507.8, 508.0-508.9, 517.1, 518.89

INFECTIOUS AND PARASITIC DISEASES

√5ᵗʰ 115.1 Infection by Histoplasma duboisii [CC] [HIV]
  African histoplasmosis
  Large form histoplasmosis
  CC Excl: For code 115.10: 115.10, 115.19, 115.90, 115.99, 117.9, 139.8;
  CC Excl: For code 115.11: 003.21, 013.00-013.16, 036.0, 047.0-047.9, 049.0-049.1, 053.0, 054.72, 072.1, 090.42, 091.81, 094.2, 098.89, 100.81, 112.83, 114.2, 115.01, 115.10-115.11, 115.19, 115.90-115.91, 115.99, 117.9, 130.0, 139.8, 320.0-320.9, 321.0-321.8, 322.0-322.9, 349.89, 349.9, 357.0; **CC Excl: For code 115.12:** 115.10, 115.12, 115.19, 115.90, 115.92, 115.99, 117.9, 139.8; **CC Excl: For code 115.13:** 115.10, 115.13, 115.19, 115.90, 115.93, 115.99, 117.9, 139.8; **CC Excl: For code 115.14:** 115.10, 115.14, 115.19, 115.90, 115.94, 115.99, 117.9, 139.8; **CC Excl: For code 115.15:** 115.05, 115.10, 115.15, 115.19, 115.90, 115.95, 115.99, 117.9, 139.8, 480.0-480.9, 481, 482.0-482.7, 482.81-482.83, 482.89, 482.9, 483.0, 483.1, 483.8, 484.1-484.8, 485-486, 487.0-487.1, 494.0-494.1, 495.0-495.9, 496, 500-505, 506.0-506.9, 507.0-507.8, 508.0-508.9, 517.1, 518.89;
  CC Excl: For code 115.19: 115.10, 115.19, 115.90, 115.99, 117.9, 139.8

√5ᵗʰ 115.9 Histoplasmosis, unspecified [CC] [HIV]
  Histoplasmosis NOS
  CC Excl: For code 115.90: 115.90, 115.99, 117.9, 139.8; **CC Excl: For code 115.91:** 003.21, 013.00-013.16, 036.0, 047.0-047.9, 049.0-049.1, 053.0, 054.72, 072.1, 090.42, 091.81, 094.2, 098.89, 100.81, 112.83, 114.2, 115.01, 115.11, 115.91, 115.99, 117.9, 130.0, 139.8, 320.0-320.9, 321.0-321.8, 322.0-322.9, 349.89, 349.9, 357.0; **CC Excl: For code 115.92:** 115.92, 115.99, 117.9, 139.8; **CC Excl: For code 115.93:** 115.93, 115.99, 117.9, 139.8; **CC Excl: For code 115.94:** 115.94, 115.99, 117.9, 139.8; **CC Excl: For code 115.95:** 115.05, 115.15, 115.95, 115.99, 117.9, 139.8; **CC Excl: For code 115.99:** 115.99, 117.9, 139.8

√4ᵗʰ 116 Blastomycotic infection

  116.0 Blastomycosis [CC]
    Blastomycotic dermatitis
    Chicago disease
    Cutaneous blastomycosis
    Disseminated blastomycosis
    Gilchrist's disease
    Infection by Blastomyces [Ajellomyces] dermatitidis
    North American blastomycosis
    Primary pulmonary blastomycosis
    CC Excl: 116.0, 117.9, 139.8

  116.1 Paracoccidioidomycosis [CC]
    Brazilian blastomycosis
    Infection by Paracoccidioides [Blastomyces] brasiliensis
    Lutz-Splendore-Almeida disease
    Mucocutaneous-lymphangitic paracoccidioidomycosis
    Pulmonary paracoccidioidomycosis
    South American blastomycosis
    Visceral paracoccidioidomycosis
    CC Excl: 116.1, 117.9, 139.8

  116.2 Lobomycosis
    Infections by Loboa [Blastomyces] loboi
    Keloidal blastomycosis
    Lobo's disease

√4ᵗʰ 117 Other mycoses

  117.0 Rhinosporidiosis
    Infection by Rhinosporidium seeberi

  117.1 Sporotrichosis
    Cutaneous sporotrichosis
    Disseminated sporotrichosis
    Infection by Sporothrix [Sporotrichum] schenckii
    Lymphocutaneous sporotrichosis
    Pulmonary sporotrichosis
    Sporotrichosis of the bones

  117.2 Chromoblastomycosis
    Chromomycosis
    Infection by Cladosporidium carrionii, Fonsecaea compactum, Fonsecaea pedrosoi, Phialophora verrucosa

  117.3 Aspergillosis [CC]
    Infection by Aspergillus species, mainly A. fumigatus, A. flavus group, A. terreus group
    CC Excl: 117.3, 117.9, 139.8
    AHA: 4Q, '97, 40

  117.4 Mycotic mycetomas [CC]
    Infection by various genera and species of Ascomycetes and Deuteromycetes, such as Acremonium [Cephalosporium] falciforme, Neotestudina rosatii, Madurella grisea, Madurella mycetomii, Pyrenochaeta romeroi, Zopfia [Leptosphaeria] senegalensis
    Madura foot, mycotic
    Maduromycosis, mycotic
    EXCLUDES actinomycotic mycetomas (039.0-039.9)
    CC Excl: 117.4, 117.9, 139.8

  117.5 Cryptococcosis [CC] [HIV]
    Busse-Buschke's disease
    European cryptococcosis
    Infection by Cryptococcus neoformans
    Pulmonary cryptococcosis
    Systemic cryptococcosis
    Torula
    CC Excl: 117.5, 117.9, 139.8

  117.6 Allescheriosis [Petriellidosis] [CC]
    Infections by Allescheria [Petriellidium] boydii [Monosporium apiospermum]
    EXCLUDES mycotic mycetoma (117.4)
    CC Excl: 117.6, 117.9, 139.8

  117.7 Zygomycosis [Phycomycosis or Mucormycosis] [CC]
    Infection by species of Absidia, Basidiobolus, Conidiobolus, Cunninghamella, Entomophthora, Mucor, Rhizopus, Saksenaea
    CC Excl: 117.7, 117.9, 139.8

  117.8 Infection by dematiacious fungi, [Phaehyphomycosis]
    Infection by dematiacious fungi, such as Cladosporium trichoides [bantianum], Dreschlera hawaiiensis, Phialophora gougerotii, Phialophora jeanselmi

  117.9 Other and unspecified mycoses

118 Opportunistic mycoses [CC] [HIV]
  Infection of skin, subcutaneous tissues, and/or organs by a wide variety of fungi generally considered to be pathogenic to compromised hosts only (e.g., infection by species of Alternaria, Dreschlera, Fusarium)
  CC Excl: 117.9, 118, 139.8

HELMINTHIASES (120-129)

√4ᵗʰ 120 Schistosomiasis [bilharziasis]
  DEF: Infection caused by *Schistosoma*, a genus of flukes or trematode parasites.

  120.0 Schistosoma haematobium
    Vesical schistosomiasis NOS

  120.1 Schistosoma mansoni
    Intestinal schistosomiasis NOS

  120.2 Schistosoma japonicum
    Asiatic schistosomiasis NOS
    Katayama disease or fever

  120.3 Cutaneous
    Cercarial dermatitis
    Infection by cercariae of Schistosoma
    Schistosome dermatitis
    Swimmers' itch

INFECTIOUS AND PARASITIC DISEASES

120.8 **Other specified schistosomiasis**
　　Infection by Schistosoma:
　　　bovis
　　　intercalatum
　　　mattheii
　　　spindale
　　Schistosomiasis chestermani

120.9 **Schistosomiasis, unspecified**
　　Blood flukes NOS
　　Hemic distomiasis

√4ᵗʰ 121 Other trematode infections

121.0 **Opisthorchiasis**
　　Infection by:
　　　cat liver fluke
　　　Opisthorchis (felineus) (tenuicollis) (viverrini)

121.1 **Clonorchiasis**
　　Biliary cirrhosis due to clonorchiasis
　　Chinese liver fluke disease
　　Hepatic distomiasis due to Clonorchis sinensis
　　Oriental liver fluke disease

121.2 **Paragonimiasis**
　　Infection by Paragonimus
　　Lung fluke disease (oriental)
　　Pulmonary distomiasis

121.3 **Fascioliasis**
　　Infection by Fasciola:
　　　gigantica
　　　hepatica
　　Liver flukes NOS
　　Sheep liver fluke infection

121.4 **Fasciolopsiasis**
　　Infection by Fasciolopsis (buski)
　　Intestinal distomiasis

121.5 **Metagonimiasis**
　　Infection by Metagonimus yokogawai

121.6 **Heterophyiasis**
　　Infection by:
　　　Heterophyes heterophyes
　　　Stellantchasmus falcatus

121.8 **Other specified trematode infections**
　　Infection by:
　　　Dicrocoelium dendriticum
　　　Echinostoma ilocanum
　　　Gastrodiscoides hominis

121.9 **Trematode infection, unspecified**
　　Distomiasis NOS
　　Fluke disease NOS

√4ᵗʰ 122 Echinococcosis
　　INCLUDES　echinococciasis
　　　　　　　　hydatid disease
　　　　　　　　hydatidosis
　　DEF: Infection caused by larval forms of tapeworms of the genus *Echinococcus*.

122.0 **Echinococcus granulosus infection of liver**
122.1 **Echinococcus granulosus infection of lung**
122.2 **Echinococcus granulosus infection of thyroid**
122.3 **Echinococcus granulosus infection, other**
122.4 **Echinococcus granulosus infection, unspecified**
122.5 **Echinococcus multilocularis infection of liver**
122.6 **Echinococcus multilocularis infection, other**
122.7 **Echinococcus multilocularis infection, unspecified**
122.8 **Echinococcosis, unspecified, of liver**
122.9 **Echinococcosis, other and unspecified**

√4ᵗʰ 123 Other cestode infection

123.0 **Taenia solium infection, intestinal form**
　　Pork tapeworm (adult) (infection)

123.1 **Cysticercosis**
　　Cysticerciasis
　　Infection by Cysticercus cellulosae [larval form of Taenia solium]
　　A: 2Q, '97, 8

123.2 **Taenia saginata infection**
　　Beef tapeworm (infection)
　　Infection by Taeniarhynchus saginatus

123.3 **Taeniasis, unspecified**

123.4 **Diphyllobothriasis, intestinal**
　　Diphyllobothrium (adult) (latum) (pacificum) infection
　　Fish tapeworm (infection)

123.5 **Sparganosis [larval diphyllobothriasis]**
　　Infection by:
　　　Diphyllobothrium larvae
　　　Sparganum (mansoni) (proliferum)
　　　Spirometra larvae

123.6 **Hymenolepiasis**
　　Dwarf tapeworm (infection)
　　Hymenolepis (diminuta) (nana) infection
　　Rat tapeworm (infection)

123.8 **Other specified cestode infection**
　　Diplogonoporus (grandis) } infection
　　Dipylidium (caninum)
　　Dog tapeworm (infection)

123.9 **Cestode infection, unspecified**
　　Tapeworm (infection) NOS

124 Trichinosis
　　Trichinella spiralis infection　　Trichiniasis
　　Trichinellosis
　　DEF: Infection by *Trichinella spiralis*, the smallest of the parasitic nematodes.

√4ᵗʰ 125 Filarial infection and dracontiasis

125.0 **Bancroftian filariasis**
　　Chyluria
　　Elephantiasis
　　Infection　　　　　} due to Wuchereria bancrofti
　　Lymphadenitis
　　Lymphangitis
　　Wuchereriasis

125.1 **Malayan filariasis**
　　Brugia filariasis
　　Chyluria
　　Elephantiasis　　} due to Brugia
　　Infection　　　　[Wuchereria]
　　Lymphadenitis　　malayi
　　Lymphangitis

125.2 **Loiasis**
　　Eyeworm disease of Africa　　Loa loa infection

125.3 **Onchocerciasis**
　　Onchocerca volvulus infection
　　Onchocercosis

125.4 **Dipetalonemiasis**
　　Infection by:
　　　Acanthocheilonema perstans
　　　Dipetalonema perstans

125.5 **Mansonella ozzardi infection**
　　Filariasis ozzardi

125.6 **Other specified filariasis**
　　Dirofilaria infection
　　Infection by:
　　　Acanthocheilonema streptocerca
　　　Dipetalonema streptocerca

125.7 **Dracontiasis**
　　Guinea-worm infection
　　Infection by Dracunculus medinensis

125.9 **Unspecified filariasis**

√4ᵗʰ 126 Ancylostomiasis and necatoriasis
　　INCLUDES　cutaneous larva migrans due to Ancylostoma
　　　　　　　　hookworm (disease) (infection)
　　　　　　　　uncinariasis

126.0 **Ancylostoma duodenale**
126.1 **Necator americanus**
126.2 **Ancylostoma braziliense**
126.3 **Ancylostoma ceylanicum**

 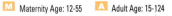

INFECTIOUS AND PARASITIC DISEASES

- **126.8** Other specified Ancylostoma
- **126.9** Ancylostomiasis and necatoriasis, unspecified
  - Creeping eruption NOS
  - Cutaneous larva migrans NOS

√4ᵗʰ **127 Other intestinal helminthiases**
- **127.0** Ascariasis
  - Ascaridiasis
  - Infection by Ascaris lumbricoides
  - Roundworm infection
- **127.1** Anisakiasis
  - Infection by Anisakis larva
- **127.2** Strongyloidiasis [HIV]
  - Infection by Strongyloides stercoralis
  - EXCLUDES trichostrongyliasis (127.6)
- **127.3** Trichuriasis
  - Infection by Trichuris trichiura
  - Trichocephaliasis
  - Whipworm (disease) (infection)
- **127.4** Enterobiasis
  - Infection by Enterobius vermicularis
  - Oxyuriasis
  - Oxyuris vermicularis infection
  - Pinworm (disease) (infection)
  - Threadworm infection
- **127.5** Capillariasis
  - Infection by Capillaria philippinensis
  - EXCLUDES infection by Capillaria hepatica (128.8)
- **127.6** Trichostrongyliasis
  - Infection by Trichostrongylus species
- **127.7** Other specified intestinal helminthiasis
  - Infection by:
    - Oesophagostomum apiostomum and related species
    - Ternidens diminutus
    - other specified intestinal helminth
  - Physalopteriasis
- **127.8** Mixed intestinal helminthiasis
  - Infection by intestinal helminths classified to more than one of the categories 120.0-127.7
  - Mixed helminthiasis NOS
- **127.9** Intestinal helminthiasis, unspecified

√4ᵗʰ **128 Other and unspecified helminthiases**
- **128.0** Toxocariasis
  - Larva migrans visceralis
  - Toxocara (canis) (cati) infection
  - Visceral larva migrans syndrome
- **128.1** Gnathostomiasis
  - Infection by Gnathostoma spinigerum and related species
- **128.8** Other specified helminthiasis
  - Infection by:
    - Angiostrongylus cantonensis
    - Capillaria hepatica
    - other specified helminth
- **128.9** Helminth infection, unspecified
  - Helminthiasis NOS   Worms NOS

129 Intestinal parasitism, unspecified

OTHER INFECTIOUS AND PARASITIC DISEASES (130–136)

√4ᵗʰ **130 Toxoplasmosis**
- INCLUDES infection by toxoplasma gondii
  - toxoplasmosis (acquired)
- EXCLUDES congenital toxoplasmosis (771.2)
- **130.0** Meningoencephalitis due to toxoplasmosis [CC] [HIV]
  - Encephalitis due to acquired toxoplasmosis
  - CC Excl: 130.0, 130.7-130.9, 139.8
- **130.1** Conjunctivitis due to toxoplasmosis [CC] [HIV]
  - CC Excl: 130.1, 130.7-130.9, 139.8
- **130.2** Chorioretinitis due to toxoplasmosis [CC] [HIV]
  - Focal retinochoroiditis due to acquired toxoplasmosis
  - CC Excl: 130.2, 130.7-130.9, 139.8
- **130.3** Myocarditis due to toxoplasmosis [CC] [HIV]
  - CC Excl: 130.3, 130.7-130.9, 139.8
- **130.4** Pneumonitis due to toxoplasmosis [CC] [HIV]
  - CC Excl: 130.4, 130.7-130.9, 139.8, 480.0-480.9, 481, 482.0-482.7, |482.81-482.83, 482.89, 482.9, 483.0, 483.1, 483.8, 484.1-484.8, 485-486, 487.0-487.1, 494.0-494.1, 495.0-495.9, 496, 500-505, 506.0-506.9, 507.0-507.8, 508.0-508.9, 517.1, 518.89
- **130.5** Hepatitis due to toxoplasmosis [CC] [HIV]
  - CC Excl: 130.5-130.9, 139.8
- **130.7** Toxoplasmosis of other specified sites [CC] [HIV]
  - CC Excl: 130.7-130.9, 139.8
- **130.8** Multisystemic disseminated toxoplasmosis [CC] [HIV]
  - Toxoplasmosis of multiple sites
  - CC Excl: See code 130.7
- **130.9** Toxoplasmosis, unspecified [HIV]

√4ᵗʰ **131 Trichomoniasis**
- INCLUDES infection due to Trichomonas (vaginalis)
- √5ᵗʰ **131.0** Urogenital trichomoniasis
  - **131.00** Urogenital trichomoniasis, unspecified
    - Fluor (vaginalis) } trichomonal or due to
    - Leukorrhea } Trichomonas
    - (vaginalis) } (vaginalis)
    - DEF: Trichomonas vaginalis infection of reproductive and urinary organs, transmitted through coitus.
  - **131.01** Trichomonal vulvovaginitis ♀
    - Vaginitis, trichomonal or due to Trichomonas (vaginalis)
    - DEF: Trichomonas vaginalis infection of vulva and vagina; often asymptomatic, transmitted through coitus.
  - **131.02** Trichomonal urethritis
    - DEF: Trichomonas vaginalis infection of the urethra.
  - **131.03** Trichomonal prostatitis ♂
    - DEF: Trichomonas vaginalis infection of the prostate.
  - **131.09** Other
- **131.8** Other specified sites
  - EXCLUDES intestinal (007.3)
- **131.9** Trichomoniasis, unspecified

√4ᵗʰ **132 Pediculosis and phthirus infestation**
- **132.0** Pediculus capitis [head louse]
- **132.1** Pediculus corporis [body louse]
- **132.2** Phthirus pubis [pubic louse]
  - Pediculus pubis
- **132.3** Mixed infestation
  - Infestation classifiable to more than one of the categories 132.0-132.2
- **132.9** Pediculosis, unspecified

√4ᵗʰ **133 Acariasis**
- **133.0** Scabies
  - Infestation by Sarcoptes scabiei   Sarcoptic itch
  - Norwegian scabies
- **133.8** Other acariasis
  - Chiggers   Infestation by:
  - Infestation by: Trombicula
    - Demodex folliculorum
- **133.9** Acariasis, unspecified
  - Infestation by mites NOS

INFECTIOUS AND PARASITIC DISEASES

✓4th 134 Other infestation

134.0 Myiasis
Infestation by:
- Dermatobia (hominis)
- fly larvae
- Gasterophilus (intestinalis)
- maggots
- Oestrus ovis

134.1 Other arthropod infestation
Infestation by:
- chigoe
- sand flea
- Tunga penetrans
- Jigger disease
- Scarabiasis
- Tungiasis

134.2 Hirudiniasis
- Hirudiniasis (external) (internal)
- Leeches (aquatic) (land)

134.8 Other specified infestations

134.9 Infestation, unspecified
- Infestation (skin) NOS
- Skin parasites NOS

135 Sarcoidosis [CC]
- Besnier-Boeck-Schaumann disease
- Lupoid (miliary) of Boeck
- Lupus pernio (Besnier)
- Lymphogranulomatosis, benign (Schaumann's)
- Sarcoid (any site):
  - NOS
  - Boeck
  - Darier-Roussy
- Uveoparotid fever

CC Excl: 135, 139.8

DEF: A chronic, granulomatous reticulosis (abnormal increase in cells), affecting any organ or tissue; acute form has high rate of remission; chronic form is progressive.

✓4th 136 Other and unspecified infectious and parasitic diseases

136.0 Ainhum
Dactylolysis spontanea

DEF: A disease affecting the toes, especially the fifth digit, and sometimes the fingers, especially seen in black adult males; it is characterized by a linear constriction around the affected digit leading to spontaneous amputation of the distal part of the digit.

136.1 Behçet's syndrome

DEF: A chronic inflammatory disorder of unknown etiology involving the small blood vessels; it is characterized by recurrent aphthous ulceration of the oral and pharyngeal mucous membranes and the genitalia, skin lesions, severe uveitis, retinal vascularitis and optic atrophy.

136.2 Specific infections by free-living amebae
Meningoencephalitis due to Naegleria

136.3 Pneumocystosis [CC] [HIV]
Pneumonia due to Pneumocystis carinii

CC Excl: 136.3, 139.8, 480.0-480.9, 481, 482.0-482.7, 482.81-482.83, 482.89, 482.9, 483.0, 483.1, 483.8, 484.1-484.8, 485-486, 487.0-487.1, 494.0-494.1, 495.0-495.9, 496, 500-505, 506.0-506.9, 507.0-507.8, 508.0-508.9, 517.1, 518.89

AHA: N-D, '87, 5, 6

DEF: Pneumocystis carinii fungus causing pneumonia in immunocompromised patients; a leading cause of death among AIDS patients.

136.4 Psorospermiasis

136.5 Sarcosporidiosis
Infection by Sarcocystis lindemanni

DEF: Sarcocystis infection causing muscle cysts of intestinal inflammation.

136.8 Other specified infectious and parasitic diseases [HIV]
Candiru infestation

136.9 Unspecified infectious and parasitic diseases
Infectious disease NOS   Parasitic disease NOS

AHA: 2Q, '91, 8

LATE EFFECTS OF INFECTIOUS AND PARASITIC DISEASES (137-139)

✓4th 137 Late effects of tuberculosis

Note: This category is to be used to indicate conditions classifiable to 010-018 as the cause of late effects, which are themselves classified elsewhere. The "late effects" include those specified as such, as sequelae, or as due to old or inactive tuberculosis, without evidence of active disease.

137.0 Late effects of respiratory or unspecified tuberculosis [CC]

CC Excl: 137.0, 139.8

137.1 Late effects of central nervous system tuberculosis [CC]

CC Excl: 137.1, 139.8

137.2 Late effects of genitourinary tuberculosis [CC]

CC Excl: 137.2, 139.8

137.3 Late effects of tuberculosis of bones and joints

137.4 Late effects of tuberculosis of other specified organs

138 Late effects of acute poliomyelitis [CC]

Note: This category is to be used to indicate conditions classifiable to 045 as the cause of late effects, which are themselves classified elsewhere. The "late effects" include conditions specified as such, or as sequelae, or as due to old or inactive poliomyelitis, without evidence of active disease.

CC Excl: 138, 139.8

✓4th 139 Late effects of other infectious and parasitic diseases

Note: This category is to be used to indicate conditions classifiable to categories 001-009, 020-041, 046-136 as the cause of late effects, which are themselves classified elsewhere. The "late effects" include conditions specified as such; they also include sequela of diseases classifiable to the above categories if there is evidence that the disease itself is no longer present.

139.0 Late effects of viral encephalitis
Late effects of conditions classifiable to 049.8-049.9, 062-064

139.1 Late effects of trachoma
Late effects of conditions classifiable to 076

139.8 Late effects of other and unspecified infectious and parasitic diseases

AHA: 4Q, '91, 15; 3Q, '90, 14; M-A, '87, 8

Tabular List — NEOPLASMS

2. NEOPLASMS (140-239)

Notes:

1. Content

This chapter contains the following broad groups:

140-195 Malignant neoplasms, stated or presumed to be primary, of specified sites, except of lymphatic and hematopoietic tissue

196-198 Malignant neoplasms, stated or presumed to be secondary, of specified sites

199 Malignant neoplasms, without specification of site

200-208 Malignant neoplasms, stated or presumed to be primary, of lymphatic and hematopoietic tissue

210-229 Benign neoplasms

230-234 Carcinoma in situ

235-238 Neoplasms of uncertain behavior [see Note, above category 235]

239 Neoplasms of unspecified nature

2. Functional activity

All neoplasms are classified in this chapter, whether or not functionally active. An additional code from Chapter 3 may be used to identify such functional activity associated with any neoplasm, e.g.:

catecholamine-producing malignant pheochromocytoma of adrenal:

code 194.0, additional code 255.6

basophil adenoma of pituitary with Cushing's syndrome:

code 227.3, additional code 255.0

3. Morphology [Histology]

For those wishing to identify the histological type of neoplasms, a comprehensive coded nomenclature, which comprises the morphology rubrics of the ICD-Oncology, is given in Appendix A.

4. Malignant neoplasms overlapping site boundaries

Categories 140-195 are for the classification of primary malignant neoplasms according to their point of origin. A malignant neoplasm that overlaps two or more subcategories within a three-digit rubric and whose point of origin cannot be determined should be classified to the subcategory .8 "Other."

For example, "carcinoma involving tip and ventral surface of tongue" should be assigned to 141.8. On the other hand, "carcinoma of tip of tongue, extending to involve the ventral surface" should be coded to 141.2, as the point of origin, the tip, is known. Three subcategories (149.8, 159.8, 165.8) have been provided for malignant neoplasms that overlap the boundaries of three-digit rubrics within certain systems.

Overlapping malignant neoplasms that cannot be classified as indicated above should be assigned to the appropriate subdivision of category 195 (Malignant neoplasm of other and ill-defined sites).

AHA: 2Q, '90, 7

DEF: An abnormal growth, such as a tumor. Morphology determines behavior, i.e., whether it will remain intact (benign) or spread to adjacent tissue (malignant). The term mass is not synonymous with neoplasm, as it is often used to describe cysts and thickenings such as those occurring with hematoma or infection.

MALIGNANT NEOPLASM OF LIP, ORAL CAVITY, AND PHARYNX (140-149)

EXCLUDES carcinoma in situ (230.0)

140 Malignant neoplasm of lip

EXCLUDES skin of lip (173.0)

140.0 Upper lip, vermilion border
Upper lip: NOS external
Upper lip: lipstick area

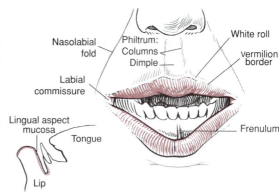

Lip

140.1 Lower lip, vermilion border
Lower lip: NOS external
Lower lip: lipstick area

140.3 Upper lip, inner aspect
Upper lip: buccal aspect frenulum
Upper lip: mucosa oral aspect

140.4 Lower lip, inner aspect
Lower lip: buccal aspect frenulum
Lower lip: mucosa oral aspect

140.5 Lip, unspecified, inner aspect
Lip, not specified whether upper or lower:
buccal aspect
frenulum
mucosa
oral aspect

140.6 Commissure of lip
Labial commissure

140.8 Other sites of lip
Malignant neoplasm of contiguous or overlapping sites of lip whose point of origin cannot be determined

140.9 Lip, unspecified, vermilion border
Lip, not specified as upper or lower:
NOS
external
lipstick area

141 Malignant neoplasm of tongue

141.0 Base of tongue
Dorsal surface of base of tongue
Fixed part of tongue NOS

141.1 Dorsal surface of tongue
Anterior two-thirds of tongue, dorsal surface
Dorsal tongue NOS
Midline of tongue
EXCLUDES dorsal surface of base of tongue (141.0)

141.2 Tip and lateral border of tongue

141.3 Ventral surface of tongue
Anterior two-thirds of tongue, ventral surface
Frenulum linguae

141.4 Anterior two-thirds of tongue, part unspecified
Mobile part of tongue NOS

141.5 Junctional zone
Border of tongue at junction of fixed and mobile parts at insertion of anterior tonsillar pillar

141.6 Lingual tonsil

141.8 Other sites of tongue
Malignant neoplasm of contiguous or overlapping sites of tongue whose point of origin cannot be determined

141.9 Tongue, unspecified
Tongue NOS

NEOPLASMS

142–146.9

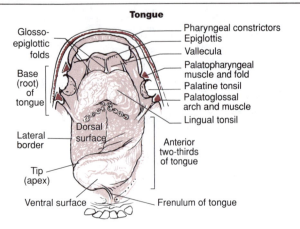

☑4th 142 Malignant neoplasm of major salivary glands
- INCLUDES: salivary ducts
- EXCLUDES: malignant neoplasm of minor salivary glands:
  - NOS (145.9)
  - buccal mucosa (145.0)
  - soft palate (145.3)
  - tongue (141.0-141.9)
  - tonsil, palatine (146.0)

- **142.0** Parotid gland
- **142.1** Submandibular gland
  - Submaxillary gland
- **142.2** Sublingual gland
- **142.8** Other major salivary glands
  - Malignant neoplasm of contiguous or overlapping sites of salivary glands and ducts whose point of origin cannot be determined
- **142.9** Salivary gland, unspecified
  - Salivary gland (major) NOS

☑4th 143 Malignant neoplasm of gum
- INCLUDES:
  - alveolar (ridge) mucosa
  - gingiva (alveolar) (marginal)
  - interdental papillae
- EXCLUDES: malignant odontogenic neoplasms (170.0-170.1)

- **143.0** Upper gum
- **143.1** Lower gum
- **143.8** Other sites of gum
  - Malignant neoplasm of contiguous or overlapping sites of gum whose point of origin cannot be determined
- **143.9** Gum, unspecified

☑4th 144 Malignant neoplasm of floor of mouth
- **144.0** Anterior portion
  - Anterior to the premolar-canine junction
- **144.1** Lateral portion
- **144.8** Other sites of floor of mouth
  - Malignant neoplasm of contiguous or overlapping sites of floor of mouth whose point of origin cannot be determined
- **144.9** Floor of mouth, part unspecified

☑4th 145 Malignant neoplasm of other and unspecified parts of mouth
- EXCLUDES: mucosa of lips (140.0-140.9)

- **145.0** Cheek mucosa
  - Buccal mucosa
  - Cheek, inner aspect
- **145.1** Vestibule of mouth
  - Buccal sulcus (upper) (lower)
  - Labial sulcus (upper) (lower)
- **145.2** Hard palate
- **145.3** Soft palate
  - EXCLUDES: nasopharyngeal [posterior] [superior] surface of soft palate (147.3)
- **145.4** Uvula
- **145.5** Palate, unspecified
  - Junction of hard and soft palate   Roof of mouth
- **145.6** Retromolar area
- **145.8** Other specified parts of mouth
  - Malignant neoplasm of contiguous or overlapping sites of mouth whose point of origin cannot be determined
- **145.9** Mouth, unspecified
  - Buccal cavity NOS
  - Minor salivary gland, unspecified site
  - Oral cavity NOS

☑4th 146 Malignant neoplasm of oropharynx
- **146.0** Tonsil
  - Tonsil:
    - NOS
    - faucial
    - palatine
  - EXCLUDES:
    - lingual tonsil (141.6)
    - pharyngeal tonsil (147.1)
  - AHA: S-O, '87, 8
- **146.1** Tonsillar fossa
- **146.2** Tonsillar pillars (anterior) (posterior)
  - Faucial pillar   Palatoglossal arch
  - Glossopalatine fold   Palatopharyngeal arch
- **146.3** Vallecula
  - Anterior and medial surface of the pharyngoepiglottic fold
- **146.4** Anterior aspect of epiglottis
  - Epiglottis, free border [margin]
  - Glossoepiglottic fold(s)
  - EXCLUDES: epiglottis:
    - NOS (161.1)
    - suprahyoid portion (161.1)
- **146.5** Junctional region
  - Junction of the free margin of the epiglottis, the aryepiglottic fold, and the pharyngoepiglottic fold
- **146.6** Lateral wall of oropharynx
- **146.7** Posterior wall of oropharynx
- **146.8** Other specified sites of oropharynx
  - Branchial cleft
  - Malignant neoplasm of contiguous or overlapping sites of oropharynx whose point of origin cannot be determined
- **146.9** Oropharynx, unspecified

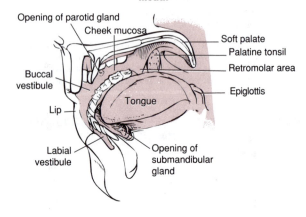

NEOPLASMS

Topical Sites in Oropharynx

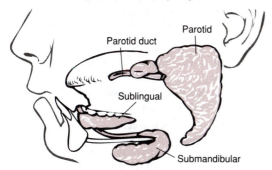

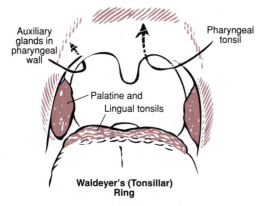

Main Salivary Glands

Waldeyer's (Tonsillar) Ring

Nasopharynx

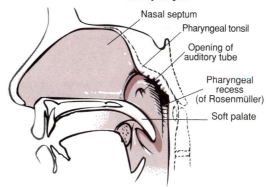

Hypopharynx

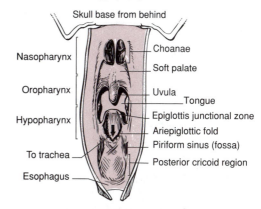

147 Malignant neoplasm of nasopharynx
- **147.0** Superior wall
  - Roof of nasopharynx
- **147.1** Posterior wall
  - Adenoid   Pharyngeal tonsil
- **147.2** Lateral wall
  - Fossa of Rosenmüller   Pharyngeal recess
  - Opening of auditory tube
- **147.3** Anterior wall
  - Floor of nasopharynx
  - Nasopharyngeal [posterior] [superior] surface of soft palate
  - Posterior margin of nasal septum and choanae
- **147.8** Other specified sites of nasopharynx
  - Malignant neoplasm of contiguous or overlapping sites of nasopharynx whose point of origin cannot be determined
- **147.9** Nasopharynx, unspecified
  - Nasopharyngeal wall NOS

148 Malignant neoplasm of hypopharynx
- **148.0** Postcricoid region
- **148.1** Pyriform sinus
  - Pyriform fossa
- **148.2** Aryepiglottic fold, hypopharyngeal aspect
  - Aryepiglottic fold or interarytenoid fold:
    - NOS
    - marginal zone
  - EXCLUDES aryepiglottic fold or interarytenoid fold, laryngeal aspect (161.1)
- **148.3** Posterior hypopharyngeal wall
- **148.8** Other specified sites of hypopharynx
  - Malignant neoplasm of contiguous or overlapping sites of hypopharynx whose point of origin cannot be determined
- **148.9** Hypopharynx, unspecified
  - Hypopharyngeal wall NOS
  - Hypopharynx NOS

149 Malignant neoplasm of other and ill-defined sites within the lip, oral cavity, and pharynx
- **149.0** Pharynx, unspecified
- **149.1** Waldeyer's ring
- **149.8** Other
  - Malignant neoplasms of lip, oral cavity, and pharynx whose point of origin cannot be assigned to any one of the categories 140-148
  - EXCLUDES "book leaf" neoplasm [ventral surface of tongue and floor of mouth] (145.8)
- **149.9** Ill-defined

MALIGNANT NEOPLASM OF DIGESTIVE ORGANS AND PERITONEUM (150-159)
EXCLUDES carcinoma in situ (230.1-230.9)

150 Malignant neoplasm of esophagus
- **150.0** Cervical esophagus
  - CC Excl: 150.0-150.9, 159.0, 159.8-159.9, 176.3, 195.8, 199.0-199.1, 239.0, 239.8-239.9
- **150.1** Thoracic esophagus
  - CC Excl: See code 150.0
- **150.2** Abdominal esophagus
  - EXCLUDES adenocarcinoma (151.0)
  - cardio-esophageal junction (151.0)
  - CC Excl: See code 150.0
- **150.3** Upper third of esophagus
  - CC Excl: See code 150.0
  - Proximal third of esophagus
- **150.4** Middle third of esophagus
  - CC Excl: See code 150.0

150.5 Lower third of esophagus [CC]
Distal third of esophagus
EXCLUDES adenocarcinoma (151.0)
cardio-esophageal junction (151.0)
CC Excl: See code 150.0

150.8 Other specified part [CC]
Malignant neoplasm of contiguous or overlapping sites of esophagus whose point of origin cannot be determined
CC Excl: See code 150.0

150.9 Esophagus, unspecified [CC]
CC Excl: See code 150.0

√4th 151 Malignant neoplasm of stomach

151.0 Cardia [CC]
Cardiac orifice
Cardio-esophageal junction
EXCLUDES squamous cell carcinoma (150.2, 150.5)
CC Excl: 151.0-151.9, 159.0, 159.8-159.9, 176.3, 195.8, 199.0-199.1, 239.0, 239.8-239.9

151.1 Pylorus [CC]
Prepylorus   Pyloric canal
CC Excl: See code 151.0

151.2 Pyloric antrum [CC]
Antrum of stomach NOS
CC Excl: See code 151.0

151.3 Fundus of stomach [CC]
CC Excl: See code 151.0

151.4 Body of stomach [CC]
CC Excl: See code 151.0

151.5 Lesser curvature, unspecified [CC]
Lesser curvature, not classifiable to 151.1-151.4
CC Excl: See code 151.0

151.6 Greater curvature, unspecified [CC]
Greater curvature, not classifiable to 151.0-151.4
CC Excl: See code 151.0

151.8 Other specified sites of stomach [CC]
Anterior wall, not classifiable to 151.0-151.4
Posterior wall, not classifiable to 151.0-151.4
Malignant neoplasm of contiguous or overlapping sites of stomach whose point of origin cannot be determined
CC Excl: See code 151.0

151.9 Stomach, unspecified [CC]
Carcinoma ventriculi   Gastric cancer
CC Excl: See code 151.0
AHA: 2Q, '01, 17

√4th 152 Malignant neoplasm of small intestine, including duodenum

152.0 Duodenum [CC]
CC Excl: 152.0, 152.8-152.9, 159.0, 159.8-159.9, 176.3, 195.8, 199.0-199.1, 239.0, 239.8-239.9

152.1 Jejunum [CC]
CC Excl: 152.1, 152.8-152.9, 159.0, 159.8-159.9, 176.3, 195.8, 199.0-199.1, 239.0, 239.8-239.9

152.2 Ileum [CC]
EXCLUDES ileocecal valve (153.4)
CC Excl: 152.2, 152.8-152.9, 159.0, 159.8-159.9, 176.3, 195.8, 199.0-199.1, 239.0, 239.8-239.9

152.3 Meckel's diverticulum [CC]
CC Excl: 152.3, 152.8-152.9, 159.0, 159.8-159.9, 176.3, 195.8, 199.0-199.1, 239.0, 239.8-239.9

152.8 Other specified sites of small intestine [CC]
Duodenojejunal junction
Malignant neoplasm of contiguous or overlapping sites of small intestine whose point of origin cannot be determined
CC Excl: 152.8-152.9, 159.0, 159.8-159.9, 176.3, 195.8, 199.0-199.1, 239.0, 239.8-239.9

152.9 Small intestine, unspecified [CC]
CC Excl: See code 152.8

√4th 153 Malignant neoplasm of colon

153.0 Hepatic flexure [CC]
CC Excl: 153.0, 153.8-153.9, 159.0, 159.8-159.9, 176.3, 195.8, 199.0-199.1, 239.0, 239.8-239.9

153.1 Transverse colon [CC]
CC Excl: 153.1, 153.8-153.9, 159.0, 159.8-159.9, 176.3, 195.8, 199.0-199.1, 239.0, 239.8-239.9

153.2 Descending colon [CC]
Left colon
CC Excl: 153.2, 153.8-153.9, 159.0, 159.8-159.9, 176.3, 195.8, 199.0-199.1, 239.0, 239.8-239.9

153.3 Sigmoid colon [CC]
Sigmoid (flexure)
EXCLUDES rectosigmoid junction (154.0)
CC Excl: 153.3, 153.8-153.9, 159.0, 159.8-159.9, 176.3, 195.8, 199.0-199.1, 239.0, 239.8-239.9

153.4 Cecum [CC]
Ileocecal valve
CC Excl: 153.4, 153.8-153.9, 159.0, 159.8-159.9, 176.3, 195.8, 199.0-199.1, 239.0, 239.8-239.9

153.5 Appendix [CC]
CC Excl: 153.5, 153.8-153.9, 159.0, 159.8-159.9, 176.3, 195.8, 199.0-199.1, 239.0, 239.8-239.9

153.6 Ascending colon [CC]
Right colon
CC Excl: 153.6, 153.8-153.9, 159.0, 159.8-159.9, 176.3, 195.8, 199.0-199.1, 239.0, 239.8-239.9

153.7 Splenic flexure [CC]
CC Excl: 153.7-153.9, 159.0, 159.8-159.9, 176.3, 195.8, 199.0-199.1, 239.0, 239.8-239.9

153.8 Other specified sites of large intestine [CC]
Malignant neoplasm of contiguous or overlapping sites of colon whose point of origin cannot be determined
EXCLUDES ileocecal valve (153.4)
rectosigmoid junction (154.0)
CC Excl: 153.8-153.9, 159.0, 159.8-159.9, 176.3, 195.8, 199.0-199.1, 239.0, 239.8-239.9

153.9 Colon, unspecified [CC]
Large intestine NOS
CC Excl: See code 153.8

√4th 154 Malignant neoplasm of rectum, rectosigmoid junction, and anus

154.0 Rectosigmoid junction [CC]
Colon with rectum
Rectosigmoid (colon)
CC Excl: 154.0, 154.8, 159.0, 159.8-159.9, 176.3, 195.8, 199.0-199.1, 239.0, 239.8-239.9

154.1 Rectum [CC]
Rectal ampulla
CC Excl: 154.1, 154.8, 159.0, 159.8-159.9, 176.3, 195.8, 199.0-199.1, 239.0, 239.8-239.9

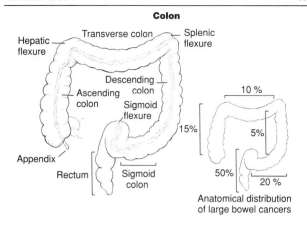

154.2 Anal canal
Anal sphincter
EXCLUDES skin of anus (172.5, 173.5)
CC Excl: 154.2-154.8, 159.0, 159.8-159.9, 176.3, 195.8, 199.0-199.1, 239.0, 239.8-239.9
AHA: 1Q, '01, 8

154.3 Anus, unspecified
EXCLUDES anus:
margin (172.5, 173.5)
skin (172.5, 173.5)
perianal skin (172.5, 173.5)
CC Excl: See code 154.2

154.8 Other
Anorectum
Cloacogenic zone
Malignant neoplasm of contiguous or overlapping sites of rectum, rectosigmoid junction, and anus whose point of origin cannot be determined
CC Excl: 154.8, 159.0, 159.8-159.9, 176.3, 195.8, 199.0-199.1, 239.0, 239.8-239.9

155 Malignant neoplasm of liver and intrahepatic bile ducts

155.0 Liver, primary
Carcinoma:
liver, specified as primary
hepatocellular
liver cell
Hepatoblastoma
CC Excl: 155.0-155.2, 159.0, 159.8-159.9, 176.3, 195.8, 199.0-199.1, 239.0, 239.8-239.9

155.1 Intrahepatic bile ducts
Canaliculi biliferi   Intrahepatic:
Interlobular: biliary passages
  bile ducts   canaliculi
  biliary canals   gall duct
EXCLUDES hepatic duct (156.1)
CC Excl: See code 155.0

155.2 Liver, not specified as primary or secondary
CC Excl: See code 155.0

156 Malignant neoplasm of gallbladder and extrahepatic bile ducts

156.0 Gallbladder
CC Excl: 156.0, 156.8-156.9, 159.0, 159.8-159.9, 176.3, 195.8, 199.0-199.1, 239.0, 239.8-239.9

156.1 Extrahepatic bile ducts
Biliary duct or passage NOS
Common bile duct
Cystic duct
Hepatic duct
Sphincter of Oddi
CC Excl: 156.1, 156.8-156.9, 159.0, 159.8-159.9, 176.3, 195.8, 199.0-199.1, 239.0, 239.8-239.9

156.2 Ampulla of Vater
CC Excl: 156.2-156.9, 159.0, 159.8-159.9, 176.3, 195.8, 199.0-199.1, 239.0, 239.8-239.9

DEF: Malignant neoplasm in the area of dilation at the juncture of the common bile and pancreatic ducts near the opening into the lumen of the duodenum.

156.8 Other specified sites of gallbladder and extrahepatic bile ducts
Malignant neoplasm of contiguous or overlapping sites of gallbladder and extrahepatic bile ducts whose point of origin cannot be determined
CC Excl: 156.8-156.9, 159.0, 159.8-159.9, 176.3, 195.8, 199.0-199.1, 239.0, 239.8-239.9

156.9 Biliary tract, part unspecified
Malignant neoplasm involving both intrahepatic and extrahepatic bile ducts
CC Excl: See code 156.8

157 Malignant neoplasm of pancreas

157.0 Head of pancreas
CC Excl: 157.0-157.9, 159.0, 159.8-159.9, 176.3, 195.8, 199.0-199.1, 239.0, 239.8-239.9
AHA: 4Q, '00, 40

157.1 Body of pancreas
CC Excl: See code 157.0

157.2 Tail of pancreas
CC Excl: See code 157.0

157.3 Pancreatic duct
Duct of:
Santorini
Wirsung
CC Excl: See code 157.0

157.4 Islets of Langerhans
Islets of Langerhans, any part of pancreas
Use additional code to identify any functional activity
CC Excl: See code 157.0

DEF: Malignant neoplasm within the structures of the pancreas that produce insulin, somatostatin and glucagon.

157.8 Other specified sites of pancreas
Ectopic pancreatic tissue
Malignant neoplasm of contiguous or overlapping sites of pancreas whose point of origin cannot be determined
CC Excl: See code 157.0

157.9 Pancreas, part unspecified
CC Excl: See code 157.0
AHA: 4Q, '89, 11

158 Malignant neoplasm of retroperitoneum and peritoneum

158.0 Retroperitoneum
Periadrenal tissue   Perirenal tissue
Perinephric tissue   Retrocecal tissue

Retroperitoneum and Peritoneum

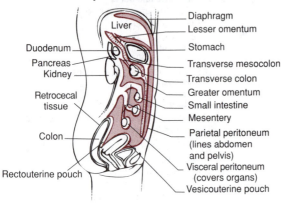

158.8 Specified parts of peritoneum
Cul-de-sac (of Douglas)
Mesentery
Mesocolon
Omentum
Peritoneum:
  parietal
  pelvic
Rectouterine pouch
Malignant neoplasm of contiguous or overlapping sites of retroperitoneum and peritoneum whose point of origin cannot be determined

158.9 Peritoneum, unspecified

✓4th **159 Malignant neoplasm of other and ill-defined sites within the digestive organs and peritoneum**

159.0 Intestinal tract, part unspecified
Intestine NOS

159.1 Spleen, not elsewhere classified
Angiosarcoma } of spleen
Fibrosarcoma

> EXCLUDES Hodgkin's disease (201.0-201.9)
> lymphosarcoma (200.1)
> reticulosarcoma (200.0)

159.8 Other sites of digestive system and intra-abdominal organs
Malignant neoplasm of digestive organs and peritoneum whose point of origin cannot be assigned to any one of the categories 150-158

> EXCLUDES anus and rectum (154.8)
> cardio-esophageal junction (151.0)
> colon and rectum (154.0)

159.9 Ill-defined
Alimentary canal or tract NOS
Gastrointestinal tract NOS

> EXCLUDES abdominal NOS (195.2)
> intra-abdominal NOS (195.2)

MALIGNANT NEOPLASM OF RESPIRATORY AND INTRATHORACIC ORGANS (160-165)

> EXCLUDES carcinoma in situ (231.0-231.9)

✓4th **160 Malignant neoplasm of nasal cavities, middle ear, and accessory sinuses**

160.0 Nasal cavities
Cartilage of nose   Septum of nose
Conchae, nasal   Vestibule of nose
Internal nose

> EXCLUDES nasal bone (170.0)
> nose NOS (195.0)
> olfactory bulb (192.0)
> posterior margin of septum and choanae (147.3)
> skin of nose (172.3, 173.3)
> turbinates (170.0)

160.1 Auditory tube, middle ear, and mastoid air cells
Antrum tympanicum   Tympanic cavity
Eustachian tube

> EXCLUDES auditory canal (external) (172.2, 173.2)
> bone of ear (meatus) (170.0)
> cartilage of ear (171.0)
> ear (external) (skin) (172.2, 173.2)

160.2 Maxillary sinus
Antrum (Highmore) (maxillary)

160.3 Ethmoidal sinus

160.4 Frontal sinus

160.5 Sphenoidal sinus

160.8 Other
Malignant neoplasm of contiguous or overlapping sites of nasal cavities, middle ear, and accessory sinuses whose point of origin cannot be determined

160.9 Accessory sinus, unspecified

✓4th **161 Malignant neoplasm of larynx**

161.0 Glottis
Intrinsic larynx
Laryngeal commissure (anterior) (posterior)
True vocal cord
Vocal cord NOS

161.1 Supraglottis
Aryepiglottic fold or interarytenoid fold, laryngeal aspect
Epiglottis (suprahyoid portion) NOS
Extrinsic larynx
False vocal cords
Posterior (laryngeal) surface of epiglottis
Ventricular bands

> EXCLUDES anterior aspect of epiglottis (146.4)
> aryepiglottic fold or interarytenoid fold:
>   NOS (148.2)
>   hypopharyngeal aspect (148.2)
>   marginal zone (148.2)

161.2 Subglottis

161.3 Laryngeal cartilages
Cartilage: Cartilage:
  arytenoid   cuneiform
  cricoid   thyroid

161.8 Other specified sites of larynx
Malignant neoplasm of contiguous or overlapping sites of larynx whose point of origin cannot be determined

161.9 Larynx, unspecified

✓4th **162 Malignant neoplasm of trachea, bronchus, and lung**

162.0 Trachea
Cartilage } of trachea
Mucosa

162.2 Main bronchus `CC`
Carina
Hilus of lung
CC Excl: 162.2, 162.8-162.9, 165.8-165.9, 176.4, 195.8, 199.0-199.1, 239.1, 239.8-239.9

162.3 Upper lobe, bronchus or lung `CC`
CC Excl: 162.3, 162.8-162.9, 165.8-165.9, 176.4, 195.8, 199.0-199.1, 239.1, 239.8-239.9

162.4 Middle lobe, bronchus or lung `CC`
CC Excl: 162.4, 162.8-162.9, 165.8-165.9, 176.4, 195.8, 199.0-199.1, 239.1, 239.8-239.9

162.5 Lower lobe, bronchus or lung `CC`
CC Excl: 162.5-162.9, 165.8-165.9, 176.4, 195.8, 199.0-199.1, 239.1, 239.8-239.9

NEOPLASMS

162.8 **Other parts of bronchus or lung** `CC`
Malignant neoplasm of contiguous or overlapping sites of bronchus or lung whose point of origin cannot be determined
CC Excl: 162.8-162.9, 165.8-165.9, 176.4, 195.8, 199.0-199.1, 239.1, 239.8-239.9

162.9 **Bronchus and lung, unspecified** `CC`
CC Excl: See code 162.8
AHA: 2Q, '97, 3; 4Q, '96, 48

✓4th 163 Malignant neoplasm of pleura

163.0 **Parietal pleura** `CC`
CC Excl: 163.0-163.9, 165.8-165.9, 195.8, 199.0-199.1, 239.1, 239.8-239.9

163.1 **Visceral pleura** `CC`
CC Excl: See code 163.0

163.8 **Other specified sites of pleura** `CC`
Malignant neoplasm of contiguous or overlapping sites of pleura whose point of origin cannot be determined
CC Excl: See code 163.0

163.9 **Pleura, unspecified** `CC`
CC Excl: See code 163.0

✓4th 164 Malignant neoplasm of thymus, heart, and mediastinum

164.0 **Thymus** `CC`
CC Excl: 164.0

164.1 **Heart** `CC`
Endocardium   Myocardium
Epicardium   Pericardium
EXCLUDES great vessels (171.4)
CC Excl: 164.1

164.2 **Anterior mediastinum** `CC`
CC Excl: 164.2-164.9, 165.8-165.9, 195.8, 199.0-199.1, 239.1, 239.8-239.9

164.3 **Posterior mediastinum** `CC`
CC Excl: See code 164.2

164.8 **Other** `CC`
Malignant neoplasm of contiguous or overlapping sites of thymus, heart, and mediastinum whose point of origin cannot be determined
CC Excl: See code 164.2

164.9 **Mediastinum, part unspecified** `CC`
CC Excl: See code 164.2

✓4th 165 Malignant neoplasm of other and ill-defined sites within the respiratory system and intrathoracic organs

165.0 **Upper respiratory tract, part unspecified**

165.8 **Other**
Malignant neoplasm of respiratory and intrathoracic organs whose point of origin cannot be assigned to any one of the categories 160-164

165.9 **Ill-defined sites within the respiratory system**
Respiratory tract NOS
EXCLUDES intrathoracic NOS (195.1)
thoracic NOS (195.1)

MALIGNANT NEOPLASM OF BONE, CONNECTIVE TISSUE, SKIN, AND BREAST (170-176)

EXCLUDES carcinoma in situ: carcinoma in situ:
breast (233.0)   skin (232.0-232.9)

✓4th 170 Malignant neoplasm of bone and articular cartilage

INCLUDES cartilage (articular) (joint)
periosteum
EXCLUDES bone marrow NOS (202.9)
cartilage:
ear (171.0)
eyelid (171.0)
larynx (161.3)
nose (160.0)
synovia (171.0-171.9)

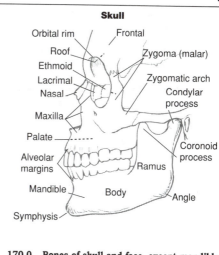

Skull

170.0 **Bones of skull and face, except mandible**
Bone: Bone:
ethmoid   sphenoid
frontal   temporal
malar   zygomatic
nasal   Maxilla (superior)
occipital   Turbinate
orbital   Upper jaw bone
parietal   Vomer
EXCLUDES carcinoma, any type except intraosseous or odontogenic:
maxilla, maxillary (sinus) (160.2)
upper jaw bone (143.0)
jaw bone (lower) (170.1)

170.1 **Mandible**
Inferior maxilla
Jaw bone NOS
Lower jaw bone
EXCLUDES carcinoma, any type except intraosseous or odontogenic:
jaw bone NOS (143.9)
lower (143.1)
upper jaw bone (170.0)

170.2 **Vertebral column, excluding sacrum and coccyx**
Spinal column   Vertebra
Spine
EXCLUDES sacrum and coccyx (170.6)

170.3 **Ribs, sternum, and clavicle**
Costal cartilage
Costovertebral joint
Xiphoid process

170.4 **Scapula and long bones of upper limb**
Acromion   Radius
Bones NOS of upper limb Ulna
Humerus
AHA: 2Q, '99, 9

170.5 **Short bones of upper limb**
Carpal   Scaphoid (of hand)
Cuneiform, wrist   Semilunar or lunate
Metacarpal   Trapezium
Navicular, of hand Trapezoid
Phalanges of hand   Unciform
Pisiform

170.6 **Pelvic bones, sacrum, and coccyx**
Coccygeal vertebra Pubic bone
Ilium   Sacral vertebra
Ischium

170.7 **Long bones of lower limb**
Bones NOS of lower limb
Femur
Fibula
Tibia

✓4th Additional Digit Required Nonspecific PDx Unacceptable PDx Manifestation Code MSP Medicare Secondary Payer ▶◀ Revised Text ● New Code ▲ Revis

2002 Ingenix, Inc.

170.8–173.5 NEOPLASMS Tabular List

170.8 Short bones of lower limb
- Astragalus [talus]
- Calcaneus
- Cuboid
- Cuneiform, ankle
- Metatarsal
- Navicular (of ankle)
- Patella
- Phalanges of foot
- Tarsal

170.9 Bone and articular cartilage, site unspecified

√4th 171 Malignant neoplasm of connective and other soft tissue

INCLUDES:
- blood vessel
- bursa
- fascia
- fat
- ligament, except uterine
- muscle
- peripheral, sympathetic, and parasympathetic nerves and ganglia
- synovia
- tendon (sheath)

EXCLUDES:
- cartilage (of):
  - articular (170.0-170.9)
  - larynx (161.3)
  - nose (160.0)
- connective tissue:
  - breast (174.0-175.9)
  - internal organs—code to malignant neoplasm of the site [e.g., leiomyosarcoma of stomach, 151.9]
- heart (164.1)
- uterine ligament (183.4)

171.0 Head, face, and neck
- Cartilage of: ear
- Cartilage of: eyelid

AHA: 2Q, '99, 6

171.2 Upper limb, including shoulder
- Arm
- Finger
- Forearm
- Hand

171.3 Lower limb, including hip
- Foot
- Leg
- Popliteal space
- Thigh
- Toe

171.4 Thorax
- Axilla
- Diaphragm
- Great vessels

EXCLUDES:
- heart (164.1)
- mediastinum (164.2-164.9)
- thymus (164.0)

171.5 Abdomen
- Abdominal wall
- Hypochondrium

EXCLUDES:
- peritoneum (158.8)
- retroperitoneum (158.0)

171.6 Pelvis
- Buttock
- Groin
- Inguinal region
- Perineum

EXCLUDES:
- pelvic peritoneum (158.8)
- retroperitoneum (158.0)
- uterine ligament, any (183.3-183.5)

171.7 Trunk, unspecified
- Back NOS
- Flank NOS

171.8 Other specified sites of connective and other soft tissue

Malignant neoplasm of contiguous or overlapping sites of connective tissue whose point of origin cannot be determined

171.9 Connective and other soft tissue, site unspecified

√4th 172 Malignant melanoma of skin

INCLUDES:
- melanocarcinoma
- melanoma (skin) NOS

EXCLUDES:
- skin of genital organs (184.0-184.9, 187.1-187.9)
- sites other than skin—code to malignant neoplasm of the site

neoplasm of melanocytes; most common in skin, may involve ...agus, anal canal, vagina, leptomeninges, conjunctiva of the

172.0 Lip

EXCLUDES: vermilion border of lip (140.0-140.1, 140.9)

172.1 Eyelid, including canthus

172.2 Ear and external auditory canal
- Auricle (ear)
- Auricular canal, external
- External [acoustic] meatus
- Pinna

172.3 Other and unspecified parts of face
- Cheek (external)
- Chin
- Eyebrow
- Forehead
- Nose, external
- Temple

172.4 Scalp and neck

172.5 Trunk, except scrotum
- Axilla
- Breast
- Buttock
- Groin
- Perianal skin
- Perineum
- Umbilicus

EXCLUDES:
- anal canal (154.2)
- anus NOS (154.3)
- scrotum (187.7)

172.6 Upper limb, including shoulder
- Arm
- Finger
- Forearm
- Hand

172.7 Lower limb, including hip
- Ankle
- Foot
- Heel
- Knee
- Leg
- Popliteal area
- Thigh
- Toe

172.8 Other specified sites of skin

Malignant melanoma of contiguous or overlapping sites of skin whose point of origin cannot be determined

172.9 Melanoma of skin, site unspecified

√4th 173 Other malignant neoplasm of skin

INCLUDES: malignant neoplasm of:
- sebaceous glands
- sudoriferous, sudoriparous glands
- sweat glands

EXCLUDES:
- Kaposi's sarcoma (176.0-176.9)
- malignant melanoma of skin (172.0-172.9)
- skin of genital organs (184.0-184.9, 187.1-187.9)

AHA: 1Q, '00, 18; 2Q, '96, 12

173.0 Skin of lip

EXCLUDES: vermilion border of lip (140.0-140.1, 140.9)

173.1 Eyelid, including canthus

EXCLUDES: cartilage of eyelid (171.0)

173.2 Skin of ear and external auditory canal
- Auricle (ear)
- Auricular canal, external
- External meatus
- Pinna

EXCLUDES: cartilage of ear (171.0)

173.3 Skin of other and unspecified parts of face
- Cheek, external
- Chin
- Eyebrow
- Forehead
- Nose, external
- Temple

AHA: 1Q, '00, 3

173.4 Scalp and skin of neck

173.5 Skin of trunk, except scrotum
- Axillary fold
- Perianal skin
- Skin of:
  - abdominal wall
  - anus
  - back
  - breast
- Skin of:
  - buttock
  - chest wall
  - groin
  - perineum
  - Umbilicus

EXCLUDES:
- anal canal (154.2)
- anus NOS (154.3)
- skin of scrotum (187.7)

AHA: 1Q, '01, 8

 Pediatric Age: 0-17   Maternity Age: 12-55   Adult Age: 15-124   CC Condition   MC Major Complication   CD Complex Dx   HIV HIV Related Dx

2002 Ingenix, Inc.

Tabular List — NEOPLASMS — 173.6–183.9

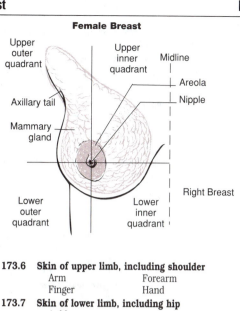

Female Breast: Upper outer quadrant, Upper inner quadrant, Midline, Areola, Nipple, Axillary tail, Mammary gland, Lower outer quadrant, Lower inner quadrant, Right Breast

173.6 Skin of upper limb, including shoulder
Arm   Forearm
Finger   Hand

173.7 Skin of lower limb, including hip
Ankle   Leg
Foot   Popliteal area
Heel   Thigh
Knee   Toe

173.8 Other specified sites of skin
Malignant neoplasm of contiguous or overlapping sites of skin whose point of origin cannot be determined

173.9 Skin, site unspecified

√4th **174 Malignant neoplasm of female breast**
INCLUDES: breast (female)   Paget's disease of:
connective tissue   breast
soft parts   nipple
EXCLUDES: skin of breast (172.5, 173.5)
AHA: 3Q, '97, 8; 4Q, '89, 11

174.0 Nipple and areola ♀
174.1 Central portion ♀
174.2 Upper-inner quadrant ♀
174.3 Lower-inner quadrant ♀
174.4 Upper-outer quadrant ♀
174.5 Lower-outer quadrant ♀
174.6 Axillary tail ♀
174.8 Other specified sites of female breast ♀
Ectopic sites   Midline of breast
Inner breast   Outer breast
Lower breast   Upper breast
Malignant neoplasm of contiguous or overlapping sites of breast whose point of origin cannot be determined

174.9 Breast (female), unspecified ♀

√4th **175 Malignant neoplasm of male breast**
EXCLUDES: skin of breast (172.5, 173.5)

175.0 Nipple and areola ♂
175.9 Other and unspecified sites of male breast ♂
Ectopic breast tissue, male

√4th **176 Kaposi's sarcoma**
AHA: 4Q, '91, 24

176.0 Skin [HIV]
176.1 Soft tissue [HIV]
INCLUDES: blood vessel
connective tissue
fascia
ligament
lymphatic(s) NEC
muscle
EXCLUDES: lymph glands and nodes (176.5)

176.2 Palate [HIV]
176.3 Gastrointestinal sites [HIV]
176.4 Lung [CC] [HIV]
CC Excl: 162.8-162.9, 165.8-165.9, 176.4, 195.8, 199.0-199.1, 239.1, 239.8-239.9

176.5 Lymph nodes [CC] [HIV]
CC Excl: 176.5, 195.8, 196.0-196.9, 199.0-199.1, 239.8-239.9

176.8 Other specified sites [HIV]
INCLUDES: oral cavity NEC

176.9 Unspecified [HIV]
Viscera NOS

MALIGNANT NEOPLASM OF GENITOURINARY ORGANS (179-189)
EXCLUDES: carcinoma in situ (233.1-233.9)

179 Malignant neoplasm of uterus, part unspecified ♀

√4th **180 Malignant neoplasm of cervix uteri**
INCLUDES: invasive malignancy [carcinoma]
EXCLUDES: carcinoma in situ (233.1)

180.0 Endocervix ♀
Cervical canal NOS   Endocervical gland
Endocervical canal

180.1 Exocervix ♀
180.8 Other specified sites of cervix ♀
Cervical stump
Squamocolumnar junction of cervix
Malignant neoplasm of contiguous or overlapping sites of cervix uteri whose point of origin cannot be determined

180.9 Cervix uteri, unspecified ♀

181 Malignant neoplasm of placenta ♀
Choriocarcinoma NOS
Chorioepithelioma NOS
EXCLUDES: chorioadenoma (destruens) (236.1)
hydatidiform mole (630)
malignant (236.1)
invasive mole (236.1)
male choriocarcinoma NOS (186.0-186.9)

√4th **182 Malignant neoplasm of body of uterus**
EXCLUDES: carcinoma in situ (233.2)

182.0 Corpus uteri, except isthmus ♀
Cornu   Fundus
Endometrium   Myometrium

182.1 Isthmus ♀
Lower uterine segment

182.8 Other specified sites of body of uterus ♀
Malignant neoplasm of contiguous or overlapping sites of body of uterus whose point of origin cannot be determined
EXCLUDES: uterus NOS (179)

√4th **183 Malignant neoplasm of ovary and other uterine adnexa**
EXCLUDES: Douglas' cul-de-sac (158.8)

183.0 Ovary ♀
Use additional code to identify any functional activity

183.2 Fallopian tube ♀
Oviduct   Uterine tube

183.3 Broad ligament ♀
Mesovarium   Parovarian region

183.4 Parametrium ♀
Uterine ligament NOS   Uterosacral ligament

183.5 Round ligament ♀
AHA: 3Q, '99, 5

183.8 Other specified sites of uterine adnexa ♀
Tubo-ovarian
Utero-ovarian
Malignant neoplasm of contiguous or overlapping sites of ovary and other uterine adnexa whose point of origin cannot be determined

183.9 Uterine adnexa, unspecified ♀

NEOPLASMS

✓4th 184 Malignant neoplasm of other and unspecified female genital organs
EXCLUDES carcinoma in situ (233.3)
- 184.0 Vagina ♀
  - Gartner's duct
  - Vaginal vault
- 184.1 Labia majora ♀
  - Greater vestibular [Bartholin's] gland
- 184.2 Labia minora ♀
- 184.3 Clitoris ♀
- 184.4 Vulva, unspecified ♀
  - External female genitalia NOS
  - Pudendum
- 184.8 Other specified sites of female genital organs ♀
  - Malignant neoplasm of contiguous or overlapping sites of female genital organs whose point of origin cannot be determined
- 184.9 Female genital organ, site unspecified ♀
  - Female genitourinary tract NOS

185 Malignant neoplasm of prostate ♂
EXCLUDES seminal vesicles (187.8)
AHA: 3Q, '99, 5; 3Q, '92, 7

✓4th 186 Malignant neoplasm of testis
Use additional code to identify any functional activity
- 186.0 Undescended testis ♂
  - Ectopic testis
  - Retained testis
- 186.9 Other and unspecified testis ♂
  - Testis: NOS
  - descended
  - Testis: scrotal

✓4th 187 Malignant neoplasm of penis and other male genital organs
- 187.1 Prepuce ♂
  - Foreskin
- 187.2 Glans penis ♂
- 187.3 Body of penis ♂
  - Corpus cavernosum
- 187.4 **Penis, part unspecified** ♂
  - Skin of penis NOS
- 187.5 Epididymis ♂
- 187.6 Spermatic cord ♂
  - Vas deferens
- 187.7 Scrotum ♂
  - Skin of scrotum
- 187.8 Other specified sites of male genital organs ♂
  - Seminal vesicle
  - Tunica vaginalis
  - Malignant neoplasm of contiguous or overlapping sites of penis and other male genital organs whose point of origin cannot be determined
- 187.9 **Male genital organ, site unspecified** ♂
  - Male genital organ or tract NOS

✓4th 188 Malignant neoplasm of bladder
EXCLUDES carcinoma in situ (233.7)
- 188.0 Trigone of urinary bladder
- 188.1 Dome of urinary bladder
- 188.2 Lateral wall of urinary bladder
- 188.3 Anterior wall of urinary bladder
- 188.4 Posterior wall of urinary bladder
- 188.5 Bladder neck
  - Internal urethral orifice
- 188.6 Ureteric orifice
- 188.7 Urachus
- 188.8 Other specified sites of bladder
  - Malignant neoplasm of contiguous or overlapping sites of bladder whose point of origin cannot be determined
- 188.9 **, part unspecified**
  - dder wall NOS
  - Q, '00, 5

✓4th 189 Malignant neoplasm of kidney and other and unspecified urinary organs
- 189.0 Kidney, except pelvis [CC]
  - Kidney NOS
  - Kidney parenchyma
  - CC Excl: 189.0-189.1, 189.8-189.9, 195.8, 199.0-199.1, 239.5, 239.8-239.9
- 189.1 Renal pelvis [CC]
  - Renal calyces
  - Ureteropelvic junction
  - CC Excl: See code 189.0
- 189.2 Ureter [CC]
  - **EXCLUDES** ureteric orifice of bladder (188.6)
  - CC Excl: 189.2, 189.8-189.9, 195.8, 199.0-199.1, 239.5, 239.8-239.9
- 189.3 Urethra
  - **EXCLUDES** urethral orifice of bladder (188.5)
- 189.4 Paraurethral glands
- 189.8 Other specified sites of urinary organs
  - Malignant neoplasm of contiguous or overlapping sites of kidney and other urinary organs whose point of origin cannot be determined
- 189.9 **Urinary organ, site unspecified**
  - Urinary system NOS

MALIGNANT NEOPLASM OF OTHER AND UNSPECIFIED SITES (190-199)
EXCLUDES carcinoma in situ (234.0-234.9)

✓4th 190 Malignant neoplasm of eye
EXCLUDES carcinoma in situ (234.0)
- eyelid (skin) (172.1, 173.1)
- cartilage (171.0)
- optic nerve (192.0)
- orbital bone (170.0)

- 190.0 Eyeball, except conjunctiva, cornea, retina, and choroid
  - Ciliary body
  - Crystalline lens
  - Iris
  - Sclera
  - Uveal tract
- 190.1 Orbit
  - Connective tissue of orbit
  - Extraocular muscle
  - Retrobulbar
  - **EXCLUDES** bone of orbit (170.0)
- 190.2 Lacrimal gland
- 190.3 Conjunctiva
- 190.4 Cornea
- 190.5 Retina
- 190.6 Choroid
- 190.7 Lacrimal duct
  - Lacrimal sac
  - Nasolacrimal duct
- 190.8 Other specified sites of eye
  - Malignant neoplasm of contiguous or overlapping sites of eye whose point of origin cannot be determined
- 190.9 **Eye, part unspecified**

✓4th 191 Malignant neoplasm of brain
EXCLUDES cranial nerves (192.0)
- retrobulbar area (190.1)

- 191.0 Cerebrum, except lobes and ventricles [CC]
  - Basal ganglia
  - Cerebral cortex
  - Corpus striatum
  - Globus pallidus
  - Hypothalamus
  - Thalamus
  - CC Excl: 191.0-191.9, 192.0-192.1, 192.8-192.9, 195.8, 199.0-199.1, 239.6-239.9
- 191.1 Frontal lobe [CC]
  - CC Excl: See code 191.0
- 191.2 Temporal lobe [CC]
  - Hippocampus
  - Uncus
  - CC Excl: See code 191.0
- 191.3 Parietal lobe [CC]
  - CC Excl: See code 191.0

NEOPLASMS

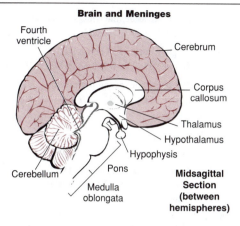

Brain and Meninges — Midsagittal Section (between hemispheres)
Labels: Fourth ventricle, Cerebrum, Corpus callosum, Thalamus, Hypothalamus, Hypophysis, Pons, Medulla oblongata, Cerebellum

191.4 Occipital lobe [CC]
CC Excl: See code 191.0

191.5 Ventricles [CC]
Choroid plexus   Floor of ventricle
CC Excl: See code 191.0

191.6 Cerebellum NOS [CC]
Cerebellopontine angle
CC Excl: See code 191.0

191.7 Brain stem [CC]
Cerebral peduncle   Midbrain
Medulla oblongata   Pons
CC Excl: See code 191.0

191.8 Other parts of brain [CC]
Corpus callosum
Tapetum
Malignant neoplasm of contiguous or overlapping sites of brain whose point of origin cannot be determined
CC Excl: See code 191.0

191.9 Brain, unspecified [CC]
Cranial fossa NOS
CC Excl: See code 191.0

√4th **192 Malignant neoplasm of other and unspecified parts of nervous system**
EXCLUDES peripheral, sympathetic, and parasympathetic nerves and ganglia (171.0-171.9)

192.0 Cranial nerves [CC]
Olfactory bulb
CC Excl: 192.0, 192.8-192.9, 195.8, 199.0-199.1, 239.6-239.9

192.1 Cerebral meninges [CC]
Dura (mater)   Meninges NOS
Falx (cerebelli) (cerebri)   Tentorium
CC Excl: 192.1, 192.8-192.9, 195.8, 199.0-199.1, 239.6-239.9

192.2 Spinal cord [CC]
Cauda equina
CC Excl: 192.2, 192.8-192.9, 195.8, 199.0-199.1, 239.6-239.9

192.3 Spinal meninges [CC]
CC Excl: 192.3-192.9, 195.8, 199.0-199.1, 239.6-239.9

192.8 Other specified sites of nervous system [CC]
Malignant neoplasm of contiguous or overlapping sites of other parts of nervous system whose point of origin cannot be determined
CC Excl: 191.0-191.9, 192.0-192.9, 195.8, 199.0-199.1, 239.6-239.9

192.9 Nervous system, part unspecified
Nervous system (central) NOS
EXCLUDES meninges NOS (192.1)

193 Malignant neoplasm of thyroid gland
Sipple's syndrome
Thyroglossal duct
Use additional code to identify any functional activity

√4th **194 Malignant neoplasm of other endocrine glands and related structures**
Use additional code to identify any functional activity
EXCLUDES islets of Langerhans (157.4)
ovary (183.0)
testis (186.0-186.9)
thymus (164.0)

194.0 Adrenal gland
Adrenal cortex   Suprarenal gland
Adrenal medulla

194.1 Parathyroid gland

194.3 Pituitary gland and craniopharyngeal duct
Craniobuccal pouch   Rathke's pouch
Hypophysis   Sella turcica
AHA: J-A, '85, 9

194.4 Pineal gland

194.5 Carotid body

194.6 Aortic body and other paraganglia
Coccygeal body   Para-aortic body
Glomus jugulare

194.8 Other
Pluriglandular involvement NOS
Note: If the sites of multiple involvements are known, they should be coded separately.

194.9 Endocrine gland, site unspecified

√4th **195 Malignant neoplasm of other and ill-defined sites**
INCLUDES malignant neoplasms of contiguous sites, not elsewhere classified, whose point of origin cannot be determined
EXCLUDES malignant neoplasm:
lymphatic and hematopoietic tissue (200.0-208.9)
secondary sites (196.0-198.8)
unspecified site (199.0-199.1)

195.0 Head, face, and neck
Cheek NOS   Nose NOS
Jaw NOS   Supraclavicular region NOS

195.1 Thorax
Axilla   Intrathoracic NOS
Chest (wall) NOS

195.2 Abdomen
Intra-abdominal NOS
AHA: 2Q, '97, 3

195.3 Pelvis
Groin
Inguinal region NOS
Presacral region
Sacrococcygeal region
Sites overlapping systems within pelvis, as:
rectovaginal (septum)
rectovesical (septum)

195.4 Upper limb
195.5 Lower limb
195.8 Other specified sites
Back NOS   Trunk NOS
Flank NOS

√4th **196 Secondary and unspecified malignant neoplasm of lymph nodes**
EXCLUDES any malignant neoplasm of lymph nodes, specified as primary (200.0-202.9)
Hodgkin's disease (201.0-201.9)
lymphosarcoma (200.1)
other forms of lymphoma (202.0-202.9)
reticulosarcoma (200.0)
AHA: 2Q, '92, 3; M-J, '85, 3

NEOPLASMS

196.0–199.0

Lymph Nodes

- Head, neck, and face
- Thoracic ducts empty into
- Left subclavian vein
- Intrathoracic
- Axillary and upper limb
- Intraabdominal
- Thoracic duct (transmits lymph through diaphragm using one-way valves)
- Cisterna chyli — Nodes generally accompany large blood vessels
- Intrapelvic
- Inguinal and lower limb

196.0   Lymph nodes of head, face, and neck CC
    Cervical   Scalene
    Cervicofacial Supraclavicular
    CC Excl: 176.5, 195.8, 196.0-196.9, 199.0-199.1, 239.8-239.9

196.1   Intrathoracic lymph nodes CC
    Bronchopulmonary   Mediastinal
    Intercostal   Tracheobronchial
    CC Excl: See code 196.0

196.2   Intra-abdominal lymph nodes CC
    Intestinal   Retroperitoneal
    Mesenteric
    CC Excl: See code 196.0

196.3   Lymph nodes of axilla and upper limb CC
    Brachial   Infraclavicular
    Epitrochlear   Pectoral
    CC Excl: See code 196.0

196.5   Lymph nodes of inguinal region and lower limb CC
    Femoral   Popliteal
    Groin   Tibial
    CC Excl: See code 196.0

196.6   Intrapelvic lymph nodes CC
    Hypogastric   Obturator
    Iliac   Parametrial
    CC Excl: See code 196.0

196.8   Lymph nodes of multiple sites CC
    CC Excl: See code 196.0

196.9   Site unspecified CC
    Lymph nodes NOS
    CC Excl: See code 196.0

✓4th **197 Secondary malignant neoplasm of respiratory and digestive systems**
    EXCLUDES   lymph node metastasis (196.0-196.9)
    AHA: M-J, '85, 3

197.0   Lung CC
    Bronchus
    CC Excl: 195.8, 197.0, 197.3, 198.89, 199.0-199.1, 239.8-239.9
    AHA: 2Q, '99, 9

197.1   Mediastinum CC
    CC Excl: 195.8, 197.1, 197.3, 198.89, 199.0-199.1, 239.8-239.9

197.2   Pleura CC
    CC Excl: 195.8, 197.2-197.3, 198.89, 199.0-199.1, 239.8-239.9
    '89, 11

197.3   ...respiratory organs CC
    ...chea
    CC Excl: 195.8, 197.0-197.3, 198.89, 199.0-199.1, 239.8-239.9

197.4   Small intestine, including duodenum CC
    CC Excl: 195.8, 197.4, 197.8, 198.89, 199.0-199.1, 239.8-239.9

197.5   Large intestine and rectum CC
    CC Excl: 195.8, 197.5, 197.8, 198.89, 199.0-199.1, 239.8-239.9

197.6   Retroperitoneum and peritoneum CC
    CC Excl: 195.8, 197.6, 197.8, 198.89, 199.0-199.1, 239.8-239.9
    AHA: 4Q, '89, 11

197.7   Liver, specified as secondary CC
    CC Excl: 195.8, 197.7-197.8, 198.89, 199.0-199.1, 239.8-239.9

197.8   Other digestive organs and spleen CC
    CC Excl: 195.8, 197.4-197.8, 198.89, 199.0-199.1, 239.8-239.9
    AHA: 2Q, '97, 3; 2Q, '92, 3

✓4th **198 Secondary malignant neoplasm of other specified sites**
    EXCLUDES   lymph node metastasis (196.0-196.9)
    AHA: M-J, '85, 3

198.0   Kidney CC
    CC Excl: 195.8, 198.0-198.1, 198.89, 199.0-199.1, 239.8-239.9

198.1   Other urinary organs CC
    CC Excl: See code 198.0

198.2   Skin CC
    Skin of breast
    CC Excl: 195.8, 198.2, 198.89, 199.0-199.1, 239.8-239.9

198.3   Brain and spinal cord CC
    CC Excl: 195.8, 198.3, 198.89, 199.0-199.1, 239.8-239.9
    AHA: 3Q, '99, 7

198.4   Other parts of nervous system CC
    Meninges (cerebral) (spinal)
    CC Excl: 195.8, 198.4, 198.89, 199.0-199.1, 239.8-239.9
    AHA: J-F, '87, 7

198.5   Bone and bone marrow CC
    CC Excl: 195.8, 198.5, 198.89, 199.0-199.1, 239.8-239.9
    AHA: 3Q, '99, 5; 2Q, '92, 3; 1Q, '91, 16; 4Q, '89, 10
    DRG 239

198.6   Ovary CC ♀
    CC Excl: 195.8, 198.6, 198.89, 199.0-199.1, 239.8-239.9

198.7   Adrenal gland CC
    Suprarenal gland
    CC Excl: 195.8, 198.7, 198.89, 199.0-199.1, 239.8-239.9

✓5th **198.8   Other specified sites**
    198.81   Breast CC
        EXCLUDES   skin of breast (198.2)
        CC Excl: 195.8, 198.81, 198.89, 199.0-199.1, 239.8-239.9

    198.82   Genital organs CC
        CC Excl: 195.8, 198.82, 198.89, 199.0-199.1, 239.8-239.9

    198.89   Other CC
        EXCLUDES   retroperitoneal lymph nodes (196.2)
        CC Excl: 195.8, 198.89, 199.0-199.1, 239.8-239.9
        AHA: 2Q, '97, 4

✓4th **199 Malignant neoplasm without specification of site**
    199.0   Disseminated CC
        Carcinomatosis
        Generalized:
            cancer   } unspecified site
            malignancy   }   (primary)
        Multiple cancer   }   (secondary)
        CC Excl: See code 198.89
        AHA: 4Q, '89, 10

199.1 Other

Cancer ⎫ unspecified site
Carcinoma ⎬ (primary)
Malignancy ⎭ (secondary)

MALIGNANT NEOPLASM OF LYMPHATIC AND HEMATOPOIETIC TISSUE (200-208)

EXCLUDES secondary neoplasm of:
  bone marrow (198.5)
  spleen (197.8)
  secondary and unspecified neoplasm of lymph nodes (196.0-196.9)

The following fifth-digit subclassification is for use with categories 200-202:
  0 unspecified site, extranodal and solid organ sites
  1 lymph nodes of head, face, and neck
  2 intrathoracic lymph nodes
  3 intra-abdominal lymph nodes
  4 lymph nodes of axilla and upper limb
  5 lymph nodes of inguinal region and lower limb
  6 intrapelvic lymph nodes
  7 spleen
  8 lymph nodes of multiple sites

200 Lymphosarcoma and reticulosarcoma
AHA: 2Q, '92, 3; N-D, '86, 5

200.0 Reticulosarcoma
Lymphoma (malignant):
  histiocytic (diffuse):
    nodular
    pleomorphic cell type
    reticulum cell type
Reticulum cell sarcoma:
  NOS
  pleomorphic cell type

CC Excl: For code 200.00: 200.00-200.08, 239.8-239.9; **For code 200.01:** 200.00, 200.01, 200.08, 239.8-239.9; **For code 200.02:** 200.00, 200.02, 200.08, 239.8-239.9; **For code 200.03:** 200.00, 200.03, 200.08, 239.8-239.9; **For code 200.04:** 200.00, 200.04, 200.08, 239.8-239.9; **For code 200.05:** 200.00, 200.05, 200.08, 239.8-239.9; **For code 200.06:** 200.00, 200.06, 200.08, 239.8-239.9; **For code 200.07:** 200.00, 200.07-200.08, 239.8-239.9; **For code 200.08:** 200.00-200.08, 239.8-239.9

AHA: For Code 200.03: ▶3Q, '01, 12◀

DEF: Malignant lymphoma of primarily histolytic cells; commonly originates in reticuloendothelium of lymph nodes.

200.1 Lymphosarcoma
Lymphoblastoma (diffuse)   Lymphosarcoma:
Lymphoma (malignant):   NOS
  lymphoblastic (diffuse)   diffuse NOS
  lymphocytic (cell type)   lymphoblastic (diffuse)
    (diffuse)   lymphocytic (diffuse)
  lymphosarcoma type   prolymphocytic
EXCLUDES lymphosarcoma:
  follicular or nodular (202.0)
  mixed cell type (200.8)
  lymphosarcoma cell leukemia (207.8)

CC Excl: For code 200.10: 200.10-200.18, 239.8-239.9; **For code 200.11:** 200.10, 200.11, 200.18, 239.8-239.9; **For code 200.12:** 200.10, 200.12, 200.18, 239.8-239.9; **For code 200.13:** 200.10, 200.13, 200.18, 239.8-239.9; **For code 200.14:** 200.10, 200.14, 200.18, 239.8-239.9; **For code 200.15:** 200.10, 200.15, 200.18, 239.8-239.9; **For code 200.16:** 200.10, 200.16, 200.18, 239.8-239.9; **For code 200.17:** 200.10, 200.17-200.18, 239.8-239.9; **For code 200.18:** 200.10-200.18, 239.8-239.9

DEF: Malignant lymphoma created from anaplastic lymphoid cells resembling lymphocytes or lymphoblasts.

200.2 Burkitt's tumor or lymphoma
Malignant lymphoma, Burkitt's type

CC Excl: For code 200.20: 200.20-200.28, 239.8-239.9; **For code 200.21:** 200.20, 200.21, 200.28, 239.8-239.9; **For code 200.22:** 200.20, 200.22, 200.28, 239.8-239.9; **For code 200.23:** 200.20, 200.23, 200.28, 239.8-239.9; **For code 200.24:** 200.20, 200.24, 200.28, 239.8-239.9; **For code 200.25:** 200.20, 200.25, 200.28, 239.8-239.9; **For code 200.26:** 200.20, 200.26, 200.28, 239.8-239.9; **For code 200.27:** 200.20, 200.27-200.28, 239.8-239.9; **For code 200.28:** 200.20-200.28, 239.8-239.9

DEF: Large osteolytic lesion most common in jaw or as abdominal mass; usually found in central Africa but reported elsewhere.

200.8 Other named variants
Lymphoma (malignant):
  lymphoplasmacytoid type
  mixed lymphocytic-histiocytic (diffuse)
Lymphosarcoma, mixed cell type (diffuse)
Reticulolymphosarcoma (diffuse)

CC Excl: For code 200.80: 200.80-200.88, 239.8-239.9; **For code 200.81:** 200.80, 200.81, 200.88, 239.8-239.9; **For code 200.82:** 200.80, 200.82, 200.88, 239.8-239.9; **For code 200.83:** 200.80, 200.83, 200.88, 239.8-239.9; **For code 200.84:** 200.80, 200.84, 200.88, 239.8-239.9; **For code 200.85:** 200.80, 200.85, 200.88, 239.8-239.9; **For code 200.86:** 200.80, 200.86, 200.88, 239.8-239.9; **For code 200.87:** 200.80, 200.87-200.88, 239.8-239.9; **For code 200.88:** 200.80-200.88, 239.8-239.9

201 Hodgkin's disease
AHA: 2Q, '92, 3; N-D, '86, 5

DEF: Painless, progressive enlargement of lymph nodes, spleen and general lymph tissue; symptoms include anorexia, lassitude, weight loss, fever, pruritis, night sweats, anemia.

201.0 Hodgkin's paragranuloma
CC Excl: For code 201.00: 201.00-201.08, 201.90, 239.8-239.9; **For code 201.01:** 201.00, 201.01, 201.08, 201.90-201.91, 239.8-239.9; **For code 201.02:** 201.00, 201.02, 201.08, 201.90, 201.92, 239.8-239.9; **For code 201.03:** 201.00, 201.03, 201.08, 201.90, 201.93, 239.8-239.9; **For code 201.04:** 201.00, 201.04, 201.08, 201.90, 201.94, 239.8-239.9; **For code 201.05:** 201.00, 201.05, 201.08, 201.90, 201.95, 239.8-239.9; **For code 201.06:** 201.00, 201.06, 201.08, 201.90, 201.96, 239.8-239.9; **For code 201.07:** 201.00, 201.07-201.08, 201.90, 201.97, 239.8-239.9; **For code 201.08:** 201.00-201.08, 201.90, 201.98, 239.8-239.9

201.1 Hodgkin's granuloma
CC Excl: For code 201.10: 201.10-201.18, 201.90, 201.98, 239.8-239.9; **For code 201.11:** 201.10, 201.11, 201.18, 201.90-201.91, 201.98, 239.8-239.9; **For code 201.12:** 201.10, 201.12, 201.18, 201.90, 201.92, 201.98, 239.8-239.9; **For code 201.13:** 201.10, 201.13, 201.18, 201.90, 201.93, 201.98, 239.8-239.9; **For code 201.14:** 201.10, 201.14, 201.18, 201.90, 201.94, 201.98, 239.8-239.9; **For code 201.15:** 201.10, 201.15, 201.18, 201.90, 201.95, 201.98, 239.8-239.9; **For code 201.16:** 201.10, 201.16, 201.18, 201.90, 201.96, 201.98, 239.8-239.9; **For code 201.17:** 201.10, 201.17-201.18, 201.90, 201.97-201.98, 239.8-239.9; **For code 201.18:** 201.10-201.18, 201.90, 201.98, 239.8-239.9

AHA: 2Q, '99, 7

201.2 Hodgkin's sarcoma
CC Excl: For code 201.20: 201.20-201.28, 201.90, 201.98, 239.8-239.9; **For code 201.21:** 201.20, 201.21, 201.28, 201.90-201.91, 201.98, 239.8-239.9; **For code 201.22:** 201.20, 201.22, 201.28, 201.90, 201.92, 201.98, 239.8-239.9; **For code 201.23:** 201.20, 201.23, 201.28, 201.90, 201.93, 201.98, 239.8-239.9; **For code 201.24:** 201.20, 201.24, 201.28, 201.90, 201.94, 201.98, 239.8-239.9; **For code 201.25:** 201.20, 201.25, 201.28, 201.90, 201.95, 201.98, 239.8-239.9; **For code 201.26:** 201.20, 201.26, 201.28, 201.90, 201.96, 201.98, 239.8-239.9; **For code 201.27:** 201.20, 201.27-201.28, 201.90, 201.97-201.98, 239.8-239.9; **For code 201.28:** 201.20-201.28, 201.90, 201.98, 239.8-239.9

§ Requires fifth-digit. See beginning of section 200–208 for codes and definitions.

NEOPLASMS

201.4 Lymphocytic-histiocytic predominance
CC Excl: For code 201.40: 201.40-201.48, 201.90, 201.98, 239.8-239.9;
For code 201.41: 201.40, 201.41, 201.48, 201.90-201.91, 201.98, 239.8-239.9; For code 201.42: 201.40, 201.42, 201.48, 201.90, 201.92, 201.98, 239.8-239.9; For code 201.43: 201.40, 201.43, 201.48, 201.90, 201.93, 201.98, 239.8-239.9; For code 201.44: 201.40, 201.44, 201.48, 201.90, 201.94, 201.98, 239.8-239.9; For code 201.45: 201.40, 201.45, 201.48, 201.90, 201.95, 201.98, 239.8-239.9; For code 201.46: 201.40, 201.46, 201.48, 201.90, 201.96, 201.98, 239.8-239.9; For code 201.47: 201.40, 201.47-201.48, 201.90, 201.97-201.98, 239.8-239.9; For code 201.48: 201.40-201.48, 201.90, 201.98, 239.8-239.9

201.5 Nodular sclerosis
Hodgkin's disease, nodular sclerosis:
  NOS
  cellular phase

CC Excl: For code 201.50: 201.50-201.58, 201.90, 201.98, 239.8-239.9; For code 201.51: 201.50, 201.51, 201.58, 201.90-201.91, 201.98, 239.8-239.9; For code 201.52: 201.50, 201.52, 201.58, 201.90, 201.92, 201.98, 239.8-239.9; For code 201.53: 201.50, 201.53, 201.58, 201.90, 201.93, 201.98, 239.8-239.9; For code 201.54: 201.50, 201.54, 201.58, 201.90, 201.94, 201.98, 239.8-239.9; For code 201.55: 201.50, 201.55, 201.58, 201.90, 201.95, 201.98, 239.8-239.9; For code 201.56: 201.50, 201.56, 201.58, 201.90, 201.96, 201.98, 239.8-239.9; For code 201.57: 201.50, 201.57-201.58, 201.90, 201.97-201.98, 239.8-239.9; For code 201.58: 201.50-201.58, 201.90, 201.98, 239.8-239.9

201.6 Mixed cellularity
CC Excl: For code 201.60: 201.60-201.68, 201.90, 201.98, 239.8-239.9; For code 201.61: 201.60, 201.61, 201.68, 201.90-201.91, 201.98, 239.8-239.9; For code 201.62: 201.60, 201.62, 201.68, 201.90, 201.92, 201.98, 239.8-239.9; For code 201.63: 201.60, 201.63, 201.68, 201.90, 201.93, 201.98, 239.8-239.9; For code 201.64: 201.60, 201.64, 201.68, 201.90, 201.94, 201.98, 239.8-239.9; For code 201.65: 201.60, 201.65, 201.68, 201.90, 201.95, 201.98, 239.8-239.9; For code 201.66: 201.60, 201.66, 201.68, 201.90, 201.96, 201.98, 239.8-239.9; For code 201.67: 201.60, 201.67-201.68, 201.90, 201.97-201.98, 239.8-239.9; For code 201.68: 201.60-201.68, 201.90, 201.98, 239.8-239.9

201.7 Lymphocytic depletion
Hodgkin's disease, lymphocytic depletion:
  NOS
  diffuse fibrosis
  reticular type

CC Excl: For code 201.70: 201.70-201.78, 201.90, 201.98, 239.8-239.9; For code 201.71: 201.70, 201.71, 201.78, 201.91, 201.98, 239.8-239.9; For code 201.72: 201.70, 201.72, 201.78, 201.92, 201.98, 239.8-239.9; For code 201.73: 201.70, 201.73, 201.78, 201.93, 201.98, 239.8-239.9; For code 201.74: 201.70, 201.74, 201.78, 201.94, 201.98, 239.8-239.9; For code 201.75: 201.70, 201.75, 201.78, 201.95, 201.98, 239.8-239.9; For code 201.76: 201.70, 201.76, 201.78, 201.96, 201.98, 239.8-239.9; For code 201.77: 201.70, 201.77-201.78, 201.97-201.98, 239.8-239.9; For code 201.78: 201.70-201.78, 201.98, 239.8-239.9

201.9 Hodgkin's disease, unspecified
Hodgkin's:
  disease NOS
  lymphoma NOS
Malignant:
  lymphogranuloma
  lymphogranulomatosis

CC Excl: For code 201.90: 201.90-201.98, 239.8-239.9; For code 201.91: 201.90, 201.91, 201.98, 239.8-239.9; For code 201.92: 201.90, 201.92, 201.98, 239.8-239.9; For code 201.93: 201.90, 201.93, 201.98, 239.8-239.9; For code 201.94: 201.90, 201.94, 201.98, 239.8-239.9; For code 201.95: 201.90, 201.95, 201.98, 239.8-239.9; For code 201.96: 201.90, 201.96, 201.98, 239.8-239.9; For code 201.97: 201.90, 201.97-201.98, 239.8-239.9; For code 201.98: 201.90-201.98, 239.8-239.9

202 Other malignant neoplasms of lymphoid and histiocytic tissue
AHA: 2Q, '92, 3; N-D, '86, 5

202.0 Nodular lymphoma
Brill-Symmers disease
Lymphoma:
  follicular (giant)
  lymphocytic, nodular
Lymphosarcoma:
  follicular (giant)
  nodular
Reticulosarcoma, follicular or nodular

CC Excl: For code 202.00: 202.00-202.08, 202.80, 202.90, 239.8-239.9; For code 202.01: 202.00, 202.01, 202.08, 202.81, 202.91, 239.8-239.9; For code 202.02: 202.00, 202.02, 202.08, 202.82, 202.92, 239.8-239.9; For code 202.03: 202.00, 202.03, 202.08, 202.83, 202.93, 239.8-239.9; For code 202.04: 202.00, 202.04, 202.08, 202.84, 202.94, 239.8-239.9; For code 202.05: 202.00, 202.05, 202.08, 202.85, 202.95, 239.8-239.9; For code 202.06: 202.00, 202.06, 202.08, 202.86, 202.96, 239.8-239.9; For code 202.07: 202.00, 202.07-202.08, 202.87, 202.97, 239.8-239.9; For code 202.08: 202.00-202.08, 202.88, 202.98, 239.8-239.9

DEF: Lymphomatous cells clustered into nodules within the lymph node; usually occurs in older adults and may involve all nodes and possibly extranodal sites.

202.1 Mycosis fungoides
CC Excl: For code 202.10: 202.10-202.18, 202.80, 202.90, 239.8-239.9; For code 202.11: 202.10, 202.11, 202.18, 202.81, 202.91, 239.8-239.9; For code 202.12: 202.10, 202.12, 202.18, 202.82, 202.92, 239.8-239.9; For code 202.13: 202.10, 202.13, 202.18, 202.83, 202.93, 239.8-239.9; For code 202.14: 202.10, 202.14, 202.18, 202.84, 202.94, 239.8-239.9; For code 202.15: 202.10, 202.15, 202.18, 202.85, 202.95, 239.8-239.9; For code 202.16: 202.10, 202.16, 202.18, 202.86, 202.96, 239.8-239.9; For code 202.17: 202.10, 202.17-202.18, 202.87, 202.97, 239.8-239.9; For code 202.18: 202.10-202.18, 202.88, 202.98, 239.8-239.9

AHA: 2Q, '92, 4

DEF: Type of cutaneous T-cell lymphoma; may evolve into generalized lymphoma; formerly thought to be of fungoid origin.

202.2 Sézary's disease
CC Excl: For code 202.20: 202.20-202.28, 202.80, 202.90, 239.8-239.9; For code 202.21: 202.20, 202.21, 202.28, 202.81, 202.91, 239.8-239.9; For code 202.22: 202.20, 202.22, 202.28, 202.82, 202.92, 239.8-239.9; For code 202.23: 202.20, 202.23, 202.28, 202.83, 202.93, 239.8-239.9; For code 202.24: 202.20, 202.24, 202.28, 202.84, 202.94, 239.8-239.9; For code 202.25: 202.20, 202.25, 202.28, 202.85, 202.95, 239.8-239.9; For code 202.26: 202.20, 202.26, 202.28, 202.86, 202.96, 239.8-239.9; For code 202.27: 202.20, 202.27-202.28, 202.87, 202.97, 239.8-239.9; For code 202.28: 202.20-202.28, 202.88, 202.98, 239.8-239.9

AHA: 2Q, '99, 7

DEF: Type of cutaneous T-cell lymphoma with erythroderma, intense pruritus, peripheral lymphadenopathy, abnormal hyperchromatic mononuclear cells in skin, lymph nodes and peripheral blood.

202.3 Malignant histiocytosis
Histiocytic medullary reticulosis
Malignant:
  reticuloendotheliosis
  reticulosis

CC Excl: For code 202.30: 202.30-202.38, 202.80, 202.90, 239.8-239.9; For code 202.31: 202.30, 202.31, 202.38, 202.81, 202.91, 239.8-239.9; For code 202.32: 202.30, 202.32, 202.38, 202.82, 202.92, 239.8-239.9; For code 202.33: 202.30, 202.33, 202.38, 202.83, 202.93, 239.8-239.9; For code 202.34: 202.30, 202.34, 202.38, 202.84, 202.94, 239.8-239.9; For code 202.35: 202.30, 202.35, 202.38, 202.85, 202.95, 239.8-239.9; For code 202.36: 202.30, 202.36, 202.38, 202.86, 202.96, 239.8-239.9; For code 202.37: 202.30, 202.37-202.38, 202.87, 202.97, 239.8-239.9; For code 202.38: 202.30-202.38, 202.88, 202.98, 239.8-239.9

NEOPLASMS

§ ✓5th 202.4 Leukemic reticuloendotheliosis [CC]
Hairy-cell leukemia

CC Excl: For code 202.40: 202.40-202.48, 202.80, 202.90, 239.8-239.9;
For code 202.41: 202.40, 202.41, 202.48, 202.81, 202.91, 239.8-239.9;
For code 202.42: 202.40, 202.42, 202.48, 202.82, 202.92, 239.8-239.9;
For code 202.43: 202.40, 202.43, 202.48, 202.83, 202.93, 239.8-239.9;
For code 202.44: 202.40, 202.44, 202.48, 202.84, 202.94, 239.8-239.9;
For code 202.45: 202.40, 202.45, 202.48, 202.85, 202.95, 239.8-239.9;
For code 202.46: 202.40, 202.46, 202.48, 202.86, 202.96, 239.8-239.9;
For code 202.47: 202.40, 202.47-202.48, 202.87, 202.97, 239.8-239.9;
For code 202.48: 202.40-202.48, 202.88, 202.98, 239.8-239.9

DEF: Chronic leukemia with large, mononuclear cells with "hairy" appearance in marrow, spleen, liver, blood.

§ ✓5th 202.5 Letterer-Siwe disease [CC]
Acute:
  differentiated progressive histiocytosis
  histiocytosis X (progressive)
  infantile reticuloendotheliosis
  reticulosis of infancy

EXCLUDES Hand-Schüller-Christian disease (277.8)
          histiocytosis (acute) (chronic) (277.8)
          histiocytosis X (chronic) (277.8)

CC Excl: For code 202.50: 202.50-202.58, 202.80, 202.90, 239.8-239.9;
For code 202.51: 202.50, 202.51, 202.58, 202.81, 202.91, 239.8-239.9;
For code 202.52: 202.50, 202.52, 202.58, 202.82, 202.92, 239.8-239.9;
For code 202.53: 202.50, 202.53, 202.58, 202.83, 202.93, 239.8-239.9;
For code 202.54: 202.50, 202.54, 202.58, 202.84, 202.94, 239.8-239.9;
For code 202.55: 202.50, 202.55, 202.58, 202.85, 202.95, 239.8-239.9;
For code 202.56: 202.50, 202.56, 202.58, 202.86, 202.96, 239.8-239.9;
For code 202.57: 202.50, 202.57-202.58, 202.87, 202.97, 239.8-239.9;
For code 202.58: 202.50-202.58, 202.88, 202.98, 239.8-239.9

DEF: A recessive reticuloendotheliosis of early childhood, with a hemorrhagic tendency, eczema-like skin eruption, hepatosplenomegaly, including lymph node enlargement, and progressive anemia; it is often a fatal disease with no established cause.

§ ✓5th 202.6 Malignant mast cell tumors [CC]
Malignant: Mast cell sarcoma
  mastocytoma   Systemic tissue mast
  mastocytosis   cell disease

EXCLUDES mast cell leukemia (207.8)

CC Excl: For code 202.60: 202.60-202.68, 202.80, 202.90, 239.8-239.9;
For code 202.61: 202.60, 202.61, 202.68, 202.81, 202.91, 239.8-239.9;
For code 202.62: 202.60, 202.62, 202.68, 202.82, 202.92, 239.8-239.9;
For code 202.63: 202.60, 202.63, 202.68, 202.83, 202.93, 239.8-239.9;
For code 202.64: 202.60, 202.64, 202.68, 202.84, 202.94, 239.8-239.9;
For code 202.65: 202.60, 202.65, 202.68, 202.85, 202.95, 239.8-239.9;
For code 202.66: 202.60, 202.66, 202.68, 202.86, 202.96, 239.8-239.9;
For code 202.67: 202.60, 202.67-202.68, 202.87, 202.97, 239.8-239.9;
For code 202.68: 202.60-202.68, 202.88, 202.98, 239.8-239.9

§ ✓5th 202.8 Other lymphomas [CC] [HIV]
Lymphoma (malignant):
  NOS
  diffuse

EXCLUDES benign lymphoma (229.0)

CC Excl: For code 202.80: 202.80-202.88, 202.90, 239.8-239.9;
For code 202.81: 202.80, 202.81, 202.88, 202.91, 239.8-239.9; For code 202.82: 202.80, 202.82, 202.88, 202.92, 239.8-239.9; For code 202.83: 202.80, 202.83, 202.88, 202.93, 239.8-239.9; For code 202.84: 202.80, 202.84, 202.88, 202.94, 239.8-239.9; For code 202.85: 202.80, 202.85, 202.88, 202.95, 239.8-239.9; For code 202.86: 202.80, 202.86, 202.88, 202.96, 239.8-239.9; For code 202.87: 202.80, 202.87-202.88, 202.97, 239.8-239.9; For code 202.88: 202.80-202.88, 202.98, 239.8-239.9

AHA: 2Q, '92, 4

§ ✓5th 202.9 Other and unspecified malignant neoplasms of lymphoid and histiocytic tissue [CC]
Malignant neoplasm of bone marrow NOS

CC Excl: For code 202.90: 202.90-202.98, 239.8-239.9; For code 202.91: 202.90, 202.91, 202.98, 239.8-239.9; For code 202.92: 202.90, 202.92, 202.98, 239.8-239.9; For code 202.93: 202.90, 202.93, 202.98, 239.8-239.9; For code 202.94: 202.90, 202.94, 202.98, 239.8-239.9; For code 202.95: 202.90, 202.95, 202.98, 239.8-239.9; For code 202.96: 202.90, 202.96, 202.98, 239.8-239.9; For code 202.97: 202.90, 202.97-202.98, 239.8-239.9; For code 202.98: 202.90-202.98, 239.8-239.9

✓4th 203 Multiple myeloma and immunoproliferative neoplasms
AHA: 4Q, '91, 26

The following fifth-digit subclassification is for use with category 203:
  0 without mention of remission
  1 in remission

✓5th 203.0 Multiple myeloma [CC]
Kahler's disease   Myelomatosis
EXCLUDES solitary myeloma (238.6)

CC Excl: 203.00-203.81, 204.00-204.91, 205.00-205.91, 206.00-206.91, 207.00-207.81, 208.00-208.91, 239.8-239.9

AHA: 1Q, '96, 16; 4Q, '89, 10

✓5th 203.1 Plasma cell leukemia [CC]
Plasmacytic leukemia
CC Excl: See code 203.0

AHA: 4Q, '90, 26; S-O, '86, 12

✓5th 203.8 Other immunoproliferative neoplasms [CC]
CC Excl: See code 203.0

AHA: 4Q, '90, 26; S-O, '86, 12

✓4th 204 Lymphoid leukemia
INCLUDES leukemia:
            lymphatic
            lymphoblastic
            lymphocytic
            lymphogenous

AHA: 3Q, '93, 4

The following fifth-digit subclassification is for use with category 204:
  0 without mention of remission
  1 in remission

✓5th 204.0 Acute [CC]
EXCLUDES acute exacerbation of chronic lymphoid leukemia (204.1)

CC Excl: See code 203.0

AHA: 3Q, '99, 6

✓5th 204.1 Chronic [CC]
CC Excl: See code 203.0

✓5th 204.2 Subacute [CC]
CC Excl: See code 203.0

✓5th 204.8 Other lymphoid leukemia [CC]
Aleukemic leukemia: Aleukemic leukemia:
  lymphatic   lymphoid
  lymphocytic
CC Excl: See code 203.0

✓5th 204.9 Unspecified lymphoid leukemia [CC]
CC Excl: See code 203.0

---

§ Requires fifth-digit. See beginning of section 200–208 for codes and definitions.

NEOPLASMS

205 Myeloid leukemia
INCLUDES leukemia:
- granulocytic
- myeloblastic
- myelocytic
- myelogenous
- myelomonocytic
- myelosclerotic
- myelosis

AHA: 3Q, '93, 3; 4Q, '91, 26; 4Q, '90, 3; M-J, '85, 18

The following fifth-digit subclassification is for use with category 205:
- 0 without mention of remission
- 1 in remission

√5th 205.0 Acute CC
Acute promyelocytic leukemia
EXCLUDES acute exacerbation of chronic myeloid leukemia (205.1)
CC Excl: See code 203.0

√5th 205.1 Chronic CC
Eosinophilic leukemia   Neutrophilic leukemia
CC Excl: See code 203.0

AHA: 1Q, 00, 6; J-A, '85, 13

√5th 205.2 Subacute CC
CC Excl: See code 203.0

√5th 205.3 Myeloid sarcoma CC
Chloroma   Granulocytic sarcoma
CC Excl: See code 203.0

√5th 205.8 Other myeloid leukemia CC
Aleukemic leukemia: Aleukemic leukemia:
- granulocytic   myeloid
- myelogenous   Aleukemic myelosis

CC Excl: See code 203.0

√5th 205.9 Unspecified myeloid leukemia CC
CC Excl: See code 203.0

206 Monocytic leukemia
INCLUDES leukemia:
- histiocytic
- monoblastic
- monocytoid

The following fifth-digit subclassification is for use with category 206:
- 0 without mention of remission
- 1 in remission

√5th 206.0 Acute CC
EXCLUDES acute exacerbation of chronic monocytic leukemia (206.1)
CC Excl: See code 203.0

√5th 206.1 Chronic CC
CC Excl: See code 203.0

√5th 206.2 Subacute CC
CC Excl: See code 203.0

√5th 206.8 Other monocytic leukemia CC
Aleukemic:
- monocytic leukemia
- monocytoid leukemia
CC Excl: See code 203.0

√5th 206.9 Unspecified monocytic leukemia CC
CC Excl: See code 203.0

207 Other specified leukemia
EXCLUDES leukemic reticuloendotheliosis (202.4)
plasma cell leukemia (203.1)

The following fifth-digit subclassification is for use with category 207:
- 0 without mention of remission
- 1 in remission

√5th 207.0 Acute erythremia and erythroleukemia CC
Acute erythremic myelosis
Di Guglielmo's disease
Erythremic myelosis
CC Excl: See code 203.0

DEF: Erythremia: polycythemia vera.

DEF: Erythroleukemia: a malignant blood dyscrasia (a myeloproliferative disorder).

√5th 207.1 Chronic erythremia CC
Heilmeyer-Schöner disease
CC Excl: See code 203.0

√5th 207.2 Megakaryocytic leukemia CC
Megakaryocytic myelosis   Thrombocytic leukemia
CC Excl: See code 203.0

√5th 207.8 Other specified leukemia CC
Lymphosarcoma cell leukemia
CC Excl: See code 203.0

208 Leukemia of unspecified cell type
The following fifth-digit subclassification is for use with category 208:
- 0 without mention of remission
- 1 in remission

√5th 208.0 Acute CC
Acute leukemia NOS   Stem cell leukemia
Blast cell leukemia
EXCLUDES acute exacerbation of chronic unspecified leukemia (208.1)
CC Excl: See code 203.0

√5th 208.1 Chronic CC
Chronic leukemia NOS
CC Excl: See code 203.0

√5th 208.2 Subacute CC
Subacute leukemia NOS
CC Excl: See code 203.0

√5th 208.8 Other leukemia of unspecified cell type CC
CC Excl: See code 203.0

√5th 208.9 Unspecified leukemia CC
Leukemia NOS
CC Excl: See code 203.0

BENIGN NEOPLASMS (210-229)

210 Benign neoplasm of lip, oral cavity, and pharynx
EXCLUDES cyst (of):
- jaw (526.0-526.2, 526.89)
- oral soft tissue (528.4)
- radicular (522.8)

210.0 Lip
Frenulum labii
Lip (inner aspect) (mucosa) (vermilion border)
EXCLUDES labial commissure (210.4)
skin of lip (216.0)

210.1 Tongue
Lingual tonsil

2002 Ingenix, Inc.

NEOPLASMS

210.2 **Major salivary glands**
Gland:
 parotid
 sublingual
Gland:
 submandibular
EXCLUDES benign neoplasms of minor salivary glands:
 NOS (210.4)
 buccal mucosa (210.4)
 lips (210.0)
 palate (hard) (soft) (210.4)
 tongue (210.1)
 tonsil, palatine (210.5)

210.3 **Floor of mouth**

210.4 **Other and unspecified parts of mouth**
Gingiva
Gum (upper) (lower)
Labial commissure
Oral cavity NOS
Oral mucosa
Palate (hard) (soft)
Uvula
EXCLUDES benign odontogenic neoplasms of bone (213.0-213.1)
developmental odontogenic cysts (526.0)
mucosa of lips (210.0)
nasopharyngeal [posterior] [superior] surface of soft palate (210.7)

210.5 **Tonsil**
Tonsil (faucial) (palatine)
EXCLUDES lingual tonsil (210.1)
pharyngeal tonsil (210.7)
tonsillar:
 fossa (210.6)
 pillars (210.6)

210.6 **Other parts of oropharynx**
Branchial cleft or vestiges
Epiglottis, anterior aspect
Fauces NOS
Mesopharynx NOS
Tonsillar:
 fossa
 pillars
Vallecula
EXCLUDES epiglottis:
 NOS (212.1)
 suprahyoid portion (212.1)

210.7 **Nasopharynx**
Adenoid tissue
Lymphadenoid tissue
Pharyngeal tonsil
Posterior nasal septum

210.8 **Hypopharynx**
Arytenoid fold
Laryngopharynx
Postcricoidregion
Pyriform fossa

210.9 **Pharynx, unspecified**
Throat NOS

211 **Benign neoplasm of other parts of digestive system**

211.0 **Esophagus**

211.1 **Stomach**
Body
Cardia } of stomach
Fundus
Cardiac orifice
Pylorus

211.2 **Duodenum, jejunum, and ileum**
Small intestine NOS
EXCLUDES ampulla of Vater (211.5)
ileocecal valve (211.3)

211.3 **Colon**
Appendix
Cecum
Ileocecal valve
Large intestine NOS
EXCLUDES rectosigmoid junction (211.4)
AHA: ▶4Q, '01, 56◀

211.4 **Rectum and anal canal**
Anal canal or sphincter
Anus NOS
Rectosigmoid junction
EXCLUDES anus:
 margin (216.5)
 skin (216.5)
 perianal skin (216.5)

211.5 **Liver and biliary passages**
Ampulla of Vater
Common bile duct
Cystic duct
Gallbladder
Hepatic duct
Sphincter of Oddi

211.6 **Pancreas, except islets of Langerhans**

211.7 **Islets of Langerhans**
Islet cell tumor
Use additional code to identify any functional activity

211.8 **Retroperitoneum and peritoneum**
Mesentery
Mesocolon
Omentum
Retroperitoneal tissue

211.9 **Other and unspecified site**
Alimentary tract NOS
Digestive system NOS
Gastrointestinal tract NOS
Intestinal tract NOS
Intestine NOS
Spleen, not elsewhere classified

212 **Benign neoplasm of respiratory and intrathoracic organs**

212.0 **Nasal cavities, middle ear, and accessory sinuses**
Cartilage of nose
Eustachian tube
Nares
Septum of nose
Sinus:
 ethmoidal
 frontal
 maxillary
 sphenoidal
EXCLUDES auditory canal (external) (216.2)
bone of:
 ear (213.0)
 nose [turbinates] (213.0)
cartilage of ear (215.0)
ear (external) (skin) (216.2)
nose NOS (229.8)
 skin (216.3)
olfactory bulb (225.1)
polyp of:
 accessory sinus (471.8)
 ear (385.30-385.35)
 nasal cavity (471.0)
 posterior margin of septum and choanae (210.7)

212.1 **Larynx**
Cartilage:
 arytenoid
 cricoid
 cuneiform
 thyroid
Epiglottis (suprahyoid portion) NOS
Glottis
Vocal cords (false) (true)
EXCLUDES epiglottis, anterior aspect (210.6)
polyp of vocal cord or larynx (478.4)

212.2 **Trachea**

212.3 **Bronchus and lung**
Carina
Hilus of lung

212.4 **Pleura**

212.5 **Mediastinum**

212.6 **Thymus**

212.7 **Heart**
EXCLUDES great vessels (215.4)

212.8 **Other specified sites**

212.9 **Site unspecified**
Respiratory organ NOS
Upper respiratory tract NOS
EXCLUDES intrathoracic NOS (229.8)
thoracic NOS (229.8)

213 **Benign neoplasm of bone and articular cartilage**
INCLUDES cartilage (articular) (joint)
periosteum
EXCLUDES cartilage of:
 ear (215.0)
 eyelid (215.0)
 larynx (212.1)
cartilage of:
 nose (212.0)
 exostosis NOS (726.91)
 synovia (215.0-215.9)

213.0 **Bones of skull and face**
EXCLUDES lower jaw bone (213.1)

NEOPLASMS

213.1 Lower jaw bone
213.2 Vertebral column, excluding sacrum and coccyx
213.3 Ribs, sternum, and clavicle
213.4 Scapula and long bones of upper limb
213.5 Short bones of upper limb
213.6 Pelvic bones, sacrum, and coccyx
213.7 Long bones of lower limb
213.8 Short bones of lower limb
213.9 Bone and articular cartilage, site unspecified

√4th 214 Lipoma
INCLUDES:
- angiolipoma
- fibrolipoma
- hibernoma
- lipoma (fetal) (infiltrating) (intramuscular)
- myelolipoma
- myxolipoma

DEF: Benign tumor frequently composed of mature fat cells; may occasionally be composed of fetal fat cells.

214.0 Skin and subcutaneous tissue of face
214.1 Other skin and subcutaneous tissue
214.2 Intrathoracic organs
214.3 Intra-abdominal organs
214.4 Spermatic cord ♂
214.8 Other specified sites
   AHA: 3Q, '94, 7
214.9 Lipoma, unspecified site

√4th 215 Other benign neoplasm of connective and other soft tissue
INCLUDES:
- blood vessel
- bursa
- fascia
- ligament
- muscle
- peripheral, sympathetic, and parasympathetic nerves and ganglia
- synovia
- tendon (sheath)

EXCLUDES:
- cartilage:
  - articular (213.0-213.9)
  - larynx (212.1)
  - nose (212.0)
- connective tissue of:
  - breast (217)
  - internal organ, except lipoma and hemangioma—code to benign neoplasm of the site
- lipoma (214.0-214.9)

215.0 Head, face, and neck
215.2 Upper limb, including shoulder
215.3 Lower limb, including hip
215.4 Thorax
   EXCLUDES: heart (212.7)
   mediastinum (212.5)
   thymus (212.6)
215.5 Abdomen
   Abdominal wall   Hypochondrium
215.6 Pelvis
   Buttock   Inguinal region
   Groin   Perineum
   EXCLUDES: uterine:
     leiomyoma (218.0-218.9)
     ligament, any (221.0)
215.7 Trunk, unspecified
   Back NOS   Flank NOS
215.8 Other specified sites
215.9 Site unspecified

√4th 216 Benign neoplasm of skin
INCLUDES:
- blue nevus   pigmented nevus
- dermatofibroma   syringoadenoma
- hydrocystoma   syringoma

EXCLUDES: skin of genital organs (221.0-222.9)
AHA: 1Q, '00, 21

216.0 Skin of lip
   EXCLUDES: vermilion border of lip (210.0)
216.1 Eyelid, including canthus
   EXCLUDES: cartilage of eyelid (215.0)
216.2 Ear and external auditory canal
   Auricle (ear)   External meatus
   Auricular canal, external Pinna
   EXCLUDES: cartilage of ear (215.0)
216.3 Skin of other and unspecified parts of face
   Cheek, external   Nose, external
   Eyebrow   Temple
216.4 Scalp and skin of neck
   AHA: 3Q, '91, 12
216.5 Skin of trunk, except scrotum
   Axillary fold   Skin of:
   Perianal skin   buttock
   Skin of: chest wall
     abdominal wall   groin
     anus   perineum
     back   Umbilicus
     breast
   EXCLUDES: anal canal (211.4)
     anus NOS (211.4)
     skin of scrotum (222.4)
216.6 Skin of upper limb, including shoulder
216.7 Skin of lower limb, including hip
216.8 Other specified sites of skin
216.9 Skin, site unspecified

217 Benign neoplasm of breast
Breast (male) (female):   Breast (male) (female):
  connective tissue   soft parts
  glandular tissue
EXCLUDES: adenofibrosis (610.2)
  benign cyst of breast (610.0)
  fibrocystic disease (610.1)
  skin of breast (216.5)
AHA: 1Q, '00, 4

√4th 218 Uterine leiomyoma
INCLUDES: fibroid (bleeding) (uterine)
  uterine:
    fibromyoma
    myoma

DEF: Benign tumor primarily derived from uterine smooth muscle tissue; may contain fibrous, fatty, or epithelial tissue; also called uterine fibroid or myoma.

218.0 Submucous leiomyoma of uterus ♀
218.1 Intramural leiomyoma of uterus ♀
   Interstitial leiomyoma of uterus
218.2 Subserous leiomyoma of uterus ♀

Types of Uterine Fibroids

Cornual — Pedunculated
Uterine cavity — Intramural
Subserosal — Submucosal
Cervical

Tabular List — NEOPLASMS — 218.9–226

- **218.9** Leiomyoma of uterus, unspecified ♀
- √4th **219** Other benign neoplasm of uterus
  - **219.0** Cervix uteri ♀
  - **219.1** Corpus uteri ♀
    - Endometrium   Myometrium
    - Fundus
  - **219.8** Other specified parts of uterus ♀
  - **219.9** Uterus, part unspecified ♀
- **220** Benign neoplasm of ovary
  - Use additional code to identify any functional activity (256.0-256.1)
  - EXCLUDES cyst:
    - corpus albicans (620.2)
    - corpus luteum (620.1)
    - endometrial (617.1)
    - follicular (atretic) (620.0)
    - graafian follicle (620.0)
    - ovarian NOS (620.2)
    - retention (620.2)
- √4th **221** Benign neoplasm of other female genital organs
  - INCLUDES adenomatous polyp
    - benign teratoma
  - EXCLUDES cyst:
    - epoophoron (752.11)
    - fimbrial (752.11)
    - Gartner's duct (752.11)
    - parovarian (752.11)
  - **221.0** Fallopian tube and uterine ligaments ♀
    - Oviduct
    - Parametruim
    - Uterine ligament (broad) (round) (uterosacral)
    - Uterine tube
  - **221.1** Vagina ♀
  - **221.2** Vulva ♀
    - Clitoris
    - External female genitalia NOS
    - Greater vestibular [Bartholin's] gland
    - Labia (majora) (minora)
    - Pudendum
    - EXCLUDES Bartholin's (duct) (gland) cyst (616.2)
  - **221.8** Other specified sites of female genital organs ♀
  - **221.9** Female genital organ, site unspecified ♀
    - Female genitourinary tract NOS
- √4th **222** Benign neoplasm of male genital organs
  - **222.0** Testis ♂
    - Use additional code to identify any functional activity
  - **222.1** Penis ♂
    - Corpus cavernosum   Prepuce
    - Glans penis
  - **222.2** Prostate ♂
    - EXCLUDES adenomatous hyperplasia of prostate (600.2)
      - prostatic:
        - adenoma (600.2)
        - enlargement (600.0)
        - hypertrophy (600.0)
  - **222.3** Epididymis ♂
  - **222.4** Scrotum ♂
    - Skin of scrotum
  - **222.8** Other specified sites of male genital organs ♂
    - Seminal vesicle
    - Spermatic cord
  - **222.9** Male genital organ, site unspecified ♂
    - Male genitourinary tract NOS
- √4th **223** Benign neoplasm of kidney and other urinary organs
  - **223.0** Kidney, except pelvis
    - Kidney NOS
    - EXCLUDES renal:
      - calyces (223.1)
      - pelvis (223.1)
  - **223.1** Renal pelvis
  - **223.2** Ureter
    - EXCLUDES ureteric orifice of bladder (223.3)
  - **223.3** Bladder
  - √5th **223.8** Other specified sites of urinary organs
    - **223.81** Urethra
      - EXCLUDES urethral orifice of bladder (223.3)
    - **223.89** Other
      - Paraurethral glands
  - **223.9** Urinary organ, site unspecified
    - Urinary system NOS
- √4th **224** Benign neoplasm of eye
  - EXCLUDES cartilage of eyelid (215.0)
    - eyelid (skin) (216.1)
    - optic nerve (225.1)
    - orbital bone (213.0)
  - **224.0** Eyeball, except conjunctiva, cornea, retina, and choroid
    - Ciliary body   Sclera
    - Iris   Uveal tract
  - **224.1** Orbit
    - EXCLUDES bone of orbit (213.0)
  - **224.2** Lacrimal gland
  - **224.3** Conjunctiva
  - **224.4** Cornea
  - **224.5** Retina
    - EXCLUDES hemangioma of retina (228.03)
  - **224.6** Choroid
  - **224.7** Lacrimal duct
    - Lacrimal sac   Nasolacrimal duct
  - **224.8** Other specified parts of eye
  - **224.9** Eye, part unspecified
- √4th **225** Benign neoplasm of brain and other parts of nervous system
  - EXCLUDES hemangioma (228.02)
    - neurofibromatosis (237.7)
    - peripheral, sympathetic, and parasympathetic nerves and ganglia (215.0-215.9)
    - retrobulbar (224.1)
  - **225.0** Brain
  - **225.1** Cranial nerves
  - **225.2** Cerebral meninges
    - Meninges NOS   Meningioma (cerebral)
  - **225.3** Spinal cord
    - Cauda equina
  - **225.4** Spinal meninges
    - Spinal meningioma
  - **225.8** Other specified sites of nervous system
  - **225.9** Nervous system, part unspecified
    - Nervous system (central) NOS
    - EXCLUDES meninges NOS (225.2)
- **226** Benign neoplasm of thyroid glands
  - Use additional code to identify any functional activity

NEOPLASMS

227 Benign neoplasm of other endocrine glands and related structures
Use additional code to identify any functional activity
EXCLUDES ovary (220)
testis (222.0)
pancreas (211.6)

- **227.0** Adrenal gland
  Suprarenal gland
- **227.1** Parathyroid gland
- **227.3** Pituitary gland and craniopharyngeal duct (pouch)
  Craniobuccal pouch Rathke's pouch
  Hypophysis Sella turcica
- **227.4** Pineal gland
  Pineal body
- **227.5** Carotid body
- **227.6** Aortic body and other paraganglia
  Coccygeal body Para-aortic body
  Glomus jugulare
  AHA: N-D, '84, 17
- **227.8** Other
- **227.9** Endocrine gland, site unspecified

228 Hemangioma and lymphangioma, any site
INCLUDES angioma (benign) (cavernous) (congenital) NOS
cavernous nevus
glomus tumor
hemangioma (benign) (congenital)
EXCLUDES benign neoplasm of spleen, except hemangioma and lymphangioma (211.9)
glomus jugulare (227.6)
nevus:
  NOS (216.0-216.9)
  blue or pigmented (216.0-216.9)
  vascular (757.32)

AHA: 1Q, '00, 21

- **228.0** Hemangioma, any site
  AHA: J-F, '85, 19

  DEF: A common benign tumor usually occurring in infancy; composed of newly formed blood vessels due to malformation of angioblastic tissue.

  - **228.00** Of unspecified site
  - **228.01** Of skin and subcutaneous tissue
  - **228.02** Of intracranial structures
  - **228.03** Of retina
  - **228.04** Of intra-abdominal structures
    Peritoneum Retroperitoneal tissue
  - **228.09** Of other sites
    Systemic angiomatosis
    AHA: 3Q, '91, 20

- **228.1** Lymphangioma, any site
  Congenital lymphangioma
  Lymphatic nevus

229 Benign neoplasm of other and unspecified sites
- **229.0** Lymph nodes
  EXCLUDES lymphangioma (228.1)
- **229.8** Other specified sites
  Intrathoracic NOS Thoracic NOS
- **229.9** Site unspecified

CARCINOMA IN SITU (230-234)
INCLUDES Bowen's disease
erythroplasia
Queyrat's erythroplasia
EXCLUDES leukoplakia—see Alphabetic Index

DEF: A neoplastic type; with tumor cells confined to epithelium of origin; without further invasion.

230 Carcinoma in situ of digestive organs
- **230.0** Lip, oral cavity, and pharynx
  Gingiva Oropharynx
  Hypopharynx Salivary gland or duct
  Mouth [any part] Tongue
  Nasopharynx
  EXCLUDES aryepiglottic fold or interarytenoid fold, laryngeal aspect (231.0)
  epiglottis:
    NOS (231.0)
    suprahyoid portion (231.0)
  skin of lip (232.0)
- **230.1** Esophagus
- **230.2** Stomach
  Body
  Cardia } of stomach
  Fundus
  Cardiac orifice Pylorus
- **230.3** Colon
  Appendix Ileocecal valve
  Cecum Large intestine NOS
  EXCLUDES rectosigmoid junction (230.4)
- **230.4** Rectum
  Rectosigmoid junction
- **230.5** Anal canal
  Anal sphincter
- **230.6** Anus, unspecified
  EXCLUDES anus:
    margin (232.5)
    skin (232.5)
    perianal skin (232.5)
- **230.7** Other and unspecified parts of intestine
  Duodenum Jejunum
  Ileum Small intestine NOS
  EXCLUDES ampulla of Vater (230.8)
- **230.8** Liver and biliary system
  Ampulla of Vater Gallbladder
  Common bile duct Hepatic duct
  Cystic duct Sphincter of Oddi
- **230.9** Other and unspecified digestive organs
  Digestive organ NOS Pancreas
  Gastrointestinal tract NOS Spleen

231 Carcinoma in situ of respiratory system
- **231.0** Larynx
  Cartilage: Epiglottis:
    arytenoid NOS
    cricoid posterior surface
    cuneiform suprahyoid portion
    thyroid Vocal cords (false) (true)
  EXCLUDES aryepiglottic fold or interarytenoid fold:
    NOS (230.0)
    hypopharyngeal aspect (230.0)
    marginal zone (230.0)
- **231.1** Trachea
- **231.2** Bronchus and lung
  Carina
  Hilus of lung
- **231.8** Other specified parts of respiratory system
  Accessory sinuses Nasal cavities
  Middle ear Pleura
  EXCLUDES ear (external) (skin) (232.2)
  nose NOS (234.8)
  skin (232.3)
- **231.9** Respiratory system, part unspecified
  Respiratory organ NOS

NEOPLASMS

✓4th 232 Carcinoma in situ of skin
  INCLUDES pigment cells
  - **232.0 Skin of lip**
    EXCLUDES vermilion border of lip (230.0)
  - **232.1 Eyelid, including canthus**
  - **232.2 Ear and external auditory canal**
  - **232.3 Skin of other and unspecified parts of face**
  - **232.4 Scalp and skin of neck**
  - **232.5 Skin of trunk, except scrotum**
    Anus, margin   Skin of:
    Axillary fold   breast
    Perianal skin   buttock
    Skin of: chest wall
      abdominal wall   groin
      anus   perineum
      back   Umbilicus
    EXCLUDES anal canal (230.5)
              anus NOS (230.6)
              skin of genital organs (233.3, 233.5-233.6)
  - **232.6 Skin of upper limb, including shoulder**
  - **232.7 Skin of lower limb, including hip**
  - **232.8 Other specified sites of skin**
  - **232.9 Skin, site unspecified**

✓4th 233 Carcinoma in situ of breast and genitourinary system
  - **233.0 Breast**
    EXCLUDES Paget's disease (174.0-174.9)
              skin of breast (232.5)
  - **233.1 Cervix uteri** ♀
    AHA: 3Q, '92, 7; 3Q, '92, 8; 1Q, '91, 11
  - **233.2 Other and unspecified parts of uterus** ♀
  - **233.3 Other and unspecified female genital organs** ♀
  - **233.4 Prostate** ♂
  - **233.5 Penis** ♂
  - **233.6 Other and unspecified male genital organs** ♂
  - **233.7 Bladder**
  - **233.9 Other and unspecified urinary organs**

✓4th 234 Carcinoma in situ of other and unspecified sites
  - **234.0 Eye**
    EXCLUDES cartilage of eyelid (234.8)
              eyelid (skin) (232.1)
              optic nerve (234.8)
              orbital bone (234.8)
  - **234.8 Other specified sites**
    Endocrine gland [any]
  - **234.9 Site unspecified**
    Carcinoma in situ NOS

NEOPLASMS OF UNCERTAIN BEHAVIOR (235-238)
Note: Categories 235–238 classify by site certain histomorphologically well-defined neoplasms, the subsequent behavior of which cannot be predicted from the present appearance.

✓4th 235 Neoplasm of uncertain behavior of digestive and respiratory systems
  - **235.0 Major salivary glands**
    Gland: Gland:
      parotid   submandibular
      sublingual
    EXCLUDES minor salivary glands (235.1)
  - **235.1 Lip, oral cavity, and pharynx**
    Gingiva   Nasopharynx
    Hypopharynx   Oropharynx
    Minor salivary glands Tongue
    Mouth
    EXCLUDES aryepiglottic fold or interarytenoid fold, laryngeal aspect (235.6)
              epiglottis:
                NOS (235.6)
                suprahyoid portion (235.6)
              skin of lip (238.2)
  - **235.2 Stomach, intestines, and rectum**
  - **235.3 Liver and biliary passages**
    Ampulla of Vater   Gallbladder
    Bile ducts [any]   Liver
  - **235.4 Retroperitoneum and peritoneum**
  - **235.5 Other and unspecified digestive organs**
    Anal: Esophagus
      canal   Pancreas
      sphincter   Spleen
    Anus NOS
    EXCLUDES anus:
                margin (238.2)
                skin (238.2)
              perianal skin (238.2)
  - **235.6 Larynx**
    EXCLUDES aryepiglottic fold or interarytenoid fold:
                NOS (235.1)
                hypopharyngeal aspect (235.1)
                marginal zone (235.1)
  - **235.7 Trachea, bronchus, and lung**
  - **235.8 Pleura, thymus, and mediastinum**
  - **235.9 Other and unspecified respiratory organs**
    Accessory sinuses   Nasal cavities
    Middle ear   Respiratory organ NOS
    EXCLUDES ear (external) (skin) (238.2)
              nose (238.8)
              skin (238.2)

✓4th 236 Neoplasm of uncertain behavior of genitourinary organs
  - **236.0 Uterus** ♀
  - **236.1 Placenta** ♀
    Chorioadenoma (destruens)
    Invasive mole
    Malignant hydatid(iform) mole
  - **236.2 Ovary** ♀
    Use additional code to identify any functional activity
  - **236.3 Other and unspecified female genital organs** ♀
  - **236.4 Testis** ♂
    Use additional code to identify any functional activity
  - **236.5 Prostate** ♂
  - **236.6 Other and unspecified male genital organs** ♂
  - **236.7 Bladder**
  - **✓5th 236.9 Other and unspecified urinary organs**
    - **236.90 Urinary organ, unspecified**
    - **236.91 Kidney and ureter**
    - **236.99 Other**

✓4th 237 Neoplasm of uncertain behavior of endocrine glands and nervous system
  - **237.0 Pituitary gland and craniopharyngeal duct**
    Use additional code to identify any functional activity
  - **237.1 Pineal gland**
  - **237.2 Adrenal gland**
    Suprarenal gland
    Use additional code to identify any functional activity
  - **237.3 Paraganglia**
    Aortic body   Coccygeal body
    Carotid body   Glomus jugulare
    AHA: N-D, '84, 17
  - **237.4 Other and unspecified endocrine glands**
    Parathyroid gland   Thyroid gland
  - **237.5 Brain and spinal cord**
  - **237.6 Meninges**
    Meninges: Meninges:
      NOS   spinal
      cerebral

✓4th Additional Digit Required   Nonspecific PDx   Unacceptable PDx   Manifestation Code   MSP Medicare Secondary Payer   ▶◀ Revised Text   ● New Code

NEOPLASMS

√5th 237.7 Neurofibromatosis
von Recklinghausen's disease
DEF: An inherited condition with developmental changes in the nervous system, muscles, bones and skin; multiple soft tumors (neurofibromas) distributed over the entire body.

- 237.70 Neurofibromatosis, unspecified
- 237.71 Neurofibromatosis, type 1 [von Recklinghausen's disease]
- 237.72 Neurofibromatosis, type 2 [acoustic neurofibromatosis]
  DEF: Inherited condition with cutaneous lesions, benign tumors of peripheral nerves and bilateral 8th nerve masses.

237.9 Other and unspecified parts of nervous system
Cranial nerves
EXCLUDES peripheral, sympathetic, and parasympathetic nerves and ganglia (238.1)

√4th 238 Neoplasm of uncertain behavior of other and unspecified sites and tissues

- 238.0 Bone and articular cartilage
  EXCLUDES cartilage:
  ear (238.1)
  eyelid (238.1)
  larynx (235.6)
  nose (235.9)
  synovia (238.1)

- 238.1 Connective and other soft tissue
  Peripheral, sympathetic, and parasympathetic nerves and ganglia
  EXCLUDES cartilage (of):
  articular (238.0)
  larynx (235.6)
  nose (235.9)
  connective tissue of breast (238.3)

- 238.2 Skin
  EXCLUDES anus NOS (235.5)
  skin of genital organs (236.3, 236.6)
  vermilion border of lip (235.1)

- 238.3 Breast
  EXCLUDES skin of breast (238.2)

- 238.4 Polycythemia vera
  DEF: Abnormal proliferation of all bone marrow elements, increased red cell mass and total blood volume; unknown etiology, frequently associated with splenomegaly, leukocytosis, and thrombocythemia.

- 238.5 Histiocytic and mast cells
  Mast cell tumor NOS   Mastocytoma NOS

- 238.6 Plasma cells
  Plasmacytoma NOS   Solitary myeloma

- 238.7 Other lymphatic and hematopoietic tissues
  Disease:
  lymphoproliferative (chronic) NOS
  myeloproliferative (chronic) NOS
  Idiopathic thrombocythemia
  Megakaryocytic myelosclerosis
  Myelodysplastic syndrome
  Myelosclerosis with myeloid metaplasia
  Panmyelosis (acute)
  EXCLUDES myelfibrosis (289.8)
  myelosclerosis NOS (289.8)
  myelosis:
  NOS (205.9)
  megakaryocytic (207.2)
  1Q, '97, 5; 2Q, '89, 8

- 238.8 Other specified sites
  Eye   Heart
  EXCLUDES eyelid (skin) (238.2)
  cartilage (238.1)

- 238.9 Site unspecified

NEOPLASMS OF UNSPECIFIED NATURE (239)

√4th 239 Neoplasms of unspecified nature
Note: Category 239 classifies by site neoplasms of unspecified morphology and behavior. The term "mass," unless otherwise stated, is not to be regarded as a neoplastic growth.
INCLUDES "growth" NOS   new growth NOS
neoplasm NOS   tumor NOS

- 239.0 Digestive system
  EXCLUDES anus:
  margin (239.2)
  skin (239.2)
  perianal skin (239.2)

- 239.1 Respiratory system

- 239.2 Bone, soft tissue, and skin
  EXCLUDES anal canal (239.0)
  anus NOS (239.0)
  bone marrow (202.9)
  cartilage:
  larynx (239.1)
  nose (239.1)
  connective tissue of breast (239.3)
  skin of genital organs (239.5)
  vermilion border of lip (239.0)

- 239.3 Breast
  EXCLUDES skin of breast (239.2)

- 239.4 Bladder
- 239.5 Other genitourinary organs
- 239.6 Brain
  EXCLUDES cerebral meninges (239.7)
  cranial nerves (239.7)

- 239.7 Endocrine glands and other parts of nervous system
  EXCLUDES peripheral, sympathetic, and parasympathetic nerves and ganglia (239.2)

- 239.8 Other specified sites
  EXCLUDES eyelid (skin) (239.2)
  cartilage (239.2)
  great vessels (239.2)
  optic nerve (239.7)

- 239.9 Site unspecified

Tabular List — ENDOCRINE, NUTRITIONAL, METABOLIC, IMMUNITY — 240–244.1

3. ENDOCRINE, NUTRITIONAL AND METABOLIC DISEASES, AND IMMUNITY DISORDERS (240-279)

EXCLUDES endocrine and metabolic disturbances specific to the fetus and newborn (775.0-775.9)

Note: All neoplasms, whether functionally active or not, are classified in Chapter 2. Codes in Chapter 3 (i.e., 242.8, 246.0, 251-253, 255-259) may be used to identify such functional activity associated with any neoplasm, or by ectopic endocrine tissue.

DISORDERS OF THYROID GLAND (240-246)

√4ᵗʰ 240 Simple and unspecified goiter
DEF: An enlarged thyroid gland often caused by an inadequate dietary intake of iodine.

240.0 Goiter, specified as simple
Any condition classifiable to 240.9, specified as simple

240.9 Goiter, unspecified
Enlargement of thyroid
Goiter or struma:
  NOS
  diffuse colloid
  endemic
Goiter or struma:
  hyperplastic
  nontoxic (diffuse)
  parenchymatous
  sporadic
EXCLUDES congenital (dyshormonogenic) goiter (246.1)

√4ᵗʰ 241 Nontoxic nodular goiter
EXCLUDES adenoma of thyroid (226)
cystadenoma of thyroid (226)

241.0 Nontoxic uninodular goiter
Thyroid nodule   Uninodular goiter (nontoxic)
DEF: Enlarged thyroid, commonly due to decreased thyroid production, with single nodule; no clinical hypothyroidism.

241.1 Nontoxic multinodular goiter
Multinodular goiter (nontoxic)
DEF: Enlarged thyroid, commonly due to decreased thyroid production with multiple nodules; no clinical hypothyroidism.

241.9 Unspecified nontoxic nodular goiter
Adenomatous goiter
Nodular goiter (nontoxic) NOS
Struma nodosa (simplex)

√4ᵗʰ 242 Thyrotoxicosis with or without goiter
EXCLUDES neonatal thyrotoxicosis (775.3)
DEF: A condition caused by excess quantities of thyroid hormones being introduced into the tissues

The following fifth-digit subclassification is for use with category 242:
  0 without mention of thyrotoxic crisis or storm
  1 with mention of thyrotoxic crisis or storm

√5ᵗʰ 242.0 Toxic diffuse goiter [CC]
Basedow's disease
Exophthalmic or toxic goiter NOS
Graves' disease
Primary thyroid hyperplasia
CC Excl: 017.50-017.56, 017.90-017.96, 240.0, 240.9, 241.0-241.9, 242.00-242.91, 243, 244.0-244.9, 245.0-245.9, 246.0-246.9, 259.8-259.9
DEF: Diffuse thyroid enlargement accompanied by hyperthyroidism, bulging eyes, and dermopathy.

√5ᵗʰ 242.1 Toxic uninodular goiter [CC]
Thyroid nodule } toxic or with
Uninodular goiter } hyperthyroidism
CC Excl: See code 242.0
DEF: Symptomatic hyperthyroidism with a single nodule on the enlarged thyroid gland. Abrupt onset of symptoms; including extreme nervousness, insomnia, weight loss, tremors, and psychosis or coma.

√5ᵗʰ 242.2 Toxic multinodular goiter [CC]
Secondary thyroid hyperplasia
CC Excl: See code 242.0
DEF: Symptomatic hyperthyroidism with multiple nodules on the enlarged thyroid gland. Abrupt onset of symptoms; including extreme nervousness, insomnia, weight loss, tremors, and psychosis or coma

√5ᵗʰ 242.3 Toxic nodular goiter, unspecified [CC]
Adenomatous goiter
Nodular goiter } toxic or with
Struma nodosa } hyperthyroidism
Any condition classifiable to 241.9 specified as toxic or with hyperthyroidism
CC Excl: See code 242.0

√5ᵗʰ 242.4 Thyrotoxicosis from ectopic thyroid nodule [CC]
CC Excl: See code 242.0

√5ᵗʰ 242.8 Thyrotoxicosis of other specified origin [CC]
Overproduction of thyroid-stimulating hormone [TSH]
Thyrotoxicosis:
  factitia from ingestion of excessive thyroid material
Use additional E code to identify cause, if drug-induced
CC Excl: See code 242.0

√5ᵗʰ 242.9 Thyrotoxicosis without mention of goiter or other cause [CC]
Hyperthyroidism NOS
Thyrotoxicosis NOS
CC Excl: See code 242.0

243 Congenital hypothyroidism
Congenital thyroid insufficiency
Cretinism (athyrotic) (endemic)
Use additional code to identify associated mental retardation
EXCLUDES congenital (dyshormonogenic) goiter (246.1)
DEF: Underproduction of thyroid hormone present from birth.

√4ᵗʰ 244 Acquired hypothyroidism
INCLUDES athyroidism (acquired)
hypothyroidism (acquired)
myxedema (adult) (juvenile)
thyroid (gland) insufficiency (acquired)

244.0 Postsurgical hypothyroidism
DEF: Underproduction of thyroid hormone due to surgical removal of all or part of the thyroid gland.

244.1 Other postablative hypothyroidism
Hypothyroidism following therapy, such as irradiation

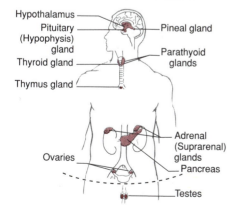

The Endocrine System

ENDOCRINE, NUTRITIONAL, METABOLIC, IMMUNITY

244.2 Iodine hypothyroidism
Hypothyroidism resulting from administration or ingestion of iodide
Use additional E code to identify drug

244.3 Other iatrogenic hypothyroidism
Hypothyroidism resulting from:
P-aminosalicylic acid [PAS]
Phenylbutazone
Resorcinol
Iatrogenic hypothyroidism NOS
Use additional E code to identify drug

244.8 Other specified acquired hypothyroidism
Secondary hypothyroidism NEC
AHA: J-A, '85, 9

244.9 Unspecified hypothyroidism
Hypothyroidism } primary or NOS
Myxedema
AHA: 3Q, '99, 19; 4Q, '96, 29

✓4th 245 Thyroiditis

245.0 Acute thyroiditis
Abscess of thyroid
Thyroiditis:
  nonsuppurative, acute
Thyroiditis:
  pyogenic
  suppurative
Use additional code to identify organism
DEF: Inflamed thyroid caused by infection, with abscess and liquid puris.

245.1 Subacute thyroiditis
Thyroiditis:
  de Quervain's
  giant cell
Thyroiditis:
  granulomatous
  viral
DEF: Inflammation of the thyroid, characterized by fever and painful enlargement of the thyroid gland, with granulomas in the gland.

245.2 Chronic lymphocytic thyroiditis
Hashimoto's disease
Struma lymphomatosa
Thyroiditis:
  autoimmune
  lymphocytic (chronic)
DEF: Autoimmune disease of thyroid; lymphocytes infiltrate the gland and thyroid antibodies are produced; women more often affected.

245.3 Chronic fibrous thyroiditis
Struma fibrosa
Thyroiditis:
  invasive (fibrous)
Thyroiditis:
  ligneous
  Riedel's
DEF: Persistent fibrosing inflammation of thyroid with adhesions to nearby structures; rare condition

245.4 Iatrogenic thyroiditis
Use additional code to identify cause
DEF: Thyroiditis resulting from treatment or intervention by physician or in a patient intervention setting.

245.8 Other and unspecified chronic thyroiditis
Chronic thyroiditis:
  NOS
  nonspecific

245.9 Thyroiditis, unspecified
Thyroiditis NOS

✓4th 246 Other disorders of thyroid

246.0 Disorders of thyrocalcitonin secretion
Hypersecretion of calcitonin or thyrocalcitonin

246.1 Dyshormonogenic goiter
Congenital (dyshormonogenic) goiter
Goiter due to enzyme defect in synthesis of thyroid hormone
Goitrous cretinism (sporadic)

246.2 Cyst of thyroid
EXCLUDES cystadenoma of thyroid (226)

246.3 Hemorrhage and infarction of thyroid

246.8 Other specified disorders of thyroid
Abnormality of thyroid-binding globulin
Atrophy of thyroid
Hyper-TBG-nemia
Hypo-TBG-nemia

246.9 Unspecified disorder of thyroid

DISEASES OF OTHER ENDOCRINE GLANDS (250-259)

✓4th 250 Diabetes mellitus
EXCLUDES gestational diabetes (648.8)
hyperglycemia NOS (790.6)
neonatal diabetes mellitus (775.1)
nonclinical diabetes (790.2)

The following fifth-digit subclassification is for use with category 250:

0 type II [non-insulin dependent type] [NIDDM type] [adult-onset type] or unspecified type, not stated as uncontrolled
   Fifth-digit 0 is for use for type II, adult-onset diabetic patients, even if the patient requires insulin

1 type I [insulin dependent type] [IDDM] [juvenile type], not stated as uncontrolled

2 type II [non-insulin dependent type] [NIDDM type] [adult-onset type] or unspecified type, uncontrolled
   Fifth-digit 2 is for use for type II, adult-onset diabetic patients, even if the patient requires insulin

3 type I [insulin dependent type] [IDDM] [juvenile type], uncontrolled

AHA: 2Q,'01, 16; 2Q,'98, 15; 4Q, '97, 32; 2Q, '97, 14; 3Q, '96, 5; 4Q, '93, 19; 2Q, '92, 5; 3Q, '91, 3; 2Q, '90, 22; N-D, '85, 11

✓5th 8 250.0 Diabetes mellitus without mention of complication CC 1-3
Diabetes mellitus without mention of complication or manifestation classifiable to 250.1-250.9
Diabetes (mellitus) NOS
CC Excl: For code 250.01-250.03: 250.00-250.93, 251.0-251.3, 259.8-259.9
AHA: 4Q, '97, 32; 3Q, '91, 3, 12; N-D, '85, 11; For code 250.00: ▶1Q, '02, 7, 11◀

✓5th 250.1 Diabetes with ketoacidosis CC 1-3
Diabetic:
  acidosis } without mention of coma
  ketosis
CC Excl: For code 250.11-250.13: 250.00-250.93, 251.0-251.3, 259.8-259.9
AHA: 3Q, '91, 6
DEF: Diabetic hyperglycemic crisis causing ketone presence in body fluids.

✓5th 250.2 Diabetes with hyperosmolarity CC 1-3
Hyperosmolar (nonketotic) coma
CC Excl: For code 250.21-250.23: 250.00-250.93, 251.0-251.3, 259.8-259.9
AHA: 4Q, '93, 19; 3Q, '91, 7

---

8 Questionable admission = 0

ENDOCRINE, NUTRITIONAL, METABOLIC, IMMUNITY

✓5th 250.3 Diabetes with other coma [CC 1-3]
Diabetic coma (with ketoacidosis)
Diabetic hypoglycemic coma
Insulin coma NOS

EXCLUDES *diabetes with hyperosmolar coma (250.2)*

CC Excl: For code 250.31-250.33: See code 250.01

AHA: 3Q, '91, 7,12

DEF: Coma (not hyperosmolar) caused by hyperglycemia or hypoglycemia as complication of diabetes.

✓5th 250.4 Diabetes with renal manifestations [CC 1-3]
Use additional code to identify manifestation, as:
diabetic:
nephropathy NOS (583.81)
nephrosis (581.81)
intercapillary glomerulosclerosis (581.81)
Kimmelstiel-Wilson syndrome (581.81)

CC Excl: For code 250.41-250.43: See code 250.01

AHA: 3Q, '91, 8,12; S-O, '87, 9; S-O, '84, 3

✓5th 250.5 Diabetes with ophthalmic manifestations [CC 1-3]
Use additional code to identify manifestation, as:
diabetic:
blindness (369.00-369.9)
cataract (366.41)
glaucoma (365.44)
retinal edema (362.83)
retinopathy (362.01-362.02)

CC Excl: For code 250.51-250.53: See code 250.01

AHA: 3Q, '91, 8; S-O, '85, 11

✓5th 250.6 Diabetes with neurological manifestations [CC 1-3]
Use additional code to identify manifestation, as:
diabetic:
amyotrophy (358.1)
mononeuropathy (354.0-355.9)
neurogenic arthropathy (713.5)
peripheral autonomic neuropathy (337.1)
polyneuropathy (357.2)

CC Excl: For code 250.61-250.63: See code 250.01

AHA: 2Q, '93, 6; 2Q, '92, 15; 3Q, '91, 9; N-D, '84, 9

✓5th 250.7 Diabetes with peripheral circulatory disorders [CC 1-3]
Use additional code to identify manifestation, as:
diabetic:
gangrene (785.4)
peripheral angiopathy (443.81)

CC Excl: For code 250.71-250.73: See code 250.01

AHA: 1Q, '96, 10; 3Q, '94, 5; 2Q, '94, 17; 3Q, '91, 10, 12; 3Q, '90, 15

DEF: Blood vessel damage or disease, usually in the feet, legs, or hands, as a complication of diabetes.

✓5th 250.8 Diabetes with other specified manifestations [CC 1-3]
Diabetic hypoglycemia
Hypoglycemic shock
Use additional code to identify manifestation, as:
any associated ulceration (707.10-707.9)
diabetic bone changes (731.8)
Use additional E code to identify cause, if drug-induced

CC Excl: For code 250.81-250.83: See code 250.01

AHA: 4Q, '00, 44; 4Q, '97, 43; 2Q, '97, 16; 4Q, '93, 20; 3Q, '91, 10

✓5th 250.9 Diabetes with unspecified complication [CC 1-3]
CC Excl: For code 250.91-250.93: See code 250.01

AHA: 2Q, '92, 15; 3Q, '91, 7, 12

✓4th 251 Other disorders of pancreatic internal secretion

251.0 Hypoglycemic coma [CC]
Iatrogenic hyperinsulinism
Non-diabetic insulin coma
Use additional E code to identify cause, if drug-induced

EXCLUDES *hypoglycemic coma in diabetes mellitus (250.3)*

CC Excl: 250.00-250.93, 251.0-251.3, 259.8-259.9

AHA: M-A, '85, 8

DEF: Coma induced by low blood sugar in non-diabetic patient.

251.1 Other specified hypoglycemia
Hyperinsulinism: Hyperplasia of pancreatic
NOS   islet beta cells NOS
ectopic
functional

EXCLUDES *hypoglycemia:*
in diabetes mellitus (250.8)
in infant of diabetic mother (775.0)
hypoglycemic coma (251.0)
neonatal hypoglycemia (775.6)

Use additional E code to identify cause, if drug-induced.

DEF: Excessive production of insulin by the pancreas; associated with obesity and insulin-producing tumors.

251.2 Hypoglycemia, unspecified
Hypoglycemia: Hypoglycemia:
NOS   spontaneous
reactive

EXCLUDES *hypoglycemia:*
with coma (251.0)
in diabetes mellitus (250.8)
leucine-induced (270.3)

AHA: M-A, '85, 7

251.3 Postsurgical hypoinsulinemia [CC]
Hypoinsulinemia following complete or partial pancreatectomy
Postpancreatectomy hyperglycemia

CC Excl: See code 251.0

AHA: 3Q, '91, 6

251.4 Abnormality of secretion of glucagon
Hyperplasia of pancreatic islet alpha cells with glucagon excess

DEF: Production malfunction of a pancreatic hormone secreted by cells of the islets of Langerhans.

251.5 Abnormality of secretion of gastrin
Hyperplasia of pancreatic alpha cells with gastrin excess
Zollinger-Ellison syndrome

ENDOCRINE, NUTRITIONAL, METABOLIC, IMMUNITY

251.8–254.0

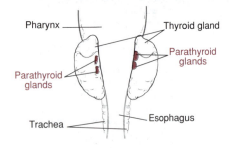

Dorsal View of Parathyroid Glands

Parathyroid glands → Parathyroid hormone (PTH) → Calcium in bones / Calcium in blood

251.8 Other specified disorders of pancreatic internal secretion
AHA: 2Q, '98, 15; 3Q, '91, 6

251.9 Unspecified disorder of pancreatic internal secretion
Islet cell hyperplasia NOS

√4th 252 Disorders of parathyroid gland

252.0 Hyperparathyroidism
Hyperplasia of parathyroid
Osteitis fibrosa cystica generalisata
von Recklinghausen's disease of bone
  EXCLUDES ectopic hyperparathyroidism (259.3)
           secondary hyperparathyroidism (of renal origin) (588.8)
DEF: Abnormally high secretion of parathyroid hormones causing bone deterioration, reduced renal function, kidney stones.

252.1 Hypoparathyroidism CC
Parathyroiditis (autoimmune)
Tetany:
  parathyroid
  parathyroprival
  EXCLUDES pseudohypoparathyroidism (275.4)
           pseudopseudohypoparathyroidism (275.4)
           tetany NOS (781.7)
           transitory neonatal hypoparathyroidism (775.4)
CC Excl: 252.0-252.9, 259.8-259.9
DEF: Abnormally low secretion of parathyroid hormones which causes decreased calcium and increased phosphorus in the blood. Resulting in muscle cramps, tetany, urinary frequency and cataracts.

252.8 Other specified disorders of parathyroid gland
Cyst } of parathyroid gland
Hemorrhage

252.9 Unspecified disorder of parathyroid gland

√4th 253 Disorders of the pituitary gland and its hypothalamic control
INCLUDES the listed conditions whether the disorder is in the pituitary or the hypothalamus
EXCLUDES Cushing's syndrome (255.0)

253.0 Acromegaly and gigantism
Overproduction of growth hormone
DEF: Acromegaly: chronic, beginning in middle age; caused by hypersecretion of the pituitary growth hormone; produces enlarged parts of skeleton, especially the nose, ears, jaws, fingers and toes.
DEF: Gigantism: pituitary gigantism caused by excess growth of short flat bones; men may grow 78 to 80 inches tall.

253.1 Other and unspecified anterior pituitary hyperfunction
Forbes-Albright syndrome
  EXCLUDES overproduction of:
           ACTH (255.3)
           thyroid-stimulating hormone [TSH] (242.8)
AHA: J-A, '85, 9
DEF: Spontaneous galactorrhea-amenorrhea syndrome unrelated to pregnancy; usually related to presence of pituitary tumor.

253.2 Panhypopituitarism CC
Cachexia, pituitary
Necrosis of pituitary (postpartum)
Pituitary insufficiency NOS
Sheehan's syndrome
Simmonds' disease
  EXCLUDES iatrogenic hypopituitarism (253.7)
CC Excl: 253.0-253.9, 259.8-259.9
DEF: Damage to or absence of pituitary gland leading to impaired sexual function, weight loss, fatigue, bradycardia, hypotension, pallor, depression, and impaired growth in children; called Simmonds' disease if cachexia is prominent.

253.3 Pituitary dwarfism
Isolated deficiency of (human) growth hormone [HGH]
Lorain-Levi dwarfism
DEF: Dwarfism with infantile physical characteristics due to abnormally low secretion of growth hormone and gonadotropin deficiency.

253.4 Other anterior pituitary disorders
Isolated or partial deficiency of an anterior pituitary hormone, other than growth hormone
Prolactin deficiency
AHA: J-A, '85, 9

253.5 Diabetes insipidus CC
Vasopressin deficiency
  EXCLUDES nephrogenic diabetes insipidus (588.1)
CC Excl: 253.1-253.2, 253.4-253.9, 259.8-259.9
DEF: Metabolic disorder causing insufficient antidiuretic hormone release; symptoms include frequent urination, thirst, ravenous hunger, loss of weight, fatigue.

253.6 Other disorders of neurohypophysis
Syndrome of inappropriate secretion of antidiuretic hormone [ADH]
  EXCLUDES ectopic antidiuretic hormone secretion (259.3)

253.7 Iatrogenic pituitary disorders
Hypopituitarism: Hypopituitarism:
  hormone-induced   postablative
  hypophysectomy-induced   radiotherapy-induced
Use additional E code to identify cause
DEF: Pituitary dysfunction that results from drug therapy, radiation therapy, or surgery, causing mild to severe symptom.

253.8 Other disorders of the pituitary and other syndromes of diencephalohypophyseal origin
Abscess of pituitary   Cyst of Rathke's pouch
Adiposogenital dystrophy   Fröhlich's syndrome
  EXCLUDES craniopharyngioma (237.0)

253.9 Unspecified
Dyspituitarism

√4th 254 Diseases of thymus gland
EXCLUDES aplasia or dysplasia with immunodeficiency (279.2)
         hypoplasia with immunodeficiency (279.2)
         myasthenia gravis (358.0)

254.0 Persistent hyperplasia of thymus
Hypertrophy of thymus
DEF: Continued abnormal growth of the twin lymphoid lobes that produce T lymphocytes.

ENDOCRINE, NUTRITIONAL, METABOLIC, IMMUNITY

254.1 Abscess of thymus `CC`
CC Excl: 254.0–254.1, 254.8–254.9, 259.8–259.9

254.8 Other specified diseases of thymus gland
Atrophy } of thymus
Cyst
EXCLUDES thymoma (212.6)

254.9 Unspecified disease of thymus gland

255 Disorders of adrenal glands
INCLUDES the listed conditions whether the basic disorder is in the adrenals or is pituitary-induced

255.0 Cushing's syndrome `CC`
Adrenal hyperplasia due to excess ACTH
Cushing's syndrome:
  NOS
  iatrogenic
  idiopathic
  pituitary-dependent
Ectopic ACTH syndrome
Iatrogenic syndrome of excess cortisol
Overproduction of cortisol
Use additional E code to identify cause, if drug-induced
EXCLUDES congenital adrenal hyperplasia (255.2)
CC Excl: 255.0-255.2, 259.8-259.9

DEF: Due to adrenal cortisol oversecretion or glucocorticoid medications; may cause fatty tissue of the face, neck and body; osteoporosis and curvature of spine, hypertension, diabetes mellitus, female genitourinary problems, male impotence, degeneration of muscle tissues, weakness.

255.1 Hyperaldosteronism
Aldosteronism (primary) (secondary)
Bartter's syndrome
Conn's syndrome

DEF: Oversecretion of aldosterone causing fluid retention, hypertension.

255.2 Adrenogenital disorders
Achard-Thiers syndrome
Adrenogenital syndromes, virilizing or feminizing, whether acquired or associated with congenital adrenal hyperplasia consequent on inborn enzyme defects in hormone synthesis
Congenital adrenal hyperplasia
Female adrenal pseudohermaphroditism
Male:
  macrogenitosomia praecox
  sexual precocity with adrenal hyperplasia
Virilization (female) (suprarenal)
EXCLUDES adrenal hyperplasia due to excess ACTH (255.0)
isosexual virilization (256.4)

255.3 Other corticoadrenal overactivity `CC`
Acquired benign adrenal androgenic overactivity
Overproduction of ACTH
CC Excl: 017.60-017.66, 017.90-017.96, 255.3-255.9, 259.8-259.9

255.4 Corticoadrenal insufficiency `CC`
Addisonian crisis   Adrenal:
Addison's disease NOS   crisis
Adrenal: hemorrhage
  atrophy (autoimmune)   infarction
  calcification   insufficiency NOS
EXCLUDES tuberculous Addison's disease (017.6)
CC Excl: See code 255.3

DEF: Underproduction of adrenal hormones causing low blood pressure.

255.5 Other adrenal hypofunction `CC`
Adrenal medullary insufficiency
EXCLUDES Waterhouse-Friderichsen syndrome (meningococcal) (036.3)
CC Excl: See code 255.3

255.6 Medulloadrenal hyperfunction `CC`
Catecholamine secretion by pheochromocytoma
CC Excl: See code 255.3

255.8 Other specified disorders of adrenal glands
Abnormality of cortisol-binding globulin

255.9 Unspecified disorder of adrenal glands

256 Ovarian dysfunction
AHA: 4Q, '00, 51

256.0 Hyperestrogenism ♀
DEF: Excess secretion of estrogen by the ovaries; characterized by ovaries containing multiple follicular cysts filled with serous fluid.

256.1 Other ovarian hyperfunction ♀
Hypersecretion of ovarian androgens
AHA: 3Q, '95, 15

256.2 Postablative ovarian failure ♀
Ovarian failure: Ovarian failure:
  iatrogenic   postsurgical
  postirradiation
▶Use additional code for states associated with artificial menopause (627.4)◀
EXCLUDES acquired absence of ovary (V45.77)
asymptomatic age-related (natural) postmenopausal status (V49.81)

DEF: Failed ovarian function after medical or surgical intervention.

256.3 Other ovarian failure
Use additional code for states associated with ▶natural menopause (627.2)◀
EXCLUDES asymptomatic age-related (natural) postmenopausal status (V49.81)
AHA: 4Q, '01, 41

256.31 Premature menopause ♀
DEF: Permanent cessation of ovarian function before the age of 40 occuring naturally of unknown cause.

256.39 Other ovarian failure ♀
Delayed menarche
Ovarian hypofunction
Primary ovarian failure NOS

256.4 Polycystic ovaries ♀
Isosexual virilization   Stein-Leventhal syndrome
DEF: Multiple serous filled cysts of ovary; symptoms of infertility, hirsutism, oligomenorrhea or amenorrhea.

256.8 Other ovarian dysfunction ♀
256.9 Unspecified ovarian dysfunction ♀

257 Testicular dysfunction

257.0 Testicular hyperfunction ♂
Hypersecretion of testicular hormones

257.1 Postablative testicular hypofunction ♂
Testicular hypofunction: Testicular hypofunction:
  iatrogenic   postsurgical
  postirradiation

257.2 Other testicular hypofunction ♂
Defective biosynthesis of testicular androgen
Eunuchoidism:
  NOS
  hypogonadotropic
Failure:
  Leydig's cell, adult
  seminiferous tubule, adult
Testicular hypogonadism
EXCLUDES azoospermia (606.0)

257.8 Other testicular dysfunction ♂
Goldberg-Maxwell syndrome
Male pseudohermaphroditism with testicular feminization
Testicular feminization

257.9 Unspecified testicular dysfunction ♂

ENDOCRINE, NUTRITIONAL, METABOLIC, IMMUNITY

√4th **258 Polyglandular dysfunction and related disorders**

258.0 Polyglandular activity in multiple endocrine adenomatosis [CC]
  Wermer's syndrome
  CC Excl: 240.0, 240.9, 241.0-241.9, 242.00-242.91, 243, 244.0-244.9, 245.0-245.9, 246.0-246.9, 250.00-250.93, 251.0-251.9, 252.0-252.9, 253.0-253.9, 254.0-254.9, 255.0-255.9, 256.0-256.2, 256.31-256.39, 256.4-256.9, 257.0-257.9, 258.0-258.9, 259.0-259.9

  DEF: Wermer's syndrome: A rare hereditary condition characterized by the presence of adenomas or hyperplasia in more than one endocrine gland causing premature aging.

258.1 Other combinations of endocrine dysfunction [CC]
  Lloyd's syndrome
  Schmidt's syndrome
  CC Excl: See code 258.0

258.8 Other specified polyglandular dysfunction [CC]
  CC Excl: See code 258.0

258.9 Polyglandular dysfunction, unspecified [CC]
  CC Excl: See code 258.0

√4th **259 Other endocrine disorders**

259.0 Delay in sexual development and puberty, not elsewhere classified
  Delayed puberty

259.1 Precocious sexual development and puberty, not elsewhere classified [P]
  Sexual precocity: Sexual precocity:
    NOS   cryptogenic
    constitutional   idiopathic

259.2 Carcinoid syndrome [CC]
  Hormone secretion by carcinoid tumors
  CC Excl: 259.2-259.3, 259.8-259.9

  DEF: Presence of carcinoid tumors that spread to liver; characterized by cyanotic flushing of skin, diarrhea, bronchospasm, acquired tricuspid and pulmonary stenosis, sudden drops in blood pressure, edema, ascites.

259.3 Ectopic hormone secretion, not elsewhere classified
  Ectopic:
    antidiuretic hormone secretion [ADH]
    hyperparathyroidism
  EXCLUDES ectopic ACTH syndrome (255.0)
  AHA: N-D, '85, 4

259.4 Dwarfism, not elsewhere classified
  Dwarfism:
    NOS
    constitutional
  EXCLUDES dwarfism:
              achondroplastic (756.4)
              intrauterine (759.7)
              nutritional (263.2)
              pituitary (253.3)
              renal (588.0)
              progeria (259.8)

259.8 Other specified endocrine disorders
  Pineal gland dysfunction   Werner's syndrome
  Progeria

259.9 Unspecified endocrine disorder
  Disturbance: Infantilism NOS
    endocrine NOS
    hormone NOS

NUTRITIONAL DEFICIENCIES (260-269)
EXCLUDES deficiency anemias (280.0-281.9)

260 Kwashiorkor [CC]
  Nutritional edema with dyspigmentation of skin and hair
  CC Excl: 260-262, 263.0-263.9

  DEF: Syndrome, particularly children; excessive carbohydrate with inadequate protein intake, inhibited growth potential, anomalies in skin and hair pigmentation, edema and liver disease.

261 Nutritional marasmus [CC]
  Nutritional atrophy
  Severe calorie deficiency
  Severe malnutrition NOS
  CC Excl: See code 260

  DEF: Protein-calorie malabsorption or malnutrition of children; characterized by tissue wasting, dehydration, and subcutaneous fat depletion; may occur with infectious disease; also called infantile atrophy.

262 Other severe, protein-calorie malnutrition [CC]
  Nutritional edema without mention of dyspigmentation of skin and hair
  CC Excl: See code 260
  AHA: 4Q, '92, 24; J-A, '85, 12

√4th **263 Other and unspecified protein-calorie malnutrition**
  AHA: 4Q, '92, 24

263.0 Malnutrition of moderate degree [CC]
  CC Excl: See code 260
  AHA: J-A, '85, 1

  DEF: Malnutrition characterized by biochemical changes in electrolytes, lipids, blood plasma.

263.1 Malnutrition of mild degree [CC]
  CC Excl: See code 260
  AHA: J-A, '85, 1

263.2 Arrested development following protein-calorie malnutrition [CC]
  Nutritional dwarfism
  Physical retardation due to malnutrition
  CC Excl: See code 260

263.8 Other protein-calorie malnutrition [CC]
  CC Excl: See code 260

263.9 Unspecified protein-calorie malnutrition [CC]
  Dystrophy due to malnutrition
  Malnutrition (calorie) NOS
  EXCLUDES nutritional deficiency NOS (269.9)
  CC Excl: See code 260
  AHA: N-D, '84, 19

√4th **264 Vitamin A deficiency**

264.0 With conjunctival xerosis
  DEF: Vitamin A deficiency with conjunctival dryness.

264.1 With conjunctival xerosis and Bitot's spot
  Bitot's spot in the young child
  DEF: Vitamin A deficiency with conjunctival dryness, superficial spots of keratinized epithelium.

264.2 With corneal xerosis
  DEF: Vitamin A deficiency with corneal dryness.

264.3 With corneal ulceration and xerosis
  DEF: Vitamin A deficiency with corneal dryness, epithelial ulceration.

264.4 With keratomalacia
  DEF: Vitamin A deficiency creating corneal dryness; progresses to corneal insensitivity, softness, necrosis; usually bilateral.

264.5 With night blindness
  DEF: Vitamin A deficiency causing vision failure in dim light.

ENDOCRINE, NUTRITIONAL, METABOLIC, IMMUNITY

264.6 With xerophthalmic scars of cornea
DEF: Vitamin A deficiency with corneal scars from dryness.

264.7 Other ocular manifestations of vitamin A deficiency
Xerophthalmia due to vitamin A deficiency

264.8 Other manifestations of vitamin A deficiency
Follicular keratosis ⎱ due to vitamin A
Xeroderma ⎰ deficiency

264.9 Unspecified vitamin A deficiency
Hypovitaminosis A NOS

√4th 265 Thiamine and niacin deficiency states

265.0 Beriberi
DEF: Inadequate vitamin B_1 (thiamine) intake, affects heart and peripheral nerves; individual may become edematous and develop cardiac disease due to the excess fluid; alcoholics and people with a diet of excessive polished rice prone to the disease.

265.1 Other and unspecified manifestations of thiamine deficiency
Other vitamin B_1 deficiency states

265.2 Pellagra
Deficiency: Deficiency:
  niacin (-tryptophan)   vitamin PP
  nicotinamide   Pellagra (alcoholic)
  nicotinic acid
DEF: Niacin deficiency causing dermatitis, inflammation of mucous membranes, diarrhea, and psychic disturbances.

√4th 266 Deficiency of B-complex components

266.0 Ariboflavinosis
Riboflavin [vitamin B_2] deficiency
AHA: S-O, '86, 10
DEF: Vitamin B_2 (riboflavin) deficiency marked by swollen lips and tongue fissures, corneal vascularization, scaling lesions, and anemia.

266.1 Vitamin B_6 deficiency
Deficiency: Deficiency:
  pyridoxal   pyridoxine
  pyridoxamine   Vitamin B_6 deficiency syndrome
EXCLUDES vitamin B_6-responsive sideroblastic anemia (285.0)
DEF: Vitamin B_6 deficiency causing skin, lip, and tongue disturbances, peripheral neuropathy; and convulsions in infants.

266.2 Other B-complex deficiencies
Deficiency: Deficiency:
  cyanocobalamin   vitamin B_{12}
  folic acid
EXCLUDES combined system disease with anemia (281.0-281.1)
          deficiency anemias (281.0-281.9)
          subacute degeneration of spinal cord with anemia (281.0-281.1)

266.9 Unspecified vitamin B deficiency

267 Ascorbic acid deficiency
Deficiency of vitamin C
Scurvy
EXCLUDES scorbutic anemia (281.8)
DEF: Vitamin C deficiency causing swollen gums, myalgia, weight loss, and weakness.

√4th 268 Vitamin D deficiency
EXCLUDES vitamin D-resistant:
            osteomalacia (275.3)
            rickets (275.3)

268.0 Rickets, active
EXCLUDES celiac rickets (579.0)
          renal rickets (588.0)
DEF: Inadequate vitamin D intake, usually in pediatrics, that affects bones most involved with muscular action; may cause nodules on ends and sides of bones; delayed closure of fontanels in infants; symptoms may include muscle soreness, and profuse sweating.

268.1 Rickets, late effect
Any condition specified as due to rickets and stated to be a late effect or sequela of rickets
Use additional code to identify the nature of late effect
DEF: Distorted or demineralized bones as a result of vitamin D deficiency.

268.2 Osteomalacia, unspecified
DEF: Softening of bones due to decrease in calcium; marked by pain, tenderness, muscular weakness, anorexia, and weight loss.

268.9 Unspecified vitamin D deficiency
Avitaminosis D

√4th 269 Other nutritional deficiencies

269.0 Deficiency of vitamin K   CC
EXCLUDES deficiency of coagulation factor due to vitamin K deficiency (286.7)
          vitamin K deficiency of newborn (776.0)
CC Excl: 269.0

269.1 Deficiency of other vitamins
Deficiency: Deficiency:
  vitamin E   vitamin P

269.2 Unspecified vitamin deficiency
Multiple vitamin deficiency NOS

269.3 Mineral deficiency, not elsewhere classified
Deficiency: Deficiency:
  calcium, dietary   iodine
EXCLUDES deficiency:
            calcium NOS (275.4)
            potassium (276.8)
            sodium (276.1)

269.8 Other nutritional deficiency
EXCLUDES adult failure to thrive (783.7)
          failure to thrive in childhood (783.41)
          feeding problems (783.3)
          newborn (779.3)

269.9 Unspecified nutritional deficiency

OTHER METABOLIC AND IMMUNITY DISORDERS (270-279)
Use additional code to identify any associated mental retardation

√4th 270 Disorders of amino-acid transport and metabolism
EXCLUDES abnormal findings without manifest disease (790.0-796.9)
          disorders of purine and pyrimidine metabolism (277.1-277.2)
          gout (274.0-274.9)

270.0 Disturbances of amino-acid transport
Cystinosis   Glycinuria (renal)
Cystinuria   Hartnup disease
Fanconi (-de Toni) (-Debré) syndrome

270.1 Phenylketonuria [PKU]
Hyperphenylalaninemia
DEF: Inherited metabolic condition causing excess phenylpyruvic and other acids in urine; results in mental retardation, neurological manifestations, including spasticity and tremors, light pigmentation, eczema, and mousy odor.

270.2 Other disturbances of aromatic amino-acid metabolism
Albinism   Hypertyrosinemia
Alkaptonuria   Indicanuria
Alkaptonuric ochronosis   Kynureninase defects
Disturbances of metabolism   Oasthouse urine disease
  of tyrosine and   Ochronosis
  tryptophan   Tyrosinosis
Homogentisic acid defects   Tyrosinuria
Hydroxykynureninuria   Waardenburg syndrome
EXCLUDES vitamin B_6-deficiency syndrome (266.1)
AHA: 3Q, '99, 20

ENDOCRINE, NUTRITIONAL, METABOLIC, IMMUNITY

270.3 **Disturbances of branched-chain amino-acid metabolism**
Disturbances of metabolism of leucine, isoleucine, and valine
Hypervalinemia
Intermittent branched-chain ketonuria
Leucine-induced hypoglycemia
Leucinosis
Maple syrup urine disease
AHA: 3Q, '00, 8

270.4 **Disturbances of sulphur-bearing amino-acid metabolism**
Cystathioninemia
Cystathioninuria
Disturbances of metabolism of methionine, homocystine, and cystathionine
Homocystinuria
Hypermethioninemia
Methioninemia

270.5 **Disturbances of histidine metabolism**
Carnosinemia
Histidinemia
Hyperhistidinemia
Imidazole aminoaciduria

270.6 **Disorders of urea cycle metabolism**
Argininosuccinic aciduria
Citrullinemia
Disorders of metabolism of ornithine, citrulline, argininosuccinic acid, arginine, and ammonia
Hyperammonemia
Hyperomithinemia

270.7 **Other disturbances of straight-chain amino-acid metabolism**
Glucoglycinuria
Glycinemia (with methyl-malonic acidemia)
Hyperglycinemia
Hyperlysinemia
Other disturbances of metabolism of glycine, threonine, serine, glutamine, and lysine
Pipecolic acidemia
Saccharopinuria
AHA: 3Q, '00, 8

270.8 **Other specified disorders of amino-acid metabolism**
Alaninemia   Iminoacidopathy
Ethanolaminuria   Prolinemia
Glycoprolinuria   Prolinuria
Hydroxyprolinemia   Sarcosinemia
Hyperprolinemia

270.9 **Unspecified disorder of amino-acid metabolism**

✓4th 271 Disorders of carbohydrate transport and metabolism
EXCLUDES abnormality of secretion of glucagon (251.4)
diabetes mellitus (250.0-250.9)
hypoglycemia NOS (251.2)
mucopolysaccharidosis (277.5)

271.0 **Glycogenosis**
Amylopectinosis
Glucose-6-phosphatase deficiency
Glycogen storage disease
McArdle's disease
Pompe's disease
von Gierke's disease
AHA: 1Q, '98, 5

271.1 **Galactosemia**
Galactose-1-phosphate uridyl transferase deficiency
Galactosuria
DEF: Any of three genetic disorders due to defective galactose metabolism; symptoms include failure to thrive in infancy, jaundice, liver and spleen damage, cataracts, and mental retardation.

271.2 **Hereditary fructose intolerance**
Essential benign fructosuria   Fructosemia
DEF: Chromosome recessive disorder of carbohydrate metabolism; in infants, occurs after dietary sugar introduced; characterized by enlarged spleen, yellowish cast to skin, and progressive inability to thrive.

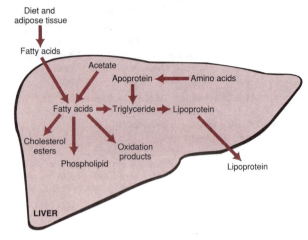
Lipid Metabolism

271.3 **Intestinal disaccharidase deficiencies and disaccharide malabsorption**
Intolerance or malabsorption (congenital) (of):
glucose-galactose
lactose
sucrose-isomaltose

271.4 **Renal glycosuria**
Renal diabetes
DEF: Persistent abnormal levels of glucose in urine, with normal blood glucose levels; caused by failure of the renal tubules to reabsorb glucose.

271.8 **Other specified disorders of carbohydrate transport and metabolism**
Essential benign pentosuria   Mannosidosis
Fucosidosis   Oxalosis
Glycolic aciduria   Xylosuria
Hyperoxaluria (primary)   Xylulosuria

271.9 **Unspecified disorder of carbohydrate transport and metabolism**

✓4th 272 Disorders of lipoid metabolism
EXCLUDES localized cerebral lipidoses (330.1)

272.0 **Pure hypercholesterolemia**
Familial hypercholesterolemia
Fredrickson Type IIa hyperlipoproteinemia
Hyperbetalipoproteinemia
Hyperlipidemia, Group A
Low-density-lipoid-type [LDL] hyperlipoproteinemia

272.1 **Pure hyperglyceridemia**
Endogenous hyperglyceridemia
Fredrickson Type IV hyperlipoproteinemia
Hyperlipidemia, Group B
Hyperprebetalipoproteinemia
Hypertriglyceridemia, essential
Very-low-density-lipoid-type [VLDL] hyperlipoproteinemia

272.2 **Mixed hyperlipidemia**
Broad- or floating-betalipoproteinemia
Fredrickson Type IIb or III hyperlipoproteinemia
Hypercholesterolemia with endogenous hyperglyceridemia
Hyperbetalipoproteinemia with prebetalipoproteinemia
Tubo-eruptive xanthoma
Xanthoma tuberosum
DEF: Elevated levels of lipoprotein, a complex of fats and proteins, in blood due to inherited metabolic disorder.

272.3 **Hyperchylomicronemia**
Bürger-Grütz syndrome
Fredrickson type I or V hyperlipoproteinemia
Hyperlipidemia, Group D
Mixed hyperglyceridemia

N Newborn Age: 0   P Pediatric Age: 0-17   M Maternity Age: 12-55   A Adult Age: 15-124   CC CC Condition   MC Major Complication   CD Complex Dx   HIV HIV Related Dx

Tabular List — **ENDOCRINE, NUTRITIONAL, METABOLIC, IMMUNITY** — 272.4–275.41

272.4 Other and unspecified hyperlipidemia
Alpha-lipoproteinemia
Combined hyperlipidemia
Hyperlipidemia NOS
Hyperlipoproteinemia NOS

DEF: Hyperlipoproteinemia: elevated levels of transient chylomicrons in the blood which are a form of lipoproteins which transport dietary cholesterol and triglycerides from the small intestine to the blood.

272.5 Lipoprotein deficiencies
Abetalipoproteinemia
Bassen-Kornzweig syndrome
High-density lipoid deficiency
Hypoalphalipoproteinemia
Hypobetalipoproteinemia (familial)

DEF: Abnormally low levels of lipoprotein, a complex of fats and protein, in the blood.

272.6 Lipodystrophy
Barraquer-Simons disease
Progressive lipodystrophy
Use additional E code to identify cause, if iatrogenic
EXCLUDES intestinal lipodystrophy (040.2)

DEF: Disturbance of fat metabolism resulting in loss of fatty tissue in some areas of the body.

272.7 Lipidoses
Chemically-induced lipidosis
Disease:
   Anderson's
   Fabry's
   Gaucher's
   I cell [mucolipidosis I]
   lipoid storage NOS
   Niemann-Pick
   pseudo-Hurler's or mucolipidosis III
   triglyceride storage, Type I or II
   Wolman's or triglyceride storage, Type III
Mucolipidosis II
Primary familial xanthomatosis
EXCLUDES cerebral lipidoses (330.1)
Tay-Sachs disease (330.1)

DEF: Lysosomal storage diseases marked by an abnormal amount of lipids in reticuloendothelial cells.

272.8 Other disorders of lipoid metabolism
Hoffa's disease or liposynovitis prepatellaris
Launois-Bensaude's lipomatosis
Lipoid dermatoarthritis

272.9 Unspecified disorder of lipoid metabolism

√4th **273 Disorders of plasma protein metabolism**
EXCLUDES agammaglobulinemia and hypogammaglobulinemia (279.0-279.2)
coagulation defects (286.0-286.9)
hereditary hemolytic anemias (282.0-282.9)

273.0 Polyclonal hypergammaglobulinemia
Hypergammaglobulinemic purpura:
   benign primary
   Waldenström's

DEF: Elevated blood levels of gamma globulins, frequently found in patients with chronic infectious diseases.

273.1 Monoclonal paraproteinemia
Benign monoclonal hypergammaglobulinemia [BMH]
Monoclonal gammopathy:
   NOS
   associated with lymphoplasmacytic dyscrasias
   benign
Paraproteinemia:
   benign (familial)
   secondary to malignant or inflammatory disease

273.2 Other paraproteinemias
Cryoglobulinemic: Mixed cryoglobulinemia
   purpura
   vasculitis

273.3 Macroglobulinemia CC
Macroglobulinemia (idiopathic) (primary)
Waldenström's macroglobulinemia
CC Excl: 273.0-273.9

DEF: Elevated blood levels of macroglobulins (plasma globulins of high weight); characterized by malignant neoplasms of bone marrow, spleen, liver, or lymph nodes; symptoms include weakness, fatigue, bleeding disorders, and vision problems.

273.8 Other disorders of plasma protein metabolism
Abnormality of transport protein
Bisalbuminemia
AHA: 2Q, '98, 11

273.9 Unspecified disorder of plasma protein metabolism

√4th **274 Gout**
EXCLUDES lead gout (984.0-984.9)
AHA: 2Q, '95, 4

DEF: Purine and pyrimidine metabolic disorders; manifested by hyperuricemia and recurrent acute inflammatory arthritis; monosodium urate or monohydrate crystals may be deposited in and around the joints, leading to joint destruction, and severe crippling.

274.0 Gouty arthropathy
√5th **274.1 Gouty nephropathy**
  274.10 Gouty nephropathy, unspecified
  AHA: N-D, '85, 15

  274.11 Uric acid nephrolithiasis
  DEF: Sodium urate stones in the kidney.

  274.19 Other

√5th **274.8 Gout with other specified manifestations**
  274.81 Gouty tophi of ear
  DEF: Chalky sodium urate deposit in the ear due to gout; produces chronic inflammation of external ear.

  274.82 Gouty tophi of other sites
  Gouty tophi of heart

  274.89 Other
  Use additional code to identify manifestations, as:
  gouty:
    iritis (364.11)   neuritis (357.4)

274.9 Gout, unspecified

√4th **275 Disorders of mineral metabolism**
EXCLUDES abnormal findings without manifest disease (790.0-796.9)

275.0 Disorders of iron metabolism
Bronzed diabetes   Pigmentary cirrhosis (of liver)
Hemochromatosis
EXCLUDES anemia:
   iron deficiency (280.0-280.9)
   sideroblastic (285.0)
AHA: 2Q, '97, 11

275.1 Disorders of copper metabolism
Hepatolenticular degeneration
Wilson's disease

275.2 Disorders of magnesium metabolism
Hypermagnesemia   Hypomagnesemia

275.3 Disorders of phosphorus metabolism
Familial hypophosphatemia Vitamin D-resistant:
Hypophosphatasia   osteomalacia
                              rickets

√5th **275.4 Disorders of calcium metabolism**
EXCLUDES parathyroid disorders (252.0-252.9)
vitamin D deficiency (268.0-268.9)
AHA: 4Q, '97, 33

  275.40 Unspecified disorder of calcium metabolism
  275.41 Hypocalcemia
  DEF: Abnormally decreased blood calcium level; symptoms include hyperactive deep tendon reflexes, muscle, abdominal cramps, and carpopedal spasm.

√4th Additional Digit Required   Nonspecific PDx   Unacceptable PDx   Manifestation Code   MSP Medicare Secondary Payer   ▶◀ Revised Text   ● New Code   ▲ Revised Code Title

2002 Ingenix, Inc.   Volume 1 — 57

275.42 Hypercalcemia
  DEF: Abnormally increased blood calcium level; symptoms include muscle weakness, fatigue, nausea, depression, and constipation.

275.49 Other disorders of calcium metabolism
  Nephrocalcinosis
  Pseudohypoparathyroidism
  Pseudopseudohypoparathyroidism
  DEF: Nephrocalcinosis: calcium phosphate deposits in the tubules of the kidney with resultant renal insufficiency.
  DEF: Pseudohypoparathyroidism: inherited disorder with signs and symptoms of hypoparathyroidism; caused by inadequate response to parathyroid hormone, not hormonal deficiency. Symptoms include muscle cramps, tetany, urinary frequency, blurred vision due to cataracts, and dry scaly skin.
  DEF: Pseudopseudohypoparathyroidism: clinical manifestations of hypoparathyroidism without affecting blood calcium levels.

275.8 Other specified disorders of mineral metabolism

275.9 Unspecified disorder of mineral metabolism

✓4th **276 Disorders of fluid, electrolyte, and acid-base balance**
  EXCLUDES diabetes insipidus (253.5)
            familial periodic paralysis (359.3)

276.0 Hyperosmolality and/or hypernatremia CC
  Sodium [Na] excess   Sodium [Na] overload
  CC Excl: 276.0-276.9

276.1 Hyposmolality and/or hyponatremia CC
  Sodium [Na] deficiency
  CC Excl: See code 276.0
  DRG 296

276.2 Acidosis CC
  Acidosis: Acidosis:
    NOS   metabolic
    lactic   respiratory
  EXCLUDES diabetic acidosis (250.1)
  CC Excl: See code 276.0
  AHA: J-F, '87, 15
  DEF: Disorder involves decrease of pH (hydrogen ion) concentration in blood and cellular tissues; caused by increase in acid and decrease in bicarbonate.

276.3 Alkalosis CC
  Alkalosis: Alkalosis:
    NOS   respiratory
    metabolic
  CC Excl: See code 276.0
  DEF: Accumulation of base (non-acid part of salt), or loss of acid without relative loss of base in body fluids; caused by increased arterial plasma bicarbonate concentration or loss of carbon dioxide due to hyperventilation.

276.4 Mixed acid-base balance disorder CC
  Hypercapnia with mixed acid-base disorder
  CC Excl: See code 276.0

276.5 Volume depletion CC
  Dehydration
  Depletion of volume of plasma or extracellular fluid
  Hypovolemia
  EXCLUDES hypovolemic shock:
              postoperative (998.0)
              traumatic (958.4)
  CC Excl: See code 276.0
  AHA: 4Q, '97, 30; 2Q, '88, 9
  DRG 296

276.6 Fluid overload CC
  Fluid retention
  EXCLUDES ascites (789.5)
            localized edema (782.3)
  CC Excl: See code 276.0

276.7 Hyperpotassemia CC
  Hyperkalemia   Potassium [K]:
  Potassium [K]:   intoxication
    excess   overload
  CC Excl: See code 276.0
  AHA: 2Q, '01, 12
  DEF: Elevated blood levels of potassium; symptoms include abnormal EKG readings, weakness; related to defective renal excretion.

276.8 Hypopotassemia
  Hypokalemia   Potassium [K] deficiency
  DEF: Decreased blood levels of potassium; symptoms include neuromuscular disorders.

276.9 Electrolyte and fluid disorders not elsewhere classified CC
  Electrolyte imbalance   Hypochloremia
  Hyperchloremia
  EXCLUDES electrolyte imbalance:
              associated with hyperemesis gravidarum (643.1)
              complicating labor and delivery (669.0)
              following abortion and ectopic or molar pregnancy (634-638 with .4, 639.4)
  CC Excl: See code 276.0
  AHA: J-F, '87, 15

✓4th **277 Other and unspecified disorders of metabolism**

✓5th **277.0 Cystic fibrosis**
  Fibrocystic disease of the pancreas
  Mucoviscidosis
  AHA: 4Q, '90, 16; 3Q, '90, 18
  DEF: Generalized, genetic disorder of infants, children, and young adults marked by exocrine gland dysfunction; characterized by chronic pulmonary disease with excess mucus production, pancreatic deficiency, high levels of electrolytes in the sweat.

  277.00 Without mention of meconium ileus CC
    ▶Cystic fibrosis NOS◀
    CC Excl: ▶277.00-277.09◀

  277.01 With meconium ileus CC N
    Meconium:
      ileus (of newborn)
      obstruction of intestine in mucoviscidosis
    CC Excl: See code 277.00

  277.02 With pulmonary manifestations CC
    Cystic fibrosis with pulmonary exacerbation
    Use additional code to identify any infectious organism present, such as: pseudomonas (041.7)
    CC Excl: See code 277.00

  277.03 With gastrointestinal manifestations CC
    EXCLUDES with meconium ileus (277.01)
    CC Excl: See code 277.00

  277.09 With other manifestations CC
    CC Excl: See code 277.00

277.1 Disorders of porphyrin metabolism
  Hematoporphyria   Porphyrinuria
  Hematoporphyrinuria   Protocoproporphyria
  Hereditary coproporphyria Protoporphyria
  Porphyria   Pyrroloporphyria

ENDOCRINE, NUTRITIONAL, METABOLIC, IMMUNITY

277.2 Other disorders of purine and pyrimidine metabolism
  Hypoxanthine-guanine-phosphoribosyltransferase deficiency [HG-PRT deficiency]
  Lesch-Nyhan syndrome
  Xanthinuria
  EXCLUDES gout (274.0-274.9)
  orotic aciduric anemia (281.4)

277.3 Amyloidosis
  Amyloidosis:
    NOS
    inherited systemic
    nephropathic
    neuropathic (Portuguese)
    secondary
  Benign paroxysmal peritonitis
  Familial Mediterranean fever
  Hereditary cardiac amyloidosis (Swiss)
  Syndrome:

  AHA: 1Q, '96, 16

  DEF: Conditions of diverse etiologies characterized by the accumulation of insoluble fibrillar proteins (amyloid) in various organs and tissues of the body, compromising vital functions.

277.4 Disorders of bilirubin excretion
  Hyperbilirubinemia:
    congenital
    constitutional
  Syndrome:
    Crigler-Najjar
  Syndrome:
    Dubin-Johnson
    Gilbert's
    Rotor's
  EXCLUDES hyperbilirubinemias specific to the perinatal period (774.0-774.7)

277.5 Mucopolysaccharidosis
  Gargoylism
  Hunter's syndrome
  Hurler's syndrome
  Lipochondrodystrophy
  Maroteaux-Lamy syndrome
  Morquio-Brailsford disease
  Osteochondrodystrophy
  Sanfilippo's syndrome
  Scheie's syndrome

  DEF: Metabolism disorders evidenced by excretion of various mucopolysaccharides in urine and infiltration of these substances into connective tissue, with resulting various defects of bone, cartilage and connective tissue.

277.6 Other deficiencies of circulating enzymes
  Alpha 1-antitrypsin deficiency
  Hereditary angioedema

277.7 Dysmetabolic syndrome X ▲
  Use additional code for associated manifestations, such as:
    cardiovascular disease ▶(414.00-414.06)◀
    obesity (278.00-278.01)

  AHA: 4Q, '01, 42

  DEF: A specific group of metabolic disorders that are related to the state of insulin resistance (decreased cellular response to insulin) without elevated blood sugars; often related to elevated cholesterol and triglycerides, obesity, cardiovascular disease, and high blood pressure.

277.8 Other specified disorders of metabolism
  Hand-Schüller-Christian disease
  Histiocytosis (acute) (chronic)
  Histiocytosis X (chronic)
  EXCLUDES histiocytosis:
    acute differentiated progressive (202.5)
    X, acute (progressive) (202.5)

  AHA: 2Q, '01, 18; S-O, '87, 9

277.9 Unspecified disorder of metabolism
  Enzymopathy NOS

✓4th **278 Obesity and other hyperalimentation**
  EXCLUDES hyperalimentation NOS (783.6)
  poisoning by vitamins NOS (963.5)
  polyphagia (783.6)

✓5th **278.0 Obesity**
  EXCLUDES adiposogenital dystrophy (253.8)
  obesity of endocrine origin NOS (259.9)

  278.00 Obesity, unspecified
    Obesity NOS
    AHA: 4Q, '01, 42;1Q, '99, 5, 6

  278.01 Morbid obesity
    DEF: Increased weight beyond limits of skeletal and physical requirements (125 percent or more over ideal body weight), as a result of excess fat in subcutaneous connective tissues.

278.1 Localized adiposity
  Fat pad

278.2 Hypervitaminosis A

278.3 Hypercarotinemia
  DEF: Elevated blood carotene level due to ingesting excess carotenoids or the inability to convert carotenoids to vitamin A.

278.4 Hypervitaminosis D
  DEF: Weakness, fatigue, loss of weight, and other symptoms resulting from ingesting excessive amounts of vitamin D.

278.8 Other hyperalimentation

✓4th **279 Disorders involving the immune mechanism**

✓5th **279.0 Deficiency of humoral immunity**
  DEF: Inadequate immune response to bacterial infections with potential reinfection by viruses due to lack of circulating immunoglobulins (acquired antibodies).

  279.00 Hypogammaglobulinemia, unspecified
    Agammaglobulinemia NOS

  279.01 Selective IgA immunodeficiency

  279.02 Selective IgM immunodeficiency CC
    CC Excl: 279.02-279.9

  279.03 Other selective immunoglobulin deficiencies CC
    Selective deficiency of IgG
    CC Excl: See code 279.02

  279.04 Congenital hypogammaglobulinemia CC
    Agammaglobulinemia:
      Bruton's type
      X-linked
    CC Excl: See code 279.02

  279.05 Immunodeficiency with increased IgM CC
    Immunodeficiency with hyper-IgM:
      autosomal recessive
      X-linked
    CC Excl: See code 279.02

  279.06 Common variable immunodeficiency CC
    Dysgammaglobulinemia (acquired) (congenital) (primary)
    Hypogammaglobulinemia:
      acquired primary
      congenital non-sex-linked
      sporadic
    CC Excl: See code 279.02

  279.09 Other CC
    Transient hypogammaglobulinemia of infancy
    CC Excl: See code 279.02

✓5th **279.1 Deficiency of cell-mediated immunity**

  279.10 Immunodeficiency with predominant T-cell defect, unspecified CC
    CC Excl: See code 279.02

    AHA: S-O, '87, 10

  279.11 DiGeorge's syndrome CC
    Pharyngeal pouch syndrome
    Thymic hypoplasia
    CC Excl: See code 279.02

    DEF: Congenital disorder due to defective development of the third and fourth pharyngeal pouches; results in hypoplasia or aplasia of the thymus, parathyroid glands; related to congenital heart defects, anomalies of the great vessels, esophageal atresia, and abnormalities of facial structures.

279.12 Wiskott-Aldrich syndrome `cc`
CC Excl: See code 279.02

DEF: A disease characterized by chronic conditions, such as eczema, suppurative otitis media and anemia; it results from an X-linked recessive gene and is classified as an immune deficiency syndrome.

279.13 Nezelof's syndrome `cc`
Cellular immunodeficiency with abnormal immunoglobulin deficiency
CC Excl: See code 279.02

DEF: Immune system disorder characterized by a pathological deficiency in cellular immunity and humoral antibodies resulting in inability to fight infectious diseases.

279.19 Other `cc`
EXCLUDES ataxia-telangiectasia (334.8)
CC Excl: See code 279.02

279.2 Combined immunity deficiency `cc`
Agammaglobulinemia:
  autosomal recessive
  Swiss-type
  x-linked recessive
Severe combined immunodeficiency [SCID]
Thymic:
  alymophoplasia
  aplasia or dysplasia with immunodeficiency
EXCLUDES thymic hypoplasia (279.11)
CC Excl: See code 279.02

DEF: Agammaglobulinemia: No immunoglobulins in the blood.

DEF: Thymic alymphoplasia: Severe combined immunodeficiency; result of failed lymphoid tissue development.

279.3 Unspecified immunity deficiency `cc`
CC Excl: See code 279.02

279.4 Autoimmune disease, not elsewhere classified `cc`
Autoimmune disease NOS
EXCLUDES transplant failure or rejection (996.80-996.89)
CC Excl: See code 279.02

279.8 Other specified disorders involving the immune mechanism `cc`
Single complement [C_1-C_9] deficiency or dysfunction
CC Excl: See code 279.02

279.9 Unspecified disorder of immune mechanism `cc`
CC Excl: See code 279.02

AHA: 3Q, '92, 13

BLOOD AND BLOOD-FORMING ORGANS

4. DISEASES OF THE BLOOD AND BLOOD-FORMING ORGANS (280-289)

EXCLUDES anemia complicating pregnancy or the puerperium (648.2)

280 Iron deficiency anemias
INCLUDES anemia:
- asiderotic
- hypochromic-microcytic
- sideropenic

EXCLUDES familial microcytic anemia (282.4)

280.0 Secondary to blood loss (chronic)
Normocytic anemia due to blood loss
EXCLUDES acute posthemorrhagic anemia (285.1)
CC Excl: 280.0-280.9, 281.0-281.9, 282.0-282.9, 283.0-283.9, 284.0-284.9, 285.0-285.9, 289.8-289.9

AHA: 4Q, '93, 34

280.1 Secondary to inadequate dietary iron intake

280.8 Other specified iron deficiency anemias
- Paterson-Kelly syndrome
- Plummer-Vinson syndrome
- Sideropenic dysphagia

280.9 Iron deficiency anemia, unspecified
Anemia:
- achlorhydric
- chlorotic
- idiopathic hypochromic
- iron [Fe] deficiency NOS

281 Other deficiency anemias

281.0 Pernicious anemia
Anemia:
- Addison's
- Biermer's
- congenital pernicious
Congenital intrinsic factor [Castle's] deficiency
EXCLUDES combined system disease without mention of anemia (266.2)
subacute degeneration of spinal cord without mention of anemia (266.2)

AHA: N-D, '84, 1; S-O, '84, 16

DEF: Chronic progressive anemia due to Vitamin B_{12} malabsorption; caused by lack of a secretion known as intrinsic factor, which is produced by the gastric mucosa of the stomach.

281.1 Other vitamin B_{12} deficiency anemia
Anemia:
- vegan's
- vitamin B_{12} deficiency (dietary)
- due to selective vitamin B_{12} malabsorption with proteinuria
Syndrome:
- Imerslund's
- Imerslund-Gräsbeck
EXCLUDES combined system disease without mention of anemia (266.2)
subacute degeneration of spinal cord without mention of anemia (266.2)

281.2 Folate-deficiency anemia
Congenital folate malabsorption
Folate or folic acid deficiency anemia:
- NOS
- dietary
- drug-induced
Goat's milk anemia
Nutritional megaloblastic anemia (of infancy)
Use additional E code to identify drug

DEF: Macrocytic anemia resembles pernicious anemia but without absence of hydrochloric acid secretions; responsive to folic acid therapy.

281.3 Other specified megaloblastic anemias not elsewhere classified
Combined B_{12} and folate-deficiency anemia
Refractory megaloblastic anemia

DEF: Megaloblasts predominant in bone marrow with few normoblasts; rare familial type associated with proteinuria and genitourinary tract anomalies.

281.4 Protein-deficiency anemia
Amino-acid-deficiency anemia
CC Excl: See code 280.0

281.8 Anemia associated with other specified nutritional deficiency
Scorbutic anemia
CC Excl: See code 280.0

281.9 Unspecified deficiency anemia
Anemia:
- dimorphic
- macrocytic
- megaloblastic NOS

Anemia:
- nutritional NOS
- simple chronic

282 Hereditary hemolytic anemias
DEF: Escalated rate of erythrocyte destruction; similar to all anemias, occurs when imbalance exists between blood loss and blood production.

282.0 Hereditary spherocytosis
Acholuric (familial) jaundice
Congenital hemolytic anemia (spherocytic)
Congenital spherocytosis
Minkowski-Chauffard syndrome
Spherocytosis (familial)
EXCLUDES hemolytic anemia of newborn (773.0-773.5)

DEF: Hereditary, chronic illness marked by abnormal red blood cell membrane; symptoms include enlarged spleen, jaundice; and anemia in severe cases.

282.1 Hereditary elliptocytosis
Elliptocytosis (congenital)
Ovalocytosis (congenital) (hereditary)

DEF: Genetic hemolytic anemia characterized by malformed, elliptical erythrocytes; there is increased destruction of red cells with resulting anemia.

282.2 Anemias due to disorders of glutathione metabolism
Anemia:
- 6-phosphogluconic dehydrogenase deficiency
- enzyme deficiency, drug-induced
- erythrocytic glutathione deficiency
- glucose-6-phosphate dehydrogenase [G-6-PD] deficiency
- glutathione-reductase deficiency
- hemolytic nonspherocytic (hereditary), type I
Disorder of pentose phosphate pathway
Favism

282.3 Other hemolytic anemias due to enzyme deficiency
Anemia:
- hemolytic nonspherocytic (hereditary), type II
- hexokinase deficiency
- pyruvate kinase [PK] deficiency
- triosephosphate isomerase deficiency

BLOOD AND BLOOD-FORMING ORGANS

282.4 Thalassemias [CC]
Cooley's anemia
Hereditary leptocytosis
Mediterranean anemia (with other hemoglobinopathy)
Microdrepanocytosis
Sickle-cell thalassemia
Thalassemia (alpha) (beta) (intermedia) (major) (minima) (minor) (mixed) (trait) (with other hemoglobinopathy)
Thalassemia-Hb-S disease
> EXCLUDES   sickle-cell:
>   anemia (282.60-282.69)
>   trait (282.5)

CC Excl: See code 280.0

282.5 Sickle-cell trait
Hb-AS genotype
Hemoglobin S [Hb-S] trait
Heterozygous:
    hemoglobin S
    Hb-S
> EXCLUDES   that with other hemoglobinopathy (282.60-282.69)
>   that with thalassemia (282.4)

DEF: Heterozygous genetic makeup characterized by one gene for normal hemoglobin and one for sickle-cell hemoglobin; clinical disease rarely present.

√5th 282.6 Sickle-cell anemia
> EXCLUDES   sickle-cell thalassemia (282.4)
>   sickle-cell trait (282.5)

DEF: Inherited blood disorder; sickle-shaped red blood cells are hard and pointed, clogging blood flow; anemia characterized by, periodic episodes of pain, acute abdominal discomfort, skin ulcerations of the legs, increased infections; occurs primarily in persons of African descent.

282.60 Sickle-cell anemia, unspecified [CC]
CC Excl: See code 280.0
AHA: 2Q, '97, 11

282.61 Hb-S disease without mention of crisis [CC]
CC Excl: See code 280.0

282.62 Hb-S disease with mention of crisis [CC]
Sickle-cell crisis NOS
CC Excl: See code 280.0
AHA: 2Q, '98, 8; 2Q, '91, 15

282.63 Sickle-cell/Hb-C disease [CC]
Hb-S/Hb-C disease
CC Excl: See code 280.0

282.69 Other [CC]
Disease:
    Hb-S/Hb-D
    Hb-S/Hb-E
Disease:
    sickle-cell/Hb-D
    sickle-cell/Hb-E
CC Excl: See code 280.0

282.7 Other hemoglobinopathies
Abnormal hemoglobin NOS
Congenital Heinz-body anemia
Disease:
    Hb-Bart's
    hemoglobin C [Hb-C]
    hemoglobin D [Hb-D]
    hemoglobin E [Hb-E]
    hemoglobin Zurich [Hb-Zurich]
Hemoglobinopathy NOS
Hereditary persistence of fetal hemoglobin [HPFH]
Unstable hemoglobin hemolytic disease
> EXCLUDES   familial polycythemia (289.6)
>   hemoglobin M [Hb-M] disease (289.7)
>   high-oxygen-affinity hemoglobin (289.0)

DEF: Any disorder of hemoglobin due to alteration of molecular structure; may include overt anemia.

282.8 Other specified hereditary hemolytic anemias
Stomatocytosis

282.9 Hereditary hemolytic anemia, unspecified
Hereditary hemolytic anemia NOS

√4th 283 Acquired hemolytic anemias
DEF: Non-hereditary anemia characterized by premature destruction of red blood cells; caused by infectious organisms, poisons, and physical agents
AHA: N-D, '84, 1

283.0 Autoimmune hemolytic anemias [CC]
Autoimmune hemolytic disease (cold type) (warm type)
Chronic cold hemagglutinin disease
Cold agglutinin disease or hemoglobinuria
Hemolytic anemia:
    cold type (secondary) (symptomatic)
    drug-induced
    warm type (secondary) (symptomatic)
Use additional E code to identify cause, if drug-induced
> EXCLUDES   Evans' syndrome (287.3)
>   hemolytic disease of newborn (773.0-773.5)

CC Excl: See code 280.0

√5th 283.1 Non-autoimmune hemolytic anemias
Use additional E code to identify cause
DEF: Hemolytic anemia and thrombocytopenia with acute renal failure; relatively rare condition; 50 percent of patients require renal dialysis.
AHA: 4Q, '93, 25

283.10 Non-autoimmune hemolytic anemia, unspecified [CC]
CC Excl: See code 280.0

283.11 Hemolytic-uremic syndrome [CC]
CC Excl: See code 280.0

283.19 Other non-autoimmune hemolytic anemias [CC]
Hemolytic anemia:
    mechanical
    microangiopathic
Hemolytic anemia:
    toxic
CC Excl: See code 280.0

283.2 Hemoglobinuria due to hemolysis from external causes [CC]
Acute intravascular hemolysis
Hemoglobinuria:
    from exertion
    march
    paroxysmal (cold) (nocturnal)
    due to other hemolysis
Marchiafava-Micheli syndrome
Use additional E code to identify cause
CC Excl: See code 280.0

283.9 Acquired hemolytic anemia, unspecified [CC]
Acquired hemolytic anemia NOS
Chronic idiopathic hemolytic anemia
CC Excl: See code 280.0

√4th 284 Aplastic anemia
AHA: 1Q, '91, 14; N-D, '84, 1; S-0, '84, 16
DEF: Bone marrow failure to produce the normal amount of blood components; generally non-responsive to usual therapy.

BLOOD AND BLOOD-FORMING ORGANS

284.0 Constitutional aplastic anemia [CC]
Aplasia, (pure) red cell:
  congenital
  of infants
  primary
Blackfan-Diamond syndrome
Familial hypoplastic anemia
Fanconi's anemia
Pancytopenia with malformations

CC Excl: See code 280.0

AHA: 1Q, '91, 14

284.8 Other specified aplastic anemias [CC]
Aplastic anemia (due to):
  chronic systemic disease
  drugs
  infection
  radiation
  toxic (paralytic)
Pancytopenia (acquired)
Red cell aplasia (acquired) (adult) (pure) (with thymoma)
Use additional E code to identify cause

CC Excl: See code 280.0

AHA: 1Q, '97, 5; 1Q, '92, 15; 1Q, '91, 14

284.9 Aplastic anemia, unspecified [CC]
Anemia:
  aplastic (idiopathic) NOS
  aregenerative
  hypoplastic NOS
Anemia:
  nonregenerative
  refractory
Medullary hypoplasia

CC Excl: See code 280.0

DEF: Group of hereditary anemias occurring in the Mediterranean and Southeast Asia; characterized by impaired hemoglobin synthesis; homozygous form may cause death in utero; mild red blood cell anomalies in heterozygous.

✓4th 285 Other and unspecified anemias
AHA: 1Q, '91, 14; N-D, '84, 1

285.0 Sideroblastic anemia [CC]
Anemia:
  hypochromic with iron loading
  sideroachrestic
  sideroblastic
    acquired
    congenital
    hereditary
    primary
    refractory
    secondary (drug-induced) (due to disease)
    sex-linked hypochromic
    vitamin B_6-responsive
Pyridoxine-responsive (hypochromic) anemia
Use additional E code to identify cause, if drug induced

CC Excl: See code 280.0

DEF: Characterized by a disruption of final heme synthesis; results in iron overload of reticuloendothelial tissues.

285.1 Acute posthemorrhagic anemia [CC]
Anemia due to acute blood loss
  EXCLUDES anemia due to chronic blood loss (280.0)
  blood loss anemia NOS (280.0)

CC Excl: 280.0-280.9, 281.0-281.9, 282.0-282.9, 283.0-283.9, 284.0, 284.8, 285.0-285.9, 289.8-289.9, 958.2

AHA: 2Q, '92, 15

✓5th 285.2 Anemia in chronic illness
AHA: 4Q, '00, 39

285.21 Anemia in end-stage renal disease
285.22 Anemia in neoplastic disease
285.29 Anemia of other chronic illness

285.8 Other specified anemias
Anemia:
  dyserythropoietic (congenital)
  dyshematopoietic (congenital)
  leukoerythroblastic
  von Jaksch's
Infantile pseudoleukemia

AHA: 1Q, '91, 16

285.9 Anemia, unspecified
Anemia:
  NOS
  essential
  normocytic, not due to blood loss
Anemia:
  profound
  progressive
  secondary
Oligocythemia

EXCLUDES anemia (due to):
  blood loss:
    acute (285.1)
    chronic or unspecified (280.0)
  iron deficiency (280.0-280.9)

AHA: ▶1Q, '02, 14;◀ 2Q, '92, 16; M-A, '85, 13; N-D, '84, 1

✓4th 286 Coagulation defects

286.0 Congenital factor VIII disorder [CC]
Antihemophilic globulin [AHG] deficiency
Factor VIII (functional) deficiency
Hemophilia:
  NOS
Hemophilia:
  A
  classical
  familial
  hereditary
Subhemophilia

EXCLUDES factor VIII deficiency with vascular defect (286.4)

CC Excl: 286.0-286.9, 287.0-287.9, 289.8-289.9

DEF: Hereditary, sex-linked, results in missing antihemophilic globulin (AHG) (factor VIII); causes abnormal coagulation characterized by increased tendency to bleeding, large bruises of skin, soft tissue; may also be bleeding in mouth, nose, gastrointestinal tract; after childhood, hemorrhages in joints, resulting in swelling and impaired function.

286.1 Congenital factor IX disorder [CC]
Christmas disease
Deficiency:
  factor IX (functional)
  plasma thromboplastin component [PTC]
Hemophilia B

CC Excl: See code 286.0

DEF: Deficiency of plasma thromboplastin component (PTC) (factor IX) and plasma thromboplastin antecedent (PTA); PTC deficiency clinically indistinguishable from classical hemophilia; PTA deficiency found in both sexes.

286.2 Congenital factor XI deficiency [CC]
Hemophilia C
Plasma thromboplastin antecedent [PTA] deficiency
Rosenthal's disease

CC Excl: See code 286.0

286.3–287.0 BLOOD AND BLOOD-FORMING ORGANS — Tabular List

286.3 Congenital deficiency of other clotting factors [CC]
Congenital afibrinogenemia
Deficiency:
AC globulin factor:
I [fibrinogen]
II [prothrombin]
V [labile]
VII [stable]
X [Stuart-Prower]
XII [Hageman]
XIII [fibrin stabilizing]
Laki-Lorand factor
proaccelerin
Disease
Owren's
Stuart-Prower
Dysfibrinogenemia (congenital)
Dysprothrombinemia (constitutional)
Hypoproconvertinemia
Hypoprothrmbinemia (hereditary)
Parahemophilia
CC Excl: See code 286.0

286.4 Von Willebrand's disease [CC]
Angiohemophilia (A) (B)
Constitutional thrombopathy
Factor VIII deficiency with vascular defect
Pseudohemophilia type B
Vascular hemophilia
von Willebrand's (-Jürgens') disease
EXCLUDES factor VIII deficiency:
NOS (286.0)
with functional defect (286.0)
hereditary capillary fragility (287.8)
CC Excl: See code 286.0

DEF: Abnormal blood coagulation caused by deficient blood Factor VII; congenital; symptoms include excess or prolonged bleeding, such as hemorrhage during menstruation, following birthing, or after surgical procedure.

286.5 Hemorrhagic disorder due to circulating anticoagulants [CC]
Antithrombinemia
Antithromboplastinemia
Antithromboplastino-genemia
Hyperheparinemia
Increase in:
anti-VIIIa
anti-IXa
anti-Xa
anti-XIa
antithrombin
Systemic lupus erythematosus [SLE] inhibitor
Use additional E code to identify cause, if drug induced
CC Excl: See code 286.0
AHA: 3Q, '92, 15; 3Q, '90, 14

286.6 Defibrination syndrome [CC]
Afibrinogenemia, acquired
Consumption coagulopathy
Diffuse or disseminated intravascular coagulation [DIC syndrome]
Fibrinolytic hemorrhage, acquired
Hemorrhagic fibrinogenolysis
Pathologic fibrinolysis
Purpura:
fibrinolytic
fulminans
EXCLUDES that complicating:
abortion (634-638 with .1, 639.1)
pregnancy or the puerperium (641.3, 666.3)
disseminated intravascular coagulation in newborn (776.2)
CC Excl: See code 286.0
AHA: 4Q, '93, 29

DEF: Characterized by destruction of circulating fibrinogen; often precipitated by other conditions, such as injury, causing release of thromboplastic particles in blood stream.

286.7 Acquired coagulation factor deficiency [CC]
Deficiency of coagulation factor due to:
liver disease
vitamin K deficiency
Hypoprothrombinemia, acquired
Use additional E code to identify cause, if drug induced
EXCLUDES vitamin K deficiency of newborn (776.0)
CC Excl: See code 286.0
AHA: 4Q, '93, 29

286.9 Other and unspecified coagulation defects [CC]
Defective coagulation NOS
Deficiency, coagulation factor NOS
Delay, coagulation
Disorder:
coagulation
hemostasis
EXCLUDES abnormal coagulation profile (790.92)
hemorrhagic disease of newborn (776.0)
that complicating:
abortion (634-638 with .1, 639.1)
pregnancy or the puerperium (641.3, 666.3)
CC Excl: See code 286.0
AHA: 4Q, '99, 22; 4Q, '93, 29

287 Purpura and other hemorrhagic conditions ✓4th
EXCLUDES hemorrhagic thrombocythemia (238.7)
purpura fulminans (286.6)
AHA: 1Q, '91, 14

287.0 Allergic purpura [CC]
Peliosis rheumatica   Purpura:
Purpura: rheumatica
anaphylactoid   Schönlein-Henoch
autoimmune   vascular
Henoch's   Vasculitis, allergic
nonthrombocytopenic:
hemorrhagic
idiopathic
EXCLUDES hemorrhagic purpura (287.3)
purpura annularis telangiectodes (709.1)
CC Excl: See code 286.0

DEF: Any hemorrhagic condition, thrombocytic or nonthrombocytopenic in origin, caused by a presumed allergic reaction.

BLOOD AND BLOOD-FORMING ORGANS

287.1 Qualitative platelet defects `CC`
  Thrombasthenia (hemorrhagic) (hereditary)
  Thrombocytasthenia
  Thrombocytopathy (dystrophic)
  Thrombopathy (Bernard-Soulier)
  EXCLUDES von Willebrand's disease (286.4)
  CC Excl: See code 286.0

287.2 Other nonthrombocytopenic purpuras `CC`
  Purpura: Purpura:
    NOS   simplex
    senile
  CC Excl: See code 286.0

287.3 Primary thrombocytopenia `CC`
  Evans' syndrome   Throbocytopenia:
  Megakaryocytic hypoplasia   congenital
  Purpura, thrombocytopenic   hereditary
    congenital   primary
    hereditary   Tidal platelet dysgenesis
    idiopathic
  EXCLUDES thrombotic thrombocytopenic purpura (446.6)
            transient thrombocytopenia of newborn (776.1)
  CC Excl: See code 286.0
  DEF: Decrease in number of blood platelets in circulating blood and purpural skin hemorrhages.

287.4 Secondary thrombocytopenia `CC`
  Posttransfusion purpura
  Thrombocytopenia (due to):
    dilutional
    drugs
    extracorporeal circulation of blood
    massive blood transfusion
    platelet alloimmunization
  Use additional E code to identify cause
  EXCLUDES transient thrombocytopenia of newborn (776.1)
  CC Excl: See code 286.0
  AHA: M-A, '85, 14
  DEF: Reduced number of platelets in circulating blood as consequence of an underlying disease or condition.

287.5 Thrombocytopenia, unspecified `CC`
  CC Excl: See code 286.0

287.8 Other specified hemorrhagic conditions `CC`
  Capillary fragility (hereditary)
  Vascular pseudohemophilia
  CC Excl: See code 286.0

287.9 Unspecified hemorrhagic conditions `CC`
  Hemorrhagic diathesis (familial)
  CC Excl: See code 286.0

✓4th 288 Diseases of white blood cells
  EXCLUDES leukemia (204.0-208.9)
  AHA: 1Q, '91, 14

288.0 Agranulocytosis `CC`
  Infantile genetic agranulocytosis   Neutropenia:
  Kostmann's syndrome   immune
  Neutropenia: periodic
    NOS   toxic
    cyclic   Neutropenic
    drug-induced   splenomegaly
  Use additional E code to identify drug or other cause
  EXCLUDES transitory neonatal neutropenia (776.7)
  CC Excl: 288.0-288.9, 289.8-289.9
  AHA: 3Q, '99, 6; 2Q, '99, 9; 3Q, '96, 16; 2Q, '96, 6
  DEF: Sudden, severe condition characterized by reduced number of white blood cells; results in sores in the throat, stomach or skin; symptoms include chills, fever; some drugs can bring on condition.

288.1 Functional disorders of polymorphonuclear neutrophils `CC`
  Chronic (childhood) granulomatous disease
  Congenital dysphagocytosis
  Job's syndrome
  Lipochrome histiocytosis (familial)
  Progressive septic granulomatosis
  CC Excl: See code 288.0

288.2 Genetic anomalies of leukocytes
  Anomaly (granulation) (granulocyte) or syndrome:
    Alder's (-Reilly)
    Chédiak-Steinbrinck (-Higashi)
    Jordan's
    May-Hegglin
    Pelger-Huet
  Hereditary:
    hypersegmentation
    hyposegmentation
    leukomelanopathy

288.3 Eosinophilia
  Eosinophilia   Eosinophilia
    allergic   secondary
    hereditary   Eosinophilic leukocytosis
    idiopathic
  EXCLUDES Löffler's syndrome (518.3)
            pulmonary eosinophilia (518.3)
  AHA: 3Q, '00, 11
  DEF: Elevated number of eosinophils in the blood; characteristic of allergic states and various parasitic infections.

288.8 Other specified disease of white blood cells
  Leukemoid reaction   Lymphocytopenia
    lymphocytic   Lymphocytosis (symptomatic)
    monocytic   Lymphopenia
    myelocytic   Monocytosis (symptomatic)
  Leukocytosis   Plasmacytosis
  EXCLUDES immunity disorders (279.0-279.9)
  AHA: M-A, '87, 12

288.9 Unspecified disease of white blood cells

✓4th 289 Other diseases of blood and blood-forming organs

289.0 Polycythemia, secondary
  High-oxygen-affinity hemoglobin
  Polycythemia:
    acquired
    benign
    due to:
      fall in plasma volume
      high altitude
    emotional
    erythropoietin
    hypoxemic
    nephrogenous
    relative
    spurious
    stress
  EXCLUDES polycythemia:
              neonatal (776.4)
              primary (238.4)
              vera (238.4)
  DEF: Elevated number of red blood cells in circulating blood as result of reduced oxygen supply to the tissues.

289.1 Chronic lymphadenitis
  Chronic:
    adenitis   } any lymph node, except
    lymphadenitis }   mesenteric
  EXCLUDES acute lymphadenitis (683)
            mesenteric (289.2)
            enlarged glands NOS (785.6)
  DEF: Persistent inflammation of lymph node tissue; origin of infection is usually elsewhere.

BLOOD AND BLOOD-FORMING ORGANS

289.2 Nonspecific mesenteric lymphadenitis
Mesenteric lymphadenitis (acute) (chronic)
DEF: Inflammation of the lymph nodes in peritoneal fold that encases abdominal organs; disease resembles acute appendicitis; unknown etiology.

289.3 Lymphadenitis, unspecified, except mesenteric
AHA: 2Q, '92, 8

289.4 Hypersplenism
"Big spleen" syndrome   Hypersplenia
Dyssplenism
EXCLUDES primary splenic neutropenia (288.0)
DEF: An overactive spleen; it causes a deficiency of the peripheral blood components, an increase in bone marrow cells and sometimes a notable increase in the size of the spleen.

√5ᵗʰ 289.5 Other diseases of spleen
   289.50 Disease of spleen, unspecified
   289.51 Chronic congestive splenomegaly
   289.59 Other
      Lien migrans   Splenic:
      Perisplenitis   fibrosis
      Splenic: infarction
        abscess   rupture, nontraumatic
        atrophy   Splenitis
        cyst   Wandering spleen
      EXCLUDES bilharzial splenic fibrosis (120.0-120.9)
                 hepatolienal fibrosis (571.5)
                 splenomegaly NOS (789.2)

289.6 Familial polycythemia
Familial:
  benign polycythemia
  erythrocytosis
DEF: Elevated number of red blood cells.

289.7 Methemoglobinemia
Congenital NADH [DPNH]-methemoglobin-reductase deficiency
Hemoglobin M [Hb-M] disease
Methemoglobinemia:
  NOS
  acquired (with sulfhemoglobinemia)
  hereditary
  toxic
Stokvis' disease
Sulfhemoglobinemia
Use additional E code to identify cause
DEF: Presence in the blood of methemoglobin, a chemically altered form of hemoglobin; causes cyanosis, headache, dizziness, ataxia dyspnea, tachycardia, nausea, stupor, coma, and, rarely, death.

289.8 Other specified diseases of blood and blood-forming organs
Hypergammaglobulinemia
Myelofibrosis
Pseudocholinesterase deficiency
AHA: ▶1Q, '02, 16;◀ 2Q, '89, 8; M-A, '87, 12

289.9 Unspecified diseases of blood and blood-forming organs
Blood dyscrasia NOS
Erythroid hyperplasia
AHA: M-A, '85, 14

5. MENTAL DISORDERS (290-319)

In the International Classification of Diseases, 9th Revision (ICD-9), the corresponding Chapter V, "Mental Disorders," includes a glossary which defines the contents of each category. The introduction to Chapter V in ICD-9 indicates that the glossary is intended so that psychiatrists can make the diagnosis based on the descriptions provided rather than from the category titles. Lay coders are instructed to code whatever diagnosis the physician records.

Chapter 5, "Mental Disorders," in ICD-9-CM uses the standard classification format with inclusion and exclusion terms, omitting the glossary as part of the main text.

The mental disorders section of ICD-9-CM has been expanded to incorporate additional psychiatric disorders not listed in ICD-9. The glossary from ICD-9 does not contain all these terms. It now appears in Appendix B, which also contains descriptions and definitions for the terms added in ICD-9-CM. Some of these were provided by the American Psychiatric Association's Task Force on Nomenclature and Statistics who are preparing the Diagnostic and Statistical Manual, Third Edition (DSM-III), and others from A Psychiatric Glossary.

The American Psychiatric Association provided invaluable assistance in modifying Chapter 5 of ICD-9-CM to incorporate detail useful to American clinicians and gave permission to use material from the aforementioned sources.

1. Manual of the *International Statistical Classification of Diseases, Injuries, and Causes of Death*, 9th Revision, World Health Organization, Geneva, Switzerland, 1975.
2. American Psychiatric Association, Task Force on Nomenclature and Statistics, Robert L. Spitzer, M.D., Chairman.
3. *A Psychiatric Glossary*, Fourth Edition, American Psychiatric Association, Washington, D.C., 1975.

PSYCHOSES (290-299)
EXCLUDES mental retardation (317-319)

ORGANIC PSYCHOTIC CONDITIONS (290-294)
INCLUDES psychotic organic brain syndrome
EXCLUDES nonpsychotic syndromes of organic etiology (310.0-310.9)
psychoses classifiable to 295-298 and without impairment of orientation, comprehension, calculation, learning capacity, and judgment, but associated with physical disease, injury, or condition affecting the brain [eg., following childbirth] (295.0-298.8)

AHA: 1Q, '88, 3

✓4th 290 Senile and presenile organic psychotic conditions
Code first the associated neurological condition
EXCLUDES dementia not classified as senile, presenile, or arteriosclerotic (294.10-294.11)
psychoses classifiable to 295-298 occurring in the senium without dementia or delirium (295.0-298.8)
senility with mental changes of nonpsychotic severity (310.1)
transient organic psychotic conditions (293.0-293.9)

290.0 Senile dementia, uncomplicated
Senile dementia:
 NOS
 simple type
EXCLUDES mild memory disturbances, not amounting to dementia, associated with senile brain disease (310.1)
senile dementia with:
 delirium or confusion (290.3)
 delusional [paranoid] features (290.20)
 depressive features (290.21)

AHA: 4Q, '99, 4

✓5th 290.1 Presenile dementia
Brain syndrome with presenile brain disease
EXCLUDES arteriosclerotic dementia (290.40-290.43)
dementia associated with other cerebral conditions (294.10-294.11)

AHA: N-D, '84, 20

290.10 Presenile dementia, uncomplicated
Presenile dementia: Presenile dementia:
 NOS simple type

290.11 Presenile dementia with delirium
Presenile dementia with acute confusional state

AHA: 1Q, '88, 3

290.12 Presenile dementia with delusional features
Presenile dementia, paranoid type

290.13 Presenile dementia with depressive features
Presenile dementia, depressed type

✓5th 290.2 Senile dementia with delusional or depressive features
EXCLUDES senile dementia:
 NOS (290.0)
 with delirium and/or confusion (290.3)

290.20 Senile dementia with delusional features
Senile dementia, paranoid type
Senile psychosis NOS

290.21 Senile dementia with depressive features

290.3 Senile dementia with delirium
Senile dementia with acute confusional state
EXCLUDES senile:
 dementia NOS (290.0)
 psychosis NOS (290.20)

✓5th 290.4 Arteriosclerotic dementia
Multi-infarct dementia or psychosis
Use additional code to identify cerebral atherosclerosis (437.0)
EXCLUDES suspected cases with no clear evidence of arteriosclerosis (290.9)

290.40 Arteriosclerotic dementia, uncomplicated
Arteriosclerotic dementia:
 NOS
 simple type

290.41 Arteriosclerotic dementia with delirium
Arteriosclerotic dementia with acute confusional state

290.42 Arteriosclerotic dementia with delusional features
Arteriosclerotic dementia, paranoid type

290.43 Arteriosclerotic dementia with depressive features
Arteriosclerotic dementia, depressed type

290.8 Other specified senile psychotic conditions
Presbyophrenic psychosis

290.9 Unspecified senile psychotic condition

✓4th 291 Alcoholic psychoses
EXCLUDES alcoholism without psychosis (303.0-303.9)

AHA: S-O, '86, 3

291.0 Alcohol withdrawal delirium
Alcoholic delirium Delirium tremens
EXCLUDES alcohol withdrawal (291.81)
CC Excl: 291.0-291.9, 292.0-292.9, 293.0-293.9, 294.0-294.9, 303.00-303.93, 304.00-304.91, 305.00-305.03, 305.20-305.93, 790.3

AHA: 2Q, '91, 11

291.1 Alcohol amnestic syndrome [CC]
Alcoholic polyneuritic psychosis
Korsakoff's psychosis, alcoholic
Wernicke-Korsakoff syndrome (alcoholic)

CC Excl: See code 291.0

AHA: 1Q, '88, 3

DEF: Prominent and lasting reduced memory span, disordered time appreciation and confabulation, occurring in alcoholics, as sequel to acute alcoholic psychosis.

291.2 Other alcoholic dementia [CC]
Alcoholic dementia NOS
Alcoholism associated with dementia NOS
Chronic alcoholic brain syndrome

CC Excl: See code 291.0

291.3 Alcohol withdrawal hallucinosis [CC]
Alcoholic: hallucinosis (acute)
Alcoholic: psychosis with hallucinosis

EXCLUDES alcohol withdrawal with delirium (291.0)
schizophrenia (295.0-295.9) and paranoid states (297.0-297.9) taking the form of chronic hallucinosis with clear consciousness in an alcoholic

CC Excl: See code 291.0

AHA: 2Q, '91, 11

DEF: Psychosis lasting less than six months with slight or no clouding of consciousness in which auditory hallucinations predominate.

291.4 Idiosyncratic alcohol intoxication [CC]
Pathologic: alcohol intoxication
Pathologic: drunkenness

EXCLUDES acute alcohol intoxication (305.0)
in alcoholism (303.0)
simple drunkenness (305.0)

CC Excl: See code 291.0

DEF: Unique behavioral patterns, like belligerence, after intake of relatively small amounts of alcohol; behavior not due to excess consumption.

291.5 Alcoholic jealousy
Alcoholic: paranoia
Alcoholic: psychosis, paranoid type

EXCLUDES nonalcoholic paranoid states (297.0-297.9)
schizophrenia, paranoid type (295.3)

√5th 291.8 Other specified alcoholic psychosis
AHA: 3Q, '94, 13; J-A, '85, 10

291.81 Alcohol withdrawal [CC]
Alcohol: abstinence syndrome or symptoms
withdrawal syndrome or symptoms

EXCLUDES alcohol withdrawal: delirium (291.0)
hallucinosis (291.3)
delirium tremens (291.0)

CC Excl: 291.0-291.9, 292.0-292.9, 293.0-293.9, 294.0-294.9, 303.00-303.93, 304.00-304.93, 305.00-305.03, 305.20-305.93, 790.3

AHA: 4Q, '96, 28; 2Q, '91, 11

291.89 Other [CC]
CC Excl: See code 291.81

291.9 Unspecified alcoholic psychosis [CC]
Alcoholic: mania NOS
psychosis NOS
Alcoholism (chronic) with psychosis

CC Excl: See code 291.0

√4th 292 Drug psychoses
INCLUDES drug-induced mental disorders
organic brain syndrome associated with consumption of drugs

Use additional code for any associated drug dependence (304.0-304.9)
Use additional E code to identify drug

AHA: 2Q, '91, 11; S-O, '86, 3

292.0 Drug withdrawal syndrome [CC]
Drug: abstinence syndrome or symptoms
withdrawal syndrome or symptoms

CC Excl: See code 291.0

AHA: 1Q, '97, 12

√5th 292.1 Paranoid and/or hallucinatory states induced by drugs

292.11 Drug-induced organic delusional syndrome [CC]
Paranoid state induced by drugs

CC Excl: See code 291.0

292.12 Drug-induced hallucinosis [CC]
Hallucinatory state induced by drugs

EXCLUDES states following LSD or other hallucinogens, lasting only a few days or less ["bad trips"] (305.3)

CC Excl: See code 291.0

292.2 Pathological drug intoxication [CC]
Drug reaction: NOS / idiosyncratic / pathologic } resulting in brief psychotic states

EXCLUDES expected brief psychotic reactions to hallucinogens ["bad trips"] (305.3)
physiological side-effects of drugs (e.g., dystonias)

CC Excl: See code 291.0

√5th 292.8 Other specified drug-induced mental disorders

292.81 Drug-induced delirium [CC]
CC Excl: See code 291.0

AHA: 1Q, '88, 3

292.82 Drug-induced dementia [CC]
CC Excl: See code 291.0

292.83 Drug-induced amnestic syndrome [CC]
CC Excl: See code 291.0

292.84 Drug-induced organic affective syndrome [CC]
Depressive state induced by drugs

CC Excl: See code 291.0

292.89 Other [CC]
Drug-induced organic personality syndrome

CC Excl: See code 291.0

292.9 Unspecified drug-induced mental disorder [CC]
Organic psychosis NOS due to or associated with drugs

CC Excl: See code 291.0

MENTAL DISORDERS

√4th 293 Transient organic psychotic conditions
INCLUDES transient organic mental disorders not associated with alcohol or drugs
Code first the associated physical or neurological condition
EXCLUDES confusional state or delirium superimposed on senile dementia (290.3)
dementia due to:
alcohol (291.0-291.9)
arteriosclerosis (290.40-290.43)
drugs (292.82)
senility (290.0)

293.0 Acute delirium
Acute:
confusional state
infective psychosis
organic reaction
posttraumatic organic psychosis
psycho-organic syndrome
Acute psychosis associated with endocrine, metabolic, or cerebrovascular disorder
Epileptic:
confusional state
twilight state
AHA: 1Q, '88, 3

293.1 Subacute delirium
Subacute:
confusional state
infective psychosis
organic reaction
posttraumatic organic psychosis
psycho-organic syndrome
psychosis associated with endocrine or metabolic disorder
AHA: 1Q, '88, 3

√5th 293.8 Other specified transient organic mental disorders

293.81 Organic delusional syndrome `CC`
Transient organic psychotic condition, paranoid type
CC Excl: 291.0-291.7, 291.81, 291.89, 291.9, 292.0-292.9, 293.0, 293.9, 294.0-294.9, 303.00-303.93, 304.00-304.93, 305.00-305.03, 305.20-305.93, 790.3

293.82 Organic hallucinosis syndrome `CC`
Transient organic psychotic condition, hallucinatory type
CC Excl: See code 293.81

293.83 Organic affective syndrome `CC`
Transient organic psychotic condition, depressive type
CC Excl: See code 293.81

293.84 Organic anxiety syndrome `CC`
CC Excl: See code 293.81

AHA: 4Q, '96, 29

293.89 Other

293.9 Unspecified transient organic mental disorder
Organic psychosis:
infective NOS
posttraumatic NOS
Organic psychosis:
transient NOS
Psycho-organic syndrome

√4th 294 Other organic psychotic conditions (chronic)
INCLUDES organic psychotic brain syndromes (chronic), not elsewhere classified
AHA: M-A, '85, 12

294.0 Amnestic syndrome
Korsakoff's psychosis or syndrome (nonalcoholic)
EXCLUDES alcoholic:
amnestic syndrome (291.1)
Korsakoff's psychosis (291.1)

√5th 294.1 Dementia in conditions classified elsewhere
Code first any underlying physical condition, as:
dementia in:
Alzheimer's disease (331.0)
cerebral lipidoses (330.1)
epilepsy (345.0-345.9)
general paresis [syphilis] (094.1)
hepatolenticular degeneration (275.1)
Huntington's chorea (333.4)
Jakob-Creutzfeldt disease (046.1)
multiple sclerosis (340)
Pick's disease of the brain (331.1)
polyarteritis nodosa (446.0)
syphilis (094.1)
EXCLUDES dementia:
arteriosclerotic (290.40-290.43)
presenile (290.10-290.13)
senile (290.0)
epileptic psychosis NOS (294.8)
AHA: 4Q, '00, 40; 1Q, '99, 14; N-D, '85, 5

294.10 Dementia in conditions classified elsewhere without behavioral disturbance
Dementia in conditions classified elsewhere NOS

294.11 Dementia in conditions classified elsewhere with behavioral disturbance
Aggressive behavior
Combative behavior
Violent behavior
Wandering off
AHA: 4Q, '00, 41

294.8 Other specified organic brain syndromes (chronic)
Epileptic psychosis NOS
Mixed paranoid and affective organic psychotic states
Use additional code for associated epilepsy (345.0-345.9)
EXCLUDES mild memory disturbances, not amounting to dementia (310.1)
AHA: 1Q, '88, 5

294.9 Unspecified organic brain syndrome (chronic) `HIV`
Organic psychosis (chronic)

OTHER PSYCHOSES (295-299)
Use additional code to identify any associated physical disease, injury, or condition affecting the brain with psychoses classifiable to 295-298

√4th 295 Schizophrenic disorders
INCLUDES schizophrenia of the types described in 295.0-295.9 occurring in children
EXCLUDES childhood type schizophrenia (299.9)
infantile autism (299.0)

The following fifth-digit subclassification is for use with category 295:
0 unspecified
1 subchronic
2 chronic
3 subchronic with acute exacerbation
4 chronic with acute exacerbation
5 in remission

DEF: Group of disorders with disturbances in thought (delusions, hallucinations), mood (blunted, flattened, inappropriate affect), sense of self, relationship to world; also bizarre, purposeless behavior, repetitious activity, or inactivity.

MENTAL DISORDERS

295.0 Simple type
Schizophrenia simplex
EXCLUDES latent schizophrenia (295.5)

CC Excl: For codes 295.00-295.04: 295.00-295.95, 296.00-296.99, 297.0-297.9, 298.0-298.9, 299.00-299.91, 300.00-300.9, 301.0-301.9, 306.0-306.9, 307.0-307.9, 308.0-308.9, 309.0-309.9, 310.0-310.9, 311, 312.00-312.9, 313.0-313.9, 314.00-314.9, 315.00-315.9, 316-317, 318.0-318.2, 319

295.1 Disorganized type
Hebephrenia
Hebephrenic type schizophrenia

CC Excl: For codes 295.10-295.14: See code 295.0

DEF: Inappropriate behavior; results in extreme incoherence and disorganization of time, place and sense of social appropriateness; withdrawal from routine social interaction may occur.

295.2 Catatonic type
Catatonic (schizophrenia):
  agitation
  excitation
  excited type
  stupor
  withdrawn type
Schizophrenic:
  catalepsy
  catatonia
  flexibilitas cerea

CC Excl: For codes 295.21-295.24: See code 295.0

DEF: Extreme changes in motor activity; one extreme is decreased response or reaction to the environment and the other is spontaneous activity.

295.3 Paranoid type
Paraphrenic schizophrenia
EXCLUDES involutional paranoid state (297.2)
  paranoia (297.1)
  paraphrenia (297.2)

CC Excl: For codes 295.30-295.34: See code 295.0

DEF: Preoccupied with delusional suspicions and auditory hallucinations related to single theme; usually hostile, grandiose, overly religious, occasionally hypochondriacal.

295.4 Acute schizophrenic episode
Oneirophrenia
Schizophreniform:
  attack
Schizophreniform:
  disorder
  psychosis, confusional type
EXCLUDES acute forms of schizophrenia of:
  catatonic type (295.2)
  hebephrenic type (295.1)
  paranoid type (295.3)
  simple type (295.0)
  undifferentiated type (295.8)

CC Excl: For codes 295.40-295.44: See code 295.0

295.5 Latent schizophrenia
Latent schizophrenic reaction
Schizophrenia:
  borderline
  incipient
  prepsychotic
  prodromal
  pseudoneurotic
  pseudopsychopathic
EXCLUDES schizoid personality (301.20-301.22)

295.6 Residual schizophrenia
Chronic undifferentiated schizophrenia
Restzustand (schizophrenic)
Schizophrenic residual state

CC Excl: For codes 295.60-295.64: See code 295.0

295.7 Schizo-affective type
Cyclic schizophrenia
Mixed schizophrenic and affective psychosis
Schizo-affective psychosis
Schizophreniform psychosis, affective type

CC Excl: For codes 295.70-295.74: See code 295.0

295.8 Other specified types of schizophrenia
Acute (undifferentiated) schizophrenia
Atypical schizophrenia
Cenesthopathic schizophrenia
EXCLUDES infantile autism (299.0)

CC Excl: For codes 295.80-295.84: See code 295.0

295.9 Unspecified schizophrenia
Schizophrenia:
  NOS
  mixed NOS
  undifferentiated NOS
Schizophrenic reaction NOS
Schizophreniform psychosis NOS

CC Excl: For codes 295.90-295.94: See code 295.0

AHA: 3Q, '95, 6

DRG 430 For code 295.90

296 Affective psychoses
INCLUDES episodic affective disorders
EXCLUDES neurotic depression (300.4)
  reactive depressive psychosis (298.0)
  reactive excitation (298.1)

The following fifth-digit subclassification is for use with categories 296.0-296.6:
  0 unspecified
  1 mild
  2 moderate
  3 severe, without mention of psychotic behavior
  4 severe, specified as with psychotic behavior
  5 in partial or unspecified remission
  6 in full remission

AHA: M-A, '85, 14

296.0 Manic disorder, single episode
Hypomania (mild) NOS
Hypomanic psychosis
Mania (monopolar) NOS
Manic-depressive psychosis or reaction:
  hypomanic
  manic
} single episode or unspecified

EXCLUDES circular type, if there was a previous attack of depression (296.4)

CC Excl: For code 296.04: See code 295.0

DEF: Mood disorder identified by hyperactivity; may show extreme agitation or exaggerated excitability; speech and thought processes may be accelerated.

296.1 Manic disorder, recurrent episode
Any condition classifiable to 296.0, stated to be recurrent

EXCLUDES circular type, if there was a previous attack of depression (296.4)

CC Excl: For code 296.14: See code 295.0

296.2 Major depressive disorder, single episode
Depressive psychosis
Endogenous depression
Involutional melancholia
Manic-depressive psychosis or reaction, depressed type
Monopolar depression
Psychotic depression
} single episode or unspecified

EXCLUDES circular type, if previous attack was of manic type (296.5)
  depression NOS (311)
  reactive depression (neurotic) (300.4)
  psychotic (298.0)

DRG 430 For code 296.20

DEF: Mood disorder that produces depression; may exhibit as sadness, low self-esteem, or guilt feelings; other manifestations may be withdrawal from friends and family; interrupted sleep.

§ Requires fifth-digit. See category 295 for codes and definitions.

MENTAL DISORDERS

§ ✓5th 296.3 Major depressive disorder, recurrent episode CC 4
Any condition classifiable to 296.2, stated to be recurrent
- EXCLUDES: circular type, if previous attack was of manic type (296.5)
  depression NOS (311)
  reactive depression (neurotic) (300.4)
  psychotic (298.0)

CC Excl: For code 296.34: See code 295.0

DRG 430 For code 296.30, 296.33 and 296.34

§ ✓5th 296.4 Bipolar affective disorder, manic CC 4
Bipolar disorder, now manic
Manic-depressive psychosis, circular type but currently manic
- EXCLUDES: brief compensatory or rebound mood swings (296.99)

CC Excl: For code 296.44: See code 295.0

§ ✓5th 296.5 Bipolar affective disorder, depressed CC 4
Bipolar disorder, now depressed
Manic-depressive psychosis, circular type but currently depressed
- EXCLUDES: brief compensatory or rebound mood swings (296.99)

CC Excl: For code 296.54: See code 295.0

§ ✓5th 296.6 Bipolar affective disorder, mixed CC 4
Manic-depressive psychosis, circular type, mixed

CC Excl: For code 296.64: See code 295.0

296.7 Bipolar affective disorder, unspecified
Atypical bipolar affective disorder NOS
Manic-depressive psychosis, circular type, current condition not specified as either manic or depressive

DEF: Manic-depressive disorder referred to as bipolar because of the mood range from manic to depressive.

✓5th 296.8 Manic-depressive psychosis, other and unspecified
- **296.80 Manic-depressive psychosis, unspecified**
  Manic-depressive:
  reaction NOS
  syndrome NOS
- **296.81 Atypical manic disorder**
- **296.82 Atypical depressive disorder**
- **296.89 Other**
  Manic-depressive psychosis, mixed type

✓5th 296.9 Other and unspecified affective psychoses
- EXCLUDES: psychogenic affective psychoses (298.0-298.8)
- **296.90 Unspecified affective psychosis**
  Affective psychosis NOS
  Melancholia NOS

AHA: M-A, '85, 14

- **296.99 Other specified affective psychoses**
  Mood swings: Mood swings:
  brief compensatory   rebound

✓4th 297 Paranoid states (Delusional disorders)
- INCLUDES: paranoid disorders
- EXCLUDES: acute paranoid reaction (298.3)
  alcoholic jealousy or paranoid state (291.5)
  paranoid schizophrenia (295.3)

297.0 Paranoid state, simple

297.1 Paranoia
Chronic paranoid psychosis
Sander's disease
Systematized delusions
- EXCLUDES: paranoid personality disorder (301.0)

297.2 Paraphrenia
Involutional paranoid state
Late paraphrenia
Paraphrenia (involutional)

DEF: Paranoid schizophrenic disorder that persists over a prolonged period but does not distort personality despite persistent delusions.

297.3 Shared paranoid disorder
Folie à deux
Induced psychosis or paranoid disorder

DEF: Mental disorder two people share; first person with the delusional disorder convinces second person because of a close relationship and shared experiences to accept the delusions.

297.8 Other specified paranoid states
Paranoia querulans
Sensitiver Beziehungswahn
- EXCLUDES: acute paranoid reaction or state (298.3)
  senile paranoid state (290.20)

297.9 Unspecified paranoid state
Paranoid: Paranoid:
  disorder NOS   reaction NOS
  psychosis NOS   state NOS

AHA: J-A, '85, 9

✓4th 298 Other nonorganic psychoses
- INCLUDES: psychotic conditions due to or provoked by:
  emotional stress
  environmental factors as major part of etiology

298.0 Depressive type psychosis CC
Psychogenic depressive psychosis
Psychotic reactive depression
Reactive depressive psychosis
- EXCLUDES: manic-depressive psychosis, depressed type (296.2-296.3)
  neurotic depression (300.4)
  reactive depression NOS (300.4)

CC Excl: See code 295.0

298.1 Excitative type psychosis
Acute hysterical psychosis   Reactive excitation
Psychogenic excitation
- EXCLUDES: manic-depressive psychosis, manic type (296.0-296.1)

DEF: Affective disorder similar to manic-depressive psychosis, in the manic phase, seemingly brought on by stress.

298.2 Reactive confusion
Psychogenic confusion   Psychogenic twilight state
- EXCLUDES: acute confusional state (293.0)

DEF: Confusion, disorientation, cloudiness in consciousness; brought on by severe emotional upheaval.

298.3 Acute paranoid reaction CC
Acute psychogenic paranoid psychosis
Bouffée délirante
- EXCLUDES: paranoid states (297.0-297.9)

CC Excl: See code 295.0

298.4 Psychogenic paranoid psychosis CC
Protracted reactive paranoid psychosis

CC Excl: See code 295.0

298.8 Other and unspecified reactive psychosis
Brief reactive psychosis NOS
Hysterical psychosis
Psychogenic psychosis NOS
Psychogenic stupor
- EXCLUDES: acute hysterical psychosis (298.1)

298.9 Unspecified psychosis HIV
Atypical psychosis
Psychosis NOS

DRG 430

---

§ Requires fifth-digit. See category 296 for codes and definitions.

299 Psychoses with origin specific to childhood
INCLUDES pervasive developmental disorders
EXCLUDES adult type psychoses occurring in childhood, as:
affective disorders (296.0-296.9)
manic-depressive disorders (296.0-296.9)
schizophrenia (295.0-295.9)

The following fifth-digit subclassification is for use with category 299:
0 current or active state
1 residual state

299.0 Infantile autism
Childhood autism
Kanner's syndrome
Infantile psychosis
EXCLUDES disintegrative psychosis (299.1)
Heller's syndrome (299.1)
schizophrenic syndrome of childhood (299.9)

CC Excl: For code 299.00: See code 295.0

DEF: Severe mental disorder of children, results in impaired social behavior; abnormal development of communicative skills, appears to be unaware of the need for emotional support and offers little emotional response to family members.

299.1 Disintegrative psychosis
Heller's syndrome
Use additional code to identify any associated neurological disorder
EXCLUDES infantile autism (299.0)
schizophrenic syndrome of childhood (299.9)

CC Excl: For code 299.10: See code 295.0

DEF: Mental disease of children identified by impaired development of reciprocal social skills, verbal and nonverbal communication skills, imaginative play.

299.8 Other specified early childhood psychoses
Atypical childhood psychosis
Borderline psychosis of childhood
EXCLUDES simple stereotypes without psychotic disturbance (307.3)

CC Excl: For code 299.80: See code 295.0

299.9 Unspecified
Child psychosis NOS
Schizophrenia, childhood type NOS
Schizophrenic syndrome of childhood NOS
EXCLUDES schizophrenia of adult type occurring in childhood (295.0-295.9)

CC Excl: For code 299.90: See code 295.0

NEUROTIC DISORDERS, PERSONALITY DISORDERS, AND OTHER NONPSYCHOTIC MENTAL DISORDERS (300-316)

300 Neurotic disorders

300.0 Anxiety states
EXCLUDES anxiety in:
acute stress reaction (308.0)
transient adjustment reaction (309.24)
neurasthenia (300.5)
psychophysiological disorders (306.0-306.9)
separation anxiety (309.21)

DEF: Mental disorder characterized by anxiety and avoidance behavior not particularly related to any specific situation or stimulus; symptoms include emotional instability, apprehension, fatigue.

300.00 Anxiety state, unspecified
Anxiety:
neurosis
reaction
Anxiety:
state (neurotic)
Atypical anxiety disorder

AHA: ▶1Q, '02, 6◄

300.01 Panic disorder
Panic: attack
Panic: state

DEF: Neurotic disorder characterized by recurrent panic or anxiety, apprehension, fear or terror; symptoms include shortness of breath, palpitations, dizziness, faintness or shakiness; fear of dying may persist or fear of other morbid consequences.

300.02 Generalized anxiety disorder
300.09 Other

300.1 Hysteria
EXCLUDES adjustment reaction (309.0-309.9)
anorexia nervosa (307.1)
gross stress reaction (308.0-308.9)
hysterical personality (301.50-301.59)
psychophysiologic disorders (306.0-306.9)

300.10 Hysteria, unspecified
300.11 Conversion disorder
Astasia-abasia, hysterical
Conversion hysteria or reaction
Hysterical blindness
deafness
paralysis

AHA: N-D, '85, 15

DEF: Mental disorder that impairs physical functions with no physiological basis; sensory motor symptoms include seizures, paralysis, temporary blindness; increase in stress or avoidance of unpleasant responsibilities may precipitate.

300.12 Psychogenic amnesia
Hysterical amnesia

300.13 Psychogenic fugue
Hysterical fugue

DEF: Dissociative hysteria; identified by loss of memory, flight from familiar surroundings; conscious activity is not associated with perception of surroundings, no later memory of episode.

300.14 Multiple personality
Dissociative identity disorder

300.15 Dissociative disorder or reaction, unspecified
DEF: Hysterical neurotic episode; sudden but temporary changes in perceived identity, memory, consciousness, segregated memory patterns exist separate from dominant personality.

300.16 Factitious illness with psychological symptoms
Compensation neurosis
Ganser's syndrome, hysterical

DEF: A disorder characterized by the purposeful assumption of mental illness symptoms; the symptoms are not real, possibly representing what the patient imagines mental illness to be like, and are acted out more often when another person is present.

300.19 Other and unspecified factitious illness
Factitious illness (with physical symptoms) NOS
EXCLUDES multiple operations or hospital addiction syndrome (301.51)

300.2 Phobic disorders
EXCLUDES anxiety state not associated with a specific situation or object (300.00-300.09)
obsessional phobias (300.3)

300.20 Phobia, unspecified
Anxiety-hysteria NOS
Phobia NOS

MENTAL DISORDERS

300.21 Agoraphobia with panic attacks
Fear of:
- open spaces ⎫
- streets ⎬ with panic attacks
- travel ⎭

300.22 Agoraphobia without mention of panic attacks
Any condition classifiable to 300.21 without mention of panic attacks

300.23 Social phobia
Fear of:
- eating in public
- public speaking

Fear of:
- washing in public

300.29 Other isolated or simple phobias
- Acrophobia
- Animal phobias
- Claustrophobia
- Fear of crowds

300.3 Obsessive-compulsive disorders
- Anancastic neurosis
- Compulsive neurosis
- Obsessional phobia [any]

EXCLUDES obsessive-compulsive symptoms occurring in:
endogenous depression (296.2-296.3)
organic states (eg., encephalitis)
schizophrenia (295.0-295.9)

300.4 Neurotic depression
- Anxiety depression
- Depression with anxiety
- Depressive reaction
- Dysthymic disorder
- Neurotic depressive state
- Reactive depression

EXCLUDES adjustment reaction with depressive symptoms (309.0-309.1)
depression NOS (311)
manic-depressive psychosis, depressed type (296.2-296.3)
reactive depressive psychosis (298.0)

DEF: Depression without psychosis; less severe depression related to personal change or unexpected circumstances; also referred to as "reactional depression."

300.5 Neurasthenia
- Fatigue neurosis
- Nervous debility
- Psychogenic: asthenia

Psychogenic: general fatigue

Use additional code to identify any associated physical disorder

EXCLUDES anxiety state (300.00-300.09)
neurotic depression (300.4)
psychophysiological disorders (306.0-306.9)
specific nonpsychotic mental disorders following organic brain damage (310.0-310.9)

DEF: Physical and mental symptoms caused primarily by what is known as mental exhaustion; symptoms include chronic weakness, fatigue.

300.6 Depersonalization syndrome
- Depersonalization disorder
- Derealization (neurotic)
- Neurotic state with depersonalization episode

EXCLUDES depersonalization associated with:
anxiety (300.00-300.09)
depression (300.4)
manic-depressive disorder or psychosis (296.0-296.9)
schizophrenia (295.0-295.9)

DEF: Dissociative disorder characterized by feelings of strangeness about self or body image; symptoms include dizziness, anxiety, fear of insanity, loss of reality of surroundings.

300.7 Hypochondriasis
Body dysmorphic disorder

EXCLUDES hypochondriasis in:
hysteria (300.10-300.19)
manic-depressive psychosis, depressed type (296.2-296.3)
neurasthenia (300.5)
obsessional disorder (300.3)
schizophrenia (295.0-295.9)

300.8 Other neurotic disorders

300.81 Somatization disorder
- Briquet's disorder
- Severe somatoform disorder

300.82 Undifferentiated somatoform disorder
- Atypical somatoform disorder
- Somatoform disorder NOS

AHA: 4Q, '96, 29

DEF: Disorders in which patients have symptoms that suggest an organic disease but no evidence of physical disorder after repeated testing.

300.89 Other
- Occupational neurosis, including writers' cramp
- Psychasthenia
- Psychasthenic neurosis

300.9 Unspecified neurotic disorder
- Neurosis NOS
- Psychoneurosis NOS

301 Personality disorders

INCLUDES character neurosis

Use additional code to identify any associated neurosis or psychosis, or physical condition

EXCLUDES nonpsychotic personality disorder associated with organic brain syndromes (310.0-310.9)

301.0 Paranoid personality disorder
- Fanatic personality
- Paranoid personality (disorder)
- Paranoid traits

EXCLUDES acute paranoid reaction (298.3)
alcoholic paranoia (291.5)
paranoid schizophrenia (295.3)
paranoid states (297.0-297.9)

AHA: J-A, '85, 9

301.1 Affective personality disorder

EXCLUDES affective psychotic disorders (296.0-296.9)
neurasthenia (300.5)
neurotic depression (300.4)

301.10 Affective personality disorder, unspecified

301.11 Chronic hypomanic personality disorder
- Chronic hypomanic disorder
- Hypomanic personality

301.12 Chronic depressive personality disorder
- Chronic depressive disorder
- Depressive character or personality

301.13 Cyclothymic disorder
- Cycloid personality
- Cyclothymia
- Cyclothymic personality

301.2 Schizoid personality disorder

EXCLUDES schizophrenia (295.0-295.9)

301.20 Schizoid personality disorder, unspecified

301.21 Introverted personality

301.22 Schizotypal personality

301.3 Explosive personality disorder
- Aggressive:
  - personality
  - reaction
- Aggressiveness
- Emotional instability (excessive)
- Pathological emotionality
- Quarrelsomeness

EXCLUDES dyssocial personality (301.7)
hysterical neurosis (300.10-300.19)

MENTAL DISORDERS

301.4 Compulsive personality disorder
Anancastic personality
Obsessional personality
EXCLUDES obsessive-compulsive disorder (300.3)
phobic state (300.20-300.29)

√5th **301.5 Histrionic personality disorder**
EXCLUDES hysterical neurosis (300.10-300.19)
DEF: Extreme emotional behavior, often theatrical; often concerned about own appeal; may demand attention, exhibit seductive behavior.

301.50 Histrionic personality disorder, unspecified
Hysterical personality NOS

301.51 Chronic factitious illness with physical symptoms
Hospital addiction syndrome
Multiple operations syndrome
Munchausen syndrome

301.59 Other histrionic personality disorder
Personality:
  emotionally unstable
  labile
Personality:
  psychoinfantile

301.6 Dependent personality disorder
Asthenic personality
Inadequate personality
Passive personality
EXCLUDES neurasthenia (300.5)
passive-aggressive personality (301.84)
DEF: Overwhelming feeling of helplessness; fears of abandonment may persist; difficulty in making personal decisions without confirmation by others; low self-esteem due to irrational sensitivity to criticism.

301.7 Antisocial personality disorder
Amoral personality
Asocial personality
Dyssocial personality
Personality disorder with predominantly sociopathic or asocial manifestation
EXCLUDES disturbance of conduct without specifiable personality disorder (312.0-312.9)
explosive personality (301.3)
AHA: S-0, '84, 16
DEF: Continuous antisocial behavior that violates rights of others; social traits include extreme aggression, total disregard for traditional social rules.

√5th **301.8 Other personality disorders**

301.81 Narcissistic personality
DEF: Grandiose fantasy or behavior, lack of social empathy, hypersensitive to the lack of others' judgment, exploits others; also sense of entitlement to have expectations met, need for continual admiration.

301.82 Avoidant personality
DEF: Personality disorder marked by feelings of social inferiority; sensitivity to criticism, emotionally restrained due to fear of rejection.

301.83 Borderline personality
DEF: Personality disorder characterized by unstable moods, self-image, and interpersonal relationships; uncontrolled anger, impulsive and self-destructive acts, fears of abandonment, feelings of emptiness and boredom, recurrent suicide threats or self-mutilation.

301.84 Passive-aggressive personality
DEF: Pattern of procrastination and refusal to meet standards; introduce own obstacles to success and exploit failure.

301.89 Other
Personality:
  eccentric
  "haltlose" type
  immature
Personality:
  masochistic
  psychoneurotic
EXCLUDES psychoinfantile personality (301.59)

301.9 Unspecified personality disorder
Pathological personality NOS
Personality disorder NOS
Psychopathic:
  constitutional state
  personality (disorder)

√4th **302 Sexual deviations and disorders**
EXCLUDES sexual disorder manifest in:
organic brain syndrome (290.0-294.9, 310.0-310.9)
psychosis (295.0-298.9)

302.0 Ego-dystonic homosexuality
Ego-dystonic lesbianism
Homosexual conflict disorder
EXCLUDES homosexual pedophilia (302.2)

302.1 Zoophilia
Bestiality
DEF: A sociodeviant disorder marked by engaging in sexual intercourse with animals.

302.2 Pedophilia
DEF: A sociodeviant condition of adults characterized by sexual activity with children.

302.3 Transvestism
EXCLUDES trans-sexualism (302.5)
DEF: The desire to dress in clothing of opposite sex.

302.4 Exhibitionism
DEF: Sexual deviant behavior; exposure of genitals to strangers; behavior prompted by intense sexual urges and fantasies.

√5th **302.5 Trans-sexualism**
EXCLUDES transvestism (302.3)
DEF: Gender identity disturbance; overwhelming desire to change anatomic sex, due to belief that individual is a member of the opposite sex.

302.50 With unspecified sexual history
302.51 With asexual history
302.52 With homosexual history
302.53 With heterosexual history

302.6 Disorders of psychosexual identity
Feminism in boys
Gender identity disorder of childhood
EXCLUDES gender identity disorder in adult (302.85)
homosexuality (302.0)
trans-sexualism (302.50-302.53)
transvestism (302.3)

√5th **302.7 Psychosexual dysfunction**
EXCLUDES impotence of organic origin (607.84)
normal transient symptoms from ruptured hymen
transient or occasional failures of erection due to fatigue, anxiety, alcohol, or drugs

302.70 Psychosexual dysfunction, unspecified
302.71 With inhibited sexual desire
302.72 With inhibited sexual excitement
Frigidity   Impotence
302.73 With inhibited female orgasm ♀
302.74 With inhibited male orgasm ♂
302.75 With premature ejaculation ♂

MENTAL DISORDERS

302.76 With functional dyspareunia ♀
Dyspareunia, psychogenic
DEF: Difficult or painful sex due to psychosomatic state.

302.79 With other specified psychosexual dysfunctions

√5th **302.8 Other specified psychosexual disorders**

302.81 Fetishism
DEF: Psychosexual disorder noted for intense sexual urges and arousal precipitated by fantasies; use of inanimate objects, such as clothing, to stimulate sexual arousal, orgasm.

302.82 Voyeurism
DEF: Psychosexual disorder characterized by uncontrollable impulse to observe others, without their knowledge, who are nude or engaged in sexual activity.

302.83 Sexual masochism
DEF: Psychosexual disorder noted for need to achieve sexual gratification through humiliating or hurtful acts inflicted on self.

302.84 Sexual sadism
DEF: Psychosexual disorder noted for need to achieve sexual gratification through humiliating or hurtful acts inflicted on someone else.

302.85 Gender identity disorder of adolescent or adult life

302.89 Other
Nymphomania   Satyriasis

302.9 Unspecified psychosexual disorder
Pathologic sexuality NOS
Sexual deviation NOS

√4th **303 Alcohol dependence syndrome**
Use additional code to identify any associated condition, as:
  alcoholic psychoses (291.0-291.9)
  drug dependence (304.0-304.9)
  physical complications of alcohol, such as:
    cerebral degeneration (331.7)
    cirrhosis of liver (571.2)
    epilepsy (345.0-345.9)
    gastritis (535.3)
    hepatitis (571.1)
    liver damage NOS (571.3)
  EXCLUDES   drunkenness NOS (305.0)

The following fifth-digit subclassification is for use with category 303:
  0 unspecified
  1 continuous
  2 episodic
  3 in remission

AHA: 3Q, '95, 6; 2Q, '91, 9; 4Q, '88, 8; S-O, '86, 3

√5th **303.0 Acute alcoholic intoxication**   CC 0-2
Acute drunkenness in alcoholism
CC Excl: For codes 303.00-303.02: 291.0-291.9, 292.0-292.9, 303.00-303.93, 304.00-304.91, 305.00-305.03, 305.20-305.93, 790.3

√5th **303.9 Other and unspecified alcohol dependence**   CC 0-2
Chronic alcoholism   Dipsomania
CC Excl: For codes 303.90-303.92: See code 303.0

AHA: 2Q, '89, 9

√4th **304 Drug dependence**
  EXCLUDES   nondependent abuse of drugs (305.1-305.9)

The following fifth-digit subclassification is for use with category 304:
  0 unspecified
  1 continuous
  2 episodic
  3 in remission

AHA: 2Q, '91, 10; 4Q, '88, 8; S-O, '86, 3

√5th **304.0 Opioid type dependence**   CC 0-2
Heroin   Opium alkaloids and their
Meperidine   derivatives
Methadone   Synthetics with morphine-like
Morphine   effects
Opium
CC Excl: For codes 304.00-304.02: See code 303.0

√5th **304.1 Barbiturate and similarly acting sedative or hypnotic dependence**   CC 0-2
Barbiturates
Nonbarbiturate sedatives and tranquilizers with a similar effect:
  chlordiazepoxide   meprobamate
  diazepam   methaqualone
  glutethimide
CC Excl: For codes 304.10-304.12: See code 303.0

√5th **304.2 Cocaine dependence**   CC 0-2
Coca leaves and derivatives
CC Excl: For codes 304.20-304.22: See code 303.0

√5th **304.3 Cannabis dependence**
Hashish   Marihuana
Hemp

√5th **304.4 Amphetamine and other psychostimulant dependence**   CC 0-2
Methylphenidate   Phenmetrazine
CC Excl: For codes 304.40-304.42: See code 303.0

√5th **304.5 Hallucinogen dependence**   CC 0-2
Dimethyltryptamine [DMT]
Lysergic acid diethylamide [LSD] and derivatives
Mescaline
Psilocybin
CC Excl: For codes 304.50-304.52: See code 303.0

√5th **304.6 Other specified drug dependence**   CC 0-2
Absinthe addiction   Glue sniffing
  EXCLUDES   tobacco dependence (305.1)
CC Excl: For codes 304.60-304.62: See code 303.0

√5th **304.7 Combinations of opioid type drug with any other**   CC 0-2
CC Excl: For codes 304.70-304.72: See code 303.0
AHA: M-A, '86, 12

√5th **304.8 Combinations of drug dependence excluding opioid type drug**   CC 0-2
CC Excl: For codes 304.80-304.82: See code 303.0
AHA: M-A, '86, 12

√5th **304.9 Unspecified drug dependence**   CC 0-2
Drug addiction NOS   Drug dependence NOS
CC Excl: For codes 304.90-304.92: See code 303.0

√4th **305 Nondependent abuse of drugs**
Note: Includes cases where a person, for whom no other diagnosis is possible, has come under medical care because of the maladaptive effect of a drug on which he is not dependent and that he has taken on his own initiative to the detriment of his health or social functioning.
  EXCLUDES   alcohol dependence syndrome (303.0-303.9)
              drug dependence (304.0-304.9)
              drug withdrawal syndrome (292.0)
              poisoning by drugs or medicinal substances (960.0-979.9)

The following fifth-digit subclassification is for use with codes 305.0, 305.2-305.9:
  0 unspecified
  1 continuous
  2 episodic
  3 in remission

AHA: 2Q, '91, 10; 4Q, '88, 8; S-O, '86, 3

305.0–306.7 MENTAL DISORDERS

§ ✓5th 305.0 Alcohol abuse [CC 0-2]
Drunkenness NOS
Excessive drinking of alcohol NOS
"Hangover" (alcohol)
Inebriety NOS
EXCLUDES acute alcohol intoxication in alcoholism (303.0)
alcoholic psychoses (291.0-291.9)
CC Excl: For codes 305.00-305.02: See code 303.0
AHA: 3Q, '96, 16

305.1 Tobacco use disorder
Tobacco dependence
EXCLUDES history of tobacco use (V15.82)
AHA: 2Q, '96, 10; N-D, '84, 12

§ ✓5th 305.2 Cannabis abuse

§ ✓5th 305.3 Hallucinogen abuse [CC 0-2]
Acute intoxication from hallucinogens ["bad trips"]
LSD reaction
CC Excl: For codes 305.30-305.32: See code 303.0

§ ✓5th 305.4 Barbiturate and similarly acting sedative or hypnotic abuse [CC 0-2]
CC Excl: For codes 305.40-305.42: See code 303.0

§ ✓5th 305.5 Opioid abuse [CC 0-2]
CC Excl: For codes 305.50-305.52: See code 303.0

§ ✓5th 305.6 Cocaine abuse [CC 0-2]
CC Excl: For codes 305.60-305.62: See code 303.0
AHA: 1Q, '93, 25

§ ✓5th 305.7 Amphetamine or related acting sympathomimetic abuse [CC 0-2]
CC Excl: For codes 305.70-305.72: See code 303.0

§ ✓5th 305.8 Antidepressant type abuse

§ ✓5th 305.9 Other, mixed, or unspecified drug abuse [CC 0-2]
"Laxative habit"
Misuse of drugs NOS
Nonprescribed use of drugs or patent medicinals
CC Excl: For codes 305.90-305.92: See code 303.0
AHA: 3Q, '99, 20

✓4th 306 Physiological malfunction arising from mental factors
INCLUDES psychogenic:
physical symptoms } not involving
physiological } tissue
manifestations } damage
EXCLUDES hysteria (300.11-300.19)
physical symptoms secondary to a psychiatric disorder classified elsewhere
psychic factors associated with physical conditions involving tissue damage classified elsewhere (316)
specific nonpsychotic mental disorders following organic brain damage (310.0-310.9)
DEF: Functional disturbances or interruptions due to mental or psychological causes; no tissue damage sustained in these conditions.

306.0 Musculoskeletal
Psychogenic paralysis
Psychogenic torticollis
EXCLUDES Gilles de la Tourette's syndrome (307.23)
paralysis as hysterical or conversion reaction (300.11)
tics (307.20-307.22)

306.1 Respiratory
Psychogenic:
air hunger
cough
hiccough
Psychogenic:
hyperventilation
yawning
EXCLUDES psychogenic asthma (316 and 493.9)

306.2 Cardiovascular
Cardiac neurosis
Cardiovascular neurosis
Neurocirculatory asthenia
Psychogenic cardiovascular disorder
EXCLUDES psychogenic paroxysmal tachycardia (316 and 427.2)
AHA: J-A, '85, 14

DEF: Neurocirculatory asthenia: functional nervous and circulatory irregularities with palpitations, dyspnea, fatigue, rapid pulse, precordial pain, fear of effort, discomfort during exercise, anxiety; also called DaCosta's syndrome, Effort syndrome, Irritable or Soldier's Heart.

306.3 Skin
Psychogenic pruritus
EXCLUDES psychogenic:
alopecia (316 and 704.00)
dermatitis (316 and 692.9)
eczema (316 and 691.8 or 692.9)
urticaria (316 and 708.0-708.9)

306.4 Gastrointestinal
Aerophagy
Cyclical vomiting, psychogenic
Diarrhea, psychogenic
Nervous gastritis
Psychogenic dyspepsia
EXCLUDES cyclical vomiting NOS (536.2)
globus hystericus (300.11)
mucous colitis (316 and 564.9)
psychogenic:
cardiospasm (316 and 530.0)
duodenal ulcer (316 and 532.0-532.9)
gastric ulcer (316 and 531.0-531.9)
peptic ulcer NOS (316 and 533.0-533.9)
vomiting NOS (307.54)
AHA: 2Q, '89, 11

DEF: Aerophagy: excess swallowing of air, usually unconscious; related to anxiety; results in distended abdomen or belching, often interpreted by the patient as a physical disorder.

✓5th 306.5 Genitourinary
EXCLUDES enuresis, psychogenic (307.6)
frigidity (302.72)
impotence (302.72)
psychogenic dyspareunia (302.76)

306.50 Psychogenic genitourinary malfunction, unspecified

306.51 Psychogenic vaginismus ♀
Functional vaginismus
DEF: Psychogenic response resulting in painful contractions of vaginal canal muscles; can be severe enough to prevent sexual intercourse.

306.52 Psychogenic dysmenorrhea ♀
306.53 Psychogenic dysuria
306.59 Other
AHA: M-A, '87, 11

306.6 Endocrine

306.7 Organs of special sense
EXCLUDES hysterical blindness or deafness (300.11)
psychophysical visual disturbances (368.16)

---

§ Requires fifth-digit. See category 305 for codes and definitions.

N Newborn Age: 0 P Pediatric Age: 0-17 M Maternity Age: 12-55 A Adult Age: 15-124 CC CC Condition MC Major Complication CD Complex Dx HIV HIV Related Dx

MENTAL DISORDERS

306.8 Other specified psychophysiological malfunction
  Bruxism   Teeth grinding

306.9 Unspecified psychophysiological malfunction
  Psychophysiologic disorder NOS
  Psychosomatic disorder NOS

√4th 307 Special symptoms or syndromes, not elsewhere classified
  Note: This category is intended for use if the psychopathology is manifested by a single specific symptom or group of symptoms which is not part of an organic illness or other mental disorder classifiable elsewhere.
  EXCLUDES: those due to mental disorders classified elsewhere
  those of organic origin

307.0 Stammering and stuttering
  EXCLUDES: dysphasia (784.5)
  lisping or lalling (307.9)
  retarded development of speech (315.31-315.39)

307.1 Anorexia nervosa CC
  EXCLUDES: eating disturbance NOS (307.50)
  feeding problem (783.3)
  of nonorganic origin (307.59)
  loss of appetite (783.0)
  of nonorganic origin (307.59)
  CC Excl: 306.4, 306.8-306.9, 307.1, 307.50-307.59, 309.22
  AHA: 4Q, '89, 11

√5th 307.2 Tics
  EXCLUDES: nail-biting or thumb-sucking (307.9)
  stereotypes occurring in isolation (307.3)
  tics of organic origin (333.3)
  DEF: Involuntary muscle response usually confined to the face, shoulders.

  307.20 Tic disorder, unspecified
  307.21 Transient tic disorder of childhood
  307.22 Chronic motor tic disorder
  307.23 Gilles de la Tourette's disorder
    Motor-verbal tic disorder
    DEF: Syndrome of facial and vocal tics in childhood; progresses to spontaneous or involuntary jerking, obscene utterances, other uncontrollable actions considered inappropriate.

307.3 Stereotyped repetitive movements
  Body-rocking   Spasmus nutans
  Head banging   Stereotypes NOS
  EXCLUDES: tics (307.20-307.23)
  of organic origin (333.3)

√5th 307.4 Specific disorders of sleep of nonorganic origin
  EXCLUDES: narcolepsy (347)
  those of unspecified cause (780.50-780.59)

  307.40 Nonorganic sleep disorder, unspecified
  307.41 Transient disorder of initiating or maintaining sleep
    Hyposomnia ⎫
    Insomnia   ⎬ associated with intermittent emotional reactions or conflicts
    Sleeplessness ⎭

  307.42 Persistent disorder of initiating or maintaining sleep
    Hyposomnia, insomnia, or sleeplessness associated with:
    anxiety
    conditioned arousal
    depression (major) (minor)
    psychosis

  307.43 Transient disorder of initiating or maintaining wakefulness
    Hypersomnia associated with acute or intermittent emotional reactions or conflicts

  307.44 Persistent disorder of initiating or maintaining wakefulness
    Hypersomnia associated with depression (major) (minor)

  307.45 Phase-shift disruption of 24-hour sleep-wake cycle
    Irregular sleep-wake rhythm, nonorganic origin
    Jet lag syndrome
    Rapid time-zone change
    Shifting sleep-work schedule

  307.46 Somnambulism or night terrors
    DEF: Sleepwalking marked by extreme terror, panic, screaming, confusion; no recall of event upon arousal; term may refer to simply the act of sleepwalking.

  307.47 Other dysfunctions of sleep stages or arousal from sleep
    Nightmares: Sleep drunkenness
    NOS
    REM-sleep type

  307.48 Repetitive intrusions of sleep
    Repetitive intrusion of sleep with:
    atypical polysomnographic features
    environmental disturbances
    repeated REM-sleep interruptions

  307.49 Other
    "Short-sleeper"
    Subjective insomnia complaint

√5th 307.5 Other and unspecified disorders of eating
  EXCLUDES: anorexia:
  nervosa (307-1)
  of unspecified cause (783.0)
  overeating, of unspecified cause (783.6)
  vomiting:
  NOS (787.0)
  cyclical (536.2)
  psychogenic (306.4)

  307.50 Eating disorder, unspecified
  307.51 Bulimia
    Overeating of nonorganic origin
    DEF: Mental disorder commonly characterized by binge eating followed by self-induced vomiting; perceptions of being fat; and fear the inability to stop eating voluntarily.

  307.52 Pica
    Perverted appetite of nonorganic origin
    DEF: Compulsive eating disorder characterized by craving for substances, other than food; such as paint chips or dirt.

  307.53 Psychogenic rumination
    Regurgitation, of nonorganic origin, of food with reswallowing
    EXCLUDES: obsessional rumination (300.3)

  307.54 Psychogenic vomiting
  307.59 Other
    Infantile feeding disturbances ⎫
    Loss of appetite   ⎬ of nonorganic origin

307.6 Enuresis
  Enuresis (primary) (secondary) of nonorganic origin
  EXCLUDES: enuresis of unspecified cause (788.3)
  DEF: Involuntary urination past age of normal control; also called bedwetting; no trace to biological problem; focus on psychological issues.

307.7 Encopresis
  Encopresis (continuous) (discontinuous) of nonorganic origin
  EXCLUDES: encopresis of unspecified cause (787.6)
  DEF: Inability to control bowel movements; cause traced to psychological, not biological, problems.

307.8–310.0 MENTAL DISORDERS

√5th 307.8 Psychalgia
- **307.80** Psychogenic pain, site unspecified
- **307.81** Tension headache
  - EXCLUDES headache:
    - NOS (784.0)
    - migraine (346.0-346.9)
  - AHA: N-D, '85, 16
- **307.89** Other
  - Psychogenic backache
  - EXCLUDES pains not specifically attributable to a psychological cause (in):
    - back (724.5)
    - joint (719.4)
    - limb (729.5)
    - lumbago (724.2)
    - rheumatic (729.0)

307.9 Other and unspecified special symptoms or syndromes, not elsewhere classified
- Hair plucking
- Lalling
- Lisping
- Masturbation
- Nail-biting
- Thumb-sucking

√4th 308 Acute reaction to stress
INCLUDES
- catastrophic stress
- combat fatigue
- gross stress reaction (acute)
- transient disorders in response to exceptional physical or mental stress which usually subside within hours or days

EXCLUDES
- adjustment reaction or disorder (309.0-309.9)
- chronic stress reaction (309.1-309.9)

- **308.0** Predominant disturbance of emotions
  - Anxiety
  - Emotional crisis } as acute reaction to exceptional [gross] stress
  - Panic state
- **308.1** Predominant disturbance of consciousness
  - Fugues as acute reaction to exceptional [gross] stress
- **308.2** Predominant psychomotor disturbance
  - Agitation states } as acute reaction to exceptional [gross] stress
  - Stupor
- **308.3** Other acute reactions to stress
  - Acute situational disturbance
  - Brief or acute posttraumatic stress disorder
  - EXCLUDES prolonged posttraumatic emotional disturbance (309.81)
- **308.4** Mixed disorders as reaction to stress
- **308.9** Unspecified acute reaction to stress

√4th 309 Adjustment reaction
INCLUDES
- adjustment disorders
- reaction (adjustment) to chronic stress

EXCLUDES
- acute reaction to major stress (308.0-308.9)
- neurotic disorders (300.0-300.9)

- **309.0** Brief depressive reaction
  - Adjustment disorder with depressed mood
  - Grief reaction
  - EXCLUDES
    - affective psychoses (296.0-296.9)
    - neurotic depression (300.4)
    - prolonged depressive reaction (309.1)
    - psychogenic depressive psychosis (298.0)
- **309.1** Prolonged depressive reaction
  - EXCLUDES
    - affective psychoses (296.0-296.9)
    - brief depressive reaction (309.0)
    - neurotic depression (300.4)
    - psychogenic depressive psychosis (298.0)

√5th 309.2 With predominant disturbance of other emotions
- **309.21** Separation anxiety disorder
  - DEF: Abnormal apprehension by a child when physically separated from support environment; byproduct of abnormal symbiotic child-parent relationship.
- **309.22** Emancipation disorder of adolescence and early adult life
  - DEF: Adjustment reaction of late adolescence; conflict over independence from parental supervision; symptoms include difficulty in making decisions, increased reliance on parental advice, deliberate adoption of values in opposition of parents.
- **309.23** Specific academic or work inhibition
- **309.24** Adjustment reaction with anxious mood
- **309.28** Adjustment reaction with mixed emotional features
  - Adjustment reaction with anxiety and depression
- **309.29** Other
  - Culture shock

309.3 With predominant disturbance of conduct
- Conduct disturbance } as adjustment reaction
- Destructiveness
- EXCLUDES
  - destructiveness in child (312.9)
  - disturbance of conduct NOS (312.9)
  - dyssocial behavior without manifest psychiatric disorder (V71.01-V71.02)
  - personality disorder with predominantly sociopathic or asocial manifestations (301.7)

309.4 With mixed disturbance of emotions and conduct

√5th 309.8 Other specified adjustment reactions
- **309.81** Prolonged posttraumatic stress disorder
  - Chronic posttraumatic stress disorder
  - Concentration camp syndrome
  - EXCLUDES posttraumatic brain syndrome:
    - nonpsychotic (310.2)
    - psychotic (293.0-293.9)
  - DEF: Preoccupation with traumatic events beyond normal experience; events such as rape, personal assault, combat, natural disasters, accidents, torture precipitate disorder; also recurring flashbacks of trauma; symptoms include difficulty remembering, sleeping, or concentrating, and guilt feelings for surviving.
- **309.82** Adjustment reaction with physical symptoms
- **309.83** Adjustment reaction with withdrawal
  - Elective mutism as adjustment reaction
  - Hospitalism (in children) NOS
- **309.89** Other

309.9 Unspecified adjustment reaction
- Adaptation reaction NOS
- Adjustment reaction NOS

√4th 310 Specific nonpsychotic mental disorders due to organic brain damage
EXCLUDES neuroses, personality disorders, or other nonpsychotic conditions occurring in a form similar to that seen with functional disorders but in association with a physical condition (300.0-300.9, 301.0-301.9)

- **310.0** Frontal lobe syndrome
  - Lobotomy syndrome
  - Postleucotomy syndrome [state]
  - EXCLUDES postcontusion syndrome (310.2)

MENTAL DISORDERS

310.1 Organic personality syndrome
Cognitive or personality change of other type, of nonpsychotic severity
Mild memory disturbance
Organic psychosyndrome of nonpsychotic severity
Presbyophrenia NOS
Senility with mental changes of nonpsychotic severity

DEF: Personality disorder caused by organic factors, such as brain lesions, head trauma, or cerebrovascular accident (CVA).

310.2 Postconcussion syndrome
Postcontusion syndrome or encephalopathy
Posttraumatic brain syndrome, nonpsychotic
Status postcommotio cerebri

EXCLUDES frontal lobe syndrome (310.0)
postencephalitic syndrome (310.8)
any organic psychotic conditions following head injury (293.0-294.0)

AHA: 4Q, '90, 24

DEF: Nonpsychotic disorder due to brain trauma, causes symptoms unrelated to any disease process; symptoms include amnesia, serial headaches, rapid heartbeat, fatigue, disrupted sleep patterns, inability to concentrate.

310.8 Other specified nonpsychotic mental disorders following organic brain damage
Postencephalitic syndrome
Other focal (partial) organic psychosyndromes

310.9 Unspecified nonpsychotic mental disorder following organic brain damage

311 Depressive disorder, not elsewhere classified
Depressive disorder NOS   Depression NOS
Depressive state NOS

EXCLUDES acute reaction to major stress with depressive symptoms (308.0)
affective personality disorder (301.10-301.13)
affective psychoses (296.0-296.9)
brief depressive reaction (309.0)
depressive states associated with stressful events (309.0-309.1)
disturbance of emotions specific to childhood and adolescence, with misery and unhappiness (313.1)
mixed adjustment reaction with depressive symptoms (309.4)
neurotic depression (300.4)
prolonged depressive adjustment reaction (309.1)
psychogenic depressive psychosis (298.0)

312 Disturbance of conduct, not elsewhere classified

EXCLUDES adjustment reaction with disturbance of conduct (309.3)
drug dependence (304.0-304.9)
dyssocial behavior without manifest psychiatric disorder (V71.01-V71.02)
personality disorder with predominantly sociopathic or asocial manifestations (301.7)
sexual deviations (302.0-302.9)

The following fifth-digit subclassification is for use with categories 312.0-312.2:
    0 unspecified
    1 mild
    2 moderate
    3 severe

312.0 Undersocialized conduct disorder, aggressive type
Aggressive outburst   Unsocialized aggressive
Anger reaction   disorder

DEF: Mental condition identified by behaviors disrespectful of others' rights and of age-appropriate social norms or rules; symptoms include bullying, vandalism, verbal and physical abusiveness, lying, stealing, defiance.

312.1 Undersocialized conduct disorder, unaggressive type
Childhood truancy, unsocialized
Solitary stealing
Tantrums

312.2 Socialized conduct disorder
Childhood truancy, socialized   Group delinquency

EXCLUDES gang activity without manifest psychiatric disorder (V71.01)

312.3 Disorders of impulse control, not elsewhere classified

312.30 Impulse control disorder, unspecified
312.31 Pathological gambling
312.32 Kleptomania
312.33 Pyromania
312.34 Intermittent explosive disorder
312.35 Isolated explosive disorder
312.39 Other

312.4 Mixed disturbance of conduct and emotions
Neurotic delinquency

EXCLUDES compulsive conduct disorder (312.3)

312.8 Other specified disturbances of conduct, not elsewhere classified

312.81 Conduct disorder, childhood onset type
312.82 Conduct disorder, adolescent onset type
312.89 Other conduct disorder

312.9 Unspecified disturbance of conduct
Delinquency (juvenile)

313 Disturbance of emotions specific to childhood and adolescence

EXCLUDES adjustment reaction (309.0-309.9)
emotional disorder of neurotic type (300.0-300.9)
masturbation, nail-biting, thumbsucking, and other isolated symptoms (307.0-307.9)

313.0 Overanxious disorder
Anxiety and fearfulness } of childhood and
Overanxious disorder   } adolescence

EXCLUDES abnormal separation anxiety (309.21)
anxiety states (300.00-300.09)
hospitalism in children (309.83)
phobic state (300.20-300.29)

313.1 Misery and unhappiness disorder

EXCLUDES depressive neurosis (300.4)

313.2 Sensitivity, shyness, and social withdrawal disorder

EXCLUDES infantile autism (299.0)
schizoid personality (301.20-301.22)
schizophrenia (295.0-295.9)

313.21 Shyness disorder of childhood
Sensitivity reaction of childhood or adolescence

313.22 Introverted disorder of childhood
Social withdrawal } of childhood or
Withdrawal reaction } adolescence

313.23 Elective mutism

EXCLUDES elective mutism as adjustment reaction (309.83)

MENTAL DISORDERS

313.3 **Relationship problems**
Sibling jealousy
EXCLUDES: relationship problems associated with aggression, destruction, or other forms of conduct disturbance (312.0-312.9)

√5th **313.8** **Other or mixed emotional disturbances of childhood or adolescence**

313.81 **Oppositional disorder**
DEF: Mental disorder of children noted for pervasive opposition, defiance of authority.

313.82 **Identity disorder**
DEF: Distress of adolescents caused by inability to form acceptable self-identity; uncertainty about career choice, sexual orientation, moral values.

313.83 **Academic underachievement disorder**

313.89 **Other** P

313.9 **Unspecified emotional disturbance of childhood or adolescence** P

√4th **314** **Hyperkinetic syndrome of childhood**
EXCLUDES: hyperkinesis as symptom of underlying disorder—code the underlying disorder

√5th **314.0** **Attention deficit disorder**
Adult
Child
DEF: A behavioral disorder usually diagnosed at an early age; characterized by the inability to focus attention for a normal period of time.

314.00 **Without mention of hyperactivity**
Predominantly inattentive type
AHA: 1Q, '97, 8

314.01 **With hyperactivity**
Combined type
Overactivity NOS
Predominantly hyperactive/impulsive type
Simple disturbance of attention with overactivity
AHA: 1Q, '97, 8

314.1 **Hyperkinesis with developmental delay**
Developmental disorder of hyperkinesis
Use additional code to identify any associated neurological disorder

314.2 **Hyperkinetic conduct disorder**
Hyperkinetic conduct disorder without developmental delay
EXCLUDES: hyperkinesis with significant delays in specific skills (314.1)

314.8 **Other specified manifestations of hyperkinetic syndrome**

314.9 **Unspecified hyperkinetic syndrome**
Hyperkinetic reaction of childhood or adolescence NOS
Hyperkinetic syndrome NOS

√4th **315** **Specific delays in development**
EXCLUDES: that due to a neurological disorder (320.0-389.9)

√5th **315.0** **Specific reading disorder**

315.00 **Reading disorder, unspecified**

315.01 **Alexia**
DEF: Lack of ability to understand written language; manifestation of aphasia.

315.02 **Developmental dyslexia**
DEF: Serious impairment of reading skills unexplained in relation to general intelligence and teaching processes; it can be inherited or congenital.

315.09 **Other**
Specific spelling difficulty

315.1 **Specific arithmetical disorder**
Dyscalculia

315.2 **Other specific learning difficulties**
EXCLUDES: specific arithmetical disorder (315.1)
specific reading disorder (315.00-315.09)

√5th **315.3** **Developmental speech or language disorder**

315.31 **Developmental language disorder**
Developmental aphasia
Expressive language disorder
Word deafness
EXCLUDES: acquired aphasia (784.3)
elective mutism (309.83, 313.0, 313.23)

315.32 **Receptive language disorder (mixed)**
Receptive expressive language disorder
AHA: 4Q, '96, 30

315.39 **Other**
Developmental articulation disorder
Dyslalia
EXCLUDES: lisping and lalling (307.9)
stammering and stuttering (307.0)

315.4 **Coordination disorder**
Clumsiness syndrome   Specific motor development
Dyspraxia syndrome   disorder

315.5 **Mixed development disorder**

315.8 **Other specified delays in development**

315.9 **Unspecified delay in development**
Developmental disorder NOS

316 **Psychic factors associated with diseases classified elsewhere**
Psychologic factors in physical conditions classified elsewhere
Use additional code to identify the associated physical condition, as:
psychogenic:
    asthma (493.9)
    dermatitis (692.9)
    duodenal ulcer (532.0-532.9)
    eczema (691.8, 692.9)
    gastric ulcer (531.0-531.9)
    mucous colitis (564.9)
    paroxysmal tachycardia (427.2)
    ulcerative colitis (556)
    urticaria (708.0-708.9)
psychosocial dwarfism (259.4)
EXCLUDES: physical symptoms and physiological malfunctions, not involving tissue damage, of mental origin (306.0-306.9)

MENTAL RETARDATION (317-319)

Use additional code(s) to identify any associated psychiatric or physical condition(s)

317 **Mild mental retardation**
High-grade defect
IQ 50-70
Mild mental subnormality

√4th **318** **Other specified mental retardation**

318.0 **Moderate mental retardation**
IQ 35-49
Moderate mental subnormality

318.1 **Severe mental retardation**
IQ 20-34   Severe mental subnormality

318.2 **Profound mental retardation**
IQ under 20   Profound mental subnormality

319 **Unspecified mental retardation**
Mental deficiency NOS   Mental subnormality NOS

6. DISEASES OF THE NERVOUS SYSTEM AND SENSE ORGANS (320-389)

INFLAMMATORY DISEASES OF THE CENTRAL NERVOUS SYSTEM (320-326)

√4th 320 Bacterial meningitis

INCLUDES:
- arachnoiditis ⎫
- leptomeningitis ⎪
- meningitis ⎬ bacterial
- meningoencephalitis ⎪
- meningomyelitis ⎪
- pachymeningitis ⎭

AHA: J-F, '87, 6

DEF: Bacterial infection causing inflammation of the lining of the brain and/or spinal cord.

320.0 Hemophilus meningitis CC
Meningitis due to Hemophilus influenzae [H. influenzae]
CC Excl: 003.21, 013.00-013.16, 036.0, 047.0-047.9, 049.0-049.1, 053.0, 054.72, 072.1, 090.42, 091.81, 094.2, 098.89, 100.81, 112.83, 114.2, 115.01, 115.11, 115.91, 130.0, 250.60-250.63, 250.80-250.93, 320.0-320.9, 321.0-321.8, 322.0-322.9, 349.89, 349.9, 357.0

320.1 Pneumococcal meningitis CC
CC Excl: See code 320.0

320.2 Streptococcal meningitis CC
CC Excl: See code 320.0

320.3 Staphylococcal meningitis CC
CC Excl: See code 320.0

320.7 Meningitis in other bacterial diseases classified elsewhere CC
Code first underlying disease, as:
- actinomycosis (039.8)
- listeriosis (027.0)
- typhoid fever (002.0)
- whooping cough (033.0-033.9)

EXCLUDES meningitis (in):
- epidemic (036.0)
- gonococcal (098.82)
- meningococcal (036.0)
- salmonellosis (003.21)
- syphilis:
  - NOS (094.2)
  - congenital (090.42)
  - meningovascular (094.2)
  - secondary (091.81)
- tuberculous (013.0)

CC Excl: See code 320.0

√5th 320.8 Meningitis due to other specified bacteria

320.81 Anaerobic meningitis CC
- Bacteroides (fragilis)
- Gram-negative anaerobes
CC Excl: See code 320.0

320.82 Meningitis due to gram-negative bacteria, not elsewhere classified CC
- Aerobacter aerogenes
- Escherichia coli [E. coli]
- Friedländer bacillus
- Klebsiella pneumoniae
- Proteus morganii
- Pseudomonas

EXCLUDES gram-negative anaerobes (320.81)

CC Excl: See code 320.0

320.89 Meningitis due to other specified bacteria CC
- Bacillus pyocyaneus
CC Excl: See code 320.0

320.9 Meningitis due to unspecified bacterium CC
Meningitis:
- bacterial NOS
- purulent NOS
Meningitis:
- pyogenic NOS
- suppurative NOS

CC Excl: See code 320.0

√4th 321 Meningitis due to other organisms
AHA: J-F, '87, 6

DEF: Infection causing inflammation of the lining of the brain and/or spinal cord, due to organisms other than bacteria.

321.0 Cryptococcal meningitis CC
Code first underlying disease (117.5)
CC Excl: See code 320.0

321.1 Meningitis in other fungal diseases CC
Code first underlying disease (110.0-118)
EXCLUDES meningitis in:
- candidiasis (112.83)
- coccidioidomycosis (114.2)
- histoplasmosis (115.01, 115.11, 115.91)

CC Excl: See code 320.0

321.2 Meningitis due to viruses not elsewhere classified CC
Code first underlying disease, as:
meningitis due to arbovirus (060.0-066.9)
EXCLUDES meningitis (due to):
- abacterial (047.0-047.9)
- adenovirus (049.1)
- aseptic NOS (047.9)
- Coxsackie (virus)(047.0)
- ECHO virus (047.1)
- enterovirus (047.0-047.9)
- herpes simplex virus (054.72)
- herpes zoster virus (053.0)
- lymphocytic choriomeningitis virus (049.0)
- mumps (072.1)
- viral NOS (047.9)
- meningo-eruptive syndrome (047.1)

CC Excl: 003.21, 013.00-013.16, 036.0, 047.0-047.9, 049.0-049.1, 053.0, 054.72, 072.1, 090.42, 091.81, 094.2, 098.89, 100.81, 112.83, 114.2, 115.01, 115.11, 115.91, 130.0, 320.0-320.9, 321.0-321.8, 322.0-322.9, 349.89, 349.9, 357.0

321.3 Meningitis due to trypanosomiasis CC
Code first underlying disease (086.0-086.9)
CC Excl: 003.21, 013.00-013.16, 036.0, 047.0-047.9, 049.0-049.1, 053.0, 054.72, 072.1, 090.42, 091.81, 094.2, 098.89, 100.81, 112.83, 114.2, 115.01, 115.11, 115.91, 130.0, 250.60-250.63, 250.80-250.93, 320.0-320.9, 321.0-321.8, 322.0-322.9, 349.89, 349.9, 357.0

321.4 Meningitis in sarcoidosis CC
Code first underlying disease (135)
CC Excl: See code 321.3

321.8 Meningitis due to other nonbacterial organisms classified elsewhere CC
Code first underlying disease
EXCLUDES leptospiral meningitis (100.81)
CC Excl: See code 321.3

√4th 322 Meningitis of unspecified cause

INCLUDES:
- arachnoiditis ⎫
- leptomeningitis ⎬ with no organism
- meningitis ⎪ specified as
- pachymeningitis ⎭ cause

AHA: J-F, '87, 6

DEF: Infection causing inflammation of the lining of the brain and/or spinal cord, due to unspecified cause.

322.0 Nonpyogenic meningitis CC
Meningitis with clear cerebrospinal fluid
CC Excl: See code 321.3

NERVOUS SYSTEM AND SENSE ORGANS

322.1 Eosinophilic meningitis `CC`
CC Excl: See code 321.3

322.2 Chronic meningitis `CC`
CC Excl: See code 321.3

322.9 Meningitis, unspecified `CC`
CC Excl: See code 321.3

√4th 323 Encephalitis, myelitis, and encephalomyelitis
  INCLUDES acute disseminated encephalomyelitis
    meningoencephalitis, except bacterial
    meningomyelitis, except bacterial
    myelitis (acute):
      ascending
      transverse
  EXCLUDES bacterial:
    meningoencephalitis (320.0-320.9)
    meningomyelitis (320.0-320.9)

DEF: Encephalitis: inflammation of brain tissues.
DEF: Myelitis: inflammation of the spinal cord.
DEF: Encephalomyelitis: inflammation of brain and spinal cord.

323.0 Encephalitis in viral diseases classified elsewhere
  Code first underlying disease, as:
    cat-scratch disease (078.3)
    infectious mononucleosis (075)
    ornithosis (073.7)
  EXCLUDES encephalitis (in):
    arthropod-borne viral (062.0-064)
    herpes simplex (054.3)
    mumps (072.2)
    poliomyelitis (045.0-045.9)
    rubella (056.01)
    slow virus infections of central nervous system (046.0-046.9)
    other viral diseases of central nervous system (049.8-049.9)
    viral NOS (049.9)

323.1 Encephalitis in rickettsial diseases classified elsewhere
  Code first underlying disease (080-083.9)
DEF: Inflammation of the brain caused by rickettsial disease carried by louse, tick, or mite.

323.2 Encephalitis in protozoal diseases classified elsewhere
  Code first underlying disease, as:
    malaria (084.0-084.9)
    trypanosomiasis (086.0-086.9)
DEF: Inflammation of the brain caused by protozoal disease carried by mosquitoes and flies.

323.4 Other encephalitis due to infection classified elsewhere
  Code first underlying disease
  EXCLUDES encephalitis (in):
    meningococcal (036.1)
    syphilis:
      NOS (094.81)
      congenital (090.41)
    toxoplasmosis (130.0)
    tuberculosis (013.6)
    meningoencephalitis due to free-living ameba [Naegleria] (136.2)

323.5 Encephalitis following immunization procedures
  Encephalitis } postimmunization or
  Encephalomyelitis } postvaccinal
  Use additional E code to identify vaccine

323.6 Postinfectious encephalitis
  Code first underlying disease
  EXCLUDES encephalitis:
    postchickenpox (052.0)
    postmeasles (055.0)
DEF: Infection, inflammation of brain several weeks following the outbreak of a systemic infection.

323.7 Toxic encephalitis
  Code first underlying cause, as:
    carbon tetrachloride (982.1)
    hydroxyquinoline derivatives (961.3)
    lead (984.0-984.9)
    mercury (985.0)
    thallium (985.8)
AHA: 2Q, '97, 8

323.8 Other causes of encephalitis `HIV`
323.9 Unspecified cause of encephalitis `HIV`

√4th 324 Intracranial and intraspinal abscess
  324.0 Intracranial abscess `CC`
    Abscess (embolic):   Abscess (embolic) of brain
      cerebellar   [any part]:
      cerebral   epidural
                                  extradural
                                  otogenic
                                  subdural
    EXCLUDES tuberculous (013.3)
  CC Excl: 006.5, 013.20-013.36, 250.60-250.63, 250.80-250.93, 324.0-324.9, 325, 348.8-348.9

  324.1 Intraspinal abscess `CC`
    Abscess (embolic) of spinal cord [any part]:
      epidural
      extradural
      subdural
    EXCLUDES tuberculous (013.5)
  CC Excl: 006.5, 013.20-013.36, 250.60-250.63, 250.80-250.93, 324.1

  324.9 Of unspecified site `CC`
    Extradural or subdural abscess NOS
  CC Excl: 006.5, 013.20-013.36, 250.60-250.63, 250.80-250.93, 324.0-324.9, 325

325 Phlebitis and thrombophlebitis of intracranial venous sinuses `CC`
  Embolism   } of cavernous, lateral, or
  Endophlebitis   } other intracranial
  Phlebitis, septic or suppurative } or unspecified
  Thrombophlebitis   } intracranial
  Thrombosis   } venous sinus
  EXCLUDES that specified as:
    complicating pregnancy, childbirth, or the puerperium (671.5)
    of nonpyogenic origin (437.6)
CC Excl: See code 324.9
DEF: Inflammation and formation of blood clot in a vein within the brain or its lining.

326 Late effects of intracranial abscess or pyogenic infection
  Note: This category is to be used to indicate conditions whose primary classification is to 320-325 [excluding 320.7, 321.0-321.8, 323.0-323.4, 323.6-323.7] as the cause of late effects, themselves classifiable elsewhere. The "late effects" include conditions specified as such, or as sequelae, which may occur at any time after the resolution of the causal condition.
  Use additional code to identify condition, as:
    hydrocephalus (331.4)
    paralysis (342.0-342.9, 344.0-344.9)

HEREDITARY AND DEGENERATIVE DISEASES OF THE CENTRAL NERVOUS SYSTEM (330-337)

EXCLUDES hepatolenticular degeneration (275.1)
multiple sclerosis (340)
other demyelinating diseases of central nervous system (341.0-341.9)

√4th 330 Cerebral degenerations usually manifest in childhood
Use additional code to identify associated mental retardation

330.0 Leukodystrophy
Krabbe's disease
Leukodystrophy NOS
globoid cell
metachromatic
sudanophilic
Pelizaeus-Merzbacher disease
Sulfatide lipidosis

DEF: Hereditary disease of arylsulfatase or cerebroside sulfatase; characterized by a diffuse loss of myelin in CNS; infantile form causes blindness, motor disturbances, rigidity, mental deterioration and, occasionally, convulsions.

330.1 Cerebral lipidoses
Amaurotic (familial) idiocy
Disease:
  Batten
  Jansky-Bielschowsky
  Kufs'
Disease:
  Spielmeyer-Vogt
  Tay-Sachs
Gangliosidosis

DEF: Genetic disorder causing abnormal lipid accumulation in the reticuloendothelial cells of the brain.

330.2 Cerebral degeneration in generalized lipidoses
Code first underlying disease, as:
  Fabry's disease (272.7)
  Gaucher's disease (272.7)
  Niemann-Pick disease (272.7)
  sphingolipidosis (272.7)

330.3 Cerebral degeneration of childhood in other diseases classified elsewhere
Code first underlying disease, as:
  Hunter's disease (277.5)
  mucopolysaccharidosis (277.5)

330.8 Other specified cerebral degenerations in childhood
Alpers' disease or gray-matter degeneration
Infantile necrotizing encephalomyelopathy
Leigh's disease
Subacute necrotizing encephalomyelopathy or encephalomyelopathy

AHA: N-D, '85, 5

330.9 Unspecified cerebral degeneration in childhood

√4th 331 Other cerebral degenerations

331.0 Alzheimer's disease
AHA: 4Q, '00, 41; 4Q, '99, 7; N-D, '84, 20

DEF: Diffuse atrophy of cerebral cortex; causing a progressive decline in intellectual and physical functions, including memory loss, personality changes and profound dementia.

331.1 Pick's disease
DEF: Rare, progressive degenerative brain disease, similar to Alzheimer's; cortical atrophy affects the frontal and temporal lobes.

331.2 Senile degeneration of brain
EXCLUDES senility NOS (797)

331.3 Communicating hydrocephalus
EXCLUDES congenital hydrocephalus (741.0, 742.3)

AHA: S-O, '85, 12

DEF: Subarachnoid hemorrhage and meningitis causing excess buildup of cerebrospinal fluid in cavities due to nonabsorption of fluid back through fluid pathways.

331.4 Obstructive hydrocephalus
Acquired hydrocephalus NOS
EXCLUDES congenital hydrocephalus (741.0, 742.3)

CC Excl: 250.60-250.63, 250.80-250.93, 331.3-331.7, 331.89, 331.9, 348.8-348.9, 741.00-741.03, 742.3-742.4, 742.59, 742.8-742.9

AHA: 1Q, '99, 9

DEF: Obstruction of cerebrospinal fluid passage from brain into spinal canal.

331.7 Cerebral degeneration in diseases classified elsewhere
Code first underlying disease, as:
  alcoholism (303.0-303.9)
  beriberi (265.0)
  cerebrovascular disease (430-438)
  congenital hydrocephalus (741.0, 742.3)
  myxedema (244.0-244.9)
  neoplastic disease (140.0-239.9)
  vitamin B_{12} deficiency (266.2)
EXCLUDES cerebral degeneration in:
  Jakob-Creutzfeldt disease (046.1)
  progressive multifocal leukoencephalopathy (046.3)
  subacute spongiform encephalopathy (046.1)

√5th 331.8 Other cerebral degeneration

331.81 Reye's syndrome
DEF: Rare childhood illness, often developed after a bout of viral upper respiratory infection; characterized by vomiting, elevated serum transaminase, changes in liver and other viscera; symptoms may be followed by an encephalopathic phase with brain swelling, disturbances of consciousness and seizures; can be fatal.

331.89 Other
Cerebral ataxia

331.9 Cerebral degeneration, unspecified

√4th 332 Parkinson's disease

332.0 Paralysis agitans
Parkinsonism or Parkinson's disease:
  NOS   primary
  idiopathic

AHA: M-A, '87, 7

DEF: Form of parkinsonism; progressive, occurs in senior years; characterized by masklike facial expression; condition affects ability to stand erect, walk smoothly; weakened muscles, also tremble and involuntarily movement.

332.1 Secondary Parkinsonism
Parkinsonism due to drugs
Use additional E code to identify drug, if drug-induced
EXCLUDES Parkinsonism (in):
  Huntington's disease (333.4)
  progressive supranuclear palsy (333.0)
  Shy-Drager syndrome (333.0)
  syphilitic (094.82)

√4th 333 Other extrapyramidal disease and abnormal movement disorders
INCLUDES other forms of extrapyramidal, basal ganglia, or striatopallidal disease
EXCLUDES abnormal movements of head NOS (781.0)

333.0 Other degenerative diseases of the basal ganglia
Atrophy or degeneration:
  olivopontocerebellar [Déjérine-Thomas syndrome]
  pigmentary pallidal [Hallervorden-Spatz disease]
  striatonigral
Parkinsonian syndrome associated with:
  idiopathic orthostatic hypotension
  symptomatic orthostatic hypotension
Progressive supranuclear ophthalmoplegia
Shy-Drager syndrome
AHA: 3Q, '96, 8

333.1 Essential and other specified forms of tremor
Benign essential tremor
Familial tremor
Use additional E code to identify drug, if drug-induced
EXCLUDES tremor NOS (781.0)

333.2 Myoclonus
Familial essential myoclonus
Progressive myoclonic epilepsy
Unverricht-Lundborg disease
Use additional E code to identify drug, if drug-induced
AHA: 3Q, '97, 4; M-A, '87, 12

DEF: Spontaneous movements or contractions of muscles.

333.3 Tics of organic origin
Use additional E code to identify drug, if drug-induced
EXCLUDES Gilles de la Tourette's syndrome (307.23)
  habit spasm (307.22)
  tic NOS (307.20)

333.4 Huntington's chorea
DEF: Genetic disease characterized by chronic progressive mental deterioration; dementia and death within 15 years of onset.

333.5 Other choreas
Hemiballism(us)
Paroxysmal choreo-athetosis
Use additional E code to identify drug, if drug-induced
EXCLUDES Sydenham's or rheumatic chorea (392.0-392.9)

333.6 Idiopathic torsion dystonia
Dystonia:
  deformans progressiva
  musculorum deformans
(Schwalbe-) Ziehen-Oppenheim disease
DEF: Sustained muscular contractions, causing twisting and repetitive movements that result in abnormal postures of trunk and limbs; etiology unknown.

333.7 Symptomatic torsion dystonia
Athetoid cerebral palsy [Vogt's disease]
Double athetosis (syndrome)
Use additional E code to identify drug, if drug-induced

√5th 333.8 Fragments of torsion dystonia
Use additional E code to identify drug, if drug-induced

333.81 Blepharospasm
DEF: Uncontrolled winking or blinking due to orbicularis oculi muscle spasm.

333.82 Orofacial dyskinesia
DEF: Uncontrolled movement of mouth or facial muscles.

333.83 Spasmodic torticollis
EXCLUDES torticollis:
  NOS (723.5)
  hysterical (300.11)
  psychogenic (306.0)
DEF: Uncontrolled movement of head due to spasms of neck muscle.

333.84 Organic writers' cramp
EXCLUDES pychogenic (300.89)

333.89 Other

√5th 333.9 Other and unspecified extrapyramidal diseases and abnormal movement disorders

333.90 Unspecified extrapyramidal disease and abnormal movement disorder

333.91 Stiff-man syndrome

333.92 Neuroleptic malignant syndrome
Use additional E code to identify drug
AHA: 4Q, '94, 37

333.93 Benign shuddering attacks
AHA: 4Q, '94, 37

333.99 Other
Restless legs
AHA: 4Q, '94, 37

√4th 334 Spinocerebellar disease
EXCLUDES olivopontocerebellar degeneration (333.0)
  peroneal muscular atrophy (356.1)

334.0 Friedreich's ataxia
DEF: Genetic recessive disease of children; sclerosis of dorsal, lateral spinal cord columns; characterized by ataxia, speech impairment, swaying and irregular movements, with muscle paralysis, especially of lower limbs.

334.1 Hereditary spastic paraplegia

334.2 Primary cerebellar degeneration
Cerebellar ataxia:
  Marie's
  Sanger-Brown
Dyssynergia cerebellaris myoclonica
Primary cerebellar degeneration:
  NOS
  hereditary
  sporadic
AHA: M-A, '87, 9

334.3 Other cerebellar ataxia
Cerebellar ataxia NOS
Use additional E code to identify drug, if drug-induced

334.4 *Cerebellar ataxia in diseases classified elsewhere*
Code first underlying disease, as:
  alcoholism (303.0-303.9)
  myxedema (244.0-244.9)
  neoplastic disease (140.0-239.9)

334.8 Other spinocerebellar diseases
Ataxia-telangiectasia [Louis-Bar syndrome]
Corticostriatal-spinal degeneration

334.9 Spinocerebellar disease, unspecified

√4th 335 Anterior horn cell disease

335.0 Werdnig-Hoffmann disease **CC**
Infantile spinal muscular atrophy
Progressive muscular atrophy of infancy
CC Excl: 250.60-250.63, 250.80-250.93, 334.8-334.9, 335.0, 335.10-335.9, 336.0-336.9, 337.0-337.9, 349.89, 349.9

DEF: Spinal muscle atrophy manifested in prenatal period or shortly after birth; symptoms include hypotonia, atrophy of skeletal muscle; death occurs in infancy.

√5th 335.1 Spinal muscular atrophy

335.10 Spinal muscular atrophy, unspecified **CC**
CC Excl: See code 335.0

335.11 Kugelberg-Welander disease **CC**
Spinal muscular atrophy:
  familial
  juvenile
CC Excl: See code 335.0

DEF: Hereditary; juvenile muscle atrophy; appears during first two decades of life; due to lesions of anterior horns of spinal cord; includes wasting, diminution of lower body muscles and twitching.

335.19 Other **CC**
Adult spinal muscular atrophy
CC Excl: See code 335.0

NERVOUS SYSTEM AND SENSE ORGANS

335.2 Motor neuron disease ✓5th

- **335.20 Amyotrophic lateral sclerosis** CC A
  - Motor neuron disease (bulbar) (mixed type)
  - CC Excl: See code 335.0
  - AHA: 4Q, '95, 81

- **335.21 Progressive muscular atrophy** CC
  - Duchenne-Aran muscular atrophy
  - Progressive muscular atrophy (pure)
  - CC Excl: See code 335.0

- **335.22 Progressive bulbar palsy** CC
  - CC Excl: See code 335.0

- **335.23 Pseudobulbar palsy** CC
  - CC Excl: See code 335.0

- **335.24 Primary lateral sclerosis** CC
  - CC Excl: See code 335.0

- **335.29 Other** CC
  - CC Excl: See code 335.0

335.8 Other anterior horn cell diseases CC
CC Excl: See code 335.0

335.9 Anterior horn cell disease, unspecified CC
CC Excl: See code 335.0

336 Other diseases of spinal cord ✓4th

336.0 Syringomyelia and syringobulbia
AHA: 1Q, '89, 10

336.1 Vascular myelopathies
Acute infarction of spinal cord (embolic) (nonembolic)
Arterial thrombosis of spinal cord
Edema of spinal cord
Hematomyelia
Subacute necrotic myelopathy

336.2 Subacute combined degeneration of spinal cord in diseases classified elsewhere
Code first underlying disease, as:
  pernicious anemia (281.0)
  other vitamin B_{12} deficiency anemia (281.1)
  vitamin B_{12} deficiency (266.2)

336.3 Myelopathy in other diseases classified elsewhere
Code first underlying disease, as:
  myelopathy in neoplastic disease (140.0-239.9)
  EXCLUDES myelopathy in:
    intervertebral disc disorder (722.70-722.73)
    spondylosis (721.1, 721.41-721.42, 721.91)
AHA: 3Q, '99, 5

336.8 Other myelopathy
Myelopathy: drug-induced
Myelopathy: radiation-induced
Use additonal E code to identify cause

336.9 Unspecified disease of spinal cord HIV
Cord compression NOS   Myelopathy NOS
EXCLUDES myelitis (323.0-323.9)
  spinal (canal) stenosis (723.0, 724.00-724.09)

337 Disorders of the autonomic nervous system ✓4th
INCLUDES disorders of peripheral autonomic, sympathetic, parasympathetic, or vegetative system
EXCLUDES familial dysautonomia [Riley-Day syndrome] (742.8)

337.0 Idiopathic peripheral autonomic neuropathy
Carotid sinus syncope or syndrome
Cervical sympathetic dystrophy or paralysis

337.1 Peripheral autonomic neuropathy in disorders classified elsewhere
Code first underlying disease, as:
  amyloidosis (277.3)
  diabetes (250.6)
AHA: 2Q, '93, 6; 3Q, '91, 9; N-D, '84, 9

337.2 Reflex sympathetic dystrophy ✓5th
AHA: 4Q, '93, 24

DEF: Disturbance of the sympathetic nervous system evidenced by sweating, pain, pallor and edema following injury to nerves or blood vessels.

- **337.20** Reflex sympathetic dystrophy, unspecified
- **337.21** Reflex sympathetic dystrophy of the upper limb
- **337.22** Reflex sympathetic dystrophy of the lower limb
- **337.29** Reflex sympathetic dystrophy of other specified site

337.3 Autonomic dysreflexia
Use additional code to identify the cause, such as:
  decubitus ulcer (707.0)
  fecal impaction (560.39)
  urinary tract infection (599.0)
AHA: 4Q, '98, 37

DEF: Noxious stimuli evokes paroxysmal hypertension, bradycardia, excess sweating, headache, pilomotor responses, facial flushing, and nasal congestion due to uncontrolled parasympathetic nerve response; usually occurs in patients with spinal cord injury above major sympathetic outflow tract (T_6).

337.9 Unspecified disorder of autonomic nervous system

OTHER DISORDERS OF THE CENTRAL NERVOUS SYSTEM (340-349)

340 Multiple sclerosis CC A
Disseminated or multiple sclerosis:
  NOS   cord
  brain stem   generalized
CC Excl: 250.60-250.63, 250.80-250.93, 340, 341.8-341.9

341 Other demyelinating diseases of central nervous system ✓4th

- **341.0 Neuromyelitis optica**
- **341.1 Schilder's disease**
  - Baló's concentric sclerosis
  - Encephalitis periaxialis concentrica [Baló's]
  - Encephalitis periaxialis diffusa [Schilder's]

  DEF: Chronic leukoencephalopathy of children and adolescents; symptoms include blindness, deafness, bilateral spasticity and progressive mental deterioration.

- **341.8 Other demyelinating diseases of central nervous system**
  - Central demyelination of corpus callosum
  - Central pontine myelinosis
  - Marchiafava (-Bignami) disease
  AHA: N-D, '87, 6

- **341.9 Demyelinating disease of central nervous system, unspecified** HIV

NERVOUS SYSTEM AND SENSE ORGANS

342 Hemiplegia and hemiparesis ✓4th

Note: This category is to be used when hemiplegia (complete) (incomplete) is reported without further specification, or is stated to be old or long-standing but of unspecified cause. The category is also for use in multiple coding to identify these types of hemiplegia resulting from any cause.

EXCLUDES congenital (343.1)
hemiplegia due to late effect of cerebrovascular accident (438.20-438.22)
infantile NOS (343.4)

The following fifth-digits are for use with codes 342.0-342.9:
- 0 affecting unspecified side
- 1 affecting dominant side
- 2 affecting nondominant side

AHA: 4Q, '94, 38

- ✓5th **342.0** Flaccid hemiplegia
- ✓5th **342.1** Spastic hemiplegia
- ✓5th **342.8** Other specified hemiplegia
- ✓5th **342.9** Hemiplegia, unspecified
    AHA: 4Q, '98, 87

343 Infantile cerebral palsy ✓4th

INCLUDES
cerebral:
  palsy NOS
  spastic infantile paralysis
congenital spastic paralysis (cerebral)
Little's disease
paralysis (spastic) due to birth injury:
  intracranial
  spinal

EXCLUDES hereditary cerebral paralysis, such as:
  hereditary spastic paraplegia (334.1)
  Vogt's disease (333.7)
spastic paralysis specified as noncongenital or noninfantile (344.0-344.9)

343.0 Diplegic
Congenital diplegia
Congenital paraplegia
DEF: Paralysis affecting both sides of the body simultaneously.

343.1 Hemiplegic
Congenital hemiplegia
EXCLUDES infantile hemiplegia NOS (343.4)

343.2 Quadriplegic CC
Tetraplegic
CC Excl: 250.60-250.63, 250.80-250.93, 342.00-342.92, 343.0-343.9, 344.00-344.61, 344.9, 348.8-348.9, 349.89, 349.9, 742.59, 742.8-742.9

343.3 Monoplegic

343.4 Infantile hemiplegia
Infantile hemiplegia (postnatal) NOS

343.8 Other specified infantile cerebral palsy

343.9 Infantile cerebral palsy, unspecified
Cerebral palsy NOS

344 Other paralytic syndromes ✓4th

Note: This category is to be used when the listed conditions are reported without further specification or are stated to be old or long-standing but of unspecified cause. The category is also for use in multiple coding to identify these conditions resulting from any cause.

INCLUDES paralysis (complete) (incomplete), except as classifiable to 342 and 343

EXCLUDES congenital or infantile cerebral palsy (343.0-343.9)
hemiplegia (342.0-342.9)
congenital or infantile (343.1, 343.4)

- ✓5th **344.0 Quadriplegia and quadriparesis**
    - **344.00 Quadriplegia unspecified** CC
        CC Excl: See code 343.2
        AHA: 4Q, '98, 38
    - **344.01 C_1-C_4 complete** CC
        CC Excl: See code 343.2
    - **344.02 C_1-C_4 incomplete** CC
        CC Excl: See code 343.2
    - **344.03 C_5-C_7 complete** CC
        CC Excl: See code 343.2
    - **344.04 C_5-C_7 incomplete** CC
        CC Excl: See code 343.2
    - **344.09 Other** CC
        CC Excl: See code 343.2
        AHA: 1Q, '01, 12; 4Q, '98, 39

- **344.1 Paraplegia**
    Paralysis of both lower limbs   Paraplegia (lower)
    AHA: M-A, '87, 10

- **344.2 Diplegia of upper limbs**
    Diplegia (upper)   Paralysis of both upper limbs

- ✓5th **344.3 Monoplegia of lower limb**
    Paralysis of lower limb
    EXCLUDES monoplegia of lower limb due to late effect of cerebrovascular accident (438.40-438.42)
    - **344.30 Affecting unspecified side**
    - **344.31 Affecting dominant side**
    - **344.32 Affecting nondominant side**

- ✓5th **344.4 Monoplegia of upper limb**
    Paralysis of upper limb
    EXCLUDES monoplegia of upper limb due to late effect of cerebrovascular accident (438.30-438.32)
    - **344.40 Affecting unspecified side**
    - **344.41 Affecting dominant side**
    - **344.42 Affecting nondominant side**

- **344.5 Unspecified monoplegia**

- ✓5th **344.6 Cauda equina syndrome**
    DEF: Dull pain and paresthesias in sacrum, perineum and bladder due to compression of spinal nerve roots; pain radiates down buttocks, back of thigh, calf of leg and into foot with prickling, burning sensations.
    - **344.60 Without mention of neurogenic bladder**
    - **344.61 With neurogenic bladder**
        Acontractile bladder
        Autonomic hyperreflexia of bladder
        Cord bladder
        Detrusor hyperreflexia
        AHA: M-J, '87, 12; M-A, '87, 10

- ✓5th **344.8 Other specified paralytic syndromes**
    - **344.81 Locked-in state**
        AHA: 4Q, '93, 24
        DEF: State of consciousness where patients are paralyzed and unable to respond to environmental stimuli; patients have eye movements, and stimuli can enter the brain but patients cannot respond to stimuli.
    - **344.89 Other specified paralytic syndrome**
        AHA: 2Q, '99, 4

- **344.9 Paralysis, unspecified**

| Tabular List | NERVOUS SYSTEM AND SENSE ORGANS | 345–348.0 |

√4th 345 Epilepsy

The following fifth-digit subclassification is for use with categories 345.0, .1, .4-.9:
- 0 without mention of intractable epilepsy
- 1 with intractable epilepsy

EXCLUDES progressive myoclonic epilepsy (333.2)

AHA: 1Q, '93, 24; 2Q, '92, 8 4Q, '92, 23

DEF: Brain disorder characterized by electrical-like disturbances; may include occasional impairment or loss of consciousness, abnormal motor phenomena and psychic or sensory disturbances.

√5th 345.0 Generalized nonconvulsive epilepsy CC 1
- Absences:
  - atonic
  - typical
- Minor epilepsy
- Petit mal
- Pykno-epilepsy
- Seizures:
  - akinetic
  - atonic

CC Excl: For code 345.01: 250.60-250.63, 345.00-345.91, 348.8-348.9, 349.89, 349.9

√5th 345.1 Generalized convulsive epilepsy CC
- Epileptic seizures:
  - clonic
  - myoclonic
  - tonic
- Epileptic seizures:
  - tonic-clonic
  - Grand mal
  - Major epilepsy

EXCLUDES convulsions:
- NOS (780.3)
- infantile (780.3)
- newborn (779.0)
- infantile spasms (345.6)

CC Excl: See code 345.01

AHA: 3Q, '97, 4

DEF: Convulsive seizures with tension of limbs (tonic) or rhythmic contractions (clonic).

345.2 Petit mal status CC
- Epileptic absence status

CC Excl: 250.60-250.63, 250.80-250.93, 345.00-345.91, 348.8-348.9, 349.89, 349.9

DEF: Minor myoclonic spasms and sudden momentary loss of consciousness in epilepsy.

345.3 Grand mal status CC
- Status epilepticus NOS

EXCLUDES epilepsia partialis continua (345.7)
- status:
  - psychomotor (345.7)
  - temporal lobe (345.7)

CC Excl: See code 345.2

DEF: Sudden loss of consciousness followed by generalized convulsions in epilepsy.

√5th 345.4 Partial epilepsy, with impairment of consciousness CC 1
- Epilepsy:
  - limbic system
  - partial:
    - secondarily generalized
    - with memory and ideational disturbances
  - psychomotor
  - psychosensory
  - temporal lobe
- Epileptic automatism

CC Excl: For code 345.41: 250.60-250.63, 345.00-345.91, 348.8-348.9, 349.89, 349.9

√5th 345.5 Partial epilepsy, without mention of impairment of consciousness CC 1
- Epilepsy:
  - Bravais-Jacksonian NOS
  - focal (motor) NOS
  - Jacksonian NOS
  - motor partial
  - partial NOS
- Epilepsy:
  - sensory-induced
  - somatomotor
  - somatosensory
  - visceral
  - visual

CC Excl: For code 345.51: See code 345.4

√5th 345.6 Infantile spasms CC 1
- Hypsarrhythmia
- Lightning spasms
- Salaam attacks

EXCLUDES salaam tic (781.0)

CC Excl: For code 345.61: See code 345.4

AHA: N-D, '84, 12

√5th 345.7 Epilepsia partialis continua CC 1
- Kojevnikov's epilepsy

CC Excl: For code 345.71: See code 345.4

DEF: Continuous muscle contractions and relaxation; result of abnormal neural discharge.

√5th 345.8 Other forms of epilepsy CC 1
- Epilepsy:
  - cursive [running]
- Epilepsy:
  - gelastic

CC Excl: For code 345.81: See code 345.4

√5th 345.9 Epilepsy, unspecified CC 1
- Epileptic convulsions, fits, or seizures NOS

EXCLUDES convulsive seizure or fit NOS (780.3)

CC Excl: For code 345.91: See code 345.4

AHA: N-D, '87, 12

√4th 346 Migraine

DEF: Benign vascular headache of extreme pain; commonly associated with irritability, nausea, vomiting and often photophobia; premonitory visual hallucination of a crescent in the visual field (scotoma).

The following fifth-digit subclassification is for use with category 346:
- 0 without mention of intractable migraine
- 1 with intractable migraine, so stated

√5th 346.0 Classical migraine
- Migraine preceded or accompanied by transient focal neurological phenomena
- Migraine with aura

√5th 346.1 Common migraine
- Atypical migraine
- Sick headache

√5th 346.2 Variants of migraine
- Cluster headache
- Histamine cephalgia
- Horton's neuralgia
- Migraine:
  - abdominal
  - basilar
- Migraine:
  - lower half
  - retinal
- Neuralgia:
  - ciliary
  - migrainous

√5th 346.8 Other forms of migraine
- Migraine:
  - hemiplegic
- Migraine:
  - ophthalmoplegic

√5th 346.9 Migraine, unspecified

AHA: N-D, '85, 16

347 Cataplexy and narcolepsy

DEF: Cataplexy: Sudden onset of muscle weakness with loss of tone and strength; caused by aggressive or spontaneous emotions.

DEF: Narcolepsy: Brief, recurrent, uncontrollable episodes of sound sleep.

√4th 348 Other conditions of brain

348.0 Cerebral cysts
- Arachnoid cyst
- Porencephalic cyst
- Porencephaly, acquired
- Pseudoporencephaly

EXCLUDES porencephaly (congenital) (742.4)

348.1–349.9 NERVOUS SYSTEM AND SENSE ORGANS

348.1 Anoxic brain damage [CC]
  EXCLUDES   that occurring in:
    abortion (634-638 with .7, 639.0)
    ectopic or molar pregnancy (639.8)
    labor or delivery (668.2, 669.4)
    that of newborn (767.0, 768.0-768.9, 772.1-772.2)
  Use additional E code to identify cause
  CC Excl: 250.60-250.63, 250.80-250.93, 348.1-348.2, 349.89, 349.9
  DEF: Brain injury due to lack of oxygen, other than birth trauma.

348.2 Benign intracranial hypertension
  Pseudotumor cerebri
  EXCLUDES   hypertensive encephalopathy (437.2)
  DEF: Elevated pressure in brain due to fluid retention in brain cavities.

348.3 Encephalopathy, unspecified [HIV]
  AHA: 3Q, '97, 4

348.4 Compression of brain
  Compression } brain (stem)
  Herniation
  Posterior fossa compression syndrome
  AHA: 4Q, '94, 37
  DEF: Elevated pressure in brain due to blood clot, tumor, fracture, abscess, other condition.

348.5 Cerebral edema
  DEF: Elevated pressure in the brain due to fluid retention in brain tissues.

348.8 Other conditions of brain
  Cerebral: Cerebral:
    calcification   fungus
  AHA: S-O, '87, 9

348.9 Unspecified condition of brain [HIV]

√4th **349 Other and unspecified disorders of the nervous system**

349.0 Reaction to spinal or lumbar puncture
  Headache following lumbar puncture
  AHA: 2Q, '99, 9; 3Q, '90, 18

349.1 Nervous system complications from surgically implanted device [CC]
  EXCLUDES   immediate postoperative complications (997.00-997.09)
    mechanical complications of nervous system device (996.2)
  CC Excl: 250.60-250.63, 250.80-250.93, 349.1, 349.89, 349.9

349.2 Disorders of meninges, not elsewhere classified
  Adhesions, meningeal (cerebral) (spinal)
  Cyst, spinal meninges
  Meningocele, acquired
  Pseudomeningocele, acquired
  AHA: 2Q, '98, 18; 3Q, '94, 4

√5th **349.8 Other specified disorders of nervous system**
  349.81 Cerebrospinal fluid rhinorrhea [CC]
    EXCLUDES   cerebrospinal fluid otorrhea (388.61)
    CC Excl: 250.60-250.63, 250.80-250.93, 349.81, 349.89, 349.9
    DEF: Cerebrospinal fluid discharging from the nose; caused by fracture of frontal bone with tearing of dura mater and arachnoid.

  349.82 Toxic encephalopathy [CC]
    Use additional E code to identify cause
    AHA: 4Q, '93, 29
    CC Excl: 013.60-013.66, 017.90-017.96, 036.1, 049.8-049.9, 052.0, 054.3, 062.0-062.9, 063.0-063.9, 072.2, 090.41, 094.81, 130.0, 250.60-250.63, 250.80-250.93, 323.0-323.9, 348.3, 348.8-348.9, 349.82-349.89, 349.9
    DEF: Brain tissue degeneration due to toxic substance.

  349.89 Other

349.9 Unspecified disorders of nervous system [HIV]
  Disorder of nervous system (central) NOS

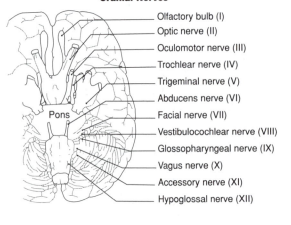

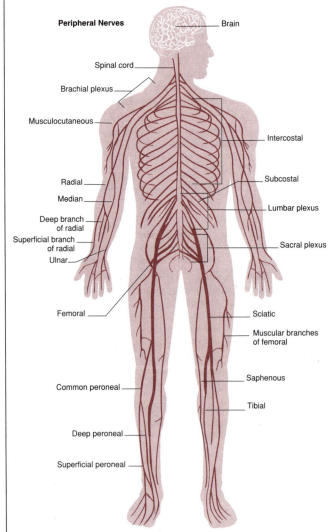

| N Newborn Age: 0 | P Pediatric Age: 0-17 | M Maternity Age: 12-55 | A Adult Age: 15-124 | CC CC Condition | MC Major Complication | CD Complex Dx | HIV HIV Related Dx |

NERVOUS SYSTEM AND SENSE ORGANS

DISORDERS OF THE PERIPHERAL NERVOUS SYSTEM (350-359)

EXCLUDES diseases of:
  acoustic [8th] nerve (388.5)
  oculomotor [3rd, 4th, 6th] nerves (378.0-378.9)
  optic [2nd] nerve (377.0-377.9)
  peripheral autonomic nerves (337.0-337.9)
  neuralgia }
  neuritis   } NOS or "rheumatic" (729.2)
  radiculitis }
  peripheral neuritis in pregnancy (646.4)

√4th **350 Trigeminal nerve disorders**
  INCLUDES disorders of 5th cranial nerve

  350.1 Trigeminal neuralgia
    Tic douloureux   Trigeminal neuralgia NOS
    Trifacial neuralgia
    EXCLUDES postherpetic (053.12)

  350.2 Atypical face pain
  350.8 Other specified trigeminal nerve disorders
  350.9 Trigeminal nerve disorder, unspecified

√4th **351 Facial nerve disorders**
  INCLUDES disorders of 7th cranial nerve
  EXCLUDES that in newborn (767.5)

  351.0 Bell's palsy
    Facial palsy
    DEF: Unilateral paralysis of face due to lesion on facial nerve; produces facial distortion.

  351.1 Geniculate ganglionitis
    Geniculate ganglionitis NOS
    EXCLUDES herpetic (053.11)
    DEF: Inflammation of tissue at bend in facial nerve.

  351.8 Other facial nerve disorders
    Facial myokymia   Melkersson's syndrome

  351.9 Facial nerve disorder, unspecified

√4th **352 Disorders of other cranial nerves**

  352.0 Disorders of olfactory [1st] nerve
  352.1 Glossopharyngeal neuralgia
    DEF: Pain between throat and ear along petrosal and jugular ganglia.

  352.2 Other disorders of glossopharyngeal [9th] nerve
  352.3 Disorders of pneumogastric [10th] nerve
    Disorders of vagal nerve
    EXCLUDES paralysis of vocal cords or larynx (478.30-478.34)
    DEF: Nerve disorder affecting ear, tongue, pharynx, larynx, esophagus, viscera and thorax.

  352.4 Disorders of accessory [11th] nerve
    DEF: Nerve disorder affecting palate, pharynx, larynx, thoracic viscera, sternocleidomastoid and trapezius muscles.

  352.5 Disorders of hypoglossal [12th] nerve
    DEF: Nerve disorder affecting tongue muscles.

  352.6 Multiple cranial nerve palsies
    Collet-Sicard syndrome
    Polyneuritis cranialis

  352.9 Unspecified disorder of cranial nerves

√4th **353 Nerve root and plexus disorders**
  EXCLUDES conditions due to:
    intervertebral disc disorders (722.0-722.9)
    spondylosis (720.0-721.9)
    vertebrogenic disorders (723.0-724.9)

  353.0 Brachial plexus lesions
    Cervical rib syndrome
    Costoclavicular syndrome
    Scalenus anticus syndrome
    Thoracic outlet syndrome
    EXCLUDES brachial neuritis or radiculitis NOS (723.4)
    that in newborn (767.6)
    DEF: Acquired disorder in tissue along nerves in shoulder; causes corresponding motor and sensory dysfunction.

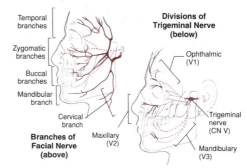

▶ Trigeminal and Facial Nerve Branches ◀

  353.1 Lumbosacral plexus lesions
    DEF: Acquired disorder in tissue along nerves in lower back; causes corresponding motor and sensory dysfunction.

  353.2 Cervical root lesions, not elsewhere classified
  353.3 Thoracic root lesions, not elsewhere classified
  353.4 Lumbosacral root lesions, not elsewhere classified
  353.5 Neuralgic amyotrophy
    Parsonage-Aldren-Turner syndrome

  353.6 Phantom limb (syndrome)
    DEF: Abnormal tingling or a burning sensation, transient aches, and intermittent or continuous pain perceived as originating in the absent limb.

  353.8 Other nerve root and plexus disorders
  353.9 Unspecified nerve root and plexus disorder

√4th **354 Mononeuritis of upper limb and mononeuritis multiplex**
  DEF: Inflammation of a single nerve; known as mononeuritis multiplex when several nerves in unrelated body areas are affected.

  354.0 Carpal tunnel syndrome
    Median nerve entrapment
    Partial thenar atrophy
    DEF: Compression of median nerve by tendons; causes pain, tingling, numbness and burning sensation in hand.

  354.1 Other lesion of median nerve
    Median nerve neuritis

  354.2 Lesion of ulnar nerve
    Cubital tunnel syndrome
    Tardy ulnar nerve palsy

  354.3 Lesion of radial nerve
    Acute radial nerve palsy
    AHA: N-D, '87, 6

  354.4 Causalgia of upper limb
    EXCLUDES causalgia:
      NOS (355.9)
      lower limb (355.71)
    DEF: Peripheral nerve damage, upper limb; usually due to injury; causes burning sensation and trophic skin changes.

  354.5 Mononeuritis multiplex
    Combinations of single conditions classifiable to 354 or 355

  354.8 Other mononeuritis of upper limb
  354.9 Mononeuritis of upper limb, unspecified

√4th **355 Mononeuritis of lower limb**

  355.0 Lesion of sciatic nerve
    EXCLUDES sciatica NOS (724.3)
    AHA: 2Q, '89, 12
    DEF: Acquired disorder of sciatic nerve; causes motor and sensory dysfunction in back, buttock and leg.

  355.1 Meralgia paresthetica
    Lateral cutaneous femoral nerve of thigh compression or syndrome
    DEF: Inguinal ligament entraps lateral femoral cutaneous nerve; causes tingling, pain and numbness along outer thigh.

  355.2 Other lesion of femoral nerve

355.3–359.0 NERVOUS SYSTEM AND SENSE ORGANS

355.3 Lesion of lateral popliteal nerve
Lesion of common peroneal nerve

355.4 Lesion of medial popliteal nerve

355.5 Tarsal tunnel syndrome
DEF: Compressed, entrapped posterior tibial nerve; causes tingling, pain and numbness in sole of foot.

355.6 Lesion of plantar nerve
Morton's metatarsalgia, neuralgia, or neuroma

√5th **355.7 Other mononeuritis of lower limb**

355.71 Causalgia of lower limb
EXCLUDES causalgia:
NOS (355.9)
upper limb (354.4)
DEF: Dysfunction of lower limb peripheral nerve, usually due to injury; causes burning pain and trophic skin changes.

355.79 Other mononeuritis of lower limb

355.8 Mononeuritis of lower limb, unspecified

355.9 Mononeuritis of unspecified site
Causalgia NOS
EXCLUDES causalgia:
lower limb (355.71)
upper limb (354.4)

√4th **356 Hereditary and idiopathic peripheral neuropathy**

356.0 Hereditary peripheral neuropathy
Déjérine-Sottas disease

356.1 Peroneal muscular atrophy
Charcôt-Marie-Tooth disease
Neuropathic muscular atrophy
DEF: Genetic disorder, in muscles innervated by peroneal nerves; symptoms include muscle wasting in lower limbs and locomotor difficulties.

356.2 Hereditary sensory neuropathy
DEF: Inherited disorder in dorsal root ganglia, optic nerve, and cerebellum, causing sensory losses, shooting pains, and foot ulcers.

356.3 Refsum's disease
Heredopathia atactica polyneuritiformis
DEF: Genetic disorder of lipid metabolism; causes persistent, painful inflammation of nerves and retinitis pigmentosa.

356.4 Idiopathic progressive polyneuropathy

356.8 Other specified idiopathic peripheral neuropathy
Supranuclear paralysis

356.9 Unspecified

√4th **357 Inflammatory and toxic neuropathy**

357.0 Acute infective polyneuritis CC
Guillain-Barré syndrome Postinfectious polyneuritis
CC Excl: 003.21, 013.00-013.16, 036.0, 036.89, 036.9, 041.81-041.89, 041.9, 047.0-047.9, 049.0-049.1, 053.0, 054.72, 072.1, 090.42, 091.81, 094.2, 098.89, 100.81, 112.83, 114.2, 115.01, 115.11, 115.91, 130.0, 139.8, 320.0-320.9, 321.0-321.8, 322.0-322.9, 349.89, 349.9, 357.0

AHA: 2Q, '98, 12

DEF: Guillain-Barré syndrome: acute demyelinatry polyneuropathy preceded by viral illness (i.e., herpes, cytomegalovirus [CMV], Epstein-Barr virus [EBV]) or a bacterial illness; areflexic motor paralysis with mild sensory disturbance and acellular rise in spinal fluid protein.

357.1 Polyneuropathy in collagen vasculardisease
Code first underlying disease, as:
disseminated lupus erythematosus (710.0)
polyarteritis nodosa (446.0)
rheumatoid arthritis (714.0)

357.2 Polyneuropathy in diabetes
Code first underlying disease (250.6)
AHA: 2Q, '92, 15; 3Q, '91, 9

357.3 Polyneuropathy in malignant disease
Code first underlying disease (140.0-208.9)

357.4 Polyneuropathy in other diseases classified elsewhere
Code first underlying disease, as:
amyloidosis (277.3)
beriberi (265.0)
deficiency of B vitamins (266.0-266.9)
diphtheria (032.0-032.9)
hypoglycemia (251.2)
pellagra (265.2)
porphyria (277.1)
sarcoidosis (135)
uremia (585)
EXCLUDES polyneuropathy in:
herpes zoster (053.13)
mumps (072.72)

AHA: 2Q, '98, 15

357.5 Alcoholic polyneuropathy

357.6 Polyneuropathy due to drugs
Use additional E code to identify drug

357.7 Polyneuropathy due to other toxic agents
Use additional E code to identify toxic agent

√5th **357.8 Other**
AHA: 2Q, '98, 12

DEF: Chronic inflammatory demyelinating polyneuritis: inflammation of peripheral nerves resulting in destruction of myelin sheath; associated with diabetes mellitus, dysproteinemias, renal failure and malnutrition; symptoms include tingling, numbness, burning pain, diminished tendon reflexes, weakness, and atrophy in lower extremities.

• **357.81 Chronic inflammatory demyelinating polyneuritis**

• **357.82 Critical illness polyneuropathy**
Acute motor neuropathy

• **357.89 Other inflammatory and toxic neuropathy**

357.9 Unspecified

√4th **358 Myoneural disorders**

358.0 Myasthenia gravis CC
CC Excl: 250.60-250.63, 250.80-250.93, 349.89, 349.9, 358.0-358.1

DEF: Autoimmune disorder of acetylcholine at neuromuscular junction; causing fatigue of voluntary muscles.

358.1 Myasthenic syndromes in diseases classified elsewhere CC

Amyotrophy
Eaton-Lambert syndrome
} from stated cause classified elsewhere

Code first underlying disease, as:
botulism (005.1)
diabetes mellitus (250.6)
hypothyroidism (244.0-244.9)
malignant neoplasm (140.0-208.9)
pernicious anemia (281.0)
thyrotoxicosis (242.0-242.9)

CC Excl: See code 358.0

358.2 Toxic myoneural disorders
Use additional E code to identify toxic agent

358.8 Other specified myoneural disorders

358.9 Myoneural disorders, unspecified

√4th **359 Muscular dystrophies and other myopathies**
EXCLUDES idiopathic polymyositis (710.4)

359.0 Congenital hereditary muscular dystrophy CC
Benign congenital myopathy   Myotubular myopathy
Central core disease   Nemaline body disease
Centronuclear myopathy
EXCLUDES arthrogryposis multiplex congenita (754.89)

CC Excl: 250.60-250.63, 250.80-250.93, 349.89, 349.9, 359.0-359.1

DEF: Genetic disorder; causing progressive or nonprogressive muscle weakness.

NERVOUS SYSTEM AND SENSE ORGANS

359.1 Hereditary progressive muscular dystrophy [CC]

Muscular dystrophy:
- NOS
- distal
- Duchenne
- Erb's
- fascioscapulohumeral

Muscular dystrophy:
- Gower's
- Landouzy-Déjérine
- limb-girdle
- ocular
- oculopharyngeal

CC Excl: See code 359.0

DEF: Genetic degenerative, muscle disease; causes progressive weakness, wasting of muscle with no nerve involvement.

359.2 Myotonic disorders

Dystrophia myotonica
Eulenburg's disease
Myotonia congenita
Paramyotonia congenita
Steinert's disease
Thomsen's disease

DEF: Impaired movement due to spasmatic, rigid muscles.

359.3 Familial periodic paralysis

Hypokalemic familial periodic paralysis

DEF: Genetic disorder; characterized by rapidly progressive flaccid paralysis; attacks often occur after exercise or exposure to cold or dietary changes.

359.4 Toxic myopathy

Use additional E code to identify toxic agent

AHA: 1Q, '88, 5

DEF: Muscle disorder caused by toxic agent.

359.5 *Myopathy in endocrine diseases classified elsewhere*

Code first underlying disease, as:
- Addison's disease (255.4)
- Cushing's syndrome (255.0)
- hypopituitarism (253.2)
- myxedema (244.0-244.9)
- thyrotoxicosis (242.0-242.9)

DEF: Muscle disorder secondary to dysfunction in hormone secretion.

359.6 *Symptomatic inflammatory myopathy in diseases classified elsewhere*

Code first underlying disease, as:
- amyloidosis (277.3)
- disseminated lupus erythematosus (710.0)
- malignant neoplasm (140.0-208.9)
- polyarteritis nodosa (446.0)
- rheumatoid arthritis (714.0)
- sarcoidosis (135)
- scleroderma (710.1)
- Sjögren's disease (710.2)

√5ᵗʰ **359.8 Other myopathies**

AHA: 3Q, '90, 17

● **359.81 Critical illness myopathy**
- Acute necrotizing myopathy
- Acute quadriplegic myopathy
- Intensive care (ICU) myopathy
- Myopathy of critical illness

● **359.89 Other myopathies**

359.9 Myopathy, unspecified

DISORDERS OF THE EYE AND ADNEXA (360-379)

√4ᵗʰ **360 Disorders of the globe**

INCLUDES: disorders affecting multiple structures of eye

√5ᵗʰ **360.0 Purulent endophthalmitis**

360.00 Purulent endophthalmitis, unspecified
360.01 Acute endophthalmitis
360.02 Panophthalmitis
360.03 Chronic endophthalmitis
360.04 Vitreous abscess

√5ᵗʰ **360.1 Other endophthalmitis**

360.11 Sympathetic uveitis

DEF: Inflammation of vascular layer of uninjured eye; follows injury to other eye.

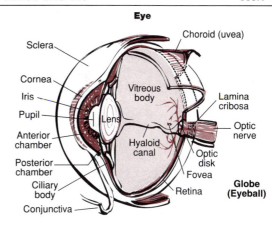
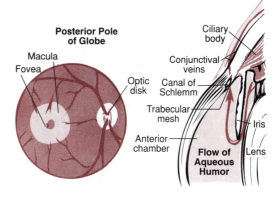

360.12 Panuveitis

DEF: Inflammation of entire vascular layer of eye, including choroid, iris and ciliary body.

360.13 Parasitic endophthalmitis NOS

DEF: Parasitic infection causing inflammation of the entire eye.

360.14 Ophthalmia nodosa

DEF: Conjunctival inflammation caused by embedded hairs.

360.19 Other

Phacoanaphylactic endophthalmitis

√5ᵗʰ **360.2 Degenerative disorders of globe**

AHA: 3Q, '91, 3

360.20 Degenerative disorder of globe, unspecified

360.21 Progressive high (degenerative) myopia

Malignant myopia

DEF: Severe, progressive nearsightedness in adults, complicated by serious disease of the choroid; leads to retinal detachment and blindness.

360.23 Siderosis

DEF: Iron pigment deposits within tissue of eyeball; caused by high iron content of blood.

360.24 Other metallosis

Chalcosis

DEF: Metal deposits, other than iron, within eyeball tissues.

360.29 Other

EXCLUDES xerophthalmia (264.7)

√5ᵗʰ **360.3 Hypotony of eye**

360.30 Hypotony, unspecified

DEF: Low osmotic pressure causing lack of tone, tension and strength.

360.31 Primary hypotony

NERVOUS SYSTEM AND SENSE ORGANS — Tabular List

360.32–361.31

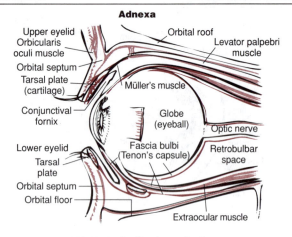

Adnexa: Upper eyelid, Orbicularis oculi muscle, Orbital septum, Tarsal plate (cartilage), Conjunctival fornix, Lower eyelid, Tarsal plate, Orbital septum, Orbital floor, Orbital roof, Levator palpebri muscle, Müller's muscle, Globe (eyeball), Optic nerve, Fascia bulbi (Tenon's capsule), Retrobulbar space, Extraocular muscle

- **360.32 Ocular fistula causing hypotony**
  - DEF: Low intraocular pressure due to leak through abnormal passage.
- **360.33 Hypotony associated with other ocular disorders**
- **360.34 Flat anterior chamber**
  - DEF: Low pressure behind cornea, causing compression.

√5th **360.4 Degenerated conditions of globe**
- **360.40 Degenerated globe or eye, unspecified**
- **360.41 Blind hypotensive eye**
  - Atrophy of globe
  - Phthisis bulbi
  - DEF: Vision loss due to extremely low intraocular pressure.
- **360.42 Blind hypertensive eye**
  - Absolute glaucoma
  - DEF: Vision loss due to painful, high intraocular pressure.
- **360.43 Hemophthalmos, except current injury**
  - EXCLUDES traumatic (871.0-871.9, 921.0-921.9)
  - DEF: Pool of blood within eyeball, not from current injury.
- **360.44 Leucocoria**
  - DEF: Whitish mass or reflex in the pupil behind lens; also called cat's eye reflex; often indicative of retinoblastoma.

√5th **360.5 Retained (old) intraocular foreign body, magnetic**
- EXCLUDES current penetrating injury with magnetic foreign body (871.5)
  - retained (old) foreign body of orbit (376.6)
- **360.50 Foreign body, magnetic, intraocular, unspecified**
- **360.51 Foreign body, magnetic, in anterior chamber**
- **360.52 Foreign body, magnetic, in iris or ciliary body**
- **360.53 Foreign body, magnetic, in lens**
- **360.54 Foreign body, magnetic, in vitreous**
- **360.55 Foreign body, magnetic, in posterior wall**
- **360.59 Foreign body, magnetic, in other or multiple sites**

√5th **360.6 Retained (old) intraocular foreign body, nonmagnetic**
- Retained (old) foreign body:
  - NOS
  - nonmagnetic
- EXCLUDES current penetrating injury with (nonmagnetic) foreign body (871.6)
  - retained (old) foreign body in orbit (376.6)
- **360.60 Foreign body, intraocular, unspecified**
- **360.61 Foreign body in anterior chamber**
- **360.62 Foreign body in iris or ciliary body**
- **360.63 Foreign body in lens**
- **360.64 Foreign body in vitreous**
- **360.65 Foreign body in posterior wall**
- **360.69 Foreign body in other or multiple sites**

√5th **360.8 Other disorders of globe**
- **360.81 Luxation of globe**
  - DEF: Displacement of eyeball.
- **360.89 Other**

360.9 Unspecified disorder of globe

√4th **361 Retinal detachments and defects**
- DEF: Light-sensitive layer at back of eye, separates from blood supply; disrupting vision.

√5th **361.0 Retinal detachment with retinal defect**
- Rhegmatogenous retinal detachment
- EXCLUDES detachment of retinal pigment epithelium (362.42-362.43)
  - retinal detachment (serous) (without defect) (361.2)
- **361.00 Retinal detachment with retinal defect, unspecified**
- **361.01 Recent detachment, partial, with single defect**
- **361.02 Recent detachment, partial, with multiple defects**
- **361.03 Recent detachment, partial, with giant tear**
- **361.04 Recent detachment, partial, with retinal dialysis**
  - Dialysis (juvenile) of retina (with detachment)
- **361.05 Recent detachment, total or subtotal**
- **361.06 Old detachment, partial**
  - Delimited old retinal detachment
- **361.07 Old detachment, total or subtotal**

√5th **361.1 Retinoschisis and retinal cysts**
- EXCLUDES juvenile retinoschisis (362.73)
  - microcystoid degeneration of retina (362.62)
  - parasitic cyst of retina (360.13)
- **361.10 Retinoschisis, unspecified**
  - DEF: Separation of retina due to degenerative process of aging; should not be confused with acute retinal detachment.
- **361.11 Flat retinoschisis**
  - DEF: Slow, progressive split of retinal sensory layers
- **361.12 Bullous retinoschisis**
  - DEF: Fluid retention between split retinal sensory layers.
- **361.13 Primary retinal cysts**
- **361.14 Secondary retinal cysts**
- **361.19 Other**
  - Pseudocyst of retina

361.2 Serous retinal detachment
- Retinal detachment without retinal defect
- EXCLUDES central serous retinopathy (362.41)
  - retinal pigment epithelium detachment (362.42-362.43)

√5th **361.3 Retinal defects without detachment**
- EXCLUDES chorioretinal scars after surgery for detachment (363.30-363.35)
  - peripheral retinal degeneration without defect (362.60-362.66)
- **361.30 Retinal defect, unspecified**
  - Retinal break(s) NOS
- **361.31 Round hole of retina without detachment**

361.32 Horseshoe tear of retina without detachment
Operculum of retina without mention of detachment

361.33 Multiple defects of retina without detachment

√5th **361.8** Other forms of retinal detachment
361.81 Traction detachment of retina
Traction detachment with vitreoretinal organization
361.89 Other
AHA: 3Q, '99, 12

361.9 Unspecified retinal detachment
AHA: N-D, '87, 10

√4th **362** Other retinal disorders
EXCLUDES chorioretinal scars (363.30-363.35)
chorioretinitis (363.0-363.2)

√5th **362.0** Diabetic retinopathy
Code first diabetes (250.5)
DEF: Retinal changes in diabetes of long duration; causes hemorrhages, microaneurysms, waxy deposits and proliferative noninflammatory degenerative disease of retina.
AHA: 3Q, '91, 8

362.01 Background diabetic retinopathy
Diabetic macular edema
Diabetic retinal edema
Diabetic retinal microaneurysms
Diabetic retinopathy NOS
362.02 Proliferative diabetic retinopathy
AHA: 3Q, '96, 5

√5th **362.1** Other background retinopathy and retinal vascular changes
362.10 Background retinopathy, unspecified
362.11 Hypertensive retinopathy
AHA: 3Q, '90, 3
DEF: Retinal irregularities caused by systemic hypertension.
362.12 Exudative retinopathy
Coats' syndrome
AHA: 3Q, '99, 12
362.13 Changes in vascular appearance
Vascular sheathing of retina
Use additional code for any associated atherosclerosis (440.8)
362.14 Retinal microaneurysms NOS
DEF: Microscopic dilation of retinal vessels in nondiabetic.
362.15 Retinal telangiectasia
DEF: Dilation of blood vessels of the retina.
362.16 Retinal neovascularization NOS
Neovascularization: Neovascularization:
  choroidal   subretinal
DEF: New and abnormal vascular growth in the retina.
362.17 Other intraretinal microvascular abnormalities
Retinal varices
362.18 Retinal vasculitis
Eales' disease   Retinal:
Retinal: perivasculitis
  arteritis   phlebitis
  endarteritis
DEF: Inflammation of retinal blood vessels.

√5th **362.2** Other proliferative retinopathy
362.21 Retrolental fibroplasia
DEF: Fibrous tissue in vitreous, from retina to lens, causing blindness; associated with premature infants requiring high amounts of oxygen.

362.29 Other nondiabetic proliferative retinopathy
AHA: 3Q, '96, 5

√5th **362.3** Retinal vascular occlusion
DEF: Obstructed blood flow to and from retina.

362.30 Retinal vascular occlusion, unspecified
362.31 Central retinal artery occlusion
362.32 Arterial branch occlusion
362.33 Partial arterial occlusion
Hollenhorst plaque
Retinal microembolism
362.34 Transient arterial occlusion
Amaurosis fugax
AHA: 1Q, '00, 16
362.35 Central retinal vein occlusion
AHA: 2Q, '93, 6
362.36 Venous tributary (branch) occlusion
362.37 Venous engorgement
Occlusion:
  incipient } of retinal vein
  partial

√5th **362.4** Separation of retinal layers
EXCLUDES retinal detachment (serous) (361.2)
rhegmatogenous (361.00-361.07)
362.40 Retinal layer separation, unspecified
362.41 Central serous retinopathy
DEF: Serous-filled blister causing detachment of retina from pigment epithelium.
362.42 Serous detachment of retinal pigment epithelium
Exudative detachment of retinal pigment epithelium
DEF: Blister of fatty fluid causing detachment of retina from pigment epithelium.
362.43 Hemorrhagic detachment of retinal pigment epithelium
DEF: Blood-filled blister causing detachment of retina from pigment epithelium.

√5th **362.5** Degeneration of macula and posterior pole
EXCLUDES degeneration of optic disc (377.21-377.24)
hereditary retinal degeneration [dystrophy] (362.70-362.77)
362.50 Macular degeneration (senile), unspecified
362.51 Nonexudative senile macular degeneration
Senile macular degeneration:
  atrophic
  dry
362.52 Exudative senile macular degeneration
Kuhnt-Junius degeneration
Senile macular degeneration:
  disciform
  wet
DEF: Leakage in macular blood vessels with loss of visual acuity.
362.53 Cystoid macular degeneration
Cystoid macular edema
DEF: Retinal swelling and cyst formation in macula.
362.54 Macular cyst, hole, or pseudohole
362.55 Toxic maculopathy
Use additional E code to identify drug, if drug induced
362.56 Macular puckering
Preretinal fibrosis
362.57 Drusen (degenerative)
DEF: White, hyaline deposits on Bruch's membrane (lamina basalis choroideae).

362.6 Peripheral retinal degenerations
EXCLUDES hereditary retinal degeneration [dystrophy] (362.70-362.77)
retinal degeneration with retinal defect (361.00-361.07)

- **362.60** Peripheral retinal degeneration, unspecified
- **362.61** Paving stone degeneration
  DEF: Degeneration of peripheral retina; causes thinning through which choroid is visible.
- **362.62** Microcystoid degeneration
  Blessig's cysts   Iwanoff's cysts
- **362.63** Lattice degeneration
  Palisade degeneration of retina
  DEF: Degeneration of retina; often bilateral, usually benign; characterized by lines intersecting at irregular intervals in peripheral retina; retinal thinning and retinal holes may occur.
- **362.64** Senile reticular degeneration
  DEF: Net-like appearance of retina; sign of degeneration.
- **362.65** Secondary pigmentary degeneration
  Pseudoretinitis pigmentosa
- **362.66** Secondary vitreoretinal degenerations

362.7 Hereditary retinal dystrophies
DEF: Genetically induced progressive changes in retina.

- **362.70** Hereditary retinal dystrophy, unspecified
- **362.71** *Retinal dystrophy in systemic or cerebroretinal lipidoses*
  Code first underlying disease, as:
    cerebroretinal lipidoses (330.1)
    systemic lipidoses (272.7)
- **362.72** *Retinal dystrophy in other systemic disorders and syndromes*
  Code first underlying disease, as:
    Bassen-Kornzweig syndrome (272.5)
    Refsum's disease (356.3)
- **362.73** Vitreoretinal dystrophies
  Juvenile retinoschisis
- **362.74** Pigmentary retinal dystrophy
  Retinal dystrophy, albipunctate
  Retinitis pigmentosa
- **362.75** Other dystrophies primarily involving the sensory retina
  Progressive cone(-rod) dystrophy
  Stargardt's disease
- **362.76** Dystrophies primarily involving the retinal pigment epithelium
  Fundus flavimaculatus
  Vitelliform dystrophy
- **362.77** Dystrophies primarily involving Bruch's membrane
  Dystrophy:
    hyaline
    pseudoinflammatory foveal
  Hereditary drusen

362.8 Other retinal disorders
EXCLUDES chorioretinal inflammations (363.0-363.2)
chorioretinal scars (363.30-363.35)

- **362.81** Retinal hemorrhage
  Hemorrhage:
    preretinal
    retinal (deep) (superficial)
    subretinal
  AHA: 4Q, '96, 43
- **362.82** Retinal exudates and deposits
- **362.83** Retinal edema
  Retinal:
    cotton wool spots
    edema (localized) (macular) (peripheral)
  DEF: Retinal swelling due to fluid accumulation.
- **362.84** Retinal ischemia
  DEF: Reduced retinal blood supply.
- **362.85** Retinal nerve fiber bundle defects
- **362.89** Other retinal disorders
- **362.9** Unspecified retinal disorder

363 Chorioretinal inflammations, scars, and other disorders of choroid

363.0 Focal chorioretinitis and focal retinochoroiditis
EXCLUDES focal chorioretinitis or retinochoroiditis in:
  histoplasmosis (115.02, 115.12, 115.92)
  toxoplasmosis (130.2)
  congenital infection (771.2)

- **363.00** Focal chorioretinitis, unspecified
  Focal:
    choroiditis or chorioretinitis NOS
    retinitis or retinochoroiditis NOS
- **363.01** Focal choroiditis and chorioretinitis, juxtapapillary
- **363.03** Focal choroiditis and chorioretinitis of other posterior pole
- **363.04** Focal choroiditis and chorioretinitis, peripheral
- **363.05** Focal retinitis and retinochoroiditis, juxtapapillary
  Neuroretinitis
- **363.06** Focal retinitis and retinochoroiditis, macular or paramacular
- **363.07** Focal retinitis and retinochoroiditis of other posterior pole
- **363.08** Focal retinitis and retinochoroiditis, peripheral

363.1 Disseminated chorioretinitis and disseminated retinochoroiditis
EXCLUDES disseminated choroiditis or chorioretinitis in secondary syphilis (091.51)
neurosyphilitic disseminated retinitis or retinochoroiditis (094.83)
retinal (peri)vasculitis (362.18)

- **363.10** Disseminated chorioretinitis, unspecified
  Disseminated:
    choroiditis or chorioretinitis NOS
    retinitis or retinochoroiditis NOS
- **363.11** Disseminated choroiditis and chorioretinitis, posterior pole
- **363.12** Disseminated choroiditis and chorioretinitis, peripheral
- **363.13** Disseminated choroiditis and chorioretinitis, generalized
  Code first any underlying disease, as:
    tuberculosis (017.3)
- **363.14** Disseminated retinitis and retinochoroiditis, metastatic
- **363.15** Disseminated retinitis and retinochoroiditis, pigment epitheliopathy
  Acute posterior multifocal placoid pigment epitheliopathy
  DEF: Widespread inflammation of retina and choroid; characterized by pigmented epithelium involvement.

363.2 Other and unspecified forms of chorioretinitis and retinochoroiditis
EXCLUDES panophthalmitis (360.02)
sympathetic uveitis (360.11)
uveitis NOS (364.3)

- **363.20** Chorioretinitis, unspecified
  Choroiditis NOS
  Retinitis NOS
  Uveitis, posterior NOS

NERVOUS SYSTEM AND SENSE ORGANS

363.21 Pars planitis
Posterior cyclitis
DEF: Inflammation of peripheral retina and ciliary body; characterized by bands of white cells.

363.22 Harada's disease
DEF: Retinal detachment and bilateral widespread exudative choroiditis; symptoms include headache, vomiting, increased lymphocytes in cerebrospinal fluid; and temporary or permanent deafness may occur.

√5th 363.3 Chorioretinal scars
Scar (postinflammatory) (postsurgical) (posttraumatic):
choroid
retina

363.30 Chorioretinal scar, unspecified
363.31 Solar retinopathy
DEF: Retinal scarring caused by solar radiation.

363.32 Other macular scars
363.33 Other scars of posterior pole
363.34 Peripheral scars
363.35 Disseminated scars

√5th 363.4 Choroidal degenerations
363.40 Choroidal degeneration, unspecified
Choroidal sclerosis NOS

363.41 Senile atrophy of choroid
DEF: Wasting away of choroid; due to aging.

363.42 Diffuse secondary atrophy of choroid
DEF: Wasting away of choroid in systemic disease.

363.43 Angioid streaks of choroid
DEF: Degeneration of choroid; characterized by dark brown steaks radiating from optic disk; occurs with pseudoxanthoma, elasticum or Paget's disease.

√5th 363.5 Hereditary choroidal dystrophies
Hereditary choroidal atrophy:
partial [choriocapillaris]
total [all vessels]

363.50 Hereditary choroidal dystrophy or atrophy, unspecified
363.51 Circumpapillary dystrophy of choroid, partial
363.52 Circumpapillary dystrophy of choroid, total
Helicoid dystrophy of choroid

363.53 Central dystrophy of choroid, partial
Dystrophy, choroidal:
central areolar
circinate

363.54 Central choroidal atrophy, total
Dystrophy, choroidal:
central gyrate
serpiginous

363.55 Choroideremia
DEF: Hereditary choroid degeneration, occurs in first decade; characterized by constricted visual field and ultimately blindness in males; less debilitating in females.

363.56 Other diffuse or generalized dystrophy, partial
Diffuse choroidal sclerosis

363.57 Other diffuse or generalized dystrophy, total
Generalized gyrate atrophy, choroid

√5th 363.6 Choroidal hemorrhage and rupture
363.61 Choroidal hemorrhage, unspecified
363.62 Expulsive choroidal hemorrhage
363.63 Choroidal rupture

√5th 363.7 Choroidal detachment
363.70 Choroidal detachment, unspecified

363.71 Serous choroidal detachment
DEF: Detachment of choroid from sclera; due to blister of serous fluid.

363.72 Hemorrhagic choroidal detachment
DEF: Detachment of choroid from sclera; due to blood-filled blister.

363.8 Other disorders of choroid
363.9 Unspecified disorder of choroid

√4th 364 Disorders of iris and ciliary body

√5th 364.0 Acute and subacute iridocyclitis
Anterior uveitis
Cyclitis } acute
Iridocyclitis } subacute
Iritis

EXCLUDES gonococcal (098.41)
herpes simplex (054.44)
herpes zoster (053.22)

364.00 Acute and subacute iridocyclitis, unspecified
364.01 Primary iridocyclitis
364.02 Recurrent iridocyclitis
364.03 Secondary iridocyclitis, infectious
364.04 Secondary iridocyclitis, noninfectious
Aqueous: Aqueous:
cells flare
fibrin

364.05 Hypopyon
DEF: Accumulation of white blood cells between cornea and lens.

√5th 364.1 Chronic iridocyclitis
EXCLUDES posterior cyclitis (363.21)

364.10 Chronic iridocyclitis, unspecified
364.11 Chronic iridocyclitis in diseases classified elsewhere
Code first underlying disease, as:
sarcoidosis (135)
tuberculosis (017.3)
EXCLUDES syphilitic iridocyclitis (091.52)
DEF: Persistent inflammation of iris and ciliary body; due to underlying disease or condition.

√5th 364.2 Certain types of iridocyclitis
EXCLUDES posterior cyclitis (363.21)
sympathetic uveitis (360.11)

364.21 Fuchs' heterochromic cyclitis
DEF: Chronic cyclitis characterized by differences in the color of the two irises; the lighter iris appears in the inflamed eye.

364.22 Glaucomatocyclitic crises
DEF: One-sided form of secondary open angle glaucoma; recurrent, uncommon and of short duration; causes high intraocular pressure, rarely damage.

364.23 Lens-induced iridocyclitis
DEF: Inflammation of iris; due to immune reaction to proteins in lens following trauma or other lens abnormality.

364.24 Vogt-Koyanagi syndrome
DEF: Uveomeningitis with exudative iridocyclitis and choroiditis; causes depigmentation of hair and skin, detached retina; tinnitus and loss of hearing may occur.

364.3 Unspecified iridocyclitis
Uveitis NOS

√5th 364.4 Vascular disorders of iris and ciliary body
364.41 Hyphema
Hemorrhage of iris or ciliary body
DEF: Hemorrhage in anterior chamber; also called hyphemia or "blood shot" eyes.

NERVOUS SYSTEM AND SENSE ORGANS

364.42 Rubeosis iridis
Neovascularization of iris or ciliary body
DEF: Blood vessel and connective tissue formation on surface of iris; symptomatic of diabetic retinopathy, central retinal vein occlusion and retinal detachment.

√5th **364.5 Degenerations of iris and ciliary body**

364.51 Essential or progressive iris atrophy

364.52 Iridoschisis
DEF: Splitting of the iris into two layers.

364.53 Pigmentary iris degeneration
Acquired heterochromia ⎫
Pigment dispersion syndrome ⎬ of iris
Translucency ⎭

364.54 Degeneration of pupillary margin
Atrophy of sphincter ⎫
Ectropion of pigment ⎬ of iris
epithelium ⎭

364.55 Miotic cysts of pupillary margin
DEF: Serous-filled sacs in pupillary margin of iris.

364.56 Degenerative changes of chamber angle

364.57 Degenerative changes of ciliary body

364.59 Other iris atrophy
Iris atrophy (generalized) (sector shaped)

√5th **364.6 Cysts of iris, ciliary body, and anterior chamber**
EXCLUDES miotic pupillary cyst (364.55)
parasitic cyst (360.13)

364.60 Idiopathic cysts
DEF: Fluid-filled sacs in iris or ciliary body; unknown etiology.

364.61 Implantation cysts
Epithelial down-growth, anterior chamber
Implantation cysts (surgical) (traumatic)

364.62 Exudative cysts of iris or anterior chamber

364.63 Primary cyst of pars plana
DEF: Fluid-filled sacs of outermost ciliary ring.

364.64 Exudative cyst of pars plana
DEF: Protein, fatty-filled sacs of outermost ciliary ring; due to fluid lead from blood vessels.

√5th **364.7 Adhesions and disruptions of iris and ciliary body**
EXCLUDES flat anterior chamber (360.34)

364.70 Adhesions of iris, unspecified
Synechiae (iris) NOS

364.71 Posterior synechiae
DEF: Adhesion binding iris to lens.

364.72 Anterior synechiae
DEF: Adhesion binding the iris to cornea.

364.73 Goniosynechiae
Peripheral anterior synechiae
DEF: Adhesion binding the iris to cornea at the angle of the anterior chamber.

364.74 Pupillary membranes
Iris bombé   Pupillary:
Pupillary: seclusion
 occlusion
DEF: Membrane traversing the pupil and blocking vision.

364.75 Pupillary abnormalities
Deformed pupil   Rupture of sphincter, pupil
Ectopic pupil

364.76 Iridodialysis
DEF: Separation of the iris from the ciliary body base; due to trauma or surgical accident.

364.77 Recession of chamber angle
DEF: Receding of anterior chamber angle of the eye; restricts vision.

364.8 Other disorders of iris and ciliary body
Prolapse of iris NOS
EXCLUDES prolapse of iris in recent wound (871.1)

364.9 Unspecified disorder of iris and ciliary body

√4th **365 Glaucoma**
EXCLUDES blind hypertensive eye [absolute glaucoma] (360.42)
congenital glaucoma (743.20-743.22)
DEF: Rise in intraocular pressure which restricts blood flow; multiple causes.

√5th **365.0 Borderline glaucoma [glaucoma suspect]**
AHA: 1Q, '90, 8

365.00 Preglaucoma, unspecified

365.01 Open angle with borderline findings
Open angle with:
  borderline intraocular pressure
  cupping of optic discs
DEF: Minor block of aqueous outflow from eye.

365.02 Anatomical narrow angle

365.03 Steroid responders

365.04 Ocular hypertension
DEF: High fluid pressure within eye; no apparent cause.

√5th **365.1 Open-angle glaucoma**

365.10 Open-angle glaucoma, unspecified
Wide-angle glaucoma NOS

365.11 Primary open angle glaucoma
Chronic simple glaucoma
DEF: High intraocular pressure, despite free flow of aqueous.

365.12 Low tension glaucoma

365.13 Pigmentary glaucoma
DEF: High intraocular pressure; due to iris pigment granules blocking aqueous flow.

365.14 Glaucoma of childhood
Infantile or juvenile glaucoma

365.15 Residual stage of open angle glaucoma

√5th **365.2 Primary angle-closure glaucoma**

365.20 Primary angle-closure glaucoma, unspecified

365.21 Intermittent angle-closure glaucoma
Angle-closure glaucoma:
  interval
  subacute
DEF: Recurring attacks of high intraocular pressure; due to blocked aqueous flow.

365.22 Acute angle-closure glaucoma
DEF: Sudden, severe rise in intraocular pressure due to blockage in aqueous drainage.

365.23 Chronic angle-closure glaucoma
AHA: 2Q, '98, 16

365.24 Residual stage of angle-closure glaucoma

√5th **365.3 Corticosteroid-induced glaucoma**
DEF: Elevated intraocular pressure; due to long-term corticosteroid therapy.

365.31 Glaucomatous stage

365.32 Residual stage

√5th **365.4 Glaucoma associated with congenital anomalies, dystrophies, and systemic syndromes**

365.41 Glaucoma associated with chamber angle anomalies
Code first associated disorder, as:
  Axenfeld's anomaly (743.44)
  Rieger's anomaly or syndrome (743.44)

365.42 Glaucoma associated with anomalies of iris
Code first associated disorder, as:
  aniridia (743.45)
  essential iris atrophy (364.51)

NERVOUS SYSTEM AND SENSE ORGANS

365.43 Glaucoma associated with other anterior segment anomalies
Code first associated disorder, as:
microcornea (743.41)

365.44 Glaucoma associated with systemic syndromes
Code first associated disease, as
neurofibromatosis (237.7)
Sturge-Weber (-Dimitri) syndrome (759.6)

√5th **365.5 Glaucoma associated with disorders of the lens**

365.51 Phacolytic glaucoma
Use additional code for associated
hypermature cataract (366.18)
DEF: Elevated intraocular pressure; due to lens protein blocking aqueous flow.

365.52 Pseudoexfoliation glaucoma
Use additional code for associated
pseudoexfoliation of capsule (366.11)
DEF: Glaucoma characterized by small grayish particles deposited on the lens.

365.59 Glaucoma associated with other lens disorders
Use additional code for associated disorder, as:
dislocation of lens (379.33-379.34)
spherophakia (743.36)

√5th **365.6 Glaucoma associated with other ocular disorders**

365.60 Glaucoma associated with unspecified ocular disorder

365.61 Glaucoma associated with pupillary block
Use additional code for associated disorder, as:
seclusion of pupil [iris bombé] (364.74)
DEF: Acute, open-angle glaucoma caused by mature cataract; aqueous flow is blocked by lens material and macrophages.

365.62 Glaucoma associated with ocular inflammations
Use additional code for associated disorder, as:
glaucomatocyclitic crises (364.22)
iridocyclitis (364.0-364.3)

365.63 Glaucoma associated with vascular disorders
Use additional code for associated disorder, as:
central retinal vein occlusion (362.35)
hyphema (364.41)

365.64 Glaucoma associated with tumors or cysts
Use additional code for associated disorder, as:
benign neoplasm (224.0-224.9)
epithelial down-growth (364.61)
malignant neoplasm (190.0-190.9)

365.65 Glaucoma associated with ocular trauma
Use additional code for associated condition, as:
contusion of globe (921.3)
recession of chamber angle (364.77)

√5th **365.8 Other specified forms of glaucoma**

365.81 Hypersecretion glaucoma
365.82 Glaucoma with increased episcleral venous pressure
365.83 Aqueous misdirection
Malignant glaucoma
365.89 Other specified glaucoma
AHA: 2Q, '98, 16

365.9 Unspecified glaucoma
AHA: 2Q, '01, 16

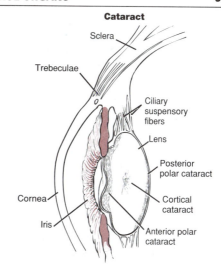

Cataract

√4th **366 Cataract**
DEF: A variety of conditions that create a cloudy, or calcified lens that obstructs vision.
EXCLUDES congenital cataract (743.30-743.34)

√5th **366.0 Infantile, juvenile, and presenile cataract**
366.00 Nonsenile cataract, unspecified
366.01 Anterior subcapsular polar cataract
DEF: Defect within the front, center lens surface.
366.02 Posterior subcapsular polar cataract
DEF: Defect within the rear, center lens surface.
366.03 Cortical, lamellar, or zonular cataract
DEF: Opacities radiating from center to edge of lens; appear as thin, concentric layers of lens.
366.04 Nuclear cataract
366.09 Other and combined forms of nonsenile cataract

√5th **366.1 Senile cataract**
AHA: 3Q, '91, 9; S-O, '85, 10

366.10 Senile cataract, unspecified ▲
366.11 Pseudoexfoliation of lens capsule ▲
366.12 Incipient cataract ▲
Cataract: Cataract:
coronary   punctate
immature NOS   Water clefts
DEF: Minor disorders of lens not affecting vision; due to aging.
366.13 Anterior subcapsular polar senile cataract ▲
366.14 Posterior subcapsular polar senile cataract ▲
366.15 Cortical senile cataract ▲
366.16 Nuclear sclerosis ▲
Cataracta brunescens
Nuclear cataract
366.17 Total or mature cataract ▲
366.18 Hypermature cataract ▲
Morgagni cataract
366.19 Other and combined forms of senile cataract ▲

√5th **366.2 Traumatic cataract**
366.20 Traumatic cataract, unspecified
366.21 Localized traumatic opacities
Vossius' ring
366.22 Total traumatic cataract
366.23 Partially resolved traumatic cataract

366.3–368.40 NERVOUS SYSTEM AND SENSE ORGANS

√5ᵗʰ 366.3 Cataract secondary to ocular disorders
- 366.30 Cataracta complicata, unspecified
- 366.31 Glaucomatous flecks (subcapsular)
  - Code first underlying glaucoma (365.0-365.9)
- 366.32 Cataract in inflammatory disorders
  - Code first underlying condition, as:
    - chronic choroiditis (363.0-363.2)
- 366.33 Cataract with neovascularization
  - Code first underlying condition, as:
    - chronic iridocyclitis (364.10)
- 366.34 Cataract in degenerative disorders
  - Sunflower cataract
  - Code first underlying condition, as:
    - chalcosis (360.24)
    - degenerative myopia (360.21)
    - pigmentary retinal dystrophy (362.74)

√5ᵗʰ 366.4 Cataract associated with other disorders
- 366.41 Diabetic cataract
  - Code first diabetes (250.5)
  - AHA: 3Q, '91, 9; S-O, '85, 11
- 366.42 Tetanic cataract
  - Code first underlying disease, as:
    - calcinosis (275.4)
    - hypoparathyroidism (252.1)
- 366.43 Myotonic cataract
  - Code first underlying disorder (359.2)
- 366.44 Cataract associated with other syndromes
  - Code first underlying condition, as:
    - craniofacial dysostosis (756.0)
    - galactosemia (271.1)
- 366.45 Toxic cataract
  - Drug-induced cataract
  - Use additional E code to identify drug or other toxic substance
- 366.46 Cataract associated with radiation and other physical influences
  - Use additional E code to identify cause

√5ᵗʰ 366.5 After-cataract
- 366.50 After-cataract, unspecified
  - Secondary cataract NOS
- 366.51 Soemmering's ring
  - DEF: A donut-shaped lens remnant and a capsule behind the pupil as a result of cataract surgery or trauma.
- 366.52 Other after-cataract, not obscuring vision
- 366.53 After-cataract, obscuring vision

366.8 Other cataract
- Calcification of lens

366.9 Unspecified cataract

√4ᵗʰ 367 Disorders of refraction and accommodation
- 367.0 Hypermetropia
  - Far-sightedness   Hyperopia
  - DEF: Refraction error, called also hyperopia, focal point is posterior to retina; abnormally short anteroposterior diameter or subnormal refractive power; causes farsightedness.
- 367.1 Myopia
  - Near-sightedness
  - DEF: Refraction error, focal point is anterior to retina; causes near-sightedness.

√5ᵗʰ 367.2 Astigmatism
- 367.20 Astigmatism, unspecified
- 367.21 Regular astigmatism
- 367.22 Irregular astigmatism

√5ᵗʰ 367.3 Anisometropia and aniseikonia
- 367.31 Anisometropia
  - DEF: Eyes with refractive powers that differ by at least one diopter.
- 367.32 Aniseikonia
  - DEF: Eyes with unequal retinal imaging; usually due to refractive error.

367.4 Presbyopia
- DEF: Loss of crystalline lens elasticity; causes errors of accommodation; due to aging.

√5ᵗʰ 367.5 Disorders of accommodation
- 367.51 Paresis of accommodation
  - Cycloplegia
  - DEF: Partial paralysis of ciliary muscle; causing focus problems.
- 367.52 Total or complete internal ophthalmoplegia
  - DEF: Total paralysis of ciliary muscle; large pupil incapable of focus.
- 367.53 Spasm of accommodation
  - DEF: Abnormal contraction of ciliary muscle; causes focus problems.

√5ᵗʰ 367.8 Other disorders of refraction and accommodation
- 367.81 Transient refractive change
- 367.89 Other
  - Drug-induced } disorders of refraction
  - Toxic   } and accommodation

367.9 Unspecified disorder of refraction and accommodation

√4ᵗʰ 368 Visual disturbances
- EXCLUDES electrophysiological disturbances (794.11-794.14)

√5ᵗʰ 368.0 Amblyopia ex anopsia
- DEF: Vision impaired due to disuse; esotropia often cause.
- 368.00 Amblyopia, unspecified
- 368.01 Strabismic amblyopia
  - Suppression amblyopia
- 368.02 Deprivation amblyopia
  - DEF: Decreased vision associated with suppressed retinal image of one eye.
- 368.03 Refractive amblyopia

√5ᵗʰ 368.1 Subjective visual disturbances
- 368.10 Subjective visual disturbance, unspecified
- 368.11 Sudden visual loss
- 368.12 Transient visual loss
  - Concentric fading   Scintillating scotoma
- 368.13 Visual discomfort
  - Asthenopia   Photophobia
  - Eye strain
- 368.14 Visual distortions of shape and size
  - Macropsia   Micropsia
  - Metamorphopsia
- 368.15 Other visual distortions and entoptic phenomena
  - Photopsia   Refractive:
  - Refractive: polyopia
  - diplopia   Visual halos
- 368.16 Psychophysical visual disturbances
  - Visual: Visual:
  - agnosia   hallucinations
  - disorientation syndrome

368.2 Diplopia
- Double vision

√5ᵗʰ 368.3 Other disorders of binocular vision
- 368.30 Binocular vision disorder, unspecified
- 368.31 Suppression of binocular vision
- 368.32 Simultaneous visual perception without fusion
- 368.33 Fusion with defective stereopsis
  - DEF: Faulty depth perception though normal ability to focus.
- 368.34 Abnormal retinal correspondence

√5ᵗʰ 368.4 Visual field defects
- 368.40 Visual field defect, unspecified

NERVOUS SYSTEM AND SENSE ORGANS — 368.41–369.16

368.41 Scotoma involving central area
Scotoma: Scotoma:
  central   paracentral
  centrocecal
DEF: Vision loss (blind spot) in central five degrees of visual field.

368.42 Scotoma of blind spot area
Enlarged: Paracecal scotoma
  angioscotoma
  blind spot

368.43 Sector or arcuate defects
Scotoma: Scotoma:
  arcuate   Seidel
  Bjerrum
DEF: Arc-shaped blind spot caused by retinal nerve damage.

368.44 Other localized visual field defect
Scotoma: Visual field defect:
  NOS   nasal step
  ring   peripheral

368.45 Generalized contraction or constriction

368.46 Homonymous bilateral field defects
Hemianopsia (altitudinal) (homonymous)
Quadrant anopia
DEF: Disorders found in the corresponding vertical halves of the visual fields of both eyes.

368.47 Heteronymous bilateral field defects
Hemianopsia: Hemianopsia:
  binasal   bitemporal
DEF: Disorders in the opposite halves of the visual fields of both eyes.

√5ᵗʰ **368.5 Color vision deficiencies**
Color blindness

368.51 Protan defect
Protanomaly   Protanopia
DEF: Mild difficulty distinguishing green and red hues with shortened spectrum; sex-linked affecting one percent of males.

368.52 Deutan defect
Deuteranomaly   Deuteranopia
DEF: Male-only disorder; difficulty in distinguishing green and red, no shortened spectrum.

368.53 Tritan defect
Tritanomaly   Tritanopia
DEF: Difficulty in distinguishing blue and yellow; occurs often due to drugs, retinal detachment and central nervous system diseases.

368.54 Achromatopsia
Monochromatism (cone) (rod)
DEF: Complete color blindness; caused by disease, injury to retina, optic nerve or pathway.

368.55 Acquired color vision deficiencies

368.59 Other color vision deficiencies

√5ᵗʰ **368.6 Night blindness**
Nyctalopia
DEF: Nyctalopia: disorder of vision in dim light or night blindness.

368.60 Night blindness, unspecified

368.61 Congenital night blindness
Hereditary night blindness
Oguchi's disease

368.62 Acquired night blindness
EXCLUDES   that due to vitamin A deficiency (264.5)

368.63 Abnormal dark adaptation curve
Abnormal threshold   } of cones or
Delayed adaptation   } rods

368.69 Other night blindness

368.8 Other specified visual disturbances
Blurred vision NOS

368.9 Unspecified visual disturbance

√4ᵗʰ **369 Blindness and low vision**

Note: Visual impairment refers to a functional limitation of the eye (e.g., limited visual acuity or visual field). It should be distinguished from visual disability, indicating a limitation of the abilities of the individual (e.g., limited reading skills, vocational skills), and from visual handicap, indicating a limitation of personal and socioeconomic independence (e.g., limited mobility, limited employability).

The levels of impairment defined in the table on the next page are based on the recommendations of the WHO Study Group on Prevention of Blindness (Geneva, November 6–10, 1972; WHO Technical Report Series 518), and of the International Council of Ophthalmology (1976).

Note that definitions of blindness vary in different settings.

For international reporting WHO defines blindness as profound impairment. This definition can be applied to blindness of one eye (369.1, 369.6) and to blindness of the individual (369.0).

For determination of benefits in the U.S.A., the definition of legal blindness as severe impairment is often used. This definition applies to blindness of the individual only.

EXCLUDES   correctable impaired vision due to refractive errors (367.0-367.9)

√5ᵗʰ **369.0 Profound impairment, both eyes**

369.00 Impairment level not further specified
Blindness:
  NOS according to WHO definition
  both eyes

369.01 Better eye: total impairment; lesser eye: total impairment

369.02 Better eye: near-total impairment; lesser eye: not further specified

369.03 Better eye: near-total impairment; lesser eye: total impairment

369.04 Better eye: near-total impairment; lesser eye: near-total impairment

369.05 Better eye: profound impairment; lesser eye: not further specified

369.06 Better eye: profound impairment; lesser eye: total impairment

369.07 Better eye: profound impairment; lesser eye: near-total impairment

369.08 Better eye: profound impairment; lesser eye: profound impairment

√4ᵗʰ **369.1 Moderate or severe impairment, better eye, profound impairment lesser eye**

369.10 Impairment level not further specified
Blindness, one eye, low vision other eye

369.11 Better eye: severe impairment; lesser eye: blind, not further specified

369.12 Better eye: severe impairment; lesser eye: total impairment

369.13 Better eye: severe impairment; lesser eye: near-total impairment

369.14 Better eye: severe impairment; lesser eye: profound impairment

369.15 Better eye: moderate impairment; lesser eye: blind, not further specified

369.16 Better eye: moderate impairment; lesser eye: total impairment

NERVOUS SYSTEM AND SENSE ORGANS

369.17 **Better eye: moderate impairment; lesser eye: near-total impairment**
369.18 **Better eye: moderate impairment; lesser eye: profound impairment**

√5th 369.2 **Moderate or severe impairment, both eyes**
    369.20 **Impairment level not further specified**
        Low vision, both eyes NOS
    369.21 **Better eye: severe impairment; lesser eye: not further specified**
    369.22 **Better eye: severe impairment; lesser eye: severe impairment**
    369.23 **Better eye: moderate impairment; lesser eye: not further specified**
    369.24 **Better eye: moderate impairment; lesser eye: severe impairment**
    369.25 **Better eye: moderate impairment; lesser eye: moderate impairment**

369.3 **Unqualified visual loss, both eyes**
    EXCLUDES   blindness NOS:
        legal [U.S.A. definition] (369.4)
        WHO definition (369.00)

369.4 **Legal blindness, as defined in U.S.A.**
    Blindness NOS according to U.S.A. definition
    EXCLUDES   legal blindness with specification of impairment level (369.01-369.08, 369.11-369.14, 369.21-369.22)

√5th 369.6 **Profound impairment, one eye**
    369.60 **Impairment level not further specified**
        Blindness, one eye
    369.61 **One eye: total impairment; other eye: not specified**
    369.62 **One eye: total impairment; other eye: near-normal vision**
    369.63 **One eye: total impairment; other eye: normal vision**
    369.64 **One eye: near-total impairment; other eye: not specified**
    369.65 **One eye: near-total impairment; other eye: near-normal vision**
    369.66 **One eye: near-total impairment; other eye: normal vision**
    369.67 **One eye: profound impairment; other eye: not specified**
    369.68 **One eye: profound impairment; other eye: near-normal vision**
    369.69 **One eye: profound impairment; other eye: normal vision**

√5th 369.7 **Moderate or severe impairment, one eye**
    369.70 **Impairment level not further specified**
        Low vision, one eye
    369.71 **One eye: severe impairment; other eye: not specified**
    369.72 **One eye: severe impairment; other eye: near-normal vision**
    369.73 **One eye: severe impairment; other eye: normal vision**
    369.74 **One eye: moderate impairment; other eye: not specified**
    369.75 **One eye: moderate impairment; other eye: near-normal vision**
    369.76 **One eye: moderate impairment; other eye: normal vision**

369.8 **Unqualified visual loss, one eye**
369.9 **Unspecified visual loss**

Classification		LEVELS OF VISUAL IMPAIRMENT	Additional descriptors which may be encountered
"legal"	WHO	Visual acuity and/or visual field limitation (whichever is worse)	
(NEAR-) NORMAL VISION		RANGE OF NORMAL VISION 20/10 20/13 20/16 20/20 20/25 2.0 1.6 1.25 1.0 0.8	
		NEAR-NORMAL VISION 20/30 20/40 20/50 20/60 0.7 0.6 0.5 0.4 0.3	
LOW VISION		MODERATE VISUAL IMPAIRMENT 20/70 20/80 20/100 20/125 20/160 0.25 0.20 0.16 0.12	Moderate low vision
		SEVERE VISUAL IMPAIRMENT 20/200 20/250 20/320 20/400 0.10 0.08 0.06 0.05 Visual field: 20 degrees or less	Severe low vision, "Legal" blindness
LEGAL BLINDNESS (U.S.A.) both eyes	BLINDNESS (WHO) one or both eyes	PROFOUND VISUAL IMPAIRMENT 20/500 20/630 20/800 20/1000 0.04 0.03 0.025 0.02 Count fingers at: less than 3m (10 ft.) Visual field: 10 degrees or less	Profound low vision, Moderate blindness
		NEAR-TOTAL VISUAL IMPAIRMENT Visual acuity: less than 0.02 (20/1000) Count fingers at: 1m (3 ft.) or less Hand movements: 5m (15 ft.) or less Light projection, light perception Visual field: 5 degrees or less	Severe blindness, Near-total blindness
		TOTAL VISUAL IMPAIRMENT No light perception (NLP)	Total blindness

Visual acuity refers to best achievable acuity with correction.
Non-listed Snellen fractions may be classified by converting to the nearest decimal equivalent, e.g. 10/200 = 0.05, 6/30 = 0.20.
CF (count fingers) without designation of distance, may be classified to profound impairment.
HM (hand motion) without designation of distance, may be classified to near-total impairment.
Visual field measurements refer to the largest field diameter for a 1/100 white test object.

√4th **370 Keratitis**
  √5th **370.0 Corneal ulcer**
    EXCLUDES   *that due to vitamin A deficiency (264.3)*
    370.00 **Corneal ulcer, unspecified**
    370.01 **Marginal corneal ulcer**
    370.02 **Ring corneal ulcer**
    370.03 **Central corneal ulcer**
    370.04 **Hypopyon ulcer**
        Serpiginous ulcer
        DEF: Corneal ulcer with an accumulation of pus in the eye's anterior chamber.
    370.05 **Mycotic corneal ulcer**
        DEF: Fungal infection causing corneal tissue loss.
    370.06 **Perforated corneal ulcer**
        DEF: Tissue loss through all layers of cornea.
    370.07 **Mooren's ulcer**
        DEF: Tissue loss, with chronic inflammation, at junction of cornea and sclera; seen in elderly.

√5th **370.2 Superficial keratitis without conjunctivitis**
    EXCLUDES   *dendritic [herpes simplex] keratitis (054.42)*

NERVOUS SYSTEM AND SENSE ORGANS 370.20–371.23

370.20 **Superficial keratitis, unspecified**
370.21 **Punctate keratitis**
  Thygeson's superficial punctate keratitis
  DEF: Formation of cellular and fibrinous deposits (keratic precipitates) on posterior surface; deposits develop after injury or iridocyclitis.

370.22 **Macular keratitis**
  Keratitis: Keratitis:
    areolar   stellate
    nummular   striate

370.23 **Filamentary keratitis**
  DEF: Keratitis characterized by twisted filaments of mucoid material on the cornea's surface.

370.24 **Photokeratitis**
  Snow blindness
  Welders' keratitis
  AHA: 3Q, '96, 6
  DEF: Painful, inflamed cornea; due to extended exposure to ultraviolet light.

√5th 370.3 **Certain types of keratoconjunctivitis**
  370.31 **Phlyctenular keratoconjunctivitis**
    Phlyctenulosis
    Use additional code for any associated tuberculosis (017.3)
    DEF: Miniature blister on conjunctiva or cornea; associated with tuberculosis and malnutrition disorders.

  370.32 **Limbar and corneal involvement in vernal conjunctivitis**
    Use additional code for vernal conjunctivitis (372.13)
    DEF: Corneal itching and inflammation in conjunctivitis; often limited to lining of eyelids.

  370.33 **Keratoconjunctivitis sicca, not specified as Sjögren's**
    EXCLUDES Sjögren's syndrome (710.2)
    DEF: Inflammation of conjunctiva and cornea; characterized by "horny" looking tissue and excess blood in these areas; decreased flow of lacrimal (tear) is a contributing factor.

  370.34 **Exposure keratoconjunctivitis**
    AHA: 3Q, '96, 6
    DEF: Incomplete closure of eyelid causing dry, inflamed eye.

  370.35 **Neurotrophic keratoconjunctivitis**

√5th 370.4 **Other and unspecified keratoconjunctivitis**
  370.40 **Keratoconjunctivitis, unspecified**
    Superficial keratitis with conjunctivitis NOS
  370.44 *Keratitis or keratoconjunctivitis in exanthema*
    Code first underlying condition (050.0-052.9)
    EXCLUDES herpes simplex (054.43)
              herpes zoster (053.21)
              measles (055.71)
  370.49 **Other**
    EXCLUDES epidemic keratoconjunctivitis (077.1)

√5th 370.5 **Interstitial and deep keratitis**
  370.50 **Interstitial keratitis, unspecified**
  370.52 **Diffuse interstitial keratitis**
    Cogan's syndrome
    DEF: Inflammation of cornea; with deposits in middle corneal layers; may obscure vision.
  370.54 **Sclerosing keratitis**
    DEF: Chronic corneal inflammation leading to opaque scarring.
  370.55 **Corneal abscess**
    DEF: Pocket of pus and inflammation on the cornea.

370.59 **Other**
  EXCLUDES disciform herpes simplex keratitis (054.43)
            syphilitic keratitis (090.3)

√5th 370.6 **Corneal neovascularization**
  370.60 **Corneal neovascularization, unspecified**
  370.61 **Localized vascularization of cornea**
    DEF: Limited infiltration of cornea by new blood vessels.
  370.62 **Pannus (corneal)**
    DEF: Buildup of superficial vascularization and granulated tissue under epithelium of cornea.
  370.63 **Deep vascularization of cornea**
    DEF: Deep infiltration of cornea by new blood vessels.
  370.64 **Ghost vessels (corneal)**

370.8 **Other forms of keratitis**
  AHA: 3Q, '94, 5

370.9 **Unspecified keratitis**

√4th 371 **Corneal opacity and other disorders of cornea**
√5th 371.0 **Corneal scars and opacities**
    EXCLUDES that due to vitamin A deficiency (264.6)
  371.00 **Corneal opacity, unspecified**
    Corneal scar NOS
  371.01 **Minor opacity of cornea**
    Corneal nebula
  371.02 **Peripheral opacity of cornea**
    Corneal macula not interfering with central vision
  371.03 **Central opacity of cornea**
    Corneal:
      leucoma } interfering with central
      macula   }   vision
  371.04 **Adherent leucoma**
    DEF: Dense, opaque corneal growth adhering to the iris; also spelled as leukoma.
  371.05 **Phthisical cornea**
    Code first underlying tuberculosis (017.3)

√5th 371.1 **Corneal pigmentations and deposits**
  371.10 **Corneal deposit, unspecified**
  371.11 **Anterior pigmentations**
    Stähli's lines
  371.12 **Stromal pigmentations**
    Hematocornea
  371.13 **Posterior pigmentations**
    Krukenberg spindle
  371.14 **Kayser-Fleischer ring**
    DEF: Copper deposits forming ring at outer edge of cornea; seen in Wilson's disease and other liver disorders.
  371.15 **Other deposits associated with metabolic disorders**
  371.16 **Argentous deposits**
    DEF: Silver deposits in cornea.

√5th 371.2 **Corneal edema**
  371.20 **Corneal edema, unspecified**
  371.21 **Idiopathic corneal edema**
    DEF: Corneal swelling and fluid retention of unknown cause.
  371.22 **Secondary corneal edema**
    DEF: Corneal swelling and fluid retention caused by an underlying disease, injury, or condition.
  371.23 **Bullous keratopathy**
    DEF: Corneal degeneration; characterized by recurring, rupturing epithelial "blisters;" ruptured blebs expose corneal nerves, cause great pain; occurs in glaucoma, iridocyclitis and Fuchs' epithelial dystrophy.

371.24–372.21 NERVOUS SYSTEM AND SENSE ORGANS — Tabular List

- **371.24 Corneal edema due to wearing of contact lenses**
- √5th **371.3 Changes of corneal membranes**
  - **371.30** Corneal membrane change, unspecified
  - **371.31** Folds and rupture of Bowman's membrane
  - **371.32** Folds in Descemet's membrane
  - **371.33** Rupture in Descemet's membrane
- √5th **371.4 Corneal degenerations**
  - **371.40** Corneal degeneration, unspecified
  - **371.41** Senile corneal changes
    - Arcus senilis   Hassall-Henle bodies
  - **371.42** Recurrent erosion of cornea
    - EXCLUDES Mooren's ulcer (370.07)
  - **371.43** Band-shaped keratopathy
    - DEF: Horizontal bands of superficial corneal calcium deposits.
  - **371.44** Other calcerous degenerations of cornea
  - **371.45** Keratomalacia NOS
    - EXCLUDES that due to vitamin A deficiency (264.4)
    - DEF: Destruction of the cornea by keratinization of the epithelium with ulceration and perforation of the cornea; seen in cases of vitamin A deficiency.
  - **371.46** Nodular degeneration of cornea
    - Salzmann's nodular dystrophy
  - **371.48** Peripheral degenerations of cornea
    - Marginal degeneration of cornea [Terrien's]
  - **371.49** Other
    - Discrete colliquative keratopathy
- √5th **371.5 Hereditary corneal dystrophies**
  - DEF: Genetic disorder; leads to opacities, edema or lesions of cornea.
  - **371.50** Corneal dystrophy, unspecified
  - **371.51** Juvenile epithelial corneal dystrophy
  - **371.52** Other anterior corneal dystrophies
    - Corneal dystrophy: microscopic cystic   Corneal dystrophy: ring-like
  - **371.53** Granular corneal dystrophy
  - **371.54** Lattice corneal dystrophy
  - **371.55** Macular corneal dystrophy
  - **371.56** Other stromal corneal dystrophies
    - Crystalline corneal dystrophy
  - **371.57** Endothelial corneal dystrophy
    - Combined corneal dystrophy
    - Cornea guttata
    - Fuchs' endothelial dystrophy
  - **371.58** Other posterior corneal dystrophies
    - Polymorphous corneal dystrophy
- √5th **371.6 Keratoconus**
  - DEF: Bilateral bulging protrusion of anterior cornea; often due to noninflammatory thinning.
  - **371.60** Keratoconus, unspecified
  - **371.61** Keratoconus, stable condition
  - **371.62** Keratoconus, acute hydrops
- √5th **371.7 Other corneal deformities**
  - **371.70** Corneal deformity, unspecified
  - **371.71** Corneal ectasia
    - DEF: Bulging protrusion of thinned, scarred cornea.
  - **371.72** Descemetocele
    - DEF: Protrusion of Descemet's membrane into cornea.
  - **371.73** Corneal staphyloma
    - DEF: Protrusion of cornea into adjacent tissue.
- √5th **371.8 Other corneal disorders**
  - **371.81** Corneal anesthesia and hypoesthesia
    - DEF: Decreased or absent sensitivity of cornea..
  - **371.82** Corneal disorder due to contact lens
    - EXCLUDES corneal edema due to contact lens (371.24)
    - DEF: Contact lens wear causing cornea disorder, excluding swelling.
  - **371.89** Other
    - AHA: 3Q, '99, 12
- **371.9 Unspecified corneal disorder**
- √4th **372 Disorders of conjunctiva**
  - EXCLUDES keratoconjunctivitis (370.3-370.4)
- √5th **372.0 Acute conjunctivitis**
  - **372.00** Acute conjunctivitis, unspecified
  - **372.01** Serous conjunctivitis, except viral
    - EXCLUDES viral conjunctivitis NOS (077.9)
  - **372.02** Acute follicular conjunctivitis
    - Conjunctival folliculosis NOS
    - EXCLUDES conjunctivitis:
      - adenoviral (acute follicular) (077.3)
      - epidemic hemorrhagic (077.4)
      - inclusion (077.0)
      - Newcastle (077.8)
      - epidemic keratoconjunctivitis (077.1)
      - pharyngoconjunctival fever (077.2)
    - DEF: Severe conjunctival inflammation with dense infiltrations of lymphoid tissues of inner eyelids; may be traced to a viral or chlamydial etiology.
  - **372.03** Other mucopurulent conjunctivitis
    - Catarrhal conjunctivitis
    - EXCLUDES blennorrhea neonatorum (gonococcal) (098.40)
      - neonatal conjunctivitis (771.6)
      - ophthalmia neonatorum NOS (771.6)
  - **372.04** Pseudomembranous conjunctivitis
    - Membranous conjunctivitis
    - EXCLUDES diphtheritic conjunctivitis (032.81)
    - DEF: Severe inflammation of conjunctiva; false membrane develops on inner surface of eyelid; membrane can be removed without harming epithelium, due to bacterial infections, toxic and allergic factors, and viral infections.
  - **372.05** Acute atopic conjunctivitis
    - DEF: Sudden, severe conjunctivitis due to allergens.
- √5th **372.1 Chronic conjunctivitis**
  - **372.10** Chronic conjunctivitis, unspecified
  - **372.11** Simple chronic conjunctivitis
  - **372.12** Chronic follicular conjunctivitis
    - DEF: Persistent conjunctival inflammation with dense, localized infiltrations of lymphoid tissues of inner eyelids.
  - **372.13** Vernal conjunctivitis
    - AHA: 3Q, '96, 8
  - **372.14** Other chronic allergic conjunctivitis
    - AHA: 3Q, '96, 8
  - **372.15** *Parasitic conjunctivitis*
    - Code first underlying disease, as:
      - filariasis (125.0-125.9)
      - mucocutaneous leishmaniasis (085.5)
- √5th **372.2 Blepharoconjunctivitis**
  - **372.20** Blepharoconjunctivitis, unspecified
  - **372.21** Angular blepharoconjunctivitis
    - DEF: Inflammation at junction of upper and lower eyelids; may block lacrimal secretions.

N Newborn Age: 0   **P** Pediatric Age: 0-17   **M** Maternity Age: 12-55   **A** Adult Age: 15-124   **CC** CC Condition   **MC** Major Complication   **CD** Complex Dx   **HIV** HIV Related Dx

372.22 Contact blepharoconjunctivitis

√5th **372.3** **Other and unspecified conjunctivitis**
- **372.30** Conjunctivitis, unspecified
- **372.31** Rosacea conjunctivitis
  Code first underlying rosacea dermatitis (695.3)
- **372.33** Conjunctivitis in mucocutaneous disease
  Code first underlying disease, as:
  erythema multiforme (695.1)
  Reiter's disease (099.3)
  EXCLUDES ocular pemphigoid (694.61)
- **372.39** Other

√5th **372.4** **Pterygium**
EXCLUDES pseudopterygium (372.52)
DEF: Wedge-shaped, conjunctival thickening that advances from the inner corner of the eye toward the cornea.
- **372.40** Pterygium, unspecified
- **372.41** Peripheral pterygium, stationary
- **372.42** Peripheral pterygium, progressive
- **372.43** Central pterygium
- **372.44** Double pterygium
- **372.45** Recurrent pterygium

√5th **372.5** **Conjunctival degenerations and deposits**
- **372.50** Conjunctival degeneration, unspecified
- **372.51** Pinguecula
  DEF: Proliferative spot on the bulbar conjunctiva located near the sclerocorneal junction, usually on the nasal side; it is seen in elderly people.
- **372.52** Pseudopterygium
  DEF: Conjunctival scar joined to the cornea; it looks like a pterygium but is not attached to the tissue.
- **372.53** Conjunctival xerosis
  EXCLUDES conjunctival xerosis due to vitamin A deficiency (264.0, 264.1, 264.7)
  DEF: Dry conjunctiva due to vitamin A deficiency; related to Bitot's spots; may develop into xerophthalmia and keratomalacia.
- **372.54** Conjunctival concretions
  DEF: Calculus or deposit on conjunctiva.
- **372.55** Conjunctival pigmentations
  Conjunctival argyrosis
  DEF: Color deposits in conjunctiva.
- **372.56** Conjunctival deposits

√5th **372.6** **Conjunctival scars**
- **372.61** Granuloma of conjunctiva
- **372.62** Localized adhesions and strands of conjunctiva
  DEF: Abnormal fibrous connections in conjunctiva.
- **372.63** Symblepharon
  Extensive adhesions of conjunctiva
  DEF: Adhesion of the eyelids to the eyeball.
- **372.64** Scarring of conjunctiva
  Contraction of eye socket (after enucleation)

√5th **372.7** **Conjunctival vascular disorders and cysts**
- **372.71** Hyperemia of conjunctiva
  DEF: Conjunctival blood vessel congestion causing eye redness.
- **372.72** Conjunctival hemorrhage
  Hyposphagma Subconjunctival hemorrhage
- **372.73** Conjunctival edema
  Chemosis of conjunctiva
  Subconjunctival edema
  DEF: Fluid retention and swelling in conjunctival tissue.
- **372.74** Vascular abnormalities of conjunctiva
  Aneurysm(ata) of conjunctiva
- **372.75** Conjunctival cysts
  DEF: Abnormal sacs of fluid in conjunctiva.

√5th **372.8** **Other disorders of conjunctiva**
- **372.81** Conjunctivochalasis
  AHA: 4Q, '00, 41
  DEF: Bilateral condition of redundant conjunctival tissue between globe and lower eyelid margin; may cover lower punctum, interferring with normal tearing.
- **372.89** Other disorders of conjunctiva

372.9 Unspecified disorder of conjunctiva

√4th **373** **Inflammation of eyelids**

√5th **373.0** **Blepharitis**
EXCLUDES blepharoconjunctivitis (372.20-372.22)
- **373.00** Blepharitis, unspecified
- **373.01** Ulcerative blepharitis
- **373.02** Squamous blepharitis

√5th **373.1** **Hordeolum and other deep inflammation of eyelid**
DEF: Purulent, localized, staphylococcal infection in sebaceous glands of eyelids.
- **373.11** Hordeolum externum
  Hordeolum NOS Stye
  DEF: Infection of the oil glands in the eyelash follicles.
- **373.12** Hordeolum internum
  Infection of meibomian gland
  DEF: Infection of the oil gland of the eyelid margin.
- **373.13** Abscess of eyelid
  Furuncle of eyelid
  DEF: Inflamed pocket of pus on the eyelid.

373.2 Chalazion
Meibomian (gland) cyst
EXCLUDES infected meibomian gland (373.12)
DEF: Chronic inflammation of the meibomian gland, causing an eyelid mass.

√5th **373.3** **Noninfectious dermatoses of eyelid**
- **373.31** Eczematous dermatitis of eyelid
- **373.32** Contact and allergic dermatitis of eyelid
- **373.33** Xeroderma of eyelid
- **373.34** Discoid lupus erythematosus of eyelid

373.4 Infective dermatitis of eyelid of types resulting in deformity
Code first underlying disease, as:
leprosy (030.0-030.9)
lupus vulgaris (tuberculous) (017.0)
yaws (102.0-102.9)

373.5 Other infective dermatitis of eyelid
Code first underlying disease, as:
actinomycosis (039.3)
impetigo (684)
mycotic dermatitis (110.0-111.9)
vaccinia (051.0)
postvaccination (999.0)
EXCLUDES herpes:
simplex (054.41)
zoster (053.20)

373.6 Parasitic infestation of eyelid
Code first underlying disease, as:
leishmaniasis (085.0-085.9)
loiasis (125.2)
onchocerciasis (125.3)
pediculosis (132.0)

373.8 Other inflammations of eyelids

373.9 Unspecified inflammation of eyelid

Entropion and Ectropion

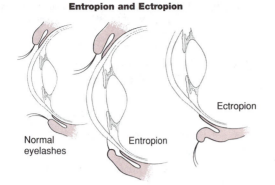

- **374 Other disorders of eyelids**
  - **374.0 Entropion and trichiasis of eyelid**
    - DEF: Entropion: turning inward of eyelid edge toward eyeball.
    - DEF: Trichiasis: ingrowing eyelashes marked by irritation with possible distortion of sight.
    - 374.00 Entropion, unspecified
    - 374.01 Senile entropion [A]
    - 374.02 Mechanical entropion
    - 374.03 Spastic entropion
    - 374.04 Cicatricial entropion
    - 374.05 Trichiasis without entropion
  - **374.1 Ectropion**
    - DEF: Turning outward (eversion) of eyelid edge; exposes palpebral conjunctiva; dryness irritation result.
    - 374.10 Ectropion, unspecified
    - 374.11 Senile ectropion [A]
    - 374.12 Mechanical ectropion
    - 374.13 Spastic ectropion
    - 374.14 Cicatricial ectropion
  - **374.2 Lagophthalmos**
    - DEF: Incomplete closure of eyes; causes dry eye and other complications.
    - 374.20 Lagophthalmos, unspecified
    - 374.21 Paralytic lagophthalmos
    - 374.22 Mechanical lagophthalmos
    - 374.23 Cicatricial lagophthalmos
  - **374.3 Ptosis of eyelid**
    - 374.30 Ptosis of eyelid, unspecified
      - AHA: 2Q, '96, 11
    - 374.31 Paralytic ptosis
      - DEF: Drooping of upper eyelid due to nerve disorder.
    - 374.32 Myogenic ptosis
      - DEF: Drooping of upper eyelid due to muscle disorder.
    - 374.33 Mechanical ptosis
      - DEF: Outside force causes drooping of upper eyelid.
    - 374.34 Blepharochalasis
      - Pseudoptosis
      - DEF: Loss of elasticity causing skin to hang over eyelid margin; due to intercellular tissue atrophy.
  - **374.4 Other disorders affecting eyelid function**
    - EXCLUDES: blepharoclonus (333.81)
      blepharospasm (333.81)
      facial nerve palsy (351.0)
      third nerve palsy or paralysis (378.51-378.52)
      tic (psychogenic) (307.20-307.23)
      organic (333.3)
    - 374.41 Lid retraction or lag
    - 374.43 Abnormal innervation syndrome
      - Jaw-blinking
      - Paradoxical facial movements
    - 374.44 Sensory disorders
    - 374.45 Other sensorimotor disorders
      - Deficient blink reflex
    - 374.46 Blepharophimosis
      - Ankyloblepharon
      - DEF: Narrowing of palpebral fissure horizontally; caused by laterally displaced inner canthi; either acquired or congenital.
  - **374.5 Degenerative disorders of eyelid and periocular area**
    - 374.50 Degenerative disorder of eyelid, unspecified
    - 374.51 Xanthelasma
      - Xanthoma (planum) (tuberosum) of eyelid
      - Code first underlying condition (272.0-272.9)
      - DEF: Fatty tumors of the eyelid linked to high fat content of blood.
    - 374.52 Hyperpigmentation of eyelid
      - Chloasma   Dyspigmentation
      - DEF: Excess pigment of eyelid.
    - 374.53 Hypopigmentation of eyelid
      - Vitiligo of eyelid
      - DEF: Lack of color pigment of the eyelid.
    - 374.54 Hypertrichosis of eyelid
      - DEF: Excessive eyelash growth.
    - 374.55 Hypotrichosis of eyelid
      - Madarosis of eyelid
      - DEF: Less than normal, or absent, eyelashes.
    - 374.56 Other degenerative disorders of skin affecting eyelid
  - **374.8 Other disorders of eyelid**
    - 374.81 Hemorrhage of eyelid
      - EXCLUDES: black eye (921.0)
    - 374.82 Edema of eyelid
      - Hyperemia of eyelid
      - DEF: Swelling and fluid retention in eyelid.
    - 374.83 Elephantiasis of eyelid
      - DEF: Filarial disease causing dermatitis and enlargement of eyelid.
    - 374.84 Cysts of eyelids
      - Sebaceous cyst of eyelid
    - 374.85 Vascular anomalies of eyelid
    - 374.86 Retained foreign body of eyelid
    - 374.87 Dermatochalasis
      - DEF: Loss of elasticity causing skin under eye to sag.
    - 374.89 Other disorders of eyelid
  - **374.9 Unspecified disorder of eyelid**
- **375 Disorders of lacrimal system**
  - **375.0 Dacryoadenitis**
    - 375.00 Dacryoadenitis, unspecified
    - 375.01 Acute dacryoadenitis
      - DEF: Severe, sudden inflammation of the lacrimal gland.
    - 375.02 Chronic dacryoadenitis
      - DEF: Persistent inflammation of the lacrimal gland.
    - 375.03 Chronic enlargement of lacrimal gland
  - **375.1 Other disorders of lacrimal gland**
    - 375.11 Dacryops
      - DEF: Overproduction and constant flow of tears; may cause distended lacrimal duct.
    - 375.12 Other lacrimal cysts and cystic degeneration
    - 375.13 Primary lacrimal atrophy

NERVOUS SYSTEM AND SENSE ORGANS

375.14 **Secondary lacrimal atrophy**
DEF: Wasting away of the lacrimal gland due to another disease.

375.15 **Tear film insufficiency, unspecified**
Dry eye syndrome
AHA: 3Q, '96, 6
DEF: Eye dryness and irritation from insufficient tear production.

375.16 **Dislocation of lacrimal gland**

√5th 375.2 **Epiphora**
DEF: Abnormal development of tears due to stricture of lacrimal passages.

375.20 **Epiphora, unspecified as to cause**

375.21 **Epiphora due to excess lacrimation**
DEF: Tear overflow due to overproduction.

375.22 **Epiphora due to insufficient drainage**
DEF: Tear overflow due to blocked drainage.

√5th 375.3 **Acute and unspecified inflammation of lacrimal passages**
EXCLUDES neonatal dacryocystitis (771.6)

375.30 **Dacryocystitis, unspecified**
375.31 **Acute canaliculitis, lacrimal**
375.32 **Acute dacryocystitis**
Acute peridacryocystitis
375.33 **Phlegmonous dacryocystitis**
DEF: Infection of the tear sac with pockets of pus.

√5th 375.4 **Chronic inflammation of lacrimal passages**
375.41 **Chronic canaliculitis**
375.42 **Chronic dacryocystitis**
375.43 **Lacrimal mucocele**

√5th 375.5 **Stenosis and insufficiency of lacrimal passages**
375.51 **Eversion of lacrimal punctum**
DEF: Abnormal turning outward of the tear duct.

375.52 **Stenosis of lacrimal punctum**
DEF: Abnormal narrowing of the tear duct.

375.53 **Stenosis of lacrimal canaliculi**
375.54 **Stenosis of lacrimal sac**
DEF: Abnormal narrowing of the tear sac.

375.55 **Obstruction of nasolacrimal duct, neonatal**
EXCLUDES congenital anomaly of nasolacrimal duct (743.65)
DEF: Acquired, abnormal obstruction of tear drainage system from the eye to the nose; in an infant.

375.56 **Stenosis of nasolacrimal duct, acquired**
375.57 **Dacryolith**
DEF: Concretion or stone anywhere in lacrimal system.

▶ **Lacrimal System** ◀

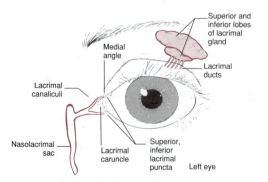

√5th 375.6 **Other changes of lacrimal passages**
375.61 **Lacrimal fistula**
DEF: Abnormal communication from the lacrimal system.

375.69 **Other**

√5th 375.8 **Other disorders of lacrimal system**
375.81 **Granuloma of lacrimal passages**
DEF: Abnormal nodules within lacrimal system.

375.89 **Other**

375.9 **Unspecified disorder of lacrimal system**

√4th 376 **Disorders of the orbit**

√5th 376.0 **Acute inflammation of orbit**
376.00 **Acute inflammation of orbit, unspecified**
376.01 **Orbital cellulitis**
Abscess of orbit
DEF: Infection of tissue between the orbital bone and eyeball.

376.02 **Orbital periostitis**
DEF: Inflammation of connective tissue covering the orbital bone.

376.03 **Orbital osteomyelitis**
DEF: Inflammation of the orbital bone.

376.04 **Tenonitis**

√5th 376.1 **Chronic inflammatory disorders of orbit**
376.10 **Chronic inflammation of orbit, unspecified**
376.11 **Orbital granuloma**
Pseudotumor (inflammatory) of orbit
DEF: Abnormal nodule between orbital bone and eyeball.

376.12 **Orbital myositis**
DEF: Painful inflammation of the muscles of the eye.

376.13 *Parasitic infestation of orbit*
Code first underlying disease, as:
hydatid infestation of orbit (122.3, 122.6, 122.9)
myiasis of orbit (134.0)

√5th 376.2 **Endocrine exophthalmos**
Code first underlying thyroid disorder (242.0-242.9)
376.21 *Thyrotoxic exophthalmos*
DEF: Painful inflammation of eye muscles.

376.22 *Exophthalmic ophthalmoplegia*
DEF: Inability to rotate eye as a result of bulging eyes.

√5th 376.3 **Other exophthalmic conditions**
376.30 **Exophthalmos, unspecified**
DEF: Abnormal protrusion of eyeball.

376.31 **Constant exophthalmos**
DEF: Continuous, abnormal protrusion or bulging of eyeball.

376.32 **Orbital hemorrhage**
DEF: Bleeding behind the eyeball, causing it to bulge forward.

376.33 **Orbital edema or congestion**
DEF: Fluid retention behind eyeball, causing forward bulge.

376.34 **Intermittent exophthalmos**
376.35 **Pulsating exophthalmos**
DEF: Bulge or protrusion; associated with a carotid-cavernous fistula.

376.36 **Lateral displacement of globe**
DEF: Abnormal displacement of the eyeball away from nose, toward temple.

√5th 376.4 **Deformity of orbit**
376.40 **Deformity of orbit, unspecified**

376.41 Hypertelorism of orbit
DEF: Abnormal increase in interorbital distance; associated with congenital facial deformities; may be accompanied by mental deficiency.

376.42 Exostosis of orbit
DEF: Abnormal bony growth of orbit.

376.43 Local deformities due to bone disease
DEF: Acquired abnormalities of orbit; due to bone disease.

376.44 Orbital deformities associated with craniofacial deformities

376.45 Atrophy of orbit
DEF: Wasting away of bone tissue of orbit.

376.46 Enlargement of orbit

376.47 Deformity due to trauma or surgery

√5th **376.5 Enophthalmos**
DEF: Recession of eyeball deep into eye socket.

376.50 Enophthalmos, unspecified as to cause

376.51 Enophthalmos due to atrophy of orbital tissue

376.52 Enophthalmos due to trauma or surgery

376.6 Retained (old) foreign body following penetrating wound of orbit
Retrobulbar foreign body

√5th **376.8 Other orbital disorders**

376.81 Orbital cysts
Encephalocele of orbit
AHA: 3Q, '99, 13

376.82 Myopathy of extraocular muscles
DEF: Disease in the muscles that control eyeball movement.

376.89 Other

376.9 Unspecified disorder of orbit

√4th **377 Disorders of optic nerve and visual pathways**

√5th **377.0 Papilledema**

377.00 Papilledema, unspecified CC
CC Excl: 017.30-017.36, 017.90-017.96, 036.81, 250.50-250.53, 250.80-250.93, 377.00-377.03, 377.14, 377.24, 379.8, 379.90, 379.99, 743.8-743.9

377.01 Papilledema associated with increased intracranial pressure CC
CC Excl: See code 377.00

377.02 Papilledema associated with decreased ocular pressure CC
CC Excl: See code 377.00

377.03 Papilledema associated with retinal disorder

377.04 Foster-Kennedy syndrome
DEF: Retrobulbar optic neuritis, central scotoma and optic atrophy; caused by tumors in frontal lobe of brain that press downward.

√5th **377.1 Optic atrophy**

377.10 Optic atrophy, unspecified

377.11 Primary optic atrophy
EXCLUDES neurosyphilitic optic atrophy (094.84)

377.12 Postinflammatory optic atrophy
DEF: : Adverse effect of inflammation causing wasting away of eye.

377.13 Optic atrophy associated with retinal dystrophies
DEF: Progressive changes in retinal tissue due to metabolic disorder causing wasting away of eye.

377.14 Glaucomatous atrophy [cupping] of optic disc

377.15 Partial optic atrophy
Temporal pallor of optic disc

377.16 Hereditary optic atrophy
Optic atrophy: dominant hereditary
Optic atrophy: Leber's

√5th **377.2 Other disorders of optic disc**

377.21 Drusen of optic disc

377.22 Crater-like holes of optic disc

377.23 Coloboma of optic disc
DEF: Ocular malformation caused by the failure of fetal fissure of optic stalk to close.

377.24 Pseudopapilledema

√5th **377.3 Optic neuritis**
EXCLUDES meningococcal optic neuritis (036.81)

377.30 Optic neuritis, unspecified

377.31 Optic papillitis
DEF: Swelling and inflammation of the optic disc.

377.32 Retrobulbar neuritis (acute)
EXCLUDES syphilitic retrobulbar neuritis (094.85)
DEF: Inflammation of optic nerve immediately behind the eyeball.

377.33 Nutritional optic neuropathy
DEF: Malnutrition causing optic nerve disorder.

377.34 Toxic optic neuropathy
Toxic amblyopia
DEF: Toxic substance causing optic nerve disorder.

377.39 Other
EXCLUDES ischemic optic neuropathy (377.41)

√5th **377.4 Other disorders of optic nerve**

377.41 Ischemic optic neuropathy
DEF: Decreased blood flow affecting optic nerve.

377.42 Hemorrhage in optic nerve sheaths
DEF: Bleeding in meningeal lining of optic nerve.

377.49 Other
Compression of optic nerve

√5th **377.5 Disorders of optic chiasm**

377.51 Associated with pituitary neoplasms and disorders
DEF: Abnormal pituitary growth causing disruption in nerve chain from retina to brain.

377.52 Associated with other neoplasms
DEF: Abnormal growth, other than pituitary, causing disruption in nerve chain from retina to brain.

377.53 Associated with vascular disorders
DEF: Vascular disorder causing disruption in nerve chain from retina to brain.

377.54 Associated with inflammatory disorders
DEF: Inflammatory disease causing disruption in nerve chain from retina to brain.

√5th **377.6 Disorders of other visual pathways**

377.61 Associated with neoplasms

377.62 Associated with vascular disorders

377.63 Associated with inflammatory disorders

√5th **377.7 Disorders of visual cortex**
EXCLUDES visual:
agnosia (368.16)
hallucinations (368.16)
halos (368.15)

377.71 Associated with neoplasms

377.72 Associated with vascular disorders

377.73 Associated with inflammatory disorders

NERVOUS SYSTEM AND SENSE ORGANS

377.75 Cortical blindness
DEF: Blindness due to brain disorder, rather than eye disorder.

377.9 Unspecified disorder of optic nerve and visual pathways

√4th **378 Strabismus and other disorders of binocular eye movements**
EXCLUDES nystagmus and other irregular eye movements (379.50-379.59)
DEF: Misalignment of the eyes due to imbalance in extraocular muscles.

√5th **378.0 Esotropia**
Convergent concomitant strabismus
EXCLUDES intermittent esotropia (378.20-378.22)
DEF: Visual axis deviation created by one eye fixing upon an image and the other eye deviating inward.

- 378.00 Esotropia, unspecified
- 378.01 Monocular esotropia
- 378.02 Monocular esotropia with A pattern
- 378.03 Monocular esotropia with V pattern
- 378.04 Monocular esotropia with other noncomitancies
  Monocular esotropia with X or Y pattern
- 378.05 Alternating esotropia
- 378.06 Alternating esotropia with A pattern
- 378.07 Alternating esotropia with V pattern
- 378.08 Alternating esotropia with other noncomitancies
  Alternating esotropia with X or Y pattern

√5th **378.1 Exotropia**
Divergent concomitant strabismus
EXCLUDES intermittent exotropia (378.20, 378.23-378.24)
DEF: Visual axis deviation created by one eye fixing upon an image and the other eye deviating outward.

- 378.10 Exotropia, unspecified
- 378.11 Monocular exotropia
- 378.12 Monocular exotropia with A pattern
- 378.13 Monocular exotropia with V pattern
- 378.14 Monocular exotropia with other noncomitancies
  Monocular exotropia with X or Y pattern
- 378.15 Alternating exotropia
- 378.16 Alternating exotropia with A pattern
- 378.17 Alternating exotropia with V pattern
- 378.18 Alternating exotropia with other noncomitancies
  Alternating exotropia with X or Y pattern

√5th **378.2 Intermittent heterotropia**
EXCLUDES vertical heterotropia (intermittent) (378.31)
DEF: Deviation of eyes seen only at intervals; it is also called strabismus.

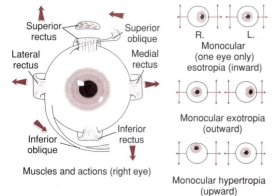

- 378.20 Intermittent heterotropia, unspecified
  Intermittent: esotropia NOS   Intermittent: exotropia NOS
- 378.21 Intermittent esotropia, monocular
- 378.22 Intermittent esotropia, alternating
- 378.23 Intermittent exotropia, monocular
- 378.24 Intermittent exotropia, alternating

√5th **378.3 Other and unspecified heterotropia**
- 378.30 Heterotropia, unspecified
- 378.31 Hypertropia
  Vertical heterotropia (constant) (intermittent)
- 378.32 Hypotropia
- 378.33 Cyclotropia
- 378.34 Monofixation syndrome
  Microtropia
- 378.35 Accommodative component in esotropia

√5th **378.4 Heterophoria**
DEF: Deviation occurring only when the other eye is covered..
- 378.40 Heterophoria, unspecified
- 378.41 Esophoria
- 378.42 Exophoria
- 378.43 Vertical heterophoria
- 378.44 Cyclophoria
- 378.45 Alternating hyperphoria

√5th **378.5 Paralytic strabismus**
DEF: Deviation of the eye due to nerve paralysis affecting muscle.
- 378.50 Paralytic strabismus, unspecified
- 378.51 Third or oculomotor nerve palsy, partial
  AHA: 3Q, '91, 9
- 378.52 Third or oculomotor nerve palsy, total
  AHA: 2Q, '89, 12
- 378.53 Fourth or trochlear nerve palsy
  AHA: 2Q, '01, 21
- 378.54 Sixth or abducens nerve palsy
  AHA: 2Q, '89, 12
- 378.55 External ophthalmoplegia
- 378.56 Total ophthalmoplegia

√5th **378.6 Mechanical strabismus**
DEF: Deviation of the eye due to an outside force upon the extraocular muscles.
- 378.60 Mechanical strabismus, unspecified
- 378.61 Brown's (tendon) sheath syndrome
  DEF: Congenital or acquired shortening of the anterior sheath of the superior oblique muscle; the eye is unable to move upward and inward; it is usually unilateral.
- 378.62 Mechanical strabismus from other musculofascial disorders
- 378.63 Limited duction associated with other conditions

√5th **378.7 Other specified strabismus**
- 378.71 Duane's syndrome
  DEF: Congenital; affects one eye; due to abnormal fibrous bands attached to rectus muscle; inability to abduct affected eye with retraction of globe.
- 378.72 Progressive external ophthalmoplegia
  DEF: Paralysis progressing from one eye muscle to another.
- 378.73 Strabismus in other neuromuscular disorders

√5th **378.8 Other disorders of binocular eye movements**
EXCLUDES nystagmus (379.50-379.56)
- 378.81 Palsy of conjugate gaze
  DEF: Paralysis progressing from one eye muscle to another.

378.82–379.50 NERVOUS SYSTEM AND SENSE ORGANS

378.82 Spasm of conjugate gaze
DEF: Muscle contractions impairing parallel movement of eye.

378.83 Convergence insufficiency or palsy
378.84 Convergence excess or spasm
378.85 Anomalies of divergence
378.86 Internuclear ophthalmoplegia
DEF: Eye movement anomaly due to brainstem lesion.

378.87 Other dissociated deviation of eye movements
Skew deviation

378.9 Unspecified disorder of eye movements
Ophthalmoplegia NOS   Strabismus NOS
AHA: 2Q, '01, 21

✓4th 379 Other disorders of eye

✓5th 379.0 Scleritis and episcleritis
EXCLUDES   syphilitic episcleritis (095.0)

379.00 Scleritis, unspecified
Episcleritis NOS

379.01 Episcleritis periodica fugax
DEF: Hyperemia (engorgement) of the sclera and overlying conjunctiva characterized by a sudden onset and short duration.

379.02 Nodular episcleritis
DEF: Inflammation of the outermost layer of the sclera, with formation of nodules.

379.03 Anterior scleritis
379.04 Scleromalacia perforans
DEF: Scleral thinning, softening and degeneration; seen with rheumatoid arthritis.

379.05 Scleritis with corneal involvement
Scleroperikeratitis

379.06 Brawny scleritis
DEF: Severe scleral inflammation with thickening corneal margins.

379.07 Posterior scleritis
Sclerotenonitis

379.09 Other
Scleral abscess

✓5th 379.1 Other disorders of sclera
EXCLUDES   blue sclera (743.47)

379.11 Scleral ectasia
Scleral staphyloma NOS
DEF: Protrusion of the contents of the eyeball where the sclera has thinned.

379.12 Staphyloma posticum
DEF: Ring-shaped protrusion or bulging of sclera and uveal tissue at posterior pole of eye.

379.13 Equatorial staphyloma
DEF: Ring-shaped protrusion or bulging of sclera and uveal tissue midway between front and back of eye.

379.14 Anterior staphyloma, localized
379.15 Ring staphyloma
379.16 Other degenerative disorders of sclera
379.19 Other

✓5th 379.2 Disorders of vitreous body
DEF: Disorder of clear gel that fills space between retina and lens.

379.21 Vitreous degeneration
Vitreous: cavitation   Vitreous: liquefaction
detachment

379.22 Crystalline deposits in vitreous
Asteroid hyalitis   Synchysis scintillans

379.23 Vitreous hemorrhage
AHA: 3Q, '91, 15

379.24 Other vitreous opacities
Vitreous floaters

379.25 Vitreous membranes and strands
379.26 Vitreous prolapse
DEF: Slipping of vitreous from normal position.

379.29 Other disorders of vitreous
EXCLUDES   vitreous abscess (360.04)
AHA: 1Q, '99, 11

✓5th 379.3 Aphakia and other disorders of lens
EXCLUDES   after-cataract (366.50-366.53)

379.31 Aphakia
EXCLUDES   cataract extraction status (V45.61)
DEF: Absence of eye's crystalline lens.

379.32 Subluxation of lens
379.33 Anterior dislocation of lens
DEF: Lens displaced toward iris.

379.34 Posterior dislocation of lens
DEF: Lens displaced backward toward vitreous.

379.39 Other disorders of lens

✓5th 379.4 Anomalies of pupillary function
379.40 Abnormal pupillary function, unspecified
379.41 Anisocoria
DEF: Unequal pupil diameter.

379.42 Miosis (persistent), not due to miotics
DEF: Abnormal contraction of pupil less than 2 millimeters.

379.43 Mydriasis (persistent), not due to mydriatics
DEF: Morbid dilation of pupil.

379.45 Argyll Robertson pupil, atypical
Argyll Robertson phenomenon or pupil, nonsyphilitic
EXCLUDES   Argyll Robertson pupil (syphilitic) (094.89)
DEF: Failure of pupil to respond to light; affects both eyes; may be caused by diseases such as syphilis of the central nervous system or miosis.

379.46 Tonic pupillary reaction
Adie's pupil or syndrome

379.49 Other
Hippus   Pupillary paralysis

✓5th 379.5 Nystagmus and other irregular eye movements
379.50 Nystagmus, unspecified
AHA: 2Q, '01, 21
DEF: Involuntary, rapid, rhythmic movement of eyeball; vertical, horizontal, rotatory or mixed; cause may be congenital, acquired, physiological, neurological, myopathic, or due to ocular diseases.

Ear and Mastoid Process

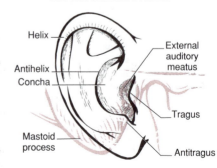

NERVOUS SYSTEM AND SENSE ORGANS

379.51 Congenital nystagmus
379.52 Latent nystagmus
379.53 Visual deprivation nystagmus
379.54 Nystagmus associated with disorders of the vestibular system
379.55 Dissociated nystagmus
379.56 Other forms of nystagmus
379.57 Deficiencies of saccadic eye movements
  Abnormal optokinetic response
  DEF: Saccadic eye movements; small, rapid, involuntary movements by both eyes simultaneously, due to changing point of fixation on visualized object.
379.58 Deficiencies of smooth pursuit movements
379.59 Other irregularities of eye movements
  Opsoclonus

379.8 Other specified disorders of eye and adnexa
√5ᵗʰ 379.9 Unspecified disorder of eye and adnexa
  379.90 Disorder of eye, unspecified
  379.91 Pain in or around eye
  379.92 Swelling or mass of eye
  379.93 Redness or discharge of eye
  379.99 Other ill-defined disorders of eye
    EXCLUDES blurred vision NOS (368.8)

DISEASES OF THE EAR AND MASTOID PROCESS (380-389)

√4ᵗʰ 380 Disorders of external ear
  √5ᵗʰ 380.0 Perichondritis of pinna
    Perichondritis of auricle
    380.00 Perichondritis of pinna, unspecified
    380.01 Acute perichondritis of pinna
    380.02 Chronic perichondritis of pinna
  √5ᵗʰ 380.1 Infective otitis externa
    380.10 Infective otitis externa, unspecified
      Otitis externa (acute):   Otitis externa (acute):
       NOS   hemorrhagica
       circumscribed   infective NOS
       diffuse
    380.11 Acute infection of pinna
      EXCLUDES furuncular otitis externa (680.0)
    380.12 Acute swimmers' ear
      Beach ear   Tank ear
      DEF: Otitis externa due to swimming.
    380.13 Other acute infections of external ear
      Code first underlying disease, as:
       erysipelas (035)
       impetigo (684)
       seborrheic dermatitis (690.10-690.18)
      EXCLUDES herpes simplex (054.73)
                herpes zoster (053.71)
    380.14 Malignant otitis externa
      DEF: Severe necrotic otitis externa; due to bacteria.
    380.15 Chronic mycotic otitis externa
      Code first underlying disease, as:
       aspergillosis (117.3)
       otomycosis NOS (111.9)
      EXCLUDES candidal otitis externa (112.82)
    380.16 Other chronic infective otitis externa
      Chronic infective otitis externa NOS
  √5ᵗʰ 380.2 Other otitis externa
    380.21 Cholesteatoma of external ear
      Keratosis obturans of external ear (canal)
      EXCLUDES cholesteatoma NOS (385.30-385.35)
                postmastoidectomy (383.32)
      DEF: Cystlike mass filled with debris, including cholesterol; rare, congenital condition.

    380.22 Other acute otitis externa
      Acute otitis externa: Acute otitis externa:
       actinic   eczematoid
       chemical   reactive
       contact
    380.23 Other chronic otitis externa
      Chronic otitis externa NOS
  √5ᵗʰ 380.3 Noninfectious disorders of pinna
    380.30 Disorder of pinna, unspecified
    380.31 Hematoma of auricle or pinna
    380.32 Acquired deformities of auricle or pinna
      EXCLUDES cauliflower ear (738.7)
    380.39 Other
      EXCLUDES gouty tophi of ear (274.81)
  380.4 Impacted cerumen
    Wax in ear
  √5ᵗʰ 380.5 Acquired stenosis of external ear canal
    Collapse of external ear canal
    380.50 Acquired stenosis of external ear canal, unspecified as to cause
    380.51 Secondary to trauma
      DEF: Narrowing of the external ear canal; due to trauma.
    380.52 Secondary to surgery
      DEF: Postsurgical narrowing of the external ear canal.
    380.53 Secondary to inflammation
      DEF: Narrowing of the external ear canal; due to chronic inflammation.
  √5ᵗʰ 380.8 Other disorders of external ear
    380.81 Exostosis of external ear canal
    380.89 Other
  380.9 Unspecified disorder of external ear
√4ᵗʰ 381 Nonsuppurative otitis media and Eustachian tube disorders
  √5ᵗʰ 381.0 Acute nonsuppurative otitis media
    Acute tubotympanic catarrh
    Otitis media, acute or subacute:
     catarrhal
     exudative
     transudative
     with effusion
    EXCLUDES otitic barotrauma (993.0)
    381.00 Acute nonsuppurative otitis media, unspecified
    381.01 Acute serous otitis media
      Acute or subacute secretory otitis media
      DEF: Sudden, severe infection of the middle ear.
    381.02 Acute mucoid otitis media
      Acute or subacute seromucinous otitis media
      Blue drum syndrome
      DEF: Sudden, severe infection of the middle ear, with mucous.
    381.03 Acute sanguinous otitis media
      DEF: Sudden, severe infection of the middle ear, with blood.
    381.04 Acute allergic serous otitis media
    381.05 Acute allergic mucoid otitis media
    381.06 Acute allergic sanguinous otitis media
  √5ᵗʰ 381.1 Chronic serous otitis media
    Chronic tubotympanic catarrh
    381.10 Chronic serous otitis media, simple or unspecified
      DEF: Persistent infection of the middle ear, without pus.
    381.19 Other
      Serosanguinous chronic otitis media

381.2 Chronic mucoid otitis media
Glue ear
EXCLUDES adhesive middle ear disease (385.10-385.19)

DEF: Chronic condition; characterized by viscous fluid in middle ear; due to obstructed Eustachian tube.

381.20 Chronic mucoid otitis media, simple or unspecified
381.29 Other
Mucosanguinous chronic otitis media

381.3 Other and unspecified chronic nonsuppurative otitis media
Otitis media, chronic:
- allergic
- exudative
- secretory

Otitis media, chronic:
- seromucinous
- transudative
- with effusion

381.4 Nonsuppurative otitis media, not specified as acute or chronic
Otitis media:
- allergic
- catarrhal
- exudative
- mucoid
- secretory

Otitis media:
- seromucinous
- serous
- transudative
- with effusion

381.5 Eustachian salpingitis
381.50 Eustachian salpingitis, unspecified
381.51 Acute Eustachian salpingitis
DEF: Sudden, severe inflammation of the Eustachian tube.
381.52 Chronic Eustachian salpingitis
DEF: Persistent inflammation of the Eustachian tube.

381.6 Obstruction of Eustachian tube
Stenosis } of Eustachian tube
Stricture
381.60 Obstruction of Eustachian tube, unspecified
381.61 Osseous obstruction of Eustachian tube
Obstruction of Eustachian tube from cholesteatoma, polyp, or other osseous lesion
381.62 Intrinsic cartilagenous obstruction of Eustachian tube
DEF: Blockage of Eustachian tube; due to cartilage overgrowth.
381.63 Extrinsic cartilagenous obstruction of Eustachian tube
Compression of Eustachian tube

381.7 Patulous Eustachian tube
DEF: Distended, oversized Eustachian tube.

381.8 Other disorders of Eustachian tube
381.81 Dysfunction of Eustachian tube
381.89 Other

381.9 Unspecified Eustachian tube disorder

382 Suppurative and unspecified otitis media
382.0 Acute suppurative otitis media
Otitis media, acute:
- necrotizing NOS

Otitis media, acute:
- purulent

382.00 Acute suppurative otitis media without spontaneous rupture of ear drum
DEF: Sudden, severe inflammation of middle ear, with pus.
382.01 Acute suppurative otitis media with spontaneous rupture of ear drum
DEF: Sudden, severe inflammation of middle ear, with pressure tearing ear drum tissue.
382.02 Acute suppurative otitis media in diseases classified elsewhere
Code first underlying disease, as:
influenza (487.8)
scarlet fever (034.1)
EXCLUDES postmeasles otitis (055.2)

382.1 Chronic tubotympanic suppurative otitis media
Benign chronic suppurative otitis media } (with anterior perforation of ear drum)
Chronic tubotympanic disease

DEF: Inflammation of tympanic cavity and auditory tube; with pus formation.

382.2 Chronic atticoantral suppurative otitis media
Chronic atticoantral disease } (with posterior or superior marginal perforation of ear drum)
Persistent mucosal disease

382.3 Unspecified chronic suppurative otitis media
Chronic purulent otitis media
EXCLUDES tuberculous otitis media (017.4)

DEF: Inflammation of upper tympanic membrane and mastoid antrum; with pus formation.

382.4 Unspecified suppurative otitis media
Purulent otitis media NOS

382.9 Unspecified otitis media
Otitis media:
- NOS
- acute NOS

Otitis media:
- chronic NOS

AHA: N-D, '84, 16

383 Mastoiditis and related conditions
383.0 Acute mastoiditis
Abscess of mastoid   Empyema of mastoid
383.00 Acute mastoiditis without complications
DEF: Sudden, severe inflammation of mastoid air cells.
383.01 Subperiosteal abscess of mastoid
CC Excl: 015.60-015.66, 017.40-017.46, 017.90-017.96, 383.00-383.9, 388.71-388.72, 388.8-388.9, 744.00, 744.02, 744.09, 744.29, 744.3

DEF: Pocket of pus within the mastoid bone.
383.02 Acute mastoiditis with other complications
Gradenigo's syndrome

383.1 Chronic mastoiditis
Caries of mastoid
Fistula of mastoid
EXCLUDES tuberculous mastoiditis (015.6)
DEF: Persistent inflammation of the mastoid air cells.

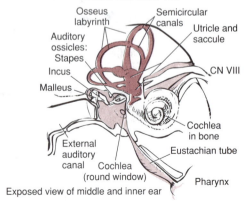

Middle and Inner Ear

Exposed view of middle and inner ear

NERVOUS SYSTEM AND SENSE ORGANS

√5th 383.2 Petrositis
  Coalescing osteitis ⎫
  Inflammation   ⎬ of petrous bone
  Osteomyelitis   ⎭

  383.20 Petrositis, unspecified
  383.21 Acute petrositis
  DEF: Sudden, severe inflammation of dense bone behind the ear.

  383.22 Chronic petrositis
  DEF: Persistent inflammation of dense bone behind the ear.

√5th 383.3 Complications following mastoidectomy
  383.30 Postmastoidectomy complication, unspecified CC
  CC Excl: See code 383.01

  383.31 Mucosal cyst of postmastoidectomy cavity
  DEF: Mucous-lined cyst cavity following removal of mastoid bone.

  383.32 Recurrent cholesteatoma of postmastoidectomy cavity
  DEF: Cystlike mass of cell debris in cavity following removal of mastoid bone.

  383.33 Granulations of postmastoidectomy cavity
  Chronic inflammation of postmastoidectomy cavity
  DEF: Granular tissue in cavity following removal of mastoid bone.

√5th 383.8 Other disorders of mastoid
  383.81 Postauricular fistula CC
  CC Excl: See code 383.01
  DEF: Abnormal passage behind mastoid cavity.

  383.89 Other

  383.9 Unspecified mastoiditis

√4th 384 Other disorders of tympanic membrane

√5th 384.0 Acute myringitis without mention of otitis media
  384.00 Acute myringitis, unspecified
  Acute tympanitis NOS
  DEF: Sudden, severe inflammation of ear drum.

  384.01 Bullous myringitis
  Myringitis bullosa hemorrhagica
  DEF: Type of viral otitis media characterized by the appearance of serous or hemorrhagic blebs on the tympanic membrane.

  384.09 Other

  384.1 Chronic myringitis without mention of otitis media
  Chronic tympanitis
  DEF: Persistent inflammation of ear drum; with no evidence of middle ear infection.

√5th 384.2 Perforation of tympanic membrane
  Perforation of ear drum: NOS persistent posttraumatic
  Perforation of ear drum: postinflammatory
  EXCLUDES otitis media with perforation of tympanic membrane (382.00-382.9)
  traumatic perforation [current injury] (872.61)

  384.20 Perforation of tympanic membrane, unspecified
  384.21 Central perforation of tympanic membrane
  384.22 Attic perforation of tympanic membrane
  Pars flaccida
  384.23 Other marginal perforation of tympanic membrane
  384.24 Multiple perforations of tympanic membrane
  384.25 Total perforation of tympanic membrane

√5th 384.8 Other specified disorders of tympanic membrane
  384.81 Atrophic flaccid tympanic membrane
  Healed perforation of ear drum
  384.82 Atrophic nonflaccid tympanic membrane

  384.9 Unspecified disorder of tympanic membrane

√4th 385 Other disorders of middle ear and mastoid
  EXCLUDES mastoiditis (383.0-383.9)

√5th 385.0 Tympanosclerosis
  385.00 Tympanosclerosis, unspecified as to involvement
  385.01 Tympanosclerosis involving tympanic membrane only
  DEF: Tough, fibrous tissue impeding functions of ear drum.

  385.02 Tympanosclerosis involving tympanic membrane and ear ossicles
  DEF: Tough, fibrous tissue impeding functions of middle ear bones (stapes, malleus, incus).

  385.03 Tympanosclerosis involving tympanic membrane, ear ossicles, and middle ear
  DEF: Tough, fibrous tissue impeding functions of ear drum, middle ear bones and middle ear canal.

  385.09 Tympanosclerosis involving other combination of structures

√5th 385.1 Adhesive middle ear disease
  Adhesive otitis   Otitis media:
  Otitis media: fibrotic
  chronic adhesive
  EXCLUDES glue ear (381.20-381.29)
  DEF: Adhesions of middle ear structures.

  385.10 Adhesive middle ear disease, unspecified as to involvement
  385.11 Adhesions of drum head to incus
  385.12 Adhesions of drum head to stapes
  385.13 Adhesions of drum head to promontorium
  385.19 Other adhesions and combinations

√5th 385.2 Other acquired abnormality of ear ossicles
  385.21 Impaired mobility of malleus
  Ankylosis of malleus
  385.22 Impaired mobility of other ear ossicles
  Ankylosis of ear ossicles, except malleus
  385.23 Discontinuity or dislocation of ear ossicles
  DEF: Disruption in auditory chain; created by malleus, incus and stapes.

  385.24 Partial loss or necrosis of ear ossicles
  DEF: Tissue loss in malleus, incus and stapes.

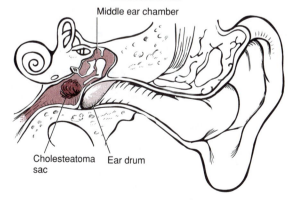

Cholesteatoma
Middle ear chamber
Cholesteatoma sac   Ear drum

385.3 Cholesteatoma of middle ear and mastoid

Cholesterosis ⎫
Epidermosis ⎬ of (middle) ear
Keratosis   ⎪
Polyp   ⎭

EXCLUDES cholesteatoma:
  external ear canal (380.21)
  recurrent of postmastoidectomy cavity (383.32)

DEF: Cystlike mass of middle ear and mastoid antrum filled with debris, including cholesterol.

- 385.30 Cholesteatoma, unspecified
- 385.31 Cholesteatoma of attic
- 385.32 Cholesteatoma of middle ear
- 385.33 Cholesteatoma of middle ear and mastoid
  AHA: 3Q, '00, 10
  DEF: Cystlike mass of cell debris in middle ear and mastoid air cells behind ear.
- 385.35 Diffuse cholesteatosis

385.8 Other disorders of middle ear and mastoid
- 385.82 Cholesterin granuloma
  DEF: Granuloma formed of fibrotic tissue; contains cholesterol crystals surrounded by foreign-body cells; found in the middle ear and mastoid area.
- 385.83 Retained foreign body of middle ear
  AHA: 3Q, '94, 7; N-D, '87, 9
- 385.89 Other

385.9 Unspecified disorder of middle ear and mastoid

386 Vertiginous syndromes and other disorders of vestibular system

EXCLUDES vertigo NOS (780.4)

AHA: M-A, '85, 12

386.0 Ménière's disease
Endolymphatic hydrops
Lermoyez's syndrome
Ménière's syndrome or vertigo

DEF: Distended membranous labyrinth of middle ear from endolymphatic hydrops; causes ischemia, failure of nerve function; hearing and balance dysfunction; symptoms include fluctuating deafness, ringing in ears and dizziness.

- 386.00 Ménière's disease, unspecified
  Ménière's disease (active)
- 386.01 Active Ménière's disease, cochleovestibular
- 386.02 Active Ménière's disease, cochlear
- 386.03 Active Ménière's disease, vestibular
- 386.04 Inactive Ménière's disease
  Ménière's disease in remission

386.1 Other and unspecified peripheral vertigo
EXCLUDES epidemic vertigo (078.81)
- 386.10 Peripheral vertigo, unspecified
- 386.11 Benign paroxysmal positional vertigo
  Benign paroxysmal positional nystagmus
- 386.12 Vestibular neuronitis
  Acute (and recurrent) peripheral vestibulopathy
  DEF: Transient benign vertigo, unknown cause; characterized by response to caloric stimulation on one side, nystagmus with rhythmic movement of eyes; normal auditory function present; occurs in young adults.
- 386.19 Other
  Aural vertigo
  Otogenic vertigo

386.2 Vertigo of central origin
Central positional nystagmus
Malignant positional vertigo

386.3 Labyrinthitis
- 386.30 Labyrinthitis, unspecified
- 386.31 Serous labyrinthitis
  Diffuse labyrinthitis
  DEF: Inflammation of labyrinth; with fluid buildup.
- 386.32 Circumscribed labyrinthitis
  Focal labyrinthitis
- 386.33 Suppurative labyrinthitis
  Purulent labyrinthitis
  DEF: Inflammation of labyrinth; with pus.
- 386.34 Toxic labyrinthitis
  DEF: Inflammation of labyrinth; due to toxic reaction.
- 386.35 Viral labyrinthitis

386.4 Labyrinthine fistula
- 386.40 Labyrinthine fistula, unspecified
- 386.41 Round window fistula
- 386.42 Oval window fistula
- 386.43 Semicircular canal fistula
- 386.48 Labyrinthine fistula of combined sites

386.5 Labyrinthine dysfunction
- 386.50 Labyrinthine dysfunction, unspecified
- 386.51 Hyperactive labyrinth, unilateral
  DEF: Oversensitivity of labyrinth to auditory signals; affecting one ear.
- 386.52 Hyperactive labyrinth, bilateral
  DEF: Oversensitivity of labyrinth to auditory signals; affecting both ears.
- 386.53 Hypoactive labyrinth, unilateral
  DEF: Reduced sensitivity of labyrinth to auditory signals; affecting one ear.
- 386.54 Hypoactive labyrinth, bilateral
  DEF: Reduced sensitivity of labyrinth to auditory signals; affecting both ears.
- 386.55 Loss of labyrinthine reactivity, unilateral
  DEF: Reduced reaction of labyrinth to auditory signals; affecting one ear.
- 386.56 Loss of labyrinthine reactivity, bilateral
  DEF: Reduced reaction of labyrinth to auditory signals; affecting both ears.
- 386.58 Other forms and combinations

386.8 Other disorders of labyrinth
386.9 Unspecified vertiginous syndromes and labyrinthine disorders

387 Otosclerosis
INCLUDES otospongiosis

DEF: Synonym for otospongiosis, spongy bone formation in the labyrinth bones of the ear; it causes progressive hearing impairment.

- 387.0 Otosclerosis involving oval window, nonobliterative
  DEF: Tough, fibrous tissue impeding functions of oval window.
- 387.1 Otosclerosis involving oval window, obliterative
  DEF: Tough, fibrous tissue blocking oval window.
- 387.2 Cochlear otosclerosis
  Otosclerosis involving: otic capsule
  Otosclerosis involving: round window
  DEF: Tough, fibrous tissue impeding functions of cochlea.
- 387.8 Other otosclerosis
- 387.9 Otosclerosis, unspecified

388 Other disorders of ear

388.0 Degenerative and vascular disorders of ear
- 388.00 Degenerative and vascular disorders, unspecified
- 388.01 Presbyacusis
  DEF: Progressive, bilateral perceptive hearing loss caused by advancing age; it is also known as presbycusis.

Tabular List — **NERVOUS SYSTEM AND SENSE ORGANS** — 388.02–389.9

- 388.02 **Transient ischemic deafness**
  DEF: Restricted blood flow to auditory organs causing temporary hearing loss.

✓5ᵗʰ 388.1 **Noise effects on inner ear**
- 388.10 Noise effects on inner ear, unspecified
- 388.11 Acoustic trauma (explosive) to ear
  Otitic blast injury
- 388.12 Noise-induced hearing loss

388.2 **Sudden hearing loss, unspecified**

✓5ᵗʰ 388.3 **Tinnitus**
DEF: Abnormal noises in ear; may be heard by others beside the affected individual; noises include ringing, clicking, roaring and buzzing.
- 388.30 Tinnitus, unspecified
- 388.31 Subjective tinnitus
- 388.32 Objective tinnitus

✓5ᵗʰ 388.4 **Other abnormal auditory perception**
- 388.40 Abnormal auditory perception, unspecified
- 388.41 Diplacusis
  DEF: Perception of a single auditory sound as two sounds at two different levels of intensity.
- 388.42 Hyperacusis
  DEF: Exceptionally acute sense of hearing caused by such conditions as Bell's palsy; this term may also refer to painful sensitivity to sounds.
- 388.43 Impairment of auditory discrimination
  DEF: Impaired ability to distinguish tone of sound.
- 388.44 Recruitment
  DEF: Perception of abnormally increased loudness caused by a slight increase in sound intensity; it is a term used in audiology.

388.5 **Disorders of acoustic nerve**
  Acoustic neuritis
  Degeneration } of acoustic or eighth nerve
  Disorder
  EXCLUDES acoustic neuroma (225.1)
            syphilitic acoustic neuritis (094.86)
  AHA: M-A, '87, 8

✓5ᵗʰ 388.6 **Otorrhea**
- 388.60 Otorrhea, unspecified
  Discharging ear NOS
- 388.61 Cerebrospinal fluid otorrhea
  EXCLUDES cerebrospinal fluid rhinorrhea (349.81)
  DEF: Spinal fluid leakage from ear.
- 388.69 Other
  Otorrhagia

✓5ᵗʰ 388.7 **Otalgia**
- 388.70 Otalgia, unspecified
  Earache NOS
- 388.71 Otogenic pain
- 388.72 Referred pain

388.8 **Other disorders of ear**

388.9 **Unspecified disorder of ear**

✓4ᵗʰ 389 **Hearing loss**

✓5ᵗʰ 389.0 **Conductive hearing loss**
  Conductive deafness
  AHA: 4Q, '89, 5
  DEF: Dysfunction in sound-conducting structures of external or middle ear causing hearing loss.
- 389.00 Conductive hearing loss, unspecified
- 389.01 Conductive hearing loss, external ear
- 389.02 Conductive hearing loss, tympanic membrane
- 389.03 Conductive hearing loss, middle ear
- 389.04 Conductive hearing loss, inner ear
- 389.08 Conductive hearing loss of combined types

✓5ᵗʰ 389.1 **Sensorineural hearing loss**
  Perceptive hearing loss or deafness
  EXCLUDES abnormal auditory perception (388.40-388.44)
            psychogenic deafness (306.7)
  AHA: 4Q, '89, 5
  DEF: Nerve conduction causing hearing loss.
- 389.10 Sensorineural hearing loss, unspecified
  AHA: 1Q, '93, 29
- 389.11 Sensory hearing loss
- 389.12 Neural hearing loss
- 389.14 Central hearing loss
- 389.18 Sensorineural hearing loss of combined types

389.2 **Mixed conductive and sensorineural hearing loss**
  Deafness or hearing loss of type classifiable to 389.0 with type classifiable to 389.1

389.7 **Deaf mutism, not elsewhere classifiable**
  Deaf, nonspeaking

389.8 **Other specified forms of hearing loss**

389.9 **Unspecified hearing loss**
  Deafness NOS

7. DISEASES OF THE CIRCULATORY SYSTEM (390-459)

ACUTE RHEUMATIC FEVER (390-392)

DEF: Febrile disease occurs mainly in children or young adults following throat infection by group A *streptococci*; symptoms include fever, joint pain, lesions of heart, blood vessels and joint connective tissue, abdominal pain, skin changes, and chorea.

390 Rheumatic fever without mention of heart involvement
Arthritis, rheumatic, acute or subacute
Rheumatic fever (active) (acute)
Rheumatism, articular, acute or subacute
EXCLUDES that with heart involvement (391.0-391.9)

✓4th **391 Rheumatic fever with heart involvement**
EXCLUDES chronic heart diseases of rheumatic origin (398.0-398.9) unless rheumatic fever is also present or there is evidence of recrudescence or activity of the rheumatic process

391.0 Acute rheumatic pericarditis
Rheumatic:
 fever (active) (acute) with pericarditis
 pericarditis (acute)
Any condition classifiable to 390 with pericarditis
EXCLUDES that not specified as rheumatic (420.0-420.9)

DEF: Sudden, severe inflammation of heart lining due to rheumatic fever.

391.1 Acute rheumatic endocarditis
Rheumatic:
 endocarditis, acute
 fever (active) (acute) with endocarditis or valvulitis
 valvulitis acute
Any condition classifiable to 390 with endocarditis or valvulitis

DEF: Sudden, severe inflammation of heart cavities due to rheumatic fever.

391.2 Acute rheumatic myocarditis
Rheumatic fever (active) (acute) with myocarditis
Any condition classifiable to 390 with myocarditis

DEF: Sudden, severe inflammation of heart muscles due to rheumatic fever.

391.8 Other acute rheumatic heart disease
Rheumatic:
 fever (active) (acute) with other or multiple types of heart involvement
 pancarditis, acute
Any condition classifiable to 390 with other or multiple types of heart involvement

391.9 Acute rheumatic heart disease, unspecified
Rheumatic:
 carditis, acute
 fever (active) (acute) with unspecified type of heart involvement
 heart disease, active or acute
Any condition classifiable to 390 with unspecified type of heart involvement

✓4th **392 Rheumatic chorea**
INCLUDES Sydenham's chorea
EXCLUDES chorea:
 NOS (333.5)
 Huntington's (333.4)

DEF: Childhood disease linked with rheumatic fever and streptococcal infections; symptoms include spasmodic, involuntary movements of limbs or facial muscles, psychic symptoms, and irritability.

392.0 With heart involvement
Rheumatic chorea with heart involvement of any type classifiable to 391

392.9 Without mention of heart involvement

CHRONIC RHEUMATIC HEART DISEASE (393-398)

393 Chronic rheumatic pericarditis
Adherent pericardium, rheumatic
Chronic rheumatic:
 mediastinopericarditis
 myopericarditis
EXCLUDES pericarditis NOS or not specified as rheumatic (423.0-423.9)

DEF: Persistent inflammation of heart lining due to rheumatic heart disease.

✓4th **394 Diseases of mitral valve**
EXCLUDES that with aortic valve involvement (396.0-396.9)

394.0 Mitral stenosis CC
Mitral (valve): Mitral (valve):
 obstruction (rheumatic) stenosis NOS
CC Excl: 390, 391.8-391.9, 394.0-394.9, 396.0-396.9, 397.9, 398.90, 398.99, 424.0, 459.89, 459.9

DEF: Narrowing, of mitral valve between left atrium and left ventricle; due to rheumatic heart disease.

394.1 Rheumatic mitral insufficiency CC
Rheumatic mitral: Rheumatic mitral:
 incompetence regurgitation
EXCLUDES that not specified as rheumatic (424.0)
CC Excl: See code 394.0

DEF: Malfunction of mitral valve between left atrium and left ventricle; due to rheumatic heart disease.

394.2 Mitral stenosis with insufficiency CC
Mitral stenosis with incompetence or regurgitation
CC Excl: See code 394.0

DEF: A narrowing or stricture of the mitral valve situated between the left atrium and left ventricle. The stenosis interferes with blood flow from the atrium into the ventricle. If the valve does not completely close, it becomes insufficient (inadequate) and cannot prevent regurgitation (abnormal backward flow) into the atrium when the left ventricle contracts. This abnormal function is also called incompetence.

394.9 Other and unspecified mitral valve diseases CC
Mitral (valve): Mitral (valve):
 disease (chronic) failure
CC Excl: See code 394.0

✓4th **395 Diseases of aortic valve**
EXCLUDES that not specified as rheumatic (424.1)
 that with mitral valve involvement (396.0-396.9)

395.0 Rheumatic aortic stenosis CC
Rheumatic aortic (valve) obstruction
CC Excl: 390, 391.8-391.9, 395.0-395.9, 396.0-396.9, 397.9, 398.90, 398.99, 424.1, 459.89, 459.9

AHA: 4Q, '88, 8

DEF: Narrowing of the aortic valve; results in backflow into ventricle; due to rheumatic heart disease.

395.1 Rheumatic aortic insufficiency CC
Rheumatic aortic: Rheumatic aortic:
 incompetence regurgitation
CC Excl: See code 395.0

DEF: Malfunction of the aortic valve; results in backflow into left ventricle; due to rheumatic heart disease.

395.2 Rheumatic aortic stenosis with insufficiency CC
Rheumatic aortic stenosis with incompetence or regurgitation
CC Excl: See code 395.0

DEF: Malfunction and narrowing, of the aortic valve; results in backflow into left ventricle; due to rheumatic heart disease.

395.9 Other and unspecified rheumatic aortic diseases CC
Rheumatic aortic (valve) disease
CC Excl: See code 395.0

CIRCULATORY SYSTEM

✓4th 396 Diseases of mitral and aortic valves
INCLUDES involvement of both mitral and aortic valves, whether specified as rheumatic or not

AHA: N-D, '87, 8

396.0 Mitral valve stenosis and aortic valve stenosis CC
Atypical aortic (valve) stenosis
Mitral and aortic (valve) obstruction (rheumatic)
CC Excl: 390, 391.8-391.9, 394.0-394.9, 395.0-395.9, 396.0-396.9, 397.9, 398.90, 398.99, 424.0-424.1, 459.89, 459.9

396.1 Mitral valve stenosis and aortic valve insufficiency CC
CC Excl: See code 396.0

396.2 Mitral valve insufficiency and aortic valve stenosis CC
CC Excl: See code 396.0
AHA: 2Q, '00, 16

396.3 Mitral valve insufficiency and aortic valve insufficiency CC
Mitral and aortic (valve): incompetence
Mitral and aortic (valve): regurgitation
CC Excl: See code 396.0

396.8 Multiple involvement of mitral and aortic valves CC
Stenosis and insufficiency of mitral or aortic valve with stenosis or insufficiency, or both, of the other valve
CC Excl: See code 396.0

396.9 Mitral and aortic valve diseases, unspecified CC
CC Excl: See code 396.0

✓4th 397 Diseases of other endocardial structures
397.0 Diseases of tricuspid valve CC
Tricuspid (valve) (rheumatic): disease, insufficiency, obstruction
Tricuspid (valve) (rheumatic): regurgitation, stenosis
CC Excl: 397.0, 398.90, 398.99, 424.2, 459.89, 459.9
AHA: 2Q, '00, 16
DEF: Malfunction of the valve between right atrium and right ventricle; due to rheumatic heart disease.

397.1 Rheumatic diseases of pulmonary valve CC
EXCLUDES that not specified as rheumatic (424.3)
CC Excl: 397.1, 398.90, 398.99, 424.3, 459.89, 459.9

397.9 Rheumatic diseases of endocardium, valve unspecified CC
Rheumatic: endocarditis (chronic), valvulitis (chronic)
EXCLUDES that not specified as rheumatic (424.90-424.99)
CC Excl: 390, 391.1, 391.8-391.9, 394.0-394.9, 395.0-395.9, 397.1, 397.9, 398.90, 398.99, 421.0-421.9, 424.0-424.99, 459.89, 459.9

✓4th 398 Other rheumatic heart disease
398.0 Rheumatic myocarditis CC
Rheumatic degeneration of myocardium
EXCLUDES myocarditis not specified as rheumatic (429.0)
CC Excl: 390, 391.2-391.9, 398.0, 398.90, 398.99, 422.0, 422.90-422.99, 429.0, 429.71, 429.79, 459.89, 459.9
DEF: Chronic inflammation of heart muscle; due to rheumatic heart disease.

✓5th 398.9 Other and unspecified rheumatic heart diseases
398.90 Rheumatic heart disease, unspecified
Rheumatic: carditis, heart disease NOS
EXCLUDES carditis not specified as rheumatic (429.89)
heart disease NOS not specified as rheumatic (429.9)

398.91 Rheumatic heart failure (congestive) CC MC
Rheumatic left ventricular failure
CC Excl: 398.90-398.99, 402.01, 402.11, 402.91, 428.0-428.9, 459.89, 459.9
AHA: 1Q, '95, 6; 3Q, '88, 3
DEF: Decreased cardiac output, edema and hypertension; due to rheumatic heart disease.

398.99 Other

HYPERTENSIVE DISEASE (401-405)
EXCLUDES that complicating pregnancy, childbirth, or the puerperium (642.0-642.9)
that involving coronary vessels (410.00-414.9)

AHA: 3Q, '90, 3; 2Q, '89, 12; S-O, '87, 9; J-A, '84, 11

✓4th 401 Essential hypertension
INCLUDES high blood pressure
hyperpiesia
hyperpiesis
hypertension (arterial) (essential) (primary) (systemic)
hypertensive vascular: degeneration, disease
EXCLUDES elevated blood pressure without diagnosis of hypertension (796.2)
pulmonary hypertension (416.0-416.9)
that involving vessels of: brain (430-438), eye (362.11)

AHA: 2Q, '92, 5
DEF: Hypertension that occurs without apparent organic cause; idiopathic.

401.0 Malignant CC
CC Excl: 401.0-401.9, 402.00-402.91, 403.00-403.91, 404.00-404.93, 405.01-405.99, 459.89, 459.9
AHA: M-J, '85, 19
DEF: Severe high arterial blood pressure; results in necrosis in kidney, retina, etc.; hemorrhages occur and death commonly due to uremia or rupture of cerebral vessel.

401.1 Benign
DEF: Mildly elevated arterial blood pressure.

401.9 Unspecified
AHA: 4Q, '97, 37

✓4th 402 Hypertensive heart disease
INCLUDES hypertensive: cardiomegaly, cardiopathy, cardiovascular disease, heart (disease) (failure)
any condition classifiable to 428, 429.0-429.3, 429.8, 429.9 due to hypertension
▶Use additional code to specify type of heart failure (428.0, 428.20-428.23, 428.30-428.33, 428.40-428.43)◀

AHA: 2Q, '93, 9; N-D, '84, 18

✓5th 402.0 Malignant
402.00 Without heart failure CC
CC Excl: See code 401.0

CIRCULATORY SYSTEM

▲   **402.01 With heart failure** `CC` `MC` `CD`
        CC Excl: 398.91, 401.0-401.9, 402.00-402.91, 403.00-403.91, 404.00-404.93, 405.01-405.99, 428.0-428.9, 459.89, 459.9

√5th **402.1 Benign**
▲   **402.10 Without heart failure**
▲   **402.11 With heart failure** `CC` `MC` `CD`
        CC Excl: See code 402.01

√5th **402.9 Unspecified**
▲   **402.90 Without heart failure**
▲   **402.91 With heart failure** `CC` `MC` `CD`
        CC Excl: See code 402.01

        AHA: 1Q, '93, 19; 2Q, '89, 12

        ▽ DRG 127

√4th **403 Hypertensive renal disease**
    INCLUDES   arteriolar nephritis
        arteriosclerosis of:
          kidney
          renal arterioles
        arteriosclerotic nephritis (chronic) (interstitial)
        hypertensive:
          nephropathy
          renal failure
          uremia (chronic)
        nephrosclerosis
        renal sclerosis with hypertension
        any condition classifiable to 585, 586, or 587
          with any condition classifiable to 401
    EXCLUDES   *acute renal failure (584.5-584.9)*
        renal disease stated as not due to hypertension
        renovascular hypertension (405.0-405.9 with fifth-digit 1)

> The following fifth-digit subclassification is for use with category 403:
>   0 without mention of renal failure
>   1 with renal failure

AHA: 4Q, '92, 22; 2Q, '92, 5

√5th **403.0 Malignant** `CC`
    CC Excl: 401.0-401.9, 402.00-402.91, 403.00-403.91, 404.00-404.93, 405.01-405.99, 459.89, 459.9

√5th **403.1 Benign** `CC 1`
    CC Excl: For code 403.11: See code 403.0

√5th **403.9 Unspecified** `CC 1`
    CC Excl: For code 403.91: See code 403.0

    AHA: For code 403.91: 2Q, '01, 11; 3Q, '91, 8

    ▽ DRG 316 For code 403.91

√4th **404 Hypertensive heart and renal disease**
    INCLUDES   disease:
        cardiorenal
        cardiovascular renal
    any condition classifiable to 402 with any condition classifiable to 403
▶Use additional code to specify type of heart failure (428.0, 428.20-428.23, 428.30-428.33, 428.40-428.43)◀

> The following fifth-digit subclassification is for use with category 404:
> ▲   0 without mention of heart failure or renal failure
> ▲   1 with heart failure
>   2 with renal failure
> ▲   3 with heart failure and renal failure

AHA: 3Q, '90, 3; J-A, '84, 14

√5th **404.0 Malignant** `CC`
    CC Excl: See code 403.0

√5th **404.1 Benign** `CC 1-3`
    CC Excl: For codes 404.11-404.13: See code 403.0

√5th **404.9 Unspecified** `CC 1-3`
    CC Excl: For codes 404.91-404.93: See code 403.0

√4th **405 Secondary hypertension**
    AHA: 3Q, '90, 3; S-O, '87, 9, 11; J-A, '84, 14

    DEF: High arterial blood pressure due to or with a variety of primary diseases, such as renal disorders, CNS disorders, endocrine, and vascular diseases.

√5th **405.0 Malignant**
     405.01 Renovascular `CC`
        CC Excl: 401.0-401.9, 402.00-402.91, 403.00-403.91, 404.00-404.93, 405.01-405.99, 459.89, 459.9

     405.09 Other `CC`
        CC Excl: See code 405.01

√5th **405.1 Benign**
     405.11 Renovascular
     405.19 Other

√5th **405.9 Unspecified**
     405.91 Renovascular
     405.99 Other
        AHA: 3Q, '00, 4

ISCHEMIC HEART DISEASE (410-414)

    INCLUDES   that with mention of hypertension
Use additional code to identify presence of hypertension (401.0-405.9)
AHA: 3Q, '91, 10; J-A, '84, 5

√4th **410 Acute myocardial infarction**
    INCLUDES   cardiac infarction
        coronary (artery):
          embolism
          occlusion
          rupture
          thrombosis
        infarction of heart, myocardium, or ventricle
        rupture of heart, myocardium, or ventricle
        any condition classifiable to 414.1-414.9
          specified as acute or with a stated duration of 8 weeks or less

> The following fifth-digit subclassification is for use with category 410:
>   0 episode of care unspecified
>   Use when the source document does not contain sufficient information for the assignment of fifth digit 1 or 2.
>   1 initial episode of care
>   Use fifth-digit 1 to designate the first episode of care (regardless of facility site) for a newly diagnosed myocardial infarction. The fifth-digit 1 is assigned regardless of the number of times a patient may be transferred during the initial episode of care.
>   2 subsequent episode of care
>   Use fifth-digit 2 to designate an episode of care following the initial episode when the patient is admitted for further observation, evaluation or treatment for a myocardial infarction that has received initial treatment, but is still less than 8 weeks old.

AHA: 3Q, '01, 21; 3Q, '98, 15; 4Q, '97, 37; 3Q, '95, 9; 4Q, '92, 24; 1Q, '92,10; 3Q, '91, 18; 1Q, '91, 14; 3Q, '89, 3

DEF: A sudden insufficiency of blood supply to an area of the heart muscle; usually due to a coronary artery occlusion.

√5th **410.0 Of anterolateral wall** `CC 1` `A`
    CC Excl: For code 410.01: 410.00-410.92, 459.89, 459.9

√4th Additional Digit Required   Nonspecific PDx   Unacceptable PDx    Manifestation Code   Medicare Secondary Payer   ▶◀ Revised Text   ● New Code   ▲ Revised Code Title

2002 Ingenix, Inc.   October 2002 • Volume 1 — 117

410.1–413.0 CIRCULATORY SYSTEM — Tabular List

Acute Myocardial Infarction

Anatomic Sites:
- Anterolateral 410.0
- Anteroseptal 410.1
- Apical 410.1
- Other lateral 410.5
- Inferoposterior 410.3
- Other and septum 410.4
- Posterobasal 410.6
- Posterolateral 410.5
- Atrium only 410.8
- Septum only
- Papillary muscle

√5th 410.1 Of other anterior wall [CC 1] [A]
Infarction:
- anterior (wall) NOS
- anteroapical
- anteroseptal

(with contiguous portion of intraventricular septum)

CC Excl: For code 410.11: See code 410.0

DRG 121 and 122 For code 410.11

√5th 410.2 Of inferolateral wall [CC 1] [A]
CC Excl: For code 410.21: See code 410.0

√5th 410.3 Of inferoposterior wall [CC 1] [A]
CC Excl: For code 410.31: See code 410.0

√5th 410.4 Of other inferior wall [CC 1] [A]
Infarction:
- diaphragmatic wall NOS
- inferior (wall) NOS

(with contiguous portion of intraventricular septum)

CC Excl: For code 410.41: See code 410.0

AHA: 1Q, '00, 7, 26; 4Q, '99, 9; 3Q, '97, 10

AHA: For code 410.41: 2Q, '01, 8, 9

DRG 121 and 122 For code 410.41

√5th 410.5 Of other lateral wall [CC 1] [A]
Infarction:
- apical-lateral
- basal-lateral
- high lateral
- posterolateral

CC Excl: For code 410.51: See code 410.0

√5th 410.6 True posterior wall infarction [CC 1] [A]
Infarction:
- posterobasal
- strictly posterior

CC Excl: For code 410.61: See code 410.0

√5th 410.7 Subendocardial infarction [CC 1] [A]
Nontransmural infarction

CC Excl: For code 410.71: See code 410.0

AHA: 1Q, '00, 7

DRG 121 and 122 For code 410.71

√5th 410.8 Of other specified sites [CC 1] [A]
Infarction of:
- atrium
- papillary muscle
- septum alone

CC Excl: For code 410.81: See code 410.0

√5th 410.9 Unspecified site [CC 1] [A]
Acute myocardial infarction NOS
Coronary occlusion NOS

CC Excl: For code 410.91: See code 410.0

AHA: 1Q, '96, 17; 1Q, '92, 9

DRG 121 and 122 For code 410.91

√4th 411 Other acute and subacute forms of ischemic heart disease
AHA: 4Q, '94, 55; 3Q, '91, 24

411.0 Postmyocardial infarction syndrome [CC] [MC] [CD] [A]
Dressler's syndrome

CC Excl: 411.0, 411.81, 411.89, 459.89, 459.9

DEF: Complication developing several days/weeks after myocardial infarction; symptoms include fever, leukocytosis, chest pain, evidence of pericarditis, pleurisy, and pneumonitis; tendency to recur.

411.1 Intermediate coronary syndrome [CC] [CD] [A]
- Impending infarction
- Preinfarction syndrome
- Preinfarction angina
- Unstable angina

EXCLUDES angina (pectoris) (413.9)
decubitus (413.0)

CC Excl: 410.00-410.92, 411.1-411.89, 413.0-413.9, 414.8-414.9, 459.89, 459.9

AHA: 3Q, '01, 15; 2Q, '01, 7, 9; 4Q, '98, 86; 2Q, '96, 10; 3Q, '91, 24; 1Q, '91, 14; 3Q, '90, 6; 4Q, '89, 10

DRG 140

DEF: A condition representing an intermediate stage between angina of effort and acute myocardial infarction. It is often documented by the physician as "unstable angina."

√5th 411.8 Other
AHA: 3Q, '91, 18; 3Q, '89, 4

411.81 Acute coronary occlusion without myocardial infarction [CC] [CD] [A]
Acute coronary (artery):
- embolism
- obstruction
- occlusion
- thrombosis

without or not resulting in myocardial infarction

EXCLUDES obstruction without infarction due to atherosclerosis ►(414.00-414.06)◄
occlusion without infarction due to atherosclerosis ►(414.00-414.06)◄

CC Excl: 410.00-410.92, 411.0-411.89, 413.0-413.9, 414.8-414.9, 459.89, 459.9

AHA: 3Q, '91, 24; 1Q, '91, 14

DEF: Interrupted blood flow to a portion of the heart; without tissue death.

411.89 Other [CC] [CD] [A]
Coronary insufficiency (acute)
Subendocardial ischemia

CC Excl: See code 411.81

AHA: 3Q, '01, 14; 1Q, '92, 9

DRG 140

412 Old myocardial infarction [A]
Healed myocardial infarction
Past myocardial infarction diagnosed on ECG [EKG] or other special investigation, but currently presenting no symptoms

AHA: 2Q, '01, 9; 3Q, '98, 15; 2Q, '91, 22; 3Q, '90, 7

√4th 413 Angina pectoris
DEF: Severe constricting pain in the chest, often radiating from the precordium to the left shoulder and down the arm, due to ischemia of the heart muscle; usually caused by coronary disease; pain is often precipitated by effort or excitement.

413.0 Angina decubitus [CC] [A]
Nocturnal angina

CC Excl: 410.00-410.92, 411.1-411.89, 413.0-413.9, 414.8-414.9, 459.89, 459.9

DEF: Angina occurring only in the recumbent position.

[N] Newborn Age: 0   [P] Pediatric Age: 0-17   [M] Maternity Age: 12-55   [A] Adult Age: 15-124   [CC] CC Condition   [MC] Major Complication   [CD] Complex Dx   [HIV] HIV Related Dx

CIRCULATORY SYSTEM

413.1 **Prinzmetal angina**
Variant angina pectoris
CC Excl: See code 413.0

DEF: Angina occurring when patient is recumbent; associated with ST-segment elevations.

413.9 **Other and unspecified angina pectoris**
Angina: Anginal syndrome
  NOS   Status anginosus
  cardiac   Stenocardia
  of effort Syncope anginosa
EXCLUDES preinfarction angina (411.1)
CC Excl: See code 413.0
AHA: 3Q, '91, 16; 3Q, '90, 6
DRG 140

√4th **414 Other forms of chronic ischemic heart disease**
EXCLUDES arteriosclerotic cardiovascular disease [ASCVD] (429.2)
cardiovascular:
  arteriosclerosis or sclerosis (429.2)
  degeneration or disease (429.2)

√5th **414.0 Coronary atherosclerosis**
Arteriosclerotic heart disease [ASHD]
Atherosclerotic heart disease
Coronary (artery):
  arteriosclerosis
  arteritis or endarteritis
  atheroma
  sclerosis
  stricture
EXCLUDES embolism of graft (996.72)
occlusion NOS of graft (996.72)
thrombus of graft (996.72)
AHA: 2Q, '97, 13; 2Q, '95, 17; 4Q, '94, 49; 2Q, '94, 13; 1Q, '94, 6; 3Q, '90, 7
DEF: A chronic condition marked by thickening and loss of elasticity of the coronary artery; caused by deposits of plaque containing cholesterol, lipoid material and lipophages.

414.00 Of unspecified type of vessel, native or graft
AHA: 3Q, '01, 15; 4Q, '99, 4; 3Q, '97, 15; 4Q, '96, 31
DRG 132

414.01 Of native coronary artery
AHA: 3Q, '01, 15; 2Q, '01, 8, 9; 3Q, '97, 15; 2Q, '96, 10; 4Q, '96, 31
DRG 132
DEF: Plaque deposits in natural heart vessels.

414.02 Of autologous vein bypass graft
DEF: Plaque deposit in grafted vein originating within patient.

414.03 Of nonautologous biological bypass graft
DEF: Plaque deposits in grafted vessel originating outside patient.

414.04 Of artery bypass graft
Internal mammary artery
AHA: 4Q, '96, 31
DEF: Plaque deposits in grafted artery originating within patient.

414.05 Of unspecified type of bypass graft
Bypass graft NOS
AHA: 3Q, '97, 15; 4Q, '96, 31

414.06 Of coronary artery of transplanted heart

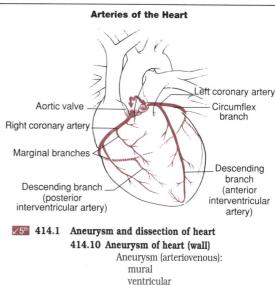
Arteries of the Heart

√5th **414.1 Aneurysm and dissection of heart**

414.10 Aneurysm of heart (wall)
Aneurysm (arteriovenous):
  mural
  ventricular

414.11 Aneurysm of coronary vessels
Aneurysm (arteriovenous) of coronary vessels
AHA: 1Q, '99, 17

414.12 Dissection of coronary artery

414.19 Other aneurysm of heart
Arteriovenous fistula, acquired, of heart

414.8 Other specified forms of chronic ischemic heart disease
Chronic coronary insufficiency
Ischemia, myocardial (chronic)
Any condition classifiable to 410 specified as chronic, or presenting with symptoms after 8 weeks from date of infarction
EXCLUDES coronary insufficiency (acute) (411.89)
AHA: 3Q, '01, 15; 1Q, '92, 10; 3Q, '90, 7, 15; 2Q, '90, 19

414.9 Chronic ischemic heart disease, unspecified
Ischemic heart disease NOS

DISEASES OF PULMONARY CIRCULATION (415-417)

√4th **415 Acute pulmonary heart disease**

415.0 Acute cor pulmonale
EXCLUDES cor pulmonale NOS (416.9)
CC Excl: 415.0, 416.8-416.9, 459.89, 459.9

DEF: A heart-lung disease marked by dilation and failure of the right side of heart; due to pulmonary embolism; ventilatory function is impaired and pulmonary hypertension results within hours.

√5th **415.1 Pulmonary embolism and infarction**
Pulmonary (artery) (vein):
  apoplexy
  embolism
  infarction (hemorrhagic)
  thrombosis
EXCLUDES that complicating:
  abortion (634-638 with .6, 639.6)
  ectopic or molar pregnancy (639.6)
  pregnancy, childbirth, or the puerperium (673.0-673.8)
AHA: 4Q, '90, 25

DEF: embolism: Closure of the pulmonary artery or branch; due to thrombosis (blood clot).

DEF: infarction: Necrosis of lung tissue; due to obstructed arterial blood supply, most often by pulmonary embolism.

415.11 Iatrogenic pulmonary embolism and infarction
CC Excl: 415.11, 415.19, 459.89, 459.9
AHA: 4Q, '95, 58

CIRCULATORY SYSTEM

415.19 Other
CC Excl: 415.11, 415.19, 459.89, 459.9

☑4th **416 Chronic pulmonary heart disease**

416.0 Primary pulmonary hypertension
Idiopathic pulmonary arteriosclerosis
Pulmonary hypertension (essential) (idiopathic) (primary)
CC Excl: 416.0, 416.8-416.9, 417.8-417.9, 459.89, 459.9
DEF: A rare increase in pulmonary circulation, often resulting in right ventricular failure or fatal syncope.

416.1 Kyphoscoliotic heart disease
DEF: High blood pressure within the lungs as a result of curvature of the spine.

416.8 Other chronic pulmonary heart diseases
Pulmonary hypertension, secondary

416.9 Chronic pulmonary heart disease, unspecified
Chronic cardiopulmonary disease
Cor pulmonale (chronic) NOS

☑4th **417 Other diseases of pulmonary circulation**

417.0 Arteriovenous fistula of pulmonary vessels
EXCLUDES: congenital arteriovenous fistula (747.3)
DEF: Abnormal communication between blood vessels within lung.

417.1 Aneurysm of pulmonary artery
EXCLUDES: congenital aneurysm (747.3)

417.8 Other specified diseases of pulmonary circulation
Pulmonary: arteritis
Pulmonary: endarteritis
Rupture } of pulmonary vessel
Stricture

417.9 Unspecified disease of pulmonary circulation

OTHER FORMS OF HEART DISEASE (420-429)

☑4th **420 Acute pericarditis**
INCLUDES: acute:
  mediastinopericarditis
  myopericarditis
  pericardial effusion
  pleuropericarditis
  pneumopericarditis
EXCLUDES: acute rheumatic pericarditis (391.0)
  postmyocardial infarction syndrome [Dressler's] (411.0)
DEF: Inflammation of the pericardium (heart sac); pericardial friction rub results from this inflammation and is heard as a scratchy or leathery sound.

420.0 Acute pericarditis in diseases classified elsewhere
Code first underlying disease, as:
  actinomycosis (039.8)
  amebiasis (006.8)
  nocardiosis (039.8)
  tuberculosis (017.9)
  uremia (585)
EXCLUDES: pericarditis (acute) (in):
  Coxsackie (virus) (074.21)
  gonococcal (098.83)
  histoplasmosis (115.0-115.9 with fifth-digit 3)
  meningococcal infection (036.41)
  syphilitic (093.81)
CC Excl: 391.0, 393, 420.0-420.99, 423.8-423.9, 459.89, 459.9

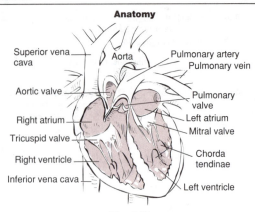

Anatomy

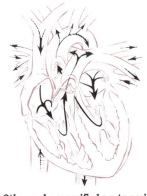

Blood Flow

☑5th **420.9 Other and unspecified acute pericarditis**

420.90 Acute pericarditis, unspecified
Pericarditis (acute): NOS
  infective NOS
Pericarditis (acute): sicca
CC Excl: See code 420.0
AHA: 2Q, '89, 12

420.91 Acute idiopathic pericarditis
Pericarditis, acute: benign
  nonspecific
Pericarditis, acute: viral
CC Excl: See code 420.0

420.99 Other
Pericarditis (acute): pneumococcal
  purulent
  staphylococcal
  streptococcal
Pericarditis (acute): suppurative
  Pneumopyopericardium
  Pyopericardium
EXCLUDES: pericarditis in diseases classified elsewhere (420.0)
CC Excl: See code 420.0

☑4th **421 Acute and subacute endocarditis**
DEF: Bacterial inflammation of the endocardium (intracardiac area); major symptoms include fever, fatigue, heart murmurs, splenomegaly, embolic episodes and areas of infarction.

421.0 Acute and subacute bacterial endocarditis
Endocarditis (acute) (chronic) (subacute):
  bacterial
  infective NOS
  lenta
  malignant
  purulent
  septic
Endocarditis (acute) (chronic) (subacute):
  ulcerative
  vegetative
  Infective aneurysm
  Subacute bacterial endocarditis [SBE]
Use additional code to identify infectious organism [e.g., Streptococcus 041.0, Staphylococcus 041.1]
CC Excl: 391.1, 397.9, 421.0-421.9, 424.90-424.99, 459.89, 459.9
AHA: 1Q, '99, 12; 1Q, '91, 15

CIRCULATORY SYSTEM

421.1 Acute and subacute infective endocarditis in diseases classified elsewhere [CC] [CD]
Code first underlying disease, as:
blastomycosis (116.0)
Q fever (083.0)
typhoid (fever) (002.0)
EXCLUDES endocarditis (in):
Coxsackie (virus) (074.22)
gonococcal (098.84)
histoplasmosis (115.0-115.9 with fifth-digit 4)
meningococcal infection (036.42)
monilial (112.81)
CC Excl: See code 421.0

421.9 Acute endocarditis, unspecified [CC] [CD] [HIV]
Endocarditis
Myoendocarditis } acute or subacute
Periendocarditis
EXCLUDES acute rheumatic endocarditis (391.1)
CC Excl: See code 421.0

√4th **422 Acute myocarditis**
EXCLUDES acute rheumatic myocarditis (391.2)
DEF: Acute inflammation of the muscular walls of the heart (myocardium).

422.0 Acute myocarditis in diseases classified elsewhere [CC] [CD]
Code first underlying disease, as:
myocarditis (acute):
influenzal (487.8)
tuberculous (017.9)
EXCLUDES myocarditis (acute) (due to):
aseptic, of newborn (074.23)
Coxsackie (virus) (074.23)
diphtheritic (032.82)
meningococcal infection (036.43)
syphilitic (093.82)
toxoplasmosis (130.3)
CC Excl: 391.2, 398.0, 422.0-422.99, 429.0, 429.71, 429.79, 459.89, 459.9

√5th **422.9 Other and unspecified acute myocarditis**

422.90 Acute myocarditis, unspecified [CC] [CD] [HIV]
Acute or subacute (interstitial) myocarditis
CC Excl: See code 422.0

422.91 Idiopathic myocarditis [CC] [CD] [HIV]
Myocarditis (acute or subacute):
Fiedler's
giant cell
isolated (diffuse) (granulomatous)
nonspecific granulomatous
CC Excl: See code 422.0

422.92 Septic myocarditis [CC] [CD] [HIV]
Myocarditis, acute or subacute:
pneumococcal
staphylococcal
Use additional code to identify infectious organism [e.g., Staphylococcus 041.1]
EXCLUDES myocarditis, acute or subacute:
in bacterial diseases classified elsewhere (422.0)
streptococcal (391.2)
CC Excl: See code 422.0

422.93 Toxic myocarditis [CC] [CD] [HIV]
CC Excl: See code 422.0
DEF: Inflammation of the heart muscle due to an adverse reaction to certain drugs or chemicals reaching the heart through the bloodstream.

422.99 Other [CC] [CD] [HIV]
CC Excl: See code 422.0

√4th **423 Other diseases of pericardium**
EXCLUDES that specified as rheumatic (393)

423.0 Hemopericardium [CC] [CD]
CC Excl: 423.0-423.9, 459.89, 459.9
DEF: Blood in the pericardial sac (pericardium).

423.1 Adhesive pericarditis [CC]
Adherent pericardium   Pericarditis:
Fibrosis of pericardium   adhesive
Milk spots   obliterative
                                 Soldiers' patches
CC Excl: See code 423.0
DEF: Two layers of serous pericardium adhere to each other by fibrous adhesions.

423.2 Constrictive pericarditis [CC]
Concato's disease   Pick's disease of heart (and liver)
CC Excl: See code 423.0
DEF: Inflammation identified by a rigid, thickened and sometimes calcified pericardium; ventricles of the heart cannot be adequately filled and congestive heart failure may result.

423.8 Other specified diseases of pericardium
Calcification } of pericardium
Fistula
AHA: 2Q, '89, 12

423.9 Unspecified disease of pericardium

√4th **424 Other diseases of endocardium**
EXCLUDES bacterial endocarditis (421.0-421.9)
rheumatic endocarditis (391.1, 394.0-397.9)
syphilitic endocarditis (093.20-093.24)

424.0 Mitral valve disorders [CC]
Mitral (valve):
incompetence
insufficiency } NOS of specified cause, except rheumatic
regurgitation
EXCLUDES mitral (valve):
disease (394.9)
failure (394.9)
stenosis (394.0)
the listed conditions:
specified as rheumatic (394.1)
unspecified as to cause but with mention of:
diseases of aortic valve (396.0-396.9)
mitral stenosis or obstruction (394.2)
CC Excl: 394.0-394.9, 396.0-396.9, 424.0, 459.89, 459.9
AHA: 2Q, '00, 16; 3Q, '98, 11; N-D, '87, 8; N-D, '84, 8

424.1 Aortic valve disorders [CC]
Aortic (valve):
incompetence
insufficiency } NOS of specified cause, except rheumatic
regurgitation
stenosis
EXCLUDES hypertrophic subaortic stenosis (425.1)
that specified as rheumatic (395.0-395.9)
that of unspecified cause but with mention of diseases of mitral valve (396.0-396.9)
CC Excl: 395.0-395.9, 396.0-396.9, 424.1, 459.89, 459.9
AHA: 4Q, '88, 8; N-D, '87, 8

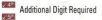 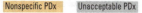 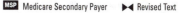

2002 Ingenix, Inc.

CIRCULATORY SYSTEM

Tabular List

424.2 **Tricuspid valve disorders, specified as nonrheumatic** [CC]
Tricuspid valve:
  incompetence
  insufficiency   } of specified cause,
  regurgitation } except rheumatic
  stenosis
  EXCLUDES rheumatic or of unspecified cause (397.0)
CC Excl: 397.0, 424.2, 459.89, 459.9

424.3 **Pulmonary valve disorders** [CC]
Pulmonic: Pulmonic:
  incompetence NOS   regurgitation NOS
  insufficiency NOS   stenosis NOS
  EXCLUDES that specified as rheumatic (397.1)
CC Excl: 397.1, 424.3, 459.89, 459.9

√5th **424.9** **Endocarditis, valve unspecified**

424.90 **Endocarditis, valve unspecified, unspecified cause** [CC] [CD]
Endocarditis (chronic):
  NOS
  nonbacterial thrombotic
Valvular:
  incompetence } of unspecified
  insufficiency } valve,
  regurgitation } unspecified
  stenosis   } cause
Valvulitis (chronic)
CC Excl: 424.90-424.99, 459.89, 459.9

424.91 **Endocarditis in diseases classified elsewhere** [CC] [CD]
Code first underlying disease as:
  atypical verrucous endocarditis [Libman-Sacks] (710.0)
  disseminated lupus erythematosus (710.0)
  tuberculosis (017.9)
  EXCLUDES syphilitic (093.20-093.24)
CC Excl: See code 424.90

424.99 **Other** [CC]
Any condition classifiable to 424.90 with specified cause, except rheumatic
  EXCLUDES endocardial fibroelastosis (425.3)
            that specified as rheumatic (397.9)
CC Excl: See code 424.90

√4th **425 Cardiomyopathy**
INCLUDES myocardiopathy
AHA: J-A, '85, 15

425.0 **Endomyocardial fibrosis** [CC]
CC Excl: 425.0-425.9, 459.89, 459.9

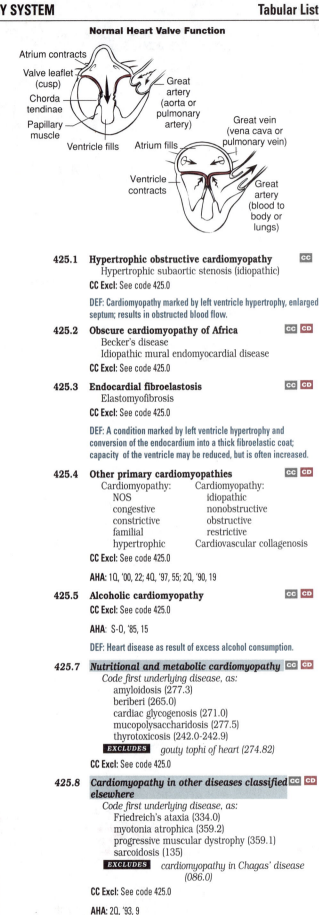

425.1 **Hypertrophic obstructive cardiomyopathy** [CC]
Hypertrophic subaortic stenosis (idiopathic)
CC Excl: See code 425.0
DEF: Cardiomyopathy marked by left ventricle hypertrophy, enlarged septum; results in obstructed blood flow.

425.2 **Obscure cardiomyopathy of Africa** [CC] [CD]
Becker's disease
Idiopathic mural endomyocardial disease
CC Excl: See code 425.0

425.3 **Endocardial fibroelastosis** [CC] [CD]
Elastomyofibrosis
CC Excl: See code 425.0
DEF: A condition marked by left ventricle hypertrophy and conversion of the endocardium into a thick fibroelastic coat; capacity of the ventricle may be reduced, but is often increased.

425.4 **Other primary cardiomyopathies** [CC] [CD]
Cardiomyopathy: Cardiomyopathy:
  NOS   idiopathic
  congestive   nonobstructive
  constrictive   obstructive
  familial   restrictive
  hypertrophic   Cardiovascular collagenosis
CC Excl: See code 425.0
AHA: 1Q, '00, 22; 4Q, '97, 55; 2Q, '90, 19

425.5 **Alcoholic cardiomyopathy** [CC] [CD]
CC Excl: See code 425.0
AHA: S-O, '85, 15
DEF: Heart disease as result of excess alcohol consumption.

425.7 **Nutritional and metabolic cardiomyopathy** [CC] [CD]
Code first underlying disease, as:
  amyloidosis (277.3)
  beriberi (265.0)
  cardiac glycogenosis (271.0)
  mucopolysaccharidosis (277.5)
  thyrotoxicosis (242.0-242.9)
  EXCLUDES gouty tophi of heart (274.82)
CC Excl: See code 425.0

425.8 **Cardiomyopathy in other diseases classified elsewhere** [CC] [CD]
Code first underlying disease, as:
  Friedreich's ataxia (334.0)
  myotonia atrophica (359.2)
  progressive muscular dystrophy (359.1)
  sarcoidosis (135)
  EXCLUDES cardiomyopathy in Chagas' disease (086.0)
CC Excl: See code 425.0
AHA: 2Q, '93, 9

425.9 **Secondary cardiomyopathy, unspecified** [CC] [CD]
CC Excl: See code 425.0

[N] Newborn Age: 0   [P] Pediatric Age: 0-17   [M] Maternity Age: 12-55   [A] Adult Age: 15-124   [CC] CC Condition   [MC] Major Complication   [CD] Complex Dx   [HIV] HIV Related Dx

122 — Volume 1   2002 Ingenix, Inc.

CIRCULATORY SYSTEM

Nerve Conduction of the Heart

[Diagram labels: Sinoatrial node (pacemaker); Internodal tracts: Anterior, Middle, Posterior; Atrioventricular node; Common bundle (of His); Atrioventricular block; Accessory bundle (of Kent); Right bundle branch; Right bundle branch block; Moderator band; Bachmann's bundle; Left bundle branch block; Left bundle branch: Anterior fascicle, Posterior fascicle; Left bundle branch hemiblock; Purkinje fibers]

426 Conduction disorders
DEF: Disruption or disturbance in the electrical impulses that regulate heartbeats.

426.0 Atrioventricular block, complete [CC MC]
Third degree atrioventricular block
CC Excl: 426.0-426.9, 427.0-427.5, 427.89, 459.89, 459.9

426.1 Atrioventricular block, other and unspecified

426.10 Atrioventricular block, unspecified [MC]
Atrioventricular [AV] block (incomplete) (partial)

426.11 First degree atrioventricular block
Incomplete atrioventricular block, first degree
Prolonged P-R interval NOS

426.12 Mobitz (type) II atrioventricular block [CC MC]
Incomplete atrioventricular block:
Mobitz (type) II
second degree, Mobitz (type) II
CC Excl: See code 426.0
DEF: Impaired conduction of excitatory impulse from cardiac atrium to ventricle through AV node.

426.13 Other second degree atrioventricular block [CC MC]
Incomplete atrioventricular block:
Mobitz (type) I [Wenckebach's]
second degree:
NOS
Mobitz (type) I
with 2:1 atrioventricular response [block]
Wenckebach's phenomenon
CC Excl: See code 426.0
DEF: Wenckebach's phenomenon: impulses generated at constant rate to sinus node, P-R interval lengthens; results in cycle of ventricular inadequacy and shortened P-R interval; second-degree A-V block commonly called "Mobitz type 1."

426.2 Left bundle branch hemiblock
Block:
left anterior fascicular
left posterior fascicular

426.3 Other left bundle branch block [MC]
Left bundle branch block:
NOS
anterior fascicular with posterior fascicular
complete
main stem

426.4 Right bundle branch block
AHA: 3Q, '00, 3

426.5 Bundle branch block, other and unspecified
426.50 Bundle branch block, unspecified
426.51 Right bundle branch block and left posterior fascicular block [MC]

426.52 Right bundle branch block and left anterior fascicular block [MC]

426.53 Other bilateral bundle branch block [CC MC]
Bifascicular block NOS
Bilateral bundle branch block NOS
Right bundle branch with left bundle branch block (incomplete) (main stem)
CC Excl: See code 426.0

426.54 Trifascicular block [CC MC]
CC Excl: See code 426.0

426.6 Other heart block [CC]
Intraventricular block: Sinoatrial block
NOS   Sinoauricular block
diffuse
myofibrillar
CC Excl: See code 426.0

426.7 Anomalous atrioventricular excitation [CC]
Atrioventricular conduction:
accelerated
accessory
pre-excitation
Ventricular pre-excitation
Wolff-Parkinson-White syndrome
CC Excl: See code 426.0
DEF: Wolff-Parkinson-White: normal conduction pathway is bypassed; results in short P-R interval on EKG; tendency to supraventricular tachycardia.

426.8 Other specified conduction disorders
426.81 Lown-Ganong-Levine syndrome [CC]
Syndrome of short P-R interval, normal QRS complexes, and supraventricular tachycardias
CC Excl: See code 426.0

426.89 Other [CC]
Dissociation:
atrioventricular [AV]
interference
isorhythmic
Nonparoxysmal AV nodal tachycardia
CC Excl: See code 426.0

426.9 Conduction disorder, unspecified [CC]
Heart block NOS   Stokes-Adams syndrome
CC Excl: See code 426.0

427 Cardiac dysrhythmias
EXCLUDES that complicating:
abortion (634-638 with .7, 639.8)
ectopic or molar pregnancy (639.8)
labor or delivery (668.1, 669.4)
AHA: J-A, '85, 15
DEF: Disruption or disturbance in the rhythm of heartbeats.

427.0 Paroxysmal supraventricular tachycardia [CC MC]
Paroxysmal tachycardia: Paroxysmal tachycardia:
atrial [PAT]   junctional
atrioventricular [AV]   nodal
CC Excl: See code 426.0
DRG 138
DEF: Rapid atrial rhythm.

427.1 Paroxysmal ventricular tachycardia [CC MC CD]
Ventricular tachycardia (paroxysmal)
CC Excl: See code 426.0
AHA: 3Q, '95, 9; M-A, '86, 11
DRG 138
DEF: Rapid ventricular rhythm.

427.2 Paroxysmal tachycardia, unspecified [CC MC]
Bouveret-Hoffmann syndrome
Paroxysmal tachycardia:
essential
NOS
CC Excl: See code 426.0

CIRCULATORY SYSTEM

427.3 Atrial fibrillation and flutter [5th]

427.31 Atrial fibrillation [CC] [MC]
CC Excl: See code 426.0
AHA: 2Q, '99, 17; 3Q, '95, 8
DRG 138
DEF: Irregular, rapid atrial contractions.

427.32 Atrial flutter [CC] [MC]
CC Excl: See code 426.0
DRG 138
DEF: Regular, rapid atrial contractions.

427.4 Ventricular fibrillation and flutter [5th]

427.41 Ventricular fibrillation [CC] [MC]
CC Excl: See code 426.0
DEF: Irregular, rapid ventricular contractions.

427.42 Ventricular flutter [CC] [MC]
CC Excl: See code 426.0
DEF: Regular, rapid, ventricular contractions.

427.5 Cardiac arrest [CC] [MC] [CD]
Cardiorespiratory arrest
CC Excl: 427.0-427.5, 459.89, 459.9
AHA: 2Q, '00, 12; 3Q, '95, 8; 2Q, '88, 8

427.6 Premature beats [5th]

427.60 Premature beats, unspecified
Ectopic beats   Premature contractions
Extrasystoles   or systoles NOS
Extrasystolic arrhythmia

427.61 Supraventricular premature beats
Atrial premature beats, contractions, or systoles

427.69 Other
Ventricular premature beats, contractions, or systoles
AHA: 4Q, '93, 42

427.8 Other specified cardiac dysrhythmias [5th]

427.81 Sinoatrial node dysfunction
Sinus bradycardia: Syndrome:
  persistent   sick sinus
  severe   tachycardia-
                      bradycardia
EXCLUDES sinus bradycardia NOS (427.89)
AHA: 3Q, '00, 8
DEF: Complex cardiac arrhythmia; appears as severe sinus bradycardia, sinus bradycardia with tachycardia, or sinus bradycardia with atrioventricular block.

427.89 Other
Rhythm disorder: Rhythm disorder:
  coronary sinus   nodal
  ectopic   Wandering (atrial)
                     pacemaker
EXCLUDES carotid sinus syncope (337.0)
▶neonatal bradycardia (779.81)◀
▶neonatal tachycardia (779.82)◀
reflex bradycardia (337.0)
tachycardia NOS (785.0)
DRG 138

427.9 Cardiac dysrhythmia, unspecified
Arrhythmia (cardiac) NOS
AHA: 2Q, '89, 10

428 Heart failure [4th]
EXCLUDES following cardiac surgery (429.4)
rheumatic (398.91)
that complicating:
  abortion (634-638 with .7, 639.8)
  ectopic or molar pregnancy (639.8)
  labor or delivery (668.1, 669.4)
▶Code, if applicable, heart failure due to hypertension first (402.0-402.9, with fifth-digit 1 or 404.0-404.9 with fifth-digit 1 or 3)◀
AHA: 3Q, '98, 5; 2Q, '90, 16; 2Q, '90, 19; 2Q, '89, 10; 3Q, '88, 3

428.0 Congestive heart failure, unspecified [CC] [MC] [CD]
Congestive heart disease
Right heart failure (secondary to left heart failure)
EXCLUDES ▶fluid overload NOS (276.6)◀
CC Excl: 398.91, 402.01, 402.11, 402.91, 428.0-428.9, 459.89, 459.9, 518.4
AHA: 2Q, '01, 13; 4Q, '00, 48; 2Q, '00, 16; 1Q, '00, 22; 4Q, '99, 4; 1Q, '99, 11; 4Q, '97, 55; 3Q, '97, 10; 3Q, '96, 9; 3Q, '91, 18; 3Q, '91, 19; 2Q, '89, 12
DRG 121 and 127
DEF: Mechanical inadequacy; caused by inability of heart to pump and circulate blood; results in fluid collection in lungs, hypertension, congestion and edema of tissue.

428.1 Left heart failure [CC] [MC] [CD]
Acute edema of lung   } with heart disease
Acute pulmonary   } NOS or heart
  edema   } failure
Cardiac asthma   Left ventricular failure
CC Excl: See code 428.0
DEF: Mechanical inadequacy of left ventricle; causing fluid in lungs.

428.2 Systolic heart failure [5th]
EXCLUDES combined systolic and diastolic heart failure (428.40-428.43)

428.20 Unspecified [CC]
CC Excl: See code 428.0

428.21 Acute [CC]
CC Excl: See code 428.0

428.22 Chronic [CC]
CC Excl: See code 428.0

428.23 Acute on chronic [CC]
CC Excl: See code 428.0

428.3 Diastolic heart failure [5th] [CC]
EXCLUDES combined systolic and diastolic heart failure (428.40-428.43)

428.30 Unspecified [CC]
CC Excl: See code 428.0

428.31 Acute [CC]
CC Excl: See code 428.0

428.32 Chronic [CC]
CC Excl: See code 428.0

428.33 Acute on chronic [CC]
CC Excl: See code 428.0

428.4 Combined systolic and diastolic heart failure [5th]

428.40 Unspecified [CC]
CC Excl: See code 428.0

428.41 Acute [CC]
CC Excl: See code 428.0

428.42 Chronic [CC]
CC Excl: See code 428.0

428.43 Acute on chronic [CC]
CC Excl: See code 428.0

428.9 Heart failure, unspecified [CC] [MC] [CD]
Cardiac failure NOS   Myocardial failure NOS
Heart failure NOS   Weak heart
CC Excl: See code 428.0
AHA: 2Q, '89, 10; N-D, '85, 14

[N] Newborn Age: 0   [P] Pediatric Age: 0-17   [M] Maternity Age: 12-55   [A] Adult Age: 15-124   [CC] CC Condition   [MC] Major Complication   [CD] Complex Dx   [HIV] HIV Related Dx

CIRCULATORY SYSTEM 429–429.9

✓4th 429 Ill-defined descriptions and complications of heart disease

429.0 Myocarditis, unspecified

Myocarditis:
- NOS
- chronic (interstitial)
- fibroid
- senile

} (with mention of arteriosclerosis)

Use additional code to identify presence of arteriosclerosis

EXCLUDES acute or subacute (422.0-422.9)
rheumatic (398.0)
acute (391.2)
that due to hypertension (402.0-402.9)

429.1 Myocardial degeneration

Degeneration of heart or myocardium:
- fatty
- mural
- muscular

Myocardial:
- degeneration
- disease

} (with mention of arteriosclerosis)

Use additional code to identify presence of arteriosclerosis

EXCLUDES that due to hypertension (402.0-402.9)

429.2 Cardiovascular disease, unspecified [A]

Arteriosclerotic cardiovascular disease [ASCVD]
Cardiovascular arteriosclerosis
Cardiovascular:
- degeneration
- disease
- sclerosis

} (with mention of arteriosclerosis)

Use additional code to identify presence of arteriosclerosis

EXCLUDES that due to hypertension (402.0-402.9)

429.3 Cardiomegaly

Cardiac: Ventricular dilatation
- dilatation
- hypertrophy

EXCLUDES that due to hypertension (402.0-402.9)

429.4 Functional disturbances following cardiac surgery [CC][CD]

Cardiac insufficiency } following cardiac surgery
Heart failure   } or due to prosthesis

Postcardiotomy syndrome
Postvalvulotomy syndrome

EXCLUDES cardiac failure in the immediate postoperative period (997.1)

CC Excl: 429.4, 429.71, 429.79, 459.89, 459.9

AHA: N-D, '85, 6

429.5 Rupture of chordae tendineae [CC][MC][CD]

CC Excl: 429.5, 429.71, 429.79, 459.89, 459.9

DEF: Torn tissue, between heart valves and papillary muscles.

429.6 Rupture of papillary muscle [CC][MC][CD]

CC Excl: 429.6, 429.71, 429.79, 429.81, 459.89, 459.9

DEF: Torn muscle, between chordae tendineae and heart wall.

✓5th 429.7 Certain sequelae of myocardial infarction, not elsewhere classified

Use additional code to identify the associated myocardial infarction:
- with onset of 8 weeks or less (410.00-410.92)
- with onset of more than 8 weeks (414.8)

EXCLUDES congenital defects of heart (745, 746)
coronary aneurysm (414.11)
disorders of papillary muscle (429.6, 429.81)
postmyocardial infarction syndrome (411.0)
rupture of chordae tendineae (429.5)

AHA: 3Q, '89, 5

Berry Aneurysms

429.71 Acquired cardiac septal defect [CC][CD][A]

EXCLUDES acute septal infarction (410.00-410.92)

CC Excl: 422.0-422.99, 429.0, 429.4-429.82, 459.89-459.9, 745.0-745.9, 746.89, 746.9, ▶747.83;◀ 747.89, 747.9, 759.7-759.89

DEF: Abnormal communication, between opposite heart chambers; due to defect of septum; not present at birth.

429.79 Other [CC][CD][A]

Mural thrombus (atrial) (ventricular), acquired, following myocardial infarction

CC Excl: See code 429.71

AHA: 1Q, '92, 10

✓5th 429.8 Other ill-defined heart diseases

429.81 Other disorders of papillary muscle [CC][MC][CD]

Papillary muscle: Papillary muscle:
- atrophy   - incompetence
- degeneration   - incoordination
- dysfunction   - scarring

CC Excl: 429.6, 429.71, 429.79, 429.81, 459.89, 459.9

429.82 Hyperkinetic heart disease [CC][CD]

CC Excl: 429.71, 429.79, 429.82, 459.89, 459.9

DEF: Condition of unknown origin in young adults; marked by increased cardiac output at rest, increased rate of ventricular ejection; may lead to heart failure.

429.89 Other

Carditis

EXCLUDES that due to hypertension (402.0-402.9)

AHA: 1Q, '92, 10

429.9 Heart disease, unspecified

Heart disease (organic) NOS   Morbus cordis NOS

EXCLUDES that due to hypertension (402.0-402.9)

AHA: 1Q, '93, 19

CEREBROVASCULAR DISEASE (430-438)

INCLUDES with mention of hypertension (conditions classifiable to 401-405)
Use additional code to identify presence of hypertension

EXCLUDES any condition classifiable to 430-434, 436, 437 occurring during pregnancy, childbirth, or the puerperium, or specified as puerperal (674.0)

▶iatrogenic cerebrovascular infarction or hemorrhage (997.02)◀

AHA: 1Q, '93, 27; 3Q, '91, 10; 3Q, '90, 3; 2Q, '89, 8; M-A, '85, 6

430 Subarachnoid hemorrhage [CC] [MC]
Meningeal hemorrhage
Ruptured:
  berry aneurysm
Ruptured:
  (congenital) cerebral aneurysm NOS

EXCLUDES syphilitic ruptured cerebral aneurysm (094.87)

CC Excl: 430, 431, 432.0-432.9, 459.89, 459.9, 780.01-780.09, 800.00-800.99, 801.00-801.99, 803.00-803.99, 804.00-804.96, 850.0-850.9, 851.00-851.99, 852.00-852.19, 852.21-852.59, 853.00-853.19, 854.00-854.19

DEF: Bleeding in space between brain and lining.

431 Intracerebral hemorrhage [CC] [MC]
Hemorrhage (of):
  basilar
  bulbar
  cerebellar
  cerebral
  cerebromeningeal
  cortical
Hemorrhage (of):
  internal capsule
  intrapontine
  pontine
  subcortical
  ventricular
Rupture of blood vessel in brain

CC Excl: See code 430

DRG 014

DEF: Bleeding within the brain.

✓4th 432 Other and unspecified intracranial hemorrhage

432.0 Nontraumatic extradural hemorrhage [CC] [MC]
Nontraumatic epidural hemorrhage
CC Excl: See code 430

DEF: Bleeding, nontraumatic, between skull and brain lining.

432.1 Subdural hemorrhage [CC] [MC]
Subdural hematoma, nontraumatic
CC Excl: See code 430

DEF: Bleeding, between outermost and other layers of brain lining.

432.9 **Unspecified intracranial hemorrhage** [MC]
Intracranial hemorrhage NOS

✓4th 433 Occlusion and stenosis of precerebral arteries

INCLUDES embolism
narrowing
obstruction
thrombosis
} of basilar, carotid, and vertebral arteries

EXCLUDES insufficiency NOS of precerebral arteries (435.0-435.9)

The following fifth-digit subclassification is for use with category 433:
0 without mention of cerebral infarction
1 with cerebral infarction

AHA: 2Q, '95, 14; 3Q, '90, 16

DEF: Blockage, stricture, arteries branching into brain.

✓5th **433.0** Basilar artery [CC 1]
CC Excl: For code 433.01: 250.70-250.93, 433.00-433.91, 435.0, 459.89, 459.9

✓5th **433.1** Carotid artery [CC 1]
CC Excl: For code 433.11: 250.70-250.93, 433.00-433.91, 459.89, 459.9
AHA: 1Q, '00, 16; For code 433.10: ▶1Q, '02, 7, 10◀

✓5th **433.2** Vertebral artery [CC 1]
CC Excl: For code 433.21: 250.70-250.93, 433.00-433.91, 435.1, 459.89, 459.9

1 Nonspecific PDx = 0

✓5th **433.3** Multiple and bilateral [CC 1]
CC Excl: For code 433.31: See code 433.11

✓5th **433.8** Other specified precerebral artery [CC 1]
CC Excl: For code 433.81: See code 433.01

✓5th 1 **433.9** Unspecified precerebral artery [CC 1]
Precerebral artery NOS
CC Excl: For code 433.91: See code 433.01

✓4th 434 Occlusion of cerebral arteries

The following fifth-digit subclassification is for use with category 433:
0 without mention of cerebral infarction
1 with cerebral infarction

AHA: 2Q, '95, 14

✓5th **434.0** Cerebral thrombosis [CC 1] [MC]
Thrombosis of cerebral arteries
CC Excl: For code 434.01: 250.70-250.93, 434.00-434.91, 436, 459.89, 459.9

✓5th **434.1** Cerebral embolism [CC 1] [MC]
CC Excl: For code 434.11: See code 434.01
AHA: 3Q, '97, 11
DRG 014 For code 434.11

✓5th 1 **434.9** Cerebral artery occlusion, unspecified [CC 1] [MC]
CC Excl: For code 434.91: See code 434.01
AHA: 4Q, '98, 87
DRG 014 For code 434.91

✓4th 435 Transient cerebral ischemia

INCLUDES cerebrovascular insufficiency (acute) with transient focal neurological signs and symptoms
insufficiency of basilar, carotid, and vertebral arteries
spasm of cerebral arteries

EXCLUDES acute cerebrovascular insufficiency NOS (437.1)
that due to any condition classifiable to 433 (433.0-433.9)

DEF: Temporary restriction of blood flow, to arteries branching into brain.

435.0 Basilar artery syndrome
435.1 Vertebral artery syndrome
435.2 Subclavian steal syndrome
DEF: Cerebrovascular insufficiency, due to occluded subclavian artery; symptoms include pain in mastoid and posterior head regions, flaccid paralysis of arm and diminished or absent radical pulse on affected side.

435.3 Vertebrobasilar artery syndrome
AHA: 4Q, '95, 60

DEF: Transient ischemic attack; due to brainstem dysfunction; symptoms include confusion, vertigo, binocular blindness, diplopia, unilateral or bilateral weakness and paresthesis of extremities.

435.8 Other specified transient cerebral ischemias [A]

CIRCULATORY SYSTEM

435.9 Unspecified transient cerebral ischemia
Impending cerebrovascular accident
Intermittent cerebral ischemia
Transient ischemic attack [TIA]
AHA: N-D, '85, 12

436 Acute, but ill-defined, cerebrovascular disease
Apoplexy, apoplectic:
  NOS
  attack
  cerebral
  seizure
Cerebral seizure
Cerebrovascular accident [CVA] NOS
Stroke

EXCLUDES any condition classifiable to categories 430-435
▶postoperative cerebrovascular accident (997.02)◀

CC Excl: 250.70-250.93, 430-431, 432.0-432.9, 434.00-434.91, 436, 459.89, 459.9, 780.01-780.09, 800.00-800.99, 801.00-801.99, 803.00-803.99, 804.00-804.96, 850.0-850.9, 851.00-851.99, 852.00-852.19, 852.21-852.59, 853.00-853.19, 854.00-854.19
AHA: 4Q, '99, 3
DRG 014

437 Other and ill-defined cerebrovascular disease

  437.0 Cerebral atherosclerosis
  Atheroma of cerebral arteries
  Cerebral arteriosclerosis

  437.1 Other generalized ischemic cerebrovascular disease
  Acute cerebrovascular insufficiency NOS
  Cerebral ischemia (chronic)

  437.2 Hypertensive encephalopathy
  CC Excl: 250.70-250.93, 437.2, 459.89, 459.9
  AHA: J-A, '84, 14
  DEF: Cerebral manifestations (such as visual disturbances and headache) due to high blood pressure.

  437.3 Cerebral aneurysm, nonruptured
  Internal carotid artery, intracranial portion
  Internal carotid artery NOS
  EXCLUDES congenital cerebral aneurysm, nonruptured (747.81)
  internal carotid artery, extracranial portion (442.81)

  437.4 Cerebral arteritis
  CC Excl: 250.70-250.93, 437.4, 459.89, 459.9
  AHA: 4Q, '99, 21
  DEF: Inflammation of a cerebral artery or arteries.

  437.5 Moyamoya disease
  CC Excl: 250.70-250.93, 437.5, 459.89, 459.9
  DEF: Cerebrovascular ischemia; vessels occlude and rupture causing tiny hemorrhages at base of brain; predominantly affects Japanese.

  437.6 Nonpyogenic thrombosis of intracranial venous sinus
  EXCLUDES pyogenic (325)
  CC Excl: 250.70-250.93, 437.6, 459.89, 459.9

  437.7 Transient global amnesia
  AHA: 4Q, '92, 20
  DEF: Episode of short-term memory loss, not often recurrent; pathogenesis unknown; with no signs or symptoms of neurological disorder.

  437.8 Other
  437.9 Unspecified
  Cerebrovascular disease or lesion NOS

438 Late effects of cerebrovascular disease
Note: This category is to be used to indicate conditions in 430-437 as the cause of late effects. The "late effects" include conditions specified as such, as sequelae, which may occur at any time after the onset of the causal condition.
AHA: 4Q, '99, 4, 6, 7; 4Q, '98, 39, 88; 4Q, '97, 35, 37; 4Q, '92, 21; N-D, '86, 12; M-A, '86, 7

  438.0 Cognitive deficits

  438.1 Speech and language deficits
    438.10 Speech and language deficit, unspecified
    438.11 Aphasia
    AHA: 4Q, '97, 36
    DEF: Impairment or absence of the ability to communicate by speech, writing or signs or to comprehend the spoken or written language due to disease or injury to the brain. Total aphasia is the loss of function of both sensory and motor areas of the brain.
    438.12 Dysphasia
    AHA: 4Q, '99, 3, 9
    DEF: Impaired speech; marked by inability to sequence language.
    438.19 Other speech and language deficits

  438.2 Hemiplegia/hemiparesis
  DEF: Paralysis of one side of the body.
    438.20 Hemiplegia affecting unspecified side
    AHA: 4Q, '99, 3, 9
    438.21 Hemiplegia affecting dominant side
    438.22 Hemiplegia affecting nondominant side
    AHA: ▶1Q, '02, 16◀

  438.3 Monoplegia of upper limb
  DEF: Paralysis of one limb or one muscle group.
    438.30 Monoplegia of upper limb affecting unspecified side
    438.31 Monoplegia of upper limb affecting dominant side
    DEF: Inability to activate learned movements; no known sensory or motor impairment.
    438.32 Monoplegia of upper limb affecting nondominant side

  438.4 Monoplegia of lower limb
    438.40 Monoplegia of lower limb affecting unspecified side
    438.41 Monoplegia of lower limb affecting dominant side
    438.42 Monoplegia of lower limb affecting nondominant side

  438.5 Other paralytic syndrome
  Use additional code to identify type of paralytic syndrome, such as:
    locked-in state (344.81)
    quadriplegia (344.00-344.09)
  EXCLUDES late effects of cerebrovascular accident with:
    hemiplegia/hemiparesis (438.20-438.22)
    monoplegia of lower limb (438.40-438.42)
    monoplegia of upper limb (438.30-438.32)
    438.50 Other paralytic syndrome affecting unspecified side
    438.51 Other paralytic syndrome affecting dominant side
    438.52 Other paralytic syndrome affecting nondominant side
    438.53 Other paralytic syndrome, bilateral
    AHA: 4Q, '98, 39

  438.6 Alterations of sensations
  Use additional code to identify the altered sensation

  438.7 Disturbances of vision
  Use additional code to identify the visual disturbance

  438.8 Other late effects of cerebrovascular disease
    438.81 Apraxia
    438.82 Dysphagia
    DEF: Inability or difficulty in swallowing.
    438.83 Facial weakness
    Facial droop

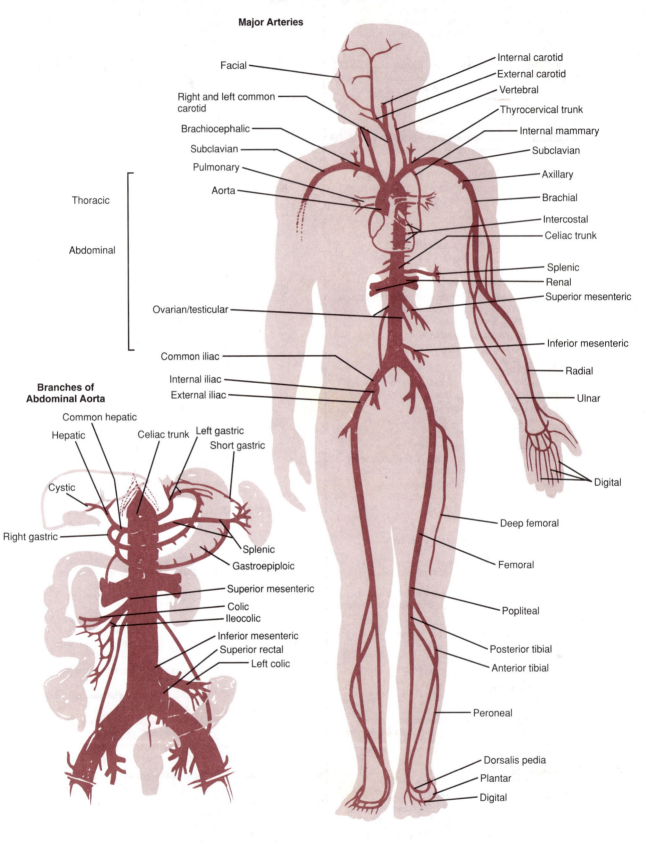

CIRCULATORY SYSTEM 438.84–441.7

- 438.84 Ataxia
- 438.85 Vertigo
- 438.89 Other late effects of cerebrovascular disease
  Use additional code to identify the late effect
  AHA: 4Q, '98, 39

438.9 Unspecified late effects of cerebrovascular disease

DISEASES OF ARTERIES, ARTERIOLES, AND CAPILLARIES (440-448)

✓4th 440 Atherosclerosis

INCLUDES
arteriolosclerosis
arteriosclerosis (obliterans) (senile)
arteriosclerotic vascular disease
atheroma
degeneration:
  arterial
  arteriovascular
  vascular
endarteritis deformans or obliterans
senile:
  arteritis
  endarteritis

EXCLUDES ▶atheroembolism (445.01-445.89)◀
atherosclerosis of bypass graft of the extremities (403.30-403.32)

DEF: Stricture and reduced elasticity of an artery; due to plaque deposits.

440.0 Of aorta
AHA: 2Q, '93, 7; 2Q, '93, 8; 4Q, '88, 8

440.1 Of renal artery
EXCLUDES atherosclerosis of renal arterioles (403.00-403.91)

✓5th 440.2 Of native arteries of the extremities
EXCLUDES atherosclerosis of bypass graft of the extremities (440.30-440.32)
AHA: 4Q, '94, 49; 4Q, '93, 27; 4Q, '92, 25; 3Q, '90, 15; M-A, '87, 6

- **440.20** Atherosclerosis of the extremities, unspecified
- **440.21** Atherosclerosis of the extremities with intermittent claudication
  DEF: Atherosclerosis; marked by pain, tension and weakness after walking; no symptoms while at rest.
- **440.22** Atherosclerosis of the extremities with rest pain
  INCLUDES any condition classifiable to 440.21
  DEF: Atherosclerosis, marked by pain, tension and weakness while at rest.
- **440.23** Atherosclerosis of the extremities with ulceration
  Use additional code for any associated ulceration (707.10-707.9)
  INCLUDES any condition classifiable to 440.21 and 440.22
  AHA: 4Q, '00, 44
- **440.24** Atherosclerosis of the extremities with gangrene
  INCLUDES any condition classifiable to 440.21, 440.22, and 440.23 with ischemic gangrene 785.4
  EXCLUDES gas gangrene (040.0)
  CC Excl: 440.24, ▶780.91-780.99,◀ 785.4, 799.8
  AHA: 4Q, '95, 54; 1Q, '95, 11
- **440.29** Other

✓5th 440.3 Of bypass graft of extremities
EXCLUDES atherosclerosis of native arteries of the extremities (440.21-440.24)
embolism [occlusion NOS] [thrombus] of graft (996.74)
AHA: 4Q, '94, 49

- **440.30** Of unspecified graft
- **440.31** Of autologous vein bypass graft
- **440.32** Of nonautologous biological bypass graft

440.8 Of other specified arteries
EXCLUDES
basilar (433.0)
carotid (433.1)
cerebral (437.0)
coronary ▶(414.00-414.06)◀
mesenteric (557.1)
precerebral (433.0-433.9)
pulmonary (416.0)
vertebral (433.2)

440.9 Generalized and unspecified atherosclerosis
Arteriosclerotic vascular disease NOS
EXCLUDES arteriosclerotic cardiovascular disease [ASCVD] (429.2)

✓4th 441 Aortic aneurysm and dissection
EXCLUDES syphilitic aortic aneurysm (093.0)
traumatic aortic aneurysm (901.0, 902.0)

✓5th 441.0 Dissection of aorta
AHA: 4Q, '89, 10
DEF: Dissection or splitting of wall of the aorta; due to blood entering through intimal tear or interstitial hemorrhage.

- **441.00** Unspecified site
  CC Excl: 250.70-250.93, 441.00-441.9, 459.89, 459.9
- **441.01** Thoracic
  CC Excl: See code 441.00
- **441.02** Abdominal
  CC Excl: See code 441.00
- **441.03** Thoracoabdominal
  CC Excl: See code 441.00

441.1 Thoracic aneurysm, ruptured
CC Excl: See code 441.00

441.2 Thoracic aneurysm without mention of rupture
AHA: 3Q, '92, 10

441.3 Abdominal aneurysm, ruptured
CC Excl: See code 441.00

441.4 Abdominal aneurysm without mention of rupture
AHA: 4Q, '00, 64; 1Q, '99, 15, 16, 17; 3Q, '92, 10

441.5 Aortic aneurysm of unspecified site, ruptured
Rupture of aorta NOS
CC Excl: See code 441.00

441.6 Thoracoabdominal aneurysm, ruptured
CC Excl: See code 441.00

441.7 Thoracoabdominal aneurysm, without mention of rupture

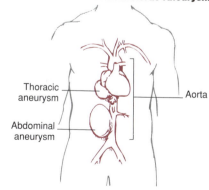

Thoracic and Abdominal Aortic Aneurysm

441.9–444.21 — CIRCULATORY SYSTEM — Tabular List

441.9 Aortic aneurysm of unspecified site without mention of rupture [A]
Aneurysm }
Dilatation } of aorta
Hyaline necrosis }

√4th **442 Other aneurysm**
  INCLUDES: aneurysm (ruptured) (cirsoid) (false) (varicose)
  aneurysmal varix
  EXCLUDES: arteriovenous aneurysm or fistula:
    acquired (447.0)
    congenital (747.60-747.69)
    traumatic (900.0-904.9)
  DEF: Dissection or splitting of arterial wall; due to blood entering through intimal tear or interstitial hemorrhage.

  442.0 Of artery of upper extremity [A]
  442.1 Of renal artery [A]
  442.2 Of iliac artery [A]
    AHA: 1Q, '99, 16, 17
  442.3 Of artery of lower extremity [A]
    Aneurysm:
      femoral } artery
      popliteal }
    AHA: 1Q, '99, 16

  √5th **442.8 Of other specified artery**
    442.81 Artery of neck [A]
      Aneurysm of carotid artery (common) (external) (internal, extracranial portion)
      EXCLUDES: internal carotid artery, intracranial portion (437.3)
    442.82 Subclavian artery [A]
    442.83 Splenic artery [A]
    442.84 Other visceral artery [A]
      Aneurysm:
        celiac
        gastroduodenal
        gastroepiploic } artery
        hepatic
        pancreaticoduodenal
        superior mesenteric
    442.89 Other [A]
      Aneurysm:
        mediastinal } artery
        spinal }
      EXCLUDES: cerebral (nonruptured) (437.3)
        congenital (747.81)
        ruptured (430)
        coronary (414.11)
        heart (414.10)
        pulmonary (417.1)
  442.9 Of unspecified site [A]

√4th **443 Other peripheral vascular disease**
  443.0 Raynaud's syndrome
    Raynaud's:
      disease
      phenomenon (secondary)
    Use additional code to identify gangrene (785.4)
    DEF: Constriction of the arteries, due to cold or stress; bilateral ischemic attacks of fingers, toes, nose or ears; symptoms include pallor, paresthesia and pain; more common in females.

  443.1 Thromboangiitis obliterans [Buerger's disease]
    Presenile gangrene
    DEF: Inflammatory disease of extremity blood vessels, mainly the lower; occurs primarily in young men and leads to tissue ischemia and gangrene.

  √5th **443.2 Other arterial dissection**
    EXCLUDES: dissection of aorta (441.00-441.03)
      dissection of coronary arteries (414.12)
    443.21 Dissection of carotid artery

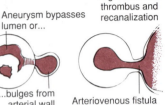

Arterial Diseases and Disorders
Lipids / Calcium deposits
Intimal proliferation
Atherosclerosis narrowing lumen
Thrombus (clot) forming in lumen
Organization of thrombus and recanalization
Embolus (from elsewhere) occluding lumen
Aneurysm bypasses lumen or...bulges from arterial wall
Arteriovenous fistula

    443.22 Dissection of iliac artery
    443.23 Dissection of renal artery
    443.24 Dissection of vertebral artery
    443.29 Dissection of other artery
  √5th **443.8 Other specified peripheral vascular diseases**
    443.81 Peripheral angiopathy in diseases classified elsewhere
      Code first underlying disease, as:
        diabetes mellitus (250.7)
      AHA: 3Q, '91, 10
    443.89 Other
      Acrocyanosis   Erythrocyanosis
      Acroparesthesia: Erythromelalgia
        simple [Schultze's type]
        vasomotor [Nothnagel's type]
      EXCLUDES: chilblains (991.5)
        frostbite (991.0-991.3)
        immersion foot (991.4)
  443.9 Peripheral vascular disease, unspecified
    Intermittent claudication NOS
    Peripheral:
      angiopathy NOS
      vascular disease NOS
    Spasm of artery
    EXCLUDES: atherosclerosis of the arteries of the extremities (440.20-440.22)
      spasm of cerebral artery (435.0-435.9)
    AHA: 4Q, '92, 25; 3Q, '91, 10

√4th **444 Arterial embolism and thrombosis**
  INCLUDES: infarction:
    embolic
    thrombotic
    occlusion
  EXCLUDES: that complicating:
    abortion (634-638 with .6, 639.6)
    ►atheroembolism (445.01-445.89)◄
    ectopic or molar pregnancy (639.6)
    pregnancy, childbirth, or the pueperium (673.0-673.8)
  AHA: 2Q, '92, 11; 4Q, '90, 27

  444.0 Of abdominal aorta [CC]
    Aortic bifurcation syndrome   Leriche's syndrome
    Aortoiliac obstruction   Saddle embolus
    CC Excl: 250.70-250.93, 444.0, 444.89, 444.9, 459.89, 459.9
    AHA: 2Q, '93, 7; 4Q, '90, 27

  444.1 Of thoracic aorta [CC]
    Embolism or thrombosis of aorta (thoracic)
    CC Excl: 250.70-250.93, 444.1, 444.89, 444.9, 459.89, 459.9

  √5th **444.2 Of arteries of the extremities**
    AHA: M-A, '87, 6

    444.21 Upper extremity [CC]
      CC Excl: 250.70-250.93, 444.21, 444.89, 444.9, 459.89, 459.9

444.22 **Lower extremity** `CC`
Arterial embolism or thrombosis:
femoral
peripheral NOS
popliteal
EXCLUDES iliofemoral (444.81)
CC Excl: 250.70-250.93, 444.22, 444.89, 444.9, 459.89, 459.9
AHA: 3Q, '90, 16

√5th **444.8** **Of other specified artery**
444.81 **Iliac artery** `CC`
CC Excl: 250.70-250.93, 444.81-444.9, 459.89, 459.9

444.89 **Other** `CC`
EXCLUDES basilar (433.0)
carotid (433.1)
cerebral (434.0-434.9)
coronary (410.00-410.92)
mesenteric (557.0)
ophthalmic (362.30-362.34)
precerebral (433.0-433.9)
pulmonary (415.19)
renal (593.81)
retinal (362.30-362.34)
vertebral (433.2)
CC Excl: 250.70-250.93, 444.89, 444.9, 459.89, 459.9

444.9 **Of unspecified artery** `CC`
CC Excl: See code 444.89

√4th **445** **Atheroembolism**
INCLUDES atherothrombotic microembolism
cholesterol embolism

√5th **445.0** **Of extremities**
445.01 **Upper extremity** `CC`
CC Excl: 250.70-250.73, 250.80-250.83, 250.90-250.93, 444.89, 444.9, 445.01, 459.89, 459.9

445.02 **Lower extremity** `CC`
CC Excl: 250.70-250.73, 250.80-250.83, 250.90-250.93, 444.89, 444.9, 445.02, 459.89, 459.9

√5th **445.8** **Of other sites**
445.81 **Kidney** `CC`
Use additional code for any associated kidney failure (584, 585)
CC Excl: 250.70-250.73, 250.80-250.83, 250.90-250.93, 444.89, 444.9, 445.81, 459.89, 459.9

445.89 **Other site** `CC`
CC Excl: 250.70-250.73, 250.80-250.83, 250.90-250.93, 444.89, 444.9, 445.89, 459.9

√4th **446** **Polyarteritis nodosa and allied conditions**
446.0 **Polyarteritis nodosa** `CC`
Disseminated necrotizing periarteritis
Necrotizing angiitis
Panarteritis (nodosa)
Periarteritis (nodosa)
CC Excl: 250.70-250.93, 446.0-446.7, 459.89, 459.9

DEF: Inflammation of small and mid-size arteries; symptoms related to involved arteries in kidneys, muscles, gastrointestinal tract and heart; results in tissue death.

446.1 **Acute febrile mucocutaneous lymph node syndrome [MCLS]**
Kawasaki disease

DEF: Acute febrile disease of children; marked by erythema of conjunctiva and mucous membranes of upper respiratory tract, skin eruptions and edema.

√5th **446.2** **Hypersensitivity angiitis**
EXCLUDES antiglomerular basement membrane disease without pulmonary hemorrhage (583.89)

446.20 **Hypersensitivity angiitis, unspecified** `CC`
CC Excl: See code 446.0

446.21 **Goodpasture's syndrome** `CC`
Antiglomerular basement membrane antibody-mediated nephritis with pulmonary hemorrhage
Use additional code to identify renal disease (583.81)
CC Excl: See code 446.0

DEF: Glomerulonephritis associated with hematuria, progresses rapidly; results in death from renal failure.

446.29 **Other specified hypersensitivity angiitis** `CC`
CC Excl: See code 446.0
AHA: 1Q, '95, 3

446.3 **Lethal midline granuloma** `CC`
Malignant granuloma of face
CC Excl: See code 446.0

DEF: Granulomatous lesion; in nose or paranasal sinuses; often fatal; occurs chiefly in males.

446.4 **Wegener's granulomatosis** `CC`
Necrotizing respiratory granulomatosis
Wegener's syndrome
CC Excl: See code 446.0
AHA: 3Q, '00, 11

DEF: A disease occurring mainly in men; marked by necrotizing granulomas and ulceration of the upper respiratory tract; underlying condition is a vasculitis affecting small vessels and is possibly due to an immune disorder.

446.5 **Giant cell arteritis** `CC`
Cranial arteritis   Temporal arteritis
Horton's disease
CC Excl: See code 446.0

DEF: Inflammation of arteries; due to giant cells affecting carotid artery branches, resulting in occlusion; symptoms include fever, headache and neurological problems; occurs in elderly.

446.6 **Thrombotic microangiopathy** `CC`
Moschcowitz's syndrome
Thrombotic thrombocytopenic purpura
CC Excl: See code 446.0

DEF: Blockage of small blood vessels; due to hyaline deposits; symptoms include purpura, CNS disorders; results in protracted disease or rapid death.

446.7 **Takayasu's disease** `CC`
Aortic arch arteritis
Pulseless disease
CC Excl: See code 446.0

DEF: Progressive obliterative arteritis of brachiocephalic trunk, left subclavian, and left common carotid arteries above aortic arch; results in ischemia in brain, heart and arm; pulses impalpable in head, neck and arms; more common in young adult females.

√4th **447** **Other disorders of arteries and arterioles**
447.0 **Arteriovenous fistula, acquired**
Arteriovenous aneurysm, acquired
EXCLUDES cerebrovascular (437.3)
coronary (414.19)
pulmonary (417.0)
surgically created arteriovenous shunt or fistula:
complication (996.1, 996.61-996.62)
status or presence (V45.1)
traumatic (900.0-904.9)

DEF: Communication between an artery and vein caused by error in healing.

447.1 **Stricture of artery**
AHA: 2Q, '93, 8; M-A, '87, 6

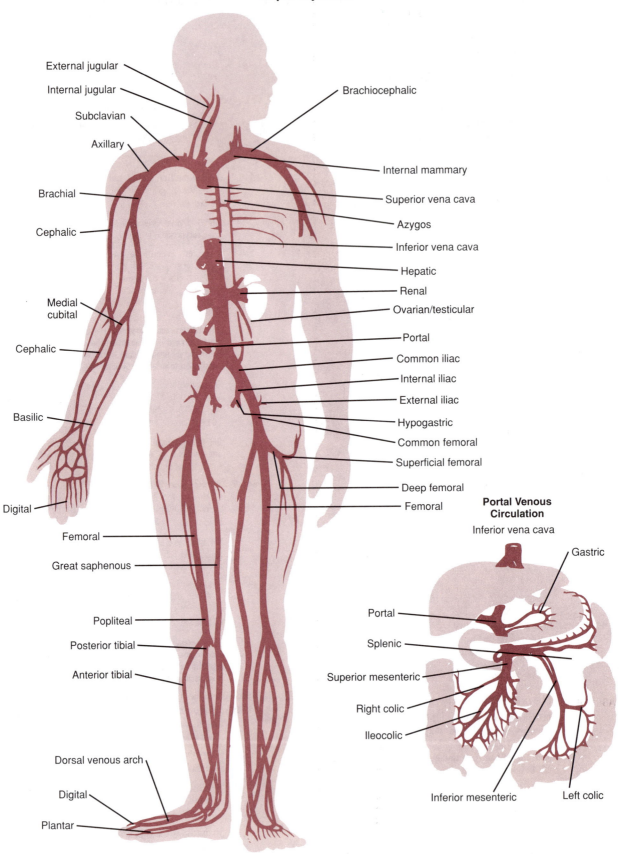

447.2 Rupture of artery
Erosion
Fistula, except arteriovenous } of artery
Ulcer

  EXCLUDES traumatic rupture of artery (900.0-904.9)

447.3 Hyperplasia of renal artery
Fibromuscular hyperplasia of renal artery
DEF: Overgrowth of cells in muscular lining of renal artery.

447.4 Celiac artery compression syndrome
Celiac axis syndrome
Marable's syndrome

447.5 Necrosis of artery

447.6 Arteritis, unspecified
Aortitis NOS
Endarteritis NOS

  EXCLUDES arteritis, endarteritis:
    aortic arch (446.7)
    cerebral (437.4)
    coronary ▶(414.00-414.06)◀
    deformans (440.0-440.9)
    obliterans (440.0-440.9)
    pulmonary (417.8)
    senile (440.0-440.9)
  polyarteritis NOS (446.0)
  syphilitic aortitis (093.1)

AHA: 1Q, '95, 3

447.8 Other specified disorders of arteries and arterioles
Fibromuscular hyperplasia of arteries, except renal

447.9 Unspecified disorders of arteries and arterioles

√4th **448 Disease of capillaries**

448.0 Hereditary hemorrhagic telangiectasia
Rendu-Osler-Weber disease
DEF: Genetic disease with onset after puberty; results in multiple telangiectases, dilated venules on skin and mucous membranes; recurrent bleeding may occur.

448.1 Nevus, non-neoplastic
Nevus:
  araneus
  senile
  spider
  stellar

  EXCLUDES neoplastic (216.0-216.9)
    port wine (757.32)
    strawberry (757.32)

DEF: Enlarged or malformed blood vessels of skin; results in reddish swelling, skin patch, or birthmark.

448.9 Other and unspecified capillary diseases
Capillary:
  hemorrhage
  hyperpermeability
  thrombosis

  EXCLUDES capillary fragility (hereditary) (287.8)

DISEASES OF VEINS AND LYMPHATICS, AND OTHER DISEASES OF CIRCULATORY SYSTEM (451-459)

√4th **451 Phlebitis and thrombophlebitis**

  INCLUDES endophlebitis   periphlebitis
    inflammation, vein   suppurative phlebitis
  Use additional E code to identify drug, if drug-induced

  EXCLUDES that complicating:
    abortion (634-638 with .7, 639.8)
    ectopic or molar pregnancy (639.8)
    pregnancy, childbirth, or the puerperium (671.0-671.9)
  that due to or following:
    implant or catheter device (996.61-996.62)
    infusion, perfusion, or transfusion (999.2)

AHA: 1Q, '92, 16

DEF: Inflammation of a vein (phlebitis) with formation of a thrombus (thrombophlebitis).

451.0 Of superficial vessels of lower extremities
Saphenous vein (greater) (lesser)
CC Excl: 250.70-250.93, 451.0-451.9, 459.89, 459.9

AHA: 3Q, '91, 16

√5th **451.1 Of deep vessels of lower extremities**
AHA: 3Q, '91, 16

451.11 Femoral vein (deep) (superficial)
CC Excl: See code 451.0

451.19 Other
Femoropopliteal vein   Tibial vein
Popliteal vein
CC Excl: See code 451.0

451.2 Of lower extremities, unspecified
CC Excl: See code 451.0

√5th **451.8 Of other sites**

  EXCLUDES intracranial venous sinus (325)
    nonpyogenic (437.6)
    portal (vein) (572.1)

451.81 Iliac vein
CC Excl: See code 451.0

451.82 Of superficial veins of upper extremities
Antecubital vein   Cephalic vein
Basilic vein

451.83 Of deep veins of upper extremities
Brachial vein   Ulnar vein
Radial vein

451.84 Of upper extremities, unspecified

451.89 Other
Axillary vein   Thrombophlebitis of
Jugular vein   breast (Mondor's
Subclavian vein   disease)

451.9 Of unspecified site

452 Portal vein thrombosis
Portal (vein) obstruction

  EXCLUDES hepatic vein thrombosis (453.0)
    phlebitis of portal vein (572.1)

CC Excl: 250.70-250.93, 452, 453.8-453.9, 459.89, 459.9

DEF: Formation of a blood clot in main vein of liver.

√4th **453 Other venous embolism and thrombosis**

  EXCLUDES that complicating:
    abortion (634-638 with .7, 639.8)
    ectopic or molar pregnancy (639.8)
    pregnancy, childbirth, or the puerperium (671.0-671.9)
    that with inflammation, phlebitis, and thrombophlebitis (451.0-451.9)

AHA: 1Q, '92, 16

453.0 Budd-Chiari syndrome
Hepatic vein thrombosis
CC Excl: 250.70-250.93, 453.0, 453.8-453.9, 459.89, 459.9

DEF: Thrombosis or other obstruction of hepatic vein; symptoms include enlarged liver, extensive collateral vessels, intractable ascites and severe portal hypertension.

453.1 Thrombophlebitis migrans
CC Excl: 250.70-250.93, 453.1, 453.8-453.9, 459.89, 459.9

DEF: Slow, advancing thrombophlebitis; appearing first in one vein then another.

453.2 Of vena cava
CC Excl: 250.70-250.93, 453.2, 453.8-453.9, 459.89, 459.9

453.3 Of renal vein
CC Excl: 250.70-250.93, 453.3, 453.8-453.9, 459.89, 459.9

CIRCULATORY SYSTEM

453.8 Of other specified veins [CC]
  EXCLUDES:
    cerebral (434.0-434.9)
    coronary (410.00-410.92)
    intracranial venous sinus (325)
      nonpyogenic (437.6)
    mesenteric (557.0)
    portal (452)
    precerebral (433.0-433.9)
    pulmonary (415.19)
  CC Excl: 250.70-250.93, 453.8-453.9, 459.89, 459.9
  AHA: 3Q, '91, 16; M-A, '87, 6
  DRG 130

453.9 Of unspecified site [CC]
  Embolism of vein   Thrombosis (vein)
  CC Excl: See code 453.8

√4th **454 Varicose veins of lower extremities**
  EXCLUDES: that complicating pregnancy, childbirth, or the puerperium (671.0)
  AHA: 2Q, '91, 20
  DEF: Dilated leg veins; due to incompetent vein valves that allow reversed blood flow and cause tissue erosion or weakness of wall; may be painful.

  454.0 With ulcer [A]
    Varicose ulcer (lower extremity, any part)
    Varicose veins with ulcer of lower extremity [any part] or of unspecified site
    Any condition classifiable to 454.9 with ulcer or specified as ulcerated
    AHA: 4Q, '99, 18

  454.1 With inflammation [A]
    Stasis dermatitis
    Varicose veins with inflammation of lower extremity [any part] or of unspecified site
    Any condition classifiable to 454.9 with inflammation or specified as inflamed

  454.2 With ulcer and inflammation [A]
    Varicose veins with ulcer and inflammation of lower extremity [any part] or of unspecified site
    Any condition classifiable to 454.9 with ulcer and inflammation

• **454.8 With other complications**
    Edema
    Pain
    Swelling

▲ **454.9 Asymptomatic varicose veins** [A]
    Phlebectasia ⎫
    Varicose veins ⎬ of lower extremity [any part] or of unspecified site
    Varix ⎭
    ▶Varicose veins NOS◀

√4th **455 Hemorrhoids**
  INCLUDES:
    hemorrhoids (anus) (rectum)
    piles
    varicose veins, anus or rectum
  EXCLUDES: that complicating pregnancy, childbirth, or the puerperium (671.8)
  DEF: Varicose condition of external hemorrhoidal veins causing painful swellings at the anus.

  455.0 Internal hemorrhoids without mention of complication
  455.1 Internal thrombosed hemorrhoids
  455.2 Internal hemorrhoids with other complication
    Internal hemorrhoids: Internal hemorrhoids:
      bleeding   strangulated
      prolapsed   ulcerated
  455.3 External hemorrhoids without mention of complication
  455.4 External thrombosed hemorrhoids
  455.5 External hemorrhoids with other complication
    External hemorrhoids: External hemorrhoids:
      bleeding   strangulated
      prolapsed   ulcerated

  455.6 Unspecified hemorrhoids without mention of complication
    Hemorrhoids NOS
  455.7 Unspecified thrombosed hemorrhoids
    Thrombosed hemorrhoids, unspecified whether internal or external
  455.8 Unspecified hemorrhoids with other complication
    Hemorrhoids, unspecified whether internal or external:
      bleeding   strangulated
      prolapsed   ulcerated
  455.9 Residual hemorrhoidal skin tags
    Skin tags, anus or rectum

√4th **456 Varicose veins of other sites**
  456.0 Esophageal varices with bleeding [CC]
    CC Excl: 251.5, 456.0, 456.20, 459.89, 459.9, 530.2, 530.7, 530.82, 531.00-531.91, 532.00-532.91, 533.00-533.91, 534.00-534.91, 535.01, 535.11, 535.21, 535.31, 535.41, 535.51, 535.61, 537.83, 562.02-562.03, 562.12-562.13, 569.3, 569.85, 578.0-578.9
    DEF: Distended, tortuous, veins of lower esophagus, usually due to portal hypertension.

  456.1 Esophageal varices without mention of bleeding

  √5th **456.2 Esophageal varices in diseases classified elsewhere**
    Code first underlying cause, as:
      cirrhosis of liver (571.0-571.9)
      portal hypertension (572.3)

    456.20 With bleeding [CC]
      CC Excl: 456.0, 456.20, 459.89, 459.9, 530.82
      AHA: N-D, '85, 14

    456.21 Without mention of bleeding

  456.3 Sublingual varices
    DEF: Distended, tortuous veins beneath tongue.

  456.4 Scrotal varices ♂
    Varicocele

  456.5 Pelvic varices
    Varices of broad ligament

  456.6 Vulval varices ♀
    Varices of perineum
    EXCLUDES: that complicating pregnancy, childbirth, or the puerperium (671.1)

  456.8 Varices of other sites
    Varicose veins of nasal septum (with ulcer)
    EXCLUDES:
      placental varices (656.7)
      retinal varices (362.17)
      varicose ulcer of unspecified site (454.0)
      varicose veins of unspecified site (454.9)

√4th **457 Noninfectious disorders of lymphatic channels**
  457.0 Postmastectomy lymphedema syndrome [A]
    Elephantiasis   ⎫
    Obliteration of lymphatic ⎬ due to mastectomy
      vessel   ⎭
    DEF: Reduced lymphatic circulation following mastectomy; symptoms include swelling of the arm on the operative side.

  457.1 Other lymphedema
    Elephantiasis   Lymphedema:
      (nonfilarial) NOS   praecox
    Lymphangiectasis   secondary
    Lymphedema: Obliteration, lymphatic vessel
      acquired (chronic)
    EXCLUDES: elephantiasis (nonfilarial):
      congenital (757.0)
      eyelid (374.83)
      vulva (624.8)
    DEF: Fluid retention due to reduced lymphatic circulation; due to other than mastectomy.

N Newborn Age: 0   P Pediatric Age: 0-17   M Maternity Age: 12-55   A Adult Age: 15-124   CC CC Condition   MC Major Complication   CD Complex Dx   HIV HIV Related Dx

CIRCULATORY SYSTEM

457.2 Lymphangitis
Lymphangitis: NOS
chronic
Lymphangitis: subacute
EXCLUDES acute lymphangitis (682.0-682.9)

457.8 Other noninfectious disorders of lymphatic channels
Chylocele (nonfilarial)
Chylous:
  ascites
  cyst
Lymph node or vessel:
  fistula
  infarction
  rupture
EXCLUDES chylocele:
  filarial (125.0-125.9)
  tunica vaginalis (nonfilarial) (608.84)

457.9 Unspecified noninfectious disorder of lymphatic channels

✓4th 458 Hypotension
INCLUDES hypopiesis
EXCLUDES cardiovascular collapse (785.50)
maternal hypotension syndrome (669.2)
shock (785.50-785.59)
Shy-Drager syndrome (333.0)

458.0 Orthostatic hypotension
Hypotension: orthostatic (chronic)
Hypotension: postural
AHA: 3Q, '00, 8; 3Q, '91, 9

DEF: Low blood pressure; occurs when standing.

458.1 Chronic hypotension
Permanent idiopathic hypotension
DEF: Persistent low blood pressure.

458.2 Iatrogenic hypotension
Postoperative hypotension
AHA: 4Q, '95, 57
DEF: Abnormally low blood pressure; due to medical treatment.

458.8 Other specified hypotension
AHA: 4Q, '97, 37

458.9 Hypotension, unspecified
Hypotension (arterial) NOS

✓4th 459 Other disorders of circulatory system

459.0 Hemorrhage, unspecified
Rupture of blood vessel NOS
Spontaneous hemorrhage NEC
EXCLUDES hemorrhage:
  gastrointestinal NOS (578.9)
  in newborn NOS (772.9)
  secondary or recurrent following trauma (958.2)
  traumatic rupture of blood vessel (900.0-904.9)
CC Excl: 459.0, 459.89, 459.9
AHA: 4Q, '90, 26

✓5th 459.1 Postphlebitic syndrome
►Chronic venous hypertension due to deep vein thrombosis◄
EXCLUDES ►chronic venous hypertension without deep vein thrombosis (459.30-459.39)◄
AHA: 2Q, '91, 20

DEF: Various conditions following deep vein thrombosis; including edema, pain, stasis dermatitis, cellulitis, varicose veins and ulceration of the lower leg.

● **459.10 Postphlebitic syndrome without complications**
Asymptomatic postphlebitic syndrome
Postphlebitic syndrome NOS

459.11 Postphlebitic syndrome with ulcer
459.12 Postphlebitic syndrome with inflammation

● **459.13 Postphlebitic syndrome with ulcer and inflammation**
● **459.19 Postphlebitic syndrome with other complication**

459.2 Compression of vein
Stricture of vein
Vena cava syndrome (inferior) (superior)

✓5th 459.3 Chronic venous hypertension (idiopathic)
Stasis edema
EXCLUDES chronic venous hypertension due to deep vein thrombosis (459.10-459.9)
varicose veins (454.0-454.9)

● **459.30 Chronic venous hypertension without complications**
Asymptomatic chronic venous hypertension
Chronic venous hypertension NOS

● **459.31 Chronic venous hypertension with ulcer**
● **459.32 Chronic venous hypertension with inflammation**
● **459.33 Chronic venous hypertension with ulcer and inflammation**
● **459.39 Chronic venous hypertension with other complication**

✓5th 459.8 Other specified disorders of circulatory system

459.81 Venous (peripheral) insufficiency, unspecified
Chronic venous insufficiency NOS
Use additional code for any associated ulceration (707.10-707.9)
AHA: 2Q, '91, 20; M-A, '87, 6

DEF: Insufficient drainage, venous blood, any part of body, results in edema or dermatosis.

459.89 Other
Collateral circulation (venous), any site
Phlebosclerosis
Venofibrosis

459.9 Unspecified circulatory system disorder

Tabular List — RESPIRATORY SYSTEM — 460–464.21

8. DISEASES OF THE RESPIRATORY SYSTEM (460-519)

Use additional code to identify infectious organism

ACUTE RESPIRATORY INFECTIONS (460-466)

EXCLUDES pneumonia and influenza (480.0-487.8)

460 Acute nasopharyngitis [common cold]
Coryza (acute)
Nasal catarrh, acute
Nasopharyngitis:
  NOS
  acute
Nasopharyngitis:
  infective NOS
Rhinitis:
  acute
  infective

EXCLUDES
nasopharyngitis, chronic (472.2)
pharyngitis:
  acute or unspecified (462)
  chronic (472.1)
rhinitis:
  allergic (477.0-477.9)
  chronic or unspecified (472.0)
sore throat:
  acute or unspecified (462)
  chronic (472.1)

AHA: 1Q, '88, 12

DEF: Acute inflammation of mucous membranes; extends from nares to pharynx.

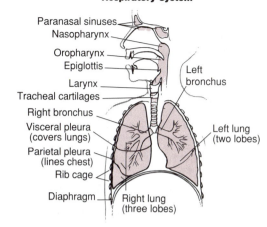

Respiratory System

✓4th 461 Acute sinusitis

INCLUDES
abscess
empyema
infection
inflammation
suppuration
  acute, of sinus
  (accessory)
  (nasal)

EXCLUDES chronic or unspecified sinusitis (473.0-473.9)

- **461.0 Maxillary**
  Acute antritis
- **461.1 Frontal**
- **461.2 Ethmoidal**
- **461.3 Sphenoidal**
- **461.8 Other acute sinusitis**
  Acute pansinusitis
- **461.9 Acute sinusitis, unspecified**
  Acute sinusitis NOS

462 Acute pharyngitis
Acute sore throat NOS
Pharyngitis (acute):
  NOS
  gangrenous
  infective
  phlegmonous
  pneumococcal
Pharyngitis (acute):
  staphylococcal
  suppurative
  ulcerative
Sore throat (viral) NOS
Viral pharyngitis

EXCLUDES
abscess:
  peritonsillar [quinsy] (475)
  pharyngeal NOS (478.29)
  retropharyngeal (478.24)
chronic pharyngitis (472.1)
infectious mononucleosis (075)
that specified as (due to):
  Coxsackie (virus) (074.0)
  gonococcus (098.6)
  herpes simplex (054.79)
  influenza (487.1)
  septic (034.0)
  streptococcal (034.0)

AHA: 4Q, '99, 26; S-O, '85, 8

463 Acute tonsillitis
Tonsillitis (acute):
  NOS
  follicular
  gangrenous
  infective
  pneumococcal
Tonsillitis (acute):
  septic
  staphylococcal
  suppurative
  ulcerative
  viral

EXCLUDES
chronic tonsillitis (474.0)
hypertrophy of tonsils (474.1)
peritonsillar abscess [quinsy] (475)
sore throat:
  acute or NOS (462)
  septic (034.0)
streptococcal tonsillitis (034.0)

AHA: N-D, '84, 16

✓4th 464 Acute laryngitis and tracheitis

EXCLUDES that associated with influenza (487.1)
that due to Streptococcus (034.0)

- **✓5th 464.0 Acute laryngitis**
  Laryngitis (acute):
    NOS
    edematous
    Hemophilus influenzae [H. influenzae]
    pneumococcal
    septic
    suppurative
    ulcerative

  EXCLUDES chronic laryngitis (476.0-476.1)
  influenzal laryngitis (487.1)

  AHA: ▶4Q, '01, 42◀

  DEF: ▶ A rapidly advancing generalized upper respiratory infection of the lingual tonsillar area, epiglottic folds, false vocal cords, and the epiglottis; seen most commonly in children, but can affect people of any age.◀

  - **464.00 Without mention of obstruction**
  - **464.01 With obstruction**

- **✓5th 464.1 Acute tracheitis**
  Tracheitis (acute):
    NOS
    catarrhal
  Tracheitis (acute):
    viral

  EXCLUDES chronic tracheitis (491.8)

  - **464.10 Without mention of obstruction**
  - **464.11 With obstruction** **CC**
    CC Excl: 012.20-012.86, 017.90-017.96, 464.10-464.31, 519.8-519.9

- **✓5th 464.2 Acute laryngotracheitis**
  Laryngotracheitis (acute)
  Tracheitis (acute) with laryngitis (acute)

  EXCLUDES chronic laryngotracheitis (476.1)

  - **464.20 Without mention of obstruction**
  - **464.21 With obstruction** **CC**
    CC Excl: See code 464.11

✓4th ✓5th Additional Digit Required | Nonspecific PDx | Unacceptable PDx | Manifestation Code | MSP Medicare Secondary Payer | ▶◀ Revised Text | ● New Code | ▲ Revised Code Title

2002 Ingenix, Inc.   January 2002 • Volume 1 — 137

464.3–472.2 RESPIRATORY SYSTEM — Tabular List

√5th **464.3 Acute epiglottitis**
Viral epiglottitis
EXCLUDES: epiglottitis, chronic (476.1)

464.30 Without mention of obstruction
464.31 With obstruction   CC
CC Excl: See code 464.11

464.4 Croup
Croup syndrome
DEF: Acute laryngeal obstruction due to allergy, foreign body or infection; symptoms include barking cough, hoarseness and harsh, persistent high-pitched respiratory sound.

√5th **464.5 Supraglottitis, unspecified**
AHA: ▶4Q, '01, 42◀
DEF: A rapidly advancing generalized upper respiratory infection of the lingual tonsillar area, epiglottic folds, false vocal cords, and the epiglottis; seen most commonly in children, but can affect people of any age.

464.50 Without mention of obstruction
AHA: ▶4Q, '01, 43◀
464.51 With obstruction

√4th **465 Acute upper respiratory infections of multiple or unspecified sites**
EXCLUDES: upper respiratory infection due to:
influenza (487.1)
Streptococcus (034.0)

465.0 Acute laryngopharyngitis
DEF: Acute infection of the vocal cords and pharynx.

465.8 Other multiple sites
Multiple URI

465.9 Unspecified site
Acute URI NOS
Upper respiratory infection (acute)

√4th **466 Acute bronchitis and bronchiolitis**
INCLUDES: that with:
bronchospasm
obstruction

466.0 Acute bronchitis
Bronchitis, acute or subacute:
 fibrinous
 membranous
 pneumococcal
 purulent
 septic
Bronchitis, acute or subacute:
 viral
 with tracheitis
Croupous bronchitis
Tracheobronchitis, acute
EXCLUDES: acute bronchitis with:
bronchiectasis (494.1)
chronic obstructive pulmonary disease (491.21)
AHA: 4Q, '96, 28; 4Q, '91, 24; 1Q, '88, 12
DEF: Acute inflammation of main branches of bronchial tree due to infectious or irritant agents; symptoms include cough with a varied production of sputum, fever, substernal soreness, and lung rales.

√5th **466.1** Acute bronchiolitis
Bronchiolitis (acute)   Capillary pneumonia
DEF: Acute inflammation of finer subdivisions of bronchial tree due to infectious or irritant agents; symptoms include cough with a varied production of sputum, fever, substernal soreness, and lung rales.

466.11 Acute bronchiolitis due to respiratory syncytial virus (RSV)
AHA: 4Q, '96, 27

466.19 Acute bronchiolitis due to other infectious organisms
Use additional code to identify organism

OTHER DISEASES OF THE UPPER RESPIRATORY TRACT (470-478)

470 Deviated nasal septum
Deflected septum (nasal) (acquired)
EXCLUDES: congenital (754.0)

√4th **471 Nasal polyps**
EXCLUDES: adenomatous polyps (212.0)

471.0 Polyp of nasal cavity
Polyp: choanal
Polyp: nasopharyngeal

471.1 Polypoid sinus degeneration
Woakes' syndrome or ethmoiditis

471.8 Other polyp of sinus
Polyp of sinus:
 accessory
 ethmoidal
 maxillary
 sphenoidal

471.9 Unspecified nasal polyp
Nasal polyp NOS

√4th **472 Chronic pharyngitis and nasopharyngitis**

472.0 Chronic rhinitis
Ozena
Rhinitis:
 NOS
 atrophic
 granulomatous
Rhinitis:
 hypertrophic
 obstructive
 purulent
 ulcerative
EXCLUDES: allergic rhinitis (477.0-477.9)
DEF: Persistent inflammation of mucous membranes of nose.

472.1 Chronic pharyngitis
Chronic sore throat
Pharyngitis: atrophic
Pharyngitis:
 granular (chronic)
 hypertrophic

472.2 Chronic nasopharyngitis
EXCLUDES: acute or unspecified nasopharyngitis (460)
DEF: Persistent inflammation of mucous membranes extending from nares to pharynx.

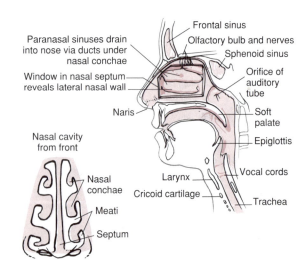

Upper Respiratory System

RESPIRATORY SYSTEM   473–478.30

Paranasal Sinuses

✓4ᵗʰ **473 Chronic sinusitis**
   INCLUDES   abscess
              empyema   (chronic) of sinus
              infection   (accessory) (nasal)
              suppuration
   EXCLUDES   acute sinusitis (461.0-461.9)

   473.0 Maxillary
      Antritis (chronic)
   473.1 Frontal
   473.2 Ethmoidal
      EXCLUDES   Woakes' ethmoiditis (471.1)
   473.3 Sphenoidal
   473.8 Other chronic sinusitis
      Pansinusitis (chronic)
   473.9 Unspecified sinusitis (chronic)
      Sinusitis (chronic) NOS

✓4ᵗʰ **474 Chronic disease of tonsils and adenoids**
   ✓5ᵗʰ **474.0 Chronic tonsillitis and adenoiditis**
      EXCLUDES   acute or unspecified tonsillitis (463)
      AHA: 4Q, '97, 38

      474.00 Chronic tonsillitis
      474.01 Chronic adenoiditis
      474.02 Chronic tonsillitis and adenoiditis
   ✓5ᵗʰ **474.1 Hypertrophy of tonsils and adenoids**
      Enlargement
      Hyperplasia   of tonsils or adenoids
      Hypertrophy
      EXCLUDES   that with:
                 adenoiditis (474.01)
                 adenoiditis and tonsillitis (474.02)
                 tonsillitis (474.00)

      474.10 Tonsils with adenoids
      474.11 Tonsils alone
      474.12 Adenoids alone
   474.2 Adenoid vegetations
      DEF: Fungus-like growth of lymph tissue between the nares and pharynx.
   474.8 Other chronic disease of tonsils and adenoids
      Amygdalolith   Tonsillar tag
      Calculus, tonsil   Ulcer, tonsil
      Cicatrix of tonsil (and adenoid)
   474.9 Unspecified chronic disease of tonsils and adenoids
      Disease (chronic) of tonsils (and adenoids)

475 Peritonsillar abscess
   Abscess of tonsil   Quinsy
   Peritonsillar cellulitis
   EXCLUDES   tonsillitis:
              acute or NOS (463)
              chronic (474.0)
   CC Excl: 475, 519.8-519.9

✓4ᵗʰ **476 Chronic laryngitis and laryngotracheitis**
   476.0 Chronic laryngitis
      Laryngitis: Laryngitis:
        catarrhal   sicca
        hypertrophic
   476.1 Chronic laryngotracheitis
      Laryngitis, chronic, with tracheitis (chronic)
      Tracheitis, chronic, with laryngitis
      EXCLUDES   chronic tracheitis (491.8)
                 laryngitis and tracheitis, acute or
                    unspecified (464.00-464.51)

✓4ᵗʰ **477 Allergic rhinitis**
   INCLUDES   allergic rhinitis (nonseasonal) (seasonal)
              hay fever
              spasmodic rhinorrhea
   EXCLUDES   allergic rhinitis with asthma (bronchial) (493.0)
   DEF: True immunoglobulin E (IgE)-mediated allergic reaction of nasal mucosa; seasonal (typical hay fever) or perennial (year-round allergens: dust, food, dander).

   477.0 Due to pollen
      Pollinosis
   477.1 Due to food
      AHA: 4Q, '00, 42
   477.8 Due to other allergen
   477.9 Cause unspecified
      AHA: 2Q, '97, 9

✓4ᵗʰ **478 Other diseases of upper respiratory tract**
   478.0 Hypertrophy of nasal turbinates
      DEF: Overgrowth, enlargement of shell-shaped bones, in nasal cavity.
   478.1 Other diseases of nasal cavity and sinuses
      Abscess
      Necrosis   of nose (septum)
      Ulcer
      Cyst or mucocele of sinus (nasal)
      Rhinolith
      EXCLUDES   varicose ulcer of nasal septum (456.8)
   ✓5ᵗʰ **478.2 Other diseases of pharynx, not elsewhere classified**
      478.20 Unspecified disease of pharynx
      478.21 Cellulitis of pharynx or nasopharynx
         CC Excl: 478.20-478.24, 519.8-519.9
      478.22 Parapharyngeal abscess
         CC Excl: See code 478.21
      478.24 Retropharyngeal abscess
         CC Excl: See code 478.21
         DEF: Purulent infection, behind pharynx and front of precerebral fascia.
      478.25 Edema of pharynx or nasopharynx
      478.26 Cyst of pharynx or nasopharynx
      478.29 Other
         Abscess of pharynx or nasopharynx
         EXCLUDES   ulcerative pharyngitis (462)
   ✓5ᵗʰ **478.3 Paralysis of vocal cords or larynx**
      DEF: Loss of motor ability of vocal cords or larynx; due to nerve or muscle damage.

      478.30 Paralysis, unspecified
         Laryngoplegia   Paralysis of glottis
         CC Excl: 478.30-478.34, 478.5, 478.70, 519.8-519.9

478.31–482.39 — **RESPIRATORY SYSTEM** — Tabular List

- **478.31** Unilateral, partial [CC]
  - CC Excl: See code 478.30
- **478.32** Unilateral, complete [CC]
  - CC Excl: See code 478.30
- **478.33** Bilateral, partial [CC]
  - CC Excl: See code 478.30
- **478.34** Bilateral, complete [CC]
  - CC Excl: See code 478.30

478.4 Polyp of vocal cord or larynx
  EXCLUDES adenomatous polyps (212.1)

478.5 Other diseases of vocal cords
  Abscess
  Cellulitis
  Granuloma   } of vocal cords
  Leukoplakia

  Chorditis (fibrinous) (nodosa) (tuberosa)
  Singers' nodes

478.6 Edema of larynx
  Edema (of):   Edema (of):
    glottis   supraglottic
    subglottic

√5th **478.7** Other diseases of larynx, not elsewhere classified
  - **478.70** Unspecified disease of larynx
  - **478.71** Cellulitis and perichondritis of larynx
    DEF: Inflammation of deep soft tissues or lining of bone of the larynx.
  - **478.74** Stenosis of larynx
  - **478.75** Laryngeal spasm
    Laryngismus (stridulus)
    DEF: Involuntary muscle contraction of the larynx.
  - **478.79** Other
    Abscess
    Necrosis
    Obstruction   } of larynx
    Pachyderma
    Ulcer
    EXCLUDES ulcerative laryngitis (464.00-464.01)
    AHA: 3Q, '91, 20

478.8 Upper respiratory tract hypersensitivity reaction, site unspecified
  EXCLUDES hypersensitivity reaction of lower respiratory tract, as:
    extrinsic allergic alveolitis (495.0-495.9)
    pneumoconiosis (500-505)

478.9 Other and unspecified diseases of upper respiratory tract
  Abscess
  Cicatrix   } of trachea

PNEUMONIA AND INFLUENZA (480-487)

EXCLUDES pneumonia:
  allergic or eosinophilic (518.3)
  aspiration:
    NOS (507.0)
    newborn (770.1)
    solids and liquids (507.0-507.8)
  congenital (770.0)
  lipoid (507.1)
  passive (514)
  rheumatic (390)

√4th **480** Viral pneumonia
  - **480.0** Pneumonia due to adenovirus
  - **480.1** Pneumonia due to respiratory syncytial virus
    AHA: 4Q, '96, 28; 1Q, '88, 12
  - **480.2** Pneumonia due to parainfluenza virus
  - **480.8** Pneumonia due to other virus not elsewhere classified [HIV]
    EXCLUDES congenital rubella pneumonitis (771.0)
    influenza with pneumonia, any form (487.0)
    pneumonia complicating viral diseases classified elsewhere (484.1-484.8)
  - **480.9** Viral pneumonia, unspecified [HIV]
    AHA: 3Q, '98, 5

481 Pneumococcal pneumonia [Streptococcus pneumoniae pneumonia] [CC MC HIV]
  Lobar pneumonia, organism unspecified
  CC Excl: 011.00-011.06, 011.10-011.16, 011.20-011.26, 011.30-011.36, 011.40-011.46, 011.50-011.56, 011.60-011.66, 011.70-011.76, 011.80-011.86, 011.90-011.96, 012.00-012.06, 012.10-012.16, 012.80-012.86, 017.90-017.96, 021.2, 031.0, 039.1, 115.05, 115.15, 115.95, 122.1, 130.4, 136.3, 480.0-480.2, 480.8-480.9, 481, 482.0-482.2, 482.30-482.32, 482.39, 482.4, 482.81-482.84, 482.89, 482.9, 483.0-483.1, 483.8, 484.1, 484.3, 484.5-484.8, 485, 486, 487.0-487.1, 494.0-494.1, 495.0-495.9, 496, 500, 501, 502, 503, 504, 505, 506.0-506.4, 506.9, 507.0-507.1, 507.8, 508.0-508.1, 508.8, 508.9, 517.1-517.8, 18.89, 519.8, 519.9, 748.61
  AHA: 2Q, '98, 7; 4Q, '92, 19; 1Q, '92, 18; 1Q, '91, 13; 1Q, '88, 13; M-A, '85, 6
  DRG 089

√4th **482** Other bacterial pneumonia
  AHA: 4Q, '93, 39
  - **482.0** Pneumonia due to Klebsiella pneumoniae [CC MC HIV]
    CC Excl: See code 481
  - **482.1** Pneumonia due to Pseudomonas [CC MC HIV]
    CC Excl: See code 481
    DRG 079
  - **482.2** Pneumonia due to Hemophilus influenzae [H. influenzae] [CC MC HIV]
    CC Excl: See code 481
  - √5th **482.3** Pneumonia due to Streptococcus
    EXCLUDES Streptococcus pneumoniae (481)
    AHA: 1Q, '88, 13
    - **482.30** Streptococcus, unspecified [CC MC HIV]
      CC Excl: See code 481
    - **482.31** Group A [CC MC HIV]
      CC Excl: See code 481
    - **482.32** Group B [CC MC HIV]
      CC Excl: See code 481
    - **482.39** Other Streptococcus [CC MC HIV]
      CC Excl: See code 481

RESPIRATORY SYSTEM

✓5ᵗʰ 482.4 Pneumonia due to Staphylococcus
AHA: 3Q, '91, 16

482.40 Pneumonia due to Staphylococcus unspecified [CC MC HIV]
CC Excl: See code 481
▽ DRG 079

482.41 Pneumonia due to Staphylococcus aureus [CC MC HIV]
CC Excl: See code 481
▽ DRG 079

482.49 Other Staphylococcus pneumonia [CC MC HIV]
CC Excl: See code 481
▽ DRG 079

✓5ᵗʰ 482.8 Pneumonia due to other specified bacteria
EXCLUDES pneumonia, complicating infectious disease classified elsewhere (484.1-484.8)

AHA: 3Q, '88, 11

482.81 Anaerobes [CC MC HIV]
Bacteroides (melaninogenicus)
Gram-negative anaerobes
CC Excl: See code 481

482.82 Escherichia coli [E. coli] [CC MC HIV]
CC Excl: See code 481

482.83 Other gram-negative bacteria [CC MC HIV]
Gram-negative pneumonia NOS
Proteus
Serratia marcescens
EXCLUDES gram-negative anaerobes (482.81)
Legionnaires' disease (482.84)
CC Excl: See code 481
AHA: 2Q, '98, 5; 3Q, '94, 9
▽ DRG 079

482.84 Legionnaires' disease [CC HIV]
CC Excl: See code 481
AHA: 4Q, '97, 38

DEF: Severe and often fatal infection by Legionella pneumophilia; symptoms include high fever, gastrointestinal pain, headache, myalgia, dry cough, and pneumonia; transmitted airborne via air conditioning systems, humidifiers, water faucets, shower heads; not person-to-person contact.

482.89 Other specified bacteria [CC MC HIV]
CC Excl: See code 481
AHA: 2Q, '97, 6

482.9 Bacterial pneumonia unspecified [CC MC HIV]
CC Excl: See code 481
AHA: 2Q, '98, 6; 2Q, '97, 6; 1Q, '94, 17

✓4ᵗʰ 483 Pneumonia due to other specified organism
AHA: N-D, '87, 5

483.0 Mycoplasma pneumoniae [CC MC]
Eaton's agent
Pleuropneumonia-like organism [PPLO]
CC Excl: See code 481

483.1 Chlamydia [CC MC]
CC Excl: See code 481
AHA: 4Q, '96, 31

483.8 Other specified organism [CC MC]
CC Excl: See code 481

✓4ᵗʰ 484 Pneumonia in infectious diseases classified elsewhere
EXCLUDES influenza with pneumonia, any form (487.0)

484.1 Pneumonia in cytomegalic inclusion disease [CC MC]
Code first underlying disease (078.5)
CC Excl: See code 481

484.3 Pneumonia in whooping cough [CC MC]
Code first underlying disease (033.0-033.9)
CC Excl: See code 481

484.5 Pneumonia in anthrax [CC MC]
Code first underlying disease (022.1)
CC Excl: See code 481

484.6 Pneumonia in aspergillosis [CC MC]
Code first underlying disease (117.3)
CC Excl: See code 481
AHA: 4Q, '97, 40

484.7 Pneumonia in other systemic mycoses [CC MC]
Code first underlying disease
EXCLUDES pneumonia in:
candidiasis (112.4)
coccidioidomycosis (114.0)
histoplasmosis (115.0-115.9 with fifth-digit 5)
CC Excl: See code 481

484.8 Pneumonia in other infectious diseases classified elsewhere [CC MC]
Code first underlying disease, as:
Q fever (083.0)
typhoid fever (002.0)
EXCLUDES pneumonia in:
actinomycosis (039.1)
measles (055.1)
nocardiosis (039.1)
ornithosis (073.0)
Pneumocystis carinii (136.3)
salmonellosis (003.22)
toxoplasmosis (130.4)
tuberculosis (011.6)
tularemia (021.2)
varicella (052.1)
CC Excl: See code 481

485 Bronchopneumonia, organism unspecified [CC MC]
Bronchopneumonia: Pneumonia:
  hemorrhagic   lobular
  terminal   segmental
Pleurobronchopneumonia
EXCLUDES bronchiolitis (acute) (466.11-466.19)
chronic (491.8)
lipoid pneumonia (507.1)
CC Excl: See code 481

RESPIRATORY SYSTEM

486 Pneumonia, organism unspecified
EXCLUDES hypostatic or passive pneumonia (514)
influenza with pneumonia, any form (487.0)
inhalation or aspiration pneumonia due to foreign materials (507.0-507.8)
pneumonitis due to fumes and vapors (506.0)

CC Excl: See code 481

AHA: 4Q, '99, 6; 3Q, '99, 9; 3Q, '98, 7; 2Q, '98, 4, 5; 1Q, '98, 8; 3Q, '97, 9; 3Q, '94, 10; 3Q, '88, 11

DRG 089 and 475

✓4th 487 Influenza
EXCLUDES Hemophilus influenzae [H. influenzae]:
infection NOS (041.5)
laryngitis (464.00-464.01)
meningitis (320.0)
pneumonia (482.2)

487.0 With pneumonia
Influenza with pneumonia, any form
Influenzal:
bronchopneumonia
pneumonia

CC Excl: See code 481

487.1 With other respiratory manifestations
Influenza NOS
Influenzal:
laryngitis
pharyngitis
respiratory infection (upper) (acute)

AHA: 4Q, '99, 26

487.8 With other manifestations
Encephalopathy due to influenza
Influenza with involvement of gastrointestinal tract
EXCLUDES "intestinal flu" [viral gastroenteritis] (008.8)

CHRONIC OBSTRUCTIVE PULMONARY DISEASE AND ALLIED CONDITIONS (490-496)
AHA: 3Q, '88, 5

490 Bronchitis, not specified as acute or chronic
Bronchitis NOS: Tracheobronchitis NOS
catarrhal
with tracheitis NOS
EXCLUDES bronchitis:
allergic NOS (493.9)
asthmatic NOS (493.9)
due to fumes and vapors (506.0)

✓4th 491 Chronic bronchitis
EXCLUDES chronic obstructive asthma (493.2)

491.0 Simple chronic bronchitis
Catarrhal bronchitis, chronic
Smokers' cough

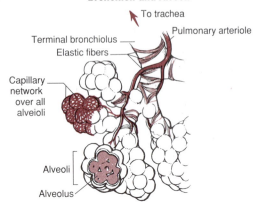

Bronchioli and Alveoli

491.1 Mucopurulent chronic bronchitis
Bronchitis (chronic) (recurrent):
fetid
mucopurulent
purulent

CC Excl: 491.1-491.9, 493.20-493.21

AHA: 3Q, '88, 12

DEF: Chronic bronchial infection characterized by both mucus and pus secretions in the bronchial tree; recurs after asymptomatic periods; signs are coughing, expectoration and secondary changes in the lung.

✓5th 491.2 Obstructive chronic bronchitis
Bronchitis:
emphysematous
obstructive (chronic) (diffuse)
Bronchitis with:
chronic airway obstruction
emphysema
EXCLUDES asthmatic bronchitis (acute) NOS (493.9)
chronic obstructive asthma (493.2)

AHA: 3Q, '97, 9; 4Q, '91, 25; 2Q, '91, 21

491.20 Without mention of acute exacerbation
Emphysema with chronic bronchitis

CC Excl: See code 491.1

AHA: 3Q, '97, 9

491.21 With acute exacerbation
Acute and chronic obstructive bronchitis
Acute bronchitis with chronic obstructive pulmonary disease [COPD]
Acute exacerbation of chronic obstructive pulmonary disease [COPD]
Emphysema with both acute and chronic bronchitis
EXCLUDES chronic obstructive asthma with acute exacerbation (493.22)

CC Excl: See code 491.1

AHA: ▶4Q, '01, 43;◀ 2Q, '96, 10

DRG 088 and 475

491.8 Other chronic bronchitis
Chronic:
tracheitis
tracheobronchitis

CC Excl: See code 491.1

491.9 Unspecified chronic bronchitis
CC Excl: See code 491.1

✓4th 492 Emphysema
AHA: 2Q, '91, 21

492.0 Emphysematous bleb
Giant bullous emphysema
Ruptured emphysematous bleb
Tension pneumatocele
Vanishing lung

AHA: 2Q, '93, 3

DEF: Formation of vesicle or bulla in emphysematous lung, more than one millimeter; contains serum or blood.

Tabular List — **RESPIRATORY SYSTEM** — 492.8–495.7

492.8 Other emphysema `CC`
  Emphysema (lung or pulmonary):
    NOS
    centriacinar
    centrilobular
    obstructive
    panacinar
    panlobular
  Emphysema (lung or pulmonary):
    unilateral
    vesicular
    MacLeod's syndrome
    Swyer-James syndrome
    Unilateral hyperlucent lung
  EXCLUDES emphysema:
    with both acute and chronic bronchitis (491.21)
    with chronic bronchitis (491.2)
    compensatory (518.2)
    due to fumes and vapors (506.4)
    interstitial (518.1)
    newborn (770.2)
    mediastinal (518.1)
    surgical (subcutaneous) (998.81)
    traumatic (958.7)

  CC Excl: 492.0, 492.8, 493.20-493.21

  AHA: 4Q, '93, 41; J-A, '84, 17

√4ᵗʰ **493 Asthma**
  EXCLUDES wheezing NOS (786.07)

  The following fifth-digit subclassification is for use with category 493:

    0 without mention of status asthmaticus or acute exacerbation or unspecified
    1 with status asthmaticus
    2 with acute exacerbation

  AHA: 4Q, '01, 43; 4Q, '00, 42; 1Q, '91, 13; 3Q, '88, 9; J-A, '85, 8; N-D, '84, 17

  DEF: Status asthmaticus: severe, intractable episode of asthma unresponsive to normal therapeutic measures.

√5ᵗʰ **493.0 Extrinsic asthma** `CC 1-2`
  Asthma:
    allergic with stated cause
    atopic
    childhood
  Asthma:
    hay
    platinum
  Hay fever with asthma
  EXCLUDES asthma:
    allergic NOS (493.9)
    detergent (507.8)
    miners' (500)
    wood (495.8)

  CC Excl: For code 493.01 and 493.02: 493.00-493.92, 517.8, 518.89, 519.8-519.9

  DEF: Transient stricture of airway diameters of bronchi; due to environmental factor; also called allergic (bronchial) asthma.

√5ᵗʰ **493.1 Intrinsic asthma** `CC 1-2`
  Late-onset asthma

  CC Excl: For code 493.11 and 493.12: See code 493.0

  AHA: 3Q, '88, 9; M-A, '85, 7

  DEF: Transient stricture, of airway diameters of bronchi; due to pathophysiological disturbances.

√5ᵗʰ **493.2 Chronic obstructive asthma** `CC`
  Asthma with chronic obstructive pulmonary disease [COPD]
  ▶Chronic asthmatic bronchitis◀
  EXCLUDES acute bronchitis (466.0)

  CC Excl: For code 493.20 and 493.21: 491.1-493.92, 517.8, 518.89, 519.8-519.9; For code 493.22: 493.00-493.92, 517.8, 518.89, 519.8-519.9

  AHA: 2Q, '91, 21; 2Q, '90, 20

  DRG 088 For code 493.20

  DEF: Persistent narrowing of airway diameters in the bronchial tree, restricting airflow and causing constant labored breathing.

√5ᵗʰ **493.9 Asthma, unspecified** `CC 1-2`
  Asthma (bronchial) (allergic NOS)
  Bronchitis:
    allergic
    asthmatic

  CC Excl: For code 493.91 and 493.92: 493.00-493.92, 517.8, 518.89, 519.8-519.9

  AHA: 4Q, '97, 40, For code 493.90: 4Q, '99, 25; 1Q, '97, 7

√4ᵗʰ **494 Bronchiectasis**
  Bronchiectasis (fusiform) (postinfectious) (recurrent)
  Bronchiolectasis
  EXCLUDES congenital (748.61)
    tuberculous bronchiectasis (current disease) (011.5)

  AHA: 4Q, '00, 42

  DEF: Dilation of bronchi; due to infection or chronic conditions; causes decreased lung capacity and recurrent infections of lungs.

  494.0 Bronchiectasis without acute exacerbation
  494.1 Bronchiectasis with acute exacerbation `CC`
    Acute bronchitis with bronchiectasis
    CC Excl: 017.90-017.96, 487.1, 494.1, 496, 506.1, 506.4, 506.9, 748.61

√4ᵗʰ **495 Extrinsic allergic alveolitis**
  INCLUDES allergic alveolitis and pneumonitis due to inhaled organic dust particles of fungal, thermophilic actinomycete, or other origin

  DEF: Pneumonitis due to particles inhaled into lung, often at workplace; symptoms include cough, chills, fever, increased heart and respiratory rates; develops within hours of exposure.

  495.0 Farmers' lung `CC`
    CC Excl: 011.00-011.96, 012.00-012.16, 012.80-012.86, 017.90-017.96, 021.2, 031.0, 039.1, 115.05, 115.15, 115.95, 122.1, 130.4, 136.3, 480.0-480.9, 481, 482.0-482.7, 482.81-482.84, 482.89, 482.9, 483.0, 483.1, 483.8, 484.1-484.8, 485-486, 487.0-487.1, 494.0-494.1, 495.0-495.9, 496, 500-505, 506.0-506.9, 507.0-507.8, 508.0-508.9, 517.1, 517.8, 518.89, 519.8-519.9, 748.61

  495.1 Bagassosis `CC`
    CC Excl: See code 495.0

  495.2 Bird-fanciers' lung `CC`
    Budgerigar-fanciers' disease or lung
    Pigeon-fanciers' disease or lung
    CC Excl: See code 495.0

  495.3 Suberosis `CC`
    Cork-handlers' disease or lung
    CC Excl: See code 495.0

  495.4 Malt workers' lung `CC`
    Alveolitis due to Aspergillus clavatus
    CC Excl: See code 495.0

  495.5 Mushroom workers' lung `CC`
    CC Excl: See code 495.0

  495.6 Maple bark-strippers' lung `CC`
    Alveolitis due to Cryptostroma corticale
    CC Excl: See code 495.0

  495.7 "Ventilation" pneumonitis `CC`
    Allergic alveolitis due to fungal, thermophilic actinomycete, and other organisms growing in ventilation [air conditioning] systems
    CC Excl: See code 495.0

RESPIRATORY SYSTEM — Tabular List

495.8 Other specified allergic alveolitis and pneumonitis [CC]
- Cheese-washers' lung
- Coffee workers' lung
- Fish-meal workers' lung
- Furriers' lung
- Grain-handlers' disease or lung
- Pituitary snuff-takers' disease
- Sequoiosis or red-cedar asthma
- Wood asthma

CC Excl: See code 495.0

495.9 Unspecified allergic alveolitis and pneumonitis [CC]
- Alveolitis, allergic (extrinsic)
- Hypersensitivity pneumonitis

CC Excl: See code 495.0

496 Chronic airway obstruction, not elsewhere classified [CC] [A]

Note: This code is not to be used with any code from categories 491-493

Chronic:
- nonspecific lung disease
- obstructive lung disease
- obstructive pulmonary disease [COPD] NOS

EXCLUDES: chronic obstructive lung disease [COPD] specified (as) (with):
- allergic alveolitis (495.0-495.9)
- asthma (493.2)
- bronchiectasis (494.0-494.1)
- bronchitis (491.20-491.21)
  - with emphysema (491.20-491.21)
- emphysema (492.0-492.8)

CC Excl: 017.90-017.96, 487.1, 494.0-494.1, 496, 506.1, 506.4, 506.9, 748.61

AHA: 2Q, '00, 15; 2Q, '92, 16; 2Q, '91, 21; 3Q, '88, 56

DRG 088

PNEUMOCONIOSES AND OTHER LUNG DISEASES DUE TO EXTERNAL AGENTS (500-508)

DEF: Permanent deposits of particulate matter, within lungs; due to occupational or environmental exposure; results in chronic induration and fibrosis. (See specific listings in 500-508 code range)

500 Coal workers' pneumoconiosis [A]
- Anthracosilicosis
- Anthracosis
- Black lung disease
- Coal workers' lung
- Miner's asthma

501 Asbestosis [A]

502 Pneumoconiosis due to other silica or silicates
- Pneumoconiosis due to talc
- Silicotic fibrosis (massive) of lung
- Silicosis (simple) (complicated)

503 Pneumoconiosis due to other inorganic dust
- Aluminosis (of lung)
- Bauxite fibrosis (of lung)
- Berylliosis
- Graphite fibrosis (of lung)
- Siderosis
- Stannosis

504 Pneumonopathy due to inhalation of other dust
- Byssinosis
- Cannabinosis
- Flax-dressers' disease

EXCLUDES:
- allergic alveolitis (495.0-495.9)
- asbestosis (501)
- bagassosis (495.1)
- farmers' lung (495.0)

505 Pneumoconiosis, unspecified

√4th 506 Respiratory conditions due to chemical fumes and vapors
Use additional E code to identify cause

506.0 Bronchitis and pneumonitis due to fumes and vapors [CC]
- Chemical bronchitis (acute)

CC Excl: 011.00-011.96, 012.10-012.16, 012.80-012.86, 017.90-017.96, 021.2, 031.0, 039.1, 115.05, 115.15, 115.95, 122.1, 130.4, 136.3, 480.0-480.9, 481, 482.0-482.7, 482.81-482.84, 482.89, 482.9, 483.0, 483.1, 483.8, 484.1-484.8, 485-486, 487.0-487.1, 494.0-494.1, 495.0-495.9, 496, 500-505, 506.0-506.9, 507.0-507.8, 508.0-508.9, 517.1, 517.8, 518.89, 519.8-519.9, 748.61

506.1 Acute pulmonary edema due to fumes and vapors [CC]
- Chemical pulmonary edema (acute)

EXCLUDES:
- acute pulmonary edema NOS (518.4)
- chronic or unspecified pulmonary edema (514)

CC Excl: See code 506.0

AHA: 3Q, '88, 4

506.2 Upper respiratory inflammation due to fumes and vapors

506.3 Other acute and subacute respiratory conditions due to fumes and vapors

506.4 Chronic respiratory conditions due to fumes and vapors
- Emphysema (diffuse) (chronic)
- Obliterative bronchiolitis (chronic) (subacute)
- Pulmonary fibrosis (chronic)

} due to inhalation of chemical fumes and vapors

506.9 Unspecified respiratory conditions due to fumes and vapors
- Silo-fillers' disease

√4th 507 Pneumonitis due to solids and liquids

EXCLUDES: fetal aspiration pneumonitis (770.1)

AHA: 3Q, '91, 16

507.0 Due to inhalation of food or vomitus [CC] [MC]
Aspiration pneumonia (due to):
- NOS
- food (regurgitated)
- gastric secretions
- milk
- saliva
- vomitus

CC Excl: See code 506.0

AHA: 1Q, '89, 10

DRG 079 and 475

507.1 Due to inhalation of oils and essences [CC] [MC]
- Lipoid pneumonia (exogenous)

EXCLUDES: endogenous lipoid pneumonia (516.8)

CC Excl: See code 506.0

507.8 Due to other solids and liquids [CC] [MC]
- Detergent asthma

CC Excl: See code 506.0

√4th 508 Respiratory conditions due to other and unspecified external agents
Use additional E code to identify cause

508.0 Acute pulmonary manifestations due to radiation [CC]
- Radiation pneumonitis

CC Excl: See code 506.0

AHA: 2Q, '88, 4

508.1 Chronic and other pulmonary manifestations due to radiation [CC]
- Fibrosis of lung following radiation

CC Excl: See code 506.0

508.8 Respiratory conditions due to other specified external agents

508.9 Respiratory conditions due to unspecified external agent

OTHER DISEASES OF RESPIRATORY SYSTEM (510-519)

✓4th 510 Empyema
Use additional code to identify infectious organism (041.0-041.9)

EXCLUDES abscess of lung (513.0)

DEF: Purulent infection, within pleural space.

510.0 With fistula
Fistula:
- bronchocutaneous
- bronchopleural
- hepatopleural
- mediastinal
- pleural
- thoracic

Any condition classifiable to 510.9 with fistula

CC Excl: 510.0, 510.9, 517.8, 518.89, 519.8-519.9

DEF: Purulent infection of respiratory cavity; with communication from cavity to another structure.

510.9 Without mention of fistula
Abscess:
- pleura
- thorax

Empyema (chest) (lung) (pleura)

Fibrinopurulent pleurisy

Pleurisy:
- purulent
- septic
- seropurulent
- suppurative

Pyopneumothorax
Pyothorax

CC Excl: See code 510.0

AHA: 3Q, '94, 6

✓4th 511 Pleurisy
EXCLUDES malignant pleural effusion (197.2)
pleurisy with mention of tuberculosis, current disease (012.0)

DEF: Inflammation of serous membrane of lungs and lining of thoracic cavity; causes exudation in cavity or membrane surface.

511.0 Without mention of effusion or current tuberculosis
Adhesion, lung or pleura
Calcification of pleura
Pleurisy (acute) (sterile):
- diaphragmatic
- fibrinous
- interlobar

Pleurisy:
- NOS
- pneumococcal
- staphylococcal
- streptococcal

Thickening of pleura

AHA: 3Q, '94, 5

511.1 With effusion, with mention of a bacterial cause other than tuberculosis
Pleurisy with effusion (exudative) (serous):
- pneumococcal
- staphylococcal
- streptococcal
- other specified nontuberculous bacterial cause

CC Excl: 011.00-011.96, 012.00-012.16, 012.80-012.86, 017.90-017.96, 511.0-511.9, 517.8, 518.89, 519.8-519.9

511.8 Other specified forms of effusion, except tuberculous
- Encysted pleurisy
- Hemopneumothorax
- Hemothorax
- Hydropneumothorax
- Hydrothorax

EXCLUDES traumatic (860.2-860.5, 862.29, 862.39)

CC Excl: See code 511.1

AHA: 1Q, '97, 10

511.9 Unspecified pleural effusion
Pleural effusion NOS
Pleurisy:
- exudative
- serofibrinous
- serous
- with effusion NOS

CC Excl: See code 511.1

AHA: 3Q, '91, 19; 4Q, '89, 11

✓4th 512 Pneumothorax
DEF: Collapsed lung; due to gas or air in pleural space.

512.0 Spontaneous tension pneumothorax
CC Excl: 512.0-512.1, 512.8, 517.8, 518.89, 519.8-519.9

AHA: 3Q, '94, 5

DEF: Leaking air from lung into lining causing collapse.

512.1 Iatrogenic pneumothorax
Postoperative pneumothorax

CC Excl: See code 512.0

AHA: 4Q, '94, 40

DEF: Air trapped in the lining of the lung following surgery.

512.8 Other spontaneous pneumothorax
Pneumothorax:
- NOS
- acute
- chronic

EXCLUDES pneumothorax:
congenital (770.2)
traumatic (860.0-860.1, 860.4-860.5)
tuberculous, current disease (011.7)

CC Excl: See code 512.0

AHA: 2Q, '93, 3

✓4th 513 Abscess of lung and mediastinum
513.0 Abscess of lung
Abscess (multiple) of lung
Gangrenous or necrotic pneumonia
Pulmonary gangrene or necrosis

CC Excl: 006.4, 011.00-011.96, 012.00-012.16, 012.80-012.86, 017.90-017.96, 513.0, 519.8-519.9

AHA: 2Q, '98, 7

513.1 Abscess of mediastinum
CC Excl: 513.1, 519.8-519.9

514 Pulmonary congestion and hypostasis
Hypostatic:
- bronchopneumonia
- pneumonia

Passive pneumonia
Pulmonary congestion (chronic) (passive)

Pulmonary edema:
- NOS
- chronic

EXCLUDES acute pulmonary edema:
NOS (518.4)
with mention of heart disease or failure (428.1)

AHA: 2Q, '98, 6; 3Q, '88, 5

DEF: Excessive retention of interstitial fluid in the lungs and pulmonary vessels; due to poor circulation.

515 Postinflammatory pulmonary fibrosis `CC`
Cirrhosis of lung
Fibrosis of lung (atrophic)
 (confluent) (massive)
 (perialveolar)
 (peribronchial) } chronic or unspecified
Induration of lung

CC Excl: 011.00-011.96, 012.00-012.16, 012.80-012.86, 017.90-017.96, 494.0-494.1, 495.0-495.9, 496, 500-505, 506.0-506.9, 507.0-507.8, 508.0-508.9, 515, 516.0-516.9, 517.2, 517.8, 518.89, 519.8-519.9, 748.61

DEF: Fibrosis and scarring of the lungs due to inflammatory reaction.

✓4th 516 Other alveolar and parietoalveolar pneumonopathy

516.0 Pulmonary alveolar proteinosis `CC`
CC Excl: See code 515
DEF: Reduced ventilation; due to proteinaceous deposits on alveoli; symptoms include dyspnea, cough, chest pain, weakness, weight loss, and hemoptysis.

516.1 Idiopathic pulmonary hemosiderosis `CC`
Code first underlying disease (275.0)
Essential brown induration of lung
CC Excl: See code 515
DEF: Fibrosis of alveolar walls; marked by abnormal amounts hemosiderin in lungs; primarily affects children; symptoms include anemia, fluid in lungs, and blood in sputum; etiology unknown.

516.2 Pulmonary alveolar microlithiasis `CC`
CC Excl: See code 515
DEF: Small calculi in pulmonary alveoli resembling sand-like particles on x-ray.

516.3 Idiopathic fibrosing alveolitis `CC`
Alveolar capillary block
Diffuse (idiopathic) (interstitial) pulmonary fibrosis
Hamman-Rich syndrome
CC Excl: See code 515

516.8 Other specified alveolar and parietoalveolar pneumonopathies `CC`
Endogenous lipoid pneumonia
Interstitial pneumonia (desquamative) (lymphoid)
EXCLUDES lipoid pneumonia, exogenous or unspecified (507.1)
CC Excl: See code 515
AHA: 1Q, '92, 12

516.9 Unspecified alveolar and parietoalveolar pneumonopathy `CC`
CC Excl: See code 515

✓4th 517 Lung involvement in conditions classified elsewhere
EXCLUDES rheumatoid lung (714.81)

517.1 Rheumatic pneumonia `CC`
Code first underlying disease (390)
CC Excl: 011.00-011.96, 012.00-012.16, 012.80-012.86, 017.90-017.96, 480.0-480.9, 481, 482.0-482.7, 482.81-482.84, 482.89, 482.9, 483.0, 483.1, 483.8, 484.1-484.8, 485-486, 487.0-487.1, 494.0-494.1, |495.0-495.9, 496, 500-505, 506.0-506.9, 507.0-507.8, 508.0-508.9, 515, 516.0-516.9, 517.1-517.8, 518.89, 519.8-519.9, 748.61

517.2 Lung involvement in systemic sclerosis `CC`
Code first underlying disease (710.1)
CC Excl: 011.00-011.96, 012.00-012.16, 012.80-012.86, 017.90-017.96, 494.0-494.1,495.0-495.9, 496, 500-505, 506.0-506.9, 507.0-507.8, 508.0-508.9, 515, 516.0-516.9, 517.2, 517.8, 518.89, 519.8-519.9, 748.61

517.8 Lung involvement in other diseases classified elsewhere `CC`
Code first underlying disease, as:
 amyloidosis (277.3)
 polymyositis (710.4)
 sarcoidosis (135)
 Sjögren's disease (710.2)
 systemic lupus erythematosus (710.0)
EXCLUDES syphilis (095.1)
CC Excl: See code 517.2

✓4th 518 Other diseases of lung

518.0 Pulmonary collapse `CC` `MC`
Atelectasis
Collapse of lung
Middle lobe syndrome
EXCLUDES atelectasis:
 congenital (partial) (770.5)
 primary (770.4)
 tuberculous, current disease (011.8)
CC Excl: 518.0, 519.8-519.9
AHA: 4Q, '90, 25

518.1 Interstitial emphysema `CC`
Mediastinal emphysema
EXCLUDES surgical (subcutaneous) emphysema (998.81)
 that in fetus or newborn (770.2)
 traumatic emphysema (958.7)
CC Excl: 518.1, 519.8-519.9
DEF: Escaped air from the alveoli trapped in the interstices of the lung; trauma or cough may cause the disease.

518.2 Compensatory emphysema
DEF: Distention of all or part of the lung caused by disease processes or surgical intervention that decreased volume in another part of the lung; overcompensation reaction to the loss of capacity in another part of the lung.

518.3 Pulmonary eosinophilia
Eosinophilic asthma
Löffler's syndrome
Pneumonia:
 allergic
 eosinophilic
Tropical eosinophilia
DEF: Infiltration, into pulmonary parenchyma of eosinophilia; results in cough, fever, and dyspnea.

518.4 Acute edema of lung, unspecified `CC`
Acute pulmonary edema NOS
Pulmonary edema, postoperative
EXCLUDES pulmonary edema:
 acute, with mention of heart disease or failure (428.1)
 chronic or unspecified (514)
 due to external agents (506.0-508.9)
CC Excl: 398.91, 428.0-428.9, 518.4, 519.8-519.9
DRG 087
DEF: Severe, sudden fluid retention within lung tissues.

RESPIRATORY SYSTEM

518.5 Pulmonary insufficiency following trauma and surgery `CC` `MC`
  Adult respiratory distress syndrome
  Pulmonary insufficiency following:
    shock
    surgery
    trauma
  Shock lung
  EXCLUDES adult respiratory distress syndrome associated with other conditions (518.82)
    pneumonia:
      aspiration (507.0)
      hypostatic (514)
    respiratory failure in other conditions (518.81, 518.83-518.84)
  CC Excl: 518.5, 519.8-519.9
  AHA: 3Q, '88, 3; 3Q, '88, 7; S-O, '87, 1

518.6 Allergic bronchopulmonary aspergillosis `CC`
  CC Excl: 518.6, 519.8-519.9
  AHA: 4Q, '97, 39
  DEF: Noninvasive hypersensitive reaction; due to allergic reaction to *Aspergillus fumigatus* (mold).

✓5ᵗʰ **518.8 Acute respiratory failure**
  518.81 Acute respiratory failure `CC` `MC`
    Respiratory failure NOS
    EXCLUDES acute and chronic respiratory failure (518.84)
      acute respiratory distress (518.82)
      chronic respiratory failure (518.83)
      respiratory arrest (799.1)
      respiratory failure, newborn ▶(770.84)◀
    CC Excl: 518.81-518.89, 519.8-519.9, 799.1
    AHA: 4Q, '98, 41; 3Q, '91, 14; 2Q, '91, 3; 4Q, '90, 25; 2Q, '90, 20; 3Q, '88, 7; 3Q, '88, 10; S-O, '87, 1
    DRG 087 and 475

  518.82 Other pulmonary insufficiency, not elsewhere classified `CC`
    Acute respiratory distress
    Acute respiratory insufficiency
    Adult respiratory distress syndrome NEC
    EXCLUDES adult respiratory distress syndrome associated with trauma and surgery (518.5)
      pulmonary insufficiency following trauma and surgery (518.5)
      respiratory distress:
        NOS (786.09)
        newborn ▶(770.89)◀
        syndrome, newborn (769)
      shock lung (518.5)
    CC Excl: See code 518.81
    AHA: 2Q, '91, 21; 3Q, '88, 7

  518.83 Chronic respiratory failure `CC` `MC`
    CC Excl: See code 518.81

  518.84 Acute and chronic respiratory failure `CC` `MC`
    Acute on chronic respiratory failure
    CC Excl: See code 518.81

  518.89 Other diseases of lung, not elsewhere classified
    Broncholithiasis   Lung disease NOS
    Calcification of lung   Pulmolithiasis
    AHA: 3Q, '90, 18; 4Q, '88, 6
    DEF: Broncholithiasis: calculi in lumen of transbronchial tree.
    DEF: Pulmolithiasis: calculi in lung.

✓4ᵗʰ **519 Other diseases of respiratory system**
  ✓5ᵗʰ **519.0 Tracheostomy complications**
    519.00 Tracheostomy complication, unspecified `CC`
      CC Excl: 519.0-519.1, 519.8-519.9

    519.01 Infection of tracheostomy `CC`
      Use additional code to identify type of infection, such as:
        abscess or cellulitis of neck (682.1)
        septicemia (038.0-038.9)
      Use additional code to identify organism (041.00-041.9)
      CC Excl: See code 519.00
      AHA: 4Q, '98, 41

    519.02 Mechanical complication of tracheostomy `CC`
      Tracheal stenosis due to tracheostomy
      CC Excl: See code 519.00

    519.09 Other tracheostomy complications `CC`
      Hemorrhage due to tracheostomy
      Tracheoesophageal fistula due to tracheostomy
      CC Excl: See code 519.00

  519.1 Other diseases of trachea and bronchus, not elsewhere classified
    Calcification }
    Stenosis   } of bronchus or trachea
    Ulcer   }
    AHA: 3Q, '88, 6

  519.2 Mediastinitis `CC`
    CC Excl: 519.2-519.3, 519.8-519.9
    DEF: Inflammation of tissue between organs behind sternum.

  519.3 Other diseases of mediastinum, not elsewhere classified
    Fibrosis   }
    Hernia   } of mediastinum
    Retraction }

  519.4 Disorders of diaphragm
    Diaphragmitis   Relaxation of diaphragm
    Paralysis of diaphragm
    EXCLUDES congenital defect of diaphragm (756.6)
      diaphragmatic hernia (551-553 with .3)
      congenital (756.6)

  519.8 Other diseases of respiratory system, not elsewhere classified
    AHA: 4Q, '89, 12

  519.9 Unspecified disease of respiratory system
    Respiratory disease (chronic) NOS

Tabular List — DIGESTIVE SYSTEM

9. DISEASES OF THE DIGESTIVE SYSTEM (520-579)

DISEASES OF ORAL CAVITY, SALIVARY GLANDS, AND JAWS (520-529)

✓4th 520 Disorders of tooth development and eruption

520.0 Anodontia
Absence of teeth (complete) (congenital) (partial)
Hypodontia
Oligodontia
EXCLUDES acquired absence of teeth (525.10-525.19)

520.1 Supernumerary teeth
Distomolar
Fourth molar
Mesiodens
Paramolar
Supplemental teeth
EXCLUDES supernumerary roots (520.2)

520.2 Abnormalities of size and form
Concrescence ⎫
Fusion   ⎬ of teeth
Gemination   ⎭

Dens evaginatus   Microdontia
Dens in dente   Peg-shaped [conical] teeth
Dens invaginatus   Supernumerary roots
Enamel pearls   Taurodontism
Macrodontia   Tuberculum paramolare
EXCLUDES that due to congenital syphilis (090.5)
tuberculum Carabelli, which is regarded as a normal variation

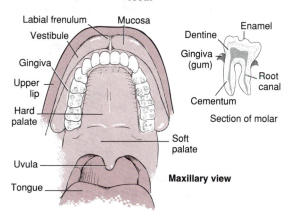
Teeth — Maxillary view; Section of molar

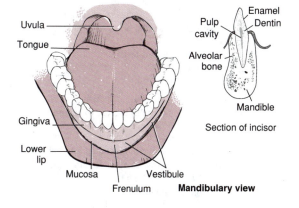
Mandibular view; Section of incisor

520.3 Mottled teeth
Mottling of enamel
Dental fluorosis   Nonfluoride enamel opacities

520.4 Disturbances of tooth formation
Aplasia and hypoplasia of cementum
Dilaceration of tooth
Enamel hypoplasia (neonatal) (postnatal) (prenatal)
Horner's teeth
Hypocalcification of teeth
Regional odontodysplasia
Turner's tooth
EXCLUDES Hutchinson's teeth and mulberry molars in congenital syphilis (090.5)
mottled teeth (520.3)

520.5 Hereditary disturbances in tooth structure, not elsewhere classified
Amelogenesis   ⎫
Dentinogenesis ⎬ imperfecta
Odontogenesis   ⎭

Dentinal dysplasia
Shell teeth

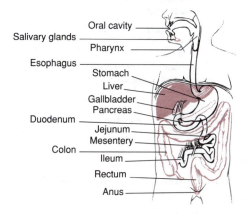
Digestive System

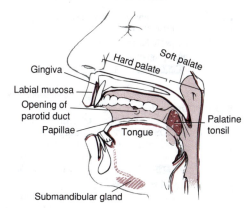
The Oral Cavity

520.6 Disturbances in tooth eruption
Teeth:
  embedded
  impacted
  natal
  neonatal
  primary [deciduous]:
    persistent
    shedding, premature
Tooth eruption:
  late
  obstructed
  premature

EXCLUDES exfoliation of teeth (attributable to disease of surrounding tissues) (525.0-525.19)
impacted or embedded teeth with abnormal position of such teeth or adjacent teeth (524.3)

520.7 Teething syndrome

520.8 Other specified disorders of tooth development and eruption
Color changes during tooth formation
Pre-eruptive color changes

EXCLUDES posteruptive color changes (521.7)

520.9 Unspecified disorder of tooth development and eruption

521 Diseases of hard tissues of teeth

521.0 Dental caries
AHA: ▶4Q, '01, 44◀

521.00 Dental caries, unspecified
521.01 Dental caries limited to enamel
Initial caries
White spot lesion
521.02 Dental caries extending into dentine
521.03 Dental caries extending into pulp
521.04 Arrested dental caries
521.05 Odontoclasia
Infantile melanodontia
Melanodontoclasia

EXCLUDES internal and external resorption of teeth (521.4)

DEF: ▶A pathological dental condition described as stained areas, loss of tooth substance, and hypoplasia linked to nutritional deficiencies during tooth development and to cariogenic oral conditions; synonyms are melanodontoclasia and infantile melanodontia.◀

521.09 Other dental caries

521.1 Excessive attrition
Approximal wear
Occlusal wear

521.2 Abrasion
Abrasion: of teeth
  dentifrice
  habitual
  occupational
  ritual
  traditional
  Wedge defect NOS

521.3 Erosion
Erosion of teeth:
  NOS
  due to:
    medicine
    persistent vomiting
Erosion of teeth:
  idiopathic
  occupational

521.4 Pathological resorption
Internal granuloma of pulp
Resorption of tooth or root (external) (internal)
DEF: Loss of dentin and cementum due to disease process.

521.5 Hypercementosis
Cementation hyperplasia
DEF: Excess deposits of cementum, on tooth root.

521.6 Ankylosis of teeth
DEF: Adhesion of tooth to surrounding bone.

521.7 Posteruptive color changes
Staining [discoloration] of teeth:
  NOS
  due to:
    drugs
    metals
    pulpal bleeding

EXCLUDES accretions [deposits] on teeth (523.6)
pre-eruptive color changes (520.8)

521.8 Other specified diseases of hard tissues of teeth
Irradiated enamel   Sensitive dentin

521.9 Unspecified disease of hard tissues of teeth

522 Diseases of pulp and periapical tissues

522.0 Pulpitis
Pulpal:
  abscess
  polyp
Pulpitis:
  acute
  chronic (hyperplastic) (ulcerative)
  suppurative

522.1 Necrosis of the pulp
Pulp gangrene
DEF: Death of pulp tissue.

522.2 Pulp degeneration
Denticles   Pulp stones
Pulp calcifications

522.3 Abnormal hard tissue formation in pulp
Secondary or irregular dentin

522.4 Acute apical periodontitis of pulpal origin
DEF: Severe inflammation of periodontal ligament due to pulpal inflammation or necrosis.

522.5 Periapical abscess without sinus
Abscess: Abscess:
  dental   dentoalveolar

EXCLUDES periapical abscess with sinus (522.7)

522.6 Chronic apical periodontitis
Apical or periapical granuloma
Apical periodontitis NOS

522.7 Periapical abscess with sinus
Fistula: Fistula:
  alveolar process   dental

522.8 Radicular cyst
Cyst: Cyst:
  apical (periodontal) residual radicular
  periapical
  radiculodental

EXCLUDES lateral developmental or lateral periodontal cyst (526.0)

DEF: Cyst in tissue around tooth apex due to chronic infection of granuloma around root.

522.9 Other and unspecified diseases of pulp and periapical tissues

523 Gingival and periodontal diseases

523.0 Acute gingivitis
EXCLUDES acute necrotizing ulcerative gingivitis (101)
herpetic gingivostomatitis (054.2)

523.1 Chronic gingivitis
Gingivitis (chronic):   Gingivitis (chronic):
  NOS   simple marginal
  desquamative   ulcerative
  hyperplastic   Gingivostomatitis

EXCLUDES herpetic gingivostomatitis (054.2)

523.2 Gingival recession
Gingival recession (generalized) (localized) (postinfective) (postoperative)

523.3 Acute periodontitis
Acute:
pericementitis
pericoronitis
Paradontal abscess
Periodontal abscess
EXCLUDES acute apical periodontitis (522.4)
periapical abscess (522.5, 522.7)
DEF: Severe inflammation, of tissues supporting teeth.

523.4 Chronic periodontitis
Alveolar pyorrhea
Chronic pericoronitis
Pericementitis (chronic)
Periodontitis:
NOS
Periodontitis:
complex
simplex
EXCLUDES chronic apical periodontitis (522.6)

523.5 Periodontosis

523.6 Accretions on teeth
Dental calculus:
subgingival
supragingival
Deposits on teeth:
betel
Deposits on teeth:
materia alba
soft
tartar
tobacco
DEF: Foreign material on tooth surface, usually plaque or calculus.

523.8 Other specified periodontal diseases
Giant cell:
epulis
peripheral granuloma
Gingival:
cysts
enlargement NOS
fibromatosis
Gingival polyp
Periodontal lesions due to traumatic occlusion
Peripheral giant cell granuloma
EXCLUDES leukoplakia of gingiva (528.6)

523.9 Unspecified gingival and periodontal disease

✓4th **524 Dentofacial anomalies, including malocclusion**

✓5th **524.0 Major anomalies of jaw size**
EXCLUDES hemifacial atrophy or hypertrophy (754.0)
unilateral condylar hyperplasia or hypoplasia of mandible (526.89)

524.00 Unspecified anomaly
DEF: Unspecified deformity of jaw size.

524.01 Maxillary hyperplasia
DEF: Overgrowth or over development of upper jaw bone.

524.02 Mandibular hyperplasia
DEF: Overgrowth or over development of lower jaw bone.

524.03 Maxillary hypoplasia
DEF: Incomplete or underdeveloped, upper jaw bone.

524.04 Mandibular hypoplasia
DEF: Incomplete or underdeveloped, lower jaw bone.

524.05 Macrogenia
DEF: Enlarged, jaw, especially chin; affects bone, soft tissue, or both.

524.06 Microgenia
DEF: Underdeveloped mandible, characterized by an extremely small chin.

524.09 Other specified anomaly

✓5th **524.1 Anomalies of relationship of jaw to cranial base**
524.10 Unspecified anomaly
Prognathism   Retrognathism
DEF: Prognathism: protrusion of lower jaw.
DEF: Retrognathism: jaw is located posteriorly to a normally positioned jaw; backward position of mandible.

524.11 Maxillary asymmetry
DEF: Absence of symmetry of maxilla.

524.12 Other jaw asymmetry
524.19 Other specified anomaly

524.2 Anomalies of dental arch relationship
Crossbite (anterior) (posterior)
Disto-occlusion
Mesio-occlusion
Midline deviation
Open bite (anterior) (posterior)
Overbite (excessive):
deep
horizontal
vertical
Overjet
Posterior lingual occlusion of mandibular teeth
Soft tissue impingement
EXCLUDES hemifacial atrophy or hypertrophy (754.0)
unilateral condylar hyperplasia or hypoplasia of mandible (526.89)

524.3 Anomalies of tooth position
Crowding
Diastema
Displacement
Rotation
Spacing, abnormal
Transposition
} of tooth, teeth

Impacted or embedded teeth with abnormal position of such teeth or adjacent teeth

524.4 Malocclusion, unspecified
DEF: Malposition of top and bottom teeth; interferes with chewing.

524.5 Dentofacial functional abnormalities
Abnormal jaw closure
Malocclusion due to:
abnormal swallowing
mouth breathing
tongue, lip, or finger habits

✓5th **524.6 Temporomandibular joint disorders**
EXCLUDES current temporomandibular joint:
dislocation (830.0-830.1)
strain (848.1)

524.60 Temporomandibular joint disorders, unspecified
Temporomandibular joint-pain-dysfunction syndrome [TMJ]

524.61 Adhesions and ankylosis (bony or fibrous)
DEF: Stiffening or union of temporomandibular joint due to bony or fibrous union across joint.

524.62 Arthralgia of temporomandibular joint
DEF: Pain in temporomandibular joint; not inflammatory in nature.

524.63 Articular disc disorder (reducing or non-reducing)

524.69 Other specified temporomandibular joint disorders

✓5th **524.7 Dental alveolar anomalies**
524.70 Unspecified alveolar anomaly
524.71 Alveolar maxillary hyperplasia
DEF: Excessive tissue formation in the dental alveoli of upper jaw.

524.72 Alveolar mandibular hyperplasia
DEF: Excessive tissue formation in the dental alveoli of lower jaw.

524.73 Alveolar maxillary hypoplasia
DEF: Incomplete or underdeveloped, alveolar tissue of upper jaw.

524.74 Alveolar mandibular hypoplasia
DEF: Incomplete or underdeveloped, alveolar tissue of lower jaw.

524.79 Other specified alveolar anomaly
524.8 Other specified dentofacial anomalies
524.9 Unspecified dentofacial anomalies

525 Other diseases and conditions of the teeth and supporting structures

525.0 Exfoliation of teeth due to systemic causes
DEF: Deterioration of teeth and surrounding structures due to systemic disease.

525.1 Loss of teeth due to trauma, extraction, or periodontal disease
AHA: 4Q, '01, 44

- **525.10** Acquired absence of teeth, unspecified
  - Edentulism
  - Tooth extraction status, NOS
- **525.11** Loss of teeth due to trauma
- **525.12** Loss of teeth due to periodontal disease
- **525.13** Loss of teeth due to caries
- **525.19** Other loss of teeth

525.2 Atrophy of edentulous alveolar ridge
525.3 Retained dental root
525.8 Other specified disorders of the teeth and supporting structures
Enlargement of alveolar ridge NOS
Irregular alveolar process

525.9 Unspecified disorder of the teeth and supporting structures

526 Diseases of the jaws

526.0 Developmental odontogenic cysts
Cyst:
- dentigerous
- eruption
- follicular
- lateral developmental
- lateral periodontal
- primordial
- Keratocyst

EXCLUDES: radicular cyst (522.8)

526.1 Fissural cysts of jaw
Cyst:
- globulomaxillary
- incisor canal
- median anterior maxillary
- median palatal
- nasopalatine
- palatine of papilla

EXCLUDES: cysts of oral soft tissues (528.4)

526.2 Other cysts of jaws
Cyst of jaw:
- NOS
- aneurysmal
- hemorrhagic
- traumatic

526.3 Central giant cell (reparative) granuloma
EXCLUDES: peripheral giant cell granuloma (523.8)

526.4 Inflammatory conditions
- Abscess
- Osteitis
- Osteomyelitis (neonatal)
- Periostitis

of jaw (acute) (chronic) (suppurative)

Sequestrum of jaw bone
EXCLUDES: alveolar osteitis (526.5)

526.5 Alveolitis of jaw
Alveolar osteitis   Dry socket
DEF: Inflammation, of alveoli or tooth socket.

526.8 Other specified diseases of the jaws

- **526.81** Exostosis of jaw
  - Torus mandibularis   Torus palatinus
  - DEF: Spur or bony outgrowth on the jaw.
- **526.89** Other
  - Cherubism
  - Fibrous dysplasia
  - Latent bone cyst
  - Osteoradionecrosis

  of jaw(s)

  Unilateral condylar hyperplasia or hypoplasia of mandible

526.9 Unspecified disease of the jaws

527 Diseases of the salivary glands

527.0 Atrophy
DEF: Wasting away, necrosis of salivary gland tissue.

527.1 Hypertrophy
DEF: Overgrowth or overdeveloped salivary gland tissue.

527.2 Sialoadenitis
Parotitis:
- NOS
- allergic
- toxic

Sialoangitis
Sialodochitis

EXCLUDES: epidemic or infectious parotitis (072.0-072.9)
uveoparotid fever (135)

DEF: Inflammation of salivary gland.

527.3 Abscess [CC]
CC Excl: 527.0-527.9, 537.89, 537.9

527.4 Fistula [CC]
EXCLUDES: congenital fistula of salivary gland (750.24)
CC Excl: See code 527.3

527.5 Sialolithiasis
Calculus
Stone
of salivary gland or duct

Sialodocholithiasis

527.6 Mucocele
Mucous:
- extravasation cyst of salivary gland
- retention cyst of salivary gland

Ranula
DEF: Dilated salivary gland cavity filled with mucous.

527.7 Disturbance of salivary secretion
- Hyposecretion
- Ptyalism
- Sialorrhea
- Xerostomia

527.8 Other specified diseases of the salivary glands
- Benign lymphoepithelial lesion of salivary gland
- Sialectasia
- Sialosis
- Stenosis
- Stricture

of salivary duct

527.9 Unspecified disease of the salivary glands

528 Diseases of the oral soft tissues, excluding lesions specific for gingiva and tongue

528.0 Stomatitis
Stomatitis:
- NOS
- ulcerative

Vesicular stomatitis

EXCLUDES: stomatitis:
- acute necrotizing ulcerative (101)
- aphthous (528.2)
- gangrenous (528.1)
- herpetic (054.2)
- Vincent's (101)

AHA: 2Q, '99, 9

DEF: Inflammation of oral mucosa; labial and buccal mucosa, tongue, plate, floor of the mouth, and gingivae.

528.1 Cancrum oris
Gangrenous stomatitis   Noma

DEF: A severely gangrenous lesion of mouth due to fusospirochetal infection; destroys buccal, labial and facial tissues; can be fatal; found primarily in debilitated and malnourished children.

528.2 Oral aphthae
- Aphthous stomatitis
- Canker sore
- Periadenitis mucosa necrotica recurrens
- Recurrent aphthous ulcer
- Stomatitis herpetiformis

EXCLUDES: herpetic stomatitis (054.2)

DEF: Small oval or round ulcers of the mouth marked by a grayish exudate and a red halo effect.

DIGESTIVE SYSTEM

528.3 Cellulitis and abscess [CC]
    Cellulitis of mouth (floor)
    Ludwig's angina
    Oral fistula
    EXCLUDES abscess of tongue (529.0)
        cellulitis or abscess of lip (528.5)
        fistula (of):
            dental (522.7)
            lip (528.5)
            gingivitis (523.0-523.1)
    CC Excl: 528.0, 528.3, 529.0, 529.2

528.4 Cysts
    Dermoid cyst
    Epidermoid cyst
    Epstein's pearl } of mouth
    Lymphoepithelial cyst
    Nasoalveolar cyst
    Nasolabial cyst
    EXCLUDES cyst: cyst:
        gingiva (523.8)   tongue (529.8)

528.5 Diseases of lips
    Abscess
    Cellulitis } of lip(s)
    Fistula
    Hypertrophy
    Cheilitis: Cheilodynia
      NOS   Cheilosis
      angular
    EXCLUDES actinic cheilitis (692.79)
        congenital fistula of lip (750.25)
        leukoplakia of lips (528.6)
    AHA: S-O, '86, 10

528.6 Leukoplakia of oral mucosa, including tongue
    Leukokeratosis of oral   Leukoplakia of:
      mucosa   lips
    Leukoplakia of: tongue
      gingiva
    EXCLUDES carcinoma in situ (230.0, 232.0)
        leukokeratosis nicotina palati (528.7)
    DEF: Thickened white patches of epithelium on mucous membranes of mouth.

528.7 Other disturbances of oral epithelium, including tongue
    Erythroplakia
    Focal epithelial hyperplasia } of mouth or tongue
    Leukoedema
    Leukokeratosis nicotina palati
    EXCLUDES carcinoma in situ (230.0, 232.0)
        leukokeratosis NOS (702)

528.8 Oral submucosal fibrosis, including of tongue

528.9 Other and unspecified diseases of the oral soft tissues
    Cheek and lip biting
    Denture sore mouth
    Denture stomatitis
    Melanoplakia
    Papillary hyperplasia of palate
    Eosinophilic granuloma
    Irritative hyperplasia } of oral mucosa
    Pyogenic granuloma
    Ulcer (traumatic)

√4th 529 Diseases and other conditions of the tongue

529.0 Glossitis
    Abscess
    Ulceration (traumatic) } of tongue
    EXCLUDES glossitis:
        benign migratory (529.1)
        Hunter's (529.4)
        median rhomboid (529.2)
        Moeller's (529.4)

529.1 Geographic tongue
    Benign migratory glossitis   Glossitis areata exfoliativa
    DEF: Chronic glossitis; marked by filiform papillae atrophy and inflammation; no known etiology.

529.2 Median rhomboid glossitis
    DEF: A noninflammatory, congenital disease characterized by rhomboid-like lesions at the middle third of the tongue's dorsal surface.

529.3 Hypertrophy of tongue papillae
    Black hairy tongue   Hypertrophy of foliate papillae
    Coated tongue   Lingua villosa nigra

529.4 Atrophy of tongue papillae
    Bald tongue   Glossitis:
    Glazed tongue   Moeller's
    Glossitis: Glossodynia exfoliativa
      Hunter's   Smooth atrophic tongue

529.5 Plicated tongue
    Fissured
    Furrowed } tongue
    Scrotal
    EXCLUDES fissure of tongue, congenital (750.13)
    DEF: Cracks, fissures or furrows, on dorsal surface of tongue.

529.6 Glossodynia
    Glossopyrosis   Painful tongue
    EXCLUDES glossodynia exfoliativa (529.4)

529.8 Other specified conditions of the tongue
    Atrophy
    Crenated
    Enlargement } (of) tongue
    Hypertrophy
    Glossocele
    Glossoptosis
    EXCLUDES erythroplasia of tongue (528.7)
        leukoplakia of tongue (528.6)
        macroglossia (congenital) (750.15)
        microglossia (congenital) (750.16)
        oral submucosal fibrosis (528.8)

529.9 Unspecified condition of the tongue

DISEASES OF ESOPHAGUS, STOMACH, AND DUODENUM (530-537)

√4th 530 Diseases of esophagus
    EXCLUDES esophageal varices (456.0-456.2)

530.0 Achalasia and cardiospasm
    Achalasia (of cardia)   Megaesophagus
    Aperistalsis of esophagus
    EXCLUDES congenital cardiospasm (750.7)
    DEF: Failure of smooth muscle fibers to relax, at gastrointestinal junctures; such as esophagogastric sphincter when swallowing.

√5th 530.1 Esophagitis
    Abscess of esophagus   Esophagitis:
    Esophagitis: peptic
      NOS   postoperative
      chemical   regurgitant
    Use additional E code to identify cause, if induced by chemical
    EXCLUDES tuberculous esophagitis (017.8)
    AHA: 4Q, '93, 27; 1Q, '92, 17; 3Q, '91, 20

530.10 Esophagitis, unspecified

530.11 Reflux esophagitis
    AHA: 4Q, '95, 82
    DEF: Inflammation of lower esophagus; due to regurgitated gastric acid.

530.12 Acute esophagitis
    AHA: ▶4Q, '01, 45◀
    DEF: ▶An acute inflammation of the mucous lining or submucosal coat of the esophagus.◀

530.19 Other esophagitis
    AHA: ▶3Q, '01, 10◀

DIGESTIVE SYSTEM

530.2 Ulcer of esophagus
Ulcer of esophagus: fungal
Ulcer of esophagus: peptic
Ulcer of esophagus due to ingestion of:
 aspirin
 chemicals
 medicines
Use additional E code to identify cause, if induced by chemical or drug

530.3 Stricture and stenosis of esophagus
Compression of esophagus
Obstruction of esophagus
EXCLUDES congenital stricture of esophagus (750.3)
AHA: 2Q, '01, 4; 2Q, '97, 3; 1Q, '88, 13

530.4 Perforation of esophagus [CC]
Rupture of esophagus
EXCLUDES traumatic perforation of esophagus (862.22, 862.32, 874.4-874.5)
CC Excl: 530.4, 530.7-530.81, 530.83-530.9

530.5 Dyskinesia of esophagus
Corkscrew esophagus   Esophagospasm
Curling esophagus   Spasm of esophagus
EXCLUDES cardiospasm (530.0)
AHA: 1Q, '88, 13; N-D, '84, 19
DEF: Difficulty performing voluntary esophageal movements.

530.6 Diverticulum of esophagus, acquired
Diverticulum, acquired: Diverticulum, acquired:
 epiphrenic   traction
 pharyngoesophageal   Zenker's
 pulsion   (hypopharyngeal)
 subdiaphragmatic   Esophageal pouch, acquired
                            Esophagocele, acquired
EXCLUDES congenital diverticulum of esophagus (750.4)
AHA: J-F, '85, 3

530.7 Gastroesophageal laceration-hemorrhage syndrome [CC]
Mallory-Weiss syndrome
CC Excl: 251.5, 456.0, 530.2, 530.4, 530.7-530.9, 531.00-531.91, 532.00-532.91, 533.00-533.91, 534.00-534.91, 535.01, 535.11, 535.21, 535.31, 535.41, 535.51, 535.61, 537.83, 562.02-562.03, 562.12-562.13, 569.3, 569.85, 578.0-578.9
DEF: Laceration of distal esophagus and proximal stomach due to vomiting, hiccups or other sustained activity.

√5th 530.8 Other specified disorders of esophagus

530.81 Esophageal reflux
Gastroesophageal reflux
EXCLUDES reflux esophagitis (530.11)
AHA: 2Q, '01, 4; 1Q, '95, 7; 4Q, '92, 27
DEF: Regurgitation of the gastric contents into esophagus and possibly pharynx; where aspiration may occur between the vocal cords and down into the trachea.

530.82 Esophageal hemorrhage [CC]
EXCLUDES hemorrhage due to esophageal varices (456.0-456.2)
CC Excl: 251.5, 456.0, 456.20, 459.89-459.9, 530.2, 530.7, 530.82, 531.00-531.21, 531.30-531.31, 531.40-531.91, 532.00-532.91, 533.00-533.91, 534.00-534.51, 534.61, 534.70-534.91, 535.01-535.11, 535.21, 535.31, 535.41, 535.51, 535.61, 537.83, 562.02-562.03, 562.12-562.13, 569.3, 569.85, 578.0-578.9

530.83 Esophageal leukoplakia

530.84 Tracheoesophageal fistula [CC]
EXCLUDES congenital tracheoesophageal fistula (750.3)
CC Excl: 530.4, 530.7, 530.81, 530.83-530.9

530.89 Other
EXCLUDES Paterson-Kelly syndrome (280.8)

530.9 Unspecified disorder of esophagus

√4th 531 Gastric ulcer
INCLUDES ulcer (peptic):
 prepyloric
 pylorus
 stomach
Use additional E code to identify drug, if drug-induced
EXCLUDES peptic ulcer NOS (533.0-533.9)

The following fifth-digit subclassification is for use with category 531:
 0 without mention of obstruction
 1 with obstruction

AHA: 1Q, '91, 15; 4Q, '90, 27

DEF: Destruction of tissue in lumen of stomach due to action of gastric acid and pepsin on gastric mucosa decreasing resistance to ulcers.

√5th 531.0 Acute with hemorrhage [CC]
CC Excl: 251.5, 456.0, 530.2, 530.7, 530.82, 531.00-531.91, 532.00-532.91, 533.00-533.91, 534.00-534.91, 535.01, 535.11, 535.21, 535.31, 535.41, 535.51, 535.61, 537.83, 537.89, 537.9, 562.02-562.03, 562.12-562.13, 569.3, 569.85, 578.0-578.9
AHA: N-D, '84, 15

√5th 531.1 Acute with perforation [CC]
CC Excl: See code 531.0

√5th 531.2 Acute with hemorrhage and perforation [CC]
CC Excl: See code 531.0

√5th 531.3 Acute without mention of hemorrhage or perforation [CC 1]
CC Excl: For code 531.31: see code 531.0

√5th 531.4 Chronic or unspecified with hemorrhage [CC]
CC Excl: See code 531.0
AHA: 4Q, '90, 22
DRG 174 For code 531.40

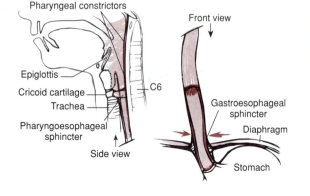

Esophagus

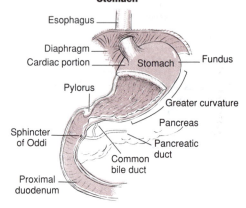

Stomach

Tabular List — DIGESTIVE SYSTEM 531.5–534

√5th **531.5 Chronic or unspecified with perforation** [CC]
CC Excl: See code 531.0

√5th **531.6 Chronic or unspecified with hemorrhage and perforation** [CC]
CC Excl: See code 531.0

√5th **531.7 Chronic without mention of hemorrhage or perforation** [CC 1]
CC Excl: For code 531.71: see code 531.0

√5th **531.9 Unspecified as acute or chronic, without mention of hemorrhage or perforation** [CC 1]
CC Excl: For code 531.91: see code 531.0

√4th **532 Duodenal ulcer**
INCLUDES   erosion (acute) of duodenum
ulcer (peptic):
  duodenum
  postpyloric
Use additional E code to identify drug, if drug-induced
EXCLUDES   peptic ulcer NOS (533.0-533.9)

The following fifth-digit subclassification is for use with category 532:
  0 without mention of obstruction
  1 with obstruction

AHA: 4Q, '90, 27; 1Q, '91, 15

DEF: Ulcers in duodenum due to action of gastric acid and pepsin on mucosa decreasing resistance to ulcers.

√5th **532.0 Acute with hemorrhage** [CC]
CC Excl: 251.5, 456.0, 530.2, 530.7, 530.82, 531.00-531.91, 532.00-532.91, 533.00-533.91, 534.00-534.91, 535.01, 535.11, 535.21, 535.31, 535.41, 535.51, 535.61, 537.3, 537.83, 537.89, 537.9, 562.02-562.03, 562.12-562.13, 569.3, 569.85, 578.0-578.9

AHA: 4Q, '90, 22

√5th **532.1 Acute with perforation** [CC]
CC Excl: See code 532.0

√5th **532.2 Acute with hemorrhage and perforation** [CC]
CC Excl: See code 532.0

√5th **532.3 Acute without mention of hemorrhage or perforation** [CC 1]
CC Excl: For code 532.31: See code 532.0

√5th **532.4 Chronic or unspecified with hemorrhage** [CC]
CC Excl: See code 532.0
DRG 174 For code 532.40

√5th **532.5 Chronic or unspecified with perforation** [CC]
CC Excl: See code 532.0

√5th **532.6 Chronic or unspecified with hemorrhage and perforation** [CC]
CC Excl: See code 532.0

√5th **532.7 Chronic without mention of hemorrhage or perforation** [CC 1]
CC Excl: For code 532.71: See code 532.0

√5th **532.9 Unspecified as acute or chronic, without mention of hemorrhage or perforation** [CC 1]
CC Excl: For code 532.91: See code 532.0

√4th **533 Peptic ulcer, site unspecified**
INCLUDES   gastroduodenal ulcer NOS   stress ulcer NOS
  peptic ulcer NOS
Use additional E code to identify drug, if drug-induced
EXCLUDES   peptic ulcer:
  duodenal (532.0-532.9)
  gastric (531.0-531.9)

The following fifth-digit subclassification is for use with category 533:
  0 without mention of obstruction
  1 with obstruction

AHA: 1Q, '91, 15; 4Q, '90, 27

DEF: Ulcer of mucous membrane of esophagus, stomach or duodenum due to gastric acid secretion.

√5th **533.0 Acute with hemorrhage** [CC]
CC Excl: See code 532.0

√5th **533.1 Acute with perforation** [CC]
CC Excl: See code 532.0

√5th **533.2 Acute with hemorrhage and perforation** [CC]
CC Excl: See code 532.0

√5th **533.3 Acute without mention of hemorrhage and perforation** [CC 1]
CC Excl: For code 533.31: See code 532.0

√5th **533.4 Chronic or unspecified with hemorrhage** [CC]
CC Excl: See code 532.0

√5th **533.5 Chronic or unspecified with perforation** [CC]
CC Excl: See code 532.0

√5th **533.6 Chronic or unspecified with hemorrhage and perforation** [CC]
CC Excl: See code 532.0

√5th **533.7 Chronic without mention of hemorrhage or perforation** [CC 1]
CC Excl: For code 533.71: See code 532.0

AHA: 2Q, '89, 16

√5th **533.9 Unspecified as acute or chronic, without mention of hemorrhage or perforation** [CC 1]
CC Excl: For code 533.91: See code 532.0

√4th **534 Gastrojejunal ulcer**
INCLUDES   ulcer (peptic) or erosion: ulcer (peptic) or erosion:
  anastomotic   jejunal
  gastrocolic   marginal
  gastrointestinal   stomal
  gastrojejunal
EXCLUDES   primary ulcer of small intestine (569.82)

The following fifth-digit subclassification is for use with category 534:
  0 without mention of obstruction
  1 with obstruction

AHA: 1Q, '91, 15; 4Q, '90, 27

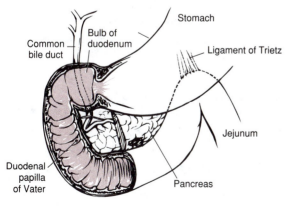

Duodenum

Additional Digit Required   Nonspecific PDx   Unacceptable PDx   Manifestation Code   [MSP] Medicare Secondary Payer   ►◄ Revised Text   ● New Code   ▲ Revised Code Title

2002 Ingenix, Inc.   Volume 1 — 155

534.0–537.0 DIGESTIVE SYSTEM

√5th **534.0 Acute with hemorrhage** [CC]
CC Excl: 251.5, 456.0, 530.2, 530.7, 530.82, 531.00-531.91, 532.00-532.91, 533.00-533.91, 534.00-534.91, 535.01, 535.11, 535.21, 535.31, 535.41, 535.51, 535.61, 537.83, 537.89, 537.9, 562.02-562.03, 562.12-562.13, 569.3, 569.85, 578.0-578.9

√5th **534.1 Acute with perforation** [CC]
CC Excl: See code 534.0

√5th **534.2 Acute with hemorrhage and perforation** [CC]
CC Excl: See code 534.0

√5th **534.3 Acute without mention of hemorrhage or perforation** [CC]
CC Excl: For code 534.31: See code 534.0

√5th **534.4 Chronic or unspecified with hemorrhage** [CC 1]
CC Excl: See code 534.0

√5th **534.5 Chronic or unspecified with perforation** [CC]
CC Excl: See code 534.0

√5th **534.6 Chronic or unspecified with hemorrhage and perforation** [CC]
CC Excl: See code 534.0

√5th **534.7 Chronic without mention of hemorrhage or perforation** [CC 1]
CC Excl: For code 534.71: See code 534.0

√5th **534.9 Unspecified as acute or chronic, without mention of hemorrhage or perforation** [CC 1]
CC Excl: For code 534.91: See code 534.0

√4th **535 Gastritis and duodenitis**

The following fifth-digit subclassification is for use with category 535:
 0 without mention of hemorrhage
 1 with hemorrhage

AHA: 2Q, '92, 9; 4Q, '91, 25

√5th **535.0 Acute gastritis** [CC 1]
CC Excl: For code 535.01: 251.5, 456.0, 530.2, 530.7, 530.82, 531.00-531.91, 532.00-532.91, 533.00-533.91, 534.00-534.91, 535.01, 535.11, 535.21, 535.31, 535.41, 535.51, 535.61, 537.83, 562.02-562.03, 562.12-562.13, 569.3, 569.85, 578.0-578.9

AHA: 2Q, '92, 8; N-D, '86, 9

√5th **535.1 Atrophic gastritis** [CC 1]
 Gastritis: Gastritis:
  atrophic-hyperplastic   chronic (atrophic)
CC Excl: For code 535.11: See code 535.01

AHA: 1Q, '94, 18

DEF: Inflammation of stomach, with mucous membrane atrophy and peptic gland destruction.

√5th **535.2 Gastric mucosal hypertrophy** [CC 1]
 Hypertrophic gastritis
CC Excl: For code 535.21: See code 535.01

√5th **535.3 Alcoholic gastritis** [CC 1]
CC Excl: For code 535.31: See code 535.01

√5th **535.4 Other specified gastritis** [CC 1]
 Gastritis:
  allergic
  bile induced
  irritant
  superficial
  toxic
CC Excl: For code 535.41: See code 535.01

AHA: 4Q, '90, 27

√5th **535.5 Unspecified gastritis and gastroduodenitis** [CC 1]
CC Excl: For code 535.51: See code 535.01

AHA: For code 535.50: 4Q, '99, 25

√5th **535.6 Duodenitis** [CC 1]
CC Excl: For code 535.61: See code 535.01

DEF: Inflammation of intestine, between pylorus and jejunum.

√4th **536 Disorders of function of stomach**
EXCLUDES functional disorders of stomach specified as psychogenic (306.4)

536.0 Achlorhydria
DEF: Absence of gastric acid due to gastric mucosa atrophy; unresponsive to histamines; also known as gastric anacidity.

536.1 Acute dilatation of stomach [CC]
 Acute distention of stomach
CC Excl: 536.1

536.2 Persistent vomiting
 Habit vomiting   Uncontrollable vomiting
 Persistent vomiting [not of pregnancy]
 EXCLUDES excessive vomiting in pregnancy (643.0-643.9)
  vomiting NOS (787.0)

536.3 Gastroparesis
AHA: 2Q, '01, 4; 4Q, '94, 42

DEF: Slight degree of paralysis within muscular coat of stomach.

√5th **536.4 Gastrostomy complications**
AHA: 4Q, '98, 42

536.40 Gastrostomy complication, unspecified [CC]
CC Excl: 536.40-536.49, 997.4, 997.71, 997.91, 997.99, 998.81, 998.83-998.9

536.41 Infection of gastrostomy [CC]
 Use additional code to specify type of infection, such as:
  abscess or cellulitis of abdomen (682.2)
  septicemia (038.0-038.9)
 Use additional code to identify organism (041.00-041.9)
CC Excl: See code 536.40

AHA: 4Q, '98, 42

536.42 Mechanical complication of gastrostomy [CC]
CC Excl: See code 536.40

536.49 Other gastrostomy complications [CC]
CC Excl: See code 536.40

AHA: 4Q, '98, 42

536.8 Dyspepsia and other specified disorders of function of stomach
 Achylia gastrica   Hyperchlorhydria
 Hourglass contraction   Hypochlorhydria
  of stomach   Indigestion
 Hyperacidity
 EXCLUDES achlorhydria (536.0)
  heartburn (787.1)

AHA: 2Q, '93, 6; 2Q, '89, 16; N-D, '84, 9

536.9 Unspecified functional disorder of stomach
 Functional gastrointestinal:
  disorder
  disturbance
  irritation

√4th **537 Other disorders of stomach and duodenum**
537.0 Acquired hypertrophic pyloric stenosis [CC]
 Constriction ⎫
 Obstruction ⎬ of pylorus, acquired or adult
 Stricture   ⎭
 EXCLUDES congenital or infantile pyloric stenosis (750.5)
CC Excl: 536.3, 536.8-536.9, 537.0, 537.3, 750.5, 750.8-750.9, 751.1, 751.5

AHA: 2Q, '01, 4; J-F, '85, 14

DIGESTIVE SYSTEM

537.1 Gastric diverticulum
  EXCLUDES congenital diverticulum of stomach (750.7)
  AHA: J-F, '85, 4
  DEF: Herniated sac or pouch, within stomach or duodenum.

537.2 Chronic duodenal ileus
  DEF: Persistent obstruction between pylorus and jejunum.

537.3 Other obstruction of duodenum CC
  Cicatrix
  Stenosis
  Stricture } of duodenum
  Volvulus
  EXCLUDES congenital obstruction of duodenum (751.1)
  CC Excl: 537.3, 750.8-750.9, 751.1, 751.5

537.4 Fistula of stomach or duodenum CC
  Gastrocolic fistula   Gastrojejunocolic fistula
  CC Excl: 537.4, 750.8-750.9, 751.5

537.5 Gastroptosis
  DEF: Downward displacement of stomach.

537.6 Hourglass stricture or stenosis of stomach
  Cascade stomach
  EXCLUDES congenital hourglass stomach (750.7)
  hourglass contraction of stomach (536.8)

✓5th **537.8 Other specified disorders of stomach and duodenum**
  AHA: 4Q, '91, 25

  537.81 Pylorospasm
    EXCLUDES congenital pylorospasm (750.5)
    DEF: Spasm of the pyloric sphincter.

  537.82 Angiodysplasia of stomach and duodenum (without mention of hemorrhage)
    AHA: 3Q, '96, 10; 4Q, '90, 4

  537.83 Angiodysplasia of stomach and duodenum with hemorrhage CC
    CC Excl: 251.5, 456.0, 530.2, 530.7, 530.82, 531.000-531.91, 532.00-532.91, 533.00-533.91, 534.00-534.91, 535.01, 535.11, 535.21, 535.31, 535.41, 535.51, 535.61, 537.83, 562.02-562.03, 562.12-562.13, 569.3, 569.85, 578.0-578.9
    DEF: Bleeding of stomach and duodenum due to vascular abnormalities.

  537.84 Dieulafoy lesion (hemorrhagic) of stomach and duodenum CC
    CC Excl: 251.5, 530.2, 530.7, 530.82, 531.00-531.91, 532.00-532.91, 533.00-533.91, 534.00-534.91, 535.01, 535.11, 535.21, 535.31, 535.41, 535.51, 535.61, 537.83-537.84, 562.02-562.03, 562.12-562.13, 569.3, 569.85-569.86, 578.0-578.1, 578.9

  537.89 Other
    Gastric or duodenal:
      prolapse
      rupture
    Intestinal metaplasia of gastric mucosa
    Passive congestion of stomach
    EXCLUDES diverticula of duodenum (562.00-562.01)
    gastrointestinal hemorrhage (578.0-578.9)
    AHA: N-D, '84, 7

537.9 Unspecified disorder of stomach and duodenum

APPENDICITIS (540-543)

✓4th **540 Acute appendicitis**
  AHA: N-D, '84, 19
  DEF: Inflammation of vermiform appendix due to fecal obstruction, neoplasm or foreign body of appendiceal lumen; causes infection, edema and infarction of appendiceal wall; may result in mural necrosis, and perforation.

  540.0 With generalized peritonitis CC
    Appendicitis (acute):
      fulminating   with:
      gangrenous   perforation
      obstructive   peritonitis (generalized)
    Cecitis (acute)   rupture
    Rupture of appendix
    EXCLUDES acute appendicitis with peritoneal abscess (540.1)
    CC Excl: 537.89, 537.9, 540.0-540.9, 541-542, 543.0, 543.9

  540.1 With peritoneal abscess CC
    With generalized peritonitis
    Abscess of appendix
    CC Excl: See code 540.0
    AHA: N-D, '84, 19

  540.9 Without mention of peritonitis CC
    Acute:
      appendicitis:
        fulminating
        gangrenous   without mention of
        inflamed   perforation,
        obstructive   peritonitis, or rupture
        cecitis
    CC Excl: See code 540.0
    AHA: 1Q, '01, 15; 4Q, '97, 52

541 Appendicitis, unqualified
  AHA: 2Q, '90, 26

542 Other appendicitis
  Appendicitis: Appendicitis:
    chronic   relapsing
    recurrent   subacute
  EXCLUDES hyperplasia (lymphoid) of appendix (543.0)
  AHA: 1Q, '01, 15

✓4th **543 Other diseases of appendix**

  543.0 Hyperplasia of appendix (lymphoid)
    DEF: Proliferation of cells in appendix tissue.

  543.9 Other and unspecified diseases of appendix
    Appendicular or appendiceal:
      colic
      concretion
      fistula
      Diverticulum
      Fecalith
      Intussusception } of appendix
      Mucocele
      Stercolith

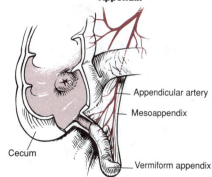
Appendix — Appendicular artery — Mesoappendix — Cecum — Vermiform appendix

HERNIA OF ABDOMINAL CAVITY (550-553)

INCLUDES hernia:
  acquired
  congenital, except diaphragmatic or hiatal

✓4th 550 Inguinal hernia

INCLUDES bubonocele
  inguinal hernia (direct) (double) (indirect)
    (oblique) (sliding)
  scrotal hernia

The following fifth-digit subclassification is for use with category 550:

0 **unilateral or unspecified (not specified as recurrent)**
   Unilateral NOS
1 **unilateral or unspecified, recurrent**
2 **bilateral (not specified as recurrent)**
   Bilateral NOS
3 **bilateral, recurrent**

AHA: N-D, '85, 12

DEF: Hernia protrusion of an abdominal organ or tissue through inguinal canal.

DEF: Indirect inguinal hernia: (external or oblique) leaves abdomen through deep inguinal ring, passes through inguinal canal lateral to the inferior epigastric artery.

DEF: Direct inguinal hernia: (internal) emerges between inferior epigastric artery and rectus muscle edge.

✓5th **550.0 Inguinal hernia, with gangrene** CC
   Inguinal hernia with gangrene (and obstruction)
   CC Excl: 537.89, 537.9, 550.00-550.93, 552.8-552.9, 553.8-553.9

✓5th **550.1 Inguinal hernia, with obstruction, without mention of gangrene** CC
   Inguinal hernia with mention of incarceration, irreducibility, or strangulation
   CC Excl: See code 550.0

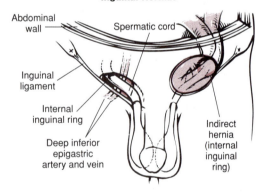

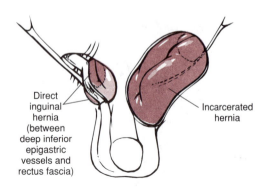

✓5th **550.9 Inguinal hernia, without mention of obstruction or gangrene**
   Inguinal hernia NOS

✓4th 551 Other hernia of abdominal cavity, with gangrene

INCLUDES that with gangrene (and obstruction)

✓5th **551.0 Femoral hernia with gangrene**

551.00 Unilateral or unspecified (not specified as recurrent) CC
   Femoral hernia NOS with gangrene
   CC Excl: 537.89, 537.9, 551.00-551.03, 552.8-552.9, 553.00-553.03, 553.8-553.9

551.01 Unilateral or unspecified, recurrent CC
   CC Excl: See code 551.0

551.02 Bilateral (not specified as recurrent) CC
   CC Excl: See code 551.0

551.03 Bilateral, recurrent CC
   CC Excl: See code 551.0

551.1 Umbilical hernia with gangrene CC
   Parumbilical hernia specified as gangrenous
   CC Excl: 537.89, 537.9, 551.1-551.29, 552.1-552.29, 552.8-552.9, 553.1-553.29, 553.8-553.9

✓5th **551.2 Ventral hernia with gangrene**

551.20 Ventral, unspecified, with gangrene CC
   CC Excl: See code 551.1

551.21 Incisional, with gangrene CC
   Hernia:
     postoperative } specified as
     recurrent, ventral } gangrenous
   CC Excl: See code 551.1

551.29 Other CC
   Epigastric hernia specified as gangrenous
   CC Excl: See code 551.1

551.3 Diaphragmatic hernia with gangrene CC
   Hernia:
     hiatal (esophageal) (sliding)
     paraesophageal } specified as
     Thoracic stomach } gangrenous

   EXCLUDES congenital diaphragmatic hernia (756.6)
   CC Excl: 551.3, 552.3, 552.8-552.9, 553.3, 553.8-553.9

551.8 Hernia of other specified sites, with gangrene CC
   Any condition classifiable to 553.8 if specified as gangrenous
   CC Excl: 537.89, 537.9, 550.00-550.93, 551.00-551.9, 552.00-552.9, 553.00-553.9

551.9 Hernia of unspecified site, with gangrene CC
   Any condition classifiable to 553.9 if specified as gangrenous
   CC Excl: See code 551.8

✓4th 552 Other hernia of abdominal cavity, with obstruction, but without mention of gangrene

EXCLUDES that with mention of gangrene (551.0-551.9)

✓5th **552.0 Femoral hernia with obstruction**
   Femoral hernia specified as incarcerated, irreducible, strangulated, or causing obstruction

552.00 Unilateral or unspecified (not specified as recurrent) CC
   CC Excl: 537.89, 537.9, 551.00-551.03, 552.00-552.03, 552.8-552.9, 553.00-553.03, 553.8-553.9

DIGESTIVE SYSTEM

552.01 Unilateral or unspecified, recurrent [CC]
CC Excl: See code 552.00

552.02 Bilateral (not specified as recurrent) [CC]
CC Excl: See code 552.00

552.03 Bilateral, recurrent [CC]
CC Excl: See code 552.00

552.1 Umbilical hernia with obstruction [CC]
Parumbilical hernia specified as incarcerated, irreducible, strangulated, or causing obstruction
CC Excl: 551.1-551.29, 552.1-552.29, 552.8-552.9, 553.8-553.9

√5th 552.2 Ventral hernia with obstruction
Ventral hernia specified as incarcerated, irreducible, strangulated, or causing obstruction

552.20 Ventral, unspecified, with obstruction [CC]
CC Excl: See code 552.1

552.21 Incisional, with obstruction [CC]
Hernia:
postoperative
recurrent, ventral } specified as incarcerated, irreducible, strangulated, or causing obstruction

CC Excl: See code 552.1

552.29 Other [CC]
Epigastric hernia specified as incarcerated, irreducible, strangulated, or causing obstruction
CC Excl: See code 552.1

552.3 Diaphragmatic hernia with obstruction [CC]
Hernia:
hiatal (esophageal)
 (sliding)
paraesophageal
Thoracic stomach
} specified as incarcerated, irreducible, strangulated, or causing obstruction

EXCLUDES congenital diaphragmatic hernia (756.6)
CC Excl: 551.3, 552.3-552.9, 553.3-553.9

552.8 Hernia of other specified sites, with obstruction [CC]
Any condition classifiable to 553.8 if specified as incarcerated, irreducible, strangulated, or causing obstruction
CC Excl: 550.00-550.93, 551.00-551.9, 552.00-552.9, 553.00-553.9

552.9 Hernia of unspecified site, with obstruction [CC]
Any condition classifiable to 553.9 if specified as incarcerated, irreducible, strangulated, or causing obstruction
CC Excl: See code 552.8

√4th 553 Other hernia of abdominal cavity without mention of obstruction or gangrene
EXCLUDES the listed conditions with mention of:
gangrene (and obstruction) (551.0-551.9)
obstruction (552.0-552.9)

√5th 553.0 Femoral hernia
553.00 Unilateral or unspecified (not specified as recurrent)
Femoral hernia NOS
553.01 Unilateral or unspecified, recurrent
553.02 Bilateral (not specified as recurrent)
553.03 Bilateral, recurrent

553.1 Umbilical hernia
Parumbilical hernia

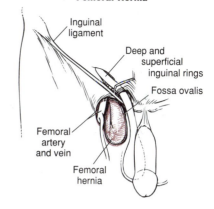

Femoral Hernia

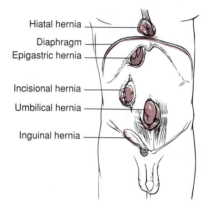

Hernias of Abdominal Cavity

√5th 553.2 Ventral hernia
553.20 Ventral, unspecified
553.21 Incisional
Hernia: Hernia:
postoperative recurrent, ventral
553.29 Other
Hernia: Hernia:
epigastric   spigelian

553.3 Diaphragmatic hernia
Hernia: Thoracic stomach
hiatal (esophageal) (sliding)
paraesophageal
EXCLUDES congenital:
diaphragmatic hernia (756.6)
hiatal hernia (750.6)
esophagocele (530.6)

AHA: 2Q, '01, 6; 1Q, '00, 6

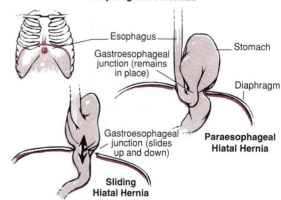

Diaphragmatic Hernias

DIGESTIVE SYSTEM

553.8 Hernia of other specified sites
Hernia:
   ischiatic
   ischiorectal
   lumbar
   obturator
   pudendal
   retroperitoneal
   sciatic
Other abdominal hernia of specified site
   EXCLUDES   *vaginal enterocele (618.6)*

553.9 Hernia of unspecified site
Enterocele
Epiplocele
Hernia:
   NOS
   interstitial
Hernia:
   intestinal
   intra-abdominal
Rupture (nontraumatic)
Sarcoepiplocele

NONINFECTIOUS ENTERITIS AND COLITIS (555-558)

√4th 555 Regional enteritis
   INCLUDES   Crohn's disease
                Granulomatous enteritis
   EXCLUDES   *ulcerative colitis (556)*
DEF: Inflammation of intestine; classified to site.

555.0 Small intestine
Ileitis:
   regional
   segmental
   terminal
Regional enteritis or Crohn's disease of:
   duodenum
   ileum
   jejunum

555.1 Large intestine
Colitis:
   granulmatous
   regional
   transmural
Regional enteritis or Crohn's disease of:
   colon
   large bowel
   rectum

AHA: 3Q, '99, 8

555.2 Small intestine with large intestine
Regional ileocolitis

555.9 Unspecified site
Crohn's disease NOS
Regional enteritis NOS
AHA: 3Q, '99, 8; 4Q, '97, 42; 2Q, '97, 3

√4th 556 Ulcerative colitis
AHA: 3Q, '99, 8

DEF: Chronic inflammation of mucosal lining of intestinal tract; may be single area or entire colon.

556.0 Ulcerative (chronic) enterocolitis
556.1 Ulcerative (chronic) ileocolitis
556.2 Ulcerative (chronic) proctitis
556.3 Ulcerative (chronic) proctosigmoiditis

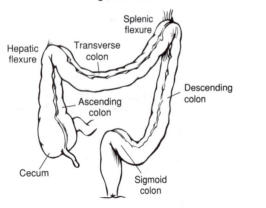

Large Intestine

556.4 Pseudopolyposis of colon
556.5 Left-sided ulcerative (chronic) colitis
556.6 Universal ulcerative (chronic) colitis
Pancolitis
556.8 Other ulcerative colitis
556.9 Ulcerative colitis, unspecified
Ulcerative enteritis NOS

√4th 557 Vascular insufficiency of intestine
   EXCLUDES   *necrotizing enterocolitis of the newborn (777.5)*
DEF: Inadequacy of intestinal vessels.

557.0 Acute vascular insufficiency of intestine   CC
Acute:
   hemorrhagic enterocolitis
   ischemic colitis, enteritis, or enterocolitis
   massive necrosis of intestine
Bowel infarction
Embolism of mesenteric artery
Fulminant enterocolitis
Hemorrhagic necrosis of intestine
Infarction of appendices epiploicae
Intestinal gangrene
Intestinal infarction (acute) (agnogenic) (hemorrhagic) (nonocclusive)
Mesenteric infarction (embolic) (thrombotic)
Necrosis of intestine
Terminal hemorrhagic enteropathy
Thrombosis of mesenteric artery

CC Excl: 557.0-557.1

DRG 188

AHA: ▶4Q, '01, 53◀

557.1 Chronic vascular insufficiency of intestine
Angina, abdominal
Chronic ischemic colitis, enteritis, or enterocolitis
Ischemic stricture of intestine
Mesenteric:
   angina
   artery syndrome (superior)
   vascular insufficiency

AHA: 3Q, '96, 9; 4Q, '90, 4; N-D, '86, 11; N-D, '84, 7

557.9 Unspecified vascular insufficiency of intestine
Alimentary pain due to vascular insufficiency
Ischemic colitis, enteritis, or enterocolitis NOS

DRG 188

√4th 558 Other and unspecified noninfectious gastroenteritis and colitis
   EXCLUDES   *infectious:*
                  colitis, enteritis, or gastroenteritis (009.0-009.1)
                  diarrhea (009.2-009.3)

558.1 Gastroenteritis and colitis due to radiation   CC
Radiation enterocolitis
CC Excl: 558.1

558.2 Toxic gastroenteritis and colitis   CC
Use additional E code to identify cause
CC Excl: 558.2

558.3 Allergic gastroenteritis and colitis
AHA: 4Q, '00, 42

DEF: True immunoglobulin E (IgE)-mediated allergic reaction of the lining of the stomach, intestines, or colon to food proteins; causes nausea, vomiting, diarrhea, and abdominal cramping.

558.9 Other and unspecified noninfectious gastroenteritis and colitis
Colitis
Enteritis
Gastroenteritis   } NOS, dietetic, or
Ileitis   noninfectious
Jejunitis
Sigmoiditis

AHA: 3Q, '99, 4, 6; N-D, '87, 7

OTHER DISEASES OF INTESTINES AND PERITONEUM (560-569)

√4th 560 Intestinal obstruction without mention of hernia
  EXCLUDES duodenum (537.2-537.3)
  inguinal hernia with obstruction (550.1)
  intestinal obstruction complicating hernia (552.0-552.9)
  mesenteric:
    embolism (557.0)
    infarction (557.0)
    thrombosis (557.0)
  neonatal intestinal obstruction (277.01, 777.1-777.2, 777.4)

560.0 Intussusception
Intussusception (colon) (intestine) (rectum)
Invagination of intestine or colon
  EXCLUDES intussusception of appendix (543.9)
CC Excl: 560.0-560.9, 569.89, 569.9

AHA: 4Q, '98, 82

DEF: Prolapse of a bowel section into adjacent section; occurs primarily in children; symptoms include paroxysmal pain, vomiting, presence of lower abdominal tumor and blood, and mucous passage from rectum.

560.1 Paralytic ileus
Adynamic ileus
Ileus (of intestine) (of bowel) (of colon)
Paralysis of intestine or colon
  EXCLUDES gallstone ileus (560.31)
CC Excl: See code 560.0

AHA: J-F, '87, 13

DEF: Obstruction of ileus due to inhibited bowel motility.

560.2 Volvulus
Knotting
Strangulation   of intestine, bowel, or
Torsion   colon
Twist
CC Excl: See code 560.0

DEF: Entanglement of bowel; causes obstruction; may compromise bowel circulation.

√5th 560.3 Impaction of intestine
560.30 Impaction of intestine, unspecified
Impaction of colon
CC Excl: See code 560.0

560.31 Gallstone ileus
Obstruction of intestine by gallstone
CC Excl: See code 560.0

Volvulus and Diverticulitis

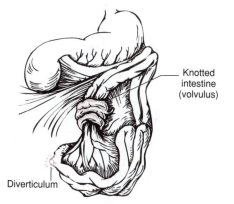

Knotted intestine (volvulus)

Diverticulum

560.39 Other
Concretion of intestine
Enterolith
Fecal impaction
CC Excl: See code 560.0

AHA: 4Q, '98, 38

√5th 560.8 Other specified intestinal obstruction
560.81 Intestinal or peritoneal adhesions with obstruction (postoperative) (postinfection)
  EXCLUDES adhesions without obstruction (568.0)
CC Excl: See code 560.0

AHA: 4Q, '95, 55; 3Q, '95, 6; N-D, '87, 9

DEF: Obstruction of peritoneum or intestine due to abnormal union of tissues.

560.89 Other
Mural thickening causing obstruction
  EXCLUDES ischemic stricture of intestine (557.1)
CC Excl: See code 560.0

AHA: 2Q, '97, 3; 1Q, '88, 6

560.9 Unspecified intestinal obstruction
Enterostenosis
Obstruction
Occlusion   of intestine or colon
Stenosis
Stricture
  EXCLUDES congenital stricture or stenosis of intestine (751.1-751.2)
CC Excl: See code 560.0

√4th 562 Diverticula of intestine
Use additional code to identify any associated: peritonitis (567.0-567.9)
  EXCLUDES congenital diverticulum of colon (751.5)
  diverticulum of appendix (543.9)
  Meckel's diverticulum (751.0)

AHA: 4Q, '91, 25; J-F, '85, 1

√5th 562.0 Small intestine
562.00 Diverticulosis of small intestine (without mention of hemorrhage)
Diverticulosis:
  duodenum
  ileum   without mention of
  jejunum   diverticulitis

DEF: Saclike herniations of mucous lining of small intestine.

562.01 Diverticulitis of small intestine (without mention of hemorrhage)
Diverticulitis (with diverticulosis):
  duodenum
  ileum
  jejunum
  small intestine

DEF: Inflamed saclike herniations of mucous lining of small intestine.

562.02 Diverticulosis of small intestine with hemorrhage
CC Excl: 251.5, 456.0, 530.2, 530.7, 530.82, 531.00-531.91, 532.00-532.91, 533.00-533.91, 534.00-534.91, 535.01, 535.11, 535.21, 535.31, 535.41, 535.51, 535.61, 537.83, 562.02-562.03, 562.12-562.13, 569.3, 569.85, 578.0-578.9

562.03 Diverticulitis of small intestine with hemorrhage
CC Excl: See code 562.02

DIGESTIVE SYSTEM

562.1 Colon ✓5th

562.10 Diverticulosis of colon (without mention of hemorrhage)
Diverticulosis:
  NOS
  intestine (large) } without mention of diverticulitis
  Diverticular disease (colon)

AHA: 4Q, '90, 21; J-F, '85, 5

DEF: Saclike herniations of mucous lining of large intestine

562.11 Diverticulitis of colon (without mention of hemorrhage)
Diverticulitis (with diverticulosis):
  NOS
  colon
  intestine (large)

AHA: 1Q, '96, 14; J-F, '85, 5

DEF: Inflamed saclike herniations of mucosal lining of large intestine.

562.12 Diverticulosis of colon with hemorrhage CC
CC Excl: See code 562.02

DRG 174

562.13 Diverticulitis of colon with hemorrhage CC
CC Excl: See code 562.02

564 Functional digestive disorders, not elsewhere classified ✓4th
EXCLUDES functional disorders of stomach (536.0-536.9)
          those specified as psychogenic (306.4)

564.0 Constipation ✓5th
AHA: ▶4Q, '01, 45◀

564.00 Constipation, unspecified
564.01 Slow transit constipation
DEF: ▶Delay in the transit of fecal material through the colon secondary to smooth muscle dysfunction or decreased peristaltic contractions along the colon: also called colonic inertia or delayed transit.◀

564.02 Outlet dysfunction constipation
DEF: ▶Failure to relax the paradoxical contractions of the striated pelvic floor muscles during the attempted defecation.◀

564.09 Other constipation

564.1 Irritable bowel syndrome
Irritable colon
Spastic colon

AHA: 1Q, '88, 6

DEF: Functional gastrointestinal disorder (FGID); symptoms following meals include diarrhea, constipation, abdominal pain; other symptoms include bloating, gas, distended abdomen, nausea, vomiting, appetite loss, emotional distress, and depression.

564.2 Postgastric surgery syndromes
Dumping syndrome   Postgastrectomy syndrome
Jejunal syndrome   Postvagotomy syndrome
EXCLUDES malnutrition following gastrointestinal surgery (579.3)
          postgastrojejunostomy ulcer (534.0-534.9)

AHA: 1Q, '95, 11

564.3 Vomiting following gastrointestinal surgery
Vomiting (bilious) following gastrointestinal surgery

564.4 Other postoperative functional disorders
Diarrhea following gastrointestinal surgery
EXCLUDES colostomy and enterostomy complications (569.60-569.69)

564.5 Functional diarrhea
EXCLUDES diarrhea:
            NOS (787.91)
            psychogenic (306.4)

DEF: Diarrhea with no detectable organic cause.

564.6 Anal spasm
Proctalgia fugax

564.7 Megacolon, other than Hirschsprung's
Dilatation of colon
EXCLUDES megacolon:
            congenital [Hirschsprung's] (751.3)
            toxic (556)

DEF: Enlarged colon; congenital or acquired; can occur acutely or become chronic.

564.8 Other specified functional disorders of intestine ✓5th
EXCLUDES malabsorption (579.0-579.9)

AHA: 1Q, '88, 6

564.81 Neurogenic bowel
AHA: 1Q, '01, 12; 4Q, '98, 45

DEF: Disorder of bowel due to spinal cord lesion above conus medullaris; symptoms include precipitous micturition, nocturia, catheter intolerance, headache, sweating, nasal obstruction and spastic contractions.

564.89 Other functional disorders of intestine
Atony of colon

564.9 Unspecified functional disorder of intestine

565 Anal fissure and fistula ✓4th

565.0 Anal fissure
Tear of anus, nontraumatic
EXCLUDES traumatic (863.89, 863.99)

DEF: Ulceration of cleft at anal mucosa; causes pain, itching, bleeding, infection, and sphincter spasm; may occur with hemorrhoids.

565.1 Anal fistula
Fistula:
  anorectal
  rectal
  rectum to skin
EXCLUDES fistula of rectum to internal organs—
            see Alphabetic Index
          ischiorectal fistula (566)
          rectovaginal fistula (619.1)

DEF: Abnormal opening on cutaneous surface near anus; may lack connection with rectum.

566 Abscess of anal and rectal regions CC
Abscess:
  ischiorectal
  perianal
  perirectal
Cellulitis:
  anal
  perirectal
  rectal
Ischiorectal fistula

CC Excl: 566

Anal Fistula and Abscess

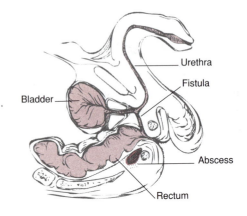

DIGESTIVE SYSTEM

✓4th 567 Peritonitis
EXCLUDES peritonitis:
  benign paroxysmal (277.3)
  pelvic, female (614.5, 614.7)
  periodic familial (277.3)
  puerperal (670)
  with or following:
    abortion (634-638 with .0, 639.0)
    appendicitis (540.0-540.1)
    ectopic or molar pregnancy (639.0)

DEF: Inflammation of the peritoneal cavity.

567.0 Peritonitis in infectious diseases classified elsewhere [CC]
Code first underlying disease
EXCLUDES peritonitis:
  gonococcal (098.86)
  syphilitic (095.2)
  tuberculous (014.0)

CC Excl: 567.0-567.9, 569.89, 569.9

567.1 Pneumococcal peritonitis [CC]
CC Excl: See code 567.0

567.2 Other suppurative peritonitis [CC]
Abscess (of):   Abscess (of):
  abdominopelvic   subhepatic
  mesenteric   subphrenic
  omentum   Peritonitis (acute):
  peritoneum   general
  retrocecal   pelvic, male
  retroperitoneal   subphrenic
  subdiaphragmatic   suppurative

CC Excl: See code 567.0

AHA: 2Q, '01, 11, 12; 3Q, '99, 9; 2Q, '98, 19

▽ DRG 188

567.8 Other specified peritonitis [CC]
Chronic proliferative   Peritonitis due to:
  peritonitis   bile
Fat necrosis of peritoneum   urine
Mesenteric saponification

CC Excl: See code 567.0

567.9 Unspecified peritonitis [CC]
Peritonitis: Peritonitis:
  NOS   of unspecified cause

CC Excl: See code 567.0

Rectum and Anus

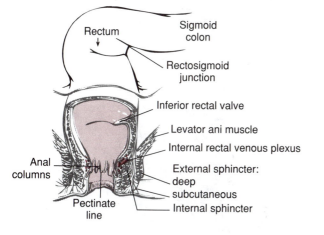

✓4th 568 Other disorders of peritoneum

568.0 Peritoneal adhesions (postoperative) (postinfection)
Adhesions (of):   Adhesions (of):
  abdominal (wall)   mesenteric
  diaphragm   omentum
  intestine   stomach
  male pelvis   Adhesive bands

EXCLUDES adhesions:
  pelvic, female (614.6)
  with obstruction:
    duodenum (537.3)
    intestine (560.81)

AHA: 4Q, '95, 55; 3Q, '95, 7; S-O, '85, 11

DEF: Abnormal union of tissues in peritoneum.

✓5th 568.8 Other specified disorders of peritoneum

568.81 Hemoperitoneum (nontraumatic) [CC]
CC Excl: 568.81

568.82 Peritoneal effusion (chronic)
EXCLUDES ascites NOS (789.5)
DEF: Persistent leakage of fluid within peritoneal cavity.

568.89 Other
Peritoneal: Peritoneal:
  cyst   granuloma

568.9 Unspecified disorder of peritoneum

✓4th 569 Other disorders of intestine

569.0 Anal and rectal polyp
Anal and rectal polyp NOS
EXCLUDES adenomatous anal and rectal polyp (211.4)

569.1 Rectal prolapse
Procidentia: Prolapse:
  anus (sphincter)   anal canal
  rectum (sphincter) rectal mucosa
Proctoptosis
EXCLUDES prolapsed hemorrhoids (455.2, 455.5)

569.2 Stenosis of rectum and anus
Stricture of anus (sphincter)

569.3 Hemorrhage of rectum and anus [CC]
EXCLUDES gastrointestinal bleeding NOS (578.9)
  melena (578.1)

CC Excl: 251.5, 456.0, 530.2, 530.7, 530.82, 531.00-531.91, 532.00-532.91, 533.00-533.91, 534.00-534.91, 535.01, 535.11, 535.21, 535.31, 535.41, 535.51, 535.61, 537.83, 562.02-562.03, 562.12-562.13, 569.3, 569.85, 578.0-578.9

✓5th 569.4 Other specified disorders of rectum and anus

569.41 Ulcer of anus and rectum
Solitary ulcer } of anus (sphincter) or
Stercoral ulcer }   rectum (sphincter)

569.42 Anal or rectal pain
AHA: 1Q, '96, 13

569.49 Other
Granuloma } of rectum (sphincter)
Rupture   }

Hypertrophy of anal papillae
Proctitis NOS

EXCLUDES fistula of rectum to:
  internal organs—see Alphabetic Index
  skin (565.1)
  hemorrhoids (455.0-455.9)
  incontinence of sphincter ani (787.6)

DIGESTIVE SYSTEM

569.5 Abscess of intestine `CC`
  EXCLUDES appendiceal abscess (540.1)
  CC Excl: 569.5

√5th **569.6 Colostomy and enterostomy complications**
  AHA: 4Q, '95, 58
  DEF: Complication in a surgically created opening, from intestine to surface skin.

  569.60 Colostomy and enterostomy complication, unspecified `CC`
    CC Excl: 569.60-569.69

  569.61 Infection of colostomy or enterostomy `CC`
    Use additional code to identify organism (041.00-041.9)
    Use additional code to specify type of infection, such as:
      abscess or cellulitis of abdomen (682.2)
      septicemia (038.0-038.9)
    CC Excl: see code 596.60

  569.62 Mechanical complication of colostomy and enterostomy `CC`
    Malfunction of colostomy and enterostomy
    CC Excl: 536.40-536.49, 569.60-569.69, 997.4, 997.71, 997.91, 997.99, 998.81, 998.83-998.9
    AHA: 4Q, '98, 44

  569.69 Other complication `CC`
    Fistula   Prolapse
    Hernia
    CC Excl: see code 596.60
    AHA: 3Q, '98, 16

√5th **569.8 Other specified disorders of intestine**
  AHA: 4Q, '91, 25

  569.81 Fistula of intestine, excluding rectum and anus
    Fistula: Fistula:
      abdominal wall   enteroenteric
      enterocolic   ileorectal
    EXCLUDES fistula of intestine to internal organs—see Alphabetic Index
      persistent postoperative fistula (998.6)
    AHA: 3Q, '99, 8

  569.82 Ulceration of intestine
    Primary ulcer of intestine
    Ulceration of colon
    EXCLUDES that with perforation (569.83)

  569.83 Perforation of intestine `CC`
    CC Excl: 569.83

  569.84 Angiodysplasia of intestine (without mention of hemorrhage)
    AHA: 3Q, '96, 10; 4Q, '90, 4; 4Q, '90, 21
    DEF: Small vascular abnormalities of the intestinal tract without bleeding problems.

  569.85 Angiodysplasia of intestine with hemorrhage `CC`
    CC Excl: 251.5, 456.0, 530.2, 530.7, 530.82, 531.00-531.91, 532.00-532.91, 533.00-533.91, 534.00-534.91, 535.01, 535.11, 535.21, 535.31, 535.41, 535.51, 535.61, 537.83, 562.02-562.03, 562.12-562.13, 569.3, 569.85, 578.0-578.9
    AHA: 3Q, '96, 9
    DEF: Small vascular abnormalities of the intestinal tract with bleeding problems.

  569.86 Dieulafoy lesion (hemorrhagic) of intestine `CC`
    CC Excl: 251.5, 530.2, 530.7, 530.82, 531.00-531.91, 532.00-532.91, 533.00-533.91, 534.00-534.91, 535.01, 535.11, 535.21, 535.31, 535.41, 535.51, 535.61, 537.83-537.84, 562.02-562.03, 562.12-562.13, 569.3, 569.85-569.86, 578.0-578.1, 578.9

  569.89 Other
    Enteroptosis
    Granuloma   } of intestine
    Prolapse
    Pericolitis
    Perisigmoiditis
    Visceroptosis
    EXCLUDES gangrene of intestine, mesentery, or omentum (557.0)
      hemorrhage of intestine NOS (578.9)
      obstruction of intestine (560.0-560.9)
    AHA: 3Q, '96, 9

569.9 Unspecified disorder of intestine

OTHER DISEASES OF DIGESTIVE SYSTEM (570-579)

570 Acute and subacute necrosis of liver `CC`
  Acute hepatic failure
  Acute or subacute hepatitis, not specified as infective
  Necrosis of liver (acute) (diffuse) (massive) (subacute)
  Parenchymatous degeneration of liver
  Yellow atrophy (liver) (acute) (subacute)
  EXCLUDES icterus gravis of newborn (773.0-773.2)
    serum hepatitis (070.2-070.3)
    that with:
      abortion (634-638 with .7, 639.8)
      ectopic or molar pregnancy (639.8)
      pregnancy, childbirth, or the puerperium (646.7)
    viral hepatitis (070.0-070.9)
  CC Excl: 570, 573.4-573.9
  AHA: 1Q, '00, 22

√4th **571 Chronic liver disease and cirrhosis**
  571.0 Alcoholic fatty liver `A`
  571.1 Acute alcoholic hepatitis `A`
    Acute alcoholic liver disease
  571.2 Alcoholic cirrhosis of liver `CC A`
    Florid cirrhosis
    Laennec's cirrhosis (alcoholic)
    CC Excl: 571.2, 573.8-573.9
    AHA: ▶1Q, '02, 3;◄ N-D, '85, 14
    DEF: Fibrosis and dysfunction, of liver; due to alcoholic liver disease.
  571.3 Alcoholic liver damage, unspecified `A`

√5th **571.4 Chronic hepatitis**
  EXCLUDES viral hepatitis (acute) (chronic) (070.0-070.9)

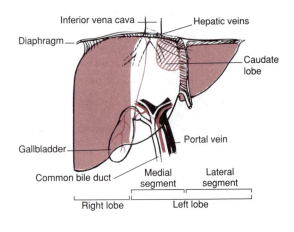

Liver

N Newborn Age: 0   P Pediatric Age: 0-17   M Maternity Age: 12-55   A Adult Age: 15-124   CC CC Condition   MC Major Complication   CD Complex Dx   HIV HIV Related Dx

164 — Volume 1 • October 2002   2002 Ingenix, Inc.

DIGESTIVE SYSTEM

571.40 Chronic hepatitis, unspecified
571.41 Chronic persistent hepatitis
571.49 Other
Chronic hepatitis:
  active
  aggressive
Recurrent hepatitis
CC Excl: 571.49, 571.5-571.9, 573.8-573.9

AHA: 3Q, '99, 19; N-D, '85, 14

571.5 Cirrhosis of liver without mention of alcohol
Cirrhosis of liver: Cirrhosis of liver:
  NOS   postnecrotic
  cryptogenic   Healed yellow atrophy
  macronodular   (liver)
  micronodular   Portal cirrhosis
  posthepatitic
CC Excl: See code 571.49

DEF: Fibrosis and dysfunction of liver; not alcohol related.

571.6 Biliary cirrhosis
Chronic nonsuppurative destructive cholangitis
Cirrhosis:
  cholangitic
  cholestatic
CC Excl: See code 571.49

571.8 Other chronic nonalcoholic liver disease
Chronic yellow atrophy (liver)
Fatty liver, without mention of alcohol
AHA: 2Q, '96, 12

571.9 Unspecified chronic liver disease without mention of alcohol

√4th **572 Liver abscess and sequelae of chronic liver disease**

572.0 Abscess of liver
EXCLUDES   amebic liver abscess (006.3)
CC Excl: 006.3, 572.0-572.1, 573.8-573.9

572.1 Portal pyemia
Phlebitis of portal vein   Pylephlebitis
Portal thrombophlebitis   Pylethrombophlebitis
CC Excl: See code 572.0

DEF: Inflammation of portal vein or branches; may be due to intestinal disease; symptoms include fever, chills, jaundice, sweating, and abscess in various body parts.

572.2 Hepatic coma
Hepatic encephalopathy
Hepatocerebral intoxication
Portal-systemic encephalopathy
CC Excl: 572.2, 573.8-573.9

AHA: ▶1Q, '02, 3;◀ 3Q, '95, 14

572.3 Portal hypertension
DEF: Abnormally high blood pressure in the portal vein.

572.4 Hepatorenal syndrome
EXCLUDES   that following delivery (674.8)
CC Excl: 572.4, 573.8-573.9

AHA: 3Q, '93, 15

DEF: Hepatic and renal failure characterized by cirrhosis with ascites or obstructive jaundice, oliguria, and low sodium concentration.

572.8 Other sequelae of chronic liver disease

√4th **573 Other disorders of liver**
EXCLUDES   amyloid or lardaceous degeneration of liver (277.3)
congenital cystic disease of liver (751.62)
glycogen infiltration of liver (271.0)
hepatomegaly NOS (789.1)
portal vein obstruction (452)

573.0 Chronic passive congestion of liver
DEF: Blood accumulation in liver tissue.

573.1 Hepatitis in viral diseases classified elswhere
Code first underlying disease as:
  Coxsackie virus disease (074.8)
  cytomegalic inclusion virus disease (078.5)
  infectious mononucleosis (075)
EXCLUDES   hepatitis (in):
  mumps (072.71)
  viral (070.0-070.9)
  yellow fever (060.0-060.9)
CC Excl: 573.1-573.3, 573.8-573.9

573.2 Hepatitis in other infectious diseases classified elsewhere
Code first underlying disease, as:
  malaria (084.9)
EXCLUDES   hepatitis in:
  late syphilis (095.3)
  secondary syphilis (091.62)
  toxoplasmosis (130.5)
CC Excl: See code 573.1

573.3 Hepatitis, unspecified
Toxic (noninfectious) hepatitis
Use additional E code to identify cause
CC Excl: See code 573.1

AHA: 3Q, '98, 3, 4; 4Q, '90, 26

573.4 Hepatic infarction
CC Excl: 570, 573.4-573.9

573.8 Other specified disorders of liver
Hepatoptosis

573.9 Unspecified disorder of liver

√4th **574 Cholelithiasis**

The following fifth-digit subclassification is for use with category 574:
  0 without mention of obstruction
  1 with obstruction

√5th **574.0** Calculus of gallbladder with acute cholecystitis
Biliary calculus ⎫
Calculus of cystic duct ⎬ with acute cholecystitis
Cholelithiasis ⎭

Any condition classifiable to 574.2 with acute cholecystitis
CC Excl: For code 574.00: 574.00-574.21, 574.40, 574.60-574.61, 574.80-574.81, 575.0, 575.10-575.12, 575.9, 576.8-576.9;
CC Excl: For code 574.01: 574.00-574.21, 574.60-574.61, 574.80-574.81, 575.0, 575.10-575.12, 575.9, 576.8-576.9

AHA: 4Q, '96, 32

√5th **574.1** Calculus of gallbladder with other cholecystitis
Biliary calculus ⎫
Calculus of cystic duct ⎬ with cholecystitis
Cholelithiasis ⎭

Cholecystitis with cholelithiasis NOS
Any condition classifiable to 574.2 with cholecystitis (chronic)
CC Excl: See code 574.01

AHA: 3Q, '99, 9; 4Q, '96, 32, 69; 2Q, '96, 13

574.2–575.4 DIGESTIVE SYSTEM — Tabular List

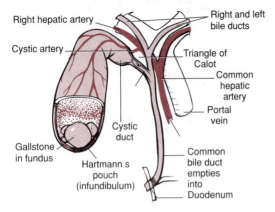

Gallbladder and Bile Ducts

✓5th **574.2 Calculus of gallbladder without mention of cholecystitis** [CC 1] [A]
Biliary:
  calculus NOS
  colic NOS
Calculus of cystic duct
Cholelithiasis NOS
Colic (recurrent) of gallbladder
Gallstone (impacted)
CC Excl: For code 574.21: See code 574.01
AHA: For code 574.20: 1Q, '88, 14

✓5th **574.3 Calculus of bile duct with acute cholecystitis** [CC] [A]
Calculus of bile duct [any] } with acute cholecystitis
Choledocholithiasis
Any condition classifiable to 574.5 with acute cholecystitis
CC Excl: 574.30-574.51, 574.60-574.61, 574.70-574.71, 574.80-574.81, 574.90-574.91, 575.0, 575.10-575.12, 576.8-576.9

✓5th **574.4 Calculus of bile duct with other cholecystitis** [CC] [A]
Calculus of bile duct [any] } with cholecystitis (chronic)
Choledocholithiasis
Any condition classifiable to 574.5 with cholecystitis (chronic)
CC Excl: See code 574.3

✓5th **574.5 Calculus of bile duct without mention of cholecystitis** [CC] [A]
Calculus of:
  bile duct [any]
  common duct
  hepatic duct
Choledocholithiasis
Hepatic:
  colic (recurrent)
  lithiasis
CC Excl: See code 574.3
AHA: 3Q, '94, 11

✓5th **574.6 Calculus of gallbladder and bile duct with acute cholecystitis** [CC] [A]
Any condition classifiable to 574.0 and 574.3
CC Excl: 574.60-574.61, 575.0, 575.10-575.12, 575.9, 576.8-576.9
AHA: 4Q, '96, 32

✓5th **574.7 Calculus of gallbladder and bile duct with other cholecystitis** [CC] [A]
Any condition classifiable to 574.1 and 574.4
CC Excl: 574.30-574.31, 574.40-574.41, 574.50-574.51, 574.60-574.61, 574.70-574.71, 574.80-574.81, 574.90-574.91, 575.0, 575.10-575.12, 576.8-576.9
AHA: 4Q, '96, 32

✓5th **574.8 Calculus of gallbladder and bile duct with acute and chronic cholecystitis** [CC] [A]
Any condition classifiable to 574.6 and 574.7
CC Excl: 574.80-574.81, 575.0, 575.10-575.12, 575.9, 576.8-576.9
AHA: 4Q, '96, 32

✓5th **574.9 Calculus of gallbladder and bile duct without cholecystitis** [CC] [A]
Any condition classifiable to 574.2 and 574.5
CC Excl: See code 574.7
AHA: 4Q, '96, 32

✓4th **575 Other disorders of gallbladder**

575.0 Acute cholecystitis [CC] [A]
Abscess of gallbladder
Angiocholecystitis
Cholecystitis:
  emphysematous (acute)
  gangrenous
  suppurative
Empyema of gallbladder
Gangrene of gallbladder
} without mention of calculus
EXCLUDES that with:
  acute and chronic cholecystitis (575.12)
  choledocholithiasis (574.3)
  choledocholithiasis and cholelithiasis (574.6)
  cholelithiasis (574.0)
CC Excl: 574.60-574.61, 574.80-574.81, 575.0, 575.10-575.12, 575.9, 576.8-576.9
AHA: 3Q, '91, 17

✓5th **575.1 Other cholecystitis**
Cholecystitis:
  NOS
  chronic
} without mention of calculus
EXCLUDES that with:
  choledocholithiasis (574.4)
  choledocholithiasis and cholelithiasis (574.8)
  cholelithiasis (574.1)
AHA: 4Q, '96, 32

575.10 Cholecystitis, unspecified [A]
Cholecystitis NOS

575.11 Chronic cholecystitis [A]

575.12 Acute and chronic cholecystitis [CC] [A]
CC Excl: 575.0, 575.10-575.12, 575.9, 576.8-576.9
AHA: 4Q, '97, 52; 4Q, '96, 32

575.2 Obstruction of gallbladder [CC] [A]
Occlusion
Stenosis
Stricture
} of cystic duct or gallbladder without mention of calculus
EXCLUDES that with calculus (574.0-574.2 with fifth-digit 1)
CC Excl: 575.2-575.9, 576.8-576.9

575.3 Hydrops of gallbladder [CC] [A]
Mucocele of gallbladder
CC Excl: See code 575.2
AHA: 2Q, '89, 13
DEF: Serous fluid accumulation in bladder.

575.4 Perforation of gallbladder [CC]
Rupture of cystic duct or gallbladder
CC Excl: See code 575.2

[N] Newborn Age: 0   [P] Pediatric Age: 0-17   [M] Maternity Age: 12-55   [A] Adult Age: 15-124   [CC] CC Condition   [MC] Major Complication   [CD] Complex Dx   [HIV] HIV Related Dx

DIGESTIVE SYSTEM

575.5 Fistula of gallbladder `cc`
Fistula: cholecystoduodenal
Fistula: cholecystoenteric
CC Excl: See code 575.2

575.6 Cholesterolosis of gallbladder
Strawberry gallbladder
AHA: 4Q, '90, 17

DEF: Cholesterol deposits in gallbladder tissue.

575.8 Other specified disorders of gallbladder
Adhesions
Atrophy
Cyst
Hypertrophy
Nonfunctioning
Ulcer
} (of) cystic duct or gallbladder

Biliary dyskinesia
EXCLUDES Hartmann's pouch of intestine (V44.3)
nonvisualization of gallbladder (793.3)
AHA: 4Q, '90, 26; 2Q, '89, 13

575.9 Unspecified disorder of gallbladder

√4ᵗʰ 576 Other disorders of biliary tract
EXCLUDES that involving the:
cystic duct (575.0-575.9)
gallbladder (575.0-575.9)

576.0 Postcholecystectomy syndrome `A`
AHA: 1Q, '88, 10

DEF: Jaundice or abdominal pain following cholecystectomy.

576.1 Cholangitis `cc`
Cholangitis:
NOS
acute
ascending
chronic
primary
Cholangitis:
recurrent
sclerosing
secondary
stenosing
suppurative
CC Excl: 576.1, 576.8-576.9
AHA: 2Q, '99, 13

576.2 Obstruction of bile duct
Occlusion
Stenosis
Stricture
} of bile duct, except cystic duct, without mention of calculus

EXCLUDES congenital (751.61)
that with calculus (574.3-574.5 with fifth-digit 1)
AHA: 1Q, '01, 8; 2Q, '99, 13

576.3 Perforation of bile duct `cc`
Rupture of bile duct, except cystic duct
CC Excl: 576.3-576.4, 576.8-576.9

576.4 Fistula of bile duct `cc`
Choledochoduodenal fistula
CC Excl: See code 576.3

576.5 Spasm of sphincter of Oddi

576.8 Other specified disorders of biliary tract
Adhesions
Atrophy
Cyst
Hypertrophy
Stasis
Ulcer
} of bile duct [any]

EXCLUDES congenital choledochal cyst (751.69)
AHA: 2Q, '99, 14

576.9 Unspecified disorder of biliary tract

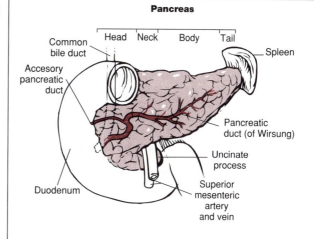

Pancreas

√4ᵗʰ 577 Diseases of pancreas

577.0 Acute pancreatitis `cc`
Abscess of pancreas
Necrosis of pancreas:
acute
infective
Pancreatitis:
NOS
Pancreatitis:
acute (recurrent)
apoplectic
hemorrhagic
subacute
suppurative
EXCLUDES mumps pancreatitis (072.3)
CC Excl: 577.0-577.1, 577.8-577.9
AHA: 3Q, '99, 9; 2Q, '98, 19; 2Q, '96, 13; 2Q, '89, 9

577.1 Chronic pancreatitis `A`
Chronic pancreatitis:
NOS
infectious
interstitial
Pancreatitis:
painless
recurrent
relapsing
AHA: 1Q, '01, 8; 2Q, '96, 13; 3Q, '94, 11

577.2 Cyst and pseudocyst of pancreas `cc`
CC Excl: 577.2, 577.8-577.9

577.8 Other specified diseases of pancreas
Atrophy
Calculus
Cirrhosis
Fibrosis
} of pancreas

Pancreatic:
infantilism
necrosis:
NOS
aseptic
Pancreatic:
necrosis:
fat
Pancreatolithiasis

EXCLUDES fibrocystic disease of pancreas
►(277.00-277.09)◄
islet cell tumor of pancreas (211.7)
pancreatic steatorrhea (579.4)
AHA: 1Q, '01, 8

577.9 Unspecified disease of pancreas

578 Gastrointestinal hemorrhage

EXCLUDES that with mention of:
   angiodysplasia of stomach and duodenum (537.83)
   angiodysplasia of intestine (569.85)
   diverticulitis, intestine:
      large (562.13)
      small (562.03)
   diverticulosis, intestine:
      large (562.12)
      small (562.02)
   gastritis and duodenitis (535.0-535.6)
   ulcer:
      duodenal, gastric, gastrojejuunal or peptic (531.00-534.91)

AHA: 2Q, '92, 9; 4Q, '90, 20

578.0 Hematemesis
Vomiting of blood

CC Excl: 251.5, 456.0, 530.2, 530.7, 530.82, 531.00-531.91, 532.00-532.91, 533.00-533.91, 534.00-534.91, 535.01, 535.11, 535.21, 535.31, 535.41, 535.51, 535.61, 537.83, 562.02-562.03, 562.12-562.13, 569.3, 569.85, 578.0-578.9

578.1 Blood in stool
Melena

EXCLUDES melena of the newborn (772.4, 777.3)
   occult blood (792.1)

CC Excl: See code 578.0

AHA: 2Q, '92, 8

DRG 174

578.9 Hemorrhage of gastrointestinal tract, unspecified
Gastric hemorrhage
Intestinal hemorrhage

CC Excl: See code 578.0

AHA: N-D, '86, 9

579 Intestinal malabsorption

579.0 Celiac disease
Celiac: Gee (-Herter) disease
   crisis   Gluten enteropathy
   infantilism   Idiopathic steatorrhea
   rickets   Nontropical sprue

DEF: Malabsorption syndrome due to gluten consumption; symptoms include fetid, bulky, frothy, oily stools; distended abdomen, gas, weight loss, asthenia, electrolyte depletion and vitamin B, D and K deficiency.

579.1 Tropical sprue
Sprue: Tropical steatorrhea
   NOS
   tropical

DEF: Diarrhea, occurs in tropics; may be due to enteric infection and malnutrition.

579.2 Blind loop syndrome
Postoperative blind loop syndrome

DEF: Obstruction or impaired passage in small intestine due to alterations, from strictures or surgery; causes stasis, abnormal bacterial flora, diarrhea, weight loss, multiple vitamin deficiency, and megaloblastic anemia.

579.3 Other and unspecified postsurgical nonabsorption
Hypoglycemia } following gastrointestinal
Malnutrition } surgery

CC Excl: 579.3-579.9

579.4 Pancreatic steatorrhea
DEF: Excess fat in feces due to absence of pancreatic juice in intestine.

579.8 Other specified intestinal malabsorption
Enteropathy: Steatorrhea (chronic)
   exudative
   protein-losing

AHA: 1Q, '88, 6

579.9 Unspecified intestinal malabsorption
Malabsorption syndrome NOS

Tabular List — GENITOURINARY SYSTEM

10. DISEASES OF THE GENITOURINARY SYSTEM (580-629)

Kidney

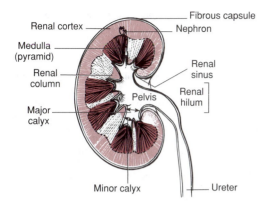

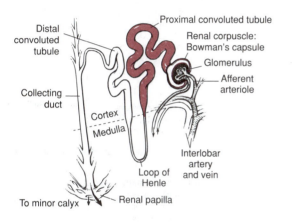

NEPHRITIS, NEPHROTIC SYNDROME, AND NEPHROSIS (580-589)

EXCLUDES hypertensive renal disease (403.00-403.91)

√4th **580 Acute glomerulonephritis**
  INCLUDES acute nephritis
  DEF: Acute, severe inflammation in tuft of capillaries that filter the kidneys.

  580.0 With lesion of proliferative glomerulonephritis CC
    Acute (diffuse) proliferative glomerulonephritis
    Acute poststreptococcal glomerulonephritis
    CC Excl: 016.00-016.06, 016.30-016.36, 016.90-016.96, 017.90-017.96, 098.10, 098.19, 098.30-098.31, 098.89, 112.2, 131.00, 131.8-131.9, 250.40-250.43, 250.80-250.93, 274.10, 274.19, 580.0-580.9, 581.0-581.9, 582.0-582.9, 583.0-583.9, 584.5-584.9, 585-587, 588.0-588.9, 589.0-589.9, 590.00-590.9, 591, 593.0-593.2, 593.89, 593.9, 599.7-599.9

  580.4 With lesion of rapidly progressive glomerulonephritis CC
    Acute nephritis with lesion of necrotizing glomerulitis
    CC Excl: See code 580.0
    DEF: Acute glomerulonephritis; progresses to ESRD with diffuse epithelial proliferation.

  √5th **580.8 With other specified pathological lesion in kidney**
    580.81 Acute glomerulonephritis in diseases classified elsewhere CC
      Code first underlying disease, as:
        infectious hepatitis (070.0-070.9)
        mumps (072.79)
        subacute bacterial endocarditis (421.0)
        typhoid fever (002.0)
      CC Excl: See code 580.0

    580.89 Other CC
      Glomerulonephritis, acute, with lesion of:
        exudative nephritis
        interstitial (diffuse) (focal) nephritis
      CC Excl: 016.00-016.06, 016.30-016.36, 016.90-016.96, 017.90-017.96, 098.10, 098.19, 098.30-098.31, 098.89, 112.2, 131.00, 131.8-131.9, 274.10, 274.19, 580.0-580.9, 581.0-581.9, 582.0-582.9, 583.0-583.9, 584.5-584.9, 585-587, 588.0-588.9, 589.0-589.9, 590.00-590.9, 591, 593.0-593.2, 593.89, 593.9, 599.7-599.9

  580.9 Acute glomerulonephritis with unspecified pathological lesion in kidney CC
    Glomerulonephritis:
      NOS
      hemorrhagic   } specified as acute
    Nephritis
    Nephropathy
    CC Excl: 016.00-016.06, 016.30-016.36, 016.90-016.96, 017.90-017.96, 098.10, 098.19, 098.30-098.31, 098.89, 112.2, 131.00, 131.8-131.9, 250.40-250.43, 250.80-250.93, 274.10, 274.19, 580.0-580.9, 581.0-581.9, 582.0-582.9, 583.0-583.9, 584.5-584.9, 585-587, 588.0-588.9, 589.0-589.9, 590.00-590.09, 591, 593.0-593.2, 593.89, 593.9, 599.7-599.9

√4th **581 Nephrotic syndrome**
  DEF: Disease process marked by symptoms such as; extensive edema, notable proteinuria, hypoalbuminemia, and susceptibility to intercurrent infections.

  581.0 With lesion of proliferative glomerulonephritis CC
    CC Excl: See code 580.9

  581.1 With lesion of membranous glomerulonephritis CC
    Epimembranous nephritis
    Idiopathic membranous glomerular disease
    Nephrotic syndrome with lesion of:
      focal glomerulosclerosis
      sclerosing membranous glomerulonephritis
      segmental hyalinosis
    CC Excl: See code 580.9

  581.2 With lesion of membranoproliferative glomerulonephritis CC
    Nephrotic syndrome with lesion (of):
      endothelial
      hypocomplementemic
      persistent
      lobular
      mesangiocapillary   } glomerulonephritis
      mixed membranous and
        proliferative
    CC Excl: See code 580.9
    DEF: Glomerulonephritis combined with clinical features of nephrotic syndrome; characterized by uneven thickening of glomerular capillary walls and mesangial cell increase; slowly progresses to ESRD.

  581.3 With lesion of minimal change glomerulonephritis CC
    Foot process disease
    Lipoid nephrosis
    Minimal change:
      glomerular disease
      glomerulitis
      nephrotic syndrome
    CC Excl: See code 580.9

581.8 With other specified pathological lesion in kidney

581.81 Nephrotic syndrome in diseases classified elsewhere [CC]
Code first underlying disease, as:
amyloidosis (277.3)
diabetes mellitus (250.4)
malaria (084.9)
polyarteritis (446.0)
systemic lupus erythematosus (710.0)

EXCLUDES nephrosis in epidemic hemorrhagic fever (078.6)

CC Excl: See code 580.9

AHA: 3Q, '91, 8,12; S-O, '85, 3

581.89 Other [CC]
Glomerulonephritis with edema and lesion of:
exudative nephritis
interstitial (diffuse) (focal) nephritis

CC Excl: See code 580.9

581.9 Nephrotic syndrome with unspecified pathological lesion in kidney [CC]
Glomerulonephritis with edema NOS
Nephritis:
nephrotic NOS
with edema NOS
Nephrosis NOS
Renal disease with edema NOS

CC Excl: See code 580.9

582 Chronic glomerulonephritis
INCLUDES chronic nephritis

DEF: Slow progressive type of nephritis characterized by inflammation of the capillary loops in the glomeruli of the kidney, which leads to renal failure.

582.0 With lesion of proliferative glomerulonephritis
Chronic (diffuse) proliferative glomerulonephritis

582.1 With lesion of membranous glomerulonephritis
Chronic glomerulonephritis:
membranous
sclerosing
Focal glomerulosclerosis
Segmental hyalinosis

AHA: S-O, '84, 16

582.2 With lesion of membranoproliferative glomerulonephritis
Chronic glomerulonephritis:
endothelial
hypocomplementemic persistent
lobular
membranoproliferative
mesangiocapillary
mixed membranous and proliferative

DEF: Chronic glomerulonephritis with mesangial cell proliferation.

582.4 With lesion of rapidly progressive glomerulonephritis
Chronic nephritis with lesion of necrotizing glomerulitis

DEF: Chronic glomerulonephritis rapidly progresses to ESRD; marked by diffuse epithelial proliferation.

582.8 With other specified pathological lesion in kidney

582.81 Chronic glomerulonephritis in diseases classified elsewhere
Code first underlying disease, as:
amyloidosis (277.3)
systemic lupus erythematosus (710.0)

582.89 Other
Chronic glomerulonephritis with lesion of:
exudative nephritis
interstitial (diffuse) (focal) nephritis

582.9 Chronic glomerulonephritis with unspecified pathological lesion in kidney
Glomerulonephritis:
NOS
hemorrhagic } specified as chronic
Nephritis
Nephropathy

AHA: 2Q, '01, 12

583 Nephritis and nephropathy, not specified as acute or chronic
INCLUDES "renal disease" so stated, not specified as acute or chronic but with stated pathology or cause

583.0 With lesion of proliferative glomerulonephritis
Proliferative: Proliferative
glomerulonephritis   nephritis NOS
(diffuse) NOS   nephropathy NOS

583.1 With lesion of membranous glomerulonephritis
Membranous:
glomerulonephritis NOS
nephritis NOS
Membranous nephropathy NOS

DEF: Kidney inflammation or dysfunction with deposits on glomerular capillary basement membranes.

583.2 With lesion of membranoproliferative glomerulonephritis
Membranoproliferative:
glomerulonephritis NOS
nephritis NOS
nephropathy NOS
Nephritis NOS, with lesion of:
hypocomplementemic
persistent
lobular
mesangiocapillary } glomerulonephritis
mixed membranous
and proliferative

DEF: Kidney inflammation or dysfunction with mesangial cell proliferation.

583.4 With lesion of rapidly progressive glomerulonephritis [CC]
Necrotizing or rapidly progressive:
glomerulitis NOS
glomerulonephritis NOS
nephritis NOS
nephropathy NOS
Nephritis, unspecified, with lesion of necrotizing glomerulitis

CC Excl: See code 580.9

DEF: Kidney inflammation or dysfunction; rapidly progresses to ESRD marked by diffuse epithelial proliferation.

583.6 With lesion of renal cortical necrosis
Nephritis NOS   } with (renal) cortical
Nephropathy NOS   }   necrosis
Renal cortical necrosis NOS

583.7 With lesion of renal medullary necrosis
Nephritis NOS   } with (renal) medullary
Nephropathy NOS   }   [papillary] necrosis

583.8 With other specified pathological lesion in kidney

583.81 Nephritis and nephropathy, not specified as acute or chronic, in diseases classified elsewhere
Code first underlying disease, as:
amyloidosis (277.3)
diabetes mellitus (250.4)
gonococcal infection (098.19)
Goodpasture's syndrome (446.21)
systemic lupus erythematosus (710.0)
tuberculosis (016.0)

EXCLUDES gouty nephropathy (274.10)
syphilitic nephritis (095.4)

AHA: 3Q, '91, 8; S-O, '85, 3

GENITOURINARY SYSTEM

583.89 Other
- Glomerulitis ⎫
- Glomerulonephritis ⎬ with lesion of:
- Nephritis ⎪ exudative nephritis
- Nephropathy ⎪ interstitial nephritis
- Renal disease ⎭

583.9 With unspecified pathological lesion in kidney
- Glomerulitis ⎫
- Glomerulonephritis ⎬ NOS
- Nephritis ⎪
- Nephropathy ⎭

EXCLUDES nephropathy complicating pregnancy, labor, or the puerperium (642.0-642.9, 646.2)
renal disease NOS with no stated cause (593.9)

✓4th 584 Acute renal failure
EXCLUDES following labor and delivery (669.3)
posttraumatic (958.5)
that complicating:
abortion (634-638 with .3, 639.3)
ectopic or molar pregnancy (639.3)

AHA: 1Q, '93, 18; 2Q, '92, 5; 4Q, '92, 22

DEF: State resulting from increasing urea and related substances from the blood (azotemia), often with urine output of less than 500 ml per day.

584.5 With lesion of tubular necrosis CC MC
Lower nephron nephrosis
Renal failure with (acute) tubular necrosis
Tubular necrosis:
  NOS
  acute

CC Excl: 250.40-250.43, 250.80-250.93, 274.10, 274.19, 580.0-580.9, 581.0-581.9, 582.0-582.9, 583.0-583.9, 584.5-584.9, 585-587, 588.0-588.9, 589.0-589.9, 590.00-590.9, 591, 593.0-593.2, 593.89, 593.9, 599.7-599.9, 753.0, 753.20-753.23, 753.29, 753.3, 753.9

DEF: Acute decline in kidney efficiency with destruction of tubules.

584.6 With lesion of renal cortical necrosis CC MC
CC Excl: See code 584.5

DEF: Acute decline in kidney efficiency with destruction of renal tissues that filter blood.

584.7 With lesion of renal medullary [papillary] necrosis CC MC
Necrotizing renal papillitis
CC Excl: See code 584.5

DEF: Acute decline in kidney efficiency with destruction of renal tissues that collect urine.

584.8 With other specified pathological lesion in kidney CC MC
CC Excl: 250.40-250.43, 250.80-250.93, 274.10, 274.19, 580.0-580.9, 581.0-581.9, 582.0-582.9, 583.0-583.9, 584.5-584.9, 585-587, 588.0-588.9, 589.0-589.9, 590.00-590.9, 591, 593.0-593.2, 593.89, 593.9, 599.7-599.9

AHA: N-D, '85, 1

584.9 Acute renal failure, unspecified CC MC
CC Excl: 250.40-250.43, 250.80-250.93, 274.10, 274.19, 580.0-580.9, 581.0-581.9, 582.0-582.9, 583.0-583.9, 584.5-584.9, 585-587, 588.0-588.9, 589.0-589.9, 590.00-590.9, 591, 593.0-593.2, 593.89, 593.9, 599.7-599.9, 753.0, 753.20-753.23, 753.29, 753.3, 753.9

AHA: 2Q, '01, 14; 1Q, '00, 22; 3Q, '96, 9; 4Q, '88, 1

DRG 316

585 Chronic renal failure CC
Chronic uremia
Use additional code to identify manifestation as:
uremic:
  neuropathy (357.4)
  pericarditis (420.0)

EXCLUDES that with any condition classifiable to 401 (403.0-403.9 with fifth-digit 1)

CC Excl: See code 584.9

AHA: 2Q, '01, 12, 13; 1Q, '01, 3; 4Q, '98, 55; 3Q, '98, 6, 7; 2Q, '98, 20; 3Q, '96, 9; 1Q, '93, 18; 3Q, '91, 8; 4Q, '89, 1; N-D, '85, 15; S-O, '84, 3

DRG 316

586 Renal failure, unspecified
Uremia NOS

EXCLUDES following labor and delivery (669.3)
posttraumatic renal failure (958.5)
that complicating:
abortion (634-638 with .3, 639.3)
ectopic or molar pregnancy (639.3)
uremia:
  extrarenal (788.9)
  prerenal (788.9)
with any condition classifiable to 401 (403.0-403.9 with fifth-digit 1)

AHA: 3Q, '98, 6; 1Q, '93, 18

DEF: Renal failure: kidney functions cease; malfunction may be due to inability to excrete metabolized substances or retain level of electrolytes.

DEF: Uremia: excess urea, creatinine and other nitrogenous products of protein and amino acid metabolism in blood due to reduced excretory function in bilateral kidney disease; also called azotemia.

587 Renal sclerosis, unspecified
Atrophy of kidney
Contracted kidney
Renal:
  cirrhosis
  fibrosis

EXCLUDES nephrosclerosis (arteriolar) (arteriosclerotic) (403.00-403.91)
with hypertension (403.00-403.92)

✓4th 588 Disorders resulting from impaired renal function

588.0 Renal osteodystrophy
Azotemic osteodystrophy
Phosphate-losing tubular disorders
Renal:
  dwarfism   infantilism
  rickets

DEF: Bone disorder that results in various bone diseases such as osteomalacia, osteoporosis or osteosclerosis; caused by impaired renal function, an abnormal level of phosphorus in the blood and impaired stimulation of the parathyroid.

588.1 Nephrogenic diabetes insipidus
EXCLUDES diabetes insipidus NOS (253.5)
DEF: Type of diabetes due to renal tubules inability to reabsorb water; not responsive to vasopressin; may develop into chronic renal insufficiency.

588.8 Other specified disorders resulting from impaired renal function
Hypokalemic nephropathy
Secondary hyperparathyroidism (of renal origin)
EXCLUDES secondary hypertension (405.0-405.9)

588.9 Unspecified disorder resulting from impaired renal function

✓4th 589 Small kidney of unknown cause
589.0 Unilateral small kidney
589.1 Bilateral small kidneys
589.9 Small kidney, unspecified

OTHER DISEASES OF URINARY SYSTEM (590-599)

✓4ᵗʰ 590 Infections of kidney
Use additional code to identify organism, such as Escherichia coli [E. coli] (041.4)

✓5ᵗʰ 590.0 Chronic pyelonephritis
Chronic pyelitis
Chronic pyonephrosis
▶Code if applicable, any casual condition first◀

590.00 Without lesion of renal medullary necrosis
590.01 With lesion of renal medullary necrosis

✓5ᵗʰ 590.1 Acute pyelonephritis
Acute pyelitis   Acute pyonephrosis

590.10 Without lesion of renal medullary necrosis CC
CC Excl: 016.00-016.06, 016.30-016.36, 016.90-016.96, 017.90-017.96, 098.10, 098.19, 098.30-098.31, 098.89, 112.2, 131.00, 131.8-131.9, 250.40-250.43, 250.80-250.93, 274.10, 274.19, 580.0-580.9, 581.0-581.9, 582.0-582.9, 583.0-583.9, 584.5-584.9, 585-587, 588.0-588.9, 589.0-589.9, 590.00-590.9, 591, 593.0-593.2, 593.89, 593.9, 599.0, 599.7-599.9

▽ DRG 320

590.11 With lesion of renal medullary necrosis CC
CC Excl: See code 590.10

590.2 Renal and perinephric abscess CC
Abscess: Abscess:
 kidney   perirenal
 nephritic   Carbuncle of kidney
CC Excl: See code 590.10

590.3 Pyeloureteritis cystica CC
Infection of renal pelvis and ureter
Ureteritis cystica
CC Excl: 016.00-016.06, 016.30-016.36, 016.90-016.96, 017.90-017.96, 098.10, 098.19, 098.30-098.31, 098.89, 112.2, 131.00, 131.8-131.9, 274.10, 274.19, 580.0-580.9, 581.0-581.9, 582.0-582.9, 583.0-583.9, 584.5-584.9, 585-587, 588.0-588.9, 589.0-589.9, 590.00-590.9, 591, 593.0-593.2, 593.89, 593.9, 599.0, 599.7-599.9

DEF: Inflammation and formation of submucosal cysts in the kidney, pelvis, and ureter.

✓5ᵗʰ 590.8 Other pyelonephritis or pyonephrosis, not specified as acute or chronic

590.80 Pyelonephritis, unspecified CC
Pyelitis NOS
Pyelonephritis NOS
CC Excl: See code 590.3
AHA: 1Q, '98, 10; 4Q, '97, 40

590.81 Pyelitis or pyelonephritis in diseases classified elsewhere CC
Code first underlying disease, as: tuberculosis (016.0)
CC Excl: See code 590.3
▽ DRG 320

590.9 Infection of kidney, unspecified CC
EXCLUDES urinary tract infection NOS (599.0)
CC Excl: See code 590.3

591 Hydronephrosis CC
Hydrocalycosis
Hydronephrosis
Hydroureteronephrosis
EXCLUDES congenital hydronephrosis (753.29)
          hydroureter (593.5)
CC Excl: See code 590.3
AHA: 2Q, '98, 9

DEF: Distention of kidney and pelvis, with urine build-up due to ureteral obstruction; pyonephrosis may result.

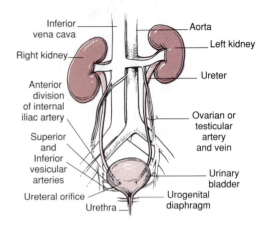

Genitourinary System

✓4ᵗʰ 592 Calculus of kidney and ureter
EXCLUDES nephrocalcinosis (275.4)

592.0 Calculus of kidney
Nephrolithiasis NOS
Renal calculus or stone
Staghorn calculus
Stone in kidney
EXCLUDES uric acid nephrolithiasis (274.11)
AHA: 1Q, '00, 4

592.1 Calculus of ureter CC
Ureteric stone
Ureterolithiasis
CC Excl: 592.0-592.9, 593.3-593.5, 593.89, 593.9, 594.0-594.9, 599.6-599.9
AHA: 2Q, '98, 9; 1Q, '98, 10; 1Q, '91, 11

592.9 Urinary calculus, unspecified
AHA: 1Q, '98, 10; 4Q, '97, 40

✓4ᵗʰ 593 Other disorders of kidney and ureter

593.0 Nephroptosis
Floating kidney
Mobile kidney

593.1 Hypertrophy of kidney

593.2 Cyst of kidney, acquired
Cyst (multiple) (solitary) of kidney, not congenital
Peripelvic (lymphatic) cyst
EXCLUDES calyceal or pyelogenic cyst of kidney (591)
          congenital cyst of kidney (753.1)
          polycystic (disease of) kidney (753.1)
AHA: 4Q, '90, 3

DEF: Abnormal, fluid-filled sac in the kidney, not present at birth.

593.3 Stricture or kinking of ureter
Angulation } of ureter (post-operative)
Constriction
Stricture of pelviureteric junction
AHA: 2Q, '98, 9

DEF: Stricture or knot in tube connecting kidney to bladder.

593.4 Other ureteric obstruction
Idiopathic retroperitoneal fibrosis
Occlusion NOS of ureter
EXCLUDES that due to calculus (592.1)
AHA: 2Q, '97, 4

GENITOURINARY SYSTEM 593.5–595.9

593.5 Hydroureter [CC]
EXCLUDES: congenital hydroureter (753.22)
hydroureteronephrosis (591)
CC Excl: 593.3-593.5, 593.89, 593.9, 595.0-595.9, 596.8-596.9, 599.0, 599.6-599.9, 753.4-753.5, 753.9

593.6 Postural proteinuria
Benign postural proteinuria   Orthostatic proteinuria
EXCLUDES: proteinuria NOS (791.0)3
DEF: Excessive amounts of serum protein in the urine caused by the body position, e.g., orthostatic and lordotic.

√5th 593.7 Vesicoureteral reflux
AHA: 4Q, '94, 42
DEF: Backflow of urine, from bladder into ureter due to obstructed bladder neck.

593.70 Unspecified or without reflux nephropathy
593.71 With reflux nephropathy, unilateral
593.72 With reflux nephropathy, bilateral
593.73 With reflux nephropathy NOS

√5th 593.8 Other specified disorders of kidney and ureter

593.81 Vascular disorders of kidney
Renal (artery):   Renal (artery):
   embolism   thrombosis
   hemorrhage   Renal infarction

593.82 Ureteral fistula
Intestinoureteral fistula
EXCLUDES: fistula between ureter and female genital tract (619.0)
DEF: Abnormal communication, between tube connecting kidney to bladder and another structure.

593.89 Other
Adhesions, kidney   Polyp of ureter
   or ureter   Pyelectasia
Periureteritis   Ureterocele
EXCLUDES: tuberculosis of ureter (016.2)
ureteritis cystica (590.3)

593.9 Unspecified disorder of kidney and ureter
Renal disease NOS
Salt-losing nephritis or syndrome
EXCLUDES: cystic kidney disease (753.1)
nephropathy, so stated (583.0-583.9)
renal disease:
   acute (580.0-580.9)
   arising in pregnancy or the puerperium (642.1-642.2, 642.4-642.7, 646.2)
   chronic (582.0-582.9)
   not specified as acute or chronic, but with stated pathology or cause (583.0-583.9)
AHA: 1Q, '93, 17

√4th 594 Calculus of lower urinary tract

594.0 Calculus in diverticulum of bladder
DEF: Stone or mineral deposit in abnormal sac on the bladder wall.

594.1 Other calculus in bladder
Urinary bladder stone
EXCLUDES: staghorn calculus (592.0)
DEF: Stone or mineral deposit in bladder.

594.2 Calculus in urethra
DEF: Stone or mineral deposit in tube that empties urine from bladder.

594.8 Other lower urinary tract calculus
AHA: J-F, '85, 16

594.9 Calculus of lower urinary tract, unspecified
EXCLUDES: calculus of urinary tract NOS (592.9)

√4th 595 Cystitis
EXCLUDES: prostatocystitis (601.3)
Use additional code to identify organism, such as Escherichia coli [E. coli] (041.4)

595.0 Acute cystitis [CC]
EXCLUDES: trigonitis (595.3)
CC Excl: 016.10-016.16, 016.30-016.36, 016.90-016.96, 017.90-017.96, 098.0, 098.11, 098.2, 098.39, 098.89, 112.2, 131.00, 131.8-131.9, 593.3-593.5, 593.89, 593.9, 595.0-595.9, 596.8-596.9, 599.0, 599.6-599.9
AHA: 2Q, '99, 15
DEF: Acute inflammation of bladder.

595.1 Chronic interstitial cystitis [CC]
Hunner's ulcer
Panmural fibrosis of bladder
Submucous cystitis
CC Excl: See code 595.0
DEF: Inflamed lesion affecting bladder wall; symptoms include urinary frequency, pain on bladder filling, nocturia, and distended bladder.

595.2 Other chronic cystitis [CC]
Chronic cystitis NOS
Subacute cystitis
EXCLUDES: trigonitis (595.3)
CC Excl: See code 595.0
DEF: Persistent inflammation of bladder.

595.3 Trigonitis
Follicular cystitis
Trigonitis (acute) (chronic)
Urethrotrigonitis
DEF: Inflammation of the triangular area of the bladder called the trigonum vesicae.

595.4 **Cystitis in diseases classified elsewhere** [CC]
Code first underlying disease, as:
   actinomycosis (039.8)
   amebiasis (006.8)
   bilharziasis (120.0-120.9)
   Echinococcus infestation (122.3, 122.6)
EXCLUDES: cystitis:
   diphtheritic (032.84)
   gonococcal (098.11, 098.31)
   monilial (112.2)
   trichomonal (131.09)
   tuberculous (016.1)
CC Excl: See code 595.0

√5th 595.8 Other specified types of cystitis

595.81 Cystitis cystica [CC]
CC Excl: See code 595.0
DEF: Inflammation of the bladder characterized by formation of multiple cysts.

595.82 Irradiation cystitis [CC]
Use additional E code to identify cause
CC Excl: See code 595.0
DEF: Inflammation of the bladder due to effects of radiation.

595.89 Other [CC]
Abscess of bladder   Cystitis:
Cystitis: emphysematous
   bullous   glandularis
CC Excl: See code 595.0

595.9 **Cystitis, unspecified** [CC]
CC Excl: See code 595.0

GENITOURINARY SYSTEM

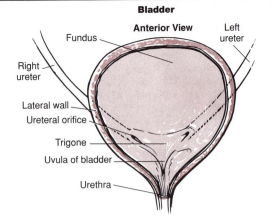

Bladder — Anterior View: Fundus, Right ureter, Left ureter, Lateral wall, Ureteral orifice, Trigone, Uvula of bladder, Urethra

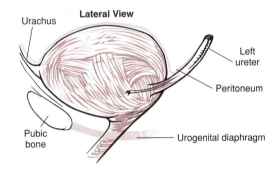

Lateral View: Urachus, Left ureter, Peritoneum, Pubic bone, Urogenital diaphragm

✓4th 596 Other disorders of bladder
Use additional code to identify urinary incontinence (625.6, 788.30-788.39).
AHA: M-A, '87, 10

596.0 Bladder neck obstruction [CC]
Contracture (acquired)
Obstruction (acquired) } of bladder neck or vesicourethral orifice
Stenosis (acquired)

EXCLUDES congenital (753.6)

CC Excl: 185, 188.0-188.9, 189.3-189.9, 596.0, 596.4, 596.51-596.59, 596.8-596.9, 600.0-600.9, 601.0-601.9, 602.0-602.9

AHA: 2Q, '01, 14; N-D, '86, 10

DEF: Bladder outlet and vesicourethral obstruction; occurs more often in males as a consequence of benign prostatic hypertrophy or prostatic cancer; may also occur in either sex due to strictures, following radiation, cystoscopy, catheterization, injury, infection, blood clots, bladder cancer, impaction or disease compressing bladder neck.

596.1 Intestinovesical fistula [CC]
Fistula:
  enterovesical
  vesicocolic
Fistula:
  vesicoenteric
  vesicorectal

CC Excl: 098.0, 098.2, 098.39, 098.89, 596.1-596.2, 596.8-596.9, 599.7-599.9, 788.1

DEF: Abnormal communication, between intestine and bladder.

596.2 Vesical fistula, not elsewhere classified [CC]
Fistula:
  bladder NOS
  urethrovesical
Fistula:
  vesicocutaneous
  vesicoperineal

EXCLUDES fistula between bladder and female genital tract (619.0)

CC Excl: See code 596.1

DEF: Abnormal communication between bladder and another structure.

596.3 Diverticulum of bladder
Diverticulitis
Diverticulum (acquired) (false) } of bladder

EXCLUDES that with calculus in diverticulum of bladder (594.0)

DEF: Abnormal pouch in bladder wall.

596.4 Atony of bladder [CC]
High compliance bladder
Hypotonicity
Inertia } of bladder

EXCLUDES neurogenic bladder (596.54)

CC Excl: 596.4, 596.51-596.59, 596.8-596.9, 599.7-599.9, 788.1

DEF: Distended, bladder with loss of expulsive force; linked to CNS disease.

✓5th 596.5 Other functional disorders of bladder
EXCLUDES cauda equina syndrome with neurogenic bladder (344.61)

596.51 Hypertonicity of bladder
Hyperactivity
Overactive bladder

DEF: Abnormal tension of muscular wall of bladder; may appear after surgery of voluntary nerve.

596.52 Low bladder compliance
DEF: Low bladder capacity; causes increased pressure and frequent urination.

596.53 Paralysis of bladder
DEF: Impaired bladder motor function due to nerve or muscle damage.

596.54 Neurogenic bladder NOS
AHA: 1Q, '01, 12

DEF: Unspecified dysfunctional bladder due to lesion of central, peripheral nervous system; may result in incontinence, residual urine retention, urinary infection, stones and renal failure.

596.55 Detrusor sphincter dyssynergia
DEF: Instability of the urinary bladder sphincter muscle associated with urinary incontinence.

596.59 Other functional disorder of bladder
Detrusor instability

DEF: Detrusor instability: instability of bladder; marked by uninhibited contractions often leading to incontinence.

596.6 Rupture of bladder, nontraumatic [CC]
CC Excl: 596.6-596.9, 599.7-599.9, 788.1

596.7 Hemorrhage into bladder wall [CC]
Hyperemia of bladder

EXCLUDES acute hemorrhagic cystitis (595.0)

CC Excl: See code 596.6

596.8 Other specified disorders of bladder
Bladder:
  calcified
  contracted
Bladder:
  hemorrhage
  hypertrophy

EXCLUDES cystocele, female (618.0, 618.2-618.4)
  hernia or prolapse of bladder, female (618.0, 618.2-618.4)

AHA: J-F, '85, 8

596.9 Unspecified disorder of bladder
AHA: J-F, '85, 8

✓4th 597 Urethritis, not sexually transmitted, and urethral syndrome
EXCLUDES nonspecific urethritis, so stated (099.4)

GENITOURINARY SYSTEM

597.0 Urethral abscess `CC`
Abscess:
    periurethral
    urethral (gland)
Abscess of:
    bulbourethral gland
Abscess of:
    Cowper's gland
    Littré's gland
    Periurethral cellulitis
EXCLUDES   urethral caruncle (599.3)

CC Excl: 098.0, 098.2, 098.39, 099.40-099.49, 112.2, 131.00, 131.02, 131.8-131.9, 597.0-597.89, 598.00-598.01, 598.8-598.9, 599.0, 599.6-599.9, 607.1-607.83, 607.89, 607.9, 608.4, 608.81, 608.85, 608.87, 608.89, 752.61-752.65, 752.69, 752.8-752.9, 753.6-753.9, 788.1

DEF: Pocket of pus in tube that empties urine from the bladder.

√5ᵗʰ **597.8 Other urethritis**
   597.80 Urethritis, unspecified
   597.81 Urethral syndrome NOS
   597.89 Other
        Adenitis, Skene's glands
        Cowperitis
        Meatitis, urethral
        Ulcer, urethra (meatus)
        Verumontanitis
        EXCLUDES   trichomonal (131.02)

√4ᵗʰ **598 Urethral stricture**
Use additional code to identify urinary incontinence (625.6, 788.30-788.39)
INCLUDES   pinhole meatus
             stricture of urinary meatus
EXCLUDES   congenital stricture of urethra and urinary meatus (753.6)

DEF: Narrowing of tube that empties urine from bladder.

√5ᵗʰ **598.0 Urethral stricture due to infection**
   598.00 Due to unspecified infection
   598.01 Due to infective diseases classified elsewhere
        Code first underlying disease, as:
            gonococcal infection (098.2)
            schistosomiasis (120.0-120.9)
            syphilis (095.8)

598.1 Traumatic urethral stricture `CC`
Stricture of urethra:
    late effect of injury
Stricture of urethra:
    postobstetric
EXCLUDES   postoperative following surgery on genitourinary tract (598.2)

CC Excl: 098.0, 098.2, 098.39, 098.89, 131.02, 598.1-598.9, 599.6-599.9, 752.61-752.65, 752.69, 753.6-753.9, 788.1

598.2 Postoperative urethral stricture `CC`
Postcatheterization stricture of urethra
CC Excl: See code 598.1
AHA: 3Q, '97, 6

598.8 Other specified causes of urethral stricture
AHA: N-D, '84, 9

598.9 Urethral stricture, unspecified

√4ᵗʰ **599 Other disorders of urethra and urinary tract**
   599.0 Urinary tract infection, site not specified `CC`
        EXCLUDES   candidiasis of urinary tract (112.2)
                   ▶urinary tract infection of newborn (771.82)◀
        Use additional code to identify organism, such as Escherichia coli [E. coli] (041.4)

CC Excl: 098.2, 098.39, 098.89, 099.40-099.49, 112.2, 131.00, 131.8-131.9, 590.10-590.9, 591, 593.89, 593.9, 595.0-595.9, 599.0, 599.6-599.9, 788.1, 996.64

AHA: 4Q, '99, 6; 2Q, '99, 15;1Q, '98, 5; 2Q, '96, 7; 4Q, '96, 33; 2Q, '95, 7; 1Q, '92, 13

▽ **DRG** 320

599.1 Urethral fistula
Fistula:
    urethroperineal
    urethrorectal
Urinary fistula NOS
EXCLUDES   fistula:
                urethroscrotal (608.89)
                urethrovaginal (619.0)
                urethrovesicovaginal (619.0)
AHA: 3Q, '97, 6

599.2 Urethral diverticulum
DEF: Abnormal pouch in urethral wall.

599.3 Urethral caruncle
Polyp of urethra

599.4 Urethral false passage `CC`
CC Excl: 597.0-597.89, 598.00-598.9, 599.1-599.9, 607.1-607.83, 607.89, 607.9, 608.4, 608.81, 608.85, 608.87, 608.89, 752.61-752.65, 752.69, 752.8-752.9, 753.9, 788.1

DEF: Abnormal opening in urethra due to surgery; trauma or disease.

599.5 Prolapsed urethral mucosa
Prolapse of urethra
Urethrocele
EXCLUDES   urethrocele, female (618.0, 618.2-618.4)

599.6 Urinary obstruction, unspecified `CC`
Obstructive uropathy NOS
Urinary (tract) obstruction NOS
Use additional code to identify urinary incontinence (625.6, 788.30-788.39)
EXCLUDES   obstructive nephropathy NOS (593.89)

CC Excl: 185, 188.0-188.9, 189.2-189.9, 274.11, 344.61, 592.1, 592.9, 593.3-593.5, 593.89, 593.9, 594.0-594.9, 595.0-595.9, 596.0, 596.51-596.59, 596.8-596.9, 597.0-597.89, 598.00-598.9, 599.0-599.9, 600.0-600.9, 601.0-601.9, 602.0-602.9, 753.0-753.9, 788.1

599.7 Hematuria `CC`
Hematuria (benign) (essential)
EXCLUDES   hemoglobinuria (791.2)
CC Excl: 592.0-592.9, 593.89, 593.9, 594.0-594.9, 596.6-596.7, 599.7-599.9

AHA: 1Q, '00, 5; 3Q, '95, 8

DEF: Blood in urine.

√5ᵗʰ **599.8 Other specified disorders of urethra and urinary tract**
Use additional code to identify urinary incontinence (625.6, 788.30-788.39), if present
EXCLUDES   symptoms and other conditions classifiable to 788.0-788.2, 788.4-788.9, 791.0-791.9

   599.81 Urethral hypermobility
        DEF: Hyperactive urethra.

   599.82 Intrinsic (urethral) spincter deficiency [ISD]
        AHA: 2Q, '96, 15
        DEF: Malfunctioning urethral sphincter.

   599.83 Urethral instability
        DEF: Inconsistent functioning of urethra.

   599.84 Other specified disorders of urethra
        Rupture of urethra (nontraumatic)
        Urethral:
            cyst
            granuloma
        DEF: Rupture of urethra due to herniation or breaking down of tissue; not due to trauma.
        DEF: Urethral cyst: abnormal sac in urethra; usually fluid filled.
        DEF: Granuloma: inflammatory cells forming small nodules in urethra.

   599.89 Other specified disorders of urinary tract

599.9–603.1 — GENITOURINARY SYSTEM — Tabular List

599.9 Unspecified disorder of urethra and urinary tract

DISEASES OF MALE GENITAL ORGANS (600–608)

√4th **600 Hyperplasia of prostate**
Use additional code to identify urinary incontinence (788.30-788.39)
AHA: 4Q, '00, 43; 3Q, '94, 12; 3Q, '92, 7; N-D, '86, 10
DEF: Fibrostromal proliferation in periurethral glands, causes blood in urine; etiology unknown.

600.0 Hypertrophy (benign) of prostate A ♂
Benign prostatic hypertrophy
Enlargement of prostate
Smooth enlarged prostate
Soft enlarged prostate
AHA: 2Q, '01, 14

600.1 Nodular prostate A ♂
Hard, firm prostate
Multinodular prostate
EXCLUDES malignant neoplasm of prostate (185)
DEF: Hard, firm nodule in prostate.

600.2 Benign localized hyperplasia of prostate A ♂
Adenofibromatous hypertrophy of prostate
Adenoma of prostate
Fibroadenoma of prostate
Fibroma of prostate
Myoma of prostate
Polyp of prostate
EXCLUDES benign neoplasms of prostate (222.2)
hypertrophy of prostate (600.0)
malignant neoplasm of prostate (185)
DEF: Benign localized hyperplasia is a clearly defined epithelial tumor. Other terms used for this condition are adenofibromatous hypertrophy of prostate, adenoma of prostate, fibroadenoma of prostate, fibroma of prostate, myoma of prostate, and polyp of prostate.

600.3 Cyst of prostate ♂
DEF: Sacs of fluid, which differentiate this from either nodular or adenomatous tumors.

600.9 Hyperplasia of prostate, unspecified ♂
Median bar
Prostatic obstruction NOS

√4th **601 Inflammatory diseases of prostate**
Use additional code to identify organism, such as Staphylococcus (041.1), or Streptococcus (041.0)

601.0 Acute prostatitis CC A ♂
CC Excl: 098.12, 098.32, 098.89, 112.2, 131.00, 131.03, 131.8-131.9, 600.0-600.9, 601.0-601.9, 602.0-602.9

601.1 Chronic prostatitis A ♂

601.2 Abscess of prostate CC A ♂
CC Excl: See code 601.0

601.3 Prostatocystitis CC A ♂
CC Excl: See code 601.0

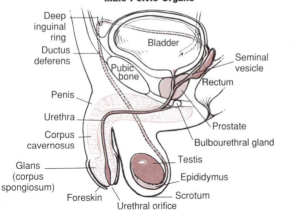
Male Pelvic Organs

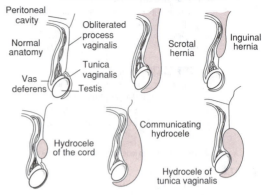
Common Inguinal Canal Anomalies

601.4 Prostatitis in diseases classified elsewhere A ♂
Code first underlying disease, as:
actinomycosis (039.8)
blastomycosis (116.0)
syphilis (095.8)
tuberculosis (016.5)
EXCLUDES prostatitis:
gonococcal (098.12, 098.32)
monilial (112.2)
trichomonal (131.03)

601.8 Other specified inflammatory diseases of prostate A ♂
Prostatitis:
cavitary
diverticular
granulomatous

601.9 Prostatitis, unspecified A ♂
Prostatitis NOS

√4th **602 Other disorders of prostate**

602.0 Calculus of prostate A ♂
Prostatic stone
DEF: Stone or mineral deposit in prostate.

602.1 Congestion or hemorrhage of prostate CC A ♂
CC Excl: See code 601.0
DEF: Bleeding or fluid collection in prostate.

602.2 Atrophy of prostate A ♂

602.3 Dysplasia of prostate ♂
Prostatic intraepithelial ▶neoplasia◀ I (PIN I)
Prostatic intraepithelial ▶neoplasia◀ II (PIN II)
EXCLUDES prostatic intraepithelial ▶neoplasia◀ III (PIN III) (233.4)
AHA: 4Q, '01, 46
DEF: Abnormality of shape and size of the intraepithelial tissues of the prostate; pre-malignant condition characterized by stalks and absence of a basilar cell layer; synonyms are intraductal dysplasia, large acinar atypical hyperplasia, atypical primary hyperplasia, hyperplasia with malignant changes, marked atypia, or duct-acinar dysplasia.

602.8 Other specified disorders of prostate A ♂
Fistula ⎫
Infarction ⎬ of prostate
Stricture ⎭
Periprostatic adhesions

602.9 Unspecified disorder of prostate A ♂

√4th **603 Hydrocele**
INCLUDES hydrocele of spermatic cord, testis, or tunica vaginalis
EXCLUDES congenital (778.6)
DEF: Circumscribed collection of fluid in tunica vaginalis, spermatic cord or testis.

603.0 Encysted hydrocele
603.1 Infected hydrocele CC
Use additional code to identify organism
CC Excl: 112.2, 131.00, 131.8-131.9, 603.0-603.9

N Newborn Age: 0   **P** Pediatric Age: 0-17   **M** Maternity Age: 12-55   **A** Adult Age: 15-124   **CC** CC Condition   **MC** Major Complication   **CD** Complex Dx   **HIV** HIV Related Dx

GENITOURINARY SYSTEM

603.8 Other specified types of hydrocele
603.9 Hydrocele, unspecified

√4th 604 Orchitis and epididymitis
Use additional code to identify organism, such as Escherichia coli [E. coli] (041.4), Staphylococcus (041.1), or Streptococcus (041.0)

604.0 Orchitis, epididymitis, and epididymo-orchitis, with abscess
Abscess of epididymis or testis
CC Excl: 072.0, 098.13-098.14, 098.33-098.34, 098.89, 112.2, 131.00, 131.8-131.9, 604.0-604.99

√5th 604.9 Other orchitis, epididymitis, and epididymo-orchitis, without mention of abscess
604.90 Orchitis and epididymitis, unspecified
604.91 Orchitis and epididymitis in diseases classified elsewhere
Code first underlying disease, as:
diphtheria (032.89)
filariasis (125.0-125.9)
syphilis (095.8)
EXCLUDES orchitis:
gonococcal (098.13, 098.33)
mumps (072.0)
tuberculous (016.5)
tuberculous epididymitis (016.4)
604.99 Other

605 Redundant prepuce and phimosis
Adherent prepuce   Phimosis (congenital)
Paraphimosis   Tight foreskin
DEF: Constriction of preputial orifice causing inability of the prepuce to be drawn back over the glans; it may be congenital or caused by infection.

√4th 606 Infertility, male
AHA: 2Q, '96, 9

606.0 Azoospermia
Absolute infertility   Infertility due to:
Infertility due to: spermatogenic arrest
  germinal (cell) aplasia   (complete)
DEF: Absence of spermatozoa in the semen or inability to produce spermatozoa.

606.1 Oligospermia
Infertility due to:
  germinal cell desquamation
  hypospermatogenesis
  incomplete spermatogenic arrest
DEF: Insufficient number of sperm in semen.

606.8 Infertility due to extratesticular causes
Infertility due to: Infertility due to:
  drug therapy   radiation
  infection   systemic disease
  obstruction of efferent
    ducts

606.9 Male infertility, unspecified

Torsion of Testes

Torsion of testis

Testes after correction showing bilateral fixation

Spermatic cord

√4th 607 Disorders of penis
EXCLUDES phimosis (605)

607.0 Leukoplakia of penis
Kraurosis of penis
EXCLUDES carcinoma in situ of penis (233.5)
erythroplasia of Queyrat (233.5)
DEF: White, thickened patches on glans penis.

607.1 Balanoposthitis
Balanitis
Use additional code to identify organism
DEF: Inflammation of glans penis and prepuce.

607.2 Other inflammatory disorders of penis
Abscess
Boil   } of corpus cavernosum
Carbuncle   } or penis
Cellulitis

Cavernitis (penis)
Use additional code to identify organism
EXCLUDES herpetic infection (054.13)

607.3 Priapism
Painful erection
DEF: Prolonged penile erection without sexual stimulation.

√5th 607.8 Other specified disorders of penis
607.81 Balanitis xerotica obliterans
Induratio penis plastica
DEF: Inflammation of the glans penis, caused by stricture of the opening of the prepuce.

607.82 Vascular disorders of penis
Embolism
Hematoma
  (nontraumatic) } of corpus cavernosum
Hemorrhage   or penis
Thrombosis

607.83 Edema of penis
DEF: Fluid retention within penile tissues.

607.84 Impotence of organic origin
EXCLUDES nonorganic or unspecified (302.72)
AHA: 3Q, '91, 11
DEF: Physiological cause interfering with erection.

607.89 Other
Atrophy
Fibrosis   } of corpus cavernosum
Hypertrophy   } or penis
Ulcer (chronic)

607.9 Unspecified disorder of penis

√4th 608 Other disorders of male genital organs
608.0 Seminal vesiculitis
Abscess   } of seminal vesicle
Cellulitis

Vesiculitis (seminal)
Use additional code to identify organism
EXCLUDES gonococcal infection (098.14, 098.34)
DEF: Inflammation of seminal vesicle.

608.1 Spermatocele
DEF: Cystic enlargement of the epididymis or the testis; the cysts contain spermatozoa.

608.2 Torsion of testis
Torsion of: Torsion of:
  epididymis   testicle
  spermatic cord
DEF: Twisted or rotated testis; may compromise blood flow.

608.3 Atrophy of testis

GENITOURINARY SYSTEM
Tabular List
608.4–614

608.4 Other inflammatory disorders of male genital organs ♂

Abscess ⎫
Boil ⎬ of scrotum, spermatic cord, testis
Carbuncle ⎪ [except abscess], tunica
Cellulitis ⎭ vaginalis, or vas deferens

Vasitis

Use additional code to identify organism

EXCLUDES abscess of testis (604.0)

√5ᵗʰ 608.8 Other specified disorders of male genital organs

608.81 Disorders of male genital organs in diseases classified elsewhere ♂

Code first underlying disease, as:
filariasis (125.0-125.9)
tuberculosis (016.5)

608.82 Hematospermia ♂

AHA: ▶4Q, '01, 46◀

DEF: ▶Presence of blood in the ejaculate; relatively common, affecting men of any age after puberty; cause is often difficult to determine since the semen originates in several organs, often the result of a viral bacterial infection and inflammation.◀

608.83 Vascular disorders ♂

Hematoma ⎫
(nontraumatic) ⎪ of seminal vesicle,
Hemorrhage ⎬ spermatic cord,
Thrombosis ⎪ testis, scrotum,
⎭ tunica vaginalis,
or vas deferens

Hematocele NOS, male

608.84 Chylocele of tunica vaginalis ♂

DEF: Chylous effusion into tunica vaginalis; due to infusion of lymphatic fluids.

608.85 Stricture ♂

Stricture of: Stricture of:
spermatic cord vas deferens
tunica vaginalis

608.86 Edema ♂

608.87 Retrograde ejaculation ♂

AHA: ▶4Q, '01, 46◀

DEF: ▶Condition where the semen travels to the bladder rather than out through the urethra due to damaged nerves causing the bladder neck to remain open during ejaculation.◀

608.89 Other ♂

Atrophy ⎫
Fibrosis ⎬ of seminal vesicle, spermatic cord, testis, scrotum, tunica vaginalis,
Hypertrophy ⎪ or vas deferens
Ulcer ⎭

EXCLUDES atrophy of testis (608.3)

608.9 Unspecified disorder of male genital organs ♂

DISORDERS OF BREAST (610-611)

√4ᵗʰ 610 Benign mammary dysplasias

610.0 Solitary cyst of breast
Cyst (solitary) of breast

610.1 Diffuse cystic mastopathy [A]
Chronic cystic mastitis   Fibrocystic disease of breast
Cystic breast

DEF: Extensive formation of nodular cysts in breast tissue; symptoms include tenderness, change in size and hyperplasia of ductal epithelium.

610.2 Fibroadenosis of breast
Fibroadenosis of breast: Fibroadenosis of breast:
NOS   diffuse
chronic   periodic
cystic   segmental

DEF: Non-neoplastic nodular condition of breast.

610.3 Fibrosclerosis of breast

DEF: Fibrous tissue in breast.

610.4 Mammary duct ectasia
Comedomastitis   Mastitis:
Duct ectasia   periductal
                       plasma cell

DEF: Atrophy of duct epithelium; causes distended collecting ducts of mammary gland; drying up of breast secretion, intraductal inflammation and periductal and interstitial chronic inflammatory reaction.

610.8 Other specified benign mammary dysplasias
Mazoplasia   Sebaceous cyst of breast

610.9 Benign mammary dysplasia, unspecified

√4ᵗʰ 611 Other disorders of breast

EXCLUDES that associated with lactation or the puerperium (675.0-676.9)

611.0 Inflammatory disease of breast
Abscess (acute) (chronic)   Mastitis (acute) (subacute)
(nonpuerperal) of: (nonpuerperal):
  areola   NOS
  breast   infective
Mammillary fistula   retromammary
                              submammary

EXCLUDES
carbuncle of breast (680.2)
chronic cystic mastitis (610.1)
neonatal infective mastitis (771.5)
thrombophlebitis of breast [Mondor's disease] (451.89)

611.1 Hypertrophy of breast
Gynecomastia
Hypertrophy of breast:
  NOS
  massive pubertal

611.2 Fissure of nipple

611.3 Fat necrosis of breast
Fat necrosis (segmental) of breast

DEF: Splitting of neutral fats in adipose tissue cells as a result of trauma; a firm circumscribed mass is then formed in the breast.

611.4 Atrophy of breast

611.5 Galactocele

611.6 Galactorrhea not associated with childbirth

√5ᵗʰ 611.7 Signs and symptoms in breast

611.71 Mastodynia
Pain in breast

611.72 Lump or mass in breast [CC]
CC Excl: 610.0-610.9, 611.0-611.9

611.79 Other
Induration of breast   Nipple discharge
Inversion of nipple   Retraction of nipple

611.8 Other specified disorders of breast
Hematoma (nontraumatic) ⎫
Infarction   ⎬ of breast

Occlusion of breast duct
Subinvolution of breast (postlactational) (postpartum)

611.9 Unspecified breast disorder

INFLAMMATORY DISEASE OF FEMALE PELVIC ORGANS (614-616)

Use additional code to identify organism, such as Staphylococcus (041.1), or Streptococcus (041.0)

EXCLUDES that associated with pregnancy, abortion, childbirth, or the puerperium (630-676.9)

√4ᵗʰ 614 Inflammatory disease of ovary, fallopian tube, pelvic cellular tissue, and peritoneum

EXCLUDES
endometritis (615.0-615.9)
major infection following delivery (670)
that complicating:
  abortion (634-638 with .0, 639.0)
  ectopic or molar pregnancy (639.0)
  pregnancy or labor (646.6)

[N] Newborn Age: 0   [P] Pediatric Age: 0-17   [M] Maternity Age: 12-55   [A] Adult Age: 15-124   [CC] CC Condition   [MC] Major Complication   [CD] Complex Dx   [HIV] HIV Related Dx

178 — Volume 1 • January 2002   2002 Ingenix, Inc.

GENITOURINARY SYSTEM

614.0 Acute salpingitis and oophoritis CC ♀
Any condition classifiable to 614.2, specified as acute or subacute
CC Excl: 016.60-016.96, 017.90-017.96, 098.15-098.17, 098.35-098.37, 098.89, 112.2, 131.00, 131.8-131.9, 614.0-614.9, 615.0-615.9, 616.8-616.9, 625.8-625.9, 629.8-629.9, 752.8-752.9

DEF: Acute inflammation, of ovary and fallopian tube.

614.1 Chronic salpingitis and oophoritis ♀
Hydrosalpinx
Salpingitis:
  follicularis
  isthmica nodosa
Any condition classifiable to 614.2, specified as chronic

DEF: Persistent inflammation of ovary and fallopian tube.

614.2 Salpingitis and oophoritis not specified as acute, subacute, or chronic ♀
Abscess (of):
  fallopian tube
  ovary
  tubo-ovarian
Oophoritis
Perioophoritis
Pyosalpinx
Perisalpingitis
Salpingitis
Salpingo-oophoritis
Tubo-ovarian inflammatory disease
EXCLUDES gonococcal infection (chronic) (098.37)
  acute (098.17)
  tuberculous (016.6)

AHA: 2Q, '91, 5

614.3 Acute parametritis and pelvic cellulitis CC ♀
Acute inflammatory pelvic disease
Any condition classifiable to 614.4, specified as acute
CC Excl: See code 614.0

DEF: Parametritis: inflammation of the parametrium; pelvic cellulitis is a synonym for parametritis.

614.4 Chronic or unspecified parametritis and pelvic cellulitis ♀
Abscess (of):
  broad ligament
  parametrium
  pelvis, female
  pouch of Douglas
} chronic or NOS

Chronic inflammatory pelvic disease
Pelvic cellulitis, female
EXCLUDES tuberculous (016.7)

614.5 Acute or unspecified pelvic peritonitis, female CC ♀
CC Excl: See code 614.0

614.6 Pelvic peritoneal adhesions, female (postoperative) (postinfection) ♀
Adhesions:
  peritubal
  tubo-ovarian
Use additional code to identify any associated infertility (628.2)

AHA: 3Q, '95, 7; 3Q, '94, 12

DEF: Fibrous scarring abnormally joining structures within abdomen.

614.7 Other chronic pelvic peritonitis, female ♀
EXCLUDES tuberculous(016.7)

614.8 Other specified inflammatory disease of female pelvic organs and tissues ♀

614.9 Unspecified inflammatory disease of female pelvic organs and tissues ♀
Pelvic infection or inflammation, female NOS
Pelvic inflammatory disease [PID]

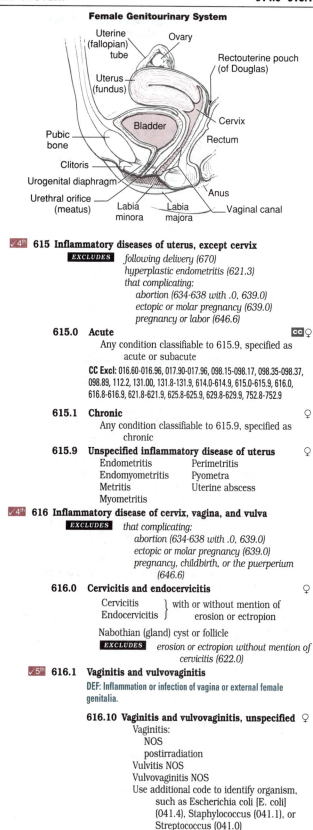

Female Genitourinary System

615 Inflammatory diseases of uterus, except cervix ✓4th
EXCLUDES following delivery (670)
  hyperplastic endometritis (621.3)
  that complicating:
    abortion (634-638 with .0, 639.0)
    ectopic or molar pregnancy (639.0)
    pregnancy or labor (646.6)

615.0 Acute CC ♀
Any condition classifiable to 615.9, specified as acute or subacute
CC Excl: 016.60-016.96, 017.90-017.96, 098.15-098.17, 098.35-098.37, 098.89, 112.2, 131.00, 131.8-131.9, 614.0-614.9, 615.0-615.9, 616.0, 616.8-616.9, 621.8-621.9, 625.8-625.9, 629.8-629.9, 752.8-752.9

615.1 Chronic ♀
Any condition classifiable to 615.9, specified as chronic

615.9 Unspecified inflammatory disease of uterus ♀
Endometritis
Endomyometritis
Metritis
Myometritis
Perimetritis
Pyometra
Uterine abscess

616 Inflammatory disease of cervix, vagina, and vulva ✓4th
EXCLUDES that complicating:
  abortion (634-638 with .0, 639.0)
  ectopic or molar pregnancy (639.0)
  pregnancy, childbirth, or the puerperium (646.6)

616.0 Cervicitis and endocervicitis ♀
Cervicitis
Endocervicitis
} with or without mention of erosion or ectropion

Nabothian (gland) cyst or follicle
EXCLUDES erosion or ectropion without mention of cervicitis (622.0)

616.1 Vaginitis and vulvovaginitis ✓5th
DEF: Inflammation or infection of vagina or external female genitalia.

616.10 Vaginitis and vulvovaginitis, unspecified ♀
Vaginitis:
  NOS
  postirradiation
Vulvitis NOS
Vulvovaginitis NOS
Use additional code to identify organism, such as Escherichia coli [E. coli] (041.4), Staphylococcus (041.1), or Streptococcus (041.0)
EXCLUDES noninfective leukorrhea (623.5)
  postmenopausal or senile vaginitis (627.3)

GENITOURINARY SYSTEM

616.11 **Vaginitis and vulvovaginitis in diseases classified elsewhere** ♀
Code first underlying disease, as:
pinworm vaginitis (127.4)
EXCLUDES herpetic vulvovaginitis (054.11)
monilial vulvovaginitis (112.1)
trichomonal vaginitis or vulvovaginitis (131.01)

616.2 **Cyst of Bartholin's gland** ♀
Bartholin's duct cyst
DEF: Fluid-filled sac within gland of vaginal orifice.

616.3 **Abscess of Bartholin's gland** CC ♀
Vulvovaginal gland abscess
CC Excl: 016.70-016.96, 017.90-017.96, 112.1-112.2, 131.00-131.01, 131.8-131.9, 616.10-616.9, 624.3-624.9, 625.8-625.9, 629.8-629.9, 752.8-752.9

616.4 **Other abscess of vulva** CC ♀
Abscess ⎫
Carbuncle ⎬ of vulva
Furuncle ⎭
CC Excl: See code 616.3

✓5th **616.5** **Ulceration of vulva**
616.50 Ulceration of vulva, unspecified ♀
Ulcer NOS of vulva
616.51 **Ulceration of vulva in diseases classified elsewhere** ♀
Code first underlying disease, as:
Behçet's syndrome (136.1)
tuberculosis (016.7)
EXCLUDES vulvar ulcer (in):
gonococcal (098.0)
herpes simplex (054.12)
syphilitic (091.0)

616.8 **Other specified inflammatory diseases of cervix, vagina, and vulva** ♀
Caruncle, vagina or labium
Ulcer, vagina
EXCLUDES noninflammatory disorders of:
cervix (622.0-622.9)
vagina (623.0-623.9)
vulva (624.0-624.9)

616.9 **Unspecified inflammatory disease of cervix, vagina, and vulva** ♀

OTHER DISORDERS OF FEMALE GENITAL TRACT (617-629)

✓4th **617 Endometriosis**
DEF: What resembles uterine mucosa (endometrial tissue) is found in the pelvic cavity.

617.0 **Endometriosis of uterus** ♀
Adenomyosis   Endometriosis:
Endometriosis: internal
cervix   myometrium
EXCLUDES stromal endometriosis (236.0)
AHA: 3Q, '92, 7
DEF: Aberrant uterine mucosal tissue; creating products of menses and inflamed uterine tissues.

617.1 **Endometriosis of ovary** ♀
Chocolate cyst of ovary
Endometrial cystoma of ovary
DEF: Aberrant uterine tissue; creating products of menses and inflamed ovarian tissues.

617.2 **Endometriosis of fallopian tube** ♀
DEF: Aberrant uterine tissue; creating products of menses and inflamed tissues of fallopian tubes.

Common Sites of Endometriosis

Common sites of endometriosis, in descending order of frequency:
(1) ovary
(2) cul de sac
(3) utersacral ligaments
(4) broad ligaments
(5) fallopian tube
(6) uterovesical fold
(7) round ligament
(8) vermiform appedix
(9) vagina
(10) rectovaginal septum

617.3 **Endometriosis of pelvic peritoneum** ♀
Endometriosis: Endometriosis:
broad ligament   parametrium
cul-de-sac (Douglas') round ligament
DEF: Aberrant uterine tissue; creating products of menses and inflamed peritoneum tissues.

617.4 **Endometriosis of rectovaginal septum and vagina** ♀
DEF: Aberrant uterine tissue; creating products of menses and inflamed tissues in and behind vagina.

617.5 **Endometriosis of intestine** ♀
Endometriosis: Endometriosis:
appendix   rectum
colon
DEF: Aberrant uterine tissue; creating products of menses and inflamed intestinal tissues.

617.6 **Endometriosis in scar of skin** ♀

617.8 **Endometriosis of other specified sites** ♀
Endometriosis: Endometriosis:
bladder   umbilicus
lung   vulva

617.9 **Endometriosis, site unspecified** ♀

✓4th **618 Genital prolapse**
Use additional code to identify urinary incontinence (625.6, 788.31, 788.33-788.39)
EXCLUDES that complicating pregnancy, labor, or delivery (654.4)

618.0 **Prolapse of vaginal walls without mention of uterine prolapse** ♀
Cystocele   Cystourethrocele
Proctocele, female ⎫
Rectocele   ⎬ without mention
Urethrocele, female ⎬ of uterine
Vaginal prolapse   ⎭ prolapse
EXCLUDES that with uterine prolapse (618.2-618.4)
enterocele (618.6)
vaginal vault prolapse following hysterectomy (618.5)

618.1 **Uterine prolapse without mention of vaginal wall prolapse** ♀
Descensus uteri   Uterine prolapse:
Uterine prolapse: first degree
NOS   second degree
complete   third degree
EXCLUDES that with mention of cystocele, urethrocele, or rectocele (618.2-618.4)

618.2 **Uterovaginal prolapse, incomplete** ♀
DEF: Downward displacement of uterus downward into vagina.

618.3 **Uterovaginal prolapse, complete** ♀
DEF: Downward displacement of uterus exposed within external genitalia.

 Newborn Age: 0   Pediatric Age: 0-17   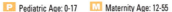 Maternity Age: 12-55   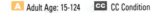 Adult Age: 15-124   CC Condition   Major Complication   Complex Dx   HIV HIV Related Dx

GENITOURINARY SYSTEM

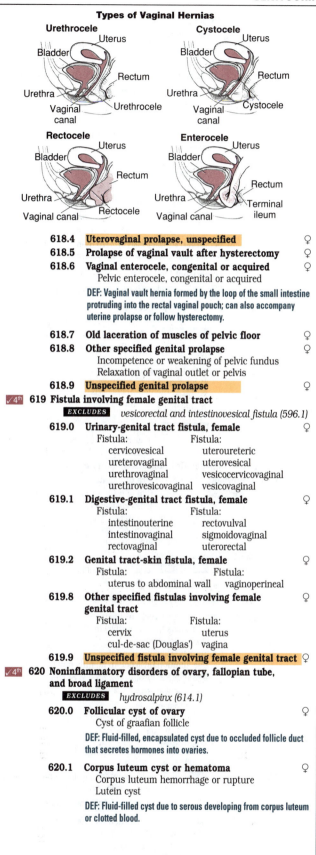

Types of Vaginal Hernias: Urethrocele, Cystocele, Rectocele, Enterocele

618.4 Uterovaginal prolapse, unspecified ♀
618.5 Prolapse of vaginal vault after hysterectomy ♀
618.6 Vaginal enterocele, congenital or acquired ♀
Pelvic enterocele, congenital or acquired
DEF: Vaginal vault hernia formed by the loop of the small intestine protruding into the rectal vaginal pouch; can also accompany uterine prolapse or follow hysterectomy.

618.7 Old laceration of muscles of pelvic floor ♀
618.8 Other specified genital prolapse ♀
Incompetence or weakening of pelvic fundus
Relaxation of vaginal outlet or pelvis

618.9 Unspecified genital prolapse ♀

√4th **619 Fistula involving female genital tract**
EXCLUDES vesicorectal and intestinovesical fistula (596.1)

619.0 Urinary-genital tract fistula, female ♀
Fistula: Fistula:
cervicovesical   uteroureteric
ureterovaginal   uterovesical
urethrovaginal   vesicocervicovaginal
urethrovesicovaginal vesicovaginal

619.1 Digestive-genital tract fistula, female ♀
Fistula: Fistula:
intestinouterine rectovulval
intestinovaginal sigmoidovaginal
rectovaginal   uterorectal

619.2 Genital tract-skin fistula, female ♀
Fistula: Fistula:
uterus to abdominal wall   vaginoperineal

619.8 Other specified fistulas involving female genital tract ♀
Fistula: Fistula:
cervix   uterus
cul-de-sac (Douglas') vagina

619.9 Unspecified fistula involving female genital tract ♀

√4th **620 Noninflammatory disorders of ovary, fallopian tube, and broad ligament**
EXCLUDES hydrosalpinx (614.1)

620.0 Follicular cyst of ovary ♀
Cyst of graafian follicle
DEF: Fluid-filled, encapsulated cyst due to occluded follicle duct that secretes hormones into ovaries.

620.1 Corpus luteum cyst or hematoma ♀
Corpus luteum hemorrhage or rupture
Lutein cyst
DEF: Fluid-filled cyst due to serous developing from corpus luteum or clotted blood.

620.2 Other and unspecified ovarian cyst ♀
Cyst:
  NOS
  corpus albicans
  retention NOS   } of ovary
  serous
  theca-lutein
Simple cystoma of ovary
EXCLUDES cystadenoma (benign) (serous) (220)
          developmental cysts (752.0)
          neoplastic cysts (220)
          polycystic ovaries (256.4)
          Stein-Leventhal syndrome (256.4)

620.3 Acquired atrophy of ovary and fallopian tube ♀
Senile involution of ovary

620.4 Prolapse or hernia of ovary and fallopian tube ♀
Displacement of ovary and fallopian tube
Salpingocele

620.5 Torsion of ovary, ovarian pedicle, or fallopian tube ♀
Torsion: Torsion:
accessory tube   hydatid of Morgagni

620.6 Broad ligament laceration syndrome ♀
Masters-Allen syndrome

620.7 Hematoma of broad ligament CC ♀
Hematocele, broad ligament
CC Excl: 620.6-620.9, 625.8-625.9, 629.8-629.9, 752.8-752.9
DEF: Blood within peritoneal fold that supports uterus.

620.8 Other noninflammatory disorders of ovary, fallopian tube, and broad ligament ♀
Cyst
Polyp } of broad ligament or fallopian tube

Infarction
Rupture } of ovary or fallopian tube

Hematosalpinx
EXCLUDES hematosalpinx in ectopic pregnancy (639.2)
          peritubal adhesions (614.6)
          torsion of ovary, ovarian pedicle, or fallopian tube (620.5)

620.9 Unspecified noninflammatory disorder of ovary, fallopian tube, and broad ligament ♀

√4th **621 Disorders of uterus, not elsewhere classified**
621.0 Polyp of corpus uteri ♀
Polyp: Polyp:
endometrium   uterus NOS
EXCLUDES cervical polyp NOS (622.7)

621.1 Chronic subinvolution of uterus ♀
EXCLUDES puerperal (674.8)
AHA: 1Q, '91, 11
DEF: Abnormal size of uterus after delivery; the uterus does not return to its normal size after the birth of a child.

621.2 Hypertrophy of uterus ♀
Bulky or enlarged uterus
EXCLUDES puerperal (674.8)

621.3 Endometrial cystic hyperplasia ♀
Hyperplasia (adenomatous) (cystic) (glandular) of endometrium
DEF: Abnormal cystic overgrowth of endometrial tissue.

621.4 Hematometra ♀
Hemometra
EXCLUDES that in congenital anomaly (752.2-752.3)
DEF: Accumulated blood in uterus.

621.5 Intrauterine synechiae ♀
Adhesions of uterus   Band(s) of uterus

GENITOURINARY SYSTEM

Uterus and Ovaries

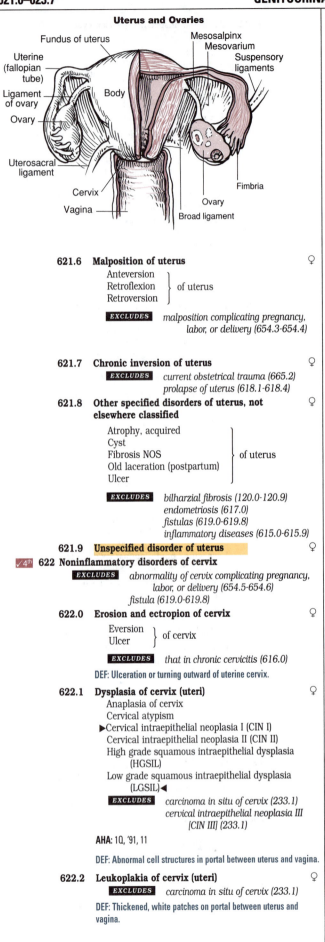

621.6 Malposition of uterus ♀
- Anteversion
- Retroflexion } of uterus
- Retroversion

EXCLUDES malposition complicating pregnancy, labor, or delivery (654.3-654.4)

621.7 Chronic inversion of uterus ♀
EXCLUDES current obstetrical trauma (665.2)
prolapse of uterus (618.1-618.4)

621.8 Other specified disorders of uterus, not elsewhere classified ♀
- Atrophy, acquired
- Cyst
- Fibrosis NOS } of uterus
- Old laceration (postpartum)
- Ulcer

EXCLUDES bilharzial fibrosis (120.0-120.9)
endometriosis (617.0)
fistulas (619.0-619.8)
inflammatory diseases (615.0-615.9)

621.9 Unspecified disorder of uterus ♀

√4th **622 Noninflammatory disorders of cervix**
EXCLUDES abnormality of cervix complicating pregnancy, labor, or delivery (654.5-654.6)
fistula (619.0-619.8)

622.0 Erosion and ectropion of cervix ♀
- Eversion
- Ulcer } of cervix

EXCLUDES that in chronic cervicitis (616.0)
DEF: Ulceration or turning outward of uterine cervix.

622.1 Dysplasia of cervix (uteri) ♀
- Anaplasia of cervix
- Cervical atypism
- ▶Cervical intraepithelial neoplasia I (CIN I)
- Cervical intraepithelial neoplasia II (CIN II)
- High grade squamous intraepithelial dysplasia (HGSIL)
- Low grade squamous intraepithelial dysplasia (LGSIL)◀

EXCLUDES carcinoma in situ of cervix (233.1)
cervical intraepithelial neoplasia III [CIN III] (233.1)

AHA: 1Q, '91, 11

DEF: Abnormal cell structures in portal between uterus and vagina.

622.2 Leukoplakia of cervix (uteri) ♀
EXCLUDES carcinoma in situ of cervix (233.1)
DEF: Thickened, white patches on portal between uterus and vagina.

622.3 Old laceration of cervix ♀
- Adhesions
- Band(s) } of cervix
- Cicatrix (postpartum)

EXCLUDES current obstetrical trauma (665.3)
DEF: Scarring or other evidence of old wound on cervix.

622.4 Stricture and stenosis of cervix ♀
- Atresia (acquired)
- Contracture } of cervix
- Occlusion

Pinpoint os uteri
EXCLUDES congenital (752.49)
that complicating labor (654.6)

622.5 Incompetence of cervix ♀
EXCLUDES complicating pregnancy (654.5)
that affecting fetus or newborn (761.0)
DEF: Inadequate functioning of cervix; marked by abnormal widening during pregnancy; causing miscarriage.

622.6 Hypertrophic elongation of cervix ♀
DEF: Overgrowth of cervix tissues extending down into vagina.

622.7 Mucous polyp of cervix ♀
Polyp NOS of cervix
EXCLUDES adenomatous polyp of cervix (219.0)

622.8 Other specified noninflammatory disorders of cervix ♀
- Atrophy (senile)
- Cyst
- Fibrosis } of cervix
- Hemorrhage

EXCLUDES endometriosis (617.0)
fistula (619.0-619.8)
inflammatory diseases (616.0)

622.9 Unspecified noninflammatory disorder of cervix ♀

√4th **623 Noninflammatory disorders of vagina**
EXCLUDES abnormality of vagina complicating pregnancy, labor, or delivery (654.7)
congenital absence of vagina (752.49)
congenital diaphragm or bands (752.49)
fistulas involving vagina (619.0-619.8)

623.0 Dysplasia of vagina ♀
EXCLUDES carcinoma in situ of vagina (233.3)

623.1 Leukoplakia of vagina ♀
DEF: Thickened white patches on vaginal canal.

623.2 Stricture or atresia of vagina ♀
- Adhesions (postoperative) (postradiation) of vagina
- Occlusion of vagina
- Stenosis, vagina
Use additional E code to identify any external cause
EXCLUDES congenital atresia or stricture (752.49)

623.3 Tight hymenal ring ♀
- Rigid hymen
- Tight hymenal ring } acquired or congenital
- Tight introitus

EXCLUDES imperforate hymen (752.42)

623.4 Old vaginal laceration ♀
EXCLUDES old laceration involving muscles of pelvic floor (618.7)
DEF: Scarring or other evidence of old wound on vagina.

623.5 Leukorrhea, not specified as infective ♀
- Leukorrhea NOS of vagina
- Vaginal discharge NOS
EXCLUDES trichomonal (131.00)
DEF: Viscid whitish discharge, from vagina.

623.6 Vaginal hematoma ♀
EXCLUDES current obstetrical trauma (665.7)

623.7 Polyp of vagina ♀

623.8 Other specified noninflammatory disorders of vagina ♀
    Cyst ⎫
    Hemorrhage ⎭ of vagina

623.9 Unspecified noninflammatory disorder of vagina ♀

✓4th **624 Noninflammatory disorders of vulva and perineum**
    EXCLUDES abnormality of vulva and perineum complicating pregnancy, labor, or delivery (654.8)
    condyloma acuminatum (078.1)
    fistulas involving:
        perineum — see Alphabetic Index
        vulva (619.0-619.8)
    vulval varices (456.6)
    vulvar involvement in skin conditions (690-709.9)

624.0 Dystrophy of vulva ♀
    Kraurosis ⎫
    Leukoplakia ⎭ of vulva
    EXCLUDES carcinoma in situ of vulva (233.3)

624.1 Atrophy of vulva ♀
624.2 Hypertrophy of clitoris ♀
    EXCLUDES that in endocrine disorders (255.2, 256.1)

624.3 Hypertrophy of labia ♀
    Hypertrophy of vulva NOS
    DEF: Overgrowth of fleshy folds on either side of vagina.

624.4 Old laceration or scarring of vulva ♀
    DEF: Scarring or other evidence of old wound on external female genitalia.

624.5 Hematoma of vulva ♀
    EXCLUDES that complicating delivery (664.5)
    DEF: Blood in tissue of external genitalia.

624.6 Polyp of labia and vulva ♀
624.8 Other specified noninflammatory disorders of vulva and perineum ♀
    Cyst ⎫
    Edema ⎬ of vulva
    Stricture ⎭
    AHA: 1Q, '95, 8

624.9 Unspecified noninflammatory disorder of vulva and perineum ♀

✓4th **625 Pain and other symptoms associated with female genital organs**

625.0 Dyspareunia ♀
    EXCLUDES psychogenic dyspareunia (302.76)
    DEF: Difficult or painful sexual intercourse.

625.1 Vaginismus ♀
    Colpospasm
    Vulvismus
    EXCLUDES psychogenic vaginismus (306.51)
    DEF: Vaginal spasms; due to involuntary contraction of musculature; prevents intercourse.

625.2 Mittelschmerz ♀
    Intermenstrual pain
    Ovulation pain
    DEF: Pain occurring between menstrual periods.

625.3 Dysmenorrhea ♀
    Painful menstruation
    EXCLUDES psychogenic dysmenorrhea (306.52)
    AHA: 2Q, '94, 12

625.4 Premenstrual tension syndromes ♀
    Menstrual:
        migraine
        molimen
    Premenstrual syndrome
    Premenstrual tension NOS

625.5 Pelvic congestion syndrome ♀
    Congestion-fibrosis syndrome Taylor's syndrome
    DEF: Excessive accumulated of blood in vessels of pelvis; may occur after orgasm; causes abnormal menstruation, lower back pain and vaginal discharge.

625.6 Stress incontinence, female ♀
    EXCLUDES mixed incontinence (788.33)
        stress incontinence, male (788.32)
    DEF: Involuntary leakage of urine due to insufficient sphincter control; occurs upon sneezing, laughing, coughing, sudden movement or lifting.

625.8 Other specified symptoms associated with female genital organs ♀
    AHA: N-D, '85, 16

625.9 Unspecified symptom associated with female genital organs ♀

✓4th **626 Disorders of menstruation and other abnormal bleeding from female genital tract**
    EXCLUDES menopausal and premenopausal bleeding (627.0)
    pain and other symptoms associated with menstrual cycle (625.2-625.4)
    postmenopausal bleeding (627.1)

626.0 Absence of menstruation ♀
    Amenorrhea (primary) (secondary)

626.1 Scanty or infrequent menstruation ♀
    Hypomenorrhea Oligomenorrhea

626.2 Excessive or frequent menstruation ♀
    Heavy periods
    Menometrorrhagia
    Menorrhagia
    Plymenorrhea
    EXCLUDES premenopausal(627.0)
        that in puberty (626.3)

626.3 Puberty bleeding ♀
    Excessive bleeding associated with onset of menstrual periods
    Pubertal menorrhagia

626.4 Irregular menstrual cycle ♀
    Irregular:
        bleeding NOS
        menstruation
        periods

626.5 Ovulation bleeding ♀
    Regular intermenstrual bleeding

626.6 Metrorrhagia ♀
    Bleeding unrelated to menstrual cycle
    Irregular intermenstrual bleeding

626.7 Postcoital bleeding ♀
    DEF: Bleeding from vagina after sexual intercourse.

626.8 Other ♀
    Dysfunctional or functional uterine hemorrhage NOS
    Menstruation:
        retained
        suppression of

626.9 Unspecified ♀

✓4th **627 Menopausal and postmenopausal disorders**
    EXCLUDES asymptomatic age-related (natural) postmenopausal status (V49.81)

627.0 Premenopausal menorrhagia ♀
    Excessive bleeding associated with onset of menopause
    Menorrhagia:
        climacteric
        menopausal
        preclimacteric

627.1 Postmenopausal bleeding ♀

627.2–629.9 GENITOURINARY SYSTEM — Tabular List

▲ **627.2 Symptomatic menopausal or female climacteric states** ♀
Symptoms, such as flushing, sleeplessness, headache, lack of concentration, associated with the menopause

627.3 Postmenopausal atrophic vaginitis ♀
Senile (atrophic) vaginitis

▲ **627.4 Symptomatic states associated with artificial menopause** ♀
Postartificial menopause syndromes
Any condition classifiable to 627.1, 627.2, or 627.3 which follows induced menopause
DEF: Conditions arising after hysterectomy.

627.8 Other specified menopausal and postmenopausal disorders ♀
EXCLUDES premature menopause NOS (256.31)

627.9 Unspecified menopausal and postmenopausal disorder ♀

√4th **628 Infertility, female**
INCLUDES primary and secondary sterility
AHA: 2Q, '96, 9; 1Q, '95, 7

DEF: Infertility: inability to conceive for at least one year with regular intercourse.

DEF: Primary infertility: occurring in patients who have never conceived.

DEF: Secondary infertility: occurring in patients who have previously conceived.

628.0 Associated with anovulation ♀
Anovulatory cycle
Use additional code for any associated Stein-Leventhal syndrome (256.4)

628.1 Of pituitary-hypothalamic origin ♀
Code first underlying cause, as:
adiposogenital dystrophy (253.8)
anterior pituitary disorder (253.0-253.4)

628.2 Of tubal origin ♀
Infertility associated with congenital anomaly of tube
Tubal:
block
occlusion
stenosis
Use additional code for any associated peritubal adhesions (614.6)

628.3 Of uterine origin ♀
Infertility associated with congenital anomaly of uterus
Nonimplantation
Use additional code for any associated tuberculous endometritis (016.7)

628.4 Of cervical or vaginal origin ♀
Infertility associated with:
anomaly of cervical mucus
congenital structural anomaly
dysmucorrhea

628.8 Of other specified origin ♀

628.9 Of unspecified origin ♀

√4th **629 Other disorders of female genital organs**

629.0 Hematocele, female, not elsewhere classified ♀
EXCLUDES hematocele or hematoma:
broad ligament (620.7)
fallopian tube (620.8)
that associated with ectopic pregnancy ▶(633.00-633.91)◀
uterus (621.4)
vagina (623.6)
vulva (624.5)

629.1 Hydrocele, canal of Nuck ♀
Cyst of canal of Nuck (acquired)
EXCLUDES congenital (752.41)

629.8 Other specified disorders of female genital organs ♀

629.9 Unspecified disorder of female genital organs ♀
Habitual aborter without current pregnancy

11. COMPLICATIONS OF PREGNANCY, CHILDBIRTH, AND THE PUERPERIUM (630-677)

ECTOPIC AND MOLAR PREGNANCY (630-633)

Use additional code from category 639 to identify any complications

630 Hydatidiform mole
Trophoblastic disease NOS   Vesicularmole
EXCLUDES chorioadenoma (destruens) (236.1)
chorionepithelioma (181)
malignant hydatidiform mole (236.1)

DEF: Abnormal product of pregnancy; marked by mass of cysts resembling bunch of grapes due to chorionic villi proliferation, and dissolution; must be surgically removed.

631 Other abnormal product of conception
Blighted ovum   Mole:
Mole: fleshy
  NOS   stone
  carneous

632 Missed abortion
Early fetal death before completion of 22 weeks' gestation with retention of dead fetus
Retained products of conception, not following spontaneous or induced abortion or delivery
EXCLUDES failed induced abortion (638.0-638.9)
fetal death (intrauterine) (late) (656.4)
missed delivery (656.4)
that with abnormal product of conception (630, 631)

AHA: 1Q, '01, 5

√4th 633 Ectopic pregnancy
INCLUDES ruptured ectopic pregnancy
DEF: Fertilized egg develops outside uterus.

  √5th 633.0 Abdominal pregnancy
  Intraperitoneal pregnancy
  • 633.00 Abdominal pregnancy without intrauterine pregnancy
  • 633.01 Abdominal pregnancy with intrauterine pregnancy

  √5th 633.1 Tubal pregnancy
  Fallopian pregnancy
  Rupture of (fallopian) tube due to pregnancy
  Tubal abortion
  AHA: 2Q, '90, 27
  • 633.10 Tubal pregnancy without intrauterine pregnancy
  • 633.11 Tubal pregnancy with intrauterine pregnancy

  √5th 633.2 Ovarian pregnancy
  • 633.20 Ovarian pregnancy without intrauterine pregnancy
  • 633.21 Ovarian pregnancy with intrauterine pregnancy

  √5th 633.8 Other ectopic pregnancy
  Pregnancy: Pregnancy:
    cervical   intraligamentous
    combined   mesometric
    cornual   mural
  • 633.80 Other ectopic pregnancy without intrauterine pregnancy
  • 633.81 Other ectopic pregnancy with intrauterine pregnancy

  √5th 633.9 Unspecified ectopic pregnancy
  • 633.90 Unspecified ectopic pregnancy without intrauterine pregnancy
  • 633.91 Unspecified ectopic pregnancy with intrauterine pregnancy

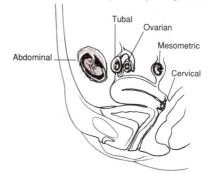

Ectopic Pregnancy Sites

OTHER PREGNANCY WITH ABORTIVE OUTCOME (634-639)

The following fourth-digit subdivisions are for use with categories 634-638:

.0 Complicated by genital tract and pelvic infection
Endometritis
Salpingo-oophoritis
Sepsis NOS
Septicemia NOS
Any condition classifiable to 639.0, with condition classifiable to 634-638
EXCLUDES urinary tract infection (634-638 with .7)

.1 Complicated by delayed or excessive hemorrhage
Afibrinogenemia
Defibrination syndrome
Intravascular hemolysis
Any condition classifiable to 639.1, with condition classifiable to 634-638
uterus

.2 Complicated by damage to pelvic organs and tissues
Laceration, perforation, or tear of:
  bladder
  uterus
Any condition classifiable to 639.2, with condition classifiable to 634-638

.3 Complicated by renal failure
Oliguria
Uremia
Any condition classifiable to 639.3, with condition classifiable to 634-638

.4 Complicated by metabolic disorder
Electrolyte imbalance with conditions classifiable to 634-638

.5 Complicated by shock
Circulatory collapse
Shock (postoperative) (septic)
Any condition classifiable to 639.5, with condition classifiable to 634-638

.6 Complicated by embolism
Embolism:
  NOS
  amniotic fluid
  pulmonary
Any condition classifiable to 639.6, with condition classifiable to 634-638

.7 With other specified complications
Cardiac arrest or failure
Urinary tract infection
Any condition classifiable to 639.8, with condition classifiable to 634-638

.8 With unspecified complication
.9 Without mention of complication

COMPLICATIONS OF PREGNANCY, CHILDBIRTH, AND THE PUERPERIUM

§ 4th 634 Spontaneous abortion

Requires fifth-digit to identify stage:
- 0 unspecified
- 1 incomplete
- 2 complete

INCLUDES miscarriage
spontaneous abortion

AHA: 2Q, '91, 16

DEF: Spontaneous premature expulsion of the products of conception from the uterus.

- **634.0** Complicated by genital tract and pelvic infection
  CC Excl: 634.00-634.92, 635.00-635.92, 636.00-636.92, 637.00-637.92, 638.0-638.9, 640.00-640.93, 641.00-641.23, 646.80-646.93, 648.90-648.94, 650, 669.40-669.44, 669.80-669.94
- **634.1** Complicated by delayed or excessive hemorrhage
  CC Excl: See code 634.0
- **634.2** Complicated by damage to pelvic organs or tissues
  CC Excl: See code 634.0
- **634.3** Complicated by renal failure
  CC Excl: See code 634.0
- **634.4** Complicated by metabolic disorder
  CC Excl: See code 634.0
- **634.5** Complicated by shock
  CC Excl: See code 634.0
- **634.6** Complicated by embolism
  CC Excl: See code 634.0
- **634.7** With other specified complications
  CC Excl: See code 634.0
- **634.8** With unspecified complication
  CC Excl: See code 634.0
- **634.9** Without mention of complication
  CC Excl: See code 634.0

§ 4th 635 Legally induced abortion

Requires fifth-digit to identify stage:
- 0 unspecified
- 1 incomplete
- 2 complete

INCLUDES abortion or termination of pregnancy:
elective
legal
therapeutic

EXCLUDES menstrual extraction or regulation (V25.3)

AHA: 2Q, '94, 14

DEF: Intentional expulsion of products of conception from uterus performed by medical professionals inside boundaries of law.

- **635.0** Complicated by genital tract and pelvic infection
- **635.1** Complicated by delayed or excessive hemorrhage
- **635.2** Complicated by damage to pelvic organs or tissues
- **635.3** Complicated by renal failure
- **635.4** Complicated by metabolic disorder
- **635.5** Complicated by shock
- **635.6** Complicated by embolism
- **635.7** With other specified complications
- **635.8** With unspecified complication
- **635.9** Without mention of complication

§ See beginning of section 634-639 for fourth-digit definitions.

§ 4th 636 Illegally induced abortion

Requires fifth-digit to identify stage:
- 0 unspecified
- 1 incomplete
- 2 complete

INCLUDES abortion:
criminal
illegal
self-induced

DEF: Intentional expulsion of products of conception from uterus; outside boundaries of law.

- **636.0** Complicated by genital tract and pelvic infection
- **636.1** Complicated by delayed or excessive hemorrhage
- **636.2** Complicated by damage to pelvic organs or tissues
- **636.3** Complicated by renal failure
- **636.4** Complicated by metabolic disorder
- **636.5** Complicated by shock
- **636.6** Complicated by embolism
- **636.7** With other specified complications
- **636.8** With unspecified complication
- **636.9** Without mention of complication

§ 4th 637 Unspecified abortion

Requires fifth-digit to identify stage:
- 0 unspecified
- 1 incomplete
- 2 complete

INCLUDES abortion NOS
retained products of conception following abortion, not classifiable elsewhere

- **637.0** Complicated by genital tract and pelvic infection
- **637.1** Complicated by delayed or excessive hemorrhage
- **637.2** Complicated by damage to pelvic organs or tissues
- **637.3** Complicated by renal failure
- **637.4** Complicated by metabolic disorder
- **637.5** Complicated by shock
- **637.6** Complicated by embolism
- **637.7** With other specified complications
- **637.8** With unspecified complication
- **637.9** Without mention of complication

§ 4th 638 Failed attempted abortion

INCLUDES failure of attempted induction of (legal) abortion

EXCLUDES incomplete abortion (634.0-637.9)

DEF: Continued pregnancy despite an attempted legal abortion.

- **638.0** Complicated by genital tract and pelvic infection
- **638.1** Complicated by delayed or excessive hemorrhage
- **638.2** Complicated by damage to pelvic organs or tissues
- **638.3** Complicated by renal failure
- **638.4** Complicated by metabolic disorder
- **638.5** Complicated by shock
- **638.6** Complicated by embolism
- **638.7** With other specified complications
- **638.8** With unspecified complication
- **638.9** Without mention of complication

COMPLICATIONS OF PREGNANCY, CHILDBIRTH, AND THE PUERPERIUM

§ ✓4th **639 Complications following abortion and ectopic and molar pregnancies**

Note: This category is provided for use when it is required to classify separately the complications classifiable to the fourth-digit level in categories 634-638; for example:

a) when the complication itself was responsible for an episode of medical care, the abortion, ectopic or molar pregnancy itself having been dealt with at a previous episode

b) when these conditions are immediate complications of ectopic or molar pregnancies classifiable to 630-633 where they cannot be identified at fourth-digit level.

639.0 Genital tract and pelvic infection
- Endometritis
- Parametritis
- Pelvic peritonitis
- Salpingitis   } following conditions classifiable to 630-638
- Salpingo-oophoritis
- Sepsis NOS
- Septicemia NOS

EXCLUDES urinary tract infection (639.8)

CC Excl: 639.0, 639.2-639.9, 640.00-640.93, 641.00-641.23, 646.80-646.93, 648.90-648.94, 650, 669.40-669.44, 669.80-669.94

639.1 Delayed or excessive hemorrhage
- Afibrinogenemia
- Defibrination syndrome } following conditions classifiable to 630-638
- Intravascular hemolysis

CC Excl: 639.1-639.9, 640.00-640.93, 641.00-641.23, 646.80-646.93, 648.90-648.94, 650, 669.40-669.44, 669.80-669.94

639.2 Damage to pelvic organs and tissues
Laceration, perforation, or tear of:
- bladder
- bowel
- broad ligament
- cervix
- periurethral tissue
- uterus
- vagina

} following conditions classifiable to 630-638

CC Excl: 639.2-639.9, 640.00-640.93, 641.00-641.23, 646.80-646.93, 648.90-648.94, 650, 669.40-669.44, 669.80-669.94

639.3 Renal failure
- Oliguria
- Renal:
  - failure (acute)
  - shutdown
  - tubular necrosis
- Uremia

} following conditions classifiable to 630-638

CC Excl: See code 639.2

639.4 Metabolic disorders
Electrolyte imbalance following conditions classifiable to 630-638

CC Excl: See code 639.2

639.5 Shock
- Circulatory collapse
- Shock (postoperative) (septic)

} following conditions classifiable to 630-638

CC Excl: See code 639.2

639.6 Embolism
Embolism:
- NOS
- air
- amniotic fluid
- blood-clot
- fat
- pulmonary
- pyemic
- septic
- soap

} following conditions classifiable to 630-638

CC Excl: See code 639.2

639.8 Other specified complications following abortion or ectopic and molar pregnancy
- Acute yellow atrophy or necrosis of liver
- Cardiac arrest or failure
- Cerebral anoxia
- Urinary tract infection

} following conditions classifiable to 630-638

CC Excl: See code 639.2

639.9 Unspecified complication following abortion or ectopic and molar pregnancy
Complication(s) not further specified following conditions classifiable to 630-638

CC Excl: See code 639.2

COMPLICATIONS MAINLY RELATED TO PREGNANCY (640-648)

INCLUDES the listed conditions even if they arose or were present during labor, delivery, or the puerperium

AHA: 2Q, '90, 11

The following fifth-digit subclassification is for use with categories 640-648 to denote the current episode of care. Valid fifth-digits are in [brackets] under each code.

0 unspecified as to episode of care or not applicable

1 delivered, with or without mention of antepartum condition
- Antepartum condition with delivery
- Delivery NOS (with mention of antepartum complication during current episode of care)
- Intrapartum obstetric condition (with mention of antepartum complication during current episode of care)
- Pregnancy, delivered (with mention of antepartum complication during current episode of care)

2 delivered, with mention of postpartum complication
- Delivery with mention of puerperal complication during current episode of care

3 antepartum condition or complication
- Antepartum obstetric condition, not delivered during the current episode of care

4 postpartum condition or complication
- Postpartum or puerperal obstetric condition or complication following delivery that occurred:
  - during previous episode of care
  - outside hospital, with subsequent admission for observation or care

✓4th **640 Hemorrhage in early pregnancy**
INCLUDES hemorrhage before completion of 22 weeks' gestation

§ ✓5th **640.0 Threatened abortion**
[0,1,3] CC Excl: 640.00-640.93, 641.00-641.13, 646.80-646.93, 648.90-648.94, 650, 669.40-669.44, 669.80-669.94

DEF: Bloody discharge during pregnancy; cervix may be dilated and pregnancy is threatened, but the pregnancy is not terminated.

§ ✓5th **640.8 Other specified hemorrhage in early pregnancy**
[0,1,3]
CC Excl: See code 640.0

§ Requires fifth-digit. Valid digits are in [brackets] under each code. See beginning of section 640-648 for codes and definitions.

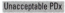 Nonspecific PDx   Unacceptable PDx   Manifestation Code 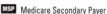 Medicare Secondary Payer ▶◀ Revised Text ● New Code ▲ Revised Code Title

COMPLICATIONS OF PREGNANCY, CHILDBIRTH, AND THE PUERPERIUM

640.9–642.5 — Tabular List

Placenta Previa: Low (marginal) implantation; Partial placenta previa; Total placenta previa

Abruptio Placentae: Partial separation (concealed bleeding); Partial separation (apparent hemorrhage); Complete separation (concealed hemorrhage)

§ √5th **640.9 Unspecified hemorrhage in early pregnancy** ♀
[0,1,3]
CC Excl: See code 640.0

√4th **641 Antepartum hemorrhage, abruptio placentae, and placenta previa**

§ √5th **641.0 Placenta previa without hemorrhage** ♀
[0,1,3]
Low impantation of placenta
Placenta previa noted: } without
   during pregnancy   } hemmorage
   before labor (and delivered
      by caesarean delivery.)

CC Excl: See code 640.0

DEF: Placenta implanted in lower segment of uterus; commonly causes hemorrhage in the last trimester of pregnancy.

§ √5th **641.1 Hemorrhage from placenta previa** ♀
[0,1,3]
Low-lying placenta
Placenta previa   } NOS or with
   incomplete   }   hemorrhage
   marginal   }   (intrapartum)
   partial
   total

EXCLUDES hemorrhage from vasa previa (663.5)
CC Excl: See code 640.0

§ √5th **641.2 Premature separation of placenta** ♀
[0,1,3]
Ablatio placentae
Abruptio placentae
Accidental antepartum hemorrhage
Couvelaire uterus
Detachment of placenta (premature)
Premature separation of normally implanted placenta

DEF: Abruptio placentae: premature detachment of the placenta, characterized by shock, oliguria and decreased fibrinogen.

§ √5th **641.3 Antepartum hemorrhage associated with coagulation defects** ♀
[0,1,3]
Antepartum or intrapartum hemorrhage associated with:
   afibrinogenemia
   hyperfibrinolysis
   hypofibrinogenemia

CC Excl: 641.30-641.93, 646.80-646.93, 648.90-648.94, 650, 669.40-669.44, 669.80-669.94

DEF: Uterine hemorrhage prior to delivery.

§ √5th **641.8 Other antepartum hemorrhage** ♀
[0,1,3]
Antepartum or intrapartum hemorrhage associated with:
   trauma
   uterine leiomyoma

CC Excl: See code 641.3

§ √5th **641.9 Unspecified antepartum hemorrhage** ♀
[0,1,3]
Hemorrhage: Hemorrhage:
   antepartum NOS   of pregnancy NOS
   intrapartum NOS

CC Excl: See code 641.3

√4th **642 Hypertension complicating pregnancy, childbirth, and the puerperium**

§ √5th **642.0 Benign essential hypertension complicating pregnancy, childbirth, and the puerperium** ♀
[0-4]
Hypertension: } specified as complicating,
   benign essential   }   or as a reason for
   chronic NOS   }   obstetric care during
   essential   }   pregnancy, childbirth,
   pre-existing NOS   }   or the puerperium

§ √5th **642.1 Hypertension secondary to renal disease, complicating pregnancy, childbirth, and the puerperium** ♀
[0-4]
Hypertension secondary to renal disease, specified as complicating, or as a reason for obstetric care during pregnancy, childbirth, or the puerperium

§ √5th **642.2 Other pre-existing hypertension complicating pregnancy, childbirth, and the puerperium** ♀
[0-4]
Hypertensive: } specified as complicating,
   heart and renal   }   or as a reason for
      disease   }   obstetric care
   heart disease   }   during pregnancy,
   renal disease   }   childbirth, or the
Malignant   }   puerperium
   hypertension   }

§ √5th **642.3 Transient hypertension of pregnancy** ♀
[0-4]
Gestational hypertension
Transient hypertension, so described, in pregnancy, childbirth, or the puerperium

AHA: 3Q, '90, 4

§ √5th **642.4 Mild or unspecified pre-eclampsia** ♀
[0-4]
Hypertension in pregnancy, childbirth, or the puerperium, not specified as pre-existing, with either albuminuria or edema, or both; mild or unspecified

Pre-eclampsia: Toxemia (pre-eclamptic):
   NOS   NOS
   mild   mild

EXCLUDES albuminuria in pregnancy, without mention of hypertension (646.2)
edema in pregnancy, without mention of hypertension (646.1)

CC Excl: 642.00-642.94, 646.10-646.14, 646.80-646.93, 648.90-648.94, 650, 669.40-669.44, 669.80-669.94

§ √5th **642.5 Severe pre-eclampsia** ♀
[0-4]
Hypertension in pregnancy, childbirth, or the puerperium, not specified as pre-existing, with either albuminuria or edema, or both; specified as severe
Pre-eclampsia, severe
Toxemia (pre-eclamptic), severe

CC Excl: See code 642.4

AHA: N-D, '85, 3

---

[1] Nonspecific PDx=0

§ Requires fifth-digit. Valid digits are in [brackets] under each code. See beginning of section 640-648 for codes and definitions.

N Newborn Age: 0 P Pediatric Age: 0-17 M Maternity Age: 12-55 A Adult Age: 15-124 CC CC Condition MC Major Complication CD Complex Dx HIV HIV Related Dx

COMPLICATIONS OF PREGNANCY, CHILDBIRTH, AND THE PUERPERIUM

§ **√5th 642.6** **Eclampsia** CC M ♀
[0-4]
Toxemia:
  eclamptic
  with convulsions
CC Excl: See code 642.4

§ **√5th 642.7** **Pre-eclampsia or eclampsia superimposed** CC M ♀
[0-4] **on pre-existing hypertension**
Conditions classifiable to 642.4-642.6, with
conditions classifiable to 642.0-642.2
CC Excl: See code 642.4

§ **√5th 642.9** **Unspecified hypertension complicating** M ♀
[0-4] **pregnancy, childbirth, or the puerperium**
Hypertension NOS, without mention of albuminuria
or edema, complicating pregnancy, childbirth,
or the puerperium

√4th 643 Excessive vomiting in pregnancy
INCLUDES hyperemesis
  vomiting:
    persistent } arising during
    vicious   pregnancy
  hyperemesis gravidarum

§ **√5th 643.0** **Mild hyperemesis gravidarum** M ♀
[0,1,3]
Hyperemesis gravidarum, mild or unspecified,
starting before the end of the 22nd week of
gestation
DEF: Detrimental vomiting and nausea.

§ **√5th 643.1** **Hyperemesis gravidarum with metabolic** M ♀
[0,1,3] **disturbance**
Hyperemesis gravidarum, starting before the end of
the 22nd week of gestation, with metabolic
disturbance, such as:
  carbohydrate depletion
  dehydration
  electrolyte imbalance

§ **√5th 643.2** **Late vomiting of pregnancy** M ♀
[0,1,3]
Excessive vomiting starting after 22 completed
weeks of gestation

§ **√5th 643.8** **Other vomiting complicating pregnancy** M ♀
[0,1,3]
Vomiting due to organic disease or other cause,
specified as complicating pregnancy, or as a
reason for obstetric care during pregnancy
Use additional code to specify cause

§ **√5th 643.9** **Unspecified vomiting of pregnancy** M ♀
[0,1,3]
Vomiting as a reason for care during pregnancy,
length of gestation unspecified

√4th 644 Early or threatened labor

§ **√5th 644.0** **Threatened premature labor** CC M ♀
[0,3]
Premature labor after 22 weeks, but before 37
completed weeks of gestation without delivery
EXCLUDES *that occurring before 22 completed
weeks of gestation (640.0)*
CC Excl: 644.00-644.21, 646.80-646.93, 648.90-648.94,
650, 669.40-669.44, 669.80-669.94

§ **√5th 644.1** **Other threatened labor** CC M ♀
[0,3]
False labor:
  NOS
  after 37 completed weeks of } without
    gestation   delivery
  Threatened labor NOS
CC Excl: See code 644.0

§ **√5th 644.2** **Early onset of delivery** M ♀
[0,1]
Onset (spontaneous) of
  delivery   } before 37 completed
Premature labor with   weeks of gestation
  onset of delivery
AHA: 2Q, '91, 16

√4th 645 Late pregnancy
AHA: 4Q, '00, 43; 4Q, '91, 26

§ **√5th 645.1** **Post term pregnancy** M ♀
[0,1,3]
Pregnancy over 40 completed weeks to 42
completed weeks gestation

§ **√5th 645.2** **Prolonged pregnancy** M ♀
[0,1,3]
Pregnancy which has advanced beyond 42
completed weeks gestation

√4th 646 Other complications of pregnancy, not elsewhere classified
Use additional code(s) to further specify complication
AHA: 4Q, '95, 59

§ **√5th 646.0** **Papyraceous fetus** M ♀
[0,1,3]
DEF: Fetus retained in the uterus beyond natural term, exhibits
parchment-like skin.

§ **√5th 646.1** **Edema or excessive weight gain in pregnancy,** M ♀
[0-4] **without mention of hypertension**
Gestational edema
Maternal obesity syndrome
EXCLUDES *that with mention of hypertension
(642.0-642.9)*

§ **√5th 646.2** **Unspecified renal disease in pregnancy,** M ♀
[0-4] **without mention of hypertension**
Albuminuria   } in pregnancy or the
Nephropathy NOS   puerperium,
Renal disease NOS   without mention
Uremia   } of hypertension
Gestational proteinuria
EXCLUDES *that with mention of hypertension
(642.0-642.9)*

§ **√5th 646.3** **Habitual aborter** M ♀
[0,1,3] EXCLUDES *with current abortion (634.0-634.9)
without current pregnancy (629.9)*
DEF: Three or more consecutive spontaneous abortions.

§ **√5th 646.4** **Peripheral neuritis in pregnancy** M ♀
[0-4]

§ **√5th 646.5** **Asymptomatic bacteriuria in pregnancy** M ♀
[0-4]

§ **√5th 646.6** **Infections of genitourinary tract in** CC M ♀
[0-4] **pregnancy**
Conditions classifiable to 590, 595, 597, 599.0, 616
complicating pregnancy, childbirth, or the
puerperium
Conditions classifiable to ▶614.0-614.5, 614.7-
614.9,◀ 615 complicating pregnancy or labor
EXCLUDES *major puerperal infection (670)*
CC Excl: 646.60-646.64, 646.80-646.93, 648.90-648.94,
650, 669.40-669.44, 669.80-669.94

§ **√5th 646.7** **Liver disorders in pregnancy** CC M ♀
[0,1,3]
Acute yellow atrophy of
  liver (obstetric) (true) }
Icterus gravis   of pregnancy
Necrosis of liver   }

EXCLUDES *hepatorenal syndrome following
delivery (674.8)
viral hepatitis (647.6)*
CC Excl: 646.70-646.93, 648.90-648.94, 650, 669.40-669.44,
669.80-669.94

§ **√5th 646.8** **Other specified complications of pregnancy** M ♀
[0-4]
Fatigue during pregnancy
Herpes gestationis
Insufficient weight gain of pregnancy
Uterine size-date discrepancy
AHA: 3Q, '98, 16; J-F, '85, 15

§ **√5th 646.9** **Unspecified complication of pregnancy** M ♀
[0,1,3]

---

[1] Nonspecific PDx=0

§ Requires fifth-digit. Valid digits are in [brackets] under each code. See beginning of section 640-648 for codes and definitions.

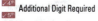 Additional Digit Required  Nonspecific PDx   Unacceptable PDx   Manifestation Code 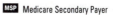 Medicare Secondary Payer 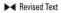 Revised Text ● New Code ▲ Revised Code Title

COMPLICATIONS OF PREGNANCY, CHILDBIRTH, AND THE PUERPERIUM

647–651.1

✓4th **647 Infectious and parasitic conditions in the mother classifiable elsewhere, but complicating pregnancy, childbirth, or the puerperium**
  INCLUDES: the listed conditions when complicating the pregnant state, aggravated by the pregnancy, or when a main reason for obstetric care
  EXCLUDES: those conditions in the mother known or suspected to have affected the fetus (655.0-655.9)
  Use additional code(s) to further specify complication

§ ✓5th **647.0 Syphilis**
  [0-4] Conditions classifiable to 090-097

§ ✓5th **647.1 Gonorrhea**
  [0-4] Conditions classifiable to 098

§ ✓5th **647.2 Other venereal diseases**
  [0-4] Conditions classifiable to 099

§ ✓5th **647.3 Tuberculosis**
  [0-4] Conditions classifiable to 010-018
  CC Excl: 646.80-646.93, 647.30-647.34, 648.90-648.94, 650, 669.40-669.44, 669.80-669.94

§ ✓5th **647.4 Malaria**
  [0-4] Conditions classifiable to 084
  CC Excl: 646.80-646.93, 647.30-647.34, 648.90-648.94, 650, 669.40-669.44, 669.80-669.94

§ ✓5th **647.5 Rubella**
  [0-4] Conditions classifiable to 056

§ ✓5th **647.6 Other viral diseases**
  [0-4] Conditions classifiable to 042 and 050-079, except 056
  AHA: J-F, '85, 15

§ ✓5th **647.8 Other specified infectious and parasitic diseases**
  [0-4]

§ ✓5th **647.9 Unspecified infection or infestation**
  [0-4]

✓4th **648 Other current conditions in the mother classifiable elsewhere, but complicating pregnancy, childbirth, or the puerperium**
  INCLUDES: the listed conditions when complicating the pregnant state, aggravated by the pregnancy, or when a main reason for obstetric care
  EXCLUDES: those conditions in the mother known or suspected to have affected the fetus (655.0-665.9)
  Use additional code(s) to identify the condition

§ ✓5th **648.0 Diabetes mellitus**
  [0-4] Conditions classifiable to 250
  EXCLUDES: gestational diabetes (648.8)
  CC Excl: 646.80-646.93, 648.00-648.04, 648.90-648.94, 650, 669.40-669.44, 669.80-669.94
  AHA: 3Q, '91, 5, 11

§ ✓5th **648.1 Thyroid dysfunction**
  [0-4] Conditions classifiable to 240-246

§ ✓5th **648.2 Anemia**
  [0-4] Conditions classifiable to 280-285
  CC Excl: 646.80-646.93, 648.20-648.24, 648.90-648.94, 650, 669.40-669.44, 669.80-669.94
  AHA: For Code 648.22: 1Q, '02, 14

§ ✓5th **648.3 Drug dependence**
  [0-4] Conditions classifiable to 304
  CC Excl: 646.80-646.93, 648.30-648.34, 648.90-648.94, 650, 669.40-669.44, 669.80-669.94
  AHA: 2Q, '98, 13; 4Q, '88, 8

§ ✓5th **648.4 Mental disorders**
  [0-4] Conditions classifiable to 290-303, 305-316, 317-319
  AHA: 2Q, '98, 13; 4Q, '95, 63

§ ✓5th **648.5 Congenital cardiovascular disorders**
  [0-4] Conditions classifiable to 745-747
  CC Excl: 646.80-646.93, 648.50-648.64, 648.90-648.94, 650, 669.40-669.44, 669.80-669.94

§ ✓5th **648.6 Other cardiovascular diseases**
  [0-4] Conditions classifiable to 390-398, 410-429
  EXCLUDES: cerebrovascular disorders in the puerperium (674.0)
  venous complications (671.0-671.9)
  CC Excl: See code 648.5
  AHA: 3Q, '98, 11

§ ✓5th **648.7 Bone and joint disorders of back, pelvis, and lower limbs**
  [0-4] Conditions classifiable to 720-724, and those classifiable to 711-719 or 725-738, specified as affecting the lower limbs

§ ✓5th **648.8 Abnormal glucose tolerance**
  [0-4] Conditions classifiable to 790.2
  Gestational diabetes
  AHA: 3Q, '91, 5
  DEF: Glucose intolerance arising in pregnancy, resolving at end of pregnancy.

§ ✓5th **648.9 Other current conditions classifiable elsewhere**
  [0-4] Conditions classifiable to 440-459
  Nutritional deficiencies [conditions classifiable to 260-269]
  AHA: N-D, '87, 10; For code 648.91: 1Q, '02, 14

NORMAL DELIVERY, AND OTHER INDICATIONS FOR CARE IN PREGNANCY, LABOR, AND DELIVERY (650-659)

The following fifth-digit subclassification is for use with categories 651-659 to denote the current episode of care. Valid fifth-digits are in [brackets] under each code.

0 unspecified as to episode of care or not applicable
1 delivered, with or without mention of antepartum condition
2 delivered, with mention of postpartum complication
3 antepartum condition or complication
4 postpartum condition or complication

650 Normal delivery
  Delivery requiring minimal or no assistance, with or without episiotomy, without fetal manipulation [e.g., rotation version] or instrumentation [forceps] of spontaneous, cephalic, vaginal, full-term, single, live-born infant. This code is for use as a single diagnosis code and is not to be used with any other code in the range 630-676.
  EXCLUDES: breech delivery (assisted) (spontaneous) NOS (652.2)
  delivery by vacuum extractor, forceps, cesarean section, or breech extraction, without specified complication (669.5-669.7)
  Use additional code to indicate outcome of delivery (V27.0)
  AHA: ▶3Q, '01, 12;◄ 3Q, '00, 5; 4Q, '95, 28, 59

✓4th **651 Multiple gestation**

§ ✓5th **651.0 Twin pregnancy**
  [0,1,3]

§ ✓5th **651.1 Triplet pregnancy**
  [0,1,3]

---

1 Nonspecific PDx=0

§ Requires fifth-digit. Valid digits are in [brackets] under each code. See beginning of section 640-648 for codes and definitions.

N Newborn Age: 0   P Pediatric Age: 0-17   M Maternity Age: 12-55   A Adult Age: 15-124   CC CC Condition   MC Major Complication   CD Complex Dx   HIV HIV Related Dx

COMPLICATIONS OF PREGNANCY, CHILDBIRTH, AND THE PUERPERIUM

651.2 Quadruplet pregnancy
[0,1,3]

651.3 Twin pregnancy with fetal loss and retention of one fetus
[0,1,3]

651.4 Triplet pregnancy with fetal loss and retention of one or more fetus(es)
[0,1,3]

651.5 Quadruplet pregnancy with fetal loss and retention of one or more fetus(es)
[0,1,3]

651.6 Other multiple pregnancy with fetal loss and retention of one or more fetus(es)
[0,1,3]

651.8 Other specified multiple gestation
[0,1,3]

651.9 Unspecified multiple gestation
[0,1,3]

652 Malposition and malpresentation of fetus
Code first any associated obstructed labor (660.0)

652.0 Unstable lie
[0,1,3]
DEF: Changing fetal position.

652.1 Breech or other malpresentation successfully converted to cephalic presentation
[0,1,3]
Cephalic version NOS

652.2 Breech presentation without mention of version
[0,1,3]
Breech delivery (assisted) (spontaneous) NOS
Buttocks presentation
Complete breech
Frank breech
EXCLUDES: *footling presentation (652.8)*
incomplete breech (652.8)
DEF: Fetal presentation of buttocks or feet at birth canal.

652.3 Transverse or oblique presentation
[0,1,3]
Oblique lie   Transverse lie
EXCLUDES: *transverse arrest of fetal head (660.3)*

652.4 Face or brow presentation
[0,1,3]
Mentum presentation

652.5 High head at term
[0,1,3]
Failure of head to enter pelvic brim

652.6 Multiple gestation with malpresentation of one fetus or more
[0,1,3]

652.7 Prolapsed arm
[0,1,3]

652.8 Other specified malposition or malpresentation
[0,1,3]
Compound presentation

652.9 Unspecified malposition or malpresentation
[0,1,3]

653 Disproportion
Code first any associated obstructed labor (660.1)

Malposition and Malpresentation

Cephalopelvic Disproportion

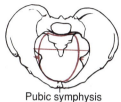

653.0 Major abnormality of bony pelvis, not further specified
[0,1,3]
Pelvic deformity NOS

653.1 Generally contracted pelvis
[0,1,3]
Contracted pelvis NOS

653.2 Inlet contraction of pelvis
[0,1,3]
Inlet contraction (pelvis)

653.3 Outlet contraction of pelvis
[0,1,3]
Outlet contraction (pelvis)

653.4 Fetopelvic disproportion
[0,1,3]
Cephalopelvic disproportion NOS
Disproportion of mixed maternal and fetal origin, with normally formed fetus

653.5 Unusually large fetus causing disproportion
[0,1,3]
Disproportion of fetal origin with normally formed fetus
Fetal disproportion NOS
EXCLUDES: *that when the reason for medical care was concern for the fetus (656.6)*

653.6 Hydrocephalic fetus causing disproportion
[0,1,3]
EXCLUDES: *that when the reason for medical care was concern for the fetus (655.0)*

653.7 Other fetal abnormality causing disproportion
[0,1,3]
Conjoined twins   Fetal:
Fetal: myelomeningocele
  ascites   sacral teratoma
  hydrops   tumor

653.8 Disproportion of other origin
[0,1,3]
EXCLUDES: *shoulder (girdle) dystocia (660.4)*

653.9 Unspecified disproportion
[0,1,3]

654 Abnormality of organs and soft tissues of pelvis
INCLUDES: the listed conditions during pregnancy, childbirth, or the puerperium
Code first any associated obstructed labor (660.2)

654.0 Congenital abnormalities of uterus
[0-4]
Double uterus   Uterus bicornis

654.1 Tumors of body of uterus
[0-4]
Uterine fibroids

654.2 Previous cesarean delivery
[0,1,3]
Uterine scar from previous cesarean delivery
AHA: 1Q, '92, 8

654.3 Retroverted and incarcerated gravid uterus
[0-4]
DEF: Retroverted: tilted back uterus; no change in angle of longitudinal axis.
DEF: Incarcerated: immobile, fixed uterus.

---

[1] Nonspecific PDx=0

§ Requires fifth-digit. Valid digits are in [brackets] under each code. See beginning of section 640-648 for codes and definitions.

COMPLICATIONS OF PREGNANCY, CHILDBIRTH, AND THE PUERPERIUM

654.4–658.1   **Tabular List**

§ ✓5th **654.4** [0-4] **Other abnormalities in shape or position of gravid uterus and of neighboring structures** MQ
     Cystocele
     Pelvic floor repair
     Pendulous abdomen
     Prolapse of gravid uterus
     Rectocele
     Rigid pelvic floor

§ ✓5th **654.5** [0-4] **Cervical incompetence** MQ
     Presence of Shirodkar suture with or without mention of cervical incompetence

DEF: Abnormal cervix; tendency to dilate in second trimester; causes premature fetal expulsion.

DEF: Shirodkar suture: purse-string suture used to artificially close incompetent cervix.

§ ✓5th **654.6** [0-4] **Other congenital or acquired abnormality of cervix** MQ
     Cicatricial cervix
     Polyp of cervix
     Previous surgery to cervix
     Rigid cervix (uteri)
     Stenosis or stricture of cervix
     Tumor of cervix

§ ✓5th **654.7** [0-4] **Congenital or acquired abnormality of vagina** MQ
     Previous surgery to vagina
     Septate vagina
     Stenosis of vagina (acquired) (congenital)
     Stricture of vagina
     Tumor of vagina

§ ✓5th **654.8** [0-4] **Congenital or acquired abnormality of vulva** MQ
     Fibrosis of perineum
     Persistent hymen
     Previous surgery to perineum or vulva
     Rigid perineum
     Tumor of vulva
     EXCLUDES varicose veins of vulva (671.1)

§ ✓5th **654.9** [0-4] **Other and unspecified** MQ
     Uterine scar NEC

✓4th **655** **Known or suspected fetal abnormality affecting management of mother**
     INCLUDES the listed conditions in the fetus as a reason for observation or obstetrical care of the mother, or for termination of pregnancy

AHA: 3Q, '90, 4

§ ✓5th **655.0** [0,1,3] **Central nervous system malformation in fetus** MQ
     Fetal or suspected fetal:
         anencephaly
         hydrocephalus
         spina bifida (with myelomeningocele)

§ ✓5th **655.1** [0,1,3] **Chromosomal abnormality in fetus** MQ

§ ✓5th **655.2** [0,1,3] **Hereditary disease in family possibly affecting fetus** MQ

§ ✓5th **655.3** [0,1,3] **Suspected damage to fetus from viral disease in the mother** MQ
     Suspected damage to fetus from maternal rubella

§ ✓5th **655.4** [0,1,3] **Suspected damage to fetus from other disease in the mother** MQ
     Suspected damage to fetus from maternal:
         alcohol addiction
         listeriosis
         toxoplasmosis

§ ✓5th **655.5** [0,1,3] **Suspected damage to fetus from drugs** MQ

§ ✓5th **655.6** [0,1,3] **Suspected damage to fetus from radiation** MQ

§ ✓5th **655.7** [0,1,3] **Decreased fetal movements** MQ

AHA: 4Q, '97, 41

§ ✓5th **655.8** [0,1,3] **Other known or suspected fetal abnormality, not elsewhere classified** MQ
     Suspected damage to fetus from:
         environmental toxins
         intrauterine contraceptive device

§ ✓5th **655.9** [0,1,3] **Unspecified** MQ

✓4th **656** **Other fetal and placental problems affecting management of mother**

§ ✓5th **656.0** [0,1,3] **Fetal-maternal hemorrhage** MQ
     Leakage (microscopic) of fetal blood into maternal circulation

§ ✓5th **656.1** [0,1,3] **Rhesus isoimmunization** MQ
     Anti-D [Rh] antibodies
     Rh incompatibility

DEF: Antibodies developing against Rh factor; mother with Rh negative develops antibodies against Rh positive fetus.

§ ✓5th **656.2** [0,1,3] **Isoimmunization from other and unspecified blood group incompatibility** MQ
     ABO isoimmunization.

§ ✓5th **656.3** [0,1,3] **Fetal distress** MQ
     Fetal metabolic acidemia
     EXCLUDES abnormal fetal acid-base balance (656.8)
                 abnormality in fetal heart rate or rhythm (659.7)
                 fetal bradycardia (659.7)
                 fetal distress NOS (656.8)
                 fetal tachycardia (659.7)
                 meconium in liquor (656.8)

DEF: Life-threatening disorder; fetal anoxia, hemolytic disease and other miscellaneous diseases cause fetal distress.

AHA: N-D, '86, 4

§ ✓5th **656.4** [0,1,3] **Intrauterine death** MQ
     Fetal death:
         NOS
         after completion of 22 weeks' gestation
         late
     Missed delivery
     EXCLUDES missed abortion (632)

§ ✓5th **656.5** [0,1,3] **Poor fetal growth** MQ
     "Light-for-dates"
     "Placental insufficiency"
     "Small-for-dates"

§ ✓5th **656.6** [0,1,3] **Excessive fetal growth** MQ
     "Large-for-dates"

§ ✓5th **656.7** [0,1,3] **Other placental conditions** MQ
     Abnormal placenta
     Placental infarct
     EXCLUDES placental polyp (674.4)
                 placentitis (658.4)

§ ✓5th **656.8** [0,1,3] **Other specified fetal and placental problems** MQ
     Abnormal acid-base balance
     Intrauterine acidosis
     Lithopedian
     Meconium in liquor

DEF: Lithopedion: Calcified fetus; not expelled by mother.

§ ✓5th **656.9** [0,1,3] **Unspecified fetal and placental problem** MQ

✓4th **657** [0,1,3] **Polyhydramnios** MQ
     Hydramnios
     § ✓5th Use 0 as fourth-digit for this category

AHA: 4Q, '91, 26

DEF: Excess amniotic fluid.

✓4th **658** **Other problems associated with amniotic cavity and membranes**
     EXCLUDES amniotic fluid embolism (673.1)

§ ✓5th **658.0** [0,1,3] **Oligohydramnios** MQ
     Oligohydramnios without mention of rupture of membranes

DEF: Deficient amount of amniotic fluid.

§ ✓5th **658.1** [0,1,3] **Premature rupture of membranes** MQ
     Rupture of amniotic sac less than 24 hours prior to the onset of labor

AHA: For code 658.13: 1Q, '01, 5; 4Q, '98, 77

---

[1] Nonspecific PDx=0
§ Requires fifth-digit. Valid digits are in [brackets] under each code. See beginning of section 640-648 for codes and definitions.

N Newborn Age: 0   P Pediatric Age: 0-17   M Maternity Age: 12-55   A Adult Age: 15-124   CC CC Condition   MC Major Complication   CD Complex Dx   HIV HIV Related Dx

COMPLICATIONS OF PREGNANCY, CHILDBIRTH, AND THE PUERPERIUM 658.2–661.2

§ ✓5th¹ **658.2** [0,1,3] **Delayed delivery after spontaneous or unspecified rupture of membranes** M ♀
  Prolonged rupture of membranes NOS
  Rupture of amniotic sac 24 hours or more prior to the onset of labor

§ ✓5th¹ **658.3** [0,1,3] **Delayed delivery after artificial rupture of membranes** M ♀

§ ✓5th¹ **658.4** [0,1,3] **Infection of amniotic cavity** M ♀
  Amnionitis   Membranitis
  Chorioamnionitis Placentitis

§ ✓5th¹ **658.8** [0,1,3] **Other** M ♀
  Amnion nodosum   Amniotic cyst

§ ✓5th¹ **658.9** [0,1,3] **Unspecified** M ♀

✓4th **659 Other indications for care or intervention related to labor and delivery, not elsewhere classified**

§ ✓5th¹ **659.0** [0,1,3] **Failed mechanical induction** M ♀
  Failure of induction of labor by surgical or other instrumental methods

§ ✓5th¹ **659.1** [0,1,3] **Failed medical or unspecified induction** M ♀
  Failed induction NOS
  Failure of induction of labor by medical methods, such as oxytocic drugs

§ ✓5th¹ **659.2** [0,1,3] **Maternal pyrexia during labor, unspecified** M ♀
  DEF: Fever during labor.

§ ✓5th¹ **659.3** [0,1,3] **Generalized infection during labor** CC M ♀
  Septicemia during labor
  CC Excl: 646.80-646.93, 648.90-648.94, 650, 659.30-659.33, 669.40-669.44, 669.80-669.94

§ ✓5th¹ **659.4** [0,1,3] **Grand multiparity** M ♀
  EXCLUDES supervision only, in pregnancy (V23.3)
  without current pregnancy (V61.5)
  DEF: Having borne six or more children previously.

§ ✓5th¹ **659.5** [0,1,3] **Elderly primigravida** M ♀
  First pregnancy in a woman who will be 35 years of age or older at expected date of delivery
  EXCLUDES supervision only, in pregnancy (V23.81)
  AHA: ▶3Q, '01, 12◀

§ ✓5th¹ **659.6** [0,1,3] **Elderly multigravida** M ♀
  Second or more pregnancy in a woman who will be 35 years of age or older at expected date of delivery
  EXCLUDES elderly primigravida 659.5
  supervision only, in pregnancy (V23.82)
  AHA: ▶3Q, '01, 12◀

§ ✓5th¹ **659.7** [0,1,3] **Abnormality in fetal heart rate or rhythm** M ♀
  Depressed fetal heart tones
  Fetal:
    bradycardia
    tachycardia
  Fetal heart rate decelerations
  Non-reassuring fetal heart rate or rhythm
  AHA: 4Q, '98, 48

§ ✓5th¹ **659.8** [0,1,3] **Other specified indications for care or intervention related to labor and delivery** M ♀
  Pregnancy in a female less than 16 years old at expected date of delivery
  Very young maternal age
  AHA: ▶3Q, '01, 12◀

§ **659.9** [0,1,3] **Unspecified indication for care or intervention related to labor and delivery** M ♀

COMPLICATIONS OCCURRING MAINLY IN THE COURSE OF LABOR AND DELIVERY (660-669)

The following fifth-digit subclassification is for use with categories 660-669 to denote the current episode of care. Valid fifth-digits are in [brackets] under each code.

0 unspecified as to episode of care or not applicable
1 delivered, with or without mention of antepartum condition
2 delivered, with mention of postpartum complication
3 antepartum condition or complication
4 postpartum condition or complication

✓4th **660 Obstructed labor**
  AHA: 3Q, '95, 10

§ ✓5th¹ **660.0** [0,1,3] **Obstruction caused by malposition of fetus at onset of labor** M ♀
  Any condition classifiable to 652, causing obstruction during labor
  Use additional code from 652.0-652.9 to identify condition

§ ✓5th¹ **660.1** [0,1,3] **Obstruction by bony pelvis** M ♀
  Any condition classifiable to 653, causing obstruction during labor
  Use additional code from 653.0-653.9 to identify condition

§ ✓5th¹ **660.2** [0,1,3] **Obstruction by abnormal pelvic soft tissues** M ♀
  Prolapse of anterior lip of cervix
  Any condition classifiable to 654, causing obstruction during labor
  Use additional code from 654.0-654.9 to identify condition

§ ✓5th¹ **660.3** [0,1,3] **Deep transverse arrest and persistent occipitoposterior position** M ♀

§ ✓5th¹ **660.4** [0,1,3] **Shoulder (girdle) dystocia** M ♀
  Impacted shoulders
  DEF: Obstructed labor due to impacted fetal shoulders.

§ ✓5th¹ **660.5** [0,1,3] **Locked twins** M ♀

§ ✓5th¹ **660.6** [0,1,3] **Failed trial of labor, unspecified** M ♀
  Failed trial of labor, without mention of condition or suspected condition

§ ✓5th¹ **660.7** [0,1,3] **Failed forceps or vacuum extractor, unspecified** M ♀
  Application of ventouse or forceps, without mention of condition

§ ✓5th¹ **660.8** [0,1,3] **Other causes of obstructed labor** M ♀

§ ✓5th¹ **660.9** [0,1,3] **Unspecified obstructed labor** M ♀
  Dystocia:
    NOS
    fetal NOS
    maternal NOS

✓4th **661 Abnormality of forces of labor**

§ ✓5th¹ **661.0** [0,1,3] **Primary uterine inertia** M ♀
  Failure of cervical dilation
  Hypotonic uterine dysfunction, primary
  Prolonged latent phase of labor
  DEF: Lack of efficient contractions during labor causing prolonged labor.

§ ✓5th¹ **661.1** [0,1,3] **Secondary uterine inertia** M ♀
  Arrested active phase of labor
  Hypotonic uterine dysfunction, secondary

§ ✓5th¹ **661.2** [0,1,3] **Other and unspecified uterine inertia** M ♀
  Desultory labor
  Irregular labor
  Poor contractions
  Slow slope active phase of labor

---

¹ Nonspecific PDx=0
§ Requires fifth-digit. Valid digits are in [brackets] under each code. See beginning of section 640-648 for codes and definitions.

COMPLICATIONS OF PREGNANCY, CHILDBIRTH, AND THE PUERPERIUM

661.3–665.5

§ ✓5th 661.3 **Precipitate labor** M ♀
[0,1,3] **DEF:** Rapid labor and delivery.

§ ✓5th 661.4 **Hypertonic, incoordinate, or prolonged** M ♀
[0,1,3] uterine contractions
　　　　Cervical spasm
　　　　Contraction ring (dystocia)
　　　　Dyscoordinate labor
　　　　Hourglass contraction of uterus
　　　　Hypertonic uterine dysfunction
　　　　Incoordinate uterine action
　　　　Retraction ring (Bandl's) (pathological)
　　　　Tetanic contractions
　　　　Uterine dystocia NOS
　　　　Uterine spasm

§ ✓5th 661.9 **Unspecified abnormality of labor** M ♀
[0,1,3]

✓4th **662 Long labor**

§ ✓5th 662.0 **Prolonged first stage** M ♀
[0,1,3]

§ ✓5th 662.1 **Prolonged labor, unspecified** M ♀
[0,1,3]

§ ✓5th 662.2 **Prolonged second stage** M ♀
[0,1,3]

§ ✓5th 662.3 **Delayed delivery of second twin, triplet, etc.** M ♀
[0,1,3]

✓4th **663 Umbilical cord complications**

§ ✓5th 663.0 **Prolapse of cord** M ♀
[0,1,3] 　　Presentation of cord
DEF: Abnormal presentation of fetus; marked by protruding umbilical cord during labor; can cause fetal death.

§ ✓5th 663.1 **Cord around neck, with compression** M ♀
[0,1,3] 　　Cord tightly around neck

§ ✓5th 663.2 **Other and unspecified cord entanglement,** M ♀
[0,1,3] with compression
　　　　Entanglement of cords of twins in mono-amniotic sac
　　　　Knot in cord (with compression)

§ ✓5th 663.3 **Other and unspecified cord entanglement,** M ♀
[0,1,3] without mention of compression

§ ✓5th 663.4 **Short cord** M ♀
[0,1,3]

§ ✓5th 663.5 **Vasa previa** M ♀
[0,1,3]
DEF: Abnormal presentation of fetus marked by blood vessels of umbilical cord in front of fetal head.

§ ✓5th 663.6 **Vascular lesions of cord** M ♀
[0,1,3] 　　Bruising of cord
　　　　Hematoma of cord
　　　　Thrombosis of vessels of cord

§ ✓5th 663.8 **Other umbilical cord complications** M ♀
[0,1,3] 　　Velamentous insertion of umbilical cord

§ ✓5th 663.9 **Unspecified umbilical cord complication** M ♀
[0,1,3]

✓4th **664 Trauma to perineum and vulva during delivery**
　　INCLUDES 　damage from instruments
　　　　　　　that from extension of episiotomy
AHA: 1Q, '92, 11; N-D, '84, 10

§ ✓5th 664.0 **First-degree perineal laceration** M ♀
[0,1,4] 　　Perineal laceration, rupture, or tear involving:
　　　　　　fourchette
　　　　　　hymen
　　　　　　labia
　　　　　　skin
　　　　　　vagina
　　　　　　vulva

Perineal Lacerations

First degree
Anus
Second degree
Third degree
Fourth degree

§ ✓5th 664.1 **Second-degree perineal laceration** M ♀
[0,1,4] 　　Perineal laceration, rupture, or tear (following episiotomy) involving:
　　　　　　pelvic floor
　　　　　　perineal muscles
　　　　　　vaginal muscles
　　EXCLUDES　that involving anal sphincter (664.2)

§ ✓5th 664.2 **Third-degree perineal laceration** M ♀
[0,1,4] 　　Perineal laceration, rupture, or tear (following episiotomy) involving:
　　　　　　anal sphincter
　　　　　　rectovaginal septum
　　　　　　sphincter NOS
　　EXCLUDES　that with anal or rectal mucosal laceration (664.3)

§ ✓5th 664.3 **Fourth-degree perineal laceration** M ♀
[0,1,4] 　　Perineal laceration, rupture, or tear as classifiable to 664.2 and involving also:
　　　　　　anal mucosa
　　　　　　rectal mucosa

§ ✓5th 664.4 **Unspecified perineal laceration** M ♀
[0,1,4] 　　Central laceration
AHA: 1Q, '92, 8

§ ✓5th 664.5 **Vulval and perineal hematoma** M ♀
[0,1,4] AHA: N-D, '84, 10

§ ✓5th 664.8 **Other specified trauma to perineum and vulva** M ♀
[0,1,4]

§ ✓5th 664.9 **Unspecified trauma to perineum and vulva** M ♀
[0,1,4]

✓4th **665 Other obstetrical trauma**
　　INCLUDES 　damage from instruments

§ ✓5th 665.0 **Rupture of uterus before onset of labor** CC M ♀
[0,1,3]
CC Excl: 646.80-646.93, 648.90-648.94, 650, 655.70-655.73, 665.00-665.11, 665.50-665.54, 665.80-665.94, 669.40-669.44, 669.80-669.94

§ ✓5th 665.1 **Rupture of uterus during labor** CC M ♀
[0,1] 　　Rupture of uterus NOS
CC Excl: See code 665.0

§ ✓5th 665.2 **Inversion of uterus** M
[0,2,4]

§ ✓5th 665.3 **Laceration of cervix** M ♀
[0,1,4]

§ ✓5th 665.4 **High vaginal laceration** M ♀
[0,1,4] 　　Laceration of vaginal wall or sulcus without mention of perineal laceration

§ ✓5th 665.5 **Other injury to pelvic organs** M ♀
[0,1,4] 　　Injury to:　　　　　Injury to:
　　　　　　bladder　　　　　urethra
AHA: M-A, '87, 10

---

1 Nonspecific PDx=0

§ Requires fifth-digit. Valid digits are in [brackets] under each code. See beginning of section 640-648 for codes and definitions.

N Newborn Age: 0 　P Pediatric Age: 0-17 　M Maternity Age: 12-55 　A Adult Age :15-124 　CC CC Condition 　MC Major Complication 　CD Complex Dx 　HIV HIV Related Dx

Tabular List
COMPLICATIONS OF PREGNANCY, CHILDBIRTH, AND THE PUERPERIUM
665.6–669.9

§ √5th 1 **665.6** **Damage to pelvic joints and ligaments** M ♀
[0,1,4]
Avulsion of inner symphyseal cartilage
Damage to coccyx
Separation of symphysis (pubis)
AHA: N-D, '84, 12

§ √5th 1 **665.7** **Pelvic hematoma** M ♀
[0,1,2,4]
Hematoma of vagina

§ √5th 1 **665.8** **Other specified obstetrical trauma** M ♀
[0-4]

§ √5th 1 **665.9** **Unspecified obstetrical trauma** M ♀
[0-4]

√4th **666** **Postpartum hemorrhage**
AHA: 1Q, '88, 14

§ √5th **666.0** **Third-stage hemorrhage** M ♀
[0,2,4]
Hemorrhage associated with retained, trapped, or adherent placenta
Retained placenta NOS

§ √5th **666.1** **Other immediate postpartum hemorrhage** M ♀
[0,2,4]
Atony of uterus
Hemorrhage within the first 24 hours following delivery of placenta
Postpartum hemorrhage (atonic) NOS

§ √5th **666.2** **Delayed and secondary postpartum hemorrhage** M ♀
[0,2,4]
Hemorrhage:
after the first 24 hours following delivery
associated with retained portions of placenta or membranes
Postpartum hemorrhage specified as delayed or secondary
Retained products of conception NOS, following delivery

§ √5th **666.3** **Postpartum coagulation defects** CC 2,4 M ♀
[0,2,4]
Postpartum: afibrinogenemia
Postpartum: fibrinolysis
CC Excl: For codes 666.32-666.34: 646.80-646.93, 648.90-648.94, 650, 666.00-666.34, 669.40-669.44, 669.80-669.94

√4th **667** **Retained placenta or membranes, without hemorrhage**
AHA: 1Q, '88, 14
DEF: Postpartum condition resulting from failure to expel placental membrane tissues due to failed contractions of uterine wall.

§ √5th **667.0** **Retained placenta without hemorrhage** M ♀
[0,2,4]
Placenta accreta
Retained placenta:
NOS
total } without hemorrhage

§ √5th **667.1** **Retained portions of placenta or membranes, Without hemorrhage** M ♀
[0,2,4]
Retained products of conception following delivery, without hemorrhage

√4th **668** **Complications of the administration of anesthetic or other sedation in labor and delivery**
INCLUDES complications arising from the administration of a general or local anesthetic, analgesic, or other sedation in labor and delivery
EXCLUDES reaction to spinal or lumbar puncture (349.0)
spinal headache (349.0)
Use additional code(s) to further specify complication

§ √5th 1 **668.0** **Pulmonary complications** CC M ♀
[0-4]
Inhalation [aspiration] of stomach contents or secretions
Mendelson's syndrome
Pressure collapse of lung } following anesthesia or other sedation in labor or delivery
CC Excl: 646.80-646.93, 648.90-648.94, 650, 668.00-668.04, 669.40-669.44, 669.80-669.94

§ √5th 1 **668.1** **Cardiac complications** CC M ♀
[0-4]
Cardiac arrest or failure following anesthesia or other sedation in labor and delivery
CC Excl: 646.80-646.93, 648.90-648.94, 650, 668.10-668.14, 669.40-669.44, 669.80-669.94

§ √5th 1 **668.2** **Central nervous system complications** CC M ♀
[0-4]
Cerebral anoxia following anesthesia or other sedation in labor and delivery
CC Excl: 646.80-646.93, 648.90-648.94, 650, 668.20-668.24, 669.40-669.44, 669.80-669.94

§ √5th 1 **668.8** **Other complications of anesthesia or other sedation in labor and delivery** CC M ♀
[0-4]
CC Excl: 646.80-646.93, 648.90-648.94, 650, 668.80-94, 668, 669.40-669.44, 669.80-669.94
AHA: 2Q, '99, 9

§ √5th 1 **668.9** **Unspecified complication of anesthesia and other sedation** CC M ♀
[0-4]
CC Excl: See code 668.8

√4th **669** **Other complications of labor and delivery, not elsewhere classified**

§ √5th 1 **669.0** **Maternal distress** M ♀
[0-4]
Metabolic disturbance in labor and delivery

§ √5th 1 **669.1** **Shock during or following labor and delivery** CC M ♀
[0-4]
Obstetric shock
CC Excl: 646.80-646.93, 648.90-648.94, 650, 669.10-669.14, 669.40-669.44, 669.80-669.94

§ √5th 1 **669.2** **Maternal hypotension syndrome** M ♀
[0-4]
DEF: Low arterial blood pressure, in mother, during labor and delivery.

§ √5th 1 **669.3** **Acute renal failure following labor and delivery** CC M ♀
[0,2,4]
CC Excl: 646.80-646.93, 648.90-648.94, 650, 669.30-669.44, 669.80-669.94

§ √5th 1 **669.4** **Other complications of obstetrical surgery and procedures** M ♀
[0-4]
Cardiac:
arrest
failure
Cerebral anoxia } following cesarean or other obstetrical surgery or procedure, including delivery NOS
EXCLUDES complications of obstetrical surgical wounds (674.1-674.3)

§ √5th 1 **669.5** **Forceps or vacuum extractor delivery without mention of indication** M ♀
[0,1]
Delivery by ventouse, without mention of indication

§ √5th 1 **669.6** **Breech extraction, without mention of indication** M ♀
[0,1]
EXCLUDES breech delivery NOS (652.2)

§ √5th 1 **669.7** **Cesarean delivery, without mention of indication** M ♀
[0,1]
AHA: For code 658.71: 1Q, '01, 11

§ √5th 1 **669.8** **Other complications of labor and delivery** M ♀
[0-4]

§ √5th 1 **669.9** **Unspecified complication of labor and delivery** M ♀
[0-4]

---

1 Nonspecific PDx=0
§ Requires fifth-digit. Valid digits are in [brackets] under each code. See beginning of section 640-648 for codes and definitions.

√4th Additional Digit Required
√5th
 Nonspecific PDx
 Unacceptable PDx
 Manifestation Code
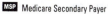 Medicare Secondary Payer
 Revised Text
● New Code
▲ Revised Code Title

2002 Ingenix, Inc.

COMPLICATIONS OF PREGNANCY, CHILDBIRTH, AND THE PUERPERIUM

COMPLICATIONS OF THE PUERPERIUM (670-677)

Note: Categories 671 and 673-676 include the listed conditions even if they occur during pregnancy or childbirth.

The following fifth-digit subclassification is for use with categories 670-676 to denote the current episode of care. Valid fifth-digits are in [brackets] under each code.

- 0 unspecified as to episode of care or not applicable
- 1 delivered, with or without mention of antepartum condition
- 2 delivered, with mention of postpartum complication
- 3 antepartum condition or complication
- 4 postpartum condition or complication

670 Major puerperal infection
[0,2,4]

§ Use 0 as fourth-digit for this category

Puerperal:
- endometritis
- fever (septic)
- pelvic:
  - cellulitis
  - sepsis

Puerperal:
- peritonitis
- pyemia
- salpingitis
- septicemia

EXCLUDES infection following abortion (639.0)
minor genital tract infection following delivery (646.6)
puerperal pyrexia NOS (672)
puerperal fever NOS (672)
puerperal pyrexia of unknown origin (672)
urinary tract infection following delivery (646.6)

CC Excl: 646.80-646.93, 648.90-648.94, 650, 669.40-669.44, 669.80-669.94, 670.00-670.04

AHA: 4Q, '91, 26; 2Q, '91, 7

DEF: Infection and inflammation, following childbirth.

671 Venous complications in pregnancy and the puerperium

§ 671.0 Varicose veins of legs
[0-4]
Varicose veins NOS

DEF: Distended, tortuous veins on legs associated with pregnancy.

§ 671.1 Varicose veins of vulva and perineum
[0-4]

DEF: Distended, tortuous veins on external female genitalia associated with pregnancy.

§ 671.2 Superficial thrombophlebitis
[0-4]
Thrombophlebitis (superficial)

CC Excl: 646.80-646.93, 648.90-648.94, 650, 669.40-669.44, 669.80-669.94, 671.20-671.94

§ 671.3 Deep phlebothrombosis, antepartum
[0,1,3]
Deep-vein thrombosis, antepartum

CC Excl: See code 671.2

§ 671.4 Deep phlebothrombosis, postpartum
[0,2,4]
Deep-vein thrombosis, postpartum
Pelvic thrombophlebitis, postpartum
Phlegmasia alba dolens (puerperal)

CC Excl: See code 671.2

§ 671.5 Other phlebitis and thrombosis
[0-4]
Cerebral venous thrombosis
Thrombosis of intracranial venous sinus

§ 671.8 Other venous complications
[0-4]
Hemorrhoids

§ 671.9 Unspecified venous complication
[0-4]
Phlebitis NOS
Thrombosis NOS

672 Pyrexia of unknown origin during the puerperium
[0,2,4]

§ Use 0 as fourth-digit for this category

Postpartum fever NOS
Puerperal fever NOS
Puerperal pyrexia NOS

AHA: 4Q, '91, 26

DEF: Fever of unknown origin experienced by the mother after childbirth.

673 Obstetrical pulmonary embolism

INCLUDES pulmonary emboli in pregnancy, childbirth, or the puerperium, or specified as puerperal
EXCLUDES embolism following abortion (639.6)

§ 673.0 Obstetrical air embolism
[0-4]

CC Excl: 646.80-646.93, 648.90-648.94, 650, 669.40-669.44, 669.80-669.94, 673.00-673.84

DEF: Sudden blocking of pulmonary artery with air or nitrogen bubbles during puerperium.

§ 673.1 Amniotic fluid embolism
[0-4]

CC Excl: See code 673.0

DEF: Sudden onset of pulmonary artery blockage from amniotic fluid entering the mother's circulation near the end of pregnancy due to strong uterine contractions.

§ 673.2 Obstetrical blood-clot embolism
[0-4]
Puerperal pulmonary embolism NOS

CC Excl: See code 673.0

DEF: Blood clot blocking artery in the lung; associated with pregnancy.

§ 673.3 Obstetrical pyemic and septic embolism
[0-4]

CC Excl: See code 673.0

§ 673.8 Other pulmonary embolism
[0-4]
Fat embolism

CC Excl: See code 673.0

674 Other and unspecified complications of the puerperium, not elsewhere classified

§ 674.0 Cerebrovascular disorders in the puerperium
[0-4]
Any condition classifiable to 430-434, 436-437 occurring during pregnancy, childbirth, or the puerperium, or specified as puerperal

EXCLUDES intracranial venous sinus thrombosis (671.5)

CC Excl: 646.80-646.93, 648.90-648.94, 650, 669.40-669.44, 669.80-669.94, 674.00-674.04

§ 674.1 Disruption of cesarean wound
[0,2,4]
Dehiscence or disruption of uterine wound

EXCLUDES uterine rupture before onset of labor (665.0)
uterine rupture during labor (665.1)

CC Excl: For Codes 674.10-674.12: 646.80-646.93, 648.90-648.94, 650, 669.40-669.44, 669.80-669.94, 674.10, 674.34

§ 674.2 Disruption of perineal wound
[0,2,4]
Breakdown of perineum
Disruption of wound of: episiotomy
Disruption of wound of: perineal laceration
Secondary perineal tear

CC Excl: See code 674.1

AHA: For code 674.24: 1Q, '97, 9

---

1 Nonspecific PDx=0
§ Requires fifth-digit. Valid digits are in [brackets] under each code. See beginning of section 640-648 for codes and definitions.

COMPLICATIONS OF PREGNANCY, CHILDBIRTH, AND THE PUERPERIUM 674.3–677

§ √5th¹ **674.3** **Other complications of obstetrical surgical wounds** M♀
[0,2,4]
  Hematoma ⎫
  Hemorrhage ⎬ of cesarean section or perineal wound
  Infection ⎭

  EXCLUDES damage from instruments in delivery (664.0-665.9)

  AHA: 2Q, '91, 7

§ √5th¹ **674.4** **Placental polyp** M♀
[0,2,4]

§ √5th¹ **674.8** **Other** M♀
[0,2,4]
  Hepatorenal syndrome, following delivery
  Postpartum:
    cardiomyopathy
    subinvolution of uterus
    uterine hypertrophy

  AHA: 3Q, '98, 16

§ √5th¹ **674.9** **Unspecified** M♀
[0,2,4]
  Sudden death of unknown cause during the puerperium

√4th **675 Infections of the breast and nipple associated with childbirth**

  INCLUDES the listed conditions during pregnancy, childbirth, or the puerperium

§ √5th¹ **675.0** **Infections of nipple** M♀
[0-4]
  Abscess of nipple

§ √5th¹ **675.1** **Abscess of breast** CC 0-2 M♀
[0-4]
  Abscess:
    mammary
    subareolar
    submammary
    purulent
    retromammary
    submammary

  CC Excl: For codes 675.10-675.12: 646.80-646.93, 648.90-648.94, 650, 669.40-669.44, 669.80-669.94, 675.00-675.94

§ √5th¹ **675.2** **Nonpurulent mastitis** M♀
[0-4]
  Lymphangitis of breast
  Mastitis:
    NOS
    interstitial
    parenchymatous

§ √5th¹ **675.8** **Other specified infections of the breast and nipple** M♀
[0-4]

§ √5th¹ **675.9** **Unspecified infection of the breast and nipple** M♀
[0-4]

√4th **676 Other disorders of the breast associated with childbirth and disorders of lactation**

  INCLUDES the listed conditions during pregnancy, the puerperium, or lactation

§ √5th¹ **676.0** **Retracted nipple** M♀
[0-4]

§ √5th¹ **676.1** **Cracked nipple** M♀
[0-4]
  Fissure of nipple

§ √5th¹ **676.2** **Engorgement of breasts** M♀
[0-4]

  DEF: Abnormal accumulation of milk in ducts of breast.

§ √5th¹ **676.3** **Other and unspecified disorder of breast** M♀
[0-4]

§ √5th¹ **676.4** **Failure of lactation** M♀
[0-4]
  Agalactia

  DEF: Abrupt ceasing of milk secretion by breast.

§ √5th¹ **676.5** **Suppressed lactation** M♀
[0-4]

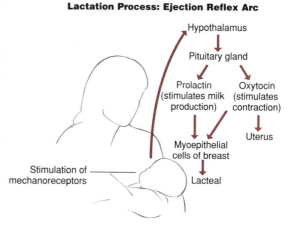
Lactation Process: Ejection Reflex Arc

§ √5th¹ **676.6** **Galactorrhea** M♀
[0-4]
  EXCLUDES galactorrhea not associated with childbirth (611.6)

  DEF: Excessive or persistent milk secretion by breast; may be in absence of nursing.

§ √5th¹ **676.8** **Other disorders of lactation** M♀
[0-4]
  Galactocele

  DEF: Galactocele: Obstructed mammary gland, creating retention cyst, results in milk-filled cysts enlarging mammary gland.

§ √5th¹ **676.9** **Unspecified disorder of lactation** M♀
[0-4]

677 Late effect of complication of pregnancy, childbirth, and the puerperium M♀
  Note: This category is to be used to indicate conditions in 632-648.9 and 651-676.9 as the cause of the late effect, themselves classifiable elsewhere. The "late effects" include conditions specified as such, or as sequelae, which may occur at any time after puerperium.
  Code first any sequelae

  AHA: 1Q, '97, 9; 4Q, '94, 42

---

¹ Nonspecific PDx=0
§ Requires fifth-digit. Valid digits are in [brackets] under each code. See beginning of section 640-648 for codes and definitions.

12. DISEASES OF THE SKIN AND SUBCUTANEOUS TISSUE
(680-709)

Skin and Subcutaneous Layer

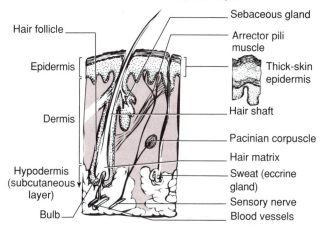

INFECTIONS OF SKIN AND SUBCUTANEOUS TISSUE (680-686)

EXCLUDES certain infections of skin classified under "Infectious and Parasitic Diseases," such as:
erysipelas (035)
erysipeloid of Rosenbach (027.1)
herpes:
  simplex (054.0-054.9)
  zoster (053.0-053.9)
molluscum contagiosum (078.0)
viral warts (078.1)

✓4th 680 Carbuncle and furuncle
  INCLUDES boil
  furunculosis

DEF: Carbuncle: necrotic boils in skin and subcutaneous tissue of neck or back mainly due to staphylococcal infection.

DEF: Furuncle: Circumscribed inflammation of corium and subcutaneous tissue due to staphylococcal infection.

680.0 Face CC
  Ear [any part]
  Face [any part, except eye]
  Nose (septum)
  Temple (region)
  EXCLUDES eyelid (373.13)
    lacrimal apparatus (375.31)
    orbit (376.01)
  CC Excl: 017.00-017.06, 017.90-017.96, ▶040.82,◀ 040.89, 041.00-041.89, 041.9, 680.0, 680.8-680.9, 686.00-686.01, 686.09, 686.1-686.9, 705.83, 709.8, V09.0-V09.91

680.1 Neck CC
  CC Excl: 017.00-017.06, 017.90-017.96, ▶040.82,◀ 040.89, 041.00-041.89, 041.9, 680.1, 680.8-680.9, 686.00-686.01, 686.09, 686.1-686.9, 705.83, 709.8, V09.0-V09.91

680.2 Trunk CC
  Abdominal wall
  Back [any part, except buttocks]
  Breast
  Chest wall
  Flank
  Groin
  Pectoral region
  Perineum
  Umbilicus
  EXCLUDES buttocks (680.5)
    external genital organs:
      female (616.4)
      male (607.2, 608.4)
  CC Excl: 017.00-017.06, 017.90-017.96, ▶040.82,◀ 040.89, 041.00-041.89, 041.9, 680.2, 680.8-680.9, 686.00-686.01, 686.09, 686.1-686.9, 705.83, 709.8, V09.0-V09.91

680.3 Upper arm and forearm CC
  Arm [any part, except hand]
  Axilla
  Shoulder
  CC Excl: 017.00-017.06, 017.90-017.96, ▶040.82,◀ 040.89, 041.00-041.89, 041.9, 680.0, 680.8-680.9, 686.00-686.01, 686.09, 686.1-686.9, 705.83, 709.8, V09.0-V09.91

680.4 Hand CC
  Finger [any]
  Thumb
  Wrist
  CC Excl: 017.00-017.06, 017.90-017.96, ▶040.82,◀ 040.89, 041.00-041.89, 041.9, 680.0, 680.8-680.9, 686.00-686.01, 686.09, 686.1-686.9, 705.83, 709.8, V09.0-V09.91

680.5 Buttock CC
  Anus
  Gluteal region
  CC Excl: 017.00-017.06, 017.90-017.96, ▶040.82,◀ 040.89, 041.00-041.89, 041.9, 680.0, 680.8-680.9, 686.00-686.01, 686.09, 686.1-686.9, 705.83, 709.8, V09.0-V09.91

680.6 Leg, except foot CC
  Ankle   Knee
  Hip   Thigh
  CC Excl: 017.00-017.06, 017.90-017.96, ▶040.82,◀ 040.89, 041.00-041.89, 041.9, 680.0, 680.8-680.9, 686.00-686.01, 686.09, 686.1-686.9, 705.83, 709.8, V09.0-V09.91

680.7 Foot CC
  Heel
  Toe
  CC Excl: 017.00-017.06, 017.90-017.96, ▶040.82,◀ 040.89, 041.00-041.89, 041.9, 680.0, 680.8-680.9, 686.00-686.01, 686.09, 686.1-686.9, 705.83, 709.8, V09.0-V09.91

680.8 Other specified sites CC
  Head [any part, except face]
  Scalp
  EXCLUDES external genital organs:
    female (616.4)
    male (607.2, 608.4)
  CC Excl: 017.00-017.06, 017.90-017.96, ▶040.82,◀ 040.89, 041.00-041.89, 041.9, 680.0, 680.8-680.9, 686.00-686.01, 686.09, 686.1-686.9, 705.83, 709.8, V09.0-V09.91

680.9 Unspecified site CC
  Boil NOS   Furuncle NOS
  Carbuncle NOS
  CC Excl: See code 680.8

✓4th 681 Cellulitis and abscess of finger and toe
  INCLUDES that with lymphangitis
  Use additional code to identify organism, such as Staphylococcus (041.1)

AHA: 2Q, '91, 5; J-F, '87, 12

DEF: Acute suppurative inflammation and edema in subcutaneous tissue or muscle of finger or toe.

✓5th 681.0 Finger
  681.00 Cellulitis and abscess, unspecified
  681.01 Felon
    Pulp abscess   Whitlow
    EXCLUDES herpetic whitlow (054.6)
    DEF: Painful abscess of fingertips caused by infection in the closed space of terminal phalanx.

  681.02 Onychia and paronychia of finger
    Panaritium } of finger
    Perionychia
    DEF: Onychia: inflammation of nail matrix; causes nail loss.
    DEF: Paronychia: inflammation of tissue folds around nail.

SKIN AND SUBCUTANEOUS TISSUE

√5th **681.1 Toe**
- **681.10** Cellulitis and abscess, unspecified
- **681.11** Onychia and paronychia of toe
  - Panaritium } of toe
  - Perionychia

681.9 Cellulitis and abscess of unspecified digit
- Infection of nail NOS

√4th **682 Other cellulitis and abscess**

INCLUDES
- abscess (acute)
- cellulitis (diffuse) } (with lymphangitis) except of finger or toe
- lymphangitis, acute

Use additional code to identify organism, such as Staphylococcus (041.1)

EXCLUDES lymphangitis (chronic) (subacute) (457.2)

AHA: 2Q, '91, 5; J-F, '87, 12; S-O, '85, 10

DEF: Cellulitis: Acute suppurative inflammation of deep subcutaneous tissue and sometimes muscle due to infection of wound, burn or other lesion.

682.0 Face
- Cheek, external
- Chin
- Forehead
- Nose, external
- Submandibular
- Temple (region)

EXCLUDES
- ear [any part] (380.10-380.16)
- eyelid (373.13)
- lacrimal apparatus (375.31)
- lip (528.5)
- mouth (528.3)
- nose (internal) (478.1)
- orbit (376.01)

CC Excl: 017.00-017.06, 017.90-017.96, 040.89, 041.00-041.89, 041.9, 682.0, 682.8-682.9, 686.00-686.01, 686.09, 686.1-686.9, 705.83, 709.8, V09.0-V09.91

682.1 Neck

CC Excl: 017.00-017.06, 017.90-017.96, 040.89, 041.00-041.89, 041.9, 682.1, 682.8-682.9, 686.00-686.01, 686.09, 686.1-686.9, 705.83, 709.8, V09.0-V09.91

682.2 Trunk
- Abdominal wall
- Back [any part, except buttock]
- Chest wall
- Flank
- Groin
- Pectoral region
- Perineum
- Umbilicus, except newborn

EXCLUDES
- anal and rectal regions (566)
- breast:
  - NOS (611.0)
  - puerperal (675.1)
- external genital organs:
  - female (616.3-616.4)
  - male (604.0, 607.2, 608.4)
- umbilicus, newborn (771.4)

CC Excl: 017.00-017.06, 017.90-017.96, 040.89, 041.00-041.89, 041.9, 682.2, 682.8-682.9, 686.00-686.01, 686.09, 686.1-686.9, 705.83, 709.8, V09.0-V09.91

AHA: 4Q, '98, 42

682.3 Upper arm and forearm
- Arm [any part, except hand]
- Axilla
- Shoulder

EXCLUDES hand (682.4)

CC Excl: 017.00-017.06, 017.90-017.96, 040.89, 041.00-041.89, 041.9, 682.3, 682.8-682.9, 686.00-686.01, 686.09, 686.1-686.9, 705.83, 709.8, V09.0-V09.91

682.4 Hand, except fingers and thumb
- Wrist

EXCLUDES finger and thumb (681.00-681.02)

682.5 Buttock
- Gluteal region

EXCLUDES anal and rectal regions (566)

CC Excl: 017.00-017.06, 017.90-017.96, 040.89, 041.00-041.89, 041.9, 682.5, 682.8-682.9, 686.00-686.01, 686.09, 686.1-686.9, 705.83, 709.8, V09.0-V09.91

682.6 Leg, except foot
- Ankle
- Hip
- Knee
- Thigh

CC Excl: 017.00-017.06, 017.90-017.96, 040.89, 041.00-041.89, 041.9, 682.6, 682.8-682.9, 686.00-686.01, 686.09, 686.1-686.9, 705.83, 709.8, V09.0-V09.91

682.7 Foot, except toes
- Heel

EXCLUDES toe (681.10-681.11)

CC Excl: 017.00-017.06, 017.90-017.96, 040.89, 041.00-041.89, 041.9, 682.7-682.9, 686.00-686.01, 686.09, 686.1-686.9, 705.83, 709.8, V09.0-V09.91

682.8 Other specified sites
- Head [except face]
- Scalp

EXCLUDES face (682.0)

CC Excl: 017.00-017.06, 017.90-017.96, 040.89, 041.00-041.89, 041.9, 682.8-682.9, 686.00-686.01, 686.09, 686.1-686.9, 705.83, 709.8, V09.0-V09.91

682.9 Unspecified site
- Abscess NOS
- Cellulitis NOS
- Lymphangitis, acute NOS

EXCLUDES lymphangitis NOS (457.2)

CC Excl: See code 682.8

683 Acute lymphadenitis
- Abscess (acute)
- Adenitis, acute } lymph gland or node, except mesenteric
- Lymphadenitis, acute

Use additional code to identify organism, such as Staphylococcus (041.1)

EXCLUDES
- enlarged glands NOS (785.6)
- lymphadenitis:
  - chronic or subacute, except mesenteric (289.1)
  - mesenteric (acute) (chronic) (subacute) (289.2)
  - unspecified (289.3)

DEF: Acute inflammation of lymph nodes due to primary infection located elsewhere in the body.

684 Impetigo
- Impetiginization of other dermatoses
- Impetigo (contagiosa) [any site] [any organism]:
  - bullous
  - circinate
  - neonatorum
  - simplex
- Pemphigus neonatorum

EXCLUDES impetigo herpetiformis (694.3)

CC Excl: 684, 686.00-686.01, 686.09, 686.1-686.9, 709.8

DEF: Infectious skin disease commonly occurring in children; caused by group A streptococci or *Staphylococcus aureus*; skin lesions usually appear on the face and consist of subcorneal vesicles and bullae that burst and form yellow crusts.

▶ **Lymphatic System of Head and Neck** ◀

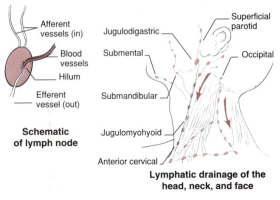

Schematic of lymph node

Lymphatic drainage of the head, neck, and face

SKIN AND SUBCUTANEOUS TISSUE 685–692.2

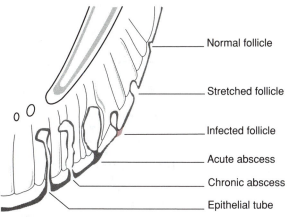

Stages of Pilonidal Disease
- Normal follicle
- Stretched follicle
- Infected follicle
- Acute abscess
- Chronic abscess
- Epithelial tube

√4th **685 Pilonidal cyst**

INCLUDES fistula } coccygeal or pilonidal
sinus

DEF: Hair-containing cyst or sinus in the tissues of the sacrococcygeal area; often drains through opening at the postanal dimple.

685.0 With abscess CC
CC Excl: 685.0-685.1, 709.8

685.1 Without mention of abscess

√4th **686 Other local infections of skin and subcutaneous tissue**
Use additional code to identify any infectious organism (041.0-041.8)

√5th **686.0 Pyoderma**
Dermatitis: Dermatitis:
  purulent   suppurative
  septic

DEF: Nonspecific purulent skin disease related most to furuncles, pustules, or possibly carbuncles.

686.00 Pyoderma, unspecified

686.01 Pyoderma gangrenosum
AHA: 4Q, '97, 42

DEF: Persistent debilitating skin disease, characterized by irregular, boggy, blue-red ulcerations, with central healing and undermined edges.

686.09 Other pyoderma

686.1 Pyogenic granuloma
Granuloma:
  septic
  suppurative
  telangiectaticum
EXCLUDES pyogenic granuloma of oral mucosa (528.9)

DEF: Solitary polypoid capillary hemangioma often asociated with local irritation, trauma, and superimposed inflammation; located on the skin and gingival or oral mucosa.

686.8 Other specified local infections of skin and subcutaneous tissue
Bacterid (pustular)   Ecthyma
Dermatitis vegetans   Perlèche
EXCLUDES dermatitis infectiosa eczematoides (690.8)
panniculitis (729.30-729.39)

686.9 Unspecified local infection of skin and subcutaneous tissue
Fistula of skin NOS
Skin infection NOS
EXCLUDES fistula to skin from internal organs — see Alphabetic Index

OTHER INFLAMMATORY CONDITIONS OF SKIN AND SUBCUTANEOUS TISSUE (690-698)
EXCLUDES panniculitis (729.30-729.39)

√4th **690 Erythematosquamous dermatosis**
EXCLUDES eczematous dermatitis of eyelid (373.31)
parakeratosis variegata (696.2)
psoriasis (696.0-696.1)
seborrheic keratosis (702.11-702.19)

√5th **690.1 Seborrheic dermatitis**
AHA: 4Q, '95, 58

690.10 Seborrheic dermatitis, unspecified
Seborrheic dermatitis NOS

690.11 Seborrhea capitis P
Cradle cap

690.12 Seborrheic infantile dermatitis P

690.18 Other seborrheic dermatitis

690.8 Other erythematosquamous dermatosis

√4th **691 Atopic dermatitis and related conditions**
DEF: Atopic dermatitis: chronic, pruritic, inflammatory skin disorder found on the face and antecubital and popliteal fossae; noted in persons with a hereditary predisposition to pruritus, and often accompanied by allergic rhinitis, hay fever, asthma, and extreme itching; also called allergic dermatitis, allergic or atopic eczema, or disseminated neurodermatitis.

691.0 Diaper or napkin rash
Ammonia dermatitis   Diaper or napkin:
Diaper or napkin: rash
  dermatitis   Psoriasiform napkin eruption
  erythema

691.8 Other atopic dermatitis and related conditions
Atopic dermatitis   Eczema:
Besnier's prurigo   intrinsic (allergic)
Eczema: Neurodermatitis:
  atopic   atopic
  flexural   diffuse (of Brocq)

√4th **692 Contact dermatitis and other eczema**
INCLUDES dermatitis: eczema (acute) (chronic):
            NOS   NOS
            contact   allergic
            occupational   erythematous
            venenata   occupational
EXCLUDES allergy NOS (995.3)
contact dermatitis of eyelids (373.32)
dermatitis due to substances taken internally (693.0-693.9)
eczema of external ear (380.22)
perioral dermatitis (695.3)
urticarial reactions (708.0-708.9, 995.1)

DEF: Contact dermatitis: acute or chronic dermatitis caused by initial irritant effect of a substance, or by prior sensitization to a substance coming once again in contact with skin.

692.0 Due to detergents
692.1 Due to oils and greases
692.2 Due to solvents
Dermatitis due to solvents of:
  chlorocompound }
  cyclohexane
  ester
  glycol   } group
  hydrocarbon
  ketone

692.3–692.83 SKIN AND SUBCUTANEOUS TISSUE

692.3 Due to drugs and medicines in contact with skin
Dermatitis (allergic) (contact) due to:
  arnica
  fungicides
  iodine
  keratolytics
  mercurials
Dermatitis (allergic) (contact) due to:
  neomycin
  pediculocides
  phenols
  scabicides
  any drug applied to skin
Dermatitis medicamentosa due to drug applied to skin
Use additional E code to identify drug
EXCLUDES allergy NOS due to drugs (995.2)
dermatitis due to ingested drugs (693.0)
dermatitis medicamentosa NOS (693.0)

692.4 Due to other chemical products
Dermatitis due to:
  acids
  adhesive plaster
  alkalis
  caustics
  dichromate
  insecticide
  nylon
  plastic
  rubber
AHA: 2Q, '89, 16

692.5 Due to food in contact with skin
Dermatitis, contact, due to:
  cereals
  fish
  flour
Dermatitis, contact, due to:
  fruit
  meat
  milk
EXCLUDES dermatitis due to:
dyes (692.89)
ingested foods (693.1)
preservatives (692.89)

692.6 Due to plants [except food]
Dermatitis due to:
  lacquer tree [Rhus verniciflua]
  poison:
    ivy [Rhus toxicodendron]
    oak [Rhus diversiloba]
    sumac [Rhus venenata]
    vine [Rhus radicans]
  primrose [Primula]
  ragweed [Senecio jacobae]
  other plants in contact with the skin
EXCLUDES allergy NOS due to pollen (477.0)
nettle rash (708.8)

✓5th 692.7 Due to solar radiation
EXCLUDES sunburn due to other ultraviolet radiation exposure (692.82)

692.70 Unspecified dermatitis due to sun

692.71 Sunburn
First degree sunburn
Sunburn NOS
AHA: ▶4Q, '01, 47◀

692.72 Acute dermatitis due to solar radiation
Berlogue dermatitis
Photoallergic response
Phototoxic response
Polymorphus light eruption
Acute solar skin damage NOS
EXCLUDES sunburn (692.71, 692.76-692.77)
Use additional E code to identify drug, if drug induced

DEF: Berloque dermatitis: Phytophotodermatitis due to sun exposure after use of a product containing bergamot oil; causes red patches, which may turn brown.

DEF: Photoallergic response: Dermatitis due to hypersensitivity to the sun; causes papulovesicular, eczematous or exudative eruptions.

DEF: Phototoxic response: Chemically induced sensitivity to sun causes burn-like reaction, occasionally vesiculation and subsequent hyperpigmentation.

DEF: Polymorphous light eruption: Inflammatory skin eruptions due to sunlight exposure; eruptions differ in size and shape.

DEF: Acute solar skin damage (NOS): Rapid, unspecified injury to skin from sun.

692.73 Actinic reticuloid and actinic granuloma
DEF: Actinic reticuloid: Dermatosis aggravated by light, causes chronic eczema-like eruption on exposed skin which extends to other unexposed surfaces; occurs in the eldery.
DEF: Actinic granuloma: Inflammatory response of skin to sun causing small nodule of microphages.

692.74 Other chronic dermatitis due to solar radiation
Chronic solar skin damage NOS
Solar elastosis
EXCLUDES actinic [solar] keratosis (702.0)

DEF: Solar elastosis: Premature aging of skin of light-skinned people; causes inelasticity, thinning or thickening, wrinkling, dryness, scaling and hyperpigmentation.

DEF: Chronic solar skin damage (NOS): Chronic skin impairment due to exposure to the sun, not otherwise specified.

692.75 Disseminated superficial actinic porokeratosis (DSAP)
DEF: Autosomal dominant skin condition occurring in skin that has been overexposed to the sun. Primarily affects women over the age of 16; characterized by numerous superficial annular, keratotic, brownish-red spots or thickenings with depressed centers and sharp, ridged borders. High risk that condition will evolve into squamous cell carcinoma.
AHA: 4Q, '00, 43

692.76 Sunburn of second degree
AHA: ▶4Q, '01, 47◀

692.77 Sunburn of third degree
AHA: ▶4Q, '01, 47◀

692.79 Other dermatitis due to solar radiation
Hydroa aestivale
Photodermatitis } (due to sun)
Photosensitiveness
Solar skin damage NOS

✓5th 692.8 Due to other specified agents

692.81 Dermatitis due to cosmetics

692.82 Dermatitis due to other radiation
Infrared rays   Tanning bed
Light, except   Ultraviolet rays, except
  from sun   from sun
Radiation NOS   X-rays
EXCLUDES solar radiation (692.70-692.79)
AHA: ▶4Q, '01, 47;◀ 3Q, '00, 5

692.83 Dermatitis due to metals
Jewelry

SKIN AND SUBCUTANEOUS TISSUE

692.89 Other
Dermatitis due to: cold weather, dyes, furs
Dermatitis due to: hot weather, preservatives
EXCLUDES allergy NOS due to animal hair, dander (animal), or dust (477.8)
sunburn (692.71, 692.76-692.77)

692.9 Unspecified cause
Dermatitis:
  NOS
  contact NOS
  venenata NOS
Eczema NOS

693 Dermatitis due to substances taken internally
EXCLUDES adverse effect NOS of drugs and medicines (995.2)
allergy NOS (995.3)
contact dermatitis (692.0-692.9)
urticarial reactions (708.0-708.9, 995.1)
DEF: Inflammation of skin due to ingested substance.

693.0 Due to drugs and medicines
Dermatitis medicamentosa NOS
Use additional E code to identify drug
EXCLUDES that due to drugs in contact with skin (692.3)

693.1 Due to food

693.8 Due to other specified substances taken internally

693.9 Due to unspecified substance taken internally
EXCLUDES dermatitis NOS (692.9)

694 Bullous dermatoses

694.0 Dermatitis herpetiformis
Dermatosis herpetiformis
Duhring's disease
Hydroa herpetiformis
EXCLUDES herpes gestationis (646.8)
dermatitis herpetiformis:
  juvenile (694.2)
  senile (694.5)
DEF: Chronic, relapsing multisystem disease manifested most in the cutaneous system; seen as an extremely pruritic eruption of various combinations of lesions that frequently heal leaving hyperpigmentation or hypopigmentation and occasionally scarring; usually associated with an asymptomatic gluten-sensitive enteropathy, and immunogenic factors are believed to play a role in its origin.

694.1 Subcorneal pustular dermatosis
Sneddon-Wilkinson disease or syndrome
DEF: Chronic relapses of sterile pustular blebs beneath the horny skin layer of the trunk and skin folds; resembles dermatitis herpetiformis.

694.2 Juvenile dermatitis herpetiformis
Juvenile pemphigoid

694.3 Impetigo herpetiformis
DEF: Rare dermatosis associated with pregnancy; marked by itching pustules in third trimester, hypocalcemia, tetany, fever and lethargy; may result in maternal or fetal death.

694.4 Pemphigus
Pemphigus:
  NOS
  erythematosus
  foliaceus
Pemphigus:
  malignant
  vegetans
  vulgaris
EXCLUDES pemphigus neonatorum (684)
CC Excl: 694.4-694.9, 709.8
DEF: Chronic, relapsing, sometimes fatal skin diseases; causes vesicles, bullae; autoantibodies against intracellular connections cause acantholysis.

694.5 Pemphigoid
Benign pemphigus NOS
Bullous pemphigoid
Herpes circinatus bullosus
Senile dermatitis herpetiformis
CC Excl: See code 694.4

694.6 Benign mucous membrane pemphigoid
Cicatricial pemphigoid
Mucosynechial atrophic bullous dermatitis
  694.60 Without mention of ocular involvement
  694.61 With ocular involvement
  Ocular pemphigus
  Mild self-limiting, subepidermal blistering of mucosa including the conjunctiva, seen predominantly in the elderly. It produces adhesions and scarring.

694.8 Other specified bullous dermatoses
EXCLUDES herpes gestationis (646.8)

694.9 Unspecified bullous dermatoses

695 Erythematous conditions

695.0 Toxic erythema
Erythema venenatum
CC Excl: 695.0-695.4, 709.8

695.1 Erythema multiforme
Erythema iris
Herpes iris
Lyell's syndrome
Scalded skin syndrome
Stevens-Johnson syndrome
Toxic epidermal necrolysis
DEF: Symptom complex with a varied skin eruption pattern of macular, bullous, papular, nodose, or vesicular lesions on the neck, face, and legs; gastritis and rheumatic pains are also noticeable, first-seen symptoms; complex is secondary to a number of factors, including infections, ingestants, physical agents, malignancy and pregnancy.

695.2 Erythema nodosum
EXCLUDES tuberculous erythema nodosum (017.1)
DEF: Panniculitis (an inflammatory reaction of the subcutaneous fat) of women, usually seen as a hypersensitivity reaction to various infections, drugs, sarcoidosis, and specific enteropathies; the acute stage is often associated with other symptoms, including fever, malaise, and arthralgia; the lesions are pink to blue in color, appear in crops as tender nodules and are found on the front of the legs below the knees.

695.3 Rosacea
Acne:
  erythematosa
  rosacea
Perioral dermatitis
Rhinophyma
DEF: Chronic skin disease, usually of the face, characterized by persistent erythema and sometimes by telangiectasis with acute episodes of edema, engorgement papules, and pustules.

695.4 Lupus erythematosus
Lupus:
  erythematodes (discoid)
  erythematosus (discoid), not disseminated
EXCLUDES lupus (vulgaris) NOS (017.0)
systemic [disseminated] lupus erythematosus (710.0)
DEF: Group of connective tissue disorders occurring as various cutaneous diseases of unknown origin; it primarily affects women between the ages of 20 and 40.

695.8 Other specified erythematous conditions
  695.81 Ritter's disease
  Dermatitis exfoliativa neonatorum
  DEF: Infectious skin disease of infants and young children marked by eruptions ranging from a localized bullous type to widespread development of easily ruptured fine vesicles and bullae; results in exfoliation of large planes of skin and leaves raw areas; also called staphylococcal scalded skin syndrome.

695.89 Other
- Erythema intertrigo
- Intertrigo
- Pityriasis rubra (Hebra)

EXCLUDES mycotic intertrigo (111.0-111.9)

AHA: S-O, '86, 10

695.9 Unspecified erythematous condition
- Erythema NOS
- Erythroderma (secondary)

√4th **696** Psoriasis and similar disorders

696.0 Psoriatic arthropathy [CC]

CC Excl: 015.80-015.96, 017.90-017.96, 036.82, 056.71, 098.50-098.51, 098.59, 098.89, 696.0, 711.00-711.99, 712.10-712.99, 713.0-713.8, 714.0, 715.00, 715.09-715.10, 715.18, 715.20-715.98, 716.00-716.99, 718.00-718.08, 719.00-719.09, 719.10, 719.18-719.19, 719.20-719.99

DEF: Psoriasis associated with inflammatory arthritis; often involves interphalangeal joints.

696.1 Other psoriasis
- Acrodermatitis continua
- Dermatitis repens
- Psoriasis: NOS
- Psoriasis: any type, except arthropathic

EXCLUDES psoriatic arthropathy (696.0)

696.2 Parapsoriasis
- Parakeratosis variegata
- Parapsoriasis lichenoides chronica
- Pityriasis lichenoides et varioliformis

DEF: Erythrodermas similar to lichen, planus and psoriasis; symptoms include redness and itching; resistant to treatment.

696.3 Pityriasis rosea
- Pityriasis circinata (et maculata)

DEF: Common, self-limited rash of unknown etiology marked by a solitary erythematous, salmon or fawn-colored herald plaque on the trunk, arms or thighs; followed by development of papular or macular lesions that tend to peel and form a scaly collarette.

696.4 Pityriasis rubra pilaris
- Devergie's disease
- Lichen ruber acuminatus

EXCLUDES pityriasis rubra (Hebra) (695.89)

DEF: Inflammatory disease of hair follicles; marked by firm, red lesions topped by horny plugs; may form patches; occurs on fingers elbows, knees.

696.5 Other and unspecified pityriasis
- Pityriasis: NOS
- Pityriasis: alba
- Pityriasis: streptogenes

EXCLUDES pityriasis:
- simplex (690.18)
- versicolor (111.0)

696.8 Other

√4th **697** Lichen

EXCLUDES lichen:
- obtusus corneus (698.3)
- pilaris (congenital) (757.39)
- ruber acuminatus (696.4)
- sclerosus et atrophicus (701.0)
- scrofulosus (017.0)
- simplex chronicus (698.3)
- spinulosus (congenital) (757.39)
- urticatus (698.2)

697.0 Lichen planus
- Lichen: planopilaris
- Lichen: ruber planus

DEF: Inflammatory, pruritic skin disease; marked by angular, flat-top, violet-colored papules; may be acute and widespread or chronic and localized.

697.1 Lichen nitidus
- Pinkus' disease

DEF: Chronic, inflammatory, usually asymptomatic skin disorder, characterized by numerous glistening, flat-topped, discrete, smooth, skin-colored micropapules most often on penis, lower abdomen, inner thighs, wrists, forearms, breasts and buttocks.

697.8 Other lichen, not elsewhere classified
- Lichen: ruber moniliforme
- Lichen: striata

697.9 Lichen, unspecified

√4th **698** Pruritus and related conditions

EXCLUDES pruritus specified as psychogenic (306.3)

DEF: Pruritus: Intense, persistent itching due to irritation of sensory nerve endings from organic or psychogenic causes.

698.0 Pruritus ani
- Perianal itch

698.1 Pruritus of genital organs

698.2 Prurigo
- Lichen urticatus
- Prurigo: NOS
- Prurigo: Hebra's
- Prurigo: mitis
- Prurigo: simplex
- Urticaria papulosa (Hebra)

EXCLUDES prurigo nodularis (698.3)

698.3 Lichenification and lichen simplex chronicus
- Hyde's disease
- Neurodermatitis (circumscripta) (local)
- Prurigo nodularis

EXCLUDES neurodermatitis, diffuse (of Brocq) (691.8)

DEF: Lichenification: thickening of skin due to prolonged rubbing or scratching.

DEF: Lichen simplex chronicus: eczematous dermatitis, of face, neck, extremities, scrotum, vulva, and perianal region due to repeated itching, rubbing and scratching; spontaneous or evolves with other dermatoses.

698.4 Dermatitis factitia [artefacta]
- Dermatitis ficta
- Neurotic excoriation
- Use additional code to identify any associated mental disorder

DEF: Various types of self-inflicted skin lesions characterized in appearance as an erythema to a gangrene.

698.8 Other specified pruritic conditions
- Pruritus: hiemalis
- Pruritus: senilis
- Winter itch

698.9 <mark>Unspecified pruritic disorder</mark>
- Itch NOS
- Pruritus NOS

OTHER DISEASES OF SKIN AND SUBCUTANEOUS TISSUE (700-709)

EXCLUDES conditions confined to eyelids (373.0-374.9)
congenital conditions of skin, hair, and nails (757.0-757.9)

700 Corns and callosities
- Callus
- Clavus

DEF: Corns: Conical or horny thickening of skin on toes, due to friction, pressure from shoes and hosiery; pain and inflammation may develop.

DEF: Callosities: Localized overgrowth (hyperplasia) of the horny epidermal layer due to pressure or friction.

√4th **701** Other hypertrophic and atrophic conditions of skin

EXCLUDES dermatomyositis (710.3)
hereditary edema of legs (757.0)
scleroderma (generalized) (710.1)

701.0 Circumscribed scleroderma
- Addison's keloid
- Dermatosclerosis, localized
- Lichen sclerosus et atrophicus
- Morphea
- Scleroderma, circumscribed or localized

DEF: Thickened, hardened, skin and subcutaneous tissue; may involve musculoskeletal system.

N Newborn Age: 0 | P Pediatric Age: 0-17 | M Maternity Age: 12-55 | A Adult Age: 15-124 | CC CC Condition | MC Major Complication | CD Complex Dx | HIV HIV Related Dx

SKIN AND SUBCUTANEOUS TISSUE

701.1 Keratoderma, acquired
Acquired:
ichthyosis
keratoderma palmaris et plantaris
Elastosis perforans serpiginosa
Hyperkeratosis:
NOS
follicularis in cutem penetrans
palmoplantaris climacterica
Keratoderma:
climactericum
tylodes, progressive
Keratosis (blennorrhagica)
EXCLUDES Darier's disease [keratosis follicularis] (congenital) (757.39)
keratosis:
arsenical (692.4)
gonococcal (098.81)
AHA: 4Q, '94, 48

701.2 Acquired acanthosis nigricans
Keratosis nigricans
DEF: Diffuse velvety hyperplasia of the spinous skin layer of the axilla and other body folds marked by gray, brown, or black pigmentation; in adult form it is often associated with an internal carcinoma (malignant acanthosis nigricans) in a benign, nevoid form it is relatively generalized; benign juvenile form with obesity is sometimes caused by an endocrine disturbance.

701.3 Striae atrophicae
Atrophic spots of skin
Atrophoderma maculatum
Atrophy blanche (of Milian)
Degenerative colloid atrophy
Senile degenerative atrophy
Striae distensae
DEF: Bands of atrophic, depressed, wrinkled skin associated with stretching of skin from pregnancy, obesity, or rapid growth during puberty.

701.4 Keloid scar
Cheloid
Hypertrophic scar
Keloid
DEF: Overgrowth of scar tissue due to excess amounts of collagen during connective tissue repair; occurs mainly on upper trunk, face.

701.5 Other abnormal granulation tissue
Excessive granulation

701.8 Other specified hypertrophic and atrophic conditions of skin
Acrodermatitis atrophicans chronica
Atrophia cutis senilis
Atrophoderma neuriticum
Confluent and reticulate papillomatosis
Cutis laxa senilis
Elastosis senilis
Folliculitis ulerythematosa reticulata
Gougerot-Carteaud syndrome or disease

701.9 Unspecified hypertrophic and atrophic conditions of skin
Atrophoderma

702 Other dermatoses
EXCLUDES carcinoma in situ (232.0-232.9)

702.0 Actinic keratosis
AHA: 1Q, '92, 18
DEF: Wart-like growth, red or skin-colored; may form a cutaneous horn.

702.1 Seborrheic keratosis
DEF: Common, benign, lightly pigmented, warty growth composed of basaloid cells.

702.11 Inflamed seborrheic keratosis
AHA: 4Q, '94, 48

702.19 Other seborrheic keratosis
Seborrheic keratosis NOS

702.8 Other specified dermatoses

703 Diseases of nail
EXCLUDES congenital anomalies (757.5)
onychia and paronychia (681.02, 681.11)

703.0 Ingrowing nail
Ingrowing nail with infection   Unguis incarnatus
EXCLUDES infection, nail NOS (681.9)

703.8 Other specified diseases of nail
Dystrophia unguium   Onychauxis
Hypertrophy of nail   Onychogryposis
Koilonychia   Onycholysis
Leukonychia (punctata) (striata)

703.9 Unspecified disease of nail

704 Diseases of hair and hair follicles
EXCLUDES congenital anomalies (757.4)

704.0 Alopecia
EXCLUDES madarosis (374.55)
syphilitic alopecia (091.82)
DEF: Lack of hair, especially on scalp; often called baldness; may be partial or total; occurs at any age.

704.00 Alopecia, unspecified
Baldness
Loss of hair

704.01 Alopecia areata
Ophiasis
DEF: Alopecia areata: usually reversible, inflammatory, patchy hair loss found in beard or scalp.
DEF: Ophiasis: alopecia areata of children; marked by band around temporal and occipital scalp margins.

704.02 Telogen effluvium
DEF: Shedding of hair from premature telogen development in follicles due to stress, including shock, childbirth, surgery, drugs or weight loss.

704.09 Other
Folliculitis decalvans
Hypotrichosis:
NOS
postinfectional NOS
Pseudopelade

704.1 Hirsutism
Hypertrichosis: Polytrichia
NOS
lanuginosa, acquired
EXCLUDES hypertrichosis of eyelid (374.54)
DEF: Excess hair growth; often in unexpected places and amounts.

704.2 Abnormalities of the hair
Atrophic hair   Trichiasis:
Clastothrix   NOS
Fragilitas crinium   cicatrical
                     Trichorrhexis (nodosa)
EXCLUDES trichiasis of eyelid (374.05)

704.3 Variations in hair color
Canities (premature)   Poliosis:
Grayness, hair (premature)   NOS
Heterochromia of hair   circumscripta, acquired

704.8 Other specified diseases of hair and hair follicles
Folliculitis: Sycosis:
NOS   NOS
abscedens et suffodiens   barbae [not parasitic]
pustular   lupoid
Perifolliculitis: vulgaris
NOS
capitis abscedens et suffodiens
scalp

704.9 Unspecified disease of hair and hair follicles

705 Disorders of sweat glands

705.0 Anhidrosis
Hypohidrosis   Oligohidrosis
DEF: Lack or deficiency of ability to sweat.

705.1–707.19 SKIN AND SUBCUTANEOUS TISSUE — Tabular List

705.1 Prickly heat
    Heat rash   Sudamina
    Miliaria rubra (tropicalis)

√5ᵗʰ **705.8 Other specified disorders of sweat glands**
  705.81 Dyshidrosis
    Cheiropompholyx   Pompholyx
    DEF: Vesicular eruption, on hands, feet causing itching and burning.

  705.82 Fox-Fordyce disease
    DEF: Chronic, usually pruritic disease chiefly of women evidenced by small follicular papular eruptions, especially in the axillary and pubic areas; develops from the closure and rupture of the affected apocrine glands' intraepidermal portion of the ducts.

  705.83 Hidradenitis
    Hidradenitis suppurativa
    DEF: Inflamed sweat glands.

  705.89 Other
    Bromhidrosis   Granulosis rubra nasi
    Chromhidrosis   Urhidrosis
    EXCLUDES hidrocystoma (216.0-216.9)
                     hyperhidrosis (780.8)
    DEF: Bromhidrosis: foul-smelling axillary sweat due to decomposed bacteria.
    DEF: Chromhidrosis: secretion of colored sweat.
    DEF: Granulosis rubra nasi: ideopathic condition of children; causes redness, sweating around nose, face and chin; tends to end by puberty.
    DEF: Urhidrosis: urinous substance, such as uric acid, in sweat; occurs in uremia.

705.9 Unspecified disorder of sweat glands
    Disorder of sweat glands NOS

√4ᵗʰ **706 Diseases of sebaceous glands**
  706.0 Acne varioliformis
    Acne: Acne:
      frontalis   necrotica
    DEF: Rare form of acne characterized by persistent brown papulopustules usually on the brow and temporoparietal part of the scalp.

  706.1 Other acne
    Acne: Acne:
      NOS   vulgaris
      conglobata   Blackhead
      cystic   Comedo
      pustular
    EXCLUDES acne rosacea (695.3)

  706.2 Sebaceous cyst
    Atheroma, skin   Wen
    Keratin cyst
    DEF: Benign epidermal cyst, contains sebum and keratin; presents as firm, circumscribed nodule.

  706.3 Seborrhea
    EXCLUDES seborrhea:
                     capitis (690.11)
                     sicca (690.18)
               seborrheic
                   dermatitis (690.10)
                   keratosis (702.11-702.19)
    DEF: Seborrheic dermatitis marked by excessive secretion of sebum; the sebum forms an oily coating, crusts, or scales on the skin; it is also called hypersteatosis.

  706.8 Other specified diseases of sebaceous glands
    Asteatosis (cutis)
    Xerosis cutis

  706.9 Unspecified disease of sebaceous glands

Six Stages of Decubitus Ulcers

 First Stage — Skin is warm, firm, or stretched

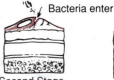 Second Stage — Bacteria enter

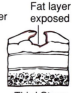 Third Stage — Fat layer exposed

 Fourth Stage — Muscle necrosis

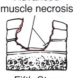 Fifth Stage — Advanced muscle necrosis

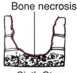 Sixth Stage — Bone necrosis

√4ᵗʰ **707 Chronic ulcer of skin**
  INCLUDES non-infected sinus of skin
               non-healing ulcer
  EXCLUDES specific infections classified under "Infectious and Parasitic Diseases" (001.0-136.9)
               varicose ulcer (454.0, 454.2)

  707.0 Decubitus ulcer [CC] [MC]
    Bed sore
    Decubitus ulcer [any site]
    Plaster ulcer
    Pressure ulcer
    CC Excl: 707.0, 707.8-707.9, 709.8
    AHA: 4Q, '99, 20; 1Q, '96, 15; 3Q, '90, 15; N-D, '87, 9

√5ᵗʰ **707.1 Ulcer of lower limbs, except decubitus**
    Ulcer, chronic:
      neurogenic } of lower limb
      trophic
    ▶Code, if applicable, any causal condition first:◀
      atherosclerosis of the extremities with ulceration (440.23)
      ▶chronic venous hypertension with ulcer (459.31)
      chronic venous hypertension with ulcer and inflammation (459.33)◀
      diabetes mellitus (250.80-250.83)
      ▶postphlebitic syndrome with ulcer (459.11)
      postphlebitic syndrome with ulcer and inflammation (459.13)◀
    AHA: 4Q, '00, 44; 4Q, '99, 15

  707.10 Ulcer of lower limb, unspecified [CC]
    CC Excl: 440.23, 707.10-707.19, 707.8-707.9, 709.8

  707.11 Ulcer of thigh [CC]
    CC Excl: See code 707.10

  707.12 Ulcer of calf [CC]
    CC Excl: See code 707.10

  707.13 Ulcer of ankle [CC]
    CC Excl: See code 707.10

  707.14 Ulcer of heel and midfoot [CC]
    Plantar surface of midfoot
    CC Excl: See code 707.10

  707.15 Ulcer of other part of foot [CC]
    Toes
    CC Excl: See code 707.10

  707.19 Ulcer of other part of lower limb [CC]
    CC Excl: See code 707.10

[N] Newborn Age: 0   [P] Pediatric Age: 0-17   [M] Maternity Age: 12-55   [A] Adult Age: 15-124   [CC] CC Condition   [MC] Major Complication   [CD] Complex Dx   [HIV] HIV Related Dx

SKIN AND SUBCUTANEOUS TISSUE

707.8 Chronic ulcer of other specified sites
Ulcer, chronic:
 neurogenic } of other specified sites
 trophic

707.9 Chronic ulcer of unspecified site
Chronic ulcer NOS
Trophic ulcer NOS
Tropical ulcer NOS
Ulcer of skin NOS

4th 708 Urticaria
EXCLUDES edema:
 angioneurotic (995.1)
 Quincke's (995.1)
 hereditary angioedema (277.6)
 urticaria:
  giant (995.1)
  papulosa (Hebra) (698.2)
  pigmentosa (juvenile) (congenital) (757.33)

DEF: Skin disorder marked by raised edematous patches of skin or mucous membrane with intense itching; also called hives.

708.0 Allergic urticaria
708.1 Idiopathic urticaria
708.2 Urticaria due to cold and heat
 Thermal urticaria
708.3 Dermatographic urticaria
 Dermatographia   Factitial urticaria
708.4 Vibratory urticaria
708.5 Cholinergic urticaria
708.8 Other specified urticaria
 Nettle rash   Urticaria:
 Urticaria: recurrent periodic
  chronic
708.9 Urticaria, unspecified
 Hives NOS

4th 709 Other disorders of skin and subcutaneous tissue
5th **709.0 Dyschromia**
EXCLUDES albinism (270.2)
 pigmented nevus (216.0-216.9)
 that of eyelid (374.52-374.53)

DEF: Pigment disorder of skin or hair.

709.00 Dyschromia, unspecified
709.01 Vitiligo
 DEF: Persistent, progressive development of nonpigmented white patches on otherwise normal skin.

709.09 Other

709.1 Vascular disorders of skin
 Angioma serpiginosum
 Purpura (primary)annularis telangiectodes

709.2 Scar conditions and fibrosis of skin
 Adherent scar (skin)   Fibrosis, skin NOS
 Cicatrix   Scar NOS
 Disfigurement (due to scar)
 EXCLUDES keloid scar (701.4)

AHA: N-D, '84, 19

Cutaneous Lesions

Surface Lesions
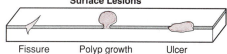
Fissure   Polyp growth   Ulcer

Solid Lesions
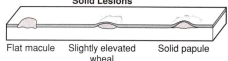
Flat macule   Slightly elevated wheal   Solid papule

Sac Lesions
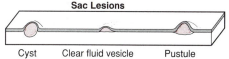
Cyst   Clear fluid vesicle   Pustule

709.3 Degenerative skin disorders
 Calcinosis: Degeneration, skin
  circumscripta   Deposits, skin
  cutis   Senile dermatosis NOS
 Colloid milium   Subcutaneous calcification

709.4 Foreign body granuloma of skin and subcutaneous tissue
 EXCLUDES residual foreign body without granuloma of skin and subcutaneous tissue (729.6)
  that of muscle (728.82)

709.8 Other specified disorders of skin
 Epithelial hyperplasia
 Menstrual dermatosis
 Vesicular eruption

AHA: N-D, '87, 6

DEF: Epithelial hyperplasia: increased number of epitheleal cells.

DEF: Vesicular eruption: liquid-filled structures appearing through skin.

709.9 Unspecified disorder of skin and subcutaneous tissue
 Dermatosis NOS

| Tabular List | MUSCULOSKELTAL SYSTEM AND CONNECTIVE TISSUE | 710–710.5 |

13. DISEASES OF THE MUSCULOSKELETAL SYSTEM AND CONNECTIVE TISSUE (710-739)

Joint Structures

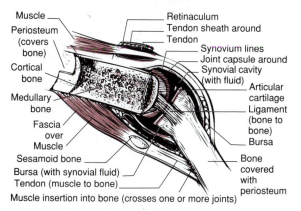

Muscle — Periosteum (covers bone) — Cortical bone — Medullary bone — Fascia over Muscle — Sesamoid bone — Bursa (with synovial fluid) — Tendon (muscle to bone) — Muscle insertion into bone (crosses one or more joints) — Retinaculum — Tendon sheath around Tendon — Synovium lines Joint capsule around Synovial cavity (with fluid) — Articular cartilage — Ligament (bone to bone) — Bursa — Bone covered with periosteum

The following fifth-digit subclassification is for use with categories 711-712, 715-716, 718-719, and 730:
- 0 site unspecified
- 1 shoulder region
  - Acromioclavicular joint(s)
  - Clavicle
  - Glenohumeral joint(s)
  - Scapula
  - Sternoclavicular joint(s)
- 2 upper arm
  - Elbow joint
  - Humerus
- 3 forearm
  - Radius
  - Ulna
  - Wrist joint
- 4 hand
  - Carpus
  - Metacarpus
  - Phalanges [fingers]
- 5 pelvic region and thigh
  - Buttock
  - Femur
  - Hip (joint)
- 6 lower leg
  - Fibula
  - Knee joint
  - Patella
  - Tibia
- 7 ankle and foot
  - Ankle joint
  - Digits [toes]
  - Metatarsus
  - Phalanges, foot
  - Tarsus
  - Other joints in foot
- 8 other specified sites
  - Head
  - Neck
  - Ribs
  - Skull
  - Trunk
  - Vertebral column
- 9 multiple sites

ARTHROPATHIES AND RELATED DISORDERS (710-719)

EXCLUDES disorders of spine (720.0-724.9)

710 Diffuse diseases of connective tissue
  INCLUDES all collagen diseases whose effects are not mainly confined to a single system
  EXCLUDES those affecting mainly the cardiovascular system, i.e., polyarteritis nodosa and allied conditions (446.0-446.7)

710.0 Systemic lupus erythematosus [CC]
  Disseminated lupus erythematosus
  Libman-Sacks disease
  Use additional code to identify manifestation, as:
    endocarditis (424.91)
    nephritis (583.81)
      chronic (582.81)
    nephrotic syndrome (581.81)
  EXCLUDES lupus erythematosus (discoid) NOS (695.4)

CC Excl: 710.0

AHA: 2Q, '97, 8

DEF: A chronic multisystemic inflammatory disease affecting connective tissue; marked by anemia, leukopenia, muscle and joint pains, fever, rash of a butterfly pattern around cheeks and forehead area; of unknown etiology.

710.1 Systemic sclerosis [CC]
  Acrosclerosis   Progressive systemic sclerosis
  CRST syndrome   Scleroderma
  EXCLUDES circumscribed scleroderma (701.0)
  ▶Use additional code to identify manifestation, as:
    lung involvement (517.8)
    myopathy (359.6)◀

CC Excl: 710.1

AHA: 1Q, '88, 6

DEF: Systemic disease, involving excess fibrotic collagen build-up; symptoms include thickened skin; fibrotic degenerative changes in various organs; and vascular abnormalities; condition occurs more often in females.

710.2 Sicca syndrome
  Keratoconjunctivitis sicca   Sjögren's disease

DEF: Autoimmune disease; associated with keratoconjunctivitis, laryngopharyngitis, rhinitis, dry mouth, enlarged parotid gland, and chronic polyarthritis.

710.3 Dermatomyositis [CC]
  Poikilodermatomyositis
  Polymyositis with skin involvement

CC Excl: 710.3

DEF: Polymyositis associated with flat-top purple papules on knuckles; marked by upper eyelid rash, edema of eyelids and orbit area, red rash on forehead, neck, shoulders, trunk and arms; symptoms include fever, weight loss aching muscles; visceral cancer (in individuals older than 40).

710.4 Polymyositis [CC]

CC Excl: 710.4

DEF: Chronic, progressive, inflammatory skeletal muscle disease; causes weakness of limb girdles, neck, pharynx; may precede or follow scleroderma, Sjogren's disease, systemic lupus erythematosus, arthritis, or malignancy.

710.5 Eosinophilia myalgia syndrome [CC]
  Toxic oil syndrome
  Use additional E code to identify drug, if drug induced

CC Excl: 292.0-292.9, 293.0-293.9, 710.5

AHA: 4Q, '92, 21

DEF: Eosinophilia myalgia syndrome (EMS): inflammatory, multisystem fibrosis; associated with ingesting elemetary L-tryptophan; symptoms include myalgia, weak limbs and bulbar muscles, distal sensory loss, areflexia, arthralgia, cough, fever, fatigue, skin rashes, myopathy, and eosinophil counts greater than 1000/microliter.

DEF: Toxic oil syndrome: syndrome silimar to EMS due to ingesting contaminated cooking oil.

MUSCULOSKELTAL SYSTEM AND CONNECTIVE TISSUE

710.8 Other specified diffuse diseases of connective tissue [CC]
Multifocal fibrosclerosis (idiopathic) NEC
Systemic fibrosclerosing syndrome

CC Excl: 710.8

AHA: M-A, '87, 12

710.9 Unspecified diffuse connective tissue disease
Collagen disease NOS

✓4th 711 Arthropathy associated with infections

INCLUDES arthritis, arthropathy, polyarthritis, polyarthropathy associated with conditions classifiable below

EXCLUDES rheumatic fever (390)

The following fifth-digit subclassification is for use with category 711; valid digits are in [brackets] under each code.

- 0 site unspecified
- 1 shoulder region
- 2 upper arm
- 3 forearm
- 4 hand
- 5 pelvic region and thigh
- 6 lower leg
- 7 ankle and foot
- 8 other specified sites
- 9 multiple sites

AHA: 1Q, '92, 17

§ ✓5th 711.0 Pyogenic arthritis [CC]
[0-9]
Arthritis or polyarthritis (due to):
coliform [Escherichia coli]
Hemophilus influenzae [H. influenzae]
pneumococcal
Pseudomonas
staphylococcal
streptococcal
Pyarthrosis
Use additional code to identify infectious organism (041.0-041.8)

CC Excl: For code 711.00: 015.80-015.96, 017.90-017.96, 036.82, 056.71, 098.50-098.51, 098.59, 098.89, 711.00-711.99, 712.10-712.99, 713.0-713.8, 714.0, 715.00, 715.09-715.10, 715.18-715.98, 716.00-716.99, 718.00-718.08, 719.00-719.10, 719.18-719.99 **For code 711.01:** 015.80-015.96, 017.90-017.96, 036.82, 056.71, 098.50-098.51, 098.59, 098.89, 711.00-711.01, 711.08-711.11, 711.18-711.21, 711.28-711.31, 711.38-711.41, 711.48-711.51, 711.58-711.61, 711.68-711.71, 711.78-711.81, 711.88-711.91, 711.98-711.99, 712.10-712.11, 712.18-712.21, 712.28-712.31, 712.38-712.81, 712.88-712.91, 712.98-712.99, 713.0-713.8, 714.0, 715.00, 715.09-715.11, 715.18-715.21, 715.28-715.31, 715.38-715.91, 715.98, 716.00-716.01, 716.08-716.11, 716.18-716.21, 716.28-716.31, 716.38-716.41, 716.48-716.51, 716.58-716.61, 716.68-716.81, 716.88-716.91, 716.98-716.99, 718.00-718.01, 718.08, 719.00-719.01, 719.11, 719.18-719.21, 719.28-719.31, 719.38-719.41, 719.48-719.51, 719.58-719.61, 719.68-719.70, 719.78-719.81, 719.88-719.91, 719.98-719.99 **For code 711.02:** 015.80-015.96, 017.90-017.96, 036.82, 056.71, 098.50-098.51, 098.59, 098.89, 711.00, 711.02, 711.08-711.10, 711.12, 711.18-711.20, 711.22, 711.28-711.30, 711.32, 711.38-711.40, 711.42, 711.48-711.50, 711.52, 711.58-711.60, 711.62, 711.68-711.70, 711.72, 711.78-711.80, 711.82, 711.88-711.90, 711.92, 711.98-711.99, 712.10, 712.12, 712.18-712.20, 712.22, 712.28-712.30, 712.32, 712.38-712.80, 712.82, 712.88-712.90, 712.92, 712.98-712.99, 713.0-713.8, 714.0, 715.00, 715.09-715.10, 715.12, 715.18, 715.20, 715.22, 715.28, 715.30, 715.32, 715.38-715.90, 715.92, 715.98, 716.00, 716.02, 716.08-716.10, 716.12, 716.18-716.20, 716.22, 716.28-716.30, 716.32, 716.38-716.40, 716.42, 716.48-716.50, 716.52, 716.58-716.60, 716.62, 716.68, 716.80, 716.82, 716.88-716.90, 716.92, 716.98-716.99, 718.00, 718.02, 718.08, 719.00, 719.02, 719.08-719.10, 719.12, 719.18-719.20, 719.22, 719.28-719.30, 719.32, 719.38-719.40, 719.42, 719.48-719.50, 719.52, 719.58-719.60, 719.62, 719.68-719.70, 719.78-719.80, 719.82, 719.88-719.90, 719.92, 719.98-719.99 **For code 711.03:** 015.80-015.96, 017.90-017.96, 036.82, 056.71, 098.50-098.51, 098.59, 098.89, 711.00, 711.03, 711.08-711.10, 711.13, 711.18-711.20, 711.23, 711.28-711.30, 711.33, 711.38-711.40, 711.43, 711.48-711.50, 711.53, 711.58-711.60, 711.63, 711.68-711.70, 711.73, 711.78-711.80, 711.83, 711.88-711.90, 711.93, 711.98-711.99, 712.10, 712.13, 712.18-712.20, 712.23, 712.28-712.30, 712.33, 712.38-712.80, 712.83, 712.88-712.90, 712.93, 712.98-712.99, 713.0-713.8, 714.0, 715.00, 715.09-715.10, 715.13, 715.18, 715.20, 715.23, 715.28, 715.30, 715.33, 715.38-715.90, 715.93, 715.98, 716.00, 716.03, 716.08-716.10, 716.13, 716.18-716.20, 716.23, 716.28-716.30, 716.33, 716.38-716.40, 716.43, 716.48-716.50, 716.53, 716.58-716.60, 716.63, 716.68, 716.80, 716.83, 716.88-716.90, 716.93, 716.98-716.99, 718.00, 718.03, 718.08, 719.00, 719.03, 719.08-719.10, 719.13, 719.18-719.20, 719.23, 719.28-719.30, 719.33, 719.38-719.40, 719.43, 719.48-719.50, 719.53, 719.58-719.60, 719.63, 719.68-719.70, 719.78-719.80, 719.83, 719.88-719.90, 719.93, 719.98-719.99 **For code 711.04:** 015.80-015.96, 017.90-017.96, 036.82, 056.71, 098.50-098.51, 098.59, 098.89, 711.00, 711.04, 711.08-711.10, 711.14, 711.18-711.20, 711.24, 711.28-711.30, 711.34, 711.38-711.40, 711.44, 711.48-711.50, 711.54, 711.58-711.60, 711.64, 711.68-711.70, 711.74, 711.78-711.80, 711.84, 711.88-711.90, 711.94, 711.98-711.99, 712.10, 712.14, 712.18-712.20, 712.24, 712.28-712.30, 712.34, 712.38-712.80, 712.84, 712.88-712.90, 712.94, 712.98-712.99, 713.0-713.8, 714.0, 715.00-715.10, 715.14, 715.18, 715.20, 715.24, 715.28, 715.30, 715.34, 715.38-715.90, 715.94, 715.98, 716.00, 716.04, 716.08-716.10, 716.14, 716.18-716.20, 716.24, 716.28-716.30, 716.34, 716.38-716.40, 716.44, 716.48-716.50, 716.54, 716.58-716.60, 716.64, 716.68, 716.80, 716.84, 716.88-716.90, 716.94, 716.98-716.99, 718.00, 718.04, 718.08, 719.00, 719.04, 719.08-719.10, 719.14, 719.18-719.20, 719.24, 719.28-719.30, 719.34, 719.38-719.40, 719.44, 719.48-719.50, 719.54, 719.58-719.60, 719.64, 719.68-719.70, 719.78-719.80, 719.84, 719.88-719.90, 719.94, 719.98-719.99 **For code 711.05:** 015.80-015.96, 017.90-017.96, 036.82, 056.71, 098.50-098.51, 098.59, 098.89, 711.00, 711.05, 711.08-711.10, 711.15, 711.18-711.20, 711.25, 711.28-711.30, 711.35, 711.38-711.40, 711.45, 711.48-711.50, 711.55, 711.58-711.60, 711.65, 711.68-711.70, 711.75, 711.78-711.80, 711.85, 711.88-711.90, 711.95, 711.98-711.99, 712.10, 712.15, 712.18-712.20, 712.25, 712.28-712.30, 712.35, 712.38-712.80, 712.85, 712.88-712.90, 712.95, 712.98-712.99, 713.0-713.8, 714.0, 715.00, 715.09-715.10, 715.15, 715.18, 715.20, 715.25, 715.28, 715.30, 715.35, 715.38-715.90, 715.95, 715.98, 716.00, 716.05, 716.08-716.10, 716.15, 716.18-716.20, 716.25, 716.28-716.30, 716.35, 716.38-716.40, 716.45, 716.48-716.50, 716.55, 716.58-716.60, 716.65, 716.68, 716.80, 716.85, 716.88-716.90, 716.95, 716.98-716.99, 718.00, 718.05, 718.08, 719.00, 719.05, 719.08-719.10, 719.15, 719.18-719.20, 719.25, 719.28-719.30, 719.35, 719.38-719.40, 719.45, 719.48-719.50, 719.55, 719.58-719.60, 719.65, 719.68-719.70, 719.78-719.80, 719.85, 719.88-719.90, 719.95, 719.98-719.99 **For code 711.06:** 015.80-015.96, 017.90-017.96, 036.82, 056.71, 098.50-098.51, 098.59, 098.89, 711.00, 711.06, 711.08-711.10, 711.16, 711.18-711.20, 711.26, 711.28-711.30, 711.36, 711.38-711.40, 711.46, 711.48-711.50, 711.56, 711.58-711.60, 711.66, 711.68-711.70, 711.76, 711.78-711.80, 711.86, 711.88-711.90, 711.96, 711.98-711.99, 712.10, 712.16, 712.18-712.20, 712.26, 712.28-712.30, 712.36, 712.38-712.80, 712.86, 712.88-712.90, 712.96, 712.98-712.99, 713.0-713.8, 714.0, 715.00, 715.09-715.10, 715.16, 715.18, 715.20, 715.26, 715.28, 715.30, 715.36, 715.38-715.90, 715.96, 715.98, 716.00, 716.06, 716.08-716.10, 716.16, 716.18-716.20, 716.26, 716.28-716.30, 716.36, 716.38-716.40, 716.46, 716.48-716.50, 716.56, 716.58-716.60, 716.66, 716.68, 716.80, 716.86, 716.88-716.90, 716.96, 716.98-716.99, 718.00, 718.08, 719.00, 719.06, 719.08-719.10, 719.16, 719.18-719.20, 719.26, 719.28-719.30, 719.36, 719.38-719.40, 719.46, 719.48-719.50, 719.56, 719.58-719.60, 719.66, 719.68-719.70, 719.76, 719.78-719.80, 719.86, 719.88-719.90, 719.96, 719.98-719.99 **For code 711.07:** 015.80-015.96, 017.90-017.96, 036.82, 056.71, 098.50-098.51, 098.59, 098.89, 711.00, 711.07-711.10, 711.17-711.20, 711.27-711.30, 711.37-711.40, 711.47-711.50, 711.57-711.60, 711.67-711.70, 711.77-711.80, 711.87-711.90, 711.97-711.99, 712.10, 712.17-712.20, 712.27-712.30, 712.37-712.80, 712.87-712.90, 712.97-712.99, 713.0-713.8, 714.0, 715.00, 715.09-715.10, 715.17-715.18, 715.20, 715.27-715.28, 715.30, 715.37-715.90, 715.97-715.98, 716.00, 716.07-716.10, 716.17-716.20, 716.27-716.30, 716.37-716.40, 716.47-716.50, 716.57-716.60, 716.67-716.68, 716.80, 716.87-716.90, 716.97-716.99, 718.00, 718.07-718.08, 719.00, 719.07-719.10, 719.17-719.20, 719.27-719.30, 719.37-719.40, 719.47-719.50, 719.57-719.60, 719.67-719.70, 719.77-719.80, 719.87-719.90, 719.97-719.99 **For code 711.08:** 015.80-015.96, 017.90-017.96, 036.82, 056.71, 098.50-098.51, 098.59, 098.89, 711.00-711.99, 712.10-712.99, 713.0-713.8, 714.0, 715.00, 715.09-715.10, 715.18-715.98, 716.00-716.99, 718.00-718.08, 719.00-719.10, 719.18-719.99 **For code 711.09:** See code 711.08

AHA: 1Q, '92, 16; 1Q, '91, 15

DEF: Infectious arthritis caused by various bacteria; marked by inflamed synovial membranes, and purulent effusion in joints.

---

§ Requires fifth-digit. Valid digits are in [brackets] under each code. See beginning of section 710-739 for codes and definitions.

MUSCULOSKELTAL SYSTEM AND CONNECTIVE TISSUE

§ ✓5th **711.1** **Arthropathy associated with Reiter's disease and nonspecific urethritis**
[0-9]
Code first underlying disease as:
nonspecific urethritis (099.4)
Reiter's disease (099.3)

DEF: Reiter's disease: joint disease marked by diarrhea, urethritis, conjunctivitis, keratosis and arthritis; of unknown etiology; affects young males.

DEF: Urethritis: inflamed urethra.

§ ✓5th **711.2** **Arthropathy in Behçet's syndrome**
[0-9]
Code first underlying disease (136.1)

DEF: Behçet's syndrome: Chronic inflammatory disorder, of unknown etiology; affects small blood vessels; causes ulcers of oral and pharyngeal mucous membranes and genitalia, skin lesions, retinal vasculitis, optic atrophy and severe uveitis.

§ ✓5th **711.3** **Postdysenteric arthropathy**
[0-9]
Code first underlying disease as:
dysentery (009.0)
enteritis, infectious (008.0-009.3)
paratyphoid fever (002.1-002.9)
typhoid fever (002.0)
EXCLUDES salmonella arthritis (003.23)

§ ✓5th **711.4** **Arthropathy associated with other bacterial diseases**
[0-9]
Code first underlying disease as:
diseases classifiable to 010-040, 090-099, except as in 711.1, 711.3, and 713.5
leprosy (030.0-030.9)
tuberculosis (015.0-015.9)
EXCLUDES gonococcal arthritis (098.50)
meningococcal arthritis (036.82)

§ ✓5th **711.5** **Arthropathy associated with other viral diseases**
[0-9]
Code first underlying disease as:
diseases classifiable to 045-049, 050-079, 480, 487
O'nyong nyong (066.3)
EXCLUDES that due to rubella (056.71)

§ ✓5th **711.6** **Arthropathy associated with mycoses** **CC**
[0-9]
Code first underlying disease (110.0-118)
CC Excl: For code 711.60: See code 711.08: **For code 711.61:** 015.80-015.96, 017.90-017.96, 036.82, 056.71, 098.50-098.51, 098.59, 098.89, 711.00-711.01, 711.08-711.11, 711.18-711.21, 711.28-711.31, 711.38-711.41, 711.48-711.51, 711.58-711.61, 711.68-711.71, 711.78-711.81, 711.88-711.91, 711.98-711.99, 712.10-712.11, 712.18-712.21, 712.28-712.31, 712.38-712.81, 712.88-712.91, 712.98-712.99, 713.0-713.8, 714.0, 715.00, 715.09-715.11, 715.18-715.21, 715.28, 715.30-715.31, 715.38-715.91, 715.98, 716.00-716.01, 716.08-716.11, 716.18-716.21, 716.28-716.31, 716.38-716.41, 716.48-716.51, 716.58-716.61, 716.68, 716.80-716.81, 716.88-716.91, 716.98-716.99, 718.00-718.01, 718.08, 719.00-719.01, 719.08-719.11, 719.18-719.21, 719.28-719.31, 719.38-719.41, 719.48-719.51, 719.58-719.61, 719.68-719.70, 719.78-719.81, 719.88-719.91, 719.98-719.99; **For code 711.62:** 015.80-015.96, 017.90-017.96, 036.82, 056.71, 098.50-098.51, 098.59, 098.89, 711.00, 711.02, 711.08-711.10, 711.12, 711.18-711.20, 711.22, 711.28-711.30, 711.32, 711.38-711.40, 711.42, 711.48-711.50, 711.52, 711.58-711.60, 711.62, 711.68-711.70, 711.72, 711.78-711.80, 711.82, 711.88-711.90, 711.92, 711.98-711.99, 712.10, 712.12, 712.18-712.20, 712.22, 712.28-712.30, 712.32, 712.38-712.80, 712.82, 712.88-712.90, 712.92, 712.98-712.99, 713.0-713.8, 714.0, 715.00, 715.09-715.10, 715.12, 715.18, 715.20, 715.22, 715.28, 715.30, 715.32, 715.38-715.90, 715.92, 715.98, 716.00, 716.02, 716.08-716.10, 716.12, 716.18-716.20, 716.22, 716.28-716.30, 716.32, 716.38-716.40, 716.42, 716.48-716.50, 716.52, 716.58-716.60, 716.62, 716.68, 716.80, 716.82, 716.88-716.90, 716.92, 716.98-716.99, 718.00, 718.02, 718.08, 719.00, 719.02, 719.08-719.10, 719.12, 719.18-719.20, 719.22, 719.28-719.30, 719.32, 719.38-719.40, 719.42, 719.48-719.50, 719.52, 719.58-719.60, 719.62, 719.68-719.70, 719.78-719.80, 719.82, 719.88-719.90, 719.92, 719.98-719.99; **For code 711.63:** 015.80-015.96, 017.90-017.96, 036.82, 056.71, 098.50-098.51, 098.59, 098.89, 711.00, 711.03, 711.08-711.10, 711.13, 711.18-711.20, 711.23, 711.28-711.30, 711.33, 711.38-711.40, 711.43, 711.48-711.50, 711.53, 711.58-711.60, 711.63, 711.68-711.70, 711.73, 711.78-711.80, 711.83, 711.88-711.90, 711.93, 711.98-711.99, 712.10, 712.13, 712.18-712.20, 712.23, 712.28-712.30, 712.33, 712.38-712.80, 712.83, 712.88-712.90, 712.93, 712.98-712.99, 713.0-713.8, 714.0, 715.00, 715.09-715.10, 715.13, 715.18, 715.20, 715.23, 715.28, 715.30, 715.33, 715.38-715.90, 715.93, 715.98, 716.00, 716.03, 716.08-716.10, 716.13, 716.18-716.20, 716.23, 716.28-716.30, 716.33, 716.38-716.40, 716.43, 716.48-716.50, 716.53, 716.58-716.60, 716.63, 716.68, 716.80, 716.83, 716.88-716.90, 716.93, 716.98-716.99, 718.00, 718.03, 718.08, 719.00, 719.03, 719.08-719.10, 719.13, 719.18-719.20, 719.23, 719.28-719.30, 719.33, 719.38-719.40, 719.43, 719.48-719.50, 719.53, 719.58-719.60, 719.63, 719.68-719.70, 719.78-719.80, 719.83, 719.88-719.90, 719.93, 719.98-719.99 **For code 711.64:** 015.80-015.96, 017.90-017.96, 036.82, 056.71, 098.50-098.51, 098.59, 098.89, 711.00, 711.04, 711.08-711.10, 711.14, 711.18-711.20, 711.24, 711.28-711.30, 711.34, 711.38-711.40, 711.44, 711.48-711.50, 711.5, 711.58-711.60, 711.64, 711.68-711.70, 711.74, 711.78-711.80, 711.84, 711.88-711.90, 711.94, 711.98-711.99, 712.10, 712.14, 712.18-712.20, 712.24, 712.28-712.30, 712.34, 712.38-712.80, 712.84, 712.88-712.90, 712.94, 712.98-712.99, 713.0-713.8, 714.0, 715.00-715.10, 715.14, 715.18, 715.20, 715.24, 715.28, 715.30, 715.34, 715.38-715.90, 715.94, 715.98, 716.00, 716.04, 716.08-716.10, 716.14, 716.18-716.20, 716.24, 716.28-716.30, 716.34, 716.38-716.40, 716.44, 716.48-716.50, 716.54, 716.58-716.60, 716.64, 716.68, 716.80, 716.84, 716.88-716.90, 716.94, 716.98-716.99, 718.00, 718.04, 718.08, 719.00, 719.04, 719.08-719.10, 719.14, 719.18-719.20, 719.24, 719.28-719.30, 719.34, 719.38-719.40, 719.44, 719.48-719.50, 719.54, 719.58-719.60, 719.64, 719.68-719.70, 719.78-719.80, 719.84, 719.88-719.90, 719.94, 719.98-719.99CC **For code 711.65:** 015.80-015.96, 017.90-017.96, 036.82, 056.71, 098.50-098.51, 098.59, 098.89, 711.00, 711.05, 711.08-711.10, 711.15, 711.18-711.20, 711.25, 711.28-711.30, 711.35, 711.38-711.40, 711.45, 711.48-711.50, 711.55, 711.58-711.60, 711.65, 711.68-711.70, 711.75, 711.78-711.80, 711.85, 711.88-711.90, 711.95, 711.98-711.99, 712.10, 712.15, 712.18-712.20, 712.25, 712.28-712.30, 712.35, 712.38-712.80, 712.85, 712.88-712.90, 712.95, 712.98-712.99, 713.0-713.8, 714.0, 715.00, 715.09-715.10, 715.15, 715.18, 715.20, 715.25, 715.28, 715.30, 715.35, 715.38-715.90, 715.95, 715.98, 716.00, 716.05, 716.08-716.10, 716.15, 716.18-716.20, 716.25, 716.28-716.30, 716.35, 716.38-716.40, 716.45, 716.48-716.50, 716.55, 716.58-716.60, 716.65, 716.68, 716.80, 716.85, 716.88-716.90, 716.95, 716.98-716.99, 718.00, 718.05, 718.08, 719.00, 719.05, 719.08-719.10, 719.15, 719.18-719.20, 719.25, 719.28-719.30, 719.35, 719.38-719.40, 719.45, 719.48-719.50, 719.55, 719.58-719.60, 719.65, 719.68-719.70, 719.75, 719.78-719.80, 719.85, 719.88-719.90, 719.95, 719.98-719.99 **For code 711.66:** 015.80-015.96, 017.90-017.96, 036.82, 056.71, 098.50-098.51, 098.59, 098.89, 711.00, 711.06, 711.08-711.10, 711.16, 711.18-711.20, 711.26, 711.28-711.30, 711.36, 711.38-711.40, 711.46, 711.48-711.50, 711.56, 711.58-711.60, 711.66, 711.68-711.70, 711.76, 711.78-711.80, 711.86, 711.88-711.90, 711.96, 711.98-711.99, 712.10, 712.16, 712.18-712.20, 712.26, 712.28-712.30, 712.36, 712.38-712.80, 712.86, 712.88-712.90, 712.96, 712.98-712.99, 713.0-713.8, 714.0, 715.00, 715.09-715.10, 715.16, 715.18, 715.20, 715.26, 715.28, 715.30, 715.36, 715.38-715.90, 715.96, 715.98, 716.00, 716.06, 716.08-716.10, 716.16, 716.18-716.20, 716.26, 716.28-716.30, 716.36, 716.38-716.40, 716.46, 716.48-716.50, 716.56, 716.58-716.60, 716.66, 716.68, 716.80, 716.86, 716.88-716.90, 716.96, 716.98-716.99, 718.00, 718.08, 719.00, 719.06, 719.08-719.10, 719.16, 719.18-719.20, 719.26, 719.28-719.30, 719.36, 719.38-719.40, 719.46, 719.48-719.50, 719.56, 719.58-719.60, 719.66, 719.68-719.70, 719.76, 719.78-719.80, 719.86, 719.88-719.90, 719.96, 719.98-719.99 **For code 711.67:** 015.80-015.96, 017.90-017.96, 036.82, 056.71, 098.50-098.51, 098.59, 098.89, 711.00, 711.07-711.10, 711.17-711.20, 711.27-711.30, 711.37-711.40, 711.47-711.50, 711.57-711.60, 711.67-711.70, 711.77-711.80, 711.87-711.90, 711.97-711.99, 712.10, 712.17-712.20, 712.27-712.30, 712.37-712.80, 712.87-712.90, 712.97-712.99, 713.0-713.8, 714.0, 715.00, 715.09-715.10, 715.17-715.18, 715.20, 715.27-715.28, 715.30, 715.37-715.90, 715.97-715.98, 716.00, 716.07-716.10, 716.17-716.20, 716.27-716.30, 716.37-716.40, 716.47-716.50, 716.57-716.60, 716.67-716.80, 716.87-716.90, 716.97-716.99, 718.00, 718.07-718.08, 719.00, 719.07-719.10, 719.17-719.20, 719.27-719.30, 719.37-719.40, 719.47-719.50, 719.57-719.60, 719.67-719.70, 719.77-719.80, 719.87-719.90, 719.97-719.99 **For code 711.68:** 015.80-015.96, 017.90-017.96, 036.82, 056.71, 098.50-098.51, 098.59, 098.89, 711.00-711.99, 712.10-712.99, 713.0-713.8, 714.0, 715.00, 715.09-715.10, 715.18-715.98, 716.00-716.99, 718.00-718.08, 719.00-719.10, 719.18-719.99 **For code 711.69:** See code 711.68

§ Requires fifth-digit. Valid digits are in [brackets] under each code. See beginning of section 710-739 for codes and definitions.

✓4th Additional Digit Required   ✓5th   Nonspecific PDx   Unacceptable PDx   Manifestation Code   **MSP** Medicare Secondary Payer   ▶◀ Revised Text   ● New Code   ▲ Revised Code Title

2002 Ingenix, Inc.

MUSCULOSKELTAL SYSTEM AND CONNECTIVE TISSUE

§ ✓5th **711.7 Arthropathy associated with helminthiasis**
[0-9]
Code first underlying disease as:
 filariasis (125.0-125.9)

§ ✓5th **711.8 Arthropathy associated with other infectious and parasitic diseases**
[0-9]
Code first underlying disease as:
 diseases classifiable to 080-088, 100-104, 130-136
EXCLUDES arthropathy associated with sarcoidosis (713.7)
AHA: 4Q, '91, 15; 3Q, '90, 14

§ ✓5th **711.9 Unspecified infective arthritis**
[0-9]
Infective arthritis or polyarthritis (acute) (chronic) (subacute) NOS

✓4th **712 Crystal arthropathies**
INCLUDES crystal-induced arthritis and synovitis
EXCLUDES gouty arthropathy (274.0)
DEF: Joint disease due to urate crystal deposit in joints or synovial membranes.

The following fifth-digit subclassification is for use with category 712; valid digits are in [brackets] under each code. See above category 710 for definitions:
 0 site unspecified
 1 shoulder region
 2 upper arm
 3 forearm
 4 hand
 5 pelvic region and thigh
 6 lower leg
 7 ankle and foot
 8 other specified sites
 9 multiple sites

§ ✓5th **712.1 Chondrocalcinosis due to dicalcium phosphate crystals**
[0-9]
Chondrocalcinosis due to dicalcium phosphate crystals (with other crystals)
Code first underlying disease (275.4)

§ ✓5th **712.2 Chondrocalcinosis due to pyrophosphate crystals**
[0-9]
Code first underlying disease (275.4)

§ ✓5th **712.3 Chondrocalcinosis, unspecified**
[0-9]
Code first underlying disease (275.4)

§ ✓5th **712.8 Other specified crystal arthropathies**
[0-9]

§ ✓5th **712.9 Unspecified crystal arthropathy**
[0-9]

✓4th **713 Arthropathy associated with other disorders classified elsewhere**
INCLUDES arthritis
 arthropathy   associated with
 polyarthritis   conditions
 polyarthropathy   classifiable below

713.0 Arthropathy associated with other endocrine and metabolic disorders
Code first underlying disease as:
 acromegaly (253.0)
 hemochromatosis (275.0)
 hyperparathyroidism (252.0)
 hypogammaglobulinemia (279.00-279.09)
 hypothyroidism (243-244.9)
 lipoid metabolism disorder (272.0-272.9)
 ochronosis (270.2)
EXCLUDES arthropathy associated with:
 amyloidosis (713.7)
 crystal deposition disorders, except gout (712.1-712.9)
 diabetic neuropathy (713.5)
 gouty arthropathy (274.0)

713.1 Arthropathy associated with gastrointestinal conditions other than infections
Code first underlying disease as:
 regional enteritis (555.0-555.9)
 ulcerative colitis (556)

713.2 Arthropathy associated with hematological disorders
Code first underlying disease as:
 hemoglobinopathy (282.4-282.7)
 hemophilia (286.0-286.2)
 leukemia (204.0-208.9)
 malignant reticulosis (202.3)
 multiple myelomatosis (203.0)
EXCLUDES arthropathy associated with Henoch-Schönlein purpura (713.6)

713.3 Arthropathy associated with dermatological disorders
Code first underlying disease as:
 erythema multiforme (695.1)
 erythema nodosum (695.2)
EXCLUDES psoriatic arthropathy (696.0)

713.4 Arthropathy associated with respiratory disorders
Code first underlying disease as:
 diseases classifiable to 490-519
EXCLUDES arthropathy associated with respiratory infections (711.0, 711.4-711.8)

713.5 Arthropathy associated with neurological disorders
Charcôt's arthropathy } associated with diseases
Neuropathic arthritis } classifiable elsewhere
Code first underlying disease as:
 neuropathic joint disease [Charcôt's joints]:
  NOS (094.0)
  diabetic (250.6)
  syringomyelic (336.0)
  tabetic [syphilitic] (094.0)

713.6 Arthropathy associated with hypersensitivity reaction
Code first underlying disease as:
 Henoch (-Schönlein) purpura (287.0)
 serum sickness (999.5)
EXCLUDES allergic arthritis NOS (716.2)

713.7 Other general diseases with articular involvement
Code first underlying disease as:
 amyloidosis (277.3)
 familial Mediterranean fever (277.3)
 sarcoidosis (135)
AHA: 2Q, '97, 12

713.8 Arthropathy associated with other condition classifiable elsewhere
Code first underlying disease as:
 conditions classifiable elsewhere except as in 711.1-711.8, 712, and 713.0-713.7

✓4th **714 Rheumatoid arthritis and other inflammatory polyarthropathies**
EXCLUDES rheumatic fever (390)
 rheumatoid arthritis of spine NOS (720.0)
AHA: 2Q, '95, 3

714.0 Rheumatoid arthritis
Arthritis or polyarthritis:
 atrophic
 rheumatic (chronic)
Use additional code to identify manifestation, as:
 myopathy (359.6)
 polyneuropathy (357.1)
EXCLUDES juvenile rheumatoid arthritis NOS (714.30)
AHA: 1Q, '90, 5
DEF: Chronic systemic disease principally of joints, manifested by inflammatory changes in articular structures and synovial membranes, atrophy, and loss in bone density.

§ Requires fifth-digit. Valid digits are in [brackets] under each code. See beginning of section 710-739 for codes and definitions.

N Newborn Age: 0   P Pediatric Age: 0-17   M Maternity Age: 12-55   A Adult Age: 15-124   CC CC Condition   MC Major Complication   CD Complex Dx   HIV HIV Related Dx

MUSCULOSKELETAL SYSTEM AND CONNECTIVE TISSUE

714.1 Felty's syndrome `CC`
Rheumatoid arthritis with splenoadenomegaly and leukopenia
CC Excl: 036.82, 056.71, 711.00-711.99, 712.10-712.99, 713.0-713.8, 714.0-714.4, 715.00, 715.09-715.10, 715.18-715.98, 716.00-716.99, 718.00-718.08, 719.00-719.10, 719.18-719.70, 719.75-719.99

DEF: Syndrome marked by rheumatoid arthritis, splenomegaly, leukopenia, pigmented spots on lower extremity skin, anemia, and thrombocytopenia.

714.2 Other rheumatoid arthritis with visceral or systemic involvement `CC`
Rheumatoid carditis
CC Excl: See code 714.1

√5th 714.3 Juvenile chronic polyarthritis
DEF: Rheumatoid arthritis of more than one joint; lasts longer than six weeks in age 17 or younger; symptoms include fever, erythematous rash, weight loss, lymphadenopathy, hepatosplenomegaly and pericarditis.

714.30 Polyarticular juvenile rheumatoid arthritis, chronic or unspecified `CC`
Juvenile rheumatoid arthritis NOS
Still's disease
CC Excl: See code 714.1

714.31 Polyarticular juvenile rheumatoid arthritis, acute `CC`
CC Excl: See code 714.1

714.32 Pauciarticular juvenile rheumatoid arthritis `CC`
CC Excl: See code 714.1

714.33 Monoarticular juvenile rheumatoid arthritis `CC`
CC Excl: See code 714.1

714.4 Chronic postrheumatic arthropathy
Chronic rheumatoid nodular fibrositis
Jaccoud's syndrome
DEF: Persistent joint disorder; follows previous rheumatic infection.

√5th 714.8 Other specified inflammatory polyarthropathies
714.81 Rheumatoid lung
Caplan's syndrome
Diffuse interstitial rheumatoid disease of lung
Fibrosing alveolitis, rheumatoid
DEF: Lung disorders associated with rheumatoid arthritis.

714.89 Other

714.9 Unspecified inflammatory polyarthropathy
Inflammatory polyarthropathy or polyarthritis NOS
EXCLUDES polyarthropathy NOS (716.5)

√4th 715 Osteoarthrosis and allied disorders
Note: Localized, in the subcategories below, includes bilateral involvement of the same site.
INCLUDES arthritis or polyarthritis:
degenerative
hypertrophic
degenerative joint disease
osteoarthritis
EXCLUDES Marie-Strümpell spondylitis (720.0)
osteoarthrosis [osteoarthritis] of spine (721.0-721.9)

The following fifth-digit subclassification is for use with category 715; valid digits are in [brackets] under each code. See definitions prior to category 710.
0 site unspecified
1 shoulder region
2 upper arm
3 forearm
4 hand
5 pelvic region and thigh
6 lower leg
7 ankle and foot
8 other specified sites
9 multiple sites

§ **√5th 715.0 Osteoarthrosis, generalized**
[0,4,9] Degenerative joint disease, involving multiple joints
Primary generalized hypertrophic osteoarthrosis
DEF: Chronic noninflammatory arthritis; marked by degenerated articular cartilage and enlarged bone; symptoms include pain and stiffness with activity; occurs among elderly.

§ **√5th 715.1 Osteoarthrosis, localized, primary**
[0-8] Localized osteoarthropathy, idiopathic

§ **√5th 715.2 Osteoarthrosis, localized, secondary**
[0-8] Coxae malum senilis

§ **√5th 715.3 Osteoarthrosis, localized, not specified whether**
[0-8] **primary or secondary**
Otto's pelvis

§ **√5th 715.8 Osteoarthrosis involving, or with mention of more**
[0,9] **than one site, but not specified as generalized**

§ **√5th¹ 715.9 Osteoarthrosis, unspecified whether generalized or**
[0-8] **localized**
AHA: For code 715.90: 2Q, '97, 12
AHA: N-D, '87, 7

√4th 716 Other and unspecified arthropathies
EXCLUDES cricoarytenoid arthropathy (478.79)

The following fifth-digit subclassification is for use with category 716; valid digits are in [brackets] under each code. See above category 710 for definitions.
0 site unspecified
1 shoulder region
2 upper arm
3 forearm
4 hand
5 pelvic region and thigh
6 lower leg
7 ankle and foot
8 other specified sites
9 multiple sites

AHA: 2Q, '95, 3

§ **√5th 716.0 Kaschin-Beck disease**
[0-9] Endemic polyarthritis
DEF: Chronic degenerative disease of spine and peripheral joints; occurs in eastern Siberian, northern Chinese, and Korean youth; may be a mycotoxicosis caused by eating cereals infected with fungus.

§ **√5th 716.1 Traumatic arthropathy**
[0-9] **AHA:** For Code 716.11: ▶1Q, '02, 9◀

---

¹ Nonspecific PDx=0
§ Requires fifth-digit. Valid digits are in [brackets] under each code. See beginning of section 710-739 for codes and definitions.

    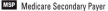

MUSCULOSKELTAL SYSTEM AND CONNECTIVE TISSUE

§ ✓5th **716.2 Allergic arthritis**
[0-9]
EXCLUDES: arthritis associated with Henoch-Schönlein purpura or serum sickness (713.6)

§ ✓5th **716.3 Climacteric arthritis** ♀
[0-9] Menopausal arthritis
DEF: Ovarian hormone deficiency; causes pain in small joints, shoulders, elbows or knees; affects females at menopause; also called arthropathia ovaripriva.

§ ✓5th **716.4 Transient arthropathy**
[0-9] EXCLUDES: palindromic rheumatism (719.3)

§ ✓5th **716.5 Unspecified polyarthropathy or polyarthritis**
[0-9]

§ ✓5th **716.6 Unspecified monoarthritis**
[0-8] Coxitis

§ ✓5th **716.8 Other specified arthropathy**
[0-9]

§ ✓5th **716.9 Arthropathy, unspecified**
[0-9]
Arthritis
Arthropathy } (acute) (chronic) (subacute)

Articular rheumatism (chronic)
Inflammation of joint NOS

✓4th **717 Internal derangement of knee**

INCLUDES: degeneration
rupture, old } of articular cartilage or meniscus of knee
tear, old

EXCLUDES: acute derangement of knee (836.0-836.6)
ankylosis (718.5)
contracture (718.4)
current injury (836.0-836.6)
deformity (736.4-736.6)
recurrent dislocation (718.3)

717.0 Old bucket handle tear of medial meniscus
Old bucket handle tear of unspecified cartilage

717.1 Derangement of anterior horn of medial meniscus

717.2 Derangement of posterior horn of medial meniscus

717.3 Other and unspecified derangement of medial meniscus
Degeneration of internal semilunar cartilage

✓5th **717.4 Derangement of lateral meniscus**

717.40 Derangement of lateral meniscus, unspecified

717.41 Bucket handle tear of lateral meniscus

717.42 Derangement of anterior horn of lateral meniscus

717.43 Derangement of posterior horn of lateral meniscus

717.49 Other

717.5 Derangement of meniscus, not elsewhere classified
Congenital discoid meniscus
Cyst of semilunar cartilage
Derangement of semilunar cartilage NOS

Disruption and Tears of Meniscus

  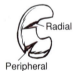
Bucket-handle Flap-type Radial Peripheral

Horizontal cleavage Vertical Congenital discoid meniscus

Internal Derangements of Knee

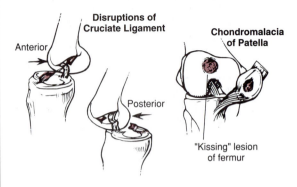

Disruptions of Cruciate Ligament — Anterior, Posterior
Chondromalacia of Patella
"Kissing" lesion of fermur

717.6 Loose body in knee
Joint mice, knee
Rice bodies, knee (joint)
DEF: The presence in the joint synovial area of a small, frequently calcified, loose body created from synovial membrane, organized fibrin fragments of articular cartilage or arthritis osteophytes.

717.7 Chondromalacia of patella
Chondromalacia patellae
Degeneration [softening] of articular cartilage of patella
AHA: M-A, '85, 14; N-D, '84, 9
DEF: Softened patella cartilage.

✓5th **717.8 Other internal derangement of knee**
717.81 Old disruption of lateral collateral ligament
717.82 Old disruption of medial collateral ligament
717.83 Old disruption of anterior cruciate ligament
717.84 Old disruption of posterior cruciate ligament
717.85 Old disruption of other ligaments of knee
Capsular ligament of knee
717.89 Other
Old disruption of ligaments NOS

717.9 Unspecified internal derangement of knee
Derangement NOS of knee

✓4th **718 Other derangement of joint**
EXCLUDES: current injury (830.0-848.9)
jaw (524.6)

The following fifth-digit subclassification is for use with category 718; valid digits are in [brackets] under each code. See above category 710 for definitions.
0 site unspecified
1 shoulder region
2 upper arm
3 forearm
4 hand
5 pelvic region and thigh
6 lower leg
7 ankle and foot
8 other specified sites
9 multiple sites

§ ✓5th **718.0 Articular cartilage disorder**
[0-5,7-9] Meniscus: Meniscus:
disorder tear, old
rupture, old Old rupture of ligament(s) of joint NOS
EXCLUDES: articular cartilage disorder:
in ochronosis (270.2)
knee (717.0-717.9)
chondrocalcinosis (275.4)
metastatic calcification (275.4)

§ Requires fifth-digit. Valid digits are in [brackets] under each code. See beginning of section 710-739 for codes and definitions.

MUSCULOSKELTAL SYSTEM AND CONNECTIVE TISSUE 718.1–720.2

§ ✓5th **718.1 Loose body in joint**
[0-5,7-9]   Joint mice
    EXCLUDES knee (717.6)
    AHA: For code 718.17: 2Q, '01, 15
    DEF: Calcified loose bodies in synovial fluid; due to arthritic osteophytes.

§ ✓5th **718.2 Pathological dislocation**
[0-9]   Dislocation or displacement of joint, not recurrent and not current injury
    Spontaneous dislocation (joint)

§ ✓5th **718.3 Recurrent dislocation of joint**
[0-9]   **AHA:** N-D, '87, 7

§ ✓5th[2] **718.4 Contracture of joint**
[0-9]   **AHA:** 4Q, '98, 40

§ ✓5th[1] **718.5 Ankylosis of joint**
[0-9]   Ankylosis of joint (fibrous) (osseous)
    EXCLUDES spine (724.9)
        stiffness of joint without mention of ankylosis (719.5)
    DEF: Immobility and solidification, of joint; due to disease, injury or surgical procedure.

§ ✓5th **718.6 Unspecified intrapelvic protrusion of acetabulum**
[0,5]   Protrusio acetabuli, unspecified
    DEF: Sinking of the floor of acetabulum; causing femoral head to protrude, limits hip movement; of unknown etiology.

§ ✓5th **718.7 Developmental dislocation of joint**
[0-9]   **EXCLUDES** ▶congenital dislocation of joint (754.0-755.8)
        traumatic dislocation of joint (830-839)◀
    AHA: 4Q, '01, 48

§ ✓5th **718.8 Other joint derangement, not elsewhere classified**
[0-9]   Flail joint (paralytic)   Instability of joint
    EXCLUDES deformities classifiable to 736 (736.0-736.9)
    AHA: For code 718.81: 2Q, '00, 14

§ ✓5th **718.9 Unspecified derangement of joint**
[0-5,7-9]   **EXCLUDES** knee (717.9)

✓4th **719 Other and unspecified disorders of joint**
    EXCLUDES jaw (524.6)

> The following fifth-digit subclassification is for use with category 719; valid digits are in [brackets] under each code. See above category 710 for definitions.
>   0 site unspecified
>   1 shoulder region
>   2 upper arm
>   3 forearm
>   4 hand
>   5 pelvic region and thigh
>   6 lower leg
>   7 ankle and foot
>   8 other specified sites
>   9 multiple sites

§ ✓5th **719.0 Effusion of joint**
[0-9]   Hydrarthrosis
    Swelling of joint, with or without pain
    EXCLUDES intermittent hydrarthrosis (719.3)

§ ✓5th **719.1 Hemarthrosis**
[0-9]   **EXCLUDES** current injury (840.0-848.9)

§ ✓5th **719.2 Villonodular synovitis**
[0-9]   **DEF:** Overgrowth of synovial tissue, especially at knee joint; due to macrophage infiltration of giant cells in synovial villi and fibrous nodules.

Joint Derangements and Disorders

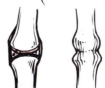

Loose body in joint   Dislocation of joint
Joint contracture   Ankylosis of joint   Synovial effusion (fluid)   Hemarthrosis (blood)

§ ✓5th **719.3 Palindromic rheumatism**
[0-9]   Hench-Rosenberg syndrome
    Intermittent hydrarthrosis
    DEF: Recurrent episodes of afebrile arthritis and periarthritis marked by their complete disappearance after a few days or hours; causes swelling, redness, and disability usually affecting only one joint; no known cause; affects adults of either sex.

§ ✓5th **719.4 Pain in joint**
[0-9]   Arthralgia
    AHA: For code 719.46: 1Q, '01, 3

§ ✓5th **719.5 Stiffness of joint, not elsewhere classified**
[0-9]

§ ✓5th **719.6 Other symptoms referable to joint**
[0-9]   Joint crepitus   Snapping hip
    AHA: 1Q, '94, 15

§ ✓5th **719.7 Difficulty in walking**
[0,5-9]   **EXCLUDES** abnormality of gait (781.2)

§ ✓5th **719.8 Other specified disorders of joint**
[0-9]   Calcification of joint   Fistula of joint
    EXCLUDES temporomandibular joint-pain-dysfunction syndrome [Costen's syndrome] (524.6)

§ ✓5th **719.9 Unspecified disorder of joint**
[0-9]

DORSOPATHIES (720-724)
    EXCLUDES curvature of spine (737.0-737.9)
        osteochondrosis of spine (juvenile) (732.0)
        adult (732.8)

✓4th **720 Ankylosing spondylitis and other inflammatory spondylopathies**

720.0 Ankylosing spondylitis
    Rheumatoid arthritis of spine NOS
    Spondylitis:
        Marie-Strümpell
        rheumatoid
    DEF: Rheumatoid arthritis of spine and sacroiliac joints; fusion and deformity in spine follows; affects mainly males; cause unknown.

720.1 Spinal enthesopathy
    Disorder of peripheral ligamentous or muscular attachments of spine
    Romanus lesion
    DEF: Tendinous or muscular vertebral bone attachment abnormality.

720.2 Sacroiliitis, not elsewhere classified
    Inflammation of sacroiliac joint NOS
    DEF: Pain due to inflammation in joint, at juncture of sacrum and hip.

---
[1] Nonspecific PDx=0
[2] Nonspecific PDx=9
§ Requires fifth-digit. Valid digits are in [brackets] under each code. See beginning of section 710-739 for codes and definitions.

MUSCULOSKELTAL SYSTEM AND CONNECTIVE TISSUE — Tabular List

- ✓5th **720.8** Other inflammatory spondylopathies
  - **720.81** *Inflammatory spondylopathies in diseases classified elsewhere*
    Code first underlying disease as:
    tuberculosis (015.0)
  - **720.89** Other
- **720.9** Unspecified inflammatory spondylopathy
  Spondylitis NOS

- ✓4th **721** Spondylosis and allied disorders
  AHA: 2Q, '89, 14
  DEF: Degenerative changes in spinal joint.
  - **721.0** Cervical spondylosis without myelopathy
    Cervical or cervicodorsal: Cervical or cervicodorsal:
    arthritis   spondylarthritis
    osteoarthritis
  - **721.1** Cervical spondylosis with myelopathy
    Anterior spinal artery compression syndrome
    Spondylogenic compression of cervical spinal cord
    Vertebral artery compression syndrome
  - **721.2** Thoracic spondylosis without myelopathy
    Thoracic: Thoracic:
    arthritis   spondylarthritis
    osteoarthritis
  - **721.3** Lumbosacral spondylosis without myelopathy
    Lumbar or lumbosacral: Lumbar or lumbosacral:
    arthritis   spondylarthritis
    osteoarthritis
  - ✓5th **721.4** Thoracic or lumbar spondylosis with myelopathy
    - **721.41** Thoracic region
      Spondylogenic compression of thoracic spinal cord
    - **721.42** Lumbar region
      Spondylogenic compression of lumbar spinal cord
  - **721.5** Kissing spine
    Baastrup's syndrome
    DEF: Compression of spinous processes of adjacent vertebrae; due to mutual contact.
  - **721.6** Ankylosing vertebral hyperostosis
  - **721.7** Traumatic spondylopathy
    Kümmell's disease or spondylitis
  - **721.8** Other allied disorders of spine
  - ✓5th **721.9** Spondylosis of unspecified site
    - **721.90** Without mention of myelopathy
      Spinal:
        arthritis (deformans) (degenerative) (hypertrophic)
        osteoarthritis NOS
      Spondylarthrosis NOS
    - **721.91** With myelopathy
      Spondylogenic compression of spinal cord NOS

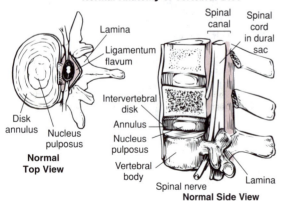

Normal Anatomy of Vertebral Disc
Normal Top View
Normal Side View

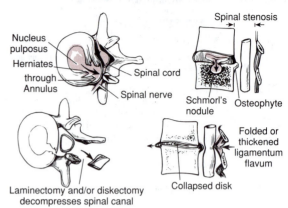

Derangement of Vertebral Disc

- ✓4th **722** Intervertebral disc disorders
  AHA: 1Q, '88, 10
  - **722.0** Displacement of cervical intervertebral disc without myelopathy [A]
    Neuritis (brachial) or radiculitis due to displacement or rupture of cervical intervertebral disc
    Any condition classifiable to 722.2 of the cervical or cervicothoracic intervertebral disc
  - ✓5th **722.1** Displacement of thoracic or lumbar intervertebral disc without myelopathy
    - **722.10** Lumbar intervertebral disc without myelopathy [A]
      Lumbago or sciatica due to displacement of intervertebral disc
      Neuritis or radiculitis due to displacement or rupture of lumbar intervertebral disc
      Any condition classifiable to 722.2 of the lumbar or lumbosacral intervertebral disc
    - **722.11** Thoracic intervertebral disc without myelopathy [A]
      Any condition classifiable to 722.2 of thoracic intervertebral disc
  - **722.2** Displacement of intervertebral disc, site unspecified, without myelopathy [A]
    Discogenic syndrome NOS
    Herniation of nucleus pulposus NOS
    Intervertebral disc NOS:
      extrusion
      prolapse
      protrusion
      rupture
    Neuritis or radiculitis due to displacement or rupture of intervertebral disc
  - ✓5th **722.3** Schmorl's nodes
    DEF: Irregular bone defect in the margin of the vertebral body; causes herniation into end plate of vertebral body.
    - **722.30** Unspecified region [A]
    - **722.31** Thoracic region [A]
    - **722.32** Lumbar region [A]
    - **722.39** Other [A]
  - **722.4** Degeneration of cervical intervertebral disc [A]
    Degeneration of cervicothoracic intervertebral disc
  - ✓5th **722.5** Degeneration of thoracic or lumbar intervertebral disc
    - **722.51** Thoracic or thoracolumbar intervertebral disc [A]
    - **722.52** Lumbar or lumbosacral intervertebral disc [A]

N Newborn Age: 0   P Pediatric Age: 0-17   M Maternity Age: 12-55   A Adult Age: 15-124   CC CC Condition   MC Major Complication   CD Complex Dx   HIV HIV Related Dx

MUSCULOSKELTAL SYSTEM AND CONNECTIVE TISSUE

722.6 **Degeneration of intervertebral disc, site unspecified**
Degenerative disc disease NOS
Narrowing of intervertebral disc or space NOS

√5th **722.7 Intervertebral disc disorder with myelopathy**
722.70 Unspecified region
722.71 Cervical region
722.72 Thoracic region
722.73 Lumbar region

√5th **722.8 Postlaminectomy syndrome**
AHA: J-F, '87, 7
DEF: Spinal disorder due to spinal laminectomy surgery.

722.80 Unspecified region
CC Excl: 722.51-722.93

722.81 Cervical region
CC Excl: See code 722.80

722.82 Thoracic region
CC Excl: See code 722.80

722.83 Lumbar region
CC Excl: See code 722.80
AHA: 2Q, '97, 15

√5th **722.9 Other and unspecified disc disorder**
Calcification of intervertebral cartilage or disc
Discitis

722.90 Unspecified region
AHA: N-D, '84, 19

722.91 Cervical region
722.92 Thoracic region
722.93 Lumbar region

√4th **723 Other disorders of cervical region**
EXCLUDES conditions due to:
intervertebral disc disorders (722.0-722.9)
spondylosis (721.0-721.9)
AHA: 3Q, '94, 14; 2Q, '89, 14

723.0 **Spinal stenosis in cervical region**
723.1 **Cervicalgia**
Pain in neck
DEF: Pain in cervical spine or neck region.

723.2 **Cervicocranial syndrome**
Barré-Liéou syndrome
Posterior cervical sympathetic syndrome
DEF: Neurologic disorder of upper cervical spine and nerve roots.

723.3 **Cervicobrachial syndrome (diffuse)**
AHA: N-D, '85, 12
DEF: Complex of symptoms due to scalenus anterior muscle compressing the brachial plexus; pain radiates from shoulder to arm or back of neck.

723.4 **Brachial neuritis or radiculitis NOS**
Cervical radiculitis
Radicular syndrome of upper limbs
CC Excl: 722.6-722.71, 722.80-722.81, 722.90-722.91, 723.0-723.9

723.5 **Torticollis, unspecified**
Contracture of neck
EXCLUDES congenital (754.1)
due to birth injury (767.8)
hysterical (300.11)
►ocular torticollis (781.93)◄
psychogenic (306.0)
spasmodic (333.83)
traumatic, current (847.0)
CC Excl: 053.71, 722.6-722.71, 722.80-722.81, 722.90-722.91, 723.0-723.9
AHA: 2Q, '01, 21; 1Q, '95, 7
DEF: Abnormally positioned neck relative to head; due to cervical muscle or fascia contractions; also called wryneck.

723.6 **Panniculitis specified as affecting neck**
DEF: Inflammation of the panniculus adiposus (subcutaneous fat) in the neck.

723.7 **Ossification of posterior longitudinal ligament in cervical region**

723.8 **Other syndromes affecting cervical region**
Cervical syndrome NEC
Klippel's disease
Occipital neuralgia
AHA: 1Q, '00, 7

723.9 **Unspecified musculoskeletal disorders and symptoms referable to neck**
Cervical (region) disorder NOS

√4th **724 Other and unspecified disorders of back**
EXCLUDES collapsed vertebra (code to cause, e.g., osteoporosis, 733.00-733.09)
conditions due to:
intervertebral disc disorders (722.0-722.9)
spondylosis (721.0-721.9)
AHA: 2Q, '89, 14

√5th **724.0 Spinal stenosis, other than cervical**
724.00 Spinal stenosis, unspecified region
724.01 Thoracic region
724.02 Lumbar region
AHA: 4Q, '99, 13

724.09 Other

724.1 **Pain in thoracic spine**
724.2 **Lumbago**
Low back pain   Lumbalgia
Low back syndrome
AHA: N-D, '85, 12

724.3 **Sciatica**
Neuralgia or neuritis of sciatic nerve
EXCLUDES specified lesion of sciatic nerve (355.0)
AHA: 2Q, '89, 12

724.4 **Thoracic or lumbosacral neuritis or radiculitis, unspecified**
Radicular syndrome of lower limbs
AHA: 2Q, '99, 3

724.5 **Backache, unspecified**
Vertebrogenic (pain) syndrome NOS

724.6 **Disorders of sacrum**
Ankylosis   } lumbosacral or sacroiliac (joint)
Instability

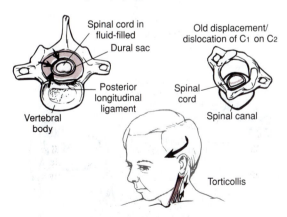

Spinal Stenosis in Cervical Region

MUSCULOSKELTAL SYSTEM AND CONNECTIVE TISSUE — Tabular List

724.7 Disorders of coccyx ✓5th
- **724.70** Unspecified disorder of coccyx
- **724.71** Hypermobility of coccyx
- **724.79** Other
  - Coccygodynia

724.8 Other symptoms referable to back
- Ossification of posterior longitudinal ligament NOS
- Panniculitis specified as sacral or affecting back

724.9 Other unspecified back disorders
- Ankylosis of spine NOS
- Compression of spinal nerve root NEC
- Spinal disorder NOS
- EXCLUDES: sacroiliitis (720.2)

RHEUMATISM, EXCLUDING THE BACK (725-729)

INCLUDES: disorders of muscles and tendons and their attachments, and of other soft tissues

725 Polymyalgia rheumatica
DEF: Joint and muscle pain, pelvis, and shoulder girdle stiffness, high sedimentation rate and temporal arteritis; occurs in elderly.

726 Peripheral enthesopathies and allied syndromes ✓4th
Note: Enthesopathies are disorders of peripheral ligamentous or muscular attachments.
EXCLUDES: spinal enthesopathy (720.1)

- **726.0** Adhesive capsulitis of shoulder
- **726.1** Rotator cuff syndrome of shoulder and allied disorders ✓5th
  - **726.10** Disorders of bursae and tendons in shoulder region, unspecified
    - Rotator cuff syndrome NOS
    - Supraspinatus syndrome NOS
    - AHA: 2Q, '01, 11
  - **726.11** Calcifying tendinitis of shoulder
  - **726.12** Bicipital tenosynovitis
  - **726.19** Other specified disorders
    - EXCLUDES: complete rupture of rotator cuff, nontraumatic (727.61)
- **726.2** Other affections of shoulder region, not elsewhere classified
  - Periarthritis of shoulder
  - Scapulohumeral fibrositis
- **726.3** Enthesopathy of elbow region ✓5th
  - **726.30** Enthesopathy of elbow, unspecified
  - **726.31** Medial epicondylitis
  - **726.32** Lateral epicondylitis
    - Epicondylitis NOS   Tennis elbow
    - Golfers' elbow
  - **726.33** Olecranon bursitis
    - Bursitis of elbow
  - **726.39** Other
- **726.4** Enthesopathy of wrist and carpus
  - Bursitis of hand or wrist
  - Periarthritis of wrist
- **726.5** Enthesopathy of hip region
  - Bursitis of hip   Psoas tendinitis
  - Gluteal tendinitis   Trochanteric tendinitis
  - Iliac crest spur
- **726.6** Enthesopathy of knee ✓5th
  - **726.60** Enthesopathy of knee, unspecified
    - Bursitis of knee NOS
  - **726.61** Pes anserinus tendinitis or bursitis
    - DEF: Inflamed tendons of sartorius, gracilis and semitendinosus muscles of medial aspect of knee.
  - **726.62** Tibial collateral ligament bursitis
    - Pellegrini-Stieda syndrome
  - **726.63** Fibular collateral ligament bursitis
  - **726.64** Patellar tendinitis
  - **726.65** Prepatellar bursitis
  - **726.69** Other
    - Bursitis:
      - infrapatellar
      - subpatellar
- **726.7** Enthesopathy of ankle and tarsus ✓5th
  - **726.70** Enthesopathy of ankle and tarsus, unspecified
    - Metatarsalgia NOS
    - EXCLUDES: Morton's metatarsalgia (355.6)
  - **726.71** Achilles bursitis or tendinitis
  - **726.72** Tibialis tendinitis
    - Tibialis (anterior) (posterior) tendinitis
  - **726.73** Calcaneal spur
    - DEF: Overgrowth of calcaneous bone; causes pain on walking; due to chronic avulsion injury of plantar fascia from calcaneus.
  - **726.79** Other
    - Peroneal tendinitis
- **726.8** Other peripheral enthesopathies
- **726.9** Unspecified enthesopathy ✓5th
  - **726.90** Enthesopathy of unspecified site
    - Capsulitis NOS
    - Periarthritis NOS
    - Tendinitis NOS
  - **726.91** Exostosis of unspecified site
    - Bone spur NOS
    - AHA: 2Q, '01, 15

727 Other disorders of synovium, tendon, and bursa ✓4th
- **727.0** Synovitis and tenosynovitis ✓5th
  - **727.00** Synovitis and tenosynovitis, unspecified
    - Synovitis NOS
    - Tenosynovitis NOS

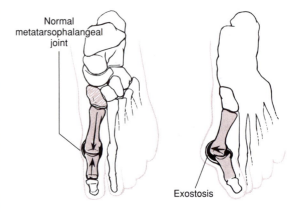

Bunion — Normal metatarsophalangeal joint; Exostosis

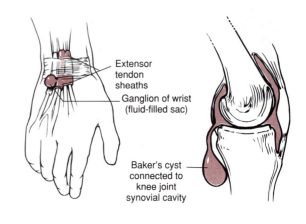

Ganglia — Extensor tendon sheaths; Ganglion of wrist (fluid-filled sac); Baker's cyst connected to knee joint synovial cavity

727.01 Synovitis and tenosynovitis in diseases classified elsewhere
Code first underlying disease as:
tuberculosis (015.0-015.9)
EXCLUDES: crystal-induced (275.4)
gonococcal (098.51)
gouty (274.0)
syphilitic (095.7)

727.02 Giant cell tumor of tendon sheath

727.03 Trigger finger (acquired)
DEF: Stenosing tenosynovitis or nodule in flexor tendon; cessation of flexion or extension movement in finger, followed by snapping into place.

727.04 Radial styloid tenosynovitis
de Quervain's disease

727.05 Other tenosynovitis of hand and wrist

727.06 Tenosynovitis of foot and ankle

727.09 Other

727.1 Bunion
DEF: Enlarged first metatarsal head due to inflamed bursa; results in laterally displaced great toe.

727.2 Specific bursitides often of occupational origin
Beat:
  elbow
  hand
  knee
Miners':
  elbow
  knee
Chronic crepitant synovitis of wrist

727.3 Other bursitis
Bursitis NOS
EXCLUDES: bursitis:
gonococcal (098.52)
subacromial (726.19)
subcoracoid (726.19)
subdeltoid (726.19)
syphilitic (095.7)
"frozen shoulder" (726.0)

✓5ᵗʰ 727.4 Ganglion and cyst of synovium, tendon, and bursa

727.40 Synovial cyst, unspecified
EXCLUDES: that of popliteal space (727.51)
AHA: 2Q, '97, 6

727.41 Ganglion of joint
727.42 Ganglion of tendon sheath
727.43 Ganglion, unspecified
727.49 Other
Cyst of bursa

✓5ᵗʰ 727.5 Rupture of synovium
727.50 Rupture of synovium, unspecified
727.51 Synovial cyst of popliteal space
Baker's cyst (knee)
727.59 Other

✓5ᵗʰ 727.6 Rupture of tendon, nontraumatic
727.60 Nontraumatic rupture of unspecified tendon
727.61 Complete rupture of rotator cuff
727.62 Tendons of biceps (long head)
727.63 Extensor tendons of hand and wrist
727.64 Flexor tendons of hand and wrist
727.65 Quadriceps tendon
727.66 Patellar tendon
727.67 Achilles tendon
727.68 Other tendons of foot and ankle
727.69 Other

✓5ᵗʰ 727.8 Other disorders of synovium, tendon, and bursa
727.81 Contracture of tendon (sheath)
Short Achilles tendon (acquired)

727.82 Calcium deposits in tendon and bursa
Calcification of tendon NOS
Calcific tendinitis NOS
EXCLUDES: peripheral ligamentous or muscular attachments (726.0-726.9)

727.83 Plica syndrome
Plica knee
AHA: 4Q, '00, 44
DEF: A fold in the synovial tissue that begins to form before birth, creating a septum between two pockets of synovial tissue; two most common plicae are the medial patellar plica and the suprapatellar plica. Plica syndrome, or plica knee, refers to symptomatic plica. Experienced by females more commonly than males.

727.89 Other
Abscess of bursa or tendon
EXCLUDES: xanthomatosis localized to tendons (272.7)
AHA: 2Q, '89, 15

727.9 Unspecified disorder of synovium, tendon, and bursa

✓4ᵗʰ 728 Disorders of muscle, ligament, and fascia
EXCLUDES: enthesopathies (726.0-726.9)
muscular dystrophies (359.0-359.1)
myoneural disorders (358.0-358.9)
myopathies (359.2-359.9)
old disruption of ligaments of knee (717.81-717.89)

728.0 Infective myositis CC
Myositis:
  purulent
  suppurative
EXCLUDES: myositis:
epidemic (074.1)
interstitial (728.81)
syphilitic (095.6)
tropical (040.81)
CC Excl: 728.0, 728.11-728.3, 728.81, 728.86
DEF: Inflamed connective septal tissue of muscle.

✓5ᵗʰ 728.1 Muscular calcification and ossification

728.10 Calcification and ossification, unspecified
Massive calcification (paraplegic)

728.11 Progressive myositis ossificans
DEF: Progressive myositic disease; marked by bony tissue formed by voluntary muscle; occurs among very young.

728.12 Traumatic myositis ossificans
Myositis ossificans (circumscripta)

728.13 Postoperative heterotopic calcification
DEF: Abnormal formation of calcium deposits in muscular tissue after surgery, marked by a corresponding loss of muscle tone and tension.

728.19 Other
Polymyositis ossificans

728.2 Muscular wasting and disuse atrophy, not elsewhere classified
Amyotrophia NOS
Myofibrosis
EXCLUDES: neuralgic amyotrophy (353.5)
progressive muscular atrophy (335.0-335.9)

728.3 Other specific muscle disorders
Arthrogryposis
Immobility syndrome (paraplegic)
EXCLUDES: arthrogryposis multiplex congenita (754.89)
stiff-man syndrome (333.91)

728.4 Laxity of ligament

728.5 Hypermobility syndrome

MUSCULOSKELTAL SYSTEM AND CONNECTIVE TISSUE

728.6 Contracture of palmar fascia
Dupuytren's contracture
DEF: Dupuytren's contracture: flexion deformity of finger, due to shortened, thickened fibrosing of palmar fascia; cause unknown; associated with long-standing epilepsy; occurs more often in males.

√5th **728.7** Other fibromatoses
728.71 Plantar fascial fibromatosis
Contracture of plantar fascia
Plantar fasciitis (traumatic)
DEF: Plantar fascia fibromatosis; causes nodular swelling and pain; not associated with contractures.

728.79 Other
Garrod's or knuckle pads
Nodular fasciitis
Pseudosarcomatous fibromatosis (proliferative) (subcutaneous)
DEF: Knuckle pads: Pea-size nodules on dorsal surface of interphalangeal joints; new growth of fibrous tissue with thickened dermis and epidermis.

√5th **728.8** Other disorders of muscle, ligament, and fascia
728.81 Interstitial myositis
DEF: Inflammation of septal connective parts of muscle tissue.

728.82 Foreign body granuloma of muscle
Talc granuloma of muscle

728.83 Rupture of muscle, nontraumatic

728.84 Diastasis of muscle
Diastasis recti (abdomen)
EXCLUDES diastasis recti complicating pregnancy, labor, and delivery (665.8)
DEF: Muscle separation, such as recti abdominis after repeated pregnancies.

728.85 Spasm of muscle

728.86 Necrotizing fasciitis
Use additional code to identify:
infectious organism (041.00-041.89)
gangrene (785.4), if applicable
CC Excl: 728.0, 728.11-728.19, 728.2, 728.3, 728.82, 728.86
AHA: 4Q, '95, 54
DEF: Fulminating infection begins with extensive cellulitis, spreads to superficial and deep fascia; causes thrombosis of subcutaneous vessels, and gangrene of underlying tissue.

728.89 Other
Eosinophilic fasciitis
Use additional E code to identify drug, if drug induced
AHA: 2Q, '01, 14, 15
DEF: Eosinophilic fasciitis: inflammation of fascia of extremities associated with eosinophilia, edema, and swelling; occurs alone or as part of myalgia syndrome.

728.9 Unspecified disorder of muscle, ligament, and fascia
AHA: 4Q, '88, 11

√4th **729** Other disorders of soft tissues
EXCLUDES acroparesthesia (443.89)
carpal tunnel syndrome (354.0)
disorders of the back (720.0-724.9)
entrapment syndromes (354.0-355.9)
palindromic rheumatism (719.3)
periarthritis (726.0-726.9)
psychogenic rheumatism (306.0)

729.0 Rheumatism, unspecified and fibrositis
DEF: General term describes diseases of muscle, tendon, nerve, joint, or bone; symptoms include pain and stiffness.

729.1 Myalgia and myositis, unspecified
Fibromyositis NOS
DEF: Myalgia: muscle pain.
DEF: Myositis: inflamed voluntary muscle.
DEF: Fibromyositis: inflamed fibromuscular tissue.

729.2 Neuralgia, neuritis, and radiculitis, unspecified
EXCLUDES brachial radiculitis (723.4)
cervical radiculitis (723.4)
lumbosacral radiculitis (724.4)
mononeuritis (354.0-355.9)
radiculitis due to intervertebral disc involvement (722.0-722.2, 722.7)
sciatica (724.3)
DEF: Neuralgia: paroxysmal pain along nerve symptoms include brief pain and tenderness at point nerve exits.
DEF: Neuritis: inflamed nerve, symptoms include paresthesia, paralysis and loss of reflexes at nerve site.
DEF: Radiculitis: inflamed nerve root.

√5th **729.3** Panniculitis, unspecified
DEF: Inflammatory reaction of subcutaneous fat; causes nodules; often develops in abdominal region.

729.30 Panniculitis, unspecified site
Weber-Christian disease
DEF: Febrile, nodular, nonsuppurative, relapsing inflammation of subcutaneous fat.

729.31 Hypertrophy of fat pad, knee
Hypertrophy of infrapatellar fat pad

729.39 Other site
EXCLUDES panniculitis specified as (affecting):
back (724.8)
neck (723.6)
sacral (724.8)

729.4 Fasciitis, unspecified
EXCLUDES necrotizing fasciitis (728.86)
nodular fasciitis (728.79)
AHA: 2Q, '94, 13

729.5 Pain in limb

729.6 Residual foreign body in soft tissue
EXCLUDES foreign body granuloma:
muscle (728.82)
skin and subcutaneous tissue (709.4)

√5th **729.8** Other musculoskeletal symptoms referable to limbs
729.81 Swelling of limb
AHA: 4Q, '88, 6

729.82 Cramp

729.89 Other
EXCLUDES abnormality of gait (781.2)
tetany (781.7)
transient paralysis of limb (781.4)
AHA: 4Q, '88, 12

729.9 Other and unspecified disorders of soft tissue
Polyalgia

MUSCULOSKELTAL SYSTEM AND CONNECTIVE TISSUE

OSTEOPATHIES, CHONDROPATHIES, AND ACQUIRED MUSCULOSKELETAL DEFORMITIES (730-739)

√4th 730 Osteomyelitis, periostitis, and other infections involving bone

EXCLUDES jaw (526.4-526.5)
petrous bone (383.2)

Use additional code to identify organism, such as Staphylococcus (041.1)

The following fifth-digit subclassification is for use with category 730; valid digits are in [brackets] under each code. See above category 710 for definitions.

    0 site unspecified
    1 shoulder region
    2 upper arm
    3 forearm
    4 hand
    5 pelvic region and thigh
    6 lower leg
    7 ankle and foot
    8 other specified sites
    9 multiple sites

AHA: 4Q, '97, 43

DEF: Osteomyelitis: bacterial inflammation of bone tissue and marrow.

DEF: Periostitis: inflammation of specialized connective tissue; causes swelling of bone and aching pain.

§ √5th 1 730.0 Acute osteomyelitis cc
[0-9]

Abscess of any bone except accessory sinus, jaw, or mastoid
Acute or subacute osteomyelitis, with or without mention of periostitis

CC Excl: For code 730.00: 015.50-015.56, 015.70-015.76, 015.90-015.96, 017.90-017.96, 730.00-730.39, 730.80-730.99 **For code 730.01:** 015.50-015.56, 015.70-015.76, 015.90-015.96, 017.90-017.96, 730.00, 730.08-730.11, 730.18-730.21, 730.28-730.31, 730.38-730.39, 730.80-730.81, 730.88-730.91, 730.98-730.99 **For code 730.02:** 015.50-015.56, 015.70-015.76, 015.90-015.96, 017.90-017.96, 730.00, 730.08-730.10, 730.12, 730.18-730.20, 730.22, 730.28-730.30, 730.32, 730.38-730.39, 730.80, 730.82, 730.88-730.90, 730.92, 730.98-730.99 **For code 730.03:** 015.50-015.56, 015.70-015.76, 015.90-015.96, 017.90-017.96, 730.00, 730.08-730.10, 730.13, 730.18-730.20, 730.23, 730.28-730.30, 730.33, 730.38-730.39, 730.80, 730.83, 730.88-730.90, 730.93, 730.98-730.99. **For code 730.04:** 015.50-015.56, 015.70-015.76, 015.90-015.96, 017.90-017.96, 730.00, 730.08-730.10, 730.14, 730.18-730.20, 730.24, 730.28-730.30, 730.34, 730.38-730.39, 730.80, 730.84, 730.88-730.90, 730.94, 730.98-730.99 **For code 730.05:** 015.10-015.16, 015.50-015.56, 015.70-015.76, 015.90-015.96, 017.90-017.96, 730.00, 730.08-730.10, 730.15, 730.18-730.20, 730.25, 730.28-730.30, 730.35, 730.38-730.39, 730.80, 730.85, 730.88-730.90, 730.95, 730.98-730.99. **For code 730.06:** 015.20-015.56, 015.70-015.76, 015.90-015.96, 017.90-017.96, 730.00, 730.08-730.10, 730.16, 730.18-730.20, 730.26, 730.28-730.30, 730.36, 730.38-730.39, 730.80, 730.86, 730.88-730.90, 730.96, 730.98-730.99 **For code 730.07:** 015.50-015.56, 015.70-015.76, 015.90-015.96, 017.90-017.96, 730.00, 730.08-730.10, 730.17-730.20, 730.27-730.30, 730.37-730.39, 730.80, 730.87-730.90, 730.97-730.99 **For code 730.08:** 015.00-015.06, 015.50-015.56, 015.70-015.76, 015.90-015.96, 017.90-017.96, 730.00-730.39, 730.80-730.99 **For code 730.09:** 015.50-015.56, 015.70-015.76, 015.90-015.96, 017.90-017.96, 730.00-730.39, 730.80-730.99

AHA: For code 730.06: ▶1Q, '02, 4◀

§ √5th 1 730.1 Chronic osteomyelitis
[0-9]

Brodie's abscess
Chronic or old osteomyelitis, with or without mention of periostitis
Sequestrum of bone
Sclerosing osteomyelitis of Garré

EXCLUDES aseptic necrosis of bone (733.40-733.49)

AHA: For code 730.17: 3Q, '00, 4

§ √5th 1 730.2 Unspecified osteomyelitis
[0-9]

Osteitis or osteomyelitis NOS, with or without mention of periostitis

§ √5th 1 730.3 Periostitis without mention of osteomyelitis
[0-9]

Abscess of periosteum } without mention of
Periostosis   } osteomyelitis

EXCLUDES that in secondary syphilis (091.61)

§ √5th 730.7 *Osteopathy resulting from poliomyelitis*
[0-9]

Code first underlying disease (045.0-045.9)

§ √5th 730.8 *Other infections involving bone in diseases classified elsewhere* cc
[0-9]

Code first underlying disease as:
tuberculosis (015.0-015.9)
typhoid fever (002.0)

EXCLUDES syphilis of bone NOS (095.5)

CC Excl: For code 730.80: See code 730.09 **CC Excl: For code 730.81:** 015.50-015.56, 015.70-015.76, 015.90-015.96, 017.90-017.96, 730.00-730.01, 730.08-730.11, 730.18-730.21, 730.28-730.31, 730.38-730.39, 730.80, 730.88-730.91, 730.98-730.99 **For code 730.82:** 015.50-015.56, 015.70-015.76, 015.90-015.96, 017.90-017.96, 730.00, 730.02, 730.08-730.10, 730.12, 730.18-730.20, 730.22, 730.28-730.30, 730.32, 730.38-730.39, 730.80, 730.88-730.90, 730.92, 730.98-730.99l **For code 730.83:** 015.50-015.56, 015.70-015.76, 015.90-015.96, 017.90-017.96, 730.00, 730.03, 730.08-730.10, 730.13, 730.18-730.20, 730.23, 730.28-730.30, 730.33, 730.38-730.39, 730.80, 730.88-730.90, 730.93, 730.98-730.99. **For code 730.84:** 015.50-015.56, 015.70-015.76, 015.90-015.96, 017.90-017.96, 730.00, 730.04, 730.08-730.10, 730.14, 730.18-730.20, 730.24, 730.28-730.30, 730.34, 730.38-730.39, 730.80, 730.88-730.90, 730.94, 730.98-730.99 **For code 730.85:** 015.10-015.16, 015.50-015.56, 015.70-015.76, 015.90-015.96, 017.90-017.96, 730.00, 730.05, 730.08-730.10, 730.15, 730.18-730.20, 730.25, 730.28-730.30, 730.35, 730.38-730.39, 730.80, 730.88-730.90, 730.95, 730.98-730.99 **For code 730.86:** 015.20-015.26, 015.50-015.56, 015.70-015.76, 015.90-015.96, 017.90-017.96, 730.00, 730.06, 730.08-730.10, 730.16, 730.18-730.20, 730.26, 730.28-730.30, 730.36, 730.38-730.39, 730.80, 730.88-730.90, 730.96, 730.98-730.99 **For code 730.87:** 015.50-015.56, 015.70-015.76, 015.90-015.96, 017.90-017.96, 730.00, 730.07-730.10, 730.17-730.20, 730.27-730.30, 730.37-730.39, 730.80, 730.88-730.90, 730.97-730.99 **For code 730.88:** 015.00-015.06, 015.50-015.56, 015.70-015.76, 015.90-015.96, 017.90-017.96, 730.00-730.39, 730.80-730.99. **For code 730.89:** 015.50-015.56, 015.70-015.76, 015.90-015.96, 017.90-017.96, 730.00-730.39, 730.80-730.99

AHA: 2Q, '97, 16; 3Q, '91, 10

§ √5th 730.9 Unspecified infection of bone cc
[0-9]

CC Excl: For code 730.90: See code 730.89 **For code 730.91:** 015.50-015.56, 015.70-015.76, 015.90-015.96, 017.90-017.96, 730.00-730.01, 730.08-730.11, 730.18-730.21, 730.28-730.31, 730.38-730.39, 730.80-730.81, 730.88-730.90, 730.98-730.99 **For code 730.92:** 015.50-015.56, 015.70-015.76, 015.90-015.96, 017.90-017.96, 730.00, 730.02, 730.08-730.10, 730.12, 730.18-730.20, 730.22, 730.28-730.30, 730.32, 730.38-730.39, 730.80, 730.82, 730.88-730.90, 730.98-730.99. **For code 730.93:** 015.50-015.56, 015.70-015.76, 015.90-015.96, 017.90-017.96, 730.00, 730.03, 730.08-730.10, 730.13, 730.18-730.20, 730.23, 730.28-730.30, 730.33, 730.38-730.39, 730.80, 730.83, 730.88-730.90, 730.98-730.99 **For code 730.94:** 015.50-015.56, 015.70-015.76, 015.90-015.96, 017.90-017.96, 730.00, 730.04, 730.08-730.10, 730.14, 730.18-730.20, 730.24, 730.28-730.30, 730.34, 730.38-730.39, 730.80, 730.84, 730.88-730.90, 730.98-730.99. **For code 730.95:** 015.10-015.16, 015.50-015.56, 015.70-015.76, 015.90-015.96, 017.90-017.96, 730.00, 730.05, 730.08-730.10, 730.15, 730.18-730.20, 730.25, 730.28-730.30, 730.35, 730.38-730.39, 730.80, 730.85, 730.88-730.90, 730.98-730.99 **For code 730.96:** 015.20-015.26, 015.50-015.56, 015.70-015.76, 015.90-015.96, 017.90-017.96, 730.00, 730.06, 730.08-730.10, 730.16, 730.18-730.20, 730.26, 730.28-730.30, 730.36, 730.38-730.39, 730.80, 730.86, 730.88-730.90, 730.98-730.99. **For code 730.97:** 015.50-015.56, 015.70-015.76, 015.90-015.96, 017.90-017.96, 730.00, 730.07-730.10, 730.17-730.20, 730.27-730.30, 730.37-730.39, 730.80, 730.87-730.90, 730.98-730.99 **For code 730.98:** 015.00-015.06, 015.50-015.56, 015.70-015.76, 015.90-015.96, 017.90-017.96, 730.00-730.39, 730.80-730.99 **For code 730.99:** 015.50-015.56, 015.70-015.76, 015.90-015.96, 017.90-017.96, 730.00-730.39, 730.80-730.99

---

[1] Nonspecific PDx=0
§ Requires fifth-digit. Valid digits are in [brackets] under each code. See beginning of section 710-739 for codes and definitions.

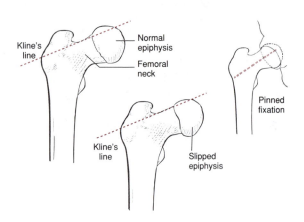

Slipped Femoral Epiphysis

✓4th **731 Osteitis deformans and osteopathies associated with other disorders classified elsewhere**

DEF: Osteitis deformans: Bone disease marked by episodes of increased bone loss, excessive repair attempts follow; causes weakened, deformed bones with increased mass, bowed long bones, deformed flat bones, pain and pathological fractures; may be fatal if associated with congestive heart failure, giant cell tumors or bone sarcoma; also called Paget's disease.

731.0 Osteitis deformans without mention of bone tumor
Paget's disease of bone

731.1 Osteitis deformans in diseases classified elsewhere
Code first underlying disease as:
  malignant neoplasm of bone (170.0-170.9)

731.2 Hypertrophic pulmonary osteoarthropathy
Bamberger-Marie disease

DEF: Clubbing, of fingers and toes; related to enlarged ends of long bones; due to chronic lung and heart disease.

731.8 Other bone involvement in diseases classified elsewhere
Code first underlying disease as:
  diabetes mellitus (250.8)
Use additional code to specify bone condition, such as:
  acute osteomyelitis (730.00-730.09)

AHA: 4Q, '97, 43; 2Q, '97, 16

✓4th **732 Osteochondropathies**

DEF: Conditions related to both bone and cartilage, or conditions in which cartilage is converted to bone (enchondral ossification).

732.0 Juvenile osteochondrosis of spine
Juvenile osteochondrosis (of):
  marginal or vertebral epiphysis (of Scheuermann)
  spine NOS
Vertebral epiphysitis
  EXCLUDES adolescent postural kyphosis (737.0)

732.1 Juvenile osteochondrosis of hip and pelvis
Coxa plana
Ischiopubic synchondrosis (of van Neck)
Osteochondrosis (juvenile) of:
  acetabulum
  head of femur (of Legg-Calvé-Perthes)
  iliac crest (of Buchanan)
  symphysis pubis (of Pierson)
Pseudocoxalgia

732.2 Nontraumatic slipped upper femoral epiphysis
Slipped upper femoral epiphysis NOS

732.3 Juvenile osteochondrosis of upper extremity
Osteochondrosis (juvenile) of:
  capitulum of humerus (of Panner)
  carpal lunate (of Kienbock)
  hand NOS
  head of humerus (of Haas)
  heads of metacarpals (of Mauclaire)
  lower ulna (of Burns)
  radial head (of Brailsford)
  upper extremity NOS

732.4 Juvenile osteochondrosis of lower extremity, excluding foot
Osteochondrosis (juvenile) of:
  lower extremity NOS
  primary patellar center (of Köhler)
  proximal tibia (of Blount)
  secondary patellar center (of Sinding-Larsen)
  tibial tubercle (of Osgood-Schlatter)
Tibia vara

732.5 Juvenile osteochondrosis of foot
Calcaneal apophysitis
Epiphysitis, os calcis
Osteochondrosis (juvenile) of:
  astragalus (of Diaz)
  calcaneum (of Sever)
  foot NOS
  metatarsal
    second (of Freiberg)
    fifth (of Iselin)
  os tibiale externum (of Haglund)
  tarsal navicular (of Köhler)

732.6 Other juvenile osteochondrosis
Apophysitis   ⎫
Epiphysitis   ⎬ specified as juvenile,
Osteochondritis   ⎪ of other site,
Osteochondrosis   ⎭ or site NOS

732.7 Osteochondritis dissecans

732.8 Other specified forms of osteochondropathy
Adult osteochondrosis of spine

732.9 Unspecified osteochondropathy
Apophysitis   ⎫ NOS
Epiphysitis   ⎬ not specified as adult
Osteochondritis   ⎪ or juvenile, of
Osteochondrosis   ⎭ unspecified site

✓4th **733 Other disorders of bone and cartilage**
  EXCLUDES bone spur (726.91)
    cartilage of, or loose body in, joint (717.0-717.9, 718.0-718.9)
    giant cell granuloma of jaw (526.3)
    osteitis fibrosa cystica generalisata (252.0)
    osteomalacia (268.2)
    polyostotic fibrous dysplasia of bone (756.54)
    prognathism, retrognathism (524.1)
    xanthomatosis localized to bone (272.7)

✓5th **733.0 Osteoporosis**

DEF: Bone mass reduction that ultimately results in fractures after minimal trauma; dorsal kyphosis or loss of height often occur.

733.00 Osteoporosis, unspecified
Wedging of vertebra NOS
AHA: ▶3Q, '01, 19;◄ 2Q, '98, 12

733.01 Senile osteoporosis
Postmenopausal osteoporosis

733.02 Idiopathic osteoporosis

733.03 Disuse osteoporosis

733.09 Other
Drug-induced osteoporosis
Use additional E code to identify drug

MUSCULOSKELETAL SYSTEM AND CONNECTIVE TISSUE

√5th 733.1 Pathologic fracture
Spontaneous fracture
EXCLUDES stress fracture (733.93-733.95)
traumatic fracture (800-829)
AHA: 4Q, '93, 25; N-D, '86, 10; N-D, '85, 16

DEF: Fracture due to bone structure weakening by pathological processes (e.g., osteoporosis, neoplasms and osteomalacia).

- **733.10** Pathologic fracture, unspecified site CC
  CC Excl: 733.10-733.19, 733.93-733.95
- **733.11** Pathologic fracture of humerus CC
  CC Excl: See code 733.10
- **733.12** Pathologic fracture of distal radius and ulna CC
  Wrist NOS
  CC Excl: See code 733.10
- **733.13** Pathologic fracture of vertebrae CC
  Collapse of vertebra NOS
  CC Excl: See code 733.10
  AHA: 3Q, '99, 5
  DRG 239
- **733.14** Pathologic fracture of neck of femur CC
  Femur NOS   Hip NOS
  CC Excl: See code 733.10
  AHA: 1Q, '01, 1; 1Q, '96, 16
- **733.15** Pathologic fracture of other specified part of femur CC
  CC Excl: See code 733.10
  AHA: 2Q, '98, 12
- **733.16** Pathologic fracture of tibia or fibula CC
  Ankle NOS
  CC Excl: See code 733.10
- **733.19** Pathologic fracture of other specified site CC
  CC Excl: See code 733.10

√4th 733.2 Cyst of bone
- **733.20** Cyst of bone (localized), unspecified
- **733.21** Solitary bone cyst
  Unicameral bone cyst
- **733.22** Aneurysmal bone cyst

DEF: Solitary bone lesion, bulges into periosteum; marked by calcified rim.

- **733.29** Other
  Fibrous dysplasia (monostotic)
  EXCLUDES cyst of jaw (526.0-526.2, 526.89)
  osteitis fibrosa cystica (252.0)
  polyostotic fibrousdyplasia of bone (756.54)

733.3 Hyperostosis of skull
Hyperostosis interna frontalis
Leontiasis ossium

DEF: Abnormal bone growth on inner aspect of cranial bones.

√5th 733.4 Aseptic necrosis of bone
EXCLUDES osteochondropathies (732.0-732.9)

DEF: Infraction of bone tissue due to a nonfectious etiology, such as a fracture, ischemic disorder or administration of immunosuppressive drugs; leads to degenerative joint disease or nonunion of fractures.

- **733.40** Aseptic necrosis of bone, site unspecified
- **733.41** Head of humerus
- **733.42** Head and neck of femur
  Femur NOS
  EXCLUDES Legg-Calvé-Perthes disease (732.1)
- **733.43** Medial femoral condyle
- **733.44** Talus
- **733.49** Other

733.5 Osteitis condensans
Piriform sclerosis of ilium

DEF: Idiopathic condition marked by low back pain; associated with oval or triangular sclerotic, opaque bone next to sacroiliac joints in the ileum.

733.6 Tietze's disease
Costochondral junction syndrome
Costochondritis

DEF: Painful, idiopathic, nonsuppurative, swollen costal cartilage sometimes confused with cardiac symptoms because the anterior chest pain resembles that of coronary artery disease.

733.7 Algoneurodystrophy
Disuse atrophy of bone   Sudeck's atrophy

DEF: Painful, idiopathic.

√5th 733.8 Malunion and nonunion of fracture
AHA: 2Q, '94, 5

- **733.81** Malunion of fracture CC
  CC Excl: 733.81-733.82
- **733.82** Nonunion of fracture CC
  Pseudoarthrosis (bone)
  CC Excl: See code 733.81

√5th 733.9 Other and unspecified disorders of bone and cartilage
- **733.90** Disorder of bone and cartilage, unspecified
- **733.91** Arrest of bone development or growth
  Epiphyseal arrest
- **733.92** Chondromalacia
  Chondromalacia:
  NOS
  localized, except patella
  systemic
  tibial plateau
  EXCLUDES chondromalacia of patella (717.7)

DEF: Articular cartilage softening.

- **733.93** Stress fracture of tibia or fibula CC
  Stress reaction of tibia or fibula
  CC Excl: 733.10-733.19, 733.93-733.95
  AHA: ▶4Q, '01, 48◀
- **733.94** Stress fracture of the metatarsals CC
  Stress reaction of metatarsals
  CC Excl: See code 733.93
  AHA: ▶4Q, '01, 48◀
- **733.95** Stress fracture of other bone CC
  Stress reaction of other bone
  CC Excl: See code 733.93
  AHA: ▶4Q, '01, 48◀
- **733.99** Other
  Diaphysitis
  Hypertrophy of bone
  Relapsing polychondritis
  AHA: J-F, '87, 14

734 Flat foot
Pes planus (acquired)
Talipes planus (acquired)
EXCLUDES congenital (754.61)
rigid flat foot (754.61)
spastic (everted) flat foot (754.61)

√4th 735 Acquired deformities of toe
EXCLUDES congenital (754.60-754.69, 755.65-755.66)

735.0 Hallux valgus (acquired)

DEF: Angled displacement of the great toe, causing it to ride over or under other toes.

Acquired Deformities of Toe

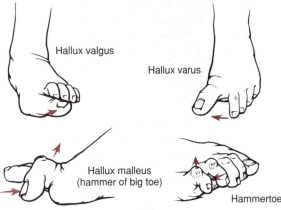

735.1 Hallux varus (acquired)
DEF: Angled displacement of the great toe toward the body midline, away from the other toes.

735.2 Hallux rigidus
DEF: Limited flexion movement at metatarsophalangeal joint of great toe; due to degenerative joint disease.

735.3 Hallux malleus
DEF: Extended proximal phalanx, flexed distal phalanges, of great toe; foot resembles claw or hammer.

735.4 Other hammer toe (acquired)

735.5 Claw toe (acquired)
DEF: Hyperextended proximal phalanges, flexed middle and distal phalanges.

735.8 Other acquired deformities of toe

735.9 Unspecified acquired deformity of toe

√4th **736 Other acquired deformities of limbs**
EXCLUDES congenital (754.3-755.9)

√5th **736.0 Acquired deformities of forearm, excluding fingers**
  736.00 Unspecified deformity
    Deformity of elbow, forearm, hand, or wrist (acquired) NOS
  736.01 Cubitus valgus (acquired)
    DEF: Deviation of the elbow away from the body midline upon extension; it occurs when the palm is turning outward.
  736.02 Cubitus varus (acquired)
    DEF: Elbow joint displacement angled laterally; when the forearm is extended, it is deviated toward the midline of the body; also called "gun stock" deformity.
  736.03 Valgus deformity of wrist (acquired)
    DEF: Abnormal angulation away from the body midline.

736.04 Varus deformity of wrist (acquired)
DEF: Abnormal angulation toward the body midline.

736.05 Wrist drop (acquired)
DEF: Inability to extend the hand at the wrist due to extensor muscle paralysis

736.06 Claw hand (acquired)
DEF: Flexion and atrophy of the hand and fingers; found in ulnar nerve lesions, syringomyelia, and leprosy.

736.07 Club hand, acquired
DEF: Twisting of the hand out of shape or position; caused by the congenital absence of the ulna or radius.

736.09 Other

736.1 Mallet finger
DEF: Permanently flexed distal phalanx.

√5th **736.2 Other acquired deformities of finger**
  736.20 Unspecified deformity
    Deformity of finger (acquired) NOS
  736.21 Boutonniere deformity
    DEF: A complete or partial protrusion of a joint finger through a defect in the extensor aponeurosis; also called buttonhole deformity.
  736.22 Swan-neck deformity
    DEF: Flexed distal and hyperextended proximal interphalangeal joint.
  736.29 Other
    EXCLUDES trigger finger (727.03)
    AHA: 2Q, '89, 13

√5th **736.3 Acquired deformities of hip**
  736.30 Unspecified deformity
    Deformity of hip (acquired) NOS
  736.31 Coxa valga (acquired)
    DEF: Increase of at least 140 degrees in the angle formed by the axis of the head and the neck of the femur, and the axis of its shaft.
  736.32 Coxa vara (acquired)
    DEF: The bending downward of the neck of the femur: causing difficulty in movement; a right angle or less may be formed by the axis of the head and neck of the femur, and the axis of its shaft.
  736.39 Other
    AHA: 2Q, '91, 18

√5th **736.4 Genu valgum or varum (acquired)**
  736.41 Genu valgum (acquired)
    DEF: Abnormally close together and an abnormally large space between the ankles; also called "knock-knees."
  736.42 Genu varum (acquired)
    DEF: Abnormally separated knees and the inward bowing of the legs; it is also called "bowlegs."

736.5 Genu recurvatum (acquired)
DEF: Hyperextended knees; also called "backknee."

736.6 Other acquired deformities of knee
Deformity of knee (acquired) NOS

Acquired Deformities of Forearm

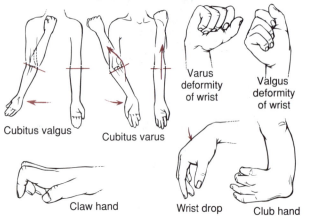

MUSCULOSKELTAL SYSTEM AND CONNECTIVE TISSUE

Acquired Deformities of Hip

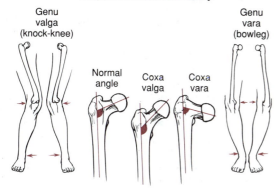

Acquired Deformities of Lower Limb

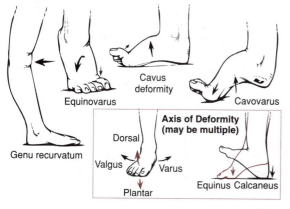

- √5th **736.7 Other acquired deformities of ankle and foot**
  EXCLUDES deformities of toe (acquired) (735.0-735.9)
  pes planus (acquired) (734)
  - **736.70 Unspecified deformity of ankle and foot, acquired**
  - 736.71 Acquired equinovarus deformity
    Clubfoot, acquired
    EXCLUDES clubfoot not specified as acquired (754.5-754.7)
  - 736.72 Equinus deformity of foot, acquired
    DEF: A plantar flexion deformity that forces people to walk on their toes.
  - 736.73 Cavus deformity of foot
    EXCLUDES that with claw foot (736.74)
    DEF: Abnormally high longitudinal arch of the foot.

Kyphosis and Lordosis

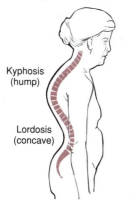

- 736.74 Claw foot, acquired
  DEF: High foot arch with hyperextended toes at metatarsophalangeal joint and flexed toes at distal joints; also called "main en griffe."
- 736.75 Cavovarus deformity of foot, acquired
  DEF: Inward turning of the heel from the midline of the leg and an abnormally high longitudinal arch.
- 736.76 Other calcaneus deformity
- 736.79 Other
  Acquired:
    pes   } not elsewhere classified
    talipes

- √5th **736.8 Acquired deformities of other parts of limbs**
  - 736.81 Unequal leg length (acquired)
  - 736.89 Other
    Deformity (acquired):
      arm or leg, not elsewhere classified
      shoulder
- **736.9 Acquired deformity of limb, site unspecified**

- √4th **737 Curvature of spine**
  EXCLUDES congenital (754.2)
  - **737.0 Adolescent postural kyphosis**
    EXCLUDES osteochondrosis of spine (juvenile) (732.0)
    adult (732.8)
  - √5th **737.1 Kyphosis (acquired)**
    - 737.10 Kyphosis (acquired) (postural)
    - 737.11 Kyphosis due to radiation
    - 737.12 Kyphosis, postlaminectomy
      AHA: J-F, '87, 7
    - 737.19 Other
      EXCLUDES that associated with conditions classifiable elsewhere (737.41)
  - √5th **737.2 Lordosis (acquired)**
    DEF: Swayback appearance created by an abnormally increased spinal curvature; it is also referred to as "hollow back" or "saddle back."
    - 737.20 Lordosis (acquired) (postural)
    - 737.21 Lordosis, postlaminectomy
    - 737.22 Other postsurgical lordosis
    - 737.29 Other
      EXCLUDES that associated with conditions classifiable elsewhere (737.42)
  - √5th **737.3 Kyphoscoliosis and scoliosis**
    DEF: Kyphoscoliosis: backward and lateral curvature of the spinal column; it is found in vertebral osteochondrosis.
    DEF: Scoliosis: an abnormal deviation of the spine to the left or right of the midline
    - 737.30 Scoliosis [and kyphoscoliosis], idiopathic
    - 737.31 Resolving infantile idiopathic scoliosis
    - 737.32 Progressive infantile idiopathic scoliosis
    - 737.33 Scoliosis due to radiation
    - 737.34 Thoracogenic scoliosis
    - 737.39 Other
      EXCLUDES that associated with conditions classifiable elsewhere (737.43)
      that in kyphoscoliotic heart disease (416.1)

MUSCULOSKELTAL SYSTEM AND CONNECTIVE TISSUE

Scoliosis and Kyphoscoliosis

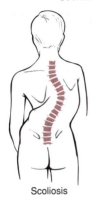
Scoliosis

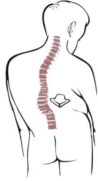
Kyphoscoliosis

737.4 Curvature of spine associated with other conditions
Code first associated condition as:
  Charcôt-Marie-Tooth disease (356.1)
  mucopolysaccharidosis (277.5)
  neurofibromatosis (237.7)
  osteitis deformans (731.0)
  osteitis fibrosa cystica (252.0)
  osteoporosis (733.00-733.09)
  poliomyelitis (138)
  tuberculosis [Pott's curvature] (015.0)

- **737.40** Curvature of spine, unspecified
- **737.41** Kyphosis
- **737.42** Lordosis
- **737.43** Scoliosis

737.8 Other curvatures of spine

737.9 Unspecified curvature of spine
Curvature of spine (acquired) (idiopathic) NOS
Hunchback, acquired
EXCLUDES deformity of spine NOS (738.5)

738 Other acquired deformity
EXCLUDES congenital (754.0-756.9, 758.0-759.9)
dentofacial anomalies (524.0-524.9)

738.0 Acquired deformity of nose
Deformity of nose (acquired)
Overdevelopment of nasal bones
EXCLUDES deflected or deviated nasal septum (470)

738.1 Other acquired deformity of head
- **738.10** Unspecified deformity
- **738.11** Zygomatic hyperplasia
  DEF: Abnormal enlargement of the zygoma (processus zygomaticus temporalis).
- **738.12** Zygomatic hypoplasia
  DEF: Underdevelopment of the zygoma (processus zygomaticus temporalis).
- **738.19** Other specified deformity

738.2 Acquired deformity of neck

738.3 Acquired deformity of chest and rib
Deformity:
  chest (acquired)   Pectus:
  rib (acquired)   carinatum, acquired
                             excavatum, acquired

738.4 Acquired spondylolisthesis
Degenerative spondylolisthesis
Spondylolysis, acquired
EXCLUDES congenital (756.12)
DEF: Vertebra displaced forward over another; due to bilateral defect in vertebral arch, eroded articular surface of posterior facts and elongated pedicle between fifth lumbar vertebra and sacrum.

738.5 Other acquired deformity of back or spine
Deformity of spine NOS
EXCLUDES curvature of spine (737.0-737.9)

738.6 Acquired deformity of pelvis
Pelvic obliquity
EXCLUDES intrapelvic protrusion of acetabulum (718.6)
that in relation to labor and delivery (653.0-653.4, 653.8-653.9)
DEF: Pelvic obliquity: slanting or inclination of the pelvis at an angle between 55 and 60 degrees between the plane of the pelvis and the horizontal plane.

738.7 Cauliflower ear
DEF: Abnormal external ear; due to injury, subsequent perichondritis.

738.8 Acquired deformity of other specified site
Deformity of clavicle
AHA: 2Q, '01, 15

738.9 Acquired deformity of unspecified site

739 Nonallopathic lesions, not elsewhere classified
INCLUDES segmental dysfunction
somatic dysfunction
DEF: Disability, loss of function or abnormality of a body part that is neither classifiable to a particular system nor brought about therapeutically to counteract another disease.

- **739.0** Head region
  Occipitocervical region
- **739.1** Cervical region
  Cervicothoracic region
- **739.2** Thoracic region
  Thoracolumbar region
- **739.3** Lumbar region
  Lumbosacral region
- **739.4** Sacral region
  Sacrococcygeal region   Sacroiliac region
- **739.5** Pelvic region
  Hip region   Pubic region
- **739.6** Lower extremities
- **739.7** Upper extremities
  Acromioclavicular region
  Sternoclavicular region
- **739.8** Rib cage
  Costochondral region   Sternochondral region
  Costovertebral region
- **739.9** Abdomen and other
  AHA: 2Q, '89, 14

CONGENITAL ANOMALIES

14. CONGENITAL ANOMALIES (740-759)

√4th 740 Anencephalus and similar anomalies

740.0 Anencephalus
Acrania
Amyelencephalus
Hemicephaly
Hemianencephaly
DEF: Fetus without cerebrum, cerebellum and flat bones of skull.

740.1 Craniorachischisis
DEF: Congenital slit in cranium and vertebral column

740.2 Iniencephaly
DEF: Spinal cord passes through enlarged occipital bone (foramen magnum); absent vertebral bone layer and spinal processes; resulting in both reduction in number and proper fusion of the vertebrae.

√4th 741 Spina bifida

EXCLUDES spina bifida occulta (756.17)

The following fifth-digit subclassification is for use with category 741:
0 unspecified region
1 cervical region
2 dorsal [thoracic] region
3 lumbar region

AHA: 3Q, '94, 7

DEF: Lack of closure of spinal cord's bony encasement; marked by cord protrusion into lumbosacral area; evident by elevated alpha-fetoprotein of amniotic fluid

√5th 741.0 With hydrocephalus CC
Arnold-Chiari syndrome, type II
Any condition classifiable to 741.9 with any condition classifiable to 742.3
Chiari malformation, type II
CC Excl: 741.00-741.93, 742.59, 742.8-742.9, 759.7-759.89
AHA: 4Q, '97, 51; 4Q, '94, 37; S-O, '87, 10

√5th 741.9 Without mention of hydrocephalus CC
Hydromeningocele (spinal)   Myelocystocele
Hydromyelocele   Rachischisis
Meningocele (spinal)   Spina bifida (aperta)
Meningomyelocele   Syringomyelocele
Myelocele
CC Excl: See code 741.0

√4th 742 Other congenital anomalies of nervous system

742.0 Encephalocele
Encephalocystocele
Encephalomyelocele
Hydroencephalocele
Hydromeningocele, cranial
Meningocele, cerebral
Meningoencephalocele
AHA: 4Q, '94, 37
DEF: Brain tissue protrudes through skull defect.

Spina Bifida

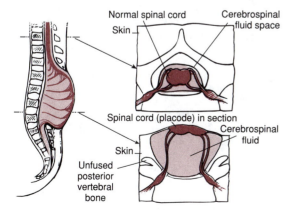

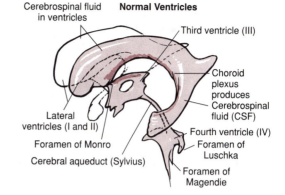

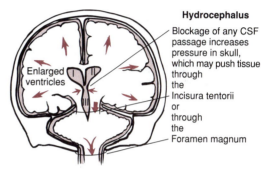

742.1 Microcephalus
Hydromicrocephaly
Micrencephaly
DEF: Extremely small head or brain.

742.2 Reduction deformities of brain
Absence
Agenesis   } of part of brain
Aplasia
Hypoplasia

Agyria   Holoprosencephaly
Arhinencephaly   Microgyria
AHA: 4Q, '94, 37

742.3 Congenital hydrocephalus
Aqueduct of Sylvius:
   anomaly
   obstruction, congenital
   stenosis
Atresia of foramina of Magendie and Luschka
Hydrocephalus in newborn
EXCLUDES hydrocephalus:
            acquired (331.3-331.4)
            due to congenital toxoplasmosis (771.2)
            with any condition classifiable to 741.9 (741.0)
DEF: Fluid accumulation within the skull; involves subarachnoid (external) or ventricular (internal) brain spaces.

742.4 Other specified anomalies of brain
Congenital cerebral cyst   Multiple anomalies of brain
Macroencephaly   NOS
Macrogyria   Porencephaly
Megalencephaly   Ulegyria
AHA: 1Q, '99, 9; 3Q, '92, 12

√5th 742.5 Other specified anomalies of spinal cord

742.51 Diastematomyelia
DEF: Congenital anomaly often associated with spina bifida; the spinal cord is separated into halves by a bony tissue resembling a "spike" (a spicule), each half surrounded by a dural sac.

CONGENITAL ANOMALIES

742.53 Hydromyelia
Hydrorhachis
DEF: Dilated central spinal cord canal; characterized by increased fluid accumulation.

742.59 Other
Amyelia
Atelomyelia
Congenital anomaly of spinal meninges
Defective development of cauda equina
Hypoplasia of spinal cord
Myelatelia
Myelodysplasia
AHA: 2Q, '91, 14; 1Q, '89, 10

742.8 Other specified anomalies of nervous system
Agenesis of nerve
Displacement of brachial plexus
Familial dysautonomia
Jaw-winking syndrome
Marcus-Gunn syndrome
Riley-Day syndrome
EXCLUDES neurofibromatosis (237.7)

742.9 Unspecified anomaly of brain, spinal cord, and nervous system
Anomaly
Congenital: disease, lesion, Deformity of: brain, nervous system, spinal cord

743 Congenital anomalies of eye

743.0 Anophthalmos
DEF: Complete absence of the eyes or the presence of vestigial eyes.

743.00 Clinical anophthalmos, unspecified
Agenesis
Congenital absence } of eye
Anophthalmos NOS

743.03 Cystic eyeball, congenital

743.06 Cryptophthalmos
DEF: Eyelids continue over eyeball, results in apparent absence of eyelids.

743.1 Microphthalmos
Dysplasia
Hypoplasia } of eye
Rudimentary eye
DEF: Abnormally small eyeballs, may be opacities of cornea and lens, scarring of choroid and retina.

743.10 Microphthalmos, unspecified
743.11 Simple microphthalmos
743.12 Microphthalmos associated with other anomalies of eye and adnexa

743.2 Buphthalmos
Glaucoma: Hydrophthalmos
  congenital
  newborn
EXCLUDES glaucoma of childhood (365.14)
traumatic glaucoma due to birth injury (767.8)
DEF: Distended, enlarged fibrous coats of eye; due to intraocular pressure of congenital glaucoma.

743.20 Buphthalmos, unspecified
743.21 Simple buphthalmos
743.22 Buphthalmos associated with other ocular anomalies
Keratoglobus, congenital
Megalocornea } associated with buphthalmos

743.3 Congenital cataract and lens anomalies
EXCLUDES infantile cataract (366.00-366.09)
DEF: Opaque eye lens.

743.30 Congenital cataract, unspecified
743.31 Capsular and subcapsular cataract
743.32 Cortical and zonular cataract
743.33 Nuclear cataract
743.34 Total and subtotal cataract, congenital
743.35 Congenital aphakia
Congenital absence of lens
743.36 Anomalies of lens shape
Microphakia   Spherophakia
743.37 Congenital ectopic lens
743.39 Other

743.4 Coloboma and other anomalies of anterior segment
DEF: Coloboma: ocular tissue defect associated with defect of ocular fetal intraocular fissure; may cause small pit on optic disk, major defects of iris, ciliary body, choroid, and retina.

743.41 Anomalies of corneal size and shape
Microcornea
EXCLUDES that associated with buphthalmos (743.22)
743.42 Corneal opacities, interfering with vision, congenital
743.43 Other corneal opacities, congenital
743.44 Specified anomalies of anterior chamber, chamber angle, and related structures
Anomaly: Anomaly:
  Axenfeld's   Rieger's
  Peters'
743.45 Aniridia
DEF: Incompletely formed or absent iris; affects both eyes; dominant trait; also called congenital hyperplasia of iris.
743.46 Other specified anomalies of iris and ciliary body
Anisocoria, congenital   Coloboma of iris
Atresia of pupil   Corectopia
743.47 Specified anomalies of sclera
743.48 Multiple and combined anomalies of anterior segment
743.49 Other

743.5 Congenital anomalies of posterior segment
743.51 Vitreous anomalies
Congenital vitreous opacity
743.52 Fundus coloboma
DEF: Absent retinal and choroidal tissue; occurs in lower fundus; a bright white ectatic zone of exposed sclera extends into and changes the optic disk.
743.53 Chorioretinal degeneration, congenital
743.54 Congenital folds and cysts of posterior segment
743.55 Congenital macular changes
743.56 Other retinal changes, congenital
AHA: 3Q, '99, 12
743.57 Specified anomalies of optic disc
Coloboma of optic disc (congenital)
743.58 Vascular anomalies
Congenital retinal aneurysm
743.59 Other

743.6 Congenital anomalies of eyelids, lacrimal system, and orbit
743.61 Congenital ptosis
DEF: Drooping of eyelid.
743.62 Congenital deformities of eyelids
Ablepharon
Absence of eyelid
Accessory eyelid
Congenital:
  ectropion
  entropion
AHA: 1Q, '00, 22

CONGENITAL ANOMALIES

743.63 Other specified congenital anomalies of eyelid
 Absence, agenesis, of cilia
743.64 Specified congenital anomalies of lacrimal gland
743.65 Specified congenital anomalies of lacrimal passages
 Absence, agenesis of:
  lacrimal apparatus
  punctum lacrimale
 Accessory lacrimal canal
743.66 Specified congenital anomalies of orbit
743.69 Other
 Accessory eye muscles

743.8 Other specified anomalies of eye
 EXCLUDES congenital nystagmus (379.51)
  ocular albinism (270.2)
  retinitis pigmentosa (362.74)

743.9 Unspecified anomaly of eye
 Congenital:
  anomaly NOS } of eye [any part]
  deformity NOS

√4th **744** Congenital anomalies of ear, face, and neck
 EXCLUDES anomaly of:
  cervical spine (754.2, 756.10-756.19)
  larynx (748.2-748.3)
  nose (748.0-748.1)
  parathyroid gland (759.2)
  thyroid gland (759.2)
  cleft lip (749.10-749.25)

√5th **744.0** Anomalies of ear causing impairment of hearing
 EXCLUDES congenital deafness without mention of cause (389.0-389.9)
 744.00 Unspecified anomaly of ear with impairment of hearing
 744.01 Absence of external ear
  Absence of:
   auditory canal (external)
   auricle (ear) (with stenosis or atresia of auditory canal)
 744.02 Other anomalies of external ear with impairment of hearing
  Atresia or stricture of auditory canal (external)
 744.03 Anomaly of middle ear, except ossicles
  Atresia or stricture of osseous meatus (ear)
 744.04 Anomalies of ear ossicles
  Fusion of ear ossicles
 744.05 Anomalies of inner ear
  Congenital anomaly of:
   membranous labyrinth
   organ of Corti
 744.09 Other
  Absence of ear, congenital

744.1 Accessory auricle
 Accessory tragus   Supernumerary:
 Polyotia   ear
 Preauricular appendage lobule
 DEF: Redundant tissue or structures of ear.

√5th **744.2** Other specified anomalies of ear
 EXCLUDES that with impairment of hearing (744.00-744.09)
 744.21 Absence of ear lobe, congenital
 744.22 Macrotia
  DEF: Abnormally large pinna of ear.
 744.23 Microtia
  DEF: Hypoplasia of pinna; associated with absent or closed auditory canal.
 744.24 Specified anomalies of Eustachian tube
  Absence of Eustachian tube
 744.29 Other
  Bat ear   Prominence of auricle
  Darwin's tubercle Ridge ear
  Pointed ear
  EXCLUDES preauricular sinus (744.46)

744.3 Unspecified anomaly of ear
 Congenital:
  anomaly NOS } of ear, not elsewhere
  deformity NOS classified

√5th **744.4** Branchial cleft cyst or fistula; preauricular sinus
 DEF: Coloboma: malclosure of the intraoccular fissure in embryo resulting in defects to optic disk, iris, ciliary body, choroid, or retina.
 744.41 Branchial cleft sinus or fistula
  Branchial:
   sinus (external) (internal)
   vestige
  DEF: Cyst due to failed closure of embryonic branchial cleft.
 744.42 Branchial cleft cyst
 744.43 Cervical auricle
 744.46 Preauricular sinus or fistula
 744.47 Preauricular cyst
 744.49 Other
  Fistula (of):   Fistula (of):
  auricle, congenital cervicoaural

744.5 Webbing of neck
 Pterygium colli
 DEF: Thick, triangular skinfold, stretches from lateral side of neck across shoulder; associated with Turner's and Noonan's syndromes.

√5th **744.8** Other specified anomalies of face and neck
 744.81 Macrocheilia
  Hypertrophy of lip, congenital
  DEF: Abnormally large lips.
 744.82 Microcheilia
  DEF: Abnormally small lips.
 744.83 Macrostomia
  DEF: Bilateral or unilateral anomaly, of mouth due to malformed maxillary and mandibular processes; results in mouth extending toward ear.
 744.84 Microstomia
  DEF: Abnormally small mouth.
 744.89 Other
  EXCLUDES congenital fistula of lip (750.25)
   musculoskeletal anomalies (754.0-754.1, 756.0)

744.9 Unspecified anomalies of face and neck
 Congenital:
  anomaly NOS } of face [any part] or
  deformity NOS neck [any part]

√4th **745** Bulbus cordis anomalies and anomalies of cardiac septal closure
 745.0 Common truncus   CC
  Absent septum } between aorta and
  Communication (abnormal) pulmonary artery
  Aortic septal defect
  Common aortopulmonary trunk
  Persistent truncus arteriosus
  CC Excl: 429.71, 429.79, 745.0-745.9, 746.89, 746.9, ▶747.83,◀ 747.89, 747.9, 759.7-759.89

√5th **745.1** Transposition of great vessels
 745.10 Complete transposition of great vessels CC
  Transposition of great vessels:
   NOS
   classical
  CC Excl: See code 745.0

Heart Defects

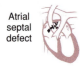
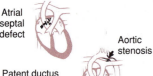

- **745.11** **Double outlet right ventricle** `CC`
  - Dextratransposition of aorta
  - Incomplete transposition of great vessels
  - Origin of both great vessels from right ventricle
  - Taussig-Bing syndrome or defect
  - **CC Excl:** See code 745.0

- **745.12** **Corrected transposition of great vessels** `CC`
  - **CC Excl:** See code 745.0

- **745.19** **Other** `CC`
  - **CC Excl:** See code 745.0

- **745.2** **Tetralogy of Fallot** `CC`
  - Fallot's pentalogy
  - Ventricular septal defect with pulmonary stenosis or atresia, dextraposition of aorta, and hypertrophy of right ventricle
  - **EXCLUDES** Fallot's triad (746.09)
  - **CC Excl:** See code 745.0
  - **DEF:** Obstructed cardiac outflow causes pulmonary stenosis, interventricular septal defect and right ventricular hypertrophy.

- **745.3** **Common ventricle** `CC`
  - Cor triloculare biatriatum
  - Single ventricle
  - **CC Excl:** See code 745.0

- **745.4** **Ventricular septal defect** `CC`
  - Eisenmenger's defect or complex
  - Gerbo dedefect
  - Interventricular septal defect
  - Left ventricular-right atrial communication
  - Roger's disease
  - **EXCLUDES** common atrioventricular canal type (745.69)
  - single ventricle (745.3)
  - **CC Excl:** See code 745.0

- **745.5** **Ostium secundum type atrial septal defect**
  - Defect: Patent or persistent:
    - atrium secundum foramen ovale
    - fossa ovalis ostium secundum
  - Lutembacher's syndrome
  - **DEF:** Opening in atrial septum due to failure of the septum secundum and the endocardial cushions to fuse; there is a rim of septum surrounding the defect.

- √5th **745.6** **Endocardial cushion defects**
  - **DEF:** Atrial and/or ventricular septa defects causing abnormal fusion of cushions in atrioventricular canal.

  - **745.60** **Endocardial cushion defect, unspecified type** `CC`
    - **CC Excl:** See code 745.0
    - **DEF:** Septal defect due to imperfect fusion of endocardial cushions.

- **745.61** **Ostium primum defect**
  - Persistent ostium primum
  - **DEF:** Opening in low, posterior septum primum; causes cleft in basal portion of atrial septum; associated with cleft mitral valve.

- **745.69** **Other** `CC`
  - Absence of atrial septum
  - Atrioventricular canal type ventricular septal defect
  - Common atrioventricular canal
  - Common atrium
  - **CC Excl:** See code 745.0

- **745.7** **Cor biloculare** `CC`
  - Absence of atrial and ventricular septa
  - **CC Excl:** See code 745.0
  - **DEF:** Atrial and ventricular septal defect; marked by heart with two cardiac chambers (one atrium, one ventricle), and one atrioventricular valve.

- **745.8** **Other**
- **745.9** **Unspecified defect of septal closure**
  - Septal defect NOS

- √4th **746** **Other congenital anomalies of heart**
  - **EXCLUDES** endocardial fibroelastosis (425.3)

- √5th **746.0** **Anomalies of pulmonary valve**
  - **EXCLUDES** infundibular or subvalvular pulmonic stenosis (746.83)
  - tetralogy of Fallot (745.2)

  - **746.00** **Pulmonary valve anomaly, unspecified**
  - **746.01** **Atresia, congenital** `CC`
    - Congenital absence of pulmonary valve
    - **CC Excl:** 746.00-746.09, 746.89, 746.9, ▶747.83,◀ 747.89, 747.9, 759.7-759.89

  - **746.02** **Stenosis, congenital** `CC`
    - **CC Excl:** See code 746.01
    - **DEF:** Stenosis of opening between pulmonary artery and right ventricle; causes obstructed blood outflow from right ventricle.

  - **746.09** **Other**
    - Congenital insufficiency of pulmonary valve
    - Fallot's triad or trilogy

- **746.1** **Tricuspid atresia and stenosis, congenital** `CC`
  - Absence of tricuspid valve
  - **CC Excl:** 746.1-746.7, 746.89, 746.9, ▶747.83,◀ 747.89, 747.9, 759.7-759.89

- **746.2** **Ebstein's anomaly** `CC`
  - **CC Excl:** See code 746.1
  - **DEF:** Malformation of the tricuspid valve characterized by septal and posterior leaflets attaching to the wall of the right ventricle; causing the right ventricle to fuse with the atrium producing a large right atrium and a small ventricle; causes a malfunction of the right ventricle with accompanying complications such as heart failure and abnormal cardiac rhythm.

- **746.3** **Congenital stenosis of aortic valve** `CC`
  - Congenital aortic stenosis
  - **EXCLUDES** congenital:
    - subaortic stenosis (746.81)
    - supravalvular aortic stenosis (747.22)
  - **CC Excl:** See code 746.1
  - **AHA:** 4Q, '88, 8
  - **DEF:** Stenosis of orifice of aortic valve; obstructs blood outflow from left ventricle.

- **746.4** **Congenital insufficiency of aortic valve** `CC`
  - Bicuspid aortic valve
  - Congenital aortic insufficiency
  - **CC Excl:** See code 746.1
  - **DEF:** Impaired functioning of aortic valve due to incomplete closure; causes backflow (regurgitation) of blood from aorta to left ventricle.

CONGENITAL ANOMALIES

746.5 **Congenital mitral stenosis** [CC]
Fused commissure
Parachute deformity } of mitral valve
Supernumerary cusps

CC Excl: See code 746.1

DEF: Stenosis of left atrioventricular orifice.

746.6 **Congenital mitral insufficiency** [CC]
CC Excl: See code 746.1

DEF: Impaired functioning of mitral valve due to incomplete closure; causes backflow of blood from left ventricle to left atrium.

746.7 **Hypoplastic left heart syndrome** [CC]
Atresia, or marked hypoplasia, of aortic orifice or valve, with hypoplasia of ascending aorta and defective development of left ventricle (with mitral valve atresia)

CC Excl: See code 746.1

√5th **746.8** **Other specified anomalies of heart**
746.81 **Subaortic stenosis** [CC]
CC Excl: 746.81-746.84, 746.89, 746.9, ▶747.83,◄ 747.89, 747.9, 759.7-759.89

DEF: Stenosis, of left ventricular outflow tract due to fibrous tissue ring or septal hypertrophy below aortic valve.

746.82 **Cor triatriatum** [CC]
CC Excl: See code 746.81

DEF: Transverse septum divides left atrium due to failed resorption of embryonic common pulmonary vein; results in three atrial chambers.

746.83 **Infundibular pulmonic stenosis** [CC]
Subvalvular pulmonic stenosis
CC Excl: See code 746.81

DEF: Stenosis of right ventricle outflow tract within infundibulum due to fibrous diaphragm below valve or long, narrow fibromuscular channel.

746.84 **Obstructive anomalies of heart, not elsewhere classified** [CC]
Uhl's disease
CC Excl: See code 746.81

746.85 **Coronary artery anomaly**
Anomalous origin or communication of coronary artery
Arteriovenous malformation of coronary artery
Coronary artery:
  absence
  arising from aorta or pulmonary trunk
  single
AHA: N-D, '85, 3

746.86 **Congenital heart block** [CC]
Complete or incomplete atrioventricular [AV] block
CC Excl: 746.86, 746.89, 746.9, ▶747.83,◄ 747.89, 747.9, 759.7-759.89

DEF: Impaired conduction of electrical impulses; due to maldeveloped junctional tissue.

746.87 **Malposition of heart and cardiac apex**
Abdominal heart   Levocardia (isolated)
Dextrocardia   Mesocardia
Ectopia cordis
EXCLUDES dextrocardia with complete transposition of viscera (759.3)

746.89 **Other**
Atresia } of cardiac vein
Hypoplasia

Congenital: Congenital:
  cardiomegaly   pericardial defect
  diverticulum,   left ventricle

AHA: 3Q, '00, 3; 1Q, '99, 11; J-F, '85, 3

746.9 **Unspecified anomaly of heart**
Congenital:
  anomaly of heart NOS
  heart disease NOS

√4th **747** **Other congenital anomalies of circulatory system**
747.0 **Patent ductus arteriosus**
Patent ductus Botalli
Persistent ductus arteriosus

DEF: Open lumen in ductus arteriosus causes arterial blood recirculation in lungs; inhibits blood supply to aorta; symptoms such as shortness of breath more noticeable upon activity.

√5th **747.1** **Coarctation of aorta**
DEF: Localized deformity of aortic media seen as a severe constriction of the vessel lumen; major symptom is high blood pressure in the arms and low pressure in the legs; a CVA, rupture of the aorta, bacterial endocarditis or congestive heart failure can follow if left untreated.

747.10 **Coarctation of aorta (preductal) (postductal)** [CC]
Hypoplasia of aortic arch
CC Excl: No Exclusions
AHA: 1Q, '99, 11; 4Q, '88, 8

747.11 **Interruption of aortic arch** [CC]
CC Excl: 747.10-747.22, ▶747.83,◄ 747.89, 747.9, 759.7-759.89

√5th **747.2** **Other anomalies of aorta**
747.20 **Anomaly of aorta, unspecified**
747.21 **Anomalies of aortic arch**
Anomalous origin, right subclavian artery
Dextraposition of aorta
Double aortic arch
Kommerell's diverticulum
Overriding aorta
Persistent:
  convolutions, aortic arch
  right aortic arch
Vascular ring
EXCLUDES hypoplasia of aortic arch (747.10)

747.22 **Atresia and stenosis of aorta** [CC]
Absence
Aplasia
Hypoplasia } of aorta
Stricture

Supra (valvular)-aortic stenosis
EXCLUDES congenital aortic (valvular) stenosis or stricture, so stated (746.3)
hypoplasia of aorta in hypoplastic left heart syndrome (746.7)

CC Excl: See code 747.11

747.29 **Other**
Aneurysm of sinus of Valsalva
Congenital:
  aneurysm } of aorta
  dilation

747.3 **Anomalies of pulmonary artery**
Agenesis
Anomaly
Atresia
Coarctation } of pulmonary artery
Hypoplasia
Stenosis

Pulmonary arteriovenous aneurysm
AHA: 1Q, '94, 15; 4Q, '88, 8

√5th **747.4** **Anomalies of great veins**
747.40 **Anomaly of great veins, unspecified**
Anomaly NOS of: Anomaly NOS of:
  pulmonary veins   vena cava

CONGENITAL ANOMALIES

747.41 Total anomalous pulmonary venous connection
  Total anomalous pulmonary venous return [TAPVR]:
    subdiaphragmatic
    supradiaphragmatic

747.42 Partial anomalous pulmonary venous connection
  Partial anomalous pulmonary venous return

747.49 Other anomalies of great veins
  Absence } of vena cava
  Congenital stenosis } (inferior) (superior)
  Persistent:
    left posterior cardinal vein
    left superior vena cava
  Scimitar syndrome
  Transposition of pulmonary veins NOS

747.5 Absence or hypoplasia of umbilical artery
  Single umbilical artery

√5th **747.6** Other anomalies of peripheral vascular system
  Absence }
  Anomaly } of artery or vein, NEC
  Atresia }
  Arteriovenous aneurysm (peripheral)
  Arteriovenous malformation of the peripheral vascular system
  Congenital:
    aneurysm (peripheral)   stricture, artery
    phlebectasia   varix
  Multiple renal arteries
  EXCLUDES anomalies of:
    cerebral vessels (747.81)
    pulmonary artery (747.3)
    congenital retinal aneurysm (743.58)
    hemangioma (228.00-228.09)
    lymphangioma (228.1)

  747.60 Anomaly of the peripheral vascular system, unspecified site

  747.61 Gastrointestinal vessel anomaly
    AHA: 3Q, '96, 10

  747.62 Renal vessel anomaly
  747.63 Upper limb vessel anomaly
  747.64 Lower limb vessel anomaly
  747.69 Anomalies of other specified sites of peripheral vascular system

√5th **747.8** Other specified anomalies of circulatory system
  747.81 Anomalies of cerebrovascular system
    Arteriovenous malformation of brain
    Cerebral arteriovenous aneurysm, congenital
    Congenital anomalies of cerebral vessels
    EXCLUDES ruptured cerebral (arteriovenous) aneurysm (430)

  747.82 Spinal vessel anomaly
    Arteriovenous malformation of spinal vessel
    AHA: 3Q, '95, 5

  747.83 Persistent fetal circulation
    Persistent pulmonary hypertension
    Primary pulmonary hypertension of newborn

  747.89 Other
    Aneurysm, congenital, specified site not elsewhere classified
    EXCLUDES congenital aneurysm:
      coronary (746.85)
      peripheral (747.6)
      pulmonary (747.3)
      retinal (743.58)

747.9 Unspecified anomaly of circulatory system

√4th **748** Congenital anomalies of respiratory system
  EXCLUDES congenital defect of diaphragm (756.6)

  748.0 Choanal atresia
    Atresia } of nares (anterior)
    Congenital stenosis } (posterior)
    DEF: Occluded posterior nares (choana), bony or membranous due to failure of embryonic bucconasal membrane to rupture.

  748.1 Other anomalies of nose
    Absent nose   Congenital:
    Accessory nose   notching of tip of nose
    Cleft nose   perforation of wall of
    Congenital: nasal sinus
      deformity of nose   Deformity of wall of nasal sinus
    EXCLUDES congenital deviation of nasal septum (754.0)

  748.2 Web of larynx
    Web of larynx: Web of larynx:
      NOS   subglottic
      glottic
    DEF: Malformed larynx; marked by thin, translucent, or thick, fibrotic spread between vocal folds; affects speech.

  748.3 Other anomalies of larynx, trachea, and bronchus
    Absence or agenesis of: Congenital:
      bronchus   dilation, trachea
      larynx   stenosis:
      trachea   larynx
    Anomaly(of):   trachea
      cricoid cartilage   tracheocele
      epiglottis   Diverticulum:
      thyroid cartilage   bronchus
      tracheal cartilage   trachea
    Atresia (of):   Fissure of epiglottis
      epiglottis   Laryngocele
      glottis   Posterior cleft of cricoid
      larynx   cartilage (congenital)
      trachea   Rudimentary tracheal
    Cleft thyroid, cartilage, bronchus
      congenital   Stridor, laryngeal, congenital
    AHA: 1Q, '99, 14

  748.4 Congenital cystic lung   CC
    Disease, lung: Honeycomb lung, congenital
      cystic, congenital
      polycystic, congenital
    EXCLUDES acquired or unspecified cystic lung (518.89)
    CC Excl: 748.4-748.9
    DEF: Enlarged air spaces of lung parenchyma.

  748.5 Agenesis, hypoplasia, and dysplasia of lung   CC
    Absence of lung (fissures) (lobe)
      (lobe)   Hypoplasia of lung
    Aplasia of lung   Sequestration of lung
    CC Excl: See code 748.4

  √5th **748.6** Other anomalies of lung
    748.60 Anomaly of lung, unspecified
    748.61 Congenital bronchiectasis   CC
      CC Excl: 494.0-494.1, 496, 506.1, 506.4, 506.9, 748.61
    748.69 Other
      Accessory lung (lobe)
      Azygos lobe (fissure), lung

  748.8 Other specified anomalies of respiratory system
    Abnormal communication between pericardial and pleural sacs
    Anomaly, pleural folds
    Atresia of nasopharynx
    Congenital cyst of mediastinum

  748.9 Unspecified anomaly of respiratory system
    Anomaly of respiratory system NOS

√4th **749** Cleft palate and cleft lip

CONGENITAL ANOMALIES

Cleft Lip and Palate

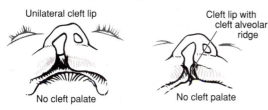

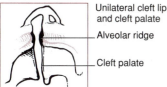

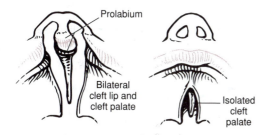

- **√5th 749.0 Cleft palate**
  - 749.00 Cleft palate, unspecified
  - 749.01 Unilateral, complete
  - 749.02 Unilateral, incomplete
    - Cleft uvula
  - 749.03 Bilateral, complete
  - 749.04 Bilateral, incomplete
- **√5th 749.1 Cleft lip**
  - Cheiloschisis   Harelip
  - Congenital fissure of lip   Labium leporinum
  - 749.10 Cleft lip, unspecified
  - 749.11 Unilateral, complete
  - 749.12 Unilateral, incomplete
  - 749.13 Bilateral, complete
  - 749.14 Bilateral, incomplete
- **√5th 749.2 Cleft palate with cleft lip**
  - Cheilopalatoschisis
  - 749.20 Cleft palate with cleft lip, unspecified
  - 749.21 Unilateral, complete
  - 749.22 Unilateral, incomplete
  - 749.23 Bilateral, complete
    - AHA: 1Q, '96, 14
  - 749.24 Bilateral, incomplete
  - 749.25 Other combinations
- **√4th 750 Other congenital anomalies of upper alimentary tract**
  - EXCLUDES dentofacial anomalies (524.0-524.9)
  - **750.0 Tongue tie**
    - Ankyloglossia
    - DEF: Restricted tongue movement due to lingual frenum extending toward tip of tongue. Tongue may be fused to mouth floor affecting speech.
  - **√5th 750.1 Other anomalies of tongue**
    - 750.10 Anomaly of tongue, unspecified
    - 750.11 Aglossia
      - DEF: Absence of tongue.
    - 750.12 Congenital adhesions of tongue
    - 750.13 Fissure of tongue
      - Bifid tongue   Double tongue
    - 750.15 Macroglossia
      - Congenital hypertrophy of tongue
    - 750.16 Microglossia
      - Hypoplasia of tongue
    - 750.19 Other
  - **√5th 750.2 Other specified anomalies of mouth and pharynx**
    - 750.21 Absence of salivary gland
    - 750.22 Accessory salivary gland
    - 750.23 Atresia, salivary duct
      - Imperforate salivary duct
    - 750.24 Congenital fistula of salivary gland
    - 750.25 Congenital fistula of lip
      - Congenital (mucus) lip pits
    - 750.26 Other specified anomalies of mouth
      - Absence of uvula
    - 750.27 Diverticulum of pharynx
      - Pharyngeal pouch
    - 750.29 Other specified anomalies of pharynx
      - Imperforate pharynx
  - **750.3 Tracheoesophageal fistula, esophageal atresia and stenosis**
    - Absent esophagus
    - Atresia of esophagus
    - Congenital:
      - esophageal ring
      - stenosis of esophagus
      - stricture of esophagus
    - Congenital fistula:
      - esophagobronchial
      - esophagotracheal
    - Imperforate esophagus
    - Webbed esophagus
  - **750.4 Other specified anomalies of esophagus**
    - Dilatation, congenital
    - Displacement, congenital
    - Diverticulum
    - Duplication
    - Giant
    } (of) esophagus
    - Esophageal pouch
    - EXCLUDES congenital hiatus hernia (750.6)
    - AHA: J-F, '85, 3
  - **750.5 Congenital hypertrophic pyloric stenosis**
    - Congenital or infantile:
      - constriction
      - hypertrophy
      - spasm
      - stenosis
      - stricture
    } of pylorus
    - DEF: Obstructed pylorus due to overgrowth of pyloric muscle.
  - **750.6 Congenital hiatus hernia**
    - Displacement of cardia through esophageal hiatus
    - EXCLUDES congenital diaphragmatic hernia (756.6)
  - **750.7 Other specified anomalies of stomach**
    - Congenital:
      - cardiospasm
      - hourglass stomach
    - Displacement of stomach
    - Diverticulum of stomach, congenital
    - Duplication of stomach
    - Megalogastria
    - Microgastria
    - Transposition of stomach
  - **750.8 Other specified anomalies of upper alimentary tract**
  - **750.9 Unspecified anomaly of upper alimentary tract**
    - Congenital:
      - anomaly NOS
      - deformity NOS
    } of upper alimentary tract [any part, except tongue]
- **√4th 751 Other congenital anomalies of digestive system**
  - **751.0 Meckel's diverticulum**
    - Meckel's diverticulum (displaced) (hypertrophic)
    - Persistent:
      - omphalomesenteric duct
      - vitelline duct
    - DEF: Malformed sacs or appendages of ileum of small intestine; can cause strangulation, volvulus and intussusception.

CONGENITAL ANOMALIES — Tabular List

751.1 Atresia and stenosis of small intestine [P]
- Atresia of:
  - duodenum
  - ileum
- Atresia of:
  - intestine NOS
- Congenital:
  - absence
  - obstruction
  - stenosis
  - stricture
  } of small intestine or intestine NOS
- Imperforate jejunum

751.2 Atresia and stenosis of large intestine, rectum, and anal canal [P]
- Absence:
  - anus (congenital)
  - appendix, congenital
  - large intestine, congenital
  - rectum
- Atresia of:
  - anus
  - colon
  - rectum
- Congenital or infantile:
  - obstruction of large intestine
  - occlusion of anus
  - stricture of anus
- Imperforate:
  - anus
  - rectum
- Stricture of rectum, congenital

AHA: 2Q, '98, 16

751.3 Hirschsprung's disease and other congenital functional disorders of colon
- Aganglionosis
- Congenital dilation of colon
- Congenital megacolon
- Macrocolon

DEF: Hirschsprung's disease: enlarged or dilated colon (megacolon), with absence of ganglion cells in the narrowed wall distally; causes inability to defecate.

751.4 Anomalies of intestinal fixation
- Congenital adhesions:
  - omental, anomalous
  - peritoneal
  - Jackson's membrane
- Malrotation of colon
- Rotation of cecum or colon:
  - failure of
  - incomplete
  - insufficient
- Universal mesentery

751.5 Other anomalies of intestine
- Congenital diverticulum, colon
- Dolichocolon
- Duplication of:
  - anus
  - appendix
  - cecum
  - intestine
- Ectopic anus
- Megaloappendix
- Megaloduodenum
- Microcolon
- Persistent cloaca
- Transposition of:
  - appendix
  - colon
  - intestine

AHA: 3Q, '01, 8

✓5th 751.6 Anomalies of gallbladder, bile ducts, and liver

751.60 Unspecified anomaly of gallbladder, bile ducts, and liver

751.61 Biliary atresia [P]
- Congenital:
  - absence
  - hypoplasia
  - obstruction
  - stricture
  } of bile duct (common) or passage

AHA: S-O, '87, 8

751.62 Congenital cystic disease of liver
- Congenital polycystic disease of liver
- Fibrocystic disease of liver

751.69 Other anomalies of gallbladder, bile ducts, and liver
- Absence of:
  - gallbladder, congenital
  - liver (lobe)
- Accessory:
  - hepatic ducts
  - liver
- Congenital:
  - choledochal cyst
  - hepatomegaly
- Duplication of:
  - biliary duct
  - cystic duct
  - gallbladder
  - liver
- Floating:
  - gallbladder
  - liver
- Intrahepatic gallbladder

AHA: S-O, '87, 8

751.7 Anomalies of pancreas
- Absence
- Accessory
- Agenesis
- Annular
- Hypoplasia
} (of) pancreas
- Ectopic pancreatic tissue
- Pancreatic heterotopia

EXCLUDES diabetes mellitus:
- congenital (250.0-250.9)
- neonatal (775.1)
- fibrocystic disease of pancreas ▶(277.00-277.09)◀

751.8 Other specified anomalies of digestive system
- Absence (complete) (partial) of alimentary tract NOS
- Duplication
- Malposition, congenital
} of digestive organs NOS

EXCLUDES congenital diaphragmatic hernia (756.6)
congenital hiatus hernia (750.6)

751.9 Unspecified anomaly of digestive system
- Congenital:
  - anomaly NOS
  - deformity NOS
} of digestive system NOS

✓4th 752 Congenital anomalies of genital organs

EXCLUDES syndromes associated with anomalies in the number and form of chromosomes (758.0-758.9)
testicular feminization syndrome (257.8)

752.0 Anomalies of ovaries ♀
- Absence, congenital
- Accessory
- Ectopic
- Streak
} (of) ovary

✓5th 752.1 Anomalies of fallopian tubes and broad ligaments

752.10 Unspecified anomaly of fallopian tubes and broad ligaments ♀

752.11 Embryonic cyst of fallopian tubes and broad ligaments ♀
- Cyst:
  - epoophoron
  - fimbrial
- Cyst:
  - Gartner's duct
  - parovarian

AHA: S-O, '85, 13

752.19 Other ♀
- Absence
- Accessory
- Atresia
} (of) fallopian tube or broad ligament

752.2 Doubling of uterus ♀
- Didelphic uterus
- Doubling of uterus [any degree] (associated with doubling of cervix and vagina)

752.3 Other anomalies of uterus ♀
- Absence, congenital
- Agenesis
- Aplasia
- Bicornuate
} (of) uterus
- Uterus unicornis
- Uterus with only one functioning horn

✓5th 752.4 Anomalies of cervix, vagina, and external female genitalia

752.40 Unspecified anomaly of cervix, vagina, and external female genitalia ♀

752.41 Embryonic cyst of cervix, vagina, and external female genitalia ♀
- Cyst of:
  - canal of Nuck, congenital
  - vagina, embryonal
  - vulva, congenital

DEF: Embryonic fluid-filled cysts, of cervix, vagina or external female genitalia.

 Newborn Age: 0   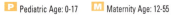 Pediatric Age: 0-17    Maternity Age: 12-55   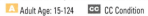 Adult Age: 15-124   CC CC Condition   MC Major Complication   Complex Dx   HIV Related Dx

CONGENITAL ANOMALIES

752.42 Imperforate hymen ♀
DEF: Complete closure of membranous fold around external opening of vagina.

752.49 Other anomalies of cervix, vagina, and external female genitalia ♀
Absence ⎫ of cervix, clitoris,
Agenesis ⎭ vagina, or vulva
Congenital stenosis or stricture of:
  cervical canal
  vagina
  EXCLUDES double vagina associated with total duplication (752.2)

√5th 752.5 Undescended and retractile testicle
AHA: 4Q, '96, 33

752.51 Undescended testis ♂
Cryptorchism
Ectopic testis

752.52 Retractile testis ♂

√5th 752.6 Hypospadias and epispadias and other penile anomalies
AHA: 4Q, '96, 34, 35

752.61 Hypospadias ♂
AHA: 3Q, '97, 6
DEF: Hypospadias: abnormal opening of urethra on the ventral surface of the penis or perineum; also a rare defect of vagina.

752.62 Epispadias ♂
Anaspadias
DEF: Epispadias: urethra opening on dorsal surface of penis; in females appears as a slit in the upper wall of urethra.

752.63 Congenital chordee ♂
DEF: Ventral bowing of penis due to fibrous band along corpus spongiosum; occurs with hypospadias.

752.64 Micropenis ♂
752.65 Hidden penis ♂
752.69 Other penile anomalies ♂

752.7 Indeterminate sex and pseudohermaphroditism
Gynandrism   Pseudohermaphroditism
Hermaphroditism   (male) (female)
Ovotestis   Pure gonadal dysgenesis
  EXCLUDES pseudohermaphroditism:
    female, with adrenocortical disorder (255.2)
    male, with gonadal disorder (257.8)
    with specified chromosomal anomaly (758.0-758.9)
    testicular feminization syndrome (257.8)
DEF: Pseudohermaphroditism: presence of gonads of one sex and external genitalia of other sex.

752.8 Other specified anomalies of genital organs
Absence of: Atresia of:
  prostate   ejaculatory duct
  spermatic cord   vas deferens
  vas deferens   Fusion of testes
Anorchism   Hypoplasia of testis
Aplasia (congenital) of: Monorchism
  prostate   Polyorchism
  round ligament
  testicle
  EXCLUDES congenital hydrocele (778.6)
    penile anomalies (752.61-752.69)
    phimosis or paraphimosis (605)

752.9 Unspecified anomaly of genital organs
Congenital:
  anomaly NOS   ⎫ of genital organ,
  deformity NOS ⎭   not elsewhere classified

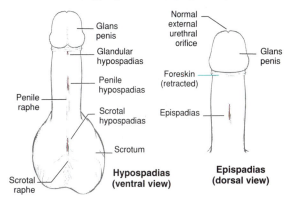

►Hypospadias and Epispadias◄

Hypospadias (ventral view) — Glans penis, Glandular hypospadias, Penile hypospadias, Scrotal hypospadias, Penile raphe, Scrotum, Scrotal raphe

Epispadias (dorsal view) — Normal external urethral orifice, Glans penis, Foreskin (retracted), Epispadias

√4th 753 Congenital anomalies of urinary system

753.0 Renal agenesis and dysgenesis
Atrophy of kidney: Atrophy of kidney:
  congenital   infantile
Congenital absence of kidney(s)
Hypoplasia of kidney(s)

√5th 753.1 Cystic kidney disease
EXCLUDES acquired cyst of kidney (593.2)
AHA: 4Q, '90, 3

753.10 Cystic kidney disease, unspecified
753.11 Congenital single renal cyst
753.12 Polycystic kidney, unspecified type
753.13 Polycystic kidney, autosomal dominant
DEF: Slow progressive disease characterized by bilateral cysts causing increased kidney size and impaired function.

753.14 Polycystic kidney, autosomal recessive
DEF: Rare disease characterized by multiple cysts involving kidneys and liver, producing renal and hepatic failure in childhood or adolescence.

753.15 Renal dysplasia
753.16 Medullary cystic kidney
Nephronopthisis
DEF: Diffuse kidney disease results in uremia onset prior to age 20.

753.17 Medullary sponge kidney
DEF: Dilated collecting tubules; usually asymptomatic but calcinosis in tubules may cause renal insufficiency.

753.19 Other specified cystic kidney disease
Multicystic kidney

√5th 753.2 Obstructive defects of renal pelvis and ureter
AHA: 4Q, '96, 35

753.20 Unspecified obstructive defect of renal pelvis and ureter
753.21 Congenital obstruction of ureteropelvic junction
DEF: Stricture at junction of ureter and renal pelvis.

753.22 Congenital obstruction of ureterovesical junction
Adynamic ureter
Congenital hydroureter
DEF: Stricture at junction of ureter and bladder.

753.23 Congenital ureterocele
753.29 Other

753.3 Other specified anomalies of kidney
Accessory kidney   Fusion of kidneys
Congenital: Giant kidney
  calculus of kidney   Horseshoe kidney
  displaced kidney   Hyperplasia of kidney
Discoid kidney   Lobulation of kidney
Double kidney with   Malrotation of kidney
  double pelvis   Trifid kidney (pelvis)
Ectopic kidney

CONGENITAL ANOMALIES

753.4 **Other specified anomalies of ureter**
    Absent ureter
    Accessory ureter
    Deviation of ureter
    Displaced ureteric orifice
    Double ureter
    Ectopic ureter
    Implantation, anomalous of ureter

753.5 **Exstrophy of urinary bladder**
    Ectopia vesicae
    Extroversion of bladder
    DEF: Absence of lower abdominal and anterior bladder walls with posterior bladder wall protrusion.

753.6 **Atresia and stenosis of urethra and bladder neck**
    Congenital obstruction:
        bladder neck
        urethra
    Congenital stricture of:
        urethra (valvular)
        urinary meatus
        vesicourethral orifice
    Imperforate urinary meatus
    Impervious urethra
    Urethral valve formation

753.7 **Anomalies of urachus**
    Cyst
    Fistula   } (of) urachussinus
    Patent
    Persistent umbilical sinus

753.8 **Other specified anomalies of bladder and urethra**
    Absence, congenital of:
        bladder
        urethra
    Accessory:
        bladder
        urethra
    Congenital:
        diverticulum of bladder
        hernia of bladder
    Congenital urethrorectal fistula
    Congenital prolapse of:
        bladder (mucosa)
        urethra
    Double:
        urethra
        urinary meatus

753.9 **Unspecified anomaly of urinary system**
    Congenital:
        anomaly NOS   } of urinary system [any part,
        deformity NOS   except urachus]

√4th **754** **Certain congenital musculoskeletal deformities**
    INCLUDES nonteratogenic deformities which are considered to be due to intrauterine malposition and pressure

754.0 **Of skull, face, and jaw**
    Asymmetry of face
    Compression facies
    Depressions in skull
    Deviation of nasal septum, congenital
    Dolichocephaly
    Plagiocephaly
    Potter's facies
    Squashed or bent nose, congenital
    EXCLUDES dentofacial anomalies (524.0-524.9)
        syphilitic saddle nose (090.5)

754.1 **Of sternocleidomastoid muscle**
    Congenital sternomastoid torticollis
    Congenital wryneck
    Contracture of sternocleidomastoid (muscle)
    Sternomastoid tumor

754.2 **Of spine**
    Congenital postural:
        lordosis
        scoliosis

√5th **754.3** **Congenital dislocation of hip**
    754.30 Congenital dislocation of hip, unilateral
        Congenital dislocation of hip NOS
    754.31 Congenital dislocation of hip, bilateral
    754.32 Congenital subluxation of hip, unilateral
        Congenital flexion deformity, hip or thigh
        Predislocation status of hip at birth
        Preluxation of hip, congenital
    754.33 Congenital subluxation of hip, bilateral
    754.35 Congenital dislocation of one hip with subluxation of other hip

√5th **754.4** **Congenital genu recurvatum and bowing of long bones of leg**

    754.40 Genu recurvatum
        DEF: Backward curving of knee joint.
    754.41 Congenital dislocation of knee (with genu recurvatum)
    754.42 Congenital bowing of femur
    754.43 Congenital bowing of tibia and fibula
    754.44 Congenital bowing of unspecified long bones of leg

√5th **754.5** **Varus deformities of feet**
    EXCLUDES acquired (736.71, 736.75, 736.79)
    754.50 Talipes varus
        Congenital varus deformity of foot, unspecified
        Pes varus
        DEF: Inverted foot marked by outer sole resting on ground.
    754.51 Talipes equinovarus
        Equinovarus (congenital)
        DEF: Elevated, outward rotation of heel; also called clubfoot.
    754.52 Metatarsus primus varus
        DEF: Malformed first metatarsal bone, with bone angled toward body.
    754.53 Metatarsus varus
    754.59 Other
        Talipes calcaneovarus

√5th **754.6** **Valgus deformities of feet**
    EXCLUDES valgus deformity of foot (acquired) (736.79)
    754.60 Talipes valgus
        Congenital valgus deformity of foot, unspecified
    754.61 Congenital pes planus
        Congenital rocker bottom flat foot
        Flat foot, congenital
        EXCLUDES pes planus (acquired) (734)
    754.62 Talipes calcaneovalgus
    754.69 Other
        Talipes: Talipes:
          equinovalgus   planovalgus

√5th **754.7** **Other deformities of feet**
    EXCLUDES acquired (736.70-736.79)
    754.70 Talipes, unspecified
        Congenital deformity of foot NOS
    754.71 Talipes cavus
        Cavus foot (congenital)
    754.79 Other
        Asymmetric talipes
        Talipes:
          calcaneus
          equinus

√5th **754.8** **Other specified nonteratogenic anomalies**
    754.81 Pectus excavatum
        Congenital funnel chest
    754.82 Pectus carinatum
        Congenital pigeon chest [breast]
    754.89 Other
        Club hand (congenital)
        Congenital:
          deformity of chest wall
          dislocation of elbow
        Generalized flexion contractures of lower limb joints, congenital
        Spade-like hand (congenital)

√4th **755** **Other congenital anomalies of limbs**
    EXCLUDES those deformities classifiable to 754.0-754.8

√5th **755.0** **Polydactyly**
    755.00 Polydactyly, unspecified digits
        Supernumerary digits
    755.01 Of fingers
        Accessory fingers

CONGENITAL ANOMALIES

755.02 Of toes
  Accessory toes

755.1 Syndactyly
  Symphalangy   Webbing of digits
  755.10 Of multiple and unspecified sites
  755.11 Of fingers without fusion of bone
  755.12 Of fingers with fusion of bone
  755.13 Of toes without fusion of bone
  755.14 Of toes with fusion of bone

755.2 Reduction deformities of upper limb
  755.20 Unspecified reduction deformity of upper limb
    Ectromelia NOS } of upper limb
    Hemimelia NOS
    Shortening of arm, congenital
  755.21 Transverse deficiency of upper limb
    Amelia of upper limb
    Congenital absence of:
      fingers, all (complete or partial)
      forearm, including hand and fingers
      upper limb, complete
    Congenital amputation of upper limb
    Transverse hemimelia of upper limb
  755.22 Longitudinal deficiency of upper limb, not elsewhere classified
    Phocomelia NOS of upper limb
    Rudimentary arm
  755.23 Longitudinal deficiency, combined, involving humerus, radius, and ulna (complete or incomplete)
    Congenital absence of arm and forearm (complete or incomplete) with or without metacarpal deficiency and/or phalangeal deficiency, incomplete
    Phocomelia, complete, of upper limb
  755.24 Longitudinal deficiency, humeral, complete or partial (with or without distal deficiencies, incomplete)
    Congenital absence of humerus (with or without absence of some [but not all] distal elements)
    Proximal phocomelia of upper limb
  755.25 Longitudinal deficiency, radioulnar, complete or partial (with or without distal deficiencies, incomplete)
    Congenital absence of radius and ulna (with or without absence of some [but not all] distal elements)
    Distal phocomelia of upper limb
  755.26 Longitudinal deficiency, radial, complete or partial (with or without distal deficiencies, incomplete)
    Agenesis of radius
    Congenital absence of radius (with or without absence of some [but not all] distal elements)
  755.27 Longitudinal deficiency, ulnar, complete or partial (with or without distal deficiencies, incomplete)
    Agenesis of ulna
    Congenital absence of ulna (with or without absence of some [but not all] distal elements)
  755.28 Longitudinal deficiency, carpals or metacarpals, complete or partial (with or without incomplete phalangeal deficiency)
  755.29 Longitudinal deficiency, phalanges, complete or partial
    Absence of finger, congenital
    Aphalangia of upper limb, terminal, complete or partial
    EXCLUDES *terminal deficiency of all five digits (755.21)*
    transverse deficiency of phalanges (755.21)

755.3 Reduction deformities of lower limb
  755.30 Unspecified reduction deformity of lower limb
    Ectromelia NOS } of lower limb
    Hemimelia NOS
    Shortening of leg, congenital
  755.31 Transverse deficiency of lower limb
    Amelia of lower limb
    Congenital absence of:
      foot
      leg, including foot and toes
      lower limb, complete
      toes, all, complete
    Transverse hemimelia of lower limb
  755.32 Longitudinal deficiency of lower limb, not elsewhere classified
    Phocomelia NOS of lower limb
  755.33 Longitudinal deficiency, combined, involving femur, tibia, and fibula (complete or incomplete)
    Congenital absence of thigh and (lower) leg (complete or incomplete) with or without metacarpal deficiency and/or phalangeal deficiency, incomplete
    Phocomelia, complete, of lower limb
  755.34 Longitudinal deficiency, femoral, complete or partial (with or without distal deficiencies, incomplete)
    Congenital absence of femur (with or without absence of some [but not all] distal elements)
    Proximal phocomelia of lower limb
  755.35 Longitudinal deficiency, tibiofibular, complete or partial (with or without distal deficiencies, incomplete)
    Congenital absence of tibia and fibula (with or without absence of some [but not all] distal elements)
    Distal phocomelia of lower limb
  755.36 Longitudinal deficiency, tibia, complete or partial (with or without distal deficiencies, incomplete)
    Agenesis of tibia
    Congenital absence of tibia (with or without absence of some [but not all] distal elements)
  755.37 Longitudinal deficiency, fibular, complete or partial (with or without distal deficiencies, incomplete)
    Agenesis of fibula
    Congenital absence of fibula (with or without absence of some [but not all] distal elements)
  755.38 Longitudinal deficiency, tarsals or metatarsals, complete or partial (with or without incomplete phalangeal deficiency)
  755.39 Longitudinal deficiency, phalanges, complete or partial
    Absence of toe, congenital
    Aphalangia of lower limb, terminal, complete or partial
    EXCLUDES *terminal deficiency of all five digits (755.31)*
    transverse deficiency of phalanges (755.31)

755.4 Reduction deformities, unspecified limb
  Absence, congenital (complete or partial) of limb NOS
  Amelia
  Ectromelia } of unspecified limb
  Hemimelia
  Phocomelia

755.5 Other anomalies of upper limb, including shoulder girdle
  755.50 Unspecified anomaly of upper limb

CONGENITAL ANOMALIES

755.51 Congenital deformity of clavicle
755.52 Congenital elevation of scapula
  Sprengel's deformity
755.53 Radioulnar synostosis
  DEF: Osseous adhesion of radius and ulna.
755.54 Madelung's deformity
  DEF: Distal ulnar overgrowth or radial shortening; also called carpus curvus.
755.55 Acrocephalosyndactyly
  Apert's syndrome
  DEF: Premature cranial suture fusion (craniostenosis); marked by cone-shaped or pointed (acrocephaly) head and webbing of the fingers (syndactyly); it is very similar to craniofacial dysostosis.
755.56 Accessory carpal bones
755.57 Macrodactylia (fingers)
  DEF: Abnormally large fingers, toes.
755.58 Cleft hand, congenital
  Lobster-claw hand
  DEF: Extended separation between fingers into metacarpus; also may refer to large fingers and absent middle fingers of hand.
755.59 Other
  Cleidocranial dysostosis
  Cubitus:
    valgus, congenital
    varus, congenital
  EXCLUDES club hand (congenital) (754.89)
    congenital dislocation of elbow (754.89)

√5th **755.6** Other anomalies of lower limb, including pelvic girdle
755.60 Unspecified anomaly of lower limb
755.61 Coxa valga, congenital
  DEF: Abnormally wide angle between the neck and shaft of the femur.
755.62 Coxa vara, congenital
  DEF: Diminished angle between neck and shaft of femur.
755.63 Other congenital deformity of hip (joint)
  Congenital anteversion of femur (neck)
  EXCLUDES congenital dislocation of hip (754.30-754.35)
  AHA: 1Q, '94, 15; S-O, '84, 15
755.64 Congenital deformity of knee (joint)
  Congenital:
    absence of patella
    genu valgum [knock-knee]
    genu varum [bowleg]
    Rudimentary patella
755.65 Macrodactylia of toes
  DEF: Abnormally large toes.
755.66 Other anomalies of toes
  Congenital: Congenital:
    hallux valgus   hammer toe
    hallux varus
755.67 Anomalies of foot, not elsewhere classified
  Astragaloscaphoid synostosis
  Calcaneonavicular bar
  Coalition of calcaneus
  Talonavicular synostosis
  Tarsal coalitions
755.69 Other
  Congenital:
    angulation of tibia
    deformity (of):
      ankle (joint)
      sacroiliac (joint)
      fusion of sacroiliac joint
755.8 Other specified anomalies of unspecified limb

755.9 **Unspecified anomaly of unspecified limb**
  Congenital:
    anomaly NOS } of unspecified limb
    deformity NOS
  EXCLUDES reduction deformity of unspecified limb (755.4)

√4th **756** Other congenital musculoskeletal anomalies
  EXCLUDES those deformities classifiable to 754.0-754.8
756.0 Anomalies of skull and face bones
  Absence of skull bones   Imperfect fusion of skull
  Acrocephaly   Oxycephaly
  Congenital deformity   Platybasia
    of forehead   Premature closure of
  Craniosynostosis   cranial sutures
  Crouzon's disease   Tower skull
  Hypertelorism   Trigonocephaly
  EXCLUDES acrocephalosyndactyly [Apert's syndrome] (755.55)
    dentofacial anomalies (524.0-524.9)
    skull defects associated with brain anomalies, such as:
      anencephalus (740.0)
      encephalocele (742.0)
      hydrocephalus (742.3)
      microcephalus (742.1)
  AHA: 3Q, '98, 9; 3Q, '96, 15

√5th **756.1** Anomalies of spine
756.10 Anomaly of spine, unspecified
756.11 Spondylolysis, lumbosacral region
  Prespondylolisthesis (lumbosacral)
  DEF: Bilateral or unilateral defect through the pars interarticularis of a vertebra causes spondylolisthesis.
756.12 Spondylolisthesis
  DEF: Downward slipping of lumbar vertebra over next vertebra; usually related to pelvic deformity.
756.13 Absence of vertebra, congenital
756.14 Hemivertebra
  DEF: Incomplete development of one side of a vertebra.
756.15 Fusion of spine [vertebra], congenital
756.16 Klippel-Feil syndrome
  DEF: Short, wide neck; limits range of motion due to abnormal number of cervical vertebra or fused hemivertebrae.
756.17 Spina bifida occulta
  EXCLUDES spina bifida (aperta) (741.0-741.9)
  DEF: Spina bifida marked by a bony spinal canal defect without a protrusion of the cord or meninges; it is diagnosed by radiography and has no symptoms.
756.19 Other
  Platyspondylia   Supernumerary vertebra
756.2 Cervical rib
  Supernumerary rib in the cervical region
  DEF: Costa cervicalis: extra rib attached to cervical vertebra.
756.3 Other anomalies of ribs and sternum
  Congenital absence of: Congenital:
    rib   fissure of sternum
    sternum   fusion of ribs
                              Sternum bifidum
  EXCLUDES nonteratogenic deformity of chest wall (754.81-754.89)
756.4 Chondrodystrophy
  Achondroplasia   Enchondromatosis
  Chondrodystrophia (fetalis) Ollier's disease
  Dyschondroplasia
  EXCLUDES lipochondrodystrophy [Hurler's syndrome] (277.5)
    Morquio's disease (277.5)
  AHA: S-O, '87, 10
  DEF: Abnormal development of cartilage.

| Tabular List | CONGENITAL ANOMALIES | 765.5–757.9 |

√5ᵗʰ **756.5 Osteodystrophies**
    756.50 Osteodystrophy, unspecified
    756.51 Osteogenesis imperfecta
        Fragilitas ossium
        Osteopsathyrosis
        DEF: A collagen disorder commonly characterized by brittle, osteoporotic, easily fractured bones, hypermobility of joints, blue sclerae, and a tendency to hemorrhage.
    756.52 Osteopetrosis
        DEF: Abnormally dense bone, optic atrophy, hepatosplenomegaly, deafness; sclerosing depletes bone marrow and nerve foramina of skull; often fatal.
    756.53 Osteopoikilosis
        DEF: Multiple sclerotic foci on ends of long bones, stippling in round, flat bones; identified by x-ray.
    756.54 Polyostotic fibrous dysplasia of bone
        DEF: Fibrous tissue displaces bone results in segmented ragged-edge café-au-lait spots; occurs in girls of early puberty.
    756.55 Chondroectodermal dysplasia
        Ellis-van Creveld syndrome
        DEF: Inadequate enchondral bone formation; impaired development of hair and teeth, polydactyly, and cardiac septum defects.
    756.56 Multiple epiphyseal dysplasia
    756.59 Other
        Albright (-McCune)-Sternberg syndrome

756.6 Anomalies of diaphragm
    Absence of diaphragm
    Congenital hernia:
        diaphragmatic
        foramen of Morgagni
    Eventration of diaphragm
    EXCLUDES congenital hiatus hernia (750.6)

√5ᵗʰ **756.7 Anomalies of abdominal wall**
    756.70 Anomaly of abdominal wall, unspecified
    756.71 Prune belly syndrome
        Eagle-Barrett syndrome
        Prolapse of bladder mucosa
        AHA: 4Q, '97, 44
        DEF: Prune belly syndrome: absence of lower rectus abdominis muscle and lower and medial oblique muscles; results in dilated bladder and ureters, dysplastic kidneys and hydronephrosis; more common in male infants with undescended testicles.
    756.79 Other congenital anomalies of abdominal wall
        Exomphalos
        Gastroschisis
        Omphalocele
        EXCLUDES umbilical hernia (551-553 with .1)
        DEF: Exomphalos: umbilical hernia prominent navel.
        DEF: Gastroschisis: fissure of abdominal wall, results in protruding small or large intestine.
        DEF: Omphalocele: hernia of umbilicus due to impaired abdominal wall; results in membrane-covered intestine protruding through peritoneum and amnion.

√5ᵗʰ **756.8 Other specified anomalies of muscle, tendon, fascia, and connective tissue**
    756.81 Absence of muscle and tendon
        Absence of muscle (pectoral)
    756.82 Accessory muscle
    756.83 Ehlers-Danlos syndrome
        DEF: Danlos syndrome: connective tissue disorder causes hyperextended skin and joints; results in fragile blood vessels with bleeding, poor wound healing and subcutaneous pseudotumors.

    756.89 Other
        Amyotrophia congenita
        Congenital shortening of tendon
        AHA: 3Q, '99, 16

756.9 Other and unspecified anomalies of musculoskeletal system
    Congenital:
        anomaly NOS } of musculoskeletal system,
        deformity NOS }   not elsewhere classified

√4ᵗʰ **757 Congenital anomalies of the integument**
    INCLUDES anomalies of skin, subcutaneous tissue, hair, nails, and breast
    EXCLUDES hemangioma (228.00-228.09)
        pigmented nevus (216.0-216.9)

757.0 Hereditary edema of legs
    Congenital lymphedema
    Hereditary trophedema
    Milroy's disease

757.1 Ichthyosis congenita
    Congenital ichthyosis
    Harlequin fetus
    Ichthyosiform erythroderma
    DEF: Overproduction of skin cells causes scaling of skin; may result in stillborn fetus or death soon after birth.

757.2 Dermatoglyphic anomalies
    Abnormal palmar creases
    DEF: Abnormal skin-line patterns of fingers, palms, toes and soles; initial finding of possible chromosomal abnormalities.

√5ᵗʰ **757.3 Other specified anomalies of skin**
    757.31 Congenital ectodermal dysplasia
        DEF: Tissues and structures originate in embryonic ectoderm; includes anhidrotic and hidrotic ectodermal dysplasia and EEC syndrome.
    757.32 Vascular hamartomas
        Birthmarks   Strawberry nevus
        Port-wine stain
        DEF: Benign tumor of blood vessels; due to malformed angioblastic tissues.
    757.33 Congenital pigmentary anomalies of skin
        Congenital poikiloderma
        Urticaria pigmentosa
        Xeroderma pigmentosum
        EXCLUDES albinism (270.2)
    757.39 Other
        Accessory skin tags, congenital
        Congenital scar
        Epidermolysis bullosa
        Keratoderma (congenital)
        EXCLUDES pilonidal cyst (685.0-685.1)

757.4 Specified anomalies of hair
    Congenital: Congenital:
      alopecia   hypertrichosis
      atrichosis   monilethrix
      beaded hair   Persistent lanugo

757.5 Specified anomalies of nails
    Anonychia   Congenital:
    Congenital: leukonychia
      clubnail   onychauxis
      koilonychia   pachyonychia

757.6 Specified anomalies of breast
    Absent
    Accessory   } breast or nipple
    Supernumerary
    Hypoplasia of breast
    EXCLUDES absence of pectoral muscle (756.81)

757.8 Other specified anomalies of the integument

757.9 Unspecified anomaly of the integument
    Congenital:
      anomaly NOS } of integument
      deformity NOS

758 Chromosomal anomalies ✓4th

INCLUDES: syndromes associated with anomalies in the number and form of chromosomes

- **758.0 Down's syndrome**
  - Mongolism
  - Translocation Down's syndrome
  - Trisomy: 21 or 22
  - G

- **758.1 Patau's syndrome**
  - Trisomy: 13
  - Trisomy: D_1

  DEF: Trisomy of 13th chromosome; characteristic failure to thrive, severe mental impairment, seizures, abnormal eyes, low-set ears and sloped forehead.

- **758.2 Edwards' syndrome**
  - Trisomy: 18
  - E_3

  DEF: Trisomy of 18th chromosome; characteristic mental and physical impairments; mainly affects females.

- **758.3 Autosomal deletion syndromes**
  - Antimongolism syndrome
  - Cri-du-chat syndrome

  DEF: Antimongolism syndrome: Deletions in 21st chromosome; characteristic oblique palpebral fissures, hypertonia, micrognathia, microcephaly, high-arched palate and impaired mental and physical growth.

  DEF: Cri-du-chat syndrome: Abnormally large distance between two organs or parts, abnormally small brain and severe mental impairment; characteristic of abnormal 5th chromosome.

- **758.4 Balanced autosomal translocation in normal individual**

- **758.5 Other conditions due to autosomal anomalies**
  - Accessory autosomes NEC

- **758.6 Gonadal dysgenesis**
  - Ovarian dysgenesis
  - Turner's syndrome
  - XO syndrome

  EXCLUDES: pure gonadal dysgenesis (752.7)

- **758.7 Klinefelter's syndrome** ♂
  - XXY syndrome

  DEF: Impaired embryonic development of seminiferous tubes; results in small testes, azoospermia, infertility and enlarged mammary glands.

- ✓5th **758.8 Other conditions due to chromosome anomalies**
  - **758.81** Other conditions due to sex chromosome anomalies
  - **758.89** Other

- **758.9 Conditions due to anomaly of unspecified chromosome**

✓4th 759 Other and unspecified congenital anomalies

- **759.0 Anomalies of spleen**
  - Aberrant } spleen
  - Absent }
  - Accessory }
  - Congenital splenomegaly
  - Ectopic spleen
  - Lobulation of spleen

- **759.1 Anomalies of adrenal gland**
  - Aberrant } adrenal gland
  - Absent }
  - Accessory }

  EXCLUDES: adrenogenital disorders (255.2)
  congenital disorders of steroid metabolism (255.2)

- **759.2 Anomalies of other endocrine glands**
  - Absent parathyroid gland
  - Accessory thyroid gland
  - Persistent thyroglossal or thyrolingual duct
  - Thyroglossal (duct) cyst

  EXCLUDES: congenital:
  goiter (246.1)
  hypothyroidism (243)

- **759.3 Situs inversus**
  - Situs inversus or transversus:
    - abdominalis
    - thoracis
  - Transposition of viscera:
    - abdominal
    - thoracic

  EXCLUDES: dextrocardia without mention of complete transposition (746.87)

  DEF: Laterally transposed thoracic and abdominal viscera.

- **759.4 Conjoined twins**
  - Craniopagus
  - Dicephalus
  - Pygopagus
  - Thoracopagus
  - Xiphopagus

- **759.5 Tuberous sclerosis**
  - Bourneville's disease
  - Epiloia

  DEF: Hamartomas of brain, retina and viscera, impaired mental ability, seizures and adenoma sebaceum.

- **759.6 Other hamartoses, not elsewhere classified**
  - Syndrome:
    - Peutz-Jeghers
    - Sturge-Weber (-Dimitri)
  - Syndrome:
    - von Hippel-Lindau

  EXCLUDES: neurofibromatosis (237.7)

  AHA: 3Q, '92, 12

  DEF: Peutz-Jeghers: hereditary syndrome characterized by hamartomas of small intestine

  DEF: Sturge-Weber: congenital syndrome characterized by unilateral port-wine stain over trigeminal nerve, underlying meninges and cerebral cortex.

  DEF: von Hipple-Lindau: hereditary syndrome of congenital angiomatosis of the retina and cerebellum.

- **759.7 Multiple congenital anomalies, so described**
  - Congenital:
    - anomaly, multiple NOS
    - deformity, multiple NOS

- ✓5th **759.8 Other specified anomalies**

  AHA: S-O, '87, 9; S-O, '85, 11

  - **759.81** Prader-Willi syndrome
  - **759.82** Marfan syndrome

    AHA: 3Q, '93, 11
  - **759.83** Fragile X syndrome

    AHA: 4Q, '94, 41
  - **759.89** Other
    - Congenital malformation syndromes affecting multiple systems, not elsewhere classified
    - Laurence-Moon-Biedl syndrome

    AHA: 1Q, '01, 3; 3Q, '99, 17, 18; 3Q, '98, 8

- **759.9 Congenital anomaly, unspecified**

15. CERTAIN CONDITIONS ORIGINATING IN THE PERINATAL PERIOD (760-779)

INCLUDES conditions which have their origin in the perinatal period even though death or morbidity occurs later

Use additional code(s) to further specify condition

MATERNAL CAUSES OF PERINATAL MORBIDITY AND MORTALITY (760-763)

AHA: 2Q, '89, 14; 3Q, '90, 5

760 Fetus or newborn affected by maternal conditions which may be unrelated to present pregnancy

INCLUDES the listed maternal conditions only when specified as a cause of mortality or morbidity of the fetus or newborn

EXCLUDES maternal endocrine and metabolic disorders affecting fetus or newborn (775.0-775.9)

AHA: 1Q, '94, 8; 2Q, '92, 12; N-D, '84, 11

- **760.0 Maternal hypertensive disorders**
  Fetus or newborn affected by maternal conditions classifiable to 642
- **760.1 Maternal renal and urinary tract diseases**
  Fetus or newborn affected by maternal conditions classifiable to 580-599
- **760.2 Maternal infections**
  Fetus or newborn affected by maternal infectious disease classifiable to 001-136 and 487, but fetus or newborn not manifesting that disease
  EXCLUDES congenital infectious diseases (771.0-771.8)
  maternal genital tract and other localized infections (760.8)
- **760.3 Other chronic maternal circulatory and respiratory diseases**
  Fetus or newborn affected by chronic maternal conditions classifiable to 390-459, 490-519, 745-748
- **760.4 Maternal nutritional disorders**
  Fetus or newborn affected by:
  maternal disorders classifiable to 260-269
  maternal malnutrition NOS
  EXCLUDES fetal malnutrition (764.10-764.29)
- **760.5 Maternal injury**
  Fetus or newborn affected by maternal conditions classifiable to 800-995
- **760.6 Surgical operation on mother**
  EXCLUDES cesarean section for present delivery (763.4)
  damage to placenta from amniocentesis, cesarean section, or surgical induction (762.1)
  previous surgery to uterus or pelvic organs (763.89)
- **760.7 Noxious influences affecting fetus via placenta or breast milk**
  Fetus or newborn affected by noxious substance transmitted via placenta or breast milk
  EXCLUDES anesthetic and analgesic drugs administered during labor and delivery (763.5)
  drug withdrawal syndrome in newborn (779.5)
  AHA: 3Q, '91, 21
  - **760.70 Unspecified noxious substance**
    Fetus or newborn affected by:
    Drug NEC
  - **760.71 Alcohol**
    Fetal alcohol syndrome
  - **760.72 Narcotics**
  - **760.73 Hallucinogenic agents**
  - **760.74 Anti-infectives**
    Antibiotics
  - **760.75 Cocaine**
    AHA: 3Q, '94, 6; 2Q, '92, 12; 4Q, '91, 26
  - **760.76 Diethylstilbestrol [DES]**
    AHA: 4Q, '94, 45
  - **760.79 Other**
    Fetus or newborn affected by:
    immune sera
    medicinal agents NEC
    toxic substance NEC
    transmitted via placenta or breast milk
- **760.8 Other specified maternal conditions affecting fetus or newborn**
  Maternal genital tract and other localized infection affecting fetus or newborn, but fetus or newborn not manifesting that disease
  EXCLUDES maternal urinary tract infection affecting fetus or newborn (760.1)
- **760.9 Unspecified maternal condition affecting fetus or newborn**

761 Fetus or newborn affected by maternal complications of pregnancy

INCLUDES the listed maternal conditions only when specified as a cause of mortality or morbidity of the fetus or newborn

- **761.0 Incompetent cervix**
  DEF: Inadequate functioning of uterine cervix.
- **761.1 Premature rupture of membranes**
- **761.2 Oligohydramnios**
  EXCLUDES that due to premature rupture of membranes (761.1)
  DEF: Deficient amniotic fluid.
- **761.3 Polyhydramnios**
  Hydramnios (acute) (chronic)
  DEF: Excess amniotic fluid.
- **761.4 Ectopic pregnancy**
  Pregnancy: abdominal intraperitoneal
  Pregnancy: tubal
- **761.5 Multiple pregnancy**
  Triplet (pregnancy)   Twin (pregnancy)
- **761.6 Maternal death**
- **761.7 Malpresentation before labor**
  Breech presentation
  External version
  Oblique lie
  Transverse lie
  Unstable lie
  } before labor
- **761.8 Other specified maternal complications of pregnancy affecting fetus or newborn**
  Spontaneous abortion, fetus
- **761.9 Unspecified maternal complication of pregnancy affecting fetus or newborn**

762 Fetus or newborn affected by complications of placenta, cord, and membranes

INCLUDES the listed maternal conditions only when specified as a cause of mortality or morbidity in the fetus or newborn

AHA: 1Q, '94, 8

- **762.0 Placenta previa**
  DEF: Placenta developed in lower segment of uterus; causes hemorrhaging in last trimester.

CONDITIONS IN THE PERINATAL PERIOD

762.1 Other forms of placental separation and hemorrhage
  Abruptio placentae
  Antepartum hemorrhage
  Damage to placenta from amniocentesis, cesarean section, or surgical induction
  Maternal blood loss
  Premature separation of placenta
  Rupture of marginal sinus

762.2 Other and unspecified morphological and functional abnormalities of placenta
  Placental: dysfunction
  Placental: insufficiency
  infarction

762.3 Placental transfusion syndromes
  Placental and cord abnormality resulting in twin-to-twin or other transplacental transfusion
  Use additional code to indicate resultant condition in fetus or newborn:
    fetal blood loss (772.0)
    polycythemia neonatorum (776.4)

762.4 Prolapsed cord
  Cord presentation

762.5 Other compression of umbilical cord
  Cord around neck   Knot in cord
  Entanglement of cord Torsion of cord

762.6 Other and unspecified conditions of umbilical cord
  Short cord
  Thrombosis
  Varices   } of umbilical cord
  Velamentous insertion
  Vasa previa
  EXCLUDES infection of umbilical cord (771.4)
               single umbilical artery (747.5)

762.7 Chorioamnionitis
  Amnionitis
  Membranitis
  Placentitis
  DEF: Inflamed fetal membrane.

762.8 Other specified abnormalities of chorion and amnion

762.9 Unspecified abnormality of chorion and amnion

√4th **763** Fetus or newborn affected by other complications of labor and delivery
  INCLUDES the listed conditions only when specified as a cause of mortality or morbidity in the fetus or newborn
  AHA: 1Q, '94, 8

763.0 Breech delivery and extraction

763.1 Other malpresentation, malposition, and disproportion during labor and delivery
  Fetus or newborn affected by:
    abnormality of bony pelvis
    contracted pelvis
    persistent occipitoposterior position
    shoulder presentation
    transverse lie
    conditions classifiable to 652, 653, and 660

763.2 Forceps delivery
  Fetus or newborn affected by forceps extraction

763.3 Delivery by vacuum extractor

763.4 Cesarean delivery
  EXCLUDES placental separation or hemorrhage from cesarean section (762.1)

763.5 Maternal anesthesia and analgesia
  Reactions and intoxications from maternal opiates and tranquilizers during labor and delivery
  EXCLUDES drug withdrawal syndrome in newborn (779.5)

763.6 Precipitate delivery
  Rapid second stage

763.7 Abnormal uterine contractions
  Fetus or newborn affected by:
    contraction ring
    hypertonic labor
    hypotonic uterine dysfunction
    uterine inertia or dysfunction
    conditions classifiable to 661, except 661.3

√5th **763.8** Other specified complications of labor and delivery affecting fetus or newborn
  AHA: 4Q, '98, 46

  763.81 Abnormality in fetal heart rate or rhythm before the onset of labor

  763.82 Abnormality in fetal heart rate or rhythm during labor
    AHA: 4Q, '98, 46

  763.83 Abnormality in fetal heart rate or rhythm, unspecified as to time of onset

  763.89 Other specified complications of labor and delivery affecting fetus or newborn
    Fetus or newborn affected by:
      abnormality of maternal soft tissues
      destructive operation on live fetus to facilitate delivery
      induction of labor (medical)
      previous surgery to uterus or pelvic organs
      other conditions classifiable to 650-669
      other procedures used in labor and delivery

763.9 Unspecified complication of labor and delivery affecting fetus or newborn

OTHER CONDITIONS ORIGINATING IN THE PERINATAL PERIOD (764-779)

The following fifth-digit subclassification is for use with ►category 764 and codes 765.0-765.1◄ to denote birthweight:
  0 unspecified [weight]
  1 less than 500 grams
  2 500-749 grams
  3 750-999 grams
  4 1,000-1,249 grams
  5 1,250-1,499 grams
  6 1,500-1,749 grams
  7 1,750-1,999 grams
  8 2,000-2,499 grams
  9 2,500 grams and over

√4th **764** Slow fetal growth and fetal malnutrition
  AHA: 1Q, '94, 8; 2Q, '91, 19; 2Q, '89, 15

√5th **764.0** "Light-for-dates" without mention of fetal malnutrition
  Infants underweight for gestational age
  "Small-for-dates"

√5th **764.1** "Light-for-dates" with signs of fetal malnutrition
  Infants "light-for-dates" classifiable to 764.0, who in addition show signs of fetal malnutrition, such as dry peeling skin and loss of subcutaneous tissue

√5th **764.2** Fetal malnutrition without mention of "light-for-dates"
  Infants, not underweight for gestational age, showing signs of fetal malnutrition, such as dry peeling skin and loss of subcutaneous tissue
  Intrauterine malnutrition

√5th **764.9** Fetal growth retardation, unspecified
  Intrauterine growth retardation
  AHA: For code 764.97: 1Q, '97, 6

CONDITIONS IN THE PERINATAL PERIOD   765–768.9

Tabular List

✓4th **765 Disorders relating to short gestation and unspecified low birthweight**
  INCLUDES: the listed conditions, without further specification, as causes of mortality, morbidity, or additional care, in fetus or newborn
  AHA: 1Q, '97, 6; 1Q, '94, 8; 2Q, '91, 19; 2Q, '89, 15

§ ✓5th **765.0 Extreme immaturity**   CC 1-8
  Note: Usually implies a birthweight of less than 1000 grams.
  ▶Use additional code for weeks of gestation (765.20-765.29)◀
  CC Excl: For codes 765.01-765.08: 764.00-764.99, 765.00-765.19, ▶765.20-765.29,◀ 767.8-767.9, 779.8, ▶779.81-779.89◀
  AHA: For code 756.03: 4Q, '01, 51

§ ✓5th **765.1 Other preterm infants**
  Note: Usually implies a birthweight of 1000-2499 grams.
  Prematurity NOS
  Prematurity or small size, not classifiable to 765.0 or as "light-for-dates" in 764
  ▶Use additional code for weeks of gestation (765.20-765.29)◀
  AHA: For code 765.10: 1Q, '94, 14
  AHA: For code 765.17: 1Q, '97, 6

✓5th **765.2 Weeks of gestation**
  765.20 Unspecified weeks of gestation
  765.21 Less than 24 completed weeks of gestation
  765.22 24 completed weeks of gestation
  765.23 25-26 completed weeks of gestation
  765.24 27-28 completed weeks of gestation
  765.25 29-30 completed weeks of gestation
  765.26 31-32 completed weeks of gestation
  765.27 33-34 completed weeks of gestation
  765.28 35-36 completed weeks of gestation
  765.29 37 or more completed weeks of gestation

✓4th **766 Disorders relating to long gestation and high birthweight**
  INCLUDES: the listed conditions, without further specification, as causes of mortality, morbidity, or additional care, in fetus or newborn

  766.0 Exceptionally large baby
  Note: Usually implies a birthweight of 4500 grams or more.

  766.1 Other "heavy-for-dates" infants
  Other fetus or infant "heavy-" or "large-for-dates" regardless of period of gestation

  766.2 Post-term infant, not "heavy-for-dates"
  Postmaturity NOS

✓4th **767 Birth trauma**
  767.0 Subdural and cerebral hemorrhage   CC
  Subdural and cerebral hemorrhage, whether described as due to birth trauma or to intrapartum anoxia or hypoxia
  Subdural hematoma (localized)
  Tentorial tear
  Use additional code to identify cause
  EXCLUDES: intraventricular hemorrhage (772.10-772.14)
  subarachnoid hemorrhage (772.2)
  CC Excl: 767.0, 767.8-767.9, ▶779.81-779.89◀

  767.1 Injuries to scalp
  Caput succedaneum
  Cephalhematoma
  Chignon (from vacuum extraction)
  Massive epicranial subaponeurotic hemorrhage

  767.2 Fracture of clavicle
  767.3 Other injuries to skeleton
  Fracture of: long bones
  Fracture of: skull
  EXCLUDES: congenital dislocation of hip (754.30-754.35)
  fracture of spine, congenital (767.4)

  767.4 Injury to spine and spinal cord
  Dislocation
  Fracture   } of spine or spinal cord
  Laceration   }   due to birth trauma
  Rupture

  767.5 Facial nerve injury
  Facial palsy

  767.6 Injury to brachial plexus
  Palsy or paralysis: brachial
  Erb (-Duchenne)
  Palsy or paralysis: Klumpke (-Déjérine)

  767.7 Other cranial and peripheral nerve injuries
  Phrenic nerve paralysis

  767.8 Other specified birth trauma
  Eye damage
  Hematoma of:
    liver (subcapsular)
    testes
    vulva
  Rupture of:
    liver
    spleen
  Scalpel wound
  Traumatic glaucoma
  EXCLUDES: hemorrhage classifiable to 772.0-772.9

  767.9 Birth trauma, unspecified
  Birth injury NOS

✓4th **768 Intrauterine hypoxia and birth asphyxia**
  Use only when associated with newborn morbidity classifiable elsewhere
  AHA: 4Q, '92, 20
  DEF: Oxygen intake insufficiency due to interrupted placental circulation or premature separation of placenta.

  768.0 Fetal death from asphyxia or anoxia before onset of labor or at unspecified time

  768.1 Fetal death from asphyxia or anoxia during labor

  768.2 Fetal distress before onset of labor, in liveborn infant
  Fetal metabolic acidemia before onset of labor, in liveborn infant

  768.3 Fetal distress first noted during labor, in liveborn infant
  Fetal metabolic acidemia first noted during labor, in liveborn infant

  768.4 Fetal distress, unspecified as to time of onset, in liveborn infant
  Fetal metabolic acidemia unspecified as to time of onset, in liveborn infant
  AHA: N-D, '86, 10

  768.5 Severe birth asphyxia   CC
  Birth asphyxia with neurologic involvement
  CC Excl: 768.5-768.9, 769, 770.0-770.9, ▶779.81-779.89◀
  AHA: N-D, '86, 3

  768.6 Mild or moderate birth asphyxia
  Birth asphyxia (without mention of neurologic involvement)
  AHA: N-D, '86, 3

  768.9 Unspecified birth asphyxia in liveborn infant
  Anoxia
  Asphyxia   } NOS, in liveborn infant
  Hypoxia

§ Requires fifth-digit. See beginning of section 764-779 for codes and definitions.

CONDITIONS IN THE PERINATAL PERIOD — Tabular List

769 Respiratory distress syndrome [CC] [N]
  Cardiorespiratory distress syndrome of newborn
  Hyaline membrane disease (pulmonary)
  Idiopathic respiratory distress syndrome [IRDS or RDS] of newborn
  Pulmonary hypoperfusion syndrome
  EXCLUDES transient tachypnea of newborn (770.6)
  CC Excl: See code 768.5
  AHA: 1Q, '89, 10; N-D, '86, 6
  DEF: Severe chest contractions upon air intake and expiratory grunting; infant appears blue due to oxygen deficiency and has rapid respiratory rate; formerly called hyaline membrane disease.

√4th **770 Other respiratory conditions of fetus and newborn**

  770.0 Congenital pneumonia [CC] [N]
    Infective pneumonia acquired prenatally
    EXCLUDES pneumonia from infection acquired after birth (480.0-486)
    CC Excl: See code 768.5

  770.1 Meconium aspiration syndrome [CC] [N]
    Aspiration of contents of birth canal NOS
    Meconium aspiration below vocal cords
    Pneumonitis:
      fetal aspiration
      meconium
    CC Excl: See code 768.5
    DEF: Aspiration of meconium by the newborn infant prior to delivery. Presence of meconium in the trachea or chest x-ray indicating patchy infiltrates in conjunction with chest hyperextension establishes this diagnosis.

  770.2 Interstitial emphysema and related conditions [CC] [N]
    Pneumomediastinum ⎫
    Pneumopericardium ⎬ originating in the perinatal period
    Pneumothorax   ⎭
    CC Excl: See code 768.5

  770.3 Pulmonary hemorrhage [CC] [N]
    Hemorrhage:
      alveolar (lung)   ⎫
      intra-alveolar (lung) ⎬ originating in the perinatal period
      massive pulmonary   ⎭
    CC Excl: See code 768.5

  770.4 Primary atelectasis [CC] [N]
    Pulmonary immaturity NOS
    CC Excl: See code 768.5
    DEF: Alveoli fail to expand causing insufficient air intake by newborn.

  770.5 Other and unspecified atelectasis [CC] [N]
    Atelectasis:
      NOS
      partial   ⎫ originating in the perinatal period
      secondary   ⎭
    Pulmonary collapse
    CC Excl: See code 768.5

  770.6 Transitory tachypnea of newborn [N]
    Idiopathic tachypnea of newborn
    Wet lung syndrome
    EXCLUDES respiratory distress syndrome (769)
    AHA: 4Q, '95, 4; 1Q, '94, 12; 3Q, '93, 7; 1Q, '89, 10; N-D, '86, 6
    DEF: Quick, shallow breathing of newborn; short-term problem.

  770.7 Chronic respiratory disease arising in the perinatal period [CC]
    Bronchopulmonary dysplasia
    Interstitial pulmonary fibrosis of prematurity
    Wilson-Mikity syndrome
    CC Excl: See code 768.5
    AHA: 2Q, '91, 19; N-D, '86, 11

  √5th **770.8 Other respiratory problems after birth**
    AHA: 2Q, '98, 10; 2Q, '96, 10

    770.81 Primary apnea of newborn [N]
      Apneic spells of newborn NOS
      Essential apnea of newborn
      Sleep apnea of newborn

    770.82 Other apnea of newborn [N]
      Obstructive apnea of newborn

    770.83 Cyanotic attacks of newborn [N]

    770.84 Respiratory failure of newborn [CC] [N]
      EXCLUDES respiratory distress syndrome (769)
      CC Excl: See code 768.5

    770.89 Other respiratory problems after birth [N]

  770.9 Unspecified respiratory condition of fetus and newborn [N]

√4th **771 Infections specific to the perinatal period**
  INCLUDES infections acquired before or during birth or via the umbilicus
  EXCLUDES congenital pneumonia (770.0)
    congenital syphilis (090.0-090.9)
    maternal infectious disease as a cause of mortality or morbidity in fetus or newborn, but fetus or newborn not manifesting the disease (760.2)
    ophthalmia neonatorum due to gonococcus (098.40)
    other infections not specifically classified to this category
  AHA: N-D, '85, 4

  771.0 Congenital rubella [CC] [N]
    Congenital rubella pneumonitis
    CC Excl: 771.0-771.2, ▶779.81-779.89◀

  771.1 Congenital cytomegalovirus infection [CC] [N]
    Congenital cytomegalic inclusion disease
    CC Excl: See code 771.0

  771.2 Other congenital infections [N]
    Congenital: Congenital:
      herpes simplex   toxoplasmosis
      listeriosis   tuberculosis
      malaria

  771.3 Tetanus neonatorum [CC] [N]
    Tetanus omphalitis
    EXCLUDES hypocalcemic tetany (775.4)
    CC Excl: 771.3, ▶779.81-779.89◀
    DEF: Severe infection of central nervous system; due to exotoxin of tetanus bacillus from navel infection prompted by nonsterile technique during umbilical ligation.

  771.4 Omphalitis of the newborn [N]
    Infection:
      navel cord
      umbilical stump
    EXCLUDES tetanus omphalitis (771.3)
    DEF: Inflamed umbilicus.

  771.5 Neonatal infective mastitis [N]
    EXCLUDES noninfective neonatal mastitis (778.7)

  771.6 Neonatal conjunctivitis and dacryocystitis [N]
    Ophthalmia neonatorum NOS
    EXCLUDES ophthalmia neonatorum due to gonococcus (098.40)

  771.7 Neonatal Candida infection [N]
    Neonatal moniliasis
    Thrush in newborn

[N] Newborn Age: 0 [P] Pediatric Age: 0-17 [M] Maternity Age: 12-55 [A] Adult Age: 15-124 [CC] CC Condition [MC] Major Complication [CD] Complex Dx [HIV] HIV Related Dx

CONDITIONS IN THE PERINATAL PERIOD

√5th **771.8 Other infection specific to the perinatal period**
▶Use additional code to identify organism◀

- **771.81 Septicemia [sepsis] of newborn**
  CC Excl: 771.4-771.89, 776.0-776.9, 779.81-779.89
- **771.82 Urinary tract infection of newborn**
- **771.83 Bacteremia of newborn**
  CC Excl: See code 771.81
- **771.89 Other infections specific to the perinatal period**
  Intra-amniotic infection of fetus NOS
  Infection of newborn NOS

√4th **772 Fetal and neonatal hemorrhage**
EXCLUDES hematological disorders of fetus and newborn (776.0-776.9)

772.0 Fetal blood loss
Fetal blood loss from:
  cut end of co-twin's cord
  placenta
  ruptured cord
  vasa previa
Fetal exsanguination
Fetal hemorrhage into:
  co-twin
  mother's circulation

√5th **772.1 Intraventricular hemorrhage**
Intraventricular hemorrhage from any perinatal cause
AHA: 4Q, '01, 49; 3Q, '92, 8; 4Q, '88, 8

- **772.10 Unspecified grade**
  CC Excl: 772.0-772.2, 772.8-772.9, 776.0-776.9, ▶779.81-779.89◀
- **772.11 Grade I**
  Bleeding into germinal matrix
  CC Excl: See code 772.10
- **772.12 Grade II**
  Bleeding into ventricle
  CC Excl: See code 772.10
- **772.13 Grade III**
  Bleeding with enlargement of ventricle
  CC Excl: See code 772.10
  AHA: 4Q, '01, 51
- **772.14 Grade IV**
  Bleeding into cerebral cortex
  CC Excl: See code 772.10

772.2 Subarachnoid hemorrhage
Subarachnoid hemorrhage from any perinatal cause
EXCLUDES subdural and cerebral hemorrhage (767.0)
CC Excl: 772.0-772.2, 772.8-772.9, 776.0-776.9, 779.7-779.89

772.3 Umbilical hemorrhage after birth
Slipped umbilical ligature

772.4 Gastrointestinal hemorrhage
EXCLUDES swallowed maternal blood (777.3)
CC Excl: 772.0, 772.4-772.5, 772.8-772.9, 776.0-776.9, ▶779.81-779.89◀

772.5 Adrenal hemorrhage
CC Excl: See code 772.4

772.6 Cutaneous hemorrhage
Bruising
Ecchymoses } in fetus or newborn
Petechiae
Superficial hematoma

772.8 Other specified hemorrhage of fetus or newborn
EXCLUDES hemorrhagic disease of newborn (776.0)
pulmonary hemorrhage (770.3)

772.9 Unspecified hemorrhage of newborn

√4th **773 Hemolytic disease of fetus or newborn, due to isoimmunization**
DEF: Hemolytic anemia of fetus or newborn due to maternal antibody formation against fetal erythrocytes; infant blood contains nonmaternal antigen.

773.0 Hemolytic disease due to Rh isoimmunization
Anemia
Erythroblastosis (fetalis)   } due to RH:
Hemolytic disease   antibodies
  (fetus) (newborn)   isoimmunization
Jaundice   maternal/fetal
                               incompatibility
Rh hemolytic disease
Rh isoimmunization
CC Excl: 773.0-773.5, ▶779.81-779.89◀

773.1 Hemolytic disease due to ABO isoimmumization
ABO hemolytic disease   ABO isoimmunization
Anemia   } due to ABO:
Erythroblastosis (fetalis) antibodies
Hemolytic disease   isoimmunization
  (fetus) (newborn)   maternal/fetal
Jaundice   incompatibility
CC Excl: See code 773.0
AHA: 3Q, '92, 8
DEF: Incompatible Rh fetal-maternal blood grouping; prematurely destroys red blood cells; detected by Coombs test.

773.2 Hemolytic disease due to other and unspecified isoimmunization
Eythroblastosis (fetalis) (neonatorum) NOS
Hemolytic disease (fetus) (newborn) NOS
Jaundice or anemia due to other and unspecified blood-group incompatibility
CC Excl: See code 773.0
AHA: 1Q, '94, 13

773.3 Hydrops fetalis due to isoimmunization
Use additional code to identify type of isoimmunization (773.0-773.2)
CC Excl: See code 773.0
DEF: Massive edema of entire body and severe anemia; may result in fetal death or stillbirth.

773.4 Kernicterus due to isoimmunization
Use additional code to identify type of isoimmunization (773.0-773.2)
CC Excl: See code 773.0
DEF: Complication of erythroblastosis fetalis associated with severe neural symptoms, high blood bilirubin levels and nerve cell destruction; results in bilirubin-pigmented gray matter of central nervous system.

773.5 Late anemia due to isoimmunization

√4th **774 Other perinatal jaundice**

774.0 *Perinatal jaundice from hereditary hemolyticanemias*
Code first underlying disease (282.0-282.9)
CC Excl: 774.0-774.7, ▶779.81-779.89◀

774.1 Perinatal jaundice from other excessive hemolysis
Fetal or neonatal jaundice from:
  bruising
  drugs or toxins transmitted from mother
  infection
  polycythemia
  swallowed maternal blood
Use additional code to identify cause
EXCLUDES jaundice due to isoimmunization (773.0-773.2)
CC Excl: See code 774.0

774.2 Neonatal jaundice associated with preterm delivery [CC] [N]
  Hyperbilirubinemia of prematurity
  Jaundice due to delayed conjugation associated with preterm delivery
  CC Excl: See code 774.0
  AHA: 3Q, '91, 21

√5th **774.3 Neonatal jaundice due to delayed conjugation from other causes**

  774.30 Neonatal jaundice due to delayed conjugation, cause unspecified [CC] [N]
  CC Excl: See code 774.0

  DEF: Jaundice of newborn with abnormal bilirubin metabolism; causes excess accumulated unconjugated bilirubin in blood.

  774.31 Neonatal jaundice due to delayed conjugation in diseases classified elsewhere [CC] [N]
  Code first underlying diseases as:
    congenital hypothyroidism (243)
    Crigler-Najjar syndrome (277.4)
    Gilbert's syndrome (277.4)
  CC Excl: See code 774.0

  774.39 Other [CC] [N]
  Jaundice due to delayed conjugation from causes, such as:
    breast milk inhibitors
    delayed development of conjugating system
  CC Excl: See code 774.0

774.4 Perinatal jaundice due to hepatocellular damage [CC] [N]
  Fetal or neonatal hepatitis
  Giant cell hepatitis
  Inspissated bile syndrome
  CC Excl: See code 774.0

774.5 Perinatal jaundice from other causes [CC] [N]
  Code first underlying cause as:
    congenital obstruction of bile duct (751.61)
    galactosemia (271.1)
    mucoviscidosis ▶(277.00-277.09)◀
  CC Excl: See code 774.0

774.6 Unspecified fetal and neonatal jaundice [N]
  Icterus neonatorum
  Neonatal hyperbilirubinemia (transient)
  Physiologic jaundice NOS in newborn
  EXCLUDES that in preterm infants (774.2)
  AHA: 1Q, '94, 13; 2Q, '89, 15

774.7 Kernicterus not due to isoimmunization [CC] [N]
  Bilirubin encephalopathy
  Kernicterus of newborn NOS
  EXCLUDES kernicterus due to isoimmunization (773.4)
  CC Excl: See code 774.0

√4th **775 Endocrine and metabolic disturbances specific to the fetus and newborn**
  INCLUDES transitory endocrine and metabolic disturbances caused by the infant's response to maternal endocrine and metabolic factors, its removal from them, or its adjustment to extrauterine existence

  775.0 Syndrome of "infant of a diabetic mother" [N]
  Maternal diabetes mellitus affecting fetus or newborn (with hypoglycemia)
  AHA: 3Q, '91, 5

  775.1 Neonatal diabetes mellitus [CC] [N]
  Diabetes mellitus syndrome in newborn infant
  CC Excl: 775.0-775.9, ▶779.81-779.89◀
  AHA: 3Q, '91, 6

  775.2 Neonatal myasthenia gravis [CC] [N]
  CC Excl: See code 775.1

  775.3 Neonatal thyrotoxicosis [CC] [N]
  Neonatal hyperthyroidism (transient)
  CC Excl: See code 775.1

  775.4 Hypocalcemia and hypomagnesemia of newborn [CC] [N]
  Cow's milk hypocalcemia
  Hypocalcemic tetany, neonatal
  Neonatal hypoparathyroidism
  Phosphate-loading hypocalcemia
  CC Excl: See code 775.1

  775.5 Other transitory neonatal electrolyte disturbances [CC] [N]
  Dehydration, neonatal
  CC Excl: See code 775.1

  775.6 Neonatal hypoglycemia [CC] [N]
  EXCLUDES infant of mother with diabetes mellitus (775.0)
  CC Excl: See code 775.1
  AHA: 1Q, '94, 8

  775.7 Late metabolic acidosis of newborn [CC] [N]
  CC Excl: See code 775.1

  775.8 Other transitory neonatal endocrine and metabolic disturbances [N]
  Amino-acid metabolic disorders described as transitory

  775.9 Unspecified endocrine and metabolic disturbances specific to the fetus and newborn [N]

√4th **776 Hematological disorders of fetus and newborn**
  INCLUDES disorders specific to the fetus or newborn

  776.0 Hemorrhagic disease of newborn [CC] [N]
  Hemorrhagic diathesis of newborn
  Vitamin K deficiency of newborn
  EXCLUDES fetal or neonatal hemorrhage (772.0-772.9)
  CC Excl: 776.0-776.9, ▶771.81-771.82, 779.81-779.89◀

  776.1 Transient neonatal thrombocytopenia [CC] [N]
  Neonatal thrombocytopenia due to:
    exchange transfusion
    idiopathic maternal thrombocytopenia
    isoimmunization
  CC Excl: See code 776.0
  DEF: Temporary decrease in blood platelets of newborn.

  776.2 Disseminated intravascular coagulation in newborn [CC] [N]
  CC Excl: See code 776.0
  DEF: Disseminated intravascular coagulation of newborn: clotting disorder due to excess thromboplastic agents in blood as a result of disease or trauma; causes blood clotting within vessels and reduces available elements necessary for blood coagulation.

  776.3 Other transient neonatal disorders of coagulation [CC] [N]
  Transient coagulation defect, newborn
  CC Excl: See code 776.0

  776.4 Polycythemia neonatorum [N]
  Plethora of newborn
  Polycythemia due to: maternal-fetal transfusion
  Polycythemia due to: donor twin transfusion
  DEF: Abnormal increase of total red blood cells of newborn.

  776.5 Congenital anemia [N]
  Anemia following fetal blood loss
  EXCLUDES anemia due to isoimmunization (773.0-773.2, 773.5)
    hereditary hemolytic anemias (282.0-282.9)

CONDITIONS IN THE PERINATAL PERIOD

776.6 Anemia of prematurity [N]

776.7 Transient neonatal neutropenia [N]
- Isoimmune neutropenia
- Maternal transfer neutropenia
- EXCLUDES: congenital neutropenia (nontransient) (288.0)
- DEF: Decreased neutrophilic leukocytes in blood of newborn.

776.8 Other specified transient hematological disorders [N]

776.9 Unspecified hematological disorder specific to fetus or newborn [N]

√4th 777 Perinatal disorders of digestive system
- INCLUDES: disorders specific to the fetus and newborn
- EXCLUDES: intestinal obstruction classifiable to 560.0-560.9

777.1 Meconium obstruction [CC][N]
- Congenital fecaliths
- Delayed passage of meconium
- Meconium ileus NOS
- Meconium plug syndrome
- EXCLUDES: meconium ileus in cystic fibrosis (277.01)
- CC Excl: 777.1-777.9, ▶779.81-779.89◀
- DEF: Meconium blocked digestive tract of newborn.

777.2 Intestinal obstruction due to inspissated milk [CC][N]
- CC Excl: See code 777.1

777.3 Hematemesis and melena due to swallowed maternal blood [N]
- Swallowed blood syndrome in newborn
- EXCLUDES: that not due to swallowed maternal blood (772.4)

777.4 Transitory ileus of newborn [N]
- EXCLUDES: Hirschsprung's disease (751.3)

777.5 Necrotizing enterocolitis in fetus or newborn [CC][N]
- Pseudomembranous enterocolitis in newborn
- CC Excl: See code 777.1
- DEF: Acute inflammation of small intestine due to pseudomembranous plaque over ulceration; may be due to aggressive antibiotic therapy.

777.6 Perinatal intestinal perforation [CC][N]
- Meconium peritonitis
- CC Excl: See code 777.1

777.8 Other specified perinatal disorders of digestive system

777.9 Unspecified perinatal disorder of digestive system [N]

√4th 778 Conditions involving the integument and temperature regulation of fetus and newborn

778.0 Hydrops fetalis not due to isoimmunization [CC][N]
- Idiopathic hydrops
- EXCLUDES: hydrops fetalis due to isoimmunization (773.3)
- CC Excl: 778.0, ▶779.81-779.89◀
- DEF: Edema of entire body, unrelated to immune response.

778.1 Sclerema neonatorum [N]
- Subcutaneous fat necrosis
- DEF: Diffuse, rapidly progressing white, waxy, nonpitting hardening of tissue, usually of legs and feet, life-threatening; found in preterm or debilitated infants; unknown etiology.

778.2 Cold injury syndrome of newborn [N]

778.3 Other hypothermia of newborn [N]

778.4 Other disturbances of temperature regulation of newborn [N]
- Dehydration fever in newborn
- Environmentally-induced pyrexia
- Hyperthermia in newborn
- Transitory fever of newborn

778.5 Other and unspecified edema of newborn [N]
- Edema neonatorum

778.6 Congenital hydrocele [N]
- Congenital hydrocele of tunica vaginalis

778.7 Breast engorgement in newborn [N]
- Noninfective mastitis of newborn
- EXCLUDES: infective mastitis of newborn (771.5)

778.8 Other specified conditions involving the integument of fetus and newborn
- Urticaria neonatorum
- EXCLUDES: impetigo neonatorum (684)
- pemphigus neonatorum (684)

778.9 Unspecified condition involving the integument and temperature regulation of fetus and newborn [N]

√4th 779 Other and ill-defined conditions originating in the perinatal period

779.0 Convulsions in newborn [CC][N]
- Fits } in newborn
- Seizures
- CC Excl: 779.0-779.1, ▶779.81-779.89◀
- AHA: N-D, '94, 11

779.1 Other and unspecified cerebral irritability in newborn [CC][N]
- CC Excl: See code 779.0

779.2 Cerebral depression, coma, and other abnormal cerebral signs [N]
- CNS dysfunction in newborn NOS

779.3 Feeding problems in newborn [CC][N]
- Regurgitation of food
- Slow feeding } in newborn
- Vomiting
- CC Excl: 779.3
- AHA: 2Q, '89, 15

779.4 Drug reactions and intoxications specific to newborn [CC][N]
- Gray syndrome from chloramphenicol administration in newborn
- EXCLUDES: fetal alcohol syndrome (760.71)
- reactions and intoxications from maternal opiates and tranquilizers (763.5)
- CC Excl: 779.4-779.5

779.5 Drug withdrawal syndrome in newborn [N]
- Drug withdrawal syndrome in infant of dependent mother
- EXCLUDES: fetal alcohol syndrome (760.71)
- AHA: 3Q, '94, 6

779.6 Termination of pregnancy (fetus) [N]
- Fetal death due to: induced abortion
- Fetal death due to: termination of pregnancy
- EXCLUDES: spontaneous abortion (fetus) (761.8)

779.7 Periventricular leukomalacia [CC][N]
- CC Excl: 772.0, 772.10-772.14, 772.2, 772.8, 772.9, 776.0-776.9, 779.7, ▶779.81-779.89◀
- AHA: 4Q, '01, 50, 51
- DEF: Necrosis of white matter adjacent to lateral ventricles with the formation of cysts; cause of PVL has not been firmly established, but thought to be related to inadequate blood flow in certain areas of the brain.

√5th 779.8 Other specified conditions originating in the perinatal period [N]
- AHA: 1Q, '94, 15

√4th Additional Digit Required | Nonspecific PDx | Unacceptable PDx | Manifestation Code | MSP Medicare Secondary Payer | ▶◀ Revised Text | ● New Code | ▲ Revised Code Title
√5th

2002 Ingenix, Inc.

- **779.81 Neonatal bradycardia**
  EXCLUDES abnormality in fetal heart rate or rhythm complicating labor and delivery (763.81-763.83)
  bradycardia due to birth asphyxia (768.5-768.9)

- **779.82 Neonatal tachycardia**
  EXCLUDES abnormality in fetal heart rate or rhythm complicating labor and delivery (763.81-763.83)

- **779.89 Other specified conditions originating in the perinatal period**

779.9 Unspecified condition originating in the perinatal period
  Congenital debility NOS
  Stillbirth NEC

16. SYMPTOMS, SIGNS, AND ILL-DEFINED CONDITIONS (780-799)

This section includes symptoms, signs, abnormal results of laboratory or other investigative procedures, and ill-defined conditions regarding which no diagnosis classifiable elsewhere is recorded.

Signs and symptoms that point rather definitely to a given diagnosis are assigned to some category in the preceding part of the classification. In general, categories 780-796 include the more ill-defined conditions and symptoms that point with perhaps equal suspicion to two or more diseases or to two or more systems of the body, and without the necessary study of the case to make a final diagnosis. Practically all categories in this group could be designated as "not otherwise specified," or as "unknown etiology," or as "transient." The Alphabetic Index should be consulted to determine which symptoms and signs are to be allocated here and which to more specific sections of the classification; the residual subcategories numbered .9 are provided for other relevant symptoms which cannot be allocated elsewhere in the classification.

The conditions and signs or symptoms included in categories 780-796 consist of: (a) cases for which no more specific diagnosis can be made even after all facts bearing on the case have been investigated; (b) signs or symptoms existing at the time of initial encounter that proved to be transient and whose causes could not be determined; (c) provisional diagnoses in a patient who failed to return for further investigation or care; (d) cases referred elsewhere for investigation or treatment before the diagnosis was made; (e) cases in which a more precise diagnosis was not available for any other reason; (f) certain symptoms which represent important problems in medical care and which it might be desired to classify in addition to a known cause.

SYMPTOMS (780-789)

AHA: 1Q, '91, 12; 2Q, '90, 3; 2Q, '90, 5; 2Q, '90, 15; M-A, '85, 3

780 General symptoms

780.0 Alteration of consciousness
EXCLUDES coma:
 diabetic (250.2-250.3)
 hepatic (572.2)
 originating in the perinatal period (779.2)

AHA: 4Q, '92, 20

780.01 Coma
CC Excl: 070.0-070.9, 250.00-250.93, 251.0-251.3, 348.8-348.9, 349.89, 349.9, 430-431, 432.0-432.9, 572.2, 780.01-780.09, 780.2, 780.4, ▶780.91-780.99,◀ 799.8, 800.00-800.99, 801.00-801.99, 803.00-803.99, 804.00-804.96, 850.0-850.9, 851.00-851.99, 852.00-852.19, 852.21-852.59, 853.00-853.19, 854.00-854.19

AHA: 3Q, '96, 16

DEF: State of unconsciousness from which the patient cannot be awakened.

780.02 Transient alteration of awareness
DEF: Temporary, recurring spells of reduced consciousness.

780.03 Persistent vegetative state
CC Excl: See code 780.01

DEF: Persistent wakefulness without consciousness due to nonfunctioning cerebral cortex.

780.09 Other
 Drowsiness Stupor
 Semicoma Unconsciousness
 Somnolence

780.1 Hallucinations
 Hallucinations: Hallucinations:
 NOS olfactory
 auditory tactile
 gustatory

EXCLUDES those associated with mental disorders, as functional psychoses (295.0-298.9)
 organic brain syndromes (290.0-294.9, 310.0-310.9)
 visual hallucinations (368.16)

CC Excl: 780.1, 780.4, ▶780.91-780.99,◀ 799.8

DEF: Perception of external stimulus in absence of stimulus; inability to distinguish between real and imagined.

780.2 Syncope and collapse
 Blackout (Near) (Pre) syncope
 Fainting Vasovagal attack

EXCLUDES carotid sinus syncope (337.0)
 heat syncope (992.1)
 neurocirculatory asthenia (306.2)
 orthostatic hypotension (458.0)
 shock NOS (785.50)

AHA: ▶1Q, '02, 6;◀ 3Q, '00, 12; 3Q, '95, 14; N-D, '85, 12

DEF: Sudden unconsciousness due to reduced blood flow to brain.

780.3 Convulsions
EXCLUDES convulsions:
 epileptic (345.10-345.91)
 in newborn (779.0)

AHA: 2Q, '97, 8; 1Q, '97, 12; 3Q, '94, 9; 1Q, '93, 24; 4Q, '92, 23; N-D, '87, 12

DEF: Sudden, involuntary contractions of the muscles.

780.31 Febrile convulsions
 Febrile seizure

CC Excl: 345.00-345.01, 345.10-345.11, 345.2-345.3, 345.40-345.41, 345.50-345.51, 345.60-345.61, 345.70-345.71, 345.80-345.81, 345.90-345.91, 348.8-348.9, 349.89, 349.9, 779.0-779.1, 780.31, 780.39, ▶780.91-780.99,◀ 799.8

AHA: 4Q, '97, 45

780.39 Other convulsions
 Convulsive disorder NOS
 Fit NOS
 Seizure NOS

CC Excl: See code 780.31

AHA: 2Q, '99, 17; 4Q, '98, 39

780.4 Dizziness and giddiness
 Light-headedness Vertigo NOS

EXCLUDES Ménière's disease and other specified vertiginous syndromes (386.0-386.9)

AHA: 3Q, '00, 12; 2Q, '97, 9; 2Q, '91, 17

DEF: Whirling sensations in head with feeling of falling.

780.5 Sleep disturbances
EXCLUDES that of nonorganic origin (307.40-307.49)

780.50 Sleep disturbance, unspecified
780.51 Insomnia with sleep apnea
DEF: Transient cessation of breathing disturbing sleep.

780.52 Other insomnia
 Insomnia NOS

DEF: Inability to maintain adequate sleep cycle.

780.53 Hypersomnia with sleep apnea
AHA: 1Q, '93, 28; N-D, '85, 4

DEF: Autonomic response inhibited during sleep; causes insufficient oxygen intake, acidosis and pulmonary hypertension.

SYMPTOMS, SIGNS, AND ILL-DEFINED CONDITIONS

780.54 Other hypersomnia
Hypersomnia NOS
DEF: Prolonged sleep cycle.

780.55 Disruptions of 24-hour sleep-wake cycle
Inversion of sleep rhythm
Irregular sleep-wake rhythm NOS
Non-24-hour sleep-wake rhythm

780.56 Dysfunctions associated with sleep stages or arousal from sleep

780.57 Other and unspecified sleep apnea
AHA: 1Q, '01, 6 ; 1Q, '97, 5; 1Q, '93, 28

780.59 Other

780.6 Fever
Chills with fever
Fever NOS
Fever of unknown origin (FUO)
Hyperpyrexia NOS
Pyrexia
Pyrexia of unknown origin
EXCLUDES pyrexia of unknown origin (during):
    in newborn (778.4)
    labor (659.2)
    the puerperium (672)
AHA: 3Q, '00,13; 4Q, '99, 26; 2Q, '91, 8

DEF: Elevated body temperature; no known cause.

780.7 Malaise and fatigue
EXCLUDES debility, unspecified (799.3)
    fatigue (during):
        combat (308.0-308.9)
        heat (992.6)
        pregnancy (646.8)
    neurasthenia (300.5)
    senile asthenia (797)
AHA: 4Q, '88, 12; M-A, '87, 8

DEF: Indefinite feeling of debility or lack of good health.

780.71 Chronic fatigue syndrome
AHA: 4Q, '98, 48

DEF: Persistent fatigue, symptoms include weak muscles, sore throat, lymphadenitis, headache, depression and mild fever; no known cause; also called chronic mononucleosis, benign myalgic encephalomyelitis, Iceland disease and neurosthenia.

780.79 Other malaise and fatigue
Asthenia NOS   Postviral (asthenic) syndrome
Lethargy   Tiredness
AHA: 1Q, '00, 6; 4Q, '99, 26

DEF: Asthenia: Any weakness, lack of strength or loss of energy, especially neuromuscular.

DEF: Lethargy: Listlessness, drowsiness, stupor and apathy.

DEF: Postviral (asthenia) syndrome: Listlessness, drowsiness, stupor and apathy; follows acute viral infection.

DEF: Tiredness: General exhaustion or fatigue.

780.8 Hyperhidrosis
Diaphoresis
Excessive sweating
DEF: Excessive sweating, appears as droplets on skin; general or localized.

780.9 Other general symptoms
EXCLUDES hypothermia:
    NOS (accidental) (991.6)
    due to anesthesia (995.89)
    of newborn (778.2-778.3)
    memory disturbance as part of a
        pattern of mental disorder
AHA: 4Q, '99, 10; 3Q, '93, 11; N-D, '85, 12

780.91 Fussy infant (baby)
780.92 Excessive crying of infant (baby)
780.99 Other general symptoms
Amnesia (retrograde)
Chill(s) NOS
Generalized pain
Hypothermia, not associated with low
    environmental temperature

781 Symptoms involving nervous and musculoskeletal systems
EXCLUDES depression NOS (311)
    disorders specifically relating to:
        back (724.0-724.9)
        hearing (388.0-389.9)
        joint (718.0-719.9)
        limb (729.0-729.9)
        neck (723.0-723.9)
        vision (368.0-369.9)
    pain in limb (729.5)

781.0 Abnormal involuntary movements
Abnormal head movements   Spasms NOS
Fasciculation   Tremor NOS
EXCLUDES abnormal reflex (796.1)
    chorea NOS (333.5)
    infantile spasms (345.60-345.61)
    spastic paralysis (342.1, 343.0-344.9)
    specified movement disorders
        classifiable to 333 (333.0-333.9)
    that of nonorganic origin (307.2-307.3)

781.1 Disturbances of sensation of smell and taste
Anosmia   Parosmia
Parageusia

DEF: Anosmia: loss of sense of smell due to organic factors, including loss of olfactory nerve conductivity, cerebral disease, nasal fossae formation and peripheral olfactory nerve diseases; can also be psychological disorder.

DEF: Parageusia: distorted sense of taste, or bad taste in mouth.

DEF: Parosmia: distorted sense of smell.

781.2 Abnormality of gait
Gait: Gait:
    ataxic   spastic
    paralytic   staggering
EXCLUDES ataxia:
    NOS (781.3)
    locomotor (progressive) (094.0)
    difficulty in walking (719.7)
DEF: Abnormal, asymmetric gait.

781.3 Lack of coordination
Ataxia NOS   Muscular incoordination
EXCLUDES ataxic gait (781.2)
    cerebellar ataxia (334.0-334.9)
    difficulty in walking (719.7)
    vertigo NOS (780.4)
AHA: 3Q, '97, 12

781.4 Transient paralysis of limb
Monoplegia, transient NOS
EXCLUDES paralysis (342.0-344.9)

781.5 Clubbing of fingers
DEF: Enlarged soft tissue of distal fingers.

SYMPTOMS, SIGNS, AND ILL-DEFINED CONDITIONS

781.6 Meningismus
Dupré's syndrome
Meningism
AHA: 3Q, '00,13; J-F, '87, 7

DEF: Condition with signs and symptoms that resemble meningeal irritation; it is associated with febrile illness and dehydration with no evidence of infection.

781.7 Tetany [CC]
Carpopedal spasm
EXCLUDES tetanus neonatorum (771.3)
tetany:
hysterical (300.11)
newborn (hypocalcemic) (775.4)
parathyroid (252.1)
psychogenic (306.0)
CC Excl: 037, 332.0-332.1, 333.0-333.99, 334.0-334.4, 342.10-342.12, 771.3, ▶780.91-780.99,◀ 781.7, 799.8

DEF: Nerve and muscle hyperexcitability; symptoms include muscle spasms, twitching, cramps, laryngospasm with inspiratory stridor, hyperreflexia and choreiform movements.

781.8 Neurologic neglect syndrome
Asomatognosia   Left-sided neglect
Hemi-akinesia   Sensory extinction
Hemi-inattention   Sensory neglect
Hemispatial neglect   Visuospatial neglect
AHA: 4Q, '94, 37

√5th 781.9 Other symptoms involving nervous and musculoskeletal systems
AHA: 4Q, '00, 45

781.91 Loss of height
EXCLUDES osteoporosis (733.00-733.09)

781.92 Abnormal posture

781.93 Ocular torticollis

781.99 Other symptoms involving nervous and musculoskeletal systems

√4th 782 Symptoms involving skin and other integumentary tissue
EXCLUDES symptoms relating to breast (611.71-611.79)

782.0 Disturbance of skin sensation
Anesthesia of skin   Numbness
Burning or prickling sensation Paresthesia
Hyperesthesia   Tingling
Hypoesthesia

782.1 Rash and other nonspecific skin eruption
Exanthem
EXCLUDES vesicular eruption (709.8)

782.2 Localized superficial swelling, mass, or lump
Subcutaneous nodules
EXCLUDES localized adiposity (278.1)

782.3 Edema
Anasarca
Dropsy
Localized edema NOS
EXCLUDES ascites (789.5)
edema of:
newborn NOS (778.5)
pregnancy (642.0-642.9, 646.1)
fluid retention (276.6)
hydrops fetalis (773.3, 778.0)
hydrothorax (511.8)
nutritional edema (260, 262)
AHA: 2Q, '00, 18

DEF: Edema: excess fluid in intercellular body tissue.
DEF: Anasarca: massive edema in all body tissues.
DEF: Dropsy: serous fluid accumulated in body cavity or cellular tissue.
DEF: Localized edema: edema in specific body areas.

782.4 Jaundice, unspecified, not of newborn
Cholemia NOS
Icterus NOS
EXCLUDES jaundice in newborn (774.0-774.7)
due to isoimmunization (773.0-773.2, 773.4)
DEF: Bilirubin deposits of skin, causing yellow cast.

782.5 Cyanosis
EXCLUDES newborn ▶(770.83)◀
DEF: Deficient oxygen of blood; causes blue cast to skin.

√5th 782.6 Pallor and flushing
782.61 Pallor
782.62 Flushing
Excessive blushing

782.7 Spontaneous ecchymoses
Petechiae
EXCLUDES ecchymosis in fetus or newborn (772.6)
purpura (287.0-287.9)
DEF: Hemorrhagic spots of skin; resemble freckles.

782.8 Changes in skin texture
Induration } of skin
Thickening

782.9 Other symptoms involving skin and integumentary tissues

√4th 783 Symptoms concerning nutrition, metabolism, and development

783.0 Anorexia
Loss of appetite
EXCLUDES anorexia nervosa (307.1)
loss of appetite of nonorganic origin (307.59)

783.1 Abnormal weight gain
EXCLUDES excessive weight gain in pregnancy (646.1)
obesity (278.00)
morbid (278.01)

√5th 783.2 Abnormal loss of weight and underweight
AHA: 4Q, '00, 45

783.21 Loss of weight
783.22 Underweight

783.3 Feeding difficulties and mismanagement
Feeding problem (elderly) (infant)
EXCLUDES feeding disturbance or problems:
in newborn (779.3)
of nonorganic origin (307.50-307.59)
AHA: 3Q, '97, 12

√5th 783.4 Lack of expected normal physiological development in childhood
EXCLUDES delay in sexual development and puberty (259.0)
gonadal dysgenesis (758.6)
pituitary dwarfism (253.3)
slow fetal growth and fetal malnutrition (764.00-764.99)
specific delays in mental development (315.0-315.9)
AHA: 4Q, '00, 45; 3Q, '97, 4

783.40 Lack of normal physiological development unspecified
Inadequate development
Lack of development

783.41 Failure to thrive [P]
Failure to gain weight
DEF: Organic failure to thrive: acute or chronic illness that interferes with nutritional intake, absorption, metabolism excretion and energy requirements. Nonorganic FTT is symptom of neglect or abuse.

783.42 Delayed milestones [P]
Late talker
Late walker

783.43–785.51 SYMPTOMS, SIGNS, AND ILL-DEFINED CONDITIONS **Tabular List**

- **783.43 Short stature**
    - Growth failure
    - Growth retardation
    - Lack of growth
    - Physical retardation
    - **DEF:** Constitutional short stature: stature inconsistent with chronological age. Genetic short stature is when skeletal maturation matches chronological age.
- **783.5 Polydipsia**
    - Excessive thirst
- **783.6 Polyphagia**
    - Excessive eating   Hyperalimentation NOS
    - **EXCLUDES** disorders of eating of nonorganic origin (307.50-307.59)
- **783.7 Adult failure to thrive** [A]
- **783.9 Other symptoms concerning nutrition, metabolism, and development**
    - Hypometabolism
    - **EXCLUDES** abnormal basal metabolic rate (794.7)
    - dehydration (276.5)
    - other disorders of fluid, electrolyte, and acid-base balance (276.0-276.9)

✓4th 784 Symptoms involving head and neck
EXCLUDES encephalopathy NOS (348.3)
specific symptoms involving neck classifiable to 723 (723.0-723.9)

- **784.0 Headache**
    - Facial pain   Pain in head NOS
    - **EXCLUDES** atypical face pain (350.2)
    - migraine (346.0-346.9)
    - tension headache (307.81)
    - **AHA:** 3Q, '00, 13; 1Q, '90, 4; 3Q, '92, 14
- **784.1 Throat pain**
    - **EXCLUDES** dysphagia (787.2)
    - neck pain (723.1)
    - sore throat (462)
    - chronic (472.1)
- **784.2 Swelling, mass, or lump in head and neck**
    - Space-occupying lesion, intracranial NOS
- **784.3 Aphasia**
    - **EXCLUDES** developmental aphasia (315.31)
    - **AHA:** 4Q, '98, 87; 3Q, '97, 12
    - **DEF:** Inability to communicate through speech, written word, or sign language.

✓5th 784.4 Voice disturbance
- **784.40 Voice disturbance, unspecified**
- **784.41 Aphonia**
    - Loss of voice
- **784.49 Other**
    - Change in voice   Hypernasality
    - Dysphonia   Hyponasality
    - Hoarseness

- **784.5 Other speech disturbance**
    - Dysarthria   Slurred speech
    - Dysphasia
    - **EXCLUDES** stammering and stuttering (307.0)
    - that of nonorganic origin (307.0, 307.9)

✓5th 784.6 Other symbolic dysfunction
EXCLUDES developmental learning delays (315.0-315.9)
- **784.60 Symbolic dysfunction, unspecified**
- **784.61 Alexia and dyslexia**
    - Alexia (with agraphia)
    - **DEF: Alexia:** Inability to understand written word due to central brain lesion.
    - **DEF: Dyslexia:** Ability to recognize letters but inability to read, spell, and write words; genetic.
- **784.69 Other**
    - Acalculia   Agraphia NOS
    - Agnosia   Apraxia

- **784.7 Epistaxis**
    - Hemorrhage from nose
    - Nosebleed
- **784.8 Hemorrhage from throat**
    - **EXCLUDES** hemoptysis (786.3)
- **784.9 Other symptoms involving head and neck**
    - Choking sensation   Mouth breathing
    - Halitosis   Sneezing

✓4th 785 Symptoms involving cardiovascular system
EXCLUDES heart failure NOS (428.9)

- **785.0 Tachycardia, unspecified**
    - Rapid heart beat
    - **EXCLUDES** ▶neonatal tachycardia (779.82)◀
    - paroxysmal tachycardia (427.0-427.2)
    - **DEF:** Excessively rapid heart rate.
- **785.1 Palpitations**
    - Awareness of heart beat
    - **EXCLUDES** specified dysrhythmias (427.0-427.9)
    - **DEF:** Shock syndrome: associated with myocardial infarction, cardiac tamponade and massive pulmonary embolism; symptoms include mental torpor, reduced blood pressure, tachycardia, pallor and cold, clammy skin.
- **785.2 Undiagnosed cardiac murmurs**
    - Heart murmurs NOS
    - **AHA:** 4Q, '92, 16
- **785.3 Other abnormal heart sounds**
    - Cardiac dullness, increased or decreased
    - Friction fremitus, cardiac
    - Precordial friction
- **785.4 Gangrene** [CC]
    - Gangrene:
        - NOS
        - spreading cutaneous
    - Gangrenous cellulitis
    - Phagedena
    - Code first any associated underlying condition:
        - diabetes (250.7)
        - Raynaud's syndrome (443.0)
    - **EXCLUDES** gangrene of certain sites — see Alphabetic Index
    - gangrene with atherosclerosis of the extremities (440.24)
    - gas gangrene (040.0)
    - **CC Excl:** 440.24, ▶780.91-780.99,◀ 785.4, 799.8
    - **AHA:** 3Q, '91, 12; 3Q, '90, 15; M-A, '86, 12
    - **DEF: Gangrene:** necrosis of skin tissue due to bacterial infection, diabetes, embolus and vascular supply loss.
    - **DEF: Gangrenous cellulitis:** group A streptococcal infection; begins with severe cellulitis, spreads to superficial and deep fascia; produces gangrene of underlying tissues.

✓5th 785.5 Shock without mention of trauma
- **785.50 Shock, unspecified** [CC] [MC] [CD]
    - Failure of peripheral circulation
    - **CC Excl:** ▶780.91-780.99,◀ 785.50-785.59, 785.9, 799.8
    - **AHA:** 2Q, '96, 10
- **785.51 Cardiogenic shock** [CC] [MC] [CD]
    - **CC Excl:** See code 785.50
    - **DEF:** Peripheral circulatory failure due to heart insufficiencies.

[N] Newborn Age: 0   [P] Pediatric Age: 0-17   [M] Maternity Age: 12-55   [A] Adult Age: 15-124   [CC] CC Condition   [MC] Major Complication   [CD] Complex Dx   [HIV] HIV Related Dx

SYMPTOMS, SIGNS, AND ILL-DEFINED CONDITIONS

785.59 Other
Shock: endotoxic, gram-negative, septic
Shock: hypovolemic

EXCLUDES shock (due to):
anesthetic (995.4)
anaphylactic (995.0)
due to serum (999.4)
electric (994.8)
following abortion (639.5)
lightning (994.0)
obstetrical (669.1)
postoperative (998.0)
traumatic (958.4)

CC Excl: see code 785.50

AHA: 2Q, '00, 3

785.6 Enlargement of lymph nodes
Lymphadenopathy   "Swollen glands"

EXCLUDES lymphadenitis (chronic) (289.1-289.3)
acute (683)

785.9 Other symptoms involving cardiovascular system
Bruit (arterial)   Weak pulse

✓4th 786 Symptoms involving respiratory system and other chest symptoms

✓5th 786.0 Dyspnea and respiratory abnormalities

786.00 Respiratory abnormality, unspecified

786.01 Hyperventilation

EXCLUDES hyperventilation, psychogenic (306.1)

DEF: Rapid breathing causes carbon dioxide loss from blood.

786.02 Orthopnea

DEF: Difficulty breathing except in upright position.

786.03 Apnea

EXCLUDES ▶apnea of newborn (770.81, 770.82)◀
sleep apnea (780.51, 780.53, 780.57)

CC Excl: 518.81-518.84, 519.8, 519.9, 786.03, 786.04, 799.1

AHA: 4Q, '98, 50

DEF: Cessation of breathing.

786.04 Cheyne-Stokes respiration

CC Excl: 518.81-518.84, 519.8, 519.9, 786.03, 786.04, 799.1

AHA: 4Q, '98, 50

DEF: Rhythmic increase of depth and frequency of breathing with apnea; occurs in frontal lobe and diencephalic dysfunction.

786.05 Shortness of breath

AHA: 4Q, '99, 25; 1Q, '99, 6; 4Q, '98, 50

DEF: Inability to take in sufficient oxygen.

786.06 Tachypnea

EXCLUDES transitory tachypnea of newborn (770.6)

AHA: 4Q, '98, 50

DEF: Abnormal rapid respiratory rate; called hyperventilation.

786.07 Wheezing

EXCLUDES asthma (493.00-493.92)

AHA: 4Q, '98, 50

DEF: Stenosis of respiratory passageway; causes whistling sound; due to asthma, coryza, croup, emphysema, hay fever, edema, and pleural effusion.

786.09 Other
Respiratory: distress, insufficiency

EXCLUDES respiratory distress:
following trauma and surgery (518.5)
newborn ▶(770.89)◀
syndrome (newborn) (769)
adult (518.5)
respiratory failure (518.81, 518.83-518.84)
newborn ▶(770.84)◀

AHA: 2Q, '98, 10; 1Q, '97, 7; 1Q, '90, 9

786.1 Stridor

EXCLUDES congenital laryngeal stridor (748.3)

DEF: Obstructed airway causes harsh sound.

786.2 Cough

EXCLUDES cough:
psychogenic (306.1)
smokers' (491.0)
with hemorrhage (786.3)

AHA: 4Q, '99, 26

786.3 Hemoptysis
Cough with hemorrhage
Pulmonary hemorrhage NOS

EXCLUDES pulmonary hemorrhage of newborn (770.3)

CC Excl: ▶780.91-780.99,◀ 786.3-786.4, 786.9, 799.8

AHA: 4Q, '90, 26

DEF: Coughing up blood or blood-stained sputum.

786.4 Abnormal sputum
Abnormal: amount, color, odor, Excessive } (of) sputum

✓5th 786.5 Chest pain

786.50 Chest pain, unspecified

AHA: ▶1Q, '02, 4;◀ 4Q, '99, 25

786.51 Precordial pain

DEF: Chest pain over heart and lower thorax.

786.52 Painful respiration
Pain: anterior chest wall, pleuritic
Pleurodynia

EXCLUDES epidemic pleurodynia (074.1)

AHA: N-D, '84, 17

786.59 Other
Discomfort, Pressure, Tightness } in chest

EXCLUDES pain in breast (611.71)

AHA: ▶1Q, '02, 6◀

786.6 Swelling, mass, or lump in chest

EXCLUDES lump in breast (611.72)

786.7 Abnormal chest sounds
Abnormal percussion, chest   Rales
Friction sounds, chest   Tympany, chest

EXCLUDES wheezing (786.07)

786.8 Hiccough

EXCLUDES psychogenic hiccough (306.1)

786.9 Other symptoms involving respiratory system and chest
Breath-holding spell

SYMPTOMS, SIGNS, AND ILL-DEFINED CONDITIONS

√4th 787 Symptoms involving digestive system
EXCLUDES constipation (564.00-564.09)
pylorospasm (537.81)
congenital (750.5)

√5th 787.0 Nausea and vomiting
Emesis
EXCLUDES hematemesis NOS (578.0)
vomiting:
bilious, following gastrointestinal surgery (564.3)
cyclical (536.2)
psychogenic (306.4)
excessive, in pregnancy (643.0-643.9)
habit (536.2)
of newborn (779.3)
psychogenic NOS (307.54)

AHA: M-A, '85, 11

787.01 Nausea with vomiting
787.02 Nausea alone
AHA: 3Q, '00, 12; 2Q, '97, 9

787.03 Vomiting alone

787.1 Heartburn
Pyrosis   Waterbrash
EXCLUDES dyspepsia or indigestion (536.8)
AHA: 2Q, '01, 6

787.2 Dysphagia
Difficulty in swallowing
AHA: 2Q, '01, 4

787.3 Flatulence, eructation, and gas pain
Abdominal distention (gaseous)
Bloating
Tympanites (abdominal) (intestinal)
EXCLUDES aerophagy (306.4)

DEF: Flatulence: Excess air or gas in intestine or stomach.
DEF: Eructation: Belching, expelling gas through mouth.
DEF: Gas pain: Gaseous pressure affecting gastrointestinal system.

787.4 Visible peristalsis
Hyperperistalsis
DEF: Increase in involuntary movements of intestines.

787.5 Abnormal bowel sounds
Absent bowel sounds
Hyperactive bowel sounds

787.6 Incontinence of feces
Encopresis NOS
Incontinence of sphincter ani
EXCLUDES that of nonorganic origin (307.7)
AHA: 1Q, '97, 9

787.7 Abnormal feces
Bulky stools
EXCLUDES abnormal stool content (792.1)
melena:
NOS (578.1)
newborn (772.4, 777.3)

√5th 787.9 Other symptoms involving digestive system
EXCLUDES gastrointestinal hemorrhage (578.0-578.9)
intestinal obstruction (560.0-560.9)
specific functional digestive disorders:
esophagus (530.0-530.9)
stomach and duodenum (536.0-536.9)
those not elsewhere classified (564.00-564.9)

787.91 Diarrhea
Diarrhea NOS
AHA: 4Q, '95, 54

787.99 Other
Change in bowel habits
Tenesmus (rectal)
DEF: Tenesmus: Painful, ineffective straining at the rectum with limited passage of fecal matter.

√4th 788 Symptoms involving urinary system
EXCLUDES hematuria (599.7)
nonspecific findings on examination of the urine (791.0-791.9)
small kidney of unknown cause (589.0-589.9)
uremia NOS (586)

788.0 Renal colic
Colic (recurrent) of: Colic (recurrent) of:
kidney   ureter
DEF: Kidney pain.

788.1 Dysuria
Painful urination   Strangury

√5th 788.2 Retention of urine
DEF: Inability to void.

788.20 Retention of urine, unspecified **CC**
CC Excl: 274.11, 344.61, 593.3-593.5, 596.0, 596.4-596.59, 596.8-596.9, 599.6, 600.1-600.9, 601.0-601.9, 602.0-602.9, 753.0, 753.1, 753.20-753.23, 753.29, 753.3-753.9, ▶780.91-780.99,◀ 788.20-788.29, 788.61-788.69, 788.9, 799.8
AHA: 3Q, '96, 10

788.21 Incomplete bladder emptying

788.29 Other specified retention of urine **CC**
CC Excl: See code 788.20

√5th 788.3 Incontinence of urine
▶Code, if applicable, any causal condition first, such as:◀
congenital ureterocele (753.23)
genital prolapse (618.0-618.9)
EXCLUDES that of nonorganic origin (307.6)
AHA: 4Q, '92, 22

788.30 Urinary incontinence, unspecified
Enuresis NOS

788.31 Urge incontinence
AHA: 1Q, '00, 19
DEF: Inability to control urination, upon urge to urinate.

788.32 Stress incontinence, male ♂
EXCLUDES stress incontinence, female (625.6)
DEF: Inability to control urination associated with weak sphincter in males.

788.33 Mixed incontinence, (male) (female)
Urge and stress
DEF: Urge, stress incontinence: involuntary discharge of urine due to anatomic displacement.

788.34 Incontinence without sensory awareness
DEF: Involuntary discharge of urine without sensory warning.

788.35 Post-void dribbling
DEF: Involuntary discharge of residual urine after voiding.

788.36 Nocturnal enuresis
DEF: Involuntary discharge of urine during the night.

788.37 Continuous leakage
DEF: Continuous, involuntary urine seepage.

788.39 Other urinary incontinence

√5th 788.4 Frequency of urination and polyuria
788.41 Urinary frequency
Frequency of micturition

SYMPTOMS, SIGNS, AND ILL-DEFINED CONDITIONS

788.42 Polyuria
DEF: Excessive urination.

788.43 Nocturia
DEF: Urination affecting sleep patterns.

788.5 Oliguria and anuria
Deficient secretion of urine
Suppression of urinary secretion
EXCLUDES that complicating:
  abortion (634-638 with .3, 639.3)
  ectopic or molar pregnancy (639.3)
  pregnancy, childbirth, or the puerperium (642.0-642.9, 646.2)

DEF: Oliguria: diminished urinary secretion related to fluid intake.
DEF: Anuria: lack of urinary secretion due to renal failure or obstructed urinary tract.

√5ᵗʰ 788.6 Other abnormality of urination
  788.61 Splitting of urinary stream
    Intermittent urinary stream
  788.62 Slowing of urinary stream
    Weak stream
  788.69 Other

788.7 Urethral discharge
  Penile discharge   Urethrorrhea

788.8 Extravasation of urine
DEF: Leaking or infiltration of urine into tissues.

788.9 Other symptoms involving urinary system
  Extrarenal uremia   Vesical:
  Vesical: tenesmus
    pain
AHA: 4Q, '88, 1

√4ᵗʰ 789 Other symptoms involving abdomen and pelvis
EXCLUDES symptoms referable to genital organs:
  female (625.0-625.9)
  male (607.0-608.9)
  psychogenic (302.70-302.79)

The following fifth-digit subclassification is to be used for codes 789.0, 789.3, 789.4, 789.6:
0 unspecified site
1 right upper quadrant
2 left upper quadrant
3 right lower quadrant
4 left lower quadrant
5 periumbilic
6 epigastric
7 generalized
9 other specified site
  Multiple sites

√5ᵗʰ 789.0 Abdominal pain
  Colic:
    NOS   infantile
  Cramps, abdominal
  EXCLUDES renal colic (788.0)
AHA: 1Q, '95, 3; For code 789.06: ▶1Q, '02, 5◀

789.1 Hepatomegaly
  Enlargement of liver

789.2 Splenomegaly
  Enlargement of spleen

√5ᵗʰ 789.3 Abdominal or pelvic swelling, mass, or lump
  Diffuse or generalized swelling or mass:
    abdominal NOS
    umbilical
  EXCLUDES abdominal distention (gaseous) (787.3)
    ascites (789.5)

√5ᵗʰ 789.4 Abdominal rigidity

789.5 Ascites CC
  Fluid in peritoneal cavity
  CC Excl: ▶780.91-780.99,◀ 789.30-789.5, 789.9, 799.8
AHA: 4Q, '89, 11
DEF: Serous fluid effusion and accumulation in abdominal cavity.

√5ᵗʰ 789.6 Abdominal tenderness
  Rebound tenderness

789.9 Other symptoms involving abdomen and pelvis
  Umbilical: Umbilical:
    bleeding   discharge

NONSPECIFIC ABNORMAL FINDINGS (790-796)
AHA: 2Q, '90, 16

√4ᵗʰ 790 Nonspecific findings on examination of blood
EXCLUDES abnormality of:
  platelets (287.0-287.9)
  thrombocytes (287.0-287.9)
  white blood cells (288.0-288.9)

√5ᵗʰ 790.0 Abnormality of red blood cells
EXCLUDES anemia:
  congenital (776.5)
  newborn, due to isoimmunization (773.0-773.2, 773.5)
  of premature infant (776.6)
  other specified types (280.0-285.9)
  hemoglobin disorders (282.5-282.7)
  polycythemia:
    familial (289.6)
    neonatorum (776.4)
    secondary (289.0)
    vera (238.4)
AHA: 4Q, '00, 46

  790.01 Precipitous drop in hematocrit
    Drop in hematocrit
  790.09 Other abnormality of red blood cells
    Abnormal red cell morphology NOS
    Abnormal red cell volume NOS
    Anisocytosis
    Poikilocytosis

790.1 Elevated sedimentation rate

790.2 Abnormal glucose tolerance test
EXCLUDES that complicating pregnancy, childbirth, or the puerperium (648.8)
AHA: 3Q, '91, 5

790.3 Excessive blood level of alcohol
  Elevated blood-alcohol
AHA: S-O, '86, 3

790.4 Nonspecific elevation of levels of transaminase or lactic acid dehydrogenase [LDH]

790.5 Other nonspecific abnormal serum enzyme levels
  Abnormal serum level of:
    acid phosphatase
    alkaline phosphatase
    amylase
    lipase
  EXCLUDES deficiency of circulating enzymes (277.6)

790.6 Other abnormal blood chemistry
  Abnormal blood level of: Abnormal blood level of:
    cobalt   magnesium
    copper   mineral
    iron   zinc
    lithium
  EXCLUDES abnormality of electrolyte or acid-base balance (276.0-276.9)
    hypoglycemia NOS (251.2)
    specific finding indicating abnormality of:
      amino-acid transport and metabolism (270.0-270.9)
      carbohydrate transport and metabolism (271.0-271.9)
      lipid metabolism (272.0-272.9)
    uremia NOS (586)
AHA: 4Q, '88, 1

SYMPTOMS, SIGNS, AND ILL-DEFINED CONDITIONS

790.7 Bacteremia `CC`
- EXCLUDES: bacteremia of newborn (771.83)
  septicemia (038)
- Use additional code to identify organism (041)
- CC Excl: 780.91-780.99, 790.7-790.99, 799.8
- AHA: 4Q, '93, 29; 3Q, '88, 12
- DEF: Bacterial infection of blood with no signs of infection.

790.8 Viremia, unspecified
- AHA: 4Q, '88, 10
- DEF: Presence of a virus in the blood stream.

√5th 790.9 Other nonspecific findings on examination of blood
- AHA: 4Q, '93, 29

790.91 Abnormal arterial blood gases

790.92 Abnormal coagulation profile
- Abnormal or prolonged:
  - bleeding time
  - coagulation time
  - partial thromboplastin time [PTT]
  - prothrombintime [PT]
- EXCLUDES: coagulation (hemorrhagic) disorders (286.0-286.9)

790.93 Elevated prostate specific antigen, (PSA) A ♂

790.94 Euthyroid sick syndrome
- AHA: 4Q, '97, 45
- DEF: Transient alteration of thyroid hormone metabolism due to nonthyroid illness or stress.

790.99 Other

√4th 791 Nonspecific findings on examination of urine
- EXCLUDES: hematuria NOS (599.7)
  specific findings indicating abnormality of:
  - amino-acid transport and metabolism (270.0-270.9)
  - carbohydrate transport and metabolism (271.0-271.9)

791.0 Proteinuria
- Albuminuria
- Bence-Jones proteinuria
- EXCLUDES: postural proteinuria (593.6)
  that arising during pregnancy or the puerperium (642.0-642.9, 646.2)
- AHA: 3Q, '91, 8
- DEF: Excess protein in urine.

791.1 Chyluria `CC`
- EXCLUDES: filarial (125.0-125.9)
- CC Excl: 780.91-780.99, 791.1, 791.9, 799.8
- DEF: Excess chyle in urine.

791.2 Hemoglobinuria
- DEF: Free hemoglobin in blood due to rapid hemolysis of red blood cells.

791.3 Myoglobinuria `CC`
- CC Excl: 780.91-780.99, 791.2-791.3, 791.9, 799.8
- DEF: Myoglobin (oxygen-transporting pigment) in urine.

791.4 Biliuria
- DEF: Bile pigments in urine.

791.5 Glycosuria
- EXCLUDES: renal glycosuria (271.4)
- DEF: Sugar in urine.

791.6 Acetonuria
- Ketonuria
- DEF: Excess acetone in urine.

791.7 Other cells and casts in urine

791.9 Other nonspecific findings on examination of urine
- Crystalluria
- Elevated urine levels of:
  - 17-ketosteroids
  - catecholamines
- Elevated urine levels of:
  - indolacetic acid
  - vanillylmandelic acid [VMA]
  - Melanuria

√4th 792 Nonspecific abnormal findings in other body substances
- EXCLUDES: that in chromosomal analysis (795.2)

792.0 Cerebrospinal fluid

792.1 Stool contents
- Abnormal stool color
- Fat in stool
- Mucus in stool
- Occult stool
- Pus in stool
- EXCLUDES: blood in stool [melena] (578.1)
  newborn (772.4, 777.3)
- AHA: 2Q, '92, 9

792.2 Semen ♂
- Abnormal spermatozoa
- EXCLUDES: azoospermia (606.0)
  oligospermia (606.1)

792.3 Amniotic fluid M♀
- AHA: N-D, '86, 4
- DEF: Nonspecific abnormal findings in amniotic fluid.

792.4 Saliva
- EXCLUDES: that in chromosomal analysis (795.2)

792.5 Cloudy (hemodialysis) (peritoneal) dialysis effluent

792.9 Other nonspecific abnormal findings in body substances
- Peritoneal fluid
- Pleural fluid
- Synovial fluid
- Vaginal fluids

√4th 793 Nonspecific abnormal findings on radiological and other examination of body structure
- INCLUDES: nonspecific abnormal findings of:
  - thermography
  - ultrasound examination [echogram]
  - x-ray examination
- EXCLUDES: abnormal results of function studies and radioisotope scans (794.0-794.9)

793.0 Skull and head
- EXCLUDES: nonspecific abnormal echoencephalogram (794.01)

793.1 Lung field
- Coin lesion } (of) lung
- Shadow
- DEF: Coin lesion of lung: coin-shaped, solitary pulmonary nodule; diagnosis includes tuberculoma, histoplasmoma, blastomycoma, coccidioidomycoma, primary carcinoma of the lung, metastatic carcinoma and benign pulmonary tumor.

793.2 Other intrathoracic organ
- Abnormal:
  - echocardiogram
  - heart shadow
- Abnormal:
  - ultrasound cardiogram
  - Mediastinal shift

793.3 Biliary tract
- Nonvisualization of gallbladder

793.4 Gastrointestinal tract

793.5 Genitourinary organs
- Filling defect:
  - bladder
  - kidney
- Filling defect:
  - ureter
- AHA: 4Q, '00, 46

793.6 Abdominal area, including retroperitoneum

793.7 Musculoskeletal system

√5th 793.8 Breast
- AHA: 4Q, '01, 51

793.80 Abnormal mammogram, unspecified

793.81 Mammographic microcalcification
- DEF: Calcium and cellular debris deposits in the breast that cannot be felt but can be detected on a mammogram; can be a sign of cancer, benign conditions, or changes in the breast tissue as a result of inflammation, injury, or obstructed duct.

SYMPTOMS, SIGNS, AND ILL-DEFINED CONDITIONS

793.89 **Other abnormal findings on radiological examination of breast**

793.9 **Other**
Abnormal:
placental finding by x-ray or ultrasound method
radiological findings in skin and subcutaneous tissue
EXCLUDES: abnormal finding by radioisotope localization of placenta (794.9)

√4th 794 **Nonspecific abnormal results of function studies**
INCLUDES: radioisotope:
scans
uptake studies
scintiphotography

√5th 794.0 **Brain and central nervous system**
794.00 **Abnormal function study, unspecified**
794.01 **Abnormal echoencephalogram**
794.02 **Abnormal electroencephalogram [EEG]**
794.09 **Other**
Abnormal brain scan

√5th 794.1 **Peripheral nervous system and special senses**
794.10 **Abnormal response to nerve stimulation, unspecified**
794.11 **Abnormal retinal function studies**
Abnormal electroretinogram [ERG]
794.12 **Abnormal electro-oculogram [EOG]**
794.13 **Abnormal visually evoked potential**
794.14 **Abnormal oculomotor studies**
794.15 **Abnormal auditory function studies**
794.16 **Abnormal vestibular function studies**
794.17 **Abnormal electromyogram [EMG]**
EXCLUDES: that of eye (794.14)
794.19 **Other**

794.2 **Pulmonary**
Abnormal lung scan
Reduced:
ventilatory capacity
vital capacity

√5th 794.3 **Cardiovascular**
794.30 **Abnormal function study, unspecified**
794.31 **Abnormal electrocardiogram [ECG] [EKG]**
794.39 **Other**
Abnormal:
ballistocardiogram
phonocardiogram
vectorcardiogram

794.4 **Kidney**
Abnormal renal function test

794.5 **Thyroid**
Abnormal thyroid:
scan
uptake

794.6 **Other endocrine function study**

794.7 **Basal metabolism**
Abnormal basal metabolic rate [BMR]

794.8 **Liver**
Abnormal liver scan

794.9 **Other**
Bladder
Pancreas
Placenta
Spleen

√4th 795 **Nonspecific abnormal histological and immunological findings**
EXCLUDES: nonspecific abnormalities of red blood cells (790.01-790.09)

√5th 795.0 **Nonspecific abnormal Papanicolaou smear of cervix** ♀
EXCLUDES: ▶carcinoma in-situ of cervix (233.1)
cervical intraepithelial neoplasia I (CIN I) (622.1)
cervical intraepithelial neoplasia II (CIN II) (622.1)
cervical intraepithelial neoplasia III (CIN III) (233.1)
dysplasia of cervix (uteri) (622.1)
high grade squamous intraepithelial dysplasia (HGSIL) (622.1)
low grade squamous intraepithelial dysplasia (LGSIL) (622.1)◀

795.00 **Nonspecific abnormal Papanicolaou smear of cervix, unspecified**
795.01 **Atypical squamous cell changes of undetermined significance favor benign (ASCUS favor benign)**
Atypical glandular cell changes of undetermined significance favor benign (AGCUS favor benign)
795.02 **Atypical squamous cell changes of undetermined significance favor dysplasia (ASCUS favor dysplasia)**
Atypical glandular cell changes of undetermined significance favor dysplasia (AGCUS favor dysplasia)
795.09 **Other nonspecific abnormal Papanicolaou smear of cervix**
Benign cellular chnages
Unsatisfactory smear

795.1 **Nonspecific abnormal Papanicolaou smear of other site**

795.2 **Nonspecific abnormal findings on chromosomal analysis**
Abnormal karyotype

√5th 795.3 **Nonspecific positive culture findings**
Positive culture findings in:
nose
sputum
throat
wound
EXCLUDES: that of:
blood (790.7-790.8)
urine (791.9)

795.31 **Nonspecific positive findings for anthrax**
Positive findings by nasal swab
795.39 **Other nonspecific positive culture findings**

795.4 **Other nonspecific abnormal histological findings**

795.5 **Nonspecific reaction to tuberculin skin test without active tuberculosis**
Abnormal result of Mantoux test
PPD positive
Tuberculin (skin test):
positive
reactor

795.6 **False positive serological test for syphilis**
False positive Wassermann reaction

√5th 795.7 **Other nonspecific immunological findings**
EXCLUDES: isoimmunization, in pregnancy (656.1-656.2)
affecting fetus or newborn (773.0-773.2)

AHA: 2Q, '93, 6

SYMPTOMS, SIGNS, AND ILL-DEFINED CONDITIONS

795.71 **Nonspecific serologic evidence of human immunodeficiency virus [HIV]**
Inclusive human immunodeficiency [HIV] test (adult) (infant)
Note: This code is **only** to be used when a test finding is reported as nonspecific. Asymptomatic positive findings are coded to V08. If any HIV infection symptom or condition is present, see code 042. Negative findings are not coded.
EXCLUDES: acquired immunodeficiency syndrome [AIDS] (042)
asymptomatic human immunodeficiency virus, [HIV] infection status (V08)
HIV infection, symptomatic (042)
human immunodeficiency virus [HIV] disease (042)
positive (status) NOS (V08)
AHA: 1Q, '93, 21; 1Q, '93, 22; 2Q, '92, 11; J-A, '87, 24

795.79 **Other and unspecified nonspecific immunological findings**
Raised antibody titer
Raised level of immunoglobulins

✓4th 796 Other nonspecific abnormal findings

796.0 **Nonspecific abnormal toxicological findings**
Abnormal levels of heavy metals or drugs in blood, urine, or other tissue
EXCLUDES: excessive blood level of alcohol (790.3)
AHA: 1Q, '97, 16

796.1 **Abnormal reflex**

796.2 **Elevated blood pressure reading without diagnosis of hypertension**
Note: This category is to be used to record an episode of elevated blood pressure in a patient in whom no formal diagnosis of hypertension has been made, or as an incidental finding.
AHA: 3Q, '90, 4; J-A, '84, 12

796.3 **Nonspecific low blood pressure reading**

796.4 **Other abnormal clinical findings**
AHA: 1Q, '97, 16

796.5 **Abnormal finding on antenatal screening** M ♀
AHA: 4Q, '97, 46

796.9 **Other**

ILL-DEFINED AND UNKNOWN CAUSES OF MORBIDITY AND MORTALITY (797-799)

797 Senility without mention of psychosis
Old age
Senescence
Senile asthenia
Senile:
  debility
  exhaustion
EXCLUDES: senile psychoses (290.0-290.9)

✓4th 798 Sudden death, cause unknown

798.0 **Sudden infant death syndrome** P
Cot death
Crib death
Sudden death of nonspecific cause in infancy
DEF: Death of infant under age one due to nonspecific cause.

798.1 **Instantaneous death**

798.2 **Death occurring in less than 24 hours from onset of symptoms, not otherwise explained**
Death known not to be violent or instantaneous, for which no cause could be discovered
Died without sign of disease

798.9 **Unattended death**
Death in circumstances where the body of the deceased was found and no cause could be discovered
Found dead

✓4th 799 Other ill-defined and unknown causes of morbidity and mortality

799.0 **Asphyxia**
EXCLUDES: asphyxia (due to):
  carbon monoxide (986)
  inhalation of food or foreign body (932-934.9)
  newborn (768.0-768.9)
  traumatic (994.7)
DEF: Lack of oxygen.

799.1 **Respiratory arrest** CC
Cardiorespiratory failure
EXCLUDES: cardiac arrest (427.5)
failure of peripheral circulation (785.50)
respiratory distress:
  NOS (786.09)
  acute (518.82)
  following trauma and surgery (518.5)
  newborn ▶(770.89)◀
  syndrome (newborn) (769)
  adult (following trauma and surgery) (518.5)
  other (518.82)
respiratory failure (518.81, 518.83-518.84)
  newborn ▶(770.84)◀
respiratory insufficiency (786.09)
  acute (518.82)
CC Excl: 518.81-518.84, ▶780.91-780.99,◀ 798.0, 799.0-799.1, 799.8

799.2 **Nervousness**
"Nerves"

799.3 **Debility, unspecified**
EXCLUDES: asthenia (780.79)
nervous debility (300.5)
neurasthenia (300.5)
senile asthenia (797)

799.4 **Cachexia** CC
Wasting disease
EXCLUDES: nutritional marasmus (261)
CC Excl: ▶780.91-780.99,◀ 799.3-799.4, 799.8
AHA: 3Q, '90, 17
DEF: General ill health and poor nutrition.

799.8 **Other ill-defined conditions**

799.9 **Other unknown and unspecified cause**
Undiagnosed disease, not specified as to site or system involved
Unknown cause of morbidity or mortality
AHA: 1Q, '98,.4; 1Q, '90, 20

Tabular List — INJURY AND POISONING

17. INJURY AND POISONING (800-999)

Use E code(s) to identify the cause and intent of the injury or poisoning (E800-E999)

Note:

1. The principle of multiple coding of injuries should be followed wherever possible. Combination categories for multiple injuries are provided for use when there is insufficient detail as to the nature of the individual conditions, or for primary tabulation purposes when it is more convenient to record a single code; otherwise, the component injuries should be coded separately.

   Where multiple sites of injury are specified in the titles, the word "with" indicates involvement of both sites, and the word "and" indicates involvement of either or both sites. The word "finger" includes thumb.

2. Categories for "late effect" of injuries are to be found at 905-909.

FRACTURES (800-829)

EXCLUDES malunion (733.81)
nonunion (733.82)
pathological or spontaneous fracture (733.10-733.19)
stress fractures (733.93-733.95)

The terms "condyle," "coronoid process," "ramus," and "symphysis" indicate the portion of the bone fractured, not the name of the bone involved.

The descriptions "closed" and "open" used in the fourth-digit subdivisions include the following terms:
  closed (with or without delayed healing):
  - comminuted
  - depressed
  - elevated
  - fissured
  - fracture NOS
  - greenstick
  - impacted
  - linear
  - simple
  - slipped epiphysis
  - spiral

  open (with or without delayed healing):
  - compound
  - infected
  - missile
  - puncture
  - with foreign body

A fracture not indicated as closed or open should be classified as closed.

AHA: 4Q, '90, 26; 3Q, '90, 5; 3Q, '90, 13; 2Q, '90, 7; 2Q, '89, 15, S-O, '85, 3

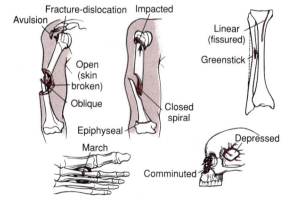

Fractures

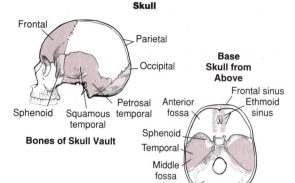

Bones of Skull Vault — Frontal, Parietal, Occipital, Sphenoid, Squamous temporal, Petrosal temporal

Base Skull from Above — Frontal sinus, Ethmoid sinus, Anterior fossa, Sphenoid, Temporal, Middle fossa, Posterior fossa, Occipital

FRACTURE OF SKULL (800-804)

The following fifth-digit subclassification is for use with the appropriate codes in categories 800, 801, 803, and 804:
- 0 unspecified state of consciousness
- 1 with no loss of consciousness
- 2 with brief [less than one hour] loss of consciousness
- 3 with moderate [1-24 hours] loss of consciousness
- 4 with prolonged [more than 24 hours] loss of consciousness and return to pre-existing conscious level
- 5 with prolonged [more than 24 hours] loss of consciousness, without return to pre-existing conscious level

Use fifth-digit 5 to designate when a patient is unconscious and dies before regaining consciousness, regardless of the duration of the loss of consciousness

- 6 with loss of consciousness of unspecified duration
- 9 with concussion, unspecified

√4th **800 Fracture of vault of skull**
  INCLUDES frontal bone
  parietal bone

  AHA: 4Q, '96, 36

  DEF: Fracture of bone that forms skull dome and protects brain.

§ √5th **800.0 Closed without mention of intracranial injury** CC MSP
  CC Excl: 800.00-801.99, 803.00-804.99, 829.0-829.1, 850.0-852.19, 852.21-854.19, 873.8-873.9, 879.8-879.9, 905.0, 925.1-925.2, 929.0-929.9, 958.8, 959.01, 959.09, 959.8-959.9

§ √5th **800.1 Closed with cerebral laceration and contusion** CC MSP
  CC Excl: See code 800.0

§ √5th **800.2 Closed with subarachnoid, subdural, and extradural hemorrhage** CC MSP
  CC Excl: See code 800.0

§ √5th **800.3 Closed with other and unspecified intracranial hemorrhage** CC MSP
  CC Excl: See code 800.0

§ √5th **800.4 Closed with intracranial injury of other and unspecified nature** CC MSP
  CC Excl: See code 800.0

§ √5th **800.5 Open without mention of intracranial injury** CC MSP
  CC Excl: See code 800.0

§ √5th **800.6 Open with cerebral laceration and contusion** CC MSP
  CC Excl: See code 800.0

§ Requires fifth-digit. See beginning of section 800-804 for codes and definitions.

INJURY AND POISONING

800.7–802.37

§ ✓5ᵗʰ **800.7 Open with subarachnoid, subdural, and extradural hemorrhage**
CC Excl: See code 800.0

§ ✓5ᵗʰ **800.8 Open with other and unspecified intracranial hemorrhage**
CC Excl: See code 800.0

§ ✓5ᵗʰ **800.9 Open with intracranial injury of other and unspecified nature**
CC Excl: See code 800.0

✓4ᵗʰ **801 Fracture of base of skull**
INCLUDES fossa:
            anterior
            middle
            posterior
            occiput bone
            orbital roof
          sinus:
            ethmoid
            frontal
            sphenoid bone
            temporal bone

AHA: 4Q, '96, 36

DEF: Fracture of bone that forms skull floor.

§ ✓5ᵗʰ **801.0 Closed without mention of intracranial injury**
CC Excl: See code 800.0

§ ✓5ᵗʰ **801.1 Closed with cerebral laceration and contusion**
CC Excl: See code 800.0
AHA: 4Q, '96, 36

§ ✓5ᵗʰ **801.2 Closed with subarachnoid, subdural, and extradural hemorrhage**
CC Excl: See code 800.0

§ ✓5ᵗʰ **801.3 Closed with other and unspecified intracranial hemorrhage**
CC Excl: See code 800.0

§ ✓5ᵗʰ **801.4 Closed with intracranial injury of other and unspecified nature**
CC Excl: See code 800.0

§ ✓5ᵗʰ **801.5 Open without mention of intracranial injury**
CC Excl: See code 800.0

§ ✓5ᵗʰ **801.6 Open with cerebral laceration and contusion**
CC Excl: See code 800.0

§ ✓5ᵗʰ **801.7 Open with subarachnoid, subdural, and extradural hemorrhage**
CC Excl: See code 800.0

§ ✓5ᵗʰ **801.8 Open with other and unspecified intracranial hemorrhage**
CC Excl: See code 800.0

§ ✓5ᵗʰ **801.9 Open with intracranial injury of other and unspecified nature**
CC Excl: See code 800.0

✓4ᵗʰ **802 Fracture of face bones**
AHA: 4Q, '96, 36

802.0 Nasal bones, closed

802.1 Nasal bones, open
CC Excl: 800.00-800.99, 801.00-801.99, 802.0-802.1, 803.00-803.99, 804.00-804.99, 829.0-829.1, 850.0-850.9, 851.00-851.99, 852.00-852.19, 852.21-852.59, 853.00-853.19, 854.00-854.19, 873.8-873.9, 879.8-879.9, 905.0, 925.1-925.2, 929.0, 929.9, 958.8, 959.01, 959.09, 959.8-959.9

Facial Fractures

LeFort Fracture Types — Frontal bone, Nasal bone, Type III, Type II, Type I, Orbital floor, Zygomatic bone (malar) and arch, Maxilla

Common Fracture Sites of Mandible — Symphysis, Parasymphysis, Body, Angle, Subcondylar

✓5ᵗʰ **802.2 Mandible, closed**
Inferior maxilla   Lower jaw (bone)

802.20 Unspecified site
CC Excl: 800.00-800.99, 801.00-801.99, 802.20-802.5, 803.00-803.99, 804.00-804.99, 829.0-829.1, 830.0-830.1, 850.0-850.9, 851.00-851.99, 852.00-852.19, 852.21-852.59, 853.00-853.19, 854.00-854.19, 873.8-873.9, 879.8-879.9, 905.0, 925.1, 925.2, 929.0, 929.9, 958.8, 959.01, 959.09, 959.8-959.9

802.21 Condylar process
CC Excl: See code 802.20

802.22 Subcondylar
CC Excl: See code 802.20

802.23 Coronoid process
CC Excl: See code 802.20

802.24 Ramus, unspecified
CC Excl: See code 802.20

802.25 Angle of jaw
CC Excl: See code 802.20

802.26 Symphysis of body
CC Excl: See code 802.20

802.27 Alveolar border of body
CC Excl: See code 802.20

802.28 Body, other and unspecified
CC Excl: See code 802.20

802.29 Multiple sites
CC Excl: See code 802.20

✓5ᵗʰ **802.3 Mandible, open**

802.30 Unspecified site
CC Excl: See code 802.20

802.31 Condylar process
CC Excl: See code 802.20

802.32 Subcondylar
CC Excl: See code 802.20

802.33 Coronoid process
CC Excl: See code 802.20

802.34 Ramus, unspecified
CC Excl: See code 802.20

802.35 Angle of jaw
CC Excl: See code 802.20

802.36 Symphysis of body
CC Excl: See code 802.20

802.37 Alveolar border of body
CC Excl: See code 802.20

§ Requires fifth-digit. See beginning of section 800-804 for codes and definitions.

N Newborn Age: 0   P Pediatric Age: 0-17   M Maternity Age: 12-55   A Adult Age: 15-124   CC CC Condition   MC Major Complication   CD Complex Dx   HIV HIV Related Dx

INJURY AND POISONING

802.38 Body, other and unspecified
CC Excl: See code 802.20

802.39 Multiple sites
CC Excl: See code 802.20

802.4 Malar and maxillary bones, closed
Superior maxilla   Zygoma
Upper jaw (bone)   Zygomatic arch
CC Excl: See code 802.20

802.5 Malar and maxillary bones, open
CC Excl: See code 802.20

802.6 Orbital floor (blow-out), closed
CC Excl: 800.00-800.99, 801.00-801.99, 802.6-802.9, 803.00-803.99, 804.00-804.99, 829.0-829.1, 850.0-850.9, 851.00-851.99, 852.00-852.19, 852.21-852.59, 853.00-853.19, 854.00-854.19, 873.8-873.9, 879.8-879.9, 905.0, 925.1-925.2, 929.0, 929.9, 958.8, 959.01, 959.09, 959.8-959.9

802.7 Orbital floor (blow-out), open
CC Excl: See code 802.6

802.8 Other facial bones, closed
Alveolus   Palate
Orbit:
  NOS
  part other than roof or floor
EXCLUDES orbital:
  floor (802.6)
  roof (801.0-801.9)
CC Excl: See code 802.6

802.9 Other facial bones, open
CC Excl: See code 802.6

803 Other and unqualified skull fractures
INCLUDES skull NOS   skull multiple NOS
AHA: 4Q, '96, 36

§ 803.0 **Closed without mention of intracranial injury**
CC Excl: 800.00-800.99, 801.00-801.99, 803.00-803.99, 804.00-804.99, 829.0-829.1, 850.0-850.9, 851.00-851.99, 852.00-852.19, 852.21-852.59, 853.00-853.19, 854.00-854.19, 873.8-873.9, 879.8-879.9, 905.0, 925.1-925.2, 929.0, 929.9, 958.8, 959.01, 959.09, 959.8-959.9

§ 803.1 **Closed with cerebral laceration and contusion**
CC Excl: See code 803.0

§ 803.2 **Closed with subarachnoid, subdural, and extradural hemorrhage**
CC Excl: See code 803.0

§ 803.3 **Closed with other and unspecified intracranial hemorrhage**
CC Excl: See code 803.0

§ 803.4 **Closed with intracranial injury of other and unspecified nature**
CC Excl: See code 803.0

§ 803.5 **Open without mention of intracranial injury**
CC Excl: See code 803.0

§ 803.6 **Open with cerebral laceration and contusion**
CC Excl: See code 803.0

§ 803.7 **Open with subarachnoid, subdural, and extradural hemorrhage**
CC Excl: See code 803.0

§ 803.8 **Open with other and unspecified intracranial hemorrhage**
CC Excl: See code 803.0

§ 803.9 **Open with intracranial injury of other and unspecified nature**
CC Excl: See code 803.0

804 Multiple fractures involving skull or face with other bones
AHA: 4Q, '96, 36

§ 804.0 **Closed without mention of intracranial injury**
CC Excl: See code 803.0

§ 804.1 **Closed with cerebral laceration and contusion**
CC Excl: See code 803.0

§ 804.2 **Closed with subarachnoid, subdural, and extradural hemorrhage**
CC Excl: See code 803.0

§ 804.3 **Closed with other and unspecified intracranial hemorrhage**
CC Excl: See code 803.0

§ 804.4 **Closed with intracranial injury of other and unspecified nature**
CC Excl: See code 803.0

§ 804.5 **Open without mention of intracranial injury**
CC Excl: See code 803.0

§ 804.6 **Open with cerebral laceration and contusion**
CC Excl: See code 803.0

§ 804.7 **Open with subarachnoid, subdural, and extradural hemorrage**
CC Excl: See code 803.0

§ 804.8 **Open with other and unspecified intracranial hemorrhage**
CC Excl: See code 803.0

§ 804.9 **Open with intracranial injury of other and unspecified nature**
CC Excl: See code 803.0

FRACTURE OF NECK AND TRUNK (805-809)

805 Fracture of vertebral column without mention of spinal cord injury
INCLUDES neural arch   transverse process
          spine   vertebra
          spinous process

The following fifth-digit subclassification is for use with codes 805.0-805.1:
0 cervical vertebra, unspecified level
1 first cervical vertebra
2 second cervical vertebra
3 third cervical vertebra
4 fourth cervical vertebra
5 fifth cervical vertebra
6 sixth cervical vertebra
7 seventh cervical vertebra
8 multiple cervical vertebrae

805.0 **Cervical, closed**
Atlas   Axis
CC Excl: 805.00-805.18, 805.8-805.9, 806.00-806.19, 806.8-806.9, 829.0-829.1, 839.00-839.18, 839.40, 839.49-839.50, 839.59, 839.69, 839.79, 839.8-839.9, 847.0, 847.9, 848.8-848.9, 879.8-879.9, 905.1, 926.11, 929.0, 929.9, 952.00-952.09, 952.8-952.9, 958.8, 959.1, 959.8-959.9

805.1 **Cervical, open**
CC Excl: See code 805.0

§ Requires fifth-digit. See beginning of section 800-804 for codes and definitions.

INJURY AND POISONING

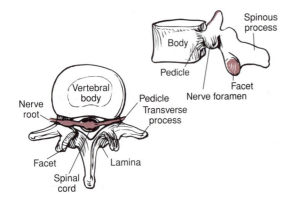

805.2 Dorsal [thoracic], closed CC MSP
CC Excl: 805.2-805.3, 805.8-805.9, 806.20-806.39, 806.8-806.9, 829.0-829.1, 839.21, 839.31, 839.40, 839.49-839.50, 839.59, 839.69, 839.79, 839.8-839.9, 847.1, 847.9, 848.8-848.9, 879.8-879.9, 905.1, 926.11, 929.0, 929.9, 952.10-952.19, 952.8-952.9, 958.8, 959.1, 959.8-959.9

805.3 Dorsal [thoracic], open CC MSP
CC Excl: See code 805.2

805.4 Lumbar, closed CC MSP
CC Excl: 805.4-805.5, 805.8-805.9, 806.4-806.5, 806.8-806.9, 829.0-829.1, 839.20, 839.30, 839.40, 839.49-839.50, 839.59, 839.69, 839.79, 839.8-839.9, 847.2, 847.9, 848.8-848.9, 879.8-879.9, 905.1, 926.11, 929.0, 929.9, 952.2, 952.8-952.9, 958.8, 959.1, 959.8-959.9

AHA: 4Q, '99, 12

805.5 Lumbar, open CC MSP
CC Excl: See code 805.4

805.6 Sacrum and coccyx, closed CC MSP
CC Excl: 805.6-805.9, 806.60-806.9, 829.0-829.1, 839.40-839.59, 839.69, 839.79, 839.8-839.9, 846.0-846.9, 847.3-847.9, 848.5-848.9, 879.8-879.9, 905.1, 926.11, 929.0, 929.9, 952.3-952.9, 958.8, 959.1, 959.8-959.9

805.7 Sacrum and coccyx, open CC MSP
CC Excl: See code 805.6

805.8 Unspecified, closed CC MSP
CC Excl: 733.10-733.19, 733.93-733.95, 805.00-805.9, 806.00-806.9, 829.0-829.1, 839.00-839.59, 839.69, 839.79, 839.8-839.9, 846.0-846.9, 847.0-847.9, 848.5-848.9, 879.8-879.9, 905.1, 926.11, 929.0, 929.9, 952.00-952.9, 958.8, 959.1, 959.8-959.9

805.9 Unspecified, open CC MSP
CC Excl: See code 805.8

√4th **806 Fracture of vertebral column with spinal cord injury**
INCLUDES any condition classifiable to 805 with:
    complete or incomplete transverse lesion (of cord)
    hematomyelia
    injury to:
        cauda equina
        nerve
    paralysis
    paraplegia
    quadriplegia
    spinal concussion

√5th **806.0 Cervical, closed**

806.00 C_1-C_4 level with unspecified spinal cord injury CC MSP
Cervical region NOS with spinal cord injury NOS
CC Excl: 733.10-733.19, 733.93-733.95, 805.00-805.18, 805.8-805.9, 806.00-806.19, 806.8-806.9, 829.0-829.1, 839.00-839.18, 839.40, 839.49-839.50, 839.59, 839.69, 839.79, 839.8-839.9, 847.9, 848.8-848.9, 879.8-879.9, 905.1, 926.11, 929.0, 929.9, 952.00-952.09, 952.8-952.9, 958.8, 959.1, 959.8-959.9

806.01 C_1-C_4 level with complete lesion of cord CC MSP
CC Excl: See code 806.00

806.02 C_1-C_4 level with anterior cord syndrome CC MSP
CC Excl: See code 806.00

806.03 C_1-C_4 level with central cord Syndrome CC MSP
CC Excl: See code 806.00

806.04 C_1-C_4 level with other specified spinal cord injury CC MSP
C_1-C_4 level with:
    incomplete spinal cord lesion NOS
    posterior cord syndrome
CC Excl: See code 806.00

806.05 C_5-C_7 level with unspecified spinal cord injury CC MSP
CC Excl: See code 806.00

806.06 C_5-C_7 level with complete lesion of cord CC MSP
CC Excl: See code 806.00

806.07 C_5-C_7 level with anterior cord syndrome CC MSP
CC Excl: See code 806.00

806.08 C_5-C_7 level with central cord syndrome CC MSP
CC Excl: See code 806.00

806.09 C_5-C_7 level with other specified spinal cord injury CC MSP
C_5-C_7 level with:
    incomplete spinal cord lesion NOS
    posterior cord syndrome
CC Excl: See code 806.00

√5th **806.1 Cervical, open**

806.10 C_1-C_4 level with unspecified spinal cord injury CC MSP
CC Excl: See code 806.00

806.11 C_1-C_4 level with complete lesion of cord CC MSP
CC Excl: See code 806.00

806.12 C_1-C_4 level with anterior cord syndrome CC MSP
CC Excl: See code 806.00

INJURY AND POISONING

806.13 C_1-C_4 level with central cord syndrome [CC] [MSP]
  CC Excl: See code 806.00

806.14 C_1-C_4 level with other specified spinal cord injury [CC] [MSP]
  C_1-C_4 level with:
    incomplete spinal cord lesion NOS
    posterior cord syndrome
  CC Excl: See code 806.00

806.15 C_5-C_7 level with unspecified spinal cord injury [CC] [MSP]
  CC Excl: See code 806.00

806.16 C_5-C_7 level with complete lesion of cord [CC] [MSP]
  CC Excl: See code 806.00

806.17 C_5-C_7 level with anterior cord syndrome [CC] [MSP]
  CC Excl: See code 806.00

806.18 C_5-C_7 level with central cord syndrome [CC] [MSP]
  CC Excl: See code 806.00

806.19 C_5-C_7 level with other specified spinal cord injury [CC] [MSP]
  C_5-C_7 level with:
    incomplete spinal cord lesion NOS
    posterior cord syndrome
  CC Excl: See code 806.00

√5th **806.2** Dorsal [thoracic], closed

806.20 T_1-T_6 level with unspecified spinal cord injury [CC] [MSP]
  Thoracic region NOS with spinal cord injury NOS
  CC Excl: 733.10-733.19, 733.93-733.95, 805.2-805.3, 805.8-805.9, 806.20-806.39, 806.8-806.9, 829.0-829.1, 839.21, 839.31, 839.40, 839.49-839.50, 839.59, 839.69, 839.79, 839.8-839.9, 847.1, 847.9, 848.8-848.9, 879.8-879.9, 905.1, 926.11, 929.0, 929.9, 952.10-952.19, 952.8-952.9, 958.8, 959.1, 959.8-959.9

806.21 T_1-T_6 level with complete lesion of cord [CC] [MSP]
  CC Excl: See code 806.20

806.22 T_1-T_6 level with anterior cord syndrome [CC] [MSP]
  CC Excl: See code 806.20

806.23 T_1-T_6 level with central cord syndrome [CC] [MSP]
  CC Excl: See code 806.20

806.24 T_1-T_6 level with other specified spinal cord injury [CC] [MSP]
  T_1-T_6 level with:
    incomplete spinal cord lesion NOS
    posterior cord syndrome
  CC Excl: See code 806.20

806.25 T_7-T_{12} level with unspecified spinal cord injury [CC] [MSP]
  CC Excl: See code 806.20

806.26 T_7-T_{12} level with complete lesion of cord [CC] [MSP]
  CC Excl: See code 806.20

806.27 T_7-T_{12} level with anterior cord syndrome [CC] [MSP]
  CC Excl: See code 806.20

806.28 T_7-T_{12} level with central cord syndrome [CC] [MSP]
  CC Excl: See code 806.20

806.29 T_7-T_{12} level with other specified spinal cord injury [CC] [MSP]
  T_7-T_{12} level with:
    incomplete spinal cord lesion NOS
    posterior cord syndrome
  CC Excl: See code 806.20

√5th **806.3** Dorsal [thoracic], open

806.30 T_1-T_6 level with unspecified spinal cord injury [CC] [MSP]
  CC Excl: See code 806.20

806.31 T_1-T_6 level with complete lesion of cord [CC] [MSP]
  CC Excl: See code 806.20

806.32 T_1-T_6 level with anteriorr cord syndrome [CC] [MSP]
  CC Excl: See code 806.20

806.33 T_1-T_6 level with centralr cord syndrome [CC] [MSP]
  CC Excl: See code 806.20

806.34 T_1-T_6 level with other specified spinal cord injury [CC] [MSP]
  T_1-T_6 level with:
    incomplete spinal cord lesion NOS
    posterior cord syndrome
  CC Excl: See code 806.20

806.35 T_7-T_{12} level with unspecified spinal cord injury [CC] [MSP]
  CC Excl: See code 806.20

806.36 T_7-T_{12} level with complete lesion of cord [CC] [MSP]
  CC Excl: See code 806.20

806.37 T_7-T_{12} level with anterior cord syndrome [CC] [MSP]
  CC Excl: See code 806.20

806.38 T_7-T_{12} level with central cord syndrome [CC] [MSP]
  CC Excl: See code 806.20

806.39 T_7-T_{12} level with other specified spinal cord injury [CC] [MSP]
  T_7-T_{12} level with:
    incomplete spinal cord lesion NOS
    posterior cord syndrome
  CC Excl: See code 806.20

806.4 Lumbar, closed [CC] [MSP]
  CC Excl: 733.10-733.19, 733.93-733.95, 805.4-805.5, 805.8-805.9, 806.4-806.5, 806.8-806.9, 829.0-829.1, 839.20, 839.30, 839.40, 839.49-839.50, 839.59, 839.69, 839.79, 839.8-839.9, 847.2, 847.9, 848.8-848.9, 879.8-879.9, 905.1, 926.11, 929.0, 929.9, 952.2, 952.8-952.9, 958.8, 959.1, 959.8-959.9
  AHA: 4Q, '99, 11, 13

806.5 Lumbar, open [CC] [MSP]
  CC Excl: See code 806.4

√5th **806.6** Sacrum and coccyx, closed

806.60 With unspecified spinal spinal cord injury [CC] [MSP]
  CC Excl: 733.10-733.19, 733.93-733.95, 805.6-805.9, 806.60-806.9, 829.0-829.1, 839.40-839.59, 839.69, 839.79, 839.8-839.9, 846.0-846.9, 847.0, 847.3-847.9, 848.5-848.9, 879.8-879.9, 905.1, 926.11, 929.0, 929.9, 952.3-952.9, 958.8, 959.1, 959.8-959.9

806.61 With complete cauda equina lesion [CC] [MSP]
  CC Excl: See code 806.60

806.62 With other cauda equina injury [CC] [MSP]
  CC Excl: See code 806.60

√4th Additional Digit Required 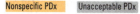Nonspecific PDx Unacceptable PDx Manifestation Code [MSP] Medicare Secondary Payer ▶◀ Revised Text ● New Code ▲ Revised Code Title

2002 Ingenix, Inc. Volume 1 — 263

INJURY AND POISONING

806.69 With other spinal cord injury [CC] [MSP]
CC Excl: See code 806.60

√5th **806.7** **Sacrum and coccyx, open**

806.70 With unspecified spinal cord injury [CC] [MSP]
CC Excl: See code 806.60

806.71 With complete cauda equina lesion [CC] [MSP]
CC Excl: See code 806.60

806.72 With other cauda equina injury [CC] [MSP]
CC Excl: See code 806.60

806.79 With other spinal cord injury [CC] [MSP]
CC Excl: See code 806.60

806.8 Unspecified, closed [CC] [MSP]
CC Excl: 733.10-733.19, 733.93-733.95, 805.00-805.09, 806.00-806.9, 829.0-829.1, 839.00-839.59, 839.69, 839.79, 839.8-839.9, 846.0-846.9, 847.0-847.9, 848.5-848.9, 879.8-879.9, 905.1, 926.11, 929.0, 929.9, 952.00-952.9, 958.8, 959.1, 959.8-959.9

806.9 Unspecified, open [CC] [MSP]
CC Excl: See code 806.8

√4th **807** **Fracture of rib(s), sternum, larynx, and trachea**

The following fifth-digit subclassification is for use with codes 807.0-807.1:
0 rib(s), unspecified
1 one rib
2 two ribs
3 three ribs
4 four ribs
5 five ribs
6 six ribs
7 seven ribs
8 eight or more ribs
9 multiple ribs, unspecified

√5th **807.0** Rib(s), closed [CC 4-9] [MSP]
CC Excl: For codes 807.04-807.09: 807.00-807.19, 807.4, 819.0-819.1, 828.0-828.1, 829.0-829.1, 848.8-848.9, 879.8-879.9, 929.0, 929.9, 958.8, 959.8-959.9

√5th **807.1** Rib(s), open [CC] [MSP]
CC Excl: See code 807.0

807.2 Sternum, closed [CC] [MSP]
CC Excl: 807.2-807.4, 829.0-829.1, 848.8-848.9, 879.8-879.9, 929.0, 929.9, 958.8, 959.8-959.9

DEF: Break in flat bone (breast bone) in anterior thorax.

807.3 Sternum, open [CC] [MSP]
CC Excl: See code 807.2

DEF: Break, with open wound, in flat bone in mid anterior thorax.

807.4 Flail chest [CC] [MSP]
CC Excl: 807.00-807.4, 829.0-829.1, 848.8-848.9, 879.8-879.9, 929.0, 929.9, 958.8, 959.8-959.9

807.5 Larynx and trachea, closed [CC] [MSP]
Hyoid bone   Trachea
Thyroid cartilage
CC Excl: 807.5-807.6, 829.0-829.1, 848.8-848.9, 879.8-879.9, 929.0, 929.9, 958.8, 959.8-959.9

807.6 Larynx and trachea, open [CC] [MSP]
CC Excl: See code 807.5

√4th **808** **Fracture of pelvis**

808.0 Acetabulum, closed [CC]
CC Excl: 733.10-733.19, 733.93-733.95, 808.0-808.1, 808.43, 808.49, 808.53, 808.59, 808.8-808.9, 809.0-809.1, 829.0-829.1, 835.00-835.13, 843.0-843.9, 846.0-846.9 848.5-848.9, 879.8-879.9, 929.0, 929.9, 958.8, 959.6, 959.8-959.9

808.1 Acetabulum, open [CC]
CC Excl: 808.0-808.1, 808.43, 808.49, 808.53, 808.59, 808.8-808.9, 809.0-809.1, 829.0-829.1, 835.00-835.13, 843.0-843.9, 846.0-846.9, 848.5-848.9, 879.8-879.9, 929.0, 929.9, 958.8, 959.6, 959.8-959.9

808.2 Pubis, closed [CC]
CC Excl: 733.10-733.19, 733.93-733.95, 808.2-808.3, 808.43, 808.49, 808.53, 808.59, 808.8-808.9, 809.0-809.1, 829.0-829.1, 835.00-835.13, 843.0-843.9, 846.0-846.9, 848.5-848.9, 879.8-879.9, 929.0, 929.9, 958.8, 959.6, 959.8-959.9

808.3 Pubis, open [CC]
CC Excl: See code 808.2

√5th **808.4** Other specified part, closed
808.41 Ilium
808.42 Ischium
808.43 Multiple pelvic fractures with disruption of pelvic circle [CC]
CC Excl: 733.10-733.19, 733.93-733.95, 808.0-808.9, 809.0-809.1, 829.0-829.1, 835.00-835.13, 843.0-843.9, 846.0-846.9, 848.5-848.9, 879.8-879.9, 929.0, 929.9, 958.8, 959.6, 959.8-959.9

808.49 Other [CC]
Innominate bone
Pelvic rim
CC Excl: See code 808.43

√5th **808.5** Other specified part, open
808.51 Ilium [CC]
CC Excl: 733.10-733.19, 733.93-733.95, 808.41, 808.43, 808.49, 808.51, 808.53, 808.59, 808.8-808.9, 809.0-809.1, 829.0-829.1, 835.00-835.13, 843.0-843.9, 846.0-846.9, 848.5-848.9, 879.8-879.9, 929.0, 929.9, 958.8, 959.6, 959.8-959.9

Tabular List — INJURY AND POISONING — 808.52–812.59

808.52 Ischium CC
CC Excl: 733.10-733.19, 733.93-733.95, 808.42-808.49, 808.52-808.59, 808.8-808.9, 809.0-809.1, 829.0-829.1, 835.00-835.13, 843.0-843.9, 846.0-846.9, 848.5-848.9, 879.8-879.9, 929.0, 929.9, 958.8, 959.6, 959.8-959.9

808.53 Multiple pelvic fractures with disruption of pelvic circle CC
CC Excl: 733.10-733.19, 733.93-733.95, 808.0-808.9 809.0-809.1, 829.0-829.1, 835.00-835.13, 843.0-843.9, 846.0-846.9, 848.5-848.9, 879.8-879.9, 929.0, 929.9, 958.8, 959.6, 959.8-959.9

808.59 Other CC
CC Excl: See code 808.53

808.8 Unspecified, closed CC
CC Excl: See code 808.53

808.9 Unspecified, open CC
CC Excl: See code 808.53

809 Ill-defined fractures of bones of trunk [4th]
INCLUDES bones of trunk with other bones except those of skull and face
multiple bones of trunk
EXCLUDES multiple fractures of:
pelvic bones alone (808.0-808.9)
ribs alone (807.0-807.1, 807.4)
ribs or sternum with limb bones (819.0-819.1, 828.0-828.1)
skull or face with other bones (804.0-804.9)

809.0 Fracture of bones of trunk, closed
809.1 Fracture of bones of trunk, open

FRACTURE OF UPPER LIMB (810-819)

810 Fracture of clavicle [4th]
INCLUDES collar bone
interligamentous part of clavicle

The following fifth-digit subclassification is for use with category 810:
0 unspecified part
  Clavicle NOS
1 sternal end of clavicle
2 shaft of clavicle
3 acromial end of clavicle

[5th] **810.0 Closed** MSP
[5th] **810.1 Open** MSP

811 Fracture of scapula [4th]
INCLUDES shoulder blade

The following fifth-digit subclassification is for use with category 811:
0 unspecified part
1 acromial process
  Acromion (process)
2 coracoid process
3 glenoid cavity and neck of scapula
9 other

[5th] **811.0 Closed** MSP
[5th] **811.1 Open** MSP

812 Fracture of humerus [4th]
[5th] **812.0 Upper end, closed**
812.00 Upper end, unspecified part
  Proximal end   Shoulder
812.01 Surgical neck
  Neck of humerus NOS
812.02 Anatomical neck
812.03 Greater tuberosity
812.09 Other
  Head   Upper epiphysis

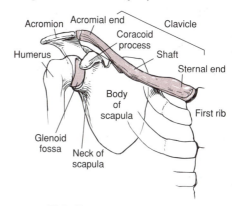
Right Clavicle and Scapula, Anterior View

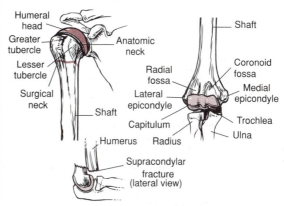
Right Humerus, Anterior View

[5th] **812.1 Upper end, open**
812.10 Upper end, unspecified part
812.11 Surgical neck
812.12 Anatomical neck
812.13 Greater tuberosity
812.19 Other

[5th] **812.2 Shaft or unspecified part, closed**
812.20 Unspecified part of humerus
  Humerus NOS   Upper arm NOS
812.21 Shaft of humerus
  AHA: 3Q, '99, 14

[5th] **812.3 Shaft or unspecified part, open**
812.30 Unspecified part of humerus
812.31 Shaft of humerus

[5th] **812.4 Lower end, closed**
  Distal end of humerus   Elbow
812.40 Lower end, unspecified part
812.41 Supracondylar fracture of humerus
812.42 Lateral condyle
  External condyle
812.43 Medial condyle
  Internal epicondyle
812.44 Condyle(s), unspecified
  Articular process NOS
  Lower epiphysis NOS
812.49 Other
  Multiple fractures of lower end
  Trochlea

[5th] **812.5 Lower end, open**
812.50 Lower end, unspecified part
812.51 Supracondylar fracture of humerus
812.52 Lateral condyle
812.53 Medial condyle
812.54 Condyle(s), unspecified
812.59 Other

813–815.1 INJURY AND POISONING **Tabular List**

Right Radius and Ulna, Anterior View

[Anatomical illustration labeled: Radius, Olecranon process, Coronoid process, Ulna, Shafts, Radial styloid process, Ulnar styloid process, Radius, Colles fracture, Humerus (lateral view), Radius dislocated, Monteggia's fracture-dislocation]

✓4th **813 Fracture of radius and ulna**

  ✓5th **813.0 Upper end, closed**
    Proximal end
    813.00 Upper end of forearm, unspecified
    813.01 Olecranon process of ulna
    813.02 Coronoid process of ulna
    813.03 Monteggia's fracture
      DEF: Fracture near the head of the ulnar shaft, causing dislocation of the radial head.
    813.04 Other and unspecified fractures of proximal end of ulna (alone)
      Multiple fractures of ulna, upper end
    813.05 Head of radius
    813.06 Neck of radius
    813.07 Other and unspecified fractures of proximal end of radius (alone)
      Multiple fractures of radius, upper end
    813.08 Radius with ulna, upper end [any part]

  ✓5th **813.1 Upper end, open**
    813.10 Upper end of forearm, unspecified
    813.11 Olecranon process of ulna
    813.12 Coronoid process of ulna
    813.13 Monteggia's fracture
    813.14 Other and unspecified fractures of proximal end of ulna (alone)
    813.15 Head of radius
    813.16 Neck of radius
    813.17 Other and unspecified fractures of proximal end of radius (alone)
    813.18 Radius with ulna, upper end [any part]

  ✓5th **813.2 Shaft, closed**
    813.20 Shaft, unspecified
    813.21 Radius (alone)
    813.22 Ulna (alone)
    813.23 Radius with ulna

  ✓5th **813.3 Shaft, open**
    813.30 Shaft, unspecified
    813.31 Radius (alone)
    813.32 Ulna (alone)
    813.33 Radius with ulna

  ✓5th **813.4 Lower end, closed**
    Distal end
    813.40 Lower end of forearm, unspecified
    813.41 Colles' fracture
      Smith's fracture
      DEF: Break of lower end of radius; associated with backward movement of the radius lower section.

    813.42 Other fractures of distal end of radius (alone)
      Dupuytren's fracture, radius
      Radius, lower end
      DEF: Dupuytren's fracture: fracture and dislocation of the forearm; the fracture is of the radius above the wrist, and the dislocation is of the ulna at the lower end.
    813.43 Distal end of ulna (alone)
      Ulna:
        head
        lower end
        lower epiphysis
        styloid process
    813.45 Torus fracture of radius
    813.44 Radius with ulna, lower end

  ✓5th **813.5 Lower end, open**
    813.50 Lower end of forearm, unspecified
    813.51 Colles' fracture
    813.52 Other fractures of distal end of radius (alone)
    813.53 Distal end of ulna (alone)
    813.54 Radius with ulna, lower end

  ✓5th **813.8 Unspecified part, closed**
    813.80 Forearm, unspecified
    813.81 Radius (alone)
      AHA: 2Q, '98, 19
    813.82 Ulna (alone)
    813.83 Radius with ulna

  ✓5th **813.9 Unspecified part, open**
    813.90 Forearm, unspecified
    813.91 Radius (alone)
    813.92 Ulna (alone)
    813.93 Radius with ulna

✓4th **814 Fracture of carpal bone(s)**
  The following fifth-digit subclassification is for use with category 814:
    0 carpal bone, unspecified
      Wrist NOS
    1 navicular [scaphoid] of wrist
    2 lunate [semilunar] bone of wrist
    3 triquetral [cuneiform] bone of wrist
    4 pisiform
    5 trapezium bone [larger multangular]
    6 trapezoid bone [smaller multangular]
    7 capitate bone [os magnum]
    8 hamate [unciform] bone
    9 other

  ✓5th **814.0 Closed**
  ✓5th **814.1 Open**

✓4th **815 Fracture of metacarpal bone(s)**
  INCLUDES hand [except finger]
    metacarpus

  The following fifth-digit subclassification is for use with category 815:
    0 metacarpal bone(s), site unspecified
    1 base of thumb [first] metacarpal
      Bennett's fracture
    2 base of other metacarpal bone(s)
    3 shaft of metacarpal bone(s)
    4 neck of metacarpal bone(s)
    9 multiple sites of metacarpus

  ✓5th **815.0 Closed**
  ✓5th **815.1 Open**

Tabular List — INJURY AND POISONING — 816–821.22

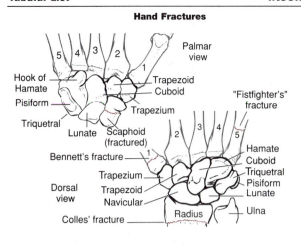

Hand Fractures

√4th **816 Fracture of one or more phalanges of hand**
INCLUDES finger(s) thumb

The following fifth-digit subclassification is for use with category 816:
0 phalanx or phalanges, unspecified
1 middle or proximal phalanx or phalanges
2 distal phalanx or phalanges
3 multiple sites

√5th 816.0 Closed
√5th 816.1 Open

√4th **817 Multiple fractures of hand bones**
INCLUDES metacarpal bone(s) with phalanx or phalanges of same hand

817.0 Closed
817.1 Open

√4th **818 Ill-defined fractures of upper limb**
INCLUDES arm NOS
multiple bones of same upper limb
EXCLUDES multiple fractures of:
metacarpal bone(s) with phalanx or phalanges (817.0-817.1)
phalanges of hand alone (816.0-816.1)
radius with ulna (813.0-813.9)

818.0 Closed
818.1 Open

√4th **819 Multiple fractures involving both upper limbs, and upper limb with rib(s) and sternum**
INCLUDES arm(s) with rib(s) or sternum
both arms [any bones]

819.0 Closed
819.1 Open

FRACTURE OF LOWER LIMB (820-829)

√4th **820 Fracture of neck of femur**
√5th 820.0 Transcervical fracture, closed
820.00 Intracapsular section, unspecified [CC]
CC Excl: 733.10-733.19, 733.93-733.95, 820.00-820.9 821.00-821.39, 827.0-827.1, 828.0-828.1, 829.0-829.1, 843.0-843.9, 848.8-848.9, 879.8-879.9, 929.0, 929.9, 958.8, 959.6, 959.8-959.9

820.01 Epiphysis (separation) (upper) [CC]
Transepiphyseal
CC Excl: See code 820.00

820.02 Midcervical section [CC]
Transcervical NOS
CC Excl: See code 820.00

820.03 Base of neck [CC]
Cervicotrochanteric section
CC Excl: See code 820.00

820.09 Other [CC]
Head of femur
Subcapital
CC Excl: See code 820.00

√5th 820.1 Transcervical fracture, open
820.10 Intracapsular section, unspecified [CC]
CC Excl: See code 820.00

820.11 Epiphysis (separation) (upper) [CC]
CC Excl: See code 820.00

820.12 Midcervical section [CC]
CC Excl: See code 820.00

820.13 Base of neck [CC]
CC Excl: See code 820.00

820.19 Other [CC]
CC Excl: See code 820.00

√5th 820.2 Pertrochanteric fracture, closed
820.20 Trochanteric section, unspecified [CC]
Trochanter: Trochanter:
NOS lesser
greater
CC Excl: See code 820.00

820.21 Intertrochanteric section [CC]
CC Excl: See code 820.00

820.22 Subtrochanteric section [CC]
CC Excl: See code 820.00

√5th 820.3 Pertrochanteric fracture, open
820.30 Trochanteric section, unspecified [CC]
CC Excl: See code 820.00

820.31 Intertrochanteric section [CC]
CC Excl: See code 820.00

820.32 Subtrochanteric section [CC]
CC Excl: See code 820.00

820.8 Unspecified part of neck of femur, closed [CC]
Hip NOS Neck of femur NOS
CC Excl: See code 820.00

820.9 Unspecified part of neck of femur, open [CC]
CC Excl: See code 820.00

√4th **821 Fracture of other and unspecified parts of femur**
√5th 821.0 Shaft or unspecified part, closed
821.00 Unspecified part of femur [CC]
Thigh Upper leg
EXCLUDES hip NOS (820.8)
CC Excl: See code 820.00

821.01 Shaft [CC]
CC Excl: See code 820.00
AHA: 1Q, '99, 5

√5th 821.1 Shaft or unspecified part, open
821.10 Unspecified part of femur [CC]
CC Excl: See code 820.00

821.11 Shaft [CC]
CC Excl: See code 820.00

√5th 821.2 Lower end, closed
Distal end
821.20 Lower end, unspecified part
821.21 Condyle, femoral
821.22 Epiphysis, lower (separation)

821.23–827 INJURY AND POISONING — Tabular List

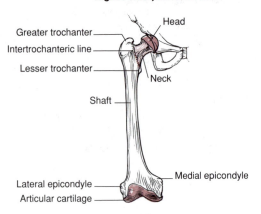

Right Femur, Anterior View

- 821.23 Supracondylar fracture of femur
- 821.29 Other
  Multiple fractures of lower end
- ✓5th 821.3 Lower end, open
  - 821.30 Lower end, unspecified part
  - 821.31 Condyle, femoral
  - 821.32 Epiphysis, lower (separation)
  - 821.33 Supracondylar fracture of femur
  - 821.39 Other
- ✓4th 822 Fracture of patella
  - 822.0 Closed
  - 822.1 Open
- ✓4th 823 Fracture of tibia and fibula
  EXCLUDES Dupuytren's fracture (824.4-824.5)
  ankle (824.4-824.5)
  radius (813.42, 813.52)
  Pott's fracture (824.4-824.5)
  that involving ankle (824.0-824.9)

  The following fifth-digit subclassification is for use with category 823:
  0 tibia alone
  1 fibula alone
  2 fibula with tibia

- ✓5th 823.0 Upper end, closed
  Head   Tibia:
  Proximal end   condyles
                       tuberosity
- ✓5th 823.1 Upper end, open
- ✓5th 823.2 Shaft, closed
- ✓5th 823.3 Shaft, open
- ✓5th 823.4 Torus fracture
- ✓5th 823.8 Unspecified part, closed
  Lower leg NOS
  AHA: For code 823.82: 1Q, '97, 8

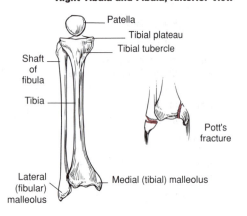

Right Tibula and Fibula, Anterior View

- ✓5th 823.9 Unspecified part, open
- ✓4th 824 Fracture of ankle
  - 824.0 Medial malleolus, closed
    Tibia involving: Tibia involving:
    ankle   malleolus
  - 824.1 Medial malleolus, open
  - 824.2 Lateral malleolus, closed
    Fibula involving:
    ankle
    malleolus
  - 824.3 Lateral malleolus, open
  - 824.4 Bimalleolar, closed
    Dupuytren's fracture, fibula   Pott's fracture
    DEF: Bimalleolar, closed: Breaking of both nodules (malleoli) on either side of ankle joint, without an open wound.
    DEF: Dupuytren's fracture (Pott's fracture): The breaking of the farthest end of the lower leg bone (fibula), with injury to the farthest end joint of the other lower leg bone (tibia).
  - 824.5 Bimalleolar, open
  - 824.6 Trimalleolar, closed
    Lateral and medial malleolus with anterior or posterior lip of tibia
  - 824.7 Trimalleolar, open
  - 824.8 Unspecified, closed
    Ankle NOS
    AHA: 3Q, '00, 12
  - 824.9 Unspecified, open
- ✓4th 825 Fracture of one or more tarsal and metatarsal bones
  - 825.0 Fracture of calcaneus, closed
    Heel bone   Os calcis
  - 825.1 Fracture of calcaneus, open
  - ✓5th 825.2 Fracture of other tarsal and metatarsal bones, closed
    - 825.20 Unspecified bone(s) of foot [except toes]
      Instep
    - 825.21 Astragalus
      Talus
    - 825.22 Navicular [scaphoid], foot
    - 825.23 Cuboid
    - 825.24 Cuneiform, foot
    - 825.25 Metatarsal bone(s)
    - 825.29 Other
      Tarsal with metatarsal bone(s) only
      EXCLUDES calcaneus (825.0)
  - ✓5th 825.3 Fracture of other tarsal and metatarsal bones, open
    - 825.30 Unspecified bone(s) of foot [except toes]
    - 825.31 Astragalus
    - 825.32 Navicular [scaphoid], foot
    - 825.33 Cuboid
    - 825.34 Cuneiform, foot
    - 825.35 Metatarsal bone(s)
    - 825.39 Other
- ✓4th 826 Fracture of one or more phalanges of foot
  INCLUDES toe(s)
  - 826.0 Closed
  - 826.1 Open
- ✓4th 827 Other, multiple, and ill-defined fractures of lower limb
  INCLUDES leg NOS
  multiple bones of same lower limb
  EXCLUDES multiple fractures of:
  ankle bones alone (824.4-824.9)
  phalanges of foot alone (826.0-826.1)
  tarsal with metatarsal bones (825.29, 825.39)
  tibia with fibula (823.0-823.9 with fifth-digit 2)

INJURY AND POISONING — 827.0–836.2

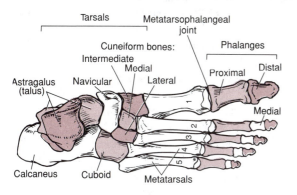
Right Foot, Dorsal — Tarsals; Metatarsophalangeal joint; Cuneiform bones: Intermediate, Medial, Lateral; Phalanges: Proximal, Distal, Medial; Astragalus (talus); Navicular; Calcaneus; Cuboid; Metatarsals

- **827.0** Closed
- **827.1** Open

✓4th **828 Multiple fractures involving both lower limbs, lower with upper limb, and lower limb(s) with rib(s) and sternum**

INCLUDES arm(s) with leg(s) [any bones]
both legs [any bones]
leg(s) with rib(s) or sternum

- **828.0** Closed MSP
- **828.1** Open MSP

✓4th **829 Fracture of unspecified bones**
- **829.0** Unspecified bone, closed
- **829.1** Unspecified bone, open

DISLOCATION (830-839)

INCLUDES displacement
subluxation

EXCLUDES congenital dislocation (754.0-755.8)
pathological dislocation (718.2)
recurrent dislocation (718.3)

The descriptions "closed" and "open," used in the fourth-digit subdivisions, include the following terms:

closed:
 complete
 dislocation NOS
 partial
 simple
 uncomplicated

open:
 compound
 infected
 with foreign body

A dislocation not indicated as closed or open should be classified as closed.

AHA: 3Q, '90, 12

✓4th **830 Dislocation of jaw**
INCLUDES jaw (cartilage) (meniscus)
mandible
maxilla (inferior)
temporomandibular (joint)

- **830.0** Closed dislocation
- **830.1** Open dislocation

✓4th **831 Dislocation of shoulder**
EXCLUDES sternoclavicular joint (839.61, 839.71)
sternum (839.61, 839.71)

The following fifth-digit subclassification is for use with category 831:
 0 shoulder, unspecified
   Humerus NOS
 1 anterior dislocation of humerus
 2 posterior dislocation of humerus
 3 inferior dislocation of humerus
 4 acromioclavicular (joint)
   Clavicle
 9 other
   Scapula

✓5th **831.0** Closed dislocation
✓5th **831.1** Open dislocation

✓4th **832 Dislocation of elbow**

The following fifth-digit subclassification is for use with category 832:
 0 elbow unspecified
 1 anterior dislocation of elbow
 2 posterior dislocation of elbow
 3 medial dislocation of elbow
 4 lateral dislocation of elbow
 9 other

✓5th **832.0** Closed dislocation
✓5th **832.1** Open dislocation

✓4th **833 Dislocation of wrist**

The following fifth-digit subclassification is for use with category 833:
 0 wrist, unspecified part
   Carpal (bone)
   Radius, distal end
 1 radioulnar (joint), distal
 2 radiocarpal (joint)
 3 midcarpal (joint)
 4 carpometacarpal (joint)
 5 metacarpal (bone), proximal end
 9 other
   Ulna, distal end

✓5th **833.0** Closed dislocation
✓5th **833.1** Open dislocation

✓4th **834 Dislocation of finger**
INCLUDES finger(s)   thumb
phalanx of hand

The following fifth-digit subclassification is for use with category 834:
 0 finger, unspecified part
 1 metacarpophalangeal (joint)
   Metacarpal (bone), distal end
 2 interphalangeal (joint), hand

✓5th **834.0** Closed dislocation
✓5th **834.1** Open dislocation

✓4th **835 Dislocation of hip**

The following fifth-digit subclassification is for use with category 835:
 0 dislocation of hip, unspecified
 1 posterior dislocation
 2 obturator dislocation
 3 other anterior dislocation

✓5th **835.0** Closed dislocation
✓5th **835.1** Open dislocation

✓4th **836 Dislocation of knee**
EXCLUDES dislocation of knee:
  old or pathological (718.2)
  recurrent (718.3)
  internal derangement of knee joint (717.0-717.5, 717.8-717.9)
  old tear of cartilage or meniscus of knee (717.0-717.5, 717.8-717.9)

- **836.0** Tear of medial cartilage or meniscus of knee, current
  Bucket handle tear:
   NOS   } current injury
   medial meniscus

- **836.1** Tear of lateral cartilage or meniscus of knee, current

- **836.2** Other tear of cartilage or meniscus of knee, current
  Tear of:
   cartilage
   (semilunar) } current injury, not specified
   meniscus   as medial or lateral

836.3–839.9 INJURY AND POISONING

- 836.3 Dislocation of patella, closed
- 836.4 Dislocation of patella, open
- ✓5th 836.5 Other dislocation of knee, closed
  - 836.50 Dislocation of knee, unspecified
  - 836.51 Anterior dislocation of tibia, proximal end
    - Posterior dislocation of femur, distal end
  - 836.52 Posterior dislocation of tibia, proximal end
    - Anterior dislocation of femur, distal end
  - 836.53 Medial dislocation of tibia, proximal end
  - 836.54 Lateral dislocation of tibia, proximal end
  - 836.59 Other
- ✓5th 836.6 Other dislocation of knee, open
  - 836.60 Dislocation of knee, unspecified
  - 836.61 Anterior dislocation of tibia, proximal end
  - 836.62 Posterior dislocation of tibia, proximal end
  - 836.63 Medial dislocation of tibia, proximal end
  - 836.64 Lateral dislocation of tibia, proximal end
  - 836.69 Other
- ✓4th 837 Dislocation of ankle
  - INCLUDES astragalus
    - fibula, distal end
    - navicular, foot
    - scaphoid, foot
    - tibia, distal end
  - 837.0 Closed dislocation
  - 837.1 Open dislocation
- ✓4th 838 Dislocation of foot

  The following fifth-digit subclassification is for use with category 838:
  - 0 foot, unspecified
  - 1 tarsal (bone), joint unspecified
  - 2 midtarsal (joint)
  - 3 tarsometatarsal (joint)
  - 4 metatarsal (bone), joint unspecified
  - 5 metatarsophalangeal (joint)
  - 6 interphalangeal (joint), foot
  - 9 other
    - Phalanx of foot
    - Toe(s)

  - ✓5th 838.0 Closed dislocation
  - ✓5th 838.1 Open dislocation **CC 9**
- ✓4th 839 Other, multiple, and ill-defined dislocations
  - ✓5th 839.0 Cervical vertebra, closed
    - Cervical spine   Neck
    - 839.00 Cervical vertebra, unspecified **CC MSP**
      - CC Excl: 805.00-805.18, 806.00-806.19, 806.8-806.9, 839.00-839.18, 847.0, 848.8-848.9, 879.8-879.9, 929.0, 929.9, 952.00-952.09, 958.8, 959.8-959.9
    - 839.01 First cervical vertebra **CC MSP**
      - CC Excl: See code 839.00
    - 839.02 Second cervical vertebra **CC MSP**
      - CC Excl: See code 839.00
    - 839.03 Third cervical vertebra **CC MSP**
      - CC Excl: See code 839.00
    - 839.04 Fourth cervical vertebra **CC MSP**
      - CC Excl: See code 839.00
    - 839.05 Fifth cervical vertebra **CC MSP**
      - CC Excl: See code 839.00
    - 839.06 Sixth cervical vertebra **CC MSP**
      - CC Excl: See code 839.00
    - 839.07 Seventh cervical vertebra **CC MSP**
      - CC Excl: See code 839.00
    - 839.08 Multiple cervical vertebrae **CC MSP**
      - CC Excl: See code 839.00
  - ✓5th 839.1 Cervical vertebra, open
    - 839.10 Cervical vertebra, unspecified **CC MSP**
      - CC Excl: See code 839.00
    - 839.11 First cervical vertebra **CC MSP**
      - CC Excl: See code 839.00
    - 839.12 Second cervical vertebra **CC MSP**
      - CC Excl: See code 839.00
    - 839.13 Third cervical vertebra **CC MSP**
      - CC Excl: See code 839.00
    - 839.14 Fourth cervical vertebra **CC MSP**
      - CC Excl: See code 839.00
    - 839.15 Fifth cervical vertebra **CC MSP**
      - CC Excl: See code 839.00
    - 839.16 Sixth cervical vertebra **CC MSP**
      - CC Excl: See code 839.00
    - 839.17 Seventh cervical vertebra **CC MSP**
      - CC Excl: See code 839.00
    - 839.18 Multiple cervical vertebrae **CC MSP**
      - CC Excl: See code 839.00
  - ✓5th 839.2 Thoracic and lumbar vertebra, closed
    - 839.20 Lumbar vertebra **MSP**
    - 839.21 Thoracic vertebra **MSP**
      - Dorsal [thoracic] vertebra
  - ✓5th 839.3 Thoracic and lumbar vertebra, open
    - 839.30 Lumbar vertebra **MSP**
    - 839.31 Thoracic vertebra **MSP**
  - ✓5th 839.4 Other vertebra, closed
    - 839.40 Vertebra, unspecified site
      - Spine NOS
    - 839.41 Coccyx
    - 839.42 Sacrum
      - Sacroiliac (joint)
    - 839.49 Other
  - ✓5th 839.5 Other vertebra, open
    - 839.50 Vertebra, unspecified site
    - 839.51 Coccyx
    - 839.52 Sacrum
    - 839.59 Other
  - ✓5th 839.6 Other location, closed
    - 839.61 Sternum
      - Sternoclavicular joint
    - 839.69 Other
      - Pelvis
  - ✓5th 839.7 Other location, open
    - 839.71 Sternum **MSP**
    - 839.79 Other **MSP**
  - 839.8 Multiple and ill-defined, closed **MSP**
    - Arm
    - Back
    - Hand
    - Multiple locations, except fingers or toes alone
    - Other ill-defined locations
    - Unspecified location
  - 839.9 Multiple and ill-defined, open **MSP**

SPRAINS AND STRAINS OF JOINTS AND ADJACENT MUSCLES
(840-848)

INCLUDES avulsion, hemarthrosis, laceration, rupture, sprain, strain, tear of: joint capsule, ligament, muscle, tendon

EXCLUDES laceration of tendon in open wounds (880-884 and 890-894 with .2)

840 Sprains and strains of shoulder and upper arm
- 840.0 Acromioclavicular (joint) (ligament)
- 840.1 Coracoclavicular (ligament)
- 840.2 Coracohumeral (ligament)
- 840.3 Infraspinatus (muscle) (tendon)
- 840.4 Rotator cuff (capsule)
  - **EXCLUDES** complete rupture of rotator cuff, nontraumatic (727.61)
- 840.5 Subscapularis (muscle)
- 840.6 Supraspinatus (muscle) (tendon)
- 840.7 Superior glenoid labrum lesion
  - SLAP lesion
  - AHA: ▶4Q,'01, 52◀
  - DEF: ▶Detachment injury of the superior aspect of the glenoid labrum which is the ring of fibrocartilage attached to the rim of the glenoid cavity of the scapula.◀
- 840.8 Other specified sites of shoulder and upper arm
- 840.9 **Unspecified site of shoulder and upper arm**
  - Arm NOS
  - Shoulder NOS

841 Sprains and strains of elbow and forearm
- 841.0 Radial collateral ligament
- 841.1 Ulnar collateral ligament
- 841.2 Radiohumeral (joint)
- 841.3 Ulnohumeral (joint)
- 841.8 Other specified sites of elbow and forearm
- 841.9 **Unspecified site of elbow and forearm**
  - Elbow NOS

842 Sprains and strains of wrist and hand
- 842.0 Wrist
  - 842.00 Unspecified site
  - 842.01 Carpal (joint)
  - 842.02 Radiocarpal (joint) (ligament)
  - 842.09 Other
    - Radioulnar joint, distal
- 842.1 Hand
  - 842.10 Unspecified site
  - 842.11 Carpometacarpal (joint)
  - 842.12 Metacarpophalangeal (joint)
  - 842.13 Interphalangeal (joint)
  - 842.19 Other
    - Midcarpal (joint)

843 Sprains and strains of hip and thigh
- 843.0 Iliofemoral (ligament)
- 843.1 Ischiocapsular (ligament)
- 843.8 Other specified sites of hip and thigh
- 843.9 **Unspecified site of hip and thigh**
  - Hip NOS
  - Thigh NOS

844 Sprains and strains of knee and leg
- 844.0 Lateral collateral ligament of knee
- 844.1 Medial collateral ligament of knee
- 844.2 Cruciate ligament of knee
- 844.3 Tibiofibular (joint) (ligament), superior
- 844.8 Other specified sites of knee and leg
- 844.9 Unspecified site of knee and leg
  - Knee NOS
  - Leg NOS

845 Sprains and strains of ankle and foot
- 845.0 Ankle
  - 845.00 Unspecified site
  - 845.01 Deltoid (ligament), ankle
    - Internal collateral (ligament), ankle
  - 845.02 Calcaneofibular (ligament)
  - 845.03 Tibiofibular (ligament), distal
  - 845.09 Other
    - Achilles tendon
- 845.1 Foot
  - 845.10 Unspecified site
  - 845.11 Tarsometatarsal (joint) (ligament)
  - 845.12 Metatarsophalangeal (joint)
  - 845.13 Interphalangeal (joint), toe
  - 845.19 Other

846 Sprains and strains of sacroiliac region
- 846.0 Lumbosacral (joint) (ligament)
- 846.1 Sacroiliac ligament
- 846.2 Sacrospinatus (ligament)
- 846.3 Sacrotuberous (ligament)
- 846.8 Other specified sites of sacroiliac region
- 846.9 **Unspecified site of sacroiliac region**

847 Sprains and strains of other and unspecified parts of back
- **EXCLUDES** lumbosacral (846.0)
- 847.0 Neck [MSP]
  - Anterior longitudinal (ligament), cervical
  - Atlanto-axial (joints)
  - Atlanto-occipital (joints)
  - Whiplash injury
  - **EXCLUDES** neck injury NOS (959.0)
    - thyroid region (848.2)
- 847.1 Thoracic
- 847.2 Lumbar
- 847.3 Sacrum
  - Sacrococcygeal (ligament)
- 847.4 Coccyx
- 847.9 **Unspecified site of back**
  - Back NOS

848 Other and ill-defined sprains and strains
- 848.0 Septal cartilage of nose
- 848.1 Jaw
  - Temporomandibular (joint) (ligament)
- 848.2 Thyroid region
  - Cricoarytenoid (joint) (ligament)
  - Cricothyroid (joint) (ligament)
  - Thyroid cartilage
- 848.3 Ribs
  - Chondrocostal (joint) } without mention of
  - Costal cartilage } injury to sternum
- 848.4 Sternum
  - 848.40 Unspecified site
  - 848.41 Sternoclavicular (joint) (ligament)
  - 848.42 Chondrosternal (joint)
  - 848.49 Other
    - Xiphoid cartilage
- 848.5 Pelvis
  - Symphysis pubis
  - **EXCLUDES** that in childbirth (665.6)
- 848.8 Other specified sites of sprains and strains
- 848.9 **Unspecified site of sprain and strain**

INTRACRANIAL INJURY, EXCLUDING THOSE WITH SKULL FRACTURE (850-854)

EXCLUDES intracranial injury with skull fracture (800-801 and 803-804, except .0 and .5)
open wound of head without intracranial injury (870.0-873.9)
skull fracture alone (800-801 and 803-804 with .0, .5)

The description "with open intracranial wound," used in the fourth-digit subdivisions, includes those specified as open or with mention of infection or foreign body.

The following fifth-digit subclassification is for use with categories 851-854:
- 0 unspecified state of consciousness
- 1 with no loss of consciousness
- 2 with brief [less than one hour] loss of consciousness
- 3 with moderate [1-24 hours] loss of consciousness
- 4 with prolonged [more than 24 hours] loss of consciousness and return to pre-existing conscious level
- 5 with prolonged [more than 24 hours] loss of consciousness, without return to pre-existing conscious level
  Use fifth-digit 5 to designate when a patient is unconscious and dies before regaining consciousness, regardless of the duration of the loss of consciousness
- 6 with loss of consciousness of unspecified duration
- 9 with concussion, unspecified

AHA: 1Q, '93, 22

√4ᵗʰ 850 Concussion

INCLUDES commotio cerebri
EXCLUDES concussion with:
cerebral laceration or contusion (851.0-851.9)
cerebral hemorrhage (852-853)
head injury NOS (959.01)

AHA: 2Q, '96, 6; 4Q, '90, 24

850.0 With no loss of consciousness [CC] [MSP]
Concussion with mental confusion or disorientation, without loss of consciousness
CC Excl: 800.00-800.99, 801.00-801.99, 803.00-803.99, 804.00-804.99, 850.0-850.9, 851.00-851.99, 852.00-852.19, 852.21-852.59, 853.00-853.19, 854.00-854.19, 873.8-873.9, 879.8-879.9, 905.0, 925.1-925.2, 929.0, 929.9, 958.8, 959.01, 959.09, 959.8-959.9

850.1 With brief loss of consciousness [CC] [MSP]
Loss of consciousness for less than one hour
CC Excl: See code 850.0
AHA: 1Q, '99, 10; 2Q, '92, 5

850.2 With moderate loss of consciousness [CC] [MSP]
Loss of consciousness for 1-24 hours
CC Excl: See code 850.0

850.3 With prolonged loss of consciousness and return to pre-existing conscious level [CC] [MSP]
Loss of consciousness for more than 24 hours with complete recovery
CC Excl: See code 850.0

850.4 With prolonged loss of consciousness, without return to pre-existing conscious level [CC] [MSP]
CC Excl: See code 850.0

850.5 With loss of consciousness of unspecified duration [CC] [MSP]
CC Excl: See code 850.0

850.9 Concussion, unspecified [CC] [MSP]
CC Excl: See code 850.0

√4ᵗʰ 851 Cerebral laceration and contusion
AHA: 4Q, '96, 36; 1Q, '93, 22; 4Q, '90, 24

§ √5ᵗʰ 851.0 Cortex (cerebral) contusion without mention of open intracranial wound [CC] [MSP]
CC Excl: See code 850.0

§ √5ᵗʰ 851.1 Cortex (cerebral) contusion with open intracranial wound [CC] [MSP]
CC Excl: See code 850.0
AHA: 1Q, '92, 9

§ √5ᵗʰ 851.2 Cortex (cerebral) laceration without mention of open intracranial wound [CC] [MSP]
CC Excl: See code 850.0

§ √5ᵗʰ 851.3 Cortex (cerebral) laceration with open intracranial wound [CC] [MSP]
CC Excl: See code 850.0

§ √5ᵗʰ 851.4 Cerebellar or brain stem contusion without mention of open intracranial wound [CC] [MSP]
CC Excl: See code 850.0

§ √5ᵗʰ 851.5 Cerebellar or brain stem contusion with open intracranial wound [CC] [MSP]
CC Excl: See code 850.0

§ √5ᵗʰ 851.6 Cerebellar or brain stem laceration without mention of open intracranial wound [CC] [MSP]
CC Excl: See code 850.0

§ √5ᵗʰ 851.7 Cerebellar or brain stem laceration with open intracranial wound [CC] [MSP]
CC Excl: See code 850.0

---

§ Requires fifth-digit. See beginning of section 850-854 for codes and definitions.

[N] Newborn Age: 0   [P] Pediatric Age: 0-17   [M] Maternity Age: 12-55   [A] Adult Age: 15-124   [CC] CC Condition   [MC] Major Complication   [CD] Complex Dx   [HIV] HIV Related Dx

INJURY AND POISONING

851.8 Other and unspecified cerebral laceration and contusion, without mention of open intracranial wound
Brain (membrane) NOS
CC Excl: See code 850.0

AHA: 4Q, '96, 37

851.9 Other and unspecified cerebral laceration and contusion, with open intracranial wound
CC Excl: See code 850.0

852 Subarachnoid, subdural, and extradural hemorrhage, following injury
EXCLUDES Cerebral contusion or laceration (with hemorrhage) (851.0-851.9)

DEF: Bleeding from lining of brain; due to injury.

852.0 Subarachnoid hemorrhage following injury without mention of open intracranial wound
Middle meningeal hemorrhage following injury
CC Excl: See code 850.0

852.1 Subarachnoid hemorrhage following injury with open intracranial wound
CC Excl: See code 850.0

852.2 Subdural hemorrhage following injury without mention of open intracranial wound
CC Excl: For code 852.20: 800.00-800.99, 801.00-801.99, 803.00-803.99, 804.00-804.99, 850.0-850.9, 851.00-851.99, 852.00-852.59, 853.00-853.19, 854.00-854.19, 873.8-873.9, 879.8-879.9, 905.0, 925.1-925.2, 929.0, 929.9, 958.8, 959.01, 959.09, 959.8-959.9 For code 852.21: 800.00-800.99, 801.00-801.99, 803.00-803.99, 804.00-804.99, 850.0-850.9, 851.00-851.99, 852.00-852.19, 852.21-852.59, 853.00-853.19, 854.00-854.19, 873.8-873.9, 879.8-879.9, 905.0, 925.1-925.2, 929.0, 929.9, 958.8, 959.01, 959.09, 959.8-959.9 For codes 852.22-852.29: See code 852.21

AHA: 4Q, '96, 43

852.3 Subdural hemorrhage following injury with open intracranial wound
CC Excl: See code 852.21

852.4 Extradural hemorrhage following injury without mention of open intracranial wound
Epidural hematoma following injury
CC Excl: See code 852.21

852.5 Extradural hemorrhage following injury with open intracranial wound
CC Excl: See code 852.21

853 Other and unspecified intracranial hemorrhage following injury

853.0 Without mention of open intracranial wound
Cerebral compression due to injury
Intracranial hematoma following injury
Traumatic cerebral hemorrhage
CC Excl: See code 852.21

AHA: 3Q, '90, 14

853.1 With open intracranial wound
CC Excl: See code 852.21

854 Intracranial injury of other and unspecified nature
INCLUDES brain injury NOS
cavernous sinus
intracranial injury
EXCLUDES any condition classifiable to 850-853
head injury NOS (959.01)

AHA: 1Q, '99, 10; 2Q, '92, 6

854.0 Without mention of open intracranial wound
CC Excl: See code 852.21

854.1 With open intracranial wound
CC Excl: See code 852.21

§ Requires fifth-digit. See beginning of section 850-854 for codes and definitions.

INTERNAL INJURY OF THORAX, ABDOMEN, AND PELVIS (860-869)
INCLUDES blast injuries
blunt trauma
bruise
concussion injuries (except cerebral)
crushing
hematoma
laceration
puncture
tear
traumatic rupture
} of internal organs

EXCLUDES concussion NOS (850.0-850.9)
flail chest (807.4)
foreign body entering through orifice (930.0-939.9)
injury to blood vessels (901.0-902.9)

The description "with open wound," used in the fourth-digit subdivisions, includes those with mention of infection or foreign body.

860 Traumatic pneumothorax and hemothorax
AHA: 2Q, '93, 4

DEF: Traumatic pneumothorax: air or gas leaking into pleural space of lung due to trauma.

DEF: Traumatic hemothorax: blood buildup in pleural space of lung due to trauma.

860.0 Pneumothorax without mention of open wound into thorax
CC Excl: 860.0-860.5, 861.20-861.32, 862.29, 862.39, 862.8-862.9, 875.0-875.1, 879.8-879.9, 929.0, 929.9, 958.7-958.8, 959.8-959.9

860.1 Pneumothorax with open wound into thorax
CC Excl: See code 860.0

860.2 Hemothorax without mention of open wound into thorax
CC Excl: See code 860.0

860.3 Hemothorax with open wound into thorax
CC Excl: See code 860.0

860.4 Pneumohemothorax without mention of open wound into thorax
CC Excl: See code 860.0

860.5 Pneumohemothorax with open wound into thorax
CC Excl: See code 860.0

861 Injury to heart and lung
EXCLUDES injury to blood vessels of thorax (901.0-901.9)

861.0 Heart, without mention of open wound into thorax
AHA: 1Q, '92, 9

861.00 Unspecified injury

861.01 Contusion
Cardiac contusion   Myocardial contusion
CC Excl: 861.00-861.13, 862.29, 862.39, 862.8-862.9, 875.0-875.1, 879.8-879.9, 929.0, 929.9, 958.7-958.8, 959.8-959.9

DEF: Bruising within the pericardium with no mention of open wound.

861.02 Laceration without penetration of heart chambers
CC Excl: See code 861.01

DEF: Tearing injury of heart tissue, without penetration of chambers; no open wound.

861.03 Laceration with penetration of heart chambers
CC Excl: See code 861.01

861.1–863.59 INJURY AND POISONING Tabular List

√5th **861.1 Heart, with open wound into thorax**
  861.10 Unspecified injury `CC` `MSP`
    CC Excl: See code 861.01
  861.11 Contusion `CC` `MSP`
    CC Excl: See code 861.01
  861.12 Laceration without penetration of heart chambers `CC` `MSP`
    CC Excl: See code 861.01
  861.13 Laceration with penetration of heart chambers `CC` `MSP`
    CC Excl: See code 861.01

√5th **861.2 Lung, without mention of open wound into thorax**
  861.20 Unspecified injury `MSP`
  861.21 Contusion `MSP`
    DEF: Bruising of lung without mention of open wound.
  861.22 Laceration `CC` `MSP`
    CC Excl: 861.20-861.32, 862.29, 862.39, 862.8-862.9, 875.0-875.1, 879.8-879.9, 929.0, 929.9, 958.7-958.8, 959.8-959.9

√5th **861.3 Lung, with open wound into thorax**
  861.30 Unspecified injury `CC` `MSP`
    CC Excl: See code 861.22
  861.31 Contusion `CC` `MSP`
    CC Excl: See code 861.22
  861.32 Laceration `CC` `MSP`
    CC Excl: See code 861.22

√4th **862 Injury to other and unspecified intrathoracic organs**
  EXCLUDES: injury to blood vessels of thorax (901.0-901.9)
  862.0 Diaphragm, without mention of open wound into cavity
  862.1 Diaphragm, with open wound into cavity `CC`
    CC Excl: 862.0-862.1, 862.29, 862.39, 862.8-862.9, 875.0-875.1, 879.8-879.9, 929.0, 929.9, 958.7-958.8, 959.8-959.9

√5th **862.2 Other specified intrathoracic organs, without mention of open wound into cavity**
  862.21 Bronchus `CC`
    CC Excl: 862.21, 862.29, 862.31, 862.39, 862.8-862.9, 875.0-875.1, 879.8-879.9, 929.0, 929.9, 958.7-958.8, 959.8-959.9
  862.22 Esophagus `CC`
    CC Excl: 862.22, 862.29, 862.32, 862.39, 862.8-862.9, 875.0-875.1, 879.8-879.9, 929.0, 929.9, 958.7-958.8, 959.8-959.9
  862.29 Other `CC`
    Pleura
    Thymus gland
    CC Excl: 862.29, 862.39, 862.8-862.9, 875.0-875.1, 879.8-879.9, 929.0, 929.9, 958.7-958.8, 959.8-959.9

√5th **862.3 Other specified intrathoracic organs, with open wound into cavity**
  862.31 Bronchus `CC`
    CC Excl: 862.21, 862.29, 862.31, 862.39, 862.8-862.9, 875.0-875.1, 879.8-879.9, 929.0, 929.9, 958.7-958.8, 959.8-959.9
  862.32 Esophagus `CC`
    CC Excl: 862.22, 862.29, 862.32, 862.39, 862.8-862.9, 875.0-875.1, 879.8-879.9, 929.0, 929.9, 958.7-958.8, 959.8-959.9
  862.39 Other `CC`
    CC Excl: 862.29, 862.39, 862.8-862.9, 875.0-875.1, 879.8-879.9, 929.0, 929.9, 958.7-958.8, 959.8-959.9

862.8 Multiple and unspecified intrathoracic organs, without mention of open wound into cavity `MSP`
  Crushed chest
  Multiple intrathoracic organs

862.9 Multiple and unspecified intrathoracic organs, with open wound into cavity `CC`
  CC Excl: See code 862.39

√4th **863 Injury to gastrointestinal tract**
  EXCLUDES: anal sphincter laceration during delivery (664.2)
    bile duct (868.0-868.1 with fifth-digit 2)
    gallbladder (868.0-868.1 with fifth-digit 2)
  863.0 Stomach, without mention of open wound into cavity `MSP`
  863.1 Stomach, with open wound into cavity `CC` `MSP`
    CC Excl: 863.0-863.1, 863.80, 863.89-863.90, 863.99, 868.00, 868.03-868.10, 868.13-868.19, 869.0-869.1, 879.2-879.9, 929.0, 929.9, 958.8, 959.8-959.9

√5th **863.2 Small intestine, without mention of open wound into cavity**
  863.20 Small intestine, unspecified site
  863.21 Duodenum
  863.29 Other

√5th **863.3 Small intestine, with open wound into cavity**
  863.30 Small intestine, unspecified site `CC` `MSP`
    CC Excl: 863.20-863.39, 863.80, 863.89-863.90, 863.99, 868.00, 868.03-868.10, 868.13-868.19, 869.0-869.1, 879.2-879.9, 929.0, 929.9, 958.8, 959.8-959.9
  863.31 Duodenum `CC` `MSP`
    CC Excl: 863.21, 863.31, 863.39, 863.80, 863.89-863.90, 863.99, 868.00, 868.03-868.10, 868.13-868.19, 869.0-869.1, 879.2-879.9, 929.0, 929.9, 958.8, 959.8-959.9
  863.39 Other `CC` `MSP`
    CC Excl: 863.20-863.39, 863.80, 863.89-863.90, 863.99, 868.00, 868.03-868.10, 868.13-868.19, 869.0-869.1, 879.2-879.9, 929.0, 929.9, 958.8, 959.8-959.9

√5th **863.4 Colon or rectum, without mention of open wound into cavity**
  863.40 Colon, unspecified site
  863.41 Ascending [right] colon
  863.42 Transverse colon
  863.43 Descending [left] colon
  863.44 Sigmoid colon
  863.45 Rectum
  863.46 Multiple sites in colon and rectum
  863.49 Other

√5th **863.5 Colon or rectum, with open wound into cavity**
  863.50 Colon, unspecified site `CC` `MSP`
    CC Excl: 863.40-863.59, 863.80, 863.89-863.90, 863.99, 868.00, 868.03-868.10, 868.13-868.19, 869.0-869.1, 879.2-879.9, 929.0, 929.9, 958.8, 959.8-959.9
  863.51 Ascending [right] colon `CC` `MSP`
    CC Excl: See code 863.50
  863.52 Transverse colon `CC` `MSP`
    CC Excl: See code 863.50
  863.53 Descending [left] colon `CC` `MSP`
    CC Excl: See code 863.50
  863.54 Sigmoid colon `CC` `MSP`
    CC Excl: See code 863.50
  863.55 Rectum `CC` `MSP`
    CC Excl: See code 863.50
  863.56 Multiple sites in colon and rectum `CC` `MSP`
    CC Excl: See code 863.50
  863.59 Other `CC` `MSP`
    CC Excl: See code 863.50

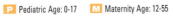

N Newborn Age: 0   **P** Pediatric Age: 0-17   **M** Maternity Age: 12-55   **A** Adult Age: 15-124   **CC** CC Condition   **MC** Major Complication   **CD** Complex Dx   **HIV** HIV Related Dx

| **Tabular List** | **INJURY AND POISONING** | **863.8–867.8** |

✓5ᵗʰ 863.8 Other and unspecified gastrointestinal sites, without mention of open wound into cavity
- 863.80 Gastrointestinal tract, unspecified site [MSP]
- 863.81 Pancreas, head [MSP]
- 863.82 Pancreas, body [MSP]
- 863.83 Pancreas, tail [MSP]
- 863.84 Pancreas, multiple and unspecified sites [MSP]
- 863.85 Appendix [MSP]
- 863.89 Other [MSP]
  - Intestine NOS

✓5ᵗʰ 863.9 Other and unspecified gastrointestinal sites, with open wound into cavity
- 863.90 Gastrointestinal tract, unspecified site [CC][MSP]
  - CC Excl: 863.80-863.84, 863.89-863.94, 863.99, 868.00, 868.03-868.10, 868.13-868.19, 869.0-869.1, 879.2-879.9, 929.0, 929.9, 958.8, 959.8-959.9
- 863.91 Pancreas, head [CC][MSP]
  - CC Excl: 863.80-863.84, 863.91-863.94, 863.99, 868.00, 868.03-868.10, 868.13-868.19, 869.0-869.1, 879.2-879.9, 929.0, 929.9, 958.8, 959.8-959.9
- 863.92 Pancreas, body [CC][MSP]
  - CC Excl: See code 863.91
- 863.93 Pancreas, tail [CC][MSP]
  - CC Excl: See code 863.91
- 863.94 Pancreas, multiple and unspecified sites [CC][MSP]
  - CC Excl: See code 863.91
- 863.95 Appendix [CC][MSP]
  - CC Excl: 863.80, 863.85, 863.95, 863.99, 868.00, 868.03-868.10, 868.13-868.19, 869.0-869.1, 879.2-879.9, 929.0, 929.9, 958.8, 959.8-959.9
- 863.99 Other [CC][MSP]
  - CC Excl: 863.80, 863.99, 868.00, 868.03-868.10, 868.13-868.19, 869.0-869.1, 879.2-879.9, 929.0, 929.9, 958.8, 959.8-959.9

✓4ᵗʰ 864 Injury to liver

The following fifth-digit subclassification is for use with category 864:
- 0 unspecified injury
- 1 hematoma and contusion
- 2 laceration, minor
  - Laceration involving capsule only, or without significant involvement of hepatic parenchyma [i.e., less than 1 cm deep]
- 3 laceration, moderate
  - Laceration involving parenchyma but without major disruption of parenchyma [i.e., less than 10 cm long and less than 3 cm deep]
- 4 laceration, major
  - Laceration with significant disruption of hepatic parenchyma [i.e., 10 cm long and 3 cm deep]
  - Multiple moderate lacerations, with or without hematoma
  - Stellate lacerations of liver
- 5 laceration, unspecified
- 9 other

✓5ᵗʰ 864.0 Without mention of open wound into cavity [CC][MSP]
- CC Excl: 863.80, 863.99, 864.00-864.19, 868.00, 868.03-868.10, 868.13-868.19, 869.0-869.1, 879.2-879.9, 929.0, 929.9, 958.8, 959.8-959.9

✓5ᵗʰ 864.1 With open wound into cavity [CC][MSP]
- CC Excl: See code 864.0

✓4ᵗʰ 865 Injury to spleen

The following fifth-digit subclassification is for use with category 865:
- 0 unspecified injury
- 1 hematoma without rupture of capsule
- 2 capsular tears, without major disruption of parenchyma
- 3 laceration extending into parenchyma
- 4 massive parenchymal disruption
- 9 other

✓5ᵗʰ 865.0 Without mention of open wound into cavity [CC][MSP]
- CC Excl: 865.00-865.19, 868.00, 868.03-868.10, 868.13-868.19, 869.0-869.1, 879.2-879.9, 929.0, 929.9, 958.8, 959.8-959.9

✓5ᵗʰ 865.1 With open wound into cavity [CC][MSP]
- CC Excl: See code 865.0

✓4ᵗʰ 866 Injury to kidney

The following fifth-digit subclassification is for use with category 866:
- 0 unspecified injury
- 1 hematoma without rupture of capsule
- 2 laceration
- 3 complete disruption of kidney parenchyma

✓5ᵗʰ 866.0 Without mention of open wound into cavity [CC][MSP]
- CC Excl: 866.00-866.13, 868.00, 868.03-868.10, 868.13-868.19, 869.0-869.1, 879.2-879.9, 929.0, 929.9, 958.8, 959.8-959.9

✓5ᵗʰ 866.1 With open wound into cavity [CC][MSP]
- CC Excl: See code 866.0

✓4ᵗʰ 867 Injury to pelvic organs
- EXCLUDES injury during delivery (664.0-665.9)

- 867.0 Bladder and urethra, without mention of open wound into cavity [CC][MSP]
  - CC Excl: 867.0-867.1, 867.6-867.9, 868.00, 868.03-868.10, 868.13-868.19, 869.0-869.1, 879.2-879.9, 929.0, 929.9, 958.8, 959.8-959.9
  - AHA: N-D, '85, 15

- 867.1 Bladder and urethra, with open wound into cavity [CC][MSP]
  - CC Excl: See code 867.0

- 867.2 Ureter, without mention of open wound into cavity [CC][MSP]
  - CC Excl: 867.2-867.3, 867.6-867.9, 868.00, 868.03-868.10, 868.13-868.19, 869.0-869.1, 879.2-879.9, 929.0, 929.9, 958.8, 959.8-959.9

- 867.3 Ureter, with open wound into cavity [CC][MSP]
  - CC Excl: See code 867.2

- 867.4 Uterus, without mention of open wound intocavity [CC][MSP][♂]
  - CC Excl: 867.4-867.9, 868.00, 868.03-868.10, 868.13-868.19, 869.0-869.1, 879.2-879.9, 929.0, 929.9, 958.8, 959.8-959.9

- 867.5 Uterus, with open wound into cavity [CC][MSP][♂]
  - CC Excl: See code 867.4

- 867.6 Other specified pelvic organs, without mention of open wound into cavity [CC][MSP]
  - Fallopian tube   Seminal vesicle
  - Ovary   Vas deferens
  - Prostate
  - CC Excl: 867.6-867.9, 868.00, 868.03-868.10, 868.13-868.19, 869.0-869.1, 879.2-879.9, 929.0, 929.9, 958.8, 959.8-959.9

- 867.7 Other specified pelvic organs, with open wound into cavity [CC][MSP]
  - CC Excl: See code 867.6

- 867.8 **Unspecified pelvic organ, without mention of open wound into cavity** [CC][MSP]
  - CC Excl: See code 867.6

✓4ᵗʰ Additional Digit Required | Nonspecific PDx | Unacceptable PDx | Manifestation Code | MSP Medicare Secondary Payer | ▶◀ Revised Text | ● New Code | ▲ Revised Code Title

2002 Ingenix, Inc.   Volume 1 — 275

INJURY AND POISONING

867.9 **Unspecified pelvic organ, with open wound into cavity** CC MSP
CC Excl: See code 867.6

✓4th **868 Injury to other intra-abdominal organs**

The following fifth-digit subclassification is for use with category 868:
- 0 unspecified intra-abdominal organ
- 1 adrenal gland
- 2 bile duct and gallbladder
- 3 peritoneum
- 4 retroperitoneum
- 9 other and multiple intra-abdominal organs

✓5th **868.0 Without mention of open wound into cavity** CC MSP
CC Excl: For code 868.00: 868.00, 868.03-868.10, 868.13-868.19, 869.0-869.1, 879.2-879.9, 929.0, 929.9, 958.8, 959.8-959.9 For code 868.01: 868.00, 868.01, 868.03-868.11, 868.13-868.19, 869.0-869.1, 879.2-879.9, 929.0, 929.9, 958.8, 959.8-959.9 For code 868.02: 868.00, 868.02-868.10, 868.13-868.19, 869.0-869.1, 879.2-879.9, 929.0, 929.9, 958.8, 959.8-959.9 For codes 868.03-868.09: 868.00, 868.03-868.10, 868.13-868.19, 869.0-869.1, 879.2-879.9, 929.0, 929.9, 958.8, 959.8-959.9

✓5th **868.1 With open wound into cavity** CC MSP
CC Excl: For code 868.10: See code 868.03 For code 868.11: 868.00, 868.01, 868.03-868.11, 868.13-868.19, 869.0-869.1, 879.2-879.9, 929.0, 929.9, 958.8, 959.8-959.9 For code 868.12: 868.00, 868.03-868.10, 868.12-868.19, 869.0-869.1, 879.2-879.9, 929.0, 929.9, 958.8, 959.8-959.9 For codes 868.13-868.19: 868.00, 868.03-868.10, 868.13-868.19, 869.0-869.1, 879.2-879.9, 929.0, 929.9, 958.8, 959.8-959.9

✓4th **869 Internal injury to unspecified or ill-defined organs**
INCLUDES: internal injury NOS
multiple internal injury NOS

869.0 Without mention of open wound into cavity CC MSP
CC Excl: See code 868.13

869.1 With open wound into cavity CC MSP
CC Excl: See code 868.13
AHA: 2Q, '89, 15

OPEN WOUND (870-897)

INCLUDES:
- animal bite
- avulsion
- cut
- laceration
- puncture wound
- traumatic amputation

EXCLUDES:
- burn (940.0-949.5)
- crushing (925-929.9)
- puncture of internal organs (860.0-869.1)
- superficial injury (910.0-919.9)
- that incidental to:
  - dislocation (830.0-839.9)
  - fracture (800.0-829.1)
  - internal injury (860.0-869.1)
  - intracranial injury (851.0-854.1)

Note: The description "complicated" used in the fourth-digit subdivisions includes those with mention of delayed healing, delayed treatment, foreign body, or infection. Use additional code to identify infection
AHA: ▶4Q, '01, 52◀

OPEN WOUND OF HEAD, NECK, AND TRUNK (870-879)

✓4th **870 Open wound of ocular adnexa**
- **870.0** Laceration of skin of eyelid and periocular area
- **870.1** Laceration of eyelid, full-thickness, not involving lacrimal passages
- **870.2** Laceration of eyelid involving lacrimal passages
- **870.3** Penetrating wound of orbit, without mention of foreign body CC
CC Excl: 870.0-870.9, 871.0-871.9, 879.8-879.9, 929.0, 929.9, 958.8, 959.8-959.9

- **870.4** Penetrating wound of orbit with foreign body CC
EXCLUDES: retained (old) foreign body in orbit (376.6)
CC Excl: See code 870.3

- **870.8** Other specified open wounds of ocular adnexa CC
CC Excl: See code 870.3

- **870.9** Unspecified open wound of ocular adnexa CC
CC Excl: See code 870.3

✓4th **871 Open wound of eyeball**
EXCLUDES: 2nd cranial nerve [optic] injury (950.0-950.9)
3rd cranial nerve [oculomotor] injury (951.0)

- **871.0** Ocular laceration without prolapse of intraocular tissue CC
CC Excl: See code 870.3
AHA: 3Q, '96, 7
DEF: Tear in ocular tissue without displacing structures.

- **871.1** Ocular laceration with prolapse or exposure of intraocular tissue CC
CC Excl: See code 870.3

- **871.2** Rupture of eye with partial loss of intraocular tissue CC
CC Excl: See code 870.3
DEF: Forcible tearing of eyeball, with tissue loss.

- **871.3** Avulsion of eye CC
Traumatic enucleation
CC Excl: See code 870.3
DEF: Traumatic extraction of eyeball from socket.

- **871.4** Unspecified laceration of eye CC
CC Excl: See code 870.3

- **871.5** Penetration of eyeball with magnetic foreign body
EXCLUDES: retained (old) magnetic foreign body in globe (360.50-360.59)

- **871.6** Penetration of eyeball with (nonmagnetic) foreign body
EXCLUDES: retained (old) (nonmagnetic) foreign body in globe (360.60-360.69)

- **871.7** Unspecified ocular penetration
- **871.9** Unspecified open wound of eyeball CC
CC Excl: See code 870.3

✓4th **872 Open wound of ear**
✓5th **872.0 External ear, without mention of complication**
- **872.00** External ear, unspecified site
- **872.01** Auricle, ear
Pinna
DEF: Open wound of fleshy, outer ear.

- **872.02** Auditory canal
DEF: Open wound of passage from external ear to eardrum.

✓5th **872.1 External ear, complicated**
- **872.10** External ear, unspecified site
- **872.11** Auricle, ear
- **872.12** Auditory canal

✓5th **872.6 Other specified parts of ear, without mention of complication**
- **872.61** Ear drum
Drumhead   Tympanic membrane
- **872.62** Ossicles
- **872.63** Eustachian tube
DEF: Open wound of channel between nasopharynx and tympanic cavity.

Tabular List — INJURY AND POISONING — 872.64–876.1

- **872.64 Cochlea**
  DEF: Open wound of snail shell shaped tube of inner ear.
- **872.69 Other and multiple sites**
- √5th **872.7 Other specified parts of ear, complicated**
  - **872.71 Ear drum**
  - **872.72 Ossicles** [CC]
    CC Excl: 872.00-872.9, 879.8-879.9, 929.0, 929.9, 958.8, 959.8-959.9
  - **872.73 Eustachian tube** [CC]
    CC Excl: See code 872.72
  - **872.74 Cochlea** [CC]
    CC Excl: See code 872.72
  - **872.79 Other and multiple sites**
- **872.8 Ear, part unspecified, without mention of complication**
  Ear NOS
- **872.9 Ear, part unspecified, complicated**

√4th **873 Other open wound of head**
- **873.0 Scalp, without mention of complication**
- **873.1 Scalp, complicated**
- √5th **873.2 Nose, without mention of complication**
  - **873.20 Nose, unspecified site**
  - **873.21 Nasal septum**
    DEF: Open wound between nasal passages.
  - **873.22 Nasal cavity**
    DEF: Open wound of nostrils.
  - **873.23 Nasal sinus**
    DEF: Open wound of mucous-lined respiratory cavities.
  - **873.29 Multiple sites**
- √5th **873.3 Nose, complicated**
  - **873.30 Nose, unspecified site**
  - **873.31 Nasal septum**
  - **873.32 Nasal cavity**
  - **873.33 Nasal sinus** [CC]
    CC Excl: 873.20-873.39, 879.8-879.9, 929.0, 929.9, 958.8, 959.8-959.9
  - **873.39 Multiple sites**
- √5th **873.4 Face, without mention of complication**
  - **873.40 Face, unspecified site**
  - **873.41 Cheek**
  - **873.42 Forehead**
    Eyebrow
    AHA: 4Q, '96, 43
  - **873.43 Lip**
  - **873.44 Jaw**
  - **873.49 Other and multiple sites**
- √5th **873.5 Face, complicated**
  - **873.50 Face, unspecified site**
  - **873.51 Cheek**
  - **873.52 Forehead**
  - **873.53 Lip**
  - **873.54 Jaw**
  - **873.59 Other and multiple sites**
- √5th **873.6 Internal structures of mouth, without mention of complication**
  - **873.60 Mouth, unspecified site**
  - **873.61 Buccal mucosa**
    DEF: Open wound of inside of cheek.
  - **873.62 Gum (alveolar process)**
  - **873.63 Tooth (broken)**
  - **873.64 Tongue and floor of mouth**
  - **873.65 Palate**
    DEF: Open wound of roof of mouth.
  - **873.69 Other and multiple sites**
- √5th **873.7 Internal structures of mouth, complicated**
  - **873.70 Mouth, unspecified site**
  - **873.71 Buccal mucosa**
  - **873.72 Gum (alveolar process)**
  - **873.73 Tooth (broken)**
  - **873.74 Tongue and floor of mouth**
  - **873.75 Palate**
  - **873.79 Other and multiple sites**
- **873.8 Other and unspecified open wound of head without mention of complication**
  Head NOS
- **873.9 Other and unspecified open wound of head, complicated** [CC]
  CC Excl: 847.0, 873.40-873.79, 873.9, 874.8-874.9, 879.8-879.9, 929.0, 929.9, 958.8, 959.8-959.9

√4th **874 Open wound of neck**
- √5th **874.0 Larynx and trachea, without mention of complication**
  - **874.00 Larynx with trachea** [CC]
    CC Excl: 847.0, 874.00-874.12, 874.8-874.9, 879.8-879.9, 929.0, 929.9, 958.8, 959.8-959.9
  - **874.01 Larynx** [CC]
    CC Excl: See code 874.00
  - **874.02 Trachea** [CC]
    CC Excl: See code 874.00
- √5th **874.1 Larynx and trachea, complicated**
  - **874.10 Larynx with trachea** [CC]
    CC Excl: See code 874.00
  - **874.11 Larynx** [CC]
    CC Excl: See code 874.00
  - **874.12 Trachea** [CC]
    CC Excl: See code 874.00
- **874.2 Thyroid gland, without mention of complication**
- **874.3 Thyroid gland, complicated** [CC]
  CC Excl: 847.0, 874.2-874.3, 874.8-874.9, 879.8-879.9, 929.0, 929.9, 958.8, 959.8-959.9
- **874.4 Pharynx, without mention of complication**
  Cervical esophagus
- **874.5 Pharynx, complicated** [CC]
  CC Excl: 847.0, 874.4-874.9, 879.8-879.9, 929.0, 929.9, 958.8, 959.8-959.9
- **874.8 Other and unspecified parts, without mention of complication**
  Nape of neck Throat NOS
  Supraclavicular region
- **874.9 Other and unspecified parts, complicated**

√4th **875 Open wound of chest (wall)**
  EXCLUDES open wound into thoracic cavity (860.0-862.9)
  traumatic pneumothorax and hemothorax (860.1, 860.3, 860.5)
  AHA: 3Q, '93, 17
- **875.0 Without mention of complication** [CC]
  CC Excl: 847.1, 862.29, 862.39, 862.8-862.9, 875.0-875.1, 879.8-879.9, 929.0, 929.9, 958.7-958.8, 959.8-959.9
- **875.1 Complicated** [CC]
  CC Excl: See code 875.0

√4th **876 Open wound of back**
  INCLUDES loin
  lumbar region
  EXCLUDES open wound into thoracic cavity (860.0-862.9)
  traumatic pneumothorax and hemothorax (860.1, 860.3, 860.5)
- **876.0 Without mention of complication**
- **876.1 Complicated**

INJURY AND POISONING

877 Open wound of buttock
INCLUDES sacroiliac region
- 877.0 Without mention of complication
- 877.1 Complicated

878 Open wound of genital organs (external), including traumatic amputation
EXCLUDES injury during delivery (664.0-665.9)
internal genital organs (867.0-867.9)
- 878.0 Penis, without mention of complication ♂
- 878.1 Penis, complicated ♂
- 878.2 Scrotum and testes, without mention of complication ♂
- 878.3 Scrotum and testes, complicated ♂
- 878.4 Vulva, without mention of complication ♀
  Labium (majus) (minus)
- 878.5 Vulva, complicated ♀
- 878.6 Vagina, without mention of complication ♀
- 878.7 Vagina, complicated ♀
- 878.8 Other and unspecified parts, without mention of complication
- 878.9 Other and unspecified parts, complicated

879 Open wound of other and unspecified sites, except limbs
- 879.0 Breast, without mention of complication
- 879.1 Breast, complicated
- 879.2 Abdominal wall, anterior, without mention of complication
  Abdominal wall NOS   Pubic region
  Epigastric region   Umbilical region
  Hypogastric region
  AHA: 2Q, '91, 22
- 879.3 Abdominal wall, anterior, complicated
- 879.4 Abdominal wall, lateral, without mention of complication
  Flank   Iliac (region)
  Groin   Inguinal region
  Hypochondrium
- 879.5 Abdominal wall, lateral, complicated
- 879.6 Other and unspecified parts of trunk, without mention of complication
  Pelvic region   Trunk NOS
  Perineum
- 879.7 Other and unspecified parts of trunk, complicated
- 879.8 Open wound(s) (multiple) of unspecified site(s) without mention of complication
  Multiple open wounds NOS   Open wound NOS
- 879.9 Open wound(s) (multiple) of unspecified site(s), complicated

OPEN WOUND OF UPPER LIMB (880-887)
AHA: N-D, '85, 5

880 Open wound of shoulder and upper arm
The following fifth-digit subclassification is for use with category 880:
0 shoulder region
1 scapular region
2 axillary region
3 upper arm
9 multiple sites

- 880.0 Without mention of complication
- 880.1 Complicated
- 880.2 With tendon involvement

881 Open wound of elbow, forearm, and wrist
The following fifth-digit subclassification is for use with category 881:
0 forearm
1 elbow
2 wrist

- 881.0 Without mention of complication
- 881.1 Complicated
- 881.2 With tendon involvement

882 Open wound of hand except finger(s) alone
- 882.0 Without mention of complication
- 882.1 Complicated
- 882.2 With tendon involvement

883 Open wound of finger(s)
INCLUDES fingernail
thumb (nail)
- 883.0 Without mention of complication
- 883.1 Complicated
- 883.2 With tendon involvement

884 Multiple and unspecified open wound of upper limb
INCLUDES arm NOS
multiple sites of one upper limb
upper limb NOS
- 884.0 Without mention of complication
- 884.1 Complicated
- 884.2 With tendon involvement

885 Traumatic amputation of thumb (complete) (partial)
INCLUDES thumb(s) (with finger(s) of either hand)
- 885.0 Without mention of complication
- 885.1 Complicated

886 Traumatic amputation of other finger(s) (complete) (partial)
INCLUDES finger(s) of one or both hands, without mention of thumb(s)
- 886.0 Without mention of complication
- 886.1 Complicated

887 Traumatic amputation of arm and hand (complete) (partial)
- 887.0 Unilateral, below elbow, without mention of complication [CC] [MSP]
  CC Excl: 880.00-880.29, 881.00-881.22, 882.0-882.2, 883.0-883.2, 884.0-884.2, 885.0-885.1, 886.0-886.1, 887.0-887.7, 929.0, 929.9, 958.8, 959.8-959.9
- 887.1 Unilateral, below elbow, complicated [CC] [MSP]
  CC Excl: See code 887.0
- 887.2 Unilateral, at or above elbow, without mention of complication [CC] [MSP]
  CC Excl: See code 887.0
- 887.3 Unilateral, at or above elbow, complicated [CC] [MSP]
  CC Excl: See code 887.0
- 887.4 Unilateral, level not specified, without mention of complication [CC] [MSP]
  CC Excl: See code 887.0
- 887.5 Unilateral, level not specified, complicated [CC] [MSP]
  CC Excl: See code 887.0
- 887.6 Bilateral [any level], without mention of complication [CC] [MSP]
  One hand and other arm
  CC Excl: See code 887.0
- 887.7 Bilateral [any level], complicated [CC] [MSP]
  CC Excl: See code 887.0

OPEN WOUND OF LOWER LIMB (890-897)
AHA: N-D, '85, 5

890 Open wound of hip and thigh
- 890.0 Without mention of complication
- 890.1 Complicated
- 890.2 With tendon involvement

Tabular List — INJURY AND POISONING

√4ᵗʰ 891 Open wound of knee, leg [except thigh], and ankle
  INCLUDES: leg NOS
    multiple sites of leg, except thigh
  EXCLUDES: that of thigh (890.0-890.2)
    with multiple sites of lower limb (894.0-894.2)
  891.0 Without mention of complication
  891.1 Complicated
  891.2 With tendon involvement

√4ᵗʰ 892 Open wound of foot except toe(s) alone
  INCLUDES: heel
  892.0 Without mention of complication
  892.1 Complicated
  892.2 With tendon involvement

√4ᵗʰ 893 Open wound of toe(s)
  INCLUDES: toenail
  893.0 Without mention of complication
  893.1 Complicated
  893.2 With tendon involvement

√4ᵗʰ 894 Multiple and unspecified open wound of lower limb
  INCLUDES: lower limb NOS
    multiple sites of one lower limb, with thigh
  894.0 Without mention of complication
  894.1 Complicated
  894.2 With tendon involvement

√4ᵗʰ 895 Traumatic amputation of toe(s) (complete) (partial)
  INCLUDES: toe(s) of one or both feet
  895.0 Without mention of complication
  895.1 Complicated

√4ᵗʰ 896 Traumatic amputation of foot (complete) (partial)
  896.0 Unilateral, without mention of complication [CC] [MSP]
    CC Excl: 890.0-890.2, 891.0-891.2, 892.0-892.2, 893.0-893.2, 894.0-894.2, 895.0-895.1, 896.0-896.3, 897.0-897.7, 929.0, 929.9, 958.8, 959.8-959.9
  896.1 Unilateral, complicated [CC] [MSP]
    CC Excl: See code 896.0
  896.2 Bilateral, without mention of complication [CC] [MSP]
    EXCLUDES: one foot and other leg (897.6-897.7)
    CC Excl: See code 896.0
  896.3 Bilateral, complicated [CC] [MSP]
    CC Excl: See code 896.0

√4ᵗʰ 897 Traumatic amputation of leg(s) (complete) (partial)
  897.0 Unilateral, below knee, without mention of complication [CC] [MSP]
    CC Excl: See code 896.0
  897.1 Unilateral, below knee, complicated [CC] [MSP]
    CC Excl: See code 896.0
  897.2 Unilateral, at or above knee, without mention of complication [CC] [MSP]
    CC Excl: See code 896.0
  897.3 Unilateral, at or above knee, complicated [CC] [MSP]
    CC Excl: See code 896.0
  897.4 Unilateral, level not specified, without mention of complication [CC] [MSP]
    CC Excl: See code 896.0
  897.5 Unilateral, level not specified, complicated [CC] [MSP]
    CC Excl: See code 896.0
  897.6 Bilateral [any level], without mention of complication [CC] [MSP]
    One foot and other leg
    CC Excl: See code 896.0
  897.7 Bilateral [any level], complicated [CC] [MSP]
    CC Excl: See code 896.0

  AHA: 3Q, '90, 5

INJURY TO BLOOD VESSELS (900-904)

INCLUDES: arterial hematoma
  avulsion
  cut
  laceration
  rupture
  traumatic aneurysm or fistula (arteriovenous)
  } of blood vessel, secondary to other injuries e.g., fracture or open wound

EXCLUDES: accidental puncture or laceration during medical procedure (998.2)
  intracranial hemorrhage following injury (851.0-854.1)

AHA: 3Q, '90, 5

√4ᵗʰ 900 Injury to blood vessels of head and neck
  √5ᵗʰ 900.0 Carotid artery
    900.00 Carotid artery, unspecified [CC] [MSP]
      CC Excl: 900.00, 900.82, 900.89, 900.9, 904.9, 929.0, 929.9, 958.8, 959.8-959.9
    900.01 Common carotid artery [CC] [MSP]
      CC Excl: See code 900.00
    900.02 External carotid artery [CC] [MSP]
      CC Excl: See code 900.00
    900.03 Internal carotid artery [CC] [MSP]
      CC Excl: See code 900.00
  900.1 Internal jugular vein [CC] [MSP]
    CC Excl: 900.82, 900.89, 900.9, 904.9, 929.0, 929.9, 958.8, 959.8-959.9
  √5ᵗʰ 900.8 Other specified blood vessels of head and neck
    900.81 External jugular vein [CC] [MSP]
      Jugular vein NOS
      CC Excl: See code 900.1
    900.82 Multiple blood vessels of head and neck [CC] [MSP]
      CC Excl: See code 900.1
    900.89 Other [CC] [MSP]
      CC Excl: See code 900.1
  900.9 **Unspecified blood vessel of head and neck** [CC] [MSP]
    CC Excl: See code 900.1

√4ᵗʰ 901 Injury to blood vessels of thorax
  EXCLUDES: traumatic hemothorax (860.2-860.5)
  901.0 Thoracic aorta [CC]
    CC Excl: 901.0, 904.9, 929.0, 929.9, 958.8, 959.8-959.9
  901.1 Innominate and subclavian arteries [CC]
    CC Excl: 901.1, 904.9, 929.0, 929.9, 958.8, 959.8-959.9
  901.2 Superior vena cava [CC]
    CC Excl: 901.2, 904.9, 929.0, 929.9, 958.8, 959.8-959.9
  901.3 Innominate and subclavian veins [CC]
    CC Excl: 901.3, 904.9, 929.0, 929.9, 958.8, 959.8-959.9
  √5ᵗʰ 901.4 Pulmonary blood vessels
    901.40 Pulmonary vessel(s), unspecified
    901.41 Pulmonary artery [CC]
      CC Excl: 901.40, 901.41, 904.9, 929.0, 929.9, 958.8, 959.8-959.9
    901.42 Pulmonary vein [CC]
      CC Excl: 901.40, 901.42, 904.9, 929.0, 929.9, 958.8, 959.8-959.9
  √5ᵗʰ 901.8 Other specified blood vessels of thorax
    901.81 Intercostal artery or vein
    901.82 Internal mammary artery or vein
    901.83 Multiple blood vessels of thorax [CC]
      CC Excl: 904.9, 929.0, 929.9, 958.8, 959.8-959.9
    901.89 Other
      Azygos vein
      Hemiazygos vein

901.9–904.1 INJURY AND POISONING

- 901.9 **Unspecified blood vessel of thorax**
- √4th 902 Injury to blood vessels of abdomen and pelvis
  - 902.0 Abdominal aorta [CC]
    - CC Excl: 902.0, 902.87, 902.89, 902.9, 904.9, 929.0, 929.9, 958.8, 959.8-959.9
  - √5th 902.1 Inferior vena cava
    - 902.10 Inferior vena cava, unspecified [CC]
      - CC Excl: 902.10, 902.87, 902.89, 902.9, 904.9, 929.0, 929.9, 958.8, 959.8-959.9
    - 902.11 Hepatic veins [CC]
      - CC Excl: 902.11, 902.87, 902.89, 902.9, 904.9, 929.0, 929.9, 958.8, 959.8-959.9
    - 902.19 Other [CC]
      - CC Excl: 902.19, 902.87, 902.89, 902.9, 904.9, 929.0, 929.9, 958.8, 959.8-959.9
  - √5th 902.2 Celiac and mesenteric arteries
    - 902.20 Celiac and mesenteric arteries, unspecified [CC]
      - CC Excl: 902.20, 902.87, 902.89, 902.9, 904.9, 929.0, 929.9, 958.8, 959.8-959.9
    - 902.21 Gastric artery
    - 902.22 Hepatic artery [CC]
      - CC Excl: 902.22, 902.87, 902.89, 902.9, 904.9, 929.0, 929.9, 958.8, 959.8-959.9
    - 902.23 Splenic artery [CC]
      - CC Excl: 902.23, 902.87, 902.89, 902.9, 904.9, 929.0, 929.9, 958.8, 959.8-959.9
    - 902.24 Other specified branches of celiac axis [CC]
      - CC Excl: 902.24, 902.87, 902.89, 902.9, 904.9, 929.0, 929.9, 958.8, 959.8-959.9
    - 902.25 Superior mesenteric artery (trunk) [CC]
      - CC Excl: 902.25, 902.87, 902.89, 902.9, 904.9, 929.0, 929.9, 958.8, 959.8-959.9
    - 902.26 Primary branches of superior mesenteric artery
      - Ileocolic artery
      - CC Excl: 902.26, 902.87, 902.89, 902.9, 904.9, 929.0, 929.9, 958.8, 959.8-959.9
    - 902.27 Inferior mesenteric artery [CC]
      - CC Excl: 902.7, 902.87, 902.89, 902.9, 904.9, 929.0, 929.9, 958.8, 959.8-959.9
    - 902.29 Other [CC]
      - CC Excl: 902.29, 902.87, 902.89, 902.9, 904.9, 929.0, 929.9, 958.8, 959.8-959.9
  - √5th 902.3 Portal and splenic veins
    - 902.31 Superior mesenteric vein and primary subdivisions [CC]
      - Ileocolic vein
      - CC Excl: 902.31, 902.87, 902.89, 902.9, 904.9, 929.0, 929.9, 958.8, 959.8-959.9
    - 902.32 Inferior mesenteric vein [CC]
      - CC Excl: 902.32, 902.87, 902.89, 902.9, 904.9, 929.0, 929.9, 958.8, 959.8-959.9
    - 902.33 Portal vein [CC]
      - CC Excl: 902.33, 902.87, 902.89, 902.9, 904.9, 929.0, 929.9, 958.8, 959.8-959.9
    - 902.34 Splenic vein [CC]
      - CC Excl: 902.34, 902.87, 902.89, 902.9, 904.9, 929.0, 929.9, 958.8, 959.8-959.9
    - 902.39 Other [CC]
      - Cystic vein   Gastric vein
      - CC Excl: 902.39, 902.87, 902.89, 902.9, 904.9, 929.0, 929.9, 958.8, 959.8-959.9
  - √5th 902.4 Renal blood vessels
    - 902.40 Renal vessel(s), unspecified [CC]
      - CC Excl: 902.40, 902.87, 902.89, 902.9, 904.9, 929.0, 929.9, 958.8, 959.8-959.9
    - 902.41 Renal artery [CC]
      - CC Excl: 902.41, 902.87, 902.89, 902.9, 904.9, 929.0, 929.9, 958.8, 959.8-959.9
    - 902.42 Renal vein [CC]
      - CC Excl: 902.42, 902.87, 902.89, 902.9, 904.9, 929.0, 929.9, 958.8, 959.8-959.9
    - 902.49 Other [CC]
      - Suprarenal arteries
      - CC Excl: 902.49, 902.87, 902.89, 902.9, 904.9, 929.0, 929.9, 958.8, 959.8-959.9
  - √5th 902.5 Iliac blood vessels
    - 902.50 Iliac vessel(s), unspecified [CC]
      - CC Excl: 902.50, 902.53-902.54, 902.59, 902.87, 902.89, 902.9, 904.9, 929.0, 929.9, 958.8, 959.8-959.9
    - 902.51 Hypogastric artery [CC]
      - CC Excl: 902.51, 902.87, 902.89, 902.9, 904.9, 929.0, 929.9, 958.8, 959.8-959.9
    - 902.52 Hypogastric vein [CC]
      - CC Excl: 902.52, 902.87, 902.89, 902.9, 904.9, 929.0, 929.9, 958.8, 959.8-959.9
    - 902.53 Iliac artery [CC]
      - CC Excl: 902.50, 902.53, 902.59, 902.87, 902.89, 902.9, 904.9, 929.0, 929.9, 958.8, 959.8-959.9
    - 902.54 Iliac vein [CC]
      - CC Excl: 902.50, 902.54, 902.59, 902.87, 902.89, 902.9, 904.9, 929.0, 929.9, 958.8, 959.8-959.9
    - 902.55 Uterine artery ♀
    - 902.56 Uterine vein ♀
    - 902.59 Other [CC]
      - CC Excl: 902.50, 902.53-902.54, 902.59, 902.87, 902.89, 902.9, 904.9, 929.0, 929.9, 958.8, 959.8-959.9
  - √5th 902.8 Other specified blood vessels of abdomen and pelvis
    - 902.81 Ovarian artery ♀
    - 902.82 Ovarian vein ♀
    - 902.87 Multiple blood vessels of abdomen and pelvis [CC]
      - CC Excl: 902.87, 902.89, 902.9, 904.9, 929.0, 929.9, 958.8, 959.8-959.9
    - 902.89 Other
  - 902.9 **Unspecified blood vessel of abdomen and pelvis**
- √4th 903 Injury to blood vessels of upper extremity
  - √5th 903.0 Axillary blood vessels
    - 903.00 Axillary vessel(s), unspecified
    - 903.01 Axillary artery
    - 903.02 Axillary vein
  - 903.1 Brachial blood vessels
  - 903.2 Radial blood vessels
  - 903.3 Ulnar blood vessels
  - 903.4 Palmar artery
  - 903.5 Digital blood vessels
  - 903.8 Other specified blood vessels of upper extremity
    - Multiple blood vessels of upper extremity
  - 903.9 **Unspecified blood vessel of upper extremity**
- √4th 904 Injury to blood vessels of lower extremity and unspecified sites
  - 904.0 Common femoral artery [CC]
    - Femoral artery above profunda origin
    - CC Excl: No exclusions
  - 904.1 Superficial femoral artery

INJURY AND POISONING

- **904.2** Femoral veins
- **904.3** Saphenous veins
  - Saphenous vein (greater) (lesser)
- ✓5th **904.4** Popliteal blood vessels
  - **904.40** Popliteal vessel(s), unspecified
  - **904.41** Popliteal artery
  - **904.42** Popliteal vein
- ✓5th **904.5** Tibial blood vessels
  - **904.50** Tibial vessel(s), unspecified
  - **904.51** Anterior tibial artery
  - **904.52** Anterior tibial vein
  - **904.53** Posterior tibial artery
  - **904.54** Posterior tibial vein
- **904.6** Deep plantar blood vessels
- **904.7** Other specified blood vessels of lower extremity
  - Multiple blood vessels of lower extremity
- **904.8** Unspecified blood vessel of lower extremity
- **904.9** Unspecified site
  - Injury to blood vessel NOS

LATE EFFECTS OF INJURIES, POISONINGS, TOXIC EFFECTS, AND OTHER EXTERNAL CAUSES (905-909)

Note: These categories are to be used to indicate conditions classifiable to 800-999 as the cause of late effects, which are themselves classified elsewhere. The "late effects" include those specified as such, or as sequelae, which may occur at any time after the acute injury.

✓4th **905** Late effects of musculoskeletal and connective tissue injuries
  AHA: 1Q, '95, 10; 2Q, '94, 3

- **905.0** Late effect of fracture of skull and face bones
  - Late effect of injury classifiable to 800-804
  - AHA: 3Q, '97, 12
- **905.1** Late effect of fracture of spine and trunk without mention of spinal cord lesion
  - Late effect of injury classifiable to 805, 807-809
- **905.2** Late effect of fracture of upper extremities
  - Late effect of injury classifiable to 810-819
- **905.3** Late effect of fracture of neck of femur
  - Late effect of injury classifiable to 820
- **905.4** Late effect of fracture of lower extremities
  - Late effect of injury classifiable to 821-827
- **905.5** Late effect of fracture of multiple and unspecified bones
  - Late effect of injury classifiable to 828-829
- **905.6** Late effect of dislocation
  - Late effect of injury classifiable to 830-839
- **905.7** Late effect of sprain and strain without mention of tendon injury
  - Late effect of injury classifiable to 840-848, except tendon injury
- **905.8** Late effect of tendon injury
  - Late effect of tendon injury due to:
    - open wound [injury classifiable to 880-884 with .2, 890-894 with .2]
    - sprain and strain [injury classifiable to 840-848]
  - AHA: 2Q, '89, 13; 2Q, '89, 15
- **905.9** Late effect of traumatic amputation
  - Late effect of injury classifiable to 885-887, 895-897
  - EXCLUDES late amputation stump complication (997.60-997.69)

✓4th **906** Late effects of injuries to skin and subcutaneous tissues

- **906.0** Late effect of open wound of head, neck, and trunk
  - Late effect of injury classifiable to 870-879
- **906.1** Late effect of open wound of extremities without mention of tendon injury
  - Late effect of injury classifiable to 880-884, 890-894 except .2
- **906.2** Late effect of superficial injury
  - Late effect of injury classifiable to 910-919
- **906.3** Late effect of contusion
  - Late effect of injury classifiable to 920-924
- **906.4** Late effect of crushing
  - Late effect of injury classifiable to 925-929
- **906.5** Late effect of burn of eye, face, head, and neck
  - Late effect of injury classifiable to 940-941
- **906.6** Late effect of burn of wrist and hand
  - Late effect of injury classifiable to 944
  - AHA: 4Q, '94, 22
- **906.7** Late effect of burn of other extremities
  - Late effect of injury classifiable to 943 or 945
  - AHA: 4Q, '94, 22
- **906.8** Late effect of burns of other specified sites
  - Late effect of injury classifiable to 942, 946-947
  - AHA: 4Q, '94, 22
- **906.9** Late effect of burn of unspecified site
  - Late effect of injury classifiable to 948-949
  - AHA: 4Q, '94, 22

✓4th **907** Late effects of injuries to the nervous system

- **907.0** Late effect of intracranial injury without mention of skull fracture
  - Late effect of injury classifiable to 850-854
  - AHA: 3Q, '90, 14
- **907.1** Late effect of injury to cranial nerve
  - Late effect of injury classifiable to 950-951
- **907.2** Late effect of spinal cord injury
  - Late effect of injury classifiable to 806, 952
  - AHA: 4Q, '98, 38
- **907.3** Late effect of injury to nerve root(s), spinal plexus(es), and other nerves of trunk
  - Late effect of injury classifiable to 953-954
- **907.4** Late effect of injury to peripheral nerve of shoulder girdle and upper limb
  - Late effect of injury classifiable to 955
- **907.5** Late effect of injury to peripheral nerve of pelvic girdle and lower limb
  - Late effect of injury classifiable to 956
- **907.9** Late effect of injury to other and unspecified nerve
  - Late effect of injury classifiable to 957

✓4th **908** Late effects of other and unspecified injuries

- **908.0** Late effect of internal injury to chest
  - Late effect of injury classifiable to 860-862
- **908.1** Late effect of internal injury to intra-abdominal organs
  - Late effect of injury classifiable to 863-866, 868
- **908.2** Late effect of internal injury to other internal organs
  - Late effect of injury classifiable to 867 or 869
- **908.3** Late effect of injury to blood vessel of head, neck, and extremities
  - Late effect of injury classifiable to 900, 903-904
- **908.4** Late effect of injury to blood vessel of thorax, abdomen, and pelvis
  - Late effect of injury classifiable to 901-902
- **908.5** Late effect of foreign body in orifice
  - Late effect of injury classifiable to 930-939
- **908.6** Late effect of certain complications of trauma
  - Late effect of complications classifiable to 958
- **908.9** Late effect of unspecified injury
  - Late effect of injury classifiable to 959
  - AHA: 3Q, '00, 4

✓4th **909** Late effects of other and unspecified external causes

- **909.0** Late effect of poisoning due to drug, medicinal or biological substance
  - Late effect of conditions classifiable to 960-979
  - EXCLUDES late effect of adverse effect of drug, medicinal or biological substance (909.5)

909.1–915.4 INJURY AND POISONING — Tabular List

909.1 Late effect of toxic effects of nonmedical substances
Late effect of conditions classifiable to 980-989

909.2 Late effect of radiation
Late effect of conditions classifiable to 990

909.3 Late effect of complications of surgical and medical care
Late effect of conditions classifiable to 996-999
AHA: 1Q, '93, 29

909.4 Late effect of certain other external causes
Late effect of conditions classifiable to 991-994

909.5 Late effect of adverse effect of drug, medical or biological substance
EXCLUDES: late effect of poisoning due to drug, medicinal or biological substance (909.0)
AHA: 4Q, '94, 48

909.9 Late effect of other and unspecified external causes

SUPERFICIAL INJURY (910-919)

EXCLUDES:
burn (blisters) (940.0-949.5)
contusion (920-924.9)
foreign body:
  granuloma (728.82)
  inadvertently left in operative wound (998.4)
  residual in soft tissue (729.6)
insect bite, venomous (989.5)
open wound with incidental foreign body (870.0-897.7)

AHA: 2Q, '89, 15

√4th 910 Superficial injury of face, neck, and scalp except eye
INCLUDES: cheek, lip, ear, nose, gum, throat
EXCLUDES: eye and adnexa (918.0-918.9)

910.0 Abrasion or friction burn without mention of infection
910.1 Abrasion or friction burn, infected
910.2 Blister without mention of infection
910.3 Blister, infected
910.4 Insect bite, nonvenomous, without mention of infection
910.5 Insect bite, nonvenomous, infected
910.6 Superficial foreign body (splinter) without major open wound and without mention of infection
910.7 Superficial foreign body (splinter) without major open wound, infected
910.8 Other and unspecified superficial injury of face, neck, and scalp without mention of infection
910.9 Other and unspecified superficial injury of face, neck, and scalp, infected

√4th 911 Superficial injury of trunk
INCLUDES: abdominal wall, interscapular region, anus, labium (majus) (minus), back, penis, breast, perineum, buttock, scrotum, chest wall, testis, flank, vagina, groin, vulva
EXCLUDES: hip (916.0-916.9)
scapular region (912.0-912.9)

911.0 Abrasion or friction burn without mention of infection
AHA: ▶3Q, '01, 10◄

911.1 Abrasion or friction burn, infected
911.2 Blister without mention of infection
911.3 Blister, infected
911.4 Insect bite, nonvenomous, without mention of infection
911.5 Insect bite, nonvenomous, infected
911.6 Superficial foreign body (splinter) without major open wound and without mention of infection
911.7 Superficial foreign body (splinter) without major open wound, infected
911.8 Other and unspecified superficial injury of trunk without mention of infection
911.9 Other and unspecified superficial injury of trunk, infected

√4th 912 Superficial injury of shoulder and upper arm
INCLUDES: axilla, scapular region

912.0 Abrasion or friction burn without mention of infection
912.1 Abrasion or friction burn, infected
912.2 Blister without mention of infection
912.3 Blister, infected
912.4 Insect bite, nonvenomous, without mention of infection
912.5 Insect bite, nonvenomous, infected
912.6 Superficial foreign body (splinter) without major open wound and without mention of infection
912.7 Superficial foreign body (splinter) without major open wound, infected
912.8 Other and unspecified superficial injury of shoulder and upper arm without mention of infection
912.9 Other and unspecified superficial injury of shoulder and upper arm, infected

√4th 913 Superficial injury of elbow, forearm, and wrist
913.0 Abrasion or friction burn without mention of infection
913.1 Abrasion or friction burn, infected
913.2 Blister without mention of infection
913.3 Blister, infected
913.4 Insect bite, nonvenomous, without mention of infection
913.5 Insect bite, nonvenomous, infected
913.6 Superficial foreign body (splinter) without major open wound and without mention of infection
913.7 Superficial foreign body (splinter) without major open wound, infected
913.8 Other and unspecified superficial injury of elbow, forearm, and wrist without mention of infection
913.9 Other and unspecified superficial injury of elbow, forearm, and wrist, infected

√4th 914 Superficial injury of hand(s) except finger(s) alone
914.0 Abrasion or friction burn without mention of infection
914.1 Abrasion or friction burn, infected
914.2 Blister without mention of infection
914.3 Blister, infected
914.4 Insect bite, nonvenomous, without mention of infection
914.5 Insect bite, nonvenomous, infected
914.6 Superficial foreign body (splinter) without major open wound and without mention of infection
914.7 Superficial foreign body (splinter) without major open wound, infected
914.8 Other and unspecified superficial injury of hand without mention of infection
914.9 Other and unspecified superficial injury of hand, infected

√4th 915 Superficial injury of finger(s)
INCLUDES: fingernail, thumb (nail)

915.0 Abrasion or friction burn without mention of infection
915.1 Abrasion or friction burn, infected
915.2 Blister without mention of infection
915.3 Blister, infected
915.4 Insect bite, nonvenomous, without mention of infection

INJURY AND POISONING

915.5 Insect bite, nonvenomous, infected
915.6 Superficial foreign body (splinter) without major open wound and without mention of infection
915.7 Superficial foreign body (splinter) without major open wound, infected
915.8 Other and unspecified superficial injury of fingers without mention of infection
   AHA: ▶3Q, '01, 10◀
915.9 Other and unspecified superficial injury of fingers, infected

√4th 916 **Superficial injury of hip, thigh, leg, and ankle**
916.0 Abrasion or friction burn without mention of infection
916.1 Abrasion or friction burn, infected
916.2 Blister without mention of infection
916.3 Blister, infected
916.4 Insect bite, nonvenomous, without mention of infection
916.5 Insect bite, nonvenomous, infected
916.6 Superficial foreign body (splinter) without major open wound and without mention of infection
916.7 Superficial foreign body (splinter) without major open wound, infected
916.8 Other and unspecified superficial injury of hip, thigh, leg, and ankle without mention of infection
916.9 Other and unspecified superficial injury of hip, thigh, leg, and ankle, infected

√4th 917 **Superficial injury of foot and toe(s)**
   INCLUDES   heel   toenail
917.0 Abrasion or friction burn without mention of infection
917.1 Abrasion or friction burn, infected
917.2 Blister without mention of infection
917.3 Blister, infected
917.4 Insect bite, nonvenomous, without mention of infection
917.5 Insect bite, nonvenomous, infected
917.6 Superficial foreign body (splinter) without major open wound and without mention of infection
917.7 Superficial foreign body (splinter) without major open wound, infected
917.8 Other and unspecified superficial injury of foot and toes without mention of infection
917.9 Other and unspecified superficial injury of foot and toes, infected

√4th 918 **Superficial injury of eye and adnexa**
   EXCLUDES   burn (940.0-940.9)
              foreign body on external eye (930.0-930.9)
918.0 Eyelids and periocular area
   Abrasion   Superficial foreign body
   Insect bite   (splinter)
918.1 Cornea
   Corneal abrasion   Superficial laceration
      EXCLUDES   corneal injury due to contact lens (371.82)
918.2 Conjunctiva
918.9 Other and unspecified superficial injuries of eye
   Eye (ball) NOS

√4th 919 **Superficial injury of other, multiple, and unspecified sites**
   EXCLUDES   multiple sites classifiable to the same three-digit category (910.0-918.9)
919.0 Abrasion or friction burn without mention of infection
919.1 Abrasion or friction burn, infected
919.2 Blister without mention of infection
919.3 Blister, infected
919.4 Insect bite, nonvenomous, without mention of infection
919.5 Insect bite, nonvenomous, infected
919.6 Superficial foreign body (splinter) without major open wound and without mention of infection
919.7 Superficial foreign body (splinter) without major open wound, infected
919.8 Other and unspecified superficial injury without mention of infection
919.9 Other and unspecified superficial injury, infected

CONTUSION WITH INTACT SKIN SURFACE (920-924)

INCLUDES   bruise   } without fracture or open
           hematoma }   wound

EXCLUDES   concussion (850.0-850.9)
           hemarthrosis (840.0-848.9)
           internal organs (860.0-869.1)
           that incidental to:
              crushing injury (925-929.9)
              dislocation (830.0-839.9)
              fracture (800.0-829.1)
              internal injury (860.0-869.1)
              intracranial injury (850.0-854.1)
              nerve injury (950.0-957.9)
              open wound (870.0-897.7)

920 **Contusion of face, scalp, and neck except eye(s)**
   Cheek   Mandibular joint area
   Ear (auricle)   Nose
   Gum   Throat
   Lip

√4th 921 **Contusion of eye and adnexa**
921.0 Black eye, not otherwise specified
921.1 Contusion of eyelids and periocular area
921.2 Contusion of orbital tissues
921.3 Contusion of eyeball
   AHA: J-A, '85, 16
921.9 Unspecified contusion of eye
   Injury of eye NOS

√4th 922 **Contusion of trunk**
922.0 Breast
922.1 Chest wall
922.2 Abdominal wall
   Flank   Groin
√5th 922.3 Back
   AHA: 4Q, '96, 39
   922.31 Back
      EXCLUDES   interscapular region (922.33)
      AHA: 3Q, '99, 14
   922.32 Buttock
   922.33 Interscapular region
922.4 Genital organs
   Labium (majus) (minus)   Vulva
   Penis   Vagina
   Perineum   Testis
   Scrotum
922.8 Multiple sites of trunk
922.9 Unspecified part
   Trunk NOS

√4th 923 **Contusion of upper limb**
√5th 923.0 Shoulder and upper arm
   923.00 Shoulder region
   923.01 Scapular region
   923.02 Axillary region
   923.03 Upper arm
   923.09 Multiple sites
√5th 923.1 Elbow and forearm
   923.10 Forearm
   923.11 Elbow
√5th 923.2 Wrist and hand(s), except finger(s) alone
   923.20 Hand(s)
   923.21 Wrist

923.3–934.8 INJURY AND POISONING

923.3 **Finger**
Fingernail   Thumb (nail)
923.8 **Multiple sites of upper limb**
923.9 **Unspecified part of upper limb**
Arm NOS

✓4th **924 Contusion of lower limb and of other and unspecified sites**
✓5th 924.0 **Hip and thigh**
924.00 Thigh
924.01 Hip
✓5th 924.1 **Knee and lower leg**
924.10 Lower leg
924.11 Knee
✓5th 924.2 **Ankle and foot, excluding toe(s)**
924.20 Foot
Heel
924.21 Ankle
924.3 **Toe**
Toenail
924.4 **Multiple sites of lower limb**
924.5 **Unspecified part of lower limb**
Leg NOS
924.8 **Multiple sites, not elsewhere classified**
924.9 **Unspecified site**

CRUSHING INJURY (925-929)

EXCLUDES concussion (850.0-850.9)
fractures (800-829)
internal organs (860.0-869.1)
that incidental to:
internal injury (860.0-869.1)
intracranial injury (850.0-854.1)

AHA: 2Q, '93, 7

✓4th **925 Crushing injury of face, scalp, and neck**
Cheek   Pharynx
Ear   Throat
Larynx
925.1 **Crushing injury of face and scalp** CC MSP
Cheek   Ear
CC Excl: 873.8-873.9, 905.0, 925.1-925.2, 929.0, 929.9, 958.8, 959.01, 959.09, 959.8-959.9
925.2 **Crushing injury of neck** CC MSP
Larynx   Throat
Pharynx
CC Excl: 873.8-873.9, 905.0, 925.1-925.2, 929.0, 929.9, 958.8, 959.01, 959.09, 959.8-959.9

✓4th **926 Crushing injury of trunk**
EXCLUDES crush injury of internal organs (860.0-869.1)
926.0 **External genitalia**
Labium (majus) (minus)   Testis
Penis   Vulva
Scrotum
✓5th 926.1 **Other specified sites**
926.11 Back
926.12 Buttock
926.19 Other
Breast
EXCLUDES crushing of chest (860.0-862.9)
926.8 **Multiple sites of trunk** MSP
926.9 **Unspecified site**
Trunk NOS

✓4th **927 Crushing injury of upper limb**
✓5th 927.0 **Shoulder and upper arm**
927.00 Shoulder region
927.01 Scapular region
927.02 Axillary region
927.03 Upper arm
927.09 Multiple sites
✓5th 927.1 **Elbow and forearm**
927.10 Forearm
927.11 Elbow
✓5th 927.2 **Wrist and hand(s), except finger(s) alone**
927.20 Hand(s)
927.21 Wrist
927.3 **Finger(s)**
927.8 **Multiple sites of upper limb**
927.9 **Unspecified site**
Arm NOS

✓4th **928 Crushing injury of lower limb**
✓5th 928.0 **Hip and thigh**
928.00 Thigh
928.01 Hip
✓5th 928.1 **Knee and lower leg**
928.10 Lower leg
928.11 Knee
✓5th 928.2 **Ankle and foot, excluding toe(s) alone**
928.20 Foot
Heel
928.21 Ankle
928.3 **Toe(s)**
928.8 **Multiple sites of lower limb**
928.9 **Unspecified site**
Leg NOS

✓4th **929 Crushing injury of multiple and unspecified sites**
EXCLUDES multiple internal injury NOS (869.0-869.1)
929.0 **Multiple sites, not elsewhere classified** CC MSP
CC Excl: 929.0, 929.9, 958.8, 959.8-959.9
929.9 **Unspecified site** MSP

EFFECTS OF FOREIGN BODY ENTERING THROUGH ORIFICE (930-939)

EXCLUDES foreign body:
granuloma (728.82)
inadvertently left in operative wound (998.4, 998.7)
in open wound (800-839, 851-897)
residual in soft tissues (729.6)
superficial without major open wound (910-919 with .6 or .7)

✓4th **930 Foreign body on external eye**
EXCLUDES foreign body in penetrating wound of:
eyeball (871.5-871.6)
retained (old) (360.5-360.6)
ocular adnexa (870.4)
retained (old) (376.6)
930.0 **Corneal foreign body**
930.1 **Foreign body in conjunctival sac**
930.2 **Foreign body in lacrimal punctum**
930.8 **Other and combined sites**
930.9 **Unspecified site**
External eye NOS

931 Foreign body in ear
Auditory canal   Auricle

932 Foreign body in nose
Nasal sinus   Nostril

✓4th **933 Foreign body in pharynx and larynx**
933.0 **Pharynx**
Nasopharynx   Throat NOS
933.1 **Larynx**
Asphyxia due to foreign body
Choking due to:
food (regurgitated)
phlegm

✓4th **934 Foreign body in trachea, bronchus, and lung**
934.0 **Trachea**
934.1 **Main bronchus**
934.8 **Other specified parts**
Bronchioles   Lung

Tabular List — INJURY AND POISONING — 934.9–944.4

- 934.9 **Respiratory tree, unspecified**
  - Inhalation of liquid or vomitus, lower respiratory tract NOS
- ✓4th 935 Foreign body in mouth, esophagus, and stomach
  - 935.0 Mouth
  - 935.1 Esophagus
    - AHA: 1Q, '88, 13
  - 935.2 Stomach
- 936 Foreign body in intestine and colon
- 937 Foreign body in anus and rectum
  - Rectosigmoid (junction)
- 938 Foreign body in digestive system, unspecified
  - Alimentary tract NOS
  - Swallowed foreign body
- ✓4th 939 Foreign body in genitourinary tract
  - 939.0 Bladder and urethra
  - 939.1 Uterus, any part ♀
    - EXCLUDES intrauterine contraceptive device:
      - complications from (996.32, 996.65)
      - presence of (V45.51)
  - 939.2 Vulva and vagina ♀
  - 939.3 Penis ♂
  - 939.9 **Unspecified site**

BURNS (940-949)

INCLUDES burns from:
- electrical heating appliance
- electricity
- flame
- hot object
- lightning
- radiation
- chemical burns (external) (internal)
- scalds

EXCLUDES friction burns (910-919 with .0, .1)
sunburn (692.71, 692.76-692.77)

AHA: 4Q, 94, 22; 2Q, '90, 7; 4Q, '88, 3; M-A, '86, 9

- ✓4th 940 Burn confined to eye and adnexa
  - 940.0 Chemical burn of eyelids and periocular area
  - 940.1 Other burns of eyelids and periocular area
  - 940.2 Alkaline chemical burn of cornea and conjunctival sac
  - 940.3 Acid chemical burn of cornea and conjunctival sac
  - 940.4 Other burn of cornea and conjunctival sac
  - 940.5 Burn with resulting rupture and destruction of eyeball
  - 940.9 Unspecified burn of eye and adnexa
- ✓4th 941 Burn of face, head, and neck
  - EXCLUDES mouth (947.0)
  - The following fifth-digit subclassification is for use with category 941:
    - 0 face and head, unspecified site
    - 1 ear [any part]
    - 2 eye (with other parts of face, head, and neck)
    - 3 lip(s)
    - 4 chin
    - 5 nose (septum)
    - 6 scalp [any part]
      - Temple (region)
    - 7 forehead and cheek
    - 8 neck
    - 9 multiple sites [except with eye] of face, head, and neck

  AHA: 4Q, '94, 22; M-A, '86, 9

  - ✓5th 941.0 **Unspecified degree**
  - ✓5th 941.1 Erythema [first degree]
  - ✓5th 941.2 Blisters, epidermal loss [second degree]
  - ✓5th 941.3 Full-thickness skin loss [third degree NOS]
  - ✓5th 941.4 Deep necrosis of underlying tissues [deep third degree] without mention of loss of a body part
  - ✓5th 941.5 Deep necrosis of underlying tissues [deep third degree] with loss of a body part
- ✓4th 942 Burn of trunk
  - EXCLUDES scapular region (943.0-943.5 with fifth-digit 6)
  - The following fifth-digit subclassification is for use with category 942:
    - 0 trunk, unspecified site
    - 1 breast
    - 2 chest wall, excluding breast and nipple
    - 3 abdominal wall
      - Flank
      - Groin
    - 4 back [any part]
      - Buttock
      - Interscapular region
    - 5 genitalia
      - Labium (majus) (minus)
      - Scrotum
      - Penis
      - Testis
      - Perineum
      - Vulva
    - 9 other and multiple sites of trunk

  AHA: 4Q, '94, 22; M-A, '86, 9

  - ✓5th 942.0 **Unspecified degree**
  - ✓5th 942.1 Erythema [first degree]
  - ✓5th 942.2 Blisters, epidermal loss [second degree]
  - ✓5th 942.3 Full-thickness skin loss [third degree NOS]
  - ✓5th 942.4 Deep necrosis of underlying tissues [deep third degree] without mention of loss of a body part
  - ✓5th 942.5 Deep necrosis of underlying tissues [deep third degree] with loss of a body part
- ✓4th 943 Burn of upper limb, except wrist and hand
  - The following fifth-digit subclassification is for use with category 943:
    - 0 upper limb, unspecified site
    - 1 forearm
    - 2 elbow
    - 3 upper arm
    - 4 axilla
    - 5 shoulder
    - 6 scapular region
    - 9 multiple sites of upper limb, except wrist and hand

  AHA: 4Q, '94, 22; M-A, '86, 9

  - ✓5th 943.0 **Unspecified degree**
  - ✓5th 943.1 Erythema [first degree]
  - ✓5th 943.2 Blisters, epidermal loss [second degree]
  - ✓5th 943.3 Full-thickness skin loss [third degree NOS]
  - ✓5th 943.4 Deep necrosis of underlying tissues [deep third degree] without mention of loss of a body part
  - ✓5th 943.5 Deep necrosis of underlying tissues [deep third degree] with loss of a body part
- ✓4th 944 Burn of wrist(s) and hand(s)
  - The following fifth-digit subclassification is for use with category 944:
    - 0 hand, unspecified site
    - 1 single digit [finger (nail)] other than thumb
    - 2 thumb (nail)
    - 3 two or more digits, not including thumb
    - 4 two or more digits including thumb
    - 5 palm
    - 6 back of hand
    - 7 wrist
    - 8 multiple sites of wrist(s) and hand(s)

  - ✓5th 944.0 **Unspecified degree**
  - ✓5th 944.1 Erythema [first degree]
  - ✓5th 944.2 Blisters, epidermal loss [second degree]
  - ✓5th 944.3 Full-thickness skin loss [third degree NOS]
  - ✓5th 944.4 Deep necrosis of underlying tissues [deep third degree] without mention of loss of a body part

944.5–949.5 INJURY AND POISONING

√5th 944.5 Deep necrosis of underlying tissues [deep third degree] with loss of a body part

√4th 945 Burn of lower limb(s)

The following fifth-digit subclassification is for use with category 945:
- 0 lower limb [leg], unspecified site
- 1 toe(s) (nail)
- 2 foot
- 3 ankle
- 4 lower leg
- 5 knee
- 6 thigh [any part]
- 9 multiple sites of lower limb(s)

AHA: 4Q, '94, 22; M-A, '86, 9

- √5th 945.0 Unspecified degree
- √5th 945.1 Erythema [first degree]
- √5th 945.2 Blisters, epidermal loss [second degree]
- √5th 945.3 Full-thickness skin loss [third degree NOS]
- √5th 945.4 Deep necrosis of underlying tissues [deep third degree] without mention of loss of a body part
- √5th 945.5 Deep necrosis of underlying tissues [deep third degree] with loss of a body part

√4th 946 Burns of multiple specified sites

INCLUDES burns of sites classifiable to more than one three-digit category in 940-945

EXCLUDES multiple burns NOS (949.0-949.5)

AHA: 4Q, '94, 22; M-A, '86, 9

- 946.0 Unspecified degree
- 946.1 Erythema [first degree]
- 946.2 Blisters, epidermal loss [second degree]
- 946.3 Full-thickness skin loss [third degree NOS]
- 946.4 Deep necrosis of underlying tissues [deep third degree] without mention of loss of a body part
- 946.5 Deep necrosis of underlying tissues [deep third degree] with loss of a body part

√4th 947 Burn of internal organs

INCLUDES burns from chemical agents (ingested)

AHA: 4Q, '94, 22; M-A, '86, 9

- 947.0 Mouth and pharynx
  - Gum
  - Tongue
- 947.1 Larynx, trachea, and lung
- 947.2 Esophagus
- 947.3 Gastrointestinal tract
  - Colon
  - Rectum
  - Small intestine
  - Stomach
- 947.4 Vagina and uterus ♀
- 947.8 Other specified sites
- 947.9 Unspecified site

√4th 948 Burns classified according to extent of body surface involved

Note: This category is to be used when the site of the burn is unspecified, or with categories 940-947 when the site is specified.

EXCLUDES sunburn (692.71, 692.76-692.77)

The following fifth-digit subclassification is for use with category 948 to indicate the percent of body surface with third degree burn; valid digits are in [brackets] under each code:
- 0 less than 10 percent or unspecified
- 1 10-19%
- 2 20-29%
- 3 30-39%
- 4 40-49%
- 5 50-59%
- 6 60-69%
- 7 70-79%
- 8 80-89%
- 9 90% or more of body surface

AHA: 4Q, '94, 22; 4Q, '88, 3; M-A, '86, 9; N-D, '84, 13

Burns

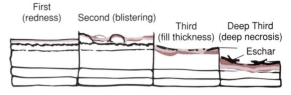

Degrees of Burns: First (redness), Second (blistering), Third (full thickness), Deep Third (deep necrosis), Eschar

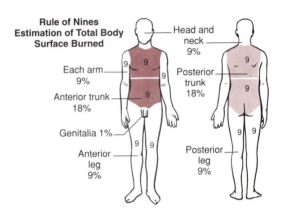

Rule of Nines Estimation of Total Body Surface Burned: Head and neck 9%, Each arm 9%, Anterior trunk 18%, Posterior trunk 18%, Genitalia 1%, Anterior leg 9%, Posterior leg 9%

- √5th 948.0 [0] Burn [any degree] involving less than 10 percent of body surface
- √5th 948.1 [0-1] 10-19 percent of body surface
- √5th 948.2 [0-2] 20-29 percent of body surface
- √5th 948.3 [0-3] 30-39 percent of body surface
- √5th 948.4 [0-4] 40-49 percent of body surface
- √5th 948.5 [0-5] 50-59 percent of body surface
- √5th 948.6 [0-6] 60-69 percent of body surface
- √5th 948.7 [0-7] 70-79 percent of body surface
- √5th 948.8 [0-8] 80-89 percent of body surface
- √5th 948.9 [0-9] 90 percent or more of body surface

√4th 949 Burn, unspecified

INCLUDES burn NOS multiple burns NOS

EXCLUDES burn of unspecified site but with statement of the extent of body surface involved (948.0-948.9)

AHA: 4Q, '94, 22; M-A, '86, 9

- 949.0 Unspecified degree
- 949.1 Erythema [first degree]
- 949.2 Blisters, epidermal loss [second degree]
- 949.3 Full-thickness skin loss [third degree NOS]
- 949.4 Deep necrosis of underlying tissues [deep third degree] without mention of loss of a body part
- 949.5 Deep necrosis of underlying tissues [deep third degree] with loss of a body part

INJURY AND POISONING

INJURY TO NERVES AND SPINAL CORD (950-957)

INCLUDES: division of nerve
lesion in continuity
traumatic neuroma
traumatic transient paralysis
(with open wound)

EXCLUDES: accidental puncture or laceration during medical procedure (998.2)

950 Injury to optic nerve and pathways
- **950.0** Optic nerve injury
  - Second cranial nerve
- **950.1** Injury to optic chiasm
- **950.2** Injury to optic pathways
- **950.3** Injury to visual cortex
- **950.9** Unspecified
  - Traumatic blindness NOS

951 Injury to other cranial nerve(s)
- **951.0** Injury to oculomotor nerve
  - Third cranial nerve
- **951.1** Injury to trochlear nerve
  - Fourth cranial nerve
- **951.2** Injury to trigeminal nerve
  - Fifth cranial nerve
- **951.3** Injury to abducens nerve
  - Sixth cranial nerve
- **951.4** Injury to facial nerve
  - Seventh cranial nerve
- **951.5** Injury to acoustic nerve
  - Auditory nerve
  - Eighth cranial nerve
  - Traumatic deafness NOS
- **951.6** Injury to accessory nerve
  - Eleventh cranial nerve
- **951.7** Injury to hypoglossal nerve
  - Twelfth cranial nerve
- **951.8** Injury to other specified cranial nerves
  - Glossopharyngeal [9th cranial] nerve
  - Olfactory [1st cranial] nerve
  - Pneumogastric [10th cranial] nerve
  - Traumatic anosmia NOS
  - Vagus [10th cranial] nerve
- **951.9** Injury to unspecified cranial nerve

952 Spinal cord injury without evidence of spinal bone injury
- **952.0** Cervical
  - **952.00** C_1-C_4 level with unspecified spinal cord injury
    - Spinal cord injury, cervical region NOS
    - CC Excl: 805.00-805.18, 805.8-805.9, 806.00-806.19, 806.8-806.9, 839.00-839.18, 839.40, 839.49-839.50, 839.59, 839.69, 839.79, 839.8-839.9, 847.9, 905.1, 926.11, 952.00-952.09, 952.8-952.9, 958.8, 959.1, 959.8-959.9

Spinal Nerve Roots

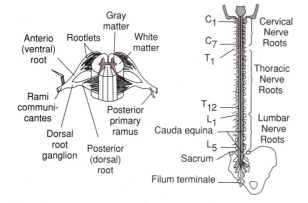

- **952.01** C_1-C_4 level with complete lesion of spinal cord
  - CC Excl: See code 952.00
- **952.02** C_1-C_4 level with anterior cord syndrome
  - CC Excl: See code 952.00
- **952.03** C_1-C_4 level with central cord syndrome
  - CC Excl: See code 952.00
- **952.04** C_1-C_4 level with other specified spinal cord injury
  - Incomplete spinal cord lesion at C_1-C_4 level: NOS
    - with posterior cord syndrome
  - CC Excl: See code 952.00
- **952.05** C_5-C_7 level with unspecified spinal cord injury
  - CC Excl: See code 952.00
- **952.06** C_5-C_7 level with complete lesion of spinal cord
  - CC Excl: See code 952.00
- **952.07** C_5-C_7 level with anterior cord syndrome
  - CC Excl: See code 952.00
- **952.08** C_5-C_7 level with central cord syndrome
  - CC Excl: See code 952.00
- **952.09** C_5-C_7 level with other specified spinal cord injury
  - Incomplete spinal cord lesion at C_5-C_7 level: NOS
    - with posterior cord syndrome
  - CC Excl: See code 952.00

- **952.1** Dorsal [thoracic]
  - **952.10** T_1-T_6 level with unspecified spinal cord injury
    - Spinal cord injury, thoracic region NOS
    - CC Excl: 805.8-805.9, 806.20-806.39, 839.40, 839.49-839.50, 839.59, 839.69, 839.79, 839.8-839.9, 847.9, 905.1, 926.11, 952.10-952.19, 952.8-952.9, 958.8, 959.1, 959.8-959.9
  - **952.11** T_1-T_6 level with complete lesion of spinal cord
    - CC Excl: See code 952.10
  - **952.12** T_1-T_6 level with anterior cord syndrome
    - CC Excl: See code 952.10
  - **952.13** T_1-T_6 level with central cord syndrome
    - CC Excl: See code 952.10
  - **952.14** T_1-T_6 level with other specified spinal cord injury
    - Incomplete spinal cord lesion at T_1-T_6 level: NOS
      - with posterior cord syndrome
    - CC Excl: See code 952.10
  - **952.15** T_7-T_{12} level with unspecified spinal cord injury
    - CC Excl: See code 952.10
  - **952.16** T_7-T_{12} level with complete lesion of spinal cord
    - CC Excl: See code 952.10
  - **952.17** T_7-T_{12} level with anterior cord syndrome
    - CC Excl: See code 952.10
  - **952.18** T_7-T_{12} level with central cord syndrome
    - CC Excl: See code 952.10

INJURY AND POISONING

952.19 T₇-T₁₂ level with other specified spinal cord injury [CC]
  Incomplete spinal cord lesion at T₇-T₁₂ level:
    NOS
    with posterior cord syndrome
  CC Excl: See code 952.10

952.2 Lumbar [CC]
  CC Excl: 805.8-805.9, 806.4-806.5, 839.40, 839.49-839.50, 839.59, 839.69, 839.79, 839.8-839.9, 847.9, 905.1, 926.11, 952.2, 952.8-952.9, 958.8, 959.1, 959.8-959.9

952.3 Sacral [CC]
  CC Excl: 805.8-805.9, 806.60-806.79, 839.40, 839.49-839.50, 839.59, 839.69, 839.79, 839.8-839.9, 847.9, 905.1, 926.11, 952.3-952.4, 952.8-952.9, 958.8, 959.1, 959.8-959.9

952.4 Cauda equina [CC]
  CC Excl: See code 952.3

952.8 Multiple sites of spinal cord [CC]
  CC Excl: 805.8-805.9, 839.40, 839.49-839.50, 839.59, 839.69, 839.79, 839.8-839.9, 847.9, 905.1, 926.11, 952.8-952.9, 958.8, 959.1, 959.8-959.9

952.9 Unspecified site of spinal cord [CC]
  CC Excl: 805.8-805.9, 839.40, 839.49-839.50, 839.59, 839.69, 839.79, 839.8-839.9, 847.9, 905.1, 926.11, 952.8-952.9, 958.8, 959.1, 959.8-959.9

✓4ᵗʰ **953** Injury to nerve roots and spinal plexus

953.0 Cervical root [CC]
  CC Excl: 953.8-953.9, 958.8, 959.8-959.9

953.1 Dorsal root [CC]
  CC Excl: See code 953.0

953.2 Lumbar root [CC]
  CC Excl: See code 953.0

953.3 Sacral root [CC]
  CC Excl: See code 953.0

953.4 Brachial plexus [CC]
  CC Excl: See code 953.0

953.5 Lumbosacral plexus [CC]
  CC Excl: See code 953.0

953.8 Multiple sites [CC]
  CC Excl: See code 953.0

953.9 Unspecified site [CC]
  CC Excl: See code 953.0

✓4ᵗʰ **954** Injury to other nerve(s) of trunk, excluding shoulder and pelvic girdles

954.0 Cervical sympathetic
954.1 Other sympathetic
  Celiac ganglion or plexus   Splanchnic nerve(s)
  Inferior mesenteric plexus Stellate ganglion
954.8 Other specified nerve(s) of trunk
954.9 Unspecified nerve of trunk

✓4ᵗʰ **955** Injury to peripheral nerve(s) of shoulder girdle and upper limb

955.0 Axillary nerve
955.1 Median nerve
955.2 Ulnar nerve
955.3 Radial nerve
955.4 Musculocutaneous nerve
955.5 Cutaneous sensory nerve, upper limb
955.6 Digital nerve
955.7 Other specified nerve(s) of shoulder girdle and upper limb
955.8 Multiple nerves of shoulder girdle and upper limb
955.9 Unspecified nerve of shoulder girdle and upper limb

✓4ᵗʰ **956** Injury to peripheral nerve(s) of pelvic girdle and lower limb

956.0 Sciatic nerve
956.1 Femoral nerve
956.2 Posterior tibial nerve
956.3 Peroneal nerve
956.4 Cutaneous sensory nerve, lower limb
956.5 Other specified nerve(s) of pelvic girdle and lower limb
956.8 Multiple nerves of pelvic girdle and lower limb
956.9 Unspecified nerve of pelvic girdle and lower limb

✓4ᵗʰ **957** Injury to other and unspecified nerves

957.0 Superficial nerves of head and neck
957.1 Other specified nerve(s)
957.8 Multiple nerves in several parts
  Multiple nerve injury NOS
957.9 Unspecified site
  Nerve injury NOS

CERTAIN TRAUMATIC COMPLICATIONS AND UNSPECIFIED INJURIES (958-959)

✓4ᵗʰ **958** Certain early complications of trauma
  EXCLUDES adult respiratory distress syndrome (518.5)
             flail chest (807.4)
             shock lung (518.5)
             that occurring during or following medical procedures (996.0-999.9)

958.0 Air embolism [CC]
  Pneumathemia
  EXCLUDES that complicating:
             abortion (634-638 with .6, 639.6)
             ectopic or molar pregnancy (639.6)
             pregnancy, childbirth, or the puerperium (673.0)
  CC Excl: 958.0, 958.8, 959.8-959.9, 997.91, 997.99, 998.81, 998.83-998.9, 999.1
  DEF: Arterial obstruction due to introduction of air bubbles into the veins following surgery or trauma.

958.1 Fat embolism [CC]
  EXCLUDES that complicating:
             abortion (634-638 with .6, 639.6)
             pregnancy, childbirth, or the puerperium (673.8)
  CC Excl: 958.1, 958.8, 959.8-959.9, 997.91, 997.99, 998.81, 998.83-998.9
  DEF: Arterial blockage due to the entrance of fat in circulatory system, after fracture of large bones or administration of corticosteroids.

958.2 Secondary and recurrent hemorrhage [CC]
  CC Excl: 958.2, 958.8, 959.8-959.9, 997.91, 997.99, 998.81, 998.83-998.9

958.3 Posttraumatic wound infection, not elsewhere classified [CC]
  EXCLUDES infected open wounds–code to complicated open wound of site
  CC Excl: 958.3, 958.8, 959.8-959.9, 997.91, 997.99, 998.81, 998.83-998.9
  AHA: ▶4Q, '01, 53;◀ S-O, '85, 10

958.4 Traumatic shock [CC] [MSP]
  Shock (immediate) (delayed) following injury
  EXCLUDES shock:
             anaphylactic (995.0)
             due to serum (999.4)
             anesthetic (995.4)
             electric (994.8)
             following abortion (639.5)
             lightning (994.0)
             nontraumatic NOS (785.50)
             obstetric (669.1)
             postoperative (998.0)
  CC Excl: 958.4, 958.8, 959.8-959.9, 997.91, 997.99, 998.81, 998.83-998.9
  DEF: Shock, immediate or delayed following injury.

[N] Newborn Age: 0   [P] Pediatric Age: 0-17   [M] Maternity Age: 12-55   [A] Adult Age: 15-124   [CC] CC Condition   [MC] Major Complication   [CD] Complex Dx   [HIV] HIV Related Dx

INJURY AND POISONING

958.5 **Traumatic anuria** `CC` `MSP`
    Crush syndrome
    Renal failure following crushing
    EXCLUDES *that due to a medical procedure (997.5)*
    CC Excl: 958.5, 958.8, 959.8-959.9, 995.4, 997.91, 997.99, 998.0, 998.11-998.13, 998.81, 998.83-998.9
    DEF: Complete suppression of urinary secretion by kidneys due to trauma.

958.6 **Volkmann's ischemic contracture**
    Posttraumatic muscle contracture
    DEF: Muscle deterioration due to loss of blood supply from injury or tourniquet; causes muscle contraction and results in inability to extend the muscles fully.

958.7 **Traumatic subcutaneous emphysema** `CC`
    EXCLUDES *subcutaneous emphysema resulting from a procedure (998.81)*
    CC Excl: 860.0-860.5, 861.20-861.32, 862.0-862.1, 862.29, 862.31-862.9, 875.0-875.1, 958.7-958.8, 959.8-959.9, 997.91, 997.99, 998.81, 998.83-998.9

958.8 **Other early complications of trauma**
    AHA: 2Q, '92, 13
    DEF: Compartmental syndrome is abnormal pressure in confined anatomical space, as in swollen muscle restricted by fascia.

√4th **959** **Injury, other and unspecified**
    INCLUDES injury NOS
    EXCLUDES injury NOS of:
        blood vessels (900.0-904.9)
        eye (921.0-921.9)
        internal organs (860.0-869.1)
        intracranial sites (854.0-854.1)
        nerves (950.0-951.9, 953.0-957.9)
        spinal cord (952.0-952.9)

√5th **959.0** **Head, face, and neck**
    959.01 **Head injury, unspecified** `MSP`
        EXCLUDES *concussion (850.1-850.9)*
            with head injury NOS (850.1-850.9)
            ▶*head injury NOS with loss of consciousness (850.1-850.5)*◀
            specified intracranial injuries (850.0-854.1)
        AHA: 4Q, '97, 46
    959.09 **Injury of face and neck** `MSP`
        Cheek   Mouth
        Ear   Nose
        Eyebrow   Throat
        Lip
        AHA: 4Q, '97, 46

959.1 **Trunk**
    Abdominal wall   External genital organs
    Back   Flank
    Breast   Groin
    Buttock   Interscapular region
    Chest wall   Perineum
    EXCLUDES *scapular region (959.2)*
    AHA: 1Q, '99, 10

959.2 **Shoulder and upper arm**
    Axilla   Scapular region

959.3 **Elbow, forearm, and wrist**
    AHA: 1Q, '97, 8

959.4 **Hand, except finger**

959.5 **Finger**
    Fingernail   Thumb (nail)

959.6 **Hip and thigh**
    Upper leg

959.7 **Knee, leg, ankle, and foot**

959.8 **Other specified sites, including multiple**
    EXCLUDES *multiple sites classifiable to the same four-digit category (959.0-959.7)*

959.9 **Unspecified site**

POISONING BY DRUGS, MEDICINAL AND BIOLOGICAL SUBSTANCES (960-979)

INCLUDES overdose of these substances
    wrong substance given or taken in error
EXCLUDES *adverse effects ["hypersensitivity," "reaction," etc.] of correct substance properly administered. Such cases are to be classified according to the nature of the adverse effect, such as:*
    adverse effect NOS (995.2)
    allergic lymphadenitis (289.3)
    aspirin gastritis (535.4)
    blood disorders (280.0-289.9)
    dermatitis:
        contact (692.0-692.9)
        due to ingestion (693.0-693.9)
    nephropathy (583.9)
    [The drug giving rise to the adverse effect may be identified by use of categories E930-E949.]
    drug dependence (304.0-304.9)
    drug reaction and poisoning affecting the newborn (760.0-779.9)
    nondependent abuse of drugs (305.0-305.9)
    pathological drug intoxication (292.2)
Use additional code to specify the effects of the poisoning
AHA: 2Q, '90, 11

√4th **960** **Poisoning by antibiotics**
    EXCLUDES *antibiotics:*
        ear, nose, and throat (976.6)
        eye (976.5)
        local (976.0)

960.0 **Penicillins**
    Ampicillin   Cloxacillin
    Carbenicillin   Penicillin G

960.1 **Antifungal antibiotics**
    Amphotericin B   Nystatin
    Griseofulvin   Trichomycin
    EXCLUDES *preparations intended for topical use (976.0-976.9)*

960.2 **Chloramphenicol group**
    Chloramphenicol   Thiamphenicol

960.3 **Erythromycin and other macrolides**
    Oleandomycin   Spiramycin

960.4 **Tetracycline group**
    Doxycycline   Oxytetracycline
    Minocycline

960.5 **Cephalosporin group**
    Cephalexin   Cephaloridine
    Cephaloglycin   Cephalothin

960.6 **Antimycobacterial antibiotics**
    Cycloserine   Rifampin
    Kanamycin   Streptomycin

960.7 **Antineoplastic antibiotics**
    Actinomycin such as:
        Bleomycin   Daunorubicin
        Cactinomycin   Mitomycin
        Dactinomycin

960.8 **Other specified antibiotics**

960.9 **Unspecified antibiotic**

√4th **961** **Poisoning by other anti-infectives**
    EXCLUDES *anti-infectives:*
        ear, nose, and throat (976.6)
        eye (976.5)
        local (976.0)

961.0 **Sulfonamides**
    Sulfadiazine   Sulfamethoxazole
    Sulfafurazole

961.1 **Arsenical anti-infectives**

961.2 **Heavy metal anti-infectives**
    Compounds of: Compounds of:
        antimony   lead
        bismuth   mercury
    EXCLUDES *mercurial diuretics (974.0)*

INJURY AND POISONING

961.3–965.6

961.3 Quinoline and hydroxyquinoline derivatives
Chiniofon
Diiodohydroxyquin
EXCLUDES antimalarial drugs (961.4)

961.4 Antimalarials and drugs acting on other blood protozoa
Chloroquine
Cycloguanil
Primaquine
Proguanil [chloroguanide]
Pyrimethamine
Quinine

961.5 Other antiprotozoal drugs
Emetine

961.6 Anthelmintics
Hexylresorcinol
Piperazine
Thiabendazole

961.7 Antiviral drugs
Methisazone
EXCLUDES amantadine (966.4)
cytarabine (963.1)
idoxuridine (976.5)

961.8 Other antimycobacterial drugs
Ethambutol
Ethionamide
Isoniazid
Para-aminosalicylic acid derivatives
Sulfones

961.9 Other and unspecified anti-infectives
Flucytosine
Nitrofuran derivatives

✓4th 962 Poisoning by hormones and synthetic substitutes
EXCLUDES oxytocic hormones (975.0)

962.0 Adrenal cortical steroids
Cortisone derivatives
Desoxycorticosterone derivatives
Fluorinated corticosteroids

962.1 Androgens and anabolic congeners
Methandriol
Nandrolone
Oxymetholone
Testosterone

962.2 Ovarian hormones and synthetic substitutes
Contraceptives, oral
Estrogens
Estrogens and progestogens, combined
Progestogens

962.3 Insulins and antidiabetic agents
Acetohexamide
Biguanide derivatives, oral
Chlorpropamide
Glucagon
Insulin
Phenformin
Sulfonylurea derivatives, oral
Tolbutamide
AHA: M-A, '85, 8

962.4 Anterior pituitary hormones
Corticotropin
Gonadotropin
Somatotropin [growth hormone]

962.5 Posterior pituitary hormones
Vasopressin
EXCLUDES oxytocic hormones (975.0)

962.6 Parathyroid and parathyroid derivatives

962.7 Thyroid and thyroid derivatives
Dextrothyroxin
Levothyroxine sodium
Liothyronine
Thyroglobulin

962.8 Antithyroid agents
Iodides
Thiouracil
Thiourea

962.9 Other and unspecified hormones and synthetic substitutes

✓4th 963 Poisoning by primarily systemic agents

963.0 Antiallergic and antiemetic drugs
Antihistamines
Chlorpheniramine
Diphenhydramine
Diphenylpyraline
Thonzylamine
Tripelennamine
EXCLUDES phenothiazine-based tranquilizers (969.1)

963.1 Antineoplastic and immunosuppressive drugs
Azathioprine
Busulfan
Chlorambucil
Cyclophosphamide
Cytarabine
Fluorouracil
Mercaptopurine
thio-TEPA
EXCLUDES antineoplastic antibiotics (960.7)

963.2 Acidifying agents

963.3 Alkalizing agents

963.4 Enzymes, not elsewhere classified
Penicillinase

963.5 Vitamins, not elsewhere classified
Vitamin A
Vitamin D
EXCLUDES nicotinic acid (972.2)
vitamin K (964.3)

963.8 Other specified systemic agents
Heavy metal antagonists

963.9 Unspecified systemic agent

✓4th 964 Poisoning by agents primarily affecting blood constituents

964.0 Iron and its compounds
Ferric salts
Ferrous sulfate and other ferrous salts

964.1 Liver preparations and other antianemic agents
Folic acid

964.2 Anticoagulants
Coumarin
Heparin
Phenindione
Warfarin sodium
AHA: 1Q, '94, 22

964.3 Vitamin K [phytonadione]

964.4 Fibrinolysis-affecting drugs
Aminocaproic acid
Streptodornase
Streptokinase
Urokinase

964.5 Anticoagulant antagonists and other coagulants
Hexadimethrine
Protamine sulfate

964.6 Gamma globulin

964.7 Natural blood and blood products
Blood plasma
Human fibrinogen
Packed red cells
Whole blood
EXCLUDES transfusion reactions (999.4-999.8)

964.8 Other specified agents affecting blood constituents
Macromolecular blood substitutes
Plasma expanders

964.9 Unspecified agent affecting blood constituents

✓4th 965 Poisoning by analgesics, antipyretics, and antirheumatics
EXCLUDES drug dependence (304.0-304.9)
nondependent abuse (305.0-305.9)

✓5th 965.0 Opiates and related narcotics

965.00 Opium (alkaloids), unspecified

965.01 Heroin
Diacetylmorphine

965.02 Methadone

965.09 Other
Codeine [methylmorphine]
Meperidine [pethidine]
Morphine

965.1 Salicylates
Acetylsalicylic acid [aspirin]
Salicylic acid salts
AHA: N-D, '94, 15

965.4 Aromatic analgesics, not elsewhere classified
Acetanilid
Paracetamol [acetaminophen]
Phenacetin [acetophenetidin]

965.5 Pyrazole derivatives
Aminophenazone [aminopyrine]
Phenylbutazone

✓5th 965.6 Antirheumatics [antiphlogistics]
EXCLUDES salicylates (965.1)
steroids (962.0-962.9)
AHA: 4Q, '98, 50

| | 965.61 | **Propionic acid derivatives**
Fenoprofen
Flurbiprofen
Ibuprofen
Ketoprofen
Naproxen
Oxaprozin
AHA: 4Q, '98, 50 |
|---|---|---|

| | 965.69 | **Other antirheumatics**
Gold salts
Indomethacin |
|---|---|---|
| | 965.7 | **Other non-narcotic analgesics**
Pyrabital |
| | 965.8 | **Other specified analgesics and antipyretics**
Pentazocine |
| | 965.9 | ==Unspecified analgesic and antipyretic== |

✓4ᵗʰ **966 Poisoning by anticonvulsants and anti-Parkinsonism drugs**

| | 966.0 | **Oxazolidine derivatives**
Paramethadione
Trimethadione |
|---|---|---|
| | 966.1 | **Hydantoin derivatives**
Phenytoin |
| | 966.2 | **Succinimides**
Ethosuximide
Phensuximide |
| | 966.3 | **Other and unspecified anticonvulsants**
Primidone
EXCLUDES *barbiturates (967.0)*
sulfonamides (961.0) |
| | 966.4 | **Anti-Parkinsonism drugs**
Amantadine
Ethopropazine [profenamine]
Levodopa [L-dopa] |

✓4ᵗʰ **967 Poisoning by sedatives and hypnotics**
EXCLUDES *drug dependence (304.0-304.9)*
nondependent abuse (305.0-305.9)

| | 967.0 | **Barbiturates**
Amobarbital [amylobarbitone]
Barbital [barbitone]
Butabarbital [butabarbitone]
Pentobarbital [pentobarbitone]
Phenobarbital [phenobarbitone]
Secobarbital [quinalbarbitone]
EXCLUDES *thiobarbiturate anesthetics (968.3)* |
|---|---|---|
| | 967.1 | **Chloral hydrate group** |
| | 967.2 | **Paraldehyde** |
| | 967.3 | **Bromine compounds**
Bromide
Carbromal (derivatives) |
	967.4	**Methaqualone compounds**
	967.5	**Glutethimide group**
	967.6	**Mixed sedatives, not elsewhere classified**
	967.8	**Other sedatives and hypnotics**
	967.9	==Unspecified sedative or hypnotic==
Sleeping:
drug ⎫
pill   ⎬ NOS
tablet ⎭

✓4ᵗʰ **968 Poisoning by other central nervous system depressants and anesthetics**
EXCLUDES *drug dependence (304.0-304.9)*
nondependent abuse (305.0-305.9)

| | 968.0 | **Central nervous system muscle-tone depressants**
Chlorphenesin (carbamate)   Methocarbamol
Mephenesin |
|---|---|---|
| | 968.1 | **Halothane** |
| | 968.2 | **Other gaseous anesthetics**
Ether
Halogenated hydrocarbon derivatives, except halothane
Nitrous oxide |
| | 968.3 | **Intravenous anesthetics**
Ketamine
Methohexital [methohexitone]
Thiobarbiturates, such as thiopental sodium |
| | 968.4 | **Other and unspecified general anesthetics** |
| | 968.5 | **Surface [topical] and infiltration anesthetics**
Cocaine   Procaine
Lidocaine [lignocaine]   Tetracaine
AHA: 1Q, '93, 25 |
	968.6	**Peripheral nerve- and plexus-blocking anesthetics**
	968.7	**Spinal anesthetics**
	968.9	**Other and unspecified local anesthetics**

✓4ᵗʰ **969 Poisoning by psychotropic agents**
EXCLUDES *drug dependence (304.0-304.9)*
nondependent abuse (305.0-305.9)

| | 969.0 | **Antidepressants**
Amitriptyline
Imipramine
Monoamine oxidase [MAO] inhibitors |
|---|---|---|
| | 969.1 | **Phenothiazine-based tranquilizers**
Chlorpromazine   Prochlorperazine
Fluphenazine   Promazine |
| | 969.2 | **Butyrophenone-based tranquilizers**
Haloperidol   Trifluperidol
Spiperone |
| | 969.3 | **Other antipsychotics, neuroleptics, and major tranquilizers** |
| | 969.4 | **Benzodiazepine-based tranquilizers**
Chlordiazepoxide   Lorazepam
Diazepam   Medazepam
Flurazepam   Nitrazepam |
| | 969.5 | **Other tranquilizers**
Hydroxyzine   Meprobamate |
| | 969.6 | **Psychodysleptics [hallucinogens]**
Cannabis (derivatives) Mescaline
Lysergide [LSD]   Psilocin
Marihuana (derivatives) Psilocybin |
| | 969.7 | **Psychostimulants**
Amphetamine
Caffeine
EXCLUDES *central appetite depressants (977.0)* |
| | 969.8 | **Other specified psychotropic agents** |
| | 969.9 | ==Unspecified psychotropic agent== |

✓4ᵗʰ **970 Poisoning by central nervous system stimulants**

| | 970.0 | **Analeptics**
Lobeline
Nikethamide |
|---|---|---|
| | 970.1 | **Opiate antagonists**
Levallorphan
Nalorphine
Naloxone |
| | 970.8 | **Other specified central nervous system stimulants** |
| | 970.9 | ==Unspecified central nervous system stimulant== |

✓4ᵗʰ **971 Poisoning by drugs primarily affecting the autonomic nervous system**

| | 971.0 | **Parasympathomimetics [cholinergics]**
Acetylcholine   Pilocarpine
Anticholinesterase:
  organophosphorus
  reversible |
|---|---|---|
| | 971.1 | **Parasympatholytics [anticholinergics and antimuscarinics] and spasmolytics**
Atropine   Quaternary ammonium
Homatropine   derivatives
Hyoscine [scopolamine]
EXCLUDES *papaverine (972.5)* |
| | 971.2 | **Sympathomimetics [adrenergics]**
Epinephrine [adrenalin] Levarterenol [noradrenalin] |
| | 971.3 | **Sympatholytics [antiadrenergics]**
Phenoxybenzamine   Tolazolinehydrochloride |
| | 971.9 | **Unspecified drug primarily affecting autonomic nervous system** |

INJURY AND POISONING 972–979.1

√4th 972 Poisoning by agents primarily affecting the cardiovascular system
- 972.0 Cardiac rhythm regulators
  - Practolol
  - Procainamide
  - Propranolol
  - Quinidine
  - EXCLUDES: lidocaine (968.5)
- 972.1 Cardiotonic glycosides and drugs of similar action
  - Digitalis glycosides
  - Digoxin
  - Strophanthins
- 972.2 Antilipemic and antiarteriosclerotic drugs
  - Clofibrate
  - Nicotinic acid derivatives
- 972.3 Ganglion-blocking agents
  - Pentamethonium bromide
- 972.4 Coronary vasodilators
  - Dipyridamole
  - Nitrates [nitroglycerin]
  - Nitrites
- 972.5 Other vasodilators
  - Cyclandelate
  - Diazoxide
  - Papaverine
  - EXCLUDES: nicotinic acid (972.2)
- 972.6 Other antihypertensive agents
  - Clonidine
  - Guanethidine
  - Rauwolfia alkaloids
  - Reserpine
- 972.7 Antivaricose drugs, including sclerosing agents
  - Sodium morrhuate
  - Zinc salts
- 972.8 Capillary-active drugs
  - Adrenochrome derivatives
  - Metaraminol
- 972.9 Other and unspecified agents primarily affecting the cardiovascular system

√4th 973 Poisoning by agents primarily affecting the gastrointestinal system
- 973.0 Antacids and antigastric secretion drugs
  - Aluminum hydroxide
  - Magnesium trisilicate
- 973.1 Irritant cathartics
  - Bisacodyl
  - Castor oil
  - Phenolphthalein
- 973.2 Emollient cathartics
  - Dioctyl sulfosuccinates
- 973.3 Other cathartics, including intestinal atonia drugs
  - Magnesium sulfate
- 973.4 Digestants
  - Pancreatin
  - Papain
  - Pepsin
- 973.5 Antidiarrheal drugs
  - Kaolin
  - Pectin
  - EXCLUDES: anti-infectives (960.0-961.9)
- 973.6 Emetics
- 973.8 Other specified agents primarily affecting the gastrointestinal system
- 973.9 **Unspecified agent primarily affecting the gastrointestinal system**

√4th 974 Poisoning by water, mineral, and uric acid metabolism drugs
- 974.0 Mercurial diuretics
  - Chlormerodrin
  - Mercaptomerin
  - Mersalyl
- 974.1 Purine derivative diuretics
  - Theobromine
  - Theophylline
  - EXCLUDES: aminophylline [theophylline ethylenediamine] (975.7)
  - caffeine (969.7)
- 974.2 Carbonic acid anhydrase inhibitors
  - Acetazolamide
- 974.3 Saluretics
  - Benzothiadiazides
  - Chlorothiazide group
- 974.4 Other diuretics
  - Ethacrynic acid
  - Furosemide
- 974.5 Electrolytic, caloric, and water-balance agents
- 974.6 Other mineral salts, not elsewhere classified
- 974.7 Uric acid metabolism drugs
  - Allopurinol
  - Colchicine
  - Probenecid

√4th 975 Poisoning by agents primarily acting on the smooth and skeletal muscles and respiratory system
- 975.0 Oxytocic agents
  - Ergot alkaloids
  - Oxytocin
  - Prostaglandins
- 975.1 Smooth muscle relaxants
  - Adiphenine
  - Metaproterenol [orciprenaline]
  - EXCLUDES: papaverine (972.5)
- 975.2 Skeletal muscle relaxants
- 975.3 Other and unspecified drugs acting on muscles
- 975.4 Antitussives
  - Dextromethorphan
  - Pipazethate
- 975.5 Expectorants
  - Acetylcysteine
  - Guaifenesin
  - Terpin hydrate
- 975.6 Anti-common cold drugs
- 975.7 Antiasthmatics
  - Aminophylline [theophylline ethylenediamine]
- 975.8 Other and unspecified respiratory drugs

√4th 976 Poisoning by agents primarily affecting skin and mucous membrane, ophthalmological, otorhinolaryngological, and dental drugs
- 976.0 Local anti-infectives and anti-inflammatory drugs
- 976.1 Antipruritics
- 976.2 Local astringents and local detergents
- 976.3 Emollients, demulcents, and protectants
- 976.4 Keratolytics, keratoplastics, other hair treatment drugs and preparations
- 976.5 Eye anti-infectives and other eye drugs
  - Idoxuridine
- 976.6 Anti-infectives and other drugs and preparations for ear, nose, and throat
- 976.7 Dental drugs topically applied
  - EXCLUDES: anti-infectives (976.0)
  - local anesthetics (968.5)
- 976.8 Other agents primarily affecting skin and mucous membrane
  - Spermicides [vaginal contraceptives]
- 976.9 **Unspecified agent primarily affecting skin and mucous membrane**

√4th 977 Poisoning by other and unspecified drugs and medicinal substances
- 977.0 Dietetics
  - Central appetite depressants
- 977.1 Lipotropic drugs
- 977.2 Antidotes and chelating agents, not elsewhere classified
- 977.3 Alcohol deterrents
- 977.4 Pharmaceutical excipients
  - Pharmaceutical adjuncts
- 977.8 Other specified drugs and medicinal substances
  - Contrast media used for diagnostic x-ray procedures
  - Diagnostic agents and kits
- 977.9 **Unspecified drug or medicinal substance**

√4th 978 Poisoning by bacterial vaccines
- 978.0 BCG
- 978.1 Typhoid and paratyphoid
- 978.2 Cholera
- 978.3 Plague
- 978.4 Tetanus
- 978.5 Diphtheria
- 978.6 Pertussis vaccine, including combinations with a pertussis component
- 978.8 Other and unspecified bacterial vaccines
- 978.9 Mixed bacterial vaccines, except combinations with a pertussis component

√4th 979 Poisoning by other vaccines and biological substances
- EXCLUDES: gamma globulin (964.6)
- 979.0 Smallpox vaccine
- 979.1 Rabies vaccine

979.2	Typhus vaccine	
979.3	Yellow fever vaccine	
979.4	Measles vaccine	
979.5	Poliomyelitis vaccine	
979.6	Other and unspecified viral and rickettsial vaccines	
	Mumps vaccine	
979.7	Mixed viral-rickettsial and bacterial vaccines, except combinations with a pertussis component	
	EXCLUDES combinations with a pertussis component (978.6)	
979.9	Other and unspecified vaccines and biological substances	

TOXIC EFFECTS OF SUBSTANCES CHIEFLY NONMEDICINAL AS TO SOURCE (980-989)

EXCLUDES burns from chemical agents (ingested) (947.0-947.9)
localized toxic effects indexed elsewhere (001.0-799.9)
respiratory conditions due to external agents (506.0-508.9)

Use additional code to specify the nature of the toxic effect

980 Toxic effect of alcohol
- 980.0 **Ethyl alcohol**
  - Denatured alcohol
  - Ethanol
  - Grain alcohol
  - Use additional code to identify any associated:
    - acute alcohol intoxication (305.0)
      - in alcoholism (303.0)
    - drunkenness (simple) (305.0)
    - pathological (291.4)

  AHA: 3Q, '96, 16

- 980.1 **Methyl alcohol**
  - Methanol
  - Wood alcohol
- 980.2 **Isopropyl alcohol**
  - Dimethyl carbinol
  - Isopropanol
  - Rubbing alcohol
- 980.3 **Fusel oil**
  - Alcohol:
    - amyl
    - butyl
  - Alcohol:
    - propyl
- 980.8 **Other specified alcohols**
- 980.9 **Unspecified alcohol**

981 Toxic effect of petroleum products
- Benzine
- Gasoline
- Kerosene
- Paraffin wax
- Petroleum:
  - ether
  - naphtha
  - spirit

982 Toxic effect of solvents other than petroleum-based
- 982.0 **Benzene and homologues**
- 982.1 **Carbon tetrachloride**
- 982.2 **Carbon disulfide**
  - Carbon bisulfide
- 982.3 **Other chlorinated hydrocarbon solvents**
  - Tetrachloroethylene
  - Trichloroethylene
  - EXCLUDES chlorinated hydrocarbon preparations other than solvents (989.2)
- 982.4 **Nitroglycol**
- 982.8 **Other nonpetroleum-based solvents**
  - Acetone

983 Toxic effect of corrosive aromatics, acids, and caustic alkalis
- 983.0 **Corrosive aromatics**
  - Carbolic acid or phenol
  - Cresol
- 983.1 **Acids**
  - Acid:
    - hydrochloric
    - nitric
  - Acid:
    - sulfuric
- 983.2 **Caustic alkalis**
  - Lye
  - Potassium hydroxide
  - Sodium hydroxide

- 983.9 **Caustic, unspecified**

984 Toxic effect of lead and its compounds (including fumes)
INCLUDES that from all sources except medicinal substances
- 984.0 **Inorganic lead compounds**
  - Lead dioxide
  - Lead salts
- 984.1 **Organic lead compounds**
  - Lead acetate
  - Tetraethyl lead
- 984.8 **Other lead compounds**
- 984.9 **Unspecified lead compound**

985 Toxic effect of other metals
INCLUDES that from all sources except medicinal substances
- 985.0 **Mercury and its compounds**
  - Minamata disease
- 985.1 **Arsenic and its compounds**
- 985.2 **Manganese and its compounds**
- 985.3 **Beryllium and its compounds**
- 985.4 **Antimony and its compounds**
- 985.5 **Cadmium and its compounds**
- 985.6 **Chromium**
- 985.8 **Other specified metals**
  - Brass fumes
  - Copper salts
  - Iron compounds
  - Nickel compounds

  AHA: 1Q, '88, 5

- 985.9 **Unspecified metal**

986 Toxic effect of carbon monoxide
Carbon monoxide from any source

987 Toxic effect of other gases, fumes, or vapors
- 987.0 **Liquefied petroleum gases**
  - Butane
  - Propane
- 987.1 **Other hydrocarbon gas**
- 987.2 **Nitrogen oxides**
  - Nitrogen dioxide
  - Nitrous fumes
- 987.3 **Sulfur dioxide**
- 987.4 **Freon**
  - Dichloromonofluoromethane
- 987.5 **Lacrimogenic gas**
  - Bromobenzyl cyanide
  - Chloroacetophenone
  - Ethyliodoacetate
- 987.6 **Chlorine gas**
- 987.7 **Hydrocyanic acid gas**
- 987.8 **Other specified gases, fumes, or vapors**
  - Phosgene
  - Polyester fumes
- 987.9 **Unspecified gas, fume, or vapor**

988 Toxic effect of noxious substances eaten as food
EXCLUDES allergic reaction to food, such as:
  gastroenteritis (558.3)
  rash (692.5, 693.1)
food poisoning (bacterial) (005.0-005.9)
toxic effects of food contaminants, such as:
  aflatoxin and other mycotoxin (989.7)
  mercury (985.0)
- 988.0 **Fish and shellfish**
- 988.1 **Mushrooms**
- 988.2 **Berries and other plants**
- 988.8 **Other specified noxious substances eaten as food**
- 988.9 **Unspecified noxious substance eaten as food**

989 Toxic effect of other substances, chiefly nonmedicinal as to source
- 989.0 **Hydrocyanic acid and cyanides**
  - Potassium cyanide
  - Sodium cyanide
  - EXCLUDES gas and fumes (987.7)
- 989.1 **Strychnine and salts**
- 989.2 **Chlorinated hydrocarbons**
  - Aldrin
  - Chlordane
  - DDT
  - Dieldrin
  - EXCLUDES chlorinated hydrocarbon solvents (982.0-982.3)

Additional Digit Required   Nonspecific PDx   Unacceptable PDx Manifestation Code MSP Medicare Secondary Payer ▶◀ Revised Text ● New Code ▲ Revised Code Title

INJURY AND POISONING

989.3 Organophosphate and carbamate
- Carbaryl
- Dichlorvos
- Malathion
- Parathion
- Phorate
- Phosdrin

989.4 Other pesticides, not elsewhere classified
- Mixtures of insecticides

989.5 Venom
- Bites of venomous snakes, lizards, and spiders
- Tick paralysis

989.6 Soaps and detergents

989.7 Aflatoxin and other mycotoxin [food contaminants]

√5th **989.8** Other substances, chiefly nonmedicinal as to source
AHA: 4Q, '95, 60

    989.81 Asbestos
        EXCLUDES asbestosis (501)
        exposure to asbestos (V15.84)

    989.82 Latex

    989.83 Silicone
        EXCLUDES silicone used in medical devices, implants and grafts (996.00-996.79)

    989.84 Tobacco
    989.89 Other

989.9 Unspecified substance, chiefly nonmedicinal as to source

OTHER AND UNSPECIFIED EFFECTS OF EXTERNAL CAUSES (990-995)

990 Effects of radiation, unspecified
- Complication of:
  - phototherapy
  - radiation therapy
- Radiation sickness

EXCLUDES specified adverse effects of radiation. Such conditions are to be classified according to the nature of the adverse effect, as:
- burns (940.0-949.5)
- dermatitis (692.7-692.8)
- leukemia (204.0-208.9)
- pneumonia (508.0)
- sunburn (692.71, 692.76-692.77)

[The type of radiation giving rise to the adverse effect may be identified by use of the E codes.]

√4th **991** Effects of reduced temperature

991.0 Frostbite of face
991.1 Frostbite of hand
991.2 Frostbite of foot
991.3 Frostbite of other and unspecified sites
991.4 Immersion foot
- Trench foot

DEF: Paresthesia, edema, blotchy cyanosis of foot, the skin is soft (macerated), pale and wrinkled, and the sole is swollen with surface ridging and following sustained immersion in water.

991.5 Chilblains
- Erythema pernio
- Perniosis

DEF: Red, swollen, itchy skin; follows damp cold exposure; also associated with pruritus and a burning feeling, in hands, feet, ears, and face in children, legs and toes in women, and hands and fingers in men.

991.6 Hypothermia
- Hypothermia (accidental)

EXCLUDES hypothermia following anesthesia (995.89)
hypothermia not associated with low environmental temperature ▶(780.99)◀

DEF: Reduced body temperature due to low environmental temperatures.

991.8 Other specified effects of reduced temperature

991.9 Unspecified effect of reduced temperature
- Effects of freezing or excessive cold NOS

√4th **992** Effects of heat and light

EXCLUDES burns (940.0-949.5)
diseases of sweat glands due to heat (705.0-705.9)
malignant hyperpyrexia following anesthesia (995.86)
sunburn (692.71, 692.76-692.77)

992.0 Heat stroke and sunstroke
- Heat apoplexy
- Heat pyrexia
- Ictus solaris
- Siriasis
- Thermoplegia

DEF: Headache, vertigo, cramps and elevated body temperature due to high environmental temperatures.

992.1 Heat syncope
- Heat collapse

992.2 Heat cramps

992.3 Heat exhaustion, anhydrotic
- Heat prostration due to water depletion

EXCLUDES that associated with salt depletion (992.4)

992.4 Heat exhaustion due to salt depletion
- Heat prostration due to salt (and water) depletion

992.5 Heat exhaustion, unspecified
- Heat prostration NOS

992.6 Heat fatigue, transient

992.7 Heat edema

DEF: Fluid retention due to high environmental temperatures.

992.8 Other specified heat effects
992.9 Unspecified

√4th **993** Effects of air pressure

993.0 Barotrauma, otitic
- Aero-otitis media
- Effects of high altitude on ears

DEF: Ringing ears, deafness, pain and vertigo due to air pressure changes.

993.1 Barotrauma, sinus
- Aerosinusitis
- Effects of high altitude on sinuses

993.2 Other and unspecified effects of high altitude
- Alpine sickness
- Andes disease
- Anoxia due to high altitude
- Hypobaropathy
- Mountain sickness

AHA: 3Q, '88, 4

993.3 Caisson disease
- Bends
- Compressed-air disease
- Decompression sickness
- Divers' palsy or paralysis

DEF: Rapid reduction in air pressure while breathing compressed air; symptoms include skin lesions, joint pains, respiratory and neurological problems.

993.4 Effects of air pressure caused by explosion
993.8 Other specified effects of air pressure
993.9 Unspecified effect of air pressure

√4th **994** Effects of other external causes

EXCLUDES certain adverse effects not elsewhere classified (995.0-995.8)

994.0 Effects of lightning
- Shock from lightning
- Struck by lightning NOS

EXCLUDES burns (940.0-949.5)

994.1 Drowning and nonfatal submersion
- Bathing cramp
- Immersion

AHA: 3Q, '88, 4

994.2 Effects of hunger
- Deprivation of food
- Starvation

994.3 Effects of thirst
- Deprivation of water

Tabular List — INJURY AND POISONING — 994.4–995.69

994.4 **Exhaustion due to exposure**

994.5 **Exhaustion due to excessive exertion**
Overexertion

994.6 **Motion sickness**
Air sickness
Seasickness
Travel sickness

994.7 **Asphyxiation and strangulation**
Suffocation (by):
bedclothes
cave-in
constriction
mechanical
plastic bag
pressure
strangulation
EXCLUDES asphyxia from:
carbon monoxide (986)
inhalation of food or foreign body (932-934.9)
other gases, fumes, and vapors (987.0-987.9)

994.8 **Electrocution and nonfatal effects of electric current**
Shock from electric current
EXCLUDES electric burns (940.0-949.5)

994.9 **Other effects of external causes**
Effects of:
abnormal gravitational [G] forces or states
weightlessness

995 Certain adverse effects not elsewhere classified
EXCLUDES complications of surgical and medical care (996.0-999.9)

995.0 **Other anaphylactic shock**
Allergic shock
Anaphylactic reaction } NOS or due to adverse effect of correct medicinal substance properly administered
Anaphylaxis

Use additional E code to identify external cause, such as:
adverse effects of correct medicinal substance properly administered [E930-E949]
EXCLUDES anaphylactic reaction to serum (999.4)
anaphylactic shock due to adverse food reaction (995.60-995.69)

AHA: 4Q, '93, 30

DEF: Immediate sensitivity response after exposure to specific antigen; results in life-threatening respiratory distress; usually followed by vascular collapse, shock, urticaria, angioedema and pruritus.

995.1 **Angioneurotic edema**
Giant urticaria
EXCLUDES urticaria:
due to serum (999.5)
other specified (698.2, 708.0-708.9, 757.33)

DEF: Circulatory response of deep dermis, subcutaneous or submucosal tissues; causes localized edema and wheals.

995.2 **Unspecified adverse effect of drug, medicinal and biological substance**
Adverse effect
Allergic reaction
Hypersensitivity
Idiosyncrasy } (due) to correct medicinal substance properly administered

Drug: hypersensitivity NOS
Drug: reaction NOS
EXCLUDES pathological drug intoxication (292.2)

AHA: 2Q, '97, 12; 3Q, '95, 13; 3Q, '92, 16

995.3 **Allergy, unspecified**
Allergic reaction NOS   Idiosyncrasy NOS
Hypersensitivity NOS
EXCLUDES allergic reaction NOS to correct medicinal substance properly administered (995.2)
specific types of allergic reaction, such as:
allergic diarrhea (558.3)
dermatitis (691.0-693.9)
hayfever (477.0-477.9)

995.4 **Shock due to anesthesia** CC
Shock due to anesthesia in which the correct substance was properly administered
EXCLUDES complications of anesthesia in labor or delivery (668.0-668.9)
overdose or wrong substance given (968.0-969.9)
postoperative shock NOS (998.0)
specified adverse effects of anesthesia classified elsewhere, such as:
anoxic brain damage (348.1)
hepatitis (070.0-070.9), etc.
unspecified adverse effect of anesthesia (995.2)

CC Excl: 958.4, 995.4, 997.91, 997.99, 998.0, 998.11-998.13, 998.81, 998.83-998.9

995.5 **Child maltreatment syndrome**
Use additional code(s), if applicable, to identify any associated injuries
Use additional E code to identify:
nature of abuse (E960-E968)
perpetrator (E967.0-E967.9)

AHA: 1Q, '98, 11

995.50 Child abuse, unspecified P

995.51 Child emotional/psychological abuse P
AHA: 4Q, '96, 38, 40

995.52 Child neglect (nutritional) P
AHA: 4Q, '96, 38, 40

995.53 Child sexual abuse P
AHA: 4Q, '96, 39, 40

995.54 Child physical abuse P
Battered baby or child syndrome
EXCLUDES shaken infant syndrome (995.55)
AHA: 3Q, '99, 14; 4Q, '96, 39, 40

995.55 Shaken infant syndrome P
Use additional code(s) to identify any associated injuries
AHA: 4Q, '96, 40, 43

995.59 Other child abuse and neglect P
Multiple forms of abuse

995.6 **Anaphylactic shock due to adverse food reaction**
Anaphylactic shock due to nonpoisonous foods
AHA: 4Q, '93, 30

995.60 Due to unspecified food
995.61 Due to peanuts
995.62 Due to crustaceans
995.63 Due to fruits and vegetables
995.64 Due to tree nuts and seeds
995.65 Due to fish
995.66 Due to food additives
995.67 Due to milk products
995.68 Due to eggs
995.69 Due to other specified food

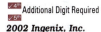 Additional Digit Required Nonspecific PDx Unacceptable PDx  Manifestation Code   **MSP** Medicare Secondary Payer   ▶◀ Revised Text   ● New Code   ▲ Revised Code Title

2002 Ingenix, Inc.

Volume 1 — 295

INJURY AND POISONING

995.7 **Other adverse food reactions, not elsewhere classified**
Use additional code to identify the type of reaction, such as:
hives (708.0)
wheezing (786.07)
EXCLUDES anaphylactic shock due to adverse food reaction (995.60-995.69)
asthma (493.0, 493.9)
dermatitis due to food (693.1)
in contact with skin (692.5)
gastroenteritis and colitis due to food (558.3)
rhinitis due to food (477.1)

√5th **995.8** **Other specified adverse effects, not elsewhere classified**

995.80 **Adult maltreatment, unspecified** A
Abused person NOS
Use additional code to identify:
any associated injury
perpetrator (E967.0-E967.9)
AHA: 4Q, '96, 41, 43

995.81 **Adult physical abuse** A
Battered:
person syndrome NEC
man
spouse
woman
Use additional code to identify:
any association injury
nature of abuse (E960-E968)
perpetrator (E967.0-E967.9)
AHA: 4Q, '96, 42, 43

995.82 **Adult emotional/psychological abuse** A
Use additional E code to identify perpetrator (E967.0-E967.9)

995.83 **Adult sexual abuse** A
Use additional code(s) to identify:
any associated injury
perpetrator (E967.0-E967.9)

995.84 **Adult neglect (nutritional)** A
Use addition code(s) to identify:
intent of neglect (E904.0, E968.4)
perpetrator (E967.0-E967.9)

995.85 **Other adult abuse and neglect** A
Multiple forms of abuse and neglect
Use additional code(s) to identify
any associated injury
intent of neglect (E904.0, E968.4)
nature of abuse (E960-E968)
perpetrator (E967.0-E967.9)

995.86 **Malignant hyperthermia** CC
Malignant hyperpyrexia due to anesthesia
CC Excl: 958.4, 995.4, 995.86, 997.91, 997.99, 998.0, 998.11-998.13, 998.81, 998.83-998.9
AHA: 4Q, '98, 51

995.89 **Other**
Hypothermia due to anesthesia

√5th **995.9** **Systemic inflammatory response syndrome (SIRS)**

995.90 **Systemic inflammatory response syndrome, unspecified** CC
SIRS NOS
CC Excl: 003.1, 020.2, 036.2, 038.0-038.9, 040.82, 040.89, 041.00-041.19, 041.2-041.7, 041.81-041.86, 041.89, 041.9, 054.5, 139.8, 995.90-995.94, V09.0-V09.91

995.91 **Systemic inflammatory response syndrome due to infectious process without organ dysfunction** CC
CC Excl: See code 995.90

995.92 **Systemic inflammatory response syndrome due to infectious process with organ dysfunction** CC
Severe sepsis
Use additional code to specify organ dysfunction, such as:
encephalopathy (348.3)
heart failure (428.0-428.9)
kidney failure (584.5-584.9, 585, 586)
CC Excl: See code 995.90

995.93 **Systemic inflammatory response syndrome due to noninfectious process without organ dysfunction** CC
CC Excl: See code 995.90

995.94 **Systemic inflammatory response syndrome due to noninfectious process with organ dysfunction** CC
Use additional code to specify organ dysfunction, such as:
encephalopathy (348.3)
heart failure (428.0-428.9)
kidney failure (584.5-584.9, 585, 586)
CC Excl: See code 995.90

COMPLICATIONS OF SURGICAL AND MEDICAL CARE, NOT ELSEWHERE CLASSIFIED (996-999)

EXCLUDES adverse effects of medicinal agents (001.0-799.9, 995.0-995.8)
burns from local applications and irradiation (940.0-949.5)
complications of:
conditions for which the procedure was performed
surgical procedures during abortion, labor, and delivery (630-676.9)
poisoning and toxic effects of drugs and chemicals (960.0-989.9)
postoperative conditions in which no complications are present, such as:
artificial opening status (V44.0-V44.9)
closure of external stoma (V55.0-V55.9)
fitting of prosthetic device (V52.0-V52.9)
specified complications classified elsewhere
anesthetic shock (995.4)
electrolyte imbalance (276.0-276.9)
postlaminectomy syndrome (722.80-722.83)
postmastectomy lymphedema syndrome (457.0)
postoperative psychosis (293.0-293.9)
any other condition classified elsewhere in the Alphabetic Index when described as due to a procedure

√4th **996** **Complications peculiar to certain specified procedures**
INCLUDES complications, not elsewhere classified, in the use of artificial substitutes [e.g., Dacron, metal, Silastic, Teflon] or natural sources [e.g., bone] involving:
anastomosis (internal)
graft (bypass) (patch)
implant
internal device:
catheter   fixation
electronic   prosthetic
reimplant
transplant
EXCLUDES accidental puncture or laceration during procedure (998.2)
complications of internal anastomosis of:
gastrointestinal tract (997.4)
urinary tract (997.5)
other specified complications classified elsewhere, such as:
hemolytic anemia (283.1)
functional cardiac disturbances (429.4)
serum hepatitis (070.2-070.3)
AHA: 1Q, '94, 3

INJURY AND POISONING

√5th 996.0 Mechanical complication of cardiac device, implant, and graft
Breakdown (mechanical)   Obstruction, mechanical
Displacement   Perforation
Leakage   Protrusion
AHA: 2Q, '93, 9

996.00 Unspecified device, implant, and graft [CC] [MSP]
CC Excl: 996.00, 996.04, 996.61-996.62, 996.70-996.74, 997.91, 997.99, 998.81, 998.83-998.9

996.01 Due to cardiac pacemaker (electrode) [CC] [MSP]
CC Excl: 996.01, 997.91, 997.99, 998.81, 998.83-998.9
AHA: 2Q, '99, 11

996.02 Due to heart valve prosthesis [CC] [MSP]
CC Excl: 996.02, 997.91, 997.99, 998.81, 998.83-998.9

996.03 Due to coronary bypass graft [CC] [MSP]
EXCLUDES atherosclerosis of graft (414.02, 414.03)
          embolism [occlusion NOS] [thrombus] of graft (996.72)
CC Excl: 996.03, 997.91, 997.99, 998.81, 998.83-998.9
AHA: 2Q, '95, 17; N-D, '86, 5

996.04 Due to automatic implantable cardiac defibrillator [CC]
CC Excl: 996.04, 997.91, 997.99, 998.81, 998.83-998.9

996.09 Other [CC] [MSP]
CC Excl: 996.09, 997.91, 997.99, 998.81, 998.83-998.9
AHA: 2Q, '93, 9

996.1 Mechanical complication of other vascular device, implant, and graft [CC] [MSP]
Mechanical complications involving:
  aortic (bifurcation) graft (replacement)
  arteriovenous:
    dialysis catheter ⎫
    fistula   ⎬ surgically created
    shunt   ⎭
  balloon (counterpulsation) device, intra-aortic
  carotid artery bypass graft
  femoral-popliteal bypass graft
  umbrella device, vena cava
EXCLUDES atherosclerosis of biological graft (440.30-440.32)
          embolism [occlusion NOS] [thrombus] of (biological) (synthetic) graft (996.74)
          peritoneal dialysis catheter (996.56)
CC Excl: 996.1, 997.91, 997.99, 998.81, 998.83-998.9
AHA: ▶1Q, '02, 13;◀ 1Q, '95, 3

996.2 Mechanical complication of nervous system device, implant, and graft [CC]
Mechanical complications involving:
  dorsal column stimulator
  electrodes implanted in brain [brain "pacemaker"]
  peripheral nerve graft
  ventricular (communicating) shunt
CC Excl: 996.2, 996.63, 996.75, 997.91, 997.99, 998.81, 998.83-998.9
AHA: 2Q, '99, 4; S-O, '87, 10

√5th 996.3 Mechanical complication of genitourinary device, implant, and graft
AHA: 3Q, '01, 13; S-O, '85, 3

996.30 Unspecified device, implant, and graft [CC] [MSP]
CC Excl: 996.30, 996.64-996.65, 996.76, 997.91, 997.99, 998.81, 998.83-998.9

996.31 Due to urethral [indwelling] catheter [MSP]

996.32 Due to intrauterine contraceptive device [MSP] ♂

996.39 Other [CC] [MSP]
Cystostomy catheter
Prosthetic reconstruction of vas deferens
Repair (graft) of ureter without mention of resection
EXCLUDES complications due to:
          external stoma of urinary tract (997.5)
          internal anastomosis of urinary tract (997.5)
CC Excl: 996.39, 996.64-996.65, 996.76, 997.91, 997.99, 998.81, 998.83-998.9

996.4 Mechanical complication of internal orthopedic device, implant, and graft [CC] [MSP]
Mechanical complications involving:
  external (fixation) device utilizing internal screw(s), pin(s) or other methods of fixation
  grafts of bone, cartilage, muscle, or tendon
  internal (fixation) device such as nail, plate, rod, etc.
EXCLUDES complications of external orthopedic device, such as:
          pressure ulcer due to cast (707.0)
CC Excl: 996.4, 996.66-996.67, 996.77-996.78, 997.91, 997.99, 998.81, 998.83-998.9
AHA: 2Q, '99, 10; 2Q, '98, 19; 2Q, '96, 11; 3Q, '95, 16; N-D, '85, 11

√5th 996.5 Mechanical complication of other specified prosthetic device, implant, and graft
Mechanical complications involving:
  prosthetic implant in:
    bile duct   chin
    breast   orbit of eye
  nonabsorbable surgical material NOS
  other graft, implant, and internal device, not elsewhere classified
AHA: 1Q, '98, 11

996.51 Due to corneal graft [CC]
CC Excl: 996.51, 997.91, 997.99

996.52 Due to graft of other tissue, not elsewhere classified [CC]
Skin graft failure or rejection
EXCLUDES failure of artificial skin graft (996.55)
          failure of decellularized allodermis (996.55)
          sloughing of temporary skin allografts or xenografts (pigskin)—omit code
CC Excl: 996.52, 996.55, 997.91, 997.99
AHA: 1Q, '96, 10

996.53 Due to ocular lens prosthesis [CC]
EXCLUDES contact lenses—code to condition
CC Excl: 996.53, 997.91, 997.99
AHA: 1Q, '00, 9

996.54 Due to breast prosthesis [CC]
Breast capsule (prosthesis)
Mammary implant
CC Excl: 996.54, 997.91, 997.99
AHA: 2Q, '98, 14; 3Q, '92, 4

996.55 Due to artificial skin graft and decellularized allodermis [CC]
Dislodgement   Non-adherence
Displacement   Poor incorporation
Failure   Shearing
CC Excl: 996.52, 996.55-996.60, 996.68-996.69, 996.70, 996.79, 997.91, 997.99
AHA: 4Q, '98, 52

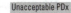 Nonspecific PDx

996.56 Due to peritoneal dialysis catheter [CC]
　　EXCLUDES *mechanical complication of arteriovenous dialysis catheter (996.1)*
　　CC Excl: 996.56, 996.59, 996.60, 996.68-996.70, 996.79, 997.91, 997.99
　　AHA: 4Q, '98, 54

996.59 Due to other implant and internal device, not elsewhere classified [CC]
　　Nonabsorbable surgical material NOS
　　Prosthetic implant in:
　　　bile duct
　　　chin
　　　orbit of eye
　　CC Excl: 996.59, 996.60, 996.68-996.70, 996.79, 997.91, 997.99
　　AHA: 2Q, '99, 13; 3Q, '94, 7

√5ᵗʰ **996.6 Infection and inflammatory reaction due to internal prosthetic device, implant, and graft**
　　Infection (causing obstruction) } due to (presence of) any device,
　　Inflammation } implant, and graft classifiable to 996.0-996.5
　　Use additional code to identify specified infections
　　AHA: 2Q, '89, 16; J-F, '87, 14

996.60 Due to unspecified device, implant, and graft [CC]
　　CC Excl: 996.00-996.30, 996.39, 996.4-996.79, 997.91, 997.99, 998.81, 998.83-998.9

996.61 Due to cardiac device, implant, and graft [CC]
　　Cardiac pacemaker or defibrillator:
　　　electrode(s), lead(s)
　　　pulse generator
　　　subcutaneous pocket
　　Coronary artery bypass graft
　　Heart valve prosthesis
　　CC Excl: 996.00-996.1, 996.52, 996.55-996.62, 996.68-996.74, 996.79, 997.91, 997.99, 998.81, 998.83-998.9

996.62 Due to other vascular device, implant, and graft [CC] [MC]
　　Arterial graft
　　Arteriovenous fistula or shunt
　　Infusion pump
　　Vascular catheter (arterial) (dialysis) (venous)
　　CC Excl: See code 996.61
　　AHA: 2Q, '94, 13

996.63 Due to nervous system device, implant, and graft [CC]
　　Electrodes implanted in brain
　　Peripheral nerve graft
　　Spinal canal catheter
　　Ventricular (communicating) shunt (catheter)
　　CC Excl: 996.2, 996.52, 996.55-996.60, 996.63, 996.68-996.70, 996.75, 996.79, 997.91, 997.99, 998.81, 998.83-998.9

996.64 Due to indwelling urinary catheter [CC]
　　Use additional code to identify specified infections, such as:
　　　Cystitis (595.0-595.9)
　　　Sepsis (038.0-038.9)
　　CC Excl: 599.0, 996.30, 996.39, 996.56-996.60, 996.64-996.65, 996.68-996.70, 996.76, 996.79, 997.91, 997.99, 998.81, 998.83-998.9

996.65 Due to other genitourinary device, implant, and graft [CC]
　　Intrauterine contraceptive device
　　CC Excl: 996.30, 996.39, 996.52, 996.55-996.60, 996.64-996.65, 996.68-996.70, 996.76, 996.79, 997.91, 997.99, 998.81, 998.83-998.9
　　AHA: 1Q, '00, 15

996.66 Due to internal joint prosthesis [CC]
　　CC Excl: 996.4, 996.52, 996.55-996.60, 996.66-996.70, 996.77-996.79, 997.91, 997.99, 998.81, 998.83-998.9
　　AHA: 2Q, '91, 18

996.67 Due to other internal orthopedic device, implant, and graft [CC]
　　Bone growth stimulator (electrode)
　　Internal fixation device (pin) (rod) (screw)
　　CC Excl: See code 996.66

996.68 Due to peritoneal dialysis catheter [CC]
　　Exit-site infection or inflammation
　　CC Excl: 996.56, 996.59, 996.60, 996.68-996.70, 996.79, 997.91, 997.99
　　AHA: 4Q, '98, 54

996.69 Due to other internal prosthetic device, implant, and graft [CC]
　　Breast prosthesis
　　Ocular lens prosthesis
　　Prosthetic orbital implant
　　CC Excl: 996.00-996.30, 996.39, 996.4-996.79, 997.91, 997.99, 998.81, 998.83-998.9
　　AHA: 4Q, '98, 52

√5ᵗʰ **996.7 Other complications of internal (biological) (synthetic) prosthetic device, implant, and graft**
　　Complication NOS }
　　　occlusion NOS }
　　Embolism } due to (presence of) any
　　Fibrosis } device, implant, and
　　Hemorrhage } graft classifiable to
　　Pain } 996.0-996.5
　　Stenosis }
　　Thrombus }
　　EXCLUDES *transplant rejection (996.8)*
　　AHA: 1Q, '89, 9; N-D, '86, 5

996.70 Due to unspecified device, implant, and graft [CC]
　　CC Excl: See code 996.69

996.71 Due to heart valve prosthesis [CC]
　　CC Excl: 996.00, 996.02, 996.09, 996.1, 996.52, 996.55-996.62, 996.68-996.74, 996.79, 997.91-997.99, 998.81, 998.83-998.9

996.72 Due to other cardiac device, implant, and graft [CC] [MC]
　　Cardiac pacemaker or defibrillator:
　　　electrode(s), lead(s)
　　　subcutaneous pocket
　　Coronary artery bypass (graft)
　　EXCLUDES *occlusion due to atherosclerosis ▶(414.02-414.06)◀*
　　CC Excl: 996.00-996.02, 996.04, 996.09, 996.1, 996.52, 996.55-996.62, 996.68-996.74, 996.79, 997.91-997.99, 998.81, 998.83-998.9
　　AHA: ▶3Q, '01, 20◀

996.73 Due to renal dialysis device, implant, and graft [CC]
　　CC Excl: 996.1, 996.52, 996.55-996.60, 996.68-996.70, 996.73, 996.79, 997.91, 997.99, 998.81, 998.83-998.9
　　AHA: 2Q, '91, 18

996.74 Due to other vascular device, implant, and graft [CC]
　　EXCLUDES *occlusion of biological graft due to atherosclerosis (440.30-440.32)*
　　CC Excl: 996.00-996.1, 996.52, 996.55-996.62, 996.68-996.74, 996.79, 997.91, 997.99, 998.81, 998.83-998.9

Tabular List — INJURY AND POISONING — 996.75–997.2

996.75 Due to nervous system device, implant, and graft CC
CC Excl: 996.2, 996.52, 996.55-996.60, 996.63, 996.68-996.70, 996.75, 996.79, 997.91, 997.99, 998.81, 998.83-998.9

996.76 Due to genitourinary device, implant, and graft CC
CC Excl: 996.30, 996.39, 996.52, 996.55-996.60, 996.64-996.65, 996.68-996.70, 996.76, 996.79, 997.91, 997.99, 998.81, 998.83-998.9

AHA: 1Q, '00, 15

996.77 Due to internal joint prosthesis CC
CC Excl: 996.4, 996.52, 996.55-996.60, 996.66-996.67, 996.69-996.70, 996.77-996.79, 997.91, 997.99, 998.81, 998.83-998.9

996.78 Due to other internal orthopedic device, implant, and graft CC
CC Excl: See code 996.77

996.79 Due to other internal prosthetic device, implant, and graft CC
CC Excl: 996.00-996.30, 996.39, 996.4-996.79, 997.91, 997.99, 998.81, 998.83-998.9

AHA: 1Q, '01, 8; 3Q, '95, 14; 3Q, '92, 4

√5th **996.8 Complications of transplanted organ**
Transplant failure or rejection
Use additional code to identify nature of complication, such as:
Cytomegalovirus (CMV) infection (078.5)
AHA: ▶3Q, '01, 12;◀ 3Q, '93, 3, 4; 2Q, '93, 11; 1Q, '93, 24

996.80 Transplanted organ, unspecified CC
CC Excl: 996.80, 996.87, 997.91, 997.99

996.81 Kidney CC
CC Excl: 996.81, 997.91, 997.99
AHA: 3Q, '98, 6, 7; 3Q, '94, 8; 2Q, '94, 9; 1Q, '93, 24

996.82 Liver CC
CC Excl: 996.82, 997.91, 997.99
AHA: 3Q, '98, 3, 4

996.83 Heart CC
CC Excl: 996.83, 997.91, 997.99
AHA: 3Q, '98, 5

996.84 Lung CC
CC Excl: 996.84, 997.91, 997.99
AHA: 3Q, '98, 5

996.85 Bone marrow CC
Graft-versus-host disease (acute) (chronic)
CC Excl: 996.85, 997.91, 997.99
AHA: 4Q, '90, 4

996.86 Pancreas CC
CC Excl: 996.86, 997.91, 997.99

996.87 Intestine CC
CC Excl: 996.80, 996.87, 997.91, 997.99

996.89 Other specified transplanted organ CC
CC Excl: 996.89, 997.91, 997.99
AHA: 3Q, '94, 5

√5th **996.9 Complications of reattached extremity or body part**
996.90 Unspecified extremity CC
CC Excl: 996.90, 997.91, 997.99, 998.81, 998.83-998.9

996.91 Forearm CC
CC Excl: 996.91, 997.91, 997.99, 998.81, 998.83-998.9

996.92 Hand CC
CC Excl: 996.92, 997.91, 997.99, 998.81, 998.83-998.9

996.93 Finger(s) CC
CC Excl: 996.93, 997.91, 997.99, 998.81, 998.83-998.9

996.94 Upper extremity, other and unspecified CC
CC Excl: 996.94, 997.91, 997.99, 998.81, 998.83-998.9

996.95 Foot and toe(s) CC
CC Excl: 996.95, 997.91, 997.99, 998.81, 998.83-998.9

996.96 Lower extremity, other and unspecified CC
CC Excl: 996.96, 997.91, 997.99, 998.81, 998.83-998.9

996.99 Other specified body part CC
CC Excl: 996.99, 997.91, 997.99, 998.81, 998.83-998.9

√4th **997 Complications affecting specified body systems, not elsewhere classified**
Use additional code to identify complications
EXCLUDES the listed conditions when specified as:
causing shock (998.0)
complications of:
anesthesia:
adverse effect (001.0-799.9, 995.0-995.8)
in labor or delivery (668.0-668.9)
poisoning (968.0-969.9)
implanted device or graft (996.0-996.9)
obstetrical procedures (669.0-669.4)
reattached extremity (996.90-996.96)
transplanted organ (996.80-996.89)

AHA: 1Q, '94, 4; 1Q, '93, 26

√5th **997.0 Nervous system complications**
CC Excl: For codes 997.00-997.09: 997.00-997.09, 997.91, 997.99, 998.81, 998.83, 998.89, 998.9

997.00 Nervous system complication, unspecified CC

997.01 Central nervous system complication CC
Anoxic brain damage
Cerebral hypoxia
EXCLUDES cerebrovascular hemorrhage or infarction (997.02)

997.02 Iatrogenic cerbrovascular infarction or hemorrhage CC
Postoperative stroke
AHA: 4Q, '95, 57

997.09 Other nervous system complications CC

997.1 Cardiac complications CC
Cardiac:
 arrest
 insufficiency   } during or resulting
Cardiorespiratory failure   from a procedure
Heart failure

EXCLUDES the listed conditions as long-term effects of cardiac surgery or due to the presence of cardiac prosthetic device (429.4)
CC Excl: 997.1, 997.91, 997.99, 998.81, 998.83-998.9

997.2 Peripheral vascular complications CC
Phlebitis or thrombophlebitis during or resulting from a procedure
EXCLUDES the listed conditions due to:
implant or catheter device (996.62)
infusion, perfusion, or transfusion (999.2)
complications affecting blood vessels (997.71-997.79)
CC Excl: 997.2, 997.79, 997.91, 997.99, 998.81, 998.83-998.9

DRG 130

√4th Additional Digit Required √5th
Nonspecific PDx   Unacceptable PDx   Manifestation Code   MSP Medicare Secondary Payer   ▶◀ Revised Text   ● New Code   ▲ Revised Code Title

2002 Ingenix, Inc.   January 2002 • Volume 1 — 299

INJURY AND POISONING

997.3 Respiratory complications [CC]
Mendelson's syndrome ⎫ resulting from a proce-
Pneumonia (aspiration) ⎭ dure

EXCLUDES iatrogenic [postoperative] pneumothorax (512.1)
iatrogenic pulmonary embolism (415.11)
Mendelson's syndrome in labor and delivery (668.0)
specified complications classified elsewhere, such as:
 adult respiratory distress syndrome (518.5)
 pulmonary edema, postoperative (518.4)
 respiratory insufficiency, acute, postoperative (518.5)
 shock lung (518.5)
 tracheostomy complications (519.00-519.09)

CC Excl: 997.3, 997.91, 997.99, 998.81, 998.83, 998.83-998.9

AHA: 1Q, '97, 10; 2Q, '93, 3; 2Q, '93, 9; 4Q, '90, 25

DEF: Mendelson's syndrome: acid pneumonitis due to aspiration of gastric acids, may occur after anesthesia or sedation.

997.4 Digestive system complications [CC]
Complications of:
 intestinal (internal) anastomosis and bypass, not elsewhere classified, except that involving urinary tract
Hepatic failure ⎫
Hepatorenal syndrome ⎬ specified as due to a procedure
Intestinal obstruction NOS ⎭

EXCLUDES gastrostomy complications (536.40-536.49)
specified gastrointestinal complications classified elsewhere, such as:
 blind loop syndrome (579.2)
 colostomy and enterostomy complications (569.60-569.69)
 gastrojejunal ulcer (534.0-534.9)
 infection of external stoma (569.61)
 pelvic peritoneal adhesions, female (614.6)
 peritoneal adhesions (568.0)
 peritoneal adhesions with obstruction (560.81)
 postcholecystectomy syndrome (576.0)
 postgastric surgery syndromes (564.2)

CC Excl: 536.40-536.49, 997.4, 997.71, 997.91, 997.99, 998.81, 998.83-998.9

AHA: 2Q, '01, 4-6; 3Q, '99, 4; 2Q, '99, 14; 3Q, '97, 7; 1Q, '97, 11; 2Q, '95, 7; 1Q, '93, 26; 3Q, '92, 15; 2Q, '89, 15; 1Q, '88, 14

DRG 188

997.5 Urinary complications [CC]
Complications of:
 external stoma of urinary tract
 internal anastomosis and bypass of urinary tract, including that involving intestinal tract
Oliguria or anuria ⎫
Renal: ⎪
 failure (acute) ⎬ specified as due to procedure
 insufficiency (acute) ⎪
Tubular necrosis (acute) ⎭

EXCLUDES specified complications classified elsewhere, such as:
postoperative stricture of:
 ureter (593.3)
 urethra (598.2)

CC Excl: 997.5, 997.72, 997.91, 997.99, 998.81, 998.83-998.9

AHA: 3Q, '96, 10, 15; 4Q, '95, 73; 1Q, '92, 13; 2Q, '89, 16; M-A, '87, 10; S-O, '85, 3

√5th 997.6 Amputation stump complication
EXCLUDES admission for treatment for a current traumatic amputation — code to complicated traumatic amputation
phantom limb (syndrome) (353.6)

AHA: 4Q, '95, 82

997.60 Unspecified complication
997.61 Neuroma of amputation stump
DEF: Hyperplasia generated nerve cell mass following amputation.

997.62 Infection (chronic) [CC]
Use additional code to identify the organism
CC Excl: 997.60, 997.62, 997.69, 997.91, 997.99, 998.81, 998.83-998.9

AHA: 4Q, '96, 46

997.69 Other

√5th 997.7 Vascular complications of other vessels
EXCLUDES peripheral vascular complications (997.2)

997.71 Vascular complications of mesenteric artery [CC]
CC Excl: 997.2, 997.71-997.79, 997.91, 997.99, 998.81, 998.83-998.9

AHA: ▶4Q, '01, 53◀

997.72 Vascular complications of renal artery [CC]
CC Excl: See code 997.71

997.79 Vascular complications of other vessels [CC]
CC Excl: See code 997.71

√5th 997.9 Complications affecting other specified body systems, not elsewhere classified [CC]
EXCLUDES specified complications classified elsewhere, such as:
 broad ligament laceration syndrome (620.6)
 postartificial menopause syndrome (627.4)
 postoperative stricture of vagina (623.2)

997.91 Hypertension
EXCLUDES essential hypertension (401.0-401.9)

AHA: 4Q, '95, 57

997.99 Other [CC]
Vitreous touch syndrome
CC Excl: 997.91, 997.99, 998.81, 998.83-998.9

AHA: 2Q, '94, 12; 1Q, '94, 17

DEF: Vitreous touch syndrome: vitreous protruding through pupil and attaches to corneal epithelium; causes aqueous fluid in vitreous body; marked by corneal edema, loss of lucidity; complication of cataract surgery.

√4th 998 Other complications of procedures, not elsewhere classified
AHA: 1Q, '94, 4

998.0 Postoperative shock [CC]
Collapse NOS ⎫ during or resulting
Shock (endotoxic) (hypo- ⎬ from a surgical
 volemic) (septic) ⎭ procedure

EXCLUDES shock:
 anaphylactic due to serum (999.4)
 anesthetic (995.4)
 electric (994.8)
 following abortion (639.5)
 obstetric (669.1)
 traumatic (958.4)

CC Excl: 958.4, 995.4, 997.91, 997.99, 998.0, 998.11-998.13, 998.81, 998.83-998.9

INJURY AND POISONING

998.1 **Hemorrhage or hematoma or seroma complicating a procedure**
  EXCLUDES hemorrhage, hematoma, or seroma:
    complicating cesarean section or puerperal perineal wound (674.3)

- **998.11 Hemorrhage complicating a procedure** CC
  CC Excl: 456.0, 456.20, 530.81-530.83, 530.89, 531.00-531.01, 531.20-531.21, 531.40-531.41, 531.60-531.61, 532.00-532.01, 532.20-532.21, 532.40-532.41, 532.60-532.61, 533.00-533.01, 533.20-533.21, 533.40-533.41, 533.60-533.61, 534.00-534.01, 534.20-534.21, 534.40-534.41, 534.60-534.61, 535.01, 535.11, 535.21, 535.31, 535.41, 535.51, 535.61, 537.83, 562.02-562.03, 562.12-562.13, 569.3, 569.85, 578.0-578.1, 578.9, 772.4, 997.91, 997.99, 998.0, 998.11-998.13, 998.81, 998.89, 998.9
  AHA: 4Q, '97, 52; 1Q, '97, 10

- **998.12 Hematoma complicating a procedure** CC
  CC Excl: see code 998.11

- **998.13 Seroma complicating a procedure** CC
  CC Excl: See code 998.11
  AHA: 4Q, '96, 46; 1Q, '93, 26; 2Q, '92, 15; S-O, '87, 8

998.2 **Accidental puncture or laceration during a procedure** CC
  Accidental perforation by catheter or other instrument during a procedure on:
    blood vessel
    nerve
    organ
  EXCLUDES iatrogenic [postoperative] pneumothorax (512.1)
    puncture or laceration caused by implanted device intentionally left in operation wound (996.0-996.5)
    specified complications classified elsewhere, such as:
      broad ligament laceration syndrome (620.6)
      trauma from instruments during delivery (664.0-665.9)
  CC Excl: 997.91, 997.99, 998.2, 998.81, 998.83-998.9
  AHA: 3Q, '94, 6; 3Q, '90, 17; 3Q, '90, 18

998.3 **Disruption of operation wound** CC
  Dehiscence } of operation wound
  Rupture
  EXCLUDES disruption of:
    cesarean wound (674.1)
    perineal wound, puerperal (674.2)
  CC Excl: 997.91, 997.99, 998.3, 998.81, 998.83-998.9
  AHA: 1Q, '93, 19

- **998.31 Disruption of internal operation wound** CC
  CC Excl: 997.91-997.99, 998.31, 998.32, 998.81-998.89, 998.9

- **998.32 Disruption of external operation wound** CC
  Disruption of operation wound NOS
  CC Excl: See code 998.31

998.4 **Foreign body accidentally left during a procedure** CC
  Adhesions   } due to foreign body accidentally left
  Obstruction } in operative wound or body
  Perforation } cavity during a procedure
  EXCLUDES obstruction or perforation caused by implanted device intentionally left in body (996.0-996.5)
  CC Excl: 997.91, 997.99, 998.4, 998.81, 998.83-998.9
  AHA: 1Q, '89, 9

998.5 **Postoperative infection**
  EXCLUDES infection due to:
    implanted device (996.60-996.69)
    infusion, perfusion, or transfusion (999.3)
    postoperative obstetrical wound infection (674.3)

- **998.51 Infected postoperative seroma** CC
  Use additional code to identify organism
  CC Excl: 997.91, 997.99, 998.51-998.59, 998.81, 998.83-998.9
  AHA: 4Q, '96, 46

- **998.59 Other postoperative infection** CC
  Abscess:
    intra-abdominal
    stitch
    subphrenic   } postoperative
    wound
  Septicemia
  Use additional code to identify infection
  CC Excl: See code 998.51
  AHA: 3Q, '98, 3; 3Q, '95, 5; 2Q, '95, 7; 3Q, '94, 6; 1Q, '93, 19; J-F, '87, 14

998.6 **Persistent postoperative fistula** CC
  CC Excl: 997.91, 997.99, 998.6, 998.81, 998.83-998.9
  AHA: J-F, '87, 14

998.7 **Acute reaction to foreign substance accidentally left during a procedure** CC
  Peritonitis: Peritonitis:
    aseptic   chemical
  CC Excl: 997.91, 997.99, 998.7, 998.81, 998.83-998.9

998.8 **Other specified complications of procedures, not elsewhere classified**
  AHA: 4Q, '94, 46; 1Q, '89, 9

- **998.81 Emphysema (subcutaneous) (surgical) resulting from a procedure**

- **998.82 Cataract fragments in eye following cataract surgery**

- **998.83 Non-healing surgical wound** CC
  CC Excl: 997.91, 997.99, 998.81, 998.83, 998.89, 998.9
  AHA: 4Q, '96, 47

- **998.89 Other specified complications** CC
  CC Excl: See code 998.83
  AHA: 3Q, '99, 13; 2Q, '98, 16

998.9 **Unspecified complication of procedure, not elsewhere classified** CC
  Postoperative complication NOS
  EXCLUDES complication NOS of obstetrical, surgery or procedure (669.4)
  CC Excl: See code 998.83
  AHA: 4Q, '93, 37

999 Complications of medical care, not elsewhere classified

INCLUDES complications, not elsewhere classified, of:
- dialysis (hemodialysis) (peritoneal) (renal)
- extracorporeal circulation
- hyperalimentation therapy
- immunization
- infusion
- inhalation therapy
- injection
- inoculation
- perfusion
- transfusion
- vaccination
- ventilation therapy

EXCLUDES specified complications classified elsewhere such as:
- complications of implanted device (996.0-996.9)
- contact dermatitis due to drugs (692.3)
- dementia dialysis (294.8)
    - transient (293.9)
- dialysis disequilibrium syndrome (276.0-276.9)
- poisoning and toxic effects of drugs and chemicals (960.0-989.9)
- postvaccinal encephalitis (323.9)
- water and electrolyte imbalance (276.0-276.9)

999.0 Generalized vaccinia
DEF: Skin eruption, self-limiting; follows vaccination; due to transient viremia with virus localized in skin.

999.1 Air embolism
Air embolism to any site following infusion, perfusion, or transfusion

EXCLUDES embolism specified as: complicating:
- abortion (634-638 with .6, 639.6)
- ectopic or molar pregnancy (639.6)
- pregnancy, childbirth, or the puerperium (673.0)
- due to implanted device (996.7)
- traumatic (958.0)

CC Excl: 958.0, 999.1

999.2 Other vascular complications
- Phlebitis
- Thromboembolism } following infusion, perfusion, or transfusion
- Thrombophlebitis

EXCLUDES the listed conditions when specified as:
- due to implanted device (996.61-996.62, 996.72-996.74)
- postoperative NOS (997.2, 997.71-997.79)

CC Excl: 999.2

AHA: 2Q, '97, 5

999.3 Other infection
- Infection
- Sepsis   } following infusion, injection, transfusion, or vaccination
- Septicemia

EXCLUDES the listed conditions when specified as:
- due to implanted device (996.60-996.69)
- postoperative NOS (998.51-998.59)

CC Excl: 999.3

AHA: 2Q, '01, 11, 12; 2Q, '97, 5; J-F, '87, 14

999.4 Anaphylactic shock due to serum
EXCLUDES shock:
- allergic NOS (995.0)
- anaphylactic:
    - NOS (995.0)
    - due to drugs and chemicals (995.0)

CC Excl: 999.4

DEF: Life-threatening hypersensitivity to foreign serum; causes respiratory distress, vascular collapse, and shock.

999.5 Other serum reaction
- Intoxication by serum
- Protein sickness
- Serum rash
- Serum sickness
- Urticaria due to serum

EXCLUDES serum hepatitis (070.2-070.3)

CC Excl: 999.5

DEF: Serum sickness: Hypersensitivity to foreign serum; causes fever, hives, swelling, and lymphadenopathy.

999.6 ABO incompatibility reaction
- Incompatible blood transfusion
- Reaction to blood group incompatibility in infusion or transfusion

CC Excl: 999.6

999.7 Rh incompatibility reaction
Reactions due to Rh factor in infusion or transfusion

CC Excl: 999.7

999.8 Other transfusion reaction
- Septic shock due to transfusion
- Transfusion reaction NOS

EXCLUDES postoperative shock (998.0)

CC Excl: 999.8

AHA: 3Q, '00, 9

999.9 Other and unspecified complications of medical care, not elsewhere classified
Complications, not elsewhere classified, of:
- electroshock
- inhalation
- ultrasound   } therapy
- ventilation

Unspecified misadventure of medical care

EXCLUDES unspecified complication of:
- phototherapy (990)
- radiation therapy (999)

AHA: 2Q, '97, 5

| Tabular List | V CODES | V01–V05.3 |

SUPPLEMENTARY CLASSIFICATION OF FACTORS INFLUENCING HEALTH STATUS AND CONTACT WITH HEALTH SERVICES (V01-V83)

This classification is provided to deal with occasions when circumstances other than a disease or injury classifiable to categories 001-999 (the main part of ICD) are recorded as "diagnoses" or "problems." This can arise mainly in three ways:

a) When a person who is not currently sick encounters the health services for some specific purpose, such as to act as a donor of an organ or tissue, to receive prophylactic vaccination, or to discuss a problem which is in itself not a disease or injury. This will be a fairly rare occurrence among hospital inpatients, but will be relatively more common among hospital outpatients and patients of family practitioners, health clinics, etc.

b) When a person with a known disease or injury, whether it is current or resolving, encounters the health care system for a specific treatment of that disease or injury (e.g., dialysis for renal disease; chemotherapy for malignancy; cast change).

c) When some circumstance or problem is present which influences the person's health status but is not in itself a current illness or injury. Such factors may be elicited during population surveys, when the person may or may not be currently sick, or be recorded as an additional factor to be borne in mind when the person is receiving care for some current illness or injury classifiable to categories 001-999.

In the latter circumstances the V code should be used only as a supplementary code and should not be the one selected for use in primary, single cause tabulations. Examples of these circumstances are a personal history of certain diseases, or a person with an artificial heart valve in situ.

AHA: J-F, '87, 8

PERSONS WITH POTENTIAL HEALTH HAZARDS RELATED TO COMMUNICABLE DISEASES (V01-V06)

EXCLUDES family history of infectious and parasitic diseases (V18.8)
personal history of infectious and parasitic diseases (V12.0)

V01 Contact with or exposure to communicable diseases
- **V01.0** Cholera
  - Conditions classifiable to 001
- **V01.1** Tuberculosis
  - Conditions classifiable to 010-018
- **V01.2** Poliomyelitis
  - Conditions classifiable to 045
- **V01.3** Smallpox
  - Conditions classifiable to 050
- **V01.4** Rubella
  - Conditions classifiable to 056
- **V01.5** Rabies
  - Conditions classifiable to 071
- **V01.6** Venereal diseases
  - Conditions classifiable to 090-099
- **V01.7** Other viral diseases
  - Conditions classifiable to 042-078 and V08, except as above
  - AHA: 2Q, '92, 11
- **V01.8** Other communicable diseases
  - Conditions classifiable to 001-136, except as above
  - AHA: J-A, '87, 24
  - • V01.81 Anthrax
  - • V01.89 Other communicable diseases
- **V01.9** Unspecified communicable disease

V02 Carrier or suspected carrier of infectious diseases
  AHA: 3Q, '95, 18; 3Q, '94, 4
- **V02.0** Cholera
- **V02.1** Typhoid
- **V02.2** Amebiasis
- **V02.3** Other gastrointestinal pathogens
- **V02.4** Diphtheria
- **V02.5** Other specified bacterial diseases
  - V02.51 Group B streptococcus
    - AHA: ▶1Q, '02, 14;◀ 4Q, '98, 56
  - V02.52 Other streptococcus
  - V02.59 Other specified bacterial diseases
    - Meningococcal
    - Staphylococcal
- **V02.6** Viral hepatitis
  - Hepatitis Australian-antigen [HAA] [SH] carrier
  - Serum hepatitis carrier
  - V02.60 Viral hepatitis carrier, unspecified
    - AHA: 4Q, '97, 47
  - V02.61 Hepatitis B carrier
    - AHA: 4Q, '97, 47
  - V02.62 Hepatitis C carrier
    - AHA: 4Q, '97, 47
  - V02.69 Other viral hepatitis carrier
    - AHA: 4Q, '97, 47
- **V02.7** Gonorrhea
- **V02.8** Other venereal diseases
- **V02.9** Other specified infectious organism
  - AHA: 3Q, '95, 18; 1Q, '93, 22; J-A, '87, 24

V03 Need for prophylactic vaccination and inoculation against bacterial diseases
  EXCLUDES vaccination not carried out because of contraindication (V64.0)
  vaccines against combinations of diseases (V06.0-V06.9)
- **V03.0** Cholera alone
- **V03.1** Typhoid-paratyphoid alone [TAB]
- **V03.2** Tuberculosis [BCG]
- **V03.3** Plague
- **V03.4** Tularemia
- **V03.5** Diphtheria alone
- **V03.6** Pertussis alone
- **V03.7** Tetanus toxoid alone
- **V03.8** Other specified vaccinations against single bacterial diseases
  - V03.81 Hemophilus influenza, type B [Hib]
  - V03.82 Streptococcus pneumoniae [pneumococcus]
  - V03.89 Other specified vaccination
    - AHA: 2Q, '00, 9
- **V03.9** Unspecified single bacterial disease

V04 Need for prophylactic vaccination and inoculation against certain viral diseases
  EXCLUDES vaccines against combinations of diseases (V06.0-V06.9)
- **V04.0** Poliomyelitis
- **V04.1** Smallpox
- **V04.2** Measles alone
- **V04.3** Rubella alone
- **V04.4** Yellow fever
- **V04.5** Rabies
- **V04.6** Mumps alone
- **V04.7** Common cold
- **V04.8** Influenza

V05 Need for other prophylactic vaccination and inoculation against single diseases
  EXCLUDES vaccines against combinations of diseases (V06.0-V06.9)
- **V05.0** Arthropod-borne viral encephalitis
- **V05.1** Other arthropod-borne viral diseases
- **V05.2** Leishmaniasis
- **V05.3** Viral hepatitis

V CODES — Tabular List

V05.4–V10.09

- **V05.4** Varicella
  - Chickenpox
- **V05.8** Other specified disease
  - AHA: 1Q, '01, 4; 3Q, '91, 20
- **V05.9** Unspecified single disease

✓4th **V06** Need for prophylactic vaccination and inoculation against combinations of diseases
  - Note: Use additional single vaccination codes from categories V03-V05 to identify any vaccinations not included in a combination code.
- **V06.0** Cholera with typhoid-paratyphoid [cholera+TAB]
- **V06.1** Diphtheria-tetanus-pertussis, combined [DTP]
  - AHA: 3Q, '98, 13
- **V06.2** Diphtheria-tetanus-pertussis with typhoid-paratyphoid [DTP+TAB]
- **V06.3** Diphtheria-tetanus-pertussis with poliomyelitis [DTP+polio]
- **V06.4** Measles-mumps-rubella [MMR]
- **V06.5** Tetanus-diphtheria [Td]
- **V06.6** Streptococcus pneumoniae [pneumococcus] and influenza
- **V06.8** Other combinations
  - EXCLUDES multiple single vaccination codes (V03.0-V05.9)
  - AHA: 1Q, '94, 19
- **V06.9** Unspecified combined vaccine

PERSONS WITH NEED FOR ISOLATION, OTHER POTENTIAL HEALTH HAZARDS AND PROPHYLACTIC MEASURES (V07-V09)

✓4th **V07** Need for isolation and other prophylactic measures
  - EXCLUDES prophylactic organ removal (V50.41-V50.49)
- ³ **V07.0** Isolation
  - Admission to protect the individual from his surroundings or for isolation of individual after contact with infectious diseases
- **V07.1** Desensitization to allergens
- **V07.2** Prophylactic immunotherapy
  - Administration of:
    - antivenin
    - immune sera [gamma globulin]
    - RhoGAM
    - tetanus antitoxin
- ✓5th **V07.3** Other prophylactic chemotherapy
  - **V07.31** Prophylactic fluoride administration
  - ³ **V07.39** Other prophylactic chemotherapy
    - EXCLUDES maintenance chemotherapy following disease (V58.1)
- **V07.4** Postmenopausal hormone replacement therapy ♀
- ³ **V07.8** Other specified prophylactic measure
  - AHA: 1Q, '92, 11
- **V07.9** Unspecified prophylactic measure

³ **V08** Asymptomatic human immunodeficiency virus [HIV] infection status
  - HIV positive NOS
  - Note: This code is *only* to be used when no HIV infection symptoms or conditions are present. If any HIV infection symptoms or conditions are present, see code 042.
  - EXCLUDES AIDS (042)
    - human immunodeficiency virus [HIV] disease (042)
    - exposure to HIV (V01.7)
    - nonspecific serologic evidence of HIV (795.71)
    - symptomatic human immunodeficiency virus [HIV] infection (042)
  - AHA: 2Q, '99, 8; 3Q, '95, 18

✓4th **V09** Infection with drug-resistant microorganisms
  - Note: This category is intended for use as an additional code for infectious conditions classified elsewhere to indicate the presence of drug-resistance of the infectious organism.
  - AHA: 3Q, '94, 4; 4Q, '93, 22
- **V09.0** Infection with microorganisms resistant to penicillins
- **V09.1** Infection with microorganisms resistant to cephalosporins and other B-lactam antibiotics
- **V09.2** Infection with microorganisms resistant to macrolides
- **V09.3** Infection with microorganisms resistant to tetracyclines
- **V09.4** Infection with microorganisms resistant to aminoglycosides
- ✓5th **V09.5** Infection with microorganisms resistant to quinolones and fluoroquinolones
  - **V09.50** Without mention of resistance to multiple quinolones and fluoroquinoles
  - **V09.51** With resistance to multiple quinolones and fluoroquinoles
- **V09.6** Infection with microorganisms resistant to sulfonamides
- ✓5th **V09.7** Infection with microorganisms resistant to other specified antimycobacterial agents
  - EXCLUDES Amikacin (V09.4)
    - Kanamycin (V09.4)
    - Streptomycin [SM] (V09.4)
  - **V09.70** Without mention of resistance to multiple antimycobacterial agents
  - **V09.71** With resistance to multiple antimycobacterial agents
- ✓5th **V09.8** Infection with microorganisms resistant to other specified drugs
  - **V09.80** Without mention of resistance to multiple drugs
  - **V09.81** With resistance to multiple drugs
- ✓5th **V09.9** Infection with drug-resistant microorganisms, unspecified
  - Drug resistance, NOS
  - **V09.90** Without mention of multiple drug resistance
  - **V09.91** With multiple drug resistance
    - Multiple drug resistance NOS

PERSONS WITH POTENTIAL HEALTH HAZARDS RELATED TO PERSONAL AND FAMILY HISTORY (V10-V19)

EXCLUDES obstetric patients where the possibility that the fetus might be affected is the reason for observation or management during pregnancy (655.0-655.9)

AHA: J-F, '87, 1

✓4th **V10** Personal history of malignant neoplasm
  - AHA: 4Q, '98, 69; 1Q, '95, 4; 3Q, '92, 5; M-J, '85, 10; 2Q, '90, 9
- ✓5th **V10.0** Gastrointestinal tract
  - History of conditions classifiable to 140-159
  - **V10.00** Gastrointestinal tract, unspecified
  - **V10.01** Tongue
  - **V10.02** Other and unspecified oral cavity and pharynx
  - **V10.03** Esophagus
  - **V10.04** Stomach
  - **V10.05** Large intestine
    - AHA: 3Q, '99, 7; 1Q, '95, 4
  - **V10.06** Rectum, rectosigmoid junction, and anus
  - **V10.07** Liver
  - **V10.09** Other

³ These V codes may be used as principal diagnosis on Medicare patients.

V CODES

√5th V10.1 Trachea, bronchus, and lung
History of conditions classifiable to 162
- V10.11 Bronchus and lung
- V10.12 Trachea

√5th V10.2 Other respiratory and intrathoracic organs
History of conditions classifiable to 160, 161, 163-165
- V10.20 Respiratory organ, unspecified
- V10.21 Larynx
- V10.22 Nasal cavities, middle ear, and accessory sinuses
- V10.29 Other

V10.3 Breast
History of conditions classifiable to 174 and 175
AHA: 4Q, '01, 66; 4Q, '98, 65; 4Q, '97, 50; 1Q, '91, 16; 1Q, '90, 21

√5th V10.4 Genital organs
History of conditions classifiable to 179-187
- V10.40 Female genital organ, unspecified ♀
- V10.41 Cervix uteri ♀
- V10.42 Other parts of uterus ♀
- V10.43 Ovary ♀
- V10.44 Other female genital organs ♀
- V10.45 Male genital organ, unspecified ♂
- V10.46 Prostate ♂
- V10.47 Testis ♂
- V10.48 Epididymis ♂
- V10.49 Other male genital organs ♂

√5th V10.5 Urinary organs
History of conditions classifiable to 188 and 189
- V10.50 Urinary organ, unspecified
- V10.51 Bladder
- V10.52 Kidney
  - EXCLUDES renal pelvis (V10.53)
- V10.53 Renal pelvis
  AHA: 4Q, '01, 55
- V10.59 Other

√5th V10.6 Leukemia
Conditions classifiable to 204-208
EXCLUDES leukemia in remission (204-208)
AHA: 2Q, '92, 13; 4Q, '91, 26; 4Q, '90, 3
- V10.60 Leukemia, unspecified
- V10.61 Lymphoid leukemia
- V10.62 Myeloid leukemia
- V10.63 Monocytic leukemia
- V10.69 Other

√5th V10.7 Other lymphatic and hematopoietic neoplasms
Conditions classifiable to 200-203
EXCLUDES listed conditions in 200-203 in remission
AHA: M-J, '85, 18
- V10.71 Lymphosarcoma and reticulosarcoma
- V10.72 Hodgkin's disease
- V10.79 Other

√5th V10.8 Personal history of malignant neoplasm of other sites
History of conditions classifiable to 170-173, 190-195
- V10.81 Bone
- V10.82 Malignant melanoma of skin
- V10.83 Other malignant neoplasm of skin
- V10.84 Eye
- V10.85 Brain
  AHA: 1Q, '01, 6
- V10.86 Other parts of nervous system
  EXCLUDES peripheral sympathetic, and parasympa-thetic nerves (V10.89)
- V10.87 Thyroid
- V10.88 Other endocrine glands and related structures
- V10.89 Other
- V10.9 Unspecified personal history of malignant neoplasm

√4th V11 Personal history of mental disorder
- V11.0 Schizophrenia
  EXCLUDES that in remission (295.0-295.9 with fifth-digit 5)
- V11.1 Affective disorders
  Personal history of manic-depressive psychosis
  EXCLUDES that in remission (296.0-296.6 with fifth-digit 5, 6)
- V11.2 Neurosis
- V11.3 Alcoholism
- V11.8 Other mental disorders
- V11.9 Unspecified mental disorder

√4th V12 Personal history of certain other diseases
AHA: 3Q, '92, 11

√5th V12.0 Infectious and parasitic diseases
- V12.00 Unspecified infectious and parasitic disease
- V12.01 Tuberculosis
- V12.02 Poliomyelitis
- V12.03 Malaria
- V12.09 Other

- V12.1 Nutritional deficiency
- V12.2 Endocrine, metabolic, and immunity disorders
  EXCLUDES history of allergy (V14.0-V14.9, V15.01-V15.09)
- V12.3 Diseases of blood and blood-forming organs

√5th V12.4 Disorders of nervous system and sense organs
- V12.40 Unspecified disorder of nervous system and sense organs
- V12.41 Benign neoplasm of the brain
  AHA: 4Q, '97, 48
- V12.49 Other disorders of nervous system and sense organs
  AHA: 4Q, '98, 59

√5th V12.5 Diseases of circulatory system
AHA: 4Q, '95, 61
EXCLUDES old myocardial infarction (412)
postmyocardial infarction syndrome (411.0)
- V12.50 Unspecified circulatory disease
- V12.51 Venous thrombosis and embolism
  Pulmonary embolism
  AHA: ▶1Q, '02, 15◀
- V12.52 Thrombophlebitis
- V12.59 Other
  AHA: 4Q, '99, 4; 4Q, '98, 88; 4Q, '97, 37

- V12.6 Diseases of respiratory system

√5th V12.7 Diseases of digestive system
AHA: 1Q, '95, 3; 2Q, '89, 16
- V12.70 Unspecified digestive disease
- V12.71 Peptic ulcer disease
- V12.72 Colonic polyps
- V12.79 Other

√4th V13 Personal history of other diseases
√5th V13.0 Disorders of urinary system
- V13.00 Unspecified urinary disorder
- V13.01 Urinary calculi
- V13.09 Other

- V13.1 Trophoblastic disease ♀
  EXCLUDES supervision during a current pregnancy (V23.1)

V CODES — Tabular List

V13.2–V16.6

- **V13.2** Other genital system and obstetric disorders
  - EXCLUDES: supervision during a current pregnancy of a woman with poor obstetric history (V23.0-V23.9)
  - habitual aborter (646.3)
  - without current pregnancy (629.9)
  - **V13.21** Personal history of pre-term labor
    - EXCLUDES: current pregnancy with history of pre-term labor (V23.41)
  - **V13.29** Other genital system and obstetric disorders
- **V13.3** Diseases of skin and subcutaneous tissue
- **V13.4** Arthritis
- **V13.5** Other musculoskeletal disorders
- **V13.6** Congenital malformations
  - AHA: 4Q, '98, 63
  - **V13.61** Hypospadias ♂
  - **V13.69** Other congenital malformations
- **V13.7** Perinatal problems
  - EXCLUDES: low birth weight status (V21.30-V21.35)
- **V13.8** Other specified diseases
- **V13.9** Unspecified disease

V14 Personal history of allergy to medicinal agents
- **V14.0** Penicillin
- **V14.1** Other antibiotic agent
- **V14.2** Sulfonamides
- **V14.3** Other anti-infective agent
- **V14.4** Anesthetic agent
- **V14.5** Narcotic agent
- **V14.6** Analgesic agent
- **V14.7** Serum or vaccine
- **V14.8** Other specified medicinal agents
- **V14.9** Unspecified medicinal agent

V15 Other personal history presenting hazards to health
- **V15.0** Allergy, other than to medicinal agents
  - EXCLUDES: allergy to food substance used as base for medicinal agent (V14.0-V14.9)
  - AHA: 4Q, '00, 42, 49
  - **V15.01** Allergy to peanuts
  - **V15.02** Allergy to milk products
    - EXCLUDES: lactose intolerance (271.3)
  - **V15.03** Allergy to eggs
  - **V15.04** Allergy to seafood
    - Seafood (octopus) (squid) ink
    - Shellfish
  - **V15.05** Allergy to other foods
    - Food additives
    - Nuts other than peanuts
  - **V15.06** Allergy to insects
    - Bugs
    - Insect bites and stings
    - Spiders
  - **V15.07** Allergy to latex
    - Latex sensitivity
  - **V15.08** Allergy to radiographic dye
    - Contrast media used for diagnostic x-ray procedures
  - **V15.09** Other allergy, other than to medicinal agents
- **V15.1** Surgery to heart and great vessels
  - EXCLUDES: replacement by transplant or other means (V42.1-V42.2, V43.2-V43.4)
- **V15.2** Surgery to other major organs
  - EXCLUDES: replacement by transplant or other means (V42.0-V43.8)
- **V15.3** Irradiation
  - Previous exposure to therapeutic or other ionizing radiation
- **V15.4** Psychological trauma
  - EXCLUDES: history of condition classifiable to 290-316 (V11.0-V11.9)
  - **V15.41** History of physical abuse
    - Rape
    - AHA: 3Q, '99, 15
  - **V15.42** History of emotional abuse
    - Neglect
    - AHA: 3Q, '99, 15
  - **V15.49** Other
    - AHA: 3Q, '99, 15
- **V15.5** Injury
- **V15.6** Poisoning
- **V15.7** Contraception
  - EXCLUDES: current contraceptive management (V25.0-V25.4)
  - presence of intrauterine contraceptive device as incidental finding (V45.5)
- **V15.8** Other specified personal history presenting hazards to health
  - AHA: 4Q, '95, 62
  - **V15.81** Noncompliance with medical treatment
    - AHA: 2Q, '01, 11; 12, 13; 2Q '99, 17; 2Q, '97, 11; 1Q, '97, 12; 3Q, '96, 9
  - **V15.82** History of tobacco use
    - EXCLUDES: tobacco dependence (305.1)
  - **V15.84** Exposure to asbestos
  - **V15.85** Exposure to potentially hazardous body fluids
  - **V15.86** Exposure to lead
  - **V15.89** Other
    - AHA: 1Q, '90, 21; N-D, '84, 12
- **V15.9** Unspecified personal history presenting hazards to health

V16 Family history of malignant neoplasm
- **V16.0** Gastrointestinal tract
  - Family history of condition classifiable to 140-159
  - AHA: 1Q, '99, 4
- **V16.1** Trachea, bronchus, and lung
  - Family history of condition classifiable to 162
- **V16.2** Other respiratory and intrathoracic organs
  - Family history of condition classifiable to 160-161, 163-165
- **V16.3** Breast
  - Family history of condition classifiable to 174
  - AHA: 2Q, '00, 8; 1Q, '92, 11
- **V16.4** Genital organs
  - Family history of condition classifiable to 179-187
  - AHA: 4Q, '97, 48
  - **V16.40** Genital organ, unspecified
  - **V16.41** Ovary
  - **V16.42** Prostate
  - **V16.43** Testis
  - **V16.49** Other
- **V16.5** Urinary organs
  - Family history of condition classifiable to 189
  - **V16.51** Kidney
  - **V16.59** Other
- **V16.6** Leukemia
  - Family history of condition classifiable to 204-208

	Tabular List	**V CODES**		**V16.7–V23.81**

V16.7	Other lymphatic and hematopoietic neoplasms	
	Family history of condition classifiable to 200-203	
V16.8	Other specified malignant neoplasm	
	Family history of other condition classifiable to 140-199	
V16.9	Unspecified malignant neoplasm	

✓4th V17 Family history of certain chronic disabling diseases
- V17.0 Psychiatric condition
  - EXCLUDES   *family history of mental retardation (V18.4)*
- V17.1 Stroke (cerebrovascular)
- V17.2 Other neurological diseases
  - Epilepsy
  - Huntington's chorea
- V17.3 Ischemic heart disease
- V17.4 Other cardiovascular diseases
- V17.5 Asthma
- V17.6 Other chronic respiratory conditions
- V17.7 Arthritis
- V17.8 Other musculoskeletal diseases

✓4th V18 Family history of certain other specific conditions
- V18.0 Diabetes mellitus
- V18.1 Other endocrine and metabolic diseases
- V18.2 Anemia
- V18.3 Other blood disorders
- V18.4 Mental retardation
- V18.5 Digestive disorders
- ✓5th V18.6 Kidney diseases
  - V18.61 Polycystic kidney
  - V18.69 Other kidney diseases
- V18.7 Other genitourinary diseases
- V18.8 Infectious and parasitic diseases

✓4th V19 Family history of other conditions
- V19.0 Blindness or visual loss
- V19.1 Other eye disorders
- V19.2 Deafness or hearing loss
- V19.3 Other ear disorders
- V19.4 Skin conditions
- V19.5 Congenital anomalies
- V19.6 Allergic disorders
- V19.7 Consanguinity
- V19.8 Other condition

PERSONS ENCOUNTERING HEALTH SERVICES IN CIRCUMSTANCES RELATED TO REPRODUCTION AND DEVELOPMENT (V20-V28)

✓4th V20 Health supervision of infant or child
- [3] V20.0 Foundling   **P**
- V20.1 Other healthy infant or child receiving care   **P**
  - Medical or nursing care supervision of healthy infant in cases of:
    - maternal illness, physical or psychiatric
    - socioeconomic adverse condition at home
    - too many children at home preventing or interfering with normal care
  - **AHA:** 1Q, '00, 25; 3Q, '89, 14
- V20.2 Routine infant or child health check   **P**
  - Developmental testing of infant or child
  - Immunizations appropriate for age
  - Routine vision and hearing testing
  - Use additional code(s) to identify:
    - special screening examination(s) performed (V73.0-V82.9)
  - EXCLUDES   *special screening for developmental handicaps (V79.3)*

✓4th V21 Constitutional states in development
- V21.0 Period of rapid growth in childhood
- V21.1 Puberty
- V21.2 Other adolescence
- ✓5th V21.3 Low birth weight status
  - EXCLUDES   *history of perinatal problems*
  - **AHA:** 4Q, '00, 51
  - V21.30 Low birth weight status, unspecified
  - V21.31 Low birth weight status, less than 500 grams
  - V21.32 Low birth weight status, 500-999 grams
  - V21.33 Low birth weight status, 1000-1499 grams
  - V21.34 Low birth weight status, 1500-1999 grams
  - V21.35 Low birth weight status, 2000-2500 grams
- V21.8 Other specified constitutional states in development
- V21.9 Unspecified constitutional state in development

✓4th V22 Normal pregnancy
  - EXCLUDES   *pregnancy examination or test, pregnancy unconfirmed (V72.4)*
- V22.0 Supervision of normal first pregnancy   ♀
  - **AHA:** 3Q, '99, 16
- V22.1 Supervision of other normal pregnancy   ♀
  - **AHA:** 3Q, '99, 16
- V22.2 Pregnant state, incidental   ♀
  - Pregnant state NOS

✓4th V23 Supervision of high-risk pregnancy
  - **AHA:** 1Q, 90, 10
- V23.0 Pregnancy with history of infertility   **M** ♀
- V23.1 Pregnancy with history of trophoblastic disease   **M** ♀
  - Pregnancy with history of:
    - hydatidiform mole
    - vesicular mole
  - EXCLUDES   *that without current pregnancy (V13.1)*
- V23.2 Pregnancy with history of abortion   **M** ♀
  - Pregnancy with history of conditions classifiable to 634-638
  - EXCLUDES   *habitual aborter:*
    - *care during pregnancy (646.3)*
    - *that without current pregnancy (629.9)*
- V23.3 Grand multiparity   **M** ♀
  - EXCLUDES   *care in relation to labor and delivery (659.4)*
    - *that without current pregnancy (V61.5)*
- ✓5th V23.4 Pregnancy with other poor obstetric history
  - Pregnancy with history of other conditions classifiable to 630-676
  - ● V23.41 Pregnancy with history of pre-term labor   **M** ♀
  - ● V23.49 Pregnancy with other poor obstetric history   **M** ♀
- V23.5 Pregnancy with other poor reproductive history   **M** ♀
  - Pregnancy with history of stillbirth or neonatal death
- V23.7 Insufficient prenatal care   **CC** **M** ♀
  - History of little or no prenatal care
  - **CC Excl:** V22.0-V22.2, V23.0-V23.9
- ✓5th V23.8 Other high-risk pregnancy
  - **AHA:** 4Q, '98, 56, 63
  - V23.81 Elderly primigravida   **CC** **M** ♀
    - First pregnancy in a woman who will be 35 years of age or older at expected date of delivery
    - EXCLUDES   *elderly primigravida complicating pregnancy (659.5)*
  - **CC Excl:** See code V23.7

---

[3] These V codes may be used as principal diagnosis on Medicare patients.

✓4th ✓5th Additional Digit Required   **Nonspecific PDx**   Unacceptable PDx   Manifestation Code   **MSP** Medicare Secondary Payer   ▶◀ Revised Text   ● New Code   ▲ Revised Code Title

2002 Ingenix, Inc.

V Codes V23.82–V27.9

V23.82 Elderly multigravida [CC] [M] ♀
Second or more pregnancy in a woman who will be 35 years of age or older at expected date of delivery
EXCLUDES: elderly multigravida complicating pregnancy (659.6)
CC Excl: See code V23.7

V23.83 Young primigravida [CC] [M] ♀
First pregnancy in a female less than 16 years old at expected date of delivery
EXCLUDES: young primigravida complicating pregnancy (659.8)
CC Excl: See code V23.7

V23.84 Young multigravida [CC] [M] ♀
Second or more pregnancy in a female less than 16 years old at expected date of delivery
EXCLUDES: young multigravida complicating pregnancy (659.8)

V23.89 Other high-risk pregnancy [CC] [M] ♀
CC Excl: See code V23.7

V23.9 Unspecified high-risk pregnancy [CC] [M] ♀
CC Excl: See code V23.7

√4th **V24 Postpartum care and examination**
  3 **V24.0 Immediately after delivery** [M] ♀
    Care and observation in uncomplicated cases
  V24.1 Lactating mother ♀
    Supervision of lactation
  V24.2 Routine postpartum follow-up ♀

√4th **V25 Encounter for contraceptive management**
AHA: 4Q, '92, 24
  √5th **V25.0 General counseling and advice**
    V25.01 Prescription of oral contraceptives ♀
    V25.02 Initiation of other contraceptive measures
      Fitting of diaphragm
      Prescription of foams, creams, or other agents
    AHA: 3Q, '97, 7
    V25.09 Other
      Family planning advice
  V25.1 Insertion of intrauterine contraceptive device ♀
  3 **V25.2 Sterilization**
    Admission for interruption of fallopian tubes or vas deferens
  3 **V25.3 Menstrual extraction** ♀
    Menstrual regulation
  √5th **V25.4 Surveillance of previously prescribed contraceptive methods**
    Checking, reinsertion, or removal of contraceptive device
    Repeat prescription for contraceptive method
    Routine examination in connection with contraceptive maintenance
    EXCLUDES: presence of intrauterine contraceptive device as incidental finding (V45.5)
    V25.40 Contraceptive surveillance, unspecified
    V25.41 Contraceptive pill ♀
    V25.42 Intrauterine contraceptive device ♀
      Checking, reinsertion, or removal of intrauterine device
    V25.43 Implantable subdermal contraceptive ♀

V25.49 Other contraceptive method
AHA: 3Q, '97, 7

V25.5 Insertion of implantable subdermal contraceptive ♀
AHA: 3Q, '92, 9

V25.8 Other specified contraceptive management
Postvasectomy sperm count
EXCLUDES: sperm count following sterilization reversal (V26.22)
  sperm count for fertility testing (V26.21)
AHA: 3Q, '96, 9

V25.9 Unspecified contraceptive management

√4th **V26 Procreative management**
  3 **V26.0 Tuboplasty or vasoplasty after previous sterilization**
    AHA: 2Q, '95, 10
  V26.1 Artificial insemination ♀
  √5th **V26.2 Investigation and testing**
    EXCLUDES: postvasectomy sperm count (V25.8)
    AHA: 4Q, '00, 56
    V26.21 Fertility testing
      Fallopian insufflation
      Sperm count for fertility testing
      EXCLUDES: genetic counseling and testing (V26.3)
    V26.22 Aftercare following sterilization reversal
      Fallopian insufflation following sterilization reversal
      Sperm count following sterilization reversal
    V26.29 Other investigation and testing
    AHA: 2Q, '96, 9; N-D, '85, 15
  V26.3 Genetic counseling and testing
    EXCLUDES: fertility testing (V26.21)
  V26.4 General counseling and advice
  √5th **V26.5 Sterilization status**
    V26.51 Tubal ligation status ♀
      EXCLUDES: infertility not due to previous tubal ligation (628.0-628.9)
    V26.52 Vasectomy status ♂
  V26.8 Other specified procreative management
  V26.9 Unspecified procreative management

√4th **V27 Outcome of delivery**
Note: This category is intended for the coding of the outcome of delivery on the mother's record.
AHA: 2Q, '91, 16
  V27.0 Single liveborn [M] ♀
    AHA: 1Q, '01, 10; 3Q, '00, 5; 4Q, '98, 77; 4Q, '95, 59; 1Q, '92, 9
  V27.1 Single stillborn [M] ♀
  V27.2 Twins, both liveborn [M] ♀
  V27.3 Twins, one liveborn and one stillborn [M] ♀
  V27.4 Twins, both stillborn [M] ♀
  V27.5 Other multiple birth, all liveborn [M] ♀
  V27.6 Other multiple birth, some liveborn [M] ♀
  V27.7 Other multiple birth, all stillborn [M] ♀
  V27.9 Unspecified outcome of delivery [M] ♀
    Single birth } outcome to infant
    Multiple birth } unspecified

---

3 These V codes may be used as principal diagnosis on Medicare patients.

  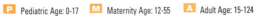

Tabular List — V CODES — V28–V42.89

- ✓4th **V28 Antenatal screening**
  - EXCLUDES: abnormal findings on screening — code to findings
    routine prenatal care (V22.0-V23.9)
  - **V28.0** Screening for chromosomal anomalies by amniocentesis ♀
  - **V28.1** Screening for raised alpha-fetoprotein levels in amniotic fluid ♀
  - **V28.2** Other screening based on amniocentesis ♀
  - **V28.3** Screening for malformation using ultrasonics ♀
  - **V28.4** Screening for fetal growth retardation using ultrasonics ♀
  - **V28.5** Screening for isoimmunization ♀
  - **V28.6** Screening for Streptococcus B ♀
    - AHA: 4Q, '97, 46
  - **V28.8** Other specified antenatal screening ♀
    - AHA: 3Q, '99, 16
  - **V28.9** Unspecified antenatal screening ♀

- ✓4th **V29 Observation and evaluation of newborns and infants for suspected condition not found**
  - Note: This category is to be used for newborns, within the neonatal period, (the first 28 days of life) who are suspected of having an abnormal condition resulting from exposure from the mother or the birth process, but without signs or symptoms, and, which after examination and observation, is found not to exist.
  - AHA: 1Q, '00, 25; 4Q, '94, 47; 1Q, '94, 9; 4Q, '92, 21
  - 3 **V29.0** Observation for suspected infectious condition N
    - AHA: 1Q, '01, 10
  - 3 **V29.1** Observation for suspected neurological condition N
  - 3 **V29.2** Observation for suspected respiratory condition N
  - 3 **V29.3** Observation for suspected genetic or metabolic condition N
    - AHA: 4Q, '98, 59, 68
  - 3 **V29.8** Observation for other specified suspected condition N
  - **V29.9** Observation for unspecified suspected condition N
    - AHA: ▶1Q, '02, 6◀

LIVEBORN INFANTS ACCORDING TO TYPE OF BIRTH (V30-V39)

Note: These categories are intended for the coding of liveborn infants who are consuming health care [e.g., crib or bassinet occupancy].

The following fourth-digit subdivisions are for use with categories V30-V39:
- ✓5th 0 Born in hospital
- 1 Born before admission to hospital
- 2 Born outside hospital and not hospitalized

The following two fifth-digits are for use with the fourth-digit .0, Born in hospital:
- 0 delivered without mention of cesarean delivery
- 1 delivered by cesarean delivery

AHA: 1Q, '01, 10

- 4 ✓4th **V30 Single liveborn**
  - AHA: 4Q, '98, 46, 59; 1Q, '94, 9
- 4 ✓4th **V31 Twin, mate liveborn**
  - AHA: 3Q, '92, 10
- 4 ✓4th **V32 Twin, mate stillborn**
- 4 ✓4th **V33 Twin, unspecified**
- 4 ✓4th **V34 Other multiple, mates all liveborn**
- 4 ✓4th **V35 Other multiple, mates all stillborn**
- 4 ✓4th **V36 Other multiple, mates live- and stillborn**
- 4 ✓4th **V37 Other multiple, unspecified**
- 5 ✓4th **V39 Unspecified**

PERSONS WITH A CONDITION INFLUENCING THEIR HEALTH STATUS (V40-V49)

Note: These categories are intended for use when these conditions are recorded as "diagnoses" or "problems."

- ✓4th **V40 Mental and behavioral problems**
  - **V40.0** Problems with learning
  - **V40.1** Problems with communication [including speech]
  - **V40.2** Other mental problems
  - **V40.3** Other behavioral problems
  - **V40.9** Unspecified mental or behavioral problem

- ✓4th **V41 Problems with special senses and other special functions**
  - **V41.0** Problems with sight
  - **V41.1** Other eye problems
  - **V41.2** Problems with hearing
  - **V41.3** Other ear problems
  - **V41.4** Problems with voice production
  - **V41.5** Problems with smell and taste
  - **V41.6** Problems with swallowing and mastication
  - **V41.7** Problems with sexual function
    - EXCLUDES: marital problems (V61.10)
      psychosexual disorders (302.0-302.9)
  - **V41.8** Other problems with special functions
  - **V41.9** Unspecified problem with special functions

- ✓4th **V42 Organ or tissue replaced by transplant**
  - INCLUDES: homologous or heterologous (animal) (human) transplant organ status
  - AHA: 3Q, '98, 3, 4
  - **V42.0** Kidney CC
    - CC Excl: 996.80-996.81, 996.87, V42.0, V42.89-V42.9
    - AHA: 3Q, '01, 12
  - **V42.1** Heart CC
    - CC Excl: 996.80, 996.83, 996.87, V42.1, V42.89-V42.9
    - AHA: 3Q, '01, 13
  - **V42.2** Heart valve CC
    - CC Excl: 996.71, V42.2, V42.89-V42.9
  - **V42.3** Skin
  - **V42.4** Bone
  - **V42.5** Cornea
  - **V42.6** Lung CC
    - CC Excl: 996.80, 996.84, 996.87, V42.6, V42.89-V42.9
  - **V42.7** Liver CC
    - CC Excl: 996.80, 996.82, 996.87, 996.87, V42.7, V42.89-V42.9
  - ✓5th **V42.8** Other specified organ or tissue
    - AHA: 4Q, '98, 64; 4Q, '97, 49
    - **V42.81** Bone marrow CC
      - CC Excl: 996.80, 996.85, 996.87, V42.9
    - **V42.82** Peripheral stem cells CC
      - CC Excl: 996.80, 996.87, V42.9
    - **V42.83** Pancreas CC
      - CC Excl: 996.80, 996.86-996.87, V42.83, V42.9
      - AHA: 2Q, '01, 16
    - **V42.84** Intestines CC
      - CC Excl: 996.80, 996.89, V42.84-V42.9
      - AHA: 4Q, '00, 48, 50
    - **V42.89** Other CC
      - CC Excl: 996.80, 996.87-996.89, V42.89-V42.9

---

3 These V codes may be used as principal diagnosis on Medicare patients.
4 These codes with the fourth digit of 0 or 1, may be used as a principal diagnosis for Medicare patients.
5 These V codes are acceptable as principal diagnosis with the fourth digit of 0.

V42.9–V45.83 — V CODES — Tabular List

- **V42.9** Unspecified organ or tissue
- ✓4th **V43** Organ or tissue replaced by other means
  - INCLUDES: replacement of organ by:
    - artificial device
    - mechanical device
    - prosthesis
  - EXCLUDES:
    - cardiac pacemaker in situ (V45.01)
    - fitting and adjustment of prosthetic device (V52.0-V52.9)
    - renal dialysis status (V45.1)
  - **V43.0** Eye globe
  - **V43.1** Lens
    - Pseudophakos
    - AHA: 4Q, '98, 65
  - **V43.2** Heart [CC]
    - CC Excl: 996.80, 996.83, 996.87, V42.1, V43.2
  - **V43.3** Heart valve
  - **V43.4** Blood vessel
  - **V43.5** Bladder
  - ✓5th **V43.6** Joint
    - **V43.60** Unspecified joint
    - **V43.61** Shoulder
    - **V43.62** Elbow
    - **V43.63** Wrist
    - **V43.64** Hip
    - **V43.65** Knee
    - **V43.66** Ankle
    - **V43.69** Other
  - **V43.7** Limb
  - ✓5th **V43.8** Organ or tissue replaced by other means
    - **V43.81** Larynx
      - AHA: 4Q, '95, 55
    - **V43.82** Breast
      - AHA: 4Q, '95, 55
    - **V43.83** Artificial skin
    - **V43.89** Other
- ✓4th **V44** Artificial opening status
  - EXCLUDES: artificial openings requiring attention or management (V55.0-V55.9)
  - **V44.0** Tracheostomy
    - AHA: 1Q, '01, 6
  - **V44.1** Gastrostomy
    - AHA: 1Q, '01, 12; 3Q, '97, 12; 1Q, '93, 26
  - **V44.2** Ileostomy
  - **V44.3** Colostomy
  - **V44.4** Other artificial opening of gastrointestinal tract
  - ✓5th **V44.5** Cystostomy
    - **V44.50** Cystostomy, unspecified
    - **V44.51** Cutaneous-vesicostomy
    - **V44.52** Appendico-vesicostomy
    - **V44.59** Other cystostomy
  - **V44.6** Other artificial opening of urinary tract
    - Nephrostomy   Urethrostomy
    - Ureterostomy
  - **V44.7** Artificial vagina
  - **V44.8** Other artificial opening status
  - **V44.9** Unspecified artificial opening status
- ✓4th **V45** Other postsurgical states
  - EXCLUDES:
    - aftercare management (V51-V58.9)
    - malfunction or other complication — code to condition
  - ✓5th **V45.0** Cardiac device in situ
    - **V45.00** Unspecified cardiac device
    - **V45.01** Cardiac pacemaker
    - **V45.02** Automatic implantable cardiac defibrillator
    - **V45.09** Other specified cardiac device
      - Carotid sinus pacemaker in situ
  - **V45.1** Renal dialysis status [CC]
    - Patient requiring intermittent renal dialysis
    - Presence of arterial-venous shunt (for dialysis)
    - EXCLUDES: admission for dialysis treatment or session (V56.0)
    - CC Excl: 996.73, V45.1
    - AHA: 2Q, '01, 12, 13
  - **V45.2** Presence of cerebrospinal fluid drainage device
    - Cerebral ventricle (communicating) shunt, valve, or device in situ
    - EXCLUDES: malfunction (996.2)
  - **V45.3** Intestinal bypass or anastomosis status
  - **V45.4** Arthrodesis status
    - AHA: N-D, '84, 18
  - ✓5th **V45.5** Presence of contraceptive device
    - EXCLUDES:
      - checking, reinsertion, or removal of device (V25.42)
      - complication from device (996.32)
      - insertion of device (V25.1)
    - **V45.51** Intrauterine contraceptive device ♀
    - **V45.52** Subdermal contraceptive implant
    - **V45.59** Other
  - ✓5th **V45.6** States following surgery of eye and adnexa
    - Cataract extraction }
    - Filtering bleb } state following eye surgery
    - Surgical eyelid adhesion }
    - EXCLUDES:
      - aphakia (379.31)
      - artificial eye globe (V43.0)
    - AHA: 4Q, '98, 65; 4Q, '97, 49
    - **V45.61** Cataract extraction status
      - Use additional code for associated artificial lens status (V43.1)
    - **V45.69** Other states following surgery of eye and adnexa
      - AHA: 2Q, '01, 16; 1Q, '98, 10; 4Q, '97, 19
  - ✓5th **V45.7** Acquired absence of organ
    - AHA: 4Q, '98, 65; 4Q, '97, 50
    - [3] **V45.71** Acquired absence of breast
      - AHA: ▶4Q, '01, 66;◀ 4Q, '97, 50
    - **V45.72** Acquired absence of intestine (large) (small)
    - **V45.73** Acquired absence of kidney
    - **V45.74** Other parts of urinary tract
      - Bladder
      - AHA: 4Q, '00, 51
    - **V45.75** Stomach
      - AHA: 4Q, '00, 51
    - **V45.76** Lung
      - AHA: 4Q, '00, 51
    - **V45.77** Genital organs
      - AHA: 4Q, '00, 51
    - **V45.78** Eye
      - AHA: 4Q, '00, 51
    - **V45.79** Other acquired absence of organ
      - AHA: 4Q, '00, 51
  - ✓5th **V45.8** Other postsurgical status
    - **V45.81** Aortocoronary bypass status
      - AHA: ▶3Q, '01, 15;◀ 3Q, '97, 16
    - **V45.82** Percutaneous transluminal coronary angioplasty status
    - **V45.83** Breast implant removal status
      - AHA: 4Q, '95, 55

[3] These V codes may be used as principal diagnosis on Medicare patients.

Tabular List — V CODES — V45.84–V50.42

V45.84 Dental restoration status
  Dental crowns status
  Dental fillings status
  AHA: 4Q, '01, 54

V45.89 Other
  Presence of neuropacemaker or other electronic device
  EXCLUDES: artificial heart valve in situ (V43.3)
  vascular prosthesis in situ (V43.4)
  AHA: 1Q, '95, 11

√4th **V46 Other dependence on machines**

  V46.0 Aspirator

  V46.1 Respirator CC
  Iron lung
  CC Excl: V46.0-V46.1, V46.8-V46.9
  AHA: 1Q, '01, 12; J-F, '87, 7 3

  ● **V46.2 Supplemental oxygen**
  Long-term oxygen therapy

  V46.8 Other enabling machines
  Hyperbaric chamber
  Possum [Patient-Operated-Selector-Mechanism]
  EXCLUDES: cardiac pacemaker (V45.0)
  kidney dialysis machine (V45.1)

  V46.9 Unspecified machine dependence

√4th **V47 Other problems with internal organs**

  V47.0 Deficiencies of internal organs

  V47.1 Mechanical and motor problems with internal organs

  V47.2 Other cardiorespiratory problems
  Cardiovascular exercise intolerance with pain (with):
    at rest
    less than ordinary activity
    ordinary activity

  V47.3 Other digestive problems

  V47.4 Other urinary problems

  V47.5 Other genital problems

  V47.9 Unspecified

√4th **V48 Problems with head, neck, and trunk**

  V48.0 Deficiencies of head
  EXCLUDES: deficiencies of ears, eyelids, and nose (V48.8)

  V48.1 Deficiencies of neck and trunk

  V48.2 Mechanical and motor problems with head

  V48.3 Mechanical and motor problems with neck and trunk

  V48.4 Sensory problem with head

  V48.5 Sensory problem with neck and trunk

  V48.6 Disfigurements of head

  V48.7 Disfigurements of neck and trunk

  V48.8 Other problems with head, neck, and trunk

  V48.9 Unspecified problem with head, neck, or trunk

√4th **V49 Other conditions influencing health status**

  V49.0 Deficiencies of limbs

  V49.1 Mechanical problems with limbs

  V49.2 Motor problems with limbs

  V49.3 Sensory problems with limbs

  V49.4 Disfigurements of limbs

  V49.5 Other problems of limbs

  √5th **V49.6 Upper limb amputation status**
  AHA: 4Q, '98, 42; 4Q, '94, 39

    V49.60 Unspecified level
    V49.61 Thumb
    V49.62 Other finger(s)
    V49.63 Hand
    V49.64 Wrist
      Disarticulation of wrist
    V49.65 Below elbow
    V49.66 Above elbow
      Disarticulation of elbow
    V49.67 Shoulder
      Disarticulation of shoulder

  √5th **V49.7 Lower limb amputation status**
  AHA: 4Q, '98, 42; 4Q, '94, 39

    V49.70 Unspecified level
    V49.71 Great toe
    V49.72 Other toe(s)
    V49.73 Foot
    V49.74 Ankle
      Disarticulation of ankle
    V49.75 Below knee
    V49.76 Above knee
      Disarticulation of knee
    V49.77 Hip
      Disarticulation of hip

  √5th **V49.8 Other specified conditions influencing health status**
  AHA: 4Q, '00, 51

    V49.81 Postmenopausal status (age-related) (natural) A ♀
    EXCLUDES: menopausal and premenopausal disorder (627.0-627.9)
    postsurgical menopause (256.2)
    premature menopause (256.31)
    symptomatic menopause (627.0-627.9)
    AHA: 4Q, '00, 54

    ▲ **V49.81 Asymptomatic postmenopausal status (age-related) (natural)**

    V49.82 Dental sealant status
    AHA: 4Q, '01, 54

    V49.89 Other specified conditions influencing health status

  V49.9 Unspecified

PERSONS ENCOUNTERING HEALTH SERVICES FOR SPECIFIC PROCEDURES AND AFTERCARE (V50-V59)

Note: Categories V51-V58 are intended for use to indicate a reason for care in patients who may have already been treated for some disease or injury not now present, or who are receiving care to consolidate the treatment, to deal with residual states, or to prevent recurrence.

EXCLUDES: follow-up examination for medical surveillance following treatment (V67.0-V67.9)

√4th **V50 Elective surgery for purposes other than remedying health states**

  ³ **V50.0 Hair transplant**

  ³ **V50.1 Other plastic surgery for unacceptable cosmetic appearance**
  Breast augmentation or reduction
  Face-lift
  EXCLUDES: plastic surgery following healed injury or operation (V51)

  ³ **V50.2 Routine or ritual circumcision** ♂
  Circumcision in the absence of significant medical indication

  V50.3 Ear piercing

  √5th **V50.4 Prophylactic organ removal**
  EXCLUDES: organ donations (V59.0-V59.9)
  therapeutic organ removal — code to condition
  AHA: 4Q, '94, 44

    ³ **V50.41 Breast**
    ³ **V50.42 Ovary** ♀

³ These V codes may be used as principal diagnosis on Medicare patients.

V50.49–V54.29 V CODES Tabular List

- ³ **V50.49** Other
- **V50.8** Other
- **V50.9** Unspecified
- ³ **V51** Aftercare involving the use of plastic surgery
  Plastic surgery following healed injury or operation
  EXCLUDES cosmetic plastic surgery (V50.1)
  plastic surgery as treatment for current injury — code to condition
  repair of scarred tissue — code to scar

- ✓4ᵗʰ **V52** Fitting and adjustment of prosthetic device and implant
  INCLUDES removal of device
  EXCLUDES malfunction or complication of prosthetic device (996.0-996.7)
  status only, without need for care (V43.0-V43.8)
  AHA: 4Q, '95, 55 ; 1Q, '90, 7
  - ³ **V52.0** Artificial arm (complete) (partial)
  - ³ **V52.1** Artificial leg (complete) (partial)
  - ³ **V52.2** Artificial eye
  - ³ **V52.3** Dental prosthetic device
  - ³ **V52.4** Breast prosthesis and implant ♀
    EXCLUDES admission for implant insertion (V50.1)
    AHA: 4Q, '95, 80, 81
  - ³ **V52.8** Other specified prosthetic device
  - **V52.9** Unspecified prosthetic device

- ✓4ᵗʰ **V53** Fitting and adjustment of other device
  INCLUDES removal of device
  replacement of device
  EXCLUDES status only, without need for care (V45.0-V45.8)
  - ✓5ᵗʰ **V53.0** Devices related to nervous system and special senses
    AHA: 4Q, '98, 66; 4Q, '97, 51
    - **V53.01** Fitting and adjustment of cerebral ventricular (communicating) shunt
      AHA: 4Q, '97, 51
    - **V53.02** Neuropacemaker (brain) (peripheral nerve) (spinal cord)
    - ³ **V53.09** Fitting and adjustment of other devices related to nervous system and special senses
      Auditory substitution device
      Visual substitution device
      AHA: 2Q '99, 4
  - **V53.1** Spectacles and contact lenses
  - **V53.2** Hearing aid
  - ✓5ᵗʰ **V53.3** Cardiac device
    Reprogramming
    AHA: 3Q, '92, 3; 1Q, '90, 7; M-J, '87, 8 ; N-D, '84, 18
    - ³ **V53.31** Cardiac pacemaker
      EXCLUDES mechanical complication of cardiac pacemaker (996.01)
      AHA: ▶1Q, '02, 3◄
    - ³ **V53.32** Automatic implantable cardiac defibrillator
    - ³ **V53.39** Other cardiac device
  - **V53.4** Orthodontic devices
  - **V53.5** Other intestinal appliance
    EXCLUDES colostomy (V55.3)
    ileostomy (V55.2)
    other artificial opening of digestive tract (V55.4)
  - **V53.6** Urinary devices
    Urinary catheter
    EXCLUDES cystostomy (V55.5)
    nephrostomy (V55.6)
    ureterostomy (V55.6)
    urethrostomy (V55.6)
  - **V53.7** Orthopedic devices
    Orthopedic: Orthopedic:
    brace   corset
    cast   shoes
    EXCLUDES other orthopedic aftercare (V54)
  - **V53.8** Wheelchair
  - **V53.9** Other and unspecified device

- ✓4ᵗʰ **V54** Other orthopedic aftercare
  EXCLUDES fitting and adjustment of orthopedic devices (V53.7)
  malfunction of internal orthopedic device (996.4)
  other complication of nonmechanical nature (996.60-996.79)
  AHA: 3Q, '95, 3
  - ³ **V54.0** Aftercare involving removal of fracture plate or other internal fixation device
    Removal of: Removal of:
    pins   rods
    plates   screws
    EXCLUDES malfunction of internal device (996.4)
    other complication of nonmechanical nature (996.60-996.79)
    removal of external fixation device ▶(V54.89)◄
  - ✓5ᵗʰ **V54.1** Aftercare for healing traumatic fracture
    - **V54.10** Aftercare for healing traumatic fracture of arm, unspecified
    - **V54.11** Aftercare for healing traumatic fracture of upper arm
    - **V54.12** Aftercare for healing traumatic fracture of lower arm
    - **V54.13** Aftercare for healing traumatic fracture of hip
    - **V54.14** Aftercare for healing traumatic fracture of leg, unspecified
    - **V54.15** Aftercare for healing traumatic fracture of upper leg
      EXCLUDES aftercare for healing traumatic fracture of hip (V54.13)
    - **V54.16** Aftercare for healing traumatic fracture of lower leg
    - **V54.17** Aftercare for healing traumatic fracture of vertebrae
    - **V54.19** Aftercare for healing traumatic fracture of other bone
  - ✓5ᵗʰ **V54.2** Aftercare for healing pathologic fracture
    - **V54.20** Aftercare for healing pathologic fracture of arm, unspecified
    - **V54.21** Aftercare for healing pathologic fracture of upper arm
    - **V54.22** Aftercare for healing pathologic fracture of lower arm
    - **V54.23** Aftercare for healing pathologic fracture of hip
    - **V54.24** Aftercare for healing pathologic fracture of leg, unspecified
    - **V54.25** Aftercare for healing pathologic fracture of upper leg
      EXCLUDES aftercare for healing pathologic fracture of hip (V54.23)
    - **V54.26** Aftercare for healing pathologic fracture of lower leg
    - **V54.27** Aftercare for healing pathologic fracture of vertebrae
    - **V54.29** Aftercare for healing pathologic fracture of other bone

³ These V codes may be used as principal diagnosis on Medicare patients.
⁶ Rehabilitation codes acceptable as a principal diagnosis when accompanied by a secondary diagnosis reflection the condition treated.

N Newborn Age: 0   **P** Pediatric Age: 0-17   **M** Maternity Age: 12-55   **A** Adult Age: 15-124   **CC** CC Condition   **MC** Major Complication   **CD** Complex Dx   **HIV** HIV Related Dx

Tabular List — V CODES — V54.8–V58.42

✓5ᵗʰ V54.8 Other orthopedic aftercare
AHA: 3Q, '01, 19; 4Q, '99, 5

● **V54.81 Aftercare following joint replacement**
Use additional code to identify joint replacement site (V43.60-V43.69)

● **V54.89 Other orthopedic aftercare**
Aftercare for healing fracture NOS

V54.9 Unspecified orthopedic aftercare

✓4ᵗʰ V55 Attention to artificial openings

INCLUDES: adjustment or repositioning of catheter
closure
passage of sounds or bougies
reforming
removal or replacement of catheter
toilet or cleansing

EXCLUDES: complications of external stoma (519.00-519.09, 569.60-569.69, 997.4, 997.5)
status only, without need for care (V44.0-V44.9)

³ **V55.0 Tracheostomy**
³ **V55.1 Gastrostomy**
AHA: 4Q, '99, 9; 3Q, '97, 7, 8; 1Q, '96, 14; 3Q, '95, 13

³ **V55.2 Ileostomy**
³ **V55.3 Colostomy**
AHA: 3Q, '97, 9

³ **V55.4 Other artificial opening of digestive tract**
³ **V55.5 Cystostomy**
³ **V55.6 Other artificial opening of urinary tract**
Nephrostomy   Urethrostomy
Ureterostomy

³ **V55.7 Artificial vagina**
³ **V55.8 Other specified artificial opening**

V55.9 Unspecified artificial opening

✓4ᵗʰ V56 Encounter for dialysis and dialysis catheter care
Use additional code to identify the associated condition
EXCLUDES: dialysis preparation — code to condition
AHA: 4Q, '98, 66; 1Q, '93, 29

³ **V56.0 Extracorporeal dialysis**
Dialysis (renal) NOS
EXCLUDES: dialysis status (V45.1)
AHA: 4Q, '00, 40; 3Q, '98, 6; 2Q, '98, 20

⁶ **V56.1 Fitting and adjustment of extracorporeal dialysis catheter**
Removal or replacement of catheter
Toilet or cleansing
Use additional code for any concurrent extracorporeal dialysis (V56.0)
AHA: 2Q, '98, 20

V56.2 Fitting and adjustment of peritoneal dialysis catheter
Use additional code for any concurrent peritoneal dialysis (V56.8)
AHA: 4Q, '98, 55

✓5ᵗʰ V56.3 Encounter for adequacy testing for dialysis
AHA: 4Q, '00, 55

V56.31 Encounter for adequacy testing for hemodialysis

V56.32 Encounter for adequacy testing for peritoneal dialysis
Peritoneal equilibration test

³ **V56.8 Other dialysis**
Peritoneal dialysis
AHA: 4Q, '98, 55

✓4ᵗʰ V57 Care involving use of rehabilitation procedures
Use additional code to identify underlying condition
AHA: ▶1Q, '02, 19;◀ 3Q, '97, 12; 1Q, '90, 6; S-O, '86, 3

V57.0 Breathing exercises

⁶ **V57.1 Other physical therapy**
Therapeutic and remedial exercises, except breathing
AHA: 4Q, '99, 5

✓5ᵗʰ V57.2 Occupational therapy and vocational rehabilitation

⁶ **V57.21 Encounter for occupational therapy**
AHA: 4Q, '99, 7

⁶ **V57.22 Encounter for vocational therapy**

⁶ **V57.3 Speech therapy**
AHA: 4Q, '97, 36

V57.4 Orthoptic training

✓5ᵗʰ V57.8 Other specified rehabilitation procedure

V57.81 Orthotic training
Gait training in the use of artificial limbs

⁶ **V57.89 Other**
Multiple training or therapy
AHA: ▶1Q, '02, 16;◀ 3Q, '01, 21; 3Q, '97, 11, 12; S-O, '86, 4

⁶ **V57.9 Unspecified rehabilitation procedure**

✓4ᵗʰ V58 Encounter for other and unspecified procedures and aftercare
EXCLUDES: convalescence and palliative care (V66)

³ **V58.0 Radiotherapy**
Encounter or admission for radiotherapy
EXCLUDES: encounter for radioactive implant — code to condition
radioactive iodine therapy — code to condition
AHA: 3Q, '92, 5; 2Q, '90, 7; J-F, '87, 13

³ **V58.1 Chemotherapy**
Encounter or admission for chemotherapy
EXCLUDES: prophylactic chemotherapy against disease which has never been present (V03.0-V07.9)
AHA: 3Q, '93, 4; 2Q, '92, 6; 2Q, '91, 17; 2Q, '90, 7; S-O, '84, 5

V58.2 Blood transfusion, without reported diagnosis

V58.3 Attention to surgical dressings and sutures
Change of dressings
Removal of sutures

✓5ᵗʰ V58.4 Other aftercare following surgery
▶Note: Codes from this subcategory should be used in conjunction with other aftercare codes to fully identify the reason for the aftercare encounter◀
EXCLUDES: aftercare following sterilization reversal surgery (V26.22)
attention to artificial openings (V55.0-V55.9)
orthopedic aftercare (V54.0-V54.9)
AHA: 4Q, '99, 9; N-D, '87, 9

³,⁷ **V58.41 Encounter for planned postoperative wound closure**
EXCLUDES: disruption of operative wound (998.3)
AHA: 4Q, '99, 15

● ⁷ **V58.42 Aftercare following surgery for neoplasm**
Conditions classifiable to 140-239

---

³ These V codes may be used as principal diagnosis on Medicare patients.
⁶ Rehabilitation codes acceptable as a principal diagnosis when accompanied by a secondary diagnosis reflection the condition treated.
⁷ These V codes are acceptable as principal diagnosis when accompanied by a diagnosis of personal history of malignancy.
These codes group to DRGs 465-466.

✓4ᵗʰ ✓5ᵗʰ Additional Digit Required | Nonspecific PDx | Unacceptable PDx | Manifestation Code | MSP Medicare Secondary Payer | ▶◀ Revised Text | ● New Code | ▲ Revised Code Title

V CODES — Tabular List

- 7 **V58.43 Aftercare following surgery for injury and trauma**
  Conditions classifiable to 800-999
  EXCLUDES *aftercare for healing traumatic fracture (V54.10-V54.19)*

- 3, 7 **V58.49 Other specified aftercare following surgery**
  AHA: 1Q, '96, 8, 9

- 7 **V58.5 Orthodontics**
  EXCLUDES *fitting and adjustment of orthodontic device (V53.4)*

- √5th **V58.6 Long-term (current) drug use**
  EXCLUDES *drug abuse (305.00-305.93)*
  drug dependence (304.00-304.93)
  AHA: 4Q, '95, 61

- 3, 7 **V58.61 Long-term (current) use of anticoagulants**
  AHA: ▶1Q, '02, 15, 16◀

- 7 **V58.62 Long-term (current) use of antibiotics**
  AHA: 4Q, '98, 59

- 3, 7 **V58.69 Long-term (current) use of other medications**
  High-risk medications
  AHA: 2Q, '00, 8; 3Q, '99, 13; 2Q, '99, 17; 1Q, '97, 12; 2Q, '96, 7

- √5th **V58.7 Aftercare following surgery to specified body systems, not elsewhere classified**
  Note: Codes from this subcategory should be used in conjunction with other aftercare codes to fully identify the reason for the aftercare encounter

- 7 **V58.71 Aftercare following surgery of the sense organs, NEC**
  Conditions classifiable to 360-379, 380-389

- 7 **V58.72 Aftercare following surgery of the nervous system, NEC**
  Conditions classifiable to 320-359
  EXCLUDES *aftercare following surgery of the sense organs, NEC (V58.71)*

- 7 **V58.73 Aftercare following surgery of the circulatory system, NEC**
  Conditions classifiable to 390-459

- 7 **V58.74 Aftercare following surgery of the respiratory system, NEC**
  Conditions classifiable to 460-519

- 7 **V58.75 Aftercare following surgery of the teeth, oral cavity and digestive system, NEC**
  Conditions classifiable to 520-579

- 7 **V58.76 Aftercare following surgery of the genitourinary system, NEC**
  Conditions classifiable to 580-629
  EXCLUDES *aftercare following sterilization reversal (V26.22)*

- 7 **V58.77 Aftercare following surgery of the skin and subcutaneous tissue, NEC**
  Conditions classifiable to 680-709

- 7 **V58.78 Aftercare following surgery of the musculoskeletal system, NEC**
  Conditions classifiable to 710-739

- √5th **V58.8 Other specified procedures and aftercare**
  AHA: 4Q, '94, 45; 2Q, '94, 8

- 7 **V58.81 Fitting and adjustment of vascular catheter**
  Removal or replacement of catheter
  Toilet or cleansing
  EXCLUDES *complication of renal dialysis (996.73)*
  complication of vascular catheter (996.74)
  dialysis preparation — code to condition
  encounter for dialysis (V56.0-V56.8)
  fitting and adjustment of dialysis catheter (V56.1)

- 7 **V58.82 Fitting and adjustment of nonvascular catheter, NEC**
  Removal or replacement of catheter
  Toilet or cleansing
  EXCLUDES *fitting and adjustment of peritoneal dialysis catheter (V56.2)*
  fitting and adjustment of urinary catheter (V53.6)

- 7 **V58.83 Encounter for therapeutic drug monitoring**
  ▶Use additional code for any associated long-term (current) drug use (V58.61-V58.69)◀
  EXCLUDES *blood-drug testing for medicolegal reasons (V70.4)*

- 3, 7 **V58.89 Other specified aftercare**
  AHA: 4Q, '98, 59

- 7 **V58.9 Unspecified aftercare**

√4th **V59 Donors**
EXCLUDES *examination of potential donor (V70.8)*
self-donation of organ or tissue — code to condition
AHA: 4Q, '95, 62; 1Q, '90, 10; N-D, '84, 8

- √5th **V59.0 Blood**
  - **V59.01** Whole blood
  - **V59.02** Stem cells
  - **V59.09** Other
- 3 **V59.1 Skin**
- 3 **V59.2 Bone**
- 3 **V59.3 Bone marrow**
- 3 **V59.4 Kidney**
- 3 **V59.5 Cornea**
- 3 **V59.6 Liver**
- 3 **V59.8 Other specified organ or tissue**
- 3 **V59.9 Unspecified organ or tissue**

PERSONS ENCOUNTERING HEALTH SERVICES IN OTHER CIRCUMSTANCES (V60-V68)

√4th **V60 Housing, household, and economic circumstances**
- **V60.0 Lack of housing**
  Hobos   Transients
  Social migrants Vagabonds
  Tramps
- **V60.1 Inadequate housing**
  Lack of heating   Technical defects in
  Restriction of space   home preventing
                       adequate care
- **V60.2 Inadequate material resources**
  Economic problem
  Poverty NOS
- **V60.3 Person living alone**

---

3 These V codes may be used as principal diagnosis on Medicare patients.
6 Rehabilitation codes acceptable as a principal diagnosis when accompanied by a secondary diagnosis reflection the condition treated.
7 These V codes are acceptable as principal diagnosis when accompanied by a diagnosis of personal history of malignancy. These codes group to DRGs 465-466.

N Newborn Age: 0   **P** Pediatric Age: 0-17   **M** Maternity Age: 12-55   **A** Adult Age: 15-124   **CC** CC Condition   **MC** Major Complication   **CD** Complex Dx   **HIV** HIV Related Dx

Tabular List — V CODES

V60.4 No other household member able to render care
Person requiring care (has) (is):
  family member too handicapped, ill, or otherwise unsuited to render care
  partner temporarily away from home
  temporarily away from usual place of abode
  EXCLUDES holiday relief care (V60.5)

V60.5 Holiday relief care
Provision of health care facilities to a person normally cared for at home, to enable relatives to take a vacation

V60.6 Person living in residential institution
Boarding school resident

V60.8 Other specified housing or economic circumstances

V60.9 Unspecified housing or economic circumstance

√4th **V61** Other family circumstances
INCLUDES when these circumstances or fear of them, affecting the person directly involved or others, are mentioned as the reason, justified or not, for seeking or receiving medical advice or care

AHA: 1Q, '90, 9

V61.0 Family disruption
Divorce
Estrangement

√5th **V61.1** Counseling for marital and partner problems
EXCLUDES problems related to:
  psychosexual disorders (302.0-302.9)
  sexual function (V41.7)

V61.10 Counseling for marital and partner problems, unspecified
Marital conflict
Partner conflict

V61.11 Counseling for victim of spousal and partner abuse
EXCLUDES encounter for treatment of current injuries due to abuse (995.80-995.85)

V61.12 Counseling for perpetrator of spousal and partner abuse

√5th **V61.2** Parent-child problems

V61.20 Counseling for parent-child problem, unspecified
Concern about behavior of child
Parent-child conflict

³ **V61.21** Counseling for victim of child abuse
Child battering   Child neglect
EXCLUDES current injuries due to abuse (995.50-995.59)

V61.22 Counseling for perpetrator of parental child abuse
EXCLUDES counseling for non-parental abuser (V62.83)

V61.29 Other
Problem concerning adopted or foster child
AHA: 3Q, '99, 16

V61.3 Problems with aged parents or in-laws

√5th **V61.4** Health problems within family
V61.41 Alcoholism in family
V61.49 Other
Care of / Presence of } sick or handicapped person in family or household

V61.5 Multiparity
V61.6 Illegitimacy or illegitimate pregnancy ♀
V61.7 Other unwanted pregnancy ♀
V61.8 Other specified family circumstances
Problems with family members NEC

V61.9 Unspecified family circumstance

√4th **V62** Other psychosocial circumstances
INCLUDES those circumstances or fear of them, affecting the person directly involved or others, mentioned as the reason, justified or not, for seeking or receiving medical advice or care
EXCLUDES previous psychological trauma (V15.41-V15.49)

V62.0 Unemployment
EXCLUDES circumstances when main problem is economic inadequacy or poverty (V60.2)

V62.1 Adverse effects of work environment

V62.2 Other occupational circumstances or maladjustment
Career choice problem
Dissatisfaction with employment

V62.3 Educational circumstances
Dissatisfaction with school environment
Educational handicap

V62.4 Social maladjustment
Cultural deprivation
Political, religious, or sex discrimination
Social:
  isolation
  persecution

V62.5 Legal circumstances
Imprisonment   Litigation
Legal investigation   Prosecution

V62.6 Refusal of treatment for reasons of religion or conscience

√5th **V62.8** Other psychological or physical stress, not elsewhere classified

V62.81 Interpersonal problems, not elsewhere classified

V62.82 Bereavement, uncomplicated
EXCLUDES bereavement as adjustment reaction (309.0)

V62.83 Counseling for perpetrator of physical/sexual abuse
EXCLUDES counseling for perpetrator of parental child abuse (V61.22)
counseling for perpetrator of spousal and partner abuse (V61.12)

V62.89 Other
Life circumstance problems
Phase of life problems

V62.9 Unspecified psychosocial circumstance

√5th **V63** Unavailability of other medical facilities for care
AHA: 1Q, '91, 21

V63.0 Residence remote from hospital or other health care facility

V63.1 Medical services in home not available
EXCLUDES no other household member able to render care (V60.4)
AHA: ►4Q, '01, 67;◄ 1Q, '01, 12

V63.2 Person awaiting admission to adequate facility elsewhere

V63.8 Other specified reasons for unavailability of medical facilities
Person on waiting list undergoing social agency investigation

V63.9 Unspecified reason for unavailability of medical facilities

√4th **V64** Persons encountering health services for specific procedures, not carried out

---

³ These V codes may be used as principal diagnosis on Medicare patients.

	V64.0	**Vaccination not carried out because of contraindication**
	V64.1	**Surgical or other procedure not carried out because of contraindication**
	V64.2	**Surgical or other procedure not carried out because of patient's decision**
		AHA: 2Q, '01, 8
	V64.3	**Procedure not carried out for other reasons**
	V64.4	**Laparoscopic surgical procedure converted to open procedure**
		AHA: 4Q, '98, 68; 4Q, '97, 52

✓4th **V65 Other persons seeking consultation without complaint or sickness**

   ³ **V65.0 Healthy person accompanying sick person**
        Boarder

   V65.1 Person consulting on behalf of another person
        Advice or treatment for nonattending third party
        EXCLUDES   concern (normal) about sick person in family (V61.41-V61.49)

   ³ **V65.2 Person feigning illness**
        Malingerer   Peregrinating patient
        AHA: 3Q, '99, 20

   V65.3 Dietary surveillance and counseling
        Dietary surveillance and counseling (in):
        NOS   gastritis
        colitis   hypercholesterolemia
        diabetes mellitus hypoglycemia
        food allergies or   obesity
          intolerance

✓5th **V65.4 Other counseling, not elsewhere classified**
        Health: Health:
          advice   instruction
          education
        EXCLUDES counseling (for):
            contraception (V25.40-V25.49)
            genetic (V26.3)
            on behalf of third party (V65.1)
            procreative management (V26.4)

       V65.40 Counseling NOS
       V65.41 Exercise counseling
       V65.42 Counseling on substance use and abuse
       V65.43 Counseling on injury prevention
       V65.44 Human immunodeficiency virus [HIV] counseling
       V65.45 Counseling on other sexually transmitted diseases
       V65.49 Other specified counseling
           AHA: 2Q, '00, 8

   V65.5 Person with feared complaint in whom no diagnosis was made
        Feared condition not demonstrated
        Problem was normal state
        "Worried well"

   V65.8 Other reasons for seeking consultation
        EXCLUDES specified symptoms
        AHA: 3Q, '92, 4

   V65.9 Unspecified reason for consultation

✓4th **V66 Convalescence and palliative care**
   ³ **V66.0 Following surgery**
   ³ **V66.1 Following radiotherapy**
   ³ **V66.2 Following chemotherapy**
   ³ **V66.3 Following psychotherapy and other treatment for mental disorder**
   ³ **V66.4 Following treatment of fracture**
     V66.5 Following other treatment
   ³ **V66.6 Following combined treatment**

   V66.7 Encounter for palliative care
        End of life care
        Hospice care
        Terminal care
        Code first underlying disease
        AHA: 1Q, '98, 11; 4Q, '96, 47, 48

   V66.9 Unspecified convalescence
        AHA: 4Q, '99, 8

✓4th **V67 Follow-up examination**
      INCLUDES surveillance only following completed treatment
      EXCLUDES surveillance of contraception (V25.40-V25.49)
   AHA: 4Q, '94, 48

✓5th **V67.0 Following surgery**
      AHA: 4Q, '00, 56; 4Q, '98, 69; 4Q, '97, 50; 2Q, '95, 8; 1Q, '95, 4; 3Q, '92, 11

   ³,⁷ **V67.00 Following surgery, unspecified**
   ³,⁷ **V67.01 Follow-up vaginal pap smear** ♀
        Vaginal pap-smear, status-post hysterectomy for malignant condition
        Use additional code to identify:
          acquired absence of uterus (V45.77)
          personal history of malignant neoplasm (V10.40-V10.44)
        EXCLUDES vaginal pap smear status-post hysterectomy for non-malignant condition (V76.47)

   ³,⁷ **V67.09 Following other surgery**
        EXCLUDES sperm count following sterilization reversal (V26.22)
            sperm count for fertility testing (V26.21)

   ³ **V67.1 Following radiotherapy**
   ³ **V67.2 Following chemotherapy**
       Cancer chemotherapy follow-up
   ³ **V67.3 Following psychotherapy and other treatment for mental disorder**
   ³,⁷ **V67.4 Following treatment of healed fracture**
       EXCLUDES current (healing) fracture aftercare (V54.0-V54.9)
      AHA: 1Q, '90, 7

✓5th **V67.5 Following other treatment**
   ³ **V67.51 Following completed treatment with high-risk medications, not elsewhere classified**
       EXCLUDES long-term (current) drug use (V58.61-V58.69)
      AHA: 1Q, '99, 5, 6; 4Q, '95, 61; 1Q, '90, 18

   ³ **V67.59 Other**
   ³ **V67.6 Following combined treatment**
   V67.9 Unspecified follow-up examination

✓4th **V68 Encounters for administrative purposes**
   V68.0 Issue of medical certificates
       Issue of medical certificate of:
         cause of death
         fitness
         incapacity
       EXCLUDES encounter for general medical examination (V70.0-V70.9)

---

³ These V codes may be used as principal diagnosis on Medicare patients.
⁷ These V codes are acceptable as principal diagnosis when accompanied by a diagnosis of personal history of malignancy. These codes group to DRGs 465-466.

Tabular List — V CODES

V68.1 Issue of repeat prescriptions
Issue of repeat prescription for:
 appliance
 glasses
 medications
 EXCLUDES: repeat prescription for contraceptives (V25.41-V25.49)

V68.2 Request for expert evidence

✓5th **V68.8 Other specified administrative purpose**

V68.81 Referral of patient without examination or treatment

V68.89 Other

V68.9 Unspecified administrative purpose

✓4th **V69 Problems related to lifestyle**
AHA: 4Q, '94, 48

V69.0 Lack of physical exercise

V69.1 Inappropriate diet and eating habits
 EXCLUDES: anorexia nervosa (307.1)
 bulimia (783.6)
 malnutrition and other nutritional deficiencies (260-269.9)
 other and unspecified eating disorders (307.50-307.59)

V69.2 High-risk sexual behavior

V69.3 Gambling and betting
 EXCLUDES: pathological gambling (312.31)

V69.8 Other problems related to lifestyle
 Self-damaging behavior

V69.9 Problem related to lifestyle, unspecified

PERSONS WITHOUT REPORTED DIAGNOSIS ENCOUNTERED DURING EXAMINATION AND INVESTIGATION OF INDIVIDUALS AND POPULATIONS ▶(V70-V83)◀

Note: Nonspecific abnormal findings disclosed at the time of these examinations are classifiable to categories 790-796.

✓4th **V70 General medical examination**
Use additional code(s) to identify any special screening examination(s) performed (V73.0-V82.9)

V70.0 Routine general medical examination at a health care facility
 Health checkup
 EXCLUDES: health checkup of infant or child (V20.2)

³ **V70.1 General psychiatric examination, requested by the authority**

V70.2 General psychiatric examination, other and unspecified

V70.3 Other medical examination for administrative purposes
 General medical examination for:
  admission to old age home
  adoption
  camp
  driving license
  immigration and naturalization
  insurance certification
  marriage
  prison
  school admission
  sports competition
 EXCLUDES: attendance for issue of medical certificates (V68.0)
  pre-employment screening (V70.5)
 AHA: 1Q, '90, 6

³ **V70.4 Examination for medicolegal reasons**
 Blood-alcohol tests
 Blood-drug tests
 Paternity testing
 EXCLUDES: examination and observation following:
  accidents (V71.3, V71.4)
  assault (V71.6)
  rape (V71.5)

³ **V70.5 Health examination of defined subpopulations**
 Armed forces personnel
 Inhabitants of institutions
 Occupational health examinations
 Pre-employment screening
 Preschool children
 Prisoners
 Prostitutes
 Refugees
 School children
 Students

V70.6 Health examination in population surveys
 EXCLUDES: special screening (V73.0-V82.9)

³ **V70.7 Examination of participant in clinical trial**
 Examination of participant or control in clinical research
 AHA: 4Q, '01, 55

V70.8 Other specified general medical examinations
 Examination of potential donor of organ or tissue

V70.9 Unspecified general medical examination

✓4th **V71 Observation and evaluation for suspected conditions not found**
 INCLUDES: This category is to be used when persons without a diagnosis are suspected of having an abnormal condition, without signs or symptoms, which requires study, but after examination and observation, is found not to exist. This category is also for use for administrative and legal observation status.
 AHA: 4Q, '94, 47; 2Q, '90, 5; M-A, '87, 1

✓5th **V71.0 Observation for suspected mental condition**

³ **V71.01 Adult antisocial behavior** A
 Dyssocial behavior or gang activity in adult without manifest psychiatric disorder

³ **V71.02 Childhood or adolescent antisocial behavior**
 Dyssocial behavior or gang activity in child or adolescent without manifest psychiatric disorder

³ **V71.09 Other suspected mental condition**

³ **V71.1 Observation for suspected malignant neoplasm**

³ **V71.2 Observation for suspected tuberculosis**

³ **V71.3 Observation following accident at work**

³ **V71.4 Observation following other accident**
 Examination of individual involved in motor vehicle traffic accident

³ **V71.5 Observation following alleged rape or seduction**
 Examination of victim or culprit

³ **V71.6 Observation following other inflicted injury**
 Examination of victim or culprit

³ **V71.7 Observation for suspected cardiovascular disease**
 AHA: 3Q, '90, 10; S-O, '87, 10

▲ ✓5th **V71.8 Observation and evaluation for other specified suspected conditions**
 AHA: 4Q, '00, 54 ; 1Q, '90, 19

³ **V71.81 Abuse and neglect**
 EXCLUDES: adult abuse and neglect (995.80-995.85)
  child abuse and neglect (995.50-995.59)
 AHA: 4Q, '00, 55

● **V71.82 Observation and evaluation for suspected exposure to anthrax**

● **V71.83 Observation and evaluation for suspected exposure to other biological agent**

³ These V codes may be used as principal diagnosis on Medicare patients.

V CODES — Tabular List

V71.89–V76.49

- ³ **V71.89** Other specified suspected conditions
- **V71.9** Observation for unspecified suspected condition
  - AHA: ▶1Q, '02, 6◀

✓4th V72 Special investigations and examinations

  INCLUDES: routine examination of specific system
  EXCLUDES: general medical examination (V70.0-V70.4)
  general screening examination of defined population groups (V70.5, V70.6, V70.7)
  routine examination of infant or child (V20.2)

  Use additional code(s) to identify any special screening examination(s) performed (V73.0-V82.9)

- ³ **V72.0** Examination of eyes and vision
- **V72.1** Examination of ears and hearing
- **V72.2** Dental examination
- ³ **V72.3** Gynecological examination ♀
  - Papanicolaou cervical smear as part of general gynecological examination
  - Pelvic examination (annual) (periodic)
  - Use additional code to identify routine vaginal Papanicolaou smear (V76.47)
  - EXCLUDES: cervical Papanicolaou smear without general gynecological examination (V76.2)
  - routine examination in contraceptive management (V25.40-V25.49)
- **V72.4** Pregnancy examination or test, pregnancy unconfirmed ♀
  - Possible pregnancy, not (yet) confirmed
  - EXCLUDES: pregnancy examination with immediate confirmation (V22.0-V22.1)
- **V72.5** Radiological examination, not elsewhere classified
  - Routine chest x-ray
  - EXCLUDES: examination for suspected tuberculosis (V71.2)
  - AHA: 1Q, '90, 19
- **V72.6** Laboratory examination
  - EXCLUDES: that for suspected disorder (V71.0-V71.9)
  - AHA: 1Q, '90, 22
- **V72.7** Diagnostic skin and sensitization tests
  - Allergy tests   Skin tests for hypersensitivity
  - EXCLUDES: diagnostic skin tests for bacterial diseases (V74.0-V74.9)
- ✓5th **V72.8** Other specified examinations
  - ³ **V72.81** Pre-operative cardiovascular examination
  - ³ **V72.82** Pre-operative respiratory examination
    - AHA: 3Q, '96, 14
  - ³ **V72.83** Other specified pre-operative examination
    - AHA: 3Q, '96, 14
  - **V72.84** Pre-operative examination, unspecified
  - **V72.85** Other specified examination
- **V72.9** Unspecified examination

✓4th V73 Special screening examination for viral and chlamydial diseases

- **V73.0** Poliomyelitis
- **V73.1** Smallpox
- **V73.2** Measles
- **V73.3** Rubella
- **V73.4** Yellow fever
- **V73.5** Other arthropod-borne viral diseases
  - Dengue fever   Viral encephalitis:
  - Hemorrhagic fever   mosquito-borne
  -     tick-borne
- **V73.6** Trachoma
- ✓5th **V73.8** Other specified viral and chlamydial diseases
  - **V73.88** Other specified chlamydial diseases
  - **V73.89** Other specified viral diseases
- ✓5th **V73.9** Unspecified viral and chlamydial disease
  - **V73.98** Unspecified chlamydial disease
  - **V73.99** Unspecified viral disease

✓4th V74 Special screening examination for bacterial and spirochetal diseases

  INCLUDES: diagnostic skin tests for these diseases

- **V74.0** Cholera
- **V74.1** Pulmonary tuberculosis
- **V74.2** Leprosy [Hansen's disease]
- **V74.3** Diphtheria
- **V74.4** Bacterial conjunctivitis
- **V74.5** Venereal disease
- **V74.6** Yaws
- **V74.8** Other specified bacterial and spirochetal diseases
  - Brucellosis   Tetanus
  - Leptospirosis   Whooping cough
  - Plague
- **V74.9** Unspecified bacterial and spirochetal disease

✓4th V75 Special screening examination for other infectious diseases

- **V75.0** Rickettsial diseases
- **V75.1** Malaria
- **V75.2** Leishmaniasis
- **V75.3** Trypanosomiasis
  - Chagas' disease
  - Sleeping sickness
- **V75.4** Mycotic infections
- **V75.5** Schistosomiasis
- **V75.6** Filariasis
- **V75.7** Intestinal helminthiasis
- **V75.8** Other specified parasitic infections
- **V75.9** Unspecified infectious disease

✓4th V76 Special screening for malignant neoplasms

- **V76.0** Respiratory organs
- ✓5th **V76.1** Breast
  - AHA: 4Q, '98, 67
  - **V76.10** Breast screening, unspecified
  - **V76.11** Screening mammogram for high-risk patient ♀
  - **V76.12** Other screening mammogram
  - **V76.19** Other screening breast examination
- **V76.2** Cervix ♀
  - Routine cervical Papanicolaou smear
  - EXCLUDES: that as part of a general gynecological examination (V72.3)
- **V76.3** Bladder
- ✓5th **V76.4** Other sites
  - **V76.41** Rectum
  - **V76.42** Oral cavity
  - **V76.43** Skin
  - **V76.44** Prostate ♂
  - **V76.45** Testis ♂
  - **V76.46** Ovary
    - AHA: 4Q, '00, 52
  - **V76.47** Vagina
    - Vaginal pap smear status-post hysterectomy for non-malignant condition
    - Use additional code to identify acquired absence of uterus (V45.77)
    - EXCLUDES: vaginal pap smear status-post hysterectomy for malignant condition (V67.01)
    - AHA: 4Q, '00, 52
  - **V76.49** Other sites
    - AHA: 1Q, '99, 4

³ These V codes may be used as principal diagnosis on Medicare patients.

 Newborn Age: 0   Pediatric Age: 0-17   Maternity Age: 12-55   Adult Age: 15-124   CC CC Condition   MC Major Complication   CD Complex Dx   HIV HIV Related Dx

V CODES

✓5ᵗʰ V76.5 Intestine
AHA: 4Q, '00, 52

    V76.50 Intestine, unspecified
    V76.51 Colon
        EXCLUDES rectum (V76.41)
        AHA: 4Q, '01, 56

    V76.52 Small intestine

✓5ᵗʰ V76.8 Other neoplasm
AHA: 4Q, '00, 52

    V76.81 Nervous system
    V76.89 Other neoplasm

V76.9 Unspecified

✓4ᵗʰ V77 Special screening for endocrine, nutritional, metabolic, and immunity disorders

    V77.0 Thyroid disorders
    V77.1 Diabetes mellitus
    V77.2 Malnutrition
    V77.3 Phenylketonuria [PKU]
    V77.4 Galactosemia
    V77.5 Gout
    V77.6 Cystic fibrosis
        Screening for mucoviscidosis
    V77.7 Other inborn errors of metabolism
    V77.8 Obesity

✓5ᵗʰ V77.9 Other and unspecified endocrine, nutritional, metabolic, and immunity disorders
AHA: 4Q, '00, 53

    V77.91 Screening for lipoid disorders
        Screening for cholesterol level
        Screening for hypercholesterolemia
        Screening for hyperlipidemia
    V77.99 Other and unspecified endocrine, nutritional, metabolic, and immunity disorders

✓4ᵗʰ V78 Special screening for disorders of blood and blood-forming organs

    V78.0 Iron deficiency anemia
    V78.1 Other and unspecified deficiency anemia
    V78.2 Sickle cell disease or trait
    V78.3 Other hemoglobinopathies
    V78.8 Other disorders of blood and blood-forming organs
    V78.9 Unspecified disorder of blood and blood-forming organs

✓4ᵗʰ V79 Special screening for mental disorders and developmental handicaps

    V79.0 Depression
    V79.1 Alcoholism
    V79.2 Mental retardation
    V79.3 Developmental handicaps in early childhood
    V79.8 Other specified mental disorders and developmental handicaps
    V79.9 Unspecified mental disorder and developmental handicap

✓4ᵗʰ V80 Special screening for neurological, eye, and ear diseases

    V80.0 Neurological conditions
    V80.1 Glaucoma
    V80.2 Other eye conditions
        Screening for:
          cataract
          congenital anomaly of eye
        Screening for:
          senile macular lesions
        EXCLUDES general vision examination (V72.0)
    V80.3 Ear diseases
        EXCLUDES general hearing examination (V72.1)

✓4ᵗʰ V81 Special screening for cardiovascular, respiratory, and genitourinary diseases

    V81.0 Ischemic heart disease
    V81.1 Hypertension
    V81.2 Other and unspecified cardiovascular conditions
    V81.3 Chronic bronchitis and emphysema
    V81.4 Other and unspecified respiratory conditions
        EXCLUDES screening for:
          lung neoplasm (V76.0)
          pulmonary tuberculosis (V74.1)
    V81.5 Nephropathy
        Screening for asymptomatic bacteriuria
    V81.6 Other and unspecified genitourinary conditions

✓4ᵗʰ V82 Special screening for other conditions

    V82.0 Skin conditions
    V82.1 Rheumatoid arthritis
    V82.2 Other rheumatic disorders
    V82.3 Congenital dislocation of hip
    V82.4 Maternal postnatal screening for chromosomal anomalies ♀
        EXCLUDES antenatal screening by amniocentesis (V28.0)
    V82.5 Chemical poisoning and other contamination
        Screening for:
          heavy metal poisoning
          ingestion of radioactive substance
          poisoning from contaminated water supply
          radiation exposure
    V82.6 Multiphasic screening

✓5ᵗʰ V82.8 Other specified conditions
AHA: 4Q, '00, 53

    V82.81 Osteoporosis
        Use additional code to identify:
          postmenopausal hormone replacement therapy status (V07.4)
          postmenopausal (age-related) (natural) status (V49.81)
        AHA: 4Q, '00, 54

    V82.89 Other specified conditions

    V82.9 Unspecified condition

✓4ᵗʰ V83 Genetic carrier status
AHA: 4Q, '01, 54

✓5ᵗʰ V83.0 Hemophilia A carrier
    V83.01 Asymptomatic hemophilia A carrier
    V83.02 Symptomatic hemophilia A carrier

✓5ᵗʰ V83.8 Other genetic carrier status
    V83.81 Cystic fibrosis gene carrier
    V83.89 Other genetic carrier status

SUPPLEMENTARY CLASSIFICATION OF EXTERNAL CAUSES OF INJURY AND POISONING (E800-E999)

This section is provided to permit the classification of environmental events, circumstances, and conditions as the cause of injury, poisoning, and other adverse effects. Where a code from this section is applicable, it is intended that it shall be used in addition to a code from one of the main chapters of ICD-9-CM, indicating the nature of the condition. Certain other conditions which may be stated to be due to external causes are classified in Chapters 1 to 16 of ICD-9-CM. For these, the "E" code classification should be used as an additional code for more detailed analysis.

Machinery accidents [other than those connected with transport] are classifiable to category E919, in which the fourth-digit allows a broad classification of the type of machinery involved. If a more detailed classification of type of machinery is required, it is suggested that the "Classification of Industrial Accidents according to Agency," prepared by the International Labor Office, be used in addition. This is reproduced in Appendix D for optional use.

Categories for "late effects" of accidents and other external causes are to be found at E929, E959, E969, E977, E989, and E999.

DEFINITIONS AND EXAMPLES RELATED TO TRANSPORT ACCIDENTS

(a) A **transport accident** (E800-E848) is any accident involving a device designed primarily for, or being used at the time primarily for, conveying persons or goods from one place to another.

INCLUDES accidents involving:
- aircraft and spacecraft (E840-E845)
- watercraft (E830-E838)
- motor vehicle (E810-E825)
- railway (E800-E807)
- other road vehicles (E826-E829)

In classifying accidents which involve more than one kind of transport, the above order of precedence of transport accidents should be used.

Accidents involving agricultural and construction machines, such as tractors, cranes, and bulldozers, are regarded as transport accidents only when these vehicles are under their own power on a highway [otherwise the vehicles are regarded as machinery]. Vehicles which can travel on land or water, such as hovercraft and other amphibious vehicles, are regarded as watercraft when on the water, as motor vehicles when on the highway, and as off-road motor vehicles when on land, but off the highway.

EXCLUDES accidents:
- in sports which involve the use of transport but where the transport vehicle itself was not involved in the accident
- involving vehicles which are part of industrial equipment used entirely on industrial premises
- occurring during transportation but unrelated to the hazards associated with the means of transportation [e.g., injuries received in a fight on board ship; transport vehicle involved in a cataclysm such as an earthquake]
- to persons engaged in the maintenance or repair of transport equipment or vehicle not in motion, unlesss injured by another vehicle in motion

(b) A **railway accident** is a transport accident involving a railway train or other railway vehicle operated on rails, whether in motion or not.

EXCLUDES accidents:
- in repair shops
- in roundhouse or on turntable
- on railway premises but not involving a train or other railway vehicle

(c) A **railway train** or **railway vehicle** is any device with or without cars coupled to it, designed for traffic on a railway.

INCLUDES interurban:
- electric car } (operated chiefly on its own right-of-way, not open to other traffic)
- streetcar
- railway train, any power [diesel] [electric] [steam]
- funicular
- monorail or two-rail
- subterranean or elevated
- other vehicle designed to run on a railway track

EXCLUDES interurban electric cars [streetcars] specified to be operating on a right-of-way that forms part of the public street or highway [definition (n)]

(d) A **railway** or **railroad** is a right-of-way designed for traffic on rails, which is used by carriages or wagons transporting passengers or freight, and by other rolling stock, and which is not open to other public vehicular traffic.

(e) A **motor vehicle accident** is a transport accident involving a motor vehicle. It is defined as a motor vehicle traffic accident or as a motor vehicle nontraffic accident according to whether the accident occurs on a public highway or elsewhere.

EXCLUDES injury or damage due to cataclysm
injury or damage while a motor vehicle, not under its own power, is being loaded on, or unloaded from, another conveyance

(f) A **motor vehicle traffic accident** is any motor vehicle accident occurring on a public highway [i.e., originating, terminating, or involving a vehicle partially on the highway]. A motor vehicle accident is assumed to have occurred on the highway unless another place is specified, except in the case of accidents involving only off-road motor vehicles which are classified as nontraffic accidents unless the contrary is stated.

(g) A **motor vehicle nontraffic accident** is any motor vehicle accident which occurs entirely in any place other than a public highway.

(h) A **public highway [trafficway]** or **street** is the entire width between property lines [or other boundary lines] of every way or place, of which any part is open to the use of the public for purposes of vehicular traffic as a matter of right or custom. A **roadway** is that part of the public highway designed, improved, and ordinarily used, for vehicular travel.

INCLUDES approaches (public) to:
- docks
- public building
- station

EXCLUDES driveway (private)
parking lot
ramp
roads in:
- airfield
- farm
- industrial premises
- mine
- private grounds
- quarry

(i) A **motor vehicle** is any mechanically or electrically powered device, not operated on rails, upon which any person or property may be transported or drawn upon a highway. Any object such as a trailer, coaster, sled, or wagon being towed by a motor vehicle is considerd a part of the motor vehicle.

> INCLUDES automobile [any type]
> bus
> construction machinery, farm and industrial machinery, steam roller, tractor, army tank, highway grader, or similar vehicle on wheels or treads, while in transport under own power
> fire engine (motorized)
> motorcycle
> motorized bicycle [moped] or scooter
> trolley bus not operating on rails
> truck
> van
>
> EXCLUDES devices used solely to move persons or materials within the confines of a building and its premises, such as:
> building elevator
> coal car in mine
> electric baggage or mail truck used solely within a railroad station
> electric truck used solely within an industrial plant
> moving overhead crane

(j) A **motorcycle** is a two-wheeled motor vehicle having one or two riding saddles and sometimes having a third wheel for the support of a sidecar. The sidecar is considered part of the motorcycle.

> INCLUDES motorized:
> bicycle [moped]
> scooter
> tricycle

(k) An **off-road motor vehicle** is a motor vehicle of special design, to enable it to negotiate rough or soft terrain or snow. Examples of special design are high construction, special wheels and tires, driven by treads, or support on a cushion of air.

> INCLUDES all terrain vehicle [ATV]
> army tank
> hovercraft, on land or swamp
> snowmobile

(l) A **driver** of a motor vehicle is the occupant of the motor vehicle operating it or intending to operate it. A **motorcyclist** is the driver of a motorcycle. Other authorized occupants of a motor vehicle are **passengers**.

(m) An **other road vehicle** is any device, except a motor vehicle, in, on, or by which any person or property may be transported on a highway.

> INCLUDES animal carrying a person or goods
> animal-drawn vehicles
> animal harnessed to conveyance
> bicycle [pedal cycle]
> streetcar
> tricycle (pedal)
>
> EXCLUDES pedestrian conveyance [definition (q)]

(n) A **streetcar** is a device designed and used primarily for transporting persons within a municipality, running on rails, usually subject to normal traffic control signals, and operated principally on a right-of-way that forms part of the traffic way. A trailer being towed by a streetcar is considered a part of the streetcar.

> INCLUDES interurban or intraurban electric or streetcar, when specified to be operating on a street or public highway
> tram (car)
> trolley (car)

(o) A **pedal cycle** is any road transport vehicle operated solely by pedals.

> INCLUDES bicycle
> pedal cycle
> tricycle
>
> EXCLUDES motorized bicycle [definition (i)]

(p) A **pedal cyclist** is any person riding on a pedal cycle or in a sidecar attached to such a vehicle.

(q) A **pedestrian conveyance** is any human powered device by which a pedestrian may move other than by walking or by which a walking person may move another pedestrian.

> INCLUDES baby carriage
> coaster wagon
> ice skates
> perambulator
> pushcart
> pushchair
> roller skates
> scooter
> skateboard
> skis
> sled
> wheelchair

(r) A **pedestrian** is any person involved in an accident who was not at the time of the accident riding in or on a motor vehicle, railroad train, streetcar, animal-drawn or other vehicle, or on a bicycle or animal.

> INCLUDES person:
> changing tire of vehicle
> in or operating a pedestrian conveyance
> making adjustment to motor of vehicle
> on foot

(s) A **watercraft** is any device for transporting passengers or goods on the water.

(t) A **small boat** is any watercraft propelled by paddle, oars, or small motor, with a passenger capacity of less than ten.

> INCLUDES boat NOS
> canoe
> coble
> dinghy
> punt
> raft
> rowboat
> rowing shell
> scull
> skiff
> small motorboat
>
> EXCLUDES barge
> lifeboat (used after abandoning ship)
> raft (anchored) being used as a diving platform
> yacht

(u) An **aircraft** is any device for transporting passengers or goods in the air.

> INCLUDES airplane [any type]
> balloon
> bomber
> dirigible
> glider (hang)
> military aircraft
> parachute

(v) A **commercial transport aircraft** is any device for collective passenger or freight transportation by air, whether run on commercial lines for profit or by government authorities, with the exception of military craft.

E CODES

RAILWAY ACCIDENTS (E800-E807)

Note: For definitions of railway accident and related terms see definitions (a) to (d).

EXCLUDES accidents involving railway train and:
aircraft (E840.0-E845.9)
motor vehicle (E810.0-E825.9)
watercraft (E830.0-E838.9)

The following fourth-digit subdivisions are for use with categories E800-E807 to identify the injured person:

.0 Railway employee
Any person who by virtue of his employment in connection with a railway, whether by the railway company or not, is at increased risk of involvement in a railway accident, such as:
catering staff of train
driver
guard
porter
postal staff on train
railway fireman
shunter
sleeping car attendant

.1 Passenger on railway
Any authorized person traveling on a train, except a railway employee.

EXCLUDES intending passenger waiting at station (.8)
unauthorized rider on railway vehicle (.8)

.2 Pedestrian
See definition (r)

.3 Pedal cyclist
See definition (p)

.8 Other specified person
Intending passenger or bystander waiting at station
Unauthorized rider on railway vehicle

.9 Unspecified person

§ ✓4th **E800 Railway accident involving collision with rolling stock**
INCLUDES collision between railway trains or railway vehicles, any kind
collision NOS on railway
derailment with antecedent collision with rolling stock or NOS

§ ✓4th **E801 Railway accident involving collision with other object**
INCLUDES collision of railway train with:
buffers
fallen tree on railway
gates
platform
rock on railway
streetcar
other nonmotor vehicle
other object

EXCLUDES collision with:
aircraft (E840.0-E842.9)
motor vehicle (E810.0-E810.9, E820.0-E822.9)

§ ✓4th **E802 Railway accident involving derailment without antecedent collision**

§ ✓4th **E803 Railway accident involving explosion, fire, or burning**
EXCLUDES explosion or fire, with antecedent derailment (E802.0-E802.9)
explosion or fire, with mention of antecedent collision (E800.0-E801.9)

§ ✓4th **E804 Fall in, on, or from railway train**
INCLUDES fall while alighting from or boarding railway train
EXCLUDES fall related to collision, derailment, or explosion of railway train (E800.0-E803.9)

§ ✓4th **E805 Hit by rolling stock**
INCLUDES crushed
injured
killed } by railway train or part
knocked down
run over

EXCLUDES pedestrian hit by object set in motion by railway train (E806.0-E806.9)

§ ✓4th **E806 Other specified railway accident**
INCLUDES hit by object falling in railway train
injured by door or window on railway train
nonmotor road vehicle or pedestrian hit by object set in motion by railway train
railway train hit by falling:
earth NOS
rock
tree
other object

EXCLUDES railway accident due to cataclysm (E908-E909)

§ ✓4th **E807 Railway accident of unspecified nature**
INCLUDES found dead } on railway right-of-way
injured } NOS

railway accident NOS

MOTOR VEHICLE TRAFFIC ACCIDENTS (E810-E819)

Note: For definitions of motor vehicle traffic accident, and related terms, see definitions (e) to (k).

EXCLUDES accidents involving motor vehicle and aircraft (E840.0-E845.9)

The following fourth-digit subdivisions are for use with categories E810-E819 to identify the injured person:

.0 Driver of motor vehicle other than motorcycle
See definition (l)

.1 Passenger in motor vehicle other than motorcycle
See definition (l)

.2 Motorcyclist
See definition (l)

.3 Passenger on motorcycle
See definition (l)

.4 Occupant of streetcar

.5 Rider of animal; occupant of animal-drawn vehicle

.6 Pedal cyclist
See definition (p)

.7 Pedestrian
See definition (r)

.8 Other specified person
Occupant of vehicle other than above
Person in railway train involved in accident
Unauthorized rider of motor vehicle

.9 Unspecified person

§§ ✓4th **E810 Motor vehicle traffic accident involving collision with train**
EXCLUDES motor vehicle collision with object set in motion by railway train (E815.0-E815.9)
railway train hit by object set in motion by motor vehicle (E818.0-E818.9)

---

§ Requires fourth-digit. See beginning of section E800-E807 for codes and definitions.
§§ Requires fourth-digit. See beginning of section E810-E819 for codes and definitions.

✓4th Fourth-digit Required ▶◀ Revised Text ● New Code ▲ Revised Code Title

2003 ICD-9-CM

§ ✓4ᵗʰ E811 Motor vehicle traffic accident involving re-entrant collision with another motor vehicle

INCLUDES collision between motor vehicle which accidentally leaves the roadway then re-enters the same roadway, or the opposite roadway on a divided highway, and another motor vehicle

EXCLUDES collision on the same roadway when none of the motor vehicles involved have left and re-entered the highway (E812.0-E812.9)

§ ✓4ᵗʰ E812 Other motor vehicle traffic accident involving collision with motor vehicle

INCLUDES collision with another motor vehicle parked, stopped, stalled, disabled, or abandoned on the highway
motor vehicle collision NOS

EXCLUDES collision with object set in motion by another motor vehicle (E815.0-E815.9)
re-entrant collision with another motor vehicle (E811.0-E811.9)

§ ✓4ᵗʰ E813 Motor vehicle traffic accident involving collision with other vehicle

INCLUDES collision between motor vehicle, any kind, and:
other road (nonmotor transport) vehicle, such as:
animal carrying a person
animal-drawn vehicle
pedal cycle
streetcar

EXCLUDES collision with:
object set in motion by nonmotor road vehicle (E815.0-E815.9)
pedestrian (E814.0-E814.9)
nonmotor road vehicle hit by object set in motion by motor vehicle (E818.0-E818.9)

§ ✓4ᵗʰ E814 Motor vehicle traffic accident involving collision with pedestrian

INCLUDES collision between motor vehicle, any kind, and pedestrian
pedestrian dragged, hit, or run over by motor vehicle, any kind

EXCLUDES pedestrian hit by object set in motion by motor vehicle (E818.0-E818.9)

§ ✓4ᵗʰ E815 Other motor vehicle traffic accident involving collision on the highway

INCLUDES collision (due to loss of control) (on highway) between motor vehicle, any kind, and:
abutment (bridge) (overpass)
animal (herded) (unattended)
fallen stone, traffic sign, tree, utility pole
guard rail or boundary fence
interhighway divider
landslide (not moving)
object set in motion by railway train or road vehicle (motor) (nonmotor)
object thrown in front of motor vehicle
other object, fixed, movable, or moving
safety island
temporary traffic sign or marker
wall of cut made for road

EXCLUDES collision with:
any object off the highway (resulting from loss of control) (E816.0-E816.9)
any object which normally would have been off the highway and is not stated to have been on it (E816.0-E816.9)
motor vehicle parked, stopped, stalled, disabled, or abandoned on highway (E812.0-E812.9)
moving landslide (E909)
motor vehicle hit by object:
set in motion by railway train or road vehicle (motor) (nonmotor) (E818.0-E818.9)
thrown into or on vehicle (E818.0-E818.9)

§ ✓4ᵗʰ E816 Motor vehicle traffic accident due to loss of control, without collision on the highway

INCLUDES motor vehicle:
failing to make curve
going out of control (due to):
blowout
burst tire
driver falling asleep
driver inattention
excessive speed
failure of mechanical part
and:
coliding with object off the highway
overturning
stopping abruptly off the highway

EXCLUDES collision on highway following loss of control (E810.0-E815.9)
loss of control of motor vehicle following collision on the highway (E810.0-E815.9)

§ ✓4ᵗʰ E817 Noncollision motor vehicle traffic accident while boarding or alighting

INCLUDES fall down stairs of motor bus
fall from car in street
injured by moving part of the vehicle
trapped by door of motor bus
while boarding or alighting

---

§ Requires fourth-digit. See beginning of section E810-E819 for codes and definitions.

✓4ᵗʰ Fourth-digit Required   ▶◀ Revised Text   ● New Code   ▲ Revised Code Title

Tabular List — E CODES — E818–E821

§§ ✓4ᵗʰ **E818 Other noncollision motor vehicle traffic accident**

INCLUDES:
accidental poisoning from exhaust gas generated by
breakage of any part of
explosion of any part of
fall, jump, or being accidentally pushed from
fire starting in
hit by object thrown into or on
injured by being thrown against some part of, or object in
injury from moving part of
object falling in or on
object thrown on
} motor vehicle while in motion

collision of railway train or road vehicle except motor vehicle, with object set in motion by motor vehicle
motor vehicle hit by object set in motion by railway train or road vehicle (motor) (nonmotor)
pedestrian, railway train, or road vehicle (motor) (nonmotor) hit by object set in motion by motor vehicle

EXCLUDES:
collision between motor vehicle and:
  object set in motion by railway train or road vehicle (motor) (nonmotor) (E815.0-E815.9)
  object thrown towards the motor vehicle (E815.0-E815.9)
person overcome by carbon monoxide generated by stationary motor vehicle off the roadway with motor running (E868.2)

§§ ✓4ᵗʰ **E819 Motor vehicle traffic accident of unspecified nature**

INCLUDES:
motor vehicle traffic accident NOS
traffic accident NOS

MOTOR VEHICLE NONTRAFFIC ACCIDENTS (E820-E825)

Note: For definitions of motor vehicle nontraffic accident and related terms see definition (a) to (k).

INCLUDES:
accidents involving motor vehicles being used in recreational or sporting activities off the highway
collision and noncollision motor vehicle accidents occurring entirely off the highway

EXCLUDES:
accidents involving motor vehicle and:
  aircraft (E840.0-E845.9)
  watercraft (E830.0-E838.9)
accidents, not on the public highway, involving agricultural and construction machinery but not involving another motor vehicle (E919.0, E919.2, E919.7)

The following fourth-digit subdivisions are for use with categories E820-E825 to identify the injured person:

- **.0 Driver of motor vehicle other than motorcycle**
  See definition (l)
- **.1 Passenger in motor vehicle other than motorcycle**
  See definition (l)
- **.2 Motorcyclist**
  See definition (l)
- **.3 Passenger on motorcycle**
  See definition (l)
- **.4 Occupant of streetcar**
- **.5 Rider of animal; occupant of animal-drawn vehicle**
- **.6 Pedal cyclist**
  See definition (p)
- **.7 Pedestrian**
  See definition (r)
- **.8 Other specified person**
  Occupant of vehicle other than above
  Person on railway train involved in accident
  Unauthorized rider of motor vehicle
- **.9 Unspecified person**

§ ✓4ᵗʰ **E820 Nontraffic accident involving motor-driven snow vehicle**

INCLUDES:
breakage of part of
fall from
hit by
overturning of
run over or dragged by
} motor-driven snow vehicle (not on public highway)

collision of motor-driven snow vehicle with:
  animal (being ridden) (-drawn vehicle)
  another off-road motor vehicle
  other motor vehicle, not on public highway
  railway train
  other object, fixed or movable
injury caused by rough landing of motor-driven snow vehicle (after leaving ground on rough terrain)

EXCLUDES:
accident on the public highway involving motor driven snow vehicle (E810.0-E819.9)

§ ✓4ᵗʰ **E821 Nontraffic accident involving other off-road motor vehicle**

INCLUDES:
breakage of part of
fall from
hit by
overturning of
run over or dragged by
thrown against some part of or object in
} off-road motor vehicle, except snow vehicle (not on public highway)

collision with:
  animal (being ridden) (-drawn vehicle)
  another off-road motor vehicle, except snow vehicle
  other motor vehicle, not on public highway
  other object, fixed or movable

EXCLUDES:
accident on public highway involving off-road motor vehicle (E810.0-E819.9)
collision between motor driven snow vehicle and other off-road motor vehicle (E820.0-E820.9)
hovercraft accident on water (E830.0-E838.9)

---

§ Requires fourth-digit. See beginning of section E820-E825 for codes and definitions.
§§ Requires fourth-digit. See beginning of section E810-E819 for codes and definitions

✓4ᵗʰ Fourth-digit Required ▶◀ Revised Text ● New Code ▲ Revised Code Title

2003 ICD-9-CM

E CODES

§§ ✓4ᵗʰ E822 Other motor vehicle nontraffic accident involving collision with moving object

INCLUDES: collision, not on public highway, between
motor vehicle, except off-road motor vehicle and:
- animal
- nonmotor vehicle
- other motor vehicle, except off-road motor vehicle
- pedestrian
- railway train
- other moving object

EXCLUDES: *collision with:*
motor-driven snow vehicle (E820.0-E820.9)
other off-road motor vehicle (E821.0-E821.9)

§§ ✓4ᵗʰ E823 Other motor vehicle nontraffic accident involving collision with stationary object

INCLUDES: collision, not on public highway, between motor vehicle, except off-road motor vehicle, and any object, fixed or movable, but not in motion

§§ ✓4ᵗʰ E824 Other motor vehicle nontraffic accident while boarding and alighting

INCLUDES:
- fall
- injury from moving part of motor vehicle
- trapped by door of motor vehicle

while boarding or alighting from motor vehicle, except off-road motor vehicle, not on public highway

§§ ✓4ᵗʰ E825 Other motor vehicle nontraffic accident of other and unspecified nature

INCLUDES:
- accidental poisoning from carbon monoxide generated by
- breakage of any part of
- explosion of any part of
- fall, jump, or being accidentally pushed from
- fire starting in
- hit by object thrown into, towards, or on
- injured by being thrown against some part of, or object in
- injury from moving part of
- object falling in or on

motor vehicle while in motion, not on public highway

motor vehicle nontraffic accident NOS

EXCLUDES: *fall from or in stationary motor vehicle (E884.9, E885.9)*
overcome by carbon monoxide or exhaust gas generated by stationary motor vehicle off the roadway with motor running (E868.2)
struck by falling object from or in stationary motor vehicle (E916)

OTHER ROAD VEHICLE ACCIDENTS (E826-E829)

Note: Other road vehicle accidents are transport accidents involving road vehicles other than motor vehicles. For definitions of other road vehicle and related terms see definitions (m) to (o).

INCLUDES: accidents involving other road vehicles being used in recreational or sporting activities

EXCLUDES: *collision of other road vehicle [any] with:*
aircraft (E840.0-E845.9)
motor vehicle (E813.0-E813.9, E820.0-E822.9)
railway train (E801.0-E801.9)

The following fourth-digit subdivisions are for use with categories E826-E829 to identify the injured person.

.0 **Pedestrian**
See definition (r)
.1 **Pedal cyclist**
See definition (p)
.2 **Rider of animal**
.3 **Occupant of animal-drawn vehicle**
.4 **Occupant of streetcar**
.8 **Other specified person**
.9 **Unspecified person**

§ ✓4ᵗʰ E826 Pedal cycle accident
[0-9]

INCLUDES:
- breakage of any part of pedal cycle
- collision between pedal cycle and:
  - animal (being ridden) (herded) (unattended)
  - another pedal cycle
  - any pedestrian
  - nonmotor road vehicle
  - other object, fixed, movable, or moving, not set in motion by motor vehicle, railway train, or aircraft
- entanglement in wheel of pedal cycle
- fall from pedal cycle
- hit by object falling or thrown on the pedal cycle
- pedal cycle accident NOS
- pedal cycle overturned

§ ✓4ᵗʰ E827 Animal-drawn vehicle accident
[0,2-4,8,9]

INCLUDES:
- breakage of any part of vehicle
- collision between animal-drawn vehicle and:
  - animal (being ridden) (herded) (unattended)
  - nonmotor road vehicle, except pedal cycle
  - pedestrian, pedestrian conveyance, or pedestrian vehicle
  - other object, fixed, movable, or moving, not set in motion by motor vehicle, railway train, or aircraft
- fall from
- knocked down by
- overturning of
- run over by
- thrown from

animal-drawn vehicle

EXCLUDES: *collision of animal-drawn vehicle with pedal cycle (E826.0-E826.9)*

---

§ Requires fourth-digit. Valid digits are in [brackets] under each code. See beginning of section E826-E829 for codes and definitions.
§§ Requires fourth-digit. See beginning of section E820-E825 for codes and definitions.

✓4ᵗʰ Fourth-digit Required   ▶◀ Revised Text   ● New Code   ▲ Revised Code Title

| Tabular List | E CODES | E828–E832 |

§§ ✓4th **E828 Accident involving animal being ridden**
[0,2,4,8,9]
  INCLUDES collision between animal being ridden and:
      another animal
      nonmotor road vehicle, except pedal cycle, and animal-drawn vehicle
      pedestrian, pedestrian conveyance, or pedestrian vehicle
      other object, fixed, movable, or moving, not set in motion by motor vehicle, railway train, or aircraft
    fall from ⎫
    knocked down by ⎬ animal being ridden
    thrown from ⎪
    trampled by ⎭
    ridden animal stumbled and fell
  EXCLUDES collision of animal being ridden with:
      animal-drawn vehicle (E827.0-E827.9)
      pedal cycle (E826.0-E826.9)

§§ ✓4th **E829 Other road vehicle accidents**
[0,4,8,9]
  INCLUDES accident while ⎫
      boarding or alighting from ⎪
      blow from object in ⎬ streetcar
      breakage of any part of ⎪ nonmotor road vehicle not classifiable to E826-E828
      caught in door of- ⎪
      derailment of ⎪
      fall in, on, or from ⎪
      fire in ⎭
    collision between streetcar or nonmotor road vehicle, except as in E826-E828, and:
      animal (not being ridden)
      another nonmotor road vehicle not classifiable to E826-E828
      pedestrian
      other object, fixed, movable, or moving, not set in motion by motor vehicle, railway train, or aircraft
    nonmotor road vehicle accident NOS
    streetcar accident NOS
  EXCLUDES collision with:
      animal being ridden (E828.0-E828.9)
      animal-drawn vehicle (E827.0-E827.9)
      pedal cycle (E826.0-E826.9)

WATER TRANSPORT ACCIDENTS (E830-E838)

Note: For definitions of water transport accident and related terms see definitions (a), (s), and (t).
  INCLUDES watercraft accidents in the course of recreational activities
  EXCLUDES accidents involving both aircraft, including objects set in motion by aircraft, and watercraft (E840.0-E845.9)

The following fourth-digit subdivisions are for use with categories E830-E838 to identify the injured person:
  .0 Occupant of small boat, unpowered
  .1 Occupant of small boat, powered
    See definition (t)
    EXCLUDES *water skier (.4)*
  .2 Occupant of other watercraft — crew
    Persons:
      engaged in operation of watercraft
      providing passenger services [cabin attendants, ship's physician, catering personnel]
      working on ship during voyage in other capacity [musician in band, operators of shops and beauty parlors]
  .3 Occupant of other watercraft — other than crew
    Passenger
    Occupant of lifeboat, other than crew, after abandoning ship
  .4 Water skier
  .5 Swimmer
  .6 Dockers, stevedores
    Longshoreman employed on the dock in loading and unloading ships
  .8 Other specified person
    Immigration and custom officials on board ship
    Person:
      accompanying passenger or member of crew visiting boat
    Pilot (guiding ship into port)
  .9 Unspecified person

§ ✓4th **E830 Accident to watercraft causing submersion**
  INCLUDES submersion and drowning due to:
      boat overturning
      boat submerging
      falling or jumping from burning ship
      falling or jumping from crushed watercraft
      ship sinking
      other accident to watercraft

§ ✓4th **E831 Accident to watercraft causing other injury**
  INCLUDES any injury, except submersion and drowning, as a result of an accident to watercraft
      burned while ship on fire
      crushed between ships in collision
      crushed by lifeboat after abandoning ship
      fall due to collision or other accident to watercraft
      hit by falling object due to accident to watercraft
      injured in watercraft accident involving collision
      struck by boat or part thereof after fall or jump from damaged boat
  EXCLUDES *burns from localized fire or explosion on board ship (E837.0-E837.9)*

§ ✓4th **E832 Other accidental submersion or drowning in water transport accident**
  INCLUDES submersion or drowning as a result of an accident other than accident to the watercraft, such as:
      fall:
        from gangplank
        from ship
        overboard
      thrown overboard by motion of ship
      washed overboard
  EXCLUDES *submersion or drowning of swimmer or diver who voluntarily jumps from boat not involved in an accident (E910.0-E910.9)*

§ Requires fourth-digit. See beginning of section E830-E838 for codes and definitions.
§§ Requires fourth-digit. Valid digits are in [brackets] under each code. See beginning of section E826-E829 for codes and definitions.

✓4th Fourth-digit Required   ▶◀ Revised Text   ● New Code   ▲ Revised Code Title

E CODES

§§ ✓4th E833 Fall on stairs or ladders in water transport
EXCLUDES *fall due to accident to watercraft (E831.0-E831.9)*

§§ ✓4th E834 Other fall from one level to another in water transport
EXCLUDES *fall due to accident to watercraft (E831.0-E831.9)*

§§ ✓4th E835 Other and unspecified fall in water transport
EXCLUDES *fall due to accident to watercraft (E831.0-E831.9)*

§§ ✓4th E836 Machinery accident in water transport
INCLUDES injuries in water transport caused by:
- deck
- engine room
- galley
- laundry
- loading

} machinery

§§ ✓4th E837 Explosion, fire, or burning in watercraft
INCLUDES
- explosion of boiler on steamship
- localized fire on ship

EXCLUDES *burning ship (due to collision or explosion) resulting in:*
submersion or drowning (E830.0-E830.9)
other injury (E831.0-E831.9)

§§ ✓4th E838 Other and unspecified water transport accident
INCLUDES
- accidental poisoning by gases or fumes on ship
- atomic power plant malfunction in watercraft
- crushed between ship and stationary object [wharf]
- crushed between ships without accident to watercraft
- crushed by falling object on ship or while loading or unloading
- hit by boat while water skiing
- struck by boat or part thereof (after fall from boat)
- watercraft accident NOS

AIR AND SPACE TRANSPORT ACCIDENTS (E840-E845)

Note: For definition of aircraft and related terms see definitions (u) and (v).

The following fourth-digit subdivisions are for use with categories E840-E845 to identify the injured person. Valid fourth digits are in [brackets] under codes E842-E845.

.0 Occupant of spacecraft

.1 Occupant of military aircraft, any
Crew in military aircraft [air force] [army] [national guard] [navy]
Passenger (civilian) (military) in military aircraft [air force] [army] [national guard] [navy]
Troops in military aircraft [air force] [army] [national guard] [navy]
EXCLUDES *occupants of aircraft operated under jurisdiction of police departments (.5)*
parachutist (.7)

.2 Crew of commercial aircraft (powered) in surface to surface transport

.3 Other occupant of commercial aircraft (powered) in surface to surface transport
Flight personnel:
 not part of crew
 on familiarization flight
Passenger on aircraft (powered) NOS

.4 Occupant of commercial aircraft (powered) in surface to air transport
Occupant [crew] [passenger] of aircraft (powered) engaged in activities, such as:
- aerial spraying (crops) (fire retardants)
- air drops of emergency supplies
- air drops of parachutists, except from military craft
- crop dusting
- lowering of construction material [bridge or telephone pole]
- sky writing

.5 Occupant of other powered aircraft
Occupant [crew] [passenger] of aircraft (powered) engaged in activities, such as:
- aerobatic flying
- aircraft racing
- rescue operation
- storm surveillance
- traffic surveillance
Occupant of private plane NOS

.6 Occupant of unpowered aircraft, except parachutist
Occupant of aircraft classifiable to E842

.7 Parachutist (military) (other)
Person making voluntary descent
EXCLUDES *person making descent after accident to aircraft (.1-.6)*

.8 Ground crew, airline employee
Persons employed at airfields (civil) (military) or launching pads, not occupants of aircraft

.9 Other person

§ ✓4th E840 Accident to powered aircraft at takeoff or landing
INCLUDES
- collision of aircraft with any object, fixed, movable, or moving
- crash
- explosion on aircraft
- fire on aircraft
- forced landing

} while taking off or landing

§ ✓4th E841 Accident to powered aircraft, other and unspecified
INCLUDES
- aircraft accident NOS
- aircraft crash or wreck NOS
- any accident to powered aircraft while in transit or when not specified whether in transit, taking off, or landing
- collision of aircraft with another aircraft, bird, or any object, while in transit
- explosion on aircraft while in transit
- fire on aircraft while in transit

§ ✓4th E842 Accident to unpowered aircraft
[6-9] **INCLUDES** any accident, except collision with powered aircraft, to:
- balloon
- glider
- hang glider
- kite carrying a person
- hit by object falling from unpowered aircraft

§ ✓4th E843 Fall in, on, or from aircraft
[0-9] **INCLUDES**
- accident in boarding or alighting from aircraft, any kind
- fall in, on, or from aircraft [any kind], while in transit, taking off, or landing, except when as a result of an accident to aircraft

---

§ Requires fourth-digit. See beginning of section E840-E845 for codes and definitions.
§§ Requires fourth-digit. See beginning of section E830-E838 for codes and definitions.

Tabular List   E CODES   E844–E849.6

§ ✓4ᵗʰ E844 Other specified air transport accidents
[0-9] INCLUDES:
    hit by:
        aircraft
        object falling from aircraft
    injury by or from:
        machinery on aircraft
        rotating propeller   } without accident to aircraft
        voluntary parachute descent
    poisoning by carbon monoxide from aircraft while in transit
    sucked into jet

    any accident involving other transport vehicle (motor) (nonmotor) due to being hit by object set in motion by aircraft (powered)

    EXCLUDES: air sickness (E903)
    effects of:
        high altitude (E902.0-E902.1)
        pressure change (E902.0-E902.1)
    injury in parachute descent due to accident to aircraft (E840.0-E842-9)

§ ✓4ᵗʰ E845 Accident involving spacecraft
[0,8,9] INCLUDES: launching pad accident
    EXCLUDES: effects of weightlessness in spacecraft (E928.0)

VEHICLE ACCIDENTS NOT ELSEWHERE CLASSIFIABLE (E846-E848)

E846 Accidents involving powered vehicles used solely within the buildings and premises of industrial or commercial establishment
Accident to, on, or involving:
    battery powered airport passenger vehicle
    battery powered trucks (baggage) (mail)
    coal car in mine
    logging car
    self propelled truck, industrial
    station baggage truck (powered)
    tram, truck, or tub (powered) in mine or quarry
Collision with:
    pedestrian
    other vehicle or object within premises
Explosion of
Fall from
Overturning of   } powered vehicle, industrial or commercial
Struck by

    EXCLUDES: accidental poisoning by exhaust gas from vehicle not elsewhere classifiable (E868.2)
    injury by crane, lift (fork), or elevator (E919.2)

E847 Accidents involving cable cars not running on rails
Accident to, on, or involving:
    cable car, not on rails
    ski chair-lift
    ski-lift with gondola
    téléférique
Breakage of cable
Caught or dragged by
Fall or jump from   } cable car, not on rails
Object thrown from or in

E848 Accidents involving other vehicles, not elsewhere classifiable
Accident to, on, or involving:
    ice yacht
    land yacht
    nonmotor, nonroad vehicle NOS

✓4ᵗʰ E849 Place of occurrence
The following category is for use to denote the place where the injury or poisoning occurred.

E849.0 Home
Apartment
Boarding house
Farm house
Home premises
House (residential)
Noninstitutional place of residence
Private:
    driveway
    garage
    garden
    home
    walk
Swimming pool in private house or garden
Yard of home

    EXCLUDES: home under construction but not yet occupied (E849.3)
    institutional place of residence (E849.7)

E849.1 Farm
Farm:
    buildings
    land under cultivation
    EXCLUDES: farm house and home premises of farm (E849.0)

E849.2 Mine and quarry
Gravel pit
Sand pit
Tunnel under construction

E849.3 Industrial place and premises
Building under construction
Dockyard
Dry dock
Factory
    building
    premises
Garage (place of work)
Industrial yard
Loading platform (factory) (store)
Plant, industrial
Railway yard
Shop (place of work)
Warehouse
Workhouse

E849.4 Place for recreation and sport
Amusement park
Baseball field
Basketball court
Beach resort
Cricket ground
Fives court
Football field
Golf course
Gymnasium
Hockey field
Holiday camp
Ice palace
Lake resort
Mountain resort
Playground, including school playground
Public park
Racecourse
Resort NOS
Riding school
Rifle range
Seashore resort
Skating rink
Sports palace
Stadium
Swimming pool, public
Tennis court
Vacation resort

    EXCLUDES: that in private house or garden (E849.0)

E849.5 Street and highway

E849.6 Public building
Building (including adjacent grounds) used by the general public or by a particular group of the public, such as:
airport
bank
café
casino
church
cinema
clubhouse
courthouse
dance hall
garage building (for car storage)
hotel
market (grocery or other commodity)
movie house
music hall
nightclub
office
office building
opera house
post office
public hall
radio broadcasting station
restaurant
school (state) (public) (private)
shop, commercial
station (bus) (railway)
store
theater

    EXCLUDES: home garage (E849.0)
    industrial building or workplace (E849.3)

---

§ Requires fourth-digit. See beginning of section E840-E845 for codes and definitions.

✓4ᵗʰ Fourth-digit Required   ▶◀ Revised Text   ● New Code   ▲ Revised Code Title

E849.7 Residential institution
- Children's home
- Dormitory
- Hospital
- Jail
- Old people's home
- Orphanage
- Prison
- Reform school

E849.8 Other specified places
- Beach NOS
- Canal
- Caravan site NOS
- Derelict house
- Desert
- Dock
- Forest
- Harbor
- Hill
- Lake NOS
- Mountain
- Parking lot
- Parking place
- Pond or pool (natural)
- Prairie
- Public place NOS
- Railway line
- Reservoir
- River
- Sea
- Seashore NOS
- Stream
- Swamp
- Trailer court
- Woods

E849.9 Unspecified place

ACCIDENTAL POISONING BY DRUGS, MEDICINAL SUBSTANCES, AND BIOLOGICALS (E850-E858)

INCLUDES accidental overdose of drug, wrong drug given or taken in error, and drug taken inadvertently
accidents in the use of drugs and biologicals in medical and surgical procedures

EXCLUDES administration with suicidal or homicidal intent or intent to harm, or in circumstances classifiable to E980-E989 (E950.0-E950.5, E962.0, E980.0-E980.5)
correct drug properly administered in therapeutic or prophylactic dosage, as the cause of adverse effect (E930.0-E949.9)

See Alphabetic Index for more complete list of specific drugs to be classified under the fourth-digit subdivisions. The American Hospital Formulary numbers can be used to classify new drugs listed by the American Hospital Formulary Service (AHFS). See Appendix C.

✓4ᵗʰ E850 Accidental poisoning by analgesics, antipyretics, and antirheumatics

E850.0 Heroin
- Diacetylmorphine

E850.1 Methadone

E850.2 Other opiates and related narcotics
- Codeine [methylmorphine]
- Meperidine [pethidine]
- Morphine
- Opium (alkaloids)

E850.3 Salicylates
- Acetylsalicylic acid [aspirin]
- Amino derivatives of salicylic acid
- Salicylic acid salts

E850.4 Aromatic analgesics, not elsewhere classified
- Acetanilid
- Paracetamol [acetaminophen]
- Phenacetin [acetophenetidin]

E850.5 Pyrazole derivatives
- Aminophenazone [amidopyrine]
- Phenylbutazone

E850.6 Antirheumatics [antiphlogistics]
- Gold salts
- Indomethacin

EXCLUDES salicylates (E850.3)
steroids (E858.0)

E850.7 Other non-narcotic analgesics
- Pyrabital

E850.8 Other specified analgesics and antipyretics
- Pentazocine

E850.9 Unspecified analgesic or antipyretic

E851 Accidental poisoning by barbiturates
- Amobarbital [amylobarbitone]
- Barbital [barbitone]
- Butabarbital [butabarbitone]
- Pentobarbital [pentobarbitone]
- Phenobarbital [phenobarbitone]
- Secobarbital [quinalbarbitone]

EXCLUDES thiobarbiturates (E855.1)

✓4ᵗʰ E852 Accidental poisoning by other sedatives and hypnotics

E852.0 Chloral hydrate group
E852.1 Paraldehyde
E852.2 Bromine compounds
- Bromides
- Carbromal (derivatives)

E852.3 Methaqualone compounds
E852.4 Glutethimide group
E852.5 Mixed sedatives, not elsewhere classified
E852.8 Other specified sedatives and hypnotics
E852.9 Unspecified sedative or hypnotic
- Sleeping:
  - drug
  - pill
  - tablet
  } NOS

✓4ᵗʰ E853 Accidental poisoning by tranquilizers

E853.0 Phenothiazine-based tranquilizers
- Chlorpromazine
- Fluphenazine
- Prochlorperazine
- Promazine

E853.1 Butyrophenone-based tranquilizers
- Haloperidol
- Spiperone
- Trifluperidol

E853.2 Benzodiazepine-based tranquilizers
- Chlordiazepoxide
- Diazepam
- Flurazepam
- Lorazepam
- Medazepam
- Nitrazepam

E853.8 Other specified tranquilizers
- Hydroxyzine
- Meprobamate

E853.9 Unspecified tranquilizer

✓4ᵗʰ E854 Accidental poisoning by other psychotropic agents

E854.0 Antidepressants
- Amitriptyline
- Imipramine
- Monoamine oxidase [MAO] inhibitors

E854.1 Psychodysleptics [hallucinogens]
- Cannabis derivatives
- Lysergide [LSD]
- Marihuana (derivatives)
- Mescaline
- Psilocin
- Psilocybin

E854.2 Psychostimulants
- Amphetamine
- Caffeine

EXCLUDES central appetite depressants (E858.8)

E854.3 Central nervous system stimulants
- Analeptics
- Opiate antagonists

E854.8 Other psychotropic agents

✓4ᵗʰ E855 Accidental poisoning by other drugs acting on central and autonomic nervous system

E855.0 Anticonvulsant and anti-Parkinsonism drugs
- Amantadine
- Hydantoin derivatives
- Levodopa [L-dopa]
- Oxazolidine derivatives [paramethadione] [trimethadione]
- Succinimides

E855.1 Other central nervous system depressants
- Ether
- Gaseous anesthetics
- Halogenated hydrocarbon derivatives
- Intravenous anesthetics
- Thiobarbiturates, such as thiopental sodium

E855.2 Local anesthetics
- Cocaine
- Lidocaine [lignocaine]
- Procaine
- Tetracaine

E CODES

E855.3 **Parasympathomimetics [cholinergics]**
  Acetylcholine Pilocarpine
  Anticholinesterase:
   organophosphorus
   reversible

E855.4 **Parasympatholytics [anticholinergics and antimuscarinics] and spasmolytics**
  Atropine
  Homatropine
  Hyoscine [scopolamine]
  Quaternary ammonium derivatives

E855.5 **Sympathomimetics [adrenergics]**
  Epinephrine [adrenalin]
  Levarterenol [noradrenalin]

E855.6 **Sympatholytics [antiadrenergics]**
  Phenoxybenzamine
  Tolazoline hydrochloride

E855.8 **Other specified drugs acting on central and autonomic nervous systems**

E855.9 **Unspecified drug acting on central and autonomic nervous systems**

E856 **Accidental poisoning by antibiotics**

E857 **Accidental poisoning by other anti-infectives**

✓4th E858 **Accidental poisoning by other drugs**
 E858.0 **Hormones and synthetic substitutes**
 E858.1 **Primarily systemic agents**
 E858.2 **Agents primarily affecting blood constituents**
 E858.3 **Agents primarily affecting cardiovascular system**
 E858.4 **Agents primarily affecting gastrointestinal system**
 E858.5 **Water, mineral, and uric acid metabolism drugs**
 E858.6 **Agents primarily acting on the smooth and skeletal muscles and respiratory system**
 E858.7 **Agents primarily affecting skin and mucous membrane, ophthalmological, otorhinolaryngological, and dental drugs**
 E858.8 **Other specified drugs**
   Central appetite depressants
 E858.9 **Unspecified drug**

ACCIDENTAL POISONING BY OTHER SOLID AND LIQUID SUBSTANCES, GASES, AND VAPORS (E860-E869)

Note: Categories in this section are intended primarily to indicate the external cause of poisoning states classifiable to 980-989. They may also be used to indicate external causes of localized effects classifiable to 001-799.

✓4th E860 **Accidental poisoning by alcohol, not elsewhere classified**
 E860.0 **Alcoholic beverages**
   Alcohol in preparations intended for consumption
 E860.1 **Other and unspecified ethyl alcohol and its products**
  Denatured alcohol Grain alcohol NOS
  Ethanol NOS Methylated spirit
 E860.2 **Methyl alcohol**
  Methanol Wood alcohol
 E860.3 **Isopropyl alcohol**
  Dimethyl carbinol Rubbing alcohol subsitute
  Isopropanol Secondary propyl alcohol
 E860.4 **Fusel oil**
  Alcohol: Alcohol:
   amyl   propyl
   butyl
 E860.8 **Other specified alcohols**
 E860.9 **Unspecified alcohol**

✓4th E861 **Accidental poisoning by cleansing and polishing agents, disinfectants, paints, and varnishes**
 E861.0 **Synthetic detergents and shampoos**
 E861.1 **Soap products**
 E861.2 **Polishes**
 E861.3 **Other cleansing and polishing agents**
   Scouring powders
 E861.4 **Disinfectants**
   Household and other disinfectants not ordinarily used on the person
   EXCLUDES *carbolic acid or phenol (E864.0)*
 E861.5 **Lead paints**
 E861.6 **Other paints and varnishes**
  Lacquers Paints, other than lead
  Oil colors White washes
 E861.9 **Unspecified**

✓4th E862 **Accidental poisoning by petroleum products, other solvents and their vapors, not elsewhere classified**
 E862.0 **Petroleum solvents**
  Petroleum: Petroleum:
   ether   naphtha
   benzine
 E862.1 **Petroleum fuels and cleaners**
  Antiknock additives to petroleum fuels
  Gas oils
  Gasoline or petrol
  Kerosene
   EXCLUDES *kerosene insecticides (E863.4)*
 E862.2 **Lubricating oils**
 E862.3 **Petroleum solids**
   Paraffin wax
 E862.4 **Other specified solvents**
   Benzene
 E862.9 **Unspecified solvent**

✓4th E863 **Accidental poisoning by agricultural and horticultural chemical and pharmaceutical preparations other than plant foods and fertilizers**
  EXCLUDES *plant foods and fertilizers (E866.5)*
 E863.0 **Insecticides of organochlorine compounds**
  Benzene hexachloride Dieldrin
  Chlordane Endrine
  DDT Toxaphene
 E863.1 **Insecticides of organophosphorus compounds**
  Demeton Parathion
  Diazinon Phenylsulphthion
  Dichlorvos Phorate
  Malathion Phosdrin
  Methyl parathion
 E863.2 **Carbamates**
  Aldicarb Propoxur
  Carbaryl
 E863.3 **Mixtures of insecticides**
 E863.4 **Other and unspecified insecticides**
   Kerosene insecticides
 E863.5 **Herbicides**
  2, 4-Dichlorophenoxyacetic acid [2, 4-D]
  2, 4, 5-Trichlorophenoxyacetic acid [2, 4, 5-T]
  Chlorates
  Diquat
  Mixtures of plant foods and fertilizers with herbicides
  Paraquat
 E863.6 **Fungicides**
  Organic mercurials (used in seed dressing)
  Pentachlorophenols
 E863.7 **Rodenticides**
  Fluoroacetates Warfarin
  Squill and derivatives Zinc phosphide
  Thallium
 E863.8 **Fumigants**
  Cyanides Phosphine
  Methyl bromide
 E863.9 **Other and unspecified**

☑4th **E864 Accidental poisoning by corrosives and caustics, not elsewhere classified**
　　EXCLUDES: those as components of disinfectants (E861.4)

E864.0 Corrosive aromatics
　　Carbolic acid or phenol

E864.1 Acids
　　Acid:
　　　　hydrochloric
　　　　nitric
　　　　sulfuric

E864.2 Caustic alkalis
　　Lye

E864.3 Other specified corrosives and caustics

E864.4 Unspecified corrosives and caustics

☑4th **E865 Accidental poisoning from poisonous foodstuffs and poisonous plants**
　　INCLUDES: any meat, fish, or shellfish
　　plants, berries, and fungi eaten as, or in mistake for, food, or by a child
　　EXCLUDES: anaphylactic shock due to adverse food reaction (995.60-995.69)
　　food poisoning (bacterial) (005.0-005.9)
　　poisoning and toxic reactions to venomous plants (E905.6-E905.7)

E865.0 Meat
E865.1 Shellfish
E865.2 Other fish
E865.3 Berries and seeds
E865.4 Other specified plants
E865.5 Mushrooms and other fungi
E865.8 Other specified foods
E865.9 Unspecified foodstuff or poisonous plant

☑4th **E866 Accidental poisoning by other and unspecified solid and liquid substances**
　　EXCLUDES: these substances as a component of:
　　medicines (E850.0-E858.9)
　　paints (E861.5-E861.6)
　　pesticides (E863.0-E863.9)
　　petroleum fuels (E862.1)

E866.0 Lead and its compounds and fumes
E866.1 Mercury and its compounds and fumes
E866.2 Antimony and its compounds and fumes
E866.3 Arsenic and its compounds and fumes
E866.4 Other metals and their compounds and fumes
　　Beryllium (compounds)　Iron (compounds)
　　Brass fumes　Manganese (compounds)
　　Cadmium (compounds)　Nickel (compounds)
　　Copper salts　Thallium (compounds)

E866.5 Plant foods and fertilizers
　　EXCLUDES: mixtures with herbicides (E863.5)

E866.6 Glues and adhesives
E866.7 Cosmetics
E866.8 Other specified solid or liquid substances
E866.9 Unspecified solid or liquid substance

E867 Accidental poisoning by gas distributed by pipeline
　　Carbon monoxide from incomplete combustion of piped gas
　　Coal gas NOS
　　Liquefied petroleum gas distributed through pipes (pure or mixed with air)
　　Piped gas (natural) (manufactured)

☑4th **E868 Accidental poisoning by other utility gas and other carbon monoxide**

E868.0 Liquefied petroleum gas distributed in mobile containers
　　Butane
　　Liquefied hydrocarbon gas NOS　} or carbon monoxide from incomplete combustion of these gases
　　Propane

E868.1 Other and unspecified utility gas
　　Acetylene
　　Gas NOS used for lighting, heating, or cooking　} or carbon monoxide from incomplete combustion of these gases
　　Water gas

E868.2 Motor vehicle exhaust gas
　　Exhaust gas from:
　　　　farm tractor, not in transit
　　　　gas engine
　　　　motor pump
　　　　motor vehicle, not in transit
　　　　any type of combustion engine not in watercraft
　　EXCLUDES: poisoning by carbon monoxide from:
　　　　aircraft while in transit (E844.0-E844.9)
　　　　motor vehicle while in transit (E818.0-E818.9)
　　　　watercraft whether or not in transit (E838.0-E838.9)

E868.3 Carbon monoxide from incomplete combustion of other domestic fuels
　　Carbon monoxide from incomplete combustion of:
　　　　coal
　　　　coke
　　　　kerosene
　　　　wood　} in domestic stove or fireplace
　　EXCLUDES: carbon monoxide from smoke and fumes due to conflagration (E890.0-E893.9)

E868.8 Carbon monoxide from other sources
　　Carbon monoxide from:
　　　　blast furnace gas
　　　　incomplete combustion of fuels in industrial use
　　　　kiln vapor

E868.9 Unspecified carbon monoxide

☑4th **E869 Accidental poisoning by other gases and vapors**
　　EXCLUDES: effects of gases used as anesthetics (E855.1, E938.2)
　　fumes from heavy metals (E866.0-E866.4)
　　smoke and fumes due to conflagration or explosion (E890.0-E899)

E869.0 Nitrogen oxides
E869.1 Sulfur dioxide
E869.2 Freon
E869.3 Lacrimogenic gas [tear gas]
　　Bromobenzyl cyanide　Ethyliodoacetate
　　Chloroacetophenone

E869.4 Second-hand tobacco smoke
E869.8 Other specified gases and vapors
　　Chlorine　Hydrocyanic acid gas

E869.9 Unspecified gases and vapors

MISADVENTURES TO PATIENTS DURING SURGICAL AND MEDICAL CARE (E870-E876)

　　EXCLUDES: accidental overdose of drug and wrong drug given in error (E850.0-E858.9)
　　surgical and medical procedures as the cause of abnormal reaction by the patient, without mention of misadventure at the time of procedure (E878.0-E879.9)

☑4th **E870 Accidental cut, puncture, perforation, or hemorrhage during medical care**

E870.0 Surgical operation
E870.1 Infusion or transfusion
E870.2 Kidney dialysis or other perfusion
E870.3 Injection or vaccination
E870.4 Endoscopic examination

E CODES

- **E870.5** Aspiration of fluid or tissue, puncture, and catheterization
  - Abdominal paracentesis
  - Aspirating needle biopsy
  - Blood sampling
  - Lumbar puncture
  - Thoracentesis
  - *EXCLUDES* heart catheterization (E870.6)
- **E870.6** Heart catheterization
- **E870.7** Administration of enema
- **E870.8** Other specified medical care
- **E870.9** Unspecified medical care

✓4th **E871 Foreign object left in body during procedure**
- **E871.0** Surgical operation
- **E871.1** Infusion or transfusion
- **E871.2** Kidney dialysis or other perfusion
- **E871.3** Injection or vaccination
- **E871.4** Endoscopic examination
- **E871.5** Aspiration of fluid or tissue, puncture, and catheterization
  - Abdominal paracentesis
  - Aspiration needle biopsy
  - Blood sampling
  - Lumbar puncture
  - Thoracentesis
  - *EXCLUDES* heart catheterization (E871.6)
- **E871.6** Heart catheterization
- **E871.7** Removal of catheter or packing
- **E871.8** Other specified procedures
- **E871.9** Unspecified procedure

✓4th **E872 Failure of sterile precautions during procedure**
- **E872.0** Surgical operation
- **E872.1** Infusion or transfusion
- **E872.2** Kidney dialysis and other perfusion
- **E872.3** Injection or vaccination
- **E872.4** Endoscopic examination
- **E872.5** Aspiration of fluid or tissue, puncture, and catheterization
  - Abdominal paracentesis
  - Aspiration needle biopsy
  - Blood sampling
  - Lumbar puncture
  - Thoracentesis
  - *EXCLUDES* heart catheterization (E872.6)
- **E872.6** Heart catheterization
- **E872.8** Other specified procedures
- **E872.9** Unspecified procedure

✓4th **E873 Failure in dosage**
  - *EXCLUDES* accidental overdose of drug, medicinal or biological substance (E850.0-E858.9)
- **E873.0** Excessive amount of blood or other fluid during transfusion or infusion
- **E873.1** Incorrect dilution of fluid during infusion
- **E873.2** Overdose of radiation in therapy
- **E873.3** Inadvertent exposure of patient to radiation during medical care
- **E873.4** Failure in dosage in electroshock or insulin-shock therapy
- **E873.5** Inappropriate [too hot or too cold] temperature in local application and packing
- **E873.6** Nonadministration of necessary drug or medicinal substance
- **E873.8** Other specified failure in dosage
- **E873.9** Unspecified failure in dosage

✓4th **E874 Mechanical failure of instrument or apparatus during procedure**
- **E874.0** Surgical operation
- **E874.1** Infusion and transfusion
  - Air in system
- **E874.2** Kidney dialysis and other perfusion
- **E874.3** Endoscopic examination
- **E874.4** Aspiration of fluid or tissue, puncture, and catheterization
  - Abdominal paracentesis
  - Aspiration needle biopsy
  - Blood sampling
  - Lumbar puncture
  - Thoracentesis
  - *EXCLUDES* heart catheterization (E874.5)
- **E874.5** Heart catheterization
- **E874.8** Other specified procedures
- **E874.9** Unspecified procedure

✓4th **E875 Contaminated or infected blood, other fluid, drug, or biological substance**
  - *INCLUDES* presence of:
    - bacterial pyrogens
    - endotoxin-producing bacteria
    - serum hepatitis-producing agent
- **E875.0** Contaminated substance transfused or infused
- **E875.1** Contaminated substance injected or used for vaccination
- **E875.2** Contaminated drug or biological substance administered by other means
- **E875.8** Other
- **E875.9** Unspecified

✓4th **E876 Other and unspecified misadventures during medical care**
- **E876.0** Mismatched blood in transfusion
- **E876.1** Wrong fluid in infusion
- **E876.2** Failure in suture and ligature during surgical operation
- **E876.3** Endotracheal tube wrongly placed during anesthetic procedure
- **E876.4** Failure to introduce or to remove other tube or instrument
  - *EXCLUDES* foreign object left in body during procedure (E871.0-E871.9)
- **E876.5** Performance of inappropriate operation
- **E876.8** Other specified misadventures during medical care
  - Performance of inappropriate treatment NEC
- **E876.9** Unspecified misadventure during medical care

SURGICAL AND MEDICAL PROCEDURES AS THE CAUSE OF ABNORMAL REACTION OF PATIENT OR LATER COMPLICATION, WITHOUT MENTION OF MISADVENTURE AT THE TIME OF PROCEDURE (E878-E879)

INCLUDES procedures as the cause of abnormal reaction, such as:
- displacement or malfunction of prosthetic device
- hepatorenal failure, postoperative
- malfunction of external stoma
- postoperative intestinal obstruction
- rejection of transplanted organ

EXCLUDES anesthetic management properly carried out as the cause of adverse effect (E937.0-E938.9)
infusion and transfusion, without mention of misadventure in the technique of procedure (E930.0-E949.9)

✓4th **E878 Surgical operation and other surgical procedures as the cause of abnormal reaction of patient, or of later complication, without mention of misadventure at the time of operation**
- **E878.0** Surgical operation with transplant of whole organ
  - Transplantation of: heart, kidney
  - Transplantation of: liver
- **E878.1** Surgical operation with implant of artificial internal device
  - Cardiac pacemaker
  - Electrodes implanted in brain
  - Heart valve prosthesis
  - Internal orthopedic device

E878.2 Surgical operation with anastomosis, bypass, or graft, with natural or artificial tissues used as implant
Anastomosis:
  arteriovenous
  gastrojejunal
Graft of blood vessel, tendon, or skin
EXCLUDES: external stoma (E878.3)

E878.3 Surgical operation with formation of external stoma
Colostomy
Cystostomy
Duodenostomy
Gastrostomy
Ureterostomy

E878.4 Other restorative surgery
E878.5 Amputation of limb(s)
E878.6 Removal of other organ (partial) (total)
E878.8 Other specified surgical operations and procedures
E878.9 Unspecified surgical operations and procedures

E879 Other procedures, without mention of misadventure at the time of procedure, as the cause of abnormal reaction of patient, or of later complication
E879.0 Cardiac catheterization
E879.1 Kidney dialysis
E879.2 Radiological procedure and radiotherapy
  EXCLUDES: radio-opaque dyes for diagnostic x-ray procedures (E947.8)
E879.3 Shock therapy
  Electroshock therapy
  Insulin-shock therapy
E879.4 Aspiration of fluid
  Lumbar puncture
  Thoracentesis
E879.5 Insertion of gastric or duodenal sound
E879.6 Urinary catheterization
E879.7 Blood sampling
E879.8 Other specified procedures
  Blood transfusion
E879.9 Unspecified procedure

ACCIDENTAL FALLS (E880-E888)

EXCLUDES: falls (in or from):
  burning building (E890.8, E891.8)
  into fire (E890.0-E899)
  into water (with submersion or drowning) (E910.0-E910.9)
  machinery (in operation) (E919.0-E919.9)
  on edged, pointed, or sharp object (E920.0-E920.9)
  transport vehicle (E800.0-E845.9)
  vehicle not elsewhere classifiable (E846-E848)

E880 Fall on or from stairs or steps
E880.0 Escalator
E880.1 Fall on or from sidewalk curb
  EXCLUDES: fall from moving sidewalk (E885.9)
E880.9 Other stairs or steps

E881 Fall on or from ladders or scaffolding
E881.0 Fall from ladder
E881.1 Fall from scaffolding

E882 Fall from or out of building or other structure
Fall from:
  balcony
  bridge
  building
  flagpole
  tower
Fall from:
  turret
  viaduct
  wall
  window
Fall through roof
  EXCLUDES: collapse of a building or structure (E916)
  fall or jump from burning building (E890.8, E891.8)

E883 Fall into hole or other opening in surface
INCLUDES: fall into:
  cavity
  dock
  hole
  pit
  quarry
fall into:
  shaft
  swimming pool
  tank
  well
EXCLUDES: fall into water NOS (E910.9)
  that resulting in drowning or submersion without mention of injury (E910.0-E910.9)

E883.0 Accident from diving or jumping into water [swimming pool]
  Strike or hit:
    against bottom when jumping or diving into water
    wall or board of swimming pool
    water surface
  EXCLUDES: diving with insufficient air supply (E913.2)
    effects of air pressure from diving (E902.2)
E883.1 Accidental fall into well
E883.2 Accidental fall into storm drain or manhole
E883.9 Fall into other hole or other opening in surface

E884 Other fall from one level to another
E884.0 Fall from playground equipment
  EXCLUDES: recreational machinery (E919.8)
E884.1 Fall from cliff
E884.2 Fall from chair
E884.3 Fall from wheelchair
E884.4 Fall from bed
E884.5 Fall from other furniture
E884.6 Fall from commode
  Toilet
E884.9 Other fall from one level to another
  Fall from:
    embankment
    haystack
    stationary vehicle
    tree

E885 Fall on same level from slipping, tripping, or stumbling
E885.0 Fall from (nonmotorized) scooter
E885.1 Fall from roller skates
  In-line skates
E885.2 Fall from skateboard
E885.3 Fall from skis
E885.4 Fall from snowboard
E885.9 Fall from other slipping, tripping, or stumbling
  Fall on moving sidewalk

E886 Fall on same level from collision, pushing, or shoving, by or with other person
  EXCLUDES: crushed or pushed by a crowd or human stampede (E917.1, E917.6)
E886.0 In sports
  Tackles in sports
  EXCLUDES: kicked, stepped on, struck by object, in sports (E917.0, E917.5)
E886.9 Other and unspecified
  Fall from collision of pedestrian (conveyance) with another pedestrian (conveyance)

E887 Fracture, cause unspecified

E888 Other and unspecified fall
Accidental fall NOS
Fall on same level NOS
E888.0 Fall resulting in striking against sharp object
  Use additional external cause code to identify object (E920)
E888.1 Fall resulting in striking against other object
E888.8 Other fall
E888.9 Unspecified fall
  Fall NOS

ACCIDENTS CAUSED BY FIRE AND FLAMES (E890-E899)

INCLUDES
  asphyxia or poisoning due to conflagration or ignition
  burning by fire
  secondary fires resulting from explosion

EXCLUDES
  arson (E968.0)
  fire in or on:
    machinery (in operation) (E919.0-E919.9)
    transport vehicle other than stationary vehicle (E800.0-E845.9)
    vehicle not elsewhere classifiable (E846-E848)

✓4th E890 Conflagration in private dwelling

INCLUDES conflagration in:
- apartment
- boarding house
- camping place
- caravan
- farmhouse
- house
- lodging house
- mobile home
- private garage
- rooming house
- tenement

conflagration originating from sources classifiable to E893-E898 in the above buildings

E890.0 Explosion caused by conflagration

E890.1 Fumes from combustion of polyvinylchloride [PVC] and similar material in conflagration

E890.2 Other smoke and fumes from conflagration
  Carbon monoxide ⎫
  Fumes NOS   ⎬ from conflagration in private building
  Smoke NOS   ⎭

E890.3 Burning caused by conflagration

E890.8 Other accident resulting from conflagration
  Collapse of ⎫
  Fall from   ⎬ burning private building
  Hit by object falling from
  Jump from ⎭

E890.9 Unspecified accident resulting from conflagration in private dwelling

✓4th E891 Conflagration in other and unspecified building or structure

Conflagration in:
- barn
- church
- convalescent and other residential home
- dormitory of educational institution
- factory
- farm outbuildings
- hospital
- hotel
- school
- store
- theater

Conflagration originating from sources classifiable to E893-E898, in the above buildings

E891.0 Explosion caused by conflagration

E891.1 Fumes from combustion of polyvinylchloride [PVC] and similar material in conflagration

E891.2 Other smoke and fumes from conflagration
  Carbon monoxide ⎫
  Fumes NOS   ⎬ from conflagration in building or structure
  Smoke NOS   ⎭

E891.3 Burning caused by conflagration

E891.8 Other accident resulting from conflagration
  Collapse of ⎫
  Fall from   ⎬ burning building or structure
  Hit by object falling from
  Jump from ⎭

E891.9 Unspecified accident resulting from conflagration of other and unspecified building or structure

E892 Conflagration not in building or structure

Fire (uncontrolled) (in) (of):
- forest
- grass
- hay
- lumber
- mine
- prairie
- transport vehicle [any], except while in transit
- tunnel

✓4th E893 Accident caused by ignition of clothing

EXCLUDES ignition of clothing:
  from highly inflammable material (E894)
  with conflagration (E890.0-E892)

E893.0 From controlled fire in private dwelling
Ignition of clothing from:
  normal fire (charcoal) (coal) (electric) (gas) (wood) in:
    brazier ⎫
    fireplace ⎬ in private dwelling (as listed in E890)
    furnace   ⎭
    stove

E893.1 From controlled fire in other building or structure
Ignition of clothing from:
  normal fire (charcoal) (coal) (electric) (gas) (wood) in:
    brazier ⎫
    fireplace ⎬ in other building or structure (as listed in E81)
    furnace   ⎭
    stove

E893.2 From controlled fire not in building or structure
Ignition of clothing from:
  bonfire (controlled)
  brazier fire (controlled), not in building or structure
  trash fire (controlled)

EXCLUDES conflagration not in building (E892)
  trash fire out of control (E892)

E893.8 From other specified sources
Ignition of clothing from:
- blowlamp
- blowtorch
- burning bedspread
- candle
- cigar
- cigarette
- lighter
- matches
- pipe
- welding torch

E893.9 Unspecified source
Ignition of clothing (from controlled fire NOS) (in building NOS) NOS

E894 Ignition of highly inflammable material

Ignition of:
- benzine
- gasoline
- fat
- kerosene   (with ignition of clothing)
- paraffin
- petrol

EXCLUDES ignition of highly inflammable material with:
  conflagration (E890.0-E892)
  explosion (E923.0-E923.9)

✓4th Fourth-digit Required   ▶◀ Revised Text   ● New Code   ▲ Revised Code Title

E895 Accident caused by controlled fire in private dwelling

Burning by (flame of) normal fire (charcoal) (coal) (electric) (gas) (wood) in:
- brazier
- fireplace
- furnace
- stove

in private dwelling (as listed in E890)

EXCLUDES burning by hot objects not producing fire or flames (E924.0-E924.9)
ignition of clothing from these sources (E893.0)
poisoning by carbon monoxide from incomplete combustion of fuel (E867-E868.9)
that with conflagration (E890.0-E890.9)

E896 Accident caused by controlled fire in other and unspecified building or structure

Burning by (flame of) normal fire (charcoal) (coal) (electric) (gas) (wood) in:
- brazier
- fireplace
- furnace
- stove

in other building or structure (as listed in E891)

EXCLUDES burning by hot objects not producing fire or flames (E924.0-E924.9)
ignition of clothing from these sources (E893.1)
poisoning by carbon monoxide from incomplete combustion of fuel (E867-E868.9)
that with conflagration (E891.0-E891.9)

E897 Accident caused by controlled fire not in building or structure

Burns from flame of:
- bonfire
- brazier fire, not in building or structure
- trash fire

controlled

EXCLUDES ignition of clothing from these sources (E893.2)
trash fire out of control (E892)
that with conflagration (E892)

✓4ᵗʰ E898 Accident caused by other specified fire and flames

EXCLUDES conflagration (E890.0-E892)
that with ignition of:
clothing (E893.0-E893.9)
highly inflammable material (E894)

E898.0 Burning bedclothes
Bed set on fire NOS

E898.1 Other

Burning by:
- blowlamp
- blowtorch
- candle
- cigar
- cigarette
- fire in room NOS

Burning by:
- lamp
- lighter
- matches
- pipe
- welding torch

E899 Accident caused by unspecified fire
Burning NOS

ACCIDENTS DUE TO NATURAL AND ENVIRONMENTAL FACTORS (E900-E909)

✓4ᵗʰ E900 Excessive heat

E900.0 Due to weather conditions
Excessive heat as the external cause of:
- ictus solaris
- siriasis
- sunstroke

E900.1 Of man-made origin

Heat (in):
- boiler room
- drying room
- factory
- furnace room

Heat (in):
- generated in transport vehicle
- kitchen

E900.9 Of unspecified origin

✓4ᵗʰ E901 Excessive cold

E901.0 Due to weather conditions
Excessive cold as the cause of:
- chilblains NOS
- immersion foot

E901.1 Of man-made origin
Contact with or inhalation of:
- dry ice
- liquid air
- liquid hydrogen
- liquid nitrogen

Prolonged exposure in:
- deep freeze unit
- refrigerator

E901.8 Other specified origin

E901.9 Of unspecified origin

✓4ᵗʰ E902 High and low air pressure and changes in air pressure

E902.0 Residence or prolonged visit at high altitude
Residence or prolonged visit at high altitude as the cause of:
- Acosta syndrome
- Alpine sickness
- altitude sickness
- Andes disease
- anoxia, hypoxia
- barotitis, barodontalgia, barosinusitis, otitic barotrauma
- hypobarism, hypobaropathy
- mountain sickness
- range disease

E902.1 In aircraft
Sudden change in air pressure in aircraft during ascent or descent as the cause of:
- aeroneurosis
- aviators' disease

E902.2 Due to diving

High air pressure from rapid descent in water
Reduction in atmospheric pressure while surfacing from deep water diving

as the cause of:
- caisson disease
- divers' disease
- divers' palsy or paralysis

E902.8 Due to other specified causes
Reduction in atmospheric pressure while surfacing from underground

E902.9 Unspecified cause

E903 Travel and motion

✓4ᵗʰ E904 Hunger, thirst, exposure, and neglect

EXCLUDES any condition resulting from homicidal intent (E968.0-E968.9)
hunger, thirst, and exposure resulting from accidents connected with transport (E800.0-E848)

E904.0 Abandonment or neglect of infants and helpless persons

Exposure to weather conditions
Hunger or thirst

resulting from abandonment or neglect

Desertion of newborn
Inattention at or after birth
Lack of care (helpless person) (infant)

EXCLUDES criminal [purposeful] neglect (E968.4)

E904.1 Lack of food
Lack of food as the cause of:
- inanition
- insufficient nourishment
- starvation

EXCLUDES hunger resulting from abandonment or neglect (E904.0)

Tabular List — E CODES — E904.2–E909.9

E904.2 Lack of water
 Lack of water as the cause of:
  dehydration
  inanition
 EXCLUDES dehydration due to acute fluid loss (276.5)

E904.3 Exposure (to weather conditions), not elsewhere classifiable
 Exposure NOS
 Humidity
 Struck by hailstones
 EXCLUDES struck by lightning (E907)

E904.9 Privation, unqualified
 Destitution

✓4th **E905 Venomous animals and plants as the cause of poisoning and toxic reactions**
 INCLUDES chemical released by animal
  insects
  release of venom through fangs, hairs, spines, tentacles, and other venom apparatus
 EXCLUDES eating of poisonous animals or plants (E865.0-E865.9)

E905.0 Venomous snakes and lizards
 Cobra   Mamba
 Copperhead snake   Rattlesnake
 Coral snake   Sea snake
 Fer de lance   Snake (venomous)
 Gila monster   Viper
 Krait   Water moccasin
 EXCLUDES bites of snakes and lizards known to be nonvenomous (E906.2)

E905.1 Venomous spiders
 Black widow spider   Tarantula (venomous)
 Brown spider

E905.2 Scorpion

E905.3 Hornets, wasps, and bees
 Yellow jacket

E905.4 Centipede and venomous millipede (tropical)

E905.5 Other venomous arthropods
 Sting of:
  ant
  caterpillar

E905.6 Venomous marine animals and plants
 Puncture by sea urchin spine
 Sting of:
  coral
  jelly fish
  nematocysts
  sea anemone
  sea cucumber
  other marine animal or plant
 EXCLUDES bites and other injuries caused by nonvenomous marine animal (E906.2-E906.8)
  bite of sea snake (venomous) (E905.0)

E905.7 Poisoning and toxic reactions caused by other plants
 Injection of poisons or toxins into or through skin by plant thorns, spines, or other mechanisms
 EXCLUDES puncture wound NOS by plant thorns or spines (E920.8)

E905.8 Other specified

E905.9 Unspecified
 Sting NOS
 Venomous bite NOS

✓4th **E906 Other injury caused by animals**
 EXCLUDES poisoning and toxic reactions caused by venomous animals and insects (E905.0-E905.9)
  road vehicle accident involving animals (E827.0-E828.9)
  tripping or falling over an animal (E885.9)

E906.0 Dog bite

E906.1 Rat bite

E906.2 Bite of nonvenomous snakes and lizards

E906.3 Bite of other animal except arthropod
 Cats   Rodents, except rats
 Moray eel   Shark

E906.4 Bite of nonvenomous arthropod
 Insect bite NOS

E906.5 Bite by unspecified animal
 Animal bite NOS

E906.8 Other specified injury caused by animal
 Butted by animal
 Fallen on by horse or other animal, not being ridden
 Gored by animal
 Implantation of quills of porcupine
 Pecked by bird
 Run over by animal, not being ridden
 Stepped on by animal, not being ridden
 EXCLUDES injury by animal being ridden (E828.0-E828.9)

E906.9 Unspecified injury caused by animal

E907 Lightning
 EXCLUDES injury from:
  fall of tree or other object caused by lightning (E916)
  fire caused by lightning (E890.0-E892)

✓4th **E908 Cataclysmic storms, and floods resulting from storms**
 EXCLUDES collapse of dam or man-made structure causing flood (E909.3)

E908.0 Hurricane
 Storm surge
 "Tidal wave" caused by storm action
 Typhoon

E908.1 Tornado
 Cyclone
 Twisters

E908.2 Floods
 Torrential rainfall
 Flash flood
 EXCLUDES collapse of dam or man-made structure causing flood (E909.3)

E908.3 Blizzard (snow) (ice)

E908.4 Dust storm

E908.8 Other cataclysmic storms

E908.9 Unspecified cataclysmic storms, and floods resulting from storms
 Storm NOS

✓4th **E909 Cataclysmic earth surface movements and eruptions**

E909.0 Earthquakes

E909.1 Volcanic eruptions
 Burns from lava
 Ash inhalation

E909.2 Avalanche, landslide, or mudslide

E909.3 Collapse of dam or man-made structure

E909.4 Tidalwave caused by earthquake
 Tidalwave NOS
 Tsunami
 EXCLUDES tidalwave caused by tropical storm (E908.0)

E909.8 Other cataclysmic earth surface movements and eruptions

E909.9 Unspecified cataclysmic earth surface movements and eruptions

ACCIDENTS CAUSED BY SUBMERSION, SUFFOCATION, AND FOREIGN BODIES (E910-E915)

✓4th E910 Accidental drowning and submersion

INCLUDES
- immersion
- swimmers' cramp

EXCLUDES
- diving accident (NOS) (resulting in injury except drowning) (E883.0)
- diving with insufficient air supply (E913.2)
- drowning and submersion due to:
  - cataclysm (E908-E909)
  - machinery accident (E919.0-E919.9)
  - transport accident (E800.0-E845.9)
- effect of high and low air pressure (E902.2)
- injury from striking against objects while in running water (E917.2)

E910.0 While water-skiing
Fall from water skis with submersion or drowning

EXCLUDES accident to water-skier involving a watercraft and resulting in submersion or other injury (E830.4, E831.4)

E910.1 While engaged in other sport or recreational activity with diving equipment
- Scuba diving NOS
- Skin diving NOS
- Underwater spear fishing NOS

E910.2 While engaged in other sport or recreational activity without diving equipment
- Fishing or hunting, except from boat or with diving equipment
- Ice skating
- Playing in water
- Surfboarding
- Swimming NOS
- Voluntarily jumping from boat, not involved in accident, for swim NOS
- Wading in water

EXCLUDES jumping into water to rescue another person (E910.3)

E910.3 While swimming or diving for purposes other than recreation or sport (with diving equipment)
- Marine salvage
- Pearl diving
- Placement of fishing nets
- Rescue (attempt) of another person
- Underwater construction or repairs

E910.4 In bathtub

E910.8 Other accidental drowning or submersion
- Drowning in: quenching tank
- Drowning in: swimming pool

E910.9 Unspecified accidental drowning or submersion
- Accidental fall into water NOS
- Drowning NOS

E911 Inhalation and ingestion of food causing obstruction of respiratory tract or suffocation
- Aspiration and inhalation of food [any] (into respiratory tract) NOS
- Asphyxia by / Choked on / Suffocation by food [including bone, seed in food, regurgitated food]
- Compression of trachea / Interruption of respiration / Obstruction of respiration by food lodged in esophagus
- Obstruction of pharynx by food (bolus)

EXCLUDES
- injury, except asphyxia and obstruction of respiratory passage, caused by food (E915)
- obstruction of esophagus by food without mention of asphyxia or obstruction of respiratory passage (E915)

E912 Inhalation and ingestion of other object causing obstruction of respiratory tract or suffocation
- Aspiration and inhalation of foreign body except food (into respiratory tract) NOS
- Foreign object [bean] [marble] in nose
- Obstruction of pharynx by foreign body
- Compression / Interruption of respiration / Obstruction of respiration by foreign body in esophagus

EXCLUDES
- injury, except asphyxia and obstruction of respiratory passage, caused by foreign body (E915)
- obstruction of esophagus by foreign body without mention of asphyxia or obstruction in respiratory passage (E915)

✓4th E913 Accidental mechanical suffocation

EXCLUDES mechanical suffocation from or by:
- accidental inhalation or ingestion of:
  - food (E911)
  - foreign object (E912)
- cataclysm (E908-E909)
- explosion (E921.0-E921.9, E923.0-E923.9)
- machinery accident (E919.0-E919.9)

E913.0 In bed or cradle
EXCLUDES suffocation by plastic bag (E913.1)

E913.1 By plastic bag

E913.2 Due to lack of air (in closed place)
- Accidentally closed up in refrigerator or other airtight enclosed space
- Diving with insufficient air supply
EXCLUDES suffocation by plastic bag (E913.1)

E913.3 By falling earth or other substance
Cave-in NOS
EXCLUDES
- cave-in caused by cataclysmic earth surface movements and eruptions (E909)
- struck by cave-in without asphyxiation or suffocation (E916)

E913.8 Other specified means
Accidental hanging, except in bed or cradle

E913.9 Unspecified means
- Asphyxia, mechanical NOS
- Suffocation NOS
- Strangulation NOS

E914 Foreign body accidentally entering eye and adnexa
EXCLUDES corrosive liquid (E924.1)

E915 Foreign body accidentally entering other orifice
EXCLUDES aspiration and inhalation of foreign body, any, (into respiratory tract) NOS (E911-E912)

OTHER ACCIDENTS (E916-E928)

E916 Struck accidentally by falling object
- Collapse of building, except on fire
- Falling:
  - rock
  - snowslide NOS
  - stone
  - tree
- Object falling from:
  - machine, not in operation
  - stationary vehicle

Code first:
- collapse of building on fire (E890.0-E891.9)
- falling object in:
  - cataclysm (E908-E909)
  - machinery accidents (E919.0-E919.9)
  - transport accidents (E800.0-E845.9)
  - vehicle accidents not elsewhere classifiable (E846-E848)
- object set in motion by:
  - explosion (E921.0-E921.9, E923.0-E923.9)
  - firearm (E922.0-E922.9)
  - projected object (E917.0-E917.9)

E917 Striking against or struck accidentally by objects or persons

INCLUDES: bumping into or against, colliding with, kicking against, stepping on, struck by — object (moving) (projected) (stationary), pedestrian conveyance, person

EXCLUDES:
fall from:
  collision with another person, except when caused by a crowd (E886.0-E886.9)
  stumbling over object (E885.9)
fall resulting in striking against object (E888.0, E888.1)
injury caused by:
  assault (E960.0-E960.1, E967.0-E967.9)
  cutting or piercing instrument (E920.0-E920.9)
  explosion (E921.0-E921.9, E923.0-E923.9)
  firearm (E922.0-E922.9)
  machinery (E919.0-E919.9)
  transport vehicle (E800.0-E845.9)
  vehicle not elsewhere classifiable (E846-E848)

E917.0 In sports without subsequent fall
Kicked or stepped on during game (football) (rugby)
Struck by hit or thrown ball
Struck by hockey stick or puck

E917.1 Caused by a crowd, by collective fear or panic without subsequent fall
Crushed
Pushed   } by crowd or human stampede
Stepped on

E917.2 In running water without subsequent fall
EXCLUDES: drowning or submersion (E910.0-E910.9)
that in sports (E917.0, E917.5)

E917.3 Furniture without subsequent fall
EXCLUDES: fall from furniture (E884.2, E884.4-E884.5)

E917.4 Other stationary object without subsequent fall
Bath tub
Fence
Lamp-post

E917.5 Object in sports with subsequent fall
Knocked down while boxing

E917.6 Caused by a crowd, by collective fear or panic with subsequent fall

E917.7 Furniture with subsequent fall
EXCLUDES: fall from furniture (E884.2, E884.4-E884.5)

E917.8 Other stationary object with subsequent fall
Bath tub
Fence
Lamp-post

E917.9 Other striking against with or without subsequent fall

E918 Caught accidentally in or between objects
Caught, crushed, jammed, or pinched in or between moving or stationary objects, such as:
escalator
folding object
hand tools, appliances, or implements
sliding door and door frame
under packing crate
washing machine wringer

EXCLUDES:
injury caused by:
  cutting or piercing instrument (E920.0-E920.9)
  machinery (E919.0-E919.9)
  transport vehicle (E800.0-E845.9)
  vehicle not elsewhere classifiable (E846-E848)
struck accidentally by:
  falling object (E916)
  object (moving) (projected) (E917.0-E917.9)

E919 Accidents caused by machinery

INCLUDES:
burned by
caught in (moving parts of)
collapse of
crushed by
cut or pierced by
drowning or submersion caused by
explosion of, on, in
fall from or into moving part of
fire starting in or on
mechanical suffocation caused by
object falling from, on, in motion by
overturning of
pinned under
run over by
struck by
thrown from
— machinery (accident)

caught between machinery and other object
machinery accident NOS

EXCLUDES:
accidents involving machinery, not in operation (E884.9, E916-E918)
injury caused by:
  electric current in connection with machinery (E925.0-E925.9)
  escalator (E880.0, E918)
  explosion of pressure vessel in connection with machinery (E921.0-E921.9)
  moving sidewalk (E885.9)
  powered hand tools, appliances, and implements (E916-E918, E920.0-E921.9, E923.0-E926.9)
  transport vehicle accidents involving machinery (E800.0-E848.9)
  poisoning by carbon monoxide generated by machine (E868.8)

E919.0 Agricultural machines
- Animal-powered agricultural machine
- Combine
- Derrick, hay
- Farm machinery NOS
- Farm tractor
- Harvester
- Hay mower or rake
- Reaper
- Thresher

EXCLUDES that in transport under own power on the highway (E810.0-E819.9)
that being towed by another vehicle on the highway (E810.0-E819.9, E827.0-E827.9, E829.0-E829.9)
that involved in accident classifiable to E820-E829 (E820.0-E829.9)

E919.1 Mining and earth-drilling machinery
- Bore or drill (land) (seabed)
- Shaft lift
- Shaft hoist
- Under-cutter

EXCLUDES coal car, tram, truck, and tub in mine (E846)

E919.2 Lifting machines and appliances
- Chain hoist
- Crane
- Derrick
- Elevator (building) (grain)
- Forklift truck
- Lift
- Pulley block
- Winch

except in agricultural or mining operations

EXCLUDES that being towed by another vehicle on the highway (E810.0-E819.9, E827.0-E827.9, E829.0-829.9)
that in transport under own power on the highway (E810.0-E819.9)
that involved in accident classifiable to E820-E829 (E820.0-E829.9)

E919.3 Metalworking machines
- Abrasive wheel
- Forging machine
- Lathe
- Mechanical shears
- Metal:
  - drilling machine
  - milling machine
  - power press
  - rolling-mill
  - sawing machine

E919.4 Woodworking and forming machines
- Band saw
- Bench saw
- Circular saw
- Molding machine
- Overhead plane
- Powered saw
- Radial saw
- Sander

EXCLUDES hand saw (E920.1)

E919.5 Prime movers, except electrical motors
- Gas turbine
- Internal combustion engine
- Steam engine
- Water driven turbine

EXCLUDES that being towed by other vehicle on the highway (E810.0-E819.9, E827.0-E827.9, E829.0-E829.9)
that in transport under own power on the highway (E810.0-E819.9)

E919.6 Transmission machinery
- Transmission:
  - belt
  - cable
  - chain
  - gear
- Transmission:
  - pinion
  - pulley
  - shaft

E919.7 Earth moving, scraping, and other excavating machines
- Bulldozer
- Road scraper
- Steam shovel

EXCLUDES that being towed by other vehicle on the highway (E810.0-E819.9, E827.0-E827.9, E829.0-E829.9)
that in transport under own power on the highway (E810.0-E819.9)

E919.8 Other specified machinery
- Machines for manufacture of:
  - clothing
  - foodstuffs and beverages
  - paper
- Printing machine
- Recreational machinery
- Spinning, weaving, and textile machines

E919.9 Unspecified machinery

☑4th **E920 Accidents caused by cutting and piercing instruments or objects**

INCLUDES accidental injury (by) object: edged, pointed, sharp

E920.0 Powered lawn mower

E920.1 Other powered hand tools
Any powered hand tool [compressed air] [electric] [explosive cartridge] [hydraulic power], such as:
- drill
- hand saw
- hedge clipper
- rivet gun
- snow blower
- staple gun

EXCLUDES band saw (E919.4)
bench saw (E919.4)

E920.2 Powered household appliances and implements
- Blender
- Electric:
  - beater or mixer
  - can opener
  - fan
  - knife
  - sewing machine
- Garbage disposal appliance

E920.3 Knives, swords, and daggers

E920.4 Other hand tools and implements
- Axe
- Can opener NOS
- Chisel
- Fork
- Hand saw
- Hoe
- Ice pick
- Needle (sewing)
- Paper cutter
- Pitchfork
- Rake
- Scissors
- Screwdriver
- Sewing machine, not powered
- Shovel

E920.5 Hypodermic needle
- Contaminated needle
- Needle stick

E920.8 Other specified cutting and piercing instruments or objects
- Arrow
- Broken glass
- Dart
- Edge of stiff paper
- Lathe turnings
- Nail
- Plant thorn
- Splinter
- Tin can lid

EXCLUDES animal spines or quills (E906.8)
flying glass due to explosion (E921.0-E923.9)

E920.9 Unspecified cutting and piercing instrument or object

| Tabular List | E CODES | E921–E926 |

☑4th **E921 Accident caused by explosion of pressure vessel**
    INCLUDES: accidental explosion of pressure vessels, whether or not part of machinery
    EXCLUDES: explosion of pressure vessel on transport vehicle (E800.0-E845.9)

    E921.0 Boilers
    E921.1 Gas cylinders
        Air tank
        Pressure gas tank
    E921.8 Other specified pressure vessels
        Aerosol can   Pressure cooker
        Automobile tire
    E921.9 Unspecified pressure vessel

☑4th **E922 Accident caused by firearm, and air gun missile**
    E922.0 Handgun
        Pistol   Revolver
        EXCLUDES: Verey pistol (E922.8)
    E922.1 Shotgun (automatic)
    E922.2 Hunting rifle
    E922.3 Military firearms
        Army rifle   Machine gun
    E922.4 Air gun
        BB gun
        Pellet gun
    ● **E922.5 Paintball gun**
    E922.8 Other specified firearm missile
        Verey pistol [flare]
    E922.9 Unspecified firearm missile
        Gunshot wound NOS
        Shot NOS

☑4th **E923 Accident caused by explosive material**
    INCLUDES: flash burns and other injuries resulting from explosion of explosive material
        ignition of highly explosive material with explosion
    EXCLUDES: explosion:
        in or on machinery (E919.0-E919.9)
        on any transport vehicle, except stationary motor vehicle (E800.0-E848)
        with conflagration (E890.0, E891.0, E892)
        secondary fires resulting from explosion (E890.0-E899)

    E923.0 Fireworks
    E923.1 Blasting materials
        Blasting cap
        Detonator
        Dynamite
        Explosive [any] used in blasting operations
    E923.2 Explosive gases
        Acetylene   Fire damp
        Butane   Gasoline fumes
        Coal gas   Methane
        Explosion in mine NOS   Propane
    E923.8 Other explosive materials
        Bomb   Torpedo
        Explosive missile   Explosion in munitions:
        Grenade   dump
        Mine   factory
        Shell
    E923.9 Unspecified explosive material
        Explosion NOS

☑4th **E924 Accident caused by hot substance or object, caustic or corrosive material, and steam**
    EXCLUDES: burning NOS (E899)
        chemical burn resulting from swallowing a corrosive substance (E860.0-E864.4)
        fire caused by these substances and objects (E890.0-E894)
        radiation burns (E926.0-E926.9)
        therapeutic misadventures (E870.0-E876.9)

    E924.0 Hot liquids and vapors, including steam
        Burning or scalding by:
            boiling water
            hot or boiling liquids not primarily caustic or corrosive
            liquid metal
            steam
            other hot vapor
        EXCLUDES: hot (boiling) tap water (E924.2)
    E924.1 Caustic and corrosive substances
        Burning by: Burning by:
          acid [any kind]   corrosive substance
          ammonia   lye
          caustic oven cleaner   vitriol
            or other substance
    E924.2 Hot (boiling) tap water
    E924.8 Other
        Burning by:
          heat from electric heating appliance
          hot object NOS
          light bulb
          steam pipe
    E924.9 Unspecified

☑4th **E925 Accident caused by electric current**
    INCLUDES: electric current from exposed wire, faulty appliance, high voltage cable, live rail, or open electric socket as the cause of:
        burn
        cardiac fibrillation
        convulsion
        electric shock
        electrocution
        puncture wound
        respiratory paralysis
    EXCLUDES: burn by heat from electrical appliance (E924.8)
        lightning (E907)

    E925.0 Domestic wiring and appliances
    E925.1 Electric power generating plants, distribution stations, transmission lines
        Broken power line
    E925.2 Industrial wiring, appliances, and electrical machinery
        Conductors
        Control apparatus
        Electrical equipment and machinery
        Transformers
    E925.8 Other electric current
        Wiring and appliances in or on:
          farm [not farmhouse]
          outdoors
          public building
          residential institutions
          schools
    E925.9 Unspecified electric current
        Burns or other injury from electric current NOS
        Electric shock NOS
        Electrocution NOS

☑4th **E926 Exposure to radiation**
    EXCLUDES: abnormal reaction to or complication of treatment without mention of misadventure (E879.2)
        atomic power plant malfunction in water transport (E838.0-E838.9)
        misadventure to patient in surgical and medical procedures (E873.2-E873.3)
        use of radiation in war operations (E996-E997.9)

☑4th Fourth-digit Required   ▶◀ Revised Text   ● New Code   ▲ Revised Code Title

E926.0 Radiofrequency radiation
Overexposure to: microwave radiation, radar radiation, radiofrequency radiation [any] from: high-powered radio and television transmitters, industrial radiofrequency induction heaters, radar installations

E926.1 Infrared heaters and lamps
Exposure to infrared radiation from heaters and lamps as the cause of:
- blistering
- burning
- charring
- inflammatory change

EXCLUDES physical contact with heater or lamp (E924.8)

E926.2 Visible and ultraviolet light sources
- Arc lamps
- Black light sources
- Electrical welding arc
- Oxygas welding torch
- Sun rays
- Tanning bed

EXCLUDES excessive heat from these sources (E900.1-E900.9)

E926.3 X-rays and other electromagnetic ionizing radiation
- Gamma rays
- X-rays (hard) (soft)

E926.4 Lasers

E926.5 Radioactive isotopes
- Radiobiologicals
- Radiopharmaceuticals

E926.8 Other specified radiation
Artificially accelerated beams of ionized particles generated by:
- betatrons
- synchrotrons

E926.9 Unspecified radiation
Radiation NOS

E927 Overexertion and strenuous movements
- Excessive physical exercise
- Overexertion (from):
  - lifting
  - pulling
  - pushing
- Strenuous movements in:
  - recreational activities
  - other activities

✓4th **E928 Other and unspecified environmental and accidental causes**

E928.0 Prolonged stay in weightless environment
Weightlessness in spacecraft (simulator)

E928.1 Exposure to noise
- Noise (pollution)
- Sound waves
- Supersonic waves

E928.2 Vibration

E928.3 Human bite

E928.8 Other

E928.9 Unspecified accident
- Accident NOS
- Blow NOS
- Casualty (not due to war)
- Decapitation
} stated as accidentally inflicted

- Knocked down
- Killed
- Injury [any part of body, or unspecified]
- Mangled
- Wound
} stated as accidentally inflicted, but not otherwise specified

EXCLUDES fracture, cause unspecified (E887)
injuries undetermined whether accidentally or purposely inflicted (E980.0-E989)

LATE EFFECTS OF ACCIDENTAL INJURY (E929)

Note: This category is to be used to indicate accidental injury as the cause of death or disability from late effects, which are themselves classifiable elsewhere. The "late effects" include conditions reported as such, or as sequelae which may occur at any time after the attempted suicide or self-inflicted injury.

✓4th **E929 Late effects of accidental injury**

EXCLUDES late effects of:
surgical and medical procedures (E870.0-E879.9)
therapeutic use of drugs and medicines (E930.0-E949.9)

E929.0 Late effects of motor vehicle accident
Late effects of accidents classifiable to E810-E825

E929.1 Late effects of other transport accident
Late effects of accidents classifiable to E800-E807, E826-E838, E840-E848

E929.2 Late effects of accidental poisoning
Late effects of accidents classifiable to E850-E858, E860-E869

E929.3 Late effects of accidental fall
Late effects of accidents classifiable to E880-E888

E929.4 Late effects of accident caused by fire
Late effects of accidents classifiable to E890-E899

E929.5 Late effects of accident due to natural and environmental factors
Late effects of accidents classifiable to E900-E909

E929.8 Late effects of other accidents
Late effects of accidents classifiable to E910-E928.8

E929.9 Late effects of unspecified accident
Late effects of accidents classifiable to E928.9

DRUGS, MEDICINAL AND BIOLOGICAL SUBSTANCES CAUSING ADVERSE EFFECTS IN THERAPEUTIC USE (E930-E949)

INCLUDES correct drug properly administered in therapeutic or prophylactic dosage, as the cause of any adverse effect including allergic or hypersensitivity reactions

EXCLUDES accidental overdose of drug and wrong drug given or taken in error (E850.0-E858.9)
accidents in the technique of administration of drug or biological substance, such as accidental puncture during injection, or contamination of drug (E870.0-E876.9)
administration with suicidal or homicidal intent or intent to harm, or in circumstances classifiable to E980-E989 (E950.0-E950.5, E962.0, E980.0-E980.5)

See Alphabetic Index for more complete list of specific drugs to be classified under the fourth-digit subdivisions. The American Hospital Formulary numbers can be used to classify new drugs listed by the American Hospital Formulary Service (AHFS). See Appendix C.

✓4th **E930 Antibiotics**

EXCLUDES that used as eye, ear, nose, and throat [ENT], and local anti-infectives (E946.0-E946.9)

E930.0 Penicillins
- Natural
- Synthetic
- Semisynthetic, such as:
  - ampicillin
  - cloxacillin
- Semisynthetic, such as:
  - nafcillin
  - oxacillin

E930.1 Antifungal antibiotics
- Amphotericin B
- Griseofulvin
- Hachimycin [trichomycin]
- Nystatin

E930.2 Chloramphenicol group
- Chloramphenicol
- Thiamphenicol

E930.3 Erythromycin and other macrolides
- Oleandomycin
- Spiramycin

Tabular List — E CODES

E930.4 Tetracycline group
- Doxycycline
- Minocycline
- Oxytetracycline

E930.5 Cephalosporin group
- Cephalexin
- Cephaloglycin
- Cephaloridine
- Cephalothin

E930.6 Antimycobacterial antibiotics
- Cycloserine
- Kanamycin
- Rifampin
- Streptomycin

E930.7 Antineoplastic antibiotics
- Actinomycins, such as:
  - Bleomycin
  - Cactinomycin
  - Dactinomycin
- Actinomycins, such as:
  - Daunorubicin
  - Mitomycin

  EXCLUDES other antineoplastic drugs (E933.1)

E930.8 Other specified antibiotics

E930.9 Unspecified antibiotic

✓4th **E931 Other anti-infectives**
EXCLUDES ENT, and local anti-infectives (E946.0-E946.9)

E931.0 Sulfonamides
- Sulfadiazine
- Sulfafurazole
- Sulfamethoxazole

E931.1 Arsenical anti-infectives

E931.2 Heavy metal anti-infectives
- Compounds of:
  - antimony
  - bismuth
- Compounds of:
  - lead
  - mercury

  EXCLUDES mercurial diuretics (E944.0)

E931.3 Quinoline and hydroxyquinoline derivatives
- Chiniofon
- Diiodohydroxyquin

  EXCLUDES antimalarial drugs (E931.4)

E931.4 Antimalarials and drugs acting on other blood protozoa
- Chloroquine phosphate
- Cycloguanil
- Primaquine
- Proguanil [chloroguanide]
- Pyrimethamine
- Quinine (sulphate)

E931.5 Other antiprotozoal drugs
- Emetine

E931.6 Anthelmintics
- Hexylresorcinol
- Male fern oleoresin
- Piperazine
- Thiabendazole

E931.7 Antiviral drugs
- Methisazone

  EXCLUDES amantadine (E936.4)
  cytarabine (E933.1)
  idoxuridine (E946.5)

E931.8 Other antimycobacterial drugs
- Ethambutol
- Ethionamide
- Isoniazid
- Para-aminosalicylic acid derivatives
- Sulfones

E931.9 Other and unspecified anti-infectives
- Flucytosine
- Nitrofuranderivatives

✓4th **E932 Hormones and synthetic substitutes**

E932.0 Adrenal cortical steroids
- Cortisone derivatives
- Desoxycorticosterone derivatives
- Fluorinated corticosteroid

E932.1 Androgens and anabolic congeners
- Nandrolone phenpropionate
- Oxymetholone
- Testosterone and preparations

E932.2 Ovarian hormones and synthetic substitutes
- Contraceptives, oral
- Estrogens
- Estrogens and progestogens combined
- Progestogens

E932.3 Insulins and antidiabetic agents
- Acetohexamide
- Biguanide derivatives, oral
- Chlorpropamide
- Glucagon
- Insulin
- Phenformin
- Sulfonylurea derivatives, oral
- Tolbutamide

  EXCLUDES adverse effect of insulin administered for shock therapy (E879.3)

E932.4 Anterior pituitary hormones
- Corticotropin
- Gonadotropin
- Somatotropin [growth hormone]

E932.5 Posterior pituitary hormones
- Vasopressin

  EXCLUDES oxytocic agents (E945.0)

E932.6 Parathyroid and parathyroid derivatives

E932.7 Thyroid and thyroid derivatives
- Dextrothyroxine
- Levothyroxine sodium
- Liothyronine
- Thyroglobulin

E932.8 Antithyroid agents
- Iodides
- Thiouracil
- Thiourea

E932.9 Other and unspecified hormones and synthetic substitutes

✓4th **E933 Primarily systemic agents**

E933.0 Antiallergic and antiemetic drugs
- Antihistamines
- Chlorpheniramine
- Diphenhydramine
- Diphenylpyraline
- Thonzylamine
- Tripelennamine

  EXCLUDES phenothiazine-based tranquilizers (E939.1)

E933.1 Antineoplastic and immunosuppressive drugs
- Azathioprine
- Busulfan
- Chlorambucil
- Cyclophosphamide
- Cytarabine
- Fluorouracil
- Mechlorethamine hydrochloride
- Mercaptopurine
- Triethylenethiophosphoramide [thio-TEPA]

  EXCLUDES antineoplastic antibiotics (E930.7)

E933.2 Acidifying agents

E933.3 Alkalizing agents

E933.4 Enzymes, not elsewhere classified
- Penicillinase

E933.5 Vitamins, not elsewhere classified
- Vitamin A
- Vitamin D

  EXCLUDES nicotinic acid (E942.2)
  vitamin K (E934.3)

E933.8 Other systemic agents, not elsewhere classified
- Heavy metal antagonists

E933.9 Unspecified systemic agent

✓4th **E934 Agents primarily affecting blood constituents**

E934.0 Iron and its compounds
- Ferric salts
- Ferrous sulphate and other ferrous salts

E934.1 Liver preparations and other antianemic agents
- Folic acid

E934.2 Anticoagulants
- Coumarin
- Heparin
- Phenindione
- Prothrombin synthesis inhibitor
- Warfarin sodium

E934.3 Vitamin K [phytonadione]

E934.4 Fibrinolysis-affecting drugs
- Aminocaproic acid
- Streptodornase
- Streptokinase
- Urokinase

✓4th Fourth-digit Required ▶◀ Revised Text ● New Code ▲ Revised Code Title

E934.5–E941.0   E CODES

- **E934.5 Anticoagulant antagonists and other coagulants**
  - Hexadimethrine bromide
  - Protamine sulfate
- **E934.6 Gamma globulin**
- **E934.7 Natural blood and blood products**
  - Blood plasma
  - Human fibrinogen
  - Packed red cells
  - Whole blood
- **E934.8 Other agents affecting blood constituents**
  - Macromolecular blood substitutes
- **E934.9 Unspecified agent affecting blood constituents**

✓4th **E935 Analgesics, antipyretics, and antirheumatics**
- **E935.0 Heroin**
  - Diacetylmorphine
- **E935.1 Methadone**
- **E935.2 Other opiates and related narcotics**
  - Codeine [methylmorphine]
  - Meperidine [pethidine]
  - Morphine
  - Opium (alkaloids)
- **E935.3 Salicylates**
  - Acetylsalicylic acid [aspirin]
  - Amino derivatives of salicylic acid
  - Salicylic acid salts
- **E935.4 Aromatic analgesics, not elsewhere classified**
  - Acetanilid
  - Paracetamol [acetaminophen]
  - Phenacetin [acetophenetidin]
- **E935.5 Pyrazole derivatives**
  - Aminophenazone [aminopyrine]
  - Phenylbutazone
- **E935.6 Antirheumatics [antiphlogistics]**
  - Gold salts
  - Indomethacin
  - EXCLUDES: salicylates (E935.3)
    steroids (E932.0)
- **E935.7 Other non-narcotic analgesics**
  - Pyrabital
- **E935.8 Other specified analgesics and antipyretics**
  - Pentazocine
- **E935.9 Unspecified analgesic and antipyretic**

✓4th **E936 Anticonvulsants and anti-Parkinsonism drugs**
- **E936.0 Oxazolidine derivatives**
  - Paramethadione
  - Trimethadione
- **E936.1 Hydantoin derivatives**
  - Phenytoin
- **E936.2 Succinimides**
  - Ethosuximide
  - Phensuximide
- **E936.3 Other and unspecified anticonvulsants**
  - Beclamide
  - Primidone
- **E936.4 Anti-Parkinsonism drugs**
  - Amantadine
  - Ethopropazine [profenamine]
  - Levodopa [L-dopa]

✓4th **E937 Sedatives and hypnotics**
- **E937.0 Barbiturates**
  - Amobarbital [amylobarbitone]
  - Barbital [barbitone]
  - Butabarbital [butabarbitone]
  - Pentobarbital [pentobarbitone]
  - Phenobarbital [phenobarbitone]
  - Secobarbital [quinalbarbitone]
  - EXCLUDES: thiobarbiturates (E938.3)
- **E937.1 Chloral hydrate group**
- **E937.2 Paraldehyde**
- **E937.3 Bromine compounds**
  - Bromide
  - Carbromal (derivatives)
- **E937.4 Methaqualone compounds**
- **E937.5 Glutethimide group**
- **E937.6 Mixed sedatives, not elsewhere classified**
- **E937.8 Other sedatives and hypnotics**
- **E937.9 Unspecified**
  - Sleeping: drug, pill, tablet } NOS

✓4th **E938 Other central nervous system depressants and anesthetics**
- **E938.0 Central nervous system muscle-tone depressants**
  - Chlorphenesin (carbamate)
  - Mephenesin
  - Methocarbamol
- **E938.1 Halothane**
- **E938.2 Other gaseous anesthetics**
  - Ether
  - Halogenated hydrocarbon derivatives, except halothane
  - Nitrous oxide
- **E938.3 Intravenous anesthetics**
  - Ketamine
  - Methohexital [methohexitone]
  - Thiobarbiturates, such as thiopental sodium
- **E938.4 Other and unspecified general anesthetics**
- **E938.5 Surface and infiltration anesthetics**
  - Cocaine
  - Lidocaine [lignocaine]
  - Procaine
  - Tetracaine
- **E938.6 Peripheral nerve- and plexus-blocking anesthetics**
- **E938.7 Spinal anesthetics**
- **E938.9 Other and unspecified local anesthetics**

✓4th **E939 Psychotropic agents**
- **E939.0 Antidepressants**
  - Amitriptyline
  - Imipramine
  - Monoamine oxidase [MAO] inhibitors
- **E939.1 Phenothiazine-based tranquilizers**
  - Chlorpromazine
  - Fluphenazine
  - Phenothiazine
  - Prochlorperazine
  - Promazine
- **E939.2 Butyrophenone-based tranquilizers**
  - Haloperidol
  - Spiperone
  - Trifluperidol
- **E939.3 Other antipsychotics, neuroleptics, and major tranquilizers**
- **E939.4 Benzodiazepine-based tranquilizers**
  - Chlordiazepoxide
  - Diazepam
  - Flurazepam
  - Lorazepam
  - Medazepam
  - Nitrazepam
- **E939.5 Other tranquilizers**
  - Hydroxyzine
  - Meprobamate
- **E939.6 Psychodysleptics [hallucinogens]**
  - Cannabis (derivatives)
  - Lysergide [LSD]
  - Marihuana (derivatives)
  - Mescaline
  - Psilocin
  - Psilocybin
- **E939.7 Psychostimulants**
  - Amphetamine
  - Caffeine
  - EXCLUDES: central appetite depressants (E947.0)
- **E939.8 Other psychotropic agents**
- **E939.9 Unspecified psychotropic agent**

✓4th **E940 Central nervous system stimulants**
- **E940.0 Analeptics**
  - Lobeline
  - Nikethamide
- **E940.1 Opiate antagonists**
  - Levallorphan
  - Nalorphine
  - Naloxone
- **E940.8 Other specified central nervous system stimulants**
- **E940.9 Unspecified central nervous system stimulant**

✓4th **E941 Drugs primarily affecting the autonomic nervous system**
- **E941.0 Parasympathomimetics [cholinergics]**
  - Acetylcholine
  - Anticholinesterase:
    - organophosphorus
    - reversible
  - Pilocarpine

✓4th Fourth-digit Required ▶◀ Revised Text ● New Code ▲ Revised Code Title

E941.1 Parasympatholytics [anticholinergics and antimuscarinics] and spasmolytics
- Atropine
- Homatropine
- Hyoscine [scopolamine]
- Quaternary ammonium derivatives

EXCLUDES papaverine (E942.5)

E941.2 Sympathomimetics [adrenergics]
- Epinephrine [adrenalin]
- Levarterenol [noradrenalin]

E941.3 Sympatholytics [antiadrenergics]
- Phenoxybenzamine
- Tolazolinehydrochloride

E941.9 Unspecified drug primarily affecting the autonomic nervous system

√4th E942 Agents primarily affecting the cardiovascular system

E942.0 Cardiac rhythm regulators
- Practolol
- Procainamide
- Propranolol
- Quinidine

E942.1 Cardiotonic glycosides and drugs of similar action
- Digitalis glycosides
- Digoxin
- Strophanthins

E942.2 Antilipemic and antiarteriosclerotic drugs
- Cholestyramine
- Clofibrate
- Nicotinic acid derivatives
- Sitosterols

EXCLUDES dextrothyroxine (E932.7)

E942.3 Ganglion-blocking agents
- Pentamethonium bromide

E942.4 Coronary vasodilators
- Dipyridamole
- Nitrates [nitroglycerin]
- Nitrites
- Prenylamine

E942.5 Other vasodilators
- Cyclandelate
- Diazoxide
- Hydralazine
- Papaverine

E942.6 Other antihypertensive agents
- Clonidine
- Guanethidine
- Rauwolfia alkaloids
- Reserpine

E942.7 Antivaricose drugs, including sclerosing agents
- Monoethanolamine
- Zinc salts

E942.8 Capillary-active drugs
- Adrenochrome derivatives
- Bioflavonoids
- Metaraminol

E942.9 Other and unspecified agents primarily affecting the cardiovascular system

√4th E943 Agents primarily affecting gastrointestinal system

E943.0 Antacids and antigastric secretion drugs
- Aluminum hydroxide
- Magnesium trisilicate

E943.1 Irritant cathartics
- Bisacodyl
- Castor oil
- Phenolphthalein

E943.2 Emollient cathartics
- Sodium dioctyl sulfosuccinate

E943.3 Other cathartics, including intestinal atonia drugs
- Magnesium sulfate

E943.4 Digestants
- Pancreatin
- Papain
- Pepsin

E943.5 Antidiarrheal drugs
- Bismuth subcarbonate
- Kaolin
- Pectin

EXCLUDES anti-infectives (E930.0-E931.9)

E943.6 Emetics

E943.8 Other specified agents primarily affecting the gastrointestinal system

E943.9 Unspecified agent primarily affecting the gastrointestinal system

√4th E944 Water, mineral, and uric acid metabolism drugs

E944.0 Mercurial diuretics
- Chlormerodrin
- Mercaptomerin
- Mercurophylline
- Mersalyl

E944.1 Purine derivative diuretics
- Theobromine
- Theophylline

EXCLUDES aminophylline [theophylline ethylenediamine] (E945.7)

E944.2 Carbonic acid anhydrase inhibitors
- Acetazolamide

E944.3 Saluretics
- Benzothiadiazides
- Chlorothiazide group

E944.4 Other diuretics
- Ethacrynic acid
- Furosemide

E944.5 Electrolytic, caloric, and water-balance agents

E944.6 Other mineral salts, not elsewhere classified

E944.7 Uric acid metabolism drugs
- Cinchophen and congeners
- Colchicine
- Phenoquin
- Probenecid

√4th E945 Agents primarily acting on the smooth and skeletal muscles and respiratory system

E945.0 Oxytocic agents
- Ergot alkaloids
- Prostaglandins

E945.1 Smooth muscle relaxants
- Adiphenine
- Metaproterenol [orciprenaline]

EXCLUDES papaverine (E942.5)

E945.2 Skeletal muscle relaxants
- Alcuronium chloride
- Suxamethonium chloride

E945.3 Other and unspecified drugs acting on muscles

E945.4 Antitussives
- Dextromethorphan
- Pipazethate hydrochloride

E945.5 Expectorants
- Acetylcysteine
- Cocillana
- Guaifenesin [glyceryl guaiacolate]
- Ipecacuanha
- Terpin hydrate

E945.6 Anti-common cold drugs

E945.7 Antiasthmatics
- Aminophylline [theophylline ethylenediamine]

E945.8 Other and unspecified respiratory drugs

√4th E946 Agents primarily affecting skin and mucous membrane, ophthalmological, otorhinolaryngological, and dental drugs

E946.0 Local anti-infectives and anti-inflammatory drugs

E946.1 Antipruritics

E946.2 Local astringents and local detergents

E946.3 Emollients, demulcents, and protectants

E946.4 Keratolytics, kerstoplastics, other hair treatment drugs and preparations

E946.5 Eye anti-infectives and other eye drugs
- Idoxuridine

E946.6 Anti-infectives and other drugs and preparations for ear, nose, and throat

E946.7 Dental drugs topically applied

E946.8 Other agents primarily affecting skin and mucous membrane
- Spermicides

E946.9 Unspecified agent primarily affecting skin and mucous membrane

√4th E947 Other and unspecified drugs and medicinal substances

E947.0 Dietetics

E947.1 Lipotropic drugs

E947.2 Antidotes and chelating agents, not elsewhere classified

E947.3 Alcohol deterrents

E947.4 Pharmaceutical excipients

E947.8 Other drugs and medicinal substances
- Contrast media used for diagnostic x-ray procedures
- Diagnostic agents and kits

E947.9 Unspecified drug or medicinal substance

✓4th **E948 Bacterial vaccines**
    E948.0 BCG vaccine
    E948.1 Typhoid and paratyphoid
    E948.2 Cholera
    E948.3 Plague
    E948.4 Tetanus
    E948.5 Diphtheria
    E948.6 Pertussis vaccine, including combinations with a pertussis component
    E948.8 Other and unspecified bacterial vaccines
    E948.9 Mixed bacterial vaccines, except combinations with a pertussis component

✓4th **E949 Other vaccines and biological substances**
    EXCLUDES: gamma globulin (E934.6)
    E949.0 Smallpox vaccine
    E949.1 Rabies vaccine
    E949.2 Typhus vaccine
    E949.3 Yellow fever vaccine
    E949.4 Measles vaccine
    E949.5 Poliomyelitis vaccine
    E949.6 Other and unspecified viral and rickettsial vaccines
        Mumps vaccine
    E949.7 Mixed viral-rickettsial and bacterial vaccines, except combinations with a pertussis component
        EXCLUDES: combinations with a pertussis component (E948.6)
    E949.9 Other and unspecified vaccines and biological substances

SUICIDE AND SELF-INFLICTED INJURY (E950-E959)

INCLUDES: injuries in suicide and attempted suicide
self-inflicted injuries specified as intentional

✓4th **E950 Suicide and self-inflicted poisoning by solid or liquid substances**
    E950.0 Analgesics, antipyretics, and antirheumatics
    E950.1 Barbiturates
    E950.2 Other sedatives and hypnotics
    E950.3 Tranquilizers and other psychotropic agents
    E950.4 Other specified drugs and medicinal substances
    E950.5 Unspecified drug or medicinal substance
    E950.6 Agricultural and horticultural chemical and pharmaceutical preparations other than plant foods and fertilizers
    E950.7 Corrosive and caustic substances
        Suicide and self-inflicted poisoning by substances classifiable to E864
    E950.8 Arsenic and its compounds
    E950.9 Other and unspecified solid and liquid substances

✓4th **E951 Suicide and self-inflicted poisoning by gases in domestic use**
    E951.0 Gas distributed by pipeline
    E951.1 Liquefied petroleum gas distributed in mobile containers
    E951.8 Other utility gas

✓4th **E952 Suicide and self-inflicted poisoning by other gases and vapors**
    E952.0 Motor vehicle exhaust gas
    E952.1 Other carbon monoxide
    E952.8 Other specified gases and vapors
    E952.9 Unspecified gases and vapors

✓4th **E953 Suicide and self-inflicted injury by hanging, strangulation, and suffocation**
    E953.0 Hanging
    E953.1 Suffocation by plastic bag
    E953.8 Other specified means
    E953.9 Unspecified means

E954 Suicide and self-inflicted injury by submersion [drowning]

✓4th **E955 Suicide and self-inflicted injury by firearms, air guns and explosives**
    E955.0 Handgun
    E955.1 Shotgun
    E955.2 Hunting rifle
    E955.3 Military firearms
    E955.4 Other and unspecified firearm
        Gunshot NOS   Shot NOS
    E955.5 Explosives
    E955.6 Air gun
        BB gun
        Pellet gun
    ● E955.7 Paintball gun
    E955.9 Unspecified

E956 Suicide and self-inflicted injury by cutting and piercing instrument

✓4th **E957 Suicide and self-inflicted injuries by jumping from high place**
    E957.0 Residential premises
    E957.1 Other man-made structures
    E957.2 Natural sites
    E957.9 Unspecified

✓4th **E958 Suicide and self-inflicted injury by other and unspecified means**
    E958.0 Jumping or lying before moving object
    E958.1 Burns, fire
    E958.2 Scald
    E958.3 Extremes of cold
    E958.4 Electrocution
    E958.5 Crashing of motor vehicle
    E958.6 Crashing of aircraft
    E958.7 Caustic substances, except poisoning
        EXCLUDES: poisoning by caustic substance (E950.7)
    E958.8 Other specified means
    E958.9 Unspecified means

E959 Late effects of self-inflicted injury
    Note: This category is to be used to indicate circumstances classifiable to E950-E958 as the cause of death or disability from late effects, which are themselves classifiable elsewhere. The "late effects" include conditions reported as such, or as sequelae which may occur at any time after the attempted suicide or self-inflicted injury.

HOMICIDE AND INJURY PURPOSELY INFLICTED BY OTHER PERSONS (E960-E969)

INCLUDES: injuries inflicted by another person with intent to injure or kill, by any means
EXCLUDES: injuries due to:
    legal intervention (E970-E978)
    operations of war (E990-E999)
    ▶terrorism (E979)◀

✓4th **E960 Fight, brawl, rape**
    E960.0 Unarmed fight or brawl
        Beatings NOS
        Brawl or fight with hands, fists, feet
        Injured or killed in fight NOS
        EXCLUDES: homicidal:
            injury by weapons (E965.0-E966, E969)
            strangulation (E963)
            submersion (E964)
    E960.1 Rape

E961 Assault by corrosive or caustic substance, except poisoning
Injury or death purposely caused by corrosive or caustic substance, such as:
acid [any]
corrosive substance
vitriol

> **EXCLUDES** burns from hot liquid (E968.3)
> chemical burns from swallowing a corrosive substance (E962.0-E962.9)

✓4th **E962 Assault by poisoning**
  E962.0 Drugs and medicinal substances
    Homicidal poisoning by any drug or medicinal substance
  E962.1 Other solid and liquid substances
  E962.2 Other gases and vapors
  E962.9 Unspecified poisoning

E963 Assault by hanging and strangulation
Homicidal (attempt):
  garrotting or ligature
  hanging
Homicidal (attempt):
  strangulation
  suffocation

E964 Assault by submersion [drowning]

✓4th **E965 Assault by firearms and explosives**
  E965.0 Handgun
    Pistol   Revolver
  E965.1 Shotgun
  E965.2 Hunting rifle
  E965.3 Military firearms
  E965.4 Other and unspecified firearm
  E965.5 Antipersonnel bomb
  E965.6 Gasoline bomb
  E965.7 Letter bomb
  E965.8 Other specified explosive
    Bomb NOS (placed in):   Dynamite
      car
      house
  E965.9 Unspecified explosive

E966 Assault by cutting and piercing instrument
Assassination (attempt), homicide (attempt) by any instrument classifiable under E920
Homicidal:
  cut
  puncture   } any part of body
  stab
  Stabbed

✓4th **E967 Perpetrator of child and adult abuse**
  Note: Selection of the correct perpetrator code is based on the relationship between the perpetrator and the victim.
  E967.0 By father, stepfather, or boyfriend
    Male partner of child's parent or guardian
  E967.1 By other specified person
  E967.2 By mother, stepmother, or girlfriend
    Female partner of child's parent or guardian
  E967.3 By spouse or partner
    Abuse of spouse or partner by ex-spouse or ex-partner
  E967.4 By child
  E967.5 By sibling
  E967.6 By grandparent
  E967.7 By other relative
  E967.8 By non-related caregiver
  E967.9 By unspecified person

✓4th **E968 Assault by other and unspecified means**
  E968.0 Fire
    Arson
    Homicidal burns NOS
    > **EXCLUDES** burns from hot liquid (E968.3)
  E968.1 Pushing from a high place
  E968.2 Striking by blunt or thrown object
  E968.3 Hot liquid
    Homicidal burns by scalding
  E968.4 Criminal neglect
    Abandonment of child, infant, or other helpless person with intent to injure or kill
  E968.5 Transport vehicle
    Being struck by other vehicle or run down with intent to injure
    Pushed in front of, thrown from, or dragged by moving vehicle with intent to injure
  E968.6 Air gun
    BB gun
    Pellet gun
  E968.7 Human bite
  E968.8 Other specified means
  E968.9 Unspecified means
    Assassination (attempt) NOS
    Homicidal (attempt):
      injury NOS
      wound NOS
    Manslaughter (nonaccidental)
    Murder (attempt) NOS
    Violence, non-accidental

E969 Late effects of injury purposely inflicted by other person
Note: This category is to be used to indicate circumstances classifiable to E960-E968 as the cause of death or disability from late effects, which are themselves classifiable elsewhere. The "late effects" include conditions reported as such, or as sequelae which may occur at any time after injury purposely inflicted by another person.

LEGAL INTERVENTION (E970-E978)

> **INCLUDES** injuries inflicted by the police or other law-enforcing agents, including military on duty, in the course of arresting or attempting to arrest lawbreakers, suppressing disturbances, maintaining order, and other legal action
> legal execution
>
> **EXCLUDES** injuries caused by civil insurrections (E990.0-E999)

E970 Injury due to legal intervention by firearms
Gunshot wound
Injury by:
  machine gun
  revolver
Injury by:
  rifle pellet or rubber bullet
  shot NOS

E971 Injury due to legal intervention by explosives
Injury by:
  dynamite
  explosive shell
Injury by:
  grenade
  mortar bomb

E972 Injury due to legal intervention by gas
Asphyxiation by gas   Poisoning by gas
Injury by tear gas

E973 Injury due to legal intervention by blunt object
Hit, struck by:
  baton (nightstick)
  blunt object
Hit, struck by:
  stave

E974 Injury due to legal intervention by cutting and piercing instrument
Cut
Incised wound
Injured by bayonet
Stab wound

E975 Injury due to legal intervention by other specified means
Blow   Manhandling

E976 Injury due to legal intervention by unspecified means

E977 Late effects of injuries due to legal intervention
Note: This category is to be used to indicate circumstances classifiable to E970-E976 as the cause of death or disability from late effects, which are themselves classifiable elsewhere. The "late effects" include conditions reported as such, or as sequelae, which may occur at any time after the injury due to legal intervention.

E978 Legal execution
All executions performed at the behest of the judiciary or ruling authority [whether permanent or temporary] as:
asphyxiation by gas
beheading, decapitation (by guillotine)
capital punishment
electrocution
hanging
poisoning
shooting
other specified means

TERRORISM (E979)

✓4ᵗʰ E979 Terrorism
Injuries resulting from the unlawful use of force or violence against persons or property to intimidate or coerce a Government, the civilian population, or any segment thereof, in furtherance of political or social objective

E979.0 Terrorism involving explosion of marine weapons
Depth-charge
Marine mine
Mine NOS, at sea or in harbour
Sea-based artillery shell
Torpedo
Underwater blast

E979.1 Terrorism involving destruction of aircraft
Aircraft used as a weapon
Aircraft:
  burned
  exploded
  shot down
Crushed by falling aircraft

E979.2 Terrorism involving other explosions and fragments
Antipersonnel bomb (fragments)
Blast NOS
Explosion (of):
  artillery shell
  breech-block
  cannon block
  mortar bomb
  munitions being used in terrorism
  NOS
Fragments from:
  artillery shell
  bomb
  grenade
  guided missile
  land-mine
  rocket
  shell
  shrapnel
Mine NOS

E979.3 Terrorism involving fires, conflagraton and hot substances
Burning building or structure:
  collapse of
  fall from
  hit by falling object in
  jump from
Conflagraton NOS
Fire (causing):
  Asphyxia
  Burns
  NOS
  Other injury
Melting of fittings and furniture in burning
Petrol bomb
Smouldering building or structure

E979.4 Terrorism involving firearms
Bullet:
  carbine
  machine gun
  pistol
  rifle
  rubber (rifle)
Pellets (shotgun)

E979.5 Terrorism involving nuclear weapons
Blast effects
Exposure to ionizing radiation from nuclear weapon
Fireball effects
Heat from nuclear weapon
Other direct and secondary effects of nuclear weapons

E979.6 Terrorism involving biological weapons
Anthrax
Cholera
Smallpox

E979.7 Terrorism involving chemical weapons
Gases, fumes, chemicals
Hydrogen cyanide
Phosgene
Sarin

E979.8 Terrorism involving other means
Drowning and submersion
Lasers
Piercing or stabbing instruments
Terrorism NOS

E979.9 Terrorism, secondary effects
Note: This code is for use to identify conditions occurring subsequent to a terrorist attack not those that are due to the initial terrorist act
EXCLUDES late effect of terrorist attack (E999.1)

INJURY UNDETERMINED WHETHER ACCIDENTALLY OR PURPOSELY INFLICTED (E980-E989)

Note: Categories E980-E989 are for use when it is unspecified or it cannot be determined whether the injuries are accidental (unintentional), suicide (attempted), or assault.

✓4ᵗʰ E980 Poisoning by solid or liquid substances, undetermined whether accidentally or purposely inflicted
E980.0 Analgesics, antipyretics, and antirheumatics
E980.1 Barbiturates
E980.2 Other sedatives and hypnotics
E980.3 Tranquilizers and other psychotropic agents
E980.4 Other specified drugs and medicinal substances
E980.5 Unspecified drug or medicinal substance
E980.6 Corrosive and caustic substances
  Poisoning, undetermined whether accidental or purposeful, by substances classifiable to E864
E980.7 Agricultural and horticultural chemical and pharmaceutical preparations other than plant foods and fertilizers
E980.8 Arsenic and its compounds
E980.9 Other and unspecified solid and liquid substances

✓4ᵗʰ E981 Poisoning by gases in domestic use, undetermined whether accidentally or purposely inflicted
E981.0 Gas distributed by pipeline
E981.1 Liquefied petroleum gas distributed in mobile containers
E981.8 Other utility gas

✓4ᵗʰ E982 Poisoning by other gases, undetermined whether accidentally or purposely inflicted
E982.0 Motor vehicle exhaust gas
E982.1 Other carbon monoxide
E982.8 Other specified gases and vapors
E982.9 Unspecified gases and vapors

✓4ᵗʰ E983 Hanging, strangulation, or suffocation, undetermined whether accidentally or purposely inflicted
E983.0 Hanging
E983.1 Suffocation by plastic bag
E983.8 Other specified means
E983.9 Unspecified means

Tabular List   **E CODES**   **E984—E999.1**

E984 Submersion [drowning], undetermined whether accidentally or purposely inflicted

✓4ᵗʰ **E985 Injury by firearms, air guns and explosives, undetermined whether accidentally or purposely inflicted**
- E985.0 Handgun
- E985.1 Shotgun
- E985.2 Hunting rifle
- E985.3 Military firearms
- E985.4 Other and unspecified firearm
- E985.5 Explosives
- E985.6 Air gun
  - BB gun
  - Pellet gun
- ● E985.7 Paintball gun

E986 Injury by cutting and piercing instruments, undetermined whether accidentally or purposely inflicted

✓4ᵗʰ **E987 Falling from high place, undetermined whether accidentally or purposely inflicted**
- E987.0 Residential premises
- E987.1 Other man-made structures
- E987.2 Natural sites
- E987.9 Unspecified site

✓4ᵗʰ **E988 Injury by other and unspecified means, undetermined whether accidentally or purposely inflicted**
- E988.0 Jumping or lying before moving object
- E988.1 Burns, fire
- E988.2 Scald
- E988.3 Extremes of cold
- E988.4 Electrocution
- E988.5 Crashing of motor vehicle
- E988.6 Crashing of aircraft
- E988.7 Caustic substances, except poisoning
- E988.8 Other specified means
- E988.9 Unspecified means

E989 Late effects of injury, undetermined whether accidentally or purposely inflicted

> Note: This category is to be used to indicate circumstances classifiable to E980-E988 as the cause of death or disability from late effects, which are themselves classifiable elsewhere. The "late effects" include conditions reported as such, or as sequelae, which may occur at any time after injury, undetermined whether accidentally or purposely inflicted.

INJURY RESULTING FROM OPERATIONS OF WAR (E990-E999)

INCLUDES   injuries to military personnel and civilians caused by war and civil insurrections and occurring during the time of war and insurrection

EXCLUDES   accidents during training of military personnel manufacture of war material and transport, unless attributable to enemy action

✓4ᵗʰ **E990 Injury due to war operations by fires and conflagrations**

INCLUDES   asphyxia, burns, or other injury originating from fire caused by a fire-producing device or indirectly by any conventional weapon

- E990.0 From gasoline bomb
- E990.9 From other and unspecified source

✓4ᵗʰ **E991 Injury due to war operations by bullets and fragments**
- E991.0 Rubber bullets (rifle)
- E991.1 Pellets (rifle)
- E991.2 Other bullets
  - Bullet [any, except rubber bullets and pellets]
    - carbine
    - machine gun
    - pistol
    - rifle
    - shotgun
- E991.3 Antipersonnel bomb (fragments)
- E991.9 Other and unspecified fragments
  - Fragments from: artillery shell, bombs, except anti-personnel grenade, guided missile
  - Fragments from: land mine, rockets, shell, Shrapnel

E992 Injury due to war operations by explosion of marine weapons
- Depth charge
- Marine mines
- Mine NOS, at sea or in harbor
- Sea-based artillery shell
- Torpedo
- Underwater blast

E993 Injury due to war operations by other explosion
- Accidental explosion of munitions being used in war
- Accidental explosion of own weapons
- Air blast NOS
- Blast NOS
- Explosion NOS
- Explosion of: artillery shell, breech block, cannon block, mortar bomb
- Injury by weapon burst

E994 Injury due to war operations by destruction of aircraft
- Airplane: burned, exploded
- Airplane: shot down
- Crushed by falling airplane

E995 Injury due to war operations by other and unspecified forms of conventional warfare
- Battle wounds
- Bayonet injury
- Drowned in war operations

E996 Injury due to war operations by nuclear weapons
- Blast effects
- Exposure to ionizing radiation from nuclear weapons
- Fireball effects
- Heat
- Other direct and secondary effects of nuclear weapons

✓4ᵗʰ **E997 Injury due to war operations by other forms of unconventional warfare**
- E997.0 Lasers
- E997.1 Biological warfare
- E997.2 Gases, fumes, and chemicals
- E997.8 Other specified forms of unconventional warfare
- E997.9 Unspecified form of unconventional warfare

E998 Injury due to war operations but occurring after cessation of hostilities
- Injuries due to operations of war but occurring after cessation of hostilities by any means classifiable under E990-E997
- Injuries by explosion of bombs or mines placed in the course of operations of war, if the explosion occurred after cessation of hostilities

▲ ✓4ᵗʰ **E999 Late effect of injury due to war operations and terrorism**

> Note: This category is to be used to indicate circumstances classifiable to ▶E979,◀ E990-E998 as the cause of death or disability from late effects, which are themselves classifiable elsewhere. The "late effects" include conditions reported as such, or as sequelae, which may occur at any time after the injury, resulting from operations of war ▶or terrorism◀.

- ● E999.0 Late effect of injury due to war operations
- ● E999.1 Late effect of injury due to terrorism

✓4ᵗʰ Fourth-digit Required   ▶◀ Revised Text   ● New Code   ▲ Revised Code Title

Official ICD·9·CM Government Appendixes

MORPHOLOGY OF NEOPLASMS

The World Health Organization has published an adaptation of the International Classification of Diseases for oncology (ICD-O). It contains a coded nomenclature for the morphology of neoplasms, which is reproduced here for those who wish to use it in conjunction with Chapter 2 of the International Classification of Diseases, 9th Revision, Clinical Modification.

The morphology code numbers consist of five digits; the first four identify the histological type of the neoplasm and the fifth indicates its behavior. The one-digit behavior code is as follows:

- /0 Benign
- /1 Uncertain whether benign or malignant
     Borderline malignancy
- /2 Carcinoma in situ
     Intraepithelial
     Noninfiltrating
     Noninvasive
- /3 Malignant, primary site
- /6 Malignant, metastatic site
     Secondary site
- /9 Malignant, uncertain whether primary or metastatic site

In the nomenclature below, the morphology code numbers include the behavior code appropriate to the histological type of neoplasm, but this behavior code should be changed if other reported information makes this necessary. For example, "chordoma (M9370/3)" is assumed to be malignant; the term "benign chordoma" should be coded M9370/0. Similarly, "superficial spreading adenocarcinoma (M8143/3)" described as "noninvasive" should be coded M8143/2 and "melanoma (M8720/3)" described as "secondary" should be coded M8720/6.

The following table shows the correspondence between the morphology code and the different sections of Chapter 2:

Morphology Code Histology/Behavior		ICD-9-CM Chapter 2
Any M8000-M8004	0	210-229 Benign neoplasms
	1	239 Neoplasms of unspecified nature
M8010+	1	235-238 Neoplasms of uncertain behavior
Any	2	230-234 Carcinoma in situ
Any	3	140-195 Malignant neoplasms, stated or presumed
		200-208 to be primary
Any	6	196-198 Malignant neoplasms, stated or presumed to be secondary

The ICD-O behavior digit /9 is inapplicable in an ICD context, since all malignant neoplasms are presumed to be primary (/3) or secondary (/6) according to other information on the medical record.

Only the first-listed term of the full ICD-O morphology nomenclature appears against each code number in the list below. The ICD-9-CM Alphabetical Index (Volume 2), however, includes all the ICD-O synonyms as well as a number of other morphological names still likely to be encountered on medical records but omitted from ICD-O as outdated or otherwise undesirable.

A coding difficulty sometimes arises where a morphological diagnosis contains two qualifying adjectives that have different code numbers. An example is "transitional cell epidermoid carcinoma." "Transitional cell carcinoma NOS" is M8120/3 and "epidermoid carcinoma NOS" is M8070/3. In such circumstances, the higher number (M8120/3 in this example) should be used, as it is usually more specific.

CODED NOMENCLATURE FOR MORPHOLOGY OF NEOPLASMS

M800 Neoplasms NOS
- M8000/0 Neoplasm, benign
- M8000/1 Neoplasm, uncertain whether benign or malignant
- M8000/3 Neoplasm, malignant
- M8000/6 Neoplasm, metastatic
- M8000/9 Neoplasm, malignant, uncertain whether primary or metastatic
- M8001/0 Tumor cells, benign
- M8001/1 Tumor cells, uncertain whether benign or malignant
- M8001/3 Tumor cells, malignant
- M8002/3 Malignant tumor, small cell type
- M8003/3 Malignant tumor, giant cell type
- M8004/3 Malignant tumor, fusiform cell type

M801-M804 Epithelial neoplasms NOS
- M8010/0 Epithelial tumor, benign
- M8010/2 Carcinoma in situ NOS
- M8010/3 Carcinoma NOS
- M8010/6 Carcinoma, metastatic NOS
- M8010/9 Carcinomatosis
- M8011/0 Epithelioma, benign
- M8011/3 Epithelioma, malignant
- M8012/3 Large cell carcinoma NOS
- M8020/3 Carcinoma, undifferentiated type NOS
- M8021/3 Carcinoma, anaplastic type NOS
- M8022/3 Pleomorphic carcinoma
- M8030/3 Giant cell and spindle cell carcinoma
- M8031/3 Giant cell carcinoma
- M8032/3 Spindle cell carcinoma
- M8033/3 Pseudosarcomatous carcinoma
- M8034/3 Polygonal cell carcinoma
- M8035/3 Spheroidal cell carcinoma
- M8040/1 Tumorlet
- M8041/3 Small cell carcinoma NOS
- M8042/3 Oat cell carcinoma
- M8043/3 Small cell carcinoma, fusiform cell type

M805-M808 Papillary and squamous cell neoplasms
- M8050/0 Papilloma NOS (except Papilloma of urinary bladder M8120/1)
- M8050/2 Papillary carcinoma in situ
- M8050/3 Papillary carcinoma NOS
- M8051/0 Verrucous papilloma
- M8051/3 Verrucous carcinoma NOS
- M8052/0 Squamous cell papilloma
- M8052/3 Papillary squamous cell carcinoma
- M8053/0 Inverted papilloma
- M8060/0 Papillomatosis NOS
- M8070/2 Squamous cell carcinoma in situ NOS
- M8070/3 Squamous cell carcinoma NOS
- M8070/6 Squamous cell carcinoma, metastatic NOS
- M8071/3 Squamous cell carcinoma, keratinizing type NOS
- M8072/3 Squamous cell carcinoma, large cell, nonkeratinizing type
- M8073/3 Squamous cell carcinoma, small cell, nonkeratinizing type
- M8074/3 Squamous cell carcinoma, spindle cell type
- M8075/3 Adenoid squamous cell carcinoma
- M8076/2 Squamous cell carcinoma in situ with questionable stromal invasion
- M8076/3 Squamous cell carcinoma, microinvasive
- M8080/2 Queyrat's erythroplasia
- M8081/2 Bowen's disease
- M8082/3 Lymphoepithelial carcinoma

M809-M811 Basal cell neoplasms
- M8090/1 Basal cell tumor
- M8090/3 Basal cell carcinoma NOS
- M8091/3 Multicentric basal cell carcinoma
- M8092/3 Basal cell carcinoma, morphea type
- M8093/3 Basal cell carcinoma, fibroepithelial type
- M8094/3 Basosquamous carcinoma
- M8095/3 Metatypical carcinoma
- M8096/0 Intraepidermal epithelioma of Jadassohn
- M8100/0 Trichoepithelioma
- M8101/0 Trichofolliculoma
- M8102/0 Tricholemmoma
- M8110/0 Pilomatrixoma

M812-M813 Transitional cell papillomas and carcinomas
- M8120/0 Transitional cell papilloma NOS
- M8120/1 Urothelial papilloma
- M8120/2 Transitional cell carcinoma in situ
- M8120/3 Transitional cell carcinoma NOS
- M8121/0 Schneiderian papilloma
- M8121/1 Transitional cell papilloma, inverted type
- M8121/3 Schneiderian carcinoma
- M8122/3 Transitional cell carcinoma, spindle cell type

APPENDIX A: MORPHOLOGY OF NEOPLASMS

M8123/3	Basaloid carcinoma
M8124/3	Cloacogenic carcinoma
M8130/3	Papillary transitional cell carcinoma

M814-M838 Adenomas and adenocarcinomas

M8140/0	Adenoma NOS
M8140/1	Bronchial adenoma NOS
M8140/2	Adenocarcinoma in situ
M8140/3	Adenocarcinoma NOS
M8140/6	Adenocarcinoma, metastatic NOS
M8141/3	Scirrhous adenocarcinoma
M8142/3	Linitis plastica
M8143/3	Superficial spreading adenocarcinoma
M8144/3	Adenocarcinoma, intestinal type
M8145/3	Carcinoma, diffuse type
M8146/0	Monomorphic adenoma
M8147/0	Basal cell adenoma
M8150/0	Islet cell adenoma
M8150/3	Islet cell carcinoma
M8151/0	Insulinoma NOS
M8151/3	Insulinoma, malignant
M8152/0	Glucagonoma NOS
M8152/3	Glucagonoma, malignant
M8153/1	Gastrinoma NOS
M8153/3	Gastrinoma, malignant
M8154/3	Mixed islet cell and exocrine adenocarcinoma
M8160/0	Bile duct adenoma
M8160/3	Cholangiocarcinoma
M8161/0	Bile duct cystadenoma
M8161/3	Bile duct cystadenocarcinoma
M8170/0	Liver cell adenoma
M8170/3	Hepatocellular carcinoma NOS
M8180/0	Hepatocholangioma, benign
M8180/3	Combined hepatocellular carcinoma and cholangiocarcinoma
M8190/0	Trabecular adenoma
M8190/3	Trabecular adenocarcinoma
M8191/0	Embryonal adenoma
M8200/0	Eccrine dermal cylindroma
M8200/3	Adenoid cystic carcinoma
M8201/3	Cribriform carcinoma
M8210/0	Adenomatous polyp NOS
M8210/3	Adenocarcinoma in adenomatous polyp
M8211/0	Tubular adenoma NOS
M8211/3	Tubular adenocarcinoma
M8220/0	Adenomatous polyposis coli
M8220/3	Adenocarcinoma in adenomatous polyposis coli
M8221/0	Multiple adenomatous polyps
M8230/3	Solid carcinoma NOS
M8231/3	Carcinoma simplex
M8240/1	Carcinoid tumor NOS
M8240/3	Carcinoid tumor, malignant
M8241/1	Carcinoid tumor, argentaffin NOS
M8241/3	Carcinoid tumor, argentaffin, malignant
M8242/1	Carcinoid tumor, nonargentaffin NOS
M8242/3	Carcinoid tumor, nonargentaffin, malignant
M8243/3	Mucocarcinoid tumor, malignant
M8244/3	Composite carcinoid
M8250/1	Pulmonary adenomatosis
M8250/3	Bronchiolo-alveolar adenocarcinoma
M8251/0	Alveolar adenoma
M8251/3	Alveolar adenocarcinoma
M8260/0	Papillary adenoma NOS
M8260/3	Papillary adenocarcinoma NOS
M8261/1	Villous adenoma NOS
M8261/3	Adenocarcinoma in villous adenoma
M8262/3	Villous adenocarcinoma
M8263/0	Tubulovillous adenoma
M8270/0	Chromophobe adenoma
M8270/3	Chromophobe carcinoma
M8280/0	Acidophil adenoma
M8280/3	Acidophil carcinoma
M8281/0	Mixed acidophil-basophil adenoma
M8281/3	Mixed acidophil-basophil carcinoma
M8290/0	Oxyphilic adenoma
M8290/3	Oxyphilic adenocarcinoma
M8300/0	Basophil adenoma
M8300/3	Basophil carcinoma
M8310/0	Clear cell adenoma
M8310/3	Clear cell adenocarcinoma NOS
M8311/1	Hypernephroid tumor
M8312/3	Renal cell carcinoma
M8313/0	Clear cell adenofibroma
M8320/3	Granular cell carcinoma
M8321/0	Chief cell adenoma
M8322/0	Water-clear cell adenoma
M8322/3	Water-clear cell adenocarcinoma
M8323/0	Mixed cell adenoma
M8323/3	Mixed cell adenocarcinoma
M8324/0	Lipoadenoma
M8330/0	Follicular adenoma
M8330/3	Follicular adenocarcinoma NOS
M8331/3	Follicular adenocarcinoma, well differentiated type
M8332/3	Follicular adenocarcinoma, trabecular type
M8333/0	Microfollicular adenoma
M8334/0	Macrofollicular adenoma
M8340/3	Papillary and follicular adenocarcinoma
M8350/3	Nonencapsulated sclerosing carcinoma
M8360/1	Multiple endocrine adenomas
M8361/1	Juxtaglomerular tumor
M8370/0	Adrenal cortical adenoma NOS
M8370/3	Adrenal cortical carcinoma
M8371/0	Adrenal cortical adenoma, compact cell type
M8372/0	Adrenal cortical adenoma, heavily pigmented variant
M8373/0	Adrenal cortical adenoma, clear cell type
M8374/0	Adrenal cortical adenoma, glomerulosa cell type
M8375/0	Adrenal cortical adenoma, mixed cell type
M8380/0	Endometrioid adenoma NOS
M8380/1	Endometrioid adenoma, borderline malignancy
M8380/3	Endometrioid carcinoma
M8381/0	Endometrioid adenofibroma NOS
M8381/1	Endometrioid adenofibroma, borderline malignancy
M8381/3	Endometrioid adenofibroma, malignant

M839-M842 Adnexal and skin appendage neoplasms

M8390/0	Skin appendage adenoma
M8390/3	Skin appendage carcinoma
M8400/0	Sweat gland adenoma
M8400/1	Sweat gland tumor NOS
M8400/3	Sweat gland adenocarcinoma
M8401/0	Apocrine adenoma
M8401/3	Apocrine adenocarcinoma
M8402/0	Eccrine acrospiroma
M8403/0	Eccrine spiradenoma
M8404/0	Hidrocystoma
M8405/0	Papillary hydradenoma
M8406/0	Papillary syringadenoma
M8407/0	Syringoma NOS
M8410/0	Sebaceous adenoma
M8410/3	Sebaceous adenocarcinoma
M8420/0	Ceruminous adenoma
M8420/3	Ceruminous adenocarcinoma

M843 Mucoepidermoid neoplasms

M8430/1	Mucoepidermoid tumor
M8430/3	Mucoepidermoid carcinoma

M844-M849 Cystic, mucinous, and serous neoplasms

M8440/0	Cystadenoma NOS
M8440/3	Cystadenocarcinoma NOS
M8441/0	Serous cystadenoma NOS
M8441/1	Serous cystadenoma, borderline malignancy
M8441/3	Serous cystadenocarcinoma NOS
M8450/0	Papillary cystadenoma NOS
M8450/1	Papillary cystadenoma, borderline malignancy
M8450/3	Papillary cystadenocarcinoma NOS
M8460/0	Papillary serous cystadenoma NOS
M8460/1	Papillary serous cystadenoma, borderline malignancy
M8460/3	Papillary serous cystadenocarcinoma
M8461/0	Serous surface papilloma NOS
M8461/1	Serous surface papilloma, borderline malignancy
M8461/3	Serous surface papillary carcinoma
M8470/0	Mucinous cystadenoma NOS
M8470/1	Mucinous cystadenoma, borderline malignancy
M8470/3	Mucinous cystadenocarcinoma NOS
M8471/0	Papillary mucinous cystadenoma NOS
M8471/1	Papillary mucinous cystadenoma, borderline malignancy
M8471/3	Papillary mucinous cystadenocarcinoma
M8480/0	Mucinous adenoma
M8480/3	Mucinous adenocarcinoma
M8480/6	Pseudomyxoma peritonei
M8481/3	Mucin-producing adenocarcinoma
M8490/3	Signet ring cell carcinoma
M8490/6	Metastatic signet ring cell carcinoma

M850-M854 Ductal, lobular, and medullary neoplasms

M8500/2	Intraductal carcinoma, noninfiltrating NOS
M8500/3	Infiltrating duct carcinoma
M8501/2	Comedocarcinoma, noninfiltrating
M8501/3	Comedocarcinoma NOS
M8502/3	Juvenile carcinoma of the breast
M8503/0	Intraductal papilloma
M8503/2	Noninfiltrating intraductal papillary adenocarcinoma
M8504/0	Intracystic papillary adenoma
M8504/2	Noninfiltrating intracystic carcinoma
M8505/0	Intraductal papillomatosis NOS
M8506/0	Subareolar duct papillomatosis
M8510/3	Medullary carcinoma NOS
M8511/3	Medullary carcinoma with amyloid stroma
M8512/3	Medullary carcinoma with lymphoid stroma
M8520/2	Lobular carcinoma in situ
M8520/3	Lobular carcinoma NOS

APPENDIX A: MORPHOLOGY OF NEOPLASMS

M8521/3	Infiltrating ductular carcinoma
M8530/3	Inflammatory carcinoma
M8540/3	Paget's disease, mammary
M8541/3	Paget's disease and infiltrating duct carcinoma of breast
M8542/3	Paget's disease, extramammary (except Paget's disease of bone)
M855	**Acinar cell neoplasms**
M8550/0	Acinar cell adenoma
M8550/1	Acinar cell tumor
M8550/3	Acinar cell carcinoma
M856-M858	**Complex epithelial neoplasms**
M8560/3	Adenosquamous carcinoma
M8561/0	Adenolymphoma
M8570/3	Adenocarcinoma with squamous metaplasia
M8571/3	Adenocarcinoma with cartilaginous and osseous metaplasia
M8572/3	Adenocarcinoma with spindle cell metaplasia
M8573/3	Adenocarcinoma with apocrine metaplasia
M8580/0	Thymoma, benign
M8580/3	Thymoma, malignant
M859-M867	**Specialized gonadal neoplasms**
M8590/1	Sex cord-stromal tumor
M8600/0	Thecoma NOS
M8600/3	Theca cell carcinoma
M8610/0	Luteoma NOS
M8620/1	Granulosa cell tumor NOS
M8620/3	Granulosa cell tumor, malignant
M8621/1	Granulosa cell-theca cell tumor
M8630/0	Androblastoma, benign
M8630/1	Androblastoma NOS
M8630/3	Androblastoma, malignant
M8631/0	Sertoli-Leydig cell tumor
M8632/1	Gynandroblastoma
M8640/0	Tubular androblastoma NOS
M8640/3	Sertoli cell carcinoma
M8641/0	Tubular androblastoma with lipid storage
M8650/0	Leydig cell tumor, benign
M8650/1	Leydig cell tumor NOS
M8650/3	Leydig cell tumor, malignant
M8660/0	Hilar cell tumor
M8670/0	Lipid cell tumor of ovary
M8671/0	Adrenal rest tumor
M868-M871	**Paragangliomas and glomus tumors**
M8680/1	Paraganglioma NOS
M8680/3	Paraganglioma, malignant
M8681/1	Sympathetic paraganglioma
M8682/1	Parasympathetic paraganglioma
M8690/1	Glomus jugulare tumor
M8691/1	Aortic body tumor
M8692/1	Carotid body tumor
M8693/1	Extra-adrenal paraganglioma NOS
M8693/3	Extra-adrenal paraganglioma, malignant
M8700/0	Pheochromocytoma NOS
M8700/3	Pheochromocytoma, malignant
M8710/3	Glomangiosarcoma
M8711/0	Glomus tumor
M8712/0	Glomangioma
M872-M879	**Nevi and melanomas**
M8720/0	Pigmented nevus NOS
M8720/3	Malignant melanoma NOS
M8721/3	Nodular melanoma
M8722/0	Balloon cell nevus
M8722/3	Balloon cell melanoma
M8723/0	Halo nevus
M8724/0	Fibrous papule of the nose
M8725/0	Neuronevus
M8726/0	Magnocellular nevus
M8730/0	Nonpigmented nevus
M8730/3	Amelanotic melanoma
M8740/0	Junctional nevus
M8740/3	Malignant melanoma in junctional nevus
M8741/2	Precancerous melanosis NOS
M8741/3	Malignant melanoma in precancerous melanosis
M8742/2	Hutchinson's melanotic freckle
M8742/3	Malignant melanoma in Hutchinson's melanotic freckle
M8743/3	Superficial spreading melanoma
M8750/0	Intradermal nevus
M8760/0	Compound nevus
M8761/1	Giant pigmented nevus
M8761/3	Malignant melanoma in giant pigmented nevus
M8770/0	Epithelioid and spindle cell nevus
M8771/3	Epithelioid cell melanoma
M8772/3	Spindle cell melanoma NOS
M8773/3	Spindle cell melanoma, type A
M8774/3	Spindle cell melanoma, type B
M8775/3	Mixed epithelioid and spindle cell melanoma
M8780/0	Blue nevus NOS
M8780/3	Blue nevus, malignant
M8790/0	Cellular blue nevus
M880	**Soft tissue tumors and sarcomas NOS**
M8800/0	Soft tissue tumor, benign
M8800/3	Sarcoma NOS
M8800/9	Sarcomatosis NOS
M8801/3	Spindle cell sarcoma
M8802/3	Giant cell sarcoma (except of bone M9250/3)
M8803/3	Small cell sarcoma
M8804/3	Epithelioid cell sarcoma
M881-M883	**Fibromatous neoplasms**
M8810/0	Fibroma NOS
M8810/3	Fibrosarcoma NOS
M8811/0	Fibromyxoma
M8811/3	Fibromyxosarcoma
M8812/0	Periosteal fibroma
M8812/3	Periosteal fibrosarcoma
M8813/0	Fascial fibroma
M8813/3	Fascial fibrosarcoma
M8814/3	Infantile fibrosarcoma
M8820/0	Elastofibroma
M8821/1	Aggressive fibromatosis
M8822/1	Abdominal fibromatosis
M8823/1	Desmoplastic fibroma
M8830/0	Fibrous histiocytoma NOS
M8830/1	Atypical fibrous histiocytoma
M8830/3	Fibrous histiocytoma, malignant
M8831/0	Fibroxanthoma NOS
M8831/1	Atypical fibroxanthoma
M8831/3	Fibroxanthoma, malignant
M8832/0	Dermatofibroma NOS
M8832/1	Dermatofibroma protuberans
M8832/3	Dermatofibrosarcoma NOS
M884	**Myxomatous neoplasms**
M8840/0	Myxoma NOS
M8840/3	Myxosarcoma
M885-M888	**Lipomatous neoplasms**
M8850/0	Lipoma NOS
M8850/3	Liposarcoma NOS
M8851/0	Fibrolipoma
M8851/3	Liposarcoma, well differentiated type
M8852/0	Fibromyxolipoma
M8852/3	Myxoid liposarcoma
M8853/3	Round cell liposarcoma
M8854/3	Pleomorphic liposarcoma
M8855/3	Mixed type liposarcoma
M8856/0	Intramuscular lipoma
M8857/0	Spindle cell lipoma
M8860/0	Angiomyolipoma
M8860/3	Angiomyoliposarcoma
M8861/0	Angiolipoma NOS
M8861/1	Angiolipoma, infiltrating
M8870/0	Myelolipoma
M8880/0	Hibernoma
M8881/0	Lipoblastomatosis
M889-M892	**Myomatous neoplasms**
M8890/0	Leiomyoma NOS
M8890/1	Intravascular leiomyomatosis
M8890/3	Leiomyosarcoma NOS
M8891/1	Epithelioid leiomyoma
M8891/3	Epithelioid leiomyosarcoma
M8892/1	Cellular leiomyoma
M8893/0	Bizarre leiomyoma
M8894/0	Angiomyoma
M8894/3	Angiomyosarcoma
M8895/0	Myoma
M8895/3	Myosarcoma
M8900/0	Rhabdomyoma NOS
M8900/3	Rhabdomyosarcoma NOS
M8901/3	Pleomorphic rhabdomyosarcoma
M8902/3	Mixed type rhabdomyosarcoma
M8903/0	Fetal rhabdomyoma
M8904/0	Adult rhabdomyoma
M8910/3	Embryonal rhabdomyosarcoma
M8920/3	Alveolar rhabdomyosarcoma
M893-M899	**Complex mixed and stromal neoplasms**
M8930/3	Endometrial stromal sarcoma
M8931/1	Endolymphatic stromal myosis
M8932/0	Adenomyoma
M8940/0	Pleomorphic adenoma
M8940/3	Mixed tumor, malignant NOS
M8950/3	Mullerian mixed tumor
M8951/3	Mesodermal mixed tumor
M8960/1	Mesoblastic nephroma
M8960/3	Nephroblastoma NOS
M8961/3	Epithelial nephroblastoma
M8962/3	Mesenchymal nephroblastoma
M8970/3	Hepatoblastoma
M8980/3	Carcinosarcoma NOS
M8981/3	Carcinosarcoma, embryonal type
M8982/0	Myoepithelioma
M8990/0	Mesenchymoma, benign
M8990/1	Mesenchymoma NOS
M8990/3	Mesenchymoma, malignant
M8991/3	Embryonal sarcoma
M900-M903	**Fibroepithelial neoplasms**
M9000/0	Brenner tumor NOS
M9000/1	Brenner tumor, borderline malignancy
M9000/3	Brenner tumor, malignant
M9010/0	Fibroadenoma NOS
M9011/0	Intracanalicular fibroadenoma NOS
M9012/0	Pericanalicular fibroadenoma
M9013/0	Adenofibroma NOS
M9014/0	Serous adenofibroma
M9015/0	Mucinous adenofibroma
M9020/0	Cellular intracanalicular fibroadenoma
M9020/1	Cystosarcoma phyllodes NOS
M9020/3	Cystosarcoma phyllodes, malignant
M9030/0	Juvenile fibroadenoma
M904	**Synovial neoplasms**
M9040/0	Synovioma, benign
M9040/3	Synovial sarcoma NOS
M9041/3	Synovial sarcoma, spindle cell type
M9042/3	Synovial sarcoma, epithelioid cell type
M9043/3	Synovial sarcoma, biphasic type
M9044/3	Clear cell sarcoma of tendons and aponeuroses

APPENDIX A: MORPHOLOGY OF NEOPLASMS

M905 **Mesothelial neoplasms**
M9050/0 Mesothelioma, benign
M9050/3 Mesothelioma, malignant
M9051/0 Fibrous mesothelioma, benign
M9051/3 Fibrous mesothelioma, malignant
M9052/0 Epithelioid mesothelioma, benign
M9052/3 Epithelioid mesothelioma, malignant
M9053/0 Mesothelioma, biphasic type, benign
M9053/3 Mesothelioma, biphasic type, malignant
M9054/0 Adenomatoid tumor NOS

M906-M909 **Germ cell neoplasms**
M9060/3 Dysgerminoma
M9061/3 Seminoma NOS
M9062/3 Seminoma, anaplastic type
M9063/3 Spermatocytic seminoma
M9064/3 Germinoma
M9070/3 Embryonal carcinoma NOS
M9071/3 Endodermal sinus tumor
M9072/3 Polyembryoma
M9073/1 Gonadoblastoma
M9080/0 Teratoma, benign
M9080/1 Teratoma NOS
M9080/3 Teratoma, malignant NOS
M9081/3 Teratocarcinoma
M9082/3 Malignant teratoma, undifferentiated type
M9083/3 Malignant teratoma, intermediate type
M9084/0 Dermoid cyst
M9084/3 Dermoid cyst with malignant transformation
M9090/0 Struma ovarii NOS
M9090/3 Struma ovarii, malignant
M9091/1 Strumal carcinoid

M910 **Trophoblastic neoplasms**
M9100/0 Hydatidiform mole NOS
M9100/1 Invasive hydatidiform mole
M9100/3 Choriocarcinoma
M9101/3 Choriocarcinoma combined with teratoma
M9102/3 Malignant teratoma, trophoblastic

M911 **Mesonephromas**
M9110/0 Mesonephroma, benign
M9110/1 Mesonephric tumor
M9110/3 Mesonephroma, malignant
M9111/1 Endosalpingioma

M912-M916 **Blood vessel tumors**
M9120/0 Hemangioma NOS
M9120/3 Hemangiosarcoma
M9121/0 Cavernous hemangioma
M9122/0 Venous hemangioma
M9123/0 Racemose hemangioma
M9124/3 Kupffer cell sarcoma
M9130/0 Hemangioendothelioma, benign
M9130/1 Hemangioendothelioma NOS
M9130/3 Hemangioendothelioma, malignant
M9131/0 Capillary hemangioma
M9132/0 Intramuscular hemangioma
M9140/3 Kaposi's sarcoma
M9141/0 Angiokeratoma
M9142/0 Verrucous keratotic hemangioma
M9150/0 Hemangiopericytoma, benign
M9150/1 Hemangiopericytoma NOS
M9150/3 Hemangiopericytoma, malignant
M9160/0 Angiofibroma NOS
M9161/1 Hemangioblastoma

M917 **Lymphatic vessel tumors**
M9170/0 Lymphangioma NOS
M9170/3 Lymphangiosarcoma
M9171/0 Capillary lymphangioma
M9172/0 Cavernous lymphangioma
M9173/0 Cystic lymphangioma
M9174/0 Lymphangiomyoma
M9174/1 Lymphangiomyomatosis
M9175/0 Hemolymphangioma

M918-M920 **Osteomas and osteosarcomas**
M9180/0 Osteoma NOS
M9180/3 Osteosarcoma NOS
M9181/3 Chondroblastic osteosarcoma
M9182/3 Fibroblastic osteosarcoma
M9183/3 Telangiectatic osteosarcoma
M9184/3 Osteosarcoma in Paget's disease of bone
M9190/3 Juxtacortical osteosarcoma
M9191/0 Osteoid osteoma NOS
M9200/0 Osteoblastoma

M921-M924 **Chondromatous neoplasms**
M9210/0 Osteochondroma
M9210/1 Osteochondromatosis NOS
M9220/0 Chondroma NOS
M9220/1 Chondromatosis NOS
M9220/3 Chondrosarcoma NOS
M9221/0 Juxtacortical chondroma
M9221/3 Juxtacortical chondrosarcoma
M9230/0 Chondroblastoma NOS
M9230/3 Chondroblastoma, malignant
M9240/3 Mesenchymal chondrosarcoma
M9241/0 Chondromyxoid fibroma

M925 **Giant cell tumors**
M9250/1 Giant cell tumor of bone NOS
M9250/3 Giant cell tumor of bone, malignant
M9251/1 Giant cell tumor of soft parts NOS
M9251/3 Malignant giant cell tumor of soft parts

M926 **Miscellaneous bone tumors**
M9260/3 Ewing's sarcoma
M9261/3 Adamantinoma of long bones
M9262/0 Ossifying fibroma

M927-M934 **Odontogenic tumors**
M9270/0 Odontogenic tumor, benign
M9270/1 Odontogenic tumor NOS
M9270/3 Odontogenic tumor, malignant
M9271/0 Dentinoma
M9272/0 Cementoma NOS
M9273/0 Cementoblastoma, benign
M9274/0 Cementifying fibroma
M9275/0 Gigantiform cementoma
M9280/0 Odontoma NOS
M9281/0 Compound odontoma
M9282/0 Complex odontoma
M9290/0 Ameloblastic fibro-odontoma
M9290/3 Ameloblastic odontosarcoma
M9300/0 Adenomatoid odontogenic tumor
M9301/0 Calcifying odontogenic cyst
M9310/0 Ameloblastoma NOS
M9310/3 Ameloblastoma, malignant
M9311/0 Odontoameloblastoma
M9312/0 Squamous odontogenic tumor
M9320/0 Odontogenic myxoma
M9321/0 Odontogenic fibroma NOS
M9330/0 Ameloblastic fibroma
M9330/3 Ameloblastic fibrosarcoma
M9340/0 Calcifying epithelial odontogenic tumor

M935-M937 **Miscellaneous tumors**
M9350/1 Craniopharyngioma
M9360/1 Pinealoma
M9361/1 Pineocytoma
M9362/3 Pineoblastoma
M9363/0 Melanotic neuroectodermal tumor
M9370/3 Chordoma

M938-M948 **Gliomas**
M9380/3 Glioma, malignant
M9381/3 Gliomatosis cerebri
M9382/3 Mixed glioma
M9383/1 Subependymal glioma
M9384/1 Subependymal giant cell astrocytoma
M9390/0 Choroid plexus papilloma NOS
M9390/3 Choroid plexus papilloma, malignant
M9391/3 Ependymoma NOS
M9392/3 Ependymoma, anaplastic type
M9393/3 Papillary ependymoma
M9394/1 Myxopapillary ependymoma
M9400/3 Astrocytoma NOS
M9401/3 Astrocytoma, anaplastic type
M9410/3 Protoplasmic astrocytoma
M9411/3 Gemistocytic astrocytoma
M9420/3 Fibrillary astrocytoma
M9421/3 Pilocytic astrocytoma
M9422/3 Spongioblastoma NOS
M9423/3 Spongioblastoma polare
M9430/3 Astroblastoma
M9440/3 Glioblastoma NOS
M9441/3 Giant cell glioblastoma
M9442/3 Glioblastoma with sarcomatous component
M9443/3 Primitive polar spongioblastoma
M9450/3 Oligodendroglioma NOS
M9451/3 Oligodendroglioma, anaplastic type
M9460/3 Oligodendroblastoma
M9470/3 Medulloblastoma NOS
M9471/3 Desmoplastic medulloblastoma
M9472/3 Medullomyoblastoma
M9480/3 Cerebellar sarcoma NOS
M9481/3 Monstrocellular sarcoma

M949-M952 **Neuroepitheliomatous neoplasms**
M9490/0 Ganglioneuroma
M9490/3 Ganglioneuroblastoma
M9491/0 Ganglioneuromatosis
M9500/3 Neuroblastoma NOS
M9501/3 Medulloepithelioma NOS
M9502/3 Teratoid medulloepithelioma
M9503/3 Neuroepithelioma NOS
M9504/3 Spongioneuroblastoma
M9505/1 Ganglioglioma
M9506/0 Neurocytoma
M9507/0 Pacinian tumor
M9510/3 Retinoblastoma NOS
M9511/3 Retinoblastoma, differentiated type
M9512/3 Retinoblastoma, undifferentiated type
M9520/3 Olfactory neurogenic tumor
M9521/3 Esthesioneurocytoma
M9522/3 Esthesioneuroblastoma
M9523/3 Esthesioneuroepithelioma

M953 **Meningiomas**
M9530/0 Meningioma NOS
M9530/1 Meningiomatosis NOS
M9530/3 Meningioma, malignant
M9531/0 Meningotheliomatous meningioma
M9532/0 Fibrous meningioma
M9533/0 Psammomatous meningioma
M9534/0 Angiomatous meningioma
M9535/0 Hemangioblastic meningioma
M9536/0 Hemangiopericytic meningioma
M9537/0 Transitional meningioma
M9538/1 Papillary meningioma
M9539/3 Meningeal sarcomatosis

M954-M957 **Nerve sheath tumor**
M9540/0 Neurofibroma NOS
M9540/1 Neurofibromatosis NOS
M9540/3 Neurofibrosarcoma
M9541/0 Melanotic neurofibroma
M9550/0 Plexiform neurofibroma
M9560/0 Neurilemmoma NOS

APPENDIX A: MORPHOLOGY OF NEOPLASMS

M9560/1	Neurinomatosis
M9560/3	Neurilemmoma, malignant
M9570/0	Neuroma NOS
M958	**Granular cell tumors and alveolar soft part sarcoma**
M9580/0	Granular cell tumor NOS
M9580/3	Granular cell tumor, malignant
M9581/3	Alveolar soft part sarcoma
M959-M963	**Lymphomas, NOS or diffuse**
M9590/0	Lymphomatous tumor, benign
M9590/3	Malignant lymphoma NOS
M9591/3	Malignant lymphoma, non Hodgkin's type
M9600/3	Malignant lymphoma, undifferentiated cell type NOS
M9601/3	Malignant lymphoma, stem cell type
M9602/3	Malignant lymphoma, convoluted cell type NOS
M9610/3	Lymphosarcoma NOS
M9611/3	Malignant lymphoma, lymphoplasmacytoid type
M9612/3	Malignant lymphoma, immunoblastic type
M9613/3	Malignant lymphoma, mixed lymphocytic-histiocytic NOS
M9614/3	Malignant lymphoma, centroblastic-centrocytic, diffuse
M9615/3	Malignant lymphoma, follicular center cell NOS
M9620/3	Malignant lymphoma, lymphocytic, well differentiated NOS
M9621/3	Malignant lymphoma, lymphocytic, intermediate differentiation NOS
M9622/3	Malignant lymphoma, centrocytic
M9623/3	Malignant lymphoma, follicular center cell, cleaved NOS
M9630/3	Malignant lymphoma, lymphocytic, poorly differentiated NOS
M9631/3	Prolymphocytic lymphosarcoma
M9632/3	Malignant lymphoma, centroblastic type NOS
M9633/3	Malignant lymphoma, follicular center cell, noncleaved NOS
M964	**Reticulosarcomas**
M9640/3	Reticulosarcoma NOS
M9641/3	Reticulosarcoma, pleomorphic cell type
M9642/3	Reticulosarcoma, nodular
M965-M966	**Hodgkin's disease**
M9650/3	Hodgkin's disease NOS
M9651/3	Hodgkin's disease, lymphocytic predominance
M9652/3	Hodgkin's disease, mixed cellularity
M9653/3	Hodgkin's disease, lymphocytic depletion NOS

M9654/3	Hodgkin's disease, lymphocytic depletion, diffuse fibrosis
M9655/3	Hodgkin's disease, lymphocytic depletion, reticular type
M9656/3	Hodgkin's disease, nodular sclerosis NOS
M9657/3	Hodgkin's disease, nodular sclerosis, cellular phase
M9660/3	Hodgkin's paragranuloma
M9661/3	Hodgkin's granuloma
M9662/3	Hodgkin's sarcoma
M969	**Lymphomas, nodular or follicular**
M9690/3	Malignant lymphoma, nodular NOS
M9691/3	Malignant lymphoma, mixed lymphocytic-histiocytic, nodular
M9692/3	Malignant lymphoma, centroblastic-centrocytic, follicular
M9693/3	Malignant lymphoma, lymphocytic, well differentiated, nodular
M9694/3	Malignant lymphoma, lymphocytic, intermediate differentiation, nodular
M9695/3	Malignant lymphoma, follicular center cell, cleaved, follicular
M9696/3	Malignant lymphoma, lymphocytic, poorly differentiated, nodular
M9697/3	Malignant lymphoma, centroblastic type, follicular
M9698/3	Malignant lymphoma, follicular center cell, noncleaved, follicular
M970	**Mycosis fungoides**
M9700/3	Mycosis fungoides
M9701/3	Sezary's disease
M971-M972	**Miscellaneous reticuloendothelial neoplasms**
M9710/3	Microglioma
M9720/3	Malignant histiocytosis
M9721/3	Histiocytic medullary reticulosis
M722/3	Letterer-Siwe's disease
M973	**Plasma cell tumors**
M9730/3	Plasma cell myeloma
M9731/0	Plasma cell tumor, benign
M9731/1	Plasmacytoma NOS
M9731/3	Plasma cell tumor, malignant
M974	**Mast cell tumors**
M9740/1	Mastocytoma NOS
M9740/3	Mast cell sarcoma
M9741/3	Malignant mastocytosis
M975	**Burkitt's tumor**
M9750/3	Burkitt's tumor
M980-M994	**Leukemias**
M980	**Leukemias NOS**
M9800/3	Leukemia NOS
M9801/3	Acute leukemia NOS

M9802/3	Subacute leukemia NOS
M9803/3	Chronic leukemia NOS
M9804/3	Aleukemic leukemia NOS
M981	**Compound leukemias**
M9810/3	Compound leukemia
M982	**Lymphoid leukemias**
M9820/3	Lymphoid leukemia NOS
M9821/3	Acute lymphoid leukemia
M9822/3	Subacute lymphoid leukemia
M9823/3	Chronic lymphoid leukemia
M9824/3	Aleukemic lymphoid leukemia
M9825/3	Prolymphocytic leukemia
M983	**Plasma cell leukemias**
M9830/3	Plasma cell leukemia
M984	**Erythroleukemias**
M9840/3	Erythroleukemia
M9841/3	Acute erythremia
M9842/3	Chronic erythremia
M985	**Lymphosarcoma cell leukemias**
M9850/3	Lymphosarcoma cell leukemia
M986	**Myeloid leukemias**
M9860/3	Myeloid leukemia NOS
M9861/3	Acute myeloid leukemia
M9862/3	Subacute myeloid leukemia
M9863/3	Chronic myeloid leukemia
M9864/3	Aleukemic myeloid leukemia
M9865/3	Neutrophilic leukemia
M9866/3	Acute promyelocytic leukemia
M987	**Basophilic leukemias**
M9870/3	Basophilic leukemia
M988	**Eosinophilic leukemias**
M9880/3	Eosinophilic leukemia
M989	**Monocytic leukemias**
M9890/3	Monocytic leukemia NOS
M9891/3	Acute monocytic leukemia
M9892/3	Subacute monocytic leukemia
M9893/3	Chronic monocytic leukemia
M9894/3	Aleukemic monocytic leukemia
M990-M994	**Miscellaneous leukemias**
M9900/3	Mast cell leukemia
M9910/3	Megakaryocytic leukemia
M9920/3	Megakaryocytic myelosis
M9930/3	Myeloid sarcoma
M9940/3	Hairy cell leukemia
M995-M997	**Miscellaneous myeloproliferative and lymphoproliferative disorders**
M9950/1	Polycythemia vera
M9951/1	Acute panmyelosis
M9960/1	Chronic myeloproliferative disease
M9961/1	Myelosclerosis with myeloid metaplasia
M9962/1	Idiopathic thrombocythemia
M9970/1	Chronic lymphoproliferative disease

APPENDIX B: GLOSSARY OF MENTAL DISORDERS

Glossary of Mental Disorders

The psychiatric terms which appear in Chapter 5, "Mental Disorders," are listed here in alphabetic sequence. Many of the glossary descriptions originally appeared in the section on Mental Disorders in the *International Classification of Diseases, 9th Revision*,[1] and others are included to define the psychiatric conditions added to ICD-9-CM. The additional definitions are based on material furnished by the *American Psychiatric Association's Task Force on Nomenclature and Statistics*[2] and from *A Psychiatric Glossary*.[3] In a few instances definitions were obtained from *Dorland's Illustrated Medical Dictionary*[4] and from *Stedman's Medical Dictionary, Illustrated*.[5]

1. *Manual of the International Classification of Diseases, Injuries, and Causes of Death*, 9th Revision. World Health Organization, Geneva, Switzerland, 1975.
2. American Psychiatric Association, Task Force on Nomenclature and Statistics, Robert L. Spitzer, Chairman.
3. *A Psychiatric Glossary*, Fourth Edition, American Psychiatric Association, Washington, D.C., 1975.
4. *Dorland's Illustrated Medical Dictionary*, Twenty-fifth Edition, W.B. Saunders Company, Philadelphia, 1974.
5. *Stedman's Medical Dictionary, Illustrated*, Twenty-third Edition, the Williams and Wilkins Company, Baltimore, 1976.

Academic underachievement disorder – Failure to achieve in most school tasks despite adequate intellectual capacity, a supportive and encouraging social environment, and apparent effort. The failure occurs in the absence of a demonstrable specific learning disability and is caused by emotional conflict not clearly associated with any other mental disorder.[2]

Adaptation reaction — *see* Adjustment reaction

Adjustment reaction or disorder – Mild or transient disorders lasting longer than acute stress reactions which occur in individuals of any age without any apparent pre-existing mental disorder. Such disorders are often relatively circumscribed or situation-specific, are generally reversible, and usually last only a few months. They are usually closely related in time and content to stresses such as bereavement, migration, or other experiences. Reactions to major stress that last longer than a few days are also included. In children such disorders are associated with no significant distortion of development.[1]

   conduct disturbance – Mild or transient disorders in which the main disturbance predominantly involves a disturbance of conduct (e.g., an adolescent grief reaction resulting in aggressive or antisocial disorder).[1]

   depressive reaction – States of depression, not specifiable as manic-depressive, psychotic, or neurotic.[1]

   brief – Generally transient, in which the depressive symptoms are usually closely related in time and content to some stressful event.[1]

   prolonged – Generally long-lasting, usually developing in association with prolonged exposure to a stressful situation.[1]

   emotional disturbance – An adjustment disorder in which the main symptoms are emotional in type (e.g., anxiety, fear, worry) but not specifically depressive.[1]

   mixed conduct and emotional disturbance – An adjustment reaction in which both emotional disturbance and disturbance of conduct are prominent features.[1]

Affective psychoses – Mental disorders, usually recurrent, in which there is a severe disturbance of mood (mostly compounded of depression and anxiety but also manifested as elation, and excitement) which is accompanied by one or more of the following – delusions, perplexity, disturbed attitude to self, disorder of perception and behavior; these are all in keeping with the individual's prevailing mood (as are hallucinations when they occur). There is a strong tendency to suicide. For practical reasons, mild disorders of mood may also be included here if the symptoms match closely the descriptions given; this applies particularly to mild hypomania.[1]

   bipolar – A manic-depressive psychosis which has appeared in both the depressive and manic form, either alternating or separated by an interval of normality.[1]

   atypical – An episode of affective psychosis with some, but not all, of the features of the one form of the disorder in individuals who have had a previous episode of the other form of the disorder.[2]

   depressed – A manic-depressive psychosis, circular type, in which the depressive form is currently present.[1]

   manic – A manic-depressive psychosis, circular type, in which the manic form is currently present.[1]

   mixed – A manic-depressive psychosis, circular type, in which both manic and depressive symptoms are present at the same time.[1]

   depressed type – A manic-depressive psychosis in which there is a widespread depressed mood of gloom and wretchedness with some degree of anxiety. There is often reduced activity but there may be restlessness and agitation. There is marked tendency to recurrence; in a few cases this may be at regular intervals.[1]

   atypical – An affective depressive disorder that cannot be classified as a manic-depressive psychosis, depressed type, or chronic depressive personality disorder, or as an adjustment disorder.[2]

   manic type – A manic-depressive psychosis characterized by states of elation or excitement out of keeping with the individual's circumstances and varying from enhanced liveliness (hypomania) to violent, almost uncontrollable, excitement. Aggression and anger, flight of ideas, distractibility, impaired judgment, and grandiose ideas are common.[1]

   mixed type – Manic-depressive psychosis syndromes corresponding to both the manic and depressed types, but which for other reasons cannot be classified more specifically.[1]

Aggressive personality — *see* Personality disorder, explosive type

Agoraphobia — *see* agoraphobia under Phobia

Alcohol dependence syndrome – A state, psychic and usually also physical, resulting from taking alcohol, characterized by behavioral and other responses that always include a compulsion to take alcohol on a continuous or periodic basis in order to experience its psychic effects, and sometimes to avoid the discomfort of its absence; tolerance may or may not be present. A person may be dependent on alcohol and other drugs; if so, also record the diagnosis of drug dependence to identify the agent. If alcohol dependence is associated with alcoholic psychosis or with physical complications, *both* diagnoses should be recorded.[1]

Alcohol intoxication

   acute – A psychic and physical state resulting from alcohol ingestion characterized by slurred speech, unsteady gait, poor coordination, flushed facies, nystagmus, sluggish reflexes, fetor alcoholica, loud speech, emotional instability (e.g., jollity followed by lugubriousness), excessive conviviality, loquacity, and poorly inhibited sexual and aggressive behavior.[2]

   idiosyncratic – Acute psychotic episodes induced by relatively small amounts of alcohol. These are regarded as individual idiosyncratic reactions to alcohol, not due to excessive consumption and without conspicuous neurological signs of intoxication.[1]

   pathological – *see* Alcohol intoxication, idiosyncratic

Alcoholic psychoses – Organic psychotic states due mainly to excessive consumption of alcohol; defects of nutrition are thought to play an important role.[1]

   alcohol abstinence syndrome — *see* alcohol withdrawal syndrome below

   alcohol amnestic syndrome – A syndrome of prominent and lasting reduction of memory span, including striking loss of recent memory, disordered time appreciation and confabulation, occurring in alcoholics as the sequel to an acute alcoholic psychosis (especially delirium tremens) or, more rarely, in the course of chronic alcoholism. It is usually accompanied by peripheral neuritis and may be associated with Wernicke's encephalopathy.[1]

   alcohol withdrawal delirium [delirium tremens] – Acute or subacute organic psychotic states in alcoholics, characterized by clouded consciousness, disorientation, fear, illusions, delusions, hallucinations of any kind, notably visual and tactile, and restlessness, tremor and sometimes fever.[1]

   alcohol withdrawal hallucinosis – A psychosis usually of less than six months' duration, with slight or no clouding of consciousness and much

APPENDIX B: GLOSSARY OF MENTAL DISORDERS

anxious restlessness in which auditory hallucinations, mostly of voices uttering insults and threats, predominate.[1]

alcohol withdrawal syndrome – Tremor of hands, tongue, and eyelids following cessation of prolonged heavy drinking of alcohol. Nausea and vomiting, dry mouth, headache, heavy perspiration, fitful sleep, acute anxiety attacks, mood depression, feelings of guilt and remorse, and irritability are associated features.[2]

alcohol delirium — see alcohol withdrawal delirium above

alcoholic dementia – Nonhallucinatory dementias occurring in association with alcoholism, but not characterized by the features of either alcohol withdrawal delirium [delirium tremens] or alcohol amnestic syndrome [Korsakoff's alcoholic psychosis].[1]

alcoholic hallucinosis — see alcohol withdrawal hallucinosis above

alcoholic jealousy – Chronic paranoid psychosis characterized by delusional jealousy and associated with alcoholism.[1]

alcoholic paranoia — see Alcoholic jealousy

alcoholic polyneuritic psychosis — see alcohol amnestic syndrome above

Alcoholism
  acute — see Alcohol intoxication, acute
  chronic — see Alcohol dependence syndrome

Alexia – Loss of a previously possessed reading facility that cannot be explained by defective visual acuity.[3]

Amnesia, psychogenic – A form of dissociative hysteria in which there is a temporary disturbance in the ability to recall important personal information which has already been registered and stored in memory. The sudden onset of this disturbance in the absence of an underlying organic mental disorder, and the extent of the disturbance being too great to be explained by ordinary forgetfulness, are the essential features.[2]

Amnestic syndrome – A syndrome of prominent and lasting reduction of memory span, including striking loss of recent memory, disordered time appreciation, and confabulation. The commonest causes are chronic alcoholism [alcohol amnestic syndrome; Korsakoff's alcoholic psychosis], chronic barbiturate dependence, and malnutrition. An amnestic syndrome may be the predominating disturbance in the early states of presenile and senile dementia, arteriosclerotic dementia, and in encephalitis and other inflammatory and degenerative diseases in which there is particular bilateral involvement of the temporal lobes, and certain temporal lobe tumors.[2]
  alcoholic — see alcohol amnestic syndrome under Alcoholic psychoses

Amoral personality — see Personality disorder, antisocial type

Anancastic [anankastic] neurosis — see Neurotic disorder, obsessive-compulsive

Anancastic [anankastic] personality — see Personality disorder, compulsive type

Anorexia nervosa – A disorder in which the main features are persistent active refusal to eat and marked loss of weight. The level of activity and alertness is characteristically high in relation to the degree of emaciation. Typically the disorder begins in teenage girls but it may sometimes begin before puberty and rarely it occurs in males. Amenorrhea is usual and there may be a variety of other physiological changes including slow pulse and respiration, low body temperature, and dependent edema. Unusual eating habits and attitudes toward food are typical and sometimes starvation follows or alternates with periods of overeating. The accompanying psychiatric symptoms are diverse.[1]

Anxiety hysteria — see phobia under Neurotic disorders

Anxiety state (neurotic) – Apprehension, tension, or uneasiness that stems from the anticipation of danger, the source of which is largely unknown or unrecognized.[3]
  atypical – An anxiety disorder that does not fulfill the criteria of generalized or panic attack anxiety. An example might be an individual with a single morbid fear.[2]
  generalized – A disorder of at least six months' duration in which the predominant feature is limited to diffuse and persistent anxiety without the specific symptoms that characterize phobic disorders, panic disorder, or obsessive-compulsive disorder.[2]
  panic attack – An episodic and often chronic, recurrent disorder in which the predominant features are anxiety attacks and nervousness. The anxiety attacks are manifested by discrete periods of sudden onset of intense apprehension, fearfulness, or terror often associated with feelings of impending doom.[2]

Aphasia, developmental – A delay in the production of spoken language. Rarely, there is also a developmental delay in the comprehension of speech sounds.[1]

Arteriosclerotic dementia – Dementia attributable, because of physical signs (on examination of the central nervous system), to degenerative arterial disease of the brain. Symptoms suggesting a focal lesion in the brain are common. There may be a fluctuating or patchy intellectual defect with insight, and an intermittent course is common. Clinical differentiation from senile or presenile dementia, which may coexist with it, may be very difficult or impossible. The diagnosis of cerebral atherosclerosis should also be recorded.[1]

Asocial personality — see Personality disorder, antisocial type

Astasia-abasia, hysterical – A form of conversion hysteria in which the individual is unable to stand or walk although the legs are otherwise under control.[4]

Asthenia, psychogenic — see neurasthenia under Neurotic disorders

Asthenic personality — see Personality disorder, dependent type

Attention deficit disorder — see Attention deficit disorder under Hyperkinetic syndrome of childhood

Autism, infantile – A syndrome present from birth or beginning almost invariably in the first 30 months. Responses to auditory and sometimes to visual stimuli are abnormal, and there are usually severe problems in the understanding of spoken language. Speech is delayed and, if it develops, is characterized by echolalia, the reversal of pronouns, immature grammatical structure, and inability to use abstract terms. There is generally an impairment in the social use of both verbal and gestural language. Problems in social relationships are most severe before the age of five years and include an impairment in the development of eye-to-eye gaze, social attachments, and cooperative play. Ritualistic behavior is usual and may include abnormal routines, resistance to change, attachment to odd objects, and stereotyped patterns of play. The capacity for abstract or symbolic thought and for imaginative play is diminished. Intelligence ranges from severely subnormal to normal or above. Performance is usually better on tasks involving rote memory or visuospatial skills than on those requiring symbolic or linguistic skills.[1]

Avoidant personality — see Personality disorder, avoidant type

"Bad trips" – Acute intoxication from hallucinogen abuse, manifested by hallucinatory states lasting only a few days or less.[1]

Barbiturate abuse – Cases where an individual has taken the drug to the detriment of his health or social functioning, in doses above or for periods beyond those normally regarded as therapeutic.[1]

Bestiality — see Zoophilia

Bipolar disorder — see Affective psychosis, bipolar
  atypical — see Affective psychosis, bipolar, atypical

Body-rocking — see Stereotyped repetitive movements

Borderline personality — see Personality disorder, borderline type

Borderline psychosis of childhood — see Psychosis, atypical childhood

Borderline schizophrenia — see Schizophrenia, latent

Bouffée délirante — see Paranoid reaction, acute

Briquet's disorder — see Somatization disorder under Neurotic disorders

Bulimia – An episodic pattern of overeating [binge eating] accompanied by an awareness of the disordered eating pattern with a fear of not being able to stop eating voluntarily. Depressive moods and self-deprecating thoughts follow the episodes of binge eating.[2]

Catalepsy schizophrenia — see Schizophrenia, catatonic type

Catastrophic stress — see Gross stress reaction

Catatonia (schizophrenic) — see Schizophrenia, catatonic type

Character neurosis — see Personality disorders

Childhood autism — see Autism, infantile

Childhood type schizophrenia — see Psychosis, child

Chronic alcoholic brain syndrome — see Alcoholic dementia under Alcoholic psychoses

Clay-eating — see Pica

APPENDIX B: GLOSSARY OF MENTAL DISORDERS

Clumsiness syndrome — *see* Coordination disorder under Developmental delay disorders, specific

Combat fatigue — *see* Posttraumatic disorder, acute

Compensation neurosis — *see* Compensation neurosis under Neurotic disorders

Compulsive conduct disorder — *see* Impulse control disorders under Conduct disorders

Compulsive neurosis — *see* Neurotic disorder, obsessive-compulsive

Compulsive personality — *see* Personality disorder, compulsive type

Concentration camp syndrome — *see* Posttraumatic stress disorder, prolonged

Conduct disorders – Disorders mainly involving aggressive and destructive behavior and disorders involving delinquency. It should be used for abnormal behavior, in individuals of any age, which gives rise to social disapproval but which is not part of any other psychiatric condition. Minor emotional disturbances may also be present. To be included, the behavior, as judged by its frequency, severity, and type of associations with other symptoms, must be abnormal in its context. Disturbances of conduct are distinguished from an adjustment reaction by a longer duration and by a lack of close relationship in time and content to some stress. They differ from a personality disorder by the absence of deeply ingrained maladaptive patterns of behavior present from adolescence or earlier.[1]

impulse control disorders – A failure to resist an impulse, drive, or temptation to perform some action which is harmful to the individual or to others. The impulse may or may not be consciously resisted, and the act may or may not be premeditated or planned. Prior to committing the act, there is an increasing sense of tension, and at the time of committing the act, there is an experience of either pleasure, gratification, or release. Immediately following the act, there may or may not be genuine regret, self-reproach, or guilt.[2] *See also* Intermittent explosive disorder, Isolated explosive disorder, Kleptomania, Pathological gambling, and Pyromania.

mixed disturbance of conduct and emotions – A disorder characterized by features of undersocialized and socialized disturbance of conduct, but in which there is also considerable emotional disturbance as shown, for example, by anxiety, misery, or obsessive manifestations.[1]

socialized conduct disorder – Conduct disorders in individuals who have acquired the values or behavior of a delinquent peer group to whom they are loyal and with whom they characteristically steal, play truant, and stay out late at night. There may also be sexual promiscuity.[1]

undersocialized conduct disturbance aggressive type – A disorder characterized by a persistent pattern of disrespect for the feelings and well-being of others (bullying, physical aggression, cruel behavior, hostility, verbal abusiveness, impudence, defiance, negativism), aggressive antisocial behavior (destructiveness, stealing, persistent lying, frequent truancy, and vandalism), and failure to develop close and stable relationships with others.[2]

unaggressive type – A disorder in which there is a lack of concern for the rights and feelings of others to a degree which indicates a failure to establish a normal degree of affection, empathy, or bond with others. There are two patterns of behavior found. In one, the child is fearful and timid, lacking self-assertiveness, resorts to self-protective and manipulative lying, indulges in whining demandingness and temper tantrums, feels rejected and unfairly treated, and is mistrustful of others. In the other pattern of the disorder, the child approaches others strictly for his own gains and acts exclusively because of exploitative and extractive goals. The child lies brazenly and steals, appearing to feel no guilt, and forms no social bonds to other individuals.[2]

Confusion, psychogenic — *see* Psychosis, reactive confusion

Confusion, reactive — *see* Psychosis, reactive confusion

Confusional state
acute — *see* Delirium, acute
epileptic — *see* Delirium, acute
subacute — *see* Delirium, subacute

Conversion hysteria — *see* Hysteria, conversion type under Neurotic disorders

Coordination disorder — *see* Coordination disorder under Developmental delay disorders, specific

Culture shock – A form of stress reaction associated with an individual's assimilation into a new culture which is vastly different from that in which he was raised.[5]

Cyclic schizophrenia — *see* Schizophrenia, schizo-affective type

Cyclothymic personality or disorder — *see* Personality disorder, cyclothymic type

Delirium – Transient organic psychotic conditions with a short course in which there is a rapidly developing onset of disorganization of higher mental processes manifested by some degree of impairment of information processing, impaired or abnormal attention, perception, memory, and thinking. Clouded consciousness, confusion, disorientation, delusions, illusions, and often vivid hallucinations predominate in the clinical picture.[1, 2]

acute – short-lived states, lasting hours or days, of the above type.[1]

subacute – states of the above type in which the symptoms, usually less florid, last for several weeks or longer, during which they may show marked fluctuations in intensity.[1]

Delirium tremens — *see* Alcohol withdrawal delirium under Alcoholic psychoses

Delusions, systematized — *see* Paranoia

Dementia – A decrement in intellectual functioning of sufficient severity to interfere with occupational or social performance, or both. There is impairment of memory and abstract thinking, the ability to learn new skills, problem solving, and judgment. There is often also personality change or impairment in impulse control. Dementia in organic psychoses may be of a chronic or progressive nature, which if untreated are usually irreversible and terminal.[1, 2]

alcoholic — *see* Alcoholic dementia under Alcoholic psychoses

arteriosclerotic — *see* Arteriosclerotic dementia

multi-infarct — *see* Arteriosclerotic dementia

presenile — *see* Presenile dementia

repeated infarct — *see* Arteriosclerotic dementia

senile — *see* Senile dementia

Depersonalization syndrome — *see* Depersonalization syndrome under Neurotic disorders

Depression – States of depression, usually of moderate but occasionally of marked intensity, which have no specifically manic-depressive or other psychotic depressive features, and which do not appear to be associated with stressful events or other features specified under neurotic depression.[1]

anxiety — *see* Depression under Neurotic disorders

endogenous — *see* Affective psychosis, depressed type

monopolar — *see* Affective psychosis, depressed type

neurotic — *see* Depression under Neurotic disorders

psychotic — *see* Affective psychosis, depressed type

psychotic reactive — *see* Psychosis, depressive

reactive — *see* Depression under Neurotic disorders

reactive psychotic — *see* Psychosis, depressive

Depressive personality or character — *see* Personality disorder, chronic depressive type

Depressive reaction — *see* Depressive reaction under Adjustment reaction

Depressive psychosis — *see* Affective psychosis, depressed type

Derealization (neurotic) — *see* Depersonalization syndrome under Neurotic disorders

Developmental delay disorders, specific – A group of disorders in which a specific delay in development is the main feature. For many the delay is not explicable in terms of general intellectual retardation or of inadequate schooling. In each case development is related to biological maturation, but it is also influenced by nonbiological factors. A diagnosis of a specific developmental delay carries no etiological implications. A diagnosis of specific delay in development should not be made if it is due to a known neurological disorder.[1]

arithmetical disorder – Disorders in which the main feature is a serious impairment in the development of arithmetical skills.[1]

articulation disorder – A delay in the development of normal word-sound production resulting in defects of articulation. Omissions or substitutions of consonants are most frequent.[1]

APPENDIX B: GLOSSARY OF MENTAL DISORDERS

coordination disorder – Disorders in which the main feature is a serious impairment in the development of motor coordination which is not explicable in terms of general intellectual retardation. The clumsiness is commonly associated with perceptual difficulties.[1]

mixed development disorder – A delay in the development of one specific skill (e.g., reading, arithmetic, speech, or coordination) is frequently associated with lesser delays in other skills. When this occurs, the diagnosis should be made according to the skill most seriously impaired. The mixed category should be used only where the mixture of delayed skills is such that no one skill is preponderantly affected.[1]

motor retardation — *see* Coordination disorder above

reading disorder or retardation – Disorders in which the main feature is a serious impairment in the development of reading or spelling skills which is not explicable in terms of general intellectual retardation or of inadequate schooling. Speech or language difficulties, impaired right-left differentiation, perceptuo-motor problems, and coding difficulties are frequently associated. Similar problems are often present in other members of the family. Adverse psychosocial factors may be present.[1]

speech or language disorder – Disorders in which the main feature is a serious impairment in the development of speech or language (syntax or semantic) which is not explicable in terms of general intellectual retardation. Most commonly there is a delay in the development of normal word-sound production resulting in defects of articulation. Omissions or substitutions of consonants are most frequent. There may also be a delay in the production of spoken language. Rarely, there is also a developmental delay in the comprehension of sounds. Includes cases in which delay is largely due to environmental privation.[1]

Dipsomania — *see* Alcohol dependence syndrome

Disorganized schizophrenia — *see* Schizophrenia, disorganized type

Dissociative hysteria — *see* Hysteria, dissociative type under Neurotic disorders

Drug abuse – Includes cases where an individual, for whom no other diagnosis is possible, has come under medical care because of the maladaptive effect of a drug on which he is not dependent (*see* Drug dependence) and that he has taken on his own initiative to the detriment of his health or social functioning. When drug abuse is secondary to a psychiatric disorder, record the disorder as an additional diagnosis.[1]

Drug dependence – A state, psychic and sometimes also physical dependence, resulting from taking a drug, characterized by behavioral and other responses that always include a compulsion to take a drug on a continuous or periodic basis in order to experience its psychic effects, and sometimes to avoid the discomfort of its absence. Tolerance may or may not be present. A person may be dependent on more than one drug.[1]

Drug psychoses – Organic mental syndromes which are due to consumption of drugs (notably amphetamines, barbiturates, and opiate and LSD groups) and solvents. Some of the syndromes in this group are not as severe as most conditions labeled "psychotic," but they are included here for practical reasons. The drug should be identified, and also a diagnosis of drug dependence should be recorded, if present.[1]

drug-induced hallucinosis – Hallucinatory states of more than a few days, but not more than a few months' duration, associated with large or prolonged intake of drugs, notably of the amphetamine and LSD groups. Auditory hallucinations usually predominate and there may be anxiety or restlessness. States following LSD or other hallucinogens lasting only a few days or less ["bad trips"] are not included.[1]

drug-induced organic delusional syndrome – Paranoid states of more than a few days, but not more than a few months' duration, associated with large or prolonged intake of drugs, notably of the amphetamine and LSD groups.[1]

drug withdrawal syndrome – States associated with drug withdrawal ranging from severe, as specified for alcohol withdrawal delirium [delirium tremens], to less severe states characterized by one or more symptoms such as convulsions, tremor, anxiety, restlessness, gastrointestinal and muscular complaints, and mild disorientation and memory disturbance.[1]

Drunkenness

acute — *see* Alcohol intoxication, acute

pathologic — *see* Alcohol intoxication, idiosyncratic

simple – A state of inebriation due to alcohol consumption without conspicuous neurological signs of intoxication.[2]

sleep – An inability to fully arouse from the sleep state characterized by failure to attain full consciousness after arousal.[2]

Dyscalculia — *see* Arithmetical disorder under Developmental delay disorders, specific

Dyslalia — *see* Articulation disorder under Developmental delay disorders, specific

Dyslexia, developmental – A disorder in which the main feature is a serious impairment of reading skills which is not explicable in terms of general intellectual retardation or of inadequate schooling. Word-blindness and strephosymbolia (tendency to reverse letters and words in reading) are included.[1,3]

Dysmenorrhea, psychogenic – Painful menstruation due to disturbance of psychic control.[4]

Dyspareunia, functional — *see* Functional dyspareunia under Psychosexual dysfunctions

Dyspraxia syndrome — *see* Coordination disorder under Developmental delay disorders, specific

Dyssocial personality — *see* Personality disorder, antisocial type

Dysuria, psychogenic – Difficulty in passing urine due to psychic factors.[4]

Eating disorders – A group of disorders characterized by a conspicuous disturbance in eating behavior.[2] *See also* Bulimia, Pica, and Rumination, psychogenic.

Eccentric personality — *see* Personality disorder, eccentric type

Elective mutism – A pervasive and persistent refusal to speak in situations not attributable to a mental disorder. In some cases the behavior may manifest a form of withdrawal reaction to a specific stressful situation, or as a predominant feature in children exhibiting shyness or social withdrawal disorders.[2]

Emancipation disorder – An adjustment reaction in adolescents or young adults in which there is symptomatic expression (e.g., difficulty in making independent decisions, increased dependence on parental advice, adoption of values deliberately oppositional to parents) of a conflict over independence following the recent assumption of a status in which the individual is more independent of parental control or supervision.[2]

Emotional disturbances specific to childhood and adolescence – Less well-differentiated emotional disorders characteristic of the childhood period. When the emotional disorder takes the form of a neurosis, the appropriate diagnosis should be made. These disorders differ from adjustment reactions in terms of longer duration and by the lack of close relationship in time and content to some stress.[1] *See also* Academic underachievement disorder, Elective mutism, Identity disorder, Introverted disorder of childhood, Misery and unhappiness disorder, Oppositional disorder, Overanxious disorder, and Shyness disorder of childhood.

Encopresis – A disorder in which the main manifestation is the persistent voluntary or involuntary passage of formed stools of normal or near-normal consistency into places not intended for that purpose in the individual's own sociocultural setting. Sometimes the child has failed to gain bowel control, and sometimes he has gained control but then later again became encopretic. There may be a variety of associated psychiatric symptoms and there may be smearing of feces. The condition would not usually be diagnosed under the age of four years.[1]

Endogenous depression — *see* Affective psychosis, depressed type

Enuresis – A disorder in which the main manifestation is a persistent involuntary voiding of urine by day or night which is considered abnormal for the age of the individual. Sometimes the child will have failed to gain bladder control and in other cases he will have gained control and then lost it. Episodic or fluctuating enuresis should be included. The disorder would not usually be diagnosed under the age of four years.[1]

Epileptic confusional or twilight state — *see* Delirium, acute

Excitation

APPENDIX B: GLOSSARY OF MENTAL DISORDERS

catatonic — see Schizophrenia, catatonic type

psychogenic — see Psychosis, excitative type

reactive — see Psychosis, excitative type

Exhaustion delirium — see Stress reaction, acute

Exhibitionism – Sexual deviation in which the main sexual pleasure and gratification is derived from exposure of the genitals to a person of the opposite sex.[1]

Explosive personality disorder — see Personality disorder, explosive type

Factitious illness – A form of hysterical neurosis in which there are physical or psychological symptoms that are not real, genuine, or natural, which are produced by the individual and are under his voluntary control.[2]

physical symptom type – The presentation of physical symptoms that may be total fabrication, self-inflicted, an exaggeration or exacerbation of a pre-existing physical condition, or any combination or variation of these.[2]

psychological symptom type – The voluntary production of symptoms suggestive of a mental disorder. Behavior may mimic psychosis or, rather, the individual's idea of psychosis.[2]

Fanatic personality — see Personality disorder, paranoid type

Fatigue neurosis — see Neurasthenia under Neurotic disorders

Feeble-minded — see Mental retardation, mild

Fetishism – A sexual deviation in which nonliving objects are utilized as a preferred or exclusive method of stimulating erotic arousal.[2]

Finger-flicking — see Stereotyped repetitive movements

Folie à deux — see Shared paranoid disorder

Frigidity – A psychosexual dysfunction in which there is partial or complete failure to attain or maintain the lubrication-swelling response of sexual excitement until completion of the sexual act.[2]

Frontal lobe syndrome – Changes in behavior following damage to the frontal areas of the brain or following interference with the connections of those areas. There is a general diminution of self-control, foresight, creativity, and spontaneity, which may be manifest as increased irritability, selfishness, restlessness, and lack of concern for others. Conscientiousness and powers of concentration are often diminished, but measurable deterioration of intellect or memory is not necessarily present. The overall picture is often one of emotional dullness, lack of drive, and slowness; but, particularly in persons previously with energetic, restless, or aggressive characteristics, there may be a change towards impulsiveness, boastfulness, temper outbursts, silly fatuous humor, and the development of unrealistic ambitions; the direction of change usually depends upon the previous personality. A considerable degree of recovery is possible and may continue over the course of several years.[1]

Fugue, psychogenic – A form of dissociative hysteria characterized by an episode of wandering with inability to recall one's prior identity. Both onset and recovery are rapid. Following recovery there is no recollection of events which took place during the fugue state.[2]

Ganser's syndrome (hysterical) – A form of factitious illness in which the patient voluntarily produces symptoms suggestive of a mental disorder.[2]

Gender identity disorder — see Gender identity disorder under Psychosexual identity disorders

Gilles de la Tourette's disorder or syndrome — see Gilles de la Tourette's disorder under Tics

Grief reaction — see Depressive reaction, brief under Adjustment reaction

Gross stress reaction — see Stress reaction, acute

Group delinquency — see Socialized conduct disorder under Conduct disorders

Habit spasm — see Chronic motor tic disorder under Tics

Hangover (alcohol) — see Drunkenness, simple

Head-banging — see Stereotyped repetitive movements

Hebephrenia — see Schizophrenia, disorganized type

Heller's syndrome — see Psychosis, disintegrative

High grade defect — see Mental retardation, mild

Homosexuality – Exclusive or predominant sexual attraction for persons of the same sex with or without physical relationship. Record homosexuality as a diagnosis whether or not it is considered as a mental disorder.[1]

Hospital addiction syndrome — see Munchausen syndrome

Hospital hoboes — see Munchausen syndrome

Hospitalism – A mild or transient adjustment reaction characterized by withdrawal seen in hospitalized patients. In young children this may be manifested by elective mutism.[1]

Hyperkinetic syndrome of childhood – Disorders in which the essential features are short attention span and distractibility. In early childhood the most striking symptom is disinhibited, poorly organized and poorly regulated extreme overactivity but in adolescence this may be replaced by underactivity. Impulsiveness, marked mood fluctuations, and aggression are also common symptoms. Delays in the development of specific skills are often present and disturbed, poor relationships are common. If the hyperkinesis is symptomatic of an underlying disorder, the diagnosis of the underlying disorder is recorded instead.[1]

attention deficit disorder – Cases of hyperkinetic syndrome in which short attention span, distractibility, and overactivity are the main manifestations without significant disturbance of conduct or delay in specific skills.[1]

hyperkinesis with developmental delay – Cases in which the hyperkinetic syndrome is associated with speech delay, clumsiness, reading difficulties, or other delays of specific skills.[1]

hyperkinetic conduct disorder – Cases in which the hyperkinetic syndrome is associated with marked conduct disturbance but not developmental delay.[1]

Hypersomnia – A disorder of initiating arousal from sleep or maintaining wakefulness.[2]

persistent – Chronic difficulty in initiating arousal from sleep or maintaining wakefulness associated with major or minor depressive mental disorders.[2]

transient – Episodes of difficulty in arousal from sleep or maintaining wakefulness associated with acute or intermittent emotional reactions or conflicts.[2]

Hypochondriasis — see Hypochondriasis under Neurotic disorders

Hypomania — see Affective psychosis, manic type

Hypomanic personality — see Personality disorder, chronic hypomanic type

Hyposomnia — see Insomnia

Hysteria — see Hysteria under Neurotic disorders

anxiety — see Phobia under Neurotic disorders

psychosis — see Psychosis, reactive

acute — see Psychosis, excitative type

Hysterical personality — see Personality disorder, histrionic type

Identity disorder – An emotional disorder caused by distress over the inability to reconcile aspects of the self into a relatively coherent and acceptable sense of self, not secondary to another mental disorder. The disturbance is manifested by intense subjective distress regarding uncertainty about a variety of issues relating to identity, including long-term goals, career choice, friendship patterns, values, and loyalties.[2]

Idiocy — see Mental retardation, profound

Imbecile — see Mental retardation, moderate

Impotence – A psychosexual dysfunction in which there is partial or complete failure to attain or maintain erection until completion of the sexual act.[2]

Impulse control disorder — see Impulse control disorders under Conduct disorders

Inadequate personality — see Personality disorder, dependent type

Induced paranoid disorder — see Shared paranoid disorder

Inebriety — see Drunkenness, simple

Infantile autism — see Autism, infantile

Insomnia – A disorder of initiating or maintaining sleep.[2]

persistent – A chronic state of sleeplessness associated with chronic anxiety, major or minor depressive disorders, or psychoses.[2]

transient – Episodes of sleeplessness associated with acute or intermittent emotional reactions or conflicts.[2]

Intermittent explosive disorder – Recurrent episodes of sudden and significant loss of control of aggressive impulses, not accounted for by any other mental disorder, which results in serious assault or destruction of property. The magnitude of the behavior during an episode is grossly out of proportion to any psychosocial stressors which may have played a role in eliciting the episode of lack of control. Following each episode

APPENDIX B: GLOSSARY OF MENTAL DISORDERS

there is genuine regret or self-reproach at the consequences of the action and the inability to control the aggressive impulse.[2]

Introverted disorder of childhood – An emotional disturbance in children chiefly manifested by a lack of interest in social relationships and indifference to social praise or criticism.[2]

Introverted personality — see Personality disorder, introverted type

Involutional melancholia — see Affective psychosis, depressed type

Involutional paranoid state — see Paraphrenia

Isolated explosive disorder – A disorder of impulse control in which there is a single discrete episode characterized by failure to resist an impulse which leads to a single, violent externally-directed act, which has a catastrophic impact on others, and for which the available information does not justify the diagnosis of another mental disorder.[2]

Isolated phobia — see Simple phobia under Phobia

Jet lag syndrome – A phase-shift disruption of the 24-hour sleep-wake cycle due to rapid time-zone changes experienced in long-distance travel.[2]

Kanner's syndrome — see Autism, infantile

Kleptomania – A disorder of impulse control characterized by a recurrent failure to resist impulses to steal objects not for immediate use or their monetary value. An increasing sense of tension is experienced prior to committing the act, with an intense experience of gratification at the time of committing the theft.[2]

Korsakoff's psychosis
  alcoholic — see Alcohol amnestic syndrome under Alcoholic psychoses
  nonalcoholic — see Amnestic syndrome

Latent schizophrenia — see Schizophrenia, latent

Lesbianism — see Homosexuality

Lobotomy syndrome — see Frontal lobe syndrome

LSD reaction – Acute intoxication from hallucinogen abuse, manifested by hallucinatory states lasting only a few days or less.[1]

Major depressive disorder — see Affective psychosis, depressed type

Malingering – A clinical picture in which the predominant feature is the presentation of fake or grossly exaggerated physical or psychiatric illness apparently under voluntary control. In contrast to factitious illness, the symptoms produced in malingering are in pursuit of a goal which, when known, is recognizable and obviously understandable in light of knowledge of the individual's circumstances. Examples of understandable goals include, but are not limited to, becoming a "patient" in order to avoid conscription or military duty, avoid work, obtain financial compensation, evade criminal prosecution, and obtain drugs.[2]

Mania (monopolar) — see Affective psychosis, manic type

Manic-depressive psychosis
  circular type — see Affective psychosis, bipolar
  depressed type — see Affective psychosis, depressed type
  manic type — see Affective psychosis, manic type
  mixed type — see Affective psychosis, mixed type

Manic disorder — see Affective psychosis, manic type
  atypical — see Affective psychosis, manic type, atypical

Masochistic personality — see Personality disorder, masochistic type

Melancholia — see Affective psychoses
  involutional — see Affective psychosis, depressed type

Mental retardation – A condition of arrested or incomplete development of mind which is especially characterized by subnormality of intelligence. The coding should be made on the individual's *current* level of functioning *without regard to its nature* or causation, such as psychosis, cultural deprivation, Down's syndrome, etc. Where there is a specific cognitive handicap — such as in speech — the diagnosis of mental retardation should be based on assessments of cognition *outside the area of specific handicap*. The assessment of intellectual level should be based on whatever information is available, including clinical evidence, adaptive behavior, and psychometric findings. The IQ levels given are based on a test with a mean of 100 and a standard deviation of 15, such as the Wechsler scales. They are provided only as a guide and should not be applied rigidly. Mental retardation often involves psychiatric disturbances and may often develop as a result of some physical disease or injury. In these cases, an additional diagnosis should be recorded to identify any associated condition, psychiatric or physical.[1]

  mild mental retardation – IQ criteria 50–70. Individuals with this level of retardation are usually educable. During the preschool period they can develop social and communication skills, have minimal retardation in sensorimotor areas, and often are not distinguished from normal children until a later age. During the school age period they can learn academic skills up to approximately the sixth-grade level. During the adult years, they can usually achieve social and vocational skills adequate for minimum self-support, but may need guidance and assistance when under social or economic stress.[1]

  moderate mental retardation – IQ criteria 35–49. Individuals with this level of retardation are usually trainable. During the preschool period they can talk or learn to communicate. They have poor social awareness and fair motor development. During the school age period they can profit from training in social and occupational skills, but they are unlikely to progress beyond the second-grade level in academic subjects. During their adult years they may achieve self-maintenance in unskilled or semi-skilled work under sheltered conditions. They need supervision and guidance when under mild social or economic stress.[2]

  severe mental retardation – IQ criteria 20–34. Individuals with this level of retardation evidence poor motor development, minimal speech, and are generally unable to profit from training and self-help during the preschool period. During the school age period they can talk or learn to communicate, can be trained in elementary health habits, and may profit from systematic habit training. During the adult years they may contribute partially to self-maintenance under complete supervision.[2]

  profound mental retardation – IQ criteria under 20. Individuals with this level of retardation evidence minimal capacity for sensorimotor functioning and need nursing care during the preschool period. During the school age period some further motor development may occur, and they may respond to minimal or limited training in self-help. During the adult years some motor and speech development may occur, and they may achieve very limited self-care and need nursing care.[2]

Merycism — see Rumination, psychogenic

Minimal brain dysfunction [MBD] — see Hyperkinetic syndrome of childhood

Misery and unhappiness disorder – An emotional disorder characteristic of childhood in which the main symptoms involve misery and unhappiness. There may also be eating and sleep disturbances.

Mood swings (brief compensatory) (rebound) – Mild disorders of mood (depression and anxiety or elation and excitement, occurring alternatingly or episodically) seen in affective psychosis.[1]

Motor tic disorders — see Tics

Motor-verbal tic disorder — see Gilles de la Tourette's disorder under Tics

Multi-infarct dementia or psychosis — see Arteriosclerotic dementia

Multiple operations syndrome — see Munchausen syndrome

Multiple personality – A form of dissociative hysteria in which there is the domination of the individual at any one time by one of two or more distinct personalities. Each personality is a fully-integrated and complex unit with memories, behavior patterns, and social friendships which determine the nature of the individual's acts when uppermost in consciousness.[2]

Munchausen syndrome – A chronic form of factitious illness in which the individual demonstrates a plausible presentation of voluntarily produced physical symptomatology of such a degree that he is able to obtain and sustain multiple hospitalizations.[2]

Narcissistic personality — see Personality disorder, narcissistic type

Nervous debility — see Neurasthenia under Neurotic disorders

Neurasthenia — see Neurasthenia under Neurotic disorders

Neurotic delinquency — see Mixed disturbance of conduct and emotions under Conduct disorders

Neurotic disorders – Neurotic disorders are mental disorders without any demonstrable organic basis in which the indi-

APPENDIX B: GLOSSARY OF MENTAL DISORDERS

vidual may have considerable insight and has unimpaired reality testing, in that he usually does not confuse his morbid subjective experiences and fantasies with external reality. Behavior may be greatly affected although usually remaining within socially acceptable limits, but personality is not disorganized. The principal manifestations include excessive anxiety, hysterical symptoms, phobias, obsessional and compulsive symptoms, and depression.[1]

anxiety states – Various combinations of physical and mental manifestations of anxiety, not attributable to real danger and occurring either in attacks [see Anxiety state, panic attacks] or as a persisting state [see Anxiety state, generalized]. The anxiety is usually diffuse and may extend to panic. Other neurotic features such as obsessional or hysterical symptoms may be present but do not dominate the clinical picture.[1]

compensation neurosis – Certain unconscious neurotic reactions in which features of secondary gain, such as a situational or financial advantage, are prominent.[3]

depersonalization – A neurotic disorder with an unpleasant state of disturbed perception in which external objects or parts of one's own body are experienced as changed in their quality, unreal, remote, or automatized. The patient is aware of the subjective nature of the change he experiences. If depersonalization occurs as a feature of anxiety, schizophrenia, or other mental disorder, the condition is classified according to the major psychiatric disorder.[1]

depression – A neurotic disorder characterized by disproportionate depression which has usually recognizably ensued on a distressing experience; it does not include among its features delusions or hallucinations, and there is often preoccupation with the psychic trauma which preceded the illness, e.g., loss of a cherished person or possession. Anxiety is also frequently present and mixed states of anxiety and depression should be included here. The distinction between depressive neurosis and psychosis should be made not only upon the degree of depression but also on the presence or absence of other neurotic and psychotic characteristics, and upon the degree of disturbance of the individual's behavior.[1]

hypochondriasis – A neurotic disorder in which the conspicuous features are excessive concern with one's health in general or the integrity and functioning of some part of one's body, or less frequently, one's mind. It is usually associated with anxiety and depression. It may occur as a feature of some other severe mental disorder (e.g., manic-depressive psychosis, depressed type, schizophrenia, hysteria) and in that case should be classified according to the corresponding major disorder.[1]

hysteria – A neurotic mental disorder in which motives, of which the patient seems unaware, produce either a restriction of the field of consciousness or disturbances of motor or sensory function which may seem to have psychological advantage or symbolic value.[1] There are three subtypes –

conversion type – The chief or only symptoms of the hysterical neurosis consist of psychogenic disturbance of function in some part of the body, e.g., paralysis, tremor, blindness, deafness, seizures.[1]

dissociative type – The most prominent feature of the hysterical neurosis is a narrowing of the field of consciousness which seems to serve an unconscious purpose and is commonly accompanied or followed by a selective amnesia. There may be dramatic but essentially superficial changes of personality [multiple personality], or sometimes the patient enters into a wandering state [fugue].[1]

factitious illness – Physical or psychological symptoms that are not real, genuine, or natural, which are produced by the individual and are under his voluntary control.[2]

neurasthenia – A neurotic disorder characterized by fatigue, irritability, headache, depression, insomnia, difficulty in concentration, and lack of capacity for enjoyment [anhedonia]. It may follow or accompany an infection or exhaustion, or arise from continued emotional stress. If neurasthenia is associated with a physical disorder, the latter should also be recorded as a diagnosis.[1]

obsessive-compulsive – States in which the outstanding symptom is a feeling of subjective compulsion, which must be resisted, to carry out some action, to dwell on an idea, to recall an experience, or to ruminate on an abstract topic. Unwanted thoughts which intrude, the insistency of words or ideas, ruminations or trains of thought are perceived by the individual to be inappropriate or nonsensical. The obsessional urge or idea is recognized as alien to the personality but as coming from within the self. Obsessional actions may be quasi-ritual performances designed to relieve anxiety, e.g., washing the hands to cope with contamination. Attempts to dispel the unwelcome thoughts or urges may lead to a severe inner struggle, with intense anxiety.[1]

occupational – A neurosis characterized by a functional disorder of a group of muscles used chiefly in one's occupation, marked by the occurrence of spasm, paresis, or incoordination on attempt to repeat the habitual movements (e.g., writer's cramp).[5]

phobic disorders – Neurotic states with abnormally intense dread of certain objects or specific situations which would not normally have that effect. If the anxiety tends to spread from a specified situation or object to a wider range of circumstances, it becomes akin to or identical with anxiety state and should be classified as such.[1] See also Phobia.

somatization disorder – A chronic, but fluctuating, neurotic disorder which begins early in life and is characterized by recurrent and multiple somatic complaints for which medical attention is sought but which are not apparently due to any physical illness. Complaints are presented in a dramatic, vague, or exaggerated way, or are part of a complicated medical history in which often many specific diagnoses have allegedly been made by other physicians. Complaints invariably refer to many organ systems (headache, fatigue, palpitations, fainting, nausea and vomiting, abdominal pains, bowel trouble, allergies, menstrual and sexual difficulties), and the individual frequently receives medical care from a number of physicians, sometimes simultaneously.[2]

Neurosis — see Neurotic disorders

Nightmares – Anxiety attacks occurring in dreams during REM sleep.[2]

Night terrors – A pathology of arousal from stage 4 sleep in which the individual experiences excessive terror and extreme panic (screaming, verbalizations), symptoms of autonomic activity, confusion, and poor recall for event.[2]

Nymphomania – Abnormal and excessive need or desire in the woman for sexual intercourse.[3]

Obsessional personality — see Personality disorder, compulsive type

Occupational neurosis — see Neurotic disorder, occupational

Oneirophrenia — see Schizophrenia, acute episode

Oppositional disorder of childhood or adolescence – A disorder characterized by pervasive opposition to all in authority regardless of self-interest, a continuous argumentativeness, and an unwillingness to respond to reasonable persuasion, not accounted for by a conduct disorder, adjustment disorder, or a psychosis of childhood. The oppositional behavior in this disorder is evoked by any demand, rule, suggestion, request, or admonishment placed on the individual.[2]

Organic affective syndrome – A clinical picture in which the predominating symptoms closely resemble those seen in either the depressive or manic affective disorders, occurring in the presence of evidence or history of a specific organic factor which is etiologically related to the disturbance, such as head trauma, endocranial tumors, and exocranial tumors secreting neurotoxic diatheses (e.g., pancreatic carcinoma). Excessive use of steroids, Cushing's syndrome, and other endocrine disorders may lead to an organic affective syndrome.[2]

Organic personality syndrome – Chronic, mild states of memory disturbance and intellectual deterioration, of nonpsychotic nature, often accompanied by increased irritability, querulousness, lassitude, and complaints of physical weakness. These states are often associated with old age, and may precede more severe states due to brain damage classifiable under senile

APPENDIX B: GLOSSARY OF MENTAL DISORDERS

or presenile dementia, dementia associated with other chronic organic psychotic brain syndromes, or delirium, delusions, hallucinosis, and depression in transient organic psychotic conditions.[1]

Organic psychosyndrome, focal (partial) – A nonpsychotic organic mental disorder resembling the postconcussion syndrome associated with localized diseases of the brain or surrounding tissues.[1]

Organic psychotic conditions – Syndromes in which there is impairment of orientation, memory, comprehension, calculation, learning capacity, and judgment. These are the essential features but there may also be shallowness or lability of affect, or a more persistent disturbance of mood, lowering of ethical standards and exaggeration or emergence of personality traits, and diminished capacity for independent decision.[1] See also Alcohol psychoses, Arteriosclerotic dementia, Drug psychoses, Presenile dementia, and Senile dementia.

  mixed paranoid and affective – Organic psychosis in which depressive and paranoid symptoms are the main features.[1]

  transient – States characterized by clouded consciousness, confusion, disorientation, illusions, and often vivid hallucinations. They are usually due to some intra- or extracerebral toxic, infectious, metabolic or other systemic disturbance and are generally reversible. Depressive and paranoid symptoms may also be present but are not the main feature. The diagnosis of the associated physical or neurological condition should also be recorded.[1]

    acute delirium – Short-lived states, lasting hours or days, of the above type.[1]

    subacute delirium – States of the above type in which the symptoms, usually less florid, last for several weeks or longer during which they may show marked fluctuations in intensity.[1]

Organic reaction — see Organic psychotic conditions, transient

Overanxious disorder – An ill-defined emotional disorder characteristic of childhood in which the main symptoms involve anxiety and fearfulness.[1]

Panic disorder — see Panic attack under Anxiety state

Paranoia – A rare chronic psychosis in which logically constructed systematized delusions have developed gradually without concomitant hallucinations or the schizophrenic type of disordered thinking. The delusions are mostly of grandeur (the paranoiac prophet or inventor), persecution, or somatic abnormality.[1]

  alcoholic — see Alcoholic jealousy under Alcoholic psychoses

  querulans – A paranoid state which, though in many ways akin to schizophrenic or affective states, differs from other paranoid states and psychogenic paranoid psychosis.[1]

  senile — see Paraphrenia

Paranoid personality — see Personality disorder, paranoid type

Paranoid reaction, acute – Paranoid states apparently provoked by some emotional stress. The stress is often misconstrued as an attack or threat. Such states are particularly prone to occur in prisoners or as acute reactions to a strange and threatening environment, e.g., in immigrants.[1]

Paranoid schizophrenia — see Schizophrenia, paranoid type

Paranoid state

  involutional — see Paraphrenia

  senile — see Paraphrenia

  simple – A psychosis, acute or chronic, not classifiable as schizophrenia or affective psychosis, in which delusions, especially of being influenced, persecuted, or treated in some special way, are the main symptoms. The delusions are of a fairly fixed, elaborate, and systematized kind.[1]

Paranoid traits — see Personality disorder, paranoid type

Paraphilia — see Sexual deviations

Paraphrenia – Paranoid psychosis in which there are conspicuous hallucinations, often in several modalities. Affective symptoms and disordered thinking, if present, do not dominate the clinical picture, and the personality is well preserved.[1]

Paraphrenic schizophrenia — see Schizophrenia, paranoid type

Passive-aggressive personality — see Personality disorder, passive-aggressive type

Passive personality — see Personality disorder, dependent type

Pathological

  alcohol intoxication — see Alcohol intoxication, idiosyncratic

  drug intoxication – Individual idiosyncratic reactions to comparatively small quantities of a drug, which take the form of acute, brief psychotic states of any type.[1]

  drunkenness — see Alcohol intoxication, idiosyncratic

  gambling – A disorder of impulse control characterized by a chronic and progressive preoccupation with gambling and urge to gamble, with subsequent gambling behavior that compromises, disrupts, or damages personal, family, and vocational pursuits.[2]

  personality — see Personality disorder

Pedophilia – Sexual deviations in which an adult engages in sexual activity with a child of the same or opposite sex.[1]

Peregrinating patient — see Malingering

Personality disorders – Deeply ingrained maladaptive patterns of behavior generally recognizable by the time of adolescence or earlier and continuing throughout most of adult life, although often becoming less obvious in middle or old age. The personality is abnormal either in the balance of its components, their quality and expression, or in its total aspect. Because of this deviation or psychopathy the patient suffers or others have to suffer, and there is an adverse effect upon the individual or on society. It includes what is sometimes called psychopathic personality, but if this is determined primarily by malfunctioning of the brain, it should be classified as one of the nonpsychotic organic brain syndromes. When the patient exhibits an anomaly of personality directly related to his neurosis or psychosis, e.g., schizoid personality and schizophrenia or anancastic personality and obsessive compulsive neurosis, the relevant neurosis or psychosis which is in evidence should be diagnosed in addition.[1]

  affective type – A chronic personality disorder characterized by lifelong predominance of a pronounced mood. The illness does not have a clear onset, and there may be intermittent periods of disturbed mood separated by periods of normal mood.[1]

  anancastic [anankastic] type — see Personality disorder, compulsive type

  antisocial type – A personality disorder characterized by disregard for social obligations, lack of feeling for others, and impetuous violence or callous unconcern. There is a gross disparity between behavior and the prevailing social norms. Behavior is not readily modifiable by experience, including punishment. People with this personality are often affectively cold, and may be abnormally aggressive or irresponsible. Their tolerance to frustration is low; they blame others or offer plausible rationalizations for the behavior which brings them into conflict with society.[1]

  asthenic type — see Personality disorder, dependent type

  avoidant type – Individuals with this disorder exhibit excessive social inhibitions and shyness, a tendency to withdraw from opportunities for developing close relationships, and a fearful expectation that they will be belittled and humiliated. Desires for affection and acceptance are strong, but they are unwilling to enter relationships unless given unusually strong guarantees that they will be uncritically accepted. Therefore, they have few close relationships and suffer from feelings of loneliness and isolation.[2]

  borderline type – Individuals with this disorder are characterized by instability in a variety of areas, including interpersonal relationships, behavior, mood, and self image. Interpersonal relationships are often intense and unstable with marked shifts of attitude over time. Frequently there is impulsive and unpredictable behavior which is potentially physically self-damaging. There may be problems tolerating being alone, and chronic feelings of emptiness or boredom.[2]

  chronic depressive type – An affective personality disorder characterized by lifelong predominance of a chronic nonpsychotic disturbance involving either intermittent or sustained periods of depressed mood (marked by worry, pessimism, low output of energy, and a sense of futility).[2]

  chronic hypomanic type – An affective personality disorder characterized by lifelong predominance of a chronic nonpsychotic disturbance involving either intermittent or sustained periods of abnormally elevated mood (unshakable optimism and an enhanced zest for life and activity).[2]

APPENDIX B: GLOSSARY OF MENTAL DISORDERS

compulsive type – A personality disorder characterized by feelings of personal insecurity, doubt, and incompleteness leading to excessive conscientiousness, checking, stubbornness, and caution. There may be insistent and unwelcome thoughts or impulses which do not attain the severity of an obsessional neurosis. There is perfectionism and meticulous accuracy and a need to check repeatedly in an attempt to ensure this. Rigidity and excessive doubt may be conspicuous.[1]

cyclothymic type – A chronic nonpsychotic disturbance involving depressed and elevated mood, lasting at least two years, separated by periods of normal mood.[2]

dependent type – A personality disorder characterized by passive compliance with the wishes of elders and others and a weak inadequate response to the demands of daily life. Lack of vigor may show itself in the intellectual or emotional spheres; there is little capacity for enjoyment.[1]

eccentric type – A personality disorder characterized by oddities of behavior which do not conform to the clinical syndromes of personality disorders described elsewhere.[2]

explosive type – A personality disorder characterized by instability of mood with liability to intemperate outbursts of anger, hate, violence, or affection. Aggression may be expressed in words or in physical violence. The outbursts cannot readily be controlled by the affected persons, who are not otherwise prone to antisocial behavior.[1]

histrionic type – A personality disorder characterized by shallow, labile affectivity, dependence on others, craving for appreciation and attention, suggestibility, and theatricality. There is often sexual immaturity, e.g., frigidity and over-responsiveness to stimuli. Under stress hysterical symptoms [neurosis] may develop.[1]

hysterical type — see Personality disorder, histrionic type

inadequate type — see Personality disorder, dependent type

introverted type – A form of schizoid personality in which the essential features are a profound defect in the ability to form social relationships and to respond to the usual forms of social reinforcements. Such patients are characteristically "loners" who do not appear distressed by their social distance and are not interested in greater social involvement.[2]

masochistic type – A personality disorder in which the individual appears to arrange life situations so as to be defeated and humiliated.[2]

narcissistic type – A personality disorder in which interpersonal difficulties are caused by an inflated sense of self-worth, and indifference to the welfare of others. Achievement deficits and social irresponsibilities are justified and sustained by a boastful arrogance, expansive fantasies, facile rationalization, and frank prevarication.[2]

paranoid type – A personality disorder in which there is excessive sensitiveness to setbacks or to what are taken to be humiliations and rebuffs, a tendency to distort experience by misconstruing the neutral or friendly actions of others as hostile or contemptuous, and a combative and tenacious sense of personal rights. There may be a proneness to jealousy or excessive self-importance. Such persons may feel helplessly humiliated and put upon; others, likewise excessively sensitive, are aggressive and insistent. In all cases there is excessive self-reference.[1]

passive-aggressive type – A personality disorder characterized by aggressive behavior manifested in passive ways, such as obstructionism, pouting, procrastination, intentional inefficiency, or stubbornness. The *aggression* often arises from resentment at failing to find gratification in a relationship with an individual or institution upon which the individual is overdependent.[3]

passive type — see Personality disorder, dependent type

schizoid type – A personality disorder in which there is withdrawal from affectional, social, and other contacts with autistic preference for fantasy and introspective reserve. Behavior may be slightly eccentric or indicate avoidance of competitive situations. Apparent coolness and detachment may mask an incapacity to express feeling.[1]

schizotypal type – A form of schizoid personality in which individuals with this disorder manifest various oddities of thinking, perception, communication, and behavior. The disturbance in thinking may be expressed as magical thinking, ideas of reference, or paranoid ideation. Perceptual disturbances may include recurrent illusions and derealization [depersonalization]. Frequently, but not invariably, the behavioral manifestations include social isolation and constricted or inappropriate affect which interferes with rapport in face-to-face interaction without any of the frank psychotic features which characterize schizophrenia.[2]

Phobia – Neurotic states with abnormally intense dread of certain objects or specific situations which would not normally have that effect. If the anxiety tends to spread from a specified situation or object to a wider range of circumstances, it becomes akin to or identical with anxiety state, and should be classified as such.[1]

acrophobia – Fear of heights[3]
agoraphobia – Fear of leaving the familiar setting of the home, and is almost always preceded by a phase during which there are recurrent panic attacks. Because of the anticipatory fear of helplessness when having a panic attack, the patient is reluctant or refuses to be alone, travel or walk alone, or to be in situations where there is no ready access to help, such as in crowds, closed or open spaces, or crowded stores.[2]
ailurophobia – Fear of cats[3]
algophobia – Fear of pain[3]
claustrophobia – Fear of closed spaces[3]
isolated phobia — see Simple phobia below
mysophobia – Fear of dirt or germs[3]
obsessional — see Neurotic disorder, obsessive-compulsive
panphobia – Fear of everything[3]
simple phobia – Fear of a discrete object or situation which is neither fear of leaving the familiar setting of the home [agoraphobia], or of being observed by others in certain situations [social phobia]. Examples of simple phobia are fear of animals, acrophobia, and claustrophobia.[2]
social phobia – Fear of situations in which the subject is exposed to possible scrutiny by others, and the possibility exists that he may act in a fashion that will be considered shameful. The most common social phobias are fears of public speaking, blushing, eating in public, writing in front of others, or using public lavatories.[2]
xenophobia – Fear of strangers[3]

Pica – Perverted appetite of nonorganic origin in which there is persistent eating of non-nutritional substances. Typically, infants ingest paint, plaster, string, hair, or cloth. Older children may have access to animal droppings, sand, bugs, leaves, or pebbles. In the adult, eating of starch or clay-earth has been observed.[2]

Postconcussion syndrome – States occurring after generalized contusion of the brain, in which the symptom picture may resemble that of the frontal lobe syndrome or that of any of the neurotic disorders, but in which in addition, headache, giddiness, fatigue, insomnia, and a subjective feeling of impaired intellectual ability are usually prominent. Mood may fluctuate, and quite ordinary stress may produce exaggerated fear and apprehension. There may be marked intolerance of mental and physical exertion, undue sensitivity to noise, and hypochondriacal preoccupation. The symptoms are more common in persons who have previously suffered from neurotic or personality disorders, or when there is a possibility of compensation. This syndrome is particularly associated with the closed type of head injury when signs of localized brain damage are slight or absent, but it may also occur in other conditions.[1]

Postcontusion syndrome or encephalopathy — see Postconcussion syndrome

Postencephalitic syndrome – A nonpsychotic organic mental disorder resembling the postconcussion syndrome associated with central nervous system infections.[1]

Postleucotomy syndrome — see Frontal lobe syndrome

Posttraumatic brain syndrome, nonpsychotic — see Postconcussion syndrome

Posttraumatic organic psychosis — see Organic psychotic conditions, transient

Posttraumatic stress disorder – The development of characteristic symptoms (re-experiencing the traumatic event,

APPENDIX B: GLOSSARY OF MENTAL DISORDERS

numbing of responsiveness to or involvement with the external world, and a variety of other autonomic, dysphoric, or cognitive symptoms) after experiencing a psychologically traumatic event or events outside the normal range of human experience (e.g., rape or assault, military combat, natural catastrophes such as flood or earthquake, or other disaster, such as airplane crash, fires, bombings).[2]

acute – Brief, episodic, or recurrent disorders lasting less than six months' duration after the onset of trauma.[2]

prolonged – Chronic disorders of the above type lasting six months or more following the trauma.[2]

Premature ejaculation — see Premature ejaculation under Psychosexual dysfunctions

Prepsychotic schizophrenia — see Schizophrenia, latent

Presbyophrenia — see Organic personality syndrome

Presenile dementia – Dementia occurring usually before the age of 65 in patients with the relatively rare forms of diffuse or lobar cerebral atrophy. The associated neurological condition (e.g., Alzheimer's disease, Pick's disease, Jakob-Creutzfeldt disease) should also be recorded as a diagnosis.[1]

Prodromal schizophrenia — see Schizophrenia, latent

Pseudoneurotic schizophrenia — see Schizophrenia, latent

Psychalgia – Pains of mental origin, e.g., headache or backache, for which a more precise medical or psychiatric diagnosis cannot be made.[1]

Psychasthenia – A functioning neurosis marked by stages of pathological fear or anxiety, obsessions, fixed ideas, tics, feelings of inadequacy, self-accusation, and peculiar feelings of strangeness, unreality, and depersonalization.[4]

Psychic shock – A sudden disturbance of mental equilibrium produced by strong emotion in response to physical or mental stress.[4]

Psychic factors associated with physical diseases – Mental disturbances or psychic factors of any type thought to have played a major part in the etiology of physical conditions, usually involving tissue damage, classified elsewhere. The mental disturbance is usually mild and nonspecific, and the psychic factors (worry, fear, conflict, etc.) may be present without any overt psychiatric disorder. Examples of these conditions are asthma, dermatitis, eczema, duodenal ulcer, ulcerative colitis, and urticaria, specified as due to psychogenic factors. Use an additional diagnosis to identify the physical condition. In the rare instance that an overt psychiatric disorder is thought to have caused the physical condition, the psychiatric diagnosis should be recorded in addition.[1]

Psychoneurosis — see Neurotic disorders

Psycho-organic syndrome — see Organic psychotic conditions, transient

Psychopathic constitutional state — see Personality disorders

Psychopathic personality — see Personality disorders

Psychophysiological disorders – A variety of physical symptoms or types of physiological malfunctions of mental origin, not involving tissue damage, and usually mediated through the autonomic nervous system. The disorders are classified according to the body system involved. If the physical symptom is secondary to a psychiatric disorder classifiable elsewhere, the physical symptom is not classified as a psychophysiological disorder. If tissue damage is involved, then the diagnosis is classified as a *Psychic factor associated with diseases classified elsewhere*.[1]

Psychosexual dysfunctions – A group of disorders in which there is recurrent and persistent dysfunction encountered during sexual activity. The dysfunction may be lifelong or acquired, generalized or situational, and total or partial.[2]

functional dyspareunia – Recurrent and persistent genital pain associated with coitus.[2]

functional vaginismus – A history of recurrent and persistent involuntary spasm of the musculature of the outer one-third of the vagina that interferes with sexual activity.[2]

inhibited female orgasm – Recurrent and persistent inhibition of the female orgasm as manifested by a delay or absence of orgasm following a normal sexual excitement phase during sexual activity.[2]

inhibited male orgasm – Recurrent and persistent inhibition of the male orgasm as manifested by a delay or absence of either the emission or ejaculation phases, or more usually, both following an adequate phase of sexual excitement.[2]

inhibited sexual desire – Persistent inhibition of desire for engaging in a particular form of sexual activity.[2]

inhibited sexual excitement – Recurrent and persistent inhibition of sexual excitement during sexual activity, manifested either by partial or complete failure to attain or maintain erection until completion of the sexual act [impotence], or partial or complete failure to attain or maintain the lubrication-swelling response of sexual excitement until completion of the sexual act [frigidity].[2]

premature ejaculation – Ejaculation occurs before the individual wishes it, because of recurrent and persistent absence of reasonable voluntary control of ejaculation and orgasm during sexual activity.[2]

Psychosexual gender identity disorders – Behavior occurring in preadolescents of immature psychosexuality, or in adults, in which there is an incongruence between the individual's anatomic sex and gender identity.[2]

gender identity disorder – In children or in adults a condition in which the individual would prefer to be of the other sex, and strongly prefers the clothes, toys, activities, and companionship of the other sex. Cross-dressing is intermittent, although it may be frequent. In children the commonest form is feminism in boys.[2]

trans-sexualism – A psychosexual identity disorder centered around fixed beliefs that the overt bodily sex is wrong. The resulting behavior is directed towards either changing the sexual organs by operation, or completely concealing the bodily sex by adopting both the dress and behavior of the opposite sex.[1]

Psychosomatic disorders — see Psychophysiological disorders

Psychosis – Mental disorders in which impairment of mental function has developed to a degree that interferes grossly with insight, ability to meet some ordinary demands of life or to maintain adequate contact with reality. It is not an exact or well defined term. Mental retardation is excluded.[1]

affective — see Affective psychoses

alcoholic — see Alcoholic psychoses

atypical childhood – A variety of atypical infantile psychoses which may show some, but not all, of the features of infantile autism. Symptoms may include stereotyped repetitive movements, hyperkinesis, self-injury, retarded speech development, echolalia, and impaired social relationships. Such disorders may occur in children of any level of intelligence but are particularly common in those with mental retardation.[1]

borderline, of childhood — see Psychosis, atypical childhood

child – A group of disorders in children, characterized by distortions in the timing, rate, and sequence of many psychological functions involving language development and social relations in which the severe qualitative abnormalities are not normal for any stage of development.[2] See also Autism, infantile, Psychosis, disintegrative, Psychosis, atypical childhood.

depressive — see Affective psychosis, depressed type

depressive type – A depressive psychosis which can be similar in its symptoms to manic-depressive psychosis, depressed type but is apparently provoked by saddening stress such as a bereavement, or a severe disappointment or frustration. There may be less diurnal variation of symptoms than in manic-depressive psychosis, depressed type, and the delusions are more often understandable in the context of the life experiences. There is usually a serious disturbance of behavior, e.g., major suicidal attempt.[1]

disintegrative – A disorder in which normal or near-normal development for the first few years is followed by a loss of social skills and of speech, together with a severe disorder of emotions, behavior, and relationships. Usually this loss of speech and of social competence takes place over a period of a few months and is accompanied by the emergence of overactivity and of stereotypies. In most cases there is intellectual impairment, but this is not a necessary part of the disorder. The condition may follow overt brain disease, such as measles

APPENDIX B: GLOSSARY OF MENTAL DISORDERS

encephalitis, but it may also occur in the absence of any known organic brain disease or damage. Any associated neurological disorder should also be recorded.[1]

epileptic – An organic psychotic condition associated with epilepsy.[1]

excitative type – An affective psychosis similar in its symptoms to manic-depressive psychosis, manic type, but apparently provoked by emotional stress.[1]

hypomanic — *see* Affective psychosis, manic type

hysterical — *see* Psychosis, reactive
  acute — *see* Psychosis, excitative type

induced — *see* Shared paranoid disorder

infantile — *see* Autism, infantile

infective — *see* Organic psychotic conditions, transient

Korsakoff's
  alcoholic — *see* alcohol amnestic syndrome under Alcoholic psychoses
  nonalcoholic — *see* Amnestic syndrome

manic-depressive — *see* Affective psychoses

multi-infarct — *see* Arteriosclerotic dementia

paranoid
  chronic — *see* Paranoia
  protracted reactive — *see* Psychosis, paranoid, psychogenic
  psychogenic – Psychogenic or reactive paranoid psychosis of any type which is more protracted than the reactions described under Paranoid reaction, acute.[1]
    acute — *see* Paranoid reaction, acute

postpartum — *see* Psychosis, puerperal

psychogenic — *see* Psychosis, reactive
  depressive — *see* Psychosis, depressive type

puerperal – Any psychosis occurring within a fixed period (approximately 90 days) after childbirth.[3] The diagnosis should be classified according to the predominant symptoms or characteristics, such as schizophrenia, affective psychosis, paranoid states, or other specified psychosis.

reactive – A psychotic condition which is largely or entirely attributable to a recent life experience. This diagnosis is not used for the wider range of psychoses in which environmental factors play some, but not the *major*, part in etiology.[1]
  brief – A florid psychosis of at least a few hours' duration but lasting no more than two weeks, with sudden onset immediately following a severe environmental stress and eventually terminating in complete recovery to the pre-psychotic state.[2]
  confusion – Mental disorders with clouded consciousness, disorientation (though less marked than in organic confusion), and diminished accessibility often accompanied by excessive activity and apparently provoked by emotional stress.[1]
  depressive — *see* Psychosis, depressive type
  schizo-affective — *see* Schizophrenia, schizo-affective type

schizophrenic — *see* Schizophrenia

schizophreniform — *see* Schizophrenia
  affective type — *see* Schizophrenia, schizo-affective type
  confusional type — *see* Schizophrenia, acute episode

senile — *see* Senile dementia, delusional type

Pyromania – A disorder of impulse control characterized by a recurrent failure to resist impulses to set fires without regard for the consequences, or with deliberate destructive intent. Invariably there is intense fascination with the setting of fires, seeing fires burn, and a satisfaction with the resultant destruction.[2]

Relationship problems of childhood – Emotional disorders characteristic of childhood in which the main symptoms involve relationship problems.[1]

Repeated infarct dementia — *see* Arteriosclerotic dementia

Residual schizophrenia — *see* Schizophrenia, residual type

Restzustand (schizophrenia) — *see* Schizophrenia, residual type

Rumination
  obsessional – The constant preoccupation with certain thoughts, with inability to dismiss them from the mind.[4] *See* Neurotic disorder, obsessive-compulsive.
  psychogenic – In children the regurgitation of food, with failure to thrive or weight loss developing after a period of normal functioning. Food is brought up without nausea, retching, or disgust. The food is then ejected from the mouth, or chewed and reswallowed.[2]

Sander's disease — *see* Paranoia

Satyriasis – Pathologic or exaggerated sexual desire or excitement in the man.[3]

Schizoid personality disorder — *see* Personality disorder, schizoid type

Schizophrenia – A group of psychoses in which there is a fundamental disturbance of personality, a characteristic distortion of thinking, often a sense of being controlled by alien forces, delusions which may be bizarre, disturbed perception, abnormal affect out of keeping with the real situation, and autism. Nevertheless, clear consciousness and intellectual capacity are usually maintained. The disturbance of personality involves its most basic functions which give the normal person his feeling of individuality, uniqueness, and self-direction. The most intimate thoughts, feelings, and acts are often felt to be known to or shared by others and explanatory delusions may develop, to the effect that natural or supernatural forces are at work to influence the schizophrenic person's thoughts and actions in ways that are often bizarre. He may see himself as the pivot of all that happens. Hallucinations, especially of hearing, are common and may comment on the patient or address him. Perception is frequently disturbed in other ways; there may be perplexity, irrelevant features may become all-important and accompanied by passivity feelings, may lead the patient to believe that everyday objects and situations possess a special, usually sinister, meaning intended for him. In the characteristic schizophrenic disturbance of thinking, peripheral and irrelevant features of a total concept, which are inhibited in normal directed mental activity, are brought to the forefront and utilized in place of the elements relevant and appropriate to the situation. Thus, thinking becomes vague, elliptical and obscure, and its expression in speech sometimes incomprehensible. Breaks and interpolations in the flow of consecutive thought are frequent, and the patient may be convinced that his thoughts are being withdrawn by some outside agency. Mood may be shallow, capricious, or incongruous. Ambivalence and disturbance of volition may appear as inertia, negativism, or stupor. Catatonia may be present. The diagnosis "schizophrenia" should not be made unless there is, or has been evident during the same illness, characteristic disturbance of thought, perception, mood, conduct, or personality — preferably in at least two of these areas. The diagnosis should not be restricted to conditions running a protracted, deteriorating, or chronic course. In addition to making the diagnosis on the criteria just given, effort should be made to specify one of the following subtypes of schizophrenia, according to the predominant symptoms.[1]

  acute (undifferentiated) – Schizophrenia of florid nature which cannot be classified as simple, catatonic, hebephrenic, paranoid, or any other types.[1]

  acute episode – Schizophrenic disorders, other than simple, hebephrenic, catatonic, and paranoid, in which there is a dream-like state with slight clouding of consciousness and perplexity. External things, people, and events may become charged with personal significance for the patient. There may be ideas of reference and emotional turmoil. In many such cases remission occurs within a few weeks or months, even without treatment.[1]

  atypical — *see* Schizophrenia, acute (undifferentiated)

  borderline — *see* Schizophrenia, latent

  catatonic type – Includes as an essential feature prominent psychomotor disturbances often alternating between extremes such as hyperkinesis and stupor, or automatic obedience and negativism. Constrained attitudes may be maintained for long periods – if the patient's limbs are put in some unnatural position, they may be held there for some time after the external force has been removed. Severe excitement may be a striking feature of the condition. Depressive or hypomanic concomitants may be present.[1]

  cenesthopathic — *see* Schizophrenia, acute (undifferentiated)

  childhood type — *see* Psychosis, child

  chronic undifferentiated — *see* Schizophrenia, residual

  cyclic — *see* Schizophrenia, schizo-affective type

  disorganized type – A form of schizophrenia in which affective changes are prominent, delusions and hallucinations fleeting and fragmentary, behav-

APPENDIX B: GLOSSARY OF MENTAL DISORDERS

ior irresponsible and unpredictable, and mannerisms common. The mood is shallow and inappropriate, accompanied by giggling or self-satisfied, self-absorbed smiling, or by a lofty manner, grimaces, mannerisms, pranks, hypochondriacal complaints, and reiterated phrases. Thought is disorganized. There is a tendency to remain solitary, and behavior seems empty of purpose and feeling. This form of schizophrenia usually starts between the ages of 15 and 25 years.[1]

hebephrenic type — *see* Schizophrenia, disorganized type

latent – It has not been possible to produce a generally acceptable description for this condition. It is not recommended for general use, but a description is provided for those who believe it to be useful – a condition of eccentric or inconsequent behavior and anomalies of affect which give the impression of schizophrenia though no definite and characteristic schizophrenic anomalies, present or past, have been manifest.[1]

paranoid type – The form of schizophrenia in which relatively stable delusions, which may be accompanied by hallucinations, dominate the clinical picture. The delusions are frequently of persecution, but may take other forms (for example, of jealousy, exalted birth, Messianic mission, or bodily change). Hallucinations and erratic behavior may occur; in some cases conduct is seriously disturbed from the outset, thought disorder may be gross, and affective flattening with fragmentary delusions and hallucinations may develop.[1]

prepsychotic — *see* Schizophrenia, latent

prodromal — *see* Schizophrenia, latent

pseudoneurotic — *see* Schizophrenia, latent

pseudopsychopathic — *see* Schizophrenia, latent

residual – A chronic form of schizophrenia in which the symptoms that persist from the acute phase have mostly lost their sharpness. Emotional response is blunted and thought disorder, even when gross, does not prevent the accomplishment of routine work.[1]

schizo-affective type – A psychosis in which pronounced manic or depressive features are intermingled with schizophrenic features and which tends towards remission without permanent defect, but which is prone to recur. The diagnosis should be made only when both the affective and schizophrenic symptoms are pronounced.[1]

simple type – A psychosis in which there is insidious development of oddities of conduct, inability to meet the demands of society, and decline in total performance. Delusions and hallucinations are not in evidence and the condition is less obviously psychotic than are the hebephrenic, catatonic, and paranoid types of schizophrenia. With increasing social impoverishment vagrancy may ensue and the patient becomes self-absorbed, idle, and aimless. Because the schizophrenic symptoms are not clear-cut, diagnosis of this form should be made sparingly, if at all.[1]

simplex — *see* Schizophrenia, simple type

Schizophrenic syndrome of childhood — *see* Psychosis, child

Schizophreniform
  attack — *see* Schizophrenia, acute episode
  disorder — *see* Schizophrenia, acute episode
  psychosis — *see* Schizophrenia
    affective type — *see* Schizophrenia, schizo-affective type
    confusional type — *see* Schizophrenia, acute episode

Schizotypal personality — *see* Personality disorder, schizotypal type

Senile dementia – Dementia occurring usually after the age of 65 in which any cerebral pathology other than that of senile atrophic change can be reasonably excluded.[1]

  delirium – Senile dementia with a superimposed reversible episode of acute confusional state.[1]

  delusional type – A type of senile dementia characterized by development in advanced old age, progressive in nature, in which delusions, varying from simple poorly formed paranoid delusions to highly formed paranoid delusional states, and hallucinations are also present.[1,2]

  depressed type – A type of senile dementia characterized by development in advanced old age, progressive in nature, in which depressive features, ranging from mild to severe forms of manic-depressive affective psychosis, are also present. Disturbance of the sleep-waking cycle and preoccupation with dead people are often particularly prominent.[1,2]

  paranoid type — *see* Senile dementia, delusional type

  simple type — *see* Senile dementia

Sensitiver Beziehungswahn – A paranoid state which, though in many ways akin to schizophrenic or affective states, differs from paranoia, simple paranoid state, shared paranoid disorder, or psychogenic psychosis.[1]

Sensitivity reaction of childhood or adolescence — *see* Shyness disorder of childhood

Separation anxiety disorder – A clinical disorder in children in which the predominant disturbance is exaggerated distress at separation from parents, home, or other familial surroundings. When separation is instituted, the child may experience anxiety to the point of panic. In adults a similar disorder is seen in agoraphobic reactions.[2]

Sexual deviations – Abnormal sexual inclinations or behavior which are part of a referral problem. The limits and features of normal sexual behavior have not been stated absolutely in different societies and cultures, but are broadly such as serve approved social and biological purposes. The sexual activity of affected persons is directed primarily either towards people not of the opposite sex, or towards sexual acts not associated with coitus normally, or towards coitus performed under abnormal circumstances. If the anomalous behavior becomes manifest only during psychosis or other mental illness the condition should be classified under the major illness. It is common for more than one anomaly to occur together in the same individual; in that case the predominant deviation is classified. It is preferable not to diagnose sexual deviation in individuals who perform deviant sexual acts when normal sexual outlets are not available to them.[1] *See also* Exhibitionism, Fetishism, Homosexuality, Nymphomania, Pedophilia, Satyriasis, Sexual masochism, Sexual sadism, Transvestism, Voyeurism, and Zoophilia. Gender identity disorder and trans-sexualism are considered to be psychosexual gender identity disorders and are not included here.

Sexual masochism – A sexual deviation in which sexual arousal and pleasure is produced in an individual by his own physical or psychological suffering, and in which there are insistent and persistent fantasies wherein sexual excitement is produced as a result of suffering.[2]

Sexual sadism – A sexual deviation in which physical or psychological suffering inflicted on another person is utilized as a method of stimulating erotic excitement and orgasm, and in which there are insistent and persistent fantasies wherein sexual excitement is produced as a result of suffering inflicted on the partner.[2]

Shared paranoid disorder – Mainly delusional psychosis, usually chronic and often without florid features, which appears to have developed as a result of a close, if not dependent, relationship with another person who already has an established similar psychosis. The delusions are at least partly shared. The rare cases in which several persons are affected should also be included here.[1]

Shifting sleep-work schedule – A sleep disorder in which the phase-shift disruption of the 24-hour sleep-wake cycle occurs due to rapid changes in the individual's work schedule.[2]

Short sleeper – Individuals who typically need only 4–6 hours of sleep within the 24-hour cycle.[2]

Shyness disorder of childhood – A persistent and excessive shrinking from familiarity or contact with all strangers of sufficient severity as to interfere with peer functioning, yet there are warm and satisfying relationships with family members. A critical feature of this disorder is that the avoidant behavior with strangers persists even after prolonged exposure or contact.[2]

Sibling jealousy or rivalry – An emotional disorder related to competition between siblings for the love of a parent or for other recognition or gain.[3]

Simple phobia — *see* Simple phobia under Phobia

Situational disturbance, acute — *see* Stress reaction, acute

Social phobia — *see* Social phobia under Phobia

APPENDIX B: GLOSSARY OF MENTAL DISORDERS

Social withdrawal of childhood — see Introverted disorder of childhood

Socialized conduct disorder — see Socialized conduct disorder under Conduct disorders

Somatization disorder — see Somatization disorder under Neurotic disorders

Somatoform disorder, atypical — see Hypochondriasis under Neurotic disorders

Spasmus nutans — see Stereotyped repetitive movements

Specific academic or work inhibition – An adjustment reaction in which a specific academic or work inhibition occurs in an individual whose intellectual capacity, skills, and previous academic or work performance have been at least adequate, and in which the inhibition occurs despite apparent effort and is not due to any other mental disorder.[2]

Stammering — see Stuttering

Starch-eating — see Pica

Status postcommotio cerebri — see Postconcussion syndrome

Stereotyped repetitive movements – Disorders in which voluntary repetitive stereotyped movements, which are not due to any psychiatric or neurological condition, constitute the main feature. Includes head-banging, spasmus nutans, rocking, twirling, finger-flicking mannerisms, and eye poking. Such movements are particularly common in cases of mental retardation with sensory impairment or with environmental monotony.[1]

Stereotypies — see Stereotyped repetitive movements

Stress reaction
  acute – Acute transient disorders of any severity and nature of emotions, consciousness, and psychomotor states (singly or in combination) which occur in individuals, without any apparent pre-existing mental disorder, in response to exceptional physical or mental stress, such as natural catastrophe or battle, and which usually subside within hours or days.[1]
  chronic — see Adjustment reaction

Stupor
  catatonic — see Schizophrenia, catatonic type
  psychogenic — see Psychosis, reactive

Stuttering – Disorders in the rhythm of speech, in which the individual knows precisely what he wishes to say, but at the time is unable to say it because of an involuntary, repetitive prolongation or cessation of a sound.[1]

Subjective insomnia complaint – A complaint of insomnia made by the individual, which has not been investigated or proven.[2]

Tension headache – Headache of mental origin for which a more precise medical or psychiatric diagnosis cannot be made.[1]

Systematized delusions — see Paranoia

Tics – Disorders of no known organic origin in which the outstanding feature consists of quick, involuntary, apparently purposeless, and frequently repeated movements which are not due to any neurological condition. Any part of the body may be involved but the face is most frequently affected. Only one form of tic may be present, or there may be a combination of tics which are carried out simultaneously, alternatively, or consecutively.[1]
  chronic motor tic disorder – A tic disorder starting in childhood and persisting into adult life. The tic is limited to no more than three motor areas, and rarely has a verbal component.[2]
  Gilles de la Tourette's disorder [motor-verbal tic disorder] – A rare disorder occurring in individuals of any level of intelligence in which facial tics and tic-like throat noises become more marked and more generalized, and in which later whole words or short sentences (often with obscene content) are ejaculated spasmodically and involuntarily. There is some overlap with other varieties of tic.[1]
  transient tic disorder of childhood – Facial or other tics beginning in childhood, but limited to one year in duration.[2]

Tobacco use disorder – Cases in which tobacco is used to the detriment of a person's health or social functioning or in which there is tobacco dependence. Dependence is included here rather than under drug dependence because tobacco differs from other drugs of dependence in its psychotoxic effects.[1]

Tranquilizer abuse – Cases where an individual has taken the drug to the detriment of his health or social functioning, in doses above or for periods beyond those normally regarded as therapeutic.[1]

Transient organic psychotic condition — see Organic psychotic conditions, transient

Trans-sexualism — see Trans-sexualism under Psychosexual identity disorders

Transvestism – Sexual deviation in which there is recurrent and persistent dressing in clothes of the opposite sex, and initially in the early stage of the illness, for the purpose of sexual arousal.[2]

Twilight state
  confusional — see Delirium, acute
  psychogenic — see Psychosis, reactive confusion

Undersocialized conduct disorder — see Undersocialized conduct disorder under Conduct disorders

Unsocialized aggressive disorder — see Undersocialized conduct disorder, aggressive type under Conduct disorders

Vaginismus, functional — see Functional vaginismus under Psychosexual dysfunctions

Vorbeireden – The symptom of the approximate answer or talking past the point, seen in the Ganser syndrome, a form of factitious illness.[2]

Voyeurism – A sexual deviation in which the individual repetitively seeks out situations in which he engages in looking at unsuspecting women who are either naked, in the act of disrobing, or engaging in sexual activity. The act of looking is accompanied by sexual excitement, frequently with orgasm. In its severe form, the act of peeping constitutes the preferred to exclusive sexual activity of the individual.[2]

Wernicke-Korsakoff syndrome — see Alcohol amnestic syndrome under Alcoholic psychoses

Withdrawal reaction of childhood or adolescence — see Introverted disorder of childhood

Word-deafness – A developmental delay in the comprehension of speech sounds.[1]

Zoophilia – Sexual or anal intercourse with animals.[1]

APPENDIX C: CLASSIFICATION OF DRUGS BY AHFS LIST

CLASSIFICATION OF DRUGS BY AMERICAN HOSPITAL FORMULARY SERVICE LIST NUMBER AND THEIR ICD-9-CM EQUIVALENTS

The coding of adverse effects of drugs is keyed to the continually revised Hospital Formulary of the American Hospital Formulary Service (AHFS) published under the direction of the American Society of Hospital Pharmacists.

The following section gives the ICD-9-CM diagnosis code for each AHFS list.

AHFS* List		ICD-9-CM Diagnosis Code
4:00	ANTIHISTAMINE DRUGS	963.0
8:00	ANTI-INFECTIVE AGENTS	
8:04	Amebacides	961.5
	hydroxyquinoline derivatives	961.3
	arsenical anti-infectives	961.1
8:08	Anthelmintics	961.6
	quinoline derivatives	961.3
8:12.04	Antifungal Antibiotics	960.1
	nonantibiotics	961.9
8:12.06	Cephalosporins	960.5
8:12.08	Chloramphenicol	960.2
8:12.12	The Erythromycins	960.3
8:12.16	The Penicillins	960.0
8:12.20	The Streptomycins	960.6
8:12.24	The Tetracyclines	960.4
8:12.28	Other Antibiotics	960.8
	antimycobacterial antibiotics	960.6
	macrolides	960.3
8:16	Antituberculars	961.8
	antibiotics	960.6
8:18	Antivirals	961.7
8:20	Plasmodicides (antimalarials)	961.4
8:24	Sulfonamides	961.0
8:26	The Sulfones	961.8
8:28	Treponemicides	961.2
8:32	Trichomonacides	961.5
	hydroxyquinoline derivatives	961.3
	nitrofuran derivatives	961.9
8:36	Urinary Germicides	961.9
	quinoline derivatives	961.3
8:40	Other Anti-Infectives	961.9
10:00	ANTINEOPLASTIC AGENTS	963.1
	antibiotics	960.7
	progestogens	962.2
12:00	AUTONOMIC DRUGS	
12:04	Parasympathomimetic (Cholinergic) Agents	971.0
12:08	Parasympatholytic (Cholinergic Blocking) Agents	971.1
12:12	Sympathomimetic (Adrenergic) Agents	971.2
12:16	Sympatholytic (Adrenergic Blocking) Agents	971.3
12:20	Skeletal Muscle Relaxants	975.2
	central nervous system muscle-tone depressants	968.0
16:00	BLOOD DERIVATIVES	964.7
20:00	BLOOD FORMATION AND COAGULATION	
20:04	Antianemia Drugs	964.1
20:04.04	Iron Preparations	964.0
20:04.08	Liver and Stomach Preparations	964.1
20:12.04	Anticoagulants	964.2
20:12.08	Antiheparin Agents	964.5
20:12.12	Coagulants	964.5
20:12.16	Hemostatics	964.5
	capillary-active drugs	972.8
	fibrinolysis-affecting agents	964.4
	natural products	964.7
24:00	CARDIOVASCULAR DRUGS	
24:04	Cardiac Drugs	972.9
	cardiotonic agents	972.1
	rhythm regulators	972.0
24:06	Antilipemic Agents	972.2
	thyroid derivatives	962.7
24:08	Hypotensive Agents	972.6
	adrenergic blocking agents	971.3
	ganglion-blocking agents	972.3
	vasodilators	972.5

AHFS* List		ICD-9-CM Diagnosis Code
24:12	Vasodilating Agents	972.5
	coronary	972.4
	nicotinic acid derivatives	972.2
24:16	Sclerosing Agents	972.7
28:00	CENTRAL NERVOUS SYSTEM DRUGS	
28:04	General Anesthetics	968.4
	gaseous anesthetics	968.2
	halothane	968.1
	intravenous anesthetics	968.3
28:08	Analgesics and Antipyretics	965.9
	antirheumatics	965.6
	aromatic analgesics	965.4
	non-narcotics NEC	965.7
	opium alkaloids	965.00
	heroin	965.01
	methadone	965.02
	specified type NEC	965.09
	pyrazole derivatives	965.5
	salicylates	965.1
	specified type NEC	965.8
28:10	Narcotic Antagonists	970.1
28:12	Anticonvulsants	966.3
	barbiturates	967.0
	benzodiazepine-based tranquilizers	969.4
	bromides	967.3
	hydantoin derivatives	966.1
	oxazolidine derivative	966.0
	succinimides	966.2
28:16.04	Antidepressants	969.0
28:16.08	Tranquilizers	969.5
	benzodiazepine-based	969.4
	butyrophenone-based	969.2
	major NEC	969.3
	phenothiazine-based	969.1
28:16.12	Other Psychotherapeutic Agents	969.8
28:20	Respiratory and Cerebral Stimulants	970.9
	analeptics	970.0
	anorexigenic agents	977.0
	psychostimulants	969.7
	specified type NEC	970.8
28:24	Sedatives and Hypnotics	967.9
	barbiturates	967.0
	benzodiazepine-based tranquilizers	969.4
	chloral hydrate group	967.1
	glutethamide group	967.5
	intravenous anesthetics	968.3
	methaqualone	967.4
	paraldehyde	967.2
	phenothiazine-based tranquilizers	969.1
	specified type NEC	967.8
	thiobarbiturates	968.3
	tranquilizer NEC	969.5
36:00	DIAGNOSTIC AGENTS	977.8
40:00	ELECTROLYTE, CALORIC, AND WATER BALANCE AGENTS NEC	974.5
40:04	Acidifying Agents	963.2
40:08	Alkalinizing Agents	963.3
40:10	Ammonia Detoxicants	974.5
40:12	Replacement Solutions NEC	974.5
	plasma volume expanders	964.8
40:16	Sodium-Removing Resins	974.5
40:18	Potassium-Removing Resins	974.5
40:20	Caloric Agents	974.5
40:24	Salt and Sugar Substitutes	974.5
40:28	Diuretics NEC	974.4
	carbonic acid anhydrase inhibitors	974.2
	mercurials	974.0
	purine derivatives	974.1
	saluretics	974.3
40:36	Irrigating Solutions	974.5
40:40	Uricosuric Agents	974.7
44:00	ENZYMES NEC	963.4
	fibrinolysis-affecting agents	964.4
	gastric agents	973.4

APPENDIX C: CLASSIFICATION OF DRUGS BY AHFS LIST

	AHFS* List	ICD-9-CM Diagnosis Code
48:00	EXPECTORANTS AND COUGH PREPARATIONS	
	antihistamine agents	963.0
	antitussives	975.4
	codeine derivatives	965.09
	expectorants	975.5
	narcotic agents NEC	965.09
52:00	EYE, EAR, NOSE, AND THROAT PREPARATIONS	
52:04	Anti-Infectives	
	ENT	976.6
	ophthalmic	976.5
52:04.04	Antibiotics	
	ENT	976.6
	ophthalmic	976.5
52:04.06	Antivirals	
	ENT	976.6
	ophthalmic	976.5
52:04.08	Sulfonamides	
	ENT	976.6
	ophthalmic	976.5
52:04.12	Miscellaneous Anti-Infectives	
	ENT	976.6
	ophthalmic	976.5
52:08	Anti-Inflammatory Agents	
	ENT	976.6
	ophthalmic	976.5
52:10	Carbonic Anhydrase Inhibitors	974.2
52:12	Contact Lens Solutions	976.5
52:16	Local Anesthetics	968.5
52:20	Miotics	971.0
52:24	Mydriatics	
	adrenergics	971.2
	anticholinergics	971.1
	antimuscarinics	971.1
	parasympatholytics	971.1
	spasmolytics	971.1
	sympathomimetics	971.2
52:28	Mouth Washes and Gargles	976.6
52:32	Vasoconstrictors	971.2
52:36	Unclassified Agents	
	ENT	976.6
	ophthalmic	976.5
56:00	GASTROINTESTINAL DRUGS	
56:04	Antacids and Absorbents	973.0
56:08	Anti-Diarrhea Agents	973.5
56:10	Antiflatulents	973.8
56:12	Cathartics NEC	973.3
	emollients	973.2
	irritants	973.1
56:16	Digestants	973.4
56:20	Emetics and Antiemetics	
	antiemetics	963.0
	emetics	973.6
56:24	Lipotropic Agents	977.1
60:00	GOLD COMPOUNDS	965.6
64:00	HEAVY METAL ANTAGONISTS	963.8
68:00	HORMONES AND SYNTHETIC SUBSTITUTES	
68:04	Adrenals	962.0
68:08	Androgens	962.1
68:12	Contraceptives	962.2
68:16	Estrogens	962.2
68:18	Gonadotropins	962.4
68:20	Insulins and Antidiabetic Agents	962.3
68:20.08	Insulins	962.3
68:24	Parathyroid	962.6
68:28	Pituitary	
	anterior	962.4
	posterior	962.5
68:32	Progestogens	962.2
68:34	Other Corpus Luteum Hormones	962.2
68:36	Thyroid and Antithyroid	
	antithyroid	962.8
	thyroid	962.7

	AHFS* List	ICD-9-CM Diagnosis Code
72:00	LOCAL ANESTHETICS NEC	968.9
	topical (surface) agents	968.5
	infiltrating agents (intradermal) (subcutaneous) (submucosal)	968.5
	nerve blocking agents (peripheral) (plexus) (regional)	968.6
	spinal	968.7
76:00	OXYTOCICS	975.0
78:00	RADIOACTIVE AGENTS	990
80:00	SERUMS, TOXOIDS, AND VACCINES	
80:04	Serums	979.9
	immune globulin (gamma) (human)	964.6
80:08	Toxoids NEC	978.8
	diphtheria	978.5
	and tetanus	978.9
	with pertussis component	978.6
	tetanus	978.4
	and diphtheria	978.9
	with pertussis component	978.6
80:12	Vaccines NEC	979.9
	bacterial NEC	978.8
	with	
	other bacterial component	978.9
	pertussis component	978.6
	viral and rickettsial component	979.7
	rickettsial NEC	979.6
	with	
	bacterial component	979.7
	pertussis component	978.6
	viral component	979.7
	viral NEC	979.6
	with	
	bacterial component	979.7
	pertussis component	978.6
	rickettsial component	979.7
84:00	SKIN AND MUCOUS MEMBRANE PREPARATIONS	
84:04	Anti-Infectives	976.0
84:04.04	Antibiotics	976.0
84:04.08	Fungicides	976.0
84:04.12	Scabicides and Pediculicides	976.0
84:04.16	Miscellaneous Local Anti-Infectives	976.0
84:06	Anti-Inflammatory Agents	976.0
84:08	Antipruritics and Local Anesthetics	
	antipruritics	976.1
	local anesthetics	968.5
84:12	Astringents	976.2
84:16	Cell Stimulants and Proliferants	976.8
84:20	Detergents	976.2
84:24	Emollients, Demulcents, and Protectants	976.3
84:28	Keratolytic Agents	976.4
84:32	Keratoplastic Agents	976.4
84:36	Miscellaneous Agents	976.8
86:00	SPASMOLYTIC AGENTS	975.1
	antiasthmatics	975.7
	papaverine	972.5
	theophyllin	974.1
88:00	VITAMINS	
88:04	Vitamin A	963.5
88:08	Vitamin B Complex	963.5
	hematopoietic vitamin	964.1
	nicotinic acid derivatives	972.2
88:12	Vitamin C	963.5
88:16	Vitamin D	963.5
88:20	Vitamin E	963.5
88:24	Vitamin K Activity	964.3
88:28	Multivitamin Preparations	963.5
92:00	UNCLASSIFIED THERAPEUTIC AGENTS	977.8

* American Hospital Formulary Service

APPENDIX D: INDUSTRIAL ACCIDENTS ACCORDING TO AGENCY

CLASSIFICATION OF INDUSTRIAL ACCIDENTS ACCORDING TO AGENCY

Annex B to the Resolution concerning Statistics of Employment Injuries adopted by the Tenth International Conference of Labor Statisticians on 12 October 1962

1 MACHINES

- **11** **Prime-Movers, except Electrical Motors**
- 111 *Steam engines*
- 112 *Internal combustion engines*
- 119 *Others*
- **12** **Transmission Machinery**
- 121 *Transmission shafts*
- 122 *Transmission belts, cables, pulleys, pinions, chains, gears*
- 129 *Others*
- **13** **Metalworking Machines**
- 131 *Power presses*
- 132 *Lathes*
- 133 *Milling machines*
- 134 *Abrasive wheels*
- 135 *Mechanical shears*
- 136 *Forging machines*
- 137 *Rolling-mills*
- 139 *Others*
- **14** **Wood and Assimilated Machines**
- 141 *Circular saws*
- 142 *Other saws*
- 143 *Molding machines*
- 144 *Overhand planes*
- 149 *Others*
- **15** **Agricultural Machines**
- 151 *Reapers (including combine reapers)*
- 152 *Threshers*
- 159 *Others*
- **16** **Mining Machinery**
- 161 *Under-cutters*
- 169 *Others*
- **19** **Other Machines Not Elsewhere Classified**
- 191 *Earth-moving machines, excavating and scraping machines, except means of transport*
- 192 *Spinning, weaving and other textile machines*
- 193 *Machines for the manufacture of foodstuffs and beverages*
- 194 *Machines for the manufacture of paper*
- 195 *Printing machines*
- 199 *Others*

2 MEANS OF TRANSPORT AND LIFTING EQUIPMENT

- **21** **Lifting Machines and Appliances**
- 211 *Cranes*
- 212 *Lifts and elevators*
- 213 *Winches*
- 214 *Pulley blocks*
- 219 *Others*
- **22** **Means of Rail Transport**
- 221 *Inter-urban railways*
- 222 *Rail transport in mines, tunnels, quarries, industrial establishments, docks, etc.*
- 229 *Others*
- **23** **Other Wheeled Means of Transport, Excluding Rail Transport**
- 231 *Tractors*
- 232 *Lorries*
- 233 *Trucks*
- 234 *Motor vehicles, not elsewhere classified*
- 235 *Animal-drawn vehicles*
- 236 *Hand-drawn vehicles*
- 239 *Others*
- **24** **Means of Air Transport**
- **25** **Means of Water Transport**
- 251 *Motorized means of water transport*
- 252 *Non-motorized means of water transport*
- **26** **Other Means of Transport**
- 261 *Cable-cars*
- 262 *Mechanical conveyors, except cable-cars*
- 269 *Others*

3 OTHER EQUIPMENT

- **31** **Pressure Vessels**
- 311 *Boilers*
- 312 *Pressurized containers*
- 313 *Pressurized piping and accessories*
- 314 *Gas cylinders*
- 315 *Caissons, diving equipment*
- 319 *Others*
- **32** **Furnaces, Ovens, Kilns**
- 321 *Blast furnaces*
- 322 *Refining furnaces*
- 323 *Other furnaces*
- 324 *Kilns*
- 325 *Ovens*
- **33** **Refrigerating Plants**
- **34** **Electrical Installations, Including Electric Motors, but Excluding Electric Hand Tools**
- 341 *Rotating machines*
- 342 *Conductors*
- 343 *Transformers*
- 344 *Control apparatus*
- 349 *Others*
- **35** **Electric Hand Tools**
- **36** **Tools, Implements, and Appliances, Except Electric Hand Tools**
- 361 *Power-driven hand tools, except electric hand tools*
- 362 *Hand tools, not power-driven*
- 369 *Others*
- **37** **Ladders, Mobile Ramps**
- **38** **Scaffolding**
- **39** **Other Equipment, Not Elsewhere Classified**

4 MATERIALS, SUBSTANCES AND RADIATIONS

- **41** **Explosives**
- **42** **Dusts, Gases, Liquids and Chemicals, Excluding Explosives**
- 421 *Dusts*
- 422 *Gases, vapors, fumes*
- 423 *Liquids, not elsewhere classified*
- 424 *Chemicals, not elsewhere classified*
- **43** **Flying Fragments**
- **44** **Radiations**
- 441 *Ionizing radiations*
- 449 *Others*
- **49** **Other Materials and Substances Not Elsewhere Classified**

5 WORKING ENVIRONMENT

- **51** **Outdoor**
- 511 *Weather*
- 512 *Traffic and working surfaces*
- 513 *Water*
- 519 *Others*
- **52** **Indoor**
- 521 *Floors*
- 522 *Confined quarters*
- 523 *Stairs*
- 524 *Other traffic and working surfaces*
- 525 *Floor openings and wall openings*
- 526 *Environmental factors (lighting, ventilation, temperature, noise, etc.)*
- 529 *Others*
- **53** **Underground**
- 531 *Roofs and faces of mine roads and tunnels, etc.*
- 532 *Floors of mine roads and tunnels, etc.*
- 533 *Working-faces of mines, tunnels, etc.*
- 534 *Mine shafts*
- 535 *Fire*
- 536 *Water*
- 539 *Others*

6 OTHER AGENCIES, NOT ELSEWHERE CLASSIFIED

- **61** **Animals**
- 611 *Live animals*
- 612 *Animal products*
- **69** **Other Agencies, Not Elsewhere Classified**

7 AGENCIES NOT CLASSIFIED FOR LACK OF SUFFICIENT DATA

APPENDIX E: LIST OF THREE-DIGIT CATEGORIES

LIST OF THREE-DIGIT CATEGORIES

1. INFECTIOUS AND PARASITIC DISEASES

Intestinal infectious diseases (001-009)
- 001 Cholera
- 002 Typhoid and paratyphoid fevers
- 003 Other salmonella infections
- 004 Shigellosis
- 005 Other food poisoning (bacterial)
- 006 Amebiasis
- 007 Other protozoal intestinal diseases
- 008 Intestinal infections due to other organisms
- 009 Ill-defined intestinal infections

Tuberculosis (010-018)
- 010 Primary tuberculous infection
- 011 Pulmonary tuberculosis
- 012 Other respiratory tuberculosis
- 013 Tuberculosis of meninges and central nervous system
- 014 Tuberculosis of intestines, peritoneum, and mesenteric glands
- 015 Tuberculosis of bones and joints
- 016 Tuberculosis of genitourinary system
- 017 Tuberculosis of other organs
- 018 Miliary tuberculosis

Zoonotic bacterial diseases (020-027)
- 020 Plague
- 021 Tularemia
- 022 Anthrax
- 023 Brucellosis
- 024 Glanders
- 025 Melioidosis
- 026 Rat-bite fever
- 027 Other zoonotic bacterial diseases

Other bacterial diseases (030-042)
- 030 Leprosy
- 031 Diseases due to other mycobacteria
- 032 Diphtheria
- 033 Whooping cough
- 034 Streptococcal sore throat and scarlatina
- 035 Erysipelas
- 036 Meningococcal infection
- 037 Tetanus
- 038 Septicemia
- 039 Actinomycotic infections
- 040 Other bacterial diseases
- 041 Bacterial infection in conditions classified elsewhere and of unspecified site

Human immunodeficiency virus (042)
- 042 Human immunodeficiency virus [HIV] disease

Poliomyelitis and other non-arthropod-borne viral diseases of central nervous system (045-049)
- 045 Acute poliomyelitis
- 046 Slow virus infection of central nervous system
- 047 Meningitis due to enterovirus
- 048 Other enterovirus diseases of central nervous system
- 049 Other non-arthropod-borne viral diseases of central nervous system

Viral diseases accompanied by exanthem (050-057)
- 050 Smallpox
- 051 Cowpox and paravaccinia
- 052 Chickenpox
- 053 Herpes zoster
- 054 Herpes simplex
- 055 Measles
- 056 Rubella
- 057 Other viral exanthemata

Arthropod-borne viral diseases (060-066)
- 060 Yellow fever
- 061 Dengue
- 062 Mosquito-borne viral encephalitis
- 063 Tick-borne viral encephalitis
- 064 Viral encephalitis transmitted by other and unspecified arthropods
- 065 Arthropod-borne hemorrhagic fever
- 066 Other arthropod-borne viral diseases

Other diseases due to viruses and Chlamydiae (070-079)
- 070 Viral hepatitis
- 071 Rabies
- 072 Mumps
- 073 Ornithosis
- 074 Specific diseases due to Coxsackievirus
- 075 Infectious mononucleosis
- 076 Trachoma
- 077 Other diseases of conjunctiva due to viruses and Chlamydiae
- 078 Other diseases due to viruses and Chlamydiae
- 079 Viral infection in conditions classified elsewhere and of unspecified site

Rickettsioses and other arthropod-borne diseases (080-088)
- 080 Louse-borne [epidemic] typhus
- 081 Other typhus
- 082 Tick-borne rickettsioses
- 083 Other rickettsioses
- 084 Malaria
- 085 Leishmaniasis
- 086 Trypanosomiasis
- 087 Relapsing fever
- 088 Other arthropod-borne diseases

Syphilis and other venereal diseases (090-099)
- 090 Congenital syphilis
- 091 Early syphilis, symptomatic
- 092 Early syphilis, latent
- 093 Cardiovascular syphilis
- 094 Neurosyphilis
- 095 Other forms of late syphilis, with symptoms
- 096 Late syphilis, latent
- 097 Other and unspecified syphilis
- 098 Gonococcal infections
- 099 Other venereal diseases

Other spirochetal diseases (100-104)
- 100 Leptospirosis
- 101 Vincent's angina
- 102 Yaws
- 103 Pinta
- 104 Other spirochetal infection

Mycoses (110-118)
- 110 Dermatophytosis
- 111 Dermatomycosis, other and unspecified
- 112 Candidiasis
- 114 Coccidioidomycosis
- 115 Histoplasmosis
- 116 Blastomycotic infection
- 117 Other mycoses
- 118 Opportunistic mycoses

Helminthiases (120-129)
- 120 Schistosomiasis [bilharziasis]
- 121 Other trematode infections
- 122 Echinococcosis
- 123 Other cestode infection
- 124 Trichinosis
- 125 Filarial infection and dracontiasis
- 126 Ancylostomiasis and necatoriasis
- 127 Other intestinal helminthiases
- 128 Other and unspecified helminthiases
- 129 Intestinal parasitism, unspecified

Other infectious and parasitic diseases (130-136)
- 130 Toxoplasmosis
- 131 Trichomoniasis
- 132 Pediculosis and phthirus infestation
- 133 Acariasis
- 134 Other infestation
- 135 Sarcoidosis
- 136 Other and unspecified infectious and parasitic diseases

Late effects of infectious and parasitic diseases (137-139)
- 137 Late effects of tuberculosis
- 138 Late effects of acute poliomyelitis
- 139 Late effects of other infectious and parasitic diseases

2. NEOPLASMS

Malignant neoplasm of lip, oral cavity, and pharynx (140-149)
- 140 Malignant neoplasm of lip
- 141 Malignant neoplasm of tongue
- 142 Malignant neoplasm of major salivary glands
- 143 Malignant neoplasm of gum
- 144 Malignant neoplasm of floor of mouth
- 145 Malignant neoplasm of other and unspecified parts of mouth
- 146 Malignant neoplasm of oropharynx
- 147 Malignant neoplasm of nasopharynx
- 148 Malignant neoplasm of hypopharynx
- 149 Malignant neoplasm of other and ill-defined sites within the lip, oral cavity, and pharynx

Malignant neoplasm of digestive organs and peritoneum (150-159)
- 150 Malignant neoplasm of esophagus
- 151 Malignant neoplasm of stomach
- 152 Malignant neoplasm of small intestine, including duodenum
- 153 Malignant neoplasm of colon
- 154 Malignant neoplasm of rectum, rectosigmoid junction, and anus
- 155 Malignant neoplasm of liver and intrahepatic bile ducts
- 156 Malignant neoplasm of gallbladder and extrahepatic bile ducts
- 157 Malignant neoplasm of pancreas
- 158 Malignant neoplasm of retroperitoneum and peritoneum
- 159 Malignant neoplasm of other and ill-defined sites within the digestive organs and peritoneum

Malignant neoplasm of respiratory and intrathoracic organs (160-165)
- 160 Malignant neoplasm of nasal cavities, middle ear, and accessory sinuses
- 161 Malignant neoplasm of larynx
- 162 Malignant neoplasm of trachea, bronchus, and lung
- 163 Malignant neoplasm of pleura
- 164 Malignant neoplasm of thymus, heart, and mediastinum
- 165 Malignant neoplasm of other and ill-defined sites within the respiratory system and intrathoracic organs

APPENDIX E: LIST OF THREE-DIGIT CATEGORIES

Malignant neoplasm of bone, connective tissue, skin, and breast (170-176)
- 170 Malignant neoplasm of bone and articular cartilage
- 171 Malignant neoplasm of connective and other soft tissue
- 172 Malignant melanoma of skin
- 173 Other malignant neoplasm of skin
- 174 Malignant neoplasm of female breast
- 175 Malignant neoplasm of male breast

Kaposi's sarcoma (176)
- 176 Kaposi's sarcoma

Malignant neoplasm of genitourinary organs (179-189)
- 179 Malignant neoplasm of uterus, part unspecified
- 180 Malignant neoplasm of cervix uteri
- 181 Malignant neoplasm of placenta
- 182 Malignant neoplasm of body of uterus
- 183 Malignant neoplasm of ovary and other uterine adnexa
- 184 Malignant neoplasm of other and unspecified female genital organs
- 185 Malignant neoplasm of prostate
- 186 Malignant neoplasm of testis
- 187 Malignant neoplasm of penis and other male genital organs
- 188 Malignant neoplasm of bladder
- 189 Malignant neoplasm of kidney and other unspecified urinary organs

Malignant neoplasm of other and unspecified sites (190-199)
- 190 Malignant neoplasm of eye
- 191 Malignant neoplasm of brain
- 192 Malignant neoplasm of other and unspecified parts of nervous system
- 193 Malignant neoplasm of thyroid gland
- 194 Malignant neoplasm of other endocrine glands and related structures
- 195 Malignant neoplasm of other and ill-defined sites
- 196 Secondary and unspecified malignant neoplasm of lymph nodes
- 197 Secondary malignant neoplasm of respiratory and digestive systems
- 198 Secondary malignant neoplasm of other specified sites
- 199 Malignant neoplasm without specification of site

Malignant neoplasm of lymphatic and hematopoietic tissue (200-208)
- 200 Lymphosarcoma and reticulosarcoma
- 201 Hodgkin's disease
- 202 Other malignant neoplasm of lymphoid and histiocytic tissue
- 203 Multiple myeloma and immunoproliferative neoplasms
- 204 Lymphoid leukemia
- 205 Myeloid leukemia
- 206 Monocytic leukemia
- 207 Other specified leukemia
- 208 Leukemia of unspecified cell type

Benign neoplasms (210-229)
- 210 Benign neoplasm of lip, oral cavity, and pharynx
- 211 Benign neoplasm of other parts of digestive system
- 212 Benign neoplasm of respiratory and intrathoracic organs
- 213 Benign neoplasm of bone and articular cartilage
- 214 Lipoma
- 215 Other benign neoplasm of connective and other soft tissue
- 216 Benign neoplasm of skin
- 217 Benign neoplasm of breast
- 218 Uterine leiomyoma
- 219 Other benign neoplasm of uterus
- 220 Benign neoplasm of ovary
- 221 Benign neoplasm of other female genital organs
- 222 Benign neoplasm of male genital organs
- 223 Benign neoplasm of kidney and other urinary organs
- 224 Benign neoplasm of eye
- 225 Benign neoplasm of brain and other parts of nervous system
- 226 Benign neoplasm of thyroid gland
- 227 Benign neoplasm of other endocrine glands and related structures
- 228 Hemangioma and lymphangioma, any site
- 229 Benign neoplasm of other and unspecified sites

Carcinoma in situ (230-234)
- 230 Carcinoma in situ of digestive organs
- 231 Carcinoma in situ of respiratory system
- 232 Carcinoma in situ of skin
- 233 Carcinoma in situ of breast and genitourinary system
- 234 Carcinoma in situ of other and unspecified sites

Neoplasms of uncertain behavior (235-238)
- 235 Neoplasm of uncertain behavior of digestive and respiratory systems
- 236 Neoplasm of uncertain behavior of genitourinary organs
- 237 Neoplasm of uncertain behavior of endocrine glands and nervous system
- 238 Neoplasm of uncertain behavior of other and unspecified sites and tissues

Neoplasms of unspecified nature (239)
- 239 Neoplasm of unspecified nature

3. ENDOCRINE, NUTRITIONAL AND METABOLIC DISEASES, AND IMMUNITY DISORDERS

Disorders of thyroid gland (240-246)
- 240 Simple and unspecified goiter
- 241 Nontoxic nodular goiter
- 242 Thyrotoxicosis with or without goiter
- 243 Congenital hypothyroidism
- 244 Acquired hypothyroidism
- 245 Thyroiditis
- 246 Other disorders of thyroid

Diseases of other endocrine glands (250-259)
- 250 Diabetes mellitus
- 251 Other disorders of pancreatic internal secretion
- 252 Disorders of parathyroid gland
- 253 Disorders of the pituitary gland and its hypothalamic control
- 254 Diseases of thymus gland
- 255 Disorders of adrenal glands
- 256 Ovarian dysfunction
- 257 Testicular dysfunction
- 258 Polyglandular dysfunction and related disorders
- 259 Other endocrine disorders

Nutritional deficiencies (260-269)
- 260 Kwashiorkor
- 261 Nutritional marasmus
- 262 Other severe protein-calorie malnutrition
- 263 Other and unspecified protein-calorie malnutrition
- 264 Vitamin A deficiency
- 265 Thiamine and niacin deficiency states
- 266 Deficiency of B-complex components
- 267 Ascorbic acid deficiency
- 268 Vitamin D deficiency
- 269 Other nutritional deficiencies

Other metabolic disorders and immunity disorders (270-279)
- 270 Disorders of amino-acid transport and metabolism
- 271 Disorders of carbohydrate transport and metabolism
- 272 Disorders of lipoid metabolism
- 273 Disorders of plasma protein metabolism
- 274 Gout
- 275 Disorders of mineral metabolism
- 276 Disorders of fluid, electrolyte, and acid-base balance
- 277 Other and unspecified disorders of metabolism
- 278 Obesity and other hyperalimentation
- 279 Disorders involving the immune mechanism

Diseases of blood and blood-forming organs (280-289)
- 280 Iron deficiency anemias
- 281 Other deficiency anemias
- 282 Hereditary hemolytic anemias
- 283 Acquired hemolytic anemias
- 284 Aplastic anemia
- 285 Other and unspecified anemias
- 286 Coagulation defects
- 287 Purpura and other hemorrhagic conditions
- 288 Diseases of white blood cells
- 289 Other diseases of blood and blood-forming organs

5. MENTAL DISORDERS

Organic psychotic conditions (290-294)
- 290 Senile and presenile organic psychotic conditions
- 291 Alcoholic psychoses
- 292 Drug psychoses
- 293 Transient organic psychotic conditions
- 294 Other organic psychotic conditions (chronic)

Other psychoses (295-299)
- 295 Schizophrenic psychoses
- 296 Affective psychoses
- 297 Paranoid states
- 298 Other nonorganic psychoses
- 299 Psychoses with origin specific to childhood

Neurotic disorders, personality disorders, and other nonpsychotic mental disorders (300-316)
- 300 Neurotic disorders
- 301 Personality disorders
- 302 Sexual deviations and disorders
- 303 Alcohol dependence syndrome
- 304 Drug dependence
- 305 Nondependent abuse of drugs
- 306 Physiological malfunction arising from mental factors

APPENDIX E: LIST OF THREE-DIGIT CATEGORIES

307 Special symptoms or syndromes, not elsewhere classified
308 Acute reaction to stress
309 Adjustment reaction
310 Specific nonpsychotic mental disorders following organic brain damage
311 Depressive disorder, not elsewhere classified
312 Disturbance of conduct, not elsewhere classified
313 Disturbance of emotions specific to childhood and adolescence
314 Hyperkinetic syndrome of childhood
315 Specific delays in development
316 Psychic factors associated with diseases classified elsewhere

Mental retardation (317-319)
317 Mild mental retardation
318 Other specified mental retardation
319 Unspecified mental retardation

6. DISEASES OF THE NERVOUS SYSTEM AND SENSE ORGANS

Inflammatory diseases of the central nervous system (320-326)
320 Bacterial meningitis
321 Meningitis due to other organisms
322 Meningitis of unspecified cause
323 Encephalitis, myelitis, and encephalomyelitis
324 Intracranial and intraspinal abscess
325 Phlebitis and thrombophlebitis of intracranial venous sinuses
326 Late effects of intracranial abscess or pyogenic infection

Hereditary and degenerative diseases of the central nervous system (330-337)
330 Cerebral degenerations usually manifest in childhood
331 Other cerebral degenerations
332 Parkinson's disease
333 Other extrapyramidal diseases and abnormal movement disorders
334 Spinocerebellar disease
335 Anterior horn cell disease
336 Other diseases of spinal cord
337 Disorders of the autonomic nervous system

Other disorders of the central nervous system (340-349)
340 Multiple sclerosis
341 Other demyelinating diseases of central nervous system
342 Hemiplegia and hemiparesis
343 Infantile cerebral palsy
344 Other paralytic syndromes
345 Epilepsy
346 Migraine
347 Cataplexy and narcolepsy
348 Other conditions of brain
349 Other and unspecified disorders of the nervous system

Disorders of the peripheral nervous system (350-359)
350 Trigeminal nerve disorders
351 Facial nerve disorders
352 Disorders of other cranial nerves
353 Nerve root and plexus disorders
354 Mononeuritis of upper limb and mononeuritis multiplex
355 Mononeuritis of lower limb
356 Hereditary and idiopathic peripheral neuropathy
357 Inflammatory and toxic neuropathy
358 Myoneural disorders
359 Muscular dystrophies and other myopathies

Disorders of the eye and adnexa (360-379)
360 Disorders of the globe
361 Retinal detachments and defects
362 Other retinal disorders
363 Chorioretinal inflammations and scars and other disorders of choroid
364 Disorders of iris and ciliary body
365 Glaucoma
366 Cataract
367 Disorders of refraction and accommodation
368 Visual disturbances
369 Blindness and low vision
370 Keratitis
371 Corneal opacity and other disorders of cornea
372 Disorders of conjunctiva
373 Inflammation of eyelids
374 Other disorders of eyelids
375 Disorders of lacrimal system
376 Disorders of the orbit
377 Disorders of optic nerve and visual pathways
378 Strabismus and other disorders of binocular eye movements
379 Other disorders of eye

Diseases of the ear and mastoid process (380-389)
380 Disorders of external ear
381 Nonsuppurative otitis media and Eustachian tube disorders
382 Suppurative and unspecified otitis media
383 Mastoiditis and related conditions
384 Other disorders of tympanic membrane
385 Other disorders of middle ear and mastoid
386 Vertiginous syndromes and other disorders of vestibular system
387 Otosclerosis
388 Other disorders of ear
389 Hearing loss

7. DISEASES OF THE CIRCULATORY SYSTEM

Acute rheumatic fever (390-392)
390 Rheumatic fever without mention of heart involvement
391 Rheumatic fever with heart involvement
392 Rheumatic chorea

Chronic rheumatic heart disease (393-398)
393 Chronic rheumatic pericarditis
394 Diseases of mitral valve
395 Diseases of aortic valve
396 Diseases of mitral and aortic valves
397 Diseases of other endocardial structures
398 Other rheumatic heart disease

Hypertensive disease (401-405)
401 Essential hypertension
402 Hypertensive heart disease
403 Hypertensive renal disease
404 Hypertensive heart and renal disease
405 Secondary hypertension

Ischemic heart disease (410-414)
410 Acute myocardial infarction
411 Other acute and subacute form of ischemic heart disease
412 Old myocardial infarction
413 Angina pectoris
414 Other forms of chronic ischemic heart disease

Diseases of pulmonary circulation (415-417)
415 Acute pulmonary heart disease
416 Chronic pulmonary heart disease
417 Other diseases of pulmonary circulation

Other forms of heart disease (420-429)
420 Acute pericarditis
421 Acute and subacute endocarditis
422 Acute myocarditis
423 Other diseases of pericardium
424 Other diseases of endocardium
425 Cardiomyopathy
426 Conduction disorders
427 Cardiac dysrhythmias
428 Heart failure
429 Ill-defined descriptions and complications of heart disease

Cerebrovascular disease (430-438)
430 Subarachnoid hemorrhage
431 Intracerebral hemorrhage
432 Other and unspecified intracranial hemorrhage
433 Occlusion and stenosis of precerebral arteries
434 Occlusion of cerebral arteries
435 Transient cerebral ischemia
436 Acute but ill-defined cerebrovascular disease
437 Other and ill-defined cerebrovascular disease
438 Late effects of cerebrovascular disease

Diseases of arteries, arterioles, and capillaries (440-448)
440 Atherosclerosis
441 Aortic aneurysm and dissection
442 Other aneurysm
443 Other peripheral vascular disease
444 Arterial embolism and thrombosis
445 Atheroembolism
446 Polyarteritis nodosa and allied conditions
447 Other disorders of arteries and arterioles
448 Diseases of capillaries

Diseases of veins and lymphatics, and other diseases of circulatory system (451-459)
451 Phlebitis and thrombophlebitis
452 Portal vein thrombosis
453 Other venous embolism and thrombosis
454 Varicose veins of lower extremities
455 Hemorrhoids
456 Varicose veins of other sites
457 Noninfective disorders of lymphatic channels
458 Hypotension
459 Other disorders of circulatory system

8. DISEASES OF THE RESPIRATORY SYSTEM

Acute respiratory infections (460-466)
460 Acute nasopharyngitis [common cold]
461 Acute sinusitis
462 Acute pharyngitis
463 Acute tonsillitis
464 Acute laryngitis and tracheitis

APPENDIX E: LIST OF THREE-DIGIT CATEGORIES

465 Acute upper respiratory infections of multiple or unspecified sites
466 Acute bronchitis and bronchiolitis

Other diseases of upper respiratory tract (470-478)
470 Deviated nasal septum
471 Nasal polyps
472 Chronic pharyngitis and nasopharyngitis
473 Chronic sinusitis
474 Chronic disease of tonsils and adenoids
475 Peritonsillar abscess
476 Chronic laryngitis and laryngotracheitis
477 Allergic rhinitis
478 Other diseases of upper respiratory tract

Pneumonia and influenza (480-487)
480 Viral pneumonia
481 Pneumococcal pneumonia [Streptococcus pneumoniae pneumonia]
482 Other bacterial pneumonia
483 Pneumonia due to other specified organism
484 Pneumonia in infectious diseases classified elsewhere
485 Bronchopneumonia, organism unspecified
486 Pneumonia, organism unspecified
487 Influenza

Chronic obstructive pulmonary disease and allied conditions (490-496)
490 Bronchitis, not specified as acute or chronic
491 Chronic bronchitis
492 Emphysema
493 Asthma
494 Bronchiectasis
495 Extrinsic allergic alveolitis
496 Chronic airways obstruction, not elsewhere classified

Pneumoconioses and other lung diseases due to external agents (500-508)
500 Coal workers' pneumoconiosis
501 Asbestosis
502 Pneumoconiosis due to other silica or silicates
503 Pneumoconiosis due to other inorganic dust
504 Pneumopathy due to inhalation of other dust
505 Pneumoconiosis, unspecified
506 Respiratory conditions due to chemical fumes and vapors
507 Pneumonitis due to solids and liquids
508 Respiratory conditions due to other and unspecified external agents

Other diseases of respiratory system (510-519)
510 Empyema
511 Pleurisy
512 Pneumothorax
513 Abscess of lung and mediastinum
514 Pulmonary congestion and hypostasis
515 Postinflammatory pulmonary fibrosis
516 Other alveolar and parietoalveolar pneumopathy
517 Lung involvement in conditions classified elsewhere
518 Other diseases of lung
519 Other diseases of respiratory system

9. DISEASES OF THE DIGESTIVE SYSTEM

Diseases of oral cavity, salivary glands, and jaws (520-529)
520 Disorders of tooth development and eruption
521 Diseases of hard tissues of teeth
522 Diseases of pulp and periapical tissues
523 Gingival and periodontal diseases
524 Dentofacial anomalies, including malocclusion
525 Other diseases and conditions of the teeth and supporting structures
526 Diseases of the jaws
527 Diseases of the salivary glands
528 Diseases of the oral soft tissues, excluding lesions specific for gingiva and tongue
529 Diseases and other conditions of the tongue

Diseases of esophagus, stomach, and duodenum (530-537)
530 Diseases of esophagus
531 Gastric ulcer
532 Duodenal ulcer
533 Peptic ulcer, site unspecified
534 Gastrojejunal ulcer
535 Gastritis and duodenitis
536 Disorders of function of stomach
537 Other disorders of stomach and duodenum

Appendicitis (540-543)
540 Acute appendicitis
541 Appendicitis, unqualified
542 Other appendicitis
543 Other diseases of appendix

Hernia of abdominal cavity (550-553)
550 Inguinal hernia
551 Other hernia of abdominal cavity, with gangrene
552 Other hernia of abdominal cavity, with obstruction, but without mention of gangrene
553 Other hernia of abdominal cavity without mention of obstruction or gangrene

Noninfective enteritis and colitis (555-558)
555 Regional enteritis
556 Ulcerative colitis
557 Vascular insufficiency of intestine
558 Other noninfective gastroenteritis and colitis

Other diseases of intestines and peritoneum (560-569)
560 Intestinal obstruction without mention of hernia
562 Diverticula of intestine
564 Functional digestive disorders, not elsewhere classified
565 Anal fissure and fistula
566 Abscess of anal and rectal regions
567 Peritonitis
568 Other disorders of peritoneum
569 Other disorders of intestine

Other diseases of digestive system (570-579)
570 Acute and subacute necrosis of liver
571 Chronic liver disease and cirrhosis
572 Liver abscess and sequelae of chronic liver disease
573 Other disorders of liver
574 Cholelithiasis
575 Other disorders of gallbladder
576 Other disorders of biliary tract
577 Diseases of pancreas
578 Gastrointestinal hemorrhage
579 Intestinal malabsorption

10. DISEASES OF THE GENITOURINARY SYSTEM

Nephritis, nephrotic syndrome, and nephrosis (580-589)
580 Acute glomerulonephritis
581 Nephrotic syndrome
582 Chronic glomerulonephritis
583 Nephritis and nephropathy, not specified as acute or chronic
584 Acute renal failure
585 Chronic renal failure
586 Renal failure, unspecified
587 Renal sclerosis, unspecified
588 Disorders resulting from impaired renal function
589 Small kidney of unknown cause

Other diseases of urinary system (590-599)
590 Infections of kidney
591 Hydronephrosis
592 Calculus of kidney and ureter
593 Other disorders of kidney and ureter
594 Calculus of lower urinary tract
595 Cystitis
596 Other disorders of bladder
597 Urethritis, not sexually transmitted, and urethral syndrome
598 Urethral stricture
599 Other disorders of urethra and urinary tract

Diseases of male genital organs (600-608)
600 Hyperplasia of prostate
601 Inflammatory diseases of prostate
602 Other disorders of prostate
603 Hydrocele
604 Orchitis and epididymitis
605 Redundant prepuce and phimosis
606 Infertility, male
607 Disorders of penis
608 Other disorders of male genital organs

Disorders of breast (610-611)
610 Benign mammary dysplasias
611 Other disorders of breast

Inflammatory disease of female pelvic organs (614-616)
614 Inflammatory disease of ovary, fallopian tube, pelvic cellular tissue, and peritoneum
615 Inflammatory diseases of uterus, except cervix
616 Inflammatory disease of cervix, vagina, and vulva

Other disorders of female genital tract (617-629)
617 Endometriosis
618 Genital prolapse
619 Fistula involving female genital tract
620 Noninflammatory disorders of ovary, fallopian tube, and broad ligament
621 Disorders of uterus, not elsewhere classified
622 Noninflammatory disorders of cervix
623 Noninflammatory disorders of vagina
624 Noninflammatory disorders of vulva and perineum

APPENDIX E: LIST OF THREE-DIGIT CATEGORIES

625 Pain and other symptoms associated with female genital organs
626 Disorders of menstruation and other abnormal bleeding from female genital tract
627 Menopausal and postmenopausal disorders
628 Infertility, female
629 Other disorders of female genital organs

11. COMPLICATIONS OF PREGNANCY, CHILDBIRTH AND THE PUERPERIUM

Ectopic and molar pregnancy and other pregnancy with abortive outcome (630-639)
630 Hydatidiform mole
631 Other abnormal product of conception
632 Missed abortion
633 Ectopic pregnancy
634 Spontaneous abortion
635 Legally induced abortion
636 Illegally induced abortion
637 Unspecified abortion
638 Failed attempted abortion
639 Complications following abortion and ectopic and molar pregnancies

Complications mainly related to pregnancy (640-648)
640 Hemorrhage in early pregnancy
641 Antepartum hemorrhage, abruptio placentae, and placenta previa
642 Hypertension complicating pregnancy, childbirth, and the puerperium
643 Excessive vomiting in pregnancy
644 Early or threatened labor
645 Prolonged pregnancy
646 Other complications of pregnancy, not elsewhere classified
647 Infective and parasitic conditions in the mother classifiable elsewhere but complicating pregnancy, childbirth, and the puerperium
648 Other current conditions in the mother classifiable elsewhere but complicating pregnancy, childbirth, and the puerperium

Normal delivery, and other indications for care in pregnancy, labor, and delivery (650-659)
650 Normal delivery
651 Multiple gestation
652 Malposition and malpresentation of fetus
653 Disproportion
654 Abnormality of organs and soft tissues of pelvis
655 Known or suspected fetal abnormality affecting management of mother
656 Other fetal and placental problems affecting management of mother
657 Polyhydramnios
658 Other problems associated with amniotic cavity and membranes
659 Other indications for care or intervention related to labor and delivery and not elsewhere classified

Complications occurring mainly in the course of labor and delivery (660-669)
660 Obstructed labor
661 Abnormality of forces of labor
662 Long labor
663 Umbilical cord complications
664 Trauma to perineum and vulva during delivery
665 Other obstetrical trauma
666 Postpartum hemorrhage
667 Retained placenta or membranes, without hemorrhage
668 Complications of the administration of anesthetic or other sedation in labor and delivery
669 Other complications of labor and delivery, not elsewhere classified

Complications of the puerperium (670-677)
670 Major puerperal infection
671 Venous complications in pregnancy and the puerperium
672 Pyrexia of unknown origin during the puerperium
673 Obstetrical pulmonary embolism
674 Other and unspecified complications of the puerperium, not elsewhere classified
675 Infections of the breast and nipple associated with childbirth
676 Other disorders of the breast associated with childbirth, and disorders of lactation
677 Late effect of complication of pregnancy, childbirth, and the puerperium

12. DISEASES OF THE SKIN AND SUBCUTANEOUS TISSUE

Infections of skin and subcutaneous tissue (680-686)
680 Carbuncle and furuncle
681 Cellulitis and abscess of finger and toe
682 Other cellulitis and abscess
683 Acute lymphadenitis
684 Impetigo
685 Pilonidal cyst
686 Other local infections of skin and subcutaneous tissue

Other inflammatory conditions of skin and subcutaneous tissue (690-698)
690 Erythematosquamous dermatosis
691 Atopic dermatitis and related conditions
692 Contact dermatitis and other eczema
693 Dermatitis due to substances taken internally
694 Bullous dermatoses
695 Erythematous conditions
696 Psoriasis and similar disorders
697 Lichen
698 Pruritus and related conditions

Other diseases of skin and subcutaneous tissue (700-709)
700 Corns and callosities
701 Other hypertrophic and atrophic conditions of skin
702 Other dermatoses
703 Diseases of nail
704 Diseases of hair and hair follicles
705 Disorders of sweat glands
706 Diseases of sebaceous glands
707 Chronic ulcer of skin
708 Urticaria
709 Other disorders of skin and subcutaneous tissue

13. DISEASES OF THE MUSCULOSKELETAL SYSTEM AND CONNECTIVE TISSUE

Arthropathies and related disorders (710-719)
710 Diffuse diseases of connective tissue
711 Arthropathy associated with infections
712 Crystal arthropathies
713 Arthropathy associated with other disorders classified elsewhere
714 Rheumatoid arthritis and other inflammatory polyarthropathies
715 Osteoarthrosis and allied disorders
716 Other and unspecified arthropathies
717 Internal derangement of knee
718 Other derangement of joint
719 Other and unspecified disorder of joint

Dorsopathies (720-724)
720 Ankylosing spondylitis and other inflammatory spondylopathies
721 Spondylosis and allied disorders
722 Intervertebral disc disorders
723 Other disorders of cervical region
724 Other and unspecified disorders of back

Rheumatism, excluding the back (725-729)
725 Polymyalgia rheumatica
726 Peripheral enthesopathies and allied syndromes
727 Other disorders of synovium, tendon, and bursa
728 Disorders of muscle, ligament, and fascia
729 Other disorders of soft tissues

Osteopathies, chondropathies, and acquired musculoskeletal deformities (730-739)
730 Osteomyelitis, periostitis, and other infections involving bone
731 Osteitis deformans and osteopathies associated with other disorders classified elsewhere
732 Osteochondropathies
733 Other disorders of bone and cartilage
734 Flat foot
735 Acquired deformities of toe
736 Other acquired deformities of limbs
737 Curvature of spine
738 Other acquired deformity
739 Nonallopathic lesions, not elsewhere classified

14. CONGENITAL ANOMALIES
740 Anencephalus and similar anomalies
741 Spina bifida
742 Other congenital anomalies of nervous system
743 Congenital anomalies of eye
744 Congenital anomalies of ear, face, and neck
745 Bulbus cordis anomalies and anomalies of cardiac septal closure
746 Other congenital anomalies of heart
747 Other congenital anomalies of circulatory system
748 Congenital anomalies of respiratory system
749 Cleft palate and cleft lip
750 Other congenital anomalies of upper alimentary tract
751 Other congenital anomalies of digestive system

APPENDIX E: LIST OF THREE-DIGIT CATEGORIES

752	Congenital anomalies of genital organs
753	Congenital anomalies of urinary system
754	Certain congenital musculoskeletal deformities
755	Other congenital anomalies of limbs
756	Other congenital musculoskeletal anomalies
757	Congenital anomalies of the integument
758	Chromosomal anomalies
759	Other and unspecified congenital anomalies

15. CERTAIN CONDITIONS ORIGINATING IN THE PERINATAL PERIOD

Maternal causes of perinatal morbidity and mortality (760-763)

760	Fetus or newborn affected by maternal conditions which may be unrelated to present pregnancy
761	Fetus or newborn affected by maternal complications of pregnancy
762	Fetus or newborn affected by complications of placenta, cord, and membranes
763	Fetus or newborn affected by other complications of labor and delivery

Other conditions originating in the perinatal period (764-779)

764	Slow fetal growth and fetal malnutrition
765	Disorders relating to short gestation and unspecified low birthweight
766	Disorders relating to long gestation and high birthweight
767	Birth trauma
768	Intrauterine hypoxia and birth asphyxia
769	Respiratory distress syndrome
770	Other respiratory conditions of fetus and newborn
771	Infections specific to the perinatal period
772	Fetal and neonatal hemorrhage
773	Hemolytic disease of fetus or newborn, due to isoimmunization
774	Other perinatal jaundice
775	Endocrine and metabolic disturbances specific to the fetus and newborn
776	Hematological disorders of fetus and newborn
777	Perinatal disorders of digestive system
778	Conditions involving the integument and temperature regulation of fetus and newborn
779	Other and ill-defined conditions originating in the perinatal period

16. SYMPTOMS, SIGNS, AND ILL-DEFINED CONDITIONS

Symptoms (780-789)

780	General symptoms
781	Symptoms involving nervous and musculoskeletal systems
782	Symptoms involving skin and other integumentary tissue
783	Symptoms concerning nutrition, metabolism, and development
784	Symptoms involving head and neck
785	Symptoms involving cardiovascular system
786	Symptoms involving respiratory system and other chest symptoms
787	Symptoms involving digestive system
788	Symptoms involving urinary system
789	Other symptoms involving abdomen and pelvis

Nonspecific abnormal findings (790-796)

790	Nonspecific findings on examination of blood
791	Nonspecific findings on examination of urine
792	Nonspecific abnormal findings in other body substances
793	Nonspecific abnormal findings on radiological and other examination of body structure
794	Nonspecific abnormal results of function studies
795	Nonspecific abnormal histological and immunological findings
796	Other nonspecific abnormal findings

Ill-defined and unknown causes of morbidity and mortality (797-799)

797	Senility without mention of psychosis
798	Sudden death, cause unknown
799	Other ill-defined and unknown causes of morbidity and mortality

17. INJURY AND POISONING

Fracture of skull (800-804)

800	Fracture of vault of skull
801	Fracture of base of skull
802	Fracture of face bones
803	Other and unqualified skull fractures
804	Multiple fractures involving skull or face with other bones

Fracture of spine and trunk (805-809)

805	Fracture of vertebral column without mention of spinal cord lesion
806	Fracture of vertebral column with spinal cord lesion
807	Fracture of rib(s), sternum, larynx, and trachea
808	Fracture of pelvis
809	Ill-defined fractures of bones of trunk

Fracture of upper limb (810-819)

810	Fracture of clavicle
811	Fracture of scapula
812	Fracture of humerus
813	Fracture of radius and ulna
814	Fracture of carpal bone(s)
815	Fracture of metacarpal bone(s)
816	Fracture of one or more phalanges of hand
817	Multiple fractures of hand bones
818	Ill-defined fractures of upper limb
819	Multiple fractures involving both upper limbs, and upper limb with rib(s) and sternum

Fracture of lower limb (820-829)

820	Fracture of neck of femur
821	Fracture of other and unspecified parts of femur
822	Fracture of patella
823	Fracture of tibia and fibula
824	Fracture of ankle
825	Fracture of one or more tarsal and metatarsal bones
826	Fracture of one or more phalanges of foot
827	Other, multiple, and ill-defined fractures of lower limb
828	Multiple fractures involving both lower limbs, lower with upper limb, and lower limb(s) with rib(s) and sternum
829	Fracture of unspecified bones

Dislocation (830-839)

830	Dislocation of jaw
831	Dislocation of shoulder
832	Dislocation of elbow
833	Dislocation of wrist
834	Dislocation of finger
835	Dislocation of hip
836	Dislocation of knee
837	Dislocation of ankle
838	Dislocation of foot
839	Other, multiple, and ill-defined dislocations

Sprains and strains of joints and adjacent muscles (840-848)

840	Sprains and strains of shoulder and upper arm
841	Sprains and strains of elbow and forearm
842	Sprains and strains of wrist and hand
843	Sprains and strains of hip and thigh
844	Sprains and strains of knee and leg
845	Sprains and strains of ankle and foot
846	Sprains and strains of sacroiliac region
847	Sprains and strains of other and unspecified parts of back
848	Other and ill-defined sprains and strains

Intracranial injury, excluding those with skull fracture (850-854)

850	Concussion
851	Cerebral laceration and contusion
852	Subarachnoid, subdural, and extradural hemorrhage, following injury
853	Other and unspecified intracranial hemorrhage following injury
854	Intracranial injury of other and unspecified nature

Internal injury of chest, abdomen, and pelvis (860-869)

860	Traumatic pneumothorax and hemothorax
861	Injury to heart and lung
862	Injury to other and unspecified intrathoracic organs
863	Injury to gastrointestinal tract
864	Injury to liver
865	Injury to spleen
866	Injury to kidney
867	Injury to pelvic organs
868	Injury to other intra-abdominal organs
869	Internal injury to unspecified or ill-defined organs

Open wound of head, neck, and trunk (870-879)

870	Open wound of ocular adnexa
871	Open wound of eyeball
872	Open wound of ear
873	Other open wound of head
874	Open wound of neck
875	Open wound of chest (wall)
876	Open wound of back
877	Open wound of buttock

APPENDIX E: LIST OF THREE-DIGIT CATEGORIES

878 Open wound of genital organs (external), including traumatic amputation
879 Open wound of other and unspecified sites, except limbs

Open wound of upper limb (880-887)
880 Open wound of shoulder and upper arm
881 Open wound of elbow, forearm, and wrist
882 Open wound of hand except finger(s) alone
883 Open wound of finger(s)
884 Multiple and unspecified open wound of upper limb
885 Traumatic amputation of thumb (complete) (partial)
886 Traumatic amputation of other finger(s) (complete) (partial)
887 Traumatic amputation of arm and hand (complete) (partial)

Open wound of lower limb (890-897)
890 Open wound of hip and thigh
891 Open wound of knee, leg [except thigh], and ankle
892 Open wound of foot except toe(s) alone
893 Open wound of toe(s)
894 Multiple and unspecified open wound of lower limb
895 Traumatic amputation of toe(s) (complete) (partial)
896 Traumatic amputation of foot (complete) (partial)
897 Traumatic amputation of leg(s) (complete) (partial)

Injury to blood vessels (900-904)
900 Injury to blood vessels of head and neck
901 Injury to blood vessels of thorax
902 Injury to blood vessels of abdomen and pelvis
903 Injury to blood vessels of upper extremity
904 Injury to blood vessels of lower extremity and unspecified sites

Late effects of injuries, poisonings, toxic effects, and other external causes (905-909)
905 Late effects of musculoskeletal and connective tissue injuries
906 Late effects of injuries to skin and subcutaneous tissues
907 Late effects of injuries to the nervous system
908 Late effects of other and unspecified injuries
909 Late effects of other and unspecified external causes

Superficial injury (910-919)
910 Superficial injury of face, neck, and scalp except eye
911 Superficial injury of trunk
912 Superficial injury of shoulder and upper arm
913 Superficial injury of elbow, forearm, and wrist
914 Superficial injury of hand(s) except finger(s) alone
915 Superficial injury of finger(s)
916 Superficial injury of hip, thigh, leg, and ankle
917 Superficial injury of foot and toe(s)
918 Superficial injury of eye and adnexa
919 Superficial injury of other, multiple, and unspecified sites

Contusion with intact skin surface (920-924)
920 Contusion of face, scalp, and neck except eye(s)
921 Contusion of eye and adnexa
922 Contusion of trunk
923 Contusion of upper limb
924 Contusion of lower limb and of other and unspecified sites

Crushing injury (925-929)
925 Crushing injury of face, scalp, and neck
926 Crushing injury of trunk
927 Crushing injury of upper limb
928 Crushing injury of lower limb
929 Crushing injury of multiple and unspecified sites

Effects of foreign body entering through orifice (930-939)
930 Foreign body on external eye
931 Foreign body in ear
932 Foreign body in nose
933 Foreign body in pharynx and larynx
934 Foreign body in trachea, bronchus, and lung
935 Foreign body in mouth, esophagus, and stomach
936 Foreign body in intestine and colon
937 Foreign body in anus and rectum
938 Foreign body in digestive system, unspecified
939 Foreign body in genitourinary tract

Burns (940-949)
940 Burn confined to eye and adnexa
941 Burn of face, head, and neck
942 Burn of trunk
943 Burn of upper limb, except wrist and hand
944 Burn of wrist(s) and hand(s)
945 Burn of lower limb(s)
946 Burns of multiple specified sites
947 Burn of internal organs
948 Burns classified according to extent of body surface involved
949 Burn, unspecified

Injury to nerves and spinal cord (950-957)
950 Injury to optic nerve and pathways
951 Injury to other cranial nerve(s)
952 Spinal cord injury without evidence of spinal bone injury
953 Injury to nerve roots and spinal plexus
954 Injury to other nerve(s) of trunk excluding shoulder and pelvic girdles
955 Injury to peripheral nerve(s) of shoulder girdle and upper limb
956 Injury to peripheral nerve(s) of pelvic girdle and lower limb
957 Injury to other and unspecified nerves

Certain traumatic complications and unspecified injuries (958-959)
958 Certain early complications of trauma
959 Injury, other and unspecified

Poisoning by drugs, medicinals and biological substances (960-979)
960 Poisoning by antibiotics
961 Poisoning by other anti-infectives
962 Poisoning by hormones and synthetic substitutes
963 Poisoning by primarily systemic agents
964 Poisoning by agents primarily affecting blood constituents
965 Poisoning by analgesics, antipyretics, and antirheumatics
966 Poisoning by anticonvulsants and anti-Parkinsonism drugs
967 Poisoning by sedatives and hypnotics
968 Poisoning by other central nervous system depressants and anesthetics
969 Poisoning by psychotropic agents
970 Poisoning by central nervous system stimulants
971 Poisoning by drugs primarily affecting the autonomic nervous system
972 Poisoning by agents primarily affecting the cardiovascular system
973 Poisoning by agents primarily affecting the gastrointestinal system
974 Poisoning by water, mineral, and uric acid metabolism drugs
975 Poisoning by agents primarily acting on the smooth and skeletal muscles and respiratory system
976 Poisoning by agents primarily affecting skin and mucous membrane, ophthalmological, otorhinolaryngological, and dental drugs
977 Poisoning by other and unspecified drugs and medicinals
978 Poisoning by bacterial vaccines
979 Poisoning by other vaccines and biological substances

Toxic effects of substances chiefly nonmedicinal as to source (980-989)
980 Toxic effect of alcohol
981 Toxic effect of petroleum products
982 Toxic effect of solvents other than petroleum-based
983 Toxic effect of corrosive aromatics, acids, and caustic alkalis
984 Toxic effect of lead and its compounds (including fumes)
985 Toxic effect of other metals
986 Toxic effect of carbon monoxide
987 Toxic effect of other gases, fumes, or vapors
988 Toxic effect of noxious substances eaten as food
989 Toxic effect of other substances, chiefly nonmedicinal as to source

Other and unspecified effects of external causes (990-995)
990 Effects of radiation, unspecified
991 Effects of reduced temperature
992 Effects of heat and light
993 Effects of air pressure
994 Effects of other external causes
995 Certain adverse effects, not elsewhere classified

Complications of surgical and medical care, not elsewhere classified (996-999)
996 Complications peculiar to certain specified procedures
997 Complications affecting specified body systems, not elsewhere classified
998 Other complications of procedures, not elsewhere classified
999 Complications of medical care, not elsewhere classified

APPENDIX E: LIST OF THREE-DIGIT CATEGORIES

SUPPLEMENTARY CLASSIFICATION OF FACTORS INFLUENCING HEALTH STATUS AND CONTACT WITH HEALTH SERVICES

Persons with potential health hazards related to communicable diseases (V01-V09)
- V01 Contact with or exposure to communicable diseases
- V02 Carrier or suspected carrier of infectious diseases
- V03 Need for prophylactic vaccination and inoculation against bacterial diseases
- V04 Need for prophylactic vaccination and inoculation against certain viral diseases
- V05 Need for other prophylactic vaccination and inoculation against single diseases
- V06 Need for prophylactic vaccination and inoculation against combinations of diseases
- V07 Need for isolation and other prophylactic measures
- V08 Asymptomatic human immunodeficiency virus [HIV] infection status
- V09 Infection with drug-resistant microorganisms

Persons with potential health hazards related to personal and family history (V10-V19)
- V10 Personal history of malignant neoplasm
- V11 Personal history of mental disorder
- V12 Personal history of certain other diseases
- V13 Personal history of other diseases
- V14 Personal history of allergy to medicinal agents
- V15 Other personal history presenting hazards to health
- V16 Family history of malignant neoplasm
- V17 Family history of certain chronic disabling diseases
- V18 Family history of certain other specific conditions
- V19 Family history of other conditions

Persons encountering health services in circumstances related to reproduction and development (V20-V29)
- V20 Health supervision of infant or child
- V21 Constitutional states in development
- V22 Normal pregnancy
- V23 Supervision of high-risk pregnancy
- V24 Postpartum care and examination
- V25 Encounter for contraceptive management
- V26 Procreative management
- V27 Outcome of delivery
- V28 Antenatal screening
- V29 Observation and evaluation of newborns and infants for suspected condition not found

Liveborn infants according to type of birth (V30-V39)
- V30 Single liveborn
- V31 Twin, mate liveborn
- V32 Twin, mate stillborn
- V33 Twin, unspecified
- V34 Other multiple, mates all liveborn
- V35 Other multiple, mates all stillborn
- V36 Other multiple, mates live- and stillborn
- V37 Other multiple, unspecified
- V39 Unspecified

Persons with a condition influencing their health status (V40-V49)
- V40 Mental and behavioral problems
- V41 Problems with special senses and other special functions
- V42 Organ or tissue replaced by transplant
- V43 Organ or tissue replaced by other means
- V44 Artificial opening status
- V45 Other postsurgical states
- V46 Other dependence on machines
- V47 Other problems with internal organs
- V48 Problems with head, neck, and trunk
- V49 Problems with limbs and other problems

Persons encountering health services for specific procedures and aftercare (V50-V59)
- V50 Elective surgery for purposes other than remedying health states
- V51 Aftercare involving the use of plastic surgery
- V52 Fitting and adjustment of prosthetic device
- V53 Fitting and adjustment of other device
- V54 Other orthopedic aftercare
- V55 Attention to artificial openings
- V56 Encounter for dialysis and dialysis catheter care
- V57 Care involving use of rehabilitation procedures
- V58 Encounter for other and unspecified procedures and aftercare
- V59 Donors

Persons encountering health services in other circumstances (V60-V69)
- V60 Housing, household, and economic circumstances
- V61 Other family circumstances
- V62 Other psychosocial circumstances
- V63 Unavailability of other medical facilities for care
- V64 Persons encountering health services for specific procedures, not carried out
- V65 Other persons seeking consultation without complaint or sickness
- V66 Convalescence and palliative care
- V67 Follow-up examination
- V68 Encounters for administrative purposes
- V69 Problems related to lifestyle

Persons without reported diagnosis encountered during examination and investigation of individuals and populations (V70-V83)
- V70 General medical examination
- V71 Observation and evaluation for suspected conditions not found
- V72 Special investigations and examinations
- V73 Special screening examination for viral and chlamydial diseases
- V74 Special screening examination for bacterial and spirochetal diseases
- V75 Special screening examination for other infectious diseases
- V76 Special screening for malignant neoplasms
- V77 Special screening for endocrine, nutritional, metabolic, and immunity disorders
- V78 Special screening for disorders of blood and blood-forming organs
- V79 Special screening for mental disorders and developmental handicaps
- V80 Special screening for neurological, eye, and ear diseases
- V81 Special screening for cardiovascular, respiratory, and genitourinary diseases
- V82 Special screening for other conditions
- V83 Genetic carrier status

SUPPLEMENTARY CLASSIFICATION OF EXTERNAL CAUSES OF INJURY AND POISONING

Railway accidents (E800-E807)
- E800 Railway accident involving collision with rolling stock
- E801 Railway accident involving collision with other object
- E802 Railway accident involving derailment without antecedent collision
- E803 Railway accident involving explosion, fire, or burning
- E804 Fall in, on, or from railway train
- E805 Hit by rolling stock
- E806 Other specified railway accident
- E807 Railway accident of unspecified nature

Motor vehicle traffic accidents (E810-E819)
- E810 Motor vehicle traffic accident involving collision with train
- E811 Motor vehicle traffic accident involving re-entrant collision with another motor vehicle
- E812 Other motor vehicle traffic accident involving collision with another motor vehicle
- E813 Motor vehicle traffic accident involving collision with other vehicle
- E814 Motor vehicle traffic accident involving collision with pedestrian
- E815 Other motor vehicle traffic accident involving collision on the highway
- E816 Motor vehicle traffic accident due to loss of control, without collision on the highway
- E817 Noncollision motor vehicle traffic accident while boarding or alighting
- E818 Other noncollision motor vehicle traffic accident
- E819 Motor vehicle traffic accident of unspecified nature

Motor vehicle nontraffic accidents (E820-E825)
- E820 Nontraffic accident involving motor-driven snow vehicle
- E821 Nontraffic accident involving other off-road motor vehicle
- E822 Other motor vehicle nontraffic accident involving collision with moving object
- E823 Other motor vehicle nontraffic accident involving collision with stationary object
- E824 Other motor vehicle nontraffic accident while boarding and alighting
- E825 Other motor vehicle nontraffic accident of other and unspecified nature

Other road vehicle accidents (E826-E829)
- E826 Pedal cycle accident
- E827 Animal-drawn vehicle accident

APPENDIX E: LIST OF THREE-DIGIT CATEGORIES

E828 Accident involving animal being ridden
E829 Other road vehicle accidents

Water transport accidents (E830-E838)
E830 Accident to watercraft causing submersion
E831 Accident to watercraft causing other injury
E832 Other accidental submersion or drowning in water transport accident
E833 Fall on stairs or ladders in water transport
E834 Other fall from one level to another in water transport
E835 Other and unspecified fall in water transport
E836 Machinery accident in water transport
E837 Explosion, fire, or burning in watercraft
E838 Other and unspecified water transport accident

Air and space transport accidents (E840-E845)
E840 Accident to powered aircraft at take-off or landing
E841 Accident to powered aircraft, other and unspecified
E842 Accident to unpowered aircraft
E843 Fall in, on, or from aircraft
E844 Other specified air transport accidents
E845 Accident involving spacecraft

Vehicle accidents, not elsewhere classifiable (E846-E849)
E846 Accidents involving powered vehicles used solely within the buildings and premises of an industrial or commercial establishment
E847 Accidents involving cable cars not running on rails
E848 Accidents involving other vehicles, not elsewhere classifiable
E849 Place of occurrence

Accidental poisoning by drugs, medicinal substances, and biologicals (E850-E858)
E850 Accidental poisoning by analgesics, antipyretics, and antirheumatics
E851 Accidental poisoning by barbiturates
E852 Accidental poisoning by other sedatives and hypnotics
E853 Accidental poisoning by tranquilizers
E854 Accidental poisoning by other psychotropic agents
E855 Accidental poisoning by other drugs acting on central and autonomic nervous systems
E856 Accidental poisoning by antibiotics
E857 Accidental poisoning by anti-infectives
E858 Accidental poisoning by other drugs

Accidental poisoning by other solid and liquid substances, gases, and vapors (E860-E869)
E860 Accidental poisoning by alcohol, not elsewhere classified
E861 Accidental poisoning by cleansing and polishing agents, disinfectants, paints, and varnishes
E862 Accidental poisoning by petroleum products, other solvents and their vapors, not elsewhere classified
E863 Accidental poisoning by agricultural and horticultural chemical and pharmaceutical preparations other than plant foods and fertilizers
E864 Accidental poisoning by corrosives and caustics, not elsewhere classified
E865 Accidental poisoning from poisonous foodstuffs and poisonous plants
E866 Accidental poisoning by other and unspecified solid and liquid substances
E867 Accidental poisoning by gas distributed by pipeline
E868 Accidental poisoning by other utility gas and other carbon monoxide
E869 Accidental poisoning by other gases and vapors

Misadventures to patients during surgical and medical care (E870-E876)
E870 Accidental cut, puncture, perforation, or hemorrhage during medical care
E871 Foreign object left in body during procedure
E872 Failure of sterile precautions during procedure
E873 Failure in dosage
E874 Mechanical failure of instrument or apparatus during procedure
E875 Contaminated or infected blood, other fluid, drug, or biological substance
E876 Other and unspecified misadventures during medical care

Surgical and medical procedures as the cause of abnormal reaction of patient or later complication, without mention of misadventure at the time of procedure (E878-E879)
E878 Surgical operation and other surgical procedures as the cause of abnormal reaction of patient, or of later complication, without mention of misadventure at the time of operation
E879 Other procedures, without mention of misadventure at the time of procedure, as the cause of abnormal reaction of patient, or of later complication

Accidental falls (E880-E888)
E880 Fall on or from stairs or steps
E881 Fall on or from ladders or scaffolding
E882 Fall from or out of building or other structure
E883 Fall into hole or other opening in surface
E884 Other fall from one level to another
E885 Fall on same level from slipping, tripping, or stumbling
E886 Fall on same level from collision, pushing or shoving, by or with other person
E887 Fracture, cause unspecified
E888 Other and unspecified fall

Accidents caused by fire and flames (E890-E899)
E890 Conflagration in private dwelling
E891 Conflagration in other and unspecified building or structure
E892 Conflagration not in building or structure
E893 Accident caused by ignition of clothing
E894 Ignition of highly inflammable material
E895 Accident caused by controlled fire in private dwelling
E896 Accident caused by controlled fire in other and unspecified building or structure
E897 Accident caused by controlled fire not in building or structure
E898 Accident caused by other specified fire and flames
E899 Accident caused by unspecified fire

Accidents due to natural and environmental factors (E900-E909)
E900 Excessive heat
E901 Excessive cold
E902 High and low air pressure and changes in air pressure
E903 Travel and motion
E904 Hunger, thirst, exposure, and neglect
E905 Venomous animals and plants as the cause of poisoning and toxic reactions
E906 Other injury caused by animals
E907 Lightning
E908 Cataclysmic storms, and floods resulting from storms
E909 Cataclysmic earth surface movements and eruptions

Accidents caused by submersion, suffocation, and foreign bodies (E910-E915)
E910 Accidental drowning and submersion
E911 Inhalation and ingestion of food causing obstruction of respiratory tract or suffocation
E912 Inhalation and ingestion of other object causing obstruction of respiratory tract or suffocation
E913 Accidental mechanical suffocation
E914 Foreign body accidentally entering eye and adnexa
E915 Foreign body accidentally entering other orifice

Other accidents (E916-E928)
E916 Struck accidentally by falling object
E917 Striking against or struck accidentally by objects or persons
E918 Caught accidentally in or between objects
E919 Accidents caused by machinery
E920 Accidents caused by cutting and piercing instruments or objects
E921 Accident caused by explosion of pressure vessel
E922 Accident caused by firearm missile
E923 Accident caused by explosive material
E924 Accident caused by hot substance or object, caustic or corrosive material, and steam
E925 Accident caused by electric current
E926 Exposure to radiation
E927 Overexertion and strenuous movements

APPENDIX E: LIST OF THREE-DIGIT CATEGORIES

E928 Other and unspecified environmental and accidental causes

Late effects of accidental injury (E929)
E929 Late effects of accidental injury

Drugs, medicinal and biological substances causing adverse effects in therapeutic use (E930-E949)
E930 Antibiotics
E931 Other anti-infectives
E932 Hormones and synthetic substitutes
E933 Primarily systemic agents
E934 Agents primarily affecting blood constituents
E935 Analgesics, antipyretics, and antirheumatics
E936 Anticonvulsants and anti-Parkinsonism drugs
E937 Sedatives and hypnotics
E938 Other central nervous system depressants and anesthetics
E939 Psychotropic agents
E940 Central nervous system stimulants
E941 Drugs primarily affecting the autonomic nervous system
E942 Agents primarily affecting the cardiovascular system
E943 Agents primarily affecting gastrointestinal system
E944 Water, mineral, and uric acid metabolism drugs
E945 Agents primarily acting on the smooth and skeletal muscles and respiratory system
E946 Agents primarily affecting skin and mucous membrane, ophthalmological, otorhinolaryngological, and dental drugs
E947 Other and unspecified drugs and medicinal substances
E948 Bacterial vaccines
E949 Other vaccines and biological substances

Suicide and self-inflicted injury (E950-E959)
E950 Suicide and self-inflicted poisoning by solid or liquid substances
E951 Suicide and self-inflicted poisoning by gases in domestic use
E952 Suicide and self-inflicted poisoning by other gases and vapors
E953 Suicide and self-inflicted injury by hanging, strangulation, and suffocation
E954 Suicide and self-inflicted injury by submersion [drowning]
E955 Suicide and self-inflicted injury by firearms and explosives
E956 Suicide and self-inflicted injury by cutting and piercing instruments
E957 Suicide and self-inflicted injuries by jumping from high place
E958 Suicide and self-inflicted injury by other and unspecified means
E959 Late effects of self-inflicted injury

Homicide and injury purposely inflicted by other persons (E960-E969)
E960 Fight, brawl, and rape
E961 Assault by corrosive or caustic substance, except poisoning
E962 Assault by poisoning
E963 Assault by hanging and strangulation
E964 Assault by submersion [drowning]
E965 Assault by firearms and explosives
E966 Assault by cutting and piercing instrument
E967 Child and adult battering and other maltreatment
E968 Assault by other and unspecified means
E969 Late effects of injury purposely inflicted by other person

Legal intervention (E970-E978)
E970 Injury due to legal intervention by firearms
E971 Injury due to legal intervention by explosives
E972 Injury due to legal intervention by gas
E973 Injury due to legal intervention by blunt object
E974 Injury due to legal intervention by cutting and piercing instruments
E975 Injury due to legal intervention by other specified means
E976 Injury due to legal intervention by unspecified means
E977 Late effects of injuries due to legal intervention
E978 Legal execution

Terrorism (E979)
E979 Terrorism

Injury undetermined whether accidentally or purposely inflicted (E980-E989)
E980 Poisoning by solid or liquid substances, undetermined whether accidentally or purposely inflicted
E981 Poisoning by gases in domestic use, undetermined whether accidentally or purposely inflicted
E982 Poisoning by other gases, undetermined whether accidentally or purposely inflicted
E983 Hanging, strangulation, or suffocation, undetermined whether accidentally or purposely inflicted
E984 Submersion [drowning], undetermined whether accidentally or purposely inflicted
E985 Injury by firearms and explosives, undetermined whether accidentally or purposely inflicted
E986 Injury by cutting and piercing instruments, undetermined whether accidentally or purposely inflicted
E987 Falling from high place, undetermined whether accidentally or purposely inflicted
E988 Injury by other and unspecified means, undetermined whether accidentally or purposely inflicted
E989 Late effects of injury, undetermined whether accidentally or purposely inflicted

Injury resulting from operations of war (E990-E999)
E990 Injury due to war operations by fires and conflagrations
E991 Injury due to war operations by bullets and fragments
E992 Injury due to war operations by explosion of marine weapons
E993 Injury due to war operations by other explosion
E994 Injury due to war operations by destruction of aircraft
E995 Injury due to war operations by other and unspecified forms of conventional warfare
E996 Injury due to war operations by nuclear weapons
E997 Injury due to war operations by other forms of unconventional warfare
E998 Injury due to war operations but occurring after cessation of hostilities
E999 Late effects of injury due to war operations

Index to Procedures

A

Abbe operation
  construction of vagina 70.61
  intestinal anastomosis — *see* Anastomosis, intestine
Abciximab, infusion 99.20
Abdominocentesis 54.91
Abdominohysterectomy 68.4
Abdominoplasty 86.83
Abdominoscopy 54.21
Abdominouterotomy 68.0
  obstetrical 74.99
Abduction, arytenoid 31.69
Ablation
  biliary tract (lesion) by ERCP 51.64
  endometrial (hysteroscopic) 68.23
  inner ear (cryosurgery) (ultrasound) 20.79
    by injection 20.72
  lesion
    esophagus 42.39
      endoscopic 42.33
    heart (ventricular) 37.33
      by cardiac catheter 37.34
    intestine
      large 45.49
        endoscopic 45.43
    large intestine 45.49
      endoscopic 45.43
  pituitary 07.69
    by
      cobalt 60 92.32
      implantation (strontium-yttrium) (Y) NEC 07.68
        transfrontal approach 07.64
        transphenoidal approach 07.65
      proton beam (Bragg peak) 92.33
  prostate
    by
      cryoablation 60.62
      laser, transurethral 60.21
      radical cryosurgery ablation (RCSA) 60.62
      radiofrequency thermotherapy 60.97
      transurethral needle ablation (TUNA) 60.97
Abortion, therapeutic 69.51
  by
    aspiration curettage 69.51
    dilation and curettage 69.01
    hysterectomy — *see* Hysterectomy
    hysterotomy 74.91
    insertion
      laminaria 69.93
      prostaglandin suppository 96.49
    intra-amniotic injection (saline) 75.0
Abrasion
  corneal epithelium 11.41
    for smear or culture 11.21
  epicardial surface 36.39
  pleural 34.6
  skin 86.25
Abscission, cornea 11.49
Absorptiometry
  photon (dual) (single) 88.98
Aburel operation (intra-amniotic injection for abortion) 75.0
Accouchement forcé 73.99
Acetabulectomy 77.85
Acetabuloplasty NEC 81.40
  with prosthetic implant 81.52
Achillorrhaphy 83.64
  delayed 83.62
Achillotenotomy 83.11
  plastic 83.85
Achillotomy 83.11
  plastic 83.85
Acid peel, skin 86.24
Acromionectomy 77.81
Acromioplasty 81.83
  for recurrent dislocation of shoulder 81.82
  partial replacement 81.81
  total replacement 81.80

Actinotherapy 99.82
Activities of daily living (ADL)
  therapy 93.83
  training for the blind 93.78
Acupuncture 99.92
  with smouldering moxa 93.35
  for anesthesia 99.91
Adams operation
  advancement of round ligament 69.22
  crushing of nasal septum 21.88
  excision of palmar fascia 82.35
Adenectomy — *see also* Excision, by site
  prostate NEC 60.69
    retropubic 60.4
Adenoidectomy (without tonsillectomy) 28.6
  with tonsillectomy 28.3
Adhesiolysis — *see also* Lysis, adhesions
  for collapse of lung 33.39
  middle ear 20.23
Adipectomy 86.83
Adjustment
  cardiac pacemaker program (reprogramming) — *omit code*
  cochlear prosthetic device (external components) 95.49
  dental 99.97
  occlusal 24.8
  spectacles 95.31
Administration (of) — *see also* Injection
  adhesion barrier substance 99.77
  antitoxins NEC 99.58
    botulism 99.57
    diphtheria 99.58
    gas gangrene 99.58
    scarlet fever 99.58
    tetanus 99.56
  Bender Visual-Motor Gestalt test 94.02
  Benton Visual Retention test 94.02
  inhaled nitric oxide 00.12
  intelligence test or scale (Stanford-Binet) (Wechsler) (adult) (children) 94.01
  Minnesota Multiphasic Personality Inventory (MMPI) 94.02
  MMPI (Minnesota Multiphasic Personality Inventory) 94.02
  neuroprotective agent 99.75
  psychologic test 94.02
  Stanford-Binet test 94.01
  toxoid
    diphtheria 99.36
      with tetanus and pertussis, combined (DTP) 99.39
    tetanus 99.38
      with diphtheria and pertussis, combined (DTP) 99.39
  vaccine — *see also* Vaccination
    BCG 99.33
    measles-mumps-rubella (MMR) 99.48
    poliomyelitis 99.41
    TAB 99.32
  Wechsler
    Intelligence Scale (adult) (children) 94.01
    Memory Scale 94.02
Adrenalectomy (unilateral) 07.22
  with partial removal of remaining gland 07.29
  bilateral 07.3
    partial 07.29
    subtotal 07.29
  complete 07.3
  partial NEC 07.29
  remaining gland 07.3
  subtotal NEC 07.29
  total 07.3
Adrenalorrhaphy 07.44
Adrenalotomy (with drainage) 07.41
Advancement
  extraocular muscle 15.12
    multiple (with resection or recession) 15.3
  eyelid muscle 08.59
  eye muscle 15.12
    multiple (with resection or recession) 15.3
  graft — *see* Graft
  leaflet (heart) 35.10

Advancement — *continued*
  pedicle (flap) 86.72
  profundus tendon (Wagner) 82.51
  round ligament 69.22
  tendon 83.71
    hand 82.51
      profundus (Wagner) 82.51
    Wagner (profundus tendon) 82.51
Albee operation
  bone peg, femoral neck 78.05
  graft for slipping patella 78.06
  sliding inlay graft, tibia 78.07
Albert operation (arthrodesis of knee) 81.22
Aldridge (-Studdiford) operation (urethral sling) 59.5
Alexander operation
  prostatectomy
    perineal 60.62
    suprapubic 60.3
  shortening of round ligaments 69.22
Alexander-Adams operation (shortening of round ligaments) 69.22
Alimentation, parenteral 99.29
Allograft — *see* Graft
Almoor operation (extrapetrosal drainage) 20.22
Altemeier operation (perineal rectal pull-through) 48.49
Alveolectomy (interradicular) (intraseptal) (radical) (simple) (with graft) (with implant) 24.5
Alveoloplasty (with graft or implant) 24.5
Alveolotomy (apical) 24.0
Ambulatory cardiac monitoring (ACM) 89.50
Ammon operation (dacryocystotomy) 09.53
Amniocentesis (transuterine) (diagnostic) 75.1
  with intra-amniotic injection of saline 75.0
Amniography 87.81
Amnioinfusion 75.37
Amnioscopy, internal 75.31
Amniotomy 73.09
  to induce labor 73.01
Amputation (cineplastic) (closed flap) (guillotine) (kineplastic) (open) 84.91
  abdominopelvic 84.19
  above-elbow 84.07
  above-knee (AK) 84.17
  ankle (disarticulation) 84.13
    through malleoli of tibia and fibula 84.14
  arm NEC 84.00
    through
      carpals 84.03
      elbow (disarticulation) 84.06
      forearm 84.05
      humerus 84.07
      shoulder (disarticulation) 84.08
      wrist (disarticulation) 84.04
    upper 84.07
  Batch-Spittler-McFaddin (knee disarticulation) 84.16
  below-knee (BK) NEC 84.15
    conversion into above-knee amputation 84.17
  Boyd (hip disarticulation) 84.18
  Callander's (knee disarticulation) 84.16
  carpals 84.03
  cervix 67.4
  Chopart's (midtarsal) 84.12
  clitoris 71.4
  Dieffenbach (hip disarticulation) 84.18
  Dupuytren's (shoulder disarticulation) 84.08
  ear, external 18.39
  elbow (disarticulation) 84.06
  finger, except thumb 84.01
    thumb 84.02
  foot (middle) 84.12
  forearm 84.05
  forefoot 84.12
  forequarter 84.09
  Gordon-Taylor (hindquarter) 84.19
  Gritti-Stokes (knee disarticulation) 84.16
  Guyon (ankle) 84.13
  hallux 84.11

Index to Procedures

Amputation — continued
- hand 84.03
- Hey's (foot) 84.12
- hindquarter 84.19
- hip (disarticulation) 84.18
- humerus 84.07
- interscapulothoracic 84.09
- interthoracoscapular 84.09
- King-Steelquist (hindquarter) 84.19
- Kirk (thigh) 84.17
- knee (disarticulation) 84.16
- Kutler (revision of current traumatic amputation of finger) 84.01
- Larry (shoulder disarticulation) 84.08
- leg NEC 84.10
  - above knee (AK) 84.17
  - below knee (BK) 84.15
  - through
    - ankle (disarticulation) 84.13
    - femur (AK) 84.17
    - foot 84.12
    - hip (disarticulation) 84.18
    - tibia and fibula (BK) 84.15
- Lisfranc
  - foot 84.12
  - shoulder (disarticulation) 84.08
- Littlewood (forequarter) 84.09
- lower limb NEC (see also Amputation, leg) 84.10
- Mazet (knee disarticulation) 84.16
- metacarpal 84.03
- metatarsal 84.11
  - head (bunionectomy) 77.59
- metatarsophalangeal (joint) 84.11
- midtarsal 84.12
- nose 21.4
- penis (circle) (complete) (flap) (partial) (radical) 64.3
- Pirogoff's (ankle amputation through malleoli of tibia and fibula) 84.14
- ray
  - finger 84.01
  - foot 84.11
  - toe (metatarsal head) 84.11
- root (tooth) (apex) 23.73
  - with root canal therapy 23.72
- shoulder (disarticulation) 84.08
- Sorondo-Ferré (hindquarter) 84.19
- S.P. Rogers (knee disarticulation) 84.16
- supracondyler, above-knee 84.17
- supramalleolar, foot 84.14
- Syme's (ankle amputation through malleoli of tibia and fibula) 84.14
- thigh 84.17
- thumb 84.02
- toe (through metatarsophalangeal joint) 84.11
- transcarpal 84.03
- transmetatarsal 84.12
- upper limb NEC (see also Amputation, arm) 84.00
- wrist (disarticulation) 84.04

Amygdalohippocampotomy 01.39

Amygdalotomy 01.39

Analysis
- character 94.03
- gastric 89.39
- psychologic 94.31
- transactional
  - group 94.44
  - individual 94.39

Anastomosis
- abdominal artery to coronary artery 36.17
- accessory-facial nerve 04.72
- accessory-hypoglossal nerve 04.73
- anus (with formation of endorectal ileal pouch) 45.95
- aorta (descending)-pulmonary (artery) 39.0
- aorta-renal artery 39.24
- aorta-subclavian artery 39.22
- aortoceliac 39.26
- aorto(ilio)femoral 39.25
- aortomesenteric 39.26
- appendix 47.99
- arteriovenous NEC 39.29
  - for renal dialysis 39.27

Anastomosis — continued
- artery (suture of distal to proximal end) 39.31
  - with
    - bypass graft 39.29
      - extracranial-intracranial [EC-IC] 39.28
    - excision or resection of vessel — see Arteriectomy, with anastomosis, by site
  - revision 39.49
- bile ducts 51.39
- bladder NEC 57.88
  - with
    - isolated segment of intestine 57.87 [45.50]
    - colon (sigmoid) 57.87 [45.52]
    - ileum 57.87 [45.51]
    - open loop of ileum 57.87 [45.51]
  - to intestine 57.88
    - ileum 57.87 [45.51]
- bowel (see also Anastomosis, intestine) 45.90
- bronchotracheal 33.48
- bronchus 33.48
- carotid-subclavian artery 39.22
- caval-mesenteric vein 39.1
- caval-pulmonary artery 39.21
- cervicoesophageal 42.59
- colohypopharyngeal (intrathoracic) 42.55
  - antesternal or antethoracic 42.65
- common bile duct 51.39
- common pulmonary trunk and left atrium (posterior wall) 35.82
- cystic bile duct 51.39
- cystocolic 57.88
- epididymis to vas deferens 63.83
- esophagocolic (intrathoracic) NEC 42.56
  - with interposition 42.55
  - antesternal or antethoracic NEC 42.66
    - with interposition 42.65
- esophagocologastric (intrathoracic) 42.55
  - antesternal or antethoracic 42.65
- esophagoduodenal (intrathoracic) NEC 42.54
  - with interposition 42.53
- esophagoenteric (intrathoracic) NEC (see also Anastomosis, esophagus, to intestinal segment) 42.54
  - antesternal or antethoracic NEC (see also Anastomosis, esophagus, antesternal, to intestinal segment) 42.64
- esophagoesophageal (intrathoracic) 42.51
  - antesternal or antethoracic 42.61
- esophagogastric (intrathoracic) 42.52
  - antesternal or antethoracic 42.62
- esophagus (intrapleural) (intrathoracic) (retrosternal) NEC 42.59
  - with
    - gastrectomy (partial) 43.5
      - complete or total 43.99
    - interposition (of) NEC 42.58
      - colon 42.55
      - jejunum 42.53
      - small bowel 42.53
  - antesternal or antethoracic NEC 42.69
    - with
      - interposition (of) NEC 42.68
        - colon 42.65
        - jejunal loop 42.63
        - small bowel 42.63
        - rubber tube 42.68
    - to intestinal segment NEC 42.64
      - with interposition 42.68
        - colon NEC 42.66
          - with interposition 42.65
        - small bowel NEC 42.64
          - with interposition 42.63
    - to intestinal segment (intrathoracic) NEC 42.54
      - with interposition 42.58
        - antesternal or antethoracic NEC 42.64
          - with interposition 42.68
        - colon (intrathoracic) NEC 42.56
          - with interposition 42.55
          - antesternal or antethoracic 42.66
            - with interposition 42.65
        - small bowel NEC 42.54
          - with interposition 42.53
          - antesternal or antethoracic 42.64
            - with interposition 42.63

Anastomosis — continued
- facial-accessory nerve 04.72
- facial-hypoglossal nerve 04.71
- fallopian tube 66.73
  - by reanastomosis 66.79
- gallbladder 51.35
  - to
    - hepatic ducts 51.31
    - intestine 51.32
    - pancreas 51.33
    - stomach 51.34
- gastroepiploic artery to coronary artery 36.17
- hepatic duct 51.39
- hypoglossal-accessory nerve 04.73
- hypoglossal-facial nerve 04.71
- ileal loop to bladder 57.87 [45.51]
- ileoanal 45.95
- ileorectal 45.93
- inferior vena cava and portal vein 39.1
- internal mammary artery (to)
  - coronary artery (single vessel) 36.15
    - double vessel 36.16
  - myocardium 36.2
- intestine 45.90
  - large-to-anus 45.95
  - large-to-large 45.94
  - large-to-rectum 45.94
  - large-to-small 45.93
  - small-to-anus 45.95
  - small-to-large 45.93
  - small-to-rectal stump 45.92
  - small-to-small 45.91
- intrahepatic 51.79
- intrathoracic vessel NEC 39.23
- kidney (pelvis) 55.86
- lacrimal sac to conjunctiva 09.82
- left-to-right (systemic-pulmonary artery) 39.0
- lymphatic (channel) (peripheral) 40.9
- mesenteric-caval 39.1
- mesocaval 39.1
- nasolacrimal 09.81
- nerve (cranial) (peripheral) NEC 04.74
  - accessory-facial 04.72
  - accessory-hypoglossal 04.73
  - hypoglossal-facial 04.71
- pancreas (duct) (to) 52.96
  - bile duct 51.39
  - gall bladder 51.33
  - intestine 52.96
  - jejunum 52.96
  - stomach 52.96
- pleurothecal (with valve) 03.79
- portacaval 39.1
- portal vein to inferior vena cava 39.1
- pulmonary-aortic (Pott's) 39.0
- pulmonary artery and superior vena cava 39.21
- pulmonary-innominate artery (Blalock) 39.0
- pulmonary-subclavian artery (Blalock-Taussig) 39.0
- pulmonary vein and azygos vein 39.23
- pyeloileocutaneous 56.51
- pyeloureterovesical 55.86
- radial artery 36.19
- rectum, rectal NEC 48.74
  - stump to small intestine 45.92
- renal (pelvis) 55.86
  - vein and splenic vein 39.1
- renoportal 39.1
- salpingothecal (with valve) 03.79
- splenic to renal veins 39.1
- splenorenal (venous) 39.1
  - arterial 39.26
- subarachnoid-peritoneal (with valve) 03.71
- subarachnoid-ureteral (with valve) 03.72
- subclavian-aortic 39.22
- superior vena cava to pulmonary artery 39.21
- systemic-pulmonary artery 39.0
- thoracic artery (to)
  - coronary artery (single) 36.15
    - double 36.16
  - myocardium 36.2
- ureter (to) NEC 56.79
  - bladder 56.74
  - colon 56.71
  - ileal pouch (bladder) 56.51
  - ileum 56.71

Anastomosis — *continued*
- ureter (to) NEC — *continued*
  - intestine 56.71
  - skin 56.61
- ureterocalyceal 55.86
- ureterocolic 56.71
- ureterovesical 56.74
- urethra (end-to-end) 58.44
- vas deferens 63.82
- veins (suture of proximal to distal end) (with bypass graft) 39.29
  - with excision or resection of vessel — *see* Phlebectomy, with anastomosis, by site
  - mesenteric to vena cava 39.1
  - portal to inferior vena cava 39.1
  - revision 39.49
  - splenic and renal 39.1
- ventricle, ventricular (intracerebral) (with valve) (*see also* Shunt, ventricular) 02.2
- ventriculoatrial (with valve) 02.32
- ventriculocaval (with valve) 02.32
- ventriculomastoid (with valve) 02.31
- ventriculopleural (with valve) 02.33
- vesicle — *see* Anastomosis, bladder

Anderson operation (tibial lengthening) 78.37

Anel operation (dilation of lacrimal duct) 09.42

Anesthesia
- acupuncture for 99.91
- cryoanalgesia, nerve (cranial) (peripheral) 04.2
- spinal — *omit code*

Aneurysmectomy 38.60
- with
  - anastomosis 38.30
    - abdominal
      - artery 38.36
      - vein 38.37
    - aorta (arch) (ascending) (descending) 38.34
    - head and neck NEC 38.32
    - intracranial NEC 38.31
    - lower limb
      - artery 38.38
      - vein 38.39
    - thoracic NEC 38.35
    - upper limb (artery) (vein) 38.33
  - graft replacement (interposition) 38.40
    - abdominal
      - aorta 38.44
      - artery 38.46
      - vein 38.47
    - aorta (arch) (ascending) (descending thoracic)
      - abdominal 38.44
      - thoracic 38.45
      - thoracoabdominal 38.45 [38.44]
    - head and neck NEC 38.42
    - intracranial NEC 38.41
    - lower limb
      - artery 38.48
      - vein 38.49
    - thoracic NEC 38.45
    - upper limb (artery) (vein) 38.43
- abdominal
  - artery 38.66
  - vein 38.67
- aorta (arch) (ascending) (descending) 38.64
- atrial, auricular 37.32
- head and neck NEC 38.62
- heart 37.32
- intracranial NEC 38.61
- lower limb
  - artery 38.68
  - vein 38.69
- sinus of Valsalva 35.39
- thoracic NEC 38.65
- upper limb (artery) (vein) 38.63
- ventricle (myocardium) 37.32

Aneurysmoplasty — *see* Aneurysmorrhaphy

Aneurysmorrhaphy NEC 39.52
- by or with
  - anastomosis — *see* Aneurysmectomy, with anastomosis, by site
  - clipping 39.51

Aneurysmorrhaphy NEC — *continued*
- by or with — *continued*
  - coagulation 39.52
  - electrocoagulation 39.52
  - endovascular graft
    - abdominal aorta 39.71
    - lower extremity artery(s) 39.79
    - thoracic aorta 39.79
    - upper extremity artery(s) 39.79
  - excision or resection — *see also* Aneurysmectomy, by site
    - with
      - anastomosis — *see* Aneurysmectomy, with anastomosis, by site
      - graft replacement — *see* Aneurysmectomy, with graft replacement, by site
  - filipuncture 39.52
  - graft replacement — *see* Aneurysmectomy, with graft replacement, by site
  - methyl methacrylate 39.52
  - suture 39.52
  - wiring 39.52
  - wrapping 39.52
- Matas' 39.52

Aneurysmotomy — *see* Aneurysmectomy

Angiectomy
- with
  - anastomosis 38.30
    - abdominal
      - artery 38.36
      - vein 38.37
    - aorta (arch) (ascending) (descending) 38.34
    - head and neck NEC 38.32
    - intracranial NEC 38.31
    - lower limb
      - artery 38.38
      - vein 38.39
    - thoracic vessel NEC 38.35
    - upper limb (artery) (vein) 38.33
  - graft replacement (interposition) 38.40
    - abdominal
      - aorta 38.44
      - artery 38.46
      - vein 38.47
    - aorta (arch) (ascending) (descending thoracic)
      - abdominal 38.44
      - thoracic 38.45
      - thoracoabdominal 38.45 [38.44]
    - head and neck NEC 38.42
    - intracranial NEC 38.41
    - lower limb
      - artery 38.48
      - vein 38.49
    - thoracic vessel NEC 38.45
    - upper limb (artery) (vein) 38.43

Angiocardiography (selective) 88.50
- carbon dioxide (negative contrast) 88.58
- combined right and left heart 88.54
- left heart (aortic valve) (atrium) (ventricle) (ventricular outflow tract) 88.53
  - combined with right heart 88.54
- right heart (atrium) (pulmonary valve) (ventricle) (ventricular outflow tract) 88.52
  - combined with left heart 88.54
- vena cava (inferior) (superior) 88.51

Angiography (arterial) (*see also* Arteriography) 88.40
- by radioisotope — *see* Scan, radioisotope, by site
- by ultrasound — *see* Ultrasonography, by site
- basilar 88.41
- brachial 88.49
- carotid (internal) 88.41
- celiac 88.47
- cerebral (posterior circulation) 88.41
- coronary NEC 88.57
- eye (fluorescein) 95.12
- femoral 88.48
- heart 88.50
- intra-abdominal NEC 88.47
- intracranial 88.41

Angiography (*see also* Arteriography) — *continued*
- intrathoracic vessels NEC 88.44
- lower extremity NEC 88.48
- neck 88.41
- placenta 88.46
- pulmonary 88.43
- renal 88.45
- specified artery NEC 88.49
- transfemoral 88.48
- upper extremity NEC 88.49
- veins — *see* Phlebography
- vertebral 88.41

Angioplasty (laser) — *see also* Repair, blood vessel
- balloon (percutaneous transluminal) NEC 39.50
  - coronary artery (single vessel) 36.01
    - with thrombolytic agent infusion 36.02
    - multiple vessels 36.05
  - other sites (femoropopliteal) (iliac) (non-coronary) (renal) (vertebral) 39.50
- coronary 36.09
  - open chest approach 36.03
  - percutaneous transluminal (balloon) (single vessel) 36.01
    - with thrombolytic agent infusion 36.02
    - multiple vessels 36.05
- percutaneous transluminal (balloon) (single vessel) 39.50
  - basilar 39.50
  - carotid 39.50
  - coronary (balloon) (single vessel) 36.01
    - with thrombolytic agent infusion 36.02
    - multiple vessels 36.05
  - femoropopliteal 39.50
  - head and neck 39.50
  - iliac 39.50
  - lower extremity NOS 39.50
  - mesenteric 39.50
  - renal 39.50
  - upper extremity NOS 39.50
  - vertebral 39.50
- specified site NEC 39.50

Angiorrhaphy 39.30
- artery 39.31
- vein 39.32

Angioscopy, percutaneous 38.22
- eye (fluorescein) 95.12

Angiotomy 38.00
- abdominal
  - artery 38.06
  - vein 38.07
- aorta (arch) (ascending) (descending) 38.04
- head and neck NEC 38.02
- intracranial NEC 38.01
- lower limb
  - artery 38.08
  - vein 38.09
- thoracic NEC 38.05
- upper limb (artery) (vein) 38.03

Angiotripsy 39.98

Ankylosis, production of — *see* Arthrodesis

Annuloplasty (heart) (posteromedial) 35.33

Anoplasty 49.79
- with hemorrhoidectomy 49.46

Anoscopy 49.21

Antibiogram — *see* Examination, microscopic

Antiembolic filter, vena cava 38.7

Antiphobic treatment 94.39

Antrectomy
- mastoid 20.49
- maxillary 22.39
  - radical 22.31
- pyloric 43.6

Antrostomy — *see* Antrotomy

Antrotomy (exploratory) (nasal sinus) 22.2
- Caldwell-Luc (maxillary sinus) 22.39
  - with removal of membrane lining 22.31
- intranasal 22.2
  - with external approach (Caldwell-Luc) 22.39
    - radical 22.31

Antrotomy — *continued*
  maxillary (simple) 22.2
    with Caldwell-Luc approach 22.39
      with removal of membrane lining 22.31
    external (Caldwell-Luc approach) 22.39
      with removal of membrane lining 22.31
    radical (with removal of membrane lining) 22.31

Antrum window operation — *see* Antrotomy, maxillary

Aorticopulmonary window operation 39.59

Aortogram, aortography (abdominal) (retrograde) (selective) (translumbar) 88.42

Aortoplasty (aortic valve) (gusset type) 35.11

Aortotomy 38.04

Apexcardiogram (with ECG lead) 89.57

Apheresis, therapeutic — *see* category 99.7 ✓4ᵗʰ

Apicectomy
  lung 32.3
  petrous pyramid 20.59
  tooth (root) 23.73
    with root canal therapy 23.72

Apicoectomy 23.73
  with root canal therapy 23.72

Apicolysis (lung) 33.39

Apicostomy, alveolar 24.0

Aponeurectomy 83.42
  hand 82.33

Aponeurorrhaphy (*see also* Suture, tendon) 83.64
  hand (*see also* Suture, tendon, hand) 82.45

Aponeurotomy 83.13
  hand 82.11

Appendectomy (with drainage) 47.09
  incidental 47.19
    laparoscopic 47.11
  laparoscopic 47.01

Appendicectomy (with drainage) 47.09
  incidental 47.19
    laparoscopic 47.11
  laparoscopic 47.01

Appendicocecostomy 47.91

Appendicoenterostomy 47.91

Appendicolysis 54.59
  with appendectomy
    laparoscopic 47.01
    other 47.09
  laparoscopic 54.51

Appendicostomy 47.91
  closure 47.92

Appendicotomy 47.2

Application
  adhesion barrier ▶substance◀ 99.77 ▲
  anti-shock trousers 93.58
  arch bars (orthodontic) 24.7
    for immobilization (fracture) 93.55
  barrier substance, adhesion 99.77 ●
  Barton's tongs (skull) (with synchronous skeletal traction) 02.94
  bone growth stimulator (surface) (transcutaneous) 99.86
  bone morphogenetic protein (recombinant) ● (rhBMP) 84.52 ●
  Bryant's traction 93.44
    with reduction of fracture or dislocation — *see* Reduction, fracture *and* Reduction, dislocation
  Buck's traction 93.46
  caliper tongs (skull) (with synchronous skeletal traction) 02.94
  cast (fiberglass) (plaster) (plastic) NEC 93.53
    with reduction of fracture or dislocation — *see* Reduction, fracture *and* Reduction, dislocation
    spica 93.51
  cervical collar 93.52
    with reduction of fracture or dislocation — *see* Reduction, fracture *and* Reduction, dislocation
  clamp, cerebral aneurysm (Crutchfield) (Silverstone) 39.51
  croupette, croup tent 93.94
  crown (artificial) 23.41

Application — *continued*
  Crutchfield tongs (skull) (with synchronous skeletal traction) 02.94
  Dunlop's traction 93.44
    with reduction of fracture or dislocation — *see* Reduction, fracture *and* Reduction, dislocation
  elastic stockings 93.59
  electronic gaiter 93.59
  external fixation device (bone) 78.10
    carpal, metacarpal 78.14
    clavicle 78.11
    femur 78.15
    fibula 78.17
    humerus 78.12
    patella 78.16
    pelvic 78.19
    phalanges (foot) (hand) 78.19
    radius 78.13
    scapula 78.11
    specified site NEC 78.19
    tarsal, metatarsal 78.18
    thorax (ribs) (sternum) 78.11
    tibia 78.17
    ulna 78.13
    vertebrae 78.19
  forceps, with delivery — *see* Delivery, forceps
  graft — *see* Graft
  gravity (G-) suit 93.59
  intermittent pressure device 93.59
  Jewett extension brace 93.59
  Jobst pumping unit (reduction of edema) 93.59
  Lyman Smith traction 93.44
    with reduction of fracture or dislocation — *see* Reduction, fracture *and* Reduction, dislocation
  MAST (military anti-shock trousers) 93.58
  Minerva jacket 93.52
  minifixator device (bone) — *see* category 78.1 ✓4ᵗʰ
  neck support (molded) 93.52
  obturator (orthodontic) 24.7
  orthodontic appliance (obturator) (wiring) 24.7
  pelvic sling 93.44
    with reduction of fracture or dislocation — *see* Reduction, fracture *and* Reduction, dislocation
  peridontal splint (orthodontic) 24.7
  plaster jacket 93.51
    Minerva 93.52
  pressure
    dressing (bandage) (Gibney) (Robert Jones') (Shanz) 93.56
    trousers (anti-shock) (MAST) 93.58
  prosthesis for missing ear 18.71
  Russell's traction 93.44
    with reduction of fracture or dislocation — *see* Reduction, fracture *and* Reduction, dislocation
  splint, for immobilization (plaster) (pneumatic) (tray) 93.54
    with fracture reduction — *see* Reduction, fracture
  stereotactic head frame 93.59
  substance, adhesion barrier 99.77 ●
  Thomas collar 93.52
    with reduction of fracture or dislocation — *see* Reduction, fracture *and* Reduction, dislocation
  traction
    with reduction of fracture or dislocation — *see* Reduction, fracture *and* Reduction, dislocation
    adhesive tape (skin) 93.46
    boot 93.46
    Bryant's 93.44
    Buck's 93.46
    Cotrel's 93.42
    Dunlop's 93.44
    gallows 93.46
    Lyman Smith 93.44
    Russell's 93.44
    skeletal NEC 93.44
      intermittent 93.43
    skin, limbs NEC 93.46

Application — *continued*
  traction — *continued*
    spinal NEC 93.42
      with skull device (halo) (caliper) (Crutchfield) (Gardner-Wells) (Vinke) (tongs) 93.41
        with synchronous insertion 02.94
    Thomas' splint 93.45
  Unna's paste boot 93.53
  vasopneumatic device 93.58
  Velpeau dressing 93.59
  Vinke tongs (skull) (with synchronous skeletal traction) 02.94
  wound dressing NEC 93.57

Arc lamp — *see* Photocoagulation

Arrest
  bone growth (epiphyseal) 78.20
    by stapling — *see* Stapling, epiphyseal plate
    femur 78.25
    fibula 78.27
    humerus 78.22
    radius 78.23
    tibia 78.27
    ulna 78.23
  cardiac, induced (anoxic) (circulatory) 39.63
  circulatory, induced (anoxic) 39.63
  hemorrhage — *see* Control, hemorrhage

Arslan operation (fenestration of inner ear) 20.61

Arteriectomy 38.60
  with
    anastomosis 38.30
      abdominal 38.36
      aorta (arch) (ascending) (descending) 38.34
      head and neck NEC 38.32
      intracranial NEC 38.31
      lower limb 38.38
      thoracic NEC 38.35
      upper limb 38.33
    graft replacement (interposition) 38.40
      abdominal
        aorta 38.44
      aorta (arch) (ascending) (descending thoracic)
        abdominal 38.44
        thoracic 38.45
        thoracoabdominal 38.45 [38.44]
      head and neck NEC 38.42
      intracranial NEC 38.41
      lower limb 38.48
      thoracic NEC 38.45
      upper limb 38.43
  abdominal 38.66
  aorta (arch) (ascending) (descending) 38.64
  head and neck NEC 38.62
  intracranial NEC 38.61
  lower limb 38.68
  thoracic NEC 38.65
  upper limb 38.63

Arteriography (contrast) (fluoroscopic) (retrograde) 88.40
  by
    radioisotope — *see* Scan, radioisotope
    ultrasound (Doppler) — *see* Ultrasonography, by site
  aorta (arch) (ascending) (descending) 88.42
  basilar 88.41
  brachial 88.49
  carotid (internal) 88.41
  cerebral (posterior circulation) 88.41
  coronary (direct) (selective) NEC 88.57
    double catheter technique (Judkins) (Ricketts and Abrams) 88.56
    single catheter technique (Sones) 88.55
  Doppler (ultrasonic) — *see* Ultrasonography, by site
  femoral 88.48
  head and neck 88.41
  intra-abdominal NEC 88.47
  intrathoracic NEC 88.44
  lower extremity 88.48
  placenta 88.46
  pulmonary 88.43
  radioisotope — *see* Scan, radioisotope
  renal 88.45

Index to Procedures

Arteriography — *continued*
  specified site NEC 88.49
  superior mesenteric artery 88.47
  transfemoral 88.48
  ultrasound — *see* Ultrasonography, by site
  upper extremity 88.49
Arterioplasty — *see* Repair, artery
Arteriorrhaphy 39.31
Arteriotomy 38.00
  abdominal 38.06
  aorta (arch) (ascending) (descending) 38.04
  head and neck NEC 38.02
  intracranial NEC 38.01
  lower limb 38.08
  thoracic NEC 38.05
  upper limb 38.03
Arteriovenostomy 39.29
  for renal dialysis 39.27
Arthrectomy 80.90
  ankle 80.97
  elbow 80.92
  foot and toe 80.98
  hand and finger 80.94
  hip 80.95
  intervertebral disc 80.5 ✓4ᵗʰ
  knee 80.96
    semilunar cartilage 80.6
  shoulder 80.91
  specified site NEC 80.99
  spine NEC 80.99
  wrist 80.93
Arthrocentesis 81.91
  for arthrography — *see* Arthrogram
Arthrodesis (compression) (extra-articular) (intra-articular) (with bone graft) (with fixation device) 81.20
  ankle 81.11
  carporadial 81.25
  cricoarytenoid 31.69
  elbow 81.24
  finger 81.28
  foot NEC 81.17
  hip 81.21
  interphalangeal
    finger 81.28
    toe NEC 77.58
      claw toe repair 77.57
      hammer toe repair 77.56
  ischiofemoral 81.21
  knee 81.22
  lumbosacral, lumbar NEC 81.08
    anterior (interbody), anterolateral technique 81.06
    lateral transverse process technique 81.07
    posterior (interbody), posterolateral technique 81.08
  McKeever (metatarsophalangeal) 81.16
  metacarpocarpal 81.26
  metacarpophalangeal 81.27
  metatarsophalangeal 81.16
  midtarsal 81.14
  plantar 81.11
  sacroiliac 81.08
  shoulder 81.23
  specified joint NEC 81.29
  spinal (*see also* Fusion, spinal) 81.00
  subtalar 81.13
  tarsometatarsal 81.15
  tibiotalar 81.11
  toe NEC 77.58
    claw toe repair 77.57
    hammer toe repair 77.56
  triple 81.12
  wrist 81.26
Arthroendoscopy — *see* Arthroscopy
Arthrogram, arthrography 88.32
  temporomandibular 87.13
Arthrolysis 93.26
Arthroplasty (with fixation device) (with traction) 81.96
  ankle 81.49
  carpals 81.75
    with prosthetic implant 81.74

Arthroplasty — *continued*
  carpocarpal, carpometacarpal 81.75
    with prosthetic implant 81.74
  Carroll and Taber (proximal interphalangeal joint) 81.72
  cup (partial hip) 81.52
  Curtis (interphalangeal joint) 81.72
  elbow 81.85
    with prosthetic replacement (total) 81.84
  femoral head NEC 81.40
    with prosthetic implant 81.52
  finger(s) 81.72
    with prosthetic implant 81.71
  foot (metatarsal) with joint replacement 81.57
  Fowler (metacarpophalangeal joint) 81.72
  hand (metacarpophalangeal) (interphalangeal) 81.72
    with prosthetic implant 81.71
  hip (with bone graft) 81.40
    cup (partial hip) 81.52
    femoral head NEC 81.40
      with prosthetic implant 81.52
        with total replacement 81.51
    partial replacement 81.52
    total replacement 81.51
  interphalangeal joint 81.72
    with prosthetic implant 81.71
  Kessler (carpometacarpal joint) 81.74
  knee (*see also* Repair, knee) 81.47
    prosthetic replacement (bicompartmental) (hemijoint) (partial) (total) (tricompartmental) (unicompartmental) 81.54
    revision 81.55
  metacarpophalangeal joint 81.72
    with prosthetic implant 81.71
  shoulder 81.83
    prosthetic replacement (partial) 81.81
      total 81.80
    for recurrent dislocation 81.82
  temporomandibular 76.5
  toe NEC 77.58
    with prosthetic replacement 81.57
    for hallux valgus repair 77.59
  wrist 81.75
    with prosthetic implant 81.74
    total replacement 81.73
Arthroscopy 80.20
  ankle 80.27
  elbow 80.22
  finger 80.24
  foot 80.28
  hand 80.24
  hip 80.25
  knee 80.26
  shoulder 80.21
  specified site NEC 80.29
  toe 80.28
  wrist 80.23
Arthrostomy (*see also* Arthrotomy) 80.10
Arthrotomy 80.10
  as operative approach — *omit code*
  with
    arthrography — *see* Arthrogram
    arthroscopy — *see* Arthroscopy
    injection of drug 81.92
    removal of prosthesis (*see also* Removal, prosthesis, joint structures) 80.00
  ankle 80.17
  elbow 80.12
  foot and toe 80.18
  hand and finger 80.14
  hip 80.15
  knee 80.16
  shoulder 80.11
  specified site NEC 80.19
  spine 80.19
  wrist 80.13
Artificial
  insemination 69.92
  kidney 39.95
  rupture of membranes 73.09
Arytenoidectomy 30.29
Arytenoidopexy 31.69

Asai operation (larynx) 31.75
Aspiration
  abscess — *see* Aspiration, by site
  anterior chamber, eye (therapeutic) 12.91
    diagnostic 12.21
  aqueous (eye) (humor) (therapeutic) 12.91
    diagnostic 12.21
  ascites 54.91
  Bartholin's gland (cyst) (percutaneous) 71.21
  biopsy — *see* Biopsy, by site
  bladder (catheter) 57.0
    percutaneous (needle) 57.11
  bone marrow (for biopsy) 41.31
    from donor for transplant 41.91
    stem cell 99.79
  branchial cleft cyst 29.0
  breast 85.91
  bronchus 96.05
    with lavage 96.56
  bursa (percutaneous) 83.94
    hand 82.92
  calculus, bladder 57.0
  cataract 13.3
    with
      phacoemulsification 13.41
      phacofragmentation 13.43
      posterior route 13.42
  chest 34.91
  cisternal 01.01
  cranial (puncture) 01.09
  craniobuccal pouch 07.72
  craniopharyngioma 07.72
  cul-de-sac (abscess) 70.0
  curettage, uterus 69.59
    after abortion or delivery 69.52
    diagnostic 69.59
    to terminate pregnancy 69.51
  cyst — *see* Aspiration, by site
  diverticulum, pharynx 29.0
  endotracheal 96.04
    with lavage 96.56
  extradural 01.09
  eye (anterior chamber) (therapeutic) 12.91
    diagnostic 12.21
  fallopian tube 66.91
  fascia 83.95
    hand 82.93
  gallbladder (percutaneous) 51.01
  hematoma — *see also* Aspiration, by site
    obstetrical 75.92
      incisional 75.91
  hydrocele, tunica vaginalis 61.91
  hygroma — *see* Aspiration, by site
  hyphema 12.91
  hypophysis 07.72
  intracranial space (epidural) (extradural) (subarachnoid) (subdural) (ventricular) 01.09
    through previously implanted catheter or reservoir (Ommaya) (Rickham) 01.02
  joint 81.91
    for arthrography — *see* Arthrogram
  kidney (cyst) (pelvis) (percutaneous) (therapeutic) 55.92
    diagnostic 55.23
  liver (percutaneous) 50.91
  lung (percutaneous) (puncture) (needle) (trocar) 33.93
  middle ear 20.09
    with intubation 20.01
  muscle 83.95
    hand 82.93
  nail 86.01
  nasal sinus 22.00
    by puncture 22.01
    through natural ostium 22.02
  nasotracheal 96.04
    with lavage 96.56
  orbit, diagnostic 16.22
  ovary 65.91
  percutaneous — *see* Aspiration, by site
  pericardium (wound) 37.0
  pituitary gland 07.72
  pleural cavity 34.91
  prostate (percutaneous) 60.91

Aspiration — *continued*
  Rathke's pouch 07.72
  seminal vesicles 60.71
  seroma — *see* Aspiration, by site
  skin 86.01
  soft tissue NEC 83.95
    hand 82.93
  spermatocele 63.91
  spinal (puncture) 03.31
  spleen (cyst) 41.1
  stem cell 99.79
  subarachnoid space (cerebral) 01.09
  subcutaneous tissue 86.01
  subdural space (cerebral) 01.09
  tendon 83.95
    hand 82.93
  testis 62.91
  thymus 07.92
  thyroid (field) (gland) 06.01
    postoperative 06.02
  trachea 96.04
    with lavage 96.56
    percutaneous 31.99
  tunica vaginalis (hydrocele) (percutaneous) 61.91
  vitreous (and replacement) 14.72
    diagnostic 14.11
Assessment
  fitness to testify 94.11
  mental status 94.11
  nutritional status 89.39
  personality 94.03
  temperament 94.02
  vocational 93.85
Assistance
  cardiac (*see also* Resuscitation, cardiac)
    extracorporeal circulation 39.61
  endotracheal respiratory — *see* category 96.7
  hepatic, extracorporeal 50.92
  respiratory (endotracheal) (mechanical) — *see* ventilation, mechanical
Astragalectomy 77.98
Asymmetrogammagram — *see* Scan, radioisotope
Atherectomy
  coronary — *see* Angioplasty
  peripheral 39.50
Atriocommissuropexy (mitral valve) 35.12
Atrioplasty NEC 37.99
  combined with repair of valvular and ventricular septal defects — *see* Repair, endocardial cushion defect
  septum (heart) NEC 35.71
Atrioseptopexy (*see also* Repair, atrial septal defect) 35.71
Atrioseptoplasty (*see also* Repair, atrial septal defect) 35.71
Atrioseptostomy (balloon) 35.41
Atriotomy 37.11
Atrioventriculostomy (cerebral-heart) 02.32
Attachment
  eye muscle
    orbicularis oculi to eyebrow 08.36
    rectus to frontalis 15.9
  pedicle (flap) graft 86.74
    hand 86.73
    lip 27.57
    mouth 27.57
  pharyngeal flap (for cleft palate repair) 27.62
    secondary or subsequent 27.63
  retina — *see* Reattachment, retina
Atticoantrostomy (ear) 20.49
Atticoantrotomy (ear) 20.49
Atticotomy (ear) 20.23
Audiometry (Békésy 5-tone) (impedance) (stapedial reflex response) (subjective) 95.41
Augmentation
  bladder 57.87
  breast — *see* Mammoplasty, augmentation
  buttock ("fanny-lift") 86.89
  chin 76.68
  genioplasty 76.68

Augmentation — *continued*
  mammoplasty — *see* Mammoplasty, augmentation
  outflow tract (pulmonary valve) (gusset type) 35.26
    in total repair of tetralogy of Fallot 35.81
  vocal cord(s) 31.0
Auriculectomy 18.39
Autograft — *see* Graft
Autologous — *see* Blood, transfusion
Autopsy 89.8
Autotransfusion (whole blood) — *see* Blood, transfusion
Autotransplant, autotransplantation — *see also* Reimplantation
  adrenal tissue (heterotopic) (orthotopic) 07.45
  kidney 55.61
  lung — *see* Transplant, transplantation, lung 33.5 ✓4ᵗʰ
  ovary 65.72
    laparoscopic 65.75
  pancreatic tissue 52.81
  parathyroid tissue (heterotopic) (orthotopic) 06.95
  thyroid tissue (heterotopic) (orthotopic) 06.94
  tooth 23.5
Avulsion, nerve (cranial) (peripheral) NEC 04.07
  acoustic 04.01
  phrenic 33.31
  sympathetic 05.29
Azygography 88.63

B

Bacterial smear — *see* Examination, microscopic
Baffes operation (interatrial transposition of venous return) 35.91
Baffle, atrial or interatrial 35.91
Balanoplasty 64.49
Baldy-Webster operation (uterine suspension) 69.22
Ballistocardiography 89.59
Balloon
  angioplasty — *see* Angioplasty, balloon
  pump, intra-aortic 37.61
  systostomy (atrial) 35.41
Ball operation
  herniorrhaphy — *see* Repair, hernia, inguinal
  undercutting 49.02
Bandage 93.57
  elastic 93.56
Banding, pulmonary artery 38.85
Bankhart operation (capsular repair into glenoid, for shoulder dislocation) 81.82
Bardenheurer operation (ligation of innominate artery) 38.85
Barium swallow 87.61
Barkan operation (goniotomy) 12.52
  with goniopuncture 12.53
Barr operation (transfer of tibialis posterior tendon) 83.75
Barsky operation (closure of cleft hand) 82.82
Basal metabolic rate 89.39
Basiotripsy 73.8
Bassett operation (vulvectomy with inguinal lymph node dissection) 71.5 *[40.3]*
Bassini operation — *see* Repair, hernia, inguinal
Batch-Spittler-McFaddin operation (knee disarticulation) 84.16
Batista operation (partial ventriculectomy) (ventricular reduction) (ventricular remodeling) 37.35
Beck operation
  aorta-coronary sinus shunt 36.39
  epicardial poudrage 36.39
Beck-Jianu operation (permanent gastrostomy) 43.19
Behavior modification 94.33

Bell-Beuttner operation (subtotal abdominal hysterectomy) 68.3
Belsey operation (esophagogastric sphincter) 44.65
Benenenti operation (rotation of bulbous urethra) 58.49
Berke operation (levator resection of eyelid) 08.33
Bicuspidization of heart valve 35.10
  aortic 35.11
  mitral 35.12
Bicycle dynamometer 93.01
Biesenberger operation (size reduction of breast, bilateral) 85.32
  unilateral 85.31
Bifurcation, bone (*see also* Osteotomy) 77.30
Bigelow operation (litholapaxy) 57.0
Bililite therapy (ultraviolet) 99.82
Billroth I operation (partial gastrectomy with gastroduodenostomy) 43.6
Billroth II operation (partial gastrectomy with gastrojejunostomy) 43.7
Binnie operation (hepatopexy) 50.69
Biofeedback, psychotherapy 94.39
Biopsy
  abdominal wall 54.22
  adenoid 28.11
  adrenal gland NEC 07.11
    closed 07.11
    open 07.12
    percutaneous (aspiration) (needle) 07.11
  alveolus 24.12
  anus 49.23
  appendix 45.26
  artery (any site) 38.21
  aspiration — *see* Biopsy, by site
  bile ducts 51.14
    closed (endoscopic) 51.14
    open 51.13
    percutaneous (needle) 51.12
  bladder 57.33
    closed 57.33
    open 57.34
    transurethral 57.33
  blood vessel (any site) 38.21
  bone 77.40
    carpal, metacarpal 77.44
    clavicle 77.41
    facial 76.11
    femur 77.45
    fibula 77.47
    humerus 77.42
    marrow 41.31
    patella 77.46
    pelvic 77.49
    phalanges (foot) (hand) 77.49
    radius 77.43
    scapula 77.41
    specified site NEC 77.49
    tarsal, metatarsal 77.48
    thorax (ribs) (sternum) 77.41
    tibia 77.47
    ulna 77.43
    vertebrae 77.49
  bowel — *see* Biopsy, intestine
  brain NEC 01.13
    closed 01.13
    open 01.14
    percutaneous (needle) 01.13
  breast 85.11
    blind 85.11
    closed 85.11
    open 85.12
    percutaneous (needle) (Vimm-Silverman) 85.11
  bronchus NEC 33.24
    brush 33.24
    closed (endoscopic) 33.24
    open 33.25
    washings 33.24
  bursa 83.21
  cardioesophageal (junction) 44.14
    closed (endoscopic) 44.14
    open 44.15

Index to Procedures

Biopsy — *continued*
- cecum 45.25
  - brush 45.25
  - closed (endoscopic) 45.25
  - open 45.26
- cerebral meninges NEC 01.11
  - closed 01.11
  - open 01.12
  - percutaneous (needle) 01.11
- cervix (punch) 67.12
  - conization (sharp) 67.2
- chest wall 34.23
- clitoris 71.11
- colon 45.25
  - brush 45.25
  - closed (endoscopic) 45.25
  - open 45.26
- conjunctiva 10.21
- cornea 11.22
- cul-de-sac 70.23
- diaphragm 34.27
- duodenum 45.14
  - brush 45.14
  - closed (endoscopic) 45.14
  - open 45.15
- ear (external) 18.12
  - middle or inner 20.32
- endocervix 67.11
- endometrium NEC 68.16
  - by
    - aspiration curettage 69.59
    - dilation and curettage 69.09
  - closed (endoscopic) 68.16
  - open 68.13
- epididymis 63.01
- esophagus 42.24
  - closed (endoscopic) 42.24
  - open 42.25
- extraocular muscle or tendon 15.01
- eye 16.23
  - muscle (oblique) (rectus) 15.01
- eyelid 08.11
- fallopian tube 66.11
- fascia 83.21
- fetus 75.33
- gallbladder 51.12
  - closed (endoscopic) 51.14
  - open 51.13
  - percutaneous (needle) 51.12
- ganglion (cranial) (peripheral) NEC 04.11
  - closed 04.11
  - open 04.12
  - percutaneous (needle) 04.11
  - sympathetic nerve 05.11
- gum 24.11
- heart 37.25
- hypophysis (*see also* Biopsy, pituitary gland) 07.15
- ileum 45.14
  - brush 45.14
  - closed (endoscopic) 45.14
  - open 45.15
- intestine NEC 45.27
  - large 45.25
    - brush 45.25
    - closed (endoscopic) 45.25
    - open 45.26
  - small 45.14
    - brush 45.14
    - closed (endoscopic) 45.14
    - open 45.15
- intra-abdominal mass 54.24
  - closed 54.24
  - percutaneous (needle) 54.24
- iris 12.22
- jejunum 45.14
  - brush 45.14
  - closed (endoscopic) 45.14
  - open 45.15
- joint structure (aspiration) 80.30
  - ankle 80.37
  - elbow 80.32
  - foot and toe 80.38
  - hand and finger 80.34
  - hip 80.35
  - knee 80.36

Biopsy — *continued*
- joint structure — *continued*
  - shoulder 80.31
  - specified site NEC 80.39
  - spine 80.39
  - wrist 80.33
- kidney 55.23
  - closed 55.23
  - open 55.24
  - percutaneous (aspiration) (needle) 55.23
- labia 71.11
- lacrimal
  - gland 09.11
  - sac 09.12
- larynx 31.43
  - brush 31.43
  - closed (endoscopic) 31.43
  - open 31.45
- lip 27.23
- liver 50.11
  - closed 50.11
  - open 50.12
  - percutaneous (aspiration) (needle) 50.11
- lung NEC 33.27
  - brush 33.24
  - closed (percutaneous) (needle) 33.26
    - brush 33.24
    - endoscopic 33.27
      - brush 33.24
  - endoscopic 33.27
    - brush 33.24
  - open 33.28
  - transbronchial 33.27
- lymphatic structure (channel) (node) (vessel) 40.11
- mediastinum NEC 34.25
  - closed 34.25
  - open 34.26
  - percutaneous (needle) 34.25
- meninges (cerebral) NEC 01.11
  - closed 01.11
  - open 01.12
  - percutaneous (needle) 01.11
  - spinal 03.32
- mesentery 54.23
- mouth NEC 27.24
- muscle 83.21
  - extraocular 15.01
  - ocular 15.01
- nasopharynx 29.12
- nerve (cranial) (peripheral) NEC 04.11
  - closed 04.11
  - open 04.12
  - percutaneous (needle) 04.11
  - sympathetic 05.11
- nose, nasal 21.22
  - sinus 22.11
    - closed (endoscopic) (needle) 22.11
    - open 22.12
- ocular muscle or tendon 15.01
- omentum
  - closed 54.24
  - open 54.23
  - percutaneous (needle) 54.24
- orbit 16.23
  - by aspiration 16.22
- ovary 65.12
  - by aspiration 65.11
  - laparoscopic 65.13
- palate (bony) 27.21
  - soft 27.22
- pancreas 52.11
  - closed (endoscopic) 52.11
  - open 52.12
  - percutaneous (aspiration) (needle) 52.11
- pancreatic duct 52.14
  - closed (endoscopic) 52.14
- parathyroid gland 06.13
- penis 64.11
- perianal tissue 49.22
- pericardium 37.24
- periprostatic 60.15
- perirectal tissue 48.26
- perirenal tissue 59.21
- peritoneal implant
  - closed 54.24

Biopsy — *continued*
- peritoneal implant — *continued*
  - open 54.23
  - percutaneous (needle) 54.24
- peritoneum
  - closed 54.24
  - open 54.23
  - percutaneous (needle) 54.24
- periurethral tissue 58.24
- perivesical tissue 59.21
- pharynx, pharyngeal 29.12
- pineal gland 07.17
- pituitary gland 07.15
  - transfrontal approach 07.13
  - transsphenoidal approach 07.14
- pleura, pleural 34.24
- prostate NEC 60.11
  - closed (transurethral) 60.11
  - open 60.12
  - percutaneous (needle) 60.11
  - transrectal 60.11
- rectum 48.24
  - brush 48.24
  - closed (endoscopic) 48.24
  - open 48.25
- retroperitoneal tissue 54.24
- salivary gland or duct 26.11
  - closed (needle) 26.11
  - open 26.12
- scrotum 61.11
- seminal vesicle NEC 60.13
  - closed 60.13
  - open 60.14
  - percutaneous (needle) 60.13
- sigmoid colon 45.25
  - brush 45.25
  - closed (endoscopic) 45.25
  - open 45.26
- sinus, nasal 22.11
  - closed (endoscopic) (needle) 22.11
  - open 22.12
- skin (punch) 86.11
- skull 01.15
- soft palate 27.22
- soft tissue NEC 83.21
- spermatic cord 63.01
- sphincter of Oddi 51.14
  - closed (endoscopic) 51.14
  - open 51.13
- spinal cord (meninges) 03.32
- spleen 41.32
  - closed 41.32
  - open 41.33
  - percutaneous (aspiration) (needle) 41.32
- stomach 44.14
  - brush 44.14
  - closed (endoscopic) 44.14
  - open 44.15
- subcutaneous tissue (punch) 86.11
- supraglottic mass 29.12
- sympathetic nerve 05.11
- tendon 83.21
  - extraocular 15.01
  - ocular 15.01
- testis NEC 62.11
  - closed 62.11
  - open 62.12
  - percutaneous (needle) 62.11
- thymus 07.16
- thyroid gland NEC 06.11
  - closed 06.11
  - open 06.12
  - percutaneous (aspiration) (needle) 06.11
- tongue 25.01
  - closed (needle) 25.01
  - open 25.02
- tonsil 28.11
- trachea 31.44
  - brush 31.44
  - closed (endoscopic) 31.44
  - open 31.45
- tunica vaginalis 61.11
- umbilicus 54.22

Biopsy

Biopsy — *continued*
- ureter 56.33
  - closed (percutaneous) 56.32
    - endoscopic 56.33
    - open 56.34
  - transurethral 56.33
- urethra 58.23
- uterus, uterine (endometrial) 68.16
  - by
    - aspiration curettage 69.59
    - dilation and curettage 69.09
  - closed (endoscopic) 68.16
  - ligaments 68.15
    - closed (endoscopic) 68.15
    - open 68.14
  - open 68.13
- uvula 27.22
- vagina 70.24
- vas deferens 63.01
- vein (any site) 38.21
- vulva 71.11

Bischoff operation (ureteroneocystostomy) 56.74

Bisection — *see also* Excision
- hysterectomy 68.3
- ovary 65.29
  - laparoscopic 65.25
- stapes foot plate 19.19
  - with incus replacement 19.11

Bischoff operation (spinal myelotomy) 03.29

Blalock operation (systemic-pulmonary anastomosis) 39.0

Blalock-Hanlon operation (creation of atrial septal defect) 35.42

Blalock-Taussig operation (sub-clavian-pulmonary anastomosis) 39.0

Blascovic operation (resection and advancement of levator palpebrae superioris) 08.33

Blepharectomy 08.20

Blepharoplasty (*see also* Reconstruction, eyelid) 08.70
- extensive 08.44

Blepharorrhaphy 08.52
- division or severing 08.02

Blepharotomy 08.09

Blind rehabilitation therapy NEC 93.78

Block
- caudal — *see* Injection, spinal
- celiac ganglion or plexus 05.31
- dissection
  - breast
    - bilateral 85.46
    - unilateral 85.45
  - bronchus 32.6
  - larynx 30.3
  - lymph nodes 40.50
  - neck 40.40
  - vulva 71.5
- epidural, spinal — *see* Injection, spinal
- gasserian ganglion 04.81
- intercostal nerves 04.81
- intrathecal — *see* Injection, spinal
- nerve (cranial) (peripheral) NEC 04.81
- paravertebral stellate ganglion 05.31
- peripheral nerve 04.81
- spinal nerve root (intrathecal) — *see* Injection, spinal
- stellate (ganglion) 05.31
- subarachnoid, spinal — *see* Injection, spinal
- sympathetic nerve 05.31
- trigeminal nerve 04.81

Blood
- flow study, Doppler-type (ultrasound) — *see* Ultrasonography
- patch, spine (epidural) 03.95
- transfusion
  - antihemophilic factor 99.06
  - autologous
    - collected prior to surgery 99.02
    - intraoperative 99.00
    - perioperative 99.00
    - postoperative 99.00
    - previously collected 99.02
    - salvage 99.00

Blood — *continued*
- transfusion — *continued*
  - blood expander 99.08
  - blood surrogate 99.09
  - coagulation factors 99.06
  - exchange 99.01
  - granulocytes 99.09
  - hemodilution 99.03
  - other substance 99.09
  - packed cells 99.04
  - plasma 99.07
  - platelets 99.05
  - serum, other 99.07
  - thrombocytes 99.05

Blount operation
- femoral shortening (with blade plate) 78.25
  - by epiphyseal stapling 78.25

Boari operation (bladder flap) 56.74

Bobb operation (cholelithotomy) 51.04

Bone
- age studies 88.33
- mineral density study 88.98

Bonney operation (abdominal hysterectomy) 68.4

Borthen operation (iridotasis) 12.63

Bost operation
- plantar dissection 80.48
- radiocarpal fusion 81.26

Bosworth operation
- arthroplasty for acromioclavicular separation 81.83
- fusion of posterior lumbar and lumbosacral spine 81.08
  - for pseudarthrosis 81.38
- resection of radial head ligaments (for tennis elbow) 80.92
- shelf procedure, hip 81.40

Bottle repair of hydrocele, tunica-vaginalis 61.2

Boyd operation (hip disarticulation) 84.18

Brachytherapy
- intravascular 92.27

Brauer operation (cardiolysis) 37.10

Breech extraction — *see* Extraction, breech

Bricker operation (ileoureterostomy) 56.51

Brisement (forcé) 93.26

Bristow operation (repair of shoulder dislocation) 81.82

Brock operation (pulmonary valvotomy) 35.03

Brockman operation (soft tissue release for clubfoot) 83.84

Bronchogram, bronchography 87.32
- endotracheal 87.31
- transcricoid 87.32

Bronchoplasty 33.48

Bronchorrhaphy 33.41

Bronchoscopy NEC 33.23
- with biopsy 33.24
  - lung 33.27
    - brush 33.24
- fiberoptic 33.22
  - with biopsy 33.24
    - lung 33.27
      - brush 33.24
- through tracheostomy 33.21
  - with biopsy 33.24
    - lung 33.27
      - brush 33.24

Bronchospirometry 89.38

Bronchostomy 33.0
- closure 33.42

Bronchotomy 33.0

Browne (-Denis) operation (hypospadias repair) 58.45

Brunschwig operation (temporary gastrostomy) 43.19

Buckling, scleral 14.49
- with
  - air tamponade 14.49
  - implant (silicone) (vitreous) 14.41
  - resection of sclera 14.49
  - vitrectomy 14.49
  - vitreous implant (silicone) 14.41

Index to Procedures

Bunionectomy (radical) 77.59
- with
  - arthrodesis 77.52
  - osteotomy of first metatarsal 77.51
  - resection of joint with prosthetic implant 77.59
  - soft tissue correction NEC 77.53

Bunnell operation (tendon transfer) 82.56

Burch procedure (retropubic urethral suspension for urinary stress incontinence) 59.5

Burgess operation (amputation of ankle) 84.14

Burn dressing 93.57

Burr holes 01.24

Bursectomy 83.5
- hand 82.31

Bursocentesis 83.94
- hand 82.92

Bursotomy 83.03
- hand 82.03

Burying of fimbriae in uterine wall 66.97

Bypass
- abdominal-coronary artery 36.17
- aortocoronary (catheter stent) (with prosthesis) (with saphenous vein graft) (with vein graft) 36.10
  - one coronary vessel 36.11
  - two coronary vessels 36.12
  - three coronary vessels 36.13
  - four coronary vessels 36.14
- arterial (graft) (mandril grown graft) (vein graft) NEC 39.29
  - carotid-cerebral 39.28
  - carotid-vertebral 39.28
  - extracranial-intracranial [EC-IC] 39.28
  - intra-abdominal NEC 39.26
  - intrathoracic NEC 39.23
  - peripheral NEC 39.29
- cardiopulmonary 39.61
  - open 39.61
  - percutaneous (closed) 39.66
- carotid-cerebral 39.28
- carotid-vertebral 39.28
- coronary (*see also* Bypass, aortocoronary) 36.10
- extracranial-intracranial [EC-IC] 39.28
- gastric 44.39
  - high 44.31
  - Printen and Mason 44.31
- gastroduodenostomy (Jaboulay's) 44.39
- gastroenterostomy 44.39
- gastroepiploic-coronary artery 36.17
- gastrogastrostomy 44.39
- heart-lung (complete) (partial) 39.61
  - open 39.61
  - percutaneous (closed) 39.66
- high gastric 44.31
- ileo-jejunal 45.91
- internal mammary-coronary artery (single) 36.15
  - double vessel 36.16
- jejunal-ileum 45.91
- pulmonary 39.61
  - open 39.61
  - percutaneous (closed) 39.66
- shunt
  - intestine
    - large-to-large 45.94
    - small-to-large 45.93
    - small-to-small 45.91
  - stomach 44.39
    - high gastric 44.31
- terminal ileum 45.93
- vascular (arterial) (graft) (mandril grown graft) (vein graft) NEC 39.29
  - aorta-carotid-brachial 39.22
  - aorta-iliac-femoral 39.25
  - aorta-renal 39.24
  - aorta-subclavian-carotid 39.22
  - aortic-superior mesenteric 39.26
  - aortocarotid 39.22
  - aortoceliac 39.26
  - aortocoronary (*see also* Bypass, aortocoronary) 36.10
  - aortofemoral 39.25

Index to Procedures

Bypass — *continued*
  vascular NEC — *continued*
    aortofemoral-popliteal 39.25
    aortoiliac 39.25
      to popliteal 39.25
    aortoiliofemoral 39.25
    aortomesenteric 39.26
    aortopopliteal 39.25
    aortorenal 39.24
    aortosubclavian 39.22
    axillary-brachial 39.29
    axillary-femoral (superficial) 39.29
    axillofemoral (superficial) 39.29
    carotid-cerebral 39.28
    carotid-vertebral 39.28
    carotid to subclavian artery 39.22
    common hepatic-common iliac-renal 39.26
    coronary (*see also* Bypass, aortocoronary) 36.10
    extracranial-intracranial [EC-IC] 39.28
    femoral-femoral 39.29
    femoroperoneal 39.29
    femoropopliteal (reversed saphenous vein) (saphenous) 39.29
    femorotibial (anterior) (posterior) 39.29
    iliofemoral 39.25
    ilioiliac 39.26
    internal mammary-coronary artery (single) 36.15
      double vessel 36.16
    intra-abdominal (arterial) NEC 39.26
      venous NEC 39.1
    intrathoracic NEC 39.23
    peripheral artery NEC 39.29
    popliteal-tibial 39.29
    renal artery 39.24
    splenorenal (venous) 39.1
      arterial 39.26
    subclavian-axillary 39.29
    subclavian-carotid 39.22
    subclavian-subclavian 39.22
    Y graft to renal arteries 39.24

C

Caldwell operation (sulcus extension) 24.91
Caldwell-Luc operation (maxillary sinusotomy) 22.39
  with removal of membrane lining 22.31
Calibration, urethra 89.29
Calicectomy (renal) 55.4
Callander operation (knee disarticulation) 84.16
Caloric test, vestibular function 95.44
Calycectomy (renal) 55.4
Calyco-ileoneocystostomy 55.86
Calycotomy (renal) 55.11
Campbell operation
  bone block, ankle 81.11
  fasciotomy (iliac crest) 83.14
  reconstruction of anterior cruciate ligament 81.45
Campimetry 95.05
Canaliculodacryocystorhinostomy 09.81
Canaliculoplasty 09.73
Canaliculorhinostomy 09.81
Canaloplasty, external auditory meatus 18.6
Cannulation — *see also* Insertion, catheter
  ampulla of Vater 51.99
  antrum 22.01
  arteriovenous 39.93
  artery 38.91
  caval-mesenteric vein 39.1
  cisterna chyli 40.61
  Eustachian tube 20.8
  lacrimal apparatus 09.42
  lymphatic duct, left (thoracic) 40.61
  nasal sinus (by puncture) 22.01
    through natural ostium 22.02
  pancreatic duct 52.92
    by retrograde endoscopy (ERP) 52.93
  renoportal 39.1

Cannulation — *see also* Insertion, catheter — *continued*
  sinus (nasal) (by puncture) 22.01
    through natural ostium 22.02
  splenorenal (venous) 39.1
    arterial 39.26
  thoracic duct (cervical approach) (thoracic approach) 40.61
Cannulization — *see* Cannulation
Canthocystostomy 09.82
Canthoplasty 08.59
Canthorrhaphy 08.52
  division or severing 08.02
Canthotomy 08.51
Capsulectomy
  joint (*see also* Arthrectomy) 80.90
  kidney 55.91
  lens 13.65
    with extraction of lens 13.51
  ovary 65.29
    laparoscopic 65.25
Capsulo-iridectomy 13.65
Capsuloplasty — *see* Arthroplasty
Capsulorrhaphy 81.96
  with arthroplasty — *see* Arthroplasty
  ankle 81.94
  foot 81.94
  lower extremity NEC 81.95
  upper extremity 81.93
Capsulotomy
  joint (*see also* Division, joint capsule) 80.40
    for claw toe repair 77.57
  lens 13.64
    with
      discission of lens 13.2
      removal of foreign body 13.02
        by magnet extraction 13.01
Cardiac
  mapping 37.27
  massage (external) (closed chest) 99.63
    open chest 37.91
  retraining 93.36
Cardiectomy (stomach) 43.5
Cardiocentesis 37.0
Cardiography (*see also* Angiocardiography) 88.50
Cardiolysis 37.10
Cardiomyopexy 36.39
Cardiomyotomy 42.7
Cardio-omentopexy 36.39
Cardiopericardiopexy 36.39
Cardioplasty (stomach and esophagus) 44.65
  stomach alone 44.66
Cardioplegia 39.63
Cardiopneumopexy 36.39
Cardiorrhaphy 37.4
Cardioschisis 37.12
Cardiosplenopexy 36.39
Cardiotomy (exploratory) 37.11
Cardiovalvulotomy — *see* Valvulotomy, heart
Cardioversion (external) 99.62
  atrial 99.61
Carotid pulse tracing with ECG lead 89.56
Carpectomy (partial) 77.84
  total 77.94
Carroll and Taber arthroplasty (proximal interphalangeal joint) 81.72
Casting (for immobilization) NEC 93.53
  with fracture-reduction — *see* Reduction, fracture
Castration
  female (oophorectomy, bilateral) 65.51
    laparoscopic 65.53
  male 62.41
C.A.T. (computerized axial tomography) (*see also* Scan, C.A.T.) 88.38
Catheterization — *see also* Insertion, catheter
  arteriovenous 39.93
  artery 38.91

Catheterization — *see also* Insertion, catheter — *continued*
  bladder, indwelling 57.94
    percutaneous (cystostomy) 57.17
    suprapubic NEC 57.18
  bronchus 96.05
    with lavage 96.56
  cardiac (right) 37.21
    combined left and right 37.23
    left 37.22
      combined with right heart 37.23
    right 37.21
      combined with left heart 37.23
  central venous NEC 38.93
    peripherally inserted central catheter (PICC) 38.93
  chest 34.04
    revision (with lysis of adhesions) 34.04
  Eustachian tube 20.8
  heart (right) 37.21
    combined left and right 37.23
    left 37.22
      combined with right heart 37.23
    right 37.21
      combined with left heart 37.23
  hepatic vein 38.93
  inferior vena cava 38.93
  intercostal space (with water seal), for drainage 34.04
    revision (with lysis of adhesions) 34.04
  lacrimonasal duct 09.44
  laryngeal 96.05
  nasolacrimal duct 09.44
  pancreatic cyst 52.01
  renal vein 38.93
  Swan-Ganz (pulmonary) 89.64
  transtracheal for oxygenation 31.99
  umbilical vein 38.92
  ureter (to kidney) 59.8
    for retrograde pyelogram 87.74
  urethra, indwelling 57.94
  vein NEC 38.93
    for renal dialysis 38.95
Cattell operation (herniorrhaphy) 53.51
Cauterization — *see also* Destruction, lesion, by site
  anus NEC 49.39
    endoscopic 49.31
  Bartholin's gland 71.24
  broad ligament 69.19
  bronchus 32.09
    endoscopic 32.01
  canaliculi 09.73
  cervix 67.32
  chalazion 08.25
  choroid plexus 02.14
  conjunctiva 10.33
    lesion 10.32
  cornea (fistula) (ulcer) 11.42
  ear, external 18.29
  endometrial implant — *see* Excision, lesion, by site
  entropion 08.41
  esophagus 42.39
    endoscopic 42.33
  eyelid 08.25
    for entropion or ectropion 08.41
  fallopian tube 66.61
    by endoscopy (hysteroscopy) (laparoscopy) 66.29
  hemorrhoids 49.43
  iris 12.41
  lacrimal
    gland 09.21
    punctum 09.72
      for eversion 09.71
    sac 09.6
  larynx 30.09
  liver 50.29
  lung 32.29
    endoscopic 32.28
  meibomian gland 08.25
  nose, for epistaxis (with packing) 21.03
  ovary 65.29
    laparoscopic 65.25

Cauterization — see also Destruction, lesion, by site — continued
  palate (bony) 27.31
  pannus (superficial) 11.42
  pharynx 29.39
  punctum, lacrimal 09.72
    for eversion 09.71
  rectum 48.32
    radical 48.31
  round ligament 69.19
  sclera 12.84
    with iridectomy 12.62
  skin 86.3
  subcutaneous tissue 86.3
  tonsillar fossa 28.7
  urethra 58.39
    endoscopic 58.31
  uterosacral ligament 69.19
  uterotubal ostia 66.61
  uterus 68.29
  vagina 70.33
  vocal cords 30.09
  vulva 71.3
Cavernoscopy 34.21
Cavernostomy 33.1
Cavernotomy, kidney 55.39
Cavography (inferior vena cava) 88.51
Cecectomy (with resection of terminal ileum) 45.72
Cecil operation (urethral reconstruction) 58.46
Cecocoloplicopexy 46.63
Cecocolostomy 45.94
Cecofixation 46.64
Ceco-ileostomy 45.93
Cecopexy 46.64
Cecoplication 46.62
Cecorrhaphy 46.75
Cecosigmoidostomy 45.94
Cecostomy (tube) (see also Colostomy) 46.10
Cecotomy 45.03
Celiocentesis 54.91
Celioscopy 54.21
Celiotomy, exploratory 54.11
Cell block and Papanicolaou smear — see Examination, microscopic
Cephalogram 87.17
  dental 87.12
  orthodontic 87.12
Cephalometry, cephalometrics 87.17
  echo 88.78
  orthodontic 87.12
  ultrasound (sonar) 88.78
  x-ray 87.81
Cephalotomy, fetus 73.8
Cerclage
  anus 49.72
  cervix 67.59
    transabdominal 67.51
    transvaginal 67.59
  isthmus uteri (cervix) 67.59
  retinal reattachment (see also Buckling, scleral) 14.49
  sclera (see also Buckling, scleral) 14.49
Cervicectomy (with synchronous colporrhaphy) 67.4
Cervicoplasty 67.69
Cesarean section 74.99
  classical 74.0
  corporeal 74.0
  extraperitoneal 74.2
  fundal 74.0
  laparotrachelotomy 74.1
  Latzko 74.2
  low cervical 74.1
  lower uterine segment 74.1
  peritoneal exclusion 74.4
  specified type NEC 74.4
  supravesical 74.2
  transperitoneal 74.4
    classical 74.0
    low cervical 74.1

Cesarean section — continued
  upper uterine segment 74.0
  vaginal 74.4
  Waters 74.2
Chandler operation (hip fusion) 81.21
Change — see also Replacement
  cast NEC 97.13
    lower limb 97.12
    upper limb 97.11
  cystostomy catheter or tube 59.94
  gastrostomy tube 97.02
  length
    bone — see either category 78.2
      Shortening, bone or category 78.3
      Lengthening, bone
    muscle 83.85
      hand 82.55
    tendon 83.85
      hand 82.55
  nephrostomy catheter or tube 55.93
  pyelostomy catheter or tube 55.94
  tracheostomy tube 97.23
  ureterostomy catheter or tube 59.93
  urethral catheter, indwelling 57.95
Character analysis, psychologic 94.03
Charles operation (correction of lymphedema) 40.9
Charnley operation (compression arthrodesis)
  ankle 81.11
  hip 81.21
  knee 81.22
Cheatle-Henry operation — see Repair, hernia, femoral
Check
  pacemaker, artificial (cardiac) (function) (rate) 89.45
    amperage threshold 89.48
    artifact wave form 89.46
    electrode impedance 89.47
    voltage threshold 89.48
  vision NEC 95.09
Cheiloplasty 27.59
Cheilorrhaphy 27.51
Cheilostomatoplasty 27.59
Cheilotomy 27.0
Chemical peel, skin 86.24
Chemocauterization — see also Destruction, lesion, by site
  corneal epithelium 11.41
  palate 27.31
Chemodectomy 39.8
Chemoembolization 99.25
Chemolysis
  nerve (peripheral) 04.2
  spinal canal structure 03.8
Chemoneurolysis 04.2
Chemonucleolysis (nucleus pulposus) 80.52
Chemopallidectomy 01.42
Chemopeel (skin) 86.24
Chemosurgery
  esophagus 42.39
    endoscopic 42.33
  Mohs' 86.24
  skin (superficial) 86.24
  stomach 43.49
    endoscopic 43.41
Chemothalamectomy 01.41
Chemotherapy — see also Immunotherapy
  Antabuse 94.25
  for cancer NEC 99.25
    brain wafer implantation 00.10
    implantation of chemotherapeutic agent 00.10
    interstitial implantation 00.10
    intracavitary implantation 00.10
    wafer chemotherapy 00.10
  lithium 94.22
  methadone 94.25
  palate (bony) 27.31
Chevalier-Jackson operation (partial laryngectomy) 30.29

Child operation (radical subtotal pancreatectomy) 52.53
Cholangiocholangiostomy 51.39
Cholangiocholecystocholedochectomy 51.22
Cholangio-enterostomy 51.39
Cholangiogastrostomy 51.39
Cholangiogram 87.54
  endoscopic retrograde (ERC) 51.11
  intraoperative 87.53
  intravenous 87.52
  percutaneous hepatic 87.51
  transhepatic 87.53
Cholangiography (see also Cholangiogram) 87.54
Cholangiojejunostomy (intrahepatic) 51.39
Cholangiopancreatography, endoscopic retrograde (ERCP) 51.10
Cholangiostomy 51.59
Cholangiotomy 51.59
Cholecystectomy (total) 51.22
  laparoscopic 51.23
  partial 51.21
    laparoscopic 51.24
Cholecystenterorrhaphy 51.91
Cholecystocecostomy 51.32
Cholecystocholangiogram 87.59
Cholecystocolostomy 51.32
Cholecystoduodenostomy 51.32
Cholecystoenterostomy (Winiwater) 51.32
Cholecystogastrostomy 51.34
Cholecystogram 87.59
Cholecystoileostomy 51.32
Cholecystojejunostomy (Roux-en-Y) (with jejunojejunostomy) 51.32
Cholecystopancreatostomy 51.33
Cholecystopexy 51.99
Cholecystorrhaphy 51.91
Cholecystostomy NEC 51.03
  by trocar 51.02
Cholecystotomy 51.04
  percutaneous 51.01
Choledochectomy 51.63
Choledochoduodenostomy 51.36
Choledochoenterostomy 51.36
Choledochojejunostomy 51.36
Choledocholithotomy 51.41
  endoscopic 51.88
Choledocholithotripsy 51.41
  endoscopic 51.88
Choledochopancreatostomy 51.39
Choledochoplasty 51.72
Choledochorrhaphy 51.71
Choledochoscopy 51.11
Choledochostomy 51.51
Choledochotomy 51.51
Cholelithotomy 51.04
Chondrectomy 80.90
  ankle 80.97
  elbow 80.92
  foot and toe 80.98
  hand and finger 80.94
  hip 80.95
  intervertebral cartilage — see category 80.5
  knee (semilunar cartilage) 80.6
  nasal (submucous) 21.5
  semilunar cartilage (knee) 80.6
  shoulder 80.91
  specified site NEC 80.99
  spine — see category 80.5
  wrist 80.93
Chondroplasty — see Arthroplasty
Chondrosternoplasty (for pectus excavatum repair) 34.74
Chondrotomy (see also Division, cartilage) 80.40
  nasal 21.1
Chopart operation (midtarsal amputation) 84.12
Chordectomy, vocal 30.22

Index to Procedures

Chordotomy (spinothalmic) (anterior) (posterior) NEC 03.29
  percutaneous 03.21
  stereotactic 03.21
Ciliarotomy 12.55
Ciliectomy (ciliary body) 12.44
  eyelid margin 08.20
Cinch, cinching
  for scleral buckling (see also Buckling, scleral) 14.49
  ocular muscle (oblique) (rectus) 15.22
    multiple (two or more muscles) 15.4
Cineangiocardiography (see also Angiocardiography) 88.50
Cineplasty, cineplastic prosthesis
  amputation — see Amputation
  arm 84.44
  biceps 84.44
  extremity 84.40
    lower 84.48
    upper 84.44
  leg 84.48
Cineradiograph — see Radiography
Cingulumotomy (brain) (percutaneous radiofrequency) 01.32
Circumcision (male) 64.0
  female 71.4
Clagett operation (closure of chest wall following open flap drainage) 34.72
Clamp and cautery, hemorrhoids 49.43
Clamping
  aneurysm (cerebral) 39.51
  blood vessel — see Ligation, blood vessel
  ventricular shunt 02.43
Clavicotomy 77.31
  fetal 73.8
Claviculectomy (partial) 77.81
  total 77.91
Clayton operation (resection of metatarsal heads and bases of phalanges) 77.88
Cleaning, wound 96.59
Clearance
  bladder (transurethral) 57.0
  pelvic
    female 68.8
    male 57.71
  prescalene fat pad 40.21
  renal pelvis (transurethral) 56.0
  ureter (transurethral) 56.0
Cleidotomy 77.31
  fetal 73.8
Clipping
  aneurysm (basilar) (carotid) (cerebellar) (cerebellopontine) (communicating artery) (vertebral) 39.51
  arteriovenous fistula 39.53
  frenulum, frenum
    labia (lips) 27.91
    lingual (tongue) 25.91
  tip of uvula 27.72
Clitoridectomy 71.4
Clitoridotomy 71.4
Clivogram 87.02
Closure — see also Repair
  abdominal wall 54.63
    delayed (granulating wound) 54.62
      secondary 54.61
      tertiary 54.62
  amputation stump, secondary 84.3
  aorticopulmonary fenestration (fistula) 39.59
  appendicostomy 47.92
  artificial opening
    bile duct 51.79
    bladder 57.82
    bronchus 33.42
    common duct 51.72
    esophagus 42.83
    gallbladder 51.92
    hepatic duct 51.79
    intestine 46.50
      large 46.52
      small 46.51

Closure — see also Repair — continued
  artificial opening — continued
    kidney 55.82
    larynx 31.62
    rectum 48.72
    stomach 44.62
    thorax 34.72
    trachea 31.72
    ureter 56.83
    urethra 58.42
  atrial septal defect (see also Repair, atrial septal defect) 35.71
    with umbrella device (King-Mills type) 35.52
    combined with repair of valvular and ventricular septal defects — see Repair, endocardial cushion defect
  bronchostomy 33.42
  cecostomy 46.52
  cholecystostomy 51.92
  cleft hand 82.82
  colostomy 46.52
  cystostomy 57.82
  diastema (alveolar) (dental) 24.8
  disrupted abdominal wall (postoperative) 54.61
  duodenostomy 46.51
  encephalocele 02.12
  endocardial cushion defect (see also Repair, endocardial cushion defect) 35.73
  enterostomy 46.50
  esophagostomy 42.83
  fenestration
    aorticopulmonary 39.59
    septal, heart (see also Repair, heart, septum) 35.70
  filtering bleb, corneoscleral (postglaucoma) 12.66
  fistula
    abdominothoracic 34.83
    anorectal 48.73
    anovaginal 70.73
    antrobuccal 22.71
    anus 49.73
    aorticopulmonary (fenestration) 39.59
    aortoduodenal 39.59
    appendix 47.92
    biliary tract 51.79
    bladder NEC 57.84
    branchial cleft 29.52
    bronchocutaneous 33.42
    bronchoesophageal 33.42
    bronchomediastinal 34.73
    bronchopleural 34.73
    bronchopleurocutaneous 34.73
    bronchopleuromediastinal 34.73
    bronchovisceral 33.42
    bronchus 33.42
    cecosigmoidal 46.76
    cerebrospinal fluid 02.12
    cervicoaural 18.79
    cervicosigmoidal 67.62
    cervicovesical 57.84
    cervix 67.62
    cholecystocolic 51.93
    cholecystoduodenal 51.93
    cholecystoenteric 51.93
    cholecystogastric 51.93
    cholecystojejunal 51.93
    cisterna chyli 40.63
    colon 46.76
    colovaginal 70.72
    common duct 51.72
    cornea 11.49
      with lamellar graft (homograft) 11.62
        autograft 11.61
    diaphragm 34.83
    duodenum 46.72
    ear, middle 19.9
    ear drum 19.4
    enterocolic 46.74
    enterocutaneous 46.74
    enterouterine 69.42
    enterovaginal 70.74
    enterovesical 57.83
    esophagobronchial 33.42
    esophagocutaneous 42.84
    esophagopleurocutaneous 34.73

Closure — see also Repair — continued
  fistula — continued
    esophagotracheal 31.73
    esophagus NEC 42.84
    fecal 46.79
    gallbladder 51.93
    gastric NEC 44.63
    gastrocolic 44.63
    gastroenterocolic 44.63
    gastroesophageal 42.84
    gastrojejunal 44.63
    gastrojejunocolic 44.63
    heart valve — see Repair, heart, valve
    hepatic duct 51.79
    hepatopleural 34.73
    hepatopulmonary 34.73
    ileorectal 46.74
    ileosigmoidal 46.74
    ileovesical 57.83
    ileum 46.74
    in ano 49.73
    intestine 46.79
      large 46.76
      small NEC 46.74
    intestinocolonic 46.74
    intestinoureteral 56.84
    intestinouterine 69.42
    intestinovaginal 70.74
    intestinovesical 57.83
    jejunum 46.74
    kidney 55.83
    lacrimal 09.99
    laryngotracheal 31.62
    larynx 31.62
    lymphatic duct, left (thoracic) 40.63
    mastoid (antrum) 19.9
    mediastinobronchial 34.73
    mediastinocutaneous 34.73
    mouth (external) 27.53
    nasal 21.82
      sinus 22.71
    nasolabial 21.82
    nasopharyngeal 21.82
    oroantral 22.71
    oronasal 21.82
    oval window (ear) 20.93
    pancreaticoduodenal 52.95
    perilymph 20.93
    perineorectal 48.73
    perineosigmoidal 46.76
    perineourethroscrotal 58.43
    perineum 71.72
    perirectal 48.93
    pharyngoesophageal 29.53
    pharynx NEC 29.53
    pleura, pleural NEC 34.93
    pleurocutaneous 34.73
    pleuropericardial 37.4
    pleuroperitoneal 34.83
    pulmonoperitoneal 34.83
    rectolabial 48.73
    rectoureteral 56.84
    rectourethral 58.43
    rectovaginal 70.73
    rectovesical 57.83
    rectovesicovaginal 57.83
    rectovulvar 48.73
    rectum NEC 48.73
    renal 55.83
    reno-intestinal 55.83
    round window 20.93
    salivary (gland) (duct) 26.42
    scrotum 61.42
    sigmoidovaginal 70.74
    sigmoidovesical 57.83
    splenocolic 41.95
    stomach NEC 44.63
    thoracic duct 40.63
    thoracoabdominal 34.83
    thoracogastric 34.83
    thoracointestinal 34.83
    thorax NEC 34.71
    trachea NEC 31.73
    tracheoesophageal 31.73
    tympanic membrane (see also Tympanoplasty) 19.4

Closure

Closure — see also Repair — continued
  fistula — continued
    umbilicourinary 57.51
    ureter 56.84
    ureterocervical 56.84
    ureterorectal 56.84
    ureterosigmoidal 56.84
    ureterovaginal 56.84
    ureterovesical 56.84
    urethra 58.43
    urethroperineal 58.43
    urethroperineovesical 57.84
    urethrorectal 58.43
    urethroscrotal 58.43
    urethrovaginal 58.43
    uteroenteric 69.42
    uterointestinal 69.42
    uterorectal 69.42
    uteroureteric 56.84
    uterovaginal 69.42
    uterovesical 57.84
    vagina 70.8
    vaginocutaneous 70.75
    vaginoenteric 70.74
    vaginoperineal 70.75
    vaginovesical 57.84
    vesicocervicovaginal 57.84
    vesicocolic 57.83
    vesicocutaneous 57.84
    vesicoenteric 57.83
    vesicometrorectal 57.83
    vesicoperineal 57.84
    vesicorectal 57.83
    vesicosigmoidal 57.83
    vesicosigmoidovaginal 57.83
    vesicoureteral 56.84
    vesicoureterovaginal 56.84
    vesicourethral 57.84
    vesicourethrorectal 57.83
    vesicouterine 57.84
    vesicovaginal 57.84
    vulva 71.72
    vulvorectal 48.73
  foramen ovale (patent) 35.71
    with
      prosthesis (open heart technique) 35.51
        closed heart technique 35.52
      tissue graft 35.61
  gastroduodenostomy 44.5
  gastrojejunostomy 44.5
  gastrostomy 44.62
  ileostomy 46.51
  jejunostomy 46.51
  laceration — see also Suture, by site
    liver 50.61
  laparotomy, delayed 54.62
  meningocele (spinal) 03.51
    cerebral 02.12
  myelomeningocele 03.52
  nephrostomy 55.82
  palmar cleft 82.82
  patent ductus arteriosus 38.85
  pelviostomy 55.82
  peptic ulcer (bleeding) (perforated) 44.40
  perforation
    ear drum (see also Tympanoplasty) 19.4
    esophagus 42.82
    nasal septum 21.88
    tympanic membrane (see also Tympanoplasty) 19.4
  proctostomy 48.72
  punctum, lacrimal (papilla) 09.91
  pyelostomy 55.82
  rectostomy 48.72
  septum defect (heart) (see also Repair, heart, septum) 35.70
  sigmoidostomy 46.52
  skin (V-Y type) 86.59
  stoma
    bile duct 51.79
    bladder 57.82
    bronchus 33.42
    common duct 51.72
    esophagus 42.83
    gallbladder 51.92
    hepatic duct 51.79

Closure — see also Repair — continued
  stoma — continued
    intestine 46.50
      large 46.52
      small 46.51
    kidney 55.82
    larynx 31.62
    rectum 48.72
    stomach 44.62
    thorax 34.72
    trachea 31.72
    ureter 56.83
    urethra 58.42
  thoracostomy 34.72
  tracheostomy 31.72
  ulcer (bleeding) (peptic) (perforated) 44.40
    duodenum 44.42
    gastric 44.41
    intestine (perforated) 46.79
    skin 86.59
    stomach 44.41
  ureterostomy 56.83
  urethrostomy 58.42
  vagina 70.4
  vascular
    percutaneous puncture — omit code
  vesicostomy 57.22
  wound — see also Suture, by site
    with graft — see Graft
    with tissue adhesive 86.59

Coagulation, electrocoagulation — see also Destruction, lesion, by site
  aneurysm (cerebral) (peripheral vessel) 39.52
  arteriovenous fistula 39.53
  brain tissue (incremental) (radio-frequency) 01.59
  broad ligament 69.19
  cervix 67.32
  ear
    external 18.29
    inner 20.79
    middle 20.51
  fallopian tube 66.61
  gasserian ganglion 04.05
  nose for epistaxis (with packing) 21.03
  ovary 65.29
    laparoscopic 65.25
  pharynx (by diathermy) 29.39
  prostatic bed 60.94
  rectum (polyp) 48.32
    radical 48.31
  retina (for)
    destruction of lesion 14.21
    reattachment 14.51
    repair of tear 14.31
  round ligament 69.19
  semicircular canals 20.79
  spinal cord (lesion) 03.4
  urethrovesical junction, transurethral 57.49
  uterosacral ligament 69.19
  uterus 68.29
  vagina 70.33
  vulva 71.3

Coating, aneurysm of brain 39.52

Cobalt-60 therapy (treatment) 92.23

Coccygectomy (partial) 77.89
  total 77.99

Coccygotomy 77.39

"Cocked hat" procedure (metacarpal lengthening and transfer of local flap) 82.69

Cockett operation (varicose vein)
  lower limb 38.59
  upper limb 38.53

Cody tack (perforation of footplate) 19.0

Coffey operation (uterine suspension) (Meig's modification) 69.22

Cole operation (anterior tarsal wedge osteotomy) 77.28

Colectomy (partial) (segmental) (subtotal) 45.79
  cecum (with terminal ileum) 45.72
  left (Hartmann) (lower) (radical) 45.75
  multiple segmental 45.71
  right (radical) 45.73
  sigmoid 45.76

Colectomy — continued
  terminal ileum with cecum 45.72
  total 45.8
  transverse 45.74

Collapse, lung, surgical 33.39
  by
    destruction of phrenic nerve 33.31
    pneumoperitoneum 33.33
    pneumothorax, artificially-induced 33.32
    thoracoplasty 33.34

Collection, sperm for artificial insemination 99.96

Collis-Nissen operation (hiatal hernia repair with esophagogastroplasty) 53.80

Colocentesis 45.03

Colocolostomy 45.94
  proximal to distal segment 45.79

Colocystoplasty 57.87 [45.52]

Colofixation 46.64

Coloileotomy 45.00

Colonna operation
  adductor tenotomy (first stage) 83.12
  hip arthroplasty (second stage) 81.40
  reconstruction of hip (second stage) 81.40

Colonoscopy 45.23
  with biopsy 45.25
    rectum 48.24
  fiberoptic (flexible) 45.23
  intraoperative 45.21
  through stoma (artificial) 45.22
  transabdominal 45.21

Colopexy 46.63

Coloplication 46.64

Coloproctostomy 45.94

Colorectosigmoidostomy 45.94

Colorectostomy 45.94

Colorrhaphy 46.75

Coloscopy — see Colonoscopy

Colosigmoidostomy 45.94

Colostomy (ileo-ascending) (ileo-transverse) (perineal) (transverse) 46.10
  with anterior rectal resection 48.62
  delayed opening 46.14
  loop 46.03
  permanent (magnetic) 46.13
  temporary 46.11

Colotomy 45.03

Colpectomy 70.4

Colpoceliocentesis 70.0

Colpocentesis 70.0

Colpocleisis (complete) (partial) 70.8

Colphysterectomy 68.59
  laparoscopically assisted (LAVH) 68.51

Colpoperineoplasty 70.79
  with repair of urethrocele 70.50

Colpoperineorrhaphy 70.71
  following delivery 75.69

Colpopexy 70.77

Colpoplasty 70.79

Colpopoiesis 70.61

Colporrhaphy 70.71
  anterior (cystocele repair) 70.51
  for repair of
    cystocele 70.51
      with rectocele 70.50
    enterocele 70.92
    rectocele 70.52
      with cystocele 70.50
    urethrocele 70.51
  posterior (rectocele repair) 70.52

Colposcopy 70.21

Colpotomy 70.14
  for pelvic peritoneal drainage 70.12

Commando operation (radical glossectomy) 25.4

Commissurotomy
  closed heart technique — see Valvulotomy, heart
  open heart technique — see Valvuloplasty, heart

Index to Procedures

Compression, trigeminal nerve 04.02
Conchectomy 21.69
Conchotomy 21.1
Conduction study, nerve 89.15
Conduitogram, ileum 87.78
Condylectomy — *see* category 77.8 ✓4ᵗʰ
  mandible 76.5
Condylotomy NEC (*see also* Division, joint capsule) 80.40
  mandible (open) 76.62
    closed 76.61
Conization
  cervix (knife) (sharp) (biopsy) 67.2
    by
      cryosurgery 67.33
      electroconization 67.32
Conjunctivocystorhinostomy 09.82
  with insertion of tube or stent 09.83
Conjunctivodacryocystorhinostomy (CDCR) 09.82
  with insertion of tube or stent 09.83
Conjunctivodacryocystostomy 09.82
  with insertion of tube or stent 09.83
Conjunctivoplasty 10.49
Conjunctivorhinostomy 09.82
  with insertion of tube or stent 09.83
Constriction of globe, for scleral buckling (*see also* Buckling, scleral) 14.49
Construction
  auricle, ear (with graft) (with implant) 18.71
  ear
    auricle (with graft) (with implant) 18.71
    meatus (osseous) (side-lined) 18.6
  endorectal ileal pouch (J-pouch) (H-pouch) (S-pouch) (with anastomosis to anus) 45.95
  esophagus, artificial — *see* Anastomosis, esophagus
  ileal bladder (open) 56.51
    closed 57.87 [45.51]
  ileal conduit 56.51
  larynx, artificial 31.75
  patent meatus (ear) 18.6
  penis (rib graft) (skin graft) (myocutaneous flap) 64.43
  pharyngeal valve, artificial 31.75
  urethra 58.46
  vagina, artificial 70.61
  venous valves (peripheral) 39.59
Consultation 89.09
  comprehensive 89.07
  limited (single organ system) 89.06
  specified type NEC 89.08
Continuous positive airway pressure (CPAP) 93.90
Control
  atmospheric pressure and composition NEC 93.98
    antigen-free air conditioning 93.98
    decompression chamber 93.97
    mountain sanatorium 93.98
  epistaxis 21.00
    by
      cauterization (and packing) 21.03
      coagulation (with packing) 21.03
      electrocoagulation (with packing) 21.03
      excision of nasal mucosa with grafting 21.07
      ligation of artery 21.09
        ethmoidal 21.04
        external carotid 21.06
        maxillary (transantral) 21.05
      packing (nasal) (anterior) 21.01
        posterior (and anterior) 21.02
      specified means NEC 21.09
  hemorrhage 39.98
    abdominal cavity 54.19
    adenoids (postoperative) 28.7
    anus (postoperative) 49.95
    bladder (postoperative) 57.93
    chest 34.09
    colon 45.49
      endoscopic 45.43

Control — *continued*
  hemorrhage — *continued*
    duodenum (ulcer) 44.49
      by
        embolization (transcatheter) 44.44
        suture (ligation) 44.42
      endoscopic 44.43
    esophagus 42.39
      endoscopic 42.33
    gastric (ulcer) 44.49
      by
        embolization (transcatheter) 44.44
        suture (ligation) 44.41
      endoscopic 44.43
    intrapleural 34.09
      postoperative (recurrent) 34.03
    laparotomy site 54.12
    nose (*see also* Control, epistaxis) 21.00
    peptic (ulcer) 44.49
      by
        embolization (transcatheter) 44.44
        suture (ligation) 44.40
      endoscopic 44.43
    pleura, pleural cavity 34.09
      postoperative (recurrent) 34.03
    postoperative NEC 39.98
    postvascular surgery 39.41
    prostate 60.94
    specified site NEC 39.98
    stomach — *see* Control, hemorrhage, gastric
    thorax NEC 34.09
      postoperative (recurrent) 34.03
    thyroid (postoperative) 06.02
    tonsils (postoperative) 28.7
Conversion
  anastomosis — *see* Revision, anastomosis
  cardiac rhythm NEC 99.69
    to sinus rhythm 99.62
  gastrostomy to jejunostomy (endoscopic) 44.32 ▲
  obstetrical position — *see* Version
Cooling, gastric 96.31
Cordectomy, vocal 30.22
Cordopexy, vocal 31.69
Cordotomy
  spinal (bilateral) NEC 03.29
    percutaneous 03.21
  vocal 31.3
Corectomy 12.12
Corelysis 12.35
Coreoplasty 12.35
Corneoconjunctivoplasty 11.53
Correction — *see also* Repair
  atresia
    esophageal 42.85
      by magnetic forces 42.99
    external meatus (ear) 18.6
    nasopharynx, nasopharyngeal 29.4
    rectum 48.0
    tricuspid 35.94
  atrial septal defect (*see also* Repair, atrial septal defect) 35.71
    combined with repair of valvular and ventricular septal defects — *see* Repair, endocardial cushion defect
  blepharoptosis (*see also* Repair, blepharoptosis) 08.36
  bunionette (with osteotomy) 77.54
  chordee 64.42
  claw toe 77.57
  cleft
    lip 27.54
    palate 27.62
  clubfoot NEC 83.84
  coarctation of aorta
    with
      anastomosis 38.34
      graft replacement 38.44
  cornea NEC 11.59
    refractive NEC 11.79
      epikeratophakia 11.76
      keratomileusis 11.71
      keratophakia 11.72
      radial keratotomy 11.75

Correction — *see also* Repair — *continued*
  esophageal atresia 42.85
    by magnetic forces 42.99
  everted lacrimal punctum 09.71
  eyelid
    ptosis (*see also* Repair, blepharoptosis) 08.36
    retraction 08.38
  fetal defect 75.36
  forcible, of musculoskeletal deformity NEC 93.29
  hammer toe 77.56
  hydraulic pressure, open surgery for penile inflatable prosthesis 64.99
    urinary artificial sphincter 58.99
  intestinal malrotation 46.80
    large 46.82
    small 46.81
  inverted uterus — *see* Repair, inverted uterus
  lymphedema (of limb) 40.9
    excision with graft 40.9
    obliteration of lymphatics 40.9
    transplantation of autogenous lymphatics 40.9
  nasopharyngeal atresia 29.4
  overlapping toes 77.58
  palate (cleft) 27.62
  prognathism NEC 76.64
  prominent ear 18.5
  punctum (everted) 09.71
  spinal pseudarthrosis — *see* Refusion, spinal
  syndactyly 86.85
  tetralogy of Fallot
    one-stage 35.81
    partial — *see* specific procedure
    total 35.81
  total anomalous pulmonary venous connection
    one-stage 35.82
    partial — *see* specific procedure
    total 35.82
  transposition, great arteries, total 35.84
  tricuspid atresia 35.94
  truncus arteriosus
    one-stage 35.83
    partial — *see* specific procedure
    total 35.83
  ureteropelvic junction 55.87
  ventricular septal defect (*see also* Repair, ventricular septal defect) 35.72
    combined with repair of valvular and atrial septal defects — *see* Repair, endocardial cushion defect
Costectomy 77.91
  with lung excision — *see* Excision, lung
  associated with thoracic operation — *omit code*
Costochondrectomy 77.91
  associated with thoracic operation — *omit code*
Costosternoplasty (pectus excavatum repair) 34.74
Costotomy 77.31
Costotransversectomy 77.91
  associated with thoracic operation — *omit code*
Counseling (for) NEC 94.49
  alcoholism 94.46
  drug addiction 94.45
  employers 94.49
  family (medical) (social) 94.49
  marriage 94.49
  ophthalmologic (with instruction) 95.36
  pastoral 94.49
Countershock, cardiac NEC 99.62
Coventry operation (tibial wedge osteotomy) 77.27
CPAP (continuous positive airway pressure) 93.90
Craniectomy 01.25
  linear (opening of cranial suture) 02.01
  reopening of site 01.23
  strip (opening of cranial suture) 02.01
Cranioclasis, fetal 73.8
Cranioplasty 02.06
  with synchronous repair of encephalocele 02.12
Craniotomy 01.24
  as operative approach — *omit code*

Craniotomy — *continued*
   fetal 73.8
   for decompression of fracture 02.02
   reopening of site 01.23

Craterization, bone (*see also* Excision, lesion, bone) 77.60

Crawford operation (tarso-frontalis sling of eyelid) 08.32

Creation — *see also* Formation
   cardiac pacemaker pocket
     with initial insertion of pacemaker — *omit code*
     new site (skin) (subcutaneous) 37.79
   conduit
     ileal (urinary) 56.51
     left ventricle and aorta 35.93
     right atrium and pulmonary artery 35.94
     right ventricle and pulmonary (distal) artery 35.92
       in repair of
         pulmonary artery atresia 35.92
         transposition of great vessels 35.92
         truncus arteriosus 35.83
   endorectal ileal pouch (J-pouch) (H-pouch) (S-pouch) (with anastomosis to anus) 45.95
   esophagogastric sphincteric competence NEC 44.66
   Hartmann pouch — *see* Colectomy, by site
   interatrial fistula 35.42
   pericardial window 37.12
   pleural window, for drainage 34.09
   pocket
     cardiac pacemaker
       with initial insertion of pacemaker — *omit code*
       new site (skin) (subcutaneous) 37.79
     loop recorder 86.09
     thalamic stimulator pulse generator
       with initial insertion of battery package — *omit code*
       new site (skin) (subcutaneous) 86.09
   shunt — *see also* Shunt
     arteriovenous fistula, for dialysis 39.93
     left-to-right (systemic to pulmonary circulation) 39.0
   subcutaneous tunnel for esophageal anastomosis 42.86
     with anastomosis — *see* Anastomosis, esophagus, antesternal
   syndactyly (finger) (toe) 86.89
   thalamic stimulator pulse generator pocket
     with initial insrtion of battery package — *omit code*
     new site (skin) (subcutaneous) 86.09
   tracheoesophageal fistula 31.95
   window
     pericardial 37.12
     pleura, for drainage 34.09

Credé maneuver 73.59

Cricoidectomy 30.29

Cricothyreotomy (for assistance in breathing) 31.1

Cricothyroidectomy 30.29

Cricothyrostomy 31.1

Cricothyrotomy (for assistance in breathing) 31.1

Cricotomy (for assistance in breathing) 31.1

Cricotracheotomy (for assistance in breathing) 31.1

Crisis intervention 94.35

Croupette, croup tent 93.94

Crown, dental (ceramic) (gold) 23.41

Crushing
   bone — *see* category 78.4 ◢4ᵗʰ
   calculus
     bile (hepatic) passage 51.49
       endoscopic 51.88
     bladder (urinary) 57.0
     pancreatic duct 52.09
       endoscopic 52.94
   fallopian tube (*see also* Ligation, fallopian tube) 66.39
   ganglion — *see* Crushing, nerve
   hemorrhoids 49.45

Crushing — *continued*
   nasal septum 21.88
   nerve (cranial) (peripheral) NEC 04.03
     acoustic 04.01
     auditory 04.01
     phrenic 04.03
       for collapse of lung 33.31
     sympathetic 05.0
     trigeminal 04.02
     vestibular 04.01
   vas deferens 63.71

Cryoablation — *see* Ablation

Cryoanalgesia
   nerve (cranial) (peripheral) 04.2

Cryoconization, cervix 67.33

Cryodestruction — *see* Destruction, lesion, by site

Cryoextraction, lens (*see also* Extraction, cataract, intracapsular) 13.19

Cryohypophysectomy (complete) (total) (*see also* Hypophysectomy) 07.69

Cryoleucotomy 01.32

Cryopexy, retinal — *see* Cryotherapy, retina

Cryoprostatectomy 60.62

Cryoretinopexy (for)
   reattachment 14.52
   repair of tear or defect 14.32

Cryosurgery — *see* Cryotherapy

Cryothalamectomy 01.41

Cryotherapy — *see also* Destruction, lesion, by site
   bladder 57.59
   brain 01.59
   cataract 13.19
   cervix 67.33
   choroid — *see* Cryotherapy, retina
   ciliary body 12.72
   corneal lesion (ulcer) 11.43
     to reshape cornea 11.79
   ear
     external 18.29
     inner 20.79
   esophagus 42.39
     endoscopic 42.33
   eyelid 08.25
   hemorrhoids 49.44
   iris 12.41
   nasal turbinates 21.61
   palate (bony) 27.31
   prostate 60.62
   retina (for)
     destruction of lesion 14.22
     reattachment 14.52
     repair of tear 14.32
   skin 86.3
   stomach 43.49
     endoscopic 43.41
   subcutaneous tissue 86.3
   turbinates (nasal) 21.61
   warts 86.3
     genital 71.3

Cryptectomy (anus) 49.39
   endoscopic 49.31

Cryptorchidectomy (unilateral) 62.3
   bilateral 62.41

Cryptotomy (anus) 49.39
   endoscopic 49.31

Cuirass 93.99

Culdocentesis 70.0

Culdoplasty 70.92

Culdoscopy (exploration) (removal of foreign body or lesion) 70.22

Culdotomy 70.12

Culp-Deweerd operation (spiral flap pyeloplasty) 55.87

Culp-Scardino operation (ureteral flap pyeloplasty) 55.87

Culture (and sensitivity) — *see* Examination, microscopic

Curettage (with packing) (with secondary closure) — *see also* Dilation and curettage
   adenoids 28.6
   anus 49.39
     endoscopic 49.31
   bladder 57.59
     transurethral 57.49
   bone (*see also* Excision, lesion, bone) 77.60
   brain 01.59
   bursa 83.39
     hand 82.29
   cartilage (*see also* Excision, lesion, joint) 80.80
   cerebral meninges 01.51
   chalazion 08.25
   conjunctiva (trachoma follicles) 10.33
   corneal epithelium 11.41
     for smear or culture 11.21
   ear, external 18.29
   eyelid 08.25
   joint (*see also* Excision, lesion, joint) 80.80
   meninges (cerebral) 01.51
     spinal 03.4
   muscle 83.32
     hand 82.22
   nerve (peripheral) 04.07
     sympathetic 05.29
   sclera 12.84
   skin 86.3
   spinal cord (meninges) 03.4
   subgingival 24.31
   tendon 83.39
     sheath 83.31
       hand 82.21
   uterus (with dilation) 69.09
     aspiration (diagnostic) NEC 69.59
       after abortion or delivery 69.52
       to terminate pregnancy 69.51
     following delivery or abortion 69.02

Curette evacuation, lens 13.2

Curtis operation (interphalangeal joint arthroplasty) 81.72

Cutaneolipectomy 86.83

Cutdown, venous 38.94

Cutting
   nerve (cranial) (peripheral) NEC 04.03
     acoustic 04.01
     auditory 04.01
     root, spinal 03.1
     sympathetic 05.0
     trigeminal 04.02
     vestibular 04.01
   pedicle (flap) graft 86.71
   pylorus (with wedge resection) 43.3
   spinal nerve root 03.1
   ureterovesical orifice 56.1
   urethral sphincter 58.5

CVP (central venous pressure monitoring) 89.62

Cyclectomy (ciliary body) 12.44
   eyelid margin 08.20

Cyclicotomy 12.55

Cycloanemization 12.74

Cyclocryotherapy 12.72

Cyclodialysis (initial) (subsequent) 12.55

Cyclodiathermy (penetrating) (surface) 12.71

Cycloelectrolysis 12.71

Cyclophotocoagulation 12.73

Cyclotomy 12.55

Cystectomy — *see also* Excision, lesion, by site
   gallbladder — *see* Cholecystectomy
   urinary (partial) (subtotal) 57.6
     complete (with urethrectomy) 57.79
     radical 57.71
       with pelvic exenteration (female) 68.8
     total (with urethrectomy) 57.79

Cystocolostomy 57.88

Cystogram, cystography NEC 87.77

Cystolitholapaxy 57.0

Cystolithotomy 57.19

Cystometrogram 89.22

Cystopexy NEC 57.89

Cystoplasty NEC 57.89

Index to Procedures

Cystoproctostomy 57.88
Cystoprostatectomy, radical 57.71
Cystopyelography 87.74
Cystorrhaphy 57.81
Cystoscopy (transurethral) 57.32
  with biopsy 57.33
  for
    control of hemorrhage
      bladder 57.93
      prostate 60.94
    retrograde pyelography 87.74
  ileal conduit 56.35
  through stoma (artificial) 57.31
Cystostomy
  closed (suprapubic) (percutaneous) 57.17
  open (suprapubic) 57.18
  percutaneous (closed) (suprapubic) 57.17
  suprapubic
    closed 57.17
    open 57.18
Cystotomy (open) (for removal of calculi) 57.19
Cystourethrogram (retrograde) (voiding) 87.76
Cystourethropexy (by) 59.79
  levator muscle sling 59.71
  retropubic suspension 59.5
  suprapubic suspension 59.4
Cystourethroplasty 57.85
Cystourethroscopy 57.32
  with biopsy
    bladder 57.33
    ureter 56.33
Cytology — *see* Examination, microscopic

D

Dacryoadenectomy 09.20
  partial 09.22
  total 09.23
Dacryoadenotomy 09.0
Dacryocystectomy (complete) (partial) 09.6
Dacryocystogram 87.05
Dacryocystorhinostomy (DCR) (by intubation) (external) (intranasal) 09.81
Dacryocystostomy 09.53
Dacryocystosyringotomy 09.53
Dacryocystotomy 09.53
Dahlman operation (excision of esophageal diverticulum) 42.31
Dana operation (posterior rhizotomy) 03.1
Danforth operation (fetal) 73.8
Darrach operation (ulnar resection) 77.83
Davis operation (intubated ureterotomy) 56.2
Deaf training 95.49
Debridement
  abdominal wall 54.3
  bone (*see also* Excision, lesion, bone) 77.60
    fracture — *see* Debridement, open fracture
  brain 01.59
  burn (skin) 86.28
    excisional 86.22
    nonexcisional 86.28
  cerebral meninges 01.51
  dental 96.54
  flap graft 86.75
  graft (flap) (pedicle) 86.75
  heart valve (calcified) — *see* Valvuloplasty, heart
  infection (skin) 86.28
    excisional 86.22
    nail bed or fold 86.27
    nonexcisional 86.28
  joint — *see* Excision, lesion, joint
  meninges (cerebral) 01.51
    spinal 03.4
  muscle 83.45
    hand 82.36
  nail 86.27
  nerve (peripheral) 04.07

Debridement — *continued*
  open fracture (compound) 79.60
    arm NEC 79.62
    carpal, metacarpal 79.63
    facial bone 76.2
    femur 79.65
    fibula 79.66
    foot NEC 79.67
    hand NEC 79.63
    humerus 79.61
    leg NEC 79.66
    phalanges
      foot 79.68
      hand 79.64
    radius 79.62
    specified site NEC 79.69
    tarsal, metatarsal 79.67
    tibia 79.66
    ulna 79.62
  patella 77.66
  pedicle graft 86.75
  skin or subcutaneous tissue (burn) (infection) (wound) 86.28
    cardioverter/defibrillator (automatic) pocket 37.99
    excisional 86.22
    graft 86.75
    nail, nail bed, or nail fold 86.27
    nonexcisional 86.28
    pacemaker pocket 37.79
    pocket
      cardiac pacemaker 37.79
      cardioverter/defibrillator (automatic) 37.99
  skull 01.25
    compound fracture 02.02
  spinal cord (meninges) 03.4
  wound (skin) 86.28
    excisional 86.22
    nonexcisional 86.28
Decapitation, fetal 73.8
Decapsulation, kidney 55.91
Declotting — *see also* Removal, thrombus
  arteriovenous cannula or shunt 39.49
Decompression
  anus (imperforate) 48.0
  biliary tract 51.49
    by intubation 51.43
      endoscopic 51.87
      percutaneous 51.98
  brain 01.24
  carpal tunnel 04.43
  cauda equina 03.09
  chamber 93.97
  colon 96.08
    by incision 45.03
    endoscopic (balloon) 46.85
  common bile duct 51.42
    by intubation 51.43
      endoscopic 51.87
      percutaneous 51.98
  cranial 01.24
    for skull fracture 02.02
  endolymphatic sac 20.79
  ganglion (peripheral) NEC 04.49
    cranial NEC 04.42
  gastric 96.07
  heart 37.0
  intestine 96.08
    by incision 45.00
    endoscopic (balloon) 46.85
  intracranial 01.24
  labyrinth 20.79
  laminectomy 03.09
  laminotomy 03.09
  median nerve 04.43
  muscle 83.02
    hand 82.02
  nerve (peripheral) NEC 04.49
    auditory 04.42
    cranial NEC 04.42
    median 04.43
    trigeminal (root) 04.41
  orbit (*see also* Orbitotomy) 16.09

Decompression — *continued*
  pancreatic duct 52.92
    endoscopic 52.93
  pericardium 37.0
  rectum 48.0
  skull fracture 02.02
  spinal cord (canal) 03.09
  tarsal tunnel 04.44
  tendon (sheath) 83.01
    hand 82.01
  thoracic outlet
    by
      myotomy (division of scalenus anticus muscle) 83.19
      tenotomy 83.13
  trigeminal (nerve root) 04.41
Decortication
  arterial 05.25
  brain 01.51
  cerebral meninges 01.51
  heart 37.31
  kidney 55.91
  lung (partial) (total) 34.51
  nasal turbinates — *see* Turbinectomy
  nose 21.89
  ovary 65.29
    laparoscopic 65.25
  periarterial 05.25
  pericardium 37.31
  ventricle, heart (complete) 37.31
Deepening
  alveolar ridge 24.5
  buccolabial sulcus 24.91
  lingual sulcus 24.91
Defatting, flap or pedicle graft 86.75
Defibrillation, electric (external) (internal) 99.62
  automatic cardioverter/defibrillator — *see* category 37.9
de Grandmont operation (tarsectomy) 08.35
Delaying of pedicle graft 86.71
Delivery (with)
  assisted spontaneous 73.59
  breech extraction (assisted) 72.52
    partial 72.52
      with forceps to aftercoming head 72.51
    total 72.54
      with forceps to aftercoming head 72.53
    unassisted (spontaneous delivery) — *omit code*
  cesarean section — *see* Cesarean section
  Credé maneuver 73.59
  De Lee maneuver 72.4
  forceps 72.9
    application to aftercoming head (Piper) 72.6
    with breech extraction
      partial 72.51
      total 72.53
    Barton's 72.4
    failed 73.3
    high 72.39
      with episiotomy 72.31
    low (outlet) 72.0
      with episiotomy 72.1
    mid 72.29
      with episiotomy 72.21
    outlet (low) 72.0
      with episiotomy 72.1
    rotation of fetal head 72.4
    trial 73.3
  instrumental NEC 72.9
    specified NEC 72.8
  key-in-lock rotation 72.4
  Kielland rotation 72.4
  Malström's extraction 72.79
    with episiotomy 72.71
  manually assisted (spontaneous) 73.59
  spontaneous (unassisted) 73.59
    assisted 73.59
  vacuum extraction 72.79
    with episiotomy 72.71
Delorme operation
  pericardiectomy 37.31
  proctopexy 48.76
  repair of prolapsed rectum 48.76

Delorme operation — *continued*
    thoracoplasty 33.34

Denervation
    aortic body 39.8
    carotid body 39.8
    facet, percutaneous (radiofrequency) 03.96
    ovarian 65.94
    paracervical uterine 69.3
    uterosacral 69.3

Denker operation (radical maxillary antrotomy) 22.31

Dennis-Barco operation — *see* Repair, hernia, femoral

Denonvillier operation (limited rhinoplasty) 21.86

Densitometry, bone (serial) (radiographic) 88.98

Depilation, skin 86.92

Derlacki operation (tympanoplasty) 19.4

Dermabond 86.59

Dermabrasion (laser) 86.25
    for wound debridement 86.28

Derotation — *see* Reduction, torsion

Desensitization
    allergy 99.12
    psychologic 94.33

Desmotomy (*see also* Division, ligament) 80.40

Destruction
    breast 85.20
    chorioretinopathy (*see also* Destruction, lesion, choroid) 14.29
    ciliary body 12.74
    epithelial downgrowth, anterior chamber 12.93
    fallopian tube 66.39
        with
            crushing (and ligation) 66.31
                by endoscopy (laparoscopy) 66.21
            division (and ligation) 66.32
                by endoscopy (culdoscopy) (hysteroscopy) (laparoscopy) (peritoneoscopy) 66.22
            ligation 66.39
                with
                    crushing 66.31
                        by endoscopy (laparoscopy) 66.21
                  division 66.32
                      by endoscopy (culdoscopy) (hysteroscopy) (laparoscopy) (peritoneoscopy) 66.22
    fetus 73.8
    hemorrhoids 49.49
        by
            cryotherapy 49.44
            sclerotherapy 49.42
    inner ear (NEC) 20.79
        by injection 20.72
    intervertebral disc (NOS) 80.50
        by injection 80.52
        by other specified method 80.59
        herniated (nucleus pulposus) 80.51
    lacrimal sac 09.6
    lesion (local)
        anus 49.39
            endoscopic 49.31
        Bartholin's gland 71.24
            by
                aspiration 71.21
                excision 71.24
                incision 71.22
                marsupialization 71.23
        biliary ducts 51.69
            endoscopic 51.64
        bladder 57.59
            transurethral 57.49
        bone — *see* Excision, lesion, bone
        bowel — *see* Destruction, lesion, intestine
        brain (transtemporal approach) NEC 01.59
            by stereotactic radiosurgery 92.40
                cobalt 60 92.32
                linear accelerator (LINAC) 92.31
                multi-source 92.32
                particle beam 92.33

Destruction — *continued*
    lesion — *continued*
        brain NEC — *continued*
            by stereotactic radiosurgery — *continued*
                particulate 92.33
                radiosurgery NEC 92.39
                single source photon 92.31
        breast NEC 85.20
        bronchus NEC 32.09
            endoscopic 32.01
        cerebral NEC 01.59
            meninges 01.51
        cervix 67.39
            by
                cauterization 67.32
                cryosurgery, cryoconization 67.33
                electroconization 67.32
        choroid 14.29
            by
                cryotherapy 14.22
                diathermy 14.21
                implantation of radiation source 14.27
                photocoagulation 14.25
                    laser 14.24
                    xenon arc 14.23
                radiation therapy 14.26
        ciliary body (nonexcisional) 12.43
            by excision 12.44
        conjunctiva 10.32
            by excision 10.31
        cornea NEC 11.49
            by
                cryotherapy 11.43
                electrocauterization 11.42
                thermocauterization 11.42
        cul-de-sac 70.32
        duodenum NEC 45.32
            by excision 45.31
            endoscopic 45.30
            endoscopic 45.30
        esophagus (chemosurgery) (cryosurgery) (electroresection) (fulguration) NEC 42.39
            by excision 42.32
            endoscopic 42.33
            endoscopic 42.33
        eye NEC 16.93
        eyebrow 08.25
        eyelid 08.25
            excisional — *see* Excision, lesion, eyelid
        heart 37.33
            by catheter ablation 37.34
        intestine (large) 45.49
            by excision 45.41
                endoscopic 45.43
                    polypectomy 45.42
            endoscopic 45.43
                polypectomy 45.42
            small 45.34
                by excision 45.33
        intranasal 21.31
        iris (nonexcisional) NEC 12.41
            by excision 12.42
        kidney 55.39
            by marsupialization 55.31
        lacrimal sac 09.6
        larynx 30.09
        liver 50.29
        lung 32.29
            endoscopic 32.28
        meninges (cerebral) 01.51
            spinal 03.4
        nerve (peripheral) 04.07
            sympathetic 05.29
        nose 21.30
            intranasal 21.31
            specified NEC 21.32
        ovary
            by
                aspiration 65.91
                excision 65.29
                    laparoscopic 65.25
            cyst by rupture (manual) 65.93
        palate (bony) (local) 27.31
            wide 27.32

Destruction — *continued*
    lesion — *continued*
        pancreas 52.22
            by marsupialization 52.3
            endoscopic 52.21
        pancreatic duct 52.22
            endoscopic 52.21
        penis 64.2
        pharynx (excisional) NEC 29.39
        pituitary gland
            by stereotactic radiosurgery 92.30
                cobalt 60 92.32
                linear accelerator (LINAC) 92.31
                multi-source 92.32
                particle beam 92.33
                particulate 92.33
                radiosurgery NEC 92.39
                single source photon 92.31
        rectum (local) 48.32
            by
                cryosurgery 48.34
                electrocoagulation 48.32
                excision 48.35
                fulguration 48.32
                laser (Argon) 48.33
            polyp 48.36
            radical 48.31
        retina 14.29
            by
                cryotherapy 14.22
                diathermy 14.21
                implantation of radiation source 14.27
                photocoagulation 14.25
                    laser 14.24
                    xenon arc 14.23
                radiation therapy 14.26
        salivary gland NEC 26.29
            by marsupialization 26.21
        sclera 12.84
        scrotum 61.3
        skin NEC 86.3
        sphincter of Oddi 51.69
            endoscopic 51.64
        spinal cord (meninges) 03.4
        spleen 41.42
            by marsupialization 41.41
        stomach 43.49
            by excision 43.42
                endoscopic 43.41
            endoscopic 43.41
        subcutaneous tissue NEC 86.3
        testis 62.2
        tongue 25.1
        urethra (excisional) 58.39
            endoscopic 58.31
        uterus 68.29
    nerve (cranial) (peripheral) (by cryoanalgesia) by radiofrequency) 04.2
        sympathetic, by injection of neurolytic agent 05.32
    neuroma
        acoustic 04.01
            by craniotomy 04.01
            by stereotactic radiosurgery 92.30
                cobalt 60 92.32
                linear accelerator (LINAC) 92.31
                multi-source 92.32
                particle beam 92.33
                particulate 92.33
                radiosurgery NEC 92.39
                single source photon 92.31
        cranial 04.07
        Morton's 04.07
        peripheral
            Morton's 04.07
    prostate (prostatic tissue)
        by
            cryotherapy 60.62
            microwave 60.96
            radiofrequency 60.97
            transurethral microwave thermotherapy (TUMT) 60.96
            transurethral needle ablation (TUNA) 60.97
            TULIP (transurethral (ultrasound) guided laser induced prostatectomy) 60.21

Index to Procedures

Destruction — *continued*
  prostate — *continued*
    TUMT (transurethral microwave thermotherapy) 60.96
    TUNA (transurethral needle ablation) 60.97
  semicircular canals, by injection 20.72
  vestibule, by injection 20.72

Detachment, uterosacral ligaments 69.3

Determination
  mental status (clinical) (medicolegal) (psychiatric) NEC 94.11
  psychologic NEC 94.09
  vital capacity (pulmonary) 89.37

Detorsion
  intestine (twisted) (volvulus) 46.80
    large 46.82
      endoscopic (balloon) 46.85
    small 46.81
  kidney 55.84
  ovary 65.95
  spermatic cord 63.52
    with orchiopexy 62.5
  testis 63.52
    with orchiopexy 62.5
  volvulus 46.80
    endoscopic (balloon) 46.85

Detoxification therapy 94.25
  alcohol 94.62
    with rehabilitation 94.63
    combined alcohol and drug 94.68
      with rehabilitation 94.69
  drug 94.65
    with rehabilitation 94.66
    combined alcohol and drug 94.68
      with rehabilitation 94.69

Devascularization, stomach 44.99

Dewebbing
  esophagus 42.01
  syndactyly (fingers) (toes) 86.85

Dextrorotation — *see* Reduction, torsion

Dialysis
  hemodiafiltration, hemofiltration (extracorporeal) 39.95
  kidney (extracorporeal) 39.95
  liver 50.92
  peritoneal 54.98
  renal (extracorporeal) 39.95

Diaphanoscopy
  nasal sinuses 89.35
  skull (newborn) 89.16

Diaphysectomy — *see* category 77.8 ✓4ᵗʰ

Diathermy 93.34
  choroid — *see* Diathermy, retina
  nasal turbinates 21.61
  retina
    for
      destruction of lesion 14.21
      reattachment 14.51
      repair of tear 14.31
  surgical — *see* Destruction, lesion, by site
  turbinates (nasal) 21.61

Dickson operation (fascial transplant) 83.82

Dickson-Diveley operation (tendon transfer and arthrodesis to correct claw toe) 77.57

Dieffenbach operation (hip disarticulation) 84.18

Dilation
  achalasia 42.92
  ampulla of Vater 51.81
    endoscopic 51.84
  anus, anal (sphincter) 96.23
  biliary duct
    endoscopic 51.84
    pancreatic duct 52.99
      endoscopic 52.98
    percutaneous (endoscopy) 51.98
    sphincter
      of Oddi 51.81
        endoscopic 51.84
      pancreatic 51.82
        endoscopic 51.85
  bladder 96.25
    neck 57.92
  bronchus 33.91

Dilation — *continued*
  cervix (canal) 67.0
    obstetrical 73.1
    to assist delivery 73.1
  choanae (nasopharynx) 29.91
  colon (endoscopic) (balloon) 46.85
  colostomy stoma 96.24
  duodenum (endoscopic) (balloon) 46.85
  endoscopic — *see* Dilation, by site
  enterostomy stoma 96.24
  esophagus (by bougie) (by sound) 42.92
  fallopian tube 66.96
  foreskin (newborn) 99.95
  frontonasal duct 96.21
  gastrojejunostomy site, endoscopic 44.22
  heart valve — *see* Valvulotomy, heart
  ileostomy stoma 96.24
  ileum (endoscopic) (balloon) 46.85
  intestinal stoma (artificial) 96.24
  intestine (endoscopic) (balloon) 46.85
  jejunum (endoscopic) (balloon) 46.85
  lacrimal
    duct 09.42
    punctum 09.41
  larynx 31.98
  lymphatic structure(s) (peripheral) 40.9
  nares 21.99
  nasolacrimal duct (retrograde) 09.43
    with insertion of tube or stent 09.44
  nasopharynx 29.91
  pancreatic duct 52.99
    endoscopic 52.98
  pharynx 29.91
  prostatic urethra (transurethral) (balloon) 60.95
  punctum, lacrimal papilla 09.41
  pylorus
    by incision 44.21
    endoscopic 44.22
  rectum 96.22
  salivary duct 26.91
  sphenoid ostia 22.52
  sphincter
    anal 96.23
    cardiac 42.92
    of Oddi 51.81
      endoscopic 51.84
    pancreatic 51.82
      endoscopic 51.85
    pylorus, endoscopic 44.22
      by incision 44.21
  Stenson's duct 26.91
  trachea 31.99
  ureter 59.8
    meatus 56.91
  ureterovesical orifice 59.8
  urethra 58.6
    prostatic (transurethral) (balloon) 60.95
  urethrovesical junction 58.6
  vagina (instrumental) (manual) NEC 96.16
  vesical neck 57.92
  Wharton's duct 26.91
  Wirsung's duct 52.99
    endoscopic 52.98

Dilation and curettage, uterus (diagnostic) 69.09
  after
    abortion 69.02
    delivery 69.02
  to terminate pregnancy 69.01

Diminution, ciliary body 12.74

Disarticulation 84.91
  ankle 84.13
  elbow 84.06
  finger, except thumb 84.01
    thumb 84.02
  hip 84.18
  knee 84.16
  shoulder 84.08
  thumb 84.02
  toe 84.11
  wrist 84.04

Discission
  capsular membrane 13.64
  cataract (Wheeler knife) (Ziegler knife) 13.2
    congenital 13.69
    secondary membrane 13.64

Discission — *continued*
  iris 12.12
  lens (capsule) (Wheeler knife) (Ziegler knife) (with capsulotomy) 13.2
  orbitomaxillary, radical 16.51
  pupillary 13.2
  secondary membrane (after cataract) 13.64
  vitreous strands (posterior approach) 14.74
    anterior approach 14.73

Discogram, diskogram 87.21

Discolysis (by injection) 80.52

Diskectomy, intervertebral 80.51
  herniated (nucleus pulposus) 80.51
  percutaneous 80.59

Dispensing (with fitting)
  contact lens 95.32
  low vision aids NEC 95.33
  spectacles 95.31

Dissection — *see also* Excision
  aneurysm 38.60
  artery-vein-nerve bundle 39.91
  branchial cleft fistula or sinus 29.52
  bronchus 32.1
  femoral hernia 53.29
  groin, radical 40.54
  larynx block (en bloc) 30.3
  mediastinum with pneumonectomy 32.5
  neck, radical 40.40
    with laryngectomy 30.4
    bilateral 40.42
    unilateral 40.41
  orbital fibrous bands 16.92
  pterygium (with reposition) 11.31
  radical neck — *see* Dissection, neck, radical
  retroperitoneal NEC 59.00
  thoracic structures (block) (en bloc) (radical) (brachial plexus, bronchus, lobe of lung, ribs, and sympathetic nerves) 32.6
  vascular bundle 39.91

Distention, bladder (therapeutic) (intermittent) 96.25

Diversion, urinary
  cutaneous 56.61
  ileal conduit 56.51
  internal NEC 56.71
  ureter to
    intestine 56.71
    skin 56.61
  uretero-ileostomy 56.51

Diversional therapy 93.81

Diverticulectomy
  bladder (suprapubic) 57.59
    transurethral approach 57.49
  duodenum 45.31
    endoscopic 45.30
  esophagus 42.31
    endoscopic 42.33
  esophagomyotomy 42.7
  hypopharyngeal (by cricopharyngeal myotomy) 29.32
  intestine
    large 45.41
      endoscopic 45.43
    small 45.33
  kidney 55.39
  Meckel's 45.33
  pharyngeal (by cricopharyngeal myotomy) 29.32
  pharyngoesophageal (by cricopharyngeal myotomy) 29.32
  stomach 43.42
    endoscopic 43.41
  urethra 58.39
    endoscopic 58.31

Division
  Achilles tendon 83.11
  adductor tendon (hip) 83.12
  adhesions — *see* Lysis, adhesions
  angle of mandible (open) 76.62
    closed 76.61
  anterior synechiae 12.32
  aponeurosis 83.13
  arcuate ligament (spine) — *omit code*
  arteriovenous fistula (with ligation) 39.53

Division

Division — *continued*
- artery (with ligation) 38.80
  - abdominal 38.86
  - aorta (arch) (ascending) (descending) 38.84
  - head and neck NEC 38.82
  - intracranial NEC 38.81
  - lower limb 38.88
  - thoracic NEC 38.85
  - upper limb 38.83
- bladder neck 57.91
- blepharorrhaphy 08.02
- blood vessels, cornea 10.1
- bone (*see also* Osteotomy) 77.30
- brain tissue 01.32
  - cortical adhesions 02.91
- canaliculus 09.52
- canthorrhaphy 08.02
- cartilage 80.40
  - ankle 80.47
  - elbow 80.42
  - foot and toe 80.48
  - hand and finger 80.44
  - hip 80.45
  - knee 80.46
  - shoulder 80.41
  - specified site NEC 80.49
  - spine 80.49
  - wrist 80.43
- cerebral tracts 01.32
- chordae tendineae 35.32
- common wall between posterior left atrium and coronary sinus (with roofing of resultant defect with patch graft) 35.82
- congenital web
  - larynx 31.98
  - pharynx 29.54
- endometrial synechiae 68.21
- fallopian tube — *see* Ligation, fallopian tube
- fascia 83.14
  - hand 82.12
- frenulum, frenum
  - labial 27.91
  - lingual 25.91
  - tongue 25.91
- ganglion, sympathetic 05.0
- glossopharyngeal nerve 29.92
- goniosynechiae 12.31
- hypophyseal stalk (*see also* Hypophysectomy, partial) 07.63
- iliotibial band 83.14
- isthmus
  - horseshoe kidney 55.85
  - thyroid 06.91
- joint capsule 80.40
  - ankle 80.47
  - elbow 80.42
  - foot and toe 80.48
  - hand and finger 80.44
  - hip 80.45
  - knee 80.46
  - shoulder 80.41
  - specified site NEC 80.49
  - wrist 80.43
- labial frenum 27.91
- lacrimal ductules 09.0
- laryngeal nerve (external) (recurrent) (superior) 31.91
- ligament 80.40
  - ankle 80.47
  - arcuate (spine) — *omit code*
  - canthal 08.36
  - elbow 80.42
  - foot and toe 80.48
  - hand and finger 80.44
  - hip 80.45
  - knee 80.46
  - palpebrae 08.36
  - shoulder 80.41
  - specified site NEC 80.49
  - spine 80.49
    - arcuate — *omit code*
    - flavum — *omit code*
  - uterosacral 69.3
  - wrist 80.43
- ligamentum flavum (spine) — *omit code*
- meninges (cerebral) 01.31

Division — *continued*
- muscle 83.19
  - hand 82.19
- nasolacrimal duct stricture (with drainage) 09.59
- nerve (cranial) (peripheral) NEC 04.03
  - acoustic 04.01
  - adrenal gland 07.42
  - auditory 04.01
  - glossopharyngeal 29.92
  - lacrimal branch 05.0
  - laryngeal (external) (recurrent) (superior) 31.91
  - phrenic 04.03
    - for collapse of lung 33.31
  - root, spinal or intraspinal 03.1
  - sympathetic 05.0
  - tracts
    - cerebral 01.32
    - spinal cord 03.29
      - percutaneous 03.21
  - trigeminal 04.02
  - vagus (*see also* Vagotomy) 44.00
  - vestibular 04.01
- otosclerotic process or material, middle ear 19.0
- papillary muscle (heart) 35.31
- patent ductus arteriosus 38.85
- penile adhesions 64.93
- posterior synechiae 12.33
- pylorus (with wedge resection) 43.3
- rectum (stricture) 48.91
- scalenus anticus muscle 83.19
- Skene's gland 71.3
- soft tissue NEC 83.19
  - hand 82.19
- sphincter
  - anal (external) (internal) 49.59
    - left lateral 49.51
    - posterior 49.52
  - cardiac 42.7
  - of Oddi 51.82
    - endoscopic 51.85
  - pancreatic 51.82
    - endoscopic 51.85
- spinal
  - cord tracts 03.29
    - percutaneous 03.21
  - nerve root 03.1
- symblepharon (with insertion of conformer) 10.5
- synechiae
  - endometrial 68.21
  - iris (posterior) 12.33
    - anterior 12.32
- tarsorrhaphy 08.02
- tendon 83.13
  - Achilles 83.11
  - adductor (hip) 83.12
  - hand 82.11
- trabeculae carneae cordis (heart) 35.35
- tympanum 20.23
- uterosacral ligaments 69.3
- vaginal septum 70.14
- vas deferens 63.71
- vein (with ligation) 38.80
  - abdominal 38.87
  - head and neck NEC 38.82
  - intracranial NEC 38.81
  - lower limb 38.89
    - varicose 38.59
  - thoracic NEC 38.85
  - upper limb 38.83
  - varicose 38.50
    - abdominal 38.57
    - head and neck NEC 38.52
    - intracranial NEC 38.51
    - lower limb 38.59
    - thoracic NEC 38.55
    - upper limb 38.53
- vitreous, cicatricial bands (posterior approach) 14.74
  - anterior approach 14.73

Doleris operation (shortening of round ligaments) 69.22

D'Ombrain operation (excision of pterygium with corneal graft) 11.32

Domestic tasks therapy 93.83

Dopplergram, Doppler flow mapping — *see also* Ultrasonography
- aortic arch 88.73
- head and neck 88.71
- heart 88.72
- thorax NEC 88.73

Dorrance operation (push-back operation for cleft palate) 27.62

Dotter operation (transluminal angioplasty) 39.59

Douche, vaginal 96.44

Douglas operation (suture of tongue to lip for micrognathia) 25.59

Doyle operation (paracervical uterine denervation) 69.3

Drainage
- by
  - anastomosis — *see* Anastomosis
  - aspiration — *see* Aspiration
  - incision — *see* Incision
- abdomen 54.19
  - percutaneous 54.91
- abscess — *see also* Drainage, by site *and* Incision, by site
  - appendix 47.2
    - with appendectomy 47.09
      - laparoscopic 47.01
  - parapharyngeal (oral) (transcervical) 28.0
  - peritonsillar (oral) (transcervical) 28.0
  - retropharyngeal (oral) (transcervical) 28.0
  - thyroid (field) (gland) 06.09
    - percutaneous (needle) 06.01
    - postoperative 06.02
  - tonsil, tonsillar (oral) (transcervical) 28.0
- antecubital fossa 86.04
- appendix 47.91
  - with appendectomy 47.09
    - laparoscopic 47.01
  - abscess 47.2
    - with appendectomy 47.09
      - laparoscopic 47.01
- axilla 86.04
- bladder (without incision) 57.0
  - by indwelling catheter 57.94
    - percutaneous suprapubic (closed) 57.17
    - suprapubic NEC 57.18
- buccal space 27.0
- bursa 83.03
  - by aspiration 83.94
    - hand 82.92
  - hand 82.03
    - by aspiration 82.92
  - radial 82.03
  - ulnar 82.03
- cerebrum, cerebral (meninges) (ventricle) (incision) (trephination) 01.39
  - by
    - anastomosis — *see* Shunt, ventricular
    - aspiration 01.09
      - through previously implanted catheter 01.02
- chest (closed) 34.04
  - open (by incision) 34.09
- cranial sinus (incision) (trephination) 01.21
  - by aspiration 01.09
- cul-de-sac 70.12
  - by aspiration 70.0
- cyst — *see also* Drainage, by site *and* Incision, by site
  - pancreas (by catheter) 52.01
    - by marsupialization 52.3
    - internal (anastomosis) 52.4
  - pilonidal 86.03
  - spleen, splenic (by marsupialization) 41.41
- duodenum (tube) 46.39
  - by incision 45.01
- ear
  - external 18.09
  - inner 20.79
  - middle (by myringotomy) 20.09
    - with intubation 20.01

Index to Procedures — Electrocoagulation

Drainage — *continued*
  epidural space cerebral (incision) (trephination) 01.24
    by aspiration 01.09
  extradural space, cerebral (incision) (trephination) 01.24
    by aspiration 01.09
  extraperitoneal 54.0
  facial region 27.0
  fascial compartments, head and neck 27.0
  fetal hydrocephalic head (needling) (trocar) 73.8
  gallbladder 51.04
    by
      anastomosis 51.35
      aspiration 51.01
      incision 51.04
  groin region (abdominal wall) (inguinal) 54.0
    skin 86.04
    subcutaneous tissue 86.04
  hematoma — *see* Drainage, by site *and* Incision, by site
  hydrocephalic head (needling) (trocar) 73.8
  hypochondrium 54.0
    intra-abdominal 54.19
  iliac fossa 54.0
  infratemporal fossa 27.0
  intracranial space (epidural) (extradural) (incision) (trephination) 01.24
    by aspiration 01.09
    subarachnoid or subdural (incision) (trephination) 01.31
      by aspiration 01.09
  intraperitoneal 54.19
    percutaneous 54.91
  kidney (by incision) 55.01
    by
      anastomosis 55.86
      catheter 59.8
    pelvis (by incision) 55.11
  liver 50.0
    by aspiration 50.91
  Ludwig's angina 27.0
  lung (by incision) 33.1
    by punch (needle) (trocar) 33.93
  midpalmar space 82.04
  mouth floor 27.0
  mucocele, nasal sinus 22.00
    by puncture 22.01
    through natural ostium 22.02
  omentum 54.19
    percutaneous 54.91
  ovary (aspiration) 65.91
    by incision 65.09
    laparoscopic 65.01
  palmar space (middle) 82.04
  pancreas (by catheter) 52.01
    by anastomosis 52.96
  parapharyngeal 28.0
  paronychia 86.04
  parotid space 27.0
  pelvic peritoneum (female) 70.12
    male 54.19
  pericardium 37.0
  perigastric 54.19
    percutaneous 54.91
  perineum
    female 71.09
    male 86.04
  perisplenic tissue 54.19
    percutaneous 54.91
  peritoneum 54.19
    pelvic (female) 70.12
    percutaneous 54.91
  peritonsillar 28.0
  pharyngeal space, lateral 27.0
  pilonidal cyst or sinus 86.03
  pleura (closed) 34.04
    open (by incision) 34.09
  popliteal space 86.04
  postural 93.99
  postzygomatic space 27.0
  pseudocyst, pancreas 52.3
    by anastomosis 52.4
  pterygopalatine fossa 27.0
  retropharyngeal 28.0
  scrotum 61.0

Drainage — *continued*
  skin 86.04
  spinal (canal) (cord) 03.09
    by anastomosis — *see* Shunt, spinal
    diagnostic 03.31
  spleen 41.2
    cyst (by marsupialization) 41.41
  subarachnoid space, cerebral (incision) (trephination) 01.31
    by aspiration 01.09
  subcutaneous tissue 86.04
  subdiaphragmatic 54.19
    percutaneous 54.91
  subdural space, cerebral (incision) (trephination) 01.31
    by aspiration 01.09
  subhepatic space 54.19
    percutaneous 54.91
  sublingual space 27.0
  submental space 27.0
  subphrenic space 54.19
    percutaneous 54.91
  supraclavicular fossa 86.04
  temporal pouches 27.0
  tendon (sheath) 83.01
    hand 82.01
  thenar space 82.04
  thorax (closed) 34.04
    open (by incision) 34.09
  thyroglossal tract (by incision) 06.09
    by aspiration 06.01
  thyroid (field) (gland) (by incision) 06.09
    by aspiration 06.01
    postoperative 06.02
  tonsil 28.0
  tunica vaginalis 61.0
  ureter (by catheter) 59.8
    by
      anastomosis NEC (*see also* Anastomosis, ureter) 56.79
      incision 56.2
  ventricle (cerebral) (incision) NEC 02.39
    by
      anastomosis — *see* Shunt, ventricular
      aspiration 01.09
        through previously implanted catheter 01.02
  vertebral column 03.09
Drawing test 94.08
Dressing
  burn 93.57
  ulcer 93.56
  wound 93.57
Drilling, bone (*see also* Incision, bone) 77.10
Ductogram, mammary 87.35
Duhamel operation (abdominoperineal pull-through) 48.65
Dührssen's
  incisions (cervix, to assist delivery) 73.93
  operation (vaginofixation of uterus) 69.22
Dunn operation (triple arthrodesis) 81.12
Duodenectomy 45.62
  with
    gastrectomy — *see* Gastrectomy
    pancreatectomy — *see* Pancreatectomy
Duodenocholedochotomy 51.51
Duodenoduodenostomy 45.91
  proximal to distal segment 45.62
Duodenoileostomy 45.91
Duodenojejunostomy 45.91
Duodenoplasty 46.79 ●
Duodenorrhaphy 46.71
Duodenoscopy 45.13
  through stoma (artificial) 45.12
  transabdominal (operative) 45.11
Duodenostomy 46.39
Duodenotomy 45.01
Dupuytren operation
  fasciectomy 82.35
  fasciotomy 82.12
    with excision 82.35
  shoulder disarticulation 84.08

Durabond 86.59
Duraplasty 02.12
Durham (-Caldwell) operation (transfer of biceps femoris tendon) 83.75
DuToit and Roux operation (staple capsulorrhaphy of shoulder) 81.82
DuVries operation (tenoplasty) 83.88
Dwyer operation
  fasciotomy 83.14
  soft tissue release NEC 83.84
  wedge osteotomy, calcaneus 77.28

E

Eagleton operation (extrapetrosal drainage) 20.22
ECG — *see* Electrocardiogram
Echocardiography 88.72
  intracardiac (ICE) 37.28
  transesophageal 88.72
    monitoring (Doppler) (ultrasound) 89.68
Echoencephalography 88.71
Echography — *see* Ultrasonography
Echogynography 88.79
Echoplacentogram 88.78
ECMO (extracorporeal membrane oxygenation) 39.65
Eden-Hybinette operation (glenoid bone block) 78.01
Educational therapy (bed-bound children) (handicapped) 93.82
EEG (electroencephalogram) 89.14
  monitoring (radiographic) (video) 89.19
Effler operation (heart) 36.2
Effleurage 93.39
EGD (esophagogastroduodenoscopy) 45.13
  with closed biopsy 45.16
Eggers operation
  tendon release (patellar retinacula) 83.13
  tendon transfer (biceps femoris tendon) (hamstring tendon) 83.75
EKG (*see also* Electrocardiogram) 89.52
Elastic hosiery 93.59
Electrocardiogram (with 12 or more leads) 89.52
  with vectorcardiogram 89.53
  fetal (scalp), intrauterine 75.32
  rhythm (with one to three leads) 89.51
Electrocautery — *see also* Cauterization
  cervix 67.32
  corneal lesion (ulcer) 11.42
  esophagus 42.39
  endoscopic 42.33
Electrocoagulation — *see also* Destruction, lesion, by site
  aneurysm (cerebral) (peripheral vessels) 39.52
  cervix 67.32
  cystoscopic 57.49
  ear
    external 18.29
    inner 20.79
    middle 20.51
  fallopian tube (lesion) 66.61
    for tubal ligation — *see* Ligation, fallopian tube
  gasserian ganglion 04.02
  nasal turbinates 21.61
  nose, for epistaxis (with packing) 21.03
  ovary 65.29
    laparoscopic 65.25
  prostatic bed 60.94
  rectum (polyp) 48.32
    radical 48.31
  retina (for)
    destruction of lesion 14.21
    reattachment 14.51
    repair of tear 14.31
  round ligament 69.19
  semicircular canals 20.79
  urethrovesical junction, transurethral 57.49

Electrocoagulation — see also Destruction, lesion, by site — *continued*
  uterine ligament 69.19
  uterosacral ligament 69.19
  uterus 68.29
  vagina 70.33
  vulva 71.3
Electrocochleography 20.31
Electroconization, cervix 67.32
Electroconvulsive therapy (ECT) 94.27
Electroencephalogram (EEG) 89.14
  monitoring (radiographic) (video) 89.19
Electrogastrogram 44.19
Electrokeratotomy 11.49
Electrolysis
  ciliary body 12.71
  hair follicle 86.92
  retina (for)
    destruction of lesion 14.21
    reattachment 14.51
    repair of tear 14.31
  skin 86.92
  subcutaneous tissue 86.92
Electromyogram, electromyography (EMG) (muscle) 93.08
  eye 95.25
  urethral sphincter 89.23
Electronarcosis 94.29
Electronic gaiter 93.59
Electronystagmogram (ENG) 95.24
Electro-oculogram (EOG) 95.22
Electroresection — *see also* Destruction, lesion, by site
  bladder neck (transurethral) 57.49
  esophagus 42.39
    endoscopic 42.33
  prostate (transurethral) 60.29
  stomach 43.49
    endoscopic 43.41
Electroretinogram (ERG) 95.21
Electroshock therapy (EST) 94.27
  subconvulsive 94.26
Elevation
  bone fragments (fractured)
    orbit 76.79
      sinus (nasal)
        frontal 22.79
        maxillary 22.79
      skull (with debridement) 02.02
      spinal 03.53
  pedicle graft 86.71
Elliot operation (scleral trephination with iridectomy) 12.61
Ellis Jones operation (repair of peroneal tendon) 83.88
Ellison operation (reinforcement of collateral ligament) 81.44
Elmslie-Cholmeley operation (tarsal wedge osteotomy) 77.28
Eloesser operation
  thoracoplasty 33.34
  thoracostomy 34.09
Elongation — *see* Lengthening
Embolectomy 38.00
  with endarterectomy — *see* Endarterectomy
  abdominal
    artery 38.06
    vein 38.07
  aorta (arch) (ascending) (descending) 38.04
  head and neck NEC 38.02
  intracranial NEC 38.01
  lower limb
    artery 38.08
    vein 38.09
  thoracic NEC 38.05
  upper limb (artery) (vein) 38.03
Embolization (transcatheter)
  adhesive (glue) 39.79
    head and neck 39.72
  arteriovenous fistula 39.53
    endovascular 39.72

Embolization — *continued*
  artery (selective) 38.80
    by
      endovascular approach 39.79
        head and neck vessels 39.72
      percutaneous transcatheter infusion 99.29
    abdominal NEC 38.86
      duodenal (transcatheter) 44.44
      gastric (transcatheter) 44.44
      renal (transcatheter) 38.86
    aorta (arch) (ascending) (descending) 38.84
    duodenal (transcatheter) 44.44
    gastric (transcatheter) 44.44
    head and neck NEC 38.82
    intracranial NEC 38.81
    lower limb 38.88
    renal (transcatheter) 38.86
    thoracic NEC 38.85
    upper limb 38.83
  AVM, intracranial, endovascular approach 39.72
  carotid cavernous fistula 39.53
  chemoembolization 99.25
  coil, endovascular 39.79
    head and neck 39.72
  vein (selective) 38.80
    abdominal NEC 38.87
      duodenal (transcatheter) 44.44
      gastric (transcatheter) 44.44
    by
      endovascular approach 39.79
        head and neck 39.72
    duodenal (transcatheter) 44.44
    gastric (transcatheter) 44.44
Embryotomy 73.8
EMG — *see* Electromyogram
Emmet operation (cervix) 67.61
Encephalocentesis (*see also* Puncture) 01.09
  fetal head, transabdominal 73.8
Encephalography (cisternal puncture) (fractional) (lumbar) (pneumoencephalogram) 87.01
Encephalopuncture 01.09
Encircling procedure — *see also* Cerclage
  sclera, for buckling 14.49
    with implant 14.41
Endarterectomy (gas) (with patch graft) 38.10
  abdominal 38.16
  aorta (arch) (ascending) (descending) 38.14
  coronary artery — *see* category 36.0
    open chest approach 36.03
  head and neck NEC 38.12
  intracranial NEC 38.11
  lower limb 38.18
  thoracic NEC 38.15
  upper limb 38.13
Endoaneurysmorrhaphy (*see also* Aneurysmorrhaphy) 39.52
  by or with
    endovascular graft
      abdominal aorta 39.71
      lower extremity artery(s) 39.79
      thoracic aorta 39.79
      upper extremity artery(s) 39.79
Endolymphatic (-subarachnoid) shunt 20.71
Endometrectomy (uterine) (internal) 68.29
  bladder 57.59
  cul-de-sac 70.32
Endoprosthesis
  bile duct 51.87
  femoral head (bipolar) 81.52
Endoscopy
  with biopsy — *see* Biopsy, by site, closed
  anus 49.21
  biliary tract (operative) 51.11
    by retrograde cholangiography (ERC) 51.11
    by retrograde cholangiopancreatography (ERCP) 51.10
    intraoperative 51.11
    percutaneous (via T-tube of other tract) 51.98
      with removal of common duct stones 51.96

Endoscopy — *continued*
  bladder 57.32
    through stoma (artificial) 57.31
  bronchus NEC 33.23
    with biopsy 33.24
    fiberoptic 33.22
    through stoma (artificial) 33.21
  colon 45.23
    through stoma (artificial) 45.22
    transabdominal (operative) 45.21
  cul-de-sac 70.22
  ear 18.11
  esophagus NEC 42.23
    through stoma (artificial) 42.22
    transabdominal (operative) 42.21
  ileum 45.13
    through stoma (artificial) 45.12
    transabdominal (operative) 45.11
  intestine NEC 45.24
    large 45.24
      fiberoptic (flexible) 45.23
      through stoma (artificial) 45.22
      transabdominal (intraoperative) 45.21
    small 45.13
      esophagogastroduodenoscopy (EGD) 45.13
        with closed biopsy 45.16
      through stoma (artificial) 45.12
      transabdominal (operative) 45.11
  jejunum 45.13
    through stoma (artificial) 45.12
    transabdominal (operative) 45.11
  kidney 55.21
  larynx 31.42
    through stoma (artificial) 31.41
  lung — *see* Bronchoscopy
  mediastinum (transpleural) 34.22
  nasal sinus 22.19
  nose 21.21
  pancreatic duct 52.13
  pelvis 55.22
  peritoneum 54.21
  pharynx 29.11
  rectum 48.23
    through stoma (artificial) 48.22
    transabdominal (operative) 48.21
  sinus, nasal 22.19
  stomach NEC 44.13
    through stoma (artificial) 44.12
    transabdominal (operative) 44.11
  thorax (transpleural) 34.21
  trachea NEC 31.42
    through stoma (artificial) 31.41
  transpleural
    mediastinum 34.22
    thorax 34.21
  ureter 56.31
  urethra 58.22
  uterus 68.12
  vagina 70.21
Enema (transanal) NEC 96.39
  for removal of impacted feces 96.38
ENG (electronystagmogram) 95.24
Enlargement
  aortic lumen, thoracic 38.14
  atrial septal defect (pre-existing) 35.41
    in repair of total anomalous pulmonary venous connection 35.82
  eye socket 16.64
  foramen ovale (pre-existing) 35.41
    in repair of total anomalous pulmonary venous connection 35.82
  intestinal stoma 46.40
    large intestine 46.43
    small intestine 46.41
  introitus 96.16
  orbit (eye) 16.64
  palpebral fissure 08.51
  punctum 09.41
  sinus tract (skin) 86.89
Enterectomy NEC 45.63
Enteroanastomosis
  large-to-large intestine 45.94
  small-to-large intestine 45.93
  small-to-small intestine 45.91

Enterocelectomy 53.9
  female 70.92
  vaginal 70.92
Enterocentesis 45.00
  duodenum 45.01
  large intestine 45.03
  small intestine NEC 45.02
Enterocholecystostomy 51.32
Enteroclysis (small bowel) 96.43
Enterocolectomy NEC 45.79
Enterocolostomy 45.93
Enteroentectropy 46.99
Enteroenterostomy 45.90
  small-to-large intestine 45.93
  small-to-small intestine 45.91
Enterogastrostomy 44.39
Enterolithotomy 45.00
Enterolysis 54.59
  laparoscopic 54.51
Enteropancreatostomy 52.96
Enterorrhaphy 46.79
  large intestine 46.75
  small intestine 46.73
Enterostomy NEC 46.39
  cecum (see also Colostomy) 46.10
  colon (transverse) (see also Colostomy) 46.10
    loop 46.03
  delayed opening 46.31
  duodenum 46.39
    loop 46.01
  feeding NEC 46.39
    percutaneous (endoscopic) 46.32
  ileum (Brooke) (Dragstedt) 46.20
    loop 46.01
  jejunum (feeding) 46.39
    loop 46.01
    percutaneous (endoscopic) 46.32
  sigmoid colon (see also Colostomy) 46.10
    loop 46.03
  transverse colon (see also Colostomy) 46.10
    loop 46.03
Enterotomy 45.00
  large intestine 45.03
  small intestine 45.02
Enucleation — see also Excision, lesion, by site
  cyst
    broad ligament 69.19
    dental 24.4
    liver 50.29
    ovarian 65.29
      laparoscopic 65.25
    parotid gland 26.29
    salivary gland 26.29
    skin 86.3
    subcutaneous tissue 86.3
  eyeball 16.49
    with implant (into Tenon's capsule) 16.42
      with attachment of muscles 16.41
EOG (electro-oculogram) 95.22
Epicardiectomy 36.39
Epididymectomy 63.4
  with orchidectomy (unilateral) 62.3
    bilateral 62.41
Epididymogram 87.93
Epididymoplasty 63.59
Epididymorrhaphy 63.81
Epididymotomy 63.92
Epididymovasostomy 63.83
Epiglottidectomy 30.21
Epikeratophakia 11.76
Epilation
  eyebrow (forceps) 08.93
    cryosurgical 08.92
    electrosurgical 08.91
  eyelid (forceps) NEC 08.93
    cryosurgical 08.92
    electrosurgical 08.91
  skin 86.92
Epiphysiodesis (see also Arrest, bone growth) —
  see category 78.2

Epiphysiolysis (see also Arrest, bone growth) —
  see category 78.2
Epiploectomy 54.4
Epiplopexy 54.74
Epiplorrhaphy 54.74
Episioperineoplasty 71.79
Episioperineorrhaphy 71.71
  obstetrical 75.69
Episioplasty 71.79
Episioproctotomy 73.6
Episiorrhaphy 71.71
  following routine episiotomy — see Episiotomy
  for obstetrical laceration 75.69
Episiotomy (with subsequent episiorrhaphy) 73.6
  high forceps 72.31
  low forceps 72.1
  mid forceps 72.21
  nonobstetrical 71.09
  outlet forceps 72.1
EPS (electrophysiologic stimulation) 37.26
Eptifibatide, infusion 99.20
Equalization, leg
  lengthening — see category 78.3
  shortening — see category 78.2
Equilibration (occlusal) 24.8
Equiloudness balance 95.43
ERC (endoscopic retrograde cholangiography) 51.11
ERCP (endoscopic retrograde cholangiopancreatography) 51.10
  cannulation of pancreatic duct 52.93
ERG (electroretinogram) 95.21
ERP (endoscopic retrograde pancreatography) 52.13
Eruption, tooth, surgical 24.6
Erythrocytapheresis, therapeutic 99.73
Escharectomy 86.22
Escharotomy 86.09
Esophageal voice training (post-laryngectomy) 93.73
Esophagectomy 42.40
  abdominothoracocervical (combined) (synchronous) 42.42
  partial or subtotal 42.41
  total 42.42
Esophagocologastrostomy (intrathoracic) 42.55
  antesternal or antethoracic 42.65
Esophagocolostomy (intrathoracic) NEC 42.56
  with interposition of colon 42.55
  antesternal or antethoracic NEC 42.66
    with interposition of colon 42.65
Esophagoduodenostomy (intrathoracic) NEC 42.54
  with
    complete gastrectomy 43.99
    interposition of small bowel 42.53
Esophagoenterostomy (intrathoracic) NEC (see also Anastomosis, esophagus, to intestinal segment) 42.54
  antesternal or antethoracic (see also Anastomosis, esophagus, antesternal, to intestinal segment) 42.64
Esophagoesophagostomy (intrathoracic) 42.51
  antesternal or antethoracic 42.61
Esophagogastrectomy 43.99
Esophagogastroduodenoscopy (EGD) 45.13
  with closed biopsy 45.16
  through stoma (artificial) 45.12
  transabdominal (operative) 45.11
Esophagogastromyotomy 42.7
Esophagogastropexy 44.65
Esophagogastroplasty 44.65
Esophagogastroscopy NEC 44.13
  through stoma (artificial) 44.12
  transabdominal (operative) 44.11
Esophagogastrostomy (intrathoracic) 42.52
  with partial gastrectomy 43.5
  antesternal or antethoracic 42.62

Esophagoileostomy (intrathoracic) NEC 42.54
  with interposition of small bowel 42.53
  antesternal or antethoracic NEC 42.64
    with interposition of small bowel 42.63
Esophagojejunostomy (intrathoracic) NEC 42.54
  with
    complete gastrectomy 43.99
    interposition of small bowel 42.53
  antesternal or antethoracic NEC 42.64
    with interposition of small bowel 42.63
Esophagomyotomy 42.7
Esophagoplasty NEC 42.89
Esophagorrhaphy 42.82
Esophagoscopy NEC 42.23
  by incision (operative) 42.21
  with closed biopsy 42.24
  through stoma (artificial) 42.22
  transabdominal (operative) 42.21
Esophagostomy 42.10
  cervical 42.11
  thoracic 42.19
Esophagotomy NEC 42.09
Estes operation (ovary) 65.72
  laparoscopic 65.75
Estlander operation (thoracoplasty) 33.34
ESWL (extracorporeal shockwave lithotripsy) NEC 98.59
  bile duct 98.52
  bladder 98.51
  gallbladder 98.52
  kidney 98.51
  Kock pouch (urinary diversion) 98.51
  renal pelvis 98.51
  specified site NEC 98.59
  ureter 98.51
Ethmoidectomy 22.63
Ethmoidotomy 22.51
Evacuation
  abscess — see Drainage, by site
  anterior chamber (eye) (aqueous) (hyphema) 12.91
  cyst — see also Excision, lesion, by site
    breast 85.91
    kidney 55.01
    liver 50.29
  hematoma — see also Incision, hematoma
    obstetrical 75.92
    incisional 75.91
  hemorrhoids (thrombosed) 49.47
  pelvic blood clot (by incision) 54.19
    by
      culdocentesis 70.0
      culdoscopy 70.22
  retained placenta
    with curettage 69.02
    manual 75.4
  streptothrix from lacrimal duct 09.42
Evaluation (of)
  audiological 95.43
  criminal responsibility, psychiatric 94.11
  functional (physical therapy) 93.01
  hearing NEC 95.49
  orthotic (for brace fitting) 93.02
  prosthetic (for artificial limb fitting) 93.03
  psychiatric NEC 94.19
    commitment 94.13
  psychologic NEC 94.08
  testimentary capacity, psychiatric 94.11
Evans operation (release of clubfoot) 83.84
Evisceration
  eyeball 16.39
    with implant (into scleral shell) 16.31
  ocular contents 16.39
    with implant (into scleral shell) 16.31
  orbit (see also Exenteration, orbit) 16.59
  pelvic (anterior) (posterior) (partial) (total) (female) 68.8
  male 57.71
Evulsion
  nail (bed) (fold) 86.23
  skin 86.3
  subcutaneous tissue 86.3

Examination

Examination (for)
  breast
    manual 89.36
    radiographic NEC 87.37
    thermographic 88.85
    ultrasonic 88.73
  cervical rib (by x-ray) 87.43
  colostomy stoma (digital) 89.33
  dental (oral mucosa) (peridontal) 89.31
    radiographic NEC 87.12
  enterostomy stoma (digital) 89.33
  eye 95.09
    color vision 95.06
    comprehensive 95.02
    dark adaptation 95.07
    limited (with prescription of spectacles) 95.01
    under anesthesia 95.04
  fetus, intrauterine 75.35
  general physical 89.7
  glaucoma 95.03
  gynecological 89.26
  hearing 95.47
  microscopic (specimen) (of) 91.9 ✓4th

Note — Use the following fourth-digit subclassification with categories 90-91 to identify type of examination:
  1 bacterial smear
  2 culture
  3 culture and sensitivity
  4 parasitology
  5 toxicology
  6 cell block and Papanicolaou smear
  9 other microscopic examination

    adenoid 90.3 ✓4th
    adrenal gland 90.1 ✓4th
    amnion 91.4 ✓4th
    anus 90.9 ✓4th
    appendix 90.9 ✓4th
    bile ducts 91.0 ✓4th
    bladder 91.3 ✓4th
    blood 90.5 ✓4th
    bone 91.5 ✓4th
      marrow 90.6 ✓4th
    brain 90.0 ✓4th
    breast 91.6 ✓4th
    bronchus 90.4 ✓4th
    bursa 91.5 ✓4th
    cartilage 91.5 ✓4th
    cervix 91.4 ✓4th
    chest wall 90.4 ✓4th
    chorion 91.4 ✓4th
    colon 90.9 ✓4th
    cul-de-sac 91.1 ✓4th
    dental 90.8 ✓4th
    diaphragm 90.4 ✓4th
    duodenum 90.8 ✓4th
    ear 90.3 ✓4th
    endocrine gland NEC 90.1 ✓4th
    esophagus 90.8 ✓4th
    eye 90.2 ✓4th
    fallopian tube 91.4 ✓4th
    fascia 91.5 ✓4th
    female genital tract 91.4 ✓4th
    fetus 91.4 ✓4th
    gallbladder 91.0 ✓4th
    hair 91.6 ✓4th
    ileum 90.9 ✓4th
    jejunum 90.9 ✓4th
    joint fluid 91.5 ✓4th
    kidney 91.2 ✓4th
    large intestine 90.9 ✓4th
    larynx 90.3 ✓4th
    ligament 91.5 ✓4th
    liver 91.0 ✓4th
    lung 90.4 ✓4th
    lymph (node) 90.7 ✓4th
    meninges 90.0 ✓4th
    mesentery 91.1 ✓4th
    mouth 90.8 ✓4th
    muscle 91.5 ✓4th
    musculoskeletal system 91.5 ✓4th
    nails 91.6 ✓4th
    nerve 90.0 ✓4th

Examination (for) — *continued*
  microscopic — *continued*
    nervous system 90.0 ✓4th
    nose 90.3 ✓4th
    omentum 91.1 ✓4th
    operative wound 91.7 ✓4th
    ovary 91.4 ✓4th
    pancreas 91.0 ✓4th
    parathyroid gland 90.1 ✓4th
    penis 91.3 ✓4th
    perirenal tissue 91.2 ✓4th
    peritoneum (fluid) 91.1 ✓4th
    periureteral tissue 91.2 ✓4th
    perivesical (tissue) 91.3 ✓4th
    pharynx 90.3 ✓4th
    pineal gland 90.1 ✓4th
    pituitary gland 90.1 ✓4th
    placenta 91.4 ✓4th
    pleura (fluid) 90.4 ✓4th
    prostate 91.3 ✓4th
    rectum 90.9 ✓4th
    retroperitoneum 91.1 ✓4th
    semen 91.3 ✓4th
    seminal vesicle 91.3 ✓4th
    sigmoid 90.9 ✓4th
    skin 91.6 ✓4th
    small intestine 90.9 ✓4th
    specified site NEC 91.8 ✓4th
    spinal fluid 90.0 ✓4th
    spleen 90.6 ✓4th
    sputum 90.4 ✓4th
    stomach 90.8 ✓4th
    stool 90.9 ✓4th
    synovial membrane 91.5 ✓4th
    tendon 91.5 ✓4th
    thorax NEC 90.4 ✓4th
    throat 90.3 ✓4th
    thymus 90.1 ✓4th
    thyroid gland 90.1 ✓4th
    tonsil 90.3 ✓4th
    trachea 90.4 ✓4th
    ureter 91.2 ✓4th
    urethra 91.3 ✓4th
    urine 91.3 ✓4th
    uterus 91.4 ✓4th
    vagina 91.4 ✓4th
    vas deferens 91.3 ✓4th
    vomitus 90.8 ✓4th
    vulva 91.4 ✓4th
  neurologic 89.13
  neuro-ophthalmology 95.03
  opthalmoscopic 16.21
  panorex, mandible 87.12
  pelvic (manual) 89.26
    instrumental (by pelvimeter) 88.25
    pelvimetric 88.25
  physical, general 89.7
  postmortem 89.8
  rectum (digital) 89.34
    endoscopic 48.23
      through stoma (artificial) 48.22
      transabdominal 48.21
  retinal disease 95.03
  specified type (manual) NEC 89.39
  thyroid field, postoperative 06.02
  uterus (digital) 68.11
    endoscopic 68.12
  vagina 89.26
    endoscopic 70.21
  visual field 95.05

Exchange transfusion 99.01
  intrauterine 75.2

Excision
  aberrant tissue — *see* Excision, lesion, by site of tissue origin
  abscess — *see* Excision, lesion, by site
  accessory tissue — *see also* Excision, lesion, by site of tissue origin
    lung 32.29
      endoscopic 32.28
    spleen 41.93
  adenoids (tag) 28.6
    with tonsillectomy 28.3
  adenoma — *see* Excision, lesion, by site
  adrenal gland (*see also* Adrenalectomy) 07.22

Excision — *continued*
  ampulla of Vater (with reimplantation of common duct) 51.62
  anal papilla 49.39
    endoscopic 49.31
  aneurysm (arteriovenous) (*see also* Aneurysmectomy) 38.60
    coronary artery 36.91
    heart 37.32
    myocardium 37.32
    sinus of Valsalva 35.39
    ventricle (heart) 37.32
  anus (complete) (partial) 49.6
  aortic subvalvular ring 35.35
  apocrine gland 86.3
  aponeurosis 83.42
    hand 82.33
  appendiceal stump 47.01-47.09
  appendices epiploicae 54.4
  appendix (*see also* Appendectomy) 47.01, 47.09
    epididymis 63.3
    testis 62.2
  arcuate ligament (spine) — *omit code*
  arteriovenous fistula (*see also* Aneurysmectomy) 38.60
  artery (*see also* Arteriectomy) 38.60
  Baker's cyst, knee 83.39
  Bartholin's gland 71.24
  basal ganglion 01.59
  bile duct 51.69
    endoscopic 51.64
  bladder — *see* Cystectomy
  bleb (emphysematous), lung 32.29
    endoscopic 32.28
  blood vessel (*see also* Angiectomy) 38.60
  bone (ends) (partial), except facial — *see category 77.8* ✓4th
    facial NEC 76.39
      total 76.45
        with reconstruction 76.44
    for graft (autograft) (homograft) — *see category 77.7* ✓4th
    fragments (chips) (*see also* Incision, bone) 77.10
    joint (*see also* Arthrotomy) 80.10
    necrotic (*see also* Sequestrectomy, bone) 77.00
    heterotopic, from
      muscle 83.32
        hand 82.22
      skin 86.3
      tendon 83.31
        hand 82.21
    mandible 76.31
      with arthrodesis — *see* Arthrodesis
      total 76.42
        with reconstruction 76.41
    spur — *see* Excision, lesion, bone
    total, except facial — *see category 77.9* ✓4th
      facial NEC 76.45
        with reconstruction 76.44
      mandible 76.42
        with reconstruction 76.41
  brain 01.59
    hemisphere 01.52
    lobe 01.53
  branchial cleft cyst or vestige 29.2
  breast (*see also* Mastectomy) 85.41
    aberrant tissue 85.24
    accessory 85.24
    ectopic 85.24
    nipple 85.25
      accessory 85.24
    segmental 85.23
    supernumerary 85.24
    wedge 85.21
  broad ligament 69.19
  bronchogenic cyst 32.09
    endoscopic 32.01
  bronchus (wide sleeve) NEC 32.1
  buccal mucosa 27.49
  bulbourethral gland 58.92
  bulbous tuberosities (mandible) (maxilla) (fibrous) (osseous) 24.31
  bunion (*see also* Bunionectomy) 77.59
  bunionette (with osteotomy) 77.54

Index to Procedures

Excision

Excision — *continued*
- bursa 83.5
  - hand 82.31
- canal of Nuck 69.19
- cardioma 37.33
- carotid body (lesion) (partial) (total) 39.8
- cartilage (*see also* Chondrectomy) 80.90
  - intervertebral — *see* category 80.5 ☑4th
  - knee (semilunar) 80.6
  - larynx 30.29
  - nasal (submucous) 21.5
- caruncle, urethra 58.39
  - endoscopic 58.31
- cataract (*see also* Extraction, cataract) 13.19
  - secondary membrane (after cataract) 13.65
- cervical
  - rib 77.91
  - stump 67.4
- cervix (stump) NEC 67.4
  - cold (knife) 67.2
  - conization 67.2
  - cryoconization 67.33
  - electroconizaton 67.32
- chalazion (multiple) (single) 08.21
- cholesteatoma — *see* Excision, lesion, by site
- choroid plexus 02.14
- cicatrix (skin) 86.3
- cilia base 08.20
- ciliary body, prolapsed 12.98
- clavicle (head) (partial) 77.81
  - total (complete) 77.91
- clitoris 71.4
- coarctation of aorta (end-to-end anastomosis) 38.64
  - with
    - graft replacement (interposition)
      - abdominal 38.44
      - thoracic 38.45
      - thoracoabdominal 38.45 [38.44]
- common
  - duct 51.63
  - wall between posterior and coronary sinus (with roofing of resultant defect with patch graft) 35.82
- condyle — *see* category 77.8 ☑4th
  - mandible 76.5
- conjunctival ring 10.31
- cornea 11.49
  - epithelium (with chemocauterization) 11.41
    - for smear or culture 11.21
- costal cartilage 80.99
- cul-de-sac (Douglas) 70.92
- cusp, heart valve 35.10
  - aortic 35.11
  - mitral 35.12
  - tricuspid 35.14
- cyst — *see also* Excision, lesion, by site
  - apical (tooth) 23.73
    - with root canal therapy 23.72
  - Baker's (popliteal) 83.39
  - breast 85.21
  - broad ligament 69.19
  - bronchogenic 32.09
    - endoscopic 32.01
  - cervix 67.39
  - dental 24.4
  - dentigerous 24.4
  - epididymis 63.2
  - fallopian tube 66.61
  - Gartner's duct 70.33
  - hand 82.29
  - labia 71.3
  - lung 32.29
    - endoscopic 32.28
  - mesonephric duct 69.19
  - Morgagni
    - female 66.61
    - male 62.2
  - müllerian duct 60.73
  - nasolabial 27.49
  - nasopalatine 27.31
    - by wide excision 27.32
  - ovary 65.29
    - laparoscopic 65.25
  - parovarian 69.19
  - pericardium 37.31

Excision — *continued*
- cyst — *see also* Excision, lesion, by site — *continued*
  - periodontal (apical) (lateral) 24.4
  - popliteal (Baker's), knee 83.39
  - radicular 24.4
  - spleen 41.42
  - synovial (membrane) 83.39
  - thyroglossal (with resection of hyoid bone) 06.7
  - urachal (bladder) 57.51
    - abdominal wall 54.3
  - vagina (Gartner's duct) 70.33
- cystic
  - duct remnant 51.61
  - hygroma 40.29
- dentinoma 24.4
- diaphragm 34.81
- disc, intervertebral (NOS) 80.50
  - herniated (nucleus pulposus) 80.51
  - other specified (diskectomy) 80.51
- diverticulum
  - ampulla of Vater 51.62
  - anus 49.39
    - endoscopic 49.31
  - bladder 57.59
    - transurethral 57.49
  - duodenum 45.31
    - endoscopic 45.30
  - esophagus (local) 42.31
    - endoscopic 42.33
  - hypopharyngeal (by cricopharyngeal myotomy) 29.32
  - intestine
    - large 45.41
      - endoscopic 45.43
    - small NEC 45.33
  - Meckel's 45.33
  - pharyngeal (by cricopharyngeal myotomy) 29.32
  - pharyngoesophageal (by cricopharyngeal myotomy) 29.32
  - stomach 43.42
    - endoscopic 43.41
  - urethra 58.39
    - endoscopic 58.31
  - ventricle, heart 37.33
- duct
  - müllerian 69.19
  - paramesonephric 69.19
  - thyroglossal (with resection of hyoid bone) 06.7
- ear, external (complete) NEC 18.39
  - partial 18.29
  - radical 18.31
- ectopic
  - abdominal fetus 74.3
  - tissue — *see also* Excision, lesion, by site of tissue origin
    - bone, from muscle 83.32
    - breast 85.24
    - lung 32.29
      - endoscopic 32.28
    - spleen 41.93
- empyema pocket, lung 34.09
- epididymis 63.4
- epiglottis 30.21
- epithelial downgrowth, anterior chamber (eye) 12.93
- epulis (gingiva) 24.31
- esophagus (*see also* Esophagectomy) 42.40
- exostosis (*see also* Excision, lesion, bone) 77.60
  - auditory canal, external 18.29
  - facial bone 76.2
  - first metatarsal (hallux valgus repair) — *see* Bunionectomy
- eye 16.49
  - with implant (into Tenon's capsule) 16.42
    - with attachment of muscles 16.41
- eyelid 08.20
  - redundant skin 08.86
- falciform ligament 54.4
- fallopian tube — *see* Salpingectomy
- fascia 83.44
  - for graft 83.43
    - hand 82.34

Excision — *continued*
- fascia — *continued*
  - hand 82.35
    - for graft 82.34
- fat pad NEC 86.3
  - knee (infrapatellar) (prepatellar) 86.3
  - scalene 40.21
- fibroadenoma, breast 85.21
- fissure, anus 49.39
  - endoscopic 49.31
- fistula — *see also* Fistulectomy
  - anal 49.12
  - arteriovenous (*see also* Aneurysmectomy) 38.60
  - ileorectal 46.74
  - lacrimal
    - gland 09.21
    - sac 09.6
  - rectal 48.73
  - vesicovaginal 57.84
- frenulum, frenum
  - labial (lip) 27.41
  - lingual (tongue) 25.92
- ganglion (hand) (tendon sheath) (wrist) 82.21
  - gasserian 04.05
  - site other than hand or nerve 83.31
  - sympathetic nerve 05.29
  - trigeminal nerve 04.05
- gastrocolic ligament 54.4
- gingiva 24.31
- glomus jugulare tumor 20.51
- goiter — *see* Thyroidectomy
- gum 24.31
- hallux valgus — *see also* Bunionectomy
  - with prosthetic implant 77.59
- hamartoma, mammary 85.21
- hematocele, tunica vaginalis 61.92
- hematoma — *see* Drainage, by site
- hemorrhoids (external) (internal) (tag) 49.46
- heterotopic bone, from
  - muscle 83.32
    - hand 82.22
  - skin 86.3
  - tendon 83.31
    - hand 82.21
- hydatid of Morgagni
  - female 66.61
  - male 62.2
- hydatid cyst, liver 50.29
- hydrocele
  - canal of Nuck (female) 69.19
  - male 63.1
  - round ligament 69.19
  - spermatic cord 63.1
  - tunica vaginalis 61.2
- hygroma, cystic 40.29
- hymen (tag) 70.31
- hymeno-urethral fusion 70.31
- intervertebral disc — *see* Excision, disc, intervertebral (NOS) 80.50
- intestine (*see also* Resection, intestine) 45.8
  - for interposition 45.50
    - large 45.52
    - small 45.51
  - large (total) 45.8
    - for interposition 45.52
    - local 45.41
      - endoscopic 45.43
    - segmental 45.79
      - multiple 45.71
  - small (total) 45.63
    - for interposition 45.51
    - local 45.33
    - partial 45.62
    - segmental 45.62
      - multiple 45.61
- intraductal papilloma 85.21
- iris prolapse 12.13
- joint (*see also* Arthrectomy) 80.90
- keloid (scar), skin 86.3
- labia — *see* Vulvectomy
- lacrimal
  - gland 09.20
    - partial 09.22
    - total 09.23
  - passage 09.6

Excision

Excision — *continued*
  lacrimal — *continued*
    sac 09.6
  lesion (local)
    abdominal wall 54.3
    accessory sinus — *see* Excision, lesion, nasal sinus
    adenoids 28.92
    adrenal gland(s) 07.21
    alveolus 24.4
    ampulla of Vater 51.62
    anterior chamber (eye) NEC 12.40
    anus 49.39
      endoscopic 49.31
    apocrine gland 86.3
    artery 38.60
      abdominal 38.66
      aorta (arch) (ascending) (descending) thoracic) 38.64
        with end-to-end anastomosis 38.45
          abdominal 38.44
          thoracic 38.45
          thoracoabdominal 38.45 [38.44]
        with graft interposition graft replacement 38.45
          abdominal 38.44
          thoracic 38.45
          thoracoabdominal 38.45 [38.44]
      head and neck NEC 38.62
      intracranial NEC 38.61
      lower limb 38.68
      thoracic NEC 38.65
      upper limb 38.63
    atrium 37.33
    auditory canal or meatus, external 18.29
      radical 18.31
    auricle, ear 18.29
      radical 18.31
    biliary ducts 51.69
      endoscopic 51.64
    bladder (transurethral) 57.49
      open 57.59
      suprapubic 57.59
    blood vessel 38.60
      abdominal
        artery 38.66
        vein 38.67
      aorta (arch) (ascending) (descending) 38.64
      head and neck NEC 38.62
      intracranial NEC 38.61
      lower limb
        artery 38.68
        vein 38.69
      thoracic NEC 38.65
      upper limb (artery) (vein) 38.63
    bone 77.60
      carpal, metacarpal 77.64
      clavicle 77.61
      facial 76.2
      femur 77.65
      fibula 77.67
      humerus 77.62
      jaw 76.2
        dental 24.4
      patella 77.66
      pelvic 77.69
      phalanges (foot) (hand) 77.69
      radius 77.63
      scapula 77.61
      skull 01.6
      specified site NEC 77.69
      tarsal, metatarsal 77.68
      thorax (ribs) (sternum) 77.61
      tibia 77.67
      ulna 77.63
      vertebrae 77.69
    brain (transtemporal approach) NEC 01.59
      by stereotactic radiosurgery 92.30
        cobalt 60 92.32
        linear accelerator (LINAC) 92.31
        multi-source 92.32
        particle beam 92.33
        particulate 92.33
        radiosurgery NEC 92.39
        single source photon 92.31

Excision — *continued*
  lesion — *continued*
    breast (segmental) (wedge) 85.21
    broad ligament 69.19
    bronchus NEC 32.09
      endoscopic 32.01
    cerebral (cortex) NEC 01.59
      meninges 01.51
    cervix (myoma) 67.39
    chest wall 34.4
    choroid plexus 02.14
    ciliary body 12.44
    colon 45.41
      endoscopic NEC 45.43
        polypectomy 45.42
    conjunctiva 10.31
    cornea 11.49
    cranium 01.6
    cul-de-sac (Douglas') 70.32
    dental (jaw) 24.4
    diaphragm 34.81
    duodenum (local) 45.31
      endoscopic 45.30
    ear, external 18.29
      radical 18.31
    endometrium 68.29
    epicardium 37.31
    epididymis 63.3
    epiglottis 30.09
    esophagus NEC 42.32
      endoscopic 42.33
    eye, eyeball 16.93
      anterior segment NEC 12.40
    eyebrow (skin) 08.20
    eyelid 08.20
      by
        halving procedure 08.24
        wedge resection 08.24
      major
        full-thickness 08.24
        partial-thickness 08.23
      minor 08.22
    fallopian tube 66.61
    fascia 83.39
      hand 82.29
    groin region (abdominal wall) (inguinal) 54.3
      skin 86.3
      subcutaneous tissue 86.3
    gum 24.31
    heart 37.33
    hepatic duct 51.69
    inguinal canal 54.3
    intestine
      large 45.41
        endoscopic NEC 45.43
          polypectomy 45.42
      small NEC 45.33
    intracranial NEC 01.59
    intranasal 21.31
    intraspinal 03.4
    iris 12.42
    jaw 76.2
      dental 24.4
    joint 80.80
      ankle 80.87
      elbow 80.82
      foot and toe 80.88
      hand and finger 80.84
      hip 80.85
      knee 80.86
      shoulder 80.81
      specified site NEC 80.89
      spine 80.89
      wrist 80.83
    kidney 55.39
      with partial nephrectomy 55.4
    labia 71.3
    lacrimal
      gland (frontal approach) 09.21
      passage 09.6
      sac 09.6
    larynx 30.09
    ligament (joint) (*see also* Excision, lesion, joint) 80.80
      broad 69.19
      round 69.19

Excision — *continued*
  lesion — *continued*
    ligament (*see also* Excision, lesion, joint) — *continued*
      uterosacral 69.19
    lip 27.43
      by wide excision 27.42
    liver 50.29
    lung NEC 32.29
      by wide excision 32.3
      endoscopic 32.28
    lymph structure(s) (channel) (vessel) NEC 40.29
      node — *see* Excision, lymph, node
    mammary duct 85.21
    mastoid (bone) 20.49
    mediastinum 34.3
    meninges (cerebral) 01.51
      spinal 03.4
    mesentery 54.4
    middle ear 20.51
    mouth NEC 27.49
    muscle 83.32
      hand 82.22
      ocular 15.13
    myocardium 37.33
    nail 86.23
    nasal sinus 22.60
      antrum 22.62
        with Caldwell-Luc approach 22.61
        specified approach NEC 22.62
      ethmoid 22.63
      frontal 22.42
      maxillary 22.62
        with Caldwell-Luc approach 22.61
        specified approach NEC 22.62
      sphenoid 22.64
    nasopharynx 29.3 ✓4ᵗʰ
    nerve (cranial) (peripheral) 04.07
      sympathetic 05.29
    nonodontogenic 24.31
    nose 21.30
      intranasal 21.31
      polyp 21.31
      skin 21.32
      specified site NEC 21.32
    odontogenic 24.4
    omentum 54.4
    orbit 16.92
    ovary 65.29
      by wedge resection 65.22
        laparoscopic 65.24
      that by laparoscope 65.25
    palate (bony) 27.31
      by wide excision 27.32
      soft 27.49
    pancreas (local) 52.22
      endoscopic 52.21
    parathyroid 06.89
    parotid gland or duct NEC 26.29
    pelvic wall 54.3
    pelvirectal tissue 48.82
    penis 64.2
    pericardium 37.31
    perineum (female) 71.3
      male 86.3
    periprostatic tissue 60.82
    perirectal tissue 48.82
    perirenal tissue 59.91
    peritoneum 54.4
    perivesical tissue 59.91
    pharynx 29.39
      diverticulum 29.32
    pineal gland 07.53
    pinna 18.29
      radical 18.31
    pituitary (gland) (*see also* Hypophysectomy, partial) 07.63
      by stereotactic radiosurgery 92.30
        cobalt 60 92.32
        linear accelerator (LINAC) 92.31
        multi-source 92.32
        particle beam 92.33
        particulate 92.33
        radiosurgery NEC 92.39
        single source photon 92.31

Index to Procedures

Excision

Excision — *continued*
  lesion — *continued*
    pleura 34.59
    pouch of Douglas 70.32
    preauricular (ear) 18.21
    presacral 54.4
    prostate (transurethral) 60.61
    pulmonary (fibrosis) 32.29
      endoscopic 32.28
    rectovaginal septum 48.82
    rectum 48.35
      polyp (endoscopic) 48.36
    retroperitoneum 54.4
    salivary gland or duct NEC 26.29
      en bloc 26.32
    sclera 12.84
    scrotum 61.3
    sinus (nasal) — *see* Excision, lesion, nasal sinus
    Skene's gland 71.3
    skin 86.3
      breast 85.21
      nose 21.32
      radical (wide) (involving underlying or adjacent structure) (with flap closure) 86.4
      scrotum 61.3
    skull 01.6
    soft tissue NEC 83.39
      hand 82.29
    spermatic cord 63.3
    sphincter of Oddi 51.62
      endoscopic 51.64
    spinal cord (meninges) 03.4
    spleen (cyst) 41.42
    stomach NEC 43.42
      endoscopic 43.41
        polyp 43.41
      polyp (endoscopic) 43.41
    subcutaneous tissue 86.3
      breast 85.21
    subgingival 24.31
    sweat gland 86.3
    tendon 83.39
      hand 82.29
      ocular 15.13
      sheath 83.31
        hand 82.21
    testis 62.2
    thorax 34.4
    thymus 07.81
    thyroid 06.31
      substernal or transsternal route 06.51
    tongue 25.1
    tonsil 28.92
    trachea 31.5
    tunica vaginalis 61.92
    ureter 56.41
    urethra 58.39
      endoscopic 58.31
    uterine ligament 69.19
    uterosacral ligament 69.19
    uterus 68.29
    vagina 70.33
    vein 38.60
      abdominal 38.67
      head and neck NEC 38.62
      intracranial NEC 38.61
      lower limb 38.69
      thoracic NEC 38.65
      upper limb 38.63
    ventricle (heart) 37.33
    vocal cords 30.09
    vulva 71.3
  ligament (*see also* Arthrectomy) 80.90
    broad 69.19
    round 69.19
    uterine 69.19
    uterosacral 69.19
  ligamentum flavum (spine) — *omit code*
  lingual tonsil 28.5
  lip 27.43
  liver (partial) 50.22
  loose body
    bone — *see* Sequestrectomy, bone
    joint 80.10

Excision — *continued*
  lung (complete) (with mediastinal dissection) 32.5
    accessory or ectopic tissue 32.29
      endoscopic 32.28
    segmental 32.3
    specified type NEC 32.29
      endoscopic 32.28
    volume reduction surgery 32.22
    wedge 32.29
  lymph, lymphatic
    drainage area 40.29
      radical — *see* Excision, lymph, node, radical
      regional (with lymph node, skin, subcutaneous tissue, and fat) 40.3
    node (simple) NEC 40.29
      with
        lymphatic drainage area (including skin, subcutaneous tissue, and fat) 40.3
        mastectomy — *see* Mastectomy, radical
        muscle and deep fascia — *see* Excision, lymph, node, radical
      axillary 40.23
        radical 40.51
        regional (extended) 40.3
      cervical (deep) (with excision of scalene fat pad) 40.21
        with laryngectomy 30.4
        radical (including muscle and deep fascia) 40.40
          bilateral 40.42
          unilateral 40.41
        regional (extended) 40.3
        superficial 40.29
      groin 40.24
        radical 40.54
        regional (extended) 40.3
      iliac 40.29
        radical 40.53
        regional (extended) 40.3
      inguinal (deep) (superficial) 40.24
        radical 40.54
        regional (extended) 40.3
      jugular — *see* Excision, lymph, node, cervical
      mammary (internal) 40.22
        external 40.29
          radical 40.59
          regional (extended) 40.3
        radical 40.59
        regional (extended) 40.3
      paratracheal — *see* Excision, lymph, node, cervical
      periaortic 40.29
        radical 40.52
        regional (extended) 40.3
      radical 40.50
        with mastectomy — *see* Mastectomy, radical
        specified site NEC 40.59
      regional (extended) 40.3
      sternal — *see* Excision, lymph, node, mammary
      structure(s) (simple) NEC 40.29
        radical 40.59
        regional (extended) 40.3
  lymphangioma (simple) — *see also* Excision, lymph, lymphatic node 40.29
  lymphocele 40.29
  mastoid (*see also* Mastoidectomy) 20.49
  median bar, transurethral approach 60.29
  meibomian gland 08.20
  meniscus (knee) 80.6
    acromioclavicular 80.91
    jaw 76.5
    sternoclavicular 80.91
    temporomandibular (joint) 76.5
    wrist 80.93
  müllerian duct cyst 60.73
  muscle 83.45
    for graft 83.43
    hand 82.34

Excision — *continued*
  muscle — *continued*
    hand 82.36
      for graft 82.34
    myositis ossificans 83.32
      hand 82.22
  nail (bed) (fold) 86.23
  nasolabial cyst 27.49
  nasopalatine cyst 27.31
    by wide excision 27.32
  neoplasm — *see* Excision, lesion, by site
  nerve (cranial) (peripheral) NEC 04.07
    sympathetic 05.29
  neuroma (Morton's) (peripheral nerve) 04.07
    acoustic 04.01
      by craniotomy 04.01
      by stereotactic radiosurgery 92.30
        cobalt 60 92.32
        linear accelerator (LINAC) 92.31
        multi-source 92.32
        particle beam 92.33
        particulate 92.33
        radiosurgery NEC 92.39
        single source photon 92.31
    sympathetic nerve 05.29
  nipple 85.25
    accessory 85.24
  odontoma 24.4
  orbital contents (*see also* Exenteration, orbit) 16.59
  osteochondritis dissecans (*see also* Excision, lesion, joint) 80.80
  ovary — *see also* Oophorectomy
    partial 65.29
      by wedge resection 65.22
        laparoscopic 65.24
      that by laparoscope 65.25
  Pancoast tumor (lung) 32.6
  pancreas (total) (with synchronous duodenectomy) 52.6
    partial NEC 52.59
      distal (tail) (with part of body) 52.52
      proximal (head) (with part of body) (with synchronous duodenectomy) 52.51
      radical subtotal 52.53
    radical (one-stage) (two-stage) 52.7
    subtotal 52.53
  paramesonephric duct 69.19
  parathyroid gland (partial) (subtotal) NEC (*see also* Parathyroidectomy) 06.89
  parotid gland (*see also* Excision, salivary gland) 26.30
  parovarian cyst 69.19
  patella (complete) 77.96
    partial 77.86
  pelvirectal tissue 48.82
  perianal tissue 49.04
    skin tags 49.03
  pericardial adhesions 37.31
  periprostatic tissue 60.82
  perirectal tissue 48.82
  perirenal tissue 59.91
  periurethral tissue 58.92
  perivesical tissue 59.91
  petrous apex cells 20.59
  pharyngeal bands 29.54
  pharynx (partial) 29.33
  pilonidal cyst or sinus (open) (with partial closure) 86.21
  pineal gland (complete) (total) 07.54
    partial 07.53
  pituitary gland (complete) (total) (*see also* Hypophysectomy) 07.69
  pleura NEC 34.59
  polyp — *see also* Excision, lesion, by site
    esophagus 42.32
      endoscopic 42.33
    large intestine 45.41
      endoscopic 45.42
    nose 21.31
    rectum (endoscopic) 48.36
    stomach (endoscopic) 43.41
  preauricular
    appendage (remnant) 18.29
    cyst, fistula, or sinus (congenital) 18.21
    remnant 18.29

Excision

Excision — *continued*
- prolapsed iris (in wound) 12.13
- prostate — *see* Prostatectomy
- pterygium (simple) 11.39
  - with corneal graft 11.32
- radius (head) (partial) 77.83
  - total 77.93
- ranula, salivary gland NEC 26.29
- rectal mucosa 48.35
- rectum — *see* Resection, rectum
- redundant mucosa
  - colostomy 45.41
    - endoscopic 45.43
  - duodenostomy 45.31
    - endoscopic 45.30
  - ileostomy 45.33
  - jejunostomy 45.33
  - perineum 71.3
  - rectum 48.35
  - vulva 71.3
- renal vessel, aberrant 38.66
- rib (cervical) 77.91
- ring of conjunctiva around cornea 10.31
- round ligament 69.19
- salivary gland 26.30
  - complete 26.32
  - partial 26.31
  - radical 26.32
- scalene fat pad 40.21
- scar — *see also* Excision, lesion, by site
  - epicardium 37.31
  - mastoid 20.92
  - pericardium 37.31
  - pleura 34.59
  - skin 86.3
  - thorax 34.4
- secondary membrane, lens 13.65
- seminal vesicle 60.73
  - with radical prostatectomy 60.5
- septum — *see also* Excision, by site
  - uterus (congenital) 68.22
  - vagina 70.33
- sinus — *see also* Excision, lesion, by site
  - nasal — *see* Sinusectomy
  - pilonidal 86.21
  - preauricular (ear) (radical) 18.21
  - tarsi 80.88
  - thyroglossal (with resection of hyoid bone) 06.7
  - urachal (bladder) 57.51
    - abdominal wall 54.3
- Skene's gland 71.3
- skin (local) 86.3
  - for graft (with closure of donor site) 86.91
    - radical (wide) (involving underlying or adjacent structure) (with flap closure) 86.4
  - tags
    - perianal 49.03
    - periauricular 18.29
- soft tissue NEC 83.49
  - hand 82.39
- spermatocele 63.2
- spinous process 77.89
- spleen (total) 41.5
  - accessory 41.93
  - partial 41.43
- stomach — *see* Gastrectomy
- sublingual gland (salivary) (*see also* Excision, salivary gland) 26.30
- submaxillary gland (*see also* Excision, salivary gland) 26.30
- supernumerary
  - breast 85.24
  - digits 86.26
- sweat gland 86.3
- synechiae — *see also* Lysis, synechiae
  - endometrial 68.21
- tarsal plate (eyelid) 08.20
  - by wedge resection 08.24
- tattoo 86.3
  - by dermabrasion 86.25
- tendon (sheath) 83.42
  - for graft 83.41
    - hand 82.32
  - hand 82.33
    - for graft 82.32

Excision — *continued*
- thymus (*see also* Thymectomy) 07.80
- thyroglossal duct or tract (with resection of hyoid bone) 06.7
- thyroid NEC (*see also* Thyroidectomy) 06.39
- tongue (complete) (total) 25.3
  - partial or subtotal 25.2
  - radical 25.4
- tonsil 28.2
  - with adenoidectomy 28.3
  - lingual 28.5
  - tag 28.4
- tooth NEC (*see also* Removal, tooth, surgical) 23.19
  - from nasal sinus 22.60
- torus
  - lingual 76.2
  - mandible, mandibularis 76.2
  - palate, palatinus 27.31
    - by wide excision 27.32
- trabeculae carneae cordis (heart) 35.35
- trochanteric lipomatosis 86.83
- tumor — *see* Excision, lesion, by site
- ulcer — *see also* Excision, lesion, by site
  - duodenum 45.31
    - endoscopic 45.30
  - stomach 43.42
    - endoscopic 43.41
- umbilicus 54.3
- urachus, urachal (cyst) (bladder) 57.51
  - abdominal wall 54.3
- ureter, ureteral 56.40
  - with nephrectomy — *see* Nephrectomy
  - partial 56.41
  - stricture 56.41
  - total 56.42
- ureterocele 56.41
- urethra, urethral 58.39
  - with complete cystectomy 57.79
  - endoscopic 58.31
  - septum 58.0
  - stricture 58.39
    - endoscopic 58.31
  - valve (congenital) 58.39
    - endoscopic (transurethral) (transvesical) 58.31
- urethrovaginal septum 70.33
- uterus (corpus) (*see also* Hysterectomy) 68.9
  - cervix 67.4
  - lesion 67.39
  - lesion 68.29
  - septum 68.22
- uvula 27.72
- vagina (total) 70.4
- varicocele, spermatic cord 63.1
- vein (*see also* Phlebectomy) 38.60
  - varicose 38.50
    - abdominal 38.57
    - head and neck NEC 38.52
    - intracranial NEC 38.51
    - lower limb 38.59
    - ovarian 38.67
    - thoracic NEC 38.55
    - upper limb 38.53
- verucca — *see also* Excision, lesion, by site
  - eyelid 08.22
- vesicovaginal septum 70.33
- vitreous opacity 14.74
  - anterior approach 14.73
- vocal cord(s) (submucous) 30.22
- vulva (bilateral) (simple) (*see also* Vulvectomy) 71.62
- wart — *see also* Excision, lesion, by site
  - eyelid 08.22
- wolffian duct 69.19
- xanthoma (tendon sheath, hand) 82.21
  - site other than hand 83.31

Excisional biopsy — *see* Biopsy

Exclusion, pyloric 44.39

Exenteration
- ethmoid air cells 22.63
- orbit 16.59
  - with
    - removal of adjacent structures 16.51
    - temporalis muscle transplant 16.59
    - therapeutic removal of bone 16.52

Exenteration — *continued*
- pelvic (organs) (female) 68.8
  - male 57.71
- petrous pyramid air cells 20.59

Exercise (physical therapy) NEC 93.19
- active musculoskeletal NEC 93.12
- assisting 93.11
  - in pool 93.31
- breathing 93.18
- musculoskeletal
  - active NEC 93.12
  - passive NEC 93.17
- neurologic 89.13
- passive musculoskeletal NEC 93.17
- resistive 93.13

Exfoliation, skin, by chemical 86.24

Exostectomy (*see also* Excision, lesion, bone) 77.60
- first metatarsal (hallux valgus repair) — *see* Bunionectomy
- hallux valgus repair (with wedge osteotomy) — *see* Bunionectomy

Expiratory flow rate 89.38

Exploration — *see also* Incision
- abdomen 54.11
- abdominal wall 54.0
- adrenal (gland) 07.41
  - field 07.00
    - bilateral 07.02
    - unilateral 07.01
- artery 38.00
  - abdominal 38.06
  - aorta (arch) (ascending) (descending) 38.04
  - head and neck NEC 38.02
  - intracranial NEC 38.01
  - lower limb 38.08
  - thoracic NEC 38.05
  - upper limb 38.03
- auditory canal, external 18.02
- axilla 86.09
- bile duct(s) 51.59
  - common duct 51.51
    - endoscopic 51.11
    - for
      - relief of obstruction 51.42
        - endoscopic 51.84
      - removal of calculus 51.41
        - endoscopic 51.88
    - laparoscopic 51.11
  - for relief of obstruction 51.49
    - endoscopic 51.84
- bladder (by incision) 57.19
  - endoscopic 57.32
  - through stoma (artificial) 57.31
- bone (*see also* Incision, bone) 77.10
- brain (tissue) 01.39
- breast 85.0
- bronchus 33.0
  - endoscopic — *see* Bronchoscopy
- bursa 83.03
  - hand 82.03
- carotid body 39.8
- carpal tunnel 04.43
- choroid 14.9
- ciliary body 12.44
- colon 45.03
- common bile duct 51.51
  - endoscopic 51.11
  - for
    - relief of obstruction 51.42
      - endoscopic 51.84
    - removal of calculus 51.41
      - endoscopic 51.88
- coronary artery 36.99
- cranium 01.24
- cul-de-sac 70.12
  - endoscopic 70.22
- disc space 03.09
- duodenum 45.01
- endoscopic — *see* Endoscopy, by site
- epididymis 63.92
- esophagus (by incision) NEC 42.09
  - endoscopic — *see* Esophagoscopy
- ethmoid sinus 22.51
- eyelid 08.09

Index to Procedures

Exploration — see also Incision — continued
  fallopian tube 66.01
  fascia 83.09
    hand 82.09
  flank 54.0
  fossa (superficial) NEC 86.09
    pituitary 07.71
  frontal sinus 22.41
  frontonasal duct 96.21
  gallbladder 51.04
  groin (region) (abdominal wall) (inguinal) 54.0
    skin and subcutaneous tissue 86.09
  heart 37.11
  hepatic duct 51.59
  hypophysis 07.72
  ileum 45.02
  inguinal canal (groin) 54.0
  intestine (by incision) NEC 45.00
    large 45.03
    small 45.02
  intrathoracic 34.02
  jejunum 45.02
  joint structures (see also Arthrotomy) 80.10
  kidney 55.01
    pelvis 55.11
  labia 71.09
  lacrimal
    gland 09.0
    sac 09.53
  laparotomy site 54.12
  larynx (by incision) 31.3
    endoscopic 31.42
  liver 50.0
  lung (by incision) 33.1
  lymphatic structure(s) (channel) (node) (vessel) 40.0
  mastoid 20.21
  maxillary antrum or sinus (Caldwell-Luc approach) 22.39
  mediastinum 34.1
    endoscopic 34.22
  middle ear (transtympanic) 20.23
  muscle 83.02
    hand 82.02
  neck (see also Exploration, thyroid) 06.09
  nerve (cranial) (peripheral) NEC 04.04
    auditory 04.01
    root (spinal) 03.09
  nose 21.1
  orbit (see also Orbitotomy) 16.09
  pancreas 52.09
    endoscopic 52.13
  pancreatic duct 52.09
    endoscopic 52.13
  pelvis (by laparotomy) 54.11
    by colpotomy 70.12
  penis 64.92
  perinephric area 59.09
  perineum (female) 71.09
    male 86.09
  peripheral vessels
    lower limb
      artery 38.08
      vein 38.09
    upper limb (artery) (vein) 38.03
  periprostatic tissue 60.81
  perirenal tissue 59.09
  perivesical tissue 59.19
  petrous pyramid air cells 20.22
  pilonidal sinus 86.03
  pineal (gland) 07.52
    field 07.51
  pituitary (gland) 07.72
    fossa 07.71
  pleura 34.09
  popliteal space 86.09
  prostate 60.0
  rectum (see also Proctoscopy) 48.23
    by incision 48.0
  retroperitoneum 54.0
  retropubic 59.19
  salivary gland 26.0
  sclera (by incision) 12.89
  scrotum 61.0

Exploration — see also Incision — continued
  shunt
    ventriculoperitoneal at
      peritoneal site 54.95
      ventricular site 02.41
  sinus
    ethmoid 22.51
    frontal 22.41
    maxillary (Caldwell-Luc approach) 22.39
    sphenoid 22.52
    tract, skin and subcutaneous tissue 86.09
  skin 86.09
  soft tissue NEC 83.09
    hand 82.09
  spermatic cord 63.93
  sphenoidal sinus 22.52
  spinal (canal) (nerve root) 03.09
  spleen 41.2
  stomach (by incision) 43.0
    endoscopic — see Gastroscopy
  subcutaneous tissue 86.09
  subdiaphragmatic space 54.11
  superficial fossa 86.09
  tarsal tunnel 04.44
  tendon (sheath) 83.01
    hand 82.01
  testes 62.0
  thymus (gland) 07.92
    field 07.91
  thyroid (field) (gland) (by incision) 06.09
    postoperative 06.02
  trachea (by incision) 31.3
    endoscopic — see Tracheoscopy
  tunica vaginalis 61.0
  tympanum 20.09
    transtympanic route 20.23
  ureter (by incision) 56.2
    endoscopic 56.31
  urethra (by incision) 58.0
    endoscopic 58.22
  uterus (corpus) 68.0
    cervix 69.95
    digital 68.11
    postpartal, manual 75.7
  vagina (by incision) 70.14
    endoscopic 70.21
  vas deferens 63.6
  vein 38.00
    abdominal 38.07
    head and neck NEC 38.02
    intracranial NEC 38.01
    lower limb 38.09
    thoracic NEC 38.05
    upper limb 38.03
  vulva (by incision) 71.09

Exposure — see also Incision, by site
  tooth (for orthodontic treatment) 24.6

Expression, trachoma follicles 10.33

Exsanguination transfusion 99.01

Extension
  buccolabial sulcus 24.91
  limb, forced 93.25
  lingual sulcus 24.91
  mandibular ridge 76.43

Exteriorization
  esophageal pouch 42.12
  intestine 46.03
    large 46.03
    small 46.01
  maxillary sinus 22.9
  pilonidal cyst or sinus (open excision) (with partial closure) 86.21

Extirpation — see also Excision, by site
  aneurysm — see Aneurysmectomy
  arteriovenous fistula — see Aneurysmectomy
  lacrimal sac 09.6
  larynx 30.3
    with radical neck dissection (with synchronous thyroidectomy)(with synchronous tracheostomy) 30.4
  nerve, tooth (see also Therapy, root canal) 23.70
  varicose vein (peripheral) (lower limb) 38.59
    upper limb 38.53

Extracorporeal
  circulation (regional), except hepatic 39.61
    hepatic 50.92
    percutaneous 39.66
  hemodialysis 39.95
  membrane oxygenation (ECMO) 39.65
  photopheresis, therapeutic 99.88
  shockwave lithotripsy (ESWL) NEC 98.59
    bile duct 98.52
    bladder 98.51
    gallbladder 98.52
    kidney 98.51
    renal pelvis 98.51
    specified site NEC 98.59
    ureter 98.51

Extracranial-intracranial bypass [EC-IC] 39.28

Extraction
  breech (partial) 72.52
    with forceps to aftercoming head 72.51
    total 72.54
      with forceps to aftercoming head 72.53
  cataract 13.19
    after cataract (by)
      capsulectomy 13.65
      capsulotomy 13.64
      discission 13.64
      excision 13.65
      iridocapsulectomy 13.65
      mechanical fragmentation 13.66
      needling 13.64
      phacofragmentation (mechanical) 13.66
    aspiration (simple) (with irrigation) 13.3
    cryoextraction (intracapsular approach) 13.19
      temporal inferior route (in presence of fistulization bleb) 13.11
    curette evacuation (extracapsular approach) 13.2
    emulsification (and aspiration) 13.41
    erysiphake (intracapsular approach) 13.19
      temporal inferior route (in presence of fistulization bleb) 13.11
    extracapsular approach (with iridectomy) NEC 13.59
      by temporal inferior route (in presence of fistulization bleb) 13.51
      aspiration (simple) (with irrigation) 13.3
      curette evacuation 13.2
      emulsification (and aspiration) 13.41
      linear extraction 13.2
      mechanical fragmentation with aspiration by
        posterior route 13.42
        specified route NEC 13.43
      phacoemulsification (ultrasonic) (with aspiration) 13.41
      phacofragmentation (mechanical)
        with aspiration by
          posterior route 13.42
          specified route NEC 13.43
        ultrasonic (with aspiration) 13.41
      rotoextraction (mechanical) with aspiration by
        posterior route 13.42
        specified route NEC 13.43
    intracapsular (combined) (simple) (with iridectomy) (with suction) (with zonulolysis) 13.19
      by temporal inferior route (in presence of fistulization bleb) 13.11
    linear extraction (extracapsular approach) 13.2
    phacoemulsification (and aspiration) 13.41
    phacofragmentation (mechanical)
      with aspiration by
        posterior route 13.42
        specified route NEC 13.43
      ultrasonic 13.41
    rotoextraction (mechanical)
      with aspiration by
        posterior route 13.42
        specified route NEC 13.43
    secondary membranous (after cataract) (by)
      capsulectomy 13.65
      capsulotomy 13.64

Extraction

Extraction — *continued*
  cataract — *continued*
    secondary membranous — *continued*
      discission 13.64
      excision 13.65
      iridocapsulectomy 13.65
      mechanical fragmentation 13.66
      needling 13.64
      phacofragmentation (mechanical) 13.66
  common duct stones (percutaneous) (through sinus tract) (with basket) 51.96
  foreign body — *see* Removal, foreign body
  kidney stone(s), percutaneous 55.03
    with fragmentation procedure 55.04
  lens (eye) (*see also* Extraction, cataract) 13.19
  Malström's 72.79
    with episiotomy 72.71
  menstrual, menses 69.6
  milk from lactating breast (manual) (pump) 99.98
  tooth (by forceps) (multiple) (single) NEC 23.09
    with mucoperiosteal flap elevation 23.19
    deciduous 23.01
    surgical NEC (*see also* Removal, tooth, surgical) 23.19
  vacuum, fetus 72.79
    with episiotomy 72.71
  vitreous (*see also* Removal, vitreous) 14.72

F

Face lift 86.82
Facetectomy 77.89
Facilitation, intraocular circulation NEC 12.59
Failed (trial) forceps 73.3
Family
  counselling (medical) (social) 94.49
  therapy 94.42
Farabeuf operation (ischiopubiotomy) 77.39
Fasanella-Servatt operation (blepharoptosis repair) 08.35
Fasciaplasty — *see* Fascioplasty
Fascia sling operation — *see* Operation, sling
Fasciectomy 83.44
  for graft 83.43
    hand 82.34
  hand 82.35
    for graft 82.34
  palmar (release of Dupuytren's contracture) 82.35
Fasciodesis 83.89
  hand 82.89
Fascioplasty (*see also* Repair, fascia) 83.89
  hand (*see also* Repair, fascia, hand) 82.89
Fasciorrhaphy — *see* Suture, fascia
Fasciotomy 83.14
  Dupuytren's 82.12
    with excision 82.35
  Dwyer 83.14
  hand 82.12
  Ober-Yount 83.14
  orbital (*see also* Orbitotomy) 16.09
  palmar (release of Dupuytren's contracture) 82.12
    with excision 82.35
Fenestration
  aneurysm (dissecting), thoracic aorta 39.54
  aortic aneurysm 39.54
  cardiac valve 35.10
  chest wall 34.01
  ear
    inner (with graft) 20.61
      revision 20.62
    tympanic 19.55
  labyrinth (with graft) 20.61
  Lempert's (endaural) 19.9
  operation (aorta) 39.54
  oval window, ear canal 19.55
  palate 27.1
  pericardium 37.12
  semicircular canals (with graft) 20.61

Fenestration — *continued*
  stapes foot plate (with vein graft) 19.19
    with incus replacement 19.11
  tympanic membrane 19.55
  vestibule (with graft) 20.61
Ferguson operation (hernia repair) 53.00
Fetography 87.81
Fetoscopy 75.31
Fiberoscopy — *see* Endoscopy, by site
Fibroidectomy, uterine 68.29
Fick operation (perforation of foot plate) 19.0
Filipuncture (aneurysm) (cerebral) 39.52
Filleting
  hammer toe 77.56
  pancreas 52.3
Filling, tooth (amalgam) (plastic) (silicate) 23.2
  root canal (*see also* therapy, root canal) 23.70
Fimbriectomy (*see also* Salpingectomy, partial) 66.69
  Uchida (with tubal ligation) 66.32
Finney operation (pyloroplasty) 44.29
Fissurectomy, anal 49.39
  endoscopic 49.31
  skin (subcutaneous tissue) 49.04
Fistulectomy — *see also* Closure, fistula, by site
  abdominothoracic 34.83
  abdominouterine 69.42
  anus 49.12
  appendix 47.92
  bile duct 51.79
  biliary tract NEC 51.79
  bladder (transurethral approach) 57.84
  bone (*see also* Excision, lesion, bone) 77.60
  branchial cleft 29.52
  bronchocutaneous 33.42
  bronchoesophageal 33.42
  bronchomediastinal 34.73
  bronchopleural 34.73
  bronchopleurocutaneous 34.73
  bronchopleuromediastinal 34.73
  bronchovisceral 33.42
  cervicosigmoidal 67.62
  cholecystogastroenteric 51.93
  cornea 11.49
  diaphragm 34.83
  enterouterine 69.42
  esophagopleurocutaneous 34.73
  esophagus NEC 42.84
  fallopian tube 66.73
  gallbladder 51.93
  gastric NEC 44.63
  hepatic duct 51.79
  hepatopleural 34.73
  hepatopulmonary 34.73
  intestine
    large 46.76
    small 46.74
  intestinouterine 69.42
  joint (*see also* Excision, lesion, joint) 80.80
  lacrimal
    gland 09.21
    sac 09.6
  laryngotracheal 31.62
  larynx 31.62
  mediastinocutaneous 34.73
  mouth NEC 27.53
  nasal 21.82
    sinus 22.71
  nasolabial 21.82
  nasopharyngeal 21.82
  oroantral 22.71
  oronasal 21.82
  pancreas 52.95
  perineorectal 71.72
  perineosigmoidal 71.72
  perirectal, not opening into rectum 48.93
  pharyngoesophageal 29.53
  pharynx NEC 29.53
  pleura 34.73
  rectolabial 71.72
  rectourethral 58.43
  rectouterine 69.42
  rectovaginal 70.73

Fistulectomy — *see also* Closure, fistula, by site — *continued*
  rectovesical 57.83
  rectovulvar 71.72
  rectum 48.73
  salivary (duct) (gland) 26.42
  scrotum 61.42
  skin 86.3
  stomach NEC 44.63
  subcutaneous tissue 86.3
  thoracoabdominal 34.83
  thoracogastric 34.83
  thoracointestinal 34.83
  thorax NEC 34.73
  trachea NEC 31.73
  tracheoesophageal 31.73
  ureter 56.84
  urethra 58.43
  uteroenteric 69.42
  uterointestinal 69.42
  uterorectal 69.42
  uterovaginal 69.42
  vagina 70.75
  vesicosigmoidovaginal 57.83
  vocal cords 31.62
  vulvorectal 71.72
Fistulization
  appendix 47.91
  arteriovenous 39.27
  cisterna chyli 40.62
  endolymphatic sac (for decompression) 20.79
  esophagus, external 42.10
    cervical 42.11
    specified technique NEC 42.19
  interatrial 35.41
  labyrinth (for decompression) 20.79
  lacrimal sac into nasal cavity 09.81
  larynx 31.29
  lymphatic duct, left (thoracic) 40.62
  orbit 16.09
  peritoneal 54.93
  salivary gland 26.49
  sclera 12.69
    by trephination 12.61
    with iridectomy 12.65
  sinus, nasal NEC 22.9
  subarachnoid space 02.2
  thoracic duct 40.62
  trachea 31.29
  tracheoesophageal 31.95
  urethrovaginal 58.0
  ventricle, cerebral (*see also* Shunt, ventricular) 02.2
Fistulogram
  abdominal wall 88.03
  chest wall 87.38
  retroperitoneum 88.14
Fistulotomy, anal 49.11
Fitting
  arch bars (orthodontic) 24.7
    for immobilization (fracture) 93.55
  artificial limb 84.40
  contact lens 95.32
  denture (total) 99.97
    bridge (fixed) 23.42
      removable 23.43
    partial (fixed) 23.42
      removable 23.43
  hearing aid 95.48
  obturator (orthodontic) 24.7
  ocular prosthetics 95.34
  orthodontic
    appliance 24.7
    obturator 24.7
    wiring 24.7
  orthotic device 93.23
  periodontal splint (orthodontic) 24.7
  prosthesis, prosthetic device
    above knee 84.45
    arm 84.43
      lower (and hand) 84.42
      upper (and shoulder) 84.41
    below knee 84.46
    hand (and lower arm) 84.42

Index to Procedures

Fitting — *continued*
  prosthesis, prosthetic device — *continued*
    leg 84.47
      above knee 84.45
      below knee 84.46
    limb NEC 84.40
    ocular 95.34
    penis (external) 64.94
    shoulder (and upper arm) 84.41
  spectacles 95.31
Five-in-one repair, knee 81.42
Fixation
  bone
    external, without reduction 93.59
      with fracture reduction — *see* Reduction, fracture
      cast immobilization NEC 93.53
      splint 93.54
      traction (skeletal) NEC 93.44
        intermittent 93.43
    internal (without fracture reduction) 78.50
      with fracture-reduction — *see* Reduction, fracture
      carpal, metacarpal 78.54
      clavicle 78.51
      femur 78.55
      fibula 78.57
      humerus 78.52
      patella 78.56
      pelvic 78.59
      phalanges (foot) (hand) 78.59
      radius 78.53
      scapula 78.51
      specified site NEC 78.59
      tarsal, metatarsal 78.58
      thorax (ribs) (sternum) 78.51
      tibia 78.57
      ulna 78.53
      vertebrae 78.59
  breast (pendulous) 85.6
  cardinal ligaments 69.22
  duodenum 46.62
    to abdominal wall 46.61
  external (without manipulation for reduction) 93.59
    with fracture-reduction — *see* Reduction, fracture
    cast immobilization NEC 93.53
    pressure dressing 93.56
    splint 93.54
    traction (skeletal) NEC 93.44
      intermittent 93.43
  hip 81.40
  ileum 46.62
    to abdominal wall 46.61
  internal
    with fracture-reduction — *see* Reduction, fracture
    without fracture-reduction — *see* Fixation, bone, internal
  intestine 46.60
    large 46.64
      to abdominal wall 46.63
    small 46.62
      to abdominal wall 46.61
      to abdominal wall 46.60
  iris (bombé) 12.11
  jejunum 46.62
    to abdominal wall 46.61
  joint — *see* Arthroplasty
  kidney 55.7
  ligament
    cardinal 69.22
    palpebrae 08.36
  omentum 54.74
  parametrial 69.22
  rectum (sling) 48.76
  spine, with fusion (*see also* Fusion, spinal) 81.00
  spleen 41.95
  tendon 83.88
    hand 82.85
  testis in scrotum 62.5
  tongue 25.59
  urethrovaginal (to Cooper's ligament) 70.77

Fixation — *continued*
  uterus (abdominal) (vaginal) (ventrofixation) 69.22
  vagina 70.77
Flooding (psychologic desensitization) 94.33
Flowmetry, Doppler (ultrasonic) — *see also* Ultrasonography
  aortic arch 88.73
  head and neck 88.71
  heart 88.72
  thorax NEC 88.73
Fluoroscopy — *see* Radiography
Fog therapy (respiratory) 93.94
Folding, eye muscle 15.22
  multiple (two or more muscles) 15.4
Foley operation (pyeloplasty) 55.87
Fontan operation (creation of conduit between right atrium and pulmonary artery) 35.94
Foraminotomy 03.09
Forced extension, limb 93.25
Forceps delivery — *see* Delivery, forceps
Formation
  adhesions
    pericardium 36.39
    pleura 34.6
  anus, artificial (*see also* Colostomy) 46.13
    duodenostomy 46.39
    ileostomy (*see also* Ileostomy) 46.23
    jejunostomy 46.39
      percutaneous (endoscopic) (PEJ) 46.32
  arteriovenous fistula (for kidney dialysis) (peripheral) (shunt) 39.27
    external cannula 39.93
  bone flap, cranial 02.03
  cardiac pacemaker pocket
    with initial insertion of pacemaker — *omit code*
    new site (skin) (subcutaneous) 37.79
  colostomy (*see also* Colostomy) 46.13
  conduit
    ileal (urinary) 56.51
    left ventricle and aorta 35.93
    right atrium and pulmonary artery 35.94
    right ventricle and pulmonary (distal) artery 35.92
      in repair of
        pulmonary artery atresia 35.92
        transposition of great vessels 35.92
        truncus arteriosus 35.83
  endorectal ileal pouch (J-pouch) (H-pouch) (S-pouch) (with anastomosis to anus) 45.95
  fistula
    arteriovenous (for kidney dialysis) (peripheral shunt) 39.27
      external cannula 39.93
    bladder to skin NEC 57.18
      with bladder flap 57.21
      percutaneous 57.17
    cutaneoperitoneal 54.93
    gastric 43.19
      percutaneous (endoscopic) (transabdominal) 43.11
    mucous (*see also* Colostomy) 46.13
    rectovaginal 48.99
    tracheoesophageal 31.95
    tubulovalvular (Beck-Jianu) (Frank's) (Janeway) (Spivack's) (Ssabanejew-Frank) 43.19
    urethrovaginal 58.0
  ileal
    bladder
      closed 57.87 [45.51]
      open 56.51
    conduit 56.51
  interatrial fistula 35.42
  mucous fistula (*see also* Colostomy) 46.13
  pericardial
    baffle, interatrial 35.91
    window 37.12
  pleural window (for drainage) 34.09
  pocket
    cardiac pacemaker
      with initial insertion of pacemaker — *omit code*

Formation — *continued*
  pocket — *continued*
    cardiac pacemaker — *continued*
      new site (skin) (subcutaneous) 37.79
    thalamic stimulator pulse generator
      with initial insertion of battery package — *omit code*
      new site (skin) (subcutaneous) 86.09
  pupil 12.39
    by iridectomy 12.14
  rectovaginal fistula 48.99
  reversed gastric tube (intrathoracic) (retrosternal) 42.58
    antesternal or antethoracic 42.68
  septal defect, interatrial 35.42
  shunt
    abdominovenous 54.94
    arteriovenous 39.93
    peritoneojugular 54.94
    peritoneo-vascular 54.94
    pleuroperitoneal 34.05
    transjugular intrahepatic portosystemic [TIPS] 39.1
  subcutaneous tunnel
    esophageal 42.86
      with anastomosis — *see* Anastomosis, esophagus, antesternal
    pulse generator lead wire 86.99
      with initial procedure — *omit code*
    thalamic stimulator pulse generator pocket
      with initial insertion of battery package — *omit code*
      new site (skin) (subcutaneous) 86.09
  syndactyly (finger) (toe) 86.89
  tracheoesophageal 31.95
  tubulovalvular fistula (Beck-Jianu) (Frank's) (Janeway) (Spivack's) (Ssabanejew-Frank) 43.19
  uretero-ileostomy, cutaneous 56.51
  ureterostomy, cutaneous 56.61
    ileal 56.51
  urethrovaginal fistula 58.0
  window
    pericardial 37.12
    pleural (for drainage) 34.09
Fothergill (-Donald) operation (uterine suspension) 69.22
Fowler operation
  arthroplasty of metacarpophalangeal joint 81.72
  release (mallet finger repair) 82.84
  tenodesis (hand) 82.85
  thoracoplasty 33.34
Fox operation (entropion repair with wedge resection) 08.43
Fracture, surgical (*see also* Osteoclasis) 78.70
  turbinates (nasal) 21.62
Fragmentation
  lithotriptor — *see* Lithotripsy
  mechanical
    cataract (with aspiration) 13.43
      posterior route 13.42
      secondary membrane 13.66
    secondary membrane (after cataract) 13.66
  ultrasonic
    cataract (with aspiration) 13.41
    stones, urinary (Kock pouch) 59.95
    urinary stones 59.95
      percutaneous nephrostomy 55.04
Franco operation (suprapubic cystotomy) 57.18
Frank operation 43.19
Frazier (-Spiller) operation (subtemporal trigeminal rhizotomy) 04.02
Fredet-Ramstedt operation (pyloromyotomy) (with wedge resection) 43.3
Freeing
  adhesions — *see* Lysis, adhesions
  anterior synechiae (with injection of air or liquid) 12.32
  artery-vein-nerve bundle 39.91
  extraocular muscle, entrapped 15.7
  goniosynechiae (with injection of air or liquid) 12.31

Freeing — continued
  intestinal segment for interposition 45.50
    large 45.52
    small 45.51
  posterior synechiae 12.33
  synechiae (posterior) 12.33
    anterior (with injection of air or liquid) 12.32
  vascular bundle 39.91
  vessel 39.91

Freezing
  gastric 96.32
  prostate 60.62

Frenckner operation (intrapetrosal drainage) 20.22

Frenectomy
  labial 27.41
  lingual 25.92
  lip 27.41
  maxillary 27.41
  tongue 25.92

Frenotomy
  labial 27.91
  lingual 25.91

Frenulumectomy — see Frenectomy

Frickman operation (abdominal proctopexy) 48.75

Frommel operation (shortening of uterosacral ligaments) 69.22

Fulguration — see also Electrocoagulation and Destruction, lesion, by site
  adenoid fossa 28.7
  anus 49.39
    endoscopic 49.31
  bladder (transurethral) 57.49
    suprapubic 57.59
  choroid 14.21
  duodenum 45.32
    endoscopic 45.30
  esophagus 42.39
    endoscopic 42.33
  large intestine 45.49
    endoscopic 45.43
      polypectomy 45.42
  penis 64.2
  perineum, female 71.3
  prostate, transurethral 60.29
  rectum 48.32
    radical 48.31
  retina 14.21
  scrotum 61.3
  Skene's gland 71.3
  skin 86.3
  small intestine NEC 45.34
    duodenum 45.32
      endoscopic 45.30
  stomach 43.49
    endoscopic 43.41
  subcutaneous tissue 86.3
  tonsillar fossa 28.7
  urethra 58.39
    endoscopic 58.31
  vulva 71.3

Function
  study — see also Scan, radioisotope
    gastric 89.39
    muscle 93.08
      ocular 95.25
    nasal 89.12
    pulmonary — see categories 89.37-89.38
    renal 92.03
    thyroid 92.01
    urethral sphincter 89.23

Fundectomy, uterine 68.3

Fundoplication (esophageal) (Nissen's) 44.66

Fundusectomy, gastric 43.89

Fusion
  atlas-axis (spine) 81.01
    for pseudarthrosis 81.31
  bone (see also Osteoplasty) 78.40
  cervical (spine) (C$_2$ level or below) NEC 81.02
    anterior (interbody), anterolateral technique 81.02

Fusion — continued
  cervical NEC — continued
    C$_1$-C$_2$ level (anterior interbody) (anterolateral) 81.01
    for pseudarthrosis 81.32
    occiput — C$_2$ 81.01
    posterior (interbody), posterolateral technique 81.03
  claw toe 77.57
  craniocervical 81.01
    for pseudarthrosis 81.31
  dorsal, dorsolumbar NEC 81.05
    anterior (interbody), anterolateral technique 81.04
      for pseudarthrosis 81.34
    for pseudarthrosis 81.35
    posterior (interbody) posterolateral technique 81.05
      for pseudarthrosis 81.35
  epiphyseal-diaphyseal (see also Arrest, bone growth) 78.20
  epiphysiodesis (see also Arrest, bone growth) 78.20
  joint (with bone graft) (see also Arthrodesis) 81.20
    ankle 81.11
    claw toe 77.57
    foot NEC 81.17
    hammer toe 77.56
    hip 81.21
    interphalangeal, finger 81.28
    ischiofemoral 81.21
    metatarsophalangeal 81.16
    midtarsal 81.14
    overlapping toe(s) 77.58
    pantalar 81.11
    spinal (see also Fusion, spinal) 81.00
    subtalar 81.13
    tarsal joints NEC 81.17
    tarsometatarsal 81.15
    tibiotalar 81.11
    toe NEC 77.58
      claw toe 77.57
      hammer toe 77.56
      overlapping toe(s) 77.58
  lip to tongue 25.59
  lumbar, lumbosacral NEC 81.08
    anterior (interbody), anterolateral technique 81.06
      for pseudarthrosis 81.36
    for pseudarthrosis 81.38
    lateral transverse process technique 81.07
      for pseudarthrosis 81.37
    posterior (interbody), posterolateral technique 81.08
      for pseudoarthrosis 81.38
  occiput — C$_2$ (spinal) 81.01
    for pseudarthrosis 81.31
  spinal (with graft) (with internal fixation) (with instrumentation) 81.00
    360 degree 81.61
    atlas-axis (anterior transoral) (posterior) 81.01
      for pseudarthrosis 81.31
    cervical (C$_2$ level or below) NEC 81.02
      anterior (interbody), anterolateral technique 81.02
        for pseudarthrosis 81.32
      C$_1$-C$_2$ level (anterior) (posterior) 81.01
        for pseudarthrosis 81.31
      for pseudarthrosis 81.32
      posterior (interbody), posterolateral technique 81.03
        for pseudarthrosis 81.33
    craniocervical (anterior) (transoral) (posterior) 81.01
      for pseudarthrosis 81.31
    dorsal, dorsolumbar NEC 81.05
      anterior (interbody), anterolateral technique 81.04
        for pseudarthrosis 81.34
      for pseudarthrosis 81.35
      posterior (interbody), posterolateral technique 81.05
        for pseudarthrosis 81.35

Fusion — continued
  spinal — continued
    lumbar, lumbosacral NEC 81.08
      anterior (interbody), anterolateral technique 81.06
        for pseudarthrosis 81.36
      for pseudarthrosis 81.38
      lateral transverse process technique 81.07
        for pseudarthrosis 81.37
      posterior (interbody), posterolateral technique 81.08
        for pseudarthrosis 81.38
    occiput — C$_2$ (anterior) (transoral) (posterior) 81.01
      for pseudarthrosis 81.31
  tongue (to lip) 25.59

G

Gait training 93.22
Galeaplasty 86.89
Galvanoionization 99.27
Games
  competitive 94.39
  organized 93.89
Gamma irradiation, stereotactic 92.32
Ganglionectomy
  gasserian 04.05
  lumbar sympathetic 05.23
  nerve (cranial) (peripheral) NEC 04.06
    sympathetic 05.29
  sphenopalatine (Meckel's) 05.21
  tendon sheath (wrist) 82.21
    site other than hand 83.31
  trigeminal 04.05
Ganglionotomy, trigeminal (radiofrequency) 04.02
Gant operation (wedge osteotomy of trochanter) 77.25
Garceau operation (tibial tendon transfer) 83.75
Gardner operation (spinal meningocele repair) 03.51
Gas endarterectomy 38.10
  abdominal 38.16
  aorta (arch) (ascending) (descending) 38.14
  coronary artery 36.09
  head and neck NEC 38.12
  intracranial NEC 38.11
  lower limb 38.18
  thoracic NEC 38.15
  upper limb 38.13
Gastrectomy (partial) (subtotal) NEC 43.89
  with
    anastomosis (to) NEC 43.89
      duodenum 43.6
      esophagus 43.5
      gastrogastric 43.89
      jejunum 43.7
    esophagogastrostomy 43.5
    gastroduodenostomy (bypass) 43.6
    gastroenterostomy (bypass) 43.7
    gastrogastrostomy (bypass) 43.89
    gastrojejunostomy (bypass) 43.7
    jejunal transposition 43.81
  complete NEC 43.99
    with intestinal interposition 43.91
  distal 43.6
  Hofmeister 43.7
  Polya 43.7
  proximal 43.5
  radical NEC 43.99
    with intestinal interposition 43.91
  total NEC 43.99
    with intestinal interposition 43.91
Gastrocamera 44.19
Gastroduodenectomy — see Gastrectomy
Gastroduodenoscopy 45.13
  through stoma (artificial) 45.12
  transabdominal (operative) 45.11

Index to Procedures

Gastroduodenostomy (bypass) (Jaboulay's) 44.39
   with partial gastrectomy 43.6
Gastroenterostomy (bypass) NEC 44.39
   with partial gastrectomy 43.7
Gastrogastrostomy (bypass) 44.39
   with partial gastrectomy 43.89
Gastrojejunostomy (bypass) 44.39
   with partial gastrectomy 43.7
   percutaneous (endoscopic) 44.32
Gastrolysis 54.59
   laparoscopic 54.51
Gastropexy 44.64
Gastroplasty NEC 44.69
Gastroplication 44.69
Gastropylorectomy 43.6
Gastrorrhaphy 44.61
Gastroscopy NEC 44.13
   through stoma (artificial) 44.12
   transabdominal (operative) 44.11
Gastrostomy (Brunschwig's) (decompression) (fine caliber tube) (Kader) (permanent) (Stamm) (Stamm-Kader) (temporary) (tube) (Witzel) 43.19
   Beck-Jianu 43.19
   Frank's 43.19
   Janeway 43.19
   percutaneous (endoscopic) (PEG) 43.11
   Spivack's 43.19
   Ssabanejew-Frank 43.19
Gastrotomy 43.0
   for control of hemorrhage 44.49
Gavage, gastric 96.35
Gelman operation (release of clubfoot) 83.84
Genioplasty (augmentation) (with graft) (with implant) 76.68
   reduction 76.67
Ghormley operation (hip fusion) 81.21
Gifford operation
   destruction of lacrimal sac 09.6
   keratotomy (delimiting) 11.1
      radial (refractive) 11.75
Gill operation
   arthrodesis of shoulder 81.23
   laminectomy 03.09
Gill-Stein operation (carporadial arthrodesis) 81.25
Gilliam operation (uterine suspension) 69.22
Gingivectomy 24.31
Gingivoplasty (with bone graft) (with soft tissue graft) 24.2
Girdlestone operation
   laminectomy with spinal fusion 81.00
   muscle transfer for claw toe repair 77.57
   resection of femoral head and neck 77.85
Girdlestone-Taylor operation (muscle transfer for claw toe repair) 77.57
Glenn operation (anastomosis of superior vena cava to right pulmonary artery) 39.21
Glenoplasty, shoulder 81.83
   with
      partial replacement 81.81
      total replacement 81.80
      for recurrent dislocation 81.82
Glomectomy
   carotid 39.8
   jugulare 20.51
Glossectomy (complete) (total) 25.3
   partial or subtotal 25.2
   radical 25.4
Glossopexy 25.59
Glossoplasty NEC 25.59
Glossorrhaphy 25.51
Glossotomy NEC 25.94
   for tongue tie 25.91
Glycoprotein IIB/IIIa inhibitor 99.20
Goebel-Frangenheim-Stoeckel operation (urethrovesical suspenion) 59.4
Goldner operation (clubfoot release) 80.48

Goldthwaite operation
   ankle stabilization 81.11
   patellar stabilization 81.44
   tendon transfer for stabilization of patella 81.44
Gonadectomy
   ovary
      bilateral 65.51
         laparoscopic 65.53
      unilateral 65.39
         laparoscopic 65.31
   testis 62.3
Goniopuncture 12.51
   with goniotomy 12.53
Gonioscopy 12.29
Goniospasis 12.59
Goniotomy (Barkan's) 12.52
   with goniopuncture 12.53
Goodal-Power operation (vagina) 70.8
Gordon-Taylor operation (hindquarter amputation) 84.19
GP IIb/IIIa inhibitor, infusion 99.20
Graber-Duvernay operation (drilling of femoral head) 77.15
Graft, grafting
   aneurysm 39.52
      endovascular
         abdominal aorta 39.71
         lower extremity artery(s) 39.79
         thoracic aorta 39.79
         upper extremity artery(s) 39.79
   artery, arterial (patch) 39.58
      with
         excision or resection of vessel — see Arteriectomy, with graft replacement
         synthetic patch (Dacron) (Teflon) 39.57
         tissue patch (vein) (autogenous) (homograft) 39.56
   blood vessel (patch) 39.58
      with
         excision or resection of vessel — see Angiectomy, with graft replacement
         synthetic patch (Dacron) (Teflon) 39.57
         tissue patch (vein) (autogenous) (homograft) 39.56
   bone (autogenous) (bone bank) (dual onlay) (heterogenous) (inlay) (massive onlay) (multiple) (osteoperiosteal) (peg) (subperiosteal) (with metallic fixation) 78.00
      with
         arthrodesis — see Arthrodesis
         arthroplasty — see Arthroplasty
         gingivoplasty 24.2
         lengthening — see Lengthening, bone
      carpals, metacarpals 78.04
      clavicle 78.01
      facial NEC 76.91
         with total ostectomy 76.44
      femur 78.05
      fibula 78.07
      humerus 78.02
      joint — see Arthroplasty
      mandible 76.91
         with total mandibulectomy 76.41
      marrow — see Transplant, bone, marrow
      nose — see Graft, nose
      patella 78.06
      pelvic 78.09
      pericranial 02.04
      phalanges (foot) (hand) 78.09
      radius 78.03
      scapula 78.01
      skull 02.04
      specified site NEC 78.09
      spine 78.09
         with fusion — see Fusion, spinal
      tarsal, metatarsal 78.08
      thorax (ribs) (sternum) 78.01
      thumb (with transfer of skin flap) 82.69
      tibia 78.07
      ulna 78.03
      vertebrae 78.09
         with fusion — see Fusion, spinal

Graft, grafting — continued
   breast (see also Mammoplasty) 85.89
   buccal sulcus 27.99
   cartilage (joint) — see also Arthroplasty
      nose — see Graft, nose
   chest wall (mesh) (silastic) 34.79
   conjunctiva (free) (mucosa) 10.44
      for symblepharon repair 10.41
   cornea (see also Keratoplasty) 11.60
   dermal-fat 86.69
   dermal regenerative 86.67
   dura 02.12
   ear
      auricle 18.79
      external auditory meatus 18.6
      inner 20.61
      pedicle preparation 86.71
   esophagus NEC 42.87
      with interposition (intrathoracic) NEC 42.58
         antesternal or antethoracic NEC 42.68
         colon (intrathoracic) 42.55
            antesternal or antethoracic 42.65
         small bowel (intrathoracic) 42.53
            antesternal or antethoracic 42.63
   eyebrow (see also Reconstruction, eyelid, with graft) 08.69
   eyelid (see also Reconstruction, eyelid, with graft) 08.69
      free mucous membrane 08.62
   eye socket (skin) (cartilage) (bone) 16.63
   fallopian tube 66.79
   fascia 83.82
      with hernia repair — see Repair, hernia
      eyelid 08.32
      hand 82.72
      tarsal cartilage 08.69
   fat pad NEC 86.89
      with skin graft — see Graft, skin, full-thickness
   flap (advanced) (rotating) (sliding) — see also Graft, skin, pedicle
      tarsoconjunctival 08.64
   hair-bearing skin 86.64
   hand
      fascia 82.72
      free skin 86.62
      muscle 82.72
      pedicle (flap) 86.73
      tendon 82.79
   heart, for revascularization — see category 36.3
   joint — see Arthroplasty
   larynx 31.69
   lip 27.56
      full-thickness 27.55
   lymphatic structure(s) (channel) (node) (vessel) 40.9
   mediastinal fat to myocardium 36.39
   meninges (cerebral) 02.12
   mouth, except palate 27.56
      full-thickness 27.55
   muscle 83.82
      hand 82.72
   myocardium, for revascularization 36.39
   nasolabial flaps 21.86
   nerve (cranial) (peripheral) 04.5
   nipple 85.86
   nose 21.89
      with
         augmentation 21.85
         rhinoplasty — see Rhinoplasty
         total reconstruction 21.83
      septum 21.88
      tip 21.86
   omentum 54.74
      to myocardium 36.39
   orbit (bone) (cartilage) (skin) 16.63
   outflow tract (patch) (pulmonary valve) 35.26
      in total repair of tetralogy of Fallot 35.81
   ovary 65.92
   palate 27.69
      for cleft palate repair 27.62
   pedicle — see Graft, skin, pedicle
   penis (rib) (skin) 64.49
   pigskin 86.65
   pinch — see Graft, skin, free

Graft, grafting
   — continued
   pocket — *see* Graft, skin, pedicle
   porcine 86.65
   postauricular (Wolff) 18.79
   razor — *see* Graft, skin, free
   rope — *see* Graft, skin, pedicle
   saphenous vein in aortocoronary bypass — *see* Bypass, aortocoronary
   scrotum 61.49
   skin (partial-thickness) (split-thickness) 86.69
     amnionic membrane 86.66
     auditory meatus (ear) 18.6
     dermal-fat 86.69
       for breast augmentation 85.50
     dermal regenerative 86.67
     ear
       auditory meatus 18.6
       postauricular 18.79
     eyelid 08.61
     flap — *see* Graft, skin, pedicle
     free (autogenous) NEC 86.60
       lip 27.56
       thumb 86.62
         for
           pollicization 82.61
           reconstruction 82.69
     full-thickness 86.63
       breast 85.83
       hand 86.61
     hair-bearing 86.64
       eyelid or eyebrow 08.63
     hand 86.62
       full-thickness 86.61
     heterograft 86.65
     homograft 86.66
     island flap 86.70
     mucous membrane 86.69
       eyelid 08.62
     nose — *see* Graft, nose
     pedicle (flap) (tube) 86.70
       advancement 86.72
       attachment to site (advanced) (double) (rotating) (sliding) 86.74
         hand (cross finger) (pocket) 86.73
         lip 27.57
         mouth 27.57
         thumb 86.73
           for
             pollicization 82.61
             reconstruction NEC 82.69
       breast 85.84
         transverse rectus abdominis musculocutaneous (TRAM) 85.7
       defatting 86.75
       delayed 86.71
       design and raising 86.71
       elevation 86.71
       preparation of (cutting) 86.71
       revision 86.75
       sculpturing 86.71
       transection 86.71
       transfer 86.74
       trimming 86.71
     postauricular 18.79
     rotation flap 86.70
     specified site NEC 86.69
       full-thickness 86.63
   tarsal cartilage 08.69
   temporalis muscle to orbit 16.63
     with exenteration of orbit 16.59
   tendon 83.81
     for joint repair — *see* Arthroplasty
     hand 82.79
   testicle 62.69
   thumb (for reconstruction) NEC 82.69
   tongue (mucosal) (skin) 25.59
   trachea 31.79
   tubular (tube) — *see* Graft, skin, pedicle
   tunnel — *see* Graft, skin, pedicle
   tympanum (*see also* Tympanoplasty) 19.4
   ureter 56.89

Graft, grafting — *continued*
   vein (patch) 39.58
     with
       excision or resection of vessel — *see* Phlebectomy, with graft replacement
       synthetic patch (Dacron) (Teflon) 39.57
       tissue patch (vein) (autogenous) (homograft) 39.56
   vermillion border (lip) 27.56
Grattage, conjunctiva 10.31
Green operation (scapulopexy) 78.41
Grice operation (subtalar arthrodesis) 81.13
Grip, strength 93.04
Gritti-Stokes operation (knee disarticulation) 84.16
Gross operation (herniorrhaphy) 53.49
Group therapy 94.44
Guttering, bone (*see also* Excision, lesion, bone) 77.60
Guyon operation (amputation of ankle) 84.13

H

Hagner operation (epididymotomy) 63.92
Halsted operation — *see* Repair, hernia, inguinal
Hampton operation (anastomosis small intestine to rectal stump) 45.92
Hanging hip operation (muscle release) 83.19
Harelip operation 27.54
Harrison-Richardson operation (vaginal suspension) 70.77
Hartmann resection (of intestine)(with pouch) — *see* Colectomy, by site
Harvesting
   bone marrow 41.91
   stem cells 99.79
Hauser operation
   achillotenotomy 83.11
   bunionectomy with adductor tendon transfer 77.53
   stabilization of patella 81.44
Heaney operation (vaginal hysterectomy) 68.59
   laparoscopically assisted (LAVH) 68.51
Hearing aid (with battery replacement) 95.49
Hearing test 95.47
Hegar operation (perineorrhaphy) 71.79
Heine operation (cyclodialysis) 12.55
Heineke-Mikulicz operation (pyloroplasty) 44.29
Heller operation (esophagomyotomy) 42.7
Hellström operation (transplantation of aberrant renal vessel) 39.55
Hemicolectomy
   left 45.75
   right (extended) 45.73
Hemicystectomy 57.6
Hemigastrectomy — *see* Gastrectomy
Hemiglossectomy 25.2
Hemilaminectomy (decompression) (exploration) 03.09
Hemilaryngectomy (anterior) (lateral) (vertical) 30.1
Hemimandibulectomy 76.31
Hemimastectomy (radical) 85.23
Hemimaxillectomy (with bone graft) (with prosthesis) 76.39
Heminephrectomy 55.4
Hemipelvectomy 84.19
Hemispherectomy (cerebral) 01.52
Hemithyroidectomy (with removal of isthmus) (with removal of portion of remaining lobe) 06.2
Hemodiafiltration (extracorporeal) 39.95
Hemodialysis (extracorporeal) 39.95
Hemodilution 99.03
Hemofiltration (extracorporeal) 39.95

Hemorrhage control — *see* Control, hemorrhage
Hemorrhoidectomy 49.46
   by
     cautery, cauterization 49.43
     crushing 49.45
     cryotherapy, cryosurgery 49.44
     excision 49.46
     injection 49.42
     ligation 49.45
Hemostasis — *see* Control, hemorrhage
Henley operation (jejunal transposition) 43.81
Hepatectomy (complete) (total) 50.4
   partial or subtotal 50.22
Hepatic assistance, extracorporeal 50.92
Hepaticocholangiojejunostomy 51.37
Hepaticocystoduodenostomy 51.37
Hepaticodochotomy 51.59
Hepaticoduodenostomy 51.37
Hepaticojejunostomy 51.37
Hepaticolithectomy 51.49
   endoscopic 51.88
Hepaticolithotomy 51.49
   endoscopic 51.88
Hepaticostomy 51.59
Hepaticotomy 51.59
Hepatocholangiocystoduodenostomy 51.37
Hepatocholedochostomy 51.43
   endoscopic 51.87
Hepatoduodenostomy 50.69
Hepatogastrostomy 50.69
Hepatojejunostomy 50.69
Hepatolithotomy
   hepatic duct 51.49
   liver 50.0
Hepatopexy 50.69
Hepatorrhaphy 50.61
Hepatostomy (external) (internal) 50.69
Hepatotomy (with packing) 50.0
Hernioplasty — *see* Repair, hernia
Herniorrhaphy — *see* Repair, hernia
Herniotomy — *see* Repair, hernia
Heterograft — *see* Graft
Heterotransplant, heterotransplan-tation — *see* Transplant
Hey operation (amputation of foot) 84.12
Hey-Groves operation (reconstruction of anterior cruciate ligament) 81.45
Heymen operation (soft tissue release for clubfoot) 83.84
Heyman-Herndon (-Strong) operation (correction of metatarsus varus) 80.48
Hibbs operation (lumbar spinal fusion) — *see* Fusion, lumbar
Higgins operation — *see* Repair, hernia, femoral
High forceps delivery 72.39
   with episiotomy 72.31
Hill-Allison operation (hiatal hernia repair, transpleural approach) 53.80
Hinging, mitral valve 35.12
His bundle recording 37.29
Hitchcock operation (anchoring tendon of biceps) 83.88
Hofmeister operation (gastrectomy) 43.7
Hoke operation
   midtarsal fusion 81.14
   triple arthrodesis 81.12
Holth operation
   iridencleisis 12.63
   sclerectomy 12.65
Homan operation (correction of lymphedema) 40.9
Homograft — *see* Graft
Homotransplant, homotransplantation — *see* Transplant
Hosiery, elastic 93.59
Hutch operation (ureteroneo-cystostomy) 56.74

Index to Procedures

Hybinette-Eden operation (glenoid bone block) 78.01
Hydrocelectomy
  canal of Nuck (female) 69.19
    male 63.1
  round ligament 69.19
  spermatic cord 63.1
  tunica vaginalis 61.2
Hydrotherapy 93.33
  assisted exercise in pool 93.31
  whirlpool 93.32
Hymenectomy 70.31
Hymenoplasty 70.76
Hymenorrhaphy 70.76
Hymenotomy 70.11
Hyperalimentation (parenteral) 99.15
Hyperbaric oxygenation 93.95
  wound 93.59
Hyperextension, joint 93.25
Hyperthermia NEC 93.35
  for cancer treatment (interstitial) (local) (radiofrequency) (regional) (ultrasound) (whole-body) 99.85
Hypnodrama, psychiatric 94.32
Hypnosis (psychotherapeutic) 94.32
  for anesthesia — *omit code*
Hypnotherapy 94.32
Hypophysectomy (complete) (total) 07.69
  partial or subtotal 07.63
    transfrontal approach 07.61
    transsphenoidal approach 07.62
  specified approach NEC 07.68
  transfrontal approach (complete) (total) 07.64
    partial 07.61
  transsphenoidal approach (complete) (total) 07.65
    partial 07.62
Hypothermia (central) (local) 99.81
  gastric (cooling) 96.31
    freezing 96.32
  systemic (in open heart surgery) 39.62
Hypotympanotomy 20.23
Hysterectomy 68.9
  abdominal 68.4
    partial or subtotal (supracervical) (supravaginal) 68.3
    radical (modified) (Wertheim's) 68.6
  vaginal (complete) (partial) (subtotal) (total) 68.59
    laparoscopically assisted (LAVH) 68.51
    radical (Schauta) 68.7
Hysterocolpectomy (radical) (vaginal) 68.7
  abdominal 68.6
Hysterogram NEC 87.85
  percutaneous 87.84
Hysterolysis 54.59
  laparoscopic 54.51
Hysteromyomectomy 68.29
Hysteropexy 69.22
Hysteroplasty 69.49
Hysterorrhaphy 69.41
Hysterosalpingography gas (contrast) 87.82
  opaque dye (contrast) 87.83
Hysterosalpingostomy 66.74
Hysteroscopy 68.12
  with
    ablation
      endometrial 68.23
    biopsy 68.16
Hysterotomy (with removal of foreign body) (with removal of hydatidiform mole) 68.0
  for intrauterine transfusion 75.2
  obstetrical 74.99
  for termination of pregnancy 74.91
Hysterotrachelectomy 67.4
Hysterotracheloplasty 69.49
Hysterotrachelorrhaphy 69.41
Hysterotrachelotomy 69.95

I

ICCE (intracapsular cataract extraction) 13.19
Ileal
  bladder
    closed 57.87 [45.51]
    open (ileoureterostomy) 56.51
  conduit (ileoureterostomy) 56.51
Ileocecostomy 45.93
Ileocolectomy 45.73
Ileocolostomy 45.93
Ileocolotomy 45.00
Ileocystoplasty (isolated segment anastomosis) (open loop) 57.87 [45.51]
Ileoduodenotomy 45.01
Ileoectomy (partial) 45.62
  with cecectomy 45.72
Ileoentectropy 46.99
Ileoesophagostomy 42.54
Ileoileostomy 45.91
  proximal to distal segment 45.62
Ileoloopogram 87.78
Ileopancreatostomy 52.96
Ileopexy 46.61
Ileoproctostomy 45.93
Ileorectostomy 45.93
Ileorrhaphy 46.73
Ileoscopy 45.13
  through stoma (artificial) 45.12
  transabdominal (operative) 45.11
Ileosigmoidostomy 45.93
Ileostomy 46.20
  continent (permanent) 46.22
    for urinary diversion 56.51
  delayed opening 46.24
  Hendon (temporary) 46.21
  loop 46.01
  Paul (temporary) 46.21
  permanent 46.23
    continent 46.22
  repair 46.41
  revision 46.41
  tangential (temporary) 46.21
  temporary 46.21
  transplantation to new site 46.23
  tube (temporary) 46.21
  ureteral
    external 56.51
    internal 56.71
Ileotomy 45.02
Ileotransversostomy 45.93
Ileoureterostomy (Bricker's) (ileal bladder) 56.51
Imaging (diagnostic)
  diagnostic, not elsewhere classified 88.90
  intraoperative (iMRI) 88.96
  magnetic resonance (nuclear) (proton) NEC 88.97
    abdomen 88.97
    bladder (urinary) 88.95
    bone marrow blood supply 88.94
    brain (brain stem) 88.91
      intraoperative (iMRI) 88.96
      real-time 88.96
    chest (hilar) (mediastinal) 88.92
    extremity (upper) (lower) 88.94
    eye orbit 88.97
    face 88.97
    head NEC 88.97
    musculoskeletal 88.94
    myocardium 88.92
    neck 88.97
    orbit of eye 88.97
    prostate 88.95
    specified site NEC 88.97
    spinal canal (cord) (spine) 88.93
Immobilization (by)
  with fracture-reduction — *see* Reduction, fracture
  bandage 93.59
  bone 93.53

Immobilization (by) — *continued*
  cast NEC 93.53
    with reduction of fracture or dislocation — *see* Reduction, fracture, *and* Reduction, dislocation
  device NEC 93.59
  pressure dressing 93.56
  splint (plaster) (tray) 93.54
    with reduction of fracture or dislocation — *see* Reduction, fracture, *and* Reduction, dislocation
  stereotactic head frame 93.59
Immunization — *see also* Vaccination
  allergy 99.12
  autoimmune disease 99.13
  BCG 99.33
  brucellosis 99.55
  cholera 99.31
  diphtheria 99.36
  DPT 99.39
  epidemic parotitis 99.46
  German measles 99.47
  Hemophilus influenzae 99.52
  influenza 99.52
  measles 99.45
  meningococcus 99.55
  mumps 99.46
  pertussis 99.37
  plague 99.34
  poliomyelitis 99.41
  rabies 99.44
  rubella 99.47
  salmonella 99.55
  smallpox 99.42
  staphylococcus 99.55
  TAB 99.32
  tetanus 99.38
  triple vaccine 99.48
  tuberculosis 99.33
  tularemia 99.35
  typhoid-paratyphoid 99.32
  typhus 99.55
  viral NEC 99.55
  whooping cough 99.37
  yellow fever 99.43
Immunoadsorption
  extracorporeal (ECI) 99.76
Immunotherapy, antineoplastic 99.28
  C-Parvum 99.28
  Interferon 99.28
  Interleukin-2 99.28
  Levamisole 99.28
  Proleukin 99.28
  Thymosin 99.28
Implant, implantation
  abdominal artery to coronary artery 36.17
  artery
    aortic branches to heart muscle 36.2
    mammary to ventricular wall (Vineberg) 36.2
  baffle, atrial or interatrial 35.91
  biliary fistulous tract into stomach or intestine 51.39
  bipolar endoprosthesis (femoral head) 81.52
  bladder sphincter, artificial (inflatable) 58.93
  blood vessels to myocardium 36.2
  bone growth stimulator (invasive) (percutaneous) (semi-invasive) — *see* category 78.9
  bone morphogenetic protein (recombinant) (rhBMP) 84.52
  breast (for augmentation) (bilateral) 85.54
    unilateral 85.53
  cardiac resynchronization device
    defibrillator (CRT-D) (total system) 00.51
      left ventricular coronary venous lead only 00.52
      pulse generator only 00.54
    pacemaker (CRT-P) (total system) 00.50
      left ventricular coronary venous lead only 00.52
      pulse generator only 00.53
  cardiomyostimulation system 37.67
  cardioverter/defibrillator (automatic) 37.94
    leads only (patch electrodes) (sensing) (pacing) 37.95

Implant, implantation

Implant, implantation — *continued*
   cardioverter/defibrillator — *continued*
      pulse generator only 37.96
      total system 37.94
   chest wall (mesh) (silastic) 34.79
   chin (polyethylene) (silastic) 76.68
   cochlear (electrode) 20.96
      prosthetic device (electrode and receiver) 20.96
         channel (single) 20.97
            multiple 20.98
         electrode only 20.99
         internal coil only 20.99
   cornea 11.73
   CRT-D (cardiac resynchronization defibrillator) 00.51 ●
      left ventricular coronary venous lead only 00.52 ●
      pulse generator only 00.54 ●
   CRT-P (cardiac resynchronization pacemaker) 00.50 ●
      left ventricular coronary venous lead only 00.52 ●
      pulse generator only 00.53 ●
   custodis eye 14.41
   dental (endosseous) (prosthetic) 23.6
   device, vascular access 86.07
   diaphragmatic pacemaker 34.85
   electrode(s)
      brain 02.93
         depth 02.93
         foramen ovale 02.93
         sphenoidal 02.96
      cardiac (initial) (transvenous) 37.70
         atrium (initial) 37.73
            replacement 37.76
         atrium and ventricle (initial) 37.72
            replacement 37.76
         epicardium (sternotomy or thoracotomy approach) 37.74
         left ventricular coronary venous system 00.52 ●
         temporary transvenous pacemaker system 37.78
            during and immediately following cardiac surgery 39.64
         ventricle (initial) 37.71
            replacement 37.76
      depth 02.93
      foramen ovale 02.96
      heart (*see also* Implant, electrode(s), cardiac) 37.70
      intracranial 02.93
      osteogenic (invasive) for bone growth stimulation — *see category* 78.9 ✓4ᵗʰ
      peripheral nerve 04.92
      sphenoidal 02.96
      spine 03.93
   electroencephalographic receiver
      brain 02.93
      intracranial 02.93
   electronic stimulator
      anus (subcutaneous) 49.92
      bladder 57.96
      bone growth (invasive) (percutaneous) (semi-invasive) 78.9 ✓4ᵗʰ
      brain 02.93
      carotid sinus 39.8
      cochlear 20.96
         channel (single) 20.97
            multiple 20.98
      intracranial 02.93
      peripheral nerve 04.92
      phrenic nerve 34.85
      skeletal muscle 83.92
      spine 03.93
      ureter 56.92
   electrostimulator — *see* Implant, electronic stimulator, by site
   endoprosthesis
      bile duct 51.87
      femoral head (bipolar) 81.52
      pancreatic duct 52.93
   endosseous (dental) 23.6
   epidural pegs 02.93
   epikeratoprosthesis 11.73

Implant, implantation — *continued*
   estradiol (pellet) 99.23
   eye (Iowa type) 16.61
      integrated 16.41
   facial bone, synthetic (alloplastic) 76.92
   fallopian tube (Mulligan hood) (silastic tube) (stent) 66.93
      into uterus 66.74
   gastroepiploic artery to coronary artery 36.17
   half-heart 37.62
   hearing device, electromagnetic 20.95
   heart
      artificial 37.62
      assist system NEC 37.62
         external (pulsatile) 37.65
         implantable (pulsatile) 37.66
         non-pulsatile 37.62
      auxiliary ventricle 37.62
      pacemaker (*see also* Implant, pacemaker, cardiac) 37.80
      valve(s)
         prosthesis or synthetic device (partial) (synthetic) (total) 35.20
            aortic 35.22
            mitral 35.24
            pulmonary 35.26
            tricuspid 35.28
         tissue graft 35.20
            aortic 35.21
            mitral 35.23
            pulmonary 35.25
            tricuspid 35.27
   inert material
      breast (for augmentation) (bilateral) 85.54
         unilateral 85.53
      larynx 31.0
      nose 21.85
      orbit (eye socket) 16.69
         reinsertion 16.62
      scleral shell (cup) (with evisceration of eyeball) 16.31
         reinsertion 16.62
      Tenon's capsule (with enucleation of eyeball) 16.42
         with attachment of muscles 16.41
         reinsertion 16.62
      urethra 59.79
      vocal cord(s) 31.0
   infusion pump 86.06
   joint (prosthesis) (silastic) (Swanson type) NEC 81.96
      ankle (total) 81.56
         revision 81.59
      carpocarpal, carpometacarpal 81.74
      elbow (total) 81.84
         revision 81.97
      extremity (bioelectric) (cineplastic) (kineplastic) 84.40
         lower 84.48
            revision 81.59
         upper 84.44
            revision 81.97
      femoral (bipolar endoprosthesis) 81.52
      finger 81.71
      hand (metacarpophalangeal) (interphalangeal) 81.71
         revision 81.97
      hip (partial) 81.52
         revision 81.53
         total 81.51
            revision 81.53
      interphalangeal 81.71
         revision 81.97
      knee (partial) (total) 81.54
         revision 81.55
      metacarpophalangeal 81.71
         revision 81.97
      shoulder (partial) 81.81
         revision 81.97
         total replacement 81.80
      toe 81.57
         for hallux valgus repair 77.59
         revision 81.59
      wrist (partial) 81.74
         revision 81.97
         total replacement 81.73

Implant, implantation — *continued*
   kidney, mechanical 55.97
   larynx 31.0
   leads (cardiac) — *see* Implant, electrode(s), cardiac
   mammary artery
      in ventricle (Vineberg) 36.2
      to coronary artery (single vessel) 36.15
         double vessel 36.16
   Mulligan hood, fallopian tube 66.93
   nerve (peripheral) 04.79
   neuropacemaker
      brain 02.93
      intracranial 02.93
      peripheral nerve 04.92
      spine 03.93
   neurostimulator
      brain 02.93
      intracranial 02.93
      peripheral nerve 04.92
      spine 03.93
   nose 21.85
   Ommaya reservoir 02.2
   orbit 16.69
      reinsertion 16.62
   outflow tract prosthesis (heart) (gusset type) in
      pulmonary valvuloplasty 35.26
      total repair of tetralogy of Fallot 35.81
   ovary into uterine cavity 65.72
      laparoscopic 65.75
   pacemaker
      brain 02.93
      cardiac (device) (initial) (permanent) (replacement) 37.80
         dual-chamber device (initial) 37.83
            replacement 37.87
         resynchronization device (CRT-P) ●
            device only (initial) (replacement) 00.53 ●
            total system 00.50 ●
            transvenous lead into left ventricular coronary venous system 00.52 ●
         single-chamber device (initial) 37.81
            rate responsive 37.82
            replacement 37.85
               rate responsive 37.86
         temporary transvenous pacemaker system 37.78
            during and immediately following cardiac surgery 39.64
      carotid sinus 39.8
      diaphragm 34.85
      intracranial 02.93
      neural
         brain 02.93
         intracranial 02.93
         peripheral nerve 04.92
         spine 03.93
      peripheral nerve 04.92
      spine 03.93
   pancreas (duct) 52.96
   penis, prosthesis (internal)
      inflatable 64.97
      non-inflatable 64.95
   port, vascular access device 86.07
   premaxilla 76.68
   progesterone (subdermal) 99.23
   prosthesis, prosthetic device
      acetabulum (Aufranc-Turner) 81.52
      ankle (total) 81.56
      arm (bioelectric) (cineplastic) (kineplastic) 84.44
      breast (Cronin) (Dow-Corning) (Perras-Pappillon) (bilateral) 85.54
         unilateral 85.53
      cochlear 20.96
         channel (single) 20.97
            multiple 20.98
      extremity (bioelectric) (cineplastic) (kineplastic) 84.40
         lower 84.48
         upper 84.44
      fallopian tube (Mulligan hood) (stent) 66.93

Index to Procedures

Implant, implantation — *continued*
  prosthesis, prosthetic device — *continued*
    femoral head (Austin-Moore) (bipolar)
      (Eicher) (Thompson) 81.52
    joint (Swanson type) NEC 81.96
      ankle (total) 81.56
      carpocarpal, carpometacarpal 81.74
      elbow (total) 81.84
      finger 81.71
      hand (metacarpophalangeal)
        (interphalangeal) 81.71
      hip (partial) 81.52
        total 81.51
      interphalangeal 81.71
      knee (partial) (total) 81.54
        revision 81.55
      metacarpophalangeal 81.71
      shoulder (partial) 81.81
        total 81.80
      toe 81.57
        for hallux valgus repair 77.59
      wrist (partial) 81.74
        total 81.73
    leg (bioelectric) (cineplastic) (kineplastic) 84.48
    outflow tract (heart) (gusset type)
      in
        pulmonary valvuloplasty 35.26
        total repair of tetralogy of Fallot 35.81
    penis (internal) (non-inflatable) 64.95
      inflatable (internal) 64.97
    skin (dermal regenerative) (matrix) 86.67
    testicular (bilateral) (unilateral) 62.7
  pulsation balloon (phase-shift) 37.61
  pump, infusion 86.06
  radial artery 36.19
  radioactive isotope 92.27
  radium (radon) 92.27
  retinal attachment 14.41
    with buckling 14.41
  Rickham reservoir 02.2
  silicone
    breast (bilateral) 85.54
      unilateral 85.53
    skin (for filling of defect) 86.02
      for augmentation NEC 86.89
  stimoceiver
    brain 02.93
    intracranial 02.93
    peripheral nerve 04.92
    spine 03.93
  subdural
    grids 02.93
    strips 02.93
  Swanson prosthesis (joint) (silastic) NEC 81.96
    carpocarpal, carpometacarpal 81.74
    finger 81.71
    hand (metacarpophalangeal)
      (interphalangeal) 81.71
    interphalangeal 81.71
    knee (partial) (total) 81.54
      revision 81.55
    metacarpophalangeal 81.71
    toe 81.57
      for hallux valgus repair 77.59
    wrist (partial) 81.74
      total 81.73
  systemic arteries into myocardium (Vineberg type operation) 36.2
  testicular prosthesis (bilateral) (unilateral) 62.7
  tissue expander (skin) NEC 86.93
    breast 85.95
  tissue mandril (for vascular graft) 39.99
    with
      blood vessel repair 39.56
      vascular bypass or shunt — *see* Bypass, vascular
  tooth (bud) (germ) 23.5
    prosthetic 23.6
  umbrella, vena cava 38.7
  ureters into
    bladder 56.74
    intestine 56.71
      external diversion 56.51
    skin 56.61

Implant, implantation — *continued*
  urethra
    for repair of urinary stress incontinence
      collagen 59.72
      fat 59.72
      polytef 59.72
  urethral sphincter, artificial (inflatable) 58.93
  urinary sphincter, artificial (inflatable) 58.93
  vascular access device 86.07
  vitreous (silicone) 14.75
    for retinal reattachment 14.41
      with buckling 14.41
  vocal cord(s) (paraglottic) 31.98
Implosion (psychologic desensitization) 94.33
Incision (and drainage)
  with
    exploration — *see* Exploration
    removal of foreign body — *see* Removal, foreign body
  abdominal wall 54.0
    as operative approach — *omit code*
  abscess — *see also* Incision, by site
    appendix 47.2
      with appendectomy 47.09
        laparoscopic 47.01
    extraperitoneal 54.0
    ischiorectal 49.01
    lip 27.0
    omental 54.19
    perianal 49.01
    perigastric 54.19
    perisplenic 54.19
    peritoneal NEC 54.19
      pelvic (female) 70.12
    retroperitoneal 54.0
    sclera 12.89
    skin 86.04
    subcutaneous tissue 86.04
    subdiaphragmatic 54.19
    subhepatic 54.19
    subphrenic 54.19
    vas deferens 63.6
  adrenal gland 07.41
  alveolus, alveolar bone 24.0
  antecubital fossa 86.09
  anus NEC 49.93
    fistula 49.11
    septum 49.91
  appendix 47.2
  artery 38.00
    abdominal 38.06
      aorta (arch) (ascending) (descending) 38.04
    head and neck NEC 38.02
    intracranial NEC 38.01
    lower limb 38.08
    thoracic NEC 38.05
    upper limb 38.03
  atrium (heart) 37.11
  auditory canal or meatus, external 18.02
  auricle 18.09
  axilla 86.09
  Bartholin's gland or cyst 71.22
  bile duct (with T or Y tube insertion) NEC 51.59
    common (exploratory) 51.51
      for
        relief of obstruction NEC 51.42
        removal of calculus 51.41
    for
      exploration 51.59
      relief of obstruction 51.49
  bladder 57.19
    neck (transurethral) 57.91
    percutaneous suprapubic (closed) 57.17
    suprapubic NEC 57.18
  blood vessel (*see also* Angiotomy) 38.00
  bone 77.10
    alveolus, alveolar 24.0
    carpals, metacarpals 77.14
    clavicle 77.11
    facial 76.09
    femur 77.15
    fibula 77.17
    humerus 77.12

Incision (and drainage) — *continued*
  bone — *continued*
    patella 77.16
    pelvic 77.19
    phalanges (foot) (hand) 77.19
    radius 77.13
    scapula 77.11
    skull 01.24
    specified site NEC 77.19
    tarsals, metatarsals 77.18
    thorax (ribs) (sternum) 77.11
    tibia 77.17
    ulna 77.13
    vertebrae 77.19
  brain 01.39
    cortical adhesions 02.91
  breast (skin) 85.0
    with removal of tissue expander 85.96
  bronchus 33.0
  buccal space 27.0
  bulbourethral gland 58.91
  bursa 83.03
    hand 82.03
    pharynx 29.0
  carotid body 39.8
  cerebral (meninges) 01.39
    epidural or extradural space 01.24
    subarachnoid or subdural space 01.31
  cerebrum 01.39
  cervix 69.95
    to
      assist delivery 73.93
      replace inverted uterus 75.93
  chalazion 08.09
    with removal of capsule 08.21
  cheek 86.09
  chest wall (for extrapleural drainage) (for removal of foreign body) 34.01
    as operative approach — *omit code*
  common bile duct (for exploration) 51.51
    for
      relief of obstruction 51.42
      removal of calculus 51.41
  common wall between posterior left atrium and coronary sinus (with roofing of resultant defect with patch graft) 35.82
  conjunctiva 10.1
  cornea 11.1
    radial (refractive) 11.75
  cranial sinus 01.21
  craniobuccal pouch 07.72
  cul-de-sac 70.12
  cyst
    dentigerous 24.0
    radicular (apical) (periapical) 24.0
  Dührssen's (cervix, to assist delivery) 73.93
  duodenum 45.01
  ear
    external 18.09
    inner 20.79
    middle 20.23
  endocardium 37.11
  endolymphatic sac 20.79
  epididymis 63.92
  epidural space, cerebral 01.24
  epigastric region 54.0
    intra-abdominal 54.19
  esophagus, esophageal NEC 42.09
    web 42.01
  exploratory — *see* Exploration
  extradural space (cerebral) 01.24
  extrapleural 34.01
  eyebrow 08.09
  eyelid 08.09
    margin (trichiasis) 08.01
  face 86.09
  fallopian tube 66.01
  fascia 83.09
    with division 83.14
      hand 82.12
    hand 82.09
      with division 82.12
  fascial compartments, head and neck 27.0
  fistula, anal 49.11
  flank 54.0
  furuncle — *see* Incision, by site

Incision

Incision (and drainage) — *continued*
  gallbladder 51.04
  gingiva 24.0
  gluteal 86.09
  groin region (abdominal wall) (inguinal) 54.0
    skin 86.09
    subcutaneous tissue 86.09
  gum 24.0
  hair follicles 86.09
  heart 37.10
    valve — *see* Valvulotomy
  hematoma — *see also* Incision, by site
    axilla 86.04
    broad ligament 69.98
    ear 18.09
    episiotomy site 75.91
    fossa (superficial) NEC 86.04
    groin region (abdominal wall) (inguinal) 54.0
      skin 86.04
      subcutaneous tissue 86.04
    laparotomy site 54.12
    mediastinum 34.1
    perineum (female) 71.09
      male 86.04
    popliteal space 86.04
    scrotum 61.0
    skin 86.04
    space of Retzius 59.19
    subcutaneous tissue 86.04
    vagina (cuff) 70.14
      episiotomy site 75.91
      obstetrical NEC 75.92
  hepatic ducts 51.59
  hordeolum 08.09
  hygroma — *see also* Incision, by site
    cystic 40.0
  hymen 70.11
  hypochondrium 54.0
    intra-abdominal 54.19
  hypophysis 07.72
  iliac fossa 54.0
  infratemporal fossa 27.0
  ingrown nail 86.09
  intestine 45.00
    large 45.03
    small 45.02
  intracerebral 01.39
  intracranial (epidural space) (extradural space) 01.24
    subarachnoid or subdural space 01.31
  intraperitoneal 54.19
  ischiorectal tissue 49.02
    abscess 49.01
  joint structures (*see also* Arthrotomy) 80.10
  kidney 55.01
    pelvis 55.11
  labia 71.09
  lacrimal
    canaliculus 09.52
    gland 09.0
    passage NEC 09.59
    punctum 09.51
    sac 09.53
  larynx NEC 31.3
  ligamentum flavum (spine) — *omit code*
  liver 50.0
  lung 33.1
  lymphangioma 40.0
  lymphatic structure (channel) (node) (vessel) 40.0
  mastoid 20.21
  mediastinum 34.1
  meibomian gland 08.09
  meninges (cerebral) 01.31
    spinal 03.09
  midpalmar space 82.04
  mouth NEC 27.92
    floor 27.0
  muscle 83.02
    with division 83.19
      hand 82.19
    hand 82.02
      with division 82.19
  myocardium 37.11
  nailbed or nailfold 86.09
  nasolacrimal duct (stricture) 09.59

Incision (and drainage) — *continued*
  neck 86.09
  nerve (cranial) (peripheral) NEC 04.04
    root (spinal) 03.1
  nose 21.1
  omentum 54.19
  orbit (*see also* Orbitotomy) 16.09
  ovary 65.09
    laparoscopic 65.01
  palate 27.1
  palmar space (middle) 82.04
  pancreas 52.09
  pancreatic sphincter 51.82
    endoscopic 51.85
  parapharyngeal (oral) (transcervical) 28.0
  paronychia 86.09
  parotid
    gland or duct 26.0
    space 27.0
  pelvirectal tissue 48.81
  penis 64.92
  perianal (skin) (tissue) 49.02
    abscess 49.01
  perigastric 54.19
  perineum (female) 71.09
    male 86.09
  peripheral vessels
    lower limb
      artery 38.08
      vein 38.09
    upper limb (artery) (vein) 38.03
  periprostatic tissue 60.81
  perirectal tissue 48.81
  perirenal tissue 59.09
  perisplenic 54.19
  peritoneum 54.95
    by laparotomy 54.19
    pelvic (female) 70.12
    male 54.19
  periureteral tissue 59.09
  periurethral tissue 58.91
  perivesical tissue 59.19
  petrous pyramid (air cells) (apex) (mastoid) 20.22
  pharynx, pharyngeal (bursa) 29.0
    space, lateral 27.0
  pilonidal sinus (cyst) 86.03
  pineal gland 07.52
  pituitary (gland) 07.72
  pleura NEC 34.09
  popliteal space 86.09
  postzygomatic space 27.0
  pouch of Douglas 70.12
  prostate (perineal approach) (transurethral approach) 60.0
  pterygopalatine fossa 27.0
  pulp canal (tooth) 24.0
  Rathke's pouch 07.72
  rectovaginal septum 48.81
  rectum 48.0
    stricture 48.91
  renal pelvis 55.11
  retroperitoneum 54.0
  retropharyngeal (oral) (transcervical) 28.0
  salivary gland or duct 26.0
  sclera 12.89
  scrotum 61.0
  sebaceous cyst 86.04
  seminal vesicle 60.72
  sinus — *see* Sinusotomy
  Skene's duct or gland 71.09
  skin 86.09
    with drainage 86.04
    breast 85.0
    cardiac pacemaker pocket, new site 37.79
    ear 18.09
    nose 21.1
    subcutaneous tunnel for pulse generator lead wire 86.99
      with initial procedure — *omit code*
    thalamic stimulator pulse generator pocket, new site 86.09
      with initial insertion of battery package — *omit code*
    tunnel, subcutaneous for pulse generator lead wire 86.99
      with initial procedure — *omit code*

Incision (and drainage) — *continued*
  skull (bone) 01.24
  soft tissue NEC 83.09
    with division 83.19
      hand 82.19
    hand 82.09
      with division 82.19
  space of Retzius 59.19
  spermatic cord 63.93
  sphincter of Oddi 51.82
    endoscopic 51.85
  spinal
    cord 03.09
    nerve root 03.1
  spleen 41.2
  stomach 43.0
  stye 08.09
  subarachnoid space, cerebral 01.31
  subcutaneous tissue 86.09
    with drainage 86.04
    tunnel
      esophageal 42.86
        with anastomosis — *see* Anastomosis, esophagus, antesternal
      pulse generator lead wire 86.99
        with initial procedure — *omit code*
  subdiaphragmatic space 54.19
  subdural space, cerebral 01.31
  sublingual space 27.0
  submandibular space 27.0
  submaxillary 86.09
    with drainage 86.04
  submental space 27.0
  subphrenic space 54.19
  supraclavicular fossa 86.09
    with drainage 86.04
  sweat glands, skin 86.04
  temporal pouches 27.0
  tendon (sheath) 83.01
    with division 83.13
      hand 82.11
    hand 82.01
      with division 82.11
  testis 62.0
  thenar space 82.04
  thymus 07.92
  thyroid (field) (gland) NEC 06.09
    postoperative 06.02
  tongue NEC 25.94
    for tongue tie 25.91
  tonsil 28.0
  trachea NEC 31.3
  tunica vaginalis 61.0
  umbilicus 54.0
  urachal cyst 54.0
  ureter 56.2
  urethra 58.0
  uterus (corpus) 68.0
    cervix 69.95
    for termination of pregnancy 74.91
    septum (congenital) 68.22
  uvula 27.71
  vagina (cuff) (septum) (stenosis) 70.14
    for
      incisional hematoma (episiotomy) 75.91
      obstetrical hematoma NEC 75.92
      pelvic abscess 70.12
  vas deferens 63.6
  vein 38.00
    abdominal 38.07
    head and neck NEC 38.02
    intracranial NEC 38.01
    lower limb 38.09
    thoracic NEC 38.05
    upper limb 38.03
  vertebral column 03.09
  vulva 71.09
    obstetrical 75.92
  web, esophageal 42.01

Incudectomy NEC 19.3
  with
    stapedectomy (*see also* Stapedectomy) 19.19
    tympanoplasty — *see* Tympanoplasty

Incudopexy 19.19

Index to Procedures

Incudostapediopexy 19.19
  with incus replacement 19.11
Indentation, sclera, for buckling (see also Buckling, scleral) 14.49
Indicator dilution flow measurement 89.68
Induction
  abortion
    by
      D and C 69.01
      insertion of prostaglandin suppository 96.49
      intra-amniotic injection (prostaglandin) (saline) 75.0
  labor
    medical 73.4
    surgical 73.01
      intra- and extra-amniotic injection 73.1
      stripping of membranes 73.1
Inflation
  belt wrap 93.99
  Eustachian tube 20.8
  fallopian tube 66.8
    with injection of therapeutic agent 66.95
Infolding, sclera, for buckling (see also Buckling, scleral) 14.49
Infraction, turbinates (nasal) 21.62
Infundibulectomy
  hypophyseal (see also Hypophysectomy, partial) 07.63
  ventricle (heart) (right) 35.34
    in total repair of tetralogy of Fallot 35.81
Infusion (intra-arterial) (intravenous)
  Abciximab 99.20
  antibiotic
    oxazolidinone class 00.14
  antineoplastic agent (chemotherapeutic) 99.25
    biological response modifier [BRM] 99.28
      high-dose interleukin-2 99.28
  biological response modifier [BRM], antineoplastic agent 99.28
    high-dose interleukin-2 99.28
  cancer chemotherapy agent NEC 99.25
  drotrecogin alfa (activated) 00.11
  electrolytes 99.18
  enzymes, thrombolytic (streptokinase) (tissue plasminogen activator) (TPA) (urokinase)
    direct coronary artery 36.04
    intravenous 99.10
  Eptifibatide 99.20
  GB IIB/IIIa inhibitor 99.20
  hormone substance NEC 99.24
  human B-type natriuretic peptide (hBNP) 00.13
  nesiritide 00.13
  neuroprotective agent 99.75
  nimodipine 99.75
  nutritional substance — see Nutrition
  platelet inhibitor
    direct coronary artery 36.04
    intravenous 99.20
  prophylactic substance NEC 99.29
  recombinant protein 00.11
  reteplase 99.10
  therapeutic substance NEC 99.29
  thrombolytic agent (enzyme) (streptokinase) 99.10
    with percutaneous transluminal angioplasty
      coronary (single vessel) 36.02
        multiple vessels 36.05
      non-coronary vessel(s) 39.50
        specified site NEC 39.50
    direct intracoronary artery 36.04
  tirofiban (HCl) 99.20
  vaccine
    tumor 99.28
Injection (into) (hypodermically) (intramuscularly) (intravenously) (acting locally or systemically)
  Actinomycin D, for cancer chemotherapy 99.25
  adhesion barrier ▶substance◀ 99.77 ▲
  alcohol
    nerve — see Injection, nerve
    spinal 03.8

Injection — continued
  anterior chamber, eye (air) (liquid) (medication) 12.92
  antibiotic 99.21
    oxazolidinone class 00.14
  anticoagulant 99.19
  anti-D (Rhesus) globulin 99.11
  antidote NEC 99.16
  anti-infective NEC 99.22
  antineoplastic agent (chemotherapeutic) NEC 99.25
    biological response modifier [BRM] 99.28
      high-dose interleukin-2 99.28
  antivenin 99.16
  barrier ▶substance,◀ adhesion 99.77 ▲
  BCG
    for chemotherapy 99.25
    vaccine 99.33
  biological response modifier [BRM], antineoplastic agent 99.28
    high-dose interleukin-2 99.28
  bone marrow 41.92
    transplant — see Transplant, bone, marrow
  breast (therapeutic agent) 85.92
    inert material (silicone) (bilateral) 85.52
      unilateral 85.51
  bursa (therapeutic agent) 83.96
    hand 82.94
  cancer chemotherapeutic agent 99.25
  caudal — see Injection, spinal
  cortisone 99.23
  costochondral junction 81.92
  dinoprost-tromethine, intraamniotic 75.0
  ear, with alcohol 20.72
  electrolytes 99.18
  enzymes, thrombolytic (streptokinase) (tissue plasminogen activator) (TPA) (urokinase)
    direct coronary artery 36.04
    intravenous 99.10
  epidural, spinal — see Injection, spinal
  esophageal varices or blood vessel (endoscopic) (sclerosing agent) 42.33
  Eustachian tube (inert material) 20.8
  eye (orbit) (retrobulbar) 16.91
    anterior chamber 12.92
    subconjunctival 10.91
  fascia 83.98
    hand 82.96
  gamma globulin 99.14
  ganglion, sympathetic 05.39
    ciliary 12.79
    paravertebral stellate 05.39
  gel, adhesion barrier ▶— see Injection, adhesion barrier substance◀
  globulin
    anti-D (Rhesus) 99.11
    gamma 99.14
    Rh immune 99.11
  heart 37.92
  heavy metal antagonist 99.16
  hemorrhoids (sclerosing agent) 49.42
  hormone NEC 99.24
  human B-type natriuretic peptide (hBNP) 00.13
  immune sera 99.14
  inert material — see Implant, inert material
  inner ear, for destruction 20.72
  insulin 99.17
  intervertebral space for herniated disc 80.52
  intra-amniotic
    for induction of
      abortion 75.0
      labor 73.1
  intrathecal — see Injection, spinal
  joint (therapeutic agent) 81.92
    temporomandibular 76.96
  kidney (cyst) (therapeutic substance) NEC 55.96
  larynx 31.0
  ligament (joint) (therapeutic substance) 81.92
  liver 50.94
  lung, for surgical collapse 33.32
  Methotrexate, for cancer chemotherapy 99.25
  nerve (cranial) (peripheral) 04.80
    agent NEC 04.89
      alcohol 04.2

Injection — continued
  nerve — continued
    agent NEC — continued
      anesthetic for analgesia 04.81
        for operative anesthesia — omit code
      neurolytic 04.2
      phenol 04.2
    laryngeal (external) (recurrent) (superior) 31.91
    optic 16.91
    sympathetic 05.39
      alcohol 05.32
      anesthetic for analgesia 05.31
      neurolytic agent 05.32
      phenol 05.32
  nesiritide 00.13
  neuroprotective agent 99.75
  nimodipine 99.75
  orbit 16.91
  pericardium 37.93
  peritoneal cavity
    air 54.96
    locally-acting therapeutic substance 54.97
  platelet inhibitor
    direct coronary artery 36.04
    intravenous 99.20
  prophylactic substance NEC 99.29
  prostate 60.92
  radioisotopes (intracavitary) (intravenous) 92.28
  renal pelvis (cyst) 55.96
  retrobulbar (therapeutic substance) 16.91
    for anesthesia — omit code
  Rh immune globulin 99.11
  RhoGAM 99.11
  sclerosing agent NEC 99.29
    esophageal varices (endoscopic) 42.33
    hemorrhoids 49.42
    pleura 34.92
      treatment of malignancy (cytotoxic agent) 34.92 [99.25]
        with tetracycline 34.92 [99.21]
    varicose vein 39.92
    vein NEC 39.92
  semicircular canals, for destruction 20.72
  silicone — see Implant, inert material
  skin (sclerosing agent) (filling material) 86.02
  soft tissue 83.98
    hand 82.96
  spinal (canal) NEC 03.92
    alcohol 03.8
    anesthetic agent for analgesia 03.91
      for operative anesthesia — omit code
    contrast material (for myelogram) 87.21
    destructive agent NEC 03.8
    neurolytic agent NEC 03.8
    phenol 03.8
    proteolytic enzyme (chemopapain) (chemodiactin) 80.52
    saline (hypothermic) 03.92
    steroid 03.92
  spinal nerve root (intrathecal) — see Injection, spinal
  steroid NEC 99.23
  subarachnoid, spinal — see Injection, spinal
  subconjunctival 10.91
  tendon 83.97
    hand 82.95
  testis 62.92
  therapeutic agent NEC 99.29
  thoracic cavity 34.92
  thrombolytic agent (enzyme) (streptokinase) 99.10
    with percutaneous transluminal angioplasty
      coronary (single vessel) 36.02
        multiple vessels 36.05
      non-coronary vessel(s) 39.50
        specified site NEC 39.50
  trachea 31.94
  tranquilizer 99.26
  tunica vaginalis (with aspiration) 61.91
  tympanum 20.94
  urethra (inert material)
    for repair of urinary stress incontinence
      collagen implant 59.72
      endoscopic injection of implant 59.72
      fat implant 59.72

Injection — *continued*
    urethra — *continued*
        for repair of urinary stress incontinence — *continued*
            polytef implant 59.72
    vaccine
        tumor 99.28
    varices, esophagus (endoscopic) (sclerosing agent) 42.33
    varicose vein (sclerosing agent) 39.92
        esophagus (endoscopic) 42.33
    vestibule, for destruction 20.72
    vitreous substitute (silicone) 14.75
        for reattachment of retina 14.59
    vocal cords 31.0

Inlay, tooth 23.3

Inoculation
    antitoxins — *see* Administration, antitoxins
    toxoids — *see* Administration, toxoids
    vaccine — *see* Administration, vaccine

Insemination, artificial 69.92

Insertion
    airway
        esophageal obturator 96.03
        nasopharynx 96.01
        oropharynx 96.02
    Allen-Brown cannula 39.93
    arch bars (orthodontic) 24.7
        for immobilization (fracture) 93.55
    atrial septal umbrella 35.52
    Austin-Moore prosthesis 81.52
    baffle, heart (atrial) (interatrial) (intra-atrial) 35.91
    bag, cervix (nonobstetrical) 67.0
        after delivery or abortion 75.8
        to assist delivery or induce labor 73.1
    Baker's (tube) (for stenting) 46.85
    balloon
        gastric 44.93
        heart (pulsation-type) (Kantrowitz) 37.61
        intestine (for decompression) (for dilation) 46.85
    Barton's tongs (skull) (with synchronous skeletal traction) 02.94
    bipolar endoprosthesis (femoral head) 81.52
    Blakemore-Sengstaken tube 96.06
    bone growth stimulator (invasive) (percutaneous) (semi-invasive) — *see* category 78.9 ✓4th
    bone morphogenetic protein (recombinant) (rhBMP) 84.52 ●
    bougie, cervix, nonobstetrical 67.0
        to assist delivery or induce labor 73.1
    breast implant (for augmentation) (bilateral) 85.54
        unilateral 85.53
    bridge (dental) (fixed) 23.42
        removable 23.43
    bubble (balloon), stomach 44.93
    caliper tongs (skull) (with synchronous skeletal traction) 02.94
    cannula
        Allen-Brown 39.93
        for extracorporeal membrane oxygenation (ECMO) — *omit code*
        nasal sinus (by puncture) 22.01
            through natural ostium 22.02
        pancreatic duct 52.92
            endoscopic 52.93
        vessel to vessel 39.93
    cardiac resynchronization device ●
        defibrillator (CRT-D) (total system) 00.51 ●
            left ventricular coronary venous lead only 00.52 ●
            pulse generator only 00.54 ●
        pacemaker (CRT-P) (total system) 00.50 ●
            left ventricular coronary venous lead only 00.52 ●
            pulse generator only 00.53 ●
    catheter
        abdomen of fetus, for intrauterine transfusion 75.2
        anterior chamber (eye), for permanent drainage (glaucoma) 12.79

Insertion — *continued*
    catheter — *continued*
        artery 38.91
        bile duct(s) 51.59
            common 51.51
                endoscopic 51.87
            endoscopic 51.87
        bladder, indwelling 57.94
            suprapubic 57.18
                percutaneous (closed) 57.17
        bronchus 96.05
            with lavage 96.56
        central venous NEC 38.93
            for
                hemodialysis 38.95
                pressure monitoring 89.62
            peripherally inserted central catheter (PICC) 38.93
        chest 34.04
            revision (with lysis of adhesions) 34.04
        esophagus (nonoperative) 96.06
            permanent tube 42.81
        intercostal (with water seal), for drainage 34.04
            revision (with lysis of adhesions) 34.04
        spinal canal space (epidural) (subarachnoid) (subdural) for infusion of therapeutic or palliative substances 03.90
        Swan-Ganz (pulmonary) 89.64
        transtracheal for oxygenation 31.99
        vein NEC 38.93
            for renal dialysis 38.95
    chest tube 34.04
    choledochohepatic tube (for decompression) 51.43
        endoscopic 51.87
    cochlear prosthetic device — *see* Implant, cochlear prosthetic device
    contraceptive device (intrauterine) 69.7
    cordis cannula 54.98
    coronary (artery)
        stent (stent graft) 36.06
    Crosby-Cooney button 54.98
    CRT-D (cardiac resynchronization defibrillator) 00.51 ●
        left ventricular coronary venous lead only 00.52 ●
        pulse generator only 00.54 ●
    CRT-P (cardiac resynchronization pacemaker) 00.50 ●
        left ventricular coronary venous lead only 00.52 ●
        pulse generator only 00.53 ●
    Crutchfield tongs (skull) (with synchronous skeletal traction) 02.94
    Davidson button 54.98
    denture (total) 99.97
    device, vascular access 86.07
    diaphragm, vagina 96.17
    drainage tube
        kidney 55.02
            pelvis 55.12
        renal pelvis 55.12
    elbow prosthesis (total) 81.84
        revision 81.97
    electrode(s)
        bone growth stimulator (invasive) (percutaneous) (semi-invasive) — *see* category 78.9 ✓4th
        brain 02.93
            depth 02.93
            foramen ovale 02.93
            sphenoidal 02.96
        heart (initial) (transvenous) 37.70
            atrium (initial) 37.73
                replacement 37.76
            atrium and ventricle (initial) 37.72
                replacement 37.76
            epicardium (sternotomy or thoracotomy approach) 37.74
            left ventricular coronary venous system 00.52 ●
            temporary transvenous pacemaker system 37.78
                during and immediately following cardiac surgery 39.64

Insertion — *continued*
    electrode(s) — *continued*
        heart — *continued*
            ventricle (initial) 37.71
                replacement 37.76
        intracranial 02.93
        osteogenic (for bone growth stimulation) — *see* category 78.9 ✓4th
        peripheral nerve 04.92
        spine 03.93
    electroencephalographic receiver — *see* Implant, electroencephalographic receiver, by site
    electronic stimulator — *see* Implant, electronic stimulator, by site
    electrostimulator — *see* Implant, electronic stimulator, by site
    endograft(s), endovascular graft(s) ●
        endovascular, head and neck vessels 39.72 ●
        endovascular, other vessels (for aneurysm) 39.79 ●
    endoprosthesis
        bile duct 51.87
        femoral head (bipolar) 81.52
        pancreatic duct 52.93
    epidural pegs 02.93
    external fixation device (bone) — *see* category 78.1 ✓4th
    facial bone implant (alloplastic) (synthetic) 76.92
    filling material, skin (filling of defect) 86.02
    filter
        vena cava (inferior) (superior) (transvenous) 38.7
    fixator, mini device (bone) — *see* category 78.1 ✓4th
    frame (stereotactic)
        for radiosurgery 93.59
    Gardner Wells tongs (skull) (with synchronous skeletal traction) 02.94
    gastric bubble (balloon) 44.93
    globe, into eye socket 16.69
    Greenfield filter 38.7
    halo device (skull) (with synchronous skeletal traction) 02.94
    Harrington rod — *see also* Fusion, spinal, by level
        with dorsal, dorsolumbar fusion 81.05
    Harris pin 79.15
    heart
        pacemaker — *see* Insertion, pacemaker, cardiac
        pump (Kantrowitz) 37.62
        valve — *see* Replacement, heart valve
    hip prosthesis (partial) 81.52
        revision 81.53
        total 81.51
            revision 81.53
    Holter valve 02.2
    Hufnagel valve — *see* Replacement, heart valve
    implant — *see* Insertion, prosthesis
    infusion pump 86.06
    intercostal catheter (with water seal) for drainage 34.04
    intra-arterial blood gas monitoring system 89.60 ●
    intrauterine
        contraceptive device 69.7
        radium (intracavitary) 69.91
        tamponade (nonobstetric) 69.91
    Kantrowitz
        heart pump 37.62
        pulsation balloon (phase-shift) 37.61
    keratoprosthesis 11.73
    King-Mills umbrella device (heart) 35.52
    Kirschner wire 93.44
        with reduction of fracture or dislocation — *see* Reduction, fracture *and* Reduction, dislocation
    laminaria, cervix 69.93
    larynx, valved tube 31.75
    leads (cardiac) — *see* Insertion, electrode(s), heart
    lens, prosthetic (intraocular) 13.70
        with cataract extraction, one-stage 13.71

Index to Procedures

Insertion — *continued*
  lens, prosthetic — *continued*
    secondary (subsequent to cataract extraction) 13.72
  loop recorder 86.09
  metal staples into epiphyseal plate (*see also* Stapling, epiphyseal plate) 78.20
  minifixator device (bone) — *see category* 78.1 ✓4ᵗʰ
  Mobitz-Uddin umbrella, vena cava 38.7
  mold, vagina 96.15
  Moore (cup) 81.52
  Myringotomy device (button) (tube) 20.01
    with intubation 20.01
  nasobiliary drainage tube (endoscopic) 51.86
  nasogastric tube
    for
      decompression, intestinal 96.07
      feeding 96.6
  naso-intestinal tube 96.08
  nasolacrimal tube or stent 09.44
  nasopancreatic drainage tube (endoscopic) 52.97
  neuropacemaker — *see* Implant, neuropacemaker, by site
  neurostimulator — *see* Implant, neurostimulator, by site
  non-coronary vessel stent(s) (stent graft) 39.90
    with angioplasty or atherectomy 39.50
    with bypass — *omit code*
  non-invasive (transcutaneous) (surface) stimulator 99.86
  obturator (orthodontic) 24.7
  ocular implant
    with synchronous
      enucleation 16.42
        with muscle attachment to implant 16.41
      evisceration 16.31
    following or secondary to enucleation 16.61
      evisceration 16.61
  Ommaya reservoir 02.2
  orbital implant (stent) (outside muscle cone) 16.69
    with orbitotomy 16.02
  orthodontic appliance (obturator) (wiring) 24.7
  outflow tract prosthesis (gusset type) (heart)
    in
      pulmonary valvuloplasty 35.26
      total repair of tetralogy of Fallot 35.81
  pacemaker
    brain 02.93
    cardiac (device) (initial) (permanent) (replacement) 37.80
      dual-chamber device (initial) 37.83
        replacement 37.87
      during and immediately following cardiac surgery 39.64
      resynchronization (CRT-P) (device)
        device only (initial) (replacement) 00.53
        total system 00.50
        transvenous lead into left ventricular coronary venous system 00.52
      single-chamber device (initial) 37.81
        rate responsive 37.82
        replacement 37.85
          rate responsive 37.86
      temporary transvenous pacemaker system 37.78
        during and immediately following cardiac surgery 39.64
    carotid 39.8
    heart — *see* Insertion, pacemaker, cardiac
    intracranial 02.93
    neural
      brain 02.93
        intracranial 02.93
      peripheral nerve 04.92
      spine 03.93
    peripheral nerve 04.92
    spine 03.93
  pacing catheter — *see* Insertion, pacemaker, cardiac

Insertion — *continued*
  pack
    auditory canal, external 96.11
    cervix (nonobstetrical) 67.0
      after delivery or abortion 75.8
      to assist delivery or induce labor 73.1
    rectum 96.19
    sella turcica 07.79
    vagina (nonobstetrical) 96.14
      after delivery or abortion 75.8
  penile prosthesis (non-inflatable) (internal) 64.95
    inflatable (internal) 64.97
  peridontal splint (orthodontic) 24.7
  peripheral blood vessel — *see* non-coronary
  pessary
    cervix 96.18
      to assist delivery or induce labor 73.1
    vagina 96.18
  pharyngeal valve, artificial 31.75
  port, vascular access 86.07
  prostaglandin suppository (for abortion) 96.49
  prosthesis, prosthetic device
    acetabulum (partial) 81.52
      revision 81.53
    ankle (total) 81.56
    arm (bioelectric) (cineplastic) (kineplastic) 84.44
    biliary tract 51.99
    breast (bilateral) 85.54
      unilateral 85.53
    chin (polyethylene) (silastic) 76.68
    elbow (total) 81.84
      revision 81.97
    extremity (bioelectric) (cineplastic) (kineplastic) 84.40
      lower 84.48
      upper 84.44
    fallopian tube 66.93
    femoral head (Austin-Moore) (bipolar) (Eicher) (Thompson) 81.52
    hip (partial) 81.52
      revision 81.53
      total 81.51
        revision 81.53
    joint — *see* Arthroplasty
    knee (partial) (total) 81.54
      revision 81.55
    leg (bioelectric) (cineplastic) (kineplastic) 84.48
    ocular (secondary) 16.61
      with orbital exenteration 16.42
    outflow tract (gusset type) (heart)
      in
        pulmonary valvuloplasty 35.26
        total repair of tetralogy of Fallot 35.81
    penis (internal) (noninflatable) 64.95
      with
        construction 64.43
        reconstruction 64.44
      inflatable (internal) 64.97
    Rosen (for urinary incontinence) 59.79
    shoulder
      partial 81.81
      revision 81.97
      total 81.80
    testicular (bilateral) (unilateral) 62.7
    toe 81.57
      hallux valgus repair 77.59
  pseudophakos (*see also* Insertion, lens) 13.70
  pump, infusion 86.06
  radioactive isotope 92.27
  radium 92.27
  radon seeds 92.27
  Reuter bobbin (with intubation) 20.01
  Rickham reservoir 02.2
  Rosen prosthesis (for urinary incontinence) 59.79
  Scribner shunt 39.93
  Sengstaken-Blakemore tube 96.06
  sensor
    intra-arterial, for continuous blood gas monitoring 89.60
  sieve, vena cava 38.7
  skeletal muscle stimulator 83.92

Insertion — *continued*
  skull
    plate 02.05
    stereotactic frame 93.59
    tongs (Barton) (caliper) (Garder Wells) (Vinke) (with synchronous skeletal traction) 02.94
  spacer (cement) in joint — *see category* 80.0 ✓4ᵗʰ
    spine 84.51
  sphenoidal electrodes 02.96
  spine
    cage (BAK) 84.51
    spacer 84.51
  Spitz-Holter valve 02.2
  Steinmann pin 93.44
    with reduction of fracture or dislocation — *see* Reduction, fracture *and* Reduction, dislocation
  stent(s) (stent graft)
    artery (bare) (bonded) (drug coated) (non-drug-eluting) 39.90
      coronary (bare) (bonded) (drug coated) (non-drug-eluting) 36.06
        drug-eluting 36.07
    bile duct 51.43
      endoscopic 51.87
      percutaneous transhepatic 51.98
    coronary (artery) 36.06
    esophagus (endoscopic) (fluoroscopic) 42.81
    non-coronary vessel 39.90
      with angioplasty or atherectomy 39.50
      with bypass — *omit code*
      drug-eluting 00.55
    pancreatic duct 52.92
      endoscopic 52.93
    peripheral vessel — *see* non-coronary vessel
    tracheobronchial 96.05
  stimoceiver — *see* Implant, stimoceiver, by site
  stimulator for bone growth — *see category* 78.9 ✓4ᵗʰ
  subdural
    grids 02.93
    strips 02.93
  suppository
    prostaglandin (for abortion) 96.49
    vagina 96.49
  Swan-Ganz catheter (pulmonary) 89.64
  tampon
    esophagus 96.06
    uterus 69.91
    vagina 96.14
      after delivery or abortion 75.8
  testicular prosthesis (bilateral) (unilateral) 62.7
  tissue expander (skin) NEC 86.93
    breast 85.95
  tissue mandril (peripheral vessel) (Dacron) (Spark's type) 39.99
    with
      blood vessel repair 39.56
      vascular bypass or shunt — *see* Bypass, vascular
  tongs, skull (with synchronous skeletal traction) 02.94
  totally implanted device for bone growth (invasive) — *see category* 78.9 ✓4ᵗʰ
  tube — *see also* Catheterization *and* Intubation
    bile duct 51.43
      endoscopic 51.87
    chest 34.04
      revision (with lysis of adhesions) 34.04
    endotracheal 96.04
    esophagus (nonoperative) (Sengstaken) 96.06
      permanent (silicone) (Souttar) 42.81
    feeding
      esophageal 42.81
      gastric 96.6
      nasogastric 96.6
    gastric
      by gastrostomy — *see category* 43.1 ✓4ᵗʰ
      for
        decompression, intestinal 96.07
        feeding 96.6
    intercostal (with water seal), for drainage 34.04

Insertion

Insertion — *continued*
- tube — *see also* Catheterization and Intubation — *continued*
  - intercostal — *continued*
    - revision (with lysis of adhesions) 34.04
  - Miller-Abbott (for intestinal decompression) 96.08
  - nasobiliary (drainage) 51.86
  - nasogastric (for intestinal decompression) NEC 96.07
  - naso-intestinal 96.08
  - nasopancreatic drainage (endoscopic) 52.97
  - pancreatic duct 52.92
    - endoscopic 52.93
  - rectum 96.09
  - stomach (nasogastric) (for intestinal decompression) NEC 96.07
    - for feeding 96.6
  - tracheobronchial 96.05
- umbrella device
  - atrial septum (King-Mills) 35.52
  - vena cava (Mobitz-Uddin) 38.7
- ureteral stent (transurethral) 59.8
  - with ureterotomy 59.8 [56.2]
- urinary sphincter, artificial (AUS) (inflatable) 58.93
- vaginal mold 96.15
- valve
  - Holter 02.2
  - Hufnagel — *see* Replacement, heart valve
  - pharyngeal (artificial) 31.75
  - Spitz-Holter 02.2
  - vas deferens 63.95
- vascular access device, totally implantable 86.07
- vena cava sieve or umbrella 38.7
- Vinke tongs (skull) (with synchronous skeletal traction) 02.94

Instillation
- bladder 96.49
- digestive tract, except gastric gavage 96.43
- genitourinary NEC 96.49
- radioisotope (intracavitary) (intravenous) 92.28

Insufflation
- Eustachian tube 20.8
- fallopian tube (air) (dye) (gas) (saline) 66.8
  - for radiography — *see* Hysterosalpingography
  - therapeutic substance 66.95
- lumbar retroperitoneal, bilateral 88.15

Intercricothyroidotomy (for assistance in breathing) 31.1

Intermittent positive pressure breathing (IPPB) 93.91

Interposition operation
- esophageal reconstruction (intrathoracic) (retrosternal) NEC (*see also* Anastomosis, esophagus, with, interposition) 42.58
- antesternal or antethoracic NEC (*see also* Anastomosis, esophagus, antesternal, with, interposition) 42.68
- uterine suspension 69.21

Interruption
- vena cava (inferior) (superior) 38.7

Interview (evaluation) (diagnostic)
- medical, except psychiatric 89.05
  - brief (abbreviated history) 89.01
  - comprehensive (history and evaluation of new problem) 89.03
  - limited (interval history) 89.02
  - specified type NEC 89.04
- psychiatric NEC 94.19
  - follow-up 94.19
  - initial 94.19
  - pre-commitment 94.13

Intimectomy 38.10
- abdominal 38.16
- aorta (arch) (ascending) (descending) 38.14
- head and neck NEC 38.12
- intracranial NEC 38.11
- lower limb 38.18
- thoracic NEC 38.15
- upper limb 38.13

Introduction
- orthodontic appliance 24.7
- therapeutic substance (acting locally or systemically) NEC 99.29
  - bursa 83.96
    - hand 82.94
  - fascia 83.98
    - hand 82.96
  - heart 37.92
  - joint 81.92
    - temporomandibular 76.96
  - ligament (joint) 81.92
  - pericardium 37.93
  - soft tissue NEC 83.98
    - hand 82.96
  - tendon 83.97
    - hand 82.95
  - vein 39.92

Intubation — *see also* Catheterization and Insertion
- bile duct(s) 51.59
  - common 51.51
    - endoscopic 51.87
  - endoscopic 51.87
- esophagus (nonoperative) (Sengstaken) 96.06
  - permanent tube (silicone) (Souttar) 42.81
- Eustachian tube 20.8
- intestine (for decompression) 96.08
- lacrimal for
  - dilation 09.42
  - tear drainage, intranasal 09.81
- larynx 96.05
- nasobiliary (drainage) 51.86
- nasogastric
  - for
    - decompression, intestinal 96.07
    - feeding 96.6
- nasolacrimal (duct) (with irrigation) 09.44
- nasopancreatic drainage (endoscopic) 52.97
- naso-intestinal 96.08
- respiratory tract NEC 96.05
- small intestine (Miller-Abbott) 96.08
- stomach (nasogastric) (for intestinal decompression) NEC 96.07
  - for feeding 96.6
- trachea 96.04
- ventriculocisternal 02.2

Invagination, diverticulum
- gastric 44.69
- pharynx 29.59
- stomach 44.69

Inversion
- appendix 47.99
- diverticulum
  - gastric 44.69
  - intestine
    - large 45.49
      - endoscopic 45.43
    - small 45.34
  - stomach 44.69
- tunica vaginalis 61.49

Ionization, medical 99.27

Iontherapy 99.27

Iontophoresis 99.27

Iridectomy (basal) (buttonhole) (optical) (peripheral) (total) 12.14
- with
  - capsulectomy 13.65
  - cataract extraction — *see* Extraction, cataract
  - filtering operation (for glaucoma) NEC 12.65
  - scleral
    - fistulization 12.65
    - thermocauterization 12.62
    - trephination 12.61

Iridencleisis 12.63
Iridesis 12.63
Irido-capsulectomy 13.65
Iridocyclectomy 12.44
Iridocystectomy 12.42
Iridodesis 12.63
Iridoplasty NEC 12.39
Iridoslerectomy 12.65

Iridosclerotomy 12.69
Iridotasis 12.63
Iridotomy 12.12
- by photocoagulation 12.12
- with transfixion 12.11
- for iris bombé 12.11
- specified type NEC 12.12

Iron lung 93.99

Irradiation
- gamma, stereotactic 92.32

Irrigation
- anterior chamber (eye) 12.91
- bronchus NEC 96.56
- canaliculus 09.42
- catheter
  - ureter 96.46
  - urinary, indwelling NEC 96.48
  - vascular 96.57
  - ventricular 02.41
  - wound 96.58
- cholecystostomy 96.41
- cornea 96.51
  - with removal of foreign body 98.21
- corpus cavernosum 64.98
- cystostomy 96.47
- ear (removal of cerumen) 96.52
- enterostomy 96.36
- eye 96.51
  - with removal of foreign body 98.21
- gastrostomy 96.36
- lacrimal
  - canaliculi 09.42
  - punctum 09.41
- muscle 83.02
  - hand 82.02
- nasal
  - passages 96.53
  - sinus 22.00
- nasolacrimal duct 09.43
  - with insertion of tube or stent 09.44
- nephrostomy 96.45
- peritoneal 54.25
- pyelostomy 96.45
- rectal 96.39
- stomach 96.33
- tendon (sheath) 83.01
  - hand 82.01
- trachea NEC 96.56
- traumatic cataract 13.3
- tube
  - biliary NEC 96.41
  - nasogastric NEC 96.34
  - pancreatic 96.42
- ureterostomy 96.46
- ventricular shunt 02.41
- wound (cleaning) NEC 96.59

Irving operation (tubal ligation) 66.32
Irwin operation (*see also* Osteotomy) 77.30
Ischiectomy (partial) 77.89
- total 77.99
Ischiopubiotomy 77.39
Isolation
- after contact with infectious disease 99.84
- ileal loop 45.51
- intestinal segment or pedicle flap
  - large 45.52
  - small 45.51

Isthmectomy, thyroid (*see also* Thyroidectomy, partial) 06.39

J

Jaboulay operation (gastroduodenostomy) 44.39
Janeway operation (permanent gastrostomy) 43.19
Jatene operation (arterial switch) 35.84
Jejunectomy 45.62
Jejunocecostomy 45.93
Jejunocholecystostomy 51.32
Jejunocolostomy 45.93

Jejunoileostomy 45.91
Jejunojejunostomy 45.91
Jejunopexy 46.61
Jejunorrhaphy 46.73
Jejunostomy (feeding) 46.39
  delayed opening 46.31
  loop 46.01
  percutaneous (endoscopic) (PEJ) 46.32
  revision 46.41
Jejunotomy 45.02
Johanson operation (urethral reconstruction) 58.46
Jones operation
  claw toe (transfer of extensor hallucis longus tendon) 77.57
    modified (with arthrodesis) 77.57
  dacryocystorhinostomy 09.81
  hammer toe (interphalangeal fusion) 77.56
    modified (tendon transfer with arthrodesis) 77.57
  repair of peroneal tendon 83.88
Joplin operation (exostectomy with tendon transfer) 77.53

K

Kader operation (temporary gastrostomy) 43.19
Kasai portoenterostomy 51.37
Kaufman operation (for urinary stress incontinence) 59.79
Kazanjiian operation (buccal vestibular sulcus extension) 24.91
Kehr operation (hepatopexy) 50.69
Keller operation (bunionectomy) 77.59
Kelly (-Kennedy) operation (urethrovesical plication) 59.3
Kelly-Stoeckel operation (urethrovesical plication) 59.3
Kelotomy 53.9
Keratectomy (complete) (partial) (superficial) 11.49
  for pterygium 11.39
    with corneal graft 11.32
Keratocentesis (for hyphema) 12.91
Keratomileusis 11.71
Keratophakia 11.72
Keratoplasty (tectonic) (with autograft) (with homograft) 11.60
  lamellar (nonpenetrating) (with homograft) 11.62
    with autograft 11.61
  penetrating (full-thickness) (with homograft) 11.64
    with autograft 11.63
  perforating — see Keratoplasty, penetrating
  refractive 11.71
  specified type NEC 11.69
Keratoprosthesis 11.73
Keratotomy (delimiting) (posterior) 11.1
  radial (refractive) 11.75
Kerr operation (low cervical cesarean section) 74.1
Kessler operation (arthroplasty, carpometacarpal joint) 81.74
Kidner operation (excision of accessory navicular bone) (with tendon transfer) 77.98
Killian operation (frontal sinusotomy) 22.41
Kineplasty — see Cineplasty
King-Steelquist operation (hind-quarter amputation) 84.19
Kirk operation (amputation through thigh) 84.17
Kock pouch
  bowel anastomosis — omit code
  continent ileostomy 46.22
  cutaneous uretero-ileostomy 56.51
    ESWL (extracorporeal shockwave lithotripsy) 98.51
  removal, calculus 57.19

Kock pouch — continued
  revision, cutaneous uretero-ileostomy 56.52
  urinary diversion procedure 56.51
Kockogram (ileal conduitogram) 87.78
Kockoscopy 45.12
Kondoleon operation (correction of lymphedema) 40.9
Krause operation (sympathetic denervation) 05.29
Kroener operation (partial salpingectomy) 66.69
Kroenlein operation (lateral orbitotomy) 16.01
Krönig operation (low cervical cesarean section) 74.1
Krukenberg operation (reconstruction of below-elbow amputation) 82.89
Kuhnt-Szymanowski operation (ectropion repair with lid reconstruction) 08.44

L

Labbe operation (gastrotomy) 43.0
Labiectomy (bilateral) 71.62
  unilateral 71.61
Labyrinthectomy (transtympanic) 20.79
Labyrinthotomy (transtympanic) 20.79
Ladd operation (mobilization of intestine) 54.95
Lagrange operation (iridosclerectomy) 12.65
Lambrinudi operation (triple arthrodesis) 81.12
Laminectomy (decompression) (for exploration) 03.09
  as operative approach — omit code
  with
    excision of herniated intervertebral disc (nucleus pulposus) 80.51
    excision of other intraspinal lesion (tumor) 03.4
  reopening of site 03.02
Laminography — see Radiography
Laminoplasty, expansile 03.09
Laminotomy (decompression) (for exploration) 03.09
  as operative approach — omit code
  reopening of site 03.02
Langenbeck operation (cleft palate repair) 27.62
Laparoamnioscopy 75.31
Laparorrhaphy 54.63
Laparoscopy 54.21
  with
    biopsy (intra-abdominal) 54.24
      uterine ligaments 68.15
      uterus 68.16
    destruction of fallopian tubes — see Destruction, fallopian tube
Laparotomy NEC 54.19
  as operative approach — omit code
  exploratory (pelvic) 54.11
  reopening of recent operative site (for control of hemorrhage) (for exploration) (for incision of hematoma) 54.12
Laparotrachelotomy 74.1
Lapidus operation (bunionectomy with metatarsal osteotomy) 77.51
Larry operation (shoulder disarticulation) 84.08
Laryngectomy
  with radical neck dissection (with synchronous thyroidectomy) (with synchronous tracheostomy) 30.4
  complete (with partial laryngectomy) (with synchronous tracheostomy) 30.3
    with radical neck dissection (with synchronous thyroidectomy) (with synchronous tracheostomy) 30.4
  frontolateral partial (extended) 30.29
  glottosupraglottic partial 30.29
  lateral partial 30.29
  partial (frontolateral) (glottosupraglottic) (lateral) (submucous) (supraglottic) (vertical) 30.29

Laryngectomy — continued
  radical (with synchronous thyroidectomy) (with synchronous tracheostomy) 30.4
  submucous (partial) 30.29
  supraglottic partial 30.29
  total (with partial pharyngectomy) (with synchronous tracheostomy) 30.3
    with radical neck dissection (with synchronous thyroidectomy) (with synchronous tracheostomy) 30.4
  vertical partial 30.29
  wide field 30.3
Laryngocentesis 31.3
Laryngoesophagectomy 30.4
Laryngofissure 30.29
Laryngogram 87.09
  contrast 87.07
Laryngopharyngectomy (with synchronous tracheostomy) 30.3
  radical (with synchronous thyroidectomy) 30.4
Laryngopharyngoesophagectomy (with synchronous tracheostomy) 30.3
  with radical neck dissection (with synchronous thyroidectomy) 30.4
Laryngoplasty 31.69
Laryngorrhaphy 31.61
Laryngoscopy (suspension) (through artificial stoma) 31.42
Laryngostomy (permanent) 31.29
  revision 31.63
  temporary (emergency) 31.1
Laryngotomy 31.3
Laryngotracheobronchoscopy 33.23
  with biopsy 33.24
Laryngotracheoscopy 31.42
Laryngotracheostomy (permanent) 31.29
  temporary (emergency) 31.1
Laryngotracheotomy (temporary) 31.1
  permanent 31.29
Laser — see also Coagulation, Destruction, and Photocoagulation by site
  angioplasty, percutaneous transluminal 39.59
  coronary — see angioplasty, coronary
Lash operation (internal cervical os repair) 67.59
Latzko operation
  cesarean section 74.2
  colpocleisis 70.4
Lavage
  antral 22.00
  bronchus NEC 96.56
    diagnostic (endoscopic) bronchoalveolar lavage (BAL) 33.24
  endotracheal 96.56
  gastric 96.33
  lung (total) (whole) 33.99
    diagnostic (endoscopic) bronchoalveolar lavage (BAL) 33.24
  nasal sinus(es) 22.00
    by puncture 22.01
    through natural ostium 22.02
  peritoneal (diagnostic) 54.25
  trachea NEC 96.56
Leadbetter operation (urethral reconstruction) 58.46
Leadbetter-Politano operation (ureteroneocystostomy) 56.74
Le Fort operation (colpocleisis) 70.8
LEEP (loop electrosurgical excision procedure) of cervix 67.32
LeMesurier operation (cleft lip repair) 27.54
Lengthening
  bone (with bone graft) 78.30
    femur 78.35
    for reconstruction of thumb 82.69
    specified site NEC (see also category 78.3) 78.39
    tibia 78.37
    ulna 78.33
  extraocular muscle NEC 15.21
    multiple (two or more muscles) 15.4

Lengthening — continued
  fascia 83.89
    hand 82.89
  hamstring NEC 83.85
  heel cord 83.85
  leg
    femur 78.35
    tibia 78.37
  levator palpebrae muscle 08.38
  muscle 83.85
    extraocular 15.21
      multiple (two or more muscles) 15.4
    hand 82.55
  palate 27.62
    secondary or subsequent 27.63
  tendon 83.85
    for claw toe repair 77.57
    hand 82.55

Leriche operation (periarterial sympathectomy) 05.25

Leucotomy, leukotomy 01.32

Leukopheresis, therapeutic 99.72

Lid suture operation (blepharoptosis) 08.31

Ligation
  adrenal vessel (artery) (vein) 07.43
  aneurysm 39.52
  appendages, dermal 86.26
  arteriovenous fistula 39.53
    coronary artery 36.99
  artery 38.80
    abdominal 38.86
    adrenal 07.43
    aorta (arch) (ascending) (descending) 38.84
    coronary (anomalous) 36.99
    ethmoidal 21.04
    external carotid 21.06
    for control of epistaxis — see Control, epistaxis
    head and neck NEC 38.82
    intracranial NEC 38.81
    lower limb 38.88
    maxillary (transantral) 21.05
    middle meningeal 02.13
    thoracic NEC 38.85
    thyroid 06.92
    upper limb 38.83
  atrium, heart 37.99
  auricle, heart 37.99
  bleeding vessel — see Control, hemorrhage
  blood vessel 38.80
    abdominal
      artery 38.86
      vein 38.87
    adrenal 07.43
    aorta (arch) (ascending) (descending) 38.84
    esophagus 42.91
      endoscopic 42.33
    head and neck NEC 38.82
    intracranial NEC 38.81
    lower limb
      artery 38.88
      vein 38.89
    meningeal (artery) (longitudinal sinus) 02.13
    thoracic NEC 38.85
    thyroid 06.92
    upper limb (artery) (vein) 38.83
  bronchus 33.92
  cisterna chyli 40.64
  coronary
    artery (anomalous) 36.99
    sinus 36.39
  dermal appendage 86.26
  ductus arteriosus, patent 38.85
  esophageal vessel 42.91
    endoscopic 42.33
  ethmoidal artery 21.04
  external carotid artery 21.06
  fallopian tube (bilateral) (remaining) (solitary) 66.39
    by endoscopy (culdoscopy) (hysteroscopy) (laparoscopy) (peritoneoscopy) 66.29
    with
      crushing 66.31
        by endoscopy (laparoscopy) 66.21

Ligation — continued
  fallopian tube — continued
    with — continued
      division 66.32
        by endoscopy (culdoscopy) (laparoscopy) (peritoneoscopy) 66.22
      Falope ring 66.39
        by endoscopy (laparoscopy) 66.29
    unilateral 66.92
  fistula, arteriovenous 39.53
    coronary artery 36.99
  gastric
    artery 38.86
    varices 44.91
      endoscopic 43.41
  hemorrhoids 49.45
  longitudinal sinus (superior) 02.13
  lymphatic (channel) (peripheral) 40.9
    thoracic duct 40.64
  maxillary artery 21.05
  meningeal vessel 02.13
  spermatic
    cord 63.72
      varicocele 63.1
    vein (high) 63.1
  splenic vessels 38.86
  subclavian artery 38.85
  superior longitudinal sinus 02.13
  supernumerary digit 86.26
  thoracic duct 40.64
  thyroid vessel (artery) (vein) 06.92
  toes (supernumerary) 86.26
  tooth 93.55
    impacted 24.6
  ulcer (peptic) (base) (bed) (bleeding vessel) 44.40
    duodenal 44.42
    gastric 44.41
  ureter 56.95
  varices
    esophageal 42.91
      endoscopic 42.33
    gastric 44.91
      endoscopic 43.41
    peripheral vein (lower limb) 38.59
      upper limb 38.53
  varicocele 63.1
  vas deferens 63.71
  vein 38.80
    abdominal 38.87
    adrenal 07.43
    head and neck NEC 38.82
    intracranial NEC 38.81
    lower limb 38.89
    spermatic, high 63.1
    thoracic NEC 38.85
    thyroid 06.92
    upper limb 38.83
    varicose 38.50
      abdominal 38.57
      esophagus 42.91
        endoscopic 42.33
      gastric 44.91
        endoscopic 43.41
      head and neck NEC 38.52
      intracranial NEC 38.51
      lower limb 38.59
      stomach 44.91
      thoracic NEC 38.55
      upper limb 38.53
  vena cava, inferior 38.7
  venous connection between anomalous vein to left innominate vein 35.82
    superior vena cava 35.82
  wart 86.26

Light coagulation — see Photocoagulation

Lindholm operation (repair of ruptured tendon) 83.88

Lingulectomy, lung 32.3

Linton operation (varicose vein) 38.59

Lipectomy (subcutaneous tissue) (abdominal) (submental) 86.83

Liposuction 86.83

Lip reading training 95.49

Lip shave 27.43

Lisfranc operation
  foot amputation 84.12
  shoulder disarticulation 84.08

Litholapaxy, bladder 57.0
  by incision 57.19

Lithotomy
  bile passage 51.49
  bladder (urinary) 57.19
  common duct 51.41
    percutaneous 51.96
  gallbladder 51.04
  hepatic duct 51.49
  kidney 55.01
    percutaneous 55.03
  ureter 56.2

Lithotripsy
  bile duct NEC 51.49
    extracorporeal shockwave (ESWL) 98.52
  bladder 57.0
    with ultrasonic fragmentation 57.0 [59.95]
    extracorporeal shockwave (ESWL) 98.51
  extracorporeal shockwave (ESWL) NEC 98.59
    bile duct 98.52
    bladder (urinary) 98.51
    gallbladder 98.52
    kidney 98.51
    Kock pouch 98.51
    renal pelvis 98.51
    specified site NEC 98.59
    ureter 98.51
  gallbladder NEC 51.04
    endoscopic 51.88
    extracorporeal shockwave (ESWL) 98.52
  kidney 56.0
    extracorporeal shockwave (ESWL) 98.51
    percutaneous nephrostomy with fragmentation (laser) (ultrasound) 55.04
  renal pelvis 56.0
    extracorporeal shockwave (ESWL) 98.51
    percutaneous nephrostomy with fragmentation (laser) (ultrasound) 55.04
  ureter 56.0
    extracorporeal shockwave (ESWL) 98.51

Littlewood operation (forequarter amputation) 84.09

LLETZ (large loop excision of the transformation zone) of cervix 67.32

Lloyd-Davies operation (abdominoperineal resection) 48.5

Lobectomy
  brain 01.53
    partial 01.59
  liver (with partial excision of adjacent lobes) 50.3
  lung (complete) 32.4
    partial 32.3
    segmental (with resection of adjacent lobes) 32.4
  thyroid (total) (unilateral) (with removal of isthmus) (with removal of portion of remaining lobe) 06.2
    partial (see also Thyroidectomy, partial) 06.39
    substernal 06.51
    subtotal (see also Thyroidectomy, partial) 06.39

Lobotomy, brain 01.32

Localization, placenta 88.78
  by RISA injection 92.17

Longmire operation (bile duct anastomosis) 51.39

Loop ileal stoma (see also Ileostomy) 46.01

Loopogram 87.78

Looposcopy (ileal conduit) 56.35

Lord operation
  dilation of anal canal for hemorrhoids 49.49
  hemorrhoidectomy 49.49
  orchidopexy 62.5

Lower GI series (x-ray) 87.64
Lucas and Murray operation (knee arthrodesis with plate) 81.22
Lumpectomy
  breast 85.21
  specified site — *see* Excision, lesion, by site
Lymphadenectomy (simple) (*see also* Excision, lymph, node) 40.29
Lymphadenotomy 40.0
Lymphangiectomy (radical) (*see also* Excision, lymph, node, by site, radical) 40.50
Lymphangiogram
  abdominal 88.04
  cervical 87.08
  intrathoracic 87.34
  lower limb 88.36
  pelvic 88.04
  upper limb 88.34
Lymphangioplasty 40.9
Lymphangiorrhaphy 40.9
Lymphangiotomy 40.0
Lymphaticostomy 40.9
  thoracic duct 40.62
Lysis
  adhesions

> Note:
> blunt — *omit code*
> digital — *omit code*
> manual — *omit code*
> mechanical — *omit code*
> without instrumentation — *omit code*

    abdominal 54.59
      laparoscopic 54.51
    appendiceal 54.59
      laparoscopic 54.51
    artery-vein-nerve bundle 39.91
    biliary tract 54.59
      laparoscopic 54.51
    bladder (neck) (intraluminal) 57.12
      external 59.11
        laparoscopic 59.12
      transurethral 57.41
    blood vessels 39.91
    bone — *see* category 78.4 ✓4ᵗʰ
    bursa 83.91
      by stretching or manipulation 93.28
      hand 82.91
    cartilage of joint 93.26
    chest wall 33.99
    choanae (nasopharynx) 29.54
    conjunctiva 10.5
    corneovitreal 12.34
    cortical (brain) 02.91
    ear, middle 20.23
    Eustachean tube 20.8
    extraocular muscle 15.7
    extrauterine 54.59
      laparoscopic 54.51
    eyelid 08.09
      and conjunctiva 10.5
    eye muscle 15.7
    fallopian tube 65.89
      laparoscopic 65.81
    fascia 83.91
      hand 82.91
        by stretching or manipulation 93.26
    gallbladder 54.59
      laparoscopic 54.51
    ganglion (peripheral) NEC 04.49
      cranial NEC 04.42
    hand 82.91
      by stretching or manipulation 93.26
    heart 37.10
    intestines 54.59
      laparoscopic 54.51
    iris (posterior) 12.33
      anterior 12.32
    joint (capsule) (structure) (*see also* Division, joint capsule) 80.40
    kidney 59.02
      laparoscopic 59.03

Lysis — *continued*
  adhesions — *continued*
    labia (vulva) 71.01
    larynx 31.92
    liver 54.59
      laparoscopic 54.51
    lung (for collapse of lung) 33.39
    mediastinum 34.99
    meninges (spinal) 03.6
      cortical 02.91
    middle ear 20.23
    muscle 83.91
      by stretching or manipulation 93.27
      extraocular 15.7
      hand 82.91
        by stretching or manipulation 93.26
    nasopharynx 29.54
    nerve (peripheral) NEC 04.49
      cranial NEC 04.42
      roots, spinal 03.6
      trigeminal 04.41
    nose, nasal 21.91
    ocular muscle 15.7
    ovary 65.89
      laparoscopic 65.81
    pelvic 54.59
      laparoscopic 54.51
    penile 64.93
    pericardium 37.12
    perineal (female) 71.01
    peripheral vessels 39.91
    perirectal 48.81
    perirenal 59.02
      laparoscopic 59.03
    peritoneum (pelvic) 54.59
      laparoscopic 54.51
    periureteral 59.02
      laparoscopic 59.03
    perivesical 59.11
      laparoscopic 59.12
    pharynx 29.54
    pleura (for collapse of lung) 33.39
    spermatic cord 63.94
    spinal (cord) (meninges) (nerve roots) 03.6
    spleen 54.59
      laparoscopic 54.51
    tendon 83.91
      by stretching or manipulation 93.27
      hand 82.91
        by stretching or manipulation 93.26
    thorax 34.99
    tongue 25.93
    trachea 31.92
    tubo-ovarian 65.89
      laparoscopic 65.81
    ureter 59.02
      with freeing or repositioning of ureter 59.02
      intraluminal 56.81
      laparoscopic 59.03
    urethra (intraluminal) 58.5
    uterus 54.59
      intraluminal 68.21
      laparoscopic 54.51
      peritoneal 54.59
        laparoscopic 54.51
    vagina (intraluminal) 70.13
    vitreous (posterior approach) 14.74
      anterior approach 14.73
    vulva 71.01
  goniosynechiae (with injection of air or liquid) 12.31
  synechiae (posterior) 12.33
    anterior (with injection of air or liquid) 12.32

M

Madlener operation (tubal ligation) 66.31
Magnet extraction
  foreign body
    anterior chamber, eye 12.01
    choroid 14.01
    ciliary body 12.01

Magnet extraction — *continued*
  foreign body — *continued*
    conjunctiva 98.22
    cornea 11.0
    eye, eyeball NEC 98.21
      anterior segment 12.01
      posterior segment 14.01
    intraocular (anterior segment) 12.01
    iris 12.01
    lens 13.01
    orbit 98.21
    retina 14.01
    sclera 12.01
    vitreous 14.01
Magnetic resonance imaging (nuclear) — *see* Imaging, magnetic resonance
Magnuson (-Stack) operation (arthroplasty for recurrent shoulder dislocation) 81.82
Malleostapediopexy 19.19
  with incus replacement 19.11
Malström's vacuum extraction 72.79
  with episiotomy 72.71
Mammaplasty — *see* Mammoplasty
Mammectomy — *see also* Mastectomy
  subcutaneous (unilateral) 85.34
    bilateral 85.36
      with synchronous implant 85.35
Mammilliplasty 85.87
Mammography NEC 87.37
Mammoplasty 85.89
  with
    full-thickness graft 85.83
    muscle flap 85.85
    pedicle graft 85.84
    split-thickness graft 85.82
  amputative (reduction) (bilateral) 85.32
    unilateral 85.31
  augmentation 85.50
    with
      breast implant (bilateral) 85.54
        unilateral 85.53
      injection into breast (bilateral) 85.52
        unilateral 85.51
  reduction (bilateral) 85.32
    unilateral 85.31
  revision 85.89
  size reduction (gynecomastia) (bilateral) 85.32
    unilateral 85.31
Mammotomy 85.0
Manchester (-Donald) (-Fothergill) operation (uterine suspension) 69.22
Mandibulectomy (partial) 76.31
  total 76.42
    with reconstruction 76.41
Maneuver (method)
  Bracht 72.52
  Credé 73.59
  De Lee (key-in-lock) 72.4
  Kristeller 72.54
  Lovset's (extraction of arms in breech birth) 72.52
  Mauriceau (-Smellie-Veit) 72.52
  Pinard (total breech extraction) 72.54
  Prague 72.52
  Ritgen 73.59
  Scanzoni (rotation) 72.4
  Van Hoorn 72.52
  Wigand-Martin 72.52
Manipulation
  with reduction of fracture or dislocation — *see* Reduction, fracture *and* Reduction, dislocation
  enterostomy stoma (with dilation) 96.24
  intestine (intra-abdominal) 46.80
    large 46.82
    small 46.81
  joint
    adhesions 93.26
      temporomandibular 76.95
    dislocation — *see* Reduction, dislocation
  lacrimal passage (tract) NEC 09.49
  muscle structures 93.27
  musculoskeletal (physical therapy) NEC 93.29

Manipulation

Manipulation — *continued*
  nasal septum, displaced 21.88
  osteopathic NEC 93.67
    for general mobilization (general articulation) 93.61
    high-velocity, low-amplitude forces (thrusting) 93.62
    indirect forces 93.65
    isotonic, isometric forces 93.64
    low-velocity, high-amplitude forces (springing) 93.63
    to move tissue fluids 93.66
  rectum 96.22
  salivary duct 26.91
  stomach, intraoperative 44.92
  temporomandibular joint NEC 76.95
  ureteral calculus by catheter
    with removal 56.0
    without removal 59.8
  uterus NEC 69.98
    gravid 75.99
    inverted
      manual replacement (following delivery) 75.94
      surgical — *see* Repair, inverted uterus

Manometry
  esophageal 89.32
  spinal fluid 89.15
  urinary 89.21

Manual arts therapy 93.81

Mapping
  cardiac (electrophysiologic) 37.27
    doppler (flow) 88.72
    electrocardiogram only 89.52

Marckwald operation (cervical os repair) 67.59

Marshall-Marchetti (-Krantz) operation (retropubic urethral suspension) 59.5

Marsupialization — *see also* Destruction, lesion, by site
  cyst
    Bartholin's 71.23
    brain 01.59
    cervical (nabothian) 67.31
    dental 24.4
    dentigerous 24.4
    kidney 55.31
    larynx 30.01
    liver 50.21
    ovary 65.21
      laparoscopic 65.23
    pancreas 52.3
    pilonidal (open excision) (with partial closure) 86.21
    salivary gland 26.21
    spinal (intraspinal) (meninges) 03.4
    spleen, splenic 41.41
  lesion
    brain 01.59
    cerebral 01.59
    liver 50.21
  pilonidal cyst or sinus (open excision) (with partial closure) 86.21
  pseudocyst, pancreas 52.3
  ranula, salivary gland 26.21

Massage
  cardiac (external) (manual) (closed) 99.63
    open 37.91
  prostatic 99.94
  rectal (for levator spasm) 99.93

MAST (military anti-shock trousers) 93.58

Mastectomy (complete) (prophylactic) (simple) (unilateral) 85.41
  with
    excision of regional lymph nodes 85.43
      bilateral 85.44
    preservation of skin and nipple 85.34
      with synchronous implant 85.33
      bilateral 85.36
        with synchronous implant 85.35
  bilateral 85.42
  extended
    radical (Urban) (unilateral) 85.47
      bilateral 85.48

Mastectomy — *continued*
  extended — *continued*
    simple (with regional lymphadenectomy) (unilateral) 85.43
      bilateral 85.44
  modified radical (unilateral) 85.43
    bilateral 85.44
  partial 85.23
  radical (Halsted) (Meyer) (unilateral) 85.45
    bilateral 85.46
    extended (Urban) (unilateral) 85.47
      bilateral 85.48
    modified (unilateral) 85.43
      bilateral 85.44
  subcutaneous 85.34
    with synchronous implant 85.33
    bilateral 85.36
      with synchronous implant 85.35
  subtotal 85.23

Masters' stress test (two-step) 89.42

Mastoidectomy (cortical) (conservative) 20.49
  complete (simple) 20.41
  modified radical 20.49
  radical 20.42
    modified 20.49
  simple (complete) 20.41

Mastoidotomy 20.21

Mastoidotympanectomy 20.42

Mastopexy 85.6

Mastoplasty — *see* Mammoplasty

Mastorrhaphy 85.81

Mastotomy 85.0

Matas operation (aneurysmorrhaphy) 39.52

Mayo operation
  bunionectomy 77.59
  herniorrhaphy 53.49
  vaginal hysterectomy 68.59
    laparoscopicaly assisted (LAVH) 68.51

Mazet operation (knee disarticulation) 84.16

McBride operation (bunionectomy with soft tissue correction) 77.53

McBurney operation — *see* Repair, hernia, inguinal

McCall operation (enterocele repair) 70.92

McCauley operation (release of clubfoot) 83.84

McDonald operation (encirclement suture, cervix) 67.59

McIndoe operation (vaginal construction) 70.61

McKeever operation (fusion of first metatarsophalangeal joint for hallux valgus repair) 77.52

McKissock operation (breast reduction) 85.33

McReynolds operation (transposition of pterygium) 11.31

McVay operation
  femoral hernia — *see* Repair, hernia, femoral
  inguinal hernia — *see* Repair, hernia, inguinal

Measurement
  airway resistance 89.38
  anatomic NEC 89.39
  arterial blood gases 89.65
    basal metabolic rate (BMR) 89.39
    blood gases
      arterial 89.65
        continuous intra-arterial 89.60 •
      venous 89.66
  body 93.07
  cardiac output (by)
    Fick method 89.67
    indicator dilution technique 89.68
    oxygen consumption technique 89.67
    thermodilution indicator 89.68
  cardiovascular NEC 89.59
  central venous pressure 89.62
  coronary blood flow 89.69
  gastric function NEC 89.39
  girth 93.07
  intelligence 94.01
  intracranial pressure 01.18
  intraocular tension or pressure 89.11
    as part of extended ophthalmologic work-up 95.03

Measurement — *continued*
  intrauterine pressure 89.62
  limb length 93.06
  lung volume 89.37
  mixed venous blood gases 89.66
  physiologic NEC 89.39
  portovenous pressure 89.62
  range of motion 93.05
  renal clearance 89.29
  respiratory NEC 89.38
  skin fold thickness 93.07
  skull circumference 93.07
  sphincter of Oddi pressure 51.15
  systemic arterial
    blood gases 89.65
      continuous intra-arterial 89.60 •
    pressure 89.61
  urine (bioassay) (chemistry) 89.29
  vascular 89.59
  venous blood gases 89.66
  vital capacity (pulmonary) 89.37

Meatoplasty
  ear 18.6
  urethra 58.47

Meatotomy
  ureter 56.1
  urethra 58.1
    internal 58.5

Mechanical ventilation — *see* Ventilation

Mediastinectomy 34.3

Mediastinoscopy (transpleural) 34.22

Mediastinotomy 34.1
  with pneumonectomy 32.5

Meloplasty, facial 86.82

Meningeorrhaphy (cerebral) 02.12
  spinal NEC 03.59
  for
    meningocele 03.51
    myelomeningocele 03.52

Meniscectomy (knee) NEC 80.6
  acromioclavicular 80.91
  sternoclavicular 80.91
  temporomandibular (joint) 76.5
  wrist 80.93

Menstrual extraction or regulation 69.6

Mentoplasty (augmentation) (with graft) (with implant) 76.68
  reduction 76.67

Mesenterectomy 54.4

Mesenteriopexy 54.75

Mesenteriplication 54.75

Mesocoloplication 54.75

Mesopexy 54.75

Metatarsectomy 77.98

Metroplasty 69.49

Mid forceps delivery 72.29

Mikulicz operation (exteriorization of intestine) (first stage) 46.03
  second stage 46.04

Miles operation (proctectomy) 48.5

Military anti-shock trousers (MAST) 93.58

Millard operation (cheiloplasty) 27.54

Miller operation
  midtarsal arthrodesis 81.14
  urethrovesical suspension 59.4

Millin-Read operation (urethrovesical suspension) 59.4

Mist therapy 93.94

Mitchell operation (hallux valgus repair) 77.51

Mobilization
  joint NEC 93.16
  mandible 76.95
  neostrophingic (mitral valve) 35.12
  spine 93.15
  stapes (transcrural) 19.0
  testis in scrotum 62.5

Mohs operation (chemosurgical excision of skin) 86.24

Molegraphy 87.81

Monitoring
  cardiac output (by)
    ambulatory (ACM) 89.50
    electrographic 89.54
      during surgery — *omit code*
    Fick method 89.67
    Holter-type device 89.50
    indicator dilution technique 89.68
    oxygen consumption technique 89.67
    specified technique NEC 89.68
    telemetry (cardiac) 89.54
    thermodilution indicator 89.68
    transesophageal (Doppler) (ultrasound) 89.68
  central venous pressure 89.62
  circulatory NEC 89.69
  continuous intra-arterial bood gas 89.60
  coronary blood flow (coincidence counting technique) 89.69
  electroencephalographic 89.19
    radio-telemetered 89.19
    video 89.19
  fetus (fetal heart)
    antepartum
      nonstress (fetal activity acceleration determinations) 75.35
      oxytocin challenge (contraction stress test) 75.35
      ultrasonography (early pregnancy) (Doppler) 88.78
    intrapartum (during labor) (extrauterine) (external) 75.34
      ausculatory (stethoscopy) — *omit code*
      internal (with contraction measurements) (ECG) 75.32
      intrauterine (direct) (ECG) 75.32
      phonocardiographic (extrauterine) 75.34
      pulsed ultrasound (Doppler) 88.78
      transcervical fetal oxygen saturation monitoring 75.38
      transcervical fetal SpO2 monitoring 75.38
  Holter-type device (cardiac) 89.50
  intracranial pressure 01.18
  pulmonary artery
    pressure 89.63
    wedge 89.64
  sleep (recording) — *see* categories 89.17-89.18
  systemic arterial pressure 89.61
  telemetry (cardiac) 89.54
  transesophageal cardiac output (Doppler) 89.68
  ventricular pressure (cardiac) 89.62
Moore operation (arthroplasty) 81.52
Moschowitz
  enterocele repair 70.92
  herniorrhaphy — *see* Repair, hernia, femoral
  sigmoidopexy 46.63
Mountain resort sanitarium 93.98
Mouth-to-mouth resuscitation 93.93
Moxibustion 93.35
MRI — *see* Imaging, magnetic resonance
Muller operation (banding of pulmonary artery) 38.85
Multiple sleep latency test (MSLT) 89.18
Mumford operation (partial claviculectomy) 77.81
Musculoplasty (*see also* Repair, muscle) 83.87
  hand (*see also* Repair, muscle, hand) 82.89
Music therapy 93.84
Mustard operation (interatrial transposition of venous return) 35.91
Myectomy 83.45
  anorectal 48.92
  eye muscle 15.13
    multiple 15.3
  for graft 83.43
    hand 82.34
  hand 82.36
    for graft 82.34
  levator palpebrae 08.33
  rectal 48.92
Myelogram, myelography (air) (gas) 87.21
  posterior fossa 87.02

Myelotomy
  spine, spinal (cord) (tract) (one-stage) (two-stage) 03.29
    percutaneous 03.21
Myocardiectomy (infarcted area) 37.33
Myocardiotomy 37.11
Myoclasis 83.99
  hand 82.99
Myomectomy (uterine) 68.29
  broad ligament 69.19
Myoplasty (*see also* Repair, muscle) 83.87
  hand (*see also* Repair, muscle, hand) 82.89
  mastoid 19.9
Myorrhaphy 83.65
  hand 82.46
Myosuture 83.65
  hand 82.46
Myotasis 93.27
Myotenontoplasty (*see also* Repair, tendon) 83.88
  hand 82.86
Myotenoplasty (*see also* Repair, tendon) 83.88
  hand 82.86
Myotenotomy 83.13
  hand 82.11
Myotomy 83.02
  with division 83.19
    hand 82.19
  colon NEC 46.92
    sigmoid 46.91
  cricopharyngeal 29.31
    that for pharyngeal (pharyngoesophageal) diverticulectomy 29.32
  esophagus 42.7
  eye (oblique) (rectus) 15.21
    multiple (two or more muscles) 15.4
  hand 82.02
    with division 82.19
  levator palpebrae 08.38
  sigmoid (colon) 46.91
Myringectomy 20.59
Myringodectomy 20.59
Myringomalleolabyrinthopexy 19.52
Myringoplasty (epitympanic, type I) (by cauterization) (by graft) 19.4
  revision 19.6
Myringostapediopexy 19.53
Myringostomy 20.01
Myringotomy (with aspiration) (with drainage) 20.09
  with insertion of tube or drainage device (button) (grommet) 20.01

N

Nailing, intramedullary — *see* Reduction, fracture with internal fixation
Narcoanalysis 94.21
Narcosynthesis 94.21
Narrowing, palpebral fissure 08.51
Nasopharyngogram 87.09
  contrast 87.06
Necropsy 89.8
Needleoscopy (fetus) 75.31
Needling
  Bartholin's gland (cyst) 71.21
  cataract (secondary) 13.64
  fallopian tube 66.91
  hydrocephalic head 73.8
  lens (capsule) 13.2
  pupillary membrane (iris) 12.35
Nephrectomy (complete) (total) (unilateral) 55.51
  bilateral 55.54
  partial (wedge) 55.4
  remaining or solitary kidney 55.52
  removal transplanted kidney 55.53
Nephrocolopexy 55.7
Nephrocystanastomosis NEC 56.73
Nephrolithotomy 55.01

Nephrolysis 59.02
  laparoscopic 59.03
Nephropexy 55.7
Nephroplasty 55.89
Nephropyeloplasty 55.87
Nephropyeloureterostomy 55.86
Nephrorrhaphy 55.81
Nephroscopy 55.21
Nephrostolithotomy, percutaneous 55.03
Nephrostomy (with drainage tube) 55.02
  closure 55.82
  percutaneous 55.03
    with fragmentation (ultrasound) 55.04
Nephrotomogram, nephrotomography NEC 87.72
Nephrotomy 55.01
Nephroureterectomy (with bladder cuff) 55.51
Nephroureterocystectomy 55.51 [57.79]
Nerve block (cranial) (peripheral) NEC (*see also* Block, by site) 04.81
Neurectasis (cranial) (peripheral) 04.91
Neurectomy (cranial) (infraorbital) (occipital) (peripheral) (spinal) NEC 04.07
  gastric (vagus) (*see also* Vagotomy) 44.00
  opticociliary 12.79
  paracervical 05.22
  presacral 05.24
  retrogasserian 04.07
  sympathetic — *see* Sympathectomy
  trigeminal 04.07
  tympanic 20.91
Neurexeresis NEC 04.07
Neuroablation
  radiofrequency 04.2
Neuroanastomosis (cranial) (peripheral) NEC 04.74
  accessory-facial 04.72
  accessory-hypoglossal 04.73
  hypoglossal-facial 04.71
Neurolysis (peripheral nerve) NEC 04.49
  carpal tunnel 04.43
  cranial nerve NEC 04.42
  spinal (cord) (nerve roots) 03.6
  tarsal tunnel 04.44
  trigeminal nerve 04.41
Neuroplasty (cranial) (peripheral) NEC 04.79
  of old injury (delayed repair) 04.76
  revision 04.75
Neurorrhaphy (cranial) (peripheral) 04.3
Neurotomy (cranial) (peripheral) (spinal) NEC 04.04
  acoustic 04.01
  glossopharyngeal 29.92
  lacrimal branch 05.0
  retrogasserian 04.02
  sympathetic 05.0
  vestibular 04.01
Neurotripsy (peripheral) NEC 04.03
  trigeminal 04.02
Nicola operation (tenodesis for recurrent dislocation of shoulder) 81.82
Nimodipine, infusion 99.75
NIPS (non-invasive programmed electrical stimulation) 37.26
Nissen operation (fundoplication of stomach) 44.66
Noble operation (plication of small intestine) 46.62
Norman Miller operation (vaginopexy) 70.77
Norton operation (extraperitoneal cesarean section) 74.2
Nuclear magnetic resonance imaging — *see* Imaging, magnetic resonance
Nutrition, concentrated substances
  enteral infusion (of) 96.6
  parenteral, total 99.15
  peripheral parenteral 99.15

Ober (-Yount) operation

O

Ober (-Yount) operation (glutealiliotibial fasciotomy) 83.14

Obliteration
  bone cavity (*see also* Osteoplasty) 78.40
  calyceal diverticulum 55.39
  canaliculi 09.6
  cerebrospinal fistula 02.12
  cul-de-sac 70.92
  frontal sinus (with fat) 22.42
  lacrimal punctum 09.91
  lumbar pseudomeningocele 03.51
  lymphatic structure(s) (peripheral) 40.9
  maxillary sinus 22.31
  meningocele (sacral) 03.51
  pelvic 68.8
  pleural cavity 34.6
  sacral meningocele 03.51
  Skene's gland 71.3
  tympanomastoid cavity 19.9
  vagina, vaginal (partial) (total) 70.4
    vault 70.8

Occlusal molds (dental) 89.31

Occlusion
  artery
    by embolization — *see* Embolization, artery
    by endovascular approach — *see* Embolization, artery
    by ligation — *see* Ligation, artery
  fallopian tube — *see* Ligation, fallopian tube
  patent ductus arteriosus (PDA) 38.85
  vein
    by embolization — *see* Embolization, vein
    by endovascular approach — *see* Embolization, vein
    by ligation — *see* Ligation, vein
  vena cava (surgical) 38.7

Occupational therapy 93.83

O'Donoghue operation (triad knee repair) 81.43

Odontectomy NEC (*see also* Removal, tooth, surgical) 23.19

Oleothorax 33.39

Olshausen operation (uterine suspension) 69.22

Omentectomy 54.4
Omentofixation 54.74
Omentopexy 54.74
Omentoplasty 54.74
Omentorrhaphy 54.74
Omentotomy 54.19
Omphalectomy 54.3
Onychectomy 86.23
Onychoplasty 86.86
Onychotomy 86.09
  with drainage 86.04

Oophorectomy (unilateral) 65.39
  with salpingectomy 65.49
    laparoscopic 65.41
  bilateral (same operative episode) 65.51
    laparoscopic 65.53
    with salpingectomy 65.61
      laparoscopic 65.63
  laparoscopic 65.31
  partial 65.29
    laparoscopic 65.25
    wedge 65.22
      that by laparoscope 65.24
  remaining ovary 65.52
    laparoscopic 65.54
    with tube 65.62
      laparoscopic 65.64

Oophorocystectomy 65.29
  laparoscopic 65.25

Oophoropexy 65.79
Oophoroplasty 65.79
Oophororrhaphy 65.71
  laparoscopic 65.74

Oophorostomy 65.09
  laparoscopic 65.01

Oophorotomy 65.09
  laparoscopic 65.01

Opening
  bony labyrinth (ear) 20.79
  cranial suture 02.01
  heart valve
    closed heart technique — *see* Valvulotomy, by site
    open heart technique — *see* Valvuloplasty, by site
  spinal dura 03.09

Operation
  Abbe
    construction of vagina 70.61
    intestinal anastomosis — *see* Anastomosis, intestine
  abdominal (region) NEC 54.99
  abdominoperineal NEC 48.5
  Aburel (intra-amniotic injection for abortion) 75.0
  Adams
    advancement of round ligament 69.22
    crushing of nasal septum 21.88
    excision of palmar fascia 82.35
  adenoids NEC 28.99
  adrenal (gland) (nerve) (vessel) NEC 07.49
  Albee
    bone peg, femoral neck 78.05
    graft for slipping patella 78.06
    sliding inlay graft, tibia 78.07
  Albert (arthrodesis, knee) 81.22
  Aldridge (-Studdiford) (urethral sling) 59.5
  Alexander
    prostatectomy
      perineal 60.62
      suprapubic 60.3
    shortening of round ligaments of uterus 69.22
  Alexander-Adams (shortening of round ligaments of uterus) 69.22
  Almoor (extrapetrosal drainage) 20.22
  Altemeier (perineal rectal pull-through) 48.49
  Ammon (dacryocystotomy) 09.53
  Anderson (tibial lengthening) 78.37
  Anel (dilation of lacrimal duct) 09.42
  anterior chamber (eye) NEC 12.99
  anti-incontinence NEC 59.79
  antrum window (nasal sinus) 22.2
    with Caldwell-Luc approach 22.39
  anus NEC 49.99
  aortic body NEC 39.8
  aorticopulmonary window 39.59
  appendix NEC 47.99
  Arslan (fenestration of inner ear) 20.61
  artery NEC 39.99
  Asai (larynx) 31.75
  Baffes (interatrial transposition of venous return) 35.91
  Baldy-Webster (uterine suspension) 69.22
  Ball
    herniorrhaphy — *see* Repair, hernia, inguinal
    undercutting 49.02
  Bankhart (capsular repair into glenoid, for shoulder dislocation) 81.82
  Bardenheurer (ligation of innominate artery) 38.85
  Barkan (goniotomy) 12.52
    with goniopuncture 12.53
  Barr (transfer of tibialis posterior tendon) 83.75
  Barsky (closure of cleft hand) 82.82
  Bassett (vulvectomy with inguinal lymph node dissection) 71.5 [40.3]
  Bassini (herniorrhaphy) — *see* Repair, hernia, inguinal
  Batch-Spittler-McFaddin (knee disarticulation) 84.16
  Batista (partial ventriculectomy) (ventricular reduction) (ventricular remodeling) 37.35
  Beck I (epicardial poudrage) 36.39
  Beck II (aorta-coronary sinus shunt) 36.39
  Beck-Jianu (permanent gastrostomy) 43.19
  Bell-Beuttner (subtotal abdominal hysterectomy) 68.3
  Belsey (esophagogastric sphincter) 44.65
  Benenenti (rotation of bulbous urethra) 58.49
  Berke (levator resection eyelid) 08.33

Operation — *continued*
  Biesenberger (size reduction of breast, bilateral) 85.32
    unilateral 85.31
  Bigelow (litholapaxy) 57.0
  biliary (duct) (tract) NEC 51.99
  Billroth I (partial gastrectomy with gastroduodenostomy) 43.6
  Billroth II (partial gastrectomy with gastrojejunostomy) 43.7
  Binnie (hepatopexy) 50.69
  Bischoff (ureteroneocystostomy) 56.74
  bisection hysterectomy 68.3
  Bishoff (spinal myelotomy) 03.29
  bladder NEC 57.99
    flap 56.74
  Blalock (systemic-pulmonary anastomosis) 39.0
  Blalock-Hanlon (creation of atrial septal defect) 35.42
  Blalock-Taussig (subclavian-pulmonary anastomosis) 39.0
  Blascovic (resection and advancement of levator palpebrae superioris) 08.33
  blood vessel NEC 39.99
  Blount
    femoral shortening (with blade plate) 78.25
    by epiphyseal stapling 78.25
  Boari (bladder flap) 56.74
  Bobb (cholelithotomy) 51.04
  bone NEC — *see* category 78.4 ▓4▓
    facial 76.99
    injury NEC — *see* category 79.9 ▓4▓
    marrow NEC 41.98
    skull NEC 02.99
  Bonney (abdominal hysterectomy) 68.4
  Borthen (iridotasis) 12.63
  Bost
    plantar dissection 80.48
    radiocarpal fusion 81.26
  Bosworth
    arthroplasty for acromioclavicular separation 81.83
    fusion of posterior lumbar spine 81.08
      for pseudarthrosis 81.38
    resection of radial head ligaments (for tennis elbow) 80.92
    shelf procedure, hip 81.40
  Bottle (repair of hydrocele of tunica vaginalis) 61.2
  Boyd (hip disarticulation) 84.18
  brain NEC 02.99
  Brauer (cardiolysis) 37.10
  breast NEC 85.99
  Bricker (ileoureterostomy) 56.51
  Bristow (repair of shoulder dislocation) 81.82
  Brock (pulmonary valvulotomy) 35.03
  Brockman (soft tissue release for clubfoot) 83.84
  bronchus NEC 33.98
  Browne (-Denis) (hypospadias repair) 58.45
  Brunschwig (temporary gastrostomy) 43.19
  buccal cavity NEC 27.99
  Bunnell (tendon transfer) 82.56
  Burch procedure (retropubic urethral suspension for urinary stress incontinence) 59.5
  Burgess (amputation of ankle) 84.14
  bursa NEC 83.99
    hand 82.99
  bypass — *see* Bypass
  Caldwell (sulcus extension) 24.91
  Caldwell-Luc (maxillary sinusotomy) 22.39
    with removal of membrane lining 22.31
  Callander (knee disarticulation) 84.16
  Campbell
    bone block, ankle 81.11
    fasciotomy (iliac crest) 83.14
    reconstruction of anterior cruciate ligaments 81.45
  canthus NEC 08.99
  cardiac NEC 37.99
    septum NEC 35.98
    valve NEC 35.99
  carotid body or gland NEC 39.8
  Carroll and Taber (arthroplasty proximal interphalangeal joint) 81.72

Index to Procedures

Operation — *continued*
Cattell (herniorrhaphy) 53.51
Cecil (urethral reconstruction) 58.46
cecum NEC 46.99
cerebral (meninges) NEC 02.99
cervix NEC 69.99
Chandler (hip fusion) 81.21
Charles (correction of lymphedema) 40.9
Charnley (compression arthrodesis)
    ankle 81.11
    hip 81.21
    knee 81.22
Cheatle-Henry — *see* Repair, hernia, femoral
chest cavity NEC 34.99
Chevalier-Jackson (partial laryngectomy) 30.29
Child (radical subtotal pancreatectomy) 52.53
Chopart (midtarsal amputation) 84.12
chordae tendineae NEC 35.32
choroid NEC 14.9
ciliary body NEC 12.98
cisterna chyli NEC 40.69
Clagett (closure of chest wall following open flap drainage) 34.72
Clayton (resection of metatarsal heads and bases of phalanges) 77.88
clitoris NEC 71.4
cocked hat (metacarpal lengthening and transfer of local flap) 82.69
Cockett (varicose vein)
    lower limb 38.59
    upper limb 38.53
Cody tack (perforation of footplate) 19.0
Coffey (uterine suspension) (Meigs' modification) 69.22
Cole (anterior tarsal wedge osteotomy) 77.28
Collis-Nissen (hiatal hernia repair) 53.80
colon NEC 46.99
Colonna
    adductor tenotomy (first stage) 83.12
    hip arthroplasty (second stage) 81.40
    reconstruction of hip (second stage) 81.40
commando (radical glossectomy) 25.4
conjunctiva NEC 10.99
    destructive NEC 10.33
cornea NEC 11.99
Coventry (tibial wedge osteotomy) 77.27
Crawford (tarso-frontalis sling of eyelid) 08.32
cul-de-sac NEC 70.92
Culp-Deweerd (spiral flap pyeloplasty) 55.87
Culp-Scardino (ureteral flap pyeloplasty) 55.87
Curtis (interphalangeal joint arthroplasty) 81.72
cystocele NEC 70.51
Dahlman (excision of esophageal diverticulum) 42.31
Dana (posterior rhizotomy) 03.1
Danforth (fetal) 73.8
Darrach (ulnar resection) 77.83
Davis (intubated ureterotomy) 56.2
de Grandmont (tarsectomy) 08.35
Delorme
    pericardiectomy 37.31
    proctopexy 48.76
    repair of prolapsed rectum 48.76
    thoracoplasty 33.34
Denker (radical maxillary antrotomy) 22.31
Dennis-Varco (herniorrhaphy) — *see* Repair, hernia, femoral
Denonvillier (limited rhinoplasty) 21.86
dental NEC 24.99
    orthodontic NEC 24.8
Derlacki (tympanoplasty) 19.4
diaphragm NEC 34.89
Dickson (fascial transplant) 83.82
Dickson-Diveley (tendon transfer and arthrodesis to correct claw toe) 77.57
Dieffenbach (hip disarticulation) 84.18
digestive tract NEC 46.99
Doléris (shortening of round ligaments) 69.22
D'Ombrain (excision of pterygium with corneal graft) 11.32
Dorrance (push-back operation for cleft palate) 27.62
Dotter (transluminal angioplasty) 39.59
Douglas (suture of tongue to lip for micrognathia) 25.59

Operation — *continued*
Doyle (paracervical uterine denervation) 69.3
Duhamel (abdominoperineal pull-through) 48.65
Dührssen (vaginofixation of uterus) 69.22
Dunn (triple arthrodesis) 81.12
duodenum NEC 46.99
Dupuytren
    fasciectomy 82.35
    fasciotomy 82.12
        with excision 82.35
    shoulder disarticulation 84.08
Durham (-Caldwell) (transfer of biceps femoris tendon) 83.75
DuToit and Roux (staple capsulorrhaphy of shoulder) 81.82
DuVries (tenoplasty) 83.88
Dwyer
    fasciotomy 83.14
    soft tissue release NEC 83.84
    wedge osteotomy, calcaneus 77.28
Eagleton (extrapetrosal drainage) 20.22
ear (external) NEC 18.9
    middle or inner NEC 20.99
Eden-Hybinette (glenoid bone block) 78.01
Effler (heart) 36.2
Eggers
    tendon release (patellar retinacula) 83.13
    tendon transfer (biceps femoris tendon) (hamstring tendon) 83.75
Elliot (scleral trephination with iridectomy) 12.61
Ellis Jones (repair of peroneal tendon) 83.88
Ellison (reinforcement of collateral ligament) 81.44
Elmslie-Cholmeley (tarsal wedge osteotomy) 77.28
Eloesser
    thoracoplasty 33.34
    thoracostomy 34.09
Emmet (cervix) 67.61
endorectal pull-through 48.41
epididymis NEC 63.99
esophagus NEC 42.99
Estes (ovary) 65.72
    laparoscopic 65.75
Estlander (thoracoplasty) 33.34
Evans (release of clubfoot) 83.84
extraocular muscle NEC 15.9
    multiple (two or more muscles) 15.4
        with temporary detachment from globe 15.3
        revision 15.6
    single 15.29
        with temporary detachment from globe 15.19
eyeball NEC 16.99
eyelid(s) NEC 08.99
face NEC 27.99
facial bone or joint NEC 76.99
fallopian tube NEC 66.99
Farabeuf (ischiopubiotomy) 77.39
Fasanella-Servatt (blepharoptosis repair) 08.35
fascia NEC 83.99
    hand 82.99
female (genital organs) NEC 71.9
    hysterectomy NEC 68.9
fenestration (aorta) 39.54
Ferguson (hernia repair) 53.00
Fick (perforation of footplate) 19.0
filtering (for glaucoma) 12.79
    with iridectomy 12.65
Finney (pyloroplasty) 44.2 ✓4ᵗʰ
fistulizing, sclera NEC 12.69
Foley (pyeloplasty) 55.87
Fontan (creation of conduit between right atrium and pulmonary artery) 35.94
Fothergill (-Donald) (uterine suspension) 69.22
Fowler
    arthroplasty of metacarpophalangeal joint 81.72
    release (mallet finger repair) 82.84
    tenodesis (hand) 82.85
    thoracoplasty 33.34
Fox (entropion repair with wedge resection) 08.43

Operation — *continued*
Franco (suprapubic cystotomy) 57.19
Frank (permanent gastrostomy) 43.19
Frazier (-Spiller) (subtemporal trigeminal rhizotomy) 04.02
Fredet-Ramstedt (pyloromyotomy) (with wedge resection) 43.3
Frenckner (intrapetrosal drainage) 20.22
Frickman (abdominal proctopexy) 48.75
Frommel (shortening of uterosacral ligaments) 69.22
Gabriel (abdominoperineal resection of rectum) 48.5
gallbladder NEC 51.99
ganglia NEC 04.99
    sympathetic 05.89
Gant (wedge osteotomy of trochanter) 77.25
Garceau (tibial tendon transfer) 83.75
Gardner (spinal meningocele repair) 03.51
gastric NEC 44.99
Gelman (release of clubfoot) 83.84
genital organ NEC
    female 71.9
    male 64.99
Ghormley (hip fusion) 81.21
Gifford
    destruction of lacrimal sac 09.6
    keratotomy (delimiting) 11.1
Gill
    arthrodesis of shoulder 81.23
    laminectomy 03.09
Gill-Stein (carporadial arthrodesis) 81.25
Gilliam (uterine suspension) 69.22
Girdlestone
    laminectomy with spinal fusion 81.00
    muscle transfer for claw toe 77.57
    resection of femoral head and neck 77.85
Girdlestone-Taylor (muscle transfer for claw toe repair) 77.57
glaucoma NEC 12.79
Glenn (anastomosis of superior vena cava to right pulmonary artery) 39.21
globus pallidus NEC 01.42
Goebel-Frangenheim-Stoeckel (urethrovesical suspension) 59.4
Goldner (clubfoot release) 80.48
Goldthwait
    ankle stabilization 81.11
    patella stabilization 81.44
    tendon transfer for patella dislocation 81.44
Goodall-Power (vagina) 70.4
Gordon-Taylor (hindquarter amputation) 84.19
Graber-Duvernay (drilling femoral head) 77.15
Green (scapulopexy) 78.41
Grice (subtalar arthrodesis) 81.13
Gritti-Stokes (knee disarticulation) 84.16
Gross (herniorrhaphy) 53.49
gum NEC 24.39
Guyon (amputation of ankle) 84.13
Hagner (epididymotomy) 63.92
Halsted — *see* Repair, hernia, inguinal
Hampton (anastomosis small intestine to rectal stump) 45.92
hanging hip (muscle release) 83.19
harelip 27.54
Harrison-Richardson (vaginal suspension) 70.77
Hartmann — *see* Colectomy, by site
Hauser
    achillotenotomy 83.11
    bunionectomy with adductor tendon transfer 77.53
    stabilization of patella 81.44
Heaney (vaginal hysterectomy) 68.59
    laparoscopically assisted (LAVH) 68.51
heart NEC 37.99
    valve NEC 35.99
    adjacent structure NEC 35.39
Hegar (perineorrhaphy) 71.79
Heine (cyclodialysis) 12.55
Heineke-Mikulicz (pyloroplasty) 44.2 ✓4ᵗʰ
Heller (esophagomyotomy) 42.7
Hellström (transplantation of aberrant renal vessel) 39.55
hemorrhoids NEC 49.49
Henley (jejunal transposition) 43.81

Operation

Operation — *continued*
- hepatic NEC 50.99
- hernia — *see* Repair, hernia
- Hey (amputation of foot) 84.12
- Hey-Groves (reconstruction of anterior cruciate ligament) 81.45
- Heyman (soft tissue release for clubfoot) 83.84
- Heyman-Herndon (-Strong) (correction of metatarsus varus) 80.48
- Hibbs (lumbar spinal fusion) — *see* Fusion, lumbar
- Higgins — *see* Repair, hernia, femoral
- Hill-Allison (hiatal hernia repair, transpleural approach) 53.80
- Hitchcock (anchoring tendon of biceps) 83.88
- Hofmeister (gastrectomy) 43.7
- Hoke
  - midtarsal fusion 81.14
  - triple arthrodesis 81.12
- Holth
  - iridencleisis 12.63
  - sclerectomy 12.65
- Homan (correction of lymphedema) 40.9
- Hutch (ureteroneocystostomy) 56.74
- Hybinette-eden (glenoid bone block) 78.01
- hymen NEC 70.91
- hypopharynx NEC 29.99
- hypophysis NEC 07.79
- ileal loop 56.51
- ileum NEC 46.99
- intestine NEC 46.99
- iris NEC 12.97
  - inclusion 12.63
- Irving (tubal ligation) 66.32
- Irwin (*see also* Osteotomy) 77.30
- Jaboulay (gastroduodenostomy) 44.39
- Janeway (permanent gastrostomy) 43.19
- Jatene (arterial switch) 35.84
- jejunum NEC 46.99
- Johanson (urethral reconstruction) 58.46
- joint (capsule) (ligament) (structure) NEC 81.99
  - facial NEC 76.99
- Jones
  - claw toe (transfer of extensor hallucis longus tendon) 77.57
    - modified (with arthrodesis) 77.57
  - dacryocystorhinostomy 09.81
  - hammer toe (interphalangeal fusion) 77.56
    - modified (tendon transfer with arthrodesis) 77.57
  - repair of peroneal tendon 83.88
- Joplin (exostectomy with tendon transfer) 77.53
- Kader (temporary gastrostomy) 43.19
- Kaufman (for urinary stress incontinence) 59.79
- Kazanjiian (buccal vestibular sulcus extension) 24.91
- Kehr (hepatopexy) 50.69
- Keller (bunionectomy) 77.59
- Kelly (-Kennedy) (urethrovesical plication) 59.3
- Kelly-Stoeckel (urethrovesical plication) 59.3
- Kerr (cesarean section) 74.1
- Kessler (arthroplasty, carpometacarpal joint) 81.74
- Kidner (excision of accessory navicular bone) (with tendon transfer) 77.98
- kidney NEC 55.99
- Killian (frontal sinusotomy) 22.41
- King-Steelquist (hindquarter amputation) 84.19
- Kirk (amputation through thigh) 84.17
- Kock pouch
  - bowel anastomosis — *omit code*
  - continent ileostomy 46.22
  - cutaneous uretero-ileostomy 56.51
  - ESWL (electrocorporeal shockwave lithotripsy) 98.51
  - removal, calculus 57.19
  - revision, cutaneous uretero-ileostomy 56.52
  - urinary diversion procedure 56.51
- Kondoleon (correction of lymphedema) 40.9
- Krause (sympathetic denervation) 05.29
- Kroener (partial salpingectomy) 66.69
- Kroenlein (lateral orbitotomy) 16.01
- Krönig (low cervical cesarean section) 74.1
- Krukenberg (reconstruction of below-elbow amputation) 82.89

Operation — *continued*
- Kuhnt-Szymanowski (ectropion repair with lid reconstruction) 08.44
- Labbe (gastrotomy) 43.0
- labia NEC 71.8
- lacrimal
  - gland 09.3
  - system NEC 09.99
- Ladd (mobilization of intestine) 54.95
- Lagrange (iridosclerectomy) 12.65
- Lambrinudi (triple arthrodesis) 81.12
- Langenbeck (cleft palate repair) 27.62
- Lapidus (bunionectomy with metatarsal osteotomy) 77.51
- Larry (shoulder disarticulation) 84.08
- larynx NEC 31.98
- Lash operation (internal cervical os repair) 67.59
- Latzko
  - cesarean section, extraperitoneal 74.2
  - colpocleisis 70.8
- Leadbetter (urethral reconstruction) 58.46
- Leadbetter-Politano (ureteroneocystostomy) 56.74
- Le Fort (colpocleisis) 70.8
- LeMesurier (cleft lip repair) 27.54
- lens NEC 13.9
- Leriche (periarterial sympathectomy) 05.25
- levator muscle sling
  - eyelid ptosis repair 08.33
  - urethrovesical suspension 59.71
  - urinary stress incontinence 59.71
- lid suture (blepharoptosis) 08.31
- ligament NEC 81.99
  - broad NEC 69.98
  - round NEC 69.98
  - uterine NEC 69.98
- Lindholm (repair of ruptured tendon) 83.88
- Linton (varicose vein) 38.59
- lip NEC 27.99
- Lisfranc
  - foot amputation 84.12
  - shoulder disarticulation 84.08
- Littlewood (forequarter amputation) 84.09
- liver NEC 50.99
- Lloyd-Davies (abdominoperineal resection) 48.5
- Longmire (bile duct anastomosis) 51.39
- Lord
  - dilation of anal canal for hemorrhoids 49.49
  - hemorrhoidectomy 49.49
  - orchidopexy 62.5
- Lucas and Murray (knee arthrodesis with plate) 81.22
- lung NEC 33.99
- lung volume reduction 32.22
- lymphatic structure(s) NEC 40.9
  - duct, left (thoracic) NEC 40.69
- Madlener (tubal ligation) 66.31
- Magnuson (-Stack) (arthroplasty for recurrent shoulder dislocation) 81.82
- male genital organs NEC 64.99
- Manchester (-Donald) (-Fothergill), (uterine suspension) 69.22
- mandible NEC 76.99
  - orthognathic 76.64
- Marckwald operation (cervical os repair) 67.59
- Marshall-Marchetti (-Krantz) (retropubic urethral suspension) 59.5
- Matas (aneurysmorrhaphy) 39.52
- Mayo
  - bunionectomy 77.59
  - herniorrhaphy 53.49
  - vaginal hysterectomy 68.59
    - laparoscopically assisted (LAVH) 68.51
- Mazet (knee disarticulation) 84.16
- McBride (bunionectomy with soft tissue correction) 77.53
- McBurney — *see* Repair, hernia, inguinal
- McCall (enterocele repair) 70.92
- McCauley (release of clubfoot) 83.84
- McDonald (encirclement suture, cervix) 67.59
- McIndoe (vaginal construction) 70.61
- McKeever (fusion of first metatarsophalangeal joint for hallux valgus repair) 77.52

Operation — *continued*
- McKissock (breast reduction) 85.33
- McReynolds (transposition of pterygium) 11.31
- McVay
  - femoral hernia — *see* Repair hernia, femoral
  - inguinal hernia — *see* Repair hernia, inguinal
- meninges (spinal) NEC 03.99
  - cerebral NEC 02.99
- mesentery NEC 54.99
- Mikulicz (exteriorization of intestine) (first stage) 46.03
  - second stage 46.04
- Miles (complete proctectomy) 48.5
- Millard (cheiloplasty) 27.54
- Miller
  - midtarsal arthrodesis 81.14
  - urethrovesical suspension 59.4
- Millin-Read (urethrovesical suspension) 59.4
- Mitchell (hallux valgus repair) 77.51
- Mohs (chemosurgical excision of skin) 86.24
- Moore (arthroplasty) 81.52
- Moschowitz
  - enterocele repair 70.92
  - herniorrhaphy — *see* Repair, hernia, femoral
  - sigmoidopexy 46.63
- mouth NEC 27.99
- Muller (banding of pulmonary artery) 38.85
- Mumford (partial claviculectomy) 77.81
- muscle NEC 83.99
  - extraocular — *see* Operation, extraocular
  - hand NEC 82.99
  - papillary heart NEC 35.31
- musculoskeletal system NEC 84.99
- Mustard (interatrial transposition of venous return) 35.91
- nail (finger) (toe) NEC 86.99
- nasal sinus NEC 22.9
- nasopharynx NEC 29.99
- nerve (cranial) (peripheral) NEC 04.99
  - adrenal NEC 07.49
  - sympathetic NEC 05.89
- nervous system NEC 05.9
- Nicola (tenodesis for recurrent dislocation of shoulder) 81.82
- nipple NEC 85.99
- Nissen (fundoplication of stomach) 44.66
- Noble (plication of small intestine) 46.62
- node (lymph) NEC 40.9
- Norman Miller (vaginopexy) 70.77
- Norton (extraperitoneal cesarean operation) 74.2
- nose, nasal NEC 21.99
  - sinus NEC 22.9
- Ober (-Yount) (gluteal-iliotibial fasciotomy) 83.14
- obstetric NEC 75.99
- ocular NEC 16.99
  - muscle — *see* Operation, extraocular muscle
- O'Donoghue (triad knee repair) 81.43
- Olshausen (uterine suspension) 69.22
- omentum NEC 54.99
- ophthalmologic NEC 16.99
- oral cavity NEC 27.99
- orbicularis muscle sling 08.36
- orbit NEC 16.98
- oropharynx NEC 29.99
- orthodontic NEC 24.8
- orthognathic NEC 76.69
- Oscar Miller (midtarsal arthrodesis) 81.14
- Osmond-Clark (soft tissue release with peroneus brevis tendon transfer) 83.75
- ovary NEC 65.99
- Oxford (for urinary incontinence) 59.4
- palate NEC 27.99
- palpebral ligament sling 08.36
- Panas (linear proctotomy) 48.0
- Pancoast (division of trigeminal nerve at foramen ovale) 04.02
- pancreas NEC 52.99
- pantaloon (revision of gastic anastomosis) 44.5
- papillary muscle (heart) NEC 35.31
- Paquin (ureteroneocystostomy) 56.74
- parathyroid gland(s) NEC 06.99
- parotid gland or duct NEC 26.99
- Partsch (marsupialization of dental cyst) 24.4

Index to Procedures

Operation — *continued*
  Pattee (auditory canal) 18.6
  Peet (splanchnic resection) 05.29
  Pemberton
    osteotomy of ilium 77.39
    rectum (mobilization and fixation for prolapse repair) 48.76
  penis NEC 64.98
  Pereyra (paraurethral suspension) 59.6
  pericardium NEC 37.99
  perineum (female) NEC 71.8
    male NEC 86.99
  perirectal tissue NEC 48.99
  perirenal tissue NEC 59.92
  peritoneum NEC 54.99
  periurethral tissue NEC 58.99
  perivesical tissue NEC 59.92
  pharyngeal flap (cleft palate repair) 27.62
    secondary or subsequent 27.63
  pharynx, pharyngeal (pouch) NEC 29.99
  pineal gland NEC 07.59
  Pinsker (obliteration of nasoseptal telangiectasia) 21.07
  Piper (forceps) 72.6
  Pirogoff (ankle amputation through malleoli of tibia and fibula) 84.14
  pituitary gland NEC 07.79
  plastic — *see* Repair, by site
  pleural cavity NEC 34.99
  Politano-Leadbetter (ureteroneocystostomy) 56.74
  pollicization (with nerves and blood supply) 82.61
  Polya (gastrectomy) 43.7
  Pomeroy (ligation and division of fallopian tubes) 66.32
  Poncet
    lengthening of Achilles tendon 83.85
    urethrostomy, perineal 58.0
  Porro (cesarean section) 74.99
  posterior chamber (eye) NEC 14.9
  Potts-Smith (descending aorta-left pulmononry artery anastomosis) 39.0
  Printen and Mason (high gastric bypass) 44.31
  prostate NEC (*see also* Prostatectomy) 60.69
    specified type 60.99
  pterygium 11.39
    with corneal graft 11.32
  Puestow (pancreaticojejunostomy) 52.96
  pull-through NEC 48.49
  pulmonary NEC 33.99
  push-back (cleft palate repair) 27.62
  Putti-Platt (capsulorrhaphy of shoulder for recurrent dislocation) 81.82
  pyloric exclusion 44.39
  pyriform sinus NEC 29.99
  "rabbit ear" (anterior urethropexy) (Tudor) 59.79
  Ramadier (intrapetrosal drainage) 20.22
  Ramstedt (pyloromyotomy) (with wedge resection) 43.3
  Rankin
    exteriorization of intestine 46.03
    proctectomy (complete) 48.5
  Rashkind (balloon septostomy) 35.41
  Rastelli (creation of conduit between right ventricle and pulmonary artery) 35.92
    in repair of
      pulmonary artery atresia 35.92
      transposition of great vessels 35.92
      truncus arteriosus 35.83
  Raz-Pereyra procedure (bladder neck suspension) 59.79
  rectal NEC 48.99
  rectocele NEC 70.52
  re-entry (aorta) 39.54
  renal NEC 55.99
  respiratory (tract) NEC 33.99
  retina NEC 14.9
  Ripstein (repair of rectal prolapse) 48.75
  Rodney Smith (radical subtotal pancreatectomy) 52.53
  Roux-en-Y
    bile duct 51.36
    cholecystojejunostomy 51.32
    esophagus (intrathoracic) 42.54

Operation — *continued*
  Roux-en-Y — *continued*
    pancreaticojejunostomy 52.96
  Roux-Goldthwait (repair of patellar dislocation) 81.44
  Roux-Herzen-Judine (jejunal loop interposition) 42.63
  Ruiz-Mora (proximal phalangectomy for hammer toe) 77.99
  Russe (bone graft of scaphoid) 78.04
  Saemisch (corneal section) 11.1
  salivary gland or duct NEC 26.99
  Salter (innominate osteotomy) 77.39
  Sauer-Bacon (abdominoperineal resection) 48.5
  Schanz (femoral osteotomy) 77.35
  Schauta (-Amreich) (radical vaginal hysterectomy) 68.7
  Schede (thoracoplasty) 33.34
  Scheie
    cautery of sclera 12.62
    sclerostomy 12.62
  Schlatter (total gastrectomy) 43.99
  Schroeder (endocervical excision) 67.39
  Schuchardt (nonobstetrical episiotomy) 71.09
  Schwartze (simple mastoidectomy) 20.41
  sclera NEC 12.89
  Scott
    intestinal bypass for obesity 45.93
    jejunocolostomy (bypass) 45.93
  scrotum NEC 61.99
  Seddon-Brooks (transfer of pectoralis major tendon) 83.75
  Semb (apicolysis of lung) 33.39
  seminal vesicle NEC 60.79
  Senning (correction of transposition of great vessels) 35.91
  Sever (division of soft tissue of arm) 83.19
  Sewell (heart) 36.2
  sex transformation NEC 64.5
  Sharrard (iliopsoas muscle transfer) 83.77
  shelf (hip arthroplasty) 81.40
  Shirodkar (encirclement suture, cervix) 67.59
  sigmoid NEC 46.99
  Silver (bunionectomy) 77.59
  Sistrunk (excision of thyroglossal cyst) 06.7
  Skene's gland NEC 71.8
  skin NEC 86.99
  skull NEC 02.99
  sling
    eyelid
      fascia lata, palpebral 08.36
      frontalis fascial 08.32
      levator muscle 08.33
      orbicularis muscle 08.36
      palpebral ligament, fascia lata 08.36
      tarsus muscle 08.35
    fascial (fascia lata)
      eye 08.32
      for facial weakness (trigeminal nerve paralysis) 86.81
      palpebral ligament 08.36
      tongue 25.59
    tongue (fascial) 25.59
    urethra (suprapubic) 59.4
      retropubic 59.5
      urethrovesical 59.5
  Slocum (pes anserinus transfer) 81.47
  Sluder (tonsillectomy) 28.2
  Smith (open osteotomy of mandible) 76.62
  Smith-Peterson (radiocarpal arthrodesis) 81.25
  Smithwick (sympathectomy) 05.29
  Soave (endorectal pull-through) 48.41
  soft tissue NEC 83.99
    hand 82.99
  Sonneberg (inferior maxillary neurectomy) 04.07
  Sorondo-Ferré (hindquarter amputation) 84.19
  Soutter (iliac crest fasciotomy) 83.14
  Spalding-Richardson (uterine suspension) 69.22
  spermatic cord NEC 63.99
  sphincter of Oddi NEC 51.89
  spinal (canal) (cord) (structures) NEC 03.99
  Spinelli (correction of inverted uterus) 75.93
  Spivack (permanent gastrostomy) 43.19

Operation — *continued*
  spleen NEC 41.99
  S.P. Rogers (knee disarticulation) 84.16
  Ssabanejew-Frank (permanent gastrostomy) 43.19
  Stacke (simple mastoidectomy) 20.41
  Stallard (conjunctivocystorhinostomy) 09.82
    with insertion of tube or stent 09.83
  Stamm (-Kader) (temporary gastrostomy) 43.19
  Steinberg 44.5
  Steindler
    fascia stripping (for cavus deformity) 83.14
    flexorplasty (elbow) 83.77
    muscle transfer 83.77
  sterilization NEC
    female (*see also* specific operation) 66.39
    male (*see also* Ligation, vas deferens) 63.70
  Stewart (renal plication with pyeloplasty) 55.87
  stomach NEC 44.99
  Stone (anoplasty) 49.79
  Strassman (metroplasty) 69.49
    metroplasty (Jones modification) 69.49
    uterus 68.22
  Strayer (gastrocnemius recession) 83.72
  stress incontinence — *see* Repair, stress incontinence
  Stromeyer-Little (hepatotomy) 50.0
  Strong (unbridling of celiac artery axis) 39.91
  Sturmdorf (conization of cervix) 67.2
  subcutaneous tissue NEC 86.99
  sublingual gland or duct NEC 26.99
  submaxillary gland or duct NEC 26.99
  Summerskill (dacryocystorhinostomy by intubation) 09.81
  Surmay (jejunostomy) 46.39
  Swenson
    bladder reconstruction 57.87
    proctectomy 48.49
  Swinney (urethral reconstruction) 58.46
  Syme
    ankle amputation through malleoli of tibia and fibula 84.14
    urethrotomy, external 58.0
  sympathetic nerve NEC 05.89
  Taarnhoj (trigeminal nerve root decompression) 04.41
  Tack (sacculotomy) 20.79
  Talma-Morison (omentopexy) 54.74
  Tanner (devascularization of stomach) 44.99
  TAPVC NEC 35.82
  tarsus NEC 08.99
    muscle sling 08.35
  tendon NEC 83.99
    extraocular NEC 15.9
    hand NEC 82.99
  testis NEC 62.99
  tetralogy of Fallot
    partial repair — *see* specific procedure
    total (one-stage) 35.81
  Thal (repair of esophageal stricture) 42.85
  thalamus 01.41
    by stereotactic radiosurgery 92.32
      cobalt 60 92.32
      linear accelerator (LINAC) 92.31
      multi-source 92.32
      particle beam 92.33
      particulate 92.33
      radiosurgery NEC 92.39
      single source photon 92.31
  Thiersch
    anus 49.79
    skin graft 86.69
      hand 86.62
  Thompson
    cleft lip repair 27.54
    correction of lymphedema 40.9
    quadricepsplasty 83.86
    thumb apposition with bone graft 82.69
  thoracic duct NEC 40.69
  thorax NEC 34.99
  Thorek (partial cholecystectomy) 51.21
  three-snip, punctum 09.51
  thymus NEC 07.99
  thyroid gland NEC 06.98
  TKP (thermokeratoplasty) 11.74
  Tomkins (metroplasty) 69.49

Operation

Operation — *continued*
  tongue NEC 25.99
    flap, palate 27.62
    tie 25.91
  tonsil NEC 28.99
  Torek (-Bevan) (orchidopexy) (first stage) (second stage) 62.5
  Torkildsen (ventriculocisternal shunt) 02.2
  Torpin (cul-de-sac resection) 70.92
  Toti (dacryocystorhinostomy) 09.81
  Touchas 86.83
  Touroff (ligation of subclavian artery) 38.85
  trabeculae corneae cordis (heart) NEC 35.35
  trachea NEC 31.99
  Trauner (lingual sulcus extension) 24.91
  truncus arteriosus NEC 35.83
  Tsuge (macrodactyly repair) 82.83
  Tudor "rabbit ear" (anterior urethropexy) 59.79
  Tuffier
    apicolysis of lung 33.39
    vaginal hysterectomy 68.59
      laparoscopically assisted (LAVH) 68.51
  tunica vaginalis NEC 61.99
  Turco (release of joint capsules in clubfoot) 80.48
  Uchida (tubal ligation with or without fimbriectomy) 66.32
  umbilicus NEC 54.99
  urachus NEC 57.51
  Urban (mastectomy) (unilateral) 85.47
    bilateral 85.48
  ureter NEC 56.99
  urethra NEC 58.99
  urinary system NEC 59.99
  uterus NEC 69.99
    supporting structures NEC 69.98
  uvula NEC 27.79
  vagina NEC 70.91
  vascular NEC 39.99
  vas deferens NFC 63.99
    ligation NEC 63.71
  vein NEC 39.99
  vena cava sieve 38.7
  vertebra NEC 78.49
  vesical (bladder) NEC 57.99
  vessel NEC 39.99
    cardiac NEC 36.99
  Vicq d'Azyr (larynx) 31.1
  Vidal (varicocele ligation) 63.1
  Vineberg (implantation of mammary artery into ventricle) 36.2
  vitreous NEC 14.79
  vocal cord NEC 31.98
  von Kraske (proctectomy) 48.64
  Voss (hanging hip operation) 83.19
  Vulpius (-Compere) (lengthening of gastrocnemius muscle) 83.85
  vulva NEC 71.8
  Ward-Mayo (vaginal hysterectomy) 68.59
    laparoscopically assisted (LAVH) 68.51
  Wardill (cleft palate) 27.62
  Waters (extraperitoneal cesarean section) 74.2
  Waterston (aorta-right pulmonary artery anastomosis) 39.0
  Watkins (-Wertheim) (uterus interposition) 69.21
  Watson-Jones
    hip arthrodesis 81.21
    reconstruction of lateral ligaments, ankle 81.49
    shoulder arthrodesis (extra-articular) 81.23
    tenoplasty 83.88
  Weir
    appendicostomy 47.91
    correction of nostrils 21.86
  Wertheim (radical hysterectomy) 68.6
  West (dacryocystorhinostomy) 09.81
  Wheeler
    entropion repair 08.44
    halving procedure (eyelid) 08.24
  Whipple (radical pancreaticoduodenectomy) 52.7
    Child modification (radical subtotal pancreatectomy) 52.53
    Rodney Smith modification (radical subtotal pancreatectomy) 52.53

Operation — *continued*
  White (lengthening of tendo calcaneus by incomplete tenotomy) 83.11
  Whitehead
    glossectomy, radical 25.4
    hemorrhoidectomy 49.46
  Whitman
    foot stabilization (talectomy) 77.98
    hip reconstruction 81.40
    repair of serratus anterior muscle 83.87
    talectomy 77.98
    trochanter wedge osteotomy 77.25
  Wier (entropion repair) 08.44
  Williams-Richardson (vaginal construction) 70.61
  Wilms (thoracoplasty) 33.34
  Wilson (angulation osteotomy for hallux valgus) 77.51
  window
    antrum (nasal sinus) — *see* Antrotomy, maxillary
    aorticopulmonary 39.59
    bone cortex (*see also* Incision, bone) 77.10
      facial 76.09
    nasoantral — *see* Antrotomy, maxillary
    pericardium 37.12
    pleural 34.09
  Winiwarter (cholecystoenterostomy) 51.32
  Witzel (temporary gastrostomy) 43.19
  Woodward (release of high riding scapula) 81.83
  Young
    epispadias repair 58.45
    tendon transfer (anterior tibialis) (repair of flat foot) 83.75
  Yount (division of iliotibial band) 83.14
  Zancolli
    capsuloplasty 81.72
    tendon transfer (biceps) 82.56
  Ziegler (iridectomy) 12.14
Operculectomy 24.6
Ophthalmectomy 16.49
  with implant (into Tenon's capsule) 16.42
    with attachment of muscles 16.41
Ophthalmoscopy 16.21
Opponensplasty (hand) 82.56
Orbitomaxillectomy, radical 16.51
Orbitotomy (anterior) (frontal) (temporofrontal) (transfrontal) NEC 16.09
  with
    bone flap 16.01
    insertion of implant 16.02
  Kroenlein (lateral) 16.01
  lateral 16.01
Orchidectomy (with epididymectomy) (unilateral) 62.3
  bilateral (radical) 62.41
  remaining or solitary testis 62.42
Orchidopexy 62.5
Orchidoplasty 62.69
Orchidorrhaphy 62.61
Orchidotomy 62.0
Orchiectomy (with epididymectomy) (unilateral) 62.3
  bilateral (radical) 62.41
  remaining or solitary testis 62.42
Orchiopexy 62.5
Orchioplasty 62.69
Orthoroentgenography — *see* Radiography
Oscar Miller operation (midtarsal arthrodesis) 81.14
Osmond-Clark operation (soft tissue release with peroneus brevis tendon transfer) 83.75
Ossiculectomy NEC 19.3
  with
    stapedectomy (*see also* Stapedectomy) 19.19
    stapes mobilization 19.0
    tympanoplasty 19.53
      revision 19.6
Ossiculotomy NEC 19.3

Ostectomy (partial), except facial — *see also* category 77.8
  facial NEC 76.39
    total 76.45
      with reconstruction 76.44
  first metatarsal head — *see* Bunionectomy
  for graft (autograft) (homograft) — *see also* category 77.7
  mandible 76.31
    total 76.42
      with reconstruction 76.41
  total, except facial — *see also* category 77.9
    facial NEC 76.45
      with reconstruction 76.44
    mandible 76.42
      with reconstruction 76.41
Osteoarthrotomy (*see also* Osteotomy) 77.30
Osteoclasis 78.70
  carpal, metacarpal 78.74
  clavicle 78.71
  ear 20.79
  femur 78.75
  fibula 78.77
  humerus 78.72
  patella 78.76
  pelvic 78.79
  phalanges (foot) (hand) 78.79
  radius 78.73
  scapula 78.71
  specified site NEC 78.79
  tarsal, metatarsal 78.78
  thorax (ribs) (sternum) 78.71
  tibia 78.77
  ulna 78.73
  vertebrae 78.79
Osteolysis — *see* category 78.4
Osteopathic manipulation (*see also* Manipulation, osteopathic) 93.67
Osteoplasty NEC — *see* category 78.4
  with bone graft — *see* Graft, bone
  for
    bone lengthening — *see* Lengthening, bone
    bone shortening — *see* Shortening, bone
    repair of malunion or nonunion of fracture — *see* Repair, fracture, malunion or nonunion
  carpal, metacarpal 78.44
  clavicle 78.41
  cranium NEC 02.06
    with
      flap (bone) 02.03
      graft (bone) 02.04
  facial bone NEC 76.69
  femur 78.45
  fibula 78.47
  humerus 78.42
  mandible, mandibular NEC 76.64
    body 76.63
    ramus (open) 76.62
      closed 76.61
  maxilla (segmental) 76.65
    total 76.66
  nasal bones 21.89
  patella 78.46
  pelvic 78.49
  phalanges (foot) (hand) 78.49
  radius 78.43
  scapula 78.41
  skull NEC 02.06
    with
      flap (bone) 02.03
      graft (bone) 02.04
  specified site NEC 78.49
  tarsal, metatarsal 78.48
  thorax (ribs) (sternum) 78.41
  tibia 78.47
  ulna 78.43
  vertebrae 78.49
Osteorrhaphy (*see also* Osteoplasty) 78.40
Osteosynthesis (fracture) — *see* Reduction, fracture
Osteotomy (adduction) (angulation) (block) (derotational) (displacement) (partial) (rotational) 77.30

Osteotomy — *continued*
  carpals, metacarpals 77.34
    wedge 77.24
  clavicle 77.31
    wedge 77.21
  facial bone NEC 76.69
  femur 77.35
    wedge 77.25
  fibula 77.37
    wedge 77.27
  humerus 77.32
    wedge 77.22
  mandible (segmental) (subapical) 76.64
    angle (open) 76.62
      closed 76.61
    body 76.63
    Gigli saw 76.61
    ramus (open) 76.62
      closed 76.61
  maxilla (segmental) 76.65
    total 76.66
  metatarsal 77.38
    wedge 77.28
      for hallux valgus repair 77.51
  patella 77.36
    wedge 77.26
  pelvic 77.39
    wedge 77.29
  phalanges (foot) (hand) 77.39
    for repair of
      bunion — *see* Bunionectomy
      bunionette 77.54
      hallux valgus — *see* Bunionectomy
    wedge 77.29
      for repair of
        bunion — *see* Bunionectomy
        bunionette 77.54
        hallux valgus — *see* Bunionectomy
  radius 77.33
    wedge 77.23
  scapula 77.31
    wedge 77.21
  specified site NEC 77.39
    wedge 77.29
  tarsal 77.38
    wedge 77.28
  thorax (ribs) (sternum) 77.31
    wedge 77.21
  tibia 77.37
    wedge 77.27
  toe 77.39
    for repair of
      bunion — *see* Bunionectomy
      bunionette 77.54
      hallux valgus — *see* Bunionectomy
    wedge 77.29
      for repair of
        bunion — *see* Bunionectomy
        bunionette 77.54
        hallux valgus — *see* Bunionectomy
  ulna 77.33
    wedge 77.23
  vertebrae 77.39
    wedge 77.29
Otonecrectomy (inner ear) 20.79
Otoplasty (external) 18.79
  auditory canal or meatus 18.6
  auricle 18.79
  cartilage 18.79
    reconstruction 18.71
  prominent or protruding 18.5
Otoscopy 18.11
Outfolding, sclera, for buckling (*see also* Buckling, scleral) 14.49
Outfracture, turbinates (nasal) 21.62
Output and clearance, circulatory 92.05
Overdistension, bladder (therapeutic) 96.25
Overlapping, sclera, for buckling (*see also* Buckling, scleral) 14.49
Oversewing
  pleural bleb 32.21
  ulcer crater (peptic) 44.40
    duodenum 44.42
    stomach 44.41

Oxford operation (for urinary incontinence) 59.4
Oximetry
  fetal pulse 75.38
Oxygenation 93.96
  extracorporeal membrane (ECMO) 39.65
  hyperbaric 93.95
  wound 93.59
Oxygen therapy (catalytic) (pump) 93.96
  hyperbaric 93.95

P

Pacemaker
  cardiac — *see also* Insertion, pacemaker, cardiac
    intraoperative (temporary) 39.64
    temporary (during and immediately following cardiac surgery) 39.64
Packing — *see also* Insertion, pack
  auditory canal 96.11
  nose, for epistaxis (anterior) 21.01
    posterior (and anterior) 21.02
  rectal 96.19
  sella turcica 07.79
  vaginal 96.14
Palatoplasty 27.69
  for cleft palate 27.62
    secondary or subsequent 27.63
Palatorrhaphy 27.61
  for cleft palate 27.62
Pallidectomy 01.42
Pallidoansotomy 01.42
Pallidotomy 01.42
  by stereotactic radiosurgery 92.32
    cobalt 60 92.32
    linear accelerator (LINAC) 92.31
    multi-source 92.32
    particle beam 92.33
    particulate 92.33
    radiosurgery NEC 92.39
    single source photon 92.31
Panas operation (linear proctotomy) 48.0
Pancoast operation (division of trigeminal nerve at foramen ovale) 04.02
Pancreatectomy (total) (with synchronous duodenectomy) 52.6
  partial NEC 52.59
    distal (tail) (with part of body) 52.52
    proximal (head) (with part of body) (with synchronous duodenectomy) 52.51
    radical 52.53
      subtotal 52.53
  radical 52.7
    subtotal 52.53
Pancreaticocystoduodenostomy 52.4
Pancreaticocystoenterostomy 52.4
Pancreaticocystogastrostomy 52.4
Pancreaticocystojejunostomy 52.4
Pancreaticoduodenectomy (total) 52.6
  partial NEC 52.59
    proximal 52.51
    radical subtotal 52.53
    radical (one-stage) (two-stage) 52.7
    subtotal 52.53
Pancreaticoduodenostomy 52.96
Pancreaticoenterostomy 52.96
Pancreaticogastrostomy 52.96
Pancreaticoileostomy 52.96
Pancreaticojejunostomy 52.96
Pancreatoduodenectomy (total) 52.6
  partial NEC 52.59
  radical (one-stage) (two-stage) 52.7
    subtotal 52.53
Pancreatogram 87.66
  endoscopic retrograde (ERP) 52.13
Pancreatolithotomy 52.09
  endoscopic 52.94
Pancreatotomy 52.09

Pancreolithotomy 52.09
  endoscopic 52.94
Panendoscopy 57.32
  specified site, other than bladder — *see* Endoscopy, by site
  through artificial stoma 57.31
Panhysterectomy (abdominal) 68.4
  vaginal 68.59
    laparoscopically assisted (LAVH) 68.51
Panniculectomy 86.83
Panniculotomy 86.83
Pantaloon operation (revision of gastric anastomosis) 44.5
Papillectomy, anal 49.39
  endoscopic 49.31
Papillotomy (pancreas) 51.82
  endoscopic 51.85
Paquin operation (ureteroneocystostomy) 56.74
Paracentesis
  abdominal (percutaneous) 54.91
  anterior chamber, eye 12.91
  bladder 57.11
  cornea 12.91
  eye (anterior chamber) 12.91
  thoracic, thoracis 34.91
  tympanum 20.09
    with intubation 20.01
Parasitology — *see* Examination, microscopic
Parathyroidectomy (partial) (subtotal) NEC 06.89
  complete 06.81
  ectopic 06.89
  global removal 06.81
  mediastinal 06.89
  total 06.81
Parenteral nutrition, total 99.15
  peripheral 99.15
Parotidectomy 26.30
  complete 26.32
  partial 26.31
  radical 26.32
Partsch operation (marsupialization of dental cyst) 24.4
Passage — *see* Insertion and Intubation
Passage of sounds, urethra 58.6
Patch
  blood, spinal (epidural) 03.95
  graft — *see* Graft
  spinal, blood (epidural) 03.95
  subdural, brain 02.12
Patellapexy 78.46
Patellaplasty NEC 78.46
Patellectomy 77.96
  partial 77.86
Pattee operation (auditory canal) 18.6
Pectenotomy (*see also* Sphincterotomy, anal) 49.59
Pedicle flap — *see* Graft, skin, pedicle
Peet operation (splanchnic resection) 05.29
PEG (percutaneous endoscopic gastrostomy) 43.11
PEJ (percutaneous endoscopic jejunostomy) 46.32
Pelvectomy, kidney (partial) 55.4
Pelvimetry 88.25
  gynecological 89.26
Pelviolithotomy 55.11
Pelvioplasty, kidney 55.87
Pelviostomy 55.12
  closure 55.82
Pelviotomy 77.39
  to assist delivery 73.94
Pelvi-ureteroplasty 55.87
Pemberton operation
  osteotomy of ilium 77.39
  rectum (mobilization and fixation for prolapse repair) 48.76
Penectomy 64.3
Pereyra operation (paraurethral suspension) 59.6
Perforation
  stapes footplate 19.0

Perfusion NEC 39.97
- carotid artery 39.97
- coronary artery 39.97
- for
  - chemotherapy NEC 99.25
  - hormone therapy NEC 99.24
- head 39.97
- hyperthermic (lymphatic), localized region or site 93.35
- intestine (large) (local) 46.96
  - small 46.95
- kidney, local 55.95
- limb (lower) (upper) 39.97
- liver, localized 50.93
- neck 39.97
- subarachnoid (spinal cord) (refrigerated saline) 03.92
- total body 39.96

Pericardiectomy 37.31
Pericardiocentesis 37.0
Pericardiolysis 37.12
Pericardioplasty 37.4
Pericardiorrhaphy 37.4
Pericardiostomy (tube) 37.12
Pericardiotomy 37.12
Peridectomy 10.31
Perilimbal suction 89.11
Perimetry 95.05
Perineoplasty 71.79
Perineorrhaphy 71.71
- obstetrical laceration (current) 75.69

Perineotomy (nonobstetrical) 71.09
- to assist delivery — see Episiotomy

Periosteotomy (see also Incision, bone) 77.10
- facial bone 76.09

Perirectofistulectomy 48.93
Peritectomy 10.31
Peritomy 10.1
Peritoneocentesis 54.91
Peritoneoscopy 54.21
Peritoneotomy 54.19
Peritoneumectomy 54.4
Phacoemulsification (ultrasonic) (with aspiration) 13.41
Phacofragmentation (mechanical) (with aspiration) 13.43
- posterior route 13.42
- ultrasonic 13.41

Phalangectomy (partial) 77.89
- claw toe 77.57
- cockup toe 77.58
- hammer toe 77.56
- overlapping toe 77.58
- total 77.99

Phalangization (fifth metacarpal) 82.81
Pharyngeal flap operation (cleft palate repair) 27.62
- secondary or subsequent 27.63

Pharyngectomy (partial) 29.33
- with laryngectomy 30.3

Pharyngogram 87.09
- contrast 87.06

Pharyngolaryngectomy 30.3
Pharyngoplasty (with silastic implant) 29.4
- for cleft palate 27.62
  - secondary or subsequent 27.63

Pharyngorrhaphy 29.51
- for cleft palate 27.62

Pharyngoscopy 29.11
Pharyngotomy 29.0
Phenopeel (skin) 86.24
Phlebectomy 38.4 ✓4ᵗʰ
- with
  - anastomosis 38.30
    - abdominal 38.37
    - head and neck NEC 38.32
    - intracranial NEC 38.31
    - lower limb 38.39
    - thoracic NEC 38.35

Phlebectomy — continued
- with — continued
  - anastomosis — continued
    - upper limb 38.33
  - graft replacement 38.4 ✓4ᵗʰ
    - abdominal 38.47
    - head and neck NEC 38.42
    - intracranial NEC 38.41
    - lower limb 38.49
    - thoracic NEC 38.45
    - upper limb 38.43
- abdominal 38.67
- head and neck NEC 38.62
- intracranial NEC 38.61
- lower limb 38.69
- thoracic NEC 38.65
- upper limb 38.63
- varicose 38.50
  - abdominal 38.57
  - head and neck NEC 38.52
  - intracranial NEC 38.51
  - lower limb 38.59
  - thoracic NEC 38.55
  - upper limb 38.53

Phlebogoniostomy 12.52
Phlebography (contrast) (retrograde) 88.60
- by radioisotope — see Scan, radioisotope, by site
- adrenal 88.65
- femoral 88.66
- head 88.61
- hepatic 88.64
- impedance 88.68
- intra-abdominal NEC 88.65
- intrathoracic NEC 88.63
- lower extremity NEC 88.66
- neck 88.61
- portal system 88.64
- pulmonary 88.62
- specified site NEC 88.67
- vena cava (inferior) (superior) 88.51

Phleborrhaphy 39.32
Phlebotomy 38.99
Phonocardiogram, with ECG lead 89.55
Photochemotherapy NEC 99.83
- extracorporeal 99.88

Photocoagulation
- ciliary body 12.73
- eye, eyeball 16.99
- iris 12.41
- macular hole — see Photocoagulation, retina
- orbital lesion 16.92
- retina
  - for
    - destruction of lesion 14.25
    - reattachment 14.55
    - repair of tear or defect 14.35
  - laser (beam)
    - for
      - destruction of lesion 14.24
      - reattachment 14.54
      - repair of tear or defect 14.34
  - xenon arc
    - for
      - destruction of lesion 14.23
      - reattachment 14.53
      - repair of tear or defect 14.33

Photography 89.39
- fundus 95.11

Photopheresis, therapeutic 99.88
Phototherapy NEC 99.83
- newborn 99.83
- ultraviolet 99.82

Phrenemphraxis 04.03
- for collapse of lung 33.31

Phrenicectomy 04.03
- for collapse of lung 33.31

Phrenicoexeresis 04.03
- for collapse of lung 33.31

Phrenicotomy 04.03
- for collapse of lung 33.31

Phrenicotripsy 04.03
- for collapse of lung 33.31

Phrenoplasty 34.84
Physical medicine — see Therapy, physical
Physical therapy — see Therapy, physical
Physiotherapy, chest 93.99
PICC (peripherally inserted central catheter) 38.93
Piercing ear, external (pinna) 18.01
Pigmenting, skin 86.02
Pilojection (aneurysm) (Gallagher) 39.52
Pinealectomy (complete) (total) 07.54
- partial 07.53

Pinealotomy (with drainage) 07.52
Pinning
- bone — see Fixation, bone, internal
- ear 18.5

Pinsker operation (obliteration of nasoseptal telangiectasia) 21.07
Piper operation (forceps) 72.6
Pirogoff operation (ankle amputation through malleoli of tibia and fibula) 84.14
Pituitectomy (complete) (total) (see also Hypophysectomy) 07.69
Placentogram, placentography 88.46
- with radioisotope (RISA) 92.17

Planing, skin 86.25
Plantation, tooth (bud) (germ) 23.5
- prosthetic 23.6

Plasma exchange 99.07
Plasmapheresis, therapeutic 99.71
Plastic repair — see Repair, by site
Plasty — see also Repair, by site
- bladder neck (V-Y) 57.85
- skin (without graft) 86.89
- subcutaneous tissue 86.89

Platelet inhibitor (GP IIb/IIIa inhibitor only), infusion 99.20
Plateletpheresis, therapeutic 99.74
Play
- psychotherapy 94.36
- therapy 93.81

Pleating
- eye muscle 15.22
  - multiple (two or more muscles) 15.4
- sclera, for buckling (see also Buckling, scleral) 14.49

Plethysmogram (carotid) 89.58
- air-filled (pneumatic) 89.58
- capacitance 89.58
- cerebral 89.58
- differential 89.58
- oculoplethysmogram 89.58
- penile 89.58
- photoelectric 89.58
- regional 89.58
- respiratory function measurement (body) 89.38
- segmental 89.58
- strain-gauge 89.58
- thoracic impedance 89.38
- venous occlusion 89.58
- water-filled 89.58

Plethysmography
- penile 89.58

Pleurectomy NEC 34.59
Pleurocentesis 34.91
Pleurodesis 34.6
- chemical 34.92
  - with cancer chemotherapy substance 34.92 [99.25]
  - tetracycline 34.92 [99.21]

Pleurolysis (for collapse of lung) 33.39
Pleuropexy 34.99
Pleurosclerosis 34.6
- chemical 34.92
  - with cancer chemotherapy substance 34.92 [99.25]
  - tetracycline 34.92 [99.21]

Pleurotomy 34.09
Plexectomy
- choroid 02.14
- hypogastric 05.24

Index to Procedures

Plication
 aneurysm
  heart 37.32
 annulus, heart valve 35.33
 bleb (emphysematous), lung 32.21
 broad ligament 69.22
 diaphragm (for hernia repair) (thoracic approach) (thoracoabdominal approach) 53.81
 eye muscle (oblique) (rectus) 15.22
  multiple (two or more muscles) 15.4
 fascia 83.89
  hand 82.89
 inferior vena cava 38.7
 intestine (jejunum) (Noble) 46.62
 Kelly (-Stoeckel) (urethrovesical junction) 59.3
 levator, for blepharoptosis 08.34
 ligament (see also Arthroplasty) 81.96
  broad 69.22
  round 69.22
  uterosacral 69.22
 mesentery 54.75
 round ligament 69.22
 sphincter, urinary bladder 57.85
 stomach 44.69
 superior vena cava 38.7
 tendon 83.85
  hand 82.55
 tricuspid valve (with repositioning) 35.14
 ureter 56.89
 urethra 58.49
 urethrovesical junction 59.3
 vein (peripheral) 39.59
 vena cava (inferior) (superior) 38.7
 ventricle (heart)
  aneurysm 37.32
Plicotomy, tympanum 20.23
Plombage, lung 33.39
Pneumocentesis 33.93
Pneumocisternogram 87.02
Pneumoencephalogram 87.01
Pneumogram, pneumography
 extraperitoneal 88.15
 mediastinal 87.33
 orbit 87.14
 pelvic 88.13
 peritoneum NEC 88.13
 presacral 88.15
 retroperitoneum 88.15
Pneumogynecography 87.82
Pneumomediastinography 87.33
Pneumonectomy (complete) (extended) (radical) (standard) (total) (with mediastinal dissection) 32.5
 partial
  complete excision, one lobe 32.4
  resection (wedge), one lobe 32.3
Pneumonolysis (for collapse of lung) 33.39
Pneumonotomy (with exploration) 33.1
Pneumoperitoneum (surgically-induced) 54.96
 for collapse of lung 33.33
 pelvic 88.12
Pneumothorax (artificial) (surgical) 33.32
 intrapleural 33.32
Pneumoventriculogram 87.02
Politano-Leadbetter operation (ureteroneocystostomy) 56.74
Politerization, Eustachian tube 20.8
Pollicization (with carry over of nerves and blood supply) 82.61
Polya operation (gastrectomy) 43.7
Polypectomy — see also Excision, lesion, by site
 esophageal 42.32
  endoscopic 42.33
 gastric (endoscopic) 43.41
 large intestine (colon) 45.42
 nasal 21.31
 rectum (endoscopic) 48.36
Polysomnogram 89.17
Pomeroy operation (ligation and division of fallopian tubes) 66.32

Poncet operation
 lengthening of Achilles tendon 83.85
 urethrostomy, perineal 58.0
Porro operation (cesarean section) 74.99
Portoenterostomy (Kasai) 51.37
Positrocephalogram 92.11
Positron emission tomography (PET) — see Scan, radioisotope
Postmortem examination 89.8
Potts-Smith operation (descending aorta-left pulmonary artery anastomosis) 39.0
Poudrage
 intrapericardial 36.39
 pleural 34.6
PPN (peripheral parenteral nutrition) 99.15
Preparation (cutting), pedicle (flap) graft 86.71
Preputiotomy 64.91
Prescription for glasses 95.31
Pressure support
 ventilation [PSV] — see category 96.7
Printen and Mason operation (high gastric bypass) 44.31
Probing
 canaliculus, lacrimal (with irrigation) 09.42
 lacrimal
  canaliculi 09.42
  punctum (with irrigation) 09.41
 nasolacrimal duct (with irrigation) 09.43
  with insertion of tube or stent 09.44
 salivary duct (for dilation of duct) (for removal of calculus) 26.91
  with incision 26.0
Procedure — see also specific procedure
 diagnostic NEC
  abdomen (region) 54.29
  adenoid 28.19
  adrenal gland 07.19
  alveolus 24.19
  amnion 75.35
  anterior chamber, eye 12.29
  anus 49.29
  appendix 45.28
  biliary tract 51.19
  bladder 57.39
  blood vessel (any site) 38.29
  bone 78.80
   carpal, metacarpal 78.84
   clavicle 78.81
   facial 76.19
   femur 78.85
   fibula 78.87
   humerus 78.82
   marrow 41.38
   patella 78.86
   pelvic 78.89
   phalanges (foot) (hand) 78.89
   radius 78.83
   scapula 78.81
   specified site NEC 78.89
   tarsal, metatarsal 78.88
   thorax (ribs) (sternum) 78.81
   tibia 78.87
   ulna 78.83
   vertebrae 78.89
  brain 01.18
  breast 85.19
  bronchus 33.29
  buccal 27.24
  bursa 83.29
  canthus 08.19
  cecum 45.28
  cerebral meninges 01.18
  cervix 67.19
  chest wall 34.28
  choroid 14.19
  ciliary body 12.29
  clitoris 71.19
  colon 45.28
  conjunctiva 10.29
  cornea 11.29
  cul-de-sac 70.29
  dental 24.19
  diaphragm 34.28

Procedure — see also specific procedure — continued
 diagnostic NEC — continued
  duodenum 45.19
  ear
   external 18.19
   inner and middle 20.39
  epididymis 63.09
  esophagus 42.29
  Eustachian tube 20.39
  extraocular muscle or tendon 15.09
  eye 16.29
   anterior chamber 12.29
   posterior chamber 14.19
  eyeball 16.29
  eyelid 08.19
  fallopian tube 66.19
  fascia (any site) 83.29
  fetus 75.35
  gallbladder 51.19
  ganglion (cranial) (peripheral) 04.19
   sympathetic 05.19
  gastric 44.19
  globus pallidus 01.18
  gum 24.19
  heart 37.29
  hepatic 50.19
  hypophysis 07.19
  ileum 45.19
  intestine 45.29
   large 45.28
   small 45.19
  iris 12.29
  jejunum 45.19
  joint (capsule) (ligament) (structure) NEC 81.98
   facial 76.19
  kidney 55.29
  labia 71.19
  lacrimal (system) 09.19
  large intestine 45.28
  larynx 31.48
  ligament 81.98
   uterine 68.19
  liver 50.19
  lung 33.29
  lymphatic structure (channel) (gland) (node) (vessel) 40.19
  mediastinum 34.29
  meninges (cerebral) 01.18
   spinal 03.39
  mouth 27.29
  muscle 83.29
   extraocular (oblique) (rectus) 15.09
   papillary (heart) 37.29
  nail 86.19
  nasopharynx 29.19
  nerve (cranial) (peripheral) NEC 04.19
   sympathetic 05.19
  nipple 85.19
  nose, nasal 21.29
   sinus 22.19
  ocular 16.29
   muscle 15.09
  omentum 54.29
  ophthalmologic 16.29
  oral (cavity) 27.29
  orbit 16.29
  orthodontic 24.19
  ovary 65.19
   laparoscopic 65.14
  palate 27.29
  pancreas 52.19
  papillary muscle (heart) 37.29
  parathyroid gland 06.19
  penis 64.19
  perianal tissue 49.29
  pericardium 37.29
  periprostatic tissue 60.18
  perirectal tissue 48.29
  perirenal tissue 59.29
  peritoneum 54.29
  periurethral tissue 58.29
  perivesical tissue 59.29
  pharynx 29.19
  pineal gland 07.19

Procedure

Procedure — see also specific procedure — continued
  diagnostic NEC — continued
    pituitary gland 07.19
    pleura 34.28
    posterior chamber, eye 14.19
    prostate 60.18
    pulmonary 33.29
    rectosigmoid 48.29
    rectum 48.29
    renal 55.29
    respiratory 33.29
    retina 14.19
    retroperitoneum 59.29
    salivary gland or duct 26.19
    sclera 12.29
    scrotum 61.19
    seminal vesicle 60.19
    sigmoid 45.28
    sinus, nasal 22.19
    skin 86.19
    skull 01.19
    soft tissue 83.29
    spermatic cord 63.09
    sphincter of Oddi 51.19
    spine, spinal (canal) (cord) (meninges) (structure) 03.39
    spleen 41.39
    stomach 44.19
    subcutaneous tissue 86.19
    sympathetic nerve 05.19
    tarsus 09.19
    tendon NEC 83.29
      extraocular 15.09
    testicle 62.19
    thalamus 01.18
    thoracic duct 40.19
    thorax 34.28
    thymus 07.19
    thyroid gland 06.19
    tongue 25.09
    tonsils 28.19
    tooth 24.19
    trachea 31.49
    tunica vaginalis 61.19
    ureter 56.39
    urethra 58.29
    uterus and supporting structures 68.19
    uvula 27.29
    vagina 70.29
    vas deferens 63.09
    vesical 57.39
    vessel (blood) (any site) 38.2
    vitreous 14.19
    vulva 71.19
  fistulizing, sclera NEC 12.69
  miscellaneous (nonoperative) NEC 99.99
  respiratory (nonoperative) NEC 93.99
  surgical — see Operation

Proctectasis 96.22
Proctectomy (partial) (see also Resection, rectum) 48.69
  abdominoperineal 48.5
  complete (Miles) (Rankin) 48.5
  pull-through 48.49
Proctoclysis 96.37
Proctolysis 48.99
Proctopexy (Delorme) 48.76
  abdominal (Ripstein) 48.75
Proctoplasty 48.79
Proctorrhaphy 48.71
Proctoscopy 48.23
  with biopsy 48.24
  through stoma (artificial) 48.22
  transabdominal approach 48.21
Proctosigmoidectomy (see also Resection, rectum) 48.69
Proctosigmoidopexy 48.76
Proctosigmoidoscopy (rigid) 48.23
  with biopsy 48.24
  flexible 45.24
  through stoma (artificial) 48.22
  transabdominal approach 48.21

Proctostomy 48.1
Proctotomy (decompression) (linear) 48.0
Production — see also Formation and Creation
  atrial septal defect 35.42
  subcutaneous tunnel for esophageal anastomosis 42.86
    with anastomosis — see Anastomosis, esophagus, antesternal
Prognathic recession 76.64
Prophylaxis, dental (scaling) (polishing) 96.54
Prostatectomy (complete) (partial) NEC 60.69
  loop 60.29
  perineal 60.62
  radical (any approach) 60.5
  retropubic (punch) (transcapsular) 60.4
  suprapubic (punch) (transvesical) 60.3
  transcapsular NEC 60.69
    retropubic 60.4
  transperineal 60.62
  transurethral 60.29
    ablation (contact) (noncontact) by laser 60.21
    electrovaporization 60.29
    enucleative 60.29
    resection of prostate (TURP) 60.29
    ultrasound guided laser induced (TULIP) 60.21
  transvesical punch (suprapubic) 60.3
Prostatocystotomy 60.0
Prostatolithotomy 60.0
Prostatotomy (perineal) 60.0
Prostatovesiculectomy 60.5
Protection (of)
  individual from his surroundings 99.84
  surroundings from individual 99.84
Psychoanalysis 94.31
Psychodrama 94.43
Psychotherapy NEC 94.39
  biofeedback 94.39
  exploratory verbal 94.37
  group 94.44
    for psychosexual dysfunctions 94.41
  play 94.36
  psychosexual dysfunctions 94.34
  supportive verbal 94.38
PTCA (percutaneous transluminal coronary angioplasty) — see Angioplasty, balloon, coronary
Ptyalectasis 26.91
Ptyalithotomy 26.0
Ptyalolithotomy 26.0
Pubiotomy 77.39
  assisting delivery 73.94
Pubococcygeoplasty 59.71
Puestow operation (pancreaticojejunostomy) 52.96
Pull-through
  abdomino-anal 48.49
  abdominoperineal 48.49
    Duhamel type 48.65
  endorectal 48.41
Pulmowrap 93.99
Pulpectomy (see also Therapy, root canal) 23.70
Pulpotomy (see also Therapy, root canal) 23.70
Pump-oxygenator, for extracorporeal circulation 39.61
  percutaneous 39.66
Punch
  operation
    bladder neck, transurethral 57.49
    prostate — see Prostatectomy
  resection, vocal cords 30.22
Puncture
  antrum (nasal) (bilateral) (unilateral) 22.01
  artery NEC 38.98
    for
      arteriography (see also Arteriography) 88.40
      coronary arteriography (see also Arteriography, coronary) 88.57
    percutanous vascular closure — omit code

Puncture — continued
  bladder, suprapubic (for drainage) NEC 57.18
    needle 57.11
    percutaneous (suprapubic) 57.17
  bursa 83.94
    hand 82.92
  cisternal 01.01
    with contrast media 87.02
  cranial 01.09
    with contrast media 87.02
  craniobuccal pouch 07.72
  craniopharyngioma 07.72
  fallopian tube 66.91
  fontanel, anterior 01.09
  heart 37.0
    for intracardiac injection 37.92
  hypophysis 07.72
  iris 12.12
  joint 81.91
  kidney (percutaneous) 55.92
  larynx 31.98
  lumbar (diagnostic) (removal of dye) 03.31
  lung (for aspiration) 33.93
  nasal sinus 22.01
  pericardium 37.0
  pituitary gland 07.72
  pleural cavity 34.91
  Rathke's pouch 07.72
  spinal 03.31
  spleen 41.1
    for biopsy 41.32
  sternal (for bone marrow biopsy) 41.31
    donor for bone marrow transplant 41.91
  vein NEC 38.99
    for
      phlebography (see also Phlebography) 88.60
      transfusion — see Transfusion
  ventricular shunt tubing 01.02
Pupillotomy 12.35
Push-back operation (cleft palate repair) 27.62
Putti-Platt operation (capsulorrhaphy of shoulder for recurrent dislocation) 81.82
Pyelogram (intravenous) 87.73
  infusion (continuous) (diuretic) 87.73
  percutaneous 87.75
  retrograde 87.74
Pyeloileostomy 56.71
Pyelolithotomy 55.11
Pyeloplasty 55.87
Pyelorrhaphy 55.81
Pyeloscopy 55.22
Pyelostolithotomy, percutaneous 55.03
Pyelostomy 55.12
  closure 55.82
Pyelotomy 55.11
Pyeloureteroplasty 55.87
Pylorectomy 43.6
Pyloroduodenotomy — see category 44.2
Pyloromyotomy (Ramstedt) (with wedge resection) 43.3
Pyloroplasty (Finney) (Heineke-Mikulicz) 44.29
  dilation, endoscopic 44.22
    by incision 44.21
  not elsewhere classified 44.29
  revision 44.29
Pylorostomy — see Gastrostomy

Q

Quadrant resection of breast 85.22
Quadricepsplasty (Thompson) 83.86
Quarantine 99.84
Quenuthoracoplasty 77.31
Quotient, respiratory 89.38

Index to Procedures

R

Rachicentesis 03.31
Rachitomy 03.09
Radiation therapy — *see also* Therapy, radiation
  teleradiotheraphy — *see* Teleradiotherapy
Radical neck dissection — *see* Dissection, neck
Radicotomy 03.1
Radiculectomy 03.1
Radiculotomy 03.1
Radiography (diagnostic) NEC 88.39
  abdomen, abdominal (flat plate) NEC 88.19
    wall (soft tissue) NEC 88.09
  adenoid 87.09
  ankle (skeletal) 88.28
    soft tissue 88.37
  bone survey 88.31
  bronchus 87.49
  chest (routine) 87.44
    wall NEC 87.39
  clavicle 87.43
  contrast (air) (gas) (radio-opaque substance) NEC
    abdominal wall 88.03
    arteries (by fluoroscopy) — *see* Arteriography
    bile ducts NEC 87.54
    bladder NEC 87.77
    brain 87.02
    breast 87.35
    bronchus NEC (transcricoid) 87.32
      endotracheal 87.31
    epididymis 87.93
    esophagus 87.61
    fallopian tubes
      gas 87.82
      opaque dye 87.83
    fistula (sinus tract) — *see also* Radiography, contrast, by site
      abdominal wall 88.03
      chest wall 87.38
    gallbladder NEC 87.59
    intervertebral disc(s) 87.21
    joints 88.32
    larynx 87.07
    lymph — *see* Lymphangiogram
    mammary ducts 87.35
    mediastinum 87.33
    nasal sinuses 87.15
    nasolacrimal ducts 87.05
    nasopharynx 87.06
    orbit 87.14
    pancreas 87.66
    pelvis
      gas 88.12
      opaque dye 88.11
    peritoneum NEC 88.13
    retroperitoneum NEC 88.15
    seminal vesicles 87.91
    sinus tract — *see also* Radiography, contrast, by site
      abdominal wall 88.03
      chest wall 87.38
      nose 87.15
    skull 87.02
    spinal disc(s) 87.21
    trachea 87.32
    uterus
      gas 87.82
      opaque dye 87.83
    vas deferens 87.94
    veins (by fluoroscopy) — *see* Phlebography
    vena cava (inferior) (superior) 88.51
  dental NEC 87.12
  diaphragm 87.49
  digestive tract NEC 87.69
    barium swallow 87.61
    lower GI series 87.64
    small bowel series 87.63
    upper GI series 87.62
  elbow (skeletal) 88.22
    soft tissue 88.35
  epididymis NEC 87.95
  esophagus 87.69
    barium-swallow 87.61
  eye 95.14

Radiography NEC — *continued*
  face, head, and neck 87.09
  facial bones 87.16
  fallopian tubes 87.85
  foot 88.28
  forearm (skeletal) 88.22
    soft tissue 88.35
  frontal area, facial 87.16
  genital organs
    female NEC 87.89
    male NEC 87.99
  hand (skeletal) 88.23
    soft tissue 88.35
  head NEC 87.09
  heart 87.49
  hip (skeletal) 88.26
    soft tissue 88.37
  intestine NEC 87.65
  kidney-ureter-bladder (KUB) 87.79
  knee (skeletal) 88.27
    soft tissue 88.37
  KUB (kidney-ureter-bladder) 87.79
  larynx 87.09
  lower leg (skeletal) 88.27
    soft tissue 88.37
  lower limb (skeletal) NEC 88.29
    soft tissue NEC 88.37
  lung 87.49
  mandible 87.16
  maxilla 87.16
  mediastinum 87.49
  nasal sinuses 87.16
  nasolacrimal duct 87.09
  nasopharynx 87.09
  neck NEC 87.09
  nose 87.16
  orbit 87.16
  pelvis (skeletal) 88.26
    pelvimetry 88.25
    soft tissue 88.19
  prostate NEC 87.92
  retroperitoneum NEC 88.16
  ribs 87.43
  root canal 87.12
  salivary gland 87.09
  seminal vesicles NEC 87.92
  shoulder (skeletal) 88.21
    soft tissue 88.35
  skeletal NEC 88.33
    series (whole or complete) 88.31
  skull (lateral, sagittal or tangential projection) NEC 87.17
  spine NEC 87.29
    cervical 87.22
    lumbosacral 87.24
    sacrococcygeal 87.24
    thoracic 87.23
  sternum 87.43
  supraorbital area 87.16
  symphysis menti 87.16
  teeth NEC 87.12
    full-mouth 87.11
  thigh (skeletal) 88.27
    soft tissue 88.37
  thyroid region 87.09
  tonsils and adenoids 87.09
  trachea 87.49
  ultrasonic — *see* Ultrasonography
  upper arm (skeletal) 88.21
    soft tissue 88.35
  upper limb (skeletal) NEC 88.24
    soft tissue NEC 88.35
  urinary system NEC 87.79
  uterus NEC 87.85
    gravid 87.81
  uvula 87.09
  vas deferens NEC 87.95
  wrist 88.23
  zygomaticomaxillary complex 87.16
Radioisotope
  scanning — *see* Scan, radioisotope
  therapy — *see* Therapy, radioisotope
Radiology
  diagnostic — *see* Radiography
  therapeutic — *see* Therapy, radiation

Radiosurgery, stereotactic 92.30
  cobalt 60 92.32
  linear accelerator (LINAC) 92.31
  multi-source 92.32
  particle beam 92.33
  particulate 92.33
  radiosurgery NEC 92.39
  single source photon 92.31
Raising, pedicle graft 86.71
Ramadier operation (intrapetrosal drainage) 20.22
Ramisection (sympathetic) 05.0
Ramstedt operation (pyeloromyotomy) (with wedge resection) 43.3
Range of motion testing 93.05
Rankin operation
  exteriorization of intestine 46.03
  proctectomy (complete) 48.5
Rashkind operation (balloon septostomy) 35.41
Rastelli operation (creation of conduit between right ventricle and pulmonary artery) 35.92
  in repair of
    pulmonary artery atresia 35.92
    transposition of great vessels 35.92
    truncus arteriosus 35.83
Raz-Pereyra procedure (Bladder neck suspension) 59.79
RCSA (radical cryosurgical ablation) of prostate 60.62
Readjustment — *see* Adjustment
Reamputation, stump 84.3
Reanastomosis — *see* Anastomosis
Reattachment
  amputated ear 18.72
  ankle 84.27
  arm (upper) NEC 84.24
  choroid and retina NEC 14.59
    by
      cryotherapy 14.52
      diathermy 14.51
      electrocoagulation 14.51
      photocoagulation 14.55
        laser 14.54
        xenon arc 14.53
  ear (amputated) 18.72
  extremity 84.29
    ankle 84.27
    arm (upper) NEC 84.24
    fingers, except thumb 84.22
      thumb 84.21
    foot 84.26
    forearm 84.23
    hand 84.23
    leg (lower) NEC 84.27
    thigh 84.28
    thumb 84.21
    toe 84.25
    wrist 84.23
  finger 84.22
    thumb 84.21
  foot 84.26
  forearm 84.23
  hand 84.23
  joint capsule (*see also* Arthroplasty) 81.96
  leg (lower) NEC 84.27
  ligament — *see also* Arthroplasty
    uterosacral 69.22
  muscle 83.74
    hand 82.54
    papillary (heart) 35.31
  nerve (peripheral) 04.79
  nose (amputated) 21.89
  papillary muscle (heart) 35.31
  penis (amputated) 64.45
  retina (and choroid) NEC 14.59
    by
      cryotherapy 14.52
      diathermy 14.51
      electrocoagulation 14.51
      photocoagulation 14.55
        laser 14.54
        xenon arc 14.53

Reattachment

Reattachment — *continued*
- tendon (to tendon) 83.73
  - hand 82.53
  - to skeletal attachment 83.88
    - hand 82.85
- thigh 84.28
- thumb 84.21
- toe 84.25
- tooth 23.5
- uterosacral ligament(s) 69.22
- vessels (peripheral) 39.59
  - renal, aberrant 39.55
- wrist 84.23

Recession
- extraocular muscle 15.11
  - multiple (two or more muscles) (with advancement or resection) 15.3
- gastrocnemius tendon (Strayer operation) 83.72
- levator palpebrae (superioris) muscle 08.38
- prognathic jaw 76.64
- tendon 83.72
  - hand 82.52

Reclosure — *see also* Closure
- disrupted abdominal wall (postoperative) 54.61

Reconstruction (plastic) — *see also* Construction and Repair, by site
- alveolus, alveolar (process) (ridge) (with graft or implant) 24.5
- artery (graft) — *see* Graft, artery
- artificial stoma, intestine 46.40
- auditory canal (external) 18.6
- auricle (ear) 18.71
- bladder 57.87
  - with
    - ileum 57.87 [45.51]
    - sigmoid 57.87 [45.52]
- bone, except facial (*see also* Osteoplasty) 78.40
  - facial NEC 76.46
    - with total ostectomy 76.44
  - mandible 76.43
    - with total mandibulectomy 76.41
- breast, total 85.7
- bronchus 33.48
- canthus (lateral) 08.59
- cardiac annulus 35.33
- chest wall (mesh) (silastic) 34.79
- cleft lip 27.54
- conjunctival cul-de-sac 10.43
  - with graft (buccal mucous membrane) (free) 10.42
- cornea NEC 11.79
- diaphragm 34.84
- ear (external) (auricle) 18.71
  - external auditory canal 18.6
  - meatus (new) (osseous skin-lined) 18.6
  - ossicles 19.3
  - prominent or protruding 18.5
- eyebrow 08.70
- eyelid 08.70
  - with graft or flap 08.69
    - hair follicle 08.63
    - mucous membrane 08.62
    - skin 08.61
    - tarsoconjunctival (one-stage) (two-stage) 08.64
  - full-thickness 08.74
    - involving lid margin 08.73
  - partial-thickness 08.72
    - involving lid margin 08.71
- eye socket 16.64
  - with graft 16.63
- fallopian tube 66.79
- foot and toes (with fixation device) 81.57
  - with prosthetic implant 81.57
- frontonasal duct 22.79
- hip (total) (with prosthesis) 81.51
- intraoral 27.59
- joint — *see* Arthroplasty
- lymphatic (by transplantation) 40.9
- mandible 76.43
  - with total mandibulectomy 76.41
- mastoid cavity 19.9
- mouth 27.59
- nipple NEC 85.87

Reconstruction (plastic) — *see also* Construction and Repair, by site — *continued*
- nose (total) (with arm flap) (with forehead flap) 21.83
- ossicles (graft) (prosthesis) NEC 19.3
  - with
    - stapedectomy 19.19
    - tympanoplasty 19.53
- pelvic floor 71.79
- penis (rib graft) (skin graft) (myocutaneous flap) 64.44
- pharynx 29.4
- scrotum (with pedicle flap) (with rotational flap) 61.49
- skin (plastic) (without graft) NEC 86.89
  - with graft — *see* Graft, skin
- subcutaneous tissue (plastic) (without skin graft) NEC 86.89
  - with graft — *see* Graft, skin
- tendon pulley —(with graft) (with local tissue) 83.83
  - for opponensplasty 82.71
  - hand 82.71
- thumb (osteoplastic) (with bone graft) (with skin graft) 82.69
- trachea (with graft) 31.75
- umbilicus 53.49
- ureteropelvic junction 55.87
- urethra 58.46
- vagina 70.62
- vas deferens, surgically divided 63.82

Recontour, gingiva 24.2

Recreational therapy 93.81

Rectectomy (*see also* Resection, rectum) 48.69

Rectopexy (Delorme) 48.76
- abdominal (Ripstein) 48.75

Rectoplasty 48.79

Rectorectostomy 48.74

Rectorrhaphy 48.71

Rectosigmoidectomy (*see also* Resection, rectum) 48.69
- transsacral 48.61

Rectosigmoidostomy 45.94

Rectostomy 48.1
- closure 48.72

Red cell survival studies 92.05

Reduction
- adipose tissue 86.83
- batwing arms 86.83
- breast (bilateral) 85.32
  - unilateral 85.31
- bulbous tuberosities (mandible) (maxilla) (fibrous) (osseous) 24.31
- buttocks 86.83
- diastasis, ankle mortise (closed) 79.77
  - open 79.87
- dislocation (of joint) (manipulation) (with cast) (with splint) (with traction device) (closed) 79.70
  - with fracture — *see* Reduction, fracture, by site
  - ankle (closed) 79.77
    - open 79.87
  - elbow (closed) 79.72
    - open 79.82
  - finger (closed) 79.74
    - open 79.84
  - foot (closed) 79.78
    - open 79.88
  - hand (closed) 79.74
    - open 79.84
  - hip (closed) 79.75
    - open 79.85
  - knee (closed) 79.76
    - open 79.86
  - open (with external fixation) (with internal fixation) 79.80
    - specified site NEC 79.89
  - shoulder (closed) 79.71
    - open 79.81
  - specified site (closed) NEC 79.79
    - open 79.89

Reduction — *continued*
- dislocation — *continued*
  - temporomandibular (closed) 76.93
    - open 76.94
  - toe (closed) 79.78
    - open 79.88
  - wrist (closed) 79.73
    - open 79.83
- elephantiasis, scrotum 61.3
- epistaxis (*see also* Control, epistaxis) 21.00
- fracture (bone) (with cast) (with splint) (with traction device) (closed) 79.00
  - with internal fixation 79.10
  - alveolar process (with stabilization of teeth)
    - mandible (closed) 76.75
      - open 76.77
    - maxilla (closed) 76.73
      - open 76.77
  - ankle — *see* Reduction, fracture, leg
  - arm (closed) NEC 79.02
    - with internal fixation 79.12
    - open 79.22
      - with internal fixation 79.32
  - blow-out — *see* Reduction, fracture, orbit
  - carpal, metacarpal (closed) 79.03
    - with internal fixation 79.13
    - open 79.23
      - with internal fixation 79.33
  - epiphysis — *see* Reduction, separation
  - facial (bone) NEC 76.70
    - closed 76.78
    - open 76.79
  - femur (closed) 79.05
    - with internal fixation 79.15
    - open 79.25
      - with internal fixation 79.35
  - fibula (closed) 79.06
    - with internal fixation 79.16
    - open 79.26
      - with internal fixation 79.36
  - foot (closed) NEC 79.07
    - with internal fixation 79.17
    - open 79.27
      - with internal fixation 79.37
  - hand (closed) NEC 79.03
    - with internal fixation 79.13
    - open 79.23
      - with internal fixation 79.33
  - humerus (closed) 79.01
    - with internal fixation 79.11
    - open 79.21
      - with internal fixation 79.31
  - jaw (lower) — *see also* Reduction, fracture, mandible
  - upper — *see* Reduction, fracture, maxilla
  - larynx 31.64
  - leg (closed) NEC 79.06
    - with internal fixation 79.16
    - open 79.26
      - with internal fixation 79.36
  - malar (closed) 76.71
    - open 76.72
  - mandible (with dental wiring) (closed) 76.75
    - open 76.76
  - maxilla (with dental wiring) (closed) 76.73
    - open 76.74
  - nasal (closed) 21.71
    - open 21.72
  - open 79.20
    - with internal fixation 79.30
    - specified site NEC 79.29
      - with internal fixation 79.39
  - orbit (rim) (wall) (closed) 76.78
    - open 76.79
  - patella (open) (with internal fixation) 79.36
  - phalanges
    - foot (closed) 79.08
      - with internal fixation 79.18
      - open 79.28
        - with internal fixation 79.38
    - hand (closed) 79.04
      - with internal fixation 79.14
      - open 79.24
        - with internal fixation 79.34

Reduction — *continued*
  fracture — *continued*
    radius (closed) 79.02
      with internal fixation 79.12
      open 79.22
        with internal fixation 79.32
    skull 02.02
    specified site (closed) NEC 79.09
      with internal fixation 79.19
      open 79.29
        with internal fixation 79.39
    spine 03.53
    tarsal, metatarsal (closed) 79.07
      with internal fixation 79.17
      open 79.27
        with internal fixation 79.37
    tibia (closed) 79.06
      with internal fixation 79.16
      open 79.26
        with internal fixation 79.36
    ulna (closed) 79.02
      with internal fixation 79.12
      open 79.22
        with internal fixation 79.32
    vertebra 03.53
    zygoma, zygomatic arch (closed) 76.71
      open 76.72
  fracture-dislocation — *see* Reduction, fracture
  heart volume 37.35
  hemorrhoids (manual) 49.41
  hernia — *see also* Repair, hernia
    manual 96.27
  intussusception (open) 46.80
    with
      fluoroscopy 96.29
      ionizing radiation enema 96.29
      ultrasonography guidance 96.29
    hydrostatic 96.29
    large intestine 46.82
      endoscopic (balloon) 46.85
    pneumatic 96.29
    small intestine 46.81
  lung volume 32.22
  malrotation, intestine (manual) (surgical) 46.80
    large 46.82
      endoscopic (balloon) 46.85
    small 46.81
  mammoplasty (bilateral) 85.32
    unilateral 85.31
  prolapse
    anus (operative) 49.94
    colostomy (manual) 96.28
    enterostomy (manual) 96.28
    ileostomy (manual) 96.28
    rectum (manual) 96.26
    uterus
      by pessary 96.18
      surgical 69.22
  ptosis overcorrection 08.37
  retroversion, uterus by pessary 96.18
  separation, epiphysis (with internal fixation) (closed) 79.40
    femur (closed) 79.45
      open 79.55
    fibula (closed) 79.46
      open 79.56
    humerus (closed) 79.41
      open 79.51
    open 79.50
    specified site (closed) NEC — *see also* category 79.4
      open — *see* category 79.5 ✓4ᵗʰ
    tibia (closed) 79.46
      open 79.56
  size
    abdominal wall (adipose) (pendulous) 86.83
    arms (adipose) (batwing) 86.83
    breast (bilateral) 85.32
      unilateral 85.31
    buttocks (adipose) 86.83
    finger (macrodactyly repair) 82.83
    skin 86.83
    subcutaneous tissue 86.83
    thighs (adipose) 86.83

Reduction — *continued*
  torsion
    intestine (manual) (surgical) 46.80
      large 46.82
        endoscopic (balloon) 46.85
      small 46.81
    kidney pedicle 55.84
    omentum 54.74
    spermatic cord 63.52
      with orchiopexy 62.5
    testis 63.52
      with orchiopexy 62.5
    uterus NEC 69.98
      gravid 75.99
    ventricular 37.35
  volvulus
    intestine 46.80
      large 46.82
        endoscopic (balloon) 46.85
      small 46.81
    stomach 44.92

Reefing, joint capsule (*see also* Arthroplasty) 81.96

Re-entry operation (aorta) 39.54

Re-establishment, continuity — *see also* Anastomosis
  bowel 46.50
  fallopian tube 66.79
  vas deferens 63.82

Referral (for)
  psychiatric aftercare (halfway house) (outpatient clinic) 94.52
  psychotherapy 94.51
  rehabilitation
    alcoholism 94.53
    drug addiction 94.54
    psychologic NEC 94.59
    vocational 94.55

Reformation
  cardiac pacemaker pocket, new site (skin) (subcutaneous) 37.79
  carioverter/defibrillator (automatic) pocket, new site (skin) (subcutaneous) 37.99
  chamber of eye 12.99

Refracture
  bone (for faulty union) (*see also* Osteoclasis) 78.70
  nasal bones 21.88

Refusion
  spinal, NOS 81.30
    atlas-axis (anterior) (transoral) (posterior) 81.31
    cervical (C_2 level or below) NEC 81.32
      anterior (interbody), anterolateral technique 81.32
      C_1-C_2 level (anterior) (posterior) 81.31
      posterior (interbody), posterolateral technique 81.33
    craniocervical (anterior) (transoral) (posterior) 81.31
    dorsal, dorsolumbar NEC 81.35
      anterior (interbody), anterolateral technique 81.34
      posterior (interbody), posterolateral technique 81.35
    lumbar, lumbosacral NEC 81.38
      anterior (interbody), anterolateral technique 81.36
      lateral transverse process technique 81.37
      posterior (interbody), posterolateral technique 81.38
    occiput — C_2 (anterior) (transoral) (posterior) 81.31
    refusion NEC 81.39

Regional blood flow study 92.05

Regulation, menstrual 69.6

Rehabilitation programs NEC 93.89
  alcohol 94.61
    with detoxification 94.63
    combined alcohol and drug 94.67
      with detoxification 94.69
  drug 94.64
    with detoxification 94.66

Rehabilitation programs NEC — *continued*
  drug — *continued*
    combined drug and alcohol 94.67
      with detoxification 94.69
  sheltered employment 93.85
  vocational 93.85

Reimplantation
  adrenal tissue (heterotopic) (orthotopic) 07.45
  artery 39.59
    renal, aberrant 39.55
  bile ducts following excision of ampulla of Vater 51.62
  extremity — *see* Reattachment, extremity
  fallopian tube into uterus 66.74
  kidney 55.61
  lung 33.5 ✓4ᵗʰ
  ovary 65.72
    laparoscopic 65.75
  pancreatic tissue 52.81
  parathyroid tissue (heterotopic) (orthotopic) 06.95
  pulmonary artery for hemitruncus repair 35.83
  renal vessel, aberrant 39.55
  testis in scrotum 62.5
  thyroid tissue (heterotopic) (orthotopic) 06.94
  tooth 23.5
  ureter into bladder 56.74

Reinforcement — *see also* Repair, by site
  sclera NEC 12.88
    with graft 12.87

Reinsertion — *see also* Insertion *or* Revision
  cystostomy tube 59.94
  fixation device (internal) (*see also* Fixation, bone, internal) 78.50
  heart valve (prosthetic) 35.95
  Holter (-Spitz) valve 02.42
  implant (expelled) (extruded)
    eyeball (with conjunctival graft) 16.62
    orbital 16.62
  nephrostomy tube 55.93
  pyelostomy tube 55.94
  ureteral stent (transurethral) 59.8
    with ureterotomy 59.8 [56.2]
  ureterostomy tube 59.93
  valve
    heart (prosthetic) 35.95
    ventricular (cerebral) 02.42

Relaxation (*see also* Release training) 94.33

Release
  carpal tunnel (for nerve decompression) 04.43
  celiac artery axis 39.91
  central slip, extensor tendon hand (mallet finger repair) 82.84
  chordee 64.42
  clubfoot NEC 83.84
  de Quervain's tenosynovitis 82.01
  Dupuytren's contracture (by palmar fasciectomy) 82.35
    by fasciotomy (subcutaneous) 82.12
      with excision 82.35
  Fowler (mallet finger repair) 82.84
  joint (capsule) (adherent) (constrictive) (*see also* Division, joint capsule) 80.40
  laryngeal 31.92
  ligament (*see also* Division, ligament) 80.40
    median arcuate 39.91
  median arcuate ligament 39.91
  muscle (division) 83.19
    hand 82.19
  nerve (peripheral) NEC 04.49
    cranial NEC 04.42
    trigeminal 04.41
  pressure, intraocular 12.79
  scar tissue
    skin 86.84
    stoma — *see* Revision, stoma
  tarsal tunnel 04.44
  tendon 83.13
    hand 82.11
      extensor, central slip (repair mallet finger) 82.84
    sheath 83.01
      hand 82.01
  tenosynovitis 83.01
    abductor pollicis longus 82.01

Release

Release — *continued*
  tenosynovitis — *continued*
    de Quervain's 82.01
    external pollicis brevis 82.01
    hand 82.01
  torsion
    intestine 46.80
      large 46.82
        endoscopic (balloon) 46.85
      small 46.81
    kidney pedicle 55.84
    ovary 65.95
    testes 63.52
  transverse carpal ligament (for nerve decompression) 04.43
  trigger finger or thumb 82.01
  urethral stricture 58.5
  Volkmann's contracture
    excision of scar, muscle 83.32
    fasciotomy 83.14
    muscle transplantation 83.77
  web contracture (skin) 86.84

Relief — *see* Release

Relocation — *see also* Revision
  cardiac pacemaker pocket, new site (skin) (subcutaneous) 37.79
  CRT-D pocket 37.99 •
  CRT-P pocket 37.79 •

Remobilization
  joint 93.16
  stapes 19.0

Remodel
  ventricle 37.35

Removal — *see also* Excision
  Abrams bar (chest wall) 34.01
  abscess — *see* Incision, by site
  adenoid tag(s) 28.6
  anal sphincter
    with revision 49.75 •
    without revision 49.76 •
  arch bars (orthodontic) 24.8
    immobilization device 97.33
  arterial graft or prosthesis 39.49
  arteriovenous shunt (device) 39.43
    with creation of new shunt 39.42
  Barton's tongs (skull) 02.95
    with synchronous replacement 02.94
  bladder sphincter, artificial 58.99
    with replacement 58.93
  blood clot — *see also* Incision, by site
    bladder (by incision) 57.19
      without incision 57.0
    kidney (without incision) 56.0
      by incision 55.01
    ureter
      by incision 56.2
  bone fragment (chip) (*see also* Incision, bone) 77.10
    joint (*see also* Arthrotomy) 80.10
    necrotic (*see also* Sequestrectomy, bone) 77.00
      joint (*see also* Arthrotomy) 80.10
    skull 01.25
      with debridement compound fracture 02.02
  bone growth stimulator — *see* category 78.6 ⬛4ᵗʰ
  bony spicules, spinal canal 03.53
  brace 97.88
  breast implant 85.94
    tissue expander 85.96
  calcareous deposit
    bursa 83.03
      hand 82.03
    tendon, intratendinous 83.39
      hand 82.29
  calcification, heart valve leaflets —*see* Valvuloplasty, heart
  calculus
    bile duct (by incision) 51.49
      endoscopic 51.88
      laparoscopic 51.88
      percutaneous 51.98
    bladder (by incision) 57.19
      without incision 57.0

Removal — *see also* Excision — *continued*
  calculus — *continued*
    common duct (by incision) 51.41
      endoscopic 51.88
      laparoscopic 51.88
      percutaneous 51.96
    gallbladder 51.04
      endoscopic 51.88
      laparoscopic 51.88
    kidney (by incision) 55.01
      without incision 56.0
      percutaneous 55.03
        with fragmentation (ultrasound) 55.04
    renal pelvis (by incision) 55.11
      percutaneous nephrostomy 55.03
        with fragmentation 55.04
      transurethral 56.0
    lacrimal
      canaliculi 09.42
        by incision 09.52
      gland 09.3
        by incision 09.0
      passage(s) 09.49
        by incision 09.59
      punctum 09.41
        by incision 09.51
      sac 09.49
        by incision 09.53
    pancreatic duct (by incision) 52.09
      endoscopic 52.94
    perirenal tissue 59.09
    pharynx 29.39
    prostate 60.0
    salivary gland (by incision) 26.0
      by probe 26.91
    ureter (by incision) 56.2
      without incision 56.0
    urethra (by incision) 58.0
      without incision 58.6
  caliper tongs (skull) 02.95
  cannula
    for extracorporeal membrane oxygenation (ECMO) — *omit code*
  cardiac pacemaker (device) (initial) (permanent)
    ▶(cardiac resynchronization device, CRT-P)◀ 37.89
    with replacement
      cardiac resynchronization pacemaker (CRT-P) •
      device only 00.53 •
      total system 00.50 •
    dual-chamber 37.87
    single-chamber device 37.85
      rate responsive 37.86
  cardioverter/defibrillator pulse generator
    without replacement ▶(cardiac resynchronization defibrillator device (CRT-D)◀ 37.99
  cast 97.88
    with reapplication 97.13
      lower limb 97.12
      upper limb 97.11
  catheter (indwelling) — *see also* Removal, tube
    bladder 97.64
    middle ear (tympanum) 20.1
    ureter 97.62
    urinary 97.64
    ventricular (cerebral) 02.43
      with synchronous replacement 02.42
  cerclage material, cervix 69.96
  cerumen, ear 96.52
  corneal epithelium 11.41
    for smear or culture 11.21
  coronary artery obstruction (thrombus) 36.09
    direct intracoronary artery infusion 36.04
    open chest approach 36.03
    percutaneous transluminal (balloon) (single vessel) 36.01
      with thrombolytic agent infusion 36.02
    multiple vessels 36.05
  Crutchfield tongs (skull) 02.95
    with synchronous replacement 02.94
  cyst — *see also* Excision, lesion, by site
    dental 24.4
    lung 32.29
      endoscopic 32.28

Index to Procedures

Removal — *see also* Excision — *continued*
  cystic duct remnant 51.61
  decidua (by)
    aspiration curettage 69.52
    curettage (D and C) 69.02
    manual 75.4
  dental wiring (immobilization device) 97.33
    orthodontic 24.8
  device (therapeutic) NEC 97.89
    abdomen NEC 97.86
    digestive system NEC 97.59
    drainage — *see* Removal, tube
    external fixation device 97.88
      mandibular NEC 97.36
      minifixator (bone) — *see* category 78.6 ⬛4ᵗʰ
    for musculoskeletal immobilization NEC 97.88
    genital tract NEC 97.79
    head and neck NEC 97.39
    intrauterine contraceptive 97.71
    thorax NEC 97.49
    trunk NEC 97.87
    urinary system NEC 97.69
  diaphragm, vagina 97.73
  drainage device — *see* Removal, tube
  dye, spinal canal 03.31
  ectopic fetus (from) 66.02
    abdominal cavity 74.3
    extraperitoneal (intraligamentous) 74.3
    fallopian tube (by salpingostomy) 66.02
      by salpingotomy 66.01
      with salpingectomy 66.62
    intraligamentous 74.3
    ovarian 74.3
    peritoneal (following uterine or tubal rupture) 74.3
    site NEC 74.3
    tubal (by salpingostomy) 66.02
      by salpingotomy 66.01
      with salpingectomy 66.62
  electrodes
    bone growth stimulator — *see* category 78.6 ⬛4ᵗʰ
    brain 01.22
      depth 01.22
        with synchronous replacement 02.93
      foramen ovale 01.22
        with synchronous replacement 02.93
      sphenoidal — *omit code*
        with synchronous replacement 02.96
    cardiac pacemaker (atrial) (transvenous) (ventricular) 37.77
      with replacement 37.76
    depth 01.22
      with synchronous replacement 02.93
    epicardial (myocardial) 37.77
      with replacement (by)
        atrial and/or ventricular lead(s) (electrode) 37.76
        epicardial lead 37.74
    epidural pegs 01.22
      with synchronous replacement 02.93
    foramen ovale 01.22
      with synchronous replacement 02.93
    intracranial 01.22
      with synchronous replacement 02.93
    peripheral nerve 04.93
      with synchronous replacement 04.92
    sphenoidal — *omit code*
      with synchronous replacement 02.96
    spinal 03.94
      with synchronous replacement 03.93
    temporary transvenous pacemaker system — *omit code*
  electroencephalographic receiver (brain) (intracranial) 01.22
    with synchronous replacement 02.93
  electronic
    stimulator
      bladder 57.98
      bone 78.6 ⬛4ᵗʰ
      brain 01.22
        with synchronous replacement 02.93
      intracranial 01.22
        with synchronous replacement 02.93

Index to Procedures

Removal — see also Excision — continued
  electronic — continued
    stimulator — continued
      peripheral nerve 04.93
        with synchronous replacement 04.92
      skeletal muscle 83.93
        with synchronous replacement 83.92
      spinal 03.94
        with synchronous replacement 03.93
      ureter 56.94
  electrostimulator — see Removal, electronic, stimulator, by site
  embolus 38.00
    with endarterectomy — see Endarterectomy
    abdominal
      artery 38.06
      vein 38.07
    aorta (arch) (ascending) (descending) 38.04
    arteriovenous shunt or cannula 39.49
    bovine graft 39.49
    head and neck vessel NEC 38.02
    intracranial vessel NEC 38.01
    lower limb
      artery 38.08
      vein 38.09
    pulmonary (artery) (vein) 38.05
    thoracic vessel NEC 38.05
    upper limb (artery) (vein) 38.03
  embryo — see Removal, ectopic fetus
  encircling tube, eye (episcleral) 14.6
  epithelial downgrowth, anterior chamber 12.93
  external fixation device 97.88
    mandibular NEC 97.36
    minifixator (bone) — see category 78.6 ✓4ᵗʰ
  extrauterine embryo — see Removal, ectopic fetus
  eyeball 16.49
    with implant 16.42
      with attachment of muscle 16.41
  fallopian tube — see Salpingectomy
  feces (impacted) (by flushing) (manual) 96.38
  fetus, ectopic — see Removal, ectopic fetus
  fingers, supernumerary 86.26
  fixation device
    external 97.88
      mandibular NEC 97.36
      minifixator (bone) — see category 78.6 ✓4ᵗʰ
    internal 78.60
      carpal, metacarpal 78.64
      clavicle 78.61
      facial (bone) 76.97
      femur 78.65
      fibula 78.67
      humerus 78.62
      patella 78.66
      pelvic 78.69
      phalanges (foot) (hand) 78.69
      radius 78.63
      scapula 78.61
      specified site NEC 78.69
      tarsal, metatarsal 78.68
      thorax (ribs) (sternum) 78.61
      tibia 78.67
      ulna 78.63
      vertebrae 78.69
  foreign body NEC (see also Incision, by site) 98.20
    abdominal (cavity) 54.92
      wall 54.0
    adenoid 98.13
      by incision 28.91
    alveolus, alveolar bone 98.22
      by incision 24.0
    antecubital fossa 98.27
      by incision 86.05
    anterior chamber 12.00
      by incision 12.02
        with use of magnet 12.01
    anus (intraluminal) 98.05
      by incision 49.93
    artifical stoma (intraluminal) 98.18
    auditory canal, external 18.02
    axilla 98.27
      by incision 86.05

Removal — see also Excision — continued
  foreign body NEC (see also Incision, by site) — continued
    bladder (without incision) 57.0
      by incision 57.19
    bone, except fixation device (see also Incision, bone) 77.10
      alveolus, alveolar 98.22
        by incision 24.0
    brain 01.39
      without incision into brain 01.24
    breast 85.0
    bronchus (intraluminal) 98.15
      by incision 33.0
    bursa 83.03
      hand 82.03
    canthus 98.22
      by incision 08.51
    cerebral meninges 01.31
    cervix (intraluminal) NEC 98.16
      penetrating 69.97
    choroid (by incision) 14.00
      with use of magnet 14.01
      without use of magnet 14.02
    ciliary body (by incision) 12.00
      with use of magnet 12.01
      without use of magnet 12.02
    conjunctiva (by magnet) 98.22
      by incision 10.0
    cornea 98.21
      by
        incision 11.1
        magnet 11.0
    duodenum 98.03
      by incision 45.01
    ear (intraluminal) 98.11
      with incision 18.09
    epididymis 63.92
    esophagus (intraluminal) 98.02
      by incision 42.09
    extrapleural (by incision) 34.01
    eye, eyeball (by magnet) 98.21
      anterior segment (by incision) 12.00
        with use of magnet 12.01
        without use of magnet 12.02
      posterior segment (by incision) 14.00
        with use of magnet 14.01
        without use of magnet 14.02
      superficial 98.21
    eyelid 98.22
      by incision 08.09
    fallopian tube
      by salpingostomy 66.02
      by salpingotomy 66.01
    fascia 83.09
      hand 82.09
    foot 98.28
    gall bladder 51.04
    groin region (abdominal wall) (inguinal) 54.0
    gum 98.22
      by incision 24.0
    hand 98.26
    head and neck NEC 98.22
    heart 37.11
    internal fixation device — see Removal, fixation device, internal
    intestine
      by incision 45.00
      large (intraluminal) 98.04
        by incision 45.03
      small (intraluminal) 98.03
        by incision 45.02
    intraocular (by incision) 12.00
      with use of magnet 12.01
      without use of magnet 12.02
    iris (by incision) 12.00
      with use of magnet 12.01
      without use of magnet 12.02
    joint structures (see also Arthrotomy) 80.10
    kidney (transurethral) (by endoscopy) 56.0
      by incision 55.01
      pelvis (transurethral) 56.0
        by incision 55.11
    labia 98.23
      by incision 71.09

Removal — see also Excision — continued
  foreign body NEC (see also Incision, by site) — continued
    lacrimal
      canaliculi 09.42
        by incision 09.52
      gland 09.3
        by incision 09.0
      passage(s) 09.49
        by incision 09.59
      punctum 09.41
        by incision 09.51
      sac 09.49
        by incision 09.53
    large intestine (intraluminal) 98.04
      by incision 45.03
    larynx (intraluminal) 98.14
      by incision 31.3
    lens 13.00
      by incision 13.02
      with use of magnet 13.01
    liver 50.0
    lower limb, except foot 98.29
      foot 98.28
    lung 33.1
    mediastinum 34.1
    meninges (cerebral) 01.31
      spinal 03.01
    mouth (intraluminal) 98.01
      by incision 27.92
    muscle 83.02
      hand 82.02
    nasal sinus 22.50
      antrum 22.2
        with Caldwell-Luc approach 22.39
      ethmoid 22.51
      frontal 22.41
      maxillary 22.2
        with Caldwell-Luc approach 22.39
      sphenoid 22.52
    nerve (cranial) (peripheral) NEC 04.04
      root 03.01
    nose (intraluminal) 98.12
      by incision 21.1
    oral cavity (intraluminal) 98.01
      by incision 27.92
    orbit (by magnet) 98.21
      by incision 16.1
    palate (penetrating) 98.22
      by incision 27.1
    pancreas 52.09
    penis 98.24
      by incision 64.92
    pericardium 37.12
    perineum (female) 98.23
      by incision 71.09
      male 98.25
        by incision 86.05
    perirenal tissue 59.09
    peritoneal cavity 54.92
    perivesical tissue 59.19
    pharynx (intraluminal) 98.13
      by pharyngotomy 29.0
    pleura (by incision) 34.09
    popliteal space 98.29
      by incision 86.05
    rectum (intraluminal) 98.05
      by incision 48.0
    renal pelvis (transurethral) 56.0
      by incision 56.1
    retina (by incision) 14.00
      with use of magnet 14.01
      without use of magnet 14.02
    retroperitoneum 54.92
    sclera (by incision) 12.00
      with use of magnet 12.01
      without use of magnet 12.02
    scrotum 98.24
      by incision 61.0
    sinus (nasal) 22.50
      antrum 22.2
        with Caldwell-Luc approach 22.39
      ethmoid 22.51
      frontal 22.41
      maxillary 22.2
        with Caldwell-Luc approach 22.39

Removal — see also Excision — continued
  foreign body NEC (see also Incision, by site) — continued
    sinus — continued
      sphenoid 22.52
    skin NEC 98.20
      by incision 86.05
    skull 01.24
      with incision into brain 01.39
    small intestine (intraluminal) 98.03
      by incision 45.02
    soft tissue NEC 83.09
      hand 82.09
    spermatic cord 63.93
    spinal (canal) (cord) (meninges) 03.01
    stomach (intraluminal) 98.03
      bubble (balloon) 44.94
      by incision 43.0
    subconjunctival (by magnet) 98.22
      by incision 10.0
    subcutaneous tissue NEC 98.20
      by incision 86.05
    supraclavicular fossa 98.27
      by incision 86.05
    tendon (sheath) 83.01
      hand 82.01
    testis 62.0
    thorax (by incision) 34.09
    thyroid (field) (gland) (by incision) 06.09
    tonsil 98.13
      by incision 28.91
    trachea (intraluminal) 98.15
      by incision 31.3
    trunk NEC 98.25
    tunica vaginalis 98.24
    upper limb, except hand 98.27
      hand 98.26
    ureter (transurethral) 56.0
      by incision 56.2
    urethra (intraluminal) 98.19
      by incision 58.0
    uterus (intraluminal) 98.16
    vagina (intraluminal) 98.17
      by incision 70.14
    vas deferens 63.6
    vitreous (by incision) 14.00
      with use of magnet 14.01
      without use of magnet 14.02
    vulva 98.23
      by incision 71.09
  gallstones
    bile duct (by incision) NEC 51.49
      endoscopic 51.88
    common duct (by incision) 51.41
      endoscopic 51.88
      percutaneous 51.96
    duodenum 45.01
    gallbladder 51.04
      endoscopic 51.88
      laparoscopic 51.88
    hepatic ducts 51.49
      endoscopic 51.88
    intestine 45.00
      large 45.03
      small NEC 45.02
    liver 50.0
  Gardner Wells tongs (skull) 02.95
    with synchronous replacement 02.94
  gastric bubble (balloon) 44.94
  granulation tissue — see also Excision, lesion, by site
    with repair — see Repair, by site
    cranial 01.6
    skull 01.6
  halo traction device (skull) 02.95
    with synchronous replacement 02.94
  heart assist system 37.64
    with replacement 37.63
    intra-aortic balloon pump (IABP) 97.44
    nonoperative 97.44
  hematoma — see Drainage, by site
  Hoffman minifixator device (bone) — see category 78.6 ✓4ᵗʰ
  hydatidiform mole 68.0
  impacted
    feces (rectum) (by flushing) (manual) 96.38

Removal — see also Excision — continued
  impacted — continued
    tooth 23.19
      from nasal sinus (maxillary) 22.61
  implant
    breast 85.94
    cochlear prosthetic device 20.99
    cornea 11.92
    lens (prosthetic) 13.8
    middle ear NEC 20.99
    ocular 16.71
      posterior segment 14.6
    orbit 16.72
    retina 14.6
    tympanum 20.1
  internal fixation device — see Removal, fixation device, internal
  intra-aortic balloon pump (IABP) 97.44
  intrauterine contraceptive device (IUD) 97.71
  joint (structure) NOS 80.90
    ankle 80.97
    elbow 80.92
    foot and toe 80.98
    hand and finger 80.94
    hip 80.95
    knee 80.96
    other specified sites 80.99
    shoulder 80.91
    spine 80.99
    toe 80.98
    wrist 80.93
  Kantrowitz heart pump 37.64
    nonoperative 97.44
  keel (tantalum plate), larynx 31.98
  kidney — see also Nephrectomy
    mechanical 55.98
    transplanted or rejected 55.53
  laminaria (tent), uterus 97.79
  leads (cardiac) — see Removal, electrodes, cardiac pacemaker
  lesion — see Excision, lesion, by site
  ligamentum flavum (spine) — omit code
  ligature
    fallopian tube 66.79
    ureter 56.86
    vas deferens 63.84
  loop recorder 86.05
  loose body
    bone — see Sequestrectomy, bone
    joint 80.10
    mesh (surgical) — see Removal, foreign body, by site
  lymph node — see Excision, lymph, node
  minifixator device (bone) — see category 78.6 ✓4ᵗʰ
    external fixation device 97.88
  Mulligan hood, fallopian tube 66.94
    with synchronous replacement 66.93
  muscle stimulator (skeletal) 83.93
    with replacement 83.92
  myringotomy device or tube 20.1
  nail (bed) (fold) 86.23
    internal fixation device — see Removal, fixation device, internal
  necrosis
    skin 86.28
      excisional 86.22
  neuropacemaker
    brain 01.22
      with synchronous replacement 02.93
    intracranial 01.22
      with synchronous replacement 02.93
    peripheral nerve 04.93
      with synchronous replacement 04.92
    spinal 03.94
      with synchronous replacement 03.93
  neurostimulator
    brain 01.22
      with synchronous replacement 02.93
    intracranial 01.22
      with synchronous replacement 02.93
    peripheral nerve 04.93
      with synchronous replacement 04.92
    spinal 03.94
      with synchronous replacement 03.93

Removal — see also Excision — continued
  nonabsorbable surgical material NEC — see Removal, foreign body, by site
  odontoma (tooth) 24.4
  orbital implant 16.72
  osteocartilagenous loose body, joint structures (see also Arthrotomy) 80.10
  outer attic wall (middle ear) 20.59
  ovo-testis (unilateral) 62.3
    bilateral 62.41
  pacemaker
    brain (intracranial) 01.22
      with synchronous replacement 02.93
    cardiac (device) (initial) (permanent) 37.89
      with replacement
        dual-chamber device 37.87
        single-chamber device 37.85
          rate responsive 37.86
      electrodes (atrial) (transvenous) (ventricular) 37.77
        with replacement 37.76
      epicardium (myocardium) 37.77
        with replacement (by)
          atrial and/or ventricular lead(s) (electrode) 37.76
          epicardial lead 37.74
      temporary transvenous pacemaker system — omit code
    intracranial 01.22
      with synchronous replacement 02.93
    neural
      brain 01.22
        with synchronous replacement 02.93
      peripheral nerve 04.93
        with synchronous replacement 04.92
      spine 03.94
        with synchronous replacement 03.93
    spinal 03.94
      with synchronous replacement 03.93
  pack, packing
    dental 97.34
    intrauterine 97.72
    nasal 97.32
    rectum 97.59
    trunk NEC 97.85
    vagina 97.75
    vulva 97.75
  pantopaque dye, spinal canal 03.31
  patella (complete) 77.96
    partial 77.86
  pectus deformity implant device 34.01
  pelvic viscera, en masse (female) 68.8
    male 57.71
  pessary, vagina NEC 97.74
  pharynx (partial) 29.33
  phlebolith — see Removal, embolus
  placenta (by)
    aspiration curettage 69.52
    D and C 69.02
    manual 75.4
  plaque, dental 96.54
  plate, skull 02.07
    with synchronous replacement 02.05
  polyp — see also Excision, lesion, by site
    esophageal 42.32
      endoscopic 42.33
    gastric (endoscopic) 43.41
    intestine 45.41
      endoscopic 45.42
    nasal 21.31
  prosthesis
    bile duct 51.95
      nonoperative 97.55
    cochlear prosthetic device 20.99
    dental 97.35
    eye 97.31
    facial bone 76.99
    fallopian tube 66.94
      with synchronous replacement 66.93
    joint structures 80.00
      ankle 80.07
      elbow 80.02
      foot and toe 80.08
      hand and finger 80.04
      hip 80.05
      knee 80.06

Index to Procedures

Removal — see also Excision — continued
 prosthesis — continued
  joint structures — continued
   shoulder 80.01
   specified site NEC 80.09
   spine 80.09
   wrist 80.03
  lens 13.8
  penis (internal) without replacement 64.96
  Rosen (urethra) 59.99
  testicular, by incision 62.0
  urinary sphincter, artificial 58.99
   with replacement 58.93
 pseudophakos 13.8
 pterygium 11.39
  with corneal graft 11.32
 pulse generator
  cardiac pacemaker 37.86
  cardioverter/defibrillator 37.99
 pump assist device, heart 37.64
  with replacement 37.63
  nonoperative 97.44
 radioactive material — see Removal, foreign body, by site
 redundant skin, eyelid 08.86
 rejected organ
  kidney 55.53
  testis 62.42
 reservoir, ventricular (Ommaya) (Rickham) 02.43
  with synchronous replacement 02.42
 retained placenta (by)
  aspiration curettage 69.52
  D and C 69.02
  manual 75.4
 retinal implant 14.6
 rhinolith 21.31
 rice bodies, tendon sheaths 83.01
  hand 82.01
 Roger-Anderson minifixator device (bone) — see category 78.6 ✓4ᵗʰ
 root, residual (tooth) (buried) (retained) 23.11
 Rosen prosthesis (urethra) 59.99
 Scribner shunt 39.43
 scleral buckle or implant 14.6
 secondary membranous cataract (with iridectomy) 13.65
 secundines (by)
  aspiration curettage 69.52
  D and C 69.02
  manual 75.4
 sequestrum — see Sequestrectomy
 seton, anus 49.93
 Shepard's tube (ear) 20.1
 Shirodkar suture, cervix 69.96
 shunt
  arteriovenous 39.43
   with creation of new shunt 39.42
  lumbar-subarachnoid NEC 03.98
  pleurothecal 03.98
  salpingothecal 03.98
  spinal (thecal) NEC 03.98
  subarachnoid-peritoneal 03.98
  subarachnoid-ureteral 03.98
 silastic tubes
  ear 20.1
  fallopian tubes 66.94
   with synchronous replacement 66.93
 skin
  necrosis or slough 86.28
   excisional 86.22
   superficial layer (by dermabrasion) 86.25
 skull tongs 02.95
  with synchronous replacement 02.94
 splint 97.88
 stent
  bile duct 97.55
  larynx 31.98
  ureteral 97.62
  urethral 97.65
 stimoceiver (brain) (intracranial) 01.22
  with synchronous replacement 02.93
 subdural
  grids 01.22
  strips 01.22
 supernumerary digit(s) 86.26

Removal — see also Excision — continued
 suture(s) NEC 97.89
  abdominal wall 97.83
  by incision — see Incision, by site
  genital tract 97.79
  head and neck 97.38
  thorax 97.43
  trunk NEC 97.84
 symblepharon — see Repair, symblepharon
 temporary transvenous pacemaker system — omit code
 testis (unilateral) 62.3
  bilateral 62.41
  remaining or solitary 62.42
 thrombus 38.00
  with endarterectomy — see Endarterectomy
  abdominal
   artery 38.06
   vein 38.07
  aorta (arch) (ascending) (descending) 38.04
  arteriovenous shunt or cannula 39.49
  bovine graft 39.49
  coronary artery 36.09
  head and neck vessel NEC 38.02
  intracranial vessel NEC 38.01
  lower limb
   artery 38.08
   vein 38.09
  pulmonary (artery) (vein) 38.05
  thoracic vessel NEC 38.05
  upper limb (artery) (vein) 38.03
 tissue expander (skin) NEC 86.05
  breast 85.96
 toes, supernumerary 86.26
 tongs, skull 02.95
  with synchronous replacement 02.94
 tonsil tag 28.4
 tooth (by forceps) (multiple) (single) NEC 23.09
  deciduous 23.01
  surgical NEC 23.19
   impacted 23.19
   residual root 23.11
   root apex 23.73
    with root canal therapy 23.72
 trachoma follicles 10.33
 T-tube (bile duct) 97.55
 tube
  appendix 97.53
  bile duct (T-tube) NEC 97.55
  cholecystostomy 97.54
  cystostomy 97.63
  ear (button) 20.1
  gastrostomy 97.51
  large intestine 97.53
  liver 97.55
  mediastinum 97.42
  nephrostomy 97.61
  pancreas 97.56
  peritoneum 97.82
  pleural cavity 97.41
  pyelostomy 97.61
  retroperitoneum 97.81
  small intestine 97.52
  thoracotomy 97.41
  tracheostomy 97.37
  tympanostomy 20.1
  tympanum 20.1
  ureterostomy 97.62
 ureteral splint (stent) 97.62
 urethral sphincter, artificial 58.99
  with replacement 58.93
 urinary sphincter, artificial 58.99
  with replacement 58.93
 utricle 20.79
 valve
  vas deferens 63.85
  ventricular (cerebral) 02.43
 vascular graft or prosthesis 39.49
 ventricular shunt or reservoir 02.43
  with synchronous replacement 02.42
 Vinke tongs (skull) 02.95
  with synchronous replacement 02.94
 vitreous (with replacement) 14.72
  anterior approach (partial) 14.71
  open sky technique 14.71

Removal — see also Excision — continued
 Wagner-Brooker minifixator device (bone) — see category 78.6 ✓4ᵗʰ
 wiring, dental (immobilization device) 97.33
  orthodontic 24.8
Renipuncture (percutaneous) 55.92
Renogram 92.03
Renotransplantation NEC 55.69
Reopening — see also Incision, by site
 blepharorrhaphy 08.02
 canthorrhaphy 08.02
 cilia base 08.71
 craniotomy or craniectomy site 01.23
 fallopian tube (divided) 66.79
 iris in anterior chambers 12.97
 laminectomy or laminotomy site 03.02
 laparotomy site 54.12
 osteotomy site (see also Incision, bone) 77.10
  facial bone 76.09
 tarsorrhaphy 08.02
 thoracotomy site (for control of hemorrhage) (for examination) (for exploration) 34.03
 thyroid field wound (for control of hemorrhage) (for examination) (for exploration) (for removal of hematoma) 06.02
Repacking — see Replacement, pack, by site
Repair
 abdominal wall 54.72
 adrenal gland 07.44
 alveolus, alveolar (process) (ridge) (with graft) (with implant) 24.5
 anal sphincter 49.79
  artificial sphincter
   implantation 49.75
   revision 49.75
  laceration (by suture) 49.71
   obstetric (current) 75.62
   old 49.79
 aneurysm (false) (true) 39.52
  by or with
   clipping 39.51
   coagulation 39.52
   coil (endovascular approach) 39.79
    head and neck 39.72
   electrocoagulation 39.52
    excision or resection of vessel — see also Aneurysmectomy, by site
    with
     anastomosis — see Aneurysmectomy, with anastomosis, by site
     graft replacement — see Aneurysmectomy, with graft replacement, by site
   endovascular graft 39.79
    abdominal aorta 39.71
    head and neck 39.72
    lower extremity artery(s) 39.79
    thoracic aorta 39.79
    upper extremity artery(s) 39.79
   filipuncture 39.52
   graft replacement — see Aneurysmectomy, with graft replacement, by site
   ligation 39.52
   liquid tissue adhesive (glue) 39.79
    endovascular approach 39.79
     head and neck 39.72
   methyl methacrylate 39.52
    endovascular approach 39.79
     head and neck 39.72
   occlusion 39.52
    endovascular approach 39.79
     head and neck 39.72
   suture 39.52
   trapping 39.52
   wiring 39.52
   wrapping (gauze) (methyl methacrylate) (plastic) 39.52
  coronary artery 36.91
  heart 37.32
  sinus of Valsalva 35.39
  thoracic aorta (dissecting), by fenestration 39.54

Repair

Repair — continued
- anomalous pulmonary venous connection (total)
  - one-stage 35.82
  - partial — see specific procedure
  - total 35.82
- anus 49.79
  - laceration (by suture) 49.71
    - obstetric (current) 75.62
      - old 49.79
- aorta 39.31
- aorticopulmonary window 39.59
- arteriovenous fistula 39.53
  - by or with
    - clipping 39.53
    - coagulation 39.53
    - coil (endovascular approach) 39.79 ●
      - head and neck vessels 39.72 ●
    - division 39.53
    - excision or resection — see also Aneurysmectomy, by site
      - with
        - anastomosis — see Aneurysmectomy, with anastomosis, by site
        - graft replacement — see Aneurysmectomy, with graft replacement, by site
    - ligation 39.53
      - coronary artery 36.99
    - occlusion 39.53
      - endovascular approach 39.79 ●
        - head and neck 39.72 ●
    - suture 39.53
- artery NEC 39.59
  - by
    - endovascular approach 39.79 ●
      - head and neck 39.72 ●
    - non-coronary percutaneous transluminal angioplasty or atherectomy
      - basilar 39.50
      - carotid 39.50
      - femoropopliteal 39.50
      - head and neck NOS 39.50
      - iliac 39.50
      - lower extremity NOS 39.50
      - mesenteric 39.50
      - renal 39.50
      - upper extremity NOS 39.50
      - vertebral 39.50
  - with
    - patch graft 39.58
      - with excision or resection of vessel — see Arteriectomy, with graft replacement, by site
      - synthetic (Dacron) (Teflon) 39.57
      - tissue (vein) (autogenous) (homograft) 39.56
    - suture 39.31
  - coronary NEC 36.99
    - by angioplasty — see Angioplasty, coronary
    - by atherectomy — see Angioplasty, coronary
- artificial opening — see Repair, stoma
- atrial septal defect 35.71
  - with
    - prosthesis (open heart technique) 35.51
      - closed heart technique 35.52
    - tissue graft 35.61
    - combined with repair of valvular and ventricular septal defects — see Repair, endocardial cushion defect
    - in total repair of total anomalous pulmonary venous connection 35.82
- atrioventricular canal defect (any type) 35.73
  - with
    - prosthesis 35.54
    - tissue graft 35.63
- bifid digit (finger) 82.89
- bile duct NEC 51.79
  - laceration (by suture) NEC 51.79
    - common bile duct 51.71
- bladder NEC 57.89
  - exstrophy 57.86
  - for stress incontinence — see Repair, stress incontinence

Repair — continued
- bladder NEC — continued
  - laceration (by suture) 57.81
    - obstetric (current) 75.61
    - old 57.89
  - neck 57.85
- blepharophimosis 08.59
- blepharoptosis 08.36
  - by
    - frontalis muscle technique (with)
      - fascial sling 08.32
      - suture 08.31
    - levator muscle technique 08.34
      - with resection or advancement 08.33
    - orbicularis oculi muscle sling 08.36
    - tarsal technique 08.35
- blood vessel NEC 39.59
  - with
    - patch graft 39.58
      - with excision or resection — see Angiectomy, with graft replacement
      - synthetic (Dacron) (Teflon) 39.57
      - tissue (vein) (autogenous) (homograft) 39.56
    - resection — see Angiectomy
    - suture 39.30
  - coronary artery NEC 36.99
    - by angioplasty — see Angioplasty, coronary
    - by atherectomy — see Angioplasty, coronary
  - peripheral vessel NEC 39.59
    - by angioplasty 39.50
    - by atherectomy 39.50
    - by endovascular approach 39.79 ●
- bone NEC (see also Osteoplasty) — see category 78.4 ✓4ᵗʰ
  - by synostosis technique — see Arthrodesis
- accessory sinus 22.79
- cranium NEC 02.06
  - with
    - flap (bone) 02.03
    - graft (bone) 02.04
  - for malunion, nonunion, or delayed union of fracture — see Repair, fracture, malunion or nonunion
- nasal 21.89
- skull NEC 02.06
  - with
    - flap (bone) 02.03
    - graft (bone) 02.04
- bottle, hydrocele of tunica vaginalis 61.2
- brain (trauma) NEC 02.92
- breast (plastic) (see also Mammoplasty) 85.89
- broad ligament 69.29
- bronchus NEC 33.48
  - laceration (by suture) 33.41
- bunionette (with osteotomy) 77.54
- canaliculus, lacrimal 09.73
- canthus (lateral) 08.59
- cardiac pacemaker NEC 37.89
  - electrode(s) (lead) NEC 37.75
- cardioverter/defibrillator (automatic) pocket (skin) (subcutaneous) 37.99
- cerebral meninges 02.12
- cervix 67.69
  - internal os 67.59
    - transabdominal 67.51
    - transvaginal 67.59
  - laceration (by suture) 67.61
    - obstetric (current) 75.51
    - old 67.69
- chest wall (mesh) (silastic) NEC 34.79
- chordae tendineae 35.32
- choroid NEC 14.9
  - with retinal repair — see Repair, retina
- cisterna chyli 40.69
- claw toe 77.57
- cleft
  - hand 82.82
  - laryngotracheal 31.69
  - lip 27.54
  - palate 27.62
    - secondary or subsequent 27.63

Repair — continued
- coarctation of aorta — see Excision, coarctation of aorta
- cochlear prosthetic device 20.99
  - external components only 95.49
- cockup toe 77.58
- colostomy 46.43
- conjunctiva NEC 10.49
  - with scleral repair 12.81
  - laceration 10.6
    - with repair of sclera 12.81
  - late effect of trachoma 10.49
- cornea NEC 11.59
  - with
    - conjunctival flap 11.53
    - transplant — see Keratoplasty
  - postoperative dehiscence 11.52
- coronary artery NEC 36.99
  - by angioplasty — see Angioplasty, coronary
  - by atherectomy — see Antioplasty, coronary
- cranium NEC 02.06
  - with
    - flap (bone) 02.03
    - graft (bone) 02.04
- cusp, valve — see Repair, heart, valve
- cystocele 70.51
  - and rectocele 70.50
- dental arch 24.8
- diaphragm NEC 34.84
- diastasis recti 83.65
- diastematomyelia 03.59
- ear (external) 18.79
  - auditory canal or meatus 18.6
  - auricle NEC 18.79
  - cartilage NEC 18.79
  - laceration (by suture) 18.4
  - lop ear 18.79
  - middle NEC 19.9
  - prominent or protruding 18.5
- ectropion 08.49
  - by or with
    - lid reconstruction 08.44
    - suture (technique) 08.42
    - thermocauterization 08.41
    - wedge resection 08.43
- encephalocele (cerebral) 02.12
- endocardial cushion defect 35.73
  - with
    - prosthesis (grafted to septa) 35.54
    - tissue graft 35.63
- enterocele (female) 70.92
  - male 53.9
- enterostomy 46.40
- entropion 08.49
  - by or with
    - lid reconstruction 08.44
    - suture (technique) 08.42
    - thermocauterization 08.41
    - wedge resection 08.43
- epicanthus (fold) 08.59
- epididymis (and spermatic cord) NEC 63.59
  - with vas deferens 63.89
- epiglottis 31.69
- episiotomy
  - routine following delivery — see Episiotomy
  - secondary 75.69
- epispadias 58.45
- esophagus, esophageal NEC 42.89
  - fistula NEC 42.84
  - stricture 42.85
- exstrophy of bladder 57.86
- eye, eyeball 16.89
  - multiple structures 16.82
  - rupture 16.82
  - socket 16.64
    - with graft 16.63
- eyebrow 08.89
  - linear 08.81
- eyelid 08.89
  - full-thickness 08.85
    - involving lid margin 08.84
  - laceration 08.81
    - full-thickness 08.85
      - involving lid margin 08.84
    - partial-thickness 08.83
      - involving lid margin 08.82

Index to Procedures

Repair — *continued*
  eyelid — *continued*
    linear 08.81
    partial-thickness 08.83
      involving lid margin 08.82
    retraction 08.38
  fallopian tube (with prosthesis) 66.79
    by
      anastomosis 66.73
      reanastomosis 66.79
      reimplantation into
        ovary 66.72
        uterus 66.74
      suture 66.71
  false aneurysm — *see* Repair, aneurysm
  fascia 83.89
    by or with
      arthroplasty — *see* Arthroplasty
      graft (fascial) (muscle) 83.82
        hand 82.72
        tendon 83.81
          hand 82.79
      suture (direct) 83.65
        hand 82.46
    hand 82.89
      by
        graft NEC 82.79
          fascial 82.72
          muscle 82.72
        suture (direct) 82.46
    joint — *see* Arthroplasty
  filtering bleb (corneal) (scleral) (by excision) 12.82
    by
      corneal graft (*see also* Keratoplasty) 11.60
      scleroplasty 12.82
      suture 11.51
      with conjunctival flap 11.53
  fistula — *see also* Closure, fistula
    anovaginal 70.73
    arteriovenous 39.53
      clipping 39.53
      coagulation 39.53
        endovascular approach 39.79 ●
          head and neck 39.72 ●
      division 39.53
      excision or resection — *see also*
        Aneurysmectomy, by site
        with
          anastomosis — *see* Aneurysmectomy,
            with anasto-mosis, by site
          graft replacement — *see*
            Aneurysmectomy, with graft
            replacement, by site
      ligation 39.53
        coronary artery 36.99
      occlusion 39.53
        endovascular approach 39.79 ●
          head and neck 39.72 ●
      suture 39.53
    cervicovesical 57.84
    cervix 67.62
    choledochoduodenal 51.72
    colovaginal 70.72
    enterovaginal 70.74
    enterovesical 57.83
    esophagocutaneous 42.84
    ileovesical 57.83
    intestinovaginal 70.74
    intestinovesical 57.83
    oroantral 22.71
    perirectal 48.93
    pleuropericardial 37.4
    rectovaginal 70.73
    rectovesical 57.83
    rectovesicovaginal 57.83
    scrotum 61.42
    sigmoidovaginal 70.74
    sinus
      nasal 22.71
      of Valsalva 35.39
    splencolic 41.95
    urethroperineovesical 57.84
    urethrovesical 57.84
    urethrovesicovaginal 57.84
    uterovesical 57.84

Repair — *continued*
  fistula — *see also* Closure, fistula — *continued*
    vagina NEC 70.75
    vaginocutaneous 70.75
    vaginoenteric NEC 70.74
    vaginoileal 70.74
    vaginoperineal 70.75
    vaginovesical 57.84
    vesicocervicovaginal 57.84
    vesicocolic 57.83
    vesicocutaneous 57.84
    vesicoenteric 57.83
    vesicointestinal 57.83
    vesicometrorectal 57.83
    vesicoperineal 57.84
    vesicorectal 57.83
    vesicosigmoidal 57.83
    vesicosigmoidovaginal 57.83
    vesicourethral 57.84
    vesicourethrorectal 57.83
    vesicouterine 57.84
    vesicovaginal 57.84
    vulva 71.72
    vulvorectal 48.73
  foramen ovale (patent) 35.71
    with
      prosthesis (open heart technique) 35.51
        closed heart technique 35.52
      tissue graft 35.61
  fracture — *see also* Reduction, fracture
    larynx 31.64
    malunion or nonunion (delayed) NEC — *see*
      category 78.4 ☑4ᵗʰ
      with
        graft — *see* Graft, bone
        insertion (of)
          bone growth stimulator (invasive) —
            see category 78.9 ☑4ᵗʰ
          internal fixation device 78.5 ☑4ᵗʰ
        manipulation for realignment — *see*
          Reduction, fracture, by site,
          closed
        osteotomy
          with
            correction of alignment — *see*
              category 77.3 ☑4ᵗʰ
            with internal fixation device
              — *see* categories
              77.3 ☑4ᵗʰ [78.5 ☑4ᵗʰ]
            with intramed-ullary rod —
              see categories
              77.3 ☑4ᵗʰ [78.5 ☑4ᵗʰ]
        replacement arthroplasty — *see*
          Arthroplasty
        sequestrectomy — *see* category
          77.0 ☑4ᵗʰ
        Sofield type procedure — *see*
          categories 77.3 ☑4ᵗʰ [78.5 ☑4ᵗʰ]
        synostosis technique — *see*
          Arthrodesis
    vertebra 03.53
  funnel chest (with implant) 34.74
  gallbladder 51.91
  gastroschisis 54.71
  great vessels NEC 39.59
    laceration (by suture) 39.30
      artery 39.31
      vein 39.32
  hallux valgus NEC 77.59
    resection of joint with prosthetic implant 77.59
  hammer toe 77.56
  hand 82.89
    with graft or implant 82.79
      fascia 82.72
      muscle 82.72
      tendon 82.79
  heart 37.4
    assist system 37.63
    septum 35.70
      with
        prosthesis 35.50
        tissue graft 35.60

Repair — *continued*
  heart — *continued*
    septum — *continued*
      atrial 35.71
        with
          prosthesis (open heart technique) 35.51
            closed heart technique 35.52
          tissue graft 35.61
        combined with repair of valvular and
          ventricular septal defects — *see*
          Repair, endocardial cushion
          defect
        in total repair of
          tetralogy of Fallot 35.81
          total anomalous pulmonary venous
            connection 35.82
          truncus arteriosus 35.83
      combined with repair of valvular defect —
        see Repair, endocardial cushion
        defect
      ventricular 35.72
        with
          prosthesis 35.53
          tissue graft 35.62
        combined with repair of valvular and
          atrial septal defects — *see*
          Repair, endocardial cushion
          defect
        in total repair of
          tetralogy of Fallot 35.81
          total anomalous pulmonary venous
            connection 35.82
          truncus arteriosus 35.83
    valve (cusps) (open heart technique) 35.10
      with prosthesis or tissue graft 35.20
      aortic (without replacement) 35.11
        with
          prosthesis 35.22
          tissue graft 35.21
        combined with repair of atrial and
          ventricular septal defects — *see*
          Repair, endocardial cushion defect
      mitral (without replacement) 35.12
        with
          prosthesis 35.24
          tissue graft 35.23
      pulmonary (without replacement) 35.13
        with
          prosthesis 35.26
            in total repair of tetralogy of
              Fallot 35.81
          tissue graft 35.25
      tricuspid (without replacement) 35.14
        with
          prosthesis 35.28
          tissue graft 35.27
  hepatic duct 51.79
  hernia NEC 53.9
    anterior abdominal wall NEC 53.59
      with prosthesis or graft 53.69
    colostomy 46.42
    crural 53.29
    cul-de-sac (Douglas') 70.92
    diaphragmatic
      abdominal approach 53.7
      thoracic, thoracoabdominal approach 53.80
    epigastric 53.59
      with prosthesis or graft 53.69
    esophageal hiatus
      abdominal approach 53.7
      thoracic, thoracoabdominal approach 53.80
    fascia 83.89
      hand 82.89
    femoral (unilateral) 53.29
      with prosthesis or graft 53.21
      bilateral 53.39
        with prosthesis or graft 53.31
    Ferguson 53.00
    Halsted 53.00
    Hill-Allison (hiatal hernia repair,
      transpleural approach) 53.80
    hypogastric 53.59
      with prosthesis or graft 53.69

☑4ᵗʰ Fourth-digit Required ▶◀ Revised Text ● New Line ▲ Revised Code

Repair

Repair — continued
- hernia NEC — continued
  - incisional 53.51
    - with prosthesis or graft 53.61
  - inguinal (unilateral) 53.00
    - with prosthesis or graft 53.05
    - bilateral 53.10
      - with prosthesis or graft 53.17
      - direct 53.11
        - with prosthesis or graft 53.14
      - direct and indirect 53.13
        - with prosthesis or graft 53.16
      - indirect 53.12
        - with prosthesis or graft 53.15
    - direct (unilateral) 53.01
      - with prosthesis or graft 53.03
      - and indirect (unilateral) 53.01
        - with prosthesis or graft 53.03
        - bilateral 53.13
          - with prosthesis or graft 53.16
        - bilateral 53.11
          - with prosthesis or graft 53.14
    - indirect (unilateral) 53.02
      - with prosthesis or graft 53.04
      - and direct (unilateral) 53.01
        - with prosthesis or graft 53.03
        - bilateral 53.13
          - with prosthesis or graft 53.16
        - bilateral 53.12
          - with prosthesis or graft 53.15
  - internal 53.9
  - ischiatic 53.9
  - ischiorectal 53.9
  - lumbar 53.9
  - manual 96.27
  - obturator 53.9
  - omental 53.9
  - paraesophageal 53.7
  - parahiatal 53.7
  - paraileostomy 46.41
  - parasternal 53.82
  - paraumbilical 53.49
    - with prosthesis 53.41
  - pericolostomy 46.42
  - perineal (enterocele) 53.9
  - preperitoneal 53.29
  - pudendal 53.9
  - retroperitoneal 53.9
  - sciatic 53.9
  - scrotal — see Repair, hernia, inguinal
  - spigelian 53.59
    - with prosthesis or graft 53.69
  - umbilical 53.49
    - with prosthesis 53.41
  - uveal 12.39
  - ventral 53.59
    - incisional 53.51
      - with prosthesis or graft 53.61
- hydrocele
  - round ligament 69.19
  - spermatic cord 63.1
  - tunica vaginalis 61.2
- hymen 70.76
- hypospadias 58.45
- ileostomy 46.41
- ingrown toenail 86.23
- intestine, intestinal NEC 46.79
  - fistula — see Closure, fistula, intestine
  - laceration
    - large intestine 46.75
    - small intestine NEC 46.73
  - stoma — see Repair, stoma
- inverted uterus NEC 69.29
  - manual
    - nonobstetric 69.94
    - obstetric 75.94
  - obstetrical
    - manual 75.94
    - surgical 75.93
  - vaginal approach 69.23
- iris (rupture) NEC 12.39
- jejunostomy 46.41
- joint (capsule) (cartilage) NEC (see also Arthroplasty) 81.96
- kidney NEC 55.89

Repair — continued
- knee (joint) NEC 81.47
  - collateral ligaments 81.46
  - cruciate ligaments 81.45
  - five-in-one 81.42
  - triad 81.43
- labia — see Repair, vulva
- laceration — see Suture, by site
- lacrimal system NEC 09.99
  - canaliculus 09.73
  - punctum 09.72
    - for eversion 09.71
- laryngostomy 31.62
- laryngotracheal cleft 31.69
- larynx 31.69
  - fracture 31.64
  - laceration 31.61
- leads (cardiac) NEC 37.75
- ligament (see also Arthroplasty) 81.96
  - broad 69.29
  - collateral, knee NEC 81.46
  - cruciate, knee NEC 81.45
  - round 69.29
  - uterine 69.29
- lip NEC 27.59
  - cleft 27.54
  - laceration (by suture) 27.51
- liver NEC 50.69
  - laceration 50.61
- lop ear 18.79
- lung NEC 33.49
- lymphatic (channel) (peripheral) NEC 40.9
  - duct, left (thoracic) NEC 40.69
- macrodactyly 82.83
- mallet finger 82.84
- mandibular ridge 76.64
- mastoid (antrum) (cavity) 19.9
- meninges (cerebral) NEC 02.12
  - spinal NEC 03.59
    - meningocele 03.51
    - myelomeningocele 03.52
- meningocele (spinal) 03.51
  - cranial 02.12
- mesentery 54.75
- mouth NEC 27.59
  - laceration NEC 27.52
- muscle NEC 83.87
  - by
    - graft or implant (fascia) (muscle) 83.82
      - hand 82.72
    - tendon 83.81
      - hand 82.79
    - suture (direct) 83.65
      - hand 82.46
    - transfer or transplantation (muscle) 83.77
      - hand 82.58
  - hand 82.89
    - by
      - graft or implant NEC 82.79
        - fascia 82.72
      - suture (direct) 82.46
      - transfer or transplantation (muscle) 82.58
- musculotendinous cuff, shoulder 83.63
- myelomeningocele 03.52
- nasal
  - septum (perforation) NEC 21.88
  - sinus NEC 22.79
    - fistula 22.71
- nasolabial flaps (plastic) 21.86
- nasopharyngeal atresia 29.4
- nerve (cranial) (peripheral) NEC 04.79
  - old injury 04.76
  - revision 04.75
  - sympathetic 05.81
- nipple NEC 85.87
- nose (external) (internal) (plastic) NEC (see also Rhinoplasty) 21.89
  - laceration (by suture) 21.81
- notched lip 27.59
- omentum 54.74
- omphalocele 53.49
  - with prosthesis 53.41
- orbit 16.89
  - wound 16.81

Repair — continued
- ostium
  - primum defect 35.73
    - with
      - prosthesis 35.54
      - tissue graft 35.63
  - secundum defect 35.71
    - with
      - prosthesis (open heart technique) 35.51
        - closed heart technique 35.52
      - tissue graft 35.61
- ovary 65.79
  - with tube 65.73
    - laparoscopic 65.76
- overlapping toe 77.58
- pacemaker
  - cardiac
    - device (permanent) 37.89
    - electrode(s) (lead) NEC 37.75
    - pocket (skin) (subcutaneous) 37.79
- palate NEC 27.69
  - cleft 27.62
    - secondary or subsequent 27.63
  - laceration (by suture) 27.61
- pancreas NEC 52.95
  - Wirsung's duct 52.99
- papillary muscle (heart) 35.31
- patent ductus arteriosus 38.85
- pectus deformity (chest) (carinatum) (excavatum) 34.74
- pelvic floor NEC 70.79
  - obstetric laceration (current) 75.69
  - old 70.79
- penis NEC 64.49
  - for epispadias or hypospadias 58.45
  - inflatable prosthesis 64.99
  - laceration 64.41
- pericardium 37.4
- perineum (female) 71.79
  - laceration (by suture) 71.71
    - obstetric (current) 75.69
    - old 71.79
  - male NEC 86.89
    - laceration (by suture) 86.59
- peritoneum NEC 54.73
  - by suture 54.64
- pharynx NEC 29.59
  - laceration (by suture) 29.51
  - plastic 29.4
- pleura NEC 34.93
- postcataract wound dehiscence 11.52
  - with conjunctival flap 11.53
- pouch of Douglas 70.52
- primum ostium defect 35.73
  - with
    - prosthesis 35.54
    - tissue graft 35.63
- prostate 60.93
- ptosis, eyelid — see Repair, blepharoptosis
- punctum, lacrimal NEC 09.72
  - for correction of eversion 09.71
- quadriceps (mechanism) 83.86
- rectocele (posterior colporrhaphy) 70.52
  - and cystocele 70.50
- rectum NEC 48.79
  - laceration (by suture) 48.71
  - prolapse NEC 48.76
    - abdominal, approach 48.75
- retina, retinal
  - detachment 14.59
    - by
      - cryotherapy 14.52
      - diathermy 14.51
      - photocoagulation 14.55
        - laser 14.54
        - xenon arc 14.53
      - scleral buckling (see also Buckling, scleral) 14.49
  - tear or defect 14.39
    - by
      - cryotherapy 14.32
      - diathermy 14.31
      - photocoagulation 14.35
        - laser 14.34
        - xenon arc 14.33

Index to Procedures

Repair — continued
  retroperitoneal tissue 54.73
  rotator cuff (suture) 83.63
  round ligament 69.29
  ruptured tendon NEC 83.88
    hand 82.86
  salivary gland or duct NEC 26.49
  sclera, scleral 12.89
    fistula 12.82
    staphyloma NEC 12.86
      with graft 12.85
  scrotum 61.49
  sinus
    nasal NEC 22.79
    of Valsalva (aneurysm) 35.39
  skin (plastic) (without graft) 86.89
    laceration (by suture) 86.59
  skull NEC 02.06
    with
      flap (bone) 02.03
      graft (bone) 02.04
  spermatic cord NEC 63.59
    laceration (by suture) 63.51
  sphincter ani 49.79
    laceration (by suture) 49.71
      obstetric (current) 75.62
      old 49.79
  spina bifida NEC 03.59
    meningocele 03.51
    myelomeningocele 03.52
  spinal (cord) (meninges) (structures) NEC 03.59
    meningocele 03.51
    myelomeningocele 03.52
  spleen 41.95
  sternal defect 78.41
  stoma
    bile duct 51.79
    bladder 57.22
    bronchus 33.42
    common duct 51.72
    esophagus 42.89
    gallbladder 51.99
    hepatic duct 51.79
    intestine 46.40
      large 46.43
      small 46.41
    kidney 55.89
    larynx 31.63
    rectum 48.79
    stomach 44.69
    thorax 34.79
    trachea 31.74
    ureter 56.62
    urethra 58.49
  stomach NEC 44.69
    laceration (by suture) 44.61
  stress incontinence (urinary) NEC 59.79
    by
      anterior urethropexy 59.79
      Burch 59.5
      cystourethropexy (with levator muscle sling) 59.71
      injection of implant (collagen) (fat) (polytef) 59.72
      paraurethral suspension (Pereyra) 59.6
      periurethral suspension 59.6
      plication of urethrovesical junction 59.3
      pubococcygeal sling 59.71
      retropubic urethral suspension 59.5
      suprapubic sling 59.4
      tension free vaginal tape 59.79
      urethrovesical suspension 59.4
        gracilis muscle transplant 59.71
        levator muscle sling 59.71
  subcutaneous tissue (plastic) (without skin graft) 86.89
    laceration (by suture) 86.59
  supracristal defect (heart) 35.72
    with
      prosthesis 35.53
      tissue graft 35.62
  symblepharon NEC 10.49
    by division (with insertion of conformer) 10.5
    with free graft 10.41
  syndactyly 86.85
  synovial membrane, joint — see Arthroplasty

Repair — continued
  telecanthus 08.59
  tendon 83.88
    by or with
      arthroplasty — see Arthroplasty
      graft or implant (tendon) 83.81
        fascia 83.82
          hand 82.72
        hand 82.79
        muscle 83.82
          hand 82.72
      suture (direct) (immediate) (primary) (see also Suture, tendon) 83.64
        hand 82.45
      transfer or transplantation (tendon) 83.75
        hand 82.56
    hand 82.86
      by
        graft or implant (tendon) 82.79
        suture (direct) (immediate) (primary) (see also Suture, tendon, hand) 82.45
        transfer or transplantation (tendon) 82.56
    rotator cuff (direct suture) 83.63
    ruptured NEC 83.88
      hand 82.86
    sheath (direct suture) 83.61
      hand 82.41
  testis NEC 62.69
  tetralogy of Fallot
    partial — see specific procedure
    total (one-stage) 35.81
  thoracic duct NEC 40.69
  thoracostomy 34.72
  thymus (gland) 07.93
  tongue NEC 25.59
  tooth NEC 23.2
    by
      crown (artificial) 23.41
      filling (amalgam) (plastic) (silicate) 23.2
      inlay 23.3
  total anomalous pulmonary venous connection
    partial — see specific procedure
    total (one-stage) 35.82
  trachea NEC 31.79
    laceration (by suture) 31.71
  tricuspid atresia 35.94
  truncus arteriosus
    partial — see specific procedure
    total (one-stage) 35.83
  tunica vaginalis 61.49
    laceration (by suture) 61.41
  tympanum — see Tympanoplasty
  ureter NEC 56.89
    laceration (by suture) 56.82
  ureterocele 56.89
  urethra NEC 58.49
    laceration (by suture) 58.41
      obstetric (current) 75.61
      old 58.49
    meatus 58.47
  urethrocele (anterior colporrhaphy) (female) 70.51
    and rectocele 70.50
  urinary sphincter, artificial (component) 58.99
  urinary stress incontinence — see Repair, stress incontinence
  uterus, uterine 69.49
    inversion — see Repair, inverted uterus
    laceration (by suture) 69.41
      obstetric (current) 75.50
      old 69.49
    ligaments 69.29
      by
        interposition 69.21
        plication 69.22
  uvula 27.73
    with synchronous cleft palate repair 27.62
  vagina, vaginal (cuff) (wall) NEC 70.79
    anterior 70.51
      with posterior repair 70.50
    cystocele 70.51
      and rectocele 70.50
    enterocele 70.92

Repair — continued
  vagina, vaginal NEC — continued
    laceration (by suture) 70.71
      obstetric (current) 75.69
      old 70.79
    posterior 70.52
      with anterior repair 70.50
    rectocele 70.52
      and cystocele 70.50
    urethrocele 70.51
      and rectocele 70.50
  varicocele 63.1
  vas deferens 63.89
    by
      anastomosis 63.82
        to epididymis 63.83
      reconstruction 63.82
    laceration (by suture) 63.81
  vein NEC 39.59
    with
      patch graft 39.58
        with excision or resection of vessel — see Phlebectomy, with graft replacement, by site
        synthetic (Dacron) (Teflon) 39.57
        tissue (vein) (autogenous) (homograft) 39.56
      suture 39.32
    by
      endovascular approach 39.79 •
      head and neck 39.72 •
  ventricular septal defect 35.72
    with
      prosthesis 35.53
        in total repair of tetralogy of Fallot 35.81
      tissue graft 35.62
    combined with repair of valvular and atrial septal defects — see Repair, endocardial cushion defect
    in total repair of
      tetralogy of Fallot 35.81
      truncus arteriosus 35.83
  vertebral arch defect (spina bifida) 03.59
  vulva NEC 71.79
    laceration (by suture) 71.71
      obstetric (current) 75.69
      old 71.79
  Wirsung's duct 52.99
  wound (skin) (without graft) 86.59
    abdominal wall 54.63
    dehiscence 54.61
    postcataract dehiscence (corneal) 11.52

Replacement
  acetabulum (with prosthesis) 81.52
  ankle, total 81.56
    revision 81.59
  aortic valve (with prosthesis) 35.22
    with tissue graft 35.21
  artery — see Graft, artery
  bag — see Replacement, pack or bag
  Barton's tongs (skull) 02.94
  bladder
    with
      ileal loop 57.87 [45.51]
      sigmoid 57.87 [45.52]
      sphincter, artificial 58.93
  caliper tongs (skull) 02.94
  cannula
    arteriovenous shunt 39.94
    pancreatic duct 97.05
    vessel-to-vessel (arteriovenous) 39.94
  cardiac resynchronization device •
    defibrillator (CRT-D) (total system) 00.51 •
      left ventricular coronary venous lead only 00.52 •
      pulse generator only 00.54 •
    pacemaker (CRT-P) (total system) 00.50 •
      left ventricular coronary venous lead only 00.52 •
      pulse generator only 00.53 •
  cardioverter/defibrillator (total system) 37.94
    leads only (electrodes) (sensing) (pacing) 37.97
    pulse generator only 37.98

Replacement

Replacement — *continued*
- cast NEC 97.13
  - lower limb 97.12
  - upper limb 97.11
- catheter
  - bladder (indwelling) 57.95
  - cystostomy 59.94
  - ventricular shunt (cerebral) 02.42
  - wound 97.15
- CRT-D (cardiac resynchronization defibrillator) 00.51
  - left ventricular coronary venous lead only 00.52
  - pulse generator only 00.54
- CRT-P (cardiac resynchronization pacemaker) 00.50
  - left ventricular coronary venous lead only 00.52
  - pulse generator only 00.53
- Crutchfield tongs (skull) 02.94
- cystostomy tube (catheter) 59.94
- diaphragm, vagina 97.24
- drain — *see also* Replacement, tube
  - vagina 97.26
  - vulva 97.26
  - wound musculoskeletal or skin 97.16
- ear (prosthetic) 18.71
- elbow (joint), total 81.84
- electrode(s) — *see* Implant, electrode or lead by site or name of device
  - brain
    - depth 02.93
    - foramen ovale 02.93
    - sphenoidal 02.96
  - depth 02.93
  - foramen ovale 02.93
  - sphenoidal 02.96
- electroencephalographic receiver (brain) (intracranial) 02.93
- electronic
  - cardioverter/defibrillator — *see* Replacement, cardioverter/defibrillator
  - leads (electrode)(s) — *see* Replacement, pacemaker, electrode(s), cardiac
  - stimulator — *see also* Implant, electronic stimulator, by site
    - bladder 57.97
    - muscle (skeletal) 83.92
    - ureter 56.93
- electrostimulator — *see* Implant, electronic stimulator by site
- enterostomy device (tube)
  - large intestine 97.04
  - small intestine 97.03
- epidural pegs 02.93
- femoral head, by prosthesis 81.52
  - revision 81.53
- Gardner Wells tongs (skull) 02.94
- graft — *see* Graft
- halo traction device (skull) 02.94
- Harrington rod (with refusion of spine) — *see* Refusion, spinal
- heart
  - artificial 37.63
  - valve (with prosthesis) (with tissue graft) 35.20
    - aortic (with prosthesis) 35.22
      - with tissue graft 35.21
    - mitral (with prosthesis) 35.24
      - with tissue graft 35.23
    - poppet (prosthetic) 35.95
    - pulmonary (with prosthesis) 35.26
      - with tissue graft 35.25
        - in total repair of tetralogy of Fallot 35.81
    - tricuspid (with prosthesis) 35.28
      - with tissue graft 35.27
- hip (partial) (with fixation device) (with prosthesis) (with traction) 81.52
  - acetabulum 81.52
    - revision 81.53
  - femoral head 81.52
    - revision 81.53
  - total 81.51
    - revision 81.53
- inverted uterus — *see* Repair, inverted uterus

Replacement — *continued*
- iris NEC 12.39
- kidney, mechanical 55.97
- knee (bicompartmental) (hemijoint) (partial) (total) (tricompartmental) (unicompartmental) 81.54
  - revision 81.55
- laryngeal stent 31.93
- leads (electrode)(s) — *see* Replacement, pacemaker, electrode(s), cardiac
- mechanical kidney 55.97
- mitral valve (with prosthesis) 35.24
  - with tissue graft 35.23
- Mulligan hood, fallopian tube 66.93
- muscle stimulator (skeletal) 83.92
- nephrostomy tube 55.93
- neuropacemaker — *see* Implant, neuropacemaker, by site
- neurostimulator — *see also* implant, neurostimulator, by site
  - peripheral nerve 04.92
  - skeletal muscle 83.92
- pacemaker
  - brain 02.93
  - cardiac device (initial) (permanent)
    - dual-chamber device 37.87
    - resynchronization — *see* Replacement, CRT-P
    - single-chamber device 37.85
      - rate responsive 37.86
  - electrode(s), cardiac (atrial) (transvenous) (ventricular) 37.76
    - epicardium (myocardium) 37.74
    - left ventricular coronary venous system 00.52
  - intracranial 02.93
  - neural
    - brain 02.93
    - intracranial 02.93
    - peripheral nerve 04.92
    - spine 03.93
  - spine 03.93
  - temporary transvenous pacemaker system 37.78
- pack or bag
  - nose 97.21
  - teeth, tooth 97.22
  - vagina 97.26
  - vulva 97.26
  - wound 97.16
- pessary, vagina NEC 97.25
- prosthesis
  - acetabulum 81.53
  - arm (bioelectric) (cineplastic) (kineplastic) 84.44
  - biliary tract 51.99
  - cochlear 20.96
    - channel (single) 20.97
      - multiple 20.98
  - elbow 81.97
  - extremity (bioelectric) (cineplastic) (kineplastic) 84.40
    - lower 84.48
    - upper 84.44
  - fallopian tube (Mulligan hood) (stent) 66.93
  - femur 81.53
  - knee 81.55
  - leg (bioelectric) (cineplastic) (kineplastic) 84.48
  - penis (internal) (non-inflatable) 64.95
    - inflatable (internal) 64.97
- pulmonary valve (with prosthesis) 35.26
  - with tissue graft 35.25
    - in total repair of tetralogy of Fallot 35.81
- pyelostomy tube 55.94
- rectal tube 96.09
- shoulder NEC 81.83
  - partial 81.81
  - total 81.80
- skull
  - plate 02.05
  - tongs 02.94
- specified appliance or device NEC 97.29
- stent
  - bile duct 97.05
  - fallopian tube 66.93

Replacement — *continued*
- stent — *continued*
  - larynx 31.93
  - pancreatic duct 97.05
  - trachea 31.93
- stimoceiver — *see* Implant, stimoceiver, by site
- subdural
  - grids 02.93
  - strips 02.93
- testis in scrotum 62.5
- tongs, skull 02.94
- tracheal stent 31.93
- tricuspid valve (with prosthesis) 35.28
  - with tissue graft 35.27
- tube
  - bile duct 97.05
  - bladder 57.95
  - cystostomy 59.94
  - esophagostomy 97.01
  - gastrostomy 97.02
  - large intestine 97.04
  - nasogastric 97.01
  - nephrostomy 55.93
  - pancreatic duct 97.05
  - pyelostomy 55.94
  - rectal 96.09
  - small intestine 97.03
  - tracheostomy 97.23
  - ureterostomy 59.93
  - ventricular (cerebral) 02.42
- umbilical cord, prolapsed 73.92
- ureter (with)
  - bladder flap 56.74
  - ileal segment implanted into bladder 56.89 [45.51]
- ureterostomy tube 59.93
- urethral sphincter, artificial 58.93
- urinary sphincter, artificial 58.93
- valve
  - heart — *see also* Replacement, heart valve
  - poppet (prosthetic) 35.95
  - ventricular (cerebral) 02.42
- ventricular shunt (catheter) (valve) 02.42
- Vinke tongs (skull) 02.94
- vitreous (silicone) 14.75
  - for retinal reattachment 14.59

Replant, replantation — *see also* Reattachment
- extremity — *see* Reattachment, extremity
- penis 64.45
- scalp 86.51
- tooth 23.5

Reposition
- cardiac pacemaker
  - electrode(s) (atrial) (transvenous) (ventricular) 37.75
  - pocket 37.79
- cardioverter/defibrillator
  - lead(s) (sensing) (pacing) (epicardial patch) 37.99
  - pocket 37.99
  - pulse generator 37.99
- cilia base 08.71
- iris 12.39
- renal vessel, aberrant 39.55
- thyroid tissue 06.94
- tricuspid valve (with plication) 35.14

Resection — *see also* Excision, by site
- abdominoendorectal (combined) 48.5
- abdominoperineal (rectum) 48.5
  - pull-through (Altmeier) (Swenson) NEC 48.49
    - Duhamel type 48.65
- alveolar process and palate (en bloc) 27.32
- aneurysm — *see* Aneurysmectomy
- aortic valve (for subvalvular stenosis) 35.11
- artery — *see* Arteriectomy
- bile duct NEC 51.69
  - common duct NEC 51.63
- bladder (partial) (segmental) (transvesical) (wedge) 57.6
  - complete or total 57.79
  - lesionNEC 57.59
    - transurethral approach 57.49
  - neck 57.59
    - transurethral approach 57.49

Index to Procedures

Resection

Resection — see also Excision, by site — continued
- blood vessel — see Angiectomy
- brain 01.59
  - by
    - stereotactic radiosurgery 92.30
      - cobalt 80 92.32
      - linear accelerator (LINAC) 92.31
      - multi-source 92.32
      - particle beam 92.33
      - particulate 92.33
      - radiosurgery NEC 92.39
      - single source photon 92.31
  - hemisphere 01.52
  - lobe 01.53
- breast — see also Mastectomy
  - quadrant 85.22
  - segmental 85.23
- broad ligament 69.19
- bronchus (sleeve) (wide sleeve) 32.1
  - block (en bloc) (with radical dissection of brachial plexus, bronchus, lobe of lung, ribs, and sympathetic nerves) 32.6
- bursa 83.5
  - hand 82.31
- cecum (and terminal ileum) 45.72
- cerebral meninges 01.51
- chest wall 34.4
- clavicle 77.81
- clitoris 71.4
- colon (partial) (segmental) 45.79
  - ascending (cecum and terminal ileum) 45.72
  - cecum (and terminal ileum) 45.72
  - complete 45.8
  - descending (sigmoid) 45.76
  - for interposition 45.52
  - Hartmann 45.75
  - hepatic flexure 45.73
  - left radical (hemicolon) 45.75
  - multiple segmental 45.71
  - right radical (hemicolon) (ileocolectomy) 45.73
  - segmental NEC 45.79
    - multiple 45.71
  - sigmoid 45.76
  - splenic flexure 45.75
  - total 45.8
  - transverse 45.74
- conjunctiva, for pterygium 11.39
- corneal graft 11.32
- cornual (fallopian tube) (unilateral) 66.69
  - bilateral 66.63
- diaphragm 34.81
- endaural 20.79
- endorectal (pull-through) (Soave) 48.41
  - combined abdominal 48.5
- esophagus (partial) (subtotal) (see also Esophagectomy) 42.41
  - total 42.42
- exteriorized intestine — see Resection, intestine, exteriorized
- fascia 83.44
  - for graft 83.43
    - hand 82.34
  - hand 82.35
    - for graft 82.34
- gallbladder (total) 51.22
- gastric (partial) (sleeve) (subtotal) NEC (see also Gastrectomy) 43.89
  - with anastomosis NEC 43.89
    - esophagogastric 43.5
    - gastroduodenal 43.6
    - gastrogastric 43.89
    - gastrojejunal 43.7
  - complete or total NEC 43.99
    - with intestinal interposition 43.91
  - radical NEC 43.99
    - with intestinal interposition 43.91
  - wedge 43.42
    - endoscopic 43.41
- hallux valgus (joint) — see also Bunionectomy
  - with prosthetic implant 77.59
- hepatic
  - duct 51.69
  - flexure (colon) 45.73

Resection — see also Excision, by site — continued
- infundibula, heart (right) 35.34
- intestine (partial) NEC 45.79
  - cecum (with terminal ileum) 45.72
  - exteriorized (large intestine) 46.04
    - small intestine 46.02
  - for interposition 45.50
    - large intestine 45.52
    - small intestine 45.51
  - hepatic flexure 45.73
  - ileum 45.62
    - with cecum 45.72
  - large (partial) (segmental) NEC 45.79
    - for interposition 45.52
    - multiple segmental 45.71
    - total 45.8
  - left hemicolon 45.75
  - multiple segmental (large intestine) 45.71
    - small intestine 45.61
  - right hemicolon 45.73
  - segmental (large intestine) 45.79
    - multiple 45.71
    - small intestine 45.62
      - multiple 45.61
  - sigmoid 45.76
  - small (partial) (segmental) NEC 45.62
    - for interposition 45.51
    - multiple segmental 45.61
    - total 45.63
  - total
    - large intestine 45.8
    - small intestine 45.63
- joint structure NEC (see also Arthrectomy) 80.90
- kidney (segmental) (wedge) 55.4
- larynx — see also Laryngectomy
  - submucous 30.29
- lesion — see Excision, lesion, by site
- levator palpebrae muscle 08.33
- ligament (see also Arthrectomy) 80.90
  - broad 69.19
  - round 69.19
  - uterine 69.19
- lip (wedge) 27.43
- liver (partial) (wedge) 50.22
  - lobe (total) 50.3
  - total 50.4
- lung (wedge) NEC 32.29
  - endoscopic 32.28
  - segmental (any part) 32.3
  - volume reduction 32.22
- meninges (cerebral) 01.51
  - spinal 03.4
- mesentery 54.4
- muscle 83.45
  - extraocular 15.13
    - with
      - advancement or recession of other eye muscle 15.3
      - suture of original insertion 15.13
    - levator palpebrae 08.33
    - Müller's, for blepharoptosis 08.35
    - orbicularis oculi 08.20
    - tarsal, for blepharoptosis 08.35
  - for graft 83.43
    - hand 82.34
  - hand 82.36
    - for graft 82.34
  - ocular — see Resection, muscle, extraocular
- myocardium 37.33
- nasal septum (submucous) 21.5
- nerve (cranial) (peripheral) NEC 04.07
  - phrenic 04.03
    - for collapse of lung 33.31
  - sympathetic 05.29
  - vagus — see Vagotomy
- nose (complete) (extended) (partial) (radical) 21.4
- omentum 54.4
- orbitomaxillary, radical 16.51
- ovary (see also Oophorectomy wedge) 65.22
  - laparoscopic 65.24
- palate (bony) (local) 27.31
  - by wide excision 27.32
  - soft 27.49

Resection — see also Excision, by site — continued
- pancreas (total) (with synchronous duodenectomy) 52.6
  - partial NEC 52.59
    - distal (tail) (with part of body) 52.52
    - proximal (head) (with part of body) (with synchronous duodenectomy) 52.51
    - radical subtotal 52.53
  - radical (one-stage) (two-stage) 52.7
  - subtotal 52.53
- pancreaticoduodenal (see also Pancreatectomy) 52.6
- pelvic viscera (en masse) (female) 68.8
  - male 57.71
- penis 64.3
- pericardium (partial) (for)
  - chronic constrictive pericarditis 37.31
  - drainage 37.12
  - removal of adhesions 37.31
- peritoneum 54.4
- pharynx (partial) 29.33
- phrenic nerve 04.03
  - for collapse of lung 33.31
- prostate — see also Prostatectomy
  - transurethral (punch) 60.29
- pterygium 11.39
- radial head 77.83
- rectosigmoid (see also Resection, rectum) 48.69
- rectum (partial) NEC 48.69
  - with
    - pelvic exenteration 68.8
    - transsacral sigmoidectomy 48.61
  - abdominoendorectal (combined) 48.5
  - abdominoperineal 48.5
    - pull-through NEC 48.49
      - Duhamel type 48.65
  - anterior 48.63
    - with colostomy (synchronous) 48.62
  - Duhamel 48.65
  - endorectal 48.41
    - combined abdominal 48.5
  - posterior 48.64
  - pull-through NEC 48.49
    - endorectal 48.41
  - submucosal (Soave) 48.41
    - combined abdominal 48.5
- rib (transaxillary) 77.91
  - as operative approach — omit code
  - incidental to thoracic operation — omit code
- right ventricle (heart), for infundibular stenosis 35.34
- root (tooth) (apex) 23.73
  - with root canal therapy 23.72
  - residual or retained 23.11
- round ligament 69.19
- sclera 12.65
  - with scleral buckling (see also Buckling, scleral) 14.49
  - lamellar (for retinal reattachment) 14.49
    - with implant 14.41
- scrotum 61.3
- soft tissue NEC 83.49
  - hand 82.39
- sphincter of Oddi 51.89
- spinal cord (meninges) 03.4
- splanchnic 05.29
- splenic flexure (colon) 45.75
- sternum 77.81
- stomach (partial) (sleeve) (subtotal) NEC (see also Gastrectomy) 43.89
  - with anastomosis NEC 43.89
    - esophagogastric 43.5
    - gastroduodenal 43.6
    - gastrogastric 43.89
    - gastrojejunal 43.7
  - complete or total NEC 43.99
    - with intestinal interposition 43.91
  - fundus 43.89
  - radical NEC 43.99
    - with intestinal interposition 43.91
  - wedge 43.42
    - endoscopic 43.41
- submucous
  - larynx 30.29
  - nasal septum 21.5

Resection — see also Excision, by site — continued
  submucous — continued
    vocal cords 30.22
  synovial membrane (complete) (partial) (see also Synovectomy) 80.70
  tarsolevator 08.33
  tendon 83.42
    hand 82.33
  thoracic structures (block) (en bloc) (radical) (brachial plexus, bronchus, lobes of lung, ribs, and sympathetic nerves) 32.6
  thorax 34.4
  tongue 25.2
    wedge 25.1
  tooth root 23.73
    with root canal therapy 23.72
      apex (abscess) 23.73
        with root canal therapy 23.72
      residual or retained 23.11
  trachea 31.5
  transurethral
    bladder NEC 57.49
    prostate 60.29
  transverse colon 45.74
  turbinates — see Turbinectomy
  ureter (partial) 56.41
    total 56.42
  uterus — see Hysterectomy
  vein — see Phlebectomy
  ventricle (heart) 37.35
    infundibula 35.34
  vesical neck 57.59
    transurethral 57.49
  vocal cords (punch) 30.22
Respirator, volume-controlled (Bennett) (Byrd) — see Ventilation
Restoration
  cardioesophageal angle 44.66
  dental NEC 23.49
    by
      application of crown (artificial) 23.41
      insertion of bridge (fixed) 23.42
        removable 23.43
  extremity — see Reattachment, extremity
  eyebrow 08.70
    with graft 08.63
  eye socket 16.64
    with graft 16.63
  tooth NEC 23.2
    by
      crown (artificial) 23.41
      filling (amalgam) (plastic) (silicate) 23.2
      inlay 23.3
Resuscitation
  artificial respiration 93.93
  cardiac 99.60
    cardioversion 99.62
      atrial 99.61
    defibrillation 99.62
    external massage 99.63
      open chest 37.91
    intracardiac injection 37.92
  cardiopulmonary 99.60
  endotracheal intubation 96.04
  manual 93.93
  mouth-to-mouth 93.93
  pulmonary 93.93
Resuture
  abdominal wall 54.61
  cardiac septum prosthesis 35.95
  chest wall 34.71
  heart valve prosthesis (poppet) 35.95
  wound (skin and subcutaneous tissue) (without graft) NEC 86.59
Retavase, infusion 99.10
Reteplase, infusion 99.10
Retinaculotomy NEC (see also Division, ligament) 80.40
  carpal tunnel (flexor) 04.43
Retraining
  cardiac 93.36
  vocational 93.85
Retrogasserian neurotomy 04.02

Revascularization
  cardiac (heart muscle) (myocardium) (direct) 36.10
    with
      bypass anastomosis
        abdominal artery to coronary artery 36.17
        aortocoronary (catheter stent) (homograft) (prosthesis) (saphenous vein graft) 36.10
          one coronary vessel 36.11
          two coronary vessels 36.12
          three coronary vessels 36.13
          four coronary vessels 36.14
        gastroepiploic artery to coronary artery 36.17
        internal mammary-coronary artery (single vessel) 36.15
          double vessel 36.16
        specified type NEC 36.19
        thoracic artery-coronary artery (single vessel) 36.15
          double vessel 36.16
      implantation of artery into heart (muscle) (myocardium) (ventricle) 36.2
    indirect 36.2
    specified type NEC 36.39
    transmyocardial open chest 36.31
      percutaneous 36.32
      specified type NEC 36.32
      thoracoscopic 36.32
Reversal, intestinal segment 45.50
  large 45.52
  small 45.51
Revision
  amputation stump 84.3
    current traumatic — see Amputation
  anastomosis
    biliary tract 51.94
    blood vessel 39.49
    gastric, gastrointestinal (with jejunal interposition) 44.5
    intestine (large) 46.94
      small 46.93
    pleurothecal 03.97
    pyelointestinal 56.72
    salpingothecal 03.97
    subarachnoid-peritoneal 03.97
    subarachnoid-ureteral 03.97
    ureterointestinal 56.72
  ankle replacement (prosthesis) 81.59
  anterior segment (eye) wound (operative) NEC 12.83
  arteriovenous shunt (cannula) (for dialysis) 39.42
  arthroplasty — see Arthroplasty
  bone flap, skull 02.06
  breast implant 85.93
  bronchostomy 33.42
  bypass graft (vascular) 39.49
    abdominal-coronary artery 36.17
    aortocoronary (catheter stent) (with prosthesis) (with saphenous vein graft) (with vein graft) 36.10
      one coronary vessel 36.11
      two coronary vessels 36.12
      three coronary vessels 36.13
      four coronary vessels 36.14
    CABG — see Revision, aortocoronary bypass graft
    chest tube — see intercostal catheter
    coronary artery bypass graft (CABG) — see Revision, aortocoronary bypass graft, abdominal-coronary artery bypass, and internal mammary-coronary artery bypass
    intercostal catheter (with lysis of adhesions) 34.04
    internal mammary-coronary artery (single) 36.15
      double vessel 36.16
  cannula, vessel-to-vessel (arteriovenous) 39.94
  canthus, lateral 08.59
  cardiac pacemaker
    device (permanent) 37.89

Revision — continued
  cardiac pacemaker — continued
    electrode(s) (atrial) (transvenous) (ventricular) 37.75
    pocket 37.79
  cardioverter/defibrillator (automatic) pocket 37.99
  cholecystostomy 51.99
  cleft palate repair 27.63
  colostomy 46.43
  conduit, urinary 56.52
  cystostomy (stoma) 57.22
  elbow replacement (prosthesis) 81.97
  enterostomy (stoma) 46.40
    large intestine 46.43
    small intestine 46.41
  enucleation socket 16.64
    with graft 16.63
  esophagostomy 42.83
  exenteration cavity 16.66
    with secondary graft 16.65
  extraocular muscle surgery 15.6
  fenestration, inner ear 20.62
  filtering bleb 12.66
  fixation device (broken) (displaced) (see also Fixation, bone, internal) 78.50
  flap or pedicle graft (skin) 86.75
  foot replacement (prosthesis) 81.59
  gastric anastomosis (with jejunal interposition) 44.5
  gastroduodenostomy (with jejunal interposition) 44.5
  gastrointestinal anastomosis (with jejunal interposition) 44.5
  gastrojejunostomy 44.5
  gastrostomy 44.69
  hand replacement (prosthesis) 81.97
  heart procedure NEC 35.95
  hip replacement (acetabulum) (femoral head) (partial) (total) 81.53
  Holter (-Spitz) valve 02.42
  ileal conduit 56.52
  ileostomy 46.41
  jejunoileal bypass 46.93
  jejunostomy 46.41
  joint replacement
    acetabulum 81.53
    ankle 81.59
    elbow 81.97
    femoral head 81.53
    foot 81.59
    hand 81.97
    hip (partial) (total) 81.53
    knee 81.55
    lower extremity NEC 81.59
    toe 81.59
    upper extremity 81.97
    wrist 81.97
  knee replacement (prosthesis) 81.55
  laryngostomy 31.63
  lateral canthus 08.59
  mallet finger 82.84
  mastoid antrum 19.9
  mastoidectomy 20.92
  nephrostomy 55.89
  neuroplasty 04.75
  ocular implant 16.62
  orbital implant 16.62
  pocket
    cardiac pacemaker
      with initial insertion of pacemaker — omit code
      new site (skin) (subcutaneous) 37.79
    thalamic stimulator pulse generator
      with initial insertion of battery package — omit code
      new site (skin) (subcutaneous) 86.09
    previous mastectomy site — see category 85.0-85.99
  proctostomy 48.79
  prosthesis
    acetabulum
      hip 81.53
    ankle 81.59
    breast 85.93
    elbow 81.97

Index to Procedures

Revision — *continued*
  prosthesis — *continued*
    femoral head 81.53
    foot 81.59
    hand 81.97
    heart valve (poppet) 35.95
    hip (partial) (total) 81.53
    knee 81.55
    lower extremity NEC 81.59
    shoulder 81.97
    toe 81.59
    upper extremity NEC 81.97
    wrist 81.97
  ptosis overcorrection 08.37
  pyelostomy 55.12
  pyloroplasty 44.29
  rhinoplasty 21.84
    scar
      skin 86.84
        with excision 86.3
  scleral fistulization 12.66
  shoulder replacement (prosthesis) 81.97
  shunt
    arteriovenous (cannula) (for dialysis) 39.42
    lumbar-subarachnoid NEC 03.97
    peritoneojugular 54.99
    peritoneovascular 54.99
    pleurothecal 03.97
    salpingothecal 03.97
    spinal (thecal) NEC 03.97
    subarachnoid-peritoneal 03.97
    subarachnoid-ureteral 03.97
    ventricular (cerebral) 02.42
    ventriculoperitoneal
      at peritoneal site 54.95
      at ventricular site 02.42
  stapedectomy NEC 19.29
    with incus replacement (homograft) (prosthesis) 19.21
  stoma
    bile duct 51.79
    bladder (vesicostomy) 57.22
    bronchus 33.42
    common duct 51.72
    esophagus 42.89
    gallbladder 51.99
    hepatic duct 51.79
    intestine 46.40
      large 46.43
      small 46.41
    kidney 55.89
    larynx 31.63
    rectum 48.79
    stomach 44.69
    thorax 34.79
    trachea 31.74
    ureter 56.62
    urethra 58.49
  tack operation 20.79
  toe replacement (prosthesis) 81.59
  tracheostomy 31.74
  tunnel
    pulse generator lead wire 86.99
      with initial procedure — *omit code*
  tympanoplasty 19.6
  uretero-ileostomy, cutaneous 56.52
  ureterostomy (cutaneous) (stoma) NEC 56.62
    ileal 56.52
  urethrostomy 58.49
  urinary conduit 56.52
  vascular procedure (previous) NEC 39.49
  ventricular shunt (cerebral) 02.42
  vesicostomy stoma 57.22
  wrist replacement (prosthesis) 81.97

Rhinectomy 21.4
Rhinocheiloplasty 27.59
  cleft lip 27.54
Rhinomanometry 89.12
Rhinoplasty (external) (internal) NEC 21.87
  augmentation (with graft) (with synthetic implant) 21.85
  limited 21.86
  revision 21.84
  tip 21.86
  twisted nose 21.84

Rhinorrhaphy (external) (internal) 21.81
  for epistaxis 21.09
Rhinoscopy 21.21
Rhinoseptoplasty 21.84
Rhinotomy 21.1
Rhizotomy (radiofrequency) (spinal) 03.1
  acoustic 04.01
  trigeminal 04.02
Rhytidectomy (facial) 86.82
  eyelid
    lower 08.86
    upper 08.87
Rhytidoplasty (facial) 86.82
Ripstein operation (repair of prolapsed rectum) 48.75
Rodney Smith operation (radical subtotal pancreatectomy) 52.53
Roentgenography — *see also* Radiography
  cardiac, negative contrast 88.58
Rolling of conjunctiva 10.33
Root
  canal (tooth) (therapy) 23.70
    with
      apicoectomy 23.72
      irrigation 23.71
    resection (tooth) (apex) 23.73
      with root canal therapy 23.72
    residual or retained 23.11
Rotation of fetal head
  forceps (instrumental) (Kielland) (Scanzoni) (key-in-lock) 72.4
  manual 73.51
Routine
  chest x-ray 87.44
  psychiatric visit 94.12
Roux-en-Y operation
  bile duct 51.36
  cholecystojejunostomy 51.32
  esophagus (intrathoracic) 42.54
  pancreaticojejunostomy 52.96
Roux-Goldthwait operation (repair of recurrent patellar dislocation) 81.44
Roux-Herzen-Judine operation (jejunal loop interposition) 42.63
Rubin test (insufflation of fallopian tube) 66.8
Ruiz-Mora operation (proximal phalangectomy for hammer toe) 77.99
Rupture
  esophageal web 42.01
  joint adhesions, manual 93.26
  membranes, artificial 73.09
    for surgical induction of labor 73.01
  ovarian cyst, manual 65.93
Russe operation (bone graft of scaphoid) 78.04

S

Sacculotomy (tack) 20.79
Sacrectomy (partial) 77.89
  total 77.99
Saemisch operation (corneal section) 11.1
Salpingectomy (bilateral) (total) (transvaginal) 66.51
  with oophorectomy 65.61
    laparoscopic 65.63
  partial (unilateral) 66.69
    with removal of tubal pregnancy 66.62
    bilateral 66.63
      for sterilization 66.39
        by endoscopy 66.29
    remaining or solitary tube 66.52
      with ovary 65.62
        laparoscopic 65.64
  unilateral (total) 66.4
    with
      oophorectomy 65.49
        laparoscopic 65.41
      removal of tubal pregnancy 66.62
    partial 66.69

Salpingography 87.85
Salpingohysterostomy 66.74
Salpingo-oophorectomy (unilateral) 65.49
  that by laparoscope 65.41
  bilateral (same operative episode) 65.61
    laparoscopic 65.63
  remaining or solitary tube and ovary 65.62
    laparoscopic 65.64
Salpingo-oophoroplasty 65.73
  laparoscopic 65.76
Salpingo-oophororrhaphy 65.79
Salpingo-oophorostomy 66.72
Salpingo-oophorotomy 65.09
  laparoscopic 65.01
Salpingoplasty 66.79
Salpingorrhaphy 66.71
Salpingosalpingostomy 66.73
Salpingostomy (for removal of non-ruptured ectopic pregnancy) 66.02
Salpingotomy 66.01
Salpingo-uterostomy 66.74
Salter operation (innominate osteotomy) 77.39
Salvage (autologous blood) (intraoperative) (perioperative) (postoperative) 99.00
Sampling, blood for genetic determination of fetus 75.33
Sandpapering (skin) 86.25
Saucerization
  bone (*see also* Excision, lesion, bone) 77.60
  rectum 48.99
Sauer-Bacon operation (abdominoperineal resection) 48.5
Scalenectomy 83.45
Scalenotomy 83.19
Scaling and polishing, dental 96.54
Scan, scanning
  C.A.T. (computerized axial tomography) 88.38
    abdomen 88.01
    bone 88.38
      mineral density 88.98
    brain 87.03
    head 87.03
    kidney 87.71
    skeletal 88.38
      mineral density 88.98
    thorax 87.41
  computerized axial tomography (C.A.T.) (*see also* Scan, C.A.T.) 88.38
  C.T. — *see* Scan, C.A.T.
  gallium — *see* Scan, radioisotope
  liver 92.02
  positron emission tomography (PET) — *see* Scan, radioisotope
  radioisotope
    adrenal 92.09
    bone 92.14
      marrow 92.05
    bowel 92.04
    cardiac output 92.05
    cardiovascular 92.05
    cerebral 92.11
    circulation time 92.05
    eye 95.16
    gastrointestinal 92.04
    head NEC 92.12
    hematopoietic 92.05
    intestine 92.04
    iodine-131 92.01
    kidney 92.03
    liver 92.02
    lung 92.15
    lymphatic system 92.16
    myocardial infarction 92.05
    pancreatic 92.04
    parathyroid 92.13
    pituitary 92.11
    placenta 92.17
    protein-bound iodine 92.01
    pulmonary 92.15
    radio-iodine uptake 92.01
    renal 92.03
    specified site NEC 92.19

Scan, scanning

Scan, scanning — *continued*
  radioisotope — *continued*
    spleen 92.05
    thyroid 92.01
    total body 92.18
    uterus 92.19
    renal 92.03
  thermal — *see* Thermography
Scapulectomy (partial) 77.81
  total 77.91
Scapulopexy 78.41
Scarification
  conjunctiva 10.33
  nasal veins (with packing) 21.03
  pericardium 36.39
  pleura 34.6
    chemical 34.92
      with cancer chemotherapy substance 34.92 [99.25]
      tetracycline 34.92 [99.21]
Schanz operation (femoral osteotomy) 77.35
Schauta (-Amreich) operation (radical vaginal hysterectomy) 68.7
Schede operation (thoracoplasty) 33.34
Scheie operation
  cautery of sclera 12.62
  sclerostomy 12.62
Schlatter operation (total gastrectomy) 43.99
Schroeder operation (endocervical excision) 67.39
Schuchardt operation (nonobstetrical episiotomy) 71.09
Schwartze operation (simple mastoidectomy) 20.41
Scintiphotography — *see* Scan, radioisotope
Scintiscan — *see* Scan, radioisotope
Sclerectomy (punch) (scissors) 12.65
  for retinal reattachment 14.49
  Holth's 12.65
  trephine 12.61
    with implant 14.41
Scleroplasty 12.89
Sclerosis — *see* Sclerotherapy
Sclerostomy (Scheie's) 12.62
Sclerotherapy
  esophageal varices (endoscopic) 42.33
  hemorrhoids 49.42
  pleura 34.92
    treatment of malignancy (cytotoxic agent) 34.92 [99.25]
    with tetracycline 34.92 [99.21]
  varicose vein 39.92
  vein NEC 39.92
Sclerotomy (exploratory) 12.89
  anterior 12.89
    with
      iridectomy 12.65
      removal of vitreous 14.71
  posterior 12.89
    with
      iridectomy 12.65
      removal of vitreous 14.72
Scott operation
  intestinal bypass for obesity 45.93
  jejunocolostomy (bypass) 45.93
Scraping
  corneal epithelium 11.41
    for smear or culture 11.21
  trachoma follicles 10.33
Scrotectomy (partial) 61.3
Scrotoplasty 61.49
Scrotorrhaphy 61.41
Scrotomy 61.0
Scrub, posterior nasal (adhesions) 21.91
Sculpturing, heart valve — *see* Valvuloplasty, heart
Section — *see also* Division *and* Incision
  cesarean — *see* Cesarean section
  ganglion, sympathetic 05.0

Section — *see also* Division *and* Incision — *continued*
  hypophyseal stalk (*see also* Hypophysectomy, partial) 07.63
  ligamentum flavum (spine) — *omit code*
  nerve (cranial) (peripheral) NEC 04.03
    acoustic 04.01
    spinal root (posterior) 03.1
    sympathetic 05.0
    trigeminal tract 04.02
  Saemisch (corneal) 11.1
  spinal ligament 80.49
    arcuate — *omit code*
    flavum — *omit code*
  tooth (impacted) 23.19
Sedden-Brooks operation (transfer of pectoralis major tendon) 83.75
Semb operation (apicolysis of lung) 33.39
Senning operation (correction of transposition of great vessels) 35.91
Separation
  twins (attached) (conjoined) (Siamese) 84.93
    asymmetrical (unequal) 84.93
    symmetrical (equal) 84.92
Septectomy
  atrial (closed) 35.41
    open 35.42
    transvenous method (balloon) 35.41
  submucous (nasal) 21.5
Septoplasty NEC 21.88
  with submucous resection of septum 21.5
Septorhinoplasty 21.84
Septostomy (atrial) (balloon) 35.41
Septotomy, nasal 21.1
Sequestrectomy
  bone 77.00
    carpals, metacarpals 77.04
    clavicle 77.01
    facial 76.01
    femur 77.05
    fibula 77.07
    humerus 77.02
    nose 21.32
    patella 77.06
    pelvic 77.09
    phalanges (foot) (hand) 77.09
    radius 77.03
    scapula 77.01
    skull 01.25
    specified site NEC 77.09
    tarsals, metatarsals 77.08
    thorax (ribs) (sternum) 77.01
    tibia 77.07
    ulna 77.03
    vertebrae 77.09
  nose 21.32
  skull 01.25
Sesamoidectomy 77.98
Setback, ear 18.5
Sever operation (division of soft tissue of arm) 83.19
Severing of blepharorrhaphy 08.02
Sewell operation (heart) 36.2
Sharrard operation (iliopsoas muscle transfer) 83.77
Shaving
  bone (*see also* Excision, lesion, bone) 77.60
  cornea (epithelium) 11.41
    for smear or culture 11.21
  patella 77.66
Shelf operation (hip arthroplasty) 81.40
Shirodkar operation (encirclement suture, cervix) 67.59
Shock therapy
  chemical 94.24
  electroconvulsive 94.27
  electrotonic 94.27
  insulin 94.24
  subconvulsive 94.26
Shortening
  bone (fusion) 78.20
    femur 78.25

Shortening — *continued*
  bone — *continued*
    specified site NEC (*see* category 78.2) ✓4ᵗʰ
    tibia 78.27
    ulna 78.23
  endopelvic fascia 69.22
  extraocular muscle NEC 15.22
    multiple (two of more muscles) 15.4
  eyelid margin 08.71
  eye muscle NEC 15.22
    multiple (two or more muscles) (with lengthening) 15.4
  finger (macrodactyly repair) 82.83
  heel cord 83.85
  levator palpebrae muscle 08.33
  ligament — *see also* Arthroplasty
    round 69.22
    uterosacral 69.22
  muscle 83.85
    extraocular 15.22
      multiple (two or more muscles) 15.4
    hand 82.55
  sclera (for repair of retinal detachment) 14.59
    by scleral buckling (*see also* Buckling, scleral) 14.49
  tendon 83.85
    hand 82.55
  ureter (with reimplantation) 56.41
Shunt — *see also* Anastomosis *and* Bypass, vascular
  abdominovenous 54.94
  aorta-coronary sinus 36.39
  aorta (descending)-pulmonary (artery) 39.0
  aortocarotid 39.22
  aortoceliac 39.26
  aortofemoral 39.25
  aortoiliac 39.25
  aortoiliofemoral 39.25
  aortomesenteric 39.26
  aorto-myocardial (graft) 36.2
  aortorenal 39.24
  aortosubclavian 39.22
  apicoaortic 35.93
  arteriovenous NEC 39.29
    for renal dialysis (by)
      anastomosis 39.27
      external cannula 39.93
  ascending aorta to pulmonary artery (Waterston) 39.0
  axillary-femoral 39.29
  carotid-carotid 39.22
  carotid-subclavian 39.22
  caval-mesenteric 39.1
  corpora cavernosa-corpus spongiosum 64.98
  corpora-saphenous 64.98
  descending aorta to pulmonary artery (Potts-Smith) 39.0
  endolymphatic (-subarachnoid) 20.71
  endolymph-perilymph 20.71
  extracranial-intracranial (EC-IC) 39.28
  femoroperoneal 39.29
  femoropopliteal 39.29
  iliofemoral 39.25
  ilioiliac 39.25
  intestinal
    large-to-large 45.94
    small-to-large 45.93
    small-to-small 45.91
  left subclavian to descending aorta (Blalock-Park) 39.0
  left-to-right (systemic-pulmonary artery) 39.0
  left ventricle (heart) (apex) and aorta 35.93
  lienorenal 39.1
  lumbar-subarachnoid (with valve) NEC 03.79
  mesocaval 39.1
  peritoneal-jugular 54.94
  peritoneo-vascular 54.94
  peritoneovenous 54.94
  pleuroperitoneal 34.05
  pleurothecal (with valve) 03.79
  portacaval (double) 39.1
  portal-systemic 39.1
  portal vein to vena cava 39.1
  pulmonary-innominate 39.0
  pulmonary vein to atrium 35.82

Shunt — see also Anastomosis and Bypass, vascular — continued
  renoportal 39.1
  right atrium and pulmonary artery 35.94
  right ventricle and pulmonary artery (distal) 35.92
    in repair of
      pulmonary artery atresia 35.92
      transposition of great vessels 35.92
      truncus arteriosus 35.83
  salpingothecal (with valve) 03.79
  semicircular-subarachnoid 20.71
  spinal (thecal) (with valve) NEC 03.79
    subarachnoid-peritoneal 03.71
    subarachnoid-ureteral 03.72
  splenorenal (venous) 39.1
    arterial 39.26
  subarachnoid-peritoneal (with valve) 03.71
  subarachnoid-ureteral (with valve) 03.72
  subclavian-pulmonary 39.0
  subdural-peritoneal (with valve) 02.34
  superior mesenteric-caval 39.1
  systemic-pulmonary artery 39.0
  transjugular intrahepatic portosystemic [TIPS] 39.1
  vena cava to pulmonary artery (Green) 39.21
  ventricular (cerebral) (with valve) 02.2
    to
      abdominal cavity or organ 02.34
      bone marrow 02.39
      cervical subarachnoid space 02.2
      circulatory system 02.32
      cisterna magna 02.2
      extracranial site NFC 02.39
      gallbladder 02.34
      head or neck structure 02.31
      intracerebral site NEC 02.2
      lumbar site 02.39
      mastoid 02.31
      nasopharynx 02.31
      thoracic cavity 02.33
      ureter 02.35
      urinary system 02.35
      venous system 02.32
  ventriculoatrial (with valve) 02.32
  ventriculocaval (with valve) 02.32
  ventriculocisternal (with valve) 02.2
  ventriculolumbar (with valve) 02.39
  ventriculomastoid (with valve) 02.31
  ventriculonasopharyngeal 02.31
  ventriculopleural (with valve) 02.33
Sialoadenectomy (parotid) (sublingual) (submaxillary) 26.30
  complete 26.32
  partial 26.31
  radical 26.32
Sialoadenolithotomy 26.0
Sialoadenotomy 26.0
Sialodochoplasty NEC 26.49
Sialogram 87.09
Sialolithotomy 26.0
Sieve, vena cava 38.7
Sigmoid bladder 57.87 [45.52]
Sigmoidectomy 45.76
Sigmoidomyotomy 46.91
Sigmoidopexy (Moschowitz) 46.63
Sigmoidoproctectomy (see also Resection, rectum) 48.69
Sigmoidoproctostomy 45.94
Sigmoidorectostomy 45.94
Sigmoidorrhaphy 46.75
Sigmoidoscopy (rigid) 48.23
  with biopsy 45.25
  flexible 45.24
  through stoma (artificial) 45.22
  transabdominal 45.21
Sigmoidosigmoidostomy 45.94
  proximal to distal segment 45.76
Sigmoidostomy (see also Colostomy) 46.10
Sigmoidotomy 45.03
Sign language 93.75
Silver operation (bunionectomy) 77.59

Sinogram
  abdominal wall 88.03
  chest wall 87.38
  retroperitoneum 88.14
Sinusectomy (nasal) (complete) (partial) (with turbinectomy) 22.60
  antrum 22.62
    with Caldwell-Luc approach 22.61
  ethmoid 22.63
  frontal 22.42
  maxillary 22.62
    with Caldwell-Luc approach 22.61
  sphenoid 22.64
Sinusotomy (nasal) 22.50
  antrum (intranasal) 22.2
    with external approach (Caldwell-Luc) 22.39
      radical (with removal of membrane lining) 22.31
  ethmoid 22.51
  frontal 22.41
  maxillary (intranasal) 22.2
    external approach (Caldwell-Luc) 22.39
      radical (with removal of membrane lining) 22.31
  multiple 22.53
  perinasal 22.50
  sphenoid 22.52
Sistrunk operation (excision of thyroglossal cyst) 06.7
Size reduction
  abdominal wall (adipose) (pendulous) 86.83
  arms (adipose) (batwing) 86.83
  breast (bilateral) 85.32
    unilateral 85.31
  buttocks (adipose) 86.83
  skin 86.83
  subcutaneous tissue 86.83
  thighs (adipose) 86.83
Skeletal series (x-ray) 88.31
Sling — see also Operation, sling
  fascial (fascia lata)
    for facial weakness (trigeminal nerve paralysis) 86.81
    mouth 86.81
    orbicularis (mouth) 86.81
    tongue 25.59
  levator muscle (urethrocystopexy) 59.71
  pubococcygeal 59.71
  rectum (puborectalis) 48.76
  tongue (fascial) 25.59
Slitting
  canaliculus for
    passage of tube 09.42
    removal of streptothrix 09.42
  lens 13.2
  prepuce (dorsal) (lateral) 64.91
Slocum operation (pes anserinus transfer) 81.47
Sluder operation (tonsillectomy) 28.2
Small bowel series (x-ray) 87.63
Smith operation (open osteotomy of mandible) 76.62
Smith-Peterson operation (radiocarpal arthrodesis) 81.25
Smithwick operation (sympathectomy) 05.29
Snaring, polyp, colon (endoscopic) 45.42
Snip, punctum (with dilation) 09.51
Soave operation (endorectal pull-through) 48.41
Somatotherapy, psychiatric NEC 94.29
Sonneberg operation (inferior maxillary neurectomy) 04.07
Sorondo-Ferrè operation (hindquarter amputation) 84.19
Soutter operation (iliac crest fasciotomy) 83.14
Spaulding-Richardson operation (uterine suspension) 69.22
Spectrophotometry NEC 89.39
  blood 89.39
  placenta 89.29
  urine 89.29
Speech therapy NEC 93.75
Spermatocelectomy 63.2

Spermatocystectomy 60.73
Spermatocystotomy 60.72
Sphenoidectomy 22.64
Sphenoidotomy 22.52
Sphincterectomy, anal 49.6
Sphincteroplasty
  anal 49.79
    obstetrical laceration (current) 75.62
    old 49.79
  bladder neck 57.85
  pancreas 51.83
  sphincter of Oddi 51.83
Sphincterorrhaphy, anal 49.71
  obstetrical laceration (current) 75.62
  old 49.79
Sphincterotomy
  anal (external) (internal) 49.59
    left lateral 49.51
    posterior 49.52
  bladder (neck) (transurethral) 57.91
  choledochal 51.82
    endoscopic 51.85
  iris 12.12
  pancreatic 51.82
    endoscopic 51.85
  sphincter of Oddi 51.82
    endoscopic 51.85
  transduodenal ampullary 51.82
    endoscopic 51.85
Spinal anesthesia — omit code
Spinelli operation (correction of inverted uterus) 75.93
Spirometry (incentive) (respiratory) 89.37
Spivack operation (permanent gastrostomy) 43.19
Splanchnicectomy 05.29
Splanchnicotomy 05.0
Splenectomy (complete) (total) 41.5
  partial 41.43
Splenogram 88.64
  radioisotope 92.05
Splenolysis 54.59
  laparoscopic 54.51
Splenopexy 41.95
Splenoplasty 41.95
Splenoportogram (by splenic arteriography) 88.64
Splenorrhaphy 41.95
Splenotomy 41.2
Splinting
  dental (for immobilization) 93.55
    orthodontic 24.7
  musculoskeletal 93.54
  ureteral 56.2
Splitting — see also Division
  canaliculus 09.52
  lacrimal papilla 09.51
  spinal cord tracts 03.29
    percutaneous 03.21
  tendon sheath 83.01
    hand 82.01
Spondylosyndesis (see also Fusion, spinal) 81.00
S.P. Rogers operation (knee disarticulation) 84.16
Ssabanejew-Frank operation (permanent gastrostomy) 43.19
Stab, intercostal 34.09
Stabilization, joint — see also Arthrodesis
  patella (for recurrent dislocation) 81.44
Stacke operation (simple mastoidectomy) 20.41
Stallard operation (conjunctivocystorhinostomy) 09.82
  with insertion of tube or stent 09.83
Stamm (-Kader) operation (temporary gastrostomy) 43.19
Stapedectomy 19.19
  with incus replacement (homograft) (prosthesis) 19.11
  revision 19.29
    with incus replacement 19.21
Stapediolysis 19.0

Stapling

Stapling
 artery 39.31
 blebs, lung (emphysematous) 32.21
 diaphysis (*see also* Stapling, epiphyseal plate) 78.20
 epiphyseal plate 78.20
  femur 78.25
  fibula 78.27
  humerus 78.22
  radius 78.23
  specified site NEC 78.29
  tibia 78.27
  ulna 78.23
 gastric varices 44.91
 graft — *see* Graft
 vein 39.32
Steinberg operation 44.5
Steindler operation
 fascia stripping (for cavus deformity) 83.14
 flexorplasty (elbow) 83.77
 muscle transfer 83.77
Stereotactic head frame application 93.59
Stereotactic radiosurgery 92.30
 cobalt 60 92.32
 linear accelerator (LINAC) 92.31
 multi-source 92.32
 particle beam 92.33
 particulate 92.33
 radiosurgery NEC 92.39
 single source photon 92.31
Sterilization
 female (*see also* specific operation) 66.39
 male NEC (*see also* Ligation, vas deferens) 63.70
Sternotomy 77.31
 as operative approach — *omit code*
 for bone marrow biopsy 41.31
Stewart operation (renal plication with pyeloplasty) 55.87
Stimulation (electronic) — *see also* Implant, electronic stimulator
 bone growth (percutaneous) — *see* category 78.9
  transcutaneous (surface) 99.86
 cardiac (external) 99.62
  internal 37.91
 carotid sinus 99.64
 defibrillator
  non-invasive programmed electrical stimulation (NIPS) 37.26
 electrophysiologic, cardiac 37.26
 nerve, peripheral or spinal cord, transcutaneous 93.39
Stitch, Kelly-Stoeckel (urethra) 59.3
Stomatoplasty 27.59
Stomatorrhaphy 27.52
Stone operation (anoplasty) 49.79
Strassman operation (metroplasty) 69.49
Strayer operation (gastrocnemius recession) 83.72
Stretching
 eyelid (with elongation) 08.71
 fascia 93.28
 foreskin 99.95
 iris 12.63
 muscle 93.27
 nerve (cranial) (peripheral) 04.91
 tendon 93.27
Stripping
 bone (*see also* Incision, bone) 77.10
 carotid sinus 39.8
 cranial suture 02.01
 fascia 83.14
  hand 82.12
 membranes for surgical induction of labor 73.1
 meninges (cerebral) 01.51
  spinal 03.4
 saphenous vein, varicose 38.59
 subdural membrane (cerebral) 01.51
  spinal 03.4
 varicose veins (lower limb) 38.59
  upper limb 38.53
 vocal cords 30.09

Stromeyer-Little operation (hepatotomy) 50.0
Strong operation (unbridling of celiac artery axis) 39.91
Stryker frame 93.59
Study
 bone mineral density 88.98
 bundle of His 37.29
 color vision 95.06
 conduction, nerve (median) 89.15
 dark adaptation, eye 95.07
 electrophysiologic stimulation and recording, cardiac 37.26
 function — *see also* Function, study
  radioisotope — *see* Scan, radioisotope
 lacrimal flow (radiographic) 87.05
 ocular motility 95.15
 pulmonary function — *see* categories 89.37-89.38
 radiographic — *see* Radiography
 radio-iodinated triolein 92.04
 renal clearance 92.03
 spirometer 89.37
 tracer — *see also* Scan, radioisotope eye (P32) 95.16
 ultrasonic — *see* Ultrasonography
 visual field 95.05
 xenon flow NEC 92.19
  cardiovascular 92.05
  pulmonary 92.15
Sturmdorf operation (conization of cervix) 67.2
Submucous resection
 larynx 30.29
 nasal septum 21.5
Summerskill operation (dacryocystorhinostomy by intubation) 09.81
Surmay operation (jejunostomy) 46.39
Suspension
 balanced, for traction 93.45
 bladder NEC 57.89
 diverticulum, pharynx 29.59
 kidney 55.7
 Olshausen (uterus) 69.22
 ovary 65.79
 paraurethral (Pereyra) 59.6
 periurethral 59.6
 urethra (retropubic) (sling) 59.5
 urethrovesical
  Goebel-Frangenheim-Stoeckel 59.4
  gracilis muscle transplant 59.71
  levator muscle sling 59.71
  Marshall-Marchetti (-Krantz) 59.5
  Millin-Read 59.4
  suprapubic 59.4
 uterus (abdominal or vaginal approach) 69.22
 vagina 70.77
Suture (laceration)
 abdominal wall 54.63
  secondary 54.61
 adenoid fossa 28.7
 adrenal (gland) 07.44
 aneurysm (cerebral) (peripheral) 39.52
 anus 49.71
  obstetric laceration (current) 75.62
  old 49.79
 aorta 39.31
 aponeurosis (*see also* Suture, tendon) 83.64
 arteriovenous fistula 39.53
 artery 39.31
  percutaneous puncture closure — *omit code*
 bile duct 51.79
 bladder 57.81
  obstetric laceration (current) 75.61
 blood vessel NEC 39.30
  artery 39.31
  percutaneous puncture closure — *omit code*
  vein 39.32
 breast (skin) 85.81
 bronchus 33.41
 bursa 83.99
  hand 82.99
 canaliculus 09.73
 cecum 46.75
 cerebral meninges 02.11

Suture — *continued*
 cervix (traumatic laceration) 67.61
  internal os, encirclement 67.59
  obstetric laceration (current) 75.51
  old 67.69
 chest wall 34.71
 cleft palate 27.62
 clitoris 71.4
 colon 46.75
 common duct 51.71
 conjunctiva 10.6
 cornea 11.51
  with conjunctival flap 11.53
 corneoscleral 11.51
  with conjunctival flap 11.53
 diaphragm 34.82
 duodenum 46.71
  ulcer (bleeding) (perforated) 44.42
   endoscopic 44.43
 dura mater (cerebral) 02.11
  spinal 03.59
 ear, external 18.4
 enterocele 70.92
 entropion 08.42
 epididymis (and)
  spermatic cord 63.51
  vas deferens 63.81
 episiotomy — *see* Episiotomy
 esophagus 42.82
 eyeball 16.89
 eyebrow 08.81
 eyelid 08.81
  with entropion or ectropion repair 08.42
 fallopian tube 66.71
 fascia 83.65
  hand 82.46
  to skeletal attachment 83.89
   hand 82.89
 gallbladder 51.91
 ganglion, sympathetic 05.81
 gingiva 24.32
 great vessel 39.30
  artery 39.31
  vein 39.32
 gum 24.32
 heart 37.4
 hepatic duct 51.79
 hymen 70.76
 ileum 46.73
 intestine 46.79
  large 46.75
  small 46.73
 jejunum 46.73
 joint capsule 81.96
  with arthroplasty — *see* Arthroplasty
  ankle 81.94
  foot 81.94
  lower extremity NEC 81.95
  upper extremity 81.93
 kidney 55.81
 labia 71.71
 laceration — *see* Suture, by site
 larynx 31.61
 ligament 81.96
  with arthroplasty — *see* Arthroplasty
  ankle 81.94
  broad 69.29
  Cooper's 54.64
  foot and toes 81.94
  gastrocolic 54.73
  knee 81.95
  lower extremity NEC 81.95
  sacrouterine 69.29
  upper extremity 81.93
  uterine 69.29
 ligation — *see* Ligation
 lip 27.51
 liver 50.61
 lung 33.43
 meninges (cerebral) 02.11
  spinal 03.59
 mesentery 54.75
 mouth 27.52
 muscle 83.65
  hand 82.46
  ocular (oblique) (rectus) 15.7

Index to Procedures

Suture — *continued*
  nerve (cranial) (peripheral) 04.3
    sympathetic 05.81
  nose (external) (internal) 21.81
    for epistaxis 21.09
  obstetric laceration NEC 75.69
    bladder 75.61
    cervix 75.51
    corpus uteri 75.52
    pelvic floor 75.69
    perineum 75.69
    rectum 75.62
    sphincter ani 75.62
    urethra 75.61
    uterus 75.50
    vagina 75.69
    vulva 75.69
  omentum 54.64
  ovary 65.71
    laparoscopic 65.74
  palate 27.61
    cleft 27.62
  palpebral fissure 08.59
  pancreas 52.95
  pelvic floor 71.71
    obstetric laceration (current) 75.69
  penis 64.41
  peptic ulcer (bleeding) (perforated) 44.40
  pericardium 37.4
  perineum (female) 71.71
    after delivery 75.69
      episiotomy repair — *see* Episiotomy
    male 86.59
  periosteum 78.20
    carpal, metacarpal 78.24
    femur 78.25
    fibula 78.27
    humerus 78.22
    pelvic 78.29
    phalanges (foot) (hand) 78.29
    radius 78.23
    specified site NEC 78.29
    tarsal, metatarsal 78.28
    tibia 78.27
    ulna 78.23
    vertebrae 78.24
  peritoneum 54.64
  periurethral tissue to symphysis pubis 59.5
  pharynx 29.51
  pleura 34.93
  rectum 48.71
    obstetric laceration (current) 75.62
  retina (for reattachment) 14.59
  sacrouterine ligament 69.29
  salivary gland 26.41
  scalp 86.59
    replantation 86.51
  sclera (with repair of conjunctiva) 12.81
  scrotum (skin) 61.41
  secondary
    abdomnninal wall 54.61
    episiotomy 75.69
    peritoneum 54.64
  sigmoid 46.75
  skin (mucous membrane) (without graft) 86.59
    with graft — *see* Graft, skin
    breast 85.81
    ear 18.4
    eyebrow 08.81
    eyelid 08.81
    nose 21.81
    penis 64.41
    scalp 86.59
      replantation 86.51
    scrotum 61.41
    vulva 71.71
  specified site NEC — *see* Repair, by site
  spermatic cord 63.51
  sphincter ani 49.71
    obstetric laceration (current) 75.62
    old 49.79
  spinal meninges 03.59
  spleen 41.95
  stomach 44.61
    ulcer (bleeding) (perforated) 44.41
      endoscopic 44.43

Suture — *continued*
  subcutaneous tissue (without skin graft) 86.59
    with graft — *see* Graft, skin
  tendon (direct) (immediate) (primary) 83.64
    delayed (secondary) 83.62
      hand NEC 82.43
        flexors 82.42
    hand NEC 82.45
      delayed (secondary) 82.43
      flexors 82.44
        delayed (secondary) 82.42
    ocular 15.7
    rotator cuff 83.63
    sheath 83.61
      hand 82.41
    supraspinatus (rotator cuff repair) 83.63
    to skeletal attachment 83.88
      hand 82.85
  Tenon's capsule 15.7
  testis 62.61
  thymus 07.93
  thyroid gland 06.93
  tongue 25.51
  tonsillar fossa 28.7
  trachea 31.71
  tunica vaginalis 61.41
  ulcer (bleeding) (perforated) (peptic) 44.40
    duodenum 44.42
      endoscopic 44.43
    gastric 44.41
      endoscopic 44.43
    intestine 46.79
    skin 86.59
    stomach 44.41
      endoscopic 44.43
  ureter 56.82
  urethra 58.41
    obstetric laceration (current) 75.61
  uterosacral ligament 69.29
  uterus 69.41
    obstetric laceration (current) 75.50
    old 69.49
  uvula 27.73
  vagina 70.71
    obstetric laceration (current) 75.69
    old 70.79
  vas deferens 63.81
  vein 39.32
  vulva 71.71
    obstetric laceration (current) 75.69
    old 71.79

Suture-ligation — *see also* Ligation
  blood vessel — *see* Ligation, blood vessel

Sweep, anterior iris 12.97

Swenson operation
  bladder reconstruction 57.87
  proctectomy 48.49

Swinney operation (urethral reconstruction) 58.46

Switch, switching
  coronary arteries 35.84
  great arteries, total 35.84

Syme operation
  ankle amputation through malleoli of tibia and fibula 84.14
  urethrotomy, external 58.0

Sympathectomy NEC 05.29
  cervical 05.22
  cervicothoracic 05.22
  lumbar 05.23
  periarterial 05.25
  presacral 05.24
  renal 05.29
  thoracolumbar 05.23
  tympanum 20.91

Sympatheticotripsy 05.0

Symphysiotomy 77.39
  assisting delivery (obstetrical) 73.94
  kidney (horseshoe) 55.85

Symphysis, pleural 34.6

Synchondrotomy (*see also* Division, cartilage) 80.40

Syndactylization 86.89

Syndesmotomy (*see also* Division, ligament) 80.40

Synechiotomy
  endometrium 68.21
  iris (posterior) 12.33
    anterior 12.32

Synovectomy (joint) (complete) (partial) 80.70
  ankle 80.77
  elbow 80.72
  foot and toe 80.78
  hand and finger 80.74
  hip 80.75
  knee 80.76
  shoulder 80.71
  specified site NEC 80.79
  spine 80.79
  tendon sheath 83.42
    hand 82.33
  wrist 80.73

Syringing
  lacrimal duct or sac 09.43
  nasolacrimal duct 09.43
    with
      dilation 09.43
      insertion of tube or stent 09.44

T

Taarnhoj operation (trigeminal nerve root decompression) 04.41

Tack operation (sacculotomy) 20.79

Take-down
  anastomosis
    arterial 39.49
    blood vessel 39.49
    gastric, gastrointestinal 44.5
    intestine 46.93
    stomach 44.5
    vascular 39.49
    ventricular 02.43
  arterial bypass 39.49
  arteriovenous shunt 39.43
    with creation of new shunt 39.42
  cecostomy 46.52
  colostomy 46.52
  duodenostomy 46.51
  enterostomy 46.50
  esophagostomy 42.83
  gastroduodenostomy 44.5
  gastrojejunostomy 44.5
  ileostomy 46.51
  intestinal stoma 46.50
    large 46.52
    small 46.51
  jejunoileal bypass 46.93
  jejunostomy 46.51
  laryngostomy 31.62
  sigmoidostomy 46.52
  stoma
    bile duct 51.79
    bladder 57.82
    bronchus 33.42
    common duct 51.72
    esophagus 42.83
    gall bladder 51.92
    hepatic duct 51.79
    intestine 46.50
      large 46.52
      small 46.51
    kidney 55.82
    larynx 31.62
    rectum 48.72
    stomach 44.62
    thorax 34.72
    trachea 31.72
    ureter 56.83
    urethra 58.42
  systemic-pulmonary artery anastomosis 39.49
    in total repair of tetralogy of Fallot 35.81
  tracheostomy 31.72
  vascular anastomosis or bypass 39.49
  ventricular shunt (cerebral) 02.43

Talectomy 77.98

Talma-Morison operation
- **Talma-Morison operation** (omentopexy) 54.74
- **Tamponade**
  - esophageal 96.06
  - intrauterine (nonobstetric) 69.91
    - after delivery or abortion 75.8
    - antepartum 73.1
  - vagina 96.14
    - after delivery or abortion 75.8
    - antepartum 73.1
- **Tanner operation** (devascularization of stomach) 44.99
- **Tap**
  - abdomen 54.91
  - chest 34.91
  - cisternal 01.01
  - cranial 01.09
  - joint 81.91
  - lumbar (diagnostic) (removal of dye) 03.31
  - perilymphatic 20.79
  - spinal (diagnostic) 03.31
  - subdural (through fontanel) 01.09
  - thorax 34.91
- **Tarsectomy** 08.20
  - de Grandmont 08.35
- **Tarsoplasty** (see also Reconstruction, eyelid) 08.70
- **Tarsorrhaphy** (lateral) 08.52
  - division or severing 08.02
- **Tattooing**
  - cornea 11.91
  - skin 86.02
- **Tautening, eyelid for entropion** 08.42
- **Telemetry** (cardiac) 89.54
- **Teleradiotherapy**
  - beta particles 92.25
  - Betatron 92.24
  - cobalt-60 92.23
  - electrons 92.25
  - iodine-125 92.23
  - linear accelerator 92.24
  - neutrons 92.26
  - particulate radiation NEC 92.26
  - photons 92.24
  - protons 92.26
  - radioactive cesium 92.23
  - radioisotopes NEC 92.23
- **Temperature gradient study** (see also Thermography) 88.89
- **Temperament assessment** 94.02
- **Tendinoplasty** — see Repair, tendon
- **Tendinosuture** (immediate) (primary) (see also Suture, tendon) 83.64
  - hand (see also Suture, tendon, hand) 82.45
- **Tendolysis** 83.91
  - hand 82.91
- **Tendoplasty** — see Repair, tendon
- **Tenectomy** 83.39
  - eye 15.13
    - levator palpebrae 08.33
    - multiple (two or more tendons) 15.3
  - hand 82.29
  - levator palpebrae 08.33
  - tendon sheath 83.31
    - hand 82.21
- **Tenodesis** (tendon fixation to skeletal attachment) 83.88
  - Fowler 82.85
  - hand 82.85
- **Tenolysis** 83.91
  - hand 82.91
- **Tenomyoplasty** (see also Repair, tendon) 83.88
  - hand (see also Repair, tendon, hand) 82.86
- **Tenomyotomy** — see Tenonectomy
- **Tenonectomy** 83.42
  - for graft 83.41
    - hand 82.32
  - hand 82.33
    - for graft 82.32
- **Tenontomyoplasty** — see Repair, tendon
- **Tenontoplasty** — see Repair, tendon

Tenoplasty (see also Repair, tendon) 83.88
- hand (see also Repair, tendon, hand) 82.86

Tenorrhaphy (see also Suture, tendon) 83.64
- hand (see also Suture, tendon, hand) 82.45
- to skeletal attachment 83.88
  - hand 82.85

Tenosuspension 83.88
- hand 82.86

Tenosuture (see also Suture, tendon) 83.64
- hand (see also Suture, tendon, hand) 82.45
- to skeletal attachment 83.88
  - hand 82.85

Tenosynovectomy 83.42
- hand 82.33

Tenotomy 83.13
- Achilles tendon 83.11
- adductor (hip) (subcutaneous) 83.12
- eye 15.12
  - levator palpebrae 08.38
  - multiple (two or more tendons) 15.4
- hand 82.11
- levator palpebrae 08.38
- pectoralis minor tendon (decompression thoracic outlet) 83.13
- stapedius 19.0
- tensor tympani 19.0

Tenovaginotomy — see Tenotomy

Tensing, orbicularis oculi 08.59

Termination of pregnancy
- by
  - aspiration curettage 69.51
  - dilation and curettage 69.01
  - hysterectomy — see Hysterectomy
  - hysterotomy 74.91
  - intra-amniotic injection (saline) 75.0

Test, testing (for)
- 14 C-Urea breath 89.39
- auditory function
  - NEC 95.46
- Bender Visual-Motor Gestalt 94.02
- Benton Visual Retention 94.02
- cardiac (vascular)
  - function NEC 89.59
  - stress 89.44
    - bicycle ergometer 89.43
    - Masters' two-step 89.42
    - treadmill 89.41
- Denver developmental (screening) 94.02
- fetus, fetal
  - nonstress (fetal activity acceleration determinations) 75.35
  - oxytocin challenge (contraction stress) 75.35
  - sensitivity (to oxytocin) — omit code
- function
  - cardiac NEC 89.59
  - hearing NEC 95.46
  - muscle (by)
    - electromyography 93.08
    - manual 93.04
  - neurologic NEC 89.15
  - vestibular 95.46
    - clinical 95.44
- glaucoma NEC 95.26
- hearing 95.47
  - clinical NEC 95.42
- intelligence 94.01
- internal jugular-subclavian venous reflux 89.62
- intracarotid amobarbital (Wada) 89.10
- Masters' two-step stress (cardiac) 89.42
- muscle function (by)
  - electromyography 93.08
  - manual 93.04
- neurologic function NEC 89.15
- nocturnal penile tumescence 89.29
- provocative, for glaucoma 95.26
- psychologic NEC 94.08
- psychometric 94.01
- radio-cobalt B_{12} Schilling 92.04
- range of motion 93.05
- rotation (Bárány chair) (hearing) 95.45
- sleep disorder function — see categories 89.17-89.18
- Stanford-Binet 94.01

Test, testing (for) — continued
- tuning fork (hearing) 95.42
- Thallium stress (transesophageal pacing) 89.44
- Urea breath, (14 C) 89.39
- vestibular function NEC 95.46
  - thermal 95.44
- Wada (hemispheric function) 89.10
- whispered speech (hearing) 95.42

TEVAP (transurethral electrovaporization of prostate) 60.29

Thalamectomy 01.41

Thalamotomy 01.41
- by stereotactic radiosurgery 92.32
  - cobalt 60 92.32
  - linear accelerator (LINAC) 92.31
  - multi-source 92.32
  - particle beam 92.33
  - particulate 92.33
  - radiosurgery NEC 92.39
  - single source photon 92.31

Thal operation (repair of esophageal stricture) 42.85

Theleplasty 85.87

Therapy
- Antabuse 94.25
- art 93.89
- aversion 94.33
- behavior 94.33
- Bennett respirator — see category 96.7 ✓4th
- blind rehabilitation NEC 93.78
- Byrd respirator — see category 96.7 ✓4th
- carbon dioxide 94.25
- cobalt-60 92.23
- conditioning, psychiatric 94.33
- continuous positive airway pressure (CPAP) 93.90
- croupette, croup tent 93.94
- daily living activities 93.83
  - for the blind 93.78
- dance 93.89
- desensitization 94.33
- detoxification 94.25
- diversional 93.81
- domestic tasks 93.83
  - for the blind 93.78
- educational (bed-bound children) (handicapped) 93.82
- electroconvulsive (ECT) 94.27
- electroshock (EST) 94.27
  - subconvulsive 94.26
- electrotonic (ETT) 94.27
- encounter group 94.44
- extinction 94.33
- family 94.42
- fog (inhalation) 93.94
- gamma ray 92.23
- group NEC 94.44
  - for psychosexual dysfunctions 94.41
- hearing NEC 95.49
- heat NEC 93.35
  - for cancer treatment 99.85
- helium 93.98
- hot pack(s) 93.35
- hyperbaric oxygen 93.95
  - wound 93.59
- hyperthermia NEC 93.35
  - for cancer treatment 99.85
- individual, psychiatric NEC 94.39
  - for psychosexual dysfunction 94.34
- industrial 93.89
- infrared irradiation 93.35
- inhalation NEC 93.96
  - nitric oxide 00.12 ●
- insulin shock 94.24
- intermittent positive pressure breathing (IPPB) 93.91
- IPPB (intermittent positive pressure breathing) 93.91
- leech 99.99 ●
- lithium 94.22
- maggot 86.28 ●
- manipulative, osteopathic (see also Manipulation, osteopathic) 93.67
- manual arts 93.81

Therapy — continued
  methadone 94.25
  mist (inhalation) 93.94
  music 93.84
  nebulizer 93.94
  neuroleptic 94.23
  nitric oxide 00.12 ▲
  occupational 93.83
  oxygen 93.96
    catalytic 93.96
    hyperbaric 93.95
      wound 93.59
      wound (hyperbaric) 93.59
  paraffin bath 93.35
  physical NEC 93.39
    combined (without mention of components) 93.38
    diagnostic NEC 93.09
  play 93.81
    psychotherapeutic 94.36
  positive and expiratory pressure — see category 96.7 ✓4ᵗʰ
  psychiatric NEC 94.39
    drug NEC 94.25
    lithium 94.22
  radiation 92.29
    contact (150 KVP or less) 92.21
    deep (200-300 KVP) 92.22
    high voltage (200-300 KVP) 92.22
    low voltage (150 KVP or less) 92.21
    megavoltage 92.24
    orthovoltage 92.22
    particle source NEC 92.26
    photon 92.24
    radioisotope (teleradiotherapy) 92.23
    retinal lesion 14.26
    superficial (150 KVP or less) 92.21
    supervoltage 92.24
  radioisotope, radioisotopic NEC 92.29
    implantation or insertion 92.27
    injection or instillation 92.28
    teleradiotherapy 92.23
  radium (radon) 92.23
  recreational 93.81
  rehabilitation NEC 93.89
  respiratory NEC 93.99
    bi-level airway pressure 93.90
    continuous positive airway pressure [CPAP] 93.90
    endotracheal respiratory assistance — see category 96.7 ✓4ᵗʰ
    intermittent mandatory ventilation [IMV] — see category 96.7 ✓4ᵗʰ
    intermittent positive pressure breathing [IPPB] 93.91
    negative pressure (continuous) [CNP] 93.99
    nitric oxide 00.12 ▲
    other continuous (unspecified duration) 96.70
      for less than 96 consecutive hours 96.71
      for 96 consecutive hours or more 96.72
    positive and expiratory pressure [PEEP] — see category 96.7 ✓4ᵗʰ
    pressure support ventilation [PSV] — see category 96.7 ✓4ᵗʰ
  root canal 23.70
    with
      apicoectomy 23.72
      irrigation 23.71
  shock
    chemical 94.24
    electric 94.27
      subconvulsive 94.26
    insulin 94.24
  speech 93.75
    for correction of defect 93.74
  ultrasound
    heat therapy 93.35 ●
    hyperthermia for cancer treatment 99.85
    physical therapy 93.35 ●
    therapeutic — see Ultrasound ●
  ultraviolet light 99.82
Thermocautery — see Cauterization
Thermography 88.89
  blood vessel 88.86

Thermography — continued
  bone 88.83
  breast 88.85
  cerebral 88.81
  eye 88.82
  lymph gland 88.89
  muscle 88.84
  ocular 88.82
  osteoarticular 88.83
  specified site NEC 88.89
  vein, deep 88.86
Thermokeratoplasty 11.74
Thermosclerectomy 12.62
Thermotherapy (hot packs) (paraffin bath) NEC 93.35
  prostate
    by
      microwave 60.96
      radiofrequency 60.97
    transurethral microwave thermotherapy (TUMT) 60.96
    transurethral needle ablation (TUNA) 60.97
    TUMT (transurethral microwave thermotherapy) 60.96
    TUNA (transurethral needle ablation) 60.97
Thiersch operation
  anus 49.79
  skin graft 86.69
    hand 86.62
Thompson operation
  cleft lip repair 27.54
  correction of lymphedema 40.9
  quadricepsplasty 83.86
  thumb apposition with bone graft 82.69
Thoracectomy 34.09
  for lung collapse 33.34
Thoracentesis 34.91
Thoracocentesis 34.91
Thoracolysis (for collapse of lung) 33.39
Thoracoplasty (anterior) (extrapleural) (paravertebral) (posterolateral) (complete) (partial) 33.34
Thoracoscopy, transpleural (for exploration) 34.21
Thoracostomy 34.09
  for lung collapse 33.32
Thoracotomy (with drainage) 34.09
  as operative approach — omit code
  exploratory 34.02
Three-snip operation, punctum 09.51
Thrombectomy 38.00
  with endarterectomy — see Endarterectomy
  abdominal
    artery 38.06
    vein 38.07
  aorta (arch) (ascending) (descending) 38.04
  bovine graft 39.49
  coronary artery 36.09
  head and neck vessel NEC 38.02
  intracranial vessel NEC 38.01
  lower limb
    artery 38.08
    vein 38.09
  pulmonary vessel 38.05
  thoracic vessel NEC 38.05
  upper limb (artery) (vein) 38.03
Thromboendarterectomy 38.10
  abdominal 38.16
  aorta (arch) (ascending) (descending) 38.14
  coronary artery 36.09
    open chest approach 36.03
  head and neck NEC 38.12
  intracranial NEC 38.11
  lower limb 38.18
  thoracic NEC 38.15
  upper limb 38.13
Thymectomy 07.80
  partial 07.81
  total 07.82
Thymopexy 07.99
Thyrochondrotomy 31.3
Thyrocricoidectomy 30.29

Thyrocricotomy (for assistance in breathing) 31.1
Thyroidectomy NEC 06.39
  by mediastinotomy (see also Thyroidectomy, substernal) 06.50
  with laryngectomy — see Laryngectomy
  complete or total 06.4
    substernal (by mediastinotomy) (transsternal route) 06.52
    transoral route (lingual) 06.6
  lingual (complete) (partial) (subtotal) (total) 06.6
  partial or subtotal NEC 06.39
    with complete removal of remaining lobe 06.2
    submental route (lingual) 06.6
    substernal (by mediastinotomy) (transsternal route) 06.51
  remaining tissue 06.4
    submental route (lingual) 06.6
    substernal (by mediastinotomy) (transsternal route) 06.50
      complete or total 06.52
      partial or subtotal 06.51
    transoral route (lingual) 06.6
    transsternal route (see also Thyroidectomy, substernal) 06.50
  unilateral (with removal of isthmus) (with removal of portion of other lobe) 06.2
Thyroidorrhaphy 06.93
Thyroidotomy (field) (gland) NEC 06.09
  postoperative 06.02
Thyrotomy 31.3
  with tantalum plate 31.69
Tirofiban (HCl), infusion 99.20
Toilette
  skin — see Debridement, skin or subcutaneous tissue
  tracheostomy 96.55
Token economy (behavior therapy) 94.33
Tomkins operation (metroplasty) 69.49
Tomography — see also Radiography
  abdomen NEC 88.02
  cardiac 87.42
  computerized axial NEC 88.38
    abdomen 88.01
    bone 88.38
      quantitative 88.98
    brain 87.03
    head 87.03
    kidney 87.71
    skeletal 88.38
      quantitative 88.98
    thorax 87.41
  head NEC 87.04
  kidney NEC 87.72
  lung 87.42
  thorax NEC 87.42
Tongue tie operation 25.91
Tonography 95.26
Tonometry 89.11
Tonsillectomy 28.2
  with adenoidectomy 28.3
Tonsillotomy 28.0
Topectomy 01.32
Torek (-Bevan) operation (orchidopexy) (first stage) (second stage) 62.5
Torkildsen operation (ventriculocisternal shunt) 02.2
Torpin operation (cul-de-sac resection) 70.92
Toti operation (dacryocystorhinostomy) 09.81
Touchas operation 86.83
Touroff operation (ligation of subclavian artery) 38.85
Toxicology — see Examination, microscopic
TPN (total parenteral nutrition) 99.15
Trabeculectomy ab externo 12.64
Trabeculodialysis 12.59
Trabeculotomy ab externo 12.54
Trachelectomy 67.4
Trachelopexy 69.22
Tracheloplasty 67.69

Trachelorrhaphy

Trachelorrhaphy (Emmet) (suture) 67.61
    obstetrical 75.51
Trachelotomy 69.95
    obstetrical 73.93
Tracheocricotomy (for assistance in breathing) 31.1
Tracheofissure 31.1
Tracheography 87.32
Tracheolaryngotomy (emergency) 31.1
    permanent opening 31.29
Tracheoplasty 31.79
    with artificial larynx 31.75
Tracheorrhaphy 31.71
Tracheoscopy NEC 31.42
    through tracheotomy (stoma) 31.41
Tracheostomy (emergency) (temporary) (for assistance in breathing) 31.1
    mediastinal 31.21
    permanent NEC 31.29
    revision 31.74
Tracheotomy (emergency) (temporary) (for assistance in breathing) 31.1
    permanent 31.29
Tracing, carotid pulse with ECG lead 89.56
Traction
    with reduction of fracture or dislocation — see Reduction, fracture and Reduction, dislocation
    adhesive tape (skin) 93.46
    boot 93.46
    Bryant's (skeletal) 93.44
    Buck's 93.46
    caliper tongs 93.41
        with synchronous insertion of device 02.94
    Cortel's (spinal) 93.42
    Crutchfield tongs 93.41
        with synchronous insertion of device 02.94
    Dunlop's (skeletal) 93.44
    gallows 93.46
    Gardner Wells 93.41
        with synchronous insertion of device 02.94
    halo device, skull 93.41
        with synchronous insertion of device 02.94
    Lyman Smith (skeletal) 93.44
    manual, intermittent 93.21
    mechanical, intermittent 93.21
    Russell's (skeletal) 93.44
    skeletal NEC 93.44
        intermittent 93.43
    skin, limbs NEC 93.46
    spinal NEC 93.42
        with skull device (halo) (caliper) (Crutchfield) (Gardner Wells) (Vinke) (tongs) 93.41
            with synchronous insertion of device 02.94
    Thomas' splint 93.45
    Vinke tongs 93.41
        with synchronous insertion of device 02.94
Tractotomy
    brain 01.32
    medulla oblongata 01.32
    mesencephalon 01.32
    percutaneous 03.21
    spinal cord (one-stage) (two-stage) 03.29
    trigeminal (percutaneous) (radiofrequency) 04.02
Training (for) (in)
    ADL (activities of daily living) 93.83
        for the blind 93.78
    ambulation 93.22
    braille 93.77
    crutch walking 93.24
    dyslexia 93.71
    dysphasia 93.72
    esophageal speech (postlaryngectomy) 93.73
    gait 93.22
    joint movements 93.14
    lip reading 93.75
    Moon (blind reading) 93.77
    orthoptic 95.35
    prenatal (natural childbirth) 93.37
    prosthetic or orthotic device usage 93.24
    relaxation 94.33

Training — continued
    speech NEC 93.75
        esophageal 93.73
        for correction of defect 93.74
    use of lead dog for the blind 93.76
    vocational 93.85
TRAM (transverse rectus abdominis musculocutaneous) flap of breast 85.7
Transactional analysis
    group 94.44
    individual 94.39
Transection — see also Division
    artery (with ligation) (see also Division, artery) 38.80
        renal, aberrant (with reimplantation) 39.55
    bone (see also Osteotomy) 77.30
    fallopian tube (bilateral) (remaining) (solitary) 66.39
        by endoscopy 66.22
        unilateral 66.92
    isthmus, thyroid 06.91
    muscle 83.19
        eye 15.13
            multiple (two or more muscles) 15.3
        hand 82.19
    nerve (cranial) (peripheral) NEC 04.03
        acoustic 04.01
        root (spinal) 03.1
        sympathetic 05.0
        tracts in spinal cord 03.29
        trigeminal 04.02
        vagus (transabdominal) (see also Vagotomy) 44.00
    pylorus (with wedge resection) 43.3
    renal vessel, aberrant (with reimplantation) 39.55
    spinal
        cord tracts 03.29
        nerve root 03.1
    tendon 83.13
        hand 82.11
    uvula 27.71
    vas deferens 63.71
    vein (with ligation) (see also Division, vein) 38.80
        renal, aberrant (with reimplantation) 39.55
        varicose (lower limb) 38.59
Transfer, transference
    bone shaft, fibula into tibia 78.47
    digital (to replace absent thumb) 82.69
        finger (to thumb) (same hand) 82.61
            to
                finger, except thumb 82.81
                opposite hand (with amputation) 82.69 [84.01]
        toe (to thumb) (with amputation) 82.69 [84.11]
            to finger, except thumb 82.81 [84.11]
    fat pad NEC 86.89
        with skin graft — see Graft, skin, full-thickness
    finger (to replace absent thumb) (same hand) 82.61
        to
            finger, except thumb 82.81
            opposite hand (with amputation) 82.69 [84.01]
    muscle origin 83.77
        hand 82.58
    nerve (cranial) (peripheral) (radial anterior) (ulnar) 04.6
    pedicle graft 86.74
    pes anserinus (tendon) (repair of knee) 81.47
    tarsoconjunctival flap, from opposing lid 08.64
    tendon 83.75
        hand 82.56
        pes anserinus (repair of knee) 81.47
    toe-to-thumb (free) (pedicle) (with amputation) 82.69 [84.11]
Transfixion — see also Fixation
    iris (bombè) 12.11
Transfusion (of) 99.03
    antihemophilic factor 99.06
    antivenin 99.16

Transfusion — continued
    autologous blood
        collected prior to surgery 99.02
        intraoperative 99.00
        perioperative 99.00
        postoperative 99.00
        previously collected 99.02
        salvage 99.00
    blood (whole) NOS 99.03
        expander 99.08
        surrogate 99.09
    bone marrow 41.00
        allogeneic 41.03
            with purging 41.02
        allograft 41.03
            with purging 41.02
        autograft 41.01
            with purging 41.09
        autologous 41.01
            with purging 41.09
    coagulation factors 99.06
    Dextran 99.08
    exchange 99.01
        intraperitoneal 75.2
        in utero (with hysterotomy) 75.2
    exsanguination 99.01
    gamma globulin 99.14
    granulocytes 99.09
    hemodilution 99.03
    intrauterine 75.2
    packed cells 99.04
    plasma 99.07
    platelets 99.05
    replacement, total 99.01
    serum NEC 99.07
    substitution 99.01
    thrombocytes 99.05
Transillumination
    nasal sinuses 89.35
    skull (newborn) 89.16
Translumbar aortogram 88.42
Transplant, transplantation
    artery 39.59
        renal, aberrant 39.55
    autotransplant — see Reimplantation
    blood vessel 39.59
        renal, aberrant 39.55
    bone (see also Graft, bone) 78.00
        marrow 41.00
            allogeneic 41.03
                with purging 41.02
            allograft 41.03
                with purging 41.02
            autograft 41.01
                with purging 41.09
            autologous 41.01
                with purging 41.09
        stem cell
            allogeneic (hematopoietic) 41.05
                with purging 41.08
            autologous (hematopoietic) 41.04
                with purging 41.07
            cord blood 41.06
    stem cell
        allogeneic (hematopoietic) 41.05
            with purging 41.08
        autologous (hematopoietic) 41.04
            with purging 41.07
        cord blood 41.06
    combined heart-lung 33.6
    conjunctiva, for pterygium 11.39
    corneal (see also Keratoplasty) 11.60
    dura 02.12
    fascia 83.82
        hand 82.72
    finger (replacing absent thumb) (same hand) 82.61
        to
            finger, except thumb 82.81
            opposite hand (with amputation) 82.69 [84.01]
    gracilis muscle (for) 83.77
        anal incontinence 49.74
        urethrovesical suspension 59.71

Transplant, transplantation — *continued*
  hair follicles
    eyebrow 08.63
    eyelid 08.63
    scalp 86.64
  heart (orthotopic) 37.5
    combined with lung 33.6
  ileal stoma to new site 46.23
  intestine 46.97
  islets of Langerhans (cells) 52.86
    allotransplantation of cells 52.85
    autotransplantation of cells 52.84
    heterotransplantation of cells 52.85
    homotransplantation of cells 52.84
  kidney NEC 55.69
  liver 50.59
    auxiliary (permanent) (temporary) (recipient's liver in situ) 50.51
    cells into spleen via percutaneous catheterization 38.91
  lung 33.50
    bilateral 33.52
    combined with heart 33.6
    double 33.52
    single 33.51
    unilateral 33.51
  lymphatic structure(s) (peripheral) 40.9
  mammary artery to myocardium or ventricular wall 36.2
  muscle 83.77
    gracilis (for) 83.77
      anal incontinence 49.74
      urethrovesical suspension 59.71
    hand 82.58
    temporalis 83.77
      with orbital exenteration 16.59
  nerve (cranial) (peripheral) 04.6
  ovary 65.92
  pancreas 52.80
    heterotransplant 52.83
    homotransplant 52.82
    islets of Langerhans (cells) 52.86
      allotransplantation of cells 52.85
      autotransplanation of cells 52.84
    islets of Langerhans — *continued*
      heterotransplantation of cells 52.85
      homotransplantation of cells 52.84
    reimplantation 52.81
  pes anserinus (tendon) (repair of knee) 81.47
  renal NEC 55.69
    vessel, aberrant 39.55
  salivary duct opening 26.49
  skin — *see* Graft skin
  spermatic cord 63.53
  spleen 41.94
  stem cell
    allogeneic (hematopoietic) 41.05
      with purging 41.08
    autologous (hematopoietic) 41.04
      with purging 41.07
    cord blood 41.06
  tendon 83.75
    hand 82.56
    pes anserinus (repair of knee) 81.47
    superior rectus (blepharoptosis) 08.36
  testis to scrotum 62.5
  thymus 07.94
  thyroid tissue 06.94
  toe (replacing absent thumb) (with amputation) 82.69 [84.11]
    to finger, except thumb 82.81 [84.11]
  tooth 23.5
  ureter to
    bladder 56.74
    ileum (external diversion) 56.51
      internal diversion only 56.71
    intestine 56.71
    skin 56.61
  vein (peripheral) 39.59
    renal, aberrant 39.55
  vitreous 14.72
    anterior approach 14.71
Transposition
  extraocular muscles 15.5

Transposition — *continued*
  eyelash flaps 08.63
    eye muscle (oblique) (rectus) 15.5
  finger (replacing absent thumb) (same hand) 82.61
    to
      finger, except thumb 82.81
      opposite hand (with ampu-tation) 82.69 [84.01]
  interatrial venous return 35.91
  jejunal (Henley) 43.81
  joint capsule (*see also* Arthroplasty) 81.96
  muscle NEC 83.79
    extraocular 15.5
    hand 82.59
  nerve (cranial) (peripheral) (radial anterior) (ulnar) 04.6
  nipple 85.86
  pterygium 11.31
  tendon NEC 83.76
    hand 82.57
  vocal cords 31.69
Transureteroureterostomy 56.75
Transversostomy (*see also* Colostomy) 46.10
Trapping, aneurysm (cerebral) 39.52
Trauner operation (lingual sulcus extension) 24.91
Trephination, trephining
  accessory sinus — *see* Sinusotomy
  corneoscleral 12.89
  cranium 01.24
  nasal sinus — *see* Sinusotomy
  sclera (with iridectomy) 12.61
Trial (failed) forceps 73.3
Trigonectomy 57.6
Trimming, amputation stump 84.3
Triple arthrodesis 81.12
Trochanterplasty 81.40
Tsuge operation (macrodactyly repair) 82.83
Tuck, tucking — *see also* Plication
  eye muscle 15.22
    multiple (two or more muscles) 15.4
  levator palpebrac, for blepharoptosis 08.34
Tudor "rabbit ear" operation (anterior urethropexy) 59.79
Tuffier operation
  apicolysis of lung 33.39
  vaginal hysterectomy 68.59
    laparoscopically assisted (LAVH) 68.51
TULIP (transurethral ultrasound guided laser induced prostatectomy) 60.21
TUMT (transurethral microwave thermotherapy) of prostate 60.96
TUNA (transurethral needle ablation) of prostate 60.97
Tunnel, subcutaneous (antethoracic) 42.86
  esophageal 42.86
    with anastomosis — *see* Anastomosis, esophagus, antesternal
  pulse generator lead wire 86.99
    with initial procedure — *omit code*
  with esophageal anastomosis 42.68
Turbinectomy (complete) (partial) NEC 21.69
  by
    cryosurgery 21.61
    diathermy 21.61
  with sinusectomy — *see* Sinusectomy
Turco operation (release of joint capsules in clubfoot) 80.48
TURP (transurethral resection of prostate) 60.29
Tylectomy (breast)(partial) 85.21
Tympanectomy 20.59
  with tympanoplasty — *see* Tympanoplasty
Tympanogram 95 .41
Tympanomastoidectomy 20.42
Tympanoplasty (type I) (with graft) 19.4
  with
    air pocket over round window 19.54
    fenestra in semicircular canal 19.55
    graft against
      incus or malleus 19.52

Tympanoplasty — *continued*
  with — *continued*
    mobile and intact stapes 19.53
    incudostapediopexy 19.52
  epitympanic, type I 19.4
  revision 19.6
  type
    II (graft against incus or malleus) 19.52
    III (graft against mobile and intact stapes) 19.53
    IV (air pocket over round window) 19.54
    V (fenestra in semicircular canal) 19.55
Tympanosympathectomy 20.91
Tympanotomy 20.09
  with intubation 20.01

U

Uchida operation (tubal ligation with or without fimbriectomy) 66.32
UFR (uroflowmetry) 89.24
Ultrasonography
  abdomen 88.76
  aortic arch 88.73
  biliary tract 88.74
  breast 88.73
  deep vein thrombosis 88.77
  digestive system 88.74
  eye 95.13
  head and neck 88.71
  heart (intravascular) 88.72
  intestine 88.74
  lung 88.73
  midline shift, brain 88.71
  multiple sites 88.79
  peripheral vascular system 88.77
  retroperitoneum 88.76
  therapeutic — *see* Ultrasound
  thorax NEC 88.73
  total body 88.79
  urinary system 88.75
  uterus 88.79
    gravid 88.78
Ultrasound
  diagnostic — *see* Ultrasonography
  fragmentation (of)
    cataract (with aspiration) 13.41
    urinary calculus, stones (Kock pouch) 59.95
  heart (intravascular) 88.72
  inner ear 20.79
  therapeutic
    head 00.01
    heart 00.02
    neck 00.01
    other therapeutic ultrasound 00.09
    peripheral vascular vessels 00.03
    vessels of head and neck 00.01
  therapy 93.35
Umbilectomy 54.3
Unbridling
  blood vessel, peripheral 39.91
  celiac artery axis 39.91
Uncovering — *see* Incision, by site
Undercutting
  hair follicle 86.09
  perianal tissue 49.02
Unroofing — *see also* Incision, by site
  external
    auditory canal 18.02
    ear NEC 18.09
  kidney cyst 55.39
UPP (urethral pressure profile) 89.25
Upper GI series (x-ray) 87.62
UPPP (uvulopalatopharyngoplasty) 27.69 [29.4]
Uranoplasty (for cleft palate repair) 27.62
Uranorrhaphy (for cleft palate repair) 27.62
Uranostaphylorrhaphy 27.62
Urban operation (mastectomy) (unilateral) 85.47
  bilateral 85.48

Ureterectomy

Ureterectomy 56.40
  with nephrectomy 55.51
  partial 56.41
  total 56.42
Ureterocecostomy 56.71
Ureterocelectomy 56.41
Ureterocolostomy 56.71
Ureterocystostomy 56.74
Ureteroenterostomy 56.71
Ureteroileostomy (internal diversion) 56.71
  external diversion 56.51
Ureterolithotomy 56.2
Ureterolysis 59.02
  with freeing or repositioning of ureter 59.02
  laparoscopic 59.03
Ureteroneocystostomy 56.74
Ureteropexy 56.85
Ureteroplasty 56.89
Ureteroplication 56.89
Ureteroproctostomy 56.71
Ureteropyelography (intravenous) (diuretic infusion) 87.73
  percutaneous 87.75
  retrograde 87.74
Ureteropyeloplasty 55.87
Ureteropyelostomy 55.86
Ureterorrhaphy 56.82
Ureteroscopy 56.31
  with biopsy 56.33
Ureterosigmoidostomy 56.71
Ureterostomy (cutaneous) (external) (tube) 56.61
  closure 56.83
  ileal 56.51
Ureterotomy 56.2
Ureteroureterostomy (crossed) 56.75
  lumbar 56.41
  resection with end-to-end anastomosis 56.41
  spatulated 56.41
Urethral catheterization, indwelling 57.94
Urethral pressure profile (UPP) 89.25
Urethrectomy (complete) (partial) (radical) 58.39
  with
    complete cystectomy 57.79
    pelvic exenteration 68.8
    radical cystectomy 57.71
Urethrocystography (retrograde) (voiding) 87.76
Urethrocystopexy (by) 59.79
  levator muscle sling 59.71
  retropubic suspension 59.5
  suprapubic suspension 59.4
Urethrolithotomy 58.0
Urethrolysis 58.5
Urethropexy 58.49
  anterior 59.79
Urethroplasty 58.49
  augmentation 59.79
  collagen implant 59.72
  fat implant 59.72
  injection (endoscopic) of implant into urethra 59.72
  polytef implant 59.72
Urethrorrhaphy 58.41
Urethroscopy 58.22
  for control of hemorrhage of prostate 60.94
  perineal 58.21
Urethrostomy (perineal) 58.0
Urethrotomy (external) 58.0
  internal (endoscopic) 58.5
Uroflowmetry (UFR) 89.24
Urography (antegrade) (excretory) (intravenous) 87.73
  retrograde 87.74
Uteropexy (abdominal approach) (vaginal approach) 69.22
UVP (uvulopalatopharyngoplasty) 27.69 [29.4]
Uvulectomy 27.72
Uvulopalatopharyngoplasty (UPPP) 27.69 [29.4]
Uvulotomy 27.71

V

Vaccination (prophylactic) (against) 99.59
  anthrax 99.55
  brucellosis 99.55
  cholera 99.31
  common cold 99.51
  disease NEC 99.55
    arthropod-borne viral NEC 99.54
  encephalitis, arthropod-borne viral 99.53
  German measles 99.47
  hydrophobia 99.44
  infectious parotitis 99.46
  influenza 99.52
  measles 99.45
  mumps 99.46
  paratyphoid fever 99.32
  pertussis 99.37
  plague 99.34
  poliomyelitis 99.41
  rabies 99.44
  Rocky Mountain spotted fever 99.55
  rubella 99.47
  rubeola 99.45
  smallpox 99.42
  Staphylococcus 99.55
  Streptococcus 99.55
  tuberculosis 99.33
  tularemia 99.35
  tumor 99.28
  typhoid 99.32
  typhus 99.55
  undulant fever 99.55
  yellow fever 99.43
Vacuum extraction, fetal head 72.79
  with episiotomy 72.71
Vagectomy (subdiaphragmatic) (see also Vagotomy) 44.00
Vaginal douche 96.44
Vaginectomy 70.4
Vaginofixation 70.77
Vaginoperineotomy 70.14
Vaginoplasty 70.79
Vaginorrhaphy 70.71
  obstetrical 75.69
Vaginoscopy 70.21
Vaginotomy 70.14
  for
    culdocentesis 70.0
    pelvic abscess 70.12
Vagotomy (gastric) 44.00
  parietal cell 44.02
  selective NEC 44.03
    highly 44.02
    Holle's 44.02
    proximal 44.02
  truncal 44.01
Valvotomy — see Valvulotomy
Valvulectomy, heart — see Valvuloplasty, heart
Valvuloplasty
  heart (open heart technique) (without valve replacement) 35.10
    with prosthesis or tissue graft — see Replacement, heart, valve, by site
    aortic valve 35.11
      percutaneous (balloon) 35.96
    combined with repair of atrial and ventricular septal defects — see Repair, endocardial cushion defect
    mitral valve 35.12
      percutaneous (balloon) 35.96
    pulmonary valve 35.13
      in total repair of tetralogy of Fallot 35.81
      percutaneous (balloon) 35.96
    tricuspid valve 35.14
Valvulotomy
  heart (closed heart technique) (transatrial) (transventricular) 35.00
    aortic valve 35.01
    mitral valve 35.02
    open heart technique — see Valvuloplasty, heart

Valvulotomy — continued
  heart — continued
    pulmonary valve 35.03
      in total repair of tetralogy of Fallot 35.81
    tricuspid valve 35.04
Varicocelectomy, spermatic cord 63.1
Varicotomy, peripheral vessels (lower limb) 38.59
  upper limb 38.53
Vascular closure, percutaneous puncture — omit code
Vascularization — see Revascularization
Vasectomy (complete) (partial) 63.73
Vasogram 87.94
Vasoligation 63.71
  gastric 38.86
Vasorrhaphy 63.81
Vasostomy 63.6
Vasotomy 63.6
Vasotripsy 63.71
Vasovasostomy 63.82
Vectorcardiogram (VCG) (with ECG) 89.53
Venectomy — see Phlebectomy
Venipuncture NEC 38.99
  for injection of contrast material — see Phlebography
Venography — see Phlebography
Venorrhaphy 39.32
Venotomy 38.00
  abdominal 38.07
  head and neck NEC 38.02
  intracranial NEC 38.01
  lower limb 38.09
  thoracic NEC 38.05
  upper limb 38.03
Venotripsy 39.98
Venovenostomy 39.29
Ventilation
  bi-level airway pressure 93.90
  continuous positive airway pressure [CPAP] 93.90
  endotracheal respiratory assistance — see category 96.7
  intermittent mandatory ventilation [IMV] — see category 96.7
  intermittent positive pressure breathing [IPPB] 93.91
  mechanical
    endotracheal respiratory assistance — see category 96.7
    intermittent mandatory ventilation [IMV] — see category 96.7
    other continuous (unspecified duration) 96.70
      for less than 96 consecutive hours 96.71
      for 96 consecutive hours or more 96.72
    positive and expiratory pressure [PEEP] — see category 96.7
    pressure support ventilation [PSV] — see category 96.7
  negative pressure (continuous) [CNP] 93.99
Ventriculectomy, heart
  partial 37.35
Ventriculocholecystostomy 02.34
Ventriculocisternostomy 02.2
Ventriculocordectomy 30.29
Ventriculogram, Ventriculography (cerebral) 87.02
  cardiac
    left ventricle (outflow tract) 88.53
      combined with right heart 88.54
    right ventricle (outflow tract) 88.52
      combined with left heart 88.54
    radionuclide cardiac 92.05
Ventriculomyocardiotomy 37.11
Ventriculoperitoneostomy 02.34
Ventriculopuncture 01.09
  through previously implanted catheter or reservoir (Ommaya) (Rickham) 01.02

Index to Procedures

Ventriculoseptopexy (see also Repair, ventricular septal defect) 35.72
Ventriculoseptoplasty (see also Repair, ventricular septal defect) 35.72
Ventriculostomy 02.2
Ventriculotomy
   cerebral 02.2
   heart 37.11
Ventriculoureterostomy 02.35
Ventriculovenostomy 02.32
Ventrofixation, uterus 69.22
Ventrohysteropexy 69.22
Ventrosuspension, uterus 69.22
VEP (visual evoked potential) 95.23
Version, obstetrical (bimanual) (cephalic) (combined) (internal) (podalic) 73.21
   with extraction 73.22
   Braxton Hicks 73.21
      with extraction 73.22
   external (bipolar) 73.91
   Potter's (podalic) 73.21
      with extraction 73.22
   Wigand's (external) 73.91
   Wright's (cephalic) 73.21
      with extraction 73.22
Vesicolithotomy (suprapubic) 57.19
Vesicostomy 57.21
Vesicourethroplasty 57.85
Vesiculectomy 60.73
   with radical prostatectomy 60.5
Vesiculogram, seminal 87.92
   contrast 87.91
Vesiculotomy 60.72
Vestibuloplasty (buccolabial) (lingual) 24.91
Vestibulotomy 20.79
Vicq D'azyr operation (larynx) 31.1
Vidal operation (varicocele ligation) 63.1
Vidianectomy 05.21
Villusectomy (see also Synovectomy) 80.70
Vision check 95.09
Visual evoked potential (VEP) 95.23
Vitrectomy (mechanical) (posterior approach) 14.74
   with scleral buckling 14.49
   anterior approach 14.73
Vocational
   assessment 93.85
   retraining 93.85
   schooling 93.82
Voice training (postlaryngectomy) 93.73
von Kraske operation (proctectomy) 48.64
Voss operation (hanging hip operation) 83.19
Vulpius (-Compere) operation (lengthening of gastrocnemius muscle) 83.85
Vulvectomy (bilateral) (simple) 71.62
   partial (unilateral) 71.61
   radical (complete) 71.5
   unilateral 71.61
V-Y operation (repair)
   bladder 57.89
      neck 57.85
   ectropion 08.44
   lip 27.59
   skin (without graft) 86.89
   subcutaneous tissue (without skin graft) 86.89
   tongue 25.59

W

Wada test (hemispheric function) 89.10
Ward-Mayo operation (vaginal hysterectomy) 68.59
   laparoscopically assisted (LAVH) 68.51
Washing — see Lavage and Irrigation
Waterston operation (aorta-right pulmonary artery anastomosis) 39.0

Watkins (-Wertheim) operation (uterus interposition) 69.21
Watson-Jones operation
   hip arthrodesis 81.21
   reconstruction of lateral ligaments, ankle 81.49
   shoulder arthrodesis (extra-articular) 81.23
   tenoplasty 83.88
Webbing (syndactylization) 86.89
Weir operation
   appendicostomy 47.91
   correction of nostrils 21.86
Wertheim operation (radical hysterectomy) 68.6
West operation (dacryocystorhinostomy) 09.81
Wheeler operation
   entropion repair 08.44
   halving procedure (eyelid) 08.24
Whipple operation (radical pancreaticoduodenectomy) 52.7
   Child modification (radical subtotal pancreatectomy) 52.53
   Rodney Smith modification (radical subtotal pancreatectomy) 52.53
White operation (lengthening of tendo calcaneus by incomplete tenotomy) 83.11
Whitehead operation
   glossectomy, radical 25.4
   hemorrhoidectomy 49.46
Whitman operation
   foot stabilization (talectomy) 77.98
   hip reconstruction 81.40
   repair of serratus anterior muscle 83.87
   talectomy 77.98
   trochanter wedge osteotomy 77.25
Wier operation (entropion repair) 08.44
Williams-Richardson operation (vaginal construction) 70.61
Wilms operation (thoracoplasty) 33.34
Wilson operation (angulation osteotomy for hallux valgus) 77.51
Window operation
   antrum (nasal sinus) — see Antrotomy, maxillary
   aorticopulmonary 39.59
   bone cortex (see also Incision, bone) 77.10
      facial 76.09
   nasoantral — see Antrotomy, maxillary
   pericardium 37.12
   pleura 34.09
Winiwarter operation (cholecystoenterostomy) 51.32
Wiring
   aneurysm 39.52
   dental (for immobilization) 93.55
      with fracture-reduction — see Reduction, fracture
   orthodontic 24.7
Wirsungojejunostomy 52.96
Witzel operation (temporary gastrostomy) 43.19
Woodward operation (release of high riding scapula) 81.83
Wrapping, aneurysm (gauze) (methyl methacrylate) (plastic) 39.52

X

Xenograft 86.65
Xerography, breast 87.36
Xeromammography 87.36
Xiphoidectomy 77.81
X-ray
   chest (routine) 87.44
      wall NEC 87.39
   contrast — see Radiography, contrast
   diagnostic — see Radiography
   injection of radio-opaque substance — see Radiography, contrast
   skeletal series, whole or complete 88.31
   therapeutic — see Therapy, radiation

Y

Young operation
   epispadias repair 58.45
   tendon transfer (anterior tibialis) (repair of flat foot) 83.75
Yount operation (division of iliotibial band) 83.14

Z

Zancolli operation
   capsuloplasty 81.72
   tendon transfer (biceps) 82.56
Ziegler operation (iridectomy) 12.14
Zonulolysis (with lens extraction) (see also Extraction, cataract, intracapsular) 13.19
Z-plasty
   epicanthus 08.59
   eyelid (see also Reconstruction, eyelid) 08.70
   hypopharynx 29.4
   skin (scar) (web contracture) 86.84
      with excision of lesion 86.3

00. PROCEDURES AND INTERVENTIONS, NOT ELSEWHERE CLASSIFIED (00)

- ✓3rd **00** Procedures and interventions, not elsewhere classified
  - ✓4th **00.0** Therapeutic ultrasound
    - **00.01** Therapeutic ultrasound of vessels of head and neck
      Anti-restenotic ultrasound
      Intravascular non-ablative ultrasound
      EXCLUDES diagnostic ultrasound of:
          eye (95.13)
          head and neck (88.71)
          that of inner ear (20.79)
      ultrasonic:
          angioplasty of non-coronary vessel (39.50)
          embolectomy (38.01, 38.02)
          endarterectomy (38.11, 38.12)
          thrombectomy (38.01, 38.02)
    - **00.02** Therapeutic ultrasound of heart
      Anti-restenotic ultrasound
      Intravascular non-ablative ultrasound
      EXCLUDES diagnostic ultrasound of heart (88.72)
      ultrasonic ablation of heart lesion (37.34)
      ultrasonic angioplasty of coronary vessels (36.01, 36.02, 36.05, 36.09)
    - **00.03** Therapeutic ultrasound of peripheral vascular vessels
      Anti-restenotic ultrasound
      Intravascular non-ablative ultrasound
      EXCLUDES diagnostic ultrasound of peripheral vascular system (88.77)
      ultrasonic angioplasty of:
          non-coronary vessel (39.50)
    - **00.09** Other therapeutic ultrasound
      EXCLUDES ultrasonic:
          fragmentation of urinary stones (59.95)
          percutaneous nephrostomy with fragmentation (55.04)
          physical therapy (93.35)
          transurethral guided laser induced prostatectomy (TULIP) (60.21)
  - ✓4th **00.1** Pharmaceuticals
    - **00.10** Implantation of chemotherapeutic agent
      Brain wafer chemotherapy
      Interstitial/intracavitary
      EXCLUDES injection or infusion of cancer chemotherapeutic substance (99.25)
    - **00.11** Infusion of drotrecogin alfa (activated)
      Infusion of recombinant protein
    - **00.12** Administration of inhaled nitric oxide
      Nitric oxide therapy
    - **00.13** Injection or infusion of nesiritide
      Human B-type natriuretic peptide (hBNP)
    - **00.14** Injection or infusion of oxazolidinone class of antibiotics
      Linezolid injection
  - ✓4th **00.5** Other cardiovascular procedures
    - **00.50** Implantation of cardiac resynchronization pacemaker without mention of defibrillation, total system [CRT-P]
      Biventricular pacing without internal cardiac defibrillator
      Implantation of cardiac resynchronization (biventricular) pulse generator pacing device, formation of pocket, transvenous leads including placement of lead into left ventricular coronary venous system, and intraoperative procedures for evaluation of lead signals
      EXCLUDES implantation of cardiac resynchronization defibrillator, total system [CRT-D] (00.51)
      insertion or replacement of any type pacemaker device (37.80-37.87)
      replacement of cardiac resynchronization:
          defibrillator, pulse generator only [CRT-D] (00.54)
          pacemaker, pulse generator only [CRT-P] (00.53)
    - **00.51** Implantation of cardiac resynchronization defibrillator, total system [CRT-D]
      Biventricular pacing with internal cardiac defibrillator
      Implantation of cardiac resynchronization (biventricular) pulse generator with defibrillator [AICD], formation of pocket, transvenous leads, including placement of lead into left ventricular coronary venous system, intraoperative procedures for evaluation of lead signals, and obtaining defibrillator threshold measurements
      EXCLUDES implantation of cardiac resynchronization pacemaker, total system [CRT-P] (00.50)
      implantation or replacement of automatic cardioverter/defibrillator, total system [AICD] (37.94)
      replacement of cardiac resynchronization defibrillator, pulse generator only [CRT-D] (00.54)
    - **00.52** Implantation or replacement of transvenous lead [electrode] into left ventricular coronary venous system
      EXCLUDES implantation of cardiac resynchronization:
          defibrillator, total system [CRT-D] (00.51)
          pacemaker, total system [CRT-P] (00.50)
      initial insertion of transvenous lead [electrode] (37.70-37.72)
      replacement of transvenous atrial and/or ventricular lead(s) [electrodes] (37.76)

PROCEDURES AND INTERVENTIONS, NEC

● **00.53** **Implantation or replacement of cardiac resynchronization pacemaker, pulse generator only [CRT-P]**
Implantation of CRT-P device with removal of any existing CRT-P or other pacemaker device
EXCLUDES *implantation of cardiac resynchronization pacemaker, total system [CRT-P] (00.50)*
implantation or replacement of cardiac resynchronization defibrillator, pulse generator only [CRT-D] (00.54)
insertion or replacement of any type pacemaker device (37.80-37.87)

● **00.54** **Implantation or replacement of cardiac resynchronization defibrillator, pulse generator device only [CRT-D]**
Implantation of CRT-D device with removal of any existing CRT-D, CRT-P, pacemaker, or defibrillator device
EXCLUDES *implantation of automatic cardioverter/defibrillator pulse generator only (37.96)*
implantation of cardiac resynchronization defibrillator, total system [CRT-D] (00.51)
implantation or replacement of cardiac resynchronization pacemaker, pulse generator only [CRT-P] (00.53)

● **00.55** **Insertion of drug-eluting non-coronary artery stent(s)**
Endograft(s)
Endovascular graft(s)
Stent graft(s)
Code also any non-coronary angioplasty or atherectomy (39.50)
EXCLUDES *drug-coated stents, e.g., heparin coated (39.90)*
insertion of drug-eluting coronary artery stent (36.07)
insertion of non-drug-eluting stent(s):
coronary artery (36.06)
non-coronary artery (39.90)
that for aneurysm repair (39.71-39.79)

Tabular List — **OPERATIONS ON THE NERVOUS SYSTEM**

1. OPERATIONS ON THE NERVOUS SYSTEM (01-05)

✓3rd 01 Incision and excision of skull, brain, and cerebral meninges

✓4th 01.0 Cranial puncture

01.01 Cisternal puncture
Cisternal tap
EXCLUDES pneumocisternogram (87.02)
DEF: Needle insertion through subarachnoid space to withdraw cerebrospinal fluid.

01.02 Ventriculopuncture through previously implanted catheter
Puncture of ventricular shunt tubing
DEF: Piercing of artificial, fluid-diverting tubing in the brain for withdrawal of cerebrospinal fluid.

01.09 Other cranial puncture
Aspiration of:
  subarachnoid space
  subdural space
Cranial aspiration NOS
Puncture of anterior fontanel
Subdural tap (through fontanel)

✓4th 01.1 Diagnostic procedures on skull, brain, and cerebral meninges

01.11 Closed [percutaneous] [needle] biopsy of cerebral meninges
Burr hole approach
DEF: Needle excision of tissue sample through skin into cerebral membranes; no other procedure performed.

01.12 Open biopsy of cerebral meninges
DEF: Open surgical excision of tissue sample from cerebral membrane.

01.13 Closed [percutaneous] [needle] biopsy of brain
Burr hole approach
Stereotactic method
AHA: M-A, '87, 9
DEF: Removal by needle of brain tissue sample through skin.

01.14 Open biopsy of brain
DEF: Open surgical excision of brain tissue sample.

01.15 Biopsy of skull

01.18 Other diagnostic procedures on brain and cerebral meninges
EXCLUDES cerebral:
    arteriography (88.41)
    thermography (88.81)
  contrast radiogram of brain (87.01-87.02)
  echoencephalogram (88.71)
  electroencephalogram (89.14)
  microscopic examination of specimen from nervous system and of spinal fluid (90.01-90.09)
  neurologic examination (89.13)
  phlebography of head and neck (88.61)
  pneumoencephalogram (87.01)
  radioisotope scan:
    cerebral (92.11)
    head NEC (92.12)
  tomography of head:
    C.A.T. scan (87.03)
    other (87.04)
AHA: 3Q, '98, 12

01.19 Other diagnostic procedures on skull
EXCLUDES transillumination of skull (89.16)
  x-ray of skull (87.17)

✓4th 01.2 Craniotomy and craniectomy
EXCLUDES decompression of skull fracture (02.02)
  exploration of orbit (16.01-16.09)
  that as operative approach — omit code
AHA: 1Q, '91, 1
DEF: Craniotomy: Incision into skull.
DEF: Craniectomy: Excision of part of skull.

01.21 Incision and drainage of cranial sinus
DEF: Incision for drainage, including drainage of air cavities in skull bones.

01.22 Removal of intracranial neurostimulator
EXCLUDES removal with synchronous replacement (02.93)

01.23 Reopening of craniotomy site
DEF: Reopening of skull incision.

01.24 Other craniotomy
Cranial: Craniotomy with
  decompression   removal of:
  exploration   epidural abscess
  trephination   extradural hematoma
Craniotomy NOS   foreign body of skull
EXCLUDES removal of foreign body with incision into brain (01.39)
AHA: 2Q, '91, 14

01.25 Other craniectomy
Debridement of skull NOS
Sequestrectomy of skull
EXCLUDES debridement of compound fracture of skull (02.02)
  strip craniectomy (02.01)

✓4th 01.3 Incision of brain and cerebral meninges

01.31 Incision of cerebral meninges
Drainage of:
  intracranial hygroma
  subarachnoid abscess (cerebral)
  subdural empyema

01.32 Lobotomy and tractotomy
Division of: Percutaneous
  brain tissue   (radiofrequency)
  cerebral tracts   cingulotomy
DEF: Lobotomy: Incision of nerve fibers of brain lobe, usually frontal.
DEF: Tractotomy: Severing of a nerve fiber group to relieve pain.

01.39 Other incision of brain
Amygdalohippocampotomy
Drainage of intracerebral hematoma
Incision of brain NOS
EXCLUDES division of cortical adhesions (02.91)

✓4th 01.4 Operations on thalamus and globus pallidus

01.41 Operations on thalamus
Chemothalamectomy Thalamotomy
EXCLUDES that by stereotactic radiosurgery (92.30-92.39)

01.42 Operations on globus pallidus
Pallidoansectomy   Pallidotomy
EXCLUDES that by stereotactic radiosurgery (92.30-92.39)

OPERATIONS ON THE NERVOUS SYSTEM

01.5 Other excision or destruction of brain and meninges
AHA: 4Q, '93, 33

01.51 Excision of lesion or tissue of cerebral meninges
Decortication
Resection } of (cerebral) meninges
Stripping of subdural membrane

EXCLUDES: biopsy of cerebral meninges (01.11-01.12)

01.52 Hemispherectomy
DEF: Removal of one half of the brain. Most often performed for malignant brain tumors or intractable epilepsy.

01.53 Lobectomy of brain
DEF: Excision of a brain lobe.

01.59 Other excision or destruction of lesion or tissue of brain
Curettage of brain
Debridement of brain
Marsupialization of brain cyst
Transtemporal (mastoid) excision of brain tumor

EXCLUDES: biopsy of brain (01.13-01.14)
that by stereotactic radiosurgery (92.30-92.39)

AHA: 3Q, '99, 7; 1Q, '99, 9; 3Q, '98, 12; 1Q, '98, 6

01.6 Excision of lesion of skull
Removal of granulation tissue of cranium

EXCLUDES: biopsy of skull (01.15)
sequestrectomy (01.25)

02 Other operations on skull, brain, and cerebral meninges

02.0 Cranioplasty
EXCLUDES: that with synchronous repair of encephalocele (02.12)

02.01 Opening of cranial suture
Linear craniectomy
Strip craniectomy
DEF: Opening of the lines of junction between the bones of the skull for removal of strips of skull bone.

02.02 Elevation of skull fracture fragments
Debridement of compound fracture of skull
Decompression of skull fracture
Reduction of skull fracture
Code also any synchronous debridement of brain (01.59)

EXCLUDES: debridement of skull NOS (01.25)
removal of granulation tissue of cranium (01.6)

02.03 Formation of cranial bone flap
Repair of skull with flap

02.04 Bone graft to skull
Pericranial graft (autogenous) (heterogenous)

02.05 Insertion of skull plate
Replacement of skull plate

02.06 Other cranial osteoplasty
Repair of skull NOS
Revision of bone flap of skull
AHA: 3Q, '98, 9

DEF: Plastic surgery repair of skull bones.

02.07 Removal of skull plate
EXCLUDES: removal with synchronous replacement (02.05)

02.1 Repair of cerebral meninges
EXCLUDES: marsupialization of cerebral lesion (01.59)

02.11 Simple suture of dura mater of brain

02.12 Other repair of cerebral meninges
Closure of fistula of cerebrospinal fluid
Dural graft
Repair of encephalocele including synchronous cranioplasty
Repair of meninges NOS
Subdural patch

02.13 Ligation of meningeal vessel
Ligation of:
longitudinal sinus
middle meningeal artery

02.14 Choroid plexectomy
Cauterization of choroid plexus
DEF: Excision or destruction of the ependymal cells that form the membrane lining in the third, fourth, and lateral ventricles of the brain and secrete cerebrospinal fluid.

02.2 Ventriculostomy
Anastomosis of ventricle to:
cervical subarachnoid space
cisterna magna
Insertion of Holter valve
Ventriculocisternal intubation
DEF: Surgical creation of an opening of ventricle; often performed to drain cerebrospinal fluid in treating hydrocephalus.

02.3 Extracranial ventricular shunt
INCLUDES: that with insertion of valve
DEF: Placement of shunt or creation of artificial passage leading from skull cavities to site outside skull to relieve excess cerebrospinal fluid created in the chorioid plexuses of the third and fourth ventricles of the brain.

02.31 Ventricular shunt to structure in head and neck
Ventricle to nasopharynx shunt
Ventriculomastoid anastomosis

02.32 Ventricular shunt to circulatory system
Ventriculoatrial anastomosis
Ventriculocaval shunt

02.33 Ventricular shunt to thoracic cavity
Ventriculopleural anastomosis

02.34 Ventricular shunt to abdominal cavity and organs
Ventriculocholecystostomy
Ventriculoperitoneostomy

02.35 Ventricular shunt to urinary system
Ventricle to ureter shunt

02.39 Other operations to establish drainage of ventricle
Ventricle to bone marrow shunt
Ventricular shunt to extracranial site NEC

02.4 Revision, removal, and irrigation of ventricular shunt
EXCLUDES: revision of distal catheter of ventricular shunt (54.95)

02.41 Irrigation and exploration of ventricular shunt
▶Exploration and ventriculoperitoneal shunt at ventricular site◀

02.42 Replacement of ventricular shunt
Reinsertion of Holter valve
Replacement of ventricular catheter
Revision of ventriculoperitoneal shunt at ventricular site
AHA: N-D, '86, 8

02.43 Removal of ventricular shunt
AHA: N-D, '86, 8

OPERATIONS ON THE NERVOUS SYSTEM

02.9 Other operations on skull, brain, and cerebral meninges

EXCLUDES operations on:
pineal gland (07.17, 07.51-07.59)
pituitary gland [hypophysis] (07.13-07.15, 07.61-07.79)

02.91 Lysis of cortical adhesions
DEF: Breaking up of fibrous structures in brain outer layer.

02.92 Repair of brain

02.93 Implantation of intracranial neurostimulator
Implantation, insertion, placement, or replacement of intracranial:
brain pacemaker [neuropacemaker]
depth electrodes
epidural pegs
electroencephalographic receiver
foramen ovale electrodes
intracranial electrostimulator
subdural grids
subdural strips
AHA: 4Q, '97, 57; 4Q, '92, 28

02.94 Insertion or replacement of skull tongs or halo traction device
AHA: 3Q, '01, 8; 3Q, '96, 14

DEF: Halo traction device: Metal or plastic band encircles the head or neck secured to the skull with four pins and attached to a metal chest plate by rods; provides support and stability for the head and neck.

DEF: Skull tongs: Device inserted into each side of the skull used to apply parallel traction to the long axis of the cervical spine.

02.95 Removal of skull tongs or halo traction device

02.96 Insertion of sphenoidal electrodes
AHA: 4Q, '92, 28

02.99 Other
EXCLUDES chemical shock therapy (94.24)
electroshock therapy:
subconvulsive (94.26)
other (94.27)

03 Operations on spinal cord and spinal canal structures
▶Code also any application or administration of an adhesion barrier substance (99.77)◀

03.0 Exploration and decompression of spinal canal structures

03.01 Removal of foreign body from spinal canal

03.02 Reopening of laminectomy site

03.09 Other exploration and decompression of spinal canal
Decompression:
laminectomy   laminotomy
▶Expansile laminoplasty◀
Exploration of spinal nerve root
Foraminotomy
EXCLUDES drainage of spinal fluid by anastomosis (03.71-03.79)
laminectomy with excision of intervertebral disc (80.51)
spinal tap (03.31)
that as operative approach — omit code
AHA: 4Q, '99, 14; 2Q, '97, 6; 2Q, '95, 9; 2Q, '95, 10; 2Q, '90, 22, S-Q, '86, 12

DEF: Decompression of spinal canal: Excision of bone pieces, hematoma or other lesion to relieve spinal cord pressure.

DEF: Foraminotomy: Removal of root opening between vertebrae to relieve nerve root pressure.

Laminotomy with Decompression

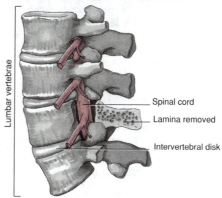

03.1 Division of intraspinal nerve root
Rhizotomy
DEF: Rhizotomy: Surgical severing of spinal nerve roots within spinal canal for pain relief.

03.2 Chordotomy
DEF: Chordotomy: Surgical cutting of lateral spinothalamic tract of spinal cord to relieve pain.

03.21 Percutaneous chordotomy
Stereotactic chordotomy
DEF: Percutaneous chordotomy: Insertion of hollow needle through skin to interrupt spinal nerve root.
DEF: Stereotactic chordotomy: Use of three-dimensional imaging to locate spinal nerve root for surgical interruption.

03.29 Other chordotomy
Chordotomy NOS
Tractotomy (one-stage) (two-stage) of spinal cord
Transection of spinal cord tracts
DEF: Tractotomy (one stage) (two stages) of the spinal cord: Surgical incision or severing of a nerve tract of spinal cord.
DEF: Transection of spinal cord tracts: Use of transverse incision to divide spinal nerve root.

03.3 Diagnostic procedures on spinal cord and spinal canal structures

03.31 Spinal tap
Lumbar puncture for removal of dye
EXCLUDES lumbar puncture for injection of dye [myelogram] (87.21)
AHA: 2Q, '90, 22
DEF: Puncture into lumbar subarachnoid space to tap cerebrospinal fluid.

03.32 Biopsy of spinal cord or spinal meninges

Lumbar Spinal Puncture

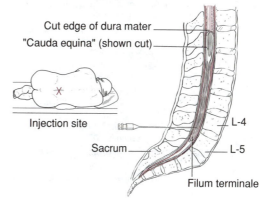

OPERATIONS ON THE NERVOUS SYSTEM

03.39 **Other diagnostic procedures on spinal cord and spinal canal structures**
  EXCLUDES: microscopic examination of specimen from nervous system or of spinal fluid (90.01-90.09)
  x-ray of spine (87.21-87.29)

03.4 **Excision or destruction of lesion of spinal cord or spinal meninges**
  Curettage
  Debridement
  Marsupialization of cyst
  Resection
  } of spinal cord or spinal meninges
  EXCLUDES: biopsy of spinal cord or meninges (03.32)
  AHA: 3Q, '95, 5

✓4th 03.5 **Plastic operations on spinal cord structures**

  03.51 **Repair of spinal meningocele**
    Repair of meningocele NOS
    DEF: Restoration of hernial protrusion of spinal meninges through defect in vertebral column.

  03.52 **Repair of spinal myelomeningocele**
    DEF: Restoration of hernial protrusion of spinal cord and meninges through defect in vertebral column.

  03.53 **Repair of vertebral fracture**
    Elevation of spinal bone fragments
    Reduction of fracture of vertebrae
    Removal of bony spicules from spinal canal
    AHA: 4Q, '99, 11, 12, 13; 3Q, '96, 14

  03.59 **Other repair and plastic operations on spinal cord structures**
    Repair of:
      diastematomyelia
      spina bifida NOS
      spinal cord NOS
      spinal meninges NOS
      vertebral arch defect

03.6 **Lysis of adhesions of spinal cord and nerve roots**
  AHA: 2Q, '98, 18

✓4th 03.7 **Shunt of spinal theca**
  INCLUDES: that with valve
  DEF: Surgical passage created from spinal cord dura mater to another channel.

  03.71 **Spinal subarachnoid-peritoneal shunt**
  03.72 **Spinal subarachnoid-ureteral shunt**
  03.79 **Other shunt of spinal theca**
    Lumbar-subarachnoid shunt NOS
    Pleurothecal anastomosis
    Salpingothecal anastomosis
    AHA: 1Q, '97, 7

03.8 **Injection of destructive agent into spinal canal**
✓4th 03.9 **Other operations on spinal cord and spinal canal structures**

  03.90 **Insertion of catheter into spinal canal for infusion of therapeutic or palliative substances**
    Insertion of catheter into epidural, subarachnoid, or subdural space of spine with intermittent or continuous infusion of drug (with creation of any reservoir)
    Code also any implantation of infusion pump (86.06)

  03.91 **Injection of anesthetic into spinal canal for analgesia**
    EXCLUDES: that for operative anesthesia — omit code
    AHA: 3Q, '00, 15; 1Q, '99, 8; 2Q, '98, 18

  03.92 **Injection of other agent into spinal canal**
    Intrathecal injection of steroid
    Subarachnoid perfusion of refrigerated saline
    EXCLUDES: injection of:
      contrast material for myelogram (87.21)
      destructive agent into spinal canal (03.8)
    AHA: 3Q, '00, 15; 2Q, '98, 18

  03.93 **Insertion or replacement of spinal neurostimulator**
    AHA: 1Q, '00, 19

  03.94 **Removal of spinal neurostimulator**
  03.95 **Spinal blood patch**
    DEF: Injection of blood into epidural space to patch hole in outer spinal membrane when blood clots.

  03.96 **Percutaneous denervation of facet**
  03.97 **Revision of spinal thecal shunt**
    AHA: 2Q, '99, 4
  03.98 **Removal of spinal thecal shunt**
  03.99 **Other**

✓3rd 04 **Operations on cranial and peripheral nerves**

✓4th 04.0 **Incision, division, and excision of cranial and peripheral nerves**
  EXCLUDES: opticociliary neurectomy (12.79)
    sympathetic ganglionectomy (05.21-05.29)

  04.01 **Excision of acoustic neuroma**
    That by craniotomy
    EXCLUDES: that by stereotactic radiosurgery (92.3)
    AHA: 2Q, '98, 20; 2Q, '95, 8; 4Q, '92, 26

  04.02 **Division of trigeminal nerve**
    Retrogasserian neurotomy
    DEF: Transection of sensory root fibers of trigeminal nerve for relief of trigeminal neuralgia.

  04.03 **Division or crushing of other cranial and peripheral nerves**
    EXCLUDES: that of:
      glossopharyngeal nerve (29.92)
      laryngeal nerve (31.91)
      nerves to adrenal glands (07.42)
      phrenic nerve for collapse of lung (33.31)
      vagus nerve (44.00-44.03)
    AHA: 2Q, '98, 20

  04.04 **Other incision of cranial and peripheral nerves**
  04.05 **Gasserian ganglionectomy**
  04.06 **Other cranial or peripheral ganglionectomy**
    EXCLUDES: sympathetic ganglionectomy (05.21-05.29)

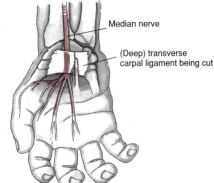

Release of Carpal Tunnel
Median nerve
(Deep) transverse carpal ligament being cut

OPERATIONS ON THE NERVOUS SYSTEM 04.07–05.9

- **04.07** Other excision or avulsion of cranial and peripheral nerves
  - Curettage ⎱
  - Debridement ⎬ of peripheral nerve
  - Resection ⎰
  - Excision of peripheral neuroma [Morton's]
  - **EXCLUDES** biopsy of cranial or peripheral nerve (04.11-04.12)
  - AHA: 2Q, '95, 8; 4Q, '92, 26

- ✓4th **04.1** Diagnostic procedures on peripheral nervous system
  - **04.11** Closed [percutaneous] [needle] biopsy of cranial or peripheral nerve or ganglion
  - **04.12** Open biopsy of cranial or peripheral nerve or ganglion
  - **04.19** Other diagnostic procedures on cranial and peripheral nerves and ganglia
    - **EXCLUDES** microscopic examination of specimen from nervous system (90.01-90.09)
      - neurologic examination (89.13)

- **04.2** Destruction of cranial and peripheral nerves
  - Destruction of cranial or peripheral nerves by:
    - cryoanalgesia
    - injection of neurolytic agent
    - radiofrequency
    - ▶Radiofrequency ablation◀
  - AHA: 4Q, '95, 74

- **04.3** Suture of cranial and peripheral nerves
- ✓4th **04.4** Lysis of adhesions and decompression of cranial and peripheral nerves
  - **04.41** Decompression of trigeminal nerve root
  - **04.42** Other cranial nerve decompression
  - **04.43** Release of carpal tunnel
  - **04.44** Release of tarsal tunnel
  - **04.49** Other peripheral nerve or ganglion decompression or lysis of adhesions
    - Peripheral nerve neurolysis NOS

- **04.5** Cranial or peripheral nerve graft
- **04.6** Transposition of cranial and peripheral nerves
  - Nerve transplantation
  - DEF: Relocation of cranial or peripheral nerves without detaching or severing them.

- ✓4th **04.7** Other cranial or peripheral neuroplasty
  - **04.71** Hypoglossal-facial anastomosis
    - DEF: Surgical connection of hypoglossal nerve to facial nerve.
  - **04.72** Accessory-facial anastomosis
    - DEF: Surgical connection of accessory nerve to facial nerve.
  - **04.73** Accessory-hypoglossal anastomosis
    - DEF: Surgical connection of accessory nerve to hypoglossal nerve.
  - **04.74** Other anastomosis of cranial or peripheral nerve
  - **04.75** Revision of previous repair of cranial and peripheral nerves
  - **04.76** Repair of old traumatic injury of cranial and peripheral nerves
  - **04.79** Other neuroplasty

- ✓4th **04.8** Injection into peripheral nerve
  - **EXCLUDES** destruction of nerve (by injection of neurolytic agent) (04.2)
  - **04.80** Peripheral nerve injection, not otherwise specified
  - **04.81** Injection of anesthetic into peripheral nerve for analgesia
    - **EXCLUDES** that for operative anesthesia — omit code
    - AHA: 1Q, '00, 7

  - **04.89** Injection of other agent, except neurolytic
    - **EXCLUDES** injection of neurolytic agent (04.2)

- ✓4th **04.9** Other operations on cranial and peripheral nerves
  - **04.91** Neurectasis
    - DEF: Surgical stretching of peripheral or cranial nerve.
  - **04.92** Implantation or replacement of peripheral neurostimulator
    - AHA: 3Q, '01, 16; 2Q, '00, 22; 3Q, '96, 12
    - DEF: Placement of or removal and replacement of test neurostimulator or permanent neurostimulator during the same episode.
  - **04.93** Removal of peripheral neurostimulator
    - AHA: 3Q, '01, 16
    - DEF: Removal of test neurostimulator or permanent neurostimulator when a permanent device is not placed during the same episode.
  - **04.99** Other

- ✓3rd **05** Operations on sympathetic nerves or ganglia
  - **EXCLUDES** paracervical uterine denervation (69.3)
  - **05.0** Division of sympathetic nerve or ganglion
    - **EXCLUDES** that of nerves to adrenal glands (07.42)
  - ✓4th **05.1** Diagnostic procedures on sympathetic nerves or ganglia
    - **05.11** Biopsy of sympathetic nerve or ganglion
    - **05.19** Other diagnostic procedures on sympathetic nerves or ganglia
  - ✓4th **05.2** Sympathectomy
    - DEF: Sympathectomy: Division of nerve pathway at a specific site of a sympathetic nerve.
    - **05.21** Sphenopalatine ganglionectomy
    - **05.22** Cervical sympathectomy
    - **05.23** Lumbar sympathectomy
      - DEF: Excision, resection of lumber chain nerve group to relieve causalgia, Raynaud's disease, or lower extremity thromboangiitis.
    - **05.24** Presacral sympathectomy
      - DEF: Excision or resection of hypogastric nerve network.
    - **05.25** Periarterial sympathectomy
      - DEF: Removal of arterial sheath containing sympathetic nerve fibers.
    - **05.29** Other sympathectomy and ganglionectomy
      - Excision or avulsion of sympathetic nerve NOS
      - Sympathetic ganglionectomy NOS
      - **EXCLUDES** biopsy of sympathetic nerve or ganglion (05.11)
        - opticociliary neurectomy (12.79)
        - periarterial sympathectomy (05.25)
        - tympanosympathectomy (20.91)

  - ✓4th **05.3** Injection into sympathetic nerve or ganglion
    - **EXCLUDES** injection of ciliary sympathetic ganglion (12.79)
    - **05.31** Injection of anesthetic into sympathetic nerve for analgesia
    - **05.32** Injection of neurolytic agent into sympathetic nerve
    - **05.39** Other injection into sympathetic nerve or ganglion

  - ✓4th **05.8** Other operations on sympathetic nerves or ganglia
    - **05.81** Repair of sympathetic nerve or ganglion
    - **05.89** Other
  - **05.9** Other operations on nervous system

2. OPERATIONS ON THE ENDOCRINE SYSTEM (06-07)

06 Operations on thyroid and parathyroid glands
- INCLUDES: incidental resection of hyoid bone

06.0 Incision of thyroid field
EXCLUDES: division of isthmus (06.91)

06.01 Aspiration of thyroid field
Percutaneous or needle drainage of thyroid field
EXCLUDES:
- aspiration biopsy of thyroid (06.11)
- drainage by incision (06.09)
- postoperative aspiration of field (06.02)

06.02 Reopening of wound of thyroid field
Reopening of wound of thyroid field for:
- control of (postoperative) hemorrhage
- examination
- exploration
- removal of hematoma

06.09 Other incision of thyroid field
- Drainage of hematoma
- Drainage of thyroglossal tract
- Exploration: neck, thyroid (field)
- Removal of foreign body
- Thyroidotomy NOS

by incision

EXCLUDES:
- postoperative exploration (06.02)
- removal of hematoma by aspiration (06.01)

06.1 Diagnostic procedures on thyroid and parathyroid glands
DEF: Insertion of needle to draw or drain fluid from around thyroid.

06.11 Closed [percutaneous] [needle] biopsy of thyroid gland
Aspiration biopsy of thyroid
DEF: Insertion of needle-type device for removal of thyroid tissue sample.

06.12 Open biopsy of thyroid gland

06.13 Biopsy of parathyroid gland

06.19 Other diagnostic procedures on thyroid and parathyroid glands
EXCLUDES:
- radioisotope scan of: parathyroid (92.13), thyroid (92.01)
- soft tissue x-ray of thyroid field (87.09)

Thyroidectomy

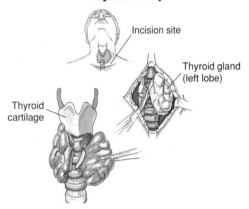

- Incision site
- Thyroid gland (left lobe)
- Thyroid cartilage

06.2 Unilateral thyroid lobectomy
Complete removal of one lobe of thyroid (with removal of isthmus or portion of other lobe)
Hemithyroidectomy
EXCLUDES: partial substernal thyroidectomy (06.51)
DEF: Excision of thyroid lobe.

06.3 Other partial thyroidectomy

06.31 Excision of lesion of thyroid
EXCLUDES: biopsy of thyroid (06.11-06.12)
DEF: Removal of growth on thyroid.

06.39 Other
Isthmectomy Partial thyroidectomy NOS
EXCLUDES: partial substernal thyroidectomy (06.51)

06.4 Complete thyroidectomy
EXCLUDES:
- complete substernal thyroidectomy (06.52)
- that with laryngectomy (30.3-30.4)

06.5 Substernal thyroidectomy
DEF: Removal of thyroid tissue below breastbone.

06.50 Substernal thyroidectomy, not otherwise specified

06.51 Partial substernal thyroidectomy

06.52 Complete substernal thyroidectomy

06.6 Excision of lingual thyroid
Excision of thyroid by:
- submental route
- transoral route

DEF: Excision of thyroid tissue at base of tongue.

06.7 Excision of thyroglossal duct or tract

06.8 Parathyroidectomy
DEF: Removal of parathyroid glands.

06.81 Complete parathyroidectomy

06.89 Other parathyroidectomy
Parathyroidectomy NOS
Partial parathyroidectomy
EXCLUDES: biopsy of parathyroid (06.13)

06.9 Other operations on thyroid (region) and parathyroid

06.91 Division of thyroid isthmus
Transection of thyroid isthmus
DEF: Cutting or division of tissue at narrowest point of thyroid.

06.92 Ligation of thyroid vessels

06.93 Suture of thyroid gland

06.94 Thyroid tissue reimplantation
Autotransplantation of thyroid tissue
DEF: Placement of thyroid tissue graft into functional site.
DEF: Autotransplantation of thyroid tissue: Tissue graft from patient thyroid tissue to another site on thyroid.

06.95 Parathyroid tissue reimplantation
Autotransplantation of parathyroid tissue
DEF: Placement of parathyroid tissue graft into functional site.
DEF: Autotransplantation of parathyroid tissue: Use of patient parathyroid tissue for graft.

06.98 Other operations on thyroid glands

06.99 Other operations on parathyroid glands

Tabular List
OPERATIONS ON THE ENDOCRINE SYSTEM

√3rd 07 Operations on other endocrine glands
INCLUDES operations on:
  adrenal glands pituitary gland
  pineal gland thymus
EXCLUDES operations on:
  aortic and carotid bodies (39.8)
  ovaries (65.0-65.99)
  pancreas (52.01-52.99)
  testes (62.0-62.99)

√4th 07.0 Exploration of adrenal field
EXCLUDES incision of adrenal (gland) (07.41)

07.00 Exploration of adrenal field, not otherwise specified

07.01 Unilateral exploration of adrenal field
DEF: Investigation of one adrenal gland for diagnostic reasons.

07.02 Bilateral exploration of adrenal field
DEF: Investigation of both adrenal glands for diagnostic reasons.

√4th 07.1 Diagnostic procedures on adrenal glands, pituitary gland, pineal gland, and thymus

07.11 Closed [percutaneous] [needle] biopsy of adrenal gland

07.12 Open biopsy of adrenal gland

07.13 Biopsy of pituitary gland, transfrontal approach
DEF: Excision of pituitary gland tissue for exam through frontal bone.

07.14 Biopsy of pituitary gland, transsphenoidal approach
DEF: Excision of pituitary gland tissue for exam through sphenoid bone.

07.15 Biopsy of pituitary gland, unspecified approach

07.16 Biopsy of thymus

07.17 Biopsy of pineal gland

07.19 Other diagnostic procedures on adrenal glands, pituitary gland, pineal gland, and thymus
EXCLUDES microscopic examination of specimen from endocrine gland (90.11-90.19)
  radioisotope scan of pituitary gland (92.11)

√4th 07.2 Partial adrenalectomy

07.21 Excision of lesion of adrenal gland
EXCLUDES biopsy of adrenal gland (07.11-07.12)

07.22 Unilateral adrenalectomy
Adrenalectomy NOS
EXCLUDES excision of remaining adrenal gland (07.3)
DEF: Excision of one adrenal gland.

07.29 Other partial adrenalectomy
Partial adrenalectomy NOS

07.3 Bilateral adrenalectomy
Excision of remaining adrenal gland
EXCLUDES bilateral partial adrenalectomy (07.29)

√4th 07.4 Other operations on adrenal glands, nerves, and vessels

07.41 Incision of adrenal gland
Adrenalotomy (with drainage)

07.42 Division of nerves to adrenal glands

07.43 Ligation of adrenal vessels

07.44 Repair of adrenal gland

07.45 Reimplantation of adrenal tissue
Autotransplantation of adrenal tissue
DEF: Placement of adrenal tissue graft into functional site.
DEF: Autotransplantation of adrenal tissue: Use of tissue graft from the patient's own body.

07.49 Other

√4th 07.5 Operations on pineal gland

07.51 Exploration of pineal field
EXCLUDES that with incision of pineal gland (07.52)

07.52 Incision of pineal gland

07.53 Partial excision of pineal gland
EXCLUDES biopsy of pineal gland (07.17)

07.54 Total excision of pineal gland
Pinealectomy (complete) (total)

07.59 Other operations on pineal gland

√4th 07.6 Hypophysectomy
DEF: Excision, destruction of pituitary gland.

07.61 Partial excision of pituitary gland, transfrontal approach
Cryohypophysectomy, partial ⎫
Division of hypophyseal stalk ⎪
Excision of lesion of pituitary [hypophysis] ⎬ transfrontal approach
Hypophysectomy, subtotal ⎪
Infundibulectomy, hypophyseal ⎭
EXCLUDES biopsy of pituitary gland, transfrontal approach (07.13)
DEF: Removal of pituitary gland, partial, through frontal bone.

07.62 Partial excision of pituitary gland, transsphenoidal approach
EXCLUDES biopsy of pituitary gland, transsphenoidal approach (07.14)
DEF: Removal of pituitary gland, partial, through sphenoid bone.

07.63 Partial excision of pituitary gland, unspecified approach
EXCLUDES biopsy of pituitary gland NOS (07.15)

07.64 Total excision of pituitary gland, transfrontal approach
Ablation of pituitary by implantation (strontium-yttrium) ⎫⎬ transfrontal approach
Cryohypophysectomy, complete ⎭
DEF: Removal of pituitary gland, total, through frontal bone.

07.65 Total excision of pituitary gland, transsphenoidal approach
DEF: Removal of pituitary gland, total, through sphenoid bone.

07.68 Total excision of pituitary gland, other specified approach
DEF: Destroy or remove pituitary gland by a specified approach, other than those listed.

OPERATIONS ON THE ENDOCRINE SYSTEM

07.69 **Total excision of pituitary gland, unspecified approach**
Hypophysectomy NOS
Pituitectomy NOS

√4th 07.7 Other operations on hypophysis

07.71 **Exploration of pituitary fossa**
EXCLUDES exploration with incision of pituitary gland (07.72)
DEF: Exploration of region of pituitary gland.

07.72 **Incision of pituitary gland**
Aspiration of:
craniobuccal pouch
craniopharyngioma
hypophysis
Aspiration of:
pituitary gland
Rathke's pouch

07.79 **Other**
Insertion of pack into sella turcica

√4th 07.8 Thymectomy
07.80 **Thymectomy, not otherwise specified**
07.81 **Partial excision of thymus**
EXCLUDES biopsy of thymus (07.16)
07.82 **Total excision of thymus**

√4th 07.9 Other operations on thymus
07.91 **Exploration of thymus field**
EXCLUDES exploration with incision of thymus (07.92)
07.92 **Incision of thymus**
07.93 **Repair of thymus**
07.94 **Transplantation of thymus**
DEF: Placement of thymus tissue grafts into functional area of gland.
07.99 **Other**
Thymopexy

3. OPERATIONS ON THE EYE (08-16)

08 Operations on eyelids
INCLUDES operations on the eyebrow

08.0 Incision of eyelid
- **08.01** Incision of lid margin
  DEF: Cutting into eyelid edge.
- **08.02** Severing of blepharorrhaphy
  DEF: Freeing of eyelids previously sutured shut.
- **08.09** Other incision of eyelid

08.1 Diagnostic procedures on eyelid
- **08.11** Biopsy of eyelid
- **08.19** Other diagnostic procedures on eyelid

08.2 Excision or destruction of lesion or tissue of eyelid
Code also any synchronous reconstruction (08.61-08.74)
EXCLUDES biopsy of eyelid (08.11)
- **08.20** Removal of lesion of eyelid, not otherwise specified
  Removal of meibomian gland NOS
- **08.21** Excision of chalazion
- **08.22** Excision of other minor lesion of eyelid
  Excision of: verruca
  Excision of: wart
- **08.23** Excision of major lesion of eyelid, partial-thickness
  Excision involving one-fourth or more of lid margin, partial-thickness
  DEF: Excision of lesion not in all eyelid layers.
- **08.24** Excision of major lesion of eyelid, full-thickness
  Excision involving one-fourth or more of lid margin, full-thickness
  Wedge resection of eyelid
  DEF: Excision of growth in all eyelid layers, full thickness.
- **08.25** Destruction of lesion of eyelid

08.3 Repair of blepharoptosis and lid retraction
- **08.31** Repair of blepharoptosis by frontalis muscle technique with suture
  DEF: Correction of drooping upper eyelid with suture of frontalis muscle.
- **08.32** Repair of blepharoptosis by frontalis muscle technique with fascial sling
  DEF: Correction of drooping upper eyelid with fascial tissue sling of frontalis muscle.
- **08.33** Repair of blepharoptosis by resection or advancement of levator muscle or aponeurosis
  DEF: Correction of drooping upper eyelid with levator muscle, extended, cut, or by expanded tendon.
- **08.34** Repair of blepharoptosis by other levator muscle techniques
- **08.35** Repair of blepharoptosis by tarsal technique
  DEF: Correction of drooping upper eyelid with tarsal muscle.
- **08.36** Repair of blepharoptosis by other techniques
  Correction of eyelid ptosis NOS
  Orbicularis oculi muscle sling for correction of blepharoptosis
- **08.37** Reduction of overcorrection of ptosis
  DEF: Correction, release of previous plastic repair of drooping eyelid.
- **08.38** Correction of lid retraction
  DEF: Fixing of withdrawn eyelid into normal position.

08.4 Repair of entropion or ectropion
- **08.41** Repair of entropion or ectropion by thermocauterization
  DEF: Restoration of eyelid margin to normal position with heat cautery.
- **08.42** Repair of entropion or ectropion by suture technique
  DEF: Restoration of eyelid margin to normal position by suture.
- **08.43** Repair of entropion or ectropion with wedge resection
  DEF: Restoration of eyelid margin to normal position by removing tissue.
- **08.44** Repair of entropion or ectropion with lid reconstruction
  DEF: Reconstruction of eyelid margin.
- **08.49** Other repair of entropion or ectropion

08.5 Other adjustment of lid position
- **08.51** Canthotomy
  DEF: Incision into outer canthus of eye.
- **08.52** Blepharorrhaphy
  Canthorrhaphy Tarsorrhaphy
  DEF: Suture together of eyelids, partial or repair; done to shorten palpebral fissure or protect cornea.
- **08.59** Other
  Canthoplasty NOS
  Repair of epicanthal fold

08.6 Reconstruction of eyelid with flaps or grafts
EXCLUDES that associated with repair of entropion and ectropion (08.44)
- **08.61** Reconstruction of eyelid with skin flap or graft
  DEF: Rebuild of eyelid by graft or flap method.
- **08.62** Reconstruction of eyelid with mucous membrane flap or graft
  DEF: Rebuild of eyelid with mucous membrane by graft or flap method.
- **08.63** Reconstruction of eyelid with hair follicle graft
  DEF: Rebuild of eyelid with hair follicle graft.
- **08.64** Reconstruction of eyelid with tarsoconjunctival flap
  Transfer of tarsoconjunctival flap from opposing lid
  DEF: Recreation of eyelid with tarsoconjunctival tissue.
- **08.69** Other reconstruction of eyelid with flaps or grafts

08.7 Other reconstruction of eyelid
EXCLUDES that associated with repair of entropion and ectropion (08.44)
- **08.70** Reconstruction of eyelid, not otherwise specified
  AHA: 2Q, '96, 11
- **08.71** Reconstruction of eyelid involving lid margin, partial-thickness
  DEF: Repair of eyelid margin not using all lid layers.
- **08.72** Other reconstruction of eyelid, partial-thickness
  DEF: Reshape of eyelid not using all lid layers.

OPERATIONS ON THE EYE

08.73 **Reconstruction of eyelid involving lid margin, full-thickness**
DEF: Repair of eyelid and margin using all tissue layers.

08.74 **Other reconstruction of eyelid, full-thickness**
DEF: Other repair of eyelid using all tissue layers.

√4th **08.8** Other repair of eyelid

08.81 **Linear repair of laceration of eyelid or eyebrow**

08.82 **Repair of laceration involving lid margin, partial-thickness**
DEF: Repair of laceration not involving all layers of eyelid margin.

08.83 **Other repair of laceration of eyelid, partial thickness**
DEF: Repair of eyelid tear not involving all eyelid layers.

08.84 **Repair of laceration involving lid margin, full-thickness**
DEF: Repair of eyelid margin tear involving all margin layers.

08.85 **Other repair of laceration of eyelid, full-thickness**
DEF: Repair of eyelid tear involving all layers.

08.86 **Lower eyelid rhytidectomy**
DEF: Removal of wrinkles from lower eyelid.

08.87 **Upper eyelid rhytidectomy**
AHA: 2Q, '96, 11
DEF: Removal of wrinkles from upper eyelid.

08.89 **Other eyelid repair**
AHA: 1Q, '00, 22

√4th **08.9** Other operations on eyelids

08.91 **Electrosurgical epilation of eyelid**
DEF: Electrical removal of eyelid hair roots.

08.92 **Cryosurgical epilation of eyelid**
DEF: Removal of eyelid hair roots by freezing.

08.93 **Other epilation of eyelid**

08.99 **Other**

√3rd **09** Operations on lacrimal system

√4th **09.0** **Incision of lacrimal gland**
Incision of lacrimal cyst (with drainage)

√4th **09.1** Diagnostic procedures on lacrimal system
09.11 **Biopsy of lacrimal gland**
09.12 **Biopsy of lacrimal sac**
09.19 **Other diagnostic procedures on lacrimal system**
EXCLUDES: contrast dacryocystogram (87.05)
soft tissue x-ray of nasolacrimal duct (87.09)

√4th **09.2** Excision of lesion or tissue of lacrimal gland
09.20 **Excision of lacrimal gland, not otherwise specified**
09.21 **Excision of lesion of lacrimal gland**
EXCLUDES: biopsy of lacrimal gland (09.11)
09.22 **Other partial dacryoadenectomy**
EXCLUDES: biopsy of lacrimal gland (09.11)
DEF: Excision, partial, of tear gland.
09.23 **Total dacryoadenectomy**
DEF: Excision, total, of tear gland.

09.3 Other operations on lacrimal gland

√4th **09.4** Manipulation of lacrimal passage
INCLUDES: removal of calculus
that with dilation
EXCLUDES: contrast dacryocystogram (87.05)

09.41 **Probing of lacrimal punctum**
DEF: Exploration of tear duct entrance with flexible rod.

09.42 **Probing of lacrimal canaliculi**
DEF: Exploration of tear duct with flexible rod.

09.43 **Probing of nasolacrimal duct**
EXCLUDES: that with insertion of tube or stent (09.44)
DEF: Exploration of passage between tear sac and nose with flexible rod.

09.44 **Intubation of nasolacrimal duct**
Insertion of stent into nasolacrimal duct
AHA: 2Q, '94, 11

09.49 **Other manipulation of lacrimal passage**

√4th **09.5** Incision of lacrimal sac and passages
09.51 **Incision of lacrimal punctum**
09.52 **Incision of lacrimal canaliculi**
09.53 **Incision of lacrimal sac**
DEF: Cutting into lacrimal pouch of tear gland.
09.59 **Other incision of lacrimal passages**
Incision (and drainage) of nasolacrimal duct NOS

09.6 **Excision of lacrimal sac and passage**
EXCLUDES: biopsy of lacrimal sac (09.12)
DEF: Removal of pouch and passage of tear gland.

09.7 Repair of canaliculus and punctum
EXCLUDES: repair of eyelid (08.81-08.89)
09.71 **Correction of everted punctum**
DEF: Repair of an outwardly turned tear duct entrance.
09.72 **Other repair of punctum**
09.73 **Repair of canaliculus**

√4th **09.8** Fistulization of lacrimal tract to nasal cavity
09.81 **Dacryocystorhinostomy [DCR]**
DEF: Creation of entrance between tear gland and nasal passage for tear flow.

09.82 **Conjunctivocystorhinostomy**
Conjunctivodacryocystorhinostomy [CDCR]
EXCLUDES: that with insertion of tube or stent (09.83)
DEF: Creation of tear drainage path from lacrimal sac to nasal cavity through conjunctiva.

09.83 **Conjunctivorhinostomy with insertion of tube or stent**
DEF: Creation of passage between eye sac membrane and nasal cavity with tube or stent.

√4th **09.9** Other operations on lacrimal system
09.91 **Obliteration of lacrimal punctum**
DEF: Destruction, total of tear gland opening in eyelid.
09.99 **Other**
AHA: 2Q, '94, 11

√3rd **10** Operations on conjunctiva

10.0 **Removal of embedded foreign body from conjunctiva by incision**
EXCLUDES: removal of:
embedded foreign body without incision (98.22)
superficial foreign body (98.21)

10.1 **Other incision of conjunctiva**

BI Bilateral Edit NC Non-covered Procedure ▶◀ Revised Text ● New Code ▲ Revised Code Title

OPERATIONS ON THE EYE

10.2 Diagnostic procedures on conjunctiva
- **10.21** Biopsy of conjunctiva
- **10.29** Other diagnostic procedures on conjunctiva

10.3 Excision or destruction of lesion or tissue of conjunctiva
- **10.31** Excision of lesion or tissue of conjunctiva
  Excision of ring of conjunctiva around cornea
  EXCLUDES biopsy of conjunctiva (10.21)
  AHA: 4Q, '00, 41; 3Q, '96, 7
  DEF: Removal of growth or tissue from eye membrane.
- **10.32** Destruction of lesion of conjunctiva
  EXCLUDES excision of lesion (10.31)
  thermocauterization for entropion (08.41)
  DEF: Destruction of eye membrane growth; not done by excision.
- **10.33** Other destructive procedures on conjunctiva
  Removal of trachoma follicles

10.4 Conjunctivoplasty
DEF: Correction of conjunctiva by plastic surgery.
- **10.41** Repair of symblepharon with free graft
  AHA: 3Q, '96, 7
- **10.42** Reconstruction of conjunctival cul-de-sac with free graft
  EXCLUDES revision of enucleation socket with graft (16.63)
  DEF: Rebuilding of eye membrane fold with graft of unattached tissue.
- **10.43** Other reconstruction of conjunctival cul-de-sac
  EXCLUDES revision of enucleation socket (16.64)
- **10.44** Other free graft to conjunctiva
- **10.49** Other conjunctivoplasty
  EXCLUDES repair of cornea with conjunctival flap (11.53)

10.5 Lysis of adhesions of conjunctiva and eyelid
Division of symblepharon (with insertion of conformer)

10.6 Repair of laceration of conjunctiva
EXCLUDES that with repair of sclera (12.81)

10.9 Other operations on conjunctiva
- **10.91** Subconjunctival injection
  AHA: 3Q, '96, 7
- **10.99** Other

11 Operations on cornea

11.0 Magnetic removal of embedded foreign body from cornea
EXCLUDES that with incision (11.1)

11.1 Incision of cornea
Incision of cornea for removal of foreign body

11.2 Diagnostic procedures on cornea
- **11.21** Scraping of cornea for smear or culture
- **11.22** Biopsy of cornea
- **11.29** Other diagnostic procedures on cornea

11.3 Excision of pterygium
- **11.31** Transposition of pterygium
  DEF: Cutting into membranous structure extending from eye membrane to cornea and suturing it in a downward position.
- **11.32** Excision of pterygium with corneal graft
  DEF: Surgical removal and repair of membranous structure extending from eye membrane to cornea using corneal tissue transplant.
- **11.39** Other excision of pterygium

11.4 Excision or destruction of tissue or other lesion of cornea
- **11.41** Mechanical removal of corneal epithelium
  That by chemocauterization
  EXCLUDES that for smear or culture (11.21)
  DEF: Removal of outer layer of cornea by mechanical means.
- **11.42** Thermocauterization of corneal lesion
  DEF: Destruction of corneal lesion by electrical cautery.
- **11.43** Cryotherapy of corneal lesion
  DEF: Destruction of corneal lesion with cold therapy.
- **11.49** Other removal or destruction of corneal lesion
  Excision of cornea NOS
  EXCLUDES biopsy of cornea (11.22)

11.5 Repair of cornea
- **11.51** Suture of corneal laceration
  AHA: 3Q, '96, 7
- **11.52** Repair of postoperative wound dehiscence of cornea
  DEF: Repair of ruptured postoperative corneal wound.
- **11.53** Repair of corneal laceration or wound with conjunctival flap
  DEF: Correction corneal wound or tear with conjunctival tissue.
- **11.59** Other repair of cornea

11.6 Corneal transplant
EXCLUDES excision of pterygium with corneal graft (11.32)
- **11.60** Corneal transplant, not otherwise specified
  Keratoplasty NOS
- **11.61** Lamellar keratoplasty with autograft
  DEF: Restoration of sight using patient's own corneal tissue, partial thickness.
- **11.62** Other lamellar keratoplasty
  AHA: S-O, '85, 6
  DEF: Restoration of sight using donor corneal tissue, partial thickness.
- **11.63** Penetrating keratoplasty with autograft
  Perforating keratoplasty with autograft
- **11.64** Other penetrating keratoplasty
  Perforating keratoplasty (with homograft)
- **11.69** Other corneal transplant

11.7 Other reconstructive and refractive surgery on cornea
- **11.71** Keratomileusis **NC**
  DEF: Restoration of corneal shape by removing portion of cornea, freezing, reshaping curve and reattaching it.
- **11.72** Keratophakia **NC**
  DEF: Correction of eye lens loss by by dissecting the central zone of the cornea and replacing it with a thickened graft of the cornea.
- **11.73** Keratoprosthesis
  DEF: Placement of corneal artificial implant.
- **11.74** Thermokeratoplasty
  DEF: Reshaping and reforming cornea by heat application.

OPERATIONS ON THE EYE

11.75 Radial keratotomy — NC
DEF: Incisions around cornea radius to correct nearsightedness.

11.76 Epikeratophakia — NC
DEF: Repair lens loss by cornea graft sutured to central corneal zone.

11.79 Other

√4th **11.9 Other operations on cornea**
- **11.91 Tattooing of cornea**
- **11.92 Removal of artificial implant from cornea**
- **11.99 Other**

√3rd **12 Operations on iris, ciliary body, sclera, and anterior chamber**
EXCLUDES: operations on cornea (11.0-11.99)

√4th **12.0 Removal of intraocular foreign body from anterior segment of eye**
- **12.00 Removal of intraocular foreign body from anterior segment of eye, not otherwise specified**
- **12.01 Removal of intraocular foreign body from anterior segment of eye with use of magnet**
- **12.02 Removal of intraocular foreign body from anterior segment of eye without use of magnet**

√4th **12.1 Iridotomy and simple iridectomy**
EXCLUDES: iridectomy associated with:
 cataract extraction (13.11-13.69)
 removal of lesion (12.41-12.42)
 scleral fistulization (12.61-12.69)
- **12.11 Iridotomy with transfixion**
- **12.12 Other iridotomy**
 Corectomy
 Discission of iris
 Iridotomy NOS
 DEF: Corectomy: Incision into iris (also called iridectomy).
- **12.13 Excision of prolapsed iris**
 DEF: Removal of downwardly placed portion of iris.
- **12.14 Other iridectomy**
 Iridectomy (basal) (peripheral) (total)
 DEF: Removal, partial or total of iris.

√4th **12.2 Diagnostic procedures on iris, ciliary body, sclera, and anterior chamber**
- **12.21 Diagnostic aspiration of anterior chamber of eye**
 DEF: Suction withdrawal of fluid from anterior eye chamber for diagnostic reasons.
- **12.22 Biopsy of iris**
- **12.29 Other diagnostic procedures on iris, ciliary body, sclera, and anterior chamber**

√4th **12.3 Iridoplasty and coreoplasty**
DEF: Correction or abnormal iris or pupil by plastic surgery.
- **12.31 Lysis of goniosynechiae**
 Lysis of goniosynechiae by injection of air or liquid
 DEF: Freeing of fibrous structures between cornea and iris by injecting air or liquid.
- **12.32 Lysis of other anterior synechiae**
 Lysis of anterior synechiae:
 NOS
 by injection of air or liquid
- **12.33 Lysis of posterior synechiae**
 Lysis of iris adhesions NOS
- **12.34 Lysis of corneovitreal adhesions**
 DEF: Release of adhesions of cornea and vitreous body.

- **12.35 Coreoplasty**
 Needling of pupillary membrane
 DEF: Correction of an iris defect.
- **12.39 Other iridoplasty**

√4th **12.4 Excision or destruction of lesion of iris and ciliary body**
- **12.40 Removal of lesion of anterior segment of eye, not otherwise specified**
- **12.41 Destruction of lesion of iris, nonexcisional**
 Destruction of lesion of iris by:
 cauterization
 cryotherapy
 photocoagulation
- **12.42 Excision of lesion of iris**
 EXCLUDES: biopsy of iris (12.22)
- **12.43 Destruction of lesion of ciliary body, nonexcisional**
- **12.44 Excision of lesion of ciliary body**

√4th **12.5 Facilitation of intraocular circulation**
- **12.51 Goniopuncture without goniotomy**
 DEF: Stab incision into anterior chamber of eye to relieve optic pressure.
- **12.52 Goniotomy without goniopuncture**
 DEF: Incision into Schlemm's canal to drain aqueous and relieve pressure.
- **12.53 Goniotomy with goniopuncture**
- **12.54 Trabeculotomy ab externo**
 DEF: Incision into supporting connective tissue strands of eye capsule, via exterior approach.
- **12.55 Cyclodialysis**
 DEF: Creation of passage between anterior chamber and suprachoroidal space.
- **12.59 Other facilitation of intraocular circulation**

√4th **12.6 Scleral fistulization**
EXCLUDES: exploratory sclerotomy (12.89)
- **12.61 Trephination of sclera with iridectomy**
 DEF: Cut around sclerocornea to remove part of the iris.
- **12.62 Thermocauterization of sclera with iridectomy**
 DEF: Destruction of outer eyeball layer with partial excision of iris using heat.
- **12.63 Iridencleisis and iridotasis**
 DEF: Creation of permanent drain in iris by transposing or stretching iris tissue.
- **12.64 Trabeculectomy ab externo**
 DEF: Excision of supporting connective tissue strands of eye capsule, via exterior approach.

Trabeculectomy Ab Externo

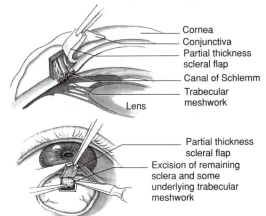

BI Bilateral Edit   NC Non-covered Procedure   ▶◀ Revised Text   ● New Code   ▲ Revised Code Title

OPERATIONS ON THE EYE

12.65 **Other scleral fistulization with iridectomy**
DEF: Creation of outer eyeball layer passage with partial excision of iris.

12.66 **Postoperative revision of scleral fistulization procedure**
Revision of filtering bleb
EXCLUDES repair of fistula (12.82)
AHA: 2Q, '01, 16

12.69 **Other fistulizing procedure**

12.7 **Other procedures for relief of elevated intraocular pressure**

12.71 **Cyclodiathermy**
DEF: Destruction of ciliary body tissue with heat.

12.72 **Cyclocryotherapy**
DEF: Destruction of ciliary body tissue by freezing.

12.73 **Cyclophotocoagulation**
DEF: Destruction of ciliary body tissue by high energy light source.

12.74 **Diminution of ciliary body, not otherwise specified**

12.79 **Other glaucoma procedures**
AHA: 2Q, '98, 16

12.8 **Operations on sclera**
EXCLUDES those associated with:
  retinal reattachment (14.41-14.59)
  scleral fistulization (12.61-12.69)

12.81 **Suture of laceration of sclera**
Suture of sclera with synchronous repair of conjunctiva

12.82 **Repair of scleral fistula**
EXCLUDES postoperative revision of scleral fistulization procedure (12.66)

12.83 **Revision of operative wound of anterior segment, not elsewhere classified**
EXCLUDES postoperative revision of scleral fistulization procedure (12.66)

12.84 **Excision or destruction of lesion of sclera**

12.85 **Repair of scleral staphyloma with graft**
DEF: Repair of protruding outer eyeball layer with a graft.

12.86 **Other repair of scleral staphyloma**

12.87 **Scleral reinforcement with graft**
DEF: Restoration of outer eyeball shape with tissue graft.

12.88 **Other scleral reinforcement**

12.89 **Other operations on sclera**
Exploratory sclerotomy

12.9 **Other operations on iris, ciliary body, and anterior chamber**

12.91 **Therapeutic evacuation of anterior chamber**
Paracentesis of anterior chamber
EXCLUDES diagnostic aspiration (12.21)

12.92 **Injection into anterior chamber**
Injection of:
  air
  liquid   } into anterior chamber
  medication
AHA: J-A, '84, 1

12.93 **Removal or destruction of epithelial downgrowth from anterior chamber**
EXCLUDES that with iridectomy (12.41-12.42)
DEF: Excision or destruction of epithelial overgrowth in anterior eye chamber.

12.97 **Other operations on iris**
12.98 **Other operations on ciliary body**
12.99 **Other operations on anterior chamber**

13 Operations on lens

13.0 **Removal of foreign body from lens**
EXCLUDES removal of pseudophakos (13.8)

13.00 **Removal of foreign body from lens, not otherwise specified**

13.01 **Removal of foreign body from lens with use of magnet**

13.02 **Removal of foreign body from lens without use of magnet**

13.1 **Intracapsular extraction of lens**
Code also any synchronous insertion of pseudophakos (13.71)
AHA: S-O, '85, 6

13.11 **Intracapsular extraction of lens by temporal inferior route**
DEF: Extraction of lens and capsule via anterior approach through outer side of eyeball.

13.19 **Other intracapsular extraction of lens**
Cataract extraction NOS
Cryoextraction of lens
Erysiphake extraction of cataract
Extraction of lens NOS

13.2 **Extracapsular extraction of lens by linear extraction technique**
AHA: S-O, '85, 6

DEF: Excision of lens without the posterior capsule at junction between the cornea and outer eyeball layer by means of a linear incision.

13.3 **Extracapsular extraction of lens by simple aspiration (and irrigation) technique**
Irrigation of traumatic cataract
AHA: S-O, '85, 6

DEF: Removal of lens without the posterior capsule by suctioning and flushing out the area.

13.4 **Extracapsular extraction of lens by fragmentation and aspiration technique**
AHA: S-O, '85, 6

DEF: Removal of lens after division into smaller pieces with posterior capsule left intact.

13.41 **Phacoemulsification and aspiration of cataract**
AHA: 3Q, '96, 4; 1Q, '94, 16

13.42 **Mechanical phacofragmentation and aspiration of cataract by posterior route**
Code also any synchronous vitrectomy (14.74)

Extraction of Lens
(with insertion of intraocular lens prosthesis)

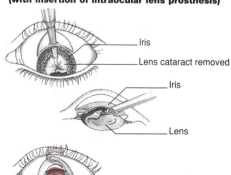

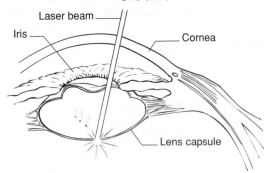

Laser Surgery (YAG)

13.43 Mechanical phacofragmentation and other aspiration of cataract

✓4th **13.5** Other extracapsular extraction of lens
Code also any synchronous insertion of pseudophakos (13.71)
AHA: S-O, '85, 6

13.51 Extracapsular extraction of lens by temporal inferior route
DEF: Removal of lens through outer eyeball with posterior capsule left intact.

13.59 Other extracapsular extraction of lens

✓4th **13.6** Other cataract extraction
Code also any synchronous insertion of pseudophakos (13.71)
AHA: S-O, '85, 6

13.64 Discission of secondary membrane [after cataract]
DEF: Breaking up of fibrotic lens capsule developed after previous lens extraction.

13.65 Excision of secondary membrane [after cataract]
Capsulectomy
DEF: Capsulectomy: Excision of lens capsule membrane after previous lens extraction.

13.66 Mechanical fragmentation of secondary membrane [after cataract]
DEF: Breaking up and removal of fibrotic lens capsule developed after previous lens extraction.

13.69 Other cataract extraction

✓4th **13.7** Insertion of prosthetic lens [pseudophakos]
AHA: J-A, '84, 1
DEF: Insertion of ocular implant, following lens extraction.

13.70 Insertion of pseudophakos, not otherwise specified

13.71 Insertion of intraocular lens prosthesis at time of cataract extraction, one-stage
Code also synchronous extraction of cataract (13.11-13.69)
AHA: 3Q, '96, 4

13.72 Secondary insertion of intraocular lens prosthesis

13.8 Removal of implanted lens
Removal of pseudophakos

13.9 Other operations on lens
AHA: 1Q, '00, 9

✓3rd **14** Operations on retina, choroid, vitreous, and posterior chamber

✓4th **14.0** Removal of foreign body from posterior segment of eye
EXCLUDES: removal of surgically implanted material (14.6)

14.00 Removal of foreign body from posterior segment of eye, not otherwise specified

14.01 Removal of foreign body from posterior segment of eye with use of magnet

14.02 Removal of foreign body from posterior segment of eye without use of magnet

✓4th **14.1** Diagnostic procedures on retina, choroid, vitreous, and posterior chamber

14.11 Diagnostic aspiration of vitreous

14.19 Other diagnostic procedures on retina, choroid, vitreous, and posterior chamber

✓4th **14.2** Destruction of lesion of retina and choroid
INCLUDES: destruction of chorioretinopathy or isolated chorioretinal lesion
EXCLUDES: that for repair of retina (14.31-14.59)
DEF: Destruction of damaged retina and choroid tissue.

14.21 Destruction of chorioretinal lesion by diathermy

14.22 Destruction of chorioretinal lesion by cryotherapy

14.23 Destruction of chorioretinal lesion by xenon arc photocoagulation

14.24 Destruction of chorioretinal lesion by laser photocoagulation

14.25 Destruction of chorioretinal lesion by photocoagulation of unspecified type

14.26 Destruction of chorioretinal lesion by radiation therapy

14.27 Destruction of chorioretinal lesion by implantation of radiation source

14.29 Other destruction of chorioretinal lesion
Destruction of lesion of retina and choroid NOS

✓4th **14.3** Repair of retinal tear
INCLUDES: repair of retinal defect
EXCLUDES: repair of retinal detachment (14.41-14.59)

14.31 Repair of retinal tear by diathermy

14.32 Repair of retinal tear by cryotherapy

14.33 Repair of retinal tear by xenon arc photocoagulation

14.34 Repair of retinal tear by laser photocoagulation
AHA: 1Q, '94, 17

14.35 Repair of retinal tear by photocoagulation of unspecified type

14.39 Other repair of retinal tear

✓4th **14.4** Repair of retinal detachment with scleral buckling and implant
DEF: Placement of material around eye to indent sclera and close a hole or tear or to reduce vitreous traction.

14.41 Scleral buckling with implant
AHA: 3Q, '96, 6

14.49 Other scleral buckling
Scleral buckling with:
air tamponade
resection of sclera
vitrectomy
AHA: 1Q, '94, 16

Tabular List
OPERATIONS ON THE EYE

√4th 14.5 Other repair of retinal detachment
  INCLUDES: that with drainage
  - **14.51 Repair of retinal detachment with diathermy**
  - **14.52 Repair of retinal detachment with cryotherapy**
  - **14.53 Repair of retinal detachment with xenon arc photocoagulation**
  - **14.54 Repair of retinal detachment with laser photocoagulation**
    AHA: N-D, '87, 10
  - **14.55 Repair of retinal detachment with photocoagulation of unspecified type**
  - **14.59 Other**

14.6 Removal of surgically implanted material from posterior segment of eye

√4th 14.7 Operations on vitreous
  - **14.71 Removal of vitreous, anterior approach**
    Open sky technique
    Removal of vitreous, anterior approach (with replacement)
    DEF: Removal of all or part of the eyeball fluid via the anterior segment of the eyeball.
  - **14.72 Other removal of vitreous**
    Aspiration of vitreous by posterior sclerotomy
  - **14.73 Mechanical vitrectomy by anterior approach**
    AHA: 3Q, '96, 4, 5
    DEF: Removal of abnormal tissue in eyeball fluid to control fibrotic overgrowth in severe intraocular injury.
  - **14.74 Other mechanical vitrectomy**
    AHA: 3Q, '96, 4, 5
  - **14.75 Injection of vitreous substitute**
    EXCLUDES: that associated with removal (14.71-14.72)
    AHA: 1Q, '98, 6; 3Q, '96, 4, 5; 1Q, '94, 17
  - **14.79 Other operations on vitreous**
    AHA: 3Q, '99, 12; 1Q, '99, 11; 1Q, '98, 6

14.9 Other operations on retina, choroid, and posterior chamber
AHA: 3Q, '96, 5

√3rd 15 Operations on extraocular muscles

√4th 15.0 Diagnostic procedures on extraocular muscles or tendons
  - **15.01 Biopsy of extraocular muscle or tendon**
  - **15.09 Other diagnostic procedures on extraocular muscles and tendons**

√4th 15.1 Operations on one extraocular muscle involving temporary detachment from globe
  - **15.11 Recession of one extraocular muscle**
    AHA: 3Q, '96, 3
    DEF: Detachment of exterior eye muscle with posterior reattachment to correct strabismus.
  - **15.12 Advancement of one extraocular muscle**
    DEF: Detachment of exterior eye muscle with forward reattachment to correct strabismus.
  - **15.13 Resection of one extraocular muscle**
  - **15.19 Other operations on one extraocular muscle involving temporary detachment from globe**
    EXCLUDES: transposition of muscle (15.5)

√4th 15.2 Other operations on one extraocular muscle
  - **15.21 Lengthening procedure on one extraocular muscle**
    DEF: Extension of exterior eye muscle length.

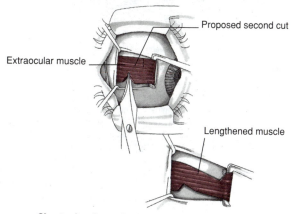

Lengthening Procedure on One Extraocular Muscle

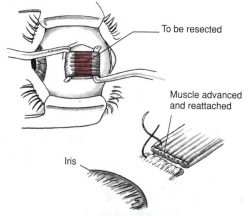

Shortening Procedure on One Extraocular Muscle

  - **15.22 Shortening procedure on one extraocular muscle**
    DEF: Shortening of exterior eye muscle.
  - **15.29 Other**

15.3 Operations on two or more extraocular muscles involving temporary detachment from globe, one or both eyes
AHA: 3Q, '96, 3

15.4 Other operations on two or more extraocular muscles, one or both eyes

15.5 Transposition of extraocular muscles
EXCLUDES: that for correction of ptosis (08.31-08.36)
DEF: Relocation of exterior eye muscle to a more functional site.

15.6 Revision of extraocular muscle surgery
DEF: Repair of previous exterior eye muscle surgery.

15.7 Repair of injury of extraocular muscle
Freeing of entrapped extraocular muscle
Lysis of adhesions of extraocular muscle
Repair of laceration of extraocular muscle, tendon, or Tenon's capsule

15.9 Other operations on extraocular muscles and tendons

√3rd 16 Operations on orbit and eyeball
EXCLUDES: reduction of fracture of orbit (76.78-76.79)

√4th 16.0 Orbitotomy
  - **16.01 Orbitotomy with bone flap**
    Orbitotomy with lateral approach
    DEF: Incision into orbital bone with insertion of small bone piece.
  - **16.02 Orbitotomy with insertion of orbital implant**
    EXCLUDES: that with bone flap (16.01)
  - **16.09 Other orbitotomy**

16.1–16.99 OPERATIONS ON THE EYE

16.1 Removal of penetrating foreign body from eye, not otherwise specified
  EXCLUDES removal of nonpenetrating foreign body (98.21)
  DEF: Removal of foreign body from an unspecified site in eye.

√4th 16.2 Diagnostic procedures on orbit and eyeball
  16.21 Ophthalmoscopy
  16.22 Diagnostic aspiration of orbit
  16.23 Biopsy of eyeball and orbit
  16.29 Other diagnostic procedures on orbit and eyeball
    EXCLUDES examination of form and structure of eye (95.11-95.16)
    general and subjective eye examination (95.01-95.09)
    microscopic examination of specimen from eye (90.21-90.29)
    objective functional tests of eye (95.21-95.26)
    ocular thermography (88.82)
    tonometry (89.11)
    x-ray of orbit (87.14, 87.16)

√4th 16.3 Evisceration of eyeball
  DEF: Removal of eyeball, leaving sclera and occasionally cornea.
  16.31 Removal of ocular contents with synchronous implant into scleral shell
    DEF: Removal of eyeball leaving outer eyeball layer with ocular implant into shell.
  16.39 Other evisceration of eyeball

√4th 16.4 Enucleation of eyeball
  DEF: Removal of entire eyeball after severing eye muscles and optic nerves.
  16.41 Enucleation of eyeball with synchronous implant into Tenon's capsule with attachment of muscles
    Integrated implant of eyeball
    DEF: Removal of eyeball with insertion of ocular implant and muscle attachment.
  16.42 Enucleation of eyeball with other synchronous implant
  16.49 Other enucleation of eyeball
    Removal of eyeball NOS

√4th 16.5 Exenteration of orbital contents
  16.51 Exenteration of orbit with removal of adjacent structures
    Radical orbitomaxillectomy
    DEF: Removal of contents of bony cavity of eye as well as related tissues and structures.
    DEF: Radical orbitomaxillectomy: Removal of contents of bony cavity of eye, related tissues and structures, and a portion of maxillary bone.
  16.52 Exenteration of orbit with therapeutic removal of orbital bone
  16.59 Other exenteration of orbit
    Evisceration of orbit NOS
    Exenteration of orbit with temporalis muscle transplant

√4th 16.6 Secondary procedures after removal of eyeball
  EXCLUDES that with synchronous:
    enucleation of eyeball (16.41-16.42)
    evisceration of eyeball (16.31)
  16.61 Secondary insertion of ocular implant
    DEF: Insertion of ocular implant after previous eye removal.
  16.62 Revision and reinsertion of ocular implant
    DEF: Reimplant or correction of ocular implant.
  16.63 Revision of enucleation socket with graft
    DEF: Implant of tissue to correct socket after eye removal.
  16.64 Other revision of enucleation socket
  16.65 Secondary graft to exenteration cavity
    DEF: Implant of tissue in place of eye after removal.
  16.66 Other revision of exenteration cavity
  16.69 Other secondary procedures after removal of eyeball

√4th 16.7 Removal of ocular or orbital implant
  16.71 Removal of ocular implant
  16.72 Removal of orbital implant

√4th 16.8 Repair of injury of eyeball and orbit
  16.81 Repair of wound of orbit
    EXCLUDES reduction of orbital fracture (76.78-76.79)
    repair of extraocular muscles (15.7)
  16.82 Repair of rupture of eyeball
    Repair of multiple structures of eye
    EXCLUDES repair of laceration of:
      cornea (11.51-11.59)
      sclera (12.81)
  16.89 Other repair of injury of eyeball or orbit

√4th 16.9 Other operations on orbit and eyeball
  EXCLUDES irrigation of eye (96.51)
    prescription and fitting of low vision aids (95.31-95.33)
    removal of:
      eye prosthesis NEC (97.31)
      nonpenetrating foreign body from eye without incision (98.21)
  16.91 Retrobulbar injection of therapeutic agent
    EXCLUDES injection of radiographic contrast material (87.14)
    opticociliary injection (12.79)
  16.92 Excision of lesion of orbit
    EXCLUDES biopsy of orbit (16.23)
  16.93 Excision of lesion of eye, unspecified structure
    EXCLUDES biopsy of eye NOS (16.23)
  16.98 Other operations on orbit
  16.99 Other operations on eyeball

OPERATIONS ON THE EAR

4. OPERATIONS ON THE EAR (18-20)

18 Operations on external ear
INCLUDES operations on:
  external auditory canal
  skin and cartilage of:
    auricle
    meatus

18.0 Incision of external ear
  EXCLUDES removal of intraluminal foreign body (98.11)

  18.01 Piercing of ear lobe
    Piercing of pinna
  18.02 Incision of external auditory canal
  18.09 Other incision of external ear

18.1 Diagnostic procedures on external ear
  18.11 Otoscopy
    DEF: Exam of the ear with instrument designed for visualization.
  18.12 Biopsy of external ear
  18.19 Other diagnostic procedures on external ear
    EXCLUDES microscopic examination of specimen from ear (90.31-90.39)

18.2 Excision or destruction of lesion of external ear
  18.21 Excision of preauricular sinus
    Radical excision of preauricular sinus or cyst
    EXCLUDES excision of preauricular remnant [appendage] (18.29)
    DEF: Excision of preauricular sinus or cyst with adjacent tissues.

  18.29 Excision or destruction of other lesion of external ear
    Cauterization
    Coagulation
    Cryosurgery   } of external ear
    Curettage
    Electrocoagulation
    Enucleation

    Excision of:
      exostosis of external auditory canal
      preauricular remnant [appendage]
    Partial excision of ear
    EXCLUDES biopsy of external ear (18.12)
      radical excision of lesion (18.31)
      removal of cerumen (96.52)

18.3 Other excision of external ear
  EXCLUDES biopsy of external ear (18.12)
  18.31 Radical excision of lesion of external ear
    EXCLUDES radical excision of preauricular sinus (18.21)
    DEF: Removal of damaged, diseased ear and adjacent tissue.
  18.39 Other
    Amputation of external ear
    EXCLUDES excision of lesion (18.21-18.29, 18.31)

18.4 Suture of laceration of external ear
18.5 Surgical correction of prominent ear
  Ear:
    pinning
    setback
  DEF: Reformation of protruding outer ear.

18.6 Reconstruction of external auditory canal
  Canaloplasty of external auditory meatus
  Construction [reconstruction] of external meatus of ear:
    osseous portion
    skin-lined portion (with skin graft)
  DEF: Repair of outer ear canal.

18.7 Other plastic repair of external ear
  18.71 Construction of auricle of ear
    Prosthetic appliance for absent ear
    Reconstruction:
      auricle
      ear
    DEF: Reformation or repair of external ear flap.
  18.72 Reattachment of amputated ear
  18.79 Other plastic repair of external ear
    Otoplasty NOS   Repair of lop ear
    Postauricular skin graft
    DEF: Postauricular skin graft: Graft repair behind ear.
    DEF: Repair of lop ear: Reconstruction of ear that is at right angle to head.

18.9 Other operations on external ear
  EXCLUDES irrigation of ear (96.52)
    packing of external auditory canal (96.11)
    removal of:
      cerumen (96.52)
      foreign body (without incision) (98.11)

19 Reconstructive operations on middle ear
  19.0 Stapes mobilization
    Division, otosclerotic:
      material
      process
    Remobilization of stapes
    Stapediolysis
    Transcrural stapes mobilization
    EXCLUDES that with synchronous stapedectomy (19.11-19.19)
    DEF: Repair of innermost bone of middle ear to enable movement and response to sound.

  19.1 Stapedectomy
    EXCLUDES revision of previous stapedectomy (19.21-19.29)
      stapes mobilization only (19.0)
    DEF: Removal of innermost bone of middle ear.
    19.11 Stapedectomy with incus replacement
      Stapedectomy with incus:
        homograft
        prosthesis
      DEF: Removal of innermost bone of middle ear with autograft or prosthesis replacement.
    19.19 Other stapedectomy

  19.2 Revision of stapedectomy
    19.21 Revision of stapedectomy with incus replacement
    19.29 Other revision of stapedectomy

  19.3 Other operations on ossicular chain
    Incudectomy NOS
    Ossiculectomy NOS
    Reconstruction of ossicles, second stage
    DEF: Incudectomy: Excision of middle bone of middle ear, not otherwise specified.
    DEF: Ossiculectomy: Excision of middle ear bones, not otherwise specified.
    DEF: Reconstruction of ossicles, second stage: Repair of middle ear bones following previous surgery.

OPERATIONS ON THE EAR

Stapedectomy with Incus Replacement

Area excised

19.4 Myringoplasty
Epitympanic, type I
Myringoplasty by:
 cauterization
Myringoplasty by:
 graft
Tympanoplasty (type I)

DEF: Epitympanic, type I: Repair over or upon eardrum.

DEF: Myringoplasty by cauterization: Plastic repair of tympanic membrane of eardrum by heat.

DEF: Graft: Plastic repair using implanted tissue.

DEF: Tympanoplasty (type I): Reconstruction of eardrum to restore hearing.

✓4th 19.5 Other tympanoplasty

19.52 Type II tympanoplasty
Closure of perforation with graft against incus or malleus

19.53 Type III tympanoplasty
Graft placed in contact with mobile and intact stapes
AHA: M-A, '85, 15

19.54 Type IV tympanoplasty
Mobile footplate left exposed with air pocket between round window and graft

19.55 Type V tympanoplasty
Fenestra in horizontal semicircular canal covered by graft

19.6 Revision of tympanoplasty
DEF: Repair or correction of previous plastic surgery on eardrum.

19.9 Other repair of middle ear
Closure of mastoid fistula
Mastoid myoplasty
Obliteration of tympanomastoid cavity

DEF: Closure of mastoid fistula: Closing of abnormal channel in mastoid.

DEF: Mastoid myoplasty: Restoration or repair of mastoid muscle.

DEF: Obliteration of tympanomastoid cavity: Removal, total, of functional elements of middle ear.

✓3rd 20 Other operations on middle and inner ear

✓4th 20.0 Myringotomy
DEF: Myringotomy: Puncture of tympanic membrane or eardrum, also called tympanocentesis

20.01 Myringotomy with insertion of tube
Myringostomy

20.09 Other myringotomy
Aspiration of middle ear NOS

20.1 Removal of tympanostomy tube

✓4th 20.2 Incision of mastoid and middle ear

20.21 Incision of mastoid

20.22 Incision of petrous pyramid air cells

20.23 Incision of middle ear
Atticotomy
Division of tympanum
Lysis of adhesions of middle ear
EXCLUDES division of otosclerotic process (19.0)
 stapediolysis (19.0)
 that with stapedectomy (19.11-19.19)

✓4th 20.3 Diagnostic procedures on middle and inner ear

20.31 Electrocochleography
DEF: Measure of electric potential of eighth cranial nerve by electrode applied sound.

20.32 Biopsy of middle and inner ear

20.39 Other diagnostic procedures on middle and inner ear
EXCLUDES auditory and vestibular function tests (89.13, 95.41-95.49)
 microscopic examination of specimen from ear (90.31-90.39)

✓4th 20.4 Mastoidectomy
Code also any:
 skin graft (18.79)
 tympanoplasty (19.4-19.55)
EXCLUDES that with implantation of cochlear prosthetic device (20.96-20.98)

DEF: Mastoidectomy: Excision of bony protrusion behind ear.

20.41 Simple mastoidectomy

20.42 Radical mastoidectomy

20.49 Other mastoidectomy
Atticoantrostomy
Mastoidectomy:
 NOS
 modified radical

DEF: Atticoantrotomy: Opening of cavity of mastoid bone and middle ear.

✓4th 20.5 Other excision of middle ear
EXCLUDES that with synchronous mastoidectomy (20.41-20.49)

20.51 Excision of lesion of middle ear
EXCLUDES biopsy of middle ear (20.32)

20.59 Other
Apicectomy of petrous pyramid
Tympanectomy

✓4th 20.6 Fenestration of inner ear

20.61 Fenestration of inner ear (initial)
Fenestration of:
 labyrinth
 semicircular canals
 vestibule
with graft (skin) (vein)

EXCLUDES that with tympanoplasty, type V (19.55)

DEF: Creation of inner ear opening.

20.62 Revision of fenestration of inner ear

✓4th 20.7 Incision, excision, and destruction of inner ear

20.71 Endolymphatic shunt
DEF: Insertion of tube to drain fluid in inner ear cavities.

20.72 Injection into inner ear
Destruction by injection (alcohol):
 inner ear
 semicircular canals
 vestibule

OPERATIONS ON THE EAR

20.79 **Other incision, excision, and destruction of inner ear**
Decompression of labyrinth
Drainage of inner ear
Fistulization:
  endolymphatic sac
  labyrinth
Incision of endolymphatic sac
Labyrinthectomy (transtympanic)
Opening of bony labyrinth
Perilymphatic tap
  EXCLUDES biopsy of inner ear (20.32)

DEF: Decompression of labyrinth: Controlled relief of pressure in cavities of inner ear.

DEF: Drainage of inner ear: Removal of fluid from inner ear.

DEF: Fistulization of endolymphatic sac: Creation of passage to fluid sac in inner ear cavities.

DEF: Fistulization of labyrinth: Creation of passage to inner ear cavities.

DEF: Incision of endolymphatic sac: Cutting into fluid sac in inner ear cavities.

DEF: Labyrinthectomy (transtympanic): Excision of cavities across eardrum.

DEF: Opening of bony labyrinth: Cutting into inner ear bony cavities.

DEF: Perilymphatic tap: Puncture or incision into fluid sac of inner ear cavities.

20.8 **Operations on Eustachian tube**
Catheterization
Inflation
Injection (Teflon paste)   } of Eustachian tube
Insufflation (boric acid-salicylic acid)
Intubation
Politzerization

DEF: Catheterization: Passing catheter into passage between pharynx and middle ear.

DEF: Inflation: Blowing air, gas or liquid into passage between pharynx and middle ear to inflate.

DEF: Injection (Teflon paste): Forcing fluid (Teflon paste) into passage between pharynx and middle ear.

DEF: Insufflation (boric acid-salicylic acid): Blowing gas or liquid into passage between pharynx and middle ear.

DEF: Intubation: Placing tube into passage between pharynx and middle ear.

DEF: Politzerization: Inflating passage between pharynx and middle ear with Politzer bag.

20.9 **Other operations on inner and middle ear**

20.91 **Tympanosympathectomy**
DEF: Excision or chemical suppression of impulses of middle ear nerves.

20.92 **Revision of mastoidectomy**
AHA: 2Q, '98, 20

DEF: Correction of previous removal of mastoid cells from temporal or mastoid bone.

20.93 **Repair of oval and round windows**
Closure of fistula: Closure of fistula:
  oval window   round window
  perilymph
DEF: Restoration of middle ear openings.

20.94 **Injection of tympanum**

20.95 **Implantation of electromagnetic hearing device**
Bone conduction hearing device
  EXCLUDES cochlear prosthetic device (20.96-20.98)

AHA: 4Q, '89, 5

20.96 **Implantation or replacement of cochlear prosthetic device, not otherwise specified**
Implantation of receiver (within skull) and insertion of electrode(s) in the cochlea
  INCLUDES mastoidectomy
  EXCLUDES electromagnetic hearing device (20.95)

AHA: 4Q, '89, 5

20.97 **Implantation or replacement of cochlear prosthetic device, single channel**
Implantation of receiver (within skull) and insertion of electrode in the cochlea
  INCLUDES mastoidectomy
  EXCLUDES electromagnetic hearing device (20.95)

AHA: 4Q, '89, 5

20.98 **Implantation or replacement of cochlear prosthetic device, multiple channel**
Implantation of receiver (within skull) and insertion of electrodes in the cochlea
  INCLUDES mastoidectomy
  EXCLUDES electromagnetic hearing device (20.95)

AHA: 4Q, '89, 5

20.99 **Other operations on middle and inner ear**
Repair or removal of cochlear prosthetic device (receiver) (electrode)
  EXCLUDES adjustment (external components) of cochlear prosthetic device (95.49)
  fitting of hearing aid (95.48)

AHA: 4Q, '89, 7

5. OPERATIONS ON THE NOSE, MOUTH, AND PHARYNX (21-29)

21 Operations on nose
  INCLUDES operations on:
  bone } of nose
  skin

  AHA: 1Q, '94, 5

21.0 Control of epistaxis
  21.00 Control of epistaxis, not otherwise specified
  21.01 Control of epistaxis by anterior nasal packing
  21.02 Control of epistaxis by posterior (and anterior) packing
  21.03 Control of epistaxis by cauterization (and packing)
  21.04 Control of epistaxis by ligation of ethmoidal arteries
  21.05 Control of epistaxis by (transantral) ligation of the maxillary artery
  21.06 Control of epistaxis by ligation of the external carotid artery
  21.07 Control of epistaxis by excision of nasal mucosa and skin grafting of septum and lateral nasal wall
  21.09 Control of epistaxis by other means

21.1 Incision of nose
  Chondrotomy   Nasal septotomy
  Incision of skin of nose

  DEF: Chondrotomy: Incision or division of nasal cartilage.

  DEF: Nasal septotomy: Incision into bone dividing nose into two chambers.

21.2 Diagnostic procedures on nose
  21.21 Rhinoscopy
    DEF: Visualization of nasal passage with nasal speculum.
  21.22 Biopsy of nose
  21.29 Other diagnostic procedures on nose
    EXCLUDES microscopic examination of specimen from nose (90.31-90.39)
    nasal:
      function study (89.12)
      x-ray (87.16)
      rhinomanometry (89.12)

21.3 Local excision or destruction of lesion of nose
  EXCLUDES biopsy of nose (21.22)
    nasal fistulectomy (21.82)
  21.30 Excision or destruction of lesion of nose, not otherwise specified
  21.31 Local excision or destruction of intranasal lesion
    Nasal polypectomy
  21.32 Local excision or destruction of other lesion of nose
    AHA: 2Q, '89, 16

21.4 Resection of nose
  Amputation of nose

21.5 Submucous resection of nasal septum
  DEF: Resection, partial, of nasal septum with mucosa reimplanted after excision.

21.6 Turbinectomy
  DEF: Removal, partial, or total of turbinate bones; inferior turbinate is most often excised.

  21.61 Turbinectomy by diathermy or cryosurgery
    DEF: Destruction of turbinate bone by heat or freezing.

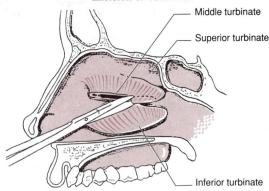

Excision of Turbinate
— Middle turbinate
— Superior turbinate
— Inferior turbinate

  21.62 Fracture of the turbinates
    DEF: Surgical breaking of turbinate bones.
  21.69 Other turbinectomy
    EXCLUDES turbinectomy associated with sinusectomy (22.31-22.39, 22.42, 22.60-22.64)

21.7 Reduction of nasal fracture
  21.71 Closed reduction of nasal fracture
  21.72 Open reduction of nasal fracture

21.8 Repair and plastic operations on the nose
  21.81 Suture of laceration of nose
  21.82 Closure of nasal fistula
    Nasolabial
    Nasopharyngeal } fistulectomy
    Oronasal

    DEF: Sealing off crack or hole between nose and lip, nose and pharynx, or nose and mouth.

  21.83 Total nasal reconstruction
    Reconstruction of nose with:
      arm flap
      forehead flap
    DEF: Reformation, plastic, of nasal structure with tissue flap from arm or forehead.

  21.84 Revision rhinoplasty
    Rhinoseptoplasty
    Twisted nose rhinoplasty
    DEF: Rhinoseptoplasty: Repair of nose and the bone dividing the nose into two chambers.
    DEF: Twisted nose rhinoplasty: Repair of nose alignment following reconstructive surgery.

  21.85 Augmentation rhinoplasty
    Augmentation rhinoplasty with:
      graft
      synthetic implant
    DEF: Implant of tissue or synthetic graft to enlarge nose.

  21.86 Limited rhinoplasty
    Plastic repair of nasolabial flaps
    Tip rhinoplasty
    DEF: Plastic repair of nasolabial flaps: Reconstruction of nasal area above lips.
    DEF: Tip rhinoplasty: Reconstruction or restoration of nasal tip.

  21.87 Other rhinoplasty
    Rhinoplasty NOS

OPERATIONS ON THE NOSE, MOUTH, AND PHARYNX

- **21.88 Other septoplasty**
  - Crushing of nasal septum
  - Repair of septal perforation
  - **EXCLUDES** septoplasty associated with submucous resection of septum (21.5)

  DEF: Crushing of nasal septum: Division and reconstruction of defects in bone dividing nasal chambers.

  DEF: Repair of septal perforation: Repair of hole in bone dividing nasal chambers with adjacent tissue.

- **21.89 Other repair and plastic operations on nose**
  - Reattachment of amputated nose

- **21.9 Other operations on nose**
  - **21.91 Lysis of adhesions of nose**
    - Posterior nasal scrub

    DEF: Posterior nasal scrub: Clearing out of abnormal adhesions in posterior nasal area.

  - **21.99 Other**
    - **EXCLUDES**
      - dilation of frontonasal duct (96.21)
      - irrigation of nasal passages (96.53)
      - removal of:
        - intraluminal foreign body without incision (98.12)
        - nasal packing (97.32)
        - replacement of nasal packing (97.21)

22 Operations on nasal sinuses

- **22.0 Aspiration and lavage of nasal sinus**
  - **22.00 Aspiration and lavage of nasal sinus, not otherwise specified**
  - **22.01 Puncture of nasal sinus for aspiration or lavage**
  - **22.02 Aspiration or lavage of nasal sinus through natural ostium**

    DEF: Withdrawal of fluid and washing of nasal cavity through natural opening.

- **22.1 Diagnostic procedures on nasal sinus**
  - **22.11 Closed [endoscopic] [needle] biopsy of nasal sinus**
  - **22.12 Open biopsy of nasal sinus**
  - **22.19 Other diagnostic procedures on nasal sinuses**
    - Endoscopy without biopsy
    - **EXCLUDES**
      - transillumination of sinus (89.35)
      - x-ray of sinus (87.15-87.16)

- **22.2 Intranasal antrotomy**
  - **EXCLUDES** antrotomy with external approach (22.31-22.39)

  DEF: Incision of intranasal sinus.

- **22.3 External maxillary antrotomy**
  - **22.31 Radical maxillary antrotomy**
    - Removal of lining membrane of maxillary sinus using Caldwell-Luc approach

    DEF: Caldwell-Luc approach: Removal of membrane lining the maxillary cavity through incision above canine teeth.

  - **22.39 Other external maxillary antrotomy**
    - Exploration of maxillary antrum with Caldwell-Luc approach

- **22.4 Frontal sinusotomy and sinusectomy**
  - **22.41 Frontal sinusotomy**
  - **22.42 Frontal sinusectomy**
    - Excision of lesion of frontal sinus
    - Obliteration of frontal sinus (with fat)
    - **EXCLUDES** biopsy of nasal sinus (22.11-22.12)

- **22.5 Other nasal sinusotomy**
  - **22.50 Sinusotomy, not otherwise specified**
  - **22.51 Ethmoidotomy**
  - **22.52 Sphenoidotomy**
  - **22.53 Incision of multiple nasal sinuses**

- **22.6 Other nasal sinusectomy**
  - **INCLUDES** that with incidental turbinectomy
  - **EXCLUDES** biopsy of nasal sinus (22.11-22.12)
  - **22.60 Sinusectomy, not otherwise specified**
  - **22.61 Excision of lesion of maxillary sinus with Caldwell-Luc approach**
  - **22.62 Excision of lesion of maxillary sinus with other approach**
  - **22.63 Ethmoidectomy**

    DEF: Removal of ethmoid cells and bone, partial or total includes excising mucosal lining, partial or total.

  - **22.64 Sphenoidectomy**

    DEF: Removal of wedge shaped sphenoid bone at base of brain.

- **22.7 Repair of nasal sinus**
  - **22.71 Closure of nasal sinus fistula**
    - Repair of oro-antral fistula
  - **22.79 Other repair of nasal sinus**
    - Reconstruction of frontonasal duct
    - Repair of bone of accessory sinus

- **22.9 Other operations on nasal sinuses**
  - Exteriorization of maxillary sinus
  - Fistulization of sinus
  - **EXCLUDES** dilation of frontonasal duct (96.21)

  DEF: Exteriorization of maxillary sinus: Creation of external maxillary cavity opening.

  DEF: Fistulization of sinus: Creation of fistula canal in nasal cavity.

23 Removal and restoration of teeth

- **23.0 Forceps extraction of tooth**
  - **23.01 Extraction of deciduous tooth**
  - **23.09 Extraction of other tooth**
    - Extraction of tooth NOS

- **23.1 Surgical removal of tooth**
  - **23.11 Removal of residual root**
  - **23.19 Other surgical extraction of tooth**
    - Odontectomy NOS
    - Removal of impacted tooth
    - Tooth extraction with elevation of mucoperiosteal flap

- **23.2 Restoration of tooth by filling**
- **23.3 Restoration of tooth by inlay**

  DEF: Restoration of tooth by cementing in a molded filling.

- **23.4 Other dental restoration**
  - **23.41 Application of crown**
  - **23.42 Insertion of fixed bridge**
  - **23.43 Insertion of removable bridge**
  - **23.49 Other**

- **23.5 Implantation of tooth**

  DEF: Insertion of a sound tooth to replace extracted tooth.

- **23.6 Prosthetic dental implant**
  - Endosseous dental implant

  DEF: Implant of artificial denture within bone covering tooth socket.

- **23.7 Apicoectomy and root canal therapy**
  - **23.70 Root canal, not otherwise specified**
  - **23.71 Root canal therapy with irrigation**

	23.72	Root canal therapy with apicoectomy
		DEF: Removal of tooth root to treat damaged root canal tissue.
	23.73	**Apicoectomy**
✓3rd **24**		**Other operations on teeth, gums, and alveoli**
	24.0	**Incision of gum or alveolar bone**
		Apical alveolotomy
✓4th **24.1**		**Diagnostic procedures on teeth, gums, and alveoli**
	24.11	Biopsy of gum
	24.12	Biopsy of alveolus
	24.19	Other diagnostic procedures on teeth, gums, and alveoli

EXCLUDES dental:
  examination (89.31)
  x-ray:
    full-mouth (87.11)
    other (87.12)
  microscopic examination of dental specimen (90.81-90.89)

24.2 **Gingivoplasty**
  Gingivoplasty with bone or soft tissue graft
  DEF: Repair of gum tissue.

✓4th **24.3** **Other operations on gum**
  24.31 Excision of lesion or tissue of gum
    EXCLUDES biopsy of gum (24.11)
      excision of odontogenic lesion (24.4)
  24.32 Suture of laceration of gum
  24.39 Other

24.4 **Excision of dental lesion of jaw**
  Excision of odontogenic lesion

24.5 **Alveoloplasty**
  Alveolectomy (interradicular) (intraseptal) (radical) (simple) (with graft or implant)
    EXCLUDES biopsy of alveolus (24.12)
      en bloc resection of alveolar process and palate (27.32)
  DEF: Repair or correction of bony tooth socket.

24.6 **Exposure of tooth**

24.7 **Application of orthodontic appliance**
  Application, insertion, or fitting of:
    arch bars   orthodontic wiring
    orthodontic obturator periodontal splint
    EXCLUDES nonorthodontic dental wiring (93.55)

24.8 **Other orthodontic operation**
  Closure of diastema   Removal of arch bars
    (alveolar) (dental)   Repair of dental arch
  Occlusal adjustment
    EXCLUDES removal of nonorthodontic wiring (97.33)

✓4th **24.9** **Other dental operations**
  24.91 Extension or deepening of buccolabial or lingual sulcus

24.99 Other
  EXCLUDES dental:
    debridement (96.54)
    examination (89.31)
    prophylaxis (96.54)
    scaling and polishing (96.54)
    wiring (93.55)
    fitting of dental appliance [denture] (99.97)
    microscopic examination of dental specimen (90.81-90.89)
    removal of dental:
      packing (97.34)
      prosthesis (97.35)
      wiring (97.33)
    replacement of dental packing (97.22)

✓3rd **25** **Operations on tongue**
  ✓4th **25.0** **Diagnostic procedures on tongue**
    25.01 Closed [needle] biopsy of tongue
    25.02 **Open biopsy of tongue**
      Wedge biopsy
    25.09 Other diagnostic procedures on tongue

  25.1 **Excision or destruction of lesion or tissue of tongue**
    EXCLUDES biopsy of tongue (25.01-25.02)
      frenumectomy:
        labial (27.41)
        lingual (25.92)

  25.2 **Partial glossectomy**
  25.3 **Complete glossectomy**
    Glossectomy NOS
    Code also any neck dissection (40.40-40.42)
  25.4 **Radical glossectomy**
    Code also any:
      neck dissection (40.40-40.42)
      tracheostomy (31.1-31.29)

  ✓4th **25.5** **Repair of tongue and glossoplasty**
    25.51 Suture of laceration of tongue
    25.59 **Other repair and plastic operations on tongue**
      Fascial sling of tongue
      Fusion of tongue (to lip)
      Graft of mucosa or skin to tongue
        EXCLUDES lysis of adhesions of tongue (25.93)
      AHA: 1Q, '97, 5

  ✓4th **25.9** **Other operations on tongue**
    25.91 Lingual frenotomy
      EXCLUDES labial frenotomy (27.91)
      DEF: Extension of groove between cheek and lips or cheek and tongue.
    25.92 **Lingual frenectomy**
      EXCLUDES labial frenectomy (27.41)
      DEF: Frenectomy: Removal of vertical membrane attaching tongue to floor mouth.
    25.93 Lysis of adhesions of tongue
    25.94 **Other glossotomy**
    25.99 **Other**

✓3rd **26** **Operations on salivary glands and ducts**
  INCLUDES operations on:
    lesser salivary ⎫
    parotid   ⎬ gland and duct
    sublingual   ⎪
    submaxillary   ⎭
  Code also any neck dissection (40.40-40.42)
  26.0 **Incision of salivary gland or duct**

OPERATIONS ON THE NOSE, MOUTH, AND PHARYNX

√4th 26.1 Diagnostic procedures on salivary glands and ducts
- 26.11 Closed [needle] biopsy of salivary gland or duct
- 26.12 Open biopsy of salivary gland or duct
- 26.19 Other diagnostic procedures on salivary glands and ducts
  - EXCLUDES: x-ray of salivary gland (87.09)

√4th 26.2 Excision of lesion of salivary gland
- 26.21 Marsupialization of salivary gland cyst
  - DEF: Creation of pouch of salivary gland cyst to drain and promote healing.
- 26.29 Other excision of salivary gland lesion
  - EXCLUDES: biopsy of salivary gland (26.11-26.12)
  - salivary fistulectomy (26.42)

√4th 26.3 Sialoadenectomy
- DEF: Removal of salivary gland.
- 26.30 Sialoadenectomy, not otherwise specified
- 26.31 Partial sialoadenectomy
- 26.32 Complete sialoadenectomy
  - En bloc excision of salivary gland lesion
  - Radical sialoadenectomy

√4th 26.4 Repair of salivary gland or duct
- 26.41 Suture of laceration of salivary gland
- 26.42 Closure of salivary fistula
  - DEF: Closing of abnormal opening in salivary gland.
- 26.49 Other repair and plastic operations on salivary gland or duct
  - Fistulization of salivary gland
  - Plastic repair of salivary gland or duct NOS
  - Transplantation of salivary duct opening

√4th 26.9 Other operations on salivary gland or duct
- 26.91 Probing of salivary duct
- 26.99 Other

√3rd 27 Other operations on mouth and face
- INCLUDES: operations on:
  - lips
  - palate
  - soft tissue of face and mouth, except tongue and gingiva
- EXCLUDES: operations on:
  - gingiva (24.0-24.99)
  - tongue (25.01-25.99)

27.0 Drainage of face and floor of mouth
- Drainage of: facial region (abscess)   Drainage of: Ludwig's angina
- fascial compartment of face
- EXCLUDES: drainage of thyroglossal tract (06.09)

27.1 Incision of palate

√4th 27.2 Diagnostic procedures on oral cavity
- 27.21 Biopsy of bony palate
- 27.22 Biopsy of uvula and soft palate
- 27.23 Biopsy of lip
- 27.24 Biopsy of mouth, unspecified structure
- 27.29 Other diagnostic procedures on oral cavity
  - EXCLUDES: soft tissue x-ray (87.09)

√4th 27.3 Excision of lesion or tissue of bony palate
- 27.31 Local excision or destruction of lesion or tissue of bony palate
  - Local excision or destruction of palate by:
    - cautery   cryotherapy
    - chemotherapy
  - EXCLUDES: biopsy of bony palate (27.21)
- 27.32 Wide excision or destruction of lesion or tissue of bony palate
  - En bloc resection of alveolar process and palate

√4th 27.4 Excision of other parts of mouth
- 27.41 Labial frenectomy
  - EXCLUDES: division of labial frenum (27.91)
  - DEF: Removal of mucous membrane fold of lip.
- 27.42 Wide excision of lesion of lip
- 27.43 Other excision of lesion or tissue of lip
- 27.49 Other excision of mouth
  - EXCLUDES: biopsy of mouth NOS (27.24)
  - excision of lesion of:
    - palate (27.31-27.32)
    - tongue (25.1)
    - uvula (27.72)
  - fistulectomy of mouth (27.53)
  - frenectomy of:
    - lip (27.41)
    - tongue (25.92)

√4th 27.5 Plastic repair of mouth
- EXCLUDES: palatoplasty (27.61-27.69)
- 27.51 Suture of laceration of lip
- 27.52 Suture of laceration of other part of mouth
- 27.53 Closure of fistula of mouth
  - EXCLUDES: fistulectomy:
    - nasolabial (21.82)
    - oro-antral (22.71)
    - oronasal (21.82)
- 27.54 Repair of cleft lip
- 27.55 Full-thickness skin graft to lip and mouth
- 27.56 Other skin graft to lip and mouth
- 27.57 Attachment of pedicle or flap graft to lip and mouth
  - AHA: 1Q, '96, 14
  - DEF: Repair of lip or mouth with tissue pedicle or flap still connected to original vascular base.
- 27.59 Other plastic repair of mouth

√4th 27.6 Palatoplasty
- 27.61 Suture of laceration of palate
- 27.62 Correction of cleft palate
  - Correction of cleft palate by push-back operation
  - EXCLUDES: revision of cleft palate repair (27.63)
- 27.63 Revision of cleft palate repair
  - Secondary:
    - attachment of pharyngeal flap
    - lengthening of palate
  - AHA: 1Q, '96, 14
- 27.69 Other plastic repair of palate
  - EXCLUDES: fistulectomy of mouth (27.53)
  - AHA: 3Q, '99, 22; 1Q, '97, 14; 3Q, '92, 18

√4th 27.7 Operations on uvula
- 27.71 Incision of uvula
- 27.72 Excision of uvula
  - EXCLUDES: biopsy of uvula (27.22)
- 27.73 Repair of uvula
  - EXCLUDES: that with synchronous cleft palate repair (27.62)
  - uranostaphylorrhaphy (27.62)
- 27.79 Other operations on uvula
  - AHA: 3Q, '92, 18

√4th 27.9 Other operations on mouth and face
- 27.91 Labial frenotomy
  - Division of labial frenum
  - EXCLUDES: lingual frenotomy (25.91)
  - DEF: Division of labial frenum: Cutting and separating mucous membrane fold of lip.

27.92–29.99 OPERATIONS ON THE NOSE, MOUTH, AND PHARYNX — Tabular List

27.92 Incision of mouth, unspecified structure
  EXCLUDES incision of:
    gum (24.0)
    palate (27.1)
    salivary gland or duct (26.0)
    tongue (25.94)
    uvula (27.71)

27.99 Other operations on oral cavity
  Graft of buccal sulcus
  EXCLUDES removal of:
    intraluminal foreign body (98.01)
    penetrating foreign body from mouth without incision (98.22)

  DEF: Graft of buccal sulcus: Implant of tissue into groove of interior cheek lining.

√3rd 28 Operations on tonsils and adenoids

28.0 Incision and drainage of tonsil and peritonsillar structures
  Drainage (oral) (transcervical) of:
    parapharyngeal
    peritonsillar
    retropharyngeal
    tonsillar } abscess

√4th 28.1 Diagnostic procedures on tonsils and adenoids
  28.11 Biopsy of tonsils and adenoids
  28.19 Other diagnostic procedures on tonsils and adenoids
    EXCLUDES soft tissue x-ray (87.09)

28.2 Tonsillectomy without adenoidectomy
  AHA: 1Q, '97, 5; 2Q, '90, 23

28.3 Tonsillectomy with adenoidectomy
28.4 Excision of tonsil tag
28.5 Excision of lingual tonsil
28.6 Adenoidectomy without tonsillectomy
  Excision of adenoid tag
28.7 Control of hemorrhage after tonsillectomy and adenoidectomy

√4th 28.9 Other operations on tonsils and adenoids
  28.91 Removal of foreign body from tonsil and adenoid by incision
    EXCLUDES that without incision (98.13)
  28.92 Excision of lesion of tonsil and adenoid
    EXCLUDES biopsy of tonsil and adenoid (28.11)
  28.99 Other

√3rd 29 Operations on pharynx
  INCLUDES operations on: operations on:
    hypopharynx   pharyngeal pouch
    nasopharynx   pyriform sinus
    oropharynx

29.0 Pharyngotomy
  Drainage of pharyngeal bursa
  EXCLUDES incision and drainage of retropharyngeal abscess (28.0)
    removal of foreign body (without incision) (98.13)

√4th 29.1 Diagnostic procedures on pharynx
  29.11 Pharyngoscopy
  29.12 Pharyngeal biopsy
    Biopsy of supraglottic mass
  29.19 Other diagnostic procedures on pharynx
    EXCLUDES x-ray of nasopharynx:
      contrast (87.06)
      other (87.09)

29.2 Excision of branchial cleft cyst or vestige
  EXCLUDES branchial cleft fistulectomy (29.52)

√4th 29.3 Excision or destruction of lesion or tissue of pharynx
  AHA: 2Q, '89, 18
  29.31 Cricopharyngeal myotomy
    EXCLUDES that with pharyngeal diverticulectomy (29.32)
    DEF: Removal of outward pouching of throat.
  29.32 Pharyngeal diverticulectomy
  29.33 Pharyngectomy (partial)
    EXCLUDES laryngopharyngectomy (30.3)
  29.39 Other excision or destruction of lesion or tissue of pharynx

29.4 Plastic operation on pharynx
  Correction of nasopharyngeal atresia
  EXCLUDES pharyngoplasty associated with cleft palate repair (27.62-27.63)
  AHA: 3Q, '99, 22; 1Q, '97, 5; 3Q, '92, 18
  DEF: Correction of nasopharyngeal atresia: Construction of normal opening for throat stricture behind nose.

√4th 29.5 Other repair of pharynx
  29.51 Suture of laceration of pharynx
  29.52 Closure of branchial cleft fistula
    DEF: Sealing off an abnormal opening of the branchial fissure in throat.
  29.53 Closure of other fistula of pharynx
    Pharyngoesophageal fistulectomy
  29.54 Lysis of pharyngeal adhesions
  29.59 Other
  AHA: 2Q, '89, 18

√4th 29.9 Other operations on pharynx
  29.91 Dilation of pharynx
    Dilation of nasopharynx
  29.92 Division of glossopharyngeal nerve
  29.99 Other
    EXCLUDES insertion of radium into pharynx and nasopharynx (92.27)
      removal of intraluminal foreign body (98.13)

6. OPERATIONS ON THE RESPIRATORY SYSTEM (30-34)

- **30 Excision of larynx**
  - **30.0 Excision or destruction of lesion or tissue of larynx**
    - **30.01 Marsupialization of laryngeal cyst**
      DEF: Incision of cyst of larynx with the edges sutured open to create pouch.
    - **30.09 Other excision or destruction of lesion or tissue of larynx**
      Stripping of vocal cords
      EXCLUDES biopsy of larynx (31.43)
      laryngeal fistulectomy (31.62)
      laryngotracheal fistulectomy (31.62)
  - **30.1 Hemilaryngectomy**
    DEF: Excision of one side (half) of larynx.
  - **30.2 Other partial laryngectomy**
    - **30.21 Epiglottidectomy**
      DEF: Placement of artificial breathing tube in windpipe through mediastinum, for long-term use.
    - **30.22 Vocal cordectomy**
      Excision of vocal cords
    - **30.29 Other partial laryngectomy**
      Excision of laryngeal cartilage
  - **30.3 Complete laryngectomy**
    Block dissection of larynx (with thyroidectomy) (with synchronous tracheostomy)
    Laryngopharyngectomy
    EXCLUDES that with radical neck dissection (30.4)
  - **30.4 Radical laryngectomy**
    Complete [total] laryngectomy with radical neck dissection (with thyroidectomy) (with synchronous tracheostomy)

- **31 Other operations on larynx and trachea**
  - **31.0 Injection of larynx**
    Injection of inert material into larynx or vocal cords
  - **31.1 Temporary tracheostomy**
    Tracheotomy for assistance in breathing
    AHA: 1Q, '97, 6
  - **31.2 Permanent tracheostomy**
    - **31.21 Mediastinal tracheostomy**
    - **31.29 Other permanent tracheostomy**
      EXCLUDES that with laryngectomy (30.3-30.4)
  - **31.3 Other incision of larynx or trachea**
    EXCLUDES that for assistance in breathing (31.1-31.29)
  - **31.4 Diagnostic procedures on larynx and trachea**
    - **31.41 Tracheoscopy through artificial stoma**
      EXCLUDES that with biopsy (31.43-31.44)
      DEF: Exam by scope of trachea through an artificial opening.

Temporary Tracheostomy

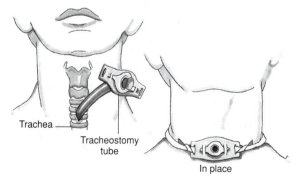

Closed Endoscopic Biopsy of Larynx

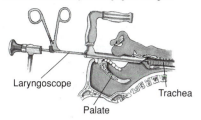

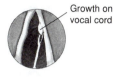

- **31.42 Laryngoscopy and other tracheoscopy**
  EXCLUDES that with biopsy (31.43-31.44)
- **31.43 Closed [endoscopic] biopsy of larynx**
- **31.44 Closed [endoscopic] biopsy of trachea**
- **31.45 Open biopsy of larynx or trachea**
- **31.48 Other diagnostic procedures on larynx**
  EXCLUDES contrast laryngogram (87.07)
  microscopic examination of specimen from larynx (90.31-90.39)
  soft tissue x-ray of larynx NEC (87.09)
- **31.49 Other diagnostic procedures on trachea**
  EXCLUDES microscopic examination of specimen from trachea (90.41-90.49)
  x-ray of trachea (87.49)
- **31.5 Local excision or destruction of lesion or tissue of trachea**
  EXCLUDES biopsy of trachea (31.44-31.45)
  laryngotracheal fistulectomy (31.62)
  tracheoesophageal fistulectomy (31.73)
- **31.6 Repair of larynx**
  - **31.61 Suture of laceration of larynx**
  - **31.62 Closure of fistula of larynx**
    Laryngotracheal fistulectomy
    Take-down of laryngostomy
    DEF: Laryngotracheal fistulectomy: Excision and closing of passage between voice box and trachea.
    DEF: Take-down of laryngostomy: Removal of laryngostomy tube and restoration of voice box.
  - **31.63 Revision of laryngostomy**
  - **31.64 Repair of laryngeal fracture**
    DEF: Alignment and positioning of harder structures of larynx such as hyoid bone; following fracture.
  - **31.69 Other repair of larynx**
    Arytenoidopexy
    Graft of larynx
    Transposition of vocal cords
    EXCLUDES construction of artificial larynx (31.75)
    DEF: Arytenoidopexy: Fixation of pitcher-shaped cartilage in voice box.
    DEF: Graft of larynx: Implant of graft tissue into voice box.
    DEF: Transposition of the vocal cords: Placement of vocal cords into more functional positions.
- **31.7 Repair and plastic operations on trachea**
  - **31.71 Suture of laceration of trachea**

OPERATIONS ON THE RESPIRATORY SYSTEM

31.72 **Closure of external fistula of trachea**
Closure of tracheotomy

31.73 **Closure of other fistula of trachea**
Tracheoesophageal fistulectomy
> **EXCLUDES** laryngotracheal fistulectomy (31.62)

DEF: Tracheoesophageal fistulectomy: Excision and closure of abnormal opening between windpipe and esophagus.

31.74 **Revision of tracheostomy**

31.75 **Reconstruction of trachea and construction of artificial larynx**
Tracheoplasty with artificial larynx

31.79 **Other repair and plastic operations on trachea**

✓4th **31.9** **Other operations on larynx and trachea**

31.91 **Division of laryngeal nerve**

31.92 **Lysis of adhesions of trachea or larynx**

31.93 **Replacement of laryngeal or tracheal stent**
DEF: Removal and substitution of tubed molding into larynx or trachea.

31.94 **Injection of locally-acting therapeutic substance into trachea**

31.95 **Tracheoesophageal fistulization**
DEF: Creation of passage between trachea and esophagus.

31.98 **Other operations on larynx**
Dilation
Division of congenital web } of larynx
Removal of keel or stent

> **EXCLUDES** removal of intraluminal foreign body from larynx without incision (98.14)

DEF: Dilation: Increasing larynx size by stretching.

DEF: Division of congenital web: Cutting and separating congenital membranes around larynx.

DEF: Removal of keel or stent: Removal of prosthetic device from larynx.

31.99 **Other operations on trachea**
> **EXCLUDES** removal of:
> intraluminal foreign body from trachea without incision (98.15)
> tracheostomy tube (97.37)
> replacement of tracheostomy tube (97.23)
> tracheostomy toilette (96.55)

AHA: 1Q, '97, 14

✓3rd **32** **Excision of lung and bronchus**
> **INCLUDES** rib resection
> sternotomy
> sternum-splitting incision } as operative approach
> thoracotomy

Code also any synchronous bronchoplasty (33.48)

DEF: Rib resection: Cutting of ribs to access operative field.

DEF: Sternotomy: Cut through breastbone as an operative approach.

DEF: Sternum-splitting incision: Breaking through breastbone to access operative field.

✓4th **32.0** **Local excision or destruction of lesion or tissue of bronchus**
> **EXCLUDES** biopsy of bronchus (33.24-33.25)
> bronchial fistulectomy (33.42)

AHA: 4Q, '88, 11

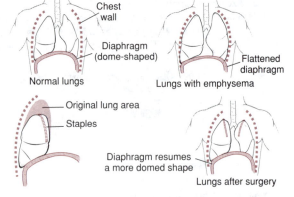

Lung Volume Reduction

32.01 **Endoscopic excision or destruction of lesion or tissue of bronchus**

32.09 **Other local excision or destruction of lesion or tissue of bronchus**
> **EXCLUDES** that by endoscopic approach (32.01)

32.1 **Other excision of bronchus**
Resection (wide sleeve) of bronchus
> **EXCLUDES** radical dissection [excision] of bronchus (32.6)

DEF: Resection (wide sleeve) of bronchus: Excision and partial, lengthwise removal of a lung branch.

✓4th **32.2** **Local excision or destruction of lesion or tissue of lung**

32.21 **Plication of emphysematous bleb**
DEF: Stitching of a swollen vesicle into folds or tuck.

32.22 **Lung volume reduction surgery** NC
AHA: 1Q, '97, 6; 3Q, '96, 20; 4Q, '95, 64

DEF: Excision of portion of lung(s) to reduce respiratory effort in moderate to severe emphysema.

32.28 **Endoscopic excision or destruction of lesion or tissue of lung**
> **EXCLUDES** biopsy of lung (33.26-33.27)

32.29 **Other local excision or destruction of lesion or tissue of lung**
Resection of lung:
  NOS
  wedge
> **EXCLUDES** biopsy of lung (33.26-33.27)
> that by endoscopic approach (32.28)
> wide excision of lesion of lung (32.3)

AHA: 3Q, '99, 3

32.3 **Segmental resection of lung**
Partial lobectomy

32.4 **Lobectomy of lung**
Lobectomy with segmental resection of adjacent lobes of lung
> **EXCLUDES** that with radical dissection [excision] of thoracic structures (32.6)

32.5 **Complete pneumonectomy**
Excision of lung NOS
Pneumonectomy (with mediastinal dissection)
AHA: 1Q, '99, 6

32.6 **Radical dissection of thoracic structures**
Block [en bloc] dissection of bronchus, lobe of lung, brachial plexus, intercostal structure, ribs (transverse process), and sympathetic nerves

OPERATIONS ON THE RESPIRATORY SYSTEM

32.9 **Other excision of lung**
  EXCLUDES: biopsy of lung and bronchus (33.24-33.27)
  pulmonary decortication (34.51)

√3rd 33 Other operations on lung and bronchus
  INCLUDES:
  rib resection
  sternotomy   } as operative
  sternum-splitting incision   approach
  thoracotomy

33.0 Incision of bronchus

33.1 Incision of lung
  EXCLUDES: puncture of lung (33.93)

√4th 33.2 Diagnostic procedures on lung and bronchus

  33.21 Bronchoscopy through artificial stoma
    EXCLUDES: that with biopsy (33.24, 33.27)
    DEF: Visual exam of lung and its branches via tube through artificial opening.

  33.22 Fiber-optic bronchoscopy
    EXCLUDES: that with biopsy (33.24, 33.27)
    DEF: Exam of lung and bronchus via flexible optical instrument for visualization.

  33.23 Other bronchoscopy
    EXCLUDES: that for:
      aspiration (96.05)
      biopsy (33.24, 33.27)
    AHA: 1Q, '99, 6

  33.24 Closed [endoscopic] biopsy of bronchus
    Bronchoscopy (fiberoptic) (rigid) with:
      brush biopsy of "lung"
      brushing or washing for specimen collection
      excision (bite) biopsy
      ▶Diagnostic bronchoalveolar lavage (BAL)◀
    EXCLUDES: closed biopsy of lung, other than brush biopsy of "lung" (33.26, 33.27)
      ▶whole lung lavage (33.99)◀
    AHA: 4Q, '92, 27; 3Q, '91, 15
    DEF: Brush biopsy: Obtaining cell or tissue samples via bristled instrument without incision.

  33.25 Open biopsy of bronchus
    EXCLUDES: open biopsy of lung (33.28)

  33.26 Closed [percutaneous] [needle] biopsy of lung
    EXCLUDES: endoscopic biopsy of lung (33.27)
    AHA: 3Q, '92, 12

  33.27 Closed endoscopic biopsy of lung
    Fiber-optic (flexible) bronchoscopy with fluoroscopic guidance with biopsy
    Transbronchial lung biopsy
    EXCLUDES: brush biopsy of "lung" (33.24)
      percutaneous biopsy of lung (33.26)
    AHA: 4Q, '92, 27; 3Q, '91, 15; S-O, '86, 11

Bronchoscopy with Bite Biopsy

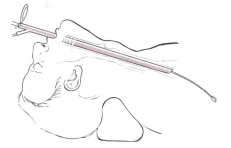

33.28 Open biopsy of lung
  AHA: 3Q, '99, 3; 3Q, '92, 12

33.29 Other diagnostic procedures on lung and bronchus
  EXCLUDES: contrast bronchogram:
    endotracheal (87.31)
    other (87.32)
    lung scan (92.15)
    magnetic resonance imaging (88.92)
    microscopic examination of specimen from bronchus or lung (90.41-90.49)
    routine chest x-ray (87.44)
    ultrasonography of lung (88.73)
    vital capacity determination (89.37)
    x-ray of bronchus or lung NOS (87.49)

√4th 33.3 Surgical collapse of lung

  33.31 Destruction of phrenic nerve for collapse of lung
    DEF: Therapeutic deadening or destruction of diaphragmatic nerve to collapse the lung.

  33.32 Artificial pneumothorax for collapse of lung
    Thoracotomy for collapse of lung
    DEF: Forcing air or gas into diaphragmatic space to achieve therapeutic collapse of lung.
    DEF: Thoracotomy for collapse of lung: Incision into chest for therapeutic collapse of lung.

  33.33 Pneumoperitoneum for collapse of lung
    DEF: Forcing air or gas into abdominal serous membrane to achieve therapeutic collapse of lung.

  33.34 Thoracoplasty
    DEF: Removal of ribs for therapeutic collapse of lungs.

  33.39 Other surgical collapse of lung
    Collapse of lung NOS

√4th 33.4 Repair and plastic operation on lung and bronchus

  33.41 Suture of laceration of bronchus

  33.42 Closure of bronchial fistula
    Closure of bronchostomy
    Fistulectomy:
      bronchocutaneous
      bronchoesophageal
      bronchovisceral
    EXCLUDES: closure of fistula:
      bronchomediastinal (34.73)
      bronchopleural (34.73)
      bronchopleuromediastinal (34.73)
    DEF: Closure of bronchostomy: Removal of bronchostomy tube and repair of surgical wound.
    DEF: Fistulectomy: Closure of abnormal passage.
    Bronchocutaneous: Between skin and lung branch.
    Bronchoesophagus: Between esophagus and lung branch.
    Bronchovisceral: Between an internal organ and lung branch.

  33.43 Closure of laceration of lung

  33.48 Other repair and plastic operations on bronchus

  33.49 Other repair and plastic operations on lung
    EXCLUDES: closure of pleural fistula (34.73)

33.5 Lung transplant
EXCLUDES combined heart-lung transplantation (33.6)

Code also cardiopulmonary bypass [extracorporeal circulation] [heart-lung machine] 39.61

AHA: 4Q, '95, 75

33.50 Lung transplantation, not otherwise specified
33.51 Unilateral lung transplantation
33.52 Bilateral lung transplantation
Double-lung transplantation
En bloc transplantation
DEF: Sequential excision and implant of both lungs.

33.6 Combined heart-lung transplantation
Code also cardiopulmonary bypass [extracorporeal circulation] [heart-lung machine] (39.61)

33.9 Other operations on lung and bronchus

33.91 Bronchial dilation
AHA: 1Q, '97, 14

33.92 Ligation of bronchus
DEF: Tying off of a lung branch.

33.93 Puncture of lung
EXCLUDES needle biopsy (33.26)
DEF: Piercing of lung with surgical instrument.

33.98 Other operations on bronchus
EXCLUDES bronchial lavage (96.56)
removal of intraluminal foreign body from bronchus without incision (98.15)

33.99 Other operations on lung
▶Whole lung lavage◀
EXCLUDES other continuous mechanical ventilation (96.70-96.72)
respiratory therapy (93.90-93.99)

34 Operations on chest wall, pleura, mediastinum, and diaphragm
EXCLUDES operations on breast (85.0-85.99)

34.0 Incision of chest wall and pleura
EXCLUDES that as operative approach — omit code

34.01 Incision of chest wall
Extrapleural drainage
EXCLUDES incision of pleura (34.09)
AHA: 3Q, '00, 12; 1Q, '92, 13

DEF: Extrapleural drainage: Incision to drain fluid from external pleura.

34.02 Exploratory thoracotomy
34.03 Reopening of recent thoracotomy site
34.04 Insertion of intercostal catheter for drainage
Chest tube
Closed chest drainage
Revision of intercostal catheter (chest tube) (with lysis of adhesions)
AHA: 1Q, '99, 10; 2Q, '99, 12; 1Q, '95, 5; 1Q, '92, 12

DEF: Insertion of catheter between ribs for drainage.

34.05 Creation of pleuroperitoneal shunt
AHA: 4Q, '94, 50

34.09 Other incision of pleura
Creation of pleural window for drainage
Intercostal stab
Open chest drainage
EXCLUDES thoracoscopy (34.21)
thoracotomy for collapse of lung (33.32)

AHA: 1Q, '94, 7; 4Q, '94, 50

DEF: Creation of pleural window: Creation of circumscribed drainage hole in serous membrane of chest.

DEF: Intercostal stab: Creation of penetrating stab wound between ribs.

DEF: Open chest drainage: Insertion of tube through ribs and serous membrane of chest for drainage.

34.1 Incision of mediastinum
EXCLUDES mediastinoscopy (34.22)
mediastinotomy associated with pneumonectomy (32.5)

34.2 Diagnostic procedures on chest wall, pleura, mediastinum, and diaphragm

34.21 Transpleural thoracoscopy
DEF: Exam of chest through serous membrane using scope.

34.22 Mediastinoscopy
Code also any lymph node biopsy (40.11)
DEF: Exam of lung cavity and heart using scope.

34.23 Biopsy of chest wall
34.24 Pleural biopsy
AHA: 1Q, '92, 14

34.25 Closed [percutaneous] [needle] biopsy of mediastinum
34.26 Open biopsy of mediastinum
34.27 Biopsy of diaphragm
34.28 Other diagnostic procedures on chest wall, pleura, and diaphragm
EXCLUDES angiocardiography (88.50-88.58)
aortography (88.42)
arteriography of:
  intrathoracic vessels NEC (88.44)
  pulmonary arteries (88.43)
microscopic examination of specimen from chest wall, pleura, and diaphragm (90.41-90.49)
phlebography of:
  intrathoracic vessels NEC (88.63)
  pulmonary veins (88.62)
radiological examinations of thorax:
  C.A.T. scan (87.41)
  diaphragmatic x-ray (87.49)
  intrathoracic lymphangiogram (87.34)
  routine chest x-ray (87.44)
  sinogram of chest wall (87.38)
  soft tissue x-ray of chest wall NEC (87.39)
  tomogram of thorax NEC (87.42)
  ultrasonography of thorax (88.73)

OPERATIONS ON THE RESPIRATORY SYSTEM

34.29 Other diagnostic procedures on mediastinum
  EXCLUDES mediastinal:
    pneumogram (87.33)
    x-ray NEC (87.49)

34.3 Excision or destruction of lesion or tissue of mediastinum
  EXCLUDES biopsy of mediastinum (34.25-34.26)
    mediastinal fistulectomy (34.73)

34.4 Excision or destruction of lesion of chest wall
  Excision of lesion of chest wall NOS (with excision of ribs)
  EXCLUDES biopsy of chest wall (34.23)
    costectomy not incidental to thoracic procedure (77.91)
    excision of lesion of:
      breast (85.20-85.25)
      cartilage (80.89)
      skin (86.2-86.3)
    fistulectomy (34.73)

√4th 34.5 Pleurectomy
  34.51 Decortication of lung
    DEF: Removal of thickened serous membrane for lung expansion.

  34.59 Other excision of pleura
    Excision of pleural lesion
    EXCLUDES biopsy of pleura (34.24)
      pleural fistulectomy (34.73)

34.6 Scarification of pleura
  Pleurosclerosis
  EXCLUDES injection of sclerosing agent (34.92)
  AHA: 1Q, '92, 12

√4th 34.7 Repair of chest wall
  DEF: Destruction of fluid-secreting serous membrane cells of chest.

  34.71 Suture of laceration of chest wall
    EXCLUDES suture of skin and subcutaneous tissue alone (86.59)

  34.72 Closure of thoracostomy
  34.73 Closure of other fistula of thorax
    Closure of:
      bronchopleural
      bronchopleurocutaneous   } fistula
      bronchopleuromediastinal

  34.74 Repair of pectus deformity
    Repair of:
      pectus carinatum } (with implant)
      pectus excavatum

    DEF: Pectus carinatum repair: Restoration of prominent chest bone defect with implant.

    DEF: Pectus excavatum: Restoration of depressed chest bone defect with implant.

  34.79 Other repair of chest wall
    Repair of chest wall NOS
    AHA: J-F, '87, 13

√4th 34.8 Operations on diaphragm
  34.81 Excision of lesion or tissue of diaphragm
    EXCLUDES biopsy of diaphragm (34.27)
  34.82 Suture of laceration of diaphragm
  34.83 Closure of fistula of diaphragm
    Thoracicoabdominal
    Thoracicogastric   } fistulectomy
    Thoracicointestinal

    DEF: Fistulectomy: Closure of abnormal passage.

  34.84 Other repair of diaphragm
    EXCLUDES repair of diaphragmatic hernia (53.7-53.82)
  34.85 Implantation of diaphragmatic pacemaker
  34.89 Other operations on diaphragm

√4th 34.9 Other operations on thorax
  34.91 Thoracentesis
    AHA: S-O, '85, 6

    DEF: Puncture of pleural cavity for fluid aspiration, also called pleurocentesis.

  34.92 Injection into thoracic cavity
    Chemical pleurodesis
    Injection of cytotoxic agent or tetracycline
    Requires additional code for any cancer chemotherapeutic substance (99.25)
    EXCLUDES that for collapse of lung (33.32)
    AHA: 1Q, '92, 12; 2Q, '89, 17

    DEF: Chemical pleurodesis: Tetracycline hydrochloride injections to create adhesions between parietal and visceral pleura for treatment of pleural effusion.

  34.93 Repair of pleura
  34.99 Other
    EXCLUDES removal of:
      mediastinal drain (97.42)
      sutures (97.43)
      thoracotomy tube (97.41)
    AHA: 1Q, '00, 17; 1Q, '88, 9

    DEF: Pleural tent: Extrapleural mobilization of parietal pleura that allows draping of membrane over visceral pleura to eliminate intrapleural dead space and seal visceral pleura.

7. OPERATIONS ON THE CARDIOVASCULAR SYSTEM (35-39)

√3rd 35 Operations on valves and septa of heart

INCLUDES: sternotomy (median) (transverse) thoracotomy } as operative approach

Code also cardiopulmonary bypass [extracorporeal circulation] [heart-lung machine] (39.61)

√4th 35.0 Closed heart valvotomy

EXCLUDES: percutaneous (balloon) valvuloplasty (35.96)

DEF: Incision into valve to restore function.

- 35.00 Closed heart valvotomy, unspecified valve
- 35.01 Closed heart valvotomy, aortic valve
- 35.02 Closed heart valvotomy, mitral valve
- 35.03 Closed heart valvotomy, pulmonary valve
- 35.04 Closed heart valvotomy, tricuspid valve

√4th 35.1 Open heart valvuloplasty without replacement

INCLUDES: open heart valvotomy
EXCLUDES: that associated with repair of:
  endocardial cushion defect (35.54, 35.63, 35.73)
  percutaneous (balloon) valvuloplasty (35.96)
  valvular defect associated with atrial and ventricular septal defects (35.54, 35.63, 35.73)

Code also cardiopulmonary bypass, if performed [extracorporeal circulation] [heart-lung machine] (39.61)

DEF: Incision into heart for plastic repair of valve without replacing valve.

- 35.10 Open heart valvuloplasty without replacement, unspecified valve
- 35.11 Open heart valvuloplasty of aortic valve without replacement
- 35.12 Open heart valvuloplasty of mitral valve without replacement
  AHA: 1Q, '97, 13
- 35.13 Open heart valvuloplasty of pulmonary valve without replacement
- 35.14 Open heart valvuloplasty of tricuspid valve without replacement

√4th 35.2 Replacement of heart valve

INCLUDES: excision of heart valve with replacement

Code also cardiopulmonary bypass [extracorporeal circulation] [heart-lung machine] (39.61)

EXCLUDES: that associated with repair of:
  endocardial cushion defect (35.54, 35.63, 35.73)
  valvular defect associated with atrial and ventricular septal defects (35.54, 35.63, 35.73)

DEF: Removal and replacement of valve with tissue from patient, animal, other human, or prosthetic (synthetic) valve.

- 35.20 Replacement of unspecified heart valve
  Repair of unspecified heart valve with tissue graft or prosthetic implant
- 35.21 Replacement of aortic valve with tissue graft
  Repair of aortic valve with tissue graft (autograft) (heterograft) (homograft)
  AHA: 2Q, '97, 8
- 35.22 Other replacement of aortic valve
  Repair of aortic valve with replacement:
    NOS
    prosthetic (partial) (synthetic) (total)
  AHA: 1Q, '96, 11
- 35.23 Replacement of mitral valve with tissue graft
  Repair of mitral valve with tissue graft (autograft) (heterograft) (homograft)
- 35.24 Other replacement of mitral valve
  Repair of mitral valve with replacement:
    NOS
    prosthetic (partial) (synthetic) (total)
  AHA: 4Q, '97, 55
- 35.25 Replacement of pulmonary valve with tissue graft
  Repair of pulmonary valve with tissue graft (autograft) (heterograft) (homograft)
  AHA: 2Q, '97, 8
- 35.26 Other replacement of pulmonary valve
  Repair of pulmonary valve with replacement:
    NOS
    prosthetic (partial) (synthetic) (total)
- 35.27 Replacement of tricuspid valve with tissue graft
  Repair of tricuspid valve with tissue graft (autograft) (heterograft) (homograft)
- 35.28 Other replacement of tricuspid valve
  Repair of tricuspid valve with replacement:
    NOS
    prosthetic (partial) (synthetic) (total)

√4th 35.3 Operations on structures adjacent to heart valves

Code also cardiopulmonary bypass [extracorporeal circulation] [heart-lung machine] (39.61)

- 35.31 Operations on papillary muscle
  Division
  Reattachment } of papillary muscle
  Repair
- 35.32 Operations on chordae tendineae
  Division } chordae tendineae
  Repair
- 35.33 Annuloplasty
  Plication of annulus
  AHA: 1Q, '97, 13; 1Q, '88, 10
  DEF: Plication of annulus: Tuck stitched in valvular ring for tightening.
- 35.34 Infundibulectomy
  Right ventricular infundibulectomy
  DEF: Infundibulectomy: Excision of funnel-shaped heart passage.
  DEF: Right ventricular infundibulectomy: Excision of funnel-shaped passage in right upper heart chamber.
- 35.35 Operations on trabeculae carneae cordis
  Division } of trabeculae carneae cordis
  Excision
  Excision of aortic subvalvular ring
- 35.39 Operations on other structures adjacent to valves of heart
  Repair of sinus of Valsalva (aneurysm)

√4th 35.4 Production of septal defect in heart

- 35.41 Enlargement of existing atrial septal defect
  Rashkind procedure
  Septostomy (atrial) (balloon)
  DEF: Enlargement of partition wall defect in lower heart chamber to improve function.
  DEF: Rashkind procedure: Enlargement of partition wall defect between the two lower heart chambers by balloon catheter.

35.42 **Creation of septal defect in heart**
Blalock-Hanlon operation
DEF: Blalock-Hanlon operation: Removal of partition wall defect in lower heart chamber.

√4th **35.5 Repair of atrial and ventricular septa with prosthesis**
INCLUDES repair of septa with synthetic implant or patch
Code also cardiopulmonary bypass [extracorporeal circulation] [heart-lung machine] (39.61)

35.50 Repair of unspecified septal defect of heart with prosthesis
EXCLUDES that associated with repair of:
endocardial cushion defect (35.54)
septal defect associated with valvular defect (35.54)

35.51 Repair of atrial septal defect with prosthesis, open technique
Atrioseptoplasty
Correction of atrial septal defect
Repair:
  foramen ovale (patent)
  ostium secundum defect
} with prosthesis

EXCLUDES that associated with repair of:
atrial septal defect associated with valvular and ventricular septal defects (35.54)
endocardial cushion defect (35.54)

DEF: Repair of opening or weakening in septum separating the atria; prosthesis implanted through heart incision.

35.52 Repair of atrial septal defect with prosthesis, closed technique
Insertion of atrial septal umbrella [King-Mills]
AHA: 3Q, '98, 11

DEF: Correction of partition wall defect in lower heart chamber with artificial material; without incision into heart.

DEF: Insertion of atrial septal umbrella (King-Mills): Correction of partition wall defect in lower heart chamber with atrial septal umbrella.

35.53 Repair of ventricular septal defect with prosthesis
Correction of ventricular septal defect
Repair of supracristal defect
} with prosthesis

EXCLUDES that associated with repair of:
endocardial cushion defect (35.54)
ventricular defect associated with valvular and atrial septal defects (35.54)

35.54 Repair of endocardial cushion defect with prosthesis
Repair:
  atrioventricular canal
  ostium primum defect
  valvular defect associated with atrial and ventricular septal defects
} with prosthesis (grafted to septa)

EXCLUDES repair of isolated:
atrial septal defect (35.51-35.52)
valvular defect (35.20, 35.22, 35.24, 35.26, 35.28)
ventricular septal defect (35.53)

√4th **35.6 Repair of atrial and ventricular septa with tissue graft**
Code also cardiopulmonary bypass [extracorporeal circulation] [heart-lung machine] (39.61)

35.60 Repair of unspecified septal defect of heart with tissue graft
EXCLUDES that associated with repair of:
endocardial cushion defect (35.63)
septal defect associated with valvular defect (35.63)

35.61 Repair of atrial septal defect with tissue graft
Atrioseptoplasty
Correction of atrial septal defect
Repair:
  foramen ovale (patent)
  ostium secundum defect
} with tissue graft

EXCLUDES that associated with repair of:
atrial septal defect associated with valvular and ventricular septal defects (35.63)
endocardial cushion defect (35.63)

35.62 Repair of ventricular septal defect with tissue graft
Correction of ventricular septal defect
Repair of supracristal defect
} with tissue graft

EXCLUDES that associated with repair of:
endocardial cushion defect (35.63)
ventricular defect associated with valvular and atrial septal defects (35.63)

35.63–35.9   OPERATIONS ON THE CARDIOVASCULAR SYSTEM   **Tabular List**

35.63 Repair of endocardial cushion defect with tissue graft
Repair of:
    atrioventricular canal
    ostium primum defect
    valvular defect associated with atrial and ventricular septal defects
} with tissue graft

EXCLUDES   repair of isolated:
    atrial septal defect (35.61)
    valvular defect (35.20-35.21, 35.23, 35.25, 35.27)
    ventricular septal defect (35.62)

√4th 35.7 Other and unspecified repair of atrial and ventricular septa
Code also cardiopulmonary bypass [extracorporeal circulation] [heart-lung machine] (39.61)

35.70 Other and unspecified repair of unspecified septal defect of heart
Repair of septal defect NOS
EXCLUDES   that associated with repair of:
    endocardial cushion defect (35.73)
    septal defect associated with valvular defect (35.73)

35.71 Other and unspecified repair of atrial septal defect
Repair NOS:
    atrial septum
    foramen ovale (patent)
    ostium secundum defect
EXCLUDES   that associated with repair of:
    atrial septal defect associated with valvular and ventricular septal defects (35.73)
    endocardial cushion defect (35.73)

35.72 Other and unspecified repair of ventricular septal defect
Repair NOS:
    supracristal defect
    ventricular septum
EXCLUDES   that associated with repair of:
    endocardial cushion defect (35.73)
    ventricular septal defect associated with valvular and atrial septal defects (35.73)

35.73 Other and unspecified repair of endocardial cushion defect
Repair NOS:
    atrioventricular canal
    ostium primum defect
    valvular defect associated with atrial and ventricular septal defects
EXCLUDES   repair of isolated:
    atrial septal defect (35.71)
    valvular defect (35.20, 35.22, 35.24, 35.26, 35.28)
    ventricular septal defect (35.72)

√4th 35.8 Total repair of certain congenital cardiac anomalies
Note: For partial repair of defect [e.g. repair of atrial septal defect in tetralogy of Fallot] — code to specific procedure

35.81 Total repair of tetralogy of Fallot
One-stage total correction of tetralogy of Fallot with or without:
    commissurotomy of pulmonary valve
    infundibulectomy
    outflow tract prosthesis
    patch graft of outflow tract
    prosthetic tube for pulmonary artery
    repair of ventricular septal defect (with prosthesis)
    take-down of previous systemic-pulmonary artery anastomosis

35.82 Total repair of total anomalous pulmonary venous connection
One-stage total correction of total anomalous pulmonary venous connection with or without:
    anastomosis between (horizontal) common pulmonary trunk and posterior wall of left atrium (side-to-side)
    enlargement of foramen ovale
    incision [excision] of common wall between posterior left atrium and coronary sinus and roofing of resultant defect with patch graft (synthetic)
    ligation of venous connection (descending anomalous vein) (to left innominate vein) (to superior vena cava)
    repair of atrial septal defect (with prosthesis)

35.83 Total repair of truncus arteriosus
One-stage total correction of truncus arteriosus with or without:
    construction (with aortic homograft) (with prosthesis) of a pulmonary artery placed from right ventricle to arteries supplying the lung
    ligation of connections between aorta and pulmonary artery
    repair of ventricular septal defect (with prosthesis)

35.84 Total correction of transposition of great vessels, not elsewhere classified
Arterial switch operation [Jatene]
Total correction of transposition of great arteries at the arterial level by switching the great arteries, including the left or both coronary arteries, implanted in the wall of the pulmonary artery
EXCLUDES   baffle operation [Mustard] [Senning] (35.91)
    creation of shunt between right ventricle and pulmonary artery [Rastelli] (35.92)

√4th 35.9 Other operations on valves and septa of heart
Code also cardiopulmonary bypass, if performed [extracorporeal circulation] [heart-lung machine] (39.61)

OPERATIONS ON THE CARDIOVASCULAR SYSTEM

35.91 Interatrial transposition of venous return
  Baffle:
    atrial
    interatrial
  Mustard's operation
  Resection of atrial septum and insertion of patch to direct systemic venous return to tricuspid valve and pulmonary venous return to mitral valve

DEF: Atrial baffle: Correction of venous flow of abnormal or deviated lower heart chamber.

DEF: Interatrial baffle: Correction of venous flow between abnormal lower heart chambers.

DEF: Mustard's operation: Creates intra-atrial baffle using pericardial tissue to correct transposition of the great vessels.

35.92 Creation of conduit between right ventricle and pulmonary artery
  Creation of shunt between right ventricle and (distal) pulmonary artery
    EXCLUDES that associated with total repair of truncus arteriosus (35.83)

35.93 Creation of conduit between left ventricle and aorta
  Creation of apicoaortic shunt
  Shunt between apex of left ventricle and aorta

35.94 Creation of conduit between atrium and pulmonary artery
  Fontan procedure

35.95 Revision of corrective procedure on heart
  Replacement of prosthetic heart valve poppet
  Resuture of prosthesis of:
    septum
    valve
    EXCLUDES complete revision — code to specific procedure
    replacement of prosthesis or graft of:
      septum (35.50-35.63)
      valve (35.20-35.28)

DEF: Replacement of prosthetic heart valve poppet: Removal and replacement of valve-supporting prosthesis.

DEF: Resuture of prosthesis of septum: Restitching of prosthesis in partition wall.

DEF: Resuture of prosthesis of valve: Restitching of prosthetic valve.

35.96 Percutaneous valvuloplasty
  Percutaneous balloon valvuloplasty
  AHA: M-J, '86, 6; N-D, '85, 10

DEF: Repair of valve with catheter.

DEF: Percutaneous balloon valvuloplasty: Repair of valve with inflatable catheter.

35.98 Other operations on septa of heart
35.99 Other operations on valves of heart

36 Operations on vessels of heart
  INCLUDES sternotomy (median) (transverse)
    thoracotomy } as operative approach

  Code also any injection or infusion of platelet inhibitor (99.20)
  Code also cardiopulmonary bypass, if performed [extracorporeal circulation] [heart-lung machine] (39.61)

36.0 Removal of coronary artery obstruction and insertion of stent(s)
AHA: 4Q, '95, 66; 2Q, '94, 13; 1Q, '94, 3; 2Q, '90, 23; N-D, '86, 8

36.01 Single vessel percutaneous transluminal coronary angioplasty [PTCA] or coronary atherectomy without mention of thrombolytic agent
  Balloon angioplasty of coronary artery
  Coronary atherectomy
  Percutaneous coronary angioplasty NOS
  PTCA NOS
    EXCLUDES multiple vessel percutaneous transluminal coronary angioplasty [PTCA] or coronary atherectomy performed during the same operation (36.05)
  Code also any insertion of coronary stent(s) (36.06)
AHA: 1Q, '01, 9; 2Q, '01, 24; 1Q, '00, 11; 1Q, '99, 17; 4Q, '98, 74, 85; 3Q, '91, 24

DEF: Balloon angioplasty: Insertion of catheter with inflation of balloon to flatten plaque and widen vessels.

36.02 Single vessel percutaneous transluminal coronary angioplasty [PTCA] or coronary atherectomy with mention of thrombolytic agent
  Balloon angioplasty of coronary artery with infusion of thrombolytic agent [streptokinase]
  Coronary atherectomy
    EXCLUDES multiple vessel percutaneous transluminal coronary angioplasty [PTCA] or coronary atherectomy performed during the same operation (36.05)
    single vessel PTCA or coronary atherectomy without mention of thrombolytic agent (36.01)
  Code also any insertion of coronary stent(s) (36.06)
AHA: 2Q, '01, 24; 1Q, '97, 3

36.03 Open chest coronary artery angioplasty
  Coronary (artery):
    endarterectomy (with patch graft)
    thromboendarterectomy (with patch graft)
  Open surgery for direct relief of coronary artery obstruction
    EXCLUDES that with coronary artery bypass graft (36.10-36.19)
  Code also any insertion of coronary stent(s) (36.06)
AHA: 2Q, '01, 24; 3Q, '93, 7

DEF: Endarterectomy (with patch graft): Excision of thickened material within coronary artery; repair with patch graft.

DEF: Thromboendarterectomy (with patch graft): Excision of blood clot and thickened material within artery; repair with patch graft.

DEF: Open surgery for direct relief of coronary artery obstruction: Removal of coronary artery obstruction through opening in chest.

OPERATIONS ON THE CARDIOVASCULAR SYSTEM

PTCA (Balloon Angioplasty)

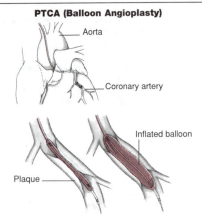

Coronary Bypass

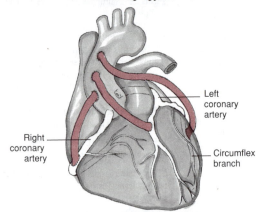

36.04 Intracoronary artery thrombolytic infusion
That by direct coronary artery injection, infusion, or catheterization
  enzyme infusion
  platelet inhibitor
  EXCLUDES infusion of platelet inhibitor (99.20)
  infusion of thrombolytic agent (99.10)
  that associated with any procedure in 36.02, 36.03

AHA: 2Q, '01, 24; 4Q, '98, 85; 1Q, '97, 3; 4Q, '95, 67

DEF: Infusion of clot breaking solution into intracoronary artery.

36.05 Multiple vessel percutaneous transluminal coronary angioplasty [PTCA] or coronary atherectomy performed during the same operation, with or without mention of thrombolytic agent
  Balloon angioplasty of multiple coronary arteries
  Coronary atherectomy
  Code also any:
    insertion of coronary artery stent(s) (36.06)
    intracoronary artery thrombolytic infusion (36.04)
  EXCLUDES single vessel [PTCA] or coronary atherectomy
    without mention of thrombolytic agent (36.01)
    with mention of thrombolytic agent (36.02)

AHA: 2Q, '01, 24; 1Q, '94, 3

36.06 Insertion of non-drug-eluting coronary artery stent(s)
  ▶Bare stent(s)
  Bonded stent(s)
  Drug-coated stent(s), e.g., heparin coated
  Endograft(s)
  Endovascular graft(s)
  Stent graft(s)◀
  Code also any:
    open chest coronary artery angioplasty (36.03)
    percutaneous transluminal coronary angioplasty [PTCA] or coronary atherectomy (36.01, 36.02, 36.05)
  EXCLUDES ▶insertion of drug-eluting coronary artery stent(s) (36.07)◀

AHA: 1Q, '01, 9; 2Q, '01, 24; 1Q, '00, 11; 1Q, '99, 17

DEF: Percutaneous implant via catheter of metal stent, to enlarge, maintain lumen size of coronary artery.

36.07 Insertion of drug-eluting coronary artery stent(s)
  Endograft(s)
  Endovascular graft(s)
  Stent graft(s)
  Code also any:
    open chest coronary artery angioplasty (36.03)
    percutaneous transluminal coronary angioplasty [PTCA] or coronary atherectomy (36.01, 36.02, 36.05)
  EXCLUDES drug-coated stents, e.g., heparin coated (36.06)
    insertion of non-drug-eluting coronary artery stent(s) (36.06)

36.09 Other removal of coronary artery obstruction
  Coronary angioplasty NOS
  EXCLUDES that by open angioplasty (36.03)
    that by percutaneous transluminal coronary angioplasty [PTCA] or coronary atherectomy (36.01-36.02, 36.05)

√4ᵗʰ 36.1 Bypass anastomosis for heart revascularization
Code also cardiopulmonary bypass [extracorporeal circulation] [heart-lung machine] (39.61)

AHA: 2Q, '96, 7; 3Q, '95, 7; 3Q, '93, 8; 1Q, '91, 7; 2Q, '90, 24; 4Q, '89, 3

DEF: Insertion of tube to bypass blocked coronary artery, correct coronary blood flow.

36.10 Aortocoronary bypass for heart revascularization, not otherwise specified
  Direct revascularization:
    cardiac
    coronary   } with catheter stent,
    heart muscle   prosthesis, or
    myocardial   vein graft
  Heart revascularization NOS

AHA: 2Q, '96, 7

36.11 Aortocoronary bypass of one coronary artery
AHA: 4Q, '89, 3

36.12 Aortocoronary bypass of two coronary arteries
AHA: 4Q, '99, 15; 2Q, '96, 7; 3Q, '97, 14; 4Q, '89, 3

36.13 Aortocoronary bypass of three coronary arteries
AHA: 2Q, '96, 7; 4Q, '89, 3

36.14 Aortocoronary bypass of four or more coronary arteries
AHA: 2Q, '96, 7; 4Q, '89, 3

OPERATIONS ON THE CARDIOVASCULAR SYSTEM

36.15 Single internal mammary-coronary artery bypass
Anastomosis (single):
mammary artery to coronary artery
thoracic artery to coronary artery
AHA: 4Q, '99, 15; 3Q, '97, 14; 2Q, '96, 7

36.16 Double internal mammary-coronary artery bypass
Anastomosis, double:
mammary artery to coronary artery
thoracic artery to coronary artery
AHA: 2Q, '96, 7

36.17 Abdominal-coronary artery bypass
Anastomosis:
gastroepiploic artery to coronary artery
AHA: 3Q, '97, 14; 4Q, '96, 64

36.19 Other bypass anastomosis for heart revascularization
AHA: 2Q, '96, 7

36.2 Heart revascularization by arterial implant
Implantation of:
aortic branches [ascending aortic branches] into heart muscle
blood vessels into myocardium
internal mammary artery [internal thoracic artery] into:
heart muscle
myocardium
ventricle
ventricular wall
Indirect heart revascularization NOS

√4th **36.3** Other heart revascularization

36.31 Open chest transmyocardial revascularization
DEF: Transmyocardial revascularization (TMR): Laser creation of channels through myocardium allows oxygenated blood flow from sinusoids to myocardial tissue.

36.32 Other transmyocardial revascularization NC
Percutaneous transmyocardial revascularization
Thoracoscopic transmyocardial revascularization
AHA: 4Q, '98, 74

36.39 Other heart revascularization
Abrasion of epicardium
Cardio-omentopexy
Intrapericardial poudrage
Myocardial graft:
mediastinal fat
omentum
pectoral muscles

DEF: Cardio-omentopexy: Suture of omentum segment to heart after drawing segment through incision in diaphragm.

DEF: Intrapericardial poudrage: Application of powder to heart lining to promote fusion.

DEF: Myocardial graft:
Mediastinal fat: Implantation in heart muscle of fat from cavity containing heart and structures.
Omentopexy: Suture of omentum to heart.

√4th **36.9** Other operations on vessels of heart
Code also cardiopulmonary bypass [extracorporeal circulation] [heart-lung machine] (39.61)

36.91 Repair of aneurysm of coronary vessel

36.99 Other operations on vessels of heart
Exploration ⎫
Incision   ⎬ of coronary artery
Ligation   ⎭
Repair of arteriovenous fistula
AHA: 1Q, '94, 3

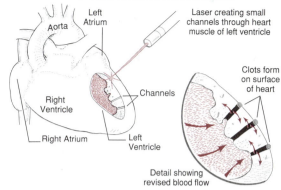
Transmyocardial Revascularization

√3rd **37** Other operations on heart and pericardium
Code also any injection or infusion of platelet inhibitor (99.20)

37.0 Pericardiocentesis
DEF: Puncture of the heart lining to withdraw fluid.

√4th **37.1** Cardiotomy and pericardiotomy
Code also cardiopulmonary bypass [extracorporeal circulation] [heart-lung machine] (39.61)

37.10 Incision of heart, not otherwise specified
Cardiolysis NOS

37.11 Cardiotomy
Incision of: Incision of:
atrium   myocardium
endocardium   ventricle

37.12 Pericardiotomy
Pericardial window   Pericardiolysis
operation   Pericardiotomy

DEF: Pericardial window operation: Incision into heart lining for drainage.
DEF: Pericardiolysis: Destruction of heart tissue lining.

√4th **37.2** Diagnostic procedures on heart and pericardium

37.21 Right heart cardiac catheterization
Cardiac catheterization NOS
EXCLUDES that with catheterization of left heart (37.23)
AHA: 2Q, '90, 23; M-J, '87, 11

37.22 Left heart cardiac catheterization
EXCLUDES that with catheterization of right heart (37.23)
AHA: 1Q, '00, 21; 2Q, '90, 23; 4Q, '88, 4; M-J, '87, 11

37.23 Combined right and left heart cardiac catheterization
AHA: 2Q, '01, 8; 1Q, '00, 20; 3Q, '98, 11; 2Q, '90, 23; M-J, '87, 11

37.24 Biopsy of pericardium

37.25 Biopsy of heart
AHA: 3Q, '94, 8

37.26 Cardiac electrophysiologic stimulation and recording studies
Electrophysiologic studies [EPS]
►Non-invasive programmed electrical stimulation (NIPS)◄
Programmed electrical stimulation
Code also any concomitant procedure
EXCLUDES His bundle recording (37.29)
AHA: ▶1Q, '02, 8, 9◄ 1Q, '99, 3; 2Q, '97, 10; 3Q, '90, 11

DEF: Diagnostic mapping and measurement of intracardiac electrical activity; requires inserting three to six catheters into heart blood vessels and positioning catheters under fluoroscopic guidance to determine site of the tachycardia or abnormal impulse pathway; may also be used to terminate arrhythmias.

OPERATIONS ON THE CARDIOVASCULAR SYSTEM

Intracardiac Echocardiography

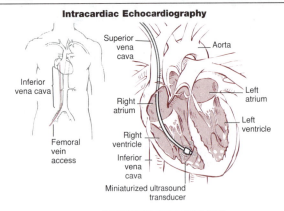

37.27 Cardiac mapping
Code also any concomitant procedure
EXCLUDES electrocardiogram (89.52)
His bundle recording (37.29)

37.28 Intracardiac echocardiography
ICE
Code also any synchronous Doppler flow mapping (88.72)

DEF: Creation of a two-dimensional graphic of heart using endoscopic echocardiographic equipment.
AHA: 4Q, '01, 62

37.29 Other diagnostic procedures on heart and pericardium
EXCLUDES angiocardiography (88.50-88.58)
cardiac function tests (89.41-89.69)
cardiovascular radioisotopic scan and function study (92.05)
coronary arteriography (88.55-88.57)
diagnostic pericardiocentesis (37.0)
diagnostic ultrasound of heart (88.72)
x-ray of heart (87.49)

AHA: S-O, '87, 3

✓4th 37.3 Pericardiectomy and excision of lesion of heart
Code also cardiopulmonary bypass [extracorporeal circulation] [heart-lung machine] (39.61)

37.31 Pericardiectomy
Excision of:
adhesions of pericardium
constricting scar of:
epicardium
pericardium

DEF: Excision of a portion of heart lining.

37.32 Excision of aneurysm of heart
Repair of aneurysm of heart

37.33 Excision or destruction of other lesion or tissue of heart
EXCLUDES catheter ablation of lesion or tissues of heart (37.34)

AHA: 2Q, '94, 12

37.34 Catheter ablation of lesion or tissues of heart

Cryoablation ⎫
Electrocurrent ⎬ of lesion or tissues of heart
Resection ⎭

AHA: 1Q, '00, 20

DEF: Destruction of heart tissue or lesion by freezing, electric current or resection.

37.35 Partial ventriculectomy [NC]
Ventricular reduction surgery
Ventricular remodeling
Code also any synchronous:
mitral valve repair (35.02, 35.12)
mitral valve replacement (35.23-35.24)

AHA: 4Q, '97, 54, 55

DEF: Removal of elliptical slice of ventricle between anterior and posterior papillary muscle; also called Batiste operation.

37.4 Repair of heart and pericardium
AHA: 2Q, '90, 24

37.5 Heart transplantation [NC]
EXCLUDES combined heart-lung transplantation (33.6)

✓4th 37.6 Implantation of heart assist system
AHA: 4Q, '95, 68

DEF: Implant of device for assisting heart in circulating blood.

37.61 Implant of pulsation balloon

37.62 Implant of other heart assist system
Insertion of centrifugal pump
Insertion of heart assist system, not specified as pulsatile
Insertion of heart assist system, NOS
Insertion of heart pump

AHA: 2Q, '90, 25

37.63 Replacement and repair of heart assist system

37.64 Removal of heart assist system
EXCLUDES that with replacement of implant (37.63)
nonoperative removal of heart assist system (97.44)

37.65 Implant of an external, pulsatile heart assist system
Note: Device not implantable (outside the body but connected to heart) with external circulation and pump
EXCLUDES implant of pulsation balloon (37.61)

DEF: Insertion of short-term circulatory support device with pump outside body.

37.66 Implant of an implantable, pulsatile heart assist system [NC]
Note: Device directly connected to the heart and implanted in the upper left quadrant of peritoneal cavity
Transportable, implantable heart assist system
EXCLUDES implant of pulsation balloon (37.61)

AHA: 1Q, '98, 8

DEF: Insertion of long-term circulatory support device with pump in body.

Ventricular Reduction Surgery

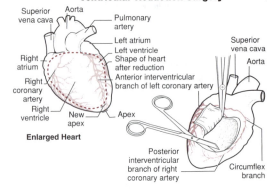

37.67 Implantation of cardiomyostimulation system

Note: Two-step open procedure consisting of tranfer of one end of the latissimus dorsi muscle; wrapping it around the heart; rib resection; implantation of epicardial cardiac pacing leads into the right ventricle; tunneling and pocket creation for the cardiomyostimulator.

AHA: 4Q, '98, 75; 1Q, '98, 8

√4th **37.7 Insertion, revision, replacement, and removal of pacemaker leads; insertion of temporary pacemaker system; or revision of pocket**

Code also any insertion and replacement of pacemaker device (37.80-37.87)

EXCLUDES ▶ implantation or replacement of transvenous lead [electrode] into left ventricular cardiac venous system (00.52) ◀

AHA: 1Q, '94, 16; 3Q, '92, 3; M-J, '87, 1

[10] **37.70 Initial insertion of lead [electrode], not otherwise specified**

EXCLUDES insertion of temporary transvenous pacemaker system (37.78)
replacement of atrial and/or ventricular lead(s) (37.76)

[10] **37.71 Initial insertion of transvenous lead [electrode] into ventricle**

EXCLUDES insertion of temporary transvenous pacemaker system (37.78)
replacement of atrial and/or ventricular lead(s) (37.76)

[11] **37.72 Initial insertion of transvenous leads [electrodes] into atrium and ventricle**

EXCLUDES insertion of temporary transvenous pacemaker system (37.78)
replacement of atrial and/or ventricular lead(s) (37.76)

AHA: 2Q, '97, 4

[10] **37.73 Initial insertion of transvenous lead [electrode] into atrium**

EXCLUDES insertion of temporary transvenous pacemaker system (37.78)
replacement of atrial and/or ventricular lead(s) (37.76)

[13] **37.74 Insertion or replacement of epicardial lead [electrode] into epicardium**

Insertion or replacement of epicardial lead by:
sternotomy
thoracotomy

EXCLUDES replacement of atrial and/or ventricular lead(s) (37.76)

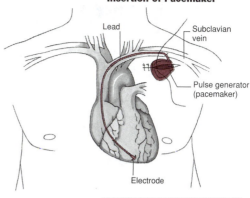

Insertion of Pacemaker

37.75 Revision of lead [electrode]

Repair of electrode [removal with re-insertion]
Repositioning of lead [electrode]
Revision of lead NOS

EXCLUDES repositioning of temporary transvenous pacemaker system — omit code

AHA: 2Q, '99, 12

[12] **37.76 Replacement of transvenous atrial and/or ventricular lead(s) [electrode]**

Removal or abandonment of existing transvenous or epicardial lead(s) with transvenous lead(s) replacement

EXCLUDES replacement of epicardial lead [electrode] (37.74)

37.77 Removal of lead(s) [electrode] without replacement

Removal:
epicardial lead (transthoracic approach)
transvenous lead(s)

EXCLUDES removal of temporary transvenous pacemaker system — omit code
that with replacement of:
atrial and/or ventricular lead(s) [electrode] (37.76)
epicardial lead [electrode] (37.74)

37.78 Insertion of temporary transvenous pacemaker system

EXCLUDES intraoperative cardiac pacemaker (39.64)

AHA: 3Q, '93, 12; 1Q, '89, 2

37.79 Revision or relocation of pacemaker pocket

Debridement and reforming pocket (skin and subcutaneous tissue)
Relocation of pocket [creation of new pocket] ▶pacemaker or CRT-P◀

√4th **37.8 Insertion, replacement, removal, and revision of pacemaker device**

Code also any lead insertion, lead replacement, lead removal and/or lead revision (37.70-37.77)

EXCLUDES ▶ implantation of cardiac resynchronization pacemaker, total system [CRT-P] (00.50)
implantation or replacement of cardiac resynchronization pacemaker pulse generator only [CRT-P] (00.53) ◀

AHA: M-J, '87, 1

37.80 Insertion of permanent pacemaker, initial or replacement, type of device not specified

---

[10] Valid OR procedure code if accompanied by one of the following codes: 37.80, 37.81, 37.82, 37.85, 37.86, 37.87
[11] Valid OR procedure code if accompanied by one of the following codes: 37.80, 37.83
[12] Valid OR procedure code if accompanied by one of the following codes: 37.80, 37.85, 37.86, 37.87
[13] Valid OR procedure code if accompanied by one of the following codes: 37.80, 37.81, 37.82, 37.83, 37.85, 37.86, 37.87

OPERATIONS ON THE CARDIOVASCULAR SYSTEM

37.81 Initial insertion of single-chamber device, not specified as rate responsive
  EXCLUDES: replacement of existing pacemaker device (37.85-37.87)

37.82 Initial insertion of a single-chamber device, rate responsive
  Rate responsive to physiologic stimuli other than atrial rate
  EXCLUDES: replacement of existing pacemaker device (37.85-37.87)

37.83 Initial insertion of dual-chamber device
  Atrial ventricular sequential device
  EXCLUDES: replacement of existing pacemaker device (37.85-37.87)
  AHA: 2Q, '97, 4

37.85 Replacement of any type pacemaker device with single-chamber device, not specified as rate responsive

37.86 Replacement of any type pacemaker device with single-chamber device, rate responsive
  Rate responsive to physiologic stimuli other than atrial rate

37.87 Replacement of any type pacemaker device with dual-chamber device
  Atrial ventricular sequential device

37.89 Revision or removal of pacemaker device
  ▶Removal without replacement of cardiac resynchronization pacemaker device [CRT-P]◀
  Repair of pacemaker device
  EXCLUDES: removal of temporary transvenous pacemaker system — omit code
  replacement of existing pacemaker device (37.85-37.87)
  ▶replacement of existing pacemaker device with CRT-P pacemaker device (00.53)◀
  AHA: N-D, '86, 1

✓4ᵗʰ 37.9 Other operations on heart and pericardium
  AHA: 3Q, '90, 11

  37.91 Open chest cardiac massage
    EXCLUDES: closed chest cardiac massage (99.63)
    AHA: 4Q, '88, 12
    DEF: Massage of heart through opening in chest wall to reinstate or maintain circulation.

  37.92 Injection of therapeutic substance into heart

Automatic Implantable Cardioverter/Defibrillator

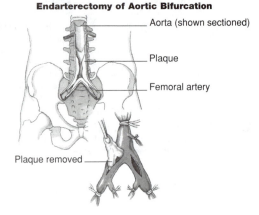

Endarterectomy of Aortic Bifurcation

37.93 Injection of therapeutic substance into pericardium

37.94 Implantation or replacement of automatic cardioverter/defibrillator, total system [AICD]
  Implantation of defibrillator with leads (epicardial patches), formation of pocket (abdominal fascia) (subcutaneous), any transvenous leads, intraoperative procedures for evaluation of lead signals, and obtaining defibrillator threshold measurements
  Techniques: lateral thoracotomy
    medial sternotomy
    subxiphoid procedure
  Code also extracorporeal circulation, if performed (39.61)
  Code also any concomitant procedure [e.g., coronary bypass] (36.01-36.19)
  EXCLUDES ▶ implantation of cardiac resynchronization defibrillator, total system [CRT-D] (00.51) ◀
  AHA: 3Q, '01, 5-7; 3Q, '99, 12; 1Q, '99, 3; 3Q, '90, 11; S-O, '87, 5
  DEF: Direct insertion, of defibrillator/cardioverter system to deliver shock and restore heart rhythm.

37.95 Implantation of automatic cardioverter/defibrillator lead(s) only
  AHA: 3Q, '90, 11

37.96 Implantation of automatic cardioverter/defibrillator pulse generator only
  EXCLUDES ▶ implantation or replacement of cardiac resynchronization defibrillator, pulse generator device only [CRT-D] (00.54)◀
  AHA: 3Q, '90, 11

37.97 Replacement of automatic cardioverter/defibrillator lead(s) only
  AHA: 3Q, '90, 11

37.98 Replacement of automatic cardioverter/defibrillator pulse generator only
  AHA: 1Q, '99, 3; 3Q, '90, 11
  EXCLUDES ▶ replacement of cardiac resynchronization defibrillator, pulse generator device only [CRT-D] (00.54)◀

---

¹⁴ Valid OR procedure code if accompanied by one of the following codes: 37.72, 37.76
¹⁵ Valid OR procedure code if accompanied by one of the following codes: 37.70, 37.71, 37.73, 37.76

OPERATIONS ON THE CARDIOVASCULAR SYSTEM

37.99 Other
Removal of cardioverter/defibrillator pulse generator only without replacement
▶Removal without replacement of cardiac resynchronization defibrillator device [CRT-D]◀
Repositioning of lead(s) (sensing) (pacing) [electrode]
Repositioning of pulse generator
Revision of cardioverter/defibrillator (automatic) pocket
▶Revision or relocation of CRT-D pocket◀
EXCLUDES cardiac retraining (93.36)
conversion of cardiac rhythm (99.60-99.69)
AHA: 1Q, '97, 12; 1Q, '94, 19; 3Q, '90, 11; 1Q, '89, 11

38 Incision, excision, and occlusion of vessels
▶Code also any application or administration of an adhesion barrier substance (99.77)◀
Code also cardiopulmonary bypass [extracorporeal circulation] [heart-lung machine] (39.61)
EXCLUDES that of coronary vessels (36.01-36.99)

The following fourth-digit subclassification is for use with appropriate categories in section 38.0, 38.1, 38.3, 38.5, 38.6, and 38.8 according to site. Valid fourth-digits are in [brackets] under each code.

0 **unspecified**
1 **intracranial vessels**
  Cerebral (anterior) (middle)
  Circle of Willis
  Posterior communicating artery
2 **other vessels of head and neck**
  Carotid artery (common) (external) (internal)
  Jugular vein (external) (internal)
3 **upper limb vessels**
  Axillary   Radial
  Brachial   Ulnar
4 **aorta**
5 **other thoracic vessels**
  Innominate   Vena cava, superior
  Pulmonary (artery) (vein)
  Subclavian
6 **abdominal arteries**
  Celiac   Mesenteric
  Gastric   Renal
  Hepatic   Splenic
  Iliac   Umbilical
  EXCLUDES abdominal aorta (4)
7 **abdominal veins**
  Iliac   Splenic
  Portal   Vena cava (inferior)
  Renal
8 **lower limb arteries**
  Femoral (common) (superficial)
  Popliteal
  Tibial
9 **lower limb veins**
  Femoral   Saphenous
  Popliteal   Tibial

38.0 Incision of vessel [0-9]
Embolectomy
Thrombectomy
EXCLUDES puncture or catheterization of any:
artery (38.91, 38.98)
vein (38.92-38.95, 38.99)
AHA: 2Q, '98, 23
DEF: Incision into vessel to remove mobile or stationary blood clot.

38.1 Endarterectomy [0-6,8]
Endarterectomy with:
  embolectomy
  patch graft
  temporary bypass during procedure
  thrombectomy
AHA: 1Q, '00, 16; 2Q, '99, 5; 2Q, '95, 16; ▶For code 38.12: 1Q, '02, 10◀
DEF: Excision of tunica intima of artery to relieve arterial walls thickened by plaque or chronic inflammation.

38.2 Diagnostic procedures on blood vessels
38.21 Biopsy of blood vessel
38.22 Percutaneous angioscopy
EXCLUDES angioscopy of eye (95.12)
38.29 Other diagnostic procedures on blood vessels
EXCLUDES blood vessel thermography (88.86)
circulatory monitoring (89.61-89.69)
contrast:
  angiocardiography (88.50-88.58)
  arteriography (88.40-88.49)
  phlebography (88.60-88.67)
impedance phlebography (88.68)
peripheral vascular ultrasonography (88.77)
plethysmogram (89.58)
AHA: 3Q, '00, 16; 1Q, '99, 7
DEF: Exam, with fiberoptic catheter inserted through peripheral artery to visualize inner lining of blood vessels.

38.3 Resection of vessel with anastomosis [0-9]
Angiectomy
Excision of:
  aneurysm (arteriovenous)   } with anastomosis
  blood vessel (lesion)
DEF: Reconstruction and reconnection of vessel after partial excision.

Methods of Vessel Anastomoses

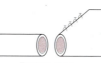
End-to-end

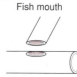
Side-to-side

Oblique cut

Fish mouth

Funnelization

End-to-side

---

§ Requires fourth-digit. Valid digits are in [brackets] under each code. See category 38 for definitions.
[16] Nonspecific OR procedure = 0

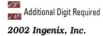

OPERATIONS ON THE CARDIOVASCULAR SYSTEM

38.4–38.94

§§ ✓4th 16 **38.4** **Resection of vessel with replacement**
[0-9]   Angiectomy
        Excision of:
            aneurysm
                (arteriovenous) or } with replacement
                blood vessel
                (lesion)

EXCLUDES endovascular repair of aneurysm (39.71-39.79)

Requires the use of one of the following fourth-digit subclassifications to identify site:

0 **unspecified site**
1 **intracranial vessels**
    Cerebral (anterior) (middle)
    Circle of Willis
    Posterior communicating artery
2 **other vessels of head and neck**
    Carotid artery (common) (external) (internal)
    Jugular vein (external) (internal)
3 **upper limb vessels**
    Axillary   Radial
    Brachial   Ulnar
4 **aorta, abdominal**
    Code also any thoracic vessel involvement
        (thoracoabdominal procedure) (38.45)
5 **thoracic vessel**
    Aorta (thoracic)
    Innominate   Subclavian
    Pulmonary (artery) (vein) Vena cava, superior
    Code also any abdominal aorta involvement
        (thoracoabdominal procedure) (38.44)
6 **abdominal arteries**
    Celiac   Mesenteric
    Gastric   Renal
    Hepatic   Splenic
    Iliac   Umbilical
    EXCLUDES abdominal aorta (4)
7 **abdominal veins**
    Iliac   Splenic
    Portal   Vena cava (inferior)
    Renal
8 **lower limb arteries**
    Femoral (common) (superficial)
    Tibial
9 **lower limb veins**
    Femoral   Saphenous
    Popliteal   Tibial

AHA: 2Q, '99, 5, 6

DEF: Excision of aneurysm (arteriovenous): Excision and replacement of segment of stretched or bulging blood vessel.

DEF: Excision of blood vessel (lesion): Excision and replacement of segment of vessel containing lesion.

§ ✓4th 16 **38.5** **Ligation and stripping of varicose veins**
[0-3,5,7,9]   **EXCLUDES** ligation of varices:
                esophageal (42.91)
                gastric (44.91)

AHA: For code 38.59: 2Q, '97, 7

DEF: Ligation of varicose veins: Typing off vein with thread or wire to eliminate blood flow; stripping involves excising length of vein.

§ ✓4th 16 **38.6** **Other excision of vessels**
[0-9]   Excision of blood vessel (lesion) NOS
        EXCLUDES excision of vessel for aortocoronary bypass (36.10-36.14)
            excision with:
                anastomosis (38.30-38.39)
                graft replacement (38.40-38.49)
                implant (38.40-38.49)

AHA: 3Q, '90, 17

38.7 **Interruption of the vena cava**
    Insertion of implant or sieve in vena cava
    Ligation of vena cava (inferior) (superior)
    Plication of vena cava

AHA: 2Q, '94, 9; S-O, '85, 5

DEF: Interruption of the blood flow through the venous heart vessels to prevent clots from reaching the chambers of the heart by means of implanting a sieve or implant, separating off a portion or by narrowing the venous blood vessels.

§ ✓4th 16 **38.8** **Other surgical occlusion of vessels**
[0-9]   Clamping
        Division
        Ligation   } of blood vessel
        Occlusion

EXCLUDES adrenal vessels (07.43)
    esophageal varices (42.91)
    gastric or duodenal vessel for ulcer (44.40-44.49)
    gastric varices (44.91)
    meningeal vessel (02.13)
    percutaneous transcatheter infusion embolization (99.29)
    spermatic vein for varicocele (63.1)
    surgical occlusion of vena cava (38.7)
    that for chemoembolization (99.25)
    that for control of (postoperative) hemorrhage:
        anus (49.95)
        bladder (57.93)
        following vascular procedure (39.41)
        nose (21.00-21.09)
        prostate (60.94)
        tonsil (28.7)
        thyroid vessel (06.92)

AHA: 2Q, '90, 23; M-A, '87, 9; For code 38.86: N-D, '87, 4

✓4th **38.9** **Puncture of vessel**
    EXCLUDES that for circulatory monitoring ▶(89.60-89.69)◀

38.91 **Arterial catheterization**
    AHA: 1Q, '97, 3; 1Q, '95, 3; 2Q, '91, 15; 2Q, '90, 23

38.92 **Umbilical vein catheterization**

38.93 **Venous catheterization, not elsewhere classified**
    EXCLUDES that for cardiac catheterization (37.21-37.23)
        that for renal dialysis (38.95)

AHA: 3Q, '00, 9; 2Q, '98, 24; 1Q, '96, 3; 2Q, '96, 15; 3Q, '91, 13; 4Q, '90, 14; 2Q, '90, 24; 3Q, '88, 13

38.94 **Venous cutdown**
    DEF: Incision of vein to place needle or catheter.

Typical Venous Cutdown

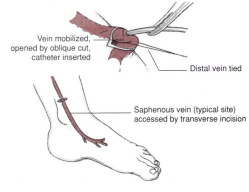

Vein mobilized, opened by oblique cut, catheter inserted

Distal vein tied

Saphenous vein (typical site) accessed by transverse incision

---

§ Requires fourth-digit. Valid digits are in [brackets] under each code. See category 38 for definitions.
§§ Requires fourth-digit. Valid digits are in [brackets] under each code. See subcategory 38.4 for definitions.
16 Nonspecific OR procedure = 0

BI Bilateral Edit   **NC** Non-covered Procedure   ▶◀ Revised Text   ● New Code   ▲ Revised Code Title

122 — Volume 3 • October 2002   2002 Ingenix, Inc.

OPERATIONS ON THE CARDIOVASCULAR SYSTEM

38.95 **Venous catheterization for renal dialysis**
  EXCLUDES: *insertion of totally implantable vascular access device [VAD] (86.07)*
  AHA: 3Q, '98, 13; 2Q, '94, 11

38.98 **Other puncture of artery**
  EXCLUDES: *that for:*
  arteriography (88.40-88.49)
  coronary arteriography (88.55-88.57)

38.99 **Other puncture of vein**
  Phlebotomy
  EXCLUDES: *that for:*
  angiography (88.60-88.68)
  extracorporeal circulation (39.61, 50.92)
  injection or infusion of:
  sclerosing solution (39.92)
  therapeutic or prophylactic substance (99.11-99.29)
  perfusion (39.96, 39.97)
  phlebography (88.60-88.68)
  transfusion (99.01-99.09)
  AHA: 4Q, '94, 50; 1Q, '88, 11

√3rd 39 Other operations on vessels
  EXCLUDES: *those on coronary vessels (36.0-36.99)*

39.0 **Systemic to pulmonary artery shunt**
  Descending aorta-pulmonary artery
  Left to right } anastomosis (graft)
  Subclavian-pulmonary

  Code also cardiopulmonary bypass [extracorporeal circulation] [heart-lung machine] (39.61)

  DEF: Descending aorta-pulmonary artery anastomosis (graft): Connection of descending main heart artery to pulmonary artery.

  DEF: Left to right anastomosis (graft): Connection of systemic arterial blood vessel to venous pulmonary system.

  DEF: Subclavian-pulmonary anastomosis (graft): Connection of subclavian artery to pulmonary artery

39.1 **Intra-abdominal venous shunt**
  Anastomosis:
    mesocaval
    portacaval
    portal vein to inferior vena cava
    splenic and renal veins
    transjugular intrahepatic portosystemic shunt [TIPS]
  EXCLUDES: *peritoneovenous shunt (54.94)*
  AHA: 4Q, '94, 50; 4Q, '93, 31; 2Q, '93, 8

  DEF: Connection of two venous blood vessels within abdominal cavity.

√4th 39.2 Other shunt or vascular bypass
  DEF: Creation of supplemental blood flow to area with inadequate blood supply due to disease or injury of vessels.

  39.21 **Caval-pulmonary artery anastomosis**
    Code also cardiopulmonary bypass (39.61)
  39.22 **Aorta-subclavian-carotid bypass**
    Bypass (arterial):
      aorta to carotid and brachial
      aorta to subclavian and carotid
      carotid to subclavian
  39.23 **Other intrathoracic vascular shunt or bypass**
    Intrathoracic (arterial) bypass graft NOS
    EXCLUDES: *coronary artery bypass (36.10-36.19)*
  39.24 **Aorta-renal bypass**

  39.25 **Aorta-iliac-femoral bypass**
    Bypass:
      aortofemoral
      aortoiliac
      aortoiliac to popliteal
      aortopopliteal
      iliofemoral [iliac-femoral]
    AHA: 4Q, '90, 27; 1Q, '88, 10

  39.26 **Other intra-abdominal vascular shunt or bypass**
    Bypass:
      aortoceliac
      aortic-superior mesenteric
      common hepatic-common iliac-renal
      Intra-abdominal arterial bypass graft NOS
    EXCLUDES: *peritoneovenous shunt (54.94)*

  39.27 **Arteriovenostomy for renal dialysis**
    Anastomosis for renal dialysis
    Formation of (peripheral) arteriovenous fistula for renal [kidney] dialysis
    Code also any renal dialysis (39.95)

  39.28 **Extracranial-intracranial (EC-IC) vascular bypass** NC
    AHA: 2Q, '92, 7; 4Q, '91, 22

  39.29 **Other (peripheral) vascular shunt or bypass**
    Bypass (graft):
      axillary-brachial
      axillary-femoral [axillofemoral] (superficial)
      brachial
      femoral-femoral
      femoroperoneal
      femoropopliteal (arteries)
      femorotibial (anterior) (posterior)
      popliteal
      vascular NOS
    EXCLUDES: *peritoneovenous shunt (54.94)*
    AHA: ▶1Q, '02, 13;◀ S-O, '85, 13

√4th 39.3 Suture of vessel
  Repair of laceration of blood vessel
  EXCLUDES: *any other vascular puncture closure device — omit code*
  suture of aneurysm (39.52)
  that for control of hemorrhage (postoperative):
    anus (49.95)
    bladder (57.93)
    following vascular procedure (39.41)
    nose (21.00-21.09)
    prostate (60.94)
    tonsil (28.7)

  39.30 **Suture of unspecified blood vessel**
  39.31 **Suture of artery**
  39.32 **Suture of vein**

√4th 39.4 Revision of vascular procedure
  39.41 **Control of hemorrhage following vascular surgery**
    EXCLUDES: *that for control of hemorrhage (postoperative):*
    anus (49.95)
    bladder (57.93)
    nose (21.00-21.09)
    prostate (60.94)
    tonsil (28.7)

OPERATIONS ON THE CARDIOVASCULAR SYSTEM — 39.42–39.59 — Tabular List

39.42 Revision of arteriovenous shunt for renal dialysis
Conversion of renal dialysis:
  end-to-end anastomosis to end-to-side
  end-to-side anastomosis to end-to-end
  vessel-to-vessel cannula to arteriovenous shunt
Removal of old arteriovenous shunt and creation of new shunt

EXCLUDES: replacement of vessel-to-vessel cannula (39.94)

AHA: 2Q, '94, 15; 4Q, '93, 33

39.43 Removal of arteriovenous shunt for renal dialysis

EXCLUDES: that with replacement [revision] of shunt (39.42)

39.49 Other revision of vascular procedure
Declotting (graft)
Revision of:
  anastomosis of blood vessel
  vascular procedure (previous)

AHA: 2Q, '98, 17; 1Q, '97, 3; 2Q, '94, 15

DEF: Declotting (graft): Removal of clot from graft.

√4th 39.5 Other repair of vessels

39.50 Angioplasty or atherectomy of non-coronary vessel
Code also any:
  Insertion of non-coronary stent(s) or stent graft(s) (39.90)
  Injection or infusion of thrombolytic agent (99.10)
Percutaneous transluminal angioplasty (PTA) of non-coronary vessels:
  head and neck arteries:
    basilar
    carotid
    vertebral
  lower extremity vessels
  mesenteric artery
  renal artery
  upper extremity vessels

AHA: 1Q, '02, 13; 2Q, '01, 23; 2Q, '00, 10; 1Q, '00, 12; 2Q, '98, 17; 1Q, '97, 3; 4Q, '96, 63; 4Q, '95, 66

39.51 Clipping of aneurysm

EXCLUDES: clipping of arteriovenous fistula (39.53)

39.52 Other repair of aneurysm
Repair of aneurysm by:
  coagulation
  electrocoagulation
  filipuncture
  methyl methacrylate
  suture
  wiring
  wrapping

EXCLUDES: endovascular repair of aneurysm (39.71-39.79)
  re-entry operation (aorta) (39.54)
  that with:
    graft replacement (38.40-38.49)
    resection (38.30-38.49, 38.60-38.69)

AHA: 1Q, '99, 15, 16, 17; 1Q, '88, 10

DEF: Application of device in abnormally stretched blood vessel to prevent movement of material collected in vessel.

DEF: Repair of aneurysm by: Coagulation: Clotting or solidifying. Electrocoagulation: Electrically produced clotting. Filipuncture: Insertion of wire or thread. Methyl methacrylate: Injection or insertion of plastic material. Suture: Stitching. Wiring: Insertion of wire. Wrapping: Compression.

39.53 Repair of arteriovenous fistula
Embolization of carotid cavernous fistula
Repair of arteriovenous fistula by:
  clipping
  coagulation
  ligation and division

EXCLUDES: repair of:
  arteriovenous shunt for renal dialysis (39.42)
  ▶head and neck vessels, endovascular approach (39.72)◀
  that with:
    graft replacement (38.40-38.49)
    resection (38.30-38.49, 38.60-38.69)

AHA: 1Q, '00, 8

DEF: Correction of arteriovenous fistula by application of clamps, causing coagulation or by tying off and dividing the connection.

39.54 Re-entry operation (aorta)
Fenestration of dissecting aneurysm of thoracic aorta
Code also cardiopulmonary bypass [extracorporeal circulation] [heart-lung machine] (39.61)

DEF: Re-entry operation: Creation of passage between stretched wall of the vessel and major arterial channel to heart.

DEF: Fenestration of dissecting aneurysm of thoracic aorta: Creation of passage between stretched arterial heart vessel and functional part of vessel.

39.55 Reimplantation of aberrant renal vessel

DEF: Reimplant of renal vessel into normal position.

39.56 Repair of blood vessel with tissue patch graft

EXCLUDES: that with resection (38.40-38.49)

39.57 Repair of blood vessel with synthetic patch graft

EXCLUDES: that with resection (38.40-38.49)

39.58 Repair of blood vessel with unspecified type of patch graft

EXCLUDES: that with resection (38.40-38.49)

39.59 Other repair of vessel
Aorticopulmonary window operation
Arterioplasty NOS
Construction of venous valves (peripheral)
Plication of vein (peripheral)
Reimplantation of artery
Code also cardiopulmonary bypass [extracorporeal circulation] [heart-lung machine] (39.61)

EXCLUDES: interruption of the vena cava (38.7)
  reimplantation of renal artery (39.55)
  that with:
    graft (39.56-39.58)
    resection (38.30-38.49, 38.60-38.69)

AHA: 4Q, '93, 31; 2Q, '89, 17; N-D, '86, 8; S-O, '85, 5; M-A, '85, 15

DEF: Aorticopulmonary window operation: Repair of abnormal opening between major heart arterial vessel above valves and pulmonary artery.

DEF: Construction of venous valves (peripheral): Reconstruction of valves within peripheral veins.

DEF: Plication of vein (peripheral): Shortening of peripheral vein.

DEF: Reimplantation of artery: Reinsertion of artery into its normal position.

OPERATIONS ON THE CARDIOVASCULAR SYSTEM 39.6–39.8

39.6 Extracorporeal circulation and procedures auxiliary to heart surgery
AHA: 1Q, '95, 5

39.61 Extracorporeal circulation auxiliary to open heart surgery
Artificial heart and lung
Cardiopulmonary bypass
Pump oxygenator

EXCLUDES
  extracorporeal hepatic assistance (50.92)
  extracorporeal membrane oxygenation [ECMO] (39.65)
  hemodialysis (39.95)
  percutaneous cardiopulmonary bypass (39.66)

AHA: 4Q, '97, 55; 3Q, '97, 14; 2Q, '97, 8; 2Q, '90, 24

39.62 Hypothermia (systemic) incidental to open heart surgery

39.63 Cardioplegia
Arrest:
  anoxic
  circulatory

DEF: Purposely inducing electromechanical cardiac arrest.

39.64 Intraoperative cardiac pacemaker
Temporary pacemaker used during and immediately following cardiac surgery

AHA: 1Q, '89, 2; M-J, '87, 3

39.65 Extracorporeal membrane oxygenation [ECMO]

EXCLUDES
  extracorporeal circulation auxiliary to open heart surgery (39.61)
  percutaneous cardiopulmonary bypass (39.66)

AHA: 2Q, '90, 23; 2Q, '89, 17; 4Q, '88, 5

DEF: Creation of closed-chest, heart-lung bypass or Bard cardiopulmonary assist system with tube insertion.

39.66 Percutaneous cardiopulmonary bypass
Closed chest

EXCLUDES
  extracorporeal circulation auxiliary to open heart surgery (39.61)
  extracorporeal hepatic assistance (50.92)
  extracorporeal membrane oxygenation [ECMO] (39.65)
  hemodialysis (39.95)

AHA: 3Q, '96, 11

DEF: Use of mechanical pump system to oxygenate and pump blood throughout the body via catheter in the femoral artery and vein.

39.7 Endovascular repair of vessel
Endoluminal repair

EXCLUDES
  angioplasty or atherectomy of non-coronary vessel (39.50)
  insertion of non-coronary stent or stents (39.90)
  other repair of aneurysm (39.52)
  resection of abdominal aorta with replacement (38.44)
  resection of lower limb arteries with replacement (38.48)
  resection of thoracic aorta with replacement (38.45)
  resection of upper limb vessels with replacement (38.43)

39.71 Endovascular implantation of graft in abdominal aorta
Endovascular repair of abdominal aortic aneurysm with graft
Stent graft(s)

AHA: ▶1Q, '02, 13;◀ 4Q, '00, 63, 64

DEF: Replacement of a section of abdominal aorta with mesh graft; via catheters inserted through femoral arteries.

39.72 Endovascular repair or occlusion of head and neck vessels
Coil embolization or occlusion
Endograft(s)
Endovascular graft(s)
Liquid tissue adhesive (glue) embolization or occlusion
Other implant or substance for repair, embolization or occlusion
That for repair of aneurysm, arteriovenous malformation [AVM] or fistula

39.79 Other endovascular repair of aneurysm of other vessels
▶Coil embolization or occlusion
Endograft(s)
Endovascular graft(s)
Liquid tissue adhesive (glue) embolization or occlusion
Other implant or substance for repair, embolization or occlusion◀

EXCLUDES ▶endovascular repair or occlusion of head and neck vessels (39.72)
  insertion of drug-eluting non-coronary artery stent(s) (00.55)
  insertion of non-coronary artery stent(s) (for other than aneurysm repair) (39.90)
  non-endovascular repair of arteriovenous fistula (39.53)
  other surgical occlusion of vessels–see category 38.8
  percutaneous transcatheter infusion (99.29)
  transcatheter embolization for gastric or duodenal bleeding (44.44)◀

AHA: 3Q, '01, 17,18; 4Q, '00, 64

39.8 Operations on carotid body and other vascular bodies
Chemodectomy   Glomectomy, carotid
Denervation of: Implantation into carotid body:
  aortic body   electronic stimulator
  carotid body   pacemaker

EXCLUDES excision of glomus jugulare (20.51)

DEF: Chemodectomy: Removal of a chemoreceptor vascular body.

DEF: Denervation of aortic body: Destruction of nerves attending the major heart blood vessels.

DEF: Destruction of carotid body: Destruction of nerves of carotid artery.

DEF: Glomectomy, carotid: Removal of the carotid artery framework.

Endovascular Repair of Abdominal Aortic Aneurysm

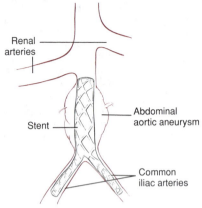

External Arteriovenous Shunt

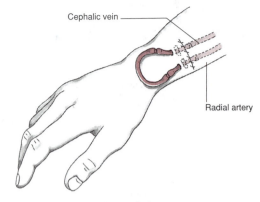

- ✓4th **39.9 Other operations on vessels**
  - **39.90 Insertion of non-drug-eluting, non-coronary artery stent(s)**
    - ▶Bare stent(s)
    - Bonded stent(s)
    - Drug-coated stent(s), i.e., heparin coated
    - Endograft(s)
    - Endovascular graft(s)◀
    - Endovascular recanalization techniques
    - Stent graft(s)
    - Code also any:
      - non-coronary angioplasty or atherectomy (39.50)
    - *EXCLUDES* ▶insertion of drug-eluting, non-coronary artery stent(s) (00.55)◀
      - *that for aneurysm repair (39.71-39.79)*
    - AHA: 1Q, '00, 12; 4Q, '96, 63

  - **39.91 Freeing of vessel**
    - Dissection and freeing of adherent tissue:
      - artery-vein-nerve bundle
      - vascular bundle

  - **39.92 Injection of sclerosing agent into vein**
    - *EXCLUDES* injection:
      - *esophageal varices (42.33)*
      - *hemorrhoids (49.42)*
    - AHA: 2Q, '92, 17

  - **39.93 Insertion of vessel-to-vessel cannula**
    - Formation of:
      - arteriovenous:
        - fistula } by external
        - shunt   } cannula
    - Code also any renal dialysis (39.95)
    - AHA: 3Q, '88, 13; S-O, '85, 5 & 12

  - **39.94 Replacement of vessel-to-vessel cannula**
    - Revision of vessel-to-vessel cannula

  - **39.95 Hemodialysis**
    - Artificial kidney   Hemodiafiltration
    - Hemofiltration   Renal dialysis
    - *EXCLUDES* *peritoneal dialysis (54.98)*
    - AHA: 2Q, '01, 2-14; 4Q, '00, 40; 2Q, '98, 20; S-O, '86, 11
    - **DEF:** Filtration process to treats acute and chronic renal failure by eliminating toxic end products of nitrogen metabolism from blood.

  - **39.96 Total body perfusion**
    - Code also substance perfused (99.21-99.29)

  - **39.97 Other perfusion**
    - Perfusion NOS   Perfusion, local
    - Perfusion, local   [regional] of:
      - [regional] of: lower limb
      - carotid artery   neck
      - coronary artery   upper limb
      - head
    - Code also substance perfused (99.21-99.29)
    - *EXCLUDES* *perfusion of:*
      - *kidney (55.95)*
      - *large intestine (46.96)*
      - *liver (50.93)*
      - *small intestine (46.95)*
    - AHA: 3Q, '96, 11

  - **39.98 Control of hemorrhage, not otherwise specified**
    - Angiotripsy
    - Control of postoperative hemorrhage NOS
    - Venotripsy
    - *EXCLUDES* *control of hemorrhage (postoperative):*
      - *anus (49.95)*
      - *bladder (57.93)*
      - *following vascular procedure (39.41)*
      - *nose (21.00-21.09)*
      - *prostate (60.94)*
      - *tonsil (28.7)*
      - *that by:*
        - *ligation (38.80-38.89)*
        - *suture (39.30-39.32)*
    - **DEF:** Angiotripsy: Clamping of tissue to stop arterial blood flow.
    - **DEF:** Venotripsy: Clamping of tissue to stop venous blood flow.

  - **39.99 Other operations on vessels**
    - *EXCLUDES* *injection or infusion of therapeutic or prophylactic substance (99.11-99.29)*
      - *transfusion of blood and blood components (99.01-99.09)*
    - AHA: 1Q, '89, 11

8. OPERATIONS ON THE HEMIC AND LYMPHATIC SYSTEM (40-41)

√3rd **40 Operations on lymphatic system**

40.0 Incision of lymphatic structures

√4th **40.1 Diagnostic procedures on lymphatic structures**

40.11 Biopsy of lymphatic structure

40.19 Other diagnostic procedures on lymphatic structures

EXCLUDES lymphangiogram:
abdominal (88.04)
cervical (87.08)
intrathoracic (87.34)
lower limb (88.36)
upper limb (88.34)
microscopic examination of specimen (90.71-90.79)
radioisotope scan (92.16)
thermography (88.89)

√4th **40.2 Simple excision of lymphatic structure**

EXCLUDES biopsy of lymphatic structure (40.11)

DEF: Removal of lymphatic structure only.

40.21 Excision of deep cervical lymph node
AHA: 4Q, '99, 16

40.22 Excision of internal mammary lymph node

40.23 Excision of axillary lymph node

40.24 Excision of inguinal lymph node

40.29 Simple excision of other lymphatic structure
Excision of:
cystic hygroma
lymphangioma
Simple lymphadenectomy
AHA: 1Q, '99, 6

DEF: Lymphangioma: Removal of benign congenital lymphatic malformation.

DEF: Simple lymphadenectomy: Removal of lymph node.

40.3 Regional lymph node excision
Extended regional lymph node excision
Regional lymph node excision with excision of lymphatic drainage area including skin, subcutaneous tissue, and fat
AHA: 2Q, '92, 7

DEF: Extended regional lymph node excision: Removal of lymph node group, including area around nodes.

√4th **40.4 Radical excision of cervical lymph nodes**
Resection of cervical lymph nodes down to muscle and deep fascia
EXCLUDES that associated with radical laryngectomy (30.4)

40.40 Radical neck dissection, not otherwise specified

40.41 Radical neck dissection, unilateral
AHA: 2Q, '99, 6

DEF: Dissection, total, of cervical lymph nodes on one side of neck.

40.42 Radical neck dissection, bilateral
DEF: Dissection, total, of cervical lymph nodes on both sides of neck.

√4th **40.5 Radical excision of other lymph nodes**
EXCLUDES that associated with radical mastectomy (85.45-85.48)

40.50 Radical excision of lymph nodes, not otherwise specified
Radical (lymph) node dissection NOS

40.51 Radical excision of axillary lymph nodes

40.52 Radical excision of periaortic lymph nodes

40.53 Radical excision of iliac lymph nodes

40.54 Radical groin dissection

40.59 Radical excision of other lymph nodes
EXCLUDES radical neck dissection (40.40-40.42)

√4th **40.6 Operations on thoracic duct**

40.61 Cannulation of thoracic duct
DEF: Placement of cannula in main lymphatic duct of chest.

40.62 Fistulization of thoracic duct
DEF: Creation of passage in main lymphatic duct of chest.

40.63 Closure of fistula of thoracic duct
DEF: Closure of fistula in main lymphatic duct of chest.

40.64 Ligation of thoracic duct
DEF: Tying off main lymphatic duct of chest.

40.69 Other operations on thoracic duct

40.9 Other operations on lymphatic structures
Anastomosis
Dilation
Ligation
Obliteration } of peripheral lymphatics
Reconstruction
Repair
Transplantation

Correction of lymphedema of limb, NOS
EXCLUDES reduction of elephantiasis of scrotum (61.3)

√3rd **41 Operations on bone marrow and spleen**

√4th **41.0 Bone marrow or hematopoietic stem cell transplant**
EXCLUDES aspiration of bone marrow from donor (41.91)
AHA: 4Q, '00, 64; 1Q, '91, 3; 4Q, '91, 26

41.00 Bone marrow transplant, not otherwise specified NC

[17] **41.01 Autologous bone marrow transplant without purging** NC
EXCLUDES that with purging (41.09)
DEF: Transplant of patient's own bone marrow.

[18] **41.02 Allogeneic bone marrow transplant with purging** NC
Allograft of bone marrow with in vitro removal (purging) of T-cells
DEF: Transplant of bone marrow from donor to patient after donor marrow purged of undesirable cells.

[18] **41.03 Allogeneic bone marrow transplant without purging** NC
Allograft of bone marrow NOS

[17] **41.04 Autologous hematopoietic stem cell transplant without purging** NC
EXCLUDES that with purging (41.07)
AHA: 4Q, '94, 52

[18] **41.05 Allogeneic hematopoietic stem cell transplant without purging** NC
EXCLUDES that with purging (41.08)
AHA: 4Q, '97, 55

---

[17] Covered procedure only when any of the following codes are present as either principal or secondary diagnosis: 200.00-202.8, 202.80-202.98, 204.01, 205.01, 206.01, 207.01, 208.01

[18] Covered procedure only when any of the following codes are present as either principal or secondary diagnosis: 204.00-208.91, 279.12, 279.2, 284.0-284.9

√3rd / √4th Additional Digit Required · Nonspecific OR Procedure · Valid OR Procedure · Non-OR Procedure

OPERATIONS ON HEMIC AND LYMPHATIC SYSTEMS

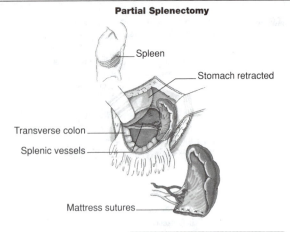

Partial Splenectomy / **Total Splenectomy**

[18] **41.06 Cord blood stem cell transplant** NC
AHA: 4Q, '97, 56

[17] **41.07 Autologous hematopoietic stem cell transplant with purging** NC
Cell depletion

[18] **41.08 Allogeneic hematopoietic stem cell transplant with purging** NC
Cell depletion

[17] **41.09 Autologous bone marrow transplant with purging** NC
With extracorporeal purging of malignant cells from marrow
Cell depletion

41.1 Puncture of spleen
EXCLUDES   aspiration biopsy of spleen (41.32)

41.2 Splenotomy

√4th **41.3 Diagnostic procedures on bone marrow and spleen**

41.31 Biopsy of bone marrow

41.32 Closed [aspiration] [percutaneous] biopsy of spleen
Needle biopsy of spleen

41.33 Open biopsy of spleen

41.38 Other diagnostic procedures on bone marrow
EXCLUDES   microscopic examination of specimen from bone marrow (90.61-90.69)
radioisotope scan (92.05)

41.39 Other diagnostic procedures on spleen
EXCLUDES   microscopic examination of specimen from spleen (90.61-90.69)
radioisotope scan (92.05)

√4th **41.4 Excision or destruction of lesion or tissue of spleen**
▶Code also any application or administration of an adhesion barrier substance (99.77)◀
EXCLUDES   excision of accessory spleen (41.93)

41.41 Marsupialization of splenic cyst
DEF: Incision of cyst of spleen with edges sutured open to create pouch.

41.42 Excision of lesion or tissue of spleen
EXCLUDES   biopsy of spleen (41.32-41.33)

41.43 Partial splenectomy
DEF: Removal of spleen, partial.

41.5 Total splenectomy
Splenectomy NOS
▶Code also any application or administration of an adhesion barrier substance (99.77)◀

√4th **41.9 Other operations on spleen and bone marrow**
▶Code also any application or administration of an adhesion barrier substance (99.77)◀

41.91 Aspiration of bone marrow from donor for transplant
EXCLUDES   biopsy of bone marrow (41.31)
AHA: 1Q, '91, 3

41.92 Injection into bone marrow
EXCLUDES   bone marrow transplant (41.00-41.03)
AHA: 3Q, '96, 17

41.93 Excision of accessory spleen
41.94 Transplantation of spleen
41.95 Repair and plastic operations on spleen
41.98 Other operations on bone marrow
41.99 Other operations on spleen

---

[17] Covered procedure only when any of the following codes are present as either principal or secondary diagnosis: 200.00-202.8, 202.80-202.98, 204.01, 205.01, 206.01, 207.01, 208.01
[18] Covered procedure only when any of the following codes are present as either principal or secondary diagnosis: 204.00-208.91, 279.12, 279.2, 284.0-284.9

9. OPERATIONS ON THE DIGESTIVE SYSTEM (42-54)

42 Operations on esophagus

42.0 Esophagotomy

42.01 Incision of esophageal web
DEF: Cutting into congenital esophageal membrane.

42.09 Other incision of esophagus
Esophagotomy NOS
EXCLUDES: *esophagomyotomy (42.7)*
esophagostomy (42.10-42.19)

42.1 Esophagostomy

42.10 Esophagostomy, not otherwise specified

42.11 Cervical esophagostomy
DEF: Creation of opening into upper region of esophagus.

42.12 Exteriorization of esophageal pouch
DEF: Transfer of section of esophageal pouch to exterior of the body.

42.19 Other external fistulization of esophagus
Thoracic esophagostomy
Code also any resection (42.40-42.42)

42.2 Diagnostic procedures on esophagus

42.21 Operative esophagoscopy by incision
DEF: Esophageal examination with an endoscope through incision.

42.22 Esophagoscopy through artificial stoma
EXCLUDES: *that with biopsy (42.24)*

42.23 Other esophagoscopy
EXCLUDES: *that with biopsy (42.24)*
AHA: 1Q, '00, 20; 3Q, '98, 11

42.24 Closed [endoscopic] biopsy of esophagus
Brushing or washing for specimen collection
Esophagoscopy with biopsy
Suction biopsy of the esophagus
EXCLUDES: *esophagogastroduodenoscopy [EGD] with closed biopsy (45.16)*
DEF: Scope passed through mouth and throat to obtain biopsy specimen, usually by brushing and swabbing.

42.25 Open biopsy of esophagus

42.29 Other diagnostic procedures on esophagus
EXCLUDES: *barium swallow (87.61)*
esophageal manometry (89.32)
microscopic examination of specimen from esophagus (90.81-90.89)
AHA: 3Q, '96, 12

42.3 Local excision or destruction of lesion or tissue of esophagus

42.31 Local excision of esophageal diverticulum

42.32 Local excision of other lesion or tissue of esophagus
EXCLUDES: *biopsy of esophagus (42.24-42.25)*
esophageal fistulectomy (42.84)

42.33 Endoscopic excision or destruction of lesion or tissue of esophagus
Ablation of esophageal neoplasm
Control of esophageal bleeding
Esophageal polypectomy
Esophageal varices
Injection of esophageal varices
} by endoscopic approach
EXCLUDES: *biopsy of esophagus (42.24-42.25)*
fistulectomy (42.84)
open ligation of esophageal varices (42.91)

42.39 Other destruction of lesion or tissue of esophagus
EXCLUDES: *that by endoscopic approach (42.33)*

42.4 Excision of esophagus
EXCLUDES: *esophagogastrectomy NOS (43.99)*

42.40 Esophagectomy, not otherwise specified

42.41 Partial esophagectomy
Code also any synchronous:
anastomosis other than end-to-end (42.51-42.69)
esophagostomy (42.10-42.19)
gastrostomy (43.11-43.19)
DEF: Surgical removal of any part of esophagus.

42.42 Total esophagectomy
Code also any synchronous:
gastrostomy (43.11-43.19)
interposition or anastomosis other than end-to-end (42.51-42.69)
EXCLUDES: *esophagogastrectomy (43.99)*
AHA: 4Q, '88, 11
DEF: Surgical removal of entire esophagus.

42.5 Intrathoracic anastomosis of esophagus
Code also any synchronous:
esophagectomy (42.40-42.42)
gastrostomy (43.1)
DEF: Connection of esophagus to conduit within chest.

42.51 Intrathoracic esophagoesophagostomy
DEF: Connection of both ends of esophagus within chest cavity.

42.52 Intrathoracic esophagogastrostomy
DEF: Connection of esophagus to stomach within chest; follows esophagogastrectomy.

42.53 Intrathoracic esophageal anastomosis with interposition of small bowel

42.54 Other intrathoracic esophagoenterostomy
Anastomosis of esophagus to intestinal segment NOS

42.55 Intrathoracic esophageal anastomosis with interposition of colon

42.56 Other intrathoracic esophagocolostomy
Esophagocolostomy NOS

42.58 Intrathoracic esophageal anastomosis with other interposition
Construction of artificial esophagus
Retrosternal formation of reversed gastric tube
DEF: Construction of artificial esophagus: Creation of artificial esophagus.
DEF: Retrosternal anastomosis of reversed gastric tube: Formation of gastric tube behind breastbone.

OPERATIONS ON THE DIGESTIVE SYSTEM

42.59 **Other intrathoracic anastomosis of esophagus**
  AHA: 4Q, '88, 11

✓4th **42.6** **Antesternal anastomosis of esophagus**
  Code also any synchronous:
    esophagectomy (42.40-42.42)
    gastrostomy (43.1)

  42.61 Antesternal esophagoesophagostomy
  42.62 Antesternal esophagogastrostomy
  42.63 Antesternal esophageal anastomosis with interposition of small bowel
  42.64 Other antesternal esophagoenterostomy
    Antethoracic:
      esophagoenterostomy
      esophagoileostomy
      esophagojejunostomy
  42.65 Antesternal esophageal anastomosis with interposition of colon
    DEF: Connection of esophagus with colon segment.
  42.66 Other antesternal esophagocolostomy
    Antethoracic esophagocolostomy
  42.68 Other antesternal esophageal anastomosis with interposition
  42.69 Other antesternal anastomosis of esophagus

42.7 **Esophagomyotomy**
  DEF: Division of esophageal muscle, usually distal.

✓4th **42.8** **Other repair of esophagus**
  42.81 Insertion of permanent tube into esophagus
    AHA: 1Q, '97, 15
  42.82 Suture of laceration of esophagus
  42.83 Closure of esophagostomy
  42.84 Repair of esophageal fistula, not elsewhere classified
    EXCLUDES repair of fistula:
              bronchoesophageal (33.42)
              esophagopleurocutaneous (34.73)
              pharyngoesophageal (29.53)
              tracheoesophageal (31.73)
  42.85 Repair of esophageal stricture
  42.86 Production of subcutaneous tunnel without esophageal anastomosis
    DEF: Surgical formation of esophageal passage, without cutting, and reconnection.
  42.87 Other graft of esophagus
    EXCLUDES antesternal esophageal anastomosis with interposition of:
              colon (42.65)
              small bowel (42.63)
              antesternal esophageal anastomosis with other interposition (42.68)
              intrathoracic esophageal anastomosis with interposition of:
              colon (42.55)
              small bowel (42.53)
              intrathoracic esophageal anastomosis with other interposition (42.58)
  42.89 Other repair of esophagus

✓4th **42.9** **Other operations on esophagus**
  42.91 Ligation of esophageal varices
    EXCLUDES that by endoscopic approach (42.33)
    DEF: Destruction of dilated veins by suture strangulation.

  42.92 Dilation of esophagus
    Dilation of cardiac sphincter
    EXCLUDES intubation of esophagus (96.03, 96.06-96.08)
    DEF: Passing of balloon or hydrostatic dilators through esophagus to enlarge esophagus and relieve obstruction.
  42.99 Other
    EXCLUDES insertion of Sengstaken tube (96.06)
              intubation of esophagus (96.03, 96.06-96.08)
              removal of intraluminal foreign body from esophagus without incision (98.02)
              tamponade of esophagus (96.06)

✓3rd **43** **Incision and excision of stomach**
  ▶Code also any application or administration of an adhesion barrier substance (99.77)◀

  43.0 **Gastrotomy**
    EXCLUDES gastrostomy (43.11-43.19)
              that for control of hemorrhage (44.49)
    AHA: 3Q, '89, 14

✓4th **43.1** **Gastrostomy**
    AHA: S-O, '85, 5

  43.11 Percutaneous [endoscopic] gastrostomy [PEG]
    Percutaneous transabdominal gastrostomy
    DEF: Endoscopic positioning of tube through abdominal wall into stomach.
  43.19 Other gastrostomy
    EXCLUDES percutaneous [endoscopic] gastrostomy [PEG] (43.11)
    AHA: 1Q, '92, 14; 3Q, '89, 14

  43.3 **Pyloromyotomy**
    DEF: Cutting into longitudinal and circular muscular membrane between stomach and small intestine.

✓4th **43.4** **Local excision or destruction of lesion or tissue of stomach**
  43.41 Endoscopic excision or destruction of lesion or tissue of stomach
    Gastric polypectomy by endoscopic approach
    Gastric varices by endoscopic approach
    EXCLUDES biopsy of stomach (44.14-44.15)
              control of hemorrhage (44.43)
              open ligation of gastric varices (44.91)
    AHA: 3Q, '96, 10
  43.42 Local excision of other lesion or tissue of stomach
    EXCLUDES biopsy of stomach (44.14-44.15)
              gastric fistulectomy (44.62-44.63)
              partial gastrectomy (43.5-43.89)
  43.49 Other destruction of lesion or tissue of stomach
    EXCLUDES that by endoscopic approach (43.41)
    AHA: N-D, '87, 5; S-O, '85, 6

  43.5 **Partial gastrectomy with anastomosis to esophagus**
    Proximal gastrectomy

OPERATIONS ON THE DIGESTIVE SYSTEM

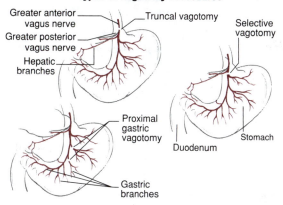
Types of Vagotomy Procedures

Billroth II Operation

- **43.6** **Partial gastrectomy with anastomosis to duodenum**
  - Billroth I operation
  - Gastropylorectomy
  - Distal gastrectomy
- **43.7** **Partial gastrectomy with anastomosis to jejunum**
  - Billroth II operation
- √4ᵗʰ **43.8** **Other partial gastrectomy**
  - **43.81** **Partial gastrectomy with jejunal transposition**
    - Henley jejunal transposition operation
    - Code also any synchronous intestinal resection (45.51)
  - **43.89** **Other**
    - Partial gastrectomy with bypass gastrogastrostomy
    - Sleeve resection of stomach
- √4ᵗʰ **43.9** **Total gastrectomy**
  - **43.91** **Total gastrectomy with intestinal interposition**
  - **43.99** **Other total gastrectomy**
    - Complete gastroduodenectomy
    - Esophagoduodenostomy with complete gastrectomy
    - Esophagogastrectomy NOS
    - Esophagojejunostomy with complete gastrectomy
    - Radical gastrectom
- √3ʳᵈ **44** **Other operations on stomach**
  - ▶Code also any application or administration of an adhesion barrier substance (99.77)◀
- √4ᵗʰ **44.0** **Vagotomy**
  - **44.00** **Vagotomy, not otherwise specified**
    - Division of vagus nerve NOS
    - **DEF:** Cutting of vagus nerve to reduce acid production.
  - **44.01** **Truncal vagotomy**
    - **DEF:** Surgical removal of vagus nerve segment near stomach branches.

Partial Gastrectomy with Anastomosis to Duodenum

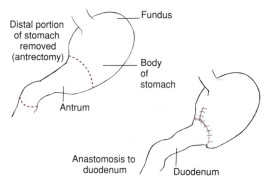

- **44.02** **Highly selective vagotomy**
  - Parietal cell vagotomy
  - Selective proximal vagotomy
  - **DEF:** Cutting select gastric branches of vagus nerve to reduce acid production and preserve other nerve functions.
- **44.03** **Other selective vagotomy**
- √4ᵗʰ **44.1** **Diagnostic procedures on stomach**
  - **44.11** **Transabdominal gastroscopy**
    - Intraoperative gastroscopy
    - **EXCLUDES** that with biopsy (44.14)
  - **44.12** **Gastroscopy through artificial stoma**
    - **EXCLUDES** that with biopsy (44.14)
  - **44.13** **Other gastroscopy**
    - **EXCLUDES** that with biopsy (44.14)
    - **AHA:** 1Q, '88, 15; N-D, '87, 5
  - **44.14** **Closed [endoscopic] biopsy of stomach**
    - Brushing or washing for specimen collection
    - **EXCLUDES** esophagogastroduodenoscopy [EGD] with closed biopsy (45.16)
    - **AHA:** 1Q, '88, 15; N-D, '87, 5
  - **44.15** **Open biopsy of stomach**
  - **44.19** **Other diagnostic procedures on stomach**
    - **EXCLUDES** gastric lavage (96.33)
      - microscopic examination of specimen from stomach (90.81-90.89)
      - upper GI series (87.62)
- √4ᵗʰ **44.2** **Pyloroplasty**
  - **44.21** **Dilation of pylorus by incision**
    - **DEF:** Cutting and suturing pylorus to relieve obstruction.
  - **44.22** **Endoscopic dilation of pylorus**
    - Dilation with balloon endoscope
    - Endoscopic dilation of gastrojejunostomy site
    - **AHA:** 2Q, '01, 17
  - **44.29** **Other pyloroplasty**
    - Pyloroplasty NOS
    - Revision of pylorus
    - **AHA:** 3Q, '99, 3
- √4ᵗʰ **44.3** **Gastroenterostomy without gastrectomy**
  - **44.31** **High gastric bypass**
    - Printen and Mason gastric bypass
    - **AHA:** M-J, '85, 17
    - **DEF:** Connection of middle part of small intestine to upper stomach to divert food passage from upper intestine.

44.32–45.12 OPERATIONS ON THE DIGESTIVE SYSTEM — Tabular List

44.32 Percutaneous [endoscopic] gastrojejunostomy
▶Endoscopic conversion of gastrostomy to jejunostomy◀
DEF: Percutaneous placement of a thin feeding tube through a gastrostomy tube and then pulling the tube into the proximal end of the jejunum.

44.39 Other gastroenterostomy
Bypass:
gastroduodenostomy
gastroenterostomy
gastrogastrostomy
Gastrojejunostomy without gastrectomy NOS
AHA: 1Q, '01, 16, 17

✓4th **44.4** Control of hemorrhage and suture of ulcer of stomach or duodenum
44.40 Suture of peptic ulcer, not otherwise specified
44.41 Suture of gastric ulcer site
EXCLUDES ligation of gastric varices (44.91)
44.42 Suture of duodenal ulcer site
AHA: J-F, '87, 11
44.43 Endoscopic control of gastric or duodenal bleeding
AHA: 2Q, '92, 17; N-D, '87, 4
44.44 Transcatheter embolization for gastric or duodenal bleeding
EXCLUDES surgical occlusion of abdominal vessels (38.86-38.87)
AHA: 1Q, '88, 15; N-D, '87, 4
DEF: Therapeutic blocking of stomach or upper small intestine blood vessel to stop hemorrhaging; accomplished by introducing various substances using a catheter.
44.49 Other control of hemorrhage of stomach or duodenum
That with gastrotomy

44.5 Revision of gastric anastomosis
Closure of: Closure of:
gastric anastomosis   gastrojejunostomy
gastroduodenostomy   Pantaloon operation

✓4th **44.6** Other repair of stomach
44.61 Suture of laceration of stomach
EXCLUDES that of ulcer site (44.41)
44.62 Closure of gastrostomy
44.63 Closure of other gastric fistula
Closure of:
gastrocolic fistula
gastrojejunocolic fistula
44.64 Gastropexy
AHA: M-J, '85, 17
DEF: Suturing of stomach into position.
44.65 Esophagogastroplasty
Belsey operation
Esophagus and stomach cardioplasty
AHA: M-J, '85, 17
44.66 Other procedures for creation of esophagogastric sphincteric competence
Fundoplication
Gastric cardioplasty
Nissen's fundoplication
Restoration of cardio-esophageal angle
AHA: 2Q, '01, 3, 5, 6; 3Q, '98, 10; M-J, '85, 17

44.69 Other
Inversion of gastric diverticulum
Repair of stomach NOS
AHA: 2Q, '01, 3; 3Q, '99, 3; M-J, '85, 17; N-D, '84, 13
DEF: Inversion of gastric diverticulum: Turning stomach inward to repair outpouch of wall.

✓4th **44.9** Other operations on stomach
44.91 Ligation of gastric varices
EXCLUDES that by endoscopic approach (43.41)
DEF: Destruction of dilated veins by suture or strangulation.
44.92 Intraoperative manipulation of stomach
Reduction of gastric volvulus
44.93 Insertion of gastric bubble (balloon) NC
44.94 Removal of gastric bubble (balloon)
44.99 Other
EXCLUDES change of gastrostomy tube (97.02)
dilation of cardiac sphincter (42.92)
gastric:
cooling (96.31)
freezing (96.32)
gavage (96.35)
hypothermia (96.31)
lavage (96.33)
insertion of nasogastric tube (96.07)
irrigation of gastrostomy (96.36)
irrigation of nasogastric tube (96.34)
removal of:
gastrostomy tube (97.51)
intraluminal foreign body from stomach without incision (98.03)
replacement of:
gastrostomy tube (97.02)
(naso-)gastric tube (97.01)

✓3rd **45** Incision, excision, and anastomosis of intestine
▶Code also any application or administration of an adhesion barrier substance (99.77)◀

✓4th **45.0** Enterotomy
EXCLUDES duodenocholedochotomy (51.41-51.42, 51.51)
that for destruction of lesion (45.30-45.34)
that of exteriorized intestine (46.14, 46.24, 46.31)
45.00 Incision of intestine not otherwise specified
45.01 Incision of duodenum
45.02 Other incision of small intestine
45.03 Incision of large intestine
EXCLUDES proctotomy (48.0)

✓4th **45.1** Diagnostic procedures on small intestine
Code also any laparotomy (54.11-54.19)
45.11 Transabdominal endoscopy of small intestine
Intraoperative endoscopy of small intestine
EXCLUDES that with biopsy (45.14)
DEF: Endoscopic exam of small intestine through abdominal wall.
DEF: Intraoperative endoscope of small intestine: Endoscopic exam of small intestine during surgery.
45.12 Endoscopy of small intestine through artificial stoma
EXCLUDES that with biopsy (45.14)
AHA: M-J, '85, 17

OPERATIONS ON THE DIGESTIVE SYSTEM 45.13–45.42

45.13 **Other endoscopy of small intestine**
Esophagogastroduodenoscopy [EGD]
EXCLUDES that with biopsy (45.14, 45.16)
AHA: N-D, '87, 5

45.14 **Closed [endoscopic] biopsy of small intestine**
Brushing or washing for specimen collection
EXCLUDES esophagogastroduodenoscopy [EGD] with closed biopsy (45.16)

45.15 **Open biopsy of small intestine**

45.16 **Esophagogastroduodenoscopy [EGD] with closed biopsy**
Biopsy of one or more sites involving esophagus, stomach, and/or duodenum
AHA: 2Q, '01, 9

45.19 **Other diagnostic procedures on small intestine**
EXCLUDES microscopic examination of specimen from small intestine (90.91-90.99)
radioisotope scan (92.04)
ultrasonography (88.74)
x-ray (87.61-87.69)

√4th **45.2** **Diagnostic procedures on large intestine**
Code also any laparotomy (54.11-54.19)

45.21 **Transabdominal endoscopy of large intestine**
Intraoperative endoscopy of large intestine
EXCLUDES that with biopsy (45.25)
DEF: Endoscopic exam of large intestine through abdominal wall.
DEF: Intraoperative endoscopy of large intestine: Endoscopic exam of large intestine during surgery.

45.22 **Endoscopy of large intestine through artificial stoma**
EXCLUDES that with biopsy (45.25)
DEF: Endoscopic exam of large intestine lining from rectum to cecum via colostomy stoma.

45.23 **Colonoscopy**
Flexible fiberoptic colonoscopy
EXCLUDES endoscopy of large intestine through artificial stoma (45.22)
flexible sigmoidoscopy (45.24)
rigid proctosigmoidoscopy (48.23)
transabdominal endoscopy of large intestine (45.21)
AHA: S-O, '85, 5
DEF: Endoscopic exam of descending colon, splenic flexure, transverse colon, hepatic flexure and cecum.

Esophagogastroduodenoscopy

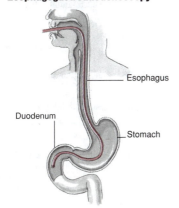

45.24 **Flexible sigmoidoscopy**
Endoscopy of descending colon
EXCLUDES rigid proctosigmoidoscopy (48.23)
DEF: Endoscopic exam of anus, rectum and sigmoid colon.

45.25 **Closed [endoscopic] biopsy of large intestine**
Biopsy, closed, of unspecified intestinal site
Brushing or washing for specimen collection
Colonoscopy with biopsy
EXCLUDES proctosigmoidoscopy with biopsy (48.24)

45.26 **Open biopsy of large intestine**

45.27 **Intestinal biopsy, site unspecified**

45.28 **Other diagnostic procedures on large intestine**

45.29 **Other diagnostic procedures on intestine, site unspecified**
EXCLUDES microscopic examination of specimen (90.91-90.99)
scan and radioisotope function study (92.04)
ultrasonography (88.74)
x-ray (87.61-87.69)

√4th **45.3** **Local excision or destruction of lesion or tissue of small intestine**

45.30 **Endoscopic excision or destruction of lesion of duodenum**
EXCLUDES biopsy of duodenum (45.14-45.15)
control of hemorrhage (44.43)
fistulectomy (46.72)

45.31 **Other local excision of lesion of duodenum**
EXCLUDES biopsy of duodenum (45.14-45.15)
fistulectomy (46.72)
multiple segmental resection (45.61)
that by endoscopic approach (45.30)

45.32 **Other destruction of lesion of duodenum**
EXCLUDES that by endoscopic approach (45.30)
AHA: N-D, '87, 5; S-O, '85, 6

45.33 **Local excision of lesion or tissue of small intestine, except duodenum**
Excision of redundant mucosa of ileostomy
EXCLUDES biopsy of small intestine (45.14-45.15)
fistulectomy (46.74)
multiple segmental resection (45.61)

45.34 **Other destruction of lesion of small intestine, except duodenum**

√4th **45.4** **Local excision or destruction of lesion or tissue of large intestine**
AHA: N-D, '87, 11

45.41 **Excision of lesion or tissue of large intestine**
Excision of redundant mucosa of colostomy
EXCLUDES biopsy of large intestine (45.25-45.27)
endoscopic polypectomy of large intestine (45.42)
fistulectomy (46.76)
multiple segmental resection (45.71)
that by endoscopic approach (45.42-45.43)

45.42 **Endoscopic polypectomy of large intestine**
EXCLUDES that by open approach (45.41)
AHA: 2Q, '90, 25
DEF: Endoscopic removal of polyp from large intestine.

45.43 Endoscopic destruction of other lesion or tissue of large intestine
Endoscopic ablation of tumor of large intestine
Endoscopic control of colonic bleeding
EXCLUDES endoscopic polypectomy of large intestine (45.42)

45.49 Other destruction of lesion of large intestine
EXCLUDES that by endoscopic approach (45.43)

√4ᵗʰ 45.5 Isolation of intestinal segment
Code also any synchronous:
anastomosis other than end-to-end (45.90-45.94)
enterostomy (46.10-46.39)

45.50 Isolation of intestinal segment, not otherwise specified
Isolation of intestinal pedicle flap
Reversal of intestinal segment
DEF: Isolation of small intestinal pedicle flap: Separation of intestinal pedicle flap.
DEF: Reversal of intestinal segment: Separation of intestinal segment.

45.51 Isolation of segment of small intestine
Isolation of ileal loop
Resection of small intestine for interposition
AHA: 3Q, '00, 7

45.52 Isolation of segment of large intestine
Resection of colon for interposition

√4ᵗʰ 45.6 Other excision of small intestine
Code also any synchronous:
anastomosis other than end-to-end (45.90-45.93, 45.95)
colostomy (46.10-46.13)
enterostomy (46.10-46.39)
EXCLUDES cecectomy (45.72)
enterocolectomy (45.79)
gastroduodenectomy (43.6-43.99)
ileocolectomy (45.73)
pancreatoduodenectomy (52.51-52.7)

45.61 Multiple segmental resection of small intestine
Segmental resection for multiple traumatic lesions of small intestine

45.62 Other partial resection of small intestine
Duodenectomy   Jejunectomy
Ileectomy
EXCLUDES duodenectomy with synchronous pancreatectomy (52.51-52.7)
resection of cecum and terminal ileum (45.72)

45.63 Total removal of small intestine

Colectomy

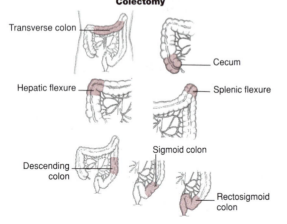

Intestinal Anastomosis

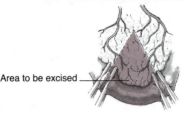

Area to be excised

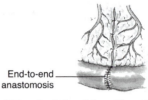

End-to-end anastomosis

√4ᵗʰ 45.7 Partial excision of large intestine
Code also any synchronous:
anastomosis other than end-to-end (45.92-45.94)
enterostomy (46.10-46.39)
AHA: 4Q, '92, 27

45.71 Multiple segmental resection of large intestine
Segmental resection for multiple traumatic lesions of large intestine

45.72 Cecectomy
Resection of cecum and terminal ileum

45.73 Right hemicolectomy
Ileocolectomy
Right radical colectomy
AHA: 3Q, '99, 10

45.74 Resection of transverse colon

45.75 Left hemicolectomy
EXCLUDES proctosigmoidectomy (48.41-48.69)
second stage Mikulicz operation (46.04)
DEF: Excision of left descending large intestine.

45.76 Sigmoidectomy
AHA: 1Q, '96, 9; 3Q, '89, 15

45.79 Other partial excision of large intestine
Enterocolectomy NEC
AHA: 3Q, '97, 9; 2Q, '91, 16

45.8 Total intra-abdominal colectomy
Excision of cecum, colon, and sigmoid
EXCLUDES coloproctectomy (48.41-48.69)

√4ᵗʰ 45.9 Intestinal anastomosis
Code also any synchronous resection (45.31-45.8, 48.41-48.69)
EXCLUDES end-to-end anastomosis — omit code

45.90 Intestinal anastomosis, not otherwise specified

45.91 Small-to-small intestinal anastomosis
AHA: M-J, '85, 17

45.92 Anastomosis of small intestine to rectal stump
Hampton procedure

45.93 Other small-to-large intestinal anastomosis
AHA: N-D, '86, 11

45.94 Large-to-large intestinal anastomosis
EXCLUDES rectorectostomy (48.74)
AHA: 3Q, '89, 15

45.95 Anastomosis to anus
Formation of endorectal ileal pouch (J-pouch) (H-pouch) (S-pouch) with anastomosis of small intestine to anus

Tabular List — OPERATIONS ON THE DIGESTIVE SYSTEM — 46–46.79

46 Other operations on intestine
▶Code also any application or administration of an adhesion barrier substance (99.77)◄

46.0 Exteriorization of intestine
INCLUDES: loop enterostomy
multiple stage resection of intestine
DEF: Bringing intestinal segment to body surface.

- **46.01 Exteriorization of small intestine**
  Loop ileostomy
- **46.02 Resection of exteriorized segment of small intestine**
- **46.03 Exteriorization of large intestine**
  Exteriorization of intestine NOS
  First stage Mikulicz exteriorization of intestine
  Loop colostomy
- **46.04 Resection of exteriorized segment of large intestine**
  Resection of exteriorized segment of intestine NOS
  Second stage Mikulicz operation

46.1 Colostomy
Code also any synchronous resection (45.49, 45.71-45.79, 45.8)
EXCLUDES: loop colostomy (46.03)
that with abdominoperineal resection of rectum (48.5)
that with synchronous anterior rectal resection (48.62)
DEF: Creation of opening from large intestine through abdominal wall to body surface.

- **46.10 Colostomy, not otherwise specified**
- **46.11 Temporary colostomy**
- **46.13 Permanent colostomy**
- **46.14 Delayed opening of colostomy**

46.2 Ileostomy
Code also any synchronous resection (45.34, 45.61-45.63)
EXCLUDES: loop ileostomy (46.01)
DEF: Creation of artificial anus by bringing ileum through abdominal wall to body surface.

- **46.20 Ileostomy, not otherwise specified**
- **46.21 Temporary ileostomy**
- **46.22 Continent ileostomy**
  AHA: M-J, '85, 17
  DEF: Creation of opening from third part of small intestine through abdominal wall, with pouch outside abdomen.
- **46.23 Other permanent ileostomy**
- **46.24 Delayed opening of ileostomy**

46.3 Other enterostomy
Code also any synchronous resection (45.61-45.8)

- **46.31 Delayed opening of other enterostomy**
- **46.32 Percutaneous (endoscopic) jejunostomy [PEJ]**
  DEF: Endoscopic placement of tube in midsection of small intestine through abdominal wall.
- **46.39 Other**
  Duodenostomy   Feeding enterostomy
  AHA: 3Q, '89, 15

46.4 Revision of intestinal stoma
DEF: Revision of opening surgically created from intestine through abdominal wall, to skin surface.

- **46.40 Revision of intestinal stoma, not otherwise specified**
  Plastic enlargement of intestinal stoma
  Reconstruction of stoma of intestine
  Release of scar tissue of intestinal stoma
  EXCLUDES: excision of redundant mucosa (45.41)
- **46.41 Revision of stoma of small intestine**
  EXCLUDES: excision of redundant mucosa (45.33)
- **46.42 Repair of pericolostomy hernia**
- **46.43 Other revision of stoma of large intestine**
  EXCLUDES: excision of redundant mucosa (45.41)

46.5 Closure of intestinal stoma
Code also any synchronous resection (45.34, 45.49, 45.61-45.8)

- **46.50 Closure of intestinal stoma, not otherwise specified**
- **46.51 Closure of stoma of small intestine**
- **46.52 Closure of stoma of large intestine**
  Closure or take-down of cecostomy
  Closure or take-down of colostomy
  Closure or take-down of sigmoidostomy
  AHA: 3Q, '97, 9; 2Q, '91, 16; N-D, '87, 8

46.6 Fixation of intestine

- **46.60 Fixation of intestine not otherwise specified**
  Fixation of intestine to abdominal wall
- **46.61 Fixation of small intestine to abdominal wall**
  Ileopexy
- **46.62 Other fixation of small intestine**
  Noble plication of small intestine
  Plication of jejunum
  DEF: Noble plication of small intestine: Fixing small intestine into place with tuck in small intestine.
  DEF: Plication of jejunum: Fixing small intestine into place with tuck in midsection.
- **46.63 Fixation of large intestine to abdominal wall**
  Cecocoloplicopexy
  Sigmoidopexy   (Moschowitz)
- **46.64 Other fixation of large intestine**
  Cecofixation   Colofixation

46.7 Other repair of intestine
EXCLUDES: closure of:
ulcer of duodenum (44.42)
vesicoenteric fistula (57.83)

- **46.71 Suture of laceration of duodenum**
- **46.72 Closure of fistula of duodenum**
- **46.73 Suture of laceration of small intestine, except duodenum**
- **46.74 Closure of fistula of small intestine, except duodenum**
  EXCLUDES: closure of:
  artificial stoma (46.51)
  vaginal fistula (70.74)
  repair of gastrojejunocolic fistula (44.63)
- **46.75 Suture of laceration of large intestine**
- **46.76 Closure of fistula of large intestine**
  EXCLUDES: closure of:
  gastrocolic fistula (44.63)
  rectal fistula (48.73)
  sigmoidovesical fistula (57.83)
  stoma (46.52)
  vaginal fistula (70.72-70.73)
  vesicocolic fistula (57.83)
  vesicosigmoidovaginal fistula (57.83)
  AHA: 3Q, '99, 8
- **46.79 Other repair of intestine**
  ▶Duodenoplasty◄

OPERATIONS ON THE DIGESTIVE SYSTEM

✓4th 46.8 Dilation and manipulation of intestine
  46.80 Intra-abdominal manipulation of intestine, not otherwise specified
    Correction of intestinal malrotation
    Reduction of:
      intestinal torsion
      intestinal volvulus
      intussusception
    EXCLUDES reduction of intussusception with:
      fluoroscopy (96.29)
      ionizing radiation enema (96.29)
      ultrasonography guidance (96.29)
    AHA: 4Q, '98, 82
    DEF: Correction of intestinal malrotation: Repair of abnormal rotation.
    DEF: Reduction of:
      Intestinal torsion: Repair of twisted segment.
      Intestinal volvulus: Repair of a knotted segment.
      Intussusception: Repair of prolapsed segment.
  46.81 Intra-abdominal manipulation of small intestine
  46.82 Intra-abdominal manipulation of large intestine
  46.85 Dilation of intestine
    Dilation (balloon) of duodenum
    Dilation (balloon) of jejunum
    Endoscopic dilation (balloon) of large intestine
    That through rectum or colostomy
    AHA: 3Q, '89, 15

✓4th 46.9 Other operations on intestines
  46.91 Myotomy of sigmoid colon
  46.92 Myotomy of other parts of colon
  46.93 Revision of anastomosis of small intestine
  46.94 Revision of anastomosis of large intestine
  46.95 Local perfusion of small intestine
    Code also substance perfused (99.21-99.29)
  46.96 Local perfusion of large intestine
    Code also substance perfused (99.21-99.29)
  46.97 Transplant of intestine NC
    AHA: 4Q, '00, 66
  46.99 Other
    Ileoentectropy
    EXCLUDES diagnostic procedures on intestine (45.11-45.29)
      dilation of enterostomy stoma (96.24)
      intestinal intubation (96.08)
      removal of:
        intraluminal foreign body from large intestine without incision (98.04)
        intraluminal foreign body from small intestine without incision (98.03)
        tube from large intestine (97.53)
        tube from small intestine (97.52)
      replacement of:
        large intestine tube or enterostomy device (97.04)
        small intestine tube or enterostomy device (97.03)
    AHA: 3Q, '99, 11; 1Q, '89, 11

✓3rd 47 Operations on appendix
  ▶Code also any application or administration of an adhesion barrier substance (99.77)◀
  INCLUDES appendiceal stump
  ✓4th 47.0 Appendectomy
    EXCLUDES incidental appendectomy, so described (47.11, 47.19)
    AHA: 4Q, '96, 64; 3Q, '92, 12
    47.01 Laparoscopic appendectomy
      AHA: 1Q, '01, 15; 4Q, '96, 64
    47.09 Other appendectomy
      AHA: 4Q, '97, 52
  ✓4th 47.1 Incidental appendectomy
    DEF: Removal of appendix during abdominal surgery as prophylactic measure, without significant appendiceal pathology.
    47.11 Laparoscopic incidental appendectomy
    47.19 Other incidental appendectomy
      AHA: 4Q, '96, 65
  47.2 Drainage of appendiceal abscess
    EXCLUDES that with appendectomy (47.0)
  ✓4th 47.9 Other operations on appendix
    47.91 Appendicostomy
    47.92 Closure of appendiceal fistula
    47.99 Other
      Anastomosis of appendix
      EXCLUDES diagnostic procedures on appendix (45.21-45.29)
      AHA: 3Q, '01, 16

✓3rd 48 Operations on rectum, rectosigmoid, and perirectal tissue
  ▶Code also any application or administration of an adhesion barrier substance (99.77)◀
  48.0 Proctotomy
    Decompression of imperforate anus
    Panas' operation [linear proctotomy]
    EXCLUDES incision of perirectal tissue (48.81)
    AHA: 3Q, '99, 8
    DEF: Incision into rectal portion of large intestine.
    DEF: Decompression of imperforate anus: opening a closed anus by means of an incision.
    DEF: Panas' operation (linear proctotomy): Linear incision into rectal portion of large intestine
  48.1 Proctostomy
  ✓4th 48.2 Diagnostic procedures on rectum, rectosigmoid, and perirectal tissue
    48.21 Transabdominal proctosigmoidoscopy
      Intraoperative proctosigmoidoscopy
      EXCLUDES that with biopsy (48.24)
    48.22 Proctosigmoidoscopy through artificial stoma
      EXCLUDES that with biopsy (48.24)
    48.23 Rigid proctosigmoidoscopy
      EXCLUDES flexible sigmoidoscopy (45.24)
      AHA: 1Q, '01, 8
    DEF: Endoscopic exam of anus, rectum and lower sigmoid colon.
    48.24 Closed [endoscopic] biopsy of rectum
      Brushing or washing for specimen collection
      Proctosigmoidoscopy with biopsy
    48.25 Open biopsy of rectum
    48.26 Biopsy of perirectal tissue

Tabular List — OPERATIONS ON THE DIGESTIVE SYSTEM 48.29–48.81

48.29 Other diagnostic procedures on rectum, rectosigmoid, and perirectal tissue
- EXCLUDES: digital examination of rectum (89.34)
  lower GI series (87.64)
  microscopic examination of specimen from rectum (90.91-90.99)

48.3 Local excision or destruction of lesion or tissue of rectum

48.31 Radical electrocoagulation of rectal lesion or tissue
- DEF: Destruction of lesion or tissue of large intestine, rectal part.

48.32 Other electrocoagulation of rectal lesion or tissue
- AHA: 2Q, '98, 18

48.33 Destruction of rectal lesion or tissue by laser

48.34 Destruction of rectal lesion or tissue by cryosurgery

48.35 Local excision of rectal lesion or tissue
- EXCLUDES: biopsy of rectum (48.24-48.25)
  [endoscopic] polypectomy of rectum (48.36)
  excision of perirectal tissue (48.82)
  hemorrhoidectomy (49.46)
  rectal fistulectomy (48.73)

48.36 [Endoscopic] polypectomy of rectum
- AHA: 4Q, '95, 65

48.4 Pull-through resection of rectum
Code also any synchronous anastomosis other than end-to-end (45.90, 45.92-45.95)

48.41 Soave submucosal resection of rectum
  Endorectal pull-through operation
- DEF: Soave submucosal resection: Resection of submucosal rectal part of large intestine by pull-through technique.
- DEF: Endorectal pull-through operation: Resection of interior large intestine by pull through technique.

48.49 Other pull-through resection of rectum
  Abdominoperineal pull-through
  Altemeier operation
  Swenson proctectomy
- EXCLUDES: Duhamel abdominoperineal pull-through (48.65)
- AHA: ▶3Q, '01, 8;◀ 2Q, '99, 13
- DEF: Abdominoperineal pull-through: Resection of large intestine, latter part, by pull-through of abdomen, scrotum or vulva and anus.
- DEF: Swenson proctatectomy: Excision of large intestine, rectal by pull-through and preserving muscles that close the anus.

48.5 Abdominoperineal resection of rectum
  Combined abdominoendorectal resection
  Complete proctectomy
  Code also any synchronous anastomosis other than end-to-end (45.90, 45.92-45.95)
- INCLUDES: with synchronous colostomy
- EXCLUDES: Duhamel abdominoperineal pull-through (48.65)
  that as part of pelvic exenteration (68.8)
- AHA: 2Q, '97, 5
- DEF: Rectal excision through cavities formed by abdomen, anus, vulva or scrotum.

48.6 Other resection of rectum
Code also any synchronous anastomosis other than end-to-end (45.90, 45.92-45.95)

48.61 Transsacral rectosigmoidectomy
- DEF: Excision through sacral bone area of sigmoid and last parts of large intestine.

48.62 Anterior resection of rectum with synchronous colostomy
- DEF: Resection of front terminal end of large intestine and creation of colostomy.

48.63 Other anterior resection of rectum
- EXCLUDES: that with synchronous colostomy (48.62)
- AHA: 1Q, '96, 9

48.64 Posterior resection of rectum

48.65 Duhamel resection of rectum
  Duhamel abdominoperineal pull-through

48.69 Other
  Partial proctectomy
  Rectal resection NOS
- AHA: J-F, '87, 11; N-D, '86, 11

48.7 Repair of rectum
- EXCLUDES: repair of:
  current obstetric laceration (75.62)
  vaginal rectocele (70.50, 70.52)

48.71 Suture of laceration of rectum

48.72 Closure of proctostomy

48.73 Closure of other rectal fistula
- EXCLUDES: fistulectomy:
  perirectal (48.93)
  rectourethral (58.43)
  rectovaginal (70.73)
  rectovesical (57.83)
  rectovesicovaginal (57.83)

48.74 Rectorectostomy
  Rectal anastomosis NOS
- DEF: Connection of two cut portions of large intestine, rectal end.

48.75 Abdominal proctopexy
  Frickman procedure
  Ripstein repair of rectal prolapse
- DEF: Fixation of rectum to adjacent abdominal structures.

48.76 Other proctopexy
  Delorme repair of prolapsed rectum
  Proctosigmoidopexy
  Puborectalis sling operation
- EXCLUDES: manual reduction of rectal prolapse (96.26)
- DEF: Delorme repair of prolapsed rectum: Fixation of collapsed large intestine, rectal part.
- DEF: Proctosigmoidopexy: Suturing of twisted large intestine, rectal part.
- DEF: Puborectalis sling operation: Fixation of large intestine, rectal part by forming puborectalis muscle into sling.

48.79 Other repair of rectum
  Repair of old obstetric laceration of rectum
- EXCLUDES: anastomosis to:
  large intestine (45.94)
  small intestine (45.92-45.93)
  repair of:
  current obstetrical laceration (75.62)
  vaginal rectocele (70.50, 70.52)

48.8 Incision or excision of perirectal tissue or lesion
- INCLUDES: pelvirectal tissue
  rectovaginal septum

48.81 Incision of perirectal tissue
  Incision of rectovaginal septum

OPERATIONS ON THE DIGESTIVE SYSTEM

48.82 **Excision of perirectal tissue**
  - EXCLUDES: perirectal biopsy (48.26)
    perirectofistulectomy (48.93)
    rectal fistulectomy (48.73)

✓4th **48.9** **Other operations on rectum and perirectal tissue**

48.91 **Incision of rectal stricture**

48.92 **Anorectal myectomy**
  - DEF: Excision of anorectal muscle.

48.93 **Repair of perirectal fistula**
  - EXCLUDES: that opening into rectum (48.73)
  - DEF: Closure of abdominal passage in tissue around large intestine, rectal part.

48.99 **Other**
  - EXCLUDES: digital examination of rectum (89.34)
    dilation of rectum (96.22)
    insertion of rectal tube (96.09)
    irrigation of rectum (96.38-96.39)
    manual reduction of rectal prolapse (96.26)
    proctoclysis (96.37)
    rectal massage (99.93)
    rectal packing (96.19)
    removal of:
      impacted feces (96.38)
      intraluminal foreign body from rectum without incision (98.05)
    rectal packing (97.59)
    transanal enema (96.39)

✓3rd **49** **Operations on anus**
  ▶Code also any application or administration of an adhesion barrier substance (99.77)◀

✓4th **49.0** **Incision or excision of perianal tissue**

49.01 **Incision of perianal abscess**

49.02 **Other incision of perianal tissue**
  Undercutting of perianal tissue
  - EXCLUDES: anal fistulotomy (49.11)

49.03 **Excision of perianal skin tags**

49.04 **Other excision of perianal tissue**
  - EXCLUDES: anal fistulectomy (49.12)
    biopsy of perianal tissue (49.22)
  - AHA: 1Q, '01, 8

✓4th **49.1** **Incision or excision of anal fistula**
  - EXCLUDES: closure of anal fistula (49.73)

49.11 **Anal fistulotomy**

49.12 **Anal fistulectomy**

✓4th **49.2** **Diagnostic procedures on anus and perianal tissue**

49.21 **Anoscopy**

49.22 **Biopsy of perianal tissue**

49.23 **Biopsy of anus**

49.29 **Other diagnostic procedures on anus and perianal tissue**
  - EXCLUDES: microscopic examination of specimen from anus (90.91-90.99)

✓4th **49.3** **Local excision or destruction of other lesion or tissue of anus**
  Anal cryptotomy
  Cauterization of lesion of anus
  - EXCLUDES: biopsy of anus (49.23)
    control of (postoperative) hemorrhage of anus (49.95)
    hemorrhoidectomy (49.46)

49.31 **Endoscopic excision or destruction of lesion or tissue of anus**

49.39 **Other local excision or destruction of lesion or tissue of anus**
  - EXCLUDES: that by endoscopic approach (49.31)
  - AHA: 1Q, '01, 8

✓4th **49.4** **Procedures on hemorrhoids**

49.41 **Reduction of hemorrhoids**
  - DEF: Manual manipulation to reduce hemorrhoids.

49.42 **Injection of hemorrhoids**

49.43 **Cauterization of hemorrhoids**
  Clamp and cautery of hemorrhoids

49.44 **Destruction of hemorrhoids by cryotherapy**

49.45 **Ligation of hemorrhoids**

49.46 **Excision of hemorrhoids**
  Hemorrhoidectomy NOS

49.47 **Evacuation of thrombosed hemorrhoids**
  - DEF: Removal of clotted material from hemorrhoid.

49.49 **Other procedures on hemorrhoids**
  Lord procedure

✓4th **49.5** **Division of anal sphincter**

49.51 **Left lateral anal sphincterotomy**

49.52 **Posterior anal sphincterotomy**

49.59 **Other anal sphincterotomy**
  Division of sphincter NOS

49.6 **Excision of anus**

✓4th **49.7** **Repair of anus**
  - EXCLUDES: repair of current obstetric laceration (75.62)

49.71 **Suture of laceration of anus**

49.72 **Anal cerclage**
  - DEF: Encircling anus with ring or sutures.

49.73 **Closure of anal fistula**
  - EXCLUDES: excision of anal fistula (49.12)

49.74 **Gracilis muscle transplant for anal incontinence**
  - DEF: Moving pubic attachment of gracilis muscle to restores anal control.

● **49.75** **Implantation or revision of artificial anal sphincter**
  Removal with subsequent replacement
  Replacement during same or subsequent operative episode

● **49.76** **Removal of artificial anal sphincter**
  Explantation or removal without replacement
  - EXCLUDES: revision with implantation during same operative episode (49.75)

49.79 **Other repair of anal sphincter**
  Repair of old obstetric laceration of anus
  - EXCLUDES: anoplasty with synchronous hemorrhoidectomy (49.46)
    repair of current obstetric laceration (75.62)
  - AHA: 2Q, '98, 16; 1Q, '97, 9

✓4th **49.9** **Other operations on anus**
  - EXCLUDES: dilation of anus (sphincter) (96.23)

49.91 **Incision of anal septum**

49.92 **Insertion of subcutaneous electrical anal stimulator**

49.93 **Other incision of anus**
  Removal of:
    foreign body from anus with incision
    seton from anus
  - EXCLUDES: anal fistulotomy (49.11)
    removal of intraluminal foreign body without incision (98.05)

OPERATIONS ON THE DIGESTIVE SYSTEM

49.94 **Reduction of anal prolapse**
    EXCLUDES: manual reduction of rectal prolapse (96.26)
    DEF: Manipulation of displaced anal tissue to normal position.

49.95 **Control of (postoperative) hemorrhage of anus**

49.99 **Other**

√3rd 50 Operations on liver
▶Code also any application or administration of an adhesion barrier substance (99.77)◀

50.0 **Hepatotomy**
    Incision of abscess of liver
    Removal of gallstones from liver
    Stromeyer-Little operation

√4th 50.1 Diagnostic procedures on liver

50.11 **Closed (percutaneous) [needle] biopsy of liver**
    Diagnostic aspiration of liver
    AHA: 4Q, '88, 12

50.12 **Open biopsy of liver**
    Wedge biopsy

50.19 Other diagnostic procedures on liver
    EXCLUDES: liver scan and radioisotope function study (92.02)
    microscopic examination of specimen from liver (91.01-91.09)

√4th 50.2 Local excision or destruction of liver tissue or lesion

50.21 **Marsupialization of lesion of liver**
    DEF: Exteriorizing lesion by incision and suturing cut edges to skin to create opening.

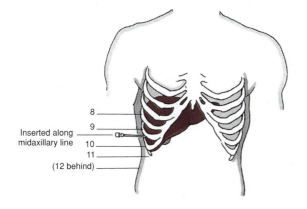

Closed Liver Biopsy
Inserted along midaxillary line 8, 9, 10, 11 (12 behind)

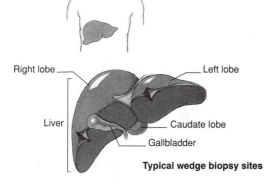

Liver Biopsy (Open, Wedge)
Right lobe — Left lobe — Liver — Caudate lobe — Gallbladder
Typical wedge biopsy sites

50.22 **Partial hepatectomy**
    Wedge resection of liver
    EXCLUDES: biopsy of liver (50.11-50.12)
    hepatic lobectomy (50.3)

50.29 **Other destruction of lesion of liver**
    Cauterization
    Enucleation   } of hepatic lesion
    Evacuation
    EXCLUDES: percutaneous aspiration of lesion (50.91)

50.3 **Lobectomy of liver**
    Total hepatic lobectomy with partial excision of other lobe

50.4 **Total hepatectomy**

√4th 50.5 Liver transplant

50.51 **Auxiliary liver transplant** NC
    Auxiliary hepatic transplantation leaving patient's own liver in situ

50.59 **Other transplant of liver** NC

√4th 50.6 Repair of liver

50.61 **Closure of laceration of liver**

50.69 **Other repair of liver**
    Hepatopexy

√4th 50.9 Other operations on liver
    EXCLUDES: lysis of adhesions (54.5)

50.91 Percutaneous aspiration of liver
    EXCLUDES: percutaneous biopsy (50.11)
    DEF: Incision into liver through body wall to withdraw fluid.

50.92 Extracorporeal hepatic assistance
    Liver dialysis
    AHA: 2Q, '01, 21
    DEF: Devices used outside body to assist liver function.

50.93 Localized perfusion of liver

50.94 Other injection of therapeutic substance into liver

50.99 Other

√3rd 51 Operations on gallbladder and biliary tract
▶Code also any application or administration of an adhesion barrier substance (99.77)◀
    INCLUDES: operations on:
        ampulla of Vater
        common bile duct
        cystic duct
        hepatic duct
        intrahepatic bile duct
        sphincter of Oddi

√4th 51.0 Cholecystotomy and cholecystostomy

51.01 **Percutaneous aspiration of gallbladder**
    ▶Percutaneous cholecystotomy for drainage
    That by: needle or catheter◀
    EXCLUDES: needle biopsy (51.12)

51.02 **Trocar cholecystostomy**
    AHA: 3Q, '89, 18
    DEF: Creating opening in gallbladder with catheter.

51.03 **Other cholecystostomy**

51.04 **Other cholecystotomy**
    Cholelithotomy NOS

√4th 51.1 Diagnostic procedures on biliary tract
    EXCLUDES: that for endoscopic procedures classifiable to 51.64, 51.84-51.88, 52.14, 52.21, 52.93-52.94, 52.97-52.98
    AHA: 2Q, '97, 7

51.10 Endoscopic retrograde cholangiopancreatography [ERCP]
EXCLUDES endoscopic retrograde:
cholangiography [ERC] (51.11)
pancreatography [ERP] (52.13)

AHA: 1Q, '01, 8; 2Q, '99, 13

DEF: Endoscopic and radioscopic exam of pancreatic and common bile ducts with contrast material injected in opposite direction of normal flow through catheter.

51.11 Endoscopic retrograde cholangiography [ERC]
Laparoscopic exploration of common bile duct
EXCLUDES endoscopic retrograde:
cholangiopancreatography [ERCP] (51.10)
pancreatography [ERP] (52.13)

AHA: 1Q, '96, 12; 3Q, '89, 18; 4Q, '88, 7

DEF: Endoscopic and radioscopic exam of common bile ducts with contrast material injected in opposite direction of normal flow through catheter.

51.12 Percutaneous biopsy of gallbladder or bile ducts
Needle biopsy of gallbladder

51.13 Open biopsy of gallbladder or bile ducts

51.14 Other closed [endoscopic] biopsy of biliary duct or sphincter of Oddi
Brushing or washing for specimen collection
Closed biopsy of biliary duct or sphincter of Oddi by procedures classifiable to 51.10-51.11, 52.13

DEF: Endoscopic biopsy of muscle tissue around pancreatic and common bile ducts.

51.15 Pressure measurement of sphincter of Oddi
Pressure measurement of sphincter by procedures classifiable to 51.10-51.11, 52.13

DEF: Pressure measurement tests of muscle tissue surrounding pancreatic and common bile ducts.

51.19 Other diagnostic procedures on biliary tract
EXCLUDES biliary tract x-ray (87.51-87.59)
microscopic examination of specimen from biliary tract (91.01-91.09)

√4th 51.2 Cholecystectomy
AHA: 1Q, '93, 17; 4Q, '91, 26; 3Q, '89, 18

51.21 Other partial cholecystectomy
Revision of prior cholecystectomy
EXCLUDES that by laparoscope (51.24)
AHA: 4Q, '96, 69

51.22 Cholecystectomy
EXCLUDES laparoscopic cholecystectomy (51.23)
AHA: 4Q, '97, 52; 2Q, '91, 16

51.23 Laparoscopic cholecystectomy
That by laser
AHA: 3Q, '98, 10; 4Q, '97, 52; 1Q, '96, 12; 2Q, '95, 11; 4Q, '91, 26

DEF: Endoscopic removal of gallbladder.

51.24 Laparoscopic partial cholecystectomy
AHA: 4Q, '96, 69

√4th 51.3 Anastomosis of gallbladder or bile duct
EXCLUDES resection with end-to-end anastomosis (51.61-51.69)

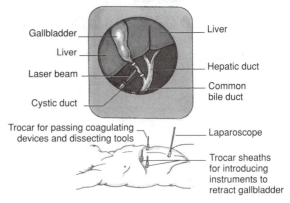

Laparoscopic Cholecystectomy by Laser

51.31 Anastomosis of gallbladder to hepatic ducts
51.32 Anastomosis of gallbladder to intestine
51.33 Anastomosis of gallbladder to pancreas
51.34 Anastomosis of gallbladder to stomach
51.35 Other gallbladder anastomosis
Gallbladder anastomosis NOS

51.36 Choledochoenterostomy
DEF: Connection of common bile duct to intestine.

51.37 Anastomosis of hepatic duct to gastrointestinal tract
▶Kasai portoenterostomy◀

51.39 Other bile duct anastomosis
Anastomosis of bile duct NOS
Anastomosis of unspecified bile duct to:
intestine   pancreas
liver   stomach

√4th 51.4 Incision of bile duct for relief of obstruction

51.41 Common duct exploration for removal of calculus
EXCLUDES percutaneous extraction (51.96)
AHA: 1Q, '96, 12; 3Q, '89, 18; 4Q, '88, 7

51.42 Common duct exploration for relief of other obstruction
AHA: 3Q, '89, 18

51.43 Insertion of choledochohepatic tube for decompression
Hepatocholedochostomy
AHA: 3Q, '89, 18; 4Q, '88, 7

51.49 Incision of other bile ducts for relief of obstruction
AHA: 3Q, '89, 18

√4th 51.5 Other incision of bile duct
EXCLUDES that for relief of obstruction (51.41-51.49)

51.51 Exploration of common duct
Incision of common bile duct
AHA: 2Q, '97, 16; 1Q, '96, 12

51.59 Incision of other bile duct
AHA: 2Q, '97, 16; 3Q, '89, 18

√4th 51.6 Local excision or destruction of lesion or tissue of biliary ducts and sphincter of Oddi
Code also anastomosis other than end-to-end (51.31, 51.36-51.39)
EXCLUDES biopsy of bile duct (51.12-51.13)

51.61 Excision of cystic duct remnant
AHA: 3Q, '89, 18

51.62 Excision of ampulla of Vater (with reimplantation of common duct)

	51.63	**Other excision of common duct**
		Choledochectomy
		EXCLUDES fistulectomy (51.72)
	51.64	**Endoscopic excision or destruction of lesion of biliary ducts or sphincter of Oddi**
		Excision or destruction of lesion of biliary duct by procedures classifiable to 51.10-51.11, 52.13
	51.69	**Excision of other bile duct**
		Excision of lesion of bile duct NOS
		EXCLUDES fistulectomy (51.79)
✓4th	**51.7**	**Repair of bile ducts**
	51.71	**Simple suture of common bile duct**
	51.72	**Choledochoplasty**
		Repair of fistula of common bile duct
	51.79	**Repair of other bile ducts**
		Closure of artificial opening of bile duct NOS
		Suture of bile duct NOS
		EXCLUDES operative removal of prosthetic device (51.95)
✓4th	**51.8**	**Other operations on biliary ducts and sphincter of Oddi**
	51.81	**Dilation of sphincter of Oddi**
		Dilation of ampulla of Vater
		EXCLUDES that by endoscopic approach (51.84)
		DEF: Dilation of muscle around common bile and pancreatic ducts; to mitigate constriction obstructing bile flow.
	51.82	**Pancreatic sphincterotomy**
		Incision of pancreatic sphincter
		Transduodenal ampullary sphincterotomy
		EXCLUDES that by endoscopic approach (51.85)
		DEF: Pancreatic sphincterotomy: Division of muscle around common bile and pancreatic ducts.
		DEF: Transduodenal ampullary sphincterotomy: Incision into muscle around common bile and pancreatic ducts; closing approach through first section of small intestine.
	51.83	**Pancreatic sphincteroplasty**
	51.84	**Endoscopic dilation of ampulla and biliary duct**
		Dilation of ampulla and biliary duct by procedures classifiable to 51.10-51.11, 52.13
	51.85	**Endoscopic sphincterotomy and papillotomy**
		Sphincterotomy and papillotomy by procedures classifiable to 51.10-51.11, 52.13
		AHA: 2Q, '97, 7
		DEF: Incision of muscle around common bile and pancreatic ducts and closing the duodenal papilla.
	51.86	**Endoscopic insertion of nasobiliary drainage tube**
		Insertion of nasobiliary tube by procedures classifiable to 51.10-51.11, 52.13
	51.87	**Endoscopic insertion of stent (tube) into bile duct**
		Endoprosthesis of bile duct
		Insertion of stent into bile duct by procedures classifiable to 51.10-51.11, 52.13
		EXCLUDES nasobiliary drainage tube (51.86)
		replacement of stent (tube) (97.05)
	51.88	**Endoscopic removal of stone(s) from biliary tract**
		Laparoscopic removal of stone(s) from biliary tract
		Removal of biliary tract stone(s) by procedures classifiable to 51.10-51.11, 52.13
		EXCLUDES percutaneous extraction of common duct stones (51.96)
		AHA: 2Q, '00, 11; 2Q, '97, 7
	51.89	**Other operations on sphincter of Oddi**
✓4th	**51.9**	**Other operations on biliary tract**
	51.91	**Repair of laceration of gallbladder**
	51.92	**Closure of cholecystostomy**
	51.93	**Closure of other biliary fistula**
		Cholecystogastroenteric fistulectomy
	51.94	**Revision of anastomosis of biliary tract**
	51.95	**Removal of prosthetic device from bile duct**
		EXCLUDES nonoperative removal (97.55)
	51.96	**Percutaneous extraction of common duct stones**
		AHA: 4Q, '88, 7
	51.98	**Other percutaneous procedures on biliary tract**
		Percutaneous biliary endoscopy via existing T-tube or other tract for:
		dilation of biliary duct stricture
		removal of stone(s) except common duct stone
		exploration (postoperative)
		Percutaneous transhepatic biliary drainage
		EXCLUDES percutaneous aspiration of gallbladder (51.01)
		percutaneous biopsy and/or collection of specimen by brushing or washing (51.12)
		percutaneous removal of common duct stone(s) (51.96)
		AHA: 1Q, '97, 14; 3Q, '89, 18; N-D, '87, 1
	51.99	**Other**
		Insertion or replacement of biliary tract prosthesis
		EXCLUDES biopsy of gallbladder (51.12-51.13)
		irrigation of cholecystostomy and other biliary tube (96.41)
		lysis of peritoneal adhesions (54.5)
		nonoperative removal of: cholecystostomy tube (97.54)
		tube from biliary tract or liver (97.55)
✓3rd	**52**	**Operations on pancreas**
		▶Code also any application or administration of an adhesion barrier substance (99.77)◀
		INCLUDES operations on pancreatic duct
✓4th	**52.0**	**Pancreatotomy**
	52.01	**Drainage of pancreatic cyst by catheter**
	52.09	**Other pancreatotomy**
		Pancreatolithotomy
		EXCLUDES drainage by anastomosis (52.4, 52.96)
		incision of pancreatic sphincter (51.82)
		marsupialization of cyst (52.3)
		DEF: Pancreatolithotomy: Incision into pancreas to remove stones.

OPERATIONS ON THE DIGESTIVE SYSTEM

52.1 ✓4th **Diagnostic procedures on pancreas**

- **52.11** Closed [aspiration] [needle] [percutaneous] biopsy of pancreas
- **52.12** Open biopsy of pancreas
- **52.13** Endoscopic retrograde pancreatography [ERP]

  EXCLUDES: endoscopic retrograde:
  cholangiography [ERC] (51.11)
  cholangiopancreatography [ERCP] (51.10)
  that for procedures classifiable to 51.14-51.15, 51.64, 51.84-51.88, 52.14, 52.21, 52.92-52.94, 52.97-52.98

- **52.14** Closed [endoscopic] biopsy of pancreatic duct

  Closed biopsy of pancreatic duct by procedures classifiable to 51.10-51.11, 52.13

- **52.19** Other diagnostic procedures on pancreas

  EXCLUDES: contrast pancreatogram (87.66)
  endoscopic retrograde pancreatography [ERP] (52.13)
  microscopic examination of specimen from pancreas (91.01-91.09)

52.2 ✓4th **Local excision or destruction of pancreas and pancreatic duct**

  EXCLUDES: biopsy of pancreas (52.11-52.12, 52.14)
  pancreatic fistulectomy (52.95)

- **52.21** Endoscopic excision or destruction of lesion or tissue of pancreatic duct

  Excision or destruction of lesion or tissue of pancreatic duct by procedures classifiable to 51.10-51.11, 52.13

- **52.22** Other excision or destruction of lesion or tissue of pancreas or pancreatic duct

52.3 Marsupialization of pancreatic cyst

  EXCLUDES: drainage of cyst by catheter (52.01)

  DEF: Incision into pancreas and suturing edges to form pocket; promotes drainage and healing.

52.4 Internal drainage of pancreatic cyst

  Pancreaticocystoduodenostomy
  Pancreaticocystogastrostomy
  Pancreaticocystojejunostomy

  DEF: Withdrawing fluid from pancreatic cyst by draining it through a created passage to another organ.

  DEF: Pancreaticocystoduodenostomy: Creation of passage from pancreatic cyst to first portion of small intestine.

  DEF: Pancreaticocystogastrostomy: Creation of passage from pancreatic cyst to stomach.

  DEF: Pancreaticocystojejunostomy: Creation of passage from pancreatic cyst to midsection of small intestine.

52.5 ✓4th **Partial pancreatectomy**

  EXCLUDES: pancreatic fistulectomy (52.95)

- **52.51** Proximal pancreatectomy

  Excision of head of pancreas (with part of body)
  Proximal pancreatectomy with synchronous duodenectomy

- **52.52** Distal pancreatectomy

  Excision of tail of pancreas (with part of body)

- **52.53** Radical subtotal pancreatectomy
- **52.59** Other partial pancreatectomy

52.6 Total pancreatectomy

  Pancreatectomy with synchronous duodenectomy

  AHA: 4Q, '96, 71

52.7 Radical pancreaticoduodenectomy

  One-stage pancreaticoduodenal resection with choledochojejunal anastomosis, pancreaticojejunal anastomosis, and gastrojejunostomy
  Two-stage pancreaticoduodenal resection (first stage) (second stage)
  Radical resection of the pancreas
  Whipple procedure

  EXCLUDES: radical subtotal pancreatectomy (52.53)

  AHA: 1Q, '01, 13

  DEF: ▶Whipple procedure: pancreaticoduodenectomy involving the removal of the head of the pancreas and part of the small intestines; pancreaticojejunostomy, choledochojejunal anastomosis, and gastrojejunostomy included in the procedure.◄

52.8 ✓4th **Transplant of pancreas**

- [19] **52.80** Pancreatic transplant, not otherwise specified [NC]
- **52.81** Reimplantation of pancreatic tissue
- [19] **52.82** Homotransplant of pancreas [NC]
- **52.83** Heterotransplant of pancreas [NC]
- **52.84** Autotransplantation of cells of islets of Langerhans

  Homotransplantation of islet cells of pancreas

  AHA: 4Q, '96, 70, 71

  DEF: Transplantation of Islet cells from pancreas to another location of same patient.

- **52.85** Allotransplantation of cells of islets of Langerhans

  Heterotransplantation of islet cells of pancreas

  AHA: 4Q, '96, 70, 71

  DEF: Transplantation of Islet cells from one individual to another.

- **52.86** Transplantation of cells of islets of Langerhans, not otherwise specified

  AHA: 4Q, '96, 70

52.9 ✓4th **Other operations on pancreas**

  DEF: Placement of tube into pancreatic duct, without an endoscope.

- **52.92** Cannulation of pancreatic duct

  EXCLUDES: that by endoscopic approach (52.93)

- **52.93** Endoscopic insertion of stent (tube) into pancreatic duct

  Insertion of cannula or stent into pancreatic duct by procedures classifiable to 51.10-51.11, 52.13

  EXCLUDES: endoscopic insertion of nasopancreatic drainage tube (52.97)
  replacement of stent (tube) (97.05)

  AHA: 2Q, '97, 7

- **52.94** Endoscopic removal of stone(s) from pancreatic duct

  Removal of stone(s) from pancreatic duct by procedures classifiable to 51.10-51.11, 52.13

- **52.95** Other repair of pancreas

  Fistulectomy } of pancreas
  Simple suture

---

[19] Covered procedure when a diagnosis code is present from 250.00-250.93 and 585, V42.0, or V42.89

BI Bilateral Edit **NC** Non-covered Procedure ▶◀ Revised Text ● New Code ▲ Revised Code Title

Indirect Repair of Hernia

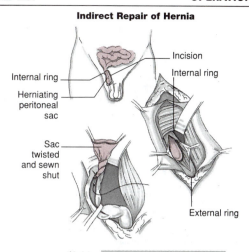

52.96 Anastomosis of pancreas
Anastomosis of pancreas (duct) to:
intestine   stomach
jejunum
EXCLUDES anastomosis to:
bile duct (51.39)
gallbladder (51.33)

52.97 Endoscopic insertion of nasopancreatic drainage tube
Insertion of nasopancreatic drainage tube by procedures classifiable to 51.10-51.11, 52.13
EXCLUDES drainage of pancreatic cyst by catheter (52.01)
replacement of stent (tube) (97.05)

52.98 Endoscopic dilation of pancreatic duct
Dilation of Wirsung's duct by procedures classifiable to 51.10-51.11, 52.13

52.99 Other
Dilation of pancreatic [Wirsung's] duct ⎫ by open
Repair of pancreatic [Wirsung's] duct ⎭ approach
EXCLUDES irrigation of pancreatic tube (96.42)
removal of pancreatic tube (97.56)

53 Repair of hernia
▶Code also any application or administration of an adhesion barrier substance (99.77)◀
INCLUDES hernioplasty   herniotomy
herniorrhaphy
EXCLUDES manual reduction of hernia (96.27)
AHA: 3Q, '94, 8

DEF: Repair of hernia: Restoration of abnormally protruding organ or tissue.
DEF: Herniorrhaphy: Repair of hernia.
DEF: Herniotomy: Division of constricted, strangulated, irreducible hernia.

53.0 Unilateral repair of inguinal hernia
- 53.00 Unilateral repair of inguinal hernia, not otherwise specified
  Inguinal herniorrhaphy NOS
- 53.01 Repair of direct inguinal hernia
  AHA: 4Q, '96, 66
- 53.02 Repair of indirect inguinal hernia
- 53.03 Repair of direct inguinal hernia with graft or prosthesis
- 53.04 Repair of indirect inguinal hernia with graft or prosthesis
- 53.05 Repair of inguinal hernia with graft or prosthesis, not otherwise specified

53.1 Bilateral repair of inguinal hernia
- 53.10 Bilateral repair of inguinal hernia, not otherwise specified
- 53.11 Bilateral repair of direct inguinal hernia
- 53.12 Bilateral repair of indirect inguinal hernia
- 53.13 Bilateral repair of inguinal hernia, one direct and one indirect
- 53.14 Bilateral repair of direct inguinal hernia with graft or prosthesis
- 53.15 Bilateral repair of indirect inguinal hernia with graft or prosthesis
- 53.16 Bilateral repair of inguinal hernia, one direct and one indirect, with graft or prosthesis
- 53.17 Bilateral inguinal hernia repair with graft or prosthesis, not otherwise specified

53.2 Unilateral repair of femoral hernia
- 53.21 Unilateral repair of femoral hernia with graft or prosthesis
- 53.29 Other unilateral femoral herniorrhaphy

53.3 Bilateral repair of femoral hernia
- 53.31 Bilateral repair of femoral hernia with graft or prosthesis
- 53.39 Other bilateral femoral herniorrhaphy

53.4 Repair of umbilical hernia
EXCLUDES repair of gastroschisis (54.71)
- 53.41 Repair of umbilical hernia with prosthesis
- 53.49 Other umbilical herniorrhaphy

53.5 Repair of other hernia of anterior abdominal wall (without graft or prosthesis)
- 53.51 Incisional hernia repair
- 53.59 Repair of other hernia of anterior abdominal wall
  Repair of hernia: Repair of hernia:
  epigastric   spigelian
  hypogastric   ventral
  AHA: 3Q, '96, 15

53.6 Repair of other hernia of anterior abdominal wall with graft or prosthesis
- 53.61 Incisional hernia repair with prosthesis
- 53.69 Repair of other hernia of anterior abdominal wall with prosthesis

53.7 Repair of diaphragmatic hernia, abdominal approach

53.8 Repair of diaphragmatic hernia, thoracic approach
DEF: Repair of diaphragmatic hernia though abdomen and thorax.
- 53.80 Repair of diaphragmatic hernia with thoracic approach, not otherwise specified
  Thoracoabdominal repair of diaphragmatic hernia
- 53.81 Plication of the diaphragm
  DEF: Tuck repair of diaphragmatic hernia.
- 53.82 Repair of parasternal hernia
  DEF: Repair of hernia protruding into breastbone area.

53.9 Other hernia repair
Repair of hernia: Repair of hernia:
ischiatic   omental
ischiorectal   retroperitoneal
lumbar   sciatic
obturator
EXCLUDES relief of strangulated hernia with exteriorization of intestine (46.01, 46.03)
repair of pericolostomy hernia (46.42)
repair of vaginal enterocele (70.92)

54 Other operations on abdominal region
▶Code also any application or administration of an adhesion barrier substance (99.77)◀

INCLUDES: operations on:
- epigastric region
- flank
- groin region
- hypochondrium
- inguinal region
- loin region
- male pelvic cavity
- mesentery
- omentum
- peritoneum
- retroperitoneal tissue space

EXCLUDES:
- female pelvic cavity (69.01-70.92)
- hernia repair (53.00-53.9)
- obliteration of cul-de-sac (70.92)
- retroperitoneal tissue dissection (59.00-59.09)
- skin and subcutaneous tissue of abdominal wall (86.01-86.99)

54.0 Incision of abdominal wall
Drainage of:
- abdominal wall
- extraperitoneal abscess
- retroperitoneal abscess

EXCLUDES:
- incision of peritoneum (54.95)
- laparotomy (54.11-54.19)

AHA: 1Q, '97, 11; N-D, '87, 12

54.1 Laparotomy
AHA: 1Q, '92, 13

DEF: Incision into abdomen.

54.11 Exploratory laparotomy
EXCLUDES: exploration incidental to intra-abdominal surgery — omit code

AHA: 3Q, '89, 14; 4Q, '88, 12

DEF: Exam of peritoneal cavity through incision into abdomen.

54.12 Reopening of recent laparotomy site
Reopening of recent laparotomy site for:
- control of hemorrhage
- exploration
- incision of hematoma

54.19 Other laparotomy
Drainage of intraperitoneal abscess or hematoma

EXCLUDES:
- culdocentesis (70.0)
- drainage of appendiceal abscess (47.2)
- exploration incidental to intra-abdominal surgery — omit code
- Ladd operation (54.95)
- percutaneous drainage of abdomen (54.91)
- removal of foreign body (54.92)

54.2 Diagnostic procedures of abdominal region

54.21 Laparoscopy
Peritoneoscopy

EXCLUDES:
- laparoscopic cholecystectomy (51.23)
- that incidental to destruction of fallopian tubes (66.21-66.29)

DEF: Endoscopic exam of peritoneal cavity through abdominal incision.

54.22 Biopsy of abdominal wall or umbilicus

54.23 Biopsy of peritoneum
Biopsy of:
- mesentery
- omentum
- peritoneal implant

EXCLUDES: closed biopsy of:
- omentum (54.24)
- peritoneum (54.24)

54.24 Closed [percutaneous] [needle] biopsy of intra-abdominal mass
Closed biopsy of:
- omentum
- peritoneal implant
- peritoneum

EXCLUDES: that of:
- fallopian tube (66.11)
- ovary (65.11)
- uterine ligaments (68.15)
- uterus (68.16)

AHA: 4Q, '97, 57

54.25 Peritoneal lavage
Diagnostic peritoneal lavage

EXCLUDES: peritoneal dialysis (54.98)

AHA: 2Q, '98, 19; 4Q, '93, 28

DEF: Irrigation of peritoneal cavity with siphoning of liquid contents for analysis.

54.29 Other diagnostic procedures on abdominal region
EXCLUDES:
- abdominal lymphangiogram (88.04)
- abdominal x-ray NEC (88.19)
- angiocardiography of venae cavae (88.51)
- C.A.T. scan of abdomen (88.01)
- contrast x-ray of abdominal cavity (88.11-88.15)
- intra-abdominal arteriography NEC (88.47)
- microscopic examination of peritoneal and retroperitoneal specimen (91.11-91.19)
- phlebography of:
  - intra-abdominal vessels NEC (88.65)
  - portal venous system (88.64)
- sinogram of abdominal wall (88.03)
- soft tissue x-ray of abdominal wall NEC (88.09)
- tomography of abdomen NEC (88.02)
- ultrasonography of abdomen and retroperitoneum (88.76)

54.3 Excision or destruction of lesion or tissue of abdominal wall or umbilicus
Debridement of abdominal wall
Omphalectomy

EXCLUDES:
- biopsy of abdominal wall or umbilicus (54.22)
- size reduction operation (86.83)
- that of skin of abdominal wall (86.22, 86.26, 86.3)

AHA: 1Q, '89, 11

54.4 Excision or destruction of peritoneal tissue
Excision of:
- appendices epiploicae
- falciform ligament
- gastrocolic ligament
- lesion of:
  - mesentery
  - omentum
  - peritoneum
- presacral lesion NOS
- retroperitoneal lesion NOS

EXCLUDES:
- biopsy of peritoneum (54.23)
- endometrectomy of cul-de-sac (70.32)

54.5 Lysis of peritoneal adhesions
Freeing of adhesions of:
    biliary tract
    intestines
    liver
    pelvic peritoneum
    peritoneum
    spleen
    uterus

EXCLUDES   lysis of adhesions of:
    bladder (59.11)
    fallopian tube and ovary (65.81, 65.89)
    kidney (59.02)
    ureter (59.02-59.03)

AHA: 3Q, '94, 8; 4Q, '90, 18

54.51 Laparoscopic lysis of peritoneal adhesions
AHA: 4Q, '96, 65

54.59 Other lysis of peritoneal adhesions
AHA: 4Q, '96, 66

54.6 Suture of abdominal wall and peritoneum

54.61 Reclosure of postoperative disruption of abdominal wall

54.62 Delayed closure of granulating abdominal wound
Tertiary subcutaneous wound closure
DEF: Closure of outer layers of abdominal wound; follows procedure to close initial layers of wound.

54.63 Other suture of abdominal wall
Suture of laceration of abdominal wall
EXCLUDES   closure of operative wound — omit code

54.64 Suture of peritoneum
Secondary suture of peritoneum
EXCLUDES   closure of operative wound — omit code

54.7 Other repair of abdominal wall and peritoneum

54.71 Repair of gastroschisis
DEF: Repair of congenital fistula of abdominal wall.

54.72 Other repair of abdominal wall

54.73 Other repair of peritoneum
Suture of gastrocolic ligament

54.74 Other repair of omentum
Epiplorrhaphy
Graft of omentum
Omentopexy
Reduction of torsion of omentum
EXCLUDES   cardio-omentopexy (36.39)

AHA: J-F, '87, 11

DEF: Epiplorrhaphy: Suture of abdominal serous membrane.

DEF: Graft of omentum: Implantation of tissue into abdominal serous membrane.

DEF: Omentopexy: Anchoring of abdominal serous membrane.

DEF: Reduction of torsion of omentum: Reduction of twisted abdominal serous membrane.

54.75 Other repair of mesentery
Mesenteric plication
Mesenteropexy
DEF: Creation of folds in mesentery for shortening.
DEF: Mesenteriopexy: Fixation of torn, incised mesentery.

54.9 Other operations of abdominal region
EXCLUDES   removal of ectopic pregnancy (74.3)

54.91 Percutaneous abdominal drainage
Paracentesis
EXCLUDES   creation of cutaneoperitoneal fistula (54.93)

AHA: 3Q, '99, 9; 2Q, '99, 14; 3Q, '98, 12; 1Q, '92, 14; 2Q, '90, 25

DEF: Puncture for removal of fluid.

54.92 Removal of foreign body from peritoneal cavity
AHA: 1Q, '89, 11

54.93 Creation of cutaneoperitoneal fistula
AHA: 2Q, '95, 10; N-D, '84, 6
DEF: Creation of opening between skin and peritoneal cavity.

54.94 Creation of peritoneovascular shunt
Peritoneovenous shunt
AHA: 1Q, '94, 7; 1Q, '88, 9; S-O, '85, 6
DEF: Construction of shunt to connect peritoneal cavity with vascular system.
DEF: Peritoneovenous shunt: Construction of shunt to connect peritoneal cavity with vein.

54.95 Incision of peritoneum
▶Exploration of ventriculoperitoneal shunt at peritoneal site◀
Ladd operation
Revision of distal catheter of ventricular shunt
Revision of ventriculoperitoneal shunt at peritoneal site
EXCLUDES   that incidental to laparotomy (54.11-54.19)

AHA: 4Q, '95, 65

DEF: Ladd operation: Peritoneal attachment of incompletely rotated cecum, obstructing duodenum.

54.96 Injection of air into peritoneal cavity
Pneumoperitoneum
EXCLUDES   that for:
    collapse of lung (33.33)
    radiography (88.12-88.13, 88.15)

54.97 Injection of locally-acting therapeutic substance into peritoneal cavity
EXCLUDES   peritoneal dialysis (54.98)

54.98 Peritoneal dialysis
EXCLUDES   peritoneal lavage (diagnostic) (54.25)

AHA: 4Q, '93, 28; N-D, '84, 6

DEF: Separation of blood elements by diffusion through membrane.

54.99 Other
EXCLUDES   removal of:
    abdominal wall sutures (97.83)
    peritoneal drainage device (97.82)
    retroperitoneal drainage device (97.81)

AHA: 1Q, '99, 4

10. OPERATIONS ON THE URINARY SYSTEM (55-59)

√3rd **55 Operations on kidney**
▶Code also any application or administration of an adhesion barrier substance (99.77)◀
  INCLUDES operations on renal pelvis
  EXCLUDES perirenal tissue (59.00-59.09, 59.21-59.29, 59.91-59.92)

√4th **55.0 Nephrotomy and nephrostomy**
  EXCLUDES drainage by:
      anastomosis (55.86)
      aspiration (55.92)

  55.01 Nephrotomy
    Evacuation of renal cyst
    Exploration of kidney
    Nephrolithotomy

  DEF: Nephrotomy: Incision into kidney.

  DEF: Evacuation of renal cyst: Draining contents of cyst.

  DEF: Exploration of kidney: Exploration through incision.

  DEF: Nephrolithotomy: Removal of kidney stone through incision.

  55.02 Nephrostomy
  AHA: 2Q, '97, 4

  55.03 Percutaneous nephrostomy without fragmentation
    Nephrostolithotomy, percutaneous (nephroscopic)
    Percutaneous removal of kidney stone(s) by:
      forceps extraction (nephroscopic)
      basket extraction
    Pyelostolithotomy, percutaneous (nephroscopic)
    With placement of catheter down ureter
    EXCLUDES percutaneous removal by fragmentation (55.04)
      repeat nephroscopic removal during current episode (55.92)

  AHA: 2Q, '96, 5

  DEF: Insertion of tube through abdominal wall without breaking up stones.

  DEF: Nephrostolithotomy: Insertion of tube through the abdominal wall to remove stones.

  DEF: Basket extraction: Removal, percutaneous of stone with grasping forceps.

  DEF: Pyelostolithotomy: Removal, percutaneous of stones from funnel-shaped portion of kidney.

  55.04 Percutaneous nephrostomy with fragmentation
    Percutaneous nephrostomy with disruption of kidney stone by ultrasonic energy and extraction (suction) through endoscope
    With placement of catheter down ureter
    With fluoroscopic guidance
    EXCLUDES repeat fragmentation during current episode (59.95)

  AHA: 1Q, '89, 1; S-O, '86, 11

  DEF: Insertion of tube through abdominal wall into kidney to break up stones.

√4th **55.1 Pyelotomy and pyelostomy**
  EXCLUDES drainage by anastomosis (55.86)
    percutaneous pyelolithotomy (55.03)
    removal of calculus without incision (56.0)

  55.11 Pyelotomy
    Exploration of renal pelvis
    Pyelolithotomy

  55.12 Pyelostomy
    Insertion of drainage tube into renal pelvis

√4th **55.2 Diagnostic procedures on kidney**

  55.21 Nephroscopy
  DEF: Endoscopic exam of renal pelvis; retrograde through ureter, percutaneous or open exposure.

  55.22 Pyeloscopy
  DEF: Fluoroscopic exam of kidney pelvis, calyces and ureters; follows IV or retrograde injection of contrast.

  55.23 Closed [percutaneous] [needle] biopsy of kidney
    Endoscopic biopsy via existing nephrostomy, nephrotomy, pyelostomy, or pyelotomy

  55.24 Open biopsy of kidney

  55.29 Other diagnostic procedures on kidney
    EXCLUDES microscopic examination of specimen from kidney (91.21-91.29)
      pyelogram:
        intravenous (87.73)
        percutaneous (87.75)
        retrograde (87.74)
      radioisotope scan (92.03)
      renal arteriography (88.45)
      tomography:
        C.A.T scan (87.71)
        other (87.72)

√4th **55.3 Local excision or destruction of lesion or tissue of kidney**

  55.31 Marsupialization of kidney lesion
  DEF: Exteriorization of lesion by incising anterior wall and suturing cut edges to create open pouch.

  55.39 Other local destruction or excision of renal lesion or tissue
    Obliteration of calyceal diverticulum
    EXCLUDES biopsy of kidney (55.23-55.24)
      partial nephrectomy (55.4)
      percutaneous aspiration of kidney (55.92)
      wedge resection of kidney (55.4)

  55.4 Partial nephrectomy
    Calycectomy
    Wedge resection of kidney
    Code also any synchronous resection of ureter (56.40-56.42)

  DEF: Surgical removal of a part of the kidney.

  DEF: Calycectomy: Removal of indentations in kidney.

√4th **55.5 Complete nephrectomy**
    Code also any synchronous excision of:
      bladder segment (57.6)
      lymph nodes (40.3, 40.52-40.59)

  55.51 Nephroureterectomy
    Nephroureterectomy with bladder cuff
    Total nephrectomy (unilateral)
    EXCLUDES removal of transplanted kidney (55.53)

  DEF: Complete removal of the kidney and all or portion of the ureter.

  DEF: Nephroureterectomy with bladder cuff: Removal of kidney, ureter, and portion of bladder attached to ureter.

  DEF: Total nephrectomy (unilateral): Complete excision of one kidney.

  55.52 Nephrectomy of remaining kidney
    Removal of solitary kidney
    EXCLUDES removal of transplanted kidney (55.53)

  55.53 Removal of transplanted or rejected kidney

OPERATIONS ON THE URINARY SYSTEM

55.54 Bilateral nephrectomy
  EXCLUDES: complete nephrectomy NOS (55.51)
  DEF: Removal of both kidneys same operative session.

√4ᵗʰ 55.6 Transplant of kidney
  55.61 Renal autotransplantation
  55.69 Other kidney transplantation
  AHA: 4Q, '96, 71

55.7 Nephropexy
  Fixation or suspension of movable [floating] kidney

√4ᵗʰ 55.8 Other repair of kidney
  55.81 Suture of laceration of kidney
  55.82 Closure of nephrostomy and pyelostomy
  DEF: Removal of tube from kidney and closure of site of tube insertion.

  55.83 Closure of other fistula of kidney
  55.84 Reduction of torsion of renal pedicle
  DEF: Restoration of twisted renal pedicle into normal position.

  55.85 Symphysiotomy for horseshoe kidney
  DEF: Division of congenitally malformed kidney into two parts.

  55.86 Anastomosis of kidney
  Nephropyeloureterostomy
  Pyeloureterovesical anastomosis
  Ureterocalyceal anastomosis
  EXCLUDES: nephrocystanastomosis NOS (56.73)
  DEF: Nephropyeloureterostomy: Creation of passage between kidney and ureter.
  DEF: Pyeloureterovesical anastomosis: Creation of passage between kidney and bladder.
  DEF: Ureterocalyceal anastomosis: Creation of passage between ureter and kidney indentations.

  55.87 Correction of ureteropelvic junction
  55.89 Other

√4ᵗʰ 55.9 Other operations on kidney
  EXCLUDES: lysis of perirenal adhesions (59.02)
  55.91 Decapsulation of kidney
  Capsulectomy } of kidney
  Decortication

  55.92 Percutaneous aspiration of kidney (pelvis)
  Aspiration of renal cyst   Renipuncture
  EXCLUDES: percutaneous biopsy of kidney (55.23)
  AHA: N-D, '84, 20
  DEF: Insertion of needle into kidney to withdraw fluid.

Symphysiostomy for Horseshoe Kidney

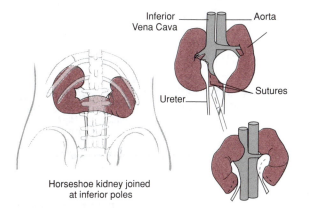

Horseshoe kidney joined at inferior poles

55.93 Replacement of nephrostomy tube
55.94 Replacement of pyelostomy tube
55.95 Local perfusion of kidney
  DEF: Fluid passage through kidney.

55.96 Other injection of therapeutic substance into kidney
  Injection into renal cyst

55.97 Implantation or replacement of mechanical kidney
55.98 Removal of mechanical kidney
55.99 Other
  EXCLUDES: removal of pyelostomy or nephrostomy tube (97.61)

√3ʳᵈ 56 Operations on ureter
  ▶Code also any application or administration of an adhesion barrier substance (99.77)◀

  56.0 Transurethral removal of obstruction from ureter and renal pelvis
  Removal of:
  blood clot
  calculus   } from ureter or renal pelvis without incision
  foreign body
  EXCLUDES: manipulation without removal of obstruction (59.8)
  that by incision (55.11, 56.2)
  transurethral insertion of ureteral stent for passage of calculus (59.8)
  AHA: 1Q, '89, 1; S-O, '86, 12
  DEF: Removal of obstruction by tube inserted through urethra to ureter.

  56.1 Ureteral meatotomy
  DEF: Incision into ureteral meatus to enlarge passage.

  56.2 Ureterotomy
  Incision of ureter for: Incision of ureter for:
  drainage   removal of calculus
  exploration
  EXCLUDES: cutting of ureterovesical orifice (56.1)
  removal of calculus without incision (56.0)
  transurethral insertion of ureteral stent for passage of calculus (59.8)
  urinary diversion (56.51-56.79)
  AHA: S-O, '86, 10

√4ᵗʰ 56.3 Diagnostic procedures on ureter
  56.31 Ureteroscopy
  56.32 Closed percutaneous biopsy of ureter
  EXCLUDES: endoscopic biopsy of ureter (56.33)
  56.33 Closed endoscopic biopsy of ureter
  Cystourethroscopy with ureteral biopsy
  Transurethral biopsy of ureter
  Ureteral endoscopy with biopsy through ureterotomy
  Ureteroscopy with biopsy
  EXCLUDES: percutaneous biopsy of ureter (56.32)
  56.34 Open biopsy of ureter
  56.35 Endoscopy (cystoscopy) (looposcopy) of ileal conduit
  DEF: Endoscopic exam of created opening between ureters and one end of small intestine; other end used to form artificial opening.

  56.39 Other diagnostic procedures on ureter
  EXCLUDES: microscopic examination of specimen from ureter (91.21-91.29)

OPERATIONS ON THE URINARY SYSTEM

✓4ᵗʰ 56.4 Ureterectomy
Code also anastomosis other than end-to-end (56.51-56.79)
EXCLUDES fistulectomy (56.84)
nephroureterectomy (55.51-55.54)

- **56.40** Ureterectomy, not otherwise specified
- **56.41** Partial ureterotomy
  - Excision of lesion of ureter
  - Shortening of ureter with reimplantation
  - **EXCLUDES** biopsy of ureter (56.32-56.34)
- **56.42** Total ureterectomy

✓4ᵗʰ 56.5 Cutaneous uretero-ileostomy
- **56.51** Formation of cutaneous uretero-ileostomy
  - Construction of ileal conduit
  - External ureteral ileostomy
  - Formation of open ileal bladder
  - Ileal loop operation
  - Ileoureterostomy (Bricker's) (ileal bladder)
  - Transplantation of ureter into ileum with external diversion
  - **EXCLUDES** closed ileal bladder (57.87)
    replacement of ureteral defect by ileal segment (56.89)
  - **DEF:** Creation of urinary passage by connecting the terminal end of small intestine to ureter then connected to opening through abdominal wall.
  - **DEF:** Construction of ileal conduit: Formation of conduit from terminal end of small intestine.
- **56.52** Revision of cutaneous uretero-ileostomy
  - **AHA:** 3Q, '96, 15; 4Q, '88, 7

✓4ᵗʰ 56.6 Other external urinary diversion
- **56.61** Formation of other cutaneous ureterostomy
  - Anastomosis of ureter to skin
  - Ureterostomy NOS
- **56.62** Revision of other cutaneous ureterostomy
  - Revision of ureterostomy stoma
  - **EXCLUDES** nonoperative removal of ureterostomy tube (97.62)

✓4ᵗʰ 56.7 Other anastomosis or bypass of ureter
EXCLUDES ureteropyelostomy (55.86)

- **56.71** Urinary diversion to intestine
  - Anastomosis of ureter to intestine
  - Internal urinary diversion NOS
  - Code also any synchronous colostomy (46.10-46.13)
  - **EXCLUDES** external ureteral ileostomy (56.51)
- **56.72** Revision of ureterointestinal anastomosis
  - **EXCLUDES** revision of external ureteral ileostomy (56.52)
- **56.73** Nephrocystanastomosis, not otherwise specified
  - **DEF:** Connection of kidney to bladder.
- **56.74** Ureteroneocystostomy
  - Replacement of ureter with bladder flap
  - Ureterovesical anastomosis
  - **DEF:** Transfer of ureter to another site in bladder.
  - **DEF:** Ureterovesical anastomosis: Implantation of ureter into bladder.
- **56.75** Transureteroureterostomy
  - **EXCLUDES** ureteroureterostomy associated with partial resection (56.41)
  - **DEF:** Separating one ureter and joining the ends to the opposite ureter.
- **56.79** Other

✓4ᵗʰ 56.8 Repair of ureter
- **56.81** Lysis of intraluminal adhesions of ureter
  - **EXCLUDES** lysis of periureteral adhesions (59.01-59.02)
    ureterolysis (59.02-59.03)
  - **DEF:** Destruction of adhesions within urethral cavity.
- **56.82** Suture of laceration of ureter
- **56.83** Closure of ureterostomy
- **56.84** Closure of other fistula of ureter
- **56.85** Ureteropexy
- **56.86** Removal of ligature from ureter
- **56.89** Other repair of ureter
  - Graft of ureter
  - Replacement of ureter with ileal segment implanted into bladder
  - Ureteroplication
  - **DEF:** Graft of ureter: Tissue from another site for graft replacement or repair of ureter.
  - **DEF:** Replacement of ureter with ileal segment implanted into bladder and ureter replacement with terminal end of small intestine.
  - **DEF:** Ureteroplication: Creation of tucks in ureter.

✓4ᵗʰ 56.9 Other operations on ureter
- **56.91** Dilation of ureteral meatus
- **56.92** Implantation of electronic ureteral stimulator
- **56.93** Replacement of electronic ureteral stimulator
- **56.94** Removal of electronic ureteral stimulator
  - **EXCLUDES** that with synchronous replacement (56.93)
- **56.95** Ligation of ureter
- **56.99** Other
  - **EXCLUDES** removal of ureterostomy tube and ureteral catheter (97.62)
    ureteral catheterization (59.8)

✓3ʳᵈ 57 Operations on urinary bladder
▶Code also any application or administration of an adhesion barrier substance (99.77)◀
EXCLUDES perivesical tissue (59.11-59.29, 59.91-59.92)
ureterovesical orifice (56.0-56.99)

- **57.0** Transurethral clearance of bladder
  - Drainage of bladder without incision
  - Removal of:
    - blood clot ⎫
    - calculus   ⎬ from bladder without incision
    - foreign body ⎭
  - **EXCLUDES** that by incision (57.19)
  - **AHA:** S-O, '86, 11
  - **DEF:** Insertion of device through urethra to cleanse bladder.

✓4ᵗʰ 57.1 Cystotomy and cystostomy
EXCLUDES cystotomy and cystostomy as operative approach — omit code
- **DEF:** Cystotomy: Incision of bladder.
- **DEF:** Cystostomy: Creation of opening into bladder.
- **57.11** Percutaneous aspiration of bladder
- **57.12** Lysis of intraluminal adhesions with incision into bladder
  - **EXCLUDES** transurethral lysis of intraluminal adhesions (57.41)
  - **DEF:** Incision into bladder to destroy lesions.

OPERATIONS ON THE URINARY SYSTEM

57.17 **Percutaneous cystostomy**
Closed cystostomy
Percutaneous suprapubic cystostomy
EXCLUDES removal of cystostomy tube (97.63)
replacement of cystostomy tube (59.94)

DEF: Incision through body wall into bladder to insert tube.

DEF: Percutaneous (closed) suprapubic cystostomy: Incision above pubic arch, through body wall, into the bladder to insert tube.

57.18 **Other suprapubic cystostomy**
EXCLUDES percutaneous cystostomy (57.17)
removal of cystostomy tube (97.63)
replacement of cystostomy tube (59.94)

57.19 **Other cystotomy**
Cystolithotomy
EXCLUDES percutaneous cystostomy (57.17)
suprapubic cystostomy (57.18)

AHA: 4Q, '95, 73; S-O, '86, 11

57.2 **Vesicostomy**
EXCLUDES percutaneous cystostomy (57.17)
suprapubic cystostomy (57.18)

57.21 **Vesicostomy**
Creation of permanent opening from bladder to skin using a bladder flap

DEF: Creation of opening from the bladder to the skin.

DEF: Creation of permanent opening from the bladder to the skin using a bladder flap to create conduit from bladder to skin using bladder tissue.

57.22 **Revision or closure of vesicostomy**
EXCLUDES closure of cystostomy (57.82)

57.3 **Diagnostic procedures on bladder**
57.31 **Cystoscopy through artificial stoma**
57.32 **Other cystoscopy**
Transurethral cystoscopy
EXCLUDES cystourethroscopy with ureteral biopsy (56.33)
retrograde pyelogram (87.74)
that for control of hemorrhage (postoperative):
bladder (57.93)
prostate (60.94)

AHA: 1Q, '01, 14

57.33 **Closed [transurethral] biopsy of bladder**
57.34 **Open biopsy of bladder**

Transurethral Cystourethroscopy

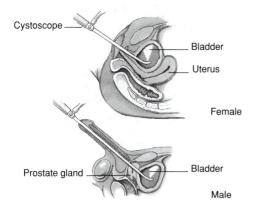

Cystoscope — Bladder
Uterus
Female

Prostate gland — Bladder
Male

57.39 **Other diagnostic procedures on bladder**
EXCLUDES cystogram NEC (87.77)
microscopic examination of specimen from bladder (91.31-91.39)
retrograde cystourethrogram (87.76)
therapeutic distention of bladder (96.25)

57.4 **Transurethral excision or destruction of bladder tissue**

DEF: Destruction of bladder tissue with instrument inserted into urethra.

57.41 **Transurethral lysis of intraluminal adhesions**
57.49 **Other transurethral excision or destruction of lesion or tissue of bladder**
Endoscopic resection of bladder lesion
EXCLUDES transurethral biopsy of bladder (57.33)
transurethral fistulectomy (57.83-57.84)

57.5 **Other excision or destruction of bladder tissue**
EXCLUDES that with transurethral approach (57.41-57.49)

57.51 **Excision of urachus**
Excision of urachal sinus of bladder
EXCLUDES excision of urachal cyst of abdominal wall (54.3)

57.59 **Open excision or destruction of other lesion or tissue of bladder**
Endometrectomy of bladder
Suprapubic excision of bladder lesion
EXCLUDES biopsy of bladder (57.33-57.34)
fistulectomy of bladder (57.83-57.84)

DEF: Endometrectomy of bladder: Removal of inner lining.

DEF: Suprapubic excision of bladder lesion: Removal of lesion by excision above suprapubic bone arch.

57.6 **Partial cystectomy**
Excision of bladder dome   Wedge resection of bladder
Trigonectomy

57.7 **Total cystectomy**
INCLUDES total cystectomy with urethrectomy

57.71 **Radical cystectomy**
Pelvic exenteration in male
Removal of bladder, prostate, seminal vesicles and fat
Removal of bladder, urethra, and fat in a female
Code also any:
lymph node dissection (40.3, 40.5)
urinary diversion (56.51-56.79)
EXCLUDES that as part of pelvic exenteration in female (68.8)

DEF: Radical cystectomy: Removal of bladder and surrounding tissue.

DEF: Pelvic exenteration in male: Excision of bladder, prostate, seminal vessels and fat.

57.79 **Other total cystectomy**

57.8 **Other repair of urinary bladder**
EXCLUDES repair of:
current obstetric laceration (75.61)
cystocele (70.50-70.51)
that for stress incontinence (59.3-59.79)

57.81 **Suture of laceration of bladder**

OPERATIONS ON THE URINARY SYSTEM

57.82 Closure of cystostomy

57.83 Repair of fistula involving bladder and intestine

Rectovesicovaginal } fistulectomy
Vesicosigmoidovaginal

57.84 Repair of other fistula of bladder

Cervicovesical
Urethroperineovesical } fistulectomy
Uterovesical
Vaginovesical

EXCLUDES vesicoureterovaginal fistulectomy (56.84)

57.85 Cystourethroplasty and plastic repair of bladder neck

Plication of sphincter of urinary bladder
V-Y plasty of bladder neck

DEF: Cystourethroplasty: Reconstruction of narrowed portion of bladder.

DEF: Plication of sphincter or urinary bladder: Creation of tuck in bladder sphincter.

DEF: V-Y plasty of bladder neck: Surgical reconstruction of the narrowed portion of bladder by V-Y technique.

57.86 Repair of bladder exstrophy

DEF: Surgical connection of a congenital bladder wall defect.

57.87 Reconstruction of urinary bladder

Anastomosis of bladder with isolated segment of ileum
Augmentation of bladder
Replacement of bladder with ileum or sigmoid [closed ileal bladder]
Code also resection of intestine (45.50-45.52)

AHA: 3Q, '00, 7

DEF: Anastomosis of bladder with isolated segment of ileum: Creation of connection between bladder and separated terminal end of small intestine.

57.88 Other anastomosis of bladder

Anastomosis of bladder to intestine NOS
Cystocolic anastomosis

EXCLUDES formation of closed ileal bladder (57.87)

57.89 Other repair of bladder

Bladder suspension, not elsewhere classified
Cystopexy NOS
Repair of old obstetric laceration of bladder

EXCLUDES repair of current obstetric laceration (75.61)

√4th **57.9** Other operations on bladder

57.91 Sphincterotomy of bladder
Division of bladder neck

AHA: 2Q, '90, 26

57.92 Dilation of bladder neck

57.93 Control of (postoperative) hemorrhage of bladder

57.94 Insertion of indwelling urinary catheter

57.95 Replacement of indwelling urinary catheter

57.96 Implantation of electronic bladder stimulator   NC

57.97 Replacement of electronic bladder stimulator   NC

57.98 Removal of electronic bladder stimulator

EXCLUDES that with synchronous replacement (57.97)

57.99 Other

EXCLUDES irrigation of:
cystostomy (96.47)
other indwelling urinary catheter (96.48)
lysis of external adhesions (59.11)
removal of:
cystostomy tube (97.63)
other urinary drainagedevice (97.64)
therapeutic distention of bladder (96.25)

√3rd **58** Operations on urethra

▶Code also any application or administration of an adhesion barrier substance (99.77)◀

INCLUDES operations on:
bulbourethral gland [Cowper's gland]
periurethral tissue

58.0 Urethrotomy

Excision of urethral septum
Formation of urethrovaginal fistula
Perineal urethrostomy
Removal of calculus from urethra by incision

EXCLUDES drainage of bulbourethral gland or periurethral tissue (58.91)
internal urethral meatotomy (58.5)
removal of urethral calculus without incision (58.6)

58.1 Urethral meatotomy

EXCLUDES internal urethral meatotomy (58.5)

DEF: Incision of urethra to enlarge passage.

√4th **58.2** Diagnostic procedures on urethra

58.21 Perineal urethroscopy

58.22 Other urethroscopy

58.23 Biopsy of urethra

58.24 Biopsy of periurethral tissue

DEF: Removal for biopsy of tissue around urethra.

58.29 Other diagnostic procedures on urethra and periurethral tissue

EXCLUDES microscopic examination of specimen from urethra (91.31-91.39)
retrograde cystourethrogram (87.76)
urethral pressure profile (89.25)
urethral sphincter electromyogram (89.23)

√4th **58.3** Excision or destruction of lesion or tissue of urethra

EXCLUDES biopsy of urethra (58.23)
excision of bulbourethral gland (58.92)
fistulectomy (58.43)
urethrectomy as part of:
complete cystectomy (57.79)
pelvic evisceration (68.8)
radical cystectomy (57.71)

58.31 Endoscopic excision or destruction of lesion or tissue of urethra
Fulguration of urethral lesion

58.39 Other local excision or destruction of lesion or tissue of urethra

Excision of:
congenital valve
lesion   } of urethra
stricture

Urethrectomy

EXCLUDES that by endoscopic appoach (58.31)

OPERATIONS ON THE URINARY SYSTEM

58.4 Repair of urethra
EXCLUDES repair of current obstetric laceration (75.61)

- **58.41** Suture of laceration of urethra
- **58.42** Closure of urethrostomy
- **58.43** Closure of other fistula of urethra
  EXCLUDES repair of urethroperineovesical fistula (57.84)
- **58.44** Reanastomosis of urethra
  Anastomosis of urethra
  DEF: Repair of severed urethra.
- **58.45** Repair of hypospadias or epispadias
  AHA: 3Q, '97, 6; 4Q, '96, 35
  DEF: Repair of abnormal urethral opening.
- **58.46** Other reconstruction of urethra
  Urethral construction
- **58.47** Urethral meatoplasty
  DEF: Reconstruction of urethral opening.
- **58.49** Other repair of urethra
  Benenenti rotation of bulbous urethra
  Repair of old obstetric laceration of urethra
  Urethral plication
  EXCLUDES repair of:
  current obstetric laceration (75.61)
  urethrocele (70.50-70.51)

58.5 Release of urethral stricture
Cutting of urethral sphincter
Internal urethral meatotomy
Urethrolysis
AHA: 1Q, '97, 13

58.6 Dilation of urethra
Dilation of urethrovesical junction
Passage of sounds through urethra
Removal of calculus from urethra without incision
EXCLUDES urethral calibration (89.29)
AHA: 1Q, '01, 14; 1Q, '97, 13

58.9 Other operations on urethra and periurethral tissue
- **58.91** Incision of periurethral tissue
  Drainage of bulbourethral gland
  DEF: Incision of tissue around urethra.
- **58.92** Excision of periurethral tissue
  EXCLUDES biopsy of periurethral tissue (58.24)
  lysis of periurethral adhesions (59.11-59.12)
- **58.93** Implantation of artificial urinary sphincter [AUS]
  Placement of inflatable:
  urethral sphincter
  bladder sphincter
  Removal with replacement of sphincter device [AUS]
  With pump and/or reservoir
- **58.99** Other
  Repair of inflatable sphincter pump and/or reservoir
  Surgical correction of hydraulic pressure of inflatable sphincter device
  Removal of inflatable urinary sphincter without replacement
  EXCLUDES removal of:
  intraluminal foreign body from urethra without incision (98.19)
  urethral stent (97.65)

59 Other operations on urinary tract
▶Code also any application or administration of an adhesion barrier substance (99.77)◀

59.0 Dissection of retroperitoneal tissue
- **59.00** Retroperitoneal dissection, not otherwise specified
- **59.02** Other lysis of perirenal or periureteral adhesions
  EXCLUDES that by laparoscope (59.03)
- **59.03** Laparoscopic lysis of perirenal or periureteral adhesions
- **59.09** Other incision of perirenal or periureteral tissue
  Exploration of perinephric area
  Incision of perirenal abscess
  DEF: Exploration of the perinephric area: Exam of tissue around the kidney by incision.
  DEF: Incision of perirenal abscess: Incising abscess in tissue around kidney.

59.1 Incision of perivesical tissue
DEF: Incising tissue around bladder.
- **59.11** Other lysis of perivesical adhesions
- **59.12** Laparoscopic lysis of perivesical adhesions
- **59.19** Other incision of perivesical tissue
  Exploration of perivesical tissue
  Incision of hematoma of space of Retzius
  Retropubic exploration

59.2 Diagnostic procedures on perirenal and perivesical tissue
- **59.21** Biopsy of perirenal or perivesical tissue
- **59.29** Other diagnostic procedures on perirenal tissue, perivesical tissue, and retroperitoneum
  EXCLUDES microscopic examination of specimen from:
  perirenal tissue (91.21-91.29)
  perivesical tissue (91.31-91.39)
  retroperitoneum NEC (91.11-91.19)
  retroperitoneal x-ray (88.14-88.16)

59.3 Plication of urethrovesical junction
Kelly-Kennedy operation on urethra
Kelly-Stoeckel urethral plication
DEF: Suturing a tuck in tissues around urethra at junction with bladder; changes angle of junction and provides support.

59.4 Suprapubic sling operation
Goebel-Frangenheim-Stoeckel urethrovesical suspension
Millin-Read urethrovesical suspension
Oxford operation for urinary incontinence
Urethrocystopexy by suprapubic suspension
DEF: Suspension of urethra from suprapubic periosteum to restore support to bladder and urethra.

59.5 Retropubic urethral suspension
Burch procedure
Marshall-Marchetti-Krantz operation
Suture of periurethral tissue to symphysis pubis
Urethral suspension NOS
AHA: 1Q, '97, 11
DEF: Suspension of urethra from pubic bone with suture placed from symphysis pubis to paraurethral tissues; elevates urethrovesical angle, restores urinary continence.

59.6 Paraurethral suspension
Pereyra paraurethral suspension
Periurethral suspension
DEF: Suspension of bladder neck from fibrous membranes of anterior abdominal wall; upward traction applied; changes angle of urethra, improves urinary control.

59.7 Other repair of urinary stress incontinence

59.71 Levator muscle operation for urethrovesical suspension
Cystourethropexy with levator muscle sling
Gracilis muscle transplant for urethrovesical suspension
Pubococcygeal sling

59.72 Injection of implant into urethra and/or bladder neck
Collagen implant
Endoscopic injection of implant
Fat implant
Polytef implant

AHA: 4Q, '95, 72, 73

DEF: Injection of collagen into submucosal tissues to increase tissue bulk and improve urinary control.

59.79 Other
Anterior urethropexy
Repair of stress incontinence NOS
Tudor "rabbit ear" urethropexy

AHA: 2Q, '01, 20; 1Q, '00, 14, 15, 19

DEF: Pubovaginal sling for treatment of stress incontinence: A strip of fascia is harvested and the vaginal epithelium is mobilized and then sutured to the midline at the urethral level to the rectus muscle to create a sling supporting the bladder.

DEF: Vaginal wall sling with bone anchors for treatment of stress incontinence: A sling for the bladder is formed by a suture attachment of vaginal wall to the abdominal wall. In addition, a suture is run from the vagina to a bone anchor placed in the pubic bone.

DEF: Transvaginal endoscopic bladder neck suspension for treatment of stress incontinence: Endoscopic surgical suturing of the vaginal epithelium and the pubocervical fascia at the bladder neck level on both sides of the urethra. Two supporting sutures are run from the vagina to an anchor placed in the pubic bone on each side.

59.8 Ureteral catheterization
Drainage of kidney by catheter
Insertion of ureteral stent
Ureterovesical orifice dilation
Code also any ureterotomy (56.2)

EXCLUDES that for:
transurethral removal of calculus or clot from ureter and renal pelvis (56.0)
retrograde pyelogram (87.74)

AHA: 3Q, '00, 7; 1Q, '89, 1; S-O, '86, 10

59.9 Other operations on urinary system

EXCLUDES nonoperative removal of therapeutic device (97.61-97.69)

59.91 Excision of perirenal or perivesical tissue
EXCLUDES biopsy of perirenal or perivesical tissue (59.21)

59.92 Other operations on perirenal or perivesical tissue

59.93 Replacement of ureterostomy tube
Change of ureterostomy tube
Reinsertion of ureterostomy tube

EXCLUDES nonoperative removal of ureterostomy tube (97.62)

59.94 Replacement of cystostomy tube
EXCLUDES nonoperative removal of cystostomy tube (97.63)

59.95 Ultrasonic fragmentation of urinary stones
Shattered urinary stones

EXCLUDES percutaneous nephrostomy with fragmentation (55.04)
shockwave disintegration (98.51)

AHA: 1Q, '89, 1; S-O, '86, 11

59.99 Other
EXCLUDES instillation of medication into urinary tract (96.49)
irrigation of urinary tract (96.45-96.48)

11. OPERATIONS ON THE MALE GENITAL ORGANS (60-64)

√3rd **60 Operations on prostate and seminal vesicles**
▶Code also any application or administration of an adhesion barrier substance (99.77)◀
INCLUDES operations on periprostatic tissue
EXCLUDES that associated with radical cystectomy (57.71)

60.0 Incision of prostate ♂
Drainage of prostatic abscess
Prostatolithotomy
EXCLUDES drainage of periprostatic tissue only (60.81)

√4th **60.1 Diagnostic procedures on prostate and seminal vesicles**

60.11 Closed [percutaneous] [needle] biopsy of prostate ♂
Approach:
  transrectal   Punch biopsy
  transurethral
DEF: Excision of prostate tissue by closed technique for biopsy.

60.12 Open biopsy of prostate ♂
60.13 Closed [percutaneous] biopsy of seminal vesicles ♂
Needle biopsy of seminal vesicles
60.14 Open biopsy of seminal vesicles ♂
60.15 Biopsy of periprostatic tissue ♂
60.18 Other diagnostic procedures on prostate and periprostatic tissue ♂
EXCLUDES microscopic examination of specimen from prostate (91.31-91.39)
  x-ray of prostate (87.92)
60.19 Other diagnostic procedures on seminal vesicles ♂
EXCLUDES microscopic examination of specimen from seminal vesicles (91.31-91.39)
  x-ray:
    contrast seminal vesiculogram (87.91)
    other (87.92)

√4th **60.2 Transurethral prostatectomy**
EXCLUDES local excision of lesion of prostate (60.61)
AHA: 2Q, '94, 9; 3Q, '92, 13

60.21 Transurethral (ultrasound) guided laser induced prostatectomy (TULIP) ♂
Ablation (contact) (noncontact) by laser
AHA: 4Q, '95, 7

60.29 Other transurethral prostatectomy ♂
Excision of median bar by transurethral approach
Transurethral electrovaporization of prostate (TEVAP)
Transurethral enucleative procedure
Transurethral prostatectomy NOS
Transurethral resection of prostate (TURP)
DEF: Excision of median bar by transurethral approach: Removal of fibrous structure of prostate.
DEF: Transurethral enucleate procedure: Transurethral prostatectomy.
AHA: 3Q, '97, 3

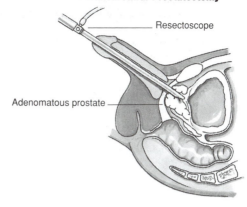
Transurethral Prostatectomy

60.3 Suprapubic prostatectomy ♂
Transvesical prostatectomy
EXCLUDES local excision of lesion of prostate (60.61)
  radical prostatectomy (60.5)
DEF: Resection of prostate through incision in abdomen above pubic arch.

60.4 Retropubic prostatectomy ♂
EXCLUDES local excision of lesion of prostate (60.61)
  radical prostatectomy (60.5)
DEF: Removal of the prostate using an abdominal approach with direct cutting into prostatic capsule.

60.5 Radical prostatectomy ♂
Prostatovesiculectomy
Radical prostatectomy by any approach
EXCLUDES cystoprostatectomy (57.71)
AHA: 3Q, '93, 12
DEF: Removal of prostate, epididymis and vas ampullae.
DEF: Prostatovesiculectomy: Removal of prostate and epididymis.

√4th **60.6 Other prostatectomy**

60.61 Local excision of lesion of prostate ♂
Excision of prostatic lesion by any approach
EXCLUDES biopsy of prostate (60.11-60.12)

60.62 Perineal prostatectomy ♂
Cryoablation of prostate
Cryoprostatectomy
Cryosurgery of prostate
Radical cryosurcial ablation of prostate (RCSA)
EXCLUDES local excision of lesion of prostate (60.61)
AHA: 4Q, '95, 71
DEF: Excision of prostate tissue through incision between scrotum and anus.

60.69 Other ♂

√4th **60.7 Operations on seminal vesicles**

60.71 Percutaneous aspiration of seminal vesicle ♂
EXCLUDES needle biopsy of seminal vesicle (60.13)
60.72 Incision of seminal vesicle ♂
60.73 Excision of seminal vesicle ♂
Excision of Müllerian duct cyst
Spermatocystectomy
EXCLUDES biopsy of seminal vesicle (60.13-60.14)
  prostatovesiculectomy (60.5)
60.79 Other operations on seminal vesicles ♂

OPERATIONS ON MALE GENITAL ORGANS

√4th **60.8 Incision or excision of periprostatic tissue**
  60.81 Incision of periprostatic tissue ♂
    Drainage of periprostatic abscess
  60.82 Excision of periprostatic tissue ♂
    Excision of lesion of periprostatic tissue
    EXCLUDES: biopsy of periprostatic tissue (60.15)

√4th **60.9 Other operations on prostate**
  60.91 Percutaneous aspiration of prostate ♂
    EXCLUDES: needle biopsy of prostate (60.11)
  60.92 Injection into prostate ♂
  60.93 Repair of prostate ♂
  60.94 Control of (postoperative) hemorrhage of prostate ♂
    Coagulation of prostatic bed
    Cystoscopy for control of prostatic hemorrhage
  60.95 Transurethral balloon dilation of the prostatic urethra ♂
    AHA: 4Q, '91, 23
    DEF: Insertion and inflation of balloon to stretch prostate passage.
  60.96 Transurethral destruction of prostate tissue by microwave thermotherapy ♂
    Transurethral microwave thermotherapy (TUMT) of prostate
    EXCLUDES: Prostatectomy:
      other (60.61-60.69)
      radical (60.5)
      retropubic (60.4)
      suprapubic (60.3)
      transurethral (60.21-60.29)
    AHA: 4Q, '00, 67
  60.97 Other transurethral destruction of prostate tissue by other thermotherapy ♂
    Radiofrequency thermotherapy
    Transurethral needle ablation (TUNA) of prostate
    EXCLUDES: Prostatectomy:
      other (60.61-60.69)
      radical (60.5)
      retropubic (60.4)
      suprapubic (60.3)
      transurethral (60.21-60.29)
    AHA: 4Q, '00, 67
  60.99 Other ♂
    EXCLUDES: prostatic massage (99.94)
    AHA: 3Q, '90, 12

√3rd **61 Operations on scrotum and tunica vaginalis**
  61.0 Incision and drainage of scrotum and tunica vaginalis ♂
    EXCLUDES: percutaneous aspiration of hydrocele (61.91)

√4th **61.1 Diagnostic procedures on scrotum and tunica vaginalis**
  61.11 Biopsy of scrotum or tunica vaginalis ♂
  61.19 Other diagnostic procedures on scrotum and tunica vaginalis ♂

  61.2 Excision of hydrocele (of tunica vaginalis) ♂
    Bottle repair of hydrocele of tunica vaginalis
    EXCLUDES: percutaneous aspiration of hydrocele (61.91)
    DEF: Removal of fluid collected in serous membrane of testes.

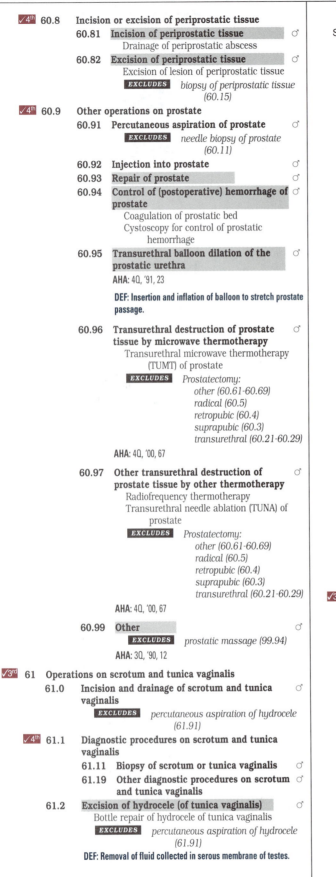

Hydrocelectomy
- Scrotal skin incised
- Sac opened
- Fluid-filled sac mobilized
- Excess tissue trimmed
- Testis
- Remaining sacular tissue folded back and sewn to itself to preclude recurrence ("bottle" procedure)

  61.3 Excision or destruction of lesion or tissue of scrotum ♂
    Fulguration of lesion
    Reduction of elephantiasis } of scrotum
    Partial scrotectomy
    EXCLUDES: biopsy of scrotum (61.11)
      scrotal fistulectomy (61.42)

√4th **61.4 Repair of scrotum and tunica vaginalis**
  61.41 Suture of laceration of scrotum and tunica vaginalis ♂
  61.42 Repair of scrotal fistula ♂
  61.49 Other repair of scrotum and tunica vaginalis ♂
    Reconstruction with rotational or pedicle flaps

√4th **61.9 Other operations on scrotum and tunica vaginalis**
  61.91 Percutaneous aspiration of tunica vaginalis ♂
    Aspiration of hydrocele of tunica vaginalis
  61.92 Excision of lesion of tunica vaginalis other than hydrocele ♂
    Excision of hematocele of tunica vaginalis
    DEF: Removal of blood collected in tunica vaginalis.
  61.99 Other ♂
    EXCLUDES: removal of foreign body from scrotum without incision (98.24)

√3rd **62 Operations on testes**
  62.0 Incision of testis ♂
√4th **62.1 Diagnostic procedures on testes**
  62.11 Closed [percutaneous] [needle] biopsy of testis ♂
  62.12 Open biopsy of testis ♂
  62.19 Other diagnostic procedures on testes ♂
  62.2 Excision or destruction of testicular lesion ♂
    Excision of appendix testis
    Excision of cyst of Morgagni in the male
    EXCLUDES: biopsy of testis (62.11-62.12)
  62.3 Unilateral orchiectomy ♂
    Orchidectomy (with epididymectomy) NOS
√4th **62.4 Bilateral orchiectomy**
    Male castration
    Radical bilateral orchiectomy (with epididymectomy)
    Code also any synchronous lymph node dissection (40.3, 40.5)
    DEF: Removal of both testes.
    DEF: Radical bilateral orchiectomy (with epididymectomy): Excision of both testes and structures that store sperm.
  62.41 Removal of both testes at same operative episode ♂
    Bilateral orchidectomy NOS

OPERATIONS ON MALE GENITAL ORGANS

62.42 **Removal of remaining testis** ♂
Removal of solitary testis

62.5 **Orchiopexy** ♂
Mobilization and replacement of testis in scrotum
Orchiopexy with detorsion of testis
Torek (-Bevan) operation (orchidopexy) (first stage) (second stage)
Transplantation to and fixation of testis in scrotum

DEF: Fixation of testis in scrotum.

DEF: Orchiopexy with detorsion of testis: Fixation and placement of testis in scrotum after correcting angle.

DEF: Torek operation (first stage) (second stage): Transfer of congenitally undescended testis from inguinal canal to scrotum.

DEF: Transplantation to and fixation of testis in scrotum: Transfer of displaced testis to scrotum.

✓4th **62.6** **Repair of testes**
EXCLUDES reduction of torsion (63.52)

62.61 **Suture of laceration of testis** ♂
62.69 **Other repair of testis** ♂
Testicular graft

62.7 **Insertion of testicular prosthesis** ♂

✓4th **62.9** Other operations on testes
62.91 Aspiration of testis ♂
EXCLUDES percutaneous biopsy of testis (62.11)

62.92 Injection of therapeutic substance into testis ♂

62.99 **Other** ♂

✓3rd **63** Operations on spermatic cord, epididymis, and vas deferens

✓4th **63.0** Diagnostic procedures on spermatic cord, epididymis, and vas deferens

63.01 **Biopsy of spermatic cord, epididymis, or vas deferens** ♂

63.09 **Other diagnostic procedures on spermatic cord, epididymis, and vas deferens** ♂
EXCLUDES contrast epididymogram (87.93)
contrast vasogram (87.94)
other x-ray of epididymis and vas deferens (87.95)

63.1 **Excision of varicocele and hydrocele of spermatic cord** ♂
High ligation of spermatic vein
Hydrocelectomy of canal of Nuck

DEF: Removal of a swollen vein and collected fluid from spermatic cord.

DEF: High ligation of spermatic vein: Tying off of spermatic vein.

DEF: Hydrocelectomy of canal of Nuck: Removal of fluid collected from serous membrane of inguinal canal.

Varicocelectomy

Ligated veins
Pampiniform plexus
Ligated veins
Vas deferens
Artery

63.2 **Excision of cyst of epididymis** ♂
Spermatocelectomy

63.3 **Excision of other lesion or tissue of spermatic cord and epididymis** ♂
Excision of appendix epididymis
EXCLUDES biopsy of spermatic cord or epididymis (63.01)

63.4 **Epididymectomy** ♂
EXCLUDES that synchronous with orchiectomy (62.3-62.42)

✓4th **63.5** Repair of spermatic cord and epididymis
63.51 **Suture of laceration of spermatic cord and epididymis** ♂
63.52 **Reduction of torsion of testis or spermatic cord** ♂
EXCLUDES that associated with orchiopexy (62.5)

DEF: Correction of twisted testicle or spermatic cord.

63.53 **Transplantation of spermatic cord** ♂
63.59 **Other repair of spermatic cord and epididymis** ♂

63.6 Vasotomy ♂
Vasostomy

DEF: Vasotomy: Incision of ducts carrying sperm from testicles.

DEF: Vasostomy: Creation of an opening into duct.

✓4th **63.7** Vasectomy and ligation of vas deferens
63.70 Male sterilization procedure, not otherwise specified NC ♂
63.71 Ligation of vas deferens NC ♂
Crushing of vas deferens
Division of vas deferens
63.72 Ligation of spermatic cord NC ♂
63.73 Vasectomy NC ♂
AHA: 2Q, '98, 13

✓4th **63.8** Repair of vas deferens and epididymis
63.81 **Suture of laceration of vas deferens and epididymis** ♂
63.82 **Reconstruction of surgically divided vas deferens** ♂
63.83 **Epididymovasostomy** ♂

DEF: Creation of new connection between vas deferens and epididymis.

63.84 **Removal of ligature from vas deferens** ♂
63.85 **Removal of valve from vas deferens** ♂
63.89 **Other repair of vas deferens and epididymis** ♂

✓4th **63.9** Other operations on spermatic cord, epididymis, and vas deferens
63.91 Aspiration of spermatocele ♂
DEF: Puncture of cystic distention of epididymis.

63.92 **Epididymotomy** ♂
DEF: Incision of epididymis.

63.93 **Incision of spermatic cord** ♂
DEF: Incision into sperm storage structure.

63.94 **Lysis of adhesions of spermatic cord** ♂
63.95 **Insertion of valve in vas deferens** ♂
63.99 **Other** ♂

✓3rd **64** Operations on penis
INCLUDES operations on:
corpora cavernosa
glans penis
prepuce

64.0 **Circumcision** ♂
DEF: Removal of penis foreskin.

OPERATIONS ON MALE GENITAL ORGANS

√4ᵗʰ 64.1 Diagnostic procedures on the penis
    64.11 Biopsy of penis ♂
    64.19 Other diagnostic procedures on penis ♂

64.2 Local excision or destruction of lesion of penis ♂
    EXCLUDES biopsy of penis (64.11)

64.3 Amputation of penis ♂

√4ᵗʰ 64.4 Repair and plastic operation on penis
    64.41 Suture of laceration of penis ♂
    64.42 Release of chordee ♂
        AHA: 4Q, '96, 34

        DEF: Correction of downward displacement of penis.

    64.43 Construction of penis ♂
    64.44 Reconstruction of penis ♂
    64.45 Replantation of penis ♂
        Reattachment of amputated penis
    64.49 Other repair of penis ♂
        EXCLUDES repair of epispadias and hypospadias (58.45)

64.5 Operations for sex transformation, not elsewhere classified [NC]♂

√4ᵗʰ 64.9 Other operations on male genital organs
    64.91 Dorsal or lateral slit of prepuce ♂
    64.92 Incision of penis ♂
    64.93 Division of penile adhesions ♂
    64.94 Fitting of external prosthesis of penis ♂
        Penile prosthesis NOS
    64.95 Insertion or replacement of non-inflatable penile prosthesis ♂
        Insertion of semi-rigid rod prosthesis into shaft of penis
        EXCLUDES external penile prosthesis (64.94)
            inflatable penile prosthesis (64.97)
            plastic repair, penis (64.43-64.49)
            that associated with:
              construction (64.43)
              reconstruction (64.44)
    64.96 Removal of internal prosthesis of penis ♂
        Removal without replacement of non-inflatable or inflatable penile prosthesis

    64.97 Insertion or replacement of inflatable penile prosthesis ♂
        Insertion of cylinders into shaft of penis and placement of pump and reservoir
        EXCLUDES external penile prosthesis (64.94)
            non-inflatable penile prosthesis (64.95)
            plastic repair, penis (64.43-64.49)

    64.98 Other operations on penis ♂
        Corpora cavernosa-corpus spongiosum shunt
        Corpora-saphenous shunt
        Irrigation of corpus cavernosum
        EXCLUDES removal of foreign body:
            intraluminal (98.19)
            without incision (98.24)
            stretching of foreskin (99.95)

    AHA: 3Q, '92, 9

    DEF: Corpora cavernosa-corpus spongiosum shunt: Insertion of shunt between erectile tissues of penis.

    DEF: Corpora-saphenous shunt: Insertion of shunt between erectile tissue and vein of penis.

    DEF: Irrigation of corpus cavernosum: Washing of erectile tissue forming dorsum and side of penis.

    64.99 Other ♂
        EXCLUDES collection of sperm for artificial insemination (99.96)

OPERATIONS ON THE FEMALE GENITAL SYSTEM

12. OPERATIONS ON THE FEMALE GENITAL ORGANS (65-71)

√3rd 65 Operations on ovary
▶Code also any application or administration of an adhesion barrier substance (99.77)◀

√4th 65.0 Oophorotomy
Salpingo-oophorotomy
DEF: Incision into ovary.
DEF: Salpingo-oophorotomy: Incision into ovary and the fallopian tube.

- 65.01 Laparoscopic oophorotomy ♀
- 65.09 Other oophorotomy ♀

√4th 65.1 Diagnostic procedures on ovaries
- 65.11 Aspiration biopsy of ovary ♀
- 65.12 Other biopsy of ovary ♀
- 65.13 Laparoscopic biopsy of ovary ♀
  AHA: 4Q, '96, 67
- 65.14 Other laparoscopic diagnostic procedures on ovaries ♀
- 65.19 Other diagnostic procedures on ovaries ♀
  EXCLUDES microscopic examination of specimen from ovary (91.41-91.49)

√4th 65.2 Local excision or destruction of ovarian lesion or tissue
- 65.21 Marsupialization of ovarian cyst ♀
  EXCLUDES that by laparoscope (65.23)
  DEF: Exteriorized cyst to outside by incising anterior wall and suturing cut edges to create open pouch.
- 65.22 Wedge resection of ovary ♀
  EXCLUDES that by laparoscope (65.24)
- 65.23 Laparoscopic marsupialization of ovarian cyst ♀
- 65.24 Laparoscopic wedge resection of ovary ♀
- 65.25 Other laparoscopic local excision or destruction of ovary ♀
- 65.29 Other local excision or destruction of ovary ♀
  Bisection ⎫
  Cauterization ⎬ of ovary
  Partial excision ⎭
  EXCLUDES biopsy of ovary (65.11-65.13)
              that by laparoscope (65.25)

√4th 65.3 Unilateral oophorectomy
- 65.31 Laparoscopic unilateral oophorectomy ♀
- 65.39 Other unilateral oophorectomy ♀
  EXCLUDES that by laparoscope (65.31)
  AHA: 4Q, '96, 66

√4th 65.4 Unilateral salpingo-oophorectomy
- 65.41 Laparoscopic unilateral salpingo-oophorectomy ♀
  AHA: 4Q, '96, 67
- 65.49 Other unilateral salpingo-oophorectomy ♀

Oophorectomy

(Illustration: Fallopian tube, Fimbria, Ovary, Ovarian cyst)

√4th 65.5 Bilateral oophorectomy
- 65.51 Other removal of both ovaries at same operative episode ♀
  Female castration
  EXCLUDES that by laparoscope (65.53)
- 65.52 Other removal of remaining ovary ♀
  Removal of solitary ovary
  EXCLUDES that by laparoscope (65.54)
- 65.53 Laparoscopic removal of both ovaries at same operative eisode ♀
- 65.54 Laparoscopic removal of remaining ovary ♀

√4th 65.6 Bilateral salpingo-oophorectomy
- 65.61 Other removal of both ovaries and tubes at same operative episode ♀
  EXCLUDES that by laparoscope (65.53)
  AHA: 4Q, '96, 65
- 65.62 Other removal of remaining ovary and tube ♀
  Removal of solitary ovary and tube
  EXCLUDES that by laparoscope (65.54)
- 65.63 Laparoscopic removal of both ovaries and tubes at the same operative episode ♀
  AHA: 4Q, '96, 68
- 65.64 Laparoscopic removal of remaining ovary and tube ♀

√4th 65.7 Repair of ovary
EXCLUDES salpingo-oophorostomy (66.72)
- 65.71 Other simple suture of ovary ♀
  EXCLUDES that by laparoscope (65.74)
- 65.72 Other reimplantation of ovary ♀
  EXCLUDES that by laparoscope (65.75)
  DEF: Grafting and repositioning of ovary at same site.
- 65.73 Other salpingo-oophoroplasty ♀
  EXCLUDES that by laparoscope (65.76)
- 65.74 Laparoscopic simple suture of ovary ♀
- 65.75 Laparoscopic reimplantation of ovary ♀
- 65.76 Laparoscopic salpingo-oophoroplasty ♀
- 65.79 Other repair of ovary ♀
  Oophoropexy

√4th 65.8 Lysis of adhesions of ovary and fallopian tube
- 65.81 Laparoscopic lysis of adhesions of ovary and fallopian tube ♀
  AHA: 4Q, '96, 67
- 65.89 Other lysis of adhesions of ovary and fallopian tube ♀
  EXCLUDES that by laparoscope (65.81)

√4th 65.9 Other operations on ovary
- 65.91 Aspiration of ovary ♀
  EXCLUDES aspiration biopsy of ovary (65.11)
- 65.92 Transplantation of ovary ♀
  EXCLUDES reimplantation of ovary (65.72, 65.75)
- 65.93 Manual rupture of ovarian cyst ♀
  DEF: Breaking up an ovarian cyst using manual technique or blunt instruments.
- 65.94 Ovarian denervation ♀
  DEF: Destruction of nerve tracts to ovary.
- 65.95 Release of torsion of ovary ♀

OPERATIONS ON THE FEMALE GENITAL SYSTEM

65.99–66.9

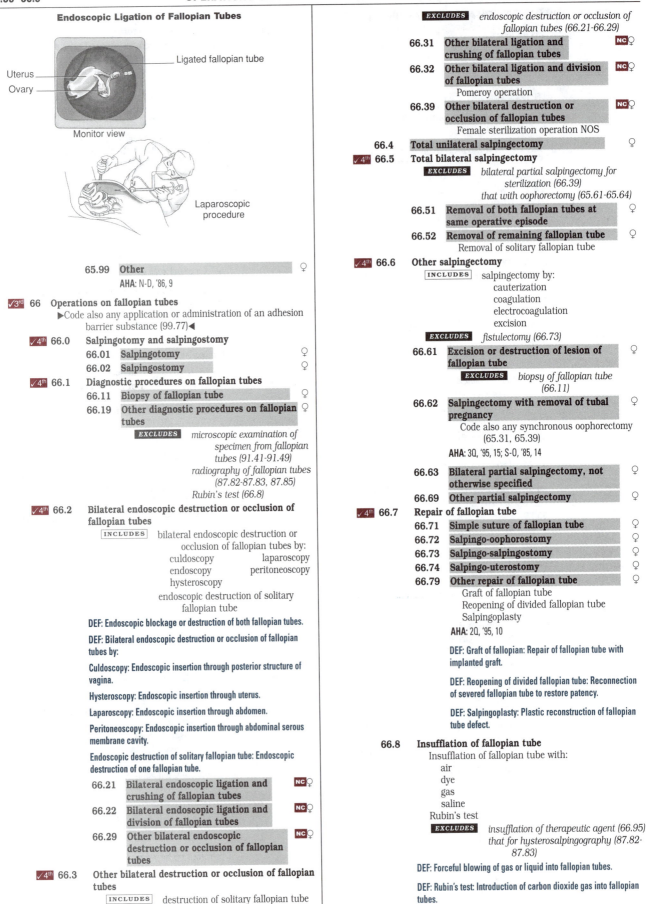

Endoscopic Ligation of Fallopian Tubes
- Uterus
- Ovary
- Ligated fallopian tube
- Monitor view
- Laparoscopic procedure

65.99 Other
AHA: N-D, '86, 9

√3rd **66 Operations on fallopian tubes**
▶Code also any application or administration of an adhesion barrier substance (99.77)◀

√4th **66.0 Salpingotomy and salpingostomy**
    66.01 Salpingotomy ♀
    66.02 Salpingostomy ♀

√4th **66.1 Diagnostic procedures on fallopian tubes**
    66.11 Biopsy of fallopian tube ♀
    66.19 Other diagnostic procedures on fallopian tubes ♀
        EXCLUDES   *microscopic examination of specimen from fallopian tubes (91.41-91.49)*
            radiography of fallopian tubes (87.82-87.83, 87.85)
            Rubin's test (66.8)

√4th **66.2 Bilateral endoscopic destruction or occlusion of fallopian tubes**
    INCLUDES   bilateral endoscopic destruction or occlusion of fallopian tubes by:
        culdoscopy   laparoscopy
        endoscopy   peritoneoscopy
        hysteroscopy
        endoscopic destruction of solitary fallopian tube

DEF: Endoscopic blockage or destruction of both fallopian tubes.
DEF: Bilateral endoscopic destruction or occlusion of fallopian tubes by:
Culdoscopy: Endoscopic insertion through posterior structure of vagina.
Hysteroscopy: Endoscopic insertion through uterus.
Laparoscopy: Endoscopic insertion through abdomen.
Peritoneoscopy: Endoscopic insertion through abdominal serous membrane cavity.
Endoscopic destruction of solitary fallopian tube: Endoscopic destruction of one fallopian tube.

    66.21 Bilateral endoscopic ligation and crushing of fallopian tubes   NC ♀
    66.22 Bilateral endoscopic ligation and division of fallopian tubes   NC ♀
    66.29 Other bilateral endoscopic destruction or occlusion of fallopian tubes   NC ♀

√4th **66.3 Other bilateral destruction or occlusion of fallopian tubes**
    INCLUDES   destruction of solitary fallopian tube

    EXCLUDES   *endoscopic destruction or occlusion of fallopian tubes (66.21-66.29)*

    66.31 Other bilateral ligation and crushing of fallopian tubes   NC ♀
    66.32 Other bilateral ligation and division of fallopian tubes   NC ♀
        Pomeroy operation
    66.39 Other bilateral destruction or occlusion of fallopian tubes   NC ♀
        Female sterilization operation NOS

66.4 Total unilateral salpingectomy ♀

√4th **66.5 Total bilateral salpingectomy**
    EXCLUDES   *bilateral partial salpingectomy for sterilization (66.39)*
            that with oophorectomy (65.61-65.64)
    66.51 Removal of both fallopian tubes at same operative episode ♀
    66.52 Removal of remaining fallopian tube ♀
        Removal of solitary fallopian tube

√4th **66.6 Other salpingectomy**
    INCLUDES   salpingectomy by:
          cauterization
          coagulation
          electrocoagulation
          excision
    EXCLUDES   *fistulectomy (66.73)*

    66.61 Excision or destruction of lesion of fallopian tube ♀
        EXCLUDES   *biopsy of fallopian tube (66.11)*
    66.62 Salpingectomy with removal of tubal pregnancy ♀
        Code also any synchronous oophorectomy (65.31, 65.39)
        AHA: 3Q, '95, 15; S-O, '85, 14
    66.63 Bilateral partial salpingectomy, not otherwise specified ♀
    66.69 Other partial salpingectomy ♀

√4th **66.7 Repair of fallopian tube**
    66.71 Simple suture of fallopian tube ♀
    66.72 Salpingo-oophorostomy ♀
    66.73 Salpingo-salpingostomy ♀
    66.74 Salpingo-uterostomy ♀
    66.79 Other repair of fallopian tube ♀
        Graft of fallopian tube
        Reopening of divided fallopian tube
        Salpingoplasty
    AHA: 2Q, '95, 10

DEF: Graft of fallopian: Repair of fallopian tube with implanted graft.
DEF: Reopening of divided fallopian tube: Reconnection of severed fallopian tube to restore patency.
DEF: Salpingoplasty: Plastic reconstruction of fallopian tube defect.

66.8 Insufflation of fallopian tube
    Insufflation of fallopian tube with:
        air
        dye
        gas
        saline
    Rubin's test
    EXCLUDES   *insufflation of therapeutic agent (66.95)*
            that for hysterosalpingography (87.82-87.83)

DEF: Forceful blowing of gas or liquid into fallopian tubes.
DEF: Rubin's test: Introduction of carbon dioxide gas into fallopian tubes.

√4th **66.9 Other operations on fallopian tubes**

OPERATIONS ON THE FEMALE GENITAL SYSTEM

66.91 Aspiration of fallopian tube

66.92 Unilateral destruction or occlusion of fallopian tube ♀
 EXCLUDES that of solitary tube (66.21-66.39)

66.93 Implantation or replacement of prosthesis of fallopian tube ♀

66.94 Removal of prosthesis of fallopian tube ♀

66.95 Insufflation of therapeutic agent into fallopian tubes ♀

66.96 Dilation of fallopian tube ♀

66.97 Burying of fimbriae in uterine wall ♀
 DEF: Implantation of fallopian tube, fringed edges into uterine wall.

66.99 Other ♀
 EXCLUDES lysis of adhesions of ovary and tube (65.81, 65.89)
 AHA: 2Q, '94, 11

√3rd 67 Operations on cervix
▶Code also any application or administration of an adhesion barrier substance (99.77)◀

67.0 Dilation of cervical canal ♀
 EXCLUDES dilation and curettage (69.01-69.09)
 that for induction of labor (73.1)

√4th 67.1 Diagnostic procedures on cervix

 67.11 Endocervical biopsy ♀
  EXCLUDES conization of cervix (67.2)

 67.12 Other cervical biopsy ♀
  Punch biopsy of cervix NOS
  EXCLUDES conization of cervix (67.2)

 67.19 Other diagnostic procedures on cervix ♀
  EXCLUDES microscopic examination of specimen from cervix (91.41-91.49)

67.2 Conization of cervix ♀
 EXCLUDES that by:
  cryosurgery (67.33)
  electrosurgery (67.32)
 DEF: Removal of cone-shaped section from distal cervix; cervical function preserved.

√4th 67.3 Other excision or destruction of lesion or tissue of cervix

 67.31 Marsupialization of cervical cyst ♀
  DEF: Incision and then suturing open of a cyst in the neck of the uterus.

 67.32 Destruction of lesion of cervix by cauterization ♀
  Electroconization of cervix
  LEEP (loop electrosurgical excision procedure)
  LLETZ (large loop excision of the transformation zone)
  AHA: 1Q, '98, 3
  DEF: Destruction of lesion of uterine neck by applying intense heat.
  DEF: Electroconization of cervix: Electrocautery excision of multilayer cone-shaped section from uterine neck.

 67.33 Destruction of lesion of cervix by cryosurgery ♀
  Cryoconization of cervix
  DEF: Destruction of lesion of uterine neck by freezing.
  DEF: Cryoconization of cervix: Excision by freezing of multilayer cone-shaped section of abnormal tissue in uterine neck.

 67.39 Other excision or destruction of lesion or tissue of cervix ♀
  EXCLUDES biopsy of cervix (67.11-67.12)
   cervical fistulectomy (67.62)
   conization of cervix (67.2)

Cerclage of Cervix
Suture material is inserted around cervix and tightened

Cervix and cervical canal

Uterus

Cervix and cervical canal

67.4 Amputation of cervix ♀
 Cervicectomy with synchronous colporrhaphy
 DEF: Excision of lower uterine neck.
 DEF: Cervicectomy with synchronous colporrhaphy: Excision of lower uterine neck with suture of vaginal stump.

√4th 67.5 Repair of internal cervical os
 AHA: 4Q, '01, 63; 3Q, '00; 11
 DEF: Repair of cervical opening defect.

 67.51 Transabdominal cerclage of cervix
 67.59 Other repair of internal cervical os
  Cerclage of isthmus uteri
  McDonald operation
  Shirodkar operation
  Transvaginal cerclage
  EXCLUDES transabdominal cerclage of cervix (67.51)
  DEF: Cerclage of isthmus uteri: Placement of encircling suture in the constricted part of the between neck and body of uterus.
  DEF: Shirodkar operation: Placement of purse-string suture in internal cervical opening.

√4th 67.6 Other repair of cervix
 EXCLUDES repair of current obstetric laceration (75.51)

 67.61 Suture of laceration of cervix ♀
 67.62 Repair of fistula of cervix ♀
  Cervicosigmoidal fistulectomy
  EXCLUDES fistulectomy:
   cervicovesical (57.84)
   ureterocervical (56.84)
   vesicocervicovaginal (57.84)
  DEF: Closure of fistula in lower uterus.
  DEF: Cervicosigmoidal fistulectomy: Excision of abnormal passage between uterine neck and torsion of large intestine.

 67.69 Other repair of cervix ♀
  Repair of old obstetric laceration of cervix

√3rd 68 Other incision and excision of uterus
▶Code also any application or administration of an adhesion barrier substance (99.77)◀

68.0 Hysterotomy ♀
 Hysterotomy with removal of hydatidiform mole
 EXCLUDES hysterotomy for termination of pregnancy (74.91)
 DEF: Incision into the uterus

√4th 68.1 Diagnostic procedures on uterus and supporting structures

OPERATIONS ON THE FEMALE GENITAL SYSTEM

68.11 Digital examination of uterus ♀
  EXCLUDES pelvic examination, so
    described (89.26)
    postpartal manual exploration
    of uterine cavity (75.7)

68.12 Hysteroscopy ♀
  EXCLUDES that with biopsy (68.16)

68.13 Open biopsy of uterus ♀
  EXCLUDES closed biopsy of uterus (68.16)

68.14 Open biopsy of uterine ligaments ♀
  EXCLUDES closed biopsy of uterine
    ligaments (68.15)

68.15 Closed biopsy of uterine ligaments ♀
  Endoscopic (laparoscopy) biopsy of uterine
    adnexa, except ovary and fallopian
    tube

68.16 Closed biopsy of uterus ♀
  Endoscopic (laparoscopy) (hysteroscopy)
    biopsy of uterus
  EXCLUDES open biopsy of uterus (68.13)

**68.19 Other diagnostic procedures on uterus
  and supporting structures** ♀
  EXCLUDES diagnostic:
    aspiration curettage (69.59)
    dilation and curettage
      (69.09)
    microscopic examination of
      specimen from uterus
      (91.41-91.49)
    pelvic examination (89.26)
    radioisotope scan of:
      placenta (92.17)
      uterus (92.19)
    ultrasonography of uterus
      (88.78-88.79)
    x-ray of uterus (87.81-87.89)

✓4th **68.2 Excision or destruction of lesion or tissue of uterus**

68.21 Division of endometrial synechiae ♀
  Lysis of intraluminal uterine adhesions
  DEF: Separation of uterine adhesions.
  DEF: Lysis of intraluminal uterine adhesion: Surgical
  destruction of adhesive, fibrous structures inside uterine
  cavity.

**68.22 Incision or excision of congenital
  septum of uterus** ♀

68.23 Endometrial ablation ♀
  Dilation and curettage
  Hysteroscopic endometrial ablation
  AHA: 4Q, '96, 68
  DEF: Removal or destruction of uterine lining; usually by
  electrocautery or loop electrosurgical excision
  procedure (LEEP).

**68.29 Other excision or destruction of lesion
  of uterus** ♀
  Uterine myomectomy
  EXCLUDES biopsy of uterus (68.13)
    uterine fistulectomy (69.42)
  AHA: 1Q, '96, 14

68.3 Subtotal abdominal hysterectomy ♀
  Supracervical hysterectomy
  DEF: Excision of uterus, except lowest part, through abdominal
  incision.

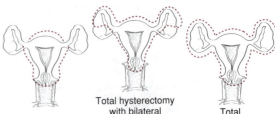

Vaginal Hysterectomy

Total hysterectomy (uterus only removed)

Total hysterectomy with bilateral salpingectomy (uterus and tubes removed)

Total hysterectomy with bilateral salpingo-oophorectomy (uterus, tubes, and ovaries removed)

68.4 Total abdominal hysterectomy ♀
  Hysterectomy:
    extended
  Code also any synchronous removal of tubes and
    ovaries (65.3-65.6)
  AHA: 4Q, '96, 65
  DEF: Complete excision of uterus and uterine neck through
  abdominal incision.

✓4th **68.5 Vaginal hysterectomy**
  Code also any synchronous:
    removal of tubes and ovaries (65.31-65.64)
    repair of cystocele or rectocele (70.50-70.52)
    repair of pelvic floor (70.79)
  DEF: Complete excision of the uterus by a vaginal approach.

**68.51 Laparoscopically assisted vaginal
  hysterectomy (LAVH)** ♀
  AHA: 4Q, '96, 68

68.59 Other vaginal hysterectomy ♀
  EXCLUDES laparoscopically assisted
    vaginal hysterectomy
    (68.51)
    radical vaginal hysterectomy
    (68.7)

68.6 Radical abdominal hysterectomy ♀
  Modified radical hysterectomy
  Wertheim's operation
  Code also any synchronous:
    lymph gland dissection (40.3, 40.5)
    removal of tubes and ovaries (65.61-65.64)
  EXCLUDES pelvic evisceration (68.8)
  DEF: Excision of uterus, loose connective tissue and smooth muscle
  around uterus and vagina via abdominal approach.

68.7 Radical vaginal hysterectomy ♀
  Schauta operation
  Code also any synchronous:
    lymph gland dissection (40.3, 40.5)
    removal of tubes and ovaries (65.61-65.64)
  DEF: Excision of uterus, loose connective tissue and smooth muscle
  around uterus and vagina via vaginal approach.

68.8 Pelvic evisceration ♀
  Removal of ovaries, tubes, uterus, vagina, bladder,
    and urethra (with removal of sigmoid colon
    and rectum)
  Code also any synchronous:
    colostomy (46.10-46.13)
    lymph gland dissection (40.3, 40.5)
    urinary diversion (56.51-56.79)

68.9 Other and unspecified hysterectomy ♀
  Hysterectomy NOS
  EXCLUDES abdominal hysterectomy, any approach
    (68.3, 68.4, 68.6)
    vaginal hysterectomy, any approach
    (68.51, 68.59, 68.7)

OPERATIONS ON THE FEMALE GENITAL SYSTEM

Dilation and Curettage

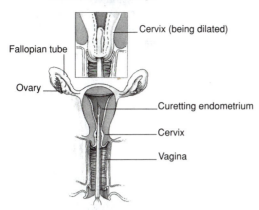

√3rd 69 Other operations on uterus and supporting structures
▶Code also any application or administration of an adhesion barrier substance (99.77)◀

√4th 69.0 Dilation and curettage of uterus
EXCLUDES: aspiration curettage of uterus (69.51-69.59)
DEF: Stretching of uterine neck to scrape tissue from walls.

- **69.01 Dilation and curettage for termination of pregnancy** ♀
  AHA: 1Q, '98, 4
- **69.02 Dilation and curettage following delivery or abortion** ♀
  AHA: 3Q, '93, 6
- **69.09 Other dilation and curettage** ♀
  Diagnostic D and C
  AHA: 1Q, '98, 4

√4th 69.1 Excision or destruction of lesion or tissue of uterus and supporting structures
- **69.19 Other excision or destruction of uterus and supporting structures** ♀
  EXCLUDES: biopsy of uterine ligament (68.14)

√4th 69.2 Repair of uterine supporting structures
- **69.21 Interposition operation** ♀
  Watkins procedure
  DEF: Repositioning or realignment of bladder and uterus.
- **69.22 Other uterine suspension** ♀
  Hysteropexy
  Manchester operation
  Plication of uterine ligament
  DEF: Hysteropexy: Fixation or anchoring of uterus.
  DEF: Manchester operation: Fixation or anchoring of uterus with suppurative banding tissue of uterine neck and vagina.
  DEF: Plication of uterine ligament: Creation of tucks in suppurative uterine banding tissue.
- **69.23 Vaginal repair of chronic inversion of uterus** ♀
  DEF: Repositioning of inverted uterus via vaginal approach.
- **69.29 Other repair of uterus and supporting structures** ♀

- **69.3 Paracervical uterine denervation** ♀

√4th 69.4 Uterine repair
EXCLUDES: repair of current obstetric laceration (75.50-75.52)
- **69.41 Suture of laceration of uterus** ♀
- **69.42 Closure of fistula of uterus** ♀
  EXCLUDES: uterovesical fistulectomy (57.84)
- **69.49 Other repair of uterus** ♀
  Repair of old obstetric laceration of uterus

√4th 69.5 Aspiration curettage of uterus
EXCLUDES: menstrual extraction (69.6)
- **69.51 Aspiration curettage of uterus for termination of pregnancy** ♀
  Therapeutic abortion NOS
- **69.52 Aspiration curettage following delivery or abortion** ♀
- **69.59 Other aspiration curettage of uterus** ♀
  AHA: 1Q, '98, 7

- **69.6 Menstrual extraction or regulation** ♀
  DEF: Induction of menstruation by low pressure suction.

- **69.7 Insertion of intrauterine contraceptive device** ♀

√4th 69.9 Other operations on uterus, cervix, and supporting structures
EXCLUDES: obstetric dilation or incision of cervix (73.1, 73.93)
- **69.91 Insertion of therapeutic device into uterus** ♀
  EXCLUDES: insertion of:
    intrauterine contraceptive device (69.7)
    laminaria (69.93)
    obstetric insertion of bag, bougie, or pack (73.1)
- **69.92 Artificial insemination** ♀
- **69.93 Insertion of laminaria** ♀
  DEF: Placement of laminaria, a sea kelp, in cervical os to induce labor; applied for six to 12 hours.
- **69.94 Manual replacement of inverted uterus** ♀
  EXCLUDES: that in immediate postpartal period (75.94)
- **69.95 Incision of cervix** ♀
  EXCLUDES: that to assist delivery (73.93)
- **69.96 Removal of cerclage material from cervix**
  DEF: Removal of ring inserted to restore uterine neck competency.
- **69.97 Removal of other penetrating foreign body from cervix** ♀
  EXCLUDES: removal of intraluminal foreign body from cervix (98.16)
- **69.98 Other operations on supporting structures of uterus** ♀
  EXCLUDES: biopsy of uterine ligament (68.14)
- **69.99 Other operations on cervix and uterus** ♀
  EXCLUDES: removal of:
    foreign body (98.16)
    intrauterine contraceptive device (97.71)
    obstetric bag, bougie, or pack (97.72)
    packing (97.72)

√3rd 70 Operations on vagina and cul-de-sac
▶Code also any application or administration of an adhesion barrier substance (99.77)◀

- **70.0 Culdocentesis** ♀
  AHA: 2Q, '90, 26
  DEF: Insertion of needle into upper vaginal vault encircling cervix to withdraw fluid.

√4th 70.1 Incision of vagina and cul-de-sac
- **70.11 Hymenotomy** ♀
- **70.12 Culdotomy** ♀
  DEF: Incision into pocket between terminal end of large intestine and posterior uterus.

OPERATIONS ON THE FEMALE GENITAL SYSTEM

70.13 Lysis of intraluminal adhesions of vagina ♀

70.14 Other vaginotomy ♀
- Division of vaginal septum
- Drainage of hematoma of vaginal cuff

DEF: Division of vaginal septum: Incision into partition of vaginal walls.

DEF: Drainage of hematoma of vaginal cuff: Incision into vaginal tissue to drain collected blood.

√4th **70.2** Diagnostic procedures on vagina and cul-de-sac
- **70.21** Vaginoscopy ♀
- **70.22** Culdoscopy ♀
  DEF: Endoscopic exam of pelvic viscera through incision in posterior vaginal wall.
- **70.23** Biopsy of cul-de-sac ♀
- **70.24** Vaginal biopsy ♀
- **70.29** Other diagnostic procedures on vagina and cul-de-sac ♀

√4th **70.3** Local excision or destruction of vagina and cul-de-sac
- **70.31** Hymenectomy ♀
- **70.32** Excision or destruction of lesion of cul-de-sac ♀
  - Endometrectomy of cul-de-sac
  - EXCLUDES biopsy of cul-de-sac (70.23)
- **70.33** Excision or destruction of lesion of vagina ♀
  - EXCLUDES biopsy of vagina (70.24)
  - vaginal fistulectomy (70.72-70.75)

70.4 Obliteration and total excision of vagina ♀
- Vaginectomy
- EXCLUDES obliteration of vaginal vault (70.8)
- DEF: Vaginectomy: Removal of vagina.

√4th **70.5** Repair of cystocele and rectocele
- **70.50** Repair of cystocele and rectocele ♀
  - DEF: Repair of anterior and posterior vaginal wall bulges.
- **70.51** Repair of cystocele ♀
  - Anterior colporrhaphy (with urethrocele repair)
  - AHA: N-D, '84, 20
- **70.52** Repair of rectocele ♀
  - Posterior colporrhaphy

√4th **70.6** Vaginal construction and reconstruction
- **70.61** Vaginal construction ♀
- **70.62** Vaginal reconstruction ♀
  - AHA: N-D, '84, 20

√4th **70.7** Other repair of vagina
- EXCLUDES lysis of intraluminal adhesions (70.13)
  - repair of current obstetric laceration (75.69)
  - that associated with cervical amputation (67.4)
- **70.71** Suture of laceration of vagina ♀
  - AHA: N-D, '84, 20
- **70.72** Repair of colovaginal fistula ♀
  - DEF: Correction of abnormal opening between midsection of large intestine and vagina.
- **70.73** Repair of rectovaginal fistula ♀
  - DEF: Correction of abnormal opening between last section of large intestine and vagina.

70.74 Repair of other vaginoenteric fistula ♀
- DEF: Correction of abnormal opening between vagina and intestine; other than mid or last sections.

70.75 Repair of other fistula of vagina ♀
- EXCLUDES repair of fistula:
  - rectovesicovaginal (57.83)
  - ureterovaginal (56.84)
  - urethrovaginal (58.43)
  - uterovaginal (69.42)
  - vesicocervicovaginal (57.84)
  - vesicosigmoidovaginal (57.83)
  - vesicoureterovaginal (56.84)
  - vesicovaginal (57.84)

70.76 Hymenorrhaphy ♀
- DEF: Closure of vagina with suture of hymenal ring or hymenal remnant flaps.

70.77 Vaginal suspension and fixation ♀
- DEF: Repair of vaginal protrusion, sinking or laxity by suturing vagina into position.

70.79 Other repair of vagina ♀
- Colpoperineoplasty
- Repair of old obstetric laceration of vagina

70.8 Obliteration of vaginal vault ♀
- LeFort operation
- DEF: LeFort operation: Uniting or sewing together vaginal walls.

√4th **70.9** Other operations on vagina and cul-de-sac
- **70.91** Other operations on vagina ♀
  - EXCLUDES insertion of:
    - diaphragm (96.17)
    - mold (96.15)
    - pack (96.14)
    - pessary (96.18)
    - suppository (96.49)
  - removal of:
    - diaphragm (97.73)
    - foreign body (98.17)
    - pack (97.75)
    - pessary (97.74)
  - replacement of:
    - diaphragm (97.24)
    - pack (97.26)
    - pessary (97.25)
  - vaginal dilation (96.16)
  - vaginal douche (96.44)
- **70.92** Other operations on cul-de-sac ♀
  - Obliteration of cul-de-sac
  - Repair of vaginal enterocele
  - AHA: 4Q, '94, 54
  - DEF: Repair of vaginal enterocele: Elimination of herniated cavity within pouch between last part of large intestine and posterior uterus.

√3rd **71** Operations on vulva and perineum
▶Code also any application or administration of an adhesion barrier substance (99.77)◀

√4th **71.0** Incision of vulva and perineum
- **71.01** Lysis of vulvar adhesions ♀
- **71.09** Other incision of vulva and perineum ♀
  - Enlargement of introitus NOS
  - EXCLUDES removal of foreign body without incision (98.23)

√4th **71.1** Diagnostic procedures on vulva
- **71.11** Biopsy of vulva ♀
- **71.19** Other diagnostic procedures on vulva ♀

√4th **71.2** Operations on Bartholin's gland
- **71.21** Percutaneous aspiration of Bartholin's gland (cyst)
- **71.22** Incision of Bartholin's gland (cyst) ♀

BI Bilateral Edit | NC Non-covered Procedure | ▶◀ Revised Text | ● New Code | ▲ Revised Code Title

162 — Volume 3 • October 2002 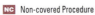 2002 Ingenix, Inc.

Marsupialization

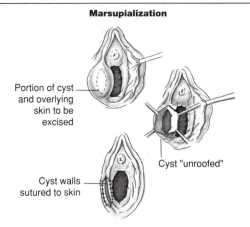

Portion of cyst and overlying skin to be excised

Cyst "unroofed"

Cyst walls sutured to skin

71.23 Marsupialization of Bartholin's gland (cyst) ♀

DEF: Incision and suturing opening of a cyst in Bartholin's gland.

71.24 Excision or other destruction of Bartholin's gland (cyst) ♀

71.29 Other operations on Bartholin's gland ♀

71.3 Other local excision or destruction of vulva and perineum ♀
Division of Skene's gland
EXCLUDES biopsy of vulva (71.11)
vulvar fistulectomy (71.72)

71.4 Operations on clitoris ♀
Amputation of clitoris
Clitoridotomy
Female circumcision

DEF: Amputation of clitoris: Removal of clitoris.

DEF: Clitoridotomy: Incision into clitoris.

DEF: Female circumcision: Incision of skin fold over clitoris.

71.5 Radical vulvectomy ♀
Code also any synchronous lymph gland dissection (40.3, 40.5)

DEF: Removal of over 80 percent of deep tissue from vulva, including tissue of abdomen, groin, labia minora, labia majora, clitoris, mons veneris, and terminal portions of urethra, vagina and other vulvar organs.

✓4th 71.6 Other vulvectomy
71.61 Unilateral vulvectomy ♀
71.62 Bilateral vulvectomy ♀
Vulvectomy NOS

✓4th 71.7 Repair of vulva and perineum
EXCLUDES repair of current obstetric laceration (75.69)

71.71 Suture of laceration of vulva or perineum ♀

71.72 Repair of fistula of vulva or perineum ♀
EXCLUDES repair of fistula:
urethroperineal (58.43)
urethroperineovesical (57.84)
vaginoperineal (70.75)

71.79 Other repair of vulva and perineum ♀
Repair of old obstetric laceration of vulva or perineum
AHA: 1Q, '97, 9

71.8 Other operations on vulva ♀
EXCLUDES removal of:
foreign body without incision (98.23)
packing (97.75)
replacement of packing (97.26)

71.9 Other operations on female genital organs ♀

13. OBSTETRICAL PROCEDURES (72-75)

√3rd 72 Forceps, vacuum, and breech delivery

- **72.0 Low forceps operation** ♀
  - Outlet forceps operation
- **72.1 Low forceps operation with episiotomy** ♀
  - Outlet forceps operation with episiotomy
- **√4th 72.2 Mid forceps operation**
  - **72.21 Mid forceps operation with episiotomy** ♀
  - **72.29 Other mid forceps operation** ♀
- **√4th 72.3 High forceps operation**
  - **72.31 High forceps operation with episiotomy** ♀
  - **72.39 Other high forceps operation** ♀
- **72.4 Forceps rotation of fetal head** ♀
  - DeLee maneuver
  - Key-in-lock rotation
  - Kielland rotation
  - Scanzoni's maneuver
  - Code also any associated forceps extraction (72.0-72.39)
- **√4th 72.5 Breech extraction**
  - **72.51 Partial breech extraction with forceps to aftercoming head** ♀
  - **72.52 Other partial breech extraction** ♀
  - **72.53 Total breech extraction with forceps to aftercoming head** ♀
  - **72.54 Other total breech extraction** ♀
- **72.6 Forceps application to aftercoming head** ♀
  - Piper forceps operation
  - **EXCLUDES** partial breech extraction with forceps to aftercoming head (72.51)
  - total breech extraction with forceps to aftercoming head (72.53)
- **√4th 72.7 Vacuum extraction**
  - **INCLUDES** Malstöm's extraction
  - **72.71 Vacuum extraction with episiotomy** ♀
  - **72.79 Other vacuum extraction** ♀
- **72.8 Other specified instrumental delivery** ♀
- **72.9 Unspecified instrumental delivery** ♀

√3rd 73 Other procedures inducing or assisting delivery

- **√4th 73.0 Artificial rupture of membranes**
  - **73.01 Induction of labor by artificial rupture of membranes** ♀
    - Surgical induction NOS
    - **EXCLUDES** artificial rupture of membranes after onset of labor (73.09)
    - **AHA:** 3Q, '00, 5
  - **73.09 Other artificial rupture of membranes** ♀
    - Artificial rupture of membranes at time of delivery

Breech Extraction

- Breech presentation
- Delivery of legs
- Baby rotated for delivery of arms
- Umbilicus

- **73.1 Other surgical induction of labor** ♀
  - Induction by cervical dilation
  - **EXCLUDES** injection for abortion (75.0)
  - insertion of suppository for abortion (96.49)
- **√4th 73.2 Internal and combined version and extraction**
  - **73.21 Internal and combined version without extraction** ♀
    - Version NOS
  - **73.22 Internal and combined version with extraction** ♀
- **73.3 Failed forceps** ♀
  - Application of forceps without delivery
  - Trial forceps
- **73.4 Medical induction of labor** ♀
  - **EXCLUDES** medication to augment active labor — omit code
- **√4th 73.5 Manually assisted delivery** ♀
  - **73.51 Manual rotation of fetal head** ♀
  - **73.59 Other manually assisted delivery** ♀
    - Assisted spontaneous delivery
    - Credé maneuver
  - **AHA:** 4Q, '98, 76
- **73.6 Episiotomy** ♀
  - Episioproctotomy
  - Episiotomy with subsequent episiorrhaphy
  - **EXCLUDES** that with:
    - high forceps (72.31)
    - low forceps (72.1)
    - mid forceps (72.21)
    - outlet forceps (72.1)
    - vacuum extraction (72.71)
  - **AHA:** 1Q, '92, 10
- **73.8 Operations on fetus to facilitate delivery** ♀
  - Clavicotomy on fetus
  - Destruction of fetus
  - Needling of hydrocephalic head
- **√4th 73.9 Other operations assisting delivery**
  - **73.91 External version** ♀
  - **73.92 Replacement of prolapsed umbilical cord** ♀
  - **73.93 Incision of cervix to assist delivery** ♀
    - Dührssen's incisions
  - **73.94 Pubiotomy to assist delivery** ♀
    - Obstetrical symphysiotomy
  - **73.99 Other** ♀
    - **EXCLUDES** dilation of cervix, obstetrical, to induce labor (73.1)
    - insertion of bag or bougie to induce labor (73.1)
    - removal of cerclage material (69.96)

√3rd 74 Cesarean section and removal of fetus

- Code also any synchronous:
  - hysterectomy (68.3-68.4, 68.6, 68.8)
  - myomectomy (68.29)
  - sterilization (66.31-66.39, 66.63)
- **74.0 Classical cesarean section** ♀
  - Transperitoneal classical cesarean section
- **74.1 Low cervical cesarean section** ♀
  - Lower uterine segment cesarean section
  - **AHA:** 1Q, '01, 11
- **74.2 Extraperitoneal cesarean section** ♀
  - Supravesical cesarean section

OBSTETRICAL PROCEDURES

74.3 Removal of extratubal ectopic pregnancy ♀
Removal of:
ectopic abdominal pregnancy
fetus from peritoneal or extraperitoneal cavity following uterine or tubal rupture
EXCLUDES that by salpingostomy (66.02)
that by salpingotomy (66.01)
that with synchronous salpingectomy (66.62)
AHA: 4Q, '92, 25; 2Q, '90, 25; 2Q, '90, 27; 1Q, '89, 11

74.4 Cesarean section of other specified type ♀
Peritoneal exclusion cesareansection
Transperitoneal cesarean section NOS
Vaginal cesarean section

✓4th 74.9 Cesarean section of unspecified type
74.91 Hysterotomy to terminate pregnancy ♀
Therapeutic abortion by hysterotomy
74.99 Other cesarean section of unspecified type ♀
Cesarean section NOS
Obstetrical abdominouterotomy
Obstetrical hysterotomy

✓3rd 75 Other obstetric operations
75.0 Intra-amniotic injection for abortion ♀
Injection of:
prostaglandin } for induction of
saline } abortion
Termination of pregnancy by intrauterine injection
EXCLUDES insertion of prostaglandin suppository for abortion (96.49)

75.1 Diagnostic amniocentesis ♀
75.2 Intrauterine transfusion ♀
Exchange transfusion in utero
Insertion of catheter into abdomen of fetus for transfusion
Code also any hysterotomy approach (68.0)

✓4th 75.3 Other intrauterine operations on fetus and amnion
Code also any hysterotomy approach (68.0)
75.31 Amnioscopy ♀
Fetoscopy
Laparoamnioscopy
75.32 Fetal EKG (scalp) ♀
75.33 Fetal blood sampling and biopsy ♀
75.34 Other fetal monitoring ♀
Fetal monitoring, not otherwise specified
EXCLUDES fetal pulse oximetry (75.38)

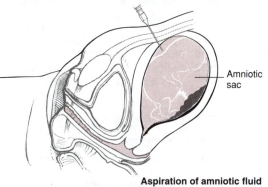

Amniocentesis
Amniotic sac
Aspiration of amniotic fluid

75.35 Other diagnostic procedures on fetus and amnion ♀
Intrauterine pressure determination
EXCLUDES amniocentesis (75.1)
diagnostic procedures on gravid uterus and placenta (87.81, 88.46, 88.78, 92.17)

75.36 Correction of fetal defect ♀
75.37 Amnioinfusion
Code also injection of antibiotic (99.21)
AHA: 4Q, '98, 76

75.38 Fetal pulse oximetry
Transcervical fetal oxygen saturation monitoring
Transcervical fetal SpO_2 monitoring
DEF: ▶Single-use sensor inserted through the birth canal and positioned to rest against the fetal cheek, forehead, or temple; infrared beam of light aimed at the fetal skin is reflected back through the sensor for analysis.◀
AHA: ▶4Q, '01, 64◀

75.4 Manual removal of retained placenta
EXCLUDES aspiration curettage (69.52)
dilation and curettage (69.02)

✓4th 75.5 Repair of current obstetric laceration of uterus
75.50 Repair of current obstetric laceration of uterus, not otherwise specified
75.51 Repair of current obstetric laceration of cervix
75.52 Repair of current obstetric laceration of corpus uteri

✓4th 75.6 Repair of other current obstetric laceration
AHA: 1Q, '92, 11
75.61 Repair of current obstetric laceration of bladder and urethra
75.62 Repair of current obstetric laceration of rectum and sphincter ani
75.69 Repair of other current obstetric laceration
Episioperineorrhaphy   Repair of:
Repair of: vagina
  pelvic floor   vulva
  perineum
Secondary repair of episiotomy
EXCLUDES repair of routine episiotomy (73.6)

75.7 Manual exploration of uterine cavity, postpartum
75.8 Obstetric tamponade of uterus or vagina
EXCLUDES antepartum tamponade (73.1)

✓4th 75.9 Other obstetric operations
75.91 Evacuation of obstetrical incisional hematoma of perineum
Evacuation of hematoma of:
episiotomy
perineorrhaphy
75.92 Evacuation of other hematoma of vulva or vagina
75.93 Surgical correction of inverted uterus
Spintelli operation
EXCLUDES vaginal repair of chronic inversion of uterus (69.23)
75.94 Manual replacement of inverted uterus
75.99 Other

14. OPERATIONS ON THE MUSCULOSKELETAL SYSTEM (76-84)

✓3rd 76 Operations on facial bones and joints
EXCLUDES: accessory sinuses (22.00-22.9)
nasal bones (21.00-21.99)
skull (01.01-02.99)

✓4th 76.0 Incision of facial bone without division

76.01 Sequestrectomy of facial bone
Removal of necrotic bone chip from facial bone

76.09 Other incision of facial bone
Reopening of osteotomy site of facial bone
EXCLUDES: osteotomy associated with orthognathic surgery (76.61-76.69)
removal of internal fixation device (76.97)

✓4th 76.1 Diagnostic procedures on facial bones and joints

76.11 Biopsy of facial bone

76.19 Other diagnostic procedures on facial bones and joints
EXCLUDES: contrast arthrogram of temporomandibular joint (87.13)
other x-ray (87.11-87.12, 87.14-87.16)

AHA: N-D, '87, 12

76.2 Local excision or destruction of lesion of facial bone
EXCLUDES: biopsy of facial bone (76.11)
excision of odontogenic lesion (24.4)

✓4th 76.3 Partial ostectomy of facial bone

76.31 Partial mandibulectomy
Hemimandibulectomy
EXCLUDES: that associated with temporomandibular arthroplasty (76.5)

DEF: Excision, partial of lower jawbone.

DEF: Hemimandibulectomy: Excision of one-half of lower jawbone.

76.39 Partial ostectomy of other facial bone
Hemimaxillectomy (with bonegraft or prosthesis)

AHA: J-F, '87, 14

DEF: Excision, partial of facial bone; other than lower jawbone.

DEF: Hemimaxillectomy (with bone graft or prosthesis): Excision of one side of upper jawbone and restoration with bone graft or prosthesis.

✓4th 76.4 Excision and reconstruction of facial bones

76.41 Total mandibulectomy with synchronous reconstruction

76.42 Other total mandibulectomy

76.43 Other reconstruction of mandible
EXCLUDES: genioplasty (76.67-76.68)
that with synchronous total mandibulectomy (76.41)

76.44 Total ostectomy of other facial bone with synchronous reconstruction

AHA: 3Q, '93, 6

DEF: Excision, facial bone, total with reconstruction during same operative session.

76.45 Other total ostectomy of other facial bone

76.46 Other reconstruction of other facial bone
EXCLUDES: that with synchronous total ostectomy (76.44)

76.5 Temporomandibular arthroplasty
AHA: 4Q, '99, 20

✓4th 76.6 Other facial bone repair and orthognathic surgery
Code also any synchronous:
bone graft (76.91)
synthetic implant (76.92)
EXCLUDES: reconstruction of facial bones (76.41-76.46)

76.61 Closed osteoplasty [osteotomy] of mandibular ramus
Gigli saw osteotomy

DEF: Reshaping and restoration of lower jawbone projection; closed surgical field.

DEF: Gigli saw osteotomy: Plastic repair using a flexible wire with saw teeth.

76.62 Open osteoplasty [osteotomy] of mandibular ramus

76.63 Osteoplasty [osteotomy] of body of mandible

76.64 Other orthognathic surgery on mandible
Mandibular osteoplasty NOS
Segmental or subapical osteotomy

76.65 Segmental osteoplasty [osteotomy] of maxilla
Maxillary osteoplasty NOS

76.66 Total osteoplasty [osteotomy] of maxilla

76.67 Reduction genioplasty
Reduction mentoplasty

DEF: Reduction of protruding chin or lower jawbone.

76.68 Augmentation genioplasty
Mentoplasty:
NOS
with graft or implant

DEF: Extension of the lower jawbone to a functional position by means of plastic surgery.

76.69 Other facial bone repair
Osteoplasty of facial bone NOS

✓4th 76.7 Reduction of facial fracture
INCLUDES: internal fixation
Code also any synchronous:
bone graft (76.91)
synthetic implant (76.92)
EXCLUDES: that of nasal bones (21.71-21.72)

76.70 Reduction of facial fracture, not otherwise specified

76.71 Closed reduction of malar and zygomatic fracture

76.72 Open reduction of malar and zygomatic fracture

76.73 Closed reduction of maxillary fracture

76.74 Open reduction of maxillary fracture

76.75 Closed reduction of mandibular fracture

76.76 Open reduction of mandibular fracture

76.77 Open reduction of alveolar fracture
Reduction of alveolar fracture with stabilization of teeth

76.78 Other closed reduction of facial fracture
Closed reduction of orbital fracture
EXCLUDES: nasal bone (21.71)

76.79 Other open reduction of facial fracture
Open reduction of orbit rim or wall
EXCLUDES: nasal bone (21.72)

✓4th 76.9 Other operations on facial bones and joints

76.91 Bone graft to facial bone
Autogenous
Bone bank } graft to facial bone
Heterogenous

76.92 Insertion of synthetic implant in facial bone
Alloplastic implant to facial bone

OPERATIONS ON THE MUSCULOSKELETAL SYSTEM

76.93 Closed reduction of temporomandibular dislocation

76.94 Open reduction of temporomandibular dislocation

76.95 Other manipulation of temporomandibular joint

76.96 Injection of therapeutic substance into temporomandibular joint

76.97 Removal of internal fixation device from facial bone
- EXCLUDES removal of:
  - dental wiring (97.33)
  - external mandibular fixation device NEC (97.36)

76.99 Other

77 Incision, excision, and division of other bones
- EXCLUDES laminectomy for decompression (03.09)
  - operations on:
    - accessory sinuses (22.00-22.9)
    - ear ossicles (19.0-19.55)
    - facial bones (76.01-76.99)
    - joint structures (80.00-81.99)
    - mastoid (19.9-20.99)
    - nasal bones (21.00-21.99)
    - skull (01.01-02.99)

The following fourth-digit subclassification is for use with appropriate categories in section 77 to identify the site. Valid fourth-digit categories are in [brackets] under each code.

- 0 unspecified site
- 1 scapula, clavicle, and thorax [ribs and sternum]
- 2 humerus
- 3 radius and ulna
- 4 carpals and metacarpals
- 5 femur
- 6 patella
- 7 tibia and fibula
- 8 tarsals and metatarsals
- 9 other
  - Pelvic bones
  - Phalanges (of foot) (of hand)
  - Vertebrae

77.0 Sequestrectomy [0-9]
- DEF: Excision and removal of dead bone.

77.1 Other incision of bone without division [0-9]
- Reopening of osteotomy site
- EXCLUDES aspiration of bone marrow, (41.31, 41.91)
  - removal of internal fixation device (78.60-78.69)
- AHA: For code 77.17: ▶1Q, '02, 3◀
- DEF: Incision into bone without division of site.

77.2 Wedge osteotomy [0-9]
- EXCLUDES that for hallux valgus (77.51)
- DEF: Removal of wedge-shaped piece of bone.

77.3 Other division of bone [0-9]
- Osteoarthrotomy
- EXCLUDES clavicotomy of fetus (73.8)
  - laminotomy or incision of vertebra (03.01-03.09)
  - pubiotomy to assist delivery (73.94)
  - sternotomy incidental to thoracic operation — omit code

77.4 Biopsy of bone [0-9]
- AHA: 2Q, '98, 12

77.5 Excision and repair of bunion and other toe deformities

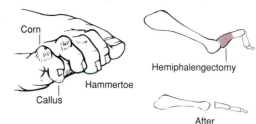

Repair of Hammertoes

77.51 Bunionectomy with soft tissue correction and osteotomy of the first metatarsal
- DEF: Incision and removal of big toe bony prominence and reconstruction with soft tissue.

77.52 Bunionectomy with soft tissue correction and arthrodesis
- DEF: Removal of big toe bony prominence and reconstruction with soft tissue and joint fixation.

77.53 Other bunionectomy with soft tissue correction

77.54 Excision or correction of bunionette
- That with osteotomy
- DEF: Resection of fifth metatarsal head via exposure of joint; includes imbrication of capsule.

77.56 Repair of hammer toe
- Fusion
- Phalangectomy (partial) } of hammer toe
- Filleting
- DEF: Repair of clawlike toe defect by joint fusion, partial removal of toe or via traction technique.

77.57 Repair of claw toe
- Fusion
- Phalangectomy (partial)
- Capsulotomy } of claw toe
- Tendon lengthening
- DEF: Repair of clawlike toe defect by joint fusion, partial removal of toe, joint capsule incision or lengthening of fibrous muscle attachment.

77.58 Other excision, fusion, and repair of toes
- Cockup toe repair
- Overlapping toe repair
- That with use of prosthetic materials

77.59 Other bunionectomy
- Resection of hallux valgus joint with insertion of prosthesis
- DEF: Resection of hallux valgus joint with insertion of prosthesis: Cutting away part of big toe with prosthesis insertion to correct bony prominence.

77.6 Local excision of lesion or tissue of bone [0-9]
- EXCLUDES biopsy of bone (77.40-77.49)
  - debridement of compound fracture (79.60-79.69)
- AHA: For code 77.61: 3Q, '01, 9; For code 77.65: S-O, '85, 4; For code 77.67: ▶1Q, '02, 3;◀ 1Q, '99, 8; For code 77.69: 2Q, '00, 18

77.7 Excision of bone for graft [0-9]
- AHA: 4Q, '99, 11, 13; For code 77.79: 2Q, '00 12, 13; 4Q, '99, 11, 13

---

§ Requires fourth-digit. Valid digits are in [brackets] under each code. See code 77 for definitions.
16 Nonspecific OR procedure=0

77.8–78.9 OPERATIONS ON THE MUSCULOSKELETAL SYSTEM — Tabular List

§ ✓4th 16 **77.8** **Other partial ostectomy**
[0-9]   Condylectomy
   EXCLUDES   amputation (84.00-84.19, 84.91)
       arthrectomy (80.90-80.99)
       excision of bone ends associated with:
           arthrodesis (81.00-81.29)
           arthroplasty (81.51-81.59, 81.71-81.81, 81.84)
       excision of cartilage (80.5-80.6, 80.80-80.99)
       excision of head of femur with synchronous replacement (81.51-81.53)
       hemilaminectomy (03.01-03.09)
       laminectomy (03.01-03.09)
       ostectomy for hallux valgus (77.51-77.59)
       partial amputation:
           finger (84.01)
           thumb (84.02)
           toe (84.11)
       resection of ribs incidental to thoracic operation — omit code
       that incidental to other operation — omit code

§ ✓4th 16 **77.9** **Total ostectomy**
[0-9]   **EXCLUDES**   amputation of limb (84.00-84.19, 84.91)
       that incidental to other operation — omit code

✓3rd **78** **Other operations on bones, except facial bones**
   EXCLUDES   operations on:
       accessory sinuses (22.00-22.9)
       facial bones (76.01-76.99)
       joint structures (80.00-81.99)
       nasal bones (21.00-21.99)
       skull (01.01-02.99)

The following fourth-digit subclassification is for use with categories in section 78 to identify the site. Valid fourth-digit categories are in [brackets] under each code.

   0 unspecified site
   1 scapula, clavicle, and thorax [ribs and sternum]
   2 humerus
   3 radius and ulna
   4 carpals and metacarpals
   5 femur
   6 patella
   7 tibia and fibula
   8 tarsals and metatarsals
   9 other
       Pelvic bones   Vertebrae
       Phalanges (of foot) (of hand)

§§ ✓4th 16 **78.0** **Bone graft**
[0-9]   Bone:
       bank graft
       graft (autogenous) (heterogenous)
   That with debridement of bone graft site (removal of sclerosed, fibrous, or necrotic bone or tissue)
   Transplantation of bone
   Code also any excision of bone for graft (77.70-77.79)
   EXCLUDES   that for bone lengthening (78.30-78.39)
   AHA: 2Q, '98, 12; 3Q, '94, 10; 1Q, '91, 3

§§ ✓4th 16 **78.1** **Application of external fixation device**
[0-9]   Minifixator with insertion of pins/wires/screws into bone
   EXCLUDES   other immobilization, pressure, and attention to wound (93.51-93.59)
   AHA: 2Q, '94, 4

§§ ✓4th 16 **78.2** **Limb shortening procedures**
[0,2-5,7-9] Epiphyseal stapling
   Open epiphysiodesis
   Percutaneous epiphysiodesis
   Resection/osteotomy

§§ ✓4th 16 **78.3** **Limb lengthening procedures**
[0,2-5,7-9] Bone graft with or without internal fixation devices or osteotomy
   Distraction technique with or without corticotomy/osteotomy
   Code also any application of an external fixation device (78.10-78.19)

§§ ✓4th 16 **78.4** **Other repair or plastic operations on bone**
[0-9]   Other operation on bone NEC
   Repair of malunion or nonunion fracture NEC
   EXCLUDES   application of external fixation device (78.10-78.19)
       limb lengthening procedures (78.30-78.39)
       limb shortening procedures (78.20-78.29)
       osteotomy (77.3)
       reconstruction of thumb (82.61-82.69)
       repair of pectus deformity (34.74)
       repair with bone graft (78.00-78.09)
   AHA: 3Q, '92, 20; 4Q, '88, 11; **For code 78.47:** 3Q, '91, 20; **For code 78.49:** 4Q, '99, 22; 1Q, '97, 5

§§ ✓4th 16 **78.5** **Internal fixation of bone without fracture reduction**
[0-9]   Internal fixation of bone (prophylactic)
   Reinsertion of internal fixation device
   Revision of displaced or broken fixation device
   EXCLUDES   arthroplasty and arthrodesis (81.00-81.85)
       bone graft (78.00-78.09)
       limb shortening procedures (78.20-78.29)
       that for fracture reduction (79.10-79.19, 79.30-79.59)
   AHA: 2Q, '99, 11; 2Q, '94, 4; **For Code 78.59:** 4Q, '99, 13

§§ ✓4th 16 **78.6** **Removal of implanted devices from bone**
[0-9]   External fixator device (invasive)
   Internal fixation device
   Removal of bone growth stimulator (invasive)
   EXCLUDES   removal of cast, splint, and traction device (Kirschner wire) (Steinmann pin) (97.88)
       removal of skull tongs or halo traction device (02.95)
   AHA: 1Q, '00, 15; For Code 78.69: 2Q, '00, 18

§§ ✓4th 16 **78.7** **Osteoclasis**
[0-9]   **DEF:** Surgical breaking or rebreaking of bone.

§§ ✓4th 16 **78.8** **Diagnostic procedures on bone, not elsewhere classified**
[0-9]   **EXCLUDES**   biopsy of bone (77.40-77.49)
       magnetic resonance imaging (88.94)
       microscopic examination of specimen from bone (91.51-91.59)
       radioisotope scan (92.14)
       skeletal x-ray (87.21-87.29, 87.43, 88.21-88.33)
       thermography (88.83)

§§ ✓4th 16 **78.9** **Insertion of bone growth stimulator**
[0-9]   Insertion of:
       bone stimulator (electrical) to aid bone healing
       osteogenic electrodes for bone growth stimulation
       totally implanted device (invasive)
   EXCLUDES   non-invasive (transcutaneous) (surface) stimulator (99.86)

---

§ Requires fourth-digit. Valid digits are in [brackets] under each code. See code 77 for definitions.
§§ Requires fourth-digit. Valid digits are in [brackets] under each code. See code 78 for definitions.
[16] Nonspecific OR procedure=0

BI Bilateral Edit   NC Non-covered Procedure   ▶◀ Revised Text   ● New Code   ▲ Revised Code Title

OPERATIONS ON THE MUSCULOSKELETAL SYSTEM

79 Reduction of fracture and dislocation
  INCLUDES: application of cast or splint
  reduction with insertion of traction device (Kirschner wire) (Steinmann pin)
  Code also any application of external fixation device (78.10-78.19)
  EXCLUDES:
   external fixation alone for immobilization of fracture (93.51-93.56, 93.59)
   internal fixation without reduction of fracture (78.50-78.59)
   operations on:
    facial bones (76.70-76.79)
    nasal bones (21.71-21.72)
    orbit (76.78-76.79)
    skull (02.02)
    vertebrae (03.53)
   removal of cast or splint (97.88)
   replacement of cast or splint (97.11-97.14)
   traction alone for reduction of fracture (93.41-93.46)

The following fourth-digit subclassification is for use with appropriate categories in section 79 to identify the site. Valid fourth-digit categories are in [brackets] under each code.
  0 unspecified site
  1 humerus
  2 radius and ulna
     Arm NOS
  3 carpals and metacarpals
     Hand NOS
  4 phalanges of hand
  5 femur
  6 tibia and fibula
     Leg NOS
  7 tarsals and metatarsals
     Foot NOS
  8 phalanges of foot
  9 other specified bone

79.0 Closed reduction of fracture without internal fixation [0-9]
  EXCLUDES: that for separation of epiphysis (79.40-79.49)
  AHA: 2Q, '94, 3; 3Q, '89, 17; 4Q, '88, 11; **For code 79.05:** 3Q, '89, 16
  DEF: Manipulative realignment of fracture; without incision or internal fixation.

79.1 Closed reduction of fracture with internal fixation [0-9]
  EXCLUDES: that for separation of epiphysis (79.40-79.49)
  AHA: 2Q, '94, 4; 4Q, '93, 35; 1Q, '93, 27
  DEF: Manipulative realignment of fracture; with internal fixation but without incision.

79.2 Open reduction of fracture without internal fixation [0-9]
  EXCLUDES: that for separation of epiphysis (79.50-79.59)
  AHA: 2Q, '94, 3

79.3 Open reduction of fracture with internal fixation [0-9]
  EXCLUDES: that for separation of epiphysis (79.50-79.59)
  AHA: 2Q, '98, 12; 3Q, '94, 10; 2Q, '94, 3; 4Q, '93, 35
  DEF: Realignment of fracture with incision and internal fixation.

79.4 Closed reduction of separated epiphysis
  [0-2,5,6,9] Reduction with or without internal fixation
  DEF: Manipulative reduction of expanded joint end of long bone to normal position without incision.

79.5 Open reduction of separated epiphysis
  [0-2,5,6,9] Reduction with or without internal fixation
  DEF: Reduction of expanded joint end of long bone with incision.

79.6 Debridement of open fracture site
  [0-9] Debridement of compound fracture
  AHA: 3Q, '95, 12; 3Q, '89, 16
  DEF: Removal of damaged tissue at fracture site.

79.7 Closed reduction of dislocation
  INCLUDES: closed reduction (with external traction device)
  EXCLUDES: closed reduction of dislocation of temporomandibular joint (76.93)
  DEF: Manipulative reduction of displaced joint without incision; with or without external traction.

  79.70 Closed reduction of dislocation of unspecified site
  79.71 Closed reduction of dislocation of shoulder
  79.72 Closed reduction of dislocation of elbow
  79.73 Closed reduction of dislocation of wrist
  79.74 Closed reduction of dislocation of hand and finger
  79.75 Closed reduction of dislocation of hip
  79.76 Closed reduction of dislocation of knee
     AHA: N-D, '86, 7
  79.77 Closed reduction of dislocation of ankle
  79.78 Closed reduction of dislocation of foot and toe
  79.79 Closed reduction of dislocation of other specified sites

79.8 Open reduction of dislocation
  INCLUDES: open reduction (with internal and external fixation devices)
  EXCLUDES: open reduction of dislocation of temporomandibular joint (76.94)
  DEF: Reduction of displaced joint via incision; with or without internal and external fixation.

  79.80 Open reduction of dislocation of unspecified site
  79.81 Open reduction of dislocation of shoulder
  79.82 Open reduction of dislocation of elbow
  79.83 Open reduction of dislocation of wrist
  79.84 Open reduction of dislocation of hand and finger
  79.85 Open reduction of dislocation of hip
  79.86 Open reduction of dislocation of knee
  79.87 Open reduction of dislocation of ankle
  79.88 Open reduction of dislocation of foot and toe
  79.89 Open reduction of dislocation of other specified sites

79.9 Unspecified operation on bone injury [0-9]

---

[16] Nonspecific OR procedure=0

80 Incision and excision of joint structures

INCLUDES operations on:
- capsule of joint
- cartilage
- condyle
- ligament
- meniscus
- synovial membrane

EXCLUDES cartilage of:
- ear (18.01-18.9)
- nose (21.00-21.99)
- temporomandibular joint (76.01-76.99)

The following fourth-digit subclassification is for use with appropriate categories in section 80 to identify the site:
- 0 unspecified site
- 1 shoulder
- 2 elbow
- 3 wrist
- 4 hand and finger
- 5 hip
- 6 knee
- 7 ankle
- 8 foot and toe
- 9 other specified sites
    Spine

80.0 Arthrotomy for removal of prosthesis
INCLUDES cement spacer

AHA: For code 80.06: 2Q, '97, 10

DEF: Incision into joint to remove prosthesis.

80.1 Other arthrotomy
Arthrostomy

EXCLUDES that for:
- arthrography (88.32)
- arthroscopy (80.20-80.29)
- injection of drug (81.92)
- operative approach — omit code

DEF: Incision into joint; other than to remove prosthesis.

DEF: Arthrostomy: Creation of opening into joint.

80.2 Arthroscopy
AHA: 3Q, '93, 5

80.3 Biopsy of joint structure
Aspiration biopsy

80.4 Division of joint capsule, ligament, or cartilage
Goldner clubfoot release
Heyman-Herndon(-Strong) correction of metatarsus varus
Release of:
- adherent or constrictive joint capsule
- joint
- ligament

EXCLUDES symphysiotomy to assist delivery (73.94)
that for:
- carpal tunnel syndrome (04.43)
- tarsal tunnel syndrome (04.44)

DEF: Incision and separation of joint tissues, including capsule, fibrous bone attachment or cartilage.

80.5 Excision or destruction of intervertebral disc

80.50 Excision or destruction of intervertebral disc, unspecified
Unspecified asto excision or destruction

80.51 Excision of intervertebral disc
Code also any concurrent spinal fusion (81.00-81.09)
Diskectomy
Level:
- cervical
- thoracic
- lumbar (lumbosacral)

Removal of herniated nucleus pulposus
That by laminotomy or hemilaminectomy
That with decompression of spinal nerve root at same level
Requires additional code for any concomitant decompression of spinal nerve root at different level from excision site

EXCLUDES intervertebral chemonucleolysis (80.52)
laminectomy for exploration of intraspinal canal (03.09)
laminotomy for decompression of spinal nerve root only (03.09)

AHA: 1Q, '96, 7; 2Q, '95, 9; 2Q, '90, 27; S-O, '86, 12

DEF: Removal of intervertebral disc.

DEF: Removal of a herniated nucleus pulposus: Removal of displaced intervertebral disc, central part.

80.52 Intervertebral chemonucleolysis
With aspiration of disc fragments
With diskography
Injection of proteolytic enzyme into intervertebral space (chymopapain)

EXCLUDES injection of anesthetic substance (03.91)
injection of other substances (03.92)

DEF: Destruction of intervertebral disc via injection of enzyme.

80.59 Other destruction of intervertebral disc
Destruction NEC
That by laser

80.6 Excision of semilunar cartilage of knee
Excision of meniscus of knee

AHA: 3Q, '00, 4; 2Q, '96, 3; 1Q, '93, 23

80.7 Synovectomy
Complete or partial resection of synovial membrane

EXCLUDES excision of Baker's cyst (83.39)

DEF: Excision of inner membrane of joint capsule.

80.8 Other local excision or destruction of lesion of joint

80.9 Other excision of joint
EXCLUDES cheilectomy of joint (77.80-77.89)
excision of bone ends (77.80-77.89)

OPERATIONS ON THE MUSCULOSKELETAL SYSTEM

✓3rd 81 Repair and plastic operations on joint structures

✓4th 81.0 Spinal fusion

▶Code also any 360 degree spinal fusion by a single incision (81.61)
Code also any insertion of interbody spinal fusion device (84.51)
Code also any insertion of recombinant bone morphogenetic protein (84.52)◀

INCLUDES arthrodesis of spine with:
  bone graft
  internal fixation

EXCLUDES corrections of pseudarthrosis of spine (81.30-81.39)
refusion of spine (81.30-81.39)

DEF: Immobilization of spinal column.

DEF: Anterior interbody fusion: Arthrodesis by excising disc and cartilage end plates with bone graft insertion between two vertebrae.

DEF: Lateral fusion: Arthrodesis by decorticating and bone grafting lateral surface of zygapophysial joint, pars interarticularis and transverse process.

DEF: Posterior fusion: Arthrodesis by decorticating and bone grafting of neural arches between right and left zygapophysial joints.

DEF: Posterolateral fusion: Arthrodesis by decorticating and bone grafting zygapophysial joint, pars interarticularis and transverse processes

81.00 Spinal fusion, not otherwise specified

81.01 Atlas-axis spinal fusion

Craniocervical fusion ⎫ by anterior
C_1-C_2 fusion   ⎬ transoral
Occiput-C_2 fusion   ⎭ or
                                   posterior
                                   technique

81.02 Other cervical fusion, anterior technique
Arthrodesis of C_2 level or below:
  anterior (interbody) technique
  anterolateral technique
AHA: 1Q, '01, 6; 1Q, '96, 7

81.03 Other cervical fusion, posterior technique
Arthrodesis of C_2 level or below:
  posterior (interbody) technique
  posterolateral technique

81.04 Dorsal and dorsolumbar fusion, anterior technique
Arthrodesis of thoracic or thoracolumbar region:
  anterior (interbody) technique
  anterolateral technique

81.05 Dorsal and dorsolumbar fusion, posterior technique
Arthrodesis of thoracic or thoracolumbar region:
  posterior (interbody) technique
  posterolateral technique
AHA: 4Q, '99, 11

81.06 Lumbar and lumbosacral fusion, anterior technique
Arthrodesis of lumbar or lumbosacral region:
  anterior (interbody) technique
  anterolateral technique
AHA: 4Q, '99, 11

81.07 Lumbar and lumbosacral fusion, lateral transverse process technique

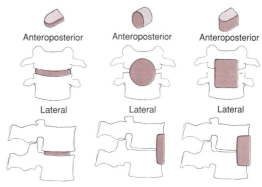

Types of Grafts for Anterior Arthrodesis
Anteroposterior   Anteroposterior   Anteroposterior
Lateral   Lateral   Lateral

81.08 Lumbar and lumbosacral fusion, posterior technique
Arthrodesis of lumbar or lumbosacral region:
  posterior (interbody) technique
  posterolateral technique
AHA: 2Q, '00, 12, 13; 4Q, '99, 13; 2Q, '95, 9

✓4th 81.1 Arthrodesis of foot and ankle

INCLUDES arthrodesis of foot and ankle with:
  bone graft
  external fixation device

DEF: Fixation of foot or ankle joints.

81.11 Ankle fusion
Tibiotalar fusion

81.12 Triple arthrodesis
Talus to calcaneus and calcaneus to cuboid and navicular

81.13 Subtalar fusion
81.14 Midtarsal fusion
81.15 Tarsometatarsal fusion
81.16 Metatarsophalangeal fusion
81.17 Other fusion of foot

✓4th 81.2 Arthrodesis of other joint

INCLUDES arthrodesis with:
  bone graft
  external fixation device
  excision of bone ends and compression

81.20 Arthrodesis of unspecified joint
81.21 Arthrodesis of hip
81.22 Arthrodesis of knee
81.23 Arthrodesis of shoulder
81.24 Arthrodesis of elbow
81.25 Carporadial fusion
81.26 Metacarpocarpal fusion
81.27 Metacarpophalangeal fusion
81.28 Interphalangeal fusion
81.29 Arthrodesis of other specified joints

✓4th 81.3 Refusion of spine

INCLUDES ▶arthrodesis of spine with:
  bone graft
  internal fixation◀
  correction of pseudarthrosis of spine

▶Code also any 360 degree spinal fusion by a single incision (81.61)
Code also any insertion of interbody spinal fusion device (84.51)
Code also any insertion of recombinant bone morphogenetic protein (84.52)◀
AHA: 4Q, '01, 64

81.30 Refusion of spine, not otherwise specified

81.31 Refusion of atlas-axis spine
Craniocervical fusion
C_1-C_2 fusion } by anterior transoral or posterior technique
Occiput C_2 fusion

81.32 Refusion of other cervical spine, anterior technique
Arthrodesis of C_2 level or below:
- anterior (interbody) technique
- anterolateral technique

81.33 Refusion of other cervical spine, posterior technique
Arthrodesis of C_2 level or below:
- posterior (interbody) technique
- posterolateral technique

81.34 Refusion of dorsal and dorsolumbar spine, anterior technique
Arthrodesis of thoracic or thoracolumbar region:
- anterior (interbody) technique
- anterolateral technique

81.35 Refusion of dorsal and dorsolumbar spine, posterior technique
Arthrodesis of thoracic or thoracolumbar region:
- posterior (interbody) technique
- posterolateral technique

81.36 Refusion of lumbar and lumbosacral spine, anterior technique
Arthrodesis of lumbar or lumbosacral region
- anterior (interbody) technique
- anterolateral technique

81.37 Refusion of lumbar and lumbosacral spine, lateral transverse process technique

81.38 Refusion of lumbar and lumbosacral spine, posterior technique
Arthrodesis of lumbar or lumbosacral region:
- posterior (interbody) technique
- posterolateral technique

81.39 Refusion of spine, not elsewhere classified

✓4th 81.4 Other repair of joint of lower extremity
INCLUDES: arthroplasty of lower extremity with:
- external traction or fixation
- graft of bone (chips) or cartilage
- internal fixation device

AHA: S-O, '85, 4

81.40 Repair of hip, not elsewhere classified

81.42 Five-in-one repair of knee
Medial meniscectomy, medial collateral ligament repair, vastus medialis advancement, semitendinosus advancement, and pes anserinus transfer

81.43 Triad knee repair
Medial meniscectomy with repair of the anterior cruciate ligament and the medial collateral ligament
O'Donoghue procedure

81.44 Patellar stabilization
Roux-Goldthwait operation for recurrent dislocation of patella

DEF: Roux-Goldthwait operation: Stabilization of patella via lateral ligament transposed at insertion beneath undisturbed medial insertion; excision of capsule ellipse and medial patella retinaculum; capsule reefed for lateral patella hold.

81.45 Other repair of the cruciate ligaments
AHA: M-A, '87, 12

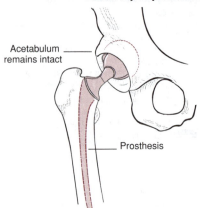

Partial Hip Replacement

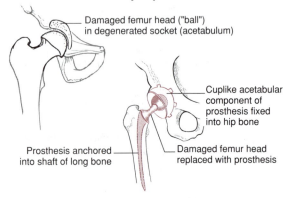

Total Hip Replacement

81.46 Other repair of the collateral ligaments

81.47 Other repair of knee
AHA: 1Q, '00, 12, 13; 1Q, '96, 3; 3Q, '93, 5

81.49 Other repair of ankle
AHA: 2Q, '01, 15; 3Q, '00, 4

✓4th 81.5 Joint replacement of lower extremity
INCLUDES: arthroplasty of lower extremity with:
- external traction or fixation
- graft of bone (chips) or cartilage
- internal fixation device or prosthesis
- removal of cement spacer

AHA: S-O, '85, 4

81.51 Total hip replacement [BI]
Replacement of both femoral head and acetabulum by prosthesis
Total reconstruction of hip

AHA: 2Q, '91, 18

DEF: Repair of both surfaces of hip joint with prosthesis.

81.52 Partial hip replacement [BI]
Bipolar endoprosthesis

AHA: 2Q, '91, 18

DEF: Repair of single surface of hip joint with prosthesis.

81.53 Revision of hip replacement [BI]
Partial
Total

AHA: 3Q, '97, 12

81.54 Total knee replacement [BI]
Bicompartmental
Tricompartmental
Unicompartmental (hemijoint)

DEF: Repair of a knee joint with prosthetic implant in one, two, or three compartments.

OPERATIONS ON THE MUSCULOSKELETAL SYSTEM

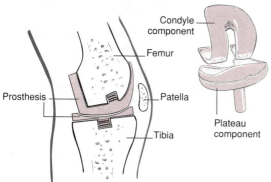

Total Knee Replacement

81.55 Revision of knee replacement
EXCLUDES: arthrodesis of knee (81.22)
AHA: 2Q, '97, 10

81.56 Total ankle replacement

81.57 Replacement of joint of foot and toe

81.59 Revision of joint replacement of lower extremity, not elsewhere classified

81.6 Other procedures on spine

81.61 360 degree spinal fusion, single incision approach
That by single incision but fusing or refusing both anterior and posterior spine
Code also refusion of spine (81.30-81.39)
Code also spinal fusion (81.00-81.08)

81.7 Arthroplasty and repair of hand, fingers, and wrist
INCLUDES: arthroplasty of hand and finger with:
external traction or fixation
graft of bone (chips) or cartilage
internal fixation device or prosthesis
EXCLUDES: operations on muscle, tendon, and fascia of hand (82.01-82.99)
DEF: Plastic surgery of hand, fingers and wrist joints.

81.71 Arthroplasty of metacarpophalangeal and interphalangeal joint with implant

81.72 Arthroplasty of metacarpophalangeal and interphalangeal joint without implant
AHA: 1Q, '93, 28

81.73 Total wrist replacement

81.74 Arthroplasty of carpocarpal or carpometacarpal joint with implant

81.75 Arthroplasty of carpocarpal or carpometacarpal joint without implant
AHA: 3Q, '93, 8

81.79 Other repair of hand, fingers, and wrist

81.8 Arthroplasty and repair of shoulder and elbow
INCLUDES: arthroplasty of upper limb NEC with:
external traction or fixation
graft of bone (chips) or cartilage
internal fixation device or prosthesis

81.80 Total shoulder replacement

81.81 Partial shoulder replacement

81.82 Repair of recurrent dislocation of shoulder
AHA: 3Q, '95, 15

81.83 Other repair of shoulder
Revision of arthroplasty of shoulder
AHA: ▶1Q, '02, 9;◀ 4Q, '01, 51; 2Q, '00, 14; 3Q, '93, 5

81.84 Total elbow replacement

81.85 Other repair of elbow

81.9 Other operations on joint structures

81.91 Arthrocentesis
Joint aspiration
EXCLUDES: that for:
arthrography (88.32)
biopsy of joint structure (80.30-80.39)
injection of drug (81.92)
DEF: Insertion of needle to withdraw fluid from joint.

81.92 Injection of therapeutic substance into joint or ligament
AHA: 2Q, '00, 14; 3Q, '89, 16

81.93 Suture of capsule or ligament of upper extremity
EXCLUDES: that associated with arthroplasty (81.71-81.75, 81.80-81.81, 81.84)

81.94 Suture of capsule or ligament of ankle and foot
EXCLUDES: that associated with arthroplasty (81.56-81.59)

81.95 Suture of capsule or ligament of other lower extremity
EXCLUDES: that associated with arthroplasty (81.51-81.55, 81.59)

81.96 Other repair of joint

81.97 Revision of joint replacement of upper extremity
Partial
Removal of cement spacer
Total

81.98 Other diagnostic procedures on joint structures
EXCLUDES: arthroscopy (80.20-80.29)
biopsy of joint structure (80.30-80.39)
microscopic examination of specimen from joint (91.51-91.59)
thermography (88.83)
x-ray (87.21-87.29, 88.21-88.33)

81.99 Other

82 Operations on muscle, tendon, and fascia of hand
INCLUDES: operations on:
aponeurosis
synovial membrane (tendon sheath)
tendon sheath

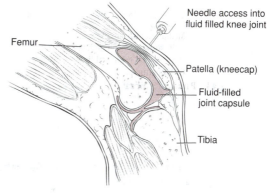

Arthrocentesis

OPERATIONS ON THE MUSCULOSKELETAL SYSTEM

✓4th 82.0 Incision of muscle, tendon, fascia, and bursa of hand

82.01 Exploration of tendon sheath of hand
Incision of } tendon sheath
Removal of rice bodies in } of hand

EXCLUDES division of tendon (82.11)

DEF: Incision into and exploring the hand's muscle and its accompanying supportive, connective tissue, bands, and sacs.

82.02 Myotomy of hand
EXCLUDES myotomy for division (82.19)
DEF: Incision into hand muscle.

82.03 Bursotomy of hand

82.04 Incision and drainage of palmar or thenar space

82.09 Other incision of soft tissue of hand
EXCLUDES incision of skin and subcutaneous tissue alone (86.01-86.09)
AHA: N-D, '87, 10

✓4th 82.1 Division of muscle, tendon, and fascia of hand

82.11 Tenotomy of hand
Division of tendon of hand

82.12 Fasciotomy of hand
Division of fascia of hand

82.19 Other division of soft tissue of hand
Division of muscle of hand

✓4th 82.2 Excision of lesion of muscle, tendon, and fascia of hand

82.21 Excision or lesion of tendon sheath of hand
Ganglionectomy of tendon sheath (wrist)

82.22 Excision of lesion of muscle of hand

82.29 Excision of other lesion of soft tissue of hand
EXCLUDES excision of lesion of skin and subcutaneous tissue (86.21-86.3)

✓4th 82.3 Other excision of soft tissue of hand
Code also any skin graft (86.61-86.62, 86.73)
EXCLUDES excision of skin and subcutaneous tissue (86.21-86.3)

82.31 Bursectomy of hand

82.32 Excision of tendon of hand for graft
DEF: Resection and excision of fibrous tissue connecting bone to hand muscle for grafting.

82.33 Other tenonectomy of hand
Tenosynovectomy of hand
EXCLUDES excision of lesion of:
tendon (82.29)
sheath (82.21)
DEF: Removal of fibrous bands connecting muscle to bone of hand.
DEF: Tenosynovectomy of hand: Excision of fibrous band connecting muscle and bone of hand and removal of coverings.

82.34 Excision of muscle or fascia of hand for graft

82.35 Other fasciectomy of hand
Release of Dupuytren's contracture
EXCLUDES excision of lesion of fascia (82.29)
DEF: Excision of fibrous connective tissue; other than for grafting or removing lesion.
DEF: Release of Dupuytren's contracture: Excision of fibrous connective tissue to correct flexion of fingers.

82.36 Other myectomy of hand
EXCLUDES excision of lesion of muscle (82.22)

82.39 Other excision of soft tissue of hand
EXCLUDES excision of skin (86.21-86.3)
excision of soft tissue lesion (82.29)

✓4th 82.4 Suture of muscle, tendon, and fascia of hand

82.41 Suture of tendon sheath of hand

82.42 Delayed suture of flexor tendon of hand
DEF: Suture of fibrous band between flexor muscle and bone; following initial repair.

82.43 Delayed suture of other tendon of hand

82.44 Other suture of flexor tendon of hand
EXCLUDES delayed suture of flexor tendon of hand (82.42)

82.45 Other suture of other tendon of hand
EXCLUDES delayed suture of other tendon of hand (82.43)

82.46 Suture of muscle or fascia of hand

✓4th 82.5 Transplantation of muscle and tendon of hand
AHA: 1Q, '93, 28

82.51 Advancement of tendon of hand
DEF: Detachment of fibrous connective muscle band and bone with reattachment at advanced point of hand.

82.52 Recession of tendon of hand
DEF: Detachment of fibrous band of muscle and bone with reattachment at drawn-back point of hand.

82.53 Reattachment of tendon of hand

82.54 Reattachment of muscle of hand

82.55 Other change in hand muscle or tendon length

82.56 Other hand tendon transfer or transplantation
EXCLUDES pollicization of thumb (82.61)
transfer of finger, except thumb (82.81)
AHA: 2Q, '99, 10; 4Q, '98, 40

82.57 Other hand tendon transposition
AHA: 1Q, '93, 28; 3Q, '93, 8

82.58 Other hand muscle transfer or transplantation

82.59 Other hand muscle transposition

✓4th 82.6 Reconstruction of thumb
INCLUDES digital transfer to act as thumb
Code also any amputation for digital transfer (84.01, 84.11)

82.61 Pollicization operation carrying over nerves and blood supply
DEF: Creation or reconstruction of a thumb with another digit, commonly the index finger.

82.69 Other reconstruction of thumb
"Cocked-hat" procedure [skin flap and bone]
Grafts:
  bone } to thumb
  skin (pedicle) }

✓4th 82.7 Plastic operation on hand with graft or implant

82.71 Tendon pulley reconstruction
Reconstruction for opponensplasty
DEF: Reconstruction of fibrous band between muscle and bone of hand.

82.72 Plastic operation on hand with graft of muscle or fascia

82.79 Plastic operation on hand with other graft or implant
Tendon graft to hand
AHA: J-F, '87, 6

OPERATIONS ON THE MUSCULOSKELETAL SYSTEM

82.8 Other plastic operations on hand
82.81 Transfer of finger, except thumb
EXCLUDES: pollicization of thumb (82.61)
82.82 Repair of cleft hand
DEF: Correction of fissure defect of hand.
82.83 Repair of macrodactyly
DEF: Reduction in size of abnormally large fingers.
82.84 Repair of mallet finger
DEF: Repair of flexed little finger.
82.85 Other tenodesis of hand
Tendon fixation of hand NOS
DEF: Fixation of fibrous connective band between muscle and bone of hand.
82.86 Other tenoplasty of hand
Myotenoplasty of hand
DEF: Myotenoplasty of hand: Plastic repair of muscle and fibrous band connecting muscle to bone.
82.89 Other plastic operations on hand
Plication of fascia
Repair of fascial hernia
EXCLUDES: that with graft or implant (82.71-82.79)

82.9 Other operations on muscle, tendon, and fascia of hand
EXCLUDES: diagnostic procedures on soft tissue of hand (83.21-83.29)
82.91 Lysis of adhesions of hand
Freeing of adhesions of fascia, muscle, and tendon of hand
EXCLUDES: decompression of carpal tunnel (04.43)
that by stretching or manipulation only (93.26)
82.92 Aspiration of bursa of hand
82.93 Aspiration of other soft tissue of hand
EXCLUDES: skin and subcutaneous tissue (86.01)
82.94 Injection of therapeutic substance into bursa of hand
82.95 Injection of therapeutic substance into tendon of hand
82.96 Other injection of locally-acting therapeutic substance into soft tissue of hand
EXCLUDES: subcutaneous or intramuscular injection (99.11-99.29)
82.99 Other operations on muscle, tendon, and fascia of hand

83 Operations on muscle, tendon, fascia, and bursa, except hand
INCLUDES: operations on:
aponeurosis
synovial membrane of bursa and tendon sheaths
tendon sheaths
EXCLUDES: diaphragm (34.81-34.89)
hand (82.01-82.99)
muscles of eye (15.01-15.9)

83.0 Incision of muscle, tendon, fascia, and bursa
83.01 Exploration of tendon sheath
Incision of tendon sheath
Removal of rice bodies from tendon sheath
DEF: Incision of external covering of fibrous cord for exam.
DEF: Removal of rice bodies from tendon sheath: Incision and removal of small bodies resembling grains of rice.
83.02 Myotomy
EXCLUDES: cricopharyngeal myotomy (29.31)
AHA: 2Q, '89, 18
83.03 Bursotomy
Removal of calcareous deposit of bursa
EXCLUDES: aspiration of bursa (percutaneous) (83.94)
83.09 Other incision of soft tissue
Incision of fascia
EXCLUDES: incision of skin and subcutaneous tissue alone (86.01-86.09)

83.1 Division of muscle, tendon, and fascia
83.11 Achillotenotomy
DEF: Incision into fibrous connective cord between adductor muscle and hip bone.
83.12 Adductor tenotomy of hip
DEF: Incision into fibrous attachment between adductor muscle and hip bone.
83.13 Other tenotomy
Aponeurotomy
Division of tendon
Tendon release
Tendon transection
Tenotomy for thoracic outlet decompression
DEF: Aponeurotomy: Incision and separation of fibrous cords attaching a muscle to bone to aid movement.
DEF: Division of tendon: Separation of fibrous band connecting muscle to bone.
DEF: Tendon release: Surgical detachment of fibrous band from muscle and/or bone.
DEF: Tendon transection: Incision across width of fibrous bands between muscle and bone.
DEF: Tenotomy for thoracic outlet decompression: Incision of fibrous muscle with separation from bone to relieve compressed thoracic outlet..
83.14 Fasciotomy
Division of fascia
Division of iliotibial band
Fascia stripping
Release of Volkmann's contracture by fasciotomy
AHA: 3Q, '98, 8
DEF: Division of fascia: Incision to separate fibrous connective tissue.
DEF: Division of iliotibial band: Incision to separate fibrous band connecting tibial bone to muscle in flank.
DEF: Fascia stripping: Incision and lengthwise separation of fibrous connective tissue.
DEF: Release of Volkmann's contracture by fasciotomy: Divisional incision of connective tissue to correct defect in flexion of finger(s).
83.19 Other division of soft tissue
Division of muscle
Muscle release
Myotomy for thoracic outlet decompression
Myotomy with division
Scalenotomy
Transection of muscle

83.2 Diagnostic procedures on muscle, tendon, fascia, and bursa, including that of hand
83.21 Biopsy of soft tissue
EXCLUDES: biopsy of chest wall (34.23)
biopsy of skin and subcutaneous tissue (86.11)

OPERATIONS ON THE MUSCULOSKELETAL SYSTEM

83.29 **Other diagnostic procedures on muscle, tendon, fascia, and bursa, including that of hand**
> **EXCLUDES** microscopic examination of specimen (91.51-91.-59)
> soft tissue x-ray (87.09, 87.38-87.39, 88.09, 88.35, 88.37)
> thermography of muscle (88.84)

✓4th 83.3 **Excision of lesion of muscle, tendon, fascia, and bursa**
> **EXCLUDES** biopsy of soft tissue (83.21)

83.31 **Excision of lesion of tendon sheath**
Excision of ganglion of tendon sheath, except of hand

83.32 **Excision of lesion of muscle**
Excision of:
heterotopic bone
muscle scar for release of Volkmann's contracture
myositis ossificans
DEF: Heterotopic bone: Bone lesion in muscle.
DEF: Muscle scar for release of Volkmann's contracture: Scarred muscle tissue interfering with finger flexion.
DEF: Myositis ossificans: Bony deposits in muscle.

83.39 **Excision of lesion of other soft tissue**
Excision of Baker's cyst
> **EXCLUDES** bursectomy (83.5)
> excision of lesion of skin and subcutaneous tissue (86.3)
> synovectomy (80.70-80.79)

AHA: 2Q, '97, 6

✓4th 83.4 **Other excision of muscle, tendon, and fascia**

83.41 **Excision of tendon for graft**

83.42 **Other tenonectomy**
Excision of:
aponeurosis
tendon sheath
Tenosynovectomy

83.43 **Excision of muscle or fascia for graft**

83.44 **Other fasciectomy**
DEF: Excision of fascia; other than for graft.

83.45 **Other myectomy**
Debridement of muscle NOS
Scalenectomy
AHA: 1Q, '99, 8
DEF: Scalenectomy: Removal of thoracic scaleni muscle tissue.

83.49 **Other excision of soft tissue**

83.5 **Bursectomy**
AHA: 2Q, '99, 11

✓4th 83.6 **Suture of muscle, tendon, and fascia**

83.61 **Suture of tendon sheath**

83.62 **Delayed suture of tendon**

83.63 **Rotator cuff repair**
AHA: 2Q, '93, 8
DEF: Repair of musculomembranous structure around shoulder joint capsule.

83.64 **Other suture of tendon**
Achillorrhaphy
Aponeurorrhaphy
> **EXCLUDES** delayed suture of tendon (83.62)

DEF: Achillorrhaphy: Suture of fibrous band connecting Achilles tendon to heel bone.

DEF: Aponeurorrhaphy: Suture of fibrous cords connecting muscle to bone.

83.65 **Other suture of muscle or fascia**
Repair of diastasis recti

✓4th 83.7 **Reconstruction of muscle and tendon**
> **EXCLUDES** reconstruction of muscle and tendon associated with arthroplasty

83.71 **Advancement of tendon**
DEF: Detaching fibrous cord between muscle and bone with reattachment at advanced point.

83.72 **Recession of tendon**
DEF: Detaching fibrous cord between muscle and bone with reattachment at drawn-back point.

83.73 **Reattachment of tendon**
83.74 **Reattachment of muscle**
83.75 **Tendon transfer or transplantation**
83.76 **Other tendon transposition**
83.77 **Muscle transfer or transplantation**
Release of Volkmann's contracture by muscle transplantation
83.79 **Other muscle transposition**

✓4th 83.8 **Other plastic operations on muscle, tendon, and fascia**
> **EXCLUDES** plastic operations on muscle, tendon, and fascia associated with arthroplasty

83.81 **Tendon graft**

83.82 **Graft of muscle or fascia**
AHA: ▶3Q, '01, 9◀

83.83 **Tendon pulley reconstruction**
DEF: Reconstruction of fibrous cord between muscle and bone; at any site other than hand.

83.84 **Release of clubfoot, not elsewhere classified**
Evans operation on clubfoot

83.85 **Other change in muscle or tendon length**
Hamstring lengthening
Heel cord shortening
Plastic achillotenotomy
Tendon plication
DEF: Plastic achillotenotomy: Increase in heel cord length.
DEF: Tendon plication: Surgical tuck of tendon.

83.86 **Quadricepsplasty**
DEF: Correction of quadriceps femoris muscle.

83.87 **Other plastic operations on muscle**
Musculoplasty   Myoplasty
AHA: 1Q, '97, 9

83.88 **Other plastic operations on tendon**
Myotenoplasty
Tendon fixation
Tenodesis
Tenoplasty

83.89 **Other plastic operations on fascia**
Fascia lengthening
Fascioplasty
Plication of fascia

✓4th 83.9 **Other operations on muscle, tendon, fascia, and bursa**
> **EXCLUDES** nonoperative:
> manipulation (93.25-93.29)
> stretching (93.27-93.29)

83.91 **Lysis of adhesions of muscle, tendon, fascia, and bursa**
> **EXCLUDES** that for tarsal tunnel syndrome (04.44)

DEF: Separation of created fibrous structures from muscle, connective tissues, bands and sacs.

OPERATIONS ON THE MUSCULOSKELETAL SYSTEM

83.92 Insertion or replacement of skeletal muscle stimulator
Implantation, insertion, placement, or replacement of skeletal muscle:
electrodes
stimulator
AHA: 2Q, '99, 10

83.93 Removal of skeletal muscle stimulator
83.94 Aspiration of bursa
83.95 Aspiration of other soft tissue
EXCLUDES that of skin and subcutaneous tissue (86.01)

83.96 Injection of therapeutic substance into bursa

83.97 Injection of therapeutic substance into tendon

83.98 Injection of locally-acting therapeutic substance into other soft tissue
EXCLUDES subcutaneous or intramuscular injection (99.11-99.29)

83.99 Other operations on muscle, tendon, fascia, and bursa
Suture of bursa

84 Other procedures on musculoskeletal system

84.0 Amputation of upper limb
EXCLUDES revision of amputation stump (84.3)

84.00 Upper limb amputation, not otherwise specified
Closed flap amputation
Kineplastic amputation
Open or guillotine amputation
Revision of current traumatic amputation
} of upper limb NOS

DEF: Closed flap amputation: Sewing a created skin flap over stump end of upper limb.

DEF: Kineplastic amputation: Amputation and preparation of stump of upper limb to permit movement.

DEF: Open or guillotine amputation: Straight incision across upper limb; used when primary closure is contraindicated.

DEF: Revision of current traumatic amputation: Reconstruction of traumatic amputation of upper limb to enable closure.

84.01 Amputation and disarticulation of finger
EXCLUDES ligation of supernumerary finger (86.26)

84.02 Amputation and disarticulation of thumb
84.03 Amputation through hand
Amputation through carpals
84.04 Disarticulation of wrist
84.05 Amputation through forearm
Forearm amputation
84.06 Disarticulation of elbow
DEF: Amputation of forearm through elbow joint.
84.07 Amputation through humerus
Upper arm amputation
84.08 Disarticulation of shoulder
DEF: Amputation of arm through shoulder joint.
84.09 Interthoracoscapular amputation
Forequarter amputation
DEF: Removal of upper arm, shoulder bone and collarbone.

84.1 Amputation of lower limb
EXCLUDES revision of amputation stump (84.3)

84.10 Lower limb amputation, not otherwise specified
Closed flap amputation
Kineplastic amputation
Open or guillotine amputation
Revision of current traumatic amputation
} of lower limb NOS

DEF: Closed flap amputation: Sewing a created skin flap over stump of lower limb.

DEF: Kineplastic amputation: Amputation and preparation of stump of lower limb to permit movement.

DEF: Open or guillotine amputation: Straight incision across lower limb; used when primary closure is contraindicated.

DEF: Revision of current traumatic amputation: Reconstruction of traumatic amputation of lower limb to enable closure.

84.11 Amputation of toe
Amputation through metatarsophalangeal joint
Disarticulation of toe
Metatarsal head amputation
Ray amputation of foot (disarticulation of the metatarsal head of the toe extending across the forefoot, just proximal to the metatarsophalangeal crease)
EXCLUDES ligation of supernumerary toe (86.26)
AHA: 4Q, '99, 19

84.12 Amputation through foot
Amputation of forefoot
Amputation through middle of foot
Chopart's amputation
Midtarsal amputation
Transmetatarsal amputation (amputation of the forefoot, including the toes)
EXCLUDES Ray amputation of foot (84.11)
AHA: 4Q, '99, 19

DEF: Amputation of forefoot: Removal of foot in front of joint between toes and body of foot.

DEF: Chopart's amputation: Removal of foot with retention of heel, ankle and other associated ankle bones.

DEF: Midtarsal amputation: Amputation of foot through tarsals.

DEF: Transmetatarsal amputation: Amputation of foot through metatarsals.

84.13 Disarticulation of ankle
DEF: Removal of foot through ankle bone.

84.14 Amputation of ankle through malleoli of tibia and fibula

84.15 Other amputation below knee
Amputation of leg through tibia and fibula NOS

84.16 Disarticulation of knee
Batch, Spitler, and McFaddin amputation
Mazet amputation
S.P. Roger's amputation
DEF: Removal of lower leg through knee joint.

84.17–84.99 OPERATIONS ON THE MUSCULOSKELETAL SYSTEM

84.17 **Amputation above knee**
Amputation of leg through femur
Amputation of thigh
Conversion of below-knee amputation into above-knee amputation
Supracondylar above-knee amputation

84.18 **Disarticulation of hip**
DEF: Removal of leg through hip joint.

84.19 **Abdominopelvic amputation**
Hemipelvectomy
Hindquarter amputation
DEF: Removal of leg and portion of pelvic bone.
DEF: Hemipelvectomy: Removal of leg and lateral pelvis.

✓4th **84.2** **Reattachment of extremity**
AHA: 1Q, '95, 8

84.21 **Thumb reattachment**
84.22 **Finger reattachment**
84.23 **Forearm, wrist, or hand reattachment**
84.24 **Upper arm reattachment**
Reattachment of arm NOS
84.25 **Toe reattachment**
84.26 **Foot reattachment**
84.27 **Lower leg or ankle reattachment**
Reattachment of leg NOS
84.28 **Thigh reattachment**
84.29 **Other reattachment**

84.3 **Revision of amputation stump**
Reamputation ⎫
Secondary closure ⎬ of stump
Trimming ⎭

EXCLUDES revision of current traumatic amputation [revision by further amputation of current injury] (84.00-84.19, 84.91)

AHA: 4Q, '99, 15; 2Q, '98, 15; 4Q, '88, 12

✓4th **84.4** **Implantation or fitting of prosthetic limb device**

84.40 **Implantation or fitting of prosthetic limb device, not otherwise specified**
84.41 **Fitting of prosthesis of upper arm and shoulder**
84.42 **Fitting of prosthesis of lower arm and hand**
84.43 **Fitting of prosthesis of arm, not otherwise specified**
84.44 **Implantation of prosthetic device of arm**
84.45 **Fitting of prosthesis above knee**
84.46 **Fitting of prosthesis below knee**
84.47 **Fitting of prosthesis of leg, not otherwise specified**
84.48 **Implantation of prosthetic device of leg**

✓4th **84.5** **Implantation of other musculoskeletal devices and substances**

● **84.51** **Insertion of interbody spinal fusion device**
Insertion of:
cages (carbon, ceramic, metal, plastic or titanium)
interbody fusion cage
synthetic cages or spacers
threaded bone dowels
Code also refusion of spine (81.30-81.39)
Code also spinal fusion (81.00-81.08)

● **84.52** **Insertion of recombinant bone morphogenetic protein rhBMP**
That via collagen sponge, coral, ceramic and other carriers
Code also primary procedure performed:
fracture repair (79.00-79.99)
spinal fusion (81.00-81.08)
spinal refusion (81.30-81.39)

✓4th **84.9** **Other operations on musculoskeletal system**
EXCLUDES nonoperative manipulation (93.25-93.29)

84.91 **Amputation, not otherwise specified**
84.92 **Separation of equal conjoined twins**
84.93 **Separation of unequal conjoined twins**
Separation of conjoined twins NOS
84.99 **Other**

15. OPERATIONS ON THE INTEGUMENTARY SYSTEM (85-86)

85 Operations on the breast

INCLUDES: operations on the skin and subcutaneous tissue of:
- breast } female or
- previous mastectomy site } male
- revision of previous mastectomy site

85.0 Mastotomys
Incision of breast (skin)
Mammotomy
EXCLUDES: aspiration of breast (85.91)
removal of implant (85.94)
AHA: 2Q, '90, 27

AHA: 2Q, '90, 27

85.1 Diagnostic procedures on breast

85.11 Closed [percutaneous] [needle] biopsy of breast
AHA: 2Q, '00, 10; 3Q, '89, 17

DEF: Mammatome biopsy: Excision of breast tissue using a needle inserted through a small incision; followed by a full cut circle of tissue surrounding the core biopsy to obtain; multiple contiguous directional sampling for definitive diagnosis and staging of cancer

85.12 Open biopsy of breast
AHA: 3Q, '89, 17; M-A, '86, 11

DEF: Excision of breast tissue for examination.

85.19 Other diagnostic procedures on breast
EXCLUDES:
- mammary ductogram (87.35)
- mammography NEC (87.37)
- manual examination (89.36)
- microscopic examination of specimen (91.61-91.69)
- thermography (88.85)
- ultrasonography (88.73)
- xerography (87.36)

85.2 Excision or destruction of breast tissue
EXCLUDES:
- mastectomy (85.41-85.48)
- reduction mammoplasty (85.31-85.32)

85.20 Excision or destruction of breast tissue, not otherwise specified

85.21 Local excision of lesion of breast
Lumpectomy
Removal of area of fibrosis from breast
EXCLUDES: biopsy of breast (85.11-85.12)
AHA: 2Q, '90, 27; 3Q, '89, 17; M-A, '86, 11

85.22 Resection of quadrant of breast

85.23 Subtotal mastectomy
EXCLUDES: quadrant resection (85.22)
AHA: 2Q, '92, 7

DEF: Excision of a large portion of breast tissue.

85.24 Excision of ectopic breast tissue
Excision of accessory nipple
DEF: Excision of breast tissue outside normal breast region.

85.25 Excision of nipple
EXCLUDES: excision of accessory nipple (85.24)

85.3 Reduction mammoplasty and subcutaneous mammectomy
AHA: 4Q, '95, 79, 80

85.31 Unilateral reduction mammoplasty
Unilateral:
- amputative mammoplasty
- size reduction mammoplasty

85.32 Bilateral reduction mammoplasty
Amputative mammoplasty
Reduction mammoplasty (for gynecomastia)

85.33 Unilateral subcutaneous mammectomy with synchronous implant
EXCLUDES: that without synchronous implant (85.34)
DEF: Removal of mammary tissue, leaving skin and nipple intact with implant of prosthesis.

85.34 Other unilateral subcutaneous mammectomy
Removal of breast tissue with preservation of skin and nipple
Subcutaneous mammectomy NOS
DEF: Excision of mammary tissue, leaving skin and nipple intact.

85.35 Bilateral subcutaneous mammectomy with synchronous implant
EXCLUDES: that without synchronous implant (85.36)
DEF: Excision of mammary tissue, both breasts, leaving skin and nipples intact; with prosthesis.

85.36 Other bilateral subcutaneous mammectomy

85.4 Mastectomy

85.41 Unilateral simple mastectomy
Mastectomy: NOS
Mastectomy: complete
DEF: Removal of one breast.

85.42 Bilateral simple mastectomy
Bilateral complete mastectomy
DEF: Removal of both breasts.

85.43 Unilateral extended simple mastectomy
Extended simple mastectomy NOS
Modified radical mastectomy
Simple mastectomy with excision of regional lymph nodes
AHA: 2Q, '92, 7; 3Q, '91, 24; 2Q, '91, 21

DEF: Removal of one breast and lymph nodes under arm.

85.44 Bilateral extended simple mastectomy
AHA: 2Q, '92, 7; 3Q, '91, 24; 2Q, '91, 21

85.45 Unilateral radical mastectomy
Excision of breast, pectoral muscles, and regional lymph nodes [axillary, clavicular, supraclavicular]
Radical mastectomy NOS
AHA: 2Q, '91, 21

DEF: Removal of one breast and regional lymph nodes, pectoral muscle and adjacent tissue.

Mastectomy

Partial mastectomy (lumpectomy): skin left intact

Simple mastectomy

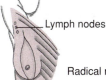

Lymph nodes

Radical mastectomy

85.46–86.05 OPERATIONS ON THE INTEGUMENTARY SYSTEM

85.46 Bilateral radical mastectomy
AHA: 2Q, '91, 21

85.47 Unilateral extended radical mastectomy
Excision of breast, muscles, and lymph nodes [axillary, clavicular, supraclavicular, internal mammary, and mediastinal]
Extended radical mastectomy NOS
DEF: Removal of one breast, regional and middle chest lymph nodes, chest muscle and adjacent tissue.

85.48 Bilateral extended radical mastectomy
DEF: Removal of both breasts, regional and middle chest lymph nodes, chest muscle and adjacent tissue.

√4th **85.5** Augmentation mammoplasty
EXCLUDES that associated with subcutaneous mammectomy (85.33, 85.35)
AHA: 3Q, '97, 12; 4Q, '95, 76, 80
DEF: Plastic surgery to increase breast size.

85.50 Augmentation mammoplasty, not otherwise specified

85.51 Unilateral injection into breast for augmentation

85.52 Bilateral injection into breast for augmentation
Injection into breast for augmentation NOS

85.53 Unilateral breast implant
AHA: 2Q, '00 18; 2Q, '98, 14

85.54 Bilateral breast implant
Breast implant NOS

85.6 Mastopexy
DEF: Anchoring of pendulous breast.

85.7 Total reconstruction of breast
AHA: 4Q, '95, 77; 1Q, '93, 27

√4th **85.8** Other repair and plastic operations on breast
EXCLUDES that for:
augmentation (85.50-85.54)
reconstruction (85.7)
reduction (85.31-85.32)
AHA: 4Q, '95, 77

85.81 Suture of laceration of breast
85.82 Split-thickness graft to breast
85.83 Full-thickness graft to breast
AHA: 4Q, '95, 77

85.84 Pedicle graft to breast
AHA: 4Q, '95, 77
DEF: Implantation of transferred muscle tissue still connected to vascular source.

85.85 Muscle flap graft to breast
AHA: 4Q, '95, 77
DEF: Relocation of nipple.

85.86 Transposition of nipple
AHA: 4Q, '95, 78

85.87 Other repair or reconstruction of nipple
AHA: 4Q, '95, 78

85.89 Other mammoplasty

√4th **85.9** Other operations on the breast
85.91 Aspiration of breast
EXCLUDES percutaneous biopsy of breast (85.11)

85.92 Injection of therapeutic agent into breast
EXCLUDES that for augmentation of breast (85.51-85.52)

85.93 Revision of implant of breast
AHA: 2Q, '98, 14; 4Q, '95, 76

85.94 Removal of implant of breast
AHA: 2Q, '98, 14; 3Q, '92, 4

85.95 Insertion of breast tissue expander
Insertion (soft tissue) of tissue expander (one or more) under muscle or platysma to develop skin flaps for donor use

85.96 Removal of breast tissue expander(s)
AHA: 2Q, '00, 18; 4Q, '95, 77

85.99 Other

√3rd **86** Operations on skin and subcutaneous tissue
INCLUDES operations on:
hair follicles
male perineum
nails
sebaceous glands
operations on:
subcutaneous fat pads
sudoriferous glands
superficial fossae

EXCLUDES those on skin of:
anus (49.01-49.99)
breast (mastectomy site) (85.0-85.99)
ear (18.01-18.9)
eyebrow (08.01-08.99)
eyelid (08.01-08.99)
female perineum (71.01-71.9)
lips (27.0-27.99)
nose (21.00-21.99)
penis (64.0-64.99)
scrotum (61.0-61.99)
vulva (71.01-71.9)

√4th **86.0** Incision of skin and subcutaneous tissue

86.01 Aspiration of skin and subcutaneous tissue
Aspiration of:
abscess
hematoma
seroma
} of nail, skin, or subcutaneous tissue
AHA: 3Q, '89, 16

86.02 Injection or tattooing of skin lesion or defect
Insertion
Injection
} of filling material
Pigmenting of skin
DEF: Pigmenting of skin: Adding color to skin.

86.03 Incision of pilonidal sinus or cyst
EXCLUDES marsupialization (86.21)

86.04 Other incision with drainage of skin and subcutaneous tissue
EXCLUDES drainage of:
fascial compartments of face and mouth (27.0)
palmar or thenar space (82.04)
pilonidal sinus or cyst (86.03)

86.05 Incision with removal of foreign body from skin and subcutaneous tissue
Removal of loop recorder
Removal of tissue expander(s) from skin or soft tissue other than breast tissue
EXCLUDES removal of foreign body without incision (98.20-98.29)
AHA: 2Q, '96, 15; N-D, '87, 10; N-D, '86, 9

OPERATIONS ON THE INTEGUMENTARY SYSTEM

86.06 **Insertion of totally implantable infusion pump**
Code also any associated catheterization
EXCLUDES   *insertion of totally implantable vascular access device (86.07)*

AHA: 2Q, '99, 4; 4Q, '90, 14

86.07 **Insertion of totally implantable vascular access device [VAD]**
Totally implanted port
EXCLUDES   *insertion of totally implantable infusion pump (86.06)*

AHA: 1Q, '01, 13; 1Q, '96, 3; 2Q, '94, 11; 3Q, '91, 13; 4Q, '90, 15

DEF: Placement of vascular access infusion catheter system under skin to allow for frequent manual infusions into blood vessel.

86.09 **Other incision of skin and subcutaneous tissue**
Creation of loop recorder pocket, new site, and insertion/relocation of device
Creation of pocket for implantable, patient-activated cardiac event recorder and insertion/relocation of device
Creation of thalamic stimulator pulse generator pocket, new site
Escharotomy
Exploration:
  sinus tract, skin
  superficial fossa
Undercutting of hair follicle
EXCLUDES   *that of:*
  cardiac pacemaker pocket, new site (37.79)
  fascial compartments of face and mouth (27.0)

AHA: 4Q, '00, 68; 4Q, '99, 21; 4Q, '97, 57; 3Q, '89, 17; N-D, '86, 1; N-D, '84, 6

✓4th **86.1** **Diagnostic procedures on skin and subcutaneous tissue**

  86.11 **Biopsy of skin and subcutaneous tissue**

  86.19 **Other diagnostic procedures on skin and subcutaneous tissue**
EXCLUDES   *microscopic examination of specimen from skin and subcutaneous tissue (91.61-91.79)*

✓4th **86.2** **Excision or destruction of lesion or tissue of skin and subcutaneous tissue**

  86.21 **Excision of pilonidal cyst or sinus**
Marsupialization of cyst
EXCLUDES   *incision of pilonidal cyst or sinus (86.03)*

DEF: Marsupialization of cyst: Incision of cyst and suturing edges to skin to open site.

86.22 **Excisional debridement of wound, infection, or burn**
Removal by excision of:
  devitalized tissue
  necrosis
  slough
EXCLUDES   *debridement of:*
  abdominal wall (wound) (54.3)
  bone (77.60-77.69)
  muscle (83.45)
    of hand (82.36)
  nail (bed) (fold) (86.27)
  nonexcisional debridement of wound, infection, or burn (86.28)
  open fracture site (79.60-79.69)
  pedicle or flap graft (86.75)

AHA: 2Q, '00, 9; 1Q, '99, 8; 2Q, '92, 17; 3Q, '91, 18; 3Q, '89, 16; 4Q, '88, 5; N-D, '86, 1

86.23 **Removal of nail, nailbed, or nail fold**

86.24 **Chemosurgery of skin**
Chemical peel of skin

DEF: Chemicals applied to destroy skin tissue.

DEF: Chemical peel of skin: Chemicals used to peel skin layers.

86.25 **Dermabrasion**
That with laser
EXCLUDES   *dermabrasion of wound to remove embedded debris (86.28)*

DEF: Removal of wrinkled or scarred skin; with fine sandpaper, wire, brushes or laser.

86.26 **Ligation of dermal appendage**
EXCLUDES   *excision of preauricular appendage (18.29)*

DEF: Tying off extra skin.

86.27 **Debridement of nail, nail bed, or nail fold**
Removal of:
  necrosis
  slough
EXCLUDES   *removal of nail, nail bed, or nail fold (86.23)*

86.28 **Nonexcisional debridement of wound, infection, or burn**
Debridement NOS
▶Maggot therapy◀
Removal of devitalized tissue, necrosis, and slough by such methods as:
  brushing
  irrigation (under pressure)
  scrubbing
  washing

AHA: 2Q, '01, 18; 3Q, '91, 18; 4Q, '88, 5

DEF: Removal of damaged skin; by methods other than excision.

86.3 **Other local excision or destruction of lesion or tissue of skin and subcutaneous tissue**
Destruction of skin by: Destruction of skin by:
  cauterization   fulguration
  cryosurgery   laser beam
That with Z-plasty
EXCLUDES   *adipectomy (86.83)*
  biopsy of skin (86.11)
  wide or radical excision of skin (86.4)
  Z-plasty without excision (86.84)

AHA: 1Q, '96, 15; 2Q, '90, 27; 1Q, '89, 12; 3Q, '89, 18; 4Q, '88, 7

86.4–86.82 OPERATIONS ON THE INTEGUMENTARY SYSTEM

86.4 **Radical excision of skin lesion**
Wide excision of skin lesion involving underlying or adjacent structure
Code also any lymph node dissection (40.3-40.5)

√4th **86.5** **Suture or other closure of skin and subcutaneous tissue**

86.51 **Replantation of scalp**

86.59 **Closure of skin and subcutaneous tissue of other sites**
Adhesives (surgical) (tissue)
Staples
Sutures
EXCLUDES: application of adhesive strips (butterfly) — omit code
AHA: 4Q, '99, 23

√4th **86.6** **Free skin graft**
INCLUDES: excision of skin for autogenous graft
EXCLUDES: construction or reconstruction of:
penis (64.43-64.44)
trachea (31.75)
vagina (70.61-70.62)
DEF: Transplantation of skin to another site.

86.60 **Free skin graft, not otherwise specified**

86.61 **Full-thickness skin graft to hand**
EXCLUDES: heterograft (86.65)
homograft (86.66)

86.62 **Other skin graft to hand**
EXCLUDES: heterograft (86.65)
homograft (86.66)

86.63 **Full-thickness skin graft to other sites**
EXCLUDES: heterograft (86.65)
homograft (86.66)

86.64 **Hair transplant**
EXCLUDES: hair follicle transplant to eyebrow or eyelash (08.63)

86.65 **Heterograft to skin**
Pigskin graft   Porcine graft
EXCLUDES: ▶application of dressing only (93.57)◀
DEF: Implantation of nonhuman tissue.

86.66 **Homograft to skin**
Graft to skin of:
amnionic membrane } from donor
skin
DEF: Implantation of tissue from human donor.

86.67 **Dermal regenerative graft**
Artificial skin, NOS
Creation of "neodermis"
Decellularized allodermis
Integumentary matrix implants
Prosthetic implant of dermal layer of skin
Regenerate dermal layer of skin
EXCLUDES: heterograft to skin (86.65)
homograft to skin (86.66)
AHA: 4Q, '98, 76, 79
DEF: Replacement of dermis and epidermal layer of skin by cultured or regenerated autologous tissue; used to treat full-thickness or deep partial-thickness burns; also called cultured epidermal autograft (CEA).

86.69 **Other skin graft to other sites**
EXCLUDES: heterograft (86.65)
homograft (86.66)
AHA: 4Q, '99, 15

√4th **86.7** **Pedicle grafts or flaps**
EXCLUDES: construction or reconstruction of:
penis (64.43-64.44)
trachea (31.75)
vagina (70.61-70.62)
DEF: Full thickness skin and subcutaneous tissue partially attached to the body by a narrow strip of tissue so that it retains its blood supply. The unattached portion is sutured to the defect.

86.70 **Pedicle or flap graft, not otherwise specified**

86.71 **Cutting and preparation of pedicle grafts or flaps**
Elevation of pedicle from its bed
Flap design and raising
Partial cutting of pedicle or tube
Pedicle delay
EXCLUDES: pollicization or digital transfer (82.61, 82.81)
revision of pedicle (86.75)
AHA: ▶4Q, '01, 66◀
DEF: Elevation and preparation of tissue still attached to vascular bed; delayed implant.
DEF: Elevation of pedicle from its bed: Separation of tissue implanted from its bed.
DEF: Flap design and raising: Planing and elevation of tissue to be implanted.

86.72 **Advancement of pedicle graft**
AHA: 3Q, '99, 9, 10

86.73 **Attachment of pedicle or flap graft to hand**
EXCLUDES: pollicization or digital transfer (82.61, 82.81)

86.74 **Attachment of pedicle or flap graft to other sites**
Attachment by   Attachment by
advanced flap   rotating flap
double pedicled flap   sliding flap
pedicle graft   tube graft
AHA: 3Q, '99, 9; 1Q, '96, 15
DEF: Fixation of tissue implant still connected to original site, other than hand.
DEF: Attachment by:
Advanced flap: Sliding tissue implant into new position.
Double pedicle flap: Implant connected to two vascular beds.
Pedicle graft: Implant connected to vascular bed.
Rotating flap: Implant rotated along curved incision.
Sliding flap: Sliding implant to site.
Tube graft: Double tissue implant to form tube with base connected to original site.

86.75 **Revision of pedicle or flap graft**
Debridement } of pedicle or flap
Defatting   }   graft
DEF: Connection of implant still attached to its vascular tissue.

√4th **86.8** **Other repair and reconstruction of skin and subcutaneous tissue**
DEF: Revision and tightening of excess, wrinkled facial skin.

86.81 **Repair for facial weakness**

86.82 **Facial rhytidectomy**
Face lift
EXCLUDES: rhytidectomy of eyelid (08.86-08.87)

86.83 **Size reduction plastic operation**
    Liposuction
    Reduction of adipose tissue of:
        abdominal wall (pendulous)
        arms (batwing)
        buttock
        thighs (trochanteric lipomatosis)
    EXCLUDES breast (85.31-85.32)
    DEF: Excision and plastic repair of excess skin and underlying tissue.

86.84 **Relaxation of scar or web contracture of skin**
    Z-plasty of skin
    EXCLUDES Z-plasty with excision of lesion (86.3)

86.85 **Correction of syndactyly**
    DEF: Plastic repair of webbed fingers or toes.

86.86 **Onychoplasty**
    DEF: Plastic repair of nail or nail bed.

86.89 **Other repair and reconstruction of skin and subcutaneous tissue**
    EXCLUDES mentoplasty (76.67-76.68)
    AHA: 1Q, '00, 26; 2Q, '98, 20; 2Q, '93, 11; 2Q, '92, 17

✓4th **86.9** **Other operations on skin and subcutaneous tissue**

86.91 **Excision of skin for graft**
    Excision of skin with closure of donor site
    EXCLUDES that with graft at same operative episode (86.60-86.69)

86.92 **Electrolysis and other epilation of skin**
    EXCLUDES epilation of eyelid (08.91-08.93)

86.93 **Insertion of tissue expander**
    Insertion (subcutaneous) (soft tissue) of expander (one or more) in scalp (subgaleal space), face, neck, trunk except breast, and upper and lower extremities for development of skin flaps for donor use
    EXCLUDES flap graft preparation (86.71)
        tissue expander, breast (85.95)

86.99 **Other**
    EXCLUDES removal of sutures from:
        abdomen (97.83)
        head and neck (97.38)
        thorax (97.43)
        trunk NEC (97.84)
        wound catheter:
            irrigation (96.58)
            replacement (97.15)

AHA: 4Q, '97, 57; N-D, '86, 1

16. MISCELLANEOUS DIAGNOSTIC AND THERAPEUTIC PROCEDURES (87-99)

✓3rd 87 Diagnostic radiology

✓4th 87.0 Soft tissue x-ray of face, head, and neck
EXCLUDES: angiography (88.40-88.68)

87.01 Pneumoencephalogram
DEF: Radiographic exam of cerebral ventricles and subarachnoid spaces; with injection of air or gas for contrast.

87.02 Other contrast radiogram of brain and skull
Pneumocisternogram
Pneumoventriculogram
Posterior fossa myelogram

DEF: Pneumocisternogram: Radiographic exam of subarachnoid spaces after injection of gas for contrast.

DEF: Pneumoventriculography: Radiographic exam of cerebral ventricles after injection of gas for contrast.

DEF: Posterior fossa myelogram: Radiographic exam of posterior channel of spinal cord after injection of gas or contrast.

87.03 Computerized axial tomography of head
C.A.T. scan of head
AHA: 3Q, '99, 7

87.04 Other tomography of head

87.05 Contrast dacryocystogram
DEF: Radiographic exam of tear sac after injection of contrast.

87.06 Contrast radiogram of nasopharynx

87.07 Contrast laryngogram

87.08 Cervical lymphangiogram
DEF: Radiographic exam of lymph vessels of neck; with or without contrast.

87.09 Other soft tissue x-ray of face, head, and neck
Noncontrast x-ray of: adenoid, larynx, nasolacrimal duct, nasopharynx
Noncontrast x-ray of: salivary gland, thyroid region, uvula
EXCLUDES: x-ray study of eye (95.14)

✓4th 87.1 Other x-ray of face, head, and neck
EXCLUDES: angiography (88.40-88.68)

87.11 Full-mouth x-ray of teeth

87.12 Other dental x-ray
Orthodontic cephalogram or cephalometrics
Panorex examination of mandible
Root canal x-ray

87.13 Temporomandibular contrast arthrogram

87.14 Contrast radiogram of orbit

87.15 Contrast radiogram of sinus

87.16 Other x-ray of facial bones
X-ray of: frontal area, mandible, maxilla, nasal sinuses, nose
X-ray of: orbit, supraorbital area, symphysis menti, zygomaticomaxillary complex

87.17 Other x-ray of skull
Lateral projection
Sagittal projection } of skull
Tangential projection

DEF: Lateral projection: Side to side view of head.

DEF: Sagittal projection: View of body in plane running midline from front to back.

DEF: Tangential projection: Views from adjacent skull surfaces.

✓4th 87.2 X-ray of spine

87.21 Contrast myelogram
DEF: Radiographic exam of space between middle and outer spinal cord coverings after injection of contrast.

87.22 Other x-ray of cervical spine

87.23 Other x-ray of thoracic spine

87.24 Other x-ray of lumbosacral spine
Sacrococcygeal x-ray

87.29 Other x-ray of spine
Spinal x-ray NOS

✓4th 87.3 Soft tissue x-ray of thorax
EXCLUDES: angiocardiography (88.50-88.58)
angiography (88.40-88.68)

87.31 Endotracheal bronchogram
DEF: Radiographic exam of lung, main branch, with contrast introduced through windpipe.

87.32 Other contrast bronchogram
Transcricoid bronchogram
DEF: Triscrichoid bronchogram: Radiographic exam of lung, main branch, with contrast introduced through cartilage of neck.

87.33 Mediastinal pneumogram
DEF: Radiographic exam of cavity containing heart, esophagus and adjacent structures.

87.34 Intrathoracic lymphangiogram
DEF: Radiographic exam of lymphatic vessels within chest; with or without contrast.

87.35 Contrast radiogram of mammary ducts
DEF: Radiographic exam of mammary ducts; with contrast.

87.36 Xerography of breast
DEF: Radiographic exam of breast via selenium-coated plates.

87.37 Other mammography
AHA: 3Q, '89, 17; 2Q, '90, 28; N-D, '87, 1

87.38 Sinogram of chest wall
Fistulogram of chest wall
DEF: Radiographic exam of chest cavity.
DEF: Fistulogram of chest wall: Radiographic exam of abnormal opening in chest.

87.39 Other soft tissue x-ray of chest wall

✓4th 87.4 Other x-ray of thorax
EXCLUDES: angiocardiography (88.50-88.58)
angiography (88.40-88.68)

87.41 Computerized axial tomography of thorax
C.A.T. scan
Crystal linea scan of x-ray beam
Electronic subtraction } of thorax
Photoelectric response
Tomography with use of computer, x-rays, and camera

Tabular List — DIAGNOSTIC AND THERAPEUTIC PROCEDURES — 87.42–88.15

- **87.42** Other tomography of thorax
  Cardiac tomogram
  DEF: Radiographic exam of chest plane.
- **87.43** X-ray of ribs, sternum, and clavicle
  Examination for:
  cervical rib
  fracture
- **87.44** Routine chest x-ray, so described
  X-ray of chest NOS
- **87.49** Other chest x-ray
  X-ray of:
  bronchus NOS
  diaphragm NOS
  heart NOS
  X-ray of:
  lung NOS
  mediastinum NOS
  trachea NOS

√4th **87.5** Biliary tract x-ray
- **87.51** Percutaneous hepatic cholangiogram
  AHA: 2Q, '90, 28; N-D, '87, 1
  DEF: Radiographic exam of bile tract of gallbladder; with needle injection of contrast into bile duct of liver.
- **87.52** Intravenous cholangiogram
  DEF: Radiographic exam of bile ducts; with intravenous contrast injection.
- **87.53** Intraoperative cholangiogram
  AHA: 1Q, '96, 12; 2Q, '90, 28; 3Q, '89, 18; 4Q, '88, 7
  DEF: Radiographic exam of bile ducts; with contrast; following gallbladder removal.
- **87.54** Other cholangiogram
- **87.59** Other biliary tract x-ray
  Cholecystogram

√4th **87.6** Other x-ray of digestive system
- **87.61** Barium swallow
- **87.62** Upper GI series
- **87.63** Small bowel series
- **87.64** Lower GI series
- **87.65** Other x-ray of intestine
- **87.66** Contrast pancreatogram
- **87.69** Other digestive tract x-ray

√4th **87.7** X-ray of urinary system
  EXCLUDES angiography of renal vessels (88.45, 88.65)
- **87.71** Computerized axial tomography of kidney
  C.A.T. scan of kidney
- **87.72** Other nephrotomogram
  DEF: Radiographic exam of kidney plane.

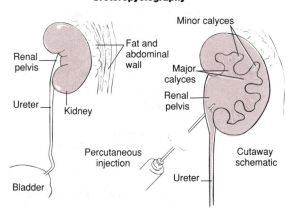

Ureteropyelography

- **87.73** Intravenous pyelogram
  Diuretic infusion pyelogram
  DEF: Radiographic exam of lower kidney, with intravenous contrast injection.
  DEF: Diuretic infusion pyelogram: Radiographic exam of lower kidney with diuretic contrast.
- **87.74** Retrograde pyelogram
- **87.75** Percutaneous pyelogram
- **87.76** Retrograde cystourethrogram
  DEF: Radiographic exam of bladder and urethra with contrast injected through catheter into bladder.
- **87.77** Other cystogram
- **87.78** Ileal conduitogram
  AHA: M-J, '87, 11
  DEF: Radiographic exam of passage created between ureter and artificial opening into abdomen.
- **87.79** Other x-ray of the urinary system
  KUB x-ray

√4th **87.8** X-ray of female genital organs
- **87.81** X-ray of gravid uterus ♀
  Intrauterine cephalometry by x-ray
- **87.82** Gas contrast hysterosalpingogram ♀
  DEF: Radiographic exam of uterus and fallopian tubes; with gas contrast.
- **87.83** Opaque dye contrast hysterosalpingogram ♀
- **87.84** Percutaneous hysterogram ♀
  DEF: Radiographic exam of uterus with contrast injected through body wall.
- **87.85** Other x-ray of fallopian tubes and uterus ♀
- **87.89** Other x-ray of female genital organs ♀

√4th **87.9** X-ray of male genital organs
- **87.91** Contrast seminal vesiculogram ♂
- **87.92** Other x-ray of prostate and seminal vesicles ♂
- **87.93** Contrast epididymogram ♂
- **87.94** Contrast vasogram ♂
- **87.95** Other x-ray of epididymis and vas deferens ♂
- **87.99** Other x-ray of male genital organs ♂

√3rd **88** Other diagnostic radiology and related techniques

√4th **88.0** Soft tissue x-ray of abdomen
  EXCLUDES angiography (88.40-88.68)
- **88.01** Computerized axial tomography of abdomen
  C.A.T. scan of abdomen
  EXCLUDES C.A.T. scan of kidney (87.71)
  AHA: 2Q, '98, 13
- **88.02** Other abdomen tomography
  EXCLUDES nephrotomogram (87.72)
- **88.03** Sinogram of abdominal wall
  Fistulogram of abdominal wall
  DEF: Radiographic exam of abnormal abdominal passage.
- **88.04** Abdominal lymphangiogram
  DEF: Radiographic exam of abdominal lymphatic vessels; with contrast.
- **88.09** Other soft tissue x-ray of abdominal wall

√4th **88.1** Other x-ray of abdomen
- **88.11** Pelvic opaque dye contrast radiography
- **88.12** Pelvic gas contrast radiography
  Pelvic pneumoperitoneum
- **88.13** Other peritoneal pneumogram
- **88.14** Retroperitoneal fistulogram
- **88.15** Retroperitoneal pneumogram

88.16 Other retroperitoneal x-ray
88.19 Other x-ray of abdomen
Flat plate of abdomen
AHA: 3Q, '99, 9

√4th 88.2 Skeletal x-ray of extremities and pelvis
EXCLUDES contrast radiogram of joint (88.32)

88.21 Skeletal x-ray of shoulder and upper arm
88.22 Skeletal x-ray of elbow and forearm
88.23 Skeletal x-ray of wrist and hand
88.24 Skeletal x-ray of upper limb, not otherwise specified
88.25 Pelvimetry
DEF: Imaging of pelvic bones to measure pelvic capacity.
88.26 Other skeletal x-ray of pelvis and hip
88.27 Skeletal x-ray of thigh, knee, and lower leg
88.28 Skeletal x-ray of ankle and foot
88.29 Skeletal x-ray of lower limb, not otherwise specified

√4th 88.3 Other x-ray
88.31 Skeletal series
X-ray of whole skeleton
88.32 Contrast arthrogram
EXCLUDES that of temporomandibular joint (87.13)
88.33 Other skeletal x-ray
EXCLUDES skeletal x-ray of:
extremities and pelvis (88.21-88.29)
face, head, and neck (87.11-87.17)
spine (87.21-87.29)
thorax (87.43)
88.34 Lymphangiogram of upper limb
88.35 Other soft tissue x-ray of upper limb
88.36 Lymphangiogram of lower limb
88.37 Other soft tissue x-ray of lower limb
EXCLUDES femoral angiography (88.48, 88.66)
88.38 Other computerized axial tomography
C.A.T. scan NOS
EXCLUDES C.A.T. scan of:
abdomen (88.01)
head (87.03)
kidney (87.71)
thorax (87.41)
88.39 X-ray, other and unspecified

√4th 88.4 Arteriography using contrast material
INCLUDES angiography of arteries
arterial puncture for injection of contrast material
radiography of arteries (by fluoroscopy)
retrograde arteriography
Note: The fourth-digit subclassification identifies the site to be viewed, not the site of injection.
EXCLUDES arteriography using:
radioisotopes or radionuclides (92.01-92.19)
ultrasound (88.71-88.79)
fluorescein angiography of eye (95.12)
AHA: N-D, '85, 14
DEF: Electromagnetic wave photography of arteries; with contrast.

88.40 Arteriography using contrast material, unspecified site

88.41 Arteriography of cerebral arteries
Angiography of:
basilar artery
carotid (internal)
posterior cerebral circulation
vertebral artery
AHA: 1Q, '00, 16; 1Q, '99, 7; 1Q, '97, 3

88.42 Aortography
Arteriography of aorta and aortic arch
AHA: 1Q, '99, 17

88.43 Arteriography of pulmonary arteries
88.44 Arteriography of other intrathoracic vessels
EXCLUDES angiocardiography (88.50-88.58)
arteriography of coronary arteries (88.55-88.57)
88.45 Arteriography of renal arteries
88.46 Arteriography of placenta
Placentogram using contrast material
88.47 Arteriography of other intra-abdominal arteries
AHA: 1Q, '00, 18; N-D, '87, 4
88.48 Arteriography of femoral and other lower extremity arteries
AHA: 2Q, '96, 6; 2Q, '89, 17
88.49 Arteriography of other specified sites

√4th 88.5 Angiocardiography using contrast material
INCLUDES arterial puncture and insertion of arterial catheter for injection of contrast material
cineangiocardiography
selective angiocardiography
Code also synchronous cardiac catheterization (37.21-37.23)
EXCLUDES angiography of pulmonary vessels (88.43, 88.62)
AHA: 3Q, '92, 10; M-J, '87, 11
DEF: Electromagnetic wave photography of heart and great vessels; with contrast.

88.50 Angiocardiography, not otherwise specified
88.51 Angiocardiography of venae cavae
Inferior vena cavography
Phlebography of vena cava (inferior) (superior)
88.52 Angiocardiography of right heart structures
Angiocardiography of:
pulmonary valve
right atrium
right ventricle (outflow tract)
EXCLUDES that combined with left heart angiocardiography (88.54)
88.53 Angiocardiography of left heart structures
Angiocardiography of:
aortic valve
left atrium
left ventricle (outflow tract)
EXCLUDES that combined with right heart angiocardiography (88.54)
AHA: 1Q, '00, 20; 4Q, '88, 4
88.54 Combined right and left heart angiocardiography

	88.55	**Coronary arteriography using a single catheter**
		Coronary arteriography by Sones technique
		Direct selective coronary arteriography using a single catheter
	88.56	**Coronary arteriography using two catheters**
		Coronary arteriography by:
		Judkins technique
		Ricketts and Abrams technique
		Direct selective coronary arteriography using two catheters
		AHA: 1Q, '00, 20; 4Q, '88, 4
	88.57	**Other and unspecified coronary arteriography**
		Coronary arteriography NOS
		AHA: 1Q, '00, 21
	88.58	**Negative-contrast cardiac roentgenography**
		Cardiac roentgenography with injection of carbon dioxide
√3rd	**88.6**	**Phlebography**
		INCLUDES angiography of veins
		radiography of veins (by fluoroscopy)
		retrograde phlebography
		venipuncture for injection of contrast material
		venography using contrast material
		Note: The fourth-digit subclassification (88.60-88.67) identifies the site to be viewed, not the site of injection.
		EXCLUDES angiography using:
		radioisotopes or radionuclides (92.01-92.19)
		ultrasound (88.71-88.79)
		fluorescein angiography of eye (95.12)
		DEF: Electromagnetic wave photography of veins; with contrast.
	88.60	**Phlebography using contrast material, unspecified site**
	88.61	**Phlebography of veins of head and neck using contrast material**
	88.62	**Phlebography of pulmonary veins using contrast material**
	88.63	**Phlebography of other intrathoracic veins using contrast material**
	88.64	**Phlebography of the portal venous system using contrast material**
		Splenoportogram (by splenic arteriography)
	88.65	**Phlebography of other intra-abdominal veins using contrast material**
	88.66	**Phlebography of femoral and other lower extremity veins using contrast material**
	88.67	**Phlebography of other specified sites using contrast material**
	88.68	**Impedance phlebography**
√4th	**88.7**	**Diagnostic ultrasound**
		INCLUDES echography
		ultrasonic angiography
		ultrasonography
		EXCLUDES ► therapeutic ultrasound (00.01-00.09) ◄
		DEF: Graphic recording of anatomical structures via high frequency, sound-wave imaging and computer graphics.
	88.71	**Diagnostic ultrasound of head and neck**
		Determination of midline shift of brain
		Echoencephalography
		EXCLUDES eye (95.13)
		AHA: ►1Q, '02, 10;◄ 1Q, '92, 11
	88.72	**Diagnostic ultrasound of heart**
		Echocardiography
		Intravascular ultrasound of heart
		AHA: 1Q, '00, 20, 21; 1Q, '99, 6; 3Q, '98, 11
	88.73	**Diagnostic ultrasound of other sites of thorax**
		Aortic arch ⎱
		Breast ⎬ ultrasonography
		Lung ⎰
	88.74	**Diagnostic ultrasound of digestive system**
	88.75	**Diagnostic ultrasound of urinary system**
	88.76	**Diagnostic ultrasound of abdomen and retroperitoneum**
		AHA: 2Q, '99, 14
	88.77	**Diagnostic ultrasound of peripheral vascular system**
		Deep vein thrombosis ultrasonic scanning
		AHA: 4Q, '99, 17; 1Q, '99, 12; 1Q, '92, 11
	88.78	**Diagnostic ultrasound of gravid uterus** ♀
		Intrauterine cephalometry:
		echo
		ultrasonic
		Placental localization by ultrasound
	88.79	**Other diagnostic ultrasound**
		Ultrasonography of:
		multiple sites
		nongravid uterus
		total body
√4th	**88.8**	**Thermography**
		DEF: Infrared photography to determine various body temperatures.
	88.81	**Cerebral thermography**
	88.82	**Ocular thermography**
	88.83	**Bone thermography**
		Osteoarticular thermography
	88.84	**Muscle thermography**
	88.85	**Breast thermography**
	88.86	**Blood vessel thermography**
		Deep vein thermography
	88.89	**Thermographay of other sites**
		Lymph gland thermography
		Thermography NOS
√4th	**88.9**	**Other diagnostic imaging**
	88.90	**Diagnostic imaging, not elsewhere classified**
	88.91	**Magnetic resonance imaging of brain and brain stem**
		EXCLUDES ► intraoperative magnetic resonance imaging (88.96)
		real-time magnetic resonance imaging (88.96) ◄
	88.92	**Magnetic resonance imaging of chest and myocardium**
		For evaluation of hilar and mediastinal lymphadenopathy
	88.93	**Magnetic resonance imaging of spinal canal**
		Spinal cord levels:
		cervical
		thoracic
		lumbar (lumbosacral)
		Spinal cord
		Spine
	88.94	**Magnetic resonance imaging of musculoskeletal**
		Bone marrow blood supply
		Extremities (upper) (lower)
	88.95	**Magnetic resonance imaging of pelvis, prostate, and bladder**
	88.96	**Other intraoperative magnetic resonance imaging**
		iMRI
		Real-time magnetic resonance imaging
	88.97	**Magnetic resonance imaging of other and unspecified sites**
		Abdomen Face
		Eye orbit Neck

DIAGNOSTIC AND THERAPEUTIC PROCEDURES

88.98 **Bone mineral density studies**
- Dual photon absorptiometry
- Quantitative computed tomography (CT) studies
- Radiographic densitometry
- Single photon absorptiometry

DEF: Dual photon absorptiometry: Measurement of bone mineral density by comparing dissipation of emission from two separate photoelectric energy peaks.

DEF: Quantitative computed tomography (CT) studies: Computer assisted analysis of x-ray absorption through bone to determine density.

DEF: Radiographic densiometry: Measurement of bone mineral density by degree of bone radiopacity.

DEF: Single photon absorptiometry: Measurement of bone mineral density by degree of dissipation of emission from one photoelectric energy peaks emitted by gadolinium 153.

89 Interview, evaluation, consultation, and examination

89.0 **Diagnostic interview, consultation, and evaluation**
> EXCLUDES: psychiatric diagnostic interview (94.11-94.19)

- **89.01** Interview and evaluation, described as brief
  - Abbreviated history and evaluation
- **89.02** Interview and evaluation, described as limited
  - Interval history and evaluation
- **89.03** Interview and evaluation, described as comprehensive
  - History and evaluation of new problem
- **89.04** Other interview and evaluation
- **89.05** Diagnostic interview and evaluation, not otherwise specified
- **89.06** Consultation, described as limited
  - Consultation on a single organ system
- **89.07** Consultation, described as comprehensive
- **89.08** Other consultation
- **89.09** Consulation, not otherwise specified

89.1 **Anatomic and physiologic measurements and manual examinations — nervous system and sense organs**
> EXCLUDES: ear examination (95.41-95.49)
> eye examination (95.01-95.26)
> the listed procedures when done as part of a general physical examination (89.7)

- **89.10** Intracarotid amobarbital test
  - Wada test
  - **DEF:** Amobarbital injections into internal carotid artery to induce hemiparalysis to determine the hemisphere that controls speech and language.
- **89.11** Tonometry
  - **DEF:** Pressure measurements inside eye.
- **89.12** Nasal function study
  - Rhinomanometry
  - **DEF:** Rhinomanometry: Measure of degree of nasal cavity obstruction.
- **89.13** Neurologic examination
- **89.14** Electroencephalogram
  > EXCLUDES: that with polysomnogram (89.17)
  - **DEF:** Recording of electrical currents in brain via electrodes to detect epilepsy, lesions and other encephalopathies.
- **89.15** Other nonoperative neurologic function tests
  - **AHA:** 3Q, '95, 5; 2Q, '91, 14; J-F, '87, 16; N-D, '84, 6

- **89.16** Transillumination of newborn skull
  - **DEF:** Light passed through newborn skull for diagnostic purposes.
- **89.17** Polysomnogram
  - Sleep recording
  - **DEF:** Graphic studies of sleep patterns.
- **89.18** Other sleep disorder function tests
  - Multiple sleep latency test [MSLT]
- **89.19** Video and radio-telemetered electroencephalographic monitoring
  - Radiographic } EEG Monitoring
  - Video
  - **AHA:** 1Q, '92, 17; 2Q, '90, 27

89.2 **Anatomic and physiologic measurements and manual examinations — genitourinary system**
> EXCLUDES: the listed procedures when done as part of a general physical examination (89.7)

AHA: 1Q, '90, 27

- **89.21** Urinary manometry
  - Manometry through:
    - indwelling ureteral catheter
    - nephrostomy
    - pyelostomy
    - ureterostomy
  - **DEF:** Measurement of urinary pressure.
  - **DEF:** Manometry through:
    - Indwelling urinary catheter: Semipermanent urinary catheter.
    - Nephrostomy: Opening into pelvis of kidney.
    - Pyelostomy: Opening in lower kidney.
    - Ureterostomy: Opening into ureter.
- **89.22** Cystometrogram
  - **DEF:** Pressure recordings at various stages of bladder filling.
- **89.23** Urethral sphincter electromyogram
- **89.24** Uroflowmetry [UFR]
  - **DEF:** Continuous recording of urine flow.
- **89.25** Urethral pressure profile [UPP]
- **89.26** Gynecological examination ♀
  - Pelvic examination
- **89.29** Other nonoperative genitourinary system measurements
  - Bioassay of urine   Urine chemistry
  - Renal clearance
  - **AHA:** N-D, '84, 6

89.3 **Other anatomic and physiologic measurements and manual examinations**
> EXCLUDES: the listed procedures when done as part of a general physical examination (89.7)

- **89.31** Dental examination
  - Oral mucosal survey
  - Periodontal survey
- **89.32** Esophageal manometry
  - **AHA:** 3Q, '96, 13
  - **DEF:** Measurement of esophageal fluid and gas pressures.
- **89.33** Digital examination of enterostomy stoma
  - Digital examination of colostomy stoma
- **89.34** Digital examination of rectum
- **89.35** Transillumination of nasal sinuses
- **89.36** Manual examination of breast

DIAGNOSTIC AND THERAPEUTIC PROCEDURES

89.37 **Vital capacity determination**
DEF: Measurement of expelled gas volume after full inhalation.

89.38 **Other nonoperative respiratory measurements**
Plethysmography for measurement of respiratory function
Thoracic impedance plethysmography
AHA: S-O, '87, 6

DEF: Plethysmography for measurement of respiratory function: Registering changes in respiratory function as noted in blood circulation.

89.39 **Other nonoperative measurements and examinations**
^{14}C-Urea breath test
Basal metabolic rate [BMR]
Gastric:
  analysis
  function NEC
EXCLUDES body measurement (93.07)
  cardiac tests (89.41-89.69)
  fundus photography (95.11)
  limb length measurement (93.06)
AHA: 2Q, '01, 9; 3Q, '00, 9; 3Q, '96, 12; 1Q, '94, 18; N-D, '84, 6

√4th **89.4** **Cardiac stress tests and pacemaker checks**

89.41 **Cardiovascular stress test using treadmill**
AHA: 1Q, '88, 11

89.42 **Masters' two-step stress test**
AHA: 1Q, '88, 11

89.43 **Cardiovascular stress test using bicycle ergometer**
AHA: 1Q, '88, 11

DEF: Electrocardiogram during exercise on bicycle with device capable of measuring muscular, metabolic and respiratory effects of exercise.

89.44 **Other cardiovascular stress test**
Thallium stress test with or without transesophageal pacing

89.45 **Artificial pacemaker rate check**
Artificial pacemaker function check NOS
AHA: ▶1Q, '02, 3◀

89.46 **Artificial pacemaker artifact wave form check**

89.47 **Artificial pacemaker electrode impedance check**

89.48 **Artificial pacemaker voltage or amperage threshold check**

√4th **89.5** **Other nonoperative cardiac and vascular diagnostic procedures**
EXCLUDES fetal EKG (75.32)

89.50 **Ambulatory cardiac monitoring**
Analog devices [Holter-type]
AHA: 4Q, '99, 21; 4Q, '91, 23

89.51 **Rhythm electrocardiogram**
Rhythm EKG (with one to three leads)

89.52 **Electrocardiogram**
ECG NOS
EKG (with 12 or more leads)
AHA: 1Q, '88, 11; S-O, '87, 6

89.53 **Vectorcardiogram (with ECG)**

89.54 **Electrographic monitoring**
Telemetry
EXCLUDES ambulatory cardiac monitoring (89.50)
  electrographic monitoring during surgery — omit code
AHA: 4Q, '91, 23; 1Q, '88, 11

DEF: Evaluation of heart electrical activity by continuous screen monitoring.

DEF: Telemetry: Evaluation of heart electrical activity; with radio signals at distance from patient.

89.55 **Phonocardiogram with ECG lead**

89.56 **Carotid pulse tracing with ECG lead**
EXCLUDES oculoplethysmography (89.58)

89.57 **Apexcardiogram (with ECG lead)**
AHA: J-F, '87, 16

89.58 **Plethysmogram**
Penile plethysmography with nerve stimulation
EXCLUDES plethysmography (for):
  measurement of respiratory function (89.38)
  thoracic impedance (89.38)
AHA: S-O, '87, 7

DEF: Determination and recording of blood variations present or passing through an organ.

89.59 **Other nonoperative cardiac and vascular measurements**
AHA: 2Q, '92, 12

DEF: Monitoring pulmonary artery pressure via catheter inserted through right lower and upper heart chambers into pulmonary artery and advancing the balloon-tip to wedge it in the distal pulmonary artery branch.

√4th **89.6** **Circulatory monitoring**
EXCLUDES electrocardiographic monitoring during surgery — omit code
AHA: M-J, '87, 11

89.60 **Continuous intra-arterial blood gas monitoring**
Insertion of blood gas monitoring system and continuous monitoring of blood gases through an intra-arterial sensor

89.61 **Systemic arterial pressure monitoring**

89.62 **Central venous pressure monitoring**

89.63 **Pulmonary artery pressure monitoring**
EXCLUDES pulmonary artery wedge monitoring (89.64)

89.64 **Pulmonary artery wedge monitoring**
Pulmonary capillary wedge [PCW] monitoring
Swan-Ganz catheterization

89.65 **Measurement of systemic arterial blood gases**
EXCLUDES ▶continuous intra-arterial blood gas monitoring (89.60)◀

89.66 **Measurement of mixed venous blood gases**

89.67 **Monitoring of cardiac output by oxygen consumption technique**
Fick method

DEF: Fick method: Indirect measure of cardiac output through blood volume flow over pulmonary capillaries; determines oxygen absorption by measure of arterial oxygen content versus venous blood content.

DIAGNOSTIC AND THERAPEUTIC PROCEDURES

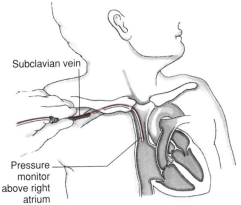

Central Venous Pressure Monitoring

89.68 Monitoring of cardiac output by other technique
Cardiac output monitor by thermodilution indicator
DEF: Cardiac output monitor by thermodilution indicator: Injection of ice cold dextrose solution into right lower heart chamber; temperature sensitive catheter monitors disappearance from beat to beat to measure expelled blood volume.

89.69 Monitoring of coronary blood flow
Coronary blood flow monitoring by coincidence counting technique

89.7 General physical examination

89.8 Autopsy

90 Microscopic examination - I
The following fourth-digit subclassification is for use with categories in section 90 to identify type of examination:
1 bacterial smear
2 culture
3 culture and sensitivity
4 parasitology
5 toxicology
6 cell block and Papanicolaou smear
9 other microscopic examination

90.0 Microscopic examination of specimen from nervous system and of spinal fluid

90.1 Microscopic examination of specimen from endocrine gland, not elsewhere classified

90.2 Microscopic examination of specimen from eye

90.3 Microscopic examination of specimen from ear, nose, throat, and larynx

90.4 Microscopic examination of specimen from trachea, bronchus, pleura, lung, and other thoracic specimen, and of sputum

90.5 Microscopic examination of blood

90.6 Microscopic examination of specimen from spleen and of bone marrow

90.7 Microscopic examination of specimen from lymph node and of lymph

90.8 Microscopic examination of specimen from upper gastrointestinal tract and of vomitus

90.9 Microscopic examination of specimen from lower gastrointestinal tract and of stool

91 Microscopic examination - II
The following fourth-digit subclassification is for use with categories in section 91 to identify type of examination:
1 bacterial smear
2 culture
3 culture and sensitivity
4 parasitology
5 toxicology
6 cell block and Papanicolaou smear
9 other microscopic examination

91.0 Microscopic examination of specimen from liver, biliary tract, and pancreas

91.1 Microscopic examination of peritoneal and retroperitoneal specimen

91.2 Microscopic examination of specimen from kidney, ureter, perirenal and periureteral tissue

91.3 Microscopic examination of specimen from bladder, urethra, prostate, seminal vesicle, perivesical tissue, and of urine and semen

91.4 Microscopic examination of specimen from female genital tract
Amnionic sac
Fetus

91.5 Microscopic examination of specimen from musculoskeletal system and of joint fluid
Microscopic examination of:
bone   ligament
bursa   muscle
cartilage   synovial membrane
fascia   tendon

91.6 Microscopic examination of specimen from skin and other integument
Microscopic examination of:
hair
nails
skin
EXCLUDES mucous membrane — code to organ site that of operative wound (91.71-91.79)

91.7 Microscopic examination of specimen from operative wound

91.8 Microscopic examination of specimen from other site

91.9 Microscopic examination of specimen from unspecified site

92 Nuclear medicine

92.0 Radioisotope scan and function study

92.01 Thyroid scan and radioisotope function studies
Iodine-131 uptake
Protein-bound iodine
Radio-iodine uptake

92.02 Liver scan and radioisotope function study

92.03 Renal scan and radioisotope function study
Renal clearance study

92.04 Gastrointestinal scan and radioisotope function study
Radio-cobalt B_{12} Schilling test
Radio-iodinated triolein study

92.05 Cardiovascular and hematopoietic scan and radioisotope function study
Bone marrow
Cardiac output
Circulation time   } scan or
Radionuclide cardiac   function
  ventriculogram   study
Spleen

AHA: 2Q, '92, 7; 1Q, '88, 11

92.09 Other radioisotope function studies

92.1 Other radioisotope scan

DIAGNOSTIC AND THERAPEUTIC PROCEDURES

- **92.11** Cerebral scan
  - Pituitary
- **92.12** Scan of other sites of head
  - EXCLUDES: eye (95.16)
- **92.13** Parathyroid scan
- **92.14** Bone scan
- **92.15** Pulmonary scan
- **92.16** Scan of lymphatic system
- **92.17** Placental scan
- **92.18** Total body scan
- **92.19** Scan of other sites

92.2 Therapeutic radiology and nuclear medicine
EXCLUDES that for:
- ablation of pituitary gland (07.64-07.69)
- destruction of chorioretinal lesion (14.26-14.27)

AHA: 3Q, '92, 5

DEF: Radiation and nuclear isotope treatment of diseased tissue.

- **92.21** Superficial radiation
  - Contact radiation [up to 150 KVP]
- **92.22** Orthovoltage radiation
  - Deep radiation [200-300 KVP]
- **92.23** Radioisotopic teleradiotherapy
  - Teleradiotherapy using:
    - cobalt-60
    - iodine-125
    - radioactive cesium
- **92.24** Teleradiotherapy using photons
  - Megavoltage NOS
  - Supervoltage NOS
  - Use of:
    - Betatron
    - linear accelerator
- **92.25** Teleradiotherapy using electrons
  - Beta particles
- **92.26** Teleradiotherapy of other particulate radiation
  - Neutrons
  - Protons NOS
- **92.27** Implantation or insertion of radioactive elements
  - Intravascular brachytherapy
  - Code also incision of site
  - AHA: 1Q, '00, 11, 12; 3Q, '94, 11; 1Q, '88, 4
- **92.28** Injection or instillation of radioisotopes
  - Intracavitary injection or
  - Intravenous instillation
- **92.29** Other radiotherapeutic procedure

92.3 Stereotactic radiosurgery
Code also stereotactic head frame application (93.59)
EXCLUDES stereotactic biopsy
AHA: 4Q, '98, 79; 4Q, '95, 70

DEF: Ablation of deep intracranial lesions; single procedure; placement of head frame for 3-D analysis of lesion, followed by radiation treatment from helmet attached to frame.

- **92.30** Stereotactic radiosurgery, not otherwise specified
- **92.31** Single source photon radiosurgery
  - High energy x-rays
  - Linear accelerator (LINAC)
- **92.32** Multi-source photon radiosurgery
  - Cobalt 60 radiation
  - Gamma irradiation
- **92.33** Particulate radiosurgery
  - Particle beam radiation (cyclotron)
  - Proton accelerator
- **92.39** Stereotactic radiosurgery, not elsewhere classified

93 Physical therapy, respiratory therapy, rehabilitation, and related procedures

93.0 Diagnostic physical therapy
AHA: N-D, '86, 7

- **93.01** Functional evaluation
- **93.02** Orthotic evaluation
- **93.03** Prosthetic evaluation
- **93.04** Manual testing of muscle function
  - AHA: J-F, '87, 16
- **93.05** Range of motion testing
  - AHA: J-F, '87, 16
- **93.06** Measurement of limb length
- **93.07** Body measurement
  - Girth measurement
  - Measurement of skull circumference
- **93.08** Electromyography
  - EXCLUDES:
    - eye EMG (95.25)
    - that with polysomnogram (89.17)
    - urethral sphincter EMG (89.23)
  - AHA: J-F, '87, 16
  - DEF: Graphic recording of electrical activity of muscle.
- **93.09** Other diagnostic physical therapy procedure

93.1 Physical therapy exercises
AHA: J-F, '87, 16; N-D, '86, 7

- **93.11** Assisting exercise
  - EXCLUDES assisted exercise in pool (93.31)
- **93.12** Other active musculoskeletal exercise
- **93.13** Resistive exercise
- **93.14** Training in joint movements
- **93.15** Mobilization of spine
- **93.16** Mobilization of other joints
  - EXCLUDES manipulation of temporomandibular joint (76.95)
- **93.17** Other passive musculoskeletal exercise
- **93.18** Breathing exercise
- **93.19** Exercise, not elsewhere classified

93.2 Other physical therapy musculoskeletal manipulation
AHA: N-D, '86, 7

- **93.21** Manual and mechanical traction
  - EXCLUDES:
    - skeletal traction (93.43-93.44)
    - skin traction (93.45-93.46)
    - spinal traction (93.41-93.42)
- **93.22** Ambulation and gait training
- **93.23** Fitting of orthotic device
- **93.24** Training in use of prosthetic or orthotic device
  - Training in crutch walking
- **93.25** Forced extension of limb
- **93.26** Manual rupture of joint adhesions
  - DEF: Therapeutic application of force to rupture adhesions restricting movement.
- **93.27** Stretching of muscle or tendon
- **93.28** Stretching of fascia
- **93.29** Other forcible correction of deformity
  - AHA: N-D, 85, 11

93.3 Other physical therapy therapeutic procedures
- **93.31** Assisted exercise in pool
- **93.32** Whirlpool treatment
- **93.33** Other hydrotherapy
- **93.34** Diathermy

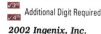

2002 Ingenix, Inc.

DIAGNOSTIC AND THERAPEUTIC PROCEDURES

93.35 **Other heat therapy**
Acupuncture with smouldering moxa
Hot packs
Hyperthermia NEC
Infrared irradiation
Moxibustion
Paraffin bath
EXCLUDES hyperthermia for treatment of cancer (99.85)

DEF: Moxibustion: Igniting moxa, a Chinese plant, for counterirritation of skin.

DEF: Paraffin bath: Hot wax treatment.

93.36 **Cardiac retraining**
DEF: Cardiac rehabilitation regimen following myocardial infarction or coronary bypass graft procedure.

93.37 **Prenatal training**
Training for natural childbirth

93.38 **Combined physical therapy without mention of the components**

93.39 **Other physical therapy**
AHA: 3Q, '97, 12; 3Q, '91, 15

✓4th **93.4** **Skeletal traction and other traction**

93.41 **Spinal traction using skull device**
Traction using: Traction using:
  caliper tongs   halo device
  Crutchfield tongs   Vinke tongs
EXCLUDES insertion of tongs or halo traction device (02.94)

AHA: ▶3Q, '01, 8;◀ 3Q, '96, 14; 2Q, '94, 3

DEF: Applying device to head to exert pulling force on spine.

93.42 **Other spinal traction**
Cotrel's traction
EXCLUDES cervical collar (93.52)
DEF: Pulling force exerted on spine without skull device.

93.43 **Intermittent skeletal traction**

93.44 **Other skeletal traction**
Bryant's ⎫
Dunlop's ⎬ traction
Lyman Smith ⎪
Russell's ⎭

93.45 **Thomas' splint traction**
DEF: Thomas splint: Placement of ring around thigh, attached to rods running length of leg for therapeutic purposes.

93.46 **Other skin traction of limbs**
Adhesive tape traction   Buck's traction
Boot traction   Gallows traction

✓4th **93.5** **Other immobilization, pressure, and attention to wound**
EXCLUDES wound cleansing (96.58-96.59)

93.51 **Application of plaster jacket**
EXCLUDES Minerva jacket (93.52)

93.52 **Application of neck support**
Application of:
  cervical collar
  Minerva jacket
  molded neck support

93.53 **Application of other cast**

93.54 **Application of splint**
Plaster splint
Tray splint
EXCLUDES periodontal splint (24.7)

93.55 **Dental wiring**
EXCLUDES that for orthodontia (24.7)

93.56 **Application of pressure dressing**
Application of:
  Gibney bandage
  Robert Jones' bandage
  Shanz dressing

93.57 **Application of other wound dressing**
▶Porcine wound dressing◀

93.58 **Application of pressure trousers**
Application of:
  anti-shock trousers
  MAST trousers
  vasopneumatic device
AHA: 3Q, '96, 13

93.59 **Other immobilization, pressure, and attention to wound**
Elastic stockings
Electronic gaiter
Intermittent pressure device
Oxygenation of wound (hyperbaric)
Stereotactic head frame application
Velpeau dressing
AHA: 3Q, '99, 7; 1Q, '99, 12, 13; 1Q, '91, 11; 1Q, '89, 12

✓4th **93.6** **Osteopathic manipulative treatment**

93.61 **Osteopathic manipulative treatment for general mobilization**
General articulatory treatment

93.62 **Osteopathic manipulative treatment using high-velocity, low-amplitude forces**
Thrusting forces

93.63 **Osteopathic manipulative treatment using low-velocity, high-amplitude forces**
Springing forces

93.64 **Osteopathic manipulative treatment using isotonic, isometric forces**

93.65 **Osteopathic manipulative treatment using indirect forces**

93.66 **Osteopathic manipulative treatment to move tissue fluids**
Lymphatic pump

93.67 **Other specified osteopathic manipulative treatment**

✓4th **93.7** **Speech and reading rehabilitation and rehabilitation of the blind**

93.71 **Dyslexia training**

93.72 **Dysphasia training**
DEF: Speech training to coordinate and arrange words in proper sequence.

93.73 **Esophageal speech training**
DEF: Speech training after voice box removal; sound is produced by vibration of air column in esophagus against the cricopharangeal sphincter.

93.74 **Speech defect training**

93.75 **Other speech training and therapy**
AHA: 4Q, '97, 36; 3Q, '97, 12

93.76 **Training in use of lead dog for the blind**

93.77 **Training in braille or Moon**

93.78 **Other rehabilitation for the blind**

✓4th **93.8** **Other rehabilitation therapy**

93.81 **Recreational therapy**
Diversional therapy
Play therapy
EXCLUDES play psychotherapy (94.36)

93.82 **Educational therapy**
Education of bed-bound children
Special schooling for the handicapped

DIAGNOSTIC AND THERAPEUTIC PROCEDURES

93.83 Occupational therapy
Daily living activities therapy
EXCLUDES: *training in activities of daily living for the blind (93.78)*
AHA: 3Q, '97, 12

93.84 Music therapy

93.85 Vocational rehabilitation
Sheltered employment
Vocational:
 assessment
 retraining
 training

93.89 Rehabilitation, not elsewhere classified

93.9 Respiratory therapy
EXCLUDES: *insertion of airway (96.01-96.05)*
other continuous mechanical ventilation (96.70-96.72)

93.90 Continuous positive airway pressure [CPAP]
AHA: ▶1Q, '02, 12, 13;◀ 3Q, '98, 14; 4Q, '91, 21
DEF: Noninvasive ventilation support system that augments the ability to breathe spontaneously without the insertion of an endotracheal tube or tracheostomy.

93.91 Intermittent positive pressure breathing [IPPB]
AHA: 4Q, '91, 21

93.93 Nonmechanical methods of resuscitation
Artificial respiration
Manual resuscitation
Mouth-to-mouth resuscitition

93.94 Respiratory medication administered by nebulizer
Mist therapy

93.95 Hyperbaric oxygenation
EXCLUDES: *oxygenation of wound (93.59)*

93.96 Other oxygen enrichment
Catalytic oxygen therapy
Cytoreductive effect
Oxygenators
Oxygen therapy
EXCLUDES: *oxygenation of wound (93.59)*

93.97 Decompression chamber

93.98 Other control of atmospheric pressure and composition
Antigen-free air conditioning
Helium therapy
EXCLUDES: ▶*inhaled nitric oxide therapy (INO) (00.12)*◀
AHA: ▶1Q, '02, 14◀

93.99 Other respiratory procedures
Continuous negative pressure ventilation [CNP]
Postural drainage
AHA: 3Q, '99, 11; 4Q, '91, 22

94 Procedures related to the psyche

94.0 Psychologic evaluation and testing

94.01 Administration of intelligence test
Administration of:
 Stanford-Binet
 Wechsler Adult Intelligence Scale
 Wechsler Intelligence Scale for Children

94.02 Administration of psychologic test
Administration of:
 Bender Visual-Motor Gestalt Test
 Benton Visual Retention Test
 Minnesota Multiphasic Personality Inventory
 Wechsler Memory Scale

94.03 Character analysis

94.08 Other psychologic evaluation and testing

94.09 Psychologic mental status determination, not otherwise specified

94.1 Psychiatric interviews, consultations, and evaluations

94.11 Psychiatric mental status determination
Clinical psychiatric mental status determination
Evaluation for criminal responsibility
Evaluation for testimentary capacity
Medicolegal mental status determination
Mental status determination NOS

94.12 Routine psychiatric visit, not otherwise specified

94.13 Psychiatric commitment evaluation
Pre-commitment interview

94.19 Other psychiatric interview and evaluation
Follow-up psychiatric interview NOS

94.2 Psychiatric somatotherapy
DEF: Biological treatment of mental disorders.

94.21 Narcoanalysis
Narcosynthesis

94.22 Lithium therapy

94.23 Neuroleptic therapy

94.24 Chemical shock therapy

94.25 Other psychiatric drug therapy
AHA: S-O, '86, 4

94.26 Subconvulsive electroshock therapy

94.27 Other electroshock therapy
Electroconvulsive therapy (ECT)
EST

94.29 Other psychiatric somatotherapy

94.3 Individual psychotherapy

94.31 Psychoanalysis

94.32 Hypnotherapy
Hypnodrome
Hypnosis

94.33 Behavior therapy
Aversion therapy
Behavior modification
Desensitization therapy
Extinction therapy
Relaxation training
Token economy

94.34 Individual therapy for psychosexual dysfunction
EXCLUDES: *that performed in group setting (94.41)*

94.35 Crisis intervention

94.36 Play psychotherapy

94.37 Exploratory verbal psychotherapy

94.38 Supportive verbal psychotherapy

94.39 Other individual psychotherapy
Biofeedback

94.4 Other psychotherapy and counselling

94.41 Group therapy for psychosexual dysfunction

94.42 Family therapy

94.43 Psychodrama

94.44 Other group therapy

94.45 Drug addiction counselling

94.46 Alcoholism counselling

94.49 Other counselling

94.5 Referral for psychologic rehabilitation

94.51 Referral for psychotherapy

94.52 Referral for psychiatric aftercare
That in:
 halfway house
 outpatient (clinic) facility

94.53–96.04 DIAGNOSTIC AND THERAPEUTIC PROCEDURES

- **94.53** Referral for alcoholism rehabilitation
- **94.54** Referral for drug addiction rehabilitation
- **94.55** Referral for vocational rehabilitation
- **94.59** Referral for other psychologic rehabilitation

√4th **94.6 Alcohol and drug rehabilitation and detoxification**
AHA: 2Q, '91, 12

- **94.61** Alcohol rehabilitation
  DEF: Program designed to restore social and physical functioning, free of the dependence of alcohol.
- **94.62** Alcohol detoxification
  DEF: Treatment of physical symptoms during withdrawal from alcohol dependence.
- **94.63** Alcohol rehabilitation and detoxification
- **94.64** Drug rehabilitation
  DEF: Program designed to restore social and physical functioning, free of the dependence of drugs.
- **94.65** Drug detoxification
  DEF: Treatment of physical symptoms during withdrawal from drug dependence.
- **94.66** Drug rehabilitation and detoxification
- **94.67** Combined alcohol and drug rehabilitation
- **94.68** Combined alcohol and drug detoxification
- **94.69** Combined alcohol and drug rehabilitation and detoxification

√3rd **95 Ophthalmologic and otologic diagnosis and treatment**

√4th **95.0 General and subjective eye examination**

- **95.01** Limited eye examination
  Eye examination with prescription of spectacles
- **95.02** Comprehensive eye examination
  Eye examination covering all aspects of the visual system
- **95.03** Extended ophthalmologic work-up
  Examination (for):
    glaucoma
    neuro-ophthalmology
    retinal disease
- **95.04** Eye examination under anesthesia
  Code also type of examination
- **95.05** Visual field study
- **95.06** Color vision study
- **95.07** Dark adaptation study
  DEF: Exam of eye's adaption to dark.
- **95.09** Eye examination, not otherwise specified
  Vision check NOS

√4th **95.1 Examinations of form and structure of eye**

- **95.11** Fundus photography
- **95.12** Fluorescein angiography or angioscopy of eye
- **95.13** Ultrasound study of eye
- **95.14** X-ray study of eye
- **95.15** Ocular motility study
- **95.16** P$_{32}$ and other tracer studies of eye

√4th **95.2 Objective functional tests of eye**
EXCLUDES   that with polysomnogram (89.17)

- **95.21** Electroretinogram [ERG]
- **95.22** Electro-oculogram [EOG]
- **95.23** Visual evoked potential [VEP]
  DEF: Measuring and recording evoked visual responses of body and senses.
- **95.24** Electronystagmogram [ENG]
  DEF: Monitoring of brain waves to record induced and spontaneous eye movements.
- **95.25** Electromyogram of eye [EMG]
- **95.26** Tonography, provocative tests, and other glaucoma testing

√4th **95.3 Special vision services**

- **95.31** Fitting and dispensing of spectacles
- **95.32** Prescription, fitting, and dispensing of contact lens
- **95.33** Dispensing of other low vision aids
- **95.34** Ocular prosthetics
- **95.35** Orthoptic training
- **95.36** Ophthalmologic counselling and instruction
  Counselling in:
    adaptation to visual loss
    use of low vision aids

√4th **95.4 Nonoperative procedures related to hearing**

- **95.41** Audiometry
  Békésy 5-tone audiometry
  Impedance audiometry
  Stapedial reflex response
  Subjective audiometry
  Tympanogram
- **95.42** Clinical test of hearing
  Tuning fork test
  Whispered speech test
- **95.43** Audiological evaluation
  Audiological evaluation by:
    Bárány noise machine
    blindfold test
    delayed feedback
    masking
    Weber lateralization
- **95.44** Clinical vestibular function tests
  Thermal test of vestibular function
- **95.45** Rotation tests
  Bárány chair
  DEF: Irrigation of ear canal with warm or cold water to evaluate vestibular function.
- **95.46** Other auditory and vestibular function tests
- **95.47** Hearing examination, not otherwise specified
- **95.48** Fitting of hearing aid
  EXCLUDES   implantation of electromagnetic hearing device (20.95)
  AHA: 4Q, '89, 5
- **95.49** Other nonoperative procedures related to hearing
  Adjustment (external components) of cochlear prosthetic device

√3rd **96 Nonoperative intubation and irrigation**

√4th **96.0 Nonoperative intubation of gastrointestinal and respiratory tracts**

- **96.01** Insertion of nasopharyngeal airway
- **96.02** Insertion of oropharyngeal airway
- **96.03** Insertion of esophageal obturator airway
- **96.04** Insertion of endotracheal tube

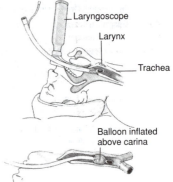

Endotracheal Intubation

DIAGNOSTIC AND THERAPEUTIC PROCEDURES

- **96.05** Other intubation of respiratory tract
  AHA: 1Q, '97, 14
- **96.06** Insertion of Sengstaken tube
  Esophageal tamponade
  DEF: Insertion of Sengstaken tube: Nonsurgical emergency measure to stop esophageal bleeding using compression exerted by inflated balloons; additional tube ports to aspirate blood and clots.
- **96.07** Insertion of other (naso-) gastric tube
  Intubation for decompression
  EXCLUDES: that for enteral infusion of nutritional substance (96.6)
- **96.08** Insertion of (naso-) intestinal tube
  Miller-Abbott tube (for decompression)
- **96.09** Insertion of rectal tube
  Replacement of rectal tube

96.1 Other nonoperative insertion
EXCLUDES: nasolacrimal intubation (09.44)
- **96.11** Packing of external auditory canal
- **96.14** Vaginal packing ♀
- **96.15** Insertion of vaginal mold ♀
- **96.16** Other vaginal dilation ♀
- **96.17** Insertion of vaginal diaphragm ♀
- **96.18** Insertion of other vaginal pessary ♀
- **96.19** Rectal packing

96.2 Nonoperative dilation and manipulation
- **96.21** Dilation of frontonasal duct
- **96.22** Dilation of rectum
- **96.23** Dilation of anal sphincter
- **96.24** Dilation and manipulation of enterostomy stoma
- **96.25** Therapeutic distention of bladder
  Intermittent distention of bladder
- **96.26** Manual reduction of rectal prolapse
- **96.27** Manual reduction of hernia
- **96.28** Manual reduction of enterostomy prolapse
  AHA: N-D, '87, 11
- **96.29** Reduction of intussusception of alimentary tract
  With:
    fluoroscopy
    ionizing radiation enema
    ultrasonography guidance
  Hydrostatic reduction
  Pneumatic reduction
  EXCLUDES: intra-abdominal manipulation of intestine, not otherwise specified (46.80)
  AHA: 4Q, '98, 82

96.3 Nonoperative alimentary tract irrigation, cleaning, and local instillation
- **96.31** Gastric cooling
  Gastric hypothermia
  DEF: Reduction of internal stomach temperature.
- **96.32** Gastric freezing
- **96.33** Gastric lavage
- **96.34** Other irrigation of (naso-)gastric tube
- **96.35** Gastric gavage
  DEF: Food forced into stomach.
- **96.36** Irrigation of gastrostomy or enterostomy
- **96.37** Proctoclysis
  DEF: Slow introduction of large amounts of fluids into lower large intestine.
- **96.38** Removal of impacted feces
  Removal of impaction:
    by flushing manually
- **96.39** Other transanal enema
  Rectal irrigation
  EXCLUDES: reduction of intussusception of alimentary tract by ionizing radiation enema (96.29)

96.4 Nonoperative irrigation, cleaning, and local instillation of other digestive and genitourinary organs
- **96.41** Irrigation of cholecystostomy and other biliary tube
- **96.42** Irrigation of pancreatic tube
- **96.43** Digestive tract instillation, except gastric gavage
- **96.44** Vaginal douche ♀
- **96.45** Irrigation of nephrostomy and pyelostomy
- **96.46** Irrigation of ureterostomy and ureteral catheter
- **96.47** Irrigation of cystostomy
- **96.48** Irrigation of other indwelling urinary catheter
- **96.49** Other genitourinary instillation
  Insertion of prostaglandin suppository
  AHA: 1Q, '01, 5

96.5 Other nonoperative irrigation and cleaning
- **96.51** Irrigation of eye
  Irrigation of cornea
  EXCLUDES: irrigation with removal of foreign body (98.21)
- **96.52** Irrigation of ear
  Irrigation with removal of cerumen
- **96.53** Irrigation of nasal passages
- **96.54** Dental scaling, polishing, and debridement
  Dental prophylaxis   Plaque removal
- **96.55** Tracheostomy toilette
- **96.56** Other lavage of bronchus and trachea
  EXCLUDES: ▶ diagnostic bronchoalveolar lavage (BAL) (33.24)
  whole lung lavage (33.99) ◀
- **96.57** Irrigation of vascular catheter
  AHA: 3Q, '93, 5
- **96.58** Irrigation of wound catheter
- **96.59** Other irrigation of wound
  Wound cleaning NOS
  EXCLUDES: debridement (86.22, 86.27-86.28)
  AHA: S-O, '85, 7

96.6 Enteral infusion of concentrated-nutritional substances

DIAGNOSTIC AND THERAPEUTIC PROCEDURES

96.7–97.43

Tabular List

√4th **96.7 Other continuous mechanical ventilation**

INCLUDES: Endotracheal respiratory assistance
Intermittent mandatory ventilation [IMV]
Positive end expiratory pressure [PEEP]
Pressure support ventilation [PSV]
That by tracheostomy
Weaning of an intubated (endotracheal tube) patient

EXCLUDES: bi-level airway pressure (93.90)
continuous negative pressure ventilation [CNP] (iron lung) (cuirass) (93.99)
continuous positive airway pressure [CPAP] (93.90)
intermittent positive pressure breathing [IPPB] (93.91)
that by face mask (93.90-93.99)
that by nasal cannula (93.90-93.99)
that by nasal catheter (93.90-93.99)

Code also any associated:
endotracheal tube insertion (96.04)
tracheostomy (31.1-31.29)

Note: **Endotracheal intubation**
To calculate the number of hours (duration) of continuous mechanical ventilation during a hospitalization, begin the count from the start of the (endotracheal) intubation. The duration ends with (endotracheal) extubation.

If a patient is intubated prior to admission, begin counting the duration from the time of the admission. If a patient is transferred (discharged) while intubated, the duration would end at the time of transfer (discharge).

For patients who begin on (endotracheal) intubation and subsequently have a tracheostomy performed for mechanical ventilation, the duration begins with the (endotracheal) intubation and ends when the mechanical ventilation is turned off (after the weaning period).

Tracheostomy
To calculate the number of hours of continuous mechanical ventilation during a hospitalization, begin counting the duration when mechanical ventilation is started. The duration ends when the mechanical ventilator is turned off (after the weaning period).

If a patient has received a tracheostomy prior to admission and is on mechanical ventilation at the time of admission, begin counting the duration from the time of admission. If a patient is transferred (discharged) while still on mechanical ventilation via tracheostomy, the duration would end at the time of the transfer (discharge).

AHA: 2Q, '92, 13; 4Q, '91, 16; 4Q, '91, 18; 4Q, '91, 21

- **96.70 Continuous mechanical ventilation of unspecified duration**
  Mechanical ventilation NOS
- **96.71 Continuous mechanical ventilation for less than 96 consecutive hours**
  AHA: ▶1Q, '02, 12;◀ 1Q, '01, 6
- **96.72 Continuous mechanical ventilation for 96 consecutive hours or more**

√3rd **97 Replacement and removal of therapeutic appliances**

√4th **97.0 Nonoperative replacement of gastrointestinal appliance**
- 97.01 Replacement of (naso-)gastric or esophagostomy tube
- 97.02 Replacement of gastrostomy tube
  AHA: 1Q, '97, 11
- 97.03 Replacement of tube or enterostomy device of small intestine
- 97.04 Replacement of tube or enterostomy device of large intestine
- 97.05 Replacement of stent (tube) in biliary or pancreatic duct
  AHA: 2Q, '99, 13

√4th **97.1 Nonoperative replacement of musculoskeletal and integumentary system appliance**
- 97.11 Replacement of cast on upper limb
- 97.12 Replacement of cast on lower limb
- 97.13 Replacement of other cast
- 97.14 Replacement of other device for musculoskeletal immobilization
- 97.15 Replacement of wound catheter
- 97.16 Replacement of wound packing or drain
  EXCLUDES: repacking of:
  dental wound (97.22)
  vulvar wound (97.26)

√4th **97.2 Other nonoperative replacement**
- 97.21 Replacement of nasal packing
- 97.22 Replacement of dental packing
- 97.23 Replacement of tracheostomy tube
  AHA: N-D, '87, 11
- 97.24 Replacement and refitting of vaginal diaphragm
- 97.25 Replacement of other vaginal pessary
- 97.26 Replacement of vaginal or vulvar packing or drain
- 97.29 Other nonoperative replacements
  AHA: 3Q, '99, 9; 3Q, '98, 12

√4th **97.3 Nonoperative removal of therapeutic device from head and neck**
- 97.31 Removal of eye prosthesis
  EXCLUDES: removal of ocular implant (16.71)
  removal of orbital implant (16.72)
- 97.32 Removal of nasal packing
- 97.33 Removal of dental wiring
- 97.34 Removal of dental packing
- 97.35 Removal of dental prosthesis
- 97.36 Removal of other external mandibular fixation device
- 97.37 Removal of tracheostomy tube
- 97.38 Removal of sutures from head and neck
- 97.39 Removal of other therapeutic device from head and neck
  EXCLUDES: removal of skull tongs (02.94)

√4th **97.4 Nonoperative removal of therapeutic device from thorax**
- 97.41 Removal of thoracotomy tube or pleural cavity drain
  AHA: 1Q, '99, 10
- 97.42 Removal of mediastinal drain
- 97.43 Removal of sutures from thorax

Intraaortic Balloon Pump

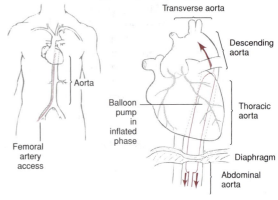

DIAGNOSTIC AND THERAPEUTIC PROCEDURES

- **97.44** Nonoperative removal of heart assist system
  Intra-aortic balloon pump (IABP)
  AHA: ▶4Q, '01, 65◀

  DEF: Non-invasive removal of ventricular assist systems, or intraaortic balloon pump, which is a balloon catheter placed into the descending thoracic aorta and timed to inflate and deflate with the patient's own heart rhythm to aid in blood circulation.

- **97.49** Removal of other device from thorax
  AHA: N-D, '86, 9

✓4th 97.5 Nonoperative removal of therapeutic device from digestive system
- **97.51** Removal of gastrostomy tube
- **97.52** Removal of tube from small intestine
- **97.53** Removal of tube from large intestine or appendix
- **97.54** Removal of cholecystostomy tube
- **97.55** Removal of T-tube, other bile duct tube, or liver tube
  Removal of bile duct stent
  AHA: 1Q, '01, 8
- **97.56** Removal of pancreatic tube or drain
- **97.59** Removal of other device from digestive system
  Removal of rectal packing

✓4th 97.6 Nonoperative removal of therapeutic device from urinary system
- **97.61** Removal of pyelostomy and nephrostomy tube
  DEF: Nonsurgical removal of tubes from lower part of kidney.
- **97.62** Removal of ureterostomy tube and ureteral catheter
- **97.63** Removal of cystostomy tube
- **97.64** Removal of other urinary drainage device
  Removal of indwelling urinary catheter
- **97.65** Removal of urethral stent
- **97.69** Removal of other device from urinary system

✓4th 97.7 Nonoperative removal of therapeutic device from genital system
- **97.71** Removal of intrauterine contraceptive device ♀
- **97.72** Removal of intrauterine pack ♀
- **97.73** Removal of vaginal diaphragm ♀
- **97.74** Removal of other vaginal pessary ♀
- **97.75** Removal of vaginal or vulvar packing ♀
- **97.79** Removal of other device from genital tract
  Removal of sutures

✓4th 97.8 Other nonoperative removal of therapeutic device
- **97.81** Removal of retroperitoneal drainage device
- **97.82** Removal of peritoneal drainage device
  AHA: 2Q, '90, 28; S-O, '86, 12
- **97.83** Removal of abdominal wall sutures
- **97.84** Removal of sutures from trunk, not elsewhere classified
- **97.85** Removal of packing from trunk, not elsewhere classified
- **97.86** Removal of other device from abdomen
- **97.87** Removal of other device from trunk
- **97.88** Removal of external immobilization device
  Removal of:
    brace
    cast
    splint
- **97.89** Removal of other therapeutic device

✓3rd 98 Nonoperative removal of foreign body or calculus

✓4th 98.0 Removal of intraluminal foreign body from digestive system without incision
  EXCLUDES removal of therapeutic device (97.51-97.59)
  DEF: Retrieval of foreign body from digestive system lining without incision.
- **98.01** Removal of intraluminal foreign body from mouth without incision
- **98.02** Removal of intraluminal foreign body from esophagus without incision
- **98.03** Removal of intraluminal foreign body from stomach and small intestine without incision
- **98.04** Removal of intraluminal foreign body from large intestine without incision
- **98.05** Removal of intraluminal foreign body from rectum and anus without incision

✓4th 98.1 Removal of intraluminal foreign body from other sites without incision
  EXCLUDES removal of therapeutic device (97.31-97.49, 97.61-97.89)
- **98.11** Removal of intraluminal foreign body from ear without incision
- **98.12** Removal of intraluminal foreign body from nose without incision
- **98.13** Removal of intraluminal foreign body from pharynx without incision
- **98.14** Removal of intraluminal foreign body from larynx without incision
- **98.15** Removal of intraluminal foreign body from trachea and bronchus without incision
- **98.16** Removal of intraluminal foreign body from uterus without incision ♀
  EXCLUDES removal of intrauterine contraceptive device (97.71)
- **98.17** Removal of intraluminal foreign body from vagina without incision ♀
- **98.18** Removal of intraluminal foreign body from artificial stoma without incision
- **98.19** Removal of intraluminal foreign body from urethra without incision

✓4th 98.2 Removal of other foreign body without incision
  EXCLUDES removal of intraluminal foreign body (98.01-98.19)
- **98.20** Removal of foreign body, not otherwise specified
- **98.21** Removal of superficial foreign body from eye without incision
- **98.22** Removal of other foreign body without incision from head and neck
  Removal of embedded foreign body from eyelid or conjunctiva without incision
- **98.23** Removal of foreign body from vulva without incision ♀
- **98.24** Removal of foreign body from scrotum or penis without incision ♂
- **98.25** Removal of other foreign body without incision from trunk except scrotum, penis, or vulva
- **98.26** Removal of foreign body from hand without incision
  AHA: N-D, '87, 10
- **98.27** Removal of foreign body without incision from upper limb, except hand
- **98.28** Removal of foreign body from foot without incision
- **98.29** Removal of foreign body without incision from lower limb, except foot

98.5–99.2 DIAGNOSTIC AND THERAPEUTIC PROCEDURES — Tabular List

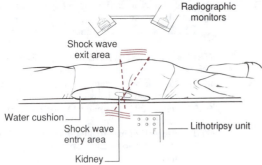

Extracorporeal Shock Wave Lithotripsy

√4th **98.5 Extracorporeal shockwave lithotripsy [ESWL]**
Lithotriptor tank procedure
Disintegration of stones by extracorporeal induced shockwaves
That with insertion of stent

DEF: Breaking of stones with high voltage condenser device synchronized with patient R waves.

98.51 Extracorporeal shockwave lithotripsy [ESWL] of the kidney, ureter and/or bladder
AHA: 4Q, '95, 73; 1Q, '89, 2

98.52 Extracorporeal shockwave lithotripsy [ESWL] of the gallbladder and/or bile duct NC

98.59 Extracorporeal shockwave lithotripsy of other sites NC

√3rd **99 Other nonoperative procedures**

√4th **99.0 Transfusion of blood and blood components**
Use additional code for that done via catheter or cutdown (38.92-38.94)

DEF: Salvaging patient blood and reinfusing it during perioperative period.

99.00 Perioperative autologous transfusion of whole blood or blood components
Intraoperative blood collection
Postoperative blood collection
Salvage
AHA: 4Q, '95, 69

99.01 Exchange transfusion
Transfusion:
  exsanguination
  replacement
AHA: 2Q, '89, 15

DEF: Repetitive withdrawal of blood, replaced by donor blood.

99.02 Transfusion of previously collected autologous blood
Blood component
AHA: 4Q, '95, 69; 1Q, '90, 10; J-A, '85, 16

DEF: Transfusion with patient's own previously withdrawn and stored blood.

99.03 Other transfusion of whole blood
Transfusion:
  blood NOS
  hemodilution
  NOS

99.04 Transfusion of packed cells

99.05 Transfusion of platelets
Transfusion of thrombocytes

99.06 Transfusion of coagulation factors
Transfusion of antihemophilic factor

99.07 Transfusion of other serum
Transfusion of plasma
EXCLUDES injection [transfusion] of:
    antivenin (99.16)
    gamma globulin (99.14)

99.08 Transfusion of blood expander
Transfusion of Dextran

99.09 Transfusion of other substance
Transfusion of:
  blood surrogate
  granulocytes
EXCLUDES transplantation [transfusion] of bone marrow (41.0)

√4th **99.1 Injection or infusion of therapeutic or prophylactic substance**
INCLUDES injection or infusion given:
  hypodermically }
  intramuscularly } acting locally or systemically
  intravenously }

99.10 Injection or infusion of thrombolytic agent
Streptokinase
Tissue plasminogen activator (TPA)
Urokinase
EXCLUDES aspirin — omit code
  GP IIB/IIIa platelet inhibitors (99.20)
  heparin (99.19)
  single vessel percutaneous transluminal coronary angioplasty [PTCA] or coronary atherectomy with mention of thrombolytic agent (36.02)
  warfarin — omit code
AHA: 2Q, '01, 7-9, 23; 4Q, '98, 83

99.11 Injection of Rh immune globulin
Injection of:
  Anti-D (Rhesus) globulin
  RhoGAM

99.12 Immunization for allergy
Desensitization

99.13 Immunization for autoimmune disease

99.14 Injection of gamma globulin
Injection of immune sera

99.15 Parenteral infusion of concentrated nutritional substances
Hyperalimentation
Total parenteral nutrition [TPN]
Peripheral parenteral nutrition [PPN]

DEF: Administration of greater than necessary amount of nutrients via other than the alimentary canal (e.g., infusion).

99.16 Injection of antidote
Injection of:
  antivenin
  heavy metal antagonist

99.17 Injection of insulin

99.18 Injection or infusion of electrolytes

99.19 Injection of anticoagulant
EXCLUDES ▶ infusion of drotrecogin alfa (activated) (00.11) ◀

√4th **99.2 Injection or infusion of other therapeutic or prophylactic substance**
INCLUDES injection or infusion given:
  hypodermically }
  intramuscularly } acting locally or systemically
  intravenously }

Use additional code for:
injection (into):
  breast (85.92)
  bursa (82.94, 83.96)
  intraperitoneal (cavity) (54.97)
  intrathecal (03.92)
  joint (76.96, 81.92)
perfusion:
  NOS (39.97)
  intestine (46.95, 46.96)
  kidney (55.95)
injection (into):
  kidney (55.96)
  liver (50.94)
  orbit (16.91)
  other sites — see Alphabetic Index
perfusion:
  liver (50.93)
  total body (39.96)

DIAGNOSTIC AND THERAPEUTIC PROCEDURES

99.20 Injection or infusion of platelet inhibitor
Glycoprotein IIB/IIIa inhibitor
GP IIB-IIIa inhibitor
GP IIB/IIIa inhibitor
EXCLUDES infusion of heparin (99.19)
injection or infusion of thrombolytic agent (99.10)
AHA: 4Q, '98, 85

99.21 Injection of antibiotic
EXCLUDES injection or infusion of oxazolidinone class of antibiotics (00.14)
AHA: 4Q, '98, 76; 2Q, '90, 24; M-A, '87, 9

99.22 Injection of other anti-infective
EXCLUDES injection or infusion of oxazolidinone class of antibiotics (00.14)

99.23 Injection of steroid
Injection of cortisone
Subdermal implantation of progesterone
AHA: 3Q, '00, 15; 1Q, '99, 8; 3Q, '96, 7; 3Q, '92, 9; S-O, '85, 7

99.24 Injection of other hormone

99.25 Injection or infusion of cancer chemotherapeutic substance
Chemoembolization
Injection or infusion of antineoplastic agent
EXCLUDES immunotherapy, antineoplastic (99.28)
implantation of chemotherapeutic agent (00.10)
injection of radioisotope (92.28)
injection or infusion of biological response modifier [BRM] as an antineoplastic agent (99.28)
AHA: 1Q, '99, 4; 1Q, '98, 6; 3Q, '96, 11; 4Q, '95, 67; 2Q, '92, 7; 1Q, '92, 12; 1Q, '88, 8; N-D, '86, 11

99.26 Injection of tranquilizer

99.27 Iontophoresis
DEF: Iontophoresis: Introduction of soluble salts into tissues via electric current.

99.28 Injection or infusion of biological response modifier [BRM] as an antineoplastic agent
High-dose interleukin-2 (IL-2) therapy
Immunotherapy, antineoplastic
Interleukin therapy
Tumor vaccine
AHA: 2Q, '99, 8; 2Q, '98, 10; 4Q, '94, 51

99.29 Injection or infusion of other therapeutic or prophylactic substance
EXCLUDES administration of neuroprotective agent (99.75)
immunization (99.31-99.59)
injection of sclerosing agent into:
esophageal varices (42.33)
hemorrhoids (49.42)
veins (39.92)
injection or infusion of:
human B-type natriuretic peptide (hBNP) (00.13)
nesiritide (00.13)
platelet inhibitor (99.20)
thrombolytic agent (99.10)
AHA: 1Q, '01, 15; 2Q, '00, 14; 1Q, '00, 8, 18, 23; 4Q, '99, 17; 3Q, '99, 21; 4Q, '98, 83; 2Q, '98, 17, 18, 23, 24; 1Q, '98, 6; 2Q, '97, 11; 1Q, '97, 3; 4Q, '95, 67; 2Q, '95, 12; 4Q, '90, 14; 2Q, '90, 23; 2Q, '89, 17; 1Q, '88, 9; N-D, '87, 4; S-O, '87, 11

√4ᵗʰ **99.3** Prophylactic vaccination and inoculation against certain bacterial diseases
DEF: Administration of a killed bacteria suspension to produce immunity.

99.31 Vaccination against cholera

99.32 Vaccination against typhoid and paratyphoid fever
Administration of TAB vaccine

99.33 Vaccination against tuberculosis
Administration of BCG vaccine

99.34 Vaccination against plague

99.35 Vaccination against tularemia

99.36 Administration of diphtheria toxoid
EXCLUDES administration of:
diphtheria antitoxin (99.58)
diphtheria-tetanus-pertussis, combined (99.39)

99.37 Vaccination against pertussis
EXCLUDES administration of diphtheria-tetanus-pertussis, combined (99.39)

99.38 Administration of tetanus toxoid
EXCLUDES administration of:
diphtheria-tetanus-pertussis, combined (99.39)
tetanus antitoxin (99.56)

99.39 Administration of diphtheria-tetanus-pertussis, combined

√4ᵗʰ **99.4** Prophylactic vaccination and inoculation against certain viral diseases
DEF: Administration of a killed virus suspension to produce immunity.

99.41 Administration of poliomyelitis vaccine

99.42 Vaccination against smallpox

99.43 Vaccination against yellow fever

99.44 Vaccination against rabies

99.45 Vaccination against measles
EXCLUDES administration of measles-mumps-rubella vaccine (99.48)

99.46 Vaccination against mumps
EXCLUDES administration of measles-mumps-rubella vaccine (99.48)

99.47 Vaccination against rubella
EXCLUDES administration of measles-mumps-rubella vaccine (99.48)

99.48 Administration of measles-mumps-rubella vaccine

√4ᵗʰ **99.5** Other vaccination and inoculation

99.51 Prophylactic vaccination against the common cold

99.52 Prophylactic vaccination against influenza

99.53 Prophylactic vaccination against arthropod-borne viral encephalitis

99.54 Prophylactic vaccination against other arthropod-borne viral diseases

99.55 Prophylactic administration of vaccine against other diseases
Vaccination against:
anthrax
brucellosis
Rocky Mountain spotted fever
Vaccination against:
Staphylococcus
Streptococcus
typhus
AHA: 2Q, '00, 9; 1Q, '94, 10

99.56 Administration of tetanus antitoxin

99.57 Administration of botulism antitoxin

DIAGNOSTIC AND THERAPEUTIC PROCEDURES

99.58 **Administration of other antitoxins**
Administration of:
- diphtheria antitoxin
- gas gangrene antitoxin
- scarlet fever antitoxin

99.59 **Other vaccination and inoculation**
Vaccination NOS
EXCLUDES injection of:
- gamma globulin (99.14)
- Rh immune globulin (99.11)
immunization for:
- allergy (99.12)
- autoimmune disease (99.13)

√4th 99.6 Conversion of cardiac rhythm
EXCLUDES open chest cardiac:
- electric stimulation (37.91)
- massage (37.91)

DEF: Correction of cardiac rhythm.

99.60 **Cardiopulmonary resuscitation, not otherwise specified**
AHA: 1Q, '94, 16

99.61 **Atrial cardioversion**
DEF: Application of electric shock to upper heart chamber to restore normal heart rhythm.

99.62 **Other electric countershock of heart**
Cardioversion:
- NOS
- external
Conversion to sinus rhythm
Defibrillation
External electrode stimulation

99.63 **Closed chest cardiac massage**
Cardiac massage NOS
Manual external cardiac massage
DEF: Application of alternating manual pressure over breastbone to restore normal heart rhythm.

99.64 **Carotid sinus stimulation**

99.69 **Other conversion of cardiac rhythm**
AHA: 4Q, '88, 11

√4th 99.7 Therapeutic apheresis or other injection, administration, or infusion of other therapeutic or prophylactic substance
DEF: Blood withdrawal from donor with desired portion removed (e.g., plasma, leukocytes, platelets, etc.) and retained; remainder transfused back into donor.

99.71 **Therapeutic plasmapheresis**
EXCLUDES ▶extracorporeal immunoadsorption [ECI] (99.76)◀

99.72 **Therapeutic leukopheresis**
Therapeutic leukocytapheresis

99.73 **Therapeutic erythrocytapheresis**
Therapeutic erythropheresis
AHA: 1Q, '94, 20

99.74 **Therapeutic plateletpheresis**

99.75 **Administration of neuroprotective agent**
AHA: 4Q, '00, 68
DEF: Direct application of neuroprotective agent (e.g., nimodipine) to miinimize ischemic injury by inhibiting toxic neurotransmitters, blocking free ions, removing free radicals, and causing vasodilation.

99.76 **Extracorporeal immunoadsorption**
Removal of antibodies from plasma with protein A columns

99.77 **Application or administration of adhesion barrier substance**

99.79 **Other**
Apheresis (harvest) of stem cells
AHA: 4Q, '97, 55

√4th 99.8 Miscellaneous physical procedures

99.81 **Hypothermia (central) (local)**
EXCLUDES
- gastric cooling (96.31)
- gastric freezing (96.32)
- that incidental to open heart surgery (39.62)

99.82 **Ultraviolet light therapy**
Actinotherapy

99.83 **Other phototherapy**
Phototherapy of the newborn
EXCLUDES
- extracorporeal photochemotherapy (99.88)
- photocoagulation of retinal lesion (14.23-14.25, 14.33-14.35, 14.53-14.55)

AHA: 2Q, '89, 15

DEF: Treating disease with light rays of various concentrations.

99.84 **Isolation**
Isolation after contact with infectious disease
Protection of individual from his surroundings
Protection of surroundings from individual

99.85 **Hyperthermia for treatment of cancer**
Hyperthermia (adjunct therapy) induced by microwave, ultrasound, low energy radio frequency, probes (interstitial), or other means in the treatment of cancer
Code also any concurrent chemotherapy or radiation therapy
AHA: 3Q, '96, 11; 3Q, '89, 17

99.86 **Non-invasive placement of bone growth stimulator**
Transcutaneous (surface) placement of pads or patches for stimulation to aid bone healing
EXCLUDES insertion of invasive or semi-invasive bone growth stimulators (device) (percutaneous electrodes) (78.90-78.99)

99.88 **Therapeutic photopheresis**
Extracorporeal photochemotherapy
Extracorporeal photopheresis
EXCLUDES
- other phototherapy (99.83)
- ultraviolet light therapy (99.82)

AHA: 2Q, '99, 7

DEF: Extracorporeal photochemotherapy: Treating disease with drugs that react to ultraviolet radiation or sunlight.

√4th 99.9 Other miscellaneous procedures

99.91 **Acupuncture for anesthesia**

99.92 **Other acupuncture**
EXCLUDES that with smouldering moxa (93.35)

99.93 **Rectal massage (for levator spasm)**

99.94 **Prostatic massage** ♂

99.95 **Stretching of foreskin** ♂

99.96 **Collection of sperm for artificial insemination** ♂

99.97 **Fitting of denture**

99.98 **Extraction of milk from lactating breast** ♀

99.99 **Other**
▶Leech therapy◀

Pharmacological Listings

Pharmacology Considerations
Medications are listed by classification and brand name for each of the chapters of ICD-9-CM. The list includes many of the common medications and should not be considered exhaustive. The pharmacology considerations that follow are presented as guidance only for the recognition of the link between implication of disease process and treatment.

Infectious and Parasitic Diseases (001-139)

AIDS Related Complex (ARC) Therapeutic Agents
Agenerase
Epivir
Hivid
Invirase
Pentam
Retrovir
Roferon-A
Videx
Vitravene
Ziagen
Crixivan
Fortovase
Intron A
Norvir
Rescriptor
Rimactane
Sustiva
Viracept
Zerit
Zovirax

Antibiotics
Achromycin-V
Amoxil
Ancef
Azactam
Bicillin
Ceclor
Cefobid
Ceftin
Cipro
Cleocin
Duricef
ERYC
Erythromycin
Fortaz
Garamycin
Levaquin
Macrobid
Maxipime
Mezlin
Monocid
Nebcin
Neo-fradin
PCE Dispertab
Penicillin G
Pfizerpen
Primaxin
Rocephin
Spectrobid
Synersid
Tazidime
Tetracycline HCl
Timentin
Trimox
Unasyn
Vancocin
Vibra-Tabs
Wycillin
Zinacef
Zosyn
Amikin
Ampicillin
Augmentin
Bactrim
Biocef
Cefizox•
Cefotan
Chloromycetin
Claforan
Cloxapen
E-Mycin
Ery-Tab
Floxin
Ganatol
Kefzol
Loribid
Maxaquin
Mefoxin
Minocin
Nallpen
NegGram
Omnipen
Penetrex
Penicillin V
Pipracil
Proloprim
Septra
Suprax
Tazicef
Terramycin
Ticar
Totacillin
Trimpex
Unipen
Vibramycin
Wyamycin S
Zefazone
Zithromx

Antiparasitics
Antiminth
Daraprim
G-Well
MepronnebuPent
Penticarinat
Protostat
Aralen
Flagyl
Helidac
Pentam 300
Pin-X
Vermox

Corticosteroids
Aristocort
Cortastat
Cortenema
Dalalone
Deltasone
Florinef acetate
Hydrocortone
Medrol
Predalone
Protocort
Solu-Medrol
Celestone
Cortef
Cortone Acetate
Decadron
Depo-Medrol
Hydeltrasol
Medralone
Orasone
Prelone
Solu-Cortef

Fungal Medications
Abelcet
Amphocin
Ancobon
Fulvicin P/G
Fungizone
Fungoid
Grisactin
Lamisil
Lotrisone
Mycelex-G
Mycostatin
Nizoral
Sporanox
AmBisome
Amphotec
Diflucan
Fungilin
Fungizone
Grifulvin
Gris-PEG
Lotrimin
Monistat
Mycolog
Nilstst
Spectazole

Tuberculosis Preparations
Capastat
Lamprene
Myambutol
Priftin
Rifadin
Rimactane
Sodium P.A.S.
Trecator-SC
INH Tablets
Laniazid
Mycobutin
Pyrazinamide
Rifamate
Seromycin
Streptomycin

Viral Agents
Agenerase
Combivir
Cytovene
Famvir
Fortovase
Herplex
Invirase
Relenza
Retrovir
Symmetrel
Valtrex
Videx
Viracept
Virazole
Vistide
Zerit
Zovirax
Alferon N
Crixivan
Epivir
Flumadine
Foscavir
HIVID
Norvir
Rescriptor
Sustiva
Tamiflu
Videx
Vira-A
Viramune
Viroptic
Vitravene
Ziagen

Neoplasms (140-239)

Adjunct
Anzemet
Compazine
Ergamisol
Leukine
Metastron
Neupogen
Prokine
Reglan
Salagen
Zinecard
Arrestin
Epogen
Kytril
Martinol
Neumega
Procrit
Quadramet
Relcomide
Sandostatin
Zofran

Androgen Inhibitor
Casodex
Lupron
Zoladex
Eulexin
Nilandron

Antibiotic Derivatives
Adriamycin
Cerubidine
Doxorubicin
Mutamycin
Blenoxane
Cosmegen
Idamycin
Mithracin

Nipent
Pacis
TheraCys
Novantrone
Rubex

Antiestrogen
Femara
Nolvadex

Antimetabolites
Adrucil
Cytosar-U
Efudex
Fludara
Fluorouracil
Intron A
Methotrexate
Roferon-A
Xeloda
Cytarabine
Droxia
Folex
Fluoroplex
FUDR
Leustatin
Purinethol
Thioguanine

Cytotoxic Agents
Adriamycin
CeeNU
Cytosar-U
Gemzar
Hydrea
Matulane
Myleran
Paraplatin
Zanosar
BiCNU
Cerubidine
Doxorubicin
Hexalen
Intron A
Mutamycin
Novantrone
Platinol

Hormones
Arimidex
Depo-Provera
Estinyl
Fareston
Megace
Teslac
Aromasin
Emcyt
Estradurin
Lupron
Stilphostrol
Zoladex

Nitrogen Mustard Derivatives
Alkeran
Leukeran
Neosar
Cytoxan
Mustargen
Thiotepa

Steroids and Combinations
Celestone Soluspan

Other
Camptosar
Elspar
Ethyol
Leucovorin
Lysodren
Navelbine
Oncovin
Photofrin
Rituxan
Taxol
TICE
Vumon
VePesid
DTIC-Dome
Ergamisol
Etopophos
Leustatin
Mesnex
Oncaspar
Phosphocol P32
Proleukin
Semzar
Taxotere
Vesanoid
Velban

Endocrine, Nutritional and Metabolic Diseases and Immunity Disorders (240-279)

Acidifier and Alkalinizers
Ammonium chloride
Sodium bicarbonate
Tham
Citrocarbonate
Sodium lactate

Antigout Agents
Anturane
Colchicine
Zyloprim
Benemid
Probalan

Antioxidants
Aquasol E
Calcium-D

Pharmacological Listing

Calcium Health Packs
Carotene Health Packs
Performance Packs
Carotene-E
Glutathione
Pure-E

Appetite Suppressants
Adipex-P
Biphetamine
Desoxyn
Fastin
Mazanor
Phentride
Pondimin
Sanorex
Adipost
Bontril
Didrex
Ionamin
Meridia
Plegine
Prelu-2
Tenuate

Diabetic Agents and Glucagon
Actos
Avandia
Diabinese
Glucophage
Glynase
Iletin II
Lispro (Humalog)
Novolin
Prandin
Rezulin
Velosulin
Amaryl
DiaBeta
Glucagon
Glucotrol
Glyset   Humulin R
Lantus
Micronase
NovoLog
Precose
Ultralente

Electrolytes and Replacement Solutions
Calcium acetate
Calcium chloride
Calcium gluconate
Calcium phosphate, dibasic
Calcium phosphate, tribasic
Dextran
Hespan
Magnesium sulfate
Potassium acetate
Potassium bicarbonate (K+ Care ET, Klor-Con/EF, K-Vescent)
Potassium chloride (Kaochlor, Kaon-Cl, Kato Powder, Kay Ciel, K-Lease, K-Lor, Klor-10%, Klor-Con, Klorvess, Klotrix, K-Lyte/Cl, K-Tab, Micro-K Extencaps, SK-Potassium Chloride, Slow-K, Ten-K)
Potassium gluconate (Glu-K, Kaon, Kayliker, K-G Elixir)
Slow-mag
Calcium carbonate
Calcium citrate
Calcium lactate
Gendex
Magnesium chloride
Phoslo
Ringer's Injection

Hormones
Anadrol-50
A.P.L.
Delatestryl
Estrace
Estratab
Factrel
Micronor
Ogen
Ortho-Novum
Pregnyl
Proscar
Testoderm
Android
Combipatch
Depo-Provers
Estraderm
Estrovis
Halotestin
Norplant
Ortho-Est
Orvette
premarin
Provera
Testred

Parathyroid-like Agents
Aredia
Calderol
Didronel
Fosamax
Osteocalcin
Salmonine
Calcimar
Cibacalcin
E-Vista
Miacalcin
Rocaltrol

Pituitary Hormones
ACTH
Cortrosyn
Genotropin
Pitressin
Stimate
Acthar
Diapid
Humatrope
Protropin

Thyroid Antagonists
Pima
Tapazole

Thyroid Hormones
Cytomel
Levothroid
Levoxyl
Synthyroid
Euthroid
Levoxine
Triostat

Vitamins
Vitamin A
Vitamin B complex (including cyanocobalamin, hydroxocobalamin, folic acid, leucovorin calcium, niacin, niacinamide, pyridoxine hydrochloride, riboflavin, thiamine hydrochloride)
Vitamin C
Vitamin D (cholecalciferol, ergocalciferol)
Vitamin E
Vitamin K analogs (menadione/menadiol sodium diphosphate, phytonadione, sodium fluoride)
Trace elements (chromium, copper, iodine, manganese, selenium, zinc)

Blood and Blood-Forming Organsl (280-289)

Coagulants
AlphaNine Coagulation Factor
Profilate OSD Antihemophilic Factor
Trasylol

Hematinics Ferrous fumarate:
Femiron
Ferrlecit
Fumerin
Hytinic
Span FF
Feostat
Fumasorb
Hemocyte
Ircon

Ferrous gluconate:
Fergon
Ferriecit

Ferrous sulfate:
Feosol
Fero-Gradumet
Ferralyn
Mol-Iron
Fer-In-Sol
Ferospace
Irospan
Slow Fe

Iron dextran:
DexFerrum
INFeD
Imferon

Others
Konyne-HT Factor IX Complex   Nu-Iron
Monoclate-P Factor VIII:C, Antihemophilic Factor

Mental Disorders (290-319)

Central Nervous System Stimulants
Cylert
Dexedrine
Provigil
Vivarin
Desoxyn
Dopram
Ritalin

Cerebral Metabolic Enhancer
Ergostat
Migranal
Hydergine

Anti-anxiety
Atarax
BuSpar
Librium
Serax
Valium
Xanax
Ativan
Libritabs
Miltown
Tranxene
Versed

Anti-depressants
Anafranil
Aventyl
Effexor
Nardil
Pamelor
Paxil
Remeron
Sinequan
Trialodine
Zoloft
Asendin
Celexa
Elavil
Norpramin
Parnate
Prozac
Serzone
Surmontil
Tofranillbutrin

Anti-psychotics
Clozaril
Haldol
Mellaril
Orap
Risperdal
Seroquel
Stelazine
Triavil
Zyprexa
Etrafon
Loxitane
Navane
Prolixin
Serentil
Serpasil
Thorazine
Trilafon

Sedatives
Ambien
Mebaral
Precedex
Restoril
Sonata
Unisom
Dalmane
Nembutal
ProSom
Seconal Sodium
Tuinal

Other Psychotrophics
Amerge
Aricept
Cognex
Eskalith
Lithane
Lithobid
Meridia
Zomig
Antabuse
Cibalith-S
Diprivan
Imitrex
Lithium Carbonate
Luvox
Methadone
Zyban

Nervous System and Sense Organs (320-389)

Antibiotics Central nervous system agents:
Amikin
Cefizox
Garamycin
Nebcin
Tazidime
Ancef
Fortaz
Kefurox
Rocephin

Optical agents:
Declomycin
Gantanol

Otics (preparations for the ear):
Augmentin
Ceclor
Gantanol
Septra
Bactrim
Ceftin
Keflex
Suprax

Anticonvulsants
Celontin
Depakene
Dilantin
Klonopin
Mebaral
Milontin
Neurontin
Phenobarbital
Tegretol
Tridione
Cerebyx
Depakote
Felbatol
Lamictal
Mesantoin
Mysoline
Peganone
Phenurone
Tranxene
Zarontin

Dopamine Receptor Agonist
Eldepryl
Parlodel
Requip
Symmetrel
Mirapex
Permax
Sinemet
Tasmar

Miscellaneous Ophthalmics
Alphagan
Emadine
Lacrisert
OptiPranolol
Propine
Trusopt
Betoptic
Iopidine
Opticrom
OPTIVAR
Timoptic
Zaditor

Migraine Agents
Amerge
Depakote
Imitrex
Isocom
Midrin
Sansert
Zomig
Cafergot
Ergostat
Inderal
Maxalt
Migranal
Wigraine

Miotics
Carboptic
Miostat
Pilostat
Miochol-E
Pilocar
Phospholine Iodide

Mydriatics
AK-Dilate
AK-Pentolate
Cyclogyl
Epinal
Homatropine
Isopto Atropine
Isopto Homatropine
Minims
Mydriacyl
AK-Nefrin
Atropisol
Epifrin
Eppy/N
Glaucon
Isopto Frin
Isopto Hyoscine
Mydfrin

Ophthalmic Antiinfectives
AK-Tracin
Chloromycetin
Garamycin
Polymyxin B Sulfate
Sodium Sulamyd
Tobrex
Bleph-10 Liqifilm
Ciloxan
Ilotycin
Oculflox
Tobradex
Vira-A

Ophthalmic Antiinflammatory Agents
Acular
Decadron Phosphate

Flarex
Maxidex
Voltarin
Fluor-Op
Ocufen

Otics
Auro-Dri
Chloromycetin Otic
Cortisporin
Murine Ear
PediOtic
Cerumex
Coly-Mycin S
LazerSporin-C
OticTridesilon

Parasympathomimetics
Duvoid
Mestinon
Tensilon
Evoxac
Prostigmin
Urecholine

Parkinsonism Agents
Akineton
Benztropine
Comtan
Eldepryl
Mirapex
Permax
Sinemet
Artane
Cogentin
Dopar
Larodopa
Parlodel
Requip
Symmetrel

Skeletal Muscle Relaxants
Dantrium
Lioresal
Zaraflex
Flexeril
Vanadom

Vertigo Agents
Antivert
Vergon

Circulatory System (390-459)
Alpha Adrenoceptor Agonists
Aldomet
Combipres
Catapres
Wytensin

Alpha Receptor Blocking Agents
Cardura
Minipress
Trandate
Hytrin
Regitine

Anginal Preparations
Calan
Cardizem
Inderal
Isordil
Nitro-Dur
Nitrogard
Papaverine
Procardia
Transderm-Nitro
Cardilate
Dilitrate-SR
Isoptin
Nitro-Bid
Nitrodisc
Nitrostat IV
Peritrate
Sorbitrate

Angiotensin Converting Enzyme Inhibitors
Accupril
Avapro
Capozide
Lotensin
Monopril
Univasc
Zestril
Altace
Capoten
Cozaar
Mavik
Prinivil
Vasotec

Antihypertensives
Aldactazide
Aldomet
Atacard
Calan
Cardizem
Catapres
Cozaar
HydroDIURIL
Hytrin
Isoptin
Lopressor
Monopril
Renese
Tenormin
Vasotec
Zestril
Aldactone
Apresoline
Avapro
Capoten
Cardura
Corlopam
Diuril
Hyperstat
Inderal
Levatol
Minipress
Procardia
Temex
Teveten
Wytensin

Arrhythmia Medications
Betapace
Cardioquin
Inderal
Mexitil
Procan
Quinaglute
Calan
Cordarone
Isoptin
Norpace
Pronestyl
Tonocard

Beta Blocking Agents
Blocadren
Cartrol

Coreg
Corzide
Kerlone
Lopressor
Sectral
Tenormin
Trandate
Zebeta
Corgard
Inderal
Levatol
Normodyne
Tenoretic
Toprol XL
Visken

Calcium Channel Blockers
Adalat
Cardene
DynaCirc
Norvasc
Posicor
Sular
Verelan
Calan
Cardizem
Isoptin
Plendil
Procardia
Vascor

Cardiac Glycosides
Lanoxin (Digoxin)

Diuretics
Aldactazide
Bumex
Demadex
Dyazide
Esidrix
HydroDIURIL
Rauzide
Zaroxolyn
Aldoril
Combipres
Diuril
Edecrin
Esimil
Lasix
Renese

Vasodilators, Cerebral
Pavabid

Vasodilators, Coronary
Cardilate
Nitro-Bid
Nitrolingual Spray
Pavabid
Sorbitrate
Isordil
Nitro-Dur
Nitrostat IV
Peritrate
Transderm-Nitro

Vasodilators, Peripheral
Apresoline
Esimil
Loniten
Dibenzyline
Hyperstat IV
Pavabid

Other
Abbokinase
Eminase
Retavase
Activase
Kabikinase

Respiratory System (460-519)
Allergy Relief Products
Anatuss
Benedrl
Brexin
Naldecon
Trimeton
Antihist-1
Bromphen
Dristan
Tavist

Antibiotics
Achromycin
Amoxicillin
Ampicillin
Augmentin
Bactrim
Bicillin
Cefizox
Cefotan
Cipro
Duricef
E-Mycin
ERYC
Floxin
Garamycin
Ilosone
Keflex
Kefurox
Levaquin
Mefoxin
Mezlin
Nebcin
PCE Dispertab
Penicillin V
Primaxin
Rocephin
Spectrobid
Tazicef
Tetracycline HCl
Timentin
Amikin
Amoxil
Ancef
Azactam
Biaxin
Ceclor
Cefobid
Ceftin
Claforan
Dynabec
Ery-Tab
Erythromycin
Fortaz
Geocillin
Iotycin
Keftab
Kefzol
Mandol
Meropen
Minocin
Netromycin
Penicillin G
Pipracil
Raxar
Septra
Suprax
Tazidime
Ticar
Trovan

Wycillin
Zefazone
Zithromax
Zagam
Zinacef

Antihistamines
Actifed
Allerest
Benadryl
Chlor-Trimeton
Coricidin
Four-Way
Tavist
Zyrtec
Allegra
Atarax
Bromphen
Claritin
Deconamine
Periactin
Triaminic

Asthma Preparations
Accolate
Alupent
Beclovent
Bronkaid
Crolom
Flovent
Maxair
Primatene
Serevent
TheoDur
Tornalate
Ventolin
AeroBid
Aminophylline
Brethine
Choledyl SA
Dilor
Intal
Metaprel
Proventil
Singulair
Tilade
Vanceril
Zyflo

Bronchial Dilators
Accolate
Aminophylline
Atrovent
Bricanyl
Bronkometer
Choledyl
Lufyllin
Maxair
Prez-D
Proventil
Quibron
Singulair
Tedral
Tornalate
Xopenex
Alupent
Asbron G
Brethaire Inhaler
Bronkephrine
Combivent
Isuprel
Marax
Medihaler-Iso
Primatene
Quadrinal
Serevent
Slo-bid
Theolair
Ventolin
Zyflo

Cold, Cough Preparations and Mucolytics
Advil Cold/Sinus
Cheracol
Dimetapp
Entex
Humibid
Naldecon
Nucofed
Quelidrine
Robitussin
Ru-Tuss
Rynatuss
Triaminic
Tussi-Organdin
Tylenol Cold/Cough
Calcidrine
Comtrex
Dimetane
Guaifed
Hycomine
Novahistine
Ornade
Quibron
Rondec
Rynatan
Sine-Aid
Tuss-Ornade
Tussionex

Corticosteroids
Aristocort
Cortone Acetate
Depo-Medrol
Hydrocortone
Solu-Cortef
Celestone
Deltasone
Hydeltrasol
Prednisone
Solu-Medrol

Nasal Preparations
Adrenalin Chloride
Beconase
Turbinaire
Otrivin
Nasalide
Privine
Vancenase
Dopram Injectable
Afrin
Decadron Phosphate
Flonase
Nasacort
Nasarel
Rhinocort
Respiratory Stimulants

Respiratory Therapy Agents
Alupent
Survanta
Arm-a-Med Isoetharine

Digestive System (520-579)
Anorectal Products
Analpram-HC
Rowasa
Proctofoam-HC

Pharmacological Listing

Antacids
- Alka-Seltzer
- Basaljel
- Gaviscon
- Mylanta
- Riopan
- Amphojel
- Di-Gel
- Maalox
- Polycitra
- Tums

Antibiotics and Antibacterials
- Amikin
- Azactam
- Cefobid
- Claforan
- Furoxone
- Mandol
- Mezlin
- Netromycin
- Primaxin
- Tazicef
- Ticar
- Vancocin
- Ancef
- Cefizox
- Cefotan
- Fortaz
- Kefzol
- Mefoxin
- Nebcin
- Pipracil
- Rocephin
- Tazidime
- Unasyn
- Zefazone

Antispasmodics and Anticholinergics
- Bentyl
- Donnatal
- Librax
- Pro-Banthine
- Reglan
- Darabid
- Levsin
- Prilosec
- Quarzan
- Robinul

Corticosteroids
- Aristocort
- Decadron
- Depo-Medrol
- Hydrocortone
- Solu-Cortef
- Cortenema
- Deltasone
- Hydeltrasol
- Prednisone
- Solu-Medrol

Diarrhea Medications
- Arco-Lase Plus
- Donnagel
- Kaopectate
- Imodium
- Mitrolan
- Pepto-Bismol
- Charcoal Plus
- Furoxone
- Kapectolin
- Lomotil
- Motofen

Digestants
- Cotazym
- Entozyme
- Lactaid
- Pancreatin
- Viokase
- Donnazyme
- Ku-Zyme
- Pancrease
- Ultrase

Flatulence Relief
- Flatulex
- Kutrase
- Phazyme
- Gas-X
- Mylicon

Gallstone Dissolution Agent
- Actigall Capsules

Gastric Acid Secretion Inhibitor
- Axid
- Zantac
- Cytotec

Gastrointestinal Antigranulomatous Disease
- Azulfidine Tablets, EN-tabs
- Mesasal
- Rowasa
- Dipentum Capsules
- Pentasa

Nausea and Vertigo Medications
- Anzemet
- Antivert
- Bucladin-S Softab
- Dramamine
- Marinol
- Tigan
- Vergon
- Anfernet
- Bonine
- Compazine
- Kytril
- Reglan
- Torecan
- Zofran

Parasympatholytics
- Bellergal-S
- Cantil
- Robinul
- Bentyl
- Levsin

Genitourinary System (580-629)

Antibiotics
- Achromycin
- Augmentin
- Azo Gantanol
- Bactrim
- Cefizox
- Cefotan
- Ceptaz
- Claforan
- E-Mycin
- Floxin
- Garamycin
- Kefurox
- Mezlin
- Nebcin
- Noroxin
- Penetrex
- Rocephin
- Sumycin
- Tazidime
- Unasyn
- Ancef
- Azactam
- Azo Gantrisin
- Ceclor
- Cefobid
- Ceftin
- Cipro
- Duricef
- Ery-tab
- Fortaz
- Keftab
- Mefoxin
- Monuril
- Netromycin
- PCE Dispertab
- Primaxin
- Septra
- Suprax
- Timentin
- Zinacef

Gonadotropin Inhibitors
- Antagon
- Synarel Nasal Solution
- Danocrine Capsules

Hormones
Androgen and estrogen combinations:
- Estratest
- Premarin with Methyltestosterone
- Premphase
- Prempro

Estrogens:
- Climara
- Estraderm
- Menest
- Premarin
- Estrace
- Estrofem
- Ogen

Gonadotropin:
- Lutrepulse
- Profasi
- Pregnyl
- Synarel

Menotropins:
- Humegon
- Repronex
- Pergonal

Progesterone:
- Cycrin
- Provera

Progestogen:
- Aygestin
- Micronor

Urinary Tract Agents
Analgesics:
- Pyridium
- Rimso-50

Antibacterials:
- Bactrim
- Furadantin
- Gantrisin
- Macrodantin
- Neosporin
- Proloprim
- Thiosulfil
- Uroqid Acid No. 2
- Cipro
- Gantanol
- Macrobid
- NegGram
- Noroxin
- Septra
- Trimpex

Antispasmodics:
- Cystospaz
- Urised
- Levsin
- Urispas

Vaginal Preparations
Antifungal agents:
- Betadine Douche
- Gyne-Lotrimin
- Mycelex
- Vagistat
- Femstat
- Monistat
- Terazol
- Yeast-X

Capsules, tablets:
- Mycelex-G
- Sultrin

Creams:
- Amino-Cerv
- Mycostatin
- Premarin
- Estrace
- Nystex
- Trysul

Inserts, suppositories:
- Terazol
- Vagisec Plus

Jellies, ointments:
- Aci-Jel

Pregnancy, Childbirth, Puerperium (630-677)

Antibiotics
- Amikin
- Azactam
- Cefizox
- Cefotan
- E-Mycin
- Ancef
- Ceclor
- Cefobid
- Claforan
- Fortaz
- Garamycin
- Kefzol
- Nebcin
- Primaxin
- Tazidime
- Timentin
- Unasyn
- Zolicef
- Keftab
- Mefoxin
- PCE Dispertab
- Rocephin
- Ticar
- Trobicin
- Zefazone
- Zyvox

Antihypertensives
- Adalat
- Aldactone
- Apresoline
- Cardizem
- Deponit
- Esidrix
- HydroDIURIL
- Hyperstat
- Inderal
- Levatol
- Midamor
- Minoxidil
- Procardia
- Tenormin
- Vasotec
- Aldactazide
- Aldomet
- Calan
- Catapres
- Diuril
- Hydralazine
- Hygroton
- Hytrin
- Isoptin
- Lopressor
- Minipress
- Nitrostat
- Renese
- Tridil
- Wytensin

Diuretics
- Aldactazide
- Bumex
- Dyazide
- Dyrenium
- Esidrix
- HydroDIURIL
- Lozol
- Rauzide
- Zaroxolyn
- AldactoneAldoril
- Demadex Diuril
- Edecrin
- Esimil
- Lasix
- Maxzide
- Renese

Galactokinetic Agents
- Syntocinon Nasal Spray

Nausea Medication
- Antivert
- Bonine
- Emetrol
- Tigan
- Arrestin
- Compazine
- Norzine
- Torecan

Oxytocics
- Hemabate
- Methergine
- Pitocin
- Cervidil
- Oxytocin
- Syntocinon

Uterine Relaxants
- Yutopar

Skin and Subcutaneous Tissue (680-709)

Abradants
- Ureacin

Acne Preparations
- Accutane Tablets
- Benzac
- Cleocin
- Desquam
- Erycette
- Persa-Gel
- Staticin
- Theramycin Z
- Azelex
- Benzamycin
- Clinda-Derm
- Emgel
- Novacet
- Retin-A
- Sulfacet-R Acne
- Xerac

Antibacterials
- Akne-Mycin
- Fungoid
- Neo-Synalar
- pHisoHex
- Cortisporin
- Furacin
- NeoDecadron
- Silvadene

Antibacterials, Antifungals and Combinations
- Benzamycin
- Lotrisone
- Nizoral
- Fungi-Nail
- Neosporin
- Sporanox

Antibiotics
- Amikin
- Azactam
- Ceclor
- Cefobid
- Ceftin
- Duricef
- Erythromycin
- Garamycin
- Ancef
- Bactroban
- Cefizox
- Cefotan
- Cipro
- ERYC
- Floxin
- Ilosone

Ilotycin
Keftab
Mandol
Mezlin
Pipracil
Rocephin
Tazidime
Timentin
Zefazone

Keflex
Kefzol
Mefoxin
Netromycin
Primaxin
Spectrobid
Ticar
Ultracef
Zinacef

Antiinflammatory Agents
Aclovate
Cortisporin
Cyclocort
Diprolene
Halog
Lidex
Mantadil
Nutracort
Synalar
Topicort
Ultravate

Aristocort
Cutivate
Decadron
Elocon
Kenalog
Lotrisone
NeoDecadron
Synacort
Temovate
Tridesilon
Westcort

Corticosteroids
Amcort
Cortef
Depo-Medrol
Solu-Cortef

Celestone
Deltasone
Hydeltrasol
Solu-Medrol

Depigmenting Agents
Benoquin Cream
Eldoquin

Eldopaque

Dermatologicals

Dermatitis Herpetiformis:
Dapsone USP

Dermatitis Relief:
Decaspray
Hytone
Mytrex

Florone
Locoid
Psorcon

Epidermal and Cellular Growth:
Lazer Cream

Fungicides:
Amphotec
BAZA Cream
Exelderm
Grisactin
Loprox
Lotrisone
Mycolog-11
Spectazole

Abelcet
Clioquinol
Fungoid Creme
Halotex
Lotrimin
Mycelex
Mycostatin

Keratolytics:
Adrucil
Keralyt Gel

Fluoroplex
Occlusal-HP

Pruritis Medications:
Alphatrex
Dermoplast
Eurax
Hytone
Locoid
Periactin
Psorcon

Betatrex
Eldecort
Florone
Hyzine-50
Mytrex
Pramosone
Vistaril

Psoriasis Agents:
Anthra-Derm
DHS Tar
Drithocreme
Folex
Pentrax
Tegison

Denorex
Dovonex
Dritho-Scalp
Neoral
Selsun
Zetar

Steroids and Combinations:
Neo-Synalar
Synalar
Vanoxide-HC

Psorcon
Synemol
Vytone

Wart Removers:
Compound W
LazerFormalyde
Podocon-25
Sal-Plant Gel
Trans-Ver-Sal
Verrex
Viranol Gel

Condylox
Occlusal
Sal-Acid Plasters
Trans-Plantar
Verr-Canth
Verrusol

Musculoskeletal System and Connective Tissue (710-739)

Analgesics
Advil
Anaprox
Ansaid
Bufferin
Clinoril
Darvon
Disalcid
Easprin
Empirin/Codeine
Esgic
Feldene
Indocin
Lortab/Lorcet
Medipren
Motrin
Naprosyn
Norgesic
Parafon Forte
Percocet
Phenaphen/Codeine
Rufen
Sarapin
Talacen
Tolectin
Tylenol
Tylox
Vicodin

Anacin
Anexsia
Ascriptin
Butazolidin
Darvocet
Datril
Dolobid
Ecotrin
Equagesic
Exedrin
Flexeril
Lodine
Meclomen
Mono-Gesic
Nalfon
Norflex
Orudis
Ponstel
Percodan
Relafen
Salflex
Synalgos-DC
Talwin
Trilisate
Tylenol/Codeine
Voltaren
Wygesic

Antibiotics (Osteomyelitis Treatments)
Amikin
Cefizox
Cipro
Floxin
Garamycin
Keftab
Kefzol
Mefoxin
Pipracil
Timentin
Zinacef

Ancef
Cefotan
Clindamycin
Fortaz
Keflex
Kefurox
Mandol
Monocid
Rocephin
Vancocin

Antiinflammatory Agents, Steroids and Combinations
Aristocort
Decadron
Hydeltra-T.B.A.
Hydrocortone
Medrol

Cortone
Deltasone Depo-Medrol
Hydeltrasol
Kenalog

Calcium Preparations
Calcium-D
Caltrate
Dical-D
Nephro-Calci
Phos-Ex

Calphosan
Citracal
Neo-Calglucon
Os-Cal
Posture

Muscle Relaxants
Flexeril
Parafon Forte
Robaxisal
Soma
Valrelease

Paraflex
Robaxin
Skelaxin
Valium

Osteoporosis Preparations
Aredia
Didronel
Fosamax
Miacalcin

Calcimar
Evista
Gerimed

Congenital Anomalies (740-759)

A pharmacological reference list cannot be presented for this chapter because most conditions listed are treatable only by surgical methods and are not affected by medications.

Conditions in the Perinatal Period (760-779)

Antibiotics
Amoxcillin
Bicillin
Dicloxacillin

Biaxin
Cloxacillin
E-Mycin

Fortaz
Kefzol
Mezlin
Rocephin
Tazicef
Ticar
Zithromax

Garamycin
Mandol
Nebcin
Spectrobid
Tazidime
Vibramycin

Bronchodilators
Aerolate Jr.
Bronkephrine
Dilor
Quadrinal
Theolair

Asbron G
Choledyl
Proventil
Somophyllin
Ventolin

Corticosteroids
Aristocort
Cortone Acetate
Deltasone
Hydeltrasol
Solu-Cortef

Celeston
Decadron
Depo-Medrol
Prednisone
Solu-Medrol

Electrolytes
Infalyte
Pedialyte

Oralyte
Rehydralyte

Galactokinetics (Milk Flow Stimulants)
Syntocinon Nasal Spray

Galactorrhea (Lactation) Inhibitors
Parlodel

Neonatal Respiratory Distress Syndrome Agents
Exosurf

Survanta

Ophthalmic Ointments, Antibiotics
Ilotycin

Rh Hemolytic Disease-Related Agents
Gamulin Rh
HypRho-D Full Dose (for baby)
HypRho-D Mini-Dose (for mother)
Win Rho-SD   Gamulin Rh
HypRho-D Full Dose (for baby)
HypRho-D Mini-Dose (for mother) Win Rho-SD

Uterine Contractants
Oxytocin

Vitamins
AquaMEPHYTON

Symptoms, Signs and Ill-Defined Conditions (780-799)

Analgesics

Acetaminophens and combinations:
Acetaminophen
Anexsia
Datril
Feverall
Midrin

Anacin—Aspirin-Free
Bufferin
Excedrin
Isocom
Tylenol

Aspirins:
Easprin
Forprin

Ecotrin

Aspirin combinations:
Anacin
Bufferin
Norgesic

Ascriptin A/D
Equagesic

Narcotics, synthetics and combinations:
Alfenta
Astramorph/PF
B&O Supprettes
Damason-P
Darvon
Dilaudid
Duramorph
Fioricet
Hydrocet
Levo-Dromoran
Lurline
Methadone-HCl
MSIR
Numorphan
Oramorph
Percodan
Phrenilin

Anexsia
Azdone
Dalgan
Darvocet-N
Demerol
Dolophine
Esgic
Fiorinal
Infumorph
Lortab
Mepergan
MS-Contin
Nubain
Oralet
Percocet
Phenaphen/Codeine
Roxanol

2002 Ingenix, Inc.

Pharmacological Listing

Roxicodone
Stadol
Sufenta
Talacen
Tylox
Sedapap
Sublimaze
Synalgos-DC
Talwin-NX
Vicodin

Nonsteroidal antiinflammatory drugs (NSAIDs):
Advil
Daypro
Feldene
Lodine
Medipren
Nalfon
Nuprin
Ponstel
Tolectin
Voltaren
Anaprox
Duract
Indocin
Meclomen
Motrin
Naprosyn
Orudis
Rufen
Toradol

Other:
Alka-Seltzer
Empirin/Codeine
Norflex
Salflex
Trilisate
Dolobid
Mono-Gesic
Parafon Forte
Sarapin

Antacids
Alka-Seltzer
Basaljel
Mylanta
Amphojel
Maalox
Riopan

Anticonvulsives
Depakane
Dilantin
Lamictal
Phenobarbital
Topamax
Depakote
Jabatril
Nurontin
Tegretol

Antiflatulents and Antigas Medications
Flatulex
Mylicon
Kutrase

Antipyretics
Acetaminophen
Feverall
Rufen
Tylenol
Ascriptin A/D
PediaProfen
Trilisate

Antispasmodics and Anticholinergics
Arco-Lase
Cantil
Donnatal
Kutrase
Levsinex
Prilosec
Quarzan
Valpin-50
Bentyl
Darabid
Kinesed
Levsin
Librax
Pro-Banthine
Robinul

Appetite Suppressants
Amphetamines:
Biphetamine
Dexedrine
Desoxyn
Didrex

Nonamphetamines:
Adipex-P
Fastin
Plegine
Prelu-2
Sanorex
Bontril
Ionamin
Pondimin
Redux
Tenuate

Digestives
Cotazym
Ku-Zyme
Pancreatin
Donnazyme
Pancrease
Viokase

Diuretics
Aldactazide
Bumex
Corzide
Diamox
Diuril
Dyrenium
Enduron
Esidrex
HydroDIURIL
Lasix
Maxzide
Moduretic
Oretic
Rauzide
Aldactone
Capozide
Demadex
Diulo
Dyazide
Edecrin
Enduronyl
Exna
Hydromox
Lozol
Midamor
Naturetin
Prinzide
Renese

Saluron
Vaseretic
Thalitone
Zestoretic

Nausea and Vertigo Agents
Antivert
Compazine
Kytril
Phenergan
Torecan
Bonine
Emetrol
Norzine
Tigan
Zofran

Sleep Aids
Ambien
Dalmane
Halcion
Valmid
Chloral hydrate
Doriden
Restoril

Hypnotics:
Butisol
Phenobarbital
Mebaral

Sedatives (barbiturates):
Benadryl
Excedrin PM
Mepergan
Tylenol PM
Versed
BufferinAF
Magonate
Phenergan
Unisom

Sedatives (nonbarbiturates):
Eldertonic
Nu-Iron
Niferex

Tonics
Inderal

Tremor Preparations
Eldertonic
Nu-Iron
Niferex
Inderal

Injury and Poisoning (800-999)
Agents Used in Poisonings
Amyl nitrate
Antizole
Benadryl
Digibind
Narcan (Naloxone)
Pralidoxime
Revex
Sodium nitrite
Antilirium
BAL
Desferal
Ipecac Syrup
Penicillamine
Protopam Chloride
Romazicon

Analgesics
Acetaminophens and combinations:
Acetaminophen
Aspirin-Free Anacin
Feverall
Midrin
Tylenol with codeine
Anexsia
Excedrin
Isocom
Tylenol

Aspirins:
Aspirin
Ecotrin
Easprin

Aspirin combinations:
Anacin
Bufferin
Norgesic
Ascriptin A/D
Equagesic

Narcotics, synthetics and combinations:
Alfenta
Astromorph/PF
B&O Supprettes
Damason-P
Darvon
Dilaudid
Duramorph
Fioricet
Hydrocet
Levo-Dromoran
Lurline
Methadone HCl
MSIR
Numorphan
Percocet
Phrenilin
Roxicodone
Stadol
Sufenta
Talacen
Tegretol
Vicodin
Zydone
Anexsia
Azdone
Dalgan
Darvocet-N
Demerol
Dolophine
Esgic
Fiorinal
Infumorph
Lortab/Lorcet
Mepergan
MS Contin
Nubain
Oramorph
Percodan
Roxanol
Sedapap
Sublimaze
Synalgos-DC
Talwin
Tylox
Wygesic

Nonsteroidal antiinflammatory drugs (NSAIDs):
Advil
Ansaid
Clinoril
Feldene
Lodine
Medipren
Nalfon
Nuprin
Ponstel
Rufen
Toradol
Anaprox
Cataflam
Daypro
Ibuprofen
Meclamen
Motrin
Naprosyn
Orudis
Relafen
Tolectin
Voltaren

Antibiotics
Achromycin
Amoxicillin
Ancef
Azactam
Cefizox
Cefotan
Claforan
Garamycin
Keftab
Kefzol
Mezlin
Netromycin
Rocephin
Timentin
Zinacef
Amikin
Amoxil
Augmentin
Ceclor
Cefobid
Cipro
Floxin
Keflex
Kefurox
Mefoxin
Nebcin
Pipracil
Tazidime
Zefazone

Anticoagulants
Calciparine
Dicumarol
Heparin Sodium
Organan
Coumadin
Fragmin
Lovenox
Panwarfin

Antihistamines
Allegra
Benadryl
Claritin
Extendryl
Optimine
Tacaryl
Zyrtec
Atarax/Vistaril
Chlor-Trimeton
Dimetap
Hismanal
Seldane
Temaril

Antivertigo Medications
Antivert
Bucladin-S
Vontrol
Bonine
Meclizine

Burn Agents
Americaine
Butesin Picrate
Collagenase Santyl
Eucerin
Panafil
Silvadine
Tronothane
Aquaphor
Chloresium
Dermoplast
Nupercainal
Prophyllin
Sween Cream

Corticosteroids
Aristocort
Decadron
Depo-Medrol
Hydrocortone
Solu-Cortef
Celestone
Deltasone
Hydeltrasol
Prednisone
Solu-Medrol

Detoxifying Agents
Mesnex Injection

Skin Wound Preparations
Betadine
DuoDERM
Debrisan

Cleansers:

Wound Dressings
Aquaphor
Critic-Aid
DuoDERM
Lazer
SSD
Chloresium
Debrisan
Granulex
Panafil

Diagnosis Code/MDC/DRG List

The following list provides the MDC and **Medical** DRG(s) to which the diagnosis code is assigned when listed as principal diagnosis with the exception of principal diagnoses in combination with secondary diagnoses causing assignment to MDC 24 or the presence of a secondary diagnosis causing assignment to MDC 25.

DX	MDC	DRG	DX	MDC	DRG	DX	MDC	DRG	DX	MDC	DRG
Infectious and Parasitic Diseases			008.46	.06	182-184	011.25	.04	.079-081	012.16	.04	.079-081
001.0	.06	182-184	008.47	.06	182-184	011.26	.04	.079-081	012.20	.04	.079-081
001.1	.06	182-184	008.49	.06	182-184	011.30	.04	.079-081	012.21	.04	.079-081
001.9	.06	182-184	008.5	.06	182-184	011.31	.04	.079-081	012.22	.04	.079-081
002.0	.18	.423	008.61	.06	182-184	011.32	.04	.079-081	012.23	.04	.079-081
002.1	.18	.423	008.62	.06	182-184	011.33	.04	.079-081	012.24	.04	.079-081
002.2	.18	.423	008.63	.06	182-184	011.34	.04	.079-081	012.25	.04	.079-081
002.3	.18	.423	008.64	.06	182-184	011.35	.04	.079-081	012.26	.04	.079-081
002.9	.18	.423	008.65	.06	182-184	011.36	.04	.079-081	012.30	.03	.073-074
003.0	.06	182-184	008.66	.06	182-184	011.40	.04	.079-081	012.31	.03	.073-074
003.1	.18	416-417	008.67	.06	182-184	011.41	.04	.079-081	012.32	.03	.073-074
003.20	.18	.423	008.69	.06	182-184	011.42	.04	.079-081	012.33	.03	.073-074
003.21	.01	.020	008.8	.06	182-184	011.43	.04	.079-081	012.34	.03	.073-074
003.22	.04	.079-081	009.0	.06	182-184	011.44	.04	.079-081	012.35	.03	.073-074
003.23	.08	.242	009.1	.06	182-184	011.45	.04	.079-081	012.36	.03	.073-074
003.24	.08	.238	009.2	.06	182-184	011.46	.04	.079-081	012.80	.04	.079-081
003.29	.18	.423	009.3	.06	182-184	011.50	.04	.079-081	012.81	.04	.079-081
003.8	.18	.423	010.00	.04	.079-081	011.51	.04	.079-081	012.82	.04	.079-081
003.9	.18	.423	010.01	.04	.079-081	011.52	.04	.079-081	012.83	.04	.079-081
004.0	.06	182-184	010.02	.04	.079-081	011.53	.04	.079-081	012.84	.04	.079-081
004.1	.06	182-184	010.03	.04	.079-081	011.54	.04	.079-081	012.85	.04	.079-081
004.2	.06	182-184	010.04	.04	.079-081	011.55	.04	.079-081	012.86	.04	.079-081
004.3	.06	182-184	010.05	.04	.079-081	011.56	.04	.079-081	013.00	.01	.020
004.8	.06	182-184	010.06	.04	.079-081	011.60	.04	.079-081	013.01	.01	.020
004.9	.06	182-184	010.10	.04	.079-081	011.61	.04	.079-081	013.02	.01	.020
005.0	.06	182-184	010.11	.04	.079-081	011.62	.04	.079-081	013.03	.01	.020
005.1	.18	.423	010.12	.04	.079-081	011.63	.04	.079-081	013.04	.01	.020
005.2	.06	182-184	010.13	.04	.079-081	011.64	.04	.079-081	013.05	.01	.020
005.3	.06	182-184	010.14	.04	.079-081	011.65	.04	.079-081	013.06	.01	.020
005.4	.06	182-184	010.15	.04	.079-081	011.66	.04	.079-081	013.10	.01	.020
005.81	.06	182-184	010.16	.04	.079-081	011.70	.04	.079-081	013.11	.01	.020
005.89	.06	182-184	010.80	.04	.079-081	011.71	.04	.079-081	013.12	.01	.020
005.9	.06	182-184	010.81	.04	.079-081	011.72	.04	.079-081	013.13	.01	.020
006.0	.06	182-184	010.82	.04	.079-081	011.73	.04	.079-081	013.14	.01	.020
006.1	.06	182-184	010.83	.04	.079-081	011.74	.04	.079-081	013.15	.01	.020
006.2	.06	182-184	010.84	.04	.079-081	011.75	.04	.079-081	013.16	.01	.020
006.3	.07	205-206	010.85	.04	.079-081	011.76	.04	.079-081	013.20	.01	.020
006.4	.04	.079-081	010.86	.04	.079-081	011.80	.04	.079-081	013.21	.01	.020
006.5	.01	.020	010.90	.04	.079-081	011.81	.04	.079-081	013.22	.01	.020
006.6	.09	283-284	010.91	.04	.079-081	011.82	.04	.079-081	013.23	.01	.020
006.8	.18	.423	010.92	.04	.079-081	011.83	.04	.079-081	013.24	.01	.020
006.9	.18	.423	010.93	.04	.079-081	011.84	.04	.079-081	013.25	.01	.020
007.0	.06	182-184	010.94	.04	.079-081	011.85	.04	.079-081	013.26	.01	.020
007.1	.06	182-184	010.95	.04	.079-081	011.86	.04	.079-081	013.30	.01	.020
007.2	.06	182-184	010.96	.04	.079-081	011.90	.04	.079-081	013.31	.01	.020
007.3	.06	182-184	011.00	.04	.079-081	011.91	.04	.079-081	013.32	.01	.020
007.4	.06	182-184	011.01	.04	.079-081	011.92	.04	.079-081	013.33	.01	.020
007.5	.06	182-184	011.02	.04	.079-081	011.93	.04	.079-081	013.34	.01	.020
007.8	.06	182-184	011.03	.04	.079-081	011.94	.04	.079-081	013.35	.01	.020
007.9	.06	182-184	011.04	.04	.079-081	011.95	.04	.079-081	013.36	.01	.020
008.00	.06	182-184	011.05	.04	.079-081	011.96	.04	.079-081	013.40	.01	.020
008.01	.06	182-184	011.06	.04	.079-081	012.00	.04	.079-081	013.41	.01	.020
008.02	.06	182-184	011.10	.04	.079-081	012.01	.04	.079-081	013.42	.01	.020
008.03	.06	182-184	011.11	.04	.079-081	012.02	.04	.079-081	013.43	.01	.020
008.04	.06	182-184	011.12	.04	.079-081	012.03	.04	.079-081	013.44	.01	.020
008.09	.06	182-184	011.13	.04	.079-081	012.04	.04	.079-081	013.45	.01	.020
008.1	.06	182-184	011.14	.04	.079-081	012.05	.04	.079-081	013.46	.01	.020
008.2	.06	182-184	011.15	.04	.079-081	012.06	.04	.079-081	013.50	.01	.020
008.3	.06	182-184	011.16	.04	.079-081	012.10	.04	.079-081	013.51	.01	.020
008.41	.06	182-184	011.20	.04	.079-081	012.11	.04	.079-081	013.52	.01	.020
008.42	.06	182-184	011.21	.04	.079-081	012.12	.04	.079-081	013.53	.01	.020
008.43	.06	182-184	011.22	.04	.079-081	012.13	.04	.079-081	013.54	.01	.020
008.44	.06	182-184	011.23	.04	.079-081	012.14	.04	.079-081	013.55	.01	.020
008.45	.06	182-184	011.24	.04	.079-081	012.15	.04	.079-081	013.56	.01	.020

Diagnosis Code/MDC/DRG List

DX	MDC	DRG
013.60	.01	.020
013.61	.01	.020
013.62	.01	.020
013.63	.01	.020
013.64	.01	.020
013.65	.01	.020
013.66	.01	.020
013.80	.01	.020
013.81	.01	.020
013.82	.01	.020
013.83	.01	.020
013.84	.01	.020
013.85	.01	.020
013.86	.01	.020
013.90	.01	.020
013.91	.01	.020
013.92	.01	.020
013.93	.01	.020
013.94	.01	.020
013.95	.01	.020
013.96	.01	.020
014.00	.06	.188-190
014.01	.06	.188-190
014.02	.06	.188-190
014.03	.06	.188-190
014.04	.06	.188-190
014.05	.06	.188-190
014.06	.06	.188-190
014.80	.06	.188-190
014.81	.06	.188-190
014.82	.06	.188-190
014.83	.06	.188-190
014.84	.06	.188-190
014.85	.06	.188-190
014.86	.06	.188-190
015.00	.08	.238
015.01	.08	.238
015.02	.08	.238
015.03	.08	.238
015.04	.08	.238
015.05	.08	.238
015.06	.08	.238
015.10	.08	.242
015.11	.08	.242
015.12	.08	.242
015.13	.08	.242
015.14	.08	.242
015.15	.08	.242
015.16	.08	.242
015.20	.08	.242
015.21	.08	.242
015.22	.08	.242
015.23	.08	.242
015.24	.08	.242
015.25	.08	.242
015.26	.08	.242
015.50	.08	.238
015.51	.08	.238
015.52	.08	.238
015.53	.08	.238
015.54	.08	.238
015.55	.08	.238
015.56	.08	.238
015.60	.03	.073-074
015.61	.03	.073-074
015.62	.03	.073-074
015.63	.03	.073-074
015.64	.03	.073-074
015.65	.03	.073-074
015.66	.03	.073-074
015.70	.08	.238
015.71	.08	.238
015.72	.08	.238
015.73	.08	.238
015.74	.08	.238
015.75	.08	.238
015.76	.08	.238
015.80	.08	.242
015.81	.08	.242
015.82	.08	.242
015.83	.08	.242
015.84	.08	.242
015.85	.08	.242
015.86	.08	.242
015.90	.08	.242
015.91	.08	.242
015.92	.08	.242
015.93	.08	.242
015.94	.08	.242
015.95	.08	.242
015.96	.08	.242
016.00	.11	.320-322
016.01	.11	.320-322
016.02	.11	.320-322
016.03	.11	.320-322
016.04	.11	.320-322
016.05	.11	.320-322
016.06	.11	.320-322
016.10	.11	.320-322
016.11	.11	.320-322
016.12	.11	.320-322
016.13	.11	.320-322
016.14	.11	.320-322
016.15	.11	.320-322
016.16	.11	.320-322
016.20	.11	.320-322
016.21	.11	.320-322
016.22	.11	.320-322
016.23	.11	.320-322
016.24	.11	.320-322
016.25	.11	.320-322
016.26	.11	.320-322
016.30	.11	.320-322
016.31	.11	.320-322
016.32	.11	.320-322
016.33	.11	.320-322
016.34	.11	.320-322
016.35	.11	.320-322
016.36	.11	.320-322
016.40	.12	.350
016.41	.12	.350
016.42	.12	.350
016.43	.12	.350
016.44	.12	.350
016.45	.12	.350
016.46	.12	.350
016.50	.12	.350
016.51	.12	.350
016.52	.12	.350
016.53	.12	.350
016.54	.12	.350
016.55	.12	.350
016.56	.12	.350
016.60	.13	.358-359,368
016.61	.13	.358-359,368
016.62	.13	.358-359,368
016.63	.13	.358-359,368
016.64	.13	.358-359,368
016.65	.13	.358-359,368
016.66	.13	.358-359,368
016.70	.13	.358-359,368
016.71	.13	.358-359,368
016.72	.13	.358-359,368
016.73	.13	.358-359,368
016.74	.13	.358-359,368
016.75	.13	.358-359,368
016.76	.13	.358-359,368
016.90	.11	.320-322
016.91	.11	.320-322
016.92	.11	.320-322
016.93	.11	.320-322
016.94	.11	.320-322
016.95	.11	.320-322
016.96	.11	.320-322
017.00	.09	.283-284
017.01	.09	.283-284
017.02	.09	.283-284
017.03	.09	.283-284
017.04	.09	.283-284
017.05	.09	.283-284
017.06	.09	.283-284
017.10	.09	.272-273
017.11	.09	.272-273
017.12	.09	.272-273
017.13	.09	.272-273
017.14	.09	.272-273
017.15	.09	.272-273
017.16	.09	.272-273
017.20	.16	.398-399
017.21	.16	.398-399
017.22	.16	.398-399
017.23	.16	.398-399
017.24	.16	.398-399
017.25	.16	.398-399
017.26	.16	.398-399
017.30	.02	.046-048
017.31	.02	.046-048
017.32	.02	.046-048
017.33	.02	.046-048
017.34	.02	.046-048
017.35	.02	.046-048
017.36	.02	.046-048
017.40	.03	.073-074
017.41	.03	.073-074
017.42	.03	.073-074
017.43	.03	.073-074
017.44	.03	.073-074
017.45	.03	.073-074
017.46	.03	.073-074
017.50	.10	.300-301
017.51	.10	.300-301
017.52	.10	.300-301
017.53	.10	.300-301
017.54	.10	.300-301
017.55	.10	.300-301
017.56	.10	.300-301
017.60	.10	.300-301
017.61	.10	.300-301
017.62	.10	.300-301
017.63	.10	.300-301
017.64	.10	.300-301
017.65	.10	.300-301
017.66	.10	.300-301
017.70	.16	.398-399
017.71	.16	.398-399
017.72	.16	.398-399
017.73	.16	.398-399
017.74	.16	.398-399
017.75	.16	.398-399
017.76	.16	.398-399
017.80	.06	.188-190
017.81	.06	.188-190
017.82	.06	.188-190
017.83	.06	.188-190
017.84	.06	.188-190
017.85	.06	.188-190
017.86	.06	.188-190
017.90	.18	.423
017.91	.18	.423
017.92	.18	.423
017.93	.18	.423
017.94	.18	.423
017.95	.18	.423
017.96	.18	.423
018.00	.18	.423
018.01	.18	.423
018.02	.18	.423
018.03	.18	.423
018.04	.18	.423
018.05	.18	.423
018.06	.18	.423
018.80	.18	.423
018.81	.18	.423
018.82	.18	.423
018.83	.18	.423
018.84	.18	.423
018.85	.18	.423
018.86	.18	.423
018.90	.18	.423
018.91	.18	.423
018.92	.18	.423
018.93	.18	.423
018.94	.18	.423
018.95	.18	.423
018.96	.18	.423
020.0	.18	.423
020.1	.18	.423
020.2	.18	.416-417
020.3	.04	.079-081
020.4	.04	.079-081
020.5	.04	.079-081
020.8	.18	.423
020.9	.18	.423
021.0	.18	.423
021.1	.06	.188-190
021.2	.04	.079-081
021.3	.18	.423
021.8	.18	.423
021.9	.18	.423
022.0	.09	.283-284
022.1	.04	.079-081
022.2	.06	.188-190
022.3	.18	.416-417
022.8	.18	.423
022.9	.18	.423
023.0	.18	.423
023.1	.18	.423
023.2	.18	.423
023.3	.18	.423
023.8	.18	.423
023.9	.18	.423
024	.18	.423
025	.18	.423
026.0	.18	.423
026.1	.18	.423
026.9	.18	.423
027.0	.18	.423
027.1	.18	.423
027.2	.18	.423
027.8	.18	.423
027.9	.18	.423
030.0	.18	.423
030.1	.18	.423
030.2	.18	.423
030.3	.18	.423
030.8	.18	.423
030.9	.18	.423
031.0	.04	.079-081
031.1	.09	.283-284
031.2	.18	.423
031.8	.18	.423
031.9	.18	.423
032.0	.03	.073-074
032.1	.03	.073-074
032.2	.03	.073-074
032.3	.03	.073-074
032.81	.02	.046-048
032.82	.05	.144-145
032.83	.06	.188-190
032.84	.11	.320-322
032.85	.09	.283-284
032.89	.18	.423
032.9	.18	.423
033.0	.04	.096-098
033.1	.04	.096-098
033.8	.04	.096-098
033.9	.04	.096-098
034.0	.03	.068-070

Diagnosis Code/MDC/DRG List

DX	MDC	DRG
034.1	18	423
035	09	277-279
036.0	01	020
036.1	01	020
036.2	18	416-417
036.3	18	416-417
036.40	05	144-145
036.41	05	144-145
036.42	05	126
036.43	05	144-145
036.81	02	045
036.82	08	242
036.89	18	416-417
036.9	18	416-417
037	18	423
038.0	18	416-417
038.10	18	416-417
038.11	18	416-417
038.19	18	416-417
038.2	18	416-417
038.3	18	416-417
038.40	18	416-417
038.41	18	416-417
038.42	18	416-417
038.43	18	416-417
038.44	18	416-417
038.49	18	416-417
038.8	18	416-417
038.9	18	416-417
039.0	09	283-284
039.1	04	079-081
039.2	06	188-190
039.3	09	283-284
039.4	09	283-284
039.8	18	423
039.9	18	423
040.0	18	423
040.1	18	423
040.2	06	188-190
040.3	18	423
040.81	08	248
040.82	18	423
040.89	18	423
041.00	18	423
041.01	18	423
041.02	18	423
041.03	18	423
041.04	18	423
041.05	18	423
041.09	18	423
041.10	18	423
041.11	18	423
041.19	18	423
041.2	18	423
041.3	18	423
041.4	18	423
041.5	18	423
041.6	18	423
041.7	18	423
041.81	18	423
041.82	18	423
041.83	18	423
041.84	18	423
041.85	18	423
041.86	18	423
041.89	18	423
041.9	18	423
042	25	489-490
045.00	01	020
045.01	01	020
045.02	01	020
045.03	01	020
045.10	01	020
045.11	01	020
045.12	01	020
045.13	01	020
045.20	18	421-422
045.21	18	421-422
045.22	18	421-422
045.23	18	421-422
045.90	01	020
045.91	01	020
045.92	01	020
045.93	01	020
046.0	01	012
046.1	01	012
046.2	01	012
046.3	01	012
046.8	01	012
046.9	01	012
047.0	01	021
047.1	01	021
047.8	01	021
047.9	01	021
048	01	021
049.0	01	021
049.1	01	021
049.8	01	020
049.9	01	020
050.0	18	421-422
050.1	18	421-422
050.2	18	421-422
050.9	18	421-422
051.0	18	421-422
051.1	09	283-284
051.2	09	283-284
051.9	18	421-422
052.0	01	020
052.1	04	079-081
052.7	18	421-422
052.8	18	421-422
052.9	18	421-422
053.0	01	021
053.10	01	018-019
053.11	01	018-019
053.12	01	018-019
053.13	01	018-019
053.19	01	018-019
053.20	02	046-048
053.21	02	046-048
053.22	02	046-048
053.29	02	046-048
053.71	03	073-074
053.79	18	421-422
053.8	18	421-422
053.9	09	272-273
054.0	09	283-284
054.10	12	350
054.10	13	358-359,368
054.11	13	358-359,368
054.12	13	358-359,368
054.13	12	350
054.19	12	350
054.19	13	358-359,368
054.2	03	185-187
054.3	01	020
054.40	02	046-048
054.41	02	046-048
054.42	02	046-048
054.43	02	046-048
054.44	02	046-048
054.49	02	046-048
054.5	18	416-417
054.6	09	283-284
054.71	06	188-190
054.72	01	021
054.73	03	073-074
054.79	18	421-422
054.8	18	421-422
054.9	09	283-284
055.0	01	020
055.1	04	079-081
055.2	03	068-070
055.71	02	046-048
055.79	18	421-422
055.8	18	421-422
055.9	18	421-422
056.00	01	018-019
056.01	01	020
056.09	01	020
056.71	08	244-245
056.79	18	421-422
056.8	18	421-422
056.9	18	421-422
057.0	18	421-422
057.8	18	421-422
057.9	18	421-422
060.0	18	421-422
060.1	18	421-422
060.9	18	421-422
061	18	421-422
062.0	01	020
062.1	01	020
062.2	01	020
062.3	01	020
062.4	01	020
062.5	01	020
062.8	01	020
062.9	01	020
063.0	01	020
063.1	01	020
063.2	01	020
063.8	01	020
063.9	01	020
064	01	020
065.0	18	421-422
065.1	18	421-422
065.2	18	421-422
065.3	18	421-422
065.4	18	421-422
065.8	18	421-422
065.9	18	421-422
066.0	18	421-422
066.1	18	421-422
066.2	01	020
066.3	18	421-422
066.4	18	421-422
066.8	18	421-422
066.9	18	421-422
070.0	07	205-206
070.1	07	205-206
070.20	07	205-206
070.21	07	205-206
070.22	07	205-206
070.23	07	205-206
070.30	07	205-206
070.31	07	205-206
070.32	07	205-206
070.33	07	205-206
070.41	07	205-206
070.42	07	205-206
070.43	07	205-206
070.44	07	205-206
070.49	07	205-206
070.51	07	205-206
070.52	07	205-206
070.53	07	205-206
070.54	07	205-206
070.59	07	205-206
070.6	07	205-206
070.9	07	205-206
071	01	020
072.0	12	350
072.1	01	021
072.2	01	020
072.3	07	204
072.71	07	205-206
072.72	01	018-019
072.79	18	421-422
072.8	18	421-422
072.9	18	421-422
073.0	04	079-081
073.7	18	421-422
073.8	18	421-422
073.9	18	421-422
074.0	03	068-070
074.1	04	089-091
074.20	05	144-145
074.21	05	144-145
074.22	05	135-137
074.23	05	144-145
074.3	18	421-422
074.8	18	421-422
075	18	421-422
076.0	02	046-048
076.1	02	046-048
076.9	02	046-048
077.0	02	046-048
077.1	02	046-048
077.2	02	046-048
077.3	02	046-048
077.4	02	046-048
077.8	02	046-048
077.98	02	046-048
077.99	02	046-048
078.0	09	283-284
078.10	09	283-284
078.11	09	283-284
078.19	09	283-284
078.2	18	421-422
078.3	16	398-399
078.4	18	421-422
078.5	18	421-422
078.6	11	320-322
078.7	18	421-422
078.81	01	034-035
078.82	06	182-184
078.88	18	421-422
078.89	18	421-422
079.0	18	421-422
079.1	18	421-422
079.2	18	421-422
079.3	18	421-422
079.4	18	421-422
079.50	18	421-422
079.51	18	421-422
079.52	18	421-422
079.53	18	421-422
079.59	18	421-422
079.6	18	421-422
079.81	18	421-422
079.88	18	421-422
079.89	18	421-422
079.98	18	421-422
079.99	18	421-422
080	18	423
081.0	18	423
081.1	18	423
081.2	18	423
081.9	18	423
082.0	18	423
082.1	18	423
082.2	18	423
082.3	18	423
082.40	18	423
082.41	18	423
082.49	18	423
082.8	18	423
082.9	18	423
083.0	18	423
083.1	18	423
083.2	18	423
083.8	18	423
083.9	18	423
084.0	18	423
084.1	18	423
084.2	18	423
084.3	18	423

Diagnosis Code/MDC/DRG List

DX	MDC	DRG
084.4	18	423
084.5	18	423
084.6	18	423
084.7	18	423
084.8	18	423
084.9	18	423
085.0	18	423
085.1	09	283-284
085.2	09	283-284
085.3	09	283-284
085.4	09	283-284
085.5	09	283-284
085.9	18	423
086.0	05	144-145
086.1	18	423
086.2	18	423
086.3	18	423
086.4	18	423
086.5	18	423
086.9	18	423
087.0	18	423
087.1	18	423
087.9	18	423
088.0	18	423
088.81	18	423
088.82	18	423
088.89	18	423
088.9	18	423
090.0	18	423
090.1	18	423
090.2	18	423
090.3	02	046-048
090.40	01	020
090.41	01	020
090.42	01	020
090.49	01	020
090.5	18	423
090.6	18	423
090.7	18	423
090.9	18	423
091.0	12	350
091.0	13	358-359,368
091.1	06	188-190
091.2	18	423
091.3	09	283-284
091.4	16	398-399
091.50	02	046-048
091.51	02	046-048
091.52	02	046-048
091.61	08	238
091.62	07	205-206
091.69	06	188-190
091.7	18	423
091.81	01	020
091.82	09	283-284
091.89	18	423
091.9	18	423
092.0	18	423
092.9	18	423
093.0	05	135-137
093.1	05	135-137
093.20	05	126
093.21	05	135-137
093.22	05	135-137
093.23	05	135-137
093.24	05	135-137
093.81	05	144-145
093.82	05	144-145
093.89	05	144-145
093.9	05	144-145
094.0	01	012
094.1	01	012
094.2	01	020
094.3	01	020
094.81	01	020
094.82	01	012
094.83	02	046-048
094.84	02	046-048
094.85	01	012
094.86	03	073-074
094.87	01	034-035
094.89	01	012
094.9	01	012
095.0	02	046-048
095.1	04	079-081
095.2	06	188-190
095.3	07	205-206
095.4	11	320-322
095.5	08	238
095.6	08	248
095.7	08	248
095.8	18	423
095.9	18	423
096	18	423
097.0	18	423
097.1	18	423
097.9	18	423
098.0	12	350
098.0	13	358-359,368
098.10	12	350
098.10	13	358-359,368
098.11	11	320-322
098.12	12	350
098.13	12	350
098.14	12	350
098.15	13	358-359,368
098.16	13	358-359,368
098.17	13	358-359,368
098.19	12	350
098.19	13	358-359,368
098.2	12	350
098.2	13	358-359,368
098.30	11	320-322
098.31	11	320-322
098.32	12	350
098.33	12	350
098.34	12	350
098.35	13	358-359,368
098.36	13	358-359,368
098.37	13	358-359,368
098.39	12	350
098.39	13	358-359,368
098.40	02	046-048
098.41	02	046-048
098.42	02	046-048
098.43	02	046-048
098.49	02	046-048
098.50	08	242
098.51	08	242
098.52	08	242
098.53	08	238
098.59	08	242
098.6	03	068-070
098.7	06	188-190
098.81	02	046-048
098.82	01	020
098.83	05	144-145
098.84	05	126
098.85	05	144-145
098.86	06	188-190
098.89	18	423
099.0	12	350
099.0	13	358-359,368
099.1	12	350
099.1	13	358-359,368
099.2	12	350
099.2	13	358-359,368
099.3	08	240-241
099.40	12	350
099.41	13	358-359,368
099.41	12	350
099.41	13	358-359,368
099.49	12	350
099.49	13	358-359,368
099.50	12	350
099.50	13	358-359,368
099.51	03	068-070
099.52	06	188-190
099.53	12	350
099.53	13	358-359,368
099.54	11	320-322
099.55	12	350
099.55	13	358-359,368
099.56	06	188-190
099.59	12	350
099.59	13	358-359,368
099.8	12	350
099.8	13	358-359,368
099.9	12	350
099.9	13	358-359,368
100.0	18	423
100.81	01	020
100.89	01	020
100.9	18	423
101	03	068-070
102.0	09	283-284
102.1	09	283-284
102.2	09	283-284
102.3	09	283-284
102.4	09	283-284
102.5	03	073-074
102.6	08	242
102.7	18	423
102.8	18	423
102.9	18	423
103.0	09	283-284
103.1	09	283-284
103.2	18	423
103.3	09	283-284
103.9	18	423
104.0	18	423
104.8	18	423
104.9	18	423
110.0	09	283-284
110.1	09	283-284
110.2	09	283-284
110.3	09	283-284
110.4	09	283-284
110.5	09	283-284
110.6	09	283-284
110.8	09	283-284
110.9	09	283-284
111.0	09	283-284
111.1	09	283-284
111.2	09	283-284
111.3	09	283-284
111.8	09	283-284
111.9	09	283-284
112.0	03	185-187
112.1	13	358-359,368
112.2	12	350
112.2	13	358-359,368
112.3	09	283-284
112.4	04	079-081
112.5	18	423
112.81	05	126
112.82	03	073-074
112.83	01	020
112.84	06	182-184
112.85	06	182-184
112.89	18	423
112.9	18	423
114.0	04	079-081
114.1	09	283-284
114.2	01	020
114.3	18	423
114.4	04	079-081
114.5	04	079-081
114.9	18	423
115.00	18	423
115.01	01	020
115.02	02	046-048
115.03	05	144-145
115.04	05	126
115.05	04	079-081
115.09	18	423
115.10	18	423
115.11	01	020
115.12	02	046-048
115.13	05	144-145
115.14	05	126
115.15	04	079-081
115.19	18	423
115.90	18	423
115.91	01	020
115.92	02	046-048
115.93	05	144-145
115.94	05	126
115.95	04	079-081
115.99	18	423
116.0	18	423
116.1	18	423
116.2	18	423
117.0	18	423
117.1	18	423
117.2	18	423
117.3	18	423
117.4	18	423
117.5	18	423
117.6	18	423
117.7	18	423
117.8	18	423
117.9	18	423
118	18	423
120.0	11	320-322
120.1	07	205-206
120.2	18	423
120.3	09	283-284
120.8	18	423
120.9	18	423
121.0	07	205-206
121.1	07	205-206
121.2	04	079-081
121.3	07	205-206
121.4	07	205-206
121.5	18	423
121.6	18	423
121.8	18	423
121.9	18	423
122.0	07	205-206
122.1	04	079-081
122.2	10	300-301
122.3	18	423
122.4	18	423
122.5	07	205-206
122.6	18	423
122.7	18	423
122.8	07	205-206
122.9	18	423
123.0	06	182-184
123.1	06	182-184
123.2	06	182-184
123.3	06	182-184
123.4	06	182-184
123.5	06	182-184
123.6	06	182-184
123.8	06	182-184
123.9	06	182-184
124	18	423
125.0	18	423
125.1	18	423
125.2	18	423
125.3	18	423
125.4	18	423
125.5	18	423
125.6	18	423
125.7	18	423
125.9	18	423

DX ....MDC ....DRG	DX ....MDC ....DRG	DX ....MDC ....DRG	DX ....MDC ....DRG
126.0 ...06 182-184	140.5 ...03 064	151.9 ...06 172-173	165.9 ...04 082
126.1 ...06 182-184	140.6 ...03 064	152.0 ...06 172-173	170.0 ...08 239
126.2 ...06 182-184	140.8 ...03 064	152.1 ...06 172-173	170.1 ...08 239
126.3 ...06 182-184	140.9 ...03 064	152.2 ...06 172-173	170.2 ...08 239
126.8 ...06 182-184	141.0 ...03 064	152.3 ...06 172-173	170.3 ...08 239
126.9 ...06 182-184	141.1 ...03 064	152.8 ...06 172-173	170.4 ...08 239
127.0 ...06 182-184	141.2 ...03 064	152.9 ...06 172-173	170.5 ...08 239
127.1 ...06 182-184	141.3 ...03 064	153.0 ...06 172-173	170.6 ...08 239
127.2 ...06 182-184	141.4 ...03 064	153.1 ...06 172-173	170.7 ...08 239
127.3 ...06 182-184	141.5 ...03 064	153.2 ...06 172-173	170.8 ...08 239
127.4 ...06 182-184	141.6 ...03 064	153.3 ...06 172-173	170.9 ...08 239
127.5 ...06 182-184	141.8 ...03 064	153.4 ...06 172-173	171.0 ...08 239
127.6 ...06 182-184	141.9 ...03 064	153.5 ...06 164-165,172-173	171.2 ...08 239
127.7 ...06 182-184	142.0 ...03 064	153.6 ...06 172-173	171.3 ...08 239
127.8 ...18 423	142.1 ...03 064	153.7 ...06 172-173	171.4 ...08 239
127.9 ...06 182-184	142.2 ...03 064	153.8 ...06 172-173	171.5 ...08 239
128.0 ...18 423	142.8 ...03 064	153.9 ...06 172-173	171.6 ...08 239
128.1 ...18 423	142.9 ...03 064	154.0 ...06 172-173	171.7 ...08 239
128.8 ...18 423	143.0 ...03 064	154.1 ...06 172-173	171.8 ...08 239
128.9 ...18 423	143.1 ...03 064	154.2 ...06 172-173	171.9 ...08 239
129 ....06 182-184	143.8 ...03 064	154.3 ...06 172-173	172.0 ...09 272-273
130.0 ...01 020	143.9 ...03 064	154.8 ...06 172-173	172.1 ...02 046-048
130.1 ...02 046-048	144.0 ...03 064	155.0 ...07 199,203	172.2 ...09 272-273
130.2 ...02 046-048	144.1 ...03 064	155.1 ...07 199,203	172.3 ...09 272-273
130.3 ...05 144-145	144.8 ...03 064	155.2 ...07 199,203	172.4 ...09 272-273
130.4 ...04 079-081	144.9 ...03 064	156.0 ...07 199,203	172.5 ...09 272-273
130.5 ...07 205-206	145.0 ...03 064	156.1 ...07 199,203	172.6 ...09 272-273
130.7 ...18 423	145.1 ...03 064	156.2 ...07 199,203	172.7 ...09 272-273
130.8 ...18 423	145.2 ...03 064	156.8 ...07 199,203	172.8 ...09 272-273
130.9 ...18 423	145.3 ...03 064	156.9 ...07 199,203	172.9 ...09 272-273
131.00 ...12 350	145.4 ...03 064	157.0 ...07 199,203	173.0 ...09 283-284
131.00 ...13 358-359,368	145.5 ...03 064	157.1 ...07 199,203	173.1 ...02 046-048
131.01 ...13 358-359,368	145.6 ...03 064	157.2 ...07 199,203	173.2 ...09 283-284
131.02 ...12 350	145.8 ...03 064	157.3 ...07 199,203	173.3 ...09 283-284
131.02 ...13 358-359,368	145.9 ...03 064	157.4 ...07 199,203	173.4 ...09 283-284
131.03 ...12 350	146.0 ...03 064	157.8 ...07 199,203	173.5 ...09 283-284
131.09 ...12 350	146.1 ...03 064	157.9 ...07 199,203	173.6 ...09 283-284
131.09 ...13 358-359,368	146.2 ...03 064	158.0 ...17 413-414	173.7 ...09 283-284
131.8 ...18 423	146.3 ...03 064	158.8 ...06 172-173	173.8 ...09 283-284
131.9 ...18 423	146.4 ...03 064	158.9 ...06 172-173	173.9 ...09 283-284
132.0 ...09 283-284	146.5 ...03 064	159.0 ...06 172-173	174.0 ...09 257-260,274-275
132.1 ...09 283-284	146.6 ...03 064	159.1 ...17 400-404	174.1 ...09 257-260,274-275
132.2 ...09 283-284	146.7 ...03 064	159.8 ...06 172-173	174.2 ...09 257-260,274-275
132.3 ...09 283-284	146.8 ...03 064	159.9 ...06 172-173	174.3 ...09 257-260,274-275
132.9 ...09 283-284	146.9 ...03 064	160.0 ...03 064	174.4 ...09 257-260,274-275
133.0 ...09 283-284	147.0 ...03 064	160.1 ...03 064	174.5 ...09 257-260,274-275
133.8 ...09 283-284	147.1 ...03 064	160.2 ...03 064	174.6 ...09 257-260,274-275
133.9 ...09 283-284	147.2 ...03 064	160.3 ...03 064	174.8 ...09 257-260,274-275
134.0 ...09 283-284	147.3 ...03 064	160.4 ...03 064	174.9 ...09 257-260,274-275
134.1 ...09 283-284	147.8 ...03 064	160.5 ...03 064	175.0 ...09 257-260,274-275
134.2 ...09 283-284	147.9 ...03 064	160.8 ...03 064	175.9 ...09 257-260,274-275
134.8 ...09 283-284	148.0 ...03 064	160.9 ...03 064	176.0 ...09 283-284
134.9 ...09 283-284	148.1 ...03 064	161.0 ...03 064	176.1 ...09 283-284
135 ....04 092-093	148.2 ...03 064	161.1 ...03 064	176.2 ...03 064
136.0 ...18 423	148.3 ...03 064	161.2 ...03 064	176.3 ...06 172-173
136.1 ...08 240-241	148.8 ...03 064	161.3 ...03 064	176.4 ...04 082
136.2 ...18 423	148.9 ...03 064	161.8 ...03 064	176.5 ...17 400-404
136.3 ...04 079-081	149.0 ...03 064	161.9 ...03 064	176.8 ...09 283-284
136.4 ...18 423	149.1 ...03 064	162.0 ...04 082	176.9 ...09 283-284
136.5 ...18 423	149.8 ...03 064	162.2 ...04 082	179 ....13 354-355,363,366-367
136.8 ...18 423	149.9 ...03 064	162.3 ...04 082	180.0 ...13 354-355,363,366-367
136.9 ...18 423	150.0 ...06 172-173	162.4 ...04 082	180.1 ...13 354-355,363,366-367
137.0 ...04 092-093	150.1 ...06 172-173	162.5 ...04 082	180.8 ...13 354-355,363,366-367
137.1 ...01 034-035	150.2 ...06 172-173	162.8 ...04 082	180.9 ...13 354-355,363,366-367
137.2 ...11 320-322	150.3 ...06 172-173	162.9 ...04 082	181. ....13 354-355,363,366-367
137.3 ...08 256	150.4 ...06 172-173	163.0 ...04 082	182.0 ...13 354-355,363,366-367
137.4 ...18 423	150.5 ...06 172-173	163.1 ...04 082	182.1 ...13 354-355,363,366-367
138 ....01 034-035	150.8 ...06 172-173	163.8 ...04 082	182.8 ...13 354-355,363,366-367
139.0 ...01 034-035	150.9 ...06 172-173	163.9 ...04 082	183.0 ...13 357,363,366-367
139.1 ...02 046-048	151.0 ...06 172-173	164.0 ...17 413-414	183.2 ...13 357,363,366-367
139.8 ...18 423	151.1 ...06 172-173	164.1 ...05 144-145	183.3 ...13 357,363,366-367
	151.2 ...06 172-173	164.2 ...04 082	183.4 ...13 357,363,366-367
Neoplasms	151.3 ...06 172-173	164.3 ...04 082	183.5 ...13 357,363,366-367
140.0 ...03 064	151.4 ...06 172-173	164.8 ...04 082	183.8 ...13 357,363,366-367
140.1 ...03 064	151.5 ...06 172-173	164.9 ...04 082	183.9 ...13 357,363,366-367
140.3 ...03 064	151.6 ...06 172-173	165.0 ...03 064	184.0 ...13 354-355,363,366-367
140.4 ...03 064	151.8 ...06 172-173	165.8 ...04 082	184.1 ...13 354-355,363,366-367

2002 Ingenix, Inc.

Diagnosis Code/MDC/DRG List

DX	MDC	DRG
184.2	13	354-355,363,366-367
184.3	13	354-355,363,366-367
184.4	13	354-355,363,366-367
184.8	13	354-355,363,366-367
184.9	13	354-355,363,366-367
185.	12	338,344,346-347
186.0	12	338,344,346-347
186.9	12	338,344,346-347
187.1	12	338,344,346-347
187.2	12	338,344,346-347
187.3	12	338,344,346-347
187.4	12	338,344,346-347
187.5	12	338,344,346-347
187.6	12	338,344,346-347
187.7	12	338,344,346-347
187.8	12	338,344,346-347
187.9	12	338,344,346-347
188.0	11	303,318-319
188.1	11	303,318-319
188.2	11	303,318-319
188.3	11	303,318-319
188.4	11	303,318-319
188.5	11	303,318-319
188.6	11	303,318-319
188.7	11	303,318-319
188.8	11	303,318-319
188.9	11	303,318-319
189.0	11	303,318-319
189.1	11	303,318-319
189.2	11	303,318-319
189.3	11	303,318-319
189.4	11	303,318-319
189.8	11	303,318-319
189.9	11	303,318-319
190.0	02	046-048
190.1	02	046-048
190.2	02	046-048
190.3	02	046-048
190.4	02	046-048
190.5	02	046-048
190.6	02	046-048
190.7	02	046-048
190.8	02	046-048
190.9	02	046-048
191.0	01	010-011
191.1	01	010-011
191.2	01	010-011
191.3	01	010-011
191.4	01	010-011
191.5	01	010-011
191.6	01	010-011
191.7	01	010-011
191.8	01	010-011
191.9	01	010-011
192.0	01	010-011
192.1	01	010-011
192.2	01	010-011
192.3	01	010-011
192.8	01	010-011
192.9	01	010-011
193	10	300-301
194.0	10	300-301
194.1	10	300-301
194.3	10	300-301
194.4	01	010-011
194.5	01	010-011
194.6	01	010-011
194.8	10	300-301
194.9	10	300-301
195.0	03	064
195.1	04	082
195.2	06	172-173
195.3	12	338,344,346-347
195.3	13	354-355,363,366-367
195.4	17	413-414
195.5	17	413-414
195.8	17	413-414
196.0	17	400-404
196.1	17	400-404
196.2	17	400-404
196.3	17	400-404
196.5	17	400-404
196.6	17	400-404
196.8	17	400-404
196.9	17	400-404
197.0	04	082
197.1	04	082
197.2	04	082
197.3	04	082
197.4	06	172-173
197.5	06	172-173
197.6	06	172-173
197.7	07	199,203
197.8	06	172-173
198.0	11	303,318-319
198.1	11	303,318-319
198.2	09	257-260,274-275
198.3	01	010-011
198.4	01	010-011
198.5	08	239
198.6	13	357,363,366-367
198.7	10	300-301
198.81	09	257-260,274-275
198.82	12	338,344,346-347
198.82	13	354-355,363,366-367
198.89	17	413-414
199.0	17	413-414
199.1	17	413-414
200.00	17	400-404
200.01	17	400-404
200.02	17	400-404
200.03	17	400-404
200.04	17	400-404
200.05	17	400-404
200.06	17	400-404
200.07	17	400-404
200.08	17	400-404
200.10	17	400-404
200.11	17	400-404
200.12	17	400-404
200.13	17	400-404
200.14	17	400-404
200.15	17	400-404
200.16	17	400-404
200.17	17	400-404
200.18	17	400-404
200.20	17	400-404
200.21	17	400-404
200.22	17	400-404
200.23	17	400-404
200.24	17	400-404
200.25	17	400-404
200.26	17	400-404
200.27	17	400-404
200.28	17	400-404
200.80	17	400-404
200.81	17	400-404
200.82	17	400-404
200.83	17	400-404
200.84	17	400-404
200.85	17	400-404
200.86	17	400-404
200.87	17	400-404
200.88	17	400-404
201.00	17	400-404
201.01	17	400-404
201.02	17	400-404
201.03	17	400-404
201.04	17	400-404
201.05	17	400-404
201.06	17	400-404
201.07	17	400-404
201.08	17	400-404
201.10	17	400-404
201.11	17	400-404
201.12	17	400-404
201.13	17	400-404
201.14	17	400-404
201.15	17	400-404
201.16	17	400-404
201.17	17	400-404
201.18	17	400-404
201.20	17	400-404
201.21	17	400-404
201.22	17	400-404
201.23	17	400-404
201.24	17	400-404
201.25	17	400-404
201.26	17	400-404
201.27	17	400-404
201.28	17	400-404
201.40	17	400-404
201.41	17	400-404
201.42	17	400-404
201.43	17	400-404
201.44	17	400-404
201.45	17	400-404
201.46	17	400-404
201.47	17	400-404
201.48	17	400-404
201.50	17	400-404
201.51	17	400-404
201.52	17	400-404
201.53	17	400-404
201.54	17	400-404
201.55	17	400-404
201.56	17	400-404
201.57	17	400-404
201.58	17	400-404
201.60	17	400-404
201.61	17	400-404
201.62	17	400-404
201.63	17	400-404
201.64	17	400-404
201.65	17	400-404
201.66	17	400-404
201.67	17	400-404
201.68	17	400-404
201.70	17	400-404
201.71	17	400-404
201.72	17	400-404
201.73	17	400-404
201.74	17	400-404
201.75	17	400-404
201.76	17	400-404
201.77	17	400-404
201.78	17	400-404
201.90	17	400-404
201.91	17	400-404
201.92	17	400-404
201.93	17	400-404
201.94	17	400-404
201.95	17	400-404
201.96	17	400-404
201.97	17	400-404
201.98	17	400-404
202.00	17	400-404
202.01	17	400-404
202.02	17	400-404
202.03	17	400-404
202.04	17	400-404
202.05	17	400-404
202.06	17	400-404
202.07	17	400-404
202.08	17	400-404
202.10	17	400-404
202.11	17	400-404
202.12	17	400-404
202.13	17	400-404
202.14	17	400-404
202.15	17	400-404
202.16	17	400-404
202.17	17	400-404
202.18	17	400-404
202.20	17	400-404
202.21	17	400-404
202.22	17	400-404
202.23	17	400-404
202.24	17	400-404
202.25	17	400-404
202.26	17	400-404
202.27	17	400-404
202.28	17	400-404
202.30	17	400-404
202.31	17	400-404
202.32	17	400-404
202.33	17	400-404
202.34	17	400-404
202.35	17	400-404
202.36	17	400-404
202.37	17	400-404
202.38	17	400-404
202.40	17	400-404
202.41	17	400-404
202.42	17	400-404
202.43	17	400-404
202.44	17	400-404
202.45	17	400-404
202.46	17	400-404
202.47	17	400-404
202.48	17	400-404
202.50	17	413-414
202.51	17	413-414
202.52	17	413-414
202.53	17	413-414
202.54	17	413-414
202.55	17	413-414
202.56	17	413-414
202.57	17	413-414
202.58	17	413-414
202.60	17	400-404
202.61	17	400-404
202.62	17	400-404
202.63	17	400-404
202.64	17	400-404
202.65	17	400-404
202.66	17	400-404
202.67	17	400-404
202.68	17	400-404
202.80	17	400-404
202.81	17	400-404
202.82	17	400-404
202.83	17	400-404
202.84	17	400-404
202.85	17	400-404
202.86	17	400-404
202.87	17	400-404
202.88	17	400-404
202.90	17	400-404
202.91	17	400-404
202.92	17	400-404
202.93	17	400-404
202.94	17	400-404
202.95	17	400-404
202.96	17	400-404
202.97	17	400-404
202.98	17	400-404
203.00	17	400-404
203.01	17	400-404
203.10	17	400-404
203.11	17	400-404
203.80	17	400-404
203.81	17	400-404
204.00	17	400,405,473
204.01	17	400,405,473
204.10	17	400-404
204.11	17	400-404
204.20	17	400-404

DX .... MDC .... DRG	DX .... MDC .... DRG	DX .... MDC .... DRG	DX .... MDC .... DRG
204.21 ..17 400-404	213.2 ...08 256	225.4 ...01 010-011	236.90 ..11 303,318-319
204.80 ..17 400-404	213.3 ...04 082	225.8 ...01 010-011	236.91 ..11 303,318-319
204.81 ..17 400-404	213.4 ...08 256	225.9 ...01 010-011	236.99 ..11 303,318-319
204.90 ..17 400-404	213.5 ...08 256	226 ....10 300-301	237.0 ...10 300-301
204.91 ..17 400-404	213.6 ...08 256	227.0 ...10 300-301	237.1 ...01 010-011
205.00 ..17 400,405,473	213.7 ...08 256	227.1 ...10 300-301	237.2 ...10 300-301
205.01 ..17 400,405,473	213.8 ...08 256	227.3 ...10 300-301	237.3 ...01 010-011
205.10 ..17 400-404	213.9 ...08 256	227.4 ...01 010-011	237.4 ...10 300-301
205.11 ..17 400-404	214.0 ...09 283-284	227.5 ...01 010-011	237.5 ...01 010-011
205.20 ..17 400-404	214.1 ...09 283-284	227.6 ...01 010-011	237.6 ...01 010-011
205.21 ..17 400-404	214.2 ...04 082	227.8 ...10 300-301	237.70 ..01 034-035
205.30 ..17 400-404	214.3 ...06 188-190	227.9 ...10 300-301	237.71 ..01 034-035
205.31 ..17 400-404	214.4 ...12 352	228.00 ..05 144-145	237.72 ..01 034-035
205.80 ..17 400-404	214.8 ...09 283-284	228.01 ..09 283-284	237.9 ...01 010-011
205.81 ..17 400-404	214.9 ...09 283-284	228.02 ..01 034-035	238.0 ...08 239
205.90 ..17 400-404	215.0 ...08 256	228.03 ..02 046-048	238.1 ...08 256
205.91 ..17 400-404	215.2 ...08 256	228.04 ..06 182-184	238.2 ...09 283-284
206.00 ..17 400,405,473	215.3 ...08 256	228.05 ..05 144-145	238.3 ...09 257-260,274-275
206.01 ..17 400,405,473	215.4 ...08 256	228.1 ...16 398-399	238.4 ...17 400-404
206.10 ..17 400-404	215.5 ...08 256	229.0 ...16 398-399	238.5 ...17 400-404
206.11 ..17 400-404	215.6 ...08 256	229.8 ...17 413-414	238.6 ...17 400-404
206.20 ..17 400-404	215.7 ...08 256	229.9 ...17 413-414	238.7 ...17 400-404
206.21 ..17 400-404	215.8 ...08 256	230.0 ...03 064	238.8 ...17 413-414
206.80 ..17 400-404	215.9 ...08 256	230.1 ...06 172-173	238.9 ...17 413-414
206.81 ..17 400-404	216.0 ...09 283-284	230.2 ...06 172-173	239.0 ...06 172-173
206.90 ..17 400-404	216.1 ...02 046-048	230.3 ...06 172-173	239.1 ...04 082
206.91 ..17 400-404	216.2 ...09 283-284	230.4 ...06 172-173	239.2 ...08 256
207.00 ..17 400,405,473	216.3 ...09 283-284	230.5 ...06 172-173	239.3 ...09 276
207.01 ..17 400,405,473	216.4 ...09 283-284	230.6 ...06 172-173	239.4 ...11 303,318-319
207.10 ..17 400-404	216.5 ...09 283-284	230.7 ...06 172-173	239.5 ...11 303,318-319
207.11 ..17 400-404	216.6 ...09 283-284	230.8 ...07 199,203	239.6 ...01 010-011
207.20 ..17 400-404	216.7 ...09 283-284	230.9 ...06 172-173	239.7 ...10 300-301
207.21 ..17 400-404	216.8 ...09 283-284	231.0 ...03 064	239.8 ...17 413-414
207.80 ..17 400-404	216.9 ...09 283-284	231.1 ...04 082	239.9 ...17 413-414
207.81 ..17 400-404	217 ....09 283-284	231.2 ...04 082	
208.00 ..17 400,405,473	218.0 ...13 358-359,369	231.8 ...04 082	**Endocrine, Nutritional and Metabolic Diseases, and Immunity Disorders**
208.01 ..17 400,405,473	218.1 ...13 358-359,369	231.9 ...04 082	
208.10 ..17 400-404	218.2 ...13 358-359,369	232.0 ...09 283-284	
208.11 ..17 400-404	218.9 ...13 358-359,369	232.1 ...02 046-048	240.0 ...10 300-301
208.20 ..17 400-404	219.0 ...13 358-359,369	232.2 ...09 283-284	240.9 ...10 300-301
208.21 ..17 400-404	219.1 ...13 358-359,369	232.3 ...09 283-284	241.0 ...10 300-301
208.80 ..17 400-404	219.8 ...13 358-359,369	232.4 ...09 283-284	241.1 ...10 300-301
208.81 ..17 400-404	219.9 ...13 358-359,369	232.5 ...09 283-284	241.9 ...10 300-301
208.90 ..17 400-404	220 ....13 358-359,369	232.6 ...09 283-284	242.00 ..10 300-301
208.91 ..17 400-404	221.0 ...13 358-359,369	232.7 ...09 283-284	242.01 ..10 300-301
210.0 ...03 185-187	221.1 ...13 358-359,369	232.8 ...09 283-284	242.10 ..10 300-301
210.1 ...03 185-187	221.2 ...13 358-359,369	232.9 ...09 283-284	242.11 ..10 300-301
210.2 ...03 073-074	221.8 ...13 358-359,369	233.0 ...09 257-260,274-275	242.20 ..10 300-301
210.3 ...03 185-187	221.9 ...13 358-359,369	233.1 ...13 354-355,363,366-367	242.21 ..10 300-301
210.4 ...03 185-187	222.0 ...12 352	233.2 ...13 354-355,363,366-367	242.30 ..10 300-301
210.5 ...03 073-074	222.1 ...12 352	233.3 ...13 354-355,363,366-367	242.31 ..10 300-301
210.6 ...03 073-074	222.2 ...12 352	233.4 ...12 338,344,346-347	242.40 ..10 300-301
210.7 ...03 073-074	222.3 ...12 352	233.5 ...12 338,344,346-347	242.41 ..10 300-301
210.8 ...03 073-074	222.4 ...12 352	233.6 ...12 338,344,346-347	242.80 ..10 300-301
210.9 ...03 073-074	222.8 ...12 352	233.7 ...11 303,318-319	242.81 ..10 300-301
211.0 ...06 188-190	222.9 ...12 352	233.9 ...11 303,318-319	242.90 ..10 300-301
211.1 ...06 188-190	223.0 ...11 303,318-319	234.0 ...02 046-048	242.91 ..10 300-301
211.2 ...06 188-190	223.1 ...11 303,318-319	234.8 ...17 413-414	243 ....10 300-301
211.3 ...06 188-190	223.2 ...11 303,318-319	234.9 ...17 413-414	244.0 ...10 300-301
211.4 ...06 188-190	223.3 ...11 303,318-319	235.0 ...03 064	244.1 ...10 300-301
211.5 ...07 205-206	223.81 ..11 303,318-319	235.1 ...03 064	244.2 ...10 300-301
211.6 ...07 204	223.89 ..11 303,318-319	235.2 ...06 172-173	244.3 ...10 300-301
211.7 ...10 300-301	223.9 ...11 303,318-319	235.3 ...07 199,203	244.8 ...10 300-301
211.8 ...06 188-190	224.0 ...02 046-048	235.4 ...06 172-173	244.9 ...10 300-301
211.9 ...06 188-190	224.1 ...02 046-048	235.5 ...06 172-173	245.0 ...10 300-301
212.0 ...03 073-074	224.2 ...02 046-048	235.6 ...03 064	245.1 ...10 300-301
212.1 ...03 073-074	224.3 ...02 046-048	235.7 ...04 082	245.2 ...10 300-301
212.2 ...04 082	224.4 ...02 046-048	235.8 ...04 082	245.3 ...10 300-301
212.3 ...04 082	224.5 ...02 046-048	235.9 ...04 082	245.4 ...10 300-301
212.4 ...04 082	224.6 ...02 046-048	236.0 ...13 354-355,363,366-367	245.8 ...10 300-301
212.5 ...04 082	224.7 ...02 046-048	236.1 ...13 354-355,363,366-367	245.9 ...10 300-301
212.6 ...16 398-399	224.8 ...02 046-048	236.2 ...13 357,363,366-367	246.0 ...10 300-301
212.7 ...05 144-145	224.9 ...02 046-048	236.3 ...13 354-355,363,366-367	246.1 ...10 300-301
212.8 ...04 082	225.0 ...01 010-011	236.4 ...12 338,344,346-347	246.2 ...10 300-301
212.9 ...04 082	225.1 ...01 010-011	236.5 ...12 338,344,346-347	246.3 ...10 300-301
213.0 ...08 256	225.2 ...01 010-011	236.6 ...12 338,344,346-347	246.8 ...10 300-301
213.1 ...03 185-187	225.3 ...01 010-011	236.7 ...11 303,318-319	246.9 ...10 300-301

DX ... MDC ... DRG	DX ... MDC ... DRG	DX ... MDC ... DRG	DX ... MDC ... DRG
250.00 ...10 294-295	256.2 ...13 358-359,369	272.2 ...10 299	279.3 ...16 398-399
250.01 ...10 294-295	256.31 ...13 358-359,369	272.3 ...10 299	279.4 ...08 240-241
250.02 ...10 294-295	256.39 ...13 358-359,369	272.4 ...10 299	279.8 ...16 398-399
250.03 ...10 294-295	256.4 ...13 358-359,369	272.5 ...10 299	279.9 ...16 398-399
250.10 ...10 294-295	256.8 ...13 358-359,369	272.6 ...10 299	
250.11 ...10 294-295	256.9 ...13 358-359,369	272.7 ...10 299	**Diseases of the Blood and Blood Forming Organs**
250.12 ...10 294-295	257.0 ...10 300-301	272.8 ...10 299	
250.13 ...10 294-295	257.1 ...10 300-301	272.9 ...10 299	280.0 ...16 395-396
250.20 ...10 294-295	257.2 ...10 300-301	273.0 ...16 398-399	280.1 ...16 395-396
250.21 ...10 294-295	257.8 ...10 300-301	273.1 ...16 398-399	280.8 ...16 395-396
250.22 ...10 294-295	257.9 ...10 300-301	273.2 ...17 400-404	280.9 ...16 395-396
250.23 ...10 294-295	258.0 ...10 300-301	273.3 ...17 400-404	281.0 ...16 395-396
250.30 ...10 294-295	258.1 ...10 300-301	273.8 ...17 413-414	281.1 ...16 395-396
250.31 ...10 294-295	258.8 ...10 300-301	273.9 ...17 413-414	281.2 ...16 395-396
250.32 ...10 294-295	258.9 ...10 300-301	274.0 ...08 244-245	281.3 ...16 395-396
250.33 ...10 294-295	259.0 ...10 300-301	274.10 ...11 331-333	281.4 ...16 395-396
250.40 ...11 331-333	259.1 ...10 300-301	274.11 ...11 323-324	281.8 ...16 395-396
250.41 ...11 331-333	259.2 ...10 300-301	274.19 ...11 331-333	281.9 ...16 395-396
250.42 ...11 331-333	259.3 ...10 300-301	274.81 ...08 244-245	282.0 ...16 395-396
250.43 ...11 331-333	259.4 ...10 300-301	274.82 ...08 244-245	282.1 ...16 395-396
250.50 ...02 046-048	259.8 ...10 300-301	274.89 ...08 244-245	282.2 ...16 395-396
250.51 ...02 046-048	259.9 ...10 300-301	274.9 ...08 244-245	282.3 ...16 395-396
250.52 ...02 046-048	260 ....10 296-298	275.0 ...10 299	282.4 ...16 395-396
250.53 ...02 046-048	261 ....10 296-298	275.1 ...10 299	282.5 ...16 395-396
250.60 ...01 018-019	262 ....10 296-298	275.2 ...10 296-298	282.60 ...16 395-396
250.61 ...01 018-019	263.0 ...10 296-298	275.3 ...10 299	282.61 ...16 395-396
250.62 ...01 018-019	263.1 ...10 296-298	275.40 ...10 296-298	282.62 ...16 395-396
250.63 ...01 018-019	263.2 ...10 296-298	275.41 ...10 296-298	282.63 ...16 395-396
250.70 ...05 130-131	263.8 ...10 296-298	275.42 ...10 296-298	282.69 ...16 395-396
250.71 ...05 130-131	263.9 ...10 296-298	275.49 ...10 296-298	282.7 ...16 395-396
250.72 ...05 130-131	264.0 ...02 046-048	275.8 ...10 299	282.8 ...16 395-396
250.73 ...05 130-131	264.1 ...02 046-048	275.9 ...10 299	282.9 ...16 395-396
250.80 ...10 294-295	264.2 ...02 046-048	276.0 ...10 296-298	283.0 ...16 395-396
250.81 ...10 294-295	264.3 ...02 046-048	276.1 ...10 296-298	283.10 ...16 395-396
250.82 ...10 294-295	264.4 ...02 046-048	276.2 ...10 296-298	283.11 ...16 395-396
250.83 ...10 294-295	264.5 ...02 046-048	276.3 ...10 296-298	283.19 ...16 395-396
250.90 ...10 294-295	264.6 ...02 046-048	276.4 ...10 296-298	283.2 ...16 395-396
250.91 ...10 294-295	264.7 ...02 046-048	276.5 ...10 296-298	283.9 ...16 395-396
250.92 ...10 294-295	264.8 ...10 296-298	276.6 ...10 296-298	284.0 ...16 395-396
250.93 ...10 294-295	264.9 ...10 296-298	276.7 ...10 296-298	284.8 ...16 395-396
251.0 ...10 296-298	265.0 ...10 296-298	276.8 ...10 296-298	284.9 ...16 395-396
251.1 ...10 300-301	265.1 ...10 296-298	276.9 ...10 296-298	285.0 ...16 395-396
251.2 ...10 296-298	265.2 ...10 296-298	277.00 ...10 296-298	285.1 ...16 395-396
251.3 ...10 296-298	266.0 ...10 296-298	277.01 ...15 387,389	285.21 ...16 395-396
251.4 ...10 300-301	266.1 ...10 296-298	277.02 ...04 ....79, 80, 81	285.22 ...16 395-396
251.5 ...06 176	266.2 ...10 296-298	277.03 ...06 188-190	285.29 ...16 395-396
251.8 ...10 300-301	266.9 ...10 296-298	277.09 ...10 296-298	285.8 ...16 395-396
251.9 ...10 300-301	267 ....10 296-298	277.1 ...10 299	285.9 ...16 395-396
252.0 ...10 300-301	268.0 ...08 244-245	277.2 ...10 299	286.0 ...16 397
252.1 ...10 300-301	268.1 ...08 244-245	277.3 ...08 240-241	286.1 ...16 397
252.8 ...10 300-301	268.2 ...08 244-245	277.4 ...07 205-206	286.2 ...16 397
252.9 ...10 300-301	268.9 ...10 296-298	277.5 ...10 299	286.3 ...16 397
253.0 ...10 300-301	269.0 ...10 296-298	277.6 ...10 299	286.4 ...16 397
253.1 ...10 300-301	269.1 ...10 296-298	277.7 ...10 299	286.5 ...16 397
253.2 ...10 300-301	269.2 ...10 296-298	277.8 ...10 299	286.6 ...16 397
253.3 ...10 300-301	269.3 ...10 296-298	277.9 ...10 299	286.7 ...16 397
253.4 ...10 300-301	269.8 ...10 296-298	278.00 ...10 296-298	286.9 ...16 397
253.5 ...10 300-301	269.9 ...10 296-298	278.01 ...10 296-298	287.0 ...16 397
253.6 ...10 300-301	270.0 ...10 299	278.1 ...10 296-298	287.1 ...16 397
253.7 ...10 300-301	270.1 ...10 299	278.2 ...10 296-298	287.2 ...16 397
253.8 ...10 300-301	270.2 ...10 299	278.3 ...10 296-298	287.3 ...16 397
253.9 ...10 300-301	270.3 ...10 299	278.4 ...10 296-298	287.4 ...16 397
254.0 ...16 398-399	270.4 ...10 299	278.8 ...10 296-298	287.5 ...16 397
254.1 ...16 398-399	270.5 ...10 299	279.00 ...16 398-399	287.8 ...16 397
254.8 ...16 398-399	270.6 ...10 299	279.01 ...16 398-399	287.9 ...16 397
254.9 ...16 398-399	270.7 ...10 299	279.02 ...16 398-399	288.0 ...16 398-399
255.0 ...10 300-301	270.8 ...10 299	279.03 ...16 398-399	288.1 ...16 398-399
255.1 ...10 300-301	270.9 ...10 299	279.04 ...16 398-399	288.2 ...16 398-399
255.2 ...10 300-301	271.0 ...10 299	279.05 ...16 398-399	288.3 ...16 398-399
255.3 ...10 300-301	271.1 ...10 299	279.06 ...16 398-399	288.8 ...16 398-399
255.4 ...10 300-301	271.2 ...06 182-184	279.09 ...16 398-399	288.9 ...16 398-399
255.5 ...10 300-301	271.3 ...06 182-184	279.10 ...16 398-399	289.0 ...16 398-399
255.6 ...10 300-301	271.4 ...10 299	279.11 ...16 398-399	289.1 ...16 398-399
255.8 ...10 300-301	271.8 ...10 299	279.12 ...16 398-399	289.2 ...06 188-190
255.9 ...10 300-301	271.9 ...10 299	279.13 ...16 398-399	289.3 ...16 398-399
256.0 ...13 358-359,369	272.0 ...10 299	279.19 ...16 398-399	289.4 ...16 398-399
256.1 ...13 358-359,369	272.1 ...10 299	279.2 ...16 398-399	289.50 ...16 398-399

DX ....MDC ....DRG	DX ....MDC ....DRG	DX ....MDC ....DRG	DX ....MDC ....DRG
289.51 ..16 398-399	295.40 ..19 430	296.56 ..19 430	301.81 ..19 428
289.59 ..16 398-399	295.41 ..19 430	296.60 ..19 430	301.82 ..19 428
289.6 ..16 398-399	295.42 ..19 430	296.61 ..19 430	301.83 ..19 428
289.7 ..16 395-396	295.43 ..19 430	296.62 ..19 430	301.84 ..19 428
289.8 ..16 398-399	295.44 ..19 430	296.63 ..19 430	301.89 ..19 428
289.9 ..16 398-399	295.45 ..19 430	296.64 ..19 430	301.9 ...19 428
	295.50 ..19 430	296.65 ..19 430	302.0 ...19 432
Mental Disorders	295.51 ..19 430	296.66 ..19 430	302.1 ...19 432
290.0 ...19 429	295.52 ..19 430	296.7 ...19 430	302.2 ...19 432
290.10 ..19 429	295.53 ..19 430	296.80 ..19 430	302.3 ...19 432
290.11 ..19 429	295.54 ..19 430	296.81 ..19 430	302.4 ...19 432
290.12 ..19 429	295.55 ..19 430	296.82 ..19 430	302.50 ..19 432
290.13 ..19 429	295.60 ..19 430	296.89 ..19 430	302.51 ..19 432
290.20 ..19 429	295.61 ..19 430	296.90 ..19 430	302.52 ..19 432
290.21 ..19 429	295.62 ..19 430	296.99 ..19 430	302.53 ..19 432
290.3 ...19 429	295.63 ..19 430	297.0 ...19 430	302.6 ...19 432
290.40 ..19 429	295.64 ..19 430	297.1 ...19 430	302.70 ..19 432
290.41 ..19 429	295.65 ..19 430	297.2 ...19 430	302.71 ..19 432
290.42 ..19 429	295.70 ..19 430	297.3 ...19 430	302.72 ..19 432
290.43 ..19 429	295.71 ..19 430	297.8 ...19 430	302.73 ..19 432
290.8 ...19 429	295.72 ..19 430	297.9 ...19 430	302.74 ..19 432
290.9 ...19 429	295.73 ..19 430	298.0 ...19 430	302.75 ..19 432
291.0 ...20 521-523	295.74 ..19 430	298.1 ...19 430	302.76 ..19 432
291.1 ...20 521-523	295.75 ..19 430	298.2 ...19 432	302.79 ..19 432
291.2 ...20 521-523	295.80 ..19 430	298.3 ...19 430	302.81 ..19 432
291.3 ...20 521-523	295.81 ..19 430	298.4 ...19 430	302.82 ..19 432
291.4 ...20 521-523	295.82 ..19 430	298.8 ...19 430	302.83 ..19 432
291.5 ...20 521-523	295.83 ..19 430	298.9 ...19 430	302.84 ..19 432
291.81 ..20 521-523	295.84 ..19 430	299.00 ..19 429	302.85 ..19 432
291.89 ..20 521-523	295.85 ..19 430	299.01 ..19 429	302.89 ..19 432
291.9 ...20 521-523	295.90 ..19 430	299.10 ..19 429	302.9 ...19 432
292.0 ...20 521-523	295.91 ..19 430	299.11 ..19 429	303.00 ..20 521-523
292.11 ..20 521-523	295.92 ..19 430	299.80 ..19 430	303.01 ..20 521-523
292.12 ..20 521-523	295.93 ..19 430	299.81 ..19 430	303.02 ..20 521-523
292.2 ...20 521-523	295.94 ..19 430	299.90 ..19 430	303.03 ..20 521-523
292.81 ..20 521-523	295.95 ..19 430	299.91 ..19 430	303.90 ..20 521-523
292.82 ..20 521-523	296.00 ..19 430	300.00 ..19 425	303.91 ..20 521-523
292.83 ..20 521-523	296.01 ..19 430	300.01 ..19 425	303.92 ..20 521-523
292.84 ..20 521-523	296.02 ..19 430	300.02 ..19 425	303.93 ..20 521-523
292.89 ..20 521-523	296.03 ..19 430	300.09 ..19 425	304.00 ..20 521-523
292.9 ...20 521-523	296.04 ..19 430	300.10 ..19 425	304.01 ..20 521-523
293.0 ...19 425	296.05 ..19 430	300.11 ..19 425	304.02 ..20 521-523
293.1 ...19 425	296.06 ..19 430	300.12 ..19 425	304.03 ..20 521-523
293.81 ..19 429	296.10 ..19 430	300.13 ..19 425	304.10 ..20 521-523
293.82 ..19 429	296.11 ..19 430	300.14 ..19 428	304.11 ..20 521-523
293.83 ..19 429	296.12 ..19 430	300.15 ..19 425	304.12 ..20 521-523
293.84 ..19 429	296.13 ..19 430	300.16 ..19 425	304.13 ..20 521-523
293.89 ..19 429	296.14 ..19 430	300.19 ..19 425	304.20 ..20 521-523
293.9 ...19 425	296.15 ..19 430	300.20 ..19 427	304.21 ..20 521-523
294.10 ..19 429	296.16 ..19 430	300.21 ..19 427	304.22 ..20 521-523
294.11 ..19 429	296.20 ..19 430	300.22 ..19 427	304.23 ..20 521-523
294.8 ...19 429	296.21 ..19 430	300.23 ..19 427	304.30 ..20 521-523
294.9 ...19 429	296.22 ..19 430	300.29 ..19 427	304.31 ..20 521-523
295.00 ..19 430	296.23 ..19 430	300.3 ...19 427	304.32 ..20 521-523
295.01 ..19 430	296.24 ..19 430	300.4 ...19 426	304.33 ..20 521-523
295.02 ..19 430	296.25 ..19 430	300.5 ...19 427	304.40 ..20 521-523
295.03 ..19 430	296.26 ..19 430	300.6 ...19 427	304.41 ..20 521-523
295.04 ..19 430	296.30 ..19 430	300.7 ...19 427	304.42 ..20 521-523
295.05 ..19 430	296.31 ..19 430	300.81 ..19 427	304.43 ..20 521-523
295.10 ..19 430	296.32 ..19 430	300.82 ..19 427	304.50 ..20 521-523
295.11 ..19 430	296.33 ..19 430	300.89 ..19 427	304.51 ..20 521-523
295.12 ..19 430	296.34 ..19 430	300.9 ...19 425	304.52 ..20 521-523
295.13 ..19 430	296.35 ..19 430	301.0 ...19 428	304.53 ..20 521-523
295.14 ..19 430	296.36 ..19 430	301.10 ..19 428	304.60 ..20 521-523
295.15 ..19 430	296.40 ..19 430	301.11 ..19 428	304.61 ..20 521-523
295.20 ..19 430	296.41 ..19 430	301.12 ..19 426	304.62 ..20 521-523
295.21 ..19 430	296.42 ..19 430	301.13 ..19 428	304.63 ..20 521-523
295.22 ..19 430	296.43 ..19 430	301.20 ..19 428	304.70 ..20 521-523
295.23 ..19 430	296.44 ..19 430	301.21 ..19 428	304.71 ..20 521-523
295.24 ..19 430	296.45 ..19 430	301.22 ..19 428	304.72 ..20 521-523
295.25 ..19 430	296.46 ..19 430	301.3 ...19 428	304.73 ..20 521-523
295.30 ..19 430	296.50 ..19 430	301.4 ...19 428	304.80 ..20 521-523
295.31 ..19 430	296.51 ..19 430	301.50 ..19 428	304.81 ..20 521-523
295.32 ..19 430	296.52 ..19 430	301.51 ..19 428	304.82 ..20 521-523
295.33 ..19 430	296.53 ..19 430	301.59 ..19 428	304.83 ..20 521-523
295.34 ..19 430	296.54 ..19 430	301.6 ...19 428	304.90 ..20 521-523
295.35 ..19 430	296.55 ..19 430	301.7 ...19 428	304.91 ..20 521-523

DX	MDC	DRG
304.92	20	521-523
304.93	20	521-523
305.00	20	521-523
305.01	20	521-523
305.02	20	521-523
305.03	20	521-523
305.1	23	467
305.20	20	521-523
305.21	20	521-523
305.22	20	521-523
305.23	20	521-523
305.30	20	521-523
305.31	20	521-523
305.32	20	521-523
305.33	20	521-523
305.40	20	521-523
305.41	20	521-523
305.42	20	521-523
305.43	20	521-523
305.50	20	521-523
305.51	20	521-523
305.52	20	521-523
305.53	20	521-523
305.60	20	521-523
305.61	20	521-523
305.62	20	521-523
305.63	20	521-523
305.70	20	521-523
305.71	20	521-523
305.72	20	521-523
305.73	20	521-523
305.80	20	521-523
305.81	20	521-523
305.82	20	521-523
305.83	20	521-523
305.90	20	521-523
305.91	20	521-523
305.92	20	521-523
305.93	20	521-523
306.0	08	248
306.1	04	101-102
306.2	05	144-145
306.3	09	283-284
306.4	06	182-184
306.50	11	331-333
306.51	13	358-359,369
306.52	13	358-359,369
306.53	11	331-333
306.59	11	331-333
306.6	10	300-301
306.7	19	427
306.8	19	432
306.9	19	427
307.0	19	432
307.1	19	428
307.20	01	034-035
307.21	01	034-035
307.22	01	034-035
307.23	01	034-035
307.3	19	432
307.40	19	432
307.41	19	432
307.42	19	432
307.43	19	432
307.44	19	432
307.45	19	432
307.46	19	432
307.47	19	432
307.48	19	432
307.49	19	432
307.50	19	432
307.51	19	432
307.52	19	431
307.53	19	427
307.54	19	427
307.59	19	432
307.6	19	431
307.7	19	431
307.80	19	427
307.81	01	024-026
307.89	19	427
307.9	19	429
308.0	19	425
308.1	19	425
308.2	19	425
308.3	19	425
308.4	19	425
308.9	19	425
309.0	19	426
309.1	19	426
309.21	19	427
309.22	19	427
309.23	19	427
309.24	19	427
309.28	19	427
309.29	19	427
309.3	19	427
309.4	19	427
309.81	19	427
309.82	19	427
309.83	19	427
309.89	19	427
309.9	19	427
310.0	19	429
310.1	19	429
310.2	01	002,024-026
310.8	19	429
310.9	19	429
311	19	426
312.00	19	431
312.01	19	431
312.02	19	431
312.03	19	431
312.10	19	431
312.11	19	431
312.12	19	431
312.13	19	431
312.20	19	431
312.21	19	431
312.22	19	431
312.23	19	431
312.30	19	431
312.31	19	428
312.32	19	428
312.33	19	431
312.34	19	428
312.35	19	428
312.39	19	428
312.4	19	431
312.81	19	431
312.82	19	431
312.89	19	431
312.9	19	431
313.0	19	427
313.1	19	427
313.21	19	431
313.22	19	431
313.23	19	431
313.3	19	431
313.81	19	431
313.82	19	431
313.83	19	431
313.89	19	431
313.9	19	431
314.00	19	431
314.01	19	431
314.1	19	431
314.2	19	431
314.8	19	431
314.9	19	431
315.00	19	431
315.01	19	431
315.02	19	431
315.09	19	431
315.1	19	431
315.2	19	431
315.31	19	431
315.32	19	431
315.39	19	431
315.4	19	431
315.5	19	431
315.8	19	431
315.9	19	431
316	19	429
317	19	429
318.0	19	429
318.1	19	429
318.2	19	429
319	19	429

Diseases of the Nervous System and Sense Organs

DX	MDC	DRG
320.0	01	020
320.1	01	020
320.2	01	020
320.3	01	020
320.7	01	020
320.81	01	020
320.82	01	020
320.89	01	020
320.9	01	020
321.0	01	020
321.1	01	020
321.2	01	020
321.3	01	020
321.4	01	020
321.8	01	020
322.0	01	020
322.1	01	020
322.2	01	020
322.9	01	020
323.0	01	020
323.1	01	020
323.2	01	020
323.4	01	020
323.5	01	020
323.6	01	020
323.7	01	034-035
323.8	01	020
323.9	01	020
324.0	01	020
324.1	01	020
324.9	01	020
325	01	034-035
326	01	034-035
330.0	01	012
330.1	01	012
330.2	01	012
330.3	01	012
330.8	01	012
330.9	01	012
331.0	01	012
331.1	01	012
331.2	01	012
331.3	01	012
331.4	01	012
331.7	01	012
331.81	01	034-035
331.89	01	012
331.9	01	012
332.0	01	012
332.1	01	012
333.0	01	012
333.1	01	034-035
333.2	01	034-035
333.3	01	034-035
333.4	01	012
333.5	01	012
333.6	01	012
333.7	01	012
333.81	02	046-048
333.82	01	034-035
333.83	01	034-035
333.84	01	034-035
333.89	01	034-035
333.90	01	012
333.91	01	034-035
333.92	01	034-035
333.93	01	034-035
333.99	01	012
334.0	01	013
334.1	01	013
334.2	01	013
334.3	01	013
334.4	01	013
334.8	01	013
334.9	01	013
335.0	01	012
335.10	01	012
335.11	01	012
335.19	01	012
335.20	01	012
335.21	01	012
335.22	01	012
335.23	01	012
335.24	01	012
335.29	01	012
335.8	01	012
335.9	01	012
336.0	01	012
336.1	01	034-035
336.2	01	034-035
336.3	01	034-035
336.8	01	034-035
336.9	01	034-035
337.0	01	018-019
337.1	01	018-019
337.20	01	018-019
337.21	01	018-019
337.22	01	018-019
337.29	01	018-019
337.3	01	018-019
337.9	01	018-019
340	01	013
341.0	01	013
341.1	01	013
341.8	01	013
341.9	01	013
342.00	01	012
342.01	01	012
342.02	01	012
342.10	01	012
342.11	01	012
342.12	01	012
342.80	01	012
342.81	01	012
342.82	01	012
342.90	01	012
342.91	01	012
342.92	01	012
343.0	01	009
343.1	01	009
343.2	01	009
343.3	01	034-035
343.4	01	009
343.8	01	034-035
343.9	01	034-035
344.00	01	009
344.01	01	009
344.02	01	009
344.03	01	009
344.04	01	009
344.09	01	009
344.1	01	009
344.2	01	009
344.30	01	034-035
344.31	01	034-035
344.32	01	034-035

DX....MDC....DRG	DX....MDC....DRG	DX....MDC....DRG	DX....MDC....DRG
344.40 ..01 034-035	353.9 ...01 018-019	360.41 ..02 046-048	362.61 ..02 046-048
344.41 ..01 034-035	354.0 ...01 018-019	360.42 ..02 046-048	362.62 ..02 046-048
344.42 ..01 034-035	354.1 ...01 018-019	360.43 ..02 046-048	362.63 ..02 046-048
344.5 ...01 034-035	354.2 ...01 018-019	360.44 ..02 046-048	362.64 ..02 046-048
344.60 ..01 018-019	354.3 ...01 018-019	360.50 ..02 046-048	362.65 ..02 046-048
344.61 ..11 331-333	354.4 ...01 018-019	360.51 ..02 046-048	362.66 ..02 046-048
344.81 ..01 034-035	354.5 ...01 018-019	360.52 ..02 046-048	362.70 ..02 046-048
344.89 ..01 034-035	354.8 ...01 018-019	360.53 ..02 046-048	362.71 ..02 046-048
344.9 ...01 034-035	354.9 ...01 018-019	360.54 ..02 046-048	362.72 ..02 046-048
345.00 ..01 024-026	355.0 ...01 018-019	360.55 ..02 046-048	362.73 ..02 046-048
345.01 ..01 024-026	355.1 ...01 018-019	360.59 ..02 046-048	362.74 ..02 046-048
345.10 ..01 024-026	355.2 ...01 018-019	360.60 ..02 046-048	362.75 ..02 046-048
345.11 ..01 024-026	355.3 ...01 018-019	360.61 ..02 046-048	362.76 ..02 046-048
345.2 ...01 024-026	355.4 ...01 018-019	360.62 ..02 046-048	362.77 ..02 046-048
345.3 ...01 024-026	355.5 ...01 018-019	360.63 ..02 046-048	362.81 ..02 046-048
345.40 ..01 024-026	355.6 ...01 018-019	360.64 ..02 046-048	362.82 ..02 046-048
345.41 ..01 024-026	355.71 ..01 018-019	360.65 ..02 046-048	362.83 ..02 046-048
345.50 ..01 024-026	355.79 ..01 018-019	360.69 ..02 046-048	362.84 ..02 046-048
345.51 ..01 024-026	355.8 ...01 018-019	360.81 ..02 046-048	362.85 ..02 046-048
345.60 ..01 024-026	355.9 ...01 018-019	360.89 ..02 046-048	362.89 ..02 046-048
345.61 ..01 024-026	356.0 ...01 018-019	360.9 ...02 046-048	362.9 ...02 046-048
345.70 ..01 024-026	356.1 ...01 018-019	361.00 ..02 046-048	363.00 ..02 046-048
345.71 ..01 024-026	356.2 ...01 018-019	361.01 ..02 046-048	363.01 ..02 046-048
345.80 ..01 024-026	356.3 ...01 034-035	361.02 ..02 046-048	363.03 ..02 046-048
345.81 ..01 024-026	356.4 ...01 018-019	361.03 ..02 046-048	363.04 ..02 046-048
345.90 ..01 024-026	356.8 ...01 018-019	361.04 ..02 046-048	363.05 ..02 046-048
345.91 ..01 024-026	356.9 ...01 018-019	361.05 ..02 046-048	363.06 ..02 046-048
346.00 ..01 024-026	357.0 ...01 020	361.06 ..02 046-048	363.07 ..02 046-048
346.01 ..01 024-026	357.1 ...01 018-019	361.07 ..02 046-048	363.08 ..02 046-048
346.10 ..01 024-026	357.2 ...01 018-019	361.10 ..02 046-048	363.10 ..02 046-048
346.11 ..01 024-026	357.3 ...01 018-019	361.11 ..02 046-048	363.11 ..02 046-048
346.20 ..01 024-026	357.4 ...01 018-019	361.12 ..02 046-048	363.12 ..02 046-048
346.21 ..01 024-026	357.5 ...01 018-019	361.13 ..02 046-048	363.13 ..02 046-048
346.80 ..01 024-026	357.6 ...01 018-019	361.14 ..02 046-048	363.14 ..02 046-048
346.81 ..01 024-026	357.7 ...01 018-019	361.19 ..02 046-048	363.15 ..02 046-048
346.90 ..01 024-026	357.8 ...01 018-019	361.2 ...02 046-048	363.20 ..02 046-048
346.91 ..01 024-026	357.81 ..01 18-19	361.30 ..02 046-048	363.21 ..02 046-048
347 ....01 034-035	357.82 ..01 18-19	361.31 ..02 046-048	363.22 ..02 046-048
348.0 ...01 034-035	357.89 ..01 18-19	361.32 ..02 046-048	363.30 ..02 046-048
348.1 ...01 034-035	359.81 ..01 34-35	361.33 ..02 046-048	363.31 ..02 046-048
348.2 ...01 024-026	359.89 ..01 34-35	361.81 ..02 046-048	363.32 ..02 046-048
348.3 ...01 016-017	357.9 ...01 018-019	361.89 ..02 046-048	363.33 ..02 046-048
348.4 ...01 023	358.0 ...01 012	361.9 ...02 046-048	363.34 ..02 046-048
348.5 ...01 023	358.1 ...01 012	362.01 ..02 046-048	363.35 ..02 046-048
348.8 ...01 016-017	358.2 ...01 018-019	362.02 ..02 046-048	363.40 ..02 046-048
348.9 ...01 016-017	358.8 ...01 018-019	362.10 ..02 046-048	363.41 ..02 046-048
349.0 ...01 024-026	358.9 ...01 018-019	362.11 ..02 046-048	363.42 ..02 046-048
349.1 ...01 034-035	359.0 ...01 034-035	362.12 ..02 046-048	363.43 ..02 046-048
349.2 ...01 034-035	359.1 ...01 034-035	362.13 ..02 046-048	363.50 ..02 046-048
349.81 ..01 034-035	359.2 ...01 034-035	362.14 ..02 046-048	363.51 ..02 046-048
349.82 ..01 034-035	359.3 ...01 034-035	362.15 ..02 046-048	363.52 ..02 046-048
349.89 ..01 016-017	359.4 ...01 034-035	362.16 ..02 046-048	363.53 ..02 046-048
349.9 ...01 016-017	359.5 ...01 034-035	362.17 ..02 046-048	363.54 ..02 046-048
350.1 ...01 018-019	359.6 ...01 034-035	362.18 ..02 046-048	363.55 ..02 046-048
350.2 ...01 018-019	359.8 ...01 034-035	362.21 ..02 046-048	363.56 ..02 046-048
350.8 ...01 018-019	359.9 ...01 034-035	362.29 ..02 046-048	363.57 ..02 046-048
350.9 ...01 018-019	360.00 ..02 044	362.30 ..02 045	363.61 ..02 046-048
351.0 ...01 018-019	360.01 ..02 044	362.31 ..02 045	363.62 ..02 046-048
351.1 ...01 018-019	360.02 ..02 044	362.32 ..02 045	363.63 ..02 046-048
351.8 ...01 018-019	360.03 ..02 046-048	362.33 ..02 045	363.70 ..02 046-048
351.9 ...01 018-019	360.04 ..02 044	362.34 ..02 045	363.71 ..02 046-048
352.0 ...01 018-019	360.11 ..02 046-048	362.35 ..02 045	363.72 ..02 046-048
352.1 ...01 018-019	360.12 ..02 046-048	362.36 ..02 045	363.8 ...02 046-048
352.2 ...01 018-019	360.13 ..02 044	362.37 ..02 045	363.9 ...02 046-048
352.3 ...01 018-019	360.14 ..02 046-048	362.40 ..02 046-048	364.00 ..02 046-048
352.4 ...01 018-019	360.19 ..02 044	362.41 ..02 046-048	364.01 ..02 046-048
352.5 ...01 018-019	360.20 ..02 046-048	362.42 ..02 046-048	364.02 ..02 046-048
352.6 ...01 018-019	360.21 ..02 046-048	362.43 ..02 046-048	364.03 ..02 046-048
352.9 ...01 018-019	360.23 ..02 046-048	362.50 ..02 046-048	364.04 ..02 046-048
353.0 ...01 018-019	360.24 ..02 046-048	362.51 ..02 046-048	364.05 ..02 046-048
353.1 ...01 018-019	360.29 ..02 046-048	362.52 ..02 046-048	364.10 ..02 046-048
353.2 ...01 018-019	360.30 ..02 046-048	362.53 ..02 046-048	364.11 ..02 046-048
353.3 ...01 018-019	360.31 ..02 046-048	362.54 ..02 046-048	364.21 ..02 046-048
353.4 ...01 018-019	360.32 ..02 046-048	362.55 ..02 046-048	364.22 ..02 046-048
353.5 ...01 018-019	360.33 ..02 046-048	362.56 ..02 046-048	364.23 ..02 046-048
353.6 ...01 018-019	360.34 ..02 046-048	362.57 ..02 046-048	364.24 ..02 046-048
353.8 ...01 018-019	360.40 ..02 046-048	362.60 ..02 046-048	364.3 ...02 046-048

Diagnosis Code/MDC/DRG List

DX	MDC	DRG
364.41	.02	.043
364.42	.02	.046-048
364.51	.02	.046-048
364.52	.02	.046-048
364.53	.02	.046-048
364.54	.02	.046-048
364.55	.02	.046-048
364.56	.02	.046-048
364.57	.02	.046-048
364.59	.02	.046-048
364.60	.02	.046-048
364.61	.02	.046-048
364.62	.02	.046-048
364.63	.02	.046-048
364.64	.02	.046-048
364.70	.02	.046-048
364.71	.02	.046-048
364.72	.02	.046-048
364.73	.02	.046-048
364.74	.02	.046-048
364.75	.02	.046-048
364.76	.02	.046-048
364.77	.02	.046-048
364.8	.02	.046-048
364.9	.02	.046-048
365.00	.02	.046-048
365.01	.02	.046-048
365.02	.02	.046-048
365.03	.02	.046-048
365.04	.02	.046-048
365.10	.02	.046-048
365.11	.02	.046-048
365.12	.02	.045
365.13	.02	.046-048
365.14	.02	.046-048
365.15	.02	.046-048
365.20	.02	.046-048
365.21	.02	.046-048
365.22	.02	.046-048
365.23	.02	.046-048
365.24	.02	.046-048
365.31	.02	.046-048
365.32	.02	.046-048
365.41	.02	.046-048
365.42	.02	.046-048
365.43	.02	.046-048
365.44	.02	.046-048
365.51	.02	.046-048
365.52	.02	.046-048
365.59	.02	.046-048
365.60	.02	.046-048
365.61	.02	.046-048
365.62	.02	.046-048
365.63	.02	.046-048
365.64	.02	.046-048
365.65	.02	.046-048
365.81	.02	.046-048
365.82	.02	.046-048
365.83	.02	.046-048
365.89	.02	.046-048
365.9	.02	.046-048
366.00	.02	.046-048
366.01	.02	.046-048
366.02	.02	.046-048
366.03	.02	.046-048
366.04	.02	.046-048
366.09	.02	.046-048
366.10	.02	.046-048
366.11	.02	.046-048
366.12	.02	.046-048
366.13	.02	.046-048
366.14	.02	.046-048
366.15	.02	.046-048
366.16	.02	.046-048
366.17	.02	.046-048
366.18	.02	.046-048
366.19	.02	.046-048
366.20	.02	.046-048
366.21	.02	.046-048
366.22	.02	.046-048
366.23	.02	.046-048
366.30	.02	.046-048
366.31	.02	.046-048
366.32	.02	.046-048
366.33	.02	.046-048
366.34	.02	.046-048
366.41	.02	.046-048
366.42	.02	.046-048
366.43	.02	.046-048
366.44	.02	.046-048
366.45	.02	.046-048
366.46	.02	.046-048
366.50	.02	.046-048
366.51	.02	.046-048
366.52	.02	.046-048
366.53	.02	.046-048
366.8	.02	.046-048
366.9	.02	.046-048
367.0	.02	.046-048
367.1	.02	.046-048
367.20	.02	.046-048
367.21	.02	.046-048
367.22	.02	.046-048
367.31	.02	.046-048
367.32	.02	.046-048
367.4	.02	.046-048
367.51	.02	.046-048
367.52	.02	.045
367.53	.02	.046-048
367.81	.02	.046-048
367.89	.02	.046-048
367.9	.02	.046-048
368.00	.02	.046-048
368.01	.02	.046-048
368.02	.02	.046-048
368.03	.02	.046-048
368.10	.02	.046-048
368.11	.02	.045
368.12	.02	.045
368.13	.02	.046-048
368.14	.02	.046-048
368.15	.02	.046-048
368.16	.02	.046-048
368.2	.02	.045
368.30	.02	.046-048
368.31	.02	.046-048
368.32	.02	.046-048
368.33	.02	.046-048
368.34	.02	.046-048
368.40	.02	.045
368.41	.02	.045
368.42	.02	.046-048
368.43	.02	.045
368.44	.02	.045
368.45	.02	.045
368.46	.02	.045
368.47	.02	.045
368.51	.02	.046-048
368.52	.02	.046-048
368.53	.02	.046-048
368.54	.02	.046-048
368.55	.02	.045
368.59	.02	.046-048
368.60	.02	.046-048
368.61	.02	.046-048
368.62	.02	.046-048
368.63	.02	.046-048
368.69	.02	.046-048
368.8	.02	.046-048
368.9	.02	.046-048
369.00	.02	.046-048
369.01	.02	.046-048
369.02	.02	.046-048
369.03	.02	.046-048
369.04	.02	.046-048
369.05	.02	.046-048
369.06	.02	.046-048
369.07	.02	.046-048
369.08	.02	.046-048
369.10	.02	.046-048
369.11	.02	.046-048
369.12	.02	.046-048
369.13	.02	.046-048
369.14	.02	.046-048
369.15	.02	.046-048
369.16	.02	.046-048
369.17	.02	.046-048
369.18	.02	.046-048
369.20	.02	.046-048
369.21	.02	.046-048
369.22	.02	.046-048
369.23	.02	.046-048
369.24	.02	.046-048
369.25	.02	.046-048
369.3	.02	.046-048
369.4	.02	.046-048
369.60	.02	.046-048
369.61	.02	.046-048
369.62	.02	.046-048
369.63	.02	.046-048
369.64	.02	.046-048
369.65	.02	.046-048
369.66	.02	.046-048
369.67	.02	.046-048
369.68	.02	.046-048
369.69	.02	.046-048
369.70	.02	.046-048
369.71	.02	.046-048
369.72	.02	.046-048
369.73	.02	.046-048
369.74	.02	.046-048
369.75	.02	.046-048
369.76	.02	.046-048
369.8	.02	.046-048
369.9	.02	.046-048
370.00	.02	.044
370.01	.02	.046-048
370.02	.02	.046-048
370.03	.02	.044
370.04	.02	.044
370.05	.02	.044
370.06	.02	.044
370.07	.02	.046-048
370.20	.02	.046-048
370.21	.02	.046-048
370.22	.02	.046-048
370.23	.02	.046-048
370.24	.02	.046-048
370.31	.02	.046-048
370.32	.02	.046-048
370.33	.02	.046-048
370.34	.02	.046-048
370.35	.02	.046-048
370.40	.02	.046-048
370.44	.02	.046-048
370.49	.02	.046-048
370.50	.02	.046-048
370.52	.02	.046-048
370.54	.02	.046-048
370.55	.02	.044
370.59	.02	.046-048
370.60	.02	.046-048
370.61	.02	.046-048
370.62	.02	.046-048
370.63	.02	.046-048
370.64	.02	.046-048
370.8	.02	.046-048
370.9	.02	.046-048
371.00	.02	.046-048
371.01	.02	.046-048
371.02	.02	.046-048
371.03	.02	.046-048
371.04	.02	.046-048
371.05	.02	.046-048
371.10	.02	.046-048
371.11	.02	.046-048
371.12	.02	.046-048
371.13	.02	.046-048
371.14	.02	.046-048
371.15	.02	.046-048
371.16	.02	.046-048
371.20	.02	.046-048
371.21	.02	.046-048
371.22	.02	.046-048
371.23	.02	.046-048
371.24	.02	.046-048
371.30	.02	.046-048
371.31	.02	.046-048
371.32	.02	.046-048
371.33	.02	.046-048
371.40	.02	.046-048
371.41	.02	.046-048
371.42	.02	.046-048
371.43	.02	.046-048
371.44	.02	.046-048
371.45	.02	.046-048
371.46	.02	.046-048
371.48	.02	.046-048
371.49	.02	.046-048
371.50	.02	.046-048
371.51	.02	.046-048
371.52	.02	.046-048
371.53	.02	.046-048
371.54	.02	.046-048
371.55	.02	.046-048
371.56	.02	.046-048
371.57	.02	.046-048
371.58	.02	.046-048
371.60	.02	.046-048
371.61	.02	.046-048
371.62	.02	.046-048
371.70	.02	.046-048
371.71	.02	.046-048
371.72	.02	.046-048
371.73	.02	.046-048
371.81	.02	.046-048
371.82	.02	.046-048
371.89	.02	.046-048
371.9	.02	.046-048
372.00	.02	.046-048
372.01	.02	.046-048
372.02	.02	.046-048
372.03	.02	.046-048
372.04	.02	.046-048
372.05	.02	.046-048
372.10	.02	.046-048
372.11	.02	.046-048
372.12	.02	.046-048
372.13	.02	.046-048
372.14	.02	.046-048
372.15	.02	.046-048
372.20	.02	.046-048
372.21	.02	.046-048
372.22	.02	.046-048
372.30	.02	.046-048
372.31	.02	.046-048
372.33	.02	.046-048
372.39	.02	.046-048
372.40	.02	.046-048
372.41	.02	.046-048
372.42	.02	.046-048
372.43	.02	.046-048
372.44	.02	.046-048
372.45	.02	.046-048
372.50	.02	.046-048
372.51	.02	.046-048
372.52	.02	.046-048
372.53	.02	.046-048

DX ... MDC ... DRG	DX ... MDC ... DRG	DX ... MDC ... DRG	DX ... MDC ... DRG
372.54 ..02 046-048	375.12 ..02 046-048	377.30 ..02 045	378.9 ..02 046-048
372.55 ..02 046-048	375.13 ..02 046-048	377.31 ..02 045	379.00 ..02 046-048
372.56 ..02 046-048	375.14 ..02 046-048	377.32 ..02 045	379.01 ..02 046-048
372.61 ..02 046-048	375.15 ..02 046-048	377.33 ..02 045	379.02 ..02 046-048
372.62 ..02 046-048	375.16 ..02 046-048	377.34 ..02 045	379.03 ..02 046-048
372.63 ..02 046-048	375.20 ..02 046-048	377.39 ..02 045	379.04 ..02 046-048
372.64 ..02 046-048	375.21 ..02 046-048	377.41 ..02 045	379.05 ..02 046-048
372.71 ..02 046-048	375.22 ..02 046-048	377.42 ..02 045	379.06 ..02 046-048
372.72 ..02 046-048	375.30 ..02 046-048	377.49 ..02 045	379.07 ..02 046-048
372.73 ..02 046-048	375.31 ..02 044	377.51 ..01 034-035	379.09 ..02 046-048
372.74 ..02 046-048	375.32 ..02 044	377.52 ..01 034-035	379.11 ..02 046-048
372.75 ..02 046-048	375.33 ..02 046-048	377.53 ..01 034-035	379.12 ..02 046-048
372.81 ..02 046-048	375.41 ..02 046-048	377.54 ..01 034-035	379.13 ..02 046-048
327.89 ..02 046-048	375.42 ..02 046-048	377.61 ..01 034-035	379.14 ..02 046-048
372.9 ..02 046-048	375.43 ..02 046-048	377.62 ..01 034-035	379.15 ..02 046-048
373.00 ..02 046-048	375.51 ..02 046-048	377.63 ..01 034-035	379.16 ..02 046-048
373.01 ..02 046-048	375.52 ..02 046-048	377.71 ..01 034-035	379.19 ..02 046-048
373.02 ..02 046-048	375.53 ..02 046-048	377.72 ..01 034-035	379.21 ..02 046-048
373.11 ..02 046-048	375.54 ..02 046-048	377.73 ..01 034-035	379.22 ..02 046-048
373.12 ..02 046-048	375.55 ..02 046-048	377.75 ..01 034-035	379.23 ..02 046-048
373.13 ..02 046-048	375.56 ..02 046-048	377.9 ..01 034-035	379.24 ..02 046-048
373.2 ..02 046-048	375.57 ..02 046-048	378.00 ..02 046-048	379.25 ..02 046-048
373.31 ..02 046-048	375.61 ..02 046-048	378.01 ..02 046-048	379.26 ..02 046-048
373.32 ..02 046-048	375.69 ..02 046-048	378.02 ..02 046-048	379.29 ..02 046-048
373.33 ..02 046-048	375.81 ..02 046-048	378.03 ..02 046-048	379.31 ..02 046-048
373.34 ..02 046-048	375.89 ..02 046-048	378.04 ..02 046-048	379.32 ..02 046-048
373.4 ..02 046-048	375.9 ..02 046-048	378.05 ..02 046-048	379.33 ..02 046-048
373.5 ..02 046-048	376.00 ..02 046-048	378.06 ..02 046-048	379.34 ..02 046-048
373.6 ..02 046-048	376.01 ..02 044	378.07 ..02 046-048	379.39 ..02 046-048
373.8 ..02 046-048	376.02 ..02 044	378.08 ..02 046-048	379.40 ..02 045
373.9 ..02 046-048	376.03 ..02 044	378.10 ..02 046-048	379.41 ..02 045
374.00 ..02 046-048	376.04 ..02 044	378.11 ..02 046-048	379.42 ..02 045
374.01 ..02 046-048	376.10 ..02 046-048	378.12 ..02 046-048	379.43 ..02 045
374.02 ..02 046-048	376.11 ..02 046-048	378.13 ..02 046-048	379.45 ..01 012
374.03 ..02 046-048	376.12 ..02 046-048	378.14 ..02 046-048	379.46 ..02 045
374.04 ..02 046-048	376.13 ..02 046-048	378.15 ..02 046-048	379.49 ..02 045
374.05 ..02 046-048	376.21 ..02 046-048	378.16 ..02 046-048	379.50 ..02 045
374.10 ..02 046-048	376.22 ..02 046-048	378.17 ..02 046-048	379.51 ..02 046-048
374.11 ..02 046-048	376.30 ..02 046-048	378.18 ..02 046-048	379.52 ..02 045
374.12 ..02 046-048	376.31 ..02 046-048	378.20 ..02 046-048	379.53 ..02 046-048
374.13 ..02 046-048	376.32 ..02 046-048	378.21 ..02 046-048	379.54 ..02 045
374.14 ..02 046-048	376.33 ..02 046-048	378.22 ..02 046-048	379.55 ..02 045
374.20 ..02 046-048	376.34 ..02 045	378.23 ..02 046-048	379.56 ..02 046-048
374.21 ..02 046-048	376.35 ..02 045	378.24 ..02 046-048	379.57 ..02 045
374.22 ..02 046-048	376.36 ..02 045	378.30 ..02 046-048	379.58 ..02 045
374.23 ..02 046-048	376.40 ..02 046-048	378.31 ..02 046-048	379.59 ..02 046-048
374.30 ..02 045	376.41 ..02 046-048	378.32 ..02 046-048	379.8 ..02 046-048
374.31 ..02 045	376.42 ..02 046-048	378.33 ..02 046-048	379.90 ..02 046-048
374.32 ..02 045	376.43 ..02 046-048	378.34 ..02 046-048	379.91 ..02 046-048
374.33 ..02 046-048	376.44 ..02 046-048	378.35 ..02 046-048	379.92 ..02 046-048
374.34 ..02 046-048	376.45 ..02 046-048	378.40 ..02 046-048	379.93 ..02 046-048
374.41 ..02 046-048	376.46 ..02 046-048	378.41 ..02 046-048	379.99 ..02 046-048
374.43 ..02 046-048	376.47 ..02 046-048	378.42 ..02 046-048	380.00 ..03 068-070
374.44 ..02 046-048	376.50 ..02 046-048	378.43 ..02 046-048	380.01 ..08 256
374.45 ..02 045	376.51 ..02 046-048	378.44 ..02 046-048	380.02 ..08 256
374.46 ..02 046-048	376.52 ..02 046-048	378.45 ..02 046-048	380.10 ..03 073-074
374.50 ..02 046-048	376.6 ..02 046-048	378.50 ..02 045	380.11 ..03 073-074
374.51 ..09 283-284	376.81 ..02 046-048	378.51 ..02 045	380.12 ..03 073-074
374.52 ..02 046-048	376.82 ..02 045	378.52 ..02 045	380.13 ..03 073-074
374.53 ..02 046-048	376.89 ..02 046-048	378.53 ..02 045	380.14 ..03 073-074
374.54 ..02 046-048	376.9 ..02 046-048	378.54 ..02 045	380.15 ..03 073-074
374.55 ..02 046-048	377.00 ..01 034-035	378.55 ..02 045	380.16 ..03 073-074
374.56 ..02 046-048	377.01 ..01 034-035	378.56 ..02 045	380.21 ..03 073-074
374.81 ..02 046-048	377.02 ..02 046-048	378.60 ..02 046-048	380.22 ..03 073-074
374.82 ..02 046-048	377.03 ..02 046-048	378.61 ..02 046-048	380.23 ..03 073-074
374.83 ..02 046-048	377.04 ..01 034-035	378.62 ..02 046-048	380.30 ..03 073-074
374.84 ..02 046-048	377.10 ..02 045	378.63 ..02 046-048	380.31 ..03 073-074
374.85 ..02 046-048	377.11 ..02 045	378.71 ..02 046-048	380.32 ..03 073-074
374.86 ..02 046-048	377.12 ..02 045	378.72 ..02 045	380.39 ..03 073-074
374.87 ..02 046-048	377.13 ..02 046-048	378.73 ..02 045	380.4 ..03 073-074
374.89 ..02 046-048	377.14 ..02 046-048	378.81 ..02 046-048	380.50 ..03 073-074
374.9 ..02 046-048	377.15 ..02 045	378.82 ..02 046-048	380.51 ..03 073-074
375.00 ..02 046-048	377.16 ..02 045	378.83 ..02 046-048	380.52 ..03 073-074
375.01 ..02 044	377.21 ..02 045	378.84 ..02 046-048	380.53 ..03 073-074
375.02 ..02 046-048	377.22 ..02 046-048	378.85 ..02 046-048	380.81 ..03 073-074
375.03 ..02 046-048	377.23 ..02 046-048	378.86 ..01 034-035	380.89 ..03 073-074
375.11 ..02 046-048	377.24 ..02 045	378.87 ..02 045	380.9 ..03 073-074

2002 Ingenix, Inc.

Diagnosis Code/MDC/DRG List

DX	MDC	DRG
381.00	.03	.068-070
381.01	.03	.068-070
381.02	.03	.068-070
381.03	.03	.068-070
381.04	.03	.068-070
381.05	.03	.068-070
381.06	.03	.068-070
381.10	.03	.068-070
381.19	.03	.068-070
381.20	.03	.068-070
381.29	.03	.068-070
381.3	.03	.068-070
381.4	.03	.068-070
381.50	.03	.068-070
381.51	.03	.068-070
381.52	.03	.068-070
381.60	.03	.073-074
381.61	.03	.073-074
381.62	.03	.073-074
381.63	.03	.073-074
381.7	.03	.073-074
381.81	.03	.073-074
381.89	.03	.073-074
381.9	.03	.073-074
382.00	.03	.068-070
382.01	.03	.068-070
382.02	.03	.068-070
382.1	.03	.068-070
382.2	.03	.068-070
382.3	.03	.068-070
382.4	.03	.068-070
382.9	.03	.068-070
383.00	.03	.068-070
383.01	.03	.068-070
383.02	.03	.068-070
383.1	.03	.068-070
383.20	.03	.068-070
383.21	.03	.068-070
383.22	.03	.068-070
383.30	.03	.073-074
383.31	.03	.073-074
383.32	.03	.073-074
383.33	.03	.073-074
383.81	.03	.073-074
383.89	.03	.073-074
383.9	.03	.068-070
384.00	.03	.068-070
384.01	.03	.068-070
384.09	.03	.068-070
384.1	.03	.068-070
384.20	.03	.073-074
384.21	.03	.073-074
384.22	.03	.073-074
384.23	.03	.073-074
384.24	.03	.073-074
384.25	.03	.073-074
384.81	.03	.073-074
384.82	.03	.073-074
384.9	.03	.073-074
385.00	.03	.073-074
385.01	.03	.073-074
385.02	.03	.073-074
385.03	.03	.073-074
385.09	.03	.073-074
385.10	.03	.073-074
385.11	.03	.073-074
385.12	.03	.073-074
385.13	.03	.073-074
385.19	.03	.073-074
385.21	.03	.073-074
385.22	.03	.073-074
385.23	.03	.073-074
385.24	.03	.073-074
385.30	.03	.073-074
385.31	.03	.073-074
385.32	.03	.073-074
385.33	.03	.073-074
385.35	.03	.073-074
385.82	.03	.073-074
385.83	.03	.073-074
385.89	.03	.073-074
385.9	.03	.073-074
386.00	.03	.065
386.01	.03	.065
386.02	.03	.065
386.03	.03	.065
386.04	.03	.065
386.10	.03	.065
386.11	.03	.065
386.12	.03	.065
386.19	.03	.065
386.2	.03	.065
386.30	.03	.065
386.31	.03	.065
386.32	.03	.065
386.33	.03	.065
386.34	.03	.065
386.35	.03	.065
386.40	.03	.073-074
386.41	.03	.073-074
386.42	.03	.073-074
386.43	.03	.073-074
386.48	.03	.073-074
386.50	.03	.065
386.51	.03	.065
386.52	.03	.065
386.53	.03	.065
386.54	.03	.065
386.55	.03	.065
386.56	.03	.065
386.58	.03	.065
386.8	.03	.065
386.9	.03	.065
387.0	.03	.073-074
387.1	.03	.073-074
387.2	.03	.073-074
387.8	.03	.073-074
387.9	.03	.073-074
388.00	.03	.073-074
388.01	.03	.073-074
388.02	.03	.073-074
388.10	.03	.073-074
388.11	.03	.073-074
388.12	.03	.073-074
388.2	.03	.073-074
388.30	.03	.073-074
388.31	.03	.073-074
388.32	.03	.073-074
388.40	.03	.073-074
388.41	.03	.073-074
388.42	.03	.073-074
388.43	.03	.073-074
388.44	.03	.073-074
388.5	.03	.073-074
388.60	.03	.073-074
388.61	.01	.034-035
388.69	.03	.073-074
388.70	.03	.073-074
388.71	.03	.073-074
388.72	.03	.073-074
388.8	.03	.073-074
388.9	.03	.073-074
389.00	.03	.073-074
389.01	.03	.073-074
389.02	.03	.073-074
389.03	.03	.073-074
389.04	.03	.073-074
389.08	.03	.073-074
389.10	.03	.073-074
389.11	.03	.073-074
389.12	.03	.073-074
389.14	.03	.073-074
389.18	.03	.073-074
389.2	.03	.073-074
389.7	.03	.073-074
389.8	.03	.073-074
389.9	.03	.073-074

Diseases of the Circulatory System

DX	MDC	DRG
390	.08	.240-241
391.0	.05	.144-145
391.1	.05	.135-137
391.2	.05	.144-145
391.8	.05	.144-145
391.9	.05	.144-145
392.0	.05	.144-145
392.9	.05	.144-145
393	.05	.144-145
394.0	.05	.135-137
394.1	.05	.135-137
394.2	.05	.135-137
394.9	.05	.135-137
395.0	.05	.135-137
395.1	.05	.135-137
395.2	.05	.135-137
395.9	.05	.135-137
396.0	.05	.135-137
396.1	.05	.135-137
396.2	.05	.135-137
396.3	.05	.135-137
396.8	.05	.135-137
396.9	.05	.135-137
397.0	.05	.135-137
397.1	.05	.135-137
397.9	.05	.135-137
398.0	.05	.144-145
398.90	.05	.144-145
398.91	.05	.115,121,127
398.99	.05	.144-145
401.0	.05	.134
401.1	.05	.134
401.9	.05	.134
402.00	.05	.134
402.01	.05	.115,121,124,127,
402.10	.05	.134
402.11	.05	.115,121,124,127,
402.90	.05	.134
402.91	.05	.115,121,124,127,
403.00	.11	.331-333
403.01	.11	.316
403.10	.11	.331-333
403.11	.11	.316
403.90	.11	.331-333
403.91	.11	.316
404.00	.05	.134
404.01	.05	.115,121,124,127,
404.02	.11	.316
404.03	.05	.115,121,124,127,
404.10	.05	.134
404.11	.05	.115,121,124,127,
404.12	.11	.316
404.13	.05	.115,121,124,127,
404.90	.05	.134
404.91	.05	.115,121,124,127,
404.92	.11	.316
404.93	.05	.115,121,124,127,
405.01	.05	.134
405.09	.05	.134
405.11	.05	.134
405.19	.05	.134
405.91	.05	.134
405.99	.05	.134
410.00	.05	.144-145
410.01	.05	.115,121-123
410.02	.05	.144-145
410.10	.05	.144-145
410.11	.05	.115,121-123
410.12	.05	.144-145
410.20	.05	.144-145
410.21	.05	.115,121-123
410.22	.05	.144-145
410.30	.05	.144-145
410.31	.05	.115,121-123
410.32	.05	.144-145
410.40	.05	.144-145
410.41	.05	.115,121-123
410.42	.05	.144-145
410.50	.05	.144-145
410.51	.05	.115,121-123
410.52	.05	.144-145
410.60	.05	.144-145
410.61	.05	.115,121-123
410.62	.05	.144-145
410.70	.05	.144-145
410.71	.05	.115,121-123
410.72	.05	.144-145
410.80	.05	.144-145
410.81	.05	.115,121-123
410.82	.05	.144-145
410.90	.05	.144-145
410.91	.05	.115,121-123
410.92	.05	.144-145
411.0	.05	.121,124,144-145
411.1	.05	.124,140
411.81	.05	.124,140
411.89	.05	.124,140
412.	.05	.132-133
413.0	.05	.140
413.1	.05	.140
413.9	.05	.140
414.00	.05	.132-133
414.01	.05	.132-133
414.02	.05	.132-133
414.03	.05	.132-133
414.04	.05	.132-133
414.05	.05	.132-133
414.06	.05	.132-133
414.10	.05	.121,144-145
414.11	.05	.121,144-145
414.12	.05	.121, 144-145
414.19	.05	.121,144-145
414.8	.05	.132-133
414.9	.05	.132-133
415.0	.05	.124,144-145
415.11	.04	.078
415.19	.04	.078
416.0	.05	.121,144-145
416.1	.05	.144-145
416.8	.05	.144-145
416.9	.05	.144-145
417.0	.05	.144-145
417.1	.05	.144-145
417.8	.05	.144-145
417.9	.05	.144-145
420.0	.05	.124,144-145
420.90	.05	.124,144-145
420.91	.05	.124,144-145
420.99	.05	.124,144-145
421.0	.05	.124,126
421.1	.05	.124,126
421.9	.05	.124,126
422.0	.05	.124,144-145
422.90	.05	.124,144-145
422.91	.05	.124,144-145
422.92	.05	.124,144-145
422.93	.05	.124,144-145
422.99	.05	.124,144-145
423.0	.05	.124,144-145
423.1	.05	.144-145
423.2	.05	.144-145
423.8	.05	.144-145
423.9	.05	.144-145
424.0	.05	.135-137
424.1	.05	.135-137
424.2	.05	.135-137
424.3	.05	.135-137
424.90	.05	.124,135-137
424.91	.05	.124,135-137

DX....MDC....DRG	DX....MDC....DRG	DX....MDC....DRG	DX....MDC....DRG
424.99 ...05 135-137	433.11 ..01 014	441.4 ...05 130-131	454.8 ...05 130-131
425.0 ...05 144-145	433.20 ..01 015	441.5 ...05 130-131	454.9 ...05 130-131
425.1 ...05 144-145	433.21 ..01 014	441.6 ...05 130-131	455.0 ...06 188-190
425.2 ...05 124,144-145	433.30 ..01 015	441.7 ...05 130-131	455.1 ...06 188-190
425.3 ...05 124,144-145	433.31 ..01 014	441.9 ...05 130-131	455.2 ...06 188-190
425.4 ...05 124,144-145	433.80 ..01 015	442.0 ...05 130-131	455.3 ...06 188-190
425.5 ...05 124,144-145	433.81 ..01 014	442.1 ...11 331-333	455.4 ...06 188-190
425.7 ...05 124,144-145	433.90 ..01 015	442.2 ...05 130-131	455.5 ...06 188-190
425.8 ...05 124,144-145	433.91 ..01 014	442.3 ...05 130-131	455.6 ...06 188-190
425.9 ...05 124,144-145	434.00 ..01 015	442.81 ..05 130-131	455.7 ...06 188-190
426.0 ...05 121,138-139	434.01 ..01 014	442.82 ..05 130-131	455.8 ...06 188-190
426.10 ..05 121,138-139	434.10 ..01 015	442.83 ..05 130-131	455.9 ...06 188-190
426.11 ..05 138-139	434.11 ..01 014	442.84 ..05 130-131	456.0 ...06 174-175
426.12 ..05 121,138-139	434.90 ..01 015	442.89 ..05 130-131	456.1 ...06 188-190
426.13 ..05 121,138-139	434.91 ..01 014	442.9 ...05 130-131	456.20 ..06 188-190
426.2 ...05 138-139	435.0 ...01 015	443.0 ...08 240-241	456.21 ..06 188-190
426.3 ...05 121,138-139	435.1 ...01 015	443.1 ...05 130-131	456.3 ...05 130-131
426.4 ...05 138-139	435.2 ...01 015	443.21 ..05 130-131	456.4 ...12 352
426.50 ..05 138-139	435.8 ...01 015	443.22 ..05 130-131	456.5 ...12 352
426.51 ..05 121,138-139	435.9 ...01 015	443.23 ..11 331-333	456.5 ...13 358-359,369
426.52 ..05 121,138-139	436 ....01 014	443.24 ..05 130-131	456.6 ...13 358-359,369
426.53 ..05 121,138-139	437.0 ...01 016-017	443.29 ..05 130-131	456.8 ...05 130-131
426.54 ..05 121,138-139	437.1 ...01 016-017	443.81 ..05 130-131	457.0 ...09 276
426.6 ...05 138-139	437.2 ...01 022	443.89 ..05 130-131	457.1 ...09 283-284
426.7 ...05 138-139	437.3 ...01 014	443.9 ...05 130-131	457.2 ...09 277-279
426.81 ..05 138-139	437.4 ...01 024-026	444.0 ...05 130-131	457.8 ...16 398-399
426.89 ..05 138-139	437.5 ...01 034-035	444.1 ...05 130-131	457.9 ...16 398-399
426.9 ...05 138-139	437.6 ...01 034-035	444.21 ..05 130-131	458.0 ...05 141-142
427.0 ...05 121,138-139	437.7 ...01 016-017	444.22 ..05 130-131	458.1 ...05 144-145
427.1 ...05 121,124,138-139	437.8 ...01 016-017	444.81 ..05 130-131	458.2 ...05 144-145
427.2 ...05 121,138-139	437.9 ...01 016-017	444.89 ..05 130-131	458.8 ...05 121,144-145
427.31 ..05 121,138-139	438.0 ...01 012	444.9 ...05 130-131	458.9 ...05 121,144-145
427.32 ..05 121,138-139	438.10 ..01 012	445.01 ..05 130-131	459.0 ...05 144-145
427.41 ..05 121,138-139	438.11 ..01 012	445.02 ..05 130-131	459.1 ...05 130-131
427.42 ..05 121,138-139	438.12 ..01 012	445.81 ..11 331-333	459.2 ...05 130-131
427.5 ...05 121,124,129	438.19 ..01 012	445.89 ..05 130-131	459.10 ..05 130-131
427.60 ..05 138-139	438.20 ..01 012	446.0 ...08 240-241	459.11 ..05 130-131
427.61 ..05 138-139	438.21 ..01 012	446.1 ...08 240-241	459.12 ..05 130-131
427.69 ..05 138-139	438.22 ..01 012	446.20 ..08 240-241	459.13 ..05 130-131
427.81 ..05 138-139	438.30 ..01 012	446.21 ..08 240-241	459.19 ..05 130-131
427.89 ..05 138-139	438.31 ..01 012	446.29 ..08 240-241	459.30 ..05 130-131
427.9 ...05 138-139	438.32 ..01 012	446.3 ...08 239	459.31 ..05 130-131
428.0 ...05 115,121,124,127	438.40 ..01 012	446.4 ...08 239	459.32 ..05 130-131
428.1 ...05 115,121,124,127	438.41 ..01 012	446.5 ...08 240-241	459.33 ..05 130-131
428.9 ...05 115,121,124,127	438.42 ..01 012	446.6 ...08 240-241	459.39 ..05 130-131
428.20 ..05 ....115, 121, 124, 127	438.50 ..01 012	446.7 ...08 240-241	459.81 ..05 130-131
428.21 ..05 ....115, 121, 124, 127	438.51 ..01 012	447.0 ...05 130-131	459.89 ..05 132-133
428.22 ..05 ....115, 121, 124, 127	438.52 ..01 012	447.1 ...05 130-131	459.9 ...05 132-133
428.23 ..05 ....115, 121, 124, 127	438.53 ..01 012	447.2 ...05 130-131	
428.30 ..05 ....115, 121, 124, 127	438.6 ...01 012	447.3 ...11 331-333	**Diseases of the Respiratory System**
428.31 ..05 ....115, 121, 124, 127	438.7 ...01 012	447.4 ...06 182-184	460 ....03 068-070
428.32 ..05 ....115, 121, 124, 127	438.81 ..01 012	447.5 ...05 130-131	461.0 ...03 068-070
428.33 ..05 ....115, 121, 124, 127	438.82 ..01 012	447.6 ...08 240-241	461.1 ...03 068-070
428.40 ..05 ....115, 121, 124, 127	438.83 ..01 012	447.8 ...05 130-131	461.2 ...03 068-070
428.41 ..05 ....115, 121, 124, 127	438.84 ..01 012	447.9 ...05 130-131	461.3 ...03 068-070
428.42 ..05 ....115, 121, 124, 127	438.85 ..01 012	448.0 ...05 130-131	461.8 ...03 068-070
428.43 ..05 ....115, 121, 124, 127	438.89 ..01 012	448.1 ...09 283-284	461.9 ...03 068-070
429.0 ...05 144-145	438.9 ...01 012	448.9 ...05 130-131	462 ....03 068-070
429.1 ...05 144-145	440.0 ...05 130-131	451.0 ...05 130-131	463 ....03 068-070
429.2 ...05 132-133	440.1 ...11 331-333	451.11 ..05 128	464.00 ..03 068-070
429.3 ...05 132-133	440.20 ..05 130-131	451.19 ..05 128	464.01 ..03 ....068.070
429.4 ...05 124,144-145	440.21 ..05 130-131	451.2 ...05 128	464.10 ..04 096-098
429.5 ...05 121,124,135-137	440.22 ..05 130-131	451.81 ..05 128	464.11 ..04 096-098
429.6 ...05 121,124,135-137	440.23 ..05 130-131	451.82 ..05 130-131	464.20 ..03 071
429.71 ..05 124,144-145	440.24 ..05 130-131	451.83 ..05 130-131	464.21 ..03 071
429.79 ..05 124,144-145	440.29 ..05 130-131	451.84 ..05 130-131	464.30 ..03 067
429.81 ..05 121,124,135-137	440.30 ..05 130-131	451.89 ..05 130-131	464.31 ..03 067
429.82 ..05 124,144-145	440.31 ..05 130-131	451.9 ...05 130-131	464.4 ...03 071
429.89 ..05 132-133	440.32 ..05 130-131	452 ....07 205-206	464.50 ..03 068-070
429.9 ...05 132-133	440.8 ...05 130-131	453.0 ...07 205-206	464.51 ..03 068-070
430 ....01 014	440.9 ...05 130-131	453.1 ...05 130-131	465.0 ...03 068-070
431 ....01 014	441.00 ..05 121,130-131	453.2 ...05 128	465.8 ...03 068-070
432.0 ...01 014	441.01 ..05 121,130-131	453.3 ...11 331-333	465.9 ...03 068-070
432.1 ...01 014	441.02 ..05 121,130-131	453.8 ...05 130-131	466.0 ...04 096-098
432.9 ...01 014	441.03 ..05 121,130-131	453.9 ...05 130-131	466.11 ..04 096-098
433.00 ..01 015	441.1 ...05 130-131	454.0 ...05 130-131	466.19 ..04 096-098
433.01 ..01 014	441.2 ...05 130-131	454.1 ...05 130-131	470 ....03 072
433.10 ..01 015	441.3 ...05 130-131	454.2 ...05 130-131	471.0 ...03 073-074

Diagnosis Code/MDC/DRG List

DX	MDC	DRG
471.1	03	073-074
471.8	03	073-074
471.9	03	073-074
472.0	03	068-070
472.1	03	068-070
472.2	03	068-070
473.0	03	068-070
473.1	03	068-070
473.2	03	068-070
473.3	03	068-070
473.8	03	068-070
473.9	03	068-070
474.00	03	068-070
474.01	03	068-070
474.02	03	068-070
474.10	03	073-074
474.11	03	073-074
474.12	03	073-074
474.2	03	073-074
474.8	03	073-074
474.9	03	073-074
475	03	068-070
476.0	03	068-070
476.1	03	068-070
477.0	03	068-070
477.1	03	068-070
477.8	03	068-070
477.9	03	068-070
478.0	03	073-074
478.1	03	073-074
478.20	03	073-074
478.21	03	068-070
478.22	03	068-070
478.24	03	068-070
478.25	03	073-074
478.26	03	073-074
478.29	03	073-074
478.30	03	073-074
478.31	03	073-074
478.32	03	073-074
478.33	03	073-074
478.34	03	073-074
478.4	03	073-074
478.5	03	073-074
478.6	03	073-074
478.70	03	073-074
478.71	03	068-070
478.74	03	073-074
478.75	03	073-074
478.79	03	073-074
478.8	03	068-070
478.9	03	068-070
480.0	04	089-091
480.1	04	089-091
480.2	04	089-091
480.8	04	089-091
480.9	04	089-091
481	04	089-091
482.0	04	079-081
482.1	04	079-081
482.2	04	089-091
482.30	04	089-091
482.31	04	089-091
482.32	04	089-091
482.39	04	089-091
482.40	04	079-081
482.40	05	121
482.40	15	387,389,489
482.41	04	079-081
482.41	05	121
482.41	15	387,389
482.49	04	079-081
482.49	05	121
482.49	15	387,389
482.49	25	489
482.81	04	079-081
482.81	15	387,389
482.81	25	489
482.82	04	079-081
482.82	15	387,389
482.82	25	489
482.83	04	079-081
482.83	15	387,389
482.83	25	489
482.84	04	079-081
482.89	04	079-081
482.89	15	387,389
482.89	25	489
482.9	04	089-091
483.0	04	089-091
483.1	04	089-091
483.1	15	387,389
483.8	04	089-091
484.1	04	079-081
484.3	04	079-081
484.5	04	079-081
484.6	04	079-081
484.7	04	079-081
484.8	04	079-081
485	04	089-091
486	04	089-091
487.0	04	089-091
487.1	03	068-070
487.8	18	421-422
490	04	096-098
491.0	04	096-098
491.1	04	088
491.20	04	088
491.21	04	088
491.8	04	088
491.9	04	088
492.0	04	088
492.8	04	088
493.00	04	096-098
493.01	04	096-098
493.02	04	096-098
493.10	04	096-098
493.11	04	096-098
493.12	04	096-098
493.20	04	088
493.21	04	088
493.22	04	088
493.90	04	096-098
493.91	04	096-098
493.92	04	096-098
494.0	04	088
494.1	04	088
495.0	04	092-093
495.1	04	092-093
495.2	04	092-093
495.3	04	092-093
495.4	04	092-093
495.5	04	092-093
495.6	04	092-093
495.7	04	092-093
495.8	04	092-093
495.9	04	092-093
496	04	088
500	04	092-093
501	04	092-093
502	04	092-093
503	04	092-093
504	04	092-093
505	04	092-093
506.0	04	101-102
506.1	04	087
506.2	04	101-102
506.3	04	101-102
506.4	04	088
506.9	04	088
507.0	04	079-081
507.1	04	079-081
507.8	04	079-081
508.0	04	101-102
508.1	04	092-093
508.8	04	101-102
508.9	04	101-102
510.0	04	079-081
510.9	04	079-081
511.0	04	089-091
511.1	04	079-081
511.8	04	085-086
511.9	04	085-086
512.0	04	094-095
512.8	04	094-095
513.0	04	079-081
513.1	04	079-081
514	04	087
515	04	092-093
516.0	04	092-093
516.1	04	092-093
516.2	04	092-093
516.3	04	092-093
516.8	04	092-093
516.9	04	092-093
517.1	04	092-093
517.2	04	092-093
517.8	04	092-093
518.0	04	101-102
518.1	04	094-095
518.2	04	101-102
518.3	04	092-093
518.4	04	087
518.5	04	087
518.6	04	092-093
518.81	04	087
518.82	04	099-100
518.83	04	087
518.84	04	087
518.84	22	506-507
518.89	04	101-102
519.00	Pre	482
519.00	04	101-102
519.01	Pre	482
519.0	04	101-102
519.02	Pre	482
519.02	04	101-102
519.09	Pre	482
519.09	04	101-102
519.1	04	096-098
519.2	04	079-081
519.3	04	101-102
519.4	04	101-102
519.8	04	101-102
519.9	04	101-102

Diseases of the Digestive System

DX	MDC	DRG
520.0	03	185-187
520.1	03	185-187
520.2	03	185-187
520.3	03	185-187
520.4	03	185-187
520.5	03	185-187
520.6	03	185-187
520.7	03	185-187
520.8	03	185-187
520.9	03	185-187
521.00	03	185-187
521.01	03	185-187
521.02	03	185-187
521.03	03	185-187
521.04	03	185-187
521.09	03	185-187
521.1	03	185-187
521.2	03	185-187
521.3	03	185-187
521.4	03	185-187
521.5	03	185-187
521.6	03	185-187
521.7	03	185-187
521.8	03	185-187
521.9	03	185-187
522.0	03	185-187
522.1	03	185-187
522.2	03	185-187
522.3	03	185-187
522.4	03	185-187
522.5	03	185-187
522.6	03	185-187
522.7	03	185-187
522.8	03	185-187
522.9	03	185-187
523.0	03	185-187
523.1	03	185-187
523.2	03	185-187
523.3	03	185-187
523.4	03	185-187
523.5	03	185-187
523.6	03	185-187
523.8	03	185-187
523.9	03	185-187
524.00	03	185-187
524.01	03	185-187
524.02	03	185-187
524.03	03	185-187
524.04	03	185-187
524.05	03	185-187
524.06	03	185-187
524.09	03	185-187
524.10	03	185-187
524.11	03	185-187
524.12	03	185-187
524.19	03	185-187
524.2	03	185-187
524.3	03	185-187
524.4	03	185-187
524.5	03	185-187
524.60	03	185-187
524.61	03	185-187
524.62	03	185-187
524.63	03	185-187
524.69	03	185-187
524.70	03	185-187
524.71	03	185-187
524.72	03	185-187
524.73	03	185-187
524.74	03	185-187
524.79	03	185-187
524.8	03	185-187
524.9	03	185-187
525.0	03	185-187
525.10	03	185-187
525.11	03	185-187
525.12	03	185-187
525.13	03	185-187
525.19	03	185-187
525.2	03	185-187
525.3	03	185-187
525.8	03	185-187
525.9	03	185-187
526.0	03	185-187
526.1	03	185-187
526.2	03	185-187
526.3	03	185-187
526.4	03	185-187
526.5	03	185-187
526.81	03	185-187
526.89	03	185-187
526.9	03	185-187
527.0	03	073-074
527.1	03	073-074
527.2	03	073-074
527.3	03	073-074
527.4	03	073-074
527.5	03	073-074
527.6	03	073-074
527.7	03	073-074
527.8	03	073-074

DX....MDC....DRG	DX....MDC....DRG	DX....MDC....DRG	DX....MDC....DRG
527.9 ...03 073-074	533.20 ..06 174-175	550.01 ..06 188-190	562.10 ..06 182-184
528.0 ...03 185-187	533.21 ..06 174-175	550.02 ..06 188-190	562.11 ..06 182-184
528.1 ...03 185-187	533.30 ..06 177-178	550.03 ..06 188-190	562.12 ..06 174-175
528.2 ...03 185-187	533.31 ..06 176	550.10 ..06 188-190	562.13 ..06 174-175
528.3 ...03 185-187	533.40 ..06 174-175	550.11 ..06 188-190	564.00 ..06 182-184
528.4 ...03 185-187	533.41 ..06 174-175	550.12 ..06 188-190	564.01 ..06 182-184
528.5 ...03 185-187	533.50 ..06 176	550.13 ..06 188-190	564.02 ..06 182-184
528.6 ...03 185-187	533.51 ..06 176	550.90 ..06 188-190	564.09 ..06 182-184
528.7 ...03 185-187	533.60 ..06 174-175	550.91 ..06 188-190	564.1 ..06 182-184
528.8 ...03 185-187	533.61 ..06 174-175	550.92 ..06 188-190	564.2 ..06 182-184
528.9 ...03 185-187	533.70 ..06 177-178	550.93 ..06 188-190	564.3 ..06 182-184
529.0 ...03 185-187	533.71 ..06 176	551.00 ..06 188-190	564.4 ..06 182-184
529.1 ...03 185-187	533.90 ..06 177-178	551.01 ..06 188-190	564.5 ..06 182-184
529.2 ...03 185-187	533.91 ..06 176	551.02 ..06 188-190	564.6 ..06 182-184
529.3 ...03 185-187	534.00 ..06 174-175	551.03 ..06 188-190	564.7 ..06 188-190
529.4 ...03 185-187	534.01 ..06 174-175	551.1 ..06 188-190	564.81 ..06 182-184
529.5 ...03 185-187	534.10 ..06 176	551.20 ..06 188-190	564.89 ..06 182-184
529.6 ...03 185-187	534.11 ..06 176	551.21 ..06 188-190	564.9 ..06 182-184
529.8 ...03 185-187	534.20 ..06 174-175	551.29 ..06 188-190	565.0 ..06 188-190
529.9 ...03 185-187	534.21 ..06 174-175	551.3 ..06 188-190	565.1 ..06 188-190
530.0 ...06 182-184	534.30 ..06 176	551.8 ..06 188-190	566 ..06 188-190
530.10 ..06 182-184	534.31 ..06 176	551.9 ..06 188-190	567.0 ..06 188-190
530.11 ..06 182-184	534.40 ..06 174-175	552.00 ..06 188-190	567.1 ..06 188-190
530.12 ..06 182-184	534.41 ..06 174-175	552.01 ..06 188-190	567.2 ..06 188-190
530.19 ..06 182-184	534.50 ..06 176	552.02 ..06 188-190	567.8 ..06 188-190
530.2 ...06 176	534.51 ..06 176	552.03 ..06 188-190	567.9 ..06 188-190
530.3 ...06 182-184	534.60 ..06 174-175	552.1 ..06 188-190	568.0 ..06 188-190
530.4 ...06 182-184	534.61 ..06 174-175	552.20 ..06 188-190	568.81 ..06 188-190
530.5 ...06 182-184	534.70 ..06 176	552.21 ..06 188-190	568.82 ..06 188-190
530.6 ...06 182-184	534.71 ..06 176	552.29 ..06 188-190	568.89 ..06 188-190
530.7 ...06 174-175	534.90 ..06 176	552.3 ..06 182-184	568.9 ..06 188-190
530.81 ..06 182-184	534.91 ..06 176	552.8 ..06 188-190	569.0 ..06 188-190
530.82 ..06 174-175	535.00 ..06 182-184	552.9 ..06 188-190	569.1 ..06 188-190
530.83 ..06 182-184	535.01 ..06 174-175	553.00 ..06 188-190	569.2 ..06 188-190
530.84 ..06 182-184	535.10 ..06 182-184	553.01 ..06 188-190	569.3 ..06 174-175
530.89 ..06 182-184	535.11 ..06 174-175	553.02 ..06 188-190	569.41 ..06 188-190
530.9 ...06 182-184	535.20 ..06 182-184	553.03 ..06 188-190	569.42 ..06 188-190
531.00 ..06 174-175	535.21 ..06 174-175	553.1 ..06 188-190	569.49 ..06 188-190
531.01 ..06 174-175	535.30 ..06 182-184	553.20 ..06 188-190	569.5 ..06 188-190
531.10 ..06 176	535.31 ..06 174-175	553.21 ..06 188-190	569.60 ..06 188-190
531.11 ..06 176	535.40 ..06 182-184	553.29 ..06 188-190	569.61 ..06 188-190
531.20 ..06 174-175	535.41 ..06 174-175	553.3 ..06 182-184	569.62 ..06 188-190
531.21 ..06 174-175	535.50 ..06 182-184	553.8 ..06 188-190	569.69 ..06 188-190
531.30 ..06 177-178	535.51 ..06 174-175	553.9 ..06 188-190	569.81 ..06 188-190
531.31 ..06 176	535.60 ..06 182-184	555.0 ..06 179	569.82 ..06 188-190
531.40 ..06 174-175	535.61 ..06 174-175	555.1 ..06 179	569.83 ..06 188-190
531.41 ..06 174-175	536.0 ..06 182-184	555.2 ..06 179	569.84 ..06 188-190
531.50 ..06 176	536.1 ..06 182-184	555.9 ..06 179	569.85 ..06 174-175
531.51 ..06 176	536.2 ..06 182-184	556.0 ..06 179	569.86 ..06 188-190
531.60 ..06 174-175	536.3 ..06 182-184	556.1 ..06 179	569.89 ..06 188-190
531.61 ..06 174-175	536.40 ..06 188-190	556.2 ..06 179	569.9 ..06 188-190
531.70 ..06 177-178	536.41 ..06 188-190	556.3 ..06 179	570 ...07 205-206
531.71 ..06 176	536.42 ..06 188-190	556.4 ..06 179	571.0 ..07 205-206
531.90 ..06 177-178	536.49 ..06 188-190	566.5 ..06 179	571.1 ..07 202
531.91 ..06 176	536.8 ..06 182-184	566.6 ..06 179	571.2 ..07 202
532.00 ..06 174-175	536.9 ..06 182-184	566.8 ..06 179	571.3 ..07 202
532.01 ..06 174-175	537.0 ..06 176	566.9 ..06 179	571.40 ..07 205-206
532.10 ..06 176	537.1 ..06 182-184	557.0 ..06 188-190	571.41 ..07 205-206
532.11 ..06 176	537.2 ..06 182-184	557.1 ..06 188-190	571.49 ..07 205-206
532.20 ..06 174-175	537.3 ..06 176	557.9 ..06 188-190	571.5 ..07 202
532.21 ..06 174-175	537.4 ..06 182-184	558.1 ..06 188-190	571.6 ..07 202
532.30 ..06 177-178	537.5 ..06 182-184	558.2 ..06 188-190	571.8 ..07 205-206
532.31 ..06 176	537.6 ..06 182-184	558.3 ..06 182-184	571.9 ..07 205-206
532.40 ..06 174-175	537.81 ..06 182-184	558.9 ..06 182-184	572.0 ..07 205-206
532.41 ..06 174-175	537.82 ..06 182-184	560.0 ..06 180-181	572.1 ..07 205-206
532.50 ..06 176	537.83 ..06 174-175	560.1 ..06 180-181	572.2 ..07 205-206
532.51 ..06 176	537.84 ..06 174-175	560.2 ..06 180-181	572.3 ..07 205-206
532.60 ..06 174-175	537.89 ..06 182-184	560.30 ..06 180-181	572.4 ..07 205-206
532.61 ..06 174-175	537.9 ..06 182-184	560.31 ..06 180-181	572.8 ..07 205-206
532.70 ..06 177-178	540.0 ..06 164-165,188-190	560.39 ..06 180-181	573.0 ..07 205-206
532.71 ..06 176	540.1 ..06 164-165,188-190	560.81 ..06 180-181	573.1 ..07 205-206
532.90 ..06 177-178	540.9 ..06 188-190	560.89 ..06 180-181	573.2 ..07 205-206
532.91 ..06 176	541 ....06 188-190	560.9 ..06 180-181	573.3 ..07 205-206
533.00 ..06 174-175	542 ....06 188-190	562.00 ..06 182-184	573.4 ..07 205-206
533.01 ..06 174-175	543.0 ..06 188-190	562.01 ..06 182-184	573.8 ..07 205-206
533.10 ..06 176	543.9 ..06 188-190	562.02 ..06 174-175	573.9 ..07 205-206
533.11 ..06 176	550.00 ..06 188-190	562.03 ..06 174-175	574.00 ..07 207-208

Diagnosis Code/MDC/DRG List

DX	MDC	DRG
574.01	07	207-208
574.10	07	207-208
574.11	07	207-208
574.20	07	207-208
574.21	07	207-208
574.30	07	207-208
574.31	07	207-208
574.40	07	207-208
574.41	07	207-208
574.50	07	207-208
574.51	07	207-208
574.60	07	207-208
574.61	07	207-208
574.70	07	207-208
574.71	07	207-208
574.80	07	207-208
574.81	07	207-208
574.90	07	207-208
574.91	07	207-208
575.0	07	207-208
575.10	07	207-208
575.11	07	207-208
575.12	07	207-208
575.2	07	207-208
575.3	07	207-208
575.4	07	207-208
575.5	07	207-208
575.6	07	207-208
575.8	07	207-208
575.9	07	207-208
576.0	07	207-208
576.1	07	207-208
576.2	07	207-208
576.3	07	207-208
576.4	07	207-208
576.5	07	207-208
576.8	07	207-208
576.9	07	207-208
577.0	07	204
577.1	07	204
577.2	07	204
577.8	07	204
577.9	07	204
578.0	06	174-175
578.1	06	174-175
578.9	06	174-175
579.0	06	182-184
579.1	06	182-184
579.2	06	182-184
579.3	06	182-184
579.4	06	182-184
579.8	06	182-184
579.9	06	182-184

Diseases of the Genitourinary System

DX	MDC	DRG
580.0	11	331-333
580.4	11	331-333
580.81	11	331-333
580.89	11	331-333
580.9	11	331-333
581.0	11	331-333
581.1	11	331-333
581.2	11	331-333
581.3	11	331-333
581.81	11	331-333
581.89	11	331-333
581.9	11	331-333
582.0	11	331-333
582.1	11	331-333
582.2	11	331-333
582.4	11	331-333
582.81	11	331-333
582.89	11	331-333
582.9	11	331-333
583.0	11	331-333
583.1	11	331-333
583.2	11	331-333
583.4	11	331-333
583.6	11	331-333
583.7	11	331-333
583.81	11	331-333
583.89	11	331-333
583.9	11	331-333
584.5	11	316
584.6	11	316
584.7	11	316
584.8	11	316
584.9	11	316
585	11	316
586	11	316
587	11	331-333
588.0	11	331-333
588.1	11	331-333
588.8	11	331-333
588.9	11	331-333
589.0	11	331-333
589.1	11	331-333
589.9	11	331-333
590.00	11	320-322
590.01	11	320-322
590.10	11	320-322
590.11	11	320-322
590.2	11	320-322
590.3	11	320-322
590.80	11	320-322
590.81	11	320-322
590.9	11	320-322
591	11	323-324
592.0	11	323-324
592.1	11	323-324
592.9	11	323-324
593.0	11	331-333
593.1	11	331-333
593.2	11	331-333
593.3	11	320-322
593.4	11	323-324
593.5	11	323-324
593.6	11	331-333
593.70	11	331-333
593.71	11	331-333
593.72	11	331-333
593.73	11	331-333
593.81	11	331-333
593.82	11	331-333
593.89	11	331-333
593.9	11	331-333
594.0	11	331-333
594.1	11	323-324
594.2	11	323-324
594.8	11	323-324
594.9	11	323-324
595.0	11	320-322
595.1	11	320-322
595.2	11	320-322
595.3	11	320-322
595.4	11	320-322
595.81	11	320-322
595.82	11	331-333
595.89	11	320-322
595.9	11	320-322
596.0	11	331-333
596.1	11	331-333
596.2	11	331-333
596.3	11	331-333
596.4	11	331-333
596.51	11	331-333
596.52	11	331-333
596.53	11	331-333
596.54	11	331-333
596.55	11	331-333
596.59	11	331-333
596.6	11	331-333
596.7	11	331-333
596.8	11	331-333
596.9	11	331-333
597.0	11	320-322
597.80	11	320-322
597.81	11	320-322
597.89	11	320-322
598.00	11	328-330
598.01	11	328-330
598.1	11	328-330
598.2	11	328-330
598.8	11	328-330
598.9	11	328-330
599.0	11	320-322
599.1	11	331-333
599.2	11	331-333
599.3	11	331-333
599.4	11	331-333
599.5	11	331-333
599.6	11	331-333
599.7	11	325-327
599.81	11	331-333
599.82	11	331-333
599.83	11	331-333
599.84	11	331-333
599.89	11	331-333
599.9	11	331-333
600.0	12	348-349
600.1	12	348-349
600.2	12	348-349
600.3	12	348-349
600.9	12	348-349
601.0	12	350
601.1	12	350
601.2	12	350
601.3	12	350
601.4	12	350
601.8	12	350
601.9	12	350
602.0	12	352
602.1	12	352
602.2	12	352
602.3	12	352
602.8	12	352
602.9	12	352
603.0	12	352
603.1	12	350
603.8	12	352
603.9	12	352
604.0	12	350
604.90	12	350
604.91	12	350
604.99	12	350
605	12	350
606.0	12	352
606.1	12	352
606.8	12	352
606.9	12	352
607.0	12	352
607.1	12	350
607.2	12	350
607.3	12	352
607.81	12	350
607.82	12	352
607.83	12	352
607.84	12	352
607.89	12	352
607.9	12	352
608.0	12	350
608.1	12	352
608.2	12	352
608.3	12	352
608.4	12	350
608.81	12	352
608.82	12	352
608.83	12	352
608.84	12	352
608.85	12	352
608.86	12	352
608.87	12	352
608.89	12	352
608.9	12	352
610.0	09	276
610.1	09	276
610.2	09	276
610.3	09	276
610.4	09	276
610.8	09	276
610.9	09	276
611.0	09	276
611.1	09	276
611.2	09	276
611.3	09	276
611.4	09	276
611.5	09	276
611.6	09	276
611.71	09	276
611.72	09	276
611.79	09	276
611.8	09	276
611.9	09	276
614.0	13	358-359,368
614.1	13	358-359,368
614.2	13	358-359,368
614.3	13	358-359,368
614.4	13	358-359,368
614.5	13	358-359,368
614.6	13	358-359,369
614.7	13	358-359,368
614.8	13	358-359,368
614.9	13	358-359,368
615.0	13	358-359,368
615.1	13	358-359,368
615.9	13	358-359,368
616.0	13	358-359,368
616.10	13	358-359,368
616.11	13	358-359,368
616.2	13	358-359,368
616.3	13	358-359,368
616.4	13	358-359,368
616.50	13	358-359,369
616.51	13	358-359,369
616.8	13	358-359,368
616.9	13	358-359,368
617.0	13	358-359,368
617.1	13	358-359,369
617.2	13	358-359,369
617.3	13	358-359,369
617.4	13	358-359,369
617.5	06	182-184
617.6	09	283-284
617.8	13	358-359,368
617.9	13	358-359,369
618.0	13	358-359,369
618.1	13	358-359,369
618.2	13	358-359,369
618.3	13	358-359,369
618.4	13	358-359,369
618.5	13	358-359,369
618.6	13	358-359,369
618.7	13	358-359,369
618.8	13	358-359,369
618.9	13	358-359,369
619.0	13	358-359,369
619.1	06	188-190
619.2	13	358-359,369
619.8	13	358-359,369
619.9	13	358-359,369
620.0	13	358-359,369
620.1	13	358-359,369
620.2	13	358-359,369
620.3	13	358-359,369
620.4	13	358-359,369
620.5	13	358-359,369
620.6	13	358-359,369

DX....MDC....DRG	DX....MDC....DRG	DX....MDC....DRG	DX....MDC....DRG
620.7 ...13 358-359,369	629.8 ...13 358-359,369	635.80 ..14 380-381	639.1 ...14 376-377
620.8 ...13 358-359,369	629.9 ...13 358-359,369	635.81 ..14 380-381	639.2 ...14 376-377
620.9 ...13 358-359,369		635.82 ..14 380-381	639.3 ...14 376-377
621.0 ...13 358-359,369	**Complications of Pregnancy,**	635.90 ..14 380-381	639.4 ...14 376-377
621.1 ...13 358-359,369	**Childbirth and the Puerperium**	635.91 ..14 380-381	639.5 ...14 376-377
621.2 ...13 358-359,369	630 ....14 383-384	635.92 ..14 380-381	639.6 ...14 376-377
621.3 ...13 358-359,369	631 ....14 383-384	636.00 ..14 380-381	639.8 ...14 376-377
621.4 ...13 358-359,369	632 ....14 380-381	636.01 ..14 380-381	639.9 ...14 376-377
621.5 ...13 358-359,369	633.00 ..14 378	636.02 ..14 380-381	640.00 ..14 379
621.6 ...13 358-359,369	633.01 ..14 378	636.10 ..14 380-381	640.01 ..14 370-375
621.7 ...13 358-359,369	633.10 ..14 378	636.11 ..14 380-381	640.03 ..14 379
621.8 ...13 358-359,369	633.11 ..14 378	636.12 ..14 380-381	640.80 ..14 379
621.9 ...13 358-359,369	633.20 ..14 378	636.20 ..14 380-381	640.81 ..14 370-375
622.0 ...13 358-359,369	633.21 ..14 378	636.21 ..14 380-381	640.83 ..14 379
622.1 ...13 358-359,369	633.80 ..14 378	636.22 ..14 380-381	640.90 ..14 379
622.2 ...13 358-359,369	633.81 ..14 378	636.30 ..14 380-381	640.91 ..14 370-375
622.3 ...13 358-359,369	633.90 ..14 378	636.31 ..14 380-381	640.93 ..14 379
622.4 ...13 358-359,369	633.91 ..14 378	636.32 ..14 380-381	641.00 ..14 469
622.5 ...13 358-359,369	633.0 ...14 378	636.40 ..14 380-381	641.01 ..14 370-372,374-375
622.6 ...13 358-359,369	633.1 ...14 378	636.41 ..14 380-381	641.03 ..14 383-384
622.7 ...13 358-359,369	633.2 ...14 378	636.42 ..14 380-381	641.10 ..14 469
622.8 ...13 358-359,369	633.8 ...14 378	636.50 ..14 380-381	641.11 ..14 370-372,374-375
622.9 ...13 358-359,369	633.9 ...14 378	636.51 ..14 380-381	641.13 ..14 383-384
623.0 ...13 358-359,369	634.00 ..14 380-381	636.52 ..14 380-381	641.20 ..14 469
623.1 ...13 358-359,369	634.01 ..14 380-381	636.60 ..14 380-381	641.21 ..14 370-372,374-375
623.2 ...13 358-359,369	634.02 ..14 380-381	636.61 ..14 380-381	641.23 ..14 383-384
623.3 ...13 358-359,369	634.10 ..14 380-381	636.62 ..14 380-381	641.30 ..14 469
623.4 ...13 358-359,369	634.11 ..14 380-381	636.70 ..14 380-381	641.31 ..14 370-372,374-375
623.5 ...13 358-359,369	634.12 ..14 380-381	636.71 ..14 380-381	641.33 ..14 383
623.6 ...13 358-359,369	634.20 ..14 380-381	636.72 ..14 380-381	641.80 ..14 469
623.7 ...13 358-359,369	634.21 ..14 380-381	636.80 ..14 380-381	641.81 ..14 370-372,374-375
623.8 ...13 358-359,369	634.22 ..14 380-381	636.81 ..14 380-381	641.83 ..14 383-384
623.9 ...13 358-359,369	634.30 ..14 380-381	636.82 ..14 380-381	641.90 ..14 469
624.0 ...13 358-359,369	634.31 ..14 380-381	636.90 ..14 380-381	641.91 ..14 370-372,374-375
624.1 ...13 358-359,369	634.32 ..14 380-381	636.91 ..14 380-381	641.93 ..14 383-384
624.2 ...13 358-359,369	634.40 ..14 380-381	636.92 ..14 380-381	642.00 ..14 469
624.3 ...13 358-359,369	634.41 ..14 380-381	637.00 ..14 380-381	642.01 ..14 370-372,374-375
624.4 ...13 358-359,369	634.42 ..14 380-381	637.01 ..14 380-381	642.02 ..14 370-372,374-375
624.5 ...13 358-359,369	634.50 ..14 380-381	637.02 ..14 380-381	642.03 ..14 383
624.6 ...13 358-359,369	634.51 ..14 380-381	637.10 ..14 380-381	642.04 ..14 376-377
624.8 ...13 358-359,369	634.52 ..14 380-381	637.11 ..14 380-381	642.10 ..14 469
624.9 ...13 358-359,369	634.60 ..14 380-381	637.12 ..14 380-381	642.11 ..14 370-372,374-375
625.0 ...13 358-359,369	634.61 ..14 380-381	637.20 ..14 380-381	642.12 ..14 370-372,374-375
625.1 ...13 358-359,369	634.62 ..14 380-381	637.21 ..14 380-381	642.13 ..14 383
625.2 ...13 358-359,369	634.70 ..14 380-381	637.22 ..14 380-381	642.14 ..14 376-377
625.3 ...13 358-359,369	634.71 ..14 380-381	637.30 ..14 380-381	642.20 ..14 469
625.4 ...13 358-359,369	634.72 ..14 380-381	637.31 ..14 380-381	642.21 ..14 370-372,374-375
625.5 ...13 358-359,369	634.80 ..14 380-381	637.32 ..14 380-381	642.22 ..14 370-372,374-375
625.6 ...13 358-359,369	634.81 ..14 380-381	637.40 ..14 380-381	642.23 ..14 383
625.8 ...13 358-359,369	634.82 ..14 380-381	637.41 ..14 380-381	642.24 ..14 376-377
625.9 ...13 358-359,369	634.90 ..14 380-381	637.42 ..14 380-381	642.30 ..14 469
626.0 ...13 358-359,369	634.91 ..14 380-381	637.50 ..14 380-381	642.31 ..14 370-375
626.1 ...13 358-359,369	634.92 ..14 380-381	637.51 ..14 380-381	642.32 ..14 370-375
626.2 ...13 358-359,369	635.00 ..14 380-381	637.52 ..14 380-381	642.33 ..14 383-384
626.3 ...13 358-359,369	635.01 ..14 380-381	637.60 ..14 380-381	642.34 ..14 376-377
626.4 ...13 358-359,369	635.02 ..14 380-381	637.61 ..14 380-381	642.40 ..14 469
626.5 ...13 358-359,369	635.10 ..14 380-381	637.62 ..14 380-381	642.41 ..14 370-372,374-375
626.6 ...13 358-359,369	635.11 ..14 380-381	637.70 ..14 380-381	642.42 ..14 370-372,374-375
626.7 ...13 358-359,369	635.12 ..14 380-381	637.71 ..14 380-381	642.43 ..14 383
626.8 ...13 358-359,369	635.20 ..14 380-381	637.72 ..14 380-381	642.44 ..14 376-377
626.9 ...13 358-359,369	635.21 ..14 380-381	637.80 ..14 380-381	642.50 ..14 469
627.0 ...13 358-359,369	635.22 ..14 380-381	637.81 ..14 380-381	642.51 ..14 370-372,374-375
627.1 ...13 358-359,369	635.30 ..14 380-381	637.82 ..14 380-381	642.52 ..14 370-372,374-375
627.2 ...13 358-359,369	635.31 ..14 380-381	637.90 ..14 380-381	642.53 ..14 383
627.3 ...13 358-359,369	635.32 ..14 380-381	637.91 ..14 380-381	642.54 ..14 376-377
627.4 ...13 358-359,369	635.40 ..14 380-381	637.92 ..14 380-381	642.60 ..14 469
627.8 ...13 358-359,369	635.41 ..14 380-381	638.0 ...14 380-381	642.61 ..14 370-372,374-375
627.9 ...13 358-359,369	635.42 ..14 380-381	638.1 ...14 380-381	642.62 ..14 370-372,374-375
628.0 ...13 358-359,369	635.50 ..14 380-381	638.2 ...14 380-381	642.63 ..14 383
628.1 ...13 358-359,369	635.51 ..14 380-381	638.3 ...14 380-381	642.64 ..14 376-377
628.2 ...13 358-359,369	635.52 ..14 380-381	638.4 ...14 380-381	642.70 ..14 469
628.3 ...13 358-359,369	635.60 ..14 380-381	638.5 ...14 380-381	642.71 ..14 370-372,374-375
628.4 ...13 358-359,369	635.61 ..14 380-381	638.6 ...14 380-381	642.72 ..14 370-372,374-375
628.8 ...13 358-359,369	635.62 ..14 380-381	638.7 ...14 380-381	642.73 ..14 383
628.9 ...13 358-359,369	635.70 ..14 380-381	638.8 ...14 380-381	642.74 ..14 376-377
629.0 ...13 358-359,369	635.71 ..14 380-381	638.9 ...14 380-381	642.90 ..14 469
629.1 ...13 358-359,369	635.72 ..14 380-381	639.0 ...14 376-377	642.91 ..14 370-372,374-375

DX....MDC....DRG	DX....MDC....DRG	DX....MDC....DRG	DX....MDC....DRG
642.92 ..14 370-372,374-375	647.10 ..14 469	648.72 ..14 ....370 -375	653.20 ..14 469
642.93 ..14 383	647.11 ..14 370-372,374-375	648.73 ..14 383	653.21 ..14 370-375
642.94 ..14 376-377	647.12 ..14 370-372,374-375	648.74 ..14 376-377	653.23 ..14 383-384
643.00 ..14 469	647.13 ..14 383	648.80 ..14 469	653.30 ..14 469
643.01 ..14 370-375	647.14 ..14 376-377	648.81 ..14 370-375	653.31 ..14 370-375
643.03 ..14 383	647.20 ..14 469	648.82 ..14 370-375	653.33 ..14 383-384
643.10 ..14 469	647.21 ..14 370-372,374-375	648.83 ..14 383	653.40 ..14 469
643.11 ..14 370-375	647.22 ..14 370-372,374-375	648.84 ..14 376-377	653.41 ..14 370-375
643.13 ..14 383	647.23 ..14 383	648.90 ..14 469	653.43 ..14 383-384
643.20 ..14 469	647.24 ..14 376-377	648.91 ..14 370-375	653.50 ..14 469
643.21 ..14 370-375	647.30 ..14 469	648.92 ..14 370-375	653.51 ..14 370-375
643.23 ..14 383	647.31 ..14 370-372,374-375	648.93 ..14 383	653.53 ..14 383-384
643.80 ..14 469	647.32 ..14 370-372,374-375	648.94 ..14 376-377	653.60 ..14 469
643.81 ..14 370-375	647.33 ..14 383	650 ..14 370-375	653.61 ..14 370-375
643.83 ..14 383	647.34 ..14 376-377	651.00 ..14 469	653.63 ..14 383-384
643.90 ..14 469	647.40 ..14 469	651.01 ..14 370-375	653.70 ..14 469
643.91 ..14 370-375	647.41 ..14 370-372,374-375	651.03 ..14 383-384	653.71 ..14 370-375
643.93 ..14 383	647.42 ..14 370-372,374-375	651.10 ..14 469	653.73 ..14 383-384
644.00 ..14 379	647.43 ..14 383	651.11 ..14 370-375	653.80 ..14 469
644.03 ..14 379	647.44 ..14 376-377	651.13 ..14 383-384	653.81 ..14 370-375
644.10 ..14 382	647.50 ..14 469	651.20 ..14 469	653.83 ..14 383-384
644.13 ..14 382	647.51 ..14 370-372,374-375	651.21 ..14 370-375	653.90 ..14 469
644.20 ..14 383-384	647.52 ..14 370-372,374-375	651.23 ..14 383-384	653.91 ..14 370-375
644.21 ..14 370-375	647.53 ..14 383	651.30 ..14 469	653.93 ..14 383-384
645.10 ..14 469	647.54 ..14 376-377	651.31 ..14 370-375	654.00 ..14 469
645.11 ..14 370-375	647.60 ..14 469	651.33 ..14 383-384	654.01 ..14 370-375
645.13 ..14 383-384	647.61 ..14 370-372,374-375	651.40 ..14 469	654.02 ..14 370-375
645.20 ..14 469	647.62 ..14 370-372,374-375	651.41 ..14 370-375	654.03 ..14 383-384
645.21 ..14 370-375	647.63 ..14 383	651.43 ..14 383-384	654.04 ..14 376-377
645.23 ..14 383-384	647.64 ..14 376-377	651.50 ..14 469	654.10 ..14 469
646.00 ..14 370-375	647.80 ..14 469	651.51 ..14 370-375	654.11 ..14 370-375
646.01 ..14 370-375	647.81 ..14 370-372,374-375	651.53 ..14 383-384	654.12 ..14 370-375
646.03 ..14 383-384	647.82 ..14 370-372,374-375	651.60 ..14 469	654.13 ..14 383-384
646.10 ..14 469	647.83 ..14 383	651.61 ..14 370-375	654.14 ..14 376-377
646.11 ..14 370-375	647.84 ..14 376-377	651.63 ..14 383-384	654.20 ..14 469
646.12 ..14 370-375	647.90 ..14 469	651.80 ..14 469	654.21 ..14 370-375
646.13 ..14 383	647.91 ..14 370-372,374-375	651.81 ..14 370-375	654.23 ..14 383-384
646.14 ..14 376-377	647.92 ..14 370-372,374-375	651.83 ..14 383-384	654.30 ..14 469
646.20 ..14 469	647.93 ..14 383	651.90 ..14 469	654.31 ..14 370-375
646.21 ..14 370-375	647.94 ..14 376-377	651.91 ..14 370-375	654.32 ..14 370-375
646.22 ..14 370-375	648.00 ..14 469	651.93 ..14 383-384	654.33 ..14 383-384
646.23 ..14 383	648.01 ..14 370-372,374-375	652.00 ..14 469	654.34 ..14 376-377
646.24 ..14 376-377	648.02 ..14 370-372,374-375	652.01 ..14 370-375	654.40 ..14 469
646.30 ..14 469	648.03 ..14 383	652.03 ..14 383-384	654.41 ..14 370-375
646.31 ..14 370-375	648.04 ..14 376-377	652.10 ..14 469	654.42 ..14 370-375
646.33 ..14 383-384	648.10 ..14 469	652.11 ..14 370-375	654.43 ..14 383-384
646.40 ..14 469	648.11 ..14 370-375	652.13 ..14 383-384	654.44 ..14 376-377
646.41 ..14 370-375	648.12 ..14 370-375	652.20 ..14 469	654.50 ..14 469
646.42 ..14 370-375	648.13 ..14 383	652.21 ..14 370-375	654.51 ..14 370-375
646.43 ..14 383	648.14 ..14 376-377	652.23 ..14 383-384	654.52 ..14 370-375
646.44 ..14 376-377	648.20 ..14 469	652.30 ..14 469	654.53 ..14 383-384
646.50 ..14 469	648.21 ..14 370-375	652.31 ..14 370-375	654.54 ..14 376-377
646.51 ..14 370-375	648.22 ..14 370-375	652.33 ..14 383-384	654.60 ..14 469
646.52 ..14 370-375	648.23 ..14 383	652.40 ..14 469	654.61 ..14 370-375
646.53 ..14 383-384	648.24 ..14 376-377	652.41 ..14 370-375	654.62 ..14 370-375
646.54 ..14 376-377	648.30 ..14 469	652.43 ..14 383-384	654.63 ..14 383-384
646.60 ..14 469	648.31 ..14 370-375	652.50 ..14 469	654.64 ..14 376-377
646.61 ..14 370-375	648.32 ..14 370-375	652.51 ..14 370-375	654.70 ..14 469
646.62 ..14 370-375	648.33 ..14 383	652.53 ..14 383-384	654.71 ..14 370-375
646.63 ..14 383	648.34 ..14 376-377	652.60 ..14 469	654.72 ..14 370-375
646.64 ..14 376-377	648.40 ..14 469	652.61 ..14 370-375	654.73 ..14 383-384
646.70 ..14 469	648.41 ..14 370-375	652.63 ..14 383-384	654.74 ..14 376-377
646.71 ..14 370-375	648.42 ..14 370-375	652.70 ..14 469	654.80 ..14 469
646.73 ..14 383	648.43 ..14 383	652.71 ..14 370-375	654.81 ..14 370-375
646.80 ..14 469	648.44 ..14 376-377	652.73 ..14 383-384	654.82 ..14 370-375
646.81 ..14 370-375	648.50 ..14 469	652.80 ..14 469	654.83 ..14 383-384
646.82 ..14 370-375	648.51 ..14 370-372,374-375	652.81 ..14 370-375	654.84 ..14 376-377
646.83 ..14 383	648.52 ..14 370-372,374-375	652.83 ..14 383-384	654.90 ..14 469
646.84 ..14 376-377	648.53 ..14 383	652.90 ..14 469	654.91 ..14 370-375
646.90 ..14 469	648.54 ..14 376-377	652.91 ..14 370-375	654.92 ..14 370-375
646.91 ..14 370-375	648.60 ..14 469	652.93 ..14 383-384	654.93 ..14 383-384
646.93 ..14 383-384	648.61 ..14 370-372,374-375	653.00 ..14 469	654.94 ..14 376-377
647.00 ..14 469	648.62 ..14 370-372,374-375	653.01 ..14 370-375	655.00 ..14 469
647.01 ..14 370-372,374-375	648.63 ..14 383	653.03 ..14 383-384	655.01 ..14 370-375
647.02 ..14 370-372,374-375	648.64 ..14 376-377	653.10 ..14 469	655.03 ..14 383-384
647.03 ..14 383	648.70 ..14 469	653.11 ..14 370-375	655.10 ..14 469
647.04 ..14 376-377	648.71 ..14 370-375	653.13 ..14 383-384	655.11 ..14 370-375

Diagnosis Code/MDC/DRG List

DX	MDC	DRG
655.13	14	383-384
655.20	14	469
655.21	14	370-375
655.23	14	383-384
655.30	14	469
655.31	14	370-375
655.33	14	383-384
655.40	14	469
655.41	14	370-375
655.43	14	383-384
655.50	14	469
655.51	14	370-375
655.53	14	383-384
655.60	14	469
655.61	14	370-375
655.63	14	383-384
655.70	14	469
655.71	14	370-375
655.73	14	383-384
655.80	14	469
655.81	14	370-375
655.83	14	383-384
655.90	14	469
655.91	14	370-375
655.93	14	383-384
656.00	14	469
656.01	14	370-375
656.03	14	383-384
656.10	14	469
656.11	14	370-375
656.13	14	383-384
656.20	14	469
656.21	14	370-375
656.23	14	383-384
656.30	14	370-375
656.31	14	370-375
656.33	14	383-384
656.40	14	370-375
656.41	14	370-375
656.43	14	383-384
656.50	14	469
656.51	14	370-375
656.53	14	383-384
656.60	14	469
656.61	14	370-375
656.63	14	383-384
656.70	14	469
656.71	14	370-375
656.73	14	383-384
656.80	14	469
656.81	14	370-375
656.83	14	383-384
656.90	14	469
656.91	14	370-375
656.93	14	383-384
657.00	14	469
657.01	14	370-375
657.03	14	383-384
658.00	14	469
658.01	14	370-375
658.03	14	383-384
658.10	14	370-375
658.11	14	370-375
658.13	14	383-384
658.20	14	370-375
658.21	14	370-375
658.23	14	383-384
658.30	14	370-375
658.31	14	370-375
658.33	14	383-384
658.40	14	370-375
658.41	14	370-375
658.43	14	383-384
658.80	14	469
658.81	14	370-375
658.83	14	383-384
658.90	14	469
658.91	14	370-375
658.93	14	383-384
659.00	14	370-375
659.01	14	370-375
659.03	14	383-384
659.10	14	370-375
659.11	14	370-375
659.13	14	383-384
659.20	14	370-375
659.21	14	370-372,374-375
659.23	14	383-384
659.30	14	370-375
659.31	14	370-372,374-375
659.33	14	383-384
659.40	14	469
659.41	14	370-375
659.43	14	383-384
659.50	14	370-375
659.51	14	370-375
659.53	14	383-384
659.60	14	370-375
659.61	14	370-375
659.63	14	383-384
659.70	14	370-375
659.71	14	370-375
659.73	14	383-384
659.80	14	370-375
659.81	14	370-375
659.83	14	383-384
659.90	14	370-375
659.91	14	370-375
659.93	14	383-384
660.00	14	370-375
660.01	14	370-375
660.03	14	383-384
660.10	14	370-375
660.11	14	370-375
660.13	14	383-384
660.20	14	370-375
660.21	14	370-375
660.23	14	383-384
660.30	14	370-375
660.31	14	370-375
660.33	14	383-384
660.40	14	370-375
660.41	14	370-375
660.43	14	383-384
660.50	14	370-375
660.51	14	370-375
660.53	14	383-384
660.60	14	370-375
660.61	14	370-375
660.63	14	383-384
660.70	14	370-375
660.71	14	370-375
660.73	14	383-384
660.80	14	370-375
660.81	14	370-375
660.83	14	383-384
660.90	14	370-375
660.91	14	370-375
660.93	14	383-384
661.00	14	370-375
661.01	14	370-375
661.03	14	383-384
661.10	14	370-375
661.11	14	370-375
661.13	14	383-384
661.20	14	370-375
661.21	14	370-375
661.23	14	383-384
661.30	14	370-375
661.31	14	370-375
661.33	14	383-384
661.40	14	370-375
661.41	14	370-375
661.43	14	383-384
661.90	14	370-375
661.91	14	370-375
661.93	14	383-384
662.00	14	370-375
662.01	14	370-375
662.03	14	383-384
662.10	14	370-375
662.11	14	370-375
662.13	14	383-384
662.20	14	370-375
662.21	14	370-375
662.23	14	383-384
662.30	14	370-375
662.31	14	370-375
662.33	14	383-384
663.00	14	370-375
663.01	14	370-375
663.03	14	383-384
663.10	14	370-375
663.11	14	370-375
663.13	14	383-384
663.20	14	370-375
663.21	14	370-375
663.23	14	383-384
663.30	14	370-375
663.31	14	370-375
663.33	14	383-384
663.40	14	370-375
663.41	14	370-375
663.43	14	383-384
663.50	14	370-375
663.51	14	370-375
663.53	14	383-384
663.60	14	370-375
663.61	14	370-375
663.63	14	383-384
663.80	14	370-375
663.81	14	370-375
663.83	14	383-384
663.90	14	370-375
663.91	14	370-375
663.93	14	383-384
664.00	14	370-375
664.01	14	370-375
664.04	14	376-377
664.10	14	370-375
664.11	14	370-375
664.14	14	376-377
664.20	14	370-375
664.21	14	370-375
664.24	14	376-377
664.30	14	370-375
664.31	14	370-375
664.34	14	376-377
664.40	14	370-375
664.41	14	370-375
664.44	14	376-377
664.50	14	370-375
664.51	14	370-375
664.54	14	376-377
664.80	14	370-375
664.81	14	370-375
664.84	14	376-377
664.90	14	370-375
664.91	14	370-375
664.94	14	376-377
665.00	14	370-375
665.01	14	370-375
665.03	14	383-384
665.10	14	370-375
665.11	14	370-375
665.20	14	370-375
665.22	14	370-375
665.24	14	376-377
665.30	14	370-375
665.31	14	370-375
665.34	14	376-377
665.40	14	370-375
665.41	14	370-375
665.44	14	376-377
665.50	14	370-375
665.51	14	370-375
665.54	14	376-377
665.60	14	370-375
665.61	14	370-375
665.64	14	376-377
665.70	14	370-375
665.71	14	370-375
665.72	14	370-375
665.74	14	376-377
665.80	14	370-375
665.81	14	370-375
665.82	14	370-375
665.83	14	383-384
665.84	14	376-377
665.90	14	370-375
665.91	14	370-375
665.92	14	370-375
665.93	14	383-384
665.94	14	376-377
666.00	14	469
666.02	14	370-375
666.04	14	376-377
666.10	14	469
666.12	14	370-372,374-375
666.14	14	376-377
666.20	14	469
666.22	14	370-372,374-375
666.24	14	376-377
666.30	14	469
666.32	14	370-372,374-375
666.34	14	376-377
667.00	14	469
667.02	14	370-372,374-375
667.04	14	376-377
667.10	14	469
667.12	14	370-372,374-375
667.14	14	376-377
668.00	14	370-375
668.01	14	370-372,374-375
668.02	14	370-372,374-375
668.03	14	383-384
668.04	14	376-377
668.10	14	370-375
668.11	14	370-372,374-375
668.12	14	370-372,374-375
668.13	14	383-384
668.14	14	376-377
668.20	14	370-375
668.21	14	370-372,374-375
668.22	14	370-372,374-375
668.23	14	383-384
668.24	14	376-377
668.80	14	370-375
668.81	14	370-372,374-375
668.82	14	370-372,374-375
668.83	14	383-384
668.84	14	376-377
668.90	14	370-375
668.91	14	370-372,374-375
668.92	14	370-372,374-375
668.93	14	383-384
668.94	14	376-377
669.00	14	370-375
669.01	14	370-375
669.02	14	370-375
669.03	14	383-384
669.04	14	376-377
669.10	14	370-375
669.11	14	370-372,374-375
669.12	14	370-372,374-375
669.13	14	383-384
669.14	14	376-377
669.20	14	370-375

Diagnosis Code/MDC/DRG List

DX	MDC	DRG	DX	MDC	DRG	DX	MDC	DRG	DX	MDC	DRG
669.21	14	370-375	673.13	14	383-384	676.22	14	370-375	690.8	09	283-284
669.22	14	370-375	673.14	14	376-377	676.23	14	383-384	691.0	09	283-284
669.23	14	383-384	673.20	14	469	676.24	14	376-377	691.8	09	283-284
669.24	14	376-377	673.21	14	370-372,374-375	676.30	14	469	692.0	09	283-284
669.30	14	370-375	673.22	14	370-372,374-375	676.31	14	370-375	692.1	09	283-284
669.32	14	370-372,374-375	673.23	14	383-384	676.32	14	370-375	692.2	09	283-284
669.34	14	376-377	673.24	14	376-377	676.33	14	383-384	692.3	09	283-284
669.40	14	370-375	673.30	14	469	676.34	14	376-377	692.4	09	283-284
669.41	14	370-372,374-375	673.31	14	370-372,374-375	676.40	14	469	692.5	09	283-284
669.42	14	370-372,374-375	673.32	14	370-372,374-375	676.41	14	370-375	692.6	09	283-284
669.44	14	376-377	673.33	14	383-384	676.42	14	370-375	692.70	09	283-284
669.50	14	370-375	673.34	14	376-377	676.43	14	383-384	692.71	09	283-284
669.51	14	370-375	673.80	14	469	676.44	14	376-377	692.72	09	283-284
669.60	14	370-375	673.81	14	370-372,374-375	676.50	14	469	692.73	09	283-284
669.61	14	370-375	673.82	14	370-372,374-375	676.51	14	370-375	692.74	09	283-284
669.70	14	370-375	673.83	14	383-384	676.52	14	370-375	692.75	09	283-284
669.71	14	370-375	673.84	14	376-377	676.53	14	383-384	692.76	09	283-284
669.80	14	370-375	674.00	14	469	676.54	14	376-377	692.77	09	283-284
669.81	14	370-375	674.01	14	370-372,374-375	676.60	14	469	692.79	09	283-284
669.82	14	370-375	674.02	14	370-372,374-375	676.61	14	370-375	692.81	09	283-284
669.83	14	383-384	674.03	14	383-384	676.62	14	370-375	692.82	09	283-284
669.84	14	376-377	674.04	14	376-377	676.63	14	383-384	692.83	09	283-284
669.90	14	370-375	674.10	14	469	676.64	14	376-377	692.89	09	283-284
669.91	14	370-375	674.12	14	370-372,374-375	676.80	14	469	692.9	09	283-284
669.92	14	370-375	674.14	14	376-377	676.81	14	370-375	693.0	09	283-284
669.93	14	383-384	674.20	14	469	676.82	14	370-375	693.1	09	283-284
669.94	14	376-377	674.22	14	370-372,374-375	676.83	14	383-384	693.8	09	283-284
670.00	14	469	674.24	14	376-377	676.84	14	376-377	693.9	09	283-284
670.02	14	370-372,374-375	674.30	14	469	676.90	14	469	694.0	09	283-284
670.04	14	376-377	674.32	14	370-372,374-375	676.91	14	370-375	694.1	09	283-284
671.00	14	469	674.34	14	376-377	676.92	14	370-375	694.2	09	283-284
671.01	14	370-375	674.40	14	469	676.93	14	383-384	694.3	09	283-284
671.02	14	370-375	674.42	14	370-375	676.94	14	376-377	694.4	09	272-273
671.03	14	383-384	674.44	14	376-377	677	14	469	694.5	09	272-273
671.04	14	376-377	674.80	14	469				694.60	09	272-273
671.10	14	469	674.82	14	370-372,374-375	**Diseases of the Skin and**			694.61	02	046-048
671.11	14	370-375	674.84	14	376-377	**Subcutaneous Tissue**			694.8	09	272-273
671.12	14	370-375	674.90	14	469	680.0	09	277-279	694.9	09	272-273
671.13	14	383-384	674.92	14	370-375	680.1	09	277-279	695.0	09	272-273
671.14	14	376-377	674.94	14	376-377	680.2	09	277-279	695.1	09	272-273
671.20	14	469	675.00	14	469	680.3	09	277-279	695.2	09	272-273
671.21	14	370-375	675.01	14	370-372,374-375	680.4	09	277-279	695.3	09	283-284
671.22	14	370-375	675.02	14	370-372,374-375	680.5	09	277-279	695.4	09	272-273
671.23	14	383-384	675.03	14	383-384	680.6	09	277-279	695.81	09	272-273
671.24	14	376-377	675.04	14	376-377	680.7	09	277-279	695.89	09	283-284
671.30	14	469	675.10	14	469	680.8	09	277-279	695.9	09	283-284
671.31	14	370-372,374-375	675.11	14	370-372,374-375	680.9	09	277-279	696.0	08	240-241
671.33	14	383-384	675.12	14	370-372,374-375	681.00	09	263-264,277-279	696.1	09	272-273
671.40	14	469	675.13	14	383-384	681.01	09	263-264,277-279	696.2	09	272-273
671.42	14	370-372,374-375	675.14	14	376-377	681.02	09	263-264,277-279	696.3	09	283-284
671.44	14	376-377	675.20	14	469	681.10	09	263-264,277-279	696.4	09	283-284
671.50	14	469	675.21	14	370-372,374-375	681.11	09	263-264,277-279	696.5	09	283-284
671.51	14	370-372,374-375	675.22	14	370-372,374-375	681.9	09	263-264,277-279	696.8	09	283-284
671.52	14	370-372,374-375	675.23	14	383-384	682.0	09	263-264,277-279	697.0	09	283-284
671.53	14	383-384	675.24	14	376-377	682.1	09	263-264,277-279	697.1	09	283-284
671.54	14	376-377	675.80	14	469	682.2	09	263-264,277-279	697.8	09	283-284
671.80	14	469	675.81	14	370-375	682.3	09	263-264,277-279	697.9	09	283-284
671.81	14	370-375	675.82	14	370-375	682.4	09	263-264,277-279	698.0	09	283-284
671.82	14	370-375	675.83	14	383-384	682.5	09	263-264,277-279	698.1	12	352
671.83	14	383-384	675.84	14	376-377	682.6	09	263-264,277-279	698.1	13	358-359,368
671.84	14	376-377	675.90	14	469	682.7	09	263-264,277-279	698.2	09	283-284
671.90	14	469	675.91	14	370-375	682.8	09	263-264,277-279	698.3	09	283-284
671.91	14	370-375	675.92	14	370-375	682.9	09	263-264,277-279	698.4	09	283-284
671.92	14	370-375	675.93	14	383-384	683	16	398-399	698.8	09	283-284
671.93	14	383-384	675.94	14	376-377	684	09	277-279	698.9	09	283-284
671.94	14	376-377	676.00	14	469	685.0	09	277-279	700	09	283-284
672.00	14	469	676.01	14	370-375	685.1	09	277-279	701.0	09	283-284
672.02	14	370-372,374-375	676.02	14	370-375	686.00	09	277-279	701.1	09	283-284
672.04	14	376-377	676.03	14	383-384	686.01	09	277-279	701.2	09	283-284
673.00	14	469	676.04	14	376-377	686.09	09	277-279	701.3	09	283-284
673.01	14	370-372,374-375	676.10	14	469	686.1	09	277-279	701.4	09	283-284
673.02	14	370-372,374-375	676.11	14	370-375	686.8	09	277-279	701.5	09	283-284
673.03	14	383-384	676.12	14	370-375	686.9	09	277-279	701.8	09	283-284
673.04	14	376-377	676.13	14	383-384	690.10	09	283-284	701.9	09	283-284
673.10	14	469	676.14	14	376-377	690.11	09	283-284	702.0	09	283-284
673.11	14	370-372,374-375	676.20	14	469	690.12	09	283-284	702.11	09	283-284
673.12	14	370-372,374-375	676.21	14	370-375	690.18	09	283-284	702.19	09	283-284

DX....MDC....DRG	DX....MDC....DRG	DX....MDC....DRG	DX....MDC....DRG
702.8...09....283-284	711.14..08....240-241	711.91..08....242	714.89..08....240-241
703.0...09....283-284	711.15..08....240-241	711.92..08....242	714.9...08....244-245
703.8...09....283-284	711.16..08....240-241	711.93..08....242	715.00..08....244-245
703.9...09....283-284	711.17..08....240-241	711.94..08....242	715.04..08....244-245
704.00..09....283-284	711.18..08....240-241	711.95..08....242	715.09..08....244-245
704.01..09....283-284	711.19..08....240-241	711.96..08....242	715.10..08....244-245
704.02..09....283-284	711.20..08....240-241	711.97..08....242	715.11..08....244-245
704.09..09....283-284	711.21..08....240-241	711.98..08....242	715.12..08....244-245
704.1...09....283-284	711.22..08....240-241	711.99..08....242	715.13..08....244-245
704.2...09....283-284	711.23..08....240-241	712.10..08....244-245	715.14..08....244-245
704.3...09....283-284	711.24..08....240-241	712.11..08....244-245	715.15..08....244-245
704.8...09....283-284	711.25..08....240-241	712.12..08....244-245	715.16..08....244-245
704.9...09....283-284	711.26..08....240-241	712.13..08....244-245	715.17..08....244-245
705.0...09....283-284	711.27..08....240-241	712.14..08....244-245	715.18..08....244-245
705.1...09....283-284	711.28..08....240-241	712.15..08....244-245	715.20..08....244-245
705.81..09....283-284	711.29..08....240-241	712.16..08....244-245	715.21..08....244-245
705.82..09....283-284	711.30..08....244-245	712.17..08....244-245	715.22..08....244-245
705.83..09....283-284	711.31..08....244-245	712.18..08....244-245	715.23..08....244-245
705.89..09....283-284	711.32..08....244-245	712.19..08....244-245	715.24..08....244-245
705.9...09....283-284	711.33..08....244-245	712.20..08....244-245	715.25..08....244-245
706.0...09....283-284	711.34..08....244-245	712.21..08....244-245	715.26..08....244-245
706.1...09....283-284	711.35..08....244-245	712.22..08....244-245	715.27..08....244-245
706.2...09....283-284	711.36..08....244-245	712.23..08....244-245	715.28..08....244-245
706.3...09....283-284	711.37..08....244-245	712.24..08....244-245	715.30..08....244-245
706.8...09....283-284	711.38..08....244-245	712.25..08....244-245	715.31..08....244-245
706.9...09....283-284	711.39..08....244-245	712.26..08....244-245	715.32..08....244-245
707.0...09....263-264,271	711.40..08....242	712.27..08....244-245	715.33..08....244-245
707.10..09....263-264,271	711.41..08....242	712.28..08....244-245	715.34..08....244-245
707.11..09....263-264,271	711.42..08....242	712.29..08....244-245	715.35..08....244-245
707.12..09....263-264,271	711.43..08....242	712.30..08....244-245	715.36..08....244-245
707.13..09....263-264,271	711.44..08....242	712.31..08....244-245	715.37..08....244-245
707.14..09....263-264,271	711.45..08....242	712.32..08....244-245	715.38..08....244-245
707.15..09....263-264,271	711.46..08....242	712.33..08....244-245	715.80..08....244-245
707.19..09....263-264,271	711.47..08....242	712.34..08....244-245	715.89..08....244-245
707.8...09....263-264,271	711.48..08....242	712.35..08....244-245	715.90..08....244-245
707.9...09....263-264,271	711.49..08....242	712.36..08....244-245	715.91..08....244-245
708.0...09....283-284	711.50..08....244-245	712.37..08....244-245	715.92..08....244-245
708.1...09....283-284	711.51..08....244-245	712.38..08....244-245	715.93..08....244-245
708.2...09....283-284	711.52..08....244-245	712.39..08....244-245	715.94..08....244-245
708.3...09....283-284	711.53..08....244-245	712.80..08....244-245	715.95..08....244-245
708.4...09....283-284	711.54..08....244-245	712.81..08....244-245	715.96..08....244-245
708.5...09....283-284	711.55..08....244-245	712.82..08....244-245	715.97..08....244-245
708.8...09....283-284	711.56..08....244-245	712.83..08....244-245	715.98..08....244-245
708.9...09....283-284	711.57..08....244-245	712.84..08....244-245	716.00..08....244-245
709.00..09....283-284	711.58..08....244-245	712.85..08....244-245	716.01..08....244-245
709.01..09....283-284	711.59..08....244-245	712.86..08....244-245	716.02..08....244-245
709.09..09....283-284	711.60..08....242	712.87..08....244-245	716.03..08....244-245
709.1...09....283-284	711.61..08....242	712.88..08....244-245	716.04..08....244-245
709.2...09....283-284	711.62..08....242	712.89..08....244-245	716.05..08....244-245
709.3...09....283-284	711.63..08....242	712.90..08....244-245	716.06..08....244-245
709.4...09....283-284	711.64..08....242	712.91..08....244-245	716.07..08....244-245
709.8...09....283-284	711.65..08....242	712.92..08....244-245	716.08..08....244-245
709.9...09....283-284	711.66..08....242	712.93..08....244-245	716.09..08....244-245
Diseases of the Musculoskeletal System and Connective Tissue	711.67..08....242	712.94..08....244-245	716.10..08....244-245
	711.68..08....242	712.95..08....244-245	716.11..08....244-245
710.0...08....240-241	711.69..08....242	712.96..08....244-245	716.12..08....244-245
710.1...08....240-241	711.70..08....242	712.97..08....244-245	716.13..08....244-245
710.2...08....240-241	711.71..08....242	712.98..08....244-245	716.14..08....244-245
710.3...08....240-241	711.72..08....242	712.99..08....244-245	716.15..08....244-245
710.4...08....240-241	711.73..08....242	713.0...08....244-245	716.16..08....244-245
710.5...08....240-241	711.74..08....242	713.1...08....244-245	716.17..08....244-245
710.8...08....240-241	711.75..08....242	713.2...08....244-245	716.18..08....244-245
710.9...08....240-241	711.76..08....242	713.3...08....244-245	716.19..08....244-245
711.00..08....242	711.77..08....242	713.4...08....244-245	716.20..08....244-245
711.01..08....242	711.78..08....242	713.5...08....244-245	716.21..08....244-245
711.02..08....242	711.79..08....242	713.6...08....244-245	716.22..08....244-245
711.03..08....242	711.80..08....242	713.7...08....244-245	716.23..08....244-245
711.04..08....242	711.81..08....242	713.8...08....244-245	716.24..08....244-245
711.05..08....242	711.82..08....242	714.0...08....240-241	716.25..08....244-245
711.06..08....242,501-502	711.83..08....242	714.1...08....240-241	716.26..08....244-245
711.07..08....242	711.84..08....242	714.2...08....240-241	716.27..08....244-245
711.08..08....242	711.85..08....242	714.30..08....240-241	716.28..08....244-245
711.09..08....242	711.86..08....242	714.31..08....240-241	716.29..08....244-245
711.10..08....240-241	711.87..08....242	714.32..08....240-241	716.30..08....244-245
711.11..08....240-241	711.88..08....242	714.33..08....240-241	716.31..08....244-245
711.12..08....240-241	711.89..08....242	714.4...08....244-245	716.32..08....244-245
711.13..08....240-241	711.90..08....242	714.81..04....092-093	716.33..08....244-245

Diagnosis Code/MDC/DRG List

DX	MDC	DRG	DX	MDC	DRG	DX	MDC	DRG	DX	MDC	DRG
716.34	08	244-245	718.03	08	250-252	718.90	08	256	719.68	08	247
716.35	08	244-245	718.04	08	250-252	718.91	08	256	719.69	08	247
716.36	08	244-245	718.05	08	256	718.92	08	256	719.70	08	247
716.37	08	244-245	718.07	08	253-255	718.93	08	256	719.75	08	247
716.38	08	244-245	718.08	08	256	718.94	08	256	719.76	08	247
716.39	08	244-245	718.09	08	256	718.95	08	256	719.77	08	247
716.40	08	246	718.10	08	256	718.97	08	256	719.78	08	247
716.41	08	246	718.11	08	256	718.98	08	256	719.79	08	247
716.42	08	246	718.12	08	256	718.99	08	256	719.80	08	247
716.43	08	246	718.13	08	256	719.00	08	256	719.81	08	247
716.44	08	246	718.14	08	256	719.01	08	256	719.82	08	247
716.45	08	246	718.15	08	256	719.02	08	256	719.83	08	247
716.46	08	246	718.17	08	256	719.03	08	256	719.84	08	247
716.47	08	246	718.18	08	256	719.04	08	256	719.85	08	247
716.48	08	246	718.19	08	256	719.05	08	256	719.86	08	247
716.49	08	246	718.20	08	250-252	719.06	08	256	719.87	08	247
716.50	08	246	718.21	08	253-255	719.07	08	256	719.88	08	247
716.51	08	246	718.22	08	253-255	719.08	08	256	719.89	08	247
716.52	08	246	718.23	08	250-252	719.09	08	256	719.90	08	247
716.53	08	246	718.24	08	250-252	719.10	08	244-245	719.91	08	247
716.54	08	246	718.25	08	256	719.11	08	244-245	719.92	08	247
716.55	08	246	718.26	08	253-255	719.12	08	244-245	719.93	08	247
716.56	08	246	718.27	08	253-255	719.13	08	244-245	719.94	08	247
716.57	08	246	718.28	08	256	719.14	08	244-245	719.95	08	247
716.58	08	246	718.29	08	256	719.15	08	244-245	719.96	08	247
716.59	08	246	718.30	08	256	719.16	08	244-245	719.97	08	247
716.60	08	246	718.31	08	253-255	719.17	08	244-245	719.98	08	247
716.61	08	246	718.32	08	253-255	719.18	08	244-245	719.99	08	247
716.62	08	246	718.33	08	250-252	719.19	08	244-245	720.0	08	240-241
716.63	08	246	718.34	08	250-252	719.20	08	244-245	720.1	08	243
716.64	08	246	718.35	08	256	719.21	08	244-245	720.2	08	243
716.65	08	246	718.36	08	253-255	719.22	08	244-245	720.81	08	243
716.66	08	246	718.37	08	253-255	719.23	08	244-245	720.89	08	243
716.67	08	246	718.38	08	256	719.24	08	244-245	720.9	08	243
716.68	08	246	718.39	08	256	719.25	08	244-245	721.0	08	243
716.80	08	246	718.40	08	256	719.26	08	244-245	721.1	08	243
716.81	08	246	718.41	08	256	719.27	08	244-245	721.2	08	243
716.82	08	246	718.42	08	256	719.28	08	244-245	721.3	08	243
716.83	08	246	718.43	08	256	719.29	08	244-245	721.41	08	243
716.84	08	246	718.44	08	256	719.30	08	244-245	721.42	08	243
716.85	08	246	718.45	08	256	719.31	08	244-245	721.5	08	243
716.86	08	246	718.46	08	256	719.32	08	244-245	721.6	08	243
716.87	08	246	718.47	08	256	719.33	08	244-245	721.7	08	243
716.88	08	246	718.48	08	256	719.34	08	244-245	721.8	08	243
716.89	08	246	718.49	08	256	719.35	08	244-245	721.90	08	243
716.90	08	246	718.50	08	244-245	719.36	08	244-245	721.91	08	243
716.91	08	246	718.51	08	244-245	719.37	08	244-245	722.0	08	243
716.92	08	246	718.52	08	244-245	719.38	08	244-245	722.10	08	243
716.93	08	246	718.53	08	244-245	719.39	08	244-245	722.11	08	243
716.94	08	246	718.54	08	244-245	719.40	08	247	722.2	08	243
716.95	08	246	718.55	08	244-245	719.41	08	247	722.30	08	243
716.96	08	246	718.56	08	244-245	719.42	08	247	722.31	08	243
716.97	08	246	718.57	08	244-245	719.43	08	247	722.32	08	243
716.98	08	246	718.58	08	244-245	719.44	08	247	722.39	08	243
716.99	08	246	718.59	08	244-245	719.45	08	247	722.4	08	243
717.0	08	253-255	718.60	08	256	719.46	08	247	722.51	08	243
717.1	08	253-255	718.65	08	256	719.47	08	247	722.52	08	243
717.2	08	253-255	718.70	08	256	719.48	08	247	722.6	08	243
717.3	08	253-255	718.71	08	256	719.49	08	247	722.70	08	243
717.40	08	253-255	718.72	08	256	719.50	08	247	722.71	08	243
717.41	08	253-255	718.73	08	256	719.51	08	247	722.72	08	243
717.42	08	253-255	718.74	08	256	719.52	08	247	722.73	08	243
717.43	08	253-255	718.75	08	256	719.53	08	247	722.80	08	243
717.49	08	253-255	718.76	08	256	719.54	08	247	722.81	08	243
717.5	08	253-255	718.77	08	256	719.55	08	247	722.82	08	243
717.6	08	256	718.78	08	256	719.56	08	247	722.83	08	243
717.7	08	253-255	718.79	08	256	719.57	08	247	722.90	08	243
717.81	08	253-255	718.80	08	256	719.58	08	247	722.91	08	243
717.82	08	253-255	718.81	08	256	719.59	08	247	722.92	08	243
717.83	08	253-255	718.82	08	256	719.60	08	247	722.93	08	243
717.84	08	253-255	718.83	08	256	719.61	08	247	723.0	08	243
717.85	08	253-255	718.84	08	256	719.62	08	247	723.1	08	243
717.89	08	253-255	718.85	08	256	719.63	08	247	723.2	01	018-019
717.9	08	253-255	718.86	08	256	719.64	08	247	723.3	01	018-019
718.00	08	256	718.87	08	256	719.65	08	247	723.4	01	018-019
718.01	08	253-255	718.88	08	256	719.66	08	247	723.5	08	243
718.02	08	253-255	718.89	08	256	719.67	08	247	723.6	09	283-284

Diagnosis Code/MDC/DRG List

DX	MDC	DRG
723.7	08	243
723.8	08	243
723.9	08	243
724.00	08	243
724.01	08	243
724.02	08	243
724.09	08	243
724.1	08	243
724.2	08	243
724.3	08	243
724.4	08	243
724.5	08	243
724.6	08	243
724.70	08	243
724.71	08	243
724.79	08	243
724.8	08	243
724.9	08	243
725.	08	240-241
726.0	08	248
726.10	08	248
726.11	08	248
726.12	08	248
726.19	08	248
726.2	08	248
726.30	08	248
726.31	08	248
726.32	08	248
726.33	08	248
726.39	08	248
726.4	08	248
726.5	08	248
726.60	08	248
726.61	08	248
726.62	08	248
726.63	08	248
726.64	08	248
726.65	08	248
726.69	08	248
726.70	08	248
726.71	08	248
726.72	08	248
726.73	08	256
726.79	08	248
726.8	08	248
726.90	08	248
726.91	08	248
727.00	08	248
727.01	08	248
727.02	08	256
727.03	08	248
727.04	08	248
727.05	08	248
727.06	08	248
727.09	08	248
727.1	08	256
727.2	08	248
727.3	08	248
727.40	08	248
727.41	08	248
727.42	08	248
727.43	08	248
727.49	08	248
727.50	08	248
727.51	08	248
727.59	08	248
727.60	08	248
727.61	08	248
727.62	08	248
727.63	08	248
727.64	08	248
727.65	08	248
727.66	08	248
727.67	08	248
727.68	08	248
727.69	08	248
727.81	08	248
727.82	08	248
727.83	08	248
727.89	08	248
727.9	08	248
728.0	08	248
728.10	08	248
728.11	08	248
728.12	08	248
728.13	08	248
728.19	08	248
728.2	08	248
728.3	08	248
728.4	08	248
728.5	08	248
728.6	08	248
728.71	08	248
728.79	08	248
728.81	08	248
728.82	08	248
728.83	08	248
728.84	08	248
728.85	08	247
728.89	08	248
728.9	08	248
729.0	08	247
729.1	08	247
729.2	01	018-019
729.30	09	283-284
729.31	09	283-284
729.39	09	283-284
729.4	08	248
729.5	08	247
729.6	08	256
729.81	08	247
729.82	08	247
729.89	08	247
729.9	08	247
730.00	08	238
730.01	08	238
730.02	08	238
730.03	08	238
730.04	08	238
730.05	08	238
730.06	08	238
730.07	08	238
730.08	08	238
730.09	08	238
730.10	08	238
730.11	08	238
730.12	08	238
730.13	08	238
730.14	08	238
730.15	08	238
730.16	08	238
730.17	08	238
730.18	08	238
730.19	08	238
730.20	08	238
730.21	08	238
730.22	08	238
730.23	08	238
730.24	08	238
730.25	08	238
730.26	08	238
730.27	08	238
730.28	08	238
730.29	08	238
730.30	08	244-245
730.31	08	244-245
730.32	08	244-245
730.33	08	244-245
730.34	08	244-245
730.35	08	244-245
730.36	08	244-245
730.37	08	256
730.38	08	256
730.39	08	256
730.70	08	256
730.71	08	256
730.72	08	256
730.73	08	256
730.74	08	256
730.75	08	256
730.76	08	256
730.77	08	256
730.78	08	256
730.79	08	256
730.80	08	238
730.81	08	238
730.82	08	238
730.83	08	238
730.84	08	238
730.85	08	238
730.86	08	238
730.87	08	238
730.88	08	238
730.89	08	238
730.90	08	238
730.91	08	238
730.92	08	238
730.93	08	238
730.94	08	238
730.95	08	238
730.96	08	238
730.97	08	238
730.98	08	238
730.99	08	238
731.0	08	244-245
731.1	08	244-245
731.2	08	244-245
731.8	08	244-245
732.0	08	244-245
732.1	08	244-245
732.2	08	244-245
732.3	08	244-245
732.4	08	244-245
732.5	08	244-245
732.6	08	244-245
732.7	08	244-245
732.8	08	244-245
732.9	08	244-245
733.00	08	244-245
733.01	08	244-245
733.02	08	244-245
733.03	08	244-245
733.09	08	244-245
733.10	08	239
733.11	08	239
733.12	08	239
733.13	08	239
733.14	08	239
733.15	08	239
733.16	08	239
733.19	08	239
733.20	08	244-245
733.21	08	244-245
733.22	08	244-245
733.29	08	244-245
733.3	08	256
733.40	08	244-245
733.41	08	244-245
733.42	08	244-245
733.43	08	244-245
733.44	08	244-245
733.49	08	244-245
733.5	08	244-245
733.6	04	101-102
733.7	08	256
733.81	08	256
733.82	08	256
733.90	08	256
733.91	08	256
733.92	08	244-245
733.93	08	239
733.94	08	239
733.95	08	239
733.99	08	256
734	08	256
735.0	08	256
735.1	08	256
735.2	08	256
735.3	08	256
735.4	08	256
735.5	08	256
735.8	08	256
735.9	08	256
736.00	08	256
736.01	08	256
736.02	08	256
736.03	08	256
736.04	08	256
736.05	01	018-019
736.06	01	018-019
736.07	01	018-019
736.09	08	256
736.1	08	256
736.20	08	256
736.21	08	256
736.22	08	256
736.29	08	256
736.30	08	256
736.31	08	256
736.32	08	256
736.39	08	256
736.41	08	256
736.42	08	256
736.5	08	256
736.6	08	256
736.70	08	256
736.71	08	256
736.72	08	256
736.73	08	256
736.74	01	018-019
736.75	08	256
736.76	08	256
736.79	08	256
736.81	08	256
736.89	08	256
736.9	08	256
737.0	08	243
737.10	08	243
737.11	08	243
737.12	08	243
737.19	08	243
737.20	08	243
737.21	08	243
737.22	08	243
737.29	08	243
737.30	08	243
737.31	08	243
737.32	08	243
737.33	08	243
737.34	08	243
737.39	08	243
737.40	08	243
737.41	08	243
737.42	08	243
737.43	08	243
737.8	08	243
737.9	08	243
738.0	03	072
738.10	08	256
738.11	08	256
738.12	08	256
738.19	08	256
738.2	08	256
738.3	08	256
738.4	08	243
738.5	08	243
738.6	08	256
738.7	03	073-074

2002 Ingenix, Inc.

Diagnosis Code/MDC/DRG List

DX	MDC	DRG
738.8	08	256
738.9	08	256
739.0	08	247
739.1	08	243
739.2	08	243
739.3	08	243
739	08	243
739.5	08	247
739.6	08	247
739.7	08	247
739.8	08	247
739.9	08	247

Congenital Anomalies

DX	MDC	DRG
740.0	01	034-035
740.1	01	034-035
740.2	01	034-035
741.00	01	034-035
741.01	01	034-035
741.02	01	034-035
741.03	01	034-035
741.90	01	034-035
741.91	01	034-035
741.92	01	034-035
741.93	01	034-035
742.0	01	034-035
742.1	01	034-035
742.2	01	034-035
742.3	01	034-035
742.4	01	034-035
742.51	01	034-035
742.53	01	034-035
742.59	01	034-035
742.8	01	034-035
742.9	01	034-035
743.00	02	046-048
743.03	02	046-048
743.06	02	046-048
743.10	02	046-048
743.11	02	046-048
743.12	02	046-048
743.20	02	046-048
743.21	02	046-048
743.22	02	046-048
743.30	02	046-048
743.31	02	046-048
743.32	02	046-048
743.33	02	046-048
743.34	02	046-048
743.35	02	046-048
743.36	02	046-048
743.37	02	046-048
743.39	02	046-048
743.41	02	046-048
743.42	02	046-048
743.43	02	046-048
743.44	02	046-048
743.45	02	046-048
743.46	02	046-048
743.47	02	046-048
743.48	02	046-048
743.49	02	046-048
743.51	02	046-048
743.52	02	046-048
743.53	02	046-048
743.54	02	046-048
743.55	02	046-048
743.56	02	046-048
743.57	02	046-048
743.58	02	046-048
743.59	02	046-048
743.61	02	046-048
743.62	02	046-048
743.63	02	046-048
743.64	02	046-048
743.65	02	046-048
743.66	02	046-048
743.69	02	046-048
743.8	02	046-048
743.9	02	046-048
744.00	03	073-074
744.01	03	073-074
744.02	03	073-074
744.03	03	073-074
744.04	03	073-074
744.05	03	073-074
744.09	03	073-074
744.1	03	073-074
744.21	03	073-074
744.22	03	073-074
744.23	03	073-074
744.24	03	073-074
744.29	03	073-074
744.3	03	073-074
744.41	03	073-074
744.42	03	073-074
744.43	03	073-074
744.46	03	073-074
744.47	03	073-074
744.49	03	073-074
744.5	09	283-284
744.81	03	185-187
744.82	03	185-187
744.83	03	185-187
744.84	03	185-187
744.89	03	073-074
744.9	09	283-284
745.0	05	135-137
745.10	05	135-137
745.11	05	135-137
745.12	05	135-137
745.19	05	135-137
745.2	05	135-137
745.3	05	135-137
745.4	05	135-137
745.5	05	135-137
745.60	05	135-137
745.61	05	135-137
745.69	05	135-137
745.7	05	135-137
745.8	05	135-137
745.9	05	135-137
746.00	05	135-137
746.01	05	135-137
746.02	05	135-137
746.09	05	135-137
746.1	05	135-137
746.2	05	135-137
746.3	05	135-137
746.4	05	135-137
746.5	05	135-137
746.6	05	135-137
746.7	05	135-137
746.81	05	135-137
746.82	05	135-137
746.83	05	135-137
746.84	05	135-137
746.85	05	135-137
746.86	05	138-139
746.87	05	135-137
746.89	05	135-137
746.9	05	135-137
747.0	05	135-137
747.10	05	135-137
747.11	05	135-137
747.20	05	135-137
747.21	05	135-137
747.22	05	135-137
747.29	05	135-137
747.3	05	135-137
747.40	05	135-137
747.41	05	135-137
747.42	05	135-137
747.49	05	135-137
747.5	05	130-131
747.60	05	130-131
747.61	05	130-131
747.62	05	130-131
747.63	05	130-131
747.64	05	130-131
747.69	05	130-131
747.81	01	034-035
747.83	15	387-389
747.89	05	130-131
747.9	05	130-131
748.0	03	073-074
748.1	03	073-074
748.2	03	073-074
748.3	03	073-074
748.4	04	101-102
748.5	04	101-102
748.60	04	101-102
748.61	04	088
748.69	04	101-102
748.8	04	101-102
748.9	04	101-102
749.00	03	185-187
749.01	03	185-187
749.02	03	185-187
749.03	03	185-187
749.04	03	185-187
749.10	03	185-187
749.11	03	185-187
749.12	03	185-187
749.13	03	185-187
749.14	03	185-187
749.20	03	185-187
749.21	03	185-187
749.22	03	185-187
749.23	03	185-187
749.24	03	185-187
749.25	03	185-187
750.0	03	185-187
750.10	03	185-187
750.11	03	185-187
750.12	03	185-187
750.13	03	185-187
750.15	03	185-187
750.16	03	185-187
750.19	03	185-187
750.21	03	073-074
750.22	03	073-074
750.23	03	073-074
750.24	03	073-074
750.25	03	185-187
750.26	03	185-187
750.27	03	073-074
750.29	03	073-074
750.3	06	188-190
750.4	06	188-190
750.5	06	188-190
750.6	06	188-190
750.7	06	188-190
750.8	06	188-190
750.9	06	188-190
751.0	06	176
751.1	06	188-190
751.2	06	188-190
751.3	06	188-190
751.4	06	188-190
751.5	06	188-190
751.60	07	207-208
751.61	07	207-208
751.62	07	205-206
751.69	07	205-206
751.7	07	204
751.8	06	188-190
751.9	06	188-190
752.0	13	358-359,369
752.10	13	358-359,369
752.11	13	358-359,369
752.19	13	358-359,369
752.2	13	358-359,369
752.3	13	358-359,369
752.40	13	358-359,369
752.41	13	358-359,369
752.42	13	358-359,369
752.49	13	358-359,369
752.51	12	352
752.52	12	352
752.61	12	352
752.62	12	352
752.63	12	352
752.64	12	352
752.65	12	352
752.69	12	352
752.7	12	352
752.7	13	358-359,369
752.8	12	352
752.8	13	358-359,369
752.9	12	352
752.9	13	358-359,369
753.0	11	331-333
753.10	11	331-333
753.11	11	331-333
753.12	11	331-333
753.13	11	331-333
753.14	11	331-333
753.15	11	331-333
753.16	11	331-333
753.17	11	331-333
753.19	11	331-333
753.20	11	331-333
753.21	11	331-333
753.22	11	331-333
753.23	11	331-333
753.29	11	331-333
753.3	11	331-333
753.4	11	331-333
753.5	11	331-333
753.6	11	331-333
753.7	11	331-333
753.8	11	331-333
753.9	11	331-333
754.0	08	256
754.1	08	256
754.2	08	256
754.30	08	256
754.31	08	256
754.32	08	256
754.33	08	256
754.35	08	256
754.40	08	256
754.41	08	253-255
754.42	08	256
754.43	08	256
754.44	08	256
754.50	08	256
754.51	08	256
754.52	08	256
754.53	08	256
754.59	08	256
754.60	08	256
754.61	08	256
754.62	08	256
754.69	08	256
754.70	08	256
754.71	08	256
754.79	08	256
754.81	04	101-102
754.82	04	101-102
754.89	08	256
755.00	08	256
755.01	08	256
755.02	08	256
755.10	08	256
755.11	08	256
755.12	08	256

DX	MDC	DRG
755.13	08	256
755.14	08	256
755.20	08	256
755.21	08	256
755.22	08	256
755.23	08	256
755.24	08	256
755.25	08	256
755.26	08	256
755.27	08	256
755.28	08	256
755.29	08	256
755.30	08	256
755.31	08	256
755.32	08	256
755.33	08	256
755.34	08	256
755.35	08	256
755.36	08	256
755.37	08	256
755.38	08	256
755.39	08	256
755.4	08	256
755.50	08	256
755.51	08	256
755.52	08	256
755.53	08	256
755.54	08	256
755.55	08	256
755.56	08	256
755.57	08	256
755.58	08	256
755.59	08	256
755.60	08	256
755.61	08	256
755.62	08	256
755.63	08	256
755.64	08	256
755.65	08	256
755.66	08	256
755.67	08	256
755.69	08	256
755.8	08	256
755.9	08	256
756.0	08	256
756.10	08	243
756.11	08	243
756.12	08	243
756.13	08	243
756.14	08	243
756.15	08	243
756.16	08	256
756.17	01	034-035
756.19	08	243
756.2	08	256
756.3	04	101-102
756.4	08	256
756.50	08	256
756.51	08	256
756.52	08	256
756.53	08	256
756.54	08	256
756.55	08	256
756.56	08	256
756.59	08	256
756.6	04	101-102
756.70	06	188-190
756.71	06	188-190
756.79	06	188-190
756.81	08	256
756.82	08	256
756.83	08	256
756.89	08	256
756.9	08	256
757.0	09	283-284
757.1	09	283-284
757.2	09	283-284
757.31	09	283-284
757.32	09	283-284
757.33	09	283-284
757.39	09	283-284
757.4	09	283-284
757.5	09	283-284
757.6	09	276
757.8	09	283-284
757.9	09	283-284
758.0	19	429
758.1	19	429
758.2	19	429
758.3	19	429
758.4	23	467
758.5	23	467
758.6	12	352
758.6	13	358-359,369
758.7	12	352
758.8	12	352
758.81	12	352
758.81	13	358-359,369
758.89	12	352
758.89	13	358-359,369
758.9	15	390
759.0	16	398-399
759.1	10	300-301
759.2	10	300-301
759.3	06	188-190
759.4	15	387,389
759.5	01	034-035
759.6	17	413-414
759.7	15	390
759.81	15	390
759.82	05	135-137
759.89	15	390
759.9	15	390

Certain Conditions Originating in the Perinatal Period

DX	MDC	DRG
760.0	15	390
760.1	15	390
760.2	15	390
760.3	15	390
760.4	15	390
760.5	15	390
760.6	15	390
760.70	15	390
760.71	15	390
760.72	15	390
760.73	15	390
760.74	15	390
760.75	15	390
760.79	15	390
760.8	15	390
760.9	15	390
761.0	15	390
761.1	15	390
761.2	15	390
761.3	15	390
761.4	15	390
761.5	15	390
761.6	15	390
761.7	15	390
761.8	15	390
761.9	15	390
762.0	15	390
762.1	15	390
762.2	15	390
762.3	15	390
762.4	15	391
762.5	15	391
762.6	15	391
762.7	15	390
762.8	15	390
762.9	15	390
763.0	15	391
763.1	15	391
763.2	15	391
763.3	15	391
763.4	15	387,389
763.5	15	390
763.6	15	391
763.7	15	390
763.81	15	390
763.82	15	390
763.83	15	390
763.89	15	390
763.9	15	391
764.00	15	390
764.01	15	390
764.02	15	390
764.03	15	390
764.04	15	390
764.05	15	390
764.06	15	390
764.07	15	390
764.08	15	390
764.09	15	391
764.10	15	390
764.11	15	387,389
764.12	15	387,389
764.13	15	387,389
764.14	15	387,389
764.15	15	387,389
764.16	15	387,389
764.17	15	387,389
764.18	15	387,389
764.19	15	390
764.20	15	390
764.21	15	387,389
764.22	15	387,389
764.23	15	387,389
764.24	15	387,389
764.25	15	387,389
764.26	15	387,389
764.27	15	387,389
764.28	15	387,389
764.29	15	390
764.90	15	390
764.91	15	390
764.92	15	390
764.93	15	390
765.17	15	387-388
765.18	15	387-388
765.19	15	387-388
765.20	15	391
765.21	15	386
765.22	15	386
765.23	15	386
765.24	15	387-388
765.25	15	387-388
765.26	15	387-388
765.27	15	387-388
765.28	15	387-388
765.29	15	391
766.0	15	391
766.1	15	391
766.2	15	391
767.0	15	387,389
767.1	15	391
767.2	15	390
767.3	15	390
767.4	15	387,389
767.5	15	390
767.6	15	390
767.7	15	387,389
767.8	15	390
767.9	15	390
768.0	15	390
768.1	15	390
768.2	15	390
768.3	15	390
768.4	15	390
768.5	15	387,389
768.6	15	391
768.9	15	390
769	15	386
770.0	15	387,389
770.1	15	387,389
770.2	15	387,389
770.3	15	387,389
770.4	15	387,389
770.5	15	390
770.6	15	390
770.7	04	92-93
770.8	15	387,389
770.81	15	390
770.82	15	390
770.83	15	390
770.84	15	387, 389
770.89	15	390
770.9	15	390
771.0	15	387,389
771.1	15	387,389
771.2	15	387,389
771.3	15	390
771.4	15	387,389
771.5	15	387,389
771.6	15	390
771.7	15	390
771.8	15	387,389
771.81	15	387, 389
771.82	15	387, 389
771.83	15	387, 389
771.89	15	387, 389
772.0	15	387,389
772.10	15	387,389
772.11	15	387,389
772.12	15	387,389
772.13	15	387,389
772.14	15	387,389
772.2	15	387,389
772.3	15	390
772.4	15	387,389
772.5	15	387,389
772.6	15	390
772.8	15	390
772.9	15	390
773.0	15	390
773.1	15	390
773.2	15	387,389
773.3	15	387,389
773.4	15	387,389
773.5	15	387,389
774.0	15	387,389
774.1	15	387,389
774.2	15	387,389
774.30	15	387,389
774.31	15	387,389
774.39	15	387,389
774.4	15	387,389
774.5	15	387,389
774.6	15	391
774.7	15	387,389
775.0	15	390
775.1	15	387,389
775.2	15	387,389
775.3	15	387,389
775.4	15	387,389
775.5	15	387,389
775.6	15	387,389
775.7	15	387,389
775.8	15	390
775.9	15	390
776.0	15	387,389
776.1	15	387,389
776.2	15	387,389
776.3	15	387,389
776.4	15	390
776.5	15	390
776.6	15	387,389

DX	MDC	DRG	DX	MDC	DRG	DX	MDC	DRG	DX	MDC	DRG
776.7	15	390	781.92	01	034-035	787.03	06	182-184	790.94	23	463-464
776.8	15	390	781.99	01	034-035	787.1	06	182-184	790.99	23	463-464
776.9	15	390	782.0	01	034-035	787.2	06	182-184	791.0	11	325-327
777.1	15	387,389	782.1	09	283-284	787.3	06	182-184	791.1	11	325-327
777.2	15	387,389	782.2	09	283-284	787.4	06	182-184	791.2	11	325-327
777.3	15	390	782.3	23	463-464	787.5	06	182-184	791.3	23	463-464
777.4	15	390	782.4	07	205-206	787.6	06	182-184	791.4	07	205-206
777.5	15	387,389	782.5	23	463-464	787.7	06	182-184	791.5	10	294-295
777.6	15	387,389	782.61	23	463-464	787.9	06	182-184	791.6	10	296-298
777.8	15	390	782.62	23	463-464	788.0	11	323-324	791.7	11	325-327
777.9	15	390	782.7	16	397	788.1	11	325-327	791.9	11	325-327
778.0	15	387,389	782.8	09	283-284	788.20	11	325-327	792.0	01	034-035
778.1	15	390	782.9	09	283-284	788.21	11	325-327	792.1	06	182-184
778.2	15	390	783.0	10	296-298	788.29	11	325-327	792.2	12	352
778.3	15	390	783.1	10	296-298	788.30	11	325-327	792.3	14	383-384
778.4	15	390	783.21	10	296-298	788.31	11	325-327	792.4	03	073-074
778.5	15	390	783.22	10	296-298	788.32	11	325-327	792.5	23	463-464
778.6	15	390	783.40	10	296-298	788.33	11	325-327	792.9	23	463-464
778.7	15	390	783.41	10	296-298	788.34	11	325-327	793.0	01	034-035
778.8	15	391	783.42	10	296-298	788.35	11	325-327	793.1	04	099-100
778.9	15	390	783.43	10	296-298	788.36	11	325-327	793.2	05	132-133
779.0	15	387,389	783.5	10	296-298	788.37	11	325-327	793.3	07	207-208
779.1	15	387,389	783.6	10	296-298	788.39	11	325-327	793.4	06	182-184
779.2	15	387,389	783.7	10	296-298	788.41	11	325-327	793.5	11	325-327
779.3	15	391	783.9	10	296-298	788.42	11	325-327	793.6	06	182-184
779.4	15	387,389	784.0	01	024-026	788.43	11	325-327	793.7	08	256
779.5	15	387,389	784.1	03	073-074	788.5	11	316	793.80	09	276
779.6	15	390	784.2	09	283-284	788.61	11	325-327	793.81	09	276
779.7	09	276	784.3	01	014	788.62	11	325-327	793.89	09	276
779.8	15	390	784.40	03	073-074	788.69	11	325-327	793.9	23	463-464
779.81	15	390	784.41	03	073-074	788.7	11	325-327	794.00	01	034-035
779.82	15	390	784.49	03	073-074	788.8	11	325-327	794.01	01	034-035
779.89	15	390	784.5	01	034-035	788.9	11	325-327	794.02	01	034-035
779.9	15	390	784.60	19	432	789.00	06	182-184	794.09	01	034-035
780.91	23	463-464	784.61	19	431	789.01	06	182-184	794.10	01	034-035
780.92	23	463-464	784.69	19	431	789.02	06	182-184	794.11	02	046-048
780.99	23	463-464	784.7	03	066	789.03	06	182-184	794.12	02	046-048
781.93	08	243	784.8	03	073-074	789.04	06	182-184	794.13	02	046-048
			784.9	03	073-074	789.05	06	182-184	794.14	02	046-048
Symptoms, Signs and Ill-defined Conditions			785.0	05	138-139	789.06	06	182-184	794.15	03	073-074
			785.1	05	138-139	789.07	06	182-184	794.16	03	073-074
780.01	01	023	785.2	05	135-137	789.09	06	182-184	794.17	08	256
780.01	15	387,389	785.3	05	144-145	789.1	07	205-206	794.19	01	034-035
780.02	01	023	785.4	05	130-131	789.2	16	398-399	794.2	04	101-102
780.09	01	023	785.50	05	115,121,124,127	789.30	06	182-184	794.30	05	144-145
780.1	19	425	785.51	05	115,121,124,127	789.31	06	182-184	794.31	05	144-145
780.2	05	141-142	785.59	18	416-417	789.32	06	182-184	794.39	05	144-145
780.31	01	024-026	785.6	16	398-399	789.33	06	182-184	794.4	11	325-327
780.31	15	387, 389	785.9	05	144-145	789.34	06	182-184	794.5	10	300-301
780.39	01	024-026	786.00	04	099-100	789.35	06	182-184	794.6	10	300-301
780.39	15	387, 389	786.01	04	099-100	789.36	06	182-184	794.7	10	300-301
780.4	03	065	786.02	04	099-100	789.37	06	182-184	794.8	07	205-206
780.50	19	432	786.03	04	099-100	789.39	06	182-184	794.9	11	325-327
780.51	01	034-035	786.03	25	490	789.40	06	182-184	795.00	13	358-359, 369
780.52	19	432	786.04	04	099-100	789.41	06	182-184	795.01	13	358-359, 369
780.53	01	034-035	786.04	25	490	789.42	06	182-184	795.02	13	358-359, 369
780.54	19	432	786.05	04	099-100	789.43	06	182-184	795.09	13	358-359, 369
780.55	19	432	786.05	25	490	789.44	06	182-184	795.0	13	358-359, 369
780.56	19	432	786.06	04	099-100	789.45	06	182-184	795.1	04	082
780.57	01	034-035	786.06	25	490	789.46	06	182-184	795.2	15	390
780.59	19	432	786.07	04	099-100	789.47	06	182-184	795.3	18	423
780.6	18	419-420,422	786.07	25	490	789.49	06	182-184	795.31	18	423
780.71	23	463-464	786.09	04	099-100	789.5	23	463-464	795.39	18	423
780.71	25	490	786.1	04	099-100	789.9	06	182-184	795.4	23	463-464
780.79	23	463-464	786.2	04	099-100	790.01	16	395-396	795.5	04	079-081
780.79	25	490	786.3	04	099-100	790.09	16	395-396	795.6	08	240-241
780.8	09	283-284	786.4	04	099-100	790.1	23	463-464	795.71	16	398-399
780.9	23	463-464	786.50	05	143	790.2	10	296-298	795.79	16	398-399
781.0	01	034-035	786.51	05	143	790.3	20	434-435, 521-523	796.0	21	454-455
781.1	01	034-035	786.52	04	099-100	790.4	23	463-464	796.1	01	034-035
781.2	01	034-035	786.59	05	143	790.5	23	463-464	796.2	05	144-145
781.3	01	034-035	786.6	04	099-100	790.6	23	463-464	796.3	05	144-145
781.4	01	034-035	786.7	04	099-100	790.7	18	416-417	796.4	23	463-464
781.5	04	101-102	786.8	04	099-100	790.8	18	421-422	796.5	14	383-384
781.6	01	034-035	786.9	04	099-100	790.91	23	463-464	796.9	23	463-464
781.7	10	296-298	787.01	06	182-184	790.92	23	463-464	797	19	429
781.91	01	034-035	787.02	06	182-184	790.93	23	463-464	798.0	01	034-035

DX....MDC....DRG	DX....MDC....DRG	DX....MDC....DRG	DX....MDC....DRG
798.1 ...05 129	800.81 ..01 002,027-030	801.76 ..01 002,027	803.39 ..01 002,027-030
798.2 ...05 129	800.82 ..01 002,027-030	801.79 ..01 002,027-030	803.40 ..01 002,027-030
798.9 ...23 467	800.83 ..01 002,027	801.80 ..01 002,027-030	803.41 ..01 002,027-030
799.0 ...04 101-102	800.84 ..01 002,027	801.81 ..01 002,027-030	803.42 ..01 002,027-030
799.1 ...04 101-102	800.85 ..01 002,027	801.82 ..01 002,027-030	803.43 ..01 002,027
799.2 ...19 425	800.86 ..01 002,027	801.83 ..01 002,027	803.44 ..01 002,027
799.3 ...23 463-464	800.89 ..01 002,027-030	801.84 ..01 002,027	803.45 ..01 002,027
799.4 ...23 463-464	800.90 ..01 002,027-030	801.85 ..01 002,027	803.46 ..01 002,027
799.8 ...23 467	800.91 ..01 002,027-030	801.86 ..01 002,027	803.49 ..01 002,027-030
799.9 ...23 467	800.92 ..01 002,027-030	801.89 ..01 002,027-030	803.50 ..01 002,027-030
	800.93 ..01 002,027	801.90 ..01 002,027-030	803.51 ..01 002,027-030
Injury and Poisoning	800.94 ..01 002,027	801.91 ..01 002,027-030	803.52 ..01 002,027-030
800.00 ..01 002,027-030	800.95 ..01 002,027	801.92 ..01 002,027-030	803.53 ..01 002,027
800.01 ..01 002,027-030	800.96 ..01 002,027	801.93 ..01 002,027	803.54 ..01 002,027
800.02 ..01 002,027-030	800.99 ..01 002,027-030	801.94 ..01 002,027	803.55 ..01 002,027
800.03 ..01 002,027	801.00 ..01 002,027-030	801.95 ..01 002,027	803.56 ..01 002,027
800.04 ..01 002,027	801.01 ..01 002,027-030	801.96 ..01 002,027	803.59 ..01 002,027-030
800.05 ..01 002,027	801.02 ..01 002,027-030	801.99 ..01 002,027-030	803.60 ..01 002,027-030
800.06 ..01 002,027	801.03 ..01 002,027	802.0 ...03 072	803.61 ..01 002,027-030
800.09 ..01 002,027-030	801.04 ..01 002,027	802.1 ...03 072	803.62 ..01 002,027-030
800.10 ..01 002,027-030	801.05 ..01 002,027	802.20 ..03 185-187	803.63 ..01 002,027
800.11 ..01 002,027-030	801.06 ..01 002,027	802.21 ..03 185-187	803.64 ..01 002,027
800.12 ..01 002,027-030	801.09 ..01 002,027-030	802.22 ..03 185-187	803.65 ..01 002,027
800.13 ..01 002,027	801.10 ..01 002,027-030	802.23 ..03 185-187	803.66 ..01 002,027
800.14 ..01 002,027	801.11 ..01 002,027-030	802.24 ..03 185-187	803.69 ..01 002,027-030
800.15 ..01 002,027	801.12 ..01 002,027-030	802.25 ..03 185-187	803.70 ..01 002,027-030
800.16 ..01 002,027	801.13 ..01 002,027	802.26 ..03 185-187	803.71 ..01 002,027-030
800.19 ..01 002,027-030	801.14 ..01 002,027	802.27 ..03 185-187	803.72 ..01 002,027-030
800.20 ..01 002,027-030	801.15 ..01 002,027	802.28 ..03 185-187	803.73 ..01 002,027
800.21 ..01 002,027-030	801.16 ..01 002,027	802.29 ..03 185-187	803.74 ..01 002,027
800.22 ..01 002,027-030	801.19 ..01 002,027-030	802.30 ..03 185-187	803.75 ..01 002,027
800.23 ..01 002,027	801.20 ..01 002,027-030	802.31 ..03 185-187	803.76 ..01 002,027
800.24 ..01 002,027	801.21 ..01 002,027-030	802.32 ..03 185-187	803.79 ..01 002,027-030
800.25 ..01 002,027	801.22 ..01 002,027-030	802.33 ..03 185-187	803.80 ..01 002,027-030
800.26 ..01 002,027	801.23 ..01 002,027	802.34 ..03 185-187	803.81 ..01 002,027-030
800.29 ..01 002,027-030	801.24 ..01 002,027	802.35 ..03 185-187	803.82 ..01 002,027-030
800.30 ..01 002,027-030	801.25 ..01 002,027	802.36 ..03 185-187	803.83 ..01 002,027
800.31 ..01 002,027-030	801.26 ..01 002,027	802.37 ..03 185-187	803.84 ..01 002,027
800.32 ..01 002,027-030	801.29 ..01 002,027-030	802.38 ..03 185-187	803.85 ..01 002,027
800.33 ..01 002,027	801.30 ..01 002,027-030	802.39 ..03 185-187	803.86 ..01 002,027
800.34 ..01 002,027	801.31 ..01 002,027-030	802.4 ...03 185-187	803.89 ..01 002,027-030
800.35 ..01 002,027	801.32 ..01 002,027-030	802.5 ...03 185-187	803.90 ..01 002,027-030
800.36 ..01 002,027	801.33 ..01 002,027	802.6 ...02 046-048	803.91 ..01 002,027-030
800.39 ..01 002,027-030	801.34 ..01 002,027	802.7 ...02 046-048	803.92 ..01 002,027-030
800.40 ..01 002,027-030	801.35 ..01 002,027	802.8 ...08 256	803.93 ..01 002,027
800.41 ..01 002,027-030	801.36 ..01 002,027	802.9 ...08 256	803.94 ..01 002,027
800.42 ..01 002,027-030	801.39 ..01 002,027-030	803.00 ..01 002,027-030	803.95 ..01 002,027
800.43 ..01 002,027	801.40 ..01 002,027-030	803.01 ..01 002,027-030	803.96 ..01 002,027
800.44 ..01 002,027	801.41 ..01 002,027-030	803.02 ..01 002,027-030	803.99 ..01 002,027-030
800.45 ..01 002,027	801.42 ..01 002,027-030	803.03 ..01 002,027	804.00 ..01 002,027-030
800.46 ..01 002,027	801.43 ..01 002,027	803.04 ..01 002,027	804.01 ..01 002,027-030
800.49 ..01 002,027-030	801.44 ..01 002,027	803.05 ..01 002,027	804.02 ..01 002,027-030
800.50 ..01 002,027-030	801.45 ..01 002,027	803.06 ..01 002,027	804.03 ..01 002,027
800.51 ..01 002,027-030	801.46 ..01 002,027	803.09 ..01 002,027-030	804.04 ..01 002,027
800.52 ..01 002,027-030	801.49 ..01 002,027-030	803.10 ..01 002,027-030	804.05 ..01 002,027
800.53 ..01 002,027	801.50 ..01 002,027-030	803.11 ..01 002,027-030	804.06 ..01 002,027
800.54 ..01 002,027	801.51 ..01 002,027-030	803.12 ..01 002,027-030	804.09 ..01 002,027-030
800.55 ..01 002,027	801.52 ..01 002,027-030	803.13 ..01 002,027	804.10 ..01 002,027-030
800.56 ..01 002,027	801.53 ..01 002,027	803.14 ..01 002,027	804.11 ..01 002,027-030
800.59 ..01 002,027-030	801.54 ..01 002,027	803.15 ..01 002,027	804.12 ..01 002,027-030
800.60 ..01 002,027-030	801.55 ..01 002,027	803.16 ..01 002,027	804.13 ..01 002,027
800.61 ..01 002,027-030	801.56 ..01 002,027	803.19 ..01 002,027-030	804.14 ..01 002,027
800.62 ..01 002,027-030	801.59 ..01 002,027-030	803.20 ..01 002,027-030	804.15 ..01 002,027
800.63 ..01 002,027	801.60 ..01 002,027-030	803.21 ..01 002,027-030	804.16 ..01 002,027
800.64 ..01 002,027	801.61 ..01 002,027-030	803.22 ..01 002,027-030	804.19 ..01 002,027-030
800.65 ..01 002,027	801.62 ..01 002,027-030	803.23 ..01 002,027	804.20 ..01 002,027-030
800.66 ..01 002,027	801.63 ..01 002,027	803.24 ..01 002,027	804.21 ..01 002,027-030
800.69 ..01 002,027-030	801.64 ..01 002,027	803.25 ..01 002,027	804.22 ..01 002,027-030
800.70 ..01 002,027-030	801.65 ..01 002,027	803.26 ..01 002,027	804.23 ..01 002,027
800.71 ..01 002,027-030	801.66 ..01 002,027	803.29 ..01 002,027-030	804.24 ..01 002,027
800.72 ..01 002,027-030	801.69 ..01 002,027-030	803.30 ..01 002,027-030	804.25 ..01 002,027
800.73 ..01 002,027	801.70 ..01 002,027-030	803.31 ..01 002,027-030	804.26 ..01 002,027
800.74 ..01 002,027	801.71 ..01 002,027-030	803.32 ..01 002,027-030	804.29 ..01 002,027-030
800.75 ..01 002,027	801.72 ..01 002,027-030	803.33 ..01 002,027	804.30 ..01 002,027-030
800.76 ..01 002,027	801.73 ..01 002,027	803.34 ..01 002,027	804.31 ..01 002,027-030
800.79 ..01 002,027-030	801.74 ..01 002,027	803.35 ..01 002,027	804.32 ..01 002,027-030
800.80 ..01 002,027-030	801.75 ..01 002,027	803.36 ..01 002,027	804.33 ..01 002,027

DX	MDC	DRG	DX	MDC	DRG	DX	MDC	DRG	DX	MDC	DRG
804.34	.01	.002,027	805.9	.08	.243	807.6	.03	.073-074	813.17	.08	.250-252
804.35	.01	.002,027	806.00	.01	.002,009	808.0	.08	.236	813.18	.08	.250-252
804.36	.01	.002,027	806.01	.01	.002,009	808.1	.08	.236	813.20	.08	.250-252
804.39	.01	.002,027-030	806.02	.01	.002,009	808.2	.08	.236	813.21	.08	.250-252
804.40	.01	.002,027-030	806.03	.01	.002,009	808.3	.08	.236	813.22	.08	.250-252
804.41	.01	.002,027-030	806.04	.01	.002,009	808.4	.08	.236	813.23	.08	.250-252
804.42	.01	.002,027-030	806.05	.01	.002,009	808.42	.08	.236	813.30	.08	.250-252
804.43	.01	.002,027	806.06	.01	.002,009	808.43	.08	.236	813.31	.08	.250-252
804.44	.01	.002,027	806.07	.01	.002,009	808.49	.08	.236	813.32	.08	.250-252
804.45	.01	.002,027	806.08	.01	.002,009	808.51	.08	.236	813.33	.08	.250-252
804.46	.01	.002,027	806.09	.01	.002,009	808.52	.08	.236	813.40	.08	.250-252
804.49	.01	.002,027-030	806.10	.01	.002,009	808.53	.08	.236	813.41	.08	.250-252
804.50	.01	.002,027-030	806.11	.01	.002,009	808.59	.08	.236	813.42	.08	.250-252
804.51	.01	.002,027-030	806.12	.01	.002,009	808.8	.08	.236	813.43	.08	.250-252
804.52	.01	.002,027-030	806.13	.01	.002,009	808.9	.08	.236	813.44	.08	.250-252
804.53	.01	.002,027	806.14	.01	.002,009	809.0	.08	.256	813.45	.08	.250-252
804.54	.01	.002,027	806.15	.01	.002,009	809.1	.08	.256	813.45	.24	.487
804.55	.01	.002,027	806.16	.01	.002,009	810.0	.08	.253-255	813.50	.08	.250-252
804.56	.01	.002,027	806.17	.01	.002,009	810.01	.08	.253-255	813.51	.08	.250-252
804.59	.01	.002,027-030	806.18	.01	.002,009	810.02	.08	.253-255	813.52	.08	.250-252
804.60	.01	.002,027-030	806.19	.01	.002,009	810.03	.08	.253-255	813.53	.08	.250-252
804.61	.01	.002,027-030	806.20	.01	.002,009	810.10	.08	.253-255	813.54	.08	.250-252
804.62	.01	.002,027-030	806.21	.01	.002,009	810.11	.08	.253-255	813.80	.08	.250-252
804.63	.01	.002,027	806.22	.01	.002,009	810.12	.08	.253-255	813.81	.08	.250-252
804.64	.01	.002,027	806.23	.01	.002,009	810.13	.08	.253-255	813.82	.08	.250-252
804.65	.01	.002,027	806.24	.01	.002,009	811.00	.08	.253-255	813.83	.08	.250-252
804.66	.01	.002,027	806.25	.01	.002,009	811.01	.08	.253-255	813.90	.08	.250-252
804.69	.01	.002,027-030	806.26	.01	.002,009	811.02	.08	.253-255	813.91	.08	.250-252
804.70	.01	.002,027-030	806.27	.01	.002,009	811.03	.08	.253-255	813.92	.08	.250-252
804.71	.01	.002,027-030	806.28	.01	.002,009	811.09	.08	.256	813.93	.08	.250-252
804.72	.01	.002,027-030	806.29	.01	.002,009	811.10	.08	.253-255	814.00	.08	.250-252
804.73	.01	.002,027	806.30	.01	.002,009	811.11	.08	.253-255	814.01	.08	.250-252
804.74	.01	.002,027	806.31	.01	.002,009	811.12	.08	.253-255	814.02	.08	.250-252
804.75	.01	.002,027	806.32	.01	.002,009	811.13	.08	.253-255	814.03	.08	.250-252
804.76	.01	.002,027	806.33	.01	.002,009	811.19	.08	.256	814.04	.08	.250-252
804.79	.01	.002,027-030	806.34	.01	.002,009	812.00	.08	.253-255	814.05	.08	.250-252
804.80	.01	.002,027-030	806.35	.01	.002,009	812.01	.08	.253-255	814.06	.08	.250-252
804.81	.01	.002,027-030	806.36	.01	.002,009	812.02	.08	.253-255	814.07	.08	.250-252
804.82	.01	.002,027-030	806.37	.01	.002,009	812.03	.08	.253-255	814.08	.08	.250-252
804.83	.01	.002,027	806.38	.01	.002,009	812.09	.08	.253-255	814.09	.08	.250-252
804.84	.01	.002,027	806.39	.01	.002,009	812.10	.08	.253-255	814.10	.08	.250-252
804.85	.01	.002,027	806.4	.01	.002,009	812.11	.08	.253-255	814.11	.08	.250-252
804.86	.01	.002,027	806.5	.01	.002,009	812.12	.08	.253-255	814.12	.08	.250-252
804.89	.01	.002,027-030	806.60	.01	.002,009	812.13	.08	.253-255	814.13	.08	.250-252
804.90	.01	.002,027-030	806.61	.01	.002,009	812.19	.08	.253-255	814.14	.08	.250-252
804.91	.01	.002,027-030	806.62	.01	.002,009	812.20	.08	.253-255	814.15	.08	.250-252
804.92	.01	.002,027-030	806.69	.01	.002,009	812.21	.08	.253-255	814.16	.08	.250-252
804.93	.01	.002,027	806.70	.01	.002,009	812.30	.08	.253-255	814.17	.08	.250-252
804.94	.01	.002,027	806.71	.01	.002,009	812.31	.08	.253-255	814.18	.08	.250-252
804.95	.01	.002,027	806.72	.01	.002,009	812.40	.08	.253-255	814.19	.08	.250-252
804.96	.01	.002,027	806.79	.01	.002,009	812.41	.08	.253-255	815.00	.08	.250-252
804.99	.01	.002,027-030	806.8	.01	.002,009	812.42	.08	.253-255	815.01	.08	.250-252
805.00	.08	.243	806.9	.01	.002,009	812.43	.08	.253-255	815.02	.08	.250-252
805.01	.08	.243	807.00	.04	.101-102	812.44	.08	.253-255	815.03	.08	.250-252
805.02	.08	.243	807.01	.04	.101-102	812.49	.08	.253-255	815.04	.08	.250-252
805.03	.08	.243	807.02	.04	.101-102	812.50	.08	.253-255	815.09	.08	.250-252
805.04	.08	.243	807.03	.04	.083-084	812.51	.08	.253-255	815.10	.08	.250-252
805.05	.08	.243	807.04	.04	.083-084	812.52	.08	.253-255	815.11	.08	.250-252
805.06	.08	.243	807.05	.04	.083-084	812.53	.08	.253-255	815.12	.08	.250-252
805.07	.08	.243	807.06	.04	.083-084	812.54	.08	.253-255	815.13	.08	.250-252
805.08	.08	.243	807.07	.04	.083-084	812.59	.08	.253-255	815.14	.08	.250-252
805.10	.08	.243	807.08	.04	.083-084	813.00	.08	.250-252	815.19	.08	.250-252
805.11	.08	.243	807.09	.04	.083-084	813.01	.08	.250-252	816.00	.08	.250-252
805.12	.08	.243	807.10	.04	.083-084	813.02	.08	.250-252	816.01	.08	.250-252
805.13	.08	.243	807.11	.04	.083-084	813.03	.08	.250-252	816.02	.08	.250-252
805.14	.08	.243	807.12	.04	.083-084	813.04	.08	.250-252	816.03	.08	.250-252
805.15	.08	.243	807.13	.04	.083-084	813.05	.08	.250-252	816.10	.08	.250-252
805.16	.08	.243	807.14	.04	.083-084	813.06	.08	.250-252	816.11	.08	.250-252
805.17	.08	.243	807.15	.04	.083-084	813.07	.08	.250-252	816.12	.08	.250-252
805.18	.08	.243	807.16	.04	.083-084	813.08	.08	.250-252	816.13	.08	.250-252
805.2	.08	.243	807.17	.04	.083-084	813.10	.08	.250-252	817.0	.08	.250-252
805.3	.08	.243	807.18	.04	.083-084	813.11	.08	.250-252	817.1	.08	.250-252
805.4	.08	.243	807.19	.04	.083-084	813.12	.08	.250-252	818.0	.08	.253-255
805.5	.08	.243	807.2	.04	.083-084	813.13	.08	.250-252	818.1	.08	.253-255
805.6	.08	.243	807.3	.04	.083-084	813.14	.08	.250-252	819.0	.21	.444-446
805.7	.08	.243	807.4	.04	.083-084	813.15	.08	.250-252	819.1	.21	.444-446
805.8	.08	.243	807.5	.03	.073-074	813.16	.08	.250-252	820.00	.08	.236

DX ... MDC ... DRG	DX ... MDC ... DRG	DX ... MDC ... DRG	DX ... MDC ... DRG
820.01 ..08 236	825.34 ..08 250-252	836.61 ..08 253-255	842.02 ..08 250-252
820.02 ..08 236	825.35 ..08 250-252	836.62 ..08 253-255	842.09 ..08 250-252
820.03 ..08 236	825.39 ..08 250-252	836.63 ..08 253-255	842.10 ..08 250-252
820.09 ..08 236	826.0 ...08 250-252	836.64 ..08 253-255	842.11 ..08 250-252
820.10 ..08 236	826.1 ...08 250-252	836.69 ..08 253-255	842.12 ..08 250-252
820.11 ..08 236	827.0 ...08 253-255	837.0 ...08 253-255	842.13 ..08 250-252
820.12 ..08 236	827.1 ...08 253-255	837.1 ...08 253-255	842.19 ..08 250-252
820.13 ..08 236	828.0 ...21 444-446	838.00 ..08 250-252	843.0 ...08 237
820.19 ..08 236	828.1 ...21 444-446	838.01 ..08 250-252	843.1 ...08 237
820.20 ..08 236	829.0 ...08 250-252	838.02 ..08 250-252	843.8 ...08 237
820.21 ..08 236	829.1 ...08 250-252	838.03 ..08 250-252	843.9 ...08 237
820.22 ..08 236	830.0 ...03 185-187	838.04 ..08 250-252	844.0 ...08 253-255
820.30 ..08 236	830.1 ...03 185-187	838.05 ..08 250-252	844.1 ...08 253-255
820.31 ..08 236	831.00 ..08 253-255	838.06 ..08 250-252	844.2 ...08 253-255
820.32 ..08 236	831.01 ..08 253-255	838.09 ..08 250-252	844.3 ...08 253-255
820.8 ...08 236	831.02 ..08 253-255	838.10 ..08 250-252	844.8 ...08 253-255
820.9 ...08 236	831.03 ..08 253-255	838.11 ..08 250-252	844.9 ...08 253-255
821.00 ..08 235	831.04 ..08 253-255	838.12 ..08 250-252	845.00 ..08 253-255
821.01 ..08 235	831.09 ..08 253-255	838.13 ..08 250-252	845.01 ..08 253-255
821.10 ..08 235	831.10 ..08 253-255	838.14 ..08 250-252	845.02 ..08 253-255
821.11 ..08 235	831.11 ..08 253-255	838.15 ..08 250-252	845.03 ..08 253-255
821.20 ..08 235	831.12 ..08 253-255	838.16 ..08 250-252	845.09 ..08 253-255
821.21 ..08 235	831.13 ..08 253-255	838.19 ..08 250-252	845.10 ..08 250-252
821.22 ..08 235	831.14 ..08 253-255	839.00 ..08 243	845.11 ..08 250-252
821.23 ..08 235	831.19 ..08 253-255	839.01 ..08 243	845.12 ..08 250-252
821.29 ..08 235	832.00 ..08 253-255	839.02 ..08 243	845.13 ..08 250-252
821.30 ..08 235	832.01 ..08 253-255	839.03 ..08 243	845.19 ..08 250-252
821.31 ..08 235	832.02 ..08 253-255	839.04 ..08 243	846.0 ...08 243
821.32 ..08 235	832.03 ..08 253-255	839.05 ..08 243	846.1 ...08 243
821.33 ..08 235	832.04 ..08 253-255	839.06 ..08 243	846.2 ...08 243
821.39 ..08 235	832.09 ..08 253-255	839.07 ..08 243	846.3 ...08 243
822.0 ...08 253-255	832.10 ..08 253-255	839.08 ..08 243	846.8 ...08 243
822.1 ...08 253-255	832.11 ..08 253-255	839.10 ..08 243	846.9 ...08 243
823.00 ..08 253-255	832.12 ..08 253-255	839.11 ..08 243	847.0 ...08 243
823.01 ..08 253-255	832.13 ..08 253-255	839.12 ..08 243	847.1 ...08 243
823.02 ..08 253-255	832.14 ..08 253-255	839.13 ..08 243	847.2 ...08 243
823.10 ..08 253-255	832.19 ..08 253-255	839.14 ..08 243	847.3 ...08 243
823.11 ..08 253-255	833.00 ..08 250-252	839.15 ..08 243	847.4 ...08 243
823.12 ..08 253-255	833.01 ..08 250-252	839.16 ..08 243	847.9 ...08 243
823.20 ..08 253-255	833.02 ..08 250-252	839.17 ..08 243	848.0 ...08 256
823.21 ..08 253-255	833.03 ..08 250-252	839.18 ..08 243	848.1 ...03 185-187
823.22 ..08 253-255	833.04 ..08 250-252	839.20 ..08 243	848.2 ...08 256
823.30 ..08 253-255	833.05 ..08 250-252	839.21 ..08 243	848.3 ...04 101-102
823.31 ..08 253-255	833.09 ..08 250-252	839.30 ..08 243	848.40 ..04 101-102
823.32 ..08 253-255	833.10 ..08 250-252	839.31 ..08 243	848.41 ..04 101-102
823.40 ..08 253-255	833.11 ..08 250-252	839.40 ..08 243	848.42 ..04 101-102
823.41 ..08 253-255	833.12 ..08 250-252	839.41 ..08 243	848.49 ..04 101-102
823.42 ..08 253-255	833.13 ..08 250-252	839.42 ..08 243	848.5 ...08 237
823.80 ..08 253-255	833.14 ..08 250-252	839.49 ..08 243	848.8 ...08 250-252
823.81 ..08 253-255	833.15 ..08 250-252	839.50 ..08 243	848.9 ...08 250-252
823.82 ..08 253-255	833.19 ..08 250-252	839.51 ..08 243	850.0 ...01 002,031-033
823.90 ..08 253-255	834.00 ..08 250-252	839.52 ..08 243	850.1 ...01 002,031-033
823.91 ..08 253-255	834.01 ..08 250-252	839.59 ..08 243	850.2 ...01 002,031-033
823.92 ..08 253-255	834.02 ..08 250-252	839.61 ..04 083-084	850.3 ...01 002,031-033
824.0 ...08 253-255	834.10 ..08 250-252	839.69 ..08 250-252	850.4 ...01 002,031-033
824.1 ...08 253-255	834.11 ..08 250-252	839.71 ..04 083-084	850.5 ...01 002,031-033
824.2 ...08 253-255	834.12 ..08 250-252	839.79 ..08 250-252	850.9 ...01 002,031-033
824.3 ...08 253-255	835.00 ..08 237	839.8 ...08 250-252	851.00 ..01 002,027-030
824.4 ...08 253-255	835.01 ..08 237	839.9 ...08 250-252	851.01 ..01 002,027-030
824.5 ...08 253-255	835.02 ..08 237	840.0 ...08 253-255	851.02 ..01 002,027-030
824.6 ...08 253-255	835.03 ..08 237	840.1 ...08 253-255	851.03 ..01 002,027
824.7 ...08 253-255	835.10 ..08 237	840.2 ...08 253-255	851.04 ..01 002,027
824.8 ...08 253-255	835.11 ..08 237	840.3 ...08 253-255	851.05 ..01 002,027
824.9 ...08 253-255	835.12 ..08 237	840.4 ...08 253-255	851.06 ..01 002,027
825.0 ...08 253-255	835.13 ..08 237	840.5 ...08 253-255	851.09 ..01 002,027-030
825.1 ...08 253-255	836.0 ...08 253-255	840.6 ...08 253-255	851.10 ..01 002,027-030
825.20 ..08 250-252	836.1 ...08 253-255	840.7 ...08 253-255	851.11 ..01 002,027-030
825.21 ..08 250-252	836.2 ...08 253-255	840.8 ...08 253-255	851.12 ..01 002,027-030
825.22 ..08 250-252	836.3 ...08 253-255	840.9 ...08 253-255	851.13 ..01 002,027
825.23 ..08 250-252	836.4 ...08 253-255	841.0 ...08 250-252	851.14 ..01 002,027
825.24 ..08 250-252	836.50 ..08 253-255	841.1 ...08 250-252	851.15 ..01 002,027
825.25 ..08 250-252	836.51 ..08 253-255	841.2 ...08 250-252	851.16 ..01 002,027
825.29 ..08 250-252	836.52 ..08 253-255	841.3 ...08 250-252	851.19 ..01 002,027-030
825.30 ..08 250-252	836.53 ..08 253-255	841.8 ...08 250-252	851.20 ..01 002,027-030
825.31 ..08 250-252	836.54 ..08 253-255	841.9 ...08 250-252	851.21 ..01 002,027-030
825.32 ..08 250-252	836.59 ..08 253-255	842.00 ..08 250-252	851.22 ..01 002,027-030
825.33 ..08 250-252	836.60 ..08 253-255	842.01 ..08 250-252	851.23 ..01 002,027

Diagnosis Code/MDC/DRG List

DX ....MDC ....DRG	DX ....MDC ....DRG	DX ....MDC ....DRG	DX ....MDC ....DRG
851.24 ..01 002,027	852.21 ..01 002,027-030	861.20 ..04 101-102	865.11 ..16 398-399
851.25 ..01 002,027	852.22 ..01 002,027-030	861.21 ..04 101-102	865.12 ..16 398-399
851.26 ..01 002,027	852.23 ..01 002,027	861.22 ..04 083-084	865.13 ..16 398-399
851.29 ..01 002,027-030	852.24 ..01 002,027	861.30 ..04 101-102	865.14 ..16 398-399
851.30 ..01 002,027-030	852.25 ..01 002,027	861.31 ..04 101-102	865.19 ..16 398-399
851.31 ..01 002,027-030	852.26 ..01 002,027	861.32 ..04 083-084	866.00 ..11 331-333
851.32 ..01 002,027-030	852.29 ..01 002,027-030	862.0 ...04 083-084	866.01 ..11 331-333
851.33 ..01 002,027	852.30 ..01 002,027-030	862.1 ...04 083-084	866.02 ..11 331-333
851.34 ..01 002,027	852.31 ..01 002,027-030	862.21 ..04 083-084	866.03 ..11 331-333
851.35 ..01 002,027	852.32 ..01 002,027-030	862.22 ..06 188-190	866.10 ..11 331-333
851.36 ..01 002,027	852.33 ..01 002,027	862.29 ..04 101-102	866.11 ..11 331-333
851.39 ..01 002,027-030	852.34 ..01 002,027	862.31 ..04 083-084	866.12 ..11 331-333
851.40 ..01 002,027-030	852.35 ..01 002,027	862.32 ..06 188-190	866.13 ..11 331-333
851.41 ..01 002,027-030	852.36 ..01 002,027	862.39 ..04 101-102	867.0 ...11 331-333
851.42 ..01 002,027-030	852.39 ..01 002,027-030	862.8 ...21 444-446	867.1 ...11 331-333
851.43 ..01 002,027	852.40 ..01 002,027-030	862.9 ...21 444-446	867.2 ...11 331-333
851.44 ..01 002,027	852.41 ..01 002,027-030	863.0 ...06 188-190	867.3 ...11 331-333
851.45 ..01 002,027	852.42 ..01 002,027-030	863.1 ...06 188-190	867.4 ...13 358-359,369
851.46 ..01 002,027	852.43 ..01 002,027	863.20 ..06 188-190	867.5 ...13 358-359,369
851.49 ..01 002,027-030	852.44 ..01 002,027	863.21 ..06 188-190	867.6 ...12 352
851.50 ..01 002,027-030	852.45 ..01 002,027	863.29 ..06 188-190	867.6 ...13 358-359,369
851.51 ..01 002,027-030	852.46 ..01 002,027	863.30 ..06 188-190	867.7 ...12 352
851.52 ..01 002,027-030	852.49 ..01 002,027-030	863.31 ..06 188-190	867.7 ...13 358-359,369
851.53 ..01 002,027	852.50 ..01 002,027-030	863.39 ..06 188-190	867.8 ...12 352
851.54 ..01 002,027	852.51 ..01 002,027-030	863.40 ..06 188-190	867.8 ...13 358-359,369
851.55 ..01 002,027	852.52 ..01 002,027-030	863.41 ..06 188-190	867.9 ...12 352
851.56 ..01 002,027	852.53 ..01 002,027	863.42 ..06 188-190	867.9 ...13 358-359,369
851.59 ..01 002,027-030	852.54 ..01 002,027	863.43 ..06 188-190	868.00 ..06 188-190
851.60 ..01 002,027-030	852.55 ..01 002,027	863.44 ..06 188-190	868.01 ..10 300-301
851.61 ..01 002,027-030	852.56 ..01 002,027	863.45 ..06 188-190	868.02 ..07 207-208
851.62 ..01 002,027-030	852.59 ..01 002,027-030	863.46 ..06 188-190	868.03 ..06 188-190
851.63 ..01 002,027	853.00 ..01 002,027-030	863.49 ..06 188-190	868.04 ..11 331-333
851.64 ..01 002,027	853.01 ..01 002,027-030	863.50 ..06 188-190	868.09 ..21 444-446
851.65 ..01 002,027	853.02 ..01 002,027-030	863.51 ..06 188-190	868.10 ..06 188-190
851.66 ..01 002,027	853.03 ..01 002,027	863.52 ..06 188-190	868.11 ..10 300-301
851.69 ..01 002,027-030	853.04 ..01 002,027	863.53 ..06 188-190	868.12 ..07 207-208
851.70 ..01 002,027-030	853.05 ..01 002,027	863.54 ..06 188-190	868.13 ..06 188-190
851.71 ..01 002,027-030	853.06 ..01 002,027	863.55 ..06 188-190	868.14 ..11 331-333
851.72 ..01 002,027-030	853.09 ..01 002,027-030	863.56 ..06 188-190	868.19 ..21 444-446
851.73 ..01 002,027	853.10 ..01 002,027-030	863.59 ..06 188-190	869.0 ...21 444-446
851.74 ..01 002,027	853.11 ..01 002,027-030	863.80 ..06 188-190	869.1 ...21 444-446
851.75 ..01 002,027	853.12 ..01 002,027-030	863.81 ..07 204	870.0 ...02 046-048
851.76 ..01 002,027	853.13 ..01 002,027	863.82 ..07 204	870.1 ...02 046-048
851.79 ..01 002,027-030	853.14 ..01 002,027	863.83 ..07 204	870.2 ...02 046-048
851.80 ..01 002,027-030	853.15 ..01 002,027	863.84 ..07 204	870.3 ...02 046-048
851.81 ..01 002,027-030	853.16 ..01 002,027	863.85 ..06 188-190	870.4 ...02 046-048
851.82 ..01 002,027-030	853.19 ..01 002,027-030	863.89 ..06 188-190	870.8 ...02 046-048
851.83 ..01 002,027	854.00 ..01 002,027-030	863.90 ..06 188-190	870.9 ...02 046-048
851.84 ..01 002,027	854.01 ..01 002,027-030	863.91 ..07 204	871.0 ...02 046-048
851.85 ..01 002,027	854.02 ..01 002,027-030	863.92 ..07 204	871.1 ...02 046-048
851.86 ..01 002,027	854.03 ..01 002,027	863.93 ..07 204	871.2 ...02 046-048
851.89 ..01 002,027-030	854.04 ..01 002,027	863.94 ..07 204	871.3 ...02 046-048
851.90 ..01 002,027-030	854.05 ..01 002,027	863.95 ..06 188-190	871.4 ...02 046-048
851.91 ..01 002,027-030	854.06 ..01 002,027	863.99 ..06 188-190	871.5 ...02 046-048
851.92 ..01 002,027-030	854.09 ..01 002,027-030	864.00 ..07 205-206	871.6 ...02 046-048
851.93 ..01 002,027	854.10 ..01 002,027-030	864.01 ..07 205-206	871.7 ...02 046-048
851.94 ..01 002,027	854.11 ..01 002,027-030	864.02 ..07 205-206	871.9 ...02 046-048
851.95 ..01 002,027	854.12 ..01 002,027-030	864.03 ..07 205-206	872.00 ..03 073-074
851.96 ..01 002,027	854.13 ..01 002,027	864.04 ..07 205-206	872.01 ..03 073-074
851.99 ..01 002,027-030	854.14 ..01 002,027	864.05 ..07 205-206	872.02 ..03 073-074
852.00 ..01 002,027-030	854.15 ..01 002,027	864.05 ..24 487	872.10 ..03 073-074
852.01 ..01 002,027-030	854.16 ..01 002,027	864.09 ..07 205-206	872.11 ..03 073-074
852.02 ..01 002,027-030	854.19 ..01 002,027-030	864.10 ..07 205-206	872.12 ..03 073-074
852.03 ..01 002,027	860.0 ...04 094-095	864.11 ..07 205-206	872.61 ..03 073-074
852.04 ..01 002,027	860.1 ...04 094-095	864.12 ..07 205-206	872.62 ..03 073-074
852.05 ..01 002,027	860.2 ...04 094-095	864.13 ..07 205-206	872.63 ..03 073-074
852.06 ..01 002,027	860.3 ...04 094-095	864.14 ..07 205-206	872.64 ..03 073-074
852.09 ..01 002,027-030	860.4 ...04 094-095	864.15 ..07 205-206	872.69 ..03 073-074
852.10 ..01 002,027-030	860.5 ...04 094-095	864.15 ..24 487	872.71 ..03 073-074
852.11 ..01 002,027-030	861.00 ..05 144-145	864.19 ..07 205-206	872.72 ..03 073-074
852.12 ..01 002,027-030	861.01 ..05 144-145	865.00 ..16 398-399	872.73 ..03 073-074
852.13 ..01 002,027	861.02 ..05 144-145	865.01 ..16 398-399	872.74 ..03 073-074
852.14 ..01 002,027	861.03 ..05 144-145	865.02 ..16 398-399	872.79 ..03 073-074
852.15 ..01 002,027	861.10 ..05 144-145	865.03 ..16 398-399	872.8 ...03 073-074
852.16 ..01 002,027	861.11 ..05 144-145	865.04 ..16 398-399	872.9 ...03 073-074
852.19 ..01 002,027-030	861.12 ..05 144-145	865.09 ..16 398-399	873.0 ...09 280-282
852.20 ..01 002,027-030	861.13 ..05 144-145	865.10 ..16 398-399	873.1 ...09 280-282

DX	MDC	DRG	DX	MDC	DRG	DX	MDC	DRG	DX	MDC	DRG
873.20	.03	.072	879.9	.21	.444-446	900.02	.21	.444-446	904.7	.21	.444-446
873.21	.03	.073-074	880.00	.09	.280-282	900.03	.21	.444-446	904.8	.21	.444-446
873.22	.03	.073-074	880.01	.09	.280-282	900.1	.21	.444-446	904.9	.21	.444-446
873.23	.03	.073-074	880.02	.09	.280-282	900.81	.21	.444-446	905.0	.01	.034-035
873.29	.03	.073-074	880.03	.09	.280-282	900.82	.21	.444-446	905.1	.08	.243
873.30	.03	.073-074	880.09	.09	.280-282	900.89	.21	.444-446	905.2	.08	.249
873.31	.03	.073-074	880.10	.21	.444-446	900.9	.21	.444-446	905.3	.08	.249
873.32	.03	.073-074	880.11	.21	.444-446	901.0	.21	.444-446	905.4	.08	.249
873.33	.03	.073-074	880.12	.21	.444-446	901.1	.21	.444-446	905.5	.08	.249
873.39	.03	.073-074	880.13	.21	.444-446	901.2	.21	.444-446	905.6	.08	.250-252
873.40	.09	.280-282	880.19	.21	.444-446	901.3	.21	.444-446	905.7	.08	.250-252
873.41	.09	.280-282	880.20	.08	.256	901.40	.21	.444-446	905.8	.08	.249
873.42	.09	.280-282	880.21	.08	.256	901.41	.21	.444-446	905.9	.08	.249
873.43	.03	.185-187	880.22	.08	.256	901.42	.21	.444-446	906.0	.09	.280-282
873.44	.03	.185-187	880.23	.08	.256	901.81	.21	.444-446	906.1	.09	.280-282
873.49	.09	.280-282	880.29	.08	.256	901.82	.21	.444-446	906.2	.09	.280-282
873.50	.09	.280-282	881.00	.09	.280-282	901.83	.21	.444-446	906.3	.09	.280-282
873.51	.09	.280-282	881.01	.09	.280-282	901.89	.21	.444-446	906.4	.09	.280-282
873.52	.09	.280-282	881.02	.09	.280-282	901.9	.21	.444-446	906.5	.09	.280-282
873.53	.03	.185-187	881.10	.21	.444-446	902.0	.21	.444-446	906.6	.09	.280-282
873.54	.03	.185-187	881.11	.21	.444-446	902.10	.21	.444-446	906.7	.09	.280-282
873.59	.09	.280-282	881.12	.21	.444-446	902.11	.21	.444-446	906.8	.09	.280-282
873.60	.03	.185-187	881.20	.08	.256	902.19	.21	.444-446	906.9	.09	.280-282
873.61	.03	.185-187	881.21	.08	.256	902.20	.21	.444-446	907.0	.01	.034-035
873.62	.03	.185-187	881.22	.08	.256	902.21	.21	.444-446	907.1	.01	.034-035
873.63	.03	.185-187	882.0	.09	.280-282	902.22	.21	.444-446	907.2	.01	.009
873.64	.03	.185-187	882.1	.21	.444-446	902.23	.21	.444-446	907.3	.01	.034-035
873.65	.03	.185-187	882.2	.08	.256	902.24	.21	.444-446	907.4	.01	.034-035
873.69	.03	.185-187	883.0	.09	.280-282	902.25	.21	.444-446	907.5	.01	.034-035
873.70	.03	.185-187	883.1	.21	.444-446	902.26	.21	.444-446	907.9	.01	.034-035
873.71	.03	.185-187	883.2	.08	.256	902.27	.21	.444-446	908.0	.04	.101-102
873.72	.03	.185-187	884.0	.09	.280-282	902.29	.21	.444-446	908.1	.06	.188-190
873.73	.03	.185-187	884.1	.21	.444-446	902.31	.21	.444-446	908.2	.12	.352
873.74	.03	.185-187	884.2	.08	.256	902.32	.21	.444-446	908.2	.13	.358-359,369
873.75	.03	.185-187	885.0	.21	.444-446	902.33	.21	.444-446	908.3	.05	.130-131
873.79	.03	.185-187	885.1	.21	.444-446	902.34	.21	.444-446	908.4	.05	.130-131
873.8	.09	.280-282	886.0	.21	.444-446	902.39	.21	.444-446	908.5	.21	.444-446
873.9	.09	.280-282	886.1	.21	.444-446	902.40	.21	.444-446	908.6	.21	.444-446
874.00	.03	.073-074	887.0	.21	.444-446	902.41	.21	.444-446	908.9	.21	.444-446
874.01	.03	.073-074	887.1	.21	.444-446	902.42	.21	.444-446	909.0	.21	.454-455
874.02	.04	.083-084	887.2	.21	.444-446	902.49	.21	.444-446	909.1	.21	.454-455
874.10	.03	.073-074	887.3	.21	.444-446	902.50	.21	.444-446	909.2	.21	.454-455
874.11	.03	.073-074	887.4	.21	.444-446	902.51	.21	.444-446	909.3	.21	.454-455
874.12	.04	.083-084	887.5	.21	.444-446	902.52	.21	.444-446	909.4	.21	.454-455
874.2	.10	.300-301	887.6	.21	.444-446	902.53	.21	.444-446	909.9	.21	.454-455
874.3	.10	.300-301	887.7	.21	.444-446	902.54	.21	.444-446	910.0	.09	.280-282
874.4	.03	.073-074	890.0	.09	.280-282	902.55	.21	.444-446	910.1	.09	.277-279
874.5	.03	.073-074	890.1	.21	.444-446	902.56	.21	.444-446	910.2	.09	.283-284
874.8	.09	.280-282	890.2	.08	.256	902.59	.21	.444-446	910.3	.09	.283-284
874.9	.09	.280-282	891.0	.09	.280-282	902.81	.21	.444-446	910.4	.09	.283-284
875.0	.09	.280-282	891.1	.21	.444-446	902.82	.21	.444-446	910.5	.09	.277-279
875.1	.21	.444-446	891.2	.08	.256	902.87	.21	.444-446	910.6	.09	.280-282
876.0	.09	.280-282	892.0	.09	.280-282	902.89	.21	.444-446	910.7	.09	.277-279
876.1	.09	.280-282	892.1	.21	.444-446	902.9	.21	.444-446	910.8	.09	.280-282
877.0	.09	.280-282	892.2	.08	.256	903.00	.21	.444-446	910.9	.09	.277-279
877.1	.09	.280-282	893.0	.09	.280-282	903.01	.21	.444-446	911.0	.09	.280-282
878.0	.12	.352	893.1	.21	.444-446	903.02	.21	.444-446	911.1	.09	.277-279
878.1	.12	.352	893.2	.08	.256	903.1	.21	.444-446	911.2	.09	.283-284
878.2	.12	.352	894.0	.09	.280-282	903.2	.21	.444-446	911.3	.09	.277-279
878.3	.12	.352	894.1	.21	.444-446	903.3	.21	.444-446	911.4	.09	.283-284
878.4	.13	.358-359,369	894.2	.08	.256	903.4	.21	.444-446	911.5	.09	.277-279
878.5	.13	.358-359,369	895.0	.21	.444-446	903.5	.21	.444-446	911.6	.09	.280-282
878.6	.13	.358-359,369	895.1	.21	.444-446	903.8	.21	.444-446	911.7	.09	.277-279
878.7	.13	.358-359,369	896.0	.21	.444-446	903.9	.21	.444-446	911.8	.09	.280-282
878.8	.12	.352	896.1	.21	.444-446	904.0	.21	.444-446	911.9	.09	.277-279
878.8	.13	.358-359,369	896.2	.21	.444-446	904.1	.21	.444-446	912.0	.09	.280-282
878.9	.12	.352	896.3	.21	.444-446	904.2	.21	.444-446	912.1	.09	.277-279
878.9	.13	.358-359,369	897.0	.21	.444-446	904.3	.21	.444-446	912.2	.09	.280-282
879.0	.09	.280-282	897.1	.21	.444-446	904.40	.21	.444-446	912.3	.09	.277-279
879.1	.09	.280-282	897.2	.21	.444-446	904.41	.21	.444-446	912.4	.09	.283-284
879.2	.09	.280-282	897.3	.21	.444-446	904.42	.21	.444-446	912.5	.09	.277-279
879.3	.21	.444-446	897.4	.21	.444-446	904.50	.21	.444-446	912.6	.09	.280-282
879.4	.09	.280-282	897.5	.21	.444-446	904.51	.21	.444-446	912.7	.09	.277-279
879.5	.21	.444-446	897.6	.21	.444-446	904.52	.21	.444-446	912.8	.09	.280-282
879.6	.09	.280-282	897.7	.21	.444-446	904.53	.21	.444-446	912.9	.09	.277-279
879.7	.21	.444-446	900.00	.21	.444-446	904.54	.21	.444-446	913.0	.09	.280-282
879.8	.09	.280-282	900.01	.21	.444-446	904.6	.21	.444-446	913.1	.09	.277-279

Diagnosis Code/MDC/DRG List

DX	MDC	DRG		DX	MDC	DRG		DX	MDC	DRG		DX	MDC	DRG
913.2	09	283-284		922.4	12	352		938	06	188-190		942.04	22	510-511
913.3	09	277-279		922.4	13	358-359,369		939.0	11	331-333		942.05	22	510-511
913.4	09	283-284		922.8	09	280-282		939.1	13	358-359,369		942.09	22	510-511
913.5	09	277-279		922.9	09	280-282		939.2	13	358-359,369		942.10	22	510-511
913.6	09	280-282		923.00	09	280-282		939.3	12	352		942.11	22	510-511
913.7	09	277-279		923.01	09	280-282		939.9	11	331-333		942.12	22	510-511
913.8	09	280-282		923.02	09	280-282		940.0	02	046-048		942.13	22	510-511
913.9	09	277-279		923.03	09	280-282		940.1	02	046-048		942.14	22	510-511
914.0	09	280-282		923.09	09	280-282		940.2	02	046-048		942.15	22	510-511
914.1	09	277-279		923.10	09	280-282		940.3	02	046-048		942.19	22	510-511
914.2	09	283-284		923.11	09	280-282		940.4	02	046-048		942.20	22	510-511
914.3	09	277-279		923.20	09	280-282		940.5	02	046-048		942.21	22	510-511
914.4	09	283-284		923.21	09	280-282		940.9	02	046-048		942.22	22	510-511
914.5	09	277-279		923.3	09	280-282		941.00	22	510-511		942.23	22	510-511
914.6	09	280-282		923.8	09	280-282		941.01	22	510-511		942.24	22	510-511
914.7	09	277-279		923.9	09	280-282		941.02	02	046-048		942.25	22	510-511
914.8	09	280-282		924.00	09	280-282		941.03	22	510-511		942.29	22	510-511
914.9	09	277-279		924.01	09	280-282		941.04	22	510-511		942.30	22	506-509
915.0	09	280-282		924.10	09	280-282		941.05	22	510-511		942.31	22	506-509
915.1	09	277-279		924.11	09	280-282		941.06	22	510-511		942.32	22	506-509
915.2	09	283-284		924.20	09	280-282		941.07	22	510-511		942.33	22	506-509
915.3	09	277-279		924.21	09	280-282		941.08	22	510-511		942.34	22	506-509
915.4	09	283-284		924.3	09	280-282		941.09	22	510-511		942.35	22	506-509
915.5	09	277-279		924.4	09	280-282		941.10	22	510-511		942.39	22	506-509
915.6	09	280-282		924.5	09	280-282		941.11	22	510-511		942.40	22	506-509
915.7	09	277-279		924.8	09	280-282		941.12	02	046-048		942.41	22	506-509
915.8	09	280-282		924.9	09	280-282		941.13	22	510-511		942.42	22	506-509
915.9	09	277-279		925.1	21	444-446		941.14	22	510-511		942.43	22	506-509
916.0	09	280-282		925.2	21	444-446		941.15	22	510-511		942.44	22	506-509
916.1	09	277-279		926.0	12	352		941.16	22	510-511		942.45	22	506-509
916.2	09	283-284		926.0	13	358-359,369		941.17	22	510-511		942.49	22	506-509
916.3	09	277-279		926.11	21	444-446		941.18	22	510-511		942.50	22	506-509
916.4	09	283-284		926.12	21	444-446		941.19	22	510-511		942.51	22	506-509
916.5	09	277-279		926.19	21	444-446		941.20	22	510-511		942.52	22	506-509
916.6	09	280-282		926.8	21	444-446		941.21	22	510-511		942.53	22	506-509
916.7	09	277-279		926.9	21	444-446		941.22	02	046-048		942.54	22	506-509
916.8	09	280-282		927.00	21	444-446		941.23	22	510-511		942.55	22	506-509
916.9	09	277-279		927.01	21	444-446		941.24	22	510-511		942.59	22	506-509
917.0	09	280-282		927.02	21	444-446		941.25	22	510-511		943.00	22	510-511
917.1	09	277-279		927.03	21	444-446		941.26	22	510-511		943.01	22	510-511
917.2	09	283-284		927.09	21	444-446		941.27	22	510-511		943.02	22	510-511
917.3	09	277-279		927.10	21	444-446		941.28	22	510-511		943.03	22	510-511
917.4	09	283-284		927.11	21	444-446		941.29	22	510-511		943.04	22	510-511
917.5	09	277-279		927.20	21	444-446		941.30	22	506-509		943.05	22	510-511
917.6	09	280-282		927.21	21	444-446		941.31	22	506-509		943.06	22	510-511
917.7	09	277-279		927.3	21	444-446		941.32	02	046-048		943.09	22	510-511
917.8	09	280-282		927.8	21	444-446		941.33	22	506-509		943.10	22	510-511
917.9	09	277-279		927.9	21	444-446		941.34	22	506-509		943.11	22	510-511
918.0	02	046-048		928.00	21	444-446		941.35	22	506-509		943.12	22	510-511
918.1	02	046-048		928.01	21	444-446		941.36	22	506-509		943.13	22	510-511
918.2	02	046-048		928.10	21	444-446		941.37	22	506-509		943.14	22	510-511
918.9	02	046-048		928.11	21	444-446		941.38	22	506-509		943.15	22	510-511
919.0	09	280-282		928.20	21	444-446		941.39	22	506-509		943.16	22	510-511
919.1	09	277-279		928.21	21	444-446		941.40	22	506-509		943.19	22	510-511
919.2	09	283-284		928.3	21	444-446		941.41	22	506-509		943.20	22	510-511
919.3	09	277-279		928.8	21	444-446		941.42	02	046-048		943.21	22	510-511
919.4	09	283-284		928.9	21	444-446		941.43	22	506-509		943.22	22	510-511
919.5	09	277-279		929.0	21	444-446		941.44	22	506-509		943.23	22	510-511
919.6	09	280-282		929.9	21	444-446		941.45	22	506-509		943.24	22	510-511
919.7	09	277-279		930.0	02	046-048		941.46	22	506-509		943.25	22	510-511
919.8	09	280-282		930.1	02	046-048		941.47	22	506-509		943.26	22	510-511
919.9	09	277-279		930.2	02	046-048		941.48	22	506-509		943.29	22	510-511
920.	09	280-282		930.8	02	046-048		941.49	22	506-509		943.30	22	506-509
921.0	02	046-048		930.9	02	046-048		941.50	22	506-509		943.31	22	506-509
921.1	02	043		931	03	073-074		941.51	22	506-509		943.32	22	506-509
921.2	02	046-048		932	03	072		941.52	02	046-048		943.33	22	506-509
921.3	02	043		933.0	03	073-074		941.53	22	506-509		943.34	22	506-509
921.9	02	046-048		933.1	03	073-074		941.54	22	506-509		943.35	22	506-509
922.0	09	280-282		934.0	04	101-102		941.55	22	506-509		943.36	22	506-509
922.1	09	280-282		934.1	04	101-102		941.56	22	506-509		943.39	22	506-509
922.2	09	280-282		934.8	04	101-102		941.57	22	506-509		943.40	22	506-509
922.31	09	280-282		934.9	04	101-102		941.58	22	506-509		943.41	22	506-509
922.31	24	484-487		935.0	03	185-187		941.59	22	506-509		943.42	22	506-509
922.32	09	280-282		935.1	06	188-190		942.00	22	510-511		943.43	22	506-509
922.32	24	484-487		935.2	06	188-190		942.01	22	510-511		943.44	22	506-509
922.33	09	280-282		936	06	188-190		942.02	22	510-511		943.45	22	506-509
922.33	24	484-487		937	06	188-190		942.03	22	510-511		943.46	22	506-509

DX....MDC....DRG	DX....MDC....DRG	DX....MDC....DRG	DX....MDC....DRG
943.49 ..22 506-509	945.16 ..22 510-511	948.72 ..22 504-505	953.8 ...01 018-019
943.50 ..22 506-509	945.19 ..22 510-511	948.73 ..22 504-505	953.9 ...01 018-019
943.51 ..22 506-509	945.20 ..22 510-511	948.74 ..22 504-505	954.0 ...01 018-019
943.52 ..22 506-509	945.21 ..22 510-511	948.75 ..22 504-505	954.1 ...01 018-019
943.53 ..22 506-509	945.22 ..22 510-511	948.76 ..22 504-505	954.8 ...01 018-019
943.54 ..22 506-509	945.23 ..22 510-511	948.77 ..22 504-505	954.9 ...01 018-019
943.55 ..22 506-509	945.24 ..22 510-511	948.80 ..22 510-511	955.0 ...01 018-019
943.56 ..22 506-509	945.25 ..22 510-511	948.81 ..22 504-505	955.1 ...01 018-019
943.59 ..22 506-509	945.26 ..22 510-511	948.82 ..22 504-505	955.2 ...01 018-019
944.00 ..22 510-511	945.29 ..22 510-511	948.83 ..22 504-505	955.3 ...01 018-019
944.01 ..22 510-511	945.30 ..22 506-509	948.84 ..22 504-505	955.4 ...01 018-019
944.02 ..22 510-511	945.31 ..22 506-509	948.85 ..22 504-505	955.5 ...01 018-019
944.03 ..22 510-511	945.32 ..22 506-509	948.86 ..22 504-505	955.6 ...01 018-019
944.04 ..22 510-511	945.33 ..22 506-509	948.87 ..22 504-505	955.7 ...01 018-019
944.05 ..22 510-511	945.34 ..22 506-509	948.88 ..22 504-505	955.8 ...01 018-019
944.06 ..22 510-511	945.35 ..22 506-509	948.90 ..22 510-511	955.9 ...01 018-019
944.07 ..22 510-511	945.36 ..22 506-509	948.91 ..22 504-505	956.0 ...01 018-019
944.08 ..22 510-511	945.39 ..22 506-509	948.92 ..22 504-505	956.1 ...01 018-019
944.10 ..22 510-511	945.40 ..22 506-509	948.93 ..22 504-505	956.2 ...01 018-019
944.11 ..22 510-511	945.41 ..22 506-509	948.94 ..22 504-505	956.3 ...01 018-019
944.12 ..22 510-511	945.42 ..22 506-509	948.95 ..22 504-505	956.4 ...01 018-019
944.13 ..22 510-511	945.43 ..22 506-509	948.96 ..22 504-505	956.5 ...01 018-019
944.14 ..22 510-511	945.44 ..22 506-509	948.97 ..22 504-505	956.8 ...01 018-019
944.15 ..22 510-511	945.45 ..22 506-509	948.98 ..22 504-505	956.9 ...01 018-019
944.16 ..22 510-511	945.46 ..22 506-509	948.99 ..22 504-505	957.0 ...01 018-019
944.17 ..22 510-511	945.49 ..22 506-509	949.0 ...22 510-511	957.1 ...01 018-019
944.18 ..22 510-511	945.50 ..22 506-509	949.1 ...22 510-511	957.8 ...01 018-019
944.20 ..22 510-511	945.51 ..22 506-509	949.2 ...22 510-511	957.9 ...01 018-019
944.21 ..22 510-511	945.52 ..22 506-509	949.3 ...22 506-509	958.0 ...04 078
944.22 ..22 510-511	945.53 ..22 506-509	949.4 ...22 506-509	958.1 ...04 078
944.23 ..22 510-511	945.54 ..22 506-509	949.5 ...22 506-509	958.2 ...21 454-455
944.24 ..22 510-511	945.55 ..22 506-509	950.0 ...02 046-048	958.3 ...18 418
944.25 ..22 510-511	945.56 ..22 506-509	950.1 ...01 034-035	958.4 ...21 454-455
944.26 ..22 510-511	945.59 ..22 506-509	950.2 ...01 034-035	958.5 ...11 316
944.27 ..22 510-511	946.0 ...22 510-511	950.3 ...01 034-035	958.6 ...08 256
944.28 ..22 510-511	946.1 ...22 510-511	950.9 ...01 034-035	958.7 ...04 094-095
944.30 ..22 506-509	946.2 ...22 510-511	951.0 ...01 018-019	958.8 ...21 454-455
944.31 ..22 506-509	946.3 ...22 506-509	951.1 ...01 018-019	959.01 ..21 444-446
944.32 ..22 506-509	946.4 ...22 506-509	951.2 ...01 018-019	959.09 ..21 444-446
944.33 ..22 506-509	946.5 ...22 506-509	951.3 ...01 002,018-019	959.1 ...21 444-446
944.34 ..22 506-509	947.0 ...03 073-074	951.4 ...01 018-019	959.2 ...21 444-446
944.35 ..22 506-509	947.1 ...04 101-102	951.5 ...03 073-074	959.3 ...21 444-446
944.36 ..22 506-509	947.2 ...06 188-190	951.6 ...01 018-019	959.4 ...21 444-446
944.37 ..22 506-509	947.3 ...06 188-190	951.7 ...01 018-019	959.5 ...21 444-446
944.38 ..22 506-509	947.4 ...13 358-359,369	951.8 ...01 018-019	959.6 ...21 444-446
944.40 ..22 506-509	947.8 ...22 510-511	951.9 ...01 018-019	959.7 ...21 444-446
944.41 ..22 506-509	947.9 ...22 510-511	952.00 ..01 009	959.8 ...21 444-446
944.42 ..22 506-509	948.00 ..22 510-511	952.01 ..01 009	959.9 ...21 444-446
944.43 ..22 506-509	948.10 ..22 510-511	952.02 ..01 009	960.0 ...21 449-451
944.44 ..22 506-509	948.11 ..22 506-509	952.03 ..01 009	960.1 ...21 449-451
944.45 ..22 506-509	948.20 ..22 510-511	952.04 ..01 009	960.2 ...21 449-451
944.46 ..22 506-509	948.21 ..22 504-505	952.05 ..01 009	960.3 ...21 449-451
944.47 ..22 506-509	948.22 ..22 504-505	952.06 ..01 009	960.4 ...21 449-451
944.48 ..22 506-509	948.30 ..22 510-511	952.07 ..01 009	960.5 ...21 449-451
944.50 ..22 506-509	948.31 ..22 504-505	952.08 ..01 009	960.6 ...21 449-451
944.51 ..22 506-509	948.32 ..22 504-505	952.09 ..01 009	960.7 ...21 449-451
944.52 ..22 506-509	948.33 ..22 504-505	952.10 ..01 009	960.8 ...21 449-451
944.53 ..22 506-509	948.40 ..22 510-511	952.11 ..01 009	960.9 ...21 449-451
944.54 ..22 506-509	948.41 ..22 506-509	952.12 ..01 009	961.0 ...21 449-451
944.55 ..22 506-509	948.42 ..22 504-505	952.13 ..01 009	961.1 ...21 449-451
944.56 ..22 506-509	948.43 ..22 504-505	952.14 ..01 009	961.2 ...21 449-451
944.57 ..22 506-509	948.44 ..22 504-505	952.15 ..01 009	961.3 ...21 449-451
944.58 ..22 506-509	948.50 ..22 510-511	952.16 ..01 009	961.4 ...21 449-451
945.00 ..22 510-511	948.51 ..22 504-505	952.17 ..01 009	961.5 ...21 449-451
945.01 ..22 510-511	948.52 ..22 504-505	952.18 ..01 009	961.6 ...21 449-451
945.02 ..22 510-511	948.53 ..22 504-505	952.19 ..01 009	961.7 ...21 449-451
945.03 ..22 510-511	948.54 ..22 504-505	952.2 ...01 009	961.8 ...21 449-451
945.04 ..22 510-511	948.55 ..22 504-505	952.3 ...01 009	961.9 ...21 449-451
945.05 ..22 510-511	948.60 ..22 510-511	952.4 ...01 009	962.0 ...21 449-451
945.06 ..22 510-511	948.61 ..22 504-505	952.8 ...01 009	962.1 ...21 449-451
945.09 ..22 510-511	948.62 ..22 504-505	952.9 ...01 009	962.2 ...21 449-451
945.10 ..22 510-511	948.63 ..22 504-505	953.0 ...01 018-019	962.3 ...21 449-451
945.11 ..22 510-511	948.64 ..22 504-505	953.1 ...01 018-019	962.4 ...21 449-451
945.12 ..22 510-511	948.65 ..22 504-505	953.2 ...01 018-019	962.5 ...21 449-451
945.13 ..22 510-511	948.66 ..22 504-505	953.3 ...01 018-019	962.6 ...21 449-451
945.14 ..22 510-511	948.70 ..22 510-511	953.4 ...01 018-019	962.7 ...21 449-451
945.15 ..22 510-511	948.71 ..22 504-505	953.5 ...01 002,018-019	962.8 ...21 449-451

Diagnosis Code/MDC/DRG List

DX	MDC	DRG	DX	MDC	DRG	DX	MDC	DRG	DX	MDC	DRG
962.9	21	449-451	972.4	21	449-451	982.3	21	449-451	994.4	21	454-455
963.0	21	449-451	972.5	21	449-451	982.4	21	449-451	994.5	21	454-455
963.1	21	449-451	972.6	21	449-451	982.8	21	449-451	994.6	03	065
963.2	21	449-451	972.7	21	449-451	983.0	21	449-451	994.7	21	454-455
963.3	21	449-451	972.8	21	449-451	983.1	21	449-451	994.8	21	454-455
963.4	21	449-451	972.9	21	449-451	983.2	21	449-451	994.9	21	454-455
963.5	21	449-451	973.0	21	449-451	983.9	21	449-451	995.0	21	447-448
963.8	21	449-451	973.1	21	449-451	984.0	21	449-451	995.1	21	447-448
963.9	21	449-451	973.2	21	449-451	984.1	21	449-451	995.2	21	449-451
964.0	21	449-451	973.3	21	449-451	984.8	21	449-451	995.3	21	447-448
964.1	21	449-451	973.4	21	449-451	984.9	21	449-451	995.4	21	454-455
964.2	21	449-451	973.5	21	449-451	985.0	21	449-451	995.50	21	454-455
964.3	21	449-451	973.6	21	449-451	985.1	21	449-451	995.51	21	454-455
964.4	21	449-451	973.8	21	449-451	985.2	21	449-451	995.52	21	454-455
964.5	21	449-451	973.9	21	449-451	985.3	21	449-451	995.53	21	454-455
964.6	21	449-451	974.0	21	449-451	985.4	21	449-451	995.54	21	454-455
964.7	21	449-451	974.1	21	449-451	985.5	21	449-451	995.55	21	454-455
964.8	21	449-451	974.2	21	449-451	985.6	21	449-451	995.59	21	454-455
964.9	21	449-451	974.3	21	449-451	985.8	21	449-451	995.7	21	454-455
965.00	21	449-451	974.4	21	449-451	985.9	21	449-451	995.80	21	454-455
965.01	21	449-451	974.5	21	449-451	986	21	449-451	995.81	21	454-455
965.02	21	449-451	974.6	21	449-451	987.0	21	449-451	995.82	21	454-455
965.09	21	449-451	974.7	21	449-451	987.1	21	449-451	995.83	21	454-455
965.1	21	449-451	975.0	21	449-451	987.2	21	449-451	995.84	21	454-455
965.4	21	449-451	975.1	21	449-451	987.3	21	449-451	995.85	21	454-455
965.5	21	449-451	975.2	21	449-451	987.4	21	449-451	995.86	21	454-455
965.61	21	449-451	975.3	21	449-451	987.5	21	449-451	995.89	21	454-455
965.69	21	449-451	975.4	21	449-451	987.6	21	449-451	995.90	18	416-417
965.7	21	449-451	975.5	21	449-451	987.7	21	449-451	995.91	18	416-417
965.8	21	449-451	975.6	21	449-451	987.8	21	449-451	995.92	18	416-417
965.9	21	449-451	975.7	21	449-451	987.9	21	449-451	995.93	18	416-417
966.0	21	449-451	975.8	21	449-451	988.0	21	449-451	995.94	18	416-417
966.1	21	449-451	976.0	21	449-451	988.1	21	449-451	996.00	05	144-145
966.2	21	449-451	976.1	21	449-451	988.2	21	449-451	996.01	05	138-139
966.3	21	449-451	976.2	21	449-451	988.8	21	449-451	996.02	05	135-137
966.4	21	449-451	976.3	21	449-451	988.9	21	449-451	996.03	05	144-145
967.0	21	449-451	976.4	21	449-451	989.0	21	449-451	996.09	05	144-145
967.1	21	449-451	976.5	02	046-048	989.1	21	449-451	996.1	05	144-145
967.2	21	449-451	976.6	21	449-451	989.2	21	449-451	996.2	01	034-035
967.3	21	449-451	976.7	21	449-451	989.3	21	449-451	996.30	11	331-333
967.4	21	449-451	976.8	21	449-451	989.4	21	449-451	996.31	11	331-333
967.5	21	449-451	976.9	21	449-451	989.5	21	449-451	996.32	13	358-359,369
967.6	21	449-451	977.0	21	449-451	989.6	21	449-451	996.39	11	331-333
967.8	21	449-451	977.1	21	449-451	989.7	21	449-451	996.4	08	249
967.9	21	449-451	977.2	21	449-451	989.8	21	449-451	996.51	02	046-048
968.0	21	449-451	977.3	21	449-451	989.9	21	449-451	996.52	21	452-453
968.1	21	449-451	977.4	21	449-451	990	21	454-455	996.53	02	046-048
968.2	21	449-451	977.8	21	449-451	991.0	21	454-455	996.54	09	276
968.3	21	449-451	977.9	21	449-451	991.1	21	454-455	996.55	21	452-453
968.4	21	449-451	978.0	21	449-451	991.2	21	454-455	996.56	21	452-453
968.5	21	449-451	978.1	21	449-451	991.3	21	454-455	996.59	21	452-453
968.6	21	449-451	978.2	21	449-451	991.4	21	454-455	996.60	21	452-453
968.7	21	449-451	978.3	21	449-451	991.5	21	454-455	996.61	05	144-145
968.9	21	449-451	978.4	21	449-451	991.6	21	454-455	996.62	05	144-145
969.0	21	449-451	978.5	21	449-451	991.8	21	454-455	996.63	01	034-035
969.1	21	449-451	978.6	21	449-451	991.9	21	454-455	996.64	11	331-333
969.2	21	449-451	978.8	21	449-451	992.0	21	454-455	996.65	11	331-333
969.3	21	449-451	978.9	21	449-451	992.1	21	454-455	996.66	08	249
969.4	21	449-451	979.0	21	449-451	992.2	21	454-455	996.67	08	249
969.5	21	449-451	979.1	21	449-451	992.3	21	454-455	996.68	21	452-453
969.6	21	449-451	979.2	21	449-451	992.4	21	454-455	996.69	21	452-453
969.7	21	449-451	979.3	21	449-451	992.5	21	454-455	996.70	21	452-453
969.8	21	449-451	979.4	21	449-451	992.6	21	454-455	996.71	05	144-145
969.9	21	449-451	979.5	21	449-451	992.7	21	454-455	996.72	05	144-145
970.0	21	449-451	979.6	21	449-451	992.8	21	454-455	996.73	05	144-145
970.1	21	449-451	979.7	21	449-451	992.9	21	454-455	996.74	05	144-145
970.8	21	449-451	979.9	21	449-451	993.0	03	068-070	996.75	01	034-035
970.9	21	449-451	980.0	21	449-451	993.1	03	068-070	996.76	11	331-333
971.0	21	449-451	980.1	21	449-451	993.2	21	454-455	996.77	08	249
971.1	21	449-451	980.2	21	449-451	993.3	21	454-455	996.78	08	249
971.2	21	449-451	980.3	21	449-451	993.4	21	454-455	996.79	21	452-453
971.3	21	449-451	980.8	21	449-451	993.8	21	454-455	996.80	21	452-453
971.9	21	449-451	980.9	21	449-451	993.9	21	454-455	996.81	11	331-333
972.0	21	449-451	981	21	449-451	994.0	21	454-455	996.82	07	205-206
972.1	21	449-451	982.0	21	449-451	994.1	21	454-455	996.83	05	144-145
972.2	21	449-451	982.1	21	449-451	994.2	21	454-455	996.84	04	101-102
972.3	21	449-451	982.2	21	449-451	994.3	21	454-455	996.85	16	398-399

DX....MDC....DRG	DX....MDC....DRG	DX....MDC....DRG	DX....MDC....DRG
996.86 ..07 204	V01.9 ...23 467	V10.44 ..17 411-412	V15.01 ..23 467
996.87 ..21 452-453	V02.0 ...23 467	V10.45 ..17 411-412	V15.02 ..23 467
996.89 ..21 452-453	V02.1 ...23 467	V10.46 ..17 411-412	V15.03 ..23 467
996.90 ..08 249	V02.2 ...23 467	V10.47 ..17 411-412	V15.04 ..23 467
996.91 ..08 249	V02.3 ...23 467	V10.48 ..17 411-412	V15.05 ..23 467
996.92 ..08 249	V02.4 ...23 467	V10.49 ..17 411-412	V15.06 ..23 467
996.93 ..08 249	V02.51 ..23 467	V10.50 ..17 411-412	V15.07 ..23 467
996.94 ..08 249	V02.52 ..23 467	V10.51 ..17 411-412	V15.08 ..23 467
996.95 ..08 249	V02.59 ..23 467	V10.52 ..17 411-412	V15.09 ..23 467
996.96 ..08 249	V02.60 ..07 205-206	V10.53 ..17 411-412	V15.1 ...23 467
996.99 ..08 249	V02.61 ..07 205-206	V10.59 ..17 411-412	V15.2 ...23 467
997.0 ...01 034-035	V02.62 ..07 205-206	V10.60 ..17 411-412	V15.3 ...23 467
997.1 ...05 144-145	V02.69 ..07 205-206	V10.61 ..17 411-412	V15.41 ..23 467
997.2 ...05 130-131	V02.7 ...23 467	V10.62 ..17 411-412	V15.42 ..23 467
997.3 ...04 101-102	V02.8 ...23 467	V10.63 ..17 411-412	V15.49 ..23 467
997.4 ...06 188-190	V02.9 ...23 467	V10.69 ..17 411-412	V15.5 ...23 467
997.5 ...11 331-333	V03.0 ...23 467	V10.71 ..17 411-412	V15.6 ...23 467
997.60 ..08 256	V03.1 ...23 467	V10.72 ..17 411-412	V15.7 ...23 467
997.61 ..08 256	V03.2 ...23 467	V10.79 ..17 411-412	V15.81 ..23 467
997.62 ..08 256	V03.3 ...23 467	V10.81 ..17 411-412	V15.89 ..23 467
997.69 ..08 256	V03.4 ...23 467	V10.82 ..17 411-412	V15.9 ...23 467
997.71 ..06 188-190	V03.5 ...23 467	V10.83 ..17 411-412	V16.0 ...23 467
997.71 ..15 ....387, 389	V03.6 ...23 467	V10.84 ..17 411-412	V16.1 ...23 467
997.72 ..11 331-333	V03.7 ...23 467	V10.85 ..17 411-412	V16.2 ...23 467
997.72 ..15 ....387, 389	V03.81 ..23 467	V10.86 ..17 411-412	V16.3 ...23 467
997.79 ..05 130-131	V03.82 ..23 467	V10.87 ..17 411-412	V16.40 ..23 467
997.79 ..15 ....387, 389	V03.89 ..23 467	V10.88 ..17 411-412	V16.41 ..23 467
997.9 ...21 452-453	V03.9 ...23 467	V10.89 ..17 411-412	V16.42 ..23 467
998.0 ...21 452-453	V04.0 ...23 467	V10.9 ...17 411-412	V16.43 ..23 467
998.11 ..15 ....387, 389	V04.1 ...23 467	V11.0 ...23 467	V16.49 ..23 467
998.11 ..21 452-453	V04.2 ...23 467	V11.1 ...23 467	V16.51 ..23 467
998.12 ..21 452-453	V04.3 ...23 467	V11.2 ...23 467	V16.59 ..23 467
998.13 ..15 ....387, 389	V04.4 ...23 467	V11.3 ...23 467	V16.6 ...23 467
998.13 ..21 452-453	V04.5 ...23 467	V11.8 ...23 467	V16.7 ...23 467
998.2 ...21 452-453	V04.6 ...23 467	V11.9 ...23 467	V16.8 ...23 467
998.3 ...21 452-453	V04.7 ...23 467	V12.00 ..23 467	V16.9 ...23 467
998.31 ..21 452-453	V04.8 ...23 467	V12.01 ..23 467	V17.0 ...23 467
998.32 ..21 452-453	V05.0 ...23 467	V12.02 ..23 467	V17.1 ...23 467
998.4 ...21 452-453	V05.1 ...23 467	V12.03 ..23 467	V17.2 ...23 467
998.51 ..15 ....387, 389	V05.2 ...23 467	V12.09 ..23 467	V17.3 ...23 467
998.51 ..18 418	V05.8 ...23 467	V12.1 ...23 467	V17.4 ...23 467
998.59 ..15 ....387, 389	V05.9 ...23 467	V12.2 ...23 467	V17.5 ...23 467
998.59 ..18 418	V06.0 ...23 467	V12.3 ...23 467	V17.6 ...23 467
998.6 ...21 452-453	V06.1 ...23 467	V12.40 ..23 467	V17.7 ...23 467
998.7 ...21 452-453	V06.2 ...23 467	V12.41 ..23 467	V17.8 ...23 467
998.81 ..21 452-453	V06.3 ...23 467	V12.49 ..23 467	V18.0 ...23 467
998.82 ..02 046-048	V06.4 ...23 467	V12.5 ...23 467	V18.1 ...23 467
998.83 ..21 452-453	V06.8 ...23 467	V12.6 ...23 467	V18.2 ...23 467
998.89 ..21 452-453	V06.9 ...23 467	V12.70 ..23 467	V18.3 ...23 467
998.9 ...21 452-453	V07.0 ...23 467	V12.71 ..23 467	V18.4 ...23 467
999.0 ...18 421-422	V07.1 ...23 467	V12.72 ..23 467	V18.5 ...23 467
999.1 ...04 078	V07.2 ...23 467	V12.79 ..23 467	V18.61 ..23 467
999.2 ...05 144-145	V07.31 ..23 467	V13.00 ..23 467	V18.69 ..23 467
999.3 ...18 423	V07.39 ..23 467	V13.01 ..23 467	V18.7 ...23 467
999.4 ...21 447-448	V07.4 ...23 467	V13.09 ..23 467	V18.8 ...23 467
999.5 ...21 447-448	V07.8 ...23 467	V13.1 ...23 467	V19.0 ...23 467
999.6 ...16 395-396	V07.9 ...23 467	V13.2 ...23 467	V19.1 ...23 467
999.7 ...16 395-396	V10.00 ..17 411-412	V13.21 ..23 467	V19.2 ...23 467
999.8 ...16 395-396	V10.01 ..17 411-412	V13.29 ..23 467	V19.3 ...23 467
999.9 ...21 452	V10.02 ..17 411-412	V13.3 ...23 467	V19.4 ...23 467
	V10.03 ..17 411-412	V13.4 ...23 467	V19.5 ...23 467
Supplementary Classification of Factors Influencing Health Status and Contact with Health Services	V10.04 ..17 411-412	V13.5 ...23 467	V19.6 ...23 467
	V10.05 ..17 411-412	V13.61 ..23 467	V19.7 ...23 467
	V10.06 ..17 411-412	V13.69 ..23 467	V19.8 ...23 467
V01.0 ...23 467	V10.07 ..17 411-412	V13.7 ...23 467	V20.0 ...23 467
V01.1 ...23 467	V10.09 ..17 411-412	V13.8 ...23 467	V20.1 ...23 467
V01.2 ...23 467	V10.11 ..17 411-412	V13.9 ...23 467	V20.2 ...23 467
V01.3 ...23 467	V10.12 ..17 411-412	V14.0 ...23 467	V21.0 ...23 467
V01.4 ...23 467	V10.20 ..17 411-412	V14.1 ...23 467	V21.1 ...23 467
V01.5 ...23 467	V10.21 ..17 411-412	V14.2 ...23 467	V21.2 ...23 467
V01.6 ...23 467	V10.22 ..17 411-412	V14.3 ...23 467	V21.30 ..23 467
V01.7 ...23 467	V10.29 ..17 411-412	V14.4 ...23 467	V21.31 ..23 467
V01.8 ...23 467	V10.3 ...17 411-412	V14.5 ...23 467	V21.32 ..23 467
V01.81 ..15 391	V10.40 ..17 411-412	V14.6 ...23 467	V21.33 ..23 467
V01.81 ..23 467	V10.41 ..17 411-412	V14.7 ...23 467	V21.34 ..23 467
V01.89 ..15 391	V10.42 ..17 411-412	V14.8 ...23 467	V21.35 ..23 467
V01.89 ..23 467	V10.43 ..17 411-412	V14.9 ...23 467	V21.8 ...23 467

Diagnosis Code/MDC/DRG List

DX	MDC	DRG
V21.9	23	467
V22.0	23	467
V22.1	23	467
V22.2	23	467
V23.0	14	469
V23.1	14	469
V23.2	14	469
V23.3	14	469
V23.41	14	469
V23.49	14	469
V23.5	14	469
V23.7	14	469
V23.81	14	469
V23.82	14	469
V23.83	14	469
V23.84	14	469
V23.89	14	469
V23.9	14	469
V24.0	14	376-377
V24.1	23	467
V24.2	23	467
V25.01	23	467
V25.02	23	467
V25.09	23	467
V25.1	23	467
V25.2	12	351
V25.2	13	358-359,369
V25.3	13	358-359,369
V25.40	23	467
V25.41	23	467
V25.42	23	467
V25.43	23	467
V25.49	23	467
V25.5	23	467
V25.8	23	467
V25.9	23	467
V26.0	12	352
V26.0	13	358-359,369
V26.1	23	467
V26.21	23	467
V26.22	23	467
V26.29	23	467
V26.3	23	467
V26.4	23	467
V26.51	23	467
V26.52	23	467
V26.8	23	467
V26.9	23	467
V27.0	23	467
V27.1	23	467
V27.2	23	467
V27.3	23	467
V27.4	23	467
V27.5	23	467
V27.6	23	467
V27.7	23	467
V27.9	23	467
V28.0	14	383-384
V28.1	14	383-384
V28.2	14	383-384
V28.3	23	467
V28.4	23	467
V28.5	23	467
V28.6	23	467
V28.8	23	467
V28.9	23	467
V29.0	23	467
V29.1	23	467
V29.2	23	467
V29.3	23	467
V29.8	23	467
V29.9	23	467
V30.00	15	391
V30.01	15	391
V30.1	15	391
V30.2	15	469
V31.00	15	391
V31.01	15	391
V31.1	15	391
V31.2	15	469
V32.00	15	391
V32.01	15	391
V32.1	15	391
V32.2	15	469
V33.00	15	391
V33.01	15	391
V33.1	15	391
V33.2	15	469
V34.00	15	391
V34.01	15	391
V34.1	15	391
V34.2	15	469
V35.00	15	391
V35.01	15	391
V35.1	15	391
V35.2	15	469
V36.00	15	391
V36.01	15	391
V36.1	15	391
V36.2	15	469
V37.00	15	391
V37.01	15	391
V37.1	15	391
V37.2	15	469
V39.00	15	391
V39.01	15	391
V39.1	15	391
V39.2	15	469
V40.0	23	467
V40.1	23	467
V40.2	23	467
V40.3	23	467
V40.9	23	467
V41.0	23	467
V41.1	23	467
V41.2	23	467
V41.3	23	467
V41.4	23	467
V41.5	23	467
V41.6	23	467
V41.7	23	467
V41.8	23	467
V41.9	23	467
V42.0	11	331-333
V42.1	05	144-145
V42.2	05	144-145
V42.3	09	283-284
V42.4	08	256
V42.5	02	046-048
V42.6	04	101-102
V42.7	07	205-206
V42.81	16	398-399
V42.82	16	398-399
V42.83	07	467
V42.84	07	467
V42.89	23	467
V42.9	23	467
V43.0	02	046-048
V43.1	02	046-048
V43.2	05	144-145
V43.3	05	144-145
V43.4	05	144-145
V43.5	11	331-333
V43.60	08	256
V43.61	08	256
V43.62	08	256
V43.63	08	256
V43.64	08	256
V43.65	08	256
V43.66	08	256
V43.69	08	256
V43.7	08	256
V43.83	23	467
V43.89	23	467
V44.0	23	467
V44.1	23	467
V44.2	23	467
V44.3	23	467
V44.4	23	467
V44.50	23	467
V44.51	23	467
V44.52	23	467
V44.59	23	467
V44.6	23	467
V44.7	23	467
V44.8	23	467
V44.9	23	467
V45.00	23	467
V45.01	23	467
V45.02	23	467
V45.09	23	467
V45.1	23	467
V45.2	23	467
V45.3	23	467
V45.4	23	467
V45.51	23	467
V45.52	23	467
V45.59	23	467
V45.61	23	467
V45.69	23	467
V45.71	23	467
V45.72	23	467
V45.73	23	467
V45.74	11	331-333
V45.75	23	467
V45.76	04	101-102
V45.77	12,13	352,358-359,369
V45.78	02	46-48
V45.79	23	467
V45.81	23	467
V45.84	23	467
V45.89	23	467
V46.0	23	467
V46.1	23	467
V46.2	23	467
V46.8	23	467
V46.9	23	467
V47.0	23	467
V47.1	23	467
V47.2	23	467
V47.3	23	467
V47.4	23	467
V47.5	23	467
V47.9	23	467
V48.0	23	467
V48.1	23	467
V48.2	23	467
V48.3	23	467
V48.4	23	467
V48.5	23	467
V48.6	23	467
V48.7	23	467
V48.8	23	467
V48.9	23	467
V49.0	23	467
V49.1	23	467
V49.2	23	467
V49.3	23	467
V49.4	23	467
V49.5	23	467
V49.81	23	467
V49.82	23	467
V49.89	23	467
V50.0	09	283-284
V50.1	09	283-284
V50.2	12	350
V50.3	23	467
V50.8	23	467
V50.9	23	467
V51	09	283-284
V52.0	08	249
V52.1	08	249
V52.2	23	467
V52.3	23	467
V52.4	23	467
V52.8	23	462
V52.9	23	462
V53.01	23	467
V53.02	23	467
V53.09	23	467
V53.1	23	467
V53.2	23	467
V53.31	05	144-145
V53.32	05	144-145
V53.39	05	144-145
V53.4	23	467
V53.5	06	188-190
V53.6	11	331-333
V53.7	08	249
V53.8	23	467
V53.9	23	467
V54.0	08	249
V54.8	08	249
V54.9	08	249
V54.10	08	249
V54.11	08	249
V54.12	08	249
V54.13	08	249
V54.14	08	249
V54.15	08	249
V54.16	08	249
V54.17	08	249
V54.19	08	249
V54.20	08	249
V54.21	08	249
V54.22	08	249
V54.23	08	249
V54.24	08	249
V54.25	08	249
V54.26	08	249
V54.27	08	249
V54.29	08	249
V54.81	08	249
V54.89	08	249
V55.0	04	101-102
V55.1	06	188-190
V55.2	06	188-190
V55.3	06	188-190
V55.4	06	188-190
V55.5	11	331-333
V55.6	11	331-333
V55.7	13	358-359,369
V55.8	23	467
V55.9	23	467
V56.0	11	317
V56.2	11	317
V56.31	11	317
V56.32	11	317
V56.8	11	317
V57.0	23	467
V57.1	23	462
V57.21	23	462
V57.22	23	462
V57.3	23	462
V57.4	23	467
V57.81	23	467
V57.89	23	462
V57.9	23	462
V58.0	17	409
V58.1	17	410,492
V58.2	23	467
V58.3	23	467
V58.41	23	465-466
V58.42	23	465,466
V58.43	23	465,466
V58.49	23	465-466
V58.5	23	465-466
V58.62	23	465-466

DX....MDC....DRG	DX....MDC....DRG	DX....MDC....DRG	DX....MDC....DRG
V58.71 ..23 465,466	V64.0 ...23 467	V71.5 ...23 467	V76.44 ..23 467
V58.72 ..23 465,466	V64.1 ...23 467	V71.6 ...21 454-455	V76.45 ..23 467
V58.73 ..23 465,466	V64.2 ...23 467	V71.7 ...05 143	V76.46 ..23 467
V58.74 ..23 465,466	V64.3 ...23 467	V71.81 ..23 467	V76.47 ..23 467
V58.75 ..23 465,466	V64.4 ...23 467	V71.82 ..23 467	V76.49 ..23 467
V58.76 ..23 465,466	V65.0 ...23 467	V71.83 ..23 467	V76.50 ..23 467
V58.77 ..23 465,466	V65.1 ...23 467	V71.89 ..23 467	V76.51 ..23 467
V58.78 ..23 465,466	V65.2 ...23 467	V71.9 ...23 467	V76.52 ..23 467
V58.81 ..23 465-466	V65.3 ...23 467	V72.0 ...23 467	V76.81 ..23 467
V58.83 ..23 465-466	V65.40 ..23 467	V72.1 ...23 467	V76.89 ..23 467
V58.89 ..23 465-466	V65.41 ..23 467	V72.2 ...23 467	V76.9 ...23 467
V58.9 ...23 465-466	V65.42 ..23 467	V72.3 ...23 467	V77.0 ...23 467
V59.0 ...23 467	V65.43 ..23 467	V72.4 ...23 467	V77.1 ...23 467
V59.1 ...09 283-284	V65.44 ..23 467	V72.5 ...23 467	V77.2 ...23 467
V59.2 ...08 256	V65.45 ..23 467	V72.6 ...23 467	V77.3 ...23 467
V59.3 ...23 467	V65.5 ...23 467	V72.7 ...23 467	V77.4 ...23 467
V59.4 ...11 331-333	V65.8 ...23 467	V72.81 ..23 467	V77.5 ...23 467
V59.5 ...23 467	V65.9 ...23 467	V72.82 ..23 467	V77.6 ...23 467
V59.8 ...23 467	V66.0 ...23 467	V72.83 ..23 467	V77.7 ...23 467
V59.9 ...23 467	V66.1 ...23 467	V72.84 ..23 467	V77.8 ...23 467
V60.0 ...23 467	V66.2 ...23 467	V72.85 ..23 467	V77.91 ..23 467
V60.1 ...23 467	V66.3 ...23 467	V72.9 ...23 467	V77.99 ..23 467
V60.2 ...23 467	V66.4 ...23 467	V73.0 ...23 467	V78.0 ...23 467
V60.3 ...23 467	V66.5 ...23 467	V73.1 ...23 467	V78.1 ...23 467
V60.4 ...23 467	V66.6 ...23 467	V73.2 ...23 467	V78.2 ...23 467
V60.5 ...23 467	V66.7 ...23 467	V73.3 ...23 467	V78.3 ...23 467
V60.6 ...23 467	V66.9 ...23 467	V73.4 ...23 467	V78.8 ...23 467
V60.8 ...23 467	V67.00 ..23 465-466	V73.5 ...23 467	V78.9 ...23 467
V60.9 ...23 467	V67.01 ..23 465-466	V73.6 ...23 467	V79.0 ...23 467
V61.0 ...23 467	V67.09 ..23 465-466	V73.88 ..23 467	V79.1 ...23 467
V61.10 ..23 467	V67.1 ...17 409	V73.89 ..23 467	V79.2 ...23 467
V61.11 ..23 467	V67.2 ...17 410,492	V73.98 ..23 467	V79.3 ...23 467
V61.12 ..23 467	V67.3 ...23 467	V73.99 ..23 467	V79.8 ...23 467
V61.20 ..23 467	V67.4 ...23 465-466	V74.0 ...23 467	V79.9 ...23 467
V61.21 ..23 467	V67.51 ..23 467	V74.1 ...23 467	V80.0 ...23 467
V61.22 ..23 467	V67.59 ..23 467	V74.2 ...23 467	V80.1 ...23 467
V61.29 ..23 467	V67.6 ...23 467	V74.3 ...23 467	V80.2 ...23 467
V61.3 ...23 467	V67.9 ...23 467	V74.4 ...23 467	V80.3 ...23 467
V61.41 ..23 467	V68.0 ...23 467	V74.5 ...23 467	V81.0 ...23 467
V61.49 ..23 467	V68.1 ...23 467	V74.6 ...23 467	V81.1 ...23 467
V61.5 ...13 358-359,369	V68.2 ...23 467	V74.8 ...23 467	V81.2 ...23 467
V61.6 ...14 383-384	V68.81 ..23 467	V74.9 ...23 467	V81.3 ...23 467
V61.7 ...14 380-381	V68.89 ..23 467	V75.0 ...23 467	V81.4 ...23 467
V61.8 ...23 467	V68.9 ...23 467	V75.1 ...23 467	V81.5 ...23 467
V61.9 ...23 467	V70.0 ...23 467	V75.2 ...23 467	V81.6 ...23 467
V62.0 ...23 467	V70.1 ...23 467	V75.3 ...23 467	V82.0 ...23 467
V62.1 ...23 467	V70.2 ...23 467	V75.4 ...23 467	V82.1 ...23 467
V62.2 ...23 467	V70.3 ...23 467	V75.5 ...23 467	V82.2 ...23 467
V62.3 ...23 467	V70.4 ...23 467	V75.6 ...23 467	V82.3 ...23 467
V62.4 ...23 467	V70.5 ...23 467	V75.7 ...23 467	V82.4 ...23 467
V62.5 ...23 467	V70.6 ...23 467	V75.8 ...23 467	V82.5 ...23 467
V62.6 ...23 467	V70.7 ...23 467	V75.9 ...23 467	V82.6 ...23 467
V62.81 ..23 467	V70.81 ..23 467	V76.0 ...23 467	V82.81 ..23 467
V62.82 ..23 467	V70.89 ..23 467	V76.10 ..23 467	V82.89 ..23 467
V62.83 ..23 467	V70.9 ...23 467	V76.11 ..23 467	V82.9 ...23 467
V62.89 ..23 467	V71.01 ..19 425	V76.12 ..23 467	V83.01 ..23 467
V62.9 ...23 467	V71.02 ..19 425	V76.19 ..23 467	V83.02 ..23 467
V63.0 ...23 467	V71.09 ..19 432	V76.2 ...23 467	V83.81 ..23 467
V63.1 ...23 467	V71.1 ...17 411-412	V76.3 ...23 467	V83.89 ..23 467
V63.2 ...23 467	V71.2 ...04 079-081	V76.41 ..23 467	
V63.8 ...23 467	V71.3 ...21 454-455	V76.42 ..23 467	
V63.9 ...23 467	V71.4 ...21 454-455	V76.43 ..23 467	

Complication & Comorbidity (CC) Code List

The following is a standard list of conditions considered to be complications and comorbidities that when present as a secondary diagnosis may affect DRG assignment. An asterisk (*) indicates a code range is represented.

*008.4	112.83	192.3	*282.6	295.92	305.61	404.91	434.91
*011	112.84	192.8	*283	295.93	305.62	404.92	436
*012.0	112.85	*196	*284	295.94	305.70	404.93	437.2
*012.1	114.0	*197	285.0	296.04	305.71	405.01	437.4
*013	114.2	*198	285.1	296.14	305.72	405.09	437.5
*014	114.3	199.0	*286	296.34	305.90	410.01	437.6
*016	114.9	*200	*287	296.44	305.91	410.11	440.24
*017.2	115.00	*201	288.0	296.54	305.92	410.21	*441.0
*017.3	115.01	*202	288.1	296.64	307.1	410.31	441.1
*017.4	115.02	*203	291.0	298.0	*320	410.41	441.3
*017.5	115.03	*204	291.1	298.3	*321	410.51	441.5
*017.6	115.04	*205	291.2	298.4	*322	410.61	441.6
*017.7	115.05	*206	291.3	299.00	*324	410.71	*444
*017.8	*115.1	*207	291.4	299.10	325	410.81	*445.0
*017.9	*115.9	*208	*291.8	299.80	331.4	410.91	445.81
*018	116.0	*242	291.9	299.90	*335	*411	446.0
031.0	116.1	*250	*292	303.00	340	*413	*446.2
*036	117.3	251.0	293.81	303.01	343.2	*415	446.3
037	117.4	251.3	293.82	303.02	*344.0	416.0	446.4
*038	117.5	252.1	293.83	303.90	345.01	*420	446.5
040.0	117.6	253.2	293.84	303.91	345.10	*421	446.6
040.82	117.7	253.5	295.00	303.92	345.11	*422	446.7
042	118	254.1	295.01	304.00	345.2	423.0	451.0
046.2	130.0	255.0	295.02	304.01	345.3	423.1	451.11
*052	130.1	255.3	295.03	304.02	345.41	423.2	451.19
*053.0	130.2	255.4	295.04	304.10	345.51	*424	451.2
*053.1	130.3	255.5	295.10	304.11	345.61	*425	451.81
053.79	130.4	255.6	295.11	304.12	345.71	426.0	452
053.8	130.5	*258	295.12	304.20	345.81	426.12	*453
054.3	130.7	259.2	295.13	304.21	345.91	426.13	456.0
054.5	130.8	260	295.14	304.22	348.1	426.53	456.20
054.71	135	261	295.21	304.40	349.1	426.54	459.0
054.72	136.3	262	295.22	304.41	349.81	426.6	464.11
054.79	137.0	*263	295.23	304.42	349.82	426.7	464.21
054.8	137.1	269.0	295.24	304.50	357.0	426.81	464.31
*055	137.2	273.3	295.30	304.51	358.0	426.89	475
*056	138	276.0	295.31	304.52	358.1	426.9	478.21
070.2	*150	276.1	295.32	304.60	359.0	427.0	478.22
070.3	*151	276.2	295.33	304.61	359.1	427.1	478.24
070.4	*152	276.3	295.34	304.62	377.00	427.2	*478.3
070.5	*153	276.4	295.40	304.70	377.01	*427.3	481
070.6	*154	276.5	295.41	304.71	377.02	*427.4	*482
070.9	*155	276.6	295.42	304.72	383.01	427.5	*483
*072	*156	276.7	295.43	304.80	383.30	*428	*484
086.0	*157	276.9	295.44	304.81	383.81	429.4	485
*090.4	162.2	*277.0	295.60	304.82	*394	429.5	486
*093	162.3	279.02	295.61	304.90	*395	429.6	487.0
094.0	162.4	279.03	295.62	304.91	*396	*429.7	491.1
094.1	162.5	279.04	295.63	304.92	*397	429.81	*491.2
094.2	162.8	279.05	295.64	305.00	398.0	429.82	491.8
094.3	162.9	279.06	295.70	305.01	398.91	430	491.9
094.81	*163	279.09	295.71	305.02	401.0	431	492.8
094.87	*164	279.1	295.72	305.30	*402.0	432.0	493.01
094.89	176.4	279.2	295.73	305.31	402.11	432.1	493.02
094.9	176.5	279.3	295.74	305.32	402.91	433.01	493.11
098.0	189.0	279.4	295.80	305.40	*403.0	433.11	493.12
*098.1	189.1	279.8	295.81	305.41	403.11	433.21	493.20
112.0	189.2	279.9	295.82	305.42	403.91	433.31	493.21
112.4	*191	280.0	295.83	305.50	*404.0	433.81	493.22
112.5	192.0	281.4	295.84	305.51	404.11	433.91	493.91
112.81	192.1	281.8	295.90	305.52	404.12	434.01	493.92
112.82	192.2	282.4	295.91	305.60	404.13	434.11	494.1

*495	535.11	580.4	*648.3	745.7	777.2	*852	902.59
496	535.21	*580.8	*648.5	746.01	777.5	*853	902.87
506.0	535.31	580.9	*648.6	746.02	777.6	*854	904.0
506.1	535.41	*581	*659.3	746.1	778.0	*860	*925
*507	535.51	583.4	*665.0	746.2	779.0	861.01	929.0
508.0	535.61	584.5	*665.1	746.3	779.1	861.02	*952
508.1	536.1	584.6	666.32	746.4	779.3	861.03	*953
510.0	*536.4	584.7	666.34	746.5	779.4	*861.1	958.0
510.9	537.0	584.8	*668	746.6	779.7	861.22	958.1
511.1	537.3	584.9	*669.1	746.7	780.01	*861.3	958.2
511.8	537.4	585	*669.3	746.81	780.03	862.1	958.3
511.9	537.83	*590.1	*670	746.82	780.1	*862.2	958.4
*512	537.84	590.2	*671.2	746.83	780.31	*862.3	958.5
*513	*540	590.3	*671.3	746.84	780.39	862.9	958.7
515	*550.0	*590.8	*671.4	746.86	781.7	863.1	995.4
*516	*550.1	590.9	*673	*747.1	785.4	*863.3	995.86
*517	*551	591	*674.0	747.22	*785.5	*863.5	*995.9
518.0	*552	592.1	674.10	748.4	786.03	*863.9	*996.0
518.1	557.0	593.5	674.12	748.5	786.04	*864	996.1
518.4	558.1	595.0	*674.2	748.61	786.3	*865	996.2
518.5	558.2	595.1	675.10	765.01	788.20	*866	996.30
518.6	*560	595.2	675.11	765.02	788.29	*867	996.39
518.81	562.02	595.4	675.12	765.03	789.5	*868	996.4
518.82	562.03	*595.8	*680	765.04	790.7	*869	*996.5
518.83	562.12	595.9	682.0	765.05	791.1	870.3	*996.6
518.84	562.13	596.0	682.1	765.06	791.3	870.4	*996.7
*519.0	566	596.1	682.2	765.07	799.1	870.8	*996.8
519.2	*567	596.2	682.3	765.08	799.4	870.9	*996.9
527.3	568.81	596.4	682.5	767.0	*800	871.0	*997.0
527.4	569.3	596.6	682.6	768.5	*801	871.1	997.1
528.3	569.5	596.7	682.8	769	802.1	871.2	997.2
530.4	*569.6	597.0	682.9	770.0	*802.2	871.3	997.3
530.7	569.83	598.1	684	770.1	*802.3	871.4	997.4
530.82	569.85	598.2	685.0	770.2	802.4	871.9	997.5
530.84	569.86	599.0	694.4	770.3	802.5	872.72	997.62
*531.0	570	599.4	694.5	770.4	802.6	872.73	997.7
*531.1	571.2	599.6	695.0	770.5	802.7	872.74	997.99
*531.2	571.49	599.7	696.0	770.7	802.8	873.33	998.0
531.31	571.5	601.0	707.0	770.84	802.9	873.9	*998.1
*531.4	571.6	601.2	*707.1	771.0	*803	*874.0	998.2
*531.5	572.0	601.3	710.0	771.1	*804	*874.1	*998.3
*531.6	572.1	602.1	710.1	771.3	*805	874.3	998.4
531.71	572.2	603.1	710.3	771.81	*806	874.5	*998.5
531.91	572.4	604.0	710.4	771.83	807.04	*875	998.6
*532.0	573.1	611.72	710.5	*772.1	807.05	*887	998.7
*532.1	573.2	614.0	710.8	772.2	807.06	*896	998.83
*532.2	573.3	614.3	*711.0	772.4	807.07	*897	998.89
532.31	573.4	614.5	*711.6	772.5	807.08	*900	998.9
*532.4	*574.0	615.0	714.1	773.0	807.09	901.0	999.1
*532.5	*574.1	616.3	714.2	773.1	*807.1	901.1	999.2
*532.6	574.21	616.4	*714.3	773.2	807.2	901.2	999.3
532.71	*574.3	620.7	*722.8	773.3	807.3	901.3	999.4
532.91	*574.4	*634	723.4	773.4	807.4	901.41	999.5
*533.0	*574.5	*639	723.5	*774.0	807.5	901.42	999.6
*533.1	*574.6	*640	728.0	774.1	807.6	901.83	999.7
*533.2	*574.7	*641.0	728.86	774.2	808.0	902.0	999.8
533.31	*574.8	*641.1	*730.0	*774.3	808.1	*902.1	V23.7
*533.4	*574.9	*641.3	*730.8	774.4	808.2	902.20	*V23.8
*533.5	575.0	*641.8	*730.9	774.5	808.3	902.22	V23.9
*533.6	575.12	*641.9	*733.1	774.7	808.43	902.23	V42.0
533.71	575.2	*642.4	*733.8	775.1	808.49	902.24	V42.1
533.91	575.3	*642.5	733.93	775.2	*808.5	902.25	V42.2
*534.0	575.4	*642.6	733.94	775.3	808.8	902.26	V42.6
*534.1	575.5	*642.7	733.95	775.4	808.9	902.27	V42.7
*534.2	576.1	*644.0	*741	775.5	*820	902.29	*V42.8
534.31	576.3	*644.1	745.0	775.6	*821.0	*902.3	V43.2
*534.4	576.4	*646.6	*745.1	775.7	*821.1	*902.4	V45.1
*534.5	577.0	*646.7	745.2	776.0	838.19	902.50	V46.1
*534.6	577.2	*647.3	745.3	776.1	*839.0	902.51	
534.71	*578	*647.4	745.4	776.2	*839.1	902.52	
534.91	579.3	*648.0	745.60	776.3	*850	902.53	
535.01	580.0	*648.2	745.69	777.1	*851	902.54	

2002 Ingenix, Inc.

Valid Three-digit ICD•9•CM Codes

Three-digit ICD-9-CM codes are used to identify a condition or disease only when a fourth or fifth digit is not available. The following are the only ICD-9-CM codes that are valid without further specificity.

024 Glanders
025 Melioidosis
035 Erysipelas
037 Tetanus
042 Human Immunodeficiency Virus (HIV) Infection
048 Other enterovirus diseases of central nervous system
061 Dengue
064 Viral encephalitis transmitted by other and unspecified arthropods
071 Rabies
075 Infectious mononucleosis
080 Louse-borne [epidemic] typhus
096 Late syphilis, latent
101 Vincent's angina
118 Opportunistic mycoses
124 Trichinosis
129 Intestinal parasitism, unspecified
135 Sarcoidosis
138 Late effects of acute poliomyelitis
179 Malignant neoplasm of uterus, part unspecified
181 Malignant neoplasm of placenta
185 Malignant neoplasm of prostate
193 Malignant neoplasm of thyroid gland
217 Benign neoplasm of breast
220 Benign neoplasm of ovary
226 Benign neoplasm of thyroid gland
243 Congenital hypothyroidism
260 Kwashiorkor
261 Nutritional marasmus
262 Other severe protein-calorie malnutrition
267 Ascorbic acid deficiency

311 Depressive disorder, not elsewhere classified
316 Psychic factors associated with diseases classified elsewhere
317 Mild mental retardation
319 Unspecified mental retardation
325 Phlebitis and thrombophlebitis of intracranial venous sinuses
326 Late effects of intracranial abscess or pyogenic infection
340 Multiple sclerosis
347 Cataplexy and narcolepsy
390 Rheumatic fever without mention of heart involvement
393 Chronic rheumatic pericarditis
412 Old myocardial infarction
430 Subarachnoid hemorrhage
431 Intracerebral hemorrhage
436 Acute, but ill-defined, cerebrovascular disease
438 Late effects of cerebrovascular disease
452 Portal vein thrombosis
460 Acute nasopharyngitis [common cold]
462 Acute pharyngitis
463 Acute tonsillitis
470 Deflected nasal septum
475 Peritonsillar abscess
481 Pneumococcal pneumonia
485 Bronchopneumonia, organism unspecified
486 Pneumonia, organism unspecified
490 Bronchitis, not specified as acute or chronic
494 Bronchiectasis
496 Chronic airway obstruction, not elsewhere classified
500 Coal workers' pneumoconiosis
501 Asbestosis
502 Pneumoconiosis due to other silica or silicates
503 Pneumoconiosis due to other inorganic dust

504 Pneumoconopathy due to inhalation of other dust
505 Pneumoconiosis, unspecified
514 Pulmonary congestion and hypostasis
515 Postinflammatory pulmonary fibrosis
541 Appendicitis, unqualified
542 Other appendicitis
566 Abscess of anal and rectal regions
570 Acute and subacute necrosis of liver
585 Chronic renal failure
586 Renal failure, unspecified
587 Renal sclerosis, unspecified
591 Hydronephrosis
605 Redundant prepuce and phimosis
630 Hydatidiform mole
631 Other abnormal product of conception
632 Missed abortion
650 Delivery in a completely normal case
677 Late effect of complication of pregnancy, childbirth, and the puerperium
683 Acute lymphadenitis
684 Impetigo
700 Corns and callosities
725 Polymyalgia rheumatica
734 Flat foot
769 Respiratory distress syndrome
797 Senility without mention of psychosis
920 Contusion of face, scalp, and neck except eye(s)
931 Foreign body in ear
932 Foreign body in nose
936 Foreign body in intestine and colon
937 Foreign body in anus and rectum
938 Foreign body in digestive system, unspecified
981 Toxic effect of petroleum products
986 Toxic effect of carbon monoxide
990 Effects of radiation, unspecified
V08 Asymptomatic HIV infection status
V51 Aftercare involving the use of plastic surgery